BMA

Infectious Diseases

Infectious Diseases

Fourth Edition

Edited by

**Jonathan Cohen,
MB, FRCP, FRCPE,
FRCPath, FMedSci**

Emeritus Professor of Infectious Diseases
Brighton and Sussex Medical School
Brighton, UK

**William G. Powderly,
MD, FRCPI**

J. William Campbell Professor of Medicine
Larry J Shapiro Director, Institute for
Public Health
Co-director, Division of Infectious Diseases
Washington University in St Louis
St Louis, MO, USA

Steven M. Opal, MD

Professor of Medicine
Infectious Disease Division
Alpert Medical School of Brown University
Providence, RI, USA

Section Editors

Thierry Calandra, MD, PhD

Chairman, Department of Medicine
Head, Infectious Diseases Service
CHUV (Centre Hospitalier
Universitaire Vaudois)
Lausanne, Switzerland

Nathan Clumeck, MD, PhD

Professor of Infectious Diseases
Honorary Head, Department of
Infectious Diseases
Saint-Pierre University Hospital
Brussels, Belgium

**Jeremy Day, MA, DTM&H,
PhD, FRCP**

Head, CNS–HIV Infections Research Group
Oxford University Clinical Research Unit
Wellcome Trust Major Overseas
Programme Vietnam
Ho Chi Minh City, Vietnam
Associate Professor
Centre for Tropical Medicine
Nuffield Department of Medicine
University of Oxford
Oxford, UK

**Jeremy Farrar, FRS, FRCP,
FMedSci, DPhil, OBE**

Director, The Wellcome Trust
London, UK

Roy M. Gulick, MD, MPH

Rochelle Belfer Professor in Medicine
Chief, Division of Infectious Diseases
Department of Medicine
Weill Cornell Medical College
New York, NY, USA

**Andy I.M. Hoepelman,
MD, PhD**

Professor in Medicine, Infectious
Diseases Specialist
Head, Department of Internal Medicine and
Infectious Diseases
University Medical Center
Utrecht, The Netherlands

Kieren A. Marr, MD

Professor of Medicine and Oncology
Director, Transplant and Oncology Infectious
Diseases Program
Johns Hopkins University School of Medicine
Baltimore, MD, USA

**Jeanne Marrazzo, MD,
MPH, FACP, FIDSA**

Director, Division of Infectious Diseases
Professor of Medicine
University of Alabama at Birmingham
School of Medicine
Birmingham, AL, USA

Didier Raoult, MD, PhD

Professor, Faculté de Médecine, Director of
the Foundation Mediterranee Infection
Unité des Rickettsies
WHO Collaborative Center for Rickettsial
Reference and Research
Marseille, France

Robert T. Schooley, MD

Professor and Head
Division of Infectious Diseases
Academic Vice Chair
Department of Medicine
University of California San Diego
San Diego, CA, USA

**Jos W.M. van der Meer,
MD, PhD, FRCP,
FRCP(Edin), FIDSA, MAE**

Emeritus Professor of Medicine
Radboud University Medical Center
Nijmegen, The Netherlands

Richard J. Whitley, MD

Distinguished Professor
Loeb Chair in Pediatrics
Professor of Pediatrics, Microbiology,
Medicine and Neurosurgery
University of Alabama
Birmingham, AL, USA

Associate Editors (Educational Content)

Courtney D. Chrisler, MD

Instructor in Medicine
Division of Infectious Diseases
Washington University in St Louis
St Louis, MO, USA

**Bethany Davies, MRCP,
FRCPath**

Specialist Registrar in Infectious Diseases and
Medical Microbiology
Brighton and Sussex University Hospitals
NHS Trust
Brighton, East Sussex, UK

For additional online content visit expertconsult.com

ELSEVIER

ELSEVIER

ISBN: 978-0-7020-6285-8
E-book: 978-0-7020-6338-1
Inkling: 978-0-7020-6339-8

Content Strategist: Belinda Kuhn
Content Development Specialist: Sharon Nash
Content Coordinator: Trinity Hutton
Project Manager: Joanna Souch
Design: Miles Hitchen
Illustration Manager: Brett MacNaughton
Marketing Manager: Melissa Fogarty

Printed in China

Last digit is the print number: 9 8 7 6 5 4 3 2 1

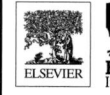

Working together
to grow libraries in
developing countries

www.elsevier.com • www.bookaid.org

CONTENTS

Preface to the Fourth Edition   xiv
List of Contributors   xv
Dedication   xxxvii

VOLUME 1

SECTION 1 Introduction to Infectious Diseases

1 The Evolution of Koch's Postulates   1
JONATHAN COHEN

2 Nature and Pathogenicity of Micro-organisms   4
JOSHUA FIERER | DAVID LOONEY | JEAN-CLAUDE PECHÈRE†

3 Host Responses to Infection   26
CARA C. WILSON | ROBERT T. SCHOOLEY

4 Emerging and Re-emerging Pathogens and Diseases, and Health Consequences of a Changing Climate   40
PHILIP M. POLGREEN | EVELYN L. POLGREEN

5 Mathematical Models in Infectious Disease Epidemiology   49
PETER J. WHITE

6 Infection Prevention and Control, and Antimicrobial Stewardship   54
RANDY A. TAPLITZ | MICHELE L. RITTER | FRANCESCA J. TORRIANI

7 Bacterial Genomes   62
PIERRE-EDOUARD FOURNIER | DIDIER RAOULT

8 The Microbiome in Infectious Diseases   68
MAKEDONKA MITREVA

SECTION 2 Syndromes by Body System

Skin and Soft Tissue   75

9 Viral Exanthems   75
ADILIA WARRIS | FRANK P. KROON

10 Cellulitis, Pyoderma, Abscesses, and Other Skin and Subcutaneous Infections   84
DENNIS L. STEVENS

11 Necrotizing Fasciitis, Gas Gangrene, Myositis and Myonecrosis   95
DENNIS L. STEVENS | MICHAEL J. ALDAPE | AMY E. BRYANT

12 Arthropod Vectors of Medical Importance   104
JEAN-MICHEL BERENGER | PHILIPPE PAROLA

13 Dermatologic Manifestations of Systemic Infections   113
CHANTAL P. BLEEKER-ROVERS | HENRY J.C. DE VRIES

14 Superficial Fungal Infections   122
DAVID W. WARNOCK | TOM M. CHILLER

PP1 Management of Infected Diabetic Foot Ulcers   130
EDGAR J.G. PETERS | BENJAMIN A. LIPSKY

PP2 Managing the Patient with Recurring Skin Infections   133
THUSHAN I. DE SILVA | STEPHEN T. GREEN

The Lymphatic System   136

15 Lymphadenopathy   136
ETHAN RUBINSTEIN† | YOAV KEYNAN

PP3 Evaluation and Management of the Solitary Enlarged Lymph Node   146
YOAV KEYNAN | ETHAN RUBINSTEIN†

The Eye   150

16 Conjunctivitis, Keratitis and Infections of Periorbital Structures   150
MICHEL DRANCOURT | MARIE BOULZE PANKERT | LOUIS HOFFART

17 Endophthalmitis   158
MICHEL DRANCOURT | FRÉDÉRIC MATONTI

18 Infectious Retinitis and Uveitis   165
MICHEL DRANCOURT

PP4 Management of Red Eye   175
MICHEL DRANCOURT | LOUIS HOFFART

The Central Nervous System   177

19 Acute and Chronic Meningitis   177
MATTHIJS C. BROUWER | DIEDERIK VAN DE BEEK

†Deceased

v

20 Encephalitis and Myelitis 189
KAREN C. BLOCH | CAROL A. GLASER | ALLAN R. TUNKEL

21 Brain Abscess and Other Focal Pyogenic Infections of the Central Nervous System 198
ITZHAK BROOK

22 Tetanus and Botulism 208
AIMEE C. HODOWANEC | THOMAS P. BLECK

23 Transmissible Spongiform Encephalopathies of Humans and Animals 214
SIMON MEAD | JOHN COLLINGE | SARAH J. TABRIZI

24 Infections in Hydrocephalus Shunts 221
ROGER BAYSTON | IVAN PELEGRIN

PP5 Role of Rapid Viral Detection in Meningitis 225
REMI N. CHARREL

PP6 Investigation of Psychiatric Manifestations of Encephalitis 227
DAVID B. CLIFFORD

The Respiratory System 229

25 Laryngitis, Epiglottitis and Pharyngitis 229
LUU-LY PHAM | RAFIK BOURAYOU | VALÉRIE MAGHRAOUI-SLIM | ISABELLE KONÉ-PAUT

26 Otitis, Sinusitis and Related Conditions 236
LUU-LY PHAM | RAFIK BOURAYOU | VALÉRIE MAGHRAOUI-SLIM | ISABELLE KONÉ-PAUT

27 Bronchitis, Bronchiectasis 243
MARCUS W. BUTLER | MICHAEL P. KEANE

28 Community-Acquired Pneumonia 251
RICHARD G. WUNDERINK

29 Hospital-Acquired, Healthcare-Associated and Ventilator-Associated Pneumonia 258
ANTOINE ROCH | GUILLEMETTE THOMAS | SAMI HRAIECH | LAURENT PAPAZIAN | WILLIAM G. POWDERLY

30 Lung Abscesses and Pleural Abscesses 263
CHRISTINA LISCYNESKY | JULIE E. MANGINO

31 Tuberculosis 271
REINOUT VAN CREVEL | PHILIP C. HILL

32 Nontuberculous Mycobacterial Diseases 285
JAKKO VAN INGEN

33 Fungal Pneumonias 292
CAROL A. KAUFFMAN

34 Management of the Infected Cystic Fibrosis Patient 300
HEATHER STRAH | DANIEL ROSENBLUTH

PP7 Investigation of Pleural Discharge/Fluid 303
SAMI HRAIECH | BENOIT D'JOURNO | LAURENT PAPAZIAN

PP8 When to Use Corticosteroids in Noncentral Nervous System Tuberculosis 306
GUY THWAITES

PP9 How to Manage a Patient on Anti-TB Therapy with Abnormal Liver Enzymes 308
L. PETER ORMEROD | THOMAS C. BAILEY

PP10 Use of Antibiotics for Exacerbations of COPD 310
JOHANNES M.A. DANIELS | MENNO M. VAN DER EERDEN

The Gastrointestinal System 312

35 Orocervical Infection 312
ROBERT C. READ

36 Gastritis, Peptic Ulceration and Related Conditions 321
JONATHAN R. WHITE | RICHARD J.M. INGRAM | JOHN C. ATHERTON

37 Food-Borne Diarrheal Illness 328
CHRISTOPHER P. CONLON

38 Acute Diarrhea 335
MICHEL DRANCOURT

39 Chronic Diarrhea 341
FLORENCE FENOLLAR

40 *Clostridium difficile* Infections in Hospitals and Community 351
MARTIJIN P. BAUER | ED J. KUIJPER

41 Intra-abdominal Sepsis, Peritonitis, Pancreatitis, Hepatobiliary and Focal Splenic Infection 355
P. RONAN O'CONNELL | GERARD SHEEHAN

42 Clinical Manifestations of Acute and Chronic Hepatitis 363
DAVID WYLES | JENNIFER LIN

PP11 Travelers' Diarrhea 375
PHILIPPE GAUTRET | PHILIPPE PAROLA

PP12 Febrile Transaminitis of Viral Etiology 377
STEVEN J. LAWRENCE

PP13 Management of CAPD Peritonitis 380
CARLOS A.Q. SANTOS

Bone and Joints 382

43 Infective and Reactive Arthritis 382
ARJUN GUPTA | ELIE F. BERBARI | JAMES M. STECKELBERG |
DOUGLAS R. OSMON

44 Acute and Chronic Osteomyelitis 388
SHIREESHA DHANIREDDY | SANTIAGO NEME

45 Infections of Prosthetic Joints and Related
Problems 399
SHADI PARSAEI | JAMES KEENEY | JONAS MARSCHALL

46 Lyme Disease 405
JOHN N. AUCOTT | BENJAMIN J. LUFT

Bloodstream, Heart and Vessels 415

47 Sepsis 415
TOM VAN DER POLL | WILLEM JOOST WIERSINGA

48 Infections Associated with Intravascular
Lines and Grafts 427
WINFRIED V. KERN

49 Systemic Candidiasis 439
BENOIT PILMIS | ZHI-TAO YANG | FANNY LANTERNIER |
OLIVIER LORTHOLARY

50 Myocarditis and Pericarditis 446
ADAM Z. BANKS | G. RALPH COREY

51 Endocarditis 456
FRANCK THUNY | GILBERT HABIB | DIDIER RAOULT |
PIERRE-EDOUARD FOURNIER

52 Rheumatic Fever 471
ABBY DOUGLAS | KUMAR VISVANATHAN

PP14 Management of Pericardial Effusion 478
FREDERIQUE GOURIET | PIERRE-YVES LEVY

PP15 Mediastinitis and Sternal
Osteomyelitis 481
CHRISTOPH SCHIMMER | RAINER G. LEYH

Obstetric and Gynecologic Infections 483

53 Vaginitis, Vulvitis, Cervicitis and Cutaneous
Vulval Lesions 483
JACK D. SOBEL

54 Infections of the Female Pelvis, Including
Septic Abortion 492
PAUL NYIRJESY | K. ASHLEY BRANDT

55 Complications of Pregnancy: Maternal
Perspectives 498
GUILLAUME DURAND | FLORENCE BRETELLE |
FLORENCE FENOLLAR

56 Fetal Implications of Maternal Infections in
Pregnancy 505
ARI BITNUN | HYTHEM AL-SUM | GREG RYAN

PP16 Treatment of a Positive *Toxoplasma* Titer in
Pregnancy 517
RONALD A. NICHOLS | THEODORE B. JONES

PP17 A Pregnant Patient with a Previous
Pregnancy Complicated by Group B
Streptococcal Disease in the Infant 520
UPTON D. ALLEN

Urinary Tract 523

57 Cystitis and Urethral Syndromes 523
STEPHEN T. CHAMBERS | SARAH C. METCALF

58 Prostatitis, Epididymitis and Orchitis 532
FLORIAN M.E. WAGENLEHNER | ADRIAN PILATZ |
WOLFGANG WEIDNER | KURT G. NABER

59 Complicated Urinary Infection, Including
Postsurgical and Catheter-Related
Infections 539
LINDSAY E. NICOLLE

60 Pyelonephritis and Abscesses of the
Kidney 547
ELODI J. DIELUBANZA | RICHARD S. MATULEWICZ |
ANTHONY J. SCHAEFFER

PP18 Tuberculosis of the Urogenital Tract 555
DAVID J. HORNE | ELIZABETH ANN MISCH

PP19 Urinary Tract Infections in Kidney Transplant
Recipients 557
KATHLEEN G. JULIAN | EMILY A. BLUMBERG

Sexually Transmitted Diseases 559

61 Syphilis 559
KHALIL G. GHANEM

62 Genital Herpes 567
CHRISTINE JOHNSTON | ANNA WALD

63 Human Papillomavirus Infections 575
VIKRANT V. SAHASRABUDDHE | STEN H. VERMUND

64 Lymphogranuloma Venereum, Chancroid
and Granuloma Inguinale 585
PAUL A. MACPHERSON | D. WILLIAM CAMERON

65 Management of Gonorrhea 592
JEANNE MARRAZZO

66 *Chlamydia trachomatis* Infection 597
STEPHEN J. JORDAN | WILLIAM M. GEISLER

PP20 Persistent and Recurrent Nongonococcal
Urethritis 603
REBECCA A. LILLIS | DAVID H. MARTIN

SECTION 3 Special Problems in Infectious Disease Practice

Fever 605

67 Pathogenesis of Fever 605
MOHAMMAD M. SAJADI | PHILIP A. MACKOWIAK

68 Fever of Unknown Origin (FUO) 611
CHESTON B. CUNHA | BURKE A. CUNHA

69 The Potential Role of Infectious
Agents in Diseases of Unknown
Etiology 625
STEVEN M. OPAL

70 Chronic Fatigue Syndrome 631
JOS W.M. VAN DER MEER | GIJS BLEIJENBERG

PP21 Factitious and Fraudulent Fever 636
ALICE CHIJIOKE EZIEFULA

PP22 Infection-Related Hemophagocytic
Syndromes 638
DENNIS W. SIMON | JOSEPH A. CARCILLO

PP23 Kawasaki Disease 640
KARI A. SIMONSEN

Environmental and Occupational Factors 643

71 Recreational Infections 643
PAVITHRA NATARAJAN | ALASTAIR MILLER

72 Occupational Infections 647
TAR-CHING AW | IAIN BLAIR | HILARY M. BABCOCK

73 Infections from Pets 656
ELLIE J.C. GOLDSTEIN | FREDRICK M. ABRAHAMIAN

74 Infections Acquired from Animals Other
Than Pets 663
DANIEL S. SHAPIRO

75 Bioterrorism and Biodefense 670
ANDREW W. ARTENSTEIN

PP24 Infections Associated with Drowning 680
ALASTAIR MILLER

PP25 Management of Human Bites 682
ELENI PATROZOU

Nosocomial Issues 684

76 Infectious Complications Following Surgery
and Trauma 684
HEATHER L. EVANS | EILEEN M. BULGER

77 Controlling Transmission of Antibiotic-
Resistant Bacteria in ICU Settings 693
MARC J.M. BONTEN

PP26 Infection in Burns 698
DAVID J. BARILLO | KEVIN K. CHUNG | CLINTON K. MURRAY

PP27 Transfusion-Related Infections 701
NAJAM A. ZAIDI

SECTION 4 Infections in the Immunocompromised Host

78 Immunodeficiencies 705
STEVEN M. HOLLAND | SERGIO D. ROSENZWEIG |
RICHARD F. SCHUMACHER | LUIGI D. NOTARANGELO

79 Infections in the Cancer Patient 723
OSCAR MARCHETTI | FREDERIC TISSOT |
THIERRY CALANDRA

80 Infections in Hematopoietic Stem Cell
Transplant Recipients 739
KIEREN A. MARR

81 Heart, Lung and Heart–Lung
Transplantation 746
PATRICIA MUÑOZ | MADDALENA GIANNELLA |
EMILIO BOUZA

82 Liver Transplantation 751
RAYMUND R. RAZONABLE

83 Intestinal Transplantation 756
KLARA M. POSFAY-BARBE | MARIAN G. MICHAELS |
MICHAEL D. GREEN

84 Kidney and Pancreas Transplant
Recipients 762
ORIOL MANUEL | CHRISTIAN TOSO |
MANUEL A. PASCUAL

85 Vasculitis and Other Immunologically
    Mediated Diseases 770
    JONATHAN COHEN

86 Splenectomy and Splenic Dysfunction 775
    STEVEN M. OPAL

87 Vaccination of the Immunocompromised
    Patient 780
    BERNARD P. VAUDAUX | SILJA BÜHLER |
    CHRISTIAN VAN DELDEN | CHRISTOPH BERGER

88 Infections Associated with
    Immunobiologics 796
    JULIE DELALOYE | CURDIN CONRAD | MICHEL GILLIET |
    GIUSEPPE PANTALEO | CAMILLO RIBI

PP28 Infectious Diseases Transmitted by
      Grafts 805
      ANDREA J. ZIMMER | LORA D. THOMAS

PP29 Evaluation of the HIV-Uninfected Adult with
      Suspected Immunodeficiency 808
      SARAH K. BROWNE

VOLUME 2

SECTION 5 HIV and AIDS

89 Epidemiology of HIV Infection 812
    RENNATUS MDODO | ANDREA A. KIM | KEVIN M. DE COCK

Prevention 824

90 Bio-behavioral Interventions to Prevent HIV
    Transmission 824
    KENNETH H. MAYER | MATTHEW J. MIMIAGA |
    STEVEN A. SAFREN

91 HIV Vaccines: Past Failures and Future
    Scientific Challenges 829
    BRUCE L. GILLIAM | ROBERT R. REDFIELD | BARRY S. PETERS

PP30 HIV Postexposure Prophylaxis 835
      ERNIE-PAUL BARRETTE | GEROME V. ESCOTA | RUPA PATEL

Pathogenesis 837

92 The Immunopathogenesis of HIV-1
    Infection 837
    RACHEL PRESTI | GIUSEPPE PANTALEO

Clinical Presentation 846

93 Primary HIV Infection 846
    BERNARD HIRSCHEL

94 Opportunistic Infections: Management and
    Prevention 850
    STÉPHANE DE WIT | NATHAN CLUMECK

95 Immune Reconstitution Disorders in Patients
    with HIV Infection 859
    MARTYN A. FRENCH | GRAEME MEINTJES

96 Tuberculosis in HIV 865
    STEPHEN D. LAWN | ROBIN WOOD

97 Neoplastic Disease 874
    CHRISTIAN HOFFMANN

98 Dermatologic Manifestations of HIV
    Infection/AIDS 879
    MISHA M. MUTIZWA | MILAN J. ANADKAT

99 HIV/AIDS-Related Problems in Low- and
    Middle-Income Countries 888
    STEVEN J. REYNOLDS | ALEXANDER C. BILLIOUX |
    THOMAS C. QUINN

PP31 How to Manage Hepatitis B Virus in the HIV
      Coinfected Patient 896
      JÜRGEN KURT ROCKSTROH | KARINE LACOMBE

PP32 How to Manage Hepatitis C Virus in the HIV
      Coinfected Patient 898
      JÜRGEN KURT ROCKSTROH | KARINE LACOMBE

AIDS in Women and Infants 900

100 HIV Infection in Children 900
     STÉPHANE BLANCHE

101 Special Problems in Women Who Have HIV
     Disease 905
     BEVERLY E. SHA | CONSTANCE A. BENSON

HIV Therapy 912

102 Principles of Management of HIV in the
     Industrialized World 912
     MARK W. HULL | MARIANNE HARRIS |
     JULIO S.G. MONTANER

103 Antiviral Therapy 918
     JOSE I. BERNARDINO | JOSE R. ARRIBAS

104 Issues in the Aging HIV-Positive
     Patient 927
     PATRICK W. MALLON | WILLIAM G. POWDERLY

105 Eradication and Cure of HIV 931
     STEPHEN J. KENT

PP33 Antiretroviral Management in Low- and Middle-Income Countries   936
SOMNUEK SUNGKANUPARPH

SECTION 6   International Medicine

Principles of International Health   938

106 Geography of Infectious Diseases   938
MARY ELIZABETH WILSON

107 Travel Medicine   948
JANE N. ZUCKERMAN

Major Tropical Syndromes: Skin and Soft Tissue   954

108 Leprosy   954
WARWICK J. BRITTON

109 Endemic Treponematoses   961
NICK J. BEECHING

Major Tropical Syndromes: The Central Nervous System   966

110 Human African Trypanosomiasis   966
CHRISTIAN BURRI | JOHANNES BLUM

111 Eosinophilic Meningitis   971
BRIAN JOHN ANGUS

112 Eye Infections in the Tropics   979
ROBIN BAILEY

Major Tropical Syndromes: The Gastrointestinal Tract   984

113 Approach to Eosinophilia in a Traveler from the Tropics   984
ANDREW P. USTIANOWSKI | JOOP E. ARENDS

114 Parasitic Infections of the Gastrointestinal Tract   989
PAUL KELLY | MABLE MUTENGO

115 Typhoid Fever and Other Enteric Fevers   1002
CHRISTIANE DOLECEK

116 Amebic Infections   1008
DAVID C. WARHURST

Major Tropical Syndromes: Systemic Infections   1014

117 Malaria   1014
ARJEN M. DONDORP | LORENZ VON SEIDLEIN

118 Schistosomiasis   1026
ALAN FENWICK

119 Cestode and Trematode Infections   1032
DAVID J. DIEMERT

120 Echinococcosis   1038
BRUNO GOTTSTEIN | GUIDO BELDI

121 Filarial Infections   1046
THOMAS B. NUTMAN

122 Infections and the Common Inherited Hemoglobin Disorders   1053
THOMAS N. WILLIAMS | DAVID J. WEATHERALL

123 Leishmaniasis   1059
ROBERT N. DAVIDSON

124 Chagas Disease (American Trypanosomiasis)   1065
MICHAEL A. MILES

125 Melioidosis   1073
SHARON J. PEACOCK | DIREK LIMMATHUROTSAKUL

126 Plague   1078
KENNETH L. GAGE | C. BEN BEARD

127 Tularemia   1085
JEANNINE M. PETERSEN | DAVID T. DENNIS | C. BEN BEARD

128 Scrub Typhus and Other Tropical Rickettsioses   1091
NICHOLAS P.J. DAY | PAUL N. NEWTON

129 Brucellosis   1098
NICK J. BEECHING | HAKAN ERDEM

130 Leptospirosis   1102
NICHOLAS P.J. DAY

131 Relapsing Fevers   1105
DAVID A. WARRELL

132 Viral Hemorrhagic Fevers   1110
AMANDA ROJEK | GAIL CARSON | YASUYUKI KATO | PETER W. HORBY | HAKAN LEBLEBICIOGLU

133 Dengue and Chikungunya 1119
CAMERON P. SIMMONS | JAMES WHITEHORN | KATHERINE ANDERS | VINH CHAU VAN NGUYEN

134 Anthrax 1123
MEHMET DOGANAY

135 The Patient Returning from the Tropics with Fever 1129
CHRISTOPHER J.M. WHITTY

PP34 Respiratory Tract Infection in a Traveler Returning from the Hajj 1132
SHRUTI SRIDHAR | JEAN-CHRISTOPHE LAGIER | PHILIPPE GAUTRET

PP35 Jaundice in the Traveler Returning from Nepal 1134
JUSTIN BEARDSLEY

PP36 Sexually Transmitted Infection in a Traveler Returning from South Africa 1137
A. WILLEM STURM

PP37 Lymphadenopathy, Splenomegaly and Anemia in a Traveler Returning from Sudan 1139
TOM DOHERTY

PP38 What are the Treatment Options for a Pregnant Patient with Malaria? 1141
ROSE MCGREADY | FRANÇOIS NOSTEN

SECTION 7 Anti-infective Therapy

136 Principles of Anti-infective Therapy and Surgical Prophylaxis 1145
EVELINA TACCONELLI | FEDERICO FOSCHI | CHRISTINA FORSTNER | ROGER G. FINCH | MATHIAS W. PLETZ

137 Mechanisms of Action 1162
FRANÇOISE VAN BAMBEKE | MARIE-PAULE MINGEOT-LECLERCQ | YOURI GLUPCZYNSKI | PAUL M. TULKENS

138 Mechanisms of Antibacterial Resistance 1181
GIAN MARIA ROSSOLINI | FABIO ARENA | TOMMASO GIANI

139 Optimizing the Use of Antimicrobial Agents: Antimicrobial Stewardship and Outpatient Parenteral Antimicrobial Therapy (OPAT) 1197
MATTHEW S. SIMON | DAVID P. CALFEE

140 β-Lactam Antibiotics 1203
RICHARD R. WATKINS | ROBERT A. BONOMO

141 Macrolides, Ketolides, Lincosamides and Streptogramins 1217
JENNIE H. KWON

142 Oxazolidinones 1230
FRANKLIN D. LOWY

143 Aminoglycosides 1233
JAMES E. LEGGETT

144 Quinolones 1239
ETHAN RUBINSTEIN† | PHILIPPE LAGACÉ-WIENS

145 Glycopeptides 1249
DIANE M. PARENTE | KERRY L. LAPLANTE

146 Tetracyclines and Chloramphenicol 1256
JASON M. POGUE | MICHAEL N. DUDLEY | AMBIKA ERANKI | KEITH S. KAYE

147 Nitroimidazoles, Metronidazole, Ornidazole and Tinidazole; and Fidaxomicin 1261
MARK H. WILCOX

148 Antituberculosis Agents 1264
GIOVANNI BATTISTA MIGLIORI | ALIMUDDIN ZUMLA

149 Miscellaneous Agents: Fusidic Acid, Nitrofurantoin and Fosfomycin 1277
ANGELA HUTTNER | STEPHAN HARBARTH

150 Folate Inhibitors 1280
EIRINI CHRISTAKI

151 Polymyxins 1285
MICHAEL J. SATLIN | STEPHEN G. JENKINS

PP39 Management Strategies for Drug-Resistant Infections 1289
GEORGE L. DAIKOS | MARIA SOULI | ANASTASIA ANTONIADOU

152 Drugs for HIV Infection 1293
BENJAMIN J. ECKHARDT | ROY M. GULICK

153 Drugs for Herpesvirus Infections 1309
MICHELLE R. SALVAGGIO | JOHN W. GNANN, JR.

154 Antiviral Agents Against Respiratory Viruses 1318
MICHAEL G. ISON | FREDERICK G. HAYDEN

155 Drugs to Treat Viral Hepatitis 1327
LEAH A. BURKE | KRISTEN M. MARKS

†Deceased

156 Systemic Antifungal Agents 1333
SHMUEL SHOHAM | ANDREAS H. GROLL |
VIDMANTAS PETRAITIS | THOMAS J. WALSH

157 Antiparasitic Agents 1345
F. MATTHEW KUHLMANN | JAMES M. FLECKENSTEIN

158 Probiotics 1373
JASMIN ISLAM

159 Infections Associated with
Biologics 1377
RUSSELL J. McCULLOH

160 Antibacterial Drugs: Looking Ahead From
the Past 1382
DAVID M. SHLAES

SECTION 8 Clinical Microbiology

General Principles 1386

161 Advances in Diagnostic Microbiology 1386
GRÉGORY DUBOURG | PIERRE-EDOUARD FOURNIER

Viruses 1390

162 Acute Gastroenteritis Viruses 1390
ARTURO S. GASTAÑADUY | RODOLFO E. BÉGUÉ

163 Measles, Mumps and Rubella Viruses 1399
SCOTT H. JAMES

164 Human Enteroviruses 1406
JOSÉ R. ROMERO

165 Hepatitis Viruses 1417
STÉPHANE CHEVALIEZ | JEAN-MICHEL PAWLOTSKY

166 Herpesviruses 1426
TYREL T. SMITH | RICHARD J. WHITLEY

167 Papillomaviruses 1439
RAPHAEL P. VISCIDI | PATTI E. GRAVITT

168 Polyomaviruses 1445
RAPHAEL P. VISCIDI | CHEN SABRINA TAN

169 Parvoviruses 1449
ALOYS C.M. KROES

170 Poxviruses 1452
R. MARK L. BULLER

171 Rabies and Rabies-Related
Viruses 1458
MARY J. WARRELL | DAVID A. WARRELL

172 Influenza Viruses 1465
SCOTT H. JAMES | RICHARD J. WHITLEY

173 Noninfluenza Respiratory Viruses 1472
MICHAEL G. ISON | NELSON LEE

174 Retroviruses and Retroviral Infections 1483
GEORGE B. KYEI | WILLIAM G. POWDERLY

175 Zoonotic Viruses 1493
LYLE R. PETERSEN | THOMAS G. KSIAZEK

Bacteria 1509

176 Staphylococci and Micrococci 1509
DAVID J. HETEM | SUZAN H.M. ROOIJAKKERS |
MIQUEL B. EKKELENKAMP

177 Streptococci and Enterococci 1523
ANDROULLA EFSTRATIOU | THERESA LAMAGNI |
CLAIRE E. TURNER

178 Aerobic Gram-Positive Bacilli 1537
GUY PROD'HOM | JACQUES BILLE

179 Neisseria 1553
TONE TØNJUM | JOS VAN PUTTEN

180 Enterobacteriaceae 1565
CLAIRE JENKINS | ROB J. RENTENAAR |
LUCE LANDRAUD | SYLVAIN BRISSE

181 Pseudomonas spp., Acinetobacter spp.
and Miscellaneous Gram-Negative
Bacilli 1579
HILMAR WISPLINGHOFF

182 Curved and Spiral Bacilli 1600
FRANCIS MÉGRAUD | DIDIER MUSSO |
MICHEL DRANCOURT | PHILIPPE LEHOURS

183 Gram-Negative Coccobacilli 1611
FIONA J. COOKE | MARY P.E. SLACK

184 Anaerobic Bacteria 1628
ITZHAK BROOK

185 Mycobacteria 1645
JAKKO VAN INGEN

186 Mycoplasma and Ureaplasma 1660
JØRGEN SKOV JENSEN

187 Rickettsia and Rickettsia-Like
Organisms 1666
EMMANOUIL ANGELAKIS | DIDIER RAOULT

188 Chlamydia 1676
MIRJA PUOLAKKAINEN | PEKKA A.I. SAIKKU

Fungi 1681

189 Opportunistic and Systemic
Fungi 1681
CHRIS KOSMIDIS | DAVID W. DENNING

190 Superficial and Subcutaneous Fungal
Pathogens 1710
MALCOLM D. RICHARDSON | CAROLINE B. MOORE

Parasites 1725

191 Protozoa: Intestinal and Urogenital Amebae,
Flagellates and Ciliates 1725
LYNNE S. GARCIA

192 Intestinal Coccidia and Microsporidia 1734
RAINER WEBER

193 Protozoa: Free-Living Amebae 1744
JENNIFER RITTENHOUSE COPE | JONATHAN S. YODER |
GOVINDA S. VISVESVARA

194 Blood and Tissue Protozoa 1751
MARÍA-JESÚS PINAZO | EDELWEISS ALDASORO |
ANTONIA CALVO-CANO | ALBERT PICADO |
JOSE MUÑOZ | JOAQUIM GASCON

195 Helminths 1763
H.D. ALAN LINDQUIST | JOHN H. CROSS[†]

Index I1

[†]Deceased

PREFACE TO THE FOURTH EDITION

We live in interesting times. The discipline of infectious diseases has rarely faced so much promise, and yet such peril. The possibility of an AIDS-free world within the next generation is now seriously contemplated, based on the intelligent use of combinations of antiretroviral agents and selected use of pre-exposure prophylaxis, and even without the benefit of a vaccine that induces sterilizing immunity against human immunodeficiency virus (HIV). This would not have seemed possible even 25 years ago. Similarly, the remarkable success story of possibly curing hepatitis C virus (HCV) with safe, oral, directly acting, antiviral agents is now well within our grasp. Only 30 years ago the cause of non-A non-B post-transfusion hepatitis was unknown and no serologic test was available to detect carriers and prevent transmission. Real progress in developing a multistage malaria vaccine has recently been made, and a vaccine for dengue is on the horizon. Promising and innovative vaccine strategies using reverse genetic approaches are now in development, targeting recalcitrant bacterial, fungal and parasitic pathogens. Rapid molecular diagnostics are finally making huge inroads in the clinical microbiology laboratory. Such advances are essential if we are to be able to make accurate diagnoses within hours and provide optimal care for our patients in this era of precision medicine.

Yet despite these advances, we are constantly reminded of just how fragile our dominion over the microbial world really is. The human population has swelled to over 7 billion inhabitants; most now reside in crowded cities, often without the benefits of adequate sanitation or reliable nutrition. As Paul Farmer has written, physicians 'need to think hard about poverty and inequality, which influence any population's morbidity and mortality', and this is no more so than in the case of infectious diseases. The global spread of antimicrobial resistance now poses the very real threat of infection for which there are no effective treatments. Novel resistance mechanisms in gram-negative bacteria have emerged and spread rapidly across the world, challenging the foundations of the modern era of medicine. Drug-resistant tuberculosis, including infection with organisms that are extensively resistant (XDR-TB), continues to challenge global efforts at control. Despite the extensive efforts to provide global access to antiretroviral therapy, new cases of HIV continue in epidemic numbers, and many continue to die from AIDS. The spread of vector-borne pathogens, especially dengue, chikungunya and Zika, continues and corona virus-related Middle Eastern respiratory syndrome has emerged as yet another unexpected challenge. Zika-induced microcephaly is hugely important and clearly demonstrates our continued vulnerability to new microbial threats. However, nothing has demonstrated our collective vulnerability to pathogenic infection more than the West African outbreak of Ebola which showed the world the devastating effects of a lethal infection. Although ultimately controlled by effective infection prevention, this outbreak reminded us of the continued importance of understanding, preventing and treating infectious diseases.

It is against this background that we have prepared this fourth edition of *Infectious Diseases*. In doing this we have been conscious not only of the extraordinary developments in the science and practice of infection, but also in the evolving needs of our readers. Scientists and practitioners turn to books like this both for specific information on unfamiliar subjects but also as a source for further education and training. Mindful of this, we have introduced a variety of exciting new elements to the book. Alongside our widely acclaimed Practice Points offering pithy, practical advice on common management problems we have now added several new features designed to assist our readers. These include online mannequins providing a ready reference to pharmacokinetic data on antimicrobial agents, which are traditionally difficult to access in an easily useful form, and also a portfolio of online multiple choice questions, fully supported by reference material, as a resource for postgraduate education. We are grateful to our two new Associate Editors in Medical Education, Bethany Davies and Courtney Chrisler, for their help with this important new addition to the book. As ever, we are indebted to the extraordinary commitment and expertise of our Section Editor colleagues and to the very many expert contributors who have so graciously agreed to undertake comprehensive revision of their chapters from the previous edition, and, in many cases, write completely new chapters. We also wish to express our profound thanks to the team at Elsevier who have cajoled, supported and encouraged us to get this done, in particular Sharon Nash, Jo Souch and Belinda Kuhn, and last but by no means least, we thank the Section Editors from the previous edition, Jack Sobel, Roger Finch, Scott Hammer, Tim Kiehn and Keith McAdam, without whom we would never have been in a position to prepare this new edition of the book. We hope that you, the reader, will find what you are looking for and we welcome feedback on how we can continue to improve *Infectious Diseases*.

Jon Cohen
William Powderly
Steven Opal

The editors would like to acknowledge and offer grateful thanks for the input of all previous editions' contributors, without whom this new edition would not have been possible.

Fredrick M. Abrahamian, DO, FACEP, FIDSA
Clinical Professor of Medicine
David Geffen School of Medicine at UCLA
Los Angeles, CA, USA
Director of Education
Department of Emergency Medicine
Olive View-UCLA Medical Center
Sylmar, CA, USA

Michael J. Aldape, PhD
Research Investigator
Infectious Disease Section
Department of Research and Development
Veterans Affairs Medical Center
Boise, ID, USA

Edelweiss Aldasoro, MD
Medical Research Fellow
ISGlobal, Barcelona Ctr. Int. Health Res. (CRESIB), Hospital
   Clínic-Universitat de Barcelona
Barcelona, Spain

Upton D. Allen, MBBS, MSc, FAAP, FRCPC, Hon FRCP(UK), FIDSA
Professor of Paediatrics
Division of Infectious Diseases
Department of Paediatrics
Hospital for Sick Children
University of Toronto
Toronto, ON, Canada

Hythem Al-Sum, MD
Clinical Fellow
Maternal-Fetal Medicine Division
Department of Obstetrics and Gynaecology
Mount Sinai Hospital-University of Toronto
Toronto, ON, Canada

Milan J. Anadkat, MD
Associate Professor of Medicine
Division of Dermatology
Washington University School of Medicine in St Louis
St Louis, MO, USA

Katherine Anders, MSc, PhD
Epidemiologist and Data Manager
Eliminate Dengue Program
Monash University
Melbourne, Australia

Emmanouil Angelakis, MD, PhD
Assistant Unité de Recherche sur les Maladies Infectieuses et
   Tropicales Emergentes
Aix–Marseille Université
Marseille, France

Brian John Angus, MBChB, MD, DTM&H, FRCP
Associate Professor and Reader in Infectious Diseases
Nuffield Department of Medicine
University of Oxford
Oxford, UK

Anastasia Antoniadou, MD
Associate Professor of Medicine and Infectious Diseases
Fourth Department of Medicine
National and Kapodistrian University of Athens
Athens, Greece

Fabio Arena, MD
Senior Research Fellow in Clinical Microbiology
Department of Medical Biotechnologies
University of Siena
Siena, Italy

Joop E. Arends, MD, PhD
Infectious Diseases Physician
Internal Medicine and Infectious Diseases
University Medical Center Utrecht (UMCU)
Utrecht, The Netherlands

Jose R. Arribas, MD
Head, Infectious Diseases Unit, Internal Medicine
Hospital La Paz
Madrid, Spain

Andrew W. Artenstein, MD
Chair, Department of Medicine
Baystate Health
Tufts University School of Medicine Chair of Medicine at Baystate
   Medical Center
Professor of Medicine
Tufts University School of Medicine
Springfield, MA, USA

John C. Atherton, MD, FRCP
Professor of Gastroenterology, Pro-Vice Chancellor and Dean of the
   Faculty of Medicine and Health Sciences
NIHR Biomedical Research Unit in Gastrointestinal and Liver
   Diseases
Nottingham University Hospitals NHS Trust
University of Nottingham, Queen's Medical Centre
Nottingham, UK

John N. Aucott, MD
Assistant Professor of Medicine
Division of Rheumatology
Johns Hopkins University School of Medicine
Baltimore, MD, USA

Tar-Ching Aw, MB, PhD, FRCPC, FFOM
Professor (EVP)
PAPRSB Institute of Health Sciences
Universiti Brunei Darussalam
Adjunct Professor
Herbert Wertheim College of Medicine
Florida International University
Miami, FL, USA

Hilary M. Babcock, MD, MPH
Medical Director
BJC Infection Prevention and Epidemiology Consortium
Medical Director of Occupational Health (Infectious Diseases)
Barnes-Jewish and St Louis Children's Hospitals
Associate Professor of Medicine
Infectious Disease Division
Department of Medicine
Washington University School of Medicine in St Louis
St Louis, MO, USA

Robin Bailey, BA, BM, FRCP, PhD, DTMH
Professor of Tropical Medicine
Department of Clinical Research
Faculty of Infectious and Tropical Diseases
London School of Hygiene and Tropical Medicine
London, UK

Thomas C. Bailey, MD
Professor of Medicine
Infectious Diseases Division
Department of Medicine
Washington University School of Medicine in St Louis
St Louis, MO, USA

Adam Z. Banks, MD
Resident, PGY-3
Department of Internal Medicine
Duke University Medical Center
Durham, NC, USA

David J. Barillo, MD, FACS, FCCM
Colonel (retired)
US Army Reserve
Disaster Response/Critical Care Consultants, LLC
Mount Pleasant, SC, USA

Ernie-Paul Barrette, MD, FACP
Associate Professor of Medicine
Department of Internal Medicine
Division of Infectious Diseases
Washington University School of Medicine in St Louis
St Louis, MO, USA

Martijn P. Bauer, MD, PhD
Senior Medical Specialist, Infectious Diseases
Center of Infectious Disease
Leiden University Medical Centre
Leiden, The Netherlands

Roger Bayston, MMedSci, MSc, PhD, FRCPath
Professor of Surgical Infection
School of Medicine
University of Nottingham
Nottingham, UK

C. Ben Beard, MS, PhD
Chief, Bacterial Diseases Branch
Division of Vector-Borne Diseases
US Centers for Disease Control and Prevention
Fort Collins, CO, USA

Justin Beardsley, MBChB
Senior Clinical Research Fellow
Nuffield Department of Medicine
Oxford University Clinical Research Unit
Ho Chi Minh City, Vietnam

Nick J. Beeching, MA, BMBCh, FRCP, FRACP, FFTM, RCPS(Glasg), DCH, DTM&H
Senior Clinical Lecturer
Department of Clinical Sciences and NIHR Health Protection
    Research Unit in Emerging and Zoonotic Infections
Liverpool School of Tropical Medicine
Pembroke Place
Liverpool, UK

Rodolfo E. Bégué, MD
Professor of Pediatrics
Department of Pediatrics
Louisiana State University HSC School of Medicine
New Orleans, LA, USA

Guido Beldi, MD
Professor in Surgery
Department for Visceral Surgery and Medicine
Bern University Hospital
University of Bern
Bern, Switzerland

Constance A. Benson, MD, FACP, FIDSA
Professor of Medicine and Global Public Health
Infectious Diseases Training Program Director
Divisions of Infectious Diseases and Global Public Health
Department of Medicine
University of California, San Diego
San Diego, CA, USA

Elie F. Berbari, MD
Professor of Medicine
Division of Infectious Diseases
Section of Orthopedic Infectious Diseases
Mayo Clinic College of Medicine
Rochester, MN, USA

Jean-Michel Berenger, MD
Medical Entomologist
Aix–Marseille Université
URMITE
Marseille, France

Christoph Berger, MD
Associate Professor of Pediatrics and Pediatric Infectious Diseases
Division of Infectious Diseases and Hospital Epidemiology
University Children's Hospital
Zürich, Switzerland

Jose I. Bernardino, MD
Assistant Physician
HIV Unit, Department of Internal Medicine
Hospital Universitario La Paz, IdiPAZ
Madrid, Spain

Jacques Bille, MD
Honorary Professor of Medical Microbiology
Institute of Microbiology
Lausanne University Hospital Center and University of Lausanne
Lausanne, Switzerland

Alexander C. Billioux, MD, DPhil
Assistant Chief of Service, Thayer Firm
Department of Medicine
The Johns Hopkins Hospital
Baltimore, MD, USA

Ari Bitnun, MD, MSc
Associate Professor
Department of Pediatrics
Hospital for Sick Children
University of Toronto
Toronto, ON, Canada

Iain Blair, MBBChir, MA, MFCM, MRCGP
Associate Professor
Institute of Public Health
College of Medicine and Health Sciences
United Arab Emirates University
Al Ain, Abu Dhabi, United Arab Emirates

Stéphane Blanche, MD
Professor of Pediatrics
Immunology and Hematology Unit
Hôpital Necker–Enfants Malades
University René Descartes
Paris, France

Thomas P. Bleck, MD
Professor of Neurological Sciences, Neurosurgery, Medicine, and
  Anesthesiology
Rush University Medical Center
Chicago, IL, USA

Chantal P. Bleeker-Rovers, MD, PhD
Internist-Specialist in Infectious Diseases
Department of Internal Medicine
Division of Infectious Diseases
Radboud University Medical Center
Nijmegen, The Netherlands

Gijs Bleijenberg, PhD
Professor Emeritus
Expert Centre for Chronic Fatigue
Radboud University Medical Center
Nijmegen, The Netherlands

Karen C. Bloch, MD, MPH
Associate Professor
Departments of Medicine (Infectious Diseases) and Health Policy
Vanderbilt University School of Medicine
Nashville, TN, USA

Johannes Blum, MD
Professor
Department of Medical Services and Diagnostics
Swiss Tropical and Public Health Institute and University of Basel
Basel, Switzerland

Emily A. Blumberg, MD
Professor of Medicine, Director Transplant Infectious Diseases
Department of Medicine
Perelman School of Medicine at the University of Pennsylvania
Philadelphia, PA, USA

Robert A. Bonomo, MD
Chief, Medical Service
Louis Stokes Cleveland Department of Veterans Affairs Medical
  Center
Professor of Medicine, Pharmacology, Biochemistry, Molecular
  Biology and Microbiology
Case Western Reserve University School of Medicine
Cleveland, OH, USA

Marc J.M. Bonten, MD, PhD
Professor of Molecular Epidemiology of Infectious Diseases
Department of Medical Microbiology
Julius Center for Health Sciences and Primary Care
University Medical Center Utrecht
Utrecht, The Netherlands

Rafik Bourayou, MD
Hospital Practitioner
Department of Pediatrics
Bicêtre Hospital
Paris, France

Emilio Bouza, MD, PhD
Head, Clinical Microbiology and ID Division
Hospital Gregorio Marañón
Universidad Complutense de Madrid
Madrid, Spain

K. Ashley Brandt, DO
Resident Physician
Department of Obstetrics and Gynecology
Drexel University College of Medicine
Philadelphia, PA, USA

Florence Bretelle, MD, PhD
Professor of Obstetrics and Gynaecology
Department of Obstetrics and Gynaecology
University of Marseille
Marseille, France

Sylvain Brisse, PhD
Research Director
Microbial Evolutionary Genomics
Institut Pasteur
Paris, France

**Warwick J. Britton, PhD, MBBS, FAAHMS, FRACP,
FRCP, FRCPA**
Bosch Professor of Medicine and Immunology
Centenary Institute and Discipline of Medicine
Sydney Medical School
University of Sydney
Sydney, Australia

Itzhak Brook, MD
Professor of Pediatrics
Georgetown University School of Medicine
Washington DC, USA

Matthijs C. Brouwer, MD, PhD
Neurologist
Department of Neurology
Academic Medical Center
University of Amsterdam
Amsterdam, The Netherlands

Sarah K. Browne, MD
Assistant Clinical Investigator
Division of Intramural Research
National Institute of Allergy and Infectious Diseases
National Institutes of Health
Bethesda, MD, USA
Division of Vaccines and Related Product Applications
Center for Biologics Evaluation and Research, Food and Drug
  Administration
Silver Spring, MD, USA

Amy E. Bryant, PhD
Research Career Scientist
Infectious Disease Section
Research and Development Service
Veterans Affairs Medical Center
Boise, ID, USA

Silja Bühler, MD, MSc
Research Scientist
Division of Infectious Diseases
Epidemiology, Biostatistics and Prevention Institute
University of Zurich
Zurich, Switzerland

Eileen M. Bulger, MD, FACS
Professor, Chief of Trauma
Department of Surgery
Harborview Medical Center, University of Washington
Seattle, WA, USA

R. Mark L. Buller, PhD
Professor of Molecular Microbiology and Immunology
Department of Molecular Microbiology and Immunology
Saint Louis University
St Louis, MO, USA

Leah A. Burke, MD
Instructor of Medicine
Department of Medicine
Division of Infectious Diseases
Weill Cornell Medical College
New York, NY, USA

Christian Burri, PhD, MPharm
Professor
Department of Medicines Research
Swiss Tropical and Public Health Institute
University of Basel
Basel, Switzerland

Marcus W. Butler, MD, MBBCh, FRCPI
Consultant Respiratory Physician
University College Dublin
School Of Medicine
St Vincent's Hospital
Dublin, Ireland

Thierry Calandra, MD, PhD
Chairman, Department of Medicine
Head, Infectious Diseases Service
CHUV (Centre Hospitalier Universitaire Vaudois)
Lausanne, Switzerland

David P. Calfee, MD, MS
Associate Professor
Departments of Medicine and Health Policy and Research
Weill Cornell Medical College
New York, NY, USA

Antonia Calvo-Cano, MD
Medical Research Fellow
ISGlobal, Barcelona Ctr. Int. Health Res. (CRESIB), Hospital
    Clínic-Universitat de Barcelona
Barcelona, Spain

D. William Cameron, MD, FRCPC, FACP
Professor of Medicine
Divisions of Infectious Diseases and Respirology
Senior Scientist
Clinical Epidemiology Program
University of Ottawa at The Ottawa Hospital Research Institute
Ottawa, ON, Canada

Joseph A. Carcillo, MD
Professor of Critical Care Medicine and Pediatrics
University of Pittsburgh
Pittsburgh, PA, USA

Gail Carson, MBChB, MRCP, DTM&H
Clinical Coordinator and Consultant in Infectious Diseases
International Severe Acute Respiratory and Emerging Infection
    Consortium
Centre for Tropical Medicine and Global Health
Nuffield Department of Medicine
University of Oxford
Oxford, UK

Stephen T. Chambers, MBChB, MSc, MD, FRACP
Professor
Department of Pathology
University of Otago, Christchurch
Clinical Director
Department of Infectious Diseases
Christchurch Hospital
Christchurch, New Zealand

Remi N. Charrel, MD, PhD
Head, Emergence and Genomics of RNA Viruses
IRD French Institute of Research for Development, INSERM U1207
EHESP French School of Public Health,
EPV UMR190 "Emergence des Pathologies Virales"
IHU Méditerranée Infection, APHM Public Hospitals of Marseille
Aix Marseille Université
Marseille, France

Vinh Chau Van Nguyen, MD, PhD
Director of the Hospital for Tropical Diseases
Ho Chi Minh City, Vietnam
Deputy Head of Infectious Disease Division
University of Medicine and Pharmacy
Ho Chi Minh City, Vietnam

Stéphane Chevaliez, PharmD, PhD
Professor of Medicine
Department of Virology
Henri Mondor Hospital
University of Paris-Est & INSERM U955
Creteil, France

Tom M. Chiller, MD
Associate Director for Epidemiologic Science
Division of Foodborne, Waterborne and Environmental Diseases
National Center for Emerging and Zoonotic Infectious Diseases
Centers for Disease Control and Prevention
Atlanta, GA, USA

Eirini Christaki, MD
Infectious Diseases Consultant
Department of Medicine
AHEPA University Hospital
Thessaloniki, Greece
Research Associate in Medicine
Alpert Medical School of Brown University
Providence, RI, USA

Kevin K. Chung, MD, FCCM, FACP
Director of Research
US Army Institute of Surgical Research, Fort Sam
Houston, TX, USA

David B. Clifford, MD
Melba and Forest Seay Professor of
Clinical Neuropharmacology in Neurology
Washington University in St Louis
Saint Louis, MO, USA

Nathan Clumeck, MD, PhD
Professor of Infectious Diseases
Honorary Head, Department of Infectious Diseases
Saint-Pierre University Hospital
Brussels, Belgium

Jonathan Cohen, MB, FRCP, FRCPE, FRCPath, FMedSci
Emeritus Professor of Infectious Diseases
Brighton and Sussex Medical School
Brighton, UK

John Collinge, MRCP, MD, FRCPath
Professor of Neurology
Head of Department
Department of Neurodegenerative Diseases/Director
MRC Prion Unit
Institute of Neurology
University College London
London, UK

Christopher P. Conlon, MA, MD, FRCP, FRCPI
Professor of Infectious Diseases
Nuffield Department of Medicine
University of Oxford
Consultant Physician
Oxford University Hospitals NHS Foundation Trust
Oxford, UK

Curdin Conrad, MD, PD&MER
Head of the Psoriasis Center
Department of Dermatology
University Hospital of Lausanne, CHUV
Lausanne, Switzerland

Fiona J. Cooke, MA, PhD, MSc, MRCP, FRCPath, DTM&H
Consultant Medical Microbiologist
Clinical Microbiology and Public Health Laboratory
Cambridge University Hospitals NHS Foundation Trust
Cambridge, UK

Jennifer Rittenhouse Cope, MD, MPH
Medical Epidemiologist
National Center for Emerging and Zoonotic Infectious Diseases
Centers for Disease Control and Prevention
Atlanta, GA, USA

G. Ralph Corey, MD
Professor of Medicine and Pathology
Department of Medicine
Duke University Medical Center
Durham, NC, USA

The late John H. Cross, PhD
Professor
Tropical Public Health
Department of Preventive Medicine and Biometrics
Uniformed Services University of the Health Sciences
Bethesda, MD, USA

Burke A. Cunha, MD, MACP
Chief, Infectious Disease Division
Winthrop-University Hospital
Mineola, New York
Professor of Medicine
State University of New York School of Medicine
Stony Brook, NY, USA

Cheston B. Cunha, MD
Assistant Professor of Medicine
Medical Director, Antimicrobial Stewardship Program
Division of Infectious Disease
Brown University Alpert School of Medicine, Rhode Island Hospital
    and Miriam Hospital
Providence, RI, USA

Benoit D'Journo, MD, PhD
Professor
Service de Chirurgie Thoracique
Assitance Publique-Hôpitaux de Marseille
Marseille, France

George L. Daikos, MD
Professor of Medicine and Infectious Diseases
First Department of Medicine
National and Kapodistrian University of Athens
Athens, Greece

Johannes M.A. Daniels, MD, PhD
Pulmonologist
Department of Pulmonary Diseases
VU University Medical Center
Amsterdam, The Netherlands

Robert N. Davidson, MD, FRCP, DTM&H
Consultant Physician
Department of Infectious Diseases and Tropical Medicine
Northwick Park Hospital
Harrow, UK

Nicholas P.J. Day, MA, BMBCh, DM, FRCP, FMedSci
Professor of Tropical Medicine
University of Oxford
Director, Mahidol-Oxford Tropical Medicine Research Unit
Faculty of Tropical Medicine
Mahidol University
Bangkok, Thailand

Kevin M. De Cock, MD, FRCP (UK), DTM&H
Director
Division of Global HIV/AIDS-Kenya
Centers for Disease Control and Prevention
Nairobi, Kenya

Thushan I. de Silva, BSc, MBChB, MRCP, FRCPath, DTM&H, PhD
NIHR Academic Clinical Lecturer in Infectious Diseases and
    Microbiology
Department of Infection and Tropical Medicine
Royal Hallamshire Hospital
Sheffield, UK

Henry J.C. de Vries, MD, PhD
Dermatologist
Department of Dermatology
Academic Medical Center (AMC)
University of Amsterdam
Amsterdam, The Netherlands
Center for Infection and Immunology Amsterdam (CINIMA)
Academic Medical Center (AMC)
University of Amsterdam
Amsterdam, The Netherlands
STI Outpatient Clinic
Public Health Service of Amsterdam (GGD Amsterdam)
Amsterdam, The Netherlands

Stéphane de Wit, MD, PhD
Head of Department
Infectious Diseases
Saint-Pierre University Hospital
Brussels, Belgium

Julie Delaloye, MD, PhD
Infectious Disease Specialist
Centre Hospitalier Universitaire Vaudois
Lausanne, Switzerland

David W. Denning, FRCP, FRCPath, FMedSci
Professor of Infectious Diseases in Global Health
The University of Manchester
Director
National Aspergillosis Centre
University Hospital of South Manchester
Manchester, UK

David T. Dennis, MD, MPH
Medical Epidemiologist
Centers for Disease Control and Prevention (Ret.)
Fort Collins, CO, USA

Shireesha Dhanireddy, MD
Associate Professor
Division of Infectious Diseases, Department of Medicine
University of Washington
Seattle, WA, USA

Elodi J. Dielubanza, MD
Housestaff Physician
Department of Urology
Feinberg School of Medicine Northwestern University
Chicago, IL, USA

David J. Diemert, MD, FRCP(C)
Associate Professor
Department of Microbiology
Immunology and Tropical Medicine
George Washington University School of Medicine and Health
  Sciences
Washington, DC, USA

Mehmet Doganay, MD
Professor of Infectious Diseases
Department of Infectious Diseases
Faculty of Medicine, Erciyes University
Kayseri, Turkey

Tom Doherty, MD, FRCP, DTM&H
Consultant Physician
Hospital for Tropical Diseases
University College London Hospitals
London, UK

Christiane Dolecek, MD, PhD, FRCP
University Research Lecturer
Centre for Tropical Medicine and Global Health
Nuffield Department of Medicine
Spatial Ecology and Epidemiology Group
Department of Zoology
University of Oxford
Oxford, UK

Arjen M. Dondorp, MD, PhD
Professor of Tropical Medicine
University of Oxford
Oxford, UK

Abby Douglas, MBBS(Hons), BMedSci
Infectious Diseases Registrar
Department of Infectious Diseases
St Vincent's Hospital Melbourne
Melbourne, Australia

Michel Drancourt, MD, PhD
Professor
Unité de Recherches sur les Maladies Infectieuses et Tropicales
  Emergentes
Aix–Marseille Université
Marseille, France

Grégory Dubourg, PharmD
University Hospital Assistant
Unité de Recherche sur les Maladies Infectieuses et Tropicales
  Emergentes
Aix-Marseille University
Marseille, France

Michael N. Dudley, PharmD, FIDSA
Senior Vice President and Chief Scientific Officer (Rempex)
Health Sciences Lead
Infectious Diseases Global Innovation Group
The Medicines Company
San Diego, CA, USA

Guillaume Durand, MD
Medicine Resident
Unité de Recherche sur les Maladies Infectieuses et Tropicales
  Emergentes
University of Marseille
Marseille, France

Benjamin J. Eckhardt, MD
Infectious Diseases Fellow
Division of Infectious Diseases
Weill Cornell Medical College
New York, NY, USA

Androulla Efstratiou, PhD
Director
WHO Collaborating Centre for Reference and Research on
  Diphtheria and Streptococcal Infections
Reference Microbiology Division
Public Health England (PHE)
London, UK

Miquel B. Ekkelenkamp, MD, PhD
Clinical Microbiologist
Department of Medical Microbiology
University Medical Center Utrecht
Utrecht, The Netherlands

Ambika Eranki, MD, MPH
Assistant Professor
Division of Infectious Disease
Department of Medicine
State University of New York/Upstate Medical Center
Syracuse, NY, USA

Hakan Erdem, MD
Professor of Infectious Diseases and Clinical Microbiology
Gulhane Medical Academy and Infectious Diseases Department
GATA Hospital
Etlik, Ankara, Turkey

Gerome V. Escota, MD
Clinical Instructor of Medicine
Division of Infectious Disease
Washington University School of Medicine in Saint Louis
Saint Louis, MO, USA

Heather L. Evans, MD, MS, FACS
Associate Professor of Surgery
Department of Surgery
University of Washington
Seattle, WA, USA

Alice Chijioke Eziefula, MA, MBBS, MRCP, FRCPath
Specialist Registrar in Infectious Diseases and Medical Microbiology
Department of Infection
Brighton and Sussex University Hospitals NHS Trust
Brighton, UK

Florence Fenollar, MD, PhD
Professor
Institut Hospitalo-Universitaire Méditerranée-Infection
Aix–Marseille Université
Marseille, France

Alan Fenwick, PhD
Professor of Tropical Parasitology
Department of Infectious Disease Epidemiology
Imperial College London
London, UK

Joshua Fierer, MD
Chief, Infectious Disease
VA San Diego Healthcare System
Professor of Medicine and Pathology
University of California San Diego
San Diego, CA, USA

Roger G. Finch, MBBS, FRCP, FRCPath, FRCPEd, FFPM
Professor of Infectious Diseases
School of Molecular Medical Science
Division of Microbiology and Infectious Disease
Nottingham University Hospitals NHS Trust
Nottingham, UK

James M. Fleckenstein, MD
Associate Professor of Medicine and Molecular Microbiology
Department of Medicine, Division of Infectious Diseases
Washington University School of Medicine in St Louis
St Louis, MO, USA

Christina Forstner, MD
Assistant Professor
Specialist for Internal Medicine
Department of Medicine I
Division of Infectious Diseases and Tropical Medicine
Medical University of Vienna
Vienna, Austria

Federico Foschi, MD
Resident Physician
Department of Internal Medicine I
Division of Infectious Diseases
Tübingen University Hospital
Tübingen, Germany

Pierre-Edouard Fournier, MD, PhD
Professor of Clinical Microbiology
Institut Hospitalo-Universitaire Méditerranée-Infection
Aix-Marseille Université
Marseille, France

Martyn A. French, MB ChB, MD, FRCPath, FRCP, FRACP
Professor in Clinical Immunology
School of Pathology and Laboratory Medicine
University of Western Australia
Perth, Australia

Kenneth L. Gage, PhD
Chief, Entomology and Ecology Activity
Bacterial Diseases Branch
Division of Vector-Borne Diseases
Centers for Disease Control and Prevention
Fort Collins, CO, USA

Lynne S. Garcia, MS, CLS, FAAM
Director
LSG & Associates
Santa Monica, CA, USA

Joaquim Gascon, MD, PhD
Research Professor
ISGlobal, Barcelona Ctr. Int. Health Res. (CRESIB), Hospital Clínic-Universitat de Barcelona
Barcelona, Spain

Arturo S. Gastañaduy, MD
Associate Professor of Pediatrics
Department of Pediatrics
Louisiana State University HSC School of Medicine
New Orleans, LA, USA

Philippe Gautret, MD, PhD, MSc, DTM&H
Director of Travel Clinic
University Hospital Institute for Infectious Diseases and Tropical Medicine, Méditerranée Infection
Aix-Marseille University
Marseille, France

William M. Geisler, MD, MPH
Professor
Department of Medicine, Division of Infectious Diseases
The University of Alabama at Birmingham
Birmingham, AL, USA

Khalil G. Ghanem, MD, PhD
Associate Professor of Medicine
Division of Infectious Diseases
Johns Hopkins University School of Medicine
Baltimore, MD, USA

Tommaso Giani, PhD
Assistant Professor
Department of Medical Biotechnologies
University of Siena
Siena, Italy

Maddalena Giannella, MD, PhD
ID Consultant
Infectious Diseases Unit, Department of Medical and Surgical
    Sciences
Sant'Orsola Hospital, University of Bologna
Bologna, Italy

Bruce L. Gilliam, MD
Associate Professor of Medicine
Institute of Human Virology
University of Maryland School of Medicine
Baltimore, MD, USA

Michel Gilliet, MS
Chief of Service
Dermatology
Department of Medicine
Centre Hospitalier Universitaire Vaudois
Lausanne, Switzerland

Carol A. Glaser, DVM, MD
Associate Clinical Professor of Pediatrics
Division of Pediatric Infectious Diseases
University of California, San Francisco
San Francisco, CA, USA

Youri Glupczynski, MD, PhD
Professor and Head of Clinical Microbiology
Microbiology Laboratory and National Reference Laboratory for
    Monitoring of Antimicrobial Resistance in Gram-Negative
    Bacteria
CHU Dinant-Godinne, UCL Namur
Yvoir, Belgium

John W. Gnann, Jr, MD
Professor of Medicine
Department of Medicine, Division of Infectious Diseases
Medical University of South Carolina
Charleston, SC, USA

Ellie J.C. Goldstein, MD, FSHEA, FIDSA
Clinical Professor of Medicine
David Geffen School of Medicine at UCLA
Los Angeles, CA, USA
Director, R.M. Alden Research Laboratory
Santa Monica, CA, USA

Bruno Gottstein, PhD, AssEVPC
Full Professor of Medical and Veterinary Parasitology
Institute of Parasitology
Department of Infectious Diseases and Pathobiology
University of Bern
Bern, Switzerland

Frederique Gouriet, MD, PhD
Physician
Research Unit of Emerging Infectious and Tropical Diseases
Faculty of Medicine
Aix-Marseille University
Marseille, France

Patti E. Gravitt, PhD, MS
Professor
Department of Pathology
University of New Mexico Health Sciences Center
Albuquerque, NM, USA

Michael D. Green, MD, MPH
Professor of Pediatrics, Surgery and Clinical and Translational
    Science
University of Pittsburgh School of Medicine
Attending Physician
Division of Infectious Diseases
Children's Hospital of Pittsburgh of UPMC
Pittsburgh, PA, USA

**Stephen T. Green, MD, BSc, MBChB, FRCP(Lond &
Glas), FFTM, DTM&H**
Honorary Professor of International Health at Sheffield Hallam
    University
Consultant Physician in Infectious Diseases and Tropical Medicine
Department of Infection and Tropical Medicine
Royal Hallamshire Hospital
Sheffield, UK

Andreas H. Groll, MD
Professor of Pediatrics
Center for Bone Marrow Transplantation and Department of
    Pediatric Hematology/Oncology
University Children's Hospital Münster
Münster, Germany

Roy M. Gulick, MD, MPH
Rochelle Belfer Professor in Medicine
Chief, Division of Infectious Diseases
Department of Medicine
Weill Cornell Medical College
New York, NY, USA

Arjun Gupta, MBBS
Internal Medicine PGY1
University of Texas Southwestern Medical Center
Dallas, TX, USA

Gilbert Habib, MD
Cardiologist
Department of Cardiology
La Timone Hospital
Marseille, France

Stephan Harbarth, MD, MS
Associate Professor of Medicine
Infection Control Programme
Department of Medicine
Geneva University Hospitals and Faculty of Medicine
Geneva, Switzerland

Marianne Harris, MD
Clinical Assistant Professor, Department of Family Practice
Associate Member, Division of AIDS
Faculty of Medicine
University of British Columbia
Vancouver, BC, Canada

Frederick G. Hayden, MD
Stuart S. Richardson Professor of Clinical Virology and Professor of Medicine
Department of Medicine
Division of Infectious Diseases and International Health
University of Virginia
Charlottesville, VA, USA

David J. Hetem, MD, PhD
Clinical Microbiologist
Department of Medical Microbiology
University Medical Center Utrecht
Utrecht, The Netherlands

Philip C. Hill, BHB, MBChB, MPH, MD, FranceCP, FAFPHM
McAuley Professor of International Health
Centre for International Health
University of Otago,
Dunedin, New Zealand

Bernard Hirschel, MD
Professor Emeritus
Division of Infectious Disease
Geneva University Hospitals
Geneva, Switzerland

Aimee C. Hodowanec, MD
Assistant Professor
Section of Infectious Diseases
Department of Medicine
Rush University Medical Center
Chicago, IL, USA

Louis Hoffart, MD
Service d'Ophtalmologie
Hôpital de la Timone
Marseille, France

Christian Hoffmann, MD, PhD
Associate Professor
University of Schleswig Holstein
Campus Kiel Hemato-oncologist Infektionsmedizinisches Centrum Hamburg (ICH) ICH Study Center Hamburg
Hamburg, Germany

Steven M. Holland, MD
Chief
Laboratory of Clinical Infectious Diseases
National Institute of Allergy and Infectious Diseases, NIH,
Bethesda, MD, USA

Peter W. Horby, MBBS, FRCP, PhD
Associate Professor
Centre for Tropical Medicine and Global Health
University of Oxford
Oxford, UK

David J. Horne, MD, MPH
Assistant Professor of Medicine
Division of Pulmonary and Critical Care Medicine, Department of Medicine
Harborview Medical Center, University of Washington
Seattle, WA, USA

Sami Hraiech, MD, PhD
Assistance Publique–Hôpitaux de Marseille
Hôpital Nord
Réanimation des Détresses Respiratoires et des Infections Sévères
Aix–Marseille Université
Marseille, France

Mark W. Hull, MD, MHSc
Clinical Associate Professor
Division of AIDS
Department of Medicine
University of British Columbia
Vancouver, BC, Canada

Angela Huttner, MD
Instructor
Infection Control Programme
Geneva University Hospitals and Faculty of Medicine
Geneva, Switzerland

Richard J.M. Ingram, BMedSci, BMBS(Hons), MRCP
Clinical Research Fellow in Gastroenterology
NIHR Biomedical Research Unit in Gastrointestinal and Liver Diseases
Nottingham University Hospitals NHS Trust
University of Nottingham, Queen's Medical Centre
Nottingham, UK

Jasmin Islam, MBBS, PhD, MRCP
Specialist Registrar Infectious Diseases and Medical Microbiology
Department of Infection and Microbiology
Brighton and Sussex University Hospital
Brighton, UK

Michael G. Ison, MD, MS, FIDSA, FAST
Associate Professor
Divisions of Infectious Diseases and Organ Transplantation
Northwestern University Feinberg School of Medicine
Chicago, IL, USA

Scott H. James, MD
Assistant Professor of Pediatrics
Department of Pediatrics
Division of Infectious Diseases
University of Alabama at Birmingham School of Medicine
Birmingham, AL, USA

Claire Jenkins, PhD
Head of E. coli, Shigella, Yersinia & Vibrio Reference Services
Gastrointestinal Bacteria Reference Unit
Public Health England
London, UK

Stephen G. Jenkins, PhD
Adjunct Professor of Pathology and Laboratory Medicine
Adjunct Professor of Pathology in Medicine
Weill Cornell Medical College
New York, NY, USA

Jørgen Skov Jensen, MD, PhD, DMedSci
Consultant Physician
Microbiology and Infection Control
Statens Serum Institut
Copenhagen, Denmark

Christine Johnston, MD, MPH
Assistant Professor of Medicine
Division of Infectious Diseases, Department of Medicine
University of Washington
Seattle, WA, USA

Theodore B. Jones, MD, FACOG
Residency Program Director
Obstetrics and Gynecology
Department of Obstetrics and Gynecology
Beaumont Oakwood
Associate Professor
Wayne State University School of Medicine
Dearborn, MI, USA

Stephen J. Jordan, MD, PhD
Clinical Fellow
Department of Medicine, Division of Infectious Diseases
The University of Alabama at Birmingham
Birmingham, AL, USA

Kathleen G. Julian, MD
Associate Professor of Medicine
Department of Medicine
Division of Infectious Diseases
Penn State Hershey Medical Center
Hershey, PA, USA

Yasuyuki Kato, MD, MPH, DTM
Chief, Division of Preparedness and Emerging Infections
Disease Control and Prevention Centre
National Centre for Global Health and Medicine
Tokyo, Japan

Carol A. Kauffman, MD
Chief, Infectious Diseases Section
Veterans Affairs Ann Arbor Healthcare System
Professor of Internal Medicine
University of Michigan Medical School
Ann Arbor, MI, USA

Keith S. Kaye, MD, MPH
Professor of Medicine
Corporate Vice President of Quality and Patient Safety
Corporate Medical Director, Infection Prevention, Epidemiology and
    Antimicrobial Stewardship
Detroit Medical Center and Wayne State University
University Health Center
Detroit, MI, USA

Michael P. Keane, MD FRCPI
Professor of Medicine
University College Dublin
School of Medicine
St Vincent's Hospital
Dublin, Ireland

James Keeney, MD
Chief, Adult Hip and Knee Reconstructions Service
Associate Professor, Department of Orthopaedic Surgery
University of Missouri
Columbia, MO, USA

Paul Kelly, MD, FRCP
Professor of Tropical Gastroenterology
Blizard Institute
Barts & The London School of Medicine
Queen Mary University of London
London, UK

Stephen J. Kent, MBBS, MD, FRACP
Professor of Microbiology and Immunology
Department of Microbiology and Immunology
University of Melbourne
Melbourne, Australia

Winfried V. Kern, MD
Professor of Internal Medicine and Infectious Diseases
Division of Infectious Diseases
University Hospital and Medical Center
Freiburg, Germany

Yoav Keynan, MD, PhD
Assistant Professor
Department of Internal Medicine
Medical Microbiology and Community Health Sciences
University of Manitoba
Winnipeg, Canada

Andrea A. Kim, PhD, MPH
Chief, Surveillance and Epidemiology Branch
Division of Global HIV/AIDS–Kenya
Centers for Disease Control and Prevention
Nairobi, Kenya

Isabelle Koné-Paut, MD
Professor of Medicine
Department of Pediatrics
University of Paris Sud
Paris, France

Chris Kosmidis, MD, PhD
Consultant in Infectious Diseases
National Aspergillosis Centre
University Hospital of South Manchester
Hon. Senior Lecturer
The University of Manchester
Manchester, UK

Aloys C.M. Kroes, MD, PhD
Professor of Medical Microbiology and Clinical Virology
Department of Medical Microbiology
Leiden University Medical Center
Leiden, The Netherlands

Frank P. Kroon, MD PhD
Internist-Specialist in Infectious Diseases
Department of Infectious Diseases
Leiden University Medical Center
Leiden, The Netherlands

Thomas G. Ksiazek, DVM, PhD
Professor
Sealy Center for Vaccine Development
University of Texas Medical Branch
Galveston, TX, USA

F. Matthew Kuhlmann, MD
Instructor in Medicine
Division of Infectious Diseases, Department of Medicine
Washington University School of Medicine in St Louis
St Louis, MO, USA

Ed J. Kuijper, MD, PhD
Professor of Medical Microbiology
Department of Medical Microbiology
Center of Infectious Disease
Leiden University Medical Centre
Leiden, The Netherlands

Jennie H. Kwon, DO
Senior Clinical Research Fellow
Division of Infectious Diseases
Department of Internal Medicine
Washington University School of Medicine in St Louis
St Louis, MO, USA

George B. Kyei, MB ChB, PhD
Assistant Professor of Medicine
Department of Medicine
Washington University School of Medicine in St Louis
Saint Louis, MO, USA

Karine Lacombe, MD, PhD
Associate Professor
Infectious Diseases Department
Hôpital St Antoine
Paris, France

Philippe Lagacé-Wiens, MD, FRCPC, DTM&H
Professor
Department of Medical Microbiology and Infectious Diseases
University of Manitoba College of Medicine
Winnipeg, Manitoba, Canada

Jean-Christophe Lagier, MD, PhD
Associate Professor of Medicine
Institut Hospitalo-Universitaire Méditerranée-Infection
  Aix-Marseille Université
Marseille, France

Theresa Lamagni, MSc, PhD
Senior Epidemiologist
Healthcare-Associated Infections and Antimicrobial Resistance
  Department
Public Health England
London, UK

Luce Landraud, MD, PhD
Medical Doctor
Microbiology Department
Archet II-Hospital
Microbial Toxins in Host Pathogen
Interactions
Sophia Antipolis University
Nice, France

Fanny Lanternier, MD
Researcher Université Paris–Descartes
Hôpital Necker–Enfants Malades
Service des Maladies Infectieuses et Tropicales
Institut Imagine, APHP, Centre d'Infectiologie Necker–Pasteur
Paris, France

Kerry L. LaPlante, PharmD, FCCP
Professor of Pharmacy
Department of Pharmacy Practice
University of Rhode Island
Kingston, RI, USA
Adjunct Clinical Associate Professor of Medicine
Alpert Medical School of Brown University
Providence, RI, USA
Director of the Rhode Island Infectious Diseases Research Program
  (RIID) and Infectious Diseases Pharmacotherapy Specialist
Veterans Affairs Medical Center
Providence, RI, USA

Stephen D. Lawn, BMedSci MB BS, MD, FRCP, DTM&H, DiP HIV MED
Professor of Infectious Diseases
Department of Clinical Research
Faculty of Infectious and Tropical Diseases
London School of Hygiene & Tropical Medicine
London, UK

Steven J. Lawrence, MD, MSc
Assistant Professor of Medicine
Department of Medicine
Washington University School of Medicine in St Louis
St Louis, MO, USA

Hakan Leblebicioglu, MD
Head of Department of Infectious Diseases & Clinical Microbiology
Coordinator of ESCMID Study Group for Infections in Travelers
  and Migrants (ESGITM)
Ondokuz Mayis University
Samsun, Turkey

Nelson Lee, MD
Professor of Infectious Medicine and Therapeutics
The Chinese University of Hong Kong
Hong Kong, People's Republic of China

James E. Leggett, MD
Associate Professor, Department of Internal Medicine, Oregon
  Health and Sciences University
Infectious Diseases, Department of Medical Education, Providence
  Portland Medical Center
Portland, OR, USA

Philippe Lehours, PharmD, PhD
Assistant Professor in Microbiology
Department of Bacteriology
University of Bordeaux
Bordeaux, France

Pierre-Yves Levy, MD
Associate Professor of Microbiology
Institut Hospitalier Universitaire Méditerranée Infection
Marseille, France

Rainer G. Leyh, MD, PhD
Professor, Director and Chairman
Department of Thoracic and Cardiovascular Surgery
Universitätsklinikum Würzburg
Würzburg, Germany

Rebecca A. Lillis, MD
Associate Professor of Medicine
Department of Medicine, Section of Infectious Diseases
Louisiana State University School of Medicine
New Orleans, LA, USA

Direk Limmathurotsakul, MD, MSc, PhD
Assistant Professor of Epidemiology
Department of Tropical Hygiene and
Mahidol-Oxford Tropical Medicine Research Unit
Faculty of Tropical Medicine
Mahidol University
Bangkok, Thailand

Jennifer Lin, MD
Chief, Division of HIV/AIDS Medicine
Santa Clara Valley Medical Center
San Jose, CA, USA
Clinical Instructor, Affiliated
Division of Infectious Diseases
Stanford University
Stanford, CA, USA

H.D. Alan Lindquist, PhD
Biologist
Senior Advisor
Water Supply and Water Resources Division
National Risk Management Research Laboratory
Office of Research and Development
U.S. Environmental Protection Agency
Cincinnati, OH, USA

Benjamin A. Lipsky, MD, FACP, FIDSA, FRCP
Emeritus Professor
Department of Medicine
University of Washington
Visiting Professor
Department of Medicine (Infectious Diseases)
Geneva University Hospitals and Faculty of Medicine
Teaching Associate
Green Templeton College
Division of Medical Sciences
University of Oxford
Oxford, UK

Christina Liscynesky, MD
Assistant Professor of Internal Medicine
Division of Infectious Disease
The Ohio State University College of Medicine
Associate Medical Director
Clinical Epidemiology at the Ohio State University Wexner Medical
   Center
Columbus, OH, USA

David Looney, MD
Staff Physician Infectious Disease
VA San Diego Healthcare System
Associate Professor of Medicine
University of California San Diego
San Diego, CA, USA

Olivier Lortholary, MD, PhD
Professor of Infectious Diseases and Tropical Medicine
Centre d'Infectiologie Necker–Pasteur
Hospital Necker Enfants Malades
Institut Pasteur
National Reference Center for Invasive Mycoses and Antifungals
Paris, France

Franklin D. Lowy, MD
Professor of Medicine and Pathology and Cell Biology
Department of Medicine
Columbia University
College of Physicians and Surgeons
New York, NY, USA

Benjamin J. Luft, MD
Edmund D. Pellegrino Professor
Department of Medicine
State University of New York at Stony Brook
Stony Brook, NY, USA

Philip A. Mackowiak, MD, MBA, MACP
Emeritus Professor of Medicine
Carolyn Frenkil and Selvin Passen History of Medicine
   Scholar-in-Residence
University of Maryland School of Medicine
Baltimore, MD, USA

Paul A. MacPherson, PhD, MD, FRCPC
Associate Professor of Medicine
Division of Infectious Diseases
The Ottawa Hospital
Ottawa, ON, Canada

Valérie Maghraoui-Slim, MD
Hospital Practitioner
Department of Pediatrics
Bicêtre Hospital
Paris, France

Patrick W. Mallon, MBBCh, FRACP, PhD
Associate Dean for Research Innovation and Impact
School of Medicine and Medical Science
University College Dublin
Dublin, Ireland

Julie E. Mangino, MD, FSHEA
Professor of Medicine
Division of Infectious Diseases
The Ohio State University College of Medicine
Medical Director
Clinical Epidemiology at the Ohio State University Wexner Medical
   Center
Columbus, OH, USA

Oriol Manuel, MD
Associate Physician
Infectious Diseases Service and Transplantation Center
University Hospital and University of Lausanne
Lausanne, Switzerland

Oscar Marchetti, MD
Associate Professor
Infectious Diseases Service
Department of Medicine
Lausanne University Hospital (CHUV)
Lausanne, Switzerland

Kristen M. Marks, MD, MS
Assistant Professor of Medicine
Weill Cornell Medical College
New York, NY, USA

Kieren A. Marr, MD
Professor of Medicine and Oncology
Director, Transplant and Oncology Infectious
Diseases Program
Johns Hopkins University School of Medicine
Baltimore, MD, USA

Jeanne Marrazzo, MD, MPH, FACP, FIDSA
Director, Division of Infectious Diseases
Professor of Medicine
University of Alabama at Birmingham School of Medicine
Birmingham, AL, USA

Jonas Marschall, MD, MSc
Director of Infection Prevention
Department of Infectious Diseases
Bern University Hospital
Bern, Switzerland
Adjunct Assistant Professor
Division of Infectious Diseases
Washington University School of Medicine in St Louis
St Louis, MO, USA

David H. Martin, MD
Harry E. Dascomb Professor of Medicine and Professor of
   Microbiology
Chief, Section of Infectious Diseases
Department of Internal Medicine
Louisiana State University Health Sciences Center
New Orleans, LA, USA

Frédéric Matonti, MD
Ophthalmology Department
Aix–Marseille Université
APHM, Hôpital Nord
Marseille, France

Richard S. Matulewicz, MS, MD
Resident Physician
Department of Urology
Northwestern University Feinberg School of Medicine
Chicago, IL, USA

Kenneth H. Mayer, MD
Professor of Medicine and Community Health
Brown University
Director of Brown University
Infectious Diseases Division
The Miriam Hospital
Providence, RI, USA

Russell J. McCulloh, MD
Assistant Professor, Infectious Diseases
Department of Pediatrics
Department of Internal Medicine
University of Missouri-Kansas City School of Medicine
Kansas City, MO, USA

Rose McGready, MBBS, PhD
Professor of Tropical Maternal and Child Health
Maternal and Child Health
Shoklo Malaria Research Unit
Mae Sot, Tak, Thailand

Rennatus Mdodo, DrPH, MS, MPhil
Epidemiologist
Surveillance and Epidemiology Branch
Division of Global HIV/AIDS-Kenya
Centers for Disease Control and Prevention
Nairobi, Kenya

Simon Mead, MD
Honorary Consultant Neurologist and Professor of Neurology
MRC Prion Unit
Institute of Neurology
University College London
London, UK

Francis Mégraud, MD
Professor of Bacteriology
University of Bordeaux
Bordeaux, France

**Graeme Meintjes, MBChB, FRCP(UK), FCP(SA),
MPH, PhD**
Associate Professor of Medicine
Department of Medicine
University of Cape Town
Cape Town, South Africa

Sarah C. Metcalf, MBChB, FRACP, DTM&H
Consultant Infectious Diseases Physician
Department of Infectious Diseases
Christchurch Hospital
Christchurch, New Zealand

Marian G. Michaels, MD, MPH
Professor of Pediatrics and Surgery
Pediatric Infectious Diseases
Children's Hospital of Pittsburgh of UPMC University of Pittsburgh
   School of Medicine
Pittsburgh, PA, USA

Giovanni Battista Migliori, MD, FRCP(Lond), FERS
Director, WHO Collaborating Center for Tuberculosis and Lung
   Diseases
Fondazione Salvatore Maugeri, Care and Research Institute
Tradate, Italy

Michael A. Miles, MSc, PhD, DSc, FRCPath
Professor of Medical Protozoology
Department of Pathogen Molecular Biology
Faculty of Infectious and Tropical Diseases
London School of Hygiene and Tropical Medicine
London, UK

Alastair Miller, MA, FRCP, FRCP(Edin), DTM&H
Honorary Senior Lecturer
Institute of Infection and Global Health
University of Liverpool
Liverpool, UK
Deputy Medical Director
Joint Royal College of Physicians Training Board
London, UK

Matthew J. Mimiaga, ScD, MPH
Professor of Epidemiology and Behavioral & Social Health Sciences
   (tenured)
Director, Institute for Community Health Promotion (ICHP)
Brown University, School of Public Health
Adjunct Professor of Epidemiology, Harvard School of Public Health
Senior Research Scientist and Director, Epidemiology and Global
   Health Research, The Fenway Institute
Harvard Medical School
Boston, MA, USA

Marie-Paule Mingeot-Leclercq, MSc, PharmD, PhD
Professor
Pharmacologie Cellulaire et Moléculaire
Louvain Drug Research Institute
Université Catholique de Louvain
Brussels, Belgium

Elizabeth Ann Misch, MD
Clinical Assistant Professor
Division of Allergy and Infectious Diseases
Department of Medicine
University of Washington
Seattle, WA, USA

Makedonka Mitreva, PhD
Assistant Professor of Medicine Infectious Diseases Division
Assistant Director
The Genome Institute
Washington University School of Medicine in St Louis
St Louis, MO, USA

Julio S.G. Montaner, MD, DSc
Professor of Medicine
Faculty of Medicine
University of British Columbia
Vancouver, BC, Canada

Caroline B. Moore, MSc, PhD, MRSB
Principal Clinical Mycologist
Mycology Reference Centre
University Hospital of South Manchester
University of Manchester
Manchester, UK

Patricia Muñoz, MD, PhD
Clinical Microbiology and Infectious Diseases Department
Hospital General Universitario Gregorio Marañón
Instituto de Investigación Sanitaria del Hospital Gregorio Marañón
CIBER Enfermedades Respiratorias-CIBERES
Medicine Department
School of Medicine
Universidad Complutense de Madrid
Madrid, Spain

Jose Muñoz, MD, PhD
Assistant Research Professor
ISGlobal, Barcelona Ctr. Int. Health Res. (CRESIB), Hospital
   Clínic-Universitat de Barcelona
Barcelona, Spain

Clinton K. Murray, MD
Colonel, Medical Corps
Professor of Medicine
Uniformed Service University Corps Specific Branch Proponent
   Officer, Medical Corps
Army Medical Department Center and School
Houston, TX, USA

Didier Musso, MD
Laboratory Director
Unit of Emerging Infectious Diseases
Institut Louis Malardé
Tahiti, French Polynesia

Mable Mutengo, MSc
Chief Biomedical Scientist
Department of Pathology and Microbiology
University Teaching Hospital
Lusaka, Zambia

Misha M. Mutizwa, MD
Assistant Professor, Dermatology
Director, HIV Dermatology
Temple University Hospital
Philadelphia, PA, USA

Kurt G. Naber, MD, PhD
Associate Professor of Urology
Department of Urology
Technical University of Munich
Munich, Germany

**Pavithra Natarajan, BMedSci, BMBS, MCRCP,
DTM&H (Hons)**
Specialist Registrar in Infectious Diseases and Tropical Medicine
Tropical and Infectious Diseases Unit
Royal Liverpool Hospital
Liverpool, UK

Santiago Neme, MD, MPH
Medical Director
Infection Prevention and Employee Health Services
Northwest Hospital/UW Medicine
Clinical Instructor and Attending Physician
Division of Allergy and Infectious Diseases
Department of Medicine
University of Washington
Seattle, WA, USA

Paul N. Newton, DPhil, MRCP
Professor of Tropical Medicine, University of Oxford
Lao-Oxford-Mahosot Hospital-Wellcome Trust Research Unit
   (LOMWRU)
Microbiology Laboratory
Mahosot Hospital
Vientiane
Lao PDR

Ronald A. Nichols, MD, MPH FACOG
Associate Program Director
Obstetrics and Gynecology
Department of Obstetrics and Gynecology
Beaumont Oakwood
Assistant Clinical Professor
Wayne State University School of Medicine
Dearborn, MI, USA

Lindsay E. Nicolle, MD, FRCPC
Professor
Departments of Internal Medicine and Medical Microbiology
University of Manitoba
Winnipeg, Manitoba, Canada

François Nosten, MD, PhD
Professor of Tropical Medicine
Shoklo Malaria Research Unit
Mahidol–Oxford University Research Unit
Mae Sot, Thailand

Luigi D. Notarangelo, MD
Prince Turki bin Abdul Aziz al-Saud Professor of Pediatrics
Harvard Medical School
Division of Immunology
Boston Children's Hospital
Boston, MA, USA

Thomas B. Nutman, MD
Head, Helminth Immunology Section
Head, Clinical Parasitology Section
Laboratory of Parasitic Diseases
National Institute of Allergy and Infectious Diseases
National Institutes of Health
Bethesda, MD, USA

Paul Nyirjesy, MD
Professor of Obstetrics and Gynecology and of Medicine
Drexel University College of Medicine
Philadelphia, PA, USA

P. Ronan O'Connell, MD, FRCSI, FRCS (Glas), FRCS (Edin)
Professor of Surgery
Head, Section of Surgery and Surgical Specialties
School of Medicine and Medical Sciences
University College Dublin
Consultant Surgeon
St Vincent's University Hospital
Dublin, Ireland

Steven M. Opal, MD
Professor of Medicine
Infectious Disease Division
Alpert Medical School of Brown University
Providence, RI, USA

L. Peter Ormerod, BSc, MB ChB(Hons), MD, DSc(Med), FRCP
Professor of Medicine
Chest Clinic
Blackburn Royal Infirmary
Blackburn, UK

Douglas R. Osmon, MD
Consultant
Division of Infectious Diseases
Mayo Clinic
Rochester, MN, USA

Marie Boulze Pankert, MD
Maisonneuve-Rosemont Hospital Research Center
Montreal, Québec, Canada
Département d'ophtalmologie
Université d'Aix-Marseille
Marseille, France

Giuseppe Pantaleo, MD
Chief of Service
Immunology and Allergy
Department of Medicine
Centre Hospitalier Universitaire Vaudois
Lausanne, Switzerland

Laurent Papazian, MD, PhD
Assistance Publique–Hôpitaux de Marseille
Hôpital Nord
Réanimation des Détresses Respiratoires et des Infections Sévères
Aix–Marseille Université
Marseille, France

Diane M. Parente, PharmD
Clinical Pharmacist Specialist, Infectious Diseases
The Miriam Hospital
Providence, RI, USA
Adjunct Assistant Professor
Department of Pharmacy Practice
University of Rhode Island College of Pharmacy
Kingston, RI, USA

Philippe Parola, MD, PhD
Professor of Medicine
Chief of the Acute infectious Diseases Unit
University Hospital Institute For Infectious Diseases and Tropical Medicine, Méditerranée Infection
Aix-Marseille University
Marseille, France

Shadi Parsaei, DO
Instructor
Division of Infectious Diseases
Washington University School of Medicine in St Louis
St Louis, MO, USA

Manuel A. Pascual, MD
Chief and Professor
Transplantation Center
Medicine and Surgery
University Hospital of Lausanne (CHUV)
Lausanne, Switzerland

Rupa Patel, MD, MPH
Instructor
Department of Medicine
Washington University School of Medicine in St Louis
St Louis, MO, USA

Eleni Patrozou, MD
Research Associate
Department of Medicine
Alpert Medical School of Brown University
Providence, RI, USA

Jean-Michel Pawlotsky, MD, PhD
Professor of Medicine
Department of Virology
Henri Mondor Hospital, University of Paris-Est & INSERM U955
Créteil, France

Sharon J. Peacock, BM, FRCP, FRCPath, PhD
Professor of Clinical Microbiology
Department of Medicine
University of Cambridge
Cambridge, UK

The late Jean-Claude Pechère
Department of Microbiology and Molecular Medicine
University of Geneva
Geneva, Switzerland

Ivan Pelegrin, MD
Infectious Diseases Research Fellow
Infectious Diseases Department
Hospital Universitari de Bellvitge
Barcelona, Spain

Barry S. Peters, MBBS, MD, FRCP
Reader in Infectious Diseases
Department of Infectious Diseases
Kings College London
London, UK

Edgar J.G. Peters, MD, PhD
Internist-Specialist in Infectious Diseases and Acute Medicine
VU University Medical Center
Department of Internal Medicine
Amsterdam, The Netherlands

Jeannine M. Petersen, PhD
Research Microbiologist
Division of Vector-Borne Diseases
Centers for Disease Control and Prevention
Fort Collins, CO, USA

Lyle R. Petersen, MD, MPH
Director
Division of Vector-Borne Diseases
Centers for Disease Control and Prevention
Fort Collins, CO, USA

Vidmantas Petraitis, MD
Senior Research Associate
Transplantation-Oncology Infectious Diseases Program
Weill Cornell Medicine of Cornell University
New York, NY, USA

Luu-Ly Pham, MD
Former Senior Registrar
Hospital Practitioner
Department of Pediatrics
Bicêtre Hospital
University of Paris Sud
Paris, France

Albert Picado, DVM, MSc, PhD
Assistant Research Professor
ISGlobal, Barcelona Ctr. Int. Health Res. (CRESIB), Hospital
  Clínic-Universitat de Barcelona
Barcelona, Spain

Adrian Pilatz, MD
Consultant Urologist
Department of Urology, Pediatric Urology and Andrology
Justus Liebig University, Giessen
Giessen, Germany

Benoit Pilmis, MD
Hospital Practitioner
Equipe Mobile d'Infectiologie
Service de Maladies Infecteuses et Tropicales
Hôpital Necker–Enfants Malades
Paris, France

María-Jesús Pinazo, MD
Medical Doctor
International Health
ISGlobal, Barcelona Ctr. Int. Health Res. (CRESIB), Hospital
  Clínic-Universitat de Barcelona
Barcelona, Spain

Mathias W. Pletz, MD
Full Professor for Infectious Diseases
Center for Infectious Diseases and Infection Control
Jena University Hospital
Jena, Germany

Jason M. Pogue, PharmD
Clinical Pharmacist, Infectious Diseases
Department of Pharmacy Services
Sinai-Grace Hospital; Detroit Medical Center
Detroit, MI, USA

Evelyn L. Polgreen, MS
Environmental Science Consultant
Oxford, UK

Philip M. Polgreen, MD MPH
Associate Professor
Department of Internal Medicine
University of Iowa
Iowa City, IA, USA

Klara M. Posfay-Barbe, MD, MS
Professor and Head of Pediatric Infectious Diseases Unit
Department of Pediatrics
Children's Hospital of Geneva, University Hospitals of Geneva
Geneva, Switzerland

William G. Powderly, MD, FRCPI
J. William Campbell Professor of Medicine
Larry J Shapiro Director, Institute for Public Health
Co-director, Division of Infectious Diseases
Washington University in St Louis
St Louis, MO, USA

Rachel Presti, MD, PhD
Assistant Professor of Medicine
Division of Infectious Disease, Department of Medicine
Washington University School of Medicine in St Louis
St Louis, MO, USA

Guy Prod'hom, MD
Head of Bacteriology Unit
Institute of Microbiology
Lausanne University Hospital Center and University of Lausanne
Lausanne, Switzerland

Mirja Puolakkainen, MD, PhD
Adjunct Professor in Medical Microbiology
Department of Virology
University of Helsinki
Helsinki, Finland

Thomas C. Quinn, MD, MSc
Professor of Medicine and Pathology
Division of Infectious Diseases
Johns Hopkins School of Medicine
Baltimore, MD, USA

Didier Raoult, MD, PhD
Professor, Faculté de Médecine, Director of the Foundation
  Mediterranee Infection Unité des Rickettsies
WHO Collaborative Center for Rickettsial Reference and Research
Marseille, France

Raymund R. Razonable, MD, FIDSA, FAST
Professor of Medicine
Chair, Transplant Infectious Diseases
Division of Infectious Diseases
Department of Medicine
William J von Liebig Center for Transplantation and Clinical
    Regeneration
Mayo Clinic
Rochester, MN, USA

Robert C. Read, MD, FRCP, FIDSA
Professor of Infectious Diseases
University of Southampton Medical School
Southampton, UK

Robert R. Redfield, MD
Professor of Medicine
Institute of Human Virology
University of Maryland School of Medicine
Baltimore, MD, USA

Rob J. Rentenaar, MD, PhD
Clinical Microbiologist
Department of Medica Microbiology
University Medical Centre Utrecht
Utrecht, The Netherlands

Steven J. Reynolds, MD, MPH, FRCP(C)
Senior Clinician
National Institute of Allergy and Infectious Diseases
National Institutes of Health
Bethesda, MD, USA
Associate Professor of Medicine and Epidemiology
Division of Infectious Diseases
Johns Hopkins University
School of Medicine
Baltimore, MD, USA

Camillo Ribi, MD
Associated Physician
Department of Immunology and Allergy
CHUV University Hospital Lausanne
Lausanne, Switzerland

Malcolm D. Richardson, PhD, FSB, FRCPath
Professor and Director
Mycology Reference Centre
University Hospital of South Manchester
University of Manchester
Manchester, UK

Michele L. Ritter, MD
Associate Clinical Professor of Medicine
Division of Infectious Diseases
Department of Medicine
University of California
San Diego, CA, USA

Antoine Roch, MD, PhD
Professor of Medicine
Assistance Publique–Hôpitaux de Marseille
Hôpital Nord
Réanimation des Détresses Respiratoires et des Infections Sévères
Aix–Marseille Université
Marseille, France

Jürgen Kurt Rockstroh, MD, JKR
Professor of Medicine
Department of Medicine I
Bonn University Hospital
University of Bonn
Bonn, Germany

Amanda Rojek, BAppSci(Hons), MBBS, MSc
Medical Doctor
Doctor of Philosophy Candidate
Epidemic Diseases Research Group, Centre for Tropical Medicine
    and Global Health
University of Oxford
Oxford, UK

José R. Romero, MD, FAAP
Professor of Pediatrics
Horace C. Cabe Endowed Chair in Infectious Diseases
Director, Pediatric Infectious Diseases Section
University of Arkansas for Medical Sciences and Arkansas Children's
    Hospital
Little Rock, AR, USA

Suzan H.M. Rooijakkers, PhD
Associate Professor
Medical Microbiology
University Medical Center Utrecht
Utrecht, The Netherlands

Daniel Rosenbluth, MD
Tracey C. and William J. Marshall Professor of Medicine
Division of Pulmonary and Critical Care Medicine
Washington University School of Medicine in St Louis
St Louis, MO, USA

Sergio D. Rosenzweig, MD, PhD
Deputy Chief, Immunology Service
Clinical Center, NIH
Bethesda, MD, USA

Gian Maria Rossolini, MD
Professor of Microbiology and Clinical Microbiology
Department of Medical Biotechnologies
University of Siena
Siena, Italy
Department of Experimental and Clinical Medicine
University of Florence
Florence, Italy
Clinical Microbiology and Virology Unit
Florence Careggi University Hospital
Florence, Italy

The late Ethan Rubinstein, MD, LLB
Sellers Professor and Head
Section of Infectious Diseases
Faculty of Medicine, Winnipeg
Manitoba, Canada

Greg Ryan, MB, DCH, FRCOG, FRCSC
Staff Perinatologist
Director
Fetal Medicine Program
Mount Sinai Hospital
Professor
Department of Obstetrics & Gynaecology and Medical Imaging
Division of Maternal-Fetal Medicine
University of Toronto
Toronto, ON, Canada

Steven A. Safren, PhD, ABPP
Professor
Department of Psychology
University of Miami
Coral Gables, FL, USA

Vikrant V. Sahasrabuddhe, MBBS, MPH, DrPH
Program Director
Division of Cancer Prevention
National Cancer Institute
Rockville, MD, USA

Pekka A.I. Saikku, MD, PhD
Emeritus Professor of Microbiology
University of Oulu
Oulu, Finland

Mohammad M. Sajadi, MD
Associate Professor of Medicine
Institute of Human Virology
University of Maryland School of Medicine
Baltimore, MD, USA

Michelle R. Salvaggio, MD
Associate Professor
Infectious Diseases Section, Department of Internal Medicine
University of Oklahoma Health Sciences Center
Oklahoma City, OK, USA

Carlos A.Q. Santos, MD
Assistant Professor of Medicine
Division of Infectious Diseases
Washington University School of Medicine in St Louis
Saint Louis, MO, USA

Michael J. Satlin, MD, MS
Assistant Professor of Medicine
Department of Internal Medicine
Division of Infectious Diseases
Weill Cornell Medical College
New York, NY, USA

Anthony J. Schaeffer, MD
Chair, Department of Urology
Herman L. Kretschmer Professor of Urology
Professor in Urology
Northwestern University Feinberg School of Medicine
Chicago, IL, USA

Christoph Schimmer, MD
Consultant of Cardiac Surgery
Department of Cardiac Surgery
University of Würzburg
Würzburg, Germany

Robert T. Schooley, MD
Professor and Head
Division of Infectious Diseases
Academic Vice Chair
Department of Medicine
University of California San Diego
San Diego, CA, USA

Richard F. Schumacher, MD
ID Consultant in the Pediatric Hematology-Oncology Unit
Pediatric Infectious Diseases (DGPI)
Pediatric Hematology Oncology Unit
University Children's Hospital, Spedali Civili
Brescia, Italy

Beverly E. Sha, MD
Professor of Medicine
Division of Infectious Diseases
Rush University Medical Center
Chicago, IL, USA

Daniel S. Shapiro, MD
Professor of Internal Medicine
University of Nevada School of Medicine
Reno, NV, USA

Gerard Sheehan, MB, FRCPI
Senior Lecturer
School of Medicine and Medical Sciences
University College Dublin
Consultant in Infectious Diseases
Mater Misericordiae University Hospital
Dublin, Ireland

David M. Shlaes, MD, PhD
Retired (from Anti-infectives Consulting, LLC)
Stonington, CT, USA

Shmuel Shoham, MD
Associate Professor of Medicine
Division of Infectious Diseases
Johns Hopkins University School of Medicine
Baltimore, MD, USA

Cameron P. Simmons, PhD
Senior Research Fellow
Department of Microbiology and Immunology
University of Melbourne
Carlton, Victoria, Australia
Senior Research Fellow
Nuffield Department of Clinical Medicine
University of Oxford
Oxford, UK

Dennis W. Simon, MD
Assistant Professor
Department of Pediatrics and Critical Care Medicine
Children's Hospital of Pittsburgh of UPMC
Pittsburgh, PA, USA

Matthew S. Simon, MD, MS
Assistant Professor of Medicine
Department of Medicine
Weill Cornell Medical College
New York, NY, USA

Kari A. Simonsen, MD
Associate Professor of Pediatrics
Chief, Division of Pediatric Infectious Diseases
University of Nebraska Medical Center
Omaha, NE, USA

Mary P.E. Slack, MA, MBBChir, FRCPath
Professor
School of Medicine
Gold Coast Campus
Griffith University
Queensland, Australia

Tyrel T. Smith
Howard Hughes Med-Grad Fellow
Department of Pediatrics Infectious Diseases
University of Alabama at Birmingham School of Medicine
Birmingham, AL, USA

Jack D. Sobel, MD
Professor of Medicine
Division of Infectious Diseases
Wayne State University School of Medicine
Detroit, Michigan, USA

Maria Souli, MD
Assistant Professor of Medicine and Infectious Diseases
Fourth Department of Medicine
National and Kapodistrian University of Athens
Athens, Greece

Shruti Sridhar, MBBS, MSc, Public Health
Research Assistant
Department of Tropical Diseases
Aix-Marseille University
Marseille, France

James M. Steckelberg, MD
Professor of Medicine
Division of Infectious Diseases
Mayo Clinic College of Medicine
Rochester, MN, USA

Dennis L. Stevens, PhD, MD
Chief, Infectious Disease Section
Veterans Affairs Medical Center
Boise, ID, USA

Heather Strah, MD
Assistant Professor of Medicine
Division of Pulmonary, Critical Care, Sleep and Allergy
Department of Internal Medicine
University of Nebraska Medical Center
Omaha, NE, USA

A. Willem Sturm, MD, PhD
Emeritus Professor Medical Microbiology
Nelson R Mandela School of Medicine
University of KwaZulu-Natal
Congella, South Africa

Somnuek Sungkanuparph, MD
Professor of Medicine
Department of Medicine
Faculty of Medicine Ramathibodi Hospital
Mahidol University
Bangkok, Thailand

Sarah J. Tabrizi, BSc(Hons), FRCP, PhD
Professor of Neurology
Department of Neurodegenerative Diseases/MRC Prion Unit
Institute of Neurology
London, UK

Evelina Tacconelli, MD, PhD
Professor of Infectious Diseases
Division of Infectious Diseases, Department of Internal Medicine
University of Tübingen
Tübingen, Germany

Chen Sabrina Tan, MD
Assistant Professor of Medicine
Beth Israel Deaconess Medical Center
Harvard Medical School
Boston, MA, USA

Randy A. Taplitz, MD
Professor of Clinical Medicine
Division of Infectious Diseases
Department of Medicine
University of California
San Diego, CA, USA

Guillemette Thomas, MD
Assistance Publique–Hôpitaux de Marseille
Hôpital Nord
Réanimation des Détresses Respiratoires et des Infections Sévères
Aix–Marseille Université
Marseille, France

Lora D. Thomas, MD, MPH
Assistant Professor
Division of Infectious Diseases
Vanderbilt University School of Medicine
Nashville, TN, USA

Franck Thuny, MD, PhD
Professor of Cardiology
Head of Unit of Heart Failure and Valve Heart Diseases
Department of Cardiology, University Hospital Nord Aix–Marseille
   University of Marseille
Marseille, France

Guy Thwaites
Professor of Infectious Diseases
Nuffield Department of Medicine
University of Oxford, Oxford, UK
Director
Oxford University Clinical Research Unit
Ho Chi Minh City
Vietnam

Frederic Tissot, MD
Chief Resident
Infectious Diseases Service
Centre Hospitalier Universitaire Vaudois and Lausanne University
   Hospital
Lausanne, Switzerland

Tone Tønjum, MD, PhD
Professor, Chief Physician
Department of Microbiology
Oslo University Hospital
University of Oslo
Oslo, Norway

Francesca J. Torriani, MD
Professor of Clinical Medicine
Division of Infectious Diseases
Department of Medicine
University of California
San Diego, CA, USA

Christian Toso, MD, PhD
Assistant Professor
Divisions of Abdominal and Transplantation Surgery
Geneva University Hospitals and Faculty of Medicine
Geneva, Switzerland

Paul M. Tulkens, MD, PhD
Professor Emeritus
Professor Invited
Pharmacologie Cellulaire et Moléculaire
Louvain Drug Research Institute
Université Catholique de Louvain
Brussels, Belgium

Allan R. Tunkel, MD, PhD
Professor of Medicine
Associate Dean for Medical Education
Warren Alpert Medical School of Brown University
Providence, RI, USA

Claire E. Turner, PhD
Imperial College Junior Research Fellow
Department of Medicine
Imperial College London
London, UK

Andrew P. Ustianowski, FRCP, PhD
Consultant in Infectious Diseases and Tropical Medicine
NW Regional Infectious Diseases Unit
North Manchester General Hospital
Manchester, UK

Françoise van Bambeke, PharmD, PhD
Professor and Senior Research Associate
Pharmacologie Cellulaire et Moléculaire
Louvain Drug Research Institute
Université Catholique de Louvain
Brussels, Belgium

Reinout van Crevel, MD, PhD
Infectious Diseases Specialist
Department of Medicine
Radboud University Medical Centre
Nijmegen, The Netherlands

Diederik van de Beek, MD, PhD
Professor of Neurology
Department of Neurology
Academic Medical Centre
University of Amsterdam
Amsterdam, The Netherlands

Christian van Delden, MD
Associate Professor of Medicine
Service of Infectious Diseases, Department of Medical Specialties
Geneva University Hospitals and Faculty of Medicine
Geneva, Switzerland

Menno M. van der Eerden, MD, PhD
Pulmonologist
Department of Pulmonary Diseases
Erasmus Medical Center
Rotterdam, The Netherlands

Jos W.M. van der Meer, MD, PhD, FRCP, FRCP(Edin), FIDSA, MAE
Emeritus Professor of Medicine
Radboud University Medical Centre
Nijmegen, The Netherlands

Tom van der Poll, MD, PhD
Professor of Medicine
Center of Experimental and Molecular Medicine & Division of
    Infectious Diseases
Academic Medical Center
University of Amsterdam
Amsterdam, The Netherlands

Jakko van Ingen, MD, PhD
Clinical Microbiology Resident
Department of Medical Microbiology
Radboud University Medical Center
Nijmegen, The Netherlands

Jos van Putten, MD, PhD
Professor of Infection Biology
Infectious Diseases and Immunology
Utrecht University
Utrecht, The Netherlands

Bernard P. Vaudaux, MD
Former Head, Unit of Pediatric Infectious Diseases and Vaccinology
Department of Pediatrics
Centre Hospitalier Universitaire Vaudois and Hôpital de l'Enfance
    de Lausanne
Lausanne, Switzerland

Sten H. Vermund, MD, PhD
Assistant Vice Chancellor for Global Health
Amos Christie Chair and Professor of Pediatrics
Department of Pediatrics and Vanderbilt Institute for Global Health
Vanderbilt University School of Medicine
Nashville, TN, USA

Raphael P. Viscidi, MD
Professor of Pediatrics
Pediatrics
Johns Hopkins University School of Medicine
Baltimore, MD, USA

Kumar Visvanathan, MBBS, PhD
Professor of Medicine
University of Melbourne
ID Physician and Clinical Director
St Vincent's Hospital
Fizroy, Victoria, Australia

Govinda S. Visvesvara, PhD
Microbiologist
National Center for Emerging and Zoonotic Infectious Diseases
Centers for Disease Control and Prevention
Atlanta, GA, USA

Lorenz von Seidlein, MD, PhD
Project Coordinator
Mahidol-Oxford Tropical Medicine Research Unit (MORU)
Faculty of Tropical Medicine
Mahidol University
Bangkok, Thailand

Florian M.E. Wagenlehner, MD
Professor of Urology
Clinic for Urology, Pediatric Urology and Andrology
Justus-Liebig-University Giessen
Giessen, Germany

Anna Wald, MD, MPH
Professor
Department of Medicine, Epidemiology, and Laboratory Medicine
University of Washington
Member, Vaccines and Infectious Diseases Division
Fred Hutchinson Cancer Research Center
Seattle, WA, USA

Thomas J. Walsh, MD, PhD (hon), FAAM, FIDSA
Director, Transplantation-Oncology Infectious Diseases Program
Professor of Medicine, Pediatrics, and Microbiology & Immunology
Weill Cornell Medicine of Cornell University
New York, NY

David C. Warhurst, BSc, PhD, DSc
Emeritus Professor of Protozoan Chemotherapy
Department of Pathogen Molecular Biology
London School of Hygiene & Tropical Medicine
London, UK

David W. Warnock, BSc, PhD, FAAM, FRCPath
Honorary Professor of Medical Mycology
Faculty of Medical and Human Sciences
University of Manchester
Manchester, UK

David A. Warrell, DM, DSc, FRCP, FRCPE, FMedSci
International Director (Hans Sloane Fellow), Royal College of
    Physicians, London, UK
Emeritus Professor of Tropical Medicine, Nuffield Department of
    Clinical Medicine and Honorary Fellow of St Cross College,
    University of Oxford, Oxford, UK
Principal Fellow, Australian Venom Research Unit, Department of
    Pharmacology and Therapeutics, University of Melbourne,
    Melbourne, Australia
International Advisor, Australian DFAT Myanmar Snake-Bite
    Project, University of Adelaide, Adelaide, Australia

Mary J. Warrell, MB, BS, FRCP, FRCPath
Honorary Senior Researcher
Oxford Vaccine Group
Centre for Clinical Vaccinology & Tropical Medicine
University of Oxford
Oxford, UK

Adilia Warris, MD, PhD
Professor of Paediatric Infectious Diseases
Institute of Medical Sciences
University of Aberdeen
Aberdeen, UK

Richard R. Watkins, MD, MS, FACP
Associate Professor of Internal Medicine
Northeast Ohio Medical University
Rootstown, OH, USA
Division of Infectious Diseases
Akron General Medical Center
Akron, OH, USA

David J. Weatherall, MD, FRCP, FRS
Regius Professor Emeritus
Weatherall Institute of Molecular Medicine
University of Oxford
Oxford, UK

Rainer Weber, MD
Professor of Infectious Diseases
Division of Infectious Diseases and Hospital Epidemiology
University Hospital
Zurich, Switzerland

Wolfgang Weidner, MD, PhD
Professor of Urology
Clinic for Urology, Pediatric Urology and Andrology
Justus-Liebig University Giessen
Giessen, Germany

Jonathan R. White, MBChB, MRCP
Clinical Research Fellow in Gastroenterology
NIHR Biomedical Research Unit in Gastrointestinal and Liver
    Diseases
Nottingham University Hospitals NHS Trust
University of Nottingham, Queen's Medical Centre
Nottingham, UK

Peter J. White, PhD
Head, Modelling and Economics Unit
Public Health England Centre for Infectious Disease Surveillance
    and Control, London, UK
MRC Centre for Outbreak Analysis and Modelling and NIHR HPRU
    in Modelling Methodology
Department of Infectious Disease Epidemiology
Imperial College London
London, UK

James Whitehorn, PhD, MRCP
Research Fellow
Department of Clinical Research
London School of Hygiene and Tropical Medicine
London, UK
Oxford University Clinical Research Unit Vietnam
Oxford, UK

Richard J. Whitley, MD
Distinguished Professor
Loeb Chair in Pediatrics
Professor of Pediatrics, Microbiology,
Medicine and Neurosurgery
University of Alabama
Birmingham, AL, USA

Christopher J.M. Whitty, FRCP, DTM&H
Consultant Physician
The Hospital for Tropical Diseases
Professor of International Health
London School of Hygiene & Tropical Medicine
London, UK

Willem Joost Wiersinga
Consultant, Internal Medicine and Infectious Diseases
Principal Investigator
Department of Medicine
Division of Infectious Diseases and Center for Experimental
    Molecular Medicine (CEMM)
Academic Medical Center
University of Amsterdam
Amsterdam, The Netherlands

Mark H. Wilcox, BMedSci, BM, BS, MD, FRCPath
Consultant and Professor of Medical Microbiology
Department of Microbiology
Leeds Teaching Hospitals
University of Leeds & Public Health England
Leeds, UK

Thomas N. Williams, MBBS, MRCP, PhD
Professor of Haemoglobinopathy Research
Department of Medicine
Imperial College,
London, UK

Cara C. Wilson, MD
Professor
Infectious Diseases Division
University of Colorado School of Medicine
Denver, CO, USA

Mary Elizabeth Wilson, MD
Adjunct Professor
Global Health and Population
Harvard T.H. Chan School of Public Health
Boston, MA, USA
Visiting Professor of Epidemiology and Biostatistics
School of Medicine
University of California San Francisco
San Francisco, CA, USA

Hilmar Wisplinghoff, MD
Physician
Institute for Medical Microbiology, Immunology and Hygiene
University of Cologne
Cologne, Germany

Robin Wood, MD, DSC (Med)
Emeritus Professor of Medicine
Desmond Tutu HIV Centre
Institute of Infectious Disease & Molecular Medicine and
    Department of Medicine
University of Cape Town
Cape Town, South Africa

Richard G. Wunderink, MD
Professor of Medicine
Division of Pulmonary and Critical Care
Northwestern University Feinberg School of Medicine
Chicago, IL, USA

David Wyles, MD
Associate Professor of Medicine
Division of Infectious Diseases
University of California San Diego
San Diego, CA, USA

Zhi-Tao Yang, MD, PhD
Doctor in Charge of ICU
Emergency Department/Pôle Sino-Français de Recherches en Science
    du Vivant et Génomique
Ruijin Hospital
Shanghai Jiaotong University, School of Medicine
Shanghai, China

Jonathan S. Yoder, MSW, MPH
Water Preparedness and Response Coordinator
National Center for Emerging and Zoonotic Infectious Diseases
Centers for Disease Control and Prevention
Atlanta, GA, USA

Najam A. Zaidi, MD, FACP, FIDSA
Consulting Infectious Disease Attending
Division of Infectious Disease
Roger Williams Medical Center
Providence, RI, USA
Medical Director
Infection Control and Antibiotic Stewardship
St Luke's Hospital
New Bedford, MA, USA
Assistant Professor of Medicine (Clinical)
Warren Alpert School of Medicine
Brown University
Providence, RI, USA

Andrea J. Zimmer, MD
Assistant Professor of Medicine
Department of Medicine, Division of Infectious Diseases
University of Nebraska Medical Center
Omaha, NE, USA

Jane N. Zuckerman, MD, FRCP, FRCPath, FFPH, FFTM
Consultant in Travel Medicine
Department of Infection
Royal Free London NHS Foundation Trust
Honorary Senior Lecturer
Department of Infection
University College London
London, UK

Alimuddin Zumla, GCDS, FRCP(Lond), FRCP(Edin), FRCPath(UK), PhD(Lond), FSB(UK)
Professor of Infectious Diseases and International Health
Division of Infection and Immunity
University College London
Consultant Infectious Diseases Physician
University College London Hospitals NHS Foundation Trust
London, UK

We dedicate this work to our teachers, who inspired and encouraged us; our students for their enthusiasm and new ideas; and our families for putting up with us for all these years.

89

Epidemiology of HIV Infection

RENNATUS MDODO | ANDREA A. KIM | KEVIN M. DE COCK

KEY CONCEPTS

- Human immunodeficiency virus (HIV) continues to be a significant global public health problem, overwhelmingly affecting low- and middle-income countries. Sub-Saharan Africa has the highest burden of HIV compared to other regions of the world, followed by the Caribbean region.

- The global number of new HIV infections has decreased and the number of people dying of acquired immunodeficiency syndrome (AIDS)-related causes has declined following the scale-up of HIV prevention and treatment strategies including: life-saving antiretroviral therapy (ART) to treat HIV infection; prevention of mother-to-child transmission (PMTCT) of HIV; widespread HIV testing; and male circumcision.

- Reaching the goal of an AIDS-free generation is within range. Through high-impact HIV prevention tools and treatment, supported by global initiatives, such as the United States President's Emergency Plan for AIDS Relief and the Global Fund to Fight AIDS, Tuberculosis, and Malaria, promising efforts are under way for some countries to change the trajectory of their HIV epidemics towards virtual elimination of HIV infection.

- Existing surveillance systems are now being replaced globally by new improved second- and third-generation surveillance systems. These new systems are informed by the state of the epidemic in a country, address the surveillance needs of the general and key populations at high risk of HIV infection, integrate behavioral measurements to complement interpretation of biologic data, and measure coverage and quality of care for persons living with HIV.

- An HIV case-based surveillance system is considered the most ideal system to capture the key points in HIV disease. This system follows cohorts of individuals from the point of diagnosis to entry into care to the end of life. Surveillance of new HIV diagnoses through HIV case reporting is not complete in most countries.

- Heterosexual intercourse is the leading mode of HIV transmission, accounting for approximately 85% of HIV cases in low-income countries. Women, especially younger women, are biologically more susceptible to HIV infection in heterosexual relationships and are twice as likely to become infected with HIV as their male counterparts. Female sex workers are 14 times as likely to be living with HIV as other women globally.

- Male-to-male sexual transmission is an important driver of the HIV epidemic in regions with concentrated HIV epidemics such as Asia and the Pacific, Latin America and the Caribbean, the USA, Canada, Australia, Western Europe and in some generalized epidemics in Africa.

- With the expansion of PMTCT interventions, the number of new HIV infections among children in low- and middle-income countries has steadily declined since 2001 and has been nearly eliminated in high-income countries such as the USA.

Introduction

More than 30 years after the recognition of the first case of acquired immunodeficiency syndrome, HIV/AIDS continues to be one of the most significant health, social and security challenges facing the global community. At the end of 2013, 35.3 million people (range 32.2–38.8

million) were living with HIV and approximately 39 million people had died because of this disease.[1] The HIV epidemic continues to overwhelmingly affect low- and middle-income countries (LMIC), where more than 90% of all people infected with HIV live (Figure 89-1), and a large proportion of adults living with HIV are women.[1]

Despite a continuing increase in the number of people living with HIV, the global HIV prevalence rate among persons aged 15–49 years has leveled at 0.8% (range 0.7–0.8%) in 2013.[1] There were an estimated 2.1 million (range 1.9–2.4 million) new infections in 2013, down from 3.4 million (range 3.3–3.6 million) in 2001 (Figure 89-2). Moreover the number of people dying of AIDS-related causes was estimated at 1.5 million (range 1.4–1.7 million) AIDS deaths in 2013, down from 2.3 million (range 2.1–2.6 million) in 2005 (Figure 89-2). Tuberculosis remains the leading cause of death among persons infected with HIV.

Though HIV has impacted all regions of the world, historic gains in fighting the pandemic have been achieved over the past decade through the scale-up of HIV prevention and treatment strategies, including antiretroviral therapy (ART) to treat HIV infection, prevention of mother-to-child transmission (PMTCT) of HIV, extensive HIV testing and male circumcision. These interventions have necessitated the use of HIV surveillance to track these achievements while monitoring changes to epidemiologic trends.[2] Although the biology and modes of transmission are broadly the same in the developing world and in high-income countries, there are some large differences in the local epidemiology of the disease, which are due to a variety of behavioral and socioeconomic factors. This chapter describes the global distribution and transmission patterns of HIV infection and highlights the response to the HIV pandemic over the past 10 years.

Surveillance of HIV Infection

The exact magnitude of the HIV epidemic can be assessed through HIV surveillance. Since the first decade of implementing HIV surveillance activities, there have been critical data generated to monitor the global HIV pandemic. However, as HIV epidemics have matured across the globe, earlier surveillance systems have become ill-equipped to capture the diversity of HIV epidemiology and explain changes over time. Recognizing these gaps, efforts are now being made to strengthen existing systems to produce timely data that will inform programs and progress for reducing the spread of HIV.

These improved systems, also known as second-generation surveillance,[3] should be informed by the state of the epidemic in a country, address the surveillance needs of not only the general population but key populations at high risk of HIV infection, and integrate behavioral measurements to complement interpretation of biologic data. Key points in a second-generation surveillance system include behavioral surveillance in the period leading up to HIV infection, HIV incidence surveillance, HIV prevalence, behavioral and morbidity surveillance from the period of infection to death, and mortality surveillance at the point of death. Third-generation surveillance systems have recently been discussed[4] which add onto a second-generation surveillance system by measuring coverage and quality of care for persons living with HIV.

The ideal surveillance system to capture the spectrum of HIV disease is an HIV case-based surveillance system that follows cohorts of individuals to sentinel events in HIV disease progression and management, from the point of diagnosis to entry into care to the end of life. Surveillance of new HIV diagnosis through HIV case reporting, however, is not complete in most countries. Improved case reporting

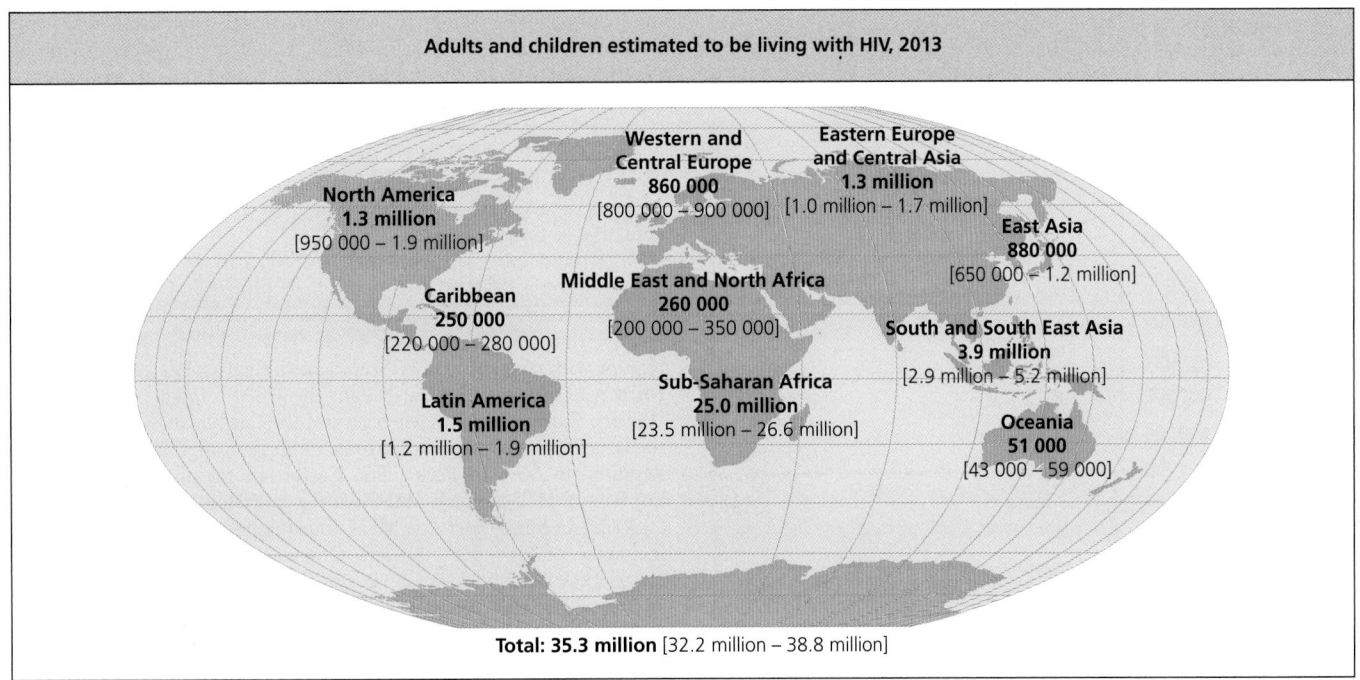

Figure 89-1 Adults and children estimated to be living with HIV, 2013. *(UNAIDS core epidemiology slides, July 2014.)*

forms and the establishment of electronic health information systems that are linked using unique identifiers to facilitate HIV case-based surveillance are needed. Furthermore, though death due to HIV/AIDS has declined in countries where ART coverage has improved, limited data are available to track trends in HIV-related mortality, challenging the ability to measure the impact of treatment programs and interpret HIV prevalence trends. Improving vital registration systems is critical to enhancing the understanding of causes of mortality, including HIV/AIDS. HIV case-based surveillance systems that are linked to civil registration systems could help in broader efforts to improve routine reporting of death.

To capture information on prevalent HIV infection in the general population, antenatal clinic (ANC) sentinel surveillance, using unlinked anonymous HIV testing (UAT) among pregnant women attending sentinel ANC sites, has been the backbone of HIV surveillance in countries with generalized HIV epidemics, where at least 1% of the adult population is living with HIV. However, the expansion of life-saving interventions, such as PMTCT and ART, has called into question the ethics of ANC sentinel surveillance where pregnant women are not provided their HIV test results due to the anonymous nature of HIV testing. Use of PMTCT programmatic data where pregnant women are routinely tested with consent and provided test results are now being evaluated for their utility for surveillance among pregnant women in lieu of UAT-based ANC sentinel surveillance. The quality of HIV testing data generated from PMTCT programs vary widely across countries and would need to demonstrate sufficiently high quality before they could be considered for use for surveillance purposes.

Both ANC- and PMTCT-based surveillance have limitations in generalizability to the broader population due to facility-based sampling and exclusion of men and women who do not attend ANC. National population-based household surveys among women and men, aimed to generate nationally representative estimates of HIV infection in the population, have been conducted since 2001, mostly in sub-Saharan Africa, and have resulted in a better understanding of HIV epidemiology in these countries. Still, there are limitations in these surveys in that they underestimate the extent of HIV infection among mobile, hidden and other vulnerable populations. Major developments in surveillance among these high-risk populations include serial integrated biologic and behavioral surveys to assess the extent to which they contribute to the broader HIV epidemic. Data from these surveys can be used for targeted prevention programs to reduce HIV transmission and improve coverage of important public health programs for these high-risk groups that are often hidden and difficult to reach.

Modes of Transmission
SEXUAL TRANSMISSION

Heterosexual transmission is the primary contributor to the scale of the HIV epidemic in low-income countries.[1] However, risk factors for heterosexual transmission can vary by setting. Most heterosexual transmission in low-income countries occurs both in the context of transactional sex, and in longer-term sexual relationships, including marriage or cohabiting relationships. Women, especially younger women, are biologically more susceptible to HIV infection in heterosexual relationships.[5] Globally, young women are twice as likely to become infected with HIV as their male counterparts, and female sex workers (FSW) are 14 times as likely to be living with HIV as other women globally.[6] Changes in sexual behavior to prevent sexual transmission of HIV, such as delayed sexual debut, condom use and reductions in sexual partners, have resulted in significant declines in high-prevalence countries. In Zimbabwe, for example, declines in new HIV infections among segments of the population were driven by behavioral shifts, notably a reduction in multiple sexual partners.[7-9]

Structural issues, including gender inequalities, restricted access to services and criminalization of high-risk behaviors, increase vulnerability to HIV. Sex workers experience high levels of exposure to HIV through behavioral risk, such as high numbers of sexual partners, often occurring concurrently, exacerbated by inconsistent condom use, and lower condom use with regular clients and with boyfriends and spouses. Based on a systematic meta-analysis conducted in 2011, the overall pooled prevalence of HIV among FSW in all regions of the world was approximately 12%, and an odds ratio for HIV infection of 13.5 compared to other women of reproductive age.[10] A recent study showed a higher global HIV prevalence among FSW, attributing 15% of HIV infections to female sex work. The greatest HIV burden among FSW is in those living in sub-Saharan Africa, with 18% of HIV prevalence attributable to this risk[11] and more than 50% of HIV prevalence

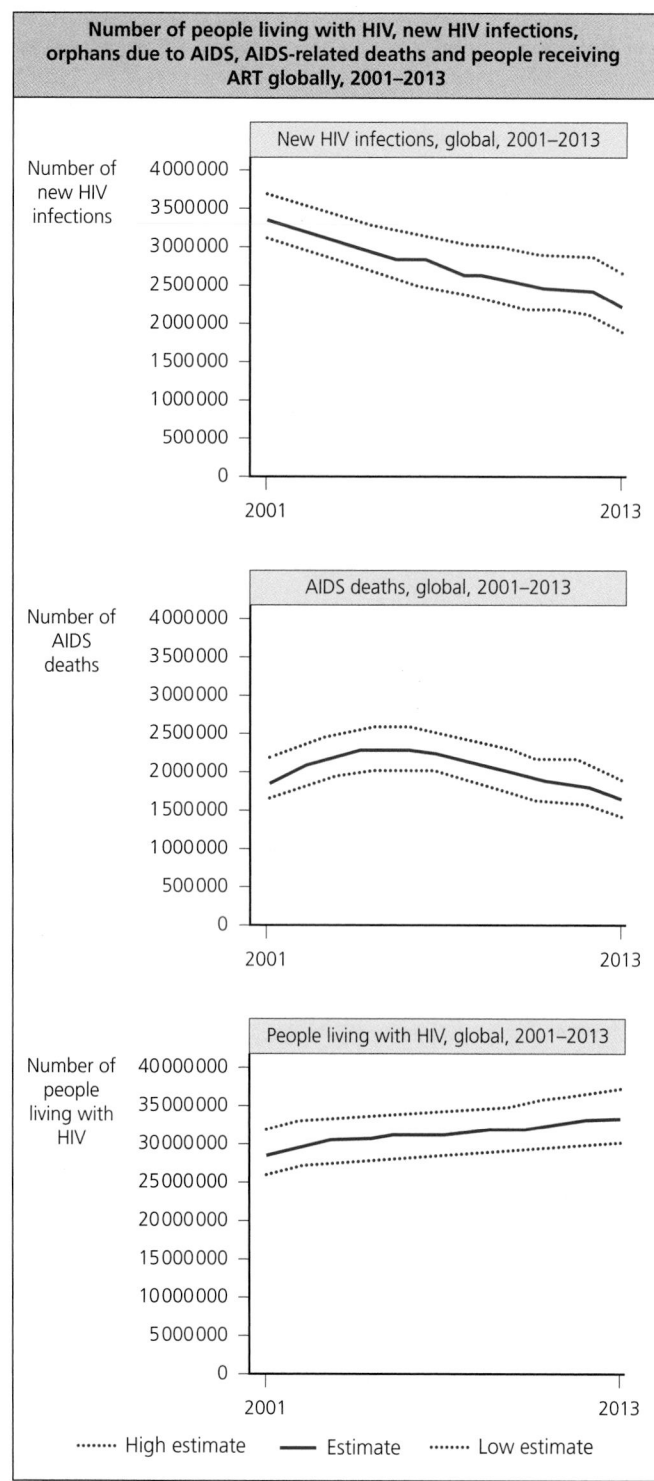

Figure 89-2   Number of people living with HIV, new HIV infections, orphans due to AIDS, AIDS-related deaths and people receiving ART globally, 2001–2013. (*UNAIDS core epidemiology slides, July 2014.*)

in sex workers globally.[12] Of the 106 000 cases of HIV attributed to FSW globally, 98 000 occur in sub-Saharan Africa.

High odds of HIV infection (between 7% and 9%) were also found in FSW in South and South East Asia, Latin America and the Caribbean regions. In East Asia, and North Africa and the Middle East, the prevalence of HIV attributable to FSW was estimated to be 3% and below 2% in Europe, North America and Oceania.[12] Based on mathematical

modeling, in West Africa 10–32% of new HIV infections were from commercial sex work. In Uganda, Swaziland and Zambia 7–11% of new infections were attributable to FSWs, their clients and clients' regular partners.[10] The proportion of new HIV infections due to sexual transmission in sex work is estimated to be a third of new infections in Ghana and 14% in Kenya.[12] To date, limited data exist on the burden of HIV among FSWs in Eastern Europe, the Middle East and North Africa to make firm conclusions on their contribution to the HIV epidemic in these regions.

Men who have sex with men (MSM) carry a disproportionate disease burden of HIV due to the high probability of transmission through receptive anal intercourse. Male-to-male sexual transmission has been an important driver of the HIV epidemic, particularly in regions with concentrated HIV epidemics such as Asia and the Pacific, Latin America and the Caribbean, the USA, Canada, Australia and Western Europe. In Latin America and the Caribbean, MSM represent the largest source of new infections, ranging from 33% in Dominican Republic to 56% in Peru.[2] The Caribbean region has the highest burden of HIV among MSM with a prevalence of 25.4% (21.4–29.5%).[11] In South East Asia MSM transmission is still significant. The incidence of HIV per 100 person-years among MSM in Thailand ranges between 5.9 (95% CI 5.2–6.8; n = 1744) and 8.2 (95% CI 3.7–18.3; n = 81). HIV prevalence among MSM in Thailand ranges from 8.2% to 68.2%. In sub-Saharan Africa, where heterosexual transmission is the predominant mode of transmission, there is increasing recognition of the role of male-to-male sex in transmission dynamics in the region.[2,11] Mostly because of criminalization of homosexuality, data on the burden of HIV among MSM in this region are limited. Since 2001, at least 14 countries in sub-Saharan Africa have conducted behavioral or HIV prevalence surveys among MSM.[12] These studies and meta-analysis reports have shown that wherever male-to-male sex has been studied in Africa, MSM carry a substantially high burden of HIV.[13–15] In Kenya HIV prevalence among MSM is between 12.3% and 43.0% and the incidence per 100 person-years ranges between 6.8 (95% CI 4.9–9.2; n=327) and 20.9 (95% CI 6.7–64.9; n=60), and HIV prevalence among MSM in South Africa ranges from 10.0% to 40.7%.[16]

PERINATAL AND POSTNATAL TRANSMISSION

Perinatal transmission of HIV can occur *in utero*, intrapartum or postnatally via breast-feeding. Most children in LMIC are infected with HIV during pregnancy, childbirth or breast-feeding by their HIV-infected mothers. In the absence of prophylaxis for mother or baby, breast-feeding by HIV-positive mothers can account for up to one-third of HIV infections among babies in sub-Saharan Africa. Without PMTCT interventions, the risk of mother-to-child transmission ranges from 20% to 45%. With specific interventions, the risk can be reduced to less than 2% in non-breast-feeding populations and to 5% or less in breast-feeding populations.[17] The additional risk of postnatal transmission attributable to breast-feeding without a maternal primary HIV intervention is estimated to be about 10–20%.[18,19] With the expansion of PMTCT interventions, the number of new HIV infections among children in LMIC has steadily declined since 2001 (Figure 89-3).

CONTAMINATED BLOOD TRANSFUSIONS

The risk of transmitting HIV infection through blood transfusion remains low globally. If a person receives a blood transfusion with HIV-infected blood, there is a 93% risk they will become infected with the virus.[20,21] Although the situation of contaminated blood is improving and most countries have blood donor screening policies[22], implementation of World Health Organization (WHO) blood safety guidelines[23] is still not universal.[24] In some low-income countries, a significant proportion of blood donations remain unscreened for HIV[25] and an estimated 5% of HIV infections may still occur through blood transfusion,[26] with women and children at greater risk because of frequent anemia requiring blood transfusion.[14] In 2014, WHO reported that 25 countries worldwide did not screen for transfusion-transmissible infections.[25]

INJECTION DRUG USE

The HIV virus can be isolated from blood-contaminated needles, syringes and injection paraphernalia, providing a biologic rationale for transmission of HIV among persons who inject drugs (PWID). PWID have twice as high a probability of HIV transmission per risky exposure compared to exposure from casual heterosexual sex.[27] Most PWID live in South East and East Asia with approximately 4.5 million PWID, followed by Eastern Europe with an estimated 3 million PWID. China is estimated to represent a majority of the PWID (2.3–2.9 million) in East Asia, followed by Japan and Indonesia. In Eastern Europe, Russia and Ukraine represent the bulk of PWID. North America has over 2.2 million PWID, Latin America and Western Europe may each have more than 1 million estimated PWID. There is little information on PWID in the Middle East, sub-Saharan Africa and in South Asia but it is estimated that in Kenya, Mauritius, and South Africa combined there may be about 300 000–350 000 PWID.[28] Of the 15.9 million (range 11.0–21.2 million) people who inject drugs globally, 3 million are living with HIV.[29] This represents a prevalence of HIV of 11.5% among PWID globally. Overall, the Russian Federation, the USA and China account for 46% of the global number of PWID that are living with HIV (21%, 15% and 10%, respectively)[29] (Figure 89-4). South East Asia and some countries in Africa, including Kenya, Tanzania, Nigeria, Mauritius and South Africa are experiencing increases in the number of PWIDs.[30] In sub-Saharan Africa 0.2% of the adult population injects drugs.[2] However, various probability-based surveys among PWID in Africa have found elevated HIV prevalence levels that range from 19% to 36% in Nairobi, Kenya,[31,32] to 16% in Zanzibar,[32] 42% in Dar es Salaam, Tanzania,[32] and 47% in Mauritius.[33]

Geographic Distribution of HIV Infection

NORTH AMERICA, AUSTRALIA AND NEW ZEALAND

From 2003 through 2010, the estimated number of people living with HIV increased by 9% in the USA. By the end of 2010, approximately 1.1 million people in the USA aged ≥13 years were living with HIV.[34] Most people (75.9%) living with HIV were men, and 68.7% of the men had infection attributed to male-to-male sexual contact. Among all people living with HIV, 15.8% were unaware of their infection.[34]

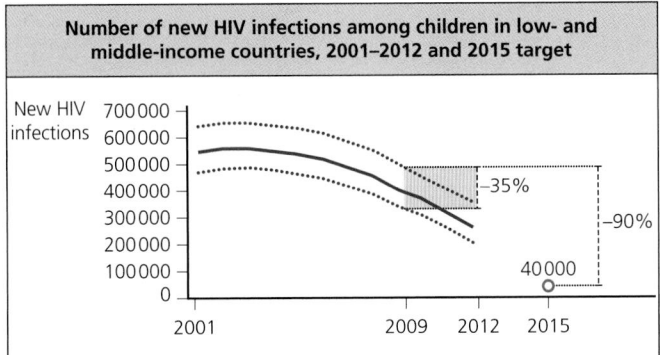

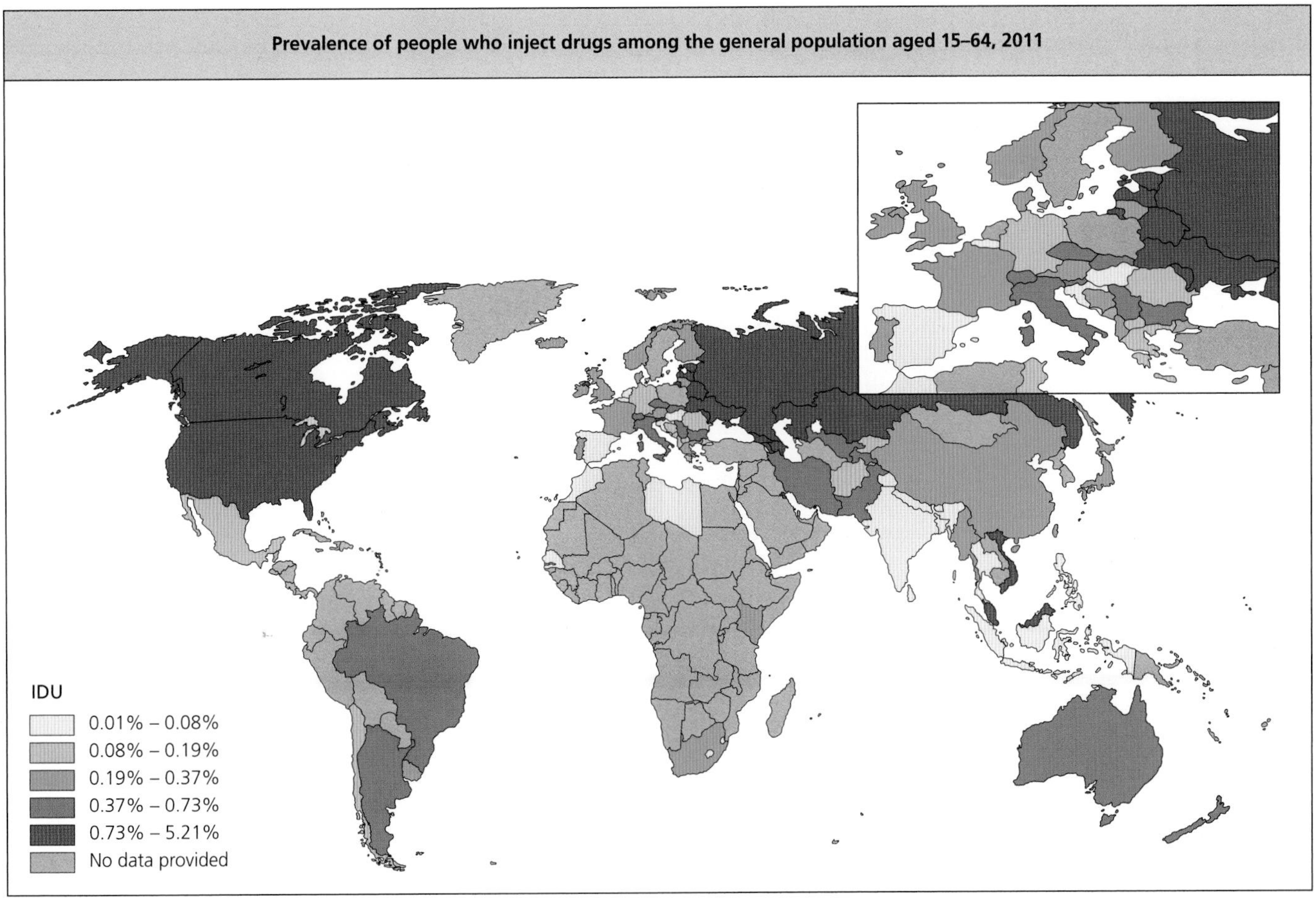

Figure 89-3 Number of new HIV infections among children in low- and middle-income countries, 2001–2012 and 2015 target. (*UNAIDS global report 2012.*)

Prevalence of people who inject drugs among the general population aged 15–64, 2011

IDU
- 0.01% – 0.08%
- 0.08% – 0.19%
- 0.19% – 0.37%
- 0.37% – 0.73%
- 0.73% – 5.21%
- No data provided

Figure 89-4 Prevalence of people who inject drugs among the general population aged 15–64, 2011 or latest year available. (*United Nations Office on Drugs and Crime.*)

Among those, the highest percentage were younger persons aged 13–24 years (58.3%), Native Hawaiians/other Pacific Islanders (26.7%) and men with infection attributed to male-to-male sexual contact (19.0%).

In 2010, the estimated number of new HIV infections in the USA was 47 500 (range: 42 000–53 000). The number of new HIV infections was highest among people aged 25–34 years (14 500; range 12 500–16 400), followed by persons aged 13–24 years (12 200; range 10 500–13 800). Among females, the number of new HIV infections decreased 21%, from 12 000 (range 10 100–13 900) in 2008 to 9500 (range 8100–10 900) in 2010. Most of the new HIV infections among females were attributed to heterosexual contact (84%).[35]

In 2010, African Americans accounted for 44% of new HIV infections in the USA, followed by Caucasians (31%) and Hispanics/Latinos (21%). Of all new HIV infections among African Americans, 51% were among MSM and 38% were attributed to heterosexual contact. Although MSM represent about 4% of the male population in the USA, in 2010 MSM accounted for 78% of the new HIV infections among males (Figure 89-5).[35]

AIDS is the leading cause of death among African Americans aged 25–44 years in the USA. Between 1981 and 2010, more than 261 000 African Americans with an AIDS diagnosis have died, including an estimated 8000 in 2010 and approximately 636 000 deaths among all races/ethnicities since the beginning of the epidemic.[36]

Since HIV reporting began in Canada in 1985 and through 2012, a cumulative total of 76 000 cases have been reported. In 2012 alone, 2000 HIV cases were reported, representing a 7.8% decrease from 2011. Approximately 23% of all cases in 2012 were among females. Over the past decade, the proportion of female cases has remained generally stable, at approximately 25%, with only slight fluctuations since 2001 and a peak of 27.8% in 2006.[37] In 2012, MSM exposure accounted for 50% of all newly diagnosed HIV cases among persons aged ≥15 years, followed by heterosexual contact (33%) and injection drug use (14%). Overall, a higher proportion of adult females than adult males acquired HIV through parenteral exposure (24% vs 12%).[37]

In Australia, since the first diagnoses in 1982, the cumulative number of people living with HIV by the fourth quarter of 2012 was approximately 33 000.[38] In 2012, there were approximately 1000 people diagnosed with HIV, a 10% increase from 2011. Of those diagnosed with HIV in 2012, 15% had been diagnosed overseas. Of all HIV diagnoses made between 2007 and 2011, 67% were among MSM and 25% were attributed to heterosexual sex.[38] In 2012 alone, of 941 cases of HIV infection newly diagnosed among adult males, the majority (80%) were attributed to MSM, with or without a history of injection drug use.[38] In New Zealand few people are infected with HIV, most of whom are MSM.[39]

EUROPE AND CENTRAL ASIA

Approximately 2.2 million people were living with HIV in the Europe and the Central Asia region in 2012.[2] The estimated adult HIV prevalence ranges from below 0.2% in parts of Central Europe to above 2%

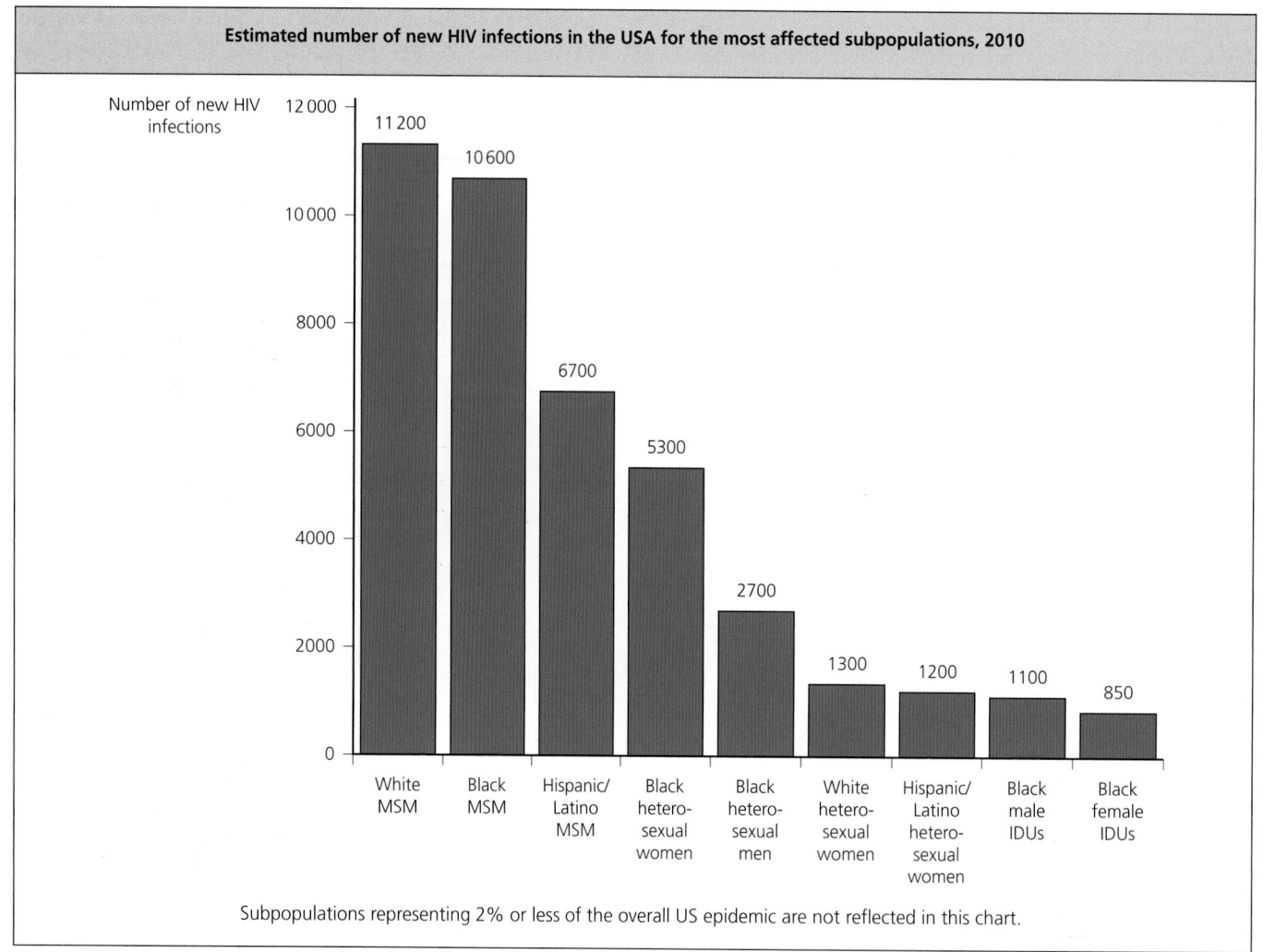

Figure 89-5 Estimated number of new HIV infections in the United States for the most affected subpopulations, 2010. (*Centers for Disease Control and Prevention HIV surveillance supplemental report 2012.*[35])

in parts of Eastern Europe.[40,41] At the end of 2011 about 900 000 people were living with HIV in Western and Central Europe.[42] Portugal had the highest HIV prevalence in Western Europe, at 0.7%, followed by Austria, France, Italy and Spain, at 0.4%.[43]

Eastern Europe and Central Asia has the world's most rapidly expanding HIV epidemics, with a 250% increase in HIV prevalence since 2001.[44] Over two-thirds of the people living with HIV in Eastern Europe are in Russia, and combined with Ukraine, these two countries accounted for about 90% of new HIV infections in the region in 2011.[44] The two countries also have the highest HIV prevalence in the region; adult HIV prevalence is 0.8% and 0.8–1.4% in Ukraine and Russia, respectively.[44]

Evidence shows increasing rates of HIV transmission in the Europe and Central Asia region. Approximately 136 000 people were newly infected with HIV in the region in 2013, an 8% rise from 2011.[45] The majority of cases were reported in Eastern Europe and Central Asia. Approximately 79 700 new HIV infections were reported in Russia alone, accounting for more than half the region's cases.[45] Cases originating from countries in sub-Saharan Africa have influenced the mode of transmission in the Europe and Central Asia region from a predominantly injection drug use-related transmission to heterosexual transmission. Among 29 000 new HIV infections reported in this region in 2012, approximately 4000 cases were migrants from countries in sub-Saharan Africa.[45]

Heterosexual transmission is the predominant mode of transmission in the Europe and Central Asia region as a whole, accounting for 31% of HIV cases in 2013, followed by injecting drug use (21%) and male-to-male transmission (10%). Male-to-male transmission is the most common mode in Western and Central Europe and transmission through injecting drug use remains significantly high in the east of the region. At the national level, injection drug use was reported as the predominant mode of transmission in Greece, Lithuania and Romania. In these three countries, transmission among PWID accounted for more than 30% of reported HIV cases (Figure 89-6).[44]

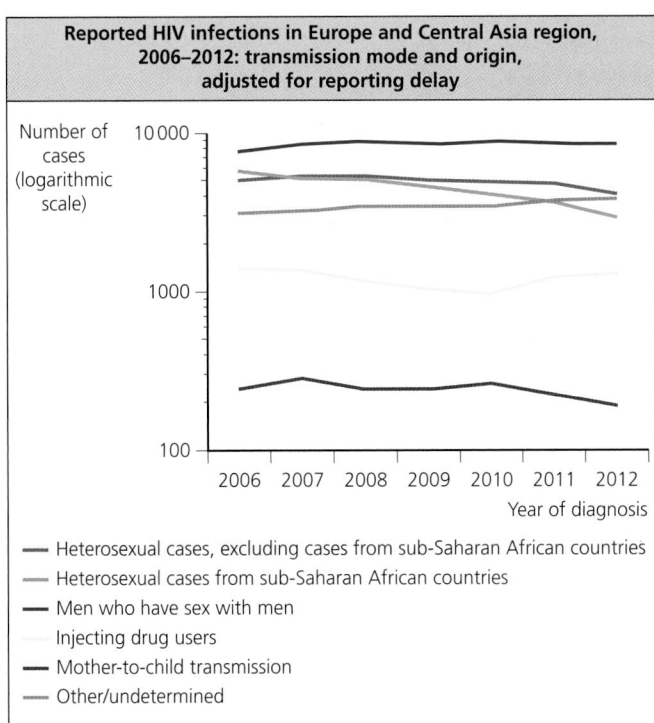

Figure 89-6   Reported HIV infections in Europe and Central Asia region, 2006–2012: transmission mode and origin, adjusted for reporting delay. *(HIV/AIDS surveillance in Europe 2012: Disease prevention and control. Stockholm: WHO Regional Office for Europe.)*

SUB-SAHARAN AFRICA

Sub-Saharan Africa has the highest burden of HIV compared to any other region of the world. Though only about 12% of the world's population live in sub-Saharan Africa, 69% of the total number of adults living with HIV and 91% of children living with HIV, live in this region.[2] The region's epidemics vary significantly in scale, with national adult HIV prevalence ranging from less than 1% in some countries of the Sahel to as high as 27% in southern Africa. Most of the region's nations have generalized HIV epidemics, where the predominant mode of transmission is through heterosexual transmission in the general population. This region has the highest burden of HIV in FSWs; 18% of HIV prevalence is attributable to this risk factor.[11] There is also a growing concern about the emerging injection drug use in Eastern and Southern Africa.[28]

An estimated 24.7 million (range 23.5–26.1 million) people were living with HIV in sub-Saharan Africa in 2013, including 2.9 million (range 2.6–3.4 million) children.[1] About 58% of all people living with HIV in this region are women and about 92% of pregnant women living with HIV reside in this region. South Africa has the highest number of people living with HIV of any country in the world (6.1 million). Swaziland has the highest HIV prevalence rate in the world, at 27%.[46] It is important to highlight that estimates of HIV prevalence and the number of persons living with HIV may differ based on the reporting organization.[1,47]

The number of new HIV infections in sub-Saharan Africa is declining. An estimated 1.5 million (range 1.3–1.6 million) people were newly infected with HIV in 2013, down from 1.7 million (range 1.6–1.9 million) in 2011. Approximately 210 000 (range 180 000–250 000) children were newly infected with HIV in 2013 – a 52% decline in infections since 2001.[1] Improved access to HIV treatment has reduced the number of people dying from AIDS-related causes, from an annual peak of 1.8 million HIV-related deaths (range 1.6–1.9 million) in 2005 to 1.1 million (range 1.0–1.3 million) in 2013. About 700 000 (39%) fewer people died from AIDS-related causes in 2013 than in 2005, with Rwanda, Eritrea, Ethiopia and Kenya reporting the highest decline in AIDS-related deaths in the region.[1] Approximately 75% of persons with HIV-associated tuberculosis live in sub-Saharan Africa,[1] emphasizing the need for integrated strategies for prevention and treatment to tackle the dual epidemics of tuberculosis and HIV.

A small proportion of the HIV epidemic in sub-Saharan Africa is attributed to HIV-2 infection. HIV-2 is primarily found in West Africa but has also been confirmed in other African countries. The highest prevalence of HIV-2 infection is found in Guinea-Bissau, with prevalence rates as high as 8% in 1990 but with a decline to 5% in 2007.[48] In contrast to the increasing spread of HIV-1, the prevalence of HIV-2 has not increased in West Africa but has been declining in several countries and shows slower progression to disease than HIV-1 infection.[49]

ASIA AND THE PACIFIC

The contribution of Asia to the HIV pandemic is relatively small. However, because of the large population sizes of China and India, the Asia and the Pacific region has the highest number of people living with HIV after sub-Saharan Africa. Overall, an estimated 4.8 million (range 4.1–5.5 million) people were living with HIV in 2013 in Asia and the Pacific, including 330 000 (range 230 000–480 000) people who were newly infected,[1] a decline of 26% since 2001.[50] In 2012, there were an estimated 1.7 million (range 1.3–2.1 million) women living with HIV in the region, accounting for approximately one-third of people living with HIV in this region. Trends in AIDS-related death are rather stable, with 270 000 persons dying of AIDS-related causes in 2012, a decline of 18% since 2005.[50]

HIV prevalence has remained highest in South East Asia since the beginning of the pandemic.[50] More than 90% of people living with HIV and more than 90% of new HIV infections in Asia and the Pacific are in 12 countries: Cambodia, China, India, Indonesia, Malaysia, Myanmar, Nepal, Pakistan, Papua New Guinea, Philippines, Thailand

and Vietnam.[50] There is evidence of emerging epidemics in some countries. Between 2001 and 2012, new HIV infections increased 2.6 times in Indonesia, eightfold in Pakistan and doubled in the Philippines (Figure 89-7).[50] In contrast, the number of new infections decreased by more than 50 percentage points since 2001 in some countries in the region, including India (51%), Myanmar (72%), Nepal (87%), Papua New Guinea (79%) and Thailand (63%).[2,50]

The HIV epidemic in Asia is concentrated among key populations at high risk of exposure to HIV infection. The prevalence of HIV infection is elevated among MSM with rates of 14% in Cambodia, 16% in India and 28% in Thailand.[51] In Indonesia, Pakistan and the Philippines, recent data suggest that injection drug use has become a

significant mode of HIV transmission. In 2012, HIV prevalence among PWID was 36% in Indonesia, 27% in Pakistan and 14% in the Philippines. The burden of HIV infection is disproportionately high among FSW in Asia and the Pacific. In China, Bangladesh and Malaysia, the odds of infection are over 50 times that of other females.[9] Though data on HIV prevalence among transgender persons are limited, there is evidence of high HIV prevalence among transgender females in Jakarta, Indonesia (31%), Port Moresby, Papua New Guinea (24%) and Maharashtra, India (19%).[51] Findings of a meta-analysis across 15 countries showed a pooled HIV prevalence of 19.1% (95% CI 17.4–20.7) for transgender women. HIV prevalence among transgender women sampled in LMIC was 17.7% (95% CI 15.6–19.8) and 21.6%

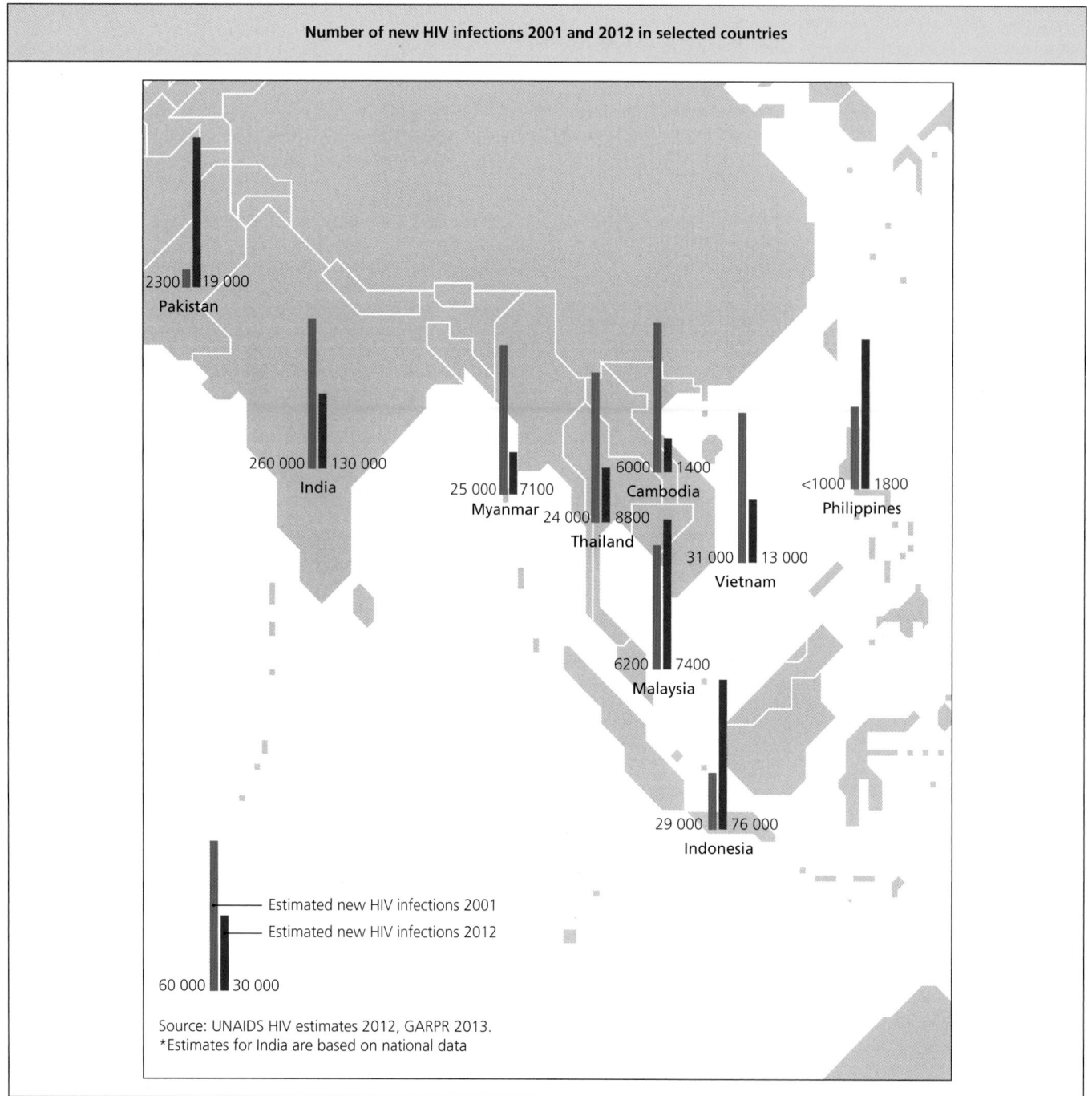

Figure 89-7 Number of new HIV infections 2001 and 2012 in selected countries. GARPR, Global AIDS Response Progress Reporting. (*UNAIDS regional report 2013: HIV in Asia and the Pacific.*)

(18.8–24.3) in high-income countries.[52] Studies from regions with generalized epidemics, such as sub-Saharan Africa, are not available.

LATIN AMERICA AND THE CARIBBEAN

The Caribbean has the second highest HIV prevalence rates in the world. Adult HIV prevalence is estimated at 1.1% (range 0.9–1.2%).[1] Approximately 96% of all people living with HIV in the Caribbean region reside in Cuba, the Dominican Republic, Haiti, Jamaica, and Trinidad and Tobago. While HIV prevalence is highest in the Bahamas (3.2% [range 3.1–3.5%]), Haiti accounts for 55% of the 250 000 (range 230 000–280 000) people living with HIV in the Caribbean in 2013.[1] More than half of people living with HIV in the region are women.

The region has seen a 52% decline in new HIV infections since 2001, from 25 000 (range 22 000–28 000) in 2001 to 12 000 (range 9400–14 000) in 2013.[1] Declining HIV incidence has also been documented in the Bahamas, Barbados, Dominican Republic, Haiti, Jamaica, and Trinidad and Tobago.[1,53] In contrast, there was an increase in new HIV infections in Cuba in 2013.[1] The primary mode of HIV transmission in this region is unprotected sex between men and women, especially between sex workers and their clients and among MSM.[1] Among FSW there is evidence of HIV prevalence rates of 5% in the Dominican Republic, 4% in Jamaica and 17% in Guyana.[54,55] HIV prevalence is high among MSM in Bahamas (26%), Belize (14%), Guyana (19%) and Haiti (18%). In Jamaica, 33% of MSM are HIV-infected[1] and HIV prevalence has risen in other marginalized groups such as the homeless, crack cocaine users and migrant laborers.[54]

Adult HIV prevalence is low in Latin American countries, at less than 1% of the general population. Still, a substantial number of people are living with HIV in the region, estimated at 1.6 million (range 1.4–2.1 million) people in 2013.[1] An estimated 83 000 were newly diagnosed cases in 2011 and an estimated 60 000 people died of AIDS in the same year. Transgender women, MSM, male and female sex workers and their clients, and PWID are the most vulnerable key populations in the Latin America region.[1] MSM transmission predominates in some countries (Mexico, Chile, Ecuador and Peru, as well as in several Central American countries), while in others (Argentina and Brazil) injection drug use accounts for about half of all infections. With approximately 10 new HIV infections occurring hourly, the epidemic in this region is concentrated in urban settings.

MIDDLE EAST AND NORTH AFRICA

In recent years, many countries in the Middle East and North Africa (MENA) region have experienced social and political unrest and conflict, which have created conditions that could exacerbate the HIV epidemic. An estimated 230 000 (range 160 000–330 000) people were living with HIV in MENA in 2013.[1]

Of concern, the HIV epidemic has grown rapidly in this region. The number of adults and children living with HIV in MENA increased by 102% from 114 000 (range 80 000–190 000) in 2001 to 230 000 (range 160 000–330 000) in 2013, and the number of new infections grew by 52% from 21 000 (range 16 000–30 000) in 2001 to 32 000 (22 000–47 000) in 2012[1] – the highest rates of increase among world regions (Figure 89-8).[56] Between 2005 and 2013, the annual number of AIDS-related deaths in MENA increased 70%, to 15,000 (range 10,000–21,000) deaths, while the worldwide number dropped by 38%.[1] The increasing AIDS-related deaths in MENA are primarily due to low levels of diagnosis and access to ART.

Regionally, heterosexual and male-to-male transmission are the most important routes of infection, followed by use of contaminated needles and syringes by PWID (e.g., in Libya PWID have an HIV prevalence of 87%[56]). The number of PWID in MENA is estimated to be 626 000 (range 335 000–1 635 000), with about one-third of them living with HIV. Iran, Pakistan and Egypt have the largest number, with a median of about 185 000, 117 000 and 89 000 PWID, respectively.[57] MSM and women engaged in transactional sex, including commercial sex work, are at highest risk of HIV infection in many countries in MENA, reflected in high prevalence among these groups. In 2013, HIV prevalence among FSW was 2% in Morocco compared

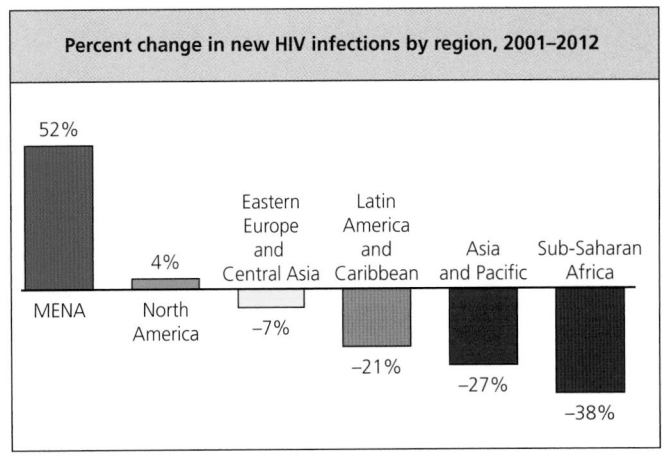

Figure 89-8 Percent change in new HIV infections by region, 2001–2012. *(UNAIDS regional report 2013: the Middle East and North Africa.)*

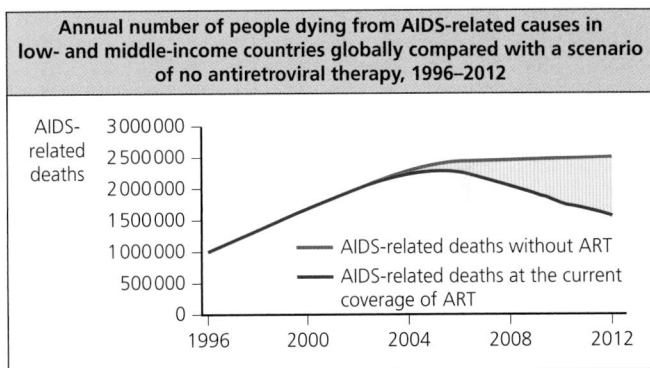

Figure 89-9 Annual number of people dying from AIDS-related causes in low- and middle-income countries globally compared with a scenario of no antiretroviral therapy, 1996–2012. *(UNAIDS global HIV/AIDS response: Epidemic update and health sector progress towards universal access. Progress report 2011.)*

to 0.1% in the general adult female population. HIV prevalence among MSM in Algeria was 13% in the same year.[1] While most nations in this region have concentrated epidemics, Djibouti and Somalia are considered to have epidemics in which HIV has spread significantly beyond key populations and into the broader general population.[56]

Global Response to HIV/AIDS

Through high-impact HIV prevention tools and treatment, supported by global initiatives, such as the US President's Emergency Plan for AIDS Relief and the Global Fund to Fight AIDS, Tuberculosis, and Malaria, promising efforts are under way for countries to change the trajectory of their HIV epidemics towards virtual elimination of HIV infection.[58] Despite progress made, the lack of political acceptance of evidence-based strategies for PWID as well as stigmatization and criminalization of MSM continue to pose a threat to the global effort against HIV/AIDS. Shifting the focus of the global response to rapid identification of HIV-infected persons, acceleration of ART for these individuals, and evidenced-based interventions designed to significantly reduce the number of new HIV infections is needed for countries to strengthen and increase the efficiency of the response to the global epidemic.[59]

TREATMENT SCALE-UP

The number of persons who were receiving ART in all regions was approximately 10 million in 2012, representing a 25-fold increase since 2003.[58] Over the past decade, an estimated 4 million deaths have been averted due to ART, with nearly 1 million averted in 2012 alone (Figure 89-9). ART coverage among treatment-eligible adults in high burden

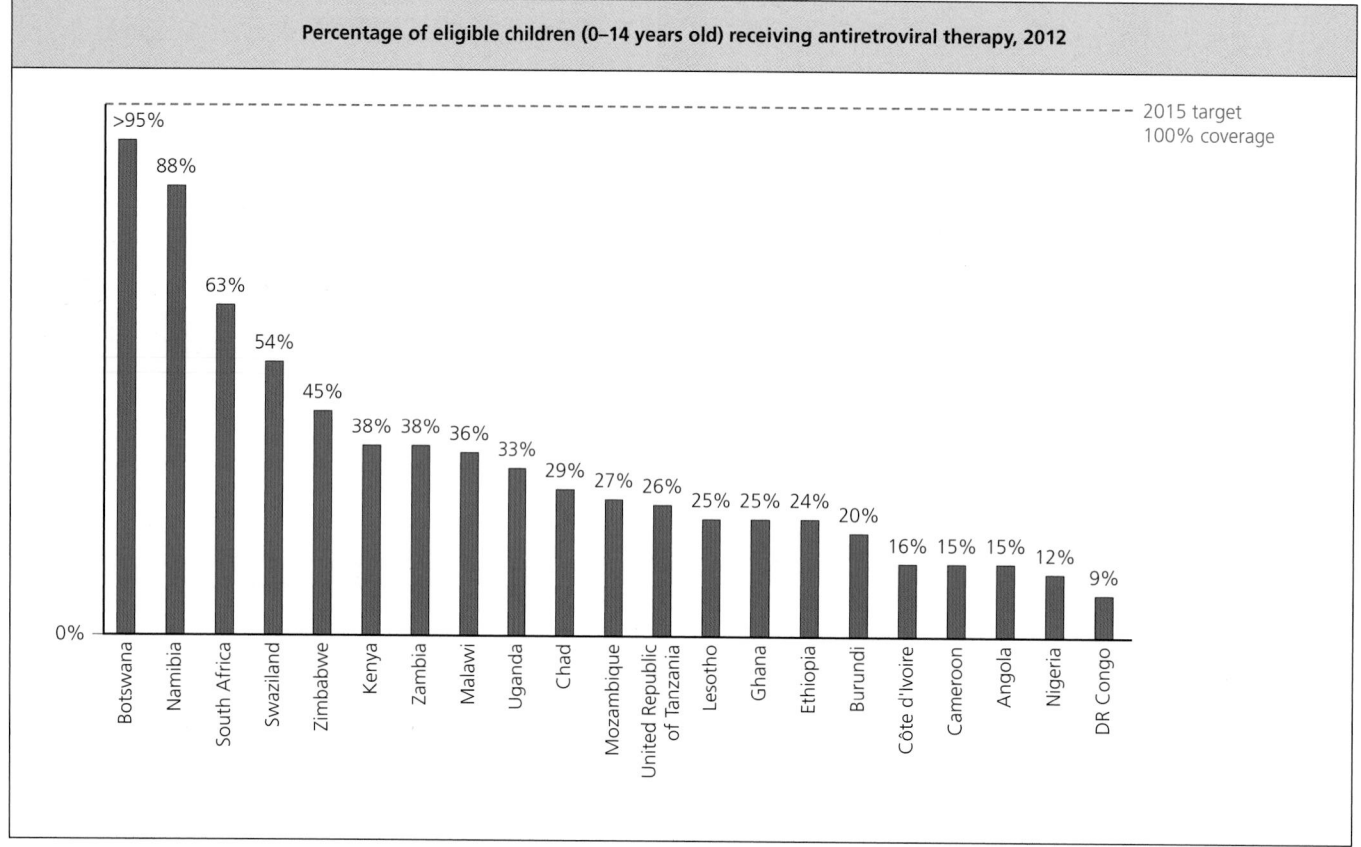

Figure 89-10   Percentage of eligible children (0–14 years old) receiving antiretroviral therapy, 2012. *(UNAIDS 2013 progress report on the global plan towards the elimination of new HIV infections among children by 2015 and keeping their mothers alive.)*

countries has reached nearly 70%. While encouraging progress, this is still below the universal access goal of 80% coverage. Among children, the situation is much worse. As of 2012, approximately 630 000 HIV-infected children were receiving ART in LMIC, representing only one-third of HIV-infected children who required treatment.[58] Substantial regional variations in ART coverage for children have been published. While Botswana and Namibia have already surpassed the universal access coverage goal for children, at greater than 95% and 88%, respectively, Côte d'Ivoire, Cameroon, Angola, Nigeria and the Democratic Republic of the Congo (DR Congo) all reported coverage rates of less than 20% of treatment-eligible children (Figure 89-10). The observed shortfall in services for children highlights the urgent need to identify children who are living with HIV and providing immediate linkages to care and treatment services.

ANTIRETROVIRAL THERAPY FOR PREVENTION AMONG HIV-POSITIVES

In 2011, the landmark HIV Prevention Trial Network 052 study provided unequivocal evidence that ART has critical prevention implications for persons living with HIV who are in sero-discordant relationships, reducing transmission by 96% to the HIV-uninfected partner with delivery of early ART.[60]

These results have had direct impact on the development of normative guidance on the use of ART for treatment and prevention, as outlined in the 2013 World Health Organization (WHO) consolidated guidelines on the use of antiretroviral drugs for treating and preventing HIV infection.[61] This guidance recommends earlier treatment – starting ART in all persons living with HIV/AIDS with a CD4 cell count of 500 cells/μL or less – and starting ART regardless of CD4 count for priority populations, including HIV-infected partners in sero-discordant couple relationships, persons with active tuberculosis disease, persons with hepatitis B virus coinfection with severe chronic

liver disease, pregnant and breast-feeding women, and children less than 5 years of age.

PRE-EXPOSURE PROPHYLAXIS FOR PREVENTION AMONG HIV-NEGATIVES

The use of antiretroviral drugs to prevent HIV transmission to HIV-negative persons has shown efficacy in concept. In 2010, results from CAPRISA 004, the first clinical trial to report on a topical gel for prevention of HIV acquisition among HIV-negative women, reported a 39% effectiveness in preventing HIV transmission.[62] The iPrex trial, also reported in 2010, reported a 44% effectiveness of daily oral pre-exposure prophylaxis (PrEP) in preventing HIV acquisition among MSM.[63] Willingness to use PrEP in this key population is low, varying globally between 40% and 70% due mainly to low effectiveness, limited awareness, side effects and cost. Concerns about accessibility, mistrust of healthcare providers and stigma are also some of the factors driving low utilization of PrEP.[64] In 2011, the TDF2 trial among heterosexual men and women in Botswana reported that the effectiveness of daily oral pre-exposure prophylaxis was 63%. Also in 2011, the Partner for PrEP trial in Kenya and Uganda reported an effectiveness of 62% among HIV-negative men and 83% among HIV-negative women in HIV sero-discordant couples.[65,66] Most recently, in 2013, daily oral pre-exposure prophylaxis was found to reduce the risk of HIV transmission by 49% in PWID in Thailand.[67]

On the basis of these results and with approval from the US Federal Drug Administration, in 2014 the US Public Health Service released clinical guidelines recommending that clinicians assess their patients who are sexually active or using illicit drugs and offer pre-exposure prophylaxis, in combination with condoms and other prevention methods, as an HIV prevention option to those who are found to have substantially high risk of acquiring HIV infection.[68]

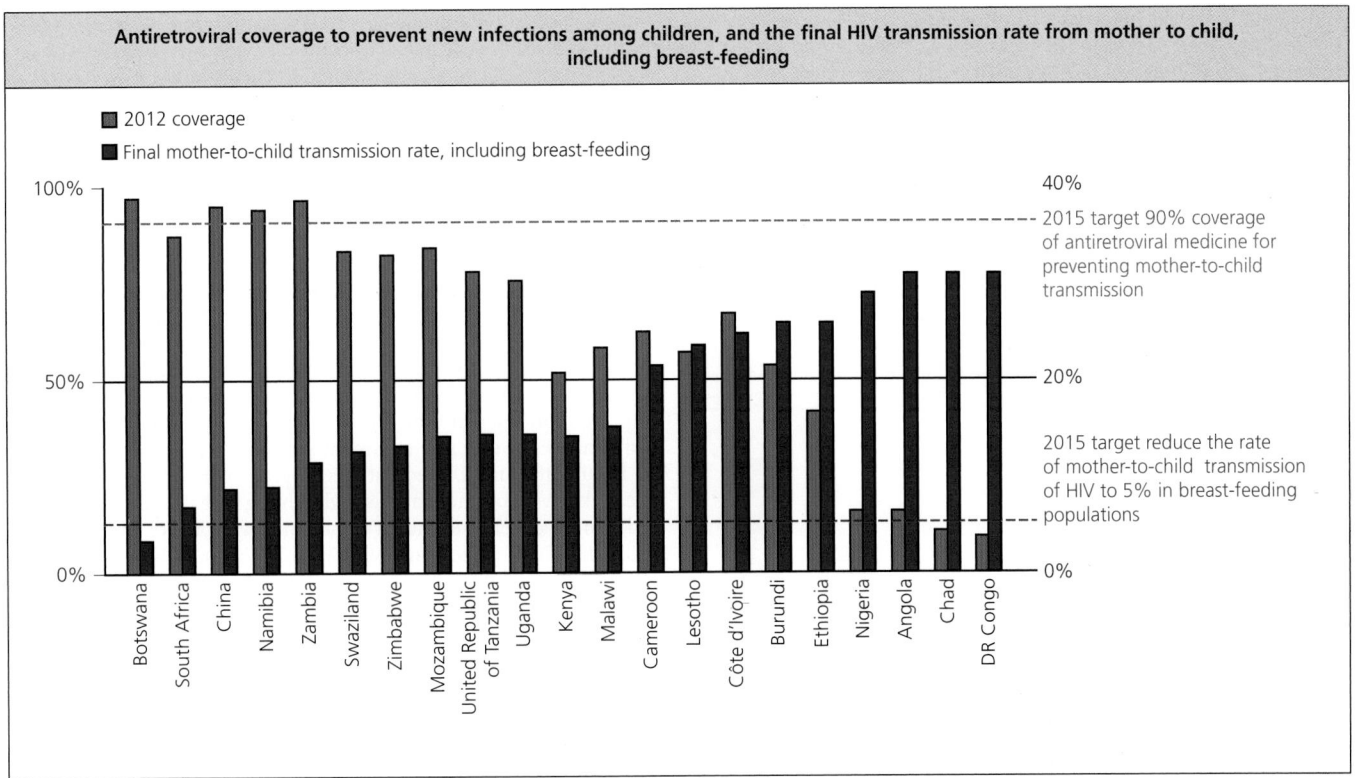

Figure 89-11 Antiretroviral coverage to prevent new infections among children, and the final HIV transmission rate from mother to child, including breast-feeding. (UNAIDS 2013 progress report on the global plan towards the elimination of new HIV infections among children by 2015 and keeping their mothers alive.)

It is important to note that evidence from clinical trials of pre-exposure prophylaxis have not all been positive. Among heterosexual women, discrepant results were found in assessments of oral pre-exposure prophylaxis in the FEM-PrEP trial and oral and topical pre-exposure prophylaxis in the VOICE trial in 2011, both of which observed low adherence to drug regimen and were stopped at interim analysis due to futility.[69,70] As evidence supporting the use of pre-exposure prophylaxis to prevent HIV transmission gains strength, resource-constrained countries should start to explore the practicalities of implementation and roll-out of pre-exposure prophylaxis services through implementation science studies which can inform future global and national guidelines for pre-exposure prophylaxis.

PREVENTION OF MOTHER-TO-CHILD TRANSMISSION OF HIV

In 2011, the United Nations launched the Global Plan towards eliminating new HIV infections among children by 2015 and keeping their mothers alive.[71] The central components of the Global Plan are to reduce the number of new infections among children by 90%, reduce the mother-to-child transmission of HIV rate to less than 5%, and reduce maternal mortality due to HIV-associated causes by 50%.

India and 21 countries in sub-Saharan Africa were identified as the priority countries for the Global Plan, accounting for approximately 90% of all HIV-infected pregnant women globally. Between 2009 and 2012, seven of the 21 priority countries in sub-Saharan Africa, including Botswana, Ethiopia, Ghana, Malawi, Namibia, Zambia and Zimbabwe, had reduced new HIV infections among children by 50% or more.[72] Mathematical modeling suggests that over 50% of the new HIV infections detected among children occurred through breast-feeding due to low coverage of prophylaxis during this period.

Between 2007 and 2010, single-dose nevirapine use decreased from 49% to 18% and more effective prophylaxis regimens increased from 13% to 57%.[73] By 2012, all 21 priority countries had phased out single-dose nevirapine prophylaxis.[72] At year-end 2012, four countries had

surpassed 90% coverage of antiretroviral prophylaxis for PMTCT, including Botswana, Ghana, Namibia and Zambia. These high coverage rates have resulted in lower rates of mother-to-child transmission of HIV compared to countries with lower PMTCT coverage rates (Figure 89-11). By 2012, Botswana was the only country that had reduced the mother-to-child transmission of HIV rate to less than 5%. Coverage rates are expected to rise over the next few years, with global recommendations on lifelong ART for pregnant and breast-feeding women regardless of immunologic status.[61]

VOLUNTARY MEDICAL MALE CIRCUMCISION

In 2007 three randomized clinical trials conducted in sub-Saharan Africa demonstrated that male circumcision could reduce the risk of male acquisition of HIV from heterosexual exposure by 60%.[74–77] These findings led to global recommendations to include male circumcision as a core component of HIV prevention strategies in settings with high HIV prevalence and low male circumcision rates and identification of 13 priority countries in eastern and southern Africa to scale-up voluntary medical male circumcision. By the end of 2013, eastern African countries had performed the largest absolute number of male circumcisions among the 13 priority countries. Kenya conducted 666 000 male circumcisions through 2013 (Figure 89-12). In contrast, scale-up of male circumcision has remained low in a number of priority countries in the southern Africa region. Cultural practices and beliefs and weak healthcare systems have been the biggest obstacles to ensuring rapid scale-up of male circumcision in these countries.

HIV TESTING AND COUNSELING

The first step in ensuring appropriate HIV prevention and treatment access is through HIV testing and counseling. Population-based surveys conducted since 2004 have found that the proportion of persons who have been tested for HIV in the past 12 months has increased in recent years (Figure 89-13). However, despite encouraging increases in the uptake of HIV testing, the situation is less optimistic in key populations at high risk of exposure to HIV. The low level of HIV testing in key populations has negative implications for both individual and population health due to lack of prevention, care and treatment interventions resulting in poor individual health outcomes as well as continued transmission of HIV between key populations and their partners.

Globally only half of all people living with HIV know their status.[1] The large proportion of persons living with HIV who remain unaware of their HIV infection presents a major obstacle to successful HIV prevention and treatment.[1] To achieve universal access to HIV testing

and counseling and knowledge of HIV status, rapid scale-up of HIV testing and counseling needs to continue, with diversification of services that enable testing to be brought to clients rather than relying on clients to seek testing on their own. Services such as provider-initiated testing and counseling have proven effective in improving the testing uptake among pregnant women attending antenatal care. Home-based testing and counseling provides an alternative option for individuals who cannot or do not access facilities for testing. New approaches such as self-testing, mobile testing and work-place testing have also been adopted as promising approaches for reaching a larger number of persons. These testing strategies should target persons at most risk of undiagnosed infection including key populations and their partners, and children of HIV-infected persons. These services, in combination, are expected to significantly increase knowledge of HIV status, including knowledge of status among couples, strengthen the broader impact of prevention interventions for the general population, and improve early linkages to care and treatment services.

In 2014, the Joint United Nations Program on HIV/AIDS (UNAIDS) released new recommendations highlighting global targets for 2020 in order to effectively end the HIV epidemic by 2030. For this goal to be realized, 90% of all persons living with HIV should be aware of their HIV-positive status; 90% of persons who are aware of their HIV-positive status should be linked into HIV care services and be receiving ART; and 90% of persons receiving ART should have achieved viral suppression. With only half of persons living with HIV aware of their status by 2014, global rates on linkage to care and ART are significantly below target, highlighting the substantial work that still needs to be done around HIV testing to successfully achieve these universal 90–90–90 targets.

These critical developments in the global response highlight the importance of scientific and programmatic evidence in guiding global efforts in responding effectively and efficiently to the HIV pandemic. The response over the past 10 years has improved health systems to deliver cost-effective and essential health services, saved millions of people's lives and has significantly changed the trajectory of

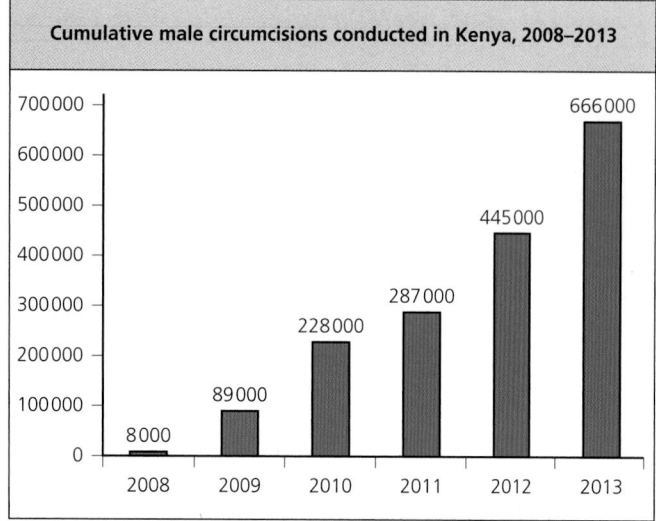

Figure 89-12 Cumulative male circumcisions conducted in Kenya, 2008–2013. *(Office of Global AIDS Coordinator, Annual progress report 2008–2013, Kenya. Estimates rounded to the nearest 1000.)*

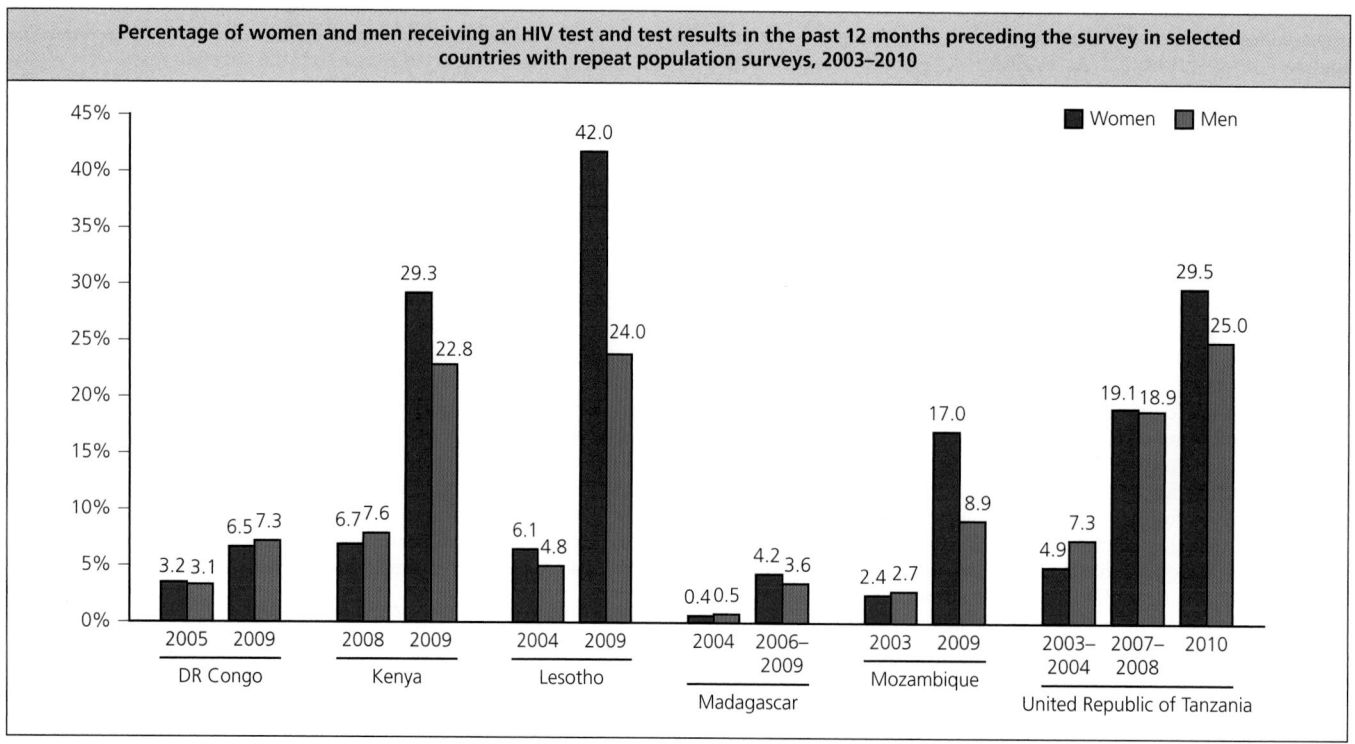

Figure 89-13 Percentage of women and men receiving an HIV test and test results in the past 12 months preceding the survey in selected countries with repeat population surveys, 2003–2010. *(UNAIDS global HIV/AIDS response: Epidemic update and health sector progress towards universal access. Progress report 2011.)*

the epidemic. As global financing for HIV is expected to fall, smart investments, informed by science and evidence, will be needed to develop targeted strategies for accelerating the identification and treatment of HIV-infected persons, with clear demonstration of population impact. This should be done in parallel with political willingness and stronger global investments in the country-led management, coordination and eventually financing of the national response to the HIV epidemic.[78]

References available online at expertconsult.com.

KEY REFERENCES

Centers for Disease Control and Prevention: *CDC trial and another major study find PrEP can reduce risk of HIV infection among heterosexuals.* Atlanta, GA: Centers for Disease Control and Prevention; 2011. Available: www.cdc.gov/nchhstp/newsroom/2011/PrEPHeterosexuals.html.

Centers for Disease Control and Prevention: *Monitoring selected national HIV prevention and care objectives by using HIV surveillance data. United States and 6 U.S. dependent areas – 2011.* HIV surveillance supplemental report 2013; 18 (No. 5). Published October 2013. Atlanta, GA: CDC; 2013.

Cohen M.S., Chen Y.Q., McCauley M., et al.: Prevention of HIV-1 infection with early antiretroviral therapy. *N Engl J Med* 2011; 265:493-505.

European Centre for Disease Prevention and Control (ECDC): *HIV/AIDS surveillance in Europe.* 2013. Stockholm: ECDC; 2014. Available: www.ecdc.europa.eu/en/publications/Publications/hiv-aids-surveillance-report-Europe-2013.pdf.

Grant R.M., Lama J.R., Anderson P.L., et al.: Preexposure chemoprophylaxis for HIV prevention in men who have sex with men. *N Engl J Med* 2010; 363:2587-2599.

Gray R.H., Kigozi G., Serwadda D., et al.: Male circumcision for HIV prevention in men in Rakai, Uganda: a randomized trial. *Lancet* 2007; 369:657-666.

Joint United Nations Programme on HIV/AIDS (UNAIDS): Regional factsheet 2012. Latin America and the Caribbean. Available: www.unaids.org/en/media/unaids/contentassets/documents/epidemiology/2012/gr2012/2012_FS_regional_la_caribbean_en.pdf.

Joint United Nations Programme on HIV/AIDS (UNAIDS): 2013 Regional report for the Middle East and North Africa. Available: www.unaidsmena.org/index_htm_files/UNAIDS_MENA_layout_30_nov.pdf.

Joint United Nations Programme on HIV/AIDS (UNAIDS): UNAIDS gap report 2014. Available: www.unaids.org/sites/default/files/en/media/unaids/contentassets/documents/unaidspublication/2014/UNAIDS_Gap_report_en.pdf.

Njeuhmeli E., Forsythe S., Reed J.: Voluntary medical male circumcision: modeling the impact and cost of expanding male circumcision for HIV prevention in eastern and southern Africa. *PLoS Med* 2011; e1001132.

World Health Organization: *Consolidated guidelines on the use of antiretroviral drugs for treating and preventing HIV infection, 2013.* Geneva: WHO; 2013. Available: http://apps.who.int/iris/bitstream/10665/85321/1/9789241505727_eng.pdf.

World Health Organization: *PMTCT strategic vision 2010–2015. Preventing mother-to-child transmission of HIV to reach the UNGASS and Millennium Development Goals.* Geneva: WHO; 2010. Available: www.who.int/hiv/pub/mtct/strategic_vision.pdf.

World Health Organization/Joint United Nations Programme on HIV/AIDS (UNAIDS)/United Nation's Children Fund (UNICEF): Global HIV/AIDS response: epidemic update and health sector progress towards universal access, progress report 2011. Available: www.afro.who.int/en/clusters-a-programmes/dpc/acquired-immune-deficiency-syndrome/features/3439-global-hivaids-response-progress-report-2011.html.

90

Bio-behavioral Interventions to Prevent HIV Transmission

KENNETH H. MAYER | MATTHEW J. MIMIAGA | STEVEN A. SAFREN

KEY CONCEPTS

- Most exposures to human immunodeficiency virus (HIV) do not result in infection.

- HIV is most often transmitted through intimate sexual contact by rapidly binding to cells that are present in the cervical, vaginal, penile, urethral and rectal mucosa.

- Adult male circumcision can decrease HIV incidence by 50%.

- Concomitant sexually transmitted infections can increase the risk of HIV transmission.

- Antiretroviral therapy is highly effective in decreasing transmission from an infected individual to an uninfected partner.

- Pre-exposure prophylaxis (PrEP) can prevent HIV transmission to at-risk sexually active individuals; however its effectiveness is highly dependent on adherence and other behavioral factors.

- Behavioral interventions to decrease HIV transmission have been successful in a wide array of settings but sustained behavior change is difficult and complex.

- Needle-exchange programs are effective in preventing HIV risk behavior and seroconversion among intravenous drug users.

HIV Transmission Dynamics

HIV transmission is a high consequence, but low probability event with the majority of relevant exposures *not* resulting in new infections.[1] There are multiple co-factors that may affect HIV transmission, which is why there is a high level of variability around estimates of the relative risk of infection for specific exposures (Table 90-1).[2] HIV may be transmitted as cell-free or cell-associated virus, and different factors may affect expression of virus concentrations in different body fluids (i.e. blood, semen or cervicovaginal secretions).[3] Lower HIV blood concentrations are associated with lower rates of HIV transmission,[4] and a recent randomized, controlled trial found that HIV-infected individuals who initiated treatment while asymptomatic were 96% less likely to transmit HIV to uninfected primary partners that those who

TABLE 90-1	Estimates of Per-Contact Risk of HIV Infection	
Type of Contact	**Risk**	
Needle sharing	60-300/10 000	
Occupational needlestick	1/300	
Receptive anal intercourse	50-300/10 000	
Receptive vaginal intercourse	10-80/10 000	
Insertive anal or vaginal intercourse	3-10/10 000	
Receptive oral intercourse	Case reports/no denominator	

were treatment-naïve.[5] Since the sexual transmission of multidrug-resistant HIV has been well documented,[6] providers need to promote safer sex and medication adherence among the patients in their care to minimize HIV spread.

Biologic Issues Related to HIV Transmission

HIV is most often transmitted through intimate sexual contact by rapidly binding to cells that are present in the cervical, vaginal, penile, urethral and rectal mucosa.[7] HIV can be found either as cell-free or cell-associated virus in blood and genital secretions, and can bind multiple cell types.[8,9] The cells that can bind HIV in the genital tract include T-helper lymphocytes, monocyte/macrophage cells and Langerhans cells, as well as follicular dendritic cells. These latter cells may be particularly important because of their mobility, since they can bind HIV on their surface membranes and/or internalize it and migrate via draining lymphatics to distal sites, where propagation in submucosal lymphoid tissue can occur, resulting in subsequent viral dissemination through the bloodstream.

Factors that are associated with increased HIV infectiousness (Table 90-2) include sexually transmitted infections[3] and noninfectious factors that can result in genital tract inflammation (e.g. douching), recruiting more white blood cells to genital mucosal surfaces.[10] Among the sexually transmitted diseases, ulcerative sexually transmitted infections such as syphilis, chancroid and genital herpes simplex virus infection afford additional portals of entry through mucosal ulcerations, but also recruit inflammatory cells that bind and propagate HIV infection.[11] Other local genital factors that are associated with increased inflammation include douching and traumatic sexual intercourse, particularly after sexual assault.

TABLE 90-2	Modifiers of the Efficiency of HIV Transmission	
	Infectiousness	**Susceptibility**
Sexually transmitted diseases	↑	↑
Genital tract inflammation (e.g. traumatic sex, douching)	↑	↑
Circumcision	↓	↓
Cervical ectopy	↑?	↑
Host genetics*	?	↓
HIV subtype†	↑	NA
Monocytotropic strain	↑	NA
Acute infection	↑	NA
Advanced infection	↑	NA
Antiretroviral therapy	↓	NA

*CCR5 mutation.
†Subtype A or C compared to B.

Different tissues in the genital tract have varying levels of susceptibility to being infected with HIV. The vaginal epithelium is stratified, and contains fewer cells with co-receptors that can bind HIV.[10] Thus, vaginal mucosa is less likely to become HIV infected than the endocervix, which has a thinner layer, is highly vascular and contains a much higher concentration of HIV-binding cells. Any physiologic event that results in ectropion (i.e. increased exposure of the endocervix), such as the use of hormonal contraceptives or occult *Chlamydia trachomatis* infection, will increase susceptibility to HIV.[12] The penile foreskin contains many cells that can readily bind and express HIV, resulting in increased HIV acquisition or transmission in uncircumcised males.[13,14] Three randomized trials of HIV-infected men in Africa have shown that adult male circumcision decreased HIV incidence by 50%.[15-17] The oropharynx contains many fewer cells that may bind HIV, which may partially explain the relative inefficiency of oral exposure to HIV as a means of transmission.[18] Moreover, salivary secretions contain several compounds that have been found to inhibit HIV transmission *in vitro*, most notably secretory leukocyte protease inhibitor (SLPI).[19] However, young rhesus macaques have been readily infected with simian immunodeficiency virus after oral challenge, with evidence of viral replication in tonsillar and adenoidal tissues.[20]

Epidemiologic Issues Related to HIV Transmission

Because of the multiple co-factors that may alter the amount of virus in the blood and genital tract, the calculation of the exact risk for infection for each type of HIV exposure is imprecise (see Tables 90-1 and 90-2). Although many people want to have a precise calculation of risk associated with specific practices, it is very difficult to determine with any certainty the precise likelihood of transmission for each specific act. It is important when patients ask questions about the likelihood of risk after an exposure to reassure them that a single, one-time exposure to HIV is unlikely to result in transmission, and that the reason why the epidemic has become so widespread is because of individuals engaging in recurrent risk-taking behavior.

Having noted the limitations of how risk calculations have been obtained, certain key principles have emerged. Direct intravenous exposure to HIV (e.g. blood transfusions) is the most efficient way of transmitting the virus, while percutaneous needlestick injuries are much less efficient in transmitting HIV (see Practice Point 30).[21] Individuals sharing needles who pull back on the syringe and have substantial blood in the syringe when passing it to their partner are more likely to transmit HIV than in a common healthcare setting where an occupational needlestick injury occurs with a solid suture needle.[22] The range of risk for individuals who share intravenous drug paraphernalia ranges from 0.6% to 3% (see Table 90-1). This range overlaps with the level of risk for individuals who engage in unprotected receptive anal or unprotected receptive vaginal intercourse, although the risk of becoming infected through unprotected receptive anal sex is 20 times greater than through unprotected vaginal sex.[23,24] One study suggested that, on average, receptive anal intercourse was more than seven times as efficient in transmitting HIV as insertive anal intercourse.[25]

For each type of exposure, many contextual variables may alter the risk of transmission. For example, variations in the prevalence of HIV in different communities may mean that the same risk behavior has a different likelihood of resulting in an infection in two different communities.[26] The amount of virus in the infected source plays a role in determining the risk of becoming HIV-infected after a relevant contact. Co-factors, like a source with a high concentration of plasma HIV RNA[27,28] or concomitant sexually transmitted infection, can greatly increase the average per-contact risk.[29,30]

In general, receptive anal intercourse is the most efficient way in which HIV is transmitted sexually, followed by receptive vaginal intercourse. Insertive penile–anal or penile–vaginal intercourse is less efficient for HIV acquisition, particularly for circumcised males, but the frequency of each behavior continues to lead to new infections. Receptive oral intercourse is a much less efficient way to acquire HIV, but

case reports have been well documented showing that oral exposure to ejaculate may result in HIV transmission.[20] In counseling patients who have concerns about the risk of acquiring HIV through oral exposure, it is important to indicate that it is less efficient than unprotected anal or vaginal intercourse, but that transmission can rarely occur. Although HIV has been found in very small concentrations in pre-ejaculatory secretions, there are no reliable case reports of HIV transmission through exposure to pre-ejaculate without semen.[31] So, HIV prevention counseling should provide education, but also assess which behaviors are important for the patient's sexual well-being, and develop prevention strategies to avoid exposure to infected secretions.

Antiretrovirals for the Prevention of HIV Transmission

HIV transmission may be decreased by biologic or behavioral means (Figure 90-1). Treating sexually transmitted infections can decrease genital tract HIV load in coinfected patients and can decrease susceptibility in at-risk persons.[19] Antiretroviral therapy can decrease genital, as well as plasma viral load and HIV transmission,[27] but the use of these drugs should be coupled with programs that encourage safer sexual behavior and optimal drug therapy adherence.

Antiretroviral drugs have also been shown to be effective when used for post-exposure prophylaxis[22] (see Practice Point 30). More recently, randomized, controlled trials have demonstrated that oral tenofovir or co-formulated tenofovir–emtricitabine can be used as pre-exposure prophylaxis (PrEP) to prevent HIV transmission to at-risk men who have sex with men and transgender women, heterosexual discordant couples, other heterosexuals and injecting drug users.[32-35] This has led to the United States Public Health Service (USPHS) issuing guidelines for the use of PrEP in the USA,[36] which state that daily oral PrEP with the fixed dose combination of tenofovir disoproxil fumarate 300 mg and emtricitabine 200 mg is recommended as one prevention option for sexually active adult men who have sex with men (MSM) who are felt to be at substantial risk of HIV acquisition. PrEP is also recommended as one prevention option for adult heterosexually active men and women, and for adult injection drug users who are at substantial risk of HIV acquisition. The USPHS recommendations also state that PrEP should be discussed with heterosexually active women and men

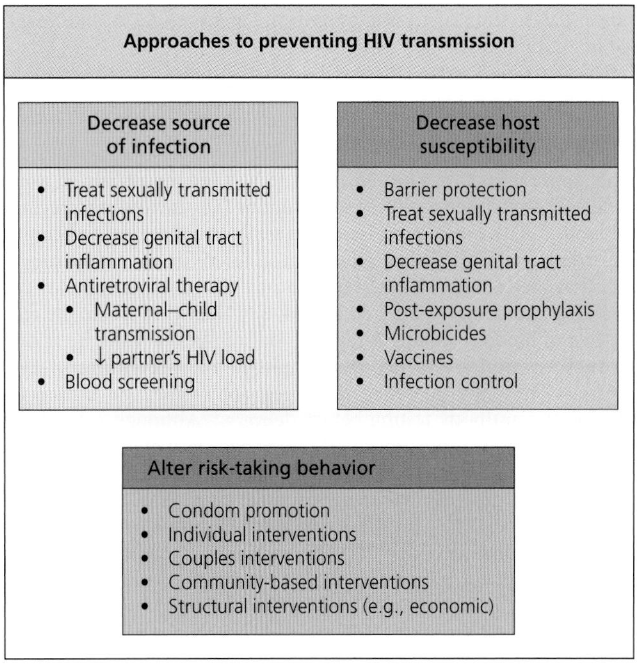

Figure 90-1 Approaches to preventing HIV transmission.

Approaches to preventing HIV transmission

Decrease source of infection
- Treat sexually transmitted infections
- Decrease genital tract inflammation
- Antiretroviral therapy
  - Maternal–child transmission
  - ↓ partner's HIV load
- Blood screening

Decrease host susceptibility
- Barrier protection
- Treat sexually transmitted infections
- Decrease genital tract inflammation
- Post-exposure prophylaxis
- Microbicides
- Vaccines
- Infection control

Alter risk-taking behavior
- Condom promotion
- Individual interventions
- Couples interventions
- Community-based interventions
- Structural interventions (e.g., economic)

whose partners are known to have HIV infection (i.e., HIV discordant couples) as one of several options to protect the uninfected partner during conception and pregnancy.

However, two studies of at-risk young African women failed to demonstrate the efficacy of the same regimens.[37,38] Assessment of drug levels in those studies as well as in some of the earlier studies[39] found that individuals who had drug levels consistent with daily pill use had significant levels of protection, approaching 99%. Thus, for any of these biologically plausible interventions to work, attention to the behavioral context in which the intervention is undertaken is essential.

Treating Sexually Transmitted Infections

There have been several studies conducted in sub-Saharan Africa to evaluate the role of treating STIs to decrease HIV transmission, with varying results. In a study in the Mwanza district of Uganda, syndromic management of STIs in an area where the epidemic was still in its early stages (i.e. 1% of the adult population were infected at the start of the study) resulted in decreasing HIV incidence in communities where the intervention was undertaken.[40] However, in a study in the Rakai district of Tanzania, periodic mass treatment of at-risk adults for STIs did not result in a decrease in HIV incidence.[29] In the latter study, the HIV epidemic was already much more advanced (i.e. 16% of the adult population were infected at the start of the study) and there was a high background rate of concomitant herpes simplex infection that was not treated in the course of the study.

Herpes simplex virus type 2 (HSV-2) seropositivity has been associated with increased risk for HIV transmission and acquisition.[41] Several studies have attempted to see whether chronic HSV-2 suppression with aciclovir or valaciclovir could decrease susceptibility to HIV acquisition.[42–44] Unfortunately, these studies did not demonstrate a protective effect when anti-HSV-2 chemoprophylaxis was used.

The findings from these studies of STI treatment suggest that this intervention may only affect HIV spread if it were to be specifically tailored to individual patients, focusing on aggressively diagnosing diseases that are common in specific communities, as opposed to using general algorithms. In addition, the benefit of STI control will be likely to have the greatest impact in areas of lower HIV prevalence. In communities where the epidemic is already more widespread, the likelihood of encountering a new partner who is HIV infected may be substantial, so the benefit of modifying a modest co-factor like an STI will be more limited.

HIV Screening as a Prevention Modality

Other approaches to the prevention of HIV in the industrialized world are so well established that they seem routine (i.e. the routine screening of blood).[21] The use of more sensitive antibody screening and careful donor history have resulted in enhanced safety in the blood supply, such that the transmission of HIV via infected blood in the past two decades is exceedingly rare. In other parts of the world where the relative cost of blood screening is high, blood supplies may not be as safe.

Another routine practice that results in the prevention of HIV transmission is the guideline that pregnant women be universally offered HIV antibody testing before delivery.[45] Although compliance with this guideline is not 100%, the rate of new perinatally transmitted infections in the USA has decreased dramatically, with fewer than 100 new infections annually in recent years (see Chapter 101).

In September 2006, the US Centers for Disease Control and Prevention recommended that HIV be routinely screened for in most medical settings for patients aged 13–64 years old because more than a quarter of the more than 1 million HIV-infected Americans were unaware of their serostatus.[46] The net effect on the HIV/AIDS epidemic in the USA remains to be seen.

Behavioral Approaches – Overview

Despite increasing access to antiretroviral therapy, blood screening and treatment of STIs, the number of new HIV infections in the USA has persisted at a plateau of approximately 56 000 new infections per year over most of this past decade.[47] The reasons why people engage in HIV risk behavior are complex, and may involve issues related to early life events, such as childhood sexual abuse, low self-esteem, contextual issues in relationships and concomitant substance use, as well as addiction to specific forms of sexual pleasure.[48] Gender-related power dynamics (e.g. the role of women in many societies) may also limit the ability to promote safer sex.[49] Thus, no single behavioral approach will invariably lead to an adaptation of consistent safer sexual or drug-using practices. Much like dieting, regular exercise and smoking cessation, no single program of HIV risk reduction will work for all at-risk individuals. However, several studies have now indicated that the provision of either individual counseling and/or small group sessions can be helpful in assisting at-risk individuals in moderating their risk.[50–54]

Good elements of risk-reduction programs include the ability of the counselor to approach the patient in a nonjudgmental manner to elicit a realistic assessment of the person's pattern of risk-taking behavior. Given the slow progress in the development of cheap, safe and effective vaccines, microbicides and other biologic approaches to the prevention of HIV transmission, the role of the provider in patient education, discussion of risk-taking behavior, initiation of risk-reduction counseling and triage to appropriate prevention services is an essential part of stopping the epidemic's further spread.

Psychosocial Models of Risk Behavior Underlying Prevention Interventions

Knowledge is one aspect of HIV prevention but ongoing risk taking is a function of many other complex psychosocial variables. The three most common models that have been employed to explain HIV risk taking are the health belief model, the theory of reasoned action and social cognitive theory (i.e. self-efficacy models).[55] Health beliefs models emphasize the role of perceived benefits and barriers to condom use and perceived severity and vulnerability to getting HIV.[56] In the theory of reasoned action, health behavior (e.g. condom use) is a function of intentions to use condoms and, in turn, intentions to use condoms are a function of variables such as attitudes and norms regarding HIV and condom use.[57] Social cognitive models (i.e. self-efficacy) explain condom use as a function of an individual's knowledge about HIV, expectation about the outcomes of using condoms (i.e. pleasure reduction versus disease prevention) and self-efficacy (i.e. that the individual will be able to use a condom in different sexual situations).[58] These psychosocial models of HIV prophylactic behavior have been tested in both cross-sectional and longitudinal studies in a variety of populations and are the basis for many of the behavioral interventions reviewed below.

Intervention models that address information, motivation and behavioral skills[59] typically take into account models of HIV risk prevention. One is the trans-theoretical model of change,[60] which posits that an intervention needs to be adaptable to an individual's current readiness to change. For example, people who are currently in a 'precontemplative' level of readiness to change do not see their behavior as problematic and do not see a reason to change; someone in a 'contemplative' level may be ambivalent about changing, and someone at a 'determination or preparation' level is ready to make a commitment. Interventions based on the trans-theoretical model try to move individuals to a more serious, higher level of readiness to change than where they are initially. Accordingly, an individual at an earlier level may benefit most from information and education, whereas someone at a mid-level or higher might benefit from more intensive motivational support and skills training.

Outcome of Large-Scale and High-Impact-for-HIV Prevention Studies in the USA

PREVENTION TRIALS DELIVERED PRIMARILY TO HETEROSEXUAL INDIVIDUALS IN STI AND PRIMARY CARE CLINICS

Two different randomized controlled trials of HIV prevention interventions have examined the efficacy of risk-reduction counseling approaches in individuals at high risk for HIV infection, by studying heterosexual individuals attending STI or primary care clinics. The first study, the US National Institute of Mental Health's Multisite HIV Prevention Trial (Project Light), recruited 3706 individuals from 37 inner-city community-based clinics in seven sites across the USA.[61]

At screening, all participants reported engaging in unprotected vaginal or anal sex within 90 days. Those in the intervention group (seven sessions of risk-reduction counseling in a group format) reported fewer unprotected sexual acts and were more likely to use condoms consistently over the follow-up period. The intervention group also reported higher overall levels of condom use.

The second large-scale study, Project RESPECT, recruited over 5787 heterosexual HIV-negative patients who presented for care at STI clinics across the USA.[62] Participants were randomized to a four-session ('enhanced counseling'), a two-session ('brief counseling') or a non-interactive ('didactic message') condition. Those assigned four-session and two-session interactive interventions had fewer new HIV infections at both 6- and 12-month intervals than those who received the non-interactive counseling. Additionally, self-reported 100% condom use was higher in both interactive counseling groups compared to the didactic message control.

Recently, Crepaz et al. evaluated the efficacy of a large number of HIV behavioral interventions in reducing unprotected sex and incident STI among African-American and Hispanic STI clinic patients.[50] HIV behavioral interventions were found to significantly reduce unprotected sex and incident STIs, providing evidence that HIV behavioral interventions provide an efficacious means of HIV/STI prevention for African-American and Hispanic patients who attend STI clinics.

As HIV risk behavior is a necessary factor for HIV infection, these studies taken together reveal that HIV risk-reduction counseling can both increase condom use and decrease sexually transmitted infections.

PREVENTION TRIALS FOR MSM
Individually Randomized Controlled Trials

One of the earlier individually randomized intervention trials[63] compared an integrated cognitive–behavioral intervention to a waiting list control among 104 homosexual men in a metropolitan area. At the post-training assessment, the experimental group had fewer high-risk sexual practices and better behavioral skills for sexual coercive situations than the wait list control.

Project EXPLORE was a large-scale randomized HIV-prevention trial among MSM conducted in six US cities, with a total of 4295 participants.[48,64] Men were randomized to receive a behavioral intervention versus standard risk-reduction counseling. Study results suggested a possible modest benefit of the intervention in reducing new HIV infections.[64] Further, the reporting of unprotected receptive anal sex with HIV-positive or unknown-status partners was significantly lower in the intervention group compared with the standard group.

Community Randomized Controlled Trials

One of the first community randomized controlled trials, the Mpowerment Project, studied a peer-outreach program for young homosexual men (aged 18–29 years).[65] To assess outcome, a cohort of 300 individuals from two communities were surveyed. In the intervention community, the proportion of participants who reported unprotected anal intercourse with non-primary partners decreased, as did the proportion of participants who reported unprotected anal intercourse. No significant changes occurred in the comparison community.

Another large-scale community randomized trial[66] involved delivering the intervention through opinion leaders (popular individuals) from the gay community in four US states. Each state randomly had both an intervention city and comparison city. In the intervention city, popular gay men were trained to spread behavior-change messages (to change norms), and in the comparison city pamphlets were placed at gay bars. Across all states, 1126 men completed baseline surveys and 1010 completed follow-up surveys. At 1-year follow-up, those in the intervention cities reported a significantly greater reduction in the frequency of unprotected anal sex during the previous 2 months, and a significantly greater increase in condom use for anal sex compared to comparison cities. Consistent with this finding, more condoms were taken from bars at the intervention cities than the comparison cities.

The community randomized trials among MSM validate the utility of providing HIV prevention, on a larger scale, to communities of MSM. From a public health perspective, raising awareness and changing norms regarding HIV prophylactic behavior can influence transmission rates at the community level.

Meta-analyses of HIV behavioral intervention studies show that HIV behavioral interventions with adult MSM result in significant reductions in self-reported sexual risk behaviors.[52,53,67] Interventions most successful in reducing risky sexual behavior are those based on theoretic models, including interpersonal skills training, incorporating several delivery methods, and being delivered over multiple sessions spanning a minimum of 3 weeks.

PREVENTION TRIALS FOR WOMEN
Individually Randomized Controlled Trials

Several large-scale multisite studies have investigated risk-reduction counseling among low-income and/or minority women. Kelly et al. randomized 197 high-risk women from an urban primary health clinic to a cognitive–behavioral risk-reduction intervention or comparison.[68] Three months later, the intervention group evidenced better sexual communication and negotiation skills (assessed by role play and self-report), and less unprotected sexual intercourse. The comparison group had no changes on these measures.

A second study of HIV risk-reduction counseling among women[69] sought to adapt models of behavioral change to social and contextual variables relevant to 128 economically disadvantaged African-American women between the ages of 18 and 29 years. At the 3-month follow-up, women in the more intensive intervention showed increased consistent condom use, sexual self-control, sexual communication and sexual assertiveness, and partner's adoption of norms supporting consistent condom use than those in the delayed educational control.

A study of 206 pregnant inner-city women randomized participants to an AIDS prevention group or to one of two controls.[70] After the intervention and after 6-month follow-up, the AIDS prevention group had increases in knowledge and safer sex behaviors in comparison with the two control groups.

Due to difficulties with retention and attrition of high-risk and hard-to-reach women in HIV prevention trials, Belcher et al. developed and tested the utility of a single-session, 2-hour one-on-one intervention using motivational interviewing and information–motivation–behavioral skills training.[71] No differences occurred in HIV knowledge, but the group that received skills training and motivational interviewing showed higher levels of HIV protective behaviors than the control group, including higher rates of condom use during vaginal intercourse, demonstrating the efficacy of a brief, minimal intervention.

Two randomized controlled trials of an HIV risk-reduction intervention using information, motivation enhancement and skills training intervention were developed for low-income, primarily African-American, women.[72,73] In both studies, the intervention consisted of four 90-minute sessions, which included personalized feedback about their HIV knowledge, risk perceptions and sexual behavior. Women who received the intervention reported stronger intentions to practice safe sex and to communicate these intentions to partners, and less unprotected intercourse and substance use near the time of sexual activity; these gains were maintained at the 3-month follow-up.

Taken together, the series of randomized controlled trials of HIV prevention counseling for high-risk women demonstrate both feasibility and efficacy of such approaches. While many of these approaches are useful, some may be difficult to disseminate. These interventions require special training and most require a significant amount of time for both the participants and the counselors. Future study of individually administered interventions should now focus on ways to implement and disseminate interventions to community-based settings.

Community Randomized Controlled Trials

To attempt to address some of the limitations of clinic-based intervention approaches for women, two studies of community-randomized trials have been undertaken. The first used nine low-income housing developments[73] and nine demographically matched control developments. The community-level intervention included workshops and community HIV prevention events implemented by popular opinion leaders within each community. The women in the housing developments ($n = 690$) were surveyed at baseline and 1 year later. This revealed that women in the intervention communities showed better decreases in unprotected sex (past 2 months) and frequency of unprotected acts.

A second community-based randomized control trial targeted low-income, primarily African-American women in four urban settings.[72] Four communities in metropolitan areas were selected: two public housing communities, a low-income neighborhood and a group of inner-city neighborhoods. The intervention consisted of distribution of HIV prevention materials, developing a peer network of community organizers and businesses, and delivering prevention messages by outreach specialists, both individually and in groups. The intervention communities evidenced increases in talking with main partners about condoms and trying to get main partners to use condoms.

HIV behavioral interventions with women have been shown to be effective in reducing overall HIV risk.[49,74] Neumann et al. conducted a meta-analysis of HIV behavioral interventions among heterosexuals and found statistically significant effects in reducing sex-related risk (OR = 0.81, 95% CI 0.53–0.90) and decreased incidence of STIs (OR = 0.74, 95% CI 0.62–0.89). Four of the 10 studies (40%) included in the behavioral analyses were individual interventions and 6 out of 10 (60%) focused exclusively on women.[49]

HIV PREVENTION INTERVENTIONS SPECIFIC TO INTRAVENOUS DRUG USERS

A review of 42 studies between 1989 and 1999 suggested that the majority found that needle-exchange programs prevent HIV risk behavior and seroconversion among intravenous drug users.[75] Most other studies of HIV prevention interventions for drug users are observational or quasi-experimental evaluation studies; however, these studies do show significant within-participant reductions in HIV risk behavior.[76]

Semaan et al. examined the efficacy of 33 intervention studies with drug users (94% intravenous drug users, 21% crack users).[77] Relative to no HIV behavioral intervention, drug users in intervention conditions significantly reduced sexual risk behaviors (OR = 0.60, 95% CI 0.43–0.85). In other words, when extrapolating results to a population with a 72% prevalence of risk behaviors, the proportion of drug users who reduced their risk behaviors was 12.6% greater in the intervention groups than in the comparison groups.

Among the studies of prevention interventions for intravenous drug users, methodologies differ and, consequently, so do the results. Sexual behavior, as shown in previous sections, is a difficult and complex behavior to change. When co-morbid with drug dependence or addiction, its complexity grows; intensive multimodal interventions currently show the most utility in this population.

Summary

Behavioral interventions to decrease HIV transmission have been successful in a wide array of settings and with diverse populations. However, in most situations, interventions were needed to sustain behavior change. Moreover, there is limited experience with these interventions in parts of the world where the epidemic is spreading most rapidly and where the social construction of reality (e.g. disempowerment of women, limited healthcare infrastructure) may limit the effectiveness of programs developed in resource-rich settings. Clearly, additional work is needed to develop culturally specific behavioral interventions, while the development of more effective biologic prevention modalities (i.e. microbicides and vaccines) is underway.

References available online at expertconsult.com.

KEY REFERENCES

Bartlett J.G., Branson B.M., Fenton K., et al.: Opt-out testing for human immunodeficiency virus in the United States: progress and challenges. *JAMA* 2008; 300(8):945-951.

Cohen M.S., Chen Y.Q., McCauley M., et al.: Prevention of HIV-1 infection with early antiretroviral therapy. *N Engl J Med* 2011; 365(6):493-505.

Crepaz N., Horn A.K., Rama S.M., et al.: The efficacy of behavioral interventions in reducing HIV risk sex behaviors and incident sexually transmitted disease in black and Hispanic sexually transmitted disease clinic patients in the United States: a meta-analytic review. *Sex Transm Dis* 2007; 34(6):319-332.

Grant R.M., Lama J.R., Anderson P.L., et al.: Preexposure chemoprophylaxis for HIV prevention in men who have sex with men. *N Engl J Med* 2010; 363(27):2587-2599.

Gray R.H., Kigozi G., Serwadda D., et al.: Male circumcision for HIV prevention in men in Rakai, Uganda: a randomised trial. *Lancet* 2007; 369(9562):657-666.

Hall H.I., Song R., Rhodes P., et al.: Estimation of HIV incidence in the United States. *JAMA* 2008; 300(5):520-529.

Herbst J.H., Beeker C., Mathew A., et al.: The effectiveness of individual-, group-, and community-level HIV behavioral risk-reduction interventions for adult men who have sex with men: a systematic review. *Am J Prev Med* 2007; 32(4):38-67.

Koblin B., Chesney M., Coates T., et al.: Effects of a behavioural intervention to reduce acquisition of HIV infection among men who have sex with men: the EXPLORE randomised controlled study. *Lancet* 2004; 364(9428):41-50.

Lavreys L., Rakwar J.P., Thompson M.L., et al.: Effect of circumcision on incidence of human immunodeficiency virus type 1 and other sexually transmitted diseases: a prospective cohort study of trucking company employees in Kenya. *J Infect Dis* 1999; 180(2):330-336.

Marazzo J., Ramjee G., Richardson B.A., et al.: Tenofovir-based preexposure prophylaxis for HIV infection among African women. *N Engl J Med* 2015; 372(6):509-518.

Quinn T.C., Wawer M.J., Sewankambo N., et al.: Viral load and heterosexual transmission of human immunodeficiency virus type 1. Rakai Project Study Group. *N Engl J Med* 2000; 342(13):921-929.

US Public Health Service/Centers for Disease Control and Prevention. Preexposure prophylaxis for the prevention of HIV infection in the United States – 2014. A clinical practice guideline. Available: www.cdc.gov/hiv/pdf/PrEPguidelines2014.pdf.

91

HIV Vaccines: Past Failures and Future Scientific Challenges

BRUCE L. GILLIAM | ROBERT R. REDFIELD | BARRY S. PETERS

KEY CONCEPTS

- Despite the increased roll out of human immunodeficiency virus (HIV) therapy in low- and middle-income countries, the large majority still do not have access to highly active antiretroviral therapy (HAART) and an HIV vaccine is needed to impact upon the epidemic.

- For the first time, an HIV vaccine study, using canarypox vector prime and gp120 envelope protein boost, showed efficacy, albeit limited.

- Even a study with limited success, the previously mentioned prime-boost study, gave new clues as to the correlates of protection.

- An improved understanding of the structure of potential neutralizing domains for HIV is likely to underpin future vaccine efforts.

- A coordinated approach among major groups working on HIV vaccine development is needed to maximize the chances of developing a strong vaccine candidate.

Introduction: Why Do We Need an HIV Vaccine?

Since 2005, the number of deaths due to acquired immune deficiency syndrome (AIDS) has decreased by 29% worldwide largely due to the increase in global access to antiretroviral therapy. However, there are still approximately 1.6 million deaths annually from HIV and AIDS and 2.3 million new infections per year. Antiretroviral therapy is currently available only to approximately 34% of those in need of treatment worldwide.[1] In addition, even in the USA only approximately 30% of those with HIV achieve complete viral suppression in plasma levels. This disparity is largely due to failure to diagnose and integrate HIV-infected individuals into effective care. Some of this can also be attributed to problems with HAART use, including adverse effects, drug interactions and the development of drug-resistant HIV strains. Measures that reduce or prevent transmission, such as condoms or male circumcision, or indeed widespread roll out of HIV therapy, are needed urgently but are often limited by social and behavioral influences. Of the various prevention measures, a prophylactic HIV vaccine is the only one likely to have a major impact on the global spread of HIV. There is, therefore, an urgent need for a safe, effective prophylactic HIV vaccine in order to improve global health. Unfortunately, as this chapter discusses, there are still significant challenges we need to overcome before reaching this goal.

The Challenge to the Development of an HIV Vaccine

When HIV was discovered in 1983, there was initially hope that a vaccine would swiftly follow. The true magnitude of the challenge in designing an HIV vaccine has only become apparent as we have gained a more thorough understanding of the complex molecular biology of HIV infection. Ancestral retroviruses have been in existence for many tens of millennia and have had a head start on us in how to evade host immune responses. Combine this with the extraordinarily rapid rate of mutation during HIV replication and it is understandable that HIV has been able to evolve superlatively effective mechanisms against vaccination. These range from the 'hiding' of potential neutralizing domains from neutralizing antibodies to the development of restriction genes whose sole purpose is to defend HIV from the host. The enormity of the scientific challenge is now apparent to all those in the field (Box 91-1).

How Would We Define a 'Successful Prophylactic HIV Vaccine'?

There has also been a re-evaluation of what might be considered a 'successful prophylactic HIV vaccine' (PHV). An ideal PHV would be one that prevents infection in almost 100% of those vaccinated; it would be cheap, easily (self-)administered, stable in all commonly encountered environmental conditions (including those found in the tropics), be completely safe and have a lifelong effect. However, a PHV would still be valuable if it did not offer protection against infection, but instead mitigated the course of the disease after infection. This would reduce morbidity and mortality from HIV. Similarly, a vaccine that reduced the infectivity of the individual would reduce the spread of the HIV epidemic (Box 91-2).

The Starting Point: Applying Approaches that Have Been Successful for Other Vaccines

It is not a prerequisite to understand how the body protects against an infective agent to develop an effective vaccine against that organism. The first successful vaccine against a viral infection was developed by Edward Jenner without any knowledge of the causative infectious agent, the way the agent was transmitted or any knowledge of how the vaccine might mediate disease. Nonetheless, a vaccine against smallpox

---

BOX 91-1 KEY DIFFICULTIES IN DEVELOPING AN HIV VACCINE

- No natural sterilizing immunity to disease.
- Huge difficulties in producing neutralizing antibodies.
- No good animal models of HIV infection.
- A pool of latently infected cells is formed early after infection.
- No good correlates of T-cell vaccine efficacy have been identified.

BOX 91-2 DEFINITIONS OF A SUCCESSFUL HIV VACCINE

- Provides protection to 70–100% and markedly slows epidemic.
- Only provides protection in 30–70% but still has significant impact on HIV epidemic.
- Does *not* prevent infection at all, but reduces the postinfection viral load, leading to:
  - slower disease progression in the individual;
  - reduced infectivity of the individual; and
  - slowing of the epidemic due to reduced transmission.

TABLE 91-1	Examples of Vaccines Used to Prevent Other Viral Illnesses		
Vaccine Type	**Diseases**	**Correlate for Protection**	**Safety Issues for HIV Vaccines**
Live attenuated	Polio (oral) Measles Mumps Rubella Varicella Yellow fever Smallpox	Antibodies	Considered too unsafe to use in HIV because of possible reversion to virulent type
Whole inactivated	Inactivated polio Hepatitis A Influenza	Antibodies	Considered to be relatively safe, although some concerns exist
Recombinant proteins	Hepatitis B Human papillomavirus	Antibodies	Considered to be relatively safe, and is the main current approach, although some viral vectors might increase the risk of infection

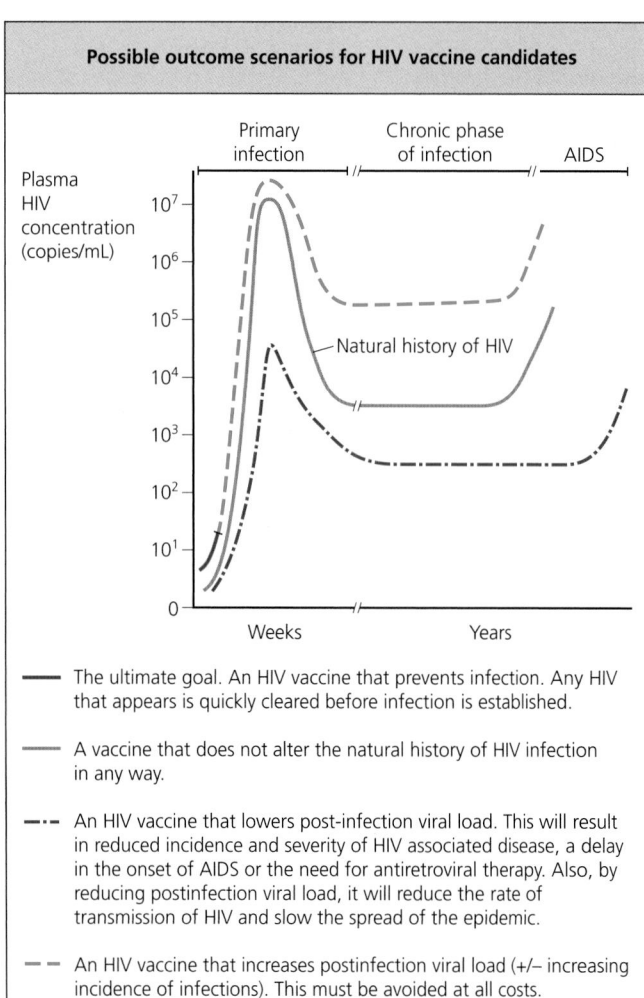

Possible outcome scenarios for HIV vaccine candidates

—— The ultimate goal. An HIV vaccine that prevents infection. Any HIV that appears is quickly cleared before infection is established.

—— A vaccine that does not alter the natural history of HIV infection in any way.

—·— An HIV vaccine that lowers post-infection viral load. This will result in reduced incidence and severity of HIV associated disease, a delay in the onset of AIDS or the need for antiretroviral therapy. Also, by reducing postinfection viral load, it will reduce the rate of transmission of HIV and slow the spread of the epidemic.

— — An HIV vaccine that increases postinfection viral load (+/− increasing incidence of infections). This must be avoided at all costs.

Figure 91-1   Possible outcome scenarios for HIV vaccine candidates.

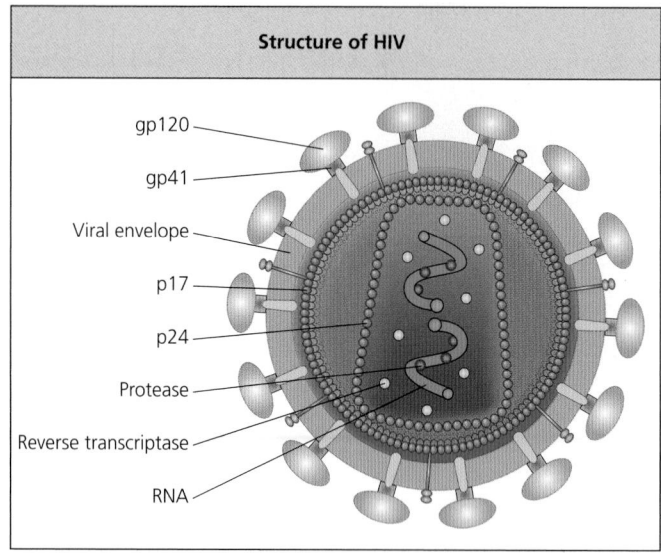

Figure 91-2   Structure of human immunodeficiency virus (HIV).

was developed.[2] Three main types of vaccine that have been successfully for the prevention of other viral illnesses are live attenuated, whole inactivated, and recombinant subunit protein vaccines (Table 91-1). All of these vaccines protect by means of antibody responses, and hence it seemed only natural in HIV vaccine development to seek vaccines that might produce neutralizing antibodies. This would tie in with our knowledge of the immune response to HIV infection (Figure 91-1). The choice of vaccine type, however, is limited by safety concerns. Live attenuated HIV vaccines have protected against infection in the nonhuman primate model but are considered too dangerous for use in humans because of the possible reversion to a more pathogenic type of virus.[3] Whole inactivated viruses seemed to offer protection in nonhuman primate models. However, this protection was found to be mediated by neutralizing antibodies (NAbs) against human cellular proteins that had been incorporated into the vaccine during production in human cell lines.[4] Hence, for reasons of safety and efficacy, most initial HIV vaccine candidates were recombinant/subunit vaccines. The first such vaccine used a recombinant envelope protein of HIV, based on gp120 (Figure 91-2). There are many other instances of viral infections for which the 'neutralizing antibody' approach has not yielded a successful vaccine, hepatitis C being one such example.

Strategies for HIV Vaccine Development

INDUCTION OF NEUTRALIZING ANTIBODIES

As noted above, neutralizing antibodies have been shown to protect against challenge from many viruses, including HIV and SHIV (chimeric SIV/HIV) in animal studies.[5] For neutralizing antibodies to be effective against HIV, they need to interfere with fusion of the virus to the host cell. HIV fuses to target cells by using a trimeric envelope complex of gp120 and gp41 subunits, which attach to CD4+ receptors and a co-receptor (usually CCR5 or CXCR4). Neutralizing antibodies of primary isolates work in one of two ways: either they prevent receptor engagement by binding to the virus surface trimer or they inhibit fusion after viral attachment has occurred.[6] The challenges lie in the

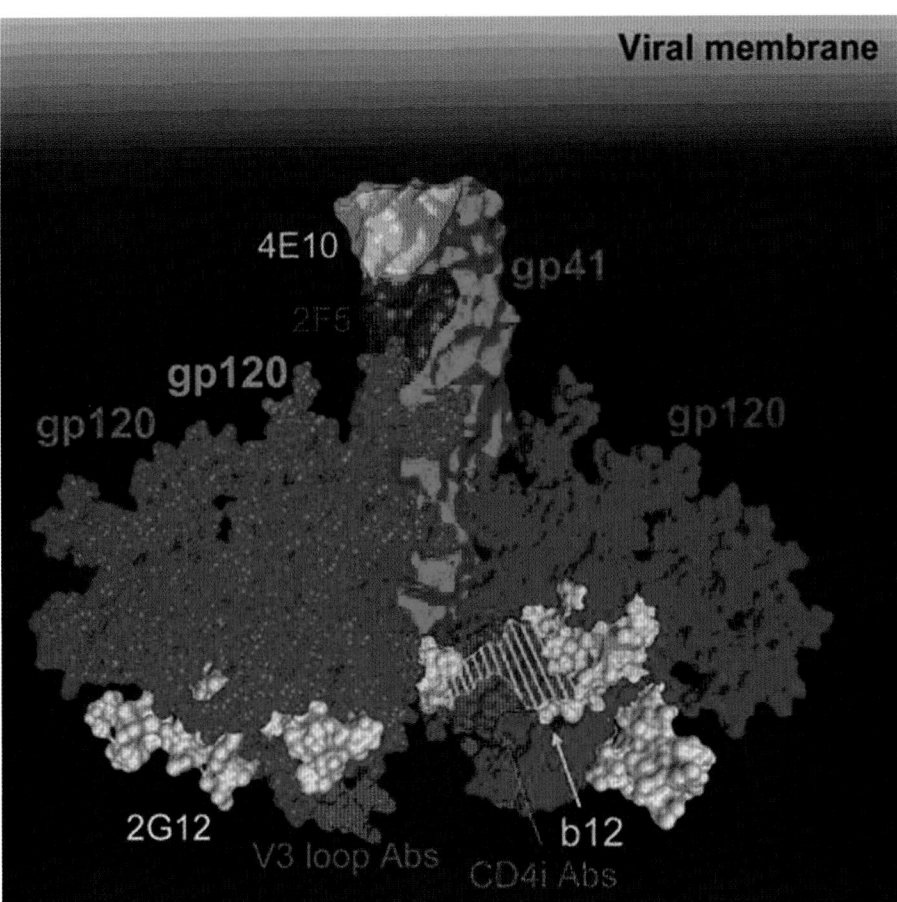

Figure 91-3   Model of HIV highlighting the mechanisms HIV uses to avoid neutralization. (*From Burton et al., Nat Immunol 2004; 5(3):233–236.*[10])

high degree of viral diversity in HIV, the fact that 'natural infection' with HIV does not prevent the occurrence of superinfection with other viral subtypes and that putative HIV vaccines have not, to date, elicited broadly neutralizing antibodies in humans. Even though neutralizing antibodies against the HIV envelope do occur naturally after infection in humans, they almost immediately select for escape mutants.[7–9] HIV has evolved a number of mechanisms to evade this neutralization (Figure 91-3).[10] The HIV envelope is heavily glycosylated. The glycans themselves are poorly immunogenic and they prevent access of antibodies to the peptides beneath them. The trimeric nature of the gp120–gp41 structure also shields the epitopes much more so than for the individual monomeric subunits.

HIV has four major conserved domains in the envelope that serve as targets for broadly neutralizing antibodies. They include the gp120 CD4-binding site region, the membrane proximal external region (MPER) of gp41, a peptide-glycan epitope in the gp120 V1V2 region and a peptide-glycan epitope in the gp120 V3 region (Figure 91-3).[11] None of them is an easy target for potential vaccine-induced antibodies for which there are several reasons (Box 91-3). Initial studies identified four broadly reactive human monoclonal antibodies which were assigned the following labels: b12, 2G12, 2F5 and 4E10. Infusion of these human monoclonal antibodies into HIV-infected patients have markedly reduced HIV viral load demonstrating their efficacy in humans.[12] Recently, in a non-human primate model, it was demonstrated that antibodies to the simian immunodeficiency virus (SIV) envelope were necessary and sufficient to prevent infection when challenged with SIV.[13] In addition, the investigators identified a 2-amino-acid sequence, similar to one which conferred resistance of HIV to neutralization by V1V2 monoclonal antibodies, that altered antigenicity and conferred resistance to neutralization. These results help to understand the results of the human clinical trials described below and provide a means of studying how best to deploy these approaches.

BOX 91-3   DIFFICULTIES IN PRODUCING NEUTRALIZING ANTIBODIES (NAbs)

- Exposed sequences on the envelope are highly variable, which rapidly leads to escape mutants.
- Exposed sequences, e.g. gp120, do not lead to NAbs of great breadth or specificity.
- The viral envelope exists as a trimer and immunogenic regions on the monomer are shielded (the envelope proteins are shielded by numerous N-linked glycans).
- The envelope protein undergoes structural changes when it binds to the CD4 receptor.
- High levels of NAbs are probably required to prevent infection.

INDUCTION OF T-CELL RESPONSES

The basis of 'T-cell vaccines' is the ability of T cells to recognize peptide sequences of HIV. CD8[+] T cells recognize peptides that are 8–11 amino acids in length that are presented on the surface of cells by major histocompatibility complex (MHC) class I antigens; CD4[+] T cells recognize peptides 10–18 amino acids in length that are presented on cells by MHC class II antigens. The disadvantage of T-cell vaccines compared to antibody vaccines is that they can only work once a cell has become infected. Thus T-cell vaccines do not prevent infection but are of potential value in controlling infections. Even with T-cell vaccines, however, there is the possibility of viral immune escape over time.[14]

As there is an incomplete understanding of the role of HIV-specific CD4[+] T cells in control of HIV infection, the problem is what responses to generate and how best to generate them. For example, T follicular helper cells play a role in B cell differentiation and affinity maturation.[15] Indeed, a subpopulation of circulating memory cells was identified that are related to germinal center T follicular helper cells and correlated with development of HIV-specific broadly neutralizing antibodies in HIV-infected individuals.[16] However, it is not yet clear how to generate T follicular helper cell responses with a vaccine and induce memory T follicular helper cells. A number of approaches are being used in order to develop T-cell responses within an HIV vaccine. Those undergoing most development at present are the use of recombinant viral vectors, DNA delivery of antigenic material using adjuvant-supported proteins and peptides, and finally a combination of more than one of these approaches.

PRIME-BOOST STRATEGY

Limitations with vaccines inducing antibodies as well as those inducing T-cell responses led the field to consider the 'prime-boost' approach. This approach uses priming with an antigen presented by one vector such as DNA or a live viral vector followed by boosting of the response by presenting the antigen by means of a different delivery system.[17,18] This 'prime-boost' approach has been extensively developed and used in clinical trials for many pathogens because it appears the most effective means of eliciting good T-cell responses. The prime-boost approach using Adenovirus5 (Ad5) and modified vaccinia Ankara (MVA) vectors has delivered some impressive results in animal models, including nonhuman primates. However, these successes have rarely carried over into trials in humans as outlined below.[19] The exception is the RV144 trial described below where the combination of ALVAC prime and AIDSVAX boost led to superior neutralization of Tier 1 viruses, viruses having high sensitivity to antibody-mediated neutralization, compared to two injections of AIDSVAX alone, clearly documenting the priming effect of the ALVAC vector.[20] The results of these human trials demonstrate the limitations of animal models in predicting the results of HIV vaccine trials in humans.

MUCOSAL HIV VACCINES

Most HIV infections are acquired by the mucosal route, vaginally, rectally or, less commonly, orally. Once HIV has gained entry via mucosa, it is transmitted quickly throughout the body. After rhesus macaques were inoculated intravaginally with SIV, the virus was detected in Langerhans cells or dendritic cells under the vaginal epithelium within 4 hours, in the internal iliac lymph nodes within 48 hours and in the blood within 5 days.[21,22] SIV was found in distant lymph nodes and bone marrow at 12 days. Once established in the lymphoid tissue, HIV undergoes massive replication in the largest mucosal-associated lymphoid tissue (MALT), the bowel, and this leads to a marked depletion of CD4+ cells in the intestinal tract.[23] HIV infection needs to be cleared before it becomes established, meaning that HIV vaccines must induce effective immune responses at the point of entry within the first few days of exposure to the virus.[24] Certainly the effective induction of mucosal immunity is thought to be one of the most important requirements for an HIV vaccine. Mucosal vaccines might offer this more than immunization by other routes[25] because of the potential for enhancement of mucosal immunity. However, not all routes of mucosal vaccination are the same. Both the quality and the quantity of antigen-specific immune responses at a mucosal site appear to be highly dependent on the exact route of mucosal vaccination. Rectal administration has been poorly studied in humans, but mice models show that vaccines can induce strong antigen-specific mucosal IgA and CTL responses in the rectum and systemically.[26,27] Nasal administration in humans induces strong antigen-specific antibody responses in salivary glands, the respiratory tract, genital tract and systemically, but not in the intestine, although this route can induce strong antigen-specific IgA and CTLs in the female genital tract.[28,29]

Lessons from the Natural History of HIV Progression

The rates of progression of HIV in the complete absence of treatment, as measured by CD4+ cell count decline, can vary enormously between patients. At one extreme are the rare 'elite non-progressors', alternatively termed 'HIV controllers', who maintain an undetectable HIV viral load in serum for long periods of time and have no discernible

CD4+ count decline during these periods. Such control has been observed for long periods, up to 25 years so far in some patients. These controllers are much more likely to have certain genetic factors, specifically certain HLA class I alleles, and also CD8+ T-cell responses generated through these alleles.[30] They are also more likely to have virus-specific, strong CD4+ T-cell responses. However, no one feature is common to all HIV controllers. Clearly there might be much to learn from these patients with regard to HIV vaccines designed to prevent or treat HIV, and this population is being studied intensively for further clues.

What Have We Learned from Human Clinical HIV Vaccine Trials to Date?

Learning from the past, most of the initial HIV vaccine candidates were subunit protein vaccines targeting the envelope protein of the virus. However, other strategies have been employed as well, including peptide vaccines, viral vector vaccines (i.e., adenovirus, alphavirus, vaccinia, canarypox, Venezuelan equine encephalitis), DNA vaccines and virus-like particles. Although several hundred phase 1/2 trials have evaluated these vaccine candidates, very few have made it to advanced phase 2 and phase 3 efficacy trials. The results of these advanced trials are discussed below.

AIDSVAX TRIALS – gP120 ENVELOPE PROTEIN VACCINE

Only one envelope protein HIV vaccine candidate has been evaluated in phase 3 trials. This candidate, a gp120 subunit vaccine called AIDSVAX, was evaluated in two large trials, VAX003 and VAX004.[31,32] VAX003 evaluated two subtype B gp120 envelope proteins in 5400 men who have sex with men (MSM) and heterosexual women at high risk whereas VAX004 evaluated a bivalent subtype B and E protein vaccine in 2500 Thai intravenous drug users. Despite the different risk groups, there were no significant reductions in HIV infections in either of the vaccinated groups.

STEP/PHAMBILI TRIALS – ADENOVIRUS VECTOR VACCINE

The STEP trial was a large phase 2b study evaluating a replication-incompetent recombinant adenovirus vaccine which was composed of three distinct vectors, one expressing HIV-1 Gag, one expressing HIV-1 Pol, and one expressing HIV-1 Nef.[33] The study randomized 3000 men and women volunteers at risk for HIV infection (1494 in the vaccine arm and 1504 in the placebo arm) in 34 study sites located in North America, South America, Australia and the Caribbean. At the first planned interim analysis the study was stopped because it met the prespecified boundaries for lack of vaccine efficacy. It is important to note that all but one infection occurred in men. Of interest, volunteers that were seropositive for Ad5 or uncircumcised had higher rates of HIV-1 infection than placebo. This higher rate was not seen in Ad5 seronegative or circumcised volunteers. Genetic sequencing of the HIV-1 strains from volunteers that acquired HIV infection demonstrated that the viruses infecting vaccine volunteers had different epitopes compared to viruses infecting placebo recipients. This divergence was limited to the epitopes encoded for by the vaccine thus indicating selective pressure of the vaccine on cytotoxic T-lymphocyte responses.[34] Immune responses as measured by ELISPOT occurred in 75% of the 25% random sample of vaccine recipients. There was no difference in the postinfection viral load set-point. The results of the STEP trial led to the halting of the Phambili (HVTN 503) Study which had been scheduled to evaluate the same adenovirus vaccine as used in the STEP trial in 3000 volunteers in South Africa.[35] At the time it was stopped, the trial had enrolled 801 volunteers, of whom 45% were women. Analysis of the data at discontinuation revealed no evidence of vaccine efficacy or change in postinfection viral load set-point. Of note, Ad5 titer, sex, age, circumcision status or herpes simplex virus 2 infection status did not have an impact on vaccine efficacy. The vaccine induced similar immunologic responses to those seen in the STEP trial.

RV144 – CANARYPOX VECTOR PRIME AND gP120 ENVELOPE PROTEIN BOOST

RV144 was a phase 3 randomized placebo-controlled trial, evaluating a prime-boost vaccine strategy using a canarypox vector (ALVAC) encoding Gag/Pro and Env antigens prime of four immunizations within 24 weeks accompanied by a boost with AIDSVAX B/E, a bivalent HIV gp120 envelope glycoprotein derived from a subtype B and subtype E envelope, given concomitantly with ALVAC at the 12- and 24-week immunizations.[36] The study enrolled 16042 volunteers primarily at heterosexual risk of acquiring HIV in Thailand. At 96 weeks using the modified intent-to-treat analysis, there were 74 HIV infections out of 7325 volunteers in the placebo group and 51 HIV infections out of 7347 volunteers in the vaccine group, offering a 31% efficacy which was statistically significant. This was the first HIV vaccine trial to demonstrate any evidence of efficacy. It is important to note that the vaccine efficacy peaked in the first 6–12 months (50–60%) only to decrease thereafter raising the important issue of durability of immune responses with this vaccine. In addition, there was not a significant broadly neutralizing antibody response. Further analysis has revealed two immune correlates of infection risk after vaccination.[37] Binding of IgG antibodies to the V1–V2 variable regions of Env inversely correlated with infection rates, while plasma IgA binding to Env directly correlated to infection rates.

HVTN 505 – DNA PRIME AND ADENOVIRUS VECTOR BOOST

This large phase 2 study evaluated a 'prime-boost strategy' with a DNA vaccine, designed to induce responses to gag, pol, nef and env proteins from subtypes A, B and C, as the prime, injections given at enrollment, week 4 and week 8, and an adenovirus vector, composed of four adenovirus vectors expressing a subtype B Gag-Pol fusion protein as well as envelope proteins from subtypes A, B and C, as the boost at week 24.[38] The study enrolled 2504 circumcised men or transgender women who have sex with men and randomized them to vaccine (1253 volunteers) or placebo (1251 volunteers). Although the vaccine had an acceptable safety profile, the study was stopped prematurely in April 2013 by the Data and Safety Monitoring Board for lack of efficacy after a planned interim analysis. HIV infection after week 28 occurred in 27 volunteers in the vaccine arm and 21 volunteers in the placebo arm. The vaccine induced both cellular and humoral immune responses but the level of responses to the V1–V2 loop were considerably lower than those seen in RV144 and the level of IgA binding antibodies was higher than those reported in RV144. The vaccine had no impact on postinfection viral load set-point compared to the placebo arm. Contrary to the STEP study, there was no evidence of an increased risk of HIV acquisition in the vaccine arm.

Correlates of Immunity

It was not until the results of the RV144 trial were reported and further investigations performed that the first evidence of potential correlates of immunity were identified. In RV144, higher plasma IgG antibody binding to a scaffolded V1–V2 antigen of the gp120 envelope correlated with lower rates of infection while direct IgA binding to an envelope panel correlated directly with a higher rate of HIV acquisition.[37] Further evaluation of RV144 and comparison with the AIDSVAX trials have demonstrated that both trials generated antibodies directed against the same V2 epitopes.[39] However, RV144 generated higher frequencies of envelope IgG3 subclass responses compared to VAX003 which correlated with a decreased risk of HIV infection in RV144.[40] In addition, the RV144 regimen generated polyfunctional Fc-mediated effector responses including ADCC through selective induction of IgG3 where as VAX003 induced mono-functional antibody responses influenced by IgG4 selection.[41] Responses to the V3 region of gp120 also correlated with HIV acquisition but only in those with lower levels of envelope specific IgA and neutralizing antibodies. These data and those of a sieve analysis have led to the hypothesis 'that IgG to linear epitopes in the V2 and V3 regions of gp120 are part of a complex interplay of immune responses that contributed to protection in RV144'.[39,42] While these studies do not provide the template for a successful vaccine, they provide a starting point to direct and inform future vaccine research.

Vaccine Strategies for the Future

There is a clear need to explore 'novel' approaches to vaccine development that are substantially, if not radically, different from anything that has preceded them. At the same time our efforts also should be directed towards advancing the knowledge of existing HIV vaccine science. We currently have a starting point as elucidated by RV144 and other vaccine trials, and from these blueprints the direction of both clinical trials and vaccine science are starting to take shape.[5,43,44] There are several key concepts and challenges within these plans. Foremost is the simultaneous pursuit of addressing basic scientific questions critical to the development of an HIV vaccine while continuing to evaluate new vaccine concepts in clinical trials. Reverse vaccinology is a concept that utilizes structural biology and vaccinology to engineer immunogens from monoclonal antibodies isolated from cases of natural infection. These immunogens are subsequently introduced as vaccines that elicit the desired or closely related protective antibodies.[45] Advances in science have allowed the elucidation of the structure of the native HIV envelope trimer as well as the identification of an increasing number of broadly neutralizing monoclonal antibodies that can serve as the basis for immunogen design.[7,46–48] This concept has recently been demonstrated with respiratory syncytial virus (RSV) where a computational protein design was demonstrated to generate protein scaffolds that accurately mimic the viral epitope structure and induce potent neutralizing antibodies.[49] Another concept that has been facilitated by the identification of monoclonal antibodies is the identification of conserved viral epitopes that occur during the host–virus interaction. An example of this is utilizing the gp120-CD4 complex, formed as HIV binds to the cell, as a vaccine target; a conformationally constrained vaccine candidate that targets this complex is currently in development.[50]

The results of RV144 provide hope for the development of a successful vaccine. Clinical HIV vaccine trials are now seeking to build on the knowledge acquired from that trial. In the first 6–12 months of the RV144 trial, vaccine efficacy was significantly higher than that noted at 3 years. Durability is therefore a key challenge in the development of a viable vaccine candidate. This has led to intensive investigation into mechanisms and strategies that might provide a solution to this problem. Adjuvants that can favorably influence the responses generated by a vaccine candidate, including interleukins and toll-like receptors, are under evaluation. Vectors such as CMV which are persistent and induce persistent effector responses have shown promise in the SIV model.[51] Another challenge is the choice of vector. Building on RV144, many trials are pursuing a prime-boost strategy while utilizing different vaccine candidates. Live vector candidates such as adenovirus, vaccinia, vesicular stomatitis virus (VSV) flavivirus and Sendai virus are being used in combination with each other, mosaic antigens and DNA vaccine candidates. With each candidate, the goal is to enhance immunogenicity (both antibody and T cell) and durability over that seen in RV144.

Key scientific, clinical and political questions remain:

- How do we identify and reproduce broadly neutralizing antibody responses in humans?
- How can we identify correlates of immunity in which to screen and select HIV vaccine candidates at an early stage?
- How can we improve upon existing animal models of HIV infection?
- How can we best identify those truly original vaccine concepts that deserve further evaluation?
- How can we maintain enthusiasm from volunteers and donors alike in the face of the lack of progress?

Advances in science and in clinical trials (RV144) have drawn a pathway to begin to provide the answers. The challenges are not all scientific: if we are to avoid delays in the development of an effective HIV vaccine, we need to facilitate a more coordinated effort of governmental, nongovernmental and academic institutions. Hopefully, we can anticipate that the key questions will be more fully addressed, that global coordination of HIV efforts will be of a higher order and that we will be closer conceptually and in terms of production and clinical testing to HIV vaccine candidates with markedly improved efficacy.

References available online at expertconsult.com.

KEY REFERENCES

Burton D.R., Poignard P., Stanfield R.L., et al.: Broadly neutralizing antibodies present new prospects to counter highly antigenically diverse viruses. *Science* 2012; 337(6091):183-186.

Correia B.E., Bates J.T., Loomis R.J., et al.: Proof of principle for epitope-focused vaccine design. *Nature* 2014; 507(7491):201-206.

DeVico A., Fouts T., Lewis G.K., et al.: Antibodies to CD4-induced sites in HIV gp120 correlate with the control of SHIV challenge in macaques vaccinated with subunit immunogens. *Proc Natl Acad Sci USA* 2007; 104(44): 17477-17482.

Fauci A.S., Marston H.D.: Ending AIDS – is an HIV vaccine necessary? *N Engl J Med* 2014; 370(6):495-498.

Hammer S.M., Sobieszczyk M.E., Janes H., et al.: Efficacy trial of a DNA/rAd5 HIV-1 preventive vaccine. *N Engl J Med* 2013; 369(22):2083-2092.

Haynes B.F., Gilbert P.B., McElrath M.J., et al.: Immune-correlates analysis of an HIV-1 vaccine efficacy trial. *N Engl J Med* 2012; 366(14):1275-1286.

Klein F., Mouquet H., Dosenovic P., et al.: Antibodies in HIV-1 vaccine development and therapy. *Science* 2013; 341(6151):1199-1204.

Montefiori D.C., Karnasuta C., Huang Y., et al.: Magnitude and breadth of the neutralizing antibody response in the RV144 and Vax003 HIV-1 vaccine efficacy trials. *J Infect Dis* 2012; 206(3):431-441.

Nabel G.J.: Designing tomorrow's vaccines. *N Engl J Med* 2013; 368(6):551-560.

Neutra M.R., Kozlowski P.A.: Mucosal vaccines: the promise and the challenge. *Nat Rev Immunol* 2006; 6:148-158.

Rerks-Ngarm S., Pitisuttithum P., Nitayaphan S., et al.: Vaccination with ALVAC and AIDSVAX to prevent HIV-1 infection in Thailand. *N Engl J Med* 2009; 361(23):2209-2220.

Roederer M., Keele B.F., Schmidt S.D., et al.: Immunological and virological mechanisms of vaccine-mediated protection against SIV and HIV. *Nature* 2014; 505(7484): 502-508.

Rolland M., Edlefsen P.T., Larsen B.B., et al.: Increased HIV-1 vaccine efficacy against viruses with genetic signatures in Env V2. *Nature* 2012; 490(7420):417-420.

Streeck H., D'Souza M.P., Littman D.R., et al.: Harnessing CD4+ T cell responses in HIV vaccine development. *Nat Med* 2013; 19(2):143-149.

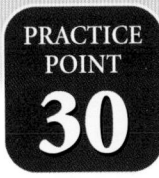

HIV Postexposure Prophylaxis

ERNIE-PAUL BARRETTE | GEROME V. ESCOTA | RUPA PATEL

Introduction

Because human immunodeficiency virus (HIV) infection is incurable, preventing HIV transmission is paramount. Exposure to HIV can occur by percutaneous, mucous membrane or non-intact skin exposure to infected blood or body fluids. It can also occur by sexual contact, trauma or needle sharing. Postexposure prophylaxis (PEP) is one method of preventing HIV transmission. PEP is the provision of antiretroviral therapy (ART) to HIV-negative persons exposed to infected materials. It should be emphasized that PEP should not replace standard infection control measures and behavioral practices that best prevent HIV exposure.

Risk of HIV Transmission

The risk of HIV transmission after an occupational exposure depends on the source material and the manner of contact (Table PP30-1). The risk is further modified by the intensity of exposure. The risk of transmission after percutaneous exposure to HIV-infected blood is estimated at 0.23–0.36%. The risk is much lower after mucous membrane exposure, estimated at 0.03–0.09%. Deep percutaneous injury, injury with a device visibly contaminated with the patient's blood, procedures involving needle placement in the source patient's vein or artery, and terminal illness in the patient are associated with higher transmission risk. Based on studies in sero-discordant couples and in mother-to-child transmission, higher viral titers may also further increase this risk. Undetectable viral load, however, does not completely eliminate the risk of HIV transmission. The risk of transmission from sources other than blood (e.g. cerebrospinal fluid) and after non-intact skin (e.g. abraded skin) exposure is unknown but considered substantially lower. Intact skin exposure is not considered a risk for HIV transmission.

The estimated per-act transmission risk during nonoccupational exposures varies by exposure type (Table PP30-1). Transmission risk can be as high as one transmission event per three penile–anal sexual encounters between a female with genital ulcerative disease and a male with AIDS. The risk of transmission after a bite injury is 0.004%.

Efficacy of HIV Postexposure Propylaxis

The best evidence for the efficacy of PEP comes from a study that enrolled healthcare workers with percutaneous exposure to HIV-infected blood. In this study, there were 33 workers who seroconverted and 665 who did not after exposure. Those who became HIV-infected were significantly less likely to have received zidovudine postexposure (OR 0.19, 95% CI 0.06–0.52, $p = 0.003$).

Observational studies conducted among men who have sex with men (MSM) and injection drug users, have shown efficacy of non-occupational PEP (nPEP). In one study, none of the 85 MSM who were offered PEP within 72 hours of HIV exposure became infected at 3 months. The PEP regimen offered was raltegravir, tenofovir and emtricitabine.

Guidelines for Providing Postexposure Prophylaxis

OCCUPATIONAL EXPOSURE

All exposures to blood and other potentially infected body fluids are considered significant. However, PEP is not recommended for exposure to body fluids not considered infectious (feces, urine, sweat, tears, saliva, sputum, vomitus) provided that these fluids are not bloody.

One should determine the HIV status of the source patient whenever possible. If unknown, a rapid HIV test should be performed. A negative test for HIV rules out HIV infection. If acute retroviral syndrome is suspected in the source patient, PEP should be initiated while testing the source for HIV RNA. If the source patient is known to be HIV-infected, information regarding HIV drug resistance and expert consultation should be obtained. However, PEP should not be delayed while gathering this information. If the source patient has a documented negative HIV test obtained near the time of exposure, PEP is not recommended. If the source patient cannot be determined, PEP maybe considered if the exposure is considered high risk.

Although PEP is most effective when administered up to 72 hours after exposure, PEP should still be considered even if delayed because the time interval after which PEP is no longer beneficial has not been determined. Expert consultation is recommended in this situation.

US Public Health Service 2013 guidelines on occupational PEP recommend a three-drug combination of antiretroviral therapy regardless of the severity of exposure.

The preferred regimen for PEP is Truvada (tenofovir/emtricitabine) plus raltegravir or dolutegravir. This regimen is chosen because of its proven effectiveness in treating HIV, minimal drug–drug interactions and its excellent tolerability. This regimen may be taken without regard for food. For alternative regimens, a consultation with an expert in antiretroviral therapy (ART) is recommended. PEP is generally prescribed for 28 days. Tenofovir is associated with worsening renal failure in persons with underlying kidney dysfunction. Although rare, severe skin hypersensitivity reaction has been reported with raltegravir. Because of the risk of serious adverse reactions with nevirapine and abacavir, these medications are contraindicated. Efavirenz should be avoided in women of childbearing age due to its potential teratogenicity.

All persons for whom PEP is prescribed should be followed up at regular intervals for HIV testing and monitoring of drug toxicity (Box PP30-1). Follow-up at 72 hours of exposure provides an opportunity to address any concerns and to assess for any adverse effects. Standard follow-up should occur at 6 weeks, and 3 and 6 months. However, with the fourth-generation combination HIV p24 antigen-HIV antibody test which allows for earlier detection of HIV, follow-up can be at 6 weeks and 4 months. Unless acute retroviral syndrome is suspected, routine testing for HIV RNA is not recommended. All persons receiving PEP should be counseled to use barrier contraception, avoid blood/tissue donation, pregnancy and breastfeeding to prevent secondary transmission, especially within the first 6–12 weeks of exposure. They should also be counseled regarding the side effects associated with the drugs used for PEP, the drug–drug interactions and the importance of adherence.

Note that the risk of transmitting hepatitis B and hepatitis C viruses after a percutaneous injury is greater than HIV. Therefore, postexposure testing for these viruses is recommended.

NONOCCUPATIONAL EXPOSURE

For those with exposure to genital secretions, blood, or other potentially infected body fluids of an HIV-infected individual, nPEP should be provided within 72 hours and continued for 28 days. It is important to contact the source person to obtain their history of ART, current

TABLE PP30-1	Risk of HIV Transmission According to Exposure	
Exposure	**HIV Transmission Risk per 10000 Exposures**
Blood transfusion	9000
Needle-sharing injection-drug use	67
Receptive anal intercourse	50
Percutaneous needle stick	30
Receptive penile–vaginal intercourse	10
Insertive anal intercourse	6.5
Insertive penile-vaginal intercourse	5
Receptive oral intercourse	1
Insertive oral intercourse	0.1

Adapted from Smith D.K., Grohskopf L.A., Black R.J., et al.: Antiretroviral postexposure prophylaxis after sexual, injection-drug use, or other nonoccupational exposure to HIV in the United States: recommendations from the U.S. Department of Health and Human Services. *MMWR Recomm Rep* 2005; 54(RR-2):7.

BOX PP30-1 LABORATORY EVALUATION FOR PERSONS WITH OCCUPATIONAL AND NONOCCUPATIONAL HIV EXPOSURE

OCCUPATIONAL EXPOSURE

HIV antibody testing at baseline and at 6 weeks, 12 weeks and 6 months after exposure.
Complete blood counts, renal and hepatic function panel at baseline and at 2 weeks after exposure; further testing is indicated if abnormalities are detected.
Testing for hepatitis B and C.*

NONOCCUPATIONAL EXPOSURE

HIV antibody testing at baseline and at 4–6 weeks, 12 weeks, and 6 months after exposure.
Complete blood counts, renal and hepatic function panel at baseline and at 4–6 weeks follow-up; further testing is indicated if abnormalities are detected.
Testing for hepatitis B and C.*
Screening for sexually transmitted diseases (gonorrhea, chlamydia, syphilis) at baseline and at 4–6 weeks or whenever clinically indicated.

*Discussed separately

viral load and drug resistance testing to guide the choice of drugs. If the exposure is from a source patient with unknown HIV status, nPEP can be initiated while waiting for the result of the HIV test in the source and discontinued if the test is negative. In cases of exposures that occurred beyond 72 hours, no firm recommendations exist. nPEP administration should be based on evaluating the exposure risk and weighing the risks and benefits of nPEP on an individual basis.

If there is ongoing exposure (e.g. sero-discordant couples, sex workers, intravenous drug users), nPEP is not recommended. In this situation, pre-exposure prophylaxis and effective risk-reduction interventions should be considered.

As in occupational PEP, the same three drug regimen is recommended in nPEP. Drug adherence should be emphasized. Administering nPEP during pregnancy is safe and potentially can prevent HIV transmission to the exposed female and from her to her newborn.

Patient evaluation after nonoccupational HIV exposure should include HIV testing at baseline, 4–6 weeks, 3 and 6 months (Box PP30-1). Follow-up visits should include assessing for acute HIV infection by history, physical examination and testing. If acute HIV infection is detected then continuation of ART is necessary beyond 28 days. HIV prevention and behavioral risk counseling should be offered during follow-up. To avoid secondary transmission, exposed individuals should be counseled on avoiding blood donation and practicing safe sex.

Further reading available online at expertconsult.com.

92

The Immunopathogenesis of HIV-1 Infection

RACHEL PRESTI | GIUSEPPE PANTALEO

KEY CONCEPTS

- HIV-1 disease is characterized by conflict between the virus and immune response.

- Many of the pathologic events in HIV-1 infection occur before the virus is detectable by clinical tests or symptoms, and before an adaptive immune response is mounted.

- Early HIV-1 infection is characterized by extremely high viral loads, a significant inflammatory response, and loss of large numbers of gut-associated lymphoid cells.

- Specific CD8+ T-cell responses appear to be able to modulate and even control HIV-1 infection. Genetic differences in the MHC1 system explain some of the variation in disease course between patients.

- HIV-1 is able to evade the immune response primarily via the generation of viral escape mutants. Continued viremia results in immune exhaustion and immune dysregulation.

- Ongoing inflammation and immune activation due to HIV replication, gut pathology, and coinfections play an important role in HIV-1 pathology and the pathogenesis of immune deficiency.

Clinical Course of Untreated HIV-1 Infection

The typical course of HIV-1 infection is defined by different phases that generally occur during a period of between 8 and 12 years.[1] Although the pattern and the course of the infection are highly variable among HIV-1-infected patients, three distinct phases can be identified (Figure 92-1):

- primary (acute) HIV-1 infection;
- chronic asymptomatic phase; and
- AIDS.

PRIMARY HIV-1 INFECTION

Primary HIV-1 infection is a transient condition, accompanied by a symptomatic illness of variable severity in 40–90% of patients, and is invariably accompanied by:

- an initial rapid rise in plasma viremia, often to levels in excess of 1 000 000 RNA copies/mL;
- a decrease in the blood CD4+ T cells and a massive decrease CD4+ T cells in tissues, particularly in the gut-associated lymphoid tissue;
- high levels of innate immune activation and inflammation; and
- a large increase in the blood CD8+ T-cell count, which correlates with resolution of symptoms.

The marked decline of plasma viremia generally coincides with resolution of the clinical syndrome.[2] The decrease in the viral load correlates with the appearance of virus-specific immune responses, particularly HIV-1-specific cytotoxic CD8+ T lymphocytes, indicating that virus-specific immune responses certainly play a crucial role in the initial downregulation of virus replication.[3-8]

The signs and symptoms of primary HIV-1 infection generally appear 2–4 weeks after virus exposure (see Figure 92-1). The duration of the clinical syndrome ranges between a few days and more than 10 weeks but generally lasts less than 14 days. The clinical presentation of the primary HIV-1 infection may mimic acute mononucleosis (see Chapter 93) as well as many other febrile acute illnesses, emphasizing the nonspecific nature of these symptoms and the difficulty of obtaining an accurate early diagnosis.

Because the acute clinical syndrome associated with primary infection is not specific for HIV-1, the diagnosis is based on laboratory tests. In this regard, it is important to underscore the fact that anti-HIV-1 antibodies are usually negative during the acute phase of illness. Early diagnosis, therefore, relies on a history of exposure, a positive p24 antigen enzyme-linked immunosorbent assay (ELISA) or the detection of plasma viral RNA (almost always >50 000 copies/mL of plasma).[2] Acute infection can be classified into stages based on the results of these tests. In Fiebig stage I, only viral RNA is detectable, p24 Ag and RNA are positive in stage II, and antibody tests become positive in stages III–V.[9,10] It is important to note that an eclipse phase of 4–11 days occurs after sexual exposure to HIV-1, during which no clinical test is positive and few symptoms occur. During this window, many of the critical events in HIV-1 pathogenesis occur, including the establishment of a reservoir of latently infected, memory CD4+ T cells.[11]

CHRONIC ASYMPTOMATIC/LATENT PHASE

Primary HIV-1 infection is followed by a long phase of clinical latency (median time of 10 years), during which neither signs nor symptoms of illness are present. Relatively stable levels of virus replication and of CD4+ T-cell counts for a variable period of time characterize this phase of infection. This 'stability' of measures of disease activity is apparent in the blood only. Virus replication in the gut and the accumulation of extracellular virus trapped in the follicular dendritic cell network are particularly active in the lymphoid tissue, where a progressive anatomic and functional deterioration occurs, impairing the ability to maintain effective specific immune responses over time.[1,12] This is reflected by the rapid increase in the levels of viremia and by a drop in CD4+ T-cell counts, which can suddenly speed up the transition from this phase to the advanced stage of the disease.

The advanced stage of HIV-1 disease is marked by low CD4+ T-cell counts (<200 cells/mL) and by the appearance of constitutional symptoms. It may be complicated by the development of AIDS-defining opportunistic infections.[1]

OVERT AIDS

Overt AIDS defines the end stage of HIV-1 infection. In the absence of antiretroviral therapy, this phase leads to death in 2–3 years. The risk for death and opportunistic infections significantly increases with CD4+ T-cell counts below 50 cells/mL. Fortunately, the advent of highly active antiretroviral therapy (HAART), including at present as many as six different classes of antiretroviral drugs administered in different combinations, significantly decreases the rate of progression, morbidity and mortality of HIV-1 infection (see Chapter 103).

PATIENT DIFFERENCES IN THE TIMELINE OF INFECTION

The clinical course of HIV-1 infection is variable. In the majority (60–70%) of HIV-1-infected patients, the median time between

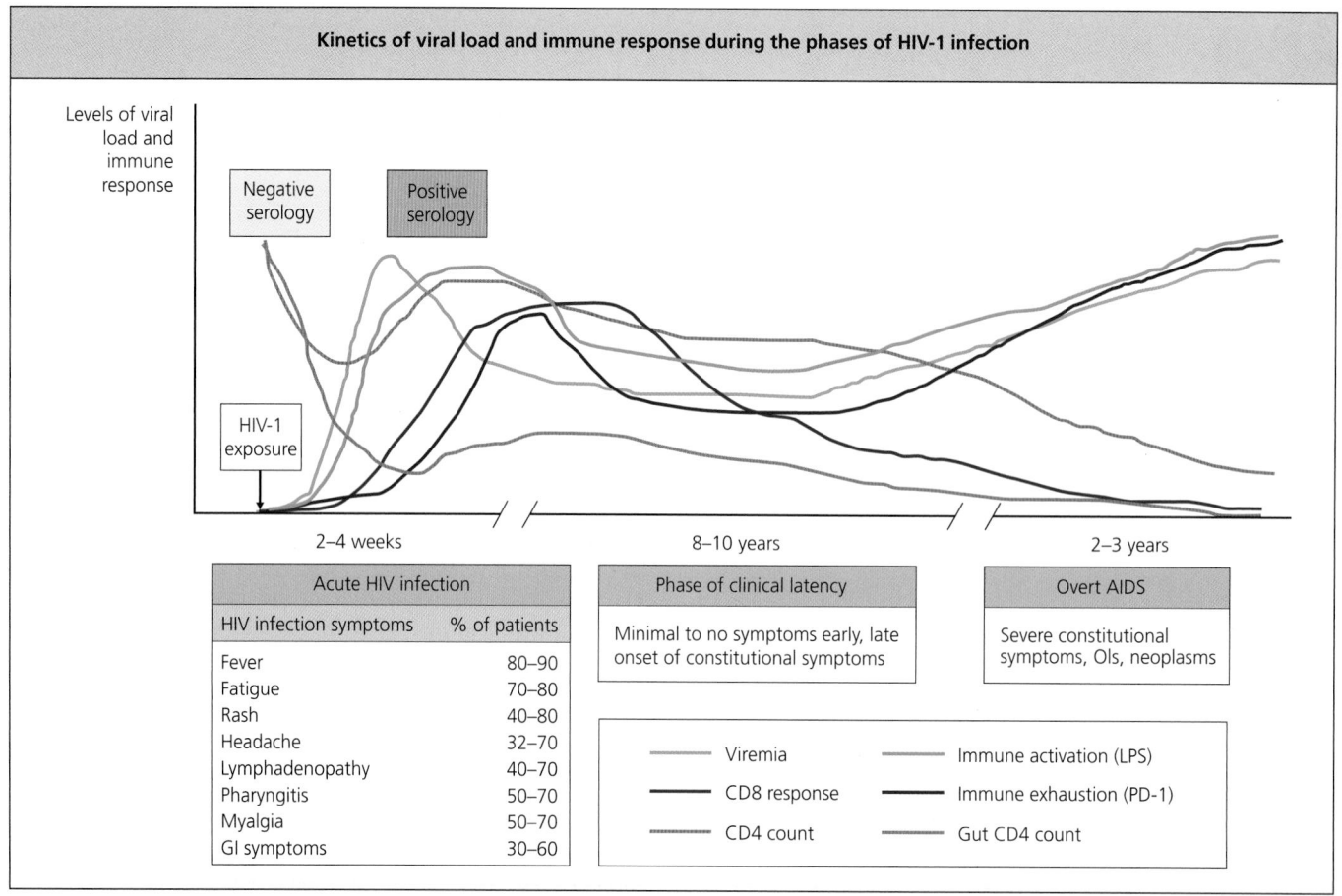

Figure 92-1   Kinetics of viral load and immune response during the phases of HIV-1 infection. After HIV-1 exposure, initial viremia is seen at ≈7 days, associated with a decline in blood and gut CD4⁺ T cells. A clinical syndrome is seen in up to 90% of HIV-1 infected persons. Downregulation of viremia and partial recovery of CD4 count is seen in conjunction with a CD8⁺ T-cell response. During the clinically latent period, a slow decline in CD4 counts and rise of viremia is associated with progressive immune activation and immune exhaustion. When CD4 counts decrease below 200 cells/mL, the clinical picture is characterized by constitutional symptoms of fatigue and weight loss as well as opportunistic infections (OIs) and AIDS-associated malignancies.

infection and development of AIDS, in the absence of therapy, is 8–10 years.[1,13,14] These HIV-1-infected persons are defined as typical progressors (Figure 92-2), and the clinical course of the infection that they generally experience is the one described above.

However, about 10–20% of subjects progress rapidly, developing AIDS in less than 5 years of infection, and they are therefore called rapid progressors (see Figure 92-2). In these patients, after the primary HIV-1 infection, plasma virus levels are often >10⁵ copies of HIV-1 RNA/mL and CD4⁺ T-cell counts start to decrease much earlier and more rapidly during the chronic asymptomatic phase, leading to the eventual development of AIDS. Furthermore, both humoral and cell-mediated HIV-1-specific immune responses are either never detected or rapidly lost after the transition from the acute to the chronic phase of infection. A longer lasting, more symptomatic acute retroviral clinical syndrome, especially if the central nervous system is involved, is also predictive of more rapid disease progression.[15-19]

At the other extreme, it is estimated that 5–15% of HIV-1-infected people will remain free of AIDS for more than 15 years; these people are termed slow progressors (see Figure 92-2). In this situation, CD4⁺ T-cell counts remain stable and they are frequently >500 cells/mL, and plasma virus levels are usually <10 000 HIV-1 RNA copies/mL. Slow progressors include a further subgroup of HIV-1-infected people, so-called long-term nonprogressors (see Figure 92-2). About 1% of HIV-1-infected subjects probably fall into this category. The definition of long-term nonprogressors should be limited to those who have had a documented infection for at least 8–10 years, are naïve to

antiretroviral therapy and have no signs of disease progression (e.g. constant high counts of CD4⁺ T cells and either low (500–1000 copies of RNA/mL) or very low (<50 copies/mL) plasma virus levels).[15-17,20]

A second group of slow progressors are able to maintain low-level viremia and high CD4 counts over a longer period, although some eventually progress to AIDS and death.[20] A subgroup of HIV-1 infected individuals with chronic infection and levels of viremia <50 copies/mL has been termed 'elite controllers'. Virologic control appears to occur early, within 1–2 years of seroconversion, and rarely happens during the chronic phase of infection.[20-22] Genome-wide association studies of elite controllers have demonstrated that the major genetic determinants of this ability affect major histocompatibility complex and implicate human leukocyte antigen (HLA) Class I peptide presentation as the primary factor explaining durable control of HIV-1 replication.[8]

This wide variability of the natural course of the disease is evidenced by the presence of different driving forces – genetic, immunologic and virologic factors – that determine the evolutionary pattern of HIV-1 infection in the individual patient.[15-18] It also underlines the need for markers of disease progression that may identify as early as possible the patients who are at risk for a more rapid disease progression. It is therefore important, first, to identify the different determinants of the rate of disease progression and, second, to elucidate how these driving forces work together. Although current guidelines have moved to recommend combination antiretroviral therapy for all patients, a better understanding of which patients are at higher risk would allow for targeted therapy directed at populations where

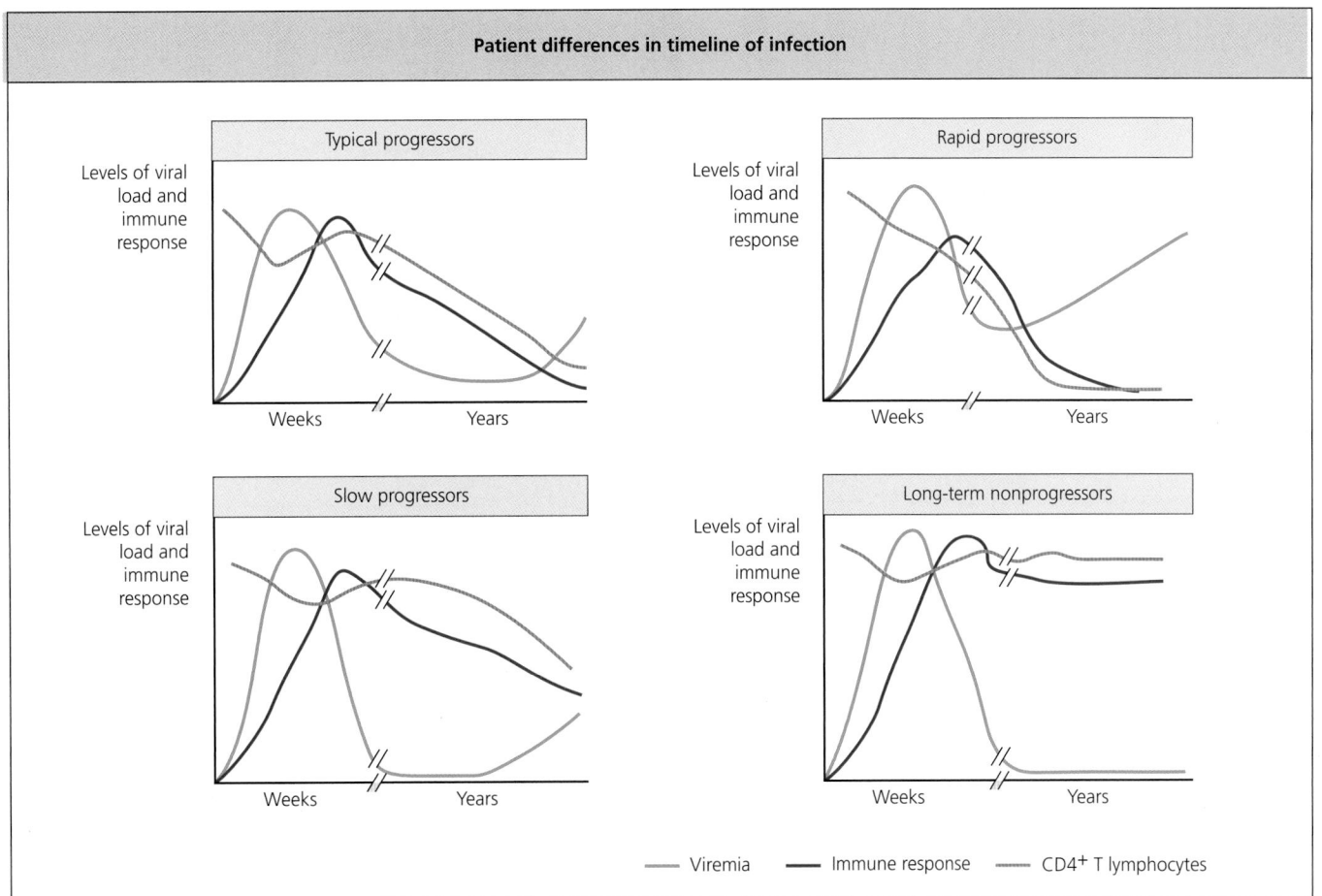

Figure 92-2   Patient differences in timeline of infection. Changes in viral load, CD4⁺ T cells and immune response in the different natural courses of HIV-1 infection.

resources are scarce, and potentially avoid some drug-induced toxicities in elite controllers.[23]

Transmission and Local Spread of HIV-1

HIV-1 can be transmitted by different routes: by sexual contact, through either genital–genital, genital–anal or genital–oral sex; by blood–blood contamination, via either transfusion of blood and infected blood-derived products or needle-sharing among intravenous drug users; and by maternal–fetal transmission. The most common route of infection is sexual transmission at the genital mucosa (Figure 92-3).[23]

FEATURES OF THE TRANSMITTED VIRUS

Individuals with chronic HIV-1 infection are infected by a genetically diverse quasispecies of HIV-1 viruses due to the sloppiness of the viral polymerase and rapid viral replication. Genetic studies of the viral envelope of HIV-1 early after transmission suggest that a limited number of viral species are transmitted,[24] although studies of the reverse-transcriptase gene revealed somewhat greater diversity.[25] Single genome amplification experiments in a well-characterized cohort of acutely infected patients showed evidence in 78 of 102 subjects of productive infection by a single virus, with the remaining subjects infected by 2–5 genetically distinct viruses.[26-28] Infections acquired via parenteral routes demonstrate somewhat more genetic diversity, likely due to surpassing the bottleneck at the mucosal barrier.[29,30] Transmitted viruses are almost universally CCR5 tropic, replicate well in CD4⁺ T cells, but not macrophages, and share other conserved features of the envelope gene.[28,29,31]

EARLY PATHOGENIC EVENTS AFTER HIV-1 ENTRY INTO THE BODY

HIV-1 can be transmitted by both cell-free virus and cell-associated virus. Although cell-associated virus may be more efficient at transmission due to concentrated virus production at points of cell contact (reviewed in reference 32), most models of infection use cell-free virus. The acute intravaginal infection of rhesus monkeys with the simian immunodeficiency virus (SIV) represents a very useful model for studying the sequence of cellular events that characterize the very early steps of infection after sexual transmission (reviewed in reference 33). In this model (see Figure 92-3), after the initial inoculum is applied, there is a fall in detectable SIV RNA in the tissue to undetectable levels, while viral DNA is present, consistent with an eclipse phase of 3–4 days. At this time point, a cluster of 40–50 CD4⁺ T cells in the endocervix and transformation zone can be identified expressing SIV RNA.[34-37] Certain features appear to increase an individual cell's susceptibility to infection. High levels of expression of CCR5, CD4, and the integrin α4β7 appear to increase susceptibility and facilitate spread of the infection, while expression of intracellular restriction factors, such as SAMHD1, may inhibit HIV replication.[38-41] Perhaps because they modulate the local inflammatory milieu and impair mucosal barriers, the risk of infection is increased by the presence of concomitant inflammatory or infectious diseases (e.g. cervicitis, urethritis, genital ulcers).

Dendritic cells (DCs) play a critically important role in early HIV-1 replication, due to their localization at mucosal surfaces and their ability to capture foreign antigens and present them via major histocompatibility complex (MHC) to T cells. DCs bind HIV-1 via C-type lectins, most notably dendritic cell-specific intercellular adhesion molecule-3-grabbing non-integrin (DC-SIGN).[42,43] DCs are poorly

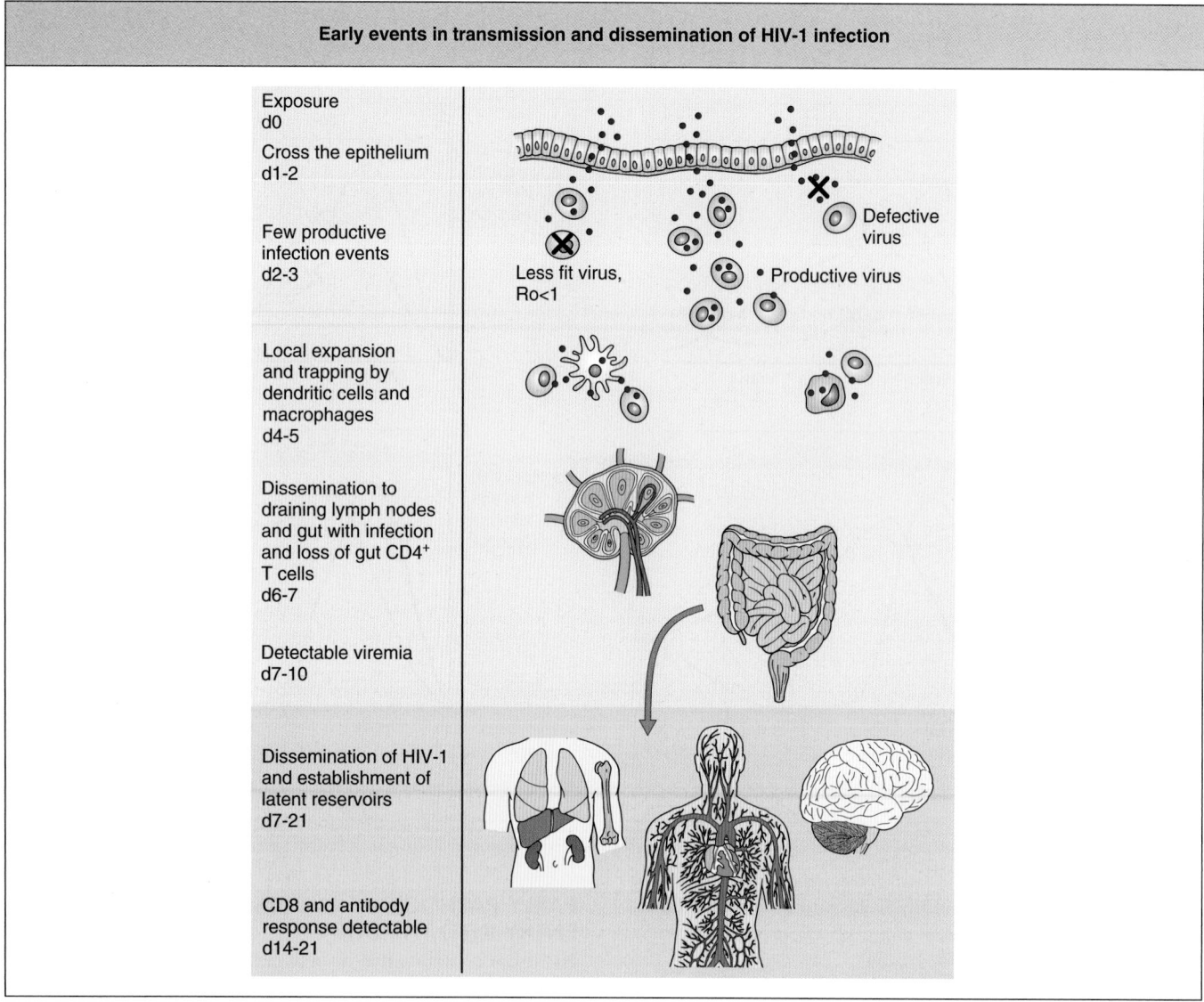

Early events in transmission and dissemination of HIV-1 infection

Exposure
d0

Cross the epithelium
d1-2

Few productive
infection events
d2-3

Less fit virus, Ro<1

Defective virus

Productive virus

Local expansion
and trapping by
dendritic cells and
macrophages
d4-5

Dissemination to
draining lymph nodes
and gut with infection
and loss of gut CD4⁺
T cells
d6-7

Detectable viremia
d7-10

Dissemination of HIV-1
and establishment of
latent reservoirs
d7-21

CD8 and antibody
response detectable
d14-21

Figure 92-3 Early events in transmission and dissemination of HIV-1 infection. After sexual exposure, few virions are able to establish a productive infection. Local expansion occurs in the first week, assisted by infection of dendritic cells and macrophages at the transmission site, and infection of the draining lymph nodes. HIV-1 rapidly disseminates to the gut, causing high levels of infection of resident CD4+ CCR5+ cells and massive depletion of lamina propria lymphocytes. Approximately 1 week after exposure, HIV-1 is detectable in the blood and rapidly causes high level viremia and symptomatic infection. HIV-1 disseminates throughout the body, establishing active infection as well as latent reservoirs. An adaptive immune response characterized by CD8 cytotoxic cells followed by antibody occurs 14–21 days after initial exposure.

infected by HIV-1, likely due to high level expression of restriction factors such as APOBEC3G/3F and TRIM-5α (see Chapter 174); however, they amplify infection via transfer of HIV-1 to CD4+CCR5+ T cells. This can be done via replication of HIV-1 in DCs, although perhaps more importantly, DC can transfer HIV-1 to T cells via the immunologic synapse or the exosome secretion pathway.[44,45]

DISSEMINATION OF HIV-1

Within 2 days of infection, HIV-1 can be detected in the draining lymphoid tissue, and it rapidly disseminates throughout the lymphoid system. Afterwards, HIV-1 enters the bloodstream, where viral replication can be detected in plasma ≈7 days after infection (see Figure 92-3). In humans, the time from mucosal infection and initial plasma viremia varies, ranging between 4 days and 11 days according to available estimates.

GASTROINTESTINAL PATHOLOGY

The study of virologic events occurring during primary infection with either HIV-1 or SIV emphasizes the key role of the gastrointestinal (GI)

tract in the establishment of infection. The majority of T cells, particularly CD4⁺ T cells, are contained within the GI tract. Memory CD4⁺ T cells within the GI tract are the earliest targets of HIV-1 during primary infection regardless of the route of infection.[46,47] The monitoring of CD4⁺ T-cell depletion following SIV infection has shown that initial decrease in CD4⁺ T cells may vary between 60% and 80% in blood and lymph nodes while the loss of CD4⁺ T cells is almost complete in the GI tract.[46-48] Studies performed in humans have also shown that, in addition to the greater depletion of CD4⁺ T cells in the gut, the proportion of HIV-1 infected CD4⁺ T cells resident in the gut is 10–100-fold higher compared to blood.[46,49] This depletion can be seen very early in acute infection, with significant loss of lamina propria CD4 cells in Fiebig stage I/II (Figure 92-4). This appears to be correlated with colonic HIV viral load, and is likely due to direct infection of these cells, which express high levels of CCR5.[50] In typical HIV-1 infection, but not nonpathogenic SIV infections or nonprogressor HIV infections, a population of CD4⁺ T cells which produce IL-17 (Th17) are preferentially depleted.[50-53] Th17 cells are critically important for maintaining epithelial integrity through the production of IL22 and for

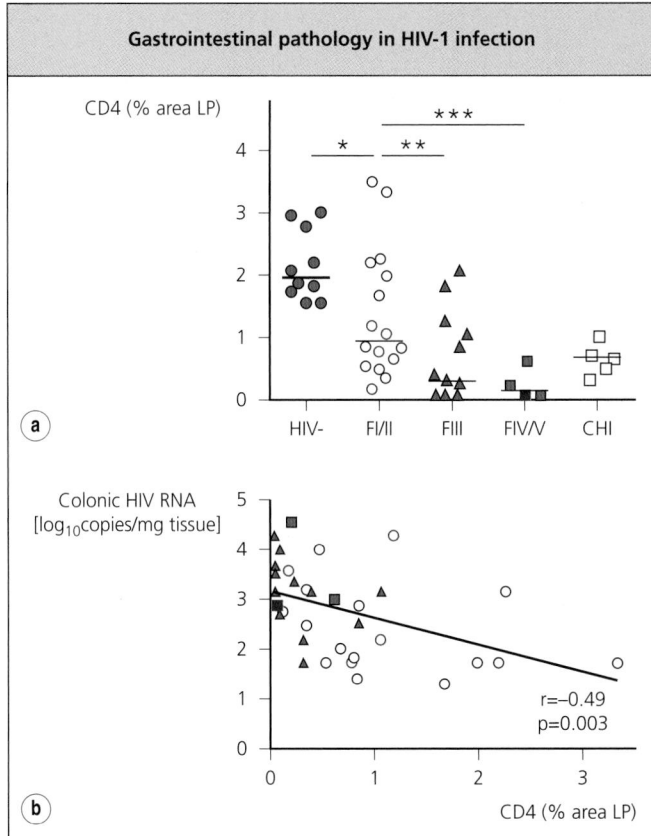

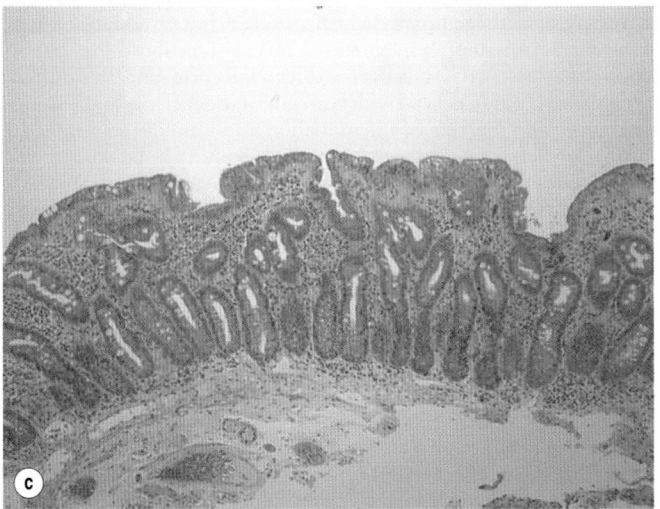

Figure 92-4   Gastrointestinal pathology in HIV-1 infection. (a) Loss of CD4⁺ T cells in the lamina propria. The percent area of lamina propria which stains for CD4⁺ T cells decreases by Fiebig stage in early infection. *p ≤0.05; **p ≤0.01; ***p ≤0.001; FI (black circle)/FII (red circle) and FIV (red square)/FV (blue square) (b) The percent area of the lamina propria which stains for CD4⁺ T cells is inversely correlated with colonic HIV-1 viral load. (c) Typical pathology seen in AIDS enteropathy with villus atrophy, decreased crypt/villus ratio and influx of lymphocytes in the lamina propria. *(a) and (b) reprinted from Schuetz A., Deleage C., Sereti I., et al.: Initiation of ART during early acute HIV Infection preserves mucosal Th17 function and reverses HIV-related immune activation. PLoS Pathog 2014; 10:(12)e1004543; (c) reprinted from Cello JP, Day LW.: Idiopathic AIDS enteropathy and treatment of gastrointestinal opportunistic pathogens. Gastroenterology 2009; 136:(6)952-65.*

mucosal defense against gut bacteria and fungi.[54] Significant intestinal pathology occurs in both acute and chronic HIV infection, including blunted villi, crypt hyperplasia, and enterocyte death[55,56] (see Figure 92-4). This enteropathy is associated with systemic circulation of bacterial byproducts, such as endotoxin and bacterial DNA,[48,57-59] which

are thought to contribute to high levels of inflammation seen in HIV-1 infection.

SYSTEMIC DISSEMINATION AND VIRAL RESERVOIRS

Once HIV-1 is present in the bloodstream, it disseminates rapidly to lymphoid tissues and throughout the body. Multiple cell types are involved in viral dissemination. HIV-1 infected CD4⁺ T cells are among the most important for this dissemination. Productively infected CD4⁺ T cells migrate robustly to lymph nodes, and spread infection to other cells via the formation of syncytia and the establishment of tethers between other cell types. They also recirculate throughout the tissues and efficiently spread HIV-1 throughout the body.[60] Recent studies have demonstrated that an important, immune privileged reservoir in HIV/SIV infection is CD4+ T follicular helper cells (Tfh) in the B-cell follicles. These cells are highly infected even in SIV-infected animals which control the infection, likely due to the fact that CD8 killer T cells are unable to access this anatomic site. Thus, these cells are an important source of latent HIV-1 in chronic infection.[61,62] Macrophages and DCs are also important for the dissemination of HIV-1, particularly to immune privileged sites such as the brain. Since myeloid lineage cells are capable of HIV-1 entry and integration, but are not robustly productively infected, they likely serve as a reservoir of virus which will be difficult to eradicate (reviewed in reference 63).

Role of the Immune Response in Determining the Setpoints for Chronic, Asymptomatic Infection

In both SIV and HIV-1 infection, the transition from primary to early chronic infection is marked by a decrease of viral RNA in plasma and the resolution of the acute clinical syndrome. Therefore, it is clear that virus-specific immune responses are not only present very early during primary infection but may also significantly affect virus distribution occurring in the early phase of both SIV and HIV-1 infection.[62]

CD8⁺ T-CELL RESPONSE TO HIV-1

The patterns of the HIV-1-specific CD8⁺ T-cell response during the chronic phase of infection generally correlate with the extent of virus control.[3,4,6-8] The critical importance of the CD8 response to infection is highlighted by the rapid loss of viral control and mortality seen after CD8 depletion in SIV-infected animals.[64,65] The appearance of CD8 cytotoxic T-cell response correlates with initial viral clearance, and the pattern of Vβ usage by selected CD8⁺ T cells is predictive of CD4 decline.[7,66] HIV-1-specific CD8⁺ T cells during primary infection are typical effector cells, i.e. IFN-γ/TNF secreting cells which also express perforin and have cytotoxic capacity. They are initially directed at HIV *Env* and *Nef* viral epitopes. Selective pressure by these immunodominant cytotoxic CD8⁺ T cells drives mutation of the virus to escape the cytotoxic response.[67,68] The HIV-1-specific CD8⁺ T-cell response remains predominantly an effector response, i.e. IFN-γ/TNF secreting cells, in association with uncontrolled virus replication. Both IL-2/IFN-γ/TNF and IFN-γ/TNF secreting CD8⁺ T cells are found in long-term nonprogressors in association with controlled virus replication.[69,70] CD8⁺ T cells from elite controllers are even more effective at secreting multiple cytokines, and are able to better proliferate and kill target HIV-1 infected cells.[71-73]

ANTIBODY RESPONSE

The antibody response to HIV-1 first appears 3–4 weeks after infection. Neutralizing antibodies against the *Env* protein appear within 3–4 months in most individuals, and are associated with escape mutations in the *Env* region.[74,75] Chronic B-cell activation and hypergammaglobulinemia due to ongoing viremia are clinical features of chronic HIV-1 infection, as is loss of recall and response to vaccination.[76,77] However, B-cell depletion in animal models does not influence disease progression, suggesting that antibody responses have limited effect in chronic infection.[78]

Broadly neutralizing antibodies, which can neutralize multiple variants of the *Env* protein, are seen in ≈20% of patients. Although they are not capable of controlling autologous infection due to selection of escape variants, they are being studied as prophylactic agents and in vaccine strategies.[79,80] Administration of neutralizing antibodies does show some efficacy against subsequent challenge, although it is dependent on a match between the antibody and SIV strain.[81,82] Slow progression and viral control has been associated with high titers of neutralizing antibodies, and broadly neutralizing antibodies are seen more often in nonprogressors.[83,84] The generation of antibodies which can generate HIV-1 specific antibody-dependent cellular cytotoxicity, appears to play a role in slower progression of HIV infection (reviewed in reference 85).

CD4+ T-CELL RESPONSE TO HIV-1

CD4+ T cells are the primary targets of HIV-1 infection, and activated HIV-specific CD4+ T cells are preferentially infected and massively depleted during infection, complicating their ability to function in the antiviral immune response.[86] Early in infection, CD4+ T cells are rapidly depleted from the blood and the gut-associated lymphoid tissue; however, CD4 Tfh cells appear to be sequestered and proliferate in the lymph nodes during early infection.[61,62,87,88] This protection of Tfh cells may in part explain the vigorous antibody response seen in chronic infection. Although chronic viremia appears to inhibit the establishment of IL-2 producing HIV-specific CD4 cells,[89] LTNP and EC maintain memory CD4+ T cells, and have strong mucosal CD4+ T-cell responses.[90,91] Preserved CD4 function in elite controllers may also allow for T-cell help, further improving the CD8 response. IL-21 has been identified as a key cytokine produced by CD4+ T cells to provide CD8+ T-cell help and control chronic viral infections.[92,93] The ability of elite controllers to suppress HIV viremia has been linked to the maintained production of IL-21 by HIV-specific CD4+ T cells.[94,95]

HIV-1 IMMUNE EVASION

HIV-1 is able to escape the immune response through a variety of mechanisms, including the following:

- preferential infection of CD4+ T cells;
- the genetic variability of HIV-1[96] allowing escape mutants to be selected;
- formation of a stable pool of latently HIV-1-infected CD4+ T cells containing virus that is capable of replicating;[11,97-99] and
- expression of viral proteins, which antagonize innate immune antiviral molecules.

As described previously, the preferential infection of HIV-specific CD4+ T cells by HIV leads to a depletion of helper T cells, especially Th1 and Th17 cells. These cells are critically important to developing and maintaining a functional immune response, as CD4 help is critically important to the induction of CD8 cytotoxic responses and antibody responses. The loss of Th17 cells results in a dysfunctional mucosal barrier, and concomitant microbial translocation and systemic immune activation.[52,54]

The high genetic variability of the virus is an efficient mechanism by which it escapes the host immune response. HIV-1 possesses the intrinsic ability to mutate very rapidly. Both during primary and established chronic infection, rapid mutations in the epitopes recognized by HIV-1-specific cytotoxic T lymphocytes (CTL) may occur. As a consequence, both humoral and cell-mediated virus-specific immune responses quickly lose their ability to control the virus efficiently.[68,75]

The rapid formation of a pool of latently HIV-1-infected CD4+ T cells is a key event in the immunopathogenesis of HIV-1 infection for several reasons. First, this event occurs very early and most probably before the appearance of the host's virus-specific immune responses. Second, the pool of latently infected CD4+ T cells contains replication-competent HIV-1 proviral DNA. The proviral DNA can be detected even in compliant HIV-1-infected persons who have been receiving HAART for a long time (i.e. for more than 2 years); moreover, the virus is wild type with respect to known drug-induced mutations in the genome. This emphasizes the fact that this pool of cells is a stable reservoir in which HIV-1 remains sheltered from the effects of host immune responses and HAART. Furthermore, it is worth noting that initiation of HAART very early during primary HIV-1 infection does not appear to have a significant impact on the size of this pool of CD4+ T cells, indicating that this pool is created very rapidly after infection. Third, the decay of this pool of infected CD4+ T lymphocytes is very slow, and the rate of decay is not much influenced by the effective suppression of virus replication obtained by antiretroviral therapy. This clearly represents a major obstacle to the goal of HIV-1 eradication and long-term control of virus replication. HIV-1 is also able to infect and integrate into myeloid cell lineages, such as DC and macrophages. Virus is trapped by the follicular DC network in lymphoid tissue, and is able to directly infect CD4 cells via the immunologic synapse without exposure to the immune response.[45,61,97]

Finally, HIV-1 encodes several proteins which impair the innate antiviral response. Cells respond to viruses and other pathogens via the sensing of pathogen-associated molecular patterns (such as viral RNA, or bacterial endotoxin) via pattern recognition receptors (Toll-like receptors or RIG-I-like receptors), leading to the production of interferon, and other antiviral molecules (reviewed in reference 100). HIV-1 is sensed by RIG-I and tetherin, which activate IRF3 to produce interferon.[101] Interferon stimulates the production of hundreds of genes, including APOBEC3G, which deaminates retroviral reverse transcription intermediate DNA.[102] HIV-1 disrupts this innate antiviral effect at multiple steps. HIV-1 *Vpu* targets tetherin and CD4 for sequestration and degradation, and prevents IRF3-driven gene induction. HIV-1 *Vif* targets APOBEC3G for degradation, and the HIV-1 protease targets RIG-I for lysosomal degradation.[103,104]

Mechanisms of Immune Deficiency

A variety of pathogenic mechanisms explain the profound immune deficiency associated with untreated HIV-1 infection. Most importantly, the loss of CD4 cells via direct infection impairs immune responses. HIV is associated with both immune deficiency and immune activation, and markers of inflammation and immune activation are strong predictors of clinical outcomes. Shifts in the microbiome and the presence of several other coinfections and opportunistic infection also contribute to disease pathogenesis.

ROLES OF CD4+ T CELLS

HIV-1 infects cells that express both the CD4 receptor and a co-receptor, which is most often CCR5 but may be CXCR4 or other chemokine receptors. While macrophages and dendritic cells are infected, they do not replicate the virus well, and the primary targets which are infected and killed are CD4+ T cells. CD4+ T cells have a central role in immunity as they provide necessary help for both cytotoxic CD8+ T cells and antibody generation and class switching.[105] Naïve CD4+ T cells will differentiate into effector and long-lived memory CD4+ T cells after stimulation by their cognate antigen. Infection of these cells is an important source of latent HIV-1 infection. Depending on the cytokine profile in the local inflammatory milieu, naïve CD4+ T cells can differentiate into a variety of distinct subsets, including Th1, Th2, Th17, Treg, Tfh, as well as Th9 and Th22 (reviewed in reference 106). There is some plasticity between these subsets, and memory T cells can acquire different traits in secondary immune responses.[107] We have previously discussed the important role of Th17 cells in mucosal immunity, the role of IL-21 production by CD4+ T cells, and the role of Tfh as an important reservoir of latent virus.

The loss of Th1 and Treg cells plays important roles in the pathogenesis of immune deficiency and explains many of the clinical features seen in late stage HIV/AIDS. Earlier studies in HIV-1 pathogenesis suggested that late stage disease was characterized by a switch from Th1 to Th2 function, with decreased production of the Th1 cytokines, IFNγ and IL-2, and increase Th2 cytokines, IL-4 and IL-10.[108] However, several studies have failed to reproduce these findings, and detailed animal studies have not shown a switch.[109,110] However, Th1 type immunity against intracellular pathogens appears to be particularly affected in late stage HIV-1 disease. Persons with genetic deficiencies that result in loss of Th1 function, such as genetic mutations in IFNγR, IL-12 or the IL-12R, present with similar diseases to those seen in late stage AIDS, such as overwhelming mycobacterial and fungal infections, and infections with gram-negative bacteria such as *Salmonella* spp.[111-114] (see Chapter 78).

The effect of HIV-1 on regulatory T cells (Treg) is even more complex (reviewed in reference 115). Treg have been identified as a subset of CD4+ T cells expressing high constitutive levels of CD25 (IL-2R), and are capable of suppressing immune functions *in vitro*.[116-118] Their function in HIV is complicated by the fact that they are commonly identified by the expression of CD4, the intracellular transcription factor FOXP3, and high CD25 expression, all of which can be seen in activated T cells such as are seen in chronic HIV infection.[119] Treg are highly susceptible to HIV-1 infection, and may be another site of persistent infection for patients on antiretroviral therapy.[120] Despite this, Treg are relatively preserved in chronic infection compared to other CD4+ T-cell subsets, possibly due to *Nef* expression.[121,122] They likely play a complex role in HIV-1 pathogenesis as they maintain suppressive functions during infection, and are able to suppress both anti-HIV immune functions and suppress chronic activation.[115,122,123] The dysregulation of Treg may explain certain features of end stage HIV-1 disease, such as intractable psoriasis and eczema.[124,125]

ROLE OF INFLAMMATION

Chronic immune activation and inflammation are characteristic of all stages of HIV-1 infection. Investigators at the beginning of the epidemic recognized that both immune deficiency and significant T-cell and B-cell activation characterize the disease now known as AIDS.[126,127] Immune activation, as measured by the expression of CD38 and HLA-DR, is a better clinical predictor of disease progression than CD4 count or viral load.[128,129] High levels of immune activation are seen very early in the acute HIV-1 infection, and are typically higher than the levels of immune activation seen during acute infection with other chronically infecting viruses, such as hepatitis B and C.

The source of this persistent activation is likely multifactorial. It has been linked to the early gastrointestinal depletion of CD4+ T cells, enteropathy and bacterial translocation, with resulting endotoxemia and high levels of soluble CD14 circulating in the blood.[57,59] Other potential sources of chronic inflammation include HIV-1 viremia, other coinfections such as HCV, reactivation of latent herpesviruses such as cytomegalovirus (CMV), and other opportunistic infections and their pathology. High levels of type I interferon (IFN), as well as several other inflammatory and coagulation parameters, are seen in chronic infection.[130,131] The major source of IFN in chronic infection is plasmacytoid DCs. IFN levels in HIV-1 infection correlate with both immune activation and other disease markers in chronic infection.[132] IFN exhibits antiviral, immune modulatory and anti-proliferative effects, and chronic high levels of IFN likely lead to a variety of immune pathologies in HIV-1 infection, including high levels of CD8 activation and CD4 depletion.

It is thought that this chronic activation eventually results in immune exhaustion and dysregulation. HIV-1 infected patients who are treated with antiretrovirals only partially reverse this chronic immune activation and inflammation.[133] Chronic high level immune activation and inflammation is thought to contribute much to the aging pathology seen in treated individuals (see Chapter 104).

IMMUNE EXHAUSTION DURING CHRONIC INFECTION

Chronic immune stimulation in the setting of uncleared viremia eventually results in a phenomenon known as immune exhaustion, wherein effector cells lose functions and proliferative capacity. Chronic antigenic stimulation causes effector cells to persist, but become unresponsive to further stimulation.[134] Recent studies have elucidated several markers of immune exhaustion, including PD-1, LAG-3, CTLA-4, and Tim-3 (reviewed in reference 135). PD-1 was the first of these

identified, initially in the lymphocytic choriomeningitis virus (LCMV) model of chronic viral infection.[136] PD-1 is a negative regulator of the immune response, and is particularly important for self-tolerance. Blocking PD-1 or its ligand, PD-L1, in chronic viral infections such as HIV-1 restores the function of exhausted CD8+ T cells.[137] Tim-3 appears to block both Th1 and Th17 type cells.[138] LAG-3 appears to coregulate exhaustion with PD-1 and Tim-3.[139] PD-1 is clearly upregulated on HIV-1 specific CD8+ T cells, and the levels correlate with viral load and CD4 counts, with lower levels seen in nonprogressors.[140] *In vitro*, blockade of PD-1 appears to restore CD8 effector functions against HIV-1[137,141], and *in vivo* in the SIV model, SIV-specific immunity is augmented by blocking PD-1.[142] PD-1 expression appears to be associated with CD38, suggesting that chronic immune activation and immune exhaustion are parallel features of the immune pathogenesis seen in HIV-1 infection.[143]

COINFECTIONS

HIV-1 infected patients are more commonly affected by several other diseases, which contribute to and complicate the ongoing pathology, immune deficiency and disease caused by HIV-1. Among the most common of these are syphilis, tuberculosis, hepatitis B and C (HBV, HCV), and cytomegalovirus (CMV). While these and other coinfections and opportunistic infections are covered elsewhere, a brief discussion of their role in HIV-1 immune pathogenesis is warranted.

Syphilis is commonly co-transmitted with HIV-1, in part due to serosorting behavior.[144,145] In many cities rates of HIV-1 infection among new cases of syphilis are as high as 60%.[146] Syphilis, and other sexually transmitted genital ulcer diseases, appear to increase the risk of HIV-1 transmission. This is likely multifactorial, and may include shared transmission routes, ulceration impairing normal skin defenses and the trafficking of activated inflammatory cells, which are highly susceptible to HIV-1 infection. Syphilis does appear to transiently increase HIV-1 viral load, further increasing transmission risks.[147,148] HIV-1 infection does not appear to significantly change the presentation or course of syphilis, although progression to neurosyphilis may be more common, especially in the setting of profound immune deficiency.[149]

Worldwide, the overlapping epidemics of tuberculosis (TB) and HIV have caused considerable morbidity and mortality. The risk of TB reactivation is ≈30-fold higher among HIV-1 infected persons. Although it has been postulated that defective macrophages may increase TB susceptibility, attack rates of household members are similar between those who are not HIV-1 infected.[150,151] The presentation of TB is dependent on the degree of immunosuppression, patients with higher CD4 counts present similarly to HIV-1 negative patients, while patients with profound immune suppression can present with normal chest radiograph (CXR), fever and weight loss.[152] Immune suppression can also impair the ability to diagnose TB as both the tuberculin skin test and IFNγ reactive assays rely on functional T-cell responses.[153] Treatment is also complicated by drug interactions between antivirals and antimycobacterial agents.[154] TB also appears to increase the risk of HIV progression and death, perhaps due to increased immune activation.[155]

HBV and HCV share many of the same routes of infection as HIV-1. With improved treatment for HIV-1 becoming available, liver disease has become a common cause of death in HIV-1 infected persons. HIV-1 infection appears to accelerate the process of liver fibrosis, cirrhosis, and progression to end stage liver disease in the setting of HBV or HCV.[156,157] Drug interactions and overlapping drug targets also complicate the treatment of HIV-1 and hepatitis.[158] Although it is not clear that coinfection with HBV or HCV has a significant effect on HIV-1 disease progression, the presence of other chronic viral infections likely increases the extent of immune activation and resultant ongoing pathology.

The role of cytomegalovirus (CMV) in AIDS pathogenesis has been suspected since before HIV-1 was identified.[159] CMV is a common latent herpes infection, which has particularly high prevalence among men who have sex with men, often reaching >90% seropositivity rates.[160] The virus is known to possess several immunosuppressive features (reviewed in reference 161). CMV reactivation causes several diseases in the setting of profound immune compromise, particularly retinitis, colitis and encephalitis, as well as undifferentiated febrile illness.[162] Reactivation of CMV has been postulated to promote further immune activation and inflammation, and in the aging population large numbers of the T-cell repertoire are devoted to anti-CMV responses.[163] CMV has also been associated with cardiovascular disease in both HIV-infected and uninfected persons, although this is complicated by the high prevalence of CMV in both communities.[164] Perhaps the best evidence that CMV contributes to chronic immune activation in HIV-1 infected patients was a trial of the anti-CMV antiviral, valganciclovir, in patients with incomplete CD4 recovery on antiretroviral therapy. In that setting, treatment with valganciclovir was associated with a reduction in immune activation.[165]

CHANGES IN THE MICROBIOME

Recent studies have revolutionized our understanding of the role that the microbiome plays in health and disease (reviewed in reference 166 and see Chapter 7). The microbiome is an aggregate of trillions of predominantly bacteria as well as viruses, fungi and other organisms which inhabit various body sites. The combined genetic material of a collection of organisms is referred to as a metagenome, and the availability of low-cost, high-throughput sequencing has allowed researchers to evaluate the human microbiome using metagenomics in a variety of states of health and disease. Numerous studies have shown that alterations in the human microbiome play important roles in disease states as varied as obesity, inflammatory and rheumatologic diseases, and mental illness.[167-169] Our understanding of HIV pathogenesis has been revolutionized by suggesting that HIV infection leads to gastrointestinal CD4 depletion and a compromised mucosal barrier, leading to microbial translocation, endotoxemia and systemic immune activation, as outlined above. To further elucidate the changes which result in pathogenesis, several studies have been performed in both HIV-infected persons and animal models to determine whether there are changes in the microbiome or metagenome which contribute to microbial translocation and pathology.[169] Most of these have focused on changes in the stool or intestinal microbiome, although significant alterations have been seen in other sites, including the oral and lung microbiome as well as the microbiome associated with genitalia. Although differences are seen between HIV+ and HIV- persons, it is still not clear whether they are due to HIV infection, to immunodeficiency, or to other environmental factors. It should be noted that significant variations exist among the healthy human population.[166,170]

Following HIV-1 infection, individuals have a shift in their gut microbiome to one that consists of a greater proportion of gram-negative bacteria with enhanced potential to induce systemic inflammation.[171] Studies have shown that both stool and mucosal microbial communities appear to shift to increased *Prevotella* and Proteobacteria family members and decreased *Bacteroides* and Firmicutes family members.[172-175] Importantly these microbiome changes, especially of mucosa-associated bacteria, have been associated with markers of microbial translocation, inflammation, and immune activation.[174,175] Increased Proteobacteria species appear to be a hallmark of inflammatory gastrointestinal diseases, such as inflammatory bowel disease. Importantly, changes in the gut bacterial microbiome have not been seen in the SIV animal model, although expansion of the virome is seen in pathogenic infection.[176] Despite this, the SIV animal model has been used to show that Proteobacteria appear to preferentially translocate systemically.[177]

Changes in the microbiome also appear to influence the risk of HIV acquisition. Bacterial vaginosis, a condition in which the normal vaginal flora changes from the acidic producing bacteria, *Lactobacillus*, to other anaerobic bacteria, especially *Gardnerella* and *Prevotella* increases susceptibility to HIV.[178] These species appear to induce a more inflammatory state which is associated with an increased risk of

acquisition and mother to child transmission.[179] Similarly, the decreased risk of HIV-1 acquisition associated with circumcision may also be due to a decrease in Clostridiales and *Prevotella*, which are uniquely abundant before circumcision.[180] In general, it is theorized that an increase in inflammatory species, such as *Prevotella*, may both bring more susceptible inflammatory cells to the transmission site as well as set up a localized inflammatory milieu which is conducive to HIV replication.

Changes in the microbiome of the oral cavity and the lung have also been described, and may account for increased pathology at both those sites in patients with HIV/AIDS. Opportunistic infections of the lung, including *Pneumocystis*, *Mycobacteria* and bacterial pneumonias are common in persons with HIV/AIDS; lung cancer is also more common. A recent study of the lung microbiome demonstrated an increase in *Tropheryma whipplei* associated with untreated HIV infection.[181] Oral pathology, especially thrush and other fungal infections, is also common in HIV infection. Similar to other sites, the oral microbiome appears to have higher proportions of *Prevotella*, *Megasphaera* and *Campylobacter* and lower proportions of the normal oral flora *Streptococcus* in the lingual microbiome.[182] Shifts in the oral fungal microbiome have identified *Pichia* abundance as a protective factor against opportunistic fungi in HIV+ subjects.[183] The extent to which these changes are pathologic or the result of immune deficiency or other exposures is unclear, and further longitudinal studies need to be conducted.

Host Genetic Factors which Modulate Disease

Recent advances in sequencing technology have allowed for multiple genome-wide association studies (GWAS) and candidate gene studies designed to understand variations in the susceptibility of individuals to HIV-1 infection as well as differences in the progression of disease once infected (reviewed in reference 184). Perhaps the strongest of these genetic factors is a homozygous deletion in a portion of the CCR5 gene, the CCR5Δ32 mutation, which confers resistance to infection, while heterozygosity has been associated with slower progression.[185-187] This genetic mutation is more common in persons of European descent. Since transmitted HIV-1 is almost universally CCR5 tropic, loss of this receptor impairs the ability of the virus to infect new cells. One patient was cured of his HIV infection after hematopoietic stem cell transplant with a donor who was homozygous for the CCR5Δ32 deletion, resulting in active efforts to understand and replicate this cure via stem cell transplant or the utilization of gene therapy techniques to create autologous CCR5 deficiency *in vivo*.[188]

The other strong association between host genetics and disease progression has been the finding that genetic variation in the MHC plays a primary role in controlling chronic HIV disease. GWAS studies have demonstrated that MHC is linked to elite control, but have not identified other genetic signatures.[8] The impact of different alleles of the HLA-B genes has a clear effect on viral setpoint and disease progression.[18] Several studies have demonstrated a negative correlation between HLA-C expression and viral load.[189,190] Other genes in the MHC have been demonstrated to be important for control of infection, although most studies suggest that the genetic signals are explained by classic HLA genes. A recent study demonstrated a potential role for the non-HLA gene, MICA, in the MHC in explaining elite control of infection.[191]

Multiple cohorts for studying HIV acquisition and virologic control have been established, and ongoing candidate gene studies, including studies of rare variation and epistatic effects should allow us to further understand the role of host genetics in influencing HIV-1 disease progression. They should be taken in the context of other studies evaluating the effects of coinfections, comorbid conditions, changes in the microbiome, and other environmental exposures on the outcome of HIV-1 infection.

Influence of Antiretroviral Therapy on Disease Pathogenesis

HAART has profound effects on reversing the immune deficiencies associated with chronic HIV infection, and patients treated early with HAART have life expectancies approaching those without HIV-1 infection.[192] However, it is clear that not all of the changes outlined in this chapter are reversed by HAART. Most importantly, the latent viral reservoir, particularly integration of HIV-1 genomic material into Tfh, DC and macrophages, appears to occur very early in the course of the disease, even before HIV-1 viral RNA is detectable in the blood.[11] This virus is protected from both the CD8+ T-cell response and HAART, and is unlikely to be eradicated with currently available strategies.[61,97,99] HAART is able to reverse many of the pathologic changes which occur in the lymph nodes and gastrointestinal tract tissues. Earlier HAART appears to be more effective at restoring full immune competence. HAART does decrease immune activation and inflammation associated with HIV-1 infection, although even in patients on long-term suppressive therapy, inflammatory markers appear to be higher than in uninfected patients.[58,133] This ongoing inflammation may be due to residual effects of the virus, medication effects, sequelae of opportunistic infections or other coinfections, or other risk factors such as smoking and alcohol use, which appear to be higher in HIV-infected patients than in control patients. This ongoing pathology has been associated with an aging phenomenon, which is described in Chapter 104.

References available online at expertconsult.com.

KEY REFERENCES

Brenchley J.M., Price D.A., Schacker T.W., et al.: Microbial translocation is a cause of systemic immune activation in chronic HIV infection. *Nat Med* 2006; 12(12):1365-1371.

Brenchley J.M., Schacker T.W., Ruff L.E., et al.: CD4+ T cell depletion during all stages of HIV disease occurs predominantly in the gastrointestinal tract. *J Exp Med* 2004; 200(6):749-759.

Day C.L., Kaufmann D.E., Kiepiela P., et al.: PD-1 expression on HIV-specific T cells is associated with T-cell exhaustion and disease progression. *Nature* 2006; 443(7109):350-354.

Eisele E., Siliciano R.F.: Redefining the viral reservoirs that prevent HIV-1 eradication. *Immunity* 2012; 37(3):377-388.

Fellay J., Shianna K.V., Ge D., et al.: A whole-genome association study of major determinants for host control of HIV-1. *Science* 2007; 317(5840):944-947.

Fukazawa Y., Lum R., Okoye A.A., et al.: B cell follicle sanctuary permits persistent productive simian immunodeficiency virus infection in elite controllers. *Nat Med* 2015; 21(2):132-139.

Giorgi J.V., Hultin L.E., McKeating J.A., et al.: Shorter survival in advanced human immunodeficiency virus type 1 infection is more closely associated with T lymphocyte activation than with plasma virus burden or virus chemokine coreceptor usage. *J Infect Dis* 1999; 179(4):859-870.

Hutter G., Nowak D., Mossner M., et al.: Long-term control of HIV by CCR5 Delta32/Delta32 stem-cell transplantation. *N Engl J Med* 2009; 360(7):692-698.

Keele B.F., Giorgi E.E., Salazar-Gonzalez J.F., et al.: Identification and characterization of transmitted and early founder virus envelopes in primary HIV-1 infection. *Proc Natl Acad Sci USA* 2008; 105(21):7552-7557.

Liao H.X., Lynch R., Zhou T., et al.: Co-evolution of a broadly neutralizing HIV-1 antibody and founder virus. *Nature* 2013; 496(7446):469-476.

Miller C.J., Alexander N.J., Sutjipto S., et al.: Genital mucosal transmission of simian immunodeficiency virus: animal model for heterosexual transmission of human immunodeficiency virus. *J Virol* 1989; 63(10):4277-4284.

Mutlu E.A., Keshavarzian A., Losurdo J., et al.: A compositional look at the human gastrointestinal microbiome and immune activation parameters in HIV infected subjects. *PLoS Pathog* 2014; 10(2):e1003829.

Okulicz J.F., Marconi V.C., Landrum M.L., et al.: Clinical outcomes of elite controllers, viremic controllers, and long-term nonprogressors in the US Department of Defense HIV natural history study. *J Infect Dis* 2009; 200(11):1714-1723.

Pereyra F., Jia X., McLaren P.J., et al.: The major genetic determinants of HIV-1 control affect HLA class I peptide presentation. *Science* 2010; 330(6010):1551-1557.

Schuetz A., Deleage C., Sereti I., et al.: Initiation of ART during early acute HIV infection preserves mucosal Th17 function and reverses HIV-related immune activation. *PLoS Pathog* 2014; 10(12):e1004543.

Veazey R.S., DeMaria M., Chalifoux L.V., et al.: Gastrointestinal tract as a major site of CD4+ T cell depletion and viral replication in SIV infection. *Science* 1998; 280(5362):427-431.

Velu V., Titanji K., Zhu B., et al.: Enhancing SIV-specific immunity in vivo by PD-1 blockade. *Nature* 2009; 458(7235):206-210.

93

Primary HIV Infection

BERNARD HIRSCHEL

KEY CONCEPTS

- Primary HIV infection (PHI) may be asymptomatic, or may cause fever, skin lesions, pharyngitis, or meningoencephalitis. It is a self-limited disease occurring within a few weeks to months after new infection with human immunodeficiency virus (HIV).

- During PHI, anti-HIV antibodies may still be absent. Diagnosis relies on measuring HIV RNA, or p24 antigen.

- Levels of HIV-RNA are typically exceedingly high (>million/mL). After the onset of the anti-HIV immune response, they decline by orders of magnitude to reach a stable plateau.

- Patients with PHI are highly infectious. One-fourth to one-half of new HIV infections originate from patients who are themselves recently infected.

- Some patients who started very early highly active antiretroviral therapy (HAART) during PHI and then stopped did not experience a viral rebound.

Introduction

Although primary HIV infection (PHI) is a rarely diagnosed, self-limiting disease, it is a topic of considerable interest, since the first encounter of HIV with the immune system sheds light on many aspects of pathogenesis. As the severity of PHI predicts progression to immunodeficiency years later,[1] it is reasonable to hope that treatment of PHI can delay or even prevent progression to AIDS. From a public health perspective, a diagnosis of PHI is important because such patients are highly infectious to others.[2,3] To miss a diagnosis of PHI is to miss an opportunity both for intervention and for prevention of further transmission.[4] Experience shows that the diagnosis is not difficult to make; education is the key.

Epidemiology

Primary HIV infection is often asymptomatic but sometimes it presents with dramatic manifestations requiring hospital admission. There is a spectrum between complete absence of symptoms during the time of seroconversion and severe disease; therefore, it is not surprising that opinions vary about the percentage of patients who have symptomatic PHI, from less than one-third to more than 90%.[5] Theoretically, the size of the inoculum, the virulence of the infecting HIV strain (including such factors as cellular tropism and cytopathogenicity) and the patient's immune status could be involved, but evidence as to whether these factors are important is lacking. One series of transfusion-associated cases found that symptomatic PHI was more frequent among those infected by people who had late-stage disease (and presumably high circulating viral loads). There is little evidence that the frequency or severity of PHI differs between transmission categories or between men and women. Symptomatic PHI can occur with HIV-2 infection and in children, although almost all cases have been reported in adults infected with HIV-1. There are theoretic reasons to believe that coinfection with other viruses, particularly from the herpes group, might enhance the proliferation of HIV, and patients who are simultaneously coinfected with cytomegalovirus have had particularly severe symptoms of PHI.

Symptoms typically start 2–4 weeks after infection, with extremes of 5 and more than 90 days. The median duration of symptoms is estimated between 12 and 28 days.[6] Moderate and subjective symptoms such as fatigue may persist for months, although almost all patients eventually enter an asymptomatic phase lasting years.

Pathogenesis and Pathology

Studies of acute simian immunodeficiency virus (SIV) infection have elucidated aspects of HIV and AIDS pathogenesis. Weeks after inoculation, SIV causes massive loss of memory CD4+ cells in many tissues,[7] but particularly in the intestinal tract. Increased permeability of the gut permits translocation of microbial products, resulting in chronic immune activation which is a hallmark of progressive HIV infection.[8]

Because PHI most often presents as a benign self-limiting disease, pathologic information is available only from easily biopsied tissues. The skin rash is caused by a dermal perivascular lymphohistiocytic infiltrate around vessels of the superficial dermis; the epidermis is normal. The inflammatory cells are predominantly of the CD4+ phenotype, and may represent a T-cell-mediated reaction to HIV and to the p24 antigen, which can be detected in Langerhans cells.

Lymph node biopsies reveal abundant HIV, including the envelope proteins gp120 and gp160 in dendritic reticulum cells, as well as in lymphocytes. The structure of the germinal centers is relatively normal and quite unlike the follicular hyperplasia of established HIV-1 infection, but extrafollicular B lymphocytes are reduced in number and the follicles are infiltrated by CD8+ T cells.[9]

Clinical Features

During PHI, HIV floods the blood with massive viremia,[10] spreading to the central nervous system[11] (CNS) and the lymphatic system, and invades a number of other tissues. Not surprisingly, PHI is a disease with protean clinical manifestations. Three main presentations have been described.

CUTANEOUS PRESENTATION

This is characterized by a maculopapular rash, 'roseola' and mucosal ulcerations (Figures 93-1 to 93-4). The rash affects the face, neck and trunk more than the limbs, although the palms and soles may be involved. Individual lesions are usually less than 1 cm in diameter and confluence is rare. Case reports have mentioned pustular eruptions, urticaria, erythema multiforme and, during the healing phase of PHI, alopecia and desquamation. Ulceration may occur on the genital and oral mucosa, including the esophagus, where differentiation from herpetic lesions or esophageal candidiasis is difficult.

PRESENTATION RESEMBLING INFECTIOUS MONONUCLEOSIS

This presentation is characterized by fever, pharyngitis, arthralgia, myalgia and lymphadenopathy. Although the expression 'mononucleosis-like illness' is firmly established, there are many differences from classic infectious mononucleosis, most notably the lack of prominent tonsillar involvement. In a large series (Table 93-1), only 20% of patients had a fever in combination with sore throat and enlarged cervical lymph nodes, whereas 10% did not have fever, sore throat or cervical lymphadenopathy.

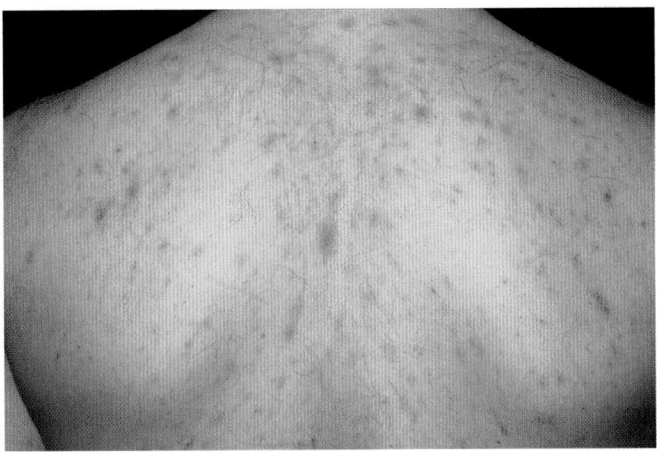

Figure 93-1 Maculopapular rash during primary HIV infection.

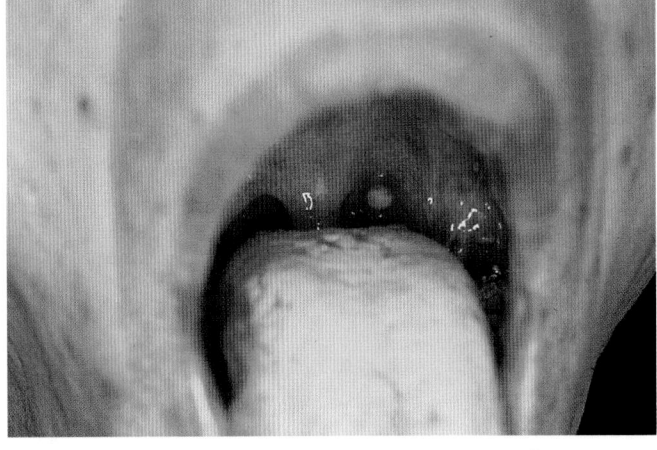

Figure 93-4 Mucosal ulcerations during primary HIV infection.

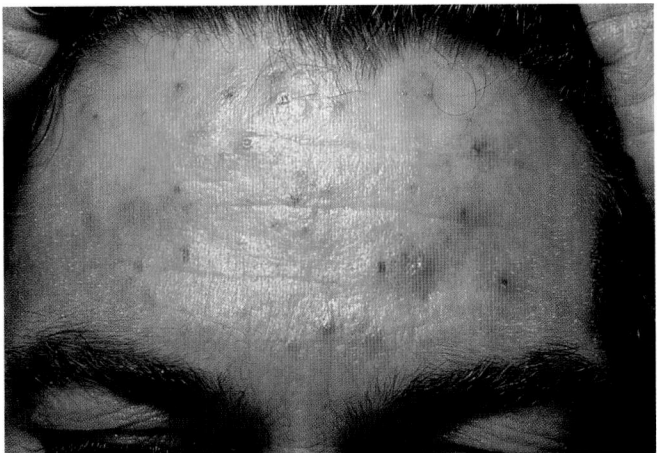

Figure 93-2 Acneiform lesions during primary HIV infection.

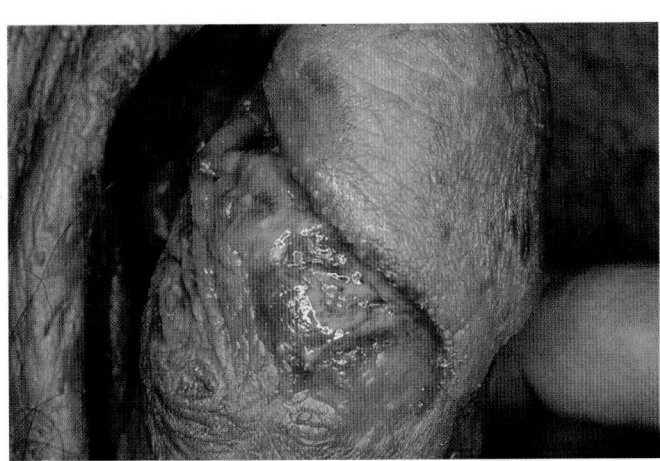

Figure 93-3 Penile ulcer during primary HIV infection.

TABLE 93-1	Signs and Symptoms of Primary HIV Infection*	
	Symptom/Sign	%
Reported by more than 50%	Fever	77
	Lethargy/fatigue	66
	Rash	56
	Myalgia	55
	Headache	51
Reported by 20–50%	Pharyngitis	44
	Cervical adenopathy	39
	Arthralgia	31
	Oral ulcer	29
	Pain on swallowing	28
	Axillary adenopathy	24
	Weight loss	24
	Nausea	24
	Diarrhea	23
	Night sweats	22
	Cough	22
	Anorexia	22
Reported by 5–20%	Abdominal pain	19
	Oral candidiasis	17
	Vomiting	12
	Photophobia	12
	Meningitis	12
	Genital ulcer	7
	Tonsillitis	7
	Depression	7
	Dizziness	6

*These signs and symptoms are reported by at least 5% of patients.[1,2]

OTHER SYMPTOMS

Table 93-1 shows the frequencies of signs and recorded symptoms in the medical charts of more than 200 patients from Switzerland and Australia. Digestive manifestations have not been well recognized in the past, but they are quite common. In exceptional cases, esophageal candidiasis (an AIDS-defining disease) may occur with a transient decline in CD4[+] lymphocyte count.

Unusual manifestations associated with PHI include:

- neurologic syndromes such as radiculopathy, peripheral facial neuropathy and Guillain–Barré syndrome, and severe encephalitis with prolonged coma and seizures; and
- pulmonary involvement, which may be more frequent in intravenous drug users where PHI can be associated with bacterial pneumonia; severe pneumonitis leading to intubation and *Pneumocystis jirovecii* pneumonia (with CD4[+] lymphocyte counts of <100/μL) has been described but is exceptional.[12]

MENINGOENCEPHALITIS

Meningoencephalitis is characterized by photophobia and neck stiffness, headaches and disordered consciousness. The headache is typically retro-orbital and exacerbated by eye movements. Depression and changes in mood are frequent and may reflect underlying encephalitis.

TABLE 93-2	Important Differential Diagnoses	
Clinical Features	**Epstein–Barr Virus Infection**	**Primary HIV Infection**
Onset	Gradual	Abrupt
Tonsil involvement	+++	+
Pharyngeal exudate	+++	–
Rash	Rare except in patients treated with antibiotics	Frequent
Jaundice	10%	Never
Diarrhea	Rare	25%
Clinical Features	**Syphilis**	**HIV Infection**
Serology	Always positive	At first negative
Chancre: timing	Before generalized rash	At the same time as rash
Chancre: pain	Painless	Painful
Clinical Features	**Enterovirus Meningitis**	**HIV Meningitis**
Population	Young adults	Young adults
Diarrhea	Rare	23%
Season	Summer–autumn	None in particular
Duration	<8 days	Often >20 days
Encephalitis	None	Frequent
Skin lesions	Rare	Frequent
Pain on swallowing	None	Frequent

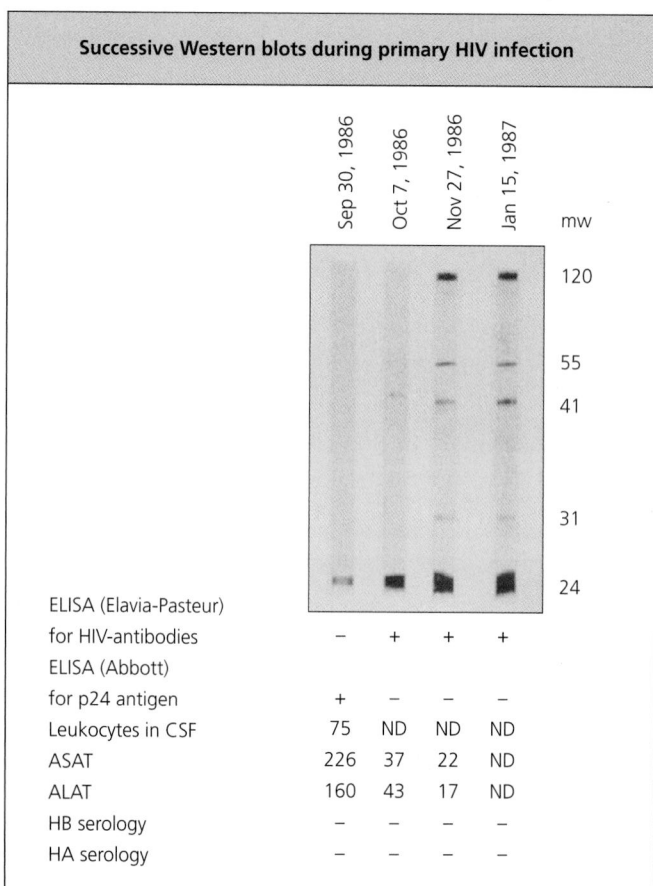

Figure 93-5 Successive Western blots during primary HIV infection. Note that on September 30, 1986, when the patient presented with fever, rash, meningitis and subclinical hepatitis, the screening enzyme-linked immunosorbent assay (ELISA) test for HIV antibodies was negative, while the Western blot showed only a single weak band corresponding to the p24 antigen. CSF, cerebrospinal fluid; ASAT, aspartate transaminase; ALAT, alanine transaminase; H, hepatitis (A or B); ND, not done.

DIFFERENTIAL DIAGNOSIS

Important differential diagnoses are listed in Table 93-2; PHI must be distinguished from Epstein–Barr virus infection (infectious mononucleosis) and enterovirus meningitis, and according to the local epidemiologic context, typhoid fever, rickettsial infections and many others. The relatively few primary HIV infections easily get lost among the multitudes who present with fever, rash and pharyngitis. For instance, an estimated 6.4 million patients seeking ambulatory care present with pharyngitis each year in the USA; of these, 8500 (0.13%) have primary HIV infection.

Diagnosis

Seroconversion (i.e. the documented first appearance of HIV antibodies in the serum) occurs days after the beginning of the symptoms of PHI. Therefore, the usual antibody tests for HIV are not entirely reliable; they are expected to be negative during the first few days of PHI (Figure 93-5). Assays differ in the duration of this 'seronegative period'; with the currently used sensitive tests, it is usually less than 1 week after the start of symptoms of PHI.

The p24 antigen is positive when the antibody test is still negative during PHI, and the same is true of HIV viremia. Whereas both tests can be used to screen for PHI, the p24 antigen test is considerably cheaper.[13] Viremia levels reach extremely high values, often in excess of 10^6 viral genomes/mL, and high titers of infectious virus have been isolated from many tissues, including seminal fluid, corroborating the epidemiologic evidence that patients who have PHI are highly infectious. Viremia decreases rapidly – at least 100-fold within days after seroconversion – but remains detectable in more than 95% of patients. Steady-state plasma viremia levels predict progression to advanced immunodeficiency and death.[14] Levels tend to remain higher in those who have symptomatic PHI.[15] Despite the relatively short duration of PHI, a substantial percentage of newly diagnosed HIV infections are acquired from patients who are themselves recently infected.[16]

Like viremia levels, lymphocyte subsets undergo rapid changes during PHI (Figure 93-6). During the first 5–10 days, lymphopenia characteristically affects both CD4[+] and CD8[+] lymphocytes, with levels[12] that may be as low as those observed in AIDS. Although opportunistic infections are rare, in vitro tests of both B and T cells show immunosuppression. Within another 2–3 weeks there is a lymphocytosis. The CD8[+] lymphocyte count expands more than the CD4[+] lymphocyte count, leading to a CD4[+]/CD8[+] lymphocyte ratio of less than 1. This low ratio persists even in patients whose CD4[+] lymphocyte count subsequently rises to normal.

Many other laboratory values may be abnormal during PHI, reflecting the acute inflammatory response (e.g. high erythrocyte sedimentation rate, increase in C-reactive protein) and involvement of the bone marrow (thrombocytopenia), the liver (increase in hepatic transaminases) and the CNS (pleocytosis of the cerebrospinal fluid).

Management

Although PHI can be severe and prolonged, it is most often a self-limiting disease. The symptoms eventually abate and the patient becomes asymptomatic. Years later, immunosuppression may appear and AIDS may develop.

FEATURES OF PRIMARY HIV INFECTION THAT MAY PREDICT THE SUBSEQUENT COURSE TOWARDS AIDS

A considerable body of evidence suggests that more severe and more prolonged PHI indicates a more unfavorable course towards AIDS.[1]

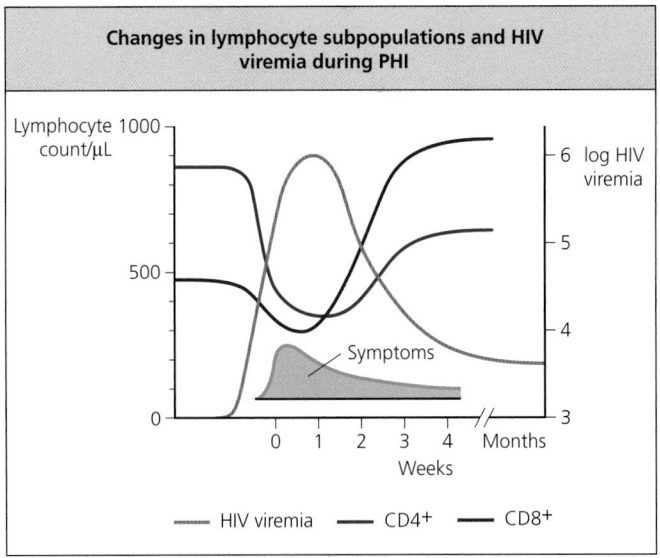

Figure 93-6 Changes in lymphocyte subpopulations and HIV viremia during primary HIV infection.

For instance, in patients who were followed after seroconversion, 58% of those who had had symptomatic PHI had developed AIDS 7 years later compared with 28% of those who had had asymptomatic PHI.[17] Another study suggested that the presence of neurologic signs at the time of PHI predicted accelerated immunosuppression,[18] although there was no specific relation to the neurologic signs of AIDS, such as AIDS-related dementia or opportunistic infections of the CNS.

DOES TREATMENT OF PRIMARY HIV INFECTION IMPROVE THE LONG-TERM OUTCOME?

This is a critically important question that regrettably remains unanswered. Arguments have shifted back and forth between advocates and opponents of treatment, but have become less acute with the availability of more effective and better tolerated antiviral drugs, and the extension of treatment indications to almost all HIV-infected patients.[19] Three different studies have enrolled patients with early infection, and randomized them between immediate and deferred treatment start:

- The 'setpoint' study recruited patients with recent, but not acute HIV infection. Patients either started therapy right away for 36 weeks and then stopped, or deferred treatment. Half of the patients in the deferred arm met criteria for ART initiation within 72 weeks, as compared to only 10% of the patients in the immediate treatment arm.[20]
- The Primo-SMH trial enrolled patients with both recent (about 2/3) and acute (1/3) HIV infection. Group 1 commenced treatment immediately and stopped after 24 weeks, group 2 stopped after 60 weeks, and group 3 did not start treatment. In comparison with group 3, viral loads were lower 36 weeks after treatment interruption in groups 1 and 2, and CD4 counts declined more slowly.[21]
- The Spartac trial included patients with early infection to either immediate treatment for 12 or 48 weeks, or deferred treatment. The time until the CD4 counts declined to less than 350/µL was longer in the 48-week group than in the other two groups.[22]

These three trials were designed at a time when there was great interest in interrupting treatment, and in limiting the exposure to antiretroviral drugs. Today, however, treatment interruptions are no longer recommended.[19]

'Setpoint', 'Primo-SMH' and 'Spartac' all show that after treatment interruption, viral RNA invariably becomes detectable again. However, the French 'Visconti' study[23] described 14 patients who started treatment 33–63 days after the probable date of infection, stopped, and did not experience a viral rebound during a median of 89 months without HAART. From a registry of patients in France who started treatment during PHI and then stopped, the authors estimated a probability of 15% of maintaining viral control 12–24 months after treatment interruption. Factors that distinguish those post-treatment-controllers from the more frequent patients who relapse are unclear at the present time, as are the reasons why post-treatment control was not observed in 'Setpoint', 'Primo-SMH' and 'Spartac'.[24] It may be relevant that the French patients commenced treatment very early.

References available online at expertconsult.com.

KEY REFERENCES

Brenchley J., Price D., Schacker T., et al.: Microbial translocation is a cause of systemic immune activation in chronic HIV infection. *Nat Med* 2006; 12:1365-1371.

Fox J., White P.J., Macdonald N., et al.: Reductions in HIV transmission risk behaviour following diagnosis of primary HIV infection: a cohort of high-risk men who have sex with men. *HIV Med* 2009; 10(7):432-438.

Lodi S.L., Fisher M., Phillips A., et al.: CASCADE Collaboration in EuroCoord. Symptomatic illness and low CD4 cell count at HIV seroconversion as markers of severe primary HIV infection. *PLoS One* 2013; 8(11):e78642.

Sáez-Cirión A.L., Bacchus C., Hocqueloux L., et al.: Post-treatment HIV-1 controllers with a long-term virological remission after the interruption of early initiated antiretroviral therapy. The ANRS VISCONTI Study. *PLoS Pathog* 2013; 9(3):e1003211.

The SPARTAC Trial Investigators.: Short-course antiretroviral therapy in primary HIV infection. *N Engl J Med* 2013; 368(3):207-217.

Tindall B., Barker S., Donovan B., et al.: Characterization of the acute clinical illness associated with human immunodeficiency virus infection. *Arch Intern Med* 1988; 148:945-949.

94

Opportunistic Infections: Management and Prevention

STÉPHANE DE WIT | NATHAN CLUMECK

KEY CONCEPTS

- The epidemiology of opportunistic infections in human immunodeficiency virus (HIV) disease has changed considerably with the introduction of effective antiretroviral drugs.

- Prevention of opportunistic infections is of prime importance to prevent morbidity and mortality from infections and to limit deterioration of the host control of HIV viral load and accelerated loss of T-cell number and function.

- Clinical features of opportunistic infections can be challenging as the degree of immune compromise can alter typical presentation of disease manifestations.

- First-choice treatments and alternative regimens for most opportunistic infections are now quite effective and the outlook for patients presenting if these HIV-associated opportunistic infections is better, particularly when combined with early institution of effective antiretroviral therapy.

- The adverse effects of immune reconstitution inflammatory syndrome (IRIS) from beginning antiretroviral therapy (ART) can be severe (e.g. initial treatment of cryptococcal meningitis with antifungal agents and ART) and this problem must be factored into the timing of treatment of opportunistic infections.

- Pre-emptive therapy and maintenance therapy against recurrence of opportunistic infections are indicated in selected patients with early HIV infection and in advanced acquired immunodeficiency syndrome (AIDS).

Introduction

The major cause of death in patients with AIDS had been the opportunistic infections (OIs) that arose as a consequence of the severe immunodeficiency characteristic of HIV infection.[1] Since the advent of the era of potent antiretroviral therapy (ART), there has been a marked decrease in the occurrence of AIDS-related opportunistic infections and a consequent increase in survival.[2] Nevertheless, there is great variability in access to ART and consequently significant AIDS-associated OIs continue. In the Western world, this is largely a consequence of delayed diagnosis, with patients presenting with an OI as the first recognition of HIV infection; in resource-poor situations, availability of ART is more of a problem. The number of circulating CD4+ T-lymphocyte count is closely correlated with the risk of developing several opportunistic infections. Once the CD4+ T-lymphocyte count falls below 200 cells/μL, the cumulative risk for developing an AIDS-defining OI is 33% by year 1 and 58% by 2 years. Therefore, CD4+ T-lymphocyte counts are the critical parameter for monitoring patients who have HIV infection because of their predictive value for both opportunistic infections and mortality. Two patterns of OI development exist – re-emergence of infections acquired early in life (often in childhood) as the CD4+ T-lymphocyte count falls, and newly acquired infection by organisms that become pathogenic in the setting of progressive immunodeficiency.

The probability of developing a given disease depends on the risk for exposure to potential pathogens, the virulence of the pathogens and the level of immunosuppression of the patient. There is a wide geographic variability in the epidemiology of opportunistic infections. In the USA and Northern Europe, pneumonia caused by *Pneumocystis jirovecii* (PJP), oropharyngeal or esophageal candidiasis, cytomegalovirus disease and infections caused by *Mycobacterium avium* complex (MAC) are common. The incidence of toxoplasmosis and tuberculosis is higher in Eastern and Southern Europe and in the low- and middle-income countries, depending on the prevalence of latent infection in the general population.

Use of Antiretroviral Therapy During Management of Acute Opportunistic Infections

Antiretroviral therapy should be initiated as soon as possible in patients with OIs for which treatment is limited or not effective and for whom the overall improvement of immune function would be beneficial. Examples of such conditions include cryptosporidiosis, microsporidiosis, progressive multifocal leukoencephalopathy and HIV-associated dementia.

For patients for whom definitive anti-infective therapy is available, the benefit of immediate initiation of ART in increasing CD4+ T-lymphocyte count and improving the patient's immunologic status must be weighed against the possibility of increased adverse effects, toxicities or drug–drug interactions. Randomized clinical trials demonstrated a clinical and survival benefit of starting ART early, within the first 2 weeks, of initiation of treatment for an acute OI.[3] The majority of OIs were PJP and serious bacterial infections, and some caution must be taken extending this recommendation to tuberculosis where the risk of immune reconstitution inflammatory syndrome (IRIS) may be higher. Cryptococcosis is the only exception to this rule, as early initiation of ART is associated with higher mortality (see section on cryptococcosis).

Prophylaxis of Opportunistic Infections

Preventive therapy for OIs was the mainstay of treatment in HIV prior to the introduction of effective ART and remains important for patients with severe immunodeficiency, even when ART-associated immune recovery can be expected.

Certain principles underlie the decision to use prophylaxis for different pathogens:

- the incidence and prevalence of specific infections in HIV-infected individuals;
- the potential severity of disease in terms of morbidity and mortality;
- the level of immunosuppression at which each disease is likely to occur;
- the feasibility and efficacy of preventive measures, and in particular their impact on quality of life and survival;

- the potential for emergence of organisms resistant to the agents used for prophylaxis;
- the risk of toxicities and drug interactions with antiretrovirals and other drugs used by HIV-infected patients;
- the issue of compliance; and
- the cost-effectiveness of prophylaxis.

As an example, PJP is very common, causes significant mortality and can be easily prevented; as a result, routine prophylaxis is recommended for all HIV-positive patients with CD4$^+$ T-lymphocyte counts less than 200 cells/μL. In contrast, candidiasis is also very common, but rarely causes mortality, is easily treated and prophylactic antifungals are associated with a significant risk of resistance, so prophylaxis is rarely given. Cryptococcal meningitis is associated with significant mortality and is preventable using fluconazole; however, prevention is not regarded as cost-effective in the West because it is relatively rare; in contrast primary prophylaxis is justified in areas such as sub-Saharan Africa and southern Asia.

Duration of Prophylaxis Against Opportunistic Infections

Susceptibility to opportunistic infections can be accurately assessed by the CD4$^+$ T-lymphocyte count. It is therefore possible to stop primary or secondary prophylaxis in patients whose immunity has improved as a consequence of highly active antiretroviral therapy (HAART) and whose T cells have risen above the threshold of increased susceptibility. This is particularly true for patients with complete viral suppression, as ongoing improvements in immune function can be expected.

By contrast, no data are available regarding the re-initiation of prophylaxis when the CD4$^+$ T-lymphocyte count decreases again to levels at which the risk for opportunistic infections exists. In particular, it is unknown whether it is better to use the threshold at which prophylaxis was stopped or the threshold below which initial prophylaxis is recommended.

Pneumocystis jirovecii Pneumonia (PJP)

Pneumocystis jirovecii (previously known as *Pneumocystis carinii*, and still often referred to as PJP for *p*neumocystis *p*neumonia) is a fungal pathogen associated with opportunistic infections, especially pneumonia, in patients with altered cell-mediated immunity. Historically, the occurrence of PJP in American gay men who had no previously known immune deficiency was the first signal of the AIDS epidemic.[4] Although the implementation of prophylaxis and the advances in ART have markedly decreased its incidence, PJP remains an important OI. Its epidemiology is uncertain; although it is generally thought to be due to reactivation of latent infection acquired during childhood or adolescence, genetic studies of *P. jirovecii* isolates suggest that recent exposure to environmental strains may be a factor in acquisition of infection. PJP typically occurs when the CD4$^+$ T-lymphocyte count is less than 200 cells/μL. The rate of relapse after a first episode of PJP is high (approximately 60% incidence within 1 year) when neither specific prophylaxis nor highly active antiretroviral therapy (HAART) is initiated.[5]

Clinical Features

Pneumocystis jirovecii infection is restricted to the lung in more than 95% of cases. The most common clinical presentation of PJP is a progressive dyspnea with dry cough, fever (often mild) and weight loss. On examination, fever and tachypnea are common, whereas lung auscultation may be normal or reveal only basal crepitations. Disseminated infection (bone marrow, spleen, liver, retina and skin) can occur spontaneously or in association with the use of aerosolized pentamidine. Chest radiography is an important step in the diagnosis, being normal in less than 5% of cases of PJP. The most common pattern is a fine bilateral interstitial and then alveolar–interstitial infiltrate

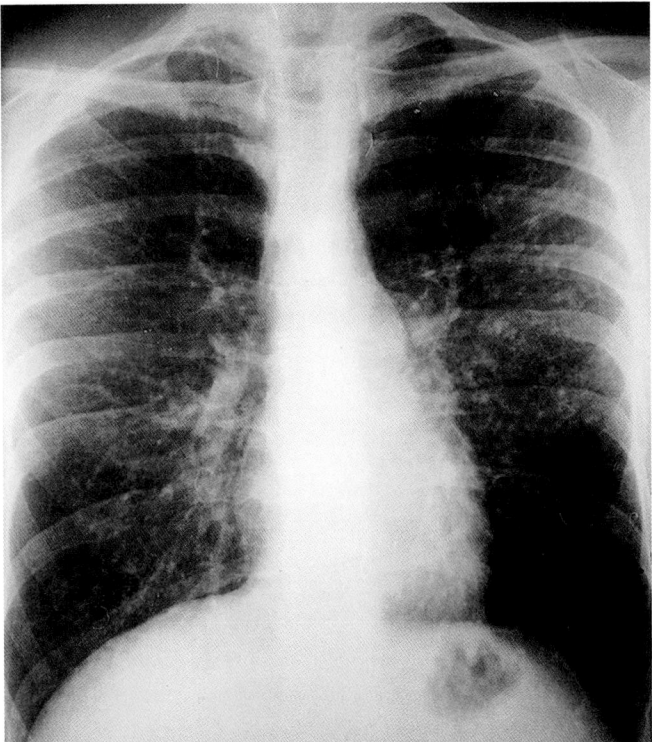

Figure 94-1 Mild *Pneumocystis jirovecii* pneumonia. There are bilateral micronodular lesions. *(Courtesy of Pierre-Marie Girard.)*

progressing from the peri-hilar to the peripheral regions (Figure 94-1). In advanced cases, progressive consolidation with air bronchograms and complete opacification of the lungs may develop (Figure 94-2). Numerous atypical patterns of PJP may occur. They include localized infiltrates, cavitary lesions, solitary lung nodules, spontaneous pneumothoraces and pleural effusions. Hilar or mediastinal lymphadenopathy is very rare.

Establishing a diagnosis of PJP requires the morphologic demonstration of the micro-organism. Arterial blood gases must be measured to assess the severity of the disease, but have no diagnostic value. Sputum examination is the least invasive procedure for collecting lower respiratory specimens. Because patients who have PJP generally do not have a productive cough, an induced sputum can be obtained after aerosolization of hypertonic saline, ideally under the supervision of a physiotherapist. In routine practice, the sensitivity of the test is approximately 50–60%. Fiberoptic bronchoscopy with bronchoalveolar lavage is the reference routine diagnostic procedure because its sensitivity is more than 95% and its specificity is 100%. When the diagnosis cannot be obtained from bronchoalveolar lavage fluid, transbronchial lung biopsy may help, although it is more invasive and is associated with a risk of bleeding and pneumothorax.

Management

The measurement of arterial gas is used routinely to define mild (PaO$_2$ ≥70 mmHg), moderate (PaO$_2$ 50–70 mmHg) and severe (PaO$_2$ <50 mmHg) PJP. Hospitalization is generally required with the exception of some cases of mild PJP, for which outpatient management with oral therapy is often possible providing no other disease is present, there is low risk of drug malabsorption, the management strategy is well understood and the patient is aware of the potential side effects of therapy. Trimethoprim–sulfamethoxazole (TMP–SMX) is the drug of choice for PJP whatever its severity, and no other drug or combination of drugs has demonstrated improved efficacy in controlled trials.[6,7] The drug is given as 15 mg/kg/day trimethoprim with 75 mg/kg/day sulfamethoxazole (in three divided doses). Side effects include rash, fever, pruritus, digestive disturbances and cytopenia, usually after 7–10

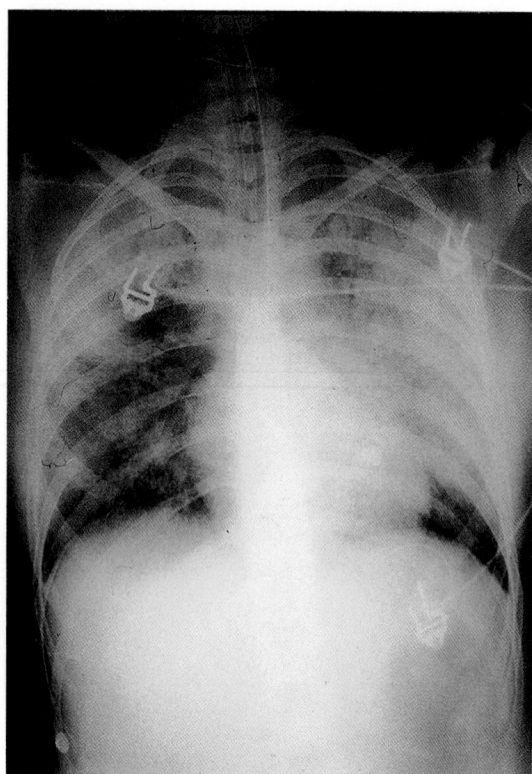

Figure 94-2 Severe *Pneumocystis jirovecii* pneumonia. This shows an extensive alveolar interstitial infiltrate with consolidation of the left lung and upper right lobe. *(Courtesy of Pierre-Marie Girard.)*

days of therapy. Approximately 10–20% of patients will need to be switched to another treatment because of TMP–SMX intolerance. It is important to determine the nature of intolerance to TMP–SMX. In practice, contraindication to reintroduction of TMP–SMX or to the use of a combination with potential cross-intolerance to sulfonamide is based on a history of anaphylaxis or exfoliative dermatitis or other life-threatening toxicity such as severe cytolytic hepatitis. Whenever possible, the first-line therapy for PJP is always TMP–SMX. For cases of mild PJP, alternates include dapsone plus trimethoprim, clindamycin plus primaquine or atovaquone. For more severe PJP, alternates include clindamycin plus primaquine or intravenous pentamidine.[7] In addition to anti-*P. jirovecii* therapy, corticosteroids are administered as soon as possible in patients who have moderate to severe disease. The use of corticosteroids is recommended in patients whose PaO_2 is less than 65 mmHg and has been shown to improve oxygenation, reduce the risk of fibrosis, decrease the need for mechanical ventilation and reduce the case fatality rate.[8] The recommended corticosteroid regimen is on days 1–5, 40 mg oral prednisone (prednisolone) q12h, on days 6–10, 40 mg oral prednisone/day and on days 11–21, 20 mg oral prednisone/day. In most cases, respiratory symptoms and oxygenation improve after 5–10 days. If a patient has been treated empirically (without definitive diagnosis), failure to improve after 5–7 days of treatment should trigger a re-evaluation, usually with bronchoscopy. Early mild deterioration is not infrequent during the first days of treatment. The duration of treatment is classically 21 days. When TMP–SMX is initiated intravenously, it can be switched to an oral formulation after a few days. Secondary prophylaxis is required after treatment of the attack.

Prevention

Prophylaxis against PJP is indicated for all HIV-infected patients with a CD4+ T-lymphocyte count less than 200 cells/µL or those with a history of oropharyngeal candidiasis or an AIDS-defining illness. TMP–SMX is the drug of choice while offering a significant reduction

in bacterial infections as well as a primary prophylaxis against toxoplasmosis. Side effects are sufficiently severe to require discontinuation of the drug in 25–50% of TMP–SMX recipients. There is good evidence that lower doses of TMP–SMX are better tolerated, and many advocate either the use of lower-dose regimens using one single-strength tablet daily or one double-strength tablet thrice weekly. Patients who have adverse reactions to TMP–SMX usually tolerate dapsone. Of note secondary prophylaxis for cerebral toxoplasmosis with pyrimethamine–sulfadiazine or a regimen including atovaquone provides an adequate primary prophylaxis for PJP.

Primary and secondary prophylaxis against PJP may be discontinued in patients treated with HAART who show an increase in CD4+ T-lymphocyte count to above 200 cells/µL for at least 3 months. Prophylaxis should be re-introduced if the CD4+ T-lymphocyte count decreases to less than 200 cells/µL.[9,10]

Of note in an observational European cohort, incidence of PJP was low and independent of prophylaxis in patients with CD4+ T-lymphocyte count between 100 and 200 cells/µL with a viral load below the limit of detection.[11]

Viral Infections

Most clinically important viral infections in HIV disease are caused by DNA viruses, the majority belonging to the Herpesviridae family. The role of viral infections such as human herpesvirus 8, Epstein–Barr virus and human papillomavirus in HIV-related neoplastic disorders is discussed elsewhere.

Cytomegalovirus Infections

Serologic evidence of cytomegalovirus (CMV) infection can be detected in approximately 60% of the adult population in the USA. The prevalence of infection is strongly influenced by socioeconomic status and sexual practices; up to 95% of men who have sex with men (MSM) are seropositive for CMV. In patients who have AIDS, CMV disease usually results from reactivation of latent infection. Progressive loss of cell-mediated immunity in patients abrogates the immunologic suppression of CMV replication. Asymptomatic excretion of CMV in urine can be detected in approximately 50% of patients who have advanced HIV disease, and over half of the patients who have CMV viremia go on to develop clinical CMV disease within 8–12 months. Cytomegalovirus end-organ disease usually occurs when the CD4+ T-lymphocyte count falls below 50 cells/µL.[12]

CYTOMEGALOVIRUS RETINITIS

Retinitis is the commonest manifestation of CMV infection in patients who have HIV infection or AIDS, accounting for 85% of CMV disease. The virus causes a relentlessly progressive, necrotizing retinitis. Cytomegalovirus retinitis is usually unilateral in the first instance, progressing to affect the contralateral eye if untreated. Patients may be initially asymptomatic but may subsequently experience blurring of vision, floaters and painless progressive visual loss. Diagnosis of CMV retinitis is made by systematic funduscopic examination by direct or indirect ophthalmoscopy. Characteristically, white, fluffy or granular lesions with perivascular white exudates associated with retinal edema and hemorrhages are seen (Figure 94-3).

GASTROINTESTINAL CYTOMEGALOVIRUS DISEASE

In the upper gastrointestinal tract, CMV causes discrete esophageal ulcers, diffuse esophagitis, gastritis, gastric ulcers, duodenal ulcers and enteritis. Esophageal CMV infection usually presents with painful dysphagia; diagnosis is established by endoscopic examination showing inflammation and ulceration, with characteristic pathologic features on tissue biopsy. Cytomegalovirus enterocolitis usually presents with abdominal pain and persistent small-volume diarrhea. Endoscopic examination of the colon typically reveals plaque-like pseudomembranes, multiple erosions and ulcers.

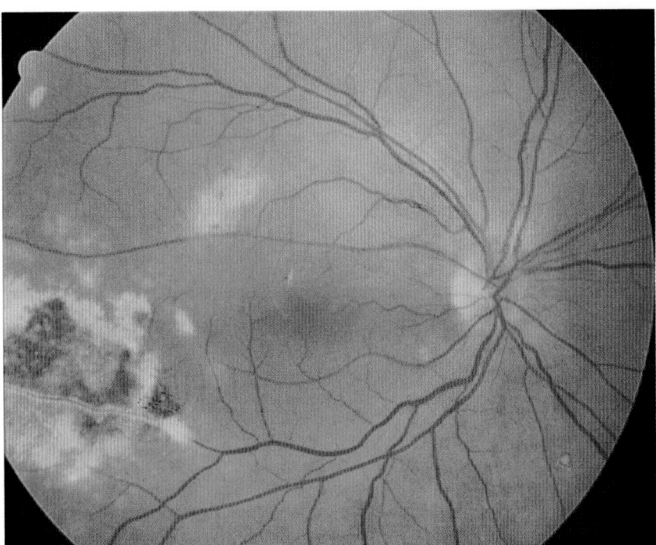

Figure 94-3 Cytomegalovirus retinitis, with characteristic perivascular hemorrhages and exudates. *(Courtesy of Maurice E. Murphy and Bruce Polsky.)*

CYTOMEGALOVIRUS DISEASE OF THE CENTRAL NERVOUS SYSTEM

The two major CMV neurologic syndromes associated with HIV disease are CMV polyradiculopathy and CMV ventriculoencephalitis. Polyradiculopathy is seen in patients who have advanced AIDS. Approximately 50% have an associated myelitis. It is characterized by lower extremity pain, sensory deficits, weakness that can rapidly progress to flaccid paralysis, and bowel and bladder dysfunction. The most marked pathologic changes in CMV polyradiculomyelitis are found in the cauda equina and lumbosacral roots. In the appropriate clinical setting, findings on MRI of diffuse enhancement of the cauda equina and the surface of the conus strongly support the diagnosis. Cerebrospinal fluid (CSF) findings include a polymorphonuclear pleocytosis, raised protein concentration and moderately low glucose concentration. Culture of CSF may be negative but CMV antigen assays and polymerase chain reaction (PCR) for CMV DNA are more sensitive techniques. Ventriculoencephalitis usually occurs in the setting of a diagnosis of CMV disease elsewhere. Patients present with fever, lethargy and confusion. Characteristic neurologic findings include nystagmus and cranial nerve palsies. MRI with gadolinium enhancement may demonstrate periventricular enhancement. Cytomegalovirus DNA can often be detected in CSF using PCR.

PULMONARY CYTOMEGALOVIRUS DISEASE

There are no particular distinguishing clinical or radiologic features to differentiate CMV pneumonitis from other causes of pneumonitis in HIV disease. Patients present with shortness of breath, dyspnea on exertion and a dry, nonproductive cough. Chest radiographs show diffuse interstitial infiltrates, and hypoxemia is usually present. Definitive diagnosis of pulmonary CMV disease in patients who have advanced HIV disease is difficult to establish because of a high incidence of asymptomatic CMV shedding – CMV can be isolated in approximately 50% of HIV-infected patients undergoing bronchoscopic examination. However, the true incidence of CMV pneumonitis is less than 10% in patients who have diagnostic bronchoscopy for evaluation of pulmonary infiltrates of unknown origin.

MANAGEMENT OF CMV DISEASE

Induction therapy is based on oral valganciclovir 900 mg twice daily for 3 weeks. Intravenous ganciclovir or forscarnet may be used in case of severe digestive dysfunction or in severe cases. Ganciclovir intravitreal injections are now rarely indicated, with the possible exception of severe central retinitis. In case of retinitis, it is recommended to continue maintenance treatment with valganciclovir, at a dose of 900 mg once daily for at least 3 months as long as CD4$^+$ T-lymphocyte count has not recovered above 100/μL. Thereafter, and subject to the favorable recovery of retinitis confirmed by an ophthalmological examination, and negative plasma CMV PCR, treatment may be discontinued. Ophthalmologic monitoring should be regularly scheduled, quarterly at first and less often as the host immunity is being reconstituted.[13] There are no recommendations for secondary prophylaxis in other localizations. There is no place for primary prophylaxis of CMV disease, but pre-emptive therapy with oral valganciclovir may be envisaged in case of plasma positive CMV PCR above 1000 copies/mL with low CD4$^+$ T-lymphocyte counts.[14,15]

Herpes Simplex Virus Infections

Reactivation of herpes simplex virus (HSV) occurs frequently in patients who have advanced HIV disease, particularly in those who have low CD4$^+$ T-lymphocyte counts (<100 cells/μL). The hallmark of herpetic lesions is painful vesicular formation at a mucocutaneous site, progressing rapidly to ulceration with an erythematous base, followed by eventual healing and re-epithelialization. As patients become more immunosuppressed, infections are characterized by prolonged viral shedding, more frequent episodes, and severe and persistent clinical disease. Recurrent genital and perirectal ulcerative lesions are the most common manifestations of HSV infection in patients who have HIV disease and are usually due to reactivation of HSV-2. Lesions may be atypical and severe in patients who have advanced disease. Prolonged new lesion formation, with continued tissue destruction, persistent viral shedding and severe local pain, is common. HSV infections can be treated either with episodic therapy when lesions occur or with daily therapy to prevent recurrences – this decision should be individualized based on the frequency and severity of recurrences. Most infections can be treated with oral valaciclovir, famciclovir or aciclovir for 5–14 days. Severe mucocutaneous HSV lesions are best treated initially with intravenous aciclovir. In case of failure or resistance, foscarnet may be used.

Varicella-Zoster Virus Infections

In the USA and Europe, most adults who have HIV disease have previously been infected with varicella-zoster virus (VZV). Owing to impaired cellular immunity, HIV-infected patients who have primary VZV are at risk of prolonged new lesion formation and are at higher risk of life-threatening visceral dissemination. Herpes zoster may be the first indication of HIV disease and can occur at any stage of HIV infection. It usually appears as a localized or segmental painful, erythematous maculopapular, then vesicular eruption along a single dermatome. In HIV-infected patients, zoster lesions may be bullous, hemorrhagic or necrotic. Patients infected with HIV are at risk of recurrent episodes of herpes zoster. Occasionally, widespread cutaneous and visceral dissemination may occur. Visceral dissemination to the lungs, the liver and the central nervous system (CNS) may cause life-threatening disease. HIV-infected patients should receive prompt antiviral therapy with oral valaciclovir, or famciclovir, for 7–10 days. More severe disease (extensive skin or visceral involvement) should be treated initially with intravenous aciclovir (10 mg/kg q8h). HIV adults who have no history of chickenpox or are seronegative for VZV should receive VZV immunoglobulin as soon as possible but within 96 hours after exposure to a patient who has chickenpox or shingles. The efficacy of aciclovir in this setting is unknown.

Progressive Multifocal Leukoencephalopathy

Progressive multifocal leukoencephalopathy (PML) is an opportunistic demyelinating infection caused by JC virus, a ubiquitous DNA papovavirus for which more than 70% of adults are seropositive. PML occurs in patients who have deficient cell-mediated immunity and is estimated to affect up to 4% of patients who have AIDS. Mortality is

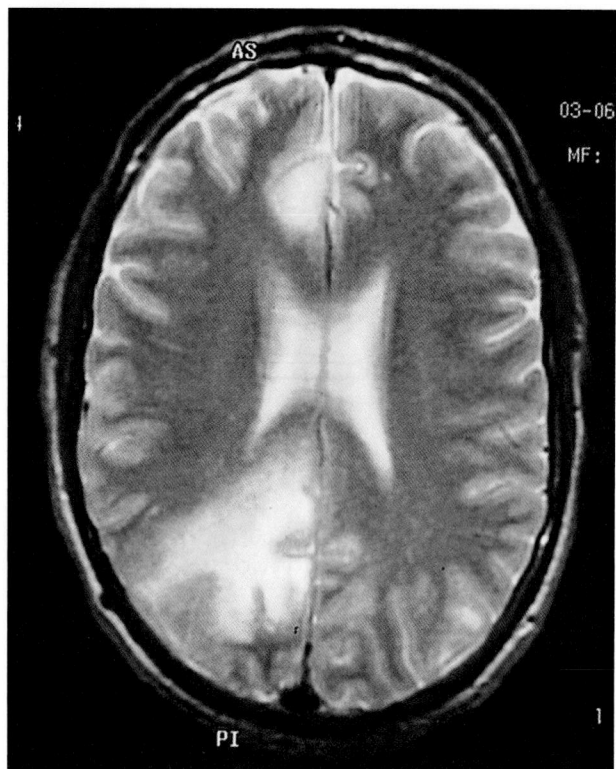

Figure 94-4 Progressive multifocal leukoencephalopathy. MRI scan showing frontal and occipital white matter lesions. (*Courtesy of Maurice E. Murphy and Bruce Polsky.*)

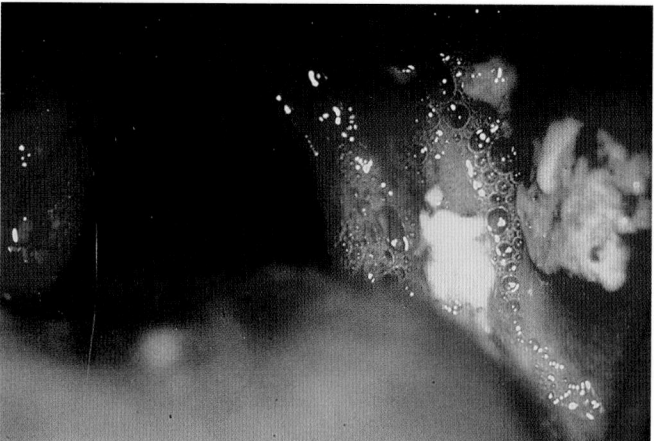

Figure 94-5 Pseudomembranous oral candidiasis ('thrush').

high, and average reported survival in AIDS patients is 2–4 months. The symptoms and characteristic radiologic findings of PML are due to virus-induced lysis of oligodendrocytes, resulting in microscopic foci of myelin breakdown that coalesce to produce larger white matter lesions (Figure 94-4). Definitive diagnosis requires tissue from brain biopsy but the identification of JC virus in the CSF by PCR has a high specificity for active disease. There is no definitive antiviral treatment for PML and optimal ART is the treatment of choice.[16] A paradoxical response to ART can be seen in some patients with PML with unexpected neurologic deterioration.

Fungal Infections

Fungi are among the most ubiquitous pathogens seen in patients who have HIV disease but are not the most common causes of mortality. Virtually all major fungal pathogens cause disease in patients who have HIV infection.

Candidiasis

Candidal infection in AIDS is almost exclusively mucosal – systemic invasion is a rare and late event. Oropharyngeal candidiasis occurs in about three-quarters of all those who have HIV infection. In about one-third it tends to be recurrent and becomes progressively more severe with increasing immunodeficiency. Esophageal involvement occurs in 20–40% of all AIDS patients, predominantly in patients who have advanced disease and severe depletion of CD4+ T-lymphocyte counts. Vulvovaginal candidiasis occurs in about 30–40% of women who have HIV infection; it appears that HIV infection *per se* is not an important risk factor for vaginal infection, although it may influence the severity and persistence of disease.

Most candidal disease, especially initial episodes, is associated with infection by *Candida albicans*. Other species, notably *C. glabrata*, *C. dubliniensis* and *C. parapsilosis*, tend to cause infection in patients who have very advanced disease and have had extensive previous exposure to antifungal agents. Most patients with oral candidiasis are symptomatic and complain of some oral discomfort. The classic presentation is of creamy-white plaques on an erythematous base – the pseudomembranous form of thrush (Figure 94-5). Other manifestations include an atrophic form that presents as erythema without plaques (often associated with patchy atrophic glossitis) and angular cheilitis, which appears as cracking, fissuring, ulceration or erythema at the corner of the mouth. Most patients who have vaginal candidiasis present with vaginal itching, burning or pain, and usually complain of a vaginal discharge. Examination of the vaginal cavity usually reveals thrush, similar to that seen in the oropharynx. Patients who have esophageal candidiasis develop ulcers and erosions of the esophagus and experience odynophagia or dysphagia. The combination of oral candidiasis and esophageal symptoms is both specific and sensitive in predicting esophageal involvement. Patients can be treated empirically with antifungal therapy. Endoscopy is reserved for those patients who fail to respond to evaluate for other diagnoses such as herpetic or cytomegalovirus esophagitis, idiopathic ulceration or resistant candidiasis. The development of oral candidiasis in an HIV-positive patient should be taken as a sign of progressive immunodeficiency. Patients should have a CD4+ T-lymphocyte count measured. If they are not currently receiving ART, it should be initiated. If they are on ART, it should be reassessed and, if necessary, changed. A number of options – both local and systemic – are available for the treatment of oral candidiasis. Initially, most patients respond well clinically to any form of antifungal therapy, although mycologic responses are less common. Esophageal disease requires systemic therapy. Fluconazole 200–400 mg q24h orally for 2–3 weeks is the therapy of choice. In case of failure or resistance, posaconazole, voriconazole or an echinocandin may be used.[17] Relapses are common if effective ART is not given and at least one-third of patients develop recurrent mucosal candidiasis. One approach to management is to treat each episode as it occurs. However, in many patients, recurrent symptomatic disease may be sufficiently severe to warrant considering chronic suppression. Fluconazole 100–200 mg q24h has proved highly successful in suppressing recurrent oropharyngeal disease and preventing esophagitis,[18] and a dose of 100 mg per week can prevent vaginal candidiasis. The major risk of this approach is the possibility of developing azole-resistant disease. However, resistant infection has become very unusual in the era of potent effective ART.

For a discussion of superficial dermatophyte infections see Chapter 98.

Cryptococcosis

Virtually all HIV-associated infection is caused by *Cryptococcus neoformans* var. *neoformans*. About 5% of patients who have advanced

HIV infection in the Western world develop disseminated cryptococcosis; the disease is more prevalent in sub-Saharan Africa and southern Asia. Most cases of infection occur in patients who have very low CD4+ lymphocyte counts (<50 cells/μL). Cryptococcosis most commonly presents as a subacute meningitis or meningoencephalitis with fever, malaise and headache. Symptoms are usually present for 2–4 weeks before diagnosis. Classic meningeal symptoms and signs (such as neck stiffness or photophobia) occur in about one-third of patients. Some patients may present with encephalopathic symptoms such as lethargy, altered mentation, personality changes and memory loss. Analysis of the CSF usually shows mildly elevated serum protein, normal or slightly low glucose, a few lymphocytes and numerous organisms. The CSF opening pressure is elevated in 25% of patients, and this has important prognostic and therapeutic implications. About one-half of patients have evidence of pulmonary involvement with cough or dyspnea and abnormal chest radiographs. Most patients who have cryptococcal meningitis have positive blood cultures. Skin involvement is common and several types of skin lesion have been described; the most common form is that resembling molluscum contagiosum.

Laboratory diagnosis is primarily mycological and is based on isolating the yeast by direct examination with India ink and culture of cerebrospinal fluid (CSF), bronchoalveolar lavage (BAL), blood, urine, pus and organs or surgical specimens. Identifying polysaccharide antigens of *C. neoformans* in serum, CSF, urine or BAL is another diagnostic tool. The reaction is very sensitive and reliable in meningoencephalitis (up to 92% of positive CSF).[19] In 2009 a new test for rapid detection of glucuronoxylomannan out of the *Cryptococcus* spp. polysaccharide capsule was developed. This easy-to-use LFA (Lateral Flow Immunoassay) dipstick test has excellent specificity and sensitivity at least equivalent (or superior) to the conventional test. Its use as a therapeutic monitoring tool also seems to be promising.[20,21] This new test also raises the value of routine screening for cryptococcosis in HIV-infected patients in endemic areas. The positivity rate is relatively high, including within asymptomatic subjects, if subjects with CD4+ T-lymphocyte count <100 or 200/μL are selected. In a retrospective South African cohort, this screening allowed identification of subjects before the development of symptomatic cryptococcal meningitis with a major impact on the prognosis, thanks to the remarkable simplicity and effectiveness of pre-emptive treatment with fluconazole. This screening is recommended, rather cautiously, by WHO, to be considered in patients with CD4+ T-lymphocyte count less than 100 μL if prevalence of symptomatic cryptococcosis is greater than 3%.[22,23]

Treatment is based on the combination of amphotericin B and 5-flucytosine. A recent study confirmed the superiority of this association (administered for 2 weeks), in terms of mortality, over the monotherapy with amphotericin B. High-dose fluconazole should be used afterwards for 10 weeks.[24] Alternative regimens are amphotericin B + fluconazole or fluconazole + 5-flucytosine. If CSF opening pressure exceeds 25 cmH$_2$O, lumbar punctures (20–30 mL) should be performed at least 2–3 times weekly to maintain pressure below 20 cmH$_2$O. Steroids or mannitol are not recommended. Secondary prophylaxis with fluconazole 200 mg daily should be provided until a stable immune reconstitution is obtained. Cryptococcosis is one of the few opportunistic infections for which early initiation of antiretroviral therapy (less than 2 weeks) is associated with increased mortality. It is generally recommended to delay ART initiation to at least 4 weeks after start of antifungal therapy to avoid severe immune reconstitution syndrome (see also Chapters 95 and 99).[25,26]

Other Endemic Mycosis (see also Chapter 189)

Histoplasmosis is caused by the dimorphic fungus *Histoplasma capsulatum*, which is endemic in the Mississippi and Ohio River valleys of North America as well as in certain parts of Central and South America, Asia, Africa and the Caribbean. *Coccidioides immitis* is a dimorphic fungus found in the soil in the desert around the south-western USA and northern Mexico, as well as focal areas of Central and South America. Penicilliosis is caused by the dimorphic fungus Talaromyces (*Penicillium marneffei*), which is endemic in South East Asia (especially northern Thailand and southern China). These fungi cause disseminated infection in patients who have AIDS in endemic areas, as well as sporadic infection among HIV-positive migrants from and visitors to endemic areas.

The most common presentation is fever and weight loss. Pneumonia is usual in coccidioidomycosis and respiratory symptoms (cough, shortness of breath) occur in about 50% of cases of histoplasmosis and penicilliosis. Local or generalized lymphadenopathy, hepatosplenomegaly, colonic lesions and skin and oral ulcers also occur. Skin involvement is more common in penicilliosis. Involvement of the gastrointestinal tract (usually as ulcers) is a feature of histoplasmosis and may present with abdominal pain or gastrointestinal bleeding. Between 5% and 10% of patients with histoplasmosis have an acute septic shock-like syndrome that includes hypotension and evidence of disseminated coagulopathy. Meningeal disease, with symptoms of lethargy, fever, headache, nausea, vomiting and/or confusion, occurs in about 10% of patients with coccidioidomycosis. Cerebrospinal fluid analysis typically reveals a lymphocytic pleocytosis with a lymphocyte count greater than 50/μL.

Diagnosis is made by culturing the organism from clinical specimens or by demonstrating it on histopathologic examination. In histoplamosis a peripheral blood smear may show intracellular organisms in white cells in many patients, and blood cultures, especially when collected using the lysis centrifugation system, are positive in over 90% of patients. Antigen detection in either urine or serum is an excellent method for diagnosing disseminated histoplasmosis.

For all infections, the management strategy is similar. Patients should receive an initial period of treatment with amphotericin B (for 1–2 weeks) until there is clinical resolution. For histoplasmosis and penicilliosis, this should be followed by itraconazole 200 mg orally q12h for at least 12 months in patients on ART with CD4+ T-lymphocyte count maintained above 150 cells/μL for 6 months. For coccidioidomycosis, fluconazole, 400–800 mg q24h orally, may be an alternative for patients who have mild disease. Complete eradication is unlikely and chronic suppressive therapy with either fluconazole 200–400 mg q24h or itraconazole 200 mg q12h is needed. Successful treatment with itraconazole or fluconazole has been reported in approximately 80% patients who have *C. immitis* meningitis.[27]

Aspergillosis

Infection with *Aspergillus* spp. is seen in patients who have advanced HIV disease. Specific risk factors that have been identified include neutropenia, use of corticosteroids and broad-spectrum antibacterial therapy and previous pneumonia, especially PJP. Typically, patients have extremely low CD4+ T-lymphocyte counts and a history of other AIDS-defining opportunistic infections. Two major syndromes predominate: respiratory tract disease and central nervous system infection.

Patients with pulmonary involvement often present with cough, shortness of breath and fever. Chest pain and hemoptysis are common. Nodular infiltrates, which may be localized or diffuse and commonly cavitate, are seen on chest radiography. Additional respiratory syndromes of pulmonary aspergilloma and localized tracheobronchial aspergillosis have been reported occasionally in patients who have AIDS. Patients who have CNS aspergillosis usually present with symptoms and signs of a mass lesion or with features of a stroke due to invasion of blood vessels. Therefore, seizures, hemiparesis and focal abnormalities are common. CT scan or MRI of the head may show single or multiple lesions, usually non-enhancing, with surrounding edema. Bony invasion is common and, because the disease may have spread from involved sinuses, the sinuses may be abnormal. Patients who have fungal sinusitis usually have the classic features of sinusitis (fever, facial pain and swelling, nasal discharge and headache). CT scan of the sinuses will usually show bony erosion, and penetration into adjacent tissues such as the brain or orbit can occur. The prognosis of aspergillosis is poor, in part because of the fungal infection itself and in part because it tends to occur in patients who have advanced AIDS and many other complications of end-stage HIV infection. There is a poorer response to therapy in patients who have AIDS than in other immunocompromised patients. Voriconazole is the treatment of choice for invasive aspergillosis.[28]

Nontuberculous Mycobacterial Infections

Mycobacterium avium complex (MAC) bacteria are ubiquitous in the environment and have been isolated from a variety of sources around the world, including soil, natural water, municipal water systems, food, house dust, and domestic and wild animals. These isolates are thought to be the source of most human infections but there is no evidence of MAC transmission from person to person. In untreated HIV-infected patients in the Western world, the incidence of MAC disease increases with falling CD4+ T-lymphocyte counts, with a cumulative probability of disseminated disease due to MAC in subjects who have CD4+ T-lymphocyte counts less than 50 cells/μL of 20–30%, and 10–20% in those who have CD4+ T-lymphocyte counts of 50–100 cells/μL.

Clinical Features

MAC infection is acquired through inhalation or ingestion of the organism, with most infections in HIV-infected patients believed to occur through colonization and invasion of the gut mucosa. Disseminated MAC disease is characterized by fever, night sweats and weight loss. The gastrointestinal tract is frequently involved and clinical manifestations include nausea, vomiting, watery diarrhea and abdominal pain. At physical examination hepatomegaly, splenomegaly and lymphadenopathy are very common, and elevations of serum alkaline phosphatase, lactate dehydrogenase and anemia are the most frequent laboratory findings. Other nontuberculous mycobacteria, including *Mycobacterium genavense*, *M. intracellulare*, *M. haemophilum*, *M. simiae*, *M. xenopi*, *M. scrofulaceum*, *M. marinum* and *M. fortuitum*, have also been described as a cause of disseminated infection in HIV-infected patients. Although MAC can commonly be isolated from sputum, pulmonary disease associated with MAC is rare. Patients should have a repeatedly positive culture in sputum, an infiltrate on chest radiograph, absence of other lung pathogens and preferably biopsy specimens showing acid-fast bacilli in abnormal lung tissue. However the isolation of MAC in the respiratory or gastrointestinal tract in those patients who have CD4+ T-lymphocyte counts less than 50 cells/μL represents a high risk for the development of MAC bacteremia. In this case prophylaxis or treatment should be considered. The most frequent nontuberculous mycobacterium isolated from sputum in HIV-infected patients is *M. kansasii*. Patients who have *M. kansasii* infection tend to have a low CD4+ T-lymphocyte count (<50 cells/μL) and the clinical and radiologic manifestations are not different from tuberculosis. The isolation of *M. kansasii* from sputum is always considered diagnostic of pulmonary disease, since colonization is uncommon.

Treatment

THERAPY FOR *MYCOBACTERIUM AVIUM* COMPLEX

Treatment regimens should include a macrolide (clarithromycin or azithromycin) plus ethambutol. The addition of rifabutin should be considered, since triple therapy has been associated with a reduction in relapses and in the emergence of resistant strains.[29] Aminoglycosides and quinolones may be useful in macrolide-resistant cases. If ART is to be used, it is important to recognize potential drug interactions between clarithromycin and both non-nucleoside reverse transcriptase inhibitors (NNRTIs) and protease inhibitors. In general, as with other opportunistic infections, therapy for disseminated MAC is for life. However, in situations where CD4+ T-lymphocyte counts remain greater than 100 cells/μL after 6–12 months of ART, patients are at low risk of recurrence of MAC and the treatment can be stopped.

TREATMENT OF OTHER NONTUBERCULOUS MYCOBACTERIA

M. kansasii is the second most frequent cause of pulmonary and disseminated nontuberculous mycobacterial disease. The treatment consists of a daily regimen of rifampin (rifampicin) or rifabutin, isoniazid and ethambutol for 12–18 months. *M. genavense* and *M. haemophilum* are resistant to isoniazid, pyrazinamide and ethambutol. *M. genavense* may be treated with a regimen similar to MAC and *M. haemophilum* with a combination of rifampin plus another active antituberculosis drug (ciprofloxacin, doxycycline, clarithromycin or amikacin). *M. simiae* and *M. xenopi* are susceptible to isoniazid, rifampin and ethambutol and should be treated for 12 months. *M. scrofulaceum* therapy requires surgery and isoniazid plus rifampin for 24 months with amikacin for 2–3 months. *M. marinum* is resistant to isoniazid and pyrazinamide. Minocycline or clarithromycin or rifampin plus ethambutol for 3 months are possible therapies. *M. fortuitum* therapy consists of amikacin plus cefoxitin plus ciprofloxacin for 1 month followed by quinolone plus clarithromycin for 3–6 months.

Prophylaxis for MAC may be provided in patients who have a CD4+ T-lymphocyte count below 50/μL with azithromycin (1200 mg weekly), but is not systematically prescribed if ART may be quickly initiated leading to immunorestoration.[30,31] Primary prophylaxis may be discontinued in patients treated with HAART who show an increase in CD4+ T-lymphocyte count to above 100/μL for at least 3 months and should be re-introduced if the CD4+ T-lymphocyte count decreases to less than 50–100/μL.[32,33]

Parasitic Infections

Toxoplasmosis

Toxoplasmosis, caused by *Toxoplasma gondii*, an obligate intracellular protozoan, is a common OI in patients with AIDS. It has a prevalence ranging from 10–40% in Europe, the Caribbean area and Africa, to 5–10% in USA. This is due to the different prevalence of *T. gondii* infection in the general population of these areas. Toxoplasmosis occurs as a result of the reactivation of latent *T. gondii* infection that has persisted in the CNS or extraneural tissues after earlier acute infection. Toxoplasmosis usually occurs late in HIV disease, when the CD4+ T-lymphocyte count is less than 100/μL. The CNS is by far the most common site of toxoplasmosis and the majority of patients have encephalitis. Retinitis, pneumonitis and myocarditis are less common manifestations. Toxoplasmic encephalitis (TE) commonly manifests as single or multiple intracerebral abscesses, with focal neurologic signs and constitutional symptoms that progress over a few days or weeks. Fever and headaches are present in 40–70% of cases, neurologic dysfunction including confusion and lethargy in 40% of cases, focal CNS deficits in 50–60% of cases, and seizures in 30–40% of cases. The constellation of fever, headaches, mild neurologic deficit or any unexplained neurologic symptoms should suggest the diagnosis of TE (Figure 94-6), and prompt computed tomography (CT) scanning or magnetic resonance imaging (MRI). MRI is more sensitive than CT scanning. Toxoplasmic abscesses are typically contrast-enhancing lesions surrounded by edema; there may be a mass effect, with displacement of the ventricles. Most patients will have specific antitoxoplasmal antibodies, indicating past infection. In most cases of encephalitis, the diagnosis of toxoplasmosis is presumptive, made on clinical–radiologic criteria and confirmed by the therapeutic response. Appropriate treatment is therefore especially important, both because the response to therapy is the main criterion for diagnosis of TE, and because early initiation of therapy gives the best prognosis. Treatment consists of initial acute therapy over 3–6 weeks followed by secondary prophylaxis to prevent reactivation. The combination of pyrimethamine 100 mg loading dose followed by 50–75 mg/day orally and

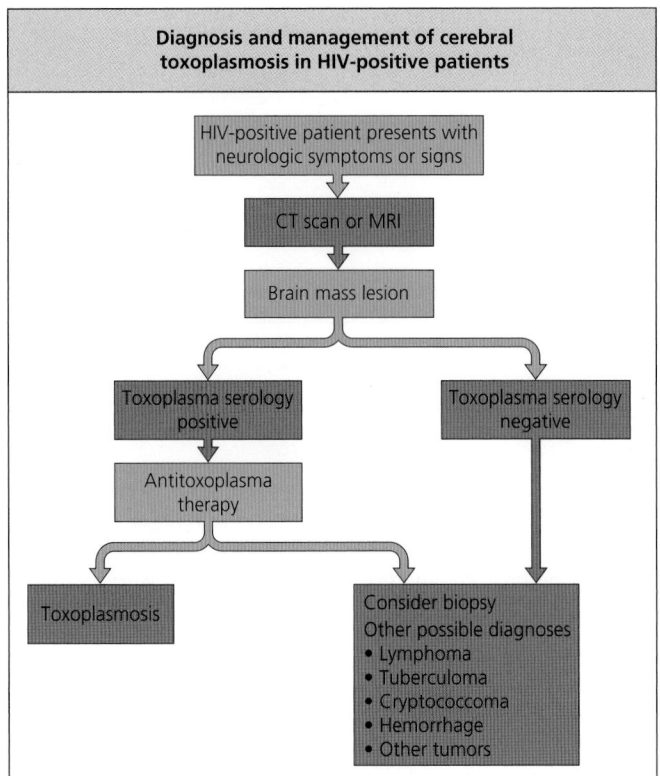

Figure 94-6 Diagnosis and management of cerebral toxoplasmosis in HIV-positive patients. *(Courtesy of Christine Katlama.)*

sulfadiazine 4–6 g/day is the first-line acute therapy.[34] These drugs act synergistically by blocking the folic acid pathway of tachyzoites, but have no effect on the cyst forms of the parasite. Folinic acid 25 mg/day orally should be given as well to prevent bone marrow toxicity. Clinical improvement occurs within 5–10 days; the diagnosis of TE is confirmed by a decrease in both neuroradiologic and clinical abnormalities. The duration of acute therapy is 6 weeks.

In case of intolerance to sulfonamides, sulfadiazine should be replaced by clindamycin (2.4 g daily in four doses), intravenously or orally. Other alternative regimens include high-dose intravenous TMP-SMX, atovaquone in association with pyrimethamine or sulfadiazine or azithromycin with pyrimethamine. Efficacy of the addition of steroids in case of perilesional edema is not established.[35] Secondary prophylaxis is with pyrimethamine 25 mg/day orally plus sulfadiazine 2 g/day orally or clindamycin 1.2–1.8 g daily until a CD4+ T-lymphocyte count of greater than 200/μL for more than 3 months is reached with ART. This combination is also effective as primary prophylaxis for PJP. If clindamycin is used, aerosolized pentamidine should be added for PJP prevention. TMP-SMZ or atovaquone are potential, poorly evaluated, alternatives.

PRIMARY PROPHYLAXIS

Toxoplasma seropositive patients who have a CD4+ T-lymphocyte count below 100/μL should receive prophylaxis against toxoplasmic encephalitis. The double-strength tablet daily dose of TMP–SMX is recommended. Alternative regimens in patients who cannot tolerate TMP–SMX include dapsone–pyrimethamine or atovaquone (with or without pyrimethamine). Prophylactic monotherapy with dapsone, clindamycin, pyrimethamine, azithromycin or clarithromycin is not recommended. Primary prophylaxis against toxoplasmic encephalitis should be discontinued in patients treated with HAART showing an increase in CD4+ T-lymphocyte count to above 200/μL for at least 3 months. Discontinuation of prophylaxis in patients where CD4+ T-lymphocyte counts have increased to 100–200 cells/μL has not been

carefully evaluated. Prophylaxis should be re-introduced if the CD4+ T-lymphocyte count decreases to below 100–200/μL.[10,36]

Intestinal Parasites

Cryptosporidiosis is a worldwide protozoan infection that is more prevalent in lower-income countries. It can affect normal hosts but is particularly severe in immunodeficient patients. Human cryptosporidiosis is generally caused by *Cryptosporidium parvum*, which is transmitted primarily by the fecal–oral route through person-to-person transmission or indirectly; outbreaks from municipal water, person-to-person transmission and animal-to-person transmission have been described. The illness is acute enteritis. Diarrhea is the main clinical symptom, ranging in severity from mild diarrhea to cholera-like, watery diarrhea. Abdominal cramps, nausea, vomiting and anorexia usually accompany the diarrhea when it is moderate or severe. Fever is uncommon and may be due to other concurrent infections. The severity of the disease is more pronounced in patients with CD4+ T-lymphocyte counts less than 50/μL. Cryptosporidiosis may rarely involve the gallbladder, the biliary tract and the pancreatic ducts (leading to cholecystitis and pancreatitis). Diagnosis is based on the identification of the parasite in feces, in tissue specimens or in other fluids, using a modified acid-fast stain such as the Ziehl–Neelsen stain.

Treatment of cryptosporidiosis is essentially symptomatic and the best option for therapy and prevention is the restoration of immune function using potent ART. The same is true for microporidiosis due to *Encephalitozoon intestinalis* or *Enterocytozoon bieneusi* and for cyclosporiasis. Isosporosis is the only infection for which effective treatment with TMP-SMX has been validated.

Bacterial Infections

Bacterial infections as a group are the most common infectious complication of HIV disease, with increased risk for infections caused by common bacterial pathogens (e.g. *Streptococcus pneumoniae*, *Haemophilus influenzae*, *Salmonella* spp.). The introduction of potent ART has been associated with a decline in the incidence of community-acquired and nosocomial bacterial pneumonia. However, the proportion of hospitalizations due to bacterial infections has increased as rates of PJP and other opportunistic infections have declined to a greater extent.

Bacterial Pneumonias

The incidence of community-acquired bacterial pneumonia is markedly higher (three- to fivefold) among HIV-infected patients than among age-matched HIV-negative persons. Risk factors for the development of bacterial pneumonia include lower CD4+ T-lymphocyte counts intravenous drug use and cigarette smoking. A previous history of pneumonia, low serum albumin and a lack of receipt of the pneumococcal vaccination when the patient had a CD4+ T-lymphocyte count greater than 200/μL are all associated with an increased risk of pneumococcal pneumonia. The clinical presentation of bacterial pneumonia in HIV-infected patients is indistinguishable from that in HIV-negative patients. The pathogens most commonly responsible for bacterial pneumonia are *Strep. pneumoniae* and *H. influenzae*. Other organisms that may cause disease include *M. catarrhalis*, *Klebsiella pneumoniae* and *Staphylococcus aureus*.[37] Empiric therapy should be based on guidelines for the general population. Bacteremia in the setting of pneumonia occurs more commonly in HIV-infected than in HIV-negative patients. Increased rates of bacteremia with pneumococcal and *H. influenzae* pneumonia have been documented. Bacteremia may also occur with other pathogens responsible for pulmonary infections (e.g. *Pseudomonas aeruginosa*).

Prevention of bacterial pneumonia should include smoking cessation and antipneumococcal vaccination in individuals with CD4+ T-lymphocyte counts above 200 cells/μL as well as annual influenza vaccination.[38,39]

Skin Infections (see also Chapter 98)

Bacterial skin infections in HIV-infected patients may vary from impetigo to folliculitis to cutaneous abscesses; cutaneous abscesses are often associated with intravenous drug use as well. Recurrences may be more frequent than in the HIV-negative population, but physical findings and responsible organisms (*Staph. aureus* and *Streptococcus* spp.) are similar. A significant increase in subcutaneous and soft-tissue abscesses associated with community-acquired methicillin-resistant *Staph. aureus* (MRSA) has been noted in the last few years in the USA among HIV-infected individuals.[40] Aggressive treatment with surgical drainage and appropriate antimicrobials is necessary.

Bacillary angiomatosis is a distinct skin infection specifically associated with HIV disease. The condition is caused either by *Bartonella henselae*, the organism also responsible for cat-scratch disease, or by *B. quintana*. The clinical appearance is of very erythematous subcutaneous nodules that may occasionally resemble Kaposi's sarcoma (Figure 94-7). Lymphadenopathy may be associated with these skin findings. Much less frequently, *B. henselae* has been identified as the cause of more deeply seated infections, including endocarditis, osteomyelitis and hepatic lesions (peliosis hepatis). Diagnosis of the skin infection may be based on the characteristic appearance, but biopsy may be carried out to rule out other causes, and it is necessary to diagnose solid organ involvement. Histology shows vascular proliferation and mixed inflammatory cells. Warthin–Starry staining reveals the organism. Treatment with azithromycin (*B. henselae*) or doxycycline (*B. quintana*) for 1–2 months for skin disease, and longer for other sites of infection is effective.

Enterocolitis

Among the bacterial pathogens causing diarrhea in HIV-infected patients are non-typhoidal *Salmonella* spp., *Shigella flexneri*, *Campylobacter jejuni* and *Clostridium difficile*. *Shigella* and *Campylobacter* spp. infections manifest similarly – patients note severe diarrhea (which may be bloody) associated with abdominal cramping, nausea and fever. Diagnosis is by stool culture. These infections may both be treated with oral quinolones, although resistance to quinolones is increasing. Non-typhoidal *Salmonella* spp. infections may present either with or without diarrhea and other symptoms of colitis. In patients without gastroin-

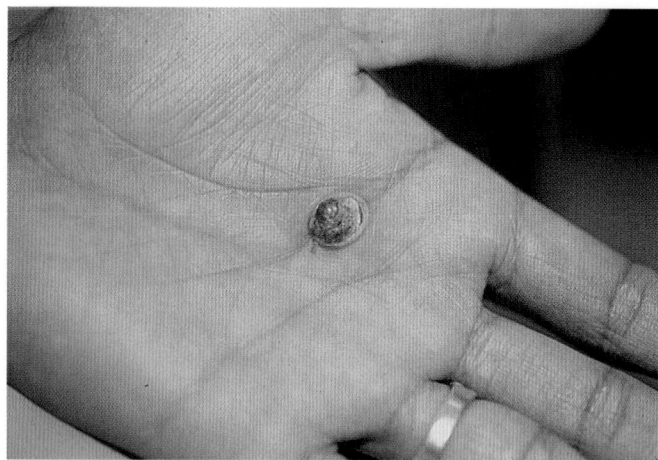

Figure 94-7 Typical appearance of bacillary angiomatosis. *(Courtesy of Christine Katlama.)*

testinal symptoms, the infection may manifest solely as fever without any localizing findings. The occurrence of *Salmonella* bacteremia is more common in patients with HIV infection than in HIV-seronegative groups. In addition, relapses of bacteremia are common. Unlike the recommendations for patients who are not immunosuppressed, even *Salmonella* infections limited to the gastrointestinal tract should be treated in HIV-infected patients. Treatment is usually with ciprofloxacin (500 mg q12h for 2–4 weeks), and suppressive therapy with ciprofloxacin is often used because of the risk of relapse.

Infection due to *C. difficile* may be more severe in HIV-infected patients, and these patients are more likely to have relapses and chronic symptoms. Antibiotic use and hospitalization are associated with the development of infection, just as they are in HIV-negative patients. *C. difficile* may also occur as a community-acquired infection in HIV-infected patients. Treatment is with oral metronidazole or vancomycin.

References available online at expertconsult.com.

KEY REFERENCES

Day J.N., Chau T.T., Wolbers M., et al.: Combination antifungal therapy for cryptococcal meningitis. *N Engl J Med* 2013; 368(14):1291-1302.

Guidelines for prevention and treatment of opportunistic infections among HIV-exposed and HIV-infected children. 2008 recommendations from the National Institutes of Health (NIH), the Centers for Disease Control and Prevention (CDC), and the HIV Medicine Association of the Infectious Diseases Society of America (HIVMA/IDSA). Available: http://aidsinfo.nih.gov/contentfiles/Adult_OI.pdf.

Jarvis J.N., Percival A., Bauman S., et al.: Evaluation of a novel point-of-care cryptococcal antigen test on serum, plasma, and urine from patients with HIV-associated cryptococcal meningitis. *Clin Infect Dis* 2011; 53(10): 1019-1023.

Kunisaki K.M., Janoff E.N.: Influenza in immunosuppressed populations: a review of infection frequency, morbidity, mortality, and vaccines responses. *Lancet Infect Dis* 2009; 12:323-333.

Lortholary O., Petrikkos G., Akova M., et al.: ESCMID guideline for the diagnosis and management of *Candida* diseases 2012: patients with HIV infection or AIDS. *Clin Microbiol Infect* 2012; 18(Suppl. 7):68-77.

Mathews W.C., Caperna J.C., Barber R.E., et al.: Incidence of and risk factors for clinically significant methicillin-resistant *Staphylococcus aureus* infection in a cohort of HIV-infected adults. *J Acquir Immune Defic Syndr* 2005; 40:155-160.

Miro J.M., Podzamczer D., Pena J.M., et al.: Discontinuation of primary and secondary *Toxoplasma gondii* prophylaxis is safe in HIV-1 infected patients after immunological recovery with HAART. Final results of the GESIDA 04/98 study. San Francisco, CA: American Society for Microbiology; 2000, abstract L16.

Mocroft A., Reiss P., Kirk O., et al.: Is it safe to discontinue primary *Pneumocystis jiroveci* pneumonia prophylaxis in patients with virologically suppressed HIV infection and a CD4 cell count <200 cells/microL? *Clin Infect Dis* 2010; 51:611-619.

Palella F.J. Jr, Delaney K.M., Moorman A.C., et al.: Declining morbidity and mortality among patients with advanced human immunodeficiency virus infection. HIV Outpatient Study Investigators. *N Engl J Med* 1998; 338: 853-860.

Pedersen R.H., Lohse N., Ostergaard L., et al.: The effectiveness of pneumococcal polysaccharide vaccination in

HIV-infected adults: a systematic review. *HIV Med* 2011; 12:323-333.

Perfect J.R., Dismukes W.E., Dromer F., et al.: Clinical practice guidelines for the management of cryptococcal disease: 2010 update by the Infectious Diseases Society of America. *Clin Infect Dis* 2010; 50(3):291-322.

Sonneville R., Schmidt M., Messika J., et al.: Neurologic outcomes and adjunctive steroids in HIV patients with severe cerebral toxoplasmosis. *Neurology* 2012; 79:1762-1766.

Tantisiriwat W., Tebas P., Clifford D., et al.: Progressive multifocal leukoencephalopathy in patients with AIDS receiving highly active antiretroviral therapy. *Clin Infect Dis* 1999; 28:1152-2124.

Wohl D.A., Kendall M.A., Andersen J., et al.: Low rate of CMV end-organ diseases in HIV-infected patients despite low CD4[+] cell counts and CMV viremia: results of ACTG protocol A5030. *HIV Clin Trials* 2009; 10:143-152.

95

Immune Reconstitution Disorders in Patients with HIV Infection

MARTYN A. FRENCH | GRAEME MEINTJES

KEY CONCEPTS

- Immune reconstitution disorders occur in up to 40% of human immunodeficiency virus (HIV) patients who start antiretroviral therapy (ART).

- An immune reconstitution inflammatory syndrome (IRIS) associated with a mycobacterial, fungal, viral or protozoal infection is the most common immune reconstitution disorder.

- An IRIS usually occurs during the first 3 months of ART in patients who commence therapy with a CD4+ T-cell count <50/μL.

- The most common manifestations of tuberculosis-associated IRIS (TB-IRIS) are fever, lymphadenitis and pulmonary disease whereas the most common manifestation of cryptococcosis-associated IRIS (C-IRIS) is recurrent meningitis.

- Central nervous system (CNS) involvement by an IRIS is potentially life-threatening.

- Most cases of IRIS are self-limiting, the median duration of TB-IRIS being 2–3 months.

- Corticosteroids may be used to treat an IRIS related to mycobacterial or fungal infection, particularly when disease is severe.

- Ceasing ART should be considered only when there is CNS involvement and a depressed level of consciousness, or if the IRIS is refractory to corticosteroid therapy.

- Flares or new presentations of infectious disease after commencing ART, such as hepatitis B virus- and hepatitis C virus-associated hepatitis, zoster, herpes and TB without exaggerated inflammation, are probably also immune reconstitution disorders.

- Other immune reconstitution disorders in HIV patients have a different immunopathogenesis to an IRIS and include Graves' disease and sarcoidosis.

Introduction

Suppression of HIV infection by combination antiretroviral therapy (ART) usually results in the reversal of HIV-induced immune defects, leading to at least partial reconstitution of the immune system and the prevention or regression of opportunistic infections and cancers. However, those patients who were very immunodeficient prior to commencing ART are susceptible to immune reconstitution disorders after ART is commenced. Three main categories of immune reconstitution disorder are recognized:

- Disease resulting from the restoration of immune responses against opportunistic pathogens. This may be indistinguishable from disease usually caused by the pathogen, such as tuberculosis (TB), herpes zoster or herpes simplex presenting in the first three months of ART, or flares of hepatitis caused by hepatitis B virus (HBV) or hepatitis C virus (HCV) infection after commencement of ART. In contrast, it may also present as an immune reconstitution inflammatory syndrome (IRIS), in which the inflammation generated by the immune response is exaggerated and/or atypical and often causes significant morbidity and sometimes mortality.

- Autoimmune disease, mainly Graves' disease.
- Immune-mediated inflammatory disease (IMID), mainly sarcoidosis.

Immune Reconstitution Inflammatory Syndromes and Related Conditions

Virtually any pathogen that can cause an opportunistic infection can provoke an IRIS when immune responses against the pathogen are restored by ART (Table 95-1). An IRIS can be differentiated from an opportunistic infection based on clinical, histopathologic and immunologic characteristics (Table 95-2).

Most patients with an IRIS present during the first 3 months of ART and usually during the first few weeks. The infection by the provoking pathogen may not be apparent before ART is commenced and is 'unmasked' by the immune response against it. Viable pathogens are usually isolated from the affected tissues of this 'unmasking' type of IRIS. In other patients, an IRIS is provoked by an infection for which the patient is receiving treatment or that has recently been treated. Pathogens are sometimes not able to be cultured, or are very difficult to culture, from specimens taken from sites of inflammation. In these cases it is likely that there is an immune response against the antigens of nonviable pathogens. In this situation, there often appears to be a paradoxical worsening of the opportunistic infection when ART is commenced (i.e. clinical deterioration on ART after initial improvement on treatment for the opportunistic infection) and, therefore, the term paradoxical IRIS is commonly used. It is important to recognize that this does not represent failure of treatment for the opportunistic infection or failure of the ART, but rather an immunopathologic reaction to residual antigens of the pathogen. As there are currently no confirmatory diagnostic tests for any type of IRIS, it is necessary to use diagnostic criteria and exclude differential diagnoses that may account for the clinical deterioration before making the diagnosis of a paradoxical IRIS (Box 95-1).

The anatomic site and clinicopathologic characteristics of the inflammation in an IRIS are largely determined by the provoking

---

BOX 95-1 KEY DIAGNOSTIC FEATURES OF AN IMMUNE RECONSTITUTION INFLAMMATORY SYNDROME

- Proven HIV infection
- Temporal relationship to antiretroviral therapy initiation
- Decrease of plasma HIV RNA level by >1log^{10}/mL
- Exaggerated and/or atypical inflammatory response
- Evidence or inference of immune recovery, for example:
  - Increase of the circulating CD4+ T-cell count
  - Evidence of increased pathogen-specific immune response, e.g. tuberculin skin test conversion
  - Evidence of an immunopathologic immune response against pathogens in affected tissues
- Exclusion of other causes for clinical deterioration, which may include:
  - Resistance of opportunistic pathogens to antimicrobial drugs
  - Another infection or malignancy
  - Adverse drug reactions
  - Poor compliance with or malabsorption of treatment for the opportunistic infection

TABLE 95-1	Pathogens that May Provoke an IRIS or Related Immune Reconstitution Disorder When Immune Responses Against the Pathogen Are Restored by Antiretroviral Therapy (ART)			
Pathogen	**Nomenclature or Disease Presentation**	**Pathogen**	**Nomenclature or Disease Presentation**	
MYCOBACTERIA		**VIRUSES**		
M. avium complex (MAC)	MAC-IRIS	Cytomegalovirus (CMV)	CMV retinitis after ART CMV immune recovery uveitis	
M. tuberculosis	TB-IRIS	Varicella-zoster virus	Cutaneous zoster after ART VZV-IRIS (usually CNS disease)	
M. leprae	Leprosy reversal reaction after commencing ART	Herpes simplex virus 1 and 2	Mucocutaneous herpes after ART (which may be necrotizing or hemorrhagic) HSV-IRIS (mainly CNS disease)	
Bacille Calmette–Guérin	BCG-IRIS			
Other nontuberculous mycobacteria (NTM)		Kaposi's sarcoma herpesvirus	KS-IRIS	
FUNGI AND YEASTS		Molluscum contagiosum virus	Inflammatory molluscum contagiosum after ART	
Cryptococcus spp.	Cryptococcal IRIS (mainly meningitis)	JC polyomavirus	PML-IRIS	
Histoplasma spp.		BK polyomavirus		
Malassezia furfur	Inflammatory seborrheic dermatitis after ART	Hepatitis B virus	Hepatitis flare after ART	
Pityrosporon spp.	Folliculitis after ART	Hepatitis C virus	Hepatitis flare after ART	
Pneumocystis jirovecii	Pneumocystis-IRIS	Parvovirus B19	Exacerbation of red cell aplasia, encephalitis after ART	
Candida				
Aspergillus		Human papillomavirus	Wart enlargement or inflammation after ART	
Penicillium		HIV	Exacerbation of HIV encephalitis after ART	
Dermatophytes	Inflammatory tinea corporis after ART	**HELMINTHS**		
PROTOZOANS		Schistosoma		
Toxoplasma gondii	Exacerbation or presentation of cerebral toxoplasmosis after ART	Strongyloides		
Leishmania spp.		**OTHER BACTERIA**		
Microsporidia		Bartonella		
Cryptosporidium parvum				

IRIS, immune reconstitution inflammatory syndrome

TABLE 95-2	Comparison of an Immune Reconstitution Inflammatory Syndrome with an Opportunistic Infection in Patients with HIV Infection	
Immune Reconstitution Inflammatory Syndrome	**Opportunistic Infection**	
Restoration of an immune response against pathogens that causes immunopathology	Failure of 'protective' immune responses to control pathogen replication	
Always associated with a decline in the plasma HIV RNA level	Usually associated with a high plasma HIV RNA level*	
Usually associated with an increasing circulating CD4+ T-cell count†	Associated with a low circulating CD4+ T-cell count	
Inflammation usually greater than in an opportunistic infection, e.g. painful tissue lesions	Tissue inflammation may be absent	
Tissue lesions exhibit changes of an immune response, e.g. scarcity of pathogens, and of immunopathology, e.g. granulomatous reaction, suppuration or necrosis	Histopathology of tissue lesions demonstrates changes of an impaired immune response, e.g. abundance of pathogens, poorly formed granulomata in mycobacterial disease	

*Persistent immune defects in patients with long-term optimal control of HIV replication on ART may rarely be complicated by opportunistic infections.
†The circulating CD4+ T-cell count may not be increased in some patients with an IRIS, e.g. about 10% of patients with MAC-IRIS do not have an increased count.[13]

pathogen. For example, TB-associated IRIS (TB-IRIS) mainly affects lymph nodes and the lungs, cryptococcal IRIS (C-IRIS) usually affects the meninges, and progressive multifocal leucoencephalopathy (PML)-associated IRIS (PML-IRIS) affects the brain. Histopathology of affected tissues often reveals evidence of an immune response against the pathogen with granulomatous inflammation or necrosis when the IRIS is associated with infection by mycobacteria, fungi or protozoa, and a CD8+ T-cell infiltrate when associated with infection by viruses, such as JC polyomavirus (the cause of PML), cytomegalovirus (CMV) and HIV.

The major risk factors for the development of a paradoxical IRIS, as exemplified by TB-IRIS, are a very low CD4+ T-cell count, disseminated infection by the provoking pathogen and a short time of therapy for the opportunistic infection before ART is commenced.[1,2] All of these risk factors are probably markers of a high pathogen load at the time of commencing ART. A low CD4+ T-cell count may also be a marker of an increased susceptibility to immunopathologic responses against pathogens during immune reconstitution. Direct evidence that a high pathogen load increases the risk of an IRIS has been obtained from studies of HIV patients with cryptococcal or tuberculous

BOX 95-2   COMMON AND IMPORTANT MANIFESTATIONS OF TB-IRIS

- Worsening or recurrence of TB symptoms
- Weight loss
- Fever and tachycardia
- Lymph node enlargement
- Abscess formation
- Respiratory manifestations
  - Progressive pulmonary infiltrates on chest radiography (several patterns described, including miliary infiltrates and consolidation)
  - Pleural effusions
  - Lymph node compression of airways
- Abdominal manifestations
  - Liver enlargement and abscesses
  - Spleen enlargement, rupture and abscesses
  - Intestinal involvement, e.g. ileocecal perforation
  - Ascites and/or peritonitis
  - Psoas and intra-abdominal abscesses
- Central nervous system manifestations
  - Tuberculoma enlargement
  - Meningitis
  - Myeloradiculitis
- Genitourinary tract manifestations
  - Renal involvement with acute renal failure
  - Ureteric compression
  - Epididymo-orchitis
- Other system involvement
  - Arthritis and osteitis
  - Pericardial effusion
  - Bone marrow involvement

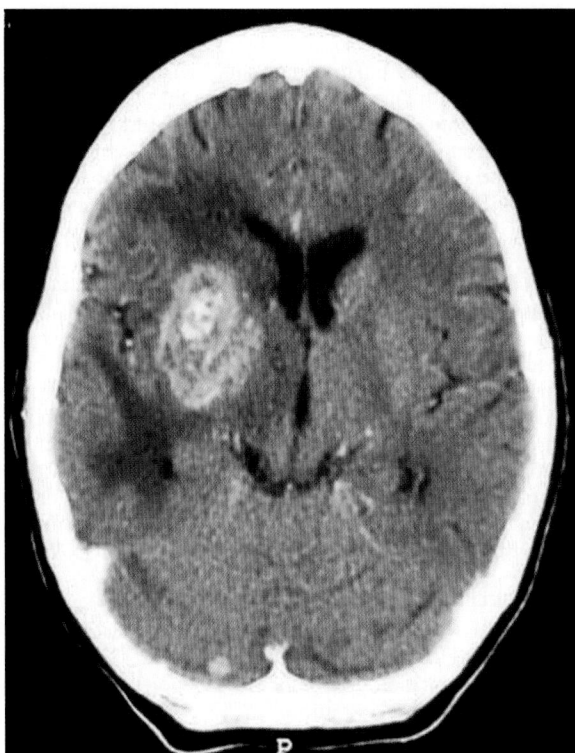

Figure 95-1   Tuberculoma with surrounding edema in TB-IRIS.

meningitis, where positive cerebrospinal fluid (CSF) cultures at the time of commencing ART significantly increased the risk of an IRIS.[3,4]

While a short interval between starting TB treatment and ART is a risk factor for TB-IRIS, this is not a reason to delay ART initiation in TB patients with low CD4[+] T-cell counts – ART within 2 weeks of TB treatment has been shown to reduce mortality in TB patients with a CD4[+] T-cell count of <50/μL.[5] In contrast, ART should be delayed in cryptococcal meningitis for 4–6 weeks as early ART is associated with excess mortality, possibly related to an IRIS mechanism.

The incidence of an IRIS among cohorts of patients initiating ART has been reported to be between 6.7% and 37.7% for those with a documented underlying opportunistic infection and between 11% and 23% among unselected patients in retrospective studies.[6] A prospective study from South Africa reported an incidence of 10.4% in an unselected cohort of 423 patients during the first 6 months of ART.[2] In this study, TB-IRIS was the commonest type of IRIS. This presents in many ways (Box 95-2) and is the most significant type of IRIS in areas where coinfection with HIV and *Mycobacterium tuberculosis* is common.[7]

CLINICAL PRESENTATION

The great majority of pathogens that cause opportunistic infections in patients with HIV infection may also be associated with an IRIS during early ART. Consequently, clinical presentations of the various types of IRIS can vary greatly.

Central Nervous System Disease

An IRIS involving the central nervous system (CNS) is potentially life-threatening and can result in permanent neurologic disability. Manifestations include new or recurrent meningitis and inflammation involving the brain parenchyma, spinal cord (myelitis) or nerve roots (radiculitis). A number of pathogens have been associated with an IRIS of the CNS but *Cryptococcus* spp. and *M. tuberculosis* are the most common. Interruption of ART should be seriously considered in these patients when they have a depressed level of consciousness and in those who do not respond to other measures, such as corticosteroid therapy.

Meningitis

Patients with cryptococcal meningitis who have been appropriately treated with antifungal therapy may experience a recurrence of

meningitis after commencing ART.[8] This occurs in up to 30% of patients and typically manifests with recurrent headaches and features of raised intracranial pressure. CSF fungal culture is usually negative, but the India ink and cryptococcal antigen tests are usually positive, reflecting persistence of nonviable organisms. The meningitis usually occurs around 4 weeks after ART is started but cases presenting months to years after ART initiation are described. The reported mortality rate has varied from 9% to 66%. Risk factors identified are disseminated disease, a shorter time between starting antifungal therapy and ART, higher CSF antigen load and persistently positive CSF cryptococcal cultures.[3] Treatment should include analgesia, therapeutic lumbar punctures to reduce raised intracranial pressure and corticosteroid therapy in severe or refractory cases. ART interruption is seldom necessary.

Similarly, patients receiving treatment for TB may present with TB meningitis (TBM) after ART initiation.[4] In some patients this will be recurrent TBM, but others will have had TB at an extraneural site and present with new TBM as an IRIS phenomenon. Treatment is with corticosteroids.

Inflammation of the Brain Parenchyma

Inflammation of the brain parenchyma due to an IRIS may manifest as focal mass lesions (granulomas, such as tuberculomas, or brain abscesses) or a diffuse process (encephalitis). Both processes may be complicated by cerebral edema. Mass lesions tend to present with focal neurologic deficits or seizures. TB-IRIS may present with the emergence or enlargement of cerebral tuberculomas (Figure 95-1). This may occur in patients already on treatment for TB. Cases of cerebral toxoplasmosis, cryptococcomas and abscesses associated with infection by nontuberculous mycobacteria (NTM), emerging or enlarging due to an IRIS, are also described. Treatment of these conditions involves appropriate treatment of the infection and corticosteroid therapy, particularly when there is significant cerebral edema and mass effect.

Encephalitis caused by an IRIS is usually associated with JC polyomavirus infection and presents with multiple focal deficits or a disturbance of higher cerebral functions.[9] In patients with severe HIV-induced immunodeficiency who are not receiving ART, JC polyomavirus infection of oligodendrocytes typically results in progressive multifocal leukoencephalopathy (PML). This is a subacute illness with progressive neurologic deterioration. Brain imaging typically does not demonstrate significant inflammation. In patients who develop PML-IRIS, associated with known or previously undiagnosed JC polyomavirus infection, after commencing ART, the clinical progression is typically accelerated and imaging demonstrates prominent inflammation (e.g. contrast enhancing lesions on computed tomography scan). Histopathology of brain biopsies in such patients often shows a perivascular mononuclear cell infiltrate consisting predominantly of CD8+ T cells.

Rare cases of encephalitis resulting from an IRIS associated with infections by varicella-zoster virus (VZV), herpes simplex virus (HSV), CMV, parvovirus B19 virus, BK virus and HIV itself have been described. In HIV-associated IRIS causing encephalitis, patients have experienced rapid deterioration of HIV dementia, which has been ascribed to an inflammatory response against HIV, or possibly auto-antigens, in the brain parenchyma that is sometimes associated with demyelination. In the few cases reported to date, histopathology on brain samples obtained by biopsy or at post-mortem showed infiltration with mononuclear cells (particularly CD8+ T cells), which in some instances was demonstrated to be associated with HIV DNA.[10]

Myelitis and Radiculitis

Myelitis caused by an IRIS has been described in association with VZV and HSV infection. The pathogen associated with the IRIS may be identified by examination of CSF for DNA by polymerase chain reaction (PCR). Spinal cord intramedullary abscess due to cryptococcal IRIS has also been reported.

Myeloradiculitis may rarely be a complication of TB-IRIS. Inflammation in the meninges results in nerve root inflammation causing neurologic fall-out in the nerve roots affected, most frequently lumbosacral nerve roots.

Eye Disease

In HIV patients with severe immunodeficiency who are not receiving ART, CMV eye disease typically manifests as necrotizing retinitis without significant inflammation. After commencing ART, retinitis may result from the unmasking of subclinical CMV infection of the eye or present as a paradoxical 'relapse' of retinitis in patients with treated CMV retinitis. Frequently, uveitis characterized by prominent inflammation also occurs in association with the retinitis.

Uveitis related to CMV may also present in patients with healed retinitis and is the most common form of ocular IRIS. There may be intense inflammation in the absence of active CMV infection and it appears that the uveitis results from an immune response against retained CMV antigens. This condition has therefore been referred to as immune recovery uveitis (IRU).[11] It may result in vitritis, papillitis, macular edema and epiretinal membranes, and can be sight-threatening. Furthermore, retinal neovascularization may be a late complication and occur over 4 years after cessation of anti-CMV therapy. The incidence of IRU is highest in patients with the largest areas of previous retinitis and may be reduced by giving therapy for CMV retinitis prior to commencing ART,[12] suggesting that the amount of residual antigen is a determinant of disease onset. Many cases are self-limiting, but orbital floor corticosteroid injections may be necessary, especially if there is declining visual acuity. The condition should be managed by an ophthalmologist.

Uveitis may also result from an IRIS associated with other pathogens including mycobacteria, *Histoplasma* spp. or *Leishmania major*. Anterior stromal keratitis resulting from an IRIS associated with VZV infection has also been described.

Lymphadenitis and Soft Tissue Abscesses

Lymphadenitis resulting from an IRIS may develop in any region of the body and is often painful (Figure 95-2). Multiple nodes that suppurate and coalesce may form inflammatory masses or abscesses, common sites being in the omentum and retroperitoneal space. The latter may form a psoas abscess. Abscesses (e.g. subcutaneous soft

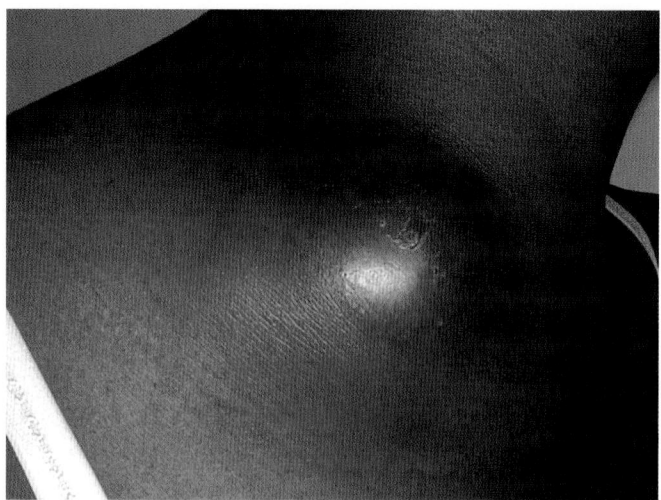

Figure 95-2 Lymphadenitis in TB-IRIS.

tissue abscesses) may also form *de novo* in soft tissues, unrelated to lymph nodes.

In low- and middle-income countries, *M. tuberculosis* is the most frequent underlying infection and lymphadenitis is the most frequent clinical manifestation of an IRIS, occurring in up to 70% of patients.[7] Patients are usually receiving treatment for TB and present with recurrent, new or worsening lymph node enlargement after starting ART (paradoxical TB-IRIS). This is most frequently in the cervical region. Nodal masses can enlarge to greater than 10 cm in diameter. Often the lymphadenitis has prominent acute inflammatory features with tenderness and red discoloration of the overlying skin and suppuration. These features would be unusual for TB lymphadenitis in a patient not receiving ART. Large amounts of pus may be aspirated from these nodes and draining sinuses may form. The pus is typically negative for *M. tuberculosis* cultures, but may be smear-positive, reflecting the presence of nonviable mycobacteria.

Lymphadenitis is also a frequent manifestation of an IRIS associated with infection by NTM, such as *M. avium* complex (MAC) and *M. scrofulaceum*. Lymphadenitis due to MAC-IRIS may persist for months or even years in some patients despite treatment for the MAC infection and corticosteroid therapy.[13] An IRIS associated with Bacille Calmette–Guérin (BCG) infection following BCG vaccination of children with HIV infection has also been described.[14] This condition manifests as an inflammatory reaction at the vaccination site as well as lymphadenitis involving the regional draining lymph nodes.

Lymphadenitis and subcutaneous abscesses have also been reported in an IRIS associated with infection by fungi, specifically cryptococci and *Histoplasma* spp. and the protozoan pathogen *Leishmania* spp.

Potential complications of lymphadenitis caused by an IRIS are airway compression, venous compression resulting in deep vein thrombosis, ureteric compression and chronic draining sinuses. Compression of airways or other vital structures is usually treated with corticosteroids.

Mucocutaneous Disease

A wide variety of skin conditions have been reported to present or worsen after ART is commenced, and probably result from restoring immune responses against skin pathogens.[15] These conditions usually cause minor morbidity and respond to specific therapy for the associated infection. An important clinical issue is the differentiation of first presentations or flares of conditions such as acne, papular pruritic eruption of AIDS and eosinophilic folliculitis after commencing ART from a drug hypersensitivity reaction involving the skin, in order to avoid unnecessary interruption of drugs.

Both herpes simplex and herpes zoster have been reported to occur with increased frequency during early ART compared to HIV-infected patients not receiving ART. In one study, herpes zoster was found to occur five times more frequently from weeks 4 to 16 after ART initiation.[16] Herpes zoster usually manifests as typical mono-dermatomal lesions that respond to antiviral therapy, but disseminated cases are reported. Herpes simplex manifests with anogenital ulceration, which may be necrotizing and hemorrhagic, and/or increased HSV shedding.[17] It typically responds to appropriate systemic antiviral therapy, although refractory cases are described.

Exacerbations of Kaposi's sarcoma (KS) due to an IRIS (paradoxical KS-IRIS) occurs in up to 15% of HIV patients starting ART[18] and may result in tumor enlargement, new lesions, inflammation and edema. Unmasking KS-IRIS may also develop after starting ART. Rapid and fatal progression of KS-IRIS is common in patients with visceral KS. It is probable that the restoration of an immune response against antigens of Kaposi's sarcoma herpesvirus (KSHV; the causative agent of KS), or possibly tumor antigens, provokes paradoxical and unmasking KS-IRIS. Resolution without treatment may occur but severe cases require treatment with systemic chemotherapy.

Mycobacterium leprae infection of the skin is recognized in the setting of HIV disease and has been documented to present as an unmasking IRIS. The reported cases have manifested with inflammatory reversal reactions involving skin lesions or neuritis.[19]

Liver Disease

Hepatotoxicity is a well-recognized complication of ART that presents as an increase in serum transaminase levels. Where a drug hypersensitivity reaction is not implicated as the cause, flares of hepatitis associated with hepatitis C virus (HCV) and hepatitis B virus (HBV) coinfection are important causes. In one study, a hepatitis flare occurred in 50% of patients with HBV and HCV coinfection, 24.3% with HBV coinfection only and 13.5% with HCV coinfection only.[20] The timing of the hepatitis flare after ART in patients with HIV and HCV or HBV coinfection is similar to that of an IRIS, suggesting that it results from restoration of immune responses against HBV or HCV in the liver. Supportive evidence is provided by changes in serologic immune markers in HIV/HBV coinfected patients with flares of hepatitis after ART.[21]

An IRIS affecting the liver usually presents with right upper quadrant pain, nausea and fever. This may be a manifestation of a severe flare of hepatitis associated with HBV or HCV infection. Infection of the liver by mycobacteria, fungi and protozoa may also provoke an inflammatory infiltrate in the liver that is characterized by granulomas or abscess formation. *M. tuberculosis* is the most common pathogen but MAC, *Leishmania* spp., *Histoplasma* spp. and *Cryptococcus neoformans* have also been implicated.

Abdominal and Renal Disease

Abdominal pain is a common manifestation of intra-abdominal lymphadenitis resulting from an IRIS, which is usually associated with mycobacterial infection. Pain may also result from hepatitis caused by an IRIS (see above). It may also be a manifestation of an IRIS associated with infections by *Histoplasma* spp. resulting in infarction of the spleen or intestinal inflammation.[22] Peritonitis due to TB-IRIS may also result in abdominal pain and even mimic a 'surgical abdomen'.

Acute kidney injury may result directly from granulomatous inflammation in the kidneys caused by TB-IRIS.

Lung Disease

Paradoxical TB-IRIS frequently presents with a recurrence of cough and other respiratory symptoms after HIV patients on treatment for TB start ART. This may be associated with new or worsening radiographic features of TB, including expanding pulmonary infiltrates, progressive cavitation, enlarging thoracic lymph nodes and enlarging pleural effusions.

In addition, patients with undiagnosed *M. tuberculosis* infection prior to ART may present with pulmonary disease soon after starting ART. This often presents in an accelerated way with prominent inflammatory features and appears to result from *M. tuberculosis* infection

being unmasked by restoration of *M. tuberculosis*-specific immune responses (unmasking TB-IRIS). This presentation may mimic that of a community-acquired bacterial pneumonia and may be associated with marked features of systemic inflammation and respiratory failure.

MAC-IRIS may manifest with thoracic involvement including pulmonary infiltrates, endobronchial lesions and thoracic node enlargement. Other NTM such as *M. celatum*, *M. xenopi* and *M. kansasii* have also been associated with focal pulmonary infiltrates due to an IRIS.

Worsening of treated *Pneumocystis jirovecii* pneumonitis (PJP) after ART is commenced may be a manifestation of an IRIS but is less common than other types of IRIS, probably because patients are often routinely given corticosteroid therapy as treatment for the PJP. Presentation has been with recurrent fever, dyspnea and cough, and chest radiography demonstrating alveolar infiltrates.[23] Bronchoscopy at the time of the IRIS typically demonstrates an unusually vigorous inflammatory response but few or no *Pneumocystis* organisms, suggesting that this is an inflammatory response to residual *P. jirovecii* antigens. Treatment is with appropriate antibiotics for PJP, usually trimethoprim–sulfamethoxazole (TMP–SMX) and corticosteroid therapy.

Cryptococcal IRIS has been reported to present as necrotizing pneumonitis and thoracic lymphadenitis.

Serous Effusions

TB-IRIS may manifest as new or enlarging serous effusions (pleural effusions, pericardial effusions and ascites). Pleural effusions may cause respiratory distress, due to compression of the underlying lung, and pericardial effusions may result in cardiac tamponade necessitating needle aspiration. Peritonitis and chylous ascites due to an IRIS associated with infection by TB and NTM have also been described.

PATHOGENESIS OF IMMUNE RECONSTITUTION INFLAMMATORY SYNDROMES

The immunopathogenesis of an IRIS may be different for different pathogens. Understanding pathogenic mechanisms, and identifying any that are common to each pathogen, is important if methods for the prevention, diagnosis and treatment of an IRIS are to be improved.

While the development of an IRIS is usually associated with an increased circulating CD4$^+$ T cell count, the role played by T cells in causing the inflammation is unclear. For example, about 10% of patients with an IRIS associated with infection by nontuberculous mycobacteria (NTM) do not experience an increased blood CD4$^+$ T-cell count[13] and several studies have not shown an association between TB-IRIS and the magnitude of the CD4$^+$ T-cell count increase. Similarly, while increased T-cell responses to mycobacterial antigens, demonstrated by T-cell production of interferon-gamma (IFN-γ), have been demonstrated in patients with TB-IRIS, a causal relationship with the IRIS has not been clearly established (reviewed in reference 24). Furthermore, using a whole blood assay of T-cell responses to cryptococcal mannoprotein (CMP) to assess recovery of cryptococcal-reactive T cells, patients who developed C-IRIS causing meningitis did not exhibit higher T-cell responses to CMP than patients who did not develop C-IRIS,[25] though increased CMP-reactive T cells localized to the CNS cannot be excluded.

An increasing amount of evidence indicates that innate immune responses contribute to the inflammation in an IRIS, particularly mediators of those responses, such as pro-inflammatory cytokines (interleukin-6 and tumor necrosis factor-alpha) and chemokines that affect the trafficking of leucocytes to sites of inflammation.[24,26] Based on a mouse model of MAC-IRIS it has been proposed that an IRIS associated with mycobacterial infection results from an accumulation of excess antigen in the context of immunosuppression, with incomplete phagocytic cell activation due to lack of T-cell help. There is then a rapid reversal of this state after commencing ART, associated with T-cell recovery, that leads to a hyper-responsive phagocytic response directed at the large amount of antigen present and exuberant inflammation mediated by pro-inflammatory cytokines[27] and probably chemokines.

MANAGEMENT OF AN IRIS

The important principles in managing an IRIS are to ensure that the patient is receiving appropriate antimicrobial therapy to suppress replication of the provoking pathogen and reduce pathogen load, continue ART unless disease is life threatening, and consider the use of anti-inflammatory therapy, such as corticosteroids, to control inflammation and provide symptom relief. Symptom relief might also require analgesics or drainage of inflammatory fluid collections.

Several characteristics of the IRIS are relevant to making decisions about treatment: most cases are self-limiting, mortality is uncommon and corticosteroid therapy has important adverse effects. In a minority of cases, an IRIS may present with severe and potentially life-threatening manifestations. This is especially the case when there is CNS involvement. Systemic corticosteroid therapy is effective in patients with TB-IRIS and has also been used in patients with an IRIS related to infection by MAC and *C. neoformans*, with several reports of a favorable response. Nonsteroidal anti-inflammatory drugs have also been used to treat an IRIS. However, other than for TB-IRIS, data from prospective controlled clinical trials of therapy for the various types of IRIS are not available and treatment guidelines are therefore informed by data from case reports.

ART is continued in most settings, but some authorities have suggested interrupting ART if an IRIS is life-threatening or unresponsive to corticosteroids. However, interruption of ART places the patient at risk of other opportunistic infections and the development of antiretroviral resistance, and an IRIS may still recur when ART is re-initiated.

Corticosteroid Therapy for TB-IRIS

Corticosteroids are often used to treat TB-IRIS and have been shown to be effective in a randomized controlled trial, through modulation of inflammation.[28] However, the risks and benefits of corticosteroid therapy are unclear and need to be carefully weighed up. Because of the immunosuppressive effect of corticosteroid therapy, its use has been associated with an excess of Kaposi's sarcoma and herpesvirus reactivations in HIV-infected patients. Also, if the diagnosis of IRIS is incorrect and the cause for deterioration is drug resistance, or an additional unrecognized infection, corticosteroids could compound the diagnostic error.

Given that most cases of TB-IRIS are self-limiting, corticosteroids are usually reserved for patients with more severe manifestations and in whom the diagnosis is certain. Such patients include those with CNS involvement, airway compression due to enlarging lymphadenopathy, refractory or debilitating lymphadenitis, or respiratory distress. The duration of corticosteroid therapy required is variable. Some patients only require a few weeks whereas a subgroup of patients with TB-IRIS may require prolonged courses to control symptoms. Prednisone is the most frequently used corticosteroid and has been used at doses varying from 10 to 120 mg daily. Usually the dose is tapered over several weeks according to clinical response.

Autoimmune Disease in HIV Patients Receiving Antiretroviral Therapy

Several types of autoimmune disease have been reported in HIV patients who have experienced immune reconstitution on ART.

However, most are single case reports and it is unclear whether their occurrence during ART is merely a coincidence. In contrast, there is compelling evidence that Graves' disease in HIV patients receiving ART is usually an immune reconstitution disorder. Thus, there are over 40 cases reported in the literature, including cases in different racial groups.[29] Graves' disease occurs predominantly in patients who had a very low CD4[+] T-cell count at the time of commencing ART and who experience a substantial increase of the count on ART. Unlike the various types of IRIS, Graves' disease in HIV patients receiving ART presents at a median time of almost 2 years after commencing ART. The immunopathogenesis therefore appears to be different from an IRIS and is probably related to an acquired defect of immune tolerance associated with higher numbers of circulating recent thymic emigrant naïve T cells.[30]

Systemic or cutaneous lupus has also been reported to present in HIV patients on ART.[31] Those cases presenting during the first 3 months of ART have had serologic evidence of lupus before treatment and it appears that the immunologic changes immediately after ART unmask clinical disease. The other cases have presented after 9 months of ART and the lupus may have resulted from an acquired disorder of immune tolerance during immune reconstitution.

The management of autoimmune disease in HIV patients receiving ART is similar to non-HIV patients but caution has to be exercised if corticosteroid and immunosuppressant therapy are used in patients with HIV infection.

Immune-Mediated Inflammatory Disease in HIV Patients Receiving Antiretroviral Therapy

Immune-mediated inflammatory disease, in which inflammation is the result of immune responses that are apparently not precipitated by infections, may also present in HIV patients responding to ART. There are many reports of sarcoidosis presenting in this context[32] and reactive arthritis, lymphoid interstitial pneumonitis, Peyronie's disease, foreign body reactions and photodermatitis have also been described. Sarcoidosis may present up to 3 years after commencement of ART. Most cases present with thoracic disease but extrathoracic disease also occurs in the skin, liver, spleen, kidneys, peripheral lymph nodes, eyes, muscle and salivary glands. In some cases, the use of IL-2 or interferon alpha (IFN-α) therapy appears to have been a precipitating factor.

The immunopathogenesis of sarcoidosis in HIV patients receiving ART is unclear but it is most likely to reflect an increased susceptibility to dysregulation of granulomatous inflammatory responses in the reconstituted immune system, which may be exacerbated by cytokine therapy that enhances type I helper T-cell (Th1) responses, such as recombinant IL-2 or IFN-α therapy.

Sarcoidosis in HIV patients receiving ART may resolve without treatment but corticosteroid therapy is sometimes necessary. It is therefore important to differentiate sarcoidosis from an IRIS associated with an infection that causes granulomatous inflammation.

References available online at expertconsult.com.

KEY REFERENCES

Barber D.L., Andrade B.B., Sereti I., et al.: Immune reconstitution inflammatory syndrome: the trouble with immunity when you had none. *Nat Rev Microbiol* 2012; 10:150-156.

Chang C.C., Crane M., Zhou J., et al.: HIV and co-infections. *Immunol Rev* 2013; 254:114-142.

Crum N.F., Ganesan A., Johns S.T., et al.: Graves' disease: an increasingly recognized immune reconstitution syndrome. *AIDS* 2006; 20:466-469.

Foulon G., Wislez M., Naccache J.-M., et al.: Sarcoidosis in HIV-infected patients in the era of highly active antiretroviral therapy. *Clin Infect Dis* 2004; 38:418-425.

Lai R.P., Nakiwala J.K., Meintjes G., et al.: The immunopathogenesis of the HIV tuberculosis immune reconstitution inflammatory syndrome. *Eur J Immunol* 2013; 43:1995-2002.

Meintjes G., Lawn S.D., Scano F., et al.: Tuberculosis-associated immune reconstitution inflammatory syndrome: case definitions for use in resource-limited settings. *Lancet Infect Dis* 2008; 8:516-523.

Meintjes G., Skolimowska K.H., Wilkinson K.A., et al.: Corticosteroids-modulated immune activation in the tuberculosis immune reconstitution inflammatory syndrome. *Am J Respir Crit Care Med* 2012; 186:369-377.

Müller M., Wandel S., Colebunders R., et al.: Immune reconstitution inflammatory syndrome in patients starting antiretroviral therapy for HIV infection: a systematic review and meta-analysis. *Lancet Infect Dis* 2010; 10:251-261.

Phillips P., Bonner S., Gataric N., et al.: Nontuberculous mycobacterial immune reconstitution syndrome in HIV-infected patients: spectrum of disease and long-term follow-up. *Clin Infect Dis* 2005; 41:1483-1497.

96

Tuberculosis in HIV

STEPHEN D. LAWN | ROBIN WOOD

KEY CONCEPTS

- Human immunodeficiency virus (HIV)-associated tuberculosis (TB) accounts for 13% of new TB cases globally and 75% occur in sub-Saharan Africa.

- TB is the leading cause of acquired immunodeficiency syndrome (AIDS)-related deaths worldwide.

- The HIV epidemic has been associated with outbreaks of multidrug-resistant TB in congregate settings.

- The interaction between HIV and TB is bi-directional.

- Combined interventions to prevent HIV-associated TB include antiretroviral therapy (ART), chemoprophylaxis, infection control and intensified case finding.

- HIV-associated TB less commonly presents with organ-specific symptoms and the risk of extrapulmonary, miliary and disseminated forms of disease increase at lower CD4 counts.

- Diagnosis of HIV-associated TB is more challenging due to an increased frequency of atypical clinical and radiographic presentations and lower bacillary burden in sputum samples.

- Management requires optimized combination of TB treatment, ART and trimethoprim–sulfamethoxazole prophylaxis.

- To minimize mortality, TB treatment must be given concurrently with ART despite pharmacokinetic interactions and risk of immune reconstitution inflammatory syndrome.

- The outcomes of the current management of HIV-associated drug-resistant TB remain poor.

Epidemiology

HIV AND TB RISK

HIV infection is a potent risk factor for the development of active tuberculosis (TB), increasing risk more than 20-fold.[1] This may potentially result from:
- high risk of reactivation of latent *Mycobacterium tuberculosis* infection;
- rapid progression of *M. tuberculosis* infection to primary active TB following recent exposure; and
- increased risk of exposure to TB.

HIV-seronegative individuals who have latent infection with *M. tuberculosis* have a lifetime risk of developing active TB of approximately 10–15%. Following HIV seroconversion, however, TB risk doubles and progressively increases with advancing immunodeficiency. The overall risk of developing active TB in HIV-infected individuals with latent *M. tuberculosis* infection is approximately 10% per year. However, the annual risk among patients with AIDS living in communities with high TB burden in sub-Saharan Africa may be as high as 30%.

HIV infection also increases the risk of progressive primary disease following recent infection with *M. tuberculosis*. Outbreaks in healthcare settings in high-income countries have been characterized by attack rates of 30–40% among HIV-infected patients, with many developing disease within 1–2 months. HIV-infected patients may be at high risk of exposure to TB in healthcare settings,[2] social mixing with high-risk groups such as intravenous drug users or living in high burden communities. However, it is not clear whether for a given exposure their susceptibility to initial infection with *M. tuberculosis* is also increased.

HIV AND THE GLOBAL BURDEN OF TB

Outbreaks of HIV-associated TB – often with multidrug-resistant (MDR) disease – in New York, USA, and other cities in higher-income countries in the early 1990s heralded a global resurgence in TB. In 1993, the World Health Organization (WHO) declared that TB was a global emergency, with HIV infection being identified as one of the key underlying drivers of the epidemic. Twenty years later, HIV-associated TB still accounted for 1.1 million (13%) of the overall global burden of 8.6 million new TB cases in 2012.[3]

In Eastern Europe, there is an important epidemiological intersection between HIV infection and TB and multidrug resistant TB (MDRTB) among intravenous drug abusers and prison populations.[4] There is also an important burden of HIV-associated TB in South and South East Asia. However, the countries of sub-Saharan Africa have borne the brunt of the epidemic (Figure 96-1).[3] Here there has been a geographical overlap between an evolving generalized HIV epidemic and the pre-existing TB epidemic in populations with poor TB control, a high prevalence of latent *M. tuberculosis* infection and high rates of TB transmission. In 2012, sub-Saharan Africa accounted for 830 000 (75%) of the 1.1 million new cases of HIV-associated TB occurring worldwide each year.[3] Incidence rates are highest towards the south and east of the continent (Figure 96-2), where HIV prevalence among new TB cases exceeds 50% in a total of nine countries. In the worst affected countries of South Africa and Swaziland, an estimated 1% or more of the national population develops TB each year, much of this disease fuelled by HIV. In impoverished South African townships, 2–3% of young adults may develop TB annually.[5]

MORTALITY AND TB TRANSMISSION RISK

Patients with HIV-associated TB have high mortality risk. In the pre-antiretroviral therapy (ART) era in sub-Saharan Africa, case fatality rates were approximately fivefold higher than in HIV-seronegative patients during the course of TB treatment (16–35% versus 4–9%).[6] A randomized trial in West Africa, however, found that mortality in HIV-coinfected patients could be halved by trimethoprim–sulfamethoxazole (TMP–SMX) prophylaxis. This indicates that many such deaths are likely to be caused by a range of other co-infections, which are prevented by TMP–SMX. These might include bacterial sepsis, toxoplasmosis and malaria, and *Pneumocystis jirovecii* pneumonia (PJP).

TB is the leading cause of HIV-related deaths worldwide, accounting for 0.32 million (20%) of the 1.6 million deaths each year.[3] Since diagnosis of TB is more difficult in HIV-infected patients, many HIV-associated TB deaths remain unascertained. Hospital-based postmortem studies over the past 20 years have found that between one-third and two-thirds of deaths among HIV-infected medical inpatients are related to TB.[7,8]

HIV-infected patients with TB are, on average, less infectious than those without HIV coinfection as they are more likely to have noninfectious extrapulmonary disease or noncavitating pulmonary disease with lower concentrations of bacilli in the sputum (Figure 96-3). In addition, debilitated patients with advanced HIV may have poor cough strength and therefore generate infectious aerosols less efficiently.[9]

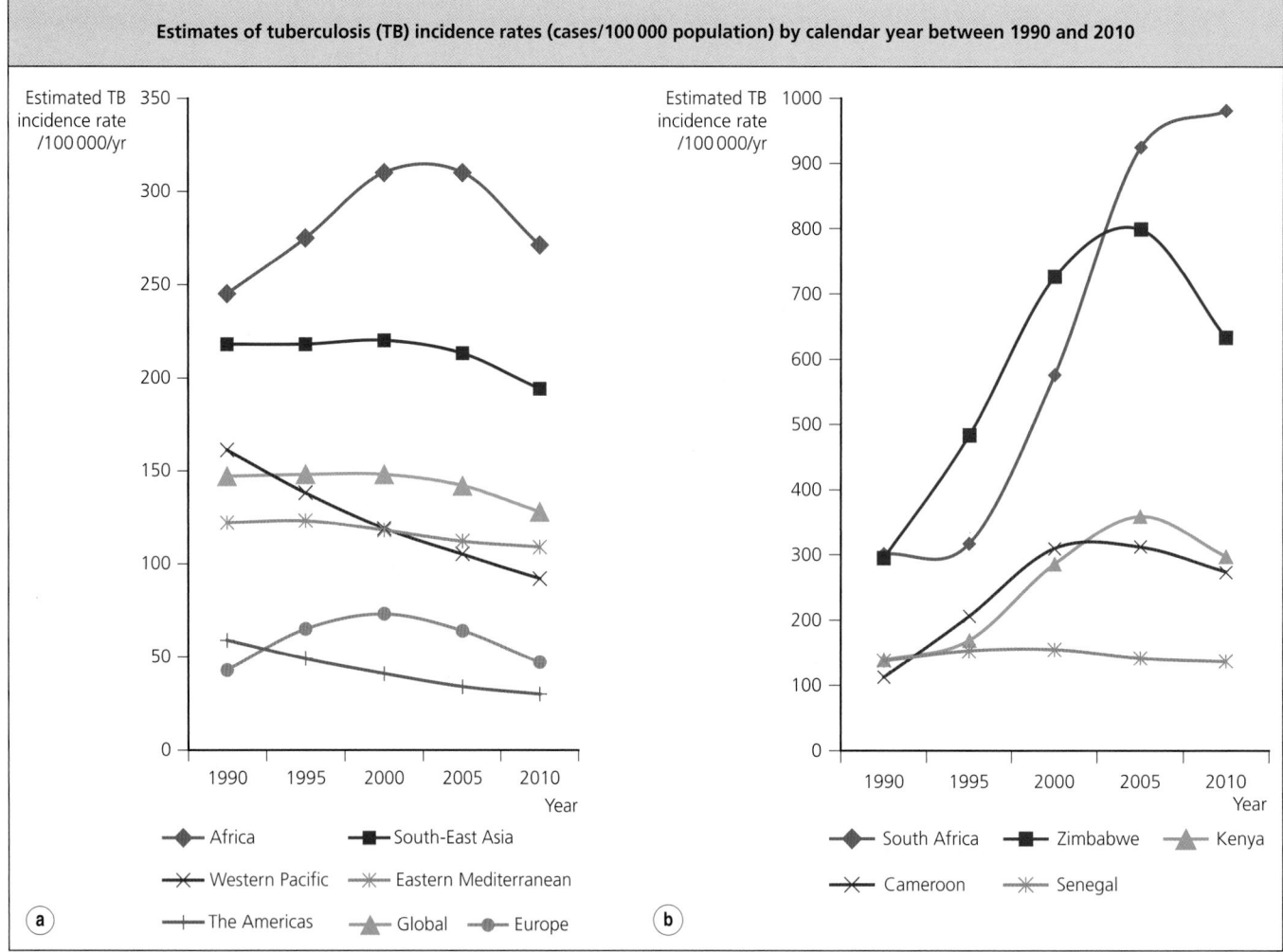

Figure 96-1   Estimates of tuberculosis (TB) incidence rates (cases/100 000 population) by calendar year between 1990 and 2010 shown (a) by World Health Organization region and (b) for selected countries in sub-Saharan Africa. Incidence rates are highest for the Africa region and increased between 1990 and 2003 due to the HIV epidemic. However, this increase has been far more marked for countries such as Zimbabwe and South Africa where HIV prevalence is much higher compared to East, Central or West Africa. (*Data from Global tuberculosis report 2013. Geneva: World Health Organization; 2013.*)

Despite this, patients with HIV-associated TB collectively constitute an important reservoir of TB transmission within the community-level and healthcare settings.

HIV AND MULTIDRUG-RESISTANT TB

Multidrug-resistant TB (MDRTB) is caused by strains of *M. tuberculosis* that are resistant to at least isoniazid and rifampin (rifampicin) and has emerged as a global epidemic, with an estimated 450 000 cases developing each year.[3] While this epidemic has largely resulted from deficiencies in TB case management and TB control programs, important synergies with the HIV epidemic are emerging. Although some data suggest that HIV may be a significant driver of MDRTB at a population level, most evidence indicates the association is closely related to environmental factors such as transmission in congregate settings.[4]

Institutional outbreaks of MDRTB have primarily affected HIV-infected patients with high attack rates and mortality.[4] These outbreaks have been linked to poor infection control practices in hospitals and prisons where patients with unrecognized TB and those with HIV infection were mixed and where diagnoses of MDRTB were often delayed. For example, a large outbreak of MDRTB and extensively drug-resistant (XDR) TB cases in 2005 was identified among HIV-infected patients attending an ART clinic at a hospital in KwaZulu Natal Province in South Africa.[10] The epidemic of HIV-associated

MDRTB in Eastern European countries of the former Soviet Union has been particularly concentrated among intravenous drug users within prisons, where infection control is poor.[4]

Several mechanisms may increase the risk of HIV-infected patients having TB caused by drug-resistant strains. These include risk of acquisition of such strains in healthcare settings and association with high-risk groups such as in prisons and intravenous drug users. They also have increased risk of recurrent TB episodes and TB drug malabsorption might also favor the development of drug resistance. In addition, TB services in some areas of sub-Saharan Africa have been overwhelmed by the escalating case load caused by HIV, thereby undermining TB treatment completion rates and cure rates. In the South African outbreak of MDR- and XDR-TB, laboratory data suggest that, in the absence of routine drug susceptibility testing, drug pressure from inappropriate treatment regimens led to sequential acquisition of resistance.[11]

Pathogenesis

CD4 T-helper cell function is central to the orchestration of cell-mediated responses to *M. tuberculosis*, culminating in the formation of epithelioid granulomas, which restrict growth of the organism. Not only are these processes fundamentally undermined by HIV-1 infection,[12] but the host response to *M. tuberculosis* at the site of disease

Estimated HIV prevalence (%) in new TB cases, 2012

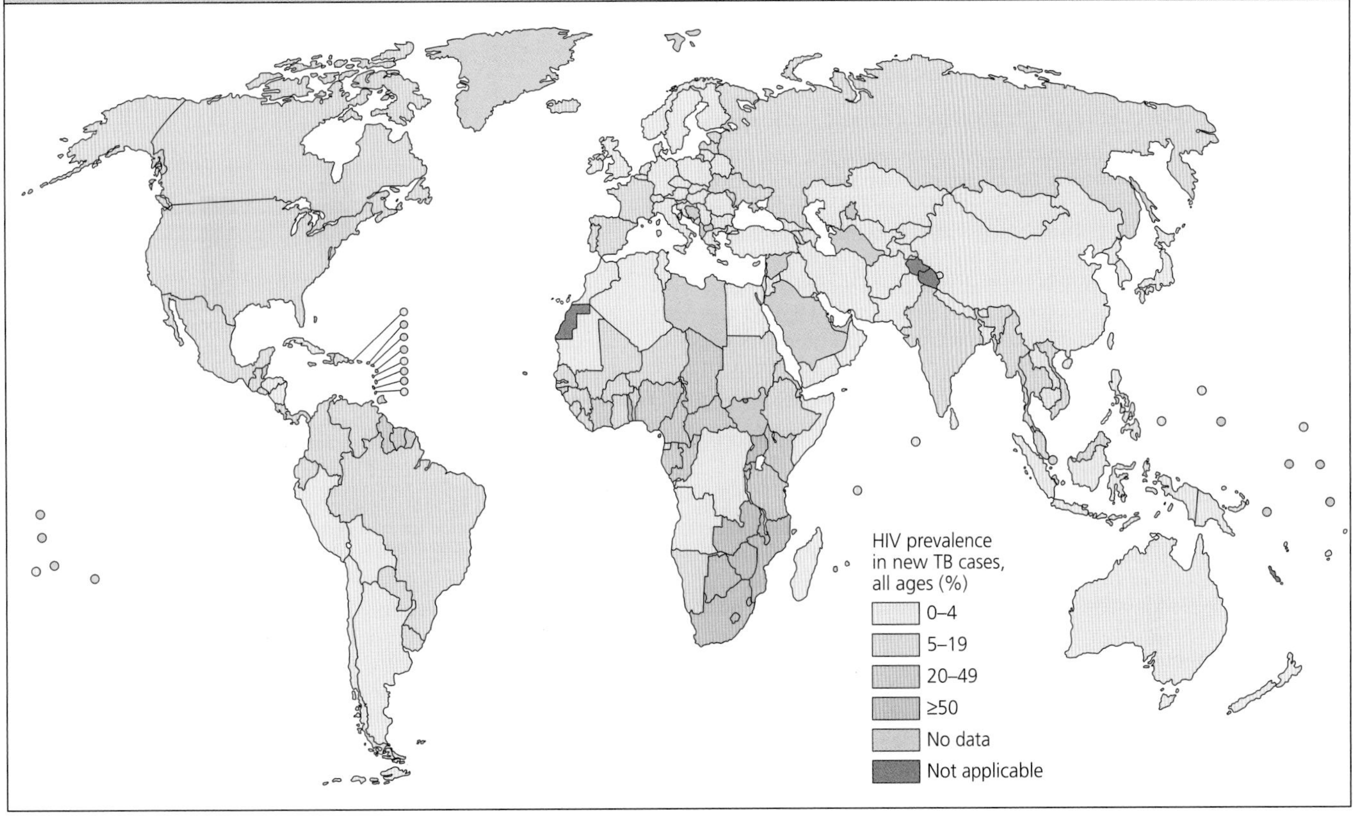

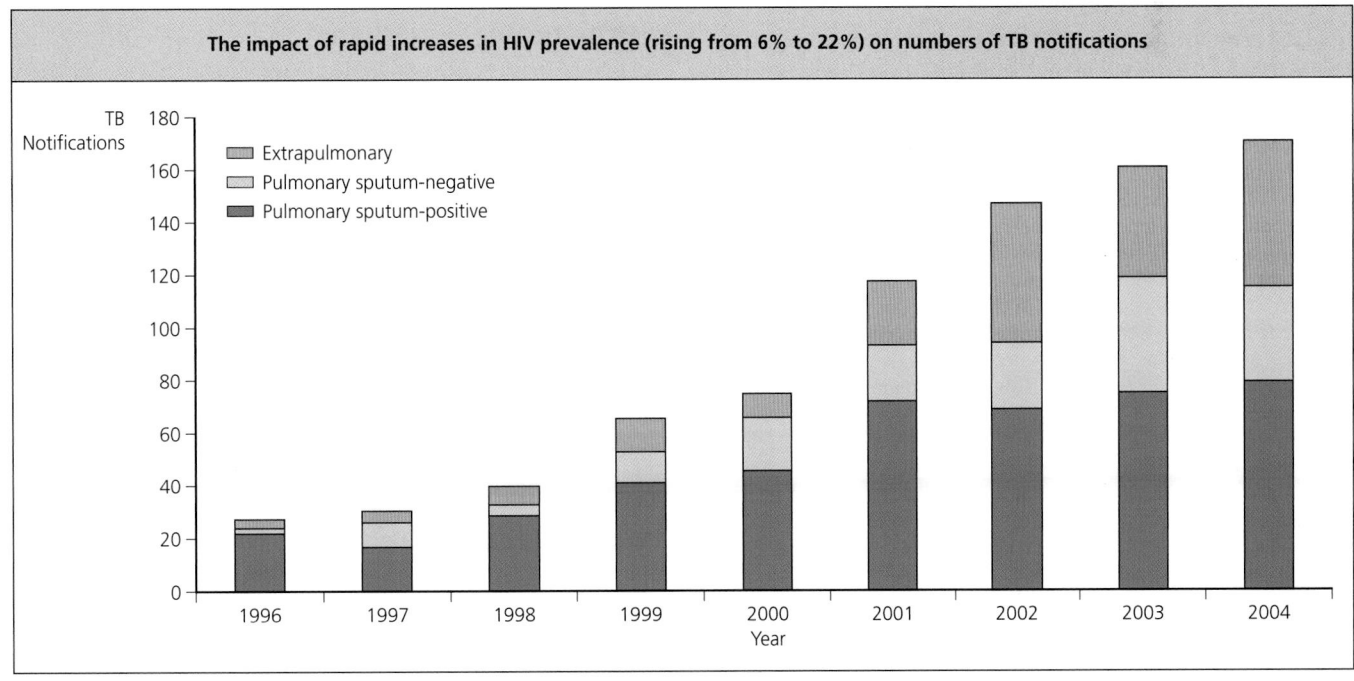

Figure 96-2 Estimated HIV infection prevalence (%) among new patients with tuberculosis (TB). *(Reproduced with permission from the World Health Organization, Global tuberculosis report 2013. Geneva: World Health Organization; 2013.)*

The impact of rapid increases in HIV prevalence (rising from 6% to 22%) on numbers of TB notifications

Figure 96-3 The impact of rapid increases in HIV prevalence (rising from 6% to 22%) on numbers of TB notifications among adults in a South African community of 13000 people between 1996 and 2004. Case numbers increased steeply as the HIV epidemic evolved, with disproportionate increases in sputum smear-negative pulmonary TB and extrapulmonary TB. *(Adapted from Lawn S.D., Bekker L.G., Middelkoop K., et al.: Impact of HIV infection on the epidemiology of tuberculosis in a peri-urban community in South Africa: the need for age-specific interventions.* Clin Infect Dis *2006; 42(7):1040-1047.)*

provides an immunologic environment that promotes HIV replication. As a result, the interaction between these diseases is bi-directional.

IMPAIRED IMMUNE RESPONSES TO *M. TUBERCULOSIS*

Following initial infection, formation of immunologically competent granulomas is essential to the containment of *M. tuberculosis* infection and prevention of reactivation of latent infection. However, HIV-1 infection impairs antigen presentation, cytokine secretion and intracellular killing of mycobacteria by mononuclear phagocytes.[12] CD4 cells are numerically depleted and functionally impaired. Inhibition of interleukin (IL)-2 signaling is associated with reduced T-cell proliferation and activation. Rates of CD4 cell loss are also greatly increased due to virus-mediated cytolysis and activation-induced apoptosis. Secretion of type 1 cytokines such as interferon-gamma (IFN-γ) and IL-12 is diminished and there is failure of recruitment of mononuclear cells to sites of *M. tuberculosis* infection. All these effects culminate in failure of granuloma formation and the host response to *M. tuberculosis*.[12]

IMPACT OF TUBERCULOSIS ON HIV-1 PATHOGENESIS

TB may serve as a co-factor that accelerates the rate of immunologic decline in coinfected patients.[13] While the laboratory data supporting this mechanism are strong, the population level impact is unclear. The HIV-1 life cycle is intimately related to the activation state of the host cell.[14] Thus, *in vitro*, *M. tuberculosis* infection increases HIV production from infected mononuclear cells and enhances the infectivity of bystander mononuclear cells for HIV.[12]

Increases in viral load have been documented in HIV-infected patients who develop TB, especially among those with relatively well-preserved CD4 cell counts.[14] HIV load is particularly increased at sites of active TB such as in the pleural space, for example. Development of TB also leads to genotypic diversification of HIV-1 and expression of new or more virulent HIV-1 quasi-species has the potential to further accelerate HIV-1 disease progression.[13]

Prevention

CHEMOPROPHYLAXIS

Isoniazid preventive therapy (IPT) is an effective intervention that can reduce risk of TB in subgroups of HIV-infected patients by preventing rapid progression of recent infection to active disease or treatment of long-standing infection, thereby reducing risk of reactivation disease. A large meta-analysis of studies examining a range of preventive regimens found an overall risk reduction of 32% in comparison with placebo.[15] The greatest reduction in TB incidence (62%) was observed among patients with a positive tuberculin skin test (TST) whereas the reduction among TST-negative individuals (11%) was not statistically significant. Isoniazid alone given for 6–12 months reduced TB incidence by 33% overall and by 64% in those with positive TST results.[15] Multidrug regimens given for 2–3 months were as effective as isoniazid alone for 6–12 months. While rates of hepatotoxicity are overall very low, rates are higher for regimens using a combination of rifampin and pyrazinamide.

The durability of the benefits of IPT is variable but is likely to depend strongly on the risk of re-infection with *M. tuberculosis* following completion of therapy and may also be affected by HIV progression. The higher the TB transmission rates, the shorter the likely duration of benefit. Data from Zambia found a sustained benefit for approximately 2.5 years whereas in South Africa and Botswana, where TB transmission rates are high, the benefit is short-lived and so more prolonged regimens are needed.[16] IPT has also been shown to be effective in reducing high TB recurrence rates following completion of TB treatment (secondary prophylaxis) in high TB prevalence settings.

IPT provides additional TB risk reduction among patients on long-term ART, as these two interventions reduce TB risk via two different

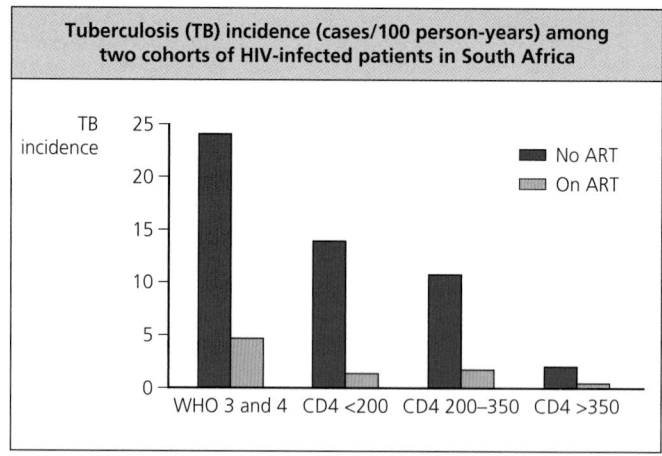

Figure 96-4 Tuberculosis (TB) incidence (cases/100 person-years) among two cohorts of HIV-infected patients in South Africa who were or were not receiving antiretroviral treatment (ART). Patients are stratified according to baseline CD4 cell count (cells/μL) and World Health Organization clinical stage. Those receiving ART had incidence rates that were approximately 80% lower than the untreated group. (*Adapted from Badri M., Wilson D., Wood R.: Effect of highly active antiretroviral therapy on incidence of tuberculosis in South Africa: a cohort study.* Lancet *2002; 359(9323):2059-2064.*)

mechanisms and are therefore complementary.[17] The former targets the organism whereas the latter restores the host immune response.

Although IPT is an effective intervention, it has not been widely implemented in resource-limited settings for several reasons, including limited healthcare capacity to deliver this intervention, difficulties in excluding active TB prior to initiating IPT, concerns about development of isoniazid resistance, logistical challenges associated with tuberculin skin testing difficulties and limited patient adherence under program conditions. Widespread scale-up of ART now provides a clinical setting where this can now be more readily implemented and uptake is increasing. Ongoing research is needed to understand how this intervention can best be utilized and implemented.

ANTIRETROVIRAL THERAPY

ART is the most effective available intervention for TB prevention in HIV-infected patients in both high-income and resource-limited settings (Figure 96-4).[18,19] TB incidence rates are reduced by two-thirds overall across a broad range of CD4 cell count strata, but with greatest benefit among those with CD4 counts lower than 200 cells/μL.[19,20] However, long-term ART does not decrease TB risk to background levels in HIV-negative individuals living in the same communities. In South Africa, rates remained approximately fourfold higher despite excellent long-term virologic responses.[21]

The persisting risk of TB during ART is largely determined by patients' absolute CD4 cell counts,[22] but it remains unclear what proportions of cases arise from reactivation of *M. tuberculosis* infection or from exogenous re-infection in healthcare settings or in the community. Defects in immune responses to *M. tuberculosis* may persist during long-term ART,[23] especially among patients with the lowest pre-ART nadir CD4 cell counts. This highlights the importance of early initiation of ART.

INFECTION CONTROL

The risk of TB transmission within health facilities has long been recognized.[2] In the 1990s a global resurgence of TB was heralded by many reports of nosocomial outbreaks of TB (mostly MDRTB) in HIV care settings in the USA and elsewhere.[4] In more recent years, rapid expansion of ART in resource-limited countries with high TB burden has paradoxically created unprecedented opportunities for HIV-infected patients and healthcare personnel to be exposed to TB in healthcare settings. This was most vividly highlighted by an outbreak of XDR-TB at a hospital in rural South Africa first reported in 2005.[10] By 2008 there had been more than 200 deaths, including some hospital staff.

Infection control within healthcare settings requires a tiered approach of:

- administrative controls, leading to prompt identification and separation of individuals with potentially infectious TB;
- environmental controls, such as adequate natural or mechanical ventilation or ultraviolet light germicidal irradiation; and
- respiratory protection using a face mask or respirator.[2]

How to implement and monitor infection control cost-effectively within healthcare facilities in resource-limited settings is a key research priority.

TB CONTROL IN SETTINGS WITH HIGH TB/HIV PREVALENCE

The World Health Organization DOTS (directly observed therapy, short course) strategy has contributed to decreases in TB notification rates in many areas of the world. However, in sub-Saharan Africa, where HIV prevalence rates are high, DOTS has failed to control the TB epidemic,[5] even in countries such as Malawi and Tanzania with well-functioning national TB control programs.

The DOTS strategy targets those with sputum smear-positive pulmonary disease who are most likely to transmit TB. DOTS does not, however, reduce the number of individuals who remain highly susceptible to TB in the community, including the large pool of those with latent *M. tuberculosis* infection who are at risk of reactivation disease. While DOTS programs need to be strengthened, a package of additional interventions is also required.[24] HIV testing among patients with newly diagnosed TB is essential to allow appropriate management and improve outcomes. Additional interventions include targeted active case-finding among HIV-infected individuals, implementation of isoniazid prophylaxis, and scale-up of ART at higher CD4 cell count thresholds. Moreover, widespread coverage of HIV testing is essential to allow those living with infection to benefit from these interventions.

While there is some evidence of a beneficial impact of ART scale-up on TB notification rates in communities in southern Africa, the long-term impact remains uncertain.[18] Since ART greatly increases life expectancy, and TB rates during long-term ART remain several-fold higher than background rates, life-time risk of developing TB remains high, thereby undermining the potential impact of ART for TB control at a population level. However, the earlier ART is started during HIV disease progression, the greater the likely population impact.[18]

Clinical Features

M. tuberculosis causes disease across the full spectrum of HIV-associated immunodeficiency and the impact of HIV on the clinical manifestations of TB is directly related to the degree of immunodeficiency. The median CD4 cell count at presentation appears to vary greatly between published series and may depend on the specific patient population and the maturity of the HIV epidemic. In San Francisco in 1990, for example, the median CD4 cell count at TB presentation was 326 cells/μL, compared to <200 cells/μL in countries of southern Africa in more recent times.[25] TB is commonly the first clinical manifestation of HIV infection, highlighting the great importance of HIV testing of all TB patients.

The spectrum of clinicopathologic manifestations of TB directly relate to blood CD4 cell counts. Features of TB in individuals with well-preserved CD4 cell counts are indistinguishable from those of HIV-seronegative individuals with TB. Progressive immunodeficiency is associated with an increasing frequency of anergic TST responses, atypical presentations of pulmonary TB and sputum smear-negative disease, and an increased frequency of extrapulmonary, miliary and disseminated disease (see Figure 96-3).

Irrespective of the site of TB, a majority of patients have systemic manifestations with fever, night sweats or weight loss. It is not uncommon for TB to present with unexplained systemic symptoms in the absence of organ-specific symptoms. In studies in Asia and sub-Saharan Africa, in which HIV-infected patient populations have been actively investigated for TB, substantial rates of subclinical TB have been documented.[26] Chronic cough has low sensitivity as a screening tool for HIV-associated TB. Thus, the WHO recommends use of a screening tool that includes one or more of the following symptoms: cough, fever, weight loss or night sweats of any duration.[27] This has much higher sensitivity but specificity is poor.

Pulmonary disease is the major manifestation of TB in both HIV-infected and non-infected patients. Symptoms and radiographic findings, however, generally have low sensitivity and specificity for diagnosis of pulmonary TB in the HIV-infected patient.[28] Radiographic appearances reveal a lower frequency of upper lobe disease, cavitation, parenchymal opacification and fibrosis, but an increased frequency of mediastinal lymphadenopathy, small pleural effusions and miliary disease. Normal radiographs may be observed in a proportion (0–30%) of patients with sputum culture-positive disease. The spectrum of appearances correlates strongly with the degree of immunodeficiency; those with high CD4 cell counts usually have a typical pattern of postprimary disease whereas those with low CD4 cell counts have a higher proportion with a primary disease pattern.[29]

Hematogenous and lymphatic dissemination of mycobacteria in HIV-infected patients increases the risk of extrapulmonary TB. This is strongly related to the degree of immunodeficiency, with the risk particularly increasing as the CD4 cell count falls below 200 cells/μL. The relative frequency of reported extrapulmonary disease also relates to the intensity of the diagnostic workup. Autopsy specimens from patients who died of TB and AIDS show a high frequency of extrapulmonary and disseminated disease with multiorgan involvement.[7]

Lymphadenitis is the most common form of extrapulmonary TB. Cervical nodes are most frequently involved, but disease also often occurs in mediastinal, mesenteric and inguinal nodes. Miliary radiographic shadowing has been reported in up to 38% of AIDS patients with extrapulmonary TB and typically presents with marked constitutional symptoms. HIV infection increases the risk of TB meningitis several-fold, but does not substantially alter the clinical and laboratory manifestations.

Pleural effusions were detected radiographically in one-fifth of a series of consecutive patients with HIV-associated TB in South Africa and were more common than disseminated or miliary TB in patients with higher CD4 cell counts. Pericardial TB is strongly associated with HIV coinfection (Figure 96-5) and is associated with a pleural effusion in up to approximately one-third of cases.

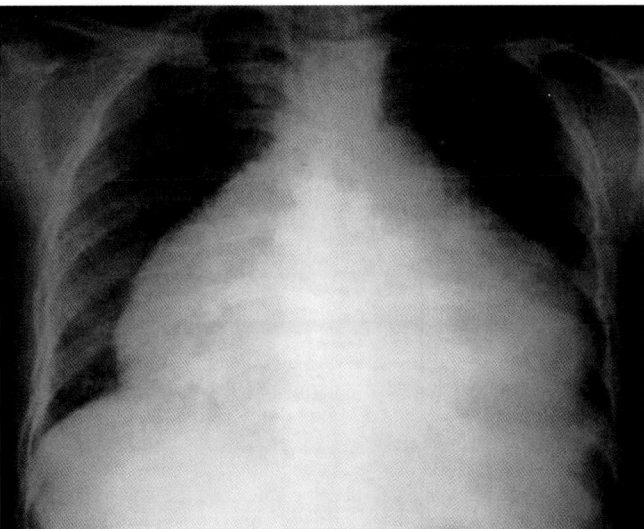

Figure 96-5 Chest radiograph of a South African patient with HIV infection and a large tuberculous pericardial effusion. *(Courtesy of Mpiko Ntsekhe, Groote Schuur Hospital, University of Cape Town.)*

TB may involve any part of the gastrointestinal tract due to either ingestion of infected sputum or hematogenous dissemination. Whereas mediastinal adenopathy is frequently detected by thoracic radiologic imaging, mesenteric TB lymphadenitis may remain undiagnosed until initiation of ART triggers the clinical presentation (see also Chapter 92). Development of abscesses in the liver, spleen and other intra-abdominal organs is also a frequent finding.

Diagnosis

The increased likelihood of atypical clinical presentations and sub-clinical TB requires a high index of suspicion for TB in the HIV-infected patient.[28] Sputum-based investigations typically have lower sensitivity among HIV coinfected patients. The frequency of atypical radiologic appearances of pulmonary TB increases with declining immune function. Histopathologic examination of tissue specimens is similarly less likely to show granulomatous inflammation typical of TB.[26] Diagnosis is highly dependent upon obtaining multiple good quality clinical samples (respiratory and non-respiratory) for myco-bacteriologic tests, which must be interpreted in the light of their known limited sensitivity.

The average sensitivity of sputum microscopy in research settings is <60% in immunocompetent patients with pulmonary TB and is reduced to 20–50% in HIV-infected patients due to lower concentrations of bacilli in the sputum. Sensitivity is approximately 10% higher when using fluorescence microscopy. Whereas positive sputum smears have low specificity in industrialized countries, they have good specificity in settings such as Africa where TB is far more common than nontuberculous mycobacterial disease.

Mycobacterial culture in selective liquid media remains the most sensitive means of detecting *M. tuberculosis* bacilli in both respiratory and nonrespiratory clinical samples and is the mainstay for confirmation of diagnoses. Due to frequent extrapulmonary disease, culture of specimens such as lymph node aspirates, urine, blood and bone marrow may provide a useful diagnostic yield. Blood cultures have been found to be positive in up to one-third of patients with advanced immunodeficiency and extrapulmonary TB. However, the time to positivity in culture is often prolonged due to the limited numbers of bacilli in samples. This is a major drawback since rapid diagnosis and treatment are key in HIV-infected patients. Moreover, due to high cost and technical complexity, culture-based diagnosis is rarely available in resource-limited settings.

Major progress has been made within the developmental pipeline for TB diagnostics over the past 10 years.[30] This includes the development of the Xpert MTB/RIF rapid molecular assay (Cepheid Inc., Sunnyvale, CA, USA). This almost fully automated, cartridge-based, 2-hour assay detects with high specificity the vast majority of smear-positive and two-thirds of smear-negative pulmonary TB cases and a variable proportion of extrapulmonary cases, depending on the sample type. It also detects >95% of mutations in the *rpoB* gene that confer rifampin resistance. Thus, this is a major breakthrough for diagnosis of HIV-associated TB and is now being widely implemented around the world.

Another development is a simple, low-cost, lateral flow assay that detects the mycobacterial cell wall glycolipid antigen, lipoarabinomannan (LAM), in urine samples, permitting a diagnosis of TB to be made with high specificity within 30 minutes.[31] Useful sensitivity is limited to adult patients with very low CD4 cell counts and so this assay is most likely to be used to accelerate the diagnosis of TB among sick HIV-infected patients prior to starting ART or among those requiring medical admission to hospital in high burden settings.

TSTs and IFN-γ release assays (IGRAs) have limited utility in the investigation of the HIV-infected patient for TB as sensitivity is limited, especially in those with low CD4 cell counts, and these tests are unable to differentiate between active disease and latent infection. Positive IGRAs may help to provide supportive evidence in a proportion of patients in low burden settings, but can neither be used as a rule-in nor a rule-out test for TB. WHO has made a specific recommendation that these assays do not have a useful role in high burden countries due to their poor predictive value in these settings.[32]

Management

Patients with HIV-associated TB should be managed with optimized antituberculosis treatment, TMP–SMX prophylaxis, and ART.[33,34]

TB TREATMENT

The first priority for patients with HIV-associated TB is to immediately start effective TB treatment using a regimen containing rifampin throughout. The incidence of relapse and/or failure among patients treated with intermittent (thrice-weekly) TB therapy throughout is 2–3 times higher than that in patients who receive a daily intensive phase. Thus, the recommended optimum standard regimen is 2 months of rifampin, isoniazid, pyrazinamide and ethambutol followed by 4 months of rifampin and isoniazid (2HRZE/4HR), with therapy administered daily throughout. Where this is not possible, an acceptable alternative is to use a thrice-weekly continuation phase. TB recurrence rates in HIV-coinfected patients are often higher than the rate of <5% typically observed in HIV-seronegative TB patients. This may be due to either relapse of incompletely cleared infection or to exogenous re-infection. Recurrence rates may be reduced by extending the duration of TB treatment (some guidelines suggest extending treatment from 6 to 9 months in patients who have evidence of slow therapeutic response) and by use of ART. In addition, secondary prophylaxis using isoniazid can be used after completion of TB treatment in settings where risk of exogenous re-infection is high.[17]

TRIMETHOPRIM–SULFAMETHOXAZOLE PROPHYLAXIS

TMP–SMX has been widely used in high-income countries for prophylaxis of HIV-infected patients against PJP, *Toxoplasma gondii* encephalitis and bacterial sepsis. Both observational and randomized controlled trials conducted in sub-Saharan Africa demonstrated that this simple intervention was associated with a substantial reduction in mortality (range, 19–46%) in patients with HIV-associated TB in the pre-ART era and that this survival benefit continues during ART.[33,34] Despite concerns over the high prevalence of bacterial resistance to this drug in some regions, survival benefit has nevertheless been demonstrated in these countries. Routine administration of TMP–SMX to patients with HIV-associated TB is recommended (480 mg twice per day or 960 mg once per day) and implementation has steadily increased over time, reaching 79% of all notified TB cases with a positive HIV test in 2012.

ANTIRETROVIRAL THERAPY

Benefits of ART

The benefits of ART for patients with HIV-associated TB are great. In observational cohort studies, ART reduces mortality risk by 64–95% in patients receiving treatment for HIV-associated TB.[35] In a randomized trial in South Africa, survival benefit was observed among those with CD4 cell counts of <200 cells/μL and 200–500 cells/μL.[36] Other reported benefits include shortening of the time to sputum smear and culture conversion and reduced TB recurrence rates. However, combined use of two multidrug regimens may be associated with drug–drug interactions, poor tolerability and higher rates of adverse drug reactions, which, for a long time led to considerable caution in managing such patients.[33,34] However, in recent years, optimum management and treatment guidelines described below have been informed by the emergence of data from observational studies and clinical trials.

Pharmacokinetic Interactions

Pharmacokinetic interactions between rifamycins (rifampin, rifapentine and rifabutin), non-nucleoside reverse transcriptase inhibitors (NNRTIs) and protease inhibitors (PIs) are mediated by the complex effects of these drug classes on the hepatic cytochrome P450 (CYP450) enzyme system. NNRTIs and PIs are substrates for these enzymes but

TABLE 96-1	Approaches to Co-treatment for HIV-Infected Patients with Rifampin-Susceptible Tuberculosis	
Combined Regimens	**Treatment Recommendations**	**Drug–Drug Interactions**
Efavirenz + rifampin-based TB treatment	No dose adjustments TDF + 3TC/FTC + EFV (WHO-recommended optimum regimen) AZT + 3TC + EFV (alternative WHO regimen)	Rifampin induces CYP2B6 but inhibition of CYP2A6 by isoniazid might account for increased efavirenz concentrations during TB treatment in those patients with slow CYP2B6 metabolizer genotype
Nevirapine + rifampin-based TB treatment	Omit 14 day lead-in phase of once-daily dose of NVP TDF + 3TC/FTC + NVP (alternative WHO regimen) AZT + 3TC + NVP (alternative WHO regimen)	Rifampin induces CYP2B6 and CYP3A4. Although TB treatment reduces nevirapine concentrations, toxicity concerns curtail increasing the dose and outcomes are acceptable (but inferior to EFV) on standard doses
Lopinavir/ritonavir + rifampin-based TB treatment	Double-dose lopinavir/ritonavir (800/200 mg 12 hourly) Or super-boost lopinavir (lopinavir/ritonavir 400/400 mg 12 hourly) Monitor alanine transaminase (ALT) closely	Rifampin induces CYP3A4, p-glycoprotein and OATP1B1. Ritonavir counteracts this effect and adjusted doses of ritonavir or lopinavir/ritonavir are used to compensate, but lopinavir concentrations may be more variable. Increased risk of hepatotoxicity, and gastrointestinal side effects
PI/ritonavir + rifabutin-based TB treatment	Reduce rifabutin dose to 150 mg daily or thrice weekly Monitor closely for rifabutin toxicity	Ritonavir-boosted PIs markedly increase rifabutin concentrations and reduce its clearance necessitating reduction in the dose of rifabutin by 50–75%. Toxicity (neutropenia, uveitis, hepatotoxicity, rash, gastrointestinal symptoms) and suboptimal rifamycin exposures with reduced dose are concerns
Triple nucleoside/tide regimen + rifampin-based TB treatment	No dose adjustments A triple nucleoside/tide regimen should include tenofovir or abacavir Monitor viral load	Triple nucleoside/tide regimens may perform adequately in patients with viral suppression who have not failed a first-line regimen, and provide alternative ART regimens in patients with contraindications to efavirenz or nevirapine, where other options are unavailable. TB treatment has minimal effect on tenofovir concentrations. Although rifampin induces the enzymes responsible for glucuronidation of abacavir and zidovudine, this effect is not thought to be clinically important

CYP, cytochrome P450; OATP, organic anion-transporting polypeptide; PI, protease inhibitor.

also act as inducers or inhibitors.[33] In contrast, the rifamycins act as potent inducers of this enzyme system, with rifampin having the greatest effect and rifabutin the least. They therefore cause reductions in plasma concentrations of the NNRTIs nevirapine and efavirenz by 30–40% and 20–25%, respectively. In addition, with the exception of ritonavir, plasma concentrations of PIs are reduced by approximately 80% due to enhanced hepatic metabolism and increased activity of the efflux multidrug transporter P-glycoprotein.

Various TB and ART regimens can be successfully combined (Table 96-1).[33] Despite reductions in concentrations of NNRTIs, excellent virologic outcomes have been reported using the standard 600 mg dose of efavirenz in combination with rifampin, and this is the first-choice recommendation in international guidelines.[37] Outcomes of nevirapine therapy may be undermined if the usual 200 mg per day lead-in dose is used in patients already receiving rifampin; preinduction of hepatic enzymes may reduce drug concentrations to subtherapeutic levels. Increased doses of nevirapine, however, are associated with greater toxicity and current WHO recommendations are to use NNRTIs at standard doses when combined with rifampin. A useful alternative strategy is to use rifabutin, which has less impact on the metabolism of NNRTIs. This agent is often used in high-income settings but availability is extremely limited in resource-limited settings.

Protease inhibitors do not achieve adequate plasma concentrations when combined with rifampin except when lopinavir or saquinavir is used in combination with ritonavir.[33] However, this frequently results in hepatotoxicity and there is substantial inter-patient variability in plasma concentrations, requiring therapeutic drug monitoring wherever possible.[33] A much better alternative is to use rifabutin, which is an effective alternative to rifampin that can be combined with most protease inhibitors. There is now increasing evidence that rifampin-based TB treatment can be successfully used in combination with integrase-inhibitor-based ART regimens.

Immune Reconstitution Inflammatory Syndrome
(see also Chapter 95)

TB treatment in HIV-negative patients may be associated with a transient worsening of clinical disease (paradoxical reactions) within the first weeks of initiation of therapy. However, the frequency of these reactions is greatly increased by concurrent use of ART. These paradoxical events, termed the TB immune reconstitution inflammatory syndrome (paradoxical TB-IRIS), result from the restoration of immune responses to mycobacterial antigens, and often occur within days or weeks of starting ART.[38] These most commonly present with fever, worsening respiratory disease and lymphadenopathy, but the possible manifestations are extremely diverse, especially in those with disseminated disease (Figure 96-6).[39] The proportion of patients affected ranges widely from 0 to over 40% depending on patient characteristics, the timing of ART initiation and case definitions used. Risk is higher the lower the baseline CD4 cell count, the greater the mycobacterial load and the shorter the delay between starting TB treatment and ART. A meta-analysis reported a summary risk estimate of 15.7%.[40] A small proportion of cases are life-threatening due, for example, to central nervous system involvement or extensive pulmonary disease. However, only approximately 3% of affected patients are estimated to die.

A second form of TB-IRIS is often referred to as 'unmasking' TB-IRIS.[38] This occurs when ART is started in patients in whom active TB remains undiagnosed. Rapid improvement in immune function leads to florid presentation of their TB during the initial weeks of ART. Effective screening for TB prior to ART is key to preventing this.

Symptoms and signs of TB-IRIS can usually be controlled by non-steroidal anti-inflammatory drugs or by use of corticosteroids in more severe cases. Doses of corticosteroid must be adjusted for rifampin interaction and tapered according to response. ART should be continued unless severe or life-threatening IRIS develops because of the ongoing risk of immunodeficiency-associated mortality. For most patients, the long-term prognosis is very good.

Optimal Timing of ART initiation

The optimum time to start ART in patients with HIV-associated TB is subject to a complex series of competing risks (Table 96-2). The high risk of morbidity and mortality in patients with very low CD4 cell counts while waiting to start ART must be balanced against the risk of

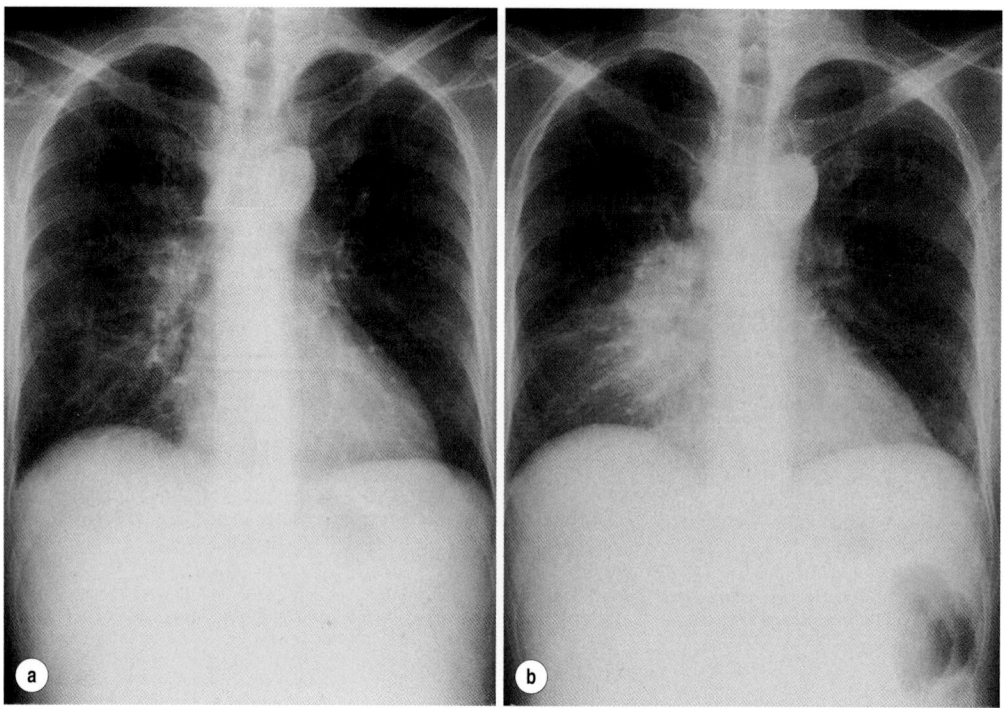

Figure 96-6 Chest radiographs illustrating tuberculosis (TB) immune reconstitution inflammatory syndrome (IRIS). This HIV-infected patient with advanced immunodeficiency had culture-confirmed drug-sensitive TB involving the right middle lobe of the lung and right hilar lymph nodes. This responded well to TB treatment with substantial resolution of the radiographic appearance over the first few weeks of treatment (a). Subsequent initiation of antiretroviral therapy resulted in a clinical and radiologic deterioration (b) and the tuberculin skin test converted from negative to strongly positive. *(Reproduced with permission from Meintjes G., Lawn S.D., Scano F., et al.: Tuberculosis-associated immune reconstitution inflammatory syndrome: case definitions for use in resource-limited settings. Lancet Infect Dis 2008; 8(8):516-23.)*

TABLE 96-2	Factors Favoring Either Early Initiation of Antiretroviral Therapy (ART) (During Intensive Phase of TB Therapy) or Delayed Initiation (During Continuation Phase)

Favors Early Initiation of ART	Favors Delayed Initiation of ART
Risk of further morbidity associated with advanced immunodeficiency Risk of mortality associated with advanced immunodeficiency Immune recovery may enhance mycobacterial clearance with the potential to shorten sputum conversion times and reduce risk of relapse	Avoids high pill burden during intensive phase of TB therapy, potentially improving tolerability and adherence Easier to diagnose and manage drug toxicities and risk of toxicity may be decreased Avoids pharmacokinetic drug interactions during intensive phase of TB therapy Lower risk of TB immune restoration disease

additive toxicities and TB-IRIS following ART initiation. Patients with baseline CD4 counts of <200 and 200–500 cells/μL have improved survival benefit from co-administered ART, and WHO recommends that ART be given to all patients concurrently with TB treatment regardless of the CD4 count.[37] Mortality is further reduced in those with CD4 cell counts <50 cells/μL if ART is started within the first 2 weeks of TB treatment. However, in those with higher CD4 cell counts, ART can be deferred until after completion of between 2 and 8 weeks of TB treatment without compromising survival but with the benefit of reducing the risk of TB-IRIS.[33] Patients with HIV-associated TB meningitis represent an important exception to this, with a randomized trial from Vietnam finding that survival was very poor regardless of the timing of ART.

DRUG-RESISTANT TUBERCULOSIS

MDRTB requires the use of a combination of a minimum of four effective drugs and XDR-TB requires the use of as many active drugs as can be achieved.[38] Mortality rates in HIV-infected and MDR- or XDR-TB patients are very high, even in specialized management programs. ART improves the prognosis of such patients. Due to slow clearance of mycobacterial antigen load, such patients may be at greater risk of developing TB-IRIS. Second line anti-TB drugs are associated with considerable adverse effects that overlap with those of ART drugs. In view of the high mortality risk, delays in initiation of ART should probably be minimized in those with MDRTB. There is a desperate need for new drug regimens for MDRTB.

References available online at expertconsult.com.

KEY REFERENCES

Abdool Karim S.S., Naidoo K., Grobler A., et al.: Timing of initiation of antiretroviral drugs during tuberculosis therapy. *N Engl J Med* 2010; 362(8):697-706.

Akolo C., Adetifa I., Shepperd S., et al.: Treatment of latent tuberculosis infection in HIV-infected persons. *Cochrane Database Syst Rev* 2010; (1):CD000171.

Getahun H., Kittikraisak W., Heilig C.M., et al.: Development of a standardized screening rule for tuberculosis in people living with HIV in resource-constrained settings: individual participant data meta-analysis of observational studies. *PLoS Med* 2011; 8(1):e1000391.

Harries A.D., Zachariah R., Corbett E.L., et al.: The HIV-associated tuberculosis epidemic – when will we act? *Lancet* 2010; 375(9729):1906-1919.

Lawn S.D., Butera S.T., Shinnick T.M.: Tuberculosis unleashed: the impact of human immunodeficiency virus infection on the host granulomatous response to *Mycobacterium tuberculosis*. *Microbes Infect* 2002;4(6):635-646.

Lawn S.D., Harries A.D., Williams B.G., et al.: Antiretroviral therapy and the control of HIV-associated tuberculosis. Will ART do it? *Int J Tuberc Lung Dis* 2011; 15(5):571-581.

Lawn S.D., Meintjes G., McIlleron H., et al.: Management of HIV-associated tuberculosis in resource-limited settings: a state-of-the-art review. *BMC Med* 2013; 11(1):253.

Lawn S.D., Mwaba P., Bates M., et al.: Advances in tuberculosis diagnostics: the Xpert MTB/RIF assay and future prospects for a point-of-care test. *Lancet Infect Dis* 2013; 13(4):349-361.

Lawn S.D., Wood R., De Cock K.M., et al.: Antiretrovirals and isoniazid preventive therapy in the prevention of HIV-associated tuberculosis in settings with limited health-care resources. *Lancet Infect Dis* 2010; 10(7): 489-498.

Lucas S.B., Hounnou A., Peacock C., et al.: The mortality and pathology of HIV infection in a West African city. *AIDS* 1993; 7(12):1569-79.

Meintjes G., Lawn S.D., Scano F., et al.: Tuberculosis-associated immune reconstitution inflammatory syndrome: case definitions for use in resource-limited settings. *Lancet Infect Dis* 2008; 8(8):516-523.

Samandari T., Agizew T.B., Nyirenda S., et al.: 6-month versus 36-month isoniazid preventive treatment for tuberculosis in adults with HIV infection in Botswana: a

randomised, double-blind, placebo-controlled trial. *Lancet* 2011; 377(9777):1588-1598.

Suthar A.B., Lawn S.D., Del Amo J., et al.: Antiretroviral therapy for prevention of tuberculosis in adults with HIV: a systematic review and meta-analysis. *PLoS Med* 2012; 9(7):e1001270.

World Health Organization: *Global tuberculosis report 2013.* Geneva: World Health Organization; 2013. Available: http://apps.who.int/iris/bitstream/10665/91355/1/9789241564656_eng.pdf.

97

Neoplastic Disease

CHRISTIAN HOFFMANN

KEY CONCEPTS

- Kaposi's sarcoma (KS) is among the most common malignancies in patients with human immunodeficiency virus (HIV) infection and has a strong association to human herpesvirus 8 (HHV-8).

- With initiation of combination antiretroviral therapy (cART), most KS lesions stabilize or even resolve completely without any other specific treatment.

- AIDS-related lymphomas (ARL) are biologically very heterogeneous and differ in their association with immune deficiency and with coinfections with oncogenic viruses.

- In contrast to ARL, the incidence of HIV-associated Hodgkin's lymphoma is not reduced with cART and it mainly occurs in patients receiving a virologically effective cART.

- Multicentric Castleman's disease (MCD) is a lymphoproliferative disease with malignant characteristics and a close association to HHV-8 which encodes a homologue of IL-6; HIV-related MCD must be considered when fever, splenomegaly and lymphadenopathy develop.

- The risk of non-AIDS-defining malignancies (non-ADM) is two to three times higher in HIV-infected patients than in the general population, with older age, smoking and low CD4+ T-cell counts as major risk factors.

- In higher-income countries, more deaths are now attributed to non-ADMs than to ADMs.

- Although there should be no difference in cancer treatment of HIV-infected and noninfected patients, interactions between antineoplastic agents and antiretroviral agents have to be considered.

Introduction

When compared with the general population, patients with human immunodeficiency virus (HIV) infection have an increased risk for the three acquired immunodeficiency syndrome (AIDS)-defining malignancies (ADMs): (1) Kaposi's sarcoma; (2) non-Hodgkin's lymphoma; and (3) cervical cancer. In addition, several non-AIDS-defining malignancies (non-ADMs), such as Hodgkin's lymphoma (HL), as well as cancers of the lung and anus, are found with increased incidence in patients living with AIDS.[1-3] With increasing age and demographic shifts of the HIV-infected population, these non-ADMs will gain further importance.[4,5] In this chapter, the epidemiology, pathogenesis, clinical features and management of the most common malignant tumors in patients with HIV infection are described.

Kaposi's Sarcoma

Kaposi's sarcoma (KS) is the most common malignancy in patients with HIV infection. Hungarian dermatologist Moritz Kaposi first described the disease in 1872. Classic KS clearly differs from HIV-associated KS, which may affect all skin and mucous membranes as well as lymph nodes and internal organs. The progression is very variable. Compared with the early years of the AIDS epidemic, the incidence of KS has fallen to less than a tenth of what it was.[6] The clinical

course of HIV-associated KS has also changed with the introduction of combination antiretroviral therapy (cART).

PATHOGENESIS

KS is characterized by abnormal neoangiogenesis, inflammation and proliferation of KS spindle cells which are considered the KS tumor cells. These cells are of endothelial cell origin, phenotypically most similar to lymphatic endothelial cells, but poorly differentiated. Since 1994, KS is known to be induced by infection with the human herpesvirus 8 (HHV-8) or Kaposi's sarcoma-associated herpesvirus (KSHV). HHV-8 can be always detected in the tumor tissue, and KS spindle cells are the predominant HHV-8-infected cells in KS.

Transmission of HHV-8 occurs predominantly via saliva, but also sexually, vertically and via blood products. The exact role of HHV-8 in the pathogenesis is not clear as infection with HHV-8 does not lead inevitably to KS. Interactions with the HIV-1 transcription activation factor Tat, possibly also with other viruses such as HHV-6 and HSV-1, change signal transduction pathways with an increased production of growth factors as well as cytokine dysregulation.[7] HHV-8 is also able to modulate pro-proliferative pathways to its advantage, while simultaneously inhibiting pro-apoptotic signaling pathways.

Among the HIV-positive population, gay men are almost the only ones affected by KS in Western countries. A severe immunodeficiency is not a prerequisite for the development of KS. Since the introduction of cART, many patients with HIV-associated KS have CD4+ T-cell counts above the level typically associated with susceptibility to opportunistic diseases.[4,5]

CLINICAL FEATURES

HIV-associated KS does not have a preferential pattern of localization. It can begin on any area of the skin, but may also appear on oral, genital, or ocular mucous membranes. Typical findings at presentation are a few asymptomatic purple macules or nodules. The tumors can remain unchanged for months to years, or grow rapidly within a few weeks and disseminate. Plaque-like and nodular KS lesions often become confluent and can be accompanied by massive lymphedema. In the oral cavity, the hard palate is frequently affected. Lesions begin with purplish erythema and progress to plaques and nodules that ulcerate easily. Regression of KS during treatment is not only indicated by reduction of the size of the lesions but also by change in color from dark to bright red.

DIAGNOSIS

Diagnosis is usually made based on clinical findings. However, in inconclusive cases a histologic diagnosis is recommended. Differential diagnosis includes other neoplasia such as cutaneous lymphomas or angiosarcoma, as well as infectious diseases such as syphilis and bacillary angiomatosis.

MANAGEMENT

If KS is newly diagnosed in an HIV-infected patient naïve to cART, cART should be initiated as a first step. Consequently, the majority of KS lesions stabilize or even resolve completely without any other specific treatment.[3,6] In patients with rapidly progressive disease or with visceral disease or lymphedema, cART should be combined with other KS therapies.

There are different treatment options, as follows (see also Table 97-1).

TABLE 97-1	Specific Therapies for Kaposi's Sarcoma When ART Alone is Not Sufficient	
Therapy	**Dosage**	**Comments**
Pegylated liposomal doxorubicin (Caelyx™ or Doxil™)	20 mg/m² iv every 2 weeks	Treatment of choice. Beware of myelotoxicity, cardiotoxicity, hand–foot syndrome
Liposomal daunorubicin (DaunoXome™)	40 mg/m² iv every 2–3 weeks	Slightly less effective than Caelyx™, seldom used but an important alternative given capacity constraints for Caelyx™
Interferon-α 2a (Roferon™)	3–6 x10⁶ IU sc 3x/week	Considerable side effects; less efficacious than with doxorubicin. Use only when CD4⁺ T cells are >200/μL and limited disease
Pegylated interferon-α 2b (PegIntron™)	50 μg sc weekly	Tolerability improved compared to conventional interferon-α. Off-label use, lack of data
Paclitaxel (Taxol™)	100 mg/m² iv every 2 weeks or 135 mg/m² iv every 3 weeks	Beware of neutropenia, peripheral neuropathy, allergic reactions, alopecia. Off-label use, caution with ART interactions

Chemotherapy

Pegylated liposomal doxorubicin hydrochloride (Caelyx™ or Doxil™) is the treatment of choice. Complete remission rates of up to 80% are possible. Usually 6–8 cycles are required to achieve a good clinical response. Beside Caelyx™, liposomal daunorubicin (DaunoXome™) or taxanes represent an alternative.

Immunotherapy

With interferons, remission rates seem to be lower than with pegylated liposomal doxorubicin. The effect mechanism of interferons on KS is not fully clarified. Apart from an immune modulating effect, interferon probably induces the apoptosis in KS cells. The effectiveness depends on the immune status.[4]

Local Therapy

Many different methods are used depending on the size and location of tumors: cosmetic camouflage, cryosurgery, intralesional injections of vinca alkaloids or interferons, soft X-ray radiation, electron beam therapy, cobalt radiation (fractionated) or imiquimod. As KS is a multifocal systemic disease, surgical treatment is limited to excisional biopsies for diagnosis and palliative removal of small tumors in cosmetically disturbing areas.

New Therapeutic Approaches

Several new therapies have been suggested, such as virustatic agents (valganciclovir), immunomodulating agents (lenalidomide, IL-12), inhibitors of angiogenesis (sirolimus, bevacizumab), new antineoplastic agents (imatinib, sorafenib) or retinoid compounds. However, these experimental compounds cannot be recommended outside clinical trials.[4,6]

Malignant Lymphomas

In comparison to the general population, HIV-infected patients are affected significantly more frequently by all types of lymphoma.[1] The incidence of lymphomas has been markedly reduced by the introduction of cART. However, this reduction overall has not been as impressive as with KS or most other opportunistic infections.[1,2,5]

Malignant lymphomas in HIV-infected patients are biologically very heterogeneous and differ in several aspects. The frequency and extent of oncogenic mutations or cytokine dysregulation differ, as does the histogenetic origin of the malignant cells. In addition, the association with Epstein–Barr virus (EBV) and other oncogenic viruses such as HHV-8 is very variable. HHV-8 is primarily linked to plasmablastic lymphoma, primary effusion lymphoma and to multicentric Castleman's disease;[8] EBV is found in almost all cases of primary central nervous system (CNS) lymphoma and HIV-associated Hodgkin's lymphoma.[9]

The extent of immunodeficiency also varies significantly. Whereas for some lymphoma subtypes, such as immunoblastic and primary CNS lymphoma, a severe immunodeficiency is required for the development of the tumor, for other lymphoma subtypes, such as Burkitt's lymphoma, chronic B-cell activation, possibly induced by even low HIV viremia, is a prerequisite. In this chapter, systemic non-Hodgkin's lymphoma (NHL), primary CNS lymphoma and Hodgkin's lymphoma will be discussed separately; multicentric Castleman's disease will also be mentioned as a distinct entity, although it is not considered a malignant lymphoma. Low-grade NHLs are very rare in HIV-infected patients, and will therefore not be discussed here.

Systemic Non-Hodgkin's Lymphomas

More than 90% of HIV-associated NHLs or AIDS-related lymphoma (ARL) are of B-cell origin. According to the WHO classification, 30–40% and 40–60% of ARL comprise Burkitt's lymphomas (BL) and diffuse large-cell B-cell lymphomas (DLBCL), respectively. Primary effusion, or body cavity-based, lymphomas are considered distinct but rare entities.

CLINICAL FEATURES

The main symptom is lymph node enlargement. B symptoms with fever, night sweats and/or weight loss are found in the majority of cases (60–80%). Extranodal involvement is common and involvement of every conceivable region of the body is possible.

DIAGNOSIS

A rapid histological diagnosis is essential. The basic pathological diagnosis should include information about the subtype of lymphoma, the proliferation rate and, if possible, the expression profile (CD20, and probably CD10, CD138, MUM-1), as these markers can have an impact on specific chemotherapy (see below).[10] All patients with suspected ARL should be staged according to the Ann Arbor classification (Table 97-2).

In advanced stages of the disease and/or cases with more than one extranodal involvement, a diagnostic lumbar puncture is advisable before initiating systemic chemotherapy to exclude meningeal involvement. However, controlled studies on the use of CNS-prophylaxis in HIV-associated DLBCL are not available and a standard procedure has not been defined.

MANAGEMENT

Every HIV-infected patient with systemic ARL should start cART, even in the setting of a preserved immune function. Some clinicians prefer to complete all six cycles due to concerns for interactions and cumulative toxicities. With the introduction of newer antiretrovirals such as raltegravir this seems no longer necessary. In Europe, diffuse large B-cell lymphomas have been treated for many years with CHOP-based regimens (usually six cycles, see Table 97-3). There are no randomized controlled trials comparing CHOP with other regimens such as CDE (cyclophosphamide/doxorubicin/etoposide) or EPOCH (etoposide/prednisone/vincristine/cyclophosphamide/doxorubicin),

TABLE 97-2	Staging According to the Updated Ann Arbor Classification
I	Involvement of a single lymph node region (I) or involvement of a single extralymphatic organ or site (IE)
II	Involvement of two or more lymph node regions on the same side of the diaphragm (II) or localized involvement of an extralymphatic organ or site plus its regional lymph nodes, with or without involvement of other lymph node regions on the same side of the diaphragm (IIE)
III	Involvement of lymph node regions on both sides of the diaphragm (III) can be accompanied by localized extralymphatic organ involvement (IIIE) or spleen involvement (IIIS) or both (IIIE+S)
IV	Diffuse or disseminated involvement of one or more extralymphatic organs with or without associated lymph node involvement; or isolated involvement of an extralymphatic organ with involvement of distal (non-regional) lymph nodes

Every Stage is Divided into Categories A and B:

A	Asymptomatic
B	General symptoms: (a) unexplained weight loss of more than 10% in the last 6 months, and/or (b) unexplained persistent or recurring fever with temperatures above 38°C, and/or (c) drenching night sweats

TABLE 97-3	CHOP Regimen*		
Cyclophosphamide	Endoxan®	750 mg/m² iv day 1
Doxorubicin	Doxo-Cell®, Adriblastin®	50 mg/m² iv day 1
Vincristine	Vincristin®	1.4 mg/m² (maximum 2 mg) iv day 1
Prednisolone	Decortin H®	2 tab. at 50 mg QD, days 1–5
Mesna	Uromitexan®	20% of cyclophosphamide dose at hours 0, 4, 8 (with reference to cyclophosphamide iv given as short infusion or orally)

*Four to six cycles of 3 weeks each; repeat on day 22.

which have been proposed by several working groups. These regimens, given for several days as infusions, are supposed to overcome the potential chemotherapy resistance of lymphoma cells.

In the case of CD20-positive B-cell lymphoma, it is not clear whether the monoclonal CD20 antibody rituximab has a similarly large clinical benefit for HIV-infected patients as it has for HIV-negative patients. Doubts were raised by a multicenter prospective and randomized US study, showing a higher incidence of severe bacterial infections in the rituximab group.[11] However, in a pooled analysis of 1546 patients from 19 prospective clinical trials, rituximab was associated with a higher overall survival.[1]

Beside DLBCL, there are special entities of ARL which require specific therapies.

Burkitt's or Burkitt-Like Lymphomas
Given the high proliferative capacity and aggressiveness of these entities, the CHOP regimen is not sufficient. There have been no randomized studies, but a modified dose-adapted protocol of the German multicenter study group for adult acute lymphoblastic leukemia (GMALL) and also a low-intensity EPOCH-R (rituximab)-based regimen may be effective in BL.

Plasmablastic Lymphomas
These lymphomas are probably DLBCL entities, but display a completely characteristic immune phenotype, which usually correlates to a post-germinal center cell. Intensive chemotherapy regimens do not seem to increase survival and the evaluation of new options such as bortezomib is urgently needed.

Primary Effusion Lymphoma
Primary effusion lymphoma (PEL), also called body cavity lymphoma, is a relatively rare entity of ARL in which a visible tumor mass is usually absent. Malignant cells can only be found in body cavities (e.g., pleural, pericardial, peritoneal), showing a non-B-, non-T phenotype. There is a close association with HHV-8, which can be detected in malignant cells.[8] The response to the CHOP regimen is usually poor.

Relapsing Disease
Given the low efficacy of different regimens in relapsed ARL, it should always be considered whether the affected patient qualifies for an autologous stem cell transplant (ASCT). The results are comparable to the HIV-negative population.[12]

Primary CNS Lymphomas
Primary CNS lymphoma (PCNSL) is defined as lymphoma presenting in the brain or spinal cord in the absence of systemic lymphoma. Histologically, findings are almost always consistent with DLBCL. An EBV-infection is found in almost 100% of cases. Due to its unique clinical, diagnostic and therapeutic features, it is discussed as a distinct entity here.

CLINICAL FEATURES
Different neurological deficits occur depending on the localization. Epileptic seizures may be the first manifestation of disease. Personality changes, changes in awareness, headaches and focal deficits such as paresis are also frequent.

DIAGNOSIS
A cranial computed tomography (CT) or magnetic resonance scan should be performed rapidly. A solitary non-encapsulated mass is usually more indicative of PCNSL. Besides cerebral toxoplasmosis, differential diagnoses include abscesses, glioblastoma and cerebral metastases of solid tumors. In the absence of increased intracranial pressure, lumbar puncture is advised. EBV DNA is commonly detected in the cerebrospinal fluid of HIV-infected patients.

MANAGEMENT
The decisive factor in PCNSL – independent of the specific therapy chosen – is the best possible immune reconstitution. With the introduction of cART, long-term remissions have become realistic.[13] All patients with PCNSL should therefore be treated intensively with cART, to achieve the best possible immune reconstitution. The prognosis for HIV-negative patients has improved in recent years due to the introduction of methotrexate-based (MTX) chemotherapies and possibly with the CD20 antibody rituximab. However, whether these results will be applicable in HIV-infected patients is not clear.[11,13]

Hodgkin's Lymphoma
The incidence of HL in HIV-infected patients is elevated by a factor of 5–15 compared to the HIV-negative population. Although it is clearly associated with immunodeficiency, HIV-related HL is not regarded as an AIDS-defining illness. There is evidence that the incidence of HIV-related HL is not reduced with cART.[2]

PATHOGENESIS
A striking difference to HL in seronegative patients is the predominance of cases with Reed–Sternberg (RS) cells, as well as the clear association with EBV infection, which is seen as an important etiologic factor. HIV-HL mainly occurs in subjects receiving a virologically effective cART.[10] Interestingly, patients whose CD4+ T-cell counts decline despite suppression of HIV replication, are at risk for HL.[2] These findings suggest altered turnover of peripheral T cells and/or trafficking into the inflammatory tumor microenvironment.

TABLE 97-4	ABVD Regimen*
Adriamycin (doxorubicin)	25 mg/m² iv days 1 + 15
Bleomycin	10 mg/m² iv days 1 + 15
Vinblastine	6 mg/m² iv days 1 + 15
Dacarbazine (DTIC)	375 mg/m² iv days 1 + 15

*Four double cycles, repeat on day 29. Due to strong emetogenicity of dacarbazine, 5HT3-receptor blocker antiemetics should always be administered, e.g., granisetron, tropisetron or ondansetron.

CLINICAL FEATURES

B symptoms occur in the majority of cases. Lymphomas are firm, immobile or hardly mobile and painless, and the distinction from NHL, HIV-related lymphadenopathy or tuberculous lymphadenitis is not possible. An advanced stage and extranodal involvement are frequent.

DIAGNOSIS

Staging is necessary as for NHL (see above). Diagnostic lymph node extirpation is even more important here than with NHL, as puncture only rarely allows diagnosis of HL. As with NHL, specimens should be sent to reference laboratories if possible.

MANAGEMENT

Risk-adapted treatment strategy in patients with HIV-related HL in accordance with standard treatment procedures established for HIV-negative patients with HL is recommended.[10] Patients with early favorable HIV-HL (Ann Arbor I–II, no risk factors) receive two to four cycles of ABVD (doxorubicin/bleomycin/vinblastine/dacarbazine) (Table 97-4) followed by 30 Gy of involved-field (IF) radiation. In patients with early unfavorable HIV-HL, four cycles of BEACOPP baseline (bleomycin/etoposide/doxorubicin/cyclophosphamide/vincristine/procarbazine/prednisone) or four cycles of ABVD + 30 Gy of IF radiation are administered. Six to eight cycles of BEACOPP baseline can be given in patients with advanced-stage HIV-HL. In patients with advanced HIV infection, BEACOPP can be replaced with ABVD. In the hitherto largest prospective trial, the complete remission rates for patients with early favorable, early unfavorable and advanced-stage HL were 96%, 100% and 86%, respectively.[10]

Multicentric Castleman's Disease

In comparison to the benign, localized hyperplasia of lymphatic tissue, first described by Benjamin Castleman in 1956, HHV-8-associated multicentric Castleman's disease (MCD), as it occurs in HIV infection, is a malignant lymphoproliferative disease. HIV-related MCD is not classified as a lymphoma or AIDS-defining illness.

PATHOGENESIS

The pathogenesis of the disease is not completely understood. However, there is a close (but not obligatory) association to HHV-8 infection. HHV-8 encodes a homologue of IL-6 that has been shown to be biologically active in several assays and whose activities mirror those of its mammalian counterparts. It also remains unclear why only a small proportion of patients with active HIV/HHV-8 coinfection develop HIV-related MCD and why many patients have a normal immune status and a low HIV plasma viremia at the time of diagnosis.[14] Progression to malignant lymphoma is frequent. However, in patients treated with rituximab, the lymphoma risk appears to be significantly lower.[13,14]

CLINICAL FEATURES

The main signs are the often significant lymph node enlargements, which are almost always combined with B symptoms, weakness and severe malaise. There is always massive splenomegaly. Hepatomegaly,

respiratory symptoms and edema are also seen in the majority of cases. The extent of symptoms may fluctuate considerably.

DIAGNOSIS

In every case of episodic flares of B symptoms and lymphadenopathy, the diagnosis of MCD must be considered. Diagnosis is made histologically after lymph node extirpation. The germinal centers of affected lymph nodes have a characteristic onion-skin appearance with vascular proliferation. C-reactive protein and HHV-8 DNA levels are useful parameters for monitoring the activity of HIV-related MCD and observing the effectiveness of MCD treatment.

MANAGEMENT

Life expectancy seems to have significantly improved with cART and the increased use of rituximab.[13,14] This monoclonal antibody against CD20-expressing cells is probably effective by eliminating or reducing the pool of HHV-8 infected B cells. Some experts advocate rituximab monotherapy in patients without organ involvement and rituximab with chemotherapy (etoposide or CHOP-based regimens) for more aggressive disease. A cART should always be given. For cases not responding to rituximab, other therapeutic approaches can be considered, among them valganciclovir or anti-IL-6 receptor antibodies such as siltuximab.

Non-AIDS-Defining Malignancies

The risk for non-ADMs overall is approximately two to three times higher in HIV-infected patients than in the non-infected population. In industrialized countries, more HIV-associated deaths are attributed to non-ADMs than to ADMs, hepatitis C or cardiovascular diseases.[5] Besides age and smoking, a low CD4+ T-cell count is a main risk factor for the development of a non-ADM. Other factors certainly play a role, such as lifestyle (mainly smoking, but also alcohol, UV exposure) or coinfections with HPV, HBV or HCV. cART seems to have little influence on the occurrence of non-ADMs. It remains controversial whether HIV-infected patients require cancer screening and preventive medical check-ups more frequently than HIV-negative patients. However, physicians should support smoking cessation, which remains the most important preventive procedure for malignant diseases. Avoidance of being overweight and ensuring a healthy lifestyle are possibly more helpful than expensive medical examinations.

Publications on different cancer entities have shown that HIV-infected patients benefit from the recent progress made in the oncological field. There should be no difference in treatment of HIV-infected and non-infected patients. This chapter discusses one entity in more detail, namely anal carcinoma.

Anal Carcinoma

Anal cancer rates are substantially higher for HIV-infected patients. According to a recent meta-analysis of 53 studies published before the end of 2011, the pooled anal cancer incidence is 46 per 100 000 men (95% CI, 31–60).[15] There seem to be marked differences in different regions of the world, with highest incidence rates in the USA and lower rates in Europe.

PATHOGENESIS

Anal carcinoma is strongly associated with infections with human papilloma virus (HPV) which infects the basal cells of the epithelium of skin and mucous membranes. HIV-infected patients commonly have coinfections with several oncogenic HPV subtypes.[15] HPV vaccines have proved protective for intraepithelial neoplasia among men who have sex with men.[16] Persistent HPV infection may lead to precancerous preliminary stages – the anal intraepithelial neoplasia (AIN). AIN is histologically graded depending on the degree of dysplasia as grade 1 (mild), grade 2 (moderate) or grade 3 (severe). Rates of progression to cancer in patients with precancerous lesions remain a matter of controversial debate. According to a recent meta-analysis, the risk seems to be substantially lower than for cervical precancerous lesions.[15]

CLINICAL FEATURES

The most common symptom in cases of anal carcinoma is rectal bleeding. Other symptoms are burning and pain during stool or pruritus. If an anal carcinoma has already developed, squamous cell carcinoma and, more seldom, transitory epithelial carcinoma are histologically present. The anal canal and sphincter can already be infiltrated at an early stage. Regional lymph nodes are affected depending upon where the anal carcinoma is localized. Deep-seated anal carcinomas infiltrate inguinal, central pelvic and high-lying mesentery. Distant metastases are rare. In addition to proctoscopy, endosonography and CT of the abdomen and the pelvis should be done if possible.

MANAGEMENT

Unfortunately, the absence of reliable evidence for any of the interventions used in AIN precludes any definitive guidance or recommendations for clinical practice.[17] With imiquimod or electrocautery, recurrence rates are substantial. If anal carcinoma manifests and the lesion is smaller than 2 cm, a continence-preserving operation is preferable. Larger lesions are treated with combined radio-chemotherapy. Although positive effects are not certain, HIV-infected patients with anal carcinoma should receive cART.

References available online at expertconsult.com.

KEY REFERENCES

Barta S.K., Xue X., Wang D., et al.: Treatment factors affecting outcomes in HIV-associated non-Hodgkin lymphomas: a pooled analysis of 1546 patients. *Blood* 2013; 122:3251-3262.

Bohlius J., Schmidlin K., Boué F., et al.: HIV-1-related Hodgkin lymphoma in the era of combination antiretroviral therapy: incidence and evolution of CD4+ T-cell lymphocytes. *Blood* 2011; 117(23):6100-6108.

Bower M., Dalla Pria A., Coyle C., et al.: Prospective stage-stratified approach to AIDS-related Kaposi's sarcoma. *J Clin Oncol* 2014; 32:409-414.

D:A:D Study Group: Factors associated with specific causes of death amongst HIV-positive individuals in the D:A:D Study. *AIDS* 2010; 24:1537-1548.

Gérard L., Michot J.M., Burcheri S., et al.: Rituximab decreases the risk of lymphoma in patients with HIV-associated multicentric Castleman disease. *Blood* 2012; 119:2228-2233.

Hentrich M., Berger M., Wyen C., et al.: Stage-adapted treatment of HIV-associated Hodgkin lymphoma: results of a prospective multicenter study. *J Clin Oncol* 2012; 30(33):4117-4123.

Kaplan L.D., Lee J.Y., Ambinder R.F., et al.: Rituximab does not improve clinical outcome in a randomized phase III trial of CHOP with or without rituximab in patients with HIV-associated non-Hodgkin's lymphoma: AIDS-malignancies consortium trial 010. *Blood* 2005; 106: 1538-1543.

Machalek D.A., Poynten M., Jin F., et al.: Anal human papillomavirus infection and associated neoplastic lesions in men who have sex with men: a systematic review and meta-analysis. *Lancet Oncol* 2012; 13:487-500.

98

Dermatologic Manifestations of HIV Infection/AIDS

MISHA M. MUTIZWA | MILAN J. ANADKAT

KEY CONCEPTS

- Nearly all individuals infected with human immunodeficiency virus (HIV) will present with a dermatologic complaint over the course of their infection.

- While patients with HIV often present with many of the commonplace dermatoses seen in the general population (e.g. psoriasis, viral warts), these conditions are more likely to be clinically atypical, severe, or treatment-refractory in the setting of immune dysregulation.

- Although antiretroviral therapy has significantly reduced the burden of HIV-associated cutaneous disease, the rare inflammatory, infectious and neoplastic dermatoses that emerged in the early years of the epidemic are still observed with surprising regularity.

- CD4 counts are still useful in compartmentalizing HIV-associated skin disease; however, epidemiologic shifts are occurring as patients are living longer with well-controlled disease.

- While newer treatment regimens are less likely to induce many of the side effects historically associated with antiretrovirals (e.g. lipodystrophy), the cutaneous manifestations of immune reconstitution are still commonly observed and have the potential to impact patient compliance.

Introduction

While antiretroviral therapy (ART) has dramatically reduced the burden of HIV-associated skin disease, HIV-infected individuals remain at considerable risk for the development of dermatologic sequelae. Indeed, the overwhelming majority of patients with HIV will present with a dermatologic complaint at some point over the course of their infection.[1] Since the start of the epidemic, it has become well-known that HIV-infected individuals can present with infectious, inflammatory and neoplastic skin conditions that are rarely seen in non-immunosuppressed cohorts. However, in the setting of HIV-induced immune dysregulation, even the commonplace dermatologic conditions seen in the general population are much more likely to be clinically atypical, severe, or treatment-refractory. Although the benefits of ART are irrefutable, all current classes of antiretrovirals also have the ability to impact the skin. Knowledge of these effects is of critical importance, as therapy-related dermatoses can be stigmatizing and can potentially impact patient compliance with medication regimens. This chapter provides a concise summary of the cutaneous manifestations of HIV infection.

Acute Exanthem of Primary HIV Infection

The acute exanthem of primary HIV infection may be seen in more than half of newly infected patients.[2] When present, it typically manifests within 6 weeks of transmission, and develops in conjunction with the fevers, myalgia, arthralgia, pharyngitis and lymphadenopathy that characterize the classic mononucleosis-like syndrome of primary HIV infection. The rash may be limited or widespread, is often asymptomatic, and is typically characterized by ill-defined erythematous maculopapules. Macular erythema or superficial erosions of the oral mucosa can also sometimes be observed.[3] The acute exanthem of primary HIV infection spontaneously resolves, typically within 2 weeks of development.

Inflammatory Dermatoses

SEBORRHEIC DERMATITIS

Seborrheic dermatitis is a chronic, inflammatory disease triggered by the presence of the ubiquitous yeast *Malassezia furfur*. While it is unknown why some people develop seborrheic dermatitis in response to *Malassezia* spp. while others do not, HIV infection is a well-established association. Indeed, the prevalence of seborrheic dermatitis is increased in all patients with HIV, although its severity tends to correlate with the degree of clinical deterioration (i.e. CD4 count).[4] Clinically, the rash presents as greasy, 'bran-like', white to yellow scaling in characteristic areas such as the scalp, ears, eyebrows, eyelids, glabella and nasal folds. Severe dermatitis can also involve areas such as the central chest and axillae, and is seen more commonly in the setting of HIV. The disease is variably symptomatic, with itch being reported by a minority of patients. Initial attempts at treatment most often involve medicated antidandruff shampoos (e.g. ketoconazole, coal tar and selenium sulfide), topical antifungals and topical steroids or calcineurin inhibitors. While the vast majority of patients respond well to topical therapies, severe or refractory cases can be treated with oral antifungals, isotretinoin or phototherapy.

ECZEMA, XEROSIS AND PRURITUS

Patients with HIV are at increased risk of both xerosis (i.e. skin dryness) and eczema/dermatitis when compared with the general population.[4] Patients with a history of childhood atopic dermatitis that has been quiescent in adulthood can commonly experience a recurrence of disease after HIV infection. Other patients with HIV can develop eczema/dermatitis for the first time in the months to years following infection. Clinically, the acute lesions of eczema classically manifest as pruritic, coalescent erythematous papules and plaques on the extremities and trunk. As patients are prone to excoriate these lesions, eventually they become chronic, with distinct morphologic features. The chronic lesions of eczema can appear as discrete, thickened, scaly plaques with accentuation of skin lines (termed lichenification), or as firm, dome-shaped, excoriated papulonodules (termed prurigo nodules).

For patients with xerosis, thorough dry skin care education is indicated, and liberal use of emollients should be advised. For those with eczema/dermatitis, treatment is similar to that in the general population, with topical steroids, calcineurin inhibitors and oral antihistamines being first line. Severe or refractory cases often respond well to phototherapy, typically narrowband UV-B (NBUVB). Thalidomide has been used with excellent results in the treatment of severe cases of HIV-associated prurigo nodularis.[5] Immunosuppressive agents should, in general, be avoided in the setting of HIV due to increased risk of severe or life-threatening infection.

While eczema and xerosis are highly associated with pruritus, it is worth noting that patients with HIV commonly itch, even in the absence of rash.[6] The reasons for this are unclear and treatment can be difficult. Over-the-counter topical preparations containing camphor and menthol, mild topical steroids and oral antihistamines can be tried. For refractory cases of pruritus, phototherapy may be beneficial.

The term pruritic papular eruption (PPE) has been applied to an intensely pruritic condition commonly seen in patients with advanced HIV disease in low- and middle-income countries, particularly in sub-Saharan Africa. Although the etiology of PPE has been extensively debated, most experts consider it to be a generalized, exuberant hypersensitivity reaction to insect bites.[7] Clinically, patients present with extensive, skin-colored to hyperpigmented excoriated papules. Although individually the lesions of PPE may resemble prurigo nodules or other eczematoid lesions, the overall presentation of PPE is distinct, and use of the term PPE should be avoided in patients living within the industrialized world.

PSORIASIS

In HIV-infected individuals, psoriasis can manifest as either new-onset psoriasis or as worsening of disease that predated infection. Although the prevalence of psoriasis, and psoriatic arthritis, is higher in all patients with HIV when compared to non-infected individuals, more severe disease is commonly seen in patients with lower CD4 counts.[8] In addition to the classic silvery scales seen in common plaque psoriasis, guttate, inverse and erythrodermic variants are commonly encountered in the setting of HIV. A reactive arthritis-like presentation of psoriasis can also be seen.[9]

Topical therapies, specifically topical steroids and vitamin D analogs, are considered first line in the treatment of psoriasis in all patients. For HIV-infected individuals with extensive or refractory disease, phototherapy (NBUVB or psoralen UV-A) or the oral retinoid acitretin should be considered (Figure 98-1). Of note, phototherapy and acitretin are therapeutically synergistic, with their combined use resulting in fewer side effects than would be expected when either is used as monotherapy. The use of systemic immunosuppressive agents in the setting of HIV is to be discouraged, as additional immunosuppression increases the risk of severe or potentially life-threatening infection. When deemed necessary, the authors would favor the use of cyclosporine or methotrexate over tumor necrosis factor-alpha inhibitors, as few data exist regarding the safety of this class of medication in HIV-infected individuals. It is important to note that antiretrovirals themselves have consistently been shown to improve psoriasis.[10] Accordingly, initiation or resumption of ART should be considered in all patients with HIV-associated psoriasis, regardless of their planned use of other therapies.

APHTHOUS STOMATITIS

Aphthous ulcers most commonly present at the oral mucosa as round-to-ovaline ulcerations of variable depth with raised, hyperemic borders. The center of each lesion is often covered with a white, grey, or yellow pseudomembrane. While aphthae are commonly encountered in the general population, HIV-infected individuals tend to have larger, more painful lesions that heal slowly and frequently recur. Lesions larger than one centimeter are termed major aphthae, and are most commonly seen in patients with CD4 counts lower than 100 cells/μL. In one large study of HIV-infected individuals, the prevalence of major aphthae was more than 3%.[11] While lesions most frequently occur on mobile, non-keratinized oral mucosal surfaces, esophageal and anogenital aphthae are not uncommon in the setting of HIV. The etiology of aphthae is unclear.

Treatment of aphthous stomatitis can be difficult. Direct application of potent topical steroids to individual lesions is often beneficial. Topical anesthetics can be helpful in managing the pain that can be associated with these lesions. Lesions not responding to topical therapy may require intralesional or systemic corticosteroids. Immunomodulating agents have also been used successfully, with thalidomide being the most consistently beneficial systemic therapy.[12] It is the authors' treatment of choice for severe or refractory disease (Figure 98-2).

EOSINOPHILIC FOLLICULITIS

Eosinophilic folliculitis is a culture-negative dermatosis characterized by an eosinophil-rich inflammatory infiltrate in or around the hair follicle. It is not commonly encountered outside the setting of HIV infection and typically presents in patients with CD4 counts below 200 cells/μL.[13] Clinically it is characterized by intensely pruritic, erythematous, follicularly based papules located on the upper trunk, face, neck and scalp. In contrast to bacterial folliculitis, with eosinophilic

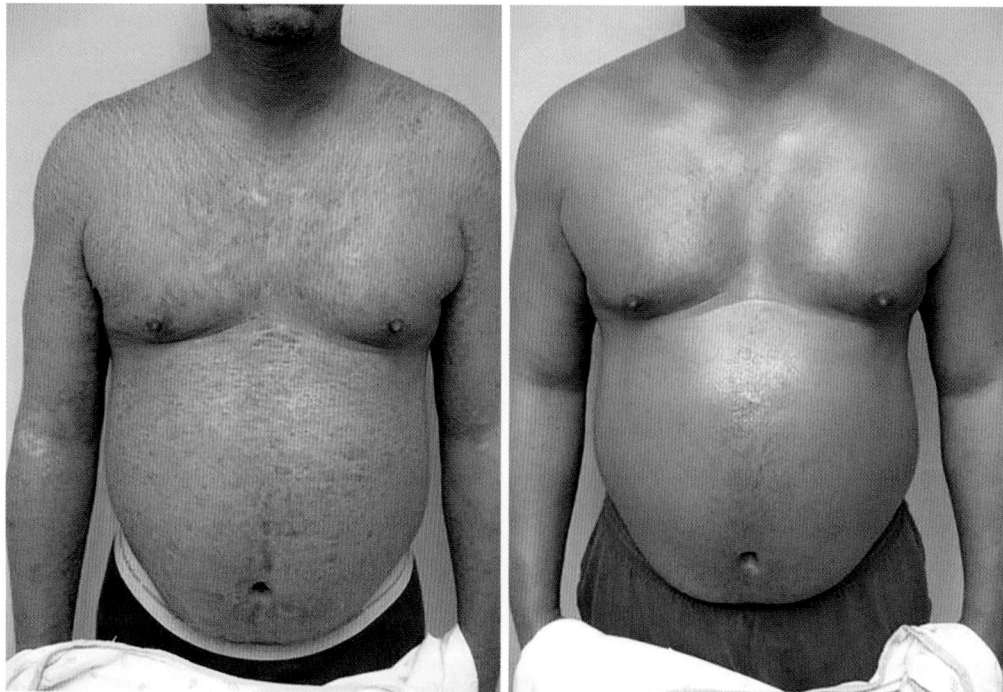

Figure 98-1 Clearance of extensive plaque psoriasis after treatment with oral acitretin and NBUVB phototherapy.

folliculitis pustules are sterile, and less commonly encountered. Often the associated pruritus is so severe that the clinician only sees follicularly based erosions, resulting from excoriation.

The clinical course of eosinophilic folliculitis is variable, and lesions tend to wax and wane in crops. Unlike in other forms of folliculitis, topical steroids and oral antihistamines are first-line treatment for mild disease. Phototherapy, tetracycline-family oral antibiotics, isotretinoin and itraconazole are common treatments for severe or refractory cases, with some experts considering itraconazole to be the treatment of choice for extensive disease. Eosinophilic folliculitis can initially present or worsen in the weeks to months following initiation or resumption of ART as a manifestation of the immune reconstitution inflammatory syndrome.[14] In these cases, ART should always be continued, with the above therapies being used as adjuncts until the disease resolves, usually after several months.

HIV PHOTODERMATITIS

HIV photodermatitis is a term used to describe a group of photodistributed rashes encountered in up to 5% of HIV-infected individuals.[15] Classically it is observed in patients with CD4 counts below 50 cells/μL. Interestingly, despite the inherent photoprotection conferred by deeply pigmented skin, HIV photodermatitis is most commonly encountered in patients of African origin, even when confounding factors like CD4 count and UV-index are controlled for.

The clinical manifestations of HIV photodermatitis are diverse, with the lichenoid morphology, characterized by violaceous papules and plaques, being most common. Eczematous, hyperpigmented and vitiliginous (i.e. depigmented) variants are also commonly seen. Regardless of morphology, the rash presents in photoexposed areas, such as the face, dorsal hands and forearms, neck and upper chest (Figure 98-3). In advanced disease, the rash can extend beyond sun-exposed areas. Exposure to certain medications, trimethoprim–sulfamethoxazole in particular, can be photosensitizing and increase the risk of HIV photodermatitis. Treatment can be difficult, and initial efforts should involve strict photoprotection and topical steroids. Thalidomide has been shown to be potentially useful in refractory cases.[16]

Infectious Dermatoses

VIRAL INFECTIONS

Human Papillomavirus (HPV)

HPV-induced lesions are extremely common in the setting of HIV infection, and represent the most common dermatologic condition for which patients seek treatment in the dedicated HIV Dermatology Clinic at one of the authors' institutions. Depending on the cutaneous site and HPV strain involved, HPV infection can manifest as common warts (HPV strains 2 and 7), plantar warts (HPV 1, 2 and 4), flat warts (HPV 3 and 10) and anogenital warts (HPV 6 and 11). In HIV-infected individuals, these lesions can be extensive, and can present in atypical locations, such as the oral mucosa. A presentation of cutaneous infection with HPV strains 5 and 8, uniquely seen in patients with HIV or

other causes of defective cell-mediated immunity, has been termed acquired epidermodysplasia verruciformis.[17] These lesions classically present as hyper- or hypopigmented macules or flat-topped papules on the face, trunk and upper extremities.

In the setting of HIV infection, benign HPV-induced lesions are often refractory to standard treatments. In general, physically destructive (e.g. cryotherapy) and anti-mitotic (e.g. intralesional bleomycin) treatment modalities are more likely to be successful than the immunologic therapies commonly employed in non-HIV-infected individuals (e.g. topical imiquimod), presumably because of HIV-associated defects in cellular immunity. Patients with anogenital and, to a lesser extent, oral mucosal lesions in particular should be managed aggressively, and screened for malignancy due to frequent coinfection with high-risk HPV strains (e.g. 16 and 18). It is the authors' opinion that all patients with anal involvement should undergo anoscopic evaluation to assess for internal extension.

Herpes Simplex Virus (HSV)

While epidemiologic studies have consistently demonstrated that HSV infection (HSV-2 in particular) is more prevalent in HIV-positive individuals, the course of HSV infection in patients with normal CD4 counts appears to be similar to that seen in the general population.[18] With advanced immunosuppression, however, HSV infection can manifest atypically with areas of extensive, chronic ulceration – most commonly perineal – or with hypertrophic lesions that can resemble tumors (Figure 98-4).[19]

Treatment of HSV should typically be initiated with either aciclovir or valaciclovir, using dosing regimens designed for use in immunosuppressed patients. In patients with extensive ulcerative or hypertrophic lesions, treatment should be continued until complete healing occurs, which may take weeks to months. Once healing does occur, suppressive therapy should generally be initiated. In patients with cutaneous lesions that are refractory to treatment, aciclovir resistance should be considered, as this is much more common in HIV-infected individuals than in those who are HIV-negative. Typically, these patients have a history of recurrent HSV infection and extensive prior treatment with aciclovir or valaciclovir. In these cases, intravenous foscarnet or cidofivir are appropriate alternatives. Topical imiquimod and compounded topical cidofivir have also been used for this indication.[20]

Cytomegalovirus (CMV)

Cutaneous CMV infection in the setting of HIV most commonly presents as chronic perineal ulceration in patients with CD4 counts <50 cells/μL.[21] While primary CMV-induced ulceration has been reported, it typically is cultured at sites of HSV-induced ulceration, and in these cases is thought to represent a secondary co-localization phenomenon and not primary infection. Accordingly, treatment should be targeted to the inciting HSV infection.

Varicella-Zoster Virus (VZV)

While the introduction of antiretroviral therapy (ART) has decreased the overall incidence of herpes zoster resulting from reactivation of

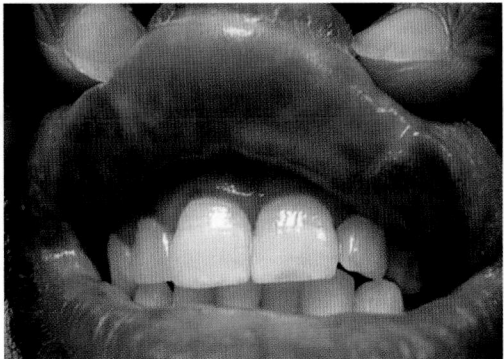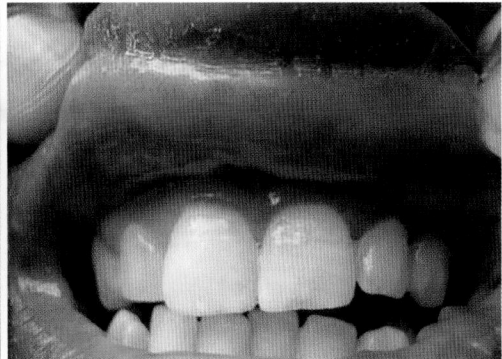

Figure 98-2 Clearance of major aphthae after treatment with thalidomide.

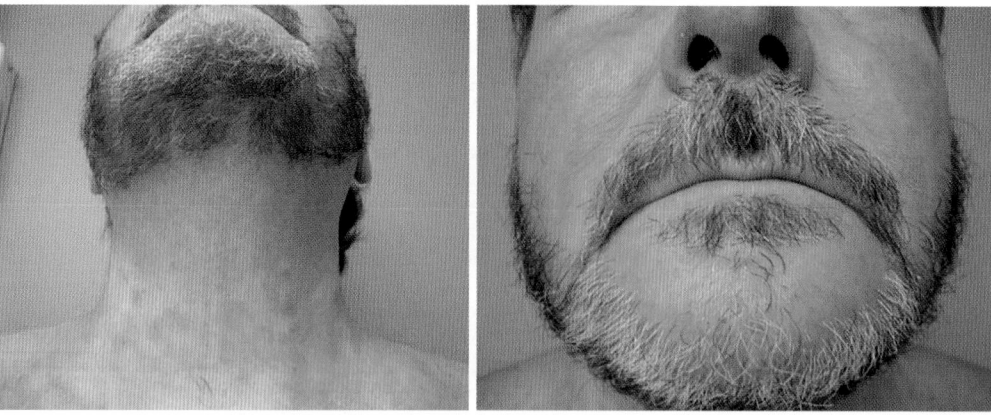

Figure 98-3 HIV photodermatitis with classic submental sparing.

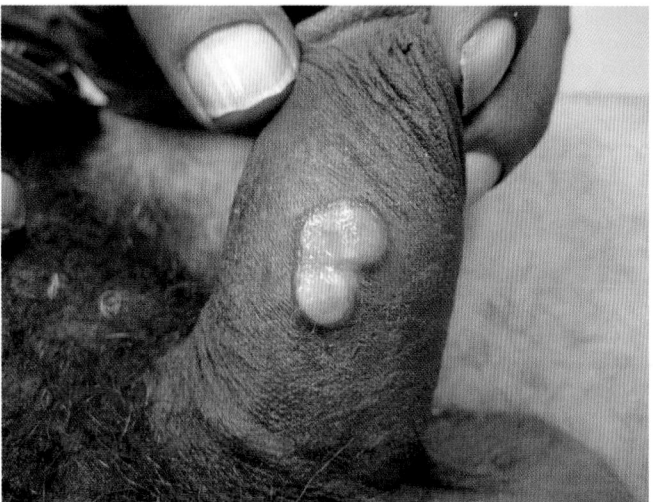

Figure 98-4 Hypertrophic herpes (herpes vegetans). While herpes lesions are rarely exophytic, the characteristic scalloped border of the lesion seen here was suggestive of HSV infection.

latent VZV infection, patients with HIV (even those who are well controlled) are up to 10 times more likely to develop zoster than the general population.[22] The increased risk for development of zoster in the weeks to months following initiation of ART is also a well-recognized phenomenon. Whether this represents an immune reconstitution inflammatory phenomenon is an area of active debate. In addition to the conventional forms of herpes zoster seen in immunocompetent patients, HIV-infected individuals have a higher incidence of atypical presentations (e.g. multidermatomal involvement, verruciform morphologies) and disseminated disease. Despite prompt initiation of appropriately dosed antivirals, clinical courses can sometimes be protracted, with increased risk of long-term sequelae, most commonly in the form of hypertrophic scarring and postherpetic neuralgia.

In HIV-positive individuals without a history of prior VZV infection or immunization, primary varicella is also a concern. The early lesions of varicella are vesicular, and the rash is preceded by a constitutional prodrome. Eventually these lesions ulcerate and form crusted scabs. The simultaneous presence of lesions at multiple stages of evolution is the hallmark of primary varicella infection (Figure 98-5). Patients with HIV are at increased risk of potentially life-threatening complications, and therapy should be initiated promptly with appropriately dosed antivirals. In the setting of immunosuppression, intravenous aciclovir is typically advised.

Molluscum Contagiosum Virus (MCV)

While MCV infection is commonly encountered in immunocompetent children and young adults, the presence of molluscum contagiosum in adults should raise suspicion for HIV infection, particularly in the setting of extensive or morphologically-atypical lesions. Molluscum contagiosum is most commonly encountered in HIV-infected individuals with CD4 counts less than 200 cells/µL.[23] In this setting, these lesions are typically encountered on the face and often lack the classic dome shape and central umbilication seen in healthy children and young adults. Lesions greater than one centimeter in diameter are termed giant molluscum, and are most commonly encountered in patients with CD4 counts less than 50 cells/µL. Treatment of molluscum contagiosum in the setting of HIV can be difficult, and most commonly involves destructive therapies (e.g. curettage and cryotherapy). Compounded topical and intravenous cidofivir has been used successfully in the treatment of extensive or refractory molluscum.[24]

Epstein–Barr Virus (EBV)

Oral hairy leukoplakia (OHL) is an EBV-induced form of benign, mucosal hyperplasia. Its development is highly associated with HIV infection. While it can occur even in well-controlled patients with HIV, it is typically seen in the setting of moderate to severe immunosuppression, with the median CD4 count of patients with OHL in one series determined to be 235 cells/µL.[25] Clinically, OHL presents as white, papillated or verrucous plaques, most commonly at the lateral tongue. Involvement of the buccal mucosa has also been reported. Unlike in oropharyngeal candidiasis, the plaques of OHL are not easily removed with physical maneuvers, such as scraping.

As OHL is generally asymptomatic, treatment beyond initiation or resumption of antiretroviral therapy is typically not indicated. In the minority of patients who report associated dysesthesias, high-dose aciclovir or valaciclovir may be beneficial. Unfortunately, once antiviral therapy is discontinued, OHL often recurs.

BACTERIAL INFECTIONS

Meticillin-Resistant Staphylococcus aureus

Compared to the general population, HIV-infected individuals have an increased prevalence of meticillin-resistant *Staphylococcus aureus* (MRSA) colonization and an accordingly increased rate of MRSA soft-tissue infections.[26] MRSA soft-tissue infections commonly present as furuncles or carbuncles, but can also be encountered as folliculitis and cellulitis. Treatment should be guided by the depth of the lesions. Superficial infections can often be treated with topical antimicrobials, such as mupirocin ointment. Antimicrobial washes (e.g. chlorhexidine and benzoyl peroxide), are extremely useful in the treatment of widespread superficial MRSA infections. Deeper lesions should be treated with appropriate systemic antimicrobials and, in the case of frank abscesses, incision and drainage is indicated. MRSA decolonization

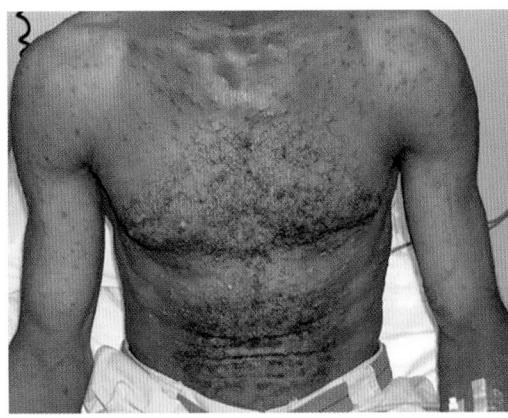
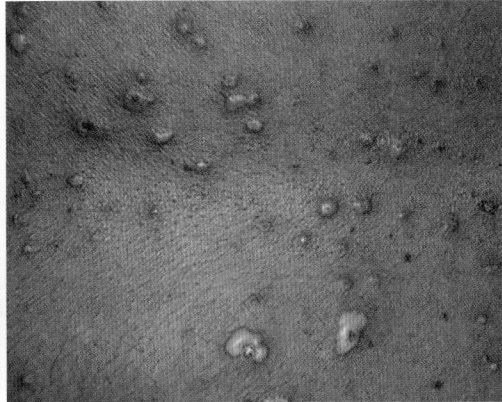

Figure 98-5 Primary varicella-zoster virus infection in a patient with HIV. Note the presence of lesions at different stages of evolution.

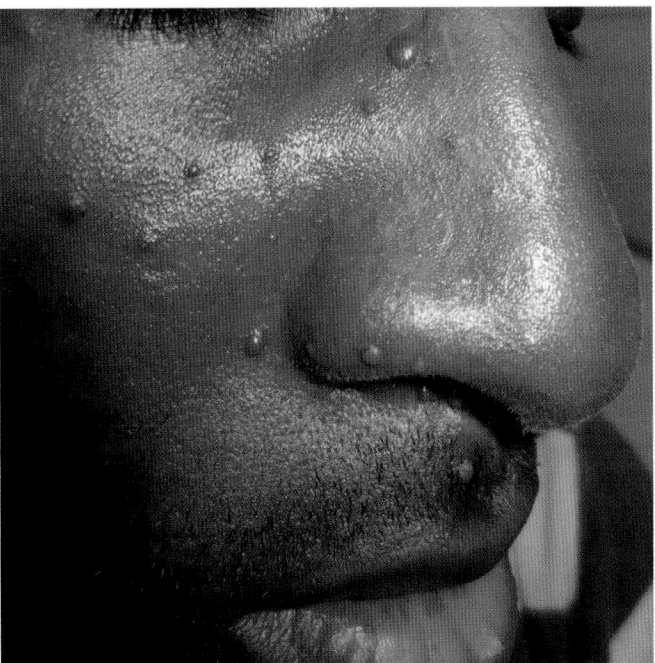

Figure 98-6 The classic dome-shaped, vascular papulonodules of bacillary angiomatosis.

efforts (e.g. cycles of mupirocin to the nares and full-body chlorhexidine washes) should be considered in patients with severe or frequently recurrent MRSA soft-tissue infection.

Bartonella

In the era of effective ART, the incidence of bacillary angiomatosis, caused by the gram-negative organisms *Bartonella hensleae* and *B. quintana*, is low. Whilst most commonly involving the skin, the lymph nodes, bone and viscera can also be affected. Cutaneous manifestations of *Bartonella* spp. infection are typically seen only in patients with CD4 counts lower than 250 cells/μL, with a median count of 21 cells/μL being reported in one case–control study.[27] Skin lesions most commonly present as dome-shaped, vascular papulonodules (Figure 98-6). More developed lesions can have a friable, eroded appearance, resembling pyogenic granulomas. Less commonly, bartonellosis can present in the skin as subcutaneous, cellulitic plaques. In these cases, skin involvement often overlies a focus of osseous involvement.

Diagnosis is made through biopsy of skin lesions, when present, with Warthin–Starry staining being used to confirm the presence of the causative organism. Indirect fluorescence antibody testing and blood culture are useful supplemental investigations. While oral erythromycin is the most commonly cited treatment in the literature, it is the authors' opinion that doxycycline is generally the most appropriate therapy for bacillary angiomatosis, given the potential interactions between macrolides and the agents used in common antiretroviral regimens. Treatment should be continued for 3–4 months.

FUNGAL INFECTIONS

Superficial Dermatophytosis

Whether superficial infection with dermatophyte species is more prevalent in patients with HIV than in the general population is unclear. Regardless, it is not uncommon to see extensive or atypically presenting superficial dermatophyte infections in HIV-positive individuals. Onychomycosis is also a commonly encountered problem, and uncommon presentations that are fairly specific to HIV-infected individuals can be seen. One such example is proximal white subungual onychomycosis, an entity characterized by infection of the proximal nail-plate with *Trichophyton rubrum*.[28] Treatment of localized, cutaneous dermatophyte infections can be achieved with topical agents, most commonly azole antifungals or terbinafine. For extensive infection or for infections involving the hair follicle (e.g. Majocchi's granuloma) or nail-plate, oral antifungals are indicated.

Candida

Oropharyngeal candidiasis (i.e. thrush) is the most common oral manifestation of HIV.[29] It is typically seen in patients with CD4 counts lower than 500 cells/μL and is frequently encountered as a presenting sign of infection. Clinically, oropharyngeal candidiasis is characterized by creamy white plaques on the oral mucosa that can be easily scraped off with a tongue blade (Figure 98-7). While *Candida albicans* is the most common species cultured from lesions of oropharyngeal candidiasis, *C. dubliniensis, C. glabrata* and *C. tropicalis* are all known causes. Treatment can be either topical (e.g. nystatin 'swish and spit' suspension, clotrimazole troches) or oral (e.g. fluconazole). Vulvovaginal candidiasis is a common problem in HIV-infected females, although it is unclear whether its prevalence is significantly increased when compared to the general population. As is the case with oropharyngeal candidiasis, both topical and oral antifungal agents can be used in the treatment of vulvovaginal candidiasis.

Disseminated Fungal Infections

In patients with severe immunosuppression, disseminated fungal infections are not uncommon, and can often present with characteristic skin findings. Disseminated fungal infections are seen almost exclusively in patients with CD4 counts of 100 cells/μL or lower.[30] The organisms associated with disseminated fungal infection in patients with HIV are summarized in Table 98-1. With the exception of sporotrichosis and, to a lesser extent, blastomycosis, primary skin involvement is exceedingly rare, and cutaneous lesions, when present, represent disseminated

TABLE 98-1	Characteristics of Disseminated Fungal Infections in HIV-Infected Individuals			
Pathologic Agent	**Geographic Distribution**	**Cutaneous Manifestations**		**Systemic Involvement**
Cryptococcus neoformans	Worldwide	Molluscum-like or erythematous papulonodules, pustules, cellulitis; oral mucosal ulceration		Pulmonary, CNS, musculoskeletal most common
Histoplasma capsulatum	Central and southeastern USA, South America	Erythematous to violaceous macules, papules, or nodules, molluscum-like papulonodules (Figure 98-8), pustules; ulceration of skin or mucosa		Pulmonary, gastrointestinal, and CNS
Coccidioides immitis	Southwestern USA, Central and South America	Molluscum-like or erythematous papulonodules; ulcers, abscesses		Pulmonary and CNS
Blastomyces dermatitidis	North America (Great Lakes region and Mississippi, Missouri and Ohio river basins)	Erythematous to violaceous papulopustules, verrucous plaques, subcutaneous nodules; abscesses, ulceration		Pulmonary, musculoskeletal, genitourinary, CNS
Paracoccidiodes brasiliensis	Central and South America	Oral or nasal erythematous to violaceous indurated plaques or ulcers		Pulmonary, gastrointestinal, musculoskeletal
Sporotrichosis schenckii	Worldwide	Fixed plaques, nodules (sometimes ulcerated) following course of lymphatics		Pulmonary, CNS, lymphoreticular, musculoskeletal
Penicillium (Talaromyces) marneffei	Asia	Molluscum-like or skin colored to erythematous papulonodules or abscesses at face, chest, extremities; orogenital exudative erosions or ulcerations		Pulmonary, lymphoreticular
Aspergillus fumigatus, Aspergillus flavus	Worldwide	Erythematous to violaceous papulonodules or plaques; necrotic ulcerations		Pulmonary, CNS, musculoskeletal

CNS, central nervous system.
Reproduced from Ramos-e-Silva M., Lima C.M., Schechtman R.C., et al.: Systemic mycoses in immunodepressed patients (AIDS). Clin Dermatol 2012; 30(6):616-627.

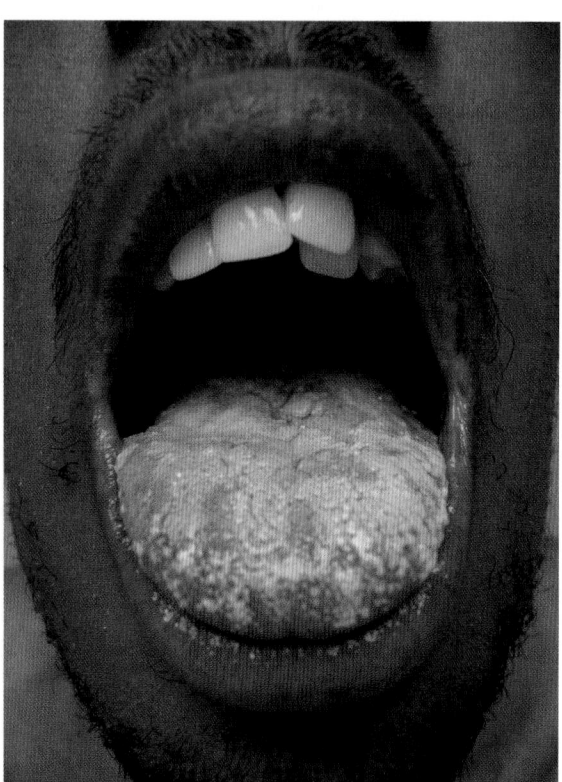

Figure 98-7 Oropharyngeal candidiasis. These creamy, white plaques are easily removed with a tongue depressor.

infection, most commonly from pulmonary inoculation. Accordingly, patients are typically ill-appearing. Treatment should be promptly initiated according to the recommendations of infectious disease specialists (see Chapter 94).

OTHER COMMON CUTANEOUS INFECTIONS AND INFESTATIONS

While they often do not represent a direct effect of HIV infection, a variety of common skin infections and infestations are seen at increased rates in HIV-infected individuals. This is likely attributable to common sociologic and behavioral risk factors. The authors believe that syphilis and scabies are particularly important for clinicians to be aware of, as atypical presentations of both entities in the setting of HIV can be seen (e.g. development of secondary syphilis symptoms prior to the resolution of the primary chancre, crusted scabies, etc.). These entities are generally treated as they would be in immunocompetent patients. However, it is important to note that in cases of crusted scabies, oral ivermectin should be used in conjunction with topical permethrin.

Cutaneous Malignancies

BASAL CELL CARCINOMA, SQUAMOUS CELL CARCINOMA AND MELANOMA

With the advent of ART, non-melanoma skin cancer (NMSC), a term used to collectively refer to basal cell carcinoma (BCC) and squamous cell carcinoma (SCC), has become the most common cutaneous malignant neoplasm encountered in patients with HIV.[31] Irrespective of CD4 count, patients with HIV are at increased risk of both NMSC and melanoma compared to non-HIV-infected individuals. The relative incidence of these entities in patients with HIV mirrors that seen in the general population, with BCC, followed by SCC, being most common. Recent data suggest that HIV infection, regardless of CD4 count, increases the risk of post-treatment recurrence, particularly with SCCs.[32] In addition to photo-induced SCCs developing in sun-exposed areas, patients with HIV are at increased risk of developing HPV-induced intraepithelial neoplasia and SCCs, most commonly of

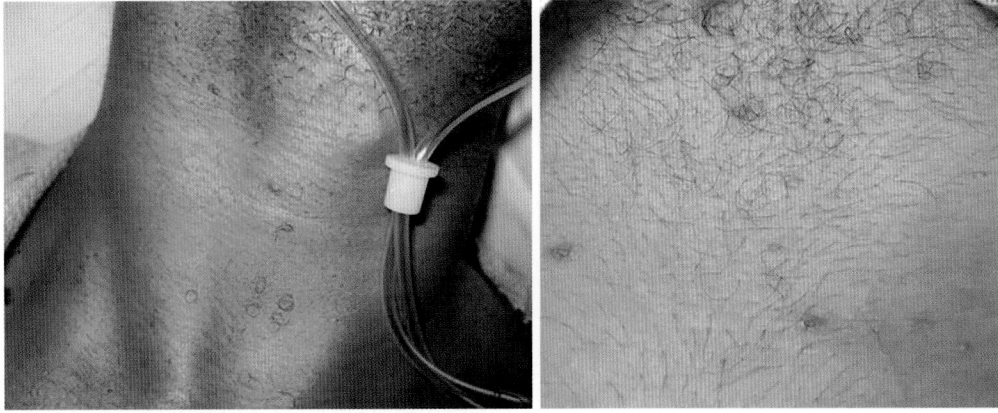

Figure 98-8   Disseminated histoplasmosis. Note the subtle umbilication of these lesions. Disseminated fungal infection should be considered in all ill-appearing HIV-infected individuals with low CD4 counts presenting with umbilicated papules.

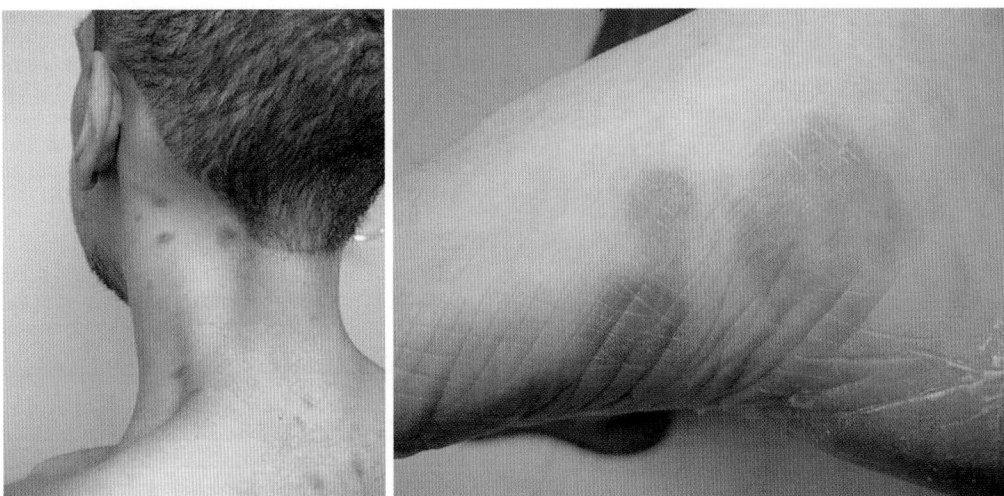

Figure 98-9   Kaposi's sarcoma. Patch and early plaque-stage lesions.

anogenital skin. Accordingly, patients with HIV should undergo regular screening for these entities.

KAPOSI'S SARCOMA

Kaposi's sarcoma (KS) is a human herpesvirus type 8-induced vascular malignancy that has the ability to affect the skin, lymph nodes, gastro-intestinal tract, lungs and, less commonly, other visceral organs.[33] Mucocutaneous lesions can present as violaceous patches, plaques, or tumors (Figure 98-9). While skin involvement most commonly involves the distal lower extremities, lesions can present anywhere on the cutaneous surface. Involvement of the oral mucosa and genitals is seen more commonly in HIV-associated KS than in other forms of the disease.

Historically, HIV-associated KS was seen almost exclusively in patients with low CD4 counts (i.e. 200 cells/µL or less). In recent years, however, an epidemiologic shift has been noted, with an increasing number of KS cases being seen in patients with well-controlled HIV. In one recent study, more than one-fifth of new cases of HIV-associated KS developed in patients with CD4 counts above 300 cells/µL.[34] The development of KS in these patients appears to be a phenomenon of accelerated immunosenescence.[35] Patients developing KS in the setting of relatively well-controlled HIV appear to have a more favorable course than those with lower CD4 counts.

Treatment of HIV-associated KS is based upon the extent and severity of the disease. In antiretroviral-naïve or recently non-compliant patients, commencement or resumption of antiretrovirals is indicated. Immune reconstitution inflammatory syndrome is a known complica-

tion of antiretroviral initiation in a minority of patients with KS, and is characterized by either the rapid development of new lesions or the progression of existing lesions within the first few months of therapy.[36] Antiretrovirals should almost always be continued in these cases, often in conjunction with systemic chemotherapy.

For patients with limited or localized disease that persists despite initiation or resumption of antiretrovirals, treatment options include observation, intralesional chemotherapy (e.g. vinblastine), cryotherapy, radiation, excisional surgery and topical retinoids (i.e. alitretinoin). Systemic chemotherapy, most commonly in the form of liposomal doxyrubicin, is indicated in patients with widespread cutaneous or lymphatic involvement and in patients with visceral disease (see Chapter 97).

Treatment-Associated Dermatoses

While antiretrovirals have resulted in the reclassification of HIV as a treatable, chronic disease, all of the current classes of ART have the ability to produce dermatologic side effects. Knowledge of these cutaneous toxicities is essential, as treatment-related dermatoses are a common reason for patient non-compliance. While most of these dermatologic side effects are mild, clinicians should be aware of the potentially life-threatening complications of ART that can initially present with cutaneous findings. Additionally, HIV-infected individuals are at increased risk of cutaneous reactions to their non-antiretroviral medications as well, most likely due to immune dysregulation. These reactions can range from mild, self-limited exanthems to life-threatening

TABLE 98-2	IRIS Events with Cutaneous Findings	
Infectious	**Inflammatory**	**Neoplastic**
HSV-1 and -2	Eosinophilic folliculitis	Kaposi's sarcoma
VZV (Herpes zoster)	Seborrheic dermatitis	
HPV	Sarcoidosis	
CMV	Acne vulgaris	
Molluscum contagiosum	Acne rosacea	
Mycobacteria (Leprosy, tuberculosis, atypical mycobacteria)	Foreign-body reactions	
Disseminated fungal (*Cryptococcus*, histoplasmosis)		
Leishmaniasis		

Reproduced from Lehloenya R., Meintjes G.: Dermatologic manifestations of the immune reconstitution inflammatory syndrome. *Dermatol Clin* 2006; 24(4):549-570.

reactions such as Stevens–Johnson syndrome and toxic epidermal necrolysis. Trimethoprim–sulfamethoxazole, in particular, is a common cause of drug reactions in HIV-positive individuals.[37]

IMMUNE RECONSTITUTION INFLAMMATORY SYNDROME

Immune reconstitution inflammatory syndrome (IRIS) is a phenomenon best described as a pathologic inflammatory response to a pre-existing antigen that develops soon after initiation of ART therapy in the setting of a decreasing viral load, with or without a corresponding increase in CD4 cell counts.[38] Specific diagnostic criteria and non-dermatologic clinical presentations are described elsewhere (Chapter 95). In some cohorts, more than half of IRIS events are dermatologic.[39] The cutaneous manifestations of IRIS include development or worsening of infectious entities, neoplastic conditions and inflammatory dermatoses (summarized in Table 98-2). With respect to these inflammatory conditions, the reasons why certain diagnoses are associated with IRIS events while other common dermatoses are not is unclear. Certain cutaneous IRIS events can be confused by patients and clinicians for drug reactions. Moreover, development or worsening of cutaneous findings due to IRIS is a common cause for patient noncompliance with ART. Regardless of the diagnosis, cutaneous IRIS events almost never require discontinuation of ART. While IRIS events are usually treated with antimicrobial, anti-inflammatory, or chemotherapeutic agents, findings will typically improve or even resolve without additional treatment after several months, as the immune system stabilizes with continued ART.

ANTIRETROVIRAL-ASSOCIATED LIPODYSTROPHY

Lipodystrophy has historically been one of the most visible and stigmatizing complications of ART, with protease inhibitors (PIs), thymidine analog nucleoside reverse transcriptase inhibitors (NRTIs) and, to a lesser extent, non-nucleoside reverse transcriptase inhibitors (NNRTIs), all being known causes.[40] Within each of these categories of antiretrovirals, the tendency towards lipodystrophy induction is agent-specific. Present day treatment regimens involving newer agents and modified dosing regimens, are much less likely to induce lipodystrophy.

Antiretroviral-associated lipodystrophy can manifest as lipoatrophy – with loss of fat in the face, extremities and buttocks – or lipohypertrophy, characterized by accumulation and redistribution of fat to the upper back, neck and abdomen.[41] The changes of lipodystrophy are typically seen within 2 years of starting therapy.[42] Clinicians should be aware of the association between lipodystrophy and metabolic abnormalities, including hyperlipidemia and insulin resistance. Patients with antiretroviral-associated lipodystrophy should be screened regularly for these abnormalities, as they may increase the risk for cardiovascular sequelae.

While studies have shown statistically significant improvement in lipodystrophy following the modification of antiretroviral regimens, these changes are often not noticeable to patients.[41] Accordingly, once lipodystrophy has developed, changes in antiretroviral regimens are generally not recommended. Two injectable dermal fillers, poly-L-lactic acid and calcium hydroxylapatite, have been approved by the FDA for the treatment of antiretroviral-associated facial lipoatrophy. Treatment of antiretroviral-associated lipohypertrophy is considerably more difficult and involves both lifestyle modifications and surgical intervention.

PIGMENTARY ALTERATION

Nail and mucocutaneous hyperpigmentation are well-recognized side effects of the NRTI zidovudine.[43] Zidovudine-associated hyperpigmentation can present either as longitudinal streaks or as diffuse hyperpigmentation of the fingernails or toenails. Mucocutaneous hyperpigmentation is less common. These pigmentary anomalies are more common and more severe in patients of color, and tend to resolve gradually with discontinuation of the medication. Zidovudine-associated hyperpigmentation is encountered less commonly today because alternative therapies are being used more frequently and because, in the instances where zidovudine is still prescribed, the doses are typically lower than those used historically.

MORBILLIFORM EXANTHEMS

While much of the literature describing the side effects of ART lumps cutaneous events together under the wastebasket term of 'rash', morbilliform exanthems seem to be the most common entity placed in this category. Clinically, morbilliform drug rashes are characterized by widespread, ill-defined maculopapular erythema. While NNRTIs in particular are well known to cause morbilliform exanthems, this side effect is common to the other classes of antiretrovirals as well.[44] Most often these reactions are mild and variably symptomatic, with pruritus being the most common complaint. In most cases of simple morbilliform drug rash, treatment with the inciting agent can be continued and the rash will resolve over the course of several weeks. Patients can be treated with topical steroids and oral antihistamines until the rash clears. However, while most antiretroviral-associated morbilliform drug rashes are mild and self-limited, clinicians must be able to distinguish these from drug-induced hypersensitivity syndrome (DISH), formerly known as drug rash with eosinophilia and systemic symptoms (DRESS), as a morbilliform exanthem is also the most common morphological presentation of this potentially life-threatening drug reaction.

DRUG-INDUCED HYPERSENSITIVITY SYNDROME (DISH)

Abacavir hypersensitivity syndrome is a well-known complication of therapy, occurring in 5–8% of patients in clinical trials.[45] This condition occurs within the first 6 weeks of abacavir therapy, with the mean onset being 9 days after initiation of therapy. While the rash associated with abacavir hypersensitivity syndrome is most commonly morbilliform, reports of urticarial, targetoid and erythrodermic presentations also exist. In addition to the rash, patients manifest with systemic symptoms, including fever and gastrointestinal disturbances, and laboratory abnormalities, most commonly transaminitis. Rechallenge in patients with a known history of abacavir hypersensitivity syndrome can result in death due to a severe, accelerated hypersensitivity reaction and is absolutely contraindicated.[46] The human leukocyte antigen (HLA) B*5701 allele has been linked with abacavir hypersensitivity syndrome, and it is recommended that all potential patients be screened for this allele prior to initiation of therapy. While abacavir is the most common antiretroviral agent to be reported to induce DISH, other antiretrovirals (e.g. lopinavir) are known but less common offenders.

Non-antiretroviral medications commonly used in HIV-infected individuals that are frequent causes of DISH include trimethoprim–sulfamethoxazole and dapsone.

RETINOID-LIKE EFFECTS

Some protease inhibitors, indinavir in particular, are associated with retinoid-like side effects, including chronic paronychia, periungual pyogenic granulomas, alopecia, chelitis and xerosis. In one study, almost a third of patients treated with indinavir developed two or more of these effects.[47] Chronic paronychia, characterized by inflamed periungual skin, should be managed with a superpotent topical steroid, often in conjunction with a topical antimicrobial agent targeted at colonizing organisms (e.g. *Candida*). Periungual pyogenic granulomas are friable, exophytic vascular lesions that develop adjacent to the nail-plate, and are best treated with topical application of silver nitrate or with surgical debulking and electrodessication of the base of the lesion.

Indinavir-associated alopecia tends to involve body hair, and in particular, hair of the lower extremities, more commonly than scalp hair.[48] Regrowth is typically seen within several months of switching to an alternative agent, even within the same antiretroviral class (e.g. ritonavir). Chelitis and xerosis associated with the use of protease inhibitors are best managed with liberal use of emollients.

INJECTION-SITE REACTIONS

Enfuvirtide, a fusion inhibitor, has been reported to result in injection-site reactions in a majority of patients.[49] These reactions include erythema, ecchymosis, induration, nodules, cysts and localized sclerosis. Despite the high incidence of injection-site reactions, the vast majority of patients are able to continue with therapy.

References available online at expertconsult.com.

KEY REFERENCES

Basarab T., Russell Jones R.: HIV-associated eosinophilic folliculitis: case report and review of the literature. *Br J Dermatol* 1996; 134(3):499-503.

Crum-Cianflone N., Hullsiek K.H., Satter E., et al.: Cutaneous malignancies among HIV-infected persons. *Arch Intern Med* 2009; 169(12);1130-1138.

Duvic M.: Papulosquamous disorders associated with human immunodeficiency virus infection. *Dermatol Clin* 1991; 9(3):523-530.

French M.A., Lenzo N., John M., et al.: Immune restoration disease after the treatment of immunodeficient HIV-infected patients with highly active antiretroviral therapy. *HIV Med* 2000; 1(2):107-115.

Gebo K.A., Kalyani R., Moore R.D., et al.: The incidence of, risk factors for, and sequelae of herpes zoster among HIV patients in the highly antiretroviral therapy era. *J Acquir Immune Defic Syndr* 2005; 40:169-174.

Introcaso C.E., Hines J.M., Kovarik C.L.: Cutaneous toxicities of antiretroviral therapy for HIV: part I.

Lipodystrophy syndrome, nucleoside reverse transcriptase inhibitors, and protease inhibitors. *J Am Acad Dermatol* 2010; 63(4):549-561.

Introcaso C.E., Hines J.M., Kovarik C.L.: Cutaneous toxicities of antiretroviral therapy for HIV: part II. Nonnucleoside reverse transcriptase inhibitors, entry and fusion inhibitors, integrase inhibitors, and immune reconstitution syndrome. *J Am Acad Dermatol* 2010; 63(4): 563-569.

Jessop S.: HIV-associated Kaposi's sarcoma. *Dermatol Clin* 2006; 24(4):509-520.

Mohle-Boetani J.C., Koehler J.E., Berger T.G., et al.: Bacillary angiomatosis and bacillary peliosis in patients infected with human immunodeficiency virus: clinical characteristics in a case–control study. *Clin Infect Dis* 1996; 22(5):794-800.

Muzyka B.C., Glick M.: Major aphthous ulcers in patients with HIV disease. *Oral Surg Oral Med Oral Pathol* 1994; 77(2):116-120.

Ramos-e-Silva M., Lima C.M., Schechtman R.C., et al.: Systemic mycoses in immunodepressed patients (AIDS). *Clin Dermatol* 2012; 30(6):616-627.

Shet A., Mathema B., Mediavilla J.R., et al.: Colonization and subsequent skin and soft tissue infection due to methicillin-resistant *Staphylococcus aureus* in a cohort of otherwise healthy adults infected with HIV type 1. *J Infect Dis* 2009; 200(1):88-93.

Sinicco A., Palestro G., Caramello P., et al.: Acute HIV-1 infection: clinical and biological study of 12 patients. *J Acquir Immune Defic Syndr* 1990; 3(3):260-265.

Strick L.B., Wald A., Celum C.: Management of herpes simplex virus type 2 infection in HIV type 1-infected persons. *Clin Infect Dis* 2006;43:347-356.

Uthayakumar S., Nandwani R., Drinkwater T., et al.: The prevalence of skin disease in HIV infection and its relationship to the degree of immunosuppression. *Br J Dermatol* 1997; 137(4):595-598.

99

HIV/AIDS-Related Problems in Low- and Middle-Income Countries

STEVEN J. REYNOLDS | ALEXANDER C. BILLIOUX | THOMAS C. QUINN

KEY CONCEPTS

- The overwhelming majority of the global burden of human immunodeficiency virus (HIV) (95% of new infections and 93% of all infected individuals) is located in low- and middle-income countries (LMIC).

- The clinical presentation of HIV in resource-limited settings is often the result of opportunistic infections resulting from endemic pathogens, behavioral and cultural practices, and access to care and treatment services.

- Tuberculosis, bacterial infections and diarrheal diseases remain the main causes of morbidity among people living with HIV in LMIC.

- Difference in HIV progression between wealthy and impoverished nations is driven by access to care, as well as coinfections such as malaria and HIV-1 subtype.

- HIV testing is critical for surveillance efforts as well as for engagement and empowerment of people living with HIV.

- Prevention and treatment programs must be efficient, integrated and well-coordinated in resource-limited settings.

- HIV continues to have far-reaching impact on healthcare systems and society in LMIC.

Introduction and Epidemiology

As of December 2012, the World Health Organization (WHO) estimated the global HIV epidemic had grown to include 35.3 million people (32 million adults and 3.3 million children). However, there are clear signs the global effort to address HIV is having an impact: the 2.3 million new infections estimated to have occurred in 2012 were down from 2.5 million the year before and 3.3 million a decade earlier. Likewise, HIV/AIDS-related deaths decreased from 2.1 million per annum in 2002 to 1.6 million by 2012. Nevertheless, the epidemic continues to disproportionately affect resource-limited settings, with 93% of people living with HIV and 95% of new HIV infections occurring in low- and middle-income countries (LMIC). The epidemic is also younger in LMIC, with the majority of incident cases occurring in young adults aged 15–24 years old. It is therefore not surprising that such a significant epidemic occurring in an economically challenged part of the world can have such a dramatic effect on social structure. Indeed, in LMIC alone, over 16.6 million children are orphaned or left vulnerable as a result of HIV.

The contrast between the impact of HIV/AIDS in the high-income countries and in LMIC is striking. Figure 99-1 illustrates the discrepancy between sub-Saharan African and global HIV prevalences. One in 300 adults aged 15–49 years is infected with HIV in the USA and Europe, while among pregnant women in some parts of sub-Saharan Africa the prevalence can reach 10–40%.[1] Compounding these differences, significant disparities in responses to the HIV epidemic exist between well- and poorly resourced nations. Although antiretroviral therapy (ART) has long been given to pregnant women and newborn infants in high-income countries to prevent transmission, until recently most HIV-positive pregnant women in LMIC received ART only at parturition or as long as the mother was breast-feeding, resulting in much higher vertical transmission of HIV in impoverished regions. Moreover, not only do differences in the supply and reliability of antiretroviral medications affect the treatment of HIV-infected individuals in LMIC, the very identification of infected individuals remains a significant problem. Over 80% of people with HIV infection are aware of their serostatus in the USA and Europe, while it is estimated that less than 40% of infected individuals in sub-Saharan Africa know their status.[2]

Recognition of these regional differences in the HIV/AIDS epidemic has motivated a global response by way of prevention and behavioral modification interventions. Widespread health education, increased use of condoms and voluntary HIV counseling and testing appear to have lowered the prevalence of HIV infection in Asia and some areas of sub-Saharan Africa. Declines in HIV prevalence in Kenya, Uganda, Zimbabwe and Haiti attributed to behavior change interventions offer encouraging support for these ongoing HIV prevention efforts. Similarly, behavior-change campaigns targeting specific 'high-risk' populations such as commercial sex workers, injection drug users, and men who have sex with men (MSM) have also demonstrated effectiveness in LMIC.

The factors responsible for the dramatic difference between the HIV epidemics in high- and low-/middle-income countries are multifactorial. Limited access to care, lack of diagnostic equipment, insufficient money to support either prevention or treatment programs, and behavioral and cultural differences all act to drive the HIV epidemic in LMIC. In turn, the high HIV prevalence in many resource-limited areas acts synergistically with high-risk sexual behaviors and the widespread prevalence of sexually transmitted diseases to propel the epidemic further. Furthermore, the coexistence of other endemic diseases in LMIC, such as tuberculosis and gastrointestinal infections, complicate the care of people with HIV infection and pose additional problems for the medical personnel caring for them.

Donor resources for HIV prevention, care and treatment have begun to break through the previous gloom in LMIC. The rapid scale-up of basic care and ART for people infected with HIV is changing the landscape and providing optimism where previously there was little hope. Figure 99-2 depicts the substantially different trends in AIDS-related deaths that would occur in LMIC with and without access to ART. However, despite consistent year-on-year growth in global spending on HIV interventions, funding will need to increase substantially in order to meet the target set by the UN General Assembly of $22–24 billion by 2015. This chapter reviews issues in the care of people living with HIV in resource-limited settings and the interventions that will shape the future of the epidemic.

Clinical Features

The diverse clinical manifestations of HIV infection in LMIC reflect the wide variety of other endemic diseases within each region. More than 100 pathogens, including viruses, bacteria, fungi, protozoa, helminths and arthropods, have been identified as causing opportunistic disease in people living with HIV, yet a relatively small number of these pathogens cause a majority of the infections and have the greatest impact on the health of infected individuals. Indeed, key differences in

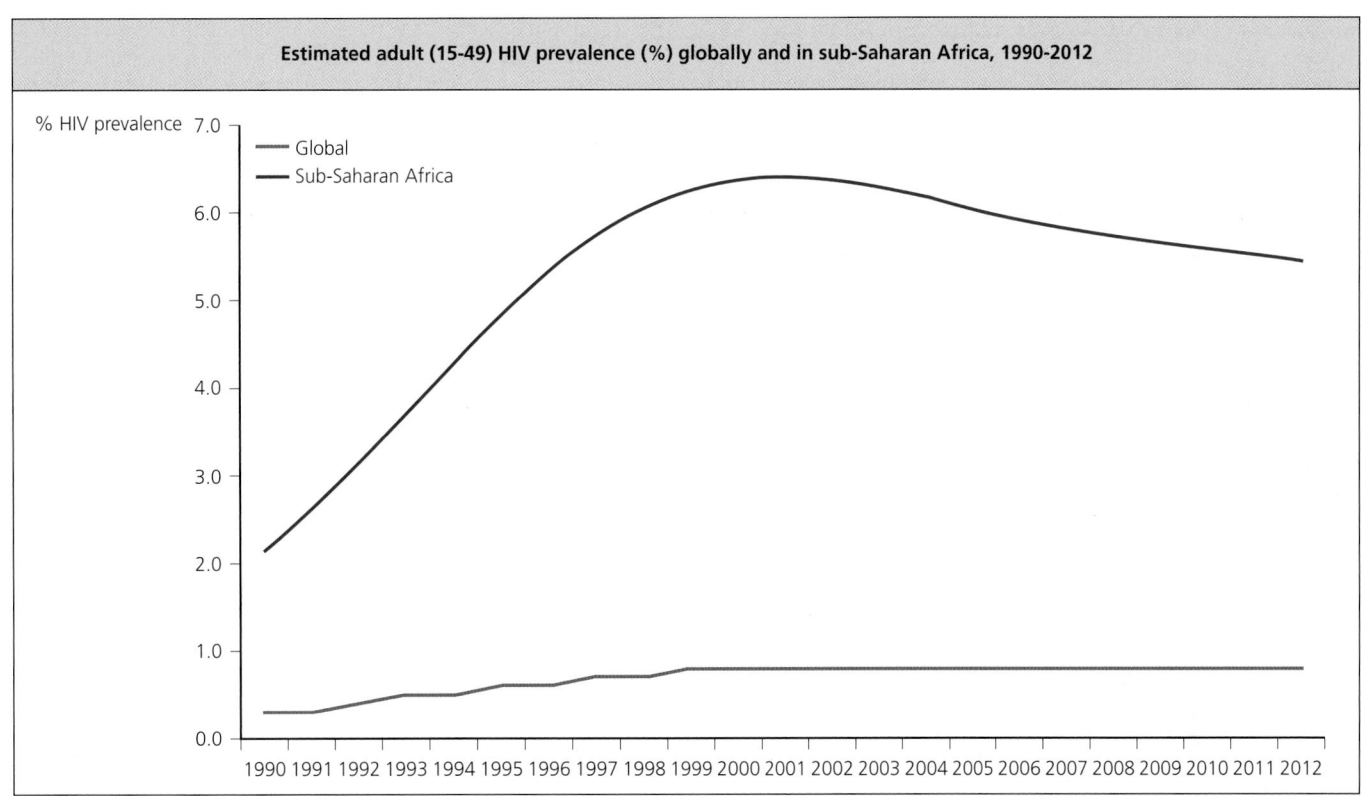

Figure 99-1   Estimated adult (15–49) HIV prevalence (%) globally and in sub-Saharan Africa, 1990–2012. *(From World Health Organization/UNAIDS:* www.unaids.org/en/dataanalysis/datatools/aidsinfo/.)

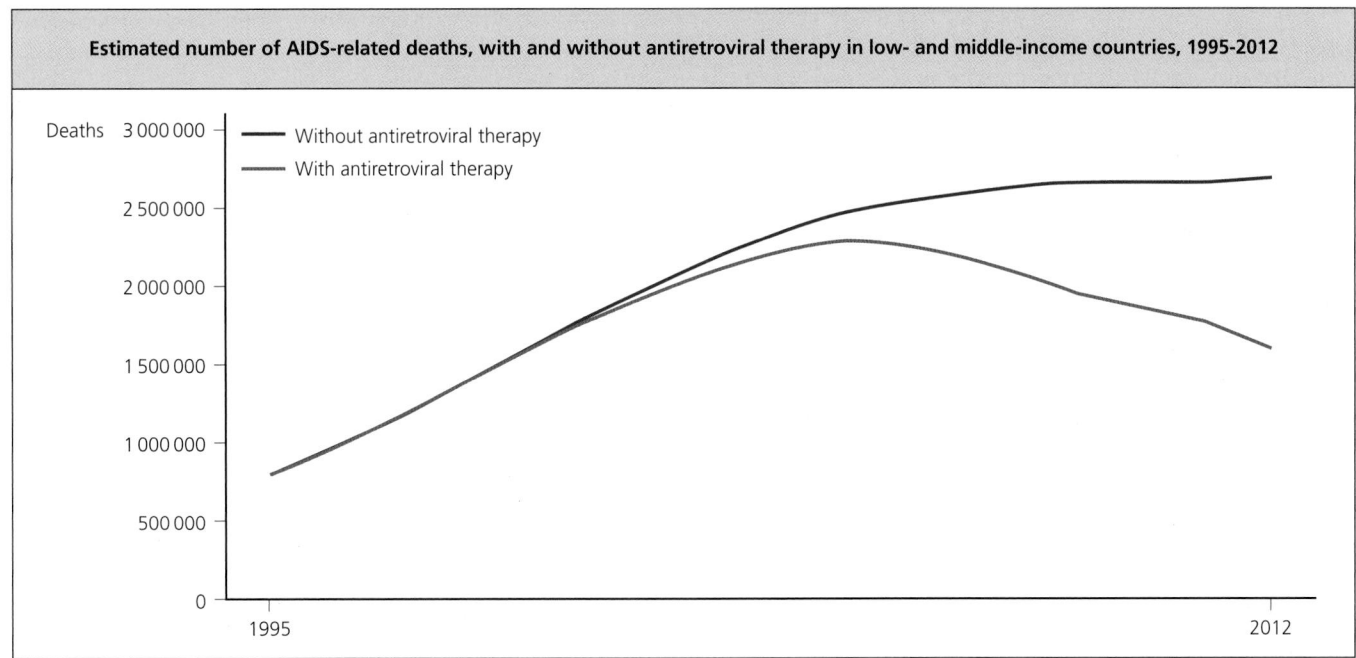

Figure 99-2   Estimated number of AIDS-related deaths, with and without antiretroviral therapy in low- and middle-income countries between 1995 and 2012. *(Source: UNAIDS 2012 estimates from Global Report: Report on the global AIDS epidemic 2013. Geneva: UNAIDS.)*

the spectrum of opportunistic infections and, by the same token, the clinical presentations of patients in LMIC and high-income countries are in part explained by factors such as the prevalence of pathogens in the environment, social behaviors and ecologic factors that result in exposure to these pathogens.

Determining the spectrum of opportunistic infections in a region requires surveillance systems and diagnostic services that may not be

available in resource-limited settings. For example, opportunistic infections that can be diagnosed with reasonable accuracy by physical examination (e.g. oral candidiasis) or inexpensive laboratory techniques (e.g. India ink stain of cerebrospinal fluid for *Cryptococcus neoformans*) may be documented more frequently than opportunistic infections requiring more expensive diagnostic technologies (e.g. *Pneumocystis jirovecii* pneumonia, disseminated *Mycobacterium avium* complex and cytomegalovirus disease). Many clinical studies and surveillance programs documenting opportunistic infections are conducted in urban centers, excluding infected individuals living in rural areas where diagnostic capabilities are more limited. Furthermore, longitudinal cohort studies are costly to maintain in resource-limited settings. Biases in diagnosing and reporting opportunistic infections may be especially important among socially disadvantaged groups with limited access to diagnostic and healthcare services. Finally, differences in clinical definitions may make comparisons between published reports difficult. For these reasons and others, much less is known about the frequency of different opportunistic infections in LMIC than in industrialized countries.

Beyond the effects of differing opportunistic infection, HIV disease itself appears to progress more rapidly in LMIC. Unfortunately, reliable data quantifying the median time from seroconversion to AIDS in resource-limited settings is limited. Early studies suggested that the time to AIDS was much shorter in sub-Saharan Africa and South East Asia; however, issues of methodology in pinpointing the time of seroconversion and reconciling different definitions of AIDS limit the interpretation of these findings. Nevertheless, one well-designed study in Uganda reported a median time from HIV seroconversion to death of 9.8 years, with time from AIDS to death of 9.3 months that varied according to AIDS-defining illness.[3] Median survival associated with wasting syndrome, Kaposi's sarcoma and esophageal candidiasis was less than 3.5 months in this study, compared with survival longer than 20 months associated with cryptosporidium diarrhea, chronic herpes simplex virus (HSV) infection and extrapulmonary tuberculosis. Evidence from Uganda also suggests that the subtype of HIV-1 affects disease progression, with subtype D progressing to AIDS more rapidly than subtype A (6.5 vs 8.0 years) due to a faster rate of $CD4^+$ decline.[4] This difference might be partially explained by earlier development of CXCR4-tropic (X4) virus among subtype D patients, as X4 virus is associated with more rapid $CD4^+$ decline than CCR5-tropic virus.[5,6]

While subtype differences may affect the rate of HIV disease progression, growing evidence indicates that opportunistic infections themselves may play a larger role in hastening $CD4^+$ decline and the development of AIDS in resource-limited settings. Analysis of cohorts containing Europeans, Europeans of African origin, and Africans found similar rates of disease progression in these populations after controlling for co-morbidities like tuberculosis.[7] Meanwhile, chronic immune activation and infections prevalent in the LMIC appear to enhance the pathogenesis of HIV, perhaps through inflammatory cytokines like tumor necrosis factor α (TNF-α) that temporarily increase the circulating pool of activated $CD4^+$ cells and subsequently increase viral replication.[8] Malaria has been demonstrated to increase transmission of HIV from pregnant mothers to their children and increases the risk of transfusion-related HIV transmission among those who develop severe anemia. Tropical infections causing genital ulcers like female genital schistosomiasis may also increase the efficiency of HIV transmission. Additionally, several drugs used to treat or prevent tropical diseases have an immunosuppressive effect and may influence susceptibility to HIV. Thus, both the rate of HIV transmission and progression may be influenced by widespread coinfections and underlying states of heightened immune activation occurring in many people in LMIC. Thus, the recent scale-up of ART access and basic HIV care including trimethoprim–sulfamethoxazole prophylaxis should ultimately have a major impact on survival in countries currently suffering high AIDS-related morbidity and death. Specific interactions between HIV and infectious diseases in LMIC are discussed briefly below.

MYCOBACTERIAL INFECTIONS

Tuberculosis (see also Chapter 96)

Tuberculosis is the most important opportunistic infection among people living with HIV in LMIC because it occurs frequently, is transmissible to both HIV-infected and non-infected individuals, and can be readily prevented and treated. Globally, tuberculosis is the leading cause of death among people with HIV infection, accounting for a quarter of deaths due to AIDS. The WHO estimates that one-third of

the world is infected with the tubercle bacillus, with one new tuberculosis infection occurring every second. Over 82% of tuberculosis infections occur in Asia, sub-Saharan Africa and Latin America, where about half of the adult population is infected. These are the same areas with growing rates of HIV, which the WHO considers to be the most important factor driving tuberculosis incidence over the past two decades.

Worldwide, an estimated 1.1 million incident cases of tuberculosis (13%) occur in the setting of HIV infection. Although the largest group of coinfected individuals lives in India, the burden of HIV coinfection per capita is highest in sub-Saharan Africa, accounting for 82% of the TB/HIV coinfected individuals globally. In 2012, nearly 40% of new TB cases in Africa were coinfected with HIV. In contrast, only 6% of AIDS patients in the USA have tuberculosis. Though rates of TB acquisition may be similar regardless of HIV serostatus, progression from latent infection to active tuberculosis disease is 20–37 times more likely among HIV-infected individuals. Indeed, the *lifetime* risk of developing active tuberculosis among latently infected people without HIV infection is 5–10%, while the *annual* risk of progression to active disease ranges from 5% to 15% among people living with HIV.

The increase in tuberculosis attributable to HIV has significantly increased the burden on tuberculosis programs in LMIC, not only because of increased prevalence but also because HIV coinfection is associated with higher morbidity and mortality related to tuberculosis. Despite accounting for only 13% of tuberculosis patients, HIV-coinfected individuals account for over 25% of tuberculosis deaths globally. A recent study of autopsies performed on patients dying of respiratory tract infections throughout Africa found tuberculosis as the most frequent cause of death in patients with HIV, accounting for over 50% of cases.[9] This was three to four times the rate of tuberculosis-related deaths found among non-HIV-infected patients. Even when not resulting in an early death, the diagnosis and treatment of HIV-associated tuberculosis can result in significant burdens on communities and individuals. Analysis of the healthcare costs throughout sub-Saharan Africa found that the expenses associated with tuberculosis were often catastrophic, especially for the most impoverished sectors of society, which are also disproportionately affected by both tuberculosis and HIV.[10]

Diagnosis, treatment and prophylaxis of HIV-associated tuberculosis are discussed in detail in Chapter 96. Given the considerable risk tuberculosis presents for individuals infected with HIV, early diagnosis and treatment of both infections are critical. However, these efforts are complicated by the atypical presentation of tuberculosis in patients with HIV, especially with advanced disease. HIV coinfected patients often have negative sputum smears and atypical findings on chest radiographs, making diagnosis challenging. Mycobacterial nucleic acid amplification assays have increased diagnostic sensitivity in this population, but the costs associated with these novel technologies are often prohibitive for LMIC. Thus, the WHO recommends low-cost symptom screening for all HIV-infected patients for the presence of cough, fevers, night sweats, or weight loss – termed intensified case finding. Patients with one or more symptoms then undergo further evaluation for tuberculosis, while patients with none of these symptoms are unlikely to have active tuberculosis disease and should be offered isoniazid preventive therapy (IPT). Several trials have demonstrated the efficacy of IPT among HIV-infected individuals in resource-limited settings, including a South African study that demonstrated an 85% reduction in the incidence of tuberculosis among HIV-infected patients treated with both IPT and ART.[11] However, a recent trial of IPT in South African miners only found reduced tuberculosis incidence while individuals were taking isoniazid, with the protective effect diminishing rapidly after discontinuation.[12] Only 14% of participants in this study were HIV-infected by self-report, indicating IPT may be of only limited use outside of HIV infection. Another method of preventing tuberculosis infection is immunization with the Bacillus Calmette–Guérin (BCG) vaccine, which over 70% of the world's children receive. Unfortunately, HIV-infected infants immunized with BCG run a small but unacceptable risk of developing disseminated BCG disease, prompting the WHO to recommend the use of IPT in these children instead of immunization.

Whether preventing or treating tuberculosis, adherence remains a critical issue among HIV-infected patients as their often larger bacillary burden increases the risk of developing resistance to tuberculosis drugs. This has emerged as a major public health problem, particularly in settings with high HIV/tuberculosis coinfection rates. Both multidrug-resistant (MDR) tuberculosis, resistant to at least both isoniazid and rifampin, and extensively drug-resistant (XDR) tuberculosis, MDR with additional resistance to all quinolones and at least one second-line injectable aminoglycoside, are found at higher rates among HIV-infected individuals. In an outbreak of tuberculosis among HIV-infected patients in South Africa, XDR cases comprised 24% of all multidrug-resistant isolates, with 52 of 53 cases dying in a median of only 16 days.[13] XDR tuberculosis has now been identified in several countries and poses a major public health threat to the fight against HIV/AIDS and tuberculosis, highlighting the need for improved diagnostic strategies, infection control measures, and newer antituberculosis drugs.

Mycobacterium avium Complex (MAC)

Although MAC is common in advanced HIV infection in the USA and Europe, it is rarely documented in LMIC. A Ugandan study found no *M. avium* among 95 blood cultures obtained from severely ill patients with advanced AIDS; nor was it recovered from 165 mycobacterial sputum cultures from both HIV-seropositive and seronegative patients at the same hospital. Similar results have been found in Côte d'Ivoire, and a survey of intestinal biopsies from 98 Ugandan, Congolese and Zambian patients who had chronic HIV-related enteropathy yielded only one case with histology suggestive of *M. avium* infection. Likewise, studies from Mexico and Brazil to Kenya and South Africa have found *M. avium* infection rates between 6% and 18% in hospitalized patients with late-stage HIV disease.

The reasons underlying the low frequency of MAC in LMIC are unclear, but possible explanations include less exposure to MAC, exposure to different variants of MAC, differences in host susceptibility, greater acquired immunity to mycobacteria, earlier death as a result of other pathogens, and diagnostic difficulties. Finally, over-reliance on the visualization of acid-fast bacilli through smear microscopy without confirmatory mycobacterial culture in many resource-limited settings may lead to misdiagnosis of nontuberculous mycobacteria as tuberculosis.[14]

Mycobacterium leprae

There is little evidence that HIV infection has a profound effect on the frequency of *M. leprae* infection (see Chapter 108). A recent analysis of leprosy trend in Zambia from 1991 to 2009 found relatively steady decline in case notification even as HIV prevalence was increasing.[15] A Ugandan study of 189 new cases of leprosy matched for age, sex and district of residence found no significant difference in overall rates of HIV seropositivity between patients with leprosy (12% HIV seropositive) and uninfected controls (18% HIV seropositive). Interestingly, studies from Kenya and Nigeria indicated that multibacillary leprosy appears to occur more frequently in HIV-infected individuals than paucibacillary disease. In addition, a Zambian study found HIV coinfected patients with active leprosy-related neuritis had poorer recovery of nerve function with corticosteroids compared to seronegative patients, indicating HIV status may lead to differences in clinical outcomes as well.

NON-MYCOBACTERIAL PULMONARY INFECTIONS

Bacterial Pneumonia

HIV-infected individuals are 25 times more likely to acquire bacterial pneumonia than the general population and are more likely to suffer subsequent bacteremia and recurrent pneumonia. Interestingly, this increased risk seems to be preserved in both high- and low-/middle-income countries, with rates of pneumonia caused by *Streptococcus*

pneumoniae and *Haemophilus influenzae* differing little globally. Overall, an individual's risk of developing pneumonia relates to their immunologic status, with higher rates of pneumonia observed at lower CD4$^+$ counts. In a study of acute respiratory illness in western Kenya, HIV-infected individuals made up only 23% of patients presenting to clinic but accounted for nearly 40% of confirmed cases. HIV-positive patients were twice as likely to have positive blood cultures and be infected with more than one bacterium compared to HIV-negative patients. The most commonly identified pathogen among HIV-positive individuals was *Strep. pneumoniae* (28%); followed by non-typhi *Salmonella* (6%), *H. influenzae* (0.4%), *Staph. aureus* (0.4%) and *Klebsiella pneumoniae* (0.4%).[16]

Pneumococcal disease is of particular concern in HIV-infected individuals. Invasive pneumococcal disease is more common in patients with HIV and causes significant morbidity and mortality. The Centers for Disease Control and Prevention recommends the pneumococcal polysaccharide vaccine to prevent infection in people with HIV in the USA, but a Ugandan trial of the 23-valent pneumococcal vaccine in HIV-infected individuals found no benefit compared to placebo, prompting the WHO to recommend the use of antibiotic prophylaxis instead of vaccination in Africa and other resource-limited contexts.[17] Nevertheless, this recommendation was based on only one study, so further studies are needed to determine the true effectiveness of pneumococcal vaccines among people living with HIV in LMIC.

Pneumocystis jirovecii Pneumonia

Pneumocystis jirovecii pneumonia (PJP) was the first presentation of the American AIDS epidemic and remains one of the most frequently encountered opportunistic infections in wealthy nations; nevertheless, it is rarely identified as a significant pathogen in LMIC. A recent meta-analysis found that a nation's gross domestic product (GDP) per capita was the strongest predictor of *Pneumocystis* infection among its citizens, with a 10% increase in the odds of *Pneumocystis* pneumonia diagnosis for every $1000 increase in GDP.[18] While some have argued that poorer diagnostic capabilities may lead to under- or misdiagnosis of *Pneumocystis* in resource-limited settings, several African studies with high-quality diagnostic methods have confirmed lower incidences. A Ugandan study of 129 HIV-infected patients with pulmonary infections and sputum smears negative for mycobacteria found *Pneumocystis jirovecii* in only 5% of patients despite the use of bronchoalveolar lavage and polymerase chain reaction-based detection.[19]

Although PJP is uncommon in Africa and Asia (7–25% prevalence in Thailand), it is encountered with similar frequency to the USA in Latin America (32–45% in Brazil) and Caribbean countries (20–24% in Mexico). A retrospective case series from the United Kingdom found a significantly higher rate of PJP in non-Africans (34%) than in Africans (17%), while a study from the Netherlands found that HIV-infected individuals of African origin were 4.8 times less likely to develop *Pneumocystis* infection than patients of Western origins. Interestingly, Haiti also has lower incidence (less than 10%) compared to other Caribbean nations, indicating possible genetic or environmental factors related to African origin that may reduce PJP incidence.

The clinical presentation of PJP in LMIC appears to be similar to that in industrialized countries. However, frequent coinfection with tuberculosis may obscure the diagnosis. The diagnosis and treatment of PJP are discussed in Chapter 94.

DIARRHEAL DISEASE

After tuberculosis, diarrheal disease is one of the most common clinical syndromes seen in persons with HIV infection in LMIC. Diarrhea lasting longer than 1 month occurs in up to 50% of patients in Africa who have AIDS, significantly more frequently than in persons with HIV infection in industrialized countries. The diarrhea is usually intermittent, not associated with blood or mucus, and is only rarely secretory in nature. In a study of Ugandan, Congolese and Zambian patients, no cause of diarrhea was found in nearly two-thirds of patients despite detailed examinations. However, other studies have identified pathogens like cryptosporidia, microsporidia, *Shigella* spp., *Salmonella* spp. and *Campylobacter* spp. with frequencies of 7–48%.

Historically, chronic diarrhea has led to a wasting syndrome known as 'slim disease'. However, not all wasting is caused by diarrhea, with 44% of patients dying with HIV wasting syndrome in Côte d'Ivoire being found to have disseminated tuberculosis at autopsy, compared to 25% of cases without wasting. Symptoms can also be similar, with chronic fever frequently associated with both tuberculosis and non-typhoid salmonellosis.

PROTOZOAN INFECTIONS

Toxoplasmosis

Toxoplasma gondii is a common opportunistic infection in both high- and low-/middle-income countries, with incidence proportional to the prevalence of latent infection in the population at risk for HIV (see Chapter 94). A higher prevalence of cerebral toxoplasmosis has been documented in Latin American patients compared to Americans, consistent with the higher prevalence of toxoplasmosis in Latin America. While up to 50% of seropositive AIDS patients in some parts of the world may develop toxoplasma encephalitis, its frequency in LMIC is unclear because of limited diagnostic capabilities. Autopsy series have suggested disease prevalence rates in late-stage AIDS patients of 15% in Abidjan, 25% in Mexico City and 36% in Kampala.

Visceral Leishmaniasis

A visceral leishmaniasis and HIV syndemic is emerging as HIV spreads from urban centers to rural settings in LMIC in which both infections exist. This was first recognized in southern Europe, where nearly 75% of adult cases of visceral leishmaniasis were related to HIV coinfection; however, the introduction of ART has significantly reduced the burden of this disease in Europe. Nevertheless, the visceral leishmaniasis/HIV syndemic continues to grow in LMIC where *Leishmania* spp. are endemic, with important clinical, diagnostic, chemotherapeutic, epidemiologic and economic implications.

The *Leishmania* spp. frequently involved in HIV infection are those that cause visceral disease, such as *Leishmania donovani* and *L. infantum* in Asia, southern Europe and Africa, and *L. chagasi* in Latin America. Indeed, HIV infection increases the risk of developing visceral leishmaniasis by 100–2320 times in endemic areas. Cutaneous leishmaniasis, on the other hand, is only rarely involved with HIV infection though it has a much wider geographic distribution. Classic visceral leishmaniasis documented in patients with HIV infection is probably caused by reactivation of latent infection because of immunosuppression. In one study, a CD4+ count less than 200 cells/μL was observed in more than 75% of the HIV-infected patients with visceral leishmaniasis, while fewer than 5% of patients had counts of 500 cells/μL or greater.

Visceral leishmaniasis presents similarly in HIV-infected and non-infected patients. Clinical features include weight loss, fever, pancytopenia and hepatosplenomegaly. Visceral locations outside the reticuloendothelial system are frequently involved during coinfection, including the blood, skin, gastrointestinal tract, lungs and central nervous system. Because of the high burden of leishmaniasis in the peripheral blood of these patients, transmission via blood or needles, particularly among intravenous drug users, is a major problem.

Diagnosis and treatment of leishmaniasis is similar in HIV-infected and uninfected individuals, but outcomes are generally poorer (see Chapter 123). A clinical trial in Ethiopia comparing individuals with and without HIV and visceral leishmaniasis found higher mortality (33.3% vs 3.6%) and relapse rates (16.7% vs 1.2%) among HIV-infected patients. Relapses of visceral leishmaniasis are frequently observed among HIV-infected individuals, raising concern for the development of resistant organisms and prompting the recommendation for the use of two-drug combination therapy to treat these patients.

Trypanosomiasis

Trypanosomiasis is almost exclusively a disease of tropical regions, with *Trypanosoma cruzi* causing Chagas disease in Latin America and *Trypanosoma brucei* causing human African trypanosomiasis, or 'sleeping sickness', in East and West Africa, leading to significant overlap with the HIV epidemic. In the 30-year period that Chagas/HIV coinfection has been studied, the majority of reported cases of Chagas disease involve reactivation of latent *T. cruzi* infection. In addition to increased risk of acquisition and reactivation of *T. cruzi* with severe immunodeficiency, clinical manifestations such as meningoencephalitis may be more frequent and more severe in those infected with HIV.

Unlike *T. cruzi* coinfection, *T. brucei* coinfection with HIV is less commonly reported. A study of African trypanosomiasis patients in Kenya found only 4 of 31 patients (13%) were HIV coinfected; by comparison, 100% of these patients had malaria coinfection. A larger study in Uganda and Tanzania comparing 16 HIV coinfected patients to 49 HIV-negative patients found no difference in clinical manifestation or mortality related to trypanosomiasis.

Malaria

Malaria is endemic to many of the regions hardest hit by the HIV epidemic: both diseases predominantly affect LMIC in the tropical regions of the globe (see Chapter 117). However, malaria and HIV often infect different subpopulations within a region, with malaria predominantly infecting children in rural areas and HIV infecting adults in urban environments. This has resulted in a smaller coinfected population than that seen with other infections like tuberculosis, perhaps explaining why initial studies examining the effect of HIV on malaria infection found no changes in the severity, incidence or successful treatment of malaria. Nevertheless, recent research reveals a complex interplay between these two infections: HIV-related immunosuppression increases the parasite burden and the risk of symptomatic malaria infection, while the malaria-related immune activation increases circulating CD4+ cells vulnerable to viral entry and results in a transient increase in viral load.

HIV-infected individuals are at increased risk of developing symptomatic malaria infections in endemic areas. Studies from both urban and rural regions of Uganda have found increased frequency of malaria episodes and greater severity of illness among HIV-infected patients.[20–22] Furthermore, vulnerability to infection and severity of malaria appeared to increase with HIV progression, with three times the risk of symptomatic malaria in patients with CD4+ counts of 200–499 cells/μL and six times the risk in patients with CD4+ counts of 199 or fewer cells/μL compared to individuals with 500 or more cells/μL. HIV infection has a particularly significant impact on children and pregnant women with malaria, both populations already at high risk for malaria infection at baseline. Among pregnant women HIV infection is associated with increased severity of malaria episodes, more profound anemia and increased maternal mortality. Placental malaria in particular is more frequently observed with HIV coinfection, resulting in increased risk of premature delivery and lower birth-weight babies. However, in holoendemic regions, HIV appears to have only a modest effect on parasitemia and clinical malaria among semi-immune adults.

Episodes of malaria parasitemia may play a role in the transmission and progression of HIV. HIV transmission may result from treatment of severe malaria-related anemia with blood transfusions in areas with suboptimal screening of the donor blood supply. Meanwhile, a study of malaria/HIV coinfected individuals in rural Malawi found that viral loads nearly doubled from baseline during episodes of acute malaria parasitemia and only returned to baseline 8–9 weeks later.[23] It is possible that malaria infection increases circulating, activated CD4+ cells that subsequently become targets for viral entry and replication, resulting in a transient increase in the circulating viral load.

Studies conducted to determine whether preventing malaria infection affects HIV progression are difficult to design because many drugs used in HIV treatment have antimalarial effects. Indeed, both co-trimoxazole and non-nucleoside reverse transcriptase inhibitors reduce the number of clinical malaria episodes in HIV-infected patients. Likewise, protease inhibitors have recently been demonstrated to reduce repeat malaria episodes by 41% among HIV-infected children in Uganda, though it remains to be established whether this was a direct effect of the protease inhibitors or because of reduced lumefantrine metabolism.[24]

Enteric Parasitic Infections

Enteric parasitic infections (e.g., isosporiasis and cryptosporidiosis) may be reported in as many as 5–10% of patients who have AIDS in the tropics, compared with 0.2% of patients who have AIDS in the USA. Isosporiasis is found more often among HIV-infected Latin American and Haitian immigrants to the USA than among native-born Americans. In Zambia, evaluation of persistent diarrhea in patients with AIDS revealed cryptosporidiosis (7%), microsporidiosis (16%), isosporiasis (37%) and no etiology (40%).[25] Treatment with albendazole resulted in a complete or partial response in 60% of those shown to have enteric parasitic infection. The prevalence of enteric parasitic infections increases as CD4+ counts decline and is reduced with restoration of the immune system through treatment with ART.

CRYPTOCOCCAL MENINGITIS

The encapsulated yeast *Cryptococcus neoformans* is an important opportunistic pathogen among people living with HIV in resource-limited settings where it causes both pulmonary cryptococcosis and cryptococcal meningitis. Within Africa and Asia, between 5 and 10% of HIV-infected individuals will develop cryptococcal infection. In sub-Saharan Africa, *Cryptococcus* spp. are the most common cause of meningitis, and, with a case fatality rate between 35 and 65% among HIV-infected patients, it accounts for 15–25% of AIDS-related deaths on the continent.

Partially underlying the high mortality rate associated with cryptococcal meningitis are challenges with diagnosis and treatment of the disease in resource-limited settings. In areas where screening programs are not in place, patients presenting with overt symptoms of meningitis often have progressed disease. Until recently, definitive diagnosis of cryptococcal meningitis required direct examination of cerebrospinal fluid with India ink or performance of latex agglutination or enzyme immunoassay studies within well-resourced laboratories. However, the advent of lateral flow immunoassays for cryptococcal antigens has both extended robust diagnostic capabilities into areas with relatively little infrastructure and made possible screening for indolent disease in endemic areas.

Treatment of cryptococcal meningitis in LMIC is complicated by limited access to the potent but expensive antifungal flucytosine, which is used in combination with amphotericin for initial clearance of the cerebrospinal fluid. Alternative treatment regimens relying on high-dose fluconazole alone are associated with reduced efficacy and poorer outcomes; however, when used in combination with amphotericin, performance is non-inferior to amphotericin plus flucytosine.[26] Patients initiating antiretroviral therapy with concomitant cryptococcal meningitis are at risk of developing severe immune reconstitution inflammatory syndrome (IRIS), but recent evidence indicates delaying ART initiation 5 weeks after treatment of cryptococcal meningitis may significantly reduce early mortality.[27]

OTHER OPPORTUNISTIC INFECTIONS

Oropharyngeal candidiasis, cytomegalovirus infection and Kaposi's sarcoma also occur in LMIC. Herpes simplex and zoster viral infections and cerebral toxoplasmosis also appear to be relatively common in most areas where diagnostic equipment is readily available, though regional variations in the frequencies of these diseases exist. *Penicillium (Talaromyces) marneffei* is a common fungal pathogen causing generalized papular skin eruptions among HIV-infected individuals in South East Asia, especially southern China and the Mekong Delta region. Mycobacterial infections apart from tuberculosis have been increasing in frequency in Southern Africa and China. Endemic Kaposi's sarcoma is most common in Central Africa, correlating with the high seroprevalence (40–60%) of HHV-8 (the virus implicated in Kaposi's sarcoma) in sub-Saharan Africa (see Chapter 166).

HIV Testing

Comprehensive testing for HIV infection is critical to addressing the HIV pandemic globally. Effective testing improves surveillance, aiding in evaluating prevention efforts, and ensures that HIV-infected individuals can be engaged in care early, avoiding preventable morbidity and mortality. Regrettably, access to testing is often inadequate in LMIC where the burden of HIV is greatest. The WHO estimates that in 2012 only half of all HIV-infected individuals in sub-Saharan Africa knew their serostatus. Fortunately, recently developed low-cost, rapid test formats capable of detecting HIV-related antibodies have helped improve access by removing the need for sophisticated laboratories and allowing same-day provision of test results.

Awareness of HIV serostatus is especially important in the high-prevalence settings of most LMIC because it offers the opportunity to access treatment – often free or low-cost through subsidization in many resource-limited settings – and to make informed, responsible decisions about child-bearing and avoiding transmission to partners. Moreover, communities throughout the world in which HIV-positive individuals from diverse backgrounds come together to support one another have demonstrated that awareness of HIV serostatus unmasks the often-invisible epidemic and permits a genuine community response, including advocacy for better national and international policies addressing the epidemic. The individual and societal benefits of HIV testing are only achievable where people feel safe in finding out their serostatus. Vulnerable communities, such as sex workers, injection drug users and men who have sex with men, are often the targets of discrimination and laws criminalizing their behaviors, resulting in low engagement in healthcare and a self-perpetuating cycle of HIV propagation. Marginalization of these high-risk groups is particularly pervasive in LMIC, hampering efforts to address the specific needs of these communities. It is therefore vital that governments and civil society make HIV testing safe by combating rejection and discrimination directed at all people living with HIV.

HIV testing is also the basis for worldwide surveillance efforts. Knowledge of the size and rate of growth of a nation's HIV epidemic is essential to plan and evaluate prevention and treatment programs. Consequently, the WHO and UNAIDS have developed national testing guidelines for HIV surveillance. These guidelines have evolved from 'first-generation' surveillance that relied on case reporting and small sentinel studies to the current 'second-generation' approach that is targeted and adaptive to the size and nature of a nation's HIV epidemic. WHO guidelines recommend different testing strategies based on three 'epidemic states':

- Low-level (<5% prevalence in all subpopulations), in which HIV has not spread widely in the population and is confined largely to high-risk individuals;
- Concentrated (>5% prevalence in any one subpopulation but <1% in pregnant women in urban areas), in which HIV has spread in at least one subpopulation but has yet to reach the general population;
- Generalized (>1% prevalence in pregnant women), in which HIV is established in the general population.

In low-level epidemics, cross-sectional studies of high-risk populations testing for HIV and other markers of high-risk activities such as other sexually transmitted infections are recommended. Generalized testing of the population is not cost-effective in these settings, so resources should be focused on vulnerable individuals and donated blood. In concentrated epidemics, countries should adopt the same practices as above with the addition of increased behavioral surveillance and monitoring of 'bridge groups' that link high-risk subpopulations with the general population. Finally, in generalized epidemics, countries should establish comprehensive surveillance systems including testing pregnant women and studying behaviors among both high-risk groups and the general population.

Most LMIC are confronted with both generalized epidemics and limited resources, making the establishment of comprehensive surveillance networks a challenge. Recognizing this, the WHO has developed three HIV testing strategies based on HIV prevalence, the objective of testing and predictive value of the test used. The first and most cost-efficient strategy involves testing of all serum specimens with one enzyme-linked immunosorbent assay (ELISA) or rapid test and considering all reactive samples as positive for HIV antibodies. This strategy is appropriate for diagnostic testing when HIV prevalence exceeds 30% in individuals with signs and symptoms of HIV, surveillance when general HIV prevalence exceeds 10%, and screening of the donor blood supply regardless of prevalence. In lower HIV prevalence settings, a second strategy in which positive ELISA or rapid tests are followed up with a second test based on a different antigen or test principle is employed. Concordant results indicate a positive or negative result, while discordant results are considered indeterminate. This strategy is recommended for diagnostic testing when HIV prevalence is 30% or less among symptomatic individuals or more than 10% among asymptomatic individuals, or for surveillance when HIV prevalence is 10% or less. Finally, when the HIV prevalence among asymptomatic individuals is less than 10%, a third strategy is recommended that adds a third test based on different antigen preparations or test principles if serum is found to be reactive on the second assay. Specimens reactive in all three assays are considered antibody-positive, while discordant results indicate the specimen is indeterminate. To further reduce the expense of HIV testing in LMIC, the WHO and UNAIDS have established an HIV test kit bulk purchase program providing assays giving the most accurate results at the lowest possible cost to AIDS control programs.

Prevention of HIV Infection

Prevention has historically been the most prominent aspect of HIV control programs in LMIC because mass-education and condom distribution are generally less expensive than large-scale provision of treatment. However, as lapsed patents and international pressure on pharmaceutical companies have reduced the cost of ART, LMIC have increasingly emphasized treatment in their national AIDS control. Nevertheless, preventive efforts combining multiple strategies remain key to limiting the magnitude of the epidemic. Therefore, prevention and treatment are more effectively seen as two complementary aspects of a unified HIV control plan, working best when both activities are coordinated. These ideas are exemplified by two recent concepts in HIV control: combination prevention and treatment as prevention.

UNAIDS defines combination prevention as 'rights-based, evidence-informed, and community-owned programs that use a mix of biomedical, behavioral, and structural interventions, prioritized to meet the current HIV prevention needs of particular individuals and communities, so as to have the greatest sustained impact on reducing new infections'.[28] This approach combines traditional programs like sexual education, abstinence and monogamy campaigns, HIV counseling and testing, and promotion of consistent condom use with more recently developed methods of prevention. Among these latter interventions are voluntary medical male circumcision, needle exchange programs, treatment of other sexually transmitted infections, and social reforms targeting vulnerable communities. Clinical trials in Uganda, Kenya and South Africa demonstrated the protective efficacy of male circumcision in reducing HIV acquisition by about 60%.[29] Several studies of needle exchange programs in LMIC have demonstrated reductions in HIV transmission from 3 to 93% among injection drug users, though some studies documented increased HIV incidence.[30] The variable efficacy of these programs reflects the importance of both high engagement in needle exchanges and consistency in the use of clean needles within communities of people injecting drugs. Data on mass treatment of sexual infections offers similarly mixed results, with one trial demonstrating 40% reduced HIV incidence and five subsequent clinical trials finding no benefit. Meanwhile, the impact of structural interventions was demonstrated in Malawi where HIV and HSV-2 incidence among girls was reduced 64% and 75%, respectively, by paying parents to keep girls in school.[31]

Another recently developed preventive strategy involves providing HIV-negative individuals in high-risk groups with antiretroviral medications prior to potential HIV exposure. This approach, termed pre-exposure prophylaxis (PrEP), has been studied in LMIC among heterosexual women, men who have sex with men and serodiscordant couples in high-prevalence settings.[32–35] Three trials found daily use of tenofovir or tenofovir–emtracitabine reduced HIV incidence by 44–75%; however, another trial involving HIV-negative women in Kenya, South Africa and Tanzania was stopped early because of lack of efficacy. These mixed results demonstrate both the potential for PrEP to dramatically reduce HIV incidence among high-risk populations, as well as the limitations of a preventive intervention reliant on consistent adherence among non-infected individuals. Additional concerns include the possibility of medication-related adverse events, propagation of resistance to first-line antiretroviral medications, and the potential for paradoxically promoting high-risk behaviors among individuals taking PrEP. While the Food and Drug Administration has approved tenofovir–emtracitabine for high-risk populations in the USA, the role of PrEP in LMIC remains to be seen.

Treatment of HIV-infected individuals with ART has also proven to be an effective preventive strategy in both high-income and resource-limited settings. The landmark HIV Prevention Trials Network 052 (HPTN 052) trial conducted in eight LMIC and the USA randomized serodiscordant couples to receive ART either at enrollment or when indicated by $CD4^+$ cell count decline below 250 or development of an AIDS-defining illness.[36] After nearly 2 years of follow-up in greater than 90% of 1763 enrolled couples, only one transmission event was observed in the early therapy group, corresponding to a 96% reduction in HIV transmission. This reduced transmission correlated with an achievement of undetectable viral loads in 89% of participants in the early treatment group compared with only 9% of the delayed group. Similarly, suppression of viral load has been demonstrated to reduce vertical transmission from mother to child. Consequently, all HIV-infected pregnant women should be initiated on ART during pregnancy and maintained on treatment at least as long as they are breast-feeding. Recently, a number of sub-Saharan African nations have established policies of retaining pregnant women on ART for life after antenatal initiation, termed 'Option B+'. This change in policy aimed at improving ART adherence among pregnant women and reducing vertical transmission brings Option B+ nations in line with most wealthy countries.

Ultimately, an effective vaccine against HIV would be the best preventive strategy. Despite a network of researchers attempting to produce such a vaccine through a variety of approaches, no successful vaccine has yet been developed. Thus, the best hope for reducing new HIV infections in LMIC involves tailoring a variety of interventions to the size and nature of each country's epidemic. Additionally, fundamental social changes, like improving the status of women and eliminating the marginalization of homosexuals, will be required if AIDS control efforts are to succeed. Implementation of such integrated prevention strategies are urgently needed given the rapid pace of HIV transmission in sub-Saharan Africa and Asia.

Prevention of Opportunistic Infections

Tuberculosis and bacteremia due to non-*typhi Salmonella* spp. and *Strep. pneumoniae* account for the greatest degree of morbidity and mortality among people living with HIV, even in the absence of profound immunosuppression.[37] Importantly, they are also both preventable and curable. Isoniazid monotherapy is a key method of primary prevention against the development of tuberculosis in earlier stages of HIV infection. Similarly, trimethoprim–sulfamethoxazole (TMP–SMX), used in high-income countries to prevent PJP and *Toxoplasma* reactivation among individuals with AIDS, has been demonstrated to reduce a number of opportunistic infections – malaria, isosporiasis and bacterial infections – in all stages of HIV infection in LMIC. A prospective cohort study conducted in Uganda demonstrated that TMP–SMX prophylaxis among HIV-positive individuals resulted in a 46% reduction in mortality, with lower rates of malaria, diarrhea and hospital admission. Beneficial effects were also seen on the rate of CD4[+] T-cell count decline and HIV viral load.[38] As a result, TMP–SMX has become an important part of HIV care in LMIC. Nevertheless, concerns regarding the large-scale use of TMP–SMX include a possible increase in antimicrobial resistance in pathogens such as non-typhoid salmonella and pneumococcus, and the potential for cross-resistance between pyrimethamine and trimethoprim, as sulfadoxine–pyrimethamine is one of the most widely used treatments against *P. falciparum*.

HIV Treatment in LMIC

Antiretroviral management in LMIC is discussed in detail in Practice Point 33. Despite the development of highly active antiretroviral therapy (HAART) nearly two decades ago, significant proportions of the world's people living with HIV remain untreated, the majority of whom live in LMIC. In 2012, only 9.7 million of the 16 million people living with HIV in LMIC eligible for treatment were receiving ART. While this represents a significant increase in coverage from just a decade ago when only 400 000 individuals received treatment, it nevertheless indicates the need for continued expansion of access to ART in much of the world. Even with significant declines in the price of ART and increases in international funding through the President's Emergency Plan for AIDS Relief (PEPFAR), the Global Fund to Fight AIDS, Tuberculosis and Malaria, and other partners, the cost of treatment remains a major obstacle to coverage. However, resource limitations are not the only reason that millions continue to lack treatment. ART coverage is also impacted by limited access to care resulting from poorly organized healthcare systems, low rates of care-seeking behavior, and the large distances rural populations must travel to reach healthcare centers in many LMIC.

Multiple studies have proved the tremendous benefit of ART in HIV-infected individuals, prompting aggressive expansion of coverage globally and dramatically reducing HIV-related morbidity and mortality. In both high-income and resource-limited settings, ART provides the only hope of survival for those with HIV infection. Moreover, the availability of ART can reinforce prevention activities by offering an incentive to seek HIV testing, preventing mother-to-child transmission, and decreasing the risk of sexual transmission.

Impact of HIV and AIDS on Healthcare Systems

The increasing number of people with HIV infection in LMIC places growing pressure on healthcare systems at all levels. Healthcare systems must not only be able to urgently treat malnutrition and opportunistic infections in patients with AIDS, but also distribute funding across population-level prevention and ART treatment programs. Each nation must use its own surveillance data to focus efforts where they can have the greatest impact. While sub-Saharan Africa allocates 66%

of funding to support treatment and care, Asia focuses this same proportion on prevention instead. AIDS prevention activities include teacher training and peer education, condom promotion and distribution, treatment of STDs, voluntary testing and counseling, transfusion screening and prevention of mother-to-child HIV transmission; while care and treatment activities involve diagnostic testing, palliative care, opportunistic infection treatment, drug costs and monitoring for ART, as well as orphanage care and living assistance. Unfortunately, the greatest need for these services exists in the nations least resourced to respond to them. Coordination of such varied activities and mobilization of the tremendous resources required by them demands a considerable commitment from both domestic and donor sources.

One significant consequence of the global effort to address the HIV epidemic has been the establishment and strengthening of primary care systems in many LMIC. Primary healthcare systems are the interface of contact between communities and national healthcare systems, bringing healthcare as close as possible to where people live and work. Whereas these programs were previously inconsistently available, underfunded and not nearly comprehensive enough in approach, recognition that the HIV pandemic cannot be addressed through vertical programs alone has led to significant investment in clinical infrastructure and health-worker training. Primary care systems not only extend the reach of healthcare systems into communities and improve individual patient outcomes, they do so at a lower cost than tertiary centers. A World Bank analysis of alternative treatment and care options concluded that community-initiated care provided at home greatly reduces the cost of care and thereby offers hope of affordability in improving the quality of the last years of life of people dying with AIDS.

The HIV epidemic has already dramatically increased the demand for medical care and reduced its supply at a given quality and price throughout resource-limited settings, and this trend will undoubtedly continue for the foreseeable future. As the number of people who have HIV infection continues to rise, access to medical care will become less available and more expensive for everyone, including people not infected with HIV, and total health expenditure per capita will rise. Meanwhile, governments in low- and middle-income countries continue to be under pressure to increase their share of healthcare spending and to provide special subsidies for the treatment of HIV infection. Unfortunately, because of the scarcity of resources and the inability or unwillingness of governments to adequately increase public health spending to offset these pressures, either of these policies may exacerbate the impact of the epidemic on the healthcare sector. Finally, governments and donors alike should recognize that HIV is unlikely to remain our chief health concern in perpetuity and thus emphasis should be placed on promoting the development of holistic, sustainable healthcare systems able to manage current and future health needs.

References available online at expertconsult.com.

KEY REFERENCES

Abu-Raddad L.J., Patnaik P., Kublin J.G.: Dual infection with HIV and malaria fuels the spread of both diseases in sub-Saharan Africa. *Science* 2006; 314(5805): 1603-1606.

Baeten J.M., Donnell D., Ndase P., et al.: Antiretroviral prophylaxis for HIV prevention in heterosexual men and women. *N Engl J Med* 2012; 367(5):399-410.

Baird S.J., Garfein R.S., McIntosh C.T., et al.: Effect of a cash transfer programme for schooling on prevalence of HIV and herpes simplex type 2 in Malawi: a cluster randomised trial. *Lancet* 2012; 379(9823):1320-1329.

Cohen M.S., Chen Y.Q., McCauley M., et al.: Prevention of HIV-1 infection with early antiretroviral therapy. *N Engl J Med* 2011; 365(6):493-505.

Golub J.E., Pronyk P., Mohapi L., et al.: Isoniazid preventive therapy, HAART and tuberculosis risk in HIV-infected

adults in South Africa: a prospective cohort. *AIDS* 2009; 23(5):631-636.

Holmes C.B., Losina E., Walensky R.P., et al.: Review of human immunodeficiency virus type 1-related opportunistic infections in sub-Saharan Africa. *Clin Infect Dis* 2003; 36(5):652-662.

Kranzer K., Govindasamy D., Ford N., et al.: Quantifying and addressing losses along the continuum of care for people living with HIV infection in sub-Saharan Africa: a systematic review. *J Int AIDS Soc* 2012; 15(2):17383.

Mermin J., Lule J., Ekwaru J.P., et al.: Effect of co-trimoxazole prophylaxis on morbidity, mortality, CD4-cell count, and viral load in HIV infection in rural Uganda. *Lancet* 2004; 364(9443):1428-1434.

Ortblad K.F., Lozano R., Murray C.J.L.: The burden of HIV. *AIDS* 2013; 27(13):2003-2017.

Pantazis N., Morrison C., Amornkul P.N., et al.: Differences in HIV natural history among African and non-African seroconverters in Europe and seroconverters in sub-Saharan Africa. *PLoS ONE* 2012; 7(3):e32369.

Quinn T.C.: Circumcision and HIV transmission. *Curr Opin Infect Dis* 2007; 20(1):33-38.

Thigpen M.C., Kebaabetswe P.M., Paxton L.A., et al.: Antiretroviral preexposure prophylaxis for heterosexual HIV transmission in Botswana. *N Engl J Med* 2012; 367(5): 423-434.

UNAIDS: *Combination HIV prevention: tailoring and coordinating biomedical, behavioural, and structural strategies to reduce new HIV infections. A UNAIDS discussion paper.* Geneva: UNAIDS; 2010.

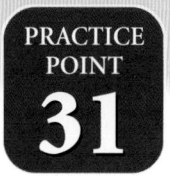

How to Manage Hepatitis B Virus in the HIV Coinfected Patient

JÜRGEN KURT ROCKSTROH | KARINE LACOMBE

Introduction

Because of shared routes of transmission and a lower response to hepatitis B virus (HBV) immunization in patients infected with human immunodeficiency virus (HIV), the prevalence of HIV/HBV coinfection ranges from 5 to 15%. In patients infected with HIV, chronic hepatitis B infection (CHB) has emerged as a major cause of morbidity and mortality, accounting for substantial rises in cirrhosis, hepatocellular carcinoma (HCC), and end-stage liver disease. Recent data also suggest that CHB might also alter the course of HIV disease by inducing a more profound immunosuppression in non-treated patients and by increasing the risk of all-cause mortality. Controlling HBV replication with anti-HIV and anti-HBV dually active drugs such as tenofovir can greatly curb the incidence of these diseases. Transplantation has a very favorable outcome in HIV/HBV coinfected patients with end-stage liver disease and referral to transplant centers should therefore be organized at an early stage.

Epidemiology

The prevalence of HIV/HBV coinfection is greatly influenced by the geographic origin of the patients, reflecting the different patterns of transmission. In countries where HBV prevalence is low (<2%, i.e. Europe, USA, Australia), HBV infection is acquired during adulthood mainly through sexual intercourse, intravenous drug use and nosocomial exposure. It affects 5–8% of HIV-infected patients, in whom HBV immunization is not performing well. Conversely, in countries where HBV prevalence is high (>8%, Africa and Asia), CHB is usually acquired perinatally or during early childhood and precedes HIV infection in most cases. The prevalence of CHB in HIV infected patients is therefore close to what is observed in the general population, ranging from 10 to 15%. In countries with intermediate HBV prevalence (2–8%, Mediterranean region, South America, Caribbean), routes of transmission are mixed and prevalence of coinfection may vary.

Pathogenesis and Pathology

Coinfection with HIV and treatment with combined antiretroviral therapy (cART) each modifies the natural history of HBV infection. Most of the liver damage associated with HBV infection stems from the immune system response to HBV. HIV infection can dampen this immunologic response. cART leads to immune system reconstitution, which in HBV-infected patients can be advantageous or deleterious. These phenomena may explain some of the effects of HIV coinfection and cART on CHB:
- higher risk of chronicity after acute HBV infection
- higher level of HBV replication and a higher rate of reactivation compared with persons without HIV coinfection
- increased liver injury (either due to immune-reconstitution hepatitis or direct hepatotoxicity) and liver disease progression in case of ART.

However, optimal control of HBV replication is more beneficial than deleterious in the long term. It induces a regression of liver fibrosis and may lead to a reduction in mortality rates to that of HIV monoinfected patients.

Some studies have also suggested that CHB may alter the evolution of HIV disease, with increased all-cause mortality, deeper immunosuppression and slower immune reconstitution after cART initiation.

Prevention

Because the risk of HBV acquisition is high in HIV-monoinfected patients, immunization should be systematically offered to anyone without any marker of resolved HBV infection. A recent clinical, randomized, multicenter trial has shown that a four double (40 µg) dose schedule provides a higher protective anti-HBs titer than the regular three 20 µg dose schedule. There is to date no clear advantage to offer immunization to patients with isolated anti-HBc antibody because apart from those who exhibit an anamnestic response, a minority of patients respond well and protection induced by immunization is of short-term duration.

Diagnosis

All patients newly diagnosed with HIV should undergo hepatitis B screening. HBV markers such as HBs antigen, anti-HBc and anti-HBs antibodies will help identify those with CHB and those in need of immunization. All anti-HBs-positive patients should also be screened for hepatitis Delta (HDV) infection because HDV considerably aggravates the prognosis of CHB. The determination of HBe status and quantification of HBV-DNA will help in providing the best therapeutic guidance. Initial liver evaluation should also contain an assessment of liver fibrosis by means of liver biopsy or noninvasive markers (particularly for identifying patients with cirrhosis who will benefit from a closer follow-up), a liver ultrasound and a biological checkup with complete liver enzymes (AST, ALT, GGT, ALP, bilirubin). Complete liver assessment should be performed annually in patients with F0–F2 fibrosis level and biannually in others. Special attention should be given to patients with isolated HBc antibody and quantification of HBV-DNA will help determine the presence of occult CHB.

Clinical Features and Management

The principal goals of anti-HBV treatment are to stop or decrease liver disease progression, prevent cirrhosis and hepatocellular carcinoma. Sustained viral control requires long-term maintenance therapy. Treatment discontinuation, especially of lamivudine, has been associated with HBV reactivation, alanine aminotransferase (ALT) flares and, in rare cases, hepatic decompensation. Following the publication of a sub-analysis of the SMART which proved that HIV-HBV coinfected patients were more at risk of liver-related events when treatment was initiated late, it is now recommended to treat all patients with dual HIV-HBV infection, regardless of the level of HBV replication or CD4 count (Figures PP31-1 and PP31-2). The only recommended drug is tenofovir because of its dual and very potent activity against HBV and HIV. After 7 years of treatment, more than 90% of patients do not exhibit HBV replication anymore. In the remaining 10%, persistence of viral replication is mainly due to non-adherence. To date, no viral resistance to tenofovir in vivo has been described, although resistant strains have been identified in vitro. The addition of lamivudine or emtricitabine is dictated by the need of also controlling HIV within an optimal antiretroviral combination. There is presently no place for pegylated-interferon because recent trials have not been able to demonstrate an impact of peg-interferon in HBe, HBs seroconversion or control of HBV-DNA in the long term, compared to nucleotide analogs, and tenofovir in particular. Patients who have an indication to treat CHB but not HIV should be offered early cART introduction.

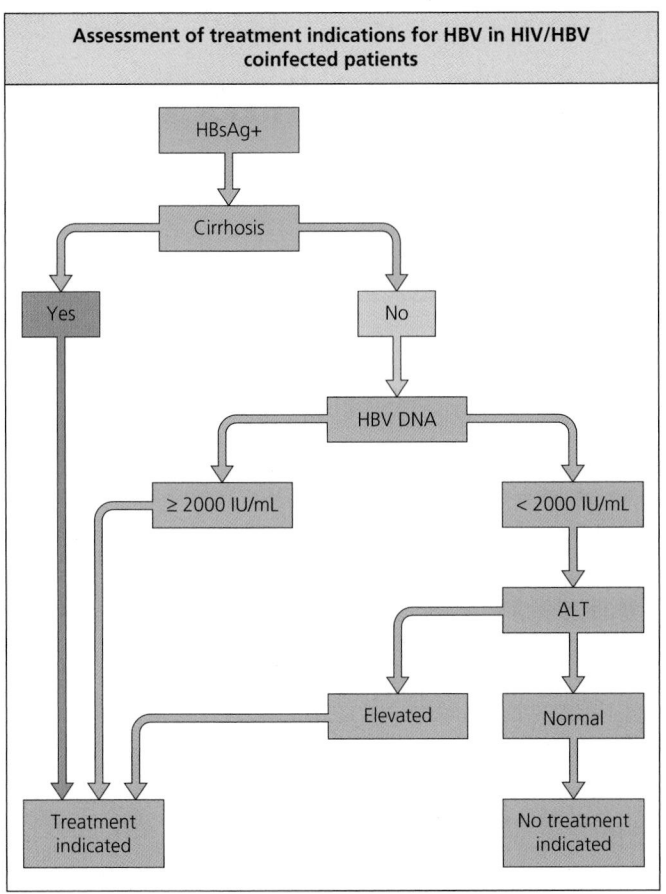

Figure PP31-1   Assessment of treatment indications for hepatitis B virus in HIV/HBV coinfected patients.

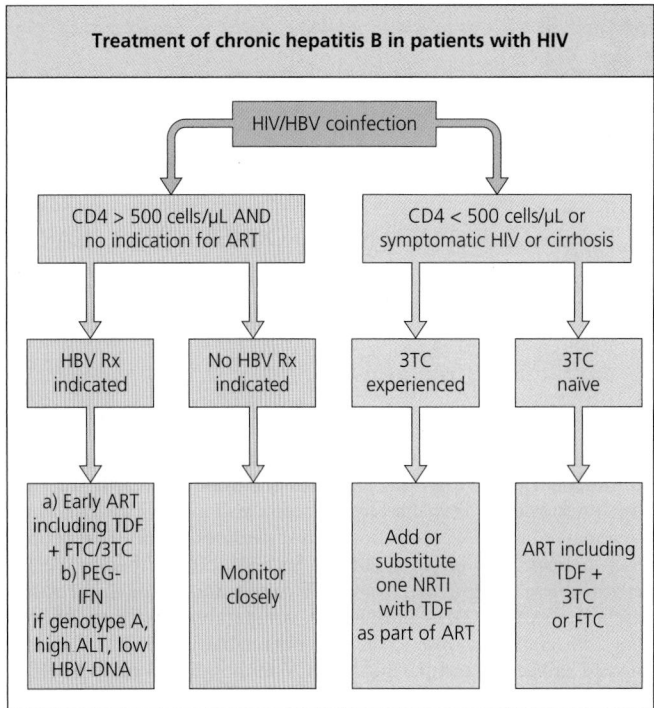

Figure PP31-2   Treatment of chronic hepatitis B in patients with HIV. TDF, tenofovir; 3TC, lamivudine; FTC, emtricitabine.

However, for those who are not keen on initiating ART, a 48-week course of peg-interferon alone or an indefinite course of adefovir + telbivudine may be offered, but the latter has not been formally evaluated in HIV/HBV infected patients. Entecavir should not be used alone because of its weak HIV antiviral activity. However, entecavir could be an option with the addition of an active cART in patients in whom tenofovir is contraindicated and who have never been exposed to lamivudine (or do not have lamivudine-associated HBV polymerase resistance).

Issues raised by the long-term treatment with tenofovir are three-fold. First, long-term tolerance of tenofovir is questionable because of its impact on renal and bone metabolism. In that perspective, the development of tenofovir alafenamide, which has the ability to reach a higher cell but lower plasma concentration, may lead to a better renal and bone profile with an equivalent antiviral efficacy. Second, although patients are virologically suppressed in the long term, they very seldom seroconvert and the risk of hepatocellular carcinoma (HCC) is low but not eliminated. Patients should therefore be screened annually (or biannually if cirrhotic) for HCC. Finally, around 10% of patients still exhibit a low level of HBV-DNA replication (ranging from 10 to 2000 IU/mL), although in most cases adherence is good. Reasons for persistent low-level replication are not clear and may be host- (immune profile) more than virus- (resistance) related.

Further reading available online at expertconsult.com.

How to Manage Hepatitis C Virus in the HIV Coinfected Patient

JÜRGEN KURT ROCKSTROH | KARINE LACOMBE

Introduction

Hepatitis C virus (HCV) coinfection can be found in 25% of all human immunodeficiency virus (HIV) patients in Europe and North America. High rates of HCV liver disease morbidity and mortality occur when accompanied by HIV coinfection; this underlines the need for proper HCV management in this setting. Successful HIV therapy delays hepatic fibrosis progression from HCV coinfection. In the direct acting antiviral (DAA) HCV treatment era, comparably high rates of sustained virologic response (SVR) are obtainable in HIV/HCV dually infected subjects in comparison to HCV monoinfected subjects. HIV/HCV coinfection always requires a careful check for drug–drug interactions between therapies for HIV, HCV and the concomitant administration of other drugs.

Epidemiology

HIV and HCV share similar routes of transmission, leading to a high rate of hepatitis C coinfection among patients with HIV. Overall around 25% of all European and North American HIV patients are estimated to have concomitant HCV coinfection. In particular, in countries where intravenous drug use is the main driver of the HIV epidemic, such as in Ukraine or Russia, up to 70% of HIV patients are dually infected with HCV. More recently, there also have been reports of an outbreak of acute HCV among HIV-seropositive men who have sex with men from Europe, Australia, Taiwan and the USA.

Clinical Features and Pathogenesis

In the natural course of hepatitis C in HIV, in the absence of antiretroviral therapy, a faster progression of hepatic fibrosis has been observed. This is particularly true in patients who exhibit CD4 counts <200 cells/μL or who develop AIDS. This enhanced fibrosis progression may be a result of the direct fibrogenic effect of HIV in the liver and a likely consequence of HIV-induced impairment of the innate and adaptive immune system leading to more inflammation, apoptosis and fibrosis. As a consequence, HCV-associated liver disease has become one of the most prominent causes of non-AIDS death in coinfected HIV subjects. Importantly, successful anti-HIV therapy can slow down the accelerated cause of fibrosis progression in HIV/HCV coinfected patients, emphasizing the importance of reducing HIV viral loads and of maintaining high CD4 counts in these patients. Interestingly, increased levels of HCV viremia which represent a hallmark of HIV/HCV coinfection have been found to decrease in a significant amount of patients in whom successful combined antiretroviral therapy has been started, again underlining the importance of controlling HIV replication in HCV-infected patients.

Management

The deleterious impact of HIV on HCV infection underlines the need for reliable anti-HCV antiviral therapies. All anti-HCV-positive, HIV-coinfected patients have to be carefully evaluated. HCV-RNA detection will delineate patients with complete recovery (HCV-RNA-negative) from those with active infection (HCV-RNA-positive). These latter patients should undergo evaluation of the liver impact of HCV infection, either by a liver biopsy or by noninvasive procedures (biochemical or morphologic by evaluation of liver stiffness).

Until recently, dual therapy with polyethylene glycol linked interferon-alfa (peg-IFN) and ribavirin (RBV) has been the gold standard for HCV therapy in HIV coinfected individuals. Overall SVR rates have been between 25 and 50%, with cure rates approaching 70–80% in HCV genotype 2 or 3 infection, but considerably lower rates (between 18 and 38%) in patients with HCV genotype 1 and 4. Treatment uptake, however, was very low, mostly due to the fear of high adverse event rates (in particular central nervous system and hematologic toxicity) associated with peg-IFN/RBV combination therapy. Comorbid medical and psychiatric conditions represent contraindications for dual HCV therapy. This issue coupled with high cost of therapy and a high proportion of genotype 1 infections with low SVR rates have limited the use of peg-IFN and RBV in these patients. However, the introduction of the first HCV protease inhibitors telaprevir and boceprevir already dramatically increased SVR rates in genotype 1 patients with HIV coinfection. In the meantime, first results of an interferon-free regimen of sofosbuvir and ribavirin in HIV/HCV dually infected individuals for 12–24 weeks have been presented from the PHOTON study demonstrating very high cure rates for genotype 2 (88% after 12 weeks of therapy) and high cure rates with genotype 1 patients after 24 weeks of treatment (76%). A somewhat lower response rate was observed in genotype 3 patients (67% after 12 weeks of therapy). In the meantime results from phase III trials for the DAA combinations sofosbuvir/ledipasvir, sofosbuvir and daclatasvir and ombitasvir, paritepravir/r, dasabuvir and ribavirin have become available with HCV cure rates on average above 95%. These impressive SVR rates were even obtained in patients with cirrhosis or prior treatment failure. In addition with availability of simeprevir also real-life data from the sofosbuvir and simeprevir combination habe been presented again demonstrating very high SVR rates which are not different from treatment reports in HCV monoinfection. All these trials strongly support the notion that in the DAA-era HCV therapy can be administered to a coinfected individual with the same chances of cure as in a patient with HCV monoinfection. The only remaining difference is the necessity for concomitant HIV therapy (unless the CD4 count is above 500/μL where one might discuss treating HCV first and then HIV) and the need to check for drug interactions between HIV and HCV drugs. As both drugs are often metabolized by the cytochrome P450 system, drug–drug interactions can be quite substantial. It is important to note that drugs such as sofosbuvir which are not metabolized by the cytochrome system can be safely co-administered with most antiretrovirals (the only exception is tipranavir/r; see also www.hep-druginteractions.org). It is however, also importnat to emphasize that drug interactions go way beyond the cytochrome p450 system and gan involve complex transporter interactions. For example ledipasvir can increase tenofovir exposure particularly in patients who are also receiving a boosted protease inhibitor. With the regulatory approval of various DAAs through the FDA, new treatment options have arisen which are summarized from the EACS guidelines (version 8 from

TABLE PP32-1	IFN-free HCV Treatment Options			
		TREATMENT DURATION & RIBAVIRIN USAGE		
HCV Genotype	**Treatment Regimen**	**Non-Cirrhotic**	**Compensated Cirrhotic**	**Decompensated Cirrhotics Child-Pugh Class B/C**
1 & 4	SOF + SMP + RBV	12 weeks without RBV	12 weeks with RBV or 24 weeks without RBV*	Not recommended
	SOF/LDV + RBV	12 weeks without RBV	12 weeks with RBV or 24 weeks without RBV in cirrhotics or pre-/post-transplant*	
	SOF + DCV + RBV	12 weeks without RBV	12 weeks with RBV or 24 weeks without RBV in cirrhotics or pre-/post-transplant*	
	OBV/PTV/r + DSV	12 weeks in GT 1b	Not Recommended	
	OBV/PTV/r + DSV + RBV	12 weeks in GT 1a	12 weeks in GT 1b 24 weeks in GT 1a	Not recommended
	OBV/PTV/r + RBV	12 weeks in GT 4	24 weeks in GT 4	Not recommended
2	SOF + DCV + RBV	12 weeks without RBV	12 weeks without RBV	12 weeks with RBV
	SOF + RBV	12 weeks	16–20 weeks[†]	
3	SOF + PEG-IFN/RBV	Not recommended	12 weeks in persons eligible for PEG-IFN	Not recommended
	SOF + RBV	24 weeks	Not recommended	
	SOF + DCV + RBV	12 weeks without RBV	24 weeks with RBV	
5	SOF/LDV	12 weeks without RBV	12 weeks without RBV	
6	In the absence of clinical data on DAAs in HCV GT 6 infection persons should be treated similarly to HCV GT 1 and 4 infection			

RBV, ribavirin; SOF, sofosbuvir; SMP, simeprevir; DCV, daclatasvir; LDV, ledipasvir; OBV, ombitasvir; PTV/r, paritaprevir/RTV; DSV, dasabuvir.
*Cirrhotic persons with negative predictors of response can be treated 24 weeks with RBV (negative predictors: treatment-experienced, platelet count < 75 × 10³/uL).
†Possible extension up to 16 weeks in treatment-naïve cirrhotics or relapsers; up to 20 weeks in treatment-experienced cirrhoticsTable is adapted from EACS guidelines version 8.0 from October 2015.

October 2015) for HIV/HCV dual-infected subjects from 2015 (Table PP32-1).

Clearly, the combination of DAAs will become highly attractive, particularly in the more difficult-to-treat patients with cirrhosis and previous non-response. In different countries and regions the respective use of combinations will depend crucially on the registered and licensed HCV drugs as well as cost coverage. Because of economic constraints, in some countries HCV therapy will remain restricted to specific inclusion criteria and compassionate use programs. Overall, however, in the setting of several available drugs and full cost coverage IFN-free regimens for all appear to be the way forward to achieve over 90% cure rates together with good tolerance of HCV therapy.

Further reading available online at expertconsult.com.

100

HIV Infection in Children

STÉPHANE BLANCHE

KEY CONCEPTS

- The risk of mother-to-child transmission of human immunodeficiency virus (HIV) is reduced to near zero thanks to antiretroviral therapy (ART) during pregnancy and – if needed – breast-feeding.

- While intrauterine transmission can occur, most transmission events from mother to infant occur during labor and delivery.

- Health of HIV-exposed but uninfected children deserves particular attention due to frequent social family vulnerability, increased risk of bacterial infection and some unresolved questions regarding the tolerance of *in utero* antiretroviral exposure.

- ART in HIV-infected children leads to a stable asymptomatic disease. Although well accepted by the vast majority, compliance to therapy sometimes needs individually tailored interventions and support.

- Transition to adult care must be anticipated and well coordinated with the young person, the family and the adult care team.

Introduction

Children become infected with human immunodeficiency virus (HIV) almost exclusively by the mother-to-child transmission route.[1] However, the risk of horizontal contamination, which has been little studied, has not completely disappeared in highly endemic, resource-poor countries.[2] Horizontal contamination may occur through unsafe blood transfusions or the use of non-sterile equipment for medical or traditional purposes. Child rape is also a significant risk. The progression of pediatric epidemics largely parallels that for infection in adults.

UNAIDS estimates that about 2.6 million children were living with HIV in 2014, with 150 000 deaths in children under 15 years of age. There were 220 000 new infections in children in 2014.[3] From 2001 to 2012, there was a 52% decline in new HIV infections among children.[4] The extremely effective prevention of mother-to-child transmission (MTCT) has greatly narrowed the gap between high- and middle- or low-income countries.[4]

Mother-to-Child Transmission

In the absence of prophylactic treatment, about 15–20% of infected mothers transmit HIV-1 to their child pre- or peripartum, with an additional risk of 10–15% associated with breast-feeding.[5] Although never strictly compared in a single cohort, the risk of MTCT appears to be similar for the different subtypes of the HIV-1 virus.[6] HIV-2 has a much lower replicative potential in humans and a lower MTCT rate than HIV-1. Even without treatment, the transmission rate of HIV-2 is only 1–2% and mostly involves women with primary infection during pregnancy or at an advanced stage of the disease.[7]

There are several pathophysiological mechanisms underlying transmission (reviewed in references 1,4). *In utero* contamination is possible, but occurs in only a minority of cases, despite possible HIV-1 replication in placental monocytes and CD4 cells. The risk of *in utero* contamination is higher in cases of chorioamniotitis and in women with very high levels of viral replication, as is observed in primary infection or in advanced stages of disease. The majority of infected children, however, are contaminated during labor, probably through mother-to-fetus microtransfusion. Transmission via breast-feeding is estimated to be 3–4% in the two first months, 1–2% in the three following months and 0.5% thereafter. The level of maternal viral replication is the major risk factor for pre-, peri- and postnatal contamination at this point, although no lower threshold for transmission in absence of antiretroviral prophylaxis has been established. The conditions of birth, particularly the duration of amniotic membrane rupture, can also increase the risk of transmission. Passage through the birth canal probably only makes a small contribution to the risk of infection: delivery by Cesarean section reduces the risk of transmission only if it is performed before labor begins. Premature birth is strongly associated with infection of the child, although it is unclear whether prematurity and its cofactors are a cause or consequence of infection. In clinical practice, viral replication detected in newborns during the first few days of life indicates *in utero* replication. By contrast, peripartum infection is detected later, generally before the age of 3 months. *In utero* infection is more frequently associated with a worse prognosis in children.[8–10] The use of antiretroviral drugs to prevent transmission has proved very effective: in optimal conditions the risk of transmission is now almost zero.[1,5,11] MTCT prophylaxis with antiretroviral drugs during pregnancy is detailed in Chapter 101.

Newborns to HIV-Infected Mothers

Most children born to HIV-infected mothers are not infected by HIV and do well, but careful management is required to optimize the postnatal phase of HIV prevention and reduce the risk of infection further. Furthermore, the child and mother are often in a situation of social, psychological and administrative vulnerability, and may be in need of appropriate support. In addition, a specific morbidity has been described in HIV-exposed but uninfected (HEU) children, some of them requiring specific evaluation.

PERINATAL CARE

The potential benefit of an antiseptic bath with a virucidal solution has not been determined; any such act should be carried out very carefully, because of the potential deleterious effects of breaks in the skin or mucous membranes in the presence of virus on these surfaces (including gastric membranes).

CHOICE OF POSTNATAL PROPHYLAXIS

The reference treatment for newborns is based on zidovudine monotherapy lasting 4–6 weeks. The contribution of this postnatal phase of prophylaxis is probably small in cases in which the mother's viral replication has been durably suppressed during the major part of the pregnancy. In contrast, a recent randomized study in children born to untreated mothers showed that an antiretroviral combination was more effective than zidovudine monotherapy alone.[12] In this study, the addition of three doses of nevirapine during the first week of life decreased the risk of intrapartum transmission to 2.4% from 4.8% for zidovudine alone. Obviously, this postnatal reinforcement only protects against intrapartum transmission and is ineffective if the newborn has already been infected *in utero*. There is currently no consensus recommendation concerning such intensification of treatment and the national guidelines in different countries propose various options; many of these options involve dual or triple therapy when such treatment can be implemented. It is important to bear in mind that our knowledge of drug tolerance and pharmacokinetics in newborns is extremely limited. Currently, a reasonable set of data is available for only three drugs: zidovudine, lamivudine and nevirapine. Based on the phase III pivotal protocol, the prophylaxis regimen proposed in US guidelines is zidovudine for 6 weeks and three doses of nevirapine during the first week of life. Other combinations are proposed elsewhere and include the addition of lamivudine for 4–6 weeks and/or nevirapine daily for 2–4 weeks. Some unexpected life-threatening events, notably cardiac dysfunction and adrenal disturbances, have been observed with ritonavir-boosted lopinavir in this particular age group. Extrapolation of such a reinforcement to all other situations of suboptimal treatment of the mother (i.e. detectable viral load near delivery, short duration of treatment, prolonged or complicated delivery) is logical but of unproven efficacy.

NUTRITION

Eliminating the risk associated with breast-feeding is currently a major issue.[13] In industrialized countries, bottle-feeding is advised, but the risk of nutritional infection associated with this type of feeding poses a major problem for most, but not all children living in middle- or low-income countries. According to WHO recommendations, bottle-feeding should be suggested only where it can be offered at a reasonable price, for a feasible duration, with reasonable acceptance rates and with sufficient food safety and precautionary measures against infection. In all other cases, maternal breast-feeding is encouraged. Several approaches to improve the safety of maternal breast-feeding are currently being implemented. The first involves the promotion of exclusive breast-feeding, given that mixed feeding methods increase the risk of child contamination. Another approach exploits the efficacy of antiretroviral drugs, either for maternal antiretroviral therapy (ART) during breast-feeding, or for 'post-exposure prophylactic' treatment of the child for the duration of breast-feeding. Both approaches are very effective although a residual risk is still observed in children. The feasibility of, and tolerance of children to this postnatal prophylactic treatment – whether given directly to the child or introduced through maternal milk – will nevertheless need to be carefully examined.[14]

HIV DIAGNOSIS IN CHILDREN

Maternal IgG antibodies cross the placenta, so the early diagnosis of infection requires a polymerase chain reaction (PCR)-based virus isolation test. PCR-based tests for DNA and those for RNA are both used and seem to give equivalent rates of diagnostic sensitivity and specificity when used for young children. These tests are ideally performed immediately after birth, but the number of infected children identified in the perinatal period is small, because most cases of contamination occur at the moment of delivery. Several weeks of viral replication are required before replication can be detected by standard methods, so screening for the virus is generally repeated at 1 and 3 months, and even at 6 months at certain centers. The sensitivity of PCR at 3 months in non breast-fed children is close to 100%.[15] Negative serological results at 18 months are often considered the endpoint in the testing process, although some centers stop follow-up after a negative PCR result at 6 months. In cases of limited access to healthcare, the first PCR test is often carried out at 5 weeks, as a compromise between reducing costs and maintaining test sensitivity. In cases of breast-feeding, the risk of infection remains until weaning, and a diagnostic test (PCR before 18 months or serological test after 18 months) must be carried out at least 4–6 weeks after the end of breast-feeding for the valid interpretation of test results. Any positive PCR result should lead to retesting without delay to confirm infection. Symptoms observed in the child may also contribute to diagnosis. Axillary adenopathies, splenomegaly and oral thrush in the first few months are highly suggestive of infection, although not disease-specific. A persistent cough, recurrent ENT (ear, nose and throat), skin and digestive infections, a state of malnutrition, neurological hypertonia or hypotonia are indicative of already advanced disease. In areas in which access to PCR is restricted, a presumptive clinical diagnosis may be sufficient for the initiation of ART in cases of suspected infection whilst awaiting confirmation by PCR-based diagnostic tests.

IMMUNIZATIONS

Vaccine schedules and the expanded immunization program (EIP) can be followed in each country as normal. The only vaccine posing a potential problem is BCG (Bacillus Calmette–Guérin), which persists in the long term, such that subsequent BCG infection is possible. Indeed, BCG vaccination is contraindicated for HIV-infected children in industrialized countries with a low incidence of tuberculosis. Elsewhere BCG vaccination is generally carried out in all HIV-exposed children, but recent WHO recommendations also advise against such vaccination in Southern hemisphere countries in which infected children are diagnosed early.[16] Other live vaccines (measles–mumps–rubella [MMR], yellow fever) do not pose the same problem of persistence and can be given normally, except to children at an advanced stage of HIV infection. Early prevention of *Pneumocystis jirovecii* infection is offered from one month until 12–18 months to children exposed to HIV, while waiting for confirmation of no infection (trimethoprim–sulfamethoxazole; 30 mg/kg sulfamethoxazole).[17] When diagnostic procedures can easily be completed and PCR results obtained in real time, this systematic prophylaxis is offered to infected children only.

HEALTH OF HIV-EXPOSED UNINFECTED CHILDREN
Susceptibility to Bacterial Infections

Several cohort studies in poor-resource countries reported a higher risk of morbidity and mortality among HIV-exposed but uninfected (HEU) children than children born to HIV-infected mothers. These cohort studies reveal two major clinical biological phenomena: an infectious risk specifically involving lower respiratory tract infections; and a link between the immune status of the mother and child morbidity and mortality.[18] Although there have not yet been similar investigations in the several large cohorts available in industrialized countries, a study reported that maternal–fetal infection with streptococcus B (Strep-agalactiae) was more frequent among HEU newborns. There are several, not mutually exclusive, possible reasons for this observed infectious susceptibility of HEU infants: a social context of poverty and limited access to care for these families; the maternal microbial ecology being unbalanced; or a true immunodeficiency in HEU children. A myriad of quantitative and qualitative immunological abnormalities have indeed been observed in these children, although some have to be confirmed.[19] They include anomalies associated with antigen presentation (altered phenotype of dendritic cells and production of IL-12) and cellular immunity (CD4/8 lymphopenia), reduction of naïve T cells or memory T cells, reduction of thymus size, increased IL-7 production and increased apoptosis of T cells. Data relevant to B-lymphocyte function and production of specific antibodies after vaccination of HEU children themselves are contradictory. Humoral immunity is in some cases considered to be impaired, but normal or even raised titers of antibodies against pertussis and pneumococcus were observed in HEU children compared to controls in a large pivotal South African study. However, the main consistent finding is the impairment of humoral immunity passively transferred from the mother to the child by placental transfer of maternal IgG.[20] The etiologies of the various intrinsic biological abnormalities observed in HEU infants other than passively transferred by maternal humoral immune deficiency remain obscure. It is difficult to dissect the role of the maternal disease itself from the potentially deleterious effects of HIV antigens to which the uninfected fetus is exposed, the effects of possible coinfections, including CMV, and even from the putative consequences of ART.

Tolerance of Antiretroviral Drugs after Exposure in utero

Fetuses and neonates generally have satisfactory tolerance to antiretroviral drugs. No evidence of teratogenesis has been found in humans for these drugs, except that efavirenz causes neural tube defects in primates and for which there are controversial data in humans. There is still some debate about the risk of prematurity associated with protease inhibitors.[21] Recent analyses suggest that prematurity could be specifically linked to ritonavir-boosted protease inhibitor treatments. The genotoxic potential of nucleoside analogs – including zidovudine, which is known to interact with both mitochondrial and nuclear DNA in humans[22] – merits particular attention. The main toxic effect of this molecule is reversible anemia, but persistent inhibition of other hematopoietic cell lines until the age of 2 years has been observed in a number of cohorts.[23,24] Dysregulation of the expression of several genes has been shown in cord blood hematopoietic stem cells from zidovudine-exposed newborns; the long-term consequences of this phenomenon are unknown.[25] An effect of zidovudine on mitochondria has been clearly demonstrated, and manifests as transient alterations to respiratory chain enzymology and as abnormally high plasma lactate concentrations in newborns and infants.[26] However, there is no consensus about the clinical significance of this transient mitochondrial injury. Quantitative and qualitative abnormalities of brain mitochondria have been demonstrated in animal models of zidovudine exposure *in utero*,[27] but again, the clinical and human relevance of these findings remains unclear. By contrast, rare cases of encephalopathy with well-documented persistent mitochondrial dysfunction have been reported among zidovudine-exposed infants.[28] The reason for the persistence of mitochondrial dysfunction for a long period after the exposure remains unknown. More recently, myocardial dysfunction in children exposed to zidovudine – more pronounced in girls – was reported.[29] The mechanism is unknown but this finding is also compatible with persistent mitochondrial dysfunction in cardiac muscle cells. Alterations to nuclear DNA are also plausible: a series of biomarkers has been observed in exposed newborns at birth, including integration of zidovudine into DNA, micronuclei, dispersed heterochromatin and aneuploidy.[19] To date, there has been only one large study on cancer incidence after *in utero* treatment with zidovudine alone or with lamivudine and it revealed no significant difference from expectations for the general population; note that the mean follow-up was only 5 years.[30] Tolerance to other nucleoside combinations must be evaluated. All available drugs of this class interact to some extent with human DNA. Fetal tolerance to other molecules of this class remains largely unknown, as does tolerance to new classes of antiintegrase drugs.

Children Infected with HIV

CLINICAL PATTERNS

In the absence of ART, disease progression differs between children in industrialized countries and those in countries with limited access to healthcare. Between 15 and 20% of infected children in Europe and North America have a risk of early and severe opportunistic infection and encephalopathy in the first 12–18 months of life.[31,32] Predictive factors for this rapid form of disease progression include the detection of *in utero* viral contamination at birth, an advanced stage of illness in the mother during pregnancy and cytomegalovirus coinfection. In low-income countries, morbidity and early death rates, mostly due to infection, are much higher. In certain child cohorts from sub-Saharan Africa, the mortality rate is 50% in the first two years of life.[33] After this, disease progression tends to be slower, close to that observed in adults, although this has not been clearly demonstrated for African children. The WHO classification of HIV-associated illnesses is provided in Box 100-1. In addition to the specific risk of encephalopathy, two other complications are more frequently observed in children than in adults. The first is lymphoid interstitial pneumonitis (Figure 100-1), leading to recurrent bacterial superinfections, the major clinical symptoms thus being those of the infections caused.[34] Unusual radiological symptoms are also observed, reflecting an interstitial syndrome of variable intensity associated with mediastinal adenopathy. This can lead to the differential diagnosis of miliary tuberculosis (especially in cases of bacterial superinfection); however, the contrast between the major abnormalities observed on radiological images and the mild symptoms can be used to exclude this diagnosis. The underlying pathophysiology remains unknown, but is often associated with

---

BOX 100-1   WHO CLASSIFICATION FOR HIV-1-INFECTED CHILDREN: CLINICAL, 1994

CLINICAL STAGE 1

- Asymptomatic
- Persistent generalized lymphadenopathy

CLINICAL STAGE 2[(I)]

- Unexplained persistent hepatosplenomegaly
- Papular pruritic eruptions
- Extensive wart virus infection
- Extensive molluscum contagiosum
- Recurrent oral ulcerations
- Unexplained persistent parotid enlargement
- Lineal gingival erythema
- Herpes zoster
- Recurrent or chronic upper respiratory tract infections (otitis media, otorrhea, sinusitis, tonsillitis)
- Fungal nail infections

CLINICAL STAGE 3[(I)]

- Unexplained moderate malnutrition not adequately responding to standard therapy
- Unexplained persistent diarrhea (14 days or more)
- Unexplained persistent fever (above 37.5 °C, intermittent or constant, for longer than one month)
- Persistent oral candidiasis (after first 6 weeks of life)
- Oral hairy leukoplakia
- Acute necrotizing ulcerative gingivitis/periodontitis
- Lymph node TB
- Pulmonary TB
- Severe recurrent bacterial pneumonia
- Symptomatic lymphoid interstitial pneumonitis
- Chronic HIV-associated lung disease including bronchiectasis
- Unexplained anemia (<8.0 g/dl), neutropenia (<0.5 x10^9/L) or chronic thrombocytopenia (<50 x10^9/L)

CLINICAL STAGE 4[(I) (II)]

- Unexplained severe wasting, stunting or severe malnutrition not responding to standard therapy
- *Pneumocystis jirovecii* pneumonia
- Recurrent severe bacterial infections (e.g. empyema, pyomyositis, bone or joint infection, meningitis, but excluding pneumonia)
- Chronic herpes simplex infection (orolabial or cutaneous of more than one month's duration, or visceral at any site)
- Extrapulmonary TB
- Kaposi's sarcoma
- Esophageal candidiasis (or *Candida* infection of trachea, bronchi or lungs)
- Central nervous system toxoplasmosis (after the neonatal period)
- HIV encephalopathy
- Cytomegalovirus (CMV) infection, retinitis or CMV infection affecting another organ, with onset at age over 1 month
- Extrapulmonary cryptococcosis (including meningitis)
- Disseminated endemic mycosis (extrapulmonary histoplasmosis, coccidioidomycosis)
- Chronic cryptosporidiosis (with diarrhea)
- Chronic isosporiasis
- Disseminated nontuberculous mycobacterial infection
- Cerebral or B-cell non-Hodgkin's lymphoma
- Progressive multifocal leukoencephalopathy
- HIV-associated cardiomyopathy or nephropathy

(I) Unexplained indicates that the condition is not explained by other causes.
(II) Some additional specific conditions may be induced in regional classifications (e.g. penicillinosis in Asia, HIV-associated rectovaginal fistula in Africa).

---

bilateral parotitis, and the biological signs include substantial CD8 hyperlymphocytosis. Coinfection may play a role, and Epstein–Barr virus (EBV) has also been implicated. Bronchoalveolar lavage, when possible, reveals hyperlymphocytosis. Another specific feature observed in children, contrasting with adults, is a higher frequency of leiomyoma or of leiomyosarcoma tumors in cases of severe immunodeficiency.[35] All organs may be affected. Here again, opportunistic EBV infection has been implicated in the pathophysiology. The proportion of children with nonprogressive disease in the long term (between 10

TABLE 100-1	WHO Classification for HIV-1-Infected Children: Immunological (2013 Revision)			
Classification of HIV-Associated Immunodeficiency	**Age-Related CD4 Values**			
	≤11mth (%)	**12–35 mth (%)**	**36–59 mth (%)**	**≥5 yr (cells/μL)**
Not significant	>35	>30	>25	>500
Mild	30–35	25–30	20–25	350–499
Advanced	25–29	20–24	15–19	200–349
Severe	<25	<20	<15	<200 (or <15%)

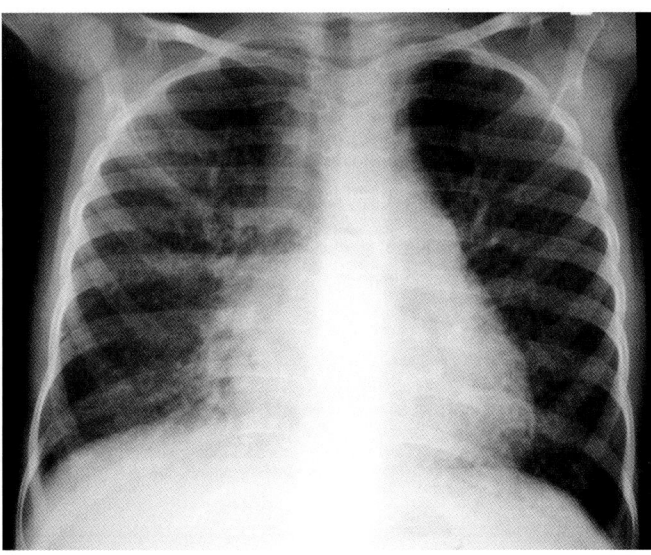

Figure 100-1 Lymphoid interstitial pneumonitis (LIP).

BOX 100-2   GUIDELINE ON WHEN TO START ANTIRETROVIRAL THERAPY AND ON PRE-EXPOSURE PROPHYLAXIS FOR HIV, 2015

WHEN TO START ART AMONG ADOLESCENTS (10–19 YEARS OF AGE)

Recommendation

ART should be initiated among all adolescents living with HIV regardless of WHO clinical stage and at any CD4 cell count (conditional recommendation, low-quality evidence).

As a priority, ART should be initiated among all adolescents with severe or advanced HIV clinical disease (WHO clinical stage 3 or 4) and adolescents with CD4 count ≤ 350 cells/mm³ (strong recommendation, moderate-quality evidence).

WHEN TO START ART AMONG CHILDREN (YOUNGER THAN 10 YEARS OF AGE)

Recommendation

ART should be initiated among all children living with HIV, regardless of WHO clinical stage or at any CD4 cell count.

- Infants diagnosed in the first year of life (strong recommendation, moderate-quality evidence).
- Children living with HIV one year old to less than 10 years old (conditional recommendation, low-quality evidence).

As a priority, ART should be initiated among all children ≤2 years old or with WHO stage 3 or 4 or CD4 count ≤750 cells/mm³ or CD percentage <25% among children younger than 5 years and CD4 count ≤350 cells/mm³ among children 5 years and older

and 15 years) has been determined in industrialized countries and found to be similar to that observed for infected adults.

PROGNOSTIC MARKERS

Predictive criteria for disease progression, in children as in adults, are CD4 levels and the viral load determined by quantitative PCR amplification of DNA. CD4 levels indicate the degree of immune deficiency and, thus, the risk of related short-term or mid-term complications.[36,37] The interpretation of CD4 levels is more difficult than in adults, because of the physiological hyperlymphocytosis observed in early life; normal adult levels are not reached until the age of 5–6 years. Counts expressed as the percentage of lymphocytes are less subject to variation and thus often preferred by pediatricians (Table 100-1). CD4 counts are nevertheless poorly predictive during the first year of life, particularly for the prediction of early-onset severe forms of disease.

TREATMENT

The prophylactic treatment of opportunistic or bacterial infections initially made a major contribution to reducing mortality rates in infected children. The preventive antibacterial efficacy of systematic administration of trimethoprim–sulfamethoxazole (TMP-SMX) has been demonstrated for all ages, starting as early as one month of age, leading to a significant decrease in mortality.[17] It is recommended for all infected children in countries in which access to healthcare is limited. Elsewhere, its prescription is more restricted: it is used either following recurrent bacterial infections despite a seemingly normal CD4 level or, more typically, following detection of CD4 lymphopenia. It is ART that has changed the outlook for children infected with HIV by greatly decreasing morbidity and mortality rates.[37] The yearly mortality in an HIV-infected cohort of children in Europe and North America decreased from 7 to 10/100 patient-years in 1994 to less than

0.5 in 2006. ART leads to chronic, stable disease in these children, compatible with balanced and satisfactory development. The toxicity profile is globally similar to that observed in adults, but with a lower drug-induced morbidity rate, probably through lower co-morbidity (alcohol, tobacco, aging).[38,39] Compliance and adherence to the treatment regimen is critical and may require specifically tailored interventions, such as individual or group support.[40,41] The risk of AIDS has now been virtually eliminated in ART-treated children, at least in the medium term, with 15 years' follow-up from the introduction of combination ART. The main issues now concern the long-term prognosis for quality of life, particularly relating to the potentially deleterious effects of the virus and/or treatment on various organs, including the vascular endothelial and central nervous systems. A large number of young adults, perinatally infected by HIV and in good health, are now followed in adult medicine centers. The passage from pediatric to adult medicine must be anticipated and carefully managed. The general principles underlying ART for children are the same as those for adults (Box 100-2). In particular, viral replication should be decreased such that levels are stable and below the detection threshold – the only guarantee of long-term efficacy and prevention of the selection of resistance mutations. In infants over the age of 2 years, indications for treatment are based on CD4 levels. Before this age, most recommendations now suggest systematic treatment, given the difficulty of predicting early and severe forms of disease. However, it is still not possible to determine how long this early treatment should last. Recently, the concept of a 'functional cure' after very early treatment has been theorized following the observation of an infected child treated at birth and who spontaneously maintained undetectable viral replication despite treatment cessation.[42] However, this encouraging finding, and the possibility of natural long-term nonprogression, must be confirmed (see Chapter 105 for detailed discussion). Recommendations concerning the choice of molecules and the threshold for starting treatment often change, and, therefore, the WHO guidelines and those of the health authorities in a number of countries should be consulted regularly.[37] In 2013, the combinations recommended are generally composed of two nucleos(t)ide analogs and either a ritonavir-boosted protease inhibitor (r-PI) or a non-nucleoside reverse transcriptase inhibitor (NNRTI). In cases of failure of a perinatal nevirapine-based prophylaxis regimen, the r-PI option should be preferred. Other than in this specific situation, both options have strengths and weaknesses. NNRTIs are generally easier to take but the 'genetic barrier to resistance' is substantially lower. The risk of early acquisition of resistance is thus high with NNRTI-based combinations, leading to a significant loss in the therapeutic reserve for the future.

Experiences from limited-resource countries are very encouraging, also showing marked decreases in mortality rates similar to those observed in the industrialized North. The main issue for the future, given the considerable number of children needing treatment, is the feasibility of implementing decentralized and long-term treatment programs on a wider scale in poor-resource countries.[43]

Transition to Adult Care

With advances in ART, most HIV-infected children survive into adulthood. Optimal healthcare for these young people includes a formal plan for the transition of care from pediatric medicine to adult healthcare provider(s). Successful transition involves the early engagement and participation of the young person and his or her family. The plan should be introduced in early adolescence and modified as the young person approaches transition. Assessment of maturity and independence is more important than chronological age to define the readiness of the young person in assuming responsibility for his or her own care before initiating the transfer. Transitional joint clinics can be useful – but not mandatory – before definitive follow-up in adult care. A close relationship and easy communication between both teams are essential. A physician dedicated to this role in the adult team is needed. The young person can have the option to go back under the pediatric team to maintain a dialogue with the adults they have known for, sometimes, the longest time of their life, but experience suggests that it is rarely needed. Although feared by families and medical teams, this transition – if well designed and conducted – is often well accepted and beneficial for the young adults.[44]

References available online at expertconsult.com.

KEY REFERENCES

Afran L., Garcia Knight M., Nduati E., et al.: HIV-exposed uninfected children: a growing population with a vulnerable immune system? *Clin Exp Immunol* 2014; 176(1): 11-22.

Bolton-Moore C., Mubiana-Mbewe M., Cantrell R.A., et al.: Clinical outcomes and CD4 cell response in children receiving antiretroviral therapy at primary health care facilities in Zambia. *JAMA* 2007; 298:1888-1899.

Chasela C.S., Hudgens M.G., Jamieson D.J., et al.: Maternal or infant antiretroviral drugs to reduce HIV-1 transmission. *N Engl J Med* 2010; 362:2271-2281.

Committee on Pediatric AIDS: Transitioning HIV-infected youth into adult health care. *Pediatrics* 2013; 132: 192-197.

Dunn D., HIV Paediatric Prognostic Markers Collaborative Study Group: Short-term risk of disease progression in HIV-1-infected children receiving no antiretroviral therapy or zidovudine monotherapy: a meta-analysis. *Lancet* 2003; 362:1605-1611.

Gray G.E., McIntyre J.A.: HIV and pregnancy. *BMJ* 2007; 334:950-953.

Kuhn L., Kasonde P., Sinkala M., et al.: Does severity of HIV disease in HIV-infected mothers affect mortality and morbidity among their uninfected infants? *Clin Infect Dis* 2005; 41:1654-1661.

Nielsen-Saines K., Watts D.H., Veloso V.G., et al.: Three postpartum antiretroviral regimens to prevent intrapartum HIV infection. *N Engl J Med* 2012; 366:2368-2379.

Persaud D., Luzuriaga K.: Absence of HIV-1 after treatment cessation in an infant. *N Engl J Med* 2014; 370:678.

Simoni J.M., Frick P.A., Pantalone D.W., et al.: Antiretroviral adherence interventions: a review of current literature and ongoing studies. *Top HIV Med* 2003; 11:185-198.

Warszawski J., Tubiana R., Le Chenadec J., et al.: Mother-to-child HIV transmission despite antiretroviral therapy in the ANRS French Perinatal Cohort. *AIDS* 2008; 22:289-299.

World Health Organization: Guideline on when to start antiretroviral therapy and on pre-exposure prophylaxis for HIV. Available: http://www.who.int/hiv/pub/guidelines/earlyrelease-arv/en/.

101

Special Problems in Women Who Have HIV Disease

BEVERLY E. SHA I CONSTANCE A. BENSON

KEY CONCEPTS

- In the USA, women currently comprise 21% of persons newly diagnosed with human immunodeficiency virus (HIV) infection. Worldwide, women comprise 51% of newly diagnosed persons.

- For women, sexually transmitted diseases, particularly genital ulcer disease, and bacterial vaginosis can increase the risk of HIV-1 acquisition and transmission.

- Antiretroviral therapy (ART) is an important tool to reduce transmission of HIV-1.

- Women generally have a lower plasma HIV-1 RNA level than men but disease progression rates are similar.

- Women with HIV-1 have higher rates of human papillomavirus infection and cervical dysplasia.

- Daily tenofovir and emtricitabine given to high-risk HIV-1 uninfected men and women can reduce their risk of acquiring HIV-1 infection.

- Maternal ART is safe and effective in reducing HIV transmission to infants.

Epidemiology

The number and proportion of women who have HIV-1 infection in the USA have been relatively stable since 2008. Of 47 352 persons estimated by the Centers for Disease Control and Prevention (CDC) to be diagnosed with HIV in 2013, 9728 (21%) were women.[1] The racial distribution of women diagnosed with HIV in 2013 was 62% African-American, 17% white and 17% Hispanic.[1]

Heterosexual transmission remains the primary route for women acquiring HIV-1 infection in the USA. For women diagnosed with HIV in 2013, estimates are that 87% acquired HIV-1 through heterosexual sex and 12% through intravenous drug use.

Worldwide, 2014 UNAIDS estimates are that, of the 34.3 million adults living with HIV-1/AIDS, 17.4 million (51%) are women.[2] Of these, 75% live in sub-Saharan Africa (see Chapter 89).

Transmission

Factors that are important in heterosexual transmission of HIV-1 infection include:
- advanced disease in the infected source partner
- measurable plasma and/or genital tract HIV-1 RNA
- presence of genital ulcers
- absence of condom use
- absence of antiretroviral therapy (ART) use[3–6]
- for HIV-1 uninfected women, receptive anal intercourse
- for HIV-1 uninfected men, heterosexual intercourse during menses.

Sexually transmitted diseases can enhance transmission and acquisition of HIV-1 by increasing genital tract HIV-1 shedding in the infected partner and reducing the integrity of mucosal tissue and recruiting immune cells that serve as targets for HIV infection in the

uninfected partner. Genital ulcer disease (herpes simplex virus [HSV], syphilis, chancroid) has been associated with an increased risk of transmission and acquisition of HIV-1 infection. In developing countries, non-ulcerative sexually transmitted diseases (gonorrhea, chlamydia, trichomoniasis) have also been associated with increased rates of HIV-1 transmission. Bacterial vaginosis has been associated with both an increased rate of HIV-1 acquisition and a 3.2-fold increased risk of HIV transmission to a male partner.[7] In HIV uninfected women, male partner circumcision has been associated with reduced risk of acquiring high-risk human papillomavirus (HPV) DNA types, cervical cancer, genital ulcer disease, bacterial vaginosis and trichomoniasis.[8] Suppression of HSV-2 infections in HIV-uninfected women does not decrease the risk of HIV acquisition or the risk of HIV transmission from herpes simplex and HIV co-infected women to their male partners.[9,10]

Some studies have suggested an increased risk of acquisition of HIV among women using progestin-only injectable contraception. Other studies have not shown this association and other forms of hormonal contraception have not increased the risk of HIV acquisition. Both the CDC and the World Health Organization (WHO) strongly encourage condom use and other preventive measures for women at high risk for HIV infection who are on progestin-only injectables.[11]

The male-to-female HIV-1 transmission rates per sex act are nearly twice those of female-to-male transmission rates, but are similar after adjusting for plasma viral load.[12] Among 2521 heterosexual serodiscordant couples in Africa, higher plasma and genital tract HIV-1 RNA levels increased the risk of heterosexual HIV-1 transmission.[13] After adjusting for plasma viral load, each 1.0 $\log_{10}$ increase in genital HIV-1 RNA was associated with a 1.67-fold ($P = 0.02$) increased risk of female-to-male transmission and 1.68-fold ($P = 0.02$) increased risk of male-to-female transmission. Early ART of 1763 HIV-infected men and women with a CD4 count between 350 and 550 cells/μL reduced the risk of transmission to their HIV-1 seronegative partners by 96% compared to delayed therapy initiated when the CD4 count fell below 350 cells/μL.[3]

Clinical Features
DISEASE MANIFESTATIONS AND PROGRESSION
Overall, there are few differences in the incidence of nongynecologic opportunistic diseases between men and women who have HIV-1 infection, except for a higher incidence of esophageal candidiasis and a lower incidence of Kaposi's sarcoma in women.[14] It is speculated that the higher incidence of candidiasis in women might be due to vaginal colonization with yeast or perhaps hormonal influences.

Several studies have now demonstrated that women have lower plasma HIV-1 RNA levels than do men after controlling for age, the interval from seroconversion, and the CD4+ lymphocyte count.[15] Another study found that this sex difference in plasma HIV-1 RNA levels disappeared 5–6 years after seroconversion. Although women may progress to AIDS with lower viral loads, the time to progression to AIDS appears to be similar for men and women. Similarly, for HIV-1-infected men and women who have adequate access to healthcare and treatment, treatment response and survival appears to be equivalent.[16]

TABLE 101-1	**Guidelines for Cervical Cancer Screening of Women with HIV-1 Infection**

Initial gynecologic examination with cervical cytology (either liquid-based Pap smear or standard Pap smear)	If normal, repeat in 6 months
	If atypical squamous cells of uncertain significance (ASCUS), three options exist for women ≥ 21 years:
	   (1) Colposcopy (ACOG and CDC prefer option 1 and 3)
	   (2) HPV (high-risk types) DNA testing; if positive proceed to colposcopy (preferred by ASCCP). If negative proceed to option 3 (ACOG, CDC) or repeat Pap smear and HPV testing in 3 years (ASCCP)
	   (3) Repeat Pap smear at 6–12 months; if abnormal proceed to colposcopy
	If atypical squamous cells cannot rule out high-grade SIL (ASC-H), proceed to colposcopy
	If low-grade SIL, proceed to colposcopy (ACOG, CDC) or obtain HPV testing, and if positive proceed to colposcopy and if negative Pap smear and HPV testing in 1 year (ASSCP)
	If high-grade SIL, immediate loop electrosurgical excision or proceed to colposcopy
	If atypical glandular cells (AGC), proceed to colposcopy

If initial two Pap smears are normal	Repeat annually as long as Pap smears remain normal

SIL, squamous intraepithelial lesion.
Compiled from ACOG Women's Health Care Physicians Practice Bulletin No. 117;[23] ASCCP 2012 updated consensus guidelines for the management of abnormal cervical cancer screening tests and cancer precursors;[24] Guidelines for the prevention and treatment of opportunistic infections in HIV-infected adults and adolescents: recommendations from the Centers for Disease Control and Prevention, the National Institutes of Health, and the HIV Medicine Association of the Infectious Diseases Society of America.[25]

GYNECOLOGIC MANIFESTATIONS

Infection

Gynecologic disorders are common in women who have HIV-1 infection.[17] Up to 50% of HIV-1-infected women develop recurrent *Candida* vaginitis, which often precedes the development of oral or esophageal candidiasis. Several longitudinal cohorts have reported that 14–18% of women who have HIV-1 infection have or develop recurrent genital HSV infection, which can be more severe or refractory to treatment than among HIV-1 seronegative women.

Genital Dysplasia

Cervicovaginal dysplasia is common in women who have HIV-1 infection.[17,18] Abnormal Papanicolaou (Pap) smears were found in 38.3% of 1713 HIV-1-infected women and 16.2% of 482 women uninfected with HIV-1 but at risk, in the Women's Interagency HIV-1 Study (WIHS) cohort.[18] In multivariate analyses, risk factors for abnormal cytology included HIV-1 infection, low CD4+ lymphocyte counts, high plasma HIV-1 RNA levels and detection of HPV. In follow-up of this cohort, HPV detection, CD4+ lymphocyte count and plasma HIV-1 RNA levels predicted regression.[19] Rates of incidence, progression and regression of abnormal cytology did not differ between the HIV-1-uninfected controls and HIV-1-infected women with CD4+ lymphocyte counts >200 cells/μL and plasma HIV-1 RNA levels below 4000 copies/mL. In another study, 20% (80/398) of HIV-1-seropositive women compared with 4% (15/357) of HIV-1-seronegative women had cervical intraepithelial neoplasia (CIN) confirmed by colposcopy.[20] The presence of CIN was found to be independently associated with:

- HPV infection (odds ratio 9.8)
- HIV-1 infection (odds ratio 3.5)
- CD4+ lymphocyte count <200/μL (odds ratio 2.7)
- age greater than 34 years (odds ratio 2.0).

The rate of CIN in women who have HIV-1 infection with <200 CD4+ lymphocytes/μL was 28% (27/95) compared with 19% (45/236) for those with higher CD4+ lymphocyte counts.

In the WIHS, both oncogenic and non-oncogenic HPV DNA types were found more frequently in cervical and anal samples from HIV-infected women than uninfected women.[21] Forty-two percent (163/386) of HIV-infected women had detectable HPV in both cervical and anal sites compared to only 8% (12/160) of HIV-uninfected women. In multivariate analysis, CD4 cell count <200 cells/μL was the strongest factor associated with HPV detection. A quadrivalent HPV vaccine (Gardasil) and a bivalent HPV vaccine (Cervarix) are approved for use in females 9–26 years of age. Both vaccines reduce the risk of high-grade dysplasia, CIN and cervical cancer. The quadrivalent HPV vaccine was shown to be highly immunogenic in HIV-1-infected

women aged 13–45 years with CD4 counts ≥200 cells/μL.[22] Women with HIV RNA plasma levels >10 000 copies/mL and/or CD4 cell counts <200 cells/μL had lower response rates.

The American College of Obstetricians and Gynecologists (ACOG), American Society for Colposcopy and Cervical Pathology (ASCCP) and CDC have each published guidelines on cervical cancer screening and the management of women who have cervical cytologic abnormalities.[23–25] ACOG and CDC recommend more frequent monitoring for HIV-infected women whereas ASCCP recommends the same management of abnormal cervical cancer screening tests as for HIV-uninfected women. Table 101-1 details these recommendations.[23–25] No national recommendations exist for routine screening of anal dysplasia. Some experts recommend anal Pap smears for women with cervical dysplasia and advanced HIV disease. Women with anal Pap smears demonstrating dysplasia should be referred for high-resolution anoscopy.[25]

Because *Candida* vaginitis, genital HSV disease, pelvic inflammatory disease (PID) and cervical dysplasia are common in women who have HIV-1 infection, these conditions, along with other common sexually transmitted diseases such as gonorrhea, chlamydial infection and syphilis, should prompt a determination of HIV-1 risk factors and appropriate HIV-1 screening as part of routine care for women.

Menstrual Cycle and Menopause

The impact of HIV-1 infection on the menstrual cycle appears to be limited. Reports of increased rates of dysmenorrhea, oligomenorrhea, amenorrhea or menorrhagia exist, but these have been discounted by other studies.[26] A combined analysis from the Women's Interagency HIV Study (WIHS) and the Heart and Estrogen/Progestin Replacement Study (HERS) with 802 HIV-infected women and 273 high-risk seronegative women found little relationship between HIV status and amenorrhea, menstrual cycle length or variability.[27]

Limited data exist on the effect of HIV infection on menopause. Some studies have suggested a slightly earlier onset of menopause among HIV-infected women (46 years vs 47 years) but this may be more related to other factors known to predict earlier onset of menopause such as substance use, tobacco smoking, low relative body weight, low socioeconomic status, depression and African-American ethnicity.

Prevention

CONTRACEPTION

Condoms are important for preventing the transmission of HIV-1 and other sexually transmitted diseases. However, alone they may not be adequate to prevent pregnancy. Reported breakage rates for male condoms are less than 2% for vaginal and anal intercourse. An evaluation of the effectiveness of the female condom at preventing pregnancy in 147 women over a 6-month period demonstrated an annual failure rate of 26%. Among 86 women who reported using the condom consistently and correctly, the annual failure rate was still 11%.[28]

Hormonal contraceptives should be considered in addition to condoms for women who have HIV-1 infection, are sexually active and wish to avoid pregnancy. Drug–drug interactions, particularly with protease inhibitors and non-nucleoside reverse transcriptase inhibitors (NNRTIs), can affect the levels of hormonal agents. Table 101-2 details these interactions and recommendations for their concomitant use.[29]

Pre-conception Counseling and Pre-exposure Prophylaxis (PrEP)

Prior to attempting to conceive, partners should be screened for genital tract infections and treated as appropriate. The infected partner should receive ART and achieve viral suppression prior to attempting conception. Artificial insemination or self-insemination timed to ovulation is the safest method for HIV-infected women who have HIV-uninfected male partners. For HIV-infected men with HIV-uninfected female partners, sperm washing techniques or *in vitro* fertilization have been safe and effective. Unfortunately these techniques are costly. More

TABLE 101-2 Drug Interactions Between Antiretrovirals and Oral Contraceptives and Recommended Adjustments

Agent	Effect on Oral Contraceptive	No Dose Adjustment	No Data	Use Alternative Agent or Second Method
Indinavir	Ethinyl estradiol AUC ↑25% Norethindrone AUC ↑26%	X		
Ritonavir	Ethinyl estradiol levels ↓40%			X
Saquinavir/r	↓Ethinyl estradiol			X
Nelfinavir	Ethinyl estradiol AUC ↓47% Norethindrone AUC ↓18%			X
Fosamprenavir	APV ↑ in ethinyl estradiol and ↑ in norethindrone Fosamprenavir with ethinyl estradiol/norethindrone APV AUC ↓22%			Use alternative method as may lead to loss of virologic response
Fosamprenavir/r	Ethinyl estradiol AUC ↓37% Norethindrone AUC ↓34%			X
Lopinavir/r	Ethinyl estradiol levels ↓42% Norethindrone AUC ↓17%			X
Atazanavir	Ethinyl estradiol AUC ↑48% Norethindrone AUC ↑110%			Use ≤ 30 µg of ethinyl estradiol
Atazanavir/r	Ethinyl estradiol AUC ↓19% Norgestimate ↑85%			Use ≥35 µg ethinyl estradiol
Atazanavir/c	Effects unknown			X
Tipranavir/r	Ethinyl estradiol AUC ↓48% Norethindrone no significant change			X
Darunavir/r	Ethinyl estradiol AUC ↓44% Norethindrone AUC ↓14%			X
Darunavir/c	Data unknown			X
Nevirapine	Ethinyl estradiol AUC ↓20% Norethindrone AUC ↓19% DMPA no significant change	X		Additional methods recommended for oral agents
Efavirenz	No effect on ethinyl estradiol levels Levonorgestrel AUC ↓83% Norelgestromin AUC ↓64% Etonogestrel (implant) ↓63%			Barrier method should be used in addition to hormone agent
Etravirine	Ethinyl estradiol AUC ↑22% Norethindrone no significant effect	X		
Rilpivirine	Ethinyl estradiol AUC ↑14% Norethindrone no significant change	X		
Maraviroc	No significant interaction	X		
Raltegravir	No significant interaction	X		
Elvitegravir/cobicistat/ emtricitabine/tenofovir	Ethinyl estradiol AUC ↓25%, C_min ↓44% Norgestimate AUC, C_max, C_min ↑ >2-fold ↑ 100%			X
Dolutegravir	No significant interaction	X		

APV, amprenavir; AUC, area under the curve; /r, ritonavir-boosted; /c, cobicistat-boosted.
Data from Panel on Antiretroviral Guidelines for Adults and Adolescents.[29]

recently, PrEP using daily tenofovir/emtricitabine in the uninfected partner has been shown to reduce the risk of heterosexual transmission by 62–75%.[30] While the addition of PrEP for the uninfected partner to treatment of the infected partner has not been studied, it seems prudent given no single intervention is fully protective against HIV transmission.

PREGNANCY

In the USA, in 1993, the rate of HIV-1 infection among women of childbearing age was 1.7 per 1000 with between 1000 and 2000 perinatally infected infants born to 6000–7000 HIV-1-infected women. CDC 2013 data indicate that fewer than 200 HIV-infected infants are born each year in the USA.[1] UNAIDS estimates for 2014 are that, worldwide, 150 000 children under 15 years of age died in 2014, and another 2.6 million children are currently living with HIV-1/AIDS, of whom 220 000 were infected in 2014.[31] From 2001 to 2012, there was a 52% decline in new HIV infections among children.[2]

Perinatal transmission can occur *in utero* and during labor and delivery, as well as postpartum, primarily through breast-feeding.[32] Excluding postpartum transmission through breast-feeding, data suggest that 75–80% of maternal–infant transmission occurs late in gestation or during labor and delivery (see Chapter 100).[33] Several studies have found that breast-feeding increases the rate of transmission by 16% over 2 years and thus breast-feeding is not recommended when safe alternatives are available.[32] Providing fully suppressive ART regimens to women during pregnancy and breast-feeding and nevirapine to their breast-fed infants reduces maternal–infant transmission.[34] Risk factors associated with transmission via breast-feeding include level of virus in the breast milk, mastitis, breast abscesses, maternal seroconversion during lactation, duration of feeding and mixed feeding.

A number of maternal and delivery factors appear to influence the risk of transmission and are listed in Table 101-3.[35] Interventions currently recommended to reduce transmission include:

- avoidance of invasive monitoring whenever possible
- avoidance of breast-feeding
- the use of ART during pregnancy and labor for the mother and in the peripartum and postpartum period for the infant
- treatment of sexually transmitted disease or vaginitis
- elective Cesarean section if plasma HIV-1 RNA level remains above 1000 copies/ml near term.

Antiretroviral Therapy to Prevent Perinatal Transmission

The landmark AIDS Clinical Trials Group (ACTG) 076 trial demonstrated a 66% reduction in maternal–infant HIV-1 transmission with zidovudine use in the mother during pregnancy, labor and delivery,

TABLE 101-3	Maternal, Labor and Delivery Factors that Increase the Risk of Maternal–Infant Transmission
Maternal Factors	**Labor and Delivery Factors**
Advanced maternal HIV disease	Chorioamnionitis
Maternal p24 antigenemia	Prolonged rupture of membranes (>4 hours)
Low maternal CD4+ lymphocyte counts	Premature delivery before 34 weeks' gestation
High maternal plasma HIV-1 RNA levels	Use of fetal scalp electrodes
Acute maternal HIV infection during pregnancy	Episiotomy with severe lacerations
Genital inflammation or maternal sexually transmitted disease at the time of delivery	Non-elective Cesarean section delivery
Detectable genital tract HIV-1 RNA near delivery	
Lack of antiretroviral therapy	
Breast-feeding	

and in the baby for the first 6 weeks of life (7.6% zidovudine vs 22.6% placebo).[36] ART diminishes maternal–infant transmission of HIV-1 through several mechanisms, including:

- decreasing maternal plasma and genital tract HIV-1 RNA levels
- decreasing exposure of the fetus to the virus *in utero*
- decreasing HIV exposure of the infant at delivery or in the neonatal period.

The end result is prevention of infection from becoming established in the fetus or infant. Transmission of HIV-1 occurs at all levels of CD4+ lymphocyte counts and even from some women who have undetectable plasma HIV-1 RNA levels, although overall the risk of transmission is greater in women who have lower CD4+ lymphocyte counts and higher plasma HIV-1 RNA levels, particularly at the time of delivery.[37] Detectable virus in the female genital tract at 38 weeks' gestation has also been independently associated with maternal–infant transmission of HIV-1.[38]

It is important to stress that even intervening late in pregnancy (including initiating therapy in the peripartum period) can diminish the risk of transmission.[39] In low- and middle-income countries, a two-dose nevirapine regimen (oral nevirapine, 200 mg as a single dose given to the mother at the onset of labor and oral nevirapine 2 mg/kg given to the infant within 72 hours of birth) was widely used based on a randomized comparison that demonstrated the two-dose nevirapine regimen reduced the risk of maternal–infant transmission by 47% compared with a truncated zidovudine regimen.[40] Follow-up data from this study, however, documented the occurrence of K103N mutations in virus recovered from up to 15% of women who were randomized to nevirapine, a mutation conferring cross-class resistance to NNRTIs (with the exception of etravirine and rilpivirine).[41] In addition, women randomized to receive nevirapine + tenofovir–emtricitabine for treatment of their HIV six or more months after receiving single-dose nevirapine for prevention of maternal–infant HIV transmission did worse than women randomized to lopinavir–ritonavir + tenofovir–emtricitabine.[42] For these reasons, WHO currently recommends the initiation of fully suppressive ART in HIV-infected pregnant women as soon as possible and to continue it lifelong wherever possible along with 6 weeks of daily nevirapine for the breast-fed HIV-exposed infant.[43]

All pregnant women should be offered HIV-1 testing. Repeat HIV antibody testing is recommended in the third trimester (preferably before 36 weeks' gestation) for women at high-risk (HIV-infected partner, community with HIV incidence in pregnant women ≥1 per 1000 per year, or incarceration) of acquiring HIV infection who have negative tests earlier in their pregnancy. Women who present to labor and delivery without prior HIV testing or are high risk and did not have their repeat testing in the third trimester should be offered a rapid HIV test to guide decisions. In general, current recommendations are to approach the treatment of the HIV-1-infected pregnant woman as if she were not pregnant and strive for maximal suppression of viral replication. Nevertheless, knowledge that limited data exist regarding toxicity of the 26 Food and Drug Administration (FDA)-approved antiretroviral agents to the developing fetus and the infant must also be taken into account. Tables 101-4 to 101-6 summarize the current information known about reverse transcriptase inhibitors, protease inhibitors, entry inhibitors and integrase inhibitors with regard to FDA approval status, placental transfer and carcinogenicity data.

To date, neither pre-term delivery nor birth defects have been clearly associated with any antiretroviral agent. Only efavirenz is listed as a class D drug with five retrospective case reports of neural tube defects ($n = 4$) and a case of Dandy–Walker malformation ($n = 1$). As of 31 January 2015, the prospective Antiretroviral Pregnancy Registry reported 20 birth defects in 852 women with first trimester efavirenz exposure.[45] This 2.3% prevalence rate falls within the expected rate of 2.72/100 live births. No specific pattern to the birth defects was seen; there was one case each of sacral myelomeningocele, anophthalmia, and cerebellar vermis abnormality. In the USA, efavirenz should be avoided when possible in the first trimester, because of evidence of teratogenicity in rhesus macaques at human doses. Because pregnancy

TABLE 101-4	Reverse Transcriptase Inhibitors					
			FDA Approved			
Agent	**Studies Showing Transmission to Fetus Prevented**	Neonates	Children	**FDA Pregnancy Category***	**Placental Transfer**	
Zidovudine	Yes	Yes	Yes	C	80%	
Didanosine	No	≥2 weeks	Yes	B	38%	
Lamivudine	Yes	Yes	Yes	C	100%	
Stavudine	No	Yes	Yes	C	50%	
Abacavir	Yes	No	≥3 months	C	High	
Emtricitabine	Yes	Yes	Yes	B	85%	
Tenofovir	No	No	≥2 years	B	60–100%	
Nevirapine	Yes	Yes	Yes	B	60–100%	
Efavirenz	No	No	≥3 months	D	49%	
Etravirine	No	No	≥6 years	B	moderate/high	
Rilpivirine	No	No	≥18 years	B	moderate/high	

*FDA pregnancy categories:
A, Adequate and well-controlled studies of pregnant women fail to demonstrate a risk to the fetus during the first trimester and no evidence of risk during later trimesters.
B, Animal studies fail to demonstrate a risk to the fetus but no adequate studies exist in pregnant women.
C, Animal studies demonstrate risk or have not been conducted and safety in human pregnancy has not yet been determined. However, the benefit of the drug may still outweigh the risk.
D, Positive evidence of human fetal risk exists based on adverse reaction data but benefits may still outweigh the risks.
Data from Panel on Antiretroviral Guidelines for Adults and Adolescents;[29] Panel on Guidelines for the Use of Antiviral Agents in Pediatric HIV Infection.[44]

TABLE 101-5	Protease Inhibitors and Pharmacokinetic (PK) Enhancer				
		FDA Approved			
Agent	**Studies Showing Transmission to Fetus Prevented**	Neonates	Children	**FDA Pregnancy Category***	**Placental Transfer**
Nelfinavir	No	No	≥2 years	B	Minimal
Indinavir	No	No	≥18 years	C	12%
Ritonavir	No	No	>1 month	B	Minimal
Saquinavir	No	No	≥2 years	B	Minimal
Fosamprenavir	No	No	≥6 months	C	24–27%
Lopinavir/r	Yes	≥2 weeks	Yes	C	20%
Atazanavir	No	No	≥3 months	B	13–21%
Tipranavir	No	No	≥2 years	C	moderate
Darunavir	No	No	≥3 years	C	24%
PK Enhancer					
Cobicistat	No	No	≥ 18 years	B	?

*FDA pregnancy categories – see Table 101-4.
Data from Panel on Antiretroviral Guidelines for Adults and Adolescents;[29] Guidelines for the Use of Antiviral Agents in Pediatric HIV Infection.[44]

is generally identified after 5–6 weeks' gestation and data to date have not identified an increased risk of teratogenicity, pregnant women on efavirenz may continue treatment.

The US Public Health Service (USPHS) has drafted the following guidelines for the treatment of HIV-1-infected pregnant women.[46]

- If the woman has had no prior ART, HIV resistance testing should be performed and treatment started as soon as possible. If the woman presents late in gestation, treatment can be started pending results of resistance testing. In the USA, one of the following 2-nucleoside reverse transcriptase inhibitor backbones is recommended (zidovudine/lamivudine, abacavir/lamivudine [if HLAB*5701 negative), tenofovir/emtricitabine or tenofovir/lamivudine) with ritonavir-boosted atazanavir or darunavir or raltegravir if resistance or toxicity do not preclude their use.[46] Consideration can be given to delaying the initiation of therapy in women with a high CD4⁺ cell count and low viral load until after 10–12 weeks' gestation, which is thought to be the critical time for fetal organogenesis.

- If the HIV-1-infected pregnant woman is already receiving ART when pregnancy is diagnosed, then therapy should be continued, even in the first trimester. Although not recommended (particularly for women with CD4⁺ lymphocyte counts <200 cells/µL), if the decision is made to stop therapy during the first trimester owing to concerns about teratogenicity, all drugs should be stopped and then restarted simultaneously in order to minimize the development of resistance.

- If zidovudine is not administered during the prepartum period or, if resistance or intolerance precludes its use, zidovudine should still be administered intravenously intrapartum if the near-term HIV RNA level is ≥1000 copies/mL and to the baby.

TABLE 101-6	Entry and Integrase Inhibitors (FDA Approved)					
Agent	Studies Showing Transmission to Fetus Prevented	Neonates	Children	FDA Pregnancy Category*	Placental Transfer
Entry Inhibitors					
Enfuvirtide	No	No	≥6 years	B	None
Maraviroc	No	No	≥16 years	B	33%
Integrase Inhibitors					
Raltegravir	No	No	≥4 weeks	C	98%
Elvitegravir/cobicistat/tenofovir/emtricitabine	No	No	≥18 years	B	?
Elvitegravir	No	No	≥18 years	B	?
Dolutegravir	No	No	≥12 years	B	?

*FDA pregnancy categories – see Table 101-4/r, ritonavir-boosted.
Data from Panel on Antiretroviral Guidelines for Adults and Adolescents;[29] Panel on Treatment of HIV-infected Pregnant Women and Prevention of Perinatal Transmission;[46] Panel on Antiretroviral Therapy and Medical Management of HIV-Infected Children.[44]

- If an HIV-1-infected woman presents in labor and no prior ART has been given, intrapartum intravenous zidovudine is recommended with consideration for Cesarean section. The newborn should receive zidovudine for 6 weeks with three doses of nevirapine at birth, 48 hours after the first dose and 96 hours after the second dose. Some experts recommend additional infant drugs in high-risk situations. The CDC's National Perinatal HIV Hotline is an excellent resource (1-888-448-8765).

Infants born to HIV-1-infected mothers who have received no ART during pregnancy or intrapartum should receive the same regimen of zidovudine and three doses of nevirapine. Consideration may also be given to treating the infant with additional antiretroviral medications. The mother's therapy should be re-evaluated after delivery in both these situations.

Resistance testing should be performed in all pregnant women with a detectable HIV-1 RNA level >500 copies/mL prior to initiating or changing therapy. While underlying resistance can affect the ability to achieve maximal viral suppression, it is not clear that the presence of mutations increases the likelihood of transmission to the infant. Resistant virus has been transmitted to infants; however, women who have zidovudine resistance mutations have not consistently transmitted infection to their infants at higher rates and, in some cases where transmission has occurred, wild-type virus was transmitted.

A meta-analysis of 15 prospective cohort studies, conducted in an era when pregnant HIV-1-infected women received no ART or zidovudine monotherapy, showed that elective Cesarean section decreased the risk of maternal–infant transmission of HIV-1 compared with other modes of delivery.[47] For women on zidovudine, transmission was 2% with elective Cesarean section and 7.3% with other modes of delivery. Because transmission rates are expected to be below 2% for women on potent ART with controlled viremia, ACOG recommends Cesarean section before the onset of labor for women who have plasma HIV-1 RNA levels above 1000 copies/mL near term. The Cesarean section should be performed at 38 weeks' gestation without amniocentesis to assess for fetal lung maturity. For a scheduled Cesarean section, intravenous zidovudine should be started 3 hours before surgery.

Duration of ruptured membranes is also associated with an increased risk of transmission. A meta-analysis of the same 15 studies used to assess the benefit of Cesarean section showed, for the first 24 hours after membrane rupture, a 2% increase in transmission for every additional hour of membrane rupture.[48] Cleansing the birth canal with a 0.25% chlorhexidine solution every 4 hours until delivery did not reduce transmission in one study, except when membranes were ruptured more than 4 hours before delivery.[49] Whether or not non-elective Cesarean section to shorten the duration of ruptured membranes or labor will further reduce transmission rates is currently unknown.

Safety monitoring guided by the pregnant woman's specific ART should be performed.[46] Routine hematologic monitoring is recommended for women on zidovudine, routine renal monitoring for women on tenofovir and liver function monitoring in all women receiving ART. Pregnant women receiving protease inhibitors and NRTIs have occasionally developed hepatic toxicity and lactic acidosis/hepatic steatosis, respectively. Women initiating nevirapine should have frequent monitoring of transaminase levels due to the risk of hepatotoxicity that can occur within the first 18 weeks. Standard glucose tolerance testing is recommended at 24–28 weeks' gestation. Some experts recommend earlier testing for women on chronic protease inhibitor therapy begun prior to pregnancy. In general, the plasma HIV-1 RNA level should be monitored 2–4 weeks after initiating or changing ART, monthly until undetectable and then every 3 months until delivery. A plasma HIV-1 RNA level should be obtained at 34–36 weeks gestation to guide decisions on mode of delivery. The CD4+ lymphocyte count should be monitored every 3 months or every 6 months if stable at the time of pregnancy. A first trimester ultrasound is recommended to guide dates. A second trimester, level II ultrasound is recommended to assess the fetus for women on combination ART.

HIV-1-infected pregnant women should be prospectively reported to the appropriate agencies that collect safety and teratogenicity data. In the USA, the Antiretroviral Pregnancy Registry can be reached at www.apregistry.com.

In general, pregnant women who have HIV-1 infection should receive prophylaxis for opportunistic infections appropriate for their stage of disease.[25] For *Pneumocystis jirovecii* pneumonia prophylaxis, some experts recommend avoiding trimethoprim–sulfamethoxazole and dapsone in the first trimester. Aerosolized pentamidine or atovaquone can be substituted during this time period. Azithromycin is preferred agent for primary *Mycobacterium avium* complex prophylaxis in pregnant women as clarithromycin is teratogenic in animals. Pregnant women who have latent tuberculosis should consider isoniazid prophylaxis during pregnancy, particularly if they have advanced disease. Pregnant women should also avoid eating raw or undercooked meat and avoid contact with cat feces to diminish the risk of toxoplasmosis. Good hand washing techniques should be employed for prevention of cytomegalovirus (CMV) disease, particularly in women who are healthcare workers or who have children in daycare settings.[25] For CMV-seronegative women who require blood transfusions, only CMV-seronegative blood products should be used.[25]

Several studies have demonstrated no adverse effect of pregnancy on the progression of HIV-1 disease for women who have CD4+ lymphocyte counts >200 cells/μL.[50] Unfortunately, women who have more advanced HIV-1 disease may not tolerate pregnancy as well and may have a higher rate of spontaneous abortion, prematurity, low birth-weight infants and other complications of pregnancy.[51]

References available online at expertconsult.com.

KEY REFERENCES

ACOG Women's Health Care Physicians Practice Bulletin: ACOG Practice Bulletin No. 117: Gynecologic care for women with human immunodeficiency virus. *Obstet Gynecol* 2010; 116:1492-1509, Reaffirmed in 2012.

Antiretroviral Pregnancy Registry Steering Committee: Antiretroviral Pregnancy Registry international interim report for 1 January 1989 through 31 January 2015, Wilmington, NC, Registry Coordinating Center, 2015. Available: www.apregistry.com.

Baeten J.M., Kahle E., Lingappa J.R., et al.: Genital HIV-1 RNA predicts risk of heterosexual HIV-1 transmission. *Sci Transpl Med* 2011; 3:77ra29.

CDC: Update to CDC's U.S. Medical Eligibility Criteria for contraceptive use, 2010. Revised recommendations for the use of hormonal contraception among women at high risk for HIV infection or infected with HIV. *MMWR Morb Mortal Wkly Rep* 2012; 61:449-452.

Cohen M.S., Chen Y.Q., McCauley M., et al.: Prevention of HIV-1 infection with early antiretroviral therapy. *N Engl J Med* 2011; 365:493-505.

International Perinatal HIV Group: Duration of ruptured membranes and vertical transmission of HIV-1: a meta-analysis from 15 prospective cohort studies. *AIDS* 2001; 15:357-368.

Jiang J., Yang X., Ye L., et al.: Pre-exposure prophylaxis for the prevention of HIV infection in high risk populations: a meta-analysis of randomized controlled trials. *PLoS ONE* 2014; 9(2):e87674.

Kojic E.M., Kang M., Cespedes M., et al.: Immunogenicity and safety of the quadrivalent human papillomavirus vaccine in HIV-1-infected women. *Clin Infect Dis* 2014; 59(1):127-135.

Kourtis A.P., Bulterys M., Nesheim S.R., et al.: Understanding the timing of HIV transmission from mother to infant. *JAMA* 2001; 285:709-712.

Massad L.S., Ahdieh L., Benning L., et al.: Evolution of cervical abnormalities among women with HIV-1: evidence from surveillance cytology in the Women's Interagency HIV Study. *J Acquir Immune Defic Syndr* 2001; 27:432-442.

Panel on Treatment of HIV-infected Pregnant Women and Prevention of Perinatal Transmission: Recommendations for use of antiretroviral drugs in pregnant HIV-1-infected women for maternal health and interventions to reduce perinatal HIV transmission in the United States. Available: http://aidsinfo.nih.gov/ContentFiles/lvguidelines/PerinatalGL.pdf.

Read JS for the International Perinatal HIV Group: The mode of delivery and the risk of vertical transmission of human immunodeficiency virus type 1: a meta-analysis of 15 prospective cohort studies. *N Engl J Med* 1999; 34:977-987.

Sterling T.R., Vlahov D., Astemborski J., et al.: Initial plasma HIV-1 RNA levels and progression to AIDS in women and men. *N Engl J Med* 2001; 344:720-725.

World Health Organization: Consolidated guidelines on the use of antiretroviral drugs for treating and preventing HIV infection: recommendations for a public health approach. Geneva: WHO; 2013. Available: www.who.int/hiv/pub/guidelines/arv2013/en/.

102

Principles of Management of HIV in the Industrialized World

MARK W. HULL | MARIANNE HARRIS | JULIO S.G. MONTANER

KEY CONCEPTS

- The primary goals of HIV management are to improve quality of life, prevent or reverse immunologic impairment, stop disease progression (by preventing opportunistic infections and cancers), and prolong survival. These are consistently achieved by suppressing viral replication with combination antiretroviral therapy (ART).

- Durable suppression of viral replication is required to prevent the emergence of drug-resistant HIV strains. To ensure this, the goal of ART is sustained undetectable plasma viral load (below the lower limit of quantification) in all patients, regardless of previous treatment experience.

- ART is most effective when taken consistently and continuously. Education, counseling and ongoing support are necessary to ensure adherence.

- Long-term ART can be associated with metabolic complications and reduced bone mineral density; however, these adverse effects are far outweighed by ART-associated decreased morbidity, prolonged survival, and significantly reduced rates of major HIV-related cardiovascular, hepatic, neurologic and renal events.

- In addition to benefits to the HIV-infected individual, immediate initiation of ART markedly reduces the risk of HIV transmission by all routes (by more than 95%).

- Criteria for treatment initiation continue to evolve; currently routine administration of ART is recommended in all individuals regardless of CD4 cell count.

Introduction

The management of HIV infection continues to evolve as a result of a better understanding of HIV pathogenesis and associated inflammation, and potential secondary benefits of antiretroviral therapy (ART). ART has advanced considerably, and regimens have become better tolerated, safer and, with the advent of fixed-dose combinations, of minimal pill burden.[1] ART-related immune reconstitution reliably prevents AIDS-related morbidity and mortality and, as a result, the life expectancy of HIV-infected individuals in the modern ART era is now measured in decades – approaching that of uninfected individuals.[2,3] Improved longevity has been associated with the emergence of new challenges, including recognized potential adverse effects of long-term exposure to ART. These include dyslipidemias, renal impairment, osteoporosis and increased risk of myocardial infarction (see Chapter 104).[4–8] Uptake of ART has also been associated with evidence of significant reduction in transmission of HIV within discordant couples and also at the population level (see Chapter 90).[9,10]

Management strategies now focus on preparing patients for early and even immediate initiation of ART, often independent of CD4 cell count levels. This is to prevent morbidity and mortality and, secondarily, HIV transmission. In addition, patients must be protected from other infectious diseases by vaccination or prophylaxis when appropriate.

Baseline Evaluation of the HIV-Infected Individual

HISTORY AND PHYSICAL EXAMINATION

The history should elicit the date of diagnosis and information regarding prior negative HIV tests in order to estimate the length of time since infection. Symptoms related to potential acute seroconversion illness, progression of chronic HIV infection, and manifestations of opportunistic infections should be explored. For patients who had previously received ART, detailed information regarding CD4 cell count nadir, opportunistic infections, previous drug regimens, prior virologic failure/drug resistance and adverse effects to previous regimens should be obtained. In addition, details regarding co-morbidities, concomitant medication, drug allergies and social factors, such as sexual practices and drug use, should be thoroughly documented.

The physical examination should emphasize clinical manifestations of HIV disease and those of AIDS-related opportunistic infections or malignancies. In patients with advanced disease (CD4 cell count <50 cells/μL), ophthalmologic assessment with a slit-lamp examination to rule out cytomegalovirus (CMV) retinitis is required. In female patients, Papanicolaou (Pap) testing should be performed to assess for cervical dysplasia. In men who have sex with men (MSM) with history of receptive anal intercourse, and in all patients with known genital warts, anal Pap testing has been recommended by some authorities.[11]

General laboratory tests to be conducted at baseline prior to the start of ART should include those listed in Table 102-1.

PROGNOSTIC LABORATORY MARKERS

The CD4 cell count and plasma HIV viral load are key prognostic markers for disease progression to AIDS or death among untreated HIV-infected individuals.[12,13] CD4 cell counts are reported in absolute numbers and as the percentage (fraction) of total lymphocytes. The CD4 cell count reflects the level of immune suppression. In adults, the CD4 cell count is normally between 400 and 1400 cells/μL. As the CD4 cell count falls below normal, and particularly once thresholds of 200 cells/μL or a CD4 percentage of 15% are reached, the risk of opportunistic infection rises.[14,15] There is diurnal variation in the CD4 cell count; it is lowest in the morning and highest in the evening. The absolute CD4 cell count can also be influenced by acute illness, co-morbidities and drugs such as systemic corticosteroids or cancer chemotherapy. Short-term CD4 fluctuations of up to 30% have been shown to occur in HIV-infected individuals who are clinically stable.[16] As a result, it is important to monitor trends in the CD4 cell count over time rather than placing too much emphasis on a single reading.

Plasma viral load has been shown to be an independent predictor of disease progression and death in untreated HIV-infected individuals, and may be a factor in deciding when to initiate ART.[17,18] Plasma viral load is also an independent predictor of the risk of HIV transmission.[19] Three assays are commonly available to quantify plasma HIV-1 viral load: the HIV RNA polymerase chain reaction (PCR), the branched-chain DNA and the nucleic acid sequence-based amplification assays (see also Chapter 174). Ultrasensitive assays have lower limits of detection of 40–50 copies/mL. The variability of the assay is approximately 0.3 $\log_{10}$ copies/mL and, as a result, a 0.5 $\log_{10}$ change in HIV RNA is regarded as a significant change in the context of ART. Among patients on ART, the plasma viral load is the primary

TABLE 102-1	Laboratory Tests for Baseline Evaluation of HIV-Infected Individuals
Test	**Comment**
HIV-SPECIFIC TESTS	
Plasma HIV RNA (viral load)	
CD4+ lymphocyte count (absolute and percentage)	
HIV resistance testing	HIV genotype
HLA-B*5701 assay	Positive result is associated with an increased risk for abacavir hypersensitivity reaction
GENERAL LABORATORY PROFILE	
Complete blood count with differential and platelet count	Evaluates baseline abnormalities such as anemia or HIV-related thrombocytopenias
Creatinine, estimated glomerular filtration rate (eGFR), urinalysis, urine albumin to creatinine or protein to creatinine ratio	Baseline renal abnormalities may require further investigation and influence choice of antiretrovirals
Liver profile (alanine aminotransferase, aspartate aminotransferase, total bilirubin, INR)	Abnormalities may require further hepatic investigations. Elevated baseline liver profile may affect antiretroviral choice (avoidance of agents associated with higher rate of hepatotoxicity)
Fasting lipid profile (total, HDL and LDL cholesterol; triglycerides; apolipoprotein B if triglycerides elevated), fasting blood sugar	Future risk of cardiac-related morbidity may require early interventions and influence the choice of antiretrovirals
Pregnancy test	
COINFECTION/OPPORTUNISTIC DISEASES ASSESSMENT	
Urine, urethral or cervical screens for sexually transmitted infections as indicated by history and examination	Ongoing screens q3 months recommended in at-risk individuals
Serologic testing for syphilis	Rapid plasma reagin (RPR) or T. pallidum EIA
Serologic testing for hepatitis A, B and C	If hepatitis B serology is in keeping with chronic infection or resolved infection, consider hepatitis B DNA screen. Vaccinate nonimmune individuals. Those with positive HCV antibody should undergo screening with HCV RNA PCR and HCV genotype
Toxoplasma and cytomegalovirus serology	
Tuberculin skin test or interferon-gamma release assay (±sputum smears and cultures for mycobacteria, as indicated by history and physical examination)	If evidence of prior exposure and no signs of active infection (latent tuberculosis infection), consider isoniazid prophylaxis
Chest radiography	
Cervical Papanicolaou smear Anal Pap	Anal Pap to be considered in MSM and history of receptive anal intercourse and in all patients with genital warts

laboratory marker of treatment efficacy, and the goal of therapy is to achieve an undetectable (below the lower limit of quantification) plasma viral load in all patients, regardless of treatment experience.

RESISTANCE TESTING AND EVALUATION OF HLA-B*5701 ALLELE STATUS

A baseline genotypic resistance test should be performed in all patients on the first available plasma viral load sample and again on a recent sample prior to selection of the first ART regimen, to evaluate for drug-resistant virus.[20] Determination of resistance at baseline (transmitted resistance) will help to guide future therapy, and resistance mutations should be taken into account even if later testing reveals wild-type virus. The HLA-B*5701 human genotypic testing should be performed in HIV-infected persons once, before starting or restarting abacavir. Positivity for this allele reliably predicts hypersensitivity to the nucleoside reverse transcriptase inhibitor (NRTI) abacavir.[11,21,22] Abacavir should be avoided in patients who are positive for the HLA-B*5701 allele. Determination of CCR-5 tropism is required prior to use of the CCR-5 antagonist, maraviroc.

COUNSELING

The need for risk reduction counseling should be assessed on an ongoing basis. This should include assessment of sexual activities, substance use and other factors that may influence adherence to ART

such as psychiatric disorders and depression. When issues are identified, patients should receive targeted counseling and appropriate referral.

Preventive Health Management

TUBERCULIN SKIN TEST

A tuberculin skin test should be performed at baseline and annually in patients at risk for exposure to tuberculosis. Induration >5 mm is considered positive, and should prompt evaluation for possible active tuberculosis prior to consideration of treatment for latent tuberculosis infection.[23] Laboratory-based interferon-gamma release assays to assess prior exposure to tuberculosis may also be available. These assays may improve assessment in individuals with prior Bacille Calmette–Guérin (BCG) vaccine or potential exposure to other mycobacteria.[11,24] A 9-month course of isoniazid in conjunction with pyridoxine is recommended as a first-line regimen, although shorter course (6-month regimen) has been used.[25]

VACCINATIONS

Standard vaccines such as diphtheria-pertussis-tetanus and measles-mumps-rubella (MMR) vaccines should be updated as necessary; live virus vaccines such as MMR and varicella should only be administered to nonpregnant individuals with CD4 counts >200 cells/μL.[26]

TABLE 102-2	Prophylaxis and Treatment for Opportunistic Infections
CD4+ Lymphocyte Cell Count	**Management Strategy**
Any	If needed, update standard diphtheria–pertussis–tetanus vaccine Annual influenza vaccine 13-valent pneumococcal conjugate vaccine followed by 23-valent pneumococcal polysaccharide vaccine. Responses may be better if CD4 >200 cells/μL. Revaccination should be considered after 5 years with the polysaccharide vaccine Hepatitis A and B vaccines Tuberculin skin test or interferon-gamma release assay (IGRA) and 9 months isoniazid prophylaxis if ≥5 mm induration or positive IGRA
<500	Any change the management strategy to say routine initiation of antiretroviral therapy recommended. Monitor CD4 cell count and viral load every 3–4 months if therapy deferred
<350	Routine initiation of antiretroviral therapy recommended in all current guidelines
<200	Initiate *Pneumocystis jirovecii* prophylaxis Trimethoprim–sulfamethoxazole 160 mg/800 mg (1 double-strength tablet) q24 h is first-line agent Alternate options: • dapsone 100 mg daily • atovaquone 1500 mg daily • inhaled pentamidine 300 mg monthly
<100	Start appropriate prophylaxis for toxoplasmosis if seropositive and if not receiving trimethoprim–sulfamethoxazole Options: • dapsone 100 mg daily with folinic acid 25 mg weekly and pyrimethamine 50 mg weekly • atovaquone 1500 mg weekly
<50	MAC prophylaxis with azithromycin 1200 mg po weekly (once baseline mycobacterial blood cultures are negative after 2–3 weeks of incubation) Ophthalmologic screening for cytomegalovirus retinitis (repeat at 6-monthly intervals)

Influenza vaccine should be administered annually at the beginning of the winter season.[27,28] Recommendations for pneumococcal vaccination have recently been updated.[29] In North America, previously unvaccinated individuals receive initially the 13-valent pneumococcal conjugate vaccine, followed sequentially by the administration of the polyvalent polysaccharide vaccine given no sooner than 8 weeks later, and repeated after 5 years. In individuals who have already received the pneumococcal vaccine, a dose of the conjugate vaccine can be administered at least 1 year following polysaccharide vaccine. Hepatitis A and B vaccines should be encouraged, particularly in at-risk individuals such as injection drug users, those with multiple sexual partners, MSM, and individuals co-infected with hepatitis C.[30] Additional vaccination strategies include the use of the human papilloma virus (HPV) vaccine in both men and women less than 26 years of age.[26]

PROPHYLAXIS

As seen in Table 102-2, as HIV disease progresses, prophylaxis for opportunistic infections becomes increasingly important (see also Chapter 94). Opportunistic infections include *Pneumocystis jirovecii* pneumonia, toxoplasmosis, *Mycobacterium avium* complex (MAC) and CMV.[25]

Both primary and secondary prophylaxis for these opportunistic infections can be discontinued in patients who experience ART-related consistent increases in their CD4 cell counts to levels >100 cells/μL for MAC, and >200 cells/μL for toxoplasmosis and *Pneumocystis jirovecii*.[31–33]

Initiation of ART

The objective of ART is to prevent disease progression and prolong survival while maintaining quality of life. Long-term non-progression (or disease remission) will be achieved by reducing plasma viral load to below the lower limit of detection of current plasma viral load assays on a sustained basis (i.e. maintaining an undetectable viral load).[2,3,34,35] In the past, treatment interruptions had been used as a clinical strategy to spare patients extended ART exposure; however, a large controlled clinical trial has shown conclusively that structured treatment interruptions are associated with both AIDS-related events and non-AIDS-related mortality.[36] Currently structured treatment interruptions are to

be strongly discouraged, and long-term (life-time) virologic suppression is the mainstay of ART.

The United States Department of Health and Human Services (DHHS) and the International Antiviral Society (IAS)–USA have produced comprehensive, and regularly updated, consensus guidelines for the management of HIV, including issues around the initiation of therapy.[1,22] These are generally consistent with guidelines published by a number of other national societies, although currently differences exist with regard to timing of initiation of ART.[37,38]

When to Start Therapy
GENERAL PRINCIPLES

ART should be commenced in patients with HIV-related symptoms or signs, opportunistic infections or cancers. For asymptomatic patients, initiation of therapy has traditionally been based primarily on CD4 cell counts as the key prognostic marker of the risk for disease progression.[12] Initial cohort studies demonstrated that a CD4 cell count of 200 cells/μL represented a critical threshold for identifying those at increased risk of AIDS-defining conditions.[39,40] As such, with concerns in the early ART era regarding ART-related toxicity, emergence of resistance and cost, therapy was often delayed until this threshold was reached in order to maximize time off ART and to intervene at a threshold of increased risk for progressive disease. However, this has become less relevant due to the recognition that HIV-infected individuals are expected to live a near-normal lifespan, with an expected survival on ART of several decades. Thus, given the projected overall ART exposure for any given HIV-infected individual, deferring therapy for a relatively brief period of time at initial diagnosis would have limited, if any, impact on these concerns. Furthermore, delaying ART may compromise the therapeutic response, tolerability and the impact on preventing HIV transmission.

Data from large cohort studies have now demonstrated that AIDS-related morbidity and mortality may occur more commonly at higher CD4 strata than previously recognized – up to 350 cells/μL.[41,42] Additionally, there is growing recognition of the deleterious consequences of chronic inflammatory states due to uncontrolled HIV replication regardless of CD4 cell count.[43,44] As such, guidelines continue to evolve with regard to the consideration of early initiation of ART at CD4 cell count strata above 500 cells/μL.[1,22,45] Data from several large collaborative cohorts and a randomized trial has demonstrated benefit from ART initiated at CD4 counts above the previously identified threshold of 350 cells/μL. In the ART Cohort Collaboration (ART-CC), deferring combination therapy until a CD4 cell count of 251–350 cells/μL was associated with higher rates of AIDS and death than starting therapy in the range 351–450 cells/μL (hazard ratio [HR] 1.28; 95% confidence interval [CI] 1.04–1.57).[46] Similarly in the HIV-CAUSAL collaboration, delaying initiation of ART until CD4 count <350 cells/μL was associated with a greater risk of AIDS-defining illness or death than initiating ART with higher CD4 count (HR 1.38; 95% CI 1.23–1.56).[42] Additional data from the North American AIDS Cohort Collaboration on Research and Design (NA-ACCORD) suggest a benefit from initiation of ART therapy above 500 cells/μL. In an analysis of individuals either initiating therapy at CD4 counts above 500 cells/μL or deferring therapy, among patients in the deferred-therapy group there was an increase in the risk of death of 94% (relative risk 1.94; 95% CI 1.37–2.79).[47]

The clinical outcomes associated with immediate use of ART within the HIV Prevention Trials Network (HPTN) 052 trial also support the use of early ART.[48] In this study, the HIV-infected members of serodiscordant couples were randomly allocated to either immediate ART (i.e. starting ART at a CD4 count of 350–550 cells/μL) or deferred ART (i.e. starting ART when the CD4 count fell below 250 cells/μL). Individuals assigned to immediate ART had fewer primary clinical events (HR 0.73; 95% CI 0.52–1.03), new-onset AIDS events (HR 0.64; 95% CI 0.43–0.96), and tuberculosis (HR 0.49; 95% CI 0.28–0.89). These data show a clear benefit to patients of starting ART early, when the CD4 count is well above 400 cells/μL. More recently, results of the START study have been published.[49] This study randomized 4685 adults with CD4 cell counts above 500 cells/μL to immediate ART or to defer ART until the CD4 count dropped below 350 cells/μL. The composite endpoint was development of an AIDS illness, a serious non-AIDS event or death. The risk of these outcomes was reduced by 57% (HR 0.43; 95% CI 0.30–0.62) in those who were randomized to start at higher CD4 cell count. Together with the secondary benefit of early ART to reduce HIV transmission (Treatment as Prevention – see below), these data have led all major guidelines, to recommend early ART to be considered in all asymptomatic individuals (in the IAS and DHHS guidelines) *regardless* of CD4 cell count.[1,22,37,38,45] It is increasingly recommended that ART should also be offered to those presenting within the seroconversion window.[1,22]

All clinical guidelines recognize that the evidence for earlier initiation of ART (i.e. above 350–500 cells/μL) is greatest in the presence of conditions that may be exacerbated by chronic HIV-related inflammatory states or ongoing uncontrolled viral replication. These conditions include underlying cardiovascular disease, hepatitis B or C coinfection (see below), and HIV-associated nephropathy.

The effectiveness of ART is critically dependent on maintaining nearly perfect levels of adherence to therapy. Incomplete adherence is a key determinant of the emergence of drug-resistant HIV,[50–52] increased risk for progression to AIDS, and death.[50,51] HIV drug resistance is typically associated with risk for cross-resistance to other members of the same drug class, limiting future treatment options. Thus, it is critical that patients be appropriately counseled, and that they have access to adherence support while initiating ART.

SPECIAL CONSIDERATIONS
Treatment as Prevention
The presence of HIV within blood and genital secretions is a critical driver of transmission events, and transmission risk has been linked to higher viral load values.[19] Results of observational cohort studies have demonstrated that ART markedly decreases HIV transmission risk within the setting of a serodiscordant relationship.[53,54] These results have been confirmed in a randomized controlled trial. HPTN052 randomized 1763 serodiscordant couples (54% from Africa, 50% male

HIV-infected partners) to receive immediate or deferred ART. Overall, 28 linked transmission events were noted, only one occurring in the early ART group (HR 0.04; 95% CI 0.01–0.27), a 96% reduction in transmission risk.[9] Recent data from the European Partners study have confirmed decreased transmission in HIV-infected MSM with documented sustained virologic suppression.[55] In an analysis of 767 serodiscordant couples, 40% of whom were MSM, there were no documented linked transmission events over approximately 44 000 condomless sex acts.[55] Mathematical models and population-based ecologic studies suggest that further expansion of antiretroviral coverage would play a major role in controlling the spread of HIV, and further support immediate initiation of ART.[10,56,57] As such, early initiation of therapy at high CD4 cell counts to prevent transmission to an uninfected partner is an additional key consideration for treatment initiation of ART in current guidelines.

Coinfection with Viral Hepatitis
Coinfection with hepatitis C and/or B virus is common among HIV-infected individuals. Coinfection with HIV may accelerate the progression of liver disease due to viral hepatitis[58,59] and conversely may enhance the risk of hepatotoxicity of some antiretroviral agents.[60,61] An additional consideration is the risk for exacerbation of hepatitis, and potentially hepatic failure, due to immune reconstitution syndrome occurring early after starting ART. Nonetheless, control of HIV replication with ART has been shown to decrease mortality due to liver disease in the setting of hepatitis C coinfection.[62,63] For a complete discussion of the management of hepatitis B and C infection, in the setting of HIV, see Practice Points 31 and 32.

Choice of Initial Antiretroviral Regimen
Current guidelines advise that regimens consist of a backbone of two NRTIs combined with either a non-nucleoside reverse transcriptase inhibitor (NNRTI), an integrase strand transfer inhibitor (INSTI) or a ritonavir-boosted protease inhibitor (PI). The choice of specific regimens and agents should be individualized, taking into account results of testing for primary resistance, patient preferences and lifestyle, coinfections (e.g. viral hepatitis), co-morbidities (e.g. diabetes, kidney disease), cardiovascular risk factors and concomitant medications. Considerations for selecting individual agents are outside the scope of this chapter. Guideline recommendations for specific preferred agents are revised regularly based on new information and the availability of new agents and fixed-dose formulations, which enhance convenience and adherence. Specific antiretroviral agents are described in detail in Chapter 103.

Monitoring Patients on Initial ART
After starting a new antiretroviral regimen, the patient should ideally have the plasma viral load checked every 4–8 weeks until a target of <50 copies/mL is achieved, a threshold typically reached within 24 weeks. Viral load monitoring can then be decreased to approximately 3–6-monthly intervals. CD4 cell counts are typically monitored in tandem with plasma viral load. However, there is no need to closely monitor CD4 cell counts if they are within or have reached the normal range in stable patients on ART. Adherence, drug intolerance, drug toxicities and clinical disease status should be re-evaluated at each visit by history, examination and regular standard laboratory monitoring of hepatic and renal function.

METABOLIC TESTING
Lipid abnormalities are common in HIV infection, with perturbations in triglyceride and high-density lipoprotein (HDL) cholesterol values.[64] Some ART regimens can lead to further abnormalities with increases in total cholesterol and triglyceride levels.[65,66] Fasting lipid profiles should be obtained at baseline, with an assessment of overall cardiovascular risk using the Framingham risk assessment score.[67] Lipid

values should be monitored every 3–4 months after initiating ART. Patients with abnormal lipid profiles should be managed according to the underlying targets set by the updated National Cholesterol Education Program guidelines.[68] Revision of the ART regimen in favor of a similarly active but more lipid-friendly option could be considered in higher-risk individuals. Alternatively, lipid-lowering strategies should be pursued.[69,70]

HIV-infected patients are at increased risk for osteopenia and osteoporosis, and resultant fractures.[71,72] This may reflect a combination of underlying HIV effects and antiretroviral drug toxicity.[6,71,73] Patients with other risk factors for bone loss should be screened using dual-energy X-ray absorptiometry (DXA). Some would advise that this test be repeated every few years, particularly in high-risk patients; however, routine use of DXA scans remains controversial (see Chapter 104).[11,74]

Changing ART

TREATMENT FAILURE

Treatment failure is defined in virologic terms as either the failure to achieve a plasma viral load <50 copies/mL or the occurrence of a *confirmed* viral load rebound (i.e. on repeat testing 2–4 weeks later) above 50 copies/mL in the absence of other obvious explanation (e.g. treatment interruption, intercurrent illness, or immunizations). It is critically important to correct the determinants of treatment failure in any given individual before a change in therapy is even considered.

If the plasma viral load rebounds despite ongoing therapy, consider imperfect adherence to the antiretroviral regimen as the most likely cause. If suboptimal adherence is identified, the reasons for missed doses should be evaluated, and the initial regimen may be salvaged if no resistance has developed. Alternative dosing regimens can often be accommodated to better suit an individual's lifestyle. Intolerance to medications may be mitigated by altering the time of dosing, administering with food and, if possible, altering dosing interval. Other issues such as depression or substance use, which can negatively impact adherence, may need to be addressed.

Another major cause of treatment failure is reduced susceptibility of the virus to one or more antiretroviral drugs in the regimen. Patients can be initially infected with drug-resistant strains of HIV. Resistant strains can also emerge when the virus is allowed to replicate in the presence of drug, as in the case of incomplete adherence, insufficiently potent regimens or suboptimal drug levels. Cross-resistance among drugs in the same class may develop and this often limits the number of fully active alternative regimens. With the currently approved first-generation NNRTIs, the risk of cross-resistance is high after an NNRTI-containing regimen fails, and in this context use of a PI-based regimen as second-line would be an option. With PI failure, intra-class cross-resistance is less predictable. Depending on the pattern of resistance, an alternative PI can often be selected. With NRTIs, the extent of class cross-resistance varies from drug to drug, with some mutations compromising multiple agents. Cross-resistance is also known to occur within newer classes of drugs. Resistance testing should be performed as soon as virologic failure is established, and the results used to design an alternative fully suppressive regimen to avoid further development of resistance.

Treatment failure may also be due to inadequate drug levels, particularly on the basis of unrecognized drug–drug interactions, either with other antiretrovirals within the regimen or with concomitant medications taken for other indications.[75] Dose adjustments may overcome some of these interactions. The use of therapeutic drug monitoring of certain antiretrovirals, particularly PIs, may be considered to establish the direction of the interaction and make appropriate adjustments.

A change in therapy in the setting of previous treatment failure should only be carried out after careful evaluation of prior drug exposure, prior response to therapies, prior tolerability and toxicity issues, as well as the results of resistance testing done on a real-time basis and on relevant stored samples, if available. Failure to address these issues effectively will invariably compromise the chances of success with the new regimen. It is critical, therefore, that the decision of when to change and what to change is arrived at under the guidance of an experienced practitioner.

When a decision is made to change therapy for confirmed virologic failure, the new regimen should be one with the highest probable effectiveness, as predicted by the patient's complete drug history and the resistance test results from both recent and archived specimens, as well as having the highest likelihood of tolerability and adherence. New regimens should contain at least two (or, if possible, three) drugs deemed to be fully active.[1,22] Maximal activity would be expected from drugs belonging to a new class to which the patient's virus has not previously been exposed and would not be expected to have any mutations conferring resistance.

TOXICITY

Tolerability issues are a frequent reason for modification of ART regimens. When the causal agent responsible for a given toxicity is known, replacing that single agent is relatively simple and usually effective. The issue is more challenging if the link between the responsible agent and the emerging toxicity is not clear. At times it is difficult to differentiate specific antiretroviral drug toxicity from a co-morbid condition or toxicity due to a concomitant medication. In such instances, other potential causes should be evaluated and managed if possible, or ruled out prior to implementing changes in the antiretroviral regimen.

Significant toxicities may also develop due to drug–drug interactions, particularly if the exposure to one agent is substantially increased in the presence of another, for example rhabdomyolysis due to increased levels of certain statins in the presence of ritonavir-boosted PIs.[75] Management of patients in a multidisciplinary setting with access to specialized pharmacists with a thorough knowledge of potential drug interactions can alleviate these problems.

If a patient experiences significant drug toxicity, brief cessation of all medications may be necessary, with consideration of an appropriate staggered stop for NNRTI-based regimens (e.g. discontinuing the NNRTI component first, and continuing with dual nucleoside therapy for an additional 7 days if the NRTI backbone is not implicated in the adverse reaction). Decreasing dosages or discontinuing a single medication is not recommended, as this will compromise the potency of the regimen and eventually promote the development of resistance. In general, as long as the antiviral potency of the regimen is preserved, exchanging an individual component of the regimen to deal with a toxicity problem is acceptable. The closer the agents are in terms of their potency and resistance profile, the easier and safer the change will be. Drug substitutions become more complicated when the patient presents with a history of prior drug exposure and/or failure of multiple regimens. In such cases, changes in therapy should only be performed under the guidance of an experienced HIV-treating physician.

MONITORING PATIENTS AFTER REGIMEN CHANGE

As with a first regimen, the patient should have the plasma viral load checked 4–8 weeks after starting a new regimen to ensure the desired early response, and followed closely until the plasma viral load is below 50 copies/mL. Adherence, drug tolerance and emerging toxicities with the new regimen will also need to be monitored as well as any changes in clinical disease status.

References available online at expertconsult.com.

KEY REFERENCES

Aberg J.A., Gallant J.E., Ghanem K.G., et al.: Primary care guidelines for the management of persons infected with HIV: 2013 update by the HIV medicine association of the Infectious Diseases Society of America. *Clin Infect Dis* 2014; 58(1):e1-e34.

Anderson J.P., Tchetgen Tchetgen E.J., Lo Re V. 3rd, et al.: Antiretroviral therapy reduces the rate of hepatic decompensation among HIV- and hepatitis C virus-coinfected veterans. *Clin Infect Dis* 2014; 58(5):719-727.

Churchill D.R., Waters L., Ahmed N., et al. British HIV Association guidelines for the treatment of HIV-1-positive adults with antiretroviral therapy 2015. Available: http://www.bhiva.org/documents/Guidelines/Treatment/2015/2015-treatment-guidelines.pdf.

Cohen M.S., Chen Y.Q., McCauley M., et al.: Prevention of HIV-1 infection with early antiretroviral therapy. *N Engl J Med* 2011; 365(6):493-505.

Emery S., Neuhaus J.A., Phillips A.N., et al.: Major clinical outcomes in antiretroviral therapy (ART)-naive participants and in those not receiving ART at baseline in the SMART study. *J Infect Dis* 2008; 197(8):1133-1144.

Grinsztejn B., Hosseinipour M.C., Ribaudo H.J., et al.: Effects of early versus delayed initiation of antiretroviral treatment on clinical outcomes of HIV-1 infection: results from the phase 3 HPTN 052 randomised controlled trial. *Lancet Infect Dis* 2014; 14(4):281-290.

Gunthard H., Aberg J.A., Eron J.J., et al.: Antiretroviral treatment of HIV infection: 2014 recommendations of the International Antiviral Society – USA panel. *JAMA* 2014; 312(4):410-425.

The INSIGHT START Study Group: *NEJM* 2015; 373(9):795-807.

Kitahata M.M., Gange S.J., Abraham A.G., et al.: Effect of early versus deferred antiretroviral therapy for HIV on survival. *N Engl J Med* 2009; 360(18):1815-1826.

Lundgren J., Gatell J., Rochstroh J., et al. European AIDS Clinical Society. Guidelines: Clinical Management and Treatment of HIV-infected adults in Europe. Version 8.0 – October 2015. Available at: http://www.eacsociety.org/files/guidelines_8_0-english_web.pdf.

Panel on Antiretroviral Guidelines for Adults and Adolescents. Guidelines for the use of antiretroviral agents in HIV-1-infected adults and adolescents. Department of Health and Human Services. February 12, 2013; 1-166. Available: http://aidsinfo.nih.gov/ContentFiles/AdultandAdolescentGL.pdf.

Panel on opportunistic infections in HIV-infected adults and adolescents. Guidelines for the prevention and treatment of opportunistic infections in HIV-infected adults and adolescents: recommendations from the Centers for Disease Control and Prevention , the National Institutes of Health, and the HIV Medicine Association of the Infectious Diseases Society of America. Available: http://aidsinfo.nih.gov/guidelines/html/4/adult-and-adolescent-oi-prevention-and-treatment-guidelines/0.

Quinn T.C., Wawer M.J., Sewankambo N., et al.: Viral load and heterosexual transmission of human immunodeficiency virus type 1. Rakai Project Study Group. *N Engl J Med* 2000; 342(13):921-929.

Samji H., Cescon A., Hogg R.S., et al.: Closing the gap: Increases in life expectancy among treated HIV-positive individuals in the United States and Canada. *PLoS ONE* 2013; 8(12):e81355.

Tanser F., Barnighausen T., Grapsa E., et al.: High coverage of ART associated with decline in risk of HIV acquisition in rural KwaZulu-Natal, South Africa. *Science* 2013; 339(6122):966-971.

World Health Organization. Consolidated guidelines on the use of antiretroviral drugs for treating and preventing HIV infection. Available: http://www.who.int/hiv/pub/guidelines/arv2013/download/en/.

103

Antiviral Therapy

JOSE I. BERNARDINO | JOSE R. ARRIBAS

KEY CONCEPTS

- There is universal consensus about when to start antiretroviral treatment. Every HIV-infected patient should be on antiretroviral treatment irrespectively of CD4 count.

- The standard of treatment is based on a backbone of two nucleoside reverse transcriptase inhibitors and either a non-nucleoside reverse transcriptase inhibitor, a protease inhibitor, boosted with low-dose ritonavir or an integrase strand transfer inhibitor.

- The primary goal of antiviral treatment is to reduce the plasma viral load (VL) to undetectable levels. With new drugs undetectability is obtained in almost 90% of the subjects.

- Virologic failure is defined as an inability to attain an undetectable VL within 24–32 weeks after commencing therapy or confirmed rebound from undetectable levels.

- Half of treated patients with detectable VL have drug resistance and around 11% have evidence of resistance mutations affecting at least three classes of antiretroviral (ARV) drugs.

- Resistance testing is recommended in all patients experiencing virologic failure while on treatment and changes in therapy should be guided by the results of resistance testing.

- Genotype-resistance testing of chronically HIV-infected, ARV-naïve patients improves clinical outcomes and is cost-effective wherever the rate of primary resistance is above 1%.

Introduction

HIV infection is a chronic disease in which, if left untreated, high-level viral replication occurs continuously for years, even during the clinically latent phase. Without optimal antiviral therapy, viral replication drives the progression of HIV disease and leads to worsening immunodeficiency as measured by decreasing CD4+ lymphocyte cell counts, which are highly predictive of the subsequent risk of opportunistic infections, malignancies and death. Suppression of HIV replication to levels in plasma below the limit of detection is the primary objective of antiretroviral (ARV) treatment as this is associated with durable clinical, virologic and immunologic responses. Inability to maintain full virologic suppression is most commonly related to suboptimal adherence but may be due to viral mutations leading to decreased drug susceptibility and resistance to the administered drug.

Decreased susceptibility to other drugs within the same class (cross-class resistance) could also occur.

Most individuals commencing ARV treatment will be expected to have successful, durable responses to treatment. In clinical trials after long periods of follow-up, virologic undetectable rates at 3–5 years greater than 80% have been reported.

There are 28 licensed drugs available for the treatment of HIV infection (Table 103-1), including six different classes acting at different sites of HIV life cycle (Figure 103-1). (See Chapter 152 for detailed discussion of antiretroviral drugs.) Several national and international guidelines have been developed in order to help in the clinical management of HIV-infected adults and adolescents, pregnant women, infants and children, those with hepatitis and tuberculosis coinfections and uninfected individuals who have occupational exposure to HIV.

When Should Antiviral Drugs Be Started?

ESTABLISHED HIV INFECTION

Until recently most guidelines recommended treatment between 350 and 500 cells/µL regardless of disease stage although some were in favour of starting treatment even for those above 500 cells/µL. Until 2015 most of the evidence recommending ARV initiation in high CD4 strata came from observational studies, which indicate that the risk of progression to clinical disease even at higher CD4 counts is high, and by the fact that earlier treatment significantly reduces this risk of HIV transmission.[1,2] The impetus for earlier therapy was also based in two additional facts: on one hand HIV-positive individuals with high CD4 counts have standardized mortality ratios that are comparable to those of the general population and on the other hand the results of the SMART study were individuals with CD4 counts > 350 cells/µL, including those not on treatment and those randomised to interrupt treatment, experiences more clinical disease than those who remained on treatment throughout.[3]

In July 2015 the results of the START trial comparing immediate ARV therapy at CD4 count > 500 cells/µL with deferred therapy until CD4 count reach less than 350 cells/µL demonstrated a clear benefit of early ARV initiation.[4] 4685 patients were followed for a mean time of 3 years and the immediate arm obtained a relative risk reduction of 57% in the composite primary endpoint including an AIDS-related event, non-AIDS related event or death from any cause. All published guidelines have incorporated the results and changed or updated the recommendations on 'when to start' (Table 103-2).

ACUTE HIV INFECTION

Overall there are no convincing data that treating patients during acute HIV infection has led to any substantial long-term benefits in terms of their immune system recovery. However, there are data suggesting that if patients were treated in the very early stages of acute HIV infection, they may preserve immune function, especially in the gut, reduce reservoir size and may also prevent dissemination of virus to sanctuary sites such as the brain. Treatment for acute HIV infection should be undertaken within a clinical trial or perhaps considered in an individual with moderate to severe symptoms, those who have a precipitous fall in CD4 count to <200 cells/µL or those with neurologic involvement (see also Chapter 93).

Which Antiretroviral Drugs to Start?

Individuals commencing ARV therapy for the first time will usually start with a combination of two nucleoside reverse transcriptase inhibitors (NRTIs) and either a non-nucleoside reverse transcriptase inhibitor (NNRTI), a protease inhibitor (PI), boosted with low-dose ritonavir or an integrase strand transfer inhibitor (INSTI) (Table 103-3). Before selecting a combination, it is important to take account of several pieces of clinical and laboratory information.

BASELINE RESISTANCE TESTING

Transmission of drug-resistant virus is well documented, with up to 15% of ARV-naïve individuals in some studies being found to harbor HIV with at least one important drug-related mutation, although this figure has important geographical differences. Studies demonstrate

TABLE 103-1	Currently Licensed Antiretroviral Drugs by Class			
NRTIs	**NNRTIs**	**Protease Inhibitors**	**Entry Inhibitors**	**Integrase Inhibitors**
Zidovudine (ZDV)	Nevirapine	Saquinavir	Enfuvirtide	Raltegravir
Stavudine	Efavirenz (EFV)	Indinavir	Maraviroc	Elvitegravir/cobicistat (EVG/c)**
Lamivudine (3TC)	Delavirdine*	Nelfinavir		Dolutegravir
Emtricitabine (FTC)	Etravirine	Fosamprenavir		
Abacavir (ABC)	Rilpivirine (RPV)	Amprenavir*		
Zalcitabine*		Lopinavir (LPV)		
Didanosine		Ritonavir (RTV)		
Tenofovir (TDF)		Atazanavir		
		Tipranavir		
		Darunavir		

Eight fixed-dose combinations are approved: ZDV + 3TC; ZDV + 3TC + ABC; ABC + 3TC; FTC + TDF; LPV + RTV; TDF + FTC + EFV; TDF + FTC + RPV; TDF + FTC + EVG/c.
*No longer commercially available.
**Cobicistat is a selective CYP3A inhibitor without any detectable antiviral activity against HIV-1.

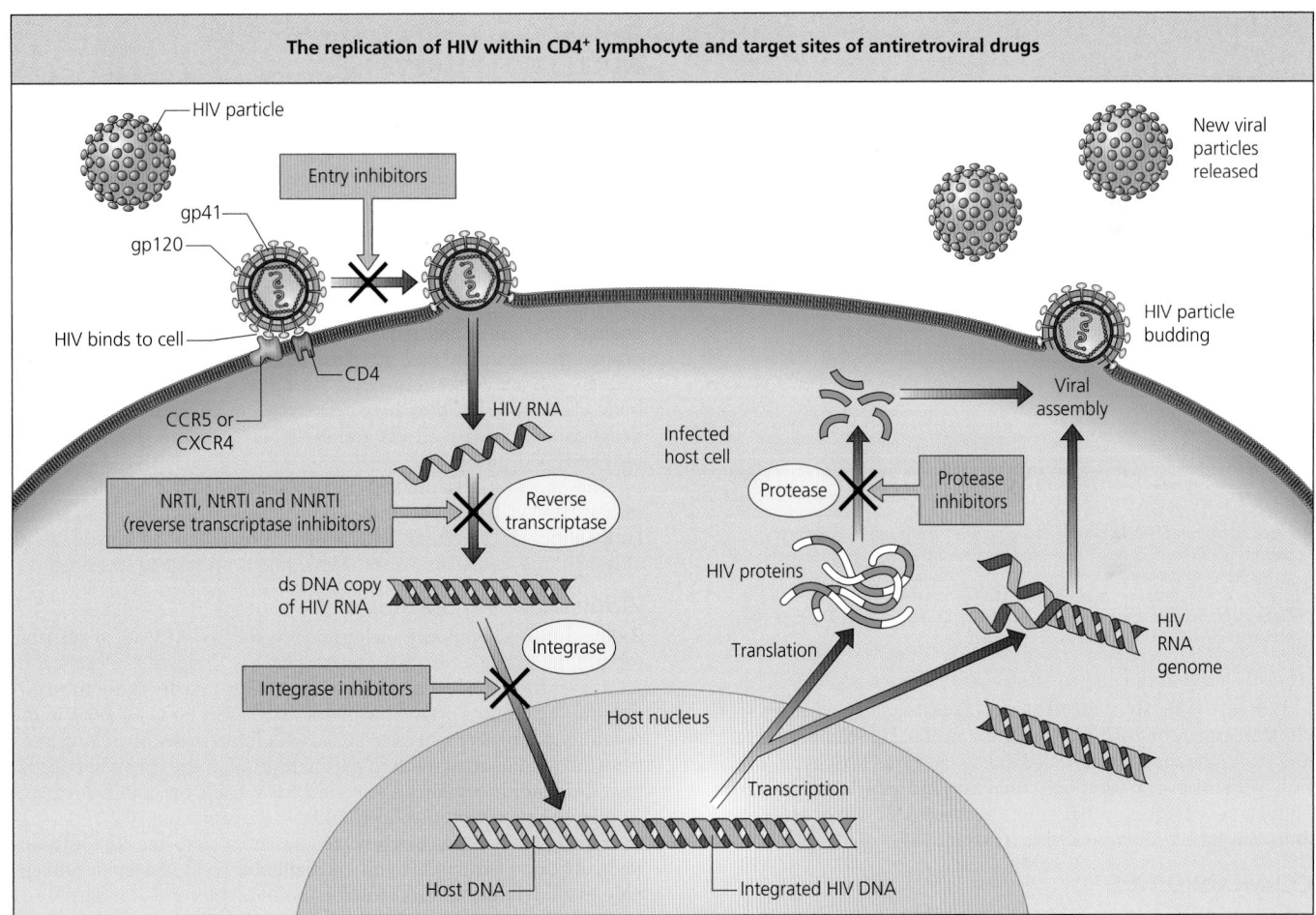

The replication of HIV within CD4+ lymphocyte and target sites of antiretroviral drugs

Figure 103-1 The replication of HIV within CD4+ lymphocyte and target sites of antiretroviral drugs. *(With permission from Bolognia J.L., Jorizzo J.L., Rapini R.P., et al., eds. Dermatology, 2nd ed. London: Mosby; 2008.)*

poorer virologic outcomes for individuals commencing combinations where transmitted resistance is present. It is widely recommended that resistance testing, where available, be performed prior to commencement of first-line therapy. With time, evidence of transmitted drug resistance may be lost due to outgrowth of wild-type virus, which is more fit, resulting in 'archiving' of resistant virus. It is recommended, therefore, that resistance testing is done on the earliest available sample following the diagnosis of HIV infection.

COINFECTIONS

It is important to establish whether an individual is coinfected with HBV or HCV before commencing ARV treatment. Coinfected patients benefit from early ARV treatment because liver fibrosis progression is reduced with HIV suppression. Tenofovir, lamivudine and emtricitabine are also active against hepatitis B and should be included in ARV combinations in HBV/HIV coinfected individuals. The usual combination is either lamivudine or emtricitabine with tenofovir. In

TABLE 103-2	Guidelines for When to Start Antiretroviral Treatment			
Guidelines	Symptomatic		Asymptomatic	Other
European AIDS Clinical Society[1]	CDC stage B or C including tuberculosis		Recommended regardless of CD4 count	Possible exception of elite controllers with high and stable CD4 count
US Department of Health and Human Sciences	Symptomatic		Recommended regardless of CD4 count	The strength and evidence for recommendation vary: strong for <500 cells/µL moderate for >500 cells/µL
International AIDS Society, USA	Symptomatic		Recommended regardless of CD4 count	The strength and evidence for recommendation vary: strong for <500 cells/µL moderate for >500 cells/µL
WHO guidelines	As a priority, ART should be initiated in all adults with WHO clinical stage 3 or 4 and individuals with CD count ≤350 cells/µL		Recommended regardless of CD4 count	Strong evidence for recommendation

TABLE 103-3	Recommended Initial Antiretroviral Regimens	
Guidelines	A	B
EACS, recommended	Rilpivirine Darunavir-ritonavir	Tenofovir–emtricitabine
	Raltegravir Elvitegravir-cobicistat	Tenofovir–emtricitabine
	Dolutegravir	Abacavir–lamivudine Tenofovir–emtricitabine
IAS–USA	Efavirenz	Tenofovir–emtricitabine Abacavir–lamivudine*
	Atazanavir–ritonavir Darunavir–ritonavir	Tenofovir–emtricitabine Abacavir–lamivudine*
	Raltegravir	Tenofovir–emtricitabine
DHHS recommended	Darunavir–ritonavir	Tenofovir–emtricitabine
	Raltegravir Elvitegravir-cobicistat	Tenofovir–emtricitabine
	Dolutegravir	Abacavir–lamivudine Tenofovir–emtricitabine

For EACS, IAS and DHHS guidelines, one drug (or ritonavir-boosted antiretroviral) from column A should be prescribed with a combination of drugs from column B.
Rilpivirine only if baseline plasma VL<100 000 copies/mL.
*Abacavir/lamivudine plus atazanavir–ritonavir or efavirenz in patients with plasma VL<100 000 copies/mL.

individuals with HCV infection an assessment of whether specific HCV treatment is required should be made. Zidovudine, didanosine and stavudine should be avoided due to increased toxicity in combination with ribavirin, although ribavirin and pegylated interferon is falling out of favor now that more effective and less toxic HCV-specific antivirals have become available (Chapter 155).

CO-MORBIDITIES

Co-morbidities, such as metabolic syndrome, heart, liver or kidney diseases, should also be considered. For example, some ritonavir-boosted PIs may increase insulin resistance and therefore make control of diabetes more difficult. PIs are also associated with increases in total cholesterol and triglycerides and in cohort studies with an increased risk of myocardial infarction. Efavirenz is associated with neuropsychiatric side effects. In some individuals, tenofovir leads to a decline in glomerular filtration rate (GFR) and may contribute to greater bone mineral density loss in high-risk patients for osteoporosis.

DRUG INTERACTIONS

NNRTIs, PIs and the boosters ritonavir or cobicistat in particular interact with numerous other medications. Interactions may lead to lower or higher levels of ARVs, risking either treatment failure or toxicity.

Furthermore, as both NNRTIs and PIs can act as inducers or inhibitors of cytochrome P450, the levels of other drugs may be affected.

Specific Antiretroviral Drugs

NUCLEOS(T)IDE REVERSE TRANSCRIPTASE INHIBITORS

Reverse transcriptase inhibitors act through one of two mechanisms. First, as 'chain terminators', they block the elongation of the DNA chain through blockage of further nucleosides. This mechanism is characteristic of the nucleoside and nucleotide analogs and depends on the intracellular phosphorylation of the drugs into the corresponding triphosphate. Second, they act by competition/binding of the reverse transcriptase in functionally essential sites. NNRTIs act only through this mechanism and not as 'chain terminators'. In general, nucleoside analogs have good oral bioavailability, are only minimally bound to plasma proteins, do not interfere with cytochrome P450 enzyme systems and are excreted through the kidneys. Because of these metabolic characteristics, they have relatively few interactions with other drugs as compared with PIs and NNRTIs. They are generally active against HIV-1 and HIV-2.

The most widely studied nucleoside/nucleotide backbones for initial ARV treatment are zidovudine–lamivudine, abacavir–lamivudine, or tenofovir with either lamivudine or emtricitabine although due to toxicity issues zidovudine is prescribed less often.

Zidovudine and Stavudine

Zidovudine is a thymidine analog and was the first ARV agent available for use. Its association with lipoatrophy has driven its relegation in guidelines to that of an alternative agent. This toxicity starts to manifest after 12 months on treatment and may affect up to 50–60% in the medium to long term. In individuals with lipoatrophy, switching away from zidovudine may result in partial reversal of the subcutaneous fat loss. Zidovudine remains a recommended agent for use in pregnant women to prevent mother-to-child HIV transmission.

Viruses resistant to currently recommended first-line NRTIs (tenofovir, abacavir, lamivudine and emtricitabine) will usually be susceptible to zidovudine and so could be useful as a second-line agent.

Stavudine is the other thymidine analog in use. It is associated with a higher incidence of lipoatrophy, the onset of which is more rapid. Stavudine can also cause peripheral neuropathy, hyperlactatemia and lactic acidosis. Stavudine has been dropped from most guidelines in higher-income countries and its widespread use in resource-poor countries, often for reasons of cost, is being widely questioned.

Abacavir and Tenofovir

Abacavir–lamivudine or tenofovir with either lamivudine or emtricitabine have become the most commonly used NRTI backbones in higher-income countries. Although both abacavir and lamivudine have plasma half-lives that do not appear to support once-daily dosing, intracellular concentrations of the active metabolites (both drugs need to be phosphorylated intracellularly) mean once-daily dosing is feasible. The CNA 30021 study demonstrated that abacavir and lamivudine given once daily (same daily dose) was not inferior to the standard twice-daily regimen.[5]

The most important adverse effect of abacavir is a hypersensitivity reaction (HSR). This syndrome appears usually 1–4 weeks after starting abacavir and includes fever, rash, abdominal pain, cough, shortness of breath and hypotension. The most serious problems, including shock and death, occur in those who continue treatment despite the development of hypersensitivity, or in those who stop drug and then are rechallenged with abacavir.

The prevalence of HSR varies widely, being seen most commonly in those of white race and is linked to HLA-B*5701 carriage. In the Predict study HLA-B*5701 screening reduced the incidence of HSR to zero.[6] HLA-B*5701 screening prior to using abacavir has become routine in clinical practice.

Two other important issues affect the use of abacavir. The first is its association seen in some cohorts with worsening cardiovascular risk although a recent meta-analysis from the FDA rules out this association. The second is that, in one large clinical trial (ACTG 5202), of poorer efficacy seen in those ARV-naïve patients who were randomized to receive abacavir and whose baseline viral load (VL) was over 100 000 copies/mL. This fact has not been confirmed in others trials, especially if the third drug is an integrase inhibitor.

Tenofovir is an NRTI that also has activity against HBV. In the GS-934 study, tenofovir, lamivudine and efavirenz were compared over 144 weeks to zidovudine, lamivudine and efavirenz. In the primary time to loss of virologic response (TLOVR) analysis, the tenofovir arm performed better. Much of the difference between the arms was related to early discontinuation in the zidovudine arm due to anemia and poorer tolerability.

Tenofovir use is associated in some patients with a reduction in renal function over time when compared to other nucleosides. Close monitoring of estimated GFR and proximal tubulopathy is recommended. Tenofovir has also been associated with a greater decline in bone mineral density than other NRTIs and a recent study has shown a link between cumulative use of tenofovir and osteoporotic fractures. Tenofovir should be used cautiously in patients who have, or are at risk of developing, renal disease and osteoporosis.

Lamivudine and Emtricitabine

Lamivudine is a cytidine analog and a component of several recommended first-line combinations. It is very well tolerated and can be given either 150 mg twice daily or 300 mg once daily. It is also available as a component of the fixed-dose combinations Combivir (zidovudine, lamivudine), Trizivir (zidovudine, abacavir, lamivudine) and Kivexa (abacavir, lamivudine). Lamivudine has a low barrier to resistance. Viruses which contain the M184V mutation are, however, less 'fit' than wild-type viruses.

Emtricitabine is a cytidine analog similar to lamivudine. These drugs should not be used together. Emtricitabine is also active against HBV and is available as part of a fixed-dose combination with tenofovir (Truvada), with both tenofovir and efavirenz (Atripla), with both tenofovir and rilpivirine (Complera/Eviplera) and with tenofovir, elvitegravir and cobicistat (Stribild).

Didanosine

Didanosine is an alternative agent for treating ARV-naïve individuals and is usually given in combination with lamivudine and either an NNRTI or a PI. It is associated with pancreatitis, lactic acidosis and peripheral neuropathy. Recent reports have linked hepatic fibrosis and portal vein thrombosis with this drug. While these adverse effects are relatively rare, their potential severity limits its use.

CHOOSING EITHER AN NNRTI- OR PI-BASED COMBINATION OR ISTI FOR FIRST-LINE THERAPY

All currently recommended first-line therapies include a drug from the NNRTI, PI or ISTI class. NNRTIs efavirenz and rilpivirine have

the benefit of low pill burden, once-daily administration and good gastrointestinal tolerance. Rilpivirine is licensed for patients with pre-antiretroviral therapy (ART) plasma VL less than 100 000 copies/mL. However, NNRTIs have a low barrier to resistance and a single mutation results in high-level resistance that impacts drugs within the same class (with the possible exception for 103N mutation and rilpivirine).

In contrast, ritonavir-boosted PIs are relatively forgiving in the face of suboptimal adherence, with high-level resistance usually requiring more than one mutation. Sequencing of PIs, even if resistance is present, may be possible. However PI-based combinations have a higher pill burden and are prone to drug–drug interactions. As a class they are more frequently associated with gastrointestinal toxicity and metabolic disturbances such as insulin resistance and dyslipidemia.

ISTI (raltegravir, elvitegravir and dolutegravir) are the newest class recommended for first-line therapy. They have an excellent tolerability profile and are noninferior, or even superior (dolutegravir), to other preferred ARV regimens. Raltegravir is dosed twice daily and elvitegravir needs boosting with cobicistat, a potent CYP3A4 inhibitor. Both drugs are susceptible to resistance mutations in case of virologic failure and have cross-resistance whereas dolutegravir has a higher genetic barrier and no emergent resistance mutation has been detected in treatment-naïve clinical trials so far.

One large strategic study (ACTG 5142) compared outcomes in those starting a two NRTI–efavirenz combination, a two NRTI-PI (lopinavir–ritonavir) and an NRTI-sparing (efavirenz–lopinavir–ritonavir) combination. This study found that at 96 weeks the two NRTI–efavirenz group was associated with fewest virologic failures.[7] The NRTI-sparing arm also performed better than the PI arm but was the arm in which most resistance was seen in those who failed.

ACTG 5257 compared three recommended first-line regimens, two PIs (atazanavir–ritonavir or darunavir–ritonavir) and one ISTI (raltegravir) all in combination with co-formulated tenofovir–emtricitabine. Equivalence in efficacy endpoint of time to virologic failure was demonstrated but raltegravir was superior in the composite endpoint of time to virologic failure or treatment failure. Darunavir-ritonavir was superior to atazanavir–ritonavir in the composite endpoint.[8]

In two recent double blind studies (GS-236-102 and 103) co-formulated elvitegravir, cobicistat, emtricitabine and tenofovir showed noninferiority at 144 weeks in comparison with co-formulated efavirenz, emtricitabine and tenofovir and atazanavir/ritonavir plus tenofovir/emtricitabine, respectively.[9,10]

The newest ISTI drug dolutegravir has shown superiority versus efavirenz in combination with abacavir–lamivudine in the double blind, double dummy SINGLE trial[11] and versus darunavir-ritonavir in combination with investigator's choice NRTIs (tenofovir–emtricitabine or abacavir–lamivudine) open label FLAMINGO trial.[12]

NNRTIs: SELECTING NEVIRAPINE, EFAVIRENZ OR RILPIVIRINE

The 2NN study compared nevirapine with efavirenz. Both drugs were given in combination with stavudine and lamivudine in treatment-naïve individuals.[13] At 48 weeks 43.7% of the nevirapine twice-daily group and 37.8% of the efavirenz group failed. This difference of 5.9% (95% CI, 0.9–12.8) just failed to reach the noninferiority margin.

To reduce the risk of hepatic toxicity and risk of Stevens–Johnson syndrome, nevirapine should be started at a dose of 200 mg once daily. Patients should be reviewed at 2 weeks and the dose increased to 200 mg twice daily if there is no evidence of toxicity. The risks of these toxicities are substantially higher in those with higher CD4 counts and in women, hence it is recommended that nevirapine is not used in men with CD4 counts >400 cells/μL and in women with CD4 counts >250 cells/μL.

While efavirenz may also be associated with both cutaneous and hepatic toxicity, the risk of serious problems is lower. However, efavirenz is associated with neuropsychiatric effects including dizziness, abnormal dreams, insomnia, hallucination and euphoria especially in the first 1–2 weeks of treatment.

Two studies compared rilpivirine with efavirenz in antiretroviral-naïve patients, one in combination with tenofovir/emtricitabine and with investigator-selected NRTIs in the other. At 48 weeks pool analysis from both studies showed a similar proportion of patients with VL < 50 copies/mL (84% with rilpivirine vs 82% with efavirenz).[14] There were more discontinuations in the efavirenz arm due to adverse events, but the rilpivirine arm showed a suboptimal response in the subgroup of patients with a baseline VL greater than 100 000 copies/mL. Rilpivirine is contraindicated with proton pump inhibitors and combination with antacids should be used with caution. Rilpivirine inhibits creatinine tubular secretion and therefore mild elevations in estimated glomerular filtration rate (eGFR) are observed.

Congenital abnormalities have been observed in cynomolgus monkeys whose mothers were treated with efavirenz during pregnancy. While prospective studies of its use in pregnant women have failed to demonstrate an excess risk of congenital abnormalities, it remains the recommendation that an alternative agent is used in women trying to conceive or in those at higher risk of unplanned pregnancy.

PROTEASE INHIBITORS

PIs act on the binding to the catalytic site of the HIV aspartic protease. This enzyme is critical in the post-translational processing of the polyprotein products of *gag* and *gag-pol* genes into the functional core proteins and viral enzymes, respectively. Its inhibition leads to the release of immature, noninfectious viral particles.

PIs are generally dependent on the cytochrome P450 3A4 hepatic isoenzyme for metabolism and can compete with other substrates of this enzyme. When the metabolism of other drugs that are dependent on the same enzyme is inhibited, the blood levels of these drugs can increase dramatically and toxic interactions may occur.

Metabolic complications have emerged in patients treated with PIs. These include glucose metabolism abnormalities (hyperglycemia or diabetes), hyperlipidemia (mainly hypertriglyceridemia, with or without associated hypercholesterolemia) and abnormal fat distribution (accumulation in the posterior neck, upper back and central abdomen).

PIs are mostly co-prescribed with ritonavir. Ritonavir even at low dose is a potent inhibitor of cytochrome P450 3A4. This results in higher drug levels of the substrate PI over the dosing period, and is associated with a lower risk of virologic failure and a lower incidence of drug resistance in those individuals who fail treatment.

Lopinavir–Ritonavir

Lopinavir is a potent inhibitor of HIV-1 protease co-formulated with ritonavir. Lopinavir is principally metabolized by the liver, and shares many of the drug interactions and contraindications common to other PIs. Two randomized controlled trials have shown better efficacy with atazanavir–ritonavir or darunavir–ritonavir when compared with lopinavir–ritonavir, partly driven by poorer tolerability of the lopinavir–ritonavir combination.

Atazanavir–Ritonavir

Atazanavir was the first licensed once-a-day PI to become available for use. While it can be given to ARV-naïve individuals without ritonavir boosting (atazanavir 400 mg once daily) it is more commonly given with ritonavir (atazanavir 300 mg/ritonavir 100 mg once daily). Studies have demonstrated that patients failing unboosted atazanavir are more likely to develop mutations not only to PIs but also to the other components of the regimen.

The most common atazanavir-related side effect is unconjugated hyperbilirubinemia due to atazanavir inhibiting glucuronosyltransferase. Atazanavir is less likely to cause both gastrointestinal side effects and lipid abnormalities than lopinavir/ritonavir. In the Castle study of ARV-naïve patients, atazanavir 300 mg/ritonavir 100 mg with tenofovir and emtricitabine once daily was found to be noninferior (in fact the data showed superiority) to lopinavir–ritonavir in combination at 96 weeks.[15]

Atazanavir has several important drug interactions:
- As it requires an acid gastric environment for optimal absorption, proton pump inhibitors are not recommended. Care must also be taken with drugs such as ranitidine.
- Efavirenz induces the metabolism of atazanavir and, if co-prescribed, atazanavir should be boosted with ritonavir and at a higher dose (atazanavir 400 mg/ritonavir 100 mg).
- Tenofovir leads to reduced atazanavir levels and, if co-prescribed, atazanavir should be given with ritonavir.

Darunavir–Ritonavir

This is the most recently licensed PI. In the Artemis study of ARV-naïve patients, darunavir 800 mg/ritonavir 100 mg with tenofovir and emtricitabine once daily was found to be superior to lopinavir–ritonavir in combination at 96 weeks.[16] Ritonavir-boosted darunavir also has substantial activity against viruses with drug-resistance mutations and therefore is an important component of salvage regimens. In patients with darunavir mutations the recommended dose is darunavir 600 mg q12h/ritonavir 100 mg q12h.

INTEGRASE STRAND TRANSFER INHIBITORS

ISTI inhibits the catalytic activity of integrase. This enzyme is critical for the irreversible integration of HIV genome into the host genome. There are three available drugs: raltegravir, elvitegravir and dolutegravir that target the strand transfer catalytic reaction through Pi-stacking with the long terminal repeats located at both endings of HIV DNA molecules.

ISTI have an excellent tolerability profile with very few side effects. All are associated with mild gastrointestinal complaints (nausea and diarrhea). Skin rash is rare after raltegravir use and in some cases CPK elevations and muscle weakness could arise. Elvitegravir needs boosting with either ritonavir or cobicistat and is associated with headache and insomnia. Dolutegravir inhibits creatinine tubular secretion and therefore mild elevations in eGFR are observed.

Raltegravir

Raltegravir was the first licensed integrase inhibitor for use in ARV-naïve patients. Raltegravir is dosed twice daily and demonstrated noninferiority versus efavirenz both co-formulated with tenofovir-emtricitabine in a double blind trial. After 5 years of follow-up, 71% of patients receiving raltegravir and 61.3% of patients receiving efavirenz maintained a VL < 50 copies/mL. It has an excellent tolerability profile and has no remarkable drug–drug interactions since it is neither a substrate nor inducer/inhibitor of CYP complex. In the recent ACTG 5257 open label trial, raltegravir demonstrated superiority in the composite endpoint of virologic or tolerability failure at 96 weeks to both atazanavir and darunavir.[8]

Elvitegravir

Two-phase 3 double blind studies demonstrated noninferiority of co-formulated tenofovir–emtricitabine–elvitegravir–cobicistat.[9,10] In the 102 study 87.6% of patients in the elvitegravir arm and 84.1% of patients in the efavirenz arm had a VL < 50 copies/mL at 48 weeks. In the 103 study 89.5% of patients with elvitegravir reached a VL < 50 copies/mL versus 86.8% with atazanavir–ritonavir. ARV initiation with co-formulated tenofovir–emtricitabine–elvitegravir–cobicistat is not recommended with an eGFR < 70 mL/min per US label and < 90 mL/min per EU label and should be changed to an alternative regimen if a patient's eGFR falls below 50 mL/min. This warning is driven by cobicistat inhibition of tubular creatinine secretion, which results in eGFR elevations. Cobicistat is a potent CYP3A4 inhibitor and has the same drug–drug interactions profile as ritonavir based regimens.

Dolutegravir

Dolutegravir is the last ISTI approved for ARV-naïve HIV patients and has a higher genetic barrier with activity against some raltegravir- and elvitegravir-resistant strains. Superiority of dolutegravir against efavirenz and darunavir–ritonavir in ARV-naïve patients has been shown. In the SINGLE trial 88% of patients with abacavir–lamivudine and dolutegravir reached a VL<50 copies/mL versus 81% with tenofovir–emtricitabine and efavirenz. In the FLAMINGO trial patients were randomized to dolutegravir or darunavir–ritonavir with investigator-selected tenofovir–emtricitabine or abacavir–lamivudine. At 48 weeks a greater proportion of patients achieved a VL<50 copies/mL with dolutegravir (90% vs 83%).

Dolutegravir has been also compared with raltegravir in the SPRING-2 trial and noninferiority was demonstrated at both 48 and 96 weeks.[17]

Monitoring First-Line Antiretroviral Treatment

VIROLOGIC AND IMMUNOLOGIC RESPONSES

The primary goal of first-line ARV treatment is to reduce the plasma VL to undetectable levels. This has been shown to minimize the risk of selecting resistant viruses and is associated with durability of treatment response. After initiating first-line ARV treatment it can take up to 24–32 weeks to reach undetectability, with the new ISTI time to reach undetectability can be as short as 8 weeks. The VL decline after treatment initiation occurs in three phases. The first phase representing the switching off of replication in productively infected cells is dramatic, with plasma VLs often declining by 2–3 log in 2 weeks. Most individuals who will fully suppress have a VL<1000 copies/mL by 8 weeks. Individuals started on ARVs should be reviewed in the first 2–4 weeks to assess for side effects, toxicity and suboptimal adherence. If available, a VL should be checked after 1 month on treatment.

CD4 responses to treatment are less predictable. In clinical trials, ARV-naïve individuals given virologically effective treatment will have average CD4 increases of 150–200 cells in 48 weeks. However, intersubject variation is large, with some having only small increases in CD4 count (so-called discordant responders).

ADHERENCE

Good adherence is critical to the success of ARV treatment. However, the minimal level of adherence necessary for success will depend on several factors, including the genetic barrier of the treatment regimen and the presence of drug resistance. Also important is the timing of nonadherence in relation to starting therapy. Poor adherence during the first few weeks when there is abundant replicating virus present is likely to be more risky than similar nonadherence when patients are fully suppressed. It has been shown that the risk of virologic failure for suboptimal adherence declines with longer duration of continuous suppression.

New Strategies

DUAL THERAPY

Although abacavir and tenofovir have an overall good toxicity profile, these NRTI are not completely exempt of important adverse events. The HSR can be virtually avoided by the use of HLA*5701 genotyping. However, there is still controversy regarding a possible increased risk of cardiovascular events in patients who have recently initiated an abacavir-based regimen. The long-term effects of tenofovir on renal and tubular function and in bone metabolism are still a source of concern especially in a progressively aging HIV-infected population. A number of clinical trials have explored nucleoside-sparing regimens in antiretroviral naïve patients. In these trials a boosted PI has been combined with an integrase transfer inhibitor, a CCR5 inhibitor (maraviroc) or with lamivudine.

The MODERN study was stopped after showing that the combination of darunavir–ritonavir plus maraviroc was inferior to darunavir–ritonavir plus tenofovir–emtricitabine.

The NEAT 001 showed that the combination of darunavir–ritonavir plus raltegravir was noninferior to darunavir–ritonavir plus tenofovir–emtricitabine. However, the raltegravir group did not meet noninferiority in patients who started therapy with a VL above 100 000 copies/mL. Also in patients with baseline CD4 cell count below 200 cells/μL, raltegravir was inferior to tenofovir–emtricitabine.[18]

The GARDEL clinical trial randomized antiretroviral naïve patients to receive dual therapy with lopinavir–ritonavir plus lamivudine 150 mg BD, or triple therapy with lopinavir–ritonavir BID plus lamivudine or emtricitabine plus a third investigator-selected NRTI in fixed-dose combinations. After 48 weeks of follow-up, dual therapy met the noninferiority end point regardless of baseline VL or CD4 cell count. Rates of resistance development were not significantly increased in the dual therapy arm.[19]

Currently no expert guideline recommends starting therapy with less than three ART drugs in treatment naïve patients. The only dual combination that holds promise to be used in naïve patients regardless of disease stage is lopinavir/ritonavir plus lamivudine.

When To Change Treatment

IN PATIENTS WITH FULLY SUPPRESSED VIRUS

In these patients switching of ARVs is usually done to improve the patient's quality of life, improve adherence, avoid or prevent long-term toxicities, preserve treatment options or decrease cost.

It is absolutely essential that any switches do not compromise antiviral efficacy. Drugs that have been previously used and have or may have been associated with prior antiviral failure and actual or potential resistance should be avoided. When a patient is infected with resistant HIV – either because of initial acquisition of drug-resistant virus or selection of resistance mutations during failure of previous regimens – careful selection of a new regimen with an adequate genetic barrier against antiretroviral resistance is very important. This issue is particularly important when switching from a high genetic barrier regimen, such as those including a PI, to a low genetic barrier regimen, such as those including NNRTI, ISTI or unboosted atazanavir.

Regimens with reduced dosing frequency and low pill burdens have higher levels of adherence. Switching to a newer agent, co-formulated drugs or a formulation with a lower pill burden and dosing frequency, or one that would be less likely to cause toxicity, are strategies used to both simplify therapy and avoid toxicity. For example, changing from zidovudine or stavudine to tenofovir or abacavir may allow a regimen with a lower dosing frequency (e.g. once daily) that is co-formulated and can prevent worsening of long-term toxicities such as lipoatrophy, dyslipidemia, or peripheral neuropathy.

Switching from one PI to another, or even to the same PI at a lower dosing frequency (e.g. once a day), can reduce dosing frequency, pill count, drug–drug or drug–food interactions and dyslipidemia, or can take advantage of co-formulation. In some cases, atazanavir can be given without ritonavir if there is ritonavir intolerance or toxicity, but not if the patient is taking tenofovir because of its lowering effect on atazanavir plasma concentrations.

The most common substitutions for regimen simplification involve a change from a PI-based to an NNRTI-based regimen or an ISTI-based regimen. Another common strategy is switching from an efavirenz-containing regimen to etravirine, rilpivirine, raltegravir or elvitegravir in patients who are experiencing central nervous system adverse effects.

In patients without history of failure on prior PI-based therapy and who have had suppressed VLs for at least 6 months and who do not have chronic hepatitis B, PI monotherapy with darunavir–ritonavir QD or lopinavir–ritonavir BID might represent an option in persons with intolerance to NRTIs or for treatment simplification.

VIROLOGIC FAILURE

Virologic failure is usually defined as an inability to attain an undetectable VL within 24–32 weeks after commencing therapy or confirmed rebound from undetectable levels. If an individual has developed resistance, the initial rebound VL is usually low, mostly less than 1000 copies/mL. In time further mutations may ensue, resulting in higher levels of replicating virus. If the initial VL rebound is high, this is usually due to periods of poor adherence. In this setting resistance mutations may also be identified on viral genotype. Significant falls in CD4 count and clinical disease are not usually seen with low-level virologic failure.

RESISTANCE

It has been estimated that 10^9 to 10^{10} virions of HIV are produced per day. Because the HIV reverse transcriptase lacks proofreading ability, mutations in the HIV genome arise spontaneously during the replication process on average once each time a viral genome is replicated. In uncontrolled HIV infection, the high HIV replication rate coupled with the mutation rate generates every possible mutation in the HIV genome each day. Thus a large pool of 'quasispecies' is created. These are genetically related but distinct HIV strains, any of which has the potential to be dominant. In most patients the dominant strain prior to any drug therapy can replicate rapidly and is termed 'wild type' based on its sequence. This wild type is usually fully susceptible to antiviral drugs. A potent ARV regimen will significantly inhibit HIV replication but an ineffective regimen or inadequate adherence by the patient will result in suboptimal inhibition of viral replication, and selection of resistant mutations. It has been calculated – and borne out in clinical practice – that the selection out of any quasispecies is highly unlikely in the presence of three drugs to which the virus is susceptible. If only one or two drugs to which the virus is sensitive are used, the selection of resistant mutants will occur. The exception to this rule are boosted PIs that by themselves are characterized by a high resilience to resistance development since multiple mutations are needed to confer resistance.

Mutations that provide a growth advantage in the presence of ARVs will allow a quasispecies to out-compete the others and become the dominant viral strain in the population, and the patient will have a 'resistant' virus.

Most mutations also reduce the viral replication rate compared with that of wild-type virus and may take a long time to emerge as the major quasispecies. Resistance to PIs usually requires the accumulation of several mutations and this may take months or even years to occur.

Mutations associated with resistance to NNRTIs (e.g. Y181C or K103N) do not appear to affect the viral replication rate and so virus can appear as the dominant quasispecies in weeks after starting nevirapine- or efavirenz-based regimens.

Without continuous pressure on the virus to maintain the dominant strain (e.g. when the drugs are stopped), the wild-type strain will re-emerge as this is usually the most efficient at replicating. The mutated strain, however, does not disappear completely but will become archived as a minority quasispecies, only to become dominant again if the drug that selected it is restarted.

Primary drug resistance develops through transmission of a resistant strain from one individual to another sexually, vertically or through infected blood. Rates of primary drug resistance vary with the methodology used, class of drug, risk behavior, geographic distribution and over time. Many centers are reporting declining rates or stable rates of primary drug resistance. Primary resistance occurs frequently enough in high-income countries to recommend baseline resistance testing prior to starting antiviral therapy for the first time. It has been shown that genotype-resistance testing of chronically HIV-infected, antiretroviral-naïve patients is likely to improve clinical outcomes and is cost-effective wherever the rate of primary resistance is above 1%.

RESISTANCE BY DRUG CLASS

The impact of various mutations alone and in combination is continuing to evolve as new drugs and new classes of these compounds are being developed.[20] There are now more than 200 mutations associated with antiretroviral resistance drugs.[21]

Nucleos(t)ide Reverse Transcriptase Inhibitors

In the NRTI class there are 50 mutations associated with resistance to thymidine analog- and nonthymidine analog-containing regimens,

as well as multi-nucleoside resistance mutations and accessory mutations.

M184V, nonthymidine analog-associated mutations such as K65R and L74V, and the multinucleoside resistance mutation Q151M act by decreasing NRTI incorporation.

By promoting a phosphorolytic reaction, thymidine analog mutations, the triple 69 insertions associated with multinucleoside resistance and many of the accessory mutations facilitate primer unblocking and enhanced removal of incorporated NRTI.

Thymidine analog mutations associated with zidovudine and stavudine accumulate in two distinct but overlapping patterns:
- type I pattern mutations M41L, D67N, L210W and T215Y; and
- type II mutations D67N, K70R, T215F and K219Q/E.

The type I pattern causes higher levels of phenotypic and clinical resistance to the thymidine analogs than the type II pattern and cross-resistance to abacavir, didanosine and tenofovir.

Non-nucleoside Reverse Transcriptase Inhibitors

NNRTIs have more than 40 reverse transcriptase mutations associated with resistance, some of which, when occurring as single mutations, can confer resistance and cross-resistance to at least three drugs in this class. The primary NNRTI resistance mutations are K103N/S, V106A/M, Y181C/I/V, Y188L/C/H and G190A/S/E. Any one of these will cause high-level resistance to nevirapine and variable levels of resistance to efavirenz. The newer NNRTI etravirine usually requires multiple mutations for resistance to be significant. It retains good activity against common single mutations (e.g. K103N.)

Protease Inhibitors

PI resistance is complex and there are more than 60 mutations associated with reducing susceptibility to these drugs. These include major protease, accessory protease and protease cleavage site mutations.

There are 17 primary resistance mutations and usually a combination of several of these is required to develop high-level resistance. The effect of these PI resistance mutations on any individual PI can be difficult to predict when many mutations are present in the same virus isolate or when mutations occur in unusual patterns. Gag cleavage site mutations and accessory compensatory mutations can all impact on the susceptibility of the virus to these drugs.

Integrase Inhibitors

There is already much known about resistance to the recently developed integrase inhibitors raltegravir and elvitegravir, with more than 30 integrase mutations found to be associated with these agents. Common mutations for raltegravir and elvitegravir include N155H and Q148H/R/K. These two mutations by themselves do not appear to confer cross-resistance to dolutegravir. Dolutegravir is the first drug outside the boosted PI family not to be associated with development of resistance in clinical trials of antiretroviral-naïve patients. In experienced patients, reduced susceptibility to dolutegravir occurs in isolates containing Q148H/R/K plus at least another mutation.

Entry Inhibitors

At least 15 gp41 mutations are associated with resistance to the fusion inhibitor enfuvirtide, the commonest occurring between positions 36 and 45. Resistance to the entry inhibitors targeting the CCR5 receptor (e.g. maraviroc) is unusual and more complex, resulting from mutations that promote gp120 binding of the virus to the CCR5 receptor, which is bound to the drug. The majority of virologic failures with this drug, however, are the outgrowth of minority species that can use the alternative CXCR4 receptor for entry.

MEASURING RESISTANCE

Most resistance tests use genomic sequencing techniques ('genotyping') that are sufficiently sensitive to pick up quasispecies which comprise at least 20% of the viral swarm as long as the VL is >1000 copies/mL. The sequences are then analyzed to produce a mutation list and this is related to whether a particular drug is predicted to be active or not. Phenotypic techniques are also available but are expensive and time consuming, and add little extra information above genotyping. There are more sensitive tests that are able to detect minority quasispecies: single genome sequencing, ultrasensitive allele specific PCR and ultra-deep sequencing that for the moment are still used for research, not for clinical practice.

RATES OF RESISTANCE

Currently, approximately half of treated patients undergoing resistance testing show evidence of drug resistance and around 11% have evidence of resistance mutations affecting at least three classes of antiretroviral drug. Primary resistance is found in around 5% of patients but varies from <1% to 15% depending on geography and how long ARV therapy has been available.

VIRAL LOAD BLIPS

Transient rises in VL levels to detectable from undetectable can occur frequently. They may represent 'noise' on the VL assay or events related to viral replication such as intercurrent systemic infection or vaccination. If low-level detectable viremia represents early virologic failure, persistently detectable VLs are usually seen, although these may remain low level for long periods despite significant development of resistance. If this is a true 'blip', a single detectable VL is followed by a return to the undetectable state. It is controversial as to whether blips are associated with a future risk of virologic failure but most are probably bursts of replication of wild-type virus from latently infected cells.

Principles of Second- and Third-Line Treatments

Individuals with virologic failure should be changed to a regimen of antiretroviral drugs based on treatment history and resistance testing, which provides two to three fully active drugs. This may result in drugs being recycled in subsequent lines of therapy if no significant resistance is present, sequencing onto new drugs in the same class if there is non-overlapping resistance or incorporating new classes of drug.

OTHER DRUGS AVAILABLE TO USE IN SECOND AND SUBSEQUENT LINES OF THERAPY

Non-nucleoside Reverse Transcriptase Inhibitors

The problems related to this class include:
- a single mutation causing high-level cross-class resistance;
- toxicity (rash and hepatotoxicity for nevirapine) and neuropsychiatric and lipid effects (efavirenz); and
- teratogenicity (central nervous system (CNS) malformations were seen in monkey studies on efavirenz).

New generation NNRTIs have to overcome these obstacles before being acceptable and becoming drugs of choice for highly active antiretroviral therapy (HAART) regimens. Etravirine was licensed for use in 2008. Etravirine it is a very attractive choice after failure of efavirenz-based regimens and development of the K103N mutation. The K103N mutation by itself does not confer resistance to etravirine. A weighted genotypic scoring algorithm is available to determine the antiviral activity of etravirine for isolates with NNRTI resistance mutations.[22]

Protease Inhibitors

Tipranavir is a nonpeptide PI which is administered with ritonavir. Tipranavir has activity against viruses that are resistant to other PI. Resistance to tipranavir itself seems to require multiple mutations. However, side effects of tipranavir are more severe than other antiretrovirals. There are also significant pharmacokinetic interactions with other antiretrovirals making tipranavir a second choice.

Darunavir–ritonavir is a boosted PI with a high genetic barrier that has a potent *in vitro* activity against both wild-type HIV-1 and HIV-2, and the majority of multiple PI-resistant HIV-1. Darunavir–ritonavir is administered daily (QD) for ARV-naïve patients and twice daily (BD) for patients infected with PI-resistant HIV.

Darunavir–ritonavir has shown remarkable activity for the treatment of patients with early virological failure and limited antiretroviral resistance in the ODIN and TITAN studies.[23,24] In addition, darunavir–ritonavir has been tested for deep salvage of multiclass-resistant HIV infection in the POWER studies.[25] Darunavir–ritonavir is a cornerstone for the treatment of antiretroviral-resistant HIV infection. Best efficacy results in clinical trials of multiclass-resistant HIV have been obtained when new drugs such as raltegravir, maraviroc and etravirine were combined with darunavir/ritonavir.

CCR5 Inhibitors

Maraviroc. Maraviroc is the first CCR5 receptor antagonist licensed for the treatment of HIV infection. Co-receptor tropism should be determined prior to using maraviroc as it is not effective against CXCR4-tropic or mixed- or dual-tropic viruses. Maraviroc is a substrate of cytochrome P450 (CYP3A) and p-glycoprotein, and has clinically significant interactions with other drugs including efavirenz and rifampin.

In the MOTIVATE 1 and 2 studies that compared maraviroc with placebo, each given in combination with an optimized background regimen to patients with advanced HIV disease and CCR5-tropic HIV-1, at 48 weeks the rates of virologic suppression to <50 copies/mL were not significant, although the mean increase in CD4 cell count was greater in the maraviroc groups. Virologic failure is usually associated with the emergence of CXCR4 virus as the development of resistance mutations is rare.

Fusion Inhibitors

Enfuvirtide blocks HIV-1 entry by inhibiting fusion. It has been used as salvage treatment of individuals with extensive, often triple class, resistance. It is expensive and needs to be given by subcutaneous injection twice daily. These factors have limited its widespread use.

Integrase Inhibitors

Raltegravir it is administered BD and has a very benign safety profile. Combined with a boosted PI it has shown high efficacy rates in patients with moderate and extensive resistance.[26]

Elvitegravir it is administered QD and needs boosting with cobicistat or ritonavir. Elvitegravir used in combination with a ritonavir-boosted PI in treatment-experienced patients has similar efficacy and safety to raltegravir.[27]

Dolutegravir is administered QD (or BD in patients with integrase mutations), and does not need boosting. Dolutegravir often remains active after failure of raltegravir or elvitegravir and has been shown to be quite efficacious in patients with moderate and extensive resistance.[28]

Other Agents in Advanced Development

THE NEED FOR NEW DRUGS?

Currently licensed drugs have short- and long-term toxicities. Convenience and ease of adherence are important in constructing regimens that are easy to tolerate. Once-a-day dosing and a low pill burden are important factors in achieving these aims. There is also active research in long-acting formulations of antiretrovirals that can be administered monthly or even bi-monthly. Moreover, patients who have developed virologic failure, often with multiple resistant mutations, need new drugs that are active against these drug-resistant strains.

Drug–Drug Interactions

Most drug interactions with ARVs are mediated through inhibition or induction of hepatic drug metabolism. For example, all PIs and NNRTIs are metabolized in the liver by the cytochrome P450 system, particularly by the CYP3A4 isoenzyme. Some PIs may also be inducers or inhibitors of other CYP isoenzymes and of p-glycoprotein or other transporters.

The inhibitory effect of ritonavir is used to advantage in boosting concentrations of the other PIs but may cause abnormally high levels of some drugs such as simvastatin. The NNRTI's CYP3A4-inducing effect can be an issue when giving atazanavir or lopinavir–ritonavir. Efavirenz can cause PI concentration to fall.

These drug interactions are not always predictable. As an example, tenofovir interacts with didanosine, increasing didanosine intracellular levels, but will decrease atazanavir plasma concentrations.

There are web-based and other resources to help identify drug–drug interactions between antiretrovirals and between other commonly prescribed drugs (http://www.hiv-druginteractions.org).

ARV and Antituberculous Therapy

There are many difficulties when it comes to managing tuberculosis (TB) and HIV coinfection. When to start antiretroviral treatment in a patient on antituberculous therapy has been an ongoing issue. Now it is clear that the fear of poor adherence, drug interactions, toxicity and development of immune reconstitution inflammatory syndrome (IRIS) is outweighed by the risk of progression and death if the HIV remains untreated in the severely immunocompromised. Randomized controlled trials[29] have shown that in patients with CD4 cell counts below 100 cells/μL, antiretroviral treatment (ART) should be started as soon as TB treatment is tolerated and wherever possible within 2 weeks. In patients with CD4 cell counts above 100 cells/μL, ART can be deferred until between 8 and 12 weeks of antituberculous treatment, especially when there are difficulties with drug–drug interactions, adherence and toxicities.

Drug interactions with the essential component of TB treatment – the rifamycins – are a problem. Rifamycins are potent inducers of drug efflux *p*-glycoprotein and of the cytochrome P450 enzyme system, especially 3A4 which is responsible for the metabolism of PIs, NNRTIs and the CCR5 inhibitor maraviroc. Rifampin also induces metabolism of the ISTI raltegravir.

This interaction limits the drugs that can be used with rifampin, leaving four nucleoside regimens thus far of unproven efficacy in HIV, or using efavirenz (600–800 mg/day) or nevirapine plus nucleosides. Efavirenz is preferred because of the better interaction profile and better efficacy seen in a cohort study from South Africa. Efavirenz doses are adjusted by some physicians to 800 mg if the patient is over 60 kg and the use of drug level monitoring can be useful in this situation. PIs boosted with ritonavir can lead to significant decreases in plasma levels and a high rate of hepatotoxicity with rifampin. If they have to be used, it is better to switch to rifabutin. Recent data have shown that it is also possible to simultaneously use rifampin and raltegravir although it is still unclear if raltegravir needs to be used at a higher dose. Pharmacokinetic data also suggest that dolutegravir can be used along with rifampin.

Chronic Hepatitis

Coinfection of chronic HBV or HCV with HIV increases the rate of progression to cirrhosis and liver cancer by four- to fivefold compared with hepatitis mono-infected individuals. The mortality rate of untreated HIV/HBV or HIV/HCV coinfected patients is approximately 10 times higher than that of patients with either infection alone.

Antiretroviral therapy may reduce the rate of progression to cirrhosis and death in these patients.

The field of therapy against hepatitis C recently underwent a revolution with the advent of direct acting antivirals that are able to cure hepatitis C in the majority of patients. In the past, the use of certain antiretrovirals, such as zidovudine and didanosine, was contraindicated if the patient also had treatment with interferon and ribavirin. With the anti-hepatitis C PIs boceprevir and telaprevir there are also relevant interactions with the anti-HIV PIs. Fortunately with the most recent anti-hepatitis C direct acting antivirals, such as sofosbuvir, interactions with antiretrovirals are much less of an issue.

Tenofovir, lamivudine and emtricitabine are agents that work against HIV; however, as they also suppress hepatitis B viral replication, they should be included in regimens given to patients coinfected with HIV and HBV. The treatment of these coinfections is discussed in Practice Point 31 and Chapters 42 and 155.

References available online at expertconsult.com.

KEY REFERENCES

Cahn P., Andrade-Villanueva J., Arribas J.R., et al.: Dual therapy with lopinavir and ritonavir plus lamivudine versus triple therapy with lopinavir and ritonavir plus two nucleoside reverse transcriptase inhibitors in antiretroviral-therapy-naive adults with HIV-1 infection: 48 week results of the randomised, open label, non-inferiority GARDEL trial. *Lancet Infect Dis* 2014; 14:572-580.

Castagna A., Maggiolo F., Penco G., et al.: Dolutegravir in antiretroviral-experienced patients with raltegravir- and/or elvitegravir-resistant HIV-1: 24-week results of the Phase III VIKING-3 Study. *J Infect Dis* 2014; 210(3): 354-362.

Clotet B., Bellos N., Molina J.-M., et al.: Efficacy and safety of darunavir-ritonavir at week 48 in treatment-experienced patients with HIV-1 infection in POWER 1 and 2: a pooled subgroup analysis of data from two randomised trials. *Lancet* 2007; 369:1169-1178.

Clotet B., Feinberg J., van Lunzen J., et al.: Once-daily dolutegravir versus darunavir plus ritonavir in antiretroviral-naïve adults with HIV-1 infection (FLAMINGO): 48 week results from the randomised open-label phase 3b study. *Lancet* 2014; 383:2222-2231.

Cohen M.S., Chen Y.Q., Mc Cauley M., et al.: Prevention of HIV-1 Infection with early antiretroviral therapy. *N Engl J Med* 2011; 365:493-505.

El-Sadr W.M., Lundgren J.D., Strategies for Management of Antiretroviral Therapy (SMART) Study Group, et al.: CD4+ count-guided interruption of antiretroviral treatment. *N Engl J Med* 2006; 355:2283-2296.

Eron J.J., Cooper D.A., Steigbigel R.T., et al.: Efficacy and safety of raltegravir for treatment of HIV for 5 years in the BENCHMRK studies: final results of two randomised, placebo-controlled trials. *Lancet Infect Dis* 2013; 13:587-596.

Grinsztejn B., Hosseinipour M.C., Ribaudo H.J., et al.: Effects of early versus delayed initiation of antiretroviral treatment on clinical outcomes of HIV-1 infection: results from the phase 3 HPTN 052 randomized controlled trial. *Lancet Infect Dis* 2014; 14(4):281-290.

The INSIGHT START Study Group: Initiation of Antiretroviral Therapy in Early Asymptomatic HIV Infection. *N Engl J Med* 2015; 373(9):795-807.

Lawn S.D., Wood R.: Timing of antiretroviral therapy for HIV-1-associated tuberculosis. *N Engl J Med* 2012; 2:474.

Lennox J.L., Landovitz R.J., Ribaudo H.J., et al.: Efficacy and tolerability of 3 nonnucleoside reverse transcriptase inhibitor-sparing antiretroviral regimens for treatment-naïve volunteers infected with HIV-1: a randomized, controlled equivalence trial. *Ann Intern Med* 2014; 161(7):461-471.

Raffi F., Babiker A.G., Richert L., et al.: Ritonavir-boosted darunavir combined with raltegravir or tenofovir-emtricitabine in antiretroviral-naïve adults infected with HIV-1: 96 week results from the NEAT001/ANRS143 randomised non-inferiority trial. *Lancet* 2014; 384(9958):1942-1951.

Riddler S.A., Haubrich R., DiRienzo A.G., et al.: AIDS Clinical Trials Group Study A5142 Team. Class-sparing regimens for initial treatment of HIV-1 infection. *N Engl J Med* 2008; 358:2095-2106.

Walmsley S., Antela A., Clumeck N., et al.: Dolutegravir plus abacavir-lamivudine for the treatment of HIV infection. *N Engl J Med* 2013; 369:1807-1818.

104

Issues in the Aging HIV-Positive Patient

PATRICK W. MALLON | WILLIAM G. POWDERLY

KEY CONCEPTS

- Non-AIDS morbidities now account for the majority of deaths in HIV-infected patients in the industrialized world.

- Morbidities of aging occur more commonly in HIV-infected patients; lifestyle issues (especially cigarette smoking), inflammation associated with chronic infection, and adverse effects of antiretroviral treatment are all believed to be associated with increased risk of co-morbidities.

- HIV-infected patients have an increased risk of atherosclerotic cardiovascular events due to inflammation associated with HIV infection, dyslipidemia from HIV protease inhibitors and through other direct effects of some antiretrovirals.

- Decreased bone mineral density is a feature of chronic HIV infection; it may be exacerbated by antiretroviral therapy and may contribute to increased risk of fractures.

- Primary and secondary prevention of co-morbidities in older HIV-infected patients should be performed according to standard guidelines for all older individuals. Antiretroviral therapy choices in older HIV-infected patients may need to be tailored according to an individual's risk of co-morbidities.

Introduction

Potent antiretroviral therapy (ART) has led to prolonged survival of individuals infected with HIV; in recent studies, the projected life expectancy of young adults who are treated early in the course of HIV infection approaches normal.[1,2] However, the aging of the HIV-infected population offers new challenges, particularly the increasing importance of age-related illnesses which contribute to the morbidity and mortality of HIV-infected individuals.

The proportion of the population living with HIV aged 50 years or over is rising every year in parallel with the prolonged survival associated with ART. In Western and Central Europe and North America almost a third of HIV-infected patients are now over the age of 50; but similar trends are occurring worldwide as access to HIV therapy becomes more available and widely implemented[3] (Figure 104-1). Illnesses traditionally seen more frequently in older individuals have assumed increasing importance as the cause of death and morbidity in HIV-infected patients, including cardiovascular disease and non-AIDS-related malignancies. HIV-infected individuals appear to be at greater risk of bone demineralization leading to osteoporosis and potentially increased fracture risk. Other areas of potential concern include renal disease, and neuro-degeneration.

HIV-infected patients have more co-morbidities than age-matched-HIV negative individuals and the overall frequency of these co-morbidities is greater in HIV-infected older adults.[4]

The *pathogenesis* of this increased risk of morbidities in older HIV-infected individuals is unclear, and somewhat controversial.[5,6] Some investigators have speculated that HIV infection may be associated with premature aging; however, the biological basis for such a hypothesis is weak. The uncertainty as to cause actually reflects, in part, the fact that the pathogenesis for each of these individual co-morbidities

is different. Indeed, it is probable that the increased likelihood of the various co-morbidities is multifactorial in origin with HIV infection, its treatment, and lifestyle/environmental factors all contributing in different ways for each of these conditions (Figure 104-2).

It has been long recognized that as we age, *lifestyle factors* play a major role in the risk of disease. Smoking, by increasing the risk of atherosclerosis and cancer, is a major cause of premature morbidity and mortality worldwide. HIV-infected patients are more likely to smoke; smoking prevalence rates are 2–3 times those of the general population in the USA and in Western Europe.[7] This undoubtedly has a significant role in the increased risk for heart and other vascular diseases in the HIV-infected population. There is an increased prevalence of drug and alcohol use among HIV-infected patients which contributes to an increased risk of many co-morbidities. Additionally, HIV-infected individuals are significantly more likely to have mental health disorders than the general population. Patients with mental health problems, especially if untreated or poorly managed, are also significantly more likely to have greater morbidity and mortality from other health issues, in part because of delayed diagnosis and nonadherence to treatment regimens.[8]

HIV infection itself may have a role in increasing risk for some of the co-morbid conditions seen in older individuals. Uncontrolled HIV infection is associated with evidence of immune activation and increased inflammation. Even in well-controlled HIV infection, there is evidence that patients have persistent inflammation greater than that seen in HIV-negative populations.[9] Ongoing inflammation is increasingly implicated in the pathogenesis of many illnesses, including atherosclerosis and bone disease. In clinical trials of treatment interruption in HIV, evidence of persistent inflammation may be associated with increased risk of non-AIDS related events such as myocardial infarction and liver disease.[10] Additionally, while antiretroviral therapy restores sufficient immune function that the risk of opportunistic infection is substantially reduced, if not eliminated, complete immune recovery does not occur in most individuals. Furthermore, immune senescence is a feature of normal aging and it is possible that the combination of prior HIV infection and aging may lead to a more accelerated loss of immune function over time as individuals get older. An additional potential factor that may be contributing to immune dysfunction and inflammation in older individuals is the increased prevalence of other viral infections among HIV-infected patients, especially persistent cytomegalovirus (CMV) infection.

Finally, *antiretroviral therapy* may influence the risk of developing several co-morbid conditions. This was first recognized in the early years of potent ART when patients presented with an increased frequency of myocardial infarction.[11] Subsequent studies have suggested that much of that risk is associated with protease inhibitor-induced hyperlipidemia (see below). Most currently used antiretroviral regimens have the potential for long-term toxicities; for example, tenofovir can cause chronic renal dysfunction and short-term increased bone demineralization.[12]

Cardiovascular Disease

Cardiovascular disease (CVD) is the commonest cause of death in the industrialized world, with incidence rates increasing as people enter their fifth decade of life. People living with chronic HIV infection are

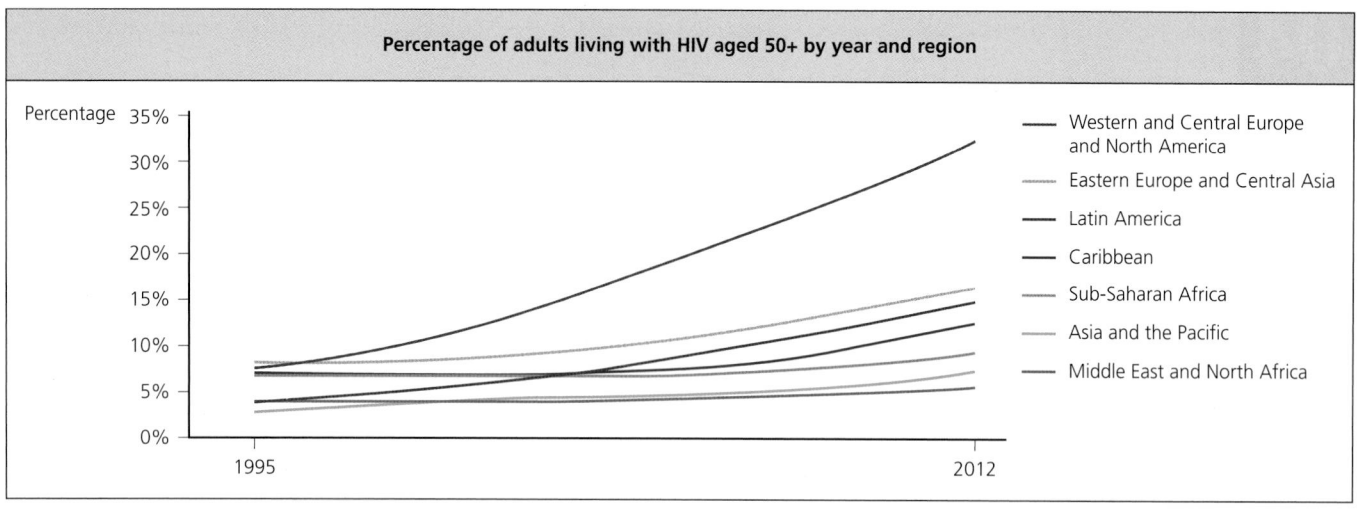

Figure 104-1   Percentage of adults living with HIV aged 50+ by year and region. *(From HIV and aging. A special supplement to the UNAIDS report on the global AIDS epidemic 2013. Figure 2. Online. Available at: http://www.unaids.org/sites/default/files/media_asset/20131101_JC2563_hiv-and-aging_en_0.pdf)*

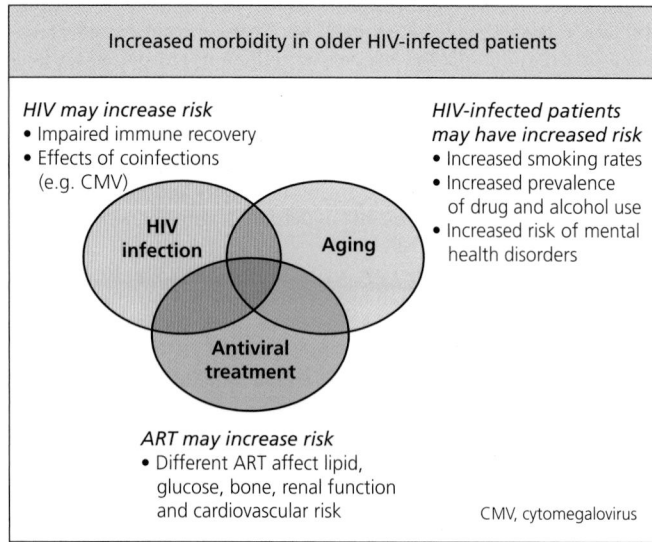

Figure 104-2   Increased morbidity in older HIV-infected patients.

at greater risk of CVD, and myocardial infarction (MI) in particular, secondary to a number of factors including lifestyle factors, effects from HIV infection itself and consequences of exposure to ART. Although approaches to minimizing CVD risk in HIV reflect those used in the general population, the unique pathogenesis of CVD observed in HIV suggests a potential role for HIV-specific interventions.

As in the general population, CVD has been identified as one of the commonest causes of death in those living with HIV, particularly in populations on effective antiretroviral therapy where the incidence of AIDS illnesses is much reduced. The **D**ata collection on **A**dverse events of anti-HIV **D**rugs (D:A:D) study, a prospective study of more than 30 000 people with HIV that examines rates of, and associations with, MI has contributed much to our understanding of the causes of MI in those with HIV.[13,14] This study has established age-related MI event rates that seem in excess of what is predicted by modelling of traditional CVD risk factors alone.[15] In addition, several large healthcare registry analyses have reported excess risk of MI in people living with HIV, with one study estimating an excess risk of MI of 50% in those with HIV when controlled for traditional CVD risk factors such as age, smoking status and hypertension.[16]

Within the D:A:D cohort, those experiencing MI are predominantly male, mean age in late 40s, most smoke and approximately one-third are classified as high CVD risk. Similar to the general population, traditional risk factors for CVD, such as smoking status, hypertension and dyslipidemia independently predict risk of MI. However, although some traditional risk factors for CVD may be over-represented in populations living with HIV, particularly smoking, which has been observed to be commoner in those with HIV in a number of studies, this imbalance in prevalence of traditional risk factors fails to fully explain the increased observed rates of MI in those with HIV. Both HIV and ART can modify dyslipidemia as well as inflammatory, endothelial and pro-coagulant pathways important in the pathogenesis of atherosclerosis and MI.[17,18] Untreated HIV infection is characterized by low total and high-density lipoprotein (HDL) cholesterol. Treatment with ART has been associated with further dyslipidemia such as increases in low-density lipoprotein (LDL) cholesterol and triglycerides; these changes were observed more with first generation protease inhibitors (PI) and were exacerbated by lipodystrophy, associated with the use of thymidine-analog nucleoside reverse transcriptase inhibitors (NRTI).[14] Those with lipodystrophy are also at greater risk of diabetes mellitus, another risk factor for CVD. Use of newer PIs and other drug classes, such as integrase strand transfer inhibitors, have been associated with much less dyslipidemia.

Untreated HIV infection is also characterized by a pro-inflammatory state, with markers of inflammation associated with development of cardiovascular events in one large prospective study. Much of this pro-inflammatory milieu is reduced by control of HIV with ART, but inflammation persists despite ART, particularly in those starting ART > 1 year since acquisition of HIV infection. In addition, exposure to some antiretrovirals has also been associated with excess risk of MI with increased MI risk seen with cumulative exposure to some PIs (lopinavir/ritonavir and indinavir but not with atazanavir) and with recent exposure to some NRTI (the guanosine analog NRTIs abacavir and didanosine). The drug associations likely reflect different pathologies, with the PI association with cumulative exposure explained at least in part by PI-induced dyslipidemia while the reversible association observed with abacavir likely related to effects on endothelial dysfunction or altered platelet reactivity.[19]

In general, the approaches to management of CVD risk and CVD events in those with HIV reflects recommendations for the general population, with a focus on primary and secondary prevention through modifying cardiovascular risk factors.[20] Among the most important is smoking cessation, which has been shown to have a positive impact on CVD events in those with HIV in the D:A:D study.[21] Screening for and treating dyslipidemia, hypertension and diabetes mellitus is also central

TABLE 104-1	Studies Summarizing Fracture Rates and HIV				
Country	N	HIV+	% Male	Fractures	Association Between Fracture and HIV
USA	119 318	33%	100	1615	HR 1.24 (1.11, 1.39)
Denmark	31 836	5306	76	806	IRR 1.5 (1.4–1.7)
Canada	540	138	0	–	OR 1.7 (1.1, 2.6)
USA	559	328	100	33	No difference in fracture rates
Spain	1 118 156	2489	–	24,457 (HIV+ 49)	HR 4.7 (2.44, 9.5) for hip fractures

Country = where study was performed. HR, hazard ration; IRR, incidence rate ratio; OR, odds ratio.

to risk reduction with management of these conditions generally reflecting what is recommended for the general population. As all of these conditions are more prevalent in older populations, this introduces issues related to medication complexity and the potential for unwanted drug interactions, particularly with the use of some HMG co-enzyme A reductase inhibitors (or statins) which have the potential for significant drug–drug interactions with both PI and NNRTI.

Osteoporosis and Fractures

Low bone mineral density (BMD) and osteoporosis is the manifestation of bone disease that raises most concern in an aging population living with HIV infection, given the propensity of low BMD to predispose to increased risk of fracture. Osteoporosis is a common condition in the general population. In HIV, low BMD and osteoporosis occur more commonly than the general population with preliminary research suggesting a link to increased fracture risk.[22] The causes of low BMD in HIV are multifactorial, with contributions from the individual, their environment, HIV infection itself and responses to ART all implicated.[23]

Many potential demographic and socioeconomic factors, such as lower body mass index (BMI), increased smoking rates and higher alcohol intake in those living with HIV, may contribute to the observed increased prevalence of low BMD and potentially fractures in this population. However, in one large cohort of subjects with and without HIV drawn from similar demographic backgrounds, HIV remained an independent predictor of low BMD even after correction for variables such as age, gender, ethnicity, BMI and level of education.[24]

Normal bone metabolism relies on a healthy equilibrium between bone formation and bone resorption, facilitating replenishment of damaged bone and maintenance of bone architecture and strength. HIV infection is characterized by a high bone turnover state, with elevations in both markers of bone formation and resorption. This high bone turnover state develops around the period of ART initiation. A number of clinical trials have identified increased bone turnover coincident with decreases in BMD in antiretroviral-naïve patients initiating ART, largely limited to the first year after ART initiation.[25] That declines in BMD have been observed regardless of the ART regimen used suggests a potential role for either viral or immune-mediated mechanisms in the development of both BMD loss and increased bone turnover. The exact mechanisms underlying these changes in bone turnover remain poorly understood. The type of ART used influences losses in BMD after initiation, with greater decreases in BMD observed in those initiating ART containing an NRTI, particularly tenofovir, and also with some PIs. Although HIV infection is associated with a high bone turnover state, there is little evidence to show that, beyond the period of ART initiation or switch, people living with HIV experience a more rapid, progressive loss of BMD than would be expected from normal age-related changes.

Vitamin D is important for normal bone health, in part through helping to maintain physiological suppression of parathyroid hormone by facilitating dietary calcium absorption. Both abnormalities in vitamin D metabolism and vitamin D deficiency (VDD) have been implicated in the low BMD observed in HIV.[26] Supplementation of high dose vitamin D and calcium for the first year of ART initiation abrogates early bone loss and is accompanied by smaller increases in bone turnover.

The principal clinical consequence of osteoporosis is fracture. In the general population, both age and extremes of body weight are associated with specific sites of osteoporotic fractures; advancing age associated more with hip, upper limb and pelvic fractures while higher body weight associated more with lower limb and ankle fractures. Several cross-sectional studies[27–31] have demonstrated higher rates of fracture in those with HIV (Table 104-1) although given the relatively young age of the HIV population the overall number of fractures contributing to these analyses is still relatively low and the association between HIV status and fracture is not consistently observed across all studies.

Fracture risk is determined by assessing bone mineral density through the use of dual energy X-ray absorptiometry (DXA), which measures BMD, combined with assessment of other risk factors that may contribute to either falls or low BMD, which provides a more accurate assessment of global fracture risk than measurement of BMD alone. The FRAX algorithm provides a country-specific framework to assess individual fracture risk based on the relative contribution of BMD and other factors such as age, gender, smoking status and secondary causes of osteoporosis, resulting in guidance on thresholds for use of bone protection therapy based on fracture risk.[32]

Most available guidance recommends screening for low BMD with DXA in those who have additional risk factors for low BMD, such as those over the age of 50, those with a history of fragility or fracture, postmenopausal women or those suffering from hypogonadism (men and women) and those with a significant history of exposure to corticosteroids. Within this patient group, DXA data should be combined with other fracture risk information to decide on the need for bone protection, where possible using country or region-specific guidelines for use.[33]

Several medications have been shown to reduce the risk of fracture in those with osteoporosis although much of the data are restricted to populations without HIV who are over 50 years old or in postmenopausal women. The bisphosphonates remain the most studied medication and are unlikely to have significant interactions with ART. All should be used with optimal vitamin D and calcium intake.

Cancer

ART has been associated with a dramatic change in cancer risk for HIV-infected individuals. The risk of developing AIDS-associated malignancies drops dramatically with the initiation of ART; the increased risk for Kaposi's sarcoma in particular, virtually disappears within 1 year of effective antiretroviral treatment. Patients remain at risk for non-Hodgkin's lymphoma for a longer period of time; however, the risk is considerably less than that of an untreated HIV-infected patient. As patients survive longer with HIV, non-AIDS cancers become increasingly prevalent.[34,35] Among HIV-infected cohorts, there is more anal and liver cancer, probably associated with the increased rates of coinfection with human papillomavirus (HPV) and hepatitis viruses respectively, although a contribution, especially for anal cancer, from prolonged ART cannot yet be excluded. There also appears to be a higher frequency of lung cancer in HIV-infected individuals, although this is largely associated with increased prevalence of smoking among HIV-infected individuals. Prostate cancer also appears to be increased in frequency. In contrast, other common cancers such as colon cancer and breast cancer, do not appear to be increased in HIV infection, nor do they appear to occur at a younger age in HIV-infected patients.

Renal Dysfunction

HIV-associated nephropathy has now become a rare cause of renal failure in patients with HIV infection with more effective ART. It is well recognized that renal function slowly declines with age, although aging-associated chronic kidney disease (CKD) occurs largely in patients over the age of 70 years. As a consequence, there are insufficient data in the HIV-infected patients at present to determine whether HIV-infected individuals are at increased risk of end-stage renal disease compared to the general population, particularly as they age. Certain antiretroviral agents have been associated with an increased risk of CKD, albeit in a small minority of individuals. Tenofovir can cause acute kidney injury in a small number of patients.[12] Increased relative risk of CKD has been associated with the use of tenofovir, ritonavir-boosted atazanavir and ritonavir-boosted lopinavir;[36] the absolute risk for renal disease remains low. Close monitoring of patients for renal disease, especially if there are other risk factors or potentially nephrotoxic therapy has to be used, is recommended.[37]

Neurocognitive Dysfunction

Advent of ART has been associated with the dramatic decline in the incidence and prevalence of AIDS-associated dementia, which is now extraordinarily rare among individuals on successful long-term ART.[38] By contrast, there appears to be no decline in the prevalence of mild HIV-associated cognitive impairment, as measured by sophisticated neuropsychological testing. This apparent paradox may be methodological but has created considerable uncertainty as to whether significant neurocognitive dysfunction will reappear as HIV-infected patients age. To this point, there is no evidence that HIV infection is associated with a greater risk of Alzheimer's disease or other aging-associated neurocognitive decline. Many experts now believe that neuropsychometric testing may not be predictive of long-term risk of specific neurodegenerative disease. However, given the increased risk of vascular disease among HIV-infected patients, especially those who smoke and have other risk factors, it is quite possible that some HIV-infected individuals will be at increased risk of vascular-associated neurocognitive conditions as they age.

Additional Management Considerations

It is very clear that as HIV-infected individuals age they are likely to develop at greater frequency, and perhaps earlier, many of the conditions that typically occur in the general population as people age. Fortunately, there is strong evidence from the general medical literature that many of these diseases can be prevented and/or mitigated with good medical care. This reinforces the need for regular screening and health maintenance among HIV-infected patients.[20,39,40] In particular, physicians should institute aggressive primary prevention for heart disease by strongly encouraging smoking cessation and controlling blood pressure and hyperlipidemia. A regular screening program for diabetes should be instituted with monitoring every 6 to 12 months. There is no evidence that HIV-infected patients should be more aggressively screened for cancer than the general population; however, such screening should be part of normal practice. (One exception to this comes from the increased prevalence of HPV-associated malignancies which may necessitate earlier and more aggressive screening for anorectal cancer.[41])

Given the potential role for uncontrolled inflammation from HIV infection in the pathogenesis of many of these conditions, there has been substantial interest in addressing the question of whether earlier use of ART might decrease the risk of these non-HIV-associated conditions. A large, randomized, controlled trial has shown a benefit to early therapy, although this was largely through a reduction in HIV-related events.[42] However, most HIV-infected individuals present relatively late in their illness and there is an immediate need to initiate ART to control their HIV infection. In such individuals, it is important to evaluate their risk for co-morbidities and to choose therapy to avoid if possible further contributing to the risk. In older patients with significant risk factors for CVD, strong consideration should be given to the avoidance of agents that significantly increase lipids (some PIs) or have other adverse cardiovascular effects (such as abacavir). In patients with significant risk for bone demineralization, consideration should be given to avoid tenofovir and ritonavir-boosted PIs. Similarly, in patients with evidence of CKD, tenofovir, atazanavir and lopinavir should be avoided if possible.

Conclusion

The morbidities of aging occur more commonly in HIV-infected patients and now account for the majority of deaths in HIV-infected patients in the industrialized world. HIV-infected patients have an increased risk of atherosclerotic cardiovascular events and decreased BMD; lifestyle issues (especially cigarette smoking), inflammation associated with chronic infection, and adverse effects of ART are all believed to be associated with this increase. As the proportion of patients living with HIV increases for many years in the near future, other long-term morbidities may emerge. In the interim, primary and secondary prevention of co-morbidities in older HIV-infected patients should be performed according to standard guidelines for all older individuals. However, ART decisions in older HIV-infected patients may need to be adjusted to account for an individual's risk of co-morbidities.

References available online at expertconsult.com.

KEY REFERENCES

Clifford D.B., Ances B.M.: HIV-associated neurocognitive disorder. *Lancet Infect Dis* 2013; 13:976-986.

Cotter A.G., Sabin C.A., Simelane S., et al.: Relative contribution of HIV infection, demographics and body mass index to bone mineral density. *AIDS* 2014; 28:2051-2060.

Deeks S.G., Phillips A.N.: HIV infection, antiretroviral treatment, ageing, and non-AIDS related morbidity. *BMJ* 2009; 338:a3172.

Duprez D.A., Neuhaus J., Kuller L.H., et al.: Inflammation, coagulation and cardiovascular disease in HIV-infected individuals. *PLoS ONE* 2012; 7(9):e44454.

European AIDS Clinical Society (EACS) Guidelines, Version 7, October 2013. Available: http://www.eacsociety.org/Portals/0/Guidelines_Online _131014.pdf.

Friis-Moller N., Reiss P., Sabin C.A., et al.: Class of antiretroviral drugs and the risk of myocardial infarction. *N Engl J Med* 2007; 356:1723-1735.

Greene M., Justice A.C., Lampiris H.W., et al.: Management of human immunodeficiency virus infection in advanced age. *JAMA* 2013; 309:1397-1405.

Lucas G.M., Ross M.J., Stock P.G., et al.: Executive Summary: Clinical Practice Guideline for the Management of Chronic Kidney Disease in Patients Infected With HIV: 2014 Update by the HIV Medicine Association of the Infectious Diseases Society of America. *Clin Infect Dis* 2014; 59:1203-1207.

Powderly W.G.: Osteoporosis and Bone Health. *Curr HIV/AIDS Rep* 2012; 9:218-222.

Smith C.J., Ryom L., Weber R., et al.: Trends in underlying causes of death in people with HIV from 1999 to 2011 (D:A:D): a multicohort collaboration. *Lancet* 2014; 384:241-248.

Worm S.W., Sabin C., Weber R., et al.: Risk of myocardial infarction in patients with HIV infection exposed to specific individual antiretroviral drugs from the 3 major drug classes: the data collection on adverse events of anti-HIV drugs (D:A:D) study. *J Infect Dis* 2010; 201:318-330.

105

Eradication and Cure of HIV

STEPHEN J. KENT

KEY CONCEPTS

- Lifelong antiretroviral therapy is expensive and has side effects; an ability to cure HIV is highly desirable.

- HIV can stably integrate and remain latent in resting CD4 T cells – this is a major barrier to cure.

- Bone marrow transplantation has been able to provide a sterilizing cure of HIV in one subject.

- Very early treatment shows promise in HIV-infected babies as a pathway to at least a transient functional cure ('remission') of HIV.

- Several antilatency drugs are being developed primarily to activate latent HIV and lead to reductions in numbers of latently infected cells.

- Gene therapy approaches to curing HIV are also under development.

- HIV may never readily be cured but there is an intense research effort ongoing to understand if curing HIV is feasible.

Introduction

Great strides have been made in the suppression of HIV infection using combination antiretroviral therapy (cART) in the last 20 years. However, the current cART paradigm has several problems. These include the need for lifelong therapy and attendant compliance problems, expense, side effects, development of drug resistance, the lack of normalization of chronic inflammatory markers, low level residual viral replication, higher rates of cardiovascular, hepatic and renal conditions, and higher rates of cancer. These issues combine to result in a suboptimal life expectancy in HIV-infected subjects. The ability to safely and inexpensively cure HIV would be a quantum advance and greatly assist in the control of the HIV epidemic.

It must be stated from the outset that HIV may never be able to be safely or inexpensively cured for reasonable numbers of subjects. Sometimes hype can exceed reality in medical research. There are, however, reasons to be hopeful, in part because a markedly increased level of research and resources is being applied to this issue in recent years.[1]

There are many barriers to the cure of HIV. HIV can stably integrate into resting CD4 T cells where it is hidden from current cART agents, which can only act on replicating virus.[2,3] Resting memory CD4 T cells have a very long lifespan since they form part of our lifelong immunological memory. The latent HIV reservoir under cART appears to have a very long half-life (decades) and does not appreciably decay.[4] Latent HIV exists in multiple tissues and organs (including the brain and the gut), although latent HIV has been most studied in blood-resting CD4 T cells. Low level HIV replication despite cART and chronic inflammation may assist in maintaining levels of the latent HIV reservoir.

There are two broad approaches to curing HIV – sterilizing and functional. A sterilizing cure is the classic infectious disease model of cure where all virus elements would be gone. A functional cure is where there may be residual virus but the virus is maintained in a quiescent state without the need for cART. A functional cure is akin to subjects with nonprogressive HIV, typically where immune responses maintain virus replication at low or undetectable levels.

There are several approaches currently in clinical trials studying aspects of cure of HIV. These can be broadly categorized as bone marrow transplant approaches, early cART therapy approaches, anti-latency drug therapy approaches, immune manipulation approaches and gene therapy approaches. They are summarized in Table 105-1.

Bone Marrow Transplantation to Cure HIV

The most celebrated case of apparent HIV cure is the 'Berlin patient'.[5] This HIV+ man developed a leukemia requiring a bone marrow transplant (BMT) and his physicians chose a donor lacking expression of CCR5, a key HIV entry receptor. His cART was stopped after the BMT and HIV viremia had not recrudesced after several years. Minimal or no HIV has been detected in both blood and other organs for many years off cART[6] (Figure 105-1). This anecdotal case of essentially sterilizing cure of HIV suggests that the primary HIV reservoir may exist in immune cells that were lost either as a result of the chemotherapy/radiotherapy induction for the BMT and/or as a result of subsequent graft-versus-host disease.

Two further cases of BMT for malignancy in the setting of HIV infection have been reported from a Boston group.[7] In these two cases the donor was not devoid of CCR5. Both subjects had low or undetectable levels of HIV after the transplantation while on cART and were subsequently taken off cART. However, after a period of a few months off cART it has recently been reported that HIV viremia was re-established. It is not yet clear if a lack of CCR5 in the donor or some other features of the BMT conditioning regimen or graft-versus-host disease will be needed to replicate the success of the Berlin patient. Although BMT is not a viable method to cure HIV, having both very high costs and very high morbidity and mortality, lessons learned from HIV+ subjects undergoing BMT may ultimately find application in safer and less expensive therapies.

Early Treatment of HIV to Control HIV off cART

The next most celebrated case of apparent HIV cure is the 'Mississippi baby'. This infant was born to a mother who found out she was HIV+ during labor (Figure 105-2). The infant had high levels of viremia at birth and was treated within hours with a triple combination of cART.[8] The infant subsequently stopped cART some 18 months later when medical care was lost. Upon subsequent testing at 24 months of age and beyond, viremia remained undetectable with minimal to no levels of residual HIV DNA detectable off cART. HIV antibodies declined and no infectious HIV could be recovered from culturing large numbers of cells. However, recent data show that HIV rebounded 27 months later and cART was re-initiated.[9] The case suggests that, at least in some cases, very early initiation of cART may substantially reduce the latent reservoir of integrated viral DNA. Although speculative, this may allow remaining immune responses or other host mechanisms to clear residual latent reservoirs. Wider studies are now planned on HIV-infected babies to evaluate whether this scenario can be replicated and the conditions needed.

Early treatment of adults with HIV infection has also been postulated to assist in the functional cure of HIV off cART.[10] A small number of subjects were studied by Walker and colleagues in the year 2000 with

TABLE 105-1	Strategies for HIV Cure				
Antilatency Strategy	**Concept**	**Advantages**	**Disadvantages**	**Current Status**	**References**
Bone marrow transplantation	Replacing bone marrow with HIV– bone marrow which lacks CCR5 both eliminates much of the reservoir and provides no new targets for new infection	One well-documented case of HIV cure (Berlin patient)	High morbidity and mortality from procedure – only done in subjects with malignancy. CCR5 negative donor may be required	Being studied on case-by-case basis	5
Early treatment of HIV	Very early treatment with cART after infection may limit size of the latent HIV reservoir such that virus recrudescence does not occur off cART	One well-documented baby transient functional cure after cART initiated early after birth	Defining subjects with very early HIV infection difficult. Treatment of adults after a few weeks of infection has modest benefit	Expanded studies of babies born to HIV+ mothers planned	8
Antilatency drug approaches	Administration of drugs to reactivate and clear latently infected cells	Trials show an increase in HIV expression after use of drug vorinostat. Multiple drugs under development	Impact of single drugs on total reservoir may be low. Safety concerns with some drugs	Multiple clinical trials underway	15
Immune manipulation	Enhancing HIV immunity to clear reactivated latently infected cells	Promising macaque-SIV studies with T cell-based vaccines and antibody infusions	No proof of concept in clinical trials	Translation to clinical trials underway	20,22
Gene therapy approaches	Eliminating CCR5 expression to render cells noninfectable	First clinical trial shows some promise in reducing viremia off cART	Small studies to date. Somewhat complex cell manipulations may be required	Expanded trials underway	24

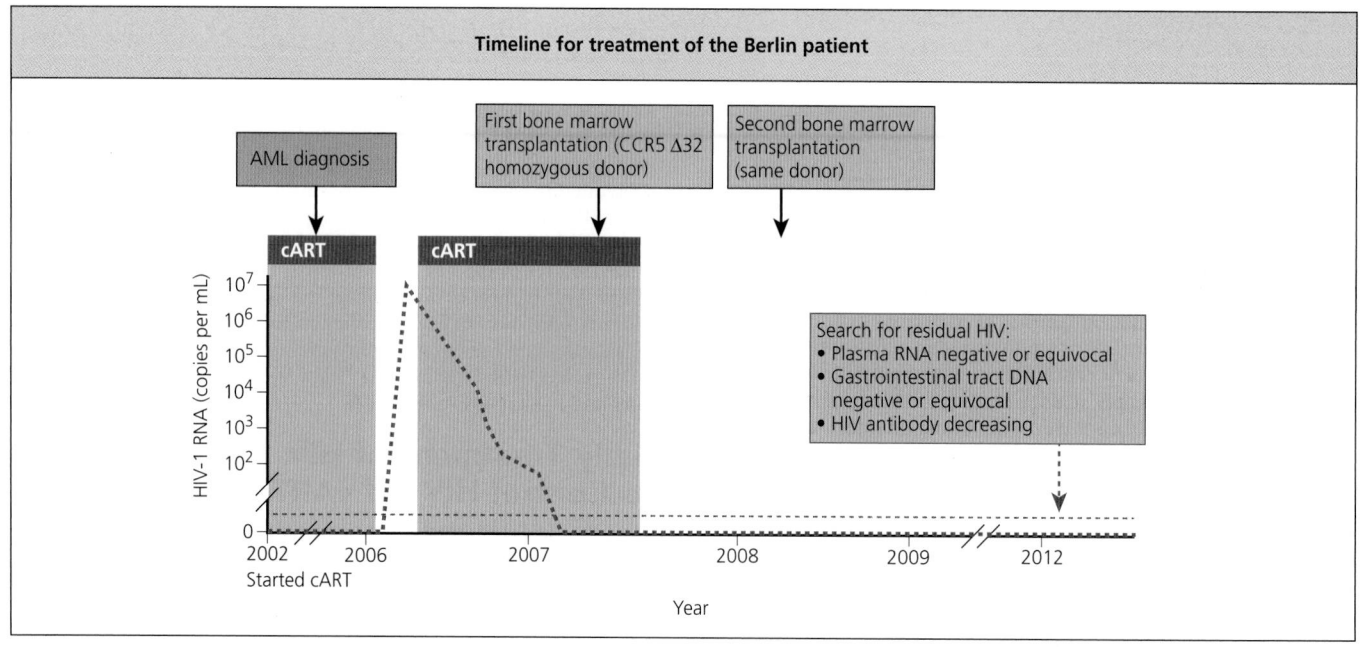

Figure 105-1 Timeline for treatment of the Berlin patient. The grey dotted line represents the limit of detection (one copy per mL) in tests used after transplantation. AML=acute myeloid leukemia; cART=combined antiretroviral therapy. (*From Kent S.J., et al.: The search for an HIV cure: tackling latent infection. Lancet Infect Dis 2013 Jul; 13(7):614-21.*)

the suggestion that early treatment facilitated improved generation of anti-HIV immunity.[11] HIV-specific CD4 T cell responses were preserved by cART since these cells are good targets for HIV infection and are often depleted. Eventual cessation of cART in this early group of subjects did not result in viral rebound. However, subsequent larger controlled trials by this group failed to confirm that early treatment resulted in significant numbers of subjects with durable control of viremia.[12] A recent large randomized trial does suggest that subsequent set point viremia levels can be lowered by early treatment, but the effect is not dramatic and uncommonly leads to a functional cure.[13] A French group has also reported on a selected set of subjects who were treated

early and control HIV off cART.[14] This group (the 'Visconti' cohort) appears to have low but detectable levels of HIV DNA. The conditions needed to replicate these findings in a controlled setting are not yet clear.

Antilatency Drug Approaches

There are several trials reported and ongoing with agents designed to activate and kill latently infected cells in subjects on cART. Drugs with the ability to inhibit histone deacetylase (HDAC) have been studied in particular. The antiepileptic drug valproate was initially studied with

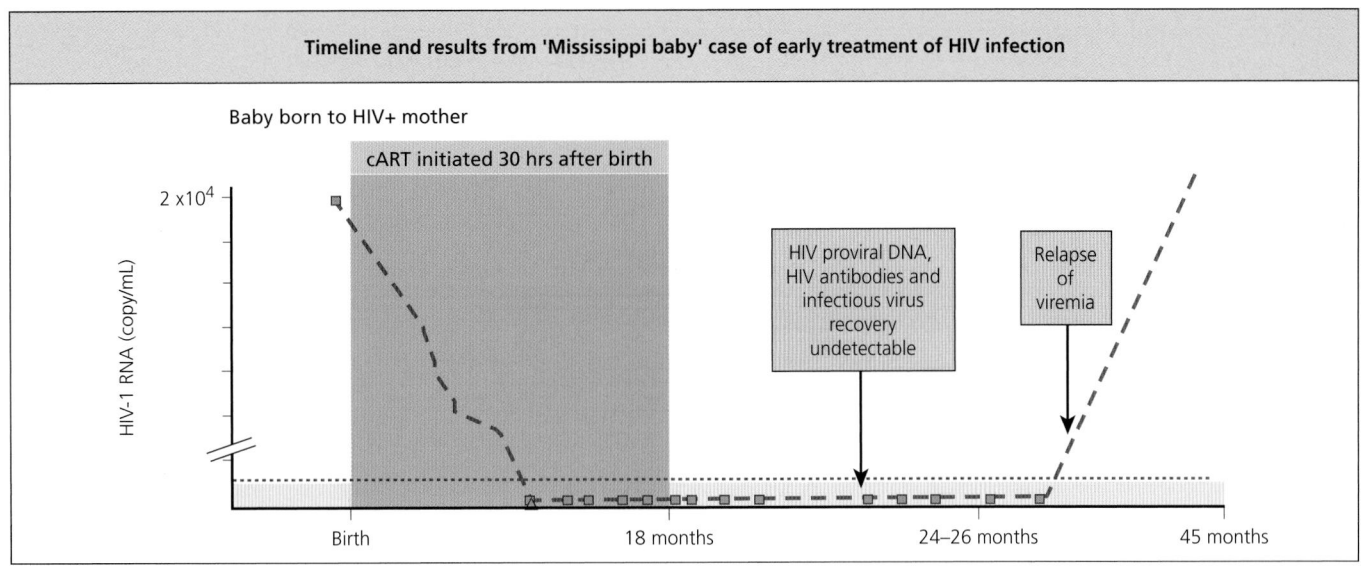

Figure 105-2   Timeline and results from the 'Mississippi baby' case of apparent HIV cure.

some promise in small studies but later found to have no effect on the reservoir size.[15] Two other HDAC inhibitors, vorinostat and panobinostat (both anticancer drugs) have been studied in three trials and have shown evidence of low levels of HIV reactivation but are likely to have only modest effects on the total latent reservoir size.[16] A small number of subjects taken off cART after panobinostat therapy had rapid rebound of viremia requiring cART. An additional HDAC inhibitor, romidepsin, is in clinical development.

There are several other potential targets by which to activate latent HIV that are also under development. The anti-alcoholism drug disulfiram activates protein kinase AKT to reactivate latent HIV and is in clinical trials in HIV-infected subjects on cART.[17] There is significant interest in developing additional antilatency drugs and additional targets under development include methylation inhibition, histone methyltransferase inhibitors, activators of NF-κB and cytokines such as IL-7. Combinations of such approaches (as is done with cART) may ultimately be needed to activate sufficient latent HIV to substantially affect the latent reservoir such that HIV viremia does not recrudesce after cART cessation.

The timing of administration of antilatency drugs has also been recently highlighted. Macaque-SIV studies have suggested that in the absence of cART the population of SIV DNA in resting CD4 T cells may be quite labile and more amenable to clearance.[18] This contrasts with the very stable and fixed population of latently infected cells on cART. This has led to the proposal of administering antilatency drugs at the initiation of cART, rather than after long-term cART, as is currently the case.[19] Combining such an approach together with studying patients during early infection (where levels of latent virus may be lower and more amenable to change) and the use of vaccine or immune therapies may result in a more substantial impact on the latent HIV reservoir.

Immune Manipulation to Reduce the Latent Reservoir

An intriguing question about some antilatency drug approaches is whether the latently infected cells actually die after reactivation or return to a latent state. It is possible that immune mechanisms will be needed to help clear the latently infected cells that are reactivated (Figure 105-3). Shan *et al.* showed *in vitro* that activated cytotoxic T cells (CTL) could recognize and kill latently infected cells reactivated with HDAC inhibitors.[20] This suggests that vaccines or other immune manipulations could act in concert with antilatency drugs to improve their efficacy. Picker and colleagues have recently shown that

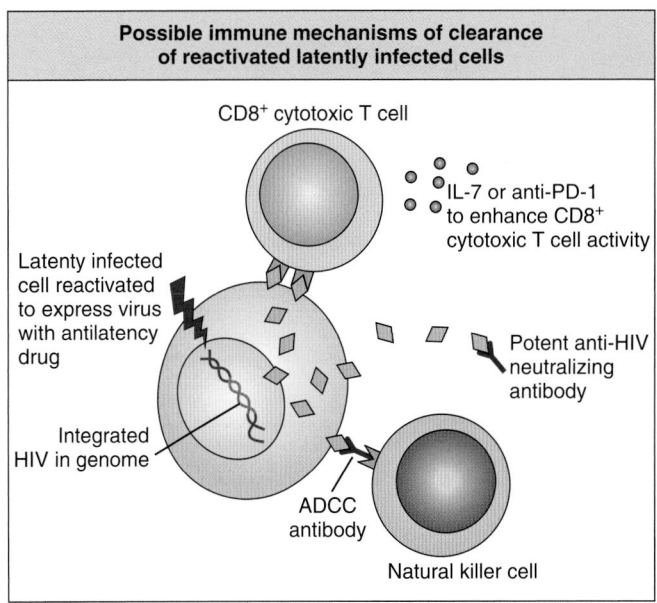

Figure 105-3   Possible immune mechanisms of clearance of reactivated latently infected cells.

CMV-based SIV vaccines can induce high levels of activated CTLs and lead to a gradual but complete clearance of both replicating and latent forms of SIV in a subset of vaccinated monkeys.[21] Improving the efficacy of T cell approaches could be achieved using cytokines such as IL-7 or blockers of the programmed cell death receptor PD-1.[22]

Neutralizing antibodies could also play some role in assisting the clearance of latently infected cells. Barouch and colleagues showed that SHIV-infected monkeys infused with the potent neutralizing antibody PGT121 had very rapid falls in SHIV viremia and reduced levels of SHIV DNA.[23] A subset of these monkeys, particularly those with low levels of viremia prior to the infusions, controlled SHIV viremia without cART after the passively-infused antibody had been cleared. Hessell and colleagues have shown that the efficacy of anti-HIV neutralizing antibodies in preventing SHIV infection of monkeys is in part dependent on the ability of the antibodies to mediate antibody-dependent cellular cytotoxicity (ADCC), typically mediated via natural killer (NK) cells.[24] Infusions of antibodies that can also kill

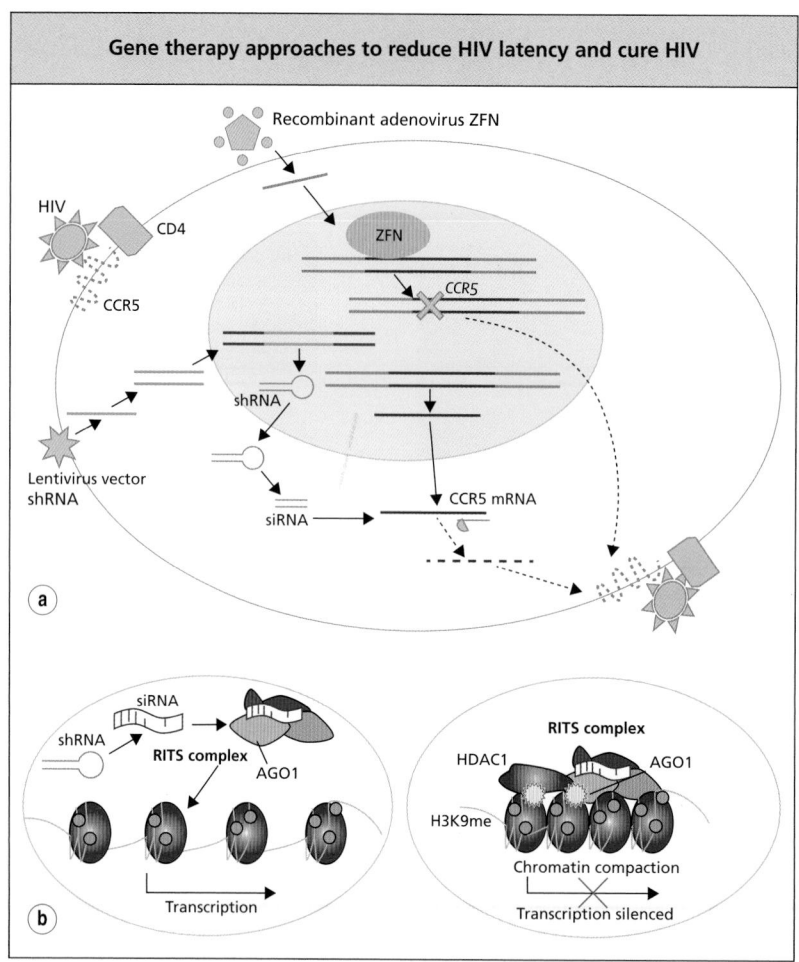

Figure 105-4   Gene therapy approaches to reduce HIV latency and cure HIV. HIV usually enters cells by use of the CCR5 and CD4 co-receptors (a). Zinc-finger nucleases (ZFN) expressed by recombinant adenoviruses can block CCR5 gene expression, rendering the cell devoid of CCR5 and resistant to HIV. Alternatively, short-hairpin RNAs (shRNAs) expressed by lentivirus vectors can degrade CCR5 RNA, also rendering the cell devoid of CCR5 and resistant to HIV, through expression of a short interfering RNA (siRNA) that binds to the CCR5 messenger RNA (mRNA). Transcription of HIV is favoured by an open chromatin structure in the nucleus, shown by widely spaced histones (b, left). siRNA can bind to the RNA-induced transcriptional silencing (RITS) complex, which can result in chromatin compaction and silencing of HIV transcription (right), potentially leading to a permanent latent state for HIV in the cell. AGO1, argonaute RISC catalytic component 1; HDAC1, histone deacetylase 1; H3K9me, trimethylation of histone H3 at lysine 9. (From Kent SJ, et al.: The search for an HIV cure: tackling latent infection. Lancet Infect Dis 2013 Jul; 13(7):614-21.)

HIV-infected cells (ADCC antibodies) should also help clear reactivated latently infected cells.

Gene Therapy Approaches to Cure HIV

Blocking the HIV co-receptor CCR5 is being studied in attempts to cure HIV. The cure of the Berlin patient administered a CCR5-defective BMT highlights the potential utility of this approach. About 1% of Caucasians are homozygous for a deletion in the *CCR5* gene that does not seem to be deleterious to their general health. These subjects who are homozygous for the common *CCR5*-deletion are naturally resistant to HIV, making CCR5 modulation an attractive target (Figure 105-4). Depletion of CCR5 expression is being attempted both through using short-hairpin RNA (shRNA) to degrade CCR5 mRNAs and through zinc-finger nucleases encoded by adenoviruses to block *CCR5* gene expression. This latter approach has been studied in a small series of subjects, with the level of reduction in CCR5 expression correlating with reduced levels of viremia off cART.[25] Wider clinical trials of these therapies with improved vectors are planned.

An alternate gene therapy approach is to enforce latency so that HIV cannot be reactivated using shRNAs that induce stable epigenetic changes in the integrated HIV DNA.[26] Such approaches, while promising *in vitro*, are not yet in clinical trials.

Conclusions

There is considerable enthusiasm amongst the community and amongst many researchers for tackling approaches to cure HIV. Several paths towards reducing or clearing cells with latent HIV infection have been developed and are in various stages of clinical studies. The recent recrudescence of viremia in two subjects who received BMT and stopped cART as well as one baby treated very early with cART does, however, provide a salutary lesson regarding the enormity of the task. Insights gained into the biology and control of latent HIV may also provide useful pathways for future HIV treatments and vaccines. Intensive research on HIV cure strategies is likely to lead to novel therapies in the coming decade.

References available online at expertconsult.com.

KEY REFERENCES

Archin N.M., Liberty A.L., Kashuba A.D., et al.: Administration of vorinostat disrupts HIV-1 latency in patients on antiretroviral therapy. *Nature* 2012; 487(7408):482-485.

Barouch D.H., Whitney J.B., Moldt B., et al.: Therapeutic efficacy of potent neutralizing HIV-1-specific monoclonal antibodies in SHIV-infected rhesus monkeys. *Nature* 2013; 7475:224-228.

Chun T.W., Fauci A.S.: HIV reservoirs: pathogenesis and obstacles to viral eradication and cure. *AIDS* 2012; 26(10):1261-1268.

Finzi D., Blankson J., Siliciano J.D., et al.: Latent infection of CD4+ T cells provides a mechanism for lifelong persistence of HIV-1, even in patients on effective combination therapy. *Nat Med* 1999; 5(5):512-517.

Hansen S.G., Piatak M. Jr, Ventura A.B., et al.: Immune clearance of highly pathogenic SIV infection. *Nature* 2013; 502(7469):100-104.

Hutter G., Nowak D., Mossner M., et al.: Long-term control of HIV by CCR5 Δ32/Δ32 stem-cell transplantation. *N Engl J Med* 2009; 360(7):692-698.

Persaud D., Gay H., Ziemniak C., et al.: Absence of detectable HIV-1 viremia after treatment cessation in an infant. *N Engl J Med* 2013; 369(19):1828-1835.

Shan L., Deng K., Shroff N.S., et al.: Stimulation of HIV-1-specific cytolytic T lymphocytes facilitates elimination of latent viral reservoir after virus reactivation. *Immunity* 2012; 36(3):491-501.

PRACTICE POINT

33

Antiretroviral Management in Low- and Middle-Income Countries

SOMNUEK SUNGKANUPARPH

Introduction

HIV/AIDS has been one of the leading causes of death in low- and middle-income countries (LMIC). The rapid scaling-up of antiretroviral therapy (ART) for the treatment of HIV infection has been remarkable in the last two decades. This progress has led to significant reductions in morbidity and mortality of HIV-infected patients in LMIC. However, significant disparities and inequities in ART coverage still persist between and within countries. The majority of HIV-infected patients in LMIC present with advanced disease. This prohibits the early initiation of ART in clinical practices. In addition, the options of antiretroviral regimens and monitoring tools are limited due to the constrained resources and large number of HIV-infected patients.

Initiation of Antiretroviral Therapy

The ultimate goal of antiretroviral therapy (ART) is to prevent morbidity and mortality from HIV infection. Effective ART with maximal and durable inhibition of HIV replication improves immune function, lowers the risk of both AIDS-defining and non-AIDS-defining complications, prolongs life and improves quality of life. Advances in ART and increasing knowledge and understanding of HIV pathogenesis in the last decade have shifted towards earlier initiation of ART. Early initiation of ART, at higher CD4 cell counts, is one of the predictors of virologic success after treatment. This also prevents disease progression, and prevents HIV transmission to sexual partners.

However, the majority of patients in LMIC usually present to healthcare facilities late. ART initiation at higher CD4 cell counts remains a challenge in LMIC. Strategic interventions to increase earlier diagnosis of HIV infection and prompt more rapid linkage to ART must be implemented. The World Health Organization (WHO) has launched global consolidated guidelines on the use of antiretroviral drugs for HIV treatment and prevention, which provide clinical, operational and programmatic guidance across the continuum of HIV diagnosis, care and treatment, covering all age groups and populations.

As a priority, ART should be initiated in all patients with severe or advanced HIV clinical disease (WHO clinical stage 3 or 4) and individuals with CD4 count ≤350 cells/μL. ART should also be initiated in all HIV-infected patients with CD4 count >350 cells/μL and ≤ 500 cells/μL regardless of WHO clinical stage. Regardless of WHO clinical stage or CD4 cell count, ART should be initiated in all HIV-infected patients with active tuberculosis, hepatitis B virus (HBV) coinfection with evidence of severe chronic liver disease, or partners with HIV in serodiscordant couples. ART should also be initiated in all HIV-infected patients at any CD4 cell count. This recommendation is based on evidence from recent clinical trials and observational studies showing that earlier use of ART results in better clinical outcomes compared with delayed treatment.

First-line ART should consist of two nucleoside reverse transcriptase inhibitors (NRTIs) plus a non-nucleoside reverse transcriptase inhibitor (NNRTI). Tenofovir (TDF) + lamivudine (3TC) (or emtricitabine, FTC) + efavirenz (EFV) as a fixed-dose combination is recommended as the preferred option to initiate ART. If TDF + 3TC (or FTC) + EFV is contraindicated or not available, one of the following options

is recommended: zidovudine (AZT) + 3TC + EFV; AZT + 3TC + nevirapine (NVP); TDF + 3TC (or FTC) + NVP. TDF + 3TC (or FTC), dually active against both HIV and HBV, is the preferred NRTI backbone for HIV-infected patients with HBV coinfection. Stavudine (d4T) use should be discontinued because of its well-recognized metabolic toxicities.

Tuberculosis (TB) is the most common opportunistic infection among HIV-infected patients in LMIC. A rifampin-based anti-TB regimen is essential. Nonetheless, rifampin induces hepatic cytochrome P-450 resulting in a significant decrease of plasma NNRTI and protease inhibitor (PI) levels. In addition, ART and anti-TB medications have overlapping toxicities, particularly cutaneous and hepatic adverse events. Simultaneous initiation of both ART and TB treatment should be avoided. Prospective studies have evaluated the optimal time for initiating ART in HIV/TB coinfected patients and demonstrated a mortality reduction among those starting ART during the early stages of TB treatment compared with those who started in the later stages or after the completion of TB treatment. Current WHO guidelines recommend that ART be initiated as soon as TB treatment is tolerated, ideally as early as 2 weeks, and not later than 8 weeks, after initiation of TB treatment. ART regimens containing EFV (600 mg per day) are less compromised by concomitant use of rifampin than are those that contained NVP (400 mg per day) (see also Chapter 96).

The full implementation of the WHO guidelines on a global scale would have a major impact on HIV-related morbidity and mortality and HIV incidence in LMIC in the near future. Achieving optimal impact would require both additional investments as well as innovation in delivery of services in each particular healthcare setting (see Chapter 99).

Management of Adverse Effects

Safe and effective antiretroviral management requires an understanding of the adverse effects associated with each antiretroviral agent. Drug-related symptoms decrease adherence, which negatively impacts virologic suppression and immunologic recovery. ART used in LMIC frequently contains older antiretroviral agents that are more likely to have adverse effects than newer, more expensive agents. Although discontinuing use of d4T has been recommended for years, it is still used in some countries. Therefore, common adverse effects associated with d4T should be well known. These include lactic acidosis, lipodystrophy, peripheral neuropathy, and other metabolic problems. Lipodystrophy has been common after rapid scale-up of ART with d4T in LMIC for the last decade. A pharmacogenetic study in Thailand has recently revealed that HLA-B*4001 is a strong genetic risk factor for d4T-associated lipodystrophy.

AZT remains on the WHO list of first-line agents and causes anemia or gastrointestinal intolerance in some patients. Although kidney adverse effects often occur in patients receiving TDF, lack of monitoring of kidney function during treatment is frequently observed in LMIC and may delay the detection of this problem. The hypersensitivity reaction to abacavir (ABC) is strongly associated with the presence of the major histocompatibility complex class I allele HLA-B*5701. Screening patients for HLA-B*5701 prior to starting treatment with ABC is strongly recommended. However, this test may not be available in some LMIC. Clinical manifestations of hypersensitivity reaction to ABC should be recognized. When hypersensitivity reaction develops, ABC must be immediately discontinued. This reaction can affect multiple organ systems in serious cases, leading to organ failure and possible death. Re-challenging with ABC following a hypersensitivity reaction is not advised since it can result in a rapid, severe, and potentially life-threatening reaction.

NVP is frequently recommended in the first-line ART in LMIC because of its efficacy and accessibility as an affordable generic combined tablet. However, NVP is not recommended for women with CD4 cell counts of >250 cells/µL and men with CD4 cell counts of >400 cells/µL at the time of NVP initiation because of a higher incidence of symptomatic, drug-induced hepatitis. NVP also frequently causes cutaneous adverse drug reactions especially during the first few weeks of treatment with an approximate incidence of 15–20%. The associations of NVP-induced skin rash and variations in major histocompatibility complex (MHC) region class I including HLA-B*3505 and single nucleotide polymorphisms (SNPs) in CCHCR1 have been reported in patients from Thailand.

Treatment Failure and HIV Drug Resistance

Viral load is recommended as the preferred monitoring approach to diagnose and confirm treatment failure. If viral load is not routinely available, CD4 cell count and clinical monitoring should be used to diagnose treatment failure. Laboratory monitoring to guide switching to second-line ART has proven to increase survival rates and is cost-effective in resource-limited settings. Viral load monitoring allows healthcare providers to detect treatment failure early with fewer HIV drug-resistance mutations and maintains options for effective second-line ART in LMIC. CD4 monitoring as the only indicator of treatment failure may lead to a premature switch to second-line ART.

Use of genotypic resistance testing to guide second-line ART has proven to be cost-effective and independently associated with improved survival in HIV-infected patients who experience treatment failure, and should be performed when the test can be accessed. However, this test may not be available or affordable in many LMIC. Strategies to make the test simple and accessible are needed to scale-up the resistance testing in LMIC. The main barriers to implementation of genotypic resistance testing are related to cost, the need for complex laboratory infrastructure, and issues with specimen transport to centralized laboratories. Dried blood spots (DBS) are easy to collect in the field, easily transported, and HIV-1 nucleic acids remain stable on DBS for long periods at ambient temperatures. Several studies have reported successful genotyping from DBS.

After rapid scale-up of ART on a wide population, continuous surveillance of transmitted HIV drug resistance is needed to inform treatment guidelines. Recent HIV drug-resistance surveillance networks have demonstrated that primary HIV drug resistance has emerged in Asia and Africa. It is of great concern that primary HIV drug resistance could limit the success of scaling-up first-line ART in the public health approach. Surveillance for transmitted HIV drug resistance is essential to assess the longer-term sustainability of currently used first-line ART regimens and program effectiveness in LMIC.

Second-Line ART

Although access to first-line ART is reasonably well established, treatment failure is inevitable in some patients. Access to second-line ART regimens in LMIC is difficult because of the expense of antiretroviral agents especially PIs. Second-line ART, even in LMIC, can achieve durable viral suppression and is associated with an increase in CD4 cell count. An increasing number of HIV-infected patients who have experienced first-line treatment failure have been observed in LMIC. Second-line options are limited, and are usually based on a ritonavir-boosted PI, which is taken in combination with two drugs in the NRTI class. In settings where the HIV drug-resistance genotypic test is available, two susceptible NRTIs according to the test results are recommended.

Third-Line ART and Beyond

National programs should develop policies for third-line ART. Third-line regimens should include new drugs with minimal risk of cross-resistance to previously used regimens, such as second-generation PIs, integrase inhibitors and second-generation NNRTIs. A study of cost-effectiveness in resource-limited settings has shown that a genotype assay to determine the resistance profile and assign an appropriate third-line regimen will increase survival rates and be cost-effective compared to the population-based approach. WHO guidelines emphasize balancing the need to develop policies for third-line ART with the need to expand access to first-line and second-line ART.

Summary

HIV/AIDS has been one of the leading causes of death in LMIC. The majority of HIV-infected patients in LMIC present with advanced disease. ART initiation at higher CD4 cell counts remains a challenge. Strategic interventions to increase earlier diagnosis of HIV infection and prompt more rapid linkage to ART must be implemented. WHO guidelines represent an important step towards achieving universal access to ART, increasing the efficiency, impact and long-term sustainability of ART programs. Viral load is recommended as the preferred monitoring approach to diagnose and confirm treatment failure. Viral load monitoring allows healthcare providers to detect treatment failure early with less HIV drug-resistance mutations and maintains options for effective second-line ART. Second-line ART can achieve durable viral suppression and is associated with an increase in CD4 cell count.

Further reading available online at expertconsult.com.

Geography of Infectious Diseases

MARY ELIZABETH WILSON

Introduction

Infectious diseases vary by geographic region and population, and they change over time. When moving from one region to another, humans are exposed to a variety of potential pathogens and also serve as part of the global dispersal process.[1] Microbes picked up at one time and in one place may manifest in disease (and potentially be transmitted) far away in time and place. Because many microbes have the capacity to persist in the human host for months, years or even decades, the relevant time frame for study of geographic exposures becomes a lifetime. Furthermore, microbes also move and change and reach humans via multiple channels.

Caring for patients requires an understanding of the basic factors that underlie the geography of human diseases and events that cause shifts in the distribution and burden of specific diseases. Current travel capacity contributes to massive population movements and rapid shifts in diseases and their distributions, but technology also provides communication channels that aid clinicians who care for patients with unfamiliar medical problems. This chapter reviews the factors that shape the global distribution of infectious diseases and the forces that are expected to shift distributions in the future. Examples illustrate the range of factors that affect the distribution and expression of infectious diseases.[2]

Many authors have traced the origins and spread of infectious diseases through history. A century and a half ago, John Snow noted that epidemics of cholera followed major routes of commerce and appeared first at seaports when entering a new region. *Yersinia pestis*, the cause of plague, accompanied trade caravans and moved across oceans with rats on ships. Exploration of the New World by Europeans introduced a range of human pathogens that killed one-third or more of the local populations in some areas of the Americas. The plants and

animals introduced as a result of this exploration have also had profound and long-lasting consequences for the ecology and economics of the new environment.[3] The speed, reach and volume of today's travel are unprecedented in human history and offer multiple potential routes to move biologic species around the globe. Pathogens of animals and plants are being transported as well, and this can affect global food security.[4] Establishment of arthropod vectors, such as mosquitoes, that are competent to transmit human pathogens in new geographic areas expands the regions that are vulnerable to outbreaks of some vector-borne infections. This chapter focuses only on pathogens that directly affect human health and on their sources (Table 106-1). When thinking about geography of human infections, it is useful to consider both the origin of the organism and the conveyor or immediate source for the human (Figure 106-1).

This chapter addresses three key issues:

- factors influencing geographic distribution: why are some infectious diseases found only in focal geographic regions or in isolated populations?
- factors influencing the burden of disease: why does the impact from widely distributed infections vary markedly from one region or one population to another? and
- factors influencing emergence of disease: what allows or facilitates the introduction, persistence and spread of an infection in a new region and what makes a region or population resistant to the introduction of an infection?

TABLE 106-1	Origins and Conveyors of Human Pathogens*	
Origin or Carrier	**Conveyor or Immediate Source**	**Examples of Disease**
Humans	Humans	HIV, syphilis, hepatitis B
Humans	Humans (airborne pathogen)	Measles, tuberculosis
Soil	Soil, airborne	Coccidioidomycosis
Soil	Food	Botulism
Animals	Water	Leptospirosis
Humans	Mosquitoes	Malaria, dengue
Humans	Soil	Hookworm, strongyloidiasis
Animals	Ticks	Lyme disease
Animals, humans	Sand flies	Leishmaniasis
Animals	Animals	Rabies
Rodents	Rodent excreta	Hantaviruses
Humans	Water, marine life	Cholera
Humans or animals (with snails as essential intermediate host)	Water	Schistosomiasis
Humans	Food, water	Typhoid fever
Animals	Water	Cryptosporidiosis, giardiasis

*Some pathogens have multiple potential sources.

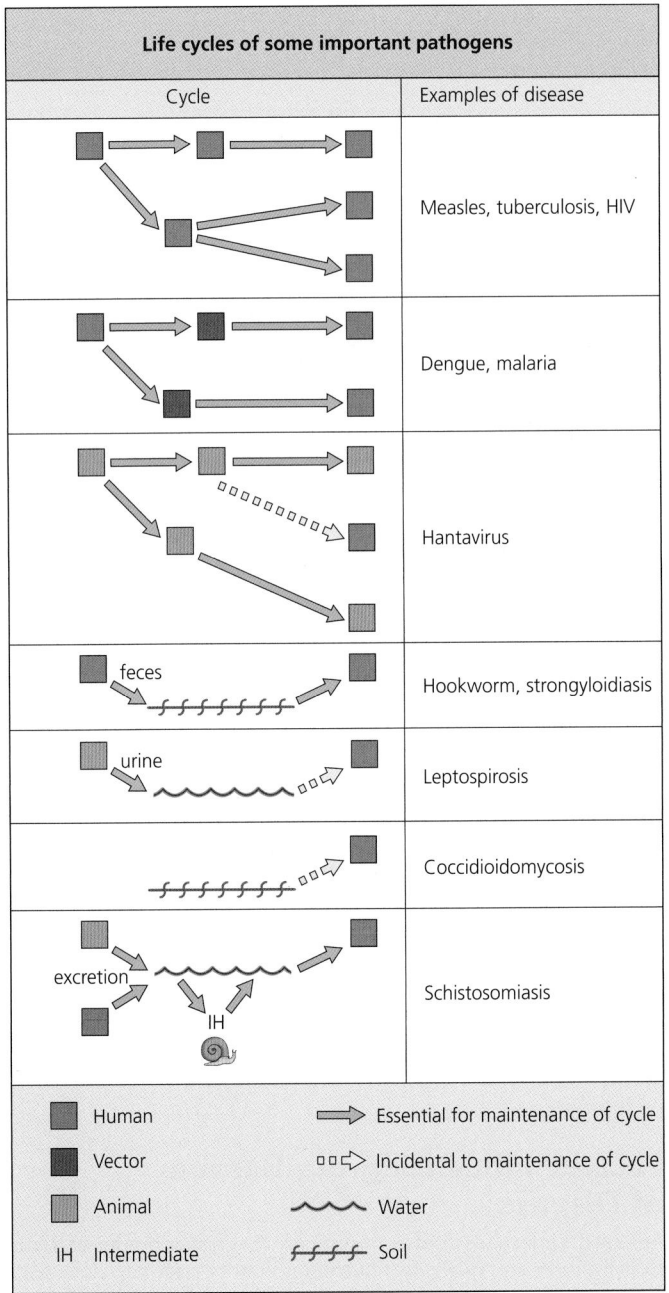

Life cycles of some important pathogens	
Cycle	Examples of disease
	Measles, tuberculosis, HIV
	Dengue, malaria
	Hantavirus
feces	Hookworm, strongyloidiasis
urine	Leptospirosis
	Coccidioidomycosis
excretion IH	Schistosomiasis

■ Human	⇨ Essential for maintenance of cycle	
■ Vector	⧈⇨ Incidental to maintenance of cycle	
■ Animal	∿∿ Water	
IH Intermediate	⌁⌁ Soil	

Figure 106-1 Life cycles of some important pathogens.

Factors Influencing Geographic Distribution

In past centuries, lack of contact with other regions could allow an infection to remain geographically isolated. Today, most infections that are found only in focal areas have biologic or geoclimatic constraints that prevent them from being introduced into other geographic regions. For example, the fungus *Coccidioides immitis*, which causes coccidioidomycosis, thrives in surface soil in arid and semiarid areas with alkaline soil, hot summers and short, moist winters; it is endemic in parts of south-western USA, Mexico and Central and South America. People become infected when they inhale arthroconidia from soil. An unusual wind storm in 1977 lifted soil from the endemic region and deposited it in northern California, outside the usual endemic region.[5] In general, infection is associated with residence in or travel through the endemic region. However, because the fungus can persist in the

human host for many years following initial infection (which may be mild and unrecognized), disease may be diagnosed far from the endemic regions. Although it is a 'place' disease, coccidioidomycosis has increased in the south-western USA in recent years, in part attributable to a large influx of susceptible humans into the endemic zone and construction and other activities that disturb the soil. Outbreaks are also linked to climatic and environmental changes.[6]

VECTORS

Many microbes require a specific arthropod vector for transmission or an animal reservoir host and hence inhabit circumscribed regions. Malaria is a vector-borne infection that cannot become established in a region unless a competent vector is present. The presence of a competent vector is a necessary but not sufficient condition for human infection. The mosquito must have a source of malarial parasites (gametocytemic human or, rarely, nonhuman primates), appropriate bioclimatic conditions and access to other humans. The ambient temperature influences the human biting rate of the mosquito, the incubation period for the parasite in the mosquito and the daily survival rate of the mosquito. Prevailing temperature and humidity must allow the mosquito to survive long enough for the malarial parasite to undergo maturation to reach an infective state for humans. Competent vectors exist in many areas with no malaria transmission, because the other conditions are not met. These areas are at risk of the introduction of malaria, as illustrated by several recent examples in the USA and elsewhere.[7,8]

An estimated 77% of the world's population lived in areas with malaria transmission in 1900. By 2002 about 48% lived in at-risk areas, but because of population growth and migration the total global population exposed to malaria had increased by 2 billion since 1900 (see Figure 106-2).[9] For example, in Africa, the population in malaria endemic zones increased by almost 200 million people between 2000 and 2010.[10] This contrasts with the situation in the USA, where malaria was endemic in many areas into the 20th century (Figure 106-3), with estimates of more than 600 000 cases in 1914. Even before extensive mosquito control programs were instituted, transmission declined. Demographic factors (population shifts from rural to urban areas), improved housing with screened doors and windows, and the availability of treatment were among the factors that contributed to this decrease.

The distribution of onchocerciasis in Africa is notable for its association with rivers.[11] The vector of this filarial parasite, the black fly (genus *Simulium*), lays her eggs on vegetation and rocks of rapidly flowing rivers and usually inhabits a region within 5–10 km on either side of a river. Another name for onchocerciasis, river blindness, describes the epidemiology as well as one consequence of infection.

Other pathogens have complex cycles of development that require one or more intermediate hosts. Distribution may remain relatively fixed, even when infected humans travel widely, if other regions do not supply the right combination and geographic proximity of hosts (Figure 106-4). Although persons with schistosomiasis visit many regions of the world, the parasite cannot be introduced into a new region unless an appropriate snail host is present, excreted eggs (in urine or feces) are released into fresh water where they reach the snail hosts, and humans subsequently have contact with the untreated water.[12] However, local ecologic changes and climate change can be associated with expansion of transmission in endemic areas or increased intensity of transmission, and this has been identified as a possible consequence of warming temperatures in China.[13] (For a more detailed consideration of the influence of climate change on the distribution of infectious diseases, see Chapter 4.)

Ebola and Marburg viruses are viruses that have focal distributions but have caused dramatic human outbreaks with high mortality. They also infect nonhuman primates and threaten the survival of great apes.[14] Recent studies suggest that bats may be the reservoir hosts.[15,16] Because these infections can be spread from person to person, secondary household and nosocomial spread in several instances has amplified what began as an isolated event. Lack of adequate resources in

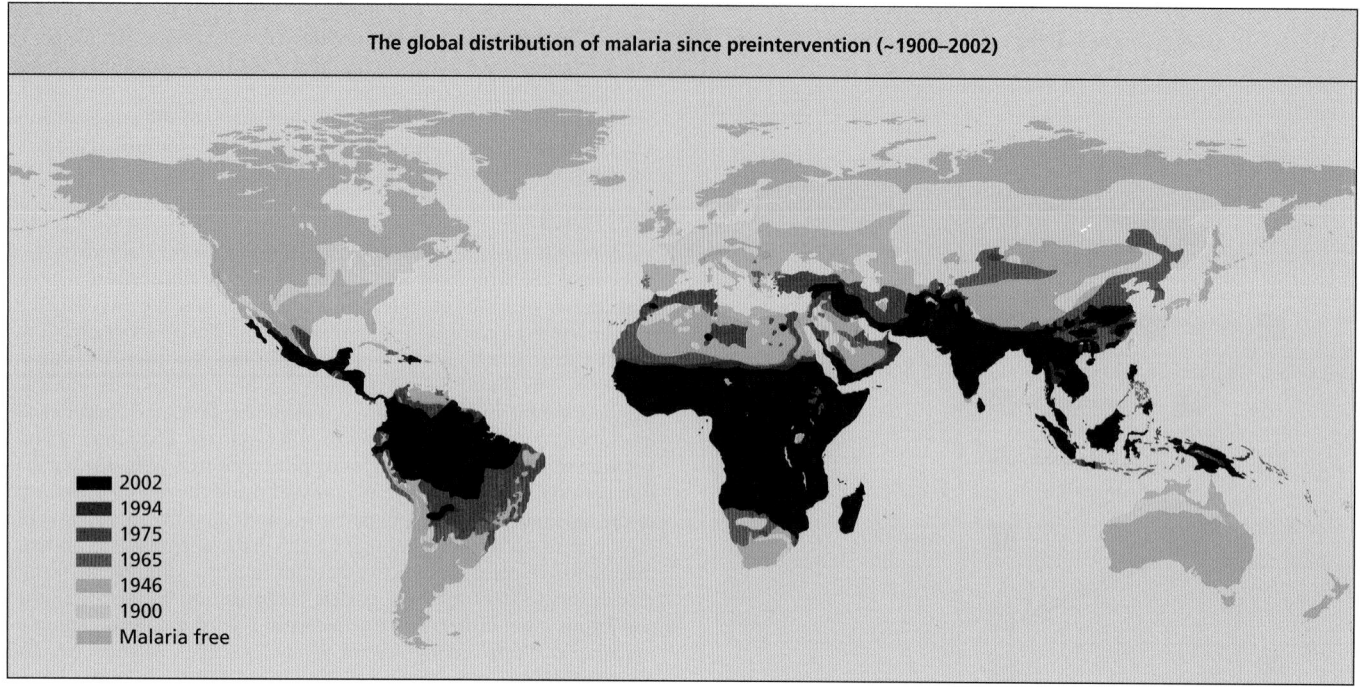

The global distribution of malaria since preintervention (~1900–2002)

- 2002
- 1994
- 1975
- 1965
- 1946
- 1900
- Malaria free

Figure 106-2 The global distribution of malaria since preintervention (~1900–2002). *(From Hay S.I., et al., Lancet Infect Dis 2004; 4(6):327–336.)*

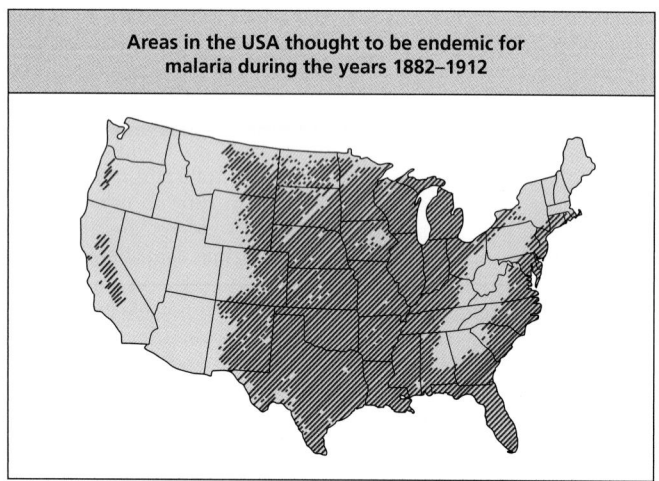

Areas in the USA thought to be endemic for malaria during the years 1882–1912

Figure 106-3 Areas of the USA thought to be endemic for malaria during the years 1882–1912. Dark blue indicate areas with malaria.

BOX 106-1 BIOLOGIC ATTRIBUTES OF ORGANISMS THAT INFLUENCE THEIR EPIDEMIOLOGY

Host range
Duration of survival in host
Route of exit from host
Route of entry into human
Inoculum needed to establish infection
Virulence
Capacity to survive outside host
Resistance to antimicrobials and chemicals

Factors Influencing the Burden of Disease

Among the infectious diseases that impose the greatest burden of death globally, most are widely distributed: respiratory tract infections (e.g. influenza, *Streptococcus pneumoniae* and others), diarrheal infections, tuberculosis, measles, AIDS and hepatitis B.[16] Most of these infections are spread from person to person. The World Health Organization estimated that about 65% of infectious diseases deaths globally in 1995 were due to infections transmitted from person to person.[17]

Burden from these diseases is unevenly distributed across populations and among different countries. Poor sanitation, lack of clean water, crowded living conditions and lack of vaccination contribute to the disproportionate burden from many of these infections in low- and middle-income countries (LMIC). In industrialized countries, pockets of high risk persist. Disadvantaged populations have higher rates of tuberculosis, HIV and many other infectious and noninfectious diseases. Rates of reported cases of tuberculosis vary widely by region and within countries (Table 106-2).[18] Figure 106-5 shows the effect of crowded living conditions on rates of tuberculosis in England and Wales in 1992.[19] Among welfare applicants and recipients addicted to drugs or alcohol in New York City, the rate of tuberculosis was 744 per 100 000 person years, or more than 70 times the overall rate for the USA.[20] The impact of an infection also derives from the access to effective therapy. Treatment of a patient with active tuberculosis can cure

---

hospitals in many developing regions contributes to the spread of infections within hospitals and clinics.

Cultural practices can lead to unusual infections in isolated areas. Residents of the highlands of Papua New Guinea developed kuru after ingestion (or percutaneous inoculation) of human tissue during the preparation of the tissues of dead relatives.

The presence of a pathogen in a region may reflect the biologic properties of the organism, its need for a certain physicochemical environment or its dependence on specific arthropods, plants or animals to provide the milieu where it can sustain its life cycle (Box 106-1). The presence of a pathogen in a region does not equate with human disease, because mechanisms must exist for the pathogen to reach a susceptible human host for human disease to occur. Exploration of new regions or changes in land use may place humans in an environment where they come into contact with microbes that were previously unrecognized as human pathogens.

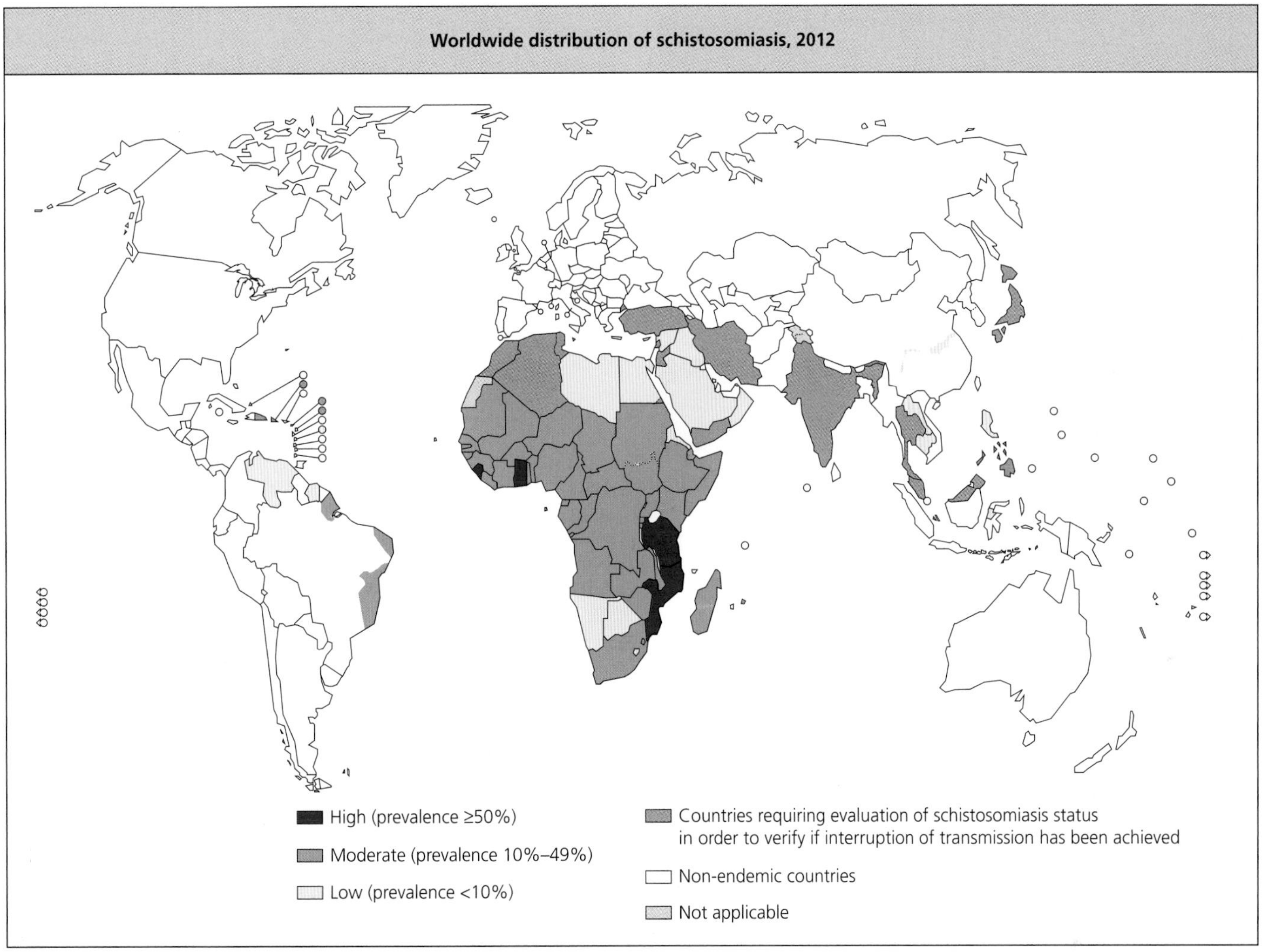

Worldwide distribution of schistosomiasis, 2012

- High (prevalence ≥50%)
- Moderate (prevalence 10%–49%)
- Low (prevalence <10%)
- Countries requiring evaluation of schistosomiasis status in order to verify if interruption of transmission has been achieved
- Non-endemic countries
- Not applicable

Figure 106-4 Worldwide distribution of schistosomiasis. *(Copyright ©World Health Organization, 2012.)*

TABLE 106-2 Rates of Reported Cases of Tuberculosis Worldwide by Region, 1990 and 2006

Region	INCIDENCE PER 100 000 POPULATION	
	1990	2013
Africa	162	3255
Americas	65	29
Eastern Mediterranean	111	109
Europe	37	40
South East Asia	200	187
Western Pacific	127	87

Data from World Health Organization: Global tuberculosis report 2013. Geneva: World Health Organization, 2013.

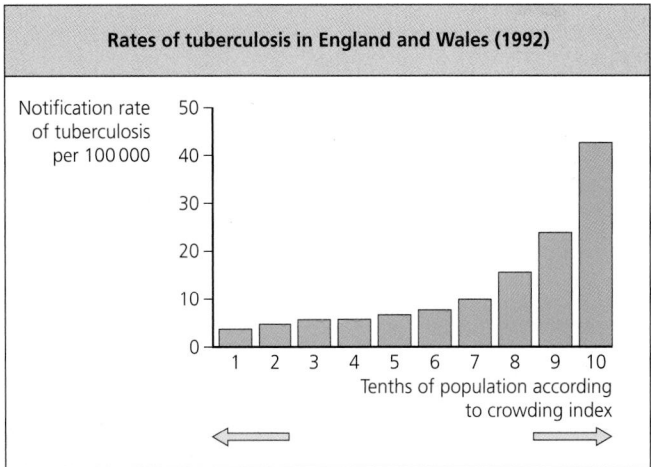

Figure 106-5 Rates of tuberculosis in England and Wales by crowding index (1992). *(Adapted from Bhatti et al. World Health Organization: Global tuberculosis report 2013. Geneva: World Health Organization, 2013.)*

the individual and eliminate a source of infection for others in the community.

Diphtheria, controlled in many parts of the world through the use of immunization, resurged in new independent states of the former Soviet Union in the 1990s, a reminder of the tenuous control over many infectious diseases.[21] Populations in other countries also felt the impact as cases related to exposures in the Russian Federation were reported in Poland, Finland, Germany and the USA. Serologic studies

in America and Europe suggest that up to 60% of adults may be susceptible to diphtheria.

Travelers to tropical and LMIC can pick up geographically focal, often vector-borne or animal-associated infections,[22] but travelers most often acquire infections with a worldwide distribution that are

BOX 106-2 FACTORS THAT INFLUENCE THE TYPES AND ABUNDANCE OF MICROBES IN A COMMUNITY

- Biogeoclimatic conditions.
- Socioeconomic conditions.
- Public health infrastructure.
- Urban versus rural environment.
- Density and mobility of population.
- Season of the year.
- Animal populations.

BOX 106-3 FACTORS THAT INFLUENCE THE PROBABILITY OF EXPOSURE TO PATHOGENS

- Living accommodation.
- Level of sanitation.
- Occupational and recreational activities.
- Food preparation and preferences.
- Sexual activities and other behavior.
- Contact with pets, other animals, vectors.
- Time spent in the area.

common in areas lacking good sanitation.[23] Food- and water-borne infections lead to travelers' diarrhea, which is caused by multiple agents, typhoid fever and hepatitis A. Respiratory tract infections may be acquired from other travelers as well as from local residents. Boxes 106-2 and 106-3 note factors that influence the types and abundance of microbes in a community and the probability of exposure to pathogens.

Hepatitis A virus remains a common cause of infection in LMIC where most persons are infected at a young age and become immune for life. Infection in young children is typically mild or inapparent. Persons living in areas of high transmission may be unaware of the presence of high levels of transmission, although nonimmune; older people (such as travelers) who enter the environment may develop severe, and occasionally fatal, infection. Countries with an improving standard of living may observe a paradoxical increase in the incidence of hepatitis A disease as the age of exposure increases, shifting the age of infection to a time when jaundice and other symptoms are more likely to occur.

Travelers also contribute to the global spread of infectious diseases.[24,25] *Neisseria meningitidis*, a global pathogen, occurs in seasonal epidemics in parts of Africa (Figure 106-6).[26] Irritation of the throat by the dry, dusty air probably contributes to invasion by colonizing bacteria.[27] Pilgrims carried an epidemic strain of *N. meningitidis* type A from southern Asia to Mecca in 1987. Other pilgrims who became colonized with the epidemic strain introduced it into sub-Saharan

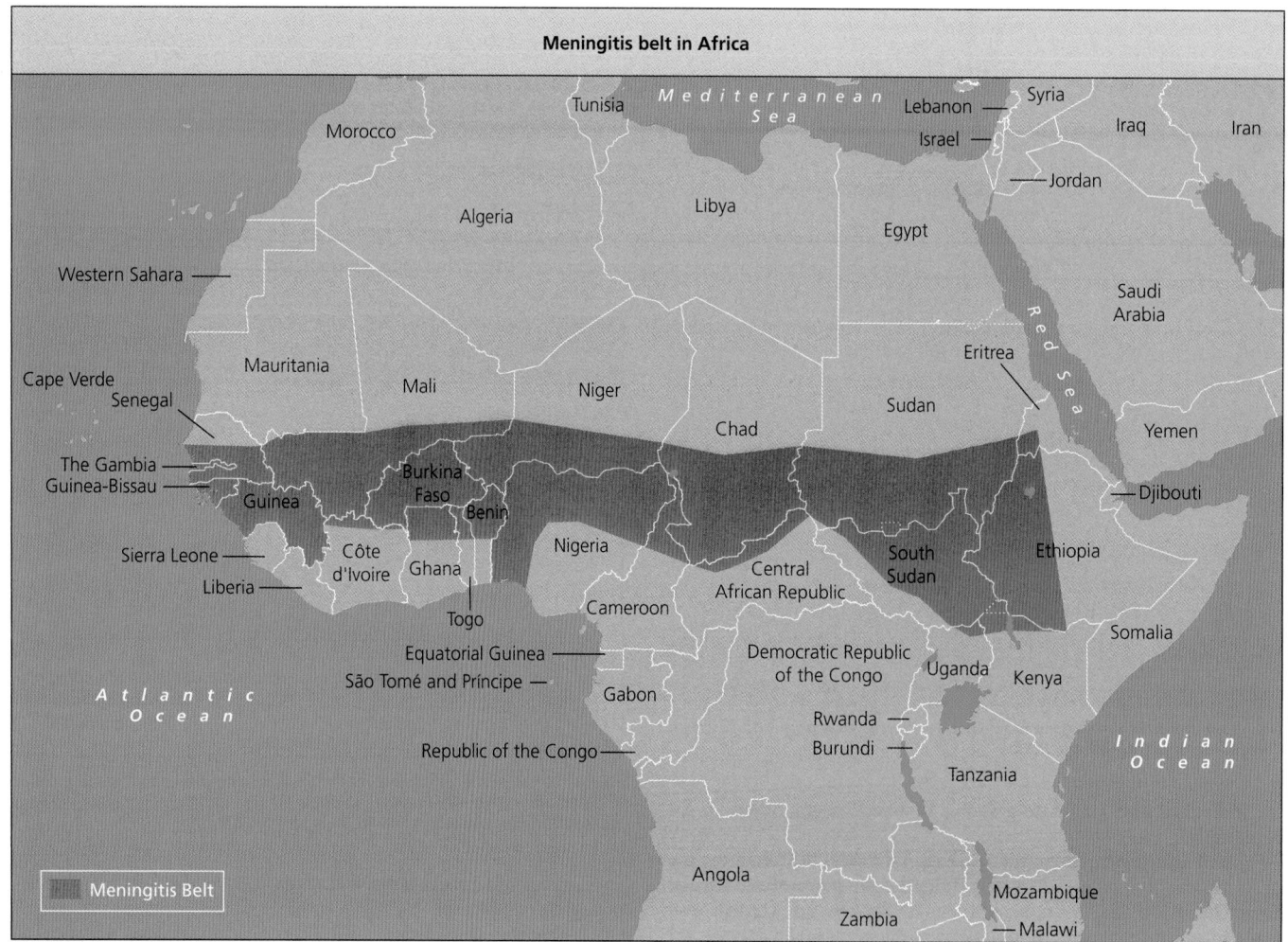

Figure 106-6 Meningitis belt in Africa. (*From Centers for Disease Control and Prevention: CDC Health information for international travel 2014. New York: Oxford University Press, 2014.*)

Africa, where it caused a wave of epidemics in 1988 and 1989. The epidemic clone spread to several countries.[28] In 1996 in Africa, major outbreaks of meningococcal meningitis occurred (>185 000 reported cases with a case fatality rate of ~10%) caused by *N. meningitidis* serogroup A, clone III-1.[29] In Canada, a virulent group C, ET-15 strain of *N. meningitidis* was associated with an increased case fatality rate.[30] In these examples, the virulence of the microbe and travel and trade acted synergistically to change the epidemiology and burden of disease. In 2000, serogroup W135 *N. meningitidis* caused an outbreak of infection in pilgrims to the Hajj and spread to their contacts and others around the world. Studies using serotyping, multilocus sequence typing, multilocus DNA fingerprints and other techniques found identical W135 isolates in multiple countries. Before this outbreak, pilgrims from many countries received a vaccine that protected against serotype A but not W135. The polysaccharide meningococcal vaccine reduces risk of disease in the vaccinated individual but does not prevent oropharyngeal carriage or transmission of *N. meningitidis*.[31]

Factors Influencing Emergence of Disease

Travel of persons from tropical regions to major urban areas throughout the world raises concerns that unusual infections could be introduced into an environment where they could spread to large populations. A key factor that determines whether a pathogen can persist and spread in a new population is its basic reproductive rate, which is the number of secondary infections produced in a susceptible population by a typical infectious individual. To become established in a new host population, a pathogen must have a basic reproductive rate that exceeds one. The basic reproductive rate for a pathogen is affected by a range of biologic, social and environmental factors, so may vary by place and population. Also critical in determining how easily an infection can be controlled is the proportion of transmission that occurs before onset of symptoms or during asymptomatic infection.[32]

Multiple factors restrict the introduction and spread or persistence of infection in a region (Box 106-4). Nutrition determines susceptibility to and severity of many infections. A substantial proportion of disease burden in LMIC can be attributed to childhood and maternal weight and micronutrient deficiencies.[33] Before measles vaccine was introduced, the epidemiology of measles exhibited marked periodicity in large populations, with peaks typically occurring every 2–3 years.[34] In small island communities (or other isolated populations), outbreaks typically occur only after periodic introductions from outside. It has been suggested that measles, as it has been known in the 20th century, could not have established itself much before 3000 BCE because before that time human populations had not achieved sufficient size to sustain the virus.

BOX 106-4 FACTORS THAT RESTRICT THE INTRODUCTION AND SPREAD OF INFECTIONS

- Geoclimatic factors that cannot support vector or intermediate host.
- Genetics of human population, making it genetically resistant or relatively resistant.
- Immunity of human population, making it not susceptible because of past infection with same or related microbe or via vaccination.
- Demographic factors (e.g. size and density of population will not support sustained transmission of diseases such as measles).
- Social and behavioral factors (e.g. absence of activities such as iv drug use and unprotected sex with multiple partners).
- Food preparation habits and local traditions (e.g. certain dishes not eaten, food always well cooked).
- High-quality housing, sanitation, public health infrastructure, good surveillance.
- High standard of living, good nutrition, lack of crowding, access to good medical care.
- Biologic characteristics of the microbe.

EXAMPLES OF EMERGING PATHOGENS

It is instructive to look at examples of infections that have recently undergone major shifts in distribution and to review the key factors that have influenced their geographic spread. A recurring theme is the movement of humans who introduce pathogens into a new region (see also Chapter 4) and human alteration of the landscape or ecology that permits contact with previously unrecognized microbes, often through interaction with animals or animal products. Many infections in humans have domestic or wild animals as their sources.[35]

Human Immunodeficiency Virus and Other Pathogens Carried by Humans

Organisms that survive primarily or entirely in the human host and are spread from person to person (e.g. by sexual or other close contact) can be carried to any part of the world. The spread of HIV in recent decades to all parts of the world is a reminder of the rapid and broad reach of travel networks. Although the infection has also spread via blood and shared needles, it has been the human host engaging in sex and reproduction who has been the origin for the majority of the infections worldwide. Person-to-person spread accounted for the rapid worldwide distribution of severe acute respiratory syndrome (SARS), a coronavirus infection, in the spring of 2003, after the virus emerged from an animal reservoir, most likely bats, and infected farmed civets.[36]

Multidrug-resistant (MDR) tuberculosis has continued to increase. The World Health Organization estimated that 450 000 cases and 170 000 deaths from MDR tuberculosis occurred in 2012.[18] Extensively drug-resistant (XDR) tuberculosis, which is virtually untreatable, has been reported by 92 countries. Almost 10% of MDR-TB cases are XDR-TB.[18] Humans also carry resistance genes and virulence factors that can be transferred to and exchanged with other microbes.[37]

Dengue Fever

Dengue fever is a mosquito-borne viral infection found in most tropical and subtropical regions globally. An estimated 96 million people have symptomatic infection each year.[38] Viremic humans regularly enter regions infested with *Aedes aegypti*, the principal vector of dengue, transporting the virus for new outbreaks. Because four serotypes of dengue virus exist and infection with one serotype does not confer lasting immunity against other serotypes, a person can be infected more than once. One study found the risk of developing severe dengue after repeat infection was 82–103 times greater than after primary infection.[39] In an outbreak in Cuba, 98.5% of cases of dengue shock syndrome (DSS) or dengue hemorrhagic fever (DHF) were in persons with a prior dengue infection.[40] Risk factors for severe dengue identified in epidemiological studies include young age, virus strain, and host genetics.[41]

Factors that have aided the spread of dengue include increasing travel to and from tropical regions; expansion of the regions infested with *Aedes aegypti* and *Aedes albopictus*; population growth and increasing urbanization in tropical areas; the use of nonbiodegradable and other containers that make ideal breeding sites for the mosquito; inadequate vector control programs and increasing resistance of vectors to insecticides.

In 2001 the vector that was implicated in an outbreak of dengue in Hawaii[42] was *Aedes albopictus*, a mosquito species that has been introduced into new regions in recent decades, probably primarily by shipping used tires and other items.[43] The virus responsible for the Hawaii outbreak was similar to dengue isolates from Tahiti, suggesting that viremic travelers introduced the virus from the South Pacific.

Although large dengue epidemics occurred in the USA in the 20th century, few cases have been acquired in the USA in recent years, despite the presence of epidemic disease in adjacent areas of Mexico and the presence of a competent vector (*Aedes aegypti*) in southeastern USA (Figure 106-7).[26] *Aedes albopictus* has even broader distribution in continental USA. The presence of screened dwellings and air conditioning may make an area relatively resistant to spread of infection, even if a competent vector infests a region. Since 2009 a few cases of local dengue transmission have occurred in Key West, Florida,[43] and

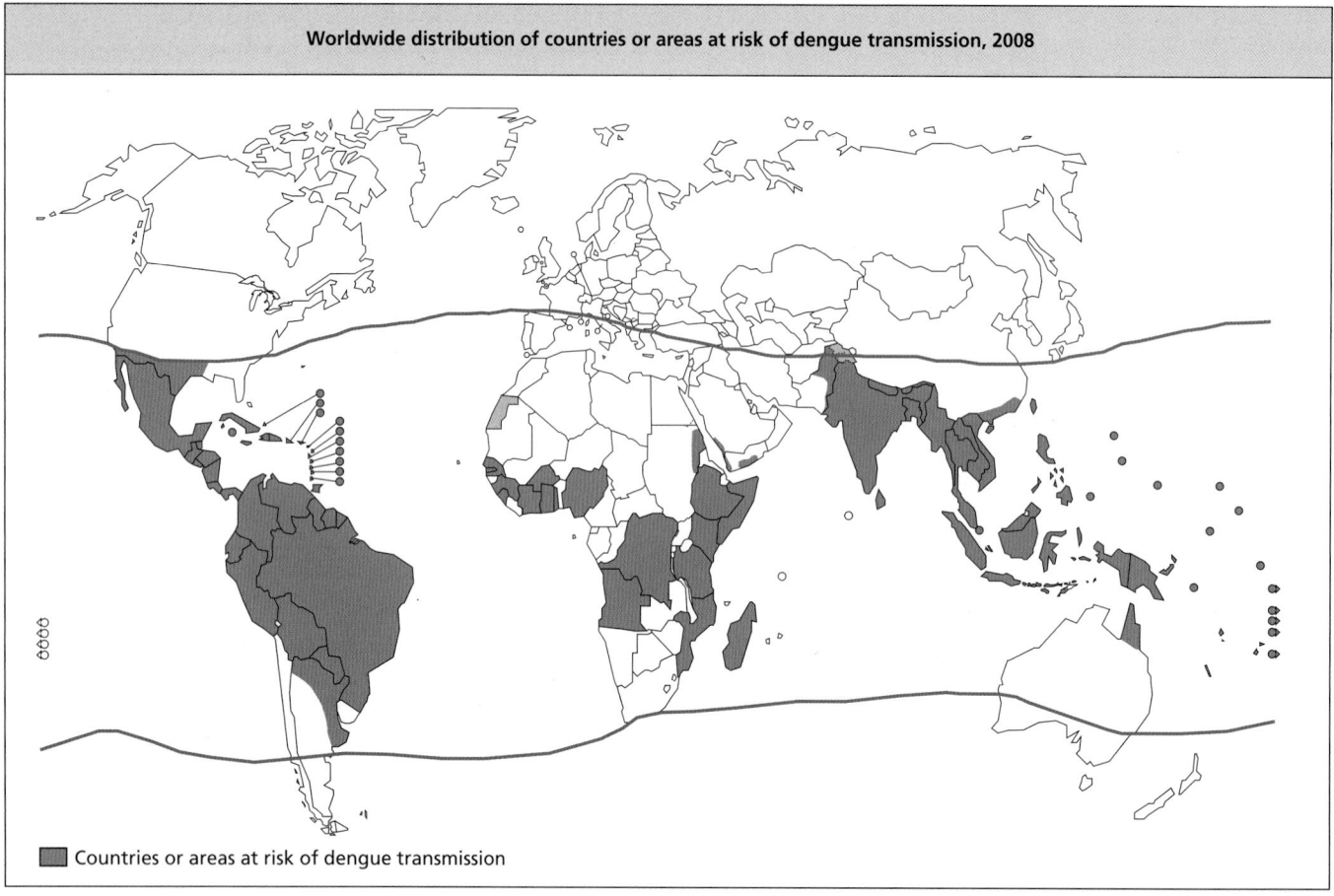

Worldwide distribution of countries or areas at risk of dengue transmission, 2008

■ Countries or areas at risk of dengue transmission

Figure 106-7   Worldwide distribution of countries or areas at risk of dengue transmission, 2008. Many areas with a competent vector do not report dengue epidemic activity. *(Copyright ©World Health Organization, 2014.)*

serologic studies have also documented that dengue infections are occurring in Texas.[44]

Chikungunya Virus

Chikungunya, a mosquito-borne alphavirus originally isolated in Tanzania in 1953, has spread from Africa, causing massive outbreaks in the Indian Ocean islands, India, and other parts of Asia since 2005. In the summer of 2007 an outbreak caused hundreds of cases (175 laboratory confirmed) in north-eastern Italy. The index case was a visitor from India. The vector implicated was *Aedes albopictus*, postulated to have been introduced via used tires.[45] Mutations in the virus may have enabled it to replicate more efficiently in *Aedes albopictus* mosquitoes, the Asian tiger mosquito, which is now widely distributed outside of Asia.[46] It can survive cooler temperatures than *Aedes aegypti*.

Beginning in late 2013 local chikungunya transmission was documented in the Caribbean islands. The virus has now spread widely in Central and South America.[47] Chikungunya virus is introduced into new areas by viremic travelers and can cause high attack rates in susceptible populations; persistent and disabling joint pain can follow acute illness, especially in older individuals.[48]

Cholera

Cholera illustrates the complex interactions between microbe, environment and host.[49] *Vibrio cholerae* lives in close association with marine life, binding to chitin in crustacean shells and colonizing surfaces of algae, phytoplankton, zooplankton and water plants. *V. cholerae* can persist within the aquatic environment for months or years, often in a viable but dormant state, noncultivable by usual techniques. Environmental factors, including temperature, salinity, pH and seawater nutrients, affect the persistence, abundance and viability of the organisms, and hence influence human epidemics.

Under conditions of population crowding, poor sanitation and lack of clean water, cholera can have a devastating impact, as was shown by the massive outbreak of El Tor cholera in Rwandan refugees in Goma, Zaire, which caused 12 000 deaths in July 1994.[50]

Toxigenic *Vibrio cholerae* O1 was introduced into Haiti in 2010 in the aftermath of the earthquake.[51] As of March 2013, it had caused >650 000 illnesses and >8000 deaths. Studies suggest that it was introduced by UN mission personnel who lacked sanitary disposal of their waste. Subsequently a tributary of the Artibonite River was contaminated with a pathogenic strain of South Asian type *Vibrio cholerae*.

The organism can be carried by humans who can introduce it into new regions. Trade probably also plays a critical role. Ballast water, picked up by boats in multiple locations and discharged at another time and place, carries a wide range of species.[52,53] In earlier studies of the ballast and bilge of cargo ships in the USA Gulf of Mexico, researchers were able to identify *V. cholerae* identical to the strains causing epidemic disease in Latin America.[54]

Food-Borne Disease

The globalized food market moves pathogens from one region to another. An outbreak of cholera in Maryland, USA, was traced to imported, contaminated commercial frozen coconut milk.[55] Alfalfa sprouts grown from contaminated seed sent to a Dutch shipper caused outbreaks of *Salmonella* spp. on two continents, the USA and Finland.[56] Commercial movement of fruits and vegetables redistributes resistance factors along with the microbes.

Travel and trade are key features in the epidemiology of the infection *Cyclospora*, a cause of gastroenteritis. For many years cases were often associated with living in or travel to areas where sanitary facilities were poor. In the summer of 1996, a large US outbreak occurred in persons who had not traveled. Over a period of a few months, 1465 cases of cyclosporiasis were reported from 20 states. The outbreak was linked to raspberries imported from Guatemala.[57]

Visceral Leishmaniasis

In the past, visceral leishmaniasis in Brazil was primarily a rural disease. Recently, however, several cities have reported large outbreaks of visceral leishmaniasis.[58] Reasons for the change in epidemiology include geoclimatic and economic factors (drought, lack of farm land, famine), leading to migration of large numbers of persons, who settle in densely populated peri-urban areas that lack basic sanitation. Domestic animals, such as dogs and chickens, are sources of blood meals for the sand fly vector of leishmaniasis. Outbreaks, affecting especially children and young adults, have occurred in many cities in Brazil. Malnutrition contributes to disease severity.

Disease–disease interactions also alter the epidemiology of infections. Visceral leishmaniasis has become an important infection in HIV-infected people in Spain and other areas where the two infections coexist.[59] The presence of HIV leads to increased risk of progression of infection; disease can also appear years after exposure.

MOVEMENT OF VECTORS AND OTHER SPECIES

Movement of nonhuman species can affect infections in humans. Importation of wild animals from Ghana into the USA led to an outbreak of monkeypox, an infection previously known to exist in Africa. Humans became infected by handling domestic prairie dogs (sold as pets) that had been housed with the imported wild animals from Africa.[60] *Aedes albopictus* introduced into the USA via used tires shipped from Asia[61] has since become established in at least 21 contiguous states of the USA and in Hawaii. *Aedes albopictus* can transmit dengue and chikungunya viruses and is a competent laboratory vector of La Crosse, yellow fever and other viruses. Multiple strains of eastern equine encephalitis virus have been isolated from *Aedes albopictus* in Florida.

Current transportation systems regularly carry all forms of life, including potential vectors, along with people and cargo. In an experiment conducted several years ago, mosquitoes, house flies and beetles in special cages were placed in the wheel bays of a Boeing 747 aircraft and carried on flights lasting up to 7 hours. Temperatures were as low as −62°F (−52°C) outside and ranged from 46°F to 77°F (8–25°C) in the wheel bays. Survival rates were greater than 99% for the beetles, 84% for the mosquitoes and 93% for the flies.[62] Occasional cases of so-called airport malaria – cases of malaria near airports in temperate regions – attest to the occasional transport and survival of an infective mosquito.

In the USA, transportation of raccoons in the late 1970s from Florida to the area between Virginia and West Virginia (in order to stock hunting clubs) unintentionally introduced a rabies virus variant into the animals of the region. From there, the rabies enzootic spread for hundreds of miles, reaching raccoons in suburban and densely populated regions of the north-east USA. Spill-over of the rabies virus variant into cats, dogs and other animal populations and direct raccoon–human interactions have had costly consequences.[63]

Highly pathogenic avian influenza A (H5N1) is a global concern.[64] It is entrenched in poultry populations in Asia and Africa and has caused outbreaks in Europe and the Middle East. Although the virus causes high mortality in infected humans, thus far H5N1 has not been able to establish sustained transmission from person to person. Most humans appear to have been infected via close contact with poultry or their products. Although the virus can be carried by migratory birds,[65] most introductions appear to have been related to movement of poultry and poultry products. In South East Asia risk was associated with duck abundance, human population and rice cropping intensity.[66]

Geographic Influences on Differential Diagnosis

Geographic exposures influence how one thinks about probable diagnoses in a given patient. In Mexico, for example, more than 50% of patients with late-onset seizures have computed tomography (CT) evidence of the parasitic infection, neurocysticercosis.[67] In Peru, 29% of persons born outside Lima who had onset of seizures after 20 years of age had serologic evidence of cysticercosis.[68] In northern Thailand, melioidosis is a common cause of sepsis, accounting for 40% of all deaths from community-acquired sepsis.[69]

In considering the consequences of exposures in other geographic regions, relevant data in assessing the probability of various infections include the duration of visit, activities and living conditions during the stay and the time lapsed since the visit. Among British travelers to West Africa, the relative risk of malaria was 80.3 times higher for persons staying for 6–12 months than among those staying 1 week.[70] In Malawi, the risk of schistosome infection increased directly with duration of stay. Seroprevalence was 11% for those present for 1 year or less, but this increased to 48% among those present for 4 years or longer.[71] In a study of persons with cysticercosis, the average time between acquisition of infection and onset of symptoms was about 7 years.[72]

For malaria, it is necessary to know not only whether infection can be acquired in a specific location but also the species of parasites present and the patterns of resistance to antimalarial agents. Figure 106-8 shows the distribution of malaria. Analysis of data from the GeoSentinel Surveillance network, a network that uses travelers as a sentinel population, finds marked differences in the spectrum of disease in relation to the place of exposure.[22,73]

Expression of disease may vary depending on age of first exposure, immunologic status of the host, genetic factors and the number and timing of subsequent exposures. Temporary residents of endemic regions have different patterns of response to a number of helminths from those of long-term residents. In cases of loiasis, temporary residents have immunologic hyperresponsiveness, high-grade eosinophilia and severe symptoms that are not seen in long-term residents of the same area.[74] Genetic factors can affect susceptibility to infection or expression of disease. Some persons, for example, are genetically resistant to infection with parvovirus because they lack appropriate receptors on their erythrocytes.[75] Persons lacking Duffy factor cannot be infected with the malarial parasite, *P. vivax*.

Conclusion

Knowledge about the geographic distribution of diseases is essential for informed evaluation and care of patients, who increasingly have had exposures in multiple geographic regions. Recent travel and trade patterns have led to more frequent contact with populations from low latitude areas, regions with greater species richness.[76] Infectious diseases are dynamic and will continue to change in distribution, and access to real time epidemiologic outbreak surveillance data such as that provided by ProMED (www.promedmail.org) is a vital tool for clinicians. Changes in virulence and shifts in resistance patterns will also require ongoing surveillance and communication to healthcare providers. Multiple factors favor even more rapid change, perhaps in unexpected ways, in the future: rapidity and volume of travel, increasing urbanization (especially in developing regions), the globalization of trade, multiple technologic changes that favor mass processing and broad dispersal, and the backdrop of ongoing microbial adaptation and change, which may be hastened by alterations in the physicochemical environment.

References available online at expertconsult.com.

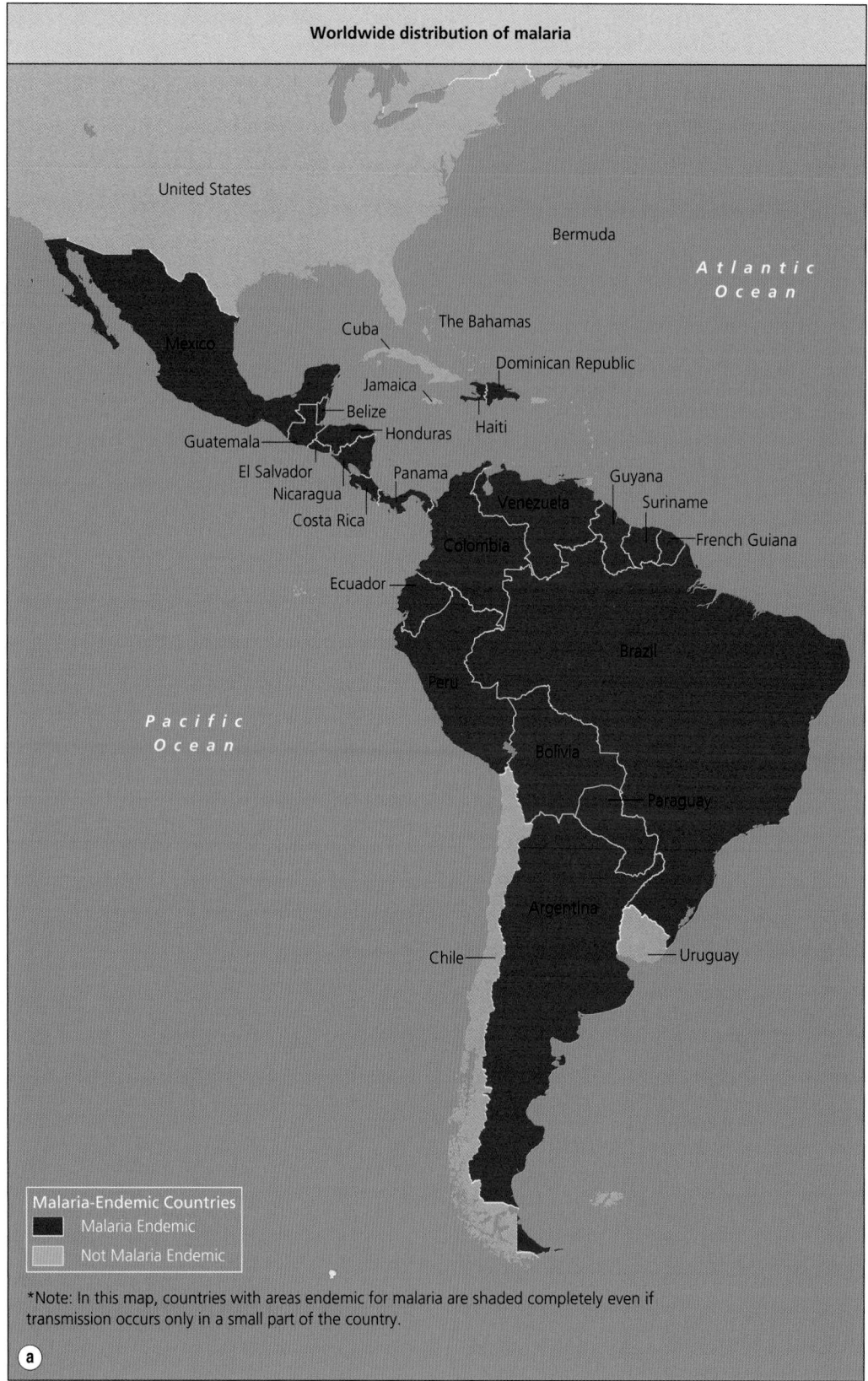

Figure 106-8   (a, b) Worldwide distribution of malaria. *(Data from Centers for Disease Control and Prevention: CDC Health information for international travel 2014.* New York: Oxford University Press, 2014.)   *Continued*

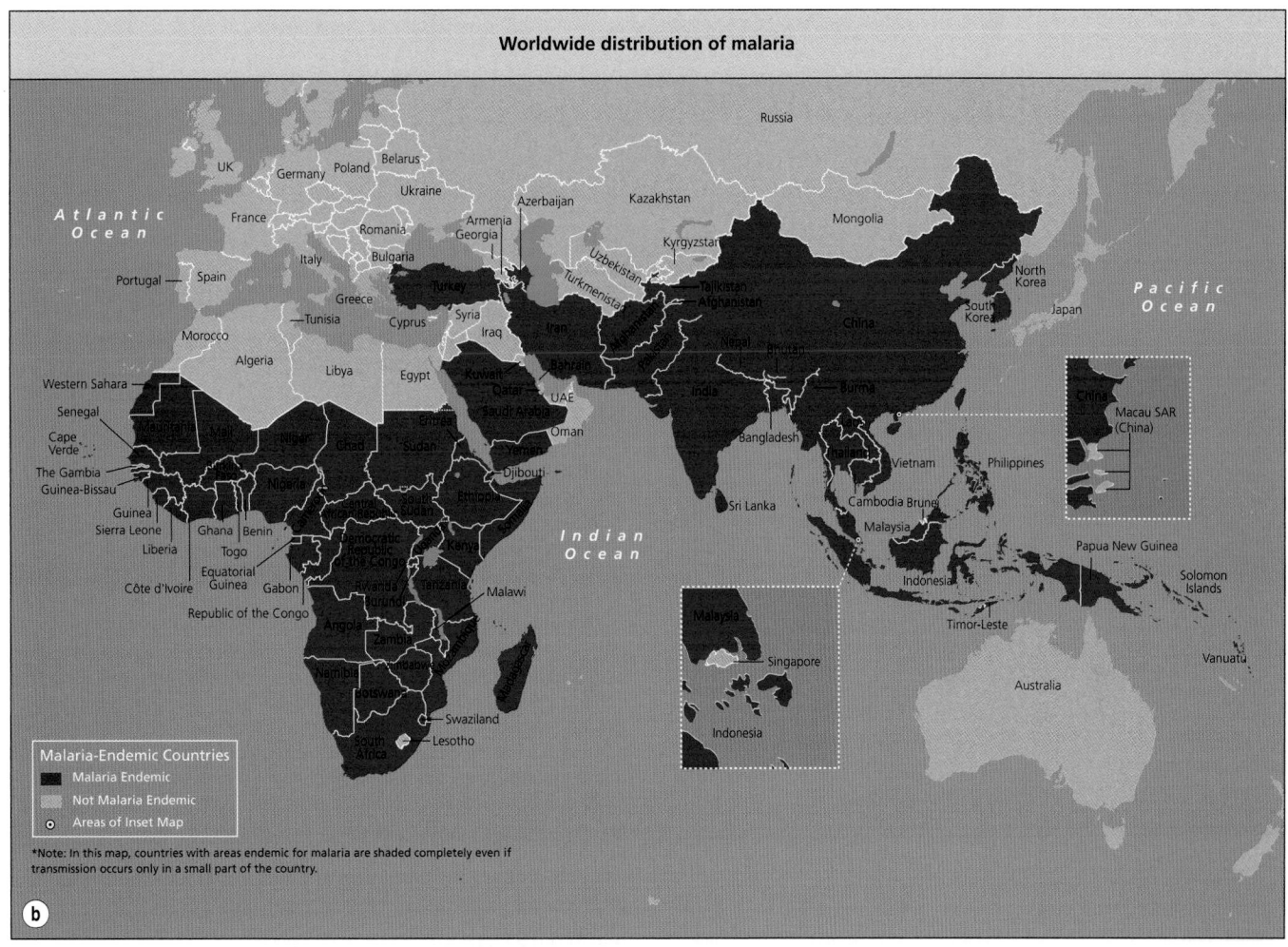

Figure 106-8, cont'd Worldwide distribution of malaria.

KEY REFERENCES

Bhatt S., Gething P.W., Brady O.J., et al.: The global distribution and burden of dengue. *Nature* 2013; 496:504-507.

Burt F.J., Rolph M.S., Mahalingam S., et al.: Chikungunya: a re-emerging virus. *Lancet* 2012; 379:662-671.

Ezzati M., Lopez A.D., Rogers A., et al.: Selected major risk factors and global and regional burden of disease. *Lancet* 2002; 360:1347-1360.

Fraser C., Riley S., Anderson R.M., et al.: Factors that make an infectious disease outbreak controllable. *PNAS* 2004; 101:6146-6151.

Freedman D.O., Weld L.H., Kozarsky P.E., et al.: Spectrum of disease and relation to place of exposure among ill returned travelers. *N Engl J Med* 2006; 354(2):119-130.

Guernier V., Hochberg M.E., Guegan J.-F.: Ecology drives the worldwide distribution of human diseases. *PLoS Biol* 2004; 2(6):740-746.

Hay S.I., Guerra C.A., Tatem A.J., et al.: The global distribution and population at risk of malaria: past, present, and future. *Lancet Infect Dis* 2004; 4(6):327-336.

Reed K.D., Melski J.W., Braham M.B., et al.: The detection of monkeypox in humans in the Western hemisphere. *N Engl J Med* 2004; 350:342-350.

Reiter P., Sprenger D.: The used tire trade: a mechanism for the worldwide dispersal of container-breeding mosquitoes. *J Am Mosq Control Assoc* 1987; 3:494-501.

Tsetsarkin K.A., Vanlandingham D.L., McGee C.E., et al.: A single mutation in chikungunya virus affects vector specificity and epidemic potential. *PLoS Pathog* 2007; 3:e201.

Weaver S.C., Lecuit M.: Chikungunya virus and the global spread of a mosquito borne disease. *N Engl J Med* 2015; 372:1-27.

Wilson M.E.: Travel and emergence of infectious diseases. *Emerg Infect Dis* 1995; 1:39-46.

Wolfe N.D., Dunavan C.P., Diamond J.: Origins of major human infectious diseases. *Nature* 2007; 447:279-283.

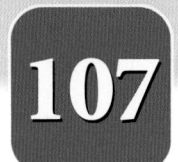

Travel Medicine

JANE N. ZUCKERMAN

KEY CONCEPTS

- With more than a million international tourists traveling around the world in 2013, and with an increasingly interconnected world, the discipline of travel medicine has never been more important in the prevention of travel-related disease in individuals and populations.

- The travel health risk assessment is an essential component of identifying the health needs and protecting the health of the individual traveler.

- The use of malaria chemoprophylaxis should be encouraged and prescribed for at risk travelers and in particular those visiting friends and relatives (VFRs).

- Bite avoidance measures are an essential adjunct to the prevention of arthropod-borne disease.

- Vaccines remain the most effective method of preventing infectious disease and influenza should be recognized as one of the most common vaccine-preventable illnesses during travel.

- Environmental hazards are an increasingly important consideration with travel to altitude in particular, being a popular pursuit.

- Accidents remain the most common cause of morbidity and mortality in travelers, with education the mainstay of prevention.

- The potential risk of importing infectious disease is likely to rise as a consequence of travel amongst such mobile populations, increasingly recognized as a real threat to global public health.

Travel medicine has become an established discipline, required to meet the health needs of ever increasing numbers of travelers to a variety of destinations. International arrivals are expected to reach nearly 1.6 billion by the year 2020, of which 1.2 billion will be intraregional and 378 million will be long-haul travelers.[1] The travel health consultation for international travelers is an example of exclusively preventive medicine and the first step is to complete a travel health risk assessment and to establish the traveler's health needs: determining the itinerary and duration of travel, the accommodation and planned activities, and the health status of the traveler.[2] In order to determine destination-specific risks, the global epidemiology of infectious disease health risks should be understood and up-to-date information should be accessed from national public health authorities.[3,4] The next step is to review the traveler's health. Although at least 25% of individuals travel with chronic medical conditions, these generally do not prevent a person from traveling. Risks can be mitigated alongside consideration of planned activities; vaccines and/or prophylactic medications should be balanced against a traveler's health requirements.

Once a travel health risk assessment has been completed, the health professional should provide the traveler with the tools to manage this risk. These usually include the administration of vaccines, self-treatment and prophylactic medications, and preventive advice. Each traveler should also be informed how to access medical care during travel and on return as many travelers will need to seek medical care during and after their trip.[5]

To take account of the constantly changing epidemiology of disease and patterns of microbial resistance, the complexity of many travel itineraries, and newly licensed vaccines and preventive medications, specialized travel clinics are available in many countries which have healthcare professionals trained in travel medicine, and which are able to provide accurate preventive advice.[6]

Immunizations

Immunizations can be divided into three categories:
- recommended as part of routine health maintenance irrespective of international travel;
- required for entry into a country under International Health Regulations (2005) or by an individual country; and
- recommended because of the potential risk of exposure during travel.

Travel-related immunizations are often the reason that an individual attends a travel clinic, although the risk of most vaccine-preventable illness is less than one case per 1000 journeys. Comprehensive travel health records should be kept: the type and dose of vaccine, date of administration, manufacturer and lot number, site of administration and administrator's signature. Prior to administration of any vaccine, patients should undergo informed consent. The use of vaccine information sheets, often available from vaccine manufacturers, will help to explain to travelers the benefits and risks of each vaccine. Full manufacturer's prescribing information should always be consulted before administration of a vaccine, as schedules, doses and products will often differ between countries.

IMMUNIZATIONS FOR ROUTINE HEALTH MAINTENANCE

The pre-travel health consultation often provides the opportunity to update routinely recommended immunizations according to age and mostly includes tetanus, diphtheria, pertussis, measles, mumps and rubella, *Haemophilus influenzae* type b, polio and pneumococcal vaccines for infants, and influenza and pneumococcal vaccines for older adults. Consideration should be given to the differences that exist between national immunization recommendations worldwide.[7,8]

Issues of inadequate coverage and waning immunity also determine the recommendation of vaccines. Measles is no longer endemic to the USA and nearly all cases are imported or linked to imported infections. Although important gains have been made in global control of measles, particularly in Africa, ongoing measles outbreaks in both low- and high-income regions threaten efforts to control the disease.[9,10] Waning immunity against pertussis has led to an increase in cases in older individuals and the introduction of adult formulations of pertussis vaccine combined with tetanus and diphtheria (Tdap).[11] Where available, this vaccine should be used to boost levels of protection for those travelers who may be at risk of exposure or, importantly, to afford protection to susceptible people encountered during travel.

Children should receive vaccines appropriate for travel and in line with the national childhood immunization program. Occasions may arise whereby the schedule of administration of a vaccine may be accelerated if a child is traveling before they would have received a scheduled vaccine and if the risk of the vaccine-preventable illness during their trip is assessed as being significant. In the case of measles, a single dose may be given from 6 to 11 months for travel to high-risk destinations, with the routine schedule still administered beginning at 12–15 months.

Older adults (those aged 65 years and over) make up an increasing proportion (as high as 15%) of international travelers. In addition, there are many travelers with chronic medical conditions such as HIV/AIDS, diabetes or chronic pulmonary, renal, hepatic or cardiac disease and it is recommended that such travelers should be vaccinated with influenza and pneumococcal vaccines. The recognition that influenza is one of the most common vaccine-preventable illnesses during travel has led to the consideration of administering vaccine to healthy travelers going to areas of seasonal influenza (year round in tropical regions, December to March in the northern hemisphere, and April to September in the southern hemisphere).[12] Outbreaks can occur out of season when persons from diverse regions of the world congregate in close quarters, such as on cruise ships or during mass gatherings, e.g. the Hajj. The practicalities of obtaining vaccine out of season or vaccine that is matched to influenza strains at the destination may be difficult. Seasonal influenza vaccine is not expected to provide protection against highly pathogenic avian influenza A (H5N1) and the role of antivirals used as self-treatment or prophylaxis has yet to be evaluated extensively.[13]

REQUIRED IMMUNIZATIONS

Vaccination may be required under International Health Regulations (IHR 2005)[14] or by an individual country as a condition of entry. The only vaccine that currently may be required under IHR (2005) is yellow fever (YF) vaccine. There is a risk of YF transmission in countries throughout the Amazon basin of South America, and in sub-Saharan Africa between 15° north and 10° south of the equator. YF is re-emerging and expanding into new regions, as has been seen in South America in 2008 with expansion of disease into new regions of Brazil, Argentina and Paraguay. Although YF disease risk maps are published by both the Centers for Disease Control and Prevention (CDC) and the World Health Organization (WHO) and national public health authorities, determining the actual risk of a traveler's journey can be challenging.[15] In general, travelers to rural regions in areas with a risk of YF transmission (either an endemic area where there are the appropriate mosquito vectors and nonhuman primate hosts for transmission, or infected areas where there are cases of YF reported) should receive vaccine. Other countries that are not at risk of YF transmission may require vaccination of travelers arriving from YF-risk countries. Country-specific requirements can be found in the CDC and WHO, National Travel Health Network and Centre (NaTHNaC) publications, and on their respective websites, amongst others.[3,16,17] Health professionals must therefore decide if the vaccine is required for entry and/or recommended because of risk. YF vaccination must be recorded in the International Certificate of Vaccination or Prophylaxis.[18] In addition to vaccine, travelers should protect themselves against the daytime-biting *Aedes* spp. mosquito through using bite avoidance measures.

In 2001, newly recognized severe adverse events, viscerotropic and neurological, were reported following administration of YF vaccine to first-time vaccine recipients. Viscerotropic reactions are reported to occur within 2 weeks following vaccination (median of 4 days) and are characterized by the dissemination of vaccine virus associated with multiorgan failure, in which approximately 50% of cases are fatal. In these cases there are high titers of circulating vaccine virus, prolonged viremia and an unregulated inflammatory response.[19,20] The neurological adverse events are characterized by a meningoencephalitis that begins up to 4 weeks following vaccination (median 14 days), with nearly all cases recovering.[21] Acute disseminated encephalomyelitis and Guillain–Barré syndrome are also associated with neurological adverse events. The risk factors do not appear to be related to mutation of vaccine virus, but rather to an alteration in the host response. Older age, particularly 60 years and older, and the absence of a thymus (a contraindication to vaccination) carry an increased risk for both viscerotropic and neurological adverse reactions.

Cholera vaccine is no longer required under IHR (2005) for international travel, and smallpox vaccine has not been required since 1982 following the global eradication of smallpox in 1977. Meningococcal vaccine is required for religious pilgrims to Saudi Arabia (see following section).

TRAVEL-RELATED IMMUNIZATIONS

Vaccines discussed in this section are recommended because there may be a risk of exposure to infectious disease during travel.

The risk of hepatitis A during travel has declined in many countries, particularly Latin America and East and South East Asia, with transition from high to lower endemicity.[22,23] Nevertheless, vaccination can be considered for most travelers as hepatitis A vaccines are well tolerated, highly effective, give long-term (perhaps lifelong) protection and are being incorporated into routine immunization schedules.[24] Hepatitis A vaccines are protective even if given shortly prior to departure and have superseded the use of immune serum globulin. Where appropriate, serological testing for previous exposure to hepatitis A can be performed in travelers with a high likelihood of previous hepatitis A infection, i.e. those born and raised in countries with high endemicity for hepatitis A and those with a history of jaundice.

Protection against both hepatitis A and B may be achieved with the use of a combined antigen vaccine, administered frequently as an accelerated primary course over a period of 3 weeks, with a booster dose a year later.

Typhoid and paratyphoid are imported diseases in most high-income countries. The highest risk of infection is in travelers to South Asia (India, Pakistan and Bangladesh); however, cases also originate from Latin America and Africa.[25,26] Multidrug-resistant *Salmonella enterica* Typhi is common. There are two vaccines with similar efficacy (60–70%): an oral live-attenuated (Ty21a) vaccine and a polysaccharide (Vi antigen) injectable vaccine.[27] The Ty21a vaccine is well-tolerated, effective in children older than 4 years and provides protection for 5 years; the Vi antigen vaccine is given in a single intramuscular dose and is effective for 2–3 years. Typhoid vaccines do not confer full protection against *S. enterica* Paratyphi, which may be more commonly imported in returning travelers than *S. enterica* Typhi.[26]

Cholera is endemic throughout Asia and Africa and parts of the Middle East; however, infection is rare in travelers. *Vibrio cholerae* 01 is endemic in all regions, whereas *V. cholerae* 0139 has circulated in Asia. More than 90% of cholera cases are reported from Africa, although some countries in Asia, such as Bangladesh where cholera is endemic, do not report cases to the WHO.[28] There is currently one cholera vaccine licensed: an oral vaccine that combines killed *V. cholerae* with the binding (B) subunit of cholera toxin. This vaccine is well tolerated and confers rates of protection between 60% and 85% against cholera depending upon the age of the recipient and the time interval measured.[29] Because of the very low risk of cholera in travelers, vaccine should be reserved for those who will be working in refugee settings or who will travel in cholera-endemic regions and will be remote from medical care. There has been interest in the use of this vaccine to protect against the syndrome of travelers' diarrhea. While there is cross protection against *Escherichia coli* expressing the heat labile enterotoxin (LT), the protection is modest and the vaccine should not generally be used for this indication.[29]

Global efforts at polio eradication have been largely successful in several WHO regions of the world (the Americas, Western Pacific and European) and in 2014, only parts of three countries in the world, Nigeria, Pakistan and Afghanistan, remain endemic for the disease, the smallest geographic area in history. Outbreaks of polio in Asia, Africa and Middle East resulting from international travel are a cause of public health concern and travelers should have completed a primary course of a polio-containing vaccine and have a booster according to their national guidelines. Saudi Arabia requires polio vaccination in travelers age 15 years and younger coming from countries reporting wild-type polio.

Other immunizations recommended because of potential exposure during travel include those against hepatitis B (administered as part of the routine childhood immunization program in more than 180 countries worldwide), Japanese B encephalitis, *Neisseria meningitidis*, rabies, tick-borne encephalitis and tuberculosis.

Japanese B encephalitis is a virus transmitted by the *Culex* spp. mosquito found in Asia. Prolonged residence in endemic areas or engaging in high-risk activities such as camping, bicycling or field work are indications for vaccination. Rural Asia, particularly where rice and pigs are farmed, is the highest risk area; pigs act as a reservoir for the virus and the rice fields as a breeding ground for the *Culex* mosquito vector. Protection is afforded following administration of a Vero cell-derived inactivated vaccine, which has replaced the mouse brain-derived vaccine.[30]

Meningococcal vaccine is recommended for travelers to areas highly endemic for meningococcal disease such as the meningitis belt of sub-Saharan Africa (particularly during the months from December to June). Following the global spread of meningococcal W135 disease, which was traced to international travel of Hajj pilgrims in 2000, Saudi Arabia requires vaccination with a quadrivalent vaccine containing serogroups A, C, Y and W135 for religious pilgrims arriving for the Hajj or Umrah.[31]

All travelers should be counseled about avoiding exposure to rabies virus. In most low-income regions of the world, rabies is transmitted to humans by the bite of a dog (see Chapters 74 and 171) although other mammals (e.g. bats, cats, foxes) can also transmit the virus. In North America, bat-transmitted rabies is most common. Pre-exposure protection against rabies should be considered for those whose risk is increased by type of activity (e.g. running, cycling), occupation (e.g. veterinarians) and longer duration of stay.[32] Children may be at increased risk as they are less likely to avoid contact with animals and to report a bite or lick. The intramuscular route of administration of the vaccine is preferred to ensure adequate development of immunity.

In order to decrease risk of transmission, all bites should be thoroughly washed with soap and water; postexposure rabies treatment should then be obtained. A traveler who has received pre-exposure vaccine will not need rabies immune globulin (RIG, either human or equine), which is difficult to obtain or unavailable in many areas of the world. If vaccine has not been received before travel, both vaccine and RIG will need to be given.[33] Regimens may differ, but if postexposure treatment is administered properly the traveler should be protected. Travelers who had an overseas rabies exposure and treatment should be evaluated upon return. They can have serology checked and postexposure treatment initiated while awaiting serologic evidence of protection (see Chapter 171).

Tick-borne encephalitis is a viral meningoencephalitis spread by *Ixodes* spp. ticks throughout forested areas of Eastern and Central Europe, and Siberia in the spring and summer months. Unpasteurized dairy products in endemic areas may also transmit the virus.[34] There are two inactivated vaccines which have limited availability outside of continental Europe and require three doses over a year to achieve full protection, which is not practical for most travelers. For rapid short-term protection of children and adults, the second dose may be given 2 weeks after the first dose and so provides at least 90% protection. Travelers to risk areas should observe bite avoidance measures against ticks by the use of protective clothing, repellents and insecticides. These measures will help to prevent Lyme disease, which is also transmitted by the bite of *Ixodes* ticks.

The risk of acquiring tuberculosis during travel is greatest in travelers to countries of high endemicity (e.g. incidence of >40 cases/100 000 population), those who will stay for a long period (>1–3 months) and those who will have close contact with potentially infectious persons (e.g. healthcare workers, and those visiting and staying with friends and relatives). The risk of infection has ranged from about 1 case/1000 persons/month in Peace Corps volunteers to 8 cases/1000 persons/month in healthcare workers.[35,36] Guidance on immunization against tuberculosis differs worldwide with countries immunizing only high risk groups or treating infection after two-step tuberculin testing. The UK has set guidelines for travelers that include children under the age of 16 and healthcare workers to high endemic regions who have not previously received BCG.[37] Travelers who are not vaccinated should be offered pre- and post-travel tuberculin (purified protein derivative) skin testing or interferon-gamma testing to check for conversion and, therefore, infection.[38] The post-travel skin test should be administered 1 month or more after return.

IMMUNIZATION IN SPECIAL GROUPS

Two important groups of travelers require special consideration before immunization – pregnant women and immunocompromised hosts (see also Chapter 87). For pregnant women, inactivated vaccines may be given but only if the risk is determined to be significant.[3,7] Live vaccines such as measles, mumps and rubella and varicella vaccine should not be administered, although data have not demonstrated clearly adverse outcomes when women have received rubella vaccine. Yellow fever vaccine should be avoided unless there is high-risk travel; seroconversion to YF virus during pregnancy may be lower, necessitating revaccination after delivery.[39]

HIV-infected patients are another group to consider separately.[3,40] All travelers should be asked about possible HIV risk factors before vaccination; the safety, immunogenicity and efficacy of the vaccine being considered, with the need being balanced against the risk of the disease. Vaccine immunogenicity decreases with advanced HIV disease; a CD4 lymphocyte count of <200–400 cells/mL or <15–25% by age-specific percentages correlates with decreased immunogenicity. Although it has not been studied clearly, this may also be a cut-off point for an increased risk of adverse consequences of live viral vaccines. If assurance of immunity is needed, then post-vaccination serology should be obtained for the appropriate antigens.

In addition to vaccination, HIV-infected travelers should consider the health risks associated with travel to low- and middle-income regions. Many enteric infections, such as *Salmonella*, *Cyclospora* and *Cryptosporidium*, and systemic infections such as leishmaniasis and tuberculosis, are more prevalent and can be prolonged and difficult to treat in HIV-infected individuals.

Travelers' Diarrhea

Travelers' diarrhea (TD) affects 30–60% of travelers and is the most common illness during visits to low-income regions of the world.[41] Illness usually begins in the first week after arrival and is typically mild, characterized by three or more loose to watery stools accompanied by another symptom of nausea, abdominal cramping or malaise. Fever is usually less than 38°C and vomiting is uncommon. In most cases, illness is self-limiting over 3–5 days and dysentery with tenesmus and bloody stools occurs in less than 10% of patients. Although most individuals can continue with their activities, about 25% will need to alter plans. Enterotoxigenic *Escherichia coli* (ETEC) accounts for 20–30% of the known causes, and a newly described *E. coli*, enteroaggregative *E. coli*, causes another 15–20%.[42,43] *Shigella*, *Salmonella* and *Campylobacter* spp. are the most common other bacteria (see Practice Point 11). Viruses (typically rotavirus and norovirus) cause 5–20% of cases and protozoa (*Giardia*, *Cryptosporidium* and, less commonly, *Cyclospora*) cause 5% or less and are usually associated with longer duration of travel. Although the overall incidence of TD does not decline with increasing time of residence in low- and middle-income areas, partial immunity will develop to ETEC diarrhea. A short course (1–3 days) of an antibiotic, such as ciprofloxacin, or where resistance to fluoroquinolones is known, azithromycin, will improve diarrhea within 20–36 hours. A full description of the prevention and treatment of TD can be found in Chapter 38 and Practice Point 11)

Malaria Prevention

Malaria is one of the most important diseases to prevent as it can be fatal. The type of malaria and the risk of acquisition vary by destination and reason for travel, but worldwide there are approximately 7500 cases each year in returned travelers. Of the five recognized species of malaria in humans (*Plasmodium falciparum*, *P. vivax*, *P. ovale*, *P. malariae* and, rarely, *P. knowlesi*), *P. falciparum* is the most severe form and is also the most frequently imported species. Over 80% of *P. falciparum* cases are acquired by travelers on trips to Africa, and especially West

Africa, where transmission can occur in both urban and rural areas. Travelers with the highest risk for acquiring malaria are those who return to their country of birth to visit friends and relatives, termed VFR travelers; they are usually traveling to West Africa where they are most likely to acquire *P. falciparum* or to South Asia where they usually acquire *P. vivax*.

BITE AVOIDANCE MEASURES

Malaria is transmitted by the female *Anopheles* mosquito, which is most active during the night-time hours from dusk to dawn. During this period travelers should wear loose-fitting cotton clothing that covers their arms and legs, apply repellents to exposed areas of skin and sleep in enclosed areas behind screens or under netting. The most effective repellents are those that contain DEET (*N,N*-diethyl-3-methylbenzamide). A concentration of 50% will provide protection lasting from 6 to 12 hours. DEET-containing repellents are safe to use in children and pregnant women, but should be applied carefully to avoid systemic absorption: they should not be applied to mucous membranes or irritated skin and should be washed off when coming indoors. Sunscreen should be applied before insect repellent. Picaridin-based repellents are also effective. Bed nets should be treated with a residual insecticide (e.g. permethrin-containing compounds). This can also be applied to clothing and will kill insects rather than only repel them. Mosquito coils and sprays containing pyrethroids can be used in enclosed sleeping areas. Bite avoidance measures, such as described above, should be used as adjuncts to the use of malaria chemoprophylaxis unless traveling in very low-risk malaria areas where medical treatment should be sought urgently if any symptoms were to develop.

CHEMOPROPHYLAXIS

Chemoprophylaxis should be taken on a regular basis during travel and for a period of time after return that depends on which medications are taken. Most cases of malaria in returned travelers occur because the traveler fails to take any chemoprophylaxis, takes incorrect prophylaxis or does not comply with their prophylaxis. The choice of a chemoprophylactic regimen should be based on risk of exposure, types of parasite prevalent in the travel destination and health conditions of the traveler. Up-to-date sources (including authoritative websites) should be consulted before prescribing any antimalarial.[3,14,16]

Chloroquine as a single agent is effective only in areas where *P. falciparum* remains sensitive or is not present: Mexico, Central America west and north of the Panama Canal, the Dominican Republic and Haiti, Egypt, most areas of the Middle East and parts of China. Travelers to all other risk areas in Africa, Asia and Latin America will need to take atovaquone–proguanil, doxycycline or mefloquine.

Atovaquone–proguanil and doxycycline are effective in treatment and prophylaxis of all malaria species, although experience using atovaquone–proguanil with non-falciparum species is limited.[44] Both drugs are started 1–2 days before exposure to malaria and then taken daily. Doxycycline is continued for 28 days after leaving the malarious area, but atovaquone–proguanil can be discontinued after 7 days because it has a causal prophylactic effect: it kills developing hepatic stage parasites, but not the dormant, hypnozoite forms of *P. vivax* or *P. ovale*. These may emerge from the liver many months after return from the place of exposure. Atovaquone–proguanil is ideally targeted for short-term travelers to areas of risk. Doxycycline cannot be given to children under the age of 8 in the USA (under 12 in the UK) or to pregnant women. It should be swallowed with water whilst in the upright position to prevent esophageal irritation. Doxycycline may predispose to vaginal yeast infection and can act as a photosensitizer.

Mefloquine is highly effective in preventing malaria, including chloroquine-resistant *P. falciparum*. When it is taken in prophylactic doses, minor gastrointestinal (GI) and neuropsychiatric events occur in 5–30% of users.[45] The neuropsychiatric side effects can include sleep disturbance, vivid dreams, mood changes, anxiety, headache and dizziness. Serious adverse events such as psychosis are rare with an occurrence of about one case per 6000–20000 users. Travelers should be screened for contraindications to mefloquine before prescribing it: a known hypersensitivity to the drug, a history of seizures or psychiatric disorder, or an underlying cardiac conduction abnormality. Some travel health consultants prescribe mefloquine 2–3 weeks before departure to assess patient tolerance and allow a switch to other agents if there is a problem. Seventy percent of adverse reactions occur during the first three doses. Loading doses of the drug are not advocated.

The combination of chloroquine plus proguanil has been recommended by practitioners in the UK for areas in which there are low levels of chloroquine-resistant *P. falciparum* malaria and only a small risk of acquisition, such as most areas of risk in India. In low-risk areas, some European experts do not recommend taking any chemoprophylaxis; rather they suggest being observant to febrile episodes and carrying stand-by self-treatment.[46] US and UK authorities do not advocate this approach. Health practitioners should consult the appropriate expert recommendations for their country.

Primaquine is an alternative chemoprophylactic in persons intolerant of other options and can be considered following specialist advice.[47] It is a causal prophylactic and will prevent the establishment of liver hypnozoites of *P. vivax* and *P. ovale*. The drug is taken daily beginning 1–2 days before exposure and can be discontinued 7 days after leaving the risk area. It is a requirement that glucose-6-phosphate dehydrogenase (G6PD) deficiency is ruled out in all persons for whom primaquine is prescribed.

Rural, forested areas of Thailand that border Burma and Cambodia, western Cambodia (including Siem Reap) and southern areas of Vietnam that border Cambodia have multidrug-resistant *P. falciparum* malaria. Travelers to these areas should take atovaquone–proguanil or doxycycline for prophylaxis.

All travelers should understand that no antimalarial is 100% protective and that they can develop malaria in spite of being compliant with prophylaxis. If they develop a fever or flu-like illness overseas that could be malaria, they should seek medical care. The evaluation needs to include a blood smear performed by a competent laboratory, because the sensitivity of symptoms or physical findings alone is low. The use of self-administered rapid diagnostic kits is not generally recommended as travelers have difficulty using and interpreting these tests; they are not currently licensed for this purpose. In circumstances where travelers cannot obtain prompt medical care, self-treatment can be considered. The self-treatment drug(s) should differ from what the traveler is taking for chemoprophylaxis. Options include atovaquone–proguanil, artemether–lumefantrine and quinine plus doxycycline.

Pregnant women should not travel to malarious areas unless absolutely necessary, because of the added risk of complications of malaria during pregnancy. Chloroquine and proguanil (with added folate) are safe. Mefloquine can be taken after the first trimester, and may be acceptable in the first trimester if there are no alternatives. Doxycycline is contraindicated and there are insufficient safety data on atovaquone–proguanil during pregnancy. Primaquine should not be given because the G6PD status of the fetus cannot be determined.

Environmental Hazards

Travel to the tropics is associated with increased heat and humidity; the effects that these changes can have on health should be taken into account. These range from a feeling of malaise and tiredness to increased loss of salt and water with resultant dehydration. Travelers should maintain hydration, limit exercise and sleep in a cool environment, particularly if they are elderly or have chronic medical problems. Excessive sun exposure should be avoided by wearing loose-fitting cotton clothing to cover exposed skin, wearing hats and using sunscreens with a sun protection factor of at least 15. If the patient is taking doxycycline for malaria prophylaxis, it is particularly important to limit sun exposure. Skin should be kept dry and clean to avoid cellulitis and dermatophyte infection.

Travelers to altitudes above 2500–3500 meters (8200–11500 feet) can experience acute mountain sickness (AMS) or the more severe and potentially fatal conditions of high-altitude pulmonary edema (HAPE) and high-altitude cerebral edema (HACE).[48,49] AMS is characterized by headache, nausea, vomiting, insomnia and lassitude and may affect up to 50% of persons who rapidly ascend above 4000 m. The risk of illness can be lessened by acclimatization: spending a few days at intermediate altitudes of 1500–3000 m and gradually ascending, sleeping at elevations no more than 300–500 m higher each night. Acetazolamide, a carbonic anhydrase inhibitor, can be taken to assist acclimatization, particularly when persons must ascend quickly. It is given at a dose of 125–250 mg orally twice daily, starting 2 days before being at altitude and for several days at altitude.[50] It has also been used to treat mild symptoms of AMS. Dexamethasone can be used to treat AMS but in severe illness the safest course is always to descend. Acetazolamide is contraindicated in persons with sulfonamide allergy.

Jet lag is a common problem, particularly when more than five time zones are crossed. It is easier to travel west and lengthen the day than to travel east and shorten the day. In order to help with jet lag, several methods have been proposed: light exposure, short-acting hypnotics and melatonin.[51] When traveling east, exposure to bright light in the late morning and early afternoon may aid in the adjustment. A short- to intermediate-acting benzodiazepine or benzodiazepine receptor agonist can facilitate and maintain sleep in the new time zone, decreasing the contribution of fatigue to the effects of time zone adjustment. Melatonin, which is secreted during the night hours, has been studied extensively. A dose of 3–8 mg taken 2–3 hours before bedtime for the first few nights in the new time zone may be helpful. However, the purity and effectiveness of over-the-counter preparations have not been documented.

Deep venous thrombosis (DVT) and pulmonary embolism are recognized complications of long-haul travel. DVTs can occur in as many as 3% of persons flying for 10–15 hours and who have cardiovascular risk factors; oral contraceptive pills, pregnancy, recent surgery, certain coagulation disorders and malignancy also contribute to risk.[52,53] Some long-haul travelers will develop a pulmonary embolism.[54] In order to decrease risk, travelers should maintain their hydration and exercise their lower extremities at regular intervals. Fitted, below-the-knee support stockings will decrease the incidence of DVT and for highest risk passengers low molecular weight heparin can be considered. Aspirin is not recommended.

Behavioral Factors

Although there is much focus on infectious illness, the most important contributors to severe morbidity and mortality, particularly in young adults, are accidents and injuries, with those related to road traffic accidents and drowning most common.[55,56] Road safety can be improved by using safety belts in vehicles, avoiding excessive speed, not driving at night or after drinking alcohol, and not riding on motorcycles and mopeds. When swimming, travelers should be aware of undercurrents and never dive into unknown waters. To prevent assault and theft, travelers should not wear jewelry and clothing that draws attention, and they should travel in groups, avoiding high-risk urban areas, particularly at night. Travel advisories are posted routinely on governmental websites.

Sexually transmitted diseases, including HIV and hepatitis B, gonorrhea, syphilis and chancroid, are prevalent in many destination countries in Africa, Asia and Latin America. Travelers should be counseled about safe sexual practices, and take condoms with them on their trip.[57,58] Postexposure prophylaxis against HIV may be necessary (see Practice Point 30),[59] and women may need emergency contraception. Tattooing, injections and dental instruments should be avoided to decrease the risk of acquiring blood-borne pathogens such as hepatitis B and C and, less likely, HIV.

Other Diseases and Considerations

Dengue fever, a viral disease (see Chapter 133) transmitted by *Aedes* mosquitoes, has seen a resurgence, particularly in Asia, the Caribbean and Latin America, and is a theoretical risk in the south-eastern USA. Dengue is characterized by the sudden onset of fever, headache, myalgias and arthralgias, abdominal discomfort, rash and mild liver abnormalities.[60] Severe disease (dengue hemorrhagic fever and dengue shock syndrome) is characterized by thrombocytopenia and vascular leak, and usually occurs in children following a second infection with a different dengue serotype. There is no vaccine available for prevention, so travelers need to exercise precaution against this daytime-feeding mosquito. Complying with bite avoidance measures will help to prevent not only dengue but a clinically similar viral infection, chikungunya virus, that in recent years has been a problem on the islands of the Indian Ocean and in countries of South and South East Asia.[61] Other less common insect-transmitted diseases such as leishmaniasis, trypanosomiasis, filariasis and rickettsial infection will also be prevented by observing insect bite avoidance measures. African trypanosomiasis has been documented in travelers to East African game parks, and African tick-bite fever caused by *Rickettsia africae* is a risk in southern Africa.[62]

Schistosoma spp. (see Chapter 118) can infect travelers who swim in fresh-water lakes and rivers, particularly in endemic areas of east and southern Africa.[63] Travelers to risk areas should avoid fresh-water swimming unless it is in a chlorinated pool. Letting water stand for 48 hours or warming it to 122°F (50°C) for 5 minutes will render it safe from the *Schistosoma* parasites. Fresh-water swimming, particularly after periods of flooding, can be a risk for acquisition of leptospirosis.

Although the viral hemorrhagic fevers, Ebola, Lassa and Marburg (see Chapter 132), garner a great deal of media attention, they are a rare risk for travelers. Current outbreaks of disease can be identified by reviewing up-to-date information on ProMED (www.promedmail .org) or by checking the disease outbreak sites of the WHO, CDC and NaTHNaC web pages. Any returning traveler who is suspected of having a viral hemorrhagic fever should be managed according to WHO guidelines.[64]

Travelers need to know how to access medical care during their trip. They should purchase a travel health insurance package that includes help in locating medical care, paying for the care upfront and, if necessary, providing for emergency evacuation. Embassies or consulates can assist in locating medical services, and mission hospitals can be a source of care. A small first-aid kit that contains analgesics, bandages, a thermometer and any frequently used over-the-counter medications is helpful as it can be difficult to find the simplest medicines overseas. All travelers should carry an extra supply of their prescription medications, and avoid putting them into checked luggage.

POST-TRAVEL ILLNESS

Travelers should report illness upon return and health practitioners should be able to recognize common syndromes: fever, diarrhea, respiratory illness and rash.[2,5,65] Although routine post-travel follow-up for short-term travelers is usually not necessary, anyone who experienced major illness overseas or new-onset illness after return should be evaluated. A differential diagnosis can be developed by considering geography (the locations visited), activities undertaken, incubation periods of disease, frequency of occurrence and preventive measures taken (e.g. immunizations, compliance with prophylaxis).[66] A more detailed discussion of individual syndromes and diseases is provided in other relevant chapters.

References available online at expertconsult.com.

KEY REFERENCES

Centers for Disease Control and Prevention: *Health information for international travel 2014*. Atlanta: US Department of Health and Human Services, Public Health Service; 2014. Available: http://wwwnc.cdc.gov/travel/page/yellowbook-home-2014.

Croft J.: *Drugs for preventing malaria in travellers (Review)*. *The Cochrane Library*, Issue 1. Chichester, UK: John Wiley; 2010.

Ericsson C.D.: Travellers' diarrhea. In: Zuckerman J.N., ed. *Principles and practice of travel medicine*. 2nd ed. Wiley-Blackwell; 2013:197-209.

Hill D.R.: Starting, organizing and marketing a travel clinic. In: Keystone J.S., Kozarsky P.E., Nothdurft H.D., et al., eds. *Travel medicine*. 3rd ed. St Louis: Mosby; 2012: 13-24.

Immunization against infectious disease. Public Health England March 2014. Available: https://www.gov.uk/government/collections/immunisation-against-infectious-disease-the-green-book.

Imray C., Booth A., Wright A., et al.: Acute altitude illnesses – Clinical Review. *BMJ* 2011; 343:d4943.

Kozarsky P.: The body of knowledge for the practice of travel medicine – 2006. *J Travel Med* 2006; 13(5): 251-254.

MacPherson D.W., Gushulak B.D., Sandhu J.: Death and international travel – the Canadian experience: 1996 to 2004. *J Travel Med* 2007; 14:77-84.

Monath T.P., Gershman M., Staples J.E., et al.: Yellow fever vaccine. In: Plotkin S.A., Orenstein W.A., Offit P.A., eds. *Vaccines*. 6th ed. Philadelphia: Saunders Elsevier; 2012:870-968.

Memish Z.A., Goubeaud A., Bröker M., et al.: Invasive meningococcal disease and travel. *J Infect Public Health* 2010; 3(4):143-151.

Ryan E.T., Wilson M.E., Kain K.C.: Illness after international travel. *N Engl J Med* 2002; 347:505-516.

Suh K.N., McCarthy A.E., Mileno M.D., et al.: High-risk travelers. In: Zuckerman J.N., ed. *Principles and practice of travel medicine*. 2nd ed. Wiley-Blackwell; 2013: 515-531.

Warrell M.J.: Current rabies vaccines and prophylaxis schedules: preventing rabies before and after exposure. *Travel Med Inf Dis* 2012; 10:1-15.

Wilder-Smith A.: Dengue infections in travelers. *Paediatr Int Child Health* 2012; 32(s1):28-32.

World Health Organization: *International travel and health, 2014*. Geneva: WHO; 2014. Available: http://www.who.int/ith/en/.

108

Leprosy

WARWICK J. BRITTON

KEY CONCEPTS

- Leprosy is a chronic infection of macrophages and Schwann cells in the skin and peripheral nerves with the noncultivable pathogen, *Mycobacterium leprae*.

- Leprosy remains endemic in many countries with a stable case detection rate of about 250 000 new cases each year, and chronic nerve function impairment from leprosy remains a significant cause of disability worldwide.

- The genome of *M. leprae* is very stable but shows a massive reduction in the number of genes compared to other mycobacteria, consistent with rigorous adaptation to intracellular growth.

- The pattern of clinical leprosy is a spectrum determined by the host cellular immune response: strong T-cell responses are associated with limited tuberculoid disease, and weak or absent T cell responses with extensive lepromatous disease.

- Fluctuations in the immune response to the pathogen are associated with two types of leprosy reactions, reversal reactions and erythema nodosum leprosum (ENL), which are major contributors to nerve impairment and disability.

- Early treatment with antibiotics is the most effective means of leprosy control and the prevention of nerve impairment.

- Multidrug therapy with defined combinations of antibiotics for multibacillary and paucibacillary leprosy is very effective with low relapse rates and is essential to prevent development of antibiotic resistance.

- Careful clinical assessment of peripheral nerves before and during therapy is an essential component of the management of leprosy patients.

- Leprosy reactions should be promptly treated with adequate dose and duration of corticosteroids to prevent further nerve impairment.

- Bacille Calmette–Guérin (BCG) immunization contributes to the prevention of leprosy.

Epidemiology

Leprosy is a chronic infection of the skin and nerves with *Mycobacterium leprae*, which, although rarely fatal, is a significant cause of disability. Over the past 20 years there have been dramatic changes in the prevalence of leprosy since the introduction of multidrug therapy (MDT).[1,2] As a result of the shorter duration of therapy and more intensive control programs, the number of registered leprosy patients receiving chemotherapy has fallen from 10–12 million to 180 618 in 2013.[3] The annual case detection rate of new cases remained high for many years, but this has fallen from 763 000 in 2001 to 215 656 in 2013. This fall represents a true decline in the incidence of leprosy worldwide; however, the case detection rate has remained at this level for some years and new measures are required to eradicate leprosy. In addition, there is a pool of 2–3 million patients with permanent nerve impairment as a consequence of leprosy.

Leprosy is widely distributed in tropical and warm temperate countries and >1 billion people live in regions where there is active transmission of *M. leprae*. The prevalence rate of new cases has fallen to <1/10 000 in almost all endemic countries, although there are pockets of high prevalence within individual countries. Currently eight countries account for 88% of new leprosy patients worldwide:

- India (59% of all new cases detected); and
- Brazil, Indonesia, Democratic Republic of Congo, Nigeria, Nepal, Bangladesh and Tanzania, in descending order.[3]

Because of the long incubation period of leprosy an individual from an endemic country may develop leprosy years after migration elsewhere. Delay in diagnosis is usually longer in non-endemic than endemic regions, and therefore leprosy should be considered as a diagnostic possibility in any person who is from an endemic country and has chronic lesions of the skin or impaired function of peripheral nerves.

Subclinical infection with *M. leprae* is far more common than overt disease.[4] Analysis of *M. leprae*-specific immune responses has demonstrated that *M. leprae* infection is common after exposure, but the majority of individuals control the infection. Currently there is no specific test to distinguish latent leprosy infection from latent tuberculosis infection, but new *M. leprae*-specific T-cell assays are being developed for epidemiological studies.

The major mechanism of transmission of *M. leprae* is thought to occur through nasal secretions, particularly from lepromatous patients.[4] Organisms probably enter through the mucosa of the upper respiratory tract and, if not controlled, disseminate to the skin and peripheral nerves. Other possible modes of transmission include breast milk from mothers with untreated lepromatous disease and uncommon cases of cutaneous inoculation. *M. leprae* infection is endemic in wild armadillos in the southern USA, and recent genetic analysis has confirmed that the identical strain of *M. leprae* infects armadillos and leprosy patients there, consistent with possible zoonotic transmission in this region.[5]

Proximity to leprosy patients is important in transmission, and the relative risk for disease for household contacts is eight- to 10-fold greater for lepromatous cases and two- to fourfold greater for tuberculoid cases.[4] Nevertheless, the majority of leprosy cases are sporadic. The incidence of leprosy peaks in two age groups (10–15 and 30–60 years of age) and there is a male predominance in most regions of about 2 : 1.[6] The incubation period varies widely from months to over 30 years, but is usually prolonged, averaging 4 years for tuberculoid and 10 years for lepromatous leprosy. In contrast to tuberculosis there is no definite evidence for increased HIV prevalence in leprosy patients or a change in the clinical spectrum of leprosy among coinfected patients.[7] Leprosy can present as an immune reconstitution syndrome in coinfected patients after starting highly active antiretroviral therapy.

Genetic factors influence both the development of leprosy and the pattern of disease. Genome-wide linkage analysis in multicase families has defined susceptibility alleles in the genes for lymphotoxin-α and the ubiquitin and proteasome-related enzymes, PARK2 and PACRG, in addition to the recognized linkage to HLA Class II and tumor necrosis factor genes.[8] The HLA locus also affects the pattern of disease: HLA-DR2 and -DR3 are associated with tuberculoid disease and HLA-DQ1 with lepromatous leprosy. Large studies in China have identified further susceptibility loci, including genes encoding the NOD2 and Toll-like receptor signaling and autophagy pathways, highlighting the importance of host immunity in pathogenesis of leprosy.[9,10] Racial and geographic factors also influence the type of leprosy, with lepromatous leprosy being less common in Africans than Indians, and most common in Chinese and Caucasians.

Pathogenesis and Pathology

Although *M. leprae* was the second bacterium to be associated with a human disease, it still cannot be cultivated *in vitro*. The organism is capable of limited multiplication in mouse footpad, with a doubling time of 11–13 days, and this has permitted drug sensitivity studies.[11] *M. leprae* is an acid-fast gram-positive bacillus and is an obligate intracellular parasite with tropism for macrophages and Schwann cells. The bacilli show preference for growth in cooler regions of the body. The unique characteristic of *M. leprae* is its predilection to infect Schwann cells. The receptor complex on the Schwann cell is the G-domain of the laminin α2 chain in the basal lamina of Schwann cells and the laminin receptor, α-dystroglycan.[12] A number of potential ligands on the surface of *M. leprae* for this complex have been identified.

Genetic and structural analyses have confirmed that *M. leprae* is a member of the family Mycobacteriaceae. Genomic analysis of four disparate isolates of *M. leprae* revealed extremely high sequence identity, with differences only in a small number of single nucleotide polymorphisms (SNP) and pseudogenes.[13,14] Recovery of ancient DNA samples from medieval leprosy patients demonstrated remarkable conservation of the genome over the last 1000 years.[15] The genome contains 1605 genes encoding proteins and 50 genes for stable RNA molecules.[13] Remarkably, half the functional genes in the *M. tuberculosis* genome are absent, being replaced by many inactivated or pseudogenes. This gene decay has removed entire metabolic pathways and regulatory genes, particularly those involved in catabolism. This may render the leprosy bacillus dependent on host metabolic products and may explain its long generation time and inability to grow in culture. Sixteen SNP subtypes were defined by genotyping *M. leprae* isolates from different continents and ancient *M. leprae* samples, and these subtypes clustered in geographical regions. This suggests that leprosy infection of humans originated in East Africa or the Near East and then spread through successive waves of human migrations.[14] Individual isolates of *M. leprae* can be distinguished by the variable number of tandem repeat sequences within their genome, but the extent of variability within individual patients for isolates collected from different sites or at different times limits the use of these repeat tandem sequences as tools for molecular epidemiologic studies.[16]

The availability of the *M. leprae* and other mycobacterial genomes has major implications for the development of new antimycobacterial drugs and *M. leprae*-specific diagnostic reagents. The complex cell wall contains important targets of the immune response, including a species-specific phenolic glycolipid-I (PGL-I) and the immunomodulatory lipoarabinomannan.[11] The cell wall biosynthetic pathways are relatively intact in *M. leprae*, despite the loss of other genes, indicating that these represent the essential genes for the formation of a minimal mycobacterial cell wall. *M. leprae* is relatively inert, and the host immune response is responsible for most of the tissue damage.

The manifestations of leprosy form a wide clinical spectrum determined by immunopathologic responses to the organism (Figure 108-1).[6,17] Patients who have the polar forms of tuberculoid (TT) and lepromatous leprosy (LL) are immunologically stable, but those who have the intermediate types of borderline-tuberculoid (BT), mid-borderline and borderline-lepromatous (BL) leprosy are immunologically unstable and subject to either a gradual decline towards the lepromatous pole or upgrading reversal reactions (RRs; see Figure 108-1). In TT a vigorous cellular response to *M. leprae* limits the disease to a few well-defined skin patches or nerve trunks.[6] The lesions are infiltrated by interferon-gamma secreting CD4+ T lymphocytes, which form well-demarcated granulomas containing epithelioid and multinucleate giant cells around dermal nerves. Few, if any, bacilli are demonstrable. Cellular immunity may be confirmed by *in vitro* lymphocyte responses to *M. leprae* antigens or skin test reactivity. Intradermal injection of heat-killed *M. leprae* causes a transient swelling at 48 hours in a sensitized subject (Fernandez reaction), followed by the development of a granulomatous nodule at 3–4 weeks (Mitsuda reaction).[6] The latter confirms an individual's capacity to mount a

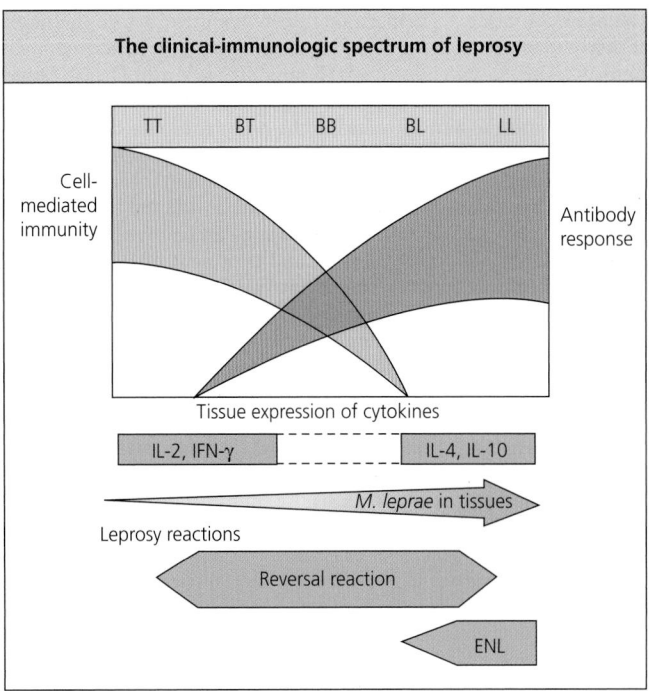

Figure 108-1 The clinical–immunologic spectrum of leprosy. This reflects the underlying host immunity as measured by the T-cell and antibody responses to *M. leprae*. Spontaneous fluctuations in the immune response are responsible for reversal reactions and erythema nodosum leprosum (ENL). TT, tuberculoid leprosy; BT, borderline-tuberculoid; BB, mid-borderline leprosy; BL, borderline-lepromatous leprosy; LL, lepromatous leprosy; IFN, interferon; IL, interleukin.

T-lymphocyte response to *M. leprae*. Antibody responses to *M. leprae* are absent or low titer.

The hallmark of LL is the absence of *M. leprae*-specific cellular immunity, and this results in uncontrolled proliferation of the bacilli with extensive infiltration of the skin and nerves and numerous lesions.[6] Histologically, the dermis contains foamy macrophages filled with multiple bacilli and a scattering of CD4+ and CD8+ lymphocytes, but no organized granulomas. There are high titers of antibodies to *M. leprae*-specific PGL and protein antigens. In borderline cases a progressive reduction in cellular responses is associated with a greater bacillary load, more frequent skin and nerve lesions, and increasing antibody levels.

The dynamic nature of the immune response to *M. leprae* is responsible for spontaneous fluctuations in the clinical pattern, termed leprosy reactions:[6,11]

- a type 1 reaction is usually an 'upgrading' RR caused by increased cellular reactivity to mycobacterial products, results in edema and acute inflammation of skin lesions and nerves, is most common in borderline patients and is a major cause of nerve damage; and
- a type 2 reaction or erythema nodosum leprosum (ENL) is a systemic inflammatory response associated with the deposition of extravascular immune complexes leading to neutrophil infiltration and activation of complement in multiple organs.[18] This is accompanied by high circulating levels of tumor necrosis factor with systemic toxicity.

Prevention

The chief means of preventing leprosy is interruption of transmission by treating those with infectious leprosy early. Multidrug therapy (MDT) was introduced because of the increasing spread of primary and secondary dapsone resistance worldwide. Its advantages are its proven efficacy[2] and improved compliance, which is related to the limited duration of therapy and its monthly observed component (see

Management, below). Furthermore, early treatment before the onset of nerve damage reduces the long-term disability associated with leprosy.[19] The effectiveness of MDT prompted a World Health Organization coordinated campaign to implement MDT in all endemic countries, with the aim of reducing the prevalence rate of leprosy to less than 1/10 000.[1,2] This has been successful at a national level, but some regions of endemic countries have yet to attain this goal. Importantly, the case detection rate has been slower to fall and has persisted around 250 000 cases per annum, indicating that leprosy control must be sustained through case detection and treatment of leprosy within integrated health programs. The recent WHO Expert Committee recommended a move from emphasizing a statistical leprosy elimination target based on case detection rates to the goal of reducing nerve function impairment and disability in leprosy patients.[2]

Meta-analysis has confirmed the significant protective effect of immunization with Bacille Calmette–Guérin (BCG) against leprosy in both clinical trials and case-control studies.[20] In a major trial in Malawi, BCG induced 50% protective efficacy against clinical leprosy, both tuberculoid and lepromatous forms. Re-immunization enhanced the protective effect by a further 50%.[21] Extensive BCG immunization of children in endemic countries has probably made a significant contribution to the decline of leprosy. The addition of heat-killed *M. leprae* to BCG did not increase the observed protective efficacy of BCG in two trials. Other experimental vaccines protect against experimental leprosy infection.[22,23]

Chemoprophylaxis may also be useful in the control of leprosy, particularly in low endemic regions. A large, randomized control trial in Bangladesh showed that a single dose of rifampin given to the close contacts of newly diagnosed leprosy patients resulted in a significant reduction of 57% (95% CI 33–72) in the incidence of leprosy in the contacts at 4 years.[24] Leprosy is commonly associated with poverty and overcrowding, and improved socioeconomic conditions have also contributed to the decline of leprosy in Europe and some Asian countries.

Clinical Features
TYPES OF LEPROSY
Indeterminate Leprosy

This is the earliest form and occurs as a single, slightly hypopigmented ill-defined macule in children, who are often contacts of leprosy patients.[6,25] The majority of these lesions are self-limiting and resolve without therapy. A minority (<25%) develop into defined lesions within the clinical spectrum.

Tuberculoid Leprosy

These lesions occur as one to three large asymmetric macules or plaques with sharply defined borders and hypopigmented anesthetic centers (Figure 108-2).[6,25] Although leprosy lesions are usually hypopigmented, in light skins the macules may appear erythematous or dyschromic. Involvement of sweat glands and hair follicles results in dryness and loss of hair. Enlarged cutaneous nerves may be palpable at the edge of the lesion, but nerve trunk involvement is minimal.

Borderline-Tuberculoid Leprosy

This is the commonest form of leprosy. The skin lesions resemble those in TT leprosy, but are more frequent and variable in appearance and their borders are less well demarcated (Figure 108-3). The outline may be irregular with adjacent 'satellite' lesions suggesting local spread. Occasionally, large patches of BT leprosy may involve a whole limb. Asymmetric enlargement of several peripheral nerves is usual and patients may present with muscle weakness or trauma secondary to sensory impairment. Progressive nerve damage is common.

Mid-borderline Leprosy

This is the most immunologically unstable form with the propensity to shift rapidly towards BT leprosy during a reversal reaction or to downgrade towards BL leprosy. The skin lesions are numerous and

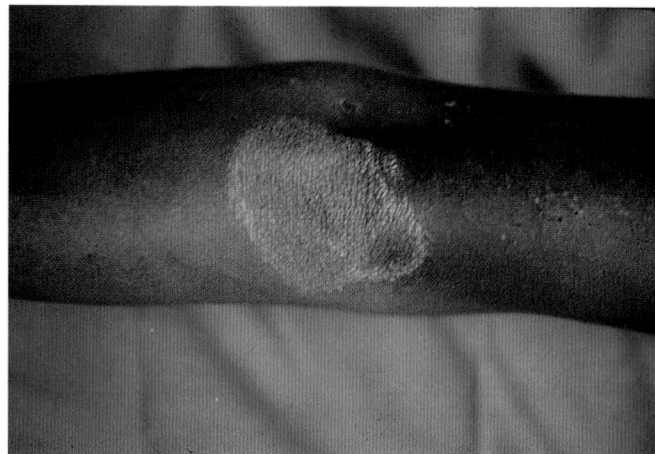

Figure 108-2 Tuberculoid leprosy. Single hypopigmented anesthetic plaque with raised border and dry surface.

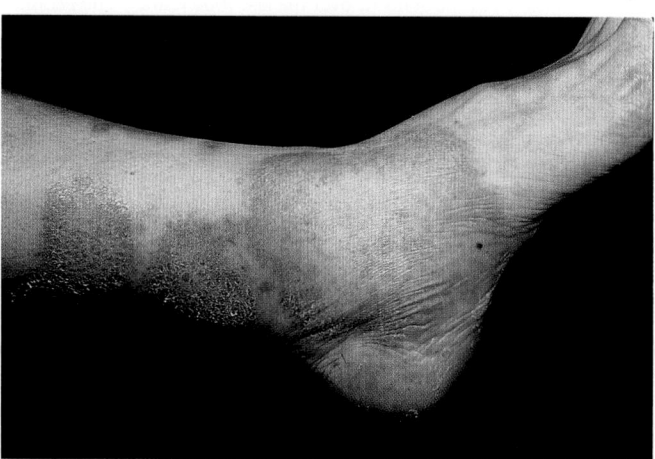

Figure 108-3 Borderline tuberculoid leprosy. Three large well-defined erythematous patches with reduced sensation, spreading borders and satellite lesions.

vary in size, shape and distribution. They may be hypopigmented or erythematous. The characteristic 'target' lesion has a broad, erythematous border with a vague outer edge and 'punched-out' pale center with sensory impairment (Figure 108-4).

Borderline-Lepromatous Leprosy

In BL leprosy there are numerous small erythematous macules, which initially may be limited in distribution but become progressively more symmetric.[6,25] Papules, nodules and succulent plaques may develop and, in contrast to tuberculoid leprosy, the lesions have normal sensation. The intervening skin is normal. Widespread nerve involvement is typical, especially if the patient has downgraded from BT leprosy.

Lepromatous Leprosy

This is a systemic disease with a generalized bacteremia leading to widespread involvement of the skin and other organs.[6,25] The first manifestation may be a diffuse infiltration of the dermis causing a smooth shiny appearance of the skin. More typically, there are numerous symmetrically distributed macules, papules or nodules, and sensation may be retained in lepromatous lesions (Figures 108-5 and 108-6). Progressive thickening of the skin results in coarsening of the facial features and nodular thickening of the ear lobes. With time the eyebrows and eyelashes become thinned.

Bacillary infiltration is responsible for gradual tissue damage in the involved organs. The nasal mucosa is infiltrated at an early stage, resulting in discharge and obstruction. Erosion of the cartilage and nasomaxillary bones results in perforation of the nasal septum,

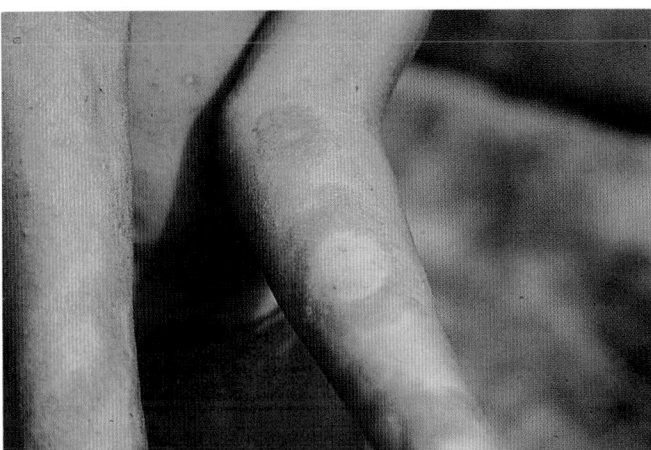

Figure 108-4 Mid-borderline leprosy. Characteristic target lesion with raised erythematous annular border and 'punched-out' central area with impaired sensation.

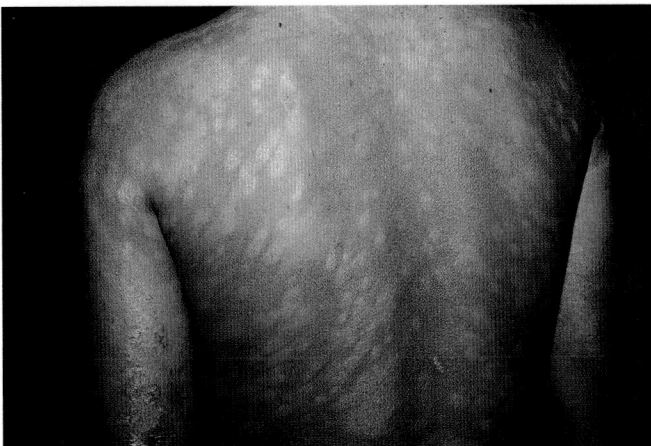

Figure 108-5 Lepromatous leprosy. Multiple, small, slightly erythematous macules with intact sensation and symmetric distribution. The skin smears of both the lesions and intervening skin are positive for acid-fast bacilli.

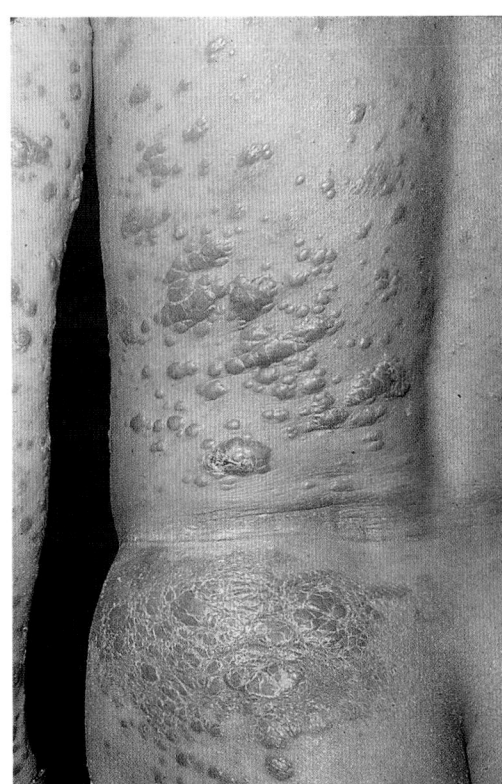

Figure 108-6 Nodular lepromatous leprosy. Diffuse infiltration of the skin by multiple nodules of varying size, each teeming with bacilli.

collapse of the nose and saddle-nose deformity. Laryngeal involvement produces hoarseness and stridor. Direct bacillary involvement of the eye causes keratitis and iritis.

Infiltration of the dermal nerves results in a peripheral sensory loss similar to that of a 'glove and stocking' neuropathy,[6] which leaves the skin susceptible to ulceration and secondary infection. Reactional episodes cause edema of the feet, shins and hands. Dactylitis develops in the hands and feet and, together with trauma and osteomyelitis, results in phalangeal erosion.

Both testicular infiltration and orchitis contribute to testicular atrophy and secondary gynecomastia. Glomerulonephritis may occur and is usually associated with ENL. Secondary amyloidosis is a consequence of recurrent ENL reactions.

PERIPHERAL NERVE INVOLVEMENT

The nerves of predilection are those at superficial sites where the nerve trunks are cooler, more readily traumatized and often anatomically constricted.[6,11] These include the:

- ulnar nerve at the medial epicondyle of the humerus;
- median nerve at the wrist;
- lateral popliteal nerve at the neck of the fibula;
- posterior tibial nerve behind and inferior to the medial malleolus; and
- radial nerve in the humeral groove posterior to the deltoid insertion.

Easily palpated superficial cutaneous nerves include the:

- superficial radial nerve at the wrist;
- greater auricular nerves;
- supraorbital nerve; and
- sural nerves.

These nerves should be examined for enlargement and associated weakness and sensory loss. The resulting muscle imbalance results in the characteristic deformities of claw hand, foot drop, claw toes and wrist drop. Autonomic nerve dysfunction contributes to impaired sweating and dry skin, which is subject to cracking, infection and poor healing. The combination of insensitive feet and claw toes leads to recurrent plantar ulceration, a major cause of disability.

In pure neural (PN) leprosy the nerve trunks are affected without any skin lesions. On biopsy the neural lesions tend to be 'lepromatous' in appearance and PN leprosy involving more than one nerve should be treated as multibacillary (MB).[6]

Before and during therapy the function of the commonly involved nerves should be assessed at regular intervals by voluntary muscle and sensory testing (preferably with nylon monofilaments) to determine whether there is ongoing nerve function impairment. This may presage the onset of a reversal reaction before nerve pain or typical skin lesions develop. Nerve conduction studies commonly detect subclinical neuropathy in BT–BL leprosy patients and these tests may become abnormal weeks before the development of clinical neuropathy.[26] Nerve function impairment may develop or worsen despite effective chemotherapy, and early recognition and therapy prevent permanent nerve damage. Patients with pre-existing nerve damage at diagnosis and MB patients are at greatest risk for new nerve function impairment and should be carefully monitored.[27]

LEPROSY REACTIONS

Reversal Reactions (RR)

These develop in about one-third of patients who have BT–BL leprosy, usually within the first year of treatment, but monitoring for new nerve function impairment should occur for 2 years.[28] They present with:

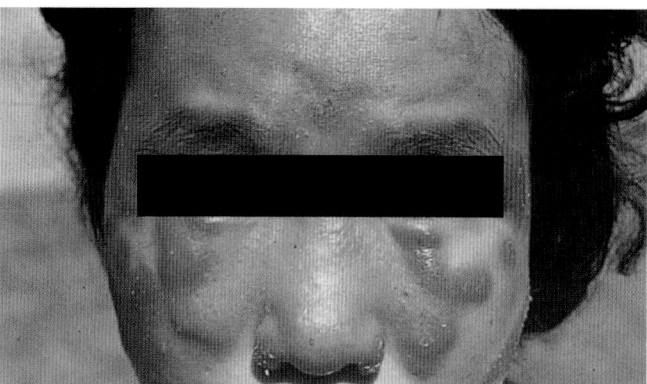

Figure 108-7 Reversal reaction. Erythema and edema in the facial lesions of a patient who has borderline-tuberculoid leprosy undergoing an upgrading reversal reaction.

- increased inflammation in established BT–BL skin lesions or new swollen lesions in BL and subpolar LL patients (Figure 108-7);
- acute neuritis with pain or tenderness in the involved nerve and loss of function; and
- recent (<6 months) or progressive nerve function impairment in the absence of painful nerves.

Silent neuritis responds to therapy for the RR. Patients at particular risk for developing RR are those who have MB leprosy involving more than two body areas, established nerve function impairment at diagnosis, facial patches or *M. leprae*-specific IgM anti-PGL antibodies.[6]

Erythema Nodosum Leprosum

This once affected 30–50% of BL and LL patients, but the frequency and severity of ENL have reduced since the regular use of clofazimine in MDT.[6] ENL may develop at any stage of therapy, but usually within the first year and is often recurrent.[29] An episode begins with fever and malaise and the rapid emergence of painful erythematous nodules, typically over the extensor surfaces of the limbs. In severe cases widespread nodules may form pustules and ulcerate (Figure 108-8). Painful neuritis is the most common complication. ENL has features of widespread immune complex deposition, including small vessel vasculitis, iridocyclitis, polyarthritis, orchitis, lymphadenitis and glomerulonephritis. Recurrent or uncontrolled ENL reactions can result in the development of secondary amyloidosis (amyloid A protein) within 3 months.

EYE INVOLVEMENT

Involvement of branches of the facial and trigeminal nerves results in lagophthalmos and corneal anesthesia, respectively, and the combination of these leads to ulceration and infection of the exposed insensitive cornea.[30] In 25–30% of patients who have LL, infiltration of the anterior segment of the eye causes a superficial punctate keratitis and iridocyclitis, which may be painless and only recognized by slit-lamp examination. Iridocyclitis is exacerbated during episodes of ENL, but can occur independently of overt reactions. The iritis may be complicated by glaucoma or cataract, both of which contribute to leprosy-associated blindness (see Chapter 18).

Diagnosis

A diagnosis of leprosy is usually straightforward if it is suspected as a cause of any skin or peripheral nerve lesion in a person from an endemic country. The cardinal signs of leprosy[6,11] are:

- skin patch with sensory loss;
- nerve enlargement; and
- acid-fast bacilli (AFB) in the skin.

The presence of one or more of these features establishes the diagnosis, which should be confirmed with a full-thickness skin biopsy.

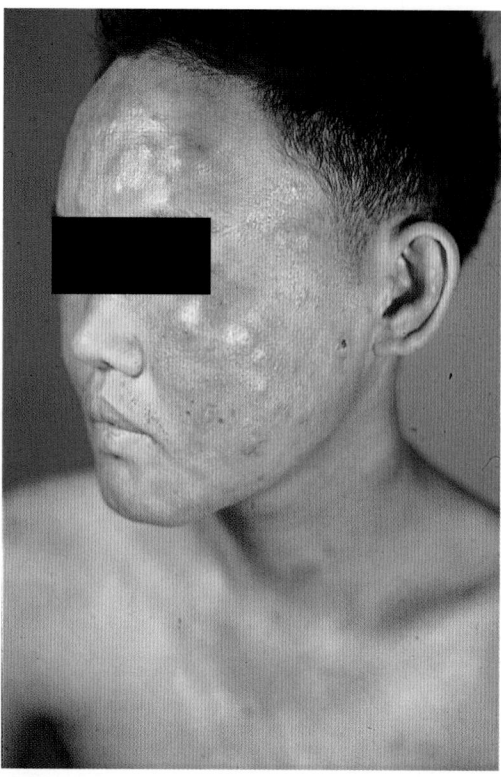

Figure 108-8 Erythema nodosum leprosum. Tender papules associated with fever, arthralgia and acute neuritis in a patient who has lepromatous leprosy.

Approximately 70% of leprosy patients have the diagnostic sign of a skin patch with sensory loss, but 30% of patients, including many MB patients, do not have sensory loss in skin lesions,[31] indicating the importance of clinical suspicion and examining for nerve enlargement for the diagnosis.

AFB are best demonstrated in slit-skin smears, which should be taken from the edges of at least two lesions and both ear lobes. If these are not available a skin biopsy should be stained for AFB with a modified Wade–Fite stain. The extent of the bacillary load can be quantitated as a bacterial index on a logarithmic scale of 1+ to 6+. The percentage of solid staining AFB in smears, the morphologic index, is an indirect measure of the viability of leprosy bacilli.[11] In PN leprosy a biopsy from a sensory nerve such as the superficial radial cutaneous nerve may be diagnostic. Polymerase chain reaction (PCR) can be used to identify *M. leprae* DNA[11] and, together with PCR-based detection of rifampin (rifampicin)-resistant strains,[32] it is a valuable tool for epidemiologic studies.

Lepromin testing and serology may be used for accurate classification of patients in research studies. Antibodies to PGL and other *M. leprae*-specific protein antigens are present in MB patients and their titer falls with effective therapy.[6,11] By contrast, patients with PB leprosy and healthy endemic controls demonstrate T cell cytokine and chemokine responses to *M. leprae*-restricted proteins.[33] In patients who have BL and LL, evidence of chronic inflammation includes anemia, hypergammaglobulinemia, elevated serum amyloid A protein and positive antinuclear and anticardiolipin autoantibodies.

Other skin diseases can be differentiated from tuberculoid leprosy by the absence of anesthesia in the lesions and the presence of nerve involvement in leprosy. Lepromatous skin lesions are not anesthetic, and biopsy may be necessary to distinguish these from those due to other systemic infections, such as leishmaniasis, secondary syphilis and other nodular or infiltrative skin conditions. Other causes of nerve enlargement, such as primary amyloidosis and familial polyneuropathy, are excluded by biopsy and family history.

Management

Successful management of leprosy requires prolonged drug treatment and careful monitoring for complications, and it is essential to enlist the patient as an ally in this process. The patient should be educated about:

- the importance of compliance;
- the first symptoms of a reaction; and
- the elements of self-care needed to prevent secondary tissue damage if there is sensory nerve impairment.

The most important step in disability prevention is the early initiation of bactericidal drug therapy.

ANTILEPROSY DRUGS

Dapsone

This is an important antileprosy drug because of its bactericidal effect at full dosage, low cost and low toxicity.[1] When used alone, stepwise dapsone resistance emerges as a major problem, owing to mutations in *folP1*, encoding dihydropteroate synthase,[34] but this is prevented by combination therapy. Mild hemolytic anemia is common, but is only severe in the presence of glucose-6-phosphate dehydrogenase deficiency, which should be excluded where possible. Dapsone hypersensitivity, with rash, fever and rarely agranulocytosis, may develop after 2–6 weeks of therapy, and dapsone should be immediately withdrawn. HLA-B*13:01, which is present in Asian but not African populations, is a major risk factor for dapsone hypersensitivity.[35] Methemoglobinemia is a potential side effect of dapsone and should be considered where patients have symptoms or signs including skin discoloration, cyanosis, headache, lightheadedness, weakness, syncope and palpitations.

Rifampin

Rifampin (rifampicin) is a key component of MDT because it is the most effective bactericidal drug against *M. leprae* when given either daily or monthly.[1,11] Toxicity is low with monthly dosage, although thrombocytopenia, hepatitis and a flu-like syndrome occasionally occur. It must be used with at least one other effective drug to prevent rifampin resistance caused by mutations in RNA polymerase.[32] Tuberculosis should always be excluded before monthly rifampin is started (see Chapters 31 and 148). Rifapentine is a long acting rifamycin-derivative, which is more bactericidal than rifampin in mice, and is currently being tested in humans.

Clofazimine

This is a fat-soluble dye that is deposited within the skin, fat stores and macrophages. It has similar bactericidal activity to dapsone and also has a significant anti-inflammatory effect.[11] It is relatively nontoxic and its only disadvantage is the associated development of a reddish skin pigmentation, which resolves after the drug has been discontinued. When used in high doses for prolonged periods clofazimine is deposited in the small intestinal wall and can cause diarrhea and pain.

Other Drugs

Three additional drugs have proven effectiveness against *M. leprae* in human and mouse studies:[2,11]

- the fluoroquinolones, ofloxacin and moxifloxacin, have moderate bactericidal activity and infrequent side effects involving the gastrointestinal tract and central nervous system;
- minocycline, the only fat-soluble tetracycline, has moderate anti-*M. leprae* activity. It is effective as an alternative drug in patients with LL or dapsone hypersensitivity and has low toxicity in adults; and
- clarithromycin has modest bactericidal activity.

MULTIDRUG THERAPY

The principle underlying MDT is the use of three drugs when the bacterial load is high in MB leprosy to treat and prevent the emergence of dapsone-resistant strains. Two drugs are sufficient for paucibacillary

disease. Since its introduction in 1982,[1,2] MDT has proved highly effective and over 15 million patients have been treated with few treatment failures and remarkably low relapse rates of about 0.1/100 patient years.

Multibacillary Multidrug Therapy

This is recommended for adult patients with mid-borderline (BB), BL, LL, smear-positive BT and PN leprosy. In leprosy control programs in endemic countries, a simplified form of classification is employed, based on the number of patches so that MB leprosy has >5 patches and paucibacillary (PB) ≤5 patches. Multibacillary MDT comprises:

- rifampin, 600 mg once a month, supervised administration;
- dapsone, 100 mg/day, self-administered; and
- clofazimine, 300 mg once a month, supervised administration; 50 mg/day, self-administered.

Originally MB-MDT was continued for at least 2 years and then until the skin smears became negative.[1] In subsequent field trials a fixed duration of MB-MDT for 2 years was as effective as 2 years with very low rates of relapse. In 1998, WHO recommended MB-MDT of 12 months duration for use in control programs, and 12-month MB-MDT is currently used in leprosy control programs in endemic countries. This duration may not be sufficient for MB leprosy patients with a high bacterial index of 4+ or more, and these patients should receive 2 years of therapy.[2] Some authorities in high-income countries prefer to use more frequent doses of rifampin, but there is no evidence that daily rifampin is more effective than when given once monthly.[11]

If clofazimine is unacceptable because of pigmentation or if dapsone hypersensitivity occurs, minocycline (100 mg daily) or ofloxacin (400 mg daily) may be substituted.[2] Patients who have rifampin intolerance require two new drugs, minocycline and ofloxacin, along with clofazimine (50 mg/day) for 6 months and then either drug with clofazimine for another 18 months.

Paucibacillary Multidrug Therapy

This is recommended for indeterminate, TT and smear-negative BT leprosy[2] and in the control programs for patients with ≤5 patches. PB-MDT comprises:

- rifampin, 600 mg once a month, supervised administration; and
- dapsone, 100 mg/day, self-administered.

This is continued for 6 months. If the skin smear is positive at any site, the patient is given MB-MDT. If an RR develops after completion of chemotherapy, MDT should be recommended while on prednisone.

TREATMENT FOR REACTIONS

Patients who have RRs, including silent nerve function impairment, require high-dose corticosteroids for a prolonged duration to permit nerve function recovery. Prednisone is started at 40 mg/day and increased to 60 mg/day if there is no response, and then to 120 mg/day if necessary. Once there is evidence of improvement on serial voluntary muscle and sensory testing, the dose is reduced over 6 weeks to 20 mg/day and this is continued for some months before gradual removal. There are few clinical trials on the therapy for RRs, but one randomized study demonstrated that outcome is improved if corticosteroids are continued for at least 5 months.[36] Longer duration therapy is often required for RRs complicating MB leprosy. It is important to maintain treatment with antimycobacterial drugs to reduce the bacillary load. Adequate analgesia is essential along with physical support during the period of active neuritis. This therapy can be successfully administered without admission if other infections and medical problems are excluded. The overall recovery rate for nerve function is 60–70%, but may be higher in RR patients who have no nerve damage at diagnosis but develop acute neuropathy during MDT.[37] Recovery is less in patients with pre-existing nerve function impairment or with chronic or recurrent reactions.[27]

Mild ENL may respond to aspirin or nonsteroidal anti-inflammatory drugs, increased clofazimine dosage and rest. However, the majority of ENL patients with moderate or severe episodes and those with neuritis require prednisone, usually starting at 40–60 mg/day. The response is rapid, but as ENL is liable to become corticosteroid-dependent, the prednisone should be withdrawn over 2–3 months. Clofazimine at a higher daily dose of 300 mg suppresses ENL after 4–6 weeks, and can be used to prevent further episodes.[6]

If the ENL is poorly controlled or recurs, it usually responds to thalidomide, 400 mg/day for 2–3 weeks, and then 100–200 mg/day as maintenance.[38] Thalidomide inhibits the release of tumor necrosis factor from macrophages and modulates T-cell function, and showed prompt efficacy for ENL in clinical trials. Its use, however, is severely limited by its teratogenicity, and thalidomide should be restricted to male and postmenopausal patients under strict supervision. Thalidomide may cause a peripheral neuropathy, but this neurotoxic effect has not been evaluated in leprosy patients.

Eye involvement is common in leprosy and particularly in ENL, and iritis requires local treatment with corticosteroid and atropine drops.[30]

OTHER THERAPIES

Prevention of disability is an important component of individual care and an increasing focus for leprosy control programs, with defined targets for disability prevention.[2] Regular monitoring of nerve function will reveal early reversible RRs. Patients with irreversible nerve function impairment must learn to care for insensitive hands and feet and be provided with appropriate footwear. Plantar ulceration requires prolonged rest for healing. Physiotherapy and reconstructive surgery for claw hands or claw feet, foot drop and lagophthalmos may prevent further tissue damage and restore appearance, and facial deformity can be corrected by plastic surgery.[39] Community-based rehabilitation is proving effective in assisting patients with persistent nerve impairment to return to full participation in their own communities.[40]

Websites

- http://www.who.int/lep/: Provides access to WHO documents on the current epidemiology, clinical features and treatment of leprosy with detailed information on MDT and leprosy control.
- https://www.leprosy-information.org/: Website providing access to current leprosy information and publications including the Global Leprosy Strategy for 2016–2020.
- http://www.lepra.org.uk/leprosy-review: Website of *Leprosy Review* – a journal contributing to the better understanding of leprosy and its control.

References available online at expertconsult.com.

KEY REFERENCES

Britton W.J., Lockwood D.N.: Leprosy. *Lancet* 2004; 363:1209-1219.

Croft R.P., Nicholls P.G., Steyerberg E.W., et al.: A clinical prediction rule for nerve-function impairment in leprosy patients. *Lancet* 2000; 355:1603-1606.

Geluk A., Bobosha K., van der Ploeg-van Schip J.J., et al.: New biomarkers with relevance to leprosy diagnosis applicable in areas hyperendemic for leprosy. *J Immunol* 2012; 188:4782-4791.

Global leprosy update, 2013: reducing disease burden. Weekly Epidemiological Record No 36, 2014, 89, 389-400.

Liu H., Irwanto A., Fu X., et al.: Discovery of six new susceptibility loci and analysis of pleiotropic effects in leprosy. *Nat Genet* 2015; 47:267-271.

Monot M., Honoré N., Garnier T., et al.: Comparative genomic and phylogeographic analysis of *Mycobacterium leprae. Nat Genet* 2009; 41:1282-1289.

Schuenemann V.J., Singh P., Mendum T.A., et al.: Genome-wide comparison of medieval and modern *Mycobacterium leprae. Science* 2013; 341:179-183.

Scollard D.M., Adams L.B., Gillis T.P., et al.: The continuing challenges of leprosy. *Clin Microbiol Rev* 2006; 19:338-381.

Setia M.S., Steinmaus C., Ho C.S., et al.: The role of BCG in prevention of leprosy: a meta-analysis. *Lancet Infect Dis* 2006; 6:162-170.

Moet F.J., Pahan D., Oskam L., et al.: Effectiveness of single dose rifampicin in preventing leprosy in close contacts of patients with newly diagnosed leprosy: cluster randomised controlled trial. *BMJ* 2008; 336:761-764.

Truman R.W., Singh P., Sharma R., et al.: Probable zoonotic leprosy in the southern United States. *N Engl J Med* 2011; 364:1626-1633.

Walker S.L., Waters M.F., Lockwood D.N.: The role of thalidomide in the management of erythema nodosum leprosum. *Lepr Rev* 2007; 78:197-215.

World Health Organization Expert Committee on Leprosy, 8th report. World Health Organization Technical Report Series No 968, 1-61. Geneva: WHO; 2012.

van Brakel W.H., Nicholls P.G., Wilder-Smith E.P., et al.: Early diagnosis of neuropathy in leprosy-comparing diagnostic tests in a large prospective study (the INFIR Cohort Study). *PLoS Negl Trop Dis* 2008; 2:e212.

Van Veen N.H., Nicholls P.G., Smith W.C., et al.: Corticosteroids for treating nerve damage in leprosy. *Cochrane Database Syst Rev* 2007; CD005491.

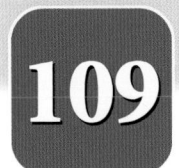

109

Endemic Treponematoses

NICK J. BEECHING

KEY CONCEPTS

- The endemic treponematoses include yaws (*Treponema pallidum* subsp. *pertenue*), endemic syphilis (*T. pallidum* subsp. *endemicum*) and pinta (*T. carateum*), which predominantly affect children in poor, rural areas of the tropics and, formerly, south east Europe.

- Although control programs have been successful in many countries since the 1940s, yaws remains a significant problem in several countries in Oceania and West Africa.

- The endemic treponematoses are transmitted by direct contact or sharing eating utensils, and do not cause venereal or congenital infections.

- They have distinct clinical presentations, with primary, secondary and late stages analogous to syphilis, with severe destructive skin, mucosal and bone lesions in late stage disease.

- Diagnosis is largely clinical, supported by the different geographical location of each disease.

- Conventional reaginic and specific treponemal tests cannot distinguish between the endemic treponematoses or syphilis. Point-of-care tests developed for syphilis are being validated for field diagnoses of the endemic treponematoses.

- Recent advances in molecular tests have yielded multiplex polymerase chain reaction (PCR) assays to support diagnosis of individual endemic treponemal infections and to monitor for possible azithromycin resistance.

- Treatment and control programs previously relied on parenteral benzathine or oral penicillin, but this has been replaced by single oral doses of azithromycin as the treatment of choice for infected individuals and contacts.

- In 2012 the World Health Organization (WHO) endorsed a new program to eliminate the endemic treponematoses by 2020.

- Clinicians in non-endemic areas should be aware of the possibility of positive 'syphilis' serology caused by endemic treponematoses in migrants from affected countries, and should consider these infections in arrivals with unusual skin or destructive gummatous lesions.

Introduction

The endemic treponematoses include yaws (also known as buba, framboesia, parangi and pian), endemic syphilis (also known as bejel, dichuchwa and sklerjevo) and pinta (also known as azul, carate and mal de pinto), all of which are chronic bacterial infections. The causative organisms (*Treponema pallidum* subsp. *pertenue*, *T. pallidum* subsp. *endemicum* and *T. carateum*, respectively) are morphologically and serologically indistinguishable from *T. pallidum* subsp. *pallidum*, which is the causative organism of venereal syphilis.[1-3]

In the 1990s, small genetic differences (single base pair changes) were identified between the organisms of the venereal and nonvenereal treponematoses but these genetic variations did not allow differentiation of one *T. pallidum* subsp. from another. Recent molecular genetic studies indicate that *T. pallidum* subsp. *pallidum*, subsp. *pertenue*, subsp. *endemicum* and a simian *T. pallidum* (Fribourg–Blanc) strain can be differentiated through subspecies-specific genetic signatures in multiple genes.[4-6]

A phylogenetic analysis indicates that *T. pallidum* subsp. *pertenue* arose first in history causing yaws in our anthropoid ancestors in the tropical belt of the Old World; it spread as yaws to the New World and as endemic syphilis to North Africa, Eastern Europe and the Middle East (through divergence of subsp. *pertenue* to subsp. *endemicum*). It finally evolved in the Americas as the modern subsp. *pallidum* strain (or a progenitor), which was introduced into the Old World as a result of the European exploration of the Americas, and disseminated as venereal syphilis all over the world.[5]

Nevertheless, in clinical practice the treponematoses (venereal and nonvenereal) continue to be diagnosed based on their distinctive clinical and epidemiologic characteristics (Table 109-1).[1,3]

Epidemiology

HISTORIC PERSPECTIVE

The endemic treponematoses, because of the disfigurement and disability they cause, were a major public health problem in the pre-antibiotic era. In 1948, the WHO and the United Nations International Children's Emergency Fund (UNICEF) sponsored a global control program. This involved 46 countries and brought these diseases under control with the help of long-acting penicillin. However, eradication was not achieved and although mandatory reporting has become patchy, yaws has increased in foci in the Pacific and West Africa. The WHO convened a meeting in 2012 and has now resolved to eliminate yaws by 2020, based on changes in programmatic approaches using single dose oral therapy with azithromycin.[7]

GEOGRAPHIC DISTRIBUTION

The endemic treponematoses are now largely confined to communities in remote rural areas living in poor, overcrowded and unhygienic conditions (Figure 109-1). Yaws occurs mainly in the warm, humid areas of Africa, South East Asia and the Pacific, the Caribbean and Central and South America. India successfully eliminated yaws in 2006; yaws now remains present only in two southeast Asian countries – Indonesia and Timor-Leste.[8] Endemic syphilis occurs mainly in the arid areas of sub-Saharan Africa and among the nomadic people of the Arabian peninsula. Pinta occurs mainly in Central and South America (among Indian tribes in the Amazon region and adjacent areas). Cases of imported yaws and endemic syphilis are sometimes encountered in the countries of the northern hemisphere, where clinicians may need to include them in the differential diagnosis.

Incidence and Prevalence

Accurate incidence and prevalence data are unavailable, with only 14 countries out of over 90 previously endemic for yaws providing recent systematic data. The last full estimate by WHO in 1995 yielded a global prevalence of 2.5 million cases, including 460 000 infectious cases. The true situation today remains unknown but in the last decade there has been a resurgence of yaws with over 20 000 cases reported annually in Papua New Guinea, the Solomon Isles and Ghana and continued transmission in Vanuatu.[7]

AGE AND SEX

Yaws and endemic syphilis usually occur in children aged 2–14 years. For pinta the range is 10–30 years. Yaws affects boys more than girls; for the other diseases there is probably no sex difference.

TABLE 109-1	Overview of Treponemal Infections					
Disease	**Organism**	**Endemic Areas**	**Primary Lesion**	**Secondary Lesions**	**Tertiary Lesions**	**Congenital Infection**
Venereal syphilis	*Treponema pallidum* subsp. *pallidum*	Worldwide	Chancre, usually in anogenital region	Mucocutaneous lesions (condylomata lata, papules, macules or maculopapules) Visceral involvement Central nervous system (CNS) involvement (usually aseptic meningitis)	Gummas, including CNS Carditis/aortitis Neurosyphilis (meningovascular, tabes, paresis)	Yes
Yaws	*Treponema pallidum* subsp. *pertenue*	Rural areas of Africa, Central and South America, the Caribbean, equatorial islands of South East Asia and remote parts of India and Thailand	Papule Papilloma Ulcer, usually on an extremity	Diffuse papules, papillomas and ulcers Osteitis Dactylitis	Destructive gummas of skin and bone	No
Pinta	*Treponema carateum*	Underdeveloped rural areas of Mexico and northern South America	Erythematous papule, usually on an extremity	Scaly papules Areas of altered skin pigmentation	Areas of altered skin pigmentation Hyperkeratosis	No
Endemic bejel	*Treponema pallidum* subsp. *endemicum*	West Africa, small foci in Zimbabwe, Botswana, Arabian peninsula and central Australia	Oral mucosal ulcer	Oral and pharyngeal ulcers Mucous patches Condyloma lata Periostitis	Gummas of skin, bone and joints	No

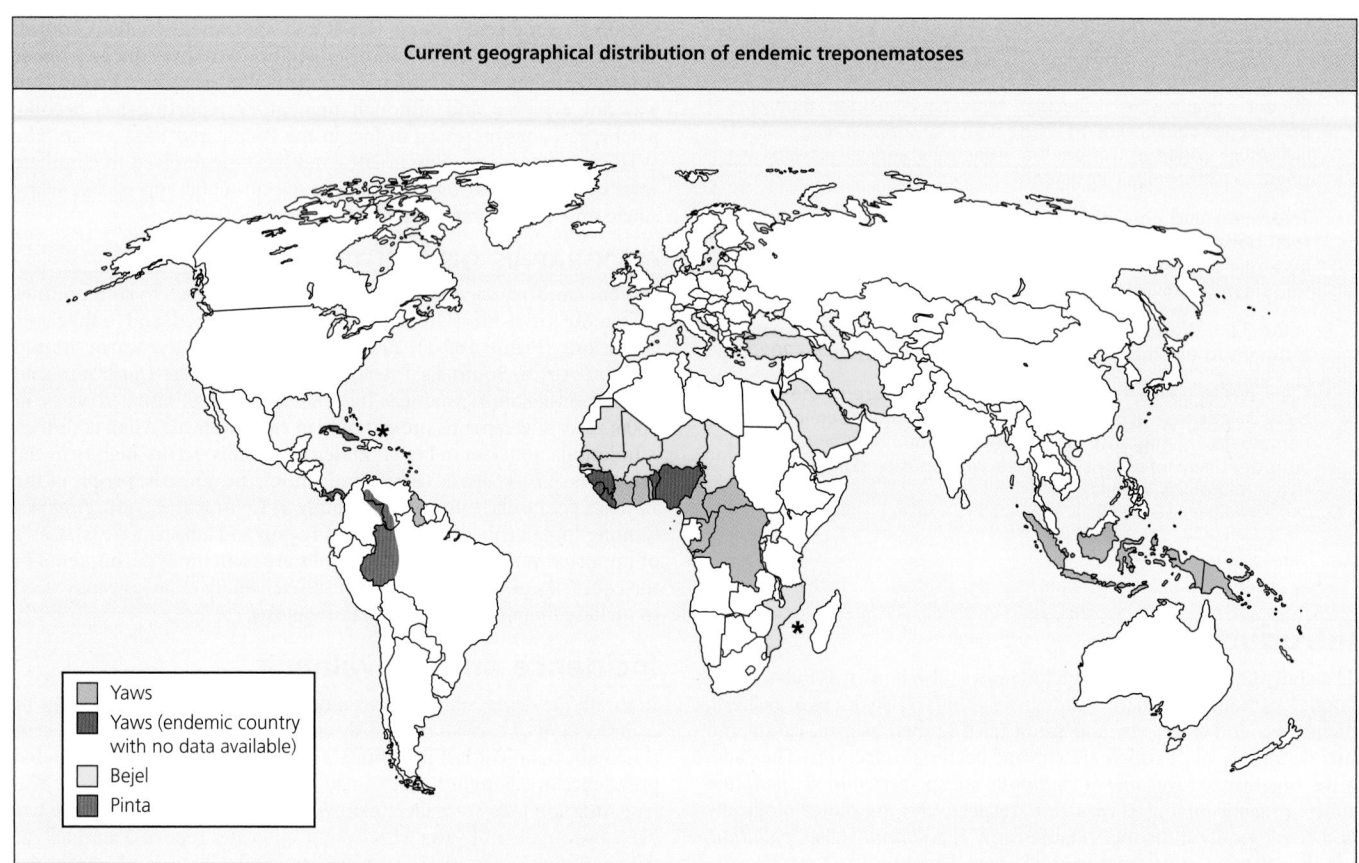

Figure 109-1 Current geographical distribution of endemic treponematoses. *Based on isolated case reports, but otherwise considered free of disease. (Adapted with permission from Giacani L., Lukehart S.A. Clin Microbiol Rev 2014; 27(1):89-115.)

MODE OF TRANSMISSION

Yaws and pinta are transmitted by direct skin-to-skin contact with infectious lesions, transmission being facilitated by a breach in the skin of the recipient. The role of nonbiting flies in the transmission is uncertain. In the case of endemic syphilis, because the initial lesions are often in or around the mouth, the infection spreads by direct contact (e.g. older children kissing their younger siblings) and by indirect contact through infected communal eating or drinking utensils.

Pathology

Yaws and endemic syphilis affect skin and bones, whereas pinta is confined to the skin.

The basic pathology in endemic treponematoses is the same as in venereal syphilis. However, the vascular changes in the endemic treponematoses are less marked. Skin biopsies from yaws patients show numerous plasma cells but few T and B cells; the treponemes are found mostly in the epidermis, whereas in venereal syphilis they are demonstrated mainly in the dermis and dermal–epidermal junction.[9] Because these differences are relative, they cannot be used to differentiate yaws from venereal syphilis.

In pinta, there is loss of melanin in basal cells, the presence of many melanophages in the dermis and the absence of inflammatory cells and treponemes in the achromic lesions.

Endemic treponematoses are not believed to be associated with congenital transmission or with involvement of the cardiovascular and nervous systems.

Prevention

It is essential not only to identify and treat clinical cases but also to recognize that the presence of clinical cases in a community necessitates an immediate search for further clinical and latent cases, which also must be treated. Treatment with penicillin or azithromycin rapidly renders patients noninfectious.

The supportive measures for control include:

- strengthening and improving accessibility of the primary health-care facilities;
- training of health workers to diagnose and treat cases, and in surveillance, health promotion and implementation of the new strategy;
- training of schoolteachers and village volunteers to recognize and refer cases, and assist in health promotion and treatment activities;
- information, education and communication, and health promotion in communities and schools;
- community engagement and involvement of chiefs and other opinion leaders;
- improvement in the standard of living and in personal and environmental hygiene; and
- provision of soap and water and clothing to children.

The current WHO approach includes an initial phase of mass azithromycin treatment of whole communities where treponematoses are endemic, to eliminate both clinical and subclinical cases. Following this, there is targeted treatment of all cases detected clinically or during follow-up serosurveys of affected communities, together with all their contacts.[7]

Clinical Features

The incubation period is 9–90 days (mean 21 days).

YAWS

Early Stage

The initial or primary lesion ('mother yaw') appears at the site of infection on an exposed part of the body. It may be a localized maculopapular eruption or a papule, which may develop into a large papilloma 2–5 cm in diameter. It is painless but itchy and may ulcerate as

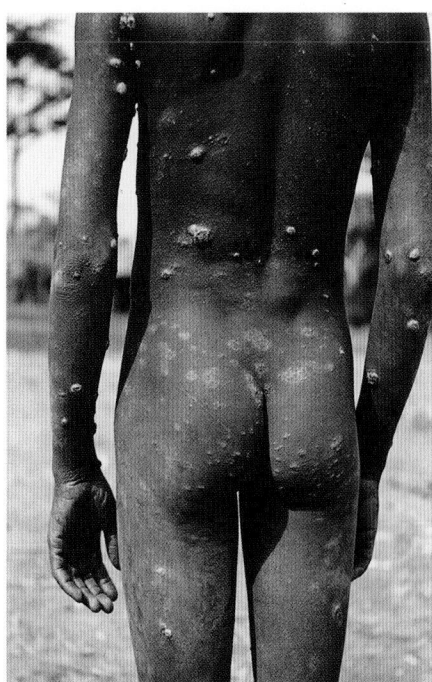

Figure 109-2 Mixed early yaws lesions: papillomata, ulceropapillomatous lesions and squamous macules. *(Courtesy of WHO, Geneva.)*

a result of scratching. It may heal in 3–6 months with or without scarring. Secondary lesions, which are the result of lymphatic and hematogenous spread of organisms, appear a few weeks to 2 years after the primary lesion. They may consist of multiple excrescences, often resembling the initial papilloma. The papillomas may ulcerate and the exudate may dry to form a yellow crust which, when removed, gives the lesion an appearance of a raspberry (hence the name 'framboesia'). The lesions may be irregular, crescentic or discoid in shape and on moist areas may mimic condylomata lata of venereal syphilis. They are rather florid and become more numerous in the rainy season (Figure 109-2). They may last up to 6 months and heal with or without scarring. Infectious relapses may occur for 5 years and, rarely, for 10 years.

Other manifestations include:
- regional lymphadenopathy;
- palmar and plantar lesions, which may be painful, resulting in a crab-like gait; and
- osteoperiostitis of the proximal phalanges of the fingers (dactylitis) or of long bones, causing nocturnal bone pains.

The patient may at any time enter latency, with only serologic evidence of the infection.

Late Stage

About 10% of patients develop late lesions after 5 years or more of untreated infection. The late stage is characterized by gummatous lesions of skin, bones and overlying tissues. The manifestations, some of which also occur in early stage disease but are now more destructive, include:
- hyperkeratosis of palms and soles with deep fissuring;
- juxta-articular subcutaneous nodules;
- more extensive osteoperiostitis of long bones (e.g. sabre tibiae);
- hyperostosis of the nasal processes of the maxillae ('goundou'); and
- ulceration of the palate and nasopharynx (rhinopharyngitis mutilans, 'gangosa'; Figure 109-3) with secondary infection resulting in foul-smelling discharge.

ENDEMIC SYPHILIS

The primary lesion is seldom seen. The early manifestations include mucous patches (i.e. shallow painless ulcers on the lips and in the

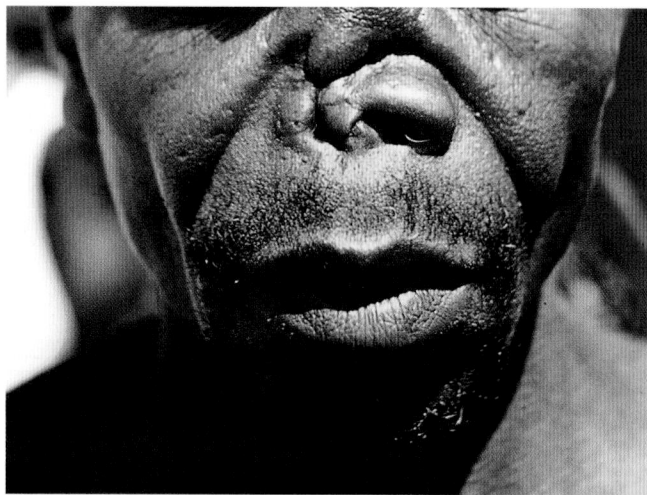

Figure 109-3 Gangosa in late stage of yaws (rhinopharyngitis mutilans; occurs also in endemic syphilis). *(Courtesy of WHO, Geneva.)*

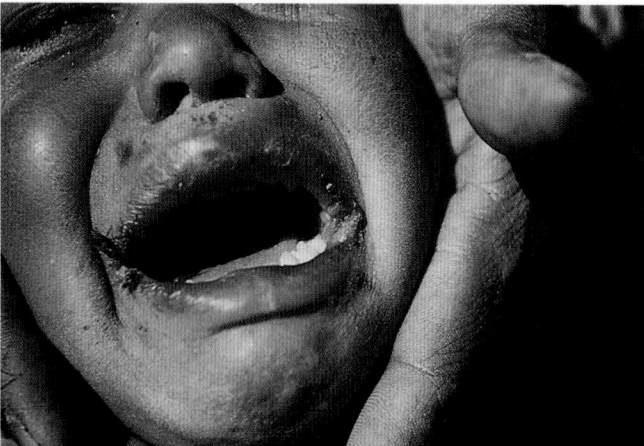

Figure 109-4 Angular stomatitis (also called split papules) of endemic syphilis; these lesions are also found in early yaws. *(Courtesy of Dr G.M. Antal.)*

oropharynx) and other mucocutaneous and bone lesions resembling those of venereal syphilis and yaws. Papillomata favor warm and moist areas and occur as split papules or angular stomatitis at the labial commissures (Figure 109-4). Later, the patient may enter the latent phase, which may be prolonged; after this some patients develop late lesions, which are similar to those seen in yaws.

PINTA

Pinta is confined to the skin and is the mildest of all treponematoses. The primary lesion, appearing at the site of entry of *T. carateum* on an exposed part of the body, is an itchy, red, scaly papule, sometimes associated with satellite lesions and regional lymphadenopathy. The secondary stage develops several months later, in other areas, with the appearance of pintids, which are similar to the initial lesions. These are also itchy. In due course, they undergo a variety of color changes from red to copper-colored, gray and bluish-black. The lesions remain infectious for many years.

The late lesions are characterized by varying degrees of hypochromia, discoloration, atrophy and achromia. Sometimes these features are seen in the same area.

ATTENUATED ENDEMIC TREPONEMATOSES

In areas of reduced transmission, the clinical expression of endemic treponematoses can be much milder (a few or even a single papilloma) or many of the infected subjects can be asymptomatic.[1,10] In the

Gambia, 9.3% of pregnant women were seropositive for a treponemal infection; children of seropositive mothers showed no signs of congenital syphilis and there was no increase in perinatal, neonatal or child deaths. No clinical signs of endemic treponematoses were found, indicating the asymptomatic nature of the infection.[11,12]

In a number of countries of West and Central Africa, high prevalence rates for syphilis have been found in pregnant women based on rapid treponemal tests; clinical cases of endemic treponematoses (yaws or bejel) are not reported or not known to exist in those areas. A serosurvey in children 2–15 years of age could help to indicate that this seroreaction is probably due to past (asymptomatic) endemic treponematoses or might be venereal (latent) syphilis.

HIV INFECTION AND ENDEMIC TREPONEMATOSES

As yet, no information is available on any interaction between HIV infection and endemic treponematoses.

Differential Diagnosis

In endemic areas, an accurate clinical diagnosis can be made in the presence of classic lesions. This will, however, necessitate appropriate training of clinicians, especially in view of the rather milder forms being encountered. The difficulties arise when there are no clinical lesions (i.e. latent cases), when venereal syphilis is also locally prevalent and when the patient is an immigrant from an endemic area presenting at a clinic in a non-endemic country. Differentiation from venereal syphilis is important because of social stigma implications. A careful and detailed history (including that of mother, father and siblings when appropriate) and thorough physical examination are always essential. Recent surveys in Vanuatu and Ghana have shown coexistence of skin lesions caused by *Haemophilus ducreyi* in communities affected by yaws, and differentiation of these is problematic without adequate diagnostic tests.[13,14]

Apart from venereal syphilis, the conditions to be considered for differential diagnosis include:

- skin sepsis, *Haemophilus ducreyi* infection, scabies, fungal infection, leprosy, lichen planus, plantar warts, psoriasis and tungiasis in a patient who has early skin lesions;
- tropical ulcer, mucocutaneous or cutaneous leishmaniasis, mycotic lesions, tuberculosis and leprosy in a patient who has gummatous ulceration; and
- tuberculosis and sickle cell disease in a patient who has dactylitis.

Pinta may need to be differentiated from pityriasis versicolor, tinea corporis, vitiligo, leprosy and chloasma.

Diagnosis

There is no test that can differentiate the treponematoses (including venereal syphilis) from one another in routine practice. The diagnosis of treponemal infection is confirmed by the demonstration of treponemes (but beware of nonpathogenic commensals) in a wet preparation of the material from early lesions by darkfield microscopy or in the biopsy material stained by the silver impregnation technique.

Serologic tests – rapid plasma reagin (RPR) or non-treponemal antibody tests, *T. pallidum* hemagglutination assay (TPHA), *T. pallidum* particle agglutination assay (TPPA) or fluorescent treponemal antibody absorption (FTA-ABS) treponemal (i.e. specific) tests – should be carried out in all cases, but their interpretation requires expertise. The treponemal tests are particularly useful to confirm a reactive non-treponemal test (exclusion of false-positives). A reactive treponemal test may indicate a current infection or a past infection ('serologic scar'). Simple and rapid point-of-care treponemal tests became recently available in the form of immunochromatographic strips; as they can use whole blood and do not require refrigeration they are extremely useful in the field.[15] While they have not been fully evaluated for diagnosis of endemic treponematoses, rapid diagnostic tests using both reaginic and specific treponemal test panels have shown excellent specificity (but reduced sensitivity) for the diagnosis of yaws in the Solomon Islands. Sensitivity is improved in individuals with higher serum RPR titers.[16] Real time quadriplex PCR assays for the four subspecies of *T. pallidum* have been used successfully to diagnose cases of yaws in Vanuatu.[17] Importantly, these assays were used successfully on samples stored on absorbed filter paper eluates (FTA Elute card), so that field surveys can be supported by specialist reference laboratories. The same team also reported on the use of a triplex PCR assay to detect mutations in the 23S rRNA genes associated with azithromycin resistance in *T. pallidum* subspecies *pallidum*. This will be important for monitoring possible emergence of azithromycin resistance in nonvenereal treponematoses, as has been seen in venereal syphilis. In the future, direct sequencing of DNA extracted from skin samples should become possible, but requires access to sophisticated laboratory support.[5]

Radiologic evidence of osteoperiostitis may assist in the diagnosis of dactylitis and tibial diseases.

If the differentiation from venereal syphilis is difficult, the patient should be managed as for venereal syphilis. This is particularly important in pregnant women, because of the severe fetal outcomes of untreated venereal syphilis in pregnancy (see Chapter 61).

Management

Until recently, parenteral penicillin was the drug of choice, using lower doses than conventionally used to treat venereal syphilis. Long-acting benzathine penicillin G, given intramuscularly in a single session, was preferred. The dose is 600 000 units for children under the age of 6 years, 1.2 million units for those aged 6–15 years and 2.4 million units for those over 15 years old. The dose may be divided, half to be given into each buttock. While it is recognized that treponematoses have remained exquisitely sensitive to penicillin, there is a report of penicillin treatment failures of yaws in Papua New Guinea.[18] A few penicillin treatment failures have also been observed in Ecuador.[19]

The distinction between relapse, re-infection or true resistance is difficult to make but these clinical failures are worrisome and should be further researched. Oral penicillin V (50 mg/kg in four divided doses) for 10 days was used in rural Guyana resulting in cure in 16 out of 17 children with yaws.[20] However, such a regimen with multiple doses has a potential adherence problem and is not suitable as an epidemiologic treatment (e.g. in elimination campaigns).

Penicillin has now been replaced by azithromycin as the drug of choice – single doses have been shown to be as effective as benzathine penicillin in treatment of yaws, although trial data are not available for the other endemic treponematoses.[21] Single dose oral therapy overcomes treatment compliance problems and obviates the difficulties of parenteral administration. It is also safe in children and in pregnant women, and there is good experience of its use in trachoma elimination campaigns. The possible emergence of azithromycin resistance should be monitored.[17] The usual azithromycin dose is 30 mg/kg, simplified to a maximum of 2 g (four tablets). For children, the regimen is simplified for field use to 500 mg for those under 6 years of age (for whom syrup is preferred), 1 g for ages 6–9, 1.5 g for those aged 10–15 and 2 g for all over 15 years old.[7]

CONTACTS

Arrangements should be made to examine and, if appropriate and after proper explanation, to treat the household contacts and other close contacts. This is equally important in the rare cases seen in nonendemic settings.

PROGNOSIS AND FOLLOW-UP

The lesions become noninfectious within 24 hours of treatment. Whereas treatment in early stages should result in cure in almost 100% of patients, it will not reverse any destructive change in late stages. RPR (or non-treponemal antibody test) titers should decline within 6–12 months, becoming negative in about 2 years. However, in a small proportion of cases, especially if treated in late stages, the RPR (or non-treponemal antibody test) may remain positive, albeit in low titer (below 1 : 8). The specific tests (i.e. TPHA, TPPA, FTA-ABS, rapid treponemal tests) will remain positive throughout life.

ACKNOWLEDGMENTS

This chapter is updated from chapters authored in previous editions by André Z. Mehues, Jai P. Narain and Kingsley B. Asiedu, and a practice point chapter previously authored by Juan Carlos Salazar.

References available online at expertconsult.com.

KEY REFERENCES

Chi K.H., Danavall D., Taleo F., et al.: Molecular differentiation of *Treponema pallidum* subspecies in skin ulceration clinically suspected as yaws in Vanuatu using real-time multiplex PCR and serological methods. *Am J Trop Med Hyg* 2015; 92(1):134-138.

Ghinai R., El-Duah P., Chi K.H., et al.: A cross-sectional study of 'yaws' in districts of Ghana which have previously undertaken azithromycin mass drug administration for trachoma control. *PLoS Negl Trop Dis* 2015; 9(1):e0003496.

Giacani L., Lukehart S.A.: The endemic treponematoses. *Clin Microbiol Rev* 2014; 27(1):89-115.

Herring A.J., Ballard R.C., Pope V., et al.: A multi-centre evaluation of nine rapid, point-of-care syphilis tests using archived sera. *Sex Transm Infect* 2006; 82(Suppl. 5):v7-v12.

Marks M., Goncalves A., Vahi V., et al.: Evaluation of a rapid diagnostic test for yaws infection in a community surveillance setting. *PLoS Negl Trop Dis* 2014; 8(9):e3156.

Marks M., Solomon A.W., Mabey D.C.: The endemic treponematoses. *Trans R Soc Trop Med Hyg* 2014; 108:601-607.

Mitjà O., Asiedu K., Mabey D.: Yaws. *Lancet* 2013; 381:763-773.

Mitjà O., Houinei W., Moses P., et al.: Mass treatment with single dose azithromycin for yaws. *N Engl J Med* 2015; 372:703-710.

Mitjà O., Šmajs D., Bassat Q.: Advances in the diagnosis of endemic treponematoses: yaws, bejel, and pinta. *PLoS Negl Trop Dis* 2013; 7(10):e2283.

Staudová B., Strouhal M., Zobaníková M., et al.: Whole genome sequence of the *Treponema pallidum* subsp. *endemicum* strain Bosnia A: the genome is related to yaws treponemes but contains few loci similar to syphilis treponemes. *PLoS Negl Trop Dis* 2014; 8(11):e3261.

World Health Organization: Summary report of a consultation on the eradication of yaws: 5–7 March 2012, Morges, Switzerland.

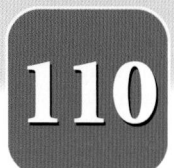

110

Human African Trypanosomiasis

CHRISTIAN BURRI | JOHANNES BLUM

KEY CONCEPTS

- Human African trypanosomiasis (HAT) (or sleeping sickness) is caused by two subspecies of the protozoan parasite *Trypanosoma brucei* transmitted by tsetse flies leading to two distinct and fatal diseases if untreated, in rural West and Central, and East and Southern Africa, respectively.

- Both forms of the disease undergo two distinct disease phases with different clinical signs and symptoms requiring different treatment: a first hemolymphatic and a second central stage after invasion by the parasite of the central nervous system (CNS).

- The diagnosis of *T.b. gambiense* HAT (Western African form) follows the pathway of serological screening, diagnostic confirmation and staging followed by treatment decision. The first step is omitted in the East African form, *T.b. rhodesiense*.

- Recently, major advances in the chemotherapy of the disease have been made and recommendations for treatment in this edition differ substantially from the previous editions.

- Nifurtimox–eflornithine combination therapy (NECT) was included in WHO's Essential Medicines List in 2009 and replaces melarsoprol as first-line treatment for second-stage *T.b. gambiense* HAT. An abridged treatment regimen for melarsoprol treatment of second-stage *T.b. rhodesiense* was recommended in 2009.

- The disease can be kept under control by passive and active surveillance of the population and identification of patients, followed by treatment, and by tsetse fly control using insecticides and traps.

Epidemiology

Human African trypanosomiasis (HAT) (or sleeping sickness) is caused by two subspecies of the extracellular protozoan parasite *Trypanosoma brucei* (Figure 110-1) which lead to diseases with distinct clinical and epidemiological patterns. *T.b. gambiense* causes a chronic form in Central and West Africa and represents >95% of all cases, while *T.b. rhodesiense* is responsible for a more acute disease form in East and Southern Africa (Figure 110-2 and Table 110-1). Thirty-one different species of tsetse flies (*Glossina* spp.) transmit the parasites while taking a blood meal.[1,2] Transmission of *T.b. gambiense* is linked to species favoring riverine vegetation (Figure 110-3) whereas *T.b. rhodesiense* is typically transmitted in woodland savanna habitats (Figure 110-4).[3] Trypanosomiasis caused by *T.b. rhodesiense* is a zoonosis with the main reservoirs either in cattle or game animals whereas *T.b. gambiense* is mainly anthroponotic.[4] The interrelationships between host, vector and parasite leads to a rural and highly focal geographical distribution of HAT.[5]

Both disease forms have a noticeable ability to break out in the absence of control measures. Systematic population screening by mobile teams followed by treatment had reduced the reported cases to 4000 by 1960; however, the collapse of health systems, environmental changes and conflicts led to resurgence to 25 000 reported cases per year and an estimated prevalence of 300 000 by 1998. Under the coordination of WHO, control measures increased significantly and the annual number of cases was brought down to a reported 6631 and 20 000 estimated in 2011.[5] In 2011 the elimination by 2020 of HAT as a public health problem was included in the WHO's roadmap of neglected tropical diseases.[6]

Pathogenesis

Sleeping sickness produces multiple pathological changes that involve most organs and systems. The damage results from a complex interplay of parasite and host factors.

A variant surface glycoprotein (VSG) coat covering the membrane of African trypanosomes protects them from lytic factors in human plasma and allows them to escape the host immune reaction.[3] In addition, trypanosomiasis is associated with general induction of immunosuppression; a recently described protein, the trypanosome suppressive immunomodulatory factor, has been postulated to play a role in immunosuppression.[5]

The second stage of infection is characterized by invasion of the central nervous system (CNS) which occurs weeks to months (*T.b. rhodesiense*) or months to years (*T.b. gambiense*) after initial infection. The invasion of the brain by trypanosomes occurs via the choroid plexus and the subsequent brain dysfunction observed in second-stage HAT is due to a complex and only partially understood interplay of parasite- and host-derived factors.[7,8] The parasites cause a lymphocytic meningoencephalitis, which particularly affects the brain stem, although cortical areas and the cerebellum are also involved. Perivascular infiltration with lymphocytes, plasma cells, macrophages and characteristic morular cells occurs; microglia and astrocytes proliferate and there is neuronal destruction and demyelination.

Prevention

Individual prophylaxis aims at preventing contact with tsetse flies or being bitten by them. Tsetse flies occur close to certain types of

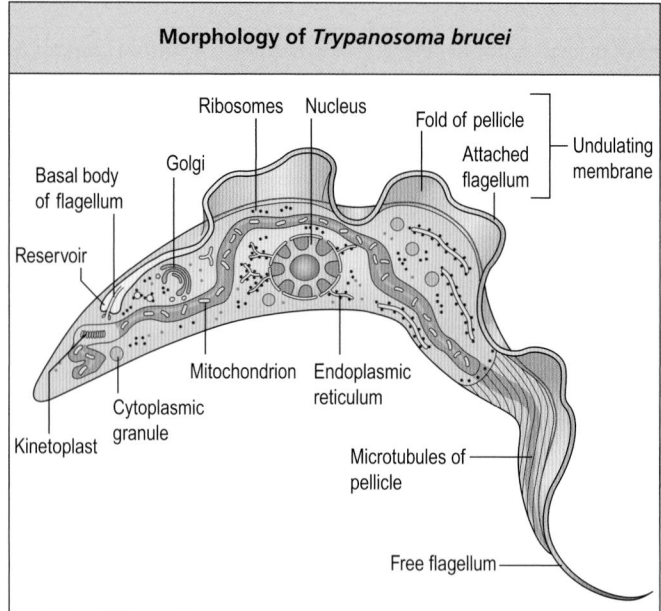

Figure 110-1 Morphology of *Trypanosoma brucei*. (*Reproduced with permission from Apted F.I.C.: Treatment of human trypanosomiasis. In: Mulligan H.W., ed. The African trypanosomiasis. London: Allen & Unwin; 1970:684–710.*)

TABLE 110-1	Differences Between *T.b. gambiense* and *T.b. rhodesiense* Sleeping Sickness	
	West African *T.b. gambiense*	East African *T.b. rhodesiense*
Parasite	*Trypanosoma brucei gambiense*	*Trypanosoma brucei rhodesiense*
Main vectors	*Glossina palpalis* group	*Glossina morsitans* group
Main habitat	Near water	Savanna, cleared bush
Highest incidence	Central African Republic, Democratic Republic of the Congo, South Sudan, north Uganda	South-east Uganda, Tanzania
Main reservoir	Humans, pig, dog	Antelope and cattle
Disease type	Chronic (years)	Acute (months)
Parasitemia	Low	Moderate
Diagnosis	Lymph node aspiration, blood (concentration methods) CSF (lumbar puncture)	Blood CSF (lumbar puncture)
Serology	CATT	None
Treatment First stage Second stage Alternative treatment	Pentamidine Nifurtimox-Eflornithine Combination Therapy (NECT) (Melarsoprol, Eflornithine)	Suramin Melarsoprol (Melarsoprol and nifurtimox)
Disease control	Active case search, treatment, tsetse trapping	Tsetse trapping, treatment

Adapted from Pepin J.: African trypanosomiasis. In: Strickland G.T., ed. *Hunter's tropical medicine and emerging infectious diseases,* 8th ed. Philadelphia: Saunders; 2000.643–654.

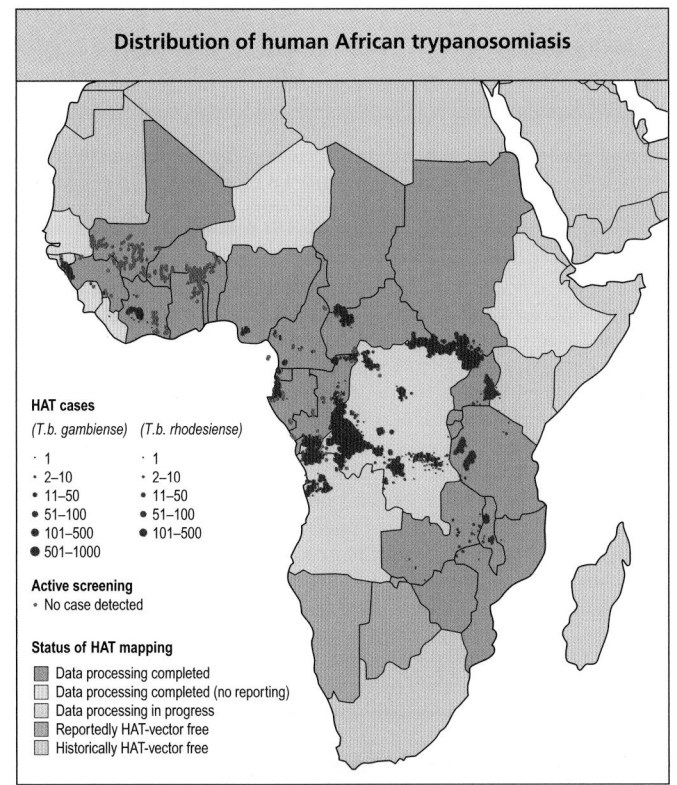

Distribution of human African trypanosomiasis

HAT cases

(T.b. gambiense) (T.b. rhodesiense)

· 1   · 1
· 2–10   · 2–10
• 11–50   • 11–50
• 51–100   • 51–100
• 101–500   • 101–500
• 501–1000

Active screening
· No case detected

Status of HAT mapping
Data processing completed
Data processing completed (no reporting)
Data processing in progress
Reportedly HAT-vector free
Historically HAT-vector free

Figure 110-2 Distribution of human African trypanosomiasis. *(Reproduced with permission from WHO: Control and surveillance of African trypanosomiasis. Geneva: WHO; 1998:1–114.)*

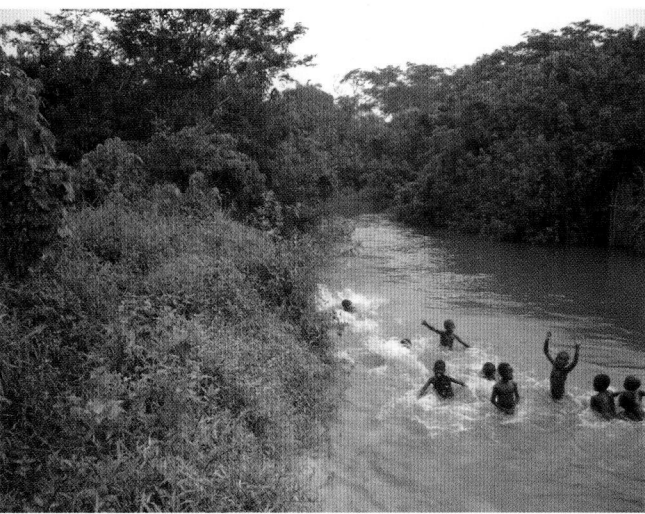

Figure 110-3 Typical place of transmission of *T.b. gambiense* where human–fly contact is high; habitat of *Glossina palpalis*. *(Source: Christian Burri [Swiss Tropical and Public Health Institute]: Kikongotanga, Democratic Republic of the Congo.)*

The most important control measure for *T.b. gambiense* trypanosomiasis is active case-finding by so-called mobile teams, followed by treatment of the infected subjects. For screening the card agglutination test for trypanosomiasis (CATT) has become a routine tool and CATT-positive patients are subjected to the full diagnostic pathways. However, in view of the low disease prevalence and need to strive for elimination, these strategies are insufficient. The newly available rapid diagnostic tests and the drugs under development provide an opportunity to extend surveillance, diagnosis and treatment to the public health system.

Reducing vector density through vector control with traps, bush clearing and spraying of pesticides is a second powerful tool in the control of HAT. Traps are made of blue and black cloth (which are the most attractive colors for tsetse flies), often treated with insecticides or complemented with baiting host odors.[5]

vegetation (e.g. *Lantana* sp.) or to water (e.g. along rivers in gallery forests). Such 'hot spots' should be avoided, thus reducing the risk of contact with the flies. The use of repellents may be considered but it is known that their protection is limited. Tsetse flies like to follow large moving objects such as cars.

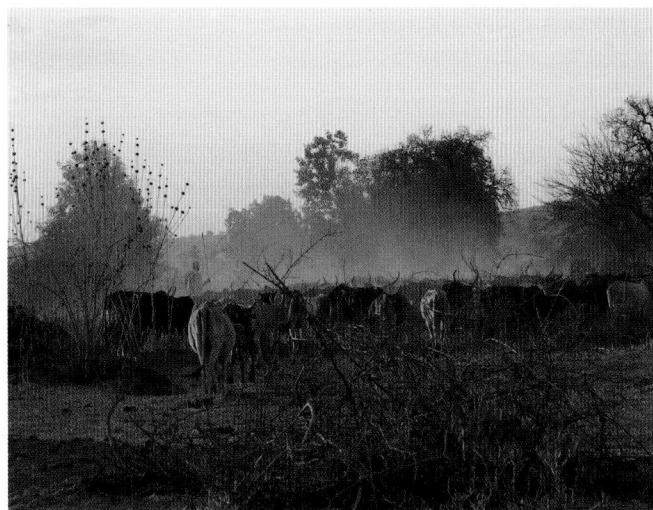

Figure 110-4   Typical place of transmission of *T.b. rhodesiense*; habitat of *Glossina morsitans*. (Source: Irene Küpfer [Swiss Tropical and Public Health Institute]: Urambo District, Tanzania.)

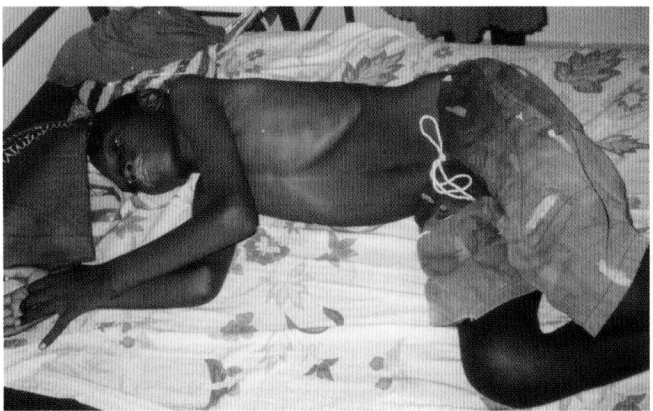

Figure 110-5   Patient with advanced second-stage *T.b. gambiense* infection. (Source: Christian Burri [Swiss Tropical and Public Health Institute]; Viana, Angola.)

Clinical Features

The clinical presentation of HAT depends on the parasite species, the stage of the disease and on the host. The signs and symptoms that characterize sleeping sickness are generally the same for both forms of the disease but differ in their frequency, severity and kinetics of appearance.

ENDEMIC COUNTRIES

T.b. gambiense *HAT*

T.b. gambiense HAT is characterized by a chronic progressive course leading to death if untreated. Fever, headache, pruritus, lymphadenopathy and, to a lesser extent, hepatosplenomegaly are the leading signs and symptoms of the first stage, but are also present to a lesser extent in the second stage. The fever is intermittent, with attacks lasting from a day to a week separated by intervals of a few days to a month or longer and is rarely seen in the second stage. Lymphadenopathy with firm, mobile, non-suppurative and painless enlargement of the posterior cervical lymph nodes is the so-called Winterbottom sign. In the second stage neuropsychiatric and sleep disturbance disorders dominate the clinical presentation (Figure 110-5).[1]

HAT causes a meningoencephalitis involving different parts of the brain. Nonspecific neurological or psychiatric symptoms such as headaches and mood or behavioral changes are commonly found in both the first and second stage, but their intensity and persistence increase

as the illness evolves.[1] The neurological symptoms include tremor, fasciculation, general motor weakness, paralysis of an extremity, epilepsy, akinesia and abnormal movements such as dyskinesia or choreoathetosis, Parkinson-like movements, unspecific movement disorders, speech disorders and abnormal primitive reflexes. Psychiatric symptoms such as irritability, psychotic reactions, aggressive behavior or inactivity with apathy may dominate the clinical picture.[9,10]

Sleep disorder is a leading symptom, hence the name 'sleeping sickness'. Somnographic studies revealed a fragmentation with frequent sleep episodes of short duration at day and night caused by a dysregulation of the circadian rhythm of the sleep–wake cycle; the total duration of sleep remains normal. Sleep structure, especially the sequence of the two types (rapid eye movement (REM) sleep and non-REM sleep) is altered and is characterized by the occurrence of sleep-onset rapid eye movement (SOREM) episodes.[11]

Cardiac involvement including QTc prolongation with risk of fatal arrhythmias, repolarization changes and low voltage, is observed in 50–70% of patients but rarely leads to clinical heart failure.[12] Endocrine disorders of the thyroid, adrenocortical and sexual function (both hypo- and hyper-function) rarely require specific treatment.[13,14]

T.b. rhodesiense *HAT*

T.b. rhodesiense HAT is classically described as an acute disease rapidly progressing to second stage and leading to death within 6 months. Recent descriptions of the clinical presentation show a high variability in different locations,[15,16] possibly due to different parasite strains. Trypanosomal chancres are the primary lesion, appearing a few days after the bite of a tsetse fly at the site of infection; they are more frequently seen in *T.b. rhodesiense* than in *T.b. gambiense*. The chancre is an erythematous and tender swelling, which later becomes indurated and eventually may ulcerate. The localization of enlarged lymph nodes is submandibular, axillary and inguinal rather than nuchal, and edema is more frequently observed.[15] Compared to *T.b. gambiense* HAT, thyroid dysfunction, adrenal insufficiency and hypogonadism are more frequent and myopericarditis may be more severe. Liver involvement with hepatomegaly is usually moderate.[15]

NON-ENDEMIC COUNTRIES

The symptomatology in Caucasians differs markedly from the textbook descriptions of African HAT patients. The disease onset is almost invariably acute and of the febrile type, regardless of the species. The incubation time of *T.b. gambiense* HAT in travelers is often shorter than 1 month, but might be as long as 7 years in immigrants. *T.b. rhodesiense* HAT has an incubation time of less than 3 weeks. It is an acute, life-threatening disease with the cardinal symptoms being high fever, headache and a trypanosomal chancre.[17]

The classic sleep disorders and neurological findings of HAT are not a hallmark in travelers, irrespective of the species. Since most travelers are detected while still in the first stage and have a short duration of the disease, sleep disorders and neuropsychiatric findings may not be present at the time of the first clinical assessment. Headache, lymphadenopathy, splenomegaly, hepatomegaly and even icterus are nonspecific findings seen in about a quarter to a half of the patients. Nonspecific gastrointestinal symptoms such as nausea, vomiting and diarrhea may dominate the clinical presentation. ECG alterations due to myopericarditis and conduction abnormalities such as transient second- and third-degree atrioventricular block, supraventricular tachycardia and ventricular premature captures have been reported. In a few travelers, HAT has been complicated by renal failure requiring hemodialysis, multiorgan failure, disseminated intravascular coagulopathy and coma with even fatal outcome.

The clinical presentation of HAT in immigrants is dominated by low grade fever and neuropsychiatric disorders.

Diagnosis

The diagnosis of *T.b. gambiense* HAT usually follows the pathway of screening, diagnostic confirmation and staging. Suspected cases detected by serological methods (usually the card agglutination test for trypanosomiasis, CATT) undergo parasitological diagnosis by investigation of the blood and/or lymph and, in case of a positive result examination of the CSF follows for stage determination. *T.b. rhodesiense* is usually directly detected in the blood.[3]

PARASITOLOGIC DIAGNOSIS

Confirmation of sleeping sickness diagnosis is dependent on finding trypanosomes in the chancre, blood, lymph gland aspirate or cerebrospinal fluid (CSF). Blood films are usually positive in *T.b. rhodesiense* infection but parasitologic diagnosis may be difficult in *T.b. gambiense* disease; repeated examination and concentration techniques improve diagnostic sensitivity. Current methods comprise microhematocrit centrifugation, the miniature anion-exchange centrifugation technique (m-AECT) and fluorescence microscopy. *T.b. gambiense* may also be diagnosed by finding parasites in aspirates from enlarged cervical lymph glands.

Determination of second-stage (CNS) disease requires examination of CSF. For concentration of parasites the modified single centrifugation of the CSF is recommended.[18] Patients with ≤5 WBC/µL and no trypanosomes in the CSF are considered to be in the first stage of the disease; those with >5 WBC/µL or trypanosomes in the CSF are defined as in the second stage and treatment should be selected accordingly.[5]

LABORATORY METHODS

For laboratory use, other methods, such as immunofluorescence (IF), indirect hemagglutination (IHA), enzyme-linked immunosorbent assay (ELISA) and different PCR methods, have been suggested.[3]

DIFFERENTIAL DIAGNOSIS

Owing to the many clinical variations of sleeping sickness, it is difficult to describe a 'typical' case of the disease; differential diagnosis from all febrile, chronic and neuropsychiatric diseases is therefore of unusual importance.

Management (Table 110-2)

Treatment of sleeping sickness has made significant progress: Nifurtimox–eflornithine combination treatment (NECT)[19,20] has replaced melarsoprol for treatment of second-stage *T.b. gambiense* HAT. *T.b. rhodesiense* treatment with melarsoprol was abridged to 10 days and pre-treatment with suramin was abandoned.[21] Phase III trials are ongoing on the oral drug fexinidazole, which has the potential to become used against the first and second stage of the disease.[22]

FIRST-LINE TREATMENT

First-Stage Gambiense HAT: Pentamidine

Pentamidine is mainly used against the first stage of Gambiense disease, albeit pharmacological evidence and reports of treated travelers indicate its effectiveness against *rhodesiense* HAT.[17,23]

The most commonly used schedule is 4 mg/kg of pentamidine isethionate for 7 days. Under field conditions, deep intramuscular injection is standard. Bolus intravenous injection must be avoided and infusions should last 60–120 minutes.

The immediate adverse drug reactions include hypotension with dizziness and sometimes collapse and shock (about 10% of patients, up to 75% after intravenous use). Nausea or vomiting, pain, sterile abscesses or necrosis at the site of intramuscular injection are occasionally observed. Systemic reactions may include azotemia due to a nephrotoxic effect, leukopenia, raised liver function enzymes, hypoglycemia and hyperglycemia.

First-Stage Rhodesiense HAT: Suramin

Suramin is effective against the first stage of both forms of the disease. The most common regimen consists of a test dose of suramin at 4–5 mg/kg on day 1, followed by five intravenous injections of 20 mg/kg every 7 days; the maximum dose per injection is 1 g.

Mild and reversible nephrotoxicity is common, the first symptoms being albuminuria, later cylinduria and hematuria; regular urine checks are advised. Other adverse drug reactions are early hypersensitivity reactions occurring in 0.1–0.3% (see test dose) causing nausea, circulatory collapse and urticaria, and rare late hypersensitivity reactions such as exfoliative dermatitis and hemolytic anemia, peripheral neuropathy and bone marrow toxicity with agranulocytosis and thrombocytopenia.

Second-Stage Gambiense HAT: NECT Combination Therapy

NECT consists of 200 mg/kg of eflornithine as an intravenous infusion over 1–2 hours every 12 hours for 7 days combined with nifurtimox at 5 mg/kg orally every 8 hours for 10 days. Adverse drug reactions include frequent nausea and vomiting (over 60%) followed by neurological disturbances, including occasional convulsions and psychiatric events like agitation; neutropenia is rare.[3,5]

NECT was included in WHO's Essential Medicines List (EML) in 2009 and 2013 for children. NECT can be considered a milestone improvement: The fatality rate during treatment is 0.5% compared to 5–6% under melarsoprol.[24] The number of infusions is reduced to 14 from 56 compared with eflornithine monotherapy, hospitalization time shortened by one-third and the relapse rate decreased to 1.4% from 5.7%.[19] However, the complexity of drug application restricts the use to second-stage disease.

Second-Stage Rhodesiense HAT: Melarsoprol

The various lengthy treatment regimens were replaced in 2009 by a short course of 2.2 mg/kg per day for 10 days with no suramin pre-treatment.[21] The potentially severe and life-threatening adverse drug reactions of melarsoprol remain. The most important is an encephalopathic syndrome occurring in 5–18% of all treated cases, which is

TABLE 110-2	Treatment of *T.b. gambiense* and *T.b. rhodesiense* Sleeping Sickness	
	West African (*T.b. gambiense*)	**East African (*T.b. rhodesiense*)**
First stage	Endemic countries: According to national legislation or guidelines Other countries: Pentamidine (pentamidine isethionate) 4 mg/kg body weight at 24-hourly intervals for 7 days im (iv infusion)	Endemic countries: According to national legislation or guidelines Other countries: Suramin Test dose of 4–5 mg/kg body weight at day 1, followed by five injections of 20 mg/kg body weight every 7 days (e.g. day 3, 10, 17, 24, 31). The maximum dose per injection is 1 g
Second stage	Endemic countries: According to national legislation or guidelines Other countries: NECT 200 mg/kg of eflornithine iv as a short infusion every 12 hours for 7 days; combined with nifurtimox 5 mg/kg orally every 8 h for 10 days	Melarsoprol 2 mg/kg body weight iv at 24-hourly intervals for 10 days

Adapted from Farrar et al., *Manson's tropical diseases*, 23rd ed, pp.606–621 Copyright © 2014, Elsevier Ltd.

fatal in 10–70%. Other frequent reactions include pyrexia, headache and general malaise, gastrointestinal problems (nausea, vomiting, diarrhea) and skin reactions (pruritus) with severe complications such as exfoliative dermatitis occurring in <1% of cases.

ALTERNATIVE TREATMENTS FOR SECOND-STAGE HAT

Eflornithine Monotherapy

Eflornithine monotherapy at a daily dosage of 400 mg/kg divided into four intravenous infusions for 14 days is an alternative to NECT when nifurtimox is not available or is contraindicated, such as in patients with epilepsy or psychosis.

Melarsoprol

The only remaining indication for melarsoprol (2.2 mg/kg per day in slow intravenous injections for 10 days) in *gambiense* HAT is for treatment of relapse after NECT.

TREATMENT IN PREGNACY

Scientific evidence on treatment during pregnancy and lactation is scarce hence recommendations are based on clinical practice.

For first-stage *gambiense* HAT, pentamidine can be given after the first trimester. For second-stage *gambiense* HAT, melarsoprol, eflornithine and nifurtimox are all contraindicated, and the timing of treatment depends on the general condition of the mother. If treatment may be postponed, pentamidine may be administered with the objective of reducing the risk for vertical transmission.

The rapid clinical evolution of *rhodesiense* HAT will generally not allow postponement of treatment with suramin (contraindicated) for first-stage or melarsoprol for second-stage disease.[5]

POST-TREATMENT FOLLOW-UP

The relapse rate after *gambiense* HAT treatment is below 5% for pentamidine (first stage) and 2% for NECT (second stage). The fixed 2 years' follow-up schedule has been replaced by a parasitological assessment, interpretation of the white blood cell count in the CSF and the clinical condition of the patient after 6 and 12 months, respectively.[5]

References available online at expertconsult.com.

KEY REFERENCES

Blum J., Schmid C., Burri C.: Clinical aspects of 2541 patients with second stage human African trypanosomiasis. *Acta Trop* 2006; 97(1):55-64.

Brun R., Blum J., Chappuis F., et al.: Human African trypanosomiasis. *Lancet* 2010; 375:148-159.

Burri C., Chappuis F., Brun R.: Human African trypanosomiasis. In: Farrar J., Hotez P., Junghanss T., et al. ed. *Manson's tropical diseases*, 23rd ed. London: Elsevier; 2013:606-621.

Kennedy P.G.: Clinical features, diagnosis, and treatment of human African trypanosomiasis (sleeping sickness). *Lancet Neurol* 2013; 12(2):186-194.

Kuepfer I., Hhary E.P., Allan M., et al.: Clinical presentation of *T.b. rhodesiense* sleeping sickness in second stage

patients from Tanzania and Uganda. *PLoS Negl Trop Dis* 2011; 5(3):e968.

Kuepfer I., Schmid C., Mpairwe A., et al.: Safety and efficacy of the 10-day melarsoprol schedule for the treatment of second stage rhodesiense sleeping sickness. *PLoS Negl Trop Dis* 2012; 6(8):e1695.

Mumba Ngoyi D., Menten J., Pyana P.P., et al.: Stage determination in sleeping sickness: comparison of two cell counting and two parasite detection techniques. *Trop Med Int Health* 2013; 18(6):778-782.

Priotto G., Kasparian S., Mutombo W., et al.: Nifurtimox–eflornithine combination therapy for second-stage African *Trypanosoma brucei gambiense* trypanosomiasis:

a multicentre, randomised, phase III, non-inferiority trial. *Lancet* 2009; 374(9683):56-64.

Simarro P.P., Cecchi G., Franco J.R., et al.: Estimating and mapping the population at risk of sleeping sickness. *PLoS Negl Trop Dis* 2012; 6(10):e1859.

Simarro P.P., Diarra A., Ruiz Postigo J.A., et al.: The human African trypanosomiasis control and surveillance programme of the World Health Organization 2000–2009: the way forward. *PLoS Negl Trop Dis* 2011; 5(2):e1007.

Urech K., Neumayr A., Blum J.: Sleeping sickness in travelers – do they really sleep? *PLoS Negl Trop Dis* 2011; 5(11):e1358.

111

Eosinophilic Meningitis

BRIAN JOHN ANGUS

KEY CONCEPTS

- Eosinophilic meningitis is defined by the presence of at least 10% eosinophils in the total cerebrospinal fluid (CSF) white cell count.

- Roundworm (nematode) infections account for most of the cases of infectious eosinophilic meningitis worldwide, especially in South East Asia.

- These are principally *Angiostrongylus cantonensis*, *Gnathostoma spinigerum* and *Baylisascaris procyonis*.

- Humans are often infected with angiostrongyloides by eating poorly cooked snails. Eating undercooked shellfish, crabs, lizards and frogs that act as transient hosts can also lead to infection.

- Neurocystercicosis (*Taenia solium*) may also present with eosinophilic meningitis. Fluke (trematode) infections occasionally occur when larvae inadvertently penetrate the central nervous system, including *Paragonimus westermani*, schistosomiasis, fascioliasis and toxocariasis.

- Treatment for eosinophilic meningitis due to parasitic infection is usually supportive and the illness is self-limiting, especially for angiostrongyloidosis.

- The use of steroids and repeated lumbar puncture is recommended to reduce inflammation and raised intracranial pressure.

- Anthelmintics such as mebendazole, albendazole and ivermectin are often used but there are concerns about paradoxical worsening of symptoms and they are unproven.

Pathogenesis and Pathology

Box 111-1 gives a summary of the main causes of eosinophilic meningitis.[1] In general, parasites invade the central nervous system (CNS) as adults, larvae or ova, through the systemic circulation or via the vertebral venous system to cause eosinophilic meningitis and often meningoencephalitis (Figure 111-1).[2] The three commonest parasitic causes of eosinophilic meningitis are the rat lungworm (*Angiostrongylus cantonensis*), gnathostomiasis (*Gnathostoma spinigerum*) and the raccoon lungworm (*Baylisascaris procyonis*). To understand the epidemiology and pathogenesis of these parasites one needs to understand the complex life cycles of the organisms and their relationships with multiple definitive, intermediate and transient (paratenic) hosts that interact with humans. An intermediate host is one that harbors the parasite only for a short transition period during which some developmental stage is completed, while the parasite does not undergo any development in a paratenic host. Humans are not natural hosts for these infections and the adult worms eventually die within the human host. As such, they are sometimes termed 'abortive zoonoses'.

Angiostrongyloidosis: Adult worms of *Angiostrongylus cantonensis* inhabit the pulmonary arteries of rats and the females lay eggs that hatch into first-stage larvae (Figure 111-2). These then migrate to the pharynx, are swallowed and passed out through the droppings. They penetrate, or are ingested by a snail or slug intermediate host where they develop into the third-stage larvae that are infective to mammals. When the snail is eaten the larvae actively penetrate the CNS and migrate to the brain where they develop into young adults. They then

travel back to the venous system and the pulmonary arteries to become sexually mature. In humans, juvenile worms migrate to the brain, or rarely the lungs, where the worms ultimately die. People can therefore acquire the infection by eating raw or undercooked snails and slugs directly but they may also acquire the infection by eating raw unwashed produce that contains a small snail. There is some question whether or not parasite larvae can survive in snail slime on vegetables.

Various animals can also act as transport hosts for *A. cantonensis*. On eating infected snails, animals such as crabs, freshwater shrimps, lizards and frogs can carry the larvae. They pause within the transient host but can then resume their development if eaten by a mammal. Therefore infection can also be acquired by ingestion of these contaminated or infected animals. *Angiostrongylus costaricensis* is found in Brazil and causes intestinal disease only.

Gnathostomiasis: The life cycle of *Gnathostoma spinigerum* (rarely *G. hispidum*, *G. doloresi* and *G. nipponicum*) (Figure 111-3) begins with eggs laid by adult worms in the stomach of the natural definitive host – pigs, cats, or dogs (it was first described in the stomach of a tiger in London Zoo). Eggs are passed in the stool and hatch in water. These first-stage larvae are ingested by small crustaceans of the genera *Cyclops* (also the intermediate host of guinea-worm *Dracunculus medinensis* and the fish tapeworm *Diphyllobothrium latum*) where second-stage larvae develop. The infected *Cyclops* is then eaten by a freshwater fish, frog, or snake which becomes the second intermediate host. There they develop into third-stage larvae to be eaten by the definitive mammalian

---

BOX 111-1   CAUSES OF EOSINOPHILIC MENINGITIS

INFECTIOUS, PARASITIC CAUSES

Roundworm (nematode) infections – commonly present as eosinophilic meningitis
Angiostrongylus cantonensis – migrating larvae are neurotropic
Gnathostoma spinigerum – migrating larvae in visceral and/or neural tissues
Baylisascaris procyonis – migrating larvae are neurotropic
Tapeworm (cestode) infections – may present as eosinophilic meningitis
Cysticercosis – cysts develop in CNS and/or visceral tissues
Fluke (trematode) infections – occasionally cause eosinophilic meningitis
Paragonimus westermani – ectopic spinal or cerebral localization
Schistosomiasis – ectopic spinal or cerebral localization
Fascioliasis – ectopic CNS localization
Other roundworm infections which occasionally cause eosinophilic meningitis
Toxocariasis — migrating larvae

NONPARASITIC, INFECTIOUS CAUSES

Coccidioidomycosis
Cryptococcosis – CSF eosinophilia rare
Myiasis – with CNS penetration
Virus and bacteria – are of uncertain causality

NONINFECTIOUS CAUSES

Idiopathic hypereosinophilic syndromes
Ventriculoperitoneal shunts
Leukemia or lymphoma with CNS involvement (Hodgkin's)
Nonsteroidal anti-inflammatory drugs
Antibiotics – ciprofloxacin, trimethoprim–sulfamethoxazole, intraventricular gentamicin or vancomycin
Myelography contrast agents
Sarcoidosis

Adapted from P.F. Weller, Semin Neurol 1993;13(2):161-168

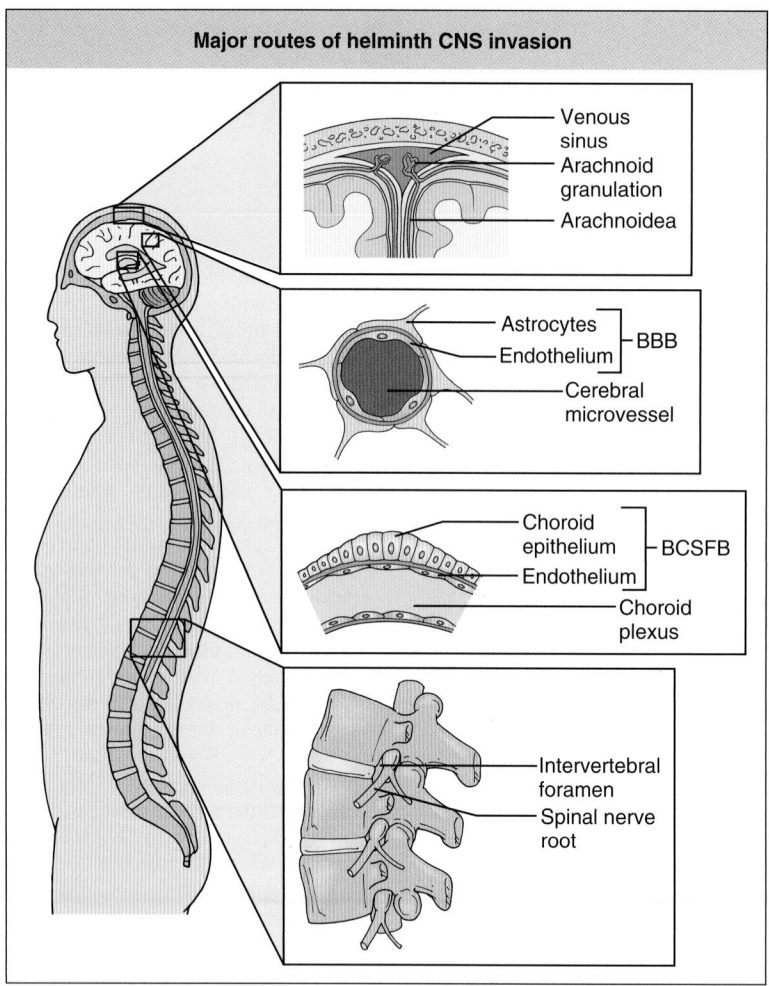

Figure 111-1 Major routes of helminth CNS invasion. Helminths can enter the CNS hematogenously through cerebral microvessels and choroid plexus, overcoming the blood–brain barrier or blood–cerebrospinal fluid barrier, respectively. Arachnoid granulations provide a site of entry through the venous system. Invasive worms can also access the CNS directly through skull and intervertebral foramina. *(From Katchanov J, Nawa Y. Parasitol Int 2010;59(4):491-6.)*

host. Alternatively, the second intermediate host may be ingested by a paratenic host such as a bird, snake, or frog, in which the larvae do not develop further but remain infective to any predator. Humans therefore can become infected by eating undercooked fish, poultry, or snake meat containing third-stage larvae, or by drinking water containing infective second-stage larvae in *Cyclops*.

Baylisascariasis: The raccoon lungworm *Baylisascaris procyonis* completes its life cycle in raccoons, with humans acquiring the infection as accidental hosts (Figure 111-4). Dogs can also serve as alternate definitive hosts, as they can harbor patent infection and shed eggs. Eggs are shed in feces, where they take 2–4 weeks to embryonate and become infective. Additionally, over 100 species of birds and mammals (especially rodents) can act as transient hosts. Eggs ingested by these hosts hatch and the larvae penetrate the gut wall and migrate into various tissues, including brain, where they encyst. The life cycle is completed when raccoons eat these hosts. Larvae then develop into egg-laying adult worms in the small intestine and eggs are eliminated in raccoon feces. Humans become accidentally infected when they ingest infective eggs from the soil, typically when young children play in the dirt. Migration of the larvae through a wide variety of tissues such as liver, heart, lungs, brain and eyes results in a visceral larva migrans syndrome similar to invasion by *Toxocara canis*. However, in contrast to *Toxocara* larvae, *Baylisascaris* larvae continue to grow during their lifetime in the human host and can cause significant tissue damage.

As well as the migrating larvae of the nematodes *A. cantonensis*, *G. spinigerum* and *B. procyonis*, other parasites can be associated with eosinophilic meningitis, including *Toxocara canis*, *Toxocara cati*, *Trichinella spiralis* and occasionally sparganosis, *Loa loa*, *Mansonella perstans*, *Ascaris lumbricoides* and *Dirofilaria immitis* (the dog heartworm).[3]

Certain trematode ova and larvae can also involve the CNS. In early schistosomiasis anomalous migration of worms to the CNS is followed by a cell-mediated response to ova deposition to form a periovular granuloma. When the subsequent humoral response to adult worms and egg antigens is excessive, Katayama fever occurs, especially in *Schistosoma japonicum* infection, with fever, eosinophilia and a self-limiting encephalopathy or myelopathy. In paragonimiasis, flukes can migrate from lung to brain through the soft tissues of the neck.

In neurocysticercosis, the larval oncospheres reach cerebral and meningeal capillaries and mature to cysticerci in the gray matter and meninges. The spinal cord is largely spared. Cysticerci survive silently for 2–10 years. Intense inflammation follows their death and antibodies appear in the cerebrospinal fluid (CSF). Healing, with fibrosis and calcification, follows. If the oncosphere enters the subarachnoid space or ventricles, then chronic eosinophilic meningitis with hydrocephalus may result. Rarely, parasites produce large cystic lesions (e.g. in paragonimiasis, hydatidosis and coenurosis).

Epidemiology

The distribution of the corresponding definitive, intermediate and transport hosts determine the epidemiology of these infections. *A. cantonensis* is found mainly in South East Asia throughout the Pacific

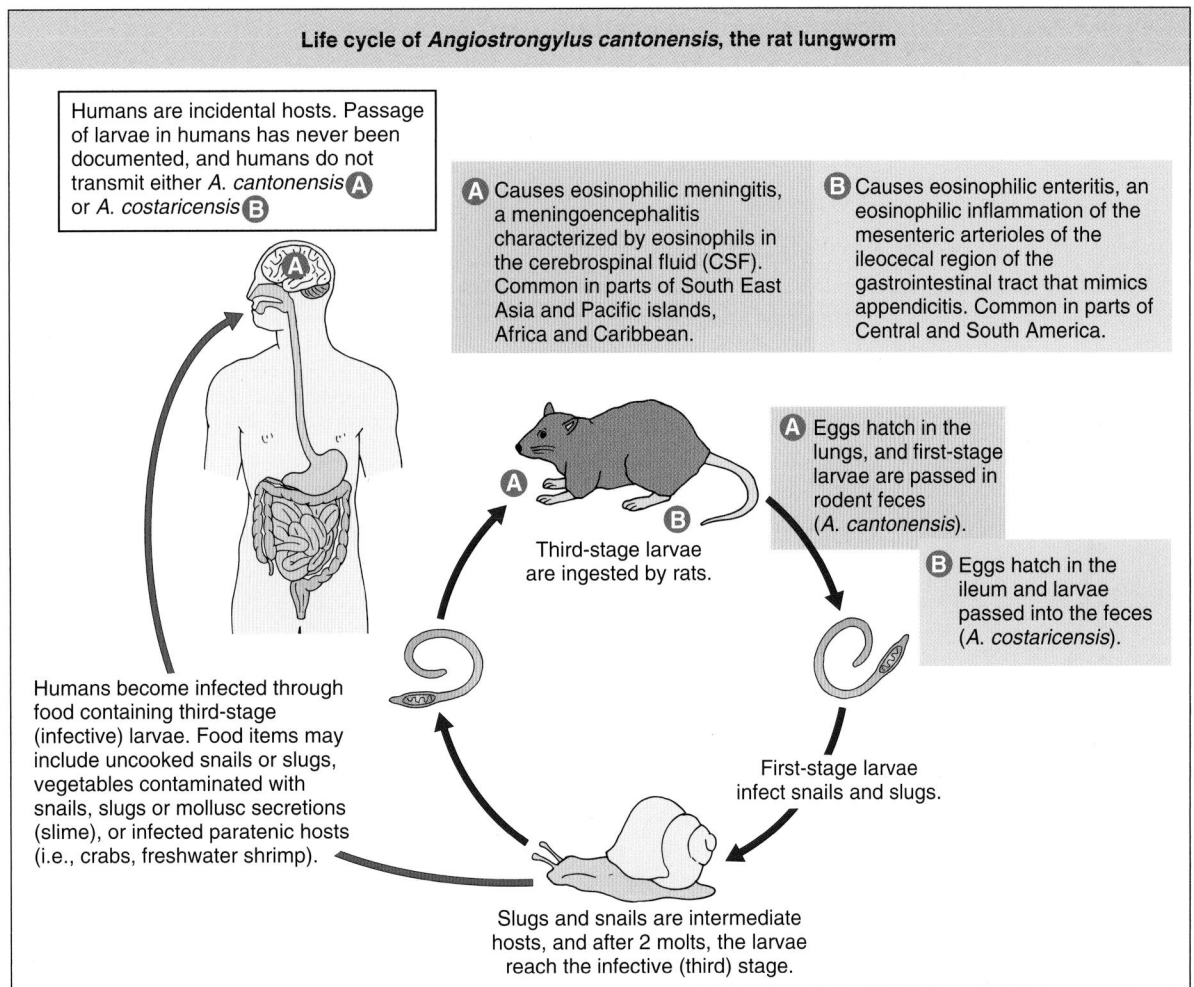

Life cycle of *Angiostrongylus cantonensis*, the rat lungworm

Humans are incidental hosts. Passage of larvae in humans has never been documented, and humans do not transmit either *A. cantonensis* Ⓐ or *A. costaricensis* Ⓑ

Ⓐ Causes eosinophilic meningitis, a meningoencephalitis characterized by eosinophils in the cerebrospinal fluid (CSF). Common in parts of South East Asia and Pacific islands, Africa and Caribbean.

Ⓑ Causes eosinophilic enteritis, an eosinophilic inflammation of the mesenteric arterioles of the ileocecal region of the gastrointestinal tract that mimics appendicitis. Common in parts of Central and South America.

Third-stage larvae are ingested by rats.

Ⓐ Eggs hatch in the lungs, and first-stage larvae are passed in rodent feces (*A. cantonensis*).

Ⓑ Eggs hatch in the ileum and larvae passed into the feces (*A. costaricensis*).

Humans become infected through food containing third-stage (infective) larvae. Food items may include uncooked snails or slugs, vegetables contaminated with snails, slugs or mollusc secretions (slime), or infected paratenic hosts (i.e., crabs, freshwater shrimp).

First-stage larvae infect snails and slugs.

Slugs and snails are intermediate hosts, and after 2 molts, the larvae reach the infective (third) stage.

Figure 111-2 Life cycle of *Angiostrongylus cantonensis*, the rat lungworm. *(Copyright © CDC. www.cdc.gov/parasites/angiostrongylus/biology.html.)*

basin, with cases particularly reported in Thailand but also Cambodia, Vietnam, Malaysia, India, Sri Lanka, Indonesia, the Philippines, Taiwan, China, Japan, Papua New Guinea, Hawaii, Tahiti and several smaller Pacific islands (Figure 111-5). It is thought that infected rats (especially *Rattus norvegicus*) traveling in ships have spread the disease into Africa, Australia and New Zealand, Cuba, Puerto Rico and Jamaica. *A. cantonensis* is now endemic in the USA, partly due to the importation of giant African land snails (*Achatina fulica*) as exotic pets, but also the spread of invasive snails, especially from South America which has been an environmental problem for many years. Angiostrongyloides have been isolated from almost all species of snails in various countries but African land snails are especially easily infected. A history of consumption of uncooked snails, *Achatina* or in Thailand *Pila* and in China the golden apple snail, *A. canaliculatus*, or freshwater prawns, frogs or lizards is often found in Thai patients.[4] There are many case reports of people eating raw snails or slugs as a 'dare' but ending up with angiostrongyloides infection.

Gnathostomiasis has a similar geographic distribution in South East Asia (Figure 111-6). Cases have been reported from Thailand, Japan, and Korea but also Ecuador and Central America. Eels are also thought to be an important route of infection in Thailand. *B. procyonis* has had a large distribution range throughout the USA in the soil of suburban neighborhoods since the 1980s (Figure 111-7).

Prevention

Prevention is by avoiding eating undercooked food, especially snails for angiostrongyloides and freshwater fish for gnathostomiasis. The spread of giant African land snails as pets highlights the importance of handwashing after handing animals as up to 25% of snails were found to be infected.

Avoidance of raccoon-contaminated soil is important and children are especially at risk of *Baylisascaris* infection. Efforts should be made to discourage children from geophagy because of the risk of toxoplasmosis and toxocariasis from cat and dog excreta, respectively.

The risk factors are summarized in Table 111-1.

Clinical Features

Fortunately these infections are uncommon even in the endemic areas. The incubation period of angiostrongyloides is 14 days (range 5–35 days). Patients usually present with symptoms and signs of meningitis over a few days and the disease is self-limiting. In a large Thai series the mortality rate was less than 0.5%.[5] Acute severe headache is the most commonly reported symptom and fever was uncommon. Neurologic findings were elicited in 42% of cases, 16% of patients had visual impairment and 12% had an abnormal fundus. There was slowly progressive impairment of sensation, which may last for a few months and weakness without localization was noted in 5% and less than 1% of patients, respectively. Cranial nerve palsies were found in 17% of patients. Electric shock-like pains (L'Hermitte's sign) may be present. Clinical signs may fluctuate markedly; the patient may have headache, confusion, severe generalized dysesthesia, neck stiffness and various focal neurologic signs but later the same day the patient may be almost symptom-free.[5]

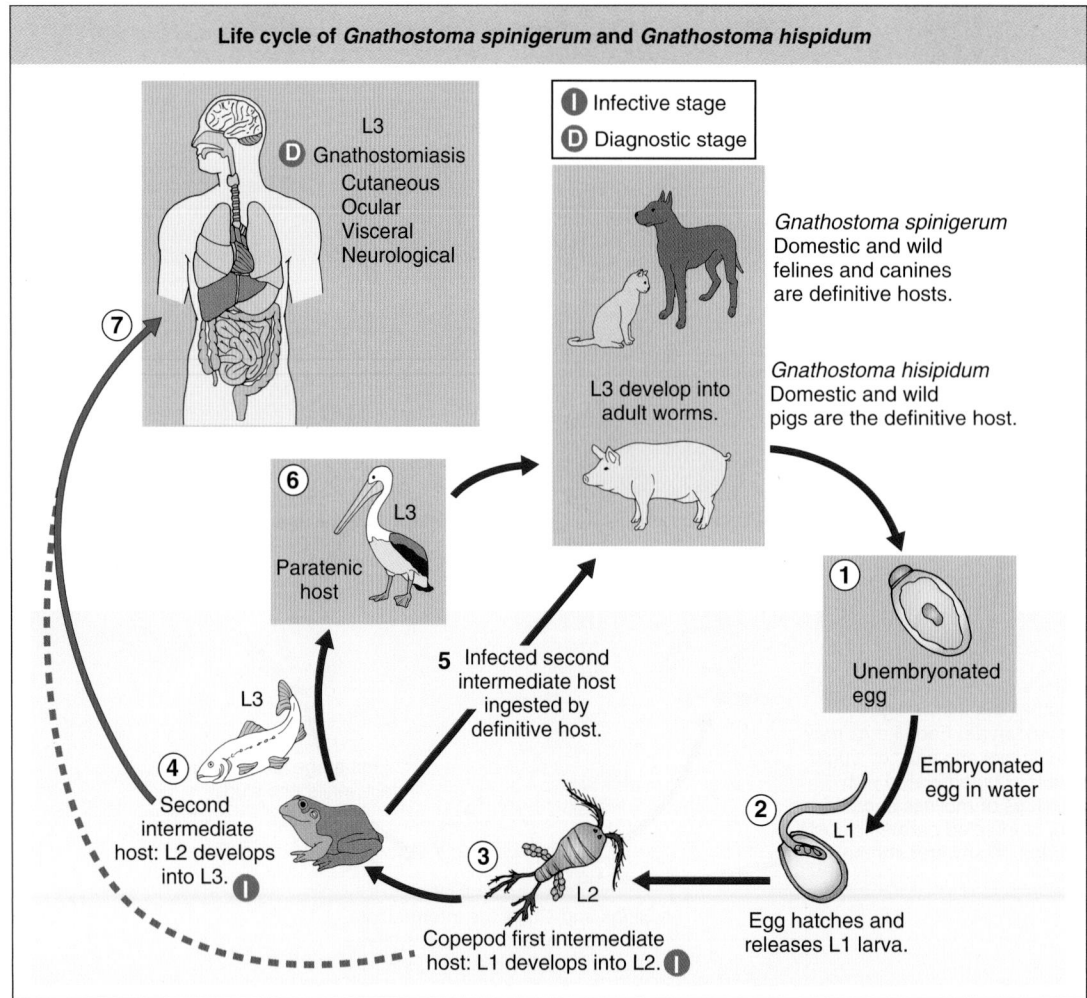

Life cycle of *Gnathostoma spinigerum* and *Gnathostoma hispidum*

L3
D Gnathostomiasis
Cutaneous
Ocular
Visceral
Neurological

I Infective stage
D Diagnostic stage

Gnathostoma spinigerum
Domestic and wild felines and canines are definitive hosts.

Gnathostoma hisipidum
Domestic and wild pigs are the definitive host.

L3 develop into adult worms.

7

6 L3
Paratenic host

5 Infected second intermediate host ingested by definitive host.

1 Unembryonated egg

L3

4 Second intermediate host: L2 develops into L3. I

3 Copepod first intermediate host: L1 develops into L2. I

L2

Embryonated egg in water

2 L1

Egg hatches and releases L1 larva.

Figure 111-3   Life cycle of *Gnathostoma spinigerum* and *Gnathostoma hispidum*. (Copyright © CDC. www.cdc.gov/parasites/gnathostoma/biology.html.)

TABLE 111-1	Main Sources of Infection for Eosinophilic Meningitis	
Source of Infection		**Disease**
FOOD	Unwashed salads	Angiostrongyliasis, cysticercosis
	Uncooked vegetables	Angiostrongyliasis, cysticercosis
	Uncooked pork	Cysticercosis, *Taenia solium*, sparganosis
	Uncooked beef	Toxoplasmosis
	Uncooked freshwater fish	Gnathostomiasis, diphyllobothriasis
	Uncooked freshwater crayfish or crabs	Paragonimiasis, angiostrongyliasis
	Uncooked snakes, frogs	Angiostrongyliasis, sparganosis
	Uncooked land molluscs (e.g. *Achatina fulica* snails)	Angiostrongyliasis
	Skin contact	Schistosomiasis
FRESH WATER	Consumption	Gnathostomiasis, sparganosis
	Geophagy (eating clay)	Toxoplasmosis, toxocariasis, ascariasis
	Soil	Baylisascariasis, strongyloidiasis
VECTORS	Mosquito (*Culex* spp.)	Bancroftian filariasis, dirofilariasis
	Blackfly (*Simulium* spp.)	Onchocerciasis
	Chrysops flies	Loiasis

Gnathostomiasis usually presents with migratory cutaneous swellings and rarely with eosinophilic meningoencephalitis or inflammatory masses in visceral organs. Gnathostoma can penetrate the spinal cord along nerve roots, causing painful radiculomyelitis. The parasite then ascends through the spinal cord to the brain. This may take several months or even years. Due to the size of the migrating larva (3.0 mm to 4.0 mm) this migration can cause direct mechanical injury including parenchymal damage from parasitic tracts and subarachnoid hemorrhage.

Baylisascariasis can be asymptomatic but the prevalence is unknown and severe cases are rare. Infection can result in visceral larva migrans or ocular larva migrans syndromes similar to toxocara. *B. procyonis* has a tendency to invade the spinal cord, brain and eye of humans, resulting in permanent neurologic damage, blindness or death.

Diagnosis

Examination of the CSF is essential but sometimes eosinophils can be mistaken for neutrophils on the slide. The total CSF white cell count is usually between 0.15 and 2 x10^9 cells/L with greater than 10% eosinophils. In the Thai series CSF on lumbar puncture was turbid with a white cell count of more than 0.5 x10^9/L in 75% of cases.[5] The protein concentration is usually raised, but the glucose is usually normal or only minimally lowered. There is usually concomitant blood eosinophilia.

Modern diagnostic methods have recently focused on antibody detection to the 29 and 31 kDa proteins of *A. cantonensis* and against the 21 and 24 kDa antigenic components of *G. spinigerum*.[6] However,

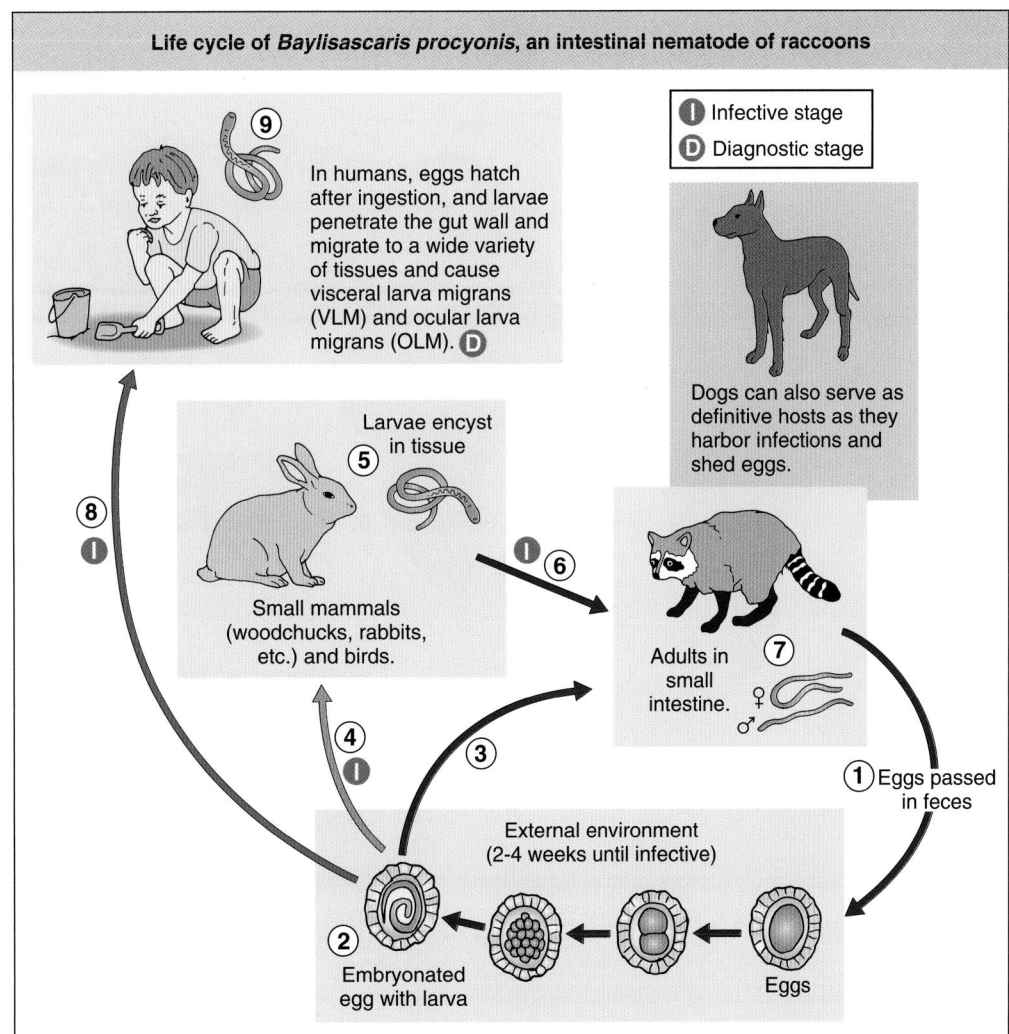

Figure 111-4   Life cycle of *Baylisascaris procyonis*, an intestinal nematode of raccoons. *(Copyright © CDC. www.cdc.gov/parasites/baylisascaris/biology.html.)*

these tests are not readily available in non-endemic areas. Antigen detection and PCR tests are in use for research but not commercially available. There are no available tests for *Baylisascaris* although the recombinant protein *B. procyonis* antigen, BpRAG1, is being developed.[7]

Computed tomography (CT) is generally unremarkable but focal lesions on scans can help to distinguish gnathostomiasis or neurocysticercosis from the more non-focal meningoencephalitis of angiostrongyloides. MRI features are nonspecific but there is an association between the presence of high brain MRI signal intensities and severity of peripheral and CSF eosinophilia in angiostrongyloides.[8] In gnathostomiasis CT scans can demonstrate areas of hemorrhage and MRI may well demonstrate abnormal enhancement and 'tracks' as well as both subarachnoid and subdural hemorrhage (Figure 111-8).[9]

Occasionally surgical exploration of the cutaneous swellings in gnathostomiasis may reveal the visible millimeter-long larvae.

Management

There are some controversies in the management of eosinophilic meningitis, especially regarding the use of anthelmintics. The mainstay treatment of cerebral angiostrongyliasis is supportive with analgesia and fluids. Migrating larvae will die over time and the acute inflammation will subside. Most patients with cerebral angiostrongyliasis have a self-limited course and recover completely. Analgesics,

corticosteroids and intermitttent lumbar puncture can relieve the symptoms of raised intracranial pressure.[10] In one randomized trial including 110 patients with eosinophilic meningitis, those who received prednisolone (60 mg daily for 2 weeks) were less likely to have persistent headache or require repeat lumbar puncture.[11] There was no additional benefit from adding albendazole in a study of 104 patients.[12] In fact there are concerns that anthelmintic treatment alone may induce an inflammatory response due to dying organisms, and clinical exacerbation of neurologic symptoms following administration has been described.[13] Surgery or laser therapy may be useful for ocular disease.[14]

The treatment of eosinophilic meningitis due to gnathostomiasis is similar to that of angiostrongyloides with the use of repeated lumbar puncture and steroids generally favoured but no randomized controlled trials. Again there are concerns that anthelmintic treatment may be harmful. In nine patients treated with albendazole, five recovered, two partially recovered and two died.[15] Recommended treatment of cutaneous gnathostomiasis is often difficult and consists of albendazole (400 mg orally twice daily for 21 days) or ivermectin (200 μg/kg/ day orally for 2 days) but there are no controlled trials and patients should be monitored closely for relapse, often needing repeated treatment. In one study of 31 patients with cutaneous gnathostomiasis in Thailand, only 41% responded clinically to a single dose of ivermectin.[16] In a study including 13 patients who developed gnathostomiasis following travel in South East Asia or Central America (including four

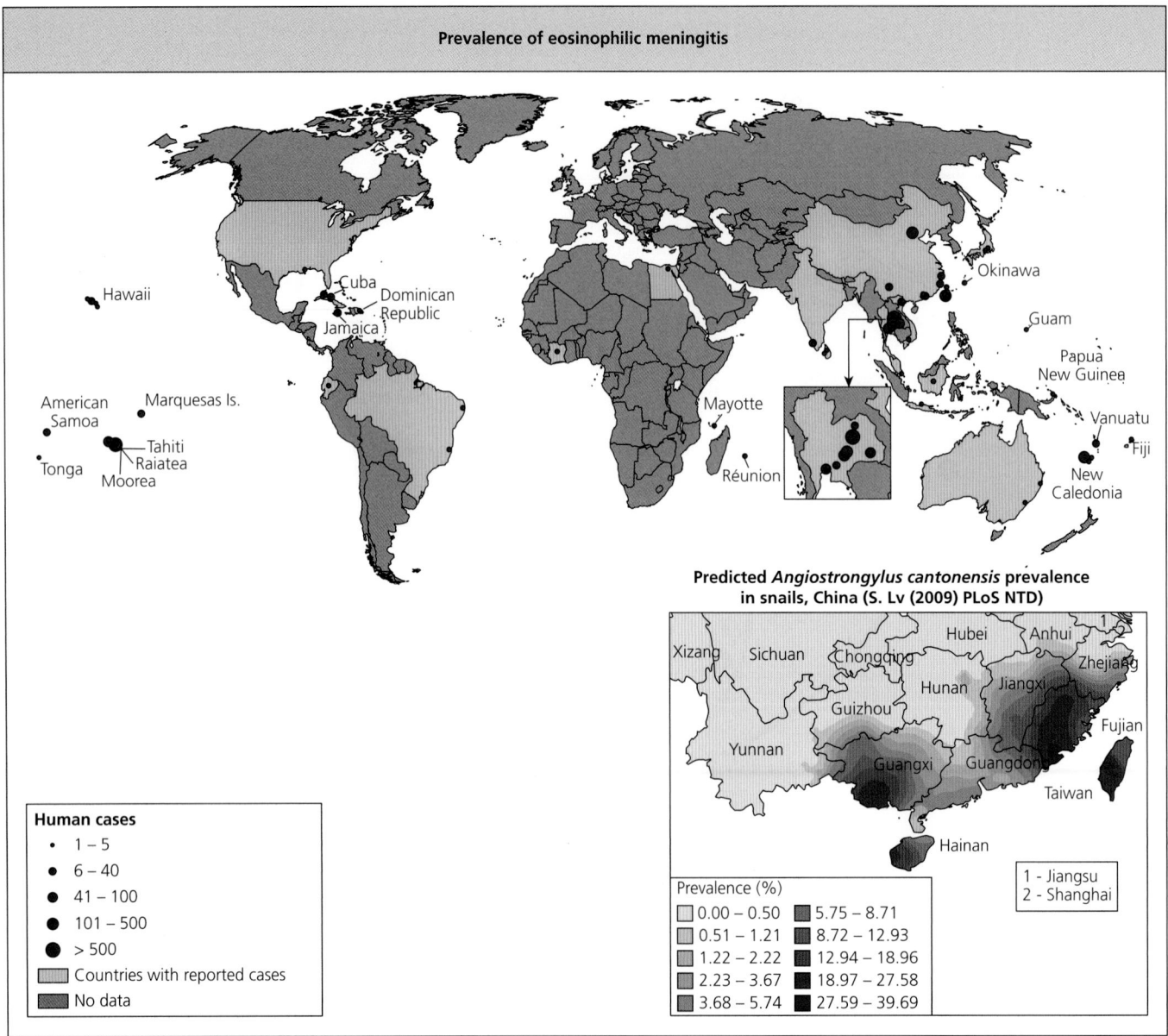

Figure 111-5 Map of prevalence of eosinophilic meningitis and predicted *Angiostrongyloides cantonensis* prevalence in snails. *(With the authors' permission; last update on 09/03/2011)*

cases of CNS disease), neither ivermectin nor albendazole was fully effective.[17] One patient treated with a single day of ivermectin and 7 of 12 patients treated with albendazole (400 mg twice a day of albendazole for 21 days) relapsed.

The effect of anthelmintic treatment of *Baylisascaris* meningoencephalitis is poor but again steroids are recommended to reduce inflammation. There is some evidence that albendazole can be an effective prophylactic if administered up to 3 days after ingestion of raccoon stool or contaminated soil.[18]

Uncommon Infective Causes of Eosinophilic Meningitis

Nonparasitic infections such as coccidioidomycosis (*Coccidioides immitis* or *Coccidioides posadasii*) and *Mycobacterium tuberculosis* can also cause eosinophilic meningitis. Many cases of viral, rickettsial and bacterial infections have been reported as being associated with eosinophilic meningitis but it is unclear if these infections were pathogenic or co-incident. Rarely, larvae of the botflies (*Dermatobia hominis*) can invade the central nervous system and cause CSF eosinophilia.

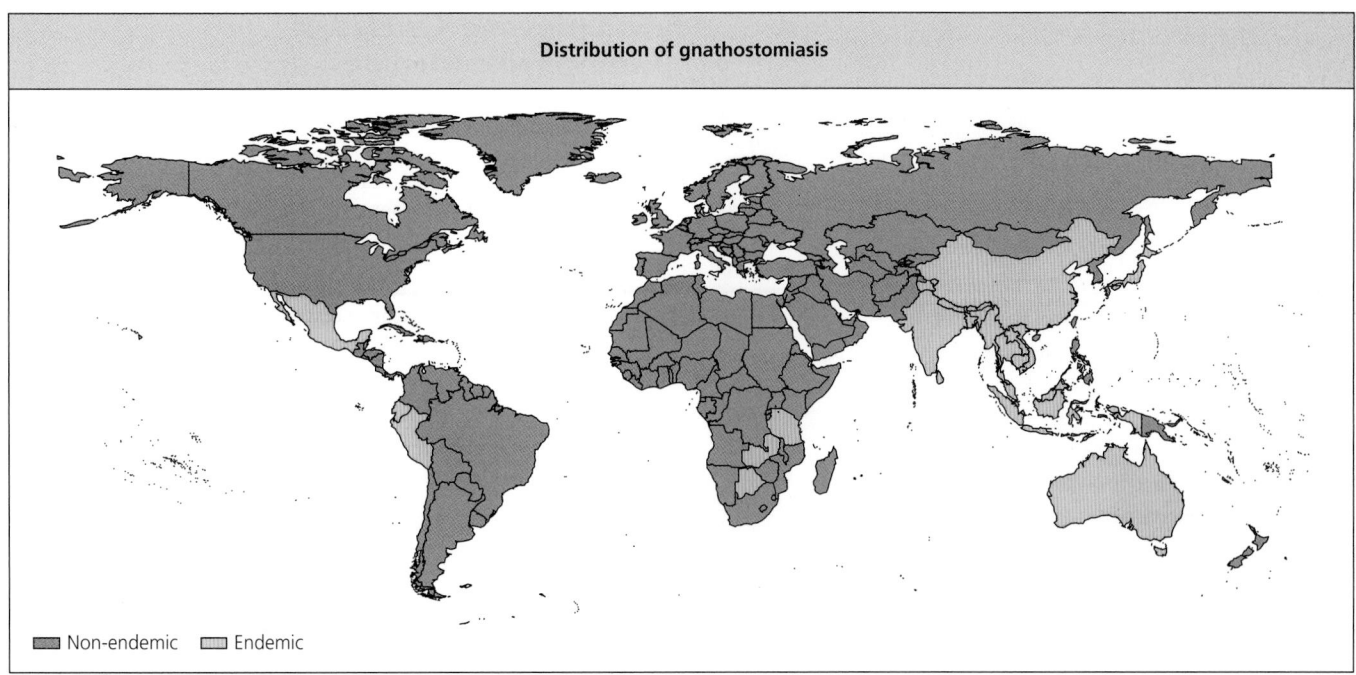

Figure 111-6   Map of distribution of gnathostomiasis. *(Source: GIDEON (1994–2011)* http://web.gideononline.com/web/epidemiology. *Copyright © GIDEON Informatics, Inc.* www.gideononline.com.)

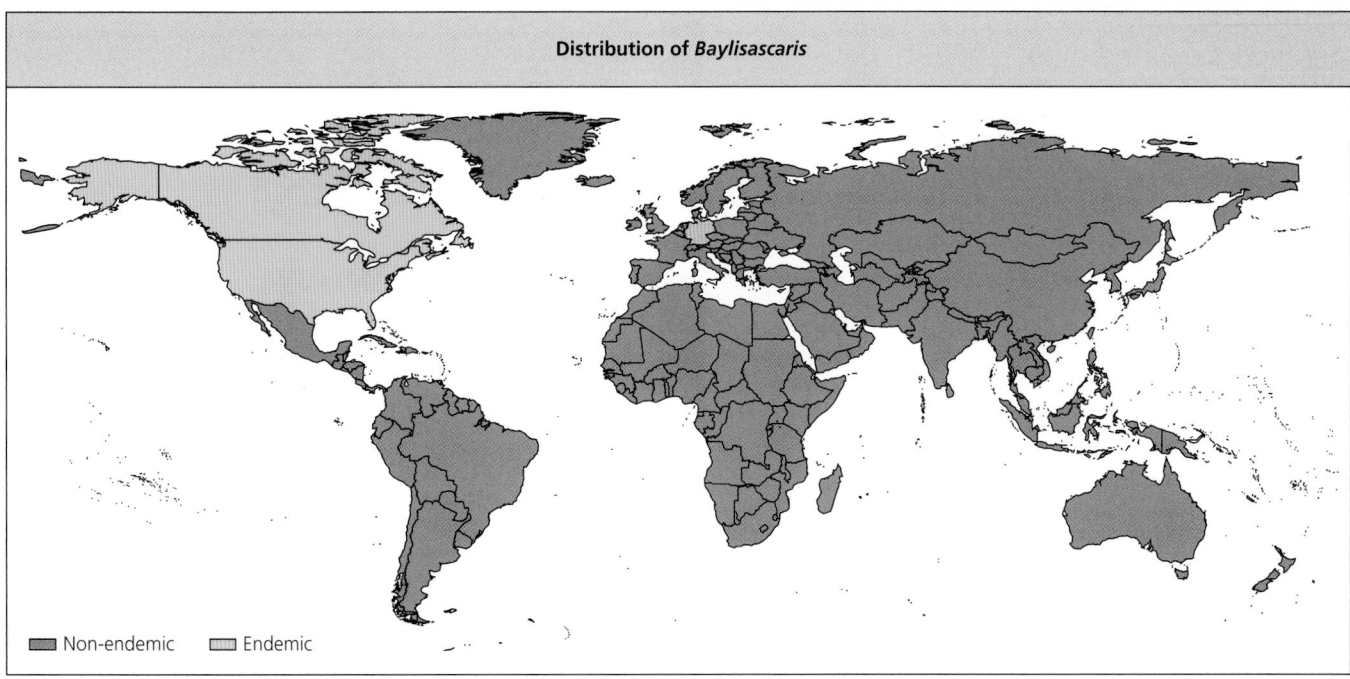

Figure 111-7   Map of distribution of *Baylisascaris*. *(Source: GIDEON (1994–2011)* http://web.gideononline.com/web/epidemiology. *Copyright © GIDEON Informatics, Inc.* www.gideononline.com.)

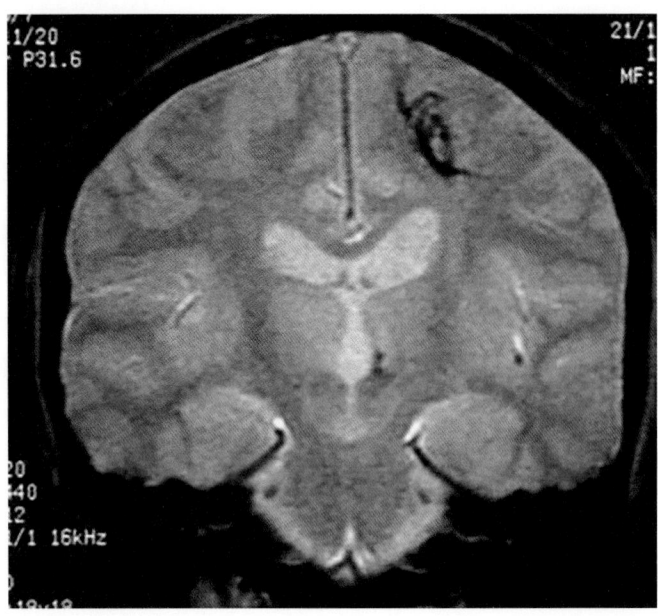

Figure 111-8 A coronal T1-weighted MRI scan showing a hemorrhagic tract from gnathostomiasis. (From Sawanyawisuth K, et al. Trans R Soc Trop Med Hyg 2009;103(1):102-4.)

Noninfective Causes of Eosinophilic Meningitis

Noninfectious causes of eosinophilic meningitis include hematologic disorders, most frequently Hodgkin's lymphoma, but also adverse drug reactions (most commonly ibuprofen and other NSAIDs), ciprofloxacin, trimethoprim-sulfamethoxazole, and intraventricular vancomycin or gentamicin). Mechanical shunt implantation, malfunction or infection can be associated with eosinophilia. It has been described as a rare complication of sarcoidosis.

There is a group of idiopathic leukoproliferative disorders characterized by blood eosinophilia in excess of 1.5×10^9/L without an apparent other cause called the hypereosinophilic syndromes, which are uncommonly complicated by eosinophilic meningitis.

CSF eosinophilia also has been found rarely in carcinoma-associated or non-Hodgkin's-associated lymphomatous meningitis, acute lymphocytic leukemia and even disseminated glioblastoma. It is also well recognized as an uncommon para-neoplastic complication of bronchogenic carcinoma and some other malignancies.

References available online at expertconsult.com.

KEY REFERENCES

Gavin P.J., Kazacos K.R., Shulman S.T.: Baylisascariasis. *Clin Microbiol Rev* 2005; 18(4):703-718.

Katchanov J., Nawa Y.: Helminthic invasion of the central nervous system: many roads lead to Rome. *Parasitol Int* 2010; 59(4):491-496.

Katchanov J., Sawanyawisuth K., Chotmongkoi V., et al.: Neurognathostomiasis, a neglected parasitosis of the central nervous system. *Emerg Infect Dis* 2011; 17(7):1174-1180.

Punyagupta S., Bunnag T., Juttijudata P.: Eosinophilic meningitis in Thailand: clinical and epidemiological characteristics of 162 patients with myeloencephalitis probably caused by *Gnathostoma spinigerum*. *J Neurol Sci* 1990; 96(2–3):241-256.

Punyagupta S., Juttijudata P., Bunnag T.: Eosinophilic meningitis in Thailand: clinical studies of 484 typical cases probably caused by *Angiostrongylus cantonensis*. *Am J Trop Med Hyg* 1975; 24(6 Pt 1):921-931.

Ramirez-Avila L., Slome S., Schuster F.L., et al.: Eosinophilic meningitis due to *Angiostrongylus* and *Gnathostoma* species. *Clin Infect Dis* 2009; 48(3):322-327.

Sawanyawisuth K., Chlebicki M.P., Pratt E., et al.: Sequential imaging studies of cerebral gnathostomiasis with subdural hemorrhage as its complication. *Trans R Soc Trop Med Hyg* 2009; 103(1):102-104.

Weller P.F.: Eosinophilic meningitis. *Am J Med* 1993; 95(3):250-253.

Wilkins P.P., Qvarnstrom Y., Whelen A.C., et al.: The current status of laboratory diagnosis of *Angiostrongylus cantonensis* infections in humans using serologic and molecular methods. *Hawaii J Med Public Health* 2013; 72(6 Suppl. 2):55-57.

Eye Infections in the Tropics

ROBIN BAILEY

This chapter discusses the contribution of infection to the major blinding diseases of the tropics and the ocular features associated with common tropical infections.

Major Blinding Infections of the Tropics

Cataract, vitamin A deficiency, trachoma and onchocerciasis are classically considered to be causes of blindness in low- and middle-income countries. Community-based surveys to identify the causes and burden of blindness have been carried out in more than 30 countries, and in many more, rapid assessment methods (rapid assessment of avoidable blindness – RAAB) have been used to generate valid prevalence estimates.[1] These show that cataract, universally, is by far the greatest cause of blindness. In 2002, trachoma and onchocerciasis were considered to account for 3.6% and 0.8 % respectively of the global burden of blindness.[2] Worldwide, infections are declining in importance, while diabetes, glaucoma and age-related macular degeneration are increasing. In trachoma, onchocerciasis, leprosy and measles, infection and host immune response play prominent and contrasting roles in the pathogenesis of blindness and ocular complications, as discussed below.

Trachoma

Trachoma is a chronic follicular keratoconjunctivitis caused by infection with *Chlamydia trachomatis*, almost exclusively of serotypes A, B, Ba and C (the 'genital' *C. trachomatis* serotypes D–K may cause disease that is indistinguishable from trachoma, but this is rare). Host tissue tropism in *C. trachomatis* is strongly related to the capacity to synthesize tryptophan, with all ocular strains having inactivating mutations in the *trpBA* tryptophan synthetase genes.[3] Trachoma is characterized by scarring sequelae in the conjunctiva after repeated infections.

EPIDEMIOLOGY

Trachoma is one of the most common infectious diseases: the World Health Organization (WHO) estimates (2012) that 241 million people live in trachoma-endemic districts and that 2.2 million people are irreversibly visually impaired due to trachoma.[4] Fifty-three countries, mainly in sub-Saharan Africa, are currently assessed as being endemic for blinding trachoma. The Global Trachoma Mapping Project (GTMP) aims to identify every district in the world with endemic disease. Trachoma is a disease of poverty, associated with poor personal and environmental hygiene, and was common in much of Europe and North America in the 19th century. The current GTMP map (www.trachomaatlas.org)[5] represents the best available information on the current distribution of active trachoma. In addition to sub-Saharan Africa, additional foci of disease occur in Asia, South America and Australia.

In trachoma-endemic communities, the main reservoir of infection is the eyes of affected children. Active trachoma is unusual among adults, and there is evidence that most transmission occurs within the family[6,7] as a result of close contact between young children and their mothers and other caregivers. Transmission is favored by poor environmental and personal hygiene, lack of water for washing, inadequate sleeping space, inadequate sanitation and the proximity of domestic animals. Fingers, fomites and flies are the main source of infection: their relative importance probably varies from one community to another.

PATHOGENESIS

There is evidence that the pathologic features of trachoma are not the result of direct tissue damage but are immunologically mediated.[8] A single infection with *C. trachomatis* usually leads to a self-limiting follicular conjunctivitis, and repeated episodes may be necessary for the development of intense inflammation and scarring sequelae. The most characteristic histologic finding in active trachoma is the presence of follicles, which resemble germinal centers in the superior tarsal conjunctiva. Subsequently subconjunctival scarring occurs and contraction of scars causes distortion of the tarsal plate, entropion and trichiasis.

Animal model data suggest that cellular immune mechanisms (specific T-helper-1 lymphocyte and gamma interferon) are of primary importance in limiting and clearing chlamydial infection.[9,10] Why some individuals clear infection without sequelae while others develop scars is unknown. There is evidence that scarred subjects have reduced capacity for interferon-gamma (IF-γ)-mediated clearance of chlamydial infection.[11] Genetic variants at the interleukin (IL)-10 locus which potentiate IL-10 transcription increase risk of scarring.[12,13] Transcriptional profiling of the conjunctiva in ocular chlamydial infection has highlighted a preponderance of molecular signatures associated with innate immunity, including natural killer (NK) cell-mediated cytotoxicity, an alternative source of IF-γ production. Other observations implicate polymorphism at the KIR and HLA-C loci (reflecting the balance between activating and suppressing NK cell responses) and matrix metalloproteases (MMPs; mediators in the extracellular matrix breakdown pathway linking inflammation and tissue remodeling) in the process by which repeated episodes of intense disease and infection lead to scarring.[14–18] Antibodies to a chlamydial heat shock protein, Hsp 60, are also associated with scarring sequelae of infection in both the eyelid and the genital tract, but it is uncertain whether these reflect a causal role for this antigen or an epiphenomenon.

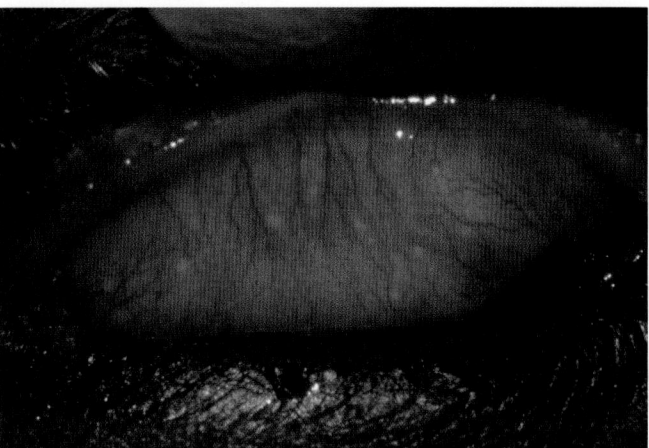

Figure 112-1   Everted eyelid showing follicular trachoma (TF).

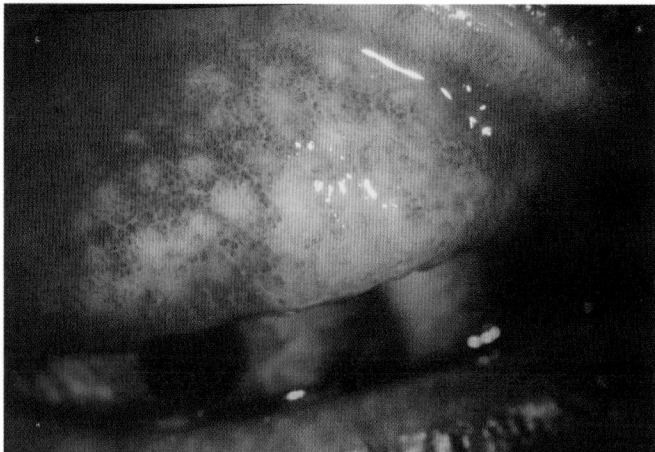

Figure 112-2   Everted eyelid showing intense inflammatory trachoma (TI). Follicles are also present.

PREVENTION

The goal of prevention is to reduce transmission to such a level that exposure to reinfection does not occur often enough to cause blinding trachoma. Measures focused on improving personal and community hygiene such as the provision of adequate water supplies, fly control and latrines are likely to reduce the incidence of trachoma, though direct evidence is lacking. A study of community education targeted at face washing showed that, with intense effort, reductions in trachoma prevalence are possible but not well sustained.[19] Treatment of active cases with antibiotics may be effective temporarily but even high coverage mass treatment may fail due to re-exposure to untreated individuals.[20] The WHO-endorsed strategy is known by the acronym SAFE: Surgery, Antibiotic treatment, Facial cleanliness and Environmental improvement. There is no vaccine at present.

CLINICAL FEATURES

In endemic communities C. trachomatis infection is usually acquired early in childhood; progressive scarring and distortion of the eyelid lead to corneal scarring and blindness, usually in late middle age. In severely affected communities signs of trachoma can be found in over 90% of children aged between 1 and 2 years and blindness rates may approach 25% in those over 60 years. In most endemic areas, there is no sex difference in prevalence or incidence until after adolescence, but both active trachoma and its scarring sequelae are more common in women, probably reflecting their closer contact with children.

Subjects with trachoma typically have few symptoms until the final stages when inturned eyelashes (trichiasis) develop. Secondary bacterial infection may play a role in progression, and in the mucopurulent conjunctivitis, nasal discharge and chronic otitis media seen in some patients.

Lymphoid follicles, the most prominent sign of active trachoma, are usually found on the superior tarsal conjunctiva, and are easily visualized by everting the upper eyelid. They may occasionally be found at the corneoscleral junction (limbal follicles). The presence of five or more of these pale off-white spots with a diameter <0.5 mm in the central area of the superior tarsal conjunctiva is needed to meet the accepted definition of trachomatous inflammation of follicular grade (Figure 112-1). Active trachoma is also associated with capillary congestion of the conjunctiva, visible as red dots of small engorged tufts (papillae) or as obscuration of the normally visible deep tarsal blood vessels by inflammatory thickening. If these blood vessels are obscured over more than half of the central area over the tarsal plate, trachomatous inflammation of intense grade (TI) is said to be present (Figure 112-2). Neovascularization of the cornea or 'pannus' is associated with active C. trachomatis infection and in trachoma typically involves the superior corneal margin.

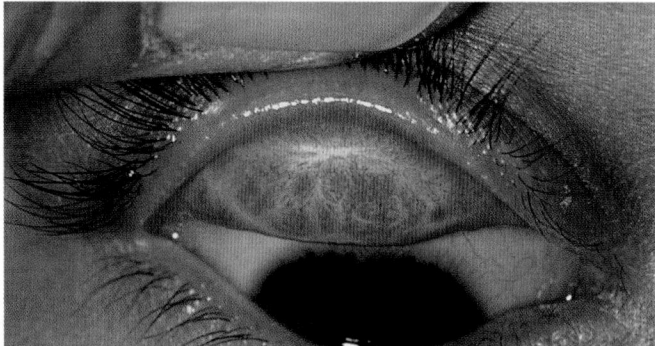

Figure 112-3   Everted eyelid showing trachomatous scarring (TS). There are also Herbert's pits visible at the corneoscleral junction. *(Courtesy of the WHO Program for the Prevention of Blindness.)*

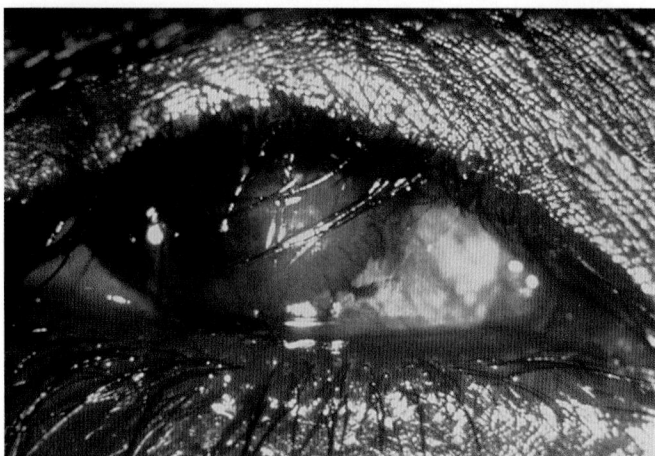

Figure 112-4   Trachomatous trichiasis (TT) and secondary corneal opacity. *(Courtesy of the WHO Program for the Prevention of Blindness.)*

Conjunctival scars (which, if clearly visible would be graded trachomatous scarring [TS]) are initially small and stellate, but eventually become broad and confluent (Figure 112-3). The scars contract, causing distortion of the tarsal plate and loss of its normal protective functions and resulting in inturning of the lashes (trichiasis, which is graded TT if any lash is in contact with the eyeball), which rub on the cornea (Figure 112-4). This can lead to corneal opacity and ultimately

TABLE 112-1	**Causes of Follicular Conjunctivitis**
Cause	**Comments**
Folliculosis	Follicles are few and occur in the inferior fornix without inflammation or hyperemia; a common finding
Viral infections	Acute, self-limiting with signs of resolution in 2 weeks
Trachoma	
'Inclusion conjunctivitis' and other ocular chlamydial infections	Also caused by ocular chlamydial infection, often with genital serotypes; frequently unilateral

'Toxic' follicular conjunctivitis:
  Molluscum contagiosum
  Drug-induced
  Eye cosmetics
	Caused by spillage of contents of molluscum lesions on eyelids
	Follows use of eye medications for months or years
	Granules of cosmetics seen in follicles

Bacterial infections: *Moraxella* spp. and others	Angular blepharitis with *Moraxella lacunata*; seen in adolescent girls who share eye make-up
Axenfeld's chronic follicular conjunctivitis	Reported in institutionalized children and native Americans, probably a mild form of trachoma[14]
Chronic follicular conjunctivitis of Thygeson	Outbreak in a Californian high school that contained trachoma cases; features compatible with mild active trachoma[14]
Parinaud's oculoglandular syndrome	Associated with pathogens invading through the conjunctivae; associated with systemic malaise and gross preauricular lymphadenopathy; some cases associated with exposure to cats and may be due to feline strains of *Chlamydia psittaci*; many other causes (e.g. syphilis, lymphogranuloma verereum, tuberculosis, tularemia, cat-scratch disease)
Vernal catarrh	Occurs in atopic subjects; characteristic appearance with giant 'cobblestone' papillae

to blindness from abrasion of the cornea. Limbal follicles may resolve to leave small depressions at the limbus known as 'Herbert's pits'.

Trachoma may be confused with other conditions producing a follicular conjunctivitis (Table 112-1). With the exception of viral conjunctivitis, which is acute and self-limiting, the other conditions in Table 112-1 are never endemic in a community. The only clinical signs unique to trachoma are limbal follicles and Herbert's pits (see Figure 112-3).[21] However, the majority of cases do not have these signs.

DIAGNOSIS

Trachoma is usually diagnosed on clinical grounds. The simplified grading scheme, including TF, TI, TS and TT, has been developed by WHO for public health purposes.[22] Several laboratory tests can be used to confirm the diagnosis, but these are rarely available in endemic areas. Chlamydial infection is characterized by blue intracytoplasmic inclusions in Giemsa-stained epithelial cell scrapings. The organism can be cultured in cell monolayers, visualized in smears using direct fluorescent antibody methods or detected by enzyme immunoassay. Nucleic acid amplification tests (NAATS) usually targeting DNA sequences in either the common plasmid pCT1 of *C. trachomatis* or the ribosomal RNA sequences which are present at high copy number,[23] are the most sensitive methods for demonstrating ocular infection.

MANAGEMENT

Individual sporadic cases may be treated with 1% tetracycline eye ointment topically q12h for 6 weeks. A single oral dose of azithromycin (20 mg/kg) is as effective.[24] Mass treatment with antibiotic is recommended by WHO for all inhabitants of any district, neighborhood or community in which the prevalence of TF exceeds 10% in children aged 1–9 years. As of 2014, over 400 million doses of azithromycin, donated by the manufacturer, have been distributed through the International Trachoma Initiative for this purpose.

Trichiasis can be treated by epilation, particularly if there only are one or a few peripheral lashes touching the eyeball,[25] and this is often a focus of traditional treatments. However, it may provide only temporary relief and lid surgery is recommended, and usually needed, to prevent corneal abrasion and blindness if entropion (in-rolling of the lid margin) is present. Bilamellar tarsal rotation[26] is the operation of choice to correct this.

Onchocerciasis

PATHOGENESIS

In the eye, as in the rest of the body, pathology results from an inflammatory reaction to microfilariae of *Onchocerca volvulus* and their *Wolbachia* endosymbionts. The most common onchocercal lesions involve the cornea, though the anterior chamber, iris, lens, retina and choroid may all be involved. Antigen-specific T-regulatory cells (Tr1), which were first described in human infections in onchocerciasis,[27] appear to induce the tolerance of high microfilarial burden that occurs in individuals with generalized onchocerciasis.[28] There is evidence that, following microfilaricidal treatment, released *Wolbachia*-derived antigens exert potent proinflammatory effects and induce neutrophil chemotaxis, both reduced by prior anti-*Wolbachia* treatment.[29]

CLINICAL FEATURES

Eye involvement in onchocerciasis is usually bilateral and (in contrast to trachoma) affects men more commonly than women. Punctate or 'snowflake' keratitis occurs as inflammatory cells accumulate around dead microfilariae and it may respond to topical corticosteroids. Sclerosing keratitis, in which neovascularization and scarring develop nasally and temporally in the cornea and then extend inwards from the inferior limbal margin to involve the whole surface in a total corneal scar, has been a common cause of blindness, particularly in savanna regions. Microfilarial movement may be visible in the anterior chamber with a slit lamp, often closely associated with the posterior corneal surface. Inflammatory reactions may produce iritis, and cataract may also contribute to reduced vision. In the posterior segment of the eye, choroidoretinal atrophy, with clumping and breaking up of the retinal pigment epithelium, and associated optic atrophy, may follow. These changes contribute further to visual loss but have no specific treatment.

Measles

PATHOGENESIS

Measles virus infection and its consequences are a major risk to sight in tropical practice. Measles remains the single leading cause of childhood blindness, with the tens of thousands of cases worldwide usually due to corneal scarring or perforation.[30] Although measles virus infects the corneal epithelium and the conjunctiva, its devastating effects on the cornea are the results of secondary processes that include infection, acute vitamin A deficiency, exposure and the effects of traditional eye medicines. Measles virus-associated immunosuppression appears to be responsible for reactivation of herpes simplex virus, which has been found in corneal ulcers after measles[31] and gut involvement appears to precipitate acute vitamin A deficiency in those with marginal reserves.

CLINICAL FEATURES

The direct effects of measles on the eye are a punctate keratitis and conjunctival lesions that are analogous to Koplik's spots, which normally resolve without sequelae. Corneal ulceration and keratomalacia with liquefaction of the cornea and the whole eye may supervene in acute vitamin A deficiency. Secondary ulceration due to herpes simplex may be typically dendritic or modified by other factors, as discussed below. If subjects are too sick or too dehydrated to close their eyes, corneal dryness and exposure ulceration may result, and in tropical practice, traditional medicines are frequently applied and may contribute to secondary infection worsening prognosis. Subjects with ocular complications of measles should be treated with vitamin A, although a recent Cochrane review suggested that the evidence to support this is still incomplete.[32] In addition, topical antibiotics and measures to avoid corneal exposure should be used. Significant progress has been made in extending measles vaccination in the last decade – in 2012 an estimated 84% of children received one dose of measles vaccine before their first birthday.[33]

Leprosy

PATHOGENESIS

Three main mechanisms in leprosy lead to eye pathology. Overwhelming bacterial infection in lepromatous leprosy can cause atrophy of the involved tissues. The eye may be involved in type I reactions (reversal reactions), in which motor and sensory nerve loss is prominent, and in type II reactions, in which inflammation within the eye is prominent. As elsewhere in the body it is the reactions that cause most damage, manifest as visual loss and blindness.

CLINICAL FEATURES (see also Chapter 108)

Lepromatous leprosy may be characterized by limbal lepromata – painless yellow or pink nodules at the corneoscleral junction. Chalky deposits may be associated with corneal invasion by *Mycobacterium leprae*. The iris can become thin and atrophic, and pathognomonic 'iris pearls' which are calcified foci of dead leprosy bacilli, appear as white nodules on the surface of the iris.[34] Type I reactions involving the fifth cranial nerve can result in corneal anesthesia, and lagophthalmos (inability to close the eyes) may occur if the seventh cranial nerve is involved. Together, they produce a cornea that is both anesthetic and exposed, and therefore requires protection. Eye health education, blinking exercises, protective spectacles and surgical procedures such as tarsorrhaphy may all be needed.[35] Type II reactions may also cause acute or chronic iritis, which requires treatment with topical corticosteroids, or scleritis that may require systemic treatment with corticosteroids and clofazimine.

Clinical Aspects of Eye Involvement in Common Tropical Infections

Bacterial Infections

TUBERCULOSIS

Primary tuberculosis may affect the conjunctiva with nodular lesions and associated chronic conjunctivitis that is not responsive to standard topical treatment. In miliary disease, tubercles may be found in the conjunctiva, the iris or the choroid. Phlyctenular conjunctivitis and granulomatous uveitis may be associated with tuberculosis but are not specific for it. Optic neuritis may complicate tuberculous basal meningitis.

SEXUALLY TRANSMITTED DISEASES

Ocular gonococcal infection, usually due to autoinoculation from the genital tract, causes an acute purulent conjunctivitis that progresses rapidly to corneal ulceration and perforation in the absence of appropriate treatment.

Gonococcal ophthalmia neonatorum, acquired by an infant passing through an infected birth canal, is similarly threatening to sight and usually presents in the first week of life as a bilateral purulent conjunctivitis.

Ocular autoinoculation from genital *C. trachomatis* infection causes a clinical picture identical to trachoma, except that it is commonly unilateral. Among infants born to infected mothers, 30% develop chlamydial ophthalmia neonatorum, which is usually a self-limiting bilateral mucopurulent conjunctivitis presenting within 2 weeks of delivery. In a small proportion of cases, pneumonia and permanent lung sequelae follow. Thus chlamydial and gonococcal ophthalmia neonatorum both require systemic and topical therapy.[36]

Iritis, retinal vasculitis, optical neuritis and disseminated chorioretinitis may be features of secondary acquired syphilis.

OTHER BACTERIAL INFECTIONS

Petechiae may be seen at the conjunctiva in meningococcal meningitis: conjunctivitis, anterior uveitis and even panophthalmitis may complicate meningococcemia. Diphtheria may present with a membranous conjunctivitis, lid edema and the local effects of exotoxin. Cholera with rapid dehydration has been associated with the acute development of cataracts. Rose spots in typhoid fever may involve the conjunctiva. The clinical picture known as Parinaud's syndrome (follicular or granulomatous conjunctivitis and preauricular lymphadenopathy, often with systemic malaise) is associated with pathogen invasion via the conjunctiva and may be seen with a number of infections, including tuberculosis, syphilis, tularemia, cat-scratch disease and lymphogranuloma venereum. Brucellosis has been associated with chronic granulomatous uveitis. Dilation of the conjunctival vessels (suffusion) and subconjunctival hemorrhages may be presenting features of leptospirosis or typhus.

Parasitic Infections

Retinal hemorrhages, and retinal whitening (Figure 112-5) are components of a specific malarial retinopathy[37] and may be the earliest sign of cerebral involvement. Unilateral edema of the eyelid (Romaña's sign) may be seen in American trypanosomiasis if the inoculation site is in the region of the eye. Chorioretinitis is the most common ocular manifestation of toxoplasmosis. An ocular larva migrans syndrome (larvae migrating within the eye) may be seen with *Toxocara* spp. and *Gnathostoma* spp., and *Loa loa* typically migrates under the conjunctiva. Egg granulomas may occur in the conjunctiva or choroid in schistosomiais. Cysticerci of *Taenia solium* may occur within the eye, often subretinally.

Viral Infections

In many tropical environments herpes simplex virus is the commonest cause of corneal ulceration, often occurring as a complication of measles or cause of high fever such as in malaria. A narrow, branching dendritic ulcer that is best seen with fluorescein staining is typical (Figure 112-6) but in tropical practice the time to presentation and inappropriate use of traditional eye medicine often modify this, leading to larger ameboid ulcers. If available, idoxuridine or aciclovir drops should be given very frequently until epithelial healing takes place.

Infection with HIV may itself cause a retinopathy with cotton wool spots, indicating damage to the retina. Cytomegalovirus retinopathy does not seem to be common in tropical practice, but syphilis, tuberculosis and herpes simplex virus and their associated ocular

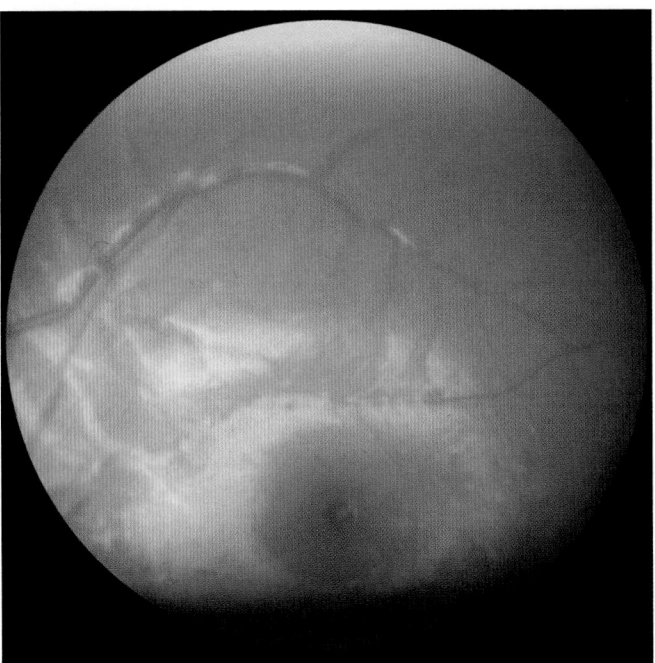

Figure 112-5 Retinal whitening in malarial retinopathy. *(Courtesy of Matthew Burton.)*

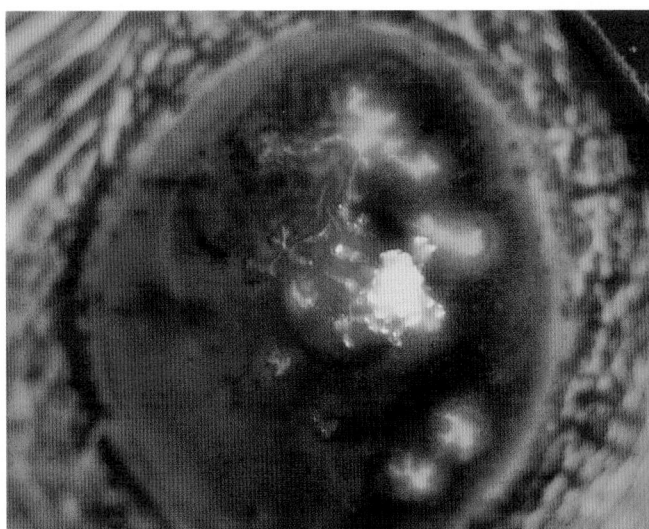

Figure 112-6 Typical dendritic ulcer caused by herpes simplex virus, visualized with fluorescein staining.

manifestations are commoner among HIV patients. Kaposi's sarcoma may involve the eyelid or conjunctiva.

Microbial Keratitis

Although contact lens use is the most important predisposing factor for microbial keratitis in industrialized country settings, in tropical practice microbial keratitis is usually the result of corneal trauma, and may have been mismanaged in the traditional sector before presentation. Patients present with a history of trauma together with photophobia, pain, loss of vision and purulent discharge, with cells and pus in the anterior chamber (hypopyon) (Figure 112-7). The corneal defect may contain bacteria (*S. aureus*, *Streptococcus*, *Proteus* or *Pseudomonas* spp. are commonly reported) or fungi (as in Figure 112-7). Fungal keratitis due to filamentous fungi such as *Aspergillus* and *Fusarium* spp. has been reported associated with trauma involving plant or organic matter. Fungal keratitis due to yeast-like fungi (particularly *Candida* spp.) is more often seen in patients with prior conditions such as deficient tear film, defective closure, or diabetes mellitus. If available, microscopy or culture of a corneal scrape, clinical features or local knowledge[38,39] may help to diagnose the cause. Medical treatment with frequent application of topical antibiotic solutions and/or antifungals may prevent corneal scarring or perforation.

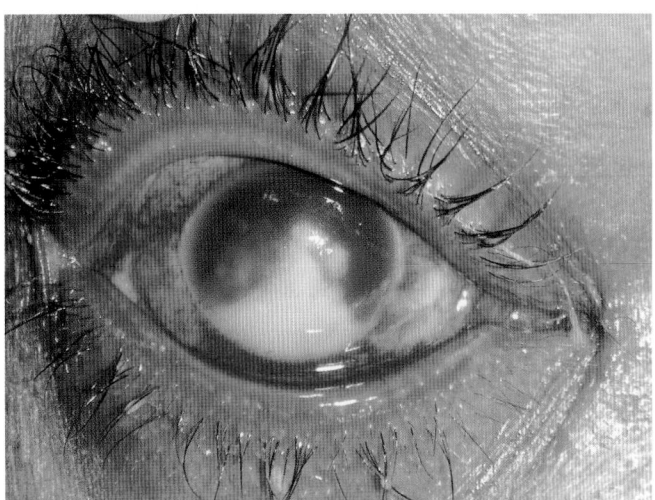

Figure 112-7 Fungal keratitis with hypopyon. *(Courtesy of Matthew Burton.)*

 References available online at expertconsult.com.

KEY REFERENCES

Beare N.A., Taylor T.E., Harding S.P., et al.: Malarial retinopathy: a newly established diagnostic sign in severe malaria. *Am J Trop Med Hyg* 2006; 75(5):790-797.

Brattig N.W.: Pathogenesis and host responses in human onchocerciasis: impact of *Onchocerca filariae* and *Wolbachia endobacteria*. *Microbes Infect* 2004; 6(1):113-128.

Gilbert C.E., Wood M., Waddel K., et al.: Causes of childhood blindness in east Africa: results in 491 pupils attending 17 schools for the blind in Malawi, Kenya and Uganda. *Ophthalmic Epidemiol* 1995; 2(2):77-84.

International Trachoma Initiative: Global atlas of trachoma: an open-access resource on the geographical distribution of trachoma. Available: www.trachomaatlas.org/.

Natividad A., Freeman T.C., Jeffries D., et al.: Human conjunctival transcriptome analysis reveals the prominence of innate defense in *Chlamydia trachomatis* infection. *Infect Immun* 2010; 78(11):4895-4911.

Rajak S.N., Habtamu E., Weiss H.A., et al.: Surgery versus epilation for the treatment of minor trichiasis in Ethiopia: a randomised controlled noninferiority trial. *PLoS Med* 2011; 8(12):e1001136.

Tamarozzi F., Halliday A., Gentil K., et al.: Onchocerciasis: the role of *Wolbachia* bacterial endosymbionts in parasite biology, disease pathogenesis, and treatment. *Clin Microbiol Rev* 2011; 24(3):459-468.

Thomas P.A., Leck A.K., Myatt M.: Characteristic clinical features as an aid to the diagnosis of suppurative keratitis caused by filamentous fungi. *Br J Ophthalmol* 2005; 89(12):1554-1558.

World Health Organization (WHO): Trachoma: situation and trends. Available: www.who.int/gho/neglected_diseases/trachoma/en/.

113

Approach to Eosinophilia in a Traveler from the Tropics

ANDREW P. USTIANOWSKI | JOOP E. ARENDS

KEY CONCEPTS

- Eosinophilia is a common finding in travelers and though most frequently related to an acquired helminth infection, other causes such as malignancies, atopy, drug hypersensitivity and autoimmune conditions need to be considered.

- A detailed travel history determining specific geographic, environmental and cultural exposures may help to narrow down the list of likely helminths; however, screening for several is often required, and screening and management algorithms have been developed.

- In an asymptomatic individual, delaying screening until several months after exposure is likely to increase the yield of the assays, and in those who are symptomatic it is common to treat on clinical suspicion, as the diagnosis may initially be difficult to confirm.

- In those with persisting eosinophilia or symptoms, expert advice should be sought because the available diagnostics are frequently suboptimal or difficult to interpret.

- It is important to confirm that eosinophilia and any symptoms resolve fully to ensure that alternative diagnoses are not missed or delayed.

Epidemiology

An elevated eosinophil count is a common, frequently under-recognized finding in travelers returning from the tropics. Although there are multiple causes of eosinophilia – from atopy, drug hypersensitivity and infections to malignancies – in a traveler it is often related to an acquired helminth infection.

In asymptomatic returning travellers, eosinophilia has been detected in 8–10%,[1–3] and of these 14–64% have been shown to have acquired worm infections.[1,3,4] However, such studies and others[5,6] have generally had methodological issues, such as retrospective designs, targeted or small patient groups, or short intervals between exposure and testing (which can significantly affect diagnostic yields). The GeoSentinel Surveillance Network has overcome some of these issues by including larger numbers of patients and has provided data on several specific helminth infections, including filariasis and schistosomiasis.[7–10] It has associated a longer time spent in the tropics to an increased chance of developing eosinophilia,[11] and has helped to determine risks of specific infections by geographic region visited. In immigrants from tropical areas eosinophilia has been detected in 12–23%,[12,13] and a large proportion of these individuals have detectable helminth infections.

The epidemiology of eosinophilia depends significantly upon the relative prevalences of helminths to which the traveler may have been exposed – which depends upon the geographic and physical exposures the individual has had.

Some helminth infections can be acquired on many continents (e.g., *Ascaris*) whereas others can be quite focal (e.g., *Loa loa*). Some are generally associated with only rural exposure (e.g., *Schistosoma*) whereas others may also be encountered in urban environments (e.g., *Gnathostoma*). They can be acquired via a variety of different routes and from differing exposures – for instance, exposure to fresh water may lead to schistosomiasis, and specific food intake may hint at

specific etiology (e.g., the consumption of water vegetation [*Fasciola*], raw or undercooked crabs/shellfish [*Paragonimus*], fish [*Anisakis* and *Gnathostoma*], snails [*Angiostrongylus cantonensis*], frog/snake [*Gnathostoma*] or pork, bear and crocodile [*Trichinella*]). A detailed travel history and inquiring into particular exposures and contact with specific vectors are therefore vital to correctly investigate and diagnose a traveler with eosinophilia.

It must be remembered that not all eosinophilia is due to such parasitic infections,[14] and therefore the full approach to such patients also relies on the exclusion of other causes (as outlined in Table 113-1), and rational diagnostic algorithms.

Pathogenesis and Pathology

Eosinophils are leukocytes derived from bone marrow via the myeloid and then granulocyte lineages. Their predominant subsequent location is within the tissues (especially gut and airway), although eosinophil levels are routinely assessed only by counting the relatively small proportion that are located within the blood. They are principally produced and activated in response to a Th2-type cytokine milieu (especially interleukin (IL)-4, IL-5, IL-13 and IgE).

Eosinophils are multifunctional proinflammatory cells that have pivotal roles in allergic responses and immunity against multicellular parasites, but also are involved in organ formation (e.g., mammary gland development) and probably many other processes. They can also be directly pathogenic – hypereosinophilia can be associated with tissue damage secondary to the effects of released granule proteins (e.g., major basic protein, eosinophilic cationic protein, eosinophil peroxidase and eosinophil-derived neurotoxin) or hyperviscosity at very high cell counts.

The upper range of normal for the eosinophil count varies with age and between laboratories. There is also marked diurnal variation in counts (with up to 40% variation coinciding with cortisol levels). However, in adults it is generally agreed that a count greater than 0.45

TABLE 113-1	Main Causes of Eosinophilia	
Category	**Main Examples**
Allergic conditions	Atopic dermatitis Asthma Allergic rhinitis Reaction to medications
Infections	Helminth infections Fungal infections (allergic bronchpulmonary aspergillosis and coccidioidomycosis)
Neoplastic and hematologic conditions	Lymphoma (esp. Hodgkin's) Leukemia Multiple malignancies Hypereosinophilic syndromes Mastocytosis
Rheumatologic and immunologic conditions	Vasculitides (esp. Churg–Strauss syndrome) Hyper-IgE syndrome Omenn syndrome
Other	Adrenal insufficiency Cholesterol embolism

$x10^9$/L is elevated. Counts greater than 1.5 $x10^9$/L are generally classified as moderate, and greater than 5 $x10^9$/L as severe. The term hypereosinophilia is sometimes used to classify counts greater than 1.5 $x10^9$/L.

There are multiple causes of eosinophilia, which may be subclassified as primary or secondary.[14] Primary eosinophilia is caused by clonal expansion of eosinophils associated with hematological malignancies, such as leukemias and myeloid disorders. Secondary eosinophilia can be due to allergies, infections, neoplastic and autoimmune conditions, and a variety of other causes (Table 113-1).

Tissue-helminth infections are often associated with eosinophilia detectable in the peripheral blood. However, some tissue helminths become effectively separated from host immune surveillance and therefore lose their propensity to induce an eosinophilia until any barriers become breached or weakened; for example, a hydatid cyst is often associated with eosinophilia only if there has been cyst leakage. Gut-lumen helminths are not usually associated with increased blood eosinophil counts, except during or soon after tissue migratory phases.

Generally, infection with unicellular parasites such as amebae and other protozoae does not cause eosinophilia. *Isospora* infection is an exception. Certain other infections, such as human immunodeficiency virus, have been associated with eosinophilia, but it is unclear whether this is directly causal or related to other undiagnosed precipitants.

While some helminth infections may be benign or self-limiting (e.g. cutaneous larva migrans due to infection with animal hookworm species) it has been estimated that between 10% and 73% of returning travelers and immigrants from tropical areas with eosinophilia have a potentially serious infection with direct health consequences for the individuals themselves or their contacts.[3,4,12,13,15–18]

It is also important to appreciate that not all individuals with helminth infection will have an elevated blood eosinophil count,[19,20] and, in those that do, the degree of eosinophilia and the associated symptoms depend on several factors. Principal amongst these are whether the individual has had prior exposure to that (or a related) helminth, the burden of infection within the individual and how long they have been infected. In general, there are higher eosinophil counts and more associated symptoms if the host is previously naïve to the parasite.

Therefore, the symptoms, clinical features and laboratory findings will frequently vary between travelers (in whom the host is generally naïve to the helminth) and immigrants or people still residing in endemic areas (where chronic heavy infections are more common).[21]

Prevention

In some environments helminths are virtually ubiquitous and preventing exposure (and therefore potential infection) is almost impossible. However certain measures can be undertaken to decrease the risks associated with specific infections.

Where helminths are transmitted via arthropod vectors, decreasing exposure to these insects may have a role – for example use of insect repellents and wearing long sleeves and trousers in the case of filariasis and *Loa loa*. Other helminths are acquired from direct cutaneous–soil exposure; avoiding walking barefoot, especially over areas that may be fecally contaminated, can prevent infections such as hookworm and strongyloidiasis. Others are acquired via poorly washed or under-cooked foodstuffs, and therefore food and water hygiene can have a role in decreasing the frequency of helminth as well as other infections.

There is some evidence supporting the application of DEET (N,N-Diethyl-m-toluamide – at concentrations found in insect repellents) to skin after exposure to fresh water potentially contaminated with *Schistosoma* to prevent the establishment of infection (by killing the larvae as they penetrate the skin layers).[22] However, few other direct methods are available to the traveler.

Clinical Features

Many travelers have asymptomatic eosinophilia. By definition they therefore have no obvious clinical symptoms or signs and their evaluation depends almost entirely on determining potential exposures (geography- or activity-based) and subsequent diagnostic algorithms.

Other travelers may be pauci-symptomatic and initially not recall or notice symptoms. An in-depth history, sometimes with leading questions (e.g. the occurrence of cutaneous lesions after exposure to fresh water – potentially the 'swimmer's itch' of schistosomiasis) is therefore required.

Others will have prominent clinical features, and in these eosinophilia will first be detected as part of their diagnostic 'work-up'. Broadly the clinical symptoms and signs can be grouped into a few major categories – cutaneous, gastrointestinal/hepatic, neurological, respiratory and 'other'.[23] Fever may also occur – either in isolation or associated with one of the above. Some helminths, and some patients, may present with a combination of such features. Clearly defining the presenting syndrome helps in arriving at the differential diagnosis. See Table 113-2 for the major causes of the specific syndromic presentations by geographic exposure.

The differential diagnosis largely revolves around those other infections and those noninfectious conditions that are associated with eosinophilia[24] (see Table 113-1). Particular attention must be paid to excluding hematological and neoplastic conditions in those patients without obvious other cause – as delays in their diagnosis may have significant impacts upon treatment and prognosis.

Diagnosis

The successful diagnosis of helminth infection, and thereby the most common causes of new-onset eosinophilia in travelers, frequently depends on the application of diagnostic algorithms – which are themselves dependent on syndromic presentation and geographic (and other) exposures.[1,23,25] As described earlier, the major helminth infections can be broadly grouped by syndromic clinical features – particularly those that cause rash, those associated with fever, those that predominantly affect the GI tract or liver, the chest, or nervous system, and those that are most commonly asymptomatic. A summary of the more common helminth causes by geographic exposure and symptomatology is given in Table 113-2. The initial investigations will depend on the most likely pathogens thus determined, and up-to-date advice on sampling and available assays (which may include nucleic acid amplification techniques) should be obtained from local and reference laboratories. Table 113-3 describes the main diagnostic investigations for commonly identified infections.

There are issues specific to parasitic infections that need to be considered in the diagnostic approach to a traveler with eosinophilia. Prominent amongst these are the prepatent period (and its relevance to the timing of investigations) and the frequency of cross-reactivity of helminth serology assays.

Many tropical diagnostics require the direct visualization of ova or the parasites themselves. Early in infection, symptoms and eosinophilia may be caused by larvae or immature parasites – which cannot yet produce ova and themselves may not be detectable by direct microscopy or other simple methods. Therefore it is possible that available diagnostic tests will be negative, and the infection can remain unconfirmed until a later date when the adult parasites or sufficient ova are produced. The time between exposure (and potentially clinical symptoms) and the ability to detect the infection with such assays is termed the prepatent period. Similar issues can occur with serologic tests; either there can be delayed antibody responses only detectable on convalescent samples, or the antibody responses assayed are those directed to antigens not yet presented by the parasite (e.g., some serologic assays for schistosomiasis detect antibodies directed toward egg antigens that will be detectable only once egg production has ensued). As a result, it is common practice in those who are asymptomatic to delay performing a tropical screen until 1–4 months after exposure, and in those with symptoms to potentially treat on clinical grounds and attempt to confirm the diagnosis only several weeks later.

TABLE 113-2	Main Helminth Causes of Eosinophilia by Geographic Exposure and Symptomatology		
Geographic Exposure	**Predominant Symptom Complex**	**Detail**	**Infection**
GLOBAL	Cutaneous	Widespread urticaria Larva currens Serpiginous, pruritic	Acute schistosomiasis *Strongyloides stercoralis* Cutaneous larva migrans*
	Gastrointestinal/hepatic	Diarrhea, pain and iron deficiency Diarrhea, pain and biliary obstruction Diarrhea, pain Pain, biliary obstruction Pain, hepatosplenomegaly	Hookworm[††]‡ *Ascaris lumbricoides*[††]‡ *Strongyloides stercoralis*‡ Liver flukes – e.g. *Fasciola hepatica* Toxocara
	Respiratory	Wheeze, dry cough, pulmonary infiltrates	Hookworm *Wuchereria bancrofti* (filariasis) *Strongyloides stercoralis* Toxocara
	Other	Lymphangitis and lymphadenitis Myalgia, periorbital cellulitis, myocarditis	*Wuchereria bancrofti* (filariasis) Trichinella
AFRICA	Cutaneous	Pruritus, dermatitis, nodules Calabar swellings, eye worm	*Onchocerca volvulus* *Loa loa*
	Gastrointestinal/hepatic	Abdominal pain, diarrhea, portal hypertension	*Schistosoma mansoni*
	Respiratory	Pain, cavitatory lesions, hemoptysis, effusions	*Paragonimus*
	Neurological	Transverse myelitis	Schistosomiaisis
	Other	Hematuria, urinary obstruction Blindness	*Schistosoma haematobium* *Onchocerca volvulus*
AMERICA – SOUTH/ CENTRAL/CARIBBEAN	Cutaneous	Migratory subcutaneous swellings	Gnathostomiasis
	Gastrointestinal/hepatic	Abdominal pain, vomiting Abdominal pain, diarrhea, portal hypertension Abdominal pain, diarrhea	*Anisakis* and *Pseudoterranova* spp. *Schistosoma mansoni* *Angiostrongylus costaricensis*
	Respiratory	Pain, cavitatory lesions, hemoptysis, effusions	*Paragonimus*
	Neurologic	Eosinophilic meningitis Meningoencephalitis, myelitis	*Angiostrongylus cantonensis* Gnathostomiasis
ASIA AND OCEANIA	Cutaneous	Migratory subcutaneous swellings	Gnathostomiasis
	Gastrointestinal/hepatic	Abdominal pain, vomiting Abdominal pain, diarrhea, portal hypertension Pain, biliary obstruction	*Anisakis* and *Pseudoterranova* spp. *Schistosoma japonicum* *Fasciola gigantica* *Clonorchis sinensis* and *Opisthorchis* spp.
	Respiratory	Wheeze, dry cough, pulmonary infiltrates Pain, cavitatory lesions, hemoptysis, effusions	*Brugia malayi* (filariasis) *Paragonimus*
	Neurologic	Eosinophilic meningitis Meningoencephalitis, myelitis	*Angiostrongylus cantonensis* Gnathostomiasis
	Other	Lymphangitis and lymphadenitis	*Brugia malayi* (filariasis)

*Usually not associated with eosinophilia.
†Usually associated with eosinophilia only during or soon after tissue migratory phase.
‡Mostly asymptomatic.

A second issue is that of serological cross-reactivity. Most diagnostics that depend on direct visualization of a parasite, its ova or cysts, allow an experienced parasitologist to make a definitive diagnosis; but those dependent on antibody responses can frequently lead to false-positive results attributable to cross-reactivity. Common examples are the cross-reactivity between filarial and *Strongyloides* serology, between schistosomiasis and *Fasciola*, and between cysticercosis and hydatid. Therefore a comparative determination of the specific titers, changes in titer as a result of specific treatment, and/or expert advice are often required to firmly establish a specific helminth diagnosis by these routes.

Management

Optimal management of eosinophilia in a traveler ideally depends on making a specific diagnosis and thence providing specific therapies and ensuring resolution. Alternatively, treating empirically once

common diagnoses have been excluded may be a possibility. Finally, in some circumstances, avoiding specific therapy and monitoring the patient to ensure spontaneous resolution may be a suitable option.

The more frequently encountered parasitic causes of eosinophilia in travelers have been summarized by geographic exposure and common symptomatology in Table 113-2. More detailed descriptions are available from a variety of sources (e.g., Checkley *et al.*[25]), and data further supporting the potential of a geographic approach are becoming more refined (e.g., GeoSentinel studies have demonstrated that the majority of filarial and 83% of *Schistosoma* infections arise in Africa, and within this continent, 73% of *Strongyloides* and *Schistosoma* infections are acquired in East or West Africa, whilst 94% of *Loa loa* and similar proportions of *Onchocerca* were diagnosed in travelers from Central Africa).

Such data have been used[4,23,25] to develop diagnostic algorithms to aid clinicians, and these can be combined with the potential use of

TABLE 113-3	Main Available Initial Diagnostics for Tropical Helminth Infections		
Helminth	**Common Diagnostic Assays**	**Helminth**	**Common Diagnostic Assays**
Angiostrongylus spp.	Serology	*Onchocerca volvulus*	Filarial serology 'Skin snips' Slit-lamp examination
Anisakis and *Pseudoterranova* spp.	Serology Visualization at endoscopy	*Paragonimus*	Stool & sputum OC&P Serology
Ascaris lumbricoides	Stool OC&P		
Filariasis and *Loa loa*	Filarial serology 'Day and night' bloods for microscopy	Schistosomiasis	Serology Stool OC&P Terminal urine microscopy
Flukes – e.g. *Fasciola hepatica, Clonorchis sinensis* and *Opisthorchis* spp.	Stool OC&P Serology	*Strongyloides stercoralis*	Serology Stool OC&P and *Strongyloides* culture
Gnathostomiasis	Serology	*Toxocara*	Serology
Hookworm	Stool OC&P Serology of little utility	*Trichinella*	Serology Histology of biopsy

OC&P, ova, cyst and parasite microscopy (after concentration steps).
For more information on specific assays and their requirements please refer to relevant sections on these infections.

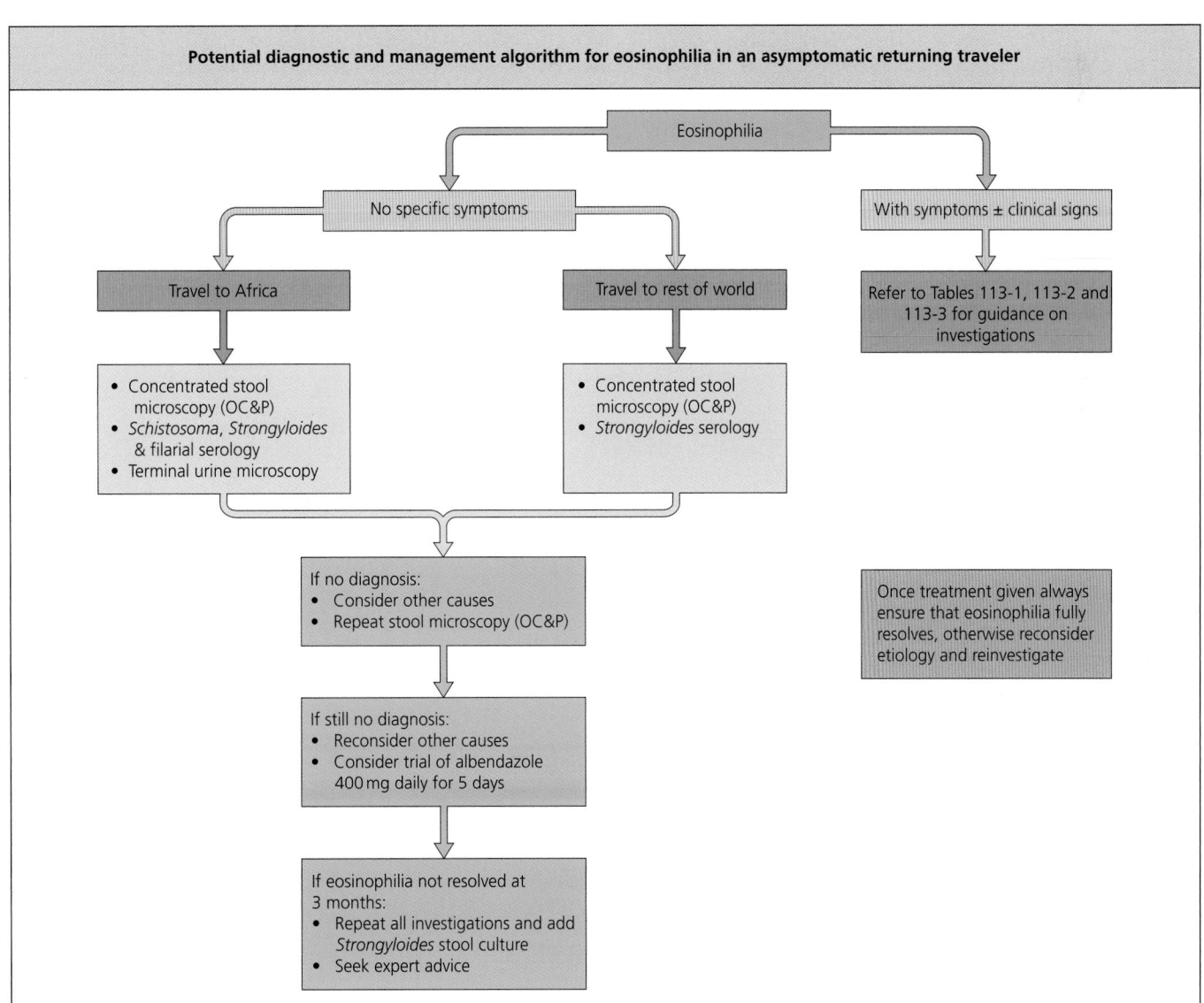

Figure 113-1   Potential diagnostic and management algorithm for eosinophilia in an asymptomatic returning traveler.

empiric broad-spectrum anthelmintic therapy or observation in pathways such as that shown in Figure 113-1.

The most commonly used empiric treatment is albendazole; however, this drug is not truly broad-spectrum, having inadequate efficacy against many helminths, and there is no consensus on suitable length of therapy. Such empiric treatment should generally be reserved for those cases of persistent eosinophilia that have remained undiagnosed despite extensive investigation, and it is vital that such treatment leads to the permanent resolution of the eosinophilia, to ensure that continuing infection or alternative causes (see Table 113-1) are not missed.

Lastly, it must be acknowledged that algorithms and tables cannot be comprehensive and that there are many rarer parasitic causes of eosinophilia (some of which are yet to have reliable diagnostics developed), so it remains important to seek expert advice should initial diagnoses be excluded.

References available online at expertconsult.com.

KEY REFERENCES

Baaten G.G., Sonder G.J., van Gool T., et al.: Travel-related schistosomiasis, strongyloidiasis, filariasis, and toxocariasis: the risk of infection and the diagnostic relevance of blood eosinophilia. *BMC Infect Dis* 2011; 11:84.

Checkley A.M., Chiodini P.L., Dockrell D.H., et al.: Eosinophilia in returning travellers and migrants from the tropics: UK recommendations for investigation and initial management. *J Infect* 2010; 60(1):1-20.

Leder K., Torresi J., Libman M.D., et al.: GeoSentinel surveillance of illness in returned travelers, 2007–2011. *Ann Intern Med* 2013; 158(6):456-468.

Lipner E.M., Law M.A., Barnett E., et al.: Filariasis in travelers presenting to the Geo-Sentinel Surveillance Network. *PLoS Negl Trop Dis* 2007; 1(3):e88.

Meltzer E., Percik R., Shatzkes J., et al.: Eosinophilia among returning travellers: a practical approach. *Am J Trop Med Hyg* 2008; 78(5):702-709.

Mendelson M., Han P.V., Vincent P., et al.: GeoSentinel Surveillance Network. Regional variation in travel-related illness acquired in Africa, March 1997–May 2011. *Emerg Infect Dis* 2014; 20(4):532-541.

Nicolls D.J., Weld L.H., Schwartz E., et al.: Characteristics of schistosomiasis in travellers reported to the GeoSentinel Surveillance Network 1997–2008. *Am J Trop Med Hyg* 2008; 79(5):729-734.

Seybolt L.M., Christiansen D., Barnett E.D.: Diagnostic evaluation of newly arrived asymptomatic refugees with eosinophilia. *Clin Infect Dis* 2006; 42(3):363-367.

Ustianowski A., Zumla A.: Eosinophilia in the returning traveler. *Infect Dis Clin North Am* 2012; 26(3):781-789.

Whetham J., Day J.N., Armstrong M., et al.: Investigation of tropical eosinophilia; assessing a strategy based on geographical area. *J Infect* 2003; 46(3):180-185.

114

Parasitic Infections of the Gastrointestinal Tract

PAUL KELLY | MABLE MUTENGO

KEY CONCEPTS

- Parasitic infections of the gastrointestinal tract are common, especially in the tropics, but occur everywhere.

- Feco-oral spread is the commonest route of infection, but other routes of infection include ground-based skin penetration and food-based contamination.

- Taxonomy is under constant revision, with recent changes in the status of *Entamoeba* spp. and microsporidia (which are now classified as fungi).

- Many infections are light and of no clinical relevance, but certain clinical syndromes need to be recognized.

- The dominant parasitic causes of diarrhea are protozoa; strongyloidiasis is also an important cause.

- Certain infections, notably amebiasis and strongyloidiasis, can disseminate to produce extraintestinal infection.

- Hookworm infection is an important cause of anemia, but it may also mask other gastrointestinal pathologies such as cancer.

- Prevention is mainly through improved hygiene; no vaccines are available.

- Mass chemotherapy may sometimes have a role in reducing the burden of consequences and rarely in reducing transmission.

Introduction

This chapter examines the parasitic causes of gastrointestinal infection in the non-immunocompromised host. The organisms involved are a very heterogeneous group of protozoa and helminths. They vary in size from coccidia, which are a few micrometers in diameter, to long multicellular organisms such as *Taenia saginata*, which can reach 25 m in length (Figure 114-1). The clinical approach is emphasized here because the parasites themselves are discussed elsewhere (see Chapters 116, 119, 120 and 191 to 195), and therapeutic agents are discussed in Chapter 157. Parasitic gastrointestinal infections in HIV infection are discussed in Chapter 94. The parasites discussed in this chapter are listed in Table 114-1.

Epidemiology

In affluent settings, parasitic infections appear to be uncommon causes of gastrointestinal illness. Certain populations are particularly likely to be affected:
- returned travelers;
- daycare workers and patients;
- children in daycare centers;
- migrant workers;
- persons with common variable immunodeficiency (CVID);
- HIV infected persons; and
- men who have sex with men.

In this setting, most common causes of parasitic gastrointestinal infection are *Giardia intestinalis* and *Cryptosporidium* spp.

In resource-poor settings the impact of parasitic infections is of great significance in terms of morbidity, mortality and economic impact. Their epidemiology is varied and their control presents a complex sociopolitical problem. Here, the most important infections

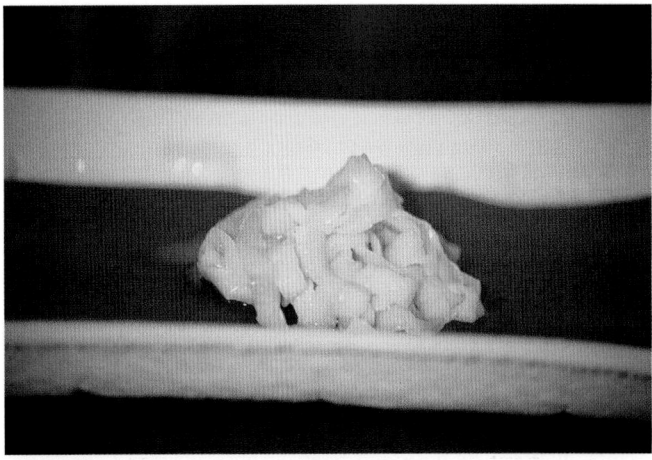

Figure 114-1 Adult beef tapeworm (*Taenia saginata*) passed in a patient's feces.

TABLE 114-1	Gastrointestinal Parasites of Pathogenic Significance
INTESTINAL PROTOZOA	
Amebae	*Entamoeba histolytica*
Bigyra	*Blastocystis hominis*
Flagellates	*Giardia intestinalis* *Dientamoeba fragilis*
Ciliate	*Balantidium coli*
Coccidia	*Cryptosporidium parvum/C. hominis* *Cyclospora cayetanensis* *Isospora belli*
INTESTINAL HELMINTHS	
Nematodes (round worms)	*Ascaris lumbricoides* Hookworms *Ancylostoma duodenale* *Necator americanus* *Trichuris trichiura* *Strongyloides stercoralis/fulleborni* *Enterobius vermicularis*
Trematodes (flukes)	*Fasciolopsis buski* *Heterophyes heterophyes*
Cestodes (tapeworms)	*Taenia solium* *Taenia saginata* *Hymenolepis nana* *Diphyllobothrium latum*

are *Entamoeba histolytica*, *G. intestinalis*, hookworms, *Ascaris* spp. and tapeworms. The burden of hepatosplenic schistosomiasis is very high in some areas (see Chapter 118).

GEOGRAPHIC DISTRIBUTION OF PARASITES

The distribution of a parasite depends upon three factors: human behavior, the physical environment and the biologic environment.

Human Behavior

Behavioral factors are often dominant but the distribution of vectors, intermediate hosts and reservoir hosts is also to some extent under human control. Some parasites are worldwide in their distribution, such as *E. histolytica* and *G. intestinalis*, whereas others are highly localized.

Physical Environment

The physical environment also affects the distribution of parasites. Temperature and humidity affect the viability of parasite ova, cysts and larvae in the external environment; viability is lost in cold or over-hot temperatures and most parasites require moist, aerobic conditions. Temperature and humidity also affect sporulation of oocysts, the rates of embryonation of nematode, cestode and trematode eggs, and the development times for hookworm and *Strongyloides* larvae. Parasites that have a soil stage are affected by the particular physical properties of the soil, including its particle size and water-holding capacity, and by factors such as rainfall. Susceptibility to anaerobic conditions is important for some parasites when 'night soil' (human feces) is used raw or after composting as a fertilizer. The aquatic environment is important in the life cycle of many parasites. In the trematodes, the cercariae of *Heterophyes* spp. must survive long enough to infect the fish or shrimp and the metacercariae of *Fasciolopsis buski* must survive long enough to infect the human or pig hosts. *Strongyloides* larvae live in the capillary water films in soil and on low vegetation.

Biologic Environment

The biologic environment also affects the epidemiology of these gastrointestinal parasites. The distribution in nature of appropriate vectors, intermediate hosts and reservoir hosts obviously affects the distribution of parasites. Examples of animal reservoirs are *F. buski* in dogs, pigs or rabbits; *Balantidium coli* in pigs; *Cryptosporidium parvum* in domestic animals, particularly cattle, *G. intestinalis* in beavers; and *Heterophyes heterophyes* in fish-eating mammals. Secondary hosts include snails for *F. buski* and freshwater fish for *H. heterophyes*.

HUMAN FACTORS

Population Density and Urbanization

The agricultural revolution in developing countries has produced large resident human populations with the potential for direct person-to-person spread of infection and greater environmental contamination by feces. In addition, animal husbandry has created other cycles for parasite transmission, for example *Cryptosporidium* spp. in calves. Rapid urbanization, especially in the tropics, is often associated with increased poverty, poor housing and unsanitary conditions. The result is that people may be living in a more fecally polluted environment than in rural areas, encouraging such diseases as amebiasis and giardiasis. Epidemics, such as outbreaks of cryptosporidiosis, may occur when public water supplies become fecally contaminated.[1] *Cyclospora cayetanensis* is transmitted via contaminated produce and contaminated drinking water. The soil-transmitted nematodes *Ascaris lumbricoides* and *Trichuris trichiura* are often more common in towns and cities. Overcrowding favors direct transmission of *Hymenolepis nana* and *Enterobius vermicularis*, especially in children when levels of hygiene and sanitation are poor.[2]

Population Movements

Population changes associated with mining, political unrest or industrialization may cause people to move into at-risk areas; travelers may also visit such areas.

Dams and Irrigation

Development programs in the tropics frequently involve irrigation projects, where contaminated water supplies reach greater numbers of people and larger water-borne outbreaks may occur. Irrigation and poor drainage facilitate the breeding of flies that may have a role in spreading fecal material.

Agriculture

Cattle raising may be complicated by bovine cysticercosis (*T. saginata*), which renders carcasses unsalable, and calves may be a source of human infection. Pigs can allow *Taenia solium*, the pork tapeworm, to be spread and *F. buski*, the intestinal fluke, to prosper. *B. coli* is also acquired from close contact with pigs. Fish farms, in which water plants such as water calthrop are grown, transmit *F. buski*, especially if human or pig feces are used as fertilizer. Foods implicated in outbreaks of cyclosporiasis in the USA include fresh raspberries, mesclun lettuce and Thai basil.[3] The use of untreated human night soil enables soil-transmitted helminths to enter the human food chain.

DOMESTIC ENVIRONMENT

Sanitation, water supplies and domestic customs in hygiene and food preparation are all very important. Children are at risk of parasitic infections because of poor hand washing after defecation, finger sucking and playing with soil. Local dietary behavior is critical for parasite transmission. Ingestion of certain fish, crustacea, molluscs and aquatic vegetation can lead to fluke infection. Tapeworms are contracted by ingestion of undercooked pork or beef (*Taenia* spp.) or certain freshwater fish (*Diphyllobothrium* spp.). Ova of hookworms penetrate skin where people walk barefoot on contaminated soil.

HOST SUSCEPTIBILITY

Host susceptibility is affected by many factors such as nutritional status, intercurrent disease, pregnancy, immunosuppressive drugs and malignancy. Previously mild or clinically inapparent infections can cause severe disease when host immunity falls, such as occurs in strongyloidiasis, in which the parasite is capable of multiplying by autoinfection within its host, and fatal amebiasis may occur if corticosteroids are administered.

Some protective immunity is usually acquired by the host but its effectiveness is variable. The absence of symptomatic giardiasis in adults in places where the infection is common is good evidence for acquired immunity. Re-infection and superinfection, possibly by different gastrointestinal parasite strains, is certainly common in areas of endemic infection. Immunodeficiency associated with HIV infection is of paramount importance in some of the more recently recognized gastrointestinal parasitic diseases such as cryptosporidiosis (see Chapter 94). While extracellular parasites (*G. intestinalis*) and certain others (*Entamoeba* spp.) are unaffected by HIV status, giardiasis is more of a problem in patients with common variable immunodeficiency (CVID) or selective IgA deficiency.

Pathogenesis and Pathology

Gastrointestinal parasites cause disease in a variety of ways. Most are present in the lumen of the gut or attached to the mucosa of the gut wall and are not capable of invasion. The coccidian parasites such as cryptosporidia can invade the epithelial cells of the small bowel. Others, such as *E. histolytica*, *Strongyloides stercoralis* and occasionally *B. coli*, do invade the mucosa (Table 114-2).

GASTROINTESTINAL PROTOZOA

Amebiasis

Amebic ulcers mostly develop in the cecum, appendix or adjacent ascending colon, although the sigmoidorectal region can be involved. Amebic ulcers are formed on the mucosa. They are usually flask-shaped with a small, raised opening and a larger area of mucosal destruction below. The mucosa between abscesses is normal but lesions can be confluent. Pathogenic amebae are able to resist

TABLE 114-2	Anatomic Location of Pathogenic Stages of Gastrointestinal Parasites		
LUMEN ONLY	Small bowel (normally)	Ascaris lumbricoides Enterobius vermicularis
MUCOSAL ATTACHMENT	Small bowel	Giardia intestinalis Tapeworm Hookworm Fasciolopsis buski Heterophyes heterophyes
	Large bowel	Trichuris trichiura
EPITHELIAL CELL INVASION	Small bowel	Isospora belli Cyclospora cayetanensis Cryptosporidium parvum/C. hominis
MUCOSAL INVASION	Small bowel	Strongyloides stercoralis
	Large bowel	Entamoeba histolytica Balantidium coli

complement-mediated lysis and they possess other virulence factors such as attachment lectins, cysteine proteases and other enzymes[4] which, it is believed, assist the trophozoites with apoptosis of mammalian intestinal cells. Amebae have tissue-lysing enzymes on their surfaces that can be released from lysosomes or after amebic rupture, and amebapores contribute to cellular pathology.[5] In a study in Bangladeshi children, acquired immunity to amebiasis was associated with the appearance of an intestinal IgA response to the parasite Gal/GalNAc lectin, the virulence factor required for attachment of E. histolytica trophozoites to human cells. An intestinal IgA response to this lectin was associated with a 70% reduction in infections in children over the 2-year study period. On the other hand, those children who developed anti-amebic IgG antibodies in the serum were more susceptible to amebiasis. Interestingly, serum anti-lectin IgG antibodies cluster in families, supporting the presence of an inherited component to susceptibility to amebic disease.[6]

Giardiasis

The histopathology of the upper small bowel varies from normal to subtotal villous atrophy in giardiasis. *Giardia* spp. seem unable to penetrate the mucosal wall in humans but are able to attach to the mucosa of the small bowel. *G. intestinalis* has multiple pathways of pathogenicity, including interruption of digestion and absorption mechanisms, effacement of the microvillous brush border, disrupted bile salt metabolism, and immune activation.

Balantidiasis

The trophozoite of *Balantidium coli* causes mucosal inflammation and ulceration, invading the distal ileal and colonic mucosa. Ulceration may be superficial or involve the full thickness of the bowel, leading to perforation.[7]

Coccidia

Cryptosporidial infection in humans is most commonly due to *Cryptosporidium parvum* and *C. hominis* (formerly *C. parvum* genotype 1) but *C. felis*, *C. muris*, *C. canis* and *C. meleagridis* have been identified in immunocompromised individuals.[8] *C. hominis* has been linked to more severe symptoms in sporadic outbreaks, in HIV-positive individuals and in Brazilian children. In a study of more than 500 Peruvian children, *C. hominis* was the predominant cryptosporidial species and subtype Ib was associated with more symptoms of nausea, vomiting and general malaise in association with diarrhea than other subtypes (Ia, Id and Ie).[9] Different subtypes of *C. hominis* have varying effects in patients with HIV-associated cryptosporidiosis.

Cryptosporidium oocysts excyst in the small intestine and the trophozoites occupy an intracellular, extracytoplasmic location in the epithelial cells of the host small intestine, inducing major cytoskeletal changes and changing its physiology.[10] Merogony amplifies the

infection, then oocysts are excreted back into the environment (Figure 114-2). Small bowel histology shows villous atrophy and crypt hyperplasia, usually with a mixed inflammatory cell infiltrate in the lamina propria, and increased apoptosis. There is impaired absorption and enhanced intestinal secretion, but the mechanism is still not completely understood.

The mechanism of diarrhea production has not been clearly established for *Cyclospora cayetanensis* or for *Isospora belli*. These organisms are found within enterocytes. As with cryptosporidiosis there is reduction in villus height with associated mucosal inflammation.[11,12]

GASTROINTESTINAL HELMINTHS

Nematode Infections

Ascariasis (Roundworm Infection). The embryonated eggs of *Ascaris lumbricoides* are ingested and hatch in the stomach and duodenum, from where the larvae penetrate the intestinal wall. They are carried to the lungs in the circulation and usually cause no symptoms unless there are a large number of larvae, in which case pneumonitis can ensue. The larvae then break out of the lung tissue and may cause some bronchial epithelial damage. Intense tissue reaction with infiltration of eosinophils, macrophages and epithelioid cells occurs. Adult worms occupy a purely luminal position with no anchorage to the gut wall (Figure 114-3).

***Anisakis* Infection.** Anisakiasis is due to infection of the stomach or intestine with one or more of several species of *Anisakis simplex* and similar nematodes. They are acquired by eating uncooked fish, usually in Japan and the Far East, and cause acute abdominal pain.

Hookworm Infection. Hookworm disease is caused by *Ancylostoma duodenale* and *Necator americanus*. Vesiculation and pustules can occur on the skin at the site of entry of the filariform larvae. In severe infections, pneumonitis occurs as larvae migrate through the lungs, with small hemorrhages into the alveoli and infiltration of eosinophils and leukocytes. Adult hookworms attach firmly to the small bowel mucosa (Figure 114-4). *A. duodenale* achieves this by means of well-developed teeth and *N. americanus* by means of cutting plates. There tends to be chronic blood loss at the site where the worm attaches.

Trichuriasis (Whip Worm Infection). Infection is acquired by ingestion of embryonated eggs through contaminated food or water. The egg of the nematode *Trichuris trichiura* hatches in the small intestine and the larva penetrates the villi causing no pathologic reaction. It re-emerges after 1 week and migrates to the cecum and colorectum. When few worms are present there is little damage, but with heavy infections there may be hemorrhage, mucopurulent stools and symptoms of dysentery, sometimes with rectal prolapse (the *Trichuris* dysentery syndrome,[13] which has an immunologic basis).

Intestinal Capillariasis. Intestinal capillariasis is caused by consumption of raw or undercooked fish containing infective stage larvae of *Capillaria philippinensis*. Worms are mainly found in the jejunum but in severe infections the entire digestive tract can be localized. Pathologic findings of intestinal capillariasis include mucosal atrophy (villus obliteration) and eosinophil and plasma cell infiltration with presence of larvae and adult worms. Due to destruction of the mucosa, there is impaired absorption of nutrients. Autoinfection is known to occur in some cases and can lead to severe infections.

Strongyloidiasis. The life cycle of *Strongyloides stercoralis* is complex (Figure 114-5). Human infection is acquired when filariform larvae in the soil penetrate the skin. This can cause petechial hemorrhages, congestion and edema at the site of entry. The larvae migrate into cutaneous blood vessels and are carried to the lungs, where they break out of the pulmonary capillaries and sequentially enter the alveoli, trachea, pharynx and then the mucosa of the duodenum and upper jejunum (Figure 114-6). There can be pathologic findings similar to those of bronchopneumonia with lobar consolidation. The females mature in the intestine (Figure 114-7), invade the tissues of the bowel wall and lay their eggs, which hatch and release first-stage (rhabditiform) larvae in the feces. In certain situations, the

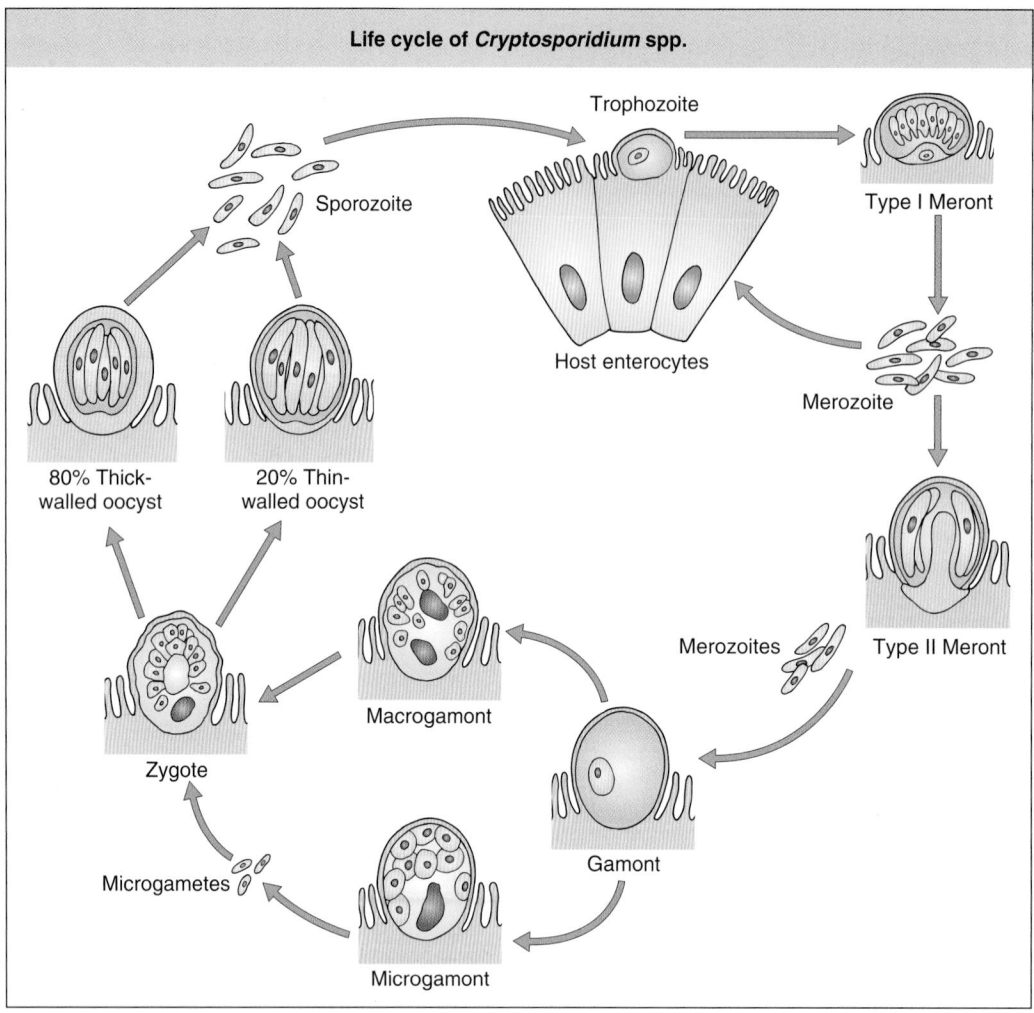

Figure 114-2 Life cycle of *Cryptosporidium* spp.

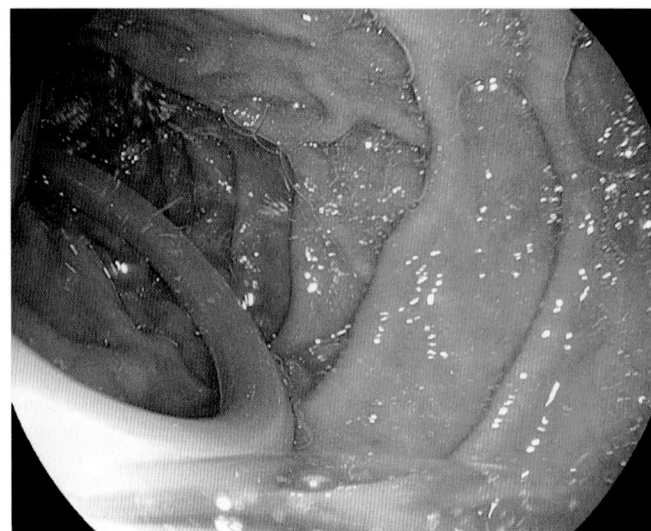

Figure 114-3 *Ascaris lumbricoides* adult worms in the duodenum seen at endoscopy.

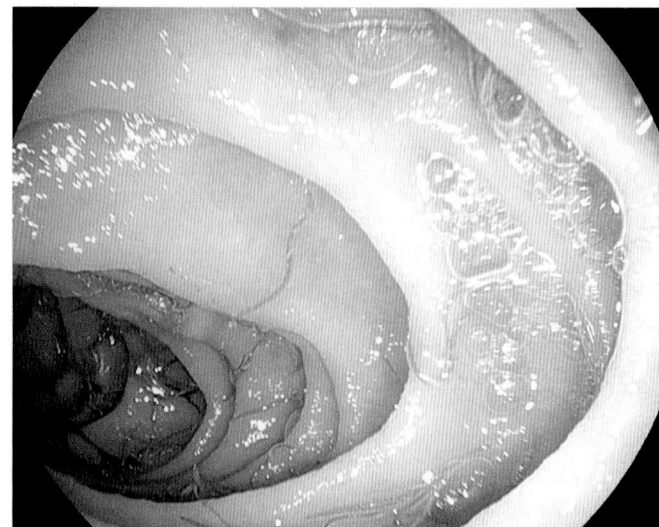

Figure 114-4 Hookworms attached to the duodenal mucosa seen at endoscopy.

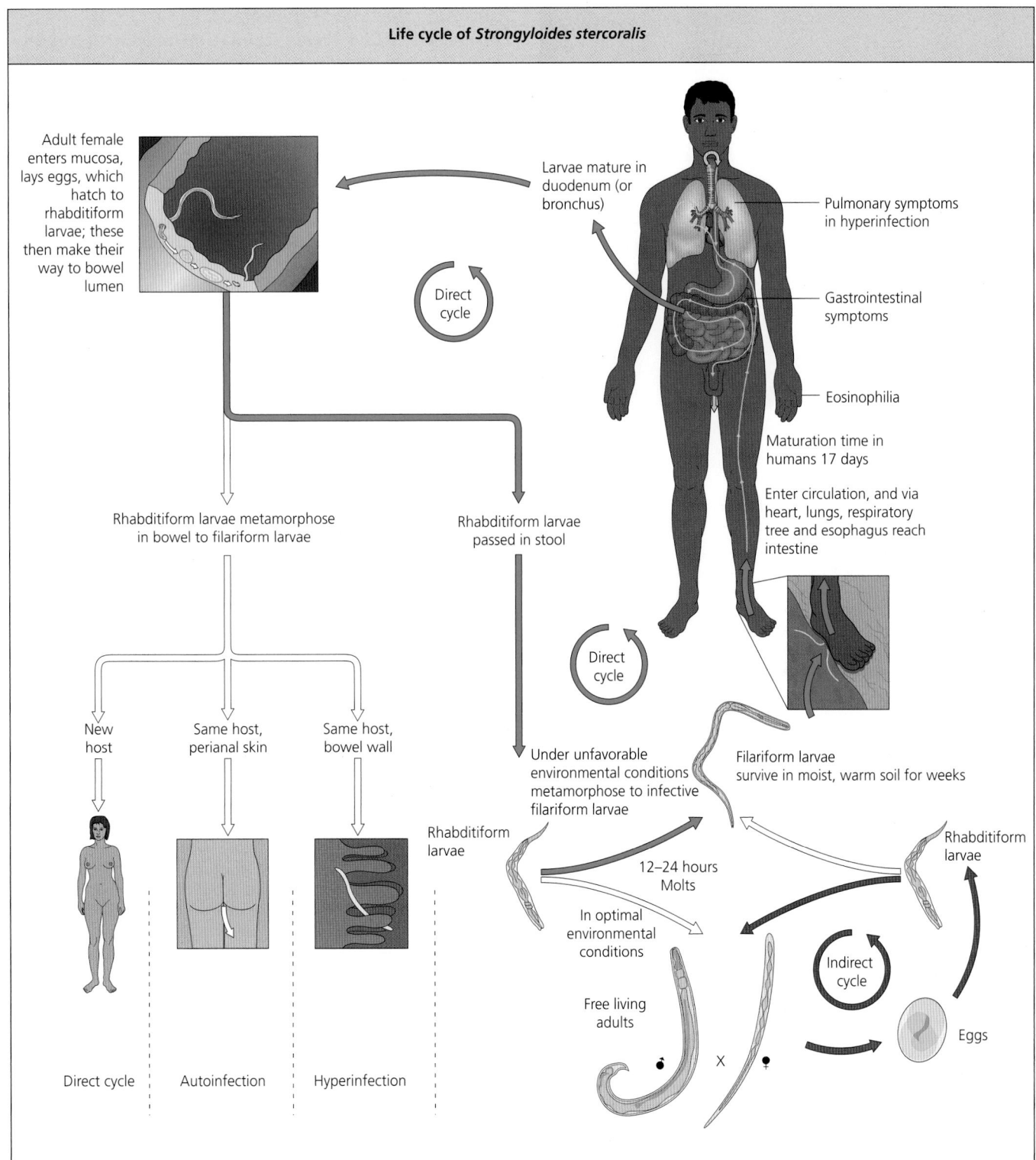

Life cycle of *Strongyloides stercoralis*

Adult female enters mucosa, lays eggs, which hatch to rhabditiform larvae; these then make their way to bowel lumen

Larvae mature in duodenum (or bronchus)

Direct cycle

Pulmonary symptoms in hyperinfection

Gastrointestinal symptoms

Eosinophilia

Maturation time in humans 17 days

Enter circulation, and via heart, lungs, respiratory tree and esophagus reach intestine

Rhabditiform larvae metamorphose in bowel to filariform larvae

Rhabditiform larvae passed in stool

New host

Same host, perianal skin

Same host, bowel wall

Direct cycle

Direct cycle

Autoinfection

Hyperinfection

Under unfavorable environmental conditions metamorphose to infective filariform larvae

Rhabditiform larvae

Filariform larvae survive in moist, warm soil for weeks

Rhabditiform larvae

12–24 hours Molts

In optimal environmental conditions

Free living adults

Indirect cycle

Eggs

X

Figure 114-5 Life cycle of *Strongyloides stercoralis*.

rhabditiform larvae mature in the intestine to the filariform stage, and these parasites bore into the wall of the duodenum and jejunum and initiate another cycle of infection, which eventually results in there being more adult worms in the small bowel. Filariform larvae that penetrate the bowel wall can spread throughout the lymphatic system to the mesenteric lymph glands and can enter the general circulation and hence the liver, lungs, kidneys and gallbladder. They can cause granulomas in the gastrointestinal tract and mesenteric glands. There

are abscesses in the lungs and there may be granuloma in the liver. Migrating larvae may cause the patient to die from sepsis arising from the normal intestinal bacterial flora.

Trematode Infections (Flukes)

***Fasciolopsis buski* Infection.** The giant intestinal fluke *F. buski* is contracted by humans and pigs through eating metacercariae attached to water plants. The parasite excysts and attaches to the mucosa of the

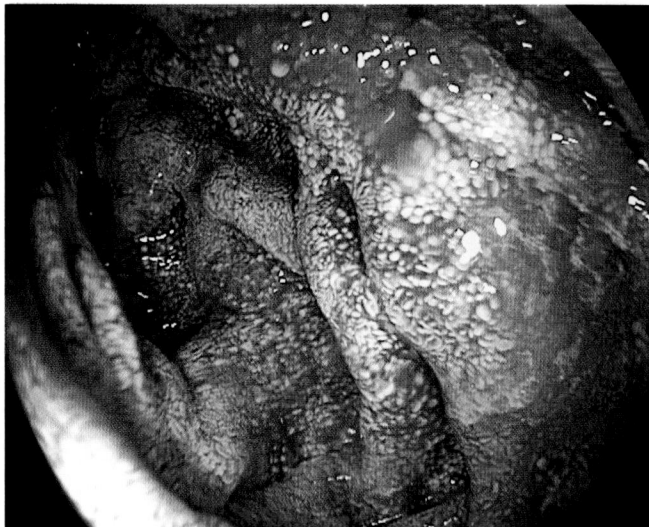

Figure 114-6   Blunting of duodenal villi due to *Strongyloides stercoralis* infection in an adult man.

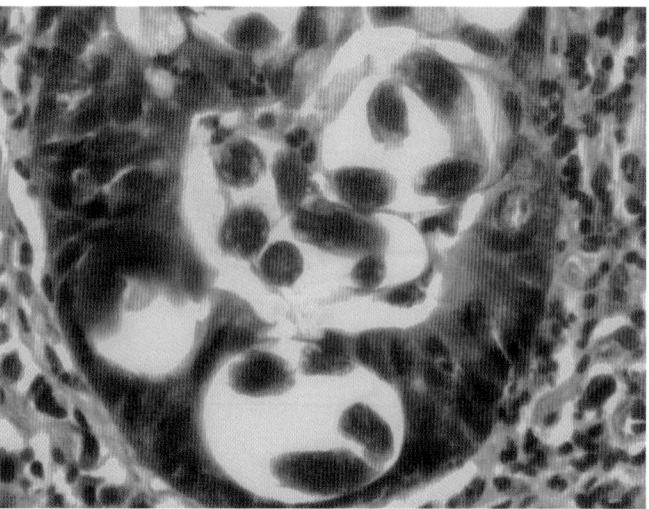

Figure 114-7   *Strongyloides stercoralis* female adult worms seen in a biopsy of the same mucosa shown in Figure 114-6.

jejunal and duodenal wall causing mechanical injury and inflammation, which can lead to ulcers, bleeding or abscesses. There may be a mild anemia and low levels of serum vitamin B12, owing to the parasite's competition for the vitamin or impairing its absorption.

Echinostomiasis. Human echinostomiasis is a food-borne infection caused by trematode parasites of the genus *Echinostoma*. Infection is acquired through consumption of raw or undercooked freshwater intermediate hosts (snails, tadpoles, fish) infected with metacercariae. Ingested metacercariae excyst in the duodenum and adult worms attach to the mucosa of the small intestine. Worms attached to the mucosa may cause ulceration and inflammation. Heavy infections can also be associated with villous atrophy and crypt hyperplasia.

Heterophyes heterophyes Infection. *H. heterophyes* is a trematode that infects humans and is found mainly in Asia. The pathology depends on the degree of infection acquired through ingestion of pickled or raw fish. The metacercariae excyst and attach to the walls of the small intestine. The adults may cause only a mild inflammatory reaction. Eggs may enter the circulation because the adults are attached deeply into the intestinal wall. Ectopic eggs can provoke granuloma formation, especially if they lodge in the heart or brain.[14]

Cestode Infections (Tapeworms)

Taenia solium and Taenia saginata Infection. The pork tapeworm (*T. solium*) and the beef tapeworm (*T. saginata*)[14] are acquired by the human host by ingestion of poorly cooked meat that contains the encysted larvae (cysticerci). The larva is digested in the stomach and the head of the tapeworm evaginates in the upper small intestine, attaches via the scolex to the intestinal mucosa and feeds by absorbing nutrients from the bowel. Very little pathology is caused by these well-adapted adult worms, which may reach 7 m and 25 m in length, respectively. The pathologically significant stage for humans is the cysticercus of *T. solium*. The eggs passed in feces are ingested and hatch when they are exposed to gastric juice. The oncospheres that are released penetrate the intestinal wall and are carried via the bloodstream and can potentially form a cysticercus in any organ. The cysticercus is an ovoid, milky-white bladder with the parasite head invaginated inside. The pathology is described in detail in Chapter 119.

Dwarf Tapeworm (Hymenolepis nana) Infection. Once the ova of the dwarf tapeworm *H. nana* are ingested they hatch in the small intestinal villus mucosa. The adult worm reaches a length of 3–4 cm and begins egg production.

Fish Tapeworm (Diphyllobothrium latum) Infection. The fish tapeworm *D. latum* has a life cycle involving a first intermediate host of tiny aquatic invertebrates, a second intermediate host of predominantly freshwater fish and a definitive host that includes humans, other terrestrial mammals and less commonly marine mammals (believed to become infected by eating anadromus fish). Infections are commonly multiple and may reach more than 100 individual worms, each measuring up to 10 m in length. The pathology is minimal from the local effects. Tapeworm anemia, due to competition for vitamin B12, has been described exclusively in Finland and has now all but died out as a result of control measures.

Prevention

The prevention and control of parasitic gastrointestinal disease can be achieved through improvement of living standards, personal hygiene and better sanitary conditions. In immunocompromised patients, different recommendations need to be considered (see Chapter 94).

PUBLIC HEALTH HYGIENE MEASURES

Disposal of human sewage and waste water is fundamental to the control of parasitic gastrointestinal infections. Fecal material contaminates agricultural food crops or water supplies if it is passed promiscuously in the fields or close to habitation or if it is deliberately used unprocessed on fields as fertilizer ('night soil'). Any of the gastrointestinal parasites can be transferred in this way.

The provision of latrines can reduce these sources of environmental contamination but, unfortunately, unless they are well constructed and maintained, latrines can themselves become important foci of infection. The prevalence of *Ascaris* infection is often higher among urban latrine users than among rural nonusers. The eggs of *A. lumbricoides* and also those of *T. trichiura* are very often resistant and can remain viable in the latrine environment for long periods. In addition, the moist soil around a latrine favors the survival of hookworm larvae[15] and the free-living cycle of *S. stercoralis*.

Sewage may enter lakes, rivers and ponds and the water then be used for drinking or irrigation. *Cryptosporidium* oocysts are particularly difficult to eliminate from water and require an efficient filtration system or boiling; chlorination does not kill the oocysts.

Composting is another reliable way of killing infective forms of parasites. This takes 3–4 months. Cysts, eggs and larvae are quite rapidly killed at temperatures of 55°C (131°F) and die within a few days at 45°C (113°F). The compost heap needs turning and good maintenance or the periphery may become an intense transmission focus. Sewage treatment removes or destroys parasites by sedimentation and the creation of completely anaerobic conditions. The eggs of *Taenia* spp. and *A. lumbricoides* are notoriously resistant and sometimes survive in the solid wastes taken from sedimentation tanks or ponds.

PERSONAL HYGIENE MEASURES

The fecal–oral route of transmission is very important, especially for intestinal protozoa. For example, infected food handlers are disseminators of *G. intestinalis* and *E. histolytica* cysts. There is high prevalence of infection in residential institutions where personal hygiene is poor. Simple hand washing before preparing and eating food prevents transmission of many infections. The soil-to-skin route of infection can be inhibited by wearing shoes. Infective forms of hookworm and *Strongyloides* larvae will be stopped from entering the skin. Persons dealing with composted human feces must use boots and gloves.

Good food hygiene is essential. Prevention of most of the parasites transferred by the fecal–oral route can be achieved by washing all salad vegetables and fruit before consumption. Kitchen utensils and hands should be washed frequently. Avoidance of wild-grown watercress and other water plants prevents *F. buski* infections. Proper cooking of meat and fish removes the risk of flesh-derived parasites such as *H. heterophyes* and tapeworms. Problems arise when cultural preferences dictate consuming these products raw, undercooked, salted, dried or pickled. The inspection of meat can detect the presence of cysticerci in the carcasses and allow infected meat to be condemned. Stopping the consumption of fish that is raw, pickled or salted is often impossible if it is part of a deep cultural tradition. Deep freezing of meat and fish at temperatures colder than $-20\,^{\circ}\mathrm{C}$ ($-4\,^{\circ}\mathrm{F}$) for 24–48 hours kills all these parasites.

PREVENTION BY CHEMOTHERAPY

Prevention by mass chemotherapy has been used against amebiasis, soil-transmitted nematodes (*A. lumbricoides*, hookworm, *T. trichiura*) and tapeworms (*T. saginata*, *T. solium*, *D. latum*). Success depends upon several factors:

- the chemotherapeutic agent used should have a broad spectrum of activity and be given annually as a single oral dose;
- the drugs should be cheap to purchase and administer; and
- the drugs should have few side effects.

F. buski infection in Indonesia has been treated by community-based praziquantel treatment but rapid re-infection followed. Selective or targeted chemotherapy may be of more use. *E. vermicularis* infection in one child requires treatment not only of that child but also all family contacts together with education in personal hygiene. In 2003 a national program of soil-transmitted hookworm control (*A. lumbricoides* and *T. trichiura*) was implemented in Uganda, which has shown a sharp reduction in intensity of infection following annual mass drug administration of albendazole to children and high-risk adults. By 2006–2007 approximately 43 million treatments had been administered.[16] Ivermectin (in two separated doses) has been used successfully as mass treatment in north-east Brazil to control both intestinal helminths (including strongyloidosis) and ectoparasites (including scabies).[17] A more recent study in Ecuador of school-age children demonstrated that treatment annually and biannually with ivermectin over a period of up to 17 years may have had a significant impact on *T. trichiura* infection.[18]

VACCINES

As yet no vaccines have been used in humans for the control of gastrointestinal parasitic diseases.

ROLE OF PROPHYLAXIS

There is no evidence for prophylactic use of chemotherapy being helpful in prevention of these gastrointestinal parasitic diseases.

Clinical Features

The symptoms produced by gastrointestinal parasites are diverse. It is important to stress that most infections are asymptomatic, and the clinical consequences of infection are determined largely by its

TABLE 114-3	Gastrointestinal Parasites Associated with Diarrhea
Acute diarrhea with or without fever	*Entamoeba histolytica* *Cryptosporidium parvum/C. hominis* *Isospora belli* *Cyclospora cayetanensis*
Diarrhea with blood in stool (dysentery), with or without fever	*Entamoeba histolytica* *Balantidium coli* *Trichuris trichiura* *Strongyloides stercoralis* (rarely)
Persistent diarrhea, often with malnutrition	*Entamoeba histolytica* *Giardia intestinalis* *Cryptosporidium parvum* *Isospora belli* *Cyclospora cayetanensis* *Trichuris trichiura* *Strongyloides stercoralis*

intensity: heavy infections can cause severe problems but light ones rarely do. Only a minority can cause diarrhea (Table 114-3). It is also important to emphasize that the identification of an infection by stool microscopy does not necessarily imply that it is the cause of a patient's symptoms, and the author frequently sees cases of anemia due to gastrointestinal cancers which have been misdiagnosed as hookworm infection with consequent delays in initiating treatment. Several helminthiases have specific clinical features.

GASTROINTESTINAL DISEASE CAUSED BY PROTOZOA

Amebiasis (Entamoeba histolytica)

It is now recognized that there are two species of amebae that were formerly termed pathogenic and nonpathogenic *E. histolytica*.[19] These are now called *Entamoeba histolytica* and *Entamoeba dispar*. Only *E. histolytica* is capable of causing disease. Confirmation that the parasite previously described as *E. histolytica* is in reality two species – *E. dispar* which is nonpathogenic and *E. histolytica* which is a pathogen – means that the natural history of amebiasis needs thorough reassessment. Haque *et al.* studied 300 preschool children in Dhaka, Bangladesh.[6] Over a 2-year period, new *E. histolytica* infections were found in half the children. Of those who were asymptomatic cyst passers, one in 10 subsequently developed diarrhea within 2 months of the start of infection; 10% of the children had diarrhea in association with *E. histolytica* and 4% were found to have amebic colitis.

Amebic Intestinal Disease

The incubation period of invasive amebiasis varies from a few days to 1–4 months. There is a good correlation with the presence of *E. histolytica* trophozoites containing ingested red blood cells. Patients may be asymptomatic or present with colicky abdominal pain, frequent bowel movements and tenesmus. Amebic dysentery is characterized by bloodstained stools with mucus occurring up to 10 times a day. The duration of the dysentery can be very variable and may last for only a few days or for several months with concomitant weight loss and debility. The symptoms may be confused with inflammatory bowel disease. In acute cases the clinical picture may mimic appendicitis, cholecystitis, intestinal obstruction or diverticulitis.

AMEBIC EXTRAINTESTINAL DISEASE

Symptoms can be gradual in onset, with right upper quadrant pain and fever. Weakness, weight loss, dry cough and sweating are less common. Tender hepatomegaly is often seen, with liver function tests that are normal or only slightly abnormal. Jaundice is very unusual, and abscesses are mostly solitary. A raised right diaphragm may be found on chest radiograph. The abscess is visualized by ultrasound, CT or MRI. Hematogenous spread to the brain (see Chapter 111), lung, pericardium and other sites is possible.

Giardiasis (Giardia intestinalis)

The clinical spectrum of giardiasis ranges from asymptomatic infection, through acute gastrointestinal infection to severe chronic diarrhea with intestinal malabsorption. The average incubation period is 9 days and the acute infection is self-limiting. Common symptoms include nausea, diarrhea, flatulence and upper abdominal cramps with distention and nausea.

Blastocystis Infection (Blastocystis hominis)

There is controversy surrounding *B. hominis*; it is unclear whether it causes gastrointestinal disease or not. When large numbers are found in stool in the absence of other parasites, bacteria or viruses it may be the cause of diarrhea, cramps, nausea, fever, vomiting and abdominal pain.

Dientamoeba fragilis Infection

Like *Blastocystis*, the pathogenicity of *D. fragilis* is uncertain. It has been associated with a wide range of symptoms. Its transmission mode is also unclear, although there are reports suggesting that it is transmitted through the eggs of *Enterobius vermicularis*.[20] Symptoms in children infected with this parasite may include intermittent diarrhea, abdominal pain, nausea, anorexia, malaise, fatigue, poor weight gain and unexplained eosinophilia.

Cryptosporidiosis (C. parvum and C. hominis)

The incubation period of *Cryptosporidium* infection averages 3–6 days. Symptoms include a flu-like illness, diarrhea, malaise, abdominal pain, anorexia, nausea, flatulence, malabsorption, vomiting, mild fever and weight loss. In the 1993 Milwaukee water-borne outbreak of cryptosporidiosis, which affected around 403 000 people, the mean duration of illness was 12 days and the median maximum number of stools per day was 12.[21] Generally the symptoms are self-limiting, and prolonged disease is uncommon. In immunocompromised patients and in malnourished children the situation is different and there can be intractable, profuse, life-threatening diarrhea.[22]

Cyclosporiasis (Cyclospora cayetanensis)

Clinical findings do not distinguish cyclosporal diarrhea from other causes of diarrhea. Other common symptoms are abdominal pain, nausea, vomiting and anorexia.[23] *Cyclospora* infection can last for 1–8 weeks.

Isosporiasis (Isospora belli)

The predominant clinical symptom is diarrhea, which may be intermittent and last for months or even years. Stools are watery, soft, foamy and offensive, which may suggest malabsorption. There is associated weight loss, abdominal pain and fever. In HIV-infected patients, chronic infection occurs.

Balantidiasis (Balantidium coli)

B. coli, the largest and least common of the human protozoan pathogens, is capable of causing an infection resembling amebic colitis. It is particularly prevalent among people living in close association with pigs in South America, Iran, Papua New Guinea and the Philippines. Up to 80% of persons carrying the organism are asymptomatic carriers. Acute diarrhea with blood and mucus begins abruptly and is associated with nausea, abdominal discomfort and marked weight loss. Peritonitis and colonic perforation can progress rapidly to death. A chronic infection occurs with intermittent diarrhea and infrequent bloody stools.

HELMINTH GASTROINTESTINAL DISEASE

Ascariasis (Ascaris lumbricoides)

Most cases of ascariasis are asymptomic; symptomatic infections are more common in children than adults. When large numbers of larvae migrate to the lungs in a short time period, *Ascaris* pneumonitis can result. This is the clinical picture of Löffler's syndrome, which is characterized by dyspnea, dry cough, wheezing or coarse rales, fever up to 40°C (104°F), transient eosinophilia and a chest radiograph that is suggestive of pneumonitis and that resolves within a couple of weeks. In addition, eosinophils, Charcot–Leyden crystals and larvae may rarely be found in the sputum. The adult worms occasionally migrate from the small bowel and cause biliary or hepatic ascariasis. Rarely, adult worms migrate into the biliary tree with secondary sepsis and abscess formation. Pancreatitis may result from migrating ascarids that obstruct the pancreatic duct. In people who have large numbers of adult worms, intestinal obstruction can occur owing to the sheer bulk of worm bodies. Adult worms migrate more in the presence of a stimulus such as a fever of over 38.9°C (102°F) or the use of a general anesthetic, and they may block the bile duct or pancreatic duct or enter the liver or peritoneal cavity.

Enterobiasis (Enterobius vermicularis)

Infection with *E. vermicularis* (threadworm or pinworm) causes few or no symptoms in the vast majority of people. The predominant symptom is nocturnal pruritus ani, caused by migration of the female worms from the anus to the perianal or perineal skin in the process of laying their eggs. In children, insomnia, loss of appetite, loss of weight, emotional instability, enuresis and irritability may also be found.

Hookworm Infection (Ancylostoma duodenale, Necator americanus)

Hookworm causes ground itch, a moderate-to-severe pruritus of the skin, usually of the feet, as the hookworm larvae penetrate. Symptoms of the intestinal phase are fatigue, nausea, vomiting, abdominal pain, diarrhea with occult bleeding, and weakness. Heavy worm burdens may have serious sequelae in young children.[24] This is particularly problematic with *A. duodenale* infection. Eosinophilia is usually present. Heavy hookworm infections can cause iron deficiency anemia[15] and hypoproteinemia with pallor, and edema of the face and feet. Iron deficiency in children is associated with impaired academic performance at school and in adults with weakness and fatigue, leading to reduced productivity.

Trichuriasis (Trichuris trichiura)

Light infections with this common, ubiquitous infection rarely cause symptoms. In heavy infections (more than 10 000 eggs per gram of feces), epigastric pain, vomiting, distention, flatulence, anorexia and weight loss may occur. Rarely the *Trichuris* dysentery syndrome may occur, with blood and mucus in the stools and, in heavy infections, prolapse of the rectum.

Intestinal Capillariasis

Symptoms of intestinal capillariasis include abdominal pain, diarrhea and weight loss. Symptoms are complicated by heavy infections emanating from autoinfection. Patients with severe diarrhea may present with hypokalemia, hypoalbuminemia and edema due to excessive fluid loss and malabsorption, with subsequent death if not properly managed.

Strongyloidiasis (Strongyloides stercoralis)

S. stercoralis largely causes asymptomatic infection of the small intestine, which can last for 30 years or longer.[25] The prepatent period from infection through the skin to the appearance of rhabditiform larvae in the stools is 1 month or more. Symptoms only develop with high intestinal worm loads, which can be the result of several factors. In people debilitated by concurrent disease or malnutrition, there may be massive invasion of the tissues by *S. stercoralis*. Treatment with immunosuppressive drugs in a patient harboring *S. stercoralis* can also lead to the same effect. Infection with human T-cell leukemia virus 1 is important in predisposing to massive infection by *S. stercoralis*. Interestingly, infection with HIV is not a common cause of the *Strongyloides* hyperinfection syndrome; this may be due to the decreased likelihood of intestinal larval migration in the presence of CD4 lymphopenia seen in HIV infection.[26] Symptoms include watery mucous diarrhea, with the severity depending on the intensity of the infection. Malabsorption of fat and vitamin B12 with a chronic diarrhea and protein-losing enteropathy has also been described and is rapidly reversed by treatment.

There are two types of skin rash. The first is larva currens, which occurs on the trunk or near the anus, and is a linear eruption in which the larvae migrate under the skin causing an itchy, nonindurated wheal with a red flare that moves rapidly and disappears in a few hours. This contrasts to the indurated and persistent track of nonhuman hookworm larvae (cutaneous larva migrans). The second type of rash is urticaria.

Features of the strongyloidiasis hyperinfection syndrome include severe diarrhea, malabsorption, edema, hepatomegaly and paralytic ileus. Gram-negative sepsis is a recognized complication. In very severe cases encephalopathy and even secondary pyogenic meningitis have been described.

Anisakiasis

Anisakiasis is commonly reported in countries where the consumption of raw seafood is practiced. The infection has been reported in Japan, Korea, the Netherlands and other Scandinavian countries. Most of the cases are due to gastric anisakiasis whereas intestinal and ectopic cases are uncommon. Symptoms associated with this infection include abrupt abdominal pain, nausea and sometimes vomiting.[27] The symptoms are not specific for anisakiasis as they are also associated with other abdominal conditions.

Fasciolopsis buski Infection

F. buski is confined to Asian countries, particularly Thailand. Symptoms are more frequent in children than adults owing to their greater exposure to water plants while at play. In heavier infections, clinical features can include diarrhea, abdominal pain, vomiting, flatulence, poor appetite, fever and eosinophilia. In very severe cases there may be ascites, edema of the face, abdomen and legs, anemia, anorexia, weakness and even intestinal obstruction.

Echinostomiasis

In light infections, symptoms are mild and most cases asymptomatic. Symptoms include abdominal pain and discomfort; nausea, vomiting, diarrhea, malnutrition and anemia occur in some cases.

Heterophyes heterophyes Infection

H. heterophyes causes few symptoms unless the infection is heavy, which is dependent on the quantities of pickled or uncooked fish eaten in endemic areas (mostly the Middle and Far East). The adult worms produce abdominal pain, diarrhea with mucus and ulceration of the intestinal wall.

Beef and Pork Tapeworm Infection (Taenia saginata and Taenia solium)

The clinical features of T. saginata, the beef tapeworm, and T. solium, the pork tapeworm, are similar. The adult worms in the gastrointestinal phase of both organisms usually cause no symptoms, but carriers can sometimes feel a proglottid emerging from the anus; the motile proglottid may be alarmingly obvious in the feces. Other associated symptoms, such as abdominal pain and distention, nausea and anorexia have been attributed to the tapeworm. There is occasionally a mild eosinophilia but there is no anemia, even in long-term infection. Cysticercosis complicates infection with T. solium only. Ingestion of T. solium eggs, from the environment or from the patient's own feces, leads to the dissemination of oncospheres in the bloodstream. These can become lodged anywhere in the subcutaneous and intramuscular tissues, where they become cysticerci. Symptoms depend on the particular body site involved, and often affect the brain (Chapter 119).

Dwarf Tapeworm Infection (Hymenolepis nana)

As with other tapeworms, there are usually few symptoms in H. nana infection. Symptoms that may occur include abdominal pain, anorexia, irritability and headache. Eosinophilia is common. Symptoms are more common in heavy infections and may cause growth retardation in children.

Fish Tapeworm Infection (Diphyllobothrium latum)

There are few if any symptoms from infection with D. latum. Symptoms including diarrhea, headache and nonspecific malaise appear to be somewhat more common than in uninfected people. Tapeworm-associated anemia is probably related to vitamin B12 deficiency caused by competition for the vitamin between the tapeworm and a genetically predisposed host; however, this is now exceedingly rare.

Diagnosis

Microscopic examination of the stool is fundamental to the diagnosis of all the gastrointestinal infections (Table 114-4). A minimum of three stool specimens, examined by trained personnel using a concentration and a permanent stain technique, should be used. Newer diagnostic approaches, based on serology, antigen detection or nucleic acid detection, are summarized in Table 114-5.

Management

GASTROINTESTINAL PROTOZOA

The management of gastrointestinal protozoa is summarized in Table 114-6. Treatment regimens are discussed in detail in Chapter 157.

Entamoeba histolytica

Treatment of E. histolytica infection is divided into two types. Luminal amebicides, such as diloxanide furoate, act on organisms in the intestinal lumen and are not effective against organisms in tissue. Tissue amebicides, such as metronidazole and tinidazole, are effective in treating invasive amebiasis but less effective in the treatment of organisms in the bowel lumen. There is some controversy about treating asymptomatic patients. Ideally, any amebic cysts should be tested to identify whether they are E. histolytica (in which case the infection should be treated to avoid the risk of developing invasive disease and to prevent secondary spread) or E. dispar (which does not require any treatment). However, until ELISA or PCR tests become widely deployed it will continue to be usual to treat asymptomatic patients in non-endemic areas with diloxanide furoate (see Table 114-6). When asymptomatic cyst carriage persists after treatment for amebic dysentery or liver abscess, further treatment with a luminal amebicide is mandatory, otherwise relapse is frequent. The treatment of asymptomatic cyst carriers in endemic areas is of questionable value because of the high rate of re-infection.

Proven amebic dysentery should always be treated. Drugs of choice are metronidazole or tinidazole followed by diloxanide furoate (see Table 114-6). Amebic liver abscess is treated with metronidazole, followed by diloxanide furoate as above. Tinidazole is an alternative; chloroquine (150 mg base q6h for 2 days, then 150 mg base q12h for 19 days) can also be used.

Giardia intestinalis

Treatment is often unnecessary because most healthy, immunocompetent patients have a self-limiting disease and recover by their own natural host defense mechanisms. Treatment of symptomatic patients reduces the duration and severity of symptoms. The treatment of asymptomatic cyst carriers is controversial in endemic areas. Generally, in a non-endemic area, asymptomatic Giardia cyst carriers are treated. The 5-nitroimidazole derivatives metronidazole or tinidazole are the treatment of choice and can be used in short courses (Table 114-6). In vitro and in vivo resistance of G. intestinalis has been demonstrated, although rarely, to conventional therapy, particularly to the 5-nitroimidazoles such as metronidazole and tinidazole.

Blastocystis hominis

If B. hominis is present in the stool, the physician must not stop looking for another cause of diarrhea. Whether any treatment is required is controversial. Metronidazole seems to be the most appropriate drug.

TABLE 114-4	Laboratory Diagnosis of Intestinal Parasites

Intestinal Protozoa	Diagnostic Method
Entamoeba histolytica and nonpathogenic ameba (E. dispar, E. hartmanni, E. coli, Iodamoeba butschlii, Endolimax nana)	Fecal microscopy • Wet direct preparations for motile trophozoites • Wet concentrated Lugol's iodine preparations for cysts • Permanent trichrome stained preparations for cysts and trophozoites Microscopy of liver abscess materials • Permanent trichrome or hematoxylin/eosin-stained preparations Enzyme linked immunosorbent assay (ELISA) of fecal specimens to detect galactose-inhibitable lectin antigen Indirect fluorescent antibody (IFA) test in suspected amebic abscess (and ameboma) Culture and zymodeme pattern analysis Polymerase chain reaction (PCR) – often available in reference laboratories Note: In the absence of ingested red blood cells in E. histolytica trophozoites, it is difficult to distinguish this parasite from E. dispar. Presence of ingested red blood cells is the definitive diagnostic characteristic for E. histolytica. The IFA test is positive in over 95% of cases after 14 days but should be confirmed by the cellulose acetate precipitin test
Giardia intestinalis	Fecal microscopy • Wet iodine or saline preparation for cysts and trophozoites • Permanent trichrome preparations for cysts and trophozoites String test (enterotest), duodenal aspirate or biopsy if fecal specimens are negative • Direct wet preparations for motile trophozoites • Permanent trichrome preparations for cysts and trophozoites ELISA tests to detect antigens in fecal specimens Indirect immunofluorescence tests for fecal specimens for specific monoclonal antibodies Direct fluorescence antibody tests (Merifluor DFA) against cell wall antigens Immunochromatographic assays Serology (not very useful as cannot distinguish current from past infection)
Blastocystis hominis	Fecal microscopy • Wet iodine or saline preparation for cysts • Permanent trichrome preparations for cysts
Dietamoeba fragilis	• Fecal microscopy • Permanent trichrome stained preparations for trophozoites
Balantidium coli	Fecal microscopy • Direct wet iodine or saline preparations (fresh or concentrated specimen)
Cryptosporidium parvum/ hominis	Fecal microscopy • Direct wet concentrated preparations for cysts • Permanent stained preparations with acid-fast stains (modified Ziehl–Neelsen), or auramine Immunofluorescence using monoclonal antibodies Immunochromatographic assays PCR for species identification (PCR is still principally a reference laboratory technique) Intestinal biopsy • Permanent stained preparations with hematoxylin/eosin stain or toluidine blue
Cyclospora cayetanensis	Fecal microscopy • Permanent stained preparations with acid-fast stains (modified Ziehl–Neelsen), or auramine O (fluorescent)
Isospora belli	Fecal microscopy • Permanent stained preparations with acid-fast stains (modified Ziehl–Neelsen), or auramine O (fluorescent)
NEMATODES (ROUNDWORMS)	
Ascaris lumbricoides	Fecal microscopy • Direct or concentrated fecal specimens for ova (embryonated and unembryonated) Macroscopic examination of expelled worms
Ancylostoma duodenale and Necator americanus (hookworm)	Fecal microscopy • Direct or concentrated (Lugol's iodine-stained preparations) fecal specimens for ova or larvae Note: Differentiate hookworm larvae from strongyloides larvae by examining the mouth parts. Hookworm larvae have a long tubular buccal cavity whereas that of strongyloides is shorter. Hookworm is also 3-4 times bigger than strongyloides
Strongyloides stercoralis	Fecal microscopy • Direct or concentrated (Lugol's iodine-stained preparations) fecal specimens for rhabditiform and filariform larvae Fecal culture techniques (agar plate and Baermann) for larvae – useful in light infections Sputum microscopy for larvae in hyperinfections Intestinal biopsy • Hematoxylin and eosin stain
Trichuris trichiura	Fecal microscopy • Direct or concentrated wet fecal preparations for ova; adult worms are rarely seen
Enterobius vermicularis	Microscopic examination for ova in: • Clear cellulose tape perianal preparations or anal swabs Anal examinations for adult worms Note: • Eggs or adult worms may be found accidentally in fecal or urine specimens • Specimen collection should be done early in the morning before bathing

TABLE 114-4	Laboratory Diagnosis of Intestinal Parasites (Continued)
Intestinal Protozoa	**Diagnostic Method**
TREMATODES (FLUKES)	
Fasciolopsis buski	Fecal microscopy for ova and adult worms in direct preparations *Note:* Adult worms are rarely recovered in fecal preparations
Clonorchis sinensis	Fecal/duodenal aspirate microscopy for ova Direct wet preparations and concentrated wet preparations
Heterophyes heterophyes	Fecal microscopy for ova and adult worms in direct preparations
CESTODES (TAPEWORMS)	
Taenia solium	Fecal microscopy for ova and proglottids ELISA tests to detect parasite antigens Serologic methods for *T. solium* cysticercosis PCR to differentiate *T. solium* from *T. saginata* *Note: T. solium* and *T. saginata* can be differentiated from gravid proglottids or the scolex recovered after purgation
Taenia saginata	Fecal microscopy for ova and proglottids
Hymenolepis nana	Fecal microscopy for ova
Diphyllobothrium latum	Fecal microscopy for ova or proglottids in wet preparations

TABLE 114-5	Immunoassays for the Detection of Intestinal Parasitic Infections				
		G	**E**	**C**	**Remarks**
Triage parasite panel enzyme immunoassay (Biosite Diagnostics, CA, USA)		+	+	+	High sensitivity and specificity.[28,29] Cannot differentiate *Entamoeba coli* from *E. dispar*
Rida Quick Cryptosporidium/Giardia/Entamoeba Combi (R-Biopharm AG, Germany)		+	+	+	Rapid test with high sensitivity and specificity for all three parasites. Cannot different *E. histolytica* from *E. dispar*
Merifluor (Meridian Diagnostic, Inc.)		+	−	+	High sensitivity and specificity[30]
Tri-Combo Parasite screen (TechLab, Inc., Blacksburg, VA)		+	+	+	High sensitivity and specificity[32]
Giardia/Cryptosporidium quik chek (TechLab, Inc., Blacksburg, VA)		+	−	+	Test is specific for *E. histolytica*, does not cross-react with *E. dispar*
ProSpecT Cryptosporidium/Giardia Microplate Assay (Remel, Inc.)		+	−	+	Detects *Cryptosporidium/Giardia* antigens in fresh or preserved fecal material[30]
ColorPAC™ Giardia/Cryptosporidium Rapid Assay (Becton, Dickinson and Company, Franklin Lakes, NJ)		+	−	+	Rapid test with high sensitivity and specificity. No reactivity with other parasites
Xpect Giardia/Cryptosporidium (Remel, Inc.)		+	−	+	
Immunocard STAT (Meridian Diagnostic, Inc.)		+	−	+	High sensitivity and specificity[31,32,33]

G, *Giardia intestinalis*; E, *Entamoeba histolytica*; C, *Cryptosporidium* spp.

Dientamoeba fragilis

In adults infected with *D. fragilis*, improvement can be seen with tetracycline; in children, metronidazole is appropriate.

Balantidium coli

Tetracycline is effective against *B. coli*. Doxycycline 100 mg daily for 10–14 days is an alternative. Other drugs to which *B. coli* is sensitive are ampicillin, metronidazole and paromomycin. Surgery may be required for fulminant disease with perforation or abscess formation.

Cryptosporidium spp. (see Chapters 94 and 192)

Cryptosporidium spp. infection in immunocompetent children responds to nitazoxanide better than to placebo, but cure is not guaranteed.[34] It presents a severe problem when it occurs in patients who have AIDS, when nitazoxanide is ineffective.[35] Where available, treatment is with HAART (highly active antiretroviral therapy) alongside or after antiparasitic treatment.

Cyclospora cayetanensis

Many cases of *C. cayetanensis* infection are self-limiting. When treatment is felt to be necessary, trimethoprim–sulfamethoxazole (TMP–SMX; co-trimoxazole) has been found to be effective, eradicating the oocysts from 94% of 16 patients in 7 days compared with 12%

of 17 patients who received placebo.[36] Relapse is common in the immunocompromised but responds to a second course of treatment. Given the propensity of sulfonamide-containing drugs to cause side effects in HIV-infected individuals, an alternative agent to TMP–SMX is required. Verdier *et al.* compared the activity of TMP–SMX 160/800 mg orally twice daily for 1 week with ciprofloxacin 500 mg twice daily for 1 week in HIV-positive patients infected with *C. cayetanensis*.[37] Whilst ciprofloxacin is not as effective as TMP–SMX against *Cyclospora*, it provides an acceptable alternative for individuals who cannot tolerate a sulfonamide.

Isospora belli

Treatment of *I. belli* infection is necessary in the immunocompromised, and oral TMP–SMX eliminates the parasite in most cases; relapse is common but retreatment is usually effective. Prophylactic TMP–SMX may then be necessary. Pyrimethamine–sulfonamide combinations have also proven to be effective.[38] If the patient is intolerant to sulfonamides, furazolidone 100 mg four times daily for 10 days is an alternative. The macrolide antibiotic roxithromycin (2.5 mg/kg q12h) was reported to be successful in a single patient with AIDS and *I. belli* infection who had not responded to TMP–SMX or pyrimethamine therapy. Isosporiasis does not respond to nitazoxanide frequently enough to be clinically useful. Biliary isosporiasis may

TABLE 114-6	Treatment of Gastrointestinal Protozoal Infection*	
Condition	Drug	Dosage
Amebiasis		
Asymptomatic carrier of intestinal cysts 1st choice	Diloxanide furoate	500 mg q8h for 10 days
2nd choice	Paromomycin (aminosidine)	500 mg q8h for 10 days
Intestinal infection (amebic dysentery or ameboma)	Metronidazole or Tinidazole followed by Diloxanide furoate or Paromomycin	750–1000 mg q8h for 5 days 2 g daily for 2–3 days 500 mg q8h for 10 days 500 mg q8h for 10 days
Amebic liver abscess	Metronidazole or Tinidazole followed by Diloxanide furoate	400–500 mg q8h for 5–10 days 2 g daily for 3–5 days 500 mg q8h for 10 days
Giardiasis		
1st choice	Tinidazole or Metronidazole	2 g single dose 400–500 mg q8h for 3 days
2nd choice	Nitazoxanide	500 mg q12h for 3 days
3rd choice	Albendazole	400 mg q24h for 5 days
4th choice	Mepacrine	100 mg q8h for 5–7 days
Balantidium coli Infection		
1st choice	Tetracycline	500 mg q6h for 10 days
Alternatives	Metronidazole or Iodoquinol	750 mg TID for 5 days 650 mg TID for 20 days
Cyclospora cayetanensis Infection		
1st choice	Trimethoprim–sulfamethoxazole (co-trimoxazole)	960 mg q12h for 7 days
Alternatives	Ciprofloxacin	500 mg q12h for 7 days
Isospora belli Infection		
1st choice	Trimethoprim (TMP)–sulfamethoxazole (SMX) (co-trimoxazole)	960 mg [160 mg (TMP)/800 mg (SMX)] q12h for 7–10 days (q6h in immunosuppressed patients)
2nd choice (if intolerant of sulfonamides)	Furazolidone	100 mg q6h for 10 days

*All treatments are adult dosage and given orally unless stated otherwise.

require intravenous SMP–TMX as both oral co-trimoxazole and oral nitazoxanide have been reported to fail in the presence of malabsorption and cholangitis due to *I. belli*.

GASTROINTESTINAL HELMINTHS

The management of gastrointestinal helminths is summarized in Table 114-7 (see Chapter 157).

Ascaris lumbricoides

Treatment is effective only against the adult worm. It is usual to treat any established infection. The drugs used are albendazole, mebendazole, levamisole or piperazine in a single adult dose of 4 g of piperazine phosphate or 4.5 g of piperazine hydrate, or pyrantel pamoate. *Ascaris* pneumonitis responds dramatically to prednisolone therapy and anthelmintics should be given 2 weeks after lung involvement. Surgery is sometimes required for bowel perforation or obstruction.

Enterobius vermicularis

E. vermicularis infection is treated with mebendazole (100 mg, single dose, which is repeated if necessary after 2–3 weeks), piperazine phosphate (4 g, single adult dose repeated after 14 days) or pyrantel pamoate (10 mg/kg, single dose). The whole family should be treated simultaneously, fresh bed linen and night clothes should be provided and the nails kept short and scrubbed. Repeat treatment may be required because recurrence is common.

Hookworm

Hookworm infection is treated by eliminating the adult worms and treating anemia if present; these treatments can be carried out concur-

rently. Mebendazole and albendazole are effective against both *A. duodenale* and *N. americanus*. In a single-dose comparison of albendazole and mebendazole, albendazole gave better cure and egg reduction rates.[39] In a study from Côte d'Ivoire, Utzinger *et al.* reported a reduction in the prevalence and intensity of hookworm infections in schoolchildren receiving praziquantel for *Schistosoma mansoni* infection. If their results are replicated they will have a significant impact upon helminth control programs.[40]

Trichuris trichiura

In symptomatic patients and in asymptomatic carriers who have high numbers of eggs, trichuriasis is treated with mebendazole or albendazole. In undernourished children who have moderate infection intensities in Jamaica, albendazole treatment also resulted in improvement in some tests of cognitive ability and in school attendance and school performance, even after controlling for socioeconomic status.[41]

Strongyloides stercoralis

S. stercoralis infection should be treated in both symptomatic and asymptomatic people because of its ability to cause hyperinfection if immunosuppression occurs. Ivermectin was very effective in a prospective randomized trial comparing the efficacy of ivermectin and thiabendazole in Cambodian refugees who had symptomatic chronic strongyloidiasis, and in a prospective randomized trial comparing a 7-day course of oral albendazole with a single dose of ivermectin in 42 Thai adults with chronic *Strongyloides*.[42] Ivermectin also looks very promising in HIV-positive patients infected with *S. stercoralis*. Albendazole is also effective and can be combined with ivermectin.

TABLE 114-7 Treatment of Gastrointestinal Helminth Infection*

Condition	Drug	Dosage
NEMATODES		
Round Worms		
Ascaris lumbricoides	Albendazole	400 mg, single dose
	Mebendazole	100 mg q12h for 3 days
	Levamisole	150 mg, single dose
	Piperazine hydrate	4.5 g, single dose
Enterobius vermicularis	Mebendazole	100 mg, single dose
	Piperazine phosphate	4 g, single dose
	Pyrantel pamoate	10 mg/kg, single dose
Ancylostoma duodenale	Mebendazole	100 mg q12h for 3 days
Necator americanus	Albendazole	200 mg q24h for 3 days
	Levamisole	150 mg, single dose (less effective against *N. americanus*)
	Pyrantel pamoate	10 mg/kg, single dose
Trichuris trichiura	Mebendazole	100 mg q12h for 3 days or 600 mg, single dose
	Albendazole	400 mg, single dose
Strongyloides stercoralis	Ivermectin	200 µg/kg, daily for 2 days
	Albendazole	400 mg q12–24h for 3 days
	Thiabendazole	25 mg/kg (max 1.5 g) q12h for 3 days
TREMATODES (FLUKES)		
Fasciolopsis buski	Praziquantel	15 mg/kg, single dose
Heterophyes heterophyes	Praziquantel	10–20 mg/kg, single dose
CESTODES (TAPEWORMS)		
Taenia solium	Praziquantel	10 mg/kg, single dose
	Niclosamide	2 g, single dose
Taenia saginata	Praziquantel	10 mg/kg, single dose
	Niclosamide	2 g, single dose
Hymenolepis nana	Praziquantel	20 mg/kg, single dose
	Niclosamide	2 g on day 1 then 1 g/q24h for 6 days
Diphyllobothrium latum	Praziquantel	10 mg/kg, single dose
	Niclosamide	2 g, single dose

*All treatments are adult dosage and given orally unless stated otherwise.

Thiabendazole, orally twice daily for 3 days, is effective but often poorly tolerated. Subcutaneous ivermectin (unlicensed in humans) has proven effective in a case of life-threatening *Strongyloides* hyperinfestation.[43] Although there are no currently known minimally effective concentrations of ivermectin for *Strongyloides* treatment in humans, repeated doses subcutaneously[44] and orally[45] appear to have a cumulatively increasing antiparasitic effect.

Fasciolopsis buski

F. buski infection is treated with praziquantel which is highly effective. Niclosamide has also been used.

Heterophyes heterophyes

H. heterophyes infection is treated with a single dose of praziquantel. Niclosamide is an alternative.

Taenia solium and Taenia saginata

Patients who have *T. solium* infection should be evaluated for the presence of cerebral cysticercosis before commencing therapy against the intestinal tapeworm. Praziquantel is effective therapy for the adult worm. Niclosamide has also been widely used.

Hymenolepis nana

H. nana infection can be treated with a single oral dose of praziquantel. Niclosamide is also successful.

Diphyllobothrium latum

D. latum infections are treated with praziquantel. Niclosamide was extensively used in the past.

References available online at expertconsult.com.

KEY REFERENCES

Abubakar I., Aliyu S.H., Arumugam C., et al.: Prevention and treatment of cryptosporidiosis in immunocompromised patients. *Cochrane Database of Syst Rev* 2007; (1): CD004932.

Amadi B.C., Mwiya M., Musuku J., et al.: Effect of nitazoxanide on morbidity and mortality in Zambian children with cryptosporidiosis: a randomised controlled trial. *Lancet* 2002; 360:1375-1380.

Fayer R.: Taxonomy and species delimitation in the genus *Cryptosporidium. Exp Parasitol* 2010; 124:90-97.

Hoge C.W., Shlim D.R., Ghimire M., et al.: Placebo-controlled trial of co-trimoxazole for *Cyclospora*

infections among travellers and foreign residents in Nepal. *Lancet* 1995; 345:691-693.

Lindsay D.S., Dubey J.P., Blagburn B.L.: Biology of *Isospora* spp. from humans, non-human primates, and domestic animals. *Clin Microbiol Rev* 1997; 10:19-34.

Ogren J., Dienus O., Lofgren S., et al.: *Dientamoeba fragilis* DNA detection in *Enterobius vermicularis* eggs. *Pathog Dis* 2013; 69:157-158.

Ralston K.S., Petri W.A.: Tissue destruction and tissue invasion by *Entamoeba histolytica. Trends Parasitol* 2011; 27:253-262.

Suputtamonkol Y., Kungpanichkul N., Silpasakorn S., et al.: Efficacy and safety of a single-dose veterinary preparation of ivermectin versus 7-day high-dose albendazole for chronic strongyloidiasis. *Int J Antimicrob Agents* 2008; 31:46-49.

Verdier R.I., Fitzgerald D.W., Johnson W.D., et al.: Trimethoprim–sulfamethoxazole compared with ciprofloxacin for treatment and prophylaxis of *Isospora belli* and *Cyclospora cayetanensis* infection in HIV-infected patients. *Ann Intern Med* 2000; 132:885-888.

115

Typhoid Fever and Other Enteric Fevers

CHRISTIANE DOLECEK

KEY CONCEPTS

- The pathogen is restricted to humans (there is no animal reservoir).

- Transmission is feco-oral.

- There is gram-negative sepsis with very low bacteremia.

- Patients are commonly treated as outpatients in endemic areas.

- Diagnosis relies on blood culture. Serology is unreliable and difficult to interpret.

- There are two licensed vaccines against S. Typhi infection, but there is no vaccine against S. Paratyphi.

- Antimicrobial drug resistance is a major challenge to the control of enteric fever.

Epidemiology

Typhoid fever and paratyphoid fever are gram-negative bacteremias caused by *Salmonella enterica* serovar Typhi (*S.* Typhi) and *Salmonella enterica* serovars Paratyphi (*S.* Paratyphi) A, B and C. Typhoid and paratyphoid fever are together known as enteric fevers. Whilst *S.* Typhi and *S.* Paratyphi A and B infections are restricted to humans, *S.* Paratyphi C has been reported to also affect a variety of animals.

Enteric fever remains endemic in Africa, Asia, Central and South America.[1] Infections seen in Europe, Australia and North America are usually acquired abroad and imported by travelers, mostly from the Indian subcontinent, South East Asia and South America (Figure 115-1).

Estimates from the World Health Organization (WHO) suggested there were approximately 21 million infections and 210 000 deaths caused by typhoid fever and 5 million cases of paratyphoid fever in the year 2000.[2] A revised estimate for 2010 suggested 27 million cases of typhoid fever.[3] There is significant regional variability in the distribution and incidence of *S.* Paratyphi A in Asia and Africa.[4] A high proportion of enteric fevers in China, India and Nepal (64%, 24% and 33%, respectively) were caused by *S.* Paratyphi A,[5,6] whilst *S.* Paratyphi A infections have only rarely been reported from Africa.[4]

Population-based surveillance studies in Asia have provided robust typhoid incidence data among 5- to 15-year-olds in Indonesia, Pakistan and India, with 180, 413 and 493 infections per 100 000 persons per year, respectively.[6] In endemic areas typhoid fever has been considered to be a disease of schoolchildren and young adults; however, recent data emphasize that it is also common in children aged between 1 and 5 years.

Transmission of typhoid fever occurs via the fecal–oral route by ingesting contaminated water or food, or through direct person-to-person contact. Bacteria are shed in the stools during an acute infection. Typhoid epidemics are usually water-borne and caused by contaminated drinking water (Figure 115-2). A study from

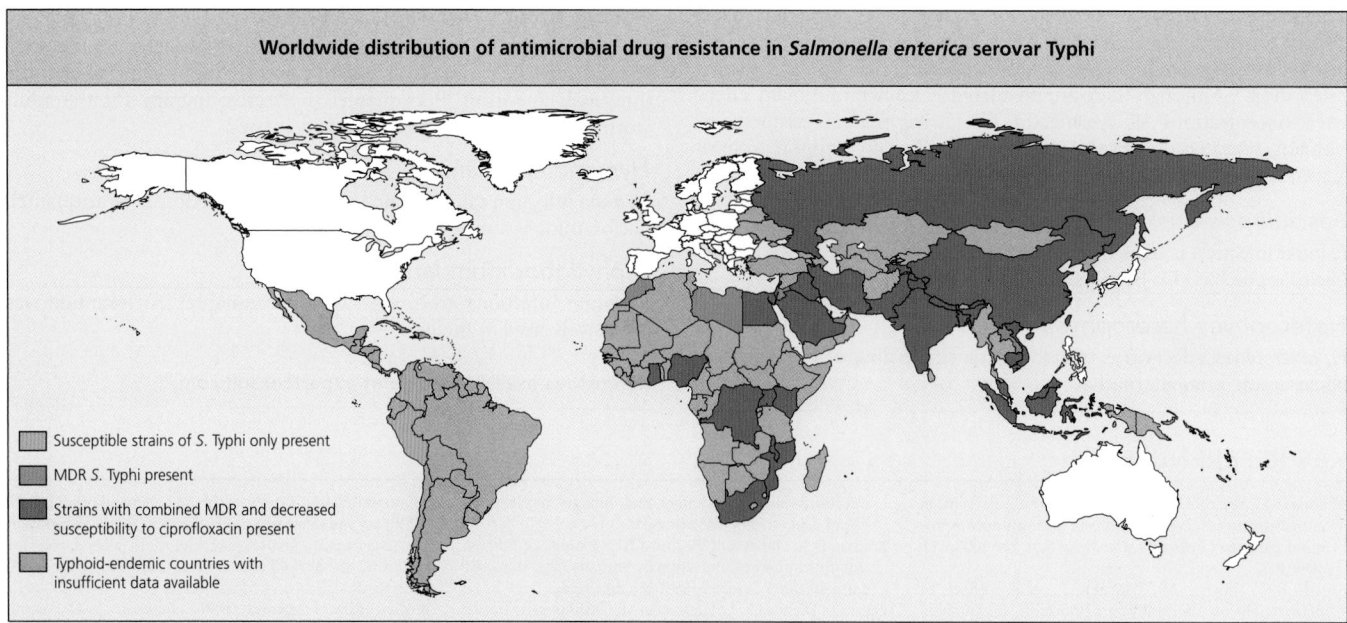

Figure 115-1 Worldwide distribution of antimicrobial drug resistance in *Salmonella enterica* serovar Typhi. Multidrug resistance (MDR) is defined as resistance to the first-line antimicrobial drugs ampicillin, trimethoprim–sulfamethoxazole and chloramphenicol. Sporadic cases of extended-spectrum β-lactamase producing *S.* Typhi isolates have been reported in India, Bangladesh, Pakistan and the Philippines. High-level ciprofloxacin resistance has been reported from India, Bangladesh, Pakistan, Nepal and the Philippines. (*Adapted from Wain et al. Lancet 2015;385(9973):1136-1145.*)

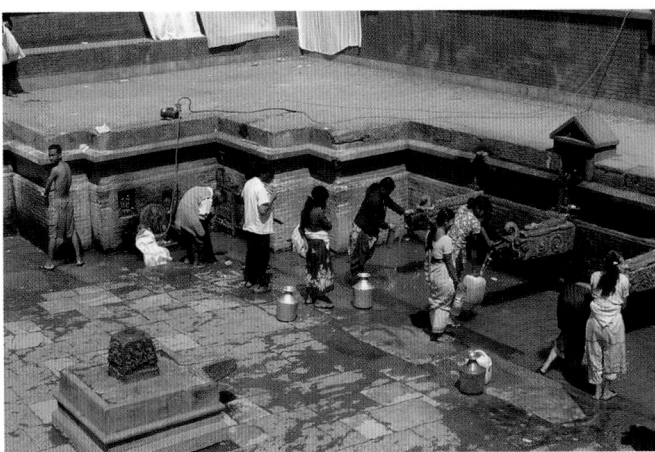

Figure 115-2 Community water spouts in Kathmandu, Nepal. Villagers, mostly women and children, are seen collecting their daily water provision from the community's stone spouts. This water is usually not boiled.

Kathmandu, Nepal, that combined spatial mapping of typhoid fever cases and high-resolution genotyping of the infecting isolates, found an extensive range of genotypes, even within individual households, suggesting indirect transmission via contaminated drinking water as the major source of infection.[7]

Additional risk factors for acquiring enteric fever are eating food prepared outside the home, shellfish from polluted water, vegetables fertilized with human waste and having a relative with a recent history of typhoid fever living in the same house. In some patients, S. Typhi or S. Paratyphi A can survive for long periods in the gallbladder without causing symptoms, and these chronic typhoid carriers are an important reservoir of infection, especially when involved in food handling.

Pathogenesis and Pathology

The species *Salmonella enterica* (see Chapter 180, *Salmonella*) is divided into six subspecies (*enterica*, *salamae*, *arizonae*, *diarizonae*, *houtenae* and *indica*) and contains more than 2400 serotypes.[8] Most of the *Salmonellae* that cause disease in humans (including S. Typhi, S. Paratyphi and S. Typhimurium) are in the subspecies *enterica*.

S. Typhi and S. Paratyphi are flagellated, non-spore-bearing, facultative anaerobic gram-negative bacilli. They are identified by a characteristic biochemical pattern and confirmed by serologic identification of their somatic lipopolysaccharide (O) and flagellar protein (H) antigens according to the Kaufmann–White scheme. S. Typhi and S. Paratyphi C sometimes possess a polysaccharide capsular Vi (virulence) antigen that coats the O antigen and potentially protects it from antibody attack.

The genome of S. Typhi is 4.8 million base pairs in length and encodes approximately 4000 genes.[9] There are several large insertions, believed to originate from bacteriophages or plasmids, termed the *Salmonella* pathogenicity islands, which encode genes that are important for survival in the host. *Salmonellae* are able to survive and multiply within the mononuclear phagocytic cells. The genomes of S. Typhi and S. Paratyphi A contain more than 200 pseudogenes. The inactivation of these genes may help explain the human host restriction of these pathogens. S. Typhi and S. Paratyphi A are clonal pathogens with very limited genetic diversity. These two pathogens are genetically distant but have converged to cause a similar clinical syndrome.

Multidrug resistance (MDR, resistance against all first-line antimicrobials, ampicillin, chloramphenicol and trimethoprim-sulfamethoxazole) of S. Typhi is mediated by an incH1 plasmid. One MDR S. Typhi lineage, haplotype 58, has become dominant and has been spreading across Asia and Africa.[10]

After ingestion in water or food, S. Typhi bacteria reach the small intestine where they adhere to the mucosal epithelial cells. They penetrate the mucosal epithelium via the M (microfold) cells and are taken up by macrophages and multiply in the mononuclear phagocytic cells of the small intestine, are drained into mesenteric lymph nodes and reach the general circulation (causing an asymptomatic primary bacteremia). During the incubation period, which varies between 7 and 14 days, the bacteria reside and multiply within the organs of the reticuloendothelial system. Bacteria are then shed into the bloodstream, marking the onset of fever and symptomatic disease. During the symptomatic stage, S. Typhi can be cultured from blood, although this is made difficult by the low bacterial load that characterizes this infection (less than one colony-forming unit per milliliter of blood).

If left untreated, the S. Typhi bacteremia persists for several weeks.[1] In this phase the organism disseminates widely to the organs of the reticuloendothelial system. S. Typhi infection produces hyperplasia of the Peyer's patches in the first week, which can resolve or progress to necrosis. Ulcers can lead to perforation and hemorrhage, usually in the third week, although these may occur earlier or later during the disease.[1] The majority of patients produce local and systemic humoral and cellular immune responses but these only protect partially against relapse or re-infection. The mortality rate of untreated typhoid used to be about 10–20%.

Prevention

Typhoid and paratyphoid fever can be prevented by the provision of safe water, safe sewage disposal and good food hygiene. Chronic typhoid carriers pose a special risk to the community, so programs to detect and treat chronic carriers need to be in place.[11]

Vaccines are another important measure to prevent enteric fever. There are two licensed vaccines for typhoid fever: the parenteral Vi polysaccharide and the oral Ty21 vaccines. The live oral Ty21 vaccine is available in enteric-coated capsules or liquid formulation. It is administered in three doses (four doses in the USA and Canada) 2 days apart and is licensed for adults and children above 6 years of age. Field studies with the oral Ty21 vaccine in the 1980s showed a protective efficacy of 96% after 3 years in Egypt, 77% in Chile after 3 years when using the liquid formulation and 53% in Indonesia after 2.5 years.[1] Herd protection was demonstrated during the field trials in Chile. Ty21a cannot be used in immune compromised patients and pregnant women, and antibiotics should be avoided 7 days before and after immunization. Booster doses are recommended every 5 years.

The injectable capsular polysaccharide Vi vaccine is given in a single dose (25 µg) and is immunogenic and licensed above 2 years of age. A single intramuscular injection conferred a protective efficacy of 55% after 3 years in South Africa and 72% after 17 months in Nepal.[1] Booster doses are recommended every 3 years. In a recent large cluster-randomized trial in slum-dwelling residents in Kolkata, the protective effectiveness for the Vi vaccine was 61%; for children between 2 and 5 years it was 80% and among unvaccinated members of the Vi vaccine cluster it was 44%, indicating strong herd protection.[12]

The novel conjugate vaccine Vi-rEPA (Vi polysaccharide coupled to recombinant exoprotein A from *Pseudomonas aeruginosa*) was immunogenic in children under 2 years and had a protective efficacy of 92% after 27 months in field trials in Vietnam,[1] but is not yet commercially available. In 2013, a novel conjugate typhoid vaccine, containing the Vi capsular polysaccharide coupled to tetanus toxoid, was licensed in India. This vaccine elicits T-cell dependent immunity and can be administered to children above 6 months.

The licensed typhoid vaccines do not protect against S. Paratyphi A, an emerging infection in Asia, and there is no licensed paratyphoid vaccine available. A polyvalent pan-enteric vaccine is urgently needed.

Clinical Features

The incubation period is approximately 7–14 days. Enteric fever presents with fever, headache, anorexia and abdominal discomfort with

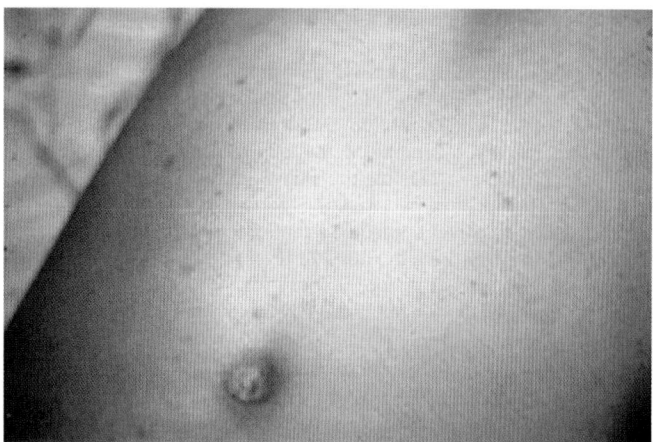

Figure 115-3 Typhoid rose spots. These are small, blanching maculopapular lesions, ~1–4 mm in size, usually seen on the trunk. They may also take on a more purpuric, nonblanching character. *(Courtesy of C.M. Parry, Liverpool, UK.)*

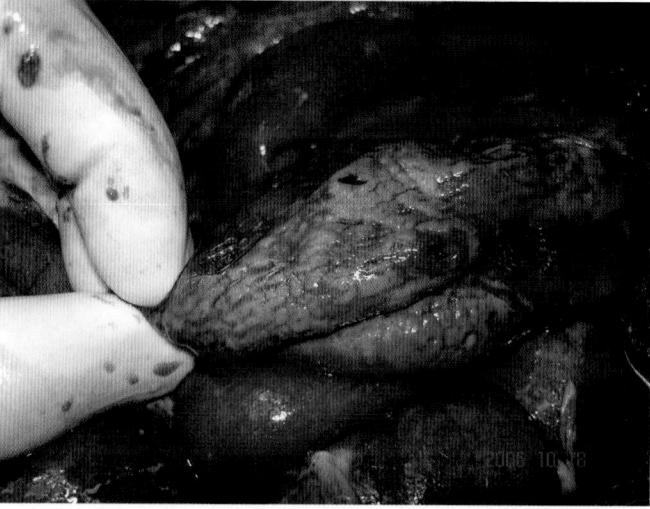

Figure 115-4 Gastrointestinal perforation, usually of the terminal ileum, is one of the most serious complications of typhoid fever. The figure shows the intraoperative picture of a patient with perforated necrotic ulcer. *(Photo credit: Pukar Maskey, Patan Hospital, Kathmandu.)*

either diarrhea or constipation.[1,13,14] This can be accompanied by nausea, vomiting and a dry cough. Often patients also experience arthralgia and myalgia. Abdominal tenderness, hepatomegaly (40–70% of patients) and splenomegaly are common. It is rare for patients with typhoid fever not to have any abdominal symptoms. Profuse diarrhea has been described in typhoid patients with HIV infection.[1]

Less than 5% of patients show rose spots, small blanching erythematous maculopapular lesions of about 2–4 mm diameter on the trunk (Figure 115-3). Hemoglobin levels, white cell counts and platelet counts are normal or reduced. Liver enzymes (aspartate aminotransferase, alanine aminotransferase) are often elevated two to three times the upper limit of normal and bilirubin is normal or slightly raised. Abdominal sonography may demonstrate enlargement of liver and spleen and prominent mesenteric lymph nodes.

Although it has been frequently cited in the literature that *S. Para-typhi* causes a milder disease, a recent prospective clinical trial has reported that enteric fever caused by *S.* Typhi and *S.* Paratyphi A are clinically indistinguishable.[5] *S.* Paratyphi A has also been described as a cause of severe enteric fever in Indonesia.[13]

COMPLICATIONS AND SEVERE TYPHOID FEVER

Complications of typhoid fever are more likely to occur in patients who have been sick for longer periods without receiving treatment and in patients with non-susceptible *S.* Typhi isolates who do not receive appropriate treatment (Box 115-1), and may develop in up to 10% of hospitalized patients.[1] Septic shock and acute respiratory distress syndrome are serious complications when treatment is delayed.

Gastrointestinal bleeding, intestinal perforation and typhoid encephalopathy are the most common severe complications. Gastrointestinal bleeding results from a necrotic Peyer's patch eroding the wall of an enteric blood vessel. Often the bleeding resolves without intervention, but in about 1–5% of cases the bleeding requires blood transfusion. Gastrointestinal perforation, usually at the terminal ileum (Figure 115-4), is the most serious complication; it occurs in about 1–3% of hospitalized cases.[1] It manifests as acute abdomen or as worsening of abdominal pain accompanied by shock. Perforation is associated with a high mortality risk and needs urgent surgical intervention.

A reduced level of consciousness or encephalopathy, often accompanied by shock, is a serious complication, associated with a mortality rate of up to 50%.[15] Typhoid encephalopathy encompasses a wide range of symptoms ranging from agitation to delirium and coma. In patients with encephalopathy, cerebrospinal fluid should be obtained and meningitis (including tuberculous meningitis) and encephalitis excluded. The prognosis of typhoid fever during pregnancy has been improved through antimicrobial treatment.

BOX 115-1 IMPORTANT COMPLICATIONS OF TYPHOID FEVER

ABDOMINAL COMPLICATIONS
Gastrointestinal bleeding
Intestinal perforation and shock
Hepatitis with/without jaundice
Cholecystitis

GENITOURINARY COMPLICATIONS
Retention of urine
Glomerulonephritis

CARDIOVASCULAR COMPLICATIONS
Asymptomatic ECG changes
Myocarditis
Sudden death

RESPIRATORY COMPLICATIONS
Pneumonia
Bronchitis

HEMATOLOGIC COMPLICATIONS
Anemia
Disseminated intravascular coagulation (DIC)

FOCAL INFECTIONS
Abscesses of brain, liver, spleen etc.

NEUROPSYCHIATRIC COMPLICATIONS
Encephalopathy – reduced consciousness levels
Meningitis
Seizures

RELAPSE

The recurrence of symptoms within 1 month after treatment has been completed and symptoms have resolved is considered a relapse. Relapse rates vary considerably (between 0% and 10%) and are related to the efficacy of the antibiotic treatment, with chloramphenicol treatment showing higher relapse rates compared to fluoroquinolone treatment.[1,13,14]

ACUTE SHEDDING AND CHRONIC CARRIAGE

During the acute illness, patients shed *S.* Typhi and *S.* Paratyphi A intermittently in their stools. In an *S.* Typhi challenge study with daily stool sampling, *S.* Typhi was identified in the stools of 18 of 24 (75%)

participants who acquired typhoid fever.[16] Between 1% and 5% of enteric fever patients become chronic carriers, harboring S. Typhi or S. Paratyphi in their gallbladder and shedding bacteria intermittently in their stools after the illness.[11] These carriers are an important reservoir of infection and are usually asymptomatic. Up to 25% of chronic carriers do not have a history of typhoid infection. The rate of carriers is higher among females and patients with cholelithiasis. Cholelithiasis and chronic carriage are risk factors for the development of gallbladder cancer. An association between urinary carriage of S. Typhi and S. Paratyphi A and schistosomiasis has been described, caused by obstructive lesions of the urinary tract.

CASE FATALITY

A recent WHO report has estimated the case fatality rate in typhoid fever at 1%.[2] There is considerable geographic variation, with high mortality of up to 30% reported in patients with severe typhoid fever in Papua New Guinea and Indonesia.[1] The most important contributor to a poor outcome is a delay in administering effective antibiotic treatment.

DIFFERENTIAL DIAGNOSIS

Typhoid fever presents with nonspecific symptoms and this makes the diagnosis difficult. Other endemic illnesses, most importantly malaria, have to be ruled out. Typhoid can occasionally present initially as gastroenteritis with vomiting and diarrhea. Differential diagnosis includes leptospirosis, typhus (rickettsial disease), tuberculosis, brucellosis, other bacterial sepsis, encephalitis, amebic liver abscesses, visceral leishmaniasis, viral diseases (dengue fever, infectious mononucleosis, hepatitis, influenza) and lymphoproliferative disease.

Antimicrobial Drug Resistance

The development of antimicrobial drug resistance is the biggest challenge for the treatment of enteric fever. Figure 115-1 gives an overview of global antimicrobial resistance patterns of S. Typhi.[17]

In 1948 the introduction of chloramphenicol revolutionized the management of typhoid fever.[13] Chloramphenicol was effective for more than 20 years, but in the 1970s independent outbreaks of chloramphenicol-resistant typhoid fever occurred in Mexico, India and Vietnam. In the late 1980s there were outbreaks of typhoid fever that were resistant against all 'first-line' antimicrobials (multidrug resistance is defined as resistance to chloramphenicol, ampicillin and trimethoprim–sulfamethoxazole).[1] These multidrug resistant (MDR) S. Typhi isolates were responsible for numerous outbreaks in countries in the Indian subcontinent, South East Asia and Africa.[9,13,14] A recent study demonstrated that there is evidence of multiple transfers of the dominant H58 S. Typhi genotype from Asia to Africa, with an ongoing epidemic of this strain in eastern and southern Africa.[10] All MDR strains so far examined have been harboring plasmids of the incHI1 incompatibility group.

The fluoroquinolone class of drugs became the treatment of choice for typhoid fever. The fluoroquinolones show excellent tissue penetration, accumulation in monocytes and macrophages and high drug levels in the gallbladder. However, relatively soon there were reports from Vietnam, India and Tajikistan of the emergence of S. Typhi isolates that responded less well to the fluoroquinolones.[1,9] In 1997, an epidemic in Tajikistan caused by those strains caused illness in more than 10 000 people and 108 deaths. These strains were resistant to nalidixic acid, the prototype quinolone, and exhibited higher minimum inhibitory concentrations (MICs) to the fluoroquinolones and were summarized as strains with decreased ciprofloxacin susceptibility (ciprofloxacin MIC between 0.12 and 1.0 µg/mL).[18,19] Although these isolates were technically still below the historical ciprofloxacin MIC resistance breakpoint of ≥4 µg/mL, patients infected with these isolates showed a poor clinical response when treated with ciprofloxacin or ofloxacin.[18]

Nalidixic acid resistance is usually caused by single point mutations in the bacterial target enzyme gyrA, either at codon 83 or 87.[18] More than 15 independent mutational events in the gyrA gene have been identified in a global selection of S. Typhi strains, selected by strong antimicrobial pressure.[10]

In 2012, the Clinical and Laboratory Standards Institute (CLSI) implemented new Salmonella-specific MIC breakpoints and disk diffusion breakpoints for ciprofloxacin (susceptible ≤0.064 µg/mL; intermediate between 0.12 to 0.5 µg/mL; and resistant ≥1.0 µg/mL).[20] In 2013, the CLSI published Salmonella-specific MIC breakpoints for ofloxacin (susceptible ≤0.125 µg/mL; intermediate between 0.25 to 1 µg/mL; and resistant ≥2 µg/mL) and levofloxacin (susceptible ≤0.125 µg/mL; intermediate between 0.25 to 1 µg/mL; and resistant ≥2 µg/mL). High-level ciprofloxacin-resistant S. Typhi and S. Paratyphi A with double mutations in gyrA and mutations in gyrB and parC from the Indian subcontinent have been described.[17] Recently there have been reports of S. Typhi isolates with reduced susceptibility to the fluoroquinolones that test nalidixic acid-sensitive,[9] suggesting another mechanism of resistance.

The re-emergence of chloramphenicol-susceptible S. Typhi has been reported in recent years from India and Nepal.[5,9] There have been worrying reports of sporadic cases of ceftriaxone-resistant S. Typhi from India, Pakistan and the Philippines, most commonly harboring plasmid-mediated extended-spectrum β-lactamase (ESBL) enzymes of the CTX-M type.[17] There has been a recent report of an azithromycin-resistant S. Paratyphi A isolate from India causing treatment failure.[17]

Diagnosis

The diagnosis of enteric fever requires the isolation of S. Typhi or S. Paratyphi from blood, bone marrow or an anatomic lesion. Blood culture is the gold standard in the diagnosis of enteric fever. This is a problem as microbiology facilities are often not available. A low bacterial load is a characteristic feature of typhoid fever, the median S. Typhi count in blood was 1 cfu/mL in a clinical study.[1] The sensitivity of blood culture is estimated to be only 50–60%; bone marrow culture is more sensitive (up to 80%), because of the higher concentration of bacteria in the bone marrow.[14] Therefore obtaining a large volume of blood – ideally 10–15 mL for schoolchildren and adults and 2-4 mL for preschool children – is recommended.

SEROLOGY

The Widal tube agglutination test, described more than 100 years ago, is based on the presence of agglutinating antibodies to the O and H antigens of Salmonella. In the original format, paired sera (acute and convalescent) were required and a fourfold increase of antibodies (to O and H antigens) supported the diagnosis of typhoid fever. However, the test is usually performed only on acute serum and lacks sensitivity and specificity. This is because not everybody mounts a detectable antibody response to S. Typhi; healthy populations in endemic areas and people who received typhoid vaccine show a high level of antibodies and there is cross-reactivity to other Salmonella serotypes. Rapid tests (Tubex, Typhidot and Typhidot M) have been developed with varying sensitivity and specificity.[14]

Management

Enteric fevers are systemic infections and antimicrobial treatment must be initiated early. It is important to provide supportive measures, such as oral and intravenous fluids, appropriate nutrition and antipyretics. More than 90% of patients are managed at home with oral antibiotics, and reliable and close medical follow-up for complications or failure to respond to therapy. Patients with persistent vomiting, severe diarrhea and abdominal distention need admission to hospital.[1]

The choice of treatment critically depends on the antimicrobial susceptibility of the isolate, but is also influenced by cost and availability, which are important factors, especially in endemic regions. Antimicrobials should be used at the highest recommended dose and the treatment course should be completed. The management of patients with enteric fever should also include blood and stool cultures

TABLE 115-1	Treatment of Uncomplicated Typhoid Fever*					
	Optimal Therapy			**Alternative Effective Drugs**		
Susceptibility	Antimicrobial	Daily dose (mg/kg)	Days	Antimicrobial	Daily dose (mg/kg)	Days
Fully sensitive	Fluoroquinolone, e.g. ofloxacin or ciprofloxacin[†]	20	7	Chloramphenicol Amoxicillin Trimethoprim–sulfamethoxazole	75 100 8/40	14–21 14 14
Multidrug resistance	Fluoroquinolone	20	7	Azithromycin[ǀ] Ceftriaxone	20 75	7 10–14
Intermediate ciprofloxacin susceptibility[‡§]	Azithromycin[ǀ] or newer fluoroquinolone, e.g. gatifloxacin[¶] (10 mg/kg/day)	20 10	7 7	Ceftriaxone	75	10–14
Ciprofloxacin resistant	Azithromycin	20	7	Ceftriaxone	75	10–14

*Based on the World Health Organization (WHO)[14] recommendations for the treatment of typhoid fever, updated with evidence from recent randomized controlled trials in typhoid fever.[21–25] Cefixime, an oral third-generation cephalosporin that was included in the WHO recommendations of 2003, should not be used and has been removed due to recent evidence.[14]

†The available fluoroquinolones (ofloxacin, ciprofloxacin, fleroxacin, pefloxacin) are all highly active and equivalent in efficacy, with the exception of norfloxacin, which has inadequate oral bioavailablity and should not be used in typhoid fever.[14]

‡Intermediate ciprofloxacin resistance (ciprofloxacin MIC of 0.12μg/mL to 0.5 μg/mL) refers to isolates with low-level resistance, which have previously been described as nalidixic acid-resistant or isolates with decreased ciprofloxacin susceptibility.

§Prolonged courses of high-dose fluoroquinolones (e.g. ofloxacin 20 mg/kg/day) have been recommended[14] and are standard treatment in many countries for nalidixic acid-resistant S. Typhi and S. Paratyphi A. In Vietnam, however, a trial using ofloxacin at 20 mg/kg/day in two divided doses for 7 days has shown treatment success in only 64% of patients and high rates of convalescent fecal (19%) carriage (at day 8),[26] whereas a trial in Nepal using ofloxacin at 20 mg/kg/day showed treatment success in 77/83 (96%) patients when evaluated on day 10.[25] In the latter trial, the medication was weighed.

ǀAzithromycin used at 20 mg/kg q24h for 7 days achieved better cure rates (91%)[22] than azithromycin 10 mg/kg q24h in multidrug-resistant and nalidixic acid-resistant typhoid fever.

¶Four published trials[21–24] (the two latter trials included monitoring for dysglycemia) show that the newer 8-methoxy-fluoroquinolone gatifloxacin is safe and efficacious in patients with typhoid fever. A retrospective study from Canada reported that gatifloxacin used in elderly patients (mean age 77 years) with type 2 diabetes has a high risk of inducing dysglycemia;[21] this was not seen in the typhoid treatment trials in young and otherwise healthy patients. However, as a consequence, gatifloxacin has been withdrawn or is not available in many countries.

after completion of treatment to check for microbiologic failure and convalescent stool carriage, as well as later follow-up to identify chronic fecal carriage.

Table 115-1 shows the recommendations of the World Health Organization for the treatment of typhoid fever, updated with evidence from recent randomized controlled trials.[14,21–25]

The fluoroquinolones have been widely used and are the most effective treatment for typhoid fever. In patients infected with nalidixic acid-susceptible isolates, fever usually resolves within 4 days, cure is achieved in 96% of patients and rates for fecal carriage and relapse are below 2%.[1] The fluoroquinolones are also recommended for the treatment of children with typhoid fever. Concerns that the fluoroquinolones might cause cartilage damage in children have led to their cautious use in many countries. However, extensive experience with the fluoroquinolones in children with cystic fibrosis, typhoid fever and bacillary dysentery has provided a body of evidence confirming that these antibiotics are safe in children.[1,14]

Nalidixic acid-resistant isolates with decreased ciprofloxacin susceptibility have recently been re-categorized as isolates with intermediate ciprofloxacin susceptibility (with a ciprofloxacin MIC of 0.12–0.5μg/mL).[20] For these isolates, azithromycin and third-generation cephalosporins (ceftriaxone) are effective. Azithromycin should be used at 20 mg/kg/day once daily for 7 days.[22] The European Committee on Antimicrobial Susceptibility Testing (EUCAST) has suggested an azithromycin MIC ≤16 μg/mL for susceptible strains that are expected to respond to treatment.[26] Ceftriaxone (2 g per day for adults, 75 mg/kg/day in children once daily) should be used for 10–14 days.[14] Ceftriaxone therapy for 7 days was associated with a relapse rate of 14%.[14] However, a recent randomized controlled trial using ceftriaxone (2 g per day for adults and 60 mg/kg/day in children under 14 years once daily) for 7 days in children and adults in Nepal showed low rates of treatment failures (4/54 patients with culture-confirmed enteric fever) with only one patient having a relapse one month after the start of treatment (Buddha Basnyat, unpublished). Although recommended in the WHO guidelines,[14] cefixime (oral third-generation cephalosporin) should not be used. A recent trial observed high treatment failure rates

of 38% and the trial was stopped early by the trial's Independent Data Safety and Monitoring Board.[23]

Despite successful trials showing that the newer generation 8-methoxy-fluoroquinolone gatifloxacin was safe and efficacious in patients infected with S. Typhi and S. Paratyphi A with decreased ciprofloxacin susceptibility,[21–24] gatifloxacin has been withdrawn or is not available in many countries because of a reported high risk of gatifloxacin-induced dysglycemia in elderly patients with type 2 diabetes.[21]

Prolonged courses of fluoroquinolones at higher doses (e.g. ofloxacin 20 mg/kg/day) have been recommended[14] and are standard treatment in many countries for S. Typhi and S. Paratyphi A with decreased ciprofloxacin susceptibilty. However, a recent trial using ofloxacin at 20 mg/kg/day for 7 days in Vietnam has shown treatment failure in 36% of patients and high rates (19%) of immediate post-treatment fecal carriage (at day 8),[25] whereas a trial in Nepal using the same regimen, but with weighed tablets, had a failure rate of 6% when evaluated on day 10.[24] However, the continued use of fluoroquinolones at suboptimal concentrations is likely to drive the step-wise accumulation of resistance mutations, leading to high-level ciprofloxacin resistance. In regions where ciprofloxacin-resistant isolates have been reported (especially India and South Asia), azithromycin and ceftriaxone are the recommended treatment options. A combination of azithromycin and ceftriaxone is increasingly used in clinical practice, especially in the Indian subcontinent and returning travellers,[27] but there are no data from randomized controlled trials.

There are few data on the treatment of typhoid fever in pregnancy. Ampicillin for fully susceptible isolates and ceftriaxone are considered safe for this indication.[14]

MANAGEMENT OF SEVERE TYPHOID FEVER

Both inpatients and outpatients should be closely monitored for the development of complications. The parenteral fluoroquinolones are probably the first choice for the treatment of severe typhoid fever in patients infected with susceptible isolates[14] and should be given for a minimum of 10 days, but there are no randomized trials to date. For patients infected with strains with intermediate ciprofloxacin susceptibility, ceftriaxone is effective.[14]

A trial conducted in the 1980s showed a dramatic beneficial effect of high-dose dexamethasone treatment (3 mg/kg for the first dose given over 30 minutes and 1 mg/kg every 6 hours for 48 hours) in severe typhoid fever patients with encephalopathy and shock, given in addition to chloramphenicol. Dexamethasone treatment reduced the mortality rate from 56% to 10% when compared to placebo.[15] Hydrocortisone at a lower dose was not effective. WHO recommend adding dexamethasone to the antimicrobial treatment of patients with confirmed or suspected enteric fever presenting with changes in mental status, if other causes of meningitis and encephalitis can be excluded.[14]

Intestinal perforation is a surgical emergency. Early intervention is crucial, and mortality rates increase as the delay between perforation and surgery lengthens, varying between 10% and 32%.[14] Metronidazole should be added to the antibiotic regimen.

Patients with intestinal hemorrhage need intensive care, monitoring and blood transfusion. Intervention is not needed unless there is significant blood loss, but cross-matched blood should be ready and the surgical team alerted.[14]

In patients presenting with a relapse, which is defined as the re-occurrence of acute illness after the patient has been treated successfully, cultures should be obtained and patients should be treated according to the susceptibility pattern of the infecting isolate.

TYPHOID CARRIERS

Chronic carriers play an important role in the transmission of typhoid and paratyphoid fever. As *S.* Typhi and *S.* Paratyphi are only shed intermittently in the feces, a series of stool cultures should be obtained to detect carriers. In order to eradicate carriage, long antimicrobial treatment courses of 6 weeks should be given according to the susceptibility of the isolates. In susceptible isolates, clearance was achieved in up to 80% with the administration of 750 mg ciprofloxacin twice daily for 28 days.[14] If cholelithiasis is present the patient may require cholecystectomy as well as antibiotic therapy.

References available online at expertconsult.com.

KEY REFERENCES

Arjyal A., Basnyat B., Koirala S., et al.: Gatifloxacin versus chloramphenicol for uncomplicated enteric fever: an open-label, randomised, controlled trial. *Lancet Infect Dis* 2011; 11(6):445-454.

Baker S., Holt K.E., Clements A.C., et al.: Combined high-resolution genotyping and geospatial analysis reveals modes of endemic urban typhoid fever transmission. *Open Biol* 2011; 1(2):110008.

Crump J.A., Luby S.P., Mintz E.D.: The global burden of typhoid fever. *Bull World Health Organ* 2004; 82(5):346-353.

Parkhill J., Dougan G., James K.D., et al.: Complete genome sequence of a multiple drug resistant *Salmonella enterica* serovar Typhi CT18. *Nature* 2001; 413(6858): 848-852.

Parry C.M., Hien T.T., Dougan G., et al.: Typhoid fever. *N Engl J Med* 2002; 347(22):1770-1782.

Wong V.K., Baker S., Pickard D.J., et al.: Phylogeographical analysis of the dominant multidrug-resistant H58 clade of *Salmonella* Typhi identifies inter- and intracontinental transmission events. *Nat Genet* 2015; 47(6):632-639.

World Health Organization: *Background document: the diagnosis, treatment and prevention of typhoid fever.* Geneva: WHO, Department of Vaccines and Biologicals; 2003. Available: www.who.int/vaccine_research/documents/en/typhoid_diagnosis.pdf.

116

Amebic Infections

DAVID C. WARHURST

- Gastrointestinal amebiasis affects 48 million people and causes 70 000 deaths each year, ranking it as the 10th most common intestinal infection globally.

- The vast majority of disease is due to infection with *Entamoeba histolytica*, but *E. moshkovskii* has more recently been identified as an important cause of disease in infants.

- It is not possible to distinguish these pathogenic species morphologically from the nonpathogenic *E. dispar*, which can inhabit the human intestine.

- The two most common forms of disease are invasive colitis and amebic liver abscess.

- Prompt diagnosis and instigation of appropriate treatment are key in determining good outcomes, and consist of initial treatment with a tissue amebicide, such as metronidazole, to kill pathogens invading tissues, followed by the use of a luminal amebicide, such as diloxanide, to kill trophozoites within the gut lumen.

Introduction

Diarrheal disease had an estimated burden of 89.5 million disability-adjusted life years (DALYs) in 2010. Intestinal parasites, particularly helminths and intestinal protozoa, play a major role as causative agents of persistent digestive symptomatologies.[1] The motile trophozoites (amebae) of *Entamoeba histolytica* live in the lumen of the large intestine, where multiplication by binary fission takes place. They can invade the colonic mucosa, producing ulceration and dysentery (Figure 116-1). Through blood-borne spread they can give rise to extraintestinal disease, usually abscesses in the liver (see Figure 116-2). Amebic dysentery is often self-limiting, but extraintestinal amebiasis is potentially fatal unless promptly diagnosed and treated, and this contributes significantly to the fact that amebiasis ranks worldwide as the fourth most common protozoan cause of death, behind malaria, African trypanosomiasis and leishmaniasis.[2]

Following multiplication in the large intestine, the trophozoites of *Entamoeba* spp. develop into cysts, a dormant stage resistant to environmental stress passed out in the feces, which serve to infect other humans after ingestion in contaminated water or food.

The organism was first observed by Lösch[3] in 1875, who reported from St Petersburg on a fatal dysentery in a patient with persistent diarrhea, fever, general weakness and tenesmus. However, it was only at the end of the 20th century that it was generally accepted that amebae termed *E. histolytica* living in the human colon comprised three distinct species, *E. histolytica*, *E. dispar* and *E. moshkovskii*, of which only *E. histolytica* was capable of causing dysentery and other disease. The separation of potentially pathogenic *E. histolytica* from morphologically similar amebae was supported by Sargeaunt and colleagues[4] in 1978 on the basis of isoenzyme patterns and on nucleic acid sequence by Diamond and Clark[5] in 1993. The World Health Organization (WHO)[6] redefined amebiasis in 1997 as infection with *E. histolytica*, with or without clinical manifestations, and noted the importance

of distinguishing it from the morphologically identical but nonpathogenic *E. dispar* described in 1925 by Emil Brumpt. It had been shown by Clark and Diamond in 1991 that *E. moshkovskii*, originally reported from Moscow sewage and capable of growing in culture at ambient temperatures (10–25 °C) as well as 37 °C, was identical to a human isolate from Laredo, Texas.[7] Found in human infections worldwide,[8,9] this was the third species in man to be morphologically identical to *E. histolytica*, and like *E. dispar* it was regarded as nonpathogenic. However the association of *E. moshkovskii* with colitis in infants in Bangladesh, and experimentally, virulence in adult C3H/HeJ, C3H/HeN and CBA/J mice have now been reported.[10] The presence of the organism in chelonians and crocodiles, possibly pointing to an infectious reservoir in animals, has also been recorded.[11]

Although epidemiologic data on prevalence of *E. histolytica* infection gained from stool examinations for '*E. histolytica*' cysts during the last century are misleading (three species with identical cysts and different pathogenicities) it is likely that mortality data from confirmed cases of invasive disease recorded then will be reliable. Similarly, prevalence data based on serology remain valuable indicators of distribution because natural infections with noninvasive species of *Entamoeba* do not elicit an antibody response.[12]

Clinically it is clearly desirable, when symptoms such as bloody diarrhea or colitis are seen and amebae are present, that:

- we should be able to confirm the presence of the pathogens, *E. histolytica* (or *E. moshkovskii* in infants or other susceptibles), ideally by reliable specific tests; and
- in the absence of a confirmed invasive infection, the true cause of the symptoms (e.g. shigellosis or similar) should be found and treated, incidentally avoiding unnecessary chemotherapy for amebiasis.

Because the three species have only recently been differentiated, it is an epidemiologic priority to understand their worldwide distribution and fully evaluate their individual significance.[13]

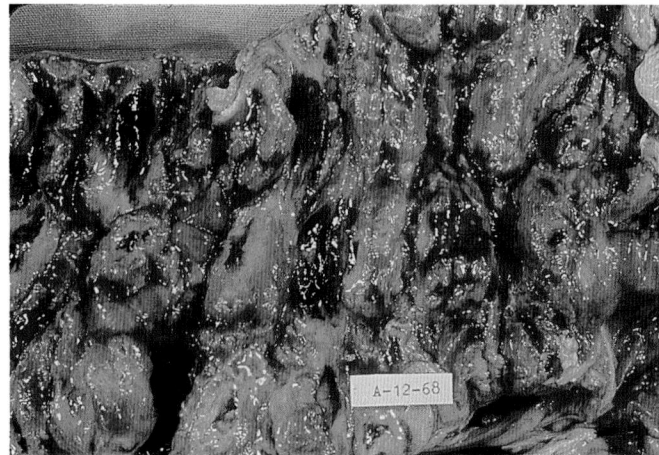

Figure 116-1 Pathology specimen from a fatal case of human amebic colitis. Deep ulcerations into the submucosa have produced abundant hemorrhages. *(Courtesy of Dr Jesús Aguirre García, Hospital General de México, Secretaria de Salud.)*

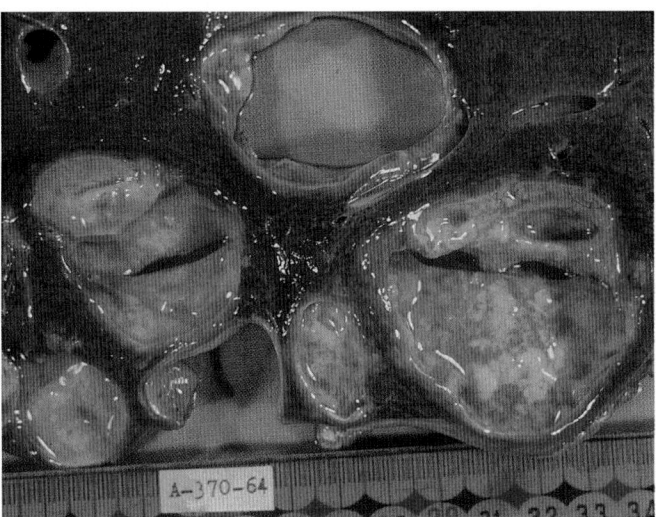

Figure 116-2 Human amebic liver abscess. Multiple abscesses, one cavitated, can be observed occupying virtually all lobes of the liver parenchyma, which is replaced by a semisolid material. *(Courtesy of Dr Jesús Aguirre García, Hospital General de México, Secretaría de Salud.)*

Epidemiology

Entamoeba histolytica (sensu lato) is one of the 10 most common intestinal infections in the world. WHO[2] estimates 48 million clinical cases per year, resulting in at least 70 000 deaths (mortality in clinical disease = 0.15%). Recent advances in molecular genetics allow the distinction of the potentially pathogenic species of *Entamoeba* from the nonpathogenic similar species. This allows scrutiny of important and previously obscure pathogen–host interactions, and is leading to a better understanding of the epidemiology of the disease, in particular the importance of *E. moshkovskii* in infant colitis.

Although invasive amebiasis is much less common in industrialized countries than in the developing world, it is still important to identify invasive *Entamoeba*, as misdiagnosis can be fatal. Disease mistaken for chronic ulcerative colitis with subsequent corticosteroid use can be disastrous. Infection rates in immigrant groups can be significant, and outbreaks can occur in institutions such as schools or psychiatric hospitals where hygiene is compromised. A major increase in intestinal amebic infections reported in men who have sex with men (MSM) in USA, Canada and England has mainly been asymptomatic, caused by the nonpathogenic *E. dispar*. The role of HIV is unclear. In 136 suspected or confirmed HIV-positive adult inpatients in Tanzania, *E. histolytica*, *E. moshkovskii* and *E. dispar* were all detected without evidence of invasive amebic disease.[9] In Japan and Taiwan, invasive amebiasis due to *E. histolytica* has been described in MSM, though there is no evidence that HIV leads to more severe disease.

Pathogenesis

Stanley[14] and Guo *et al.*[15] have reviewed amebiasis in general, and in particular the expanding knowledge of pathogenesis and invasion.

The first stage in invasive pathogenesis is attachment of the trophozoite to the human target cell, erythrocyte, enterocyte or leukocyte, which is made by a surface-located Eh-adherence lectin and is necessary for all subsequent changes. The adherence of the binding domain to target cells can be inhibited experimentally by D-galactose or N-acetyl D-galactosamine, and naturally by colonic mucin. Eh-adherence lectin is also used by the amebae for binding bacteria prior to phagocytosis. The carbohydrate recognition domain (CRD) of Eh-adherence lectin is only 89% conserved in the homologous sequence expressed by nonpathogenic *E. dispar*.[14,15] It is probable that Eh-adherence lectin responds to attachment by stimulating cytoskeletal changes in the ameba, and the transfer of cysteine proteinases

(EhCP-) and amebapores (EhAP-) from granules in the amebic cytoplasm to the membrane or external medium.

Subsequently, amebae produce a range of neutral cysteine proteinases which are expressed on the cell membrane or are secreted to the exterior. These break down matrix collagen, allowing the spread of amebae in the submucosa. Attracted (and activated) by interleukin (IL)-8 or other cytokines, neutrophils (and to a lesser extent macrophages) invade the mucosa and ease the entry of the amebae to the submucosa and deeper layers of the colonic wall.

Following binding to the intestinal mucosal cell through the adherence lectin, *E. histolytica* engulfs fragments of the cell (trogocytosis or 'nibbling'), and causes death of the cell, probably due to loss of membrane integrity. Ingestion of dead cells does not appear to be common, and the invasive process seems likely to involve the ameba moving from cell to cell over the colonic epithelium in progressive destruction of the integrity of the cell sheet.

Recent studies[16] have shed considerable light on the molecular basis of virulence in amebiasis, and genome sequencing has allowed comparison of *E. histolytica* with nonvirulent clones and related amebae.[17]

Transmission and Prevention

Although other animals can be infected, there is effectively no reservoir of *E. histolytica* other than humans. All age groups are susceptible to infection; persons with asymptomatic intestinal infection are most likely to be excreting cysts. Young children are likely to infect their carers, and healthy infected adults involved in food preparation in unsanitary conditions are also implicated. In endemic areas poor education, poverty, overcrowding, lack of sanitation and shortage of uncontaminated water supplies favor fecal–oral transmission.

Cysts passed in stool are fully developed, infective and resistant to stomach acid. Thus the direct fecal–oral transmission route is probably more important than for geohelminths (where development to the infective stage generally takes place outside the body). The inoculum size can be small ($\ll$100 cysts). However, cysts are susceptible to death by desiccation which limits persistence in the environment. Those in fecal material die within 10 minutes on the surface of the hands, but can survive under (long) fingernails for 45 minutes. Conditions of high relative humidity prolong survival. Although killed by freezing, cysts can survive in water at low temperatures for at least 3 months, and for more than 100 hours at 25 °C (77 °F) in water or moist conditions, but die rapidly in water above 50 °C (122 °F). Thus pasteurization or brief boiling is sufficient to eliminate transmission from milk or water.

Residual concentrations of chlorine sufficient to eliminate bacterial contamination from drinking water will not kill cysts: 3 mg/L is needed for 30 minutes. Cysts may be removed from water by slow filtration through biologic sand filters or rapid sand filtration after flocculation. Risk factors for infection in endemic areas have been reported to be crowding, illiteracy, lack of safe drinking water and inadequate disposal of human waste. Improving water supplies and health education should be the priority, together with early diagnosis and treatment,[18] and these should diminish the prevalence of infection and the importance of the direct fecal–oral transmission route.

The value of treatment of asymptomatic infected persons in controlling disease transmission is uncertain. In endemic areas, a high re-infection rate will likely negate any practical benefit.[19,20] In nonendemic areas recommendations for treatment of asymptomatic carriers do not usually include a tissue amebicide, which avoids major ethical objections on the grounds of side effects. Two alternatives are available:[21] paromomycin 25–35 mg/kg q8h for 7–10 days, or diloxanide furoate (if available) 500 mg q8h for 10 days.

Clinical Features

Amebic invasion more commonly remains localized in the colon but can metastasize via the portal vein to the liver and, more rarely, by extension from a liver abscess into pleura, lungs and/or pericardium. The amebae invade the colonic mucosa through small punctures in the mucosal surface and spread laterally into the submucosa, producing typical flask-shaped ulcers (see Figure 116-5). Extension may occur rarely from the colon to large abdominal vessels and other viscera including the urogenital system, or extremely rarely to the brain by hematogenous spread.

Extension to the skin can take place through rupture of an untreated liver abscess or from a perforated colonic segment. Primary infection of the skin can also be acquired by direct contact with an infected subject during vaginal or anal intercourse.

INTESTINAL AMEBIASIS (Table 116-1)

The spectrum of invasive disease ranges in severity from mild diarrhea to life-threatening fulminating necrotic colitis (see Figure 116-1) and perforation of the colon, which are the main causes of death in invasive intestinal amebiasis. Other complications include direct extension to the skin and dissemination, mainly to the liver (Figures 116-2 and 116-3). Severe intestinal amebiasis is twice as frequent in adults as in children,[21,22] where it may be associated with undernourishment.

The usual manifestation of invasive disease is an acute rectocolitis. Most patients present with a nontoxic dysenteric syndrome (a 'walking dysentery') and generalized symptoms are less prominent than in *Shigella* dysentery. The onset is usually gradual; 85% of patients develop intense abdominal pain (see Table 116-1).[21,22] Initial loose watery stools

rapidly become bloodstained and mucoid. Tenesmus associated with rectosigmoidal involvement occurs in 50% of patients. Invasive amebic colitis is an emergency that may progress to life-threatening fulminant colitis with perforation and development of amebic peritonitis. The risk of progression is influenced by nutritional factors, age and susceptibility, and, probably, inter-strain differences in virulence. Ulceration and necrosis can lead to multiple perforations and give rise to purulent peritonitis. In a series of 62 patients with fulminant amebic colitis seen by Guarner[21] from 1963 to 1970, 57.5% showed a single perforation, 28% multiple perforations and none was found in 14.5%.

Ameboma is an abnormal response, probably to prolonged infection and manifesting as a marked granuloma, mimicking colon carcinoma, except in its rapid response to metronidazole.

AMEBIC LIVER ABSCESS

Liver abscess is the most common extraintestinal form of amebiasis. It can occur in all age groups, but is 10 times more frequent in adults, with three to five times as many cases seen in men.[22] Lesions are usually single and localized to the right lobe of the liver in the posterior, external and superior portions.[21]

Amebae probably spread from the intestine to the liver through the portal circulation. While liver abscess develops after intestinal infection, patients rarely have associated amebic rectocolitis although the large intestine is colonized with *E. histolytica* in more than 70% of cases.

In most patients, particularly those under 30 years of age and children,[22] the clinical presentation and course of disease are typical (Table 116-2). The onset is abrupt, with pain in the upper abdomen and high fever. The pain is intense and constant, radiating to the scapular region and right shoulder; it increases with coughing, deep breathing or when the patient rests on the right side. When the abscess is located in the left lobe, the pain tends to be felt in the epigastrium and may radiate

TABLE 116-1	Clinical Features of Acute Amebic Colitis	
Clinical Feature		**Percentage of Cases**
Symptoms for:		
0–1 week		48
2–4 weeks		37
>4 weeks		15
Diarrhea		100
Dysentery		99
Abdominal pain		85
Lower back pain		66
Fever		38
Abdominal tenderness		83

From Adams E.B., McLeod I.N.: Invasive amebiasis. 1: Amebic dysentery and its complications. Medicine (Baltimore) 1977; 56:315-323.

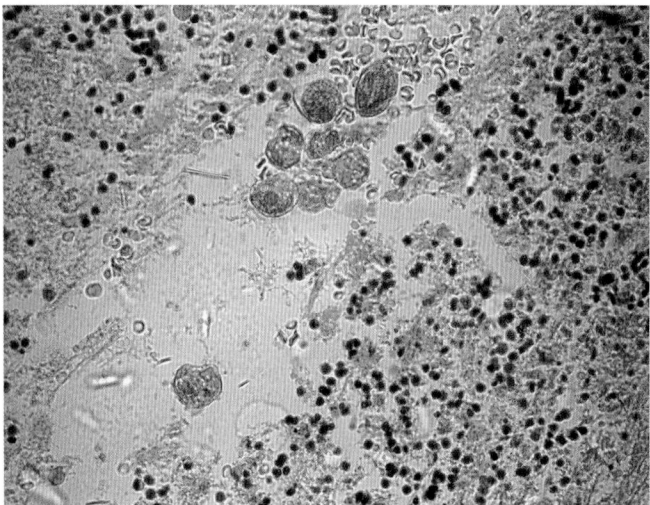

Figure 116-3 Liver abscess section stained with Ehrlich's hematoxylin and eosin. Many dark-stained nuclei of necrotic liver cells are seen around the liquid content of the abscess. A group of amebic trophozoites is seen adjacent to an area of bleeding.

TABLE 116-2	Clinical Features of Amebic Liver Abscess	
Clinical Feature		**Percentage of Cases**
Symptoms for:		
<2 weeks		37–66
2–4 weeks		20–40
4–12 weeks		16–42
>12 weeks		5–11
Fever		71–98
Abdominal pain		62–98
Diarrhea/dysentery		14–66
Cough		10–32
Weight loss		33–53
Tender liver		80–95
Hepatomegaly		43–93
Epigastric tenderness		22
Rales, rhonchi		8–47
Jaundice		10–25
White cell count >10 ×10⁹/L		63–94
Elevated transaminases		26–50
Elevated alkaline phosphatase		38–84
Elevated bilirubin		10–25
Increased erythrocyte sedimentation rate		81

Based on Martínez-Palomo A. and Ruíz-Palacios G.: Amebiasis. In: Mahmoud A.A.F., Warren K.E., ed. Tropical and geographical medicine. New York: McGraw–Hill; 1989:327-344.

to the left shoulder. Fever is present in most cases; it varies between 38°C and 40°C (100–104°F), frequently in spikes, but is sometimes constant over several days, with rigors and profuse sweating. There is anorexia and rapid weight loss; one-third of patients have nonproductive cough. Nausea and vomiting may occur and in some cases there may be diarrhea or dysentery. Physical examination reveals a pale wasted patient with tender hepatomegaly. Digital pressure in the right lower intercostal spaces produces intense pain and there is often marked tenderness on percussion over the right lower ribs in the posterior region. Movement of the right side of the chest and diaphragm is greatly restricted, as is the intensity of respiratory sounds. Older patients may present with a chronic and milder nonspecific febrile illness, hepatomegaly, anemia and abnormal liver function tests.[22]

Complications

Amebic liver abscesses commonly produce thoracic complications, particularly pleurisy with a nonpurulent pleural effusion, rupture into the bronchial tree and, less commonly, rupture into the pleural cavity or amebic pericarditis. Rupture into the abdomen occurs in approximately 8% of patients; only rarely do abscesses rupture into the gallbladder, stomach, duodenum, colon or inferior vena cava. Occasionally, an abscess may erode through the abdominal wall and reach the skin. Secondary infection of amebic abscesses is an uncommon complication, which should be suspected when the patient presents with a severe toxic state and fails to respond to anti-amebic chemotherapy.[21]

Diagnosis

AMEBIC COLITIS

Although diarrhea alone may be the presenting feature, amebic colitis, like shigellosis, classically presents with bloody diarrhea or dysentery. The infection needs to be differentiated from carcinoma, necrotizing colitis, cytomegalovirus colitis (in acquired immunodeficiency syndrome), antibiotic-associated colitis and inflammatory bowel disease (misdiagnosis and corticosteroid treatment can be fatal here). Definitive diagnosis depends upon laboratory tests. Detection of specific antibody (IgG) in serologic tests is extremely valuable for confirming invasive amebic disease.

In classic fecal microscopy, nonpathogenic *Entamoeba* spp. such as *E. coli*, *E. hartmanni*, *E. polecki*-like amebae (including *E. chattoni*[23]) and also *Iodamoeba butschlii* and *Endolimax nana* can be distinguished from *E. histolytica*, *E. dispar* and *E. moshkovskii* by the size of cysts, nuclear number and/or nature of inclusions. Cysts of the last three species are all quadrinucleate and average 12 μm in diameter (10–20 μm). Morphology of the trophozoite is usable, since to find amebae that have ingested erythrocytes in fresh samples of mucoid or bloody mucoid stools, or in a rectal scrape/rectosigmoidoscopy sample from suspected amebic colitis (Figure 116-4) is diagnostically highly predictive of *E. histolytica* infection.[24] However, the laboratory worker must be sufficiently skilled – a potential pitfall is distinguishing erythrophagocytosis in human leukocytes with densely staining polymorphic or monocytic nuclei from the generally larger, vacuolated and motile amebic trophozoites, which have difficult-to-detect poorly staining nuclei. When recognizable amebic trophozoites without ingested red blood cells are seen well away from bleeding areas, in advance of the main inflammatory response, it can also be strongly suggestive of invasive disease (Figures 116-5 and 116-6). The nonmicroscopic molecular biologic technique of nested polymerase chain reaction (PCR) and the simpler, but still expensive, technique of specific *E. histolytica* antigen detection, which can both be carried out on stool samples, are recommended[25] in preference to microscopy. Buss et al.[26] found that the TechLab® *E. histolytica* II antigen-detection test based on Eh-adherence lectin detected *E. histolytica* infections more accurately than another similarly based test. Antigen detection test kits are unfortunately not as sensitive as PCR.

AMEBIC LIVER ABSCESS

Amebic liver abscess is usually accompanied by right hypochondrial pain and tender liver. The diaphragm is often raised on chest

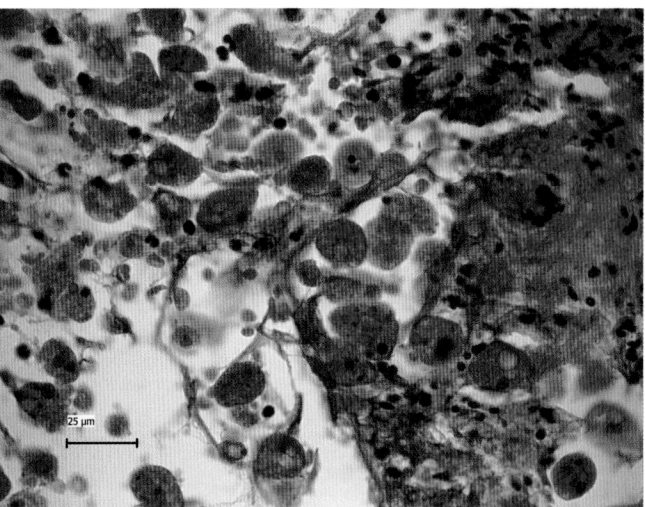

Figure 116-4 Section through bleeding colonic ulcer showing *E. histolytica* trophozoites with ingested red blood cells in human colonic submucosa and undermined mucosa. Leukocytes from the cellular reaction are visible, and they show typically strongly stained nuclei and sparse cytoplasm. The technique is Ehrlich's alum hematoxylin with eosin, which stains erythrocytes well but does not clearly show the amebic nuclei. *(Courtesy of John Williams, LSHTM.)*

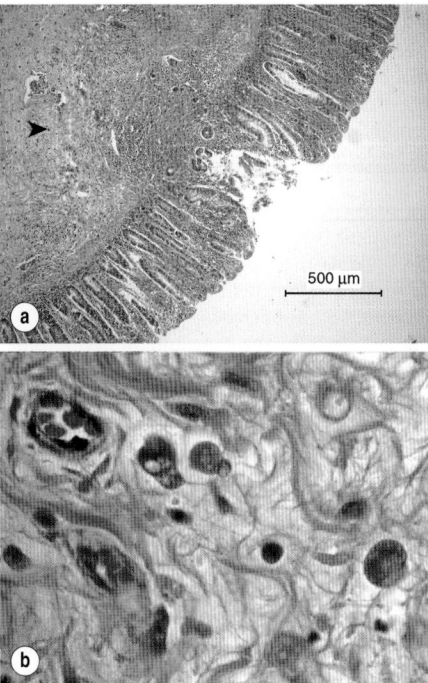

Figure 116-5 (a) Small mucosal ulcer, with early submucosal spread. Deep in the submucosa, all we see suggestive of a cellular response is in lymphatic vessels, near the blue arrow that shows the position of the advancing front of invading amebae. In the detail of this area (b) no leakage of blood or obvious damage to tissues has taken place, and the amebae have ingested no red blood cells. The technique is Ehrlich's alum hematoxylin with eosin, which stains erythrocytes well but does not clearly show the amebic nuclei. *(Courtesy of John Williams, LSHTM.)*

radiograph. A neutrophil leukocytosis (>10 x10^9/L) and a raised alkaline phosphatase may be detected (see Table 116-2). There is usually a space-occupying lesion in the liver on ultrasound and computed tomography (CT) scan. If an aspirate is done, amebic trophozoites may be detected microscopically, by antigen detection or by PCR, in the atypical 'pus' (mainly necrotic liver parenchyma with few neutrophils or macrophages). Serology for anti-amebic antibody, which is elevated in more than 90% of cases, is very helpful.[22]

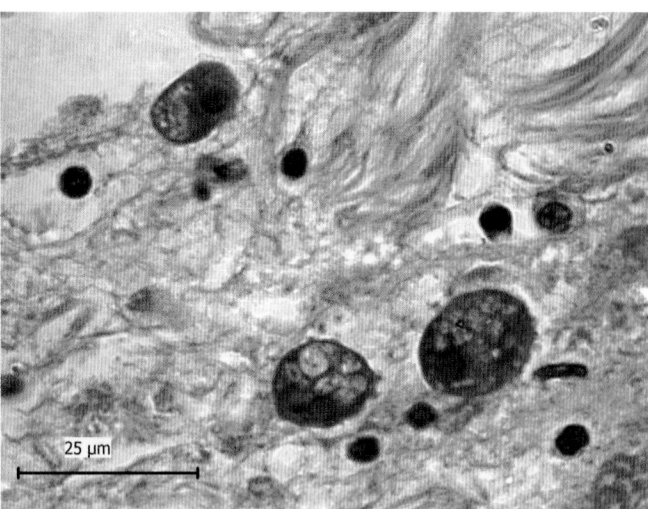

Figure 116-6 *E. histolytica* trophozoites in human colonic submucosa. A few leukocytes from the cellular reaction, with heavily stained nuclei and sparse cytoplasm, are visible. Weigert's iron hematoxylin and eosin highlights the dark staining of a chromatin ring just inside the nuclear membrane in each ameba. The abundant cytoplasm contains vacuoles with host-cell material in the process of digestion. *(Courtesy of John Williams, LSHTM.)*

DIFFERENTIAL DIAGNOSIS

Pyogenic abscess and neoplasm of the liver are the most important alternative diagnoses. Pyogenic abscess is more common in older patients with a previous history of hepatobiliary or abdominal disease. The presenting features may be jaundice, pruritus and septic shock, with no hepatomegaly or elevated diaphragm in the chest radiograph, while amebic serology is negative. Needle aspiration allows microscopy and culture in such circumstances.

Where the patient is febrile and wasted and has vague abdominal discomfort, liver neoplasm is suspected. CT imaging and tests for tumor markers such as alpha-fetoprotein and carcinoembryonic antigen will delineate the cause.[14] Stool microscopy, antigen testing or PCR should be carried out, to search for the concomitant asymptomatic intestinal ameba infection commonly found in amebic liver abscess cases.

Management

Because they are efficiently absorbed from the small intestine and reach high concentrations in the tissues, metronidazole and related 5-nitroimidazole compounds are the drugs of choice for treatment of invasive amebiasis. They are termed 'tissue amebicides'. Concentrations in the large intestinal content do not reach amebicidal levels, and only those trophozoites invading the mucosa and deeper tissues are affected. Since they do not prevent the production of infective cysts in the lumen, the tissue amebicides are often reported to be 'inactive against the cysts'. Actually, none of the available amebicides is active against the cysts themselves. The 5-nitroimidazoles have few negative features: adverse interactions are seen with alcohol (also warfarin and phenytoin) and they are known to be mutagenic against bacteria in the Ames test. Although cancer has been reported in mouse testing, no carcinogenic effects have been reported in humans. Although their effect on fetal development is unknown, it is recommended that, because of their ability to cross the placental barrier and rapidly enter the fetal circulation, they should be avoided in the first trimester and prescribed under strict supervision during the second and third trimesters. Similarly, because of secretion in breast-milk, breast-feeding should be suspended if 5-nitroimidazoles are prescribed.

The tissue amebicides emetine hydrochloride and dehydroemetine (cardiovascular and gastrointestinal adverse effects), combined with chloroquine, are seldom used now except in resistance. Despite isolated reports of failure in the treatment of amebic liver abscess with metronidazole, and even though *in vitro* studies confirm that some established and long-cultivated isolates of the organism are indeed metronidazole-resistant,[27] clinical metronidazole resistance is vanishingly rare.

USE OF LUMINAL AMEBICIDES AFTER TREATMENT WITH TISSUE AMEBICIDES

Since 5-nitroimidazole tissue amebicides are ineffective against the trophozoites in the colonic lumen, complete treatment for both intestinal and extraintestinal infection with *E. histolytica* should be followed by a course of a luminal amebicide for elimination of infection. Two alternatives are available[21] (see above): diloxanide furoate (if available) in adults, 500 mg orally q8h for 10 days, or paromomycin 25–35 mg/kg orally q8h for 7–10 days. Both these agents are poorly absorbed from the intestine and so reach optimal amebicidal concentrations within the intestinal lumen, without troublesome side effects. Paromomycin is the usual choice, as the availability of diloxanide is patchy. These have also been recommended for the treatment of asymptomatic infections in food handlers and when infection control measures are being applied within families and close associates of infected persons.

FULMINANT AMEBIC COLITIS

Guarner[21] reports on a series of 47 patients with known or suspected perforation who had surgical treatment. Of 20 who received conservative surgery (i.e. without removal of part of the colon), 16 (80%) died (7 had colostomy, 6 ileostomy, 1 exteriorization of the affected segments, 5 suture of a single perforation and 1 surgical drainage). Where the treatment included resection (i.e. removal of a damaged part or whole of the colon), mortality was 56%. Guarner stresses the importance of making an adequate evaluation of the magnitude of the colonic lesions, as well as the possibility of liver lesions: 'Surgery should be immediate and radical.' When the right colon is involved, right colectomy is indicated; when both sides are involved, total colectomy is indicated. In a total colectomy, ileostomy and suprapubic exteriorization of the rectal segment ought to be performed. Primary anastomosis is not advised; it is better to exteriorize. The patients should always be nursed in intensive care to allow maintenance of vascular tone and osmotic pressure, and to avoid respiratory problems. Antibacterial and anti-amebic therapy should be instituted at an early preoperative stage, using a broad-spectrum antibiotic and 500 mg metronidazole intravenously q8h with intravenous fluid replacement.

Further advice on amebic peritonitis supporting the above surgical approach is given by Cook,[28] who refers to case reviews by Shukla et al.[29] Gastric suction is recommended. Overall mortality may be over 50%, but resection of the necrotic area with exteriorization of both cut ends of the bowel allowed survival in six of nine cases.

AMEBOMA

An ameboma is an amebic granuloma that often localizes in the ascending colon. Guarner[21] recommends a cautious attitude to surgical intervention. In his series of 71 cases, 42 treated medically and 29 surgically, all of those medically treated were cured by chemotherapy, whereas there was 17% mortality in the surgical group. However, there may have been differences in severity between treatment groups.

AMEBIC LIVER ABSCESS

Amebic liver abscess should be treated with chemotherapy; surgery is rarely indicated. A marked reduction in amebic liver abscess mortality followed the introduction of metronidazole and reduction in surgical intervention.[21,30] Unlike in pyogenic abscesses, drainage of 'pus' is not generally recommended. Only 2% of amebic liver abscesses are reported to be contaminated with bacteria, and surgical intervention itself can be responsible. However, aspiration of the abscess may be necessary where it is more than 10 cm in diameter and also when in the left liver lobe. Percutaneous drainage is usually sufficient and safer than the open surgical approach. Surgery should be reserved for patients with ruptured abscesses, with bacterial superinfection or with abscesses that cannot be reached safely by the percutaneous route. Amebic liver abscesses are usually accompanied by asymptomatic intestinal infection and elimination of intestinal carriage using luminal amebicides should be undertaken to prevent recurrence and to protect close associates of the patient from infection.

Percutaneous Drainage

Indications for percutaneous drainage[21] of an amebic liver abscess are:

- imminent rupture of a large abscess
- as a complementary therapy to shorten the course of the disease when the response to chemotherapy has been slow
- when pyogenic or mixed infection is suspected (e.g. persisting fever on treatment).

Drainage should be carried out under ultrasound or CT guidance. Catheters should *not* be left in for drainage and should be rapidly removed to avoid contaminating the track and skin.

Surgical Drainage

Indications for surgical drainage[21] include:

- imminent rupture of an inaccessible liver abscess, especially of the left lobe
- a risk of peritoneal leakage of necrotic fluid after aspiration
- rupture of a liver abscess.

When surgical drainage is indicated in left lobe disease, with the patient lying supine, a 5–10 cm incision on the midline will isolate the drainage point. The study of Guarner[21] should be consulted in cases of pleuropulmonary involvement, amebic pericarditis or cerebral amebiasis.[21]

Conclusion

In summary, prompt diagnosis and treatment will control most cases of amebic liver abscess. In general, a full clinical recovery and disappearance of the liver lesions (confirmed by CT scanning) can be expected for uncomplicated cases. In 85% of cases liver reveals resolution of abscesses within 6 months of treatment; the remaining 15% still show imaging defects 3 years after treatment.[21]

References available online at expertconsult.com.

KEY REFERENCES

Ali I.K., Clark C.G., Petri W.A.: Molecular epidemiology of amebiasis. *Infect Genet Evol* 2008; 8:698-707.

Blessmann J., Binh H.D., Hung D.M., et al.: Treatment of amoebic liver abscess with metronidazole alone or in combination with ultrasound-guided needle aspiration: a comparative, prospective and randomized study. *Trop Med Int Health* 2003; 8:1030-1034.

Clark C.G., Diamond L.S.: The Laredo strain and other 'Entamoeba histolytica-like' amoebae are *Entamoeba moshkovskii*. *Mol Biochem Parasitol* 1991; 46:11-18.

Cook G.C.: Tropical gastroenterological problems. In: Cook G.C., Zumla A.I., eds. *Manson's tropical diseases*, 21st ed. Philadelphia: Saunders; 2003:132-133.

Diamond L.S., Clark C.G.: A redescription of *Entamoeba histolytica* Schaudinn, 1903 (emended Walker, 1911) separating it from *Entamoeba dispar* Brumpt, 1925. *J Eukaryot Microbiol* 1993; 40:340-344.

González-Ruiz A., Haque R., Aguirre A., et al.: Value of microscopy in the diagnosis of dysentery associated with invasive *Entamoeba histolytica*. *J Clin Pathol* 1994; 47:236-239.

Guarner V.: Treatment of amebiasis. In: Martínez-Palomo A., ed. *Amebiasis: human parasitic diseases*. Amsterdam: Elsevier Science; 1986:189-212.

Jackson T.F.H.G., Gathiram V., Simjee A.E.: Seroepidemiological study of antibody responses to the zymodemes of *Entamoeba histolytica*. *Lancet* 1985; 30:716-719.

Martínez-Palomo A., Ruíz-Palacios G.: Amebiasis. In: Mahmoud A.A.F., Warren K.E., eds. *Tropical and geographical medicine*. New York: McGraw-Hill; 1989: 327-344.

Ralston K.S., Solga M.D., Mackey-Lawrence N.M., et al.: Trogocytosis by *Entamoeba histolytica* contributes to cell-killing and tissue invasion. *Nature* 2014; 508(7497): 526-530.

Sepúlveda B., Treviño-García Manzo N.: Clinical manifestations and diagnosis of amebiasis. In: Martínez-Palomo A., ed. *Amebiasis: human parasitic diseases*. Amsterdam: Elsevier Science; 1986:169-188.

Shimokawa C., Kabir M., Taniuchi M., et al.: *Entamoeba moshkovskii* is associated with diarrhea in infants and causes diarrhea and colitis in mice. *J Inf Dis* 2012; 206:744-751.

Warhurst D.C.: *Entamoeba histolytica* and amebiasis. In: Feachem R.G., Bradley D.J., Garelick H., et al., eds. *Sanitation and disease: health aspects of excreta and wastewater management. World Bank Studies in Water Supply and Sanitation 3*. Chichester: Wiley; 1983: 337-347.

117

Malaria

ARJEN M. DONDORP | LORENZ VON SEIDLEIN

KEY CONCEPTS

- In terms of disease burden, malaria is the most damaging parasitic disease afflicting mankind.

- Malaria has been eliminated from many regions, including North America and Europe. Over the last decade much progress has been made to control malaria in hot tropical regions of Africa and Asia. Implementation of effective antimalarial treatment and wide deployment of insecticide-treated bed nets have contributed to this success.

- Of the five known *Plasmodium* species causing malaria in humans, *P. falciparum* is the most pathogenic, responsible for most malaria-related mortality worldwide. In contrast, *P. vivax* is the more sophisticated organism, which goes into a sleeper (hypnozoic) stage in the liver where it can be eliminated only with 8-aminoquinolines. These latent *vivax* forms are the most plausible explanation for delays in vivax malaria control compared to the more successful control of falciparum malaria.

- A critical breakthrough in the management and control of uncomplicated malaria has been the introduction of artemisinin combination therapy (ACT). ACT is now available in all malaria-endemic regions and has revolutionized the oral treatment of malaria.

- Two large clinical trials have demonstrated that parenteral artesunate is the optimal therapy for severe malaria that cannot be treated with oral drugs.

- The emergence of artemisinin and ACT partner drug resistance in *P. falciparum* is the single biggest threat to hopes to control, eliminate or even eradicate malaria.

- Decades of malaria vaccine development have yet to result in a licensed, highly protective, long-lasting vaccine candidate.

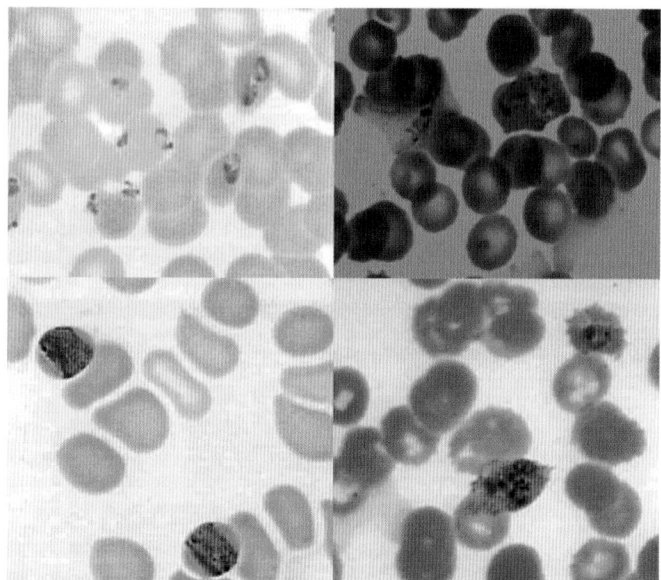

Figure 117-1 Asexual stages of (clockwise, starting left upper corner) *Plasmodium falciparum*, *P. vivax*, *P. ovale* and *P. malariae*. (Courtesy of Dr Kesinee Chotivanich.)

Introduction

Malaria is a parasitic disease caused by the coccidian protozoa of the genus *Plasmodium*, and transmitted by *Anopheles* spp. Human malaria can be caused by the four *Plasmodium* species: *P. falciparum*, *P. ovale*, *P. vivax* and *P. malariae* (Figure 117-1). In addition, clusters of malaria caused by *P. knowlesi* jumping species from long-tailed macaque monkeys to man are common in some forested regions in South East Asia.[1] The life cycle of the parasite is summarized in Figure 117-2. Although it is increasingly recognized that *P. vivax* is able to cause severe disease in humans, including severe anemia, pulmonary edema, hemoglobinuria and rarely coma,[2] the majority of severe disease is caused by *P. falciparum*. Malaria is transmitted in 108 countries (Figure 117-3) inhabited by roughly 3 billion people, and, in 2012, caused an estimated 207 million cases and 627 000 deaths (range 473 000–789 000).[3] The majority (>80%) of these casualties are children in sub-Saharan Africa, where transmission intensity is high. The total burden of malaria disease, however, is similar in Asia, where transmission is low, but the population size much larger.

Epidemiology

GEOGRAPHIC DISTRIBUTION

Malaria control efforts during the last century eliminated malaria from North America, Europe and Russia, but it has remained a major

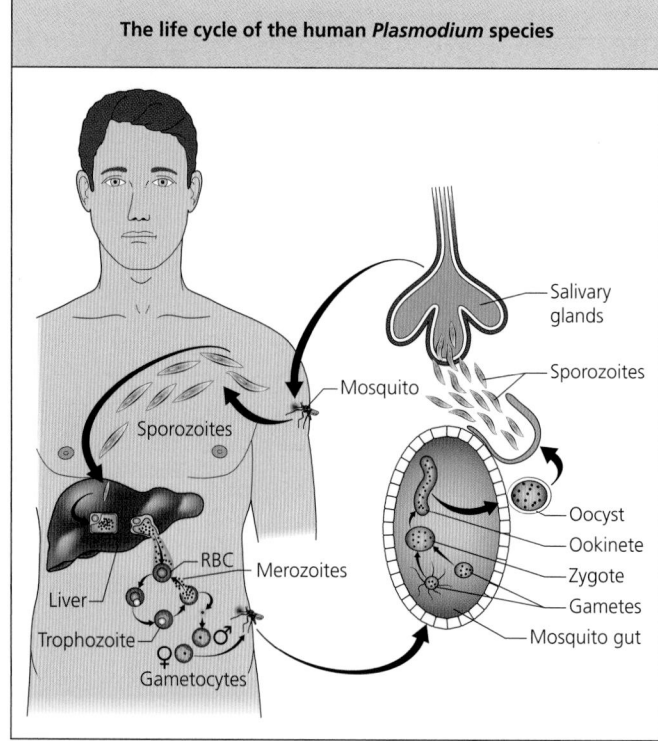

Figure 117-2 The life cycle of the human *Plasmodium* species. (Adapted from White NJ. Antimalarial drug resistance. J Clin Invest 2004;113:1084–92.)

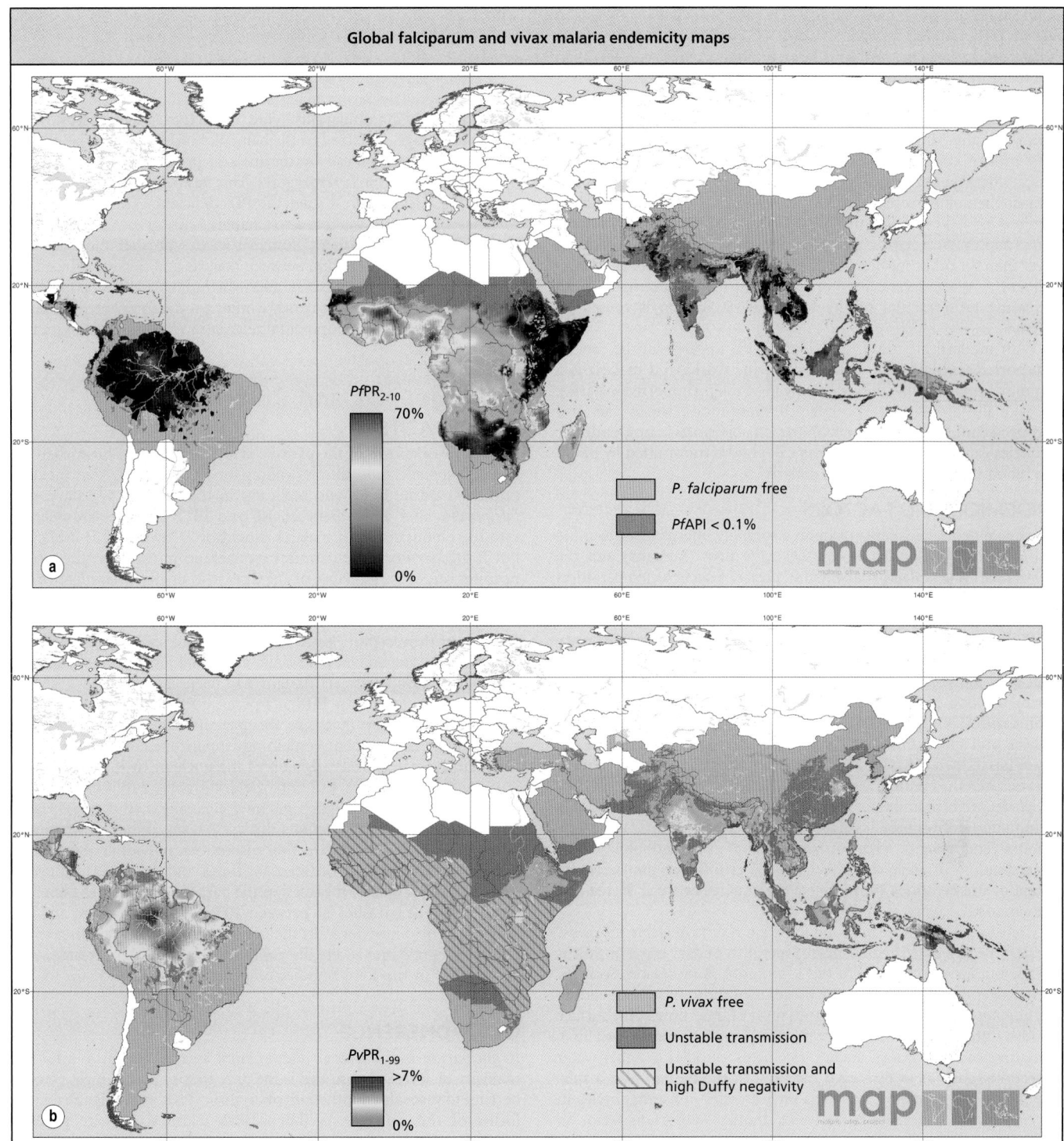

Figure 117-3   Global falciparum and vivax malaria endemicity maps. (a) Endemicity data were compiled using both prevalence data and climatologic information. The spatial distribution of *P. falciparum* malaria prevalence rates, age standardized to 2–10 years (*Pf*PR$_{2-10}$) are categorized low (blue) to high prevalence (red). The rest of the land area was defined as unstable risk (medium gray areas, where *Pf*API <0.1 per 1000 pa) or no risk (light gray). (b) The spatial distribution of *P. vivax* malaria prevalence rates, age standardized from 1–99 year, from low (blue) to higher prevalence (red). The rest of the land area was defined as no risk (light grey) or low, unstable risk (dark grey). Areas with a high proportion of Duffy-negative individuals (a blood group receptor needed for *P. vivax* invasion) are striped. (*From Hay SI, et al. PLoS Med 2009;6(3):e1000048.*)

problem throughout the tropics. At the end of the 20th century, child-hood mortality caused by malaria was on the increase. However, at the beginning of this millennium a surge in efforts towards malaria control, including the wide distribution of impregnated bed nets and the deployment of effective treatment with artemisinin-based combi-nation therapy, has reduced malaria-attributable mortality by 45% globally and by 49% in Africa.[3]

Geographic information systems help to estimate the malaria burden and distribution from a combination of case-incidence data and parasite prevalence, using plausible biologic constraints for malaria transmission by the *Anopheles* vector based on temperature data, and information on vegetation and population[4] (Figure 117-3). In large parts of sub-Saharan Africa transmission is moderate to high, with falciparum malaria prevalence rates above 50%, and the number of infectious mosquito bites (expressed as the entomologic inoculation rate or EIR) ranging between 10 and 1000 per year. Outside Africa, falciparum malaria prevalence is largely hypoendemic, with less than 10% parasite rates, corresponding to an EIR of <1 per year.

In Asia *P. vivax* is responsible for approximately half of the malaria burden, and is also common in Central and South America, North Africa and the Middle East (Figure 117-3). Mixed infection with *P. falciparum* is common in South East Asia. *P. vivax* is rare in West Africa, where the majority of people lack the erythrocyte surface Duffy-antigen/chemokine receptor (Duffy blood group negative), which is required for red cell invasion. The prevalence of malaria caused by *P. ovale* (mainly West Africa and Asia) and *P. malariae* is always much lower than the other species. Mixed infection with *P. falciparum* occurs frequently. With decreasing prevalence of falciparum malaria an increasing ratio/fraction of the total malaria burden is caused by *P. vivax*.

With modern air travel, individuals with malaria can be rapidly transported within hours to any part of the world, and malaria is a common imported infection occurring in travelers (imported malaria). Occasionally airplanes carry infected mosquitoes, which can give unexpected infections in the neighborhood of airports in non-endemic countries (airport malaria). Malaria can also be transmitted by blood and blood products (transfusion malaria).

EPIDEMIOLOGIC FACTORS

Malaria epidemiology depends upon a complex interplay between the vector (female *Anopheles* mosquitoes), the host (humans) and the malaria parasite. Malaria transmission does not occur at temperatures below 16°C (61°F) or above 33°C (91°F) ambient temperature, and at altitudes of 2000 m above sea level, because sporogony (the development of the sporozoite in the mosquito) cannot take place. Longevity of the vector, which is climate-dependent, has to be at least a week, since after the sexual forms of the parasite (gametocytes) are engulfed during a blood meal, sporogony takes 6–12 days (shorter at higher temperatures). Of the >400 species of *Anopheles*, only 80 can transmit malaria, and approximately 45 are considered important vectors. Each vector has its own behavior and blood-feeding patterns, although most bites occur in the evening, at night or in the early morning. For example *Anopheles gambiae*, an important malaria vector in Africa, feeds mainly on humans (anthropophilic), bites mainly after 23:00 hours and mostly indoors (endophagic) where it also tends to rest (endophilic). The understanding of such vector behavior is critical for the successful design of interventions to minimize the contact between vector and human host.

Constant, frequent, year-round infection is termed stable transmission. In the sub-Sahel region from Senegal to Sudan, transmission is intense but largely confined to the 3–4-month rainy season. Seasonal rainfall dramatically increases the breeding of mosquitoes. Depending on the *Anopheles* species, larvae spend most of their time at the surface of fresh water and brackish water marshes (mal-aria means 'bad air'), mangrove swamps, grassy ditches, rice fields, puddles or other water collections, such as in discarded car tires. In the human host a subpopulation of gametocytes appears after a series of asexual cycles in *P. falciparum*, but earlier in *P. vivax*, another important factor in malaria transmission. Gametocyte density is higher in patients with high parasite densities, in nonimmune individuals (children) and with the use of an antimalarial drug to which the parasite is resistant.

Certain genetic hemoglobinopathies protect against the development of severe falciparum malaria. This has led to a state of 'balanced polymorphism' in populations living in malaria-endemic areas, where the disadvantage conferred by the hemoglobinopathy, especially in the homozygotes, is balanced by the malaria protective effect, which is mainly evident in the heterozygotes. This has been most convincingly shown for sickle cell disease, G6PD deficiency, thalassemia and Melanesian ovalocytosis (see also Chapter 122).

Where malaria prospers, human societies prosper the least, and there is a striking correlation between malaria and poverty. The effects of malaria are felt on diverse areas, including fertility, population growth, savings and investments, worker productivity, medical costs, absenteeism, subtle developmental retardation in children and premature mortality.

Pathogenesis and Pathology

THE PARASITE

The sporozoite form of the parasite is injected into the host when the female *Anopheles* mosquito is probing for a blood meal. After inoculation the parasite hides and replicates in the liver for 5–7 days in *P. falciparum*, after which between 10^5 and 10^6 merozoites are released into the bloodstream. In malaria caused by *P. vivax* and *P. ovale*, but not *P. falciparum*, some parasites stay behind in the liver; these hypnozoites can cause a relapse of the disease long after treatment of the blood stage infection. The merozoites quickly invade circulating erythrocytes, where the erythrocytic cycle of the parasite begins. For *P. falciparum*, the receptors involved in merozoite invasion can be divided regarding the dependency on sialic acid residues (on glycophorins). The blood group antigen Basigin has been identified as a strain-independent receptor for PfRh5, a parasite ligand essential for blood stage growth.[5] After invasion, the parasite matures from a small ring form to the pigment-containing trophozoite, and develops into the mature schizont after division of the nucleus. In *P. falciparum*, *P. vivax* and *P. ovale* after 48 hours the erythrocyte ruptures and 6–36 merozoites are released, which will invade passing erythrocytes (Figure 117-4). In *P. knowlesi* infections this cycle takes 24 hours, whereas it takes 72 hours in *P. malariae*. In a susceptible individual, the parasite population expands by between six times and 20 times per cycle.[6] About 12–13 days after inoculation the parasite number has increased from about 10 parasites to between 10^8 and 10^{10} parasites, and the patient starts to have fever. In the nonimmune patient the disease can quickly progress into severe disease if the infection is not treated, with an increase in the total number of parasites in the body up to 10^{12} to 10^{13}.[7]

CYTOADHERENCE

P. falciparum is the human *Plasmodium* species responsible for the majority of severe disease and is the only species that induces cytoadherence to vascular endothelium of erythrocytes containing the mature forms of the parasite. As the parasite matures, parasite proteins are transported and inserted into the erythrocyte membrane. The

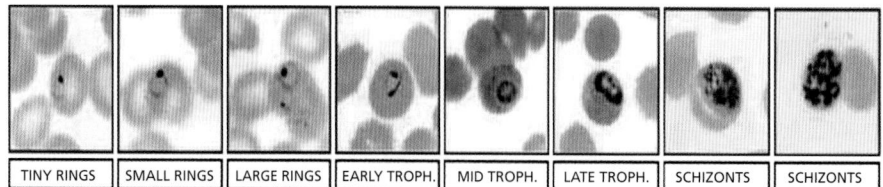

| TINY RINGS | SMALL RINGS | LARGE RINGS | EARLY TROPH. | MID TROPH. | LATE TROPH. | SCHIZONTS | SCHIZONTS |

Figure 117-4 Developmental stages of *Plasmodium falciparum* during the 48-hour asexual life cycle. Mature stages; trophozoites (troph.) and schizonts efficiently adhere to the endothelial lining in the microcirculation, so that these stages are rarely seen in the peripheral blood. If present in the peripheral blood, this denotes a large parasite biomass, associated with severe disease. (*Courtesy of Dr Kamolrat Silamut.*)

high molecular transmembrane protein *P. falciparum* erythrocyte membrane protein 1, or *Pf*EMP1, is the most important ligand for cytoadherence.[8]

Cytoadhesion begins at approximately 12 hours of parasite development, 50% of the maximum effect is obtained at 14–16 hours, and adherence is highly effective in the second half of the parasite life cycle.[9] As a result, late stages of *P. falciparum* (schizonts) are only rarely detected in peripheral blood, and when they do appear in significant numbers (>20% of the total parasites) this is a poor prognostic sign, representing a large sequestered parasite load.[10] In contrast, *P. vivax* schizonts can be frequently detected in peripheral blood slides consistent with minimal sequestration of this species.

*Pf*EMP1 is encoded by the highly variable *VAR* gene family, comprising around 60 genes. The high switch rate between these genes gives rise to a new variant *Pf*EMP1 in 2% of the parasites every new cycle, and this clonal antigenic variation helps the parasite escape the immune system.[11] *Pf*EMP1 is expressed on the surface of 'knobs', which can be identified by electron microscopy as protrusions from the erythrocyte membrane acting as points of attachment to the vascular endothelium. Other surface proteins that might play a role in cytoadherence are sequestrin, rifin and surfin. On the vascular endothelium numerous receptors that can bind *Pf*EMP1 have been identified, with different distributions in various organs and different contributions to rolling, tethering and finally stable binding of the parasitized erythrocyte. Of these, only CD36, which is constitutionally expressed on most vascular beds but remarkably absent in brain vessels, and chondroitin sulfate A (CSA), the main receptor in the placenta, are able to support firm adhesion under flow conditions.[11] The intercellular adhesion molecule 1 (ICAM-1) is the most important receptor on brain endothelium, and its expression is upregulated by the proinflammatory cytokine tumor necrosis factor (TNF).

In addition to the cytoadherence of red blood cells containing more mature parasites to endothelium, they can also stick to uninfected red blood cells (rosetting), or through platelets to other parasitized red cells (auto-agglutination). The resulting clumps of erythrocytes are thought to contribute further to defects of microvascular perfusion.

PERMEABILITY AND INTRACRANIAL PRESSURE

There is a mild generalized increase in systemic vascular permeability in severe malaria, but the blood–brain barrier (BBB) in adults with cerebral malaria is functionally grossly intact.[12] Studies in African children with cerebral malaria show an increase in BBB permeability with a disruption of endothelial intercellular tight junctions. Imaging studies reveal that most adults with cerebral malaria have no cerebral edema. A recent study conducted in children with severe malaria in Malawi found increased brain volume in children who died from cerebral malaria but was uncommon in those who did not die from the disease, a finding that suggests that raised intracranial pressure may contribute to a fatal outcome.[13] Similarly, opening pressures on lumbar puncture are usually normal in adult patients, but are elevated in over 80% of children with cerebral malaria.[14] However, the use of mannitol is not recommended in either pediatric or adult patients with cerebral malaria.[15,16] Raised intracranial pressure in children is more likely a feature developing in the later stages of cerebral malaria, rather than a primary cause for coma.

IMMUNOLOGIC FACTORS AND CYTOKINES

Despite the enormous intravascular antigenic load in malaria, with the formation and deposition of immune complexes and variable complement depletion, there is little evidence of a specific immunopathologic process in severe malaria. As in other severe infections, blood concentrations of proinflammatory cytokines like TNF, interleukin (IL)-1, interferon-gamma (IFN-γ), IL-6 and IL-18 are raised, as well as anti-inflammatory Th2 cytokines (IL-4, IL-10), but there is an imbalance in patients with a fatal course of the disease.[17]

A potent stimulator inducing proinflammatory cytokine production by leukocytes is the glycosylphosphatidylinositol (GPI) anchor of *P. falciparum*. GPI stimulates the production of TNF and possibly also the lymphokine 'lymphotoxin'. Both cytokines can upregulate the expression of ICAM-1 and vascular cell adhesion molecule 1 (VCAM-1) on endothelium cells, and could thus promote sequestration of parasitized erythrocytes in the brain, contributing to coma. High plasma concentrations of TNF in patients with falciparum malaria correlate with disease severity, including coma, hypoglycemia, hyperparasitemia and death. However, a trial using monoclonal antibodies against TNF did not show a beneficial effect on either mortality or coma duration, but was associated with a significant increase in neurologic sequelae.[18] Moreover, concentrations of TNF are also high in paroxysms of uncomplicated vivax malaria.

Further downstream in the cytokine cascade, nitric oxide (NO) production is increased via inducible NO synthase (iNOS), and iNOS expression is increased in the brain in fatal cerebral malaria. NO has been proposed as a cause for coma through interference with neurotransmission, but more recent studies have shown reduced levels of NO and its precursor, L-arginine, in severe malaria, related to endothelial dysfunction in these patients.[19]

Prevention and Malaria Control

Malaria prevention and control have currently three principal components:

- reduction of contact between vector and human host;
- prevention of disease through prophylactic or presumptive use of antimalarial drugs; and
- early diagnosis and adequate treatment (described below) of malaria episodes to minimize the risk for transmission.

MINIMIZING CONTACT BETWEEN VECTOR AND HUMAN HOST

The affluent traveler has a range of effective options to prevent mosquito bites, which include screened windows, air conditioning, protective clothing and insect repellents (topical, e.g. DEET, or spatial, e.g. insect coils). Few of these are permanently available to the majority of residents in malaria-endemic regions who depend on indoor residual insecticide spraying (IRS) and bed nets impregnated with insecticides (ITNs) to prevent mosquito bites. IRS can be highly effective against indoor resting (endophylic) *Anopheles* species, but sustaining high coverage has proven a challenge and IRS has therefore mixed popularity among malaria control experts.[20,21] Emergence and spread of mosquitoes resistant to insecticides (e.g. pyrethroids and dichlorodiphenyltrichloroethane [DDT]) is an increasing concern in sub-Saharan Africa.

A second approach to prevent mosquito bites is the use of insecticide-impregnated bed nets. A series of randomized trials has demonstrated the high effectiveness of ITNs,[22] and their wide-scale distribution has probably contributed importantly to a decrease in malaria transmission in many African countries. The effect on transmission is less in Asian countries, since the prevalent transmitting *Anopheles* vectors in these regions generally tend to bite outside sleeping hours.[23] Bed nets requiring regular dipping in insecticide solutions have been replaced by 'long-lasting insecticidal nets', which remain effective for years. Delivery of these nets through social marketing has been advocated, but free distribution of nets is probably needed to achieve impact in sub-Saharan Africa.[24] Today the large funding agencies are providing ITNs free of cost at an unprecedented scale. But just as for IRS, the emergence and spread of insecticide-resistant mosquitoes is a concern.

PREVENTION OF DISEASE THROUGH PROPHYLACTIC USE OF ANTIMALARIAL DRUGS

Travelers visiting malaria-endemic countries are frequently advised to take prophylactic antimalarial drugs. The choice of drug will depend on pharmacokinetic/dynamic properties, safety profiles and the prevailing drug resistance patterns in the area. Since these patterns change over time, the recommendations given below in Table 117-7 can serve only as a guideline. With decreasing risks to become infected some experts feel that stand-by medication for self-treatment when malaria is suspected or diagnosed is a more efficient and less costly approach.

For people living in malaria-endemic countries, targeted prophylactic use of antimalarial drugs has been popular as a measure for malaria control in the form of intermittent presumptive treatment (IPT). IPT has been mainly advocated for infants (IPTi) and pregnant women (IPTp) in sub-Saharan Africa. The experience of IPT is mostly based on use of sulfadoxine–pyrimethamine (S–P), which is increasingly losing its efficacy on the continent.[25] IPTp is still thought to be beneficial in regions with high malaria transmission. However, with the steady increase in S–P resistance there will be a need for an alternative drug regimen which is highly efficacious and which can be safely used throughout pregnancy. Recent trials have failed to identify a suitable replacement for S–P.[26,27]

IPTi has not found substantial uptake to date. Much malaria-related illness and death in Africa occurs in children aged under 5 years during 4 months of the rainy season. For this reason the World Health Organization has recommended the administration of monthly amodiaquine and S–P (maximum four doses) to all children aged 3–59 months in this region from the start of the yearly transmission season.[28] Seasonal malaria chemoprevention is effective when delivered through schools or to adults at high risk of malaria.[29]

VACCINE DEVELOPMENT

Despite the accepted need and great promises of a vaccine that can protect against malaria there is still no malaria vaccine licensed. *P. falciparum* is genetically complex and antigenic surface proteins are highly variable. Yet protective immunity can be obtained with age in populations residing in malaria-endemic areas. Immunoglobulin purified from the blood of immune adults from endemic regions can passively transfer protection against *P. falciparum*.[30] Cell-mediated immunity is thought to play an important role in the immunity against malaria but remains incompletely understood.

The vaccine candidate currently furthest in development is RTS,S, a recombinant protein pre-erythrocytic stage vaccine, based on *P. falciparum* circumsporozoite antigen combined with the ASO1E adjuvant. Large phase III trials show an adjusted vaccine efficacy of 53% (95% CI 28–69) against developing clinical malaria in children aged 5–17 months during a mean duration of 8 months follow-up, but trials in younger children showed lower protection[31] which puts into question the usefulness of administering RTS,S as part of existing childhood vaccination schemes. RTS,S was the first ever malaria vaccine to be licensed (2015). How the vaccine will be deployed and integrated with other malaria control measures is currently under discussion. There is ongoing research to combine the RTS,S antigen with other promising vaccine targets.

Alternative vaccine candidates include attenuated whole-parasite vaccines which are highly protective, but they are challenging to manufacture and to administer.[32] Cellular immunity is targeted by the prime–boost approach. Priming vectored vaccines trigger only modest responses focused on the recombinant antigen and the subsequent boosting vaccines trigger strong, nonspecific responses. This heterologous sequence of prime–boost vaccines produces strong immunologic responses to recombinant antigens. Other vaccine candidates target the blood stages of the parasite, and finally, the sexual stages of the parasite offer another target for vaccine development, which would prevent the transmission of malaria.

MALARIA ELIMINATION AND ERADICATION

After failed attempts during the 1950s and 1960s there is new enthusiasm for malaria elimination and ultimately eradication of malaria. The scaling up of the available control tools including ITNs and early diagnosis and treatment with highly effective malaria therapy would reduce and ultimately terminate malaria transmission as long as no resistant vectors and parasites emerge. Specifically the emergence of artemisinin-resistant and increasingly also partner drug resistant *P. falciparum* strains in South East Asia poses an important threat that could reverse the achievements made in malaria control since the beginning of the century and should be addressed with an immediate sense of urgency. The only reasonably promising strategy to stop the spread of resistant *P. falciparum* strains is the focal elimination of malaria in areas where resistance has been documented. Ideally the complete infected population in such areas should receive adequate treatment, including asymptomatic individuals not spontaneously seeking treatment. Novel molecular approaches can detect very low density infections and have demonstrated a large previously unknown reservoir of asymptomatic infections even in low-transmission settings, however cost and turnaround-time prevent the use of such diagnostics as public health tools. The development of rapid diagnostic tests for the detection of ultra-low HRP2 concentrations are under consideration. Presumptive treatment of populations with high sub-patent parasite prevalence might prove an essential tool for malaria elimination from those populations. Such presumptive drug administrations have an extensive record and have succeeded in terminating malaria transmission in some situations, but not in others.[33] The available drug regimens are still appropriate for such interventions but the participation of large populations and the reintroduction of parasites remain major challenges.

Clinical Features

The clinical manifestations of malaria are critically dependent on the immune status of the host. In areas of stable high transmission (sub-Saharan Africa) severe falciparum malaria occurs predominantly between 6 months and 3 years of age; mild symptoms are seen in older children and a state of partial immunity (or 'premunition') means that adults are usually asymptomatic. With transmission intensity decreasing in several African countries, the susceptible period for symptomatic disease will shift to a slightly older age. In low transmission areas, severe and symptomatic disease occurs at all ages, and will particularly affect young adults because of higher exposure of this age group, e.g. through forest work (Figure 117-5). Pregnant women are at increased risk of developing symptomatic and severe malaria in all endemic settings.

UNCOMPLICATED MALARIA

In most cases, the incubation period for falciparum and vivax malaria is around 2 weeks. The majority (>90%) of *P. falciparum* infections in travelers occur within 8 weeks of leaving an endemic area. Some *P. vivax* strains (var. *hibernans*) in a few areas of China and North and South Korea have extremely long incubation times (up to 9–12 months).

The clinical features of all four human malarias start nonspecifically and resemble influenza. Headache, muscular ache, vague abdominal discomfort, lethargy and dysphoria often precede the fever. Rising temperatures initially cause shivering, mild chills, worsening headaches, malaise and loss of appetite. If the infection is untreated, the fever in *P. vivax* and *P. ovale* regularizes to a 2-day cycle (tertian malaria; fever on the third day if the starting day is counted as number one) and *P. malaria* fever spikes occur every 3 days (quartan malaria; fever on the fourth day). The fever pattern in *P. falciparum* is more variable, since the infection tends to be less synchronized. Classic 'paroxysms' are therefore more common in tertian and quartan malaria, and consist of an abrupt steeply rising temperature to >39°C (102°F), with intense headache and highly uncomfortable 'cold chills' with peripheral vasoconstriction, and dramatic rigors with shaking limbs and teeth chatter. This is followed by a 'hot stage' during which the patient may have a temperature well over 40°C (104°F), with peripheral vasodilatation, often with restlessness and vomiting. During defervescence, the patient has profuse perspiration and feels exhausted, which can last for several days. As the infection continues, the spleen and liver enlarge and anemia develops. Mild abdominal discomfort is common in malaria. In routine clinical practice in malarious areas malaria is rarely the cause of lymphadenopathy, pharyngitis or a rash.

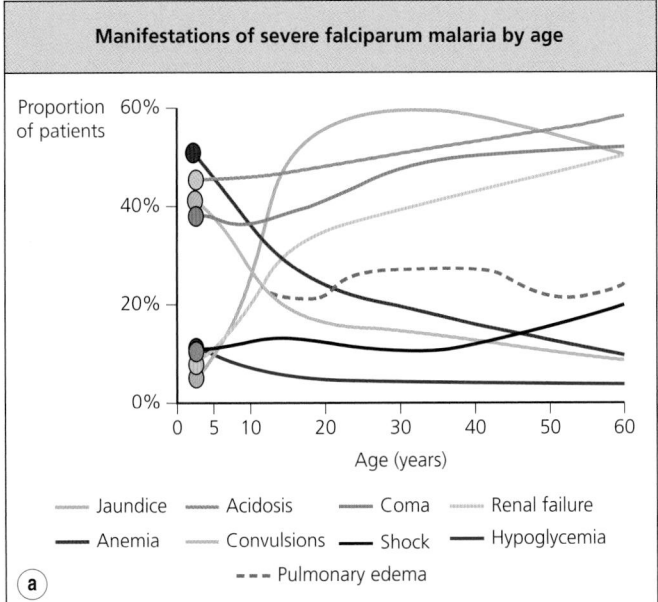

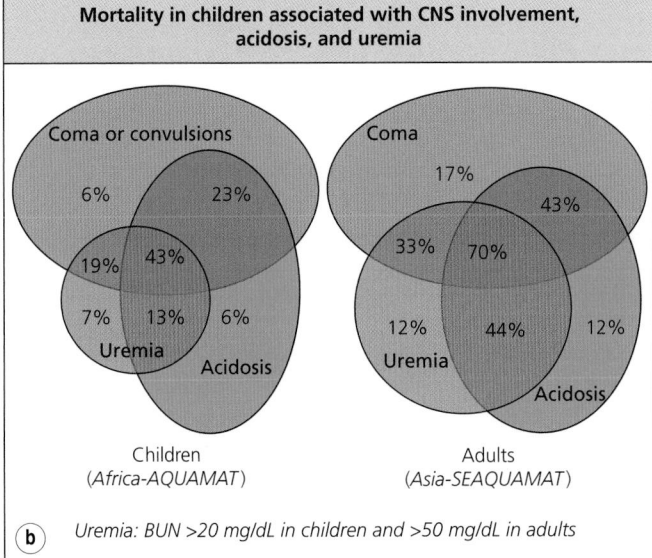

Figure 117-5 (a) Manifestations of severe falciparum malaria by age. (b) Mortality in children associated with CNS involvement, acidosis, and uremia. Data from 3228 prospectively studied African children with severe falciparum malaria.[34] Surface areas denote the relative prevalence of the different severity signs, which frequently coexist. The percentages denote the observed mortality associated with the presenting signs.

SEVERE MALARIA

The majority of severe malaria is caused by falciparum malaria in nonimmune individuals, although severe vivax malaria is increasingly recognized as a major health problem in some of the *P. vivax* endemic regions.[2] Severe malaria is a multisystem disease. In a minority of patients cerebral malaria is an isolated presentation; it is usually associated with other signs of severe disease. In areas of high transmission in sub-Saharan Africa severe malaria is mainly a pediatric disease. Important symptoms in children are severe anemia, hypoglycemia and coma with convulsions. In a very large randomized severe falciparum malaria trial in African children, base deficit, impaired consciousness, convulsions, elevated blood urea and underlying chronic illness were associated independently with death.[34] Manifestations of severe falciparum malaria by age and mortality in children associated with CNS involvement, acidosis and uremia are shown in Figure 117-5.

In low transmission areas such as South East Asia, young adults are generally the most affected group. Cerebral malaria, metabolic acidosis, renal failure, severe jaundice and acute respiratory distress syndrome (ARDS) are the most prominent complications in this group. Coma and acidosis have the strongest prognostic significance, whereas patients developing ARDS or renal failure have a high risk of dying (Figure 117-5). Definitions of the clinical manifestations of severe falciparum malaria are summarized in Table 117-1.

Cerebral Malaria

The clinical picture is that of a diffuse encephalopathy with unrousable coma; focal signs are relatively uncommon. In young children coma can develop rapidly, with a mean onset after only 2 days of fever. One or more generalized seizures, which cannot be distinguished clinically from febrile convulsions, often precede the coma. In adults the onset in usually more gradual, with high fever (mean duration of 5 days) and increasing drowsiness, but sometimes agitation. Convulsions are present in about 15% of the cases, whereas more than 50% of pediatric cases have convulsions. Convulsions are most frequently generalized, but in small children approximately 25% have subtle or subclinical convulsions, with seizure activity on electroencephalography, but only minor convulsive movements of limbs or facial muscles. These patients often have deviated eyes, excessive salivation and irregular breathing patterns. Signs of meningism are absent, although passive resistance to neck flexion is not uncommon. The eyes often show a divergent gaze. Grinding of the teeth (bruxism) and a positive pout reflex are common in cases with deep coma. Various forms of abnormal posturing can be present, with either a decorticate pattern with flexor rigidity of the arms and extension of the legs or a decerebrate pattern with abnormal extensor responses in arms and legs with or without opisthotonos.[35]

In areas of high transmission a high background prevalence of peripheral parasitemia can hamper the diagnosis of 'cerebral malaria'. A positive blood slide in a febrile comatose child in this setting does not exclude other possible diagnoses, and bacteremia can be present in up to 20% of these patients.[36] Broad-spectrum antibiotic treatment may be prudent until bacteremia can be excluded.

The presence of retinal hemorrhages on ophthalmoscopy can sometimes be useful here because of its specificity for malaria and the fact that they are present in the majority of patients with cerebral malaria[37] (Figure 117-6).

In surviving patients, the median time to full recovery of consciousness is approximately 24 hours in children, compared to 48 hours in adults. Neurologic sequelae are rare in adults recovering from cerebral malaria (<1%), but more frequent in children, with approximately 12% still having symptoms at the time of discharge, including hemiplegia, cortical blindness, aphasia and cerebellar ataxia.[38] These symptoms will completely resolve over a period from 1 to 6 months in over half of the children, but a quarter of these will be left with major residual neurologic deficits although various studies report different proportions. More subtle cognitive impairments as a late consequence of cerebral malaria are common in children, especially in those cases presenting with a combination of coma, hypoglycemia and seizures.[39]

Acidosis

Metabolic acidosis, measured as base excess, correlates closely with death in severe malaria.[34] Acidosis results from accumulation of lactic acid and other unidentified organic acids as a result of tissue ischemia, compounded by reduced hepatic clearance. Renal impairment can further aggravate the metabolic acidosis. Lactic acidosis is often associated with hypoglycemia.

Anemia

Anemia is mainly a complication in young children and its pathogenesis is multifactorial. Red cells will be destroyed at the moment of schizont rupture, but the rapid decline in hematocrit is more importantly determined by an accelerated destruction of nonparasitized red cells. Moreover, reticulocyte counts are low in the acute phase of the

TABLE 117-1	Manifestations and Complications of Severe Falciparum Malaria, Including Current Opinions About Pathophysiology and Treatment		
Manifestations and Complications	**Pathophysiology**		**Treatment**
Coma (Glasgow Coma Score <11; Blantyre Coma Score <3) and convulsions	Sequestration of parasitized red blood cells in the cerebral microcirculation and other factors		Hypoglycemia and other causes of meningo/encephalitis should be excluded Good general intensive nursing care, including close observation of breathing, eye care Give nasogastric tube, Foley catheter If feasible: intubation to protect airway Frequent monitoring of blood glucose. Treat convulsions (e.g. diazepam); prophylactic anticonvulsive treatment is not recommended
Anemia (Hct <20%, in presence of parasitemia >100 000/µL)	Loss of parasitized red blood cells, increased splenic clearance of uninfected red blood cells (decreased red cell deformability, immunologic factors?), dyserythropoiesis		General recommendation: transfusion if in distress, or Hct <20% (adults), or Hb <5 g/dL in children but cut-off is not well defined
Hyperparasitemia (>10% infected red blood cells)	Host immunologic factors and parasite virulence factors (multiplication rate, red cell selectivity)		Start parenteral antimalarial drugs promptly in effective doses (artemisinins; if quinine: give loading dose) Exchange transfusion (?)
Hypoglycemia (blood glucose <40 mg/dL)	Increased use, decreased production (?) Quinine-related hyperinsulinism		Glucose 10%, 4 mg/kg bodyweight
Acute renal failure (plasma creatinine >3 mg/dL)	Acute tubular necrosis. Prerenal component (dehydration)		Record input/output (Foley catheter). Check biochemistry (BUN, electrolytes), start or transfer for renal replacement therapy (hemofiltration or hemodialysis preferred over peritoneal dialysis)
Severe jaundice (bilirubin >3.0 mg/dL, with parasitemia >100 000/µL)	Mainly in adults; multifactorial		No specific treatment. Monitor blood glucose
Fluid/electrolyte imbalances, metabolic acidosis (venous plasma bicarbonate <15 mmol/L or lactate >4 mmol/L)	Dehydration, SIADH (?). Only minor increase in capillary permeability, compromised microcirculation by sequestration and other factors causing anaerobic glycolysis		Careful fluid resuscitation Bicarbonate administration only if pH ≤7.15 Dialysis as treatment for severe acidosis has been advocated
Respiratory distress and pulmonary edema	Acidosis-related deep breathing Pulmonary edema (ARDS) mainly in adults and pregnant women Etiology unknown; cytokine mediated (?)		See also acidosis ARDS: do not overfill, positive-pressure mechanical ventilation with PEEP etc. Do not allow 'permissive hypercapnia' (brain swelling) Distinguish from pneumonia
Blackwater fever	Related to severe malaria, quinine use and G6PD deficiency		Transfusion if needed Bicarbonate administration (?)
Circulatory shock (systolic BP <90 mmHg [80 mmHg in children] with cold extremities)	Relatively rare in malaria (nitric oxide binding by free hemoglobin?) Consider concurrent sepsis		Fluids, inotropic drugs (do not use adrenaline [epinephrine] because of lactic acidosis), antibiotics
Abnormal bleeding	Diffuse intravascular coagulation: consider concomitant sepsis Isolated thrombocytopenia (very common) not enough explanation		No specific treatment Packed red cell transfusion if indicated

Aspects of pathophysiologic mechanisms or treatment that are still controversial are marked (?).
ARDS, adult respiratory distress syndrome; G6PD, glucose-6-phosphate dehydrogenase; Hct, hematocrit; PEEP, positive end-expiratory pressure; SIADH, syndrome of inappropriate antidiuretic hormone secretion.

disease because of bone marrow dyserythropoiesis. Increased clearance of uninfected erythrocytes is associated with their increased rigidity and possibly with neomembrane antigens resulting from aborted merozoite invasion, which makes them more prone to removal in the sinusoids of the spleen.[40] Anemia in African children is only partly explained by malaria. In addition, bacteremia, hookworm, HIV infection and deficiency of vitamin A and vitamin B12 are all associated with severe anemia.[41]

Hypoglycemia

Hypoglycemia is most prominent in small children and pregnant women with severe malaria. Demand is increased because of increased anaerobic glycolysis (also causing lactic acidosis), increased metabolic demands of the febrile illness, and the malaria parasites that use glucose as their major fuel. Supply is reduced as a result of reduced oral intake, vomiting and failure of hepatic gluconeogenesis, although this has been contested. Hepatic glycogen is exhausted rapidly. The net result is hypoglycemia in 20–30% of children with severe malaria. In patients treated with quinine, this is compounded by quinine-stimulated pancreatic β-cell insulin secretion.[42] Untreated hypoglycemia can cause neurologic damage and is associated with residual neurologic deficit in survivors. The correction of hypoglycemia has therefore a high priority in the management of severe malaria.

Renal Impairment

Acute renal failure is a feared complication of adult severe malaria and most frequently results from acute tubular necrosis. Usually the patient is oliguric for a median of 4 days, but nonoliguric renal failure may also occur. Renal microvascular obstruction and cellular injury consequent upon sequestration in the kidney and the filtration of free

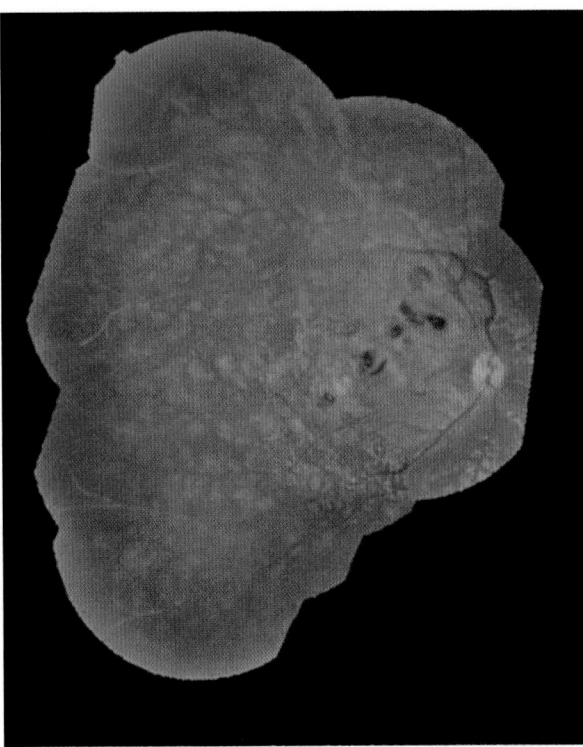

Figure 117-6 Retinal hemorrhages are found in the majority of pediatric and adult patients with cerebral malaria. Because of its specificity, it can be a useful tool to distinguish malaria from other causes of febrile illnesses with coma. *(Courtesy of Dr Richard Maude.)*

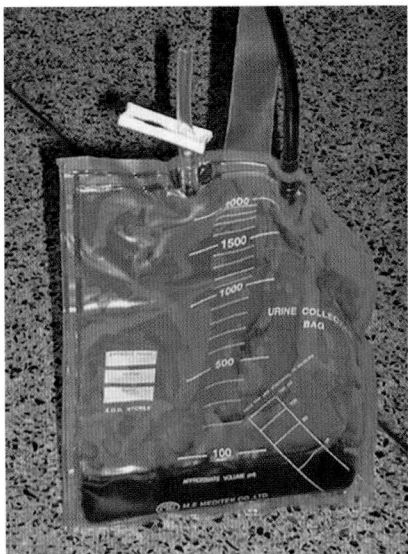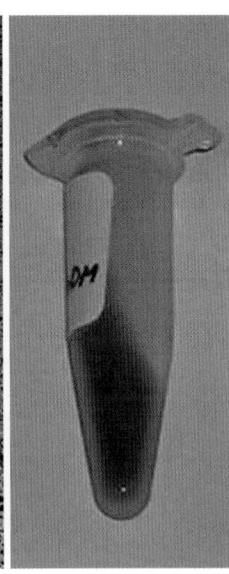

Figure 117-7 Blackwater fever in an adult patient with severe malaria. Massive intravascular hemolysis of both infected and uninfected erythrocytes causes 'Coca-Cola'-like discoloring of the urine.

hemoglobin, myoglobin and other cellular material are contributing factors.[43] Elevated plasma TNF has also been associated with renal impairment. Significant glomerulonephritis is rare, except in chronic *P. malariae* malaria which can cause an immune complex glomerulo-nephritis with a nephrotic syndrome.

Respiratory Distress

Respiratory distress manifesting as deep breathing or tachypnea is associated with poor outcome in children with severe malaria.[44] There may be intercostal recession, use of the accessory muscles of respiration and flaring of the alae nasi. Respiratory distress is often present as respiratory compensation for a profound metabolic acidosis, but can also be caused by the presence of severe anemia or a concomitant lung infection. Pulmonary edema is rare in children. Respiratory depression can be caused by an overuse of anticonvulsants, particularly phenobarbital in combination with benzodiazepines. Identification of these different causes of respiratory distress is important as each requires a different treatment modality.

In adults with severe falciparum malaria, but occasionally in severe vivax infections, ARDS with increased pulmonary capillary permeability can develop, which has a high mortality rate. Pregnant women are especially prone to this complication. Overhydration aggravates the condition, but is not the cause of the respiratory distress; the pulmonary capillary wedge pressure is usually normal.

Blackwater Fever

A minority of patients (6% in adult severe malaria) develop massive intravascular hemolysis and the passage of 'Coca-Cola'-colored urine (Figure 117-7). The pathogenesis of blackwater fever could be related to a build-up of oxidative stress in the erythrocyte membrane. Risk factors are glucose-6-phosphate dehydrogenase (G6PD) deficiency and the use of oxidative drugs such as primaquine.[45] Blackwater fever may contribute to the development of acute renal failure, although in the majority of cases renal function remains normal.

Shock

Shock or 'algid malaria' is relatively rare in severe malaria (around 10%). In most cases the blood pressure of patients with malaria is at the lower end of the normal range, probably due to vasodilation. Marked hypotension in a few cases may be the result of dehydration, but is more commonly due to concomitant sepsis, and possible sources (e.g. respiratory and urinary tract infections) should be investigated.

Bleeding

Bleeding due to the commonly occurring thrombocytopenia in malaria is rare. Bleeding is more likely to occur in the setting of disseminated intravascular coagulation, which should prompt the clinician to consider concomitant sepsis as a cause. More often there is only subtle activation of the coagulation cascade with a reduction in antithrombin III concentration, an increase in thrombin–antithrombin III complexes and a reduction in factor XII and prekallikrein activities, which do not appear to be clinically significant.[46]

MALARIA IN PREGNANCY

In areas of high transmission, the risk of low birth-weight (i.e. <2.5 kg) roughly doubles when women have placental malaria; the effect is greatest during first and second pregnancies. Lower birth-weight is associated with increased infant mortality.[47] Maternal anemia is exacerbated, but most mothers remain asymptomatic despite intense accumulation of infected erythrocytes in the placental microcirculation. Congenital malaria occurs in roughly 5% of neonates but clears spontaneously in 62% of cases.[48] Maternal HIV infection predisposes pregnant women to malaria, predisposes to congenital malaria, and exacerbates reductions in birth-weight. In areas with unstable malaria transmission, pregnant women are at increased risk of developing severe falciparum malaria with a very high mortality rate (roughly 50%). High parasitemias, severe anemia, hypoglycemia and acute pulmonary edema are all more frequent in pregnant than in nonpregnant women. In severe disease, fetal distress, premature labour, and stillbirth can occur. In *P. vivax* infections in pregnancy, severe malaria is rare. No intense placental sequestration occurs yet the average reduction in birth-weight is roughly 107 g (compared with 170 g in falciparum malaria).[49] Even oligosymptomatic, promptly treated *P. falciparum* or *P. vivax* infections increase the risks associated with having abortions and low birth-weight (all gravida). The risk of infant death is particularly high if maternal malaria occurs during late (i.e., near-term) pregnancy. Maternal death from hemorrhage at childbirth is associated to malaria-induced anemia.

Diagnosis

Because of the high prevalence of the disease in the tropics and the danger of developing severe disease, a traveler with fever who has been in a malarious area within the previous 2 months must be considered to have malaria unless proven otherwise. Similarly, in patients living in endemic countries who present with a fever, the suspicion of malaria should be high. On the other hand there tends to be overdiagnosis of malaria in high transmission malarious countries, partly because of the lack of diagnostic facilities. A clinical diagnosis of both uncomplicated and severe malaria is not reliable because of the nonspecific presentation of the disease.

The diagnosis of malaria should be confirmed by either a rapid diagnostic test or microscopy of stained thin and thick blood films, at a magnification of 1000. The intraerythrocytic parasites must be identified and counted. In severe malaria, the developmental stage of the parasites and the percentage of neutrophils containing malarial pigment have prognostic significance. A negative blood smear makes the diagnosis of clinical malaria very unlikely, unless the patient has received antimalarial treatment before presentation. If there is still uncertainty the slide should be repeated every 12 hours for 48 hours. Microscopy with fluorescent staining of the buffy coat (quantitative buffy coat analysis or QBC) has a higher sensitivity to detect low density parasitemias, but this is seldom needed.

Rapid diagnostic tests (RDTs) of the *P. falciparum* antigens *Pf*HRP2 and *p*LDH have a diagnostic sensitivity similar to that of microscopy, but do not require an experienced microscopist, have gained in popularity with donors and are now widely available in malaria-endemic regions. There are, however, drawbacks to RDTs. Parasitemia and parasite stages cannot be assessed in this way. *Pf*HRP2 remains circulating weeks after cure, which can lead to false-positive results in high transmission settings in patients with a recent malaria attack. A range of RDTs to detect *P. falciparum* as well as *P. vivax* are currently marketed. The FIND collaboration provides an ongoing independent evaluation of currently available products.[50]

The detection of parasites using molecular tools such as quantitative polymerase chain reaction (qPCR) plays a major role in research. Loop-mediated isothermal PCR (LAMP), which does not require expensive equipment, might be a useful sensitive diagnostic tool in certain settings.

DIFFERENTIAL DIAGNOSIS

Malaria is a great mimic and must enter the differential diagnosis of a number of clinical presentations.

- In the acute presentation, fever due to malaria needs to be differentiated from typhoid, viral illnesses such as dengue fever and influenza, leptospirosis, brucellosis and respiratory and urinary tract infections. Less common causes of tropical fevers include leishmaniasis, trypanosomiasis, rickettsial infections and relapsing fevers.
- In the case of cerebral malaria, it is of utmost importance to exclude the presence of hypoglycemia as a contributing factor. The principal differential diagnosis in tropical areas is of a bacterial or viral meningoencephalitis. If the patient presents with any sign of meningeal involvement a lumbar puncture should be performed. In small children this implies that in most cases a lumbar puncture will be necessary. Some African centers treating pediatric cerebral malaria postpone lumbar puncture fearing herniation related to raised intracranial pressure, which is present in a majority of their cases. These centers start empiric antibiotic coverage in all children until results of lumbar puncture become available. Other differential diagnoses include enteric fevers, trypanosomiasis, brain abscess and other causes of coma.
- The anemia of malaria can be confused with other common causes of hemolytic anemia in the tropics such as that due to the hemoglobinopathies (e.g. sickle cell disease, thalassemia), G6PD deficiency and the South East Asian form of ovalocytosis. The

anemia of malaria must be differentiated from that of iron, folate or vitamin B12 deficiency. Hookworm and HIV infection are also associated with severe anemia.
- The renal failure of malaria must be distinguished from renal impairment due to sickle cell disease, leptospirosis, use of traditional herbal medicines and chronic renal disease resulting from glomerulonephritis and hypertension.
- The jaundice and hepatomegaly of malaria must be distinguished from that of viral hepatitis (A, B and E, cytomegalovirus and Epstein–Barr virus infections), leptospirosis, yellow fever, biliary disease and drug-induced disease, including alcohol.

Management

UNCOMPLICATED MALARIA

Malaria Caused by Plasmodium falciparum

Today, resistance of *P. falciparum* against chloroquine and S–P has reached nearly all parts of the tropics. To ensure efficacy and to limit the chances of *de novo* appearance and spread of antimalarial drug resistance, falciparum malaria should be treated with combinations of two or more blood schizontocidal drugs with independent modes of action. Artemisinin combination therapy (ACT) has become the standard recommendation for treatment of uncomplicated malaria, endorsed by the WHO. The potent antimalarial capacity of the artemisinins quickly reduces the total body parasite number, which will not only relieve symptoms rapidly, but will also reduce the chance of emergence of clones resistant against the partner drug. The partner drug mutually protects the artemisinin component against resistance development.[51]

To ensure treatment courses that do not exceed 3 days, the partner drug to the artemisinin derivative should have a longer half-life in order to kill the remaining parasites (about 10^3 to 10^5 of the initial 10^8 to 10^{13}). Possible partner drugs in ACT regimens include amodiaquine, atovaquone–proguanil, clindamycin, doxycycline, lumefantrine, mefloquine, piperaquine, pyronaridine, chlorproguanil–dapsone, proguanil–dapsone, S–P and tetracyclines. Of these partner drugs, lumefantrine, mefloquine and piperaquine have proven efficacy even in areas of multidrug-resistant *P. falciparum*. The combination of an artemisinin derivative with amodiaquine or S–P has been shown to be effective only in areas where amodiaquine and S–P monotherapy failure rates do not exceed 20%. Chloroquine cannot be recommended because of widespread high-level resistance. Of these combinations, artemether–lumefantrine, dihydroartemisinin–piperaquine, artesunate–mefloquine and artesunate–amodiaquine are now available as fixed combinations. Artesunate–pyronaridine has recently been licensed and surveillance is ongoing to assure the safety of the combination in large populations. Wide deployment of fixed combinations will preclude the use of artemisinin monotherapy, which is an important strategy to reduce the spread of drug resistance.

The following ACTs are currently recommended for treatment of uncomplicated falciparum malaria:[52]

- artemether + lumefantrine
- artesunate + amodiaquine
- artesunate + mefloquine
- artesunate + S–P
- dihydroartemisinin + piperaquine.

Artesunate with pyronaridine has recently been registered in some South East Asian countries. Reduced efficacy of artesunate, characterized by an important deceleration in parasite clearance, has been conclusively proven in 2009 in western Cambodia[53] and has since emerged and spread eastward to central Vietnam and the South China sea and westward to Myanmar.[54–56] In western Cambodia and on the Thai–Myanmar border, concomitant resistance against several partner drugs have resulted in worrying high failure rates of ACTs. No cases of clinical failures of ACTs have been reported from the African continent at the time of writing but close monitoring is warranted. An effective combination therapy not containing an artemisinin derivative is atovaquone–proguanil (Malarone), which can be used in the treatment

TABLE 117-2	Dosing Schedule for Artemether-Lumefantrine	
Body Weight (kg)	**Dose (mg) of Artemether + Lumefantrine Given Twice Daily for 3 Days**	
5 to < 15	20 + 120	
15 to < 25	40 + 240	
25 to < 35	60 + 360	
≥ 35	80 + 480	

TABLE 117-3	Dosing Schedule for Artesunate Plus Amodiaquine
Body Weight (kg)	**Artesunate + Amodiaquine Dose (mg) Given Daily for 3 Days**
4.5 to < 9	25 + 67.5
9 to < 18	50 + 135
18 to < 36	100 + 270
≥ 36	200 + 540

TABLE 117-4	Dosing Schedule for Artesunate-Mefloquine
Body Weight (kg)	**Artesunate + Mefloquine Dose (mg) Given Daily for 3 Days**
5 to < 9	25 + 55
9 to < 18	50 + 110
18 to < 30	100 + 220
≥ 30	200 + 440

TABLE 117-5	Dosing Schedule for Artesunate Plus Sulfadoxin-Pyrimethamine	
Body Weight (kg)	**Artesunate Dose Given Daily for 3 Days (mg)**	**Sulfadoxine/Pyrimethamine Dose (mg) Given as a Single Dose on Day 1**
5 to < 10	25	250/12.5
10 to < 25	50	500/25
25 to < 50	100	1000/50
≥ 50	200	1500/75

TABLE 117-6	Dosing Schedule for Dihydroartemisinin-Piperaquine
Body Weight (kg)	**Dihydroartemisinin + Piperaquine Dose (mg) Given Daily for 3 Days**
5 to < 8	20 + 160
8 to < 11	30 + 240
11 to < 17	40 + 320
17 to < 25	60 + 480
25 to < 36	80 + 640
36 to < 60	120 + 960
60 < 80	160 + 1280
>80	200 + 1600

TABLE 117-7	Recommendations on the Treatment of Falciparum Malaria in Nonimmune Adult Travelers

For travelers returning to non-endemic countries

Artemether–lumefantrine (1.5 mg/12 mg/kg bd for 3 days)

If no ACT available: atovaquone–proguanil (1 g/400 mg q24h for 3 days) or quinine (10 mg/kg q8h) plus doxycycline* (3.5 mg/kg q24h) or clindamycin (10 mg/kg q12h); drugs to be given for 7 days and generally poorly tolerated

For severe malaria

The antimalarial treatment of severe malaria in travelers is the same as the general recommendation for severe malaria
Travelers with severe malaria should be managed in an intensive care unit
Hemofiltration or hemodialysis should be started early in acute renal failure
Endotracheal intubation with positive-pressure ventilation is indicated in comatose patients, and if there is respiratory insufficiency or intractable seizures

*Doxycycline should not be used in children under 8 years of age.

of imported uncomplicated falciparum malaria in returning travelers in non-endemic countries. Quinine, in combination with doxycycline, tetracycline or clindamycin, remains effective but the prolonged 7-day regimen required to cure falciparum malaria is difficult to tolerate and tends to have poor adherence. Development of new asexual blood stage antimalarials is clearly urgently needed. Promising compounds under development include ozonides (synthetic endoperoxides), spiroindolones and imidazolopiperazines. In regions with artemisinin resistance, a single low dose of primaquine (0.25 mg/kg body weight) is recommended as a gametocytocidal additional treatment in patients with falciparum malaria. Primaquine is an oxidative drug that can cause severe hemolysis in individuals with glucose-6-phosphate (G6PD) deficiency. However, this low dose is considered to be safe irrespective of the G6PD-status of the patient.

Tables 117-2 to 117-6 summarize the different drug combinations and dosing schemes for the treatment of uncomplicated falciparum malaria. Table 117-7 summarizes treatment of uncomplicated falciparum malaria in returning nonimmune adult travelers, and Table 117-8 in pregnant women. If the patient is vomiting and not tolerating oral treatment, parenteral treatment with artesunate, artemether or quinine is warranted. Hyperparasitemia above 4% is, for some authors, also an indication for parenteral treatment, even in the absence of any other severity sign. Others recommend an oral ACT under close supervision.[52] Hyperparasitemia above 10% should always be treated with parenteral antimalarials.

Malaria Caused by P. vivax, P. ovale and P. malariae

P. vivax and P. ovale form hypnozoites, parasite stages in the liver that can result in multiple relapses of infection, weeks to months after the primary infection. The interval between the primary episode and relapses is related to strain-specific characteristics. Strains circulating close to the equator (e.g. in Indonesia) tend to have a shorter relapse interval (weeks) compared to strains circulating in more northern latitudes (months).[57]

Radical cure of the infection targets both the blood stage (schizonts) and the liver stage (hypnozoites), preventing recrudescence as well as relapse. In general, P. vivax, P. ovale and P. malariae remain sensitive to chloroquine, which continues to be the treatment of choice in regions where the parasites remain sensitive due to the low cost, high tolerability and the long half-life. Important chloroquine-resistant vivax malaria has been reported, especially from Papua New Guinea and parts of Indonesia. In these settings, dihydroartemisinin–piperaquine and artemether–lumefantrine are an effective treatment for vivax malaria.[58]

In view of the increasing resistance to chloroquine in P. vivax, the potential for misdiagnosis and subsequent inadvertent use of

TABLE 117-8	Treatment of Uncomplicated Malaria in Pregnancy
FALCIPARUM MALARIA	
First trimester	Quinine (10 mg/kg q8h), preferably plus clindamycin (5 mg/kg q8h) for 7 days An artemisinin-based combination therapy (ACT) should be used if it is considered that the benefits of treating outweigh the risks of not treating when the only drug option available is an ACT
Second and third trimesters	ACT known to be effective in the country/region or artesunate (2 mg/kg q24h) plus clindamycin for 7 days, or quinine plus clindamycin for 7 days
Severe malaria	As in nonpregnant individuals (see Table 117-7) Increased risk of hypoglycemia in quinine-treated patients
VIVAX MALARIA	
Chloroquine-sensitive	Chloroquine 25 mg base/kg divided over 3 days Primaquine is contraindicated during pregnancy Chloroquine prophylaxis (300 mg base once per week) should be continued until delivery
Chloroquine-resistant	ACT in 2nd and 3rd trimesters, such as artemether lumefantrine or dihydroartemisinin–piperaquine (dosing as in falciparum malaria)

chloroquine to treat falciparum malaria, and operational advantages, artemisinin combination treatment seems a good first-line treatment for all human malarias.[59]

The radical cure of vivax (and ovale) malaria, that is the cure of the hypnozoites and hence the prevention of relapses, requires treatment with an 8-aminoquinoline. The (currently) only licensed and widely available 8-aminoquinoline is primaquine. There is insufficient evidence from treatment trials to recommend or reject one drug regimen over another. The current WHO recommended regimen is 15 mg/day for 14 days (for an adult patient). Better results may be achieved with higher doses. However primaquine dosing is limited by unacceptable tolerability. Specifically in patients with G6PD deficiency, treatment with 8-aminoquinolines can trigger hemolysis which can be severe enough to require transfusions in rare cases. Hence it is recommended to use the fluorescent spot test to determine G6PD activity prior to dosing. For patients with reduced G6PD activity the WHO recommends 45 mg/week for 8 weeks.[52] The evidence for the efficacy of this regimen is limited.

Tafenoquine, another 8-aminoquinoline, has been in development for nearly three decades. Recent promising efficacy trials suggest that a single dose of tafenoquine may be sufficient for the radical cure of vivax malaria.[60] Such single dose tafenoquine regimens could improve adherence dramatically. However, tafenoquine, like all 8-aminoquinolines, can trigger hemolysis in G6PD-deficient individuals requiring the assessment of the G6PD status prior to dosing. The licensing of tafenoquine may well depend on the availability of an appropriate co-diagnostic test marketed with the drug.

The following drug regimens are currently recommended for treatment of uncomplicated vivax malaria (Box 117-1):[52]

- chloroquine + primaquine
- ACT + primaquine.

The recommended treatment for malaria caused by *P. ovale* is the same as that given to achieve radical cure in vivax malaria, i.e. with chloroquine + primaquine or ACT + primaquine. *P. malariae* should be treated with the standard regimen of chloroquine or ACT as for vivax malaria, but does not require radical cure with primaquine. ACTs should replace chloroquine when chloroquine resistance is suspected but are more costly than chloroquine.

BOX 117-1	TREATMENT OF UNCOMPLICATED VIVAX AND OVALE MALARIA

- Chloroquine 25 mg base/kg divided over 3 days, combined with primaquine 0.25 mg base/kg, taken with food once daily for 14 days is the treatment of choice for chloroquine-sensitive infections. In Oceania and South East Asia the dose of primaquine should be 0.5 mg/kg
- An artemisinin combination therapy (artemether–lumefantrine or dihydroartemisinin–piperaquine) combined with primaquine should be given for chloroquine-resistant vivax malaria
- In moderate glucose-6-phosphate dehydrogenase (G6PD) deficiency, primaquine 0.75 mg base/kg should be given once a week for 6 weeks. In severe G6PD deficiency, primaquine should not be given
- Where artemisinin combination therapy has been adopted as the first-line treatment for *Plasmodium falciparum* malaria, it may also be used for *P. vivax* malaria in combination with primaquine for radical cure. Artesunate plus sulfadoxine–pyrimethamine (S–P) is the exception, since S–P is generally not effective against *P. vivax*

TABLE 117-9	Antimalarial Treatment of Severe Malaria
Artesunate*	2.4 mg/kg iv or im stat, at 12 and 24 h, then daily (artesunic acid (60 mg) is dissolved in 0.6 ml 5% sodium bicarbonate and injected iv as a bolus, or diluted to 5 ml with 5% dextrose for im injection; 1 ampoule = 60 mg)
Artemether	3.2 mg/kg im stat, followed by 1.6 mg/kg daily; **not** for iv administration (1 ampoule = 80 mg)
Quinine	20 mg/kg dihydrochloride salt by iv infusion over 4 h, followed by 10 mg/kg infused over 2–8 h q8h

*Parenteral artesunate is the drug of choice for the treatment of severe malaria.

SEVERE MALARIA

Antimalarial Treatment

Prompt start of parenteral antimalarial treatment in full doses is essential in this life-threatening condition. Large trials in Asia and Africa (SEAQUAMAT and AQUAMAT) have conclusively proven that parenteral artesunate for the treatment of severe malaria is superior in saving lives compared to quinine.[61,62] International treatment guidelines recommend parenteral artesunate 2.4 mg/kg intravenous or intramuscular stat, at 12 and 24 h, then daily, as treatment of choice for severe malaria in both adults and children and irrespective of the epidemiologic setting. Because of its life-saving effect on the mother, parenteral artesunate is also the first-line treatment in severe malaria during pregnancy in all trimesters. Treatment of the acute phase of severe vivax malaria is the same as for severe falciparum malaria. If the patient is recovering and able to take oral medication, parenteral treatment can be changed to oral treatment. A full course of an ACT can be chosen as follow-on oral treatment.

Artesunate and Artemether

The artemisinin derivatives are rapidly parasitocidal, and crucially unlike quinine they kill young circulating parasites before they sequester in the deep microvasculature.

Intramuscular (fat-soluble) artemether, unlike intramuscular (water-soluble) artesunate, is erratically absorbed in patients with severe disease, and might explain why trials in both adults and children have shown similar mortality in patients treated with intramuscular artemether compared to quinine. There are insufficient trials with the other parenteral fat-soluble artemisinin-derivative artemotil (artemether) to allow firm recommendations. Dosing schemes of artesunate and artemether are summarized in Table 117-9.

Quinine

In the absence of parenteral artesunate, parenteral quinine remains the drug of choice for severe malaria. Because of its cardiotoxicity, intravenous infusion should be carried out over 4 hours. Where intravenous infusion is not practical, quinine can be given by deep intramuscular injection in the upper thigh. Quinine is a relatively toxic drug with a narrow therapeutic ratio.[42] Quinine-induced hyperinsulinemic hypoglycemia is a particular problem in patients with severe malaria, especially during pregnancy, and is impossible to diagnose clinically in the already unconscious patient. Frequent monitoring of blood glucose concentrations is therefore essential. It is also important that parasitocidal drug levels are obtained as quickly as possible, so in patients who have not been given a dose of quinine <12 hours before admission an initial loading dose of 20 mg/kg should be administered.[42] In severe malaria the dose should be reduced by one-third after 48 hours if there is no clinical improvement or if there is renal failure. Dosing schemes are summarized in Table 117-9.

Since severe malaria is a multiorgan disease, appropriate supportive treatment is crucial for survival of the patient. Convulsions should be treated with rectal diazepam, intravenous lorazepam, paraldehyde or other standard anticonvulsants, after high-flow oxygen and appropriate airway management have been initiated. Severe anemia should be treated with blood transfusion. Acute renal failure is more common in adults but has likely been underrecognised in paediatric severe malaria in Africa, and has a very high untreated mortality rate. Hemofiltration, when available, is superior to peritoneal dialysis in terms of mortality and cost-effectiveness.[63]

Hemodynamic shock in severe malaria is relatively rare and should prompt a septic screen and start of appropriate broad-spectrum antibiotics to cover the possibility of bacterial sepsis. In pediatric severe malaria concomitant invasive bacterial infection is very common (around 10–20%), and co-administration of antibiotics to the antimalarial treatment is recommended. In addition, good nursing care is essential, with particular attention to fluid balance, management of the unconscious patient and detection of potentially lethal complications such as hypoglycemia. Mechanical ventilation in the unconscious patient helps to protect the airway. There is no role for aggressive fluid therapy; a large trial showed conclusively that fluid bolus therapy in pediatric severe malaria patients with compensated shock results in excess mortality.[64] In adults, severe adverse effects of liberal fluid therapy, even under stringent monitoring of fluid status, have also been documented.[65] In the absence of hypotension, a conservative fluid regimen without fluid bolus therapy is recommended.

Many resource-poor countries are at a stage where basic intensive care support in regional hospitals is becoming feasible, a development that has great potential to further reduce mortality. All adjunctive treatments to date that have been studied in randomized trials in patients with severe malaria have not been able to show additional benefits.

References available online at expertconsult.com.

KEY REFERENCES

Barnes K.I., Durrheim D.N., Little F., et al.: Effect of artemether–lumefantrine policy and improved vector control on malaria burden in KwaZulu–Natal, South Africa. *PLoS Med* 2005; 2(11):e330.

Dondorp A., Nosten F., Stepniewska K., et al.: Artesunate versus quinine for treatment of severe falciparum malaria: a randomised trial. *Lancet* 2005; 366(9487):717-725.

Dondorp A.M., Desakorn V., Pongtavornpinyo W., et al.: Estimation of the total parasite biomass in acute falciparum malaria from plasma PfHRP2. *PLoS Med* 2005; 2(8):e204.

Dondorp A.M., Fanello C.I., Hendriksen I.C., et al.: Artesunate versus quinine in the treatment of severe falciparum malaria in African children (AQUAMAT): an open-label, randomised trial. *Lancet* 2010; 376(9753): 1647-1657.

Hay S.I., Guerra C.A., Gething P.W., et al.: A world malaria map: *Plasmodium falciparum* endemicity in 2007. *PLoS Med. [Research Support, Non-U.S. Gov't]* 2009; 6(3):e1000048.

Lengeler C.: Insecticide-treated bednets and curtains for preventing malaria. *Cochrane Database Syst Rev* 2000; (2):CD000363.

Ratcliff A., Siswantoro H., Kenangalem E., et al.: Two fixed-dose artemisinin combinations for drug-resistant falciparum and vivax malaria in Papua, Indonesia: an open-label randomised comparison. *Lancet* 2007; 369(9563):757-765.

Simpson J.A., Aarons L., Collins W.E., et al.: Population dynamics of untreated *Plasmodium falciparum* malaria within the adult human host during the expansion phase of the infection. *Parasitology* 2002; 124(Pt 3):247-263.

White N.J., Imwong M.: Relapse. *Adv Parasitol* 2012; 80:113-150.

White N.J., Pukrittayakamee S., Hien T.T., et al.: Malaria. *Lancet* 2014; 383(9918):723-735.

118

Schistosomiasis

ALAN FENWICK

KEY CONCEPTS

- Schistosomiasis is a disease caused by infection with a digenetic blood-living trematode worm.

- It is a very common infection particularly in sub-Saharan Africa, with over 200 million of the rural poor estimated to be harboring worms.

- Schistosomiasis causes long-term organ damage leading to death many years after infection.

- Tourists and visitors to Africa can return with this infection, but it is a rare occurence.

- Efforts are being made to provide treatments with praziquantel throughout Africa to those infected or at risk.

- The World Health Organization are encouraging countries to aim for elimination of transmission by 2025.

Introduction

Schistosomiasis or bilharzia, caused by infection with trematode *Schistosoma* spp., is one of the most debilitating helminthic diseases among rural populations, particularly in sub-Saharan Africa. Schistosomiasis can cause a wide range of symptoms and consequences depending on the species, the worm burden and the length of time infected. There are three major species that affect humans, of which two are predominant in Africa (*Schistosoma haematobium* and *Schistosoma mansoni*) and the third is only found in the Far East, e.g. China and the Philippines (*Schistosoma japonicum*). The life cycle of schistosomiasis is shown in Figure 118-1. Another two less widespread species – *Schistosoma mekongi* in South East Asia and *Schistosoma intercalatum* in Africa – are considered to be less of a public health problem. *S. mansoni* is the only schistosome found in the Americas.

Epidemiology

Schistosomiasis is prevalent in 76 countries and territories in tropical and subtropical regions (Figure 118-2), with a minimum estimated 230 million people infected and some estimates that up to 440 million might be suffering from schistosomiasis.[1] Approximately 85% of infections are found in sub-Saharan Africa.[2] The geographic distribution of *S. haematobium* and *S. mansoni* within endemic areas is dependent on the presence of suitable aquatic intermediate host snails (*Bulinus* and *Biomphalaria* spp., respectively). Human urination and defecation lead to excretion of schistosome eggs into fresh water and subsequent infection in these snails, while exposure during activities such as swimming, fishing or irrigation leads to cercariae from snails infecting humans and completing the cycle. In the case of *S. japonicum*, a reservoir of adult worm infection exists in domestic and wild animals and the snail intermediate hosts of *S. japonicum* are amphibious *Oncomelania* species.

Schistosomiasis is a highly geographically localized disease because transmission levels are determined by snail distribution, and human cultural, social and behavioral activities (Figure 118-3). Recent irrigation projects[3] have led to increased infection in some areas and climate change could effect changes in infection rates.[4] Detailed information on geographic distribution in each endemic country/area can only be obtained through rapid epidemiologic mapping[5] or using geographical information system (GIS) technology.[6] *S. mekongi* is present only in the Mekong River basin in South East Asia, though latest research suggests that the distribution may be a little wider, with intermediate host *Neotricula aperta* snails. Finally, *S. intercalatum* is present in limited areas in Central and West Africa with *Bulinus* spp. as snail host.

In endemic areas, children may acquire infection in infancy,[7] probably through being bathed in infested water by their carers (Figure 118-4). Prevalence of infection usually increases with age, peaks at age 10–20 years and then decreases in adults, although this pattern is seen more with *S. haematobium* than *S. mansoni*. Intensity of infection, which is measured as the number of eggs excreted (a surrogate estimate of worm load) in urine (*S. haematobium*) or feces (*S. mansoni, S. japonicum, S. mekongi* and *S. intercalatum*), follows a similar pattern to prevalence: increasing with age through childhood and then decreasing in adults. Schistosomiasis does, however, result in exceptional consequences when epidemiologic conditions are extreme – for example, car washers in Kenya present a unique situation of repeated heavy infections,[8] despite frequent treatment.

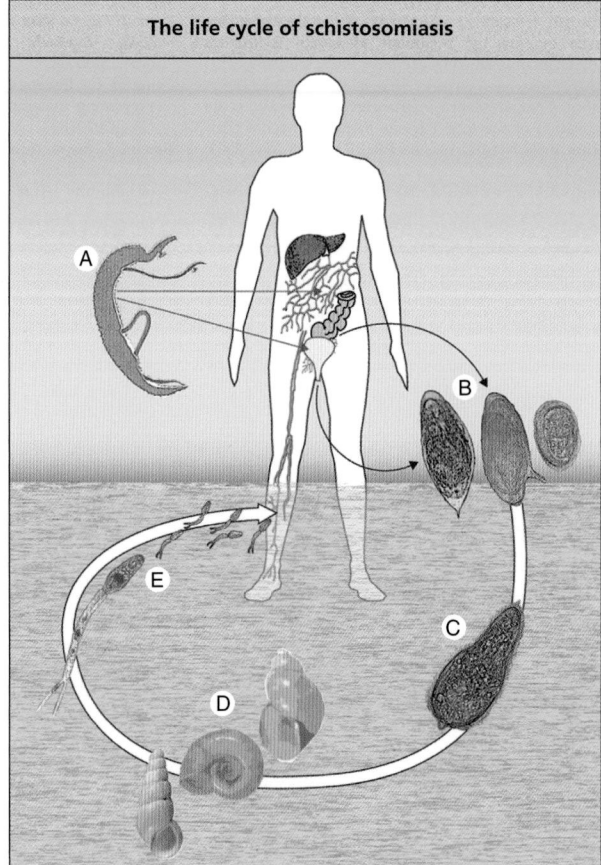

The life cycle of schistosomiasis

Figure 118-1 The life cycle of schistosomiasis. (A) Paired adult worms (larger male enfolding slender female). (B) Eggs (left to right, *S. haematobium, S. mansoni, S. japonicum*). (C) Ciliated miracidium. (D) Intermediate host snails (left to right, *Oncomelania, Biomphalaria, Bulinus*). (E) Cercariae. *(Reprinted from Colley D.G., Bustinduy A.L., Secor W.E. and King C.H. Human schistosomiasis. Lancet, 384 (9948): 20–26 September 2014, pp. 1094–1095. Figure 1.)*

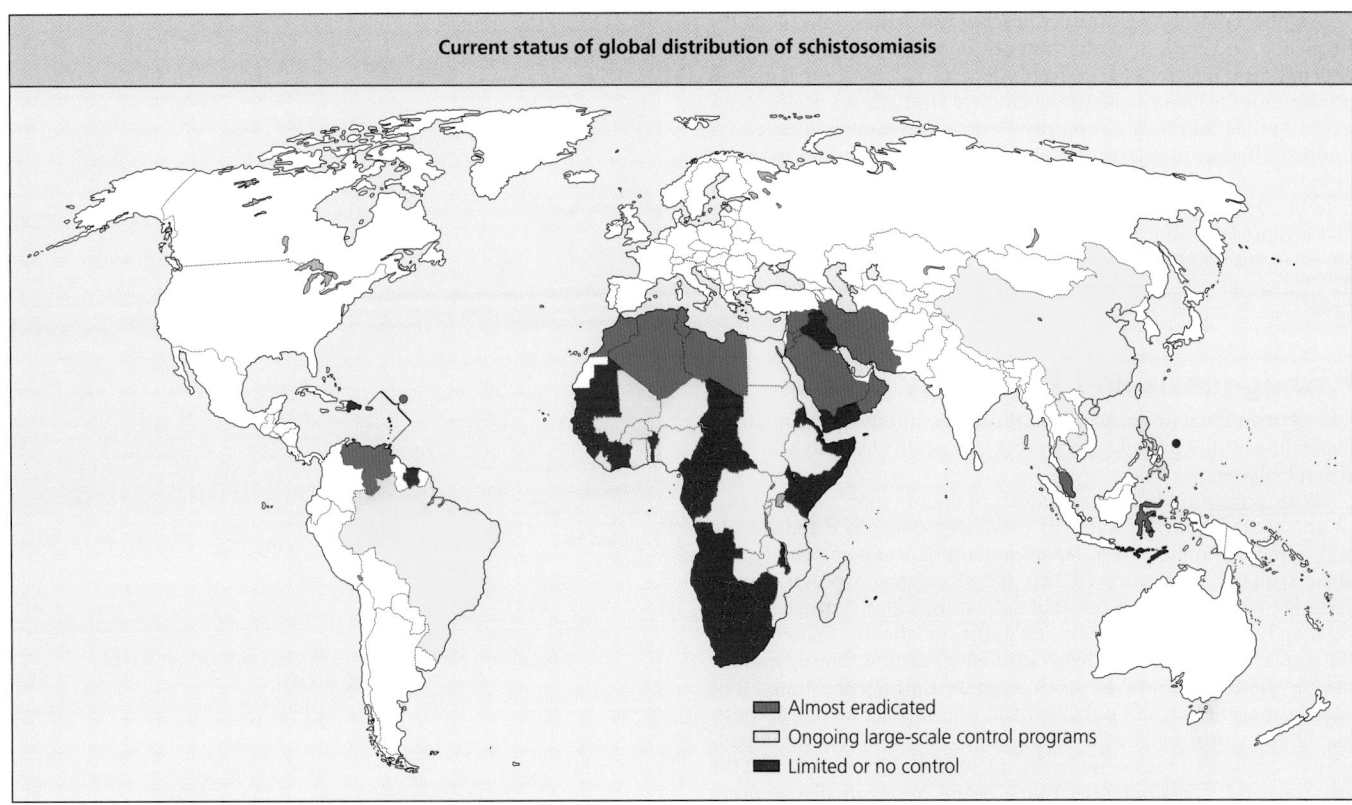

Figure 118-2   Current status of global distribution of schistosomiasis. *(From the World Health Organization, with modification.)*

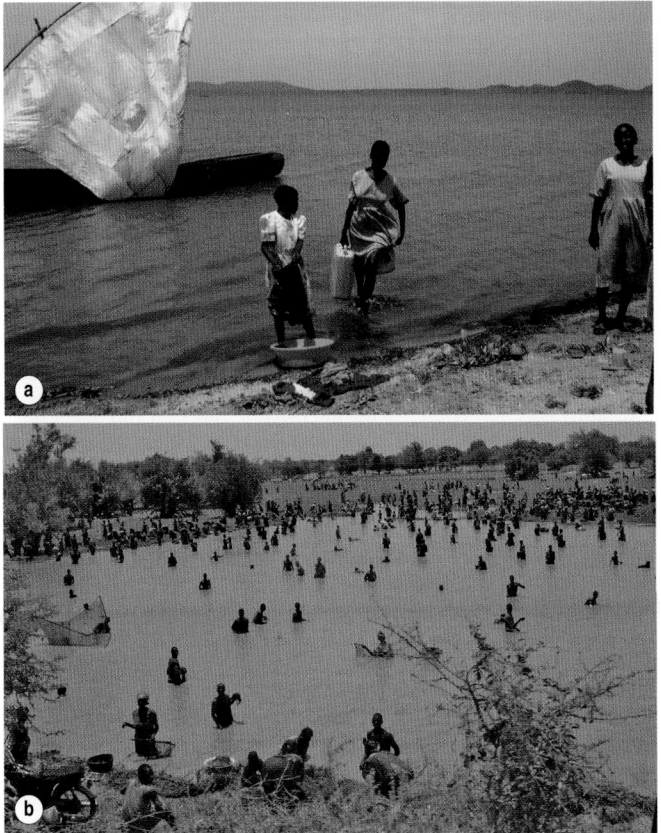

Figure 118-3   Water contact activities. (a) Girls collecting water and washing in Lake Victoria in Uganda. (b) Mass fishing activities in Burkina Faso.

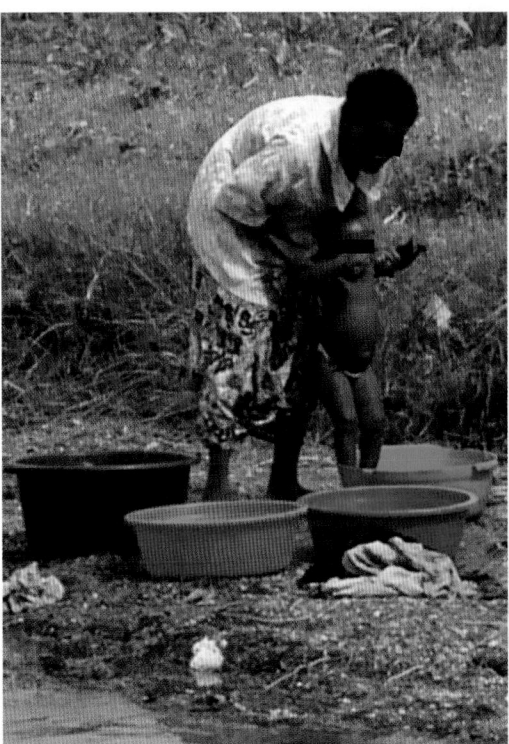

Figure 118-4   Water contact – baby bathing. A baby is being washed by the mother near Lake Victoria in Uganda. *(Courtesy of Dr J. Russell Stothard.)*

Another epidemiologic feature of schistosome infections is that the frequency distribution of the number of worms in individuals in endemic areas is aggregated or overdispersed.[9] This means that in most populations the majority of infected individuals harbor a relatively low worm burden and only a minority (5–15%) are heavily infected (as measured by eggs in stool or urine). Consequently, this minority group of individuals is most likely to show severe morbidity. Factors that may determine predisposition to heavy or light infection include age, innate and acquired immunity and/or genetic background of individuals.[10] However, it should be realized that there is probably subtle morbidity in all cases of infection even though this may not be immediately apparent.

Pathogenesis and Pathology

Disease manifestations caused by schistosome infections are multiple, depending on the parasite species, but can be divided into acute and chronic phases.

Acute schistosomiasis is seen most commonly soon after exposure to an infested body of water in previously unexposed individuals, and is more common in *S. japonicum* and *S. mansoni*. The typical acute symptoms are observed after the percutaneous penetration of cercariae which can cause cercarial dermatitis, a local hypersensitivity reaction to the penetrating parasites at the site of entry. Subsequently, Katayama fever, a systemic hypersensitivity reaction, can then occur during the next month as larvae migrate through the lungs. The exact pathogenesis is still unknown, but is probably a serum sickness-like illness caused by circulating immune complexes and proinflammatory cytokines in response to the migrating schistosomula and the egg antigens.[11] Classically, egg laying begins approximately 6 weeks after infection, and the onset of oviposition can cause severe bloody diarrhea.

In longer-term chronic schistosomiasis, caused by continued infection with mating worm pairs, pathologic lesions are mainly localized in specific sites within infected individuals, and for a long period symptoms are rarely recognized until significant organ damage has occurred. Although the adult worms are living in the blood vessels and are feeding on blood, it is the eggs and the subsequent host granulomatous reactions to the eggs trapped in tissues that cause the most damage. Through the secretion of proteolytic enzymes, and perhaps aided by urinary tract or intestinal movement, the eggs rupture capillary vessels and then pass through the tissues to the lumen of these viscera where they are carried to the outside via urine or stools. This process causes bleeding, which in the short term causes overt blood in the urine and blood in the stool (less easily visible) and in the longer term contributes to anemia. A significant proportion of parasite eggs, however, are either retained in local tissues (bladder or gut walls) or carried via venous blood to distant organs such as the liver and lung, and are trapped there due to their relatively large size (60–170 μm). As long as the worms are alive, the numbers of trapped eggs continue to accumulate in the tissues. At these sites, miracidia in the trapped eggs secrete soluble antigens that diffuse out of the egg shell, triggering a marked inflammatory and granulomatous response from the host immune system. As a result, the individual eggs (or cluster of eggs in the case of *S. japonicum*) are enclosed by the aggregated immune cells, including eosinophils, forming granulomas (Figure 118-5).

The granulomatous response is a form of delayed-type hypersensitivity reaction and is dependent predominantly on CD4$^+$ T-cell-mediated mechanisms.[12] Granulomas are tumor-like inflammatory nodules which can cause intrahepatic portal vein obstruction, leading to portal hypertension, or obstruct urine flow through the ureters, leading to hydroureters and hydronephrosis. The miracidia within the eggs, however, survive for only 6–8 weeks and then die, thus eliminating the continuous antigenic stimulation. The granulomas may then disperse and fibrous tissues form. The tissue damage caused by scattered eggs does not cause a significant problem, but when numerous eggs are trapped the damage becomes significant. Therefore, the severity of

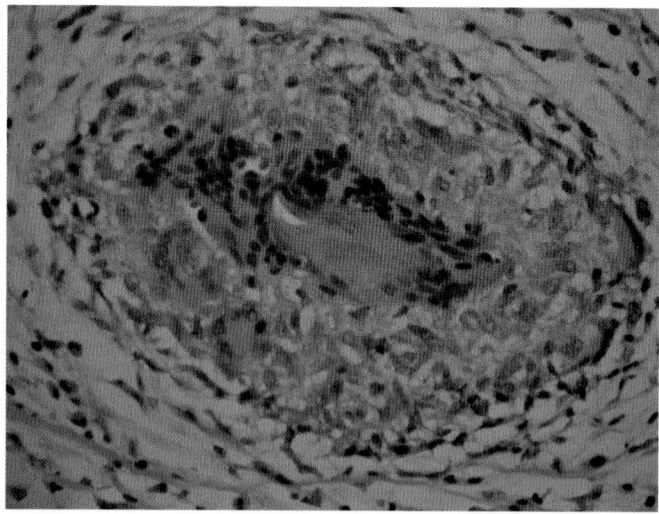

Figure 118-5   Multiple granulomata surrounding eggs. (*Courtesy of Dr Robert Goldin.*)

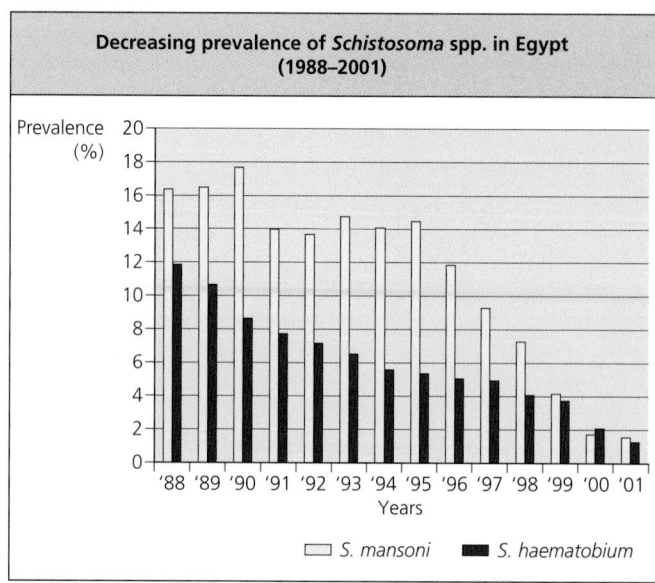

Figure 118-6   Decreasing prevalence of *Schistosoma* spp. in Egypt (1988–2001) in the course of an ongoing treatment campaign. (*Redrawn from Fenwick et al., Trends Parasitol 2003; 19(11):509-515.*)

morbidity is closely related to the intensity of infection and the passage of time.

Prevention

Prevention can be separated into prevention of infection in the millions of residents of endemic areas, and prevention of infection in the relatively few tourists and visitors to endemic countries. In poverty-stricken rural areas, prevention of infection by improved water supplies and sanitation is fundamental to the elimination of schistosomiasis, as was achieved several decades ago in Japan and more recently in Puerto Rico.[13] In the meantime, current proactive control programs in low- and middle-income countries target prevention of morbidity using MDA (mass drug administration), i.e. chemotherapy using the one drug available – praziquantel – with elimination some way in the future. The first country to embark on this strategy, Egypt, has significantly reduced the prevalence of infection and reduced the public health importance of schistosomiasis, but this took 20 years (Figure 118-6).[14]

Thus for indigenous residents in endemic areas the risks are complex and multifaceted, often reflecting the degree of education, socioeconomic status and cultural and recreational practices. In many areas in sub-Saharan Africa, the snail-infested water bodies may be the only water sources in their daily life, and for fishermen, farmers and domestic washing, contact is unavoidable. How can people with regular water contact escape infection? Strategies considered for prevention may include mollusciciding to kill intermediate host snails, chemotherapy of infected individuals to reduce transmission sources, health education to improve hygiene, provision of latrines and sewage disposal, installation of a clean water supply, and economic and social development in general. Each of these strategies has its limitations and should be used in conjunction with others in an integrated manner according to local conditions. In recent years, despite investments to develop antischistosome vaccines, and promise in laboratory studies using a mouse model, a successful vaccine and a practical vaccination strategy are still some way off.

To reduce morbidity, a preventive chemotherapy strategy has been recommended by the World Health Organization.[15] Annual treatment during school-aged years is the preferred strategy because it should prevent the devastating consequences of organ damage at a later stage of life. Since 2002, the Schistosomiasis Control Initiative (SCI) based at Imperial College London has implemented a sustainable integrated chemotherapy strategy using praziquantel against schistosomiasis and adding in albendazole to control the concurrent intestinal helminth infections,[16] and by 2014 over 100 million treatments were dispensed in 16 countries. An integrated program against neglected tropical diseases including schistosomiasis is now being implemented in most sub-Saharan African countries, and the target is to deliver 100 million treatments every year from 2016.[17]

This program has been made feasible by the annual increase in the donation of praziquantel by the pharmaceutical company Merck KGaA, which reached 105 million tablets by 2015 and will increase to 250 million tablets annually from 2016.[18,19] Without human contact with fresh water there would be no infection. For nonindigenous travelers into endemic areas, therefore, avoidance of all freshwater sources is prudent, because a single exposure to many cercariae can have severe consequences. In recent years, returning travelers who had swum in Lake Malawi has been one of the most frequently recognized sources of infection. Treatment with praziquantel 2 months after returning home provides a simple cure.

Clinical Features

The clinical manifestations of schistosomiasis are related not only to the parasite species but also to the intensity of infection, the length of time the individual has been infected and genetic make-up of the infected individuals.[10] Disease manifestations have multiple stages and also interact with other coinfections such as HIV and malaria, and nutritional conditions.

The first clinical manifestations occur as individuals are acquiring infection, as cercarial penetration of the host skin can provoke a temporary urticarial rash that can manifest within hours of exposure (contacting cercariae-infested water) and sometimes persist for days as maculopapular lesions. Such cercarial dermatitis, also called 'swimmer's itch', usually occurs in those who have not previously been exposed, e.g. tourists and migrants. The lesions are usually self-limited and often go unrecognized in endemic areas.

Early infections are mostly asymptomatic (except for blood in the urine) but in some cases of heavy naïve infections the disease starts suddenly with nonspecific symptoms, such as fever, fatigue, myalgia, malaise, nonproductive cough, eosinophilia and patchy pulmonary infiltrates on chest radiography. With *S. mansoni*, abdominal symptoms such as stomach ache, loose stools and diarrhea may develop later when egg deposition begins. Most patients recover spontaneously after 2–10 weeks, but some may develop persistent and more serious disease with weight loss, dyspnea, diarrhea, diffuse abdominal pain, bloody diarrhea, hepatosplenomegaly and widespread rash.

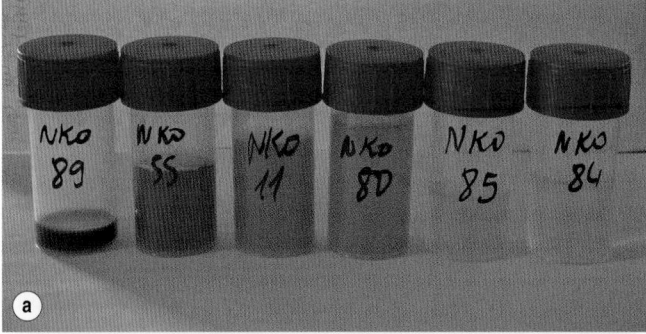

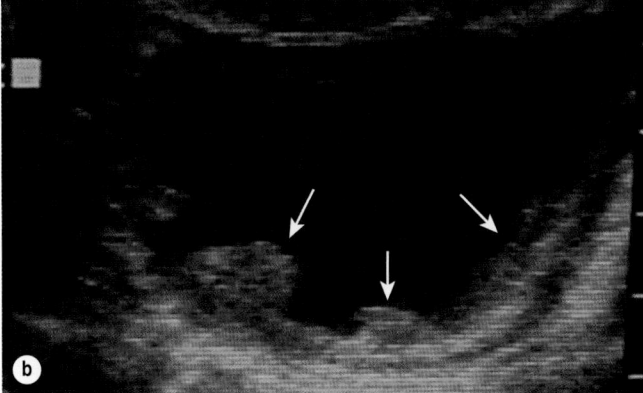

Figure 118-7 Urinary schistosomiasis. (a) Blood in urine samples collected during a school survey in Burkina Faso. (b) Ultrasound image of the bladder wall from a child infected with *S. haematobium*.

Chronic schistosomiasis and its liver and bladder sequelae may develop within months but usually takes 5–10 years after infection depending on the accumulated intensity of infection or the length of exposure to infection. Symptoms, signs and pathologic lesions are species-specific.

Urinary Schistosomiasis, Recently Renamed as Urogenital Schistosomiasis

Urogenital schistosomiasis is caused by infection with *S. haematobium*. Most infected individuals show some symptoms, the most common of which is hematuria (Figure 118-7a). Other early signs include frequency of urination, dysuria and proteinuria. Hematuria in school-aged children in sub-Saharan Africa, although usually present, is not considered important, because it is often unrecognized as a disease symptom. In girls, it may be confused with menstruation; in boys, it may be considered as a sign of puberty in local perception. The prevalence of these symptoms varies according to the degree of endemicity in each local setting but rates of almost 100% in infected children are not unusual. In contrast, hematuria may trigger returning tourists to seek treatment.

Ultrasound examination of the urinary tract in longstanding infections usually indicates thickening of the urinary bladder wall (Figure 118-7b) and granulomas; hydronephrosis and evidence of bladder and ureteric calcification can be seen. Kidney function is usually well preserved, but may be complicated by frequent urinary tract bacterial infection and bladder or ureteric stone formation. There is strong epidemiologic association with squamous bladder cancer, which occurs characteristically in older age groups, especially historically in Egypt, where there is now evidence that with the recent decline of *S. haematobium*, the cancer has decreased.[20]

Intestinal/Hepatic Schistosomiasis

Intestinal/hepatic schistosomiasis is caused by infection with *S. mansoni*, *S. japonicum*, *S. mekongi* or *S. intercalatum*, with most of the reports of the first two species. There is no definitive symptom such as blood in the urine, and so in many cases with light infections, symptoms and signs are nonspecific and unrecognized. In a relatively small proportion of individuals with heavier infections and/or with a long history of exposure, chronic or intermittent abdominal pain and discomfort, loss of appetite and diarrhea with or without blood may be common.

The serious long-term consequences of infection are liver disease that manifests as early inflammatory and late fibrotic stages. The early stage is typified as hepatomegaly due to the granulomatous response – sharp-edged enlargement of the left liver lobe and perhaps splenomegaly. At this stage liver function can be normal. Ultrasound examination may reveal mild forms of diffuse fibrosis. With the progression of the disease, massive deposition of the diffuse collagen deposits in the periportal spaces leads to pathognomonic periportal or Symmer's pipe-stem fibrosis (which is classic *S. mansoni* pathology). This in turn leads to portal hypertension, splenomegaly, collateral venous circulation and esophageal varices. The liver is not necessarily enlarged and may even be shrunk, and liver function tests remain largely unaffected, in contrast to other causes of liver disease. Ultrasonography will reveal typical fibrotic streaks and portal vein dilation. The late stage of liver disease may be associated with extensive splenomegaly, ascites and repeated episodes of hematemesis, which is often fatal (Figure 118-8).

UNUSUAL CONSEQUENCES OF SCHISTOSOMIASIS

Schistosomiasis may also appear in other forms, e.g. pulmonary, genital or neurologic. These are caused by the deposition of schistosome eggs or worms in these organs/systems and subsequent host granulomatous responses. A common and yet only recently recognized complication is female genital schistosomiasis, which is caused by *S. haematobium* infections in women, with up to 75% of those infected having schistosome eggs in the uterine cervix, vagina or vulva. It usually manifests as mucosal grainy sandy patches, mucosal bleeding and inflammation, and later as ulcerative lesions in these genital areas. Investigations have shown that genital schistosomiasis can significantly increase the chances of HIV infection.[21,22]

Another serious possible complication is neurologic schistosomiasis, which can be present in infections with all three main species.[23] Cerebral complications associated with *S. japonicum* can occur during all phases of infection from acute to chronic. These include delirium, loss of consciousness, seizures, dysphasia, visual field impairment, focal motor deficits and ataxia. Spinal complications such as myelopathy are primarily caused by *S. mansoni* but can complicate later stages of *S. haematobium* infection and occur during the acute phase of egg production (see Chapter 111). Severe myelopathy can provoke a complete flaccid paraplegia with areflexia, sphincter dysfunction and sensory disturbances.[24]

Diagnosis

Travelers with nonspecific malaise after visiting Africa need to be questioned about water contact. Apart from blood in the urine, infection with different schistosome species manifests nonspecific clinical features, and therefore a history of possible contact with infested water in endemic areas in tropical or subtropical regions is an important indicator for a suspicion of schistosomiasis.

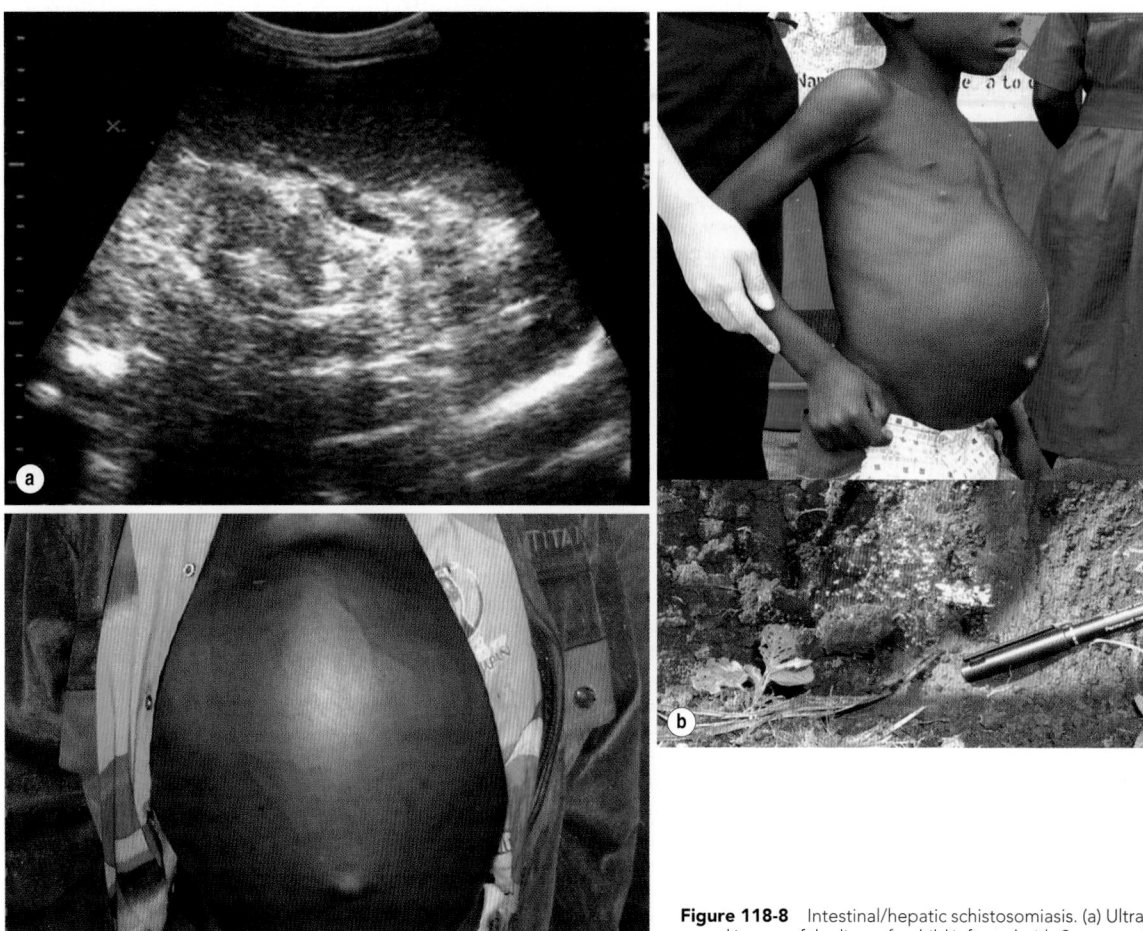

Figure 118-8 Intestinal/hepatic schistosomiasis. (a) Ultrasound image of the liver of a child infected with *S. mansoni*. (b) Advanced case of *S. mansoni* infection of a child with blood in the stool and ascites. (c) Advanced case of *S. mansoni* infection of an adult.

Parasitologic examination of urine (for distinctive eggs of *S. haematobium*) or stool (for *S. mansoni, S. japonicum, S. mekongi* and *S. intercalatum* eggs) by microscopy remains the gold standard for the diagnosis of schistosomiasis (see also Chapter 195). However, it must be noted that in some cases with advanced stage of infection eggs may not be present in urine or stools. Moreover, microscopic examination of stool has a relatively low sensitivity and repeated samples or multiple tests may be required to detect eggs in those with low intensity infections. For *S. haematobium*, urine should preferably be collected around noon, when egg passage is maximal, and generally 10 mL should be concentrated through filtration onto a nitrocellulose filter for examination under a microscope and eggs counted. A less sensitive but useful method for *S. haematobium* is detecting hematuria with a reagent strip that reacts to blood.

For intestinal schistosomes, definitive diagnosis relies on demonstrating eggs in feces; unfortunately, failure to find eggs does not necessarily mean that the individual is uninfected. The most commonly used stool examination method is the Kato–Katz thick smear, which examines 41.7 mg feces in each smear, and enables quantification of the egg load. The intensity of infection is expressed as number of eggs per gram of feces; this is assumed to be proportional to the number of worms.

Serologic tests using schistosome antigens to detect antibodies in urine are more sensitive and more pleasant than stool examination, but for people in regions endemic for schistosomiasis, serology is unable to discriminate between active infection and past exposure. Antigen detection techniques that use labeled monoclonal antibodies to detect circulating anodic antigens or circulating cathodic antigens in serum or urine have been developed. The methods are quantitative and can be used to estimate the worm burden, but they have low sensitivity for light infections.[25]

Clinical diagnosis by ultrasonography of the liver or urinary tract pathology is a valuable tool for longer-term infections. Standard protocols (Niamey protocols)[26] for ultrasound examination have been developed to classify schistosome hepatic fibrosis and urinary tract lesions. It is very useful for evaluating the treatment effect and the reversal of schistosome pathology, but requires specific expertise. In hospital settings, cystoscopy and endoscopy may be used to visualize tissue lesions. Where other methods have failed and schistosomiasis is still suspected, tissue samples may be obtained from rectal mucosa, bladder and liver biopsies, and examined for schistosome eggs.

Management

For the individual patient in the doctor's surgery, treatment of schistosomiasis is relatively inexpensive and safe using praziquantel, which is active against all adult schistosome species at a single oral dose of 40 mg/kg given after food. Praziquantel rarely causes significant side effects; however, in those with heavy worm burdens, abdominal pain, nausea and vomiting may occur.

The World Health Organization has declared that praziquantel is safe for pregnant women and young children (≤4 years of age or ≤94 cm in height). The drug is not effective against eggs and immature worms, and therefore treatment should wait until 2 months after last known exposure. Following a single treatment, 70–100% of individuals cease to excrete eggs in urine or feces; in those not cured, the intensity of infection (egg counts) should be reduced by over 90%.[27]

For acute early cases, which may occur when naïve patients are exposed for the first time to a heavy infection, treatment should be given to suppress the hypersensitivity reaction, and a combination of praziquantel and artemisinin might be given since praziquantel is effective at killing adult worms while artemesinin will kill immature worms that are unaffected by praziquantel. Praziquantel therapy in early chronic infections will result in reversal of pathologies such as hepatomegaly, bladder wall thickening or hydroureters. However, in late stage infections with severe pathologic conditions, such as portal hypertension or extensive hydronephrosis, general medical care will be required. In extreme cases, corrective surgical procedures for portal hypertension or urinary tract anatomic alterations may be necessary.

As a public health problem, in Africa in particular, the World Health Assembly in 2012 passed a resolution (65.21)[18] calling on all member states to proactively implement Mass Drug Administration to reach out to all communities in endemic areas in order to eliminate the morbidity due to schistosomiasis and then proceed to elimination of transmission. The ideal treatment strategy is expected to be annual treatment, based as much on logistics and cost as scientific evidence of speed of re-infection. Some reports of resistance have been recorded but the belief is that resistance by schistosomes to praziquantel is unlikely.[19]

References available online at expertconsult.com.

KEY REFERENCES

65th World Health Assembly: Elimination of schistosomiasis. WHA 65.21. Available: www.who.int/neglected _diseases/mediacentre/WHA_65.21_Eng.pdf.

Carod-Artal F.J.: Neurological complications of *Schistosoma* infection. *Trans R Soc Trop Med Hyg* 2008; 102(2): 107-116.

Colley D.G., Bustinduy A.L., Secor W.E., et al.: Human schistosomiasis. *Lancet* 2014; 83(9936):2253-2264.

Fenwick A., Webster J.P.: Schistosomiasis: challenges for control, treatment and drug resistance. *Curr Opin Infect Dis* 2006; 19(6):577-582.

Kjetland E.F., Leutscher P.D., Ndhlovu P.D.: A review of female genital schistosomiasis. *Trends Parasitol* 2012; 28:58-65.

Ross A.G., Vickers D., Olds G.R., et al.: Katayama syndrome. *Lancet Infect Dis* 2007; 7(3):218-224.

119

Cestode and Trematode Infections

DAVID J. DIEMERT

KEY CONCEPTS

- Cestodes (tapeworms) and trematodes (flukes) are ubiquitous flatworms that mostly cause zoonotic infections, although humans can be incidentally parasitized. The adult beef and pork tapeworms (*Taenia saginata* and *Taenia solium*, respectively) are the exception, with humans being the exclusive definitive hosts for both.

- Neurocysticercosis, caused by infection by the larval stage of *Taenia solium*, is a leading preventable cause of seizures worldwide.

- Treatment of viable intraparenchymal cysticercal cysts should include directed antiparasitic medication in combination with systemic corticosteroids. Management of extraparenchymal cysts should be referred to experienced specialists in infectious diseases and neurosurgery.

- *Clonorchis sinensis*, *Opisthorchis felineus* and *Opisthorchis viverrini* are the three most important food-borne liver flukes worldwide, affecting over 45 million people, and can induce cholangiocarcinoma as well as other hepatobiliary pathology.

- Infection with the lung fluke, *Paragonimus westermani*, occurs after ingestion of shellfish contaminated with larval forms of the parasite and is found throughout eastern Asia. It is associated with chronic pulmonary disease that can be confused with active tuberculosis.

Introduction

Cestodes (tapeworms) and trematodes (flukes) are ubiquitous flatworms that are capable of infecting both vertebrates and invertebrates. The life cycles of both types of helminth are complex and are characterized by morphologically distinct developmental stages of the parasite being harbored by different host species (see Figure 119-1 for the representative flatworm life cycle of *T. solium*). Most of these worms are restricted in the range of host species that they can infect, particularly the definitive host of the adult reproductive worms. From among the large number of parasitic flatworms, humans are the preferred host of only a few, although more are capable of causing incidental (paratenic) human infection.

Despite this variety, the life cycles of the flatworms that infect humans have several features in common:
- all trematodes undergo asexual reproduction in aquatic snails, the intermediate host, and sexual reproduction in a definitive mammalian host;
- the geographic distribution of infections with the various host flukes corresponds to the range of their intermediate snail host;
- when eggs passed in the waste products (usually feces) of a definitive host infected with an adult fluke come into contact with fresh water, they hatch to release larvae that then infect snails.

Flukes are categorized according to where they reside in the human host: blood flukes (*Schistosoma* species), intestinal flukes (*Fasciolopsis*), liver flukes (*Clonorchis*, *Opisthorchis* and *Fasciola*) and lung flukes (*Paragonimus*). In the case of schistosomiasis, larvae (referred to as cercariae) released by snails penetrate skin or mucous membranes that come into contact with infected water. Other human trematode

parasites cause infection through consumption of food – usually a form of fish or seafood – contaminated with encysted intermediate stages (metacercariae). They are mainly found throughout the tropics and subtropics, although a few species are also found in temperate climates.

Adult cestodes are tapeworms that are parasitic in the intestinal tracts of various vertebrate hosts. Intermediate hosts become infected by oral ingestion of eggs that develop into a cystic larval form in host tissues. The life cycle is completed when these infected tissues are eaten by a suitable definitive host. Tapeworms are flat, segmented worms, composed of a head (scolex) and a series of symmetric segments, known as proglottids. The scolex may be equipped with hooks, suckers or elongated grooves to facilitate attachment to the host's intestine. Each proglottid possesses a complete set of both male and female reproductive organs; sperm are typically transferred between adjacent segments, giving rise to gravid proglottids that contain thousands of embryonated eggs. Gravid segments detach from the parent worm and either exit intact via the feces, or disintegrate before leaving the host, releasing embryonated eggs. Cestodes lack a functional digestive tract; the tegument, or body covering, serves as a metabolically active layer

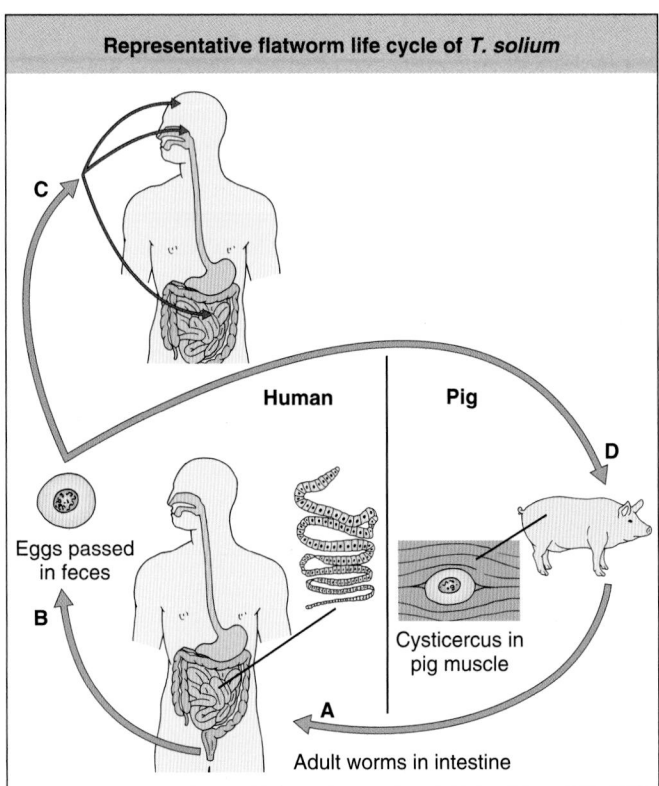

Figure 119-1 Representative flatworm life cycle of *Taenia solium*. (A) Humans ingest raw or undercooked meat from an infected pig containing cysticerci that develop into adult tapeworms in the host intestine. (B) Eggs or gravid proglottid segments are passed in feces and contaminate the environment. (C) Eggs are ingested by humans, releasing oncospheres that penetrate the intestinal wall and disseminate, especially to the brain, subcutaneous tissues and eyes where they encyst to form cysticerci. (D) Eggs can also be ingested by pigs, resulting in cysticerci in pig muscles.

through which nutrients are absorbed. Although adult tapeworms do not cause much pathology, the encysted larval forms of cestode parasites (termed cysticerci) often have serious adverse consequences for the intermediate human host, especially neurocysticercosis caused by the larval stages of the pork tapeworm, *Taenia solium*.

Schistosomiasis is discussed in Chapter 118 and echinococcosis in Chapter 120.

Cestode Infections

Tapeworm Infections

TAENIASIS

For both the beef tapeworm, *Taenia saginata* (Figure 119-2), and the pork tapeworm, *T. solium* (Figure 119-1), humans are the exclusive definitive hosts. Infection is acquired by eating raw or undercooked beef or pork, respectively, that contains living cysticerci. The clinical consequences of taeniasis are usually mild and are limited to minor abdominal symptoms, such as epigastric discomfort, nausea and vomiting with *T. saginata*, and abdominal pain, distention and diarrhea with *T. solium*. *T. saginata* proglottids may migrate spontaneously from the anus, causing considerable alarm in the host. *Taenia* spp. do not appear to have any significant nutritional effect on their host. The principal complication of infection with *T. solium* is that eggs may be passed in the feces and subsequently be ingested and cause cysticercosis (see below) either in the same host or in others living in close proximity.

DIPHYLLOBOTHRIASIS

Diphyllobothrium latum is the longest parasite that infects humans: adult worms can achieve a length of more than 10 m (33 feet) in the small intestine. Maintenance of the life cycle of *D. latum* requires that feces of infected hosts be discarded into fresh water that contains the appropriate crustacean and fish intermediate hosts and that the infected fish be eaten raw by definitive hosts. Although *D. latum* was previously a common infection in Scandinavia, the incidence there has been reduced markedly because of improved sanitation, so that most cases now occur in Russia, Brazil and Japan.[1] Humans are the most important definitive host for this tapeworm, although bears, dogs and other carnivores may serve as reservoir hosts. Adult worms cause

minimal clinical disease, although they may compete with the host for absorption of vitamin B12 from the intestinal lumen and cause megaloblastic anemia, although this is now rarely seen. Various other *Diphyllobothrium* spp. that usually occur in wild animals may infect humans incidentally, principally in the sub-Arctic and the northern Pacific areas. Clinical consequences of these infections are relatively minor.

HYMENOLEPIASIS

Infection with the dwarf tapeworm (so-called because of its small size) *Hymenolepis nana* occurs worldwide, mostly in children living in conditions with poor sanitation. Rodents are the principal animal reservoir. Infection is acquired either by ingestion of embryonated eggs (from rodents or humans) or an infected insect containing cysticercoid metacestodes. Ingested eggs hatch in the small intestine, releasing larvae that penetrate the lamina propria of the small bowel epithelium where they differentiate into cysticercoids that re-enter the intestinal lumen and attach to the surface of the villous tissue. These develop into new tapeworms approximately 4 cm in length. If an intact cysticercus is ingested, it attaches directly to the small intestinal wall and matures into an adult worm. Although most infections are asymptomatic, heavy infections may result in diarrhea.

ZOONOTIC TAPEWORMS

Several tapeworms that are not primarily adapted to humans may nevertheless cause incidental human infection after accidental exposure. *Hymenolepis diminuta* is a tapeworm of rodents that uses their fleas as an intermediate host. Similarly, *Dipylidium caninum* passes between dogs and their fleas. Both are occasional sources of human infection worldwide, principally in children, through the accidental ingestion of fleas. There are no known serious clinical consequences with either tapeworm infection.

DIAGNOSIS AND MANAGEMENT OF TAPEWORM INFECTIONS

Diagnosis of tapeworm infection is made by microscopic identification of characteristic eggs in the feces, although the species cannot be determined based on morphology since members of the genera *Taenia* and *Diphyllobothrium* produce identically shaped eggs (Figure 119-3). Speciation can be made by examination of entire proglottids which may sometimes be found in the feces. Treatment with a single dose of

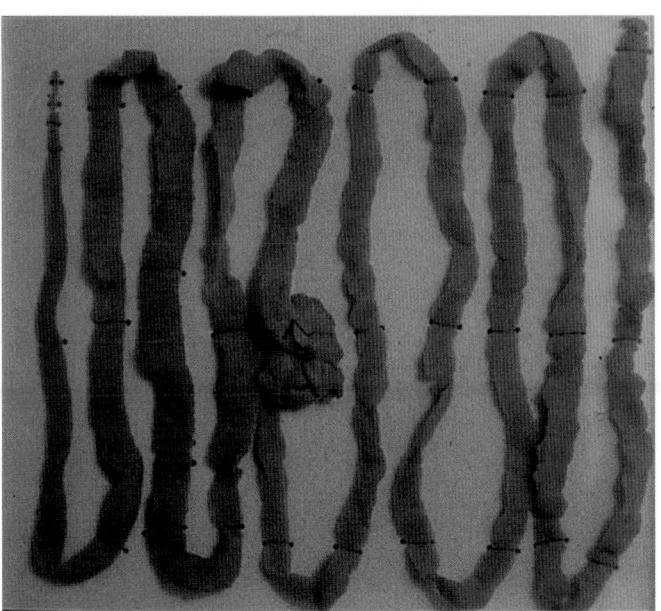

Figure 119-2 *Taenia saginata*. A mature worm may be up to 10 m (33 feet) long. *(Courtesy of Guy Baily.)*

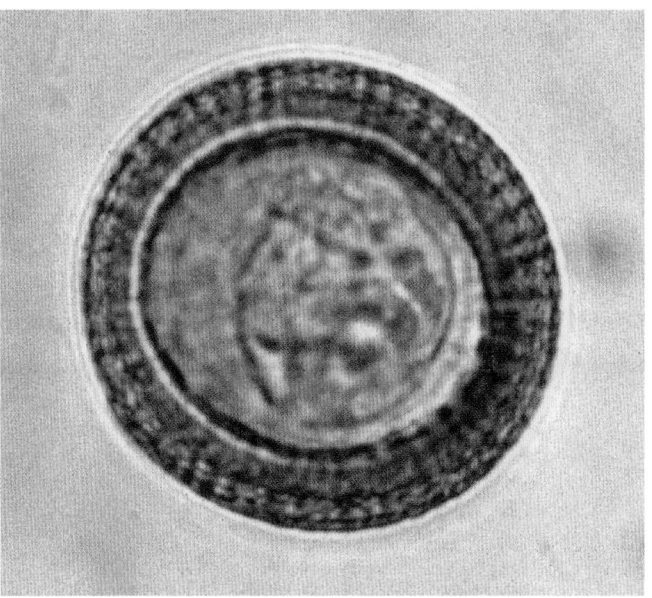

Figure 119-3 *Taenia* egg. Speciation cannot be done based on morphology. Eggs measure between 30 and 40 μm in diameter.

praziquantel at 10 mg/kg is effective for all human tapeworms except *H. nana*, for which at least 25 mg/kg should be administered.[2] Care should be taken to rule out cysticercosis, as praziquantel may induce seizures or other symptoms as a result of an inflammatory response to dying cysticerci (see below).

Cysticercosis

EPIDEMIOLOGY AND PREVENTION

Cysticercosis results from the oral ingestion of eggs of the pork tapeworm *T. solium*. Although food or water contaminated with human feces can be the source of the tapeworm eggs, evidence indicates that the most common source is an asymptomatic tapeworm carrier in the household (Figure 119-1).[3] Autoinfection may also occur in individuals harboring adult tapeworms in their intestines. Infected pigs serve to perpetuate the infection: pigs have access to contaminated human feces by their coexistence with humans in the domestic setting and the lack of adequate sanitation and sewage facilities. Cysticercosis remains endemic in most low-income countries, especially in Latin America and Asia (particularly China and South East Asia).[4] The World Health Assembly in 2003 recommended several measures to control *T. solium* infection with the aim of reducing the incidence of neurocysticercosis, including mass or selected treatment with praziquantel to reduce the prevalence of adult worm infection in endemic areas, improved pig husbandry, enforced meat inspection and control, and treatment of infected animals.[5]

PATHOGENESIS

After ingestion, *T. solium* ova hatch upon exposure to gastric acid and intestinal enzymes, releasing oncospheres (embryos) that invade the intestinal wall, enter the vasculature and migrate to host tissues where they develop into larval cysts. In most tissues, cysts are eliminated by the host's immune system, except for sites such as the central nervous system and the eye, which are immunologically privileged, and both striated and cardiac muscle where development to the cysticercus stage is rapid. Cysts are normally approximately 1 cm in diameter and consist of a larval scolex that is surrounded by a vesicle formed by extension of the parasite's tegument, all of which is encased by a host-derived capsule.

Cysts can be found in any part of the central nervous system, although the majority are located in the brain parenchyma, where they initially form viable vesicles that may remain alive for years. However, the host's immune system eventually prevails and the cysticercus dies, a process called involution. First, the vesicular fluid becomes turbid and a thick collagen capsule forms around the dying cyst together with diffuse edema (colloidal stage). The scolex then shows signs of degenerating into coarse granules (granular stage), corresponding to resolution of the surrounding edema and eventual formation of a calcified nodule that represents a dead cysticercus. The significant clinical consequences of cysticercosis are primarily related to the neurologic involvement of this infection (Figure 119-4).

CLINICAL FEATURES

Most of the morbidity and mortality due to this infection is caused by neurocysticercosis, with seizures and sequelae of raised intracranial pressure being the most common clinical manifestations. Symptomatic neurocysticercosis results from a combination of factors, including the number, stage and location of the cysts, together with the severity of the host's immune response against the parasites. As many as 70% of individuals with neurocysticercosis will present with seizures.[6] Other manifestations include those of intracranial hypertension (focal signs, altered mental status and seizures), caused primarily by hydrocephalus but also rarely by cysticercotic encephalitis due to a massive inflammatory response to multiple parenchymal cysticerci resulting in diffuse cerebral edema. Hydrocephalus occurs most commonly with cysts that are located in the ventricles or subarachnoid space. If untreated, hydrocephalus may lead to permanent loss of cerebral function with dementia and cortical blindness. Various focal neurologic

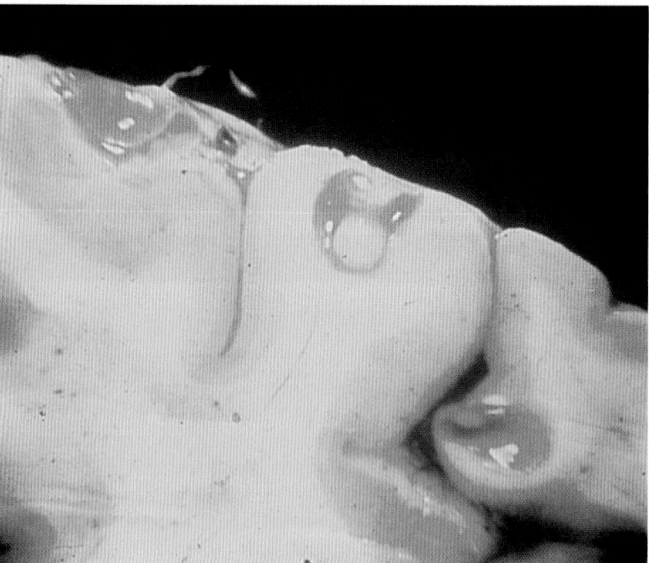

Figure 119-4 Cysticerci in the brain. *(Courtesy of Guy Baily.)*

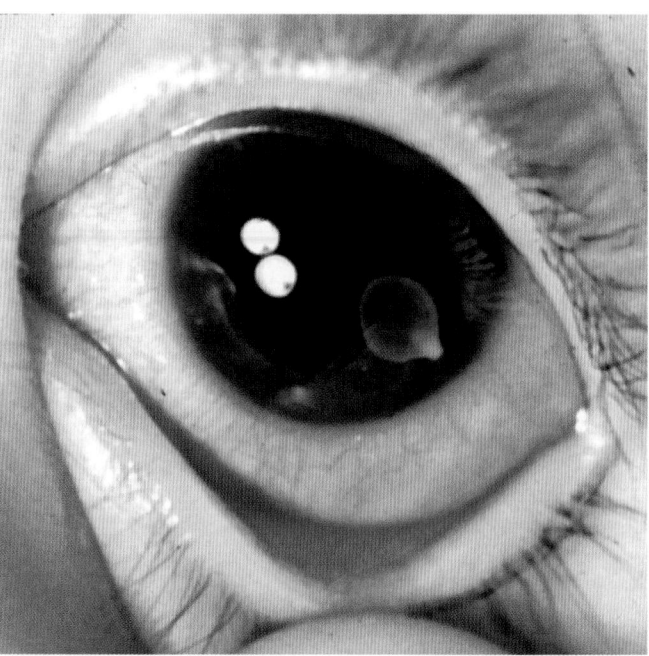

Figure 119-5 Cysticercus of *Taenia solium* floating in the anterior chamber of the eye.

findings may also occur and usually follow a subacute or chronic course, although acute signs may arise due to a stroke.

Ophthalmic cysticercosis is not uncommon and typically manifests as intraocular cysts floating freely in the vitreous or the subretinal space, where they give rise to visual field defects or scotomata (Figure 119-5). Development of uveitis or retinitis may result in permanent loss of vision.

Extraneural cysticercosis is usually asymptomatic and consists initially of nontender subcutaneous nodules or discrete swellings of particular muscles in which cysticerci have embedded. Several months after initially being noticed, the nodules may swell and become tender as the cysts begin to involute and die. Ultimately, the cysts will calcify; subcutaneous and intramuscular calcifications may persist for years after cysticercal death.

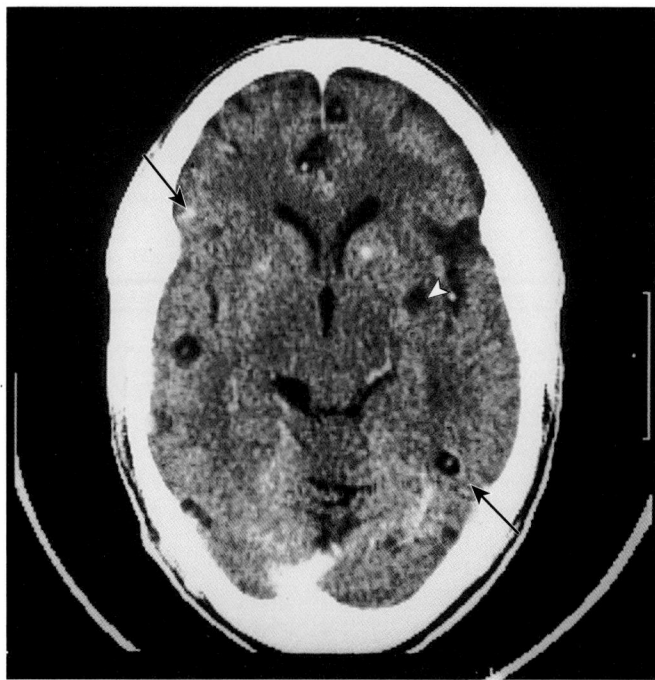

Figure 119-6   CT image of neurocysticercosis. Viable cysts appear as radiolucent defects (arrowhead). The central protoscolex may be visualized as a radiodense spot (bottom right arrow). Cysts that show ring enhancement are probably degenerating. Calcified cysts (top left arrow) are dead and will not benefit from specific therapy. *(Courtesy of Guy Baily.)*

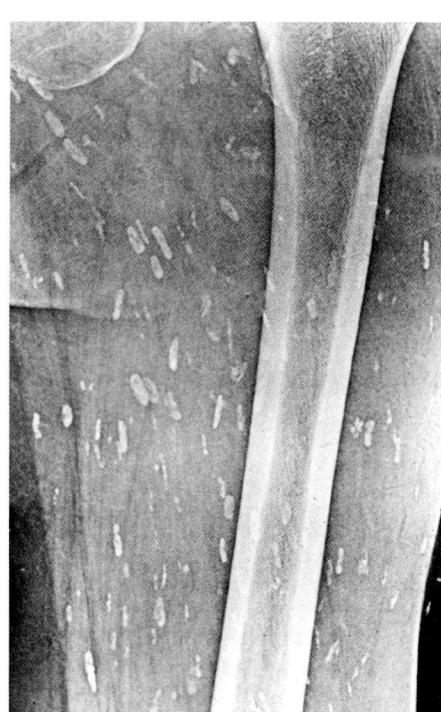

Figure 119-7   Plain radiograph of lower leg with numerous calcified cysticerci of *Taenia solium*.

DIAGNOSIS

Diagnosis of neurocysticercosis is usually made on the basis of imaging studies – computed tomography (CT) or magnetic resonance imaging (MRI) – and confirmatory serology. Although MRI has better accuracy in making a diagnosis – especially for cysts in the ventricles or basal cisterns – CT is more commonly used in most endemic areas. On CT, viable cysts appear as hypodense lesions whereas degenerating cysts appear as contrast-enhancing lesions with a surrounding ring of edema (Figure 119-6). The scolex may sometimes be visualized in the interior of viable cysts, but usually not in degenerating ones. After involution, the edema resolves, leaving a calcified nodule. The most commonly used serologic test is the enzyme-linked immunoelectrotransfer blot developed by the Centers for Disease Control and Prevention that detects antibodies reactive with glycoproteins derived from *T. solium* cysts. This assay has a specificity of 100% and reported overall sensitivity of 98%, although the sensitivity is considerably lower for individuals with only a solitary enhancing parenchymal cyst.[7]

Occasionally, evidence of extracranial cysticercosis may aid in the diagnosis, particularly direct visualization of ophthalmic cysticerci, palpation of subcutaneous cysticerci or evidence of cigar-shaped intramuscular calcifications seen on plain radiography (Figure 119-7). A set of diagnostic criteria has been formulated to aid in the diagnosis of neurocysticercosis, which permits classification as either definitive or probable disease.[8]

MANAGEMENT

Treatment of neurocysticercosis consists of a combination of antiparasitic and symptomatic modalities and should involve specialists in infectious diseases, neurology, neuroimaging and neurosurgery. Antiparasitic measures include cysticidal medications (albendazole or praziquantel) and surgical resection of cysts, whereas symptomatic interventions can include antiepileptics, analgesics and placement of ventricular shunts.[9]

There has been considerable controversy over the use of cysticidal medications, mostly because treatment-associated parasite death can lead to an acute inflammatory reaction in the surrounding brain tissue, which can result in seizures, raised intracranial pressure and even death. However, cumulative evidence has demonstrated that treatment of viable intraparenchymal cysts results in reduced numbers of seizures and faster resolution of cysts.[10] Although single enhancing lesions may resolve spontaneously,[11] studies support the value of administering cysticidal treatment.[12] Albendazole (15 mg/kg daily for 7 days, although recent data suggests improved benefit of increasing the dose to 30 mg/kg daily) is preferred over praziquantel (100 mg/kg daily in three doses for 15 days) because of its higher cysticidal effect and the fact that serum concentrations of praziquantel are decreased with concomitant use of corticosteroids. For patients with multiple viable intraparenchymal cysticerci, a recent randomized, controlled trial demonstrated a marked increased parasiticidal effect with combination albendazole and praziquantel administered at standard doses.[13] Corticosteroids should be administered together with cysticidal treatment to reduce the headache, vomiting and other complications that may result from the inflammation induced by dying intraparenchymal parasites, whether single or multiple.

Cysticercotic encephalitis should not be treated with cysticidal drugs because this may result in increased intracranial pressure. Treatment for this condition is with high-dose steroids and diuretics. Cysticidal treatment is also not indicated for individuals with calcified lesions alone since these represent degenerated parasites.

Treatment of extraparenchymal cysts is considerably more complex and should be managed by a multidisciplinary team that includes specialists in infectious diseases and neurosurgery. Subarachnoid and Sylvian fissure cysts should be treated with cysticidal drugs and high-dose steroids, although placement of a ventricular shunt should be performed first in cases with hydrocephalus. Ventricular cysts may be amenable to excision via surgery or neuroendoscopy; adjunct antiparasitic treatment is controversial.

Other Larval Cestode Infections

COENUROSIS

Humans are occasionally accidentally infected with the metacestode (juvenile stage) of *Taenia multiceps*, *T. brauni*, *T. serialis* or *T. glomerata*, the adult forms of which normally infect dogs. Intermediate

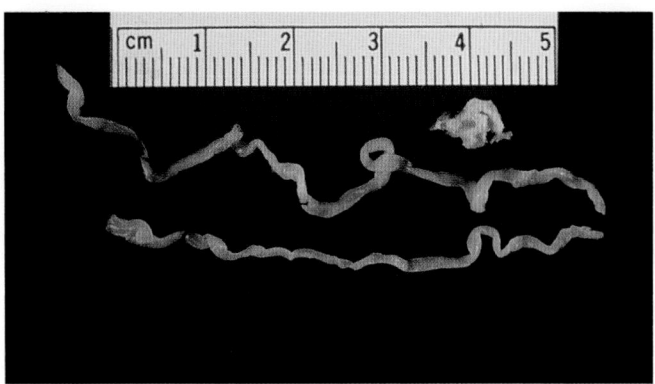

Figure 119-8 Sparganum worm dissected from an inguinal mass. (*Courtesy of Guy Baily.*)

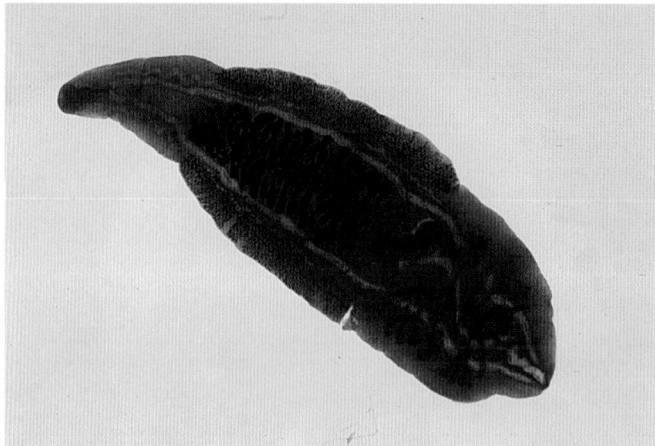

Figure 119-9 An adult liver fluke (*Clonorchis sinensis*). The worm is typically about 2 cm in length. (*Courtesy of Guy Baily.*)

hosts include cattle, sheep and rodents. Metacestodes, known as coenuri, are released from eggs ingested in contaminated water or food. These penetrate the intestinal wall and migrate to subcutaneous tissues and in the case of *T. multiceps*, to the central nervous system (CNS) where they can form large cysts, usually 2–5 cm in diameter, with multiple invaginated protoscolices. CNS disease can present with headache, seizures, hemiparesis, or hydrocephalus, and is frequently fatal.

Human cases are rare and largely occur in Africa, although infections have been reported worldwide. Diagnostic criteria include epidemiologic, clinical, radiologic and biopsy findings; serology is not available. Treatment usually involves surgical excision if the cyst is accessible, although anthelmintic therapy with albendazole and praziquantel has been successful in some patients.[14]

SPARGANOSIS

Infection by the migratory plerocercoid larvae of the cestodes *Spirometra mansonoides* and other *Spirometra* spp. is termed sparganosis. Whereas dogs and cats are the definitive hosts there are two intermediate stages, the first in small crustaceans and the second in reptiles, amphibians, birds and some mammals. Humans become infected by eating the raw or undercooked flesh of an intermediate host such as frog or snake, or from using the skin or flesh of such animals as a poultice for wounds or sore eyes, as is practiced in parts of eastern Asia. *Spirometra* cannot complete its life cycle in humans, but instead larvae remain trapped in various tissues such as the brain.

Clinically, a localized subcutaneous inflammatory swelling forms from entry of the larva into host tissue, which can slowly migrate and contains a single worm-like sparganum (Figure 119-8). If the worm enters via a dressing placed over the eye, migration into the brain may occur along the optic nerve, with devastating results. Treatment consists of surgical excision.

Trematode Infections

Liver Fluke Infections

EPIDEMIOLOGY

Clonorchis sinensis, Opisthorchis viverrini and *Opisthorchis felineus* are three closely related species that produce similar clinical manifestations in humans. *C. sinensis* (Figure 119-9) is the most common of the three, with over 35 million people infected in China, Japan, Korea, Taiwan and eastern Russia. *O. viverrini* is endemic in northern Thailand, Laos, Cambodia and southern Vietnam, whereas opisthorchiasis due to *O. felineus* occurs in Kazakhstan, Russia and Ukraine.[15] All three species are acquired by ingesting raw or undercooked freshwater fish or crab harboring metacercariae, with dogs and cats serving as the most common reservoir hosts. Adult worms living in definitive hosts produce eggs that are excreted in feces. Eggs that reach fresh water are

eaten by the intermediate aquatic snail host, in which the miracidia hatch and develop; motile cercariae subsequently released from the snails encyst under the scales of appropriate freshwater fish or crustaceae, completing the life cycle.

PATHOGENESIS AND PATHOLOGY

Ingested larvae excyst in the small intestine and transform into immature flukes that migrate into the biliary tract, where they develop into hermaphroditic adult flukes that begin producing eggs after about 4 weeks. Adult worms may survive for decades within the small bile ducts of the liver, where they feed on epithelium. Pathologic consequences arise from the mechanical injury and eosinophilic inflammatory reaction caused by adult worms present in the bile ducts. Over time, heavy infections lead to desquamation of the biliary epithelium, leading to hyperplasia, and eventual fibrosis or metaplastic changes that are a precursor to developing cholangiocarcinoma. Infection with either *C. sinensis* or *O. viverrini* is one of the strongest predictors of developing cholangiocarcinoma, with an associated fivefold increase in risk.[16]

CLINICAL FEATURES

Most individuals with liver flukes are only infected with a few worms and are asymptomatic. Heavier infections may be associated with nonspecific epigastric or right upper quadrant pain, nausea, anorexia and diarrhea.[17] Heavy infections are also associated with recurrent ascending cholangitis and pancreatitis due to secondary bacterial infection and stone formation in chronically infected, fibrosed bile ducts.

DIAGNOSIS AND MANAGEMENT

Eggs of liver flukes can be detected by microscopic examination of a concentrated sample of feces; differentiation between the eggs of the various species is often difficult. Eosinophilia and elevated levels of serum IgE are often present in heavy infections. On ultrasound, aggregates of flukes may be visualized as echogenic foci within bile ducts. Treatment with praziquantel 75 mg/kg/day in three doses for 2 days is highly effective, as is albendazole 10 mg/kg/day for 7 days.

Fascioliasis

Humans are occasionally infected with the sheep liver fluke, *Fasciola hepatica* (Figure 119-10), or the closely related cattle fluke, *F. gigantica*. Both are acquired by ingesting water or leafy wild plants that grow in standing bodies of fresh water and that are contaminated with cercariae released from the intermediate aquatic snail host. *F. hepatica* is found worldwide, with the highest prevalence reported in Bolivia and Peru, whereas *F. gigantica* is endemic in Africa and Asia.[18] After excysting in the small intestine, metacercariae penetrate the intestinal wall

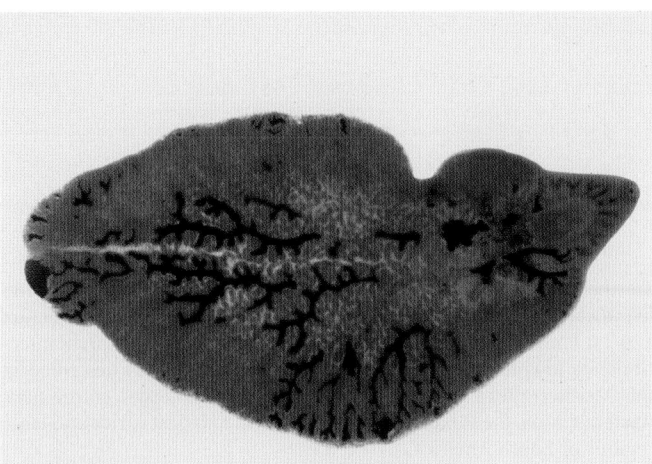

Figure 119-10   A typical adult *Fasciola hepatica*, measuring 30 × 14 μm.

and migrate to the surface of the liver which they invade to enter the parenchymal tissue. Migration of the immature worms to the liver can be associated with acute fever, eosinophilia and painful hepatomegaly that usually subside within a month. Ingested metacercariae occasionally migrate to tissues other than the liver such as the brain or kidney, where they may present as a small mass lesion. Chronic infection may be associated with features of intermittent biliary obstruction, including cholangitis, stones and pancreatitis.

Microscopic identification of eggs in the feces is the definitive method of diagnosis, although the sensitivity can be low because eggs are produced only intermittently. Imaging by ultrasound, CT, or MRI may reveal hepatic or biliary involvement. Diagnosis can also be made using serology (an ELISA), even in the acute stage of infection before the appearance of eggs in the feces, although there is some cross-reactivity with antigens of other trematodes.[19] *Fasciola* is the only human flatworm that is not effectively treated with praziquantel. Triclabendazole is the recommended treatment, and is available in the USA from the Centers for Disease Control and Prevention through an investigational protocol. It is given as a single oral dose of 10 mg/kg, although some experts recommend a second dose in cases of heavy infection. Serology should revert to normal within 6–12 months following treatment, assuming no re-infection. Fecal examination should be repeated 3 months after treatment and, if positive, a second dose of triclabendazole is recommended.[20]

Lung Fluke Infections
EPIDEMIOLOGY
The lung fluke, *Paragonimus westermani*, is found throughout eastern Asia and infects a wide variety of mammalian reservoir hosts. Numerous fresh water crustaceans such as crabs and crayfish serve as intermediate hosts and infection occurs when these are eaten raw or lightly cooked. Several other members of the *Paragonimus* genus routinely cause human infection, mostly in areas of eastern Asia, central and western Africa, and Latin America. A cluster of cases of North American paragonimiasis, caused by *Paragonimus kellicotti*, and associated with ingestion of raw crayfish has been recently described in the mid-west USA.[21]

PATHOGENESIS AND PATHOLOGY
Ingested metacercariae excyst in the small intestine and penetrate into the abdominal cavity where they develop into immature flukes before crossing the diaphragm to enter the lungs and mature into reproductive adults within 2–3 months. Pairs of *P. westermani* worms live within a host-derived fibrous capsule at the periphery of the lungs. Pathology results from the local effects of established adult worms and the surrounding inflammatory reaction characterized by eosinophilic infiltration. Occasionally, worms develop in ectopic sites such as the brain, muscle, liver or skin. Other species of *Paragonimus* can cause significant tissue damage as the larvae migrate through the viscera.

CLINICAL FEATURES
Adult *P. westermani* worms may cause progressive disease characterized by chronic cough that is productive of blood-tinged sputum. Complications include recurrent bacterial pneumonia, lung abscess, empyema and pneumothorax. Larval migration due to non-*P. westermani* species, especially in Asia, may give rise to migratory subcutaneous nodules and more seriously to an eosinophilic meningitis.[22]

DIAGNOSIS AND MANAGEMENT
Diagnosis is by microscopic identification of eggs in the sputum or feces (due to swallowed sputum). Chest radiography may reveal cavitary disease that must be distinguished from lung abscess due to other causes, especially tuberculosis. Eosinophilia is common, especially during the acute phase of infection. Serologic tests for *P. westermani* are available and may be useful in differentiating disease from tuberculosis. Praziquantel at a dose of 75 mg/kg in three divided doses for 2 days is the drug of choice and is effective against extrapulmonary disease; triclabendazole may be used as an alternative.

Intestinal Fluke Infections
Over 70 species of intestinal flukes have been reported to infect humans, but most cases are due to *Fasciolopsis buski*, *Echinostoma*, *Heterophyes* and *Metagonimus* species. All are found throughout eastern Asia, whereas *Heterophyes* is also found in the Middle East and North Africa. All are zoonoses and infect humans only incidentally; for *F. buski* the reservoir hosts include pigs and dogs. Humans acquire infection by consuming contaminated aquatic plants (especially bamboo shoots and water chestnuts for *F. buski*) or fish (*Echinostoma*, *Metagonimus* and *Heterophyes*). Infections are usually asymptomatic, although heavier infections can result in diarrhea alternating with constipation, abdominal pain, nausea and vomiting. Intestinal obstruction or malabsorption may develop in the most severe cases.

Diagnosis is based on identification of characteristic operculated eggs on microscopic examination of feces. The treatment of choice for all intestinal flukes is praziquantel 75 mg/kg in three divided doses given in one day.

References available online at expertconsult.com.

KEY REFERENCES

Baird R.A., Wiebe S., Zunt J.R., et al.: Evidence-based guideline: treatment of parenchymal neurocysticercosis: report of the Guideline Development Subcommittee of the American Academy of Neurology. *Neurology* 2013; 80:1424-1429.

Cabada M.M., White A.C. Jr: New developments in epidemiology, diagnosis, and treatment of fascioliasis. *Curr Opin Infect Dis* 2012; 25:518-522.

Dick T.A., Nelson P.A., Choudhury A.: Diphyllobothriasis: update on human cases, foci patterns and sources of human infections and future considerations. *Southeast Asian J Trop Med Public Health* 2001; 32(Suppl. 2): 59-76.

Garcia H.H., Del Brutto O.H., Cysticercosis Working Group in Peru: Neurocysticercosis: updated concepts about an old disease. *Lancet Neurol* 2005; 4:653-661.

Garcia H.H., Gonzales I., Lescano A.G., et al.: Efficacy of combined antiparasitic therapy with praziquantel and albendazole for neurocysticercosis: a double-blind, randomised controlled trial. *Lancet Infect Dis* 2014; 14:687-695.

Lescano A.G., Zunt J.: Other cestodes: sparganosis, coenurosis and *Taenia crassiceps* cysticercosis. *Handb Clin Neurol* 2013; 114:335-345.

Otte W.M., Singla M., Sander J.W., et al.: Drug therapy for solitary cysticercus granuloma: a systematic review and meta-analysis. *Neurology* 2013; 80:152-162.

Petney T.N., Andrews R.H., Saijuntha W., et al.: The zoonotic, fish-borne liver flukes *Clonorchis sinensis*, *Opisthorchis felineus* and *Opisthorchis viverrini*. *Int J Parasitol* 2013; 43:1031-1046.

Villegas F., Angles R., Barrientos R., et al.: Administration of triclabendazole is safe and effective in controlling fascioliasis in an endemic community of the Bolivian Altiplano. *PLoS Negl Trop Dis* 2012; 6:e1720.

120

Echinococcosis

BRUNO GOTTSTEIN | GUIDO BELDI

Epidemiology

Echinococcus spp. are cestode parasites, commonly known as small tapeworms, that parasitize the small intestine of animal carnivores. Their medical importance is due to the ability of the larval stages to infect humans. Within the genus, there are two species that are responsible for the majority of severe clinical problems around the world:

- *Echinococcus granulosus*, which is the causative agent of cystic echinococcosis (CE)
- *Echinococcus multilocularis*, which causes alveolar echinococcosis (AE).

In addition. *E. equinus, E. ortleppi, E. vogeli, E. oligarthrus* and *E. shiquicus* have rarely been associated with human disease. CE and AE differ profoundly in their clinical manifestations and disease progress; therefore they are described separately in the subsections below.

ECHINOCOCCUS GRANULOSUS

Infections with *E. granulosus* occur on all populated continents, predominantly in countries with large pastoral and rangeland areas. Dogs are the main definitive hosts of the G1/G2 strain *E. granulosus* and livestock, particularly sheep, are the main intermediate hosts (Figure 120-1). The G1/2 strain of the parasite accounts for most human infections worldwide. High prevalences of G1/G2 have been described in the Mediterranean basin, the Near and Middle East, central Asia, western China, the Russian Federation, North and East Africa and large regions of South America.

While other species and genotypes (e.g. *E. ortleppi*; G3-G10) previously classified as *E. granulosus* can also infect humans, they will not be further discussed in this chapter due to their rare occurrence.

The main risk factors for human infection with *E. granulosus* include: living or working in pastoral areas; dog ownership and presence of stray dogs; uncontrolled slaughtering and access of carnivores to raw inappropriately discarded viscera; and poor environmental and water hygiene.[1-5] In some countries (e.g. Kenya, China, Argentina, Peru) incidence can reach 50 CE cases per 100 000 persons/year. In highly affected areas of such countries (Turkana district in Kenya, Tibetan and Kazakh parts of China), disease prevalence can reach 5% or even more.

ECHINOCOCCUS MULTILOCULARIS

The definitive hosts of *E. multilocularis* are foxes and raccoons (Figure 120-2). Domestic dogs are also susceptible and are an important infection source for humans in highly endemic areas. In the definitive host, egg production starts as early as 28 days after infection. Eggs are infectious to intermediate hosts, and small rodents play a crucial role in maintaining the life cycle. Other intermediate hosts include animals such as beavers, pigs and dogs, and humans, where primary larval maturation of the parasite (the so-called metacestode) occurs within the liver (see Figure 120-2). Subsequent metastases can affect adjacent or distant organs, including the lungs, brain and bones. Proliferation of the metacestode occurs by exogenous budding of small conglomerated parasite vesicles. The metacestode tissue can resemble that of a progressively infiltrating tumor. Central necrosis may develop broadening the differential diagnosis.

E. multilocularis is restricted to the northern hemisphere. In North America, it occurs in the northern tundra zone of Alaska, USA and Canada. Recent reports document that the parasite now affects the southern half of three provinces in Canada (Manitoba, Saskatchewan and Alberta) and 13 contiguous states in the USA.[6] In Europe, AE has been recognized in humans in eastern France, Switzerland, Austria and southern Germany for more than 10 decades at a constant annual incidence rate. In the past 15 years, however, the European endemic area has dramatically expanded, to include the Baltic states, Poland, Slovakia, Romania and Slovenia among others.[7] This increase in wildlife prevalence has been explained by the increase of the European fox population as a result of the successful control of rabies by vaccination. In tandem, there has been an increase in the incidence of new human AE cases in several European countries.[8-10] In Asia *E. multilocularis* occurs across the tundra, from the White Sea eastward to the Bering Strait, covering large parts of Russia, Kazakhstan, Mongolia, China and northern Japan.

While AE in Europe is principally considered a rare disease, with average incidences of 0.03 to 0.30/100 000 inhabitants/year, these figures do not reflect the actual population at risk of hyperendemic regions, where far higher incidences, from 4.7 to 8.1 cases per 100 000 inhabitants/year are observed.[11] Globally, AE causes an annual loss of approximately 660 000 disability-adjusted life years.[12] The global

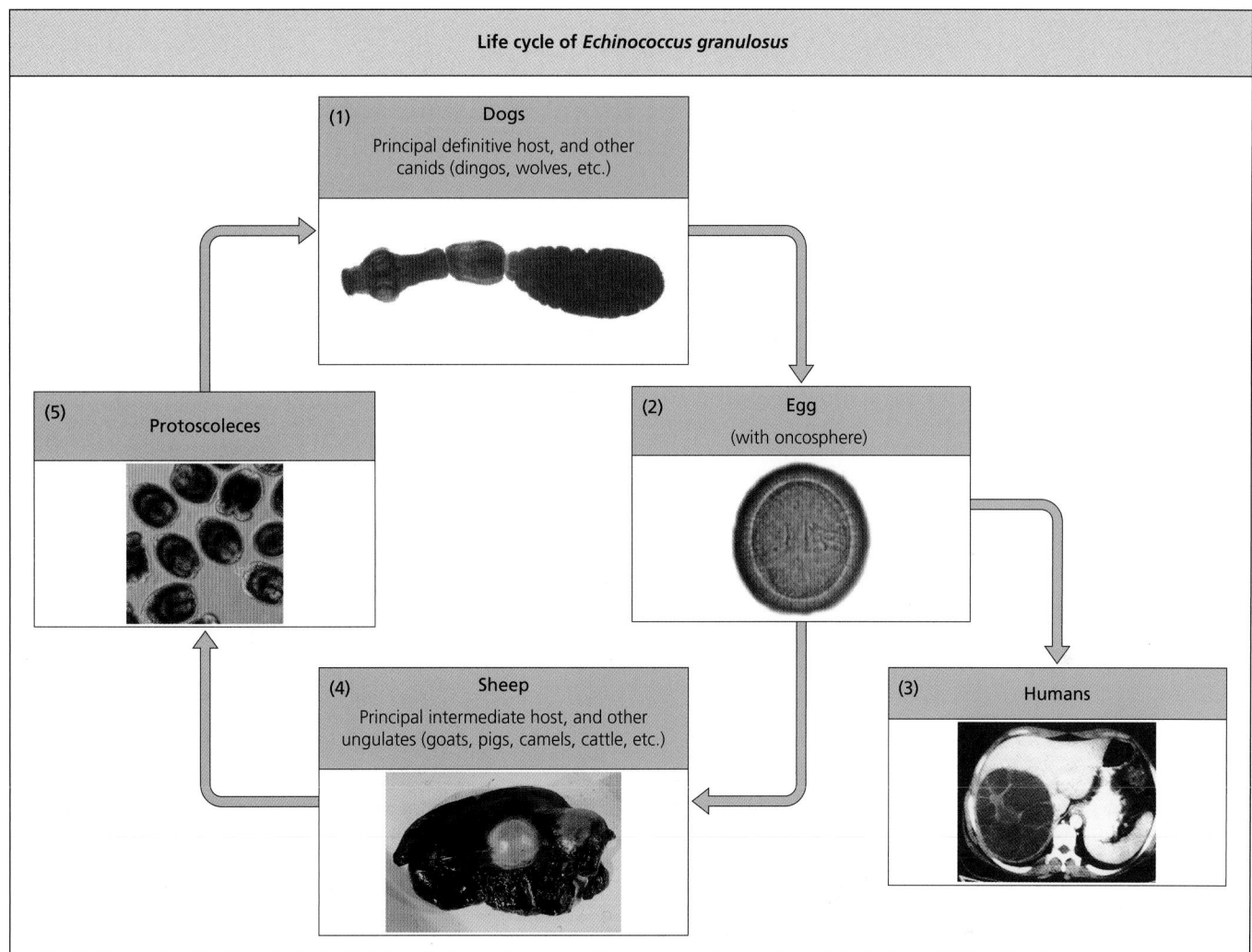

Figure 120-1 Life cycle of *Echinococcus granulosus*. Adult tapeworms (1) parasitize the small intestine of definitive hosts, mainly dogs, among other canids. Parasite proglottids and eggs are shed with the feces, such eggs (2) being infectious for intermediate hosts including humans. Hydatid cyst (4) formation occurs predominantly in the liver, but also in lungs and other organs. Imaging techniques such as CT demonstrate well-delineated, fluid-filled, usually unilocular bladder-like lesions. Internal daughter cysts may be visible in larger cysts as septated segments within the primary cyst (3). The endogenous formation of brood capsules and protoscolices (5) is a prerequisite for completion of the life cycle, which occurs when definitive hosts ingest protoscolex-containing hydatid cysts. *(Courtesy of B. Gottstein, University of Bern, Switzerland.)*

annual incidence of AE cases per year is estimated at 18 235; of these 91% (16 692) are considered to occur in China, 1180 in Russia and 426 in the rest of the world.[12]

Pathogenesis and Pathology
ECHINOCOCCUS GRANULOSUS

Accidental ingestion of *E. granulosus* eggs by humans results in the release of oncospheres that migrate to primary target organs such as liver and to some extent also lungs, and less frequently to other organs such as the kidney, spleen, brain, heart and bone. There, the oncosphere differentiates and develops into a well-delineated spherical 'hydatid cyst' over several months or years (see Figure 120-1). Tissue damage and/or organ dysfunction result from this gradual process of space-occupying displacement of vital host tissue, vessels or parts of organs. Consequently, clinical manifestations are primarily determined by the site, size and number of the cysts, and are therefore highly variable. Accidental rupture of the cysts results in a release of cyst fluid and a concomitant dissemination of protoscolices. This can lead to anaphylactic reactions and the formation of multiple secondary cysts, which grow out of the disseminated protoscolices.

Histologic characteristics of a typical hydatid include a thin spherical germinal layer as the primary site of parasite development (Figure 120-3). It is surrounded by a thick laminated layer that is composed of mucins bearing defined galactose-rich carbohydrates and accompanied by calcium inositol hexakisphosphate deposits, as recently reviewed by Diaz *et al.*[13]

The proliferating germinal layer can form protoscolices, brood capsules and occasionally also daughter cysts within the fluid-filled hydatid cyst lumen. The presence of metabolically active hydatid cysts evokes a host immune response, which is involved in the formation of a host-derived adventitious capsule that contributes to the host control of cysts growth. Conversely, the parasite is assumed to down-regulate efficient host immune reactions via immunomodulating metabolites.[14] Tamarozzi *et al.*[15] proposed that the development of a hydatid cyst is favored by a skewing of the host's immunity towards a Th2 response. While a Th1 cell activation seemed to be more related to protective immunity, disease susceptibility was associated with a Th2-oriented cytokine profile[16] and impairment of dendritic cell maturation.[17]

Efficient periparasitic immunity and/or chemotherapy can lead to cyst degeneration, which leads to an increasing calcification in the periphery of the cyst, a typical feature found on imaging. Uncontrolled cyst growth in the liver may lead to pressure atrophy of the surrounding parenchyma and cholestasis by compression of the bile ducts.

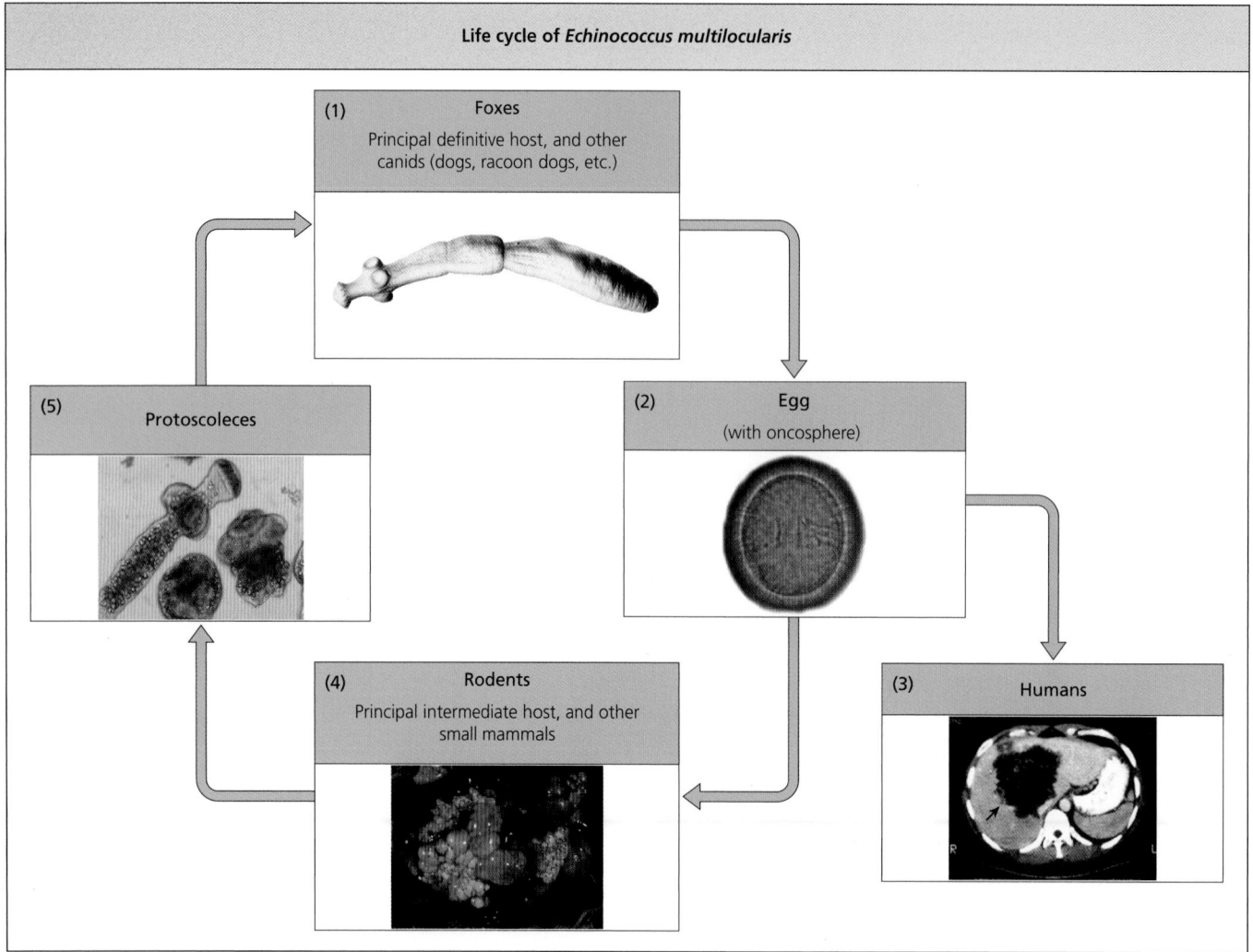

Figure 120-2   Life cycle of *Echinococcus multilocularis*. This involves predominantly foxes as definitive hosts, and occasionally other carnivores such as raccoon dogs or domestic dogs, among other canids. Egg production by the tapeworm (1) starts as early as 28 days after infection. Eggs (2) ingested by a suitable intermediate host, including humans and various small rodent species, will result in a subsequent metacestode development, (arrow) predominantly in the liver (3). Macroscopically, the typical lesion is characterized by a dispersed mass of fibrous tissue with a multitude of interconnected vesicles ranging from a few millimeters to centimeters in size (4). The lesion often contains focal necrotic zones with scattered calcifications, as demonstrated by CT. Oral ingestion of protoscolex-containing (5) metacestodes by definitive hosts completes the life cycle. *(Courtesy of B. Gottstein and A. Hemphill, University of Bern, Switzerland.)*

The appearance of CE cysts on medical imaging (most usually ultrasonography) are highly diverse[18] and have resulted in the classification of hepatic CE cysts into five stages, with a further substratification of stage CE3 into CE3a and CE3b. Parasite 'activity' levels were then assigned to these stages, with a division into active (CE1 and CE2), transitional (CE3a and CE3b) and inactive (CE4 and CE5).[18] CE cyst staging directly correlates to growth versus decay of the parasite, and is therefore of importance in clinical practice for the prognostic assessment of any treatment option that is applied to a given CE patient.

ECHINOCOCCUS MULTILOCULARIS

In infected humans the *E. multilocularis* metacestode (larva) appears macroscopically as a dispersed mass of fibrous tissue with a conglomerate of scattered vesiculated cavities with diameters ranging from a few millimeters to centimeters in size. In advanced chronic cases, a central necrotic cavity containing a viscous fluid may form; rarely bacterial superinfection occurs. The lesion often contains focal calcification, typically within the metacestode tissue rather than the periphery as in CE (Figure 120-4). A central lesion may also be surrounded by multiple scattered smaller lesions, mimicking a grape-like structure within the hepatic parenchyma.

Microscopically, the hepatic lesion is characterized by a conglomerate of small vesicles and cysts demarcated by a thin PAS-positive laminated layer with or without an inner germinated layer (Figure 120-5). Parasite proliferation is usually accompanied by a granulomatous response, including vigorous synthesis of fibrous and germinated tissue in the periphery of the metacestode, as well as central necrosis. Both reactions protect the host against larval growth but may also be deleterious.[19] In contrast to lesions in susceptible rodent hosts, lesions from infected human patients rarely show protoscolex formation within vesicles and cysts.

Genetic and immunologic host factors are responsible for the resistance shown by some patients in whom there is an early 'dying out' or 'abortion' of the metacestode[20] (Figure 120-5). Therefore, not everyone infected with *E. multilocularis* is susceptible to unlimited metacestode proliferation and thus disease (AE).[21,22] The immune response that develops against the larval stages of *E. multilocularis* accounts for a controlled parasite tissue development as well as for immunopathologic events. Varying innate and immunologic host factors proved responsible for the occurrence of principally three different outcomes of infection: (1) resistance as shown by the presence of 'dying out' or 'aborted' metacestodes; (2) controlled susceptibility as shown by a

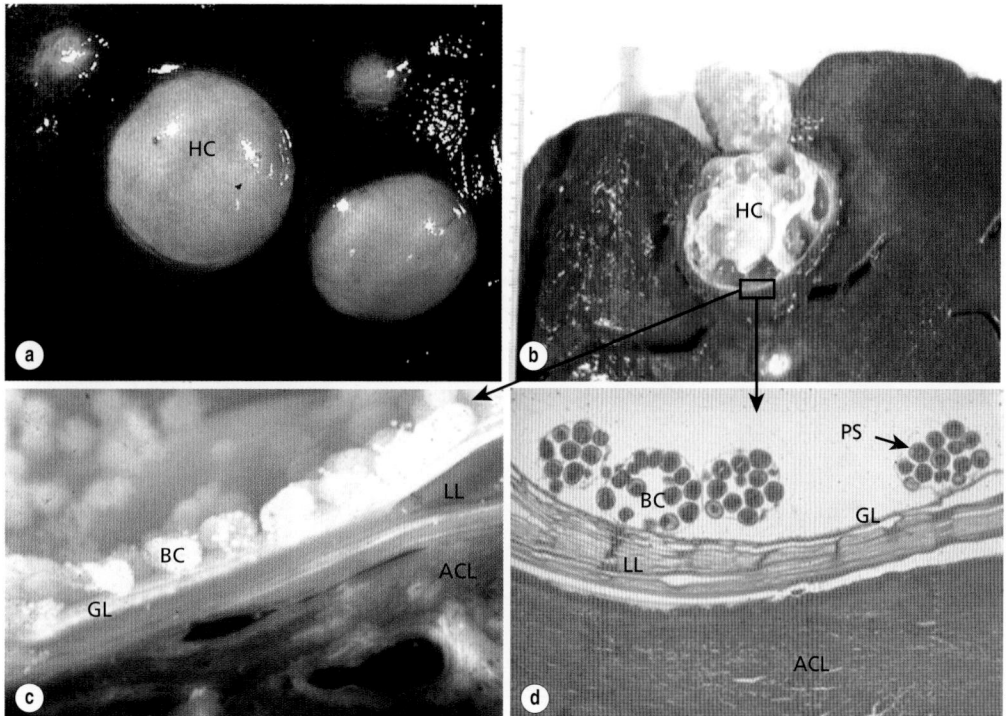

Figure 120-3   *Echinococcus granulosus* hydatid cysts (HC) affect the liver (a) in approximately 60% and lungs in 20% of cases, among other organs (20%). Well-delineated spherical cysts can be internally septated into daughter cysts, becoming visible, e.g. by CT (see Figure 120-1) or after surgical opening of such a cyst (b). (c, d) Microscopically, the cyst wall consists of a very thin inner germinal and nucleated layer (GL) with a predominantly syncytial structure. The germinal layer is externally protected by an acellular laminated layer (LL) of variable thickness. Periparasitically, the host tissue reacts with the formation of an adventitious connective tissue layer (ACL) that encapsulates the actual parasitic hydatid cysts. The germinal layer synthesizes internally brood capsules (BC) which themselves contain a collection of several protoscolices (PS). Protoscolices are infectious units of the parasite, each developing into a single tapeworm within the small intestine of definitive hosts. *(Courtesy of B. Gottstein, University of Bern, Switzerland (a); H.M. Seitz, University of Bonn, Germany (b,c); J. Eckert, University of Zurich, Switzerland (d).)*

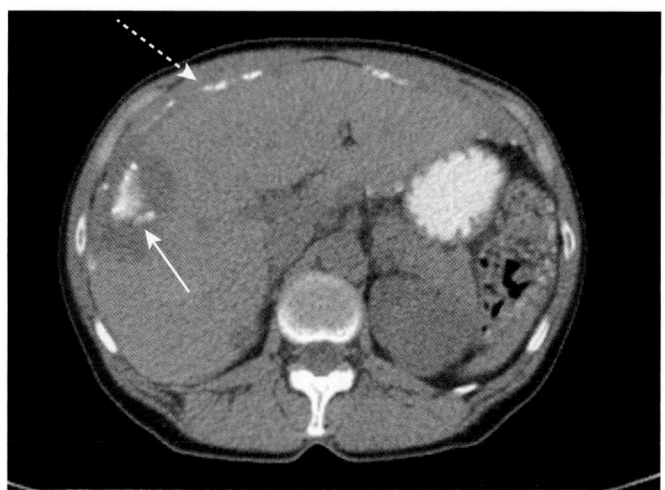

Figure 120-4   Computed tomography without vascular contrast media of a patient with AE and associated peritoneal seeding. Lesions in the liver (solid arrow) are hypodense compared to the unaffected liver and contain calcifications. Calcifications of peritoneal seeding are visible on the surface of the liver (dashed arrow).

slowly growing metacestode tissue – this group refers to the conventional AE patients where clinical signs manifest between 5 and 15 years following infection; (3) a third group is affected by an uncontrolled hyperproliferation of the metacestode due to an impaired immune response (acquired immunodeficiency syndrome [AIDS] or other immunodeficiencies, e.g. following orthotopic liver transplantation – see reference 52) (Figure 120-6). Thus, a lack or deficiency of T-helper (Th) cell activity such as in advanced AIDS is associated with a rapid

and unlimited growth and dissemination of the parasite in AE[23] (Figure 120-5), and recovery of the T cell status in AIDS is prognostically favorable.[24] Chauchet *et al.*[25] found that the more aggressive immunosuppressive treatment of malignant and inflammatory diseases performed in Europe resulted in increased AE numbers among such patients, and that AE consequently also is an emerging opportunistic disease.

Prevention

Prevention of both CE and AE focuses primarily on veterinary interventions to control the extent and intensity of infection in definitive and intermediate host populations. This includes regular deworming of dogs for *E. granulosus*, and sanitary precautions when handling domestic dogs to prevent infection and egg excretion, dog registration and control of stray dog numbers.

Regular praziquantel treatment of wildlife definitive hosts and domestic dogs in highly *E. multilocularis*-endemic areas may contribute to lowering of the prevalence of AE in affected zones. Finally, a vaccine to protect ruminant intermediate hosts from *E. granulosus* infection is available.[26]

Clinical Features

The initial phase of *Echinococcus* infection is always asymptomatic. The infection may remain asymptomatic for years or decades depending upon the size and site of the developing cyst (CE) or metacestode mass (AE). After a highly variable incubation period, the infection may become symptomatic (both CE and AE) due to a range of different events.

CYSTIC ECHINOCOCCOSIS

Echinococcus granulosus does not cause damage due to any inherent cytotoxic effect. Rather, growing cysts can result in deformation and

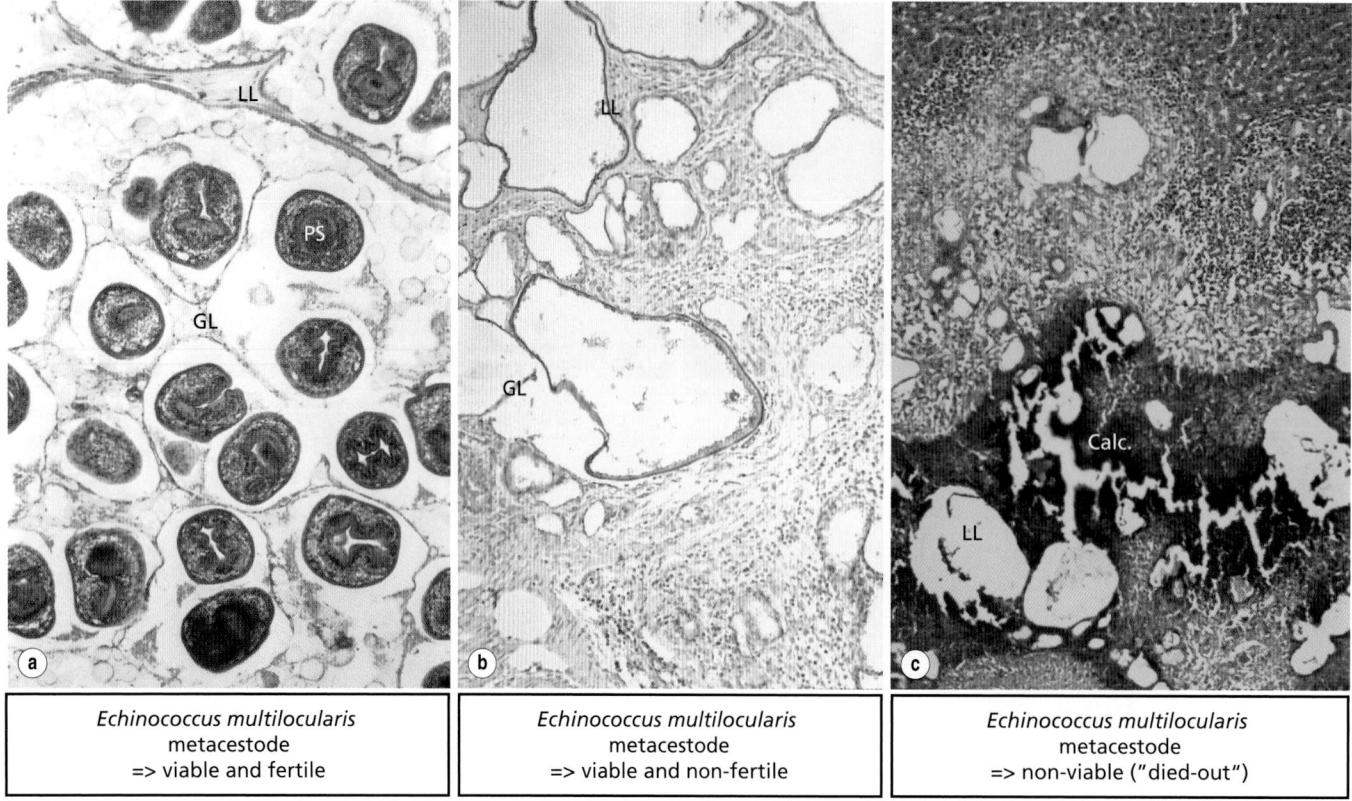

| *Echinococcus multilocularis* metacestode => viable and fertile | *Echinococcus multilocularis* metacestode => viable and non-fertile | *Echinococcus multilocularis* metacestode => non-viable ("died-out") |

Figure 120-5 Histologically, the hepatic lesion in AE is caused by the *E. multilocularis* metacestode tissue, which consists of a conglomerate of small parasitic vesicles and cysts demarcated by a thin laminated layer (LL) with or without an inner germinal layer (GL) and, predominantly upon maturation in rodents, a collection of protoscolices (PS). Such a metacestode (a) is considered as fully viable and fertile (infectious for definitive hosts such as foxes). In humans, 90% of hepatic metacestode-induced lesions do not form protoscolices; these are considered as viable but non-fertile (b). In some rodents and in many humans, the metacestode dies out after a certain infection period (c), and is thus considered as non-viable. Histologically, these lesions are characterized by the lack of a germinal layer and the presence of some laminated layer (LL), and predominately of a marked calcification process (Calc.). *(Courtesy of B. Gottstein, University of Bern, Switzerland.)*

dysfunction of adjacent organ tissues or vascular components leading to symptoms. In the case of hepatic CE (which accounts for approximately 60–70% of CE cases), signs and symptoms include hepatomegaly, right epigastric pain, nausea, vomiting and occasionally jaundice. In inoperable cases, hepatic compromise may lead to cholestatic cirrhosis. Up to 20% of hepatic CE patients develop biliary complications ranging from mild to severe.[27] Bacterial cyst infection and abscess formation is another, less frequent complication causing right upper quadrant pain.[28]

Lung disease accounts for approximately 20% of CE and presents with chronic cough, hemoptysis, pneumothorax, pleuritis, lung abscess and parasitic lung embolism. Rare but often catastrophic infestations can affect the heart or the brain. In the heart this can present as tumor, pericardial effusion including tamponade, complete heart block and sudden death. In the spine and brain presentation is as a tumor with neurologic symptoms.

A cyst may rupture and spill its contents into the adjacent site. Rupture into the biliary tree will mimic biliary colic or result in jaundice, cholangitis or obstructive pancreatitis. This is the presenting symptom in 5–25% of patients. Anaphylactic shock is an important possible consequence of rupture, and is often the initial and life-threatening manifestation. Each spilled protoscolex can develop into a secondary cyst, and this is the most frequent reason for relapse following surgical intervention.

The majority of patients with CE have single-organ involvement with solitary cysts. Simultaneous involvement of two or more organs is observed in 10–15% of patients, depending on the geographic origin of the patient and the strain of the parasite. In hepatic CE, the right lobe is more frequently affected than the left. Cyst size varies between 1 and 15 cm in diameter. Cyst growth ranges between an increase in

size of a few millimeters (1/3 of the patients) to approximately 10 mm (most of the patients) per year; 1 in 10 of the patients exhibit a rapid increase, with an annual average of 30 mm. In Europe, the average age of patients at diagnosis is 36 years. The higher endemicity is in a given area, the higher is the rate of CE-affected children. Approximately 10% of the CE cases occur in children overall (a much higher rate can occur in highly endemic areas), and the rate of lung involvement is significantly increased among this group (up to 50%).

HEPATIC ALVEOLAR ECHINOCOCCOSIS

AE patients usually become symptomatic after an incubation period of 5–15 years, with most patients between 40 and 60 years old (range of 6–80 years), with no gender predominance. In patients with hepatic AE, the size of the lesion can range from a few millimeters up to 50 cm. A classification of the different types and stages of AE was published in 2006 and has been widely adopted.[29] The disease starts frequently with nonspecific symptoms such as epigastric pain or jaundice. Clinical signs at diagnosis include hepatomegaly, jaundice, secondary biliary cirrhosis, liver abscess and portal hypertension. Imaging reveals typical calcification in 70% of cases and central or peripheral necrotic cavities (also 70%). The infiltrative, tumor-like growth of AE (average volume increase of 15 mL/year) causes a range of complications. These include: (1) jaundice due to invasion of large biliary vessels at the liver hilum, which can be complicated by (recurrent) cholangitis eventually leading to cirrhosis and portal hypertension; (2) invasion of vascular walls with hematogenous spread, vascular occlusion/thrombosis; (3) poor vascularization of AE lesions leading to necrosis and formation of necrotic cavities which are at risk of bacterial infection with abscess formation.[22] Metastatic disease occurs in approximately 20–35% of patients and has been described in brain, spine, lung and bone.[30]

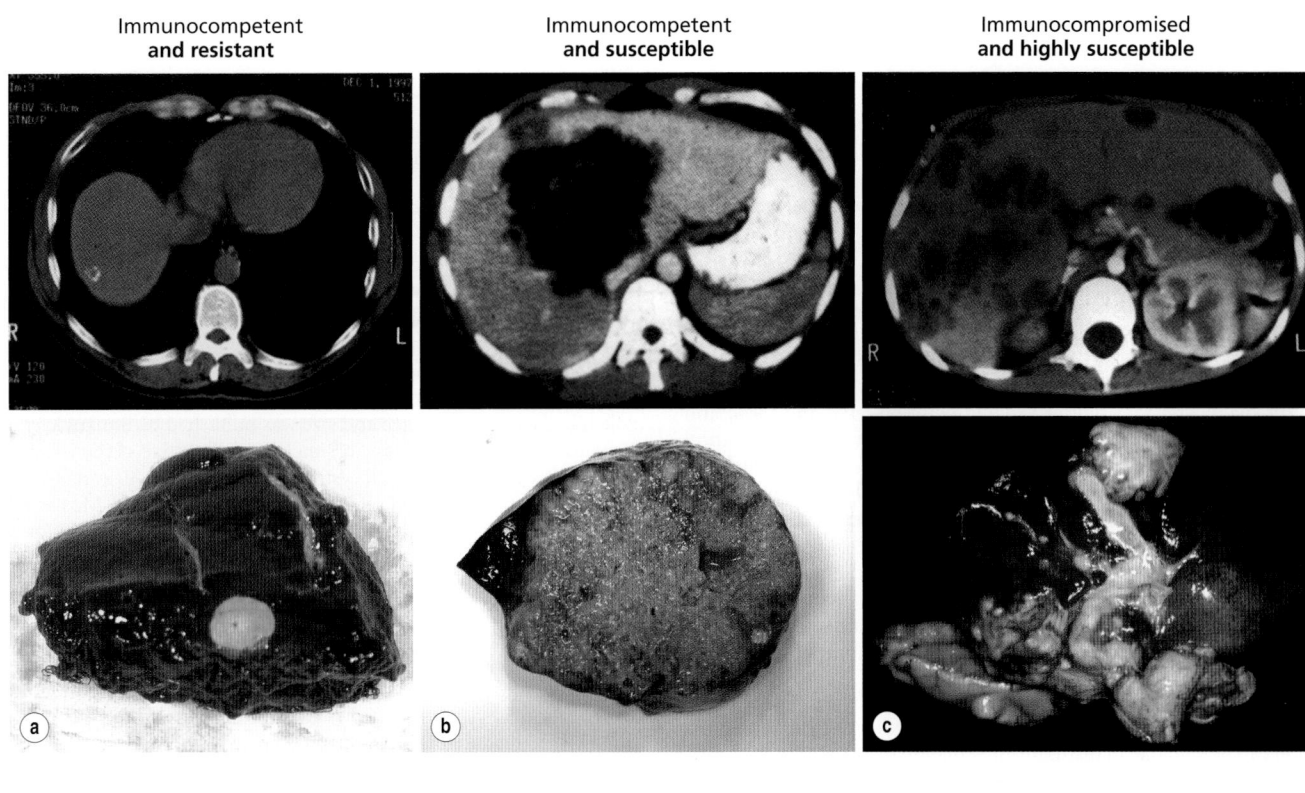

Figure 120-6 Dependent on the kind of immune response and associated immunopathologic events, three different outcomes of infection, i.e. three principally different clinical presentations, are encountered in humans infected with *E. multilocularis*: (a) resistance as shown by the presence of 'dying out' or 'aborted' metacestodes; such lesions are fully calcified, no longer contain living parasite cells, but have an inert laminated layer that can still act as an immunostimulator with a corresponding host humoral immune response; (b) controlled susceptibility as shown by a slowly growing metacestode tissue; this group refers to the conventional AE patients; periparasitic inflammatory processes as well as fibrinogenic and collagenic encapsulation partially control the metacestode growth; (c) a third group is affected by an uncontrolled hyperproliferation of the metacestode due to an impaired immune response (AIDS or other immunodeficiencies); rapid metastases formation within the liver and subsequently at other sites will occur. Lower panel of pictures shows resected lesions representative for the three groups (a–c), each characterized by typical CT-imaging. *(Courtesy of B. Gottstein, University of Bern, Switzerland; Franz Allerberger, Austrian Agency for Health, Vienna (c).)*

Diagnosis

ECHINOCOCCUS GRANULOSUS

In many cases, diagnosis is based upon history, examination and imaging findings, and serology is a complementary tool. Sonography is the primary diagnostic procedure of choice for hepatic cases, although false-positives occur in up to 10% of cases due to the presence of non-echinococcal serous cysts, abscesses or tumors. An international classification and staging of ultrasound images in CE yields relatively standardized perspectives for CE treatment.

Thus active and transitional cysts (CE1, CE2, C3a and CE3b) require treatment, whereas inactive cysts (CE4 and CE5) may result in a wait-and-watch approach. The treatment option depends also on the dichotomy between uncomplicated versus complicated cysts.

The main diagnostic features in imaging studies of cystic echinococcosis include:

- separation of the membrane from the wall
- daughter cysts
- ruptured cysts.

Computed tomography is the best investigation for detecting calcifications (up to 10%), extrahepatic disease and volumetric follow-up assessment; MRI assists in the diagnosis by identifying changes in the intra- and extrahepatic venous systems and the biliary tree. Ultrasonography is also helpful in following up treated patients as successfully treated cysts become hyperechogenic.

Aspiration cytology has the risk of spillage and associated anaphylactic shock and should be used only if imaging studies remain equivocal. It may be helpful in the detection of pulmonary, renal and other nonhepatic lesions. The viability of aspirated protoscolices can be determined by microscopic demonstration of flame cell activity and trypan blue dye exclusion. Anti-Ag5 monoclonal antibody has been used for the detection of the respective antigen in diagnostic fine-needle aspiration biopsies (FNABs) from patients with suspected CE.[31,32]

Immunodiagnostic tests to detect serum antibodies are used to support the clinical diagnosis of CE.[16] The indirect hemagglutination tests (IHAT) and the enzyme-linked immunosorbent assay (ELISA) using *E. granulosus* hydatid fluid antigen are the most sensitive for hepatic cases (85–98%), but sensitivity is much lower for pulmonary cysts and in children (50–60%). However, these tests are conventionally only used for primary screening, since their specificity is too low for definitive interpretation of findings. In consequence, sera positive with these screening tests are reinvestigated using specific confirmation tests such as immunoblotting for 8 kDa/12 kDa subunits of *E. granulosus* antigen B.[33]

ECHINOCOCCUS MULTILOCULARIS

Imaging

Ultrasonography, CT and MRI are of greatest diagnostic value, and perform similarly.[34] Ultrasonography is the preferred imaging procedure for mass screening programs in which hyperechogenic and hypoechogenic zones characterize the lesions which may reflect central necrotic cavities. CT scan is most useful to identify calcifications and lesions typically do not enhance with contrast. The lesions are heterogeneous, low attenuation masses with irregular contours and lack well-delineated walls. Magnetic resonance imaging adds to diagnosis, in particular in cases with brain involvement, and can help visualize pathologically altered microstructures in certain affected organs and identify necrosis and fibrosis.[35] However, in contrast to CT, microcalcifications are not visualized by MRI.

PNM Classification

The resemblance of AE to malignant diseases led to the introduction of a PNM classification for AE of the liver, as follows: P = parasitic mass in the liver, N = involvement of neighboring organs including lymph nodes, M = metastases. This facilitates clinical management and treatment evaluation.[18,29]

Immunodiagnosis

Serologic tests are a valuable secondary diagnostic tool and are more reliable in the diagnosis of AE than CE.[18,33] Tests based on purified *E. multilocularis* antigens such as the Em2 antigen and recombinant antigens from the family of EMR proteins (EmII/3-10, EM10, and Em18) exhibit diagnostic sensitivities ranging between 91% and 99%, and specificities of 98–100%.[18,33] These antigens allow discrimination between the alveolar and the cystic forms of disease with a reliability of 95%. Seroepidemiologic studies reveal asymptomatic preclinical cases of human AE as well as cases in which the metacestode has died out at an apparently early stage of infection.[20,21] Serologic tests are of value for assessing the efficacy of treatment and chemotherapy only when linked to appropriate imaging investigations. Prognostically, significant decline and subsequent disappearance of anti-Em18 antibody levels, coupled to PET negativity, indicates inactivation of AE.[36,37]

Histology

Where there is diagnostic uncertainty, fine-needle puncture and aspiration can be valuable in distinguishing malignancies, within the limits of the sensitivity of this method. However, modern imaging modalities in parallel with serologic testing are usually sufficient for diagnosis. Analyses of surgically resected samples or fine needle aspirates include the use of species-specific MAbs (MAbG11) or polymerase chain reaction (PCR).[32] Viability assessment can be performed with reverse transcription (RT)-PCR.[38,39]

Management

ECHINOCOCCUS GRANULOSUS

Surgery remains the mainstay in the treatment of symptomatic hepatic CE. Cystectomy, pericystectomy or complete surgical resection offer a good chance for cure and should be undertaken wherever possible.

A pragmatic approach in clinical practice is to divide newly diagnosed CE patients into two categories:[22]

- Patients with complicated CE cysts which need individualized treatment adapted to the resources of the place where the patient needs to be treated, and
- Patients with uncomplicated CE cysts, for which standardized cyst stage-specific management is appropriate.

Complicated CE Cysts

Since the liver and lungs are the two organs most frequently infected, cysto-biliary and cysto-bronchial fistulas are the most common complications. However, diagnosis of fistulas before they become patent and active is difficult. MRI with MR cholangiography (MRC) can detect fistulas before they cause complications.[40] Rupture and spillage of cyst content into the biliary tree leads rapidly to biliary obstruction and cholangitis. Clearance of the obstructing material by means of endoscopic retrograde cholangiopancreatography (ERCP) is indicated, along with immediate albendazole therapy.

Cyst rupture into a bronchus results into expectoration of hydatid fluid and cyst fragments. Benzimidazole therapy should be started immediately, and surgical removal of the cyst and fistula closure should be anticipated. Hydatid cyst fluid contains multiple allergenic components that on rupture may lead to a severe type 1 hypersensitivity reaction (anaphylaxis) requiring resuscitation.

Pressure effects on adjoining structures are managed with surgical decompression; although there is a risk of loss of organ function due to pressure atrophy.

Uncomplicated CE Cysts

Patients with uncomplicated cysts may be treated on the basis of four different principles:

1. Chemotherapeutically, with albendazole or mebendazole
2. Percutaneous sterilization technique (PAIR = Puncture – Aspiration (of cyst content) – Inoculation (of a scolicidal solution) – Reaspiration)
3. Conventional surgical procedures
4. 'Watch and wait' approach.

(1) Preferably albendazole (15 mg/kg/d [max 800 mg] per os in two divided doses, for between 1 and 6 months), but also mebendazole (dosage has to be individualized upon determination of plasma concentrations), can provide an alternative to surgery in patients with uncomplicated cysts. A retrospective analysis of data collected from six treatment centers with regard to the long-term outcome after albendazole treatment by cyst stage and size was published by Stojkovic *et al.*[41] Benzimidazoles worked best in small (≤6 cm) active cysts, where the overall effectiveness across all cyst stages was between 40 and 60%. The length of treatment with albendazole has not been defined. Most experts agreed that it should be given for at least 3 months, possibly up to 6 months. As the process of cyst involution and degeneration continues after discontinuation of treatment, final assessment of treatment should not be before 12 months after termination of chemotherapy. Hepatic toxicity is a potential side effect of albendazole. If the rise of liver enzymes is mild to moderate (2–4 times normal levels), interruption of treatment is not necessary. If the rise is more than fourfold, treatment interruption is recommended.[18] Benzimidazoles should be reintroduced with dose adaptation following normalization.

(2) Ultrasonography-guided percutaneous sterilization of cyst content (PAIR) may cure disease in a proportion of patients. This minimally invasive technique is suitable for CE1 and CE3a hepatic cysts of 5–6 cm to <10 cm in diameter in which cysto-biliary fistulas have been excluded (sclerosing cholangitis and liver failure can occur due to accidental spillage of parasitocidal agents such as 95% ethanol or 20% saline solution). PAIR should be restricted to experienced clinics with a high load of CE patients. Follow-up for several years is conventional, to detect relapses and secondary CE.[18]

(3) Conventional surgical approaches: (a) partial cystectomy: removal of the parasite-derived cyst components (endocyst plus content) and part of the pericyst (host-derived connective tissue capsule); (b) total cystectomy: removal of the parasite-derived cyst components (endocyst plus content) and the entire pericyst (host-derived connective tissue capsule); (c) additionally, removal of part of the organ in which the CE cyst is embedded – by resection – may be needed.

Approach (a) includes the following main steps: perinterventional benzimidazole metaphylaxis (therapeutic dosage) and careful prevention of spillage of hydatid fluid when the cyst is punctured and the cyst material is removed; sterilization of the cavity with 20% normal saline or 95% ethanol through the trocar after careful exclusion of cysto-biliary fistulas; closure of fistulas; filling of the residual cavity with an omentoplasty where appropriate.

Approach (b) includes total cystectomy and partial liver resection: The endocyst plus content and the entire periparasitic connective tissue capsule are fully resected; this technique may also include some portion of periparasitic liver tissue. Fistulas are closed and the residual cavity may be filled by an omentoplasty. A more radical approach consists in resection of a whole part of the organ in which the cyst is embedded, such as a liver lobe.

Since CE is usually a relatively benign disorder, preference should always be given to the surgical technique that holds the smallest risk for the patient.

(4) With the 'watch and wait' approach the cyst is allowed to progress along its natural course.[42] Starting from WHO stage CE1, the parasite steadily grows over time. At a variable time point, involution starts followed by increasing degeneration of the cyst until the final stage, CE5, is reached, where the parasite appears dead. Center-based experience suggests that for inactive CE4 and CE5 cysts, long-term

observation is a safe approach with low risk of relapse or complications. It is recommended that patients with CE4 and CE5 cysts should be followed for several years.[18] When considering the 'watch and wait' approach the regional anatomical setting of the cyst must be carefully evaluated to ensure that the space-occupying lesion does not compromise neighboring organs and structures.

ECHINOCOCCUS MULTILOCULARIS

The following strategies are commonly accepted for treatment of AE.

(1) Currently, surgery with the aim of cure is recommended if resection of the lesion including a 2 cm margin of healthy liver tissue is practicable. This is accompanied by at least 2 years of albendazole therapy.[18,43] Follow-up after surgery should probably be life-long because AE tends to grow along bile ducts that may not be visible during surgery. Recurrences have been observed almost 20 years after surgery. After successful surgery, there is rapid decline in anti-Em18 or anti-Em2+ antibodies, and seroconversion to undetectable levels correlates well with curative resection.[36,44]

(2) For patients where lesions have advanced to a stage at which curative resection appears highly unlikely or impossible, benzimidazole treatment, in most cases life-long, and interdisciplinary management of acute problems, such as obstruction of bile ducts, abscess formation and thrombosis of major blood vessels, is the therapeutic approach. Reassessment of resectability should be regularly performed. Palliative surgery should be restricted to individual cases with complications that cannot be otherwise controlled.[45]

Albendazole is the most frequently used benzimidazole compound, because of its good bioavailability and ease of administration. The recommended dose is 10–15 mg/kg/day (usually 2 x 400 mg) in two divided doses with fat-rich meals. Mebendazole 40–50 mg/kg/day split into three divided doses with fat-rich meals is an alternative. It can also be tried if albendazole is not tolerated or appears ineffective.[18]

Liver enzymes and leukocytes should be monitored initially at 2-weekly intervals, then monthly and later every 3 months. Aminotransferase levels four times above normal and low leukocyte counts require discontinuation of benzimidazoles and workup to investigate possible reasons.[18]

Monitoring of patients includes regular imaging with ultrasound at intervals that need to be adapted to circumstances and MRI/CT every 2–3 years. Albendazole sulfoxide plasma levels 4h after the intake of the morning dose should be measured 1, 4 and 12 weeks after the start of benzimidazole therapy and 2–4 weeks after each dose adjustment. The therapeutic range is 0.65–3 µmol/L.[18]

There is emerging evidence that in a small proportion of long-term-treated patients benzimidazoles may act in a parasitocidal manner.[46,47] Reliable criteria for parasite death are, however, missing. Crouzet et al.[47] recommended on the basis of their findings that patients should only be considered for discontinuation if the following combination of criteria is fulfilled: disappearance of anti-Em18 antibodies, more than 50% of the lesion calcified at initial diagnosis and a negative PET.[47]

(3) Liver transplantation is the very last resort and should be considered only in the very late stages of the disease. Re-infestation rates are high after liver transplantation.[18,48] Bresson-Hadni et al.,[49] however, concluded from a case series that residual or metastatic lesions are not necessarily a contraindication for liver transplantation since albendazole can control residual or recurrent AE. There is controversy, however, about the success of controlling accelerated growth of AE metastases under immunosuppression with benzimidazoles.

Conclusion

The ultrasound-based WHO CE cyst classification serves as a framework on which to base rational stage-specific treatment algorithms, and it is hoped that this will lead to improved and standardized treatment for all patients. However, the system has yet to be implemented by all clinical health services.

Similarly, substantial progress has been made in the diagnosis, staging and treatment of AE, enabling most patients to have a good life expectancy and quality in economically well-situated regions.

However, a significant number of patients fail to benefit from advances made, since most disease occurs in poorly resourced geographical areas, where diagnostic facilities and access to expertise are limited. Referral of patients to multidisciplinary treatment centres enhances experience and quality of care for both CE and AE.

References available online at expertconsult.com.

KEY REFERENCES

Ammann R.W., Renner E.C., Gottstein B., et al., Swiss Echinococcosis Study Group: Immunosurveillance of alveolar echinococcosis by specific humoral and cellular immune tests: prospective long-term analysis of the Swiss chemotherapy trial (1976–2001). *J Hepatol* 2004; 41:551-559.

Brunetti E., Kern P., Vuitton D.A.: Writing Panel for the WHO-IWGE: Expert consensus for the diagnosis and treatment of cystic and alveolar echinococcosis in humans. *Acta Trop* 2010; 114:1-16.

Caoduro C., Porot C., Vuitton D.A., et al.: The role of delayed 18F-FDG PET imaging in the follow-up of patients with alveolar echinococcosis. *J Nucl Med* 2013; 54(3):358-363.

Chauchet A., Grenouillet F., Knapp J., et al.: Emergence of a new opportunistic infection in Europe: hepatic alveolar echinococcosis. Fifty case-report. *J Hepatol* 2013; 58(Suppl. 11):S381.

Crouzet J., Grenouillet F., Delabrousse E., et al.: Personalized management of patients with inoperable alveolar echinococcosis undergoing treatment with albendazole: usefulness of positron-emission-tomography combined with serological and computed tomography follow-up. *Clin Microbiol Infect* 2010; 16(6):788-791.

Kern P., Wen H., Sato N., et al.: WHO classification of alveolar echinococcosis: principles and application. *Parasitol Int* 2006; 55(Suppl.):S283-S287.

Reuter S., Nüssle K., Kolokythas O., et al.: Alveolar liver echinococcosis: a comparative study of three imaging techniques. *Infection* 2001; 29:119-125.

Sailer M., Soelder B., Allerberger F., et al.: Alveolar echinococcosis in a six-year-old girl with AIDS. *J Pediatr* 1997; 130:320-323.

Stojkovic M., Gottstein B., Junghanns T.: Echinococcosis. In: Farrar J., Hotez P.J., Junghanss T., et al., eds. *Manson's tropical diseases*, 23rd ed. Philadelphia: Elsevier Saunders; 2014:795-819.

Stojkovic M., Zwahlen M., Teggi A., et al.: Treatment response of cystic echinococcosis to benzimidazoles: a systematic review. *PLoS Negl Trop Dis* 2009; 3(9):e524.

Torgerson P.R., Keller K., Magnotta M., et al.: The global burden of alveolar echinococcosis. *PLoS Negl Trop Dis* 2010; 4(6):e722.

Vuitton D.A., Wang Q., Zhou H.X., et al.: A historical view of alveolar echinococcosis, 160 years after the discovery of the first case in humans: part 1. What have we learnt on the distribution of the disease and on its parasitic agent? *Chin Med J (Engl)* 2011; 124(18):2943-2953.

121

Filarial Infections

THOMAS B. NUTMAN

KEY CONCEPTS

- Filarial infections are chronic tissue invasive nematode infections.

- The majority of filarial infections are manifested as a clinically asymptomatic (subclinical) state.

- Travelers to filarial-endemic regions present with clinical symptoms more often than those indigenous to the same regions – a reflection of an immunologically hyperresponsive state.

- Adverse events following treatment of most filarial infections are related to the numbers of circulating parasites (microfilariae).

- Pathology associated with lymphatic filariasis and onchocerciasis is primarily immune-mediated.

- All of the filarial parasites (except *Loa loa*) that infect humans contain a *Wolbachia* endosymbiont that can be targeted for therapy with specific antibiotics.

- Definitive diagnosis of the filariases is made by finding the organism or its DNA in the appropriate tissue (blood or skin).

- *Wuchereria* and *Brugia* microfilariae typically have a nocturnal periodicity whereas *Loa loa* has a diurnal periodicity. *Mansonella* spp. and *Onchocerca* microfilariae have no discernible periodicity.

Introduction

Filarial worms are nematodes that dwell in the subcutaneous tissues and the lymphatics of their human hosts. Eight filarial species infect humans (Table 121-1); of these, four – *Wuchereria bancrofti*, *Brugia malayi*, *Onchocerca volvulus* and *Loa loa* – are responsible for the majority of serious filarial infections. Filarial parasites infect an estimated 180 million persons worldwide, and are transmitted by specific species of mosquitoes or other arthropods. They have complex life cycles (Figure 121-1), including infective larval stages carried by insects, and adult worms that reside in either lymphatic or subcutaneous tissues of the definitive host – humans. The offspring of adults are microfilariae, which, depending on their species, are 200–250 μm long and 5–7 μm wide, may or may not be enveloped in a loose sheath, and either circulate in the blood or migrate through the skin (Table 121-1). Completion of the life cycle depends upon ingestion of microfilariae by the arthropod vector. Over 1–2 weeks these develop into new infective larvae. Adult worms live for many years, whereas microfilariae survive for 3–36 months. The *Rickettsia*-like obligate endosymbiont *Wolbachia* has been found intracellularly in all stages of *Brugia*, *Wuchereria*, *Mansonella* and *Onchocerca* and has become a target for anti-filarial chemotherapy.

Epidemiology

LYMPHATIC FILARIASIS

There are 120 million people in at least 72 countries of the world infected with lymphatic filarial parasites, and an estimated 1.2 billion people (20% of the world's population) are at risk of infection.[1] Of these infections, 90% are caused by *Wuchereria bancrofti*, whose only host is humans, and most of the remainder are caused by *Brugia malayi*

and *Brugia timori*. The major vectors for *W. bancrofti* are culicine mosquitoes in most urban and semiurban areas, anopheline mosquitoes in the more rural areas of Africa and elsewhere, and *Aedes* spp. in many of the endemic Pacific islands. For the *Brugia* parasites, *Mansonia* spp. serve as the major vector, but in some areas anopheline mosquitoes are responsible for transmitting infection. *Brugia* parasites are confined to areas of southern and eastern Asia, especially India, Malaysia, Indonesia, Timor-Leste and the Philippines.

ONCHOCERCIASIS

There are almost 18 million people in 37 endemic countries infected with *Onchocerca volvulus*; 99% live in sub-Saharan Africa.[2] Humans are the exclusive definitive host of *O. volvulus*; there is no non-human reservoir of infection. Blackflies of several *Simulium* species are the vectors of infection, and because the larvae of these flies require fast-flowing water for development, transmission is limited to areas within the flight range of the flies that breed in such rivers. Thus, the distribution of onchocerciasis ('river blindness') is very much determined by river systems and tributaries where the infection is endemic.

LOIASIS

Loa loa infects approximately 13 million people in the rainforest belt of western and central Africa and equatorial Sudan, where the vector – *Chrysops* flies – can easily find breeding spots.

MANSONELLA INFECTIONS

Mansonellosis

Although there are no reliable estimates of the number of people with *Mansonella ozzardi* infection, it is known that infection with this parasite is limited to parts of South America and some Caribbean islands, where it is transmitted by either midges (*Culicoides* spp.) or blackflies.

Perstans Filariasis

Mansonella perstans, distributed across the center of Africa and in northeastern South America, is transmitted by midges. The prevalence of infection is poorly understood, as is its transmission dynamics.

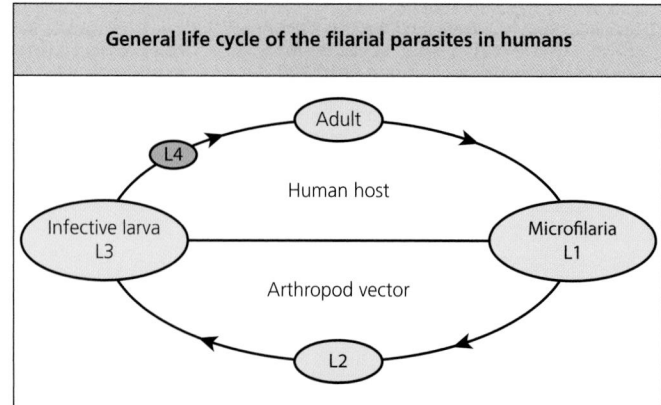

Figure 121-1 General life cycle of the filarial parasites in humans. Microfilariae (L1) are produced by the adult worms. L2 and L3 are larval development stages in the arthropod vector. L3 larval forms are infective for humans. L4 develop from the L3s within 1–2 weeks depending on the filarial species.

| TABLE 121-1 | Parasites Causing Human Filarial Infections | | | | | | | |

Parasite	Number of People Infected Worldwide	Associated Disease	Vector	Geographic Distribution	Location of Adult	Location of Microfilariae	Sheathed Microfilariae	Periodicity of Microfilariae
Wuchereria bancrofti	120 million	Lymphatic filariasis	Mosquitoes	Tropics and subtropics worldwide	Lymphatic tissue	Blood	+	Nocturnal (95%) Subperiodic (5%)
Brugia malayi	10 million	Lymphatic filariasis	Mosquitoes	Asia, India, Philippines	Lymphatic tissue	Blood	+	Nocturnal (75%) Subperiodic (25%)
Brugia timori	<0.8 million	Lymphatic filariasis	Mosquitoes	Indonesia, Timor-Leste	Lymphatic tissue	Blood	+	Nocturnal
Loa loa	12 million	Loiasis	Deerflies	Central and West Africa	Subcutaneous tissue	Blood	+	Diurnal
Onchocerca volvulus	39 million	Onchocerciasis	Blackflies	Africa (99%), Americas, Yemen	Subcutaneous tissue	Skin, eye	–	None
Mansonella ozzardi	Unknown	Mansonellosis	Midges, blackflies	South and Central America, Caribbean	Undetermined	Blood	–	None
Mansonella perstans	Unknown	*Perstans* filariasis	Midges	South and Central America, Africa	Body cavities, mesentery, perirenal tissue	Blood	–	None
Mansonella streptocerca	Unknown	Streptocerciasis	Midges	Africa	Undetermined	Skin	–	None

Streptocerciasis

Streptocerciasis, infection with the filarial nematode *Mansonella streptocerca*, is limited to the tropical rain forests of central Africa and western Uganda. Transmitted by midges (*Culicoides*), there are no good estimates of the number of people infected with this filarial parasite.

Pathogenesis and Pathology

Pathology associated with the filariases results from a complex interplay of the pathogenic potential of the parasite (and its endosymbionts), the immune response of the host and external ('complicating') bacterial and fungal infections.[3–9]

LYMPHATIC FILARIASIS

Although genital abnormalities (especially hydrocele) and lymphedema or elephantiasis are the most recognizable clinical entities associated with lymphatic filarial infections (Figure 121-2), earlier changes can be detected when lymphoscintigraphy or ultrasound techniques are used,[7] including lymphatic dilation with abnormal lymphatic function. Such subclinical changes can be seen even in young children[10] and can occur with or without a localized inflammatory response. Secondary host inflammation, including responses to bacterial and fungal superinfections of tissues with compromised lymphatic function, causes most of the progression and physical destruction associated with elephantiasis. Microbial products from the *Wolbachia* endosymbionts of the parasite may also play a role in inducing this local inflammation.

Immune-mediated pathology in lymphatic filariasis most commonly derives from the consequences of the response to dead or dying worms in the lymphatics. However, the pathogenesis of the syndrome of tropical pulmonary eosinophilia is distinctly different[11] where inflammation results from IgE- and eosinophil-mediated inflammation to the microfilarial stage parasites.

ONCHOCERCIASIS

The most significant pathology in onchocerciasis occurs in the skin (Figure 121-3) or eyes. There are both noninflammatory and

inflammatory routes to tissue damage.[9] In 'steady-state' chronic *O. volvulus* infections, though microfilariae migrate through or live in the skin they induce little inflammatory response; however, as a consequence of secreted/excreted proteins (often with enzymatic activity) there is resultant hyperpigmentation, atrophy and thinning of the skin (see Figure 121-3). Superimposed inflammatory reactions to dying microfilariae result in episodic papular dermatitis. In the eyes, these inflammatory responses result either in a characteristic punctate keratitis and, ultimately, anterior segment blindness, or in uveitis and retinal lesions that can lead to posterior segment blindness. Again, the endosymbiont bacterium (*Wolbachia* spp.) within *O. volvulus* adult worms and microfilariae may play a role in the pathogenesis of onchocerciasis skin and eye disease.[4]

LOIASIS

'Calabar' swellings, the episodic angioedematous lesions characteristic of loiasis, are not well studied. Presumably, they are the consequence of immune-mediated inflammatory responses to migrating subcutaneous adult worm antigens (Figure 121-4). Not common in untreated patients, but increasingly problematic in populations receiving ivermectin for co-endemic onchocerciasis, is a central nervous system (CNS) depression syndrome leading to coma or even death.[12] Its pathogenesis is suspected to involve inflammatory responses to dying microfilariae in cerebral vessels, but the details remain uncertain.

MANSONELLA INFECTIONS

Mansonellosis

Largely considered non-pathogenic, there are no reliable data on pathogenesis for *M. ozzardi* infection.

Perstans Filariasis

Pathology, when present, in *M. perstans* infections is largely confined to serosal surfaces and is felt to reflect eosinophil-mediated inflammation.

Streptocerciasis

Streptocerciasis affects primarily the skin. When present, disease manifestations include pruritus, dermal thickening, skin pigmentation,

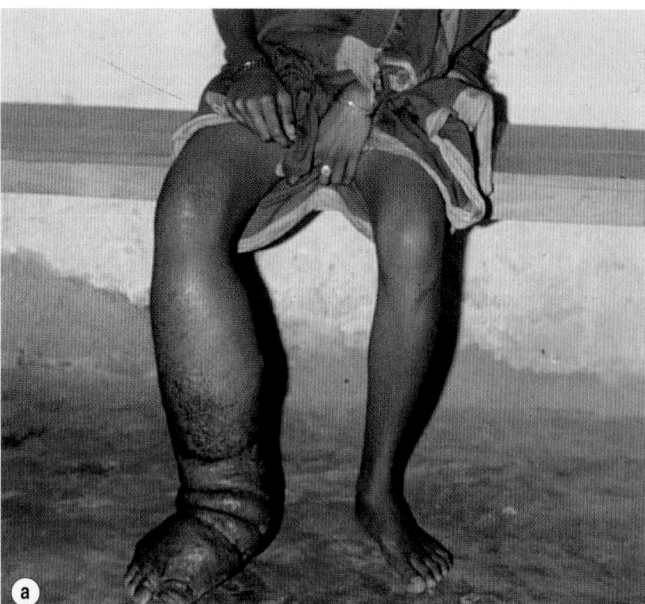

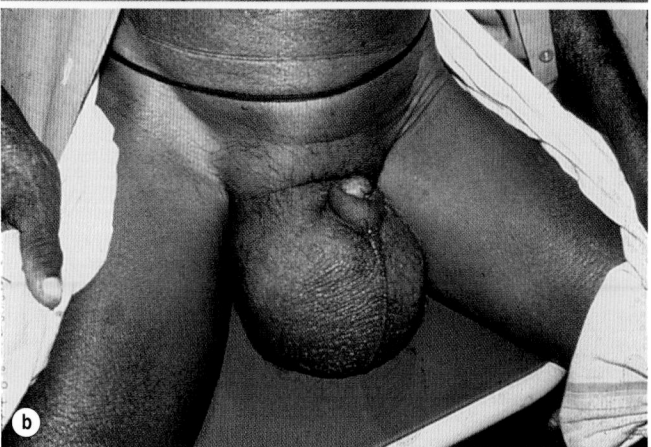

Figure 121-2 Elephantiasis. (a) Already advanced elephantiasis in a 14-year-old Indian girl who has bancroftian filariasis. Although such clinical expression of filarial disease is more commonly seen in adults, infection in endemic areas is usually established in early childhood. (b) Scrotal edema with bilateral hydroceles in an adult man who has bancroftian filariasis.

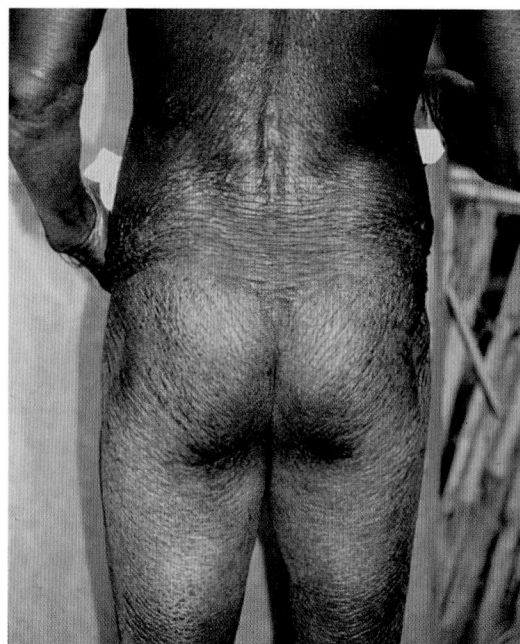

Figure 121-3 Onchocerciasis. Evidence of excoriation caused by the patient's trying to relieve the maddening pruritus caused by onchocerciasis. Note also the marked dermal atrophy associated with chronic infection.

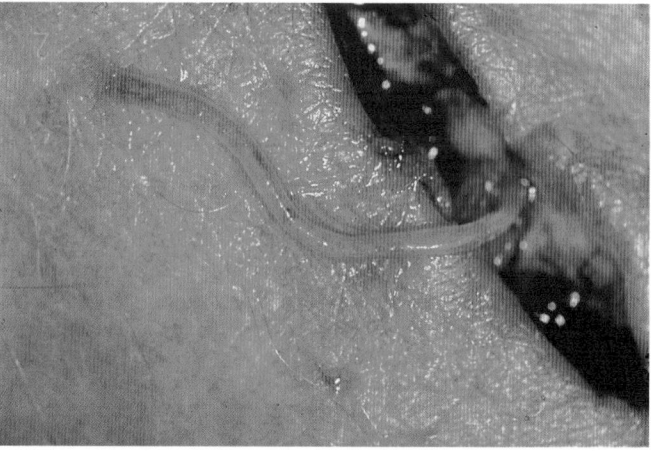

Figure 121-4 *Loa loa* adult worm. The worm has been teased from the subcutaneous tissue after incision was made through a small pruritic nodular eruption (0.5 cm in diameter) in an expatriate patient who had loiasis. Such eruptions can occur spontaneously or after treatment with DEC.

subcutaneous nodules and lymphadenitis, that can be indistinguishable from onchocerciasis. The pathogenetic mechanisms underlying disease in this infection are largely similar to those felt to be operative in *O. volvulus* infection.

Prevention

Filarial infections can be acquired only from vector-borne infective larvae. Therefore, prevention of infection can be achieved either by decreasing contact between humans and vectors, generally through vector control efforts, or by decreasing the amount of infection the vector can acquire to pass on to uninfected individuals, through treating the human host.

LYMPHATIC FILARIASIS
Population-Based Prevention

Efforts to decrease lymphatic filariasis in populations through mosquito-vector control have usually proved ineffective owing to high cost and the long lifespan of the parasite (4–8 years). With the advent of extremely effective single-dose, once-yearly, two-drug regimens (albendazole 400 mg plus either ivermectin 200–400 μg/kg or diethylcarbamazine (DEC) 6 mg/kg), the alternative approach of treating whole populations (and thereby decreasing microfilariae available to the vectors) has become the norm.[10] Indeed, it is this strategy that forms the basis of the new Global Program to Eliminate Lymphatic Filariasis undertaken by the World Health Organization (WHO) and a Global Alliance of public and private sector partners.[13,14]

Individual-Based Prevention

Contact with infected mosquitoes can be decreased through the use of personal insect repellents, bed nets and insecticide-impregnated materials. Alternatively, suggestive evidence from animal models and limited experience in human populations indicate that a prophylactic regimen of DEC (6 mg/kg/day for 2 days each month) could provide effective protection against infection.

ONCHOCERCIASIS
Population-Based Prevention

Despite its considerable expense, a highly successful program to prevent onchocerciasis based on large-scale vector control was undertaken in 11 West African countries by the WHO, the United Nations Development Program and the World Bank. In its 27 years of existence this 'Onchocerciasis Control Program' was extraordinarily successful in 'reclaiming' both land and lives of people otherwise severely compromised by onchocercal disease. However, this expensive and difficult approach to population-based prevention of onchocerciasis has been supplanted by a strategy that both treats and prevents infection through the use of once- or twice-yearly ivermectin in affected populations of all countries where onchocerciasis is endemic.[15,16]

Individual-Based Prevention

Decreased contact with infected blackflies through protective clothing and repellents is helpful in preventing infection. There are no known prophylactic treatment regimens yet defined as efficacious in humans.

LOIASIS
Population-Based Prevention

No specific prevention efforts in populations have been undertaken.

Individual-Based Prevention

There are good data that repeated use of DEC (300 mg weekly or 6 mg/kg/day for 2 days each month in adults) is effective prophylaxis against acquisition of *L. loa* infection.[17]

MANSONELLA INFECTIONS
Population-Based Prevention

No specific prevention efforts in populations have been undertaken for any of these infections.

Individual-Based Prevention

Personal protection measures to limit contact with biting midges or blackflies may provide some individual protection.

Clinical Features
LYMPHATIC FILARIASIS
Subclinical (Asymptomatic) Presentations

Of all the patients who have lymphatic filariasis, at least half appear clinically asymptomatic. Some of these have microfilariae circulating in their blood, while others have infections identifiable only by filarial antigen in the circulation. Essentially all have hidden damage to their lymphatic or renal systems.[18,19]

Acute Manifestations

There are three major acute manifestations of lymphatic filariasis, each with a different set of causative mechanisms and pathogenic implications. The first and most important is acute inflammation of the limbs or scrotum (sometimes with systemic symptoms) that is related to bacterial or fungal superinfection of tissues with already compromised lymphatic function.[20–22]

Often confused with this picture in the past, a second type of acute syndrome is characterized by initiation of inflammation in the lymph nodes (commonly the inguinal or axillary node) with 'retrograde' extension down the lymphatic tract and an accompanying 'cold' edema. Here the inflammation appears to be immune-mediated around dying parasites in the nodes; it is much less frequent than the episodes of inflammation initiated by dermal infection.[23]

A third acute filarial syndrome is tropical pulmonary eosinophilia (Weingarten's syndrome), a distinctly different syndrome caused by an immunologic hyperresponsiveness to filarial infection.[11] It is characterized by:
- extremely high levels of peripheral blood eosinophilia;
- asthma-like symptoms;
- restrictive (and often obstructive) lung disease;
- very high levels of specific antifilarial antibodies; and
- an excellent therapeutic response to appropriate antifilarial treatment with diethylcarbamazine (DEC).

While occurring with a frequency of less than 1% of all cases of lymphatic filariasis, it is nevertheless a severe condition that can lead to chronic interstitial fibrosis and pulmonary failure.[24–25]

Chronic Manifestations

Hydrocele, even though found only with *W. bancrofti* (and not *Brugia*) infections, is the most common clinical manifestation of lymphatic filariasis. It is seen principally after puberty, and there is a progressive increase in prevalence with age.[18] In some endemic communities, as many as 40–60% of all adult males have hydrocele. It often develops in the absence of overt inflammatory reactions and, indeed, many patients who have hydrocele also have microfilariae circulating in the blood. The localization of adult worms in the lymphatics of the spermatic cord leads to a thickening so that the cord is palpable on physical examination of most patients. Hydroceles can become massive but still occur in the absence of any lymphedema or elephantiasis in the penis and scrotum (see Figure 121-2).[26–27]

Although lymphedema can also develop in the absence of overt inflammatory reactions and in the early stages be associated with microfilaremia, the development of elephantiasis (either of the limbs or the genitals) is most frequently associated with a history of recurrent inflammatory episodes. Patients who have chronic lymphedema or elephantiasis are rarely microfilaremic. Very important in the progression of these lesions is the fact that the redundant skin folds, cracks and fissures of the skin provide havens for bacteria and fungi to thrive and intermittently penetrate the epidermis, leading to either local or systemic infections.

Chyluria, another of the chronic filarial syndromes, is caused by the intermittent flow of intestinal lymph (chyle) through ruptured lymphatics into the renal pelvis and subsequently into the urine. The mechanisms underlying this have not been well defined and the clinical course is known to be intermittent. Nutritional compromise can, however, be severe in patients who have chronic chyluria; special diets (low-fat and high-protein, supplemented with fluids) can often be helpful.

A variety of other syndromes coexisting with filariasis are found in filarial-endemic regions; because they sometimes show evidence of therapeutic response to DEC they have been regarded as possible manifestations of lymphatic filariasis. These include arthritis (typically monoarticular), endomyocardial fibrosis, tenosynovitis, thrombophlebitis, lateral popliteal nerve palsy and others. Although future studies may strengthen an etiologic relationship with filarial infection, such presentations cannot now be confidently attributed to lymphatic filarial infection.

ONCHOCERCIASIS
Chronic Presentations

Most damage from onchocerciasis occurs in the skin and eye. Subcutaneous nodules (generally 1–6 cm in diameter) can be palpated superficially, but most skin involvement is a waxing and waning of papular rashes, essentially always accompanied by itching (see Figure 121-3) likely because of inflammatory responses to dying microfilariae. During the long course of infection, the skin becomes extensively damaged, losing much of its elasticity and even pigmentation. Indeed, when the skin over the inguinal nodes (which are often enlarged by their continued stimulation from dying microfilariae) becomes so atrophic that it cannot support the underlying lymph nodes, the clinical presentation of 'hanging groin' occurs.

In the eye, acute changes are those associated with dying microfilariae and the local inflammatory reactions that they induce. In the cornea, 'fluffy opacities' (inflammatory cells associated with the dying microfilariae) can lead to punctate keratitis, and in prolonged and heavy infection inflammation in the cornea results in sclerosing keratitis; inflammatory responses localized elsewhere in the eye lead to iridocyclitis, choroidoretinitis or optic atrophy. Longer-term complications of these inflammatory eye processes also include glaucoma and cataracts.

LOIASIS

The two most characteristic clinical features of loiasis are the passage of an adult filarial worm across the eye ('eye worm'), often in an otherwise asymptomatic person, and Calabar swellings.[6,28] Calabar swellings are transient localized areas of episodic angioedema. If the inflammatory reaction extends to nearby joints or peripheral nerves, corresponding symptoms may develop.

MANSONELLA INFECTIONS

Mansonellosis

Although *M. ozzardi* has often been considered nonpathogenic, headache, articular pain, fever, pulmonary symptoms, adenopathy, hepatomegaly and pruritus, have been ascribed to *M. ozzardi* infection.[29]

Perstans Filariasis

The clinical features of *M. perstans* infection are poorly defined. Most patients appear to be clinically asymptomatic, but manifestations may include transient angioedema and pruritus of the arms, face, or other parts of the body (analogous to the Calabar swellings of loiasis); fever; headache; arthralgias; and right-upper-quadrant pain. Occasionally, pericarditis and hepatitis occur.[30]

Streptocerciasis

The major clinical manifestations of *M. streptocerca* infection involve the skin and include pruritus, papular rashes and pigmentation changes that are often indistinguishable from those in onchocerciasis. Many infected individuals have inguinal adenopathy, although most are clinically asymptomatic.

FILARIAL INFECTIONS IN TRAVELERS AND EXPATRIATES

Expatriate visitors to regions endemic for loiasis and other filariases often have clinical manifestations of their filarial infections that reflect either the lack of chronicity of their infection or an immune-mediated hyperresponsiveness. Indeed, these 'temporary residents' manifest prominent signs and symptoms of inflammatory reactions (including allergic reactions) to the mature or maturing parasites. In loiasis, these manifestations have included primarily Calabar swellings, urticaria, rashes and occasionally asthma.[17] In bancroftian filariasis (when military personnel or other migrants to endemic areas have acquired these infections), the manifestations have usually been lymphangitis, lymphadenitis and genital pain (from inflammation of the associated lymphatics), with hives, rashes and other 'allergic-like' manifestations, including eosinophilia.[31]

Diagnosis

Except for *W. bancrofti* infections, diagnosis of filarial infections depends principally on the direct demonstration of the parasite (almost always microfilariae) in blood or skin specimens using relatively cumbersome techniques and having to take into account the periodicity (nocturnal or diurnal) of microfilariae (see Table 121-1). Most alternative methods based on detection of antibodies by immunodiagnostic tests have proved unsatisfactory because of their failure to distinguish active and past infections and problems with specificity. However, there is now good evidence that species-specific recombinant antigens have improved the value of antibody-based immunodiagnostics.

LYMPHATIC FILARIASIS

Circulating filarial antigen detection, with its very high specificity and sensitivity, should now be regarded as the 'gold standard' for diagnosing *W. bancrofti* infections.[32] Two commercial assays are available: one is an enzyme-linked immunosorbent assay that yields semiquantitative results; the other is a simple card (immunochromatographic) test which yields only qualitative (positive or negative) answers. No such test is available for brugian filariasis.

Before the development of the circulating filarial antigen assay, the standard approach to diagnosing lymphatic filarial infection was detection of microfilariae in blood, and this is still required for both brugian filariasis and where the antigen detection test is not available for bancroftian filariasis. The optimal timing of blood draws must take into account the possible nocturnal periodicity of the parasites: namely, between 10.00 pm and 2.00 am for most brugian filariasis and bancroftian infections.[8] The simplest technique for examining blood or other fluids (e.g. hydrocele fluid or articular effusions) is to spread 20 µL evenly over a clean slide that is dried and then stained with Giemsa or a similar stain. The larger the blood volumes examined, the greater the likelihood of detecting low levels of parasitemia. Other concentration techniques are also available.

Serologic assays using recombinant *Wuchereria*- or *Brugia*-specific antigens (e.g. Bm14, Wb123, BmR1) have been developed and, in the absence of previous anthelmintic treatment, are useful in the diagnosis of an individual patient and for use in surveillance following mass drug administration campaigns.[33–35]

ONCHOCERCIASIS

Classic parasitologic techniques are most commonly used to diagnose onchocerciasis.[2] Microfilariae can be visualized directly in the anterior chamber fluid of the eye by slit-lamp examination of patients. Skin microfilariae can be visualized after a skin snip has removed the most superficial layers of skin with either a corneoscleral punch or a small needle and disposable scalpel blade to obtain approximately 1 mg of a bloodless piece of skin. This sample is then placed in saline for examination for the emergence of microfilariae after 30 minutes to 24 hours. Alternative tests rely on molecular-based detection using polymerase chain reaction-based assays on skin snip-derived DNA. Also, subcutaneous or deep nodules (generally 1–6 cm in size) can be detected by palpation or ultrasound, and the adult worms they contain can be identified histologically in specimens that have been removed surgically.

Serologic assays using recombinant *O. volvulus*-specific recombinant antigens (e.g. Ov16 and others) have been developed and, in the absence of previous anthelmintic treatment, are useful in the diagnosis of an individual patient and for use in surveillance following mass drug administration campaigns. A rapid point-of-care test measuring IgG4 antibodies to Ov16[36] is now available commercially.

LOIASIS

The diagnosis of loiasis remains dependent on direct parasitologic identification (most frequently microfilariae in the blood) or indirect serologic approaches in association with a compatible clinical presentation and exposure history. *Loa loa* microfilarial periodicity in the blood means that blood sampling must be done near midday (usually between 10.00 am and 2.00 pm). DNA-based diagnostics (polymerase chain reaction [PCR], real time PCR, loop mediated isothermal amplification [LAMP]) have been used quite successfully on whole blood but are available clinically in only a few tertiary referral centers.

Serologic assays using recombinant *L. loa* antigens have been developed, including a sensitive and specific rapid assay that uses immunoassays to detect antibodies to the recombinant *L. loa* antigen LLSXP-1.[37-38]

Management

LYMPHATIC FILARIASIS

Treatment of the Infection

Remarkable advances in treating lymphatic filarial infection have recently been achieved, but most of these have focused not on individual patients but on the community reduction of microfilaremia through once-yearly treatment, as described above. With newer definitions of clinical syndromes in lymphatic filariasis and new tools to assess clinical status (e.g., ultrasound, lymphoscintigraphy, circulating filarial antigen assays, PCR) approaches to treatment based on infection status can be considered.

Diethylcarbamazine ([DEC], 6 mg/kg daily for 12 days), which has both macro- and microfilaricidal properties, remains the drug of choice for the treatment of active lymphatic filariasis (defined by microfilaremia, antigen positivity, or adult worms on ultrasound), although albendazole (400 mg twice daily for 21 days) has also demonstrated macrofilaricidal efficacy. A 4- to 6-week course of doxycycline (targeting the intracellular *Wolbachia*) also has significant macrofilaricidal activity, as has DEC/albendazole used daily for 7 days.[39] The addition of DEC to a 3-week course of doxycycline has also been shown to be efficacious in lymphatic filariasis.[40]

Because the use of DEC in patients who have either onchocerciasis or loiasis can be unsafe (see below), it is important that individual patients who have bancroftian filariasis and who live in areas endemic for these other infections be examined for coinfection with these parasites before being treated with DEC.

Both DEC and ivermectin, given at the doses necessary to treat microfilaremic patients, cause minimal or no drug-induced side effects. However, their rapid killing of microfilariae releases enough antigen to overwhelm the modulating effects of the host's immune system and to induce a variety of post-treatment reactions.[41] These occur in proportion to the pre-treatment microfilarial levels and include headaches, fever, myalgia, lymphadenopathy and occasionally rash, itching and other symptoms. Although the most severely affected patients can also experience postural hypotension, generally these reactions are well managed through the use of antipyretics, antihistamines or, in the most severe instances, corticosteroids. In the tropical eosinophilia syndrome, as there are no microfilariae in the blood, there is no exacerbation of symptoms, but rather a steady improvement over the 2–4 weeks during which DEC is administered.

Treating the Disease

Although it is important to treat the infection, management of the consequences of these infections (particularly the lymphedema, elephantiasis and genital pathology) is what is often of greatest concern to the patient. In persons with chronic manifestations of lymphatic filariasis, treatment regimens that emphasize hygiene, prevention of secondary bacterial infections and physiotherapy have gained wide acceptance for morbidity control. These regimens are similar to those recommended for lymphedema of most non-filarial causes and known by a variety of names, including *complex decongestive physiotherapy* and *complex lymphedema therapy*. Hydroceles (Figure 121-2) can be managed surgically. With chronic manifestations of lymphatic filariasis, drug treatment should be reserved for individuals with evidence of active infection, although a 6-week course of doxycycline has been shown to provide improvement in filarial lymphedema irrespective of disease activity.[42]

Noninvasive management of chyluria relies on nutritional support, especially replacement of fat-rich diets with high-protein, high-fluid diets supplemented where possible with medium-chain triglycerides. Surgery, the sclerosing effects of lymphangiography or, often, time alone can also lead to the cessation of the leakage of lymph into the renal pelvis, collecting system and urine.

ONCHOCERCIASIS

The main goals of therapy are to prevent the development of irreversible lesions and to alleviate symptoms. Surgical excision is recommended when nodules are located on the head (because of the proximity of microfilaria-producing adult worms to the eye), but chemotherapy is the mainstay of management. Ivermectin, a semisynthetic macrocyclic lactone active against microfilariae, is the first-line agent for the treatment of onchocerciasis. It is given orally in a single dose of 150 μg/kg, either yearly or semiannually. More frequent ivermectin administration (every 3 months) has been suggested to ameliorate pruritus and skin disease.[43]

The side reactions that follow treatment of onchocerciasis with ivermectin (or, earlier, with DEC) have been termed the Mazzotti reaction. They result from the rapid killing of microfilariae and consist primarily of headache, fever, pruritus, adenopathy, rash and, occasionally, postural hypotension. Although pronounced after DEC, they are much milder after ivermectin and are self-limiting (beginning within hours of treatment and persisting as long as 4–5 days); they can be managed satisfactorily with antipyretics, analgesics, antihistamines and, if necessary, systemic corticosteroids.

Because adult worms, which are generally not killed by either ivermectin or DEC, continue to shed microfilariae for up to 12–15 years, symptoms may recur and require additional 'microfilaricidal' treatment over an extended period of time.

With the demonstration of efficacy of a 6-week course of doxycycline for the sterilization of adult female *Onchocerca* worms,[44] doxycycline has begun to be considered a macrofilaricidal (or macrofilaristatic) drug for *O. volvulus*.[45]

LOIASIS

The approach to treatment of loiasis depends on the clinical presentation. In patients who do not have microfilaremia, DEC 8–10 mg/kg/day for 3 weeks is the optimal treatment and results in cure of approximately half of the patients. Repeated courses of the drug are indicated when patients become symptomatic again and each repeated treatment results in additional patient cures.[46]

For microfilaremic patients, the approach to treatment is more difficult because the side reactions induced by the dying microfilariae can include CNS complications and even death. Such severe reactions rarely, if ever, occur in patients who have blood microfilaria counts of less than 2000/mL of blood (drawn at the time of day for peak parasitemia). However, even in a very controlled hospital setting, when highly microfilaremic loiasis patients were treated with DEC (initially at very low dosages – 0.25 mg/kg – and then increased progressively), there were still some patients in whom there was development of a post-treatment encephalopathy and death. This was not prevented even when corticosteroids were co-administered.[47]

When ivermectin is used instead of DEC, the clearance of microfilaremia from the blood is very much slower and not so complete. While it is much safer than DEC, both in terms of the systemic side reactions that it elicits (similar to those of the Mazzotti reaction) and in terms of avoiding the catastrophic neurologic complications in patients with extremely high levels of microfilaremia (especially >30 000 mf/mL), ivermectin has still led to instances of CNS deterioration, coma and death.[12,47] With optimal clinical care, the transient CNS compromise of such ivermectin-treated patients can be managed successfully and catastrophic results minimized. However, the treatment of *Loa*-endemic populations with ivermectin (usually as part of national programs linked to the African Program for Onchocerciasis Control[2] or the Global Program to Eliminate Lymphatic Filariasis) often must be rendered in remote areas without access to optimal medical management. Therefore, this potential complication of treatment provides a major challenge that must be overcome before these massive public health initiatives can be successfully implemented in the *Loa*-endemic regions of Africa.

If patients experience an adult *L. loa* crossing the eye below the conjunctiva, such worms can be removed through simple surgical incision of the conjunctiva, but because usually there are multiple parasites within the patient a single procedure may not be curative.[48]

MANSONELLA INFECTIONS

Mansonellosis

Therapy with single-dose ivermectin is the standard approach for *M. ozzardi* infection.

Perstans Filariasis

With the identification of a *Wolbachia* endosymbiont in *M. perstans*, doxycycline (200 mg twice a day) for 6 weeks has been established as the first effective treatment for this infection.[49]

Streptocerciasis

Therapy with single-dose yearly ivermectin is the standard approach for *M. streptocerca* infection. DEC is a therapeutic alternative, although it should be used with caution in heavily microfilaremic patients.

References available online at expertconsult.com.

KEY REFERENCES

Boatin B.: The Onchocerciasis Control Programme in West Africa (OCP). *Ann Trop Med Parasitol* 2008; 102(Suppl.1):13-17.

Chippaux J.P., Boussinesq M., et al.: Severe adverse reaction risks during mass treatment with ivermectin in loiasis-endemic areas. *Parasitol Today* 1996; 12:448-450.

Coulibaly Y.I., Dembele B., et al.: A randomized trial of doxycycline for *Mansonella perstans* infection. *N Engl J Med* 2009; 361:1448-1458.

Francis H., Awadzi K., et al.: The Mazzotti reaction following treatment of onchocerciasis with diethylcarbamazine: clinical severity as a function of infection intensity. *Am J Trop Med Hyg* 1985; 34:529-536.

Klion A.D., Massougbodji A., et al.: Loiasis in endemic and nonendemic populations: immunologically mediated differences in clinical presentation. *J Infect Dis* 1991; 163:1318-1325.

Mand S., Debrah A.Y., Klarmann U.L., et al.: Doxycycline improves filarial lymphedema independent of active filarial infection: a randomized controlled trial. *Clin Infect Dis* 2012; 55:621-630.

Ottesen E.A., Hooper P.J., et al.: The global programme to eliminate lymphatic filariasis: health impact after 8 years. *PLoS Negl Trop Dis* 2008; 2:e317.

Ottesen E.A., Nutman T.B.: Tropical pulmonary eosinophilia. *Annu Rev Med* 1992; 43:417-424.

Rom W.N., Vijayan V.K., et al.: Persistent lower respiratory tract inflammation associated with interstitial lung disease in patients with tropical pulmonary eosinophilia following conventional treatment with diethylcarbamazine. *Am Rev Respir Dis* 1990; 142:1088-1092.

Taylor M.J., Hoerauf A., et al.: Lymphatic filariasis and onchocerciasis. *Lancet* 2010; 376:1175-1185.

Weil G.J., Ramzy R.M.: Diagnostic tools for filariasis elimination programs. *Trends Parasitol* 2007; 23:78-82.

Infections and the Common Inherited Hemoglobin Disorders

THOMAS N. WILLIAMS | DAVID J. WEATHERALL

KEY CONCEPTS

- The inherited hemoglobin disorders are the commonest monogenic diseases. Between 300 000 and 400 000 babies are born with them each year. Eighty percent of births are in low- or middle-income countries (LMIC).

- The frequency of these diseases is likely to increase significantly in the future.

- All these diseases are associated with increased susceptibility to a wide range of infections.

- The diagnosis of infection is often complicated by underlying complications of the hemoglobin disorder.

- Blood-borne infection is still a major risk, particularly in LMIC.

- Because the pattern of infection varies between different types of hemoglobin disorders, an accurate diagnosis of the particular disorder is a vital part of the management of episodes of infection.

Classification and Epidemiology

CLASSIFICATION

Different forms of hemoglobin (Hb) are produced in embryonic, fetal and adult life, each consisting of pairs of different globin chains. Adult hemoglobin consists of a major component HbA ($\alpha_2\beta_2$) and a minor fraction HbA$_2$ ($\alpha_2\delta_2$). In fetal life the major hemoglobin is HbF ($\alpha_2\gamma_2$). The inherited disorders of hemoglobin are classified into two major groups (Box 122-1). First there are the structural hemoglobin variants. Although there are many hundreds of these variants, only three reach extremely high frequencies: Hbs S, C and E. The clinical manifestations of Hbs S and C are related to abnormal structure-function mecha-

nisms, while those of HbE result from its reduced rate of synthesis. Second are the thalassemias, which result from many different mutations that reduce the synthesis of the α- or β-globin chains.[1] As shown in Box 122-1 the compound heterozygous inheritance of both structural variants and β-thalassemia, notably HbS β-thalassemia and HbE β-thalassemia, are of considerable clinical importance; globally, HbE β-thalassemia accounts for about 50% of severe cases of β-thalassemia.

EPIDEMIOLOGY

The global distribution of Hbs S and E and of the different forms of thalassemia are shown in Figures 122-1 to 122-3 and the reasons for the remarkably high frequency of these diseases are summarized in Box 122-2. Natural selection is of key importance.[2] Carriers for the sickle cell, mild forms of α-thalassemia and HbC genes show significant protection against *Plasmodium falciparum* malaria. There is increasing evidence that the *same* applies to carriers for HbE or β-thalassemia. The complex mechanisms for this protection are not yet fully understood. It has been found recently that there is complex interplay between these protective mechanisms. For instance, although carriers of the sickle cell and mild α-thalassemia genes are protected against malaria, those that inherit both these genes lose their protection completely.[3] Such complex epistatic interactions will undoubtedly be found for other genetic polymorphisms of this type.

Other factors that maintain the high frequency of the hemoglobin disorders include a high level of consanguinity in many of the affected populations, the epidemiological transition whereby improvements in public health allow more affected babies to survive to present for treatment, and emigration from high-frequency countries to richer-resourced countries where treatment is available for these disorders.

Pathogenesis and Pathology

The increased susceptibility to certain forms of infection in patients with inherited disorders of hemoglobin is best understood by first considering their molecular pathology.

SICKLE CELL ANEMIA AND ITS VARIANTS

The substitution of valine for glutamic acid at position 6 in the β-globin chain of HbS leads to deformity of the red cells at relatively low oxygen tensions.[4] The characteristic sickle shape reflects polymerization of the globin chains and leads to a variable degree of vaso-occlusion. The latter results in reperfusion injury characterized by excessive oxidant generation and activation of the endothelium of small vessels with diminished nitric oxide availability. Vascular occlusion leads to widespread complications including early splenic atrophy,

---

BOX 122-1   A CLASSIFICATION OF THE COMMON INHERITED HEMOGLOBIN DISORDERS

Structural Hemoglobin Variants
- HbS
- HbC
- HbE
- Many rarer forms

Thalassemias
- α-thalassemia
  - α^+-thalassemia
  - α^0-thalassemia
- β-thalassemia
  - β^+-thalassemia
  - β^0-thalassemia
- $\delta\beta$-thalassemia

Common Compound Heterozygotes
- HbS β-thalassemia
- HbE β-thalassemia
- HbSC disease
- α^+/α^0-thalassemia

BOX 122-2   FACTORS RESPONSIBLE FOR THE HIGH LEVEL OF INHERITED HEMOGLOBIN DISORDERS

- Natural selection
- High frequency of consanguinity
- Epidemiological transition
- Population migration
- Increasing population size

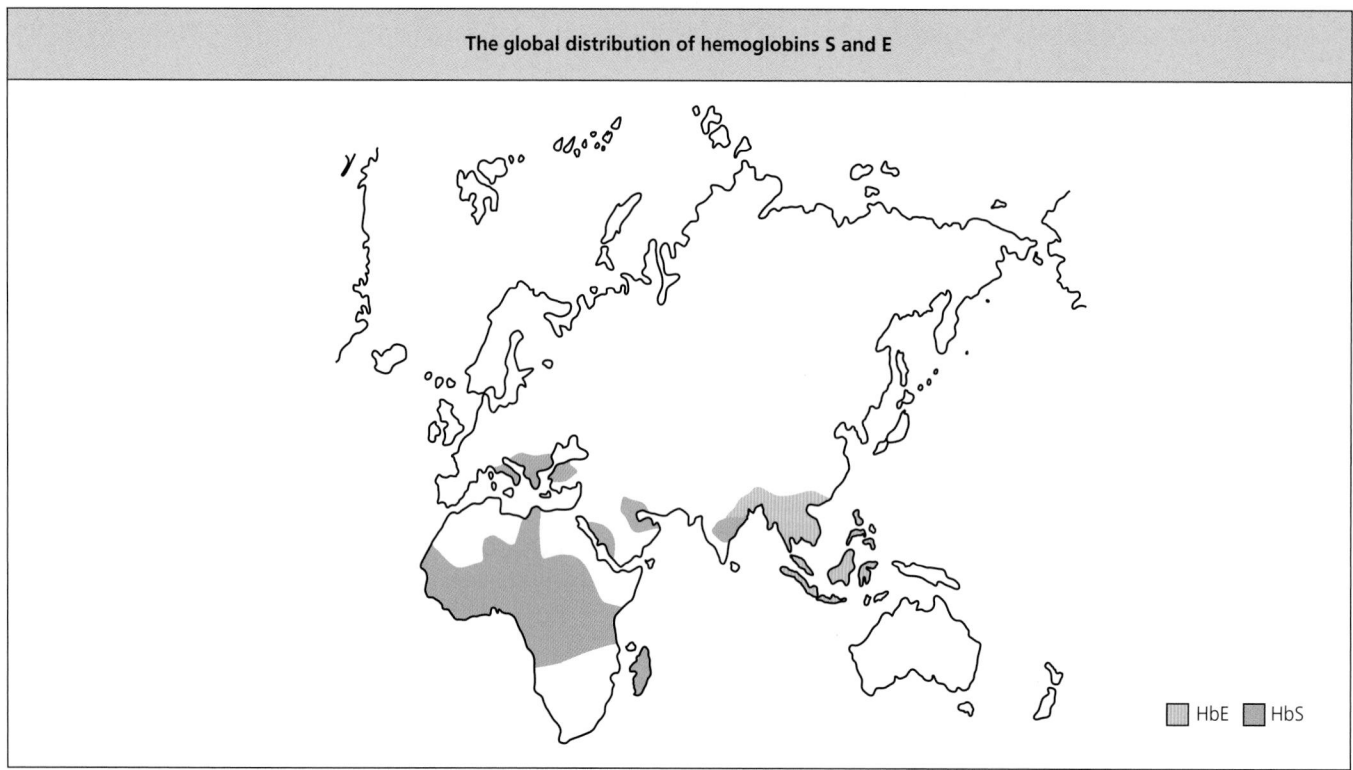

The global distribution of hemoglobins S and E

HbE   HbS

Figure 122-1 The global distribution of hemoglobins S (HbS) and E (HbE). The patchy distribution of HbS in the New World as a result of emigration from Africa is not shown. *(From Weatherall D.J., Clegg J.B.: The thalassaemia syndromes, 4th ed. Oxford: Blackwell Science; 2001. Used with permission.)*

infarction of bone marrow leading to painful crises, chronic leg ulcers, vascular complications of the brain, and many other forms of tissue damage. The deformity of the red cells is associated with a hemolytic anemia of varying severity.

By far the most important factor in proneness to infection based on the pathophysiology of sickle cell disease is the very early loss of splenic function due to damage to the spleen by the deformed sickle cells.[5] Susceptibility to invasive pneumococcal infection is the major cause of early death in babies and young children. There may also be increased proneness to other infections, notably *Haemophilus influenzae* type B (Hib). The increased frequency of *Salmonella* osteomyelitis results from infection of the marrow and overlying bone infarcts that occur during painful crises. While there is no evidence of increased susceptibility to viral infections, the aplastic crises that tend to occur in small epidemics are undoubtedly due to parvovirus infection.[6] In infections of this type in patients with sickle cell anemia, because of the extremely shortened lifespan of their red cells, profound anemia develops over a very short period. They are also prone to severe complications of influenza, including the precipitation of painful crises.[7] The hemolytic anemia results in increased bilirubin production with a high frequency of gallstone formation and associated infection of the gallbladder. There is a high frequency of the genetic mutation that results in Gilbert's syndrome in those of African origin and those affected are even more prone to this complication.[8]

THE THALASSEMIAS

The α-thalassemias result from deletions or point mutations in one or both of the linked pairs of α-globin genes (αα/αα).[1] They are divided into the α+- and α0-thalassemias. In the former a single α gene is lost by deletion or its function is suppressed by a point mutation, the so-called non-deletion (ND) form (-α/αα, αNDα/αα). Although these are the commonest genetic disorders they are not associated with severe anemia. The α0-thalassemias are characterized by deletion of both of the linked pairs of α-globin genes (–/αα). In the compound heterozygous state for α0- and α+-thalassemia (-α/–) there is significant

imbalance of globin-chain synthesis with the production of excess β-chains which form unstable tetramers called HbH. HbH disease is characterized by a hemolytic anemia of varying severity associated with splenomegaly. The homozygous state for α0-thalassemia (–/–) causes stillbirth.

The β-thalassemias result from many different mutations of the β-globin genes (β/β) which result in a variable degree of suppression of globin-chain production leading to an excess of α-chains that precipitate and cause severe damage to the red cell precursors and red cells in the circulation.[9] Depending at least in part on the severity of the β-globin gene mutation these conditions vary in their phenotype from β-thalassemia major, which requires lifelong transfusion, to a milder form of the disease called β-thalassemia intermedia. HbE thalassemia shows a wide range of phenotypic expression, from a transfusion-dependent disorder like thalassemia major to a condition that is associated with normal growth and development, albeit at a relatively low hemoglobin level.[10]

Inadequately transfused patients with severe β-thalassemia, as well as profound anemia, develop skeletal deformities due to bone marrow expansion, progressive splenomegaly, defective growth and development, and a wide range of other complications. In well-transfused patients iron loading, both from transfused blood and due to increased iron absorption, is an important complication that has to be dealt with by the administration of chelating agents.

The common symptomatic form of α-thalassemia, HbH disease, also shows wide phenotypic diversity depending, at least in part, on the molecular forms of α-thalassemia that have been inherited. Like HbE β-thalassemia, at one end of the spectrum it is a transfusion-dependent disorder, mainly due to relatively severe hemolysis.

The pattern of infection in the severe β-thalassemias is different to that in sickle cell anemia in many respects.[11] Before the days when adequate transfusion levels were achieved, progressive splenomegaly was extremely common, necessitating splenectomy. At that time there was an extremely high rate of infection after splenectomy, particularly in children aged less than 5 years. Although the situation has improved

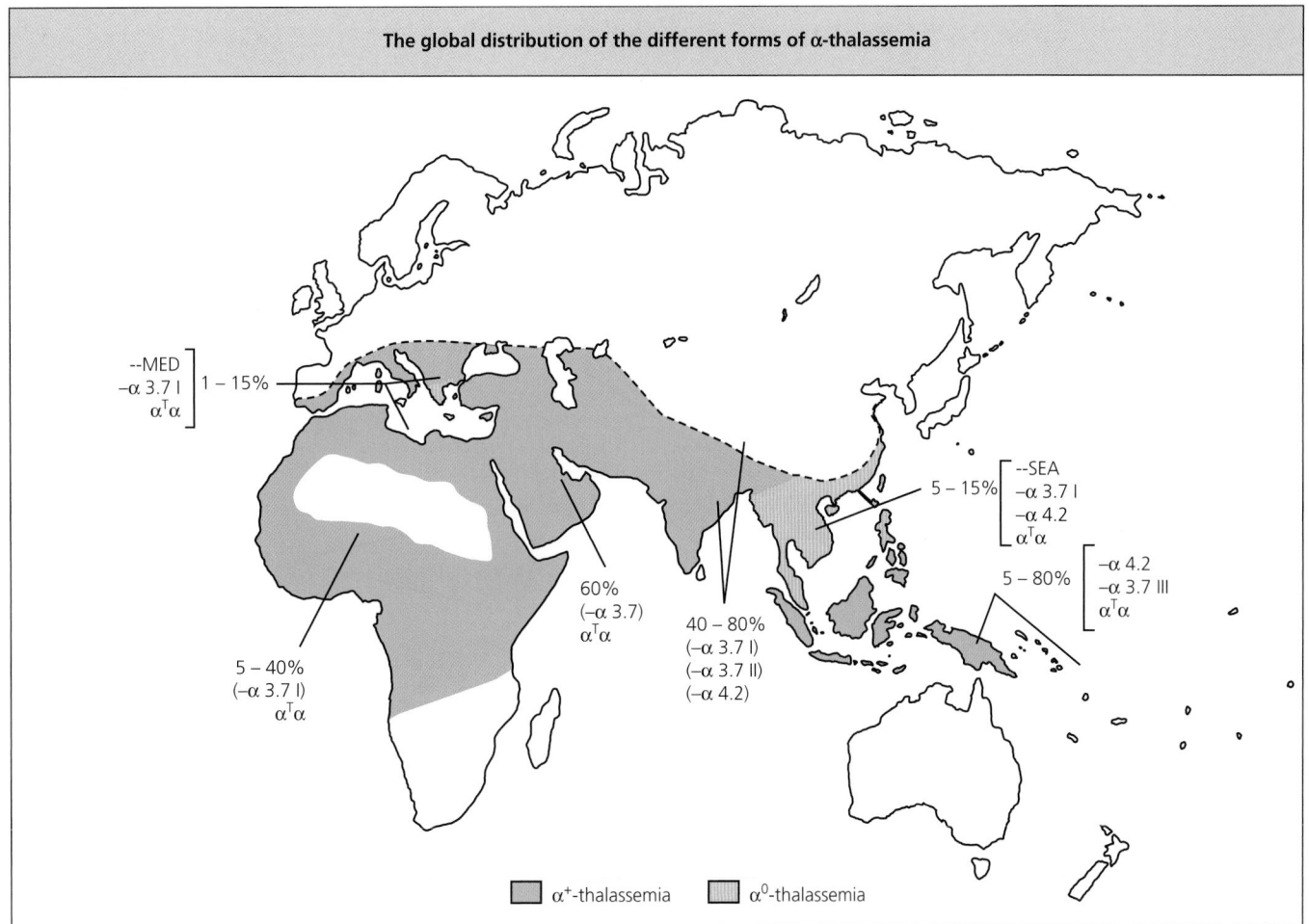

Figure 122-2 The global distribution of the different forms of α-thalassemia. The main forms of the disease that are shown are the carrier states for α+-thalassemia and its different forms, -α^{3.7 I}, -α^{3.7 II}, -α^{3.7 III}. The common forms of α⁰-thalassemia, –α^{SEA} and –α^{MED} are also shown. The very high, if approximate, gene frequencies are also shown, indicating that this is the commonest genetic disease globally. *(From Weatherall D.J., Clegg JB.: The thalassaemia syndromes, 4th ed. Oxford: Blackwell Science; 2001. Used with permission.)*

considerably following the administration of adequate transfusion and the use of iron chelating agents, progressive splenomegaly is still seen quite often and a significant number of splenectomies are still carried out with the risk of infection with similar organisms to those that occur in sickle cell anemia. Patients with β-thalassemia are also prone to a wide range of other infections.[1] Because of transfusion dependence blood-borne infections are still common, notably hepatitis B and C and human immunodeficiency viruses (HIVs). Malaria is also an important blood-borne infection in some of the developing countries in the tropics.

The only pathogens that have been shown quite unequivocally to occur with an increased frequency in iron-loaded patients with β-thalassemia are those of the *Yersinia* genus, which normally have a low rate of pathogenicity and an unusually high requirement for iron. They do not secrete sideropores but have receptors for ferrioxamine and become pathogenic in the presence of iron which is bound to the widely used chelating agent desferrioxamine.[11] There have been many reports of severe infections with this organism in patients with severe β-thalassemia. Reports have also documented the occurrence of severe, invasive fungal infections, in particular mucormycosis, in multiply-transfused patients with β-thalassemia, although the mechanism underlying this susceptibility is unclear. Patients with sickle cell anemia, while they are less prone to malaria, have severe complications and a high mortality risk if they are infected.[12] There is strong evidence that in the case of *Plasmodium vivax* malaria carriers for α-thalassemia and patients with HbE β-thalassemia are more susceptible than normal

individuals. This probably reflects the fact that the receptor for *P. vivax* is the Duffy antigen which is expressed at a higher level on relatively young red cells, which are present in all the hemoglobin disorders.

PREVENTION

Marked reduction in the births of babies with serious forms of β-thalassemia and to a lesser extent with sickle cell anemia have been achieved in many countries. Programs of this type rely on intensive public education about the nature of the inherited hemoglobin disorders, prenatal screening of parents to detect those at risk for having an infected child, prenatal diagnosis by analysis of DNA obtained by chorionic villus sampling, and termination of pregnancy in cases in which the genotype is that of sickle cell anemia or a severe form of thalassemia.[1]

In many of the higher-income countries in which prenatal diagnosis for sickle cell anemia is not yet widely applied, screening of newborn babies at risk is now carried out, either by the use of hemoglobin electrophoresis or high performance liquid chromatography (HPLC) analysis. Early administration of prophylactic penicillin has been shown to deliver a remarkable reduction in early deaths from infection.[13] Recent studies in Africa suggest that early deaths are associated with similar organisms to those in the higher-income countries and the development of neonatal diagnosis and prophylaxis of this type is likely to have a major effect in reducing early death rates.[14] Vaccination with pneumococcal, Hib and meningococcal vaccines are also being incorporated into these regimens. In the case of the severe forms of

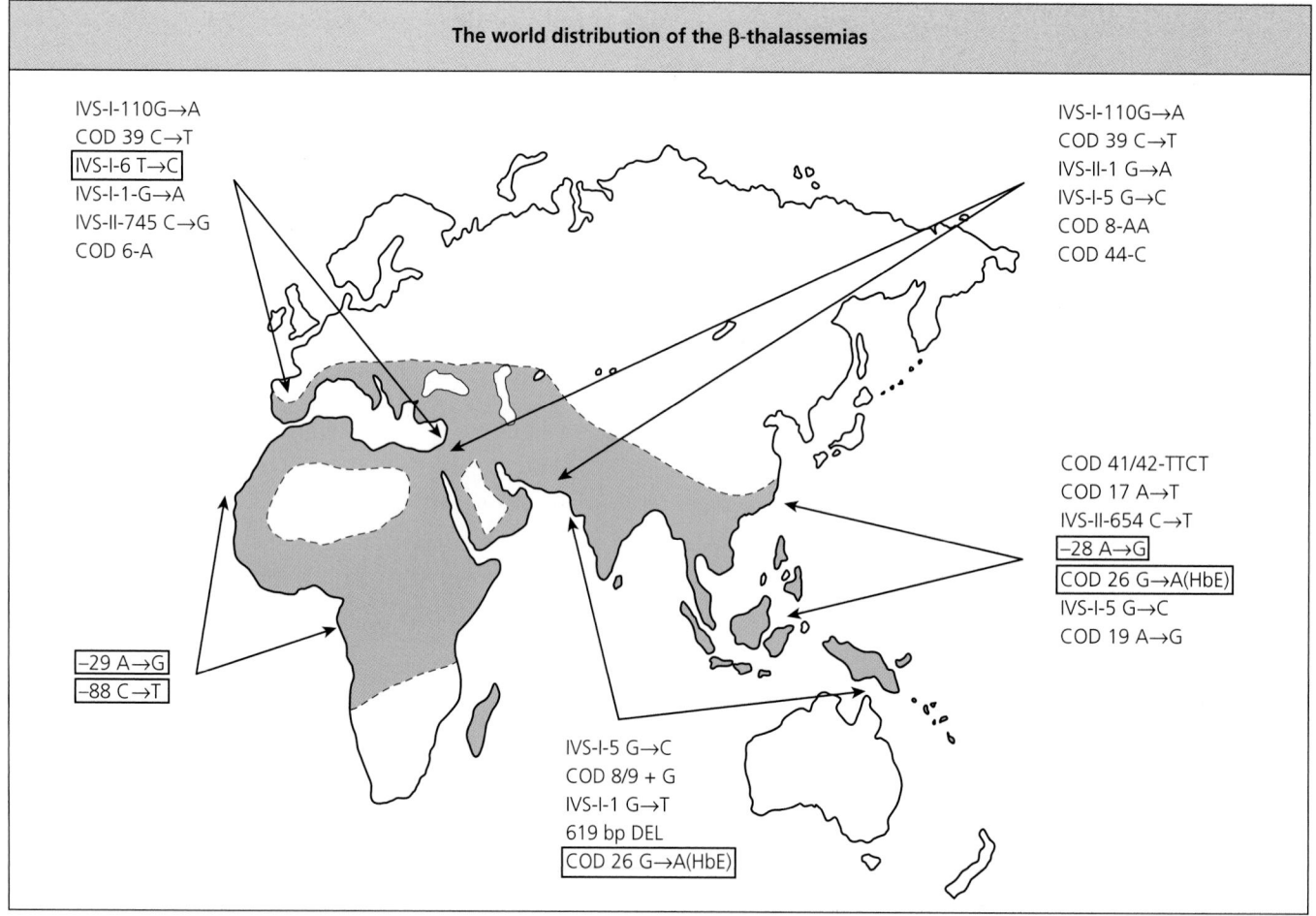

The world distribution of the β-thalassemias

IVS-I-110G→A
COD 39 C→T
IVS-I-6 T→C
IVS-I-1-G→A
IVS-II-745 C→G
COD 6-A

IVS-I-110G→A
COD 39 C→T
IVS-II-1 G→A
IVS-I-5 G→C
COD 8-AA
COD 44-C

COD 41/42-TTCT
COD 17 A→T
IVS-II-654 C→T
−28 A→G
COD 26 G→A(HbE)
IVS-I-5 G→C
COD 19 A→G

−29 A→G
−88 C→T

IVS-I-5 G→C
COD 8/9 + G
IVS-I-1 G→T
619 bp DEL
COD 26 G→A(HbE)

Figure 122-3 The world distribution of the β-thalassemias. The remarkable diversity of the different mutations that are involved in β-thalassemia in different ethnic groups are indicated. Those in boxes are the milder β-thalassemia mutations that occur in different populations, particularly in West Africa. *(From Weatherall D.J., Clegg J.B.: The thalassaemia syndromes, 4th ed. Oxford: Blackwell Science; 2001. Used with permission.)*

α- or β-thalassemia similar regimens are only indicated in those who have undergone splenectomy, regardless of their age.

Other important preventive measures for reducing the frequency of infectious complications include prophylaxis for blood-borne infection and malaria. Although the former is particularly relevant to those with transfusion-dependent forms of thalassemia it is becoming important in those with sickle cell anemia because increasing numbers are being placed on regular transfusion, particularly to reduce the frequency of neurological complications. The organisms of particular importance are hepatitis B and C viruses, HIV and malaria. Although donor screening programs have had a major effect in reducing the frequency of blood-borne infections of this type, they still remain a considerable problem in many low- and middle-income countries.

Malaria prophylaxis and the use of bednets are vital in countries with a high rate of malaria transmission.

CLINICAL FEATURES

The clinical findings of infection in patients with inherited hemoglobin disorders are particularly complex because they are often associated with symptoms and signs of complications of the underlying disorder.

Sickle Cell Anemia and its Variants[15]

The particularly high frequency of pneumococcal infection in early childhood is, unless protective action has been taken, a very common cause of mortality. Major episodes usually occur in children under 2 years of age and the disease usually has a rapid onset characterized by fever, convulsions and early coma. The condition may progress rapidly as a form of severe sepsis associated with shock and features of the Waterhouse–Friederichsen syndrome. Hemorrhagic features of disseminated intravascular coagulation may also occur. In other cases the clinical picture is dominated by the signs of bacterial meningitis or pneumonia.

Osteomyelitis, usually due to *Salmonella* infection, is characterized by localized and persistent bone pain and extreme tenderness on palpation. Aplastic crises are characterized by symptoms of infection associated with those of sudden and profound anemia. The acute chest syndrome is characterized by shortness of breath, collapse and severe hypoxia, as demonstrated by pulse oximetry and blood gas analysis. Malarial infection is often associated with profound anemia.

The Thalassemias[11]

The symptoms and signs of patients who have developed severe pneumococcal or related infections after splenectomy are similar to those described above with sickle cell anemia and splenic malfunction. However, patients with severe forms of thalassemia are prone to a wide variety of infections that are often the presenting feature. The clinical picture is characterized by fever, malaise, a worsening of the anemia and, sometimes, increasing splenomegaly. The infections that are caused by *Yersinia* spp. in iron-loaded patients receiving the chelating agent desferrioxamine are usually characterized by severe abdominal pain, diarrhea, vomiting, fever and a sore throat. Occasionally there may be an associated development of an acute abdomen due to rupture of the bowel. Blood-borne infections with hepatitis B or C viruses may later be associated with the clinical picture of chronic viral hepatitis, often complicated by associated liver damage due to excess iron.

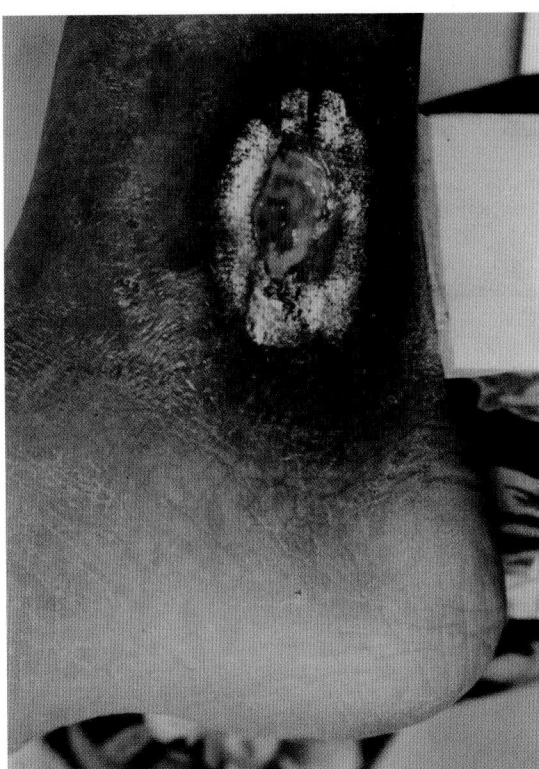

Figure 122-4 A chronic ulcer on the ankle of a patient with β-thalassemia. *(From Weatherall D.J., Clegg J.B.: The thalassaemia syndromes, 4th ed. Oxford: Blackwell Science; 2001. Used with permission.)*

Chronic leg ulcers, which usually are found on the medial side of the legs just above the ankle, are characterized by persistent pain; in those that become secondarily infected there is usually a purulent discharge (Figure 122-4).

DIAGNOSIS

For the diagnosis of the infectious complications of the hemoglobin disorders it is important first to identify the particular disease involved.

In sickle cell anemia and its related disorders the diagnosis can be easily achieved by hemoglobin electrophoresis or HPLC analysis. It is very important to also check the parents for the presence of the carrier state for either HbS or a related variant.[15] In the β-thalassemias the diagnosis is most easily made by HPLC analysis, which shows high levels of HbF and much reduced or absent levels of HbA.[1] Similarly, in HbE β-thalassemia the pattern is characterized by a predominance of HbE with varying levels of HbF, but no HbA. Again it is vital to check the parents; in the β-thalassemias both of them have a raised level of HbA$_2$ while in HbE β-thalassemia one parent has a raised level of HbA$_2$ and the other HbA with approximately 20–30% of HbE. These diagnoses are most easily carried out by HPLC analysis. The more severe form of α-thalassemia, HbH disease, is identified by the presence of variable amounts of HbH associated with HbA and normal or reduced levels of HbA$_2$, again easily identifiable by HPLC analysis.[1]

These definitive diagnostic tests must be accompanied by detailed hematological studies.[1,15] Sickle cell disease is characterized by a variable degree of anemia and the peripheral blood film often shows sickled erythrocytes; the reticulocyte count is always elevated. In all forms of β-thalassemia there is a variable degree of anemia associated with characteristic morphological changes of the red cells which show microcytosis and hypochromia with a varying percentage of target cells. In those with hemoglobin H disease, as well as it showing similar morphological changes of their red cells and a raised reticulocyte count, the presence of HbH can be demonstrated by incubating the red cells with brilliant cresyl blue dye followed by a search for red cell inclusion bodies produced by the precipitation of HbH.

An accurate diagnosis of the form of hemoglobin disorder and knowledge of the common infectious complications in the different varieties provides a valuable background to the diagnostic tests required for infectious episodes.[16,17] In cases of severe pneumococcal sepsis or related infections in babies and young children with defective splenic function in sickle cell anemia, or in those with severe β-thalassemia who have been splenectomized, urgent blood cultures are required. In cases in which the physical examination has suggested the possibility of pneumonia or meningitis urgent radiological investigation or lumbar puncture are also indicated. The diagnosis of aplastic crisis in sickle cell anemia due to parvovirus infection can be made on the hematological findings, which show a profound drop in the hemoglobin level associated with the absence of reticulocytes in the peripheral blood; the bone marrow shows marked hypoplasia of the red cell progenitors. In patients with sickle cell anemia and severe bone pain the distinction between *Salmonella* osteomyelitis and an infarct may be extremely difficult. Radiological studies may not be helpful but the addition of ultrasonography may be helpful in confirming a subperiosteal collection and in guiding aspiration to distinguish between collections of blood or pus.[18] The diagnosis is usually confirmed by culture of aspirates.

The diagnosis of blood-borne infections in the hemoglobin disorders requires analysis for the different hepatitis viruses, HIV and, in endemic areas, malarial parasites in the peripheral blood. The presence of chronic leg ulcers requires careful culture of the lesions to identify possible secondary infection. The diagnosis of *Yersinia* infections that mainly affect iron-loaded patients with β-thalassemia requires the assessment of the body iron load by measurement of the serum ferritin level or, better, using hepatic MRI measurements. Appropriate blood cultures are also required.

The most difficult differential diagnosis in infectious complications is between pneumonia and pulmonary infarction in the acute chest syndrome in sickle cell anemia.[15] Both conditions are associated with pulmonary infiltrates on the chest radiograph. Arterial blood gases may be reduced in both conditions, although the degree of hypoxia is often out of proportion to the consolidation, particularly in cases of pulmonary infarction. The occurrence of fat embolism as the cause of the condition can sometimes be diagnosed by the demonstration of fat-laden macrophages obtained by bronchial lavage.

TREATMENT

The acute infections that occur at a particularly high frequency in babies and children with sickle cell anemia during the early years of life, and those that follow splenectomy at any age in patients with severe forms of thalassemia, are treated using similar principles. These infections are medical emergencies requiring a rapid clinical evaluation, blood and urine culture, a complete blood count and a chest radiograph. Those that are severely anemic require immediate cross-match for early transfusion. Although until fairly recently it has been common practice to treat these young children with large doses of penicillin, because of the occurrence of at least partial penicillin resistance and the possibility that other organisms than the pneumococcus may be involved, it is now advised that broad-spectrum antibiotics should be administered intravenously, ceftriaxone for example.[19] If penicillin-resistant pneumococcal infection is suspected on epidemiological grounds then a second agent, either vancomycin or rifampin, should be added. Other supportive measures include adequate oxygenation, fluid replacement, the administration of plasma and platelets in cases associated with intravascular coagulation, and the control of convulsions with appropriate anticonvulsant agents. The principles of management of acute infections of this type, or other severe infections, in patients with β-thalassemia who have undergone splenectomy are similar.[20]

The management of other infectious complications of sickle cell anemia is more straightforward. Following the diagnosis of an aplastic crisis the patient should receive regular blood transfusion to maintain the hemoglobin at its usual steady-state level. Since spontaneous recovery usually takes several weeks it is very important that these patients are followed up at regular intervals. The management of *Salmonella* osteomyelitis requires therapy for at least 4–6 weeks. Chloramphenicol or ampicillin have been widely used for the management of this condition although more recently cefotaxime or ceftriaxone are also proving valuable, particularly in cases where the infection has become disseminated.

The chronic leg ulcers that are common in both sickle cell anemia and severe β-thalassemia are best managed with thorough and regular wound toilet, culture and the use of appropriate antibiotics if the lesion has become infected. In cases in which healing does not occur after a reasonable time of conservative management, skin grafts may be required.[15,21]

The infections that occur with *Yersinia* spp. are mainly restricted to patients with severe thalassemia on regular transfusion and iron chelation, although they may occur more commonly in association with sickle cell anemia now that high level transfusion is becoming more common. The iron chelation drug desferrioxamine should be stopped, stool cultures examined for *Yersinia* spp. and antibiotic treatment administered with either an aminoglycoside or co-trimoxazole.

The blood-borne and bone marrow transplant infections that occur in all forms of severe hemoglobin disorders, which are now becoming much less common due to adequate donor screening programs, require appropriate management of the different forms of viral hepatitis, HIV, malaria[22] and other viral infections.

References available online at expertconsult.com.

KEY REFERENCES

Kato G.J., Gladwin M.T.: Mechanisms and clinical complications of hemolysis in sickle cell disease and thalassemia. In: Steinberg M.H., Forget B.G., Higgs D.R., et al., eds. *Disorders of hemoglobin*. 2nd ed. Cambridge: Cambridge University Press; 2009:201-224.

Kitchen A.D., John A.J.B.: Transfusion borne infections. In: Murphy M.E., Pamphilon D.H., eds. *Practical transfusion medicine*. 2nd ed. Oxford: Blackwell; 2005:208-228.

Olivieri N.F., Weatherall D.J.: Clinical aspects of beta thalassemia and related disorders. In: Steinberg M.H., Forget B.G., Higgs D.R., et al., eds. *Disorders of hemoglobin*. 2nd ed. Cambridge: Cambridge University Press; 2009: 357-416.

Pearson H.A., Gallagher D., Chilcote R., et al.: Developmental pattern of splenic dysfunction in sickle cell disorders. *Pediatrics* 1985; 76(3):392-397.

Serjeant G.R.: *Sickle cell disease*. 2nd ed. New York: Oxford University Press; 1992.

Thein S.L., Wood W.G.: The molecular basis of β-thalassemia, δβ-thalassemia, and hereditary persistence of fetal hemoglobin. In: Steinberg M.H., Forget B.G., Higgs D.R., et al., eds. *Disorders of hemoglobin*. 2nd ed. Cambridge: Cambridge University Press; 2009:323-356.

Weatherall D.J., Clegg J.B.: *The thalassaemia syndromes*. 4th ed. Oxford: Blackwell Science; 2001.

Williams T.N., Obaro S.K.: Sickle cell disease and malaria morbidity: a tale with two tails. *Trends Parasitol* 2011; 27(7):315-320.

Williams T.N., Uyoga S., Macharia A., et al.: Bacteraemia in Kenyan children with sickle-cell anaemia: a retrospective cohort and case-control study. *Lancet* 2009; 374(9698): 1364-1370.

Williams T.N., Weatherall D.J.: World distribution, population genetics, and health burden of the hemoglobinopathies. *Cold Spring Harb Perspect Med* 2012; 2:a011692.

123

Leishmaniasis

ROBERT N. DAVIDSON

KEY CONCEPTS

- Leishmaniasis comprises several clinical syndromes: visceral, cutaneous and mucosal.

- Visceral leishmaniasis is fatal unless treated.

- It is a protozoal infection, spread by the bite of sandflies.

- Some forms are zoonotic, with animal hosts and man accidentally involved.

- Other forms are anthroponotic.

- HIV coinfection increases the risk of disease and of treatment failure.

- Treatment with antimonials has been largely superseded by liposomal amphotericin and miltefosine

Epidemiology

Leishmania may cause cutaneous (CL), mucocutaneous (MCL) or visceral (VL, kala-azar) disease. The distribution is shown in Figure 123-1; ~1.5 million cases of CL and ~50 000 cases of VL occur annually.[1] Sandflies transmit leishmaniasis from a range of infected animals (i.e. zoonotic) or from human to human (i.e. anthroponotic). Transmission varies according to climate, habitat, season and occupation (Figure 123-2).

VISCERAL LEISHMANIASIS

This is caused by *Leishmania donovani*, *L. infantum* and *L. chagasi* (see Figure 123-1); the latter two species are indistinguishable. A reduction of dichlorodiphenyltrichloroethane (DDT) spraying against mosquitoes in South Asia heralded the start of the present epidemic of *L. donovani* VL.

Population movement, famine, and civil war and climate cause epidemics of VL (*L. donovani*) in Sudan and Somalia. Coinfections of human immunodeficiency virus (HIV) and *Leishmania* are common in Ethiopia, and sporadic in India and South America. In Europe prior to effective antiretrovirals, 20–70% of cases of VL (due to *L. infantum*) were coinfected with HIV, and 1.5–9% of acquired immunodeficiency syndrome (AIDS) patients had VL.[2]

Subclinical or self-healing infection occurs frequently where *L. infantum* or *L. chagasi* is involved, and sometimes also with *L. donovani*.[3]

CUTANEOUS LEISHMANIASIS

In the Old World, *L. tropica* causes anthroponotic CL in urban environments; breakdown of infrastructure in Afghanistan has caused large outbreaks. *L. major* causes sporadic zoonotic CL in those exposed to gerbil burrows, especially where there has been irrigation. Smaller numbers of CL cases are caused by *L. infantum* in Europe and *L. aethiopica* in Ethiopia and parts of Kenya.

In the New World, CL is mainly caused by members of the *Leishmania mexicana* complex and the *Leishmania braziliensis* complex.[4]

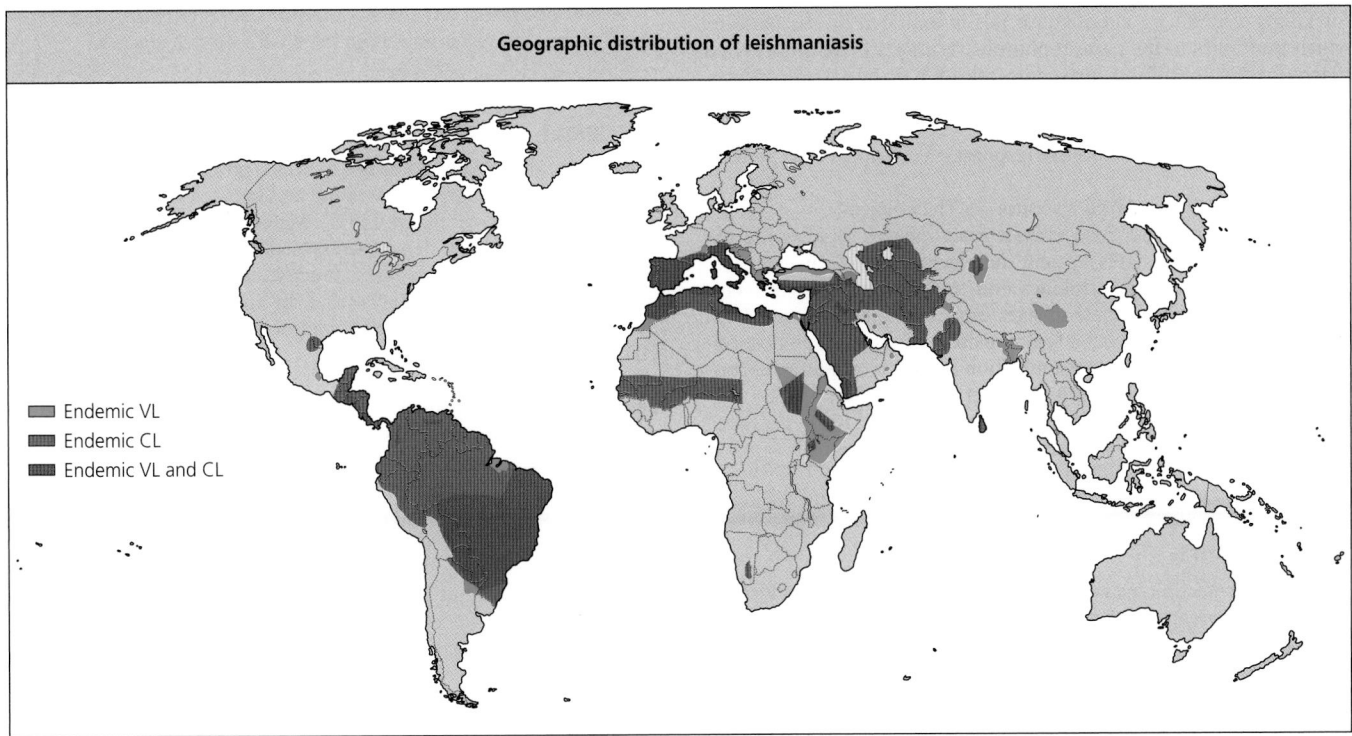

Geographic distribution of leishmaniasis

- Endemic VL
- Endemic CL
- Endemic VL and CL

Figure 123-1 Geographic distribution of leishmaniasis. More than 90% of VL cases occur in India/Nepal/Bangladesh, Sudan/Ethiopia and Brazil, and more than 90% of CL cases occur in Brazil/Peru, Algeria, Saudi Arabia and Syria/Iraq/Iran/Afghanistan. *(Courtesy of Pablo Martín-Rabadán and Emilio Bouza.)*

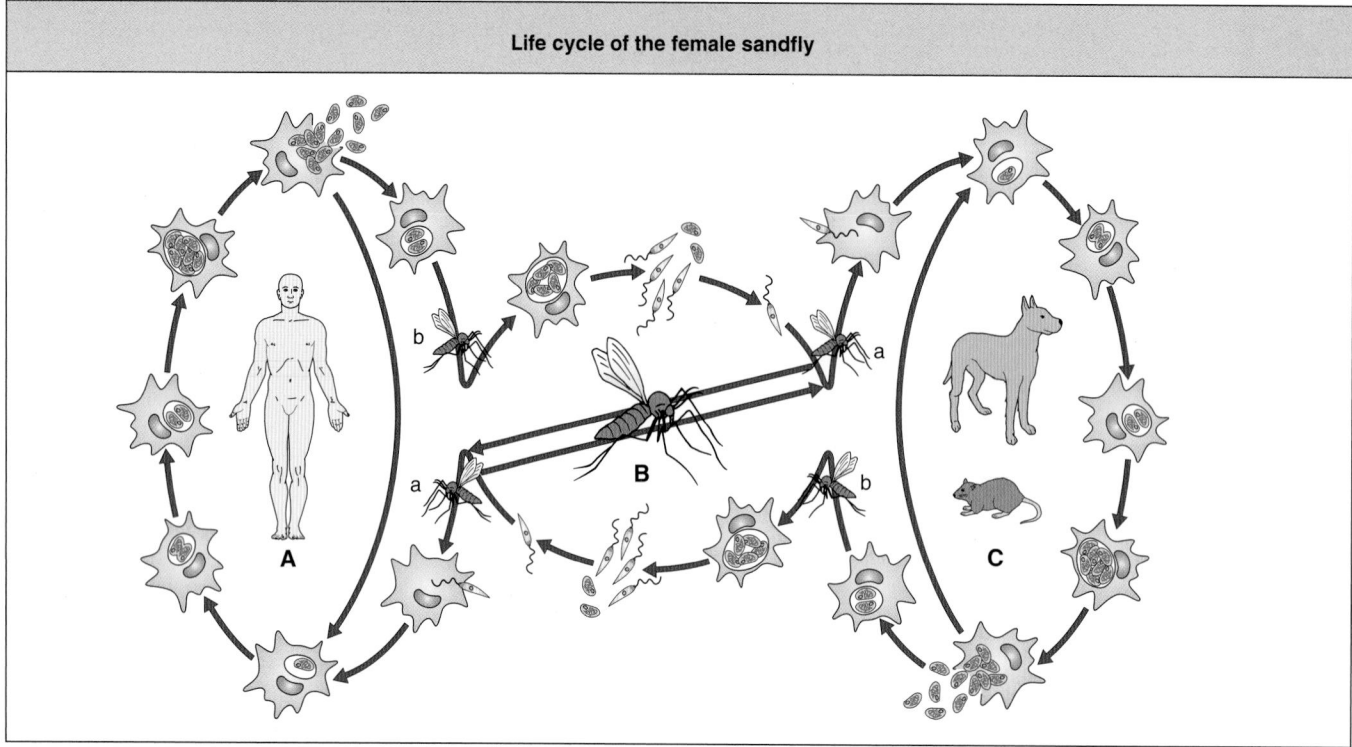

Life cycle of the female sandfly

Figure 123-2   Life cycle of the female sandfly. The female sandfly (B) inoculates promastigotes (flagelate forms) into man (A) or animal hosts (C) whilst feeding. Visceral leishmaniasis: *Leishmania infantum/L. chagasi* are zoonotic – the usual host is a canine. *L donovani* is anthroponotic, with human cases of VL or PKDL being the source of infection. Cutaneous leishmaniasis: the lesions are the source of parasites to sandflies. *L. tropica* is anthroponotic, *L. major*, *L. braziliensis* and *L. mexicana* are zoonotic, with a range of mammals being the usual hosts.

Deforestation brings humans into close contact with animal hosts and sandflies.

Pathogenesis and Pathology

Infected macrophages produce nitric oxide as an innate mechanism for killing *Leishmania* amastigotes; this is inhibited by the parasite, which multiplies in the parasitophorous vacuole. Eventually, infected macrophages rupture and amastigotes are taken up by new phagocytes. Macrophages and dendritic cells present *Leishmania* antigens to T cells and this results in either:

- an effective cellular immune response – a T-helper (Th)1 pattern; or
- an ineffective humoral response – a Th2 pattern.

In the Th1 response, T cells activate macrophages by releasing the cytokines interferon (IFN)-γ and interleukin (IL)-2. In the Th2 response, T cells release cytokines and transforming growth factor (TGF)-β, which inhibit macrophages from killing amastigotes. Each *Leishmania* species produces a typical pattern of disease, and host cellular immunity (genetic factors, nutrition and co-morbidities all contribute) at the time of infection will determine whether:

- a clinical or subclinical infection results
- the disease is visceral, cutaneous or mucocutaneous
- lesions are few or diffuse
- response to treatment is complete or partial.[5]

Prevention

Individual protection against nocturnal sandfly bites is provided by insecticide-impregnated bed nets. Long sleeves and trousers, and permethrin-impregnated clothing may also help.[6]

Animal reservoirs of *Leishmania* can be controlled, e.g. by bulldozing gerbil burrows or killing infected dogs. Domestic dogs can be given deltamethrin-impregnated collars or 65% spot-on solution of permethrin.[7] Active case finding and treatment of patients with VL and post-kala-azar dermal leishmaniasis (PKDL) caused by *L. donovani* and CL caused by *L. tropica* reduce human-to-human transmission. Early case finding is possible using serologic tests, e.g. the direct agglutination test (DAT) and rapid tests using a recombinant antigen, rK39.[8]

Sandflies are susceptible to residual insecticides; spraying homes or fogging streets reduces the density of peridomestic sandflies.

A vaccine against any forms of leishmaniasis remains to be developed; several strategies have been tried with limited success.[9]

Clinical Features

VISCERAL LEISHMANIASIS

After an incubation period of 2–8 months (range 10 days to >2 years), the patient develops pyrexia, wasting and hepatosplenomegaly, which may become massive (Figure 123-3). Males outnumber females, especially where females are denied access to early diagnosis and treatment. When treatment is provided free, or active case-finding done, the ratio of male:female cases approaches 1:1. In Europe or Brazil, VL affects mainly infants (hence the name *L. infantum*) or adults coinfected with HIV.

In India, Kenya and Somalia, VL patients often experience ill-defined symptoms for months, presenting with fever, discomfort from an enlarged spleen, abdominal swelling, weight loss, epistaxis, cough or diarrhea. Conversely, in Sudan, especially during an epidemic, there is characteristically high fever, progressing over a few weeks to prostration, weakness, dyspnea and acute anemia.

The physical signs (Table 123-1) depend upon the duration of the disease, the nutritional state of the patient and the presence of complications. Advanced cases are thin, wasted and cannot walk unaided. Hair changes and pedal edema accompany hypoalbuminemia, but ascites is rare. Hyperpigmentation of the face, hands, feet and abdomen occurs ('kala-azar' means 'black sickness'). The spleen is enlarged in >90% of cases. Though massive spleens do occur, reaching the left or right iliac fossa, the average spleen in VL only reaches 5–10 cm below the left costal margin. It is smooth, firm and nontender unless there has been a recent infarct. The liver is moderately enlarged in one-third

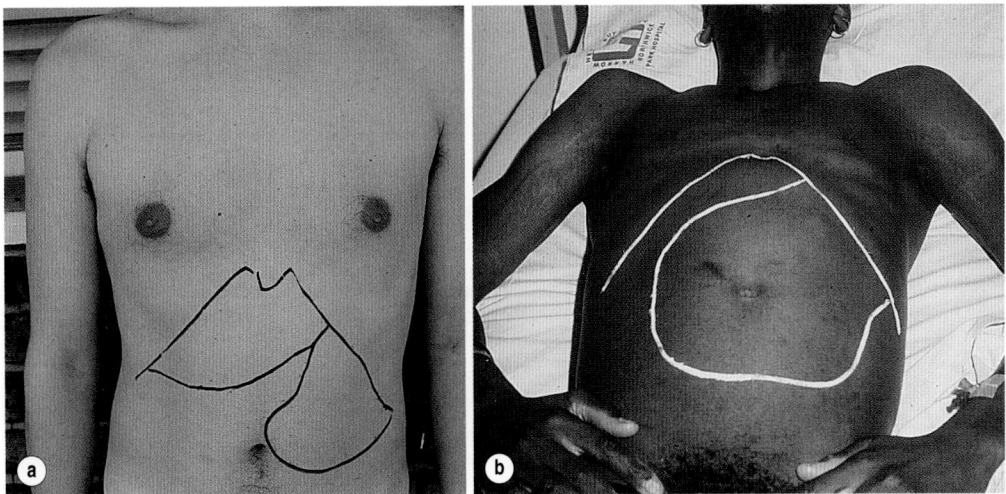

Figure 123-3   Visceral leishmaniasis. (a) Hepatosplenomegaly and pallor in a 29-year-old Italian man. (b) Splenomegaly and pallor in a 23-year-old Angolan man. Both complained of weight loss, fatigue and fever of several weeks' duration.

TABLE 123-1	Features of Visceral Leishmaniasis (*Leishmania donovani*)*
Feature	**Proportion Affected (%)**
AGE	
<9 years	22 (*L. infantum* and *L. chagasi* more commonly affect children and infants)
<15 years	44
CLINICAL FEATURES	
Fever	83–100
Wasting	70–100
Uncomfortable spleen	81–88
Cough	72–83
Epistaxis	44–55
Diarrhea	25–55
Vomiting	2–37
Splenomegaly	93 (adults), 98 (children)
Lymphadenopathy	55–86 (uncommon outside Africa)
Jaundice	2–7
Edema	2–7
LABORATORY FINDINGS	
Globulin >30 g/L	98
Anemia	61–92
Albumin <30 g/L	88
Leukopenia	84
Thrombocytopenia	73
Elevated bilirubin	17
Elevated alkaline phosphatase	40
Positive *Leishmania* serology	95
Parasitologically proven	96

*The duration of symptoms is 2–4 months but is shorter in children.

of cases. Lymphadenopathy is common in African patients, in whom 1–2 cm lymph nodes are often palpable in the groins. Jaundice, mucosal and retinal hemorrhage, and episcleritis are occasional features. Neurologic complications, such as confusion, tremor and ataxia, convulsions, foot-drop and nerve deafness, are occasionally seen. After weeks to months of illness, most VL patients die, often with bleeding (nasal, intestinal, intracranial), bacterial pneumonia, anemic heart failure, tuberculosis, dysentery, measles or other infections (e.g. cancrum oris).

Leishmaniasis in Patients Who Are Immunosuppressed or Have HIV

Visceral leishmaniasis is an AIDS-defining opportunistic infection. Currently, HIV/VL is commonest in Ethiopia, India and Brazil.[2] In southern Europe numbers of coinfected cases fell dramatically after the adoption of highly active antiretroviral treatment in 1996. VL in HIV coinfected patients in Europe characteristically occurs at very low CD4 counts, and affects injecting drug users disproportionately because shared syringes spread the infection. The clinical features of HIV/VL in Europe are often atypical: the symptoms vague, the laboratory abnormalities nonspecific and hepatosplenomegaly absent or unimpressive. *Leishmania* amastigotes may be found unexpectedly in circulating neutrophils or bone marrow aspirates of febrile HIV-positive patients, or in rectal, gastric or skin biopsies. *Leishmania* serology is negative in many such patients. During treatment, patients may experience drug toxicity (especially pancreatitis on antimonials) and even if apparently responding well they are prone to relapse. With antiretrovirals, many HIV-infected patients with *L. infantum* achieve long-term cure; the danger of relapse recedes once their CD4 count is >200 cells/µL for >3 months. A minority of HIV/VL patients never achieve a good CD4 response, despite effective HIV suppression, and relapse repeatedly, eventually becoming nonresponsive to all antileishmanial drugs.

L. donovani (especially in Sudan/Ethiopia) is more virulent than *L. infantum* in Europe, and the clinical picture of HIV/VL is indistinguishable from VL in HIV-negative patients. Those with HIV coinfection have high mortality during and after treatment, and higher rates of relapse and PKDL.[10,11] In Ethiopia, even good CD4 responses may not protect against repeated relapses. Cutaneous leishmaniasis occurs in patients who have HIV coinfection in Europe, Africa and South America. The lesions may be nondescript, or resemble those of diffuse cutaneous leishmaniasis (DCL, see below).

VL may occasionally occur in patients immunosuppressed by drugs or who have undergone organ transplantation or thymectomy. There is usually no prior history of leishmaniasis, and travel to endemic areas may have been years previously.

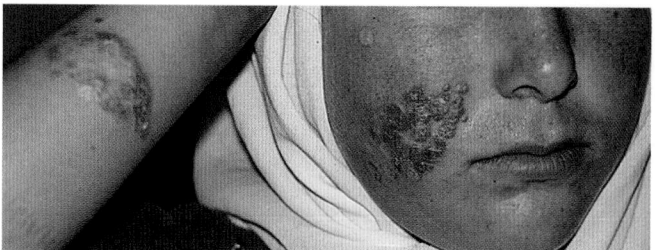

Figure 123-4 Cutaneous leishmaniasis recidivans. *Leishmania tropica* leishmaniasis lesions on the face and forearm of a Syrian girl. These had been present for 4 years with slow healing in the center and multiple recurrences despite courses of intralesional meglumine antimonate.

Post-Kala-Azar Dermal Leishmaniasis

After successful treatment for VL due to *L. donovani* (but not *L. chagasi/L. infantum*), patients may develop a prolonged inflammatory reaction in skin and/or mucosae called post-kala-azar dermal leishmaniasis (PKDL).

In Sudan, PKDL occurs toward the end of apparently successful treatment or weeks to months later. Mild PKDL affects ~55% of VL patients, including those with subclinical VL.[12] In India, PKDL is less common, and occurs months to years after VL. Occasionally, PKDL is acute and severe, resulting in desquamation of skin and mucosae. More commonly, it is characterized by the development of hypopigmented patches, nodules and plaques. Parasites are infrequent or absent from the biopsies. Patients with PKDL may transmit *L. donovani* via sandflies, and may represent a reservoir of anthroponotic infection between outbreaks.

CUTANEOUS LEISHMANIASIS

In CL (Figure 123-4) amastigotes multiply in dermal macrophages near the site of inoculation, typically on the arms, legs, face or ears. The lesions may be:

- nodular or ulcerative; and
- single or with multiple satellite nodules or lymphangitic spread.

The most typical lesion of CL is a nodule or chronic ulcer with a diameter of 2–5 cm and indurated margins. The ulcer may be covered by a fibrinous crust or exudate. It is painful if large or secondarily infected.

The histologic picture is of an intense lymphoid and monocytic infiltrate with granulomas. A 'tissue-paper' scar remains after healing. The median spontaneous healing rate differs for each species, typically:

- <5 months for *L. major*
- <8 months for *L. mexicana*
- <1 year for *L. tropica* and *L. braziliensis*.

There are two chronic forms of CL. Diffuse cutaneous leishmaniasis is rare but disfiguring. Widespread plaques containing huge numbers of amastigotes persist for decades. People with DCL are anergic to leishmanin, but do not have visceral dissemination or systemic symptoms. DCL is caused mainly by *L. aethiopica* in Africa and *L. amazonensis* in South and Central America. Leishmaniasis recidivans is a chronic, nonhealing or relapsing cutaneous infection, seen mainly with *L. tropica* infection in the Middle East. These patients are hypersensitive to leishmanin and organisms are rarely identified (see Figure 123-4).

MUCOCUTANEOUS LEISHMANIASIS

Mucocutaneous leishmaniasis (MCL; Figure 123-5) occurs in ~3–10% of cases of CL due to *L. b. braziliensis*, especially in Peru and Bolivia. MCL usually occurs months to years after CL has healed, but simultaneous CL and MCL can occur, as can MCL without previous CL. Usually the tip of the nose, nasal cartilage or upper lip are involved first with a painless induration or ulceration. The condition may remain static or may extend over months to years into the

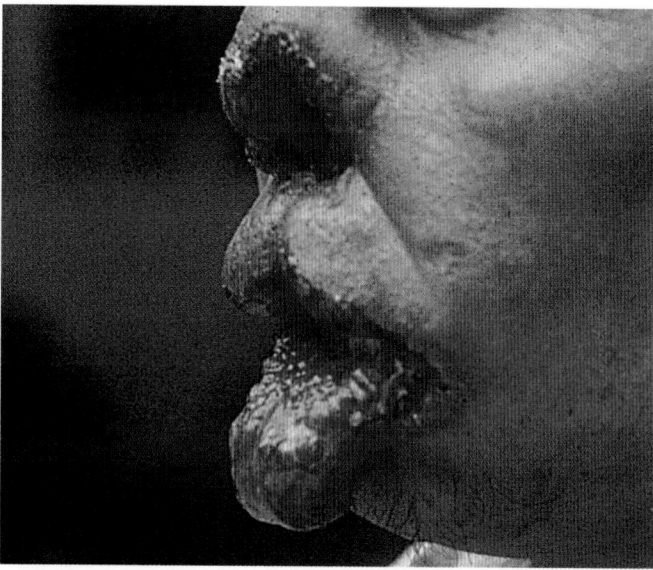

Figure 123-5 Mucocutaneous leishmaniasis. A young man from Peru who had a 2-year history of slow enlargement of the lips and ulceration of the nostrils. (*Courtesy of Professor Luis Valda Rodriguez.*)

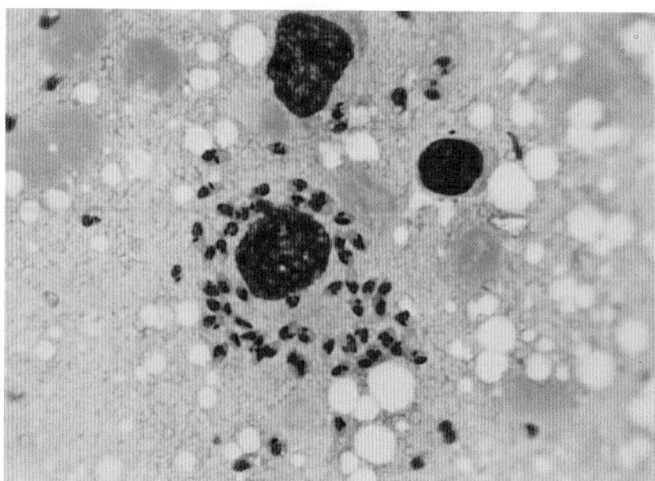

Figure 123-6 Amastigotes (Leishman–Donovan bodies) in bone marrow aspirate from a patient who had *Leishmania infantum* VL and AIDS. The nucleus and kinetoplast stain deeply with Giemsa and give the organism its characteristic appearance. *Histoplasma* spp. are the main source of mistaken identification in bone marrow smears, but lack these structures. Amastigotes measure 2–3 mm in length and are found within macrophages in tissue sections, but usually lie free in smears because infected macrophages burst as they are smeared.

nasopharynx, palate, uvula, larynx and upper airways. The nose may be destroyed.

Biopsies show a chronic inflammatory and granulomatous infiltrate with very few amastigotes. Cultures or polymerase chain reaction (PCR)-based testing of biopsies are usually positive for *L. braziliensis*. Less severe oral (e.g. tongue), nasal or laryngeal involvement occasionally occurs with other species (e.g. *L. infantum*) and this often indicates an underlying immune defect.

Diagnosis

CLASSIC PARASITOLOGIC DIAGNOSIS

Clinical leishmaniasis is ideally confirmed by isolating *Leishmania*, or obtaining a positive PCR from aspirates or biopsies of lesions. Some of the sample is smeared onto glass slides stained with Giemsa and examined for amastigotes (Figure 123-6). The rest of the sample is inoculated into suitable media and cultured at 26–28°C; a positive culture produces motile promastigotes within 2 weeks.

In VL, positive yields from smears of aspirates are of the following order: spleen, >95%; bone marrow or liver, 70–85%; lymph node (Africa), 58–65%; and buffy coat of blood (HIV/VL), ~70%.[11] Cultures yield about another 10% in good hands. The technique of splenic aspirate is shown in Figure 123-7.

In CL, DCL, PKDL and MCL, slit skin smears are taken from the raised edge of the CL ulcer or center of the CL nodule (Figure 123-8). Amastigotes are most abundant in fresh CL lesions and are very numerous in DCL. Conversely, they are infrequent in old CL lesions, in MCL and in PKDL.

MOLECULAR PARASITOLOGIC DIAGNOSIS

In VL patients, whether coinfected with HIV or not, the sensitivity of PCR on bone marrow aspirates and peripheral blood is >95%.[13,14] In PKDL or CL, 92–98% of skin samples are PCR-positive for leishmania DNA.[15,16]

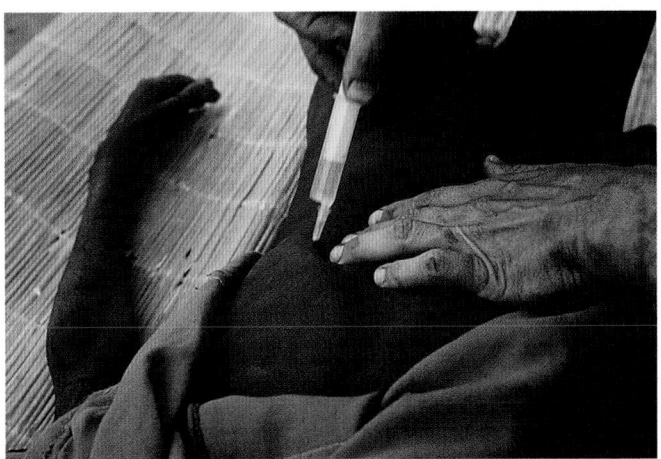

Figure 123-7 Splenic aspiration. The picture shows a splenic aspirate being performed under field conditions on a child suffering from *Leishmania donovani* kala-azar in South Sudan. The procedure is simple, painless and safe if the prothrombin time is normal and the platelet count is above 40 ×10⁹/L. Palpate the spleen and mark its outline. Using a 30 mm long 21-gauge needle attached to a 5 mL syringe, penetrate the skin over the spleen. Withdraw the plunger 1 mL and plunge the needle into the spleen upwards at an angle of 45° and withdraw immediately, maintaining suction. The tiny amount of material obtained is sufficient for culture and smear. (*Courtesy of Drs Robert Wilkinson and Jill Seaman.*)

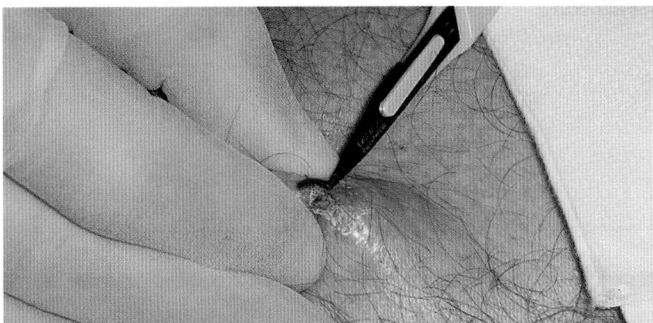

Figure 123-8 Slit skin smear. The picture shows a slit skin smear being taken from the edge of a chronic *Leishmania infantum* ulcer obtained in Malta. Smears are taken from the raised edge of the ulcer or center of the nodule, where amastigotes are most abundant. The skin is cleaned and then firmly pinched throughout the procedure to squeeze away blood. A 5 mm long and 3 mm deep incision is made and then the scalpel is turned through 90° and the blade is used to scrape the edge of the slit. A line of tissue scrapings is gently streaked on to a slide and the process is repeated until two or three lines of scrapings are present on at least two slides. Further scrapings and fluid oozing from the pinched slit are put into culture medium.

IMMUNOLOGIC DIAGNOSIS

In VL, 95% of cases have high titers of anti-*Leishmania* antibodies by the direct agglutination test (DAT), immunofluorescent antibody test (IFAT) or ELISA. A major advance is the dipstick test using the rK39 antigen, which gives sensitivity and specificity for VL of >90% in India.[8]

In Europe, ~30% of HIV/VL patients have negative serology for *Leishmania*; in Africa, *Leishmania* serology is positive in most HIV/VL patients.[11] In VL, the leishmanin skin test is invariably negative, indicating antigen-specific anergy. In CL, *Leishmania* serology may be weakly positive and the leishmanin skin test is usually positive. In MCL and PKDL, both serology and the leishmanin skin test are usually positive. In DCL, both serology and the leishmanin skin test are negative.

Management

Ideally, VL, like other life-threatening infections, should be treated with combination chemotherapy to improve cure rates, reduce duration and toxicity of treatment, reduce relapses and (in areas of anthroponotic transmission) delay the development of drug-resistant *L. donovani.*[17]

ANTILEISHMANIAL DRUGS

Pentavalent Antimonials

Pentavalent antimonials (Sb^v) have been used since the 1940s. Sodium stibogluconate contains Sb^v 100 mg/mL; meglumine antimonate contains 85 mg/mL. In the systemic treatment of VL, CL and MCL, a single daily dose of 20 mg Sb^v/kg is used for 28 days. Intravenous injections are less painful than intramuscular injections. Courses of up to 3 months are used for PKDL. Primary resistance to Sb^v is seen in ~1% of cases in Africa and up to 60% in parts of India. Relapse rates should be <5%, but secondary Sb^v resistance is likely to develop in patients who relapse unless they are re-treated very thoroughly.

Toxicity. Sb^v is reduced by parasite reductases to SbIII, and human reductases might perform a similar function. This may account for the unpredictable toxicity of Sb^v, as well as explaining why toxicity is rare in 'well' patients treated for PKDL, but common in 'ill' patients with VL, particularly those with HIV/VL. Sb^v-induced hyperamylasemia is common, and pancreatitis may be symptomatic and even fatal, especially in those coinfected with HIV.[18] Elevated liver enzymes, arthralgia and myalgia, thrombocytopenia, leukopenia, anorexia and thrombophlebitis all occur. Patients may experience symptoms indistinguishable from VL itself: lethargy, headache, nausea, vomiting. Electrocardiograph changes (ST-segment and T-wave) are common; prolongation of the corrected QT interval to >0.5 s is an indication to pause therapy.[19] Acute renal failure, thrombocytopenia, arthritis, tremors and exfoliative dermatitis occur occasionally. If toxicity occurs, treatment should be changed to another agent. If only Sb^v is available, treatment should be stopped for 1–2 days; if toxicity recurs, the daily dose should be reduced.

Before starting treatment, ideally a full blood count, biochemistry profile and electrocardiograph should be obtained. Patients should be hospitalized during systemic Sb^v therapy where possible, and biochemical and hematologic parameters monitored twice-weekly. This is usually impossible in endemic countries, where Sb^v is administered by a nurse to outpatients without the facilities for monitoring toxicity. Sudden deaths, thought to be due to arrhythmias, occur occasionally in VL patients. It is unclear what proportion of deaths in VL is due to Sb^v. However, in a randomized controlled study involving 580 VL patients, many of whom were HIV positive, the mortality rate was 10% among patients treated with Sb^v versus 2% among miltefosine recipients.[20]

Intralesional Administration. When used intralesionally, ~1 ml of undiluted Sb^v is infiltrated into the base and edges of a CL lesion, every 2–3 days for up to 2–3 weeks. There are no systemic side effects, but the injections are painful.

Amphotericin

Amphotericin deoxycholate is a powerful antileishmanial and is remarkably nontoxic in a regimen of 15 doses of 1 mg/kg on alternate days.[21] The main limitation is the need for hospitalization and slow intravenous infusions. Renal function and electrolytes should be monitored weekly. Amphotericin is the drug of choice for advanced MCL, for which Sb[v] treatment is often ineffective, and total doses of 30 mg/kg are used. Amphotericin has not been systematically assessed for CL or PKDL.

Liposomal Amphotericin. Particles of amphotericin are taken up by macrophages and target drug to the site of infection, achieving very high levels in liver and spleen. Liposomal amphotericin (AmBisome®) has lower renal and infusion toxicity than amphotericin but is more expensive. It has been extensively used, and is licensed for VL in many countries. It is rapidly effective and nontoxic for VL.[22–24] The licensed regimen is a total dose of 20–30 mg/kg, given as at least five daily doses of 3–4 mg/kg over a period of 10–21 days. Liposomal amphotericin can be dosed flexibly, since it has low toxicity and a prolonged tissue half-life in spleen and liver (and, presumably, bone marrow).

Very short courses of liposomal amphotericin (two doses of 10 mg/kg) have been used in Europe. While total doses as low as 5 mg/kg as a single dose have a high cure rate in India, liposomal amphotericin is not as effective in Sudan.[25] Regimens currently under consideration are a single dose of AmBisome 5 mg/kg plus a short course of either intramuscular paromomycin sulfate or oral miltefosine. CL can successfully be treated with ~20 mg/kg liposomal amphotericin over 10 days.[26,27]

Miltefosine

Miltefosine is an oral drug with good efficacy against VL;[28] it is licensed in several countries. Side effects include vomiting and diarrhea and elevation of liver enzymes, urea and creatinine. Miltefosine should be avoided in pregnancy, and women of child-bearing potential must use effective contraception during and for 2 months after treatment. The 28-day regimen for patients >25 kg is 100 mg/day; for children 2–12 years (8–25 kg) it is 2.5 mg/kg/day (max. 50 mg/day). Miltefosine should be taken in divided doses with meals.

Miltefosine is highly effective against *L. braziliensis* CL and MCL in South America[29,30] and against *L. major* CL in Iran.[31]

Paromomycin (Aminosidine)

Paromomycin (aminosidine) sulfate is an aminoglycoside which is a highly effective and cheap antileishmanial for VL, though it has little efficacy in CL or MCL. It is licensed in India in the dose of paromomycin sulfate 15 mg/kg/day for 21 days.[32] This dose is equivalent to paromomycin (base) 11 mg/kg/day. It is well tolerated, with little nephro- or oto-toxicity.[32]

A combination of Sb[v] and paromomycin has been used extensively in Sudan with good effect.[17,33] The regimen is sodium stibogluconate 20 mg/kg/day plus paromomycin sulfate 15 mg/kg/day, both given intramuscularly daily for 17 days.

Pentamidine

Pentamidine is not routinely used for VL, although short courses – seven doses of 2 mg/kg on alternate days, or four doses of 3 mg/kg on alternate days – are effective for New World CL.[34]

Second-Line Oral Agents

Ketoconazole is effective for CL caused by *L. major* and *L. mexicana*, but is less effective against *L. tropica*, *L. aethiopica* and *L. braziliensis*. Fluconazole[35] and itraconazole have similar efficacy and are better tolerated. Imidazoles cannot reliably cure VL or PKDL.

TOPICAL TREATMENT

Topical paromomycin in the treatment of CL has been evaluated in many studies. At best, it shows a modest benefit over placebo and is usually less effective than Sb[v].[36]

MONITORING RESPONSE TO TREATMENT

Visceral Leishmaniasis

Intercurrent infections such as malaria, tuberculosis and dysentery must be treated, and hydration and nutrition provided. Severely ill patients should receive empiric broad-spectrum antibiotics to cover sepsis; the best-tolerated treatment in very ill VL patients is liposomal amphotericin. With effective treatment, the patient will be afebrile within 1 week and clinical and laboratory abnormalities will improve within 2 weeks. After successful treatment, amastigotes will be absent from aspirates and cultures will be negative; a test-of-cure aspirate is always needed if the patient has previously relapsed or has not shown a full clinical recovery. The patient should be reviewed during 6–12 months after treatment. Slight splenomegaly may persist for several months. Most relapses occur within 6 months. Body weight, spleen size, full blood count, serum albumin concentration and ESR are all sensitive markers of recurrent VL. A relapse rate of <5% is expected for immunocompetent patients but is common among patients coinfected with HIV. Maintenance with intravenous pentamidine every 2–4 weeks or liposomal amphotericin weekly may prevent or delay relapse for patients who have HIV infection, but efficacy is unproven. HIV coinfected patients should be started on ART, irrespective of the CD4 count, since relapsing VL carries a high morbidity and mortality.

When treating a relapse of VL, a drug combination is advised, and parasite clearance should be confirmed by a test-of-cure aspirate.

Cutaneous Leishmaniasis

Treatment is necessary if the lesions are large, multiple, disfiguring or overlie a joint. Intralesional Sb[v] is cheap and usually effective but CL due to *L. braziliensis* should be treated systemically to reduce the risk of subsequent MCL. Most relapses of CL will occur within 12 months.

Mucocutaneous Leishmaniasis

Untreated MCL will slowly progress to produce extensive mutilating lesions. Early lesions respond better to treatment but the response is slow and relapses are common. Corticosteroids should be added if the larynx or airways are involved, to prevent edema complicating the start of treatment. Relapse may occur up to several years after treatment, so prolonged clinical follow-up is necessary.

References available online at expertconsult.com.

KEY REFERENCES

Balasegaram M.L., Ritmeijer K., Lima M.A., et al.: Liposomal amphotericin B as a treatment for human leishmaniasis. *Expert Opin Emerg Drugs* 2012; 17(4):493-510.

Chappuis F., Rijal S., Soto A., et al.: A meta-analysis of the diagnostic performance of the direct agglutination test and rK39 dipstick for visceral leishmaniasis. *BMJ* 2006; 333(7571):723.

Cota G.F., de Sousa M.R., Demarqui F.N., et al.: The diagnostic accuracy of serologic and molecular methods for detecting visceral leishmaniasis in HIV infected patients: meta-analysis. *PLoS Negl Trop Dis* 2012; 6(5): e1665.

den Boer M., Argaw D., Jannin J., et al.: Leishmaniasis impact and treatment access. *Clin Microbiol Infect* 2011; 17:1471-1477.

Ritmeijer K., Dejenie A., Assefa Y., et al.: A comparison of miltefosine and sodium stibogluconate for treatment of visceral leishmaniasis in an Ethiopian population with high prevalence of HIV infection. *Clin Infect Dis* 2006; 43:357-364.

Sundar S., Makharia A., More D.K., et al.: Short-course of oral miltefosine for treatment of visceral leishmaniasis. *Clin Infect Dis* 2000; 31:1110-1113.

Ter Horst R., Collin S.M., Ritmeijer K., et al.: Concordant HIV infection and visceral leishmaniasis in Ethiopia: the influence of antiretroviral treatment and other factors on outcome. *Clin Infect Dis* 2008; 46(11):1702-1709.

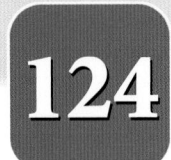

124

Chagas Disease (American Trypanosomiasis)

MICHAEL A. MILES

KEY CONCEPTS

- Chagas disease is an anthropozoonosis caused by the protozoan parasite *Trypanosoma cruzi*.

- *T. cruzi* is transmitted by contamination of mucous membranes or abraded skin with the infected feces of blood-sucking triatomine bugs.

- Other routes of infection are blood transfusion, congenital, organ donation and oral via triatomine-contaminated food, particularly plant and fruit juices.

- Once acquired, *T. cruzi* infection is usually life-long.

- *T. cruzi* is diverse, with six distinct genetic lineages – TcI to TcVI – with disparate geographic distributions.

- There are three clinical phases of Chagas disease: (1) acute, which may be asymptomatic or fatal; (2) chronic indeterminate, with normal 12-lead ECG and radiographs of thorax and abdomen, and (3) chronic symptomatic, primarily characterized by chagasic cardiomyopathy and ECG abnormalities, and which in the Southern Cone region of South America may also be associated with megaesophagus and megacolon.

- Blood parasitemia may be detectable in the acute phase but inapparent to microscopic methods in the chronic phase; commercial rapid serologic tests are available, some with high sensitivity and specificity.

- In the immunocompromised, such as those with HIV coinfection, the acute phase may be reactivated, associated with potential meningoencephalitis and a poor prognosis.

- Acute cases, congenital cases, immunocompromised cases, children, and young adults up to age 18 are treated with the oral drug benznidazole; in older adults side effects may prevent treatment; there are no reliable biomarkers of cure.

- Prevention of Chagas disease is principally by: spraying human dwellings with pyrethroid insecticides, coupled with health education and community support; screening of blood and organ donors; prenatal serology of women to facilitate prevention and treatment of congenital cases.

Epidemiology

GEOGRAPHIC DISTRIBUTION

In Latin America Chagas disease is still considered to be the most important parasitic disease and it remains a public health problem in many countries,[1] although disease control has dramatically improved in the past two decades. By the end of the 1980s an estimated 16–18 million people were infected, with 90–100 million at risk, and 450 000 new cases each year. However, transmission of *Trypanosoma cruzi* has declined substantially since the launch in 1991 of the Southern Cone Initiative (by six endemic countries – Argentina, Bolivia, Brazil, Chile, Paraguay and Uruguay) and similar initiatives in Central America and the Andean Pact countries since 1997.[2] Currently it is thought that less than 9 million people are infected, and Brazil, Uruguay and Chile have

been declared free of transmission by the domiciliated insect vector, *Triatoma infestans* (Figure 124-1). Nevertheless, around 40 million people remain at risk of infection, and transmission is still present, particularly in the Gran Chaco region of South America.[3] In the USA it is estimated that around 300 000 migrants from Latin America are infected.[4] *T. cruzi* infected triatomines and mammals, such as opossums, armadillos, raccoons and wood rats (and in some regions domestic dogs) can be found widely, although there are very few documented cases of autochthonous vector-borne transmission to humans.[5]

ETIOLOGIC AGENT AND TRANSMISSION

T. cruzi is a protozoan parasite within the order Kinetoplastida and family Trypanosomatidae. Like other kinetoplastids *T. cruzi* has mitochondrial DNA within a kinetoplast, which is a discrete organelle and important diagnostic feature, visible in stained organisms by light microscopy.

T. cruzi is remarkably diverse; six distinct genetic lineages (TcI–TcVI) or discrete typing units (DTUs) have so far been defined, with broadly different but not entirely exclusive geographic and ecologic associations.[5] Thus, TcI is the principal agent of Chagas disease in endemic countries north of the Amazon, where chagasic cardiomyopathy occurs, and TcIV is a secondary agent in Venezuela, whereas in the Southern Cone region of South America TcI is sylvatic but human TcI infections are sporadic. In contrast, TcII, TcV and TcVI are the predominant agents of Chagas disease in the Southern Cone region and may be associated with both chagasic cardiomyopathy and megasyndromes.[5] TcIII is widely distributed throughout South America in armadillos, particularly *Dasypus* species; however TcIII infections in humans and domestic dogs are, as yet, rare. TcV and TcVI are relatively recent hybrids of TcII and TcIII.[6]

More than 150 mammal species of 24 families have been recorded as infected with *T. cruzi* and all mammal species are considered susceptible. Birds and reptiles are not susceptible to *T. cruzi* infection, although some species of triatomine bug do feed on them. Dogs, rodents and cats can be important domestic hosts, and guinea pigs where bred for food, but larger domestic animals are seldom infected. Chickens are not infected but are epidemiologically important because they can sustain large triatomine populations, propagating household infestation.

Triatomine bugs acquire *T. cruzi* infection by feeding on the blood of an infected mammal or rarely by probing another bug that has recently fed. In the vector *T. cruzi* multiplies in the gut lumen as epimastigotes by binary fission. Infective (metacyclic) nondividing trypomastigotes arise in the triatomine hindgut and rectum. Transmission is not by the triatomine bite but by contamination of either mucous membranes or abraded skin with *T. cruzi* metacyclic trypomastigotes in bug feces deposited during or shortly after the blood meal; dessicated bug feces are no longer infectious. There may be a lesion at the conjunctival or cutaneous portal of entry (see below). In the mammal host, *T. cruzi* can invade a wide range of cell types, particularly heart, skeletal and smooth muscle, where transformation to the amastigote stage occurs.[7] The amastigote has no visible flagellum and multiplies by binary fission in the cell cytoplasm, as a pseudocyst. After around 5 days the amastigotes transform into trypomastigotes, which are released when the cell ruptures to invade further cells and form new

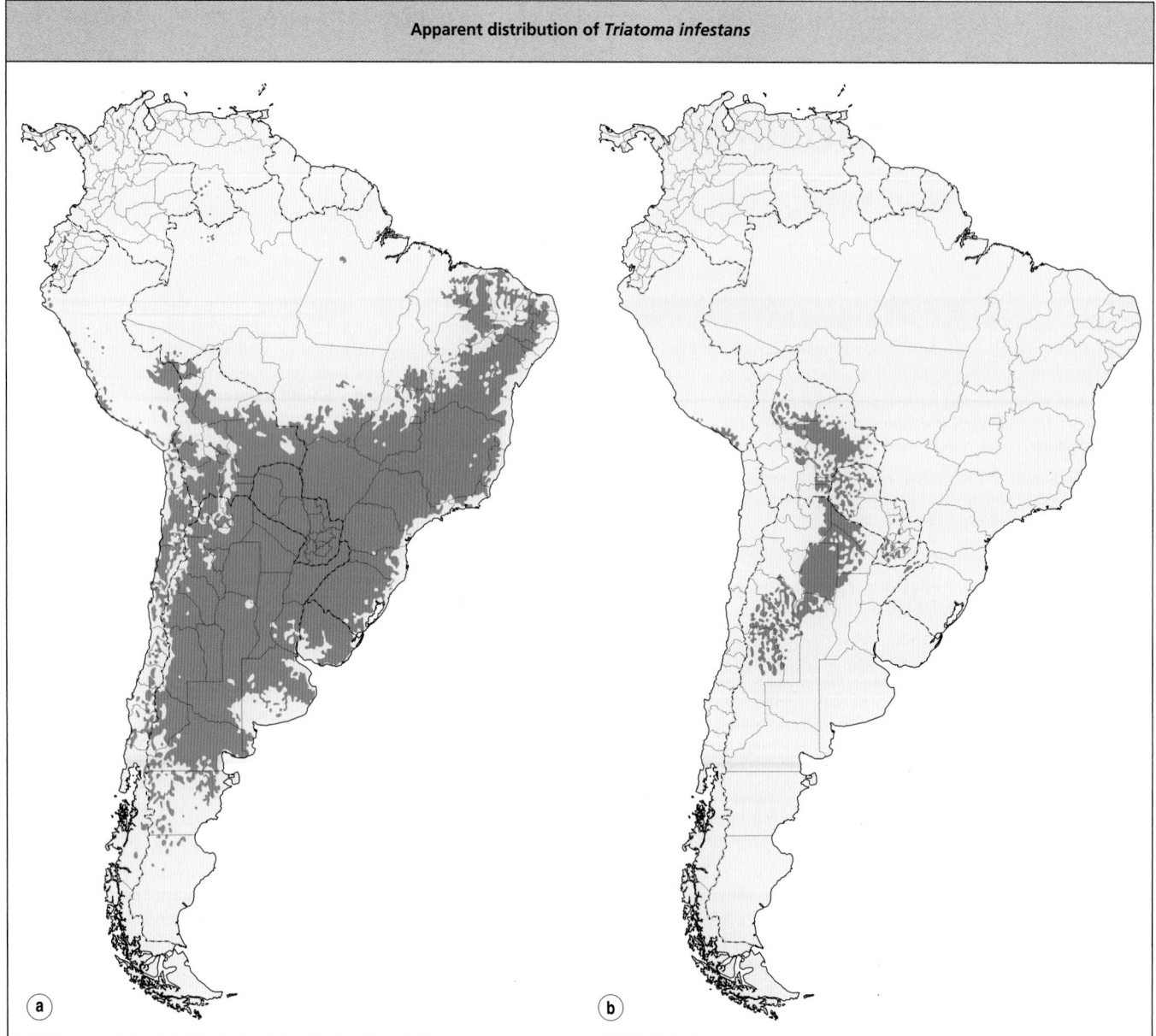

Apparent distribution of *Triatoma infestans*

(a)

(b)

Figure 124-1 Apparent distribution of *Triatoma infestans*. (a) Maximum predicted distribution in the absence of control interventions. (b) An estimate of current distribution based on report from the Intergovernment Commission for the Southern Cone Initiative. *(Reproduced with permission from Schofield et al. Trends Parasitol 2006; 22:583-588. Copyright Elsevier 2006.)*

pseudocysts or to circulate in the blood as nondividing trypomastigotes (Figure 124-2), from which they may be ingested by another feeding triatomine.

There are approximately 140 known species of triatomine bug (Hemiptera: Reduviidae: Triatominae) of which all but 13 are confined to the Americas. The most important vectors of Chagas disease are in the genera *Triatoma*, *Rhodnius* and *Panstrongylus*, because they include species that invade and colonize human dwellings, particularly, but not only, poor housing with mud walls and palm roofs.[8] *Triatoma infestans* is the main domiciliated vector species in the Southern Cone countries and in southern Peru although this triatomine species is far less widely distributed after the Southern Cone control campaign. *Rhodnius prolixus* and *Triatoma dimidiata* are vectors in northern South America and Central America, although *R. prolixus* is now considered to be virtually eliminated from Central America. *Panstrongylus megistus* is a vector in central and eastern Brazil and *Triatoma brasiliensis* in northeastern Brazil (Figure 124-3). Nevertheless, in the Americas *T. cruzi* is

recorded from the majority of triatomine species, and others, such as *Panstrongylus lignarius* and *Eratryus mucronatus*, may act as secondary vectors, invading and colonizing human dwellings.[8]

The time required for development from triatomine egg to adult is influenced by species, access to blood meals and seasonal/environmental conditions. However, the generation time may be less than 6 months. Later-stage nymphs may resist starvation for many months. Natural habitats of triatomines are anywhere that animals have their nests and refuges, including palm trees, hollow trees, burrows and rock piles (Figure 124-4).

Triatomines become infective around 20 days after ingesting an infectious blood meal; all stages are susceptible to infection. Since older bugs have had more feeds they are more likely to be infected. Important secondary routes of infection are blood and organ donation, and congenital transmission. As vector-borne transmission has declined, oral transmission has become more apparent; a recent oral outbreak in Venezuela affected 100 school children, who were believed to be

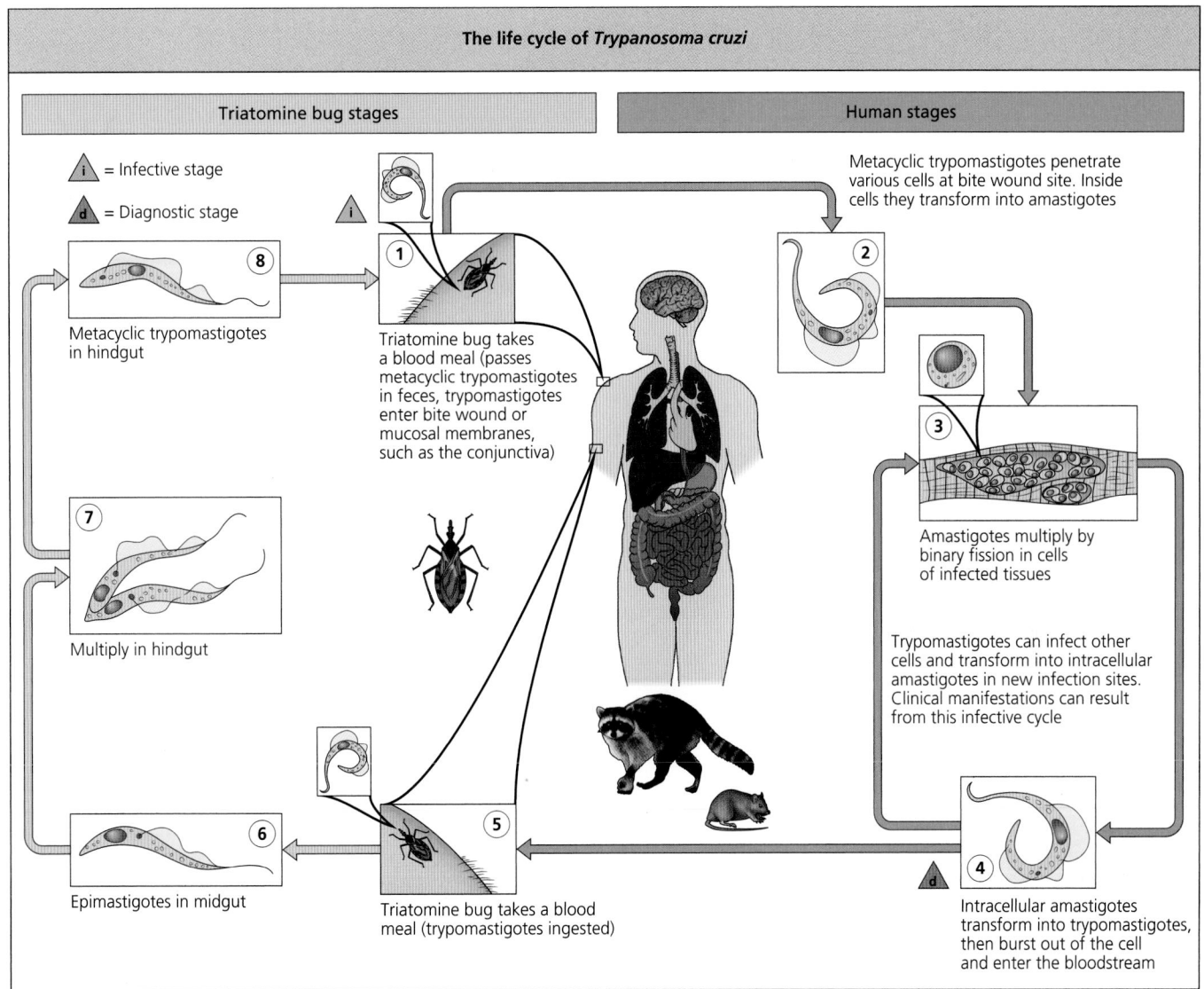

The life cycle of *Trypanosoma cruzi*

Triatomine bug stages

Human stages

i = Infective stage

d = Diagnostic stage

8 — Metacyclic trypomastigotes in hindgut

1 — Triatomine bug takes a blood meal (passes metacyclic trypomastigotes in feces, trypomastigotes enter bite wound or mucosal membranes, such as the conjunctiva)

7 — Multiply in hindgut

6 — Epimastigotes in midgut

5 — Triatomine bug takes a blood meal (trypomastigotes ingested)

2 — Metacyclic trypomastigotes penetrate various cells at bite wound site. Inside cells they transform into amastigotes

3 — Amastigotes multiply by binary fission in cells of infected tissues

Trypomastigotes can infect other cells and transform into intracellular amastigotes in new infection sites. Clinical manifestations can result from this infective cycle

4 — Intracellular amastigotes transform into trypomastigotes, then burst out of the cell and enter the bloodstream

Figure 124-2   The life cycle of *Trypanosoma cruzi. (Modified from US Centers for Disease Control and Prevention (CDC), Atlanta, GA, USA. Public Health Image Library ID#3384: www.cdc.gov/parasites/chagas/biology.html).*

infected by consumption of triatomine-contaminated fruit (guava) juice.[9,10]

Clinical Features, Pathology and Pathogenesis

ACUTE PHASE

The initial acute phase of *T. cruzi* infection may be asymptomatic, is not commonly reported and when recognized is usually in children and young adults. The incubation period may be as short as 2 weeks or up to several months. Metacyclic trypomastigotes that enter cells and produce replicating amastigotes at the portal of entry may induce a local inflammatory response. If parasites enter via the conjunctiva the local lesion may comprise unilateral conjunctivitis and periophthalmic edema (Romaña's sign) with regional lymphadenopathy (Figure 124-5); if entry is via abraded skin there may be an indurated edematous cutaneous lesion (cutaneous chagoma). Occasionally, multiple chagomas are seen in the acute phase in infants, in congenital cases, or in immunocompromised patients. Acute systemic infection can be accompanied by fever, myalgia, headache, hepatosplenomegaly, generalized lymphadenopathy, facial or generalized edema, rash, vomiting, diarrhea and anorexia. ECG abnormalities in the acute phase

include sinus tachycardia, increased P–R interval, T-wave changes and low QRS voltage. Acute phase infections are fatal in 5–10% of cases, particularly in children. If pseudocysts are numerous there may be substantial focal cardiac lesions and an extensive inflammatory response, with infiltration of lymphocytes, monocytes and/or polymorphonuclear cells, destruction of heart muscle and fibrosis.[11,12]

CHRONIC INDETERMINATE PHASE

In immunocompetent individuals surviving acute phase infection, intracellular multiplication and parasitemia in the blood subside due to the host's immune response, although in the absence of chemotherapy low level infection almost always remains. The majority of individuals stay in the asymptomatic indeterminate phase for life. ECG abnormalities typical of chronic chagasic cardiomyopathy arise in up to 30% of human infections; in some cases in the Southern Cone region this may be associated with intestinal chagasic megasyndromes.[11,12]

CHRONIC SYMPTOMATIC PHASE

Cardiac signs include dysrhythmias, palpitations, chest pain, edema, dizziness, syncope and dyspnea. The most typical ECG changes are right bundle branch block and left anterior hemiblock, but there may

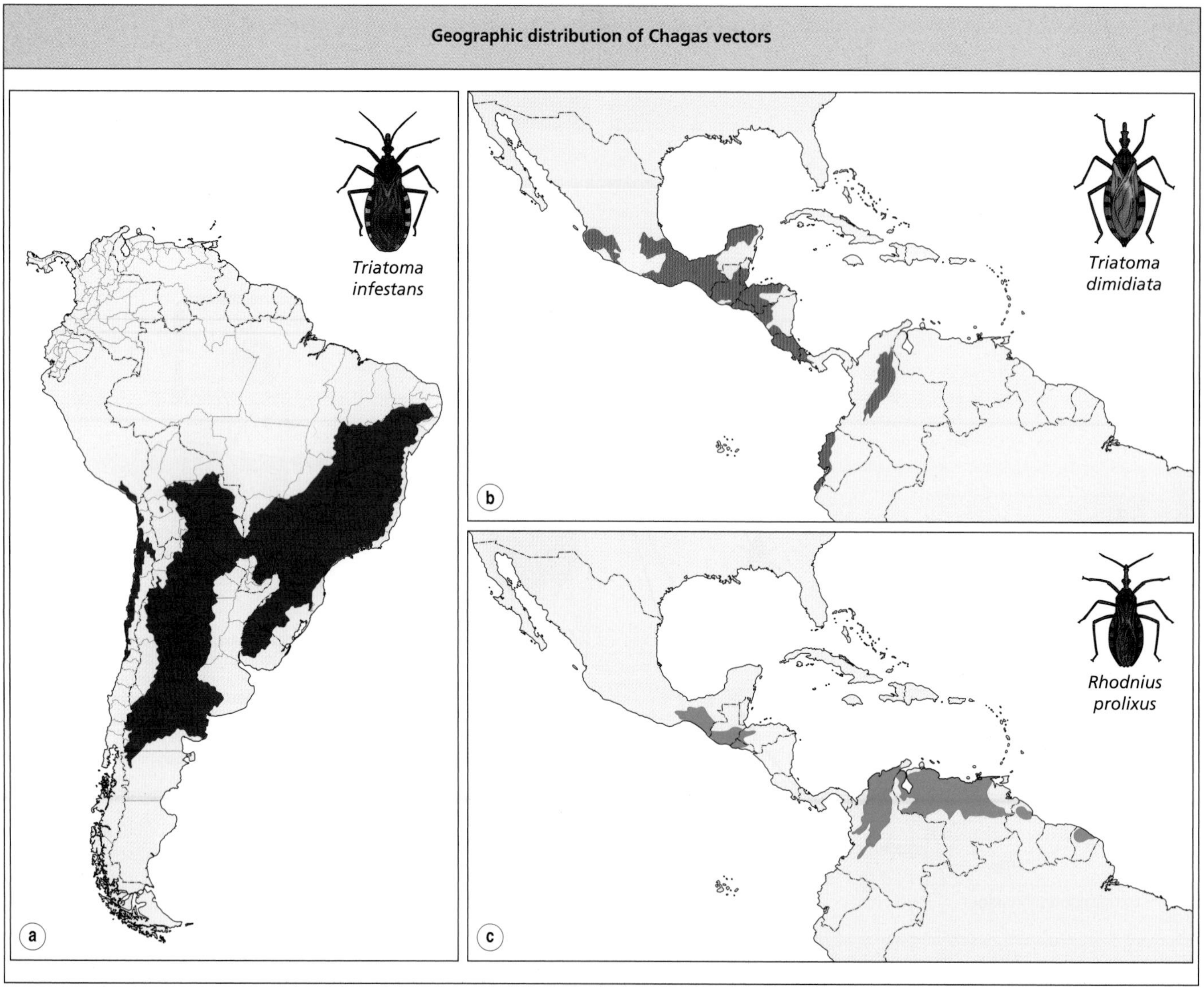

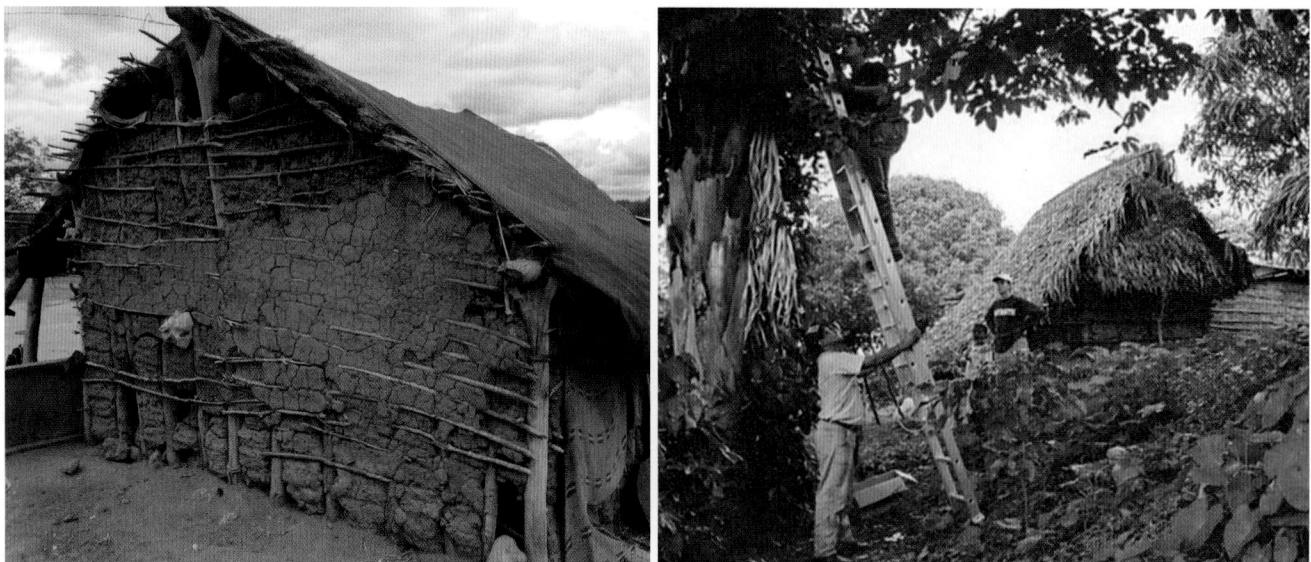

Geographic distribution of Chagas vectors

(a) *Triatoma infestans*

(b) *Triatoma dimidiata*

(c) *Rhodnius prolixus*

Figure 124-3 Distribution of Chagas vectors. Maps indicating the historical distribution of (a) *Triatoma infestans*, (b) *Triatoma dimidiata* and (c) *Rhodnius prolixus*. *(Source: Pan American Health Organization/World Health Organization. 1989. Unpublished document WHO/VBC/89.967. Geneva, Switzerland.)*

Figure 124-4 Examples of typical house constructions that favour triatomine infestation and transmission of *Trypanosoma cruzi*: left timber frame and mud wall; right house with palm roof and adjacent palm tree (courtesy of Louisa Messenger and Matthew Yeo).

also be atrioventricular (AV) conduction abnormalities, including complete AV block. Many different types of dysrhythmia may occur, including sinus bradycardia, sinoatrial block, ventricular tachycardia, primary T-wave changes and abnormal Q waves.

Associated chronic phase gastrointestinal symptoms result from denervation of hollow viscera and consequent dysfunction. Chagasic megaesophagus (Figure 124-6) is more common than chagasic megacolon (Figure 124-7). Both are associated with chagasic cardiomyopathy, and can occasionally be found in children, probably due to congenital transmission.[13] Signs of megaesophagus include loss of peristalsis, regurgitation and dysphagia. Constipation and abdominal pain are typical symptoms of megacolon. Advanced megacolon may be associated with obstruction, perforation and sepsis.

The differential diagnosis of Chagas disease includes distinction from all other types of heart disease and ECG abnormalities, but changes such as right bundle branch block and left anterior hemiblock associated with a history of exposure to *T. cruzi* infection are indicative. Megacolon due to Hirschsprung's disease is usually recognizable, in part because of its rarity in adults.[11,12]

The pathogenesis of chronic Chagas disease is still somewhat enigmatic.[14] Pathogenesis has been described as involving an inflammatory response, focal neurologic damage and, sometimes, autoimmunity. *T. cruzi* invades and replicates in macrophages, fibroblasts, Schwann cells, and smooth and striated myocytes, and parasite DNA can be found in

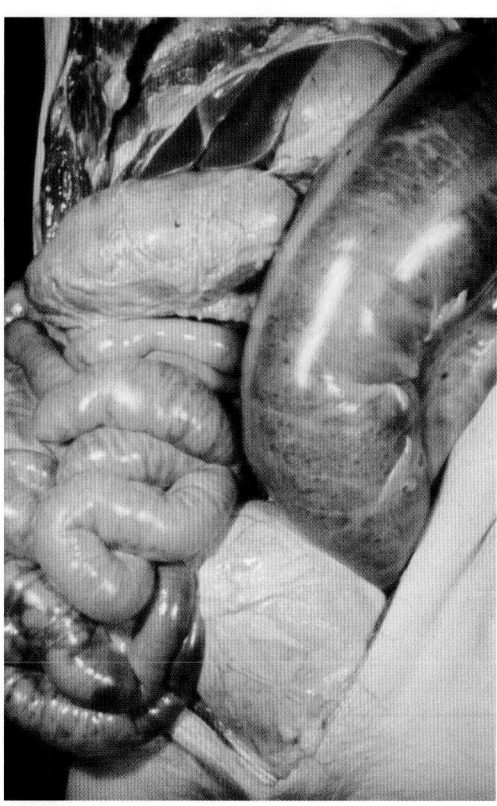

Figure 124-7   Chagasic megacolon. *(Courtesy of J.S. de Oliveira.)*

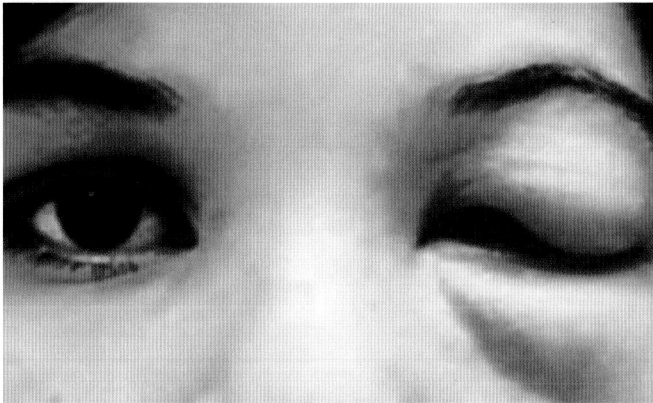

Figure 124-5   Romaña's sign. Acute Chagas disease in a young child. *(Source: Special Programme for Research and Training in Tropical Diseases (TDR). World Health Organization Image ID#9305157.)*

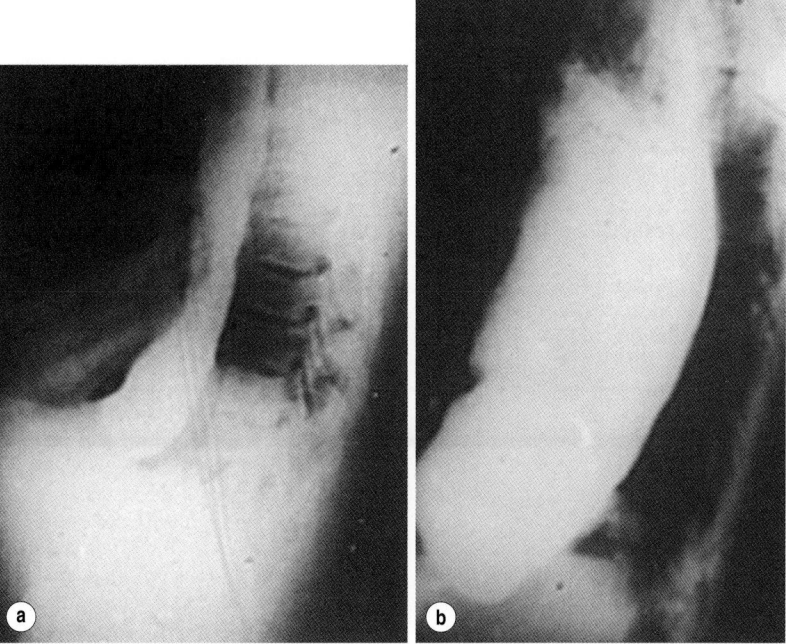

Figure 124-6   Chagasic megaesophagus. Barium contrast radiographs showing (a) megaesophagus grade III and (b) megaesophagus grade IV in a patient with chronic Chagas disease. *(Modified with permission from Coura J.R.: Chagas disease: what is known and what is needed – a background article. Mem Inst Oswaldo Cruz 2007; 102(Suppl.1):113–122.)*

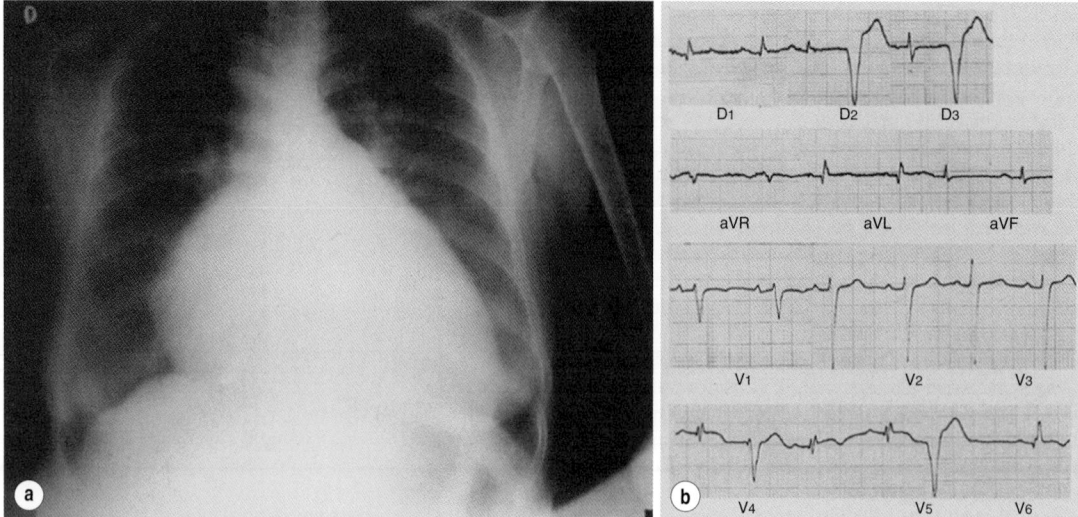

Figure 124-8   Patient with advanced Chagas cardiomyopathy. (a) Radiography showing enlargement of heart. (b) ECG showing ventricular extrasystoles, atrioventricular block, ischemia and myocardial fibrosis in chronic chagasic heart disease. *(Reproduced with permission from Coura J.R.: Chagas disease: what is known and what is needed – a background article. Mem Inst Oswaldo Cruz 2007; 102(Suppl.1):113–122.)*

heart muscle and smooth muscle of the alimentary tract in the chronic phase. It is known that antigens released from ruptured pseudocysts may spread from the immediate site of infection and be adsorbed to uninfected cells. This may lead to an extension of focal damage and the release of normally sequestered host antigens, which could precipitate autoimmunity.[14]

Focal lesions in the conducting system of the heart are associated, both clinically and experimentally, with corresponding ECG abnormalities. The pathogenesis of this 'neurogenic' form of chronic Chagas disease is thought to depend upon irreversible neuron loss in the acute phase, exacerbated by further loss with age, such that a threshold is reached beyond which organ function is perturbed. Gross pathology of the heart consists of megacardia and focal thinning of the myocardium, especially at the apex of the left ventricle, which may lead to apical aneurysm formation, considered to be pathognomonic of chronic chagasic cardiomyopathy[11,12,14] (Figure 124-8).

CONGENITAL INFECTION

Perinatal transmission of *T. cruzi* parasites occurs in 2–10% of women of child-bearing age with indeterminate or chronic Chagas disease. Characteristic signs of congenital infection are: low birth weight, hepatosplenomegaly, jaundice, anemia, interstitial pneumonia, myocarditis, neurologic signs and meningoencephalitis. The ECG in congenital cases is usually normal but there may be low-voltage complexes, decreased T-wave height and increased AV conduction time.[12]

POST-TRANSFUSION

Transfusion is the second most common form of transmission of *T. cruzi*. The risk of parasite transmission from one unit of blood of an infected donor fluctuates between 12% and 20%.[15] The appearance of symptoms such as general lymphadenopathy and splenomegaly are common and occur several months after the blood transfusion.[12]

IN IMMUNOCOMPROMISED PATIENTS

An immunocompromised state may lead to reactivation of infection in up to 40% of patients, producing symptoms typical of the acute phase. In immunocompetent adults the blood–brain barrier is seldom breached but meningoencephalitis is more common in infants and in immunocompromised adults. Chagas disease in patients infected with human immunodeficiency virus (HIV) is associated with advanced disease with CD4 counts <200 cells/μL. The central nervous system (CNS) and the heart are the most commonly affected sites in HIV, accounting for up to 75% and 44% of chagasic disease respectively.

CNS manifestations include acute fatal meningoencephalitis, tumor-like lesions or a granulomatous encephalitis. Cardiac manifestations are heart failure and arrhythmias.[16] Treatment of *T. cruzi* infection in HIV-positive individuals should be started early in the reactivation process, with meningoencephalitis requiring elevated drug doses and carrying a very poor prognosis.[16]

ORAL INFECTION

T. cruzi infective metacyclics have the capacity to cross both the oral mucosa and the wall of the stomach. Common sources of infection are plant (sugar cane) and fruit juices (acai) contaminated with triatomines but food may also theoretically be exposed to infected opossum anal gland secretions, where metacyclic trypomastigotes may develop; transmission can arise from infected mammal reservoir hosts by consumption of raw meat or blood. Such oral infections may lead to multiple simultaneous acute Chagas disease with fatalities.[9]

Diagnosis

PARASITOLOGIC DIAGNOSIS

During the acute phase of infection, parasitemia may be detectable by microscopy of: blood in unstained wet films; Giemsa-stained thick blood films; the buffy coat layer after centrifugation of hematocrit capillaries (with care to avoid exposure to infection); the sediment after centrifugation of recently separated serum (Strout's method); the centrifuged blood after lysis of red cells with 0.87% ammonium chloride. The hematocrit method is recommended for detection of congenital infection in newborn infants with seropositive mothers. All these methods may fail in the acute phase of infection if the parasitemia is low, even though amastigotes are sequestered in the tissues and replicating in pseudocysts. Parasitemia in the chronic phase of infection is almost never detectable by any of these parasitologic methods, except in immunocompromised patients with a reactivated acute phase.[12]

Xenodiagnosis is more sensitive, in which uninfected triatomine bugs from laboratory colonies fed only on birds (e.g. chickens or pigeons) are allowed to feed on the suspected patient. With *R. prolixus* there may be a localized cutaneous hypersensitivity reaction in sensitized individuals; very rarely there may be signs of anaphylactic response. The bugs are dissected about 20–25 days after feeding and the hind gut contents examined by microscopy for the presence of *T. cruzi* epimastigotes. Care must be taken to avoid exposure to infective metacyclic trypomastigotes and bugs should be dissected behind a small angled Perspex screen or in a microbiologic safety cabinet. To avoid false-positives, sterile, ciliate-free saline should be used for dissections and colony bugs of *T. infestans* should be examined periodically for infection with the monoxenous flagellate *Blastocrithidia triatomae*. In areas where *Rhodnius* spp. are vectors of *T. cruzi*, xenodiagnosis may yield the nonpathogenic human trypanosome *Trypanosoma rangeli* and its long, slender epimastigotes may be seen (up to 80 μm); infective *T. rangeli* trypomastigotes occur in the salivary glands of *Rhodnius* and transmission is by insect bite, not by contamination with bug feces.

Culture of venous blood is an alternative to xenodiagnosis but lacks sensitivity, requires aseptic procedures and is vulnerable to contamination. Blood must be centrifuged to deposit all cells and plasma discarded; antibodies in plasma impede the development of epimastigotes, which are vulnerable to complement-mediated lysis.

MOLECULAR METHODS

Detection of *T. cruzi* DNA by amplification of multicopy targets (such as the 195 base pair satellite repeat) with the polymerase chain reaction (PCR), real-time PCR or other DNA amplification methods may be sensitive adjuncts to parasitologic diagnosis. However, although immensely valuable for research and epidemiologic studies, vulnerability to DNA contamination and technical complexity means that standardized rapid diagnostic tests for routine clinical application are not yet available.[12]

SEROLOGY

Serum antibodies to *T. cruzi* are usually detectable within a few days of infection, with an initial IgM response and a sustained IgG response, which in the absence of successful chemotherapy usually persists for life. There are now numerous commercial serologic tests available, several of which are rapid tests for clinical use. Sensitivities and specificities may be 95% or greater but vary between tests. Cross-reactions may occur, for example with visceral leishmaniasis. Infants born of seropositive mothers may be seropositive for up to 9 months after birth due to transplacental transfer of IgG. *T. cruzi* lineage-specific serology using synthetic peptides is under development as a means of indirectly investigating the *T. cruzi* lineage an individual carries.[17]

Prevention

There is no vaccine for Chagas disease and prospects for vaccine development are remote due to the possible autoimmune pathogenesis and impracticality of vaccine trials. Current preventive measures are focused primarily on the elimination of triatomine colonies and the serologic screening of blood donors to prevent transfusion of contaminated blood.[1,2] In addition, prenatal serologic surveillance of women in endemic areas is recommended to facilitate diagnosis and treatment of congenital infection in the newborn, and to consider prophylactic treatment of women before pregnancy. Given adequate resources and careful clinical management, it may be possible to offer active case detection and chemotherapy to children and young adults up to the age of 15 or 18, who are less vulnerable to the side effects of drug treatment.

Chagas disease is maintained by poverty and poor housing (see Figure 124-4). Thus, prevention of triatomine infestation relies principally on residual spraying with insecticides, in conjunction with health education and community participation, and, if resources allow, improvement of housing.[1,2] Bed nets may provide personal protection only but will not eliminate bug infestation; curtain or mesh screens may be helpful where sylvatic bugs invade houses. Pyrethroids, which have low toxicity, high residual activity and to which there is little, sporadic resistance among triatomines, are the insecticides of choice. Prevention of oral infection requires health education on food hygiene, shielding of carefully collected plants and fruits from triatomines and decontamination of derived juices by heat treatment/pasteurization.[18]

TABLE 124-1	Screening of Blood Donors for *Trypanosoma cruzi* in Latin America	
	Coverage (%)	Seropositive (%)
SOUTHERN CONE COUNTRIES		
Argentina	100	4.50
Bolivia	86	9.90
Brazil	100	0.61
Chile	75*	0.47
Paraguay	99	2.80
Uruguay	100	0.47
ANDEAN PACT COUNTRIES		
Colombia	99	0.98
Ecuador	100	0.15
Peru	99	0.26
Venezuela	100	0.67
CENTRAL AMERICA		
Belize	100	0.40
Costa Rica	100	0.34
El Salvador	100	2.46
Guatemala	100	0.79
Honduras	100	1.40
Nicaragua	100	0.49
Panama	98	0.90

*98% in endemic regions.
From Schofield et al., Trends Parasitol 2006; 22:583-588. Copyright Elsevier 2006.

Blood and organ donors should be questioned to ascertain whether they or their mother were resident in an endemic region, whether they have had a blood transfusion or whether they have spent time in an endemic locality; if so they should normally not be donors unless tested and proven to be seronegative (Table 124-1). Prophylactic chemotherapy may be considered for future organ recipients who are seropositive carriers of *T. cruzi* infection and who will be immunosuppressed, and therefore potentially vulnerable to recrudescence of an acute infection.[15]

Management

There are only two drugs currently available to treat Chagas disease: benznidazole and nifurtimox, neither of which guarantees cure of adult chronic infection.[19] Benznidazole is usually considered to be the drug of choice due to its fewer side effects. Treatment is essential during the acute phase of infection because it may be life-saving. Similarly, congenital cases also demand treatment. Immunocompromised patients must also be treated and, if tolerated, double or even higher dose rates may be recommended to treat meningoencephalitis. Children under 7 years of age usually tolerate chemotherapy well, and side effects may be limited in children and young adults up to the age of 18. Nevertheless, treatment should be monitored carefully for the appearance of side effects; rare cases of Stevens–Johnson syndrome are known. In adults side effects are more severe and chemotherapy often has to be stopped due to the early appearance of dermatologic complications. Parasitologic cure is difficult to ascertain because negative parasitology is not sufficiently sensitive to prove absence of infection; there are no biomarkers for cure and reversion of conventional serology may take decades.[20] Pathogenesis and prognosis might be largely attributable to the extent of acute phase damage; the influence of sustained low-level infection is under investigation.[19] A randomized trial of benznidazole in patients with established cardiomyopathy showed no benefit in terms of clinical cardiac deterioration after 5 years of follow up.[21] Two drugs that showed potential experimentally, posoconazole and ravuconazole, have failed in clinical trials;[19,22] fexinidazole is under clinical evaluation;[23] a pediatric formulation of benznidazole has been developed and added to the WHO Essential Medicine List.[24]

Benznidazole is given orally at 5–10 mg/kg/day for adults, 10 mg/kg for children, in two divided doses for 60 days. Common adverse events, particularly in adults, are rashes, fever, nausea, peripheral polyneuritis, anorexia, weight loss, headache and insomnia, leukopenia and (rarely) agranulocytosis, with dermatologic side effects leading to discontinuation of treatment. Blood cell counts should be performed before the start of treatment and weekly during treatment to detect possible bone marrow suppression. Treatment is contraindicated during pregnancy, in hepatic or renal failure, and in cases of hematopathology or neuropathology.[12]

For nifurtimox, recommended oral doses are 15–20 mg/kg for children, 12.5–15 mg/kg for adolescents below 16 years old, 8–10 mg/kg for adults, 25 mg/kg for treatment of meningoencephalitis and 10–20 mg/kg for congenital cases, administered in three divided doses for 90 days in acute cases and for up to 120 days in chronic cases. In adults it is recommended to start treatment with low doses and increase by 2 mg/kg per week until reaching the maximal dose. Adverse events include anorexia, weight loss, nausea, vomiting and abdominal discomfort. In some patients, symptoms of central nervous system toxicity may be present, such as irritability, insomnia, disorientation, tremors, polyneuropathy, dizziness, vertigo and mood changes. Reversible psychiatric symptoms may also be present in elderly patients. Nifurtimox is not recommended during pregnancy.[12]

Supportive chemotherapy is often required for the treatment of adverse events, such as fever, vomiting, diarrhea and convulsions. Management of acute meningoencephalitis may require anticonvulsants, sedatives and intravenous mannitol. Management of chronic chagasic heart disease may be a balancing act between patient management, drug administration and use of a pacemaker.[3] Sodium intake is restricted if there is acute-phase heart failure and diuretics and digitalis may be indicated.

Vasodilation (angiotensin-converting enzyme inhibitors) and maintenance of normal serum potassium may be required initially; digitalis is advisable only as a last resort because it may aggravate dysrhythmias. Bradycardia that does not respond to atropine, atrial fibrillation with a slow ventricular response or complete AV block may necessitate a pacemaker. Surgical resection of dysrhythmic endocardial regions and of ventricular aneurysms has been suggested. Heart transplantation for end-stage chagasic cardiomyopathy has been shown to be a valuable treatment option.[15]

Megaesophagus may improve with dietary control or respond to dilation of the cardiac sphincter using probes, air or hydrostatic pressure. The surgical procedure for alleviating advanced megaesophagus involves selective removal of a portion of muscle at the junction between the esophagus and stomach. Severe megaesophagus may demand replacement of the distal esophagus with another part of the alimentary tract such as the jejunum.[25] The recommended surgical treatments for megacolon are anterior rectosigmoidectomy and the modified Duhamel–Haddad operation.[26]

References available online at expertconsult.com.

KEY REFERENCES

Bahia M.T., Nascimento A.F., Mazzeti A.L., et al.: Antitrypanosomal activity of fexnidazole metabolites, potential new drug candiates for Chagas disease. *Antimicrob Agents Chemother* 2014; 58:4362-4370.

Bern C.: Chagas disease in the immunosuppressed host. *Curr Opin Infect Dis* 2012; 25:450-457.

Bern C., Kjos S., Yabsley M.J., et al.: *Trypanosoma cruzi* and Chagas disease in the United States. *Clin Microbiol Rev* 2011; 24:655-681.

Clark E.H., Sherbuk J., Okamoto E., et al.: Hyperendemic Chagas disease and the unmet need for pacemakers in the Bolivian Chaco. *PLoS Negl Trop Dis* 2014; 8:e2801.

Kransdorf E.P., Czer L.S., Luthringer D.J., et al.: Heart transplantation for Chagas cardiomyopathy in the United States. *Am J Transplant* 2013; 13:3262-3268.

Miles M.A., Llewellyn M.S., Lewis M.D., et al.: The molecular epidemiology and phylogeography of *Trypanosoma cruzi* and parallel research on *Leishmania*: looking back and to the future. *Parasitology* 2009; 136:1509-1528.

Rassi A. Jr, Rassi A., Marin-Neto J.A.: Chagas disease. *Lancet* 2010; 375:1388-1402.

Shikanai-Yasuda M.A., Carvalho N.B.: Oral transmission of Chagas disease. *Clin Infect Dis* 2012; 54:845-852.

World Health Organization (WHO): *Control of Chagas disease: second report of the WHO Expert Committee. Technical Report Series 905.* Geneva: WHO; 2002.

Zingales B., Miles M.A., Moraes C.B., et al.: Drug discovery for Chagas disease should consider *Trypanosoma cruzi* strain diversity. *Mem Inst Oswaldo Cruz* 2014; 109:828-833.

125

Melioidosis

SHARON J. PEACOCK | DIREK LIMMATHUROTSAKUL

KEY CONCEPTS

- Melioidosis is a serious bacterial infection caused by the gram-negative bacillus *Burkholderia pseudomallei*.

- Infection results from inoculation, inhalation or ingestion of *B. pseudomallei* present in the environment.

- Most cases are diagnosed in South East Asia and northern Australia, but the disease is under-recognized in many parts of the world.

- Diabetes mellitus is the most common predisposing factor.

- Most adult cases present with acute sepsis associated with bacterial dissemination, although almost any organ or tissue can be involved.

- Microbiologic culture and identification of *B. pseudomallei* represents the diagnostic gold standard.

- Antimicrobial therapy involves a minimum of 10 days' parenteral therapy, followed by oral antibiotics for 12–20 weeks.

- Death from melioidosis occurs in 12–40% of cases, mostly as a result of sepsis and its complications.

- The most common complication in survivors is relapse from a persistent focus.

Epidemiology

The global distribution of melioidosis is shown in Figure 125-1, and reported incidence rates are summarized in Table 125-1. Most cases occur in countries where *Burkholderia pseudomallei* is present in the environment, although imported cases may present anywhere in the world and occur most frequently in immigrants, soldiers and tourists.[4] Mother-to-child and person-to-person transmission is very rare, while patient-to-patient transmission in the hospital setting has not been reported in the published literature. Rare laboratory-acquired infections have been described (reviewed in reference 5). Melioidosis is seasonal in the tropics, where most cases present during the rainy season. Males are more often affected than females, and infection can occur at any age with a peak incidence in people aged 40–60 years. Predisposing factors include diabetes mellitus, chronic lung or kidney disease, thalassemia, alcohol excess, malignancy and immunosuppressive treatment (including corticosteroids) (reviewed in reference 6). One or more predisposing factors are identified in around three-quarters of adult cases.

Pathogenesis and Pathology

Putative virulence factors include quorum sensing, a type III secretion system cluster 3 (T3SS3) that shares homology to the *inv/spa/prg* TTSS of *Salmonella enterica* serovar Typhimurium and the *ipa/mxi/spa* TTSS of *Shigella flexneri*, a type VI secretion system (T6SS), *Burkholderia* lethal factor 1 that is similar to *Escherichia coli* cytotoxic capsular polysaccharide, lipopolysaccharide and flagella (reviewed in reference 4). *B. pseudomallei* is a facultative intracellular pathogen that can invade nonphagocytic cells and persist in phagocytes. Following uptake, the organism can escape the endosome and propel itself within and between cells by polar nucleation of actin and induce cell fusion.

TTSS3 is central to this process, and BimA is required for actin-based bacterial motility.[7] Reversible colony morphology switching associated with complex alterations in protein expression has been described, and this may be associated with adaptive changes that facilitate bacterial survival *in vivo*.[8]

The cytokines interferon-gamma (IFN-γ), tumor necrosis factor (TNF) and interleukin (IL)-12 and IL-18 play an important role in early resistance against experimental *B. pseudomallei* infection. These cytokines are expressed during human melioidosis, and may contribute to pathogenesis since high plasma levels of several cytokines are correlated with mortality.

The macroscopic pathology of melioidosis is primarily one of abscess formation. These may be single or multiple, and present in one or more organs. The histopathologic appearance of infected human tissue forms a spectrum from acute to chronic granulomatous inflammation. Samples taken at post-mortem show focal or diffuse acute necrotizing inflammation with varying numbers of neutrophils, macrophages, lymphocytes and 'giant cells' of unknown cell type.[9] Intracellular bacteria have been observed within macrophages and giant cells.[9]

Prevention

In areas where *B. pseudomallei* is present in the environment, water should be boiled before consumption and protective gear (waterproof shoes or boots and protective gloves) worn when in contact with soil (e.g. during agricultural work).[10] An umbrella should be used for protection from rain where possible, and nose and mouth should be covered if caught in a dust cloud.[10] These recommendations are based on a case–control study (Box 125-1), but their efficacy has not been evaluated.[10] No *B. pseudomallei* vaccine is available for human use (reviewed in reference 11).

TABLE 125-1	Incidence of Melioidosis in Endemic Areas*		
Countries, Areas	**Year Reported**	**Incidence of Melioidosis (per 100 000 person-years)**	**Case Fatality Rate**
SOUTH EAST ASIA			
Thailand, Ubon Ratchathani	1997–2006	12.7	43%
Malaysia, Kedah[2]	2005–2008	16.4	65%
Malaysia, Pahang	2005–2006	4.3	44%
Singapore	1998–2007	1.3	16%
OCEANIA			
Australia, northern Australia[3]	2009–2010	50.2	12%
Torres Strait Islands	1995–2000	42.7	22%
Papua New Guinea, Balimo district	1994–1995 and 1998	20.0	40%
EMERGING AREAS			
Taiwan	2001–2006	0.7	Not available

*Reviewed by Limmathurotsakul and Peacock.[1]

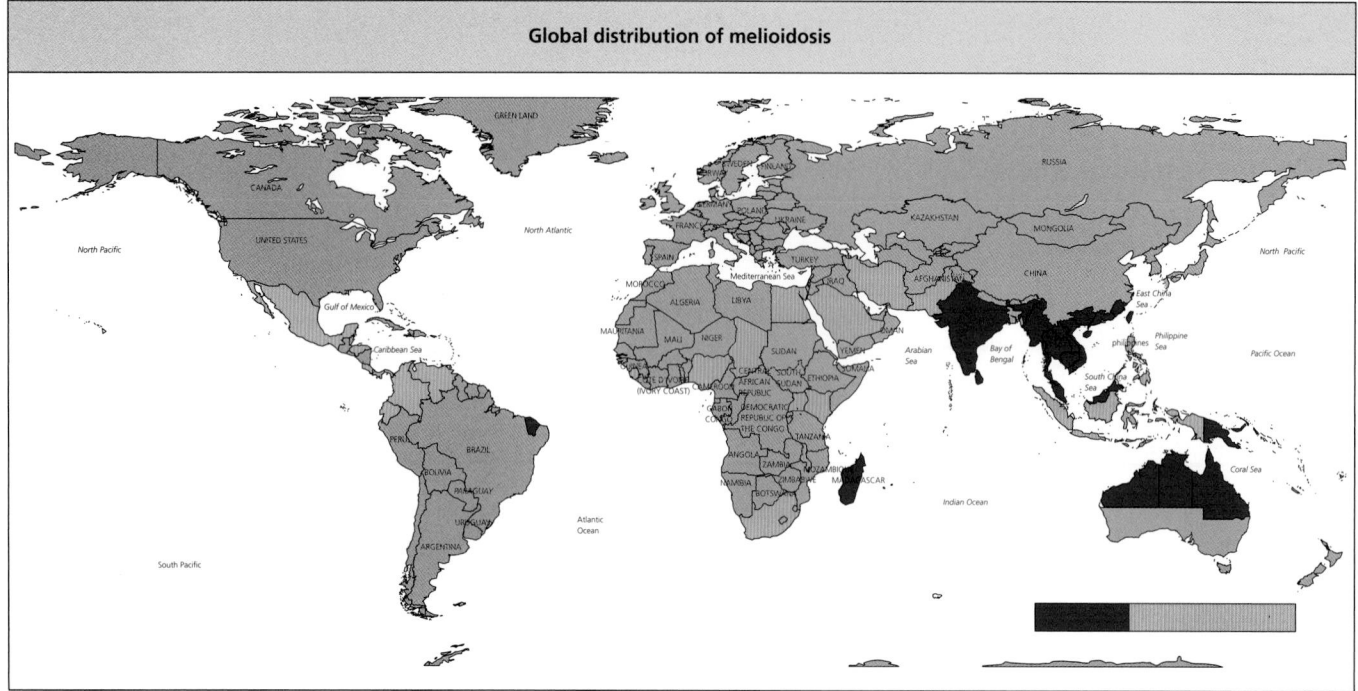

Figure 125-1 Global distribution of melioidosis. (*Reproduced from Limmathurotsakul D., Dance D.A.B., Wuthiekanun V., et al.: Systematic review and consensus guidelines for environmental sampling of* Burkholderia pseudomallei. *PLoS Negl Trop Dis 2013; 7(3):e2105.*)

BOX 125-1 RECOMMENDATIONS FOR THE PREVENTION OF MELIOIDOSIS

1. Avoid direct contact with soil or environmental water.
2. If contact with soil or environmental water is necessary, wear protective gear including rubber gloves, boots or waders, and wash with soap and clean water immediately after exposure.
3. In the event of an injury involving contamination with soil or environmental water, immediately clean the wound with soap and clean water.
4. Keep open wounds covered and avoid contact with soil or water until completely healed. Do not apply any herbal remedies or other substances to the wound. In the event that the wound comes into contact with soil or environmental water, clean the wound thoroughly with soap and clean water.
5. Always wear shoes. Do not walk barefoot.
6. Only drink bottled or boiled water. Do not drink any untreated water.
7. Do not eat food contaminated with soil or dust. If food is to be eaten without cooking, wash thoroughly using clean water. Use clean eating utensils, and wash these in clean water.
8. When outside, avoid heavy rain or dust clouds. If caught in a dust cloud, cover mouth and nose. Use an umbrella to protect yourself from the rain.
9. Do not smoke.
10. Be aware that you are at greater risk of melioidosis if you have certain conditions, including diabetes, chronic kidney disease, and diseases that require steroid therapy or medications that suppress the immune system.

Reproduced with permission from Limmathurotsakul D., Kanoksil M., Wuthiekanun V., et al.: Activities of daily living associated with acquisition of melioidosis in northeast Thailand: a matched case–control study. PLoS Negl Trop Dis 2013; 7(2): e2072.

Clinical Features

The period between an exposure event that results in melioidosis and clinical features of infection is variable and often difficult to define. In one study, 25% of cases remembered an inoculation event prior to illness, from which an incubation period of 1–21 days (mean 9 days) was derived.[6] The incubation period following a high inoculum event

such as near drowning may be as short as 24 hours. By contrast, exposure may be followed by a prolonged period of latency, the maximum recorded being 62 years. Time from onset of clinical manifestations to presentation to a medical facility is also variable. In northeast Thailand, around a third of patients had symptoms for less than 7 days, one half reported being unwell for 7–28 days, and the remainder had symptoms for more than 28 days.[12] In northern Australia, 11% of patients presenting for the first time had symptoms for more than 2 months.[13]

Severity of disease ranges from an acute fulminant bacteremia to a chronic localized infection, but most adult patients present with acute sepsis associated with bacterial dissemination.[14] Bacteremia is detected in around half of cases, and septic shock is common in this group. The lung is involved in approximately half of all cases, manifesting as pneumonia and/or lung abscess(es). Respiratory involvement may be clinically and radiologically indistinguishable from tuberculosis (Figure 125-2).[15] Solitary or multiple abscesses are detected in the liver and/or spleen in around one-quarter of cases in Thailand when abdominal imaging is performed as routine.[16] Renal abscesses are often associated with calculi and urinary tract infection. Infection involving the urinary tract is present in at least one-quarter of Thai patients based on a urine culture positive for *B. pseudomallei*.[17] Genitourinary infection is common in Australia, with prostatic abscesses occurring in 20% of male patients.[13] Many patients with hepatosplenic abscess(es), urinary tract infection, or prostatic abscesses lack signs and symptoms associated with the organ(s) infected.[13,16,17] A neurologic syndrome of meningoencephalitis with varying involvement of the brain stem, cerebellum and spinal cord has been reported in 3% of melioidosis cases in Darwin, Australia.[13] Prominent features on presentation were unilateral limb weakness, predominant cerebellar signs, mixed cerebellar and brain stem features with peripheral weakness, or flaccid paraparesis.[13] Peripheral motor weakness may mimic Guillain–Barré syndrome, and unilateral limb weakness may mimic a stroke. Focal suppurative infections involving the central nervous system (CNS) with or without meningitis have been reported. CNS infections occur in around 1.5% of melioidosis patients in Thailand,[18] but the syndrome of meningoencephalitis has not been defined in this setting. Figure 125-3 shows serial computed tomography (CT) brain scans with contrast performed on a patient with central nervous system involvement.

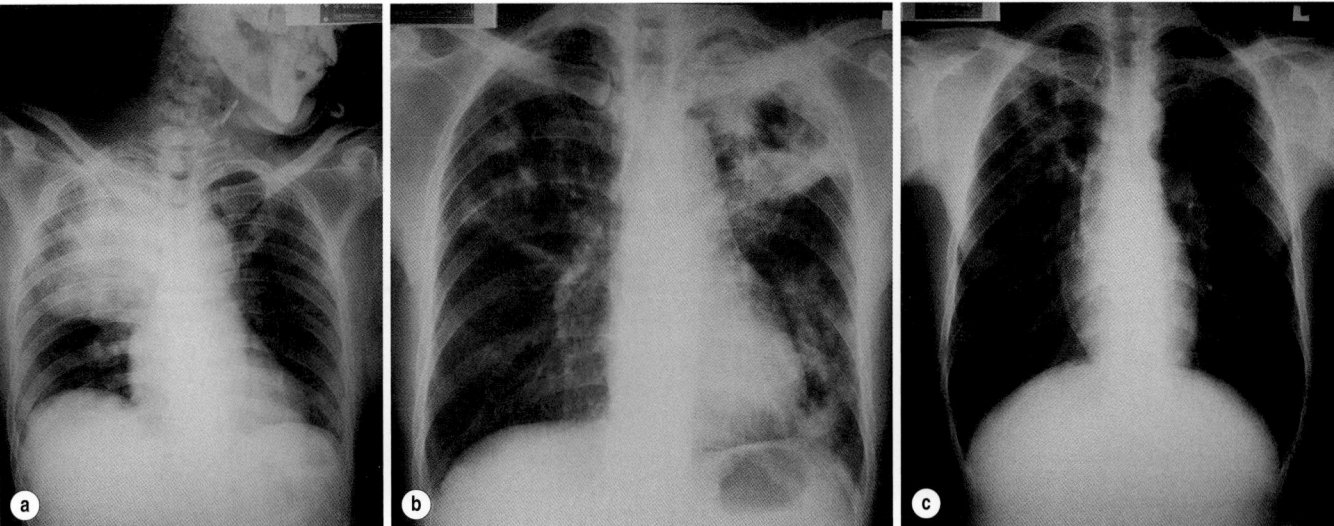

Figure 125-2   Chest radiographs of three patients with melioidosis and sputum culture-positive for *Burkholderia pseudomallei*. (a) Right upper lobe consolidation in a patient with acute pneumonia. (b) Right upper and lower lobe infiltration, and cavity in left upper lobe in a patient with chronic cough and fever for 30 days. (c) Moderately thickened wall cavity with subjacent infiltration in right upper lobe in a patient with chronic cough and fever for 30 days. *(Courtesy of Ms Pornpan Suntornsut et al., in Suntornsut P., Kasemsupat K., Silairatana S., et al.: Prevalence of melioidosis in patients with suspected pulmonary tuberculosis and sputum smear negative for acid-fast bacilli in northeast Thailand. Am J Trop Med Hyg 2013; 89(5): 983-5.)*

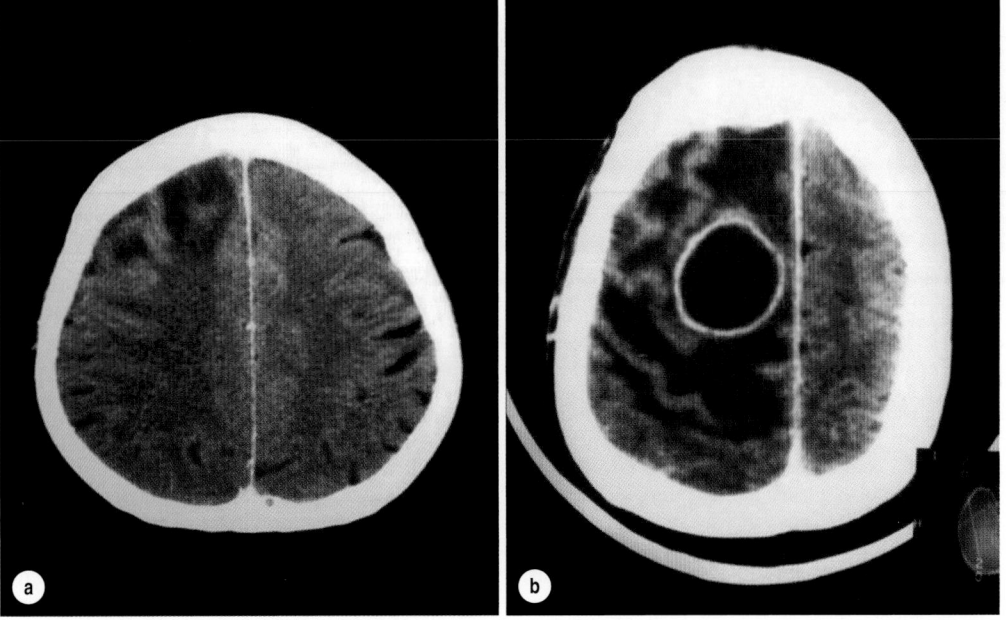

Figure 125-3   CT brain scans. (a) Hypodensity in the right frontal lobe in a patient with fever and a hemiparesis. (b) Ring-enhancing lesion with surrounding edema in the right frontoparietal lobe in the same patient re-presented 2 months later with worsening headache and hemiparesis. *(Reproduced with permission from Limmathurotsakul D., Chaowagul W., Wongsrikaew P., et al.: Variable presentation of neurological melioidosis in Northeast Thailand. Am J Trop Med Hyg 2007; 77:118-120.)*

Osteoarticular involvement is diagnosed in around one-sixth of patients in Thailand,[19] but only 4% of those affected in Australia.[13] The knee is the most common site for septic arthritis, and more than one joint is involved in a quarter of affected cases. Osteomyelitis is often secondary to infection of another organ, although localized osteomyelitis does occur. Skin and soft tissue infections are found in a quarter of cases in Thailand and one-sixth in Australia. This includes superficial pustules, subcutaneous abscesses and pyomyositis (Figure 125-4). Such foci may represent the source of systemic infection, or may result from hematogenous or local spread. Soft tissue infection may run an aggressive course similar to that seen for necrotizing fasciitis caused by other organisms. Infections involving many other sites have been described, including lymphadenitis, mycotic aneurysm, mediastinal

infection, pyopericarditis, orbital cellulitis, corneal ulcers, acute otitis media, sinusitis and abscess formation in the breast, scrotum and deep tissues of the neck.

Melioidosis in Thai children presents as acute suppurative parotitis in around one-third of cases, but this is uncommon in Thai adults and very rare in Australia. Parotitis is bilateral in 10% of cases and may be complicated by rupture into the auditory canal, facial nerve palsy and necrotizing fasciitis.

Diagnosis

Given the myriad of possible presentations, a high index of suspicion is essential for clinicians working in areas that are endemic for

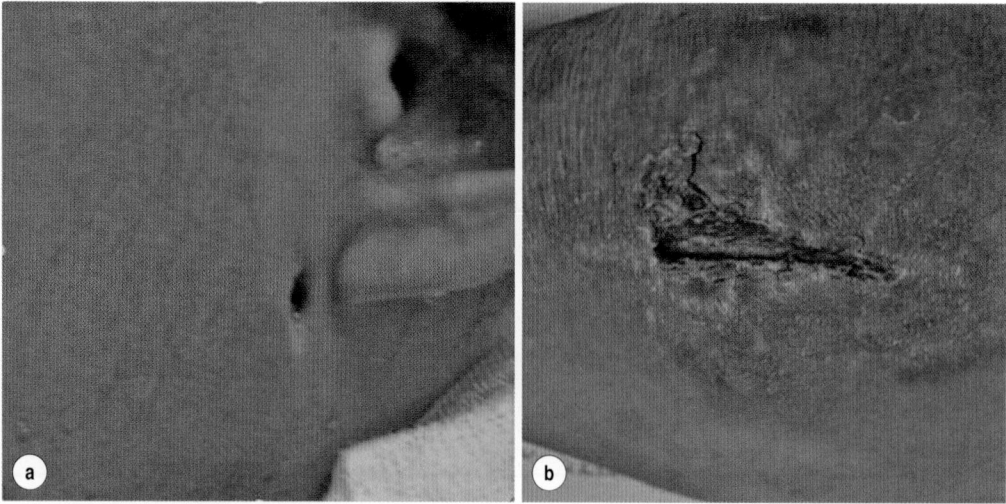

Figure 125-4 (a) Abscess affecting the pre-auricular area. (b) Infected soft tissue of the heel. *(Courtesy of Drs Rapeephan Rattanawongnara and Ekamol Tantisattamo.)*

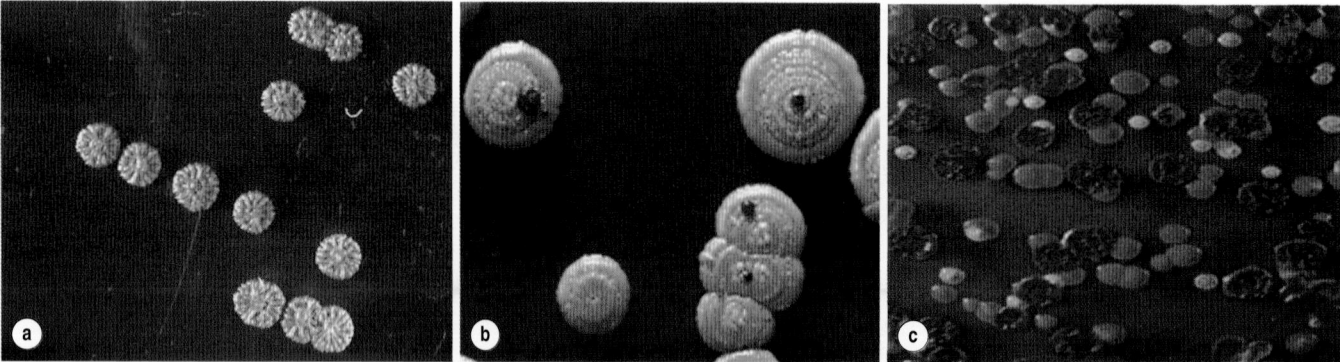

Figure 125-5 Colony variation is commonly seen during culture of clinical isolates on Ashdown agar. (a) Typical colony appearance of *B. pseudomallei* after incubation at 37 °C in air for 3 days. (b) Colony variation within a single colony in which the parental colony (pink) has given rise to a second type (red). (c) Variable colony morphology from a single sample; genotyping confirmed the presence of a single clone. *(Courtesy of Mrs Vanaporn Wuthiekanun and Dr Narisara Chantratita, reproduced from Wiersinga W.J., van der Poll T., White N.J., et al.: Melioidosis: insights into the pathogenicity of* Burkholderia pseudomallei. *Nat Rev Microbiol 2006; 4:272-282.)*

melioidosis. This infection should also be considered when investigating the cause of fever in returning travelers or army personnel who could have been exposed to a contaminated environment. Microbiologic culture and identification of *B. pseudomallei* represents the diagnostic gold standard (Figure 125-5). Unlike the investigation of many other bacterial infections, culture should be performed on all available specimens, including blood, urine, throat swab, respiratory secretions, pus and swabs from surface wounds. Growth of even a single *B. pseudomallei* colony from any sample is diagnostic for melioidosis, since the organism is not a member of the normal human flora. Because the organism can become disseminated in the host, the site of culture positivity may not necessarily reflect the major site of clinical infection. For example, a throat swab may be positive for *B. pseudomallei* in a patient who presents with a splenic abscess.

The diagnostic laboratory should be alerted to the possibility of melioidosis because the sample and culture should be handled in a biological safety cabinet,[5] and because the organism can easily be misidentified as *Pseudomonas* spp. or overlooked as a contaminant (especially in cultures of samples taken from colonized sites). Speed to blood culture positivity has prognostic significance, and the bacterial counts of *B. pseudomallei* in blood and urine are positively associated with outcome (reviewed in reference 12). An immunofluorescent microscopy assay that can be used directly on samples has been described that provides a rapid presumptive diagnosis of melioidosis, but the antibody used is not commercially available and the assay is restricted to a small number of laboratories in Thailand.

Polymerase chain reaction (PCR) has been evaluated for the diagnosis of melioidosis but is not in routine use. Serologic assays such as the indirect hemagglutination (IHA) test have no role in the diagnosis of melioidosis where infection is endemic since anti-*B. pseudomallei* antibodies are common in the general population.[12] A single IHA titer of >1:40 or a rising titer in an individual who has not previously resided in areas where melioidosis is endemic may be diagnostically useful but requires careful interpretation based on a detailed travel and medical history.

Management

Appropriate parenteral antimicrobial agents should be commenced immediately on suspicion of the diagnosis of melioidosis. Ideally, culture should be performed prior to their administration but treatment should not be delayed if culture cannot be performed rapidly, as in the case of aspiration of pus under imaging or operative procedure. Choice and duration of therapy are shown in Table 125-2. Although granulocyte colony-stimulating factor (G-CSF) is used in patients with septic shock due to melioidosis at the Royal Darwin Hospital, a randomized placebo-controlled trial of G-CSF for severe melioidosis in northeast Thailand failed to show an effect on mortality.[20] No other adjunctive therapies have been shown to improve outcome from melioidosis. Patients with severe melioidosis associated with septic shock, respiratory failure associated with severe infection or acute respiratory distress syndrome, acute renal failure and other manifestations of a

TABLE 125-2	Antimicrobial Treatment of Melioidosis		
Drug	**Dose**	**Duration**	
INITIAL PARENTERAL TREATMENT			
Ceftazidime *or* meropenem	50 mg/kg/dose (up to 2 g) q6–8h* *or* 25 mg/kg/dose (up to 1 g) q8h*	Minimum 10–14 days, or longer (4–8 weeks) for deep-seated infection, organ abscesses, osteomyelitis, septic arthritis or neurologic melioidosis	
ORAL ERADICATIVE TREATMENT			
Trimethoprim–sulfamethoxazole	Weight-based regimen for adults (q12h): 2 × 160–800 mg (960 mg) tablets if >60 kg 3 × 80–400 mg (480 mg) tablets if 40–60 kg 1 × 160–800 mg (960 mg) tablets *or* 2 × 80–400 mg (480 mg) tablets if <40 kg	Minimum 12–20 weeks	

Notes: Amoxicillin–clavulanate is an alternative treatment for pregnant women and children younger than 8 years and as an alternative to first-line therapy in other patient groups. Amoxicillin–clavulanate dosing for melioidosis is reviewed in reference 14. For intravenous-phase treatment, the recommended dose is 20/5 mg/kg q4h. Parenteral amoxicillin–clavulanate is associated with higher rates of treatment failure, so avoid if first-line drugs can be given. For oral eradicative treatment, use amoxicillin–clavulanate at a dose of 20/5 mg/kg q8h. For adult patients <60 kg a dose of 1000/250 mg q8h is suggested. For patients >60 kg, the recommended maximum dose is 1500/375 mg q8h. Oral amoxicillin–clavulanate is associated with higher rates of relapse.

Adjust drug dosages as necessary in patients with renal failure, a common complication of melioidosis.

*Consider addition of trimethoprim–sulfamethoxazole 8/40 mg/kg (up to 320/1600 mg) q12h for treatment of patients with neurologic, prostatic, bone or joint melioidosis.

severe septic illness require intensive care management where this is available. The availability of intensive care facilities is an important contributor to the marked difference in outcome for high-income versus low- or lower-middle-income countries.

Hematologic and biochemical blood tests should be performed to detect the onset of acute renal failure, abnormal liver function tests and anemia, all of which are well recognized during severe melioidosis. Arterial blood gases should be taken in patients with lung involvement and/or any evidence of respiratory impairment. Admission C-reactive protein may be normal or only mildly elevated, including in patients with severe sepsis, fatal cases and in relapsed melioidosis.

A chest radiograph should be taken in all patients with suspected melioidosis. Common radiographic patterns include localized patchy alveolar infiltrate, focal, multifocal or lobar consolidation, diffuse interstitial shadowing considered consistent with blood-borne spread of infection, pleural effusion and upper-lobe involvement which may include cavitation. The radiographic pattern may mimic tuberculosis. The development of empyema and/or lung abscess(es) is well recognized, and repeat chest radiographs are indicated for patients with respiratory involvement.

Abdominal ultrasound or CT scan should be performed on all patients with melioidosis to exclude the presence of abscesses in liver and spleen, and in the prostate in male patients. A 'Swiss cheese' appearance on ultrasound or a 'honeycomb' appearance on CT scan are characteristic for hepatosplenic melioidosis. Transrectal ultrasound findings of prostatic abscesses include solitary and multiple abscesses. Early brain CT scan may be normal in patients with neurologic melioidosis, but magnetic resonance imaging often shows dramatic changes. The need for other imaging will depend on clinical features and organ involvement.

Parenteral antibiotics are required for a minimum of 10 days or until clear clinical improvement is observed (whichever is longer). This is followed by oral antibiotics for 12–20 weeks (or more if clinically indicated), as described in Table 125-2. Melioidosis is characterized by difficulty in eradicating the causative organisms. Fever clearance is often slow (median fever clearance time of 9 days), and without evidence of clinical deterioration is not normally sufficient to indicate the need for a change in therapy. Sputum and draining abscess cultures may remain positive for several weeks in a patient who is otherwise responding to treatment. A patient who has clinical deterioration or persistently positive blood cultures should be viewed as failing treatment, at which stage the need for imaging, drainage of collections and change in antimicrobial therapy should be considered.

Death from melioidosis currently occurs in around 40% of cases in Thailand and 12% in Australia.[13,21] Most deaths are due to uncontrolled sepsis and/or organ dysfunction, including respiratory and renal failure. The single most important complication for patients who survive the first episode is recurrent melioidosis, which may occur despite prolonged appropriate oral antimicrobial treatment. Based on the latest randomized-controlled trial, culture-confirmed recurrent melioidosis occurs in around 8% of patients followed for 3 years.[22] Recurrence represents either relapse following failure to eradicate bacteria responsible for the primary infection, or re-infection with a new strain. Half of recurrent cases are due to relapse and the other half to re-infection.[22] Time to recurrence is significantly shorter for episodes due to relapse compared with those due to re-infection. Choice and duration of oral antimicrobial therapy are the most important determinants of relapse, followed by the presence of a positive blood culture and multifocal distribution.[23]

References available online at expertconsult.com.

KEY REFERENCES

Cheng A.C., Currie B.J.: Melioidosis: epidemiology, pathophysiology, and management. *Clin Microbiol Rev* 2005; 18(2):383-416.

Chetchotisakd P., Chierakul W., Chaowagul W., et al.: Trimethoprim–sulfamethoxazole versus trimethoprim–sulfamethoxazole plus doxycycline as oral eradicative treatment for melioidosis (MERTH): a multicentre, double-blind, non-inferiority, randomised controlled trial. *Lancet* 2014; 383:807-814.

Currie B.J., Ward L., Cheng A.C.: The epidemiology and clinical spectrum of melioidosis: 540 cases from the 20 year Darwin prospective study. *PLoS Negl Trop Dis* 2010; 4(11):e900.

Limmathurotsakul D., Chaowagul W., Chierakul W., et al.: Risk factors for recurrent melioidosis in northeast Thailand. *Clin Infect Dis* 2006; 43(8):979-986.

Limmathurotsakul D., Kanoksil M., Wuthiekanun V., et al.: Activities of daily living associated with acquisition of melioidosis in northeast Thailand: a matched case–control study. *PLoS Negl Trop Dis* 2013; 7(2):e2072.

Limmathurotsakul D., Peacock S.J.: Melioidosis: a clinical overview. *Br Med Bull* 2011; 99:125-139.

Peacock S.J., Limmathurotsakul D., Lubell Y., et al.: Melioidosis vaccines: a systematic review and appraisal of the potential to exploit biodefense vaccines for public health purposes. *PLoS Negl Trop Dis* 2012; 6(1):e1488.

Peacock S.J., Schweizer H.P., Dance D.A., et al.: Management of accidental laboratory exposure to *Burkholderia pseudomallei* and *B. mallei*. *Emerg Infect Dis* 2008; 14(7):e2.

Wiersinga W.J., Currie B.J., Peacock S.J.: Melioidosis. *N Engl J Med* 2012; 367(11):1035-1044.

Wiersinga W.J., van der Poll T., White N.J., et al.: Melioidosis: insights into the pathogenicity of *Burkholderia pseudomallei*. *Nat Rev Microbiol* 2006; 4(4):272-282.

Wuthiekanun V., Peacock S.J.: Management of melioidosis. *Expert Rev Anti Infect Ther* 2006; 4(3):445-455.

126

Plague

KENNETH L. GAGE | C. BEN BEARD

Introduction

Plague is an acute, life-threatening zoonosis caused by the bacterium *Yersinia pestis*.[1-4] The disease is best known for three devastating pandemics, including the 14th-century outbreak known as the Black Death. Plague is primarily a disease of rodents, and humans typically acquire infection as a result of being bitten by rodent fleas, less commonly by handling infected animals, and rarely by inhaling infectious respiratory particles. Historically, urban, rat-borne outbreaks have been responsible for most epidemics. Over the past half century, however, most outbreaks have occurred in remote, rural populations.[5] The three principal clinical forms of plague are bubonic, septic (or septicemic) and pneumonic. The most common of these is bubonic plague, an acute illness characterized by fever and enlarged tender lymph nodes (buboes) that usually appear in the groin, axillary or cervical regions proximal to the site of inoculation. Bacteremia and sepsis occur when lymphatic defenses have been breached (septic plague) and plague pneumonia can arise from inhaling infectious respiratory droplets or secondarily as a result of blood-borne invasion of the lungs. Occasionally, pneumonic plague spreads from person to person, most often in crowded, substandard living conditions.[6]

Plague is often fatal when not diagnosed and treated appropriately early in the course of infection.[1,2,4,7,8] Certain aminoglycosides, tetracyclines, chloramphenicol and fluoroquinolones can be used to treat human plague.[1,3,7,8,9] Control during outbreaks relies on prompt identification and treatment of cases, isolation of pneumonic cases and identification of their contacts, and flea control.[1,3,6] Pneumonic patients should be isolated under respiratory droplet precautions until they are no longer infectious.[1,6] Persons who have been in close contact (<2 m) with pneumonic patients should receive antimicrobial prophylaxis. Others who have more distant contact should be monitored for fever. Human plague risks can be reduced by environmental sanitation measures intended to decrease rodent populations.[1] Plague is considered to be an important potential weapon of bioterrorism.[2,7]

Epidemiology

AGENT

Y. pestis is a gram-negative, microaerophilic coccobacillus belonging to the Enterobacteriaceae.[10] Molecular studies indicate this bacterium has recently evolved from the enteric pathogen, *Y. pseudotuberculosis*.[11] *Y. pestis* is nonmotile, nonsporulating, does not ferment lactose and exhibits bipolar staining with Wayson, Wright or Giemsa stain. Growth occurs in a variety of media at a wide range of temperatures (4–40 °C; optimal 28–30 °C) and pH values (5.0–9.6; optimal 7.2–7.6).[10]

The plague bacterium produces many factors that enable it to survive in and cause disease within its mammalian hosts (virulence factors) and be transmitted by flea vectors (transmission factors) (Table 126-1).[3,10,12] Some factors are expressed selectively at temperatures and environments encountered in fleas or mammals. In mammals, plasminogen activator (Pla) degrades fibrin in blood clots and reduces inflammatory infiltrates, thereby helping *Y. pestis* escape from the site of inoculation.[13,14] *Yersinia* outer protein (Yop)M, which is resistant to Pla activity, competes for thrombin and inhibits activation of platelets, further promoting dissemination of *Y. pestis* within the host. Temperature-dependent modification of *Y. pestis* lipopolysaccharides (LPS) also appears to enhance Pla activity. Poor recognition by Toll-like receptor 4 of the tetra-acylated form of LPS produced at mammalian body temperatures further reduces early inflammatory responses. *Y. pestis* also can behave as a facultative intracellular pathogen, invading and multiplying within host macrophages.[15] Survival within host cells is made possible by a type III secretion system composed of various Yops that interfere with the production of proinflammatory cytokines, impair the cytoskeletal dynamics of phagocytes, inhibit the phagocyte's oxidative burst, and cause immune cell death by apoptosis. At mammalian host temperatures *Y. pestis* produces a capsular antigen (*caf1* or F1 antigen) that renders it resistant to phagocytosis and, along with the effects of various Yops, allows it to multiply extracellularly. A fimbrial structure (pH 6 antigen) provides additional resistance to phagocytosis, perhaps by mediating translocation of Yops into host cells. Another *Y. pestis* adhesin, Ail, also could aid in Yop translocation into phagocytes.[16] Various iron uptake systems, including one that utilizes the siderophore yersiniabactin, enable the plague bacterium to compete with its hosts for this essential nutrient.[10]

Recent molecular phylogeny studies suggest that *Y. pestis* evolved in China with later dissemination to western and central Asia and Africa as a result of natural spread among rodents and transport by human commerce.[11] Widespread dissemination of 1.ORI branch strains of *Y. pestis* occurred during the last pandemic, which began in China in the late 1800s.[11]

LIFE CYCLE

Y. pestis is maintained by flea-borne transmission between susceptible rodents and survival of infectious fleas in burrows or other suitable off-host environments (Figure 126-1).[1,4,12] Others have proposed that

TABLE 126-1 Proposed Virulence and Transmission Factors for *Yersinia pestis*

Genomic Element	Virulence or Transmission Factor	Proposed Role in Virulence or Transmission
9.5 kb plasmid (pesticin plasmid or pPCP; a 19 kb dimer of this plasmid also exists)	Pesticin sensitivity (Pst)	Loss of sensitivity to pesticin (a bacteriocin) is associated with reduced siderophore binding capability (affects iron uptake)
	Plasminogen activator (Pla)	Fibrinolytic activity (important for dissemination from the site of inoculation)
70–75 kb plasmid (low calcium response plasmid or pCD)	*Yersinia* outer proteins (Yops – encoded by genes found in the Yop virulon, a type III secretion system; includes LcrV or V antigen and other Yops)	Proposed functions vary among Yops and include: translocation of other Yops (effectors) across cell membranes; disruption of phagocyte cytoskeleton dynamics and interference with phagocytosis; immunosuppressive effects, including blocking production of proinflammatory cytokines, interfering with activation of B and T cells, promoting production of IL-10; inhibition of the oxidative burst; binding thrombin (interferes with thrombin–platelet aggregation); global depletion of natural killer (NK) cells and induction of apoptosis in macrophages
100–110 kb plasmid	Murine toxin (Ymt)	Required for survival in fleas; also has β-adrenergic antagonist activity in rats and mice but not guinea-pigs, rabbits, dogs or nonhuman primates
	F1 'capsular' antigen (Caf1)	Gelatinous capsular or envelope material associated with resistance to phagocytosis by monocytes
Chromosomal	Pigmentation (*pgm*) locus, includes genes of *hms* locus and the high pathogenicity island, including the *ybt* operon	Pigment-positive strains (Pgm+) bind hemin and appear pigmented on culture media containing Congo Red; *pgm* locus contains genes of the high pathogenicity island (HPI), which is found in other yersiniae and certain related enteric bacteria; the HPI contains the *ybt* (yersiniabactin) operon, which encodes genes of a siderophore-based iron uptake system; the *pgm* locus also contains the *hms* locus, which produces biofilm and must be functional for 'blocking' to occur in the flea vector (blocking increases efficiency of *Y. pestis* transmission by fleas)
	Endotoxin (lipopolysaccharide)	Lipopolysaccharide release associated with major pathogenic effects of plague sepsis, systemic inflammatory response syndrome and associated adult respiratory distress syndrome, cytokine activation, complement cascade, disseminated intravascular coagulation, bleeding, unresponsive shock and organ failure
	Serum resistance (lipopolysaccharide in part)	Resistance to complement-mediated lysis; proposed to be related in part to lipopolysaccharide structure
	pH 6 antigen (*psa*)	Fimbrial structure expressed best at pH 5.0–6.7; proposed to mediate attachment to host cells or promote suppression of phagocytosis by aiding entry of Yops into phagocytic cells

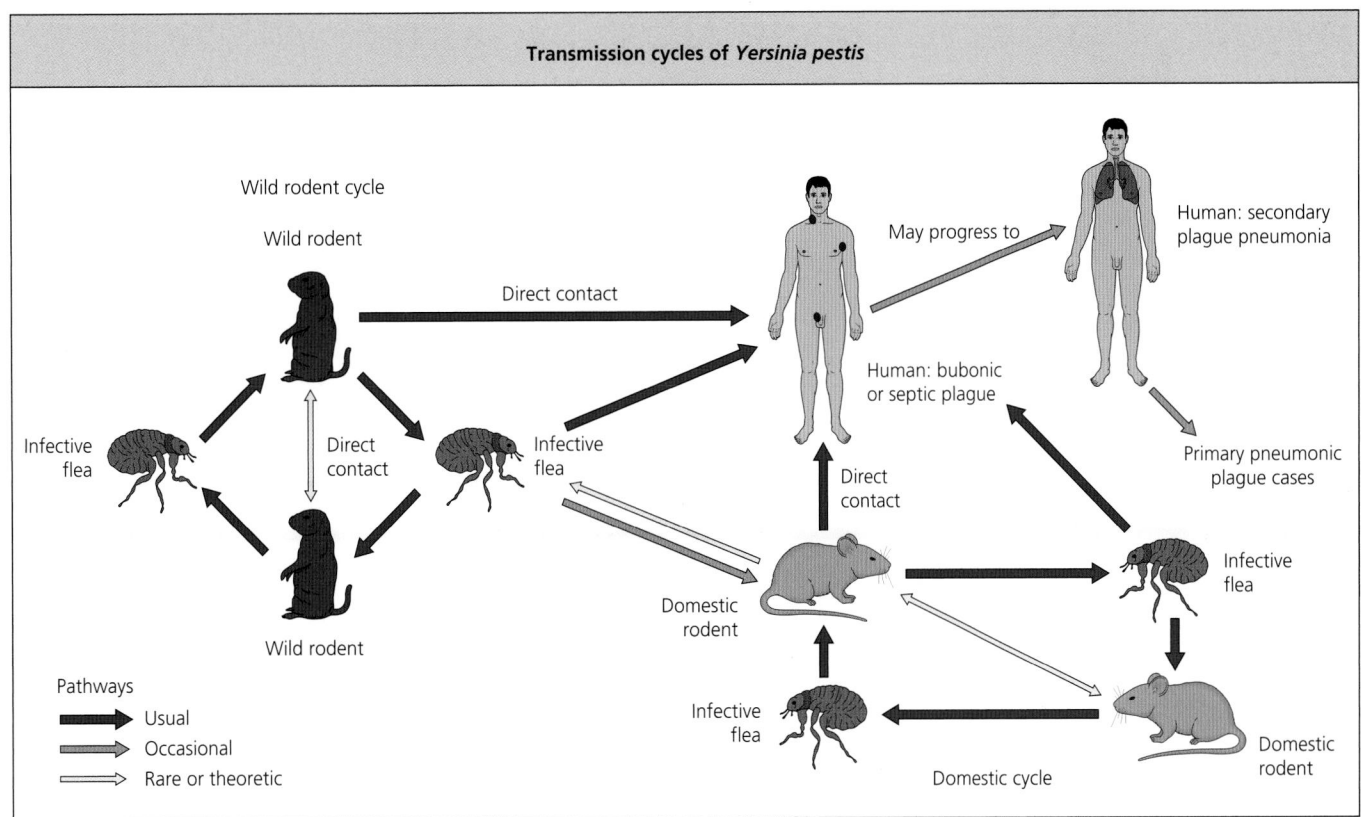

Figure 126-1 Transmission cycles of *Yersinia pestis*.

Y. pestis can survive for long periods in soils or in chronically infected rodents,[12] but evidence that either is important under natural conditions is limited. Humans and other incidental hosts of *Y. pestis* are not directly involved in plague maintenance.

Although most foci are maintained by transmission between wild rodents and their fleas, commensal rats (*Rattus rattus, R. norvegicus*, etc.) and rat fleas, especially *Xenopsylla cheopis*, are the principal sources of large epidemics. In a few areas, such as Madagascar, rats also act as the primary rodent reservoirs of *Y. pestis*.[4] Susceptible rodents play a critical role in plague cycles by serving as sources of infection for feeding fleas.[12] Although virtually any rodent can be infected with *Y. pestis*, not all succumb to plague, and the susceptibility of rodent populations and species can vary greatly. Only those fleas that feed on dying rodents with very high ($>10^6$ *Y. pestis*/mL blood) bacteremias are likely to become infected. Besides enabling infection of blood-feeding fleas by *Y. pestis*, fatal bacteremias in rodents force infected fleas to abandon their dead hosts and seek new ones, thus promoting spread of the disease.

GEOGRAPHIC DISTRIBUTION

Plague is widely distributed throughout the world, with human cases being reported from 10 or so countries each year.[5] Countries reporting significant plague outbreaks during the interval from 2000 to 2009 are shown in Figure 126-2.

POPULATIONS AFFECTED

Plague mostly affects impoverished populations of low- and middle-income countries (LMIC) living in rural villages that are heavily infested with commensal rats and their fleas. Urban rat-borne plague is now unusual, but still occasionally occurs in LMIC.[1,2,4,5] In the USA, most persons are exposed to infection around rural residences that provide shelter and food for rodents.[1] Cases also occasionally occur among campers, hikers, hunters, pet owners, veterinary staff, wildlife biologists or others exposed to plague in natural settings or through handling infected animals.[1,4,12]

In the absence of control measures, plague can spread from rural areas to population centers, either through unintended transport of infected animals, or by passage of infection between adjoining rodent populations.[1,2,4] Occasionally, persons who travel during the incubation phase later develop plague pneumonia and transmit the disease to others. Plague risks for persons visiting endemic areas for business or tourism are extremely low because these persons typically stay in relatively modern hotels and spend little time in the rural villages most likely to be affected by the disease.

DISEASE INCIDENCE

Virtually all plague cases reported to the World Health Organization (WHO) in recent decades have come from Africa, Asia and the Americas. Over the last 20–30 years there has been a striking shift in distribution of cases from Asia to the African region.[1,4,5,12] Based on the latest WHO statistics, 25 countries reported a total of 53 398 cases (mean of 2322 cases per year) and 4058 deaths (7.6% fatality rate) from 1987 to 2009.[5] During this 23-year period, countries in Africa, including Madagascar, accounted for approximately 85% of cases reported from 1987 to 2009, with the remaining cases occurring in Asia (11%) and the Americas (4%). Most African cases occurred in Madagascar (31.3%), Democratic Republic of Congo (25%) and Tanzania (12%). This trend continued from 2004 to 2009, as the African region accounted for 97.6% of the world's cases and 96.6% of all plague deaths over this interval.[5] At present, plague occurs only sporadically in Asia and the Americas, although large outbreaks remain a possibility.

Although large outbreaks have not been reported in the USA since the disease was first introduced in the early 1900s, plague remains a threat in this country[1] with nearly 500 cases of human plague reported to the CDC since 1950 (CDC unpublished data). The most recent outbreak occurred in 2006 when 17 cases were reported from seven states.[17] Although plague remains enzootic and occasionally causes epizootics in rural areas within the 17 westernmost states, about 90% of all human cases reported in the past three decades have occurred in New Mexico, Colorado, Arizona and California.

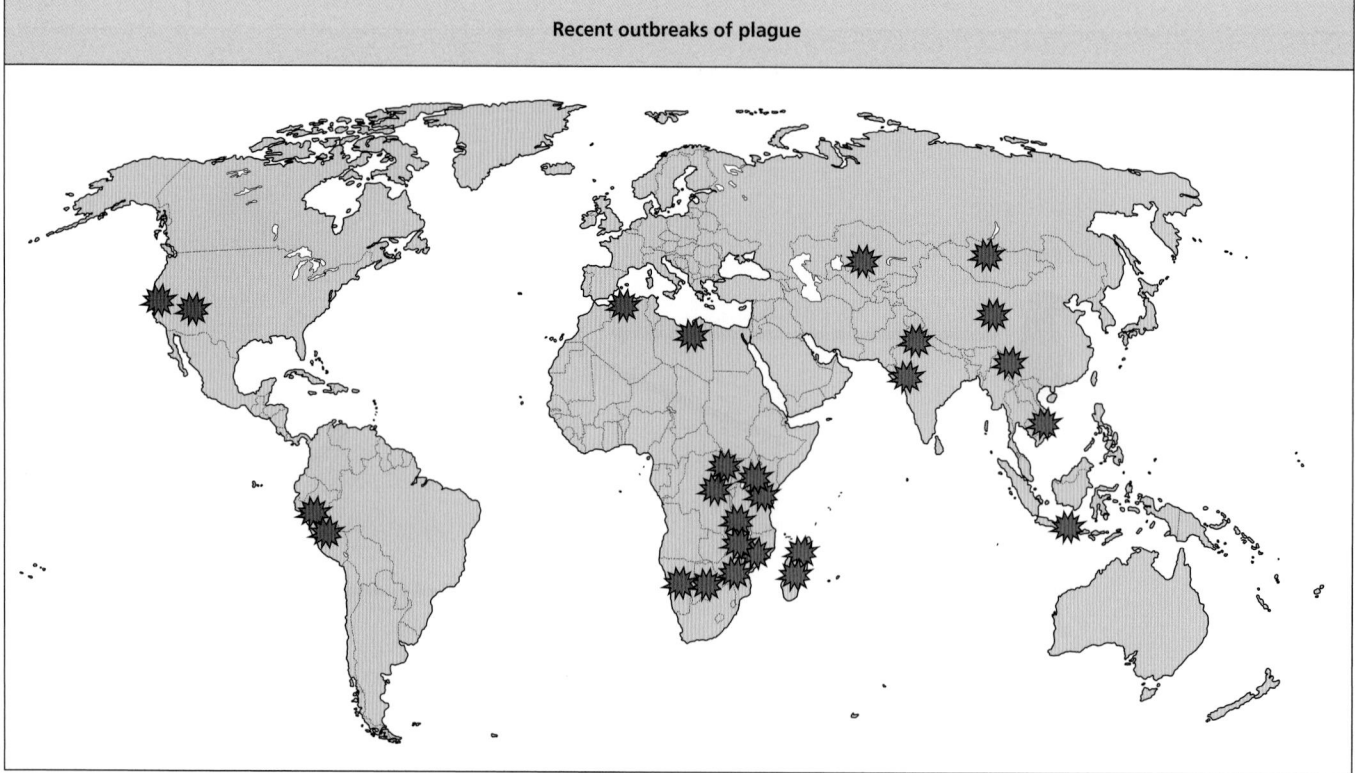

Recent outbreaks of plague

Figure 126-2   Recent outbreaks of plague. *(Compiled from sources of the World Health Organization, the Centers for Disease Control and Prevention, and the individual countries.)*

SOURCES OF INFECTION AND RISKS FOR HUMANS

Flea bites are the most common source of human *Y. pestis* infection.[1] Plague also can be acquired through handling infected animals, as occurs among marmot hunters in central Asia, and others in the USA who handle infected carcasses of prairie dogs, ground squirrels, rabbits or wild carnivores.[1,2,4,5] Guinea-pigs in plague-endemic Andean countries can acquire *Y. pestis* infections from other rodents and serve as sources of exposure for persons who skin these animals for food. Pet owners and veterinary staff may become infected with *Y. pestis* while caring for infected domestic cats.[18] Outbreaks of plague have occurred in Saudi Arabia, Libya, Jordan, Kazakhstan and Afghanistan as a result of persons handling or consuming infected camel or goat meat.[4]

Human risks of exposure are typically greatest during epizootics when *Y. pestis* spreads rapidly through rodent populations, causing high host mortality and abandonment of dead hosts by fleas. Even in the presence of efficient flea vectors, epizootics probably occur only when favorable environmental conditions cause rodent host densities to exceed certain threshold levels, resulting in increased levels of host-to-host contact and transfer of infectious fleas between hosts.

Primary pneumonic plague occurs when persons inhale infectious respiratory secretions.[1,6] This usually occurs when persons with bubonic plague develop secondary pulmonary infection and then spread the disease to others through infectious respiratory droplets, starting a chain of airborne transmission. Persons living in the same home as a pneumonic plague patient or attending the sick are especially at risk. Unfortunately, plague can be spread intentionally as an aerosol, an event that could cause severe outbreaks with many fatalities (see also Chapter 75). For these reasons *Y. pestis* is classified as a Tier 1 category A agent (highest bioterrorism risk), along with the agents of anthrax, smallpox, tularemia and viral hemorrhagic fevers.[9] *Y. pestis* strains could also be genetically modified to confer resistance to antibiotics used to treat plague.

Primary pneumonic plague comprises only a small fraction of the total number of cases in any plague-endemic region. In the USA such cases represent only about 2% of total cases, nearly all of which were associated with handling cats that had plague pneumonia and cough.[18] Human-to-human spread of plague through respiratory contact has not been documented in the USA since 1924,[6] but the likelihood of pneumonic plague outbreaks remains high in many low- and middle-income countries.

SEASONALITY

Flea-borne cases of human plague in the northern hemisphere are most likely to occur in the warmer months when epizootic transmission peaks.[1,12] In tropical and semitropical plague foci, transmission may vary between a wet, relatively cool season and another season of hotter, drier weather, with fewer cases occurring during the latter period. Occasional winter cases occur in temperate regions among hunters, trappers, pet owners or veterinary staff handling infected animals.

Pathogenesis and Pathology

Y. pestis is among the most pathogenic bacteria known, using numerous chromosomal and plasmid-encoded gene products to promote its establishment and spread within the host (see Table 126-1).[1,2,3,10,13,14,15,16]

Y. pestis organisms inoculated through the skin or mucous membranes travel to and multiply within regional lymph nodes.[1,2] In the early stages of infection, nodes are edematous and congested with minimal inflammatory infiltrates and vascular injury. Fully developed buboes are surrounded by serous fluid, contain large numbers of plague bacteria and exhibit considerable vascular damage, hemorrhagic necrosis and neutrophil infiltrates. In later stages, abscess formation and spontaneous rupture of nodes may infrequently occur.

Plague sepsis in the absence of signs of localized infection, particularly a bubo, is termed primary septic plague and can result from direct entry of *Y. pestis* through broken skin, mucous membranes or the bite of an infectious flea.[1] Septic plague can also occur secondarily to bubonic or pneumonic plague when lymphatic or pulmonary defenses are breached and *Y. pestis* enters the bloodstream and multiplies en masse, causing the systemic inflammatory response associated with gram-negative sepsis and frequently including shock, adult respiratory distress syndrome (ARDS) and disseminated intravascular coagulation (DIC). Bacteremia commonly occurs in all forms of plague, while sepsis occurs less commonly and can be immediately life-threatening.

Y. pestis can cause serious disease in almost any organ. Fatal cases commonly experience diffuse interstitial myocarditis with cardiac dilation, multifocal necrosis of the liver, diffuse hemorrhagic splenic necrosis and fibrin thrombi in renal glomeruli.[1] DIC can occur, resulting in thrombosis within the microvasculature, necrosis and bleeding, and widespread cutaneous, mucosal and serosal petechiae and ecchymoses, as well as occasional gangrene of acral parts, such as the fingers and toes (see Figure 126-4).

Primary plague pneumonia[1,6] often begins as a lobular process and then extends by confluence, becoming lobar and then multilobar. Typically, plague organisms are numerous in alveoli and pulmonary secretions. Secondary plague pneumonia arising from hematogenous spread of *Y. pestis* typically begins as a diffuse interstitial process, with plague bacilli appearing most numerous in interstitial spaces. Pathologic findings in untreated cases of plague pneumonia usually include edema, diffuse pulmonary congestion, hemorrhagic necrosis and scant infiltration by neutrophils.[1]

Prevention and Control

Rapid identification and treatment of cases is of utmost importance to limit fatalities and prevent human-to-human spread of plague.[1,2,6] In endemic regions, human and animal-based surveillance should be done to identify areas at risk. Epidemiologic investigations of human cases and threatening epizootics must also be conducted to effectively target control actions. Rapid implementation of flea control to reduce risk is also critical. Other environmental measures include reducing sources of food and shelter for rodents. Rodenticides should be used only after flea control has been completed to reduce the chances that infected fleas will leave dying hosts and feed on humans.[5]

Health providers also need appropriate education and consultation on how to help others protect themselves. Personal protective measures should be encouraged along with avoidance of sick or dead animals, use of effective insect repellents, flea control for pets, use of rubber gloves by hunters, and provision of prompt veterinary care for cats that might be ill with plague. Prophylactic antimicrobial therapy is recommended for persons who have close exposure to pneumonic plague patients, have handled *Y. pestis*-infected animals, or been bitten by rodent fleas in areas with recent epizootic activity. Recommended prophylactic antimicrobials include doxycycline, ciprofloxacin and levofloxacin. A plague vaccine is no longer available commercially, although clinical trials of recombinant vaccines containing F1 (*caf1*) and V antigens of *Y. pestis* (see Table 126-1) have been initiated.[3]

Clinical Features

BUBONIC PLAGUE

The incubation period of bubonic plague is usually 2–6 days but occasionally longer. Typically, patients experience acute onset of fever, chills, myalgias, arthralgias, headache and lethargy.[1,2] Tenderness and pain often occur within 24 hours in a lymph node(s) proximal to the initial site of inoculation. The femoral and inguinal nodes are most commonly affected, axillary and cervical nodes less so, depending on the site of inoculation and geographic location of the cases. Cervical lymph node involvement is more commonly observed in countries where individuals sleep on hut floors, presumably because of greater risk of being bitten in the neck region by floor-dwelling fleas. Buboes become progressively swollen, painful and tender, sometimes exquisitely so. Typically, the patient avoids movement, stretching and

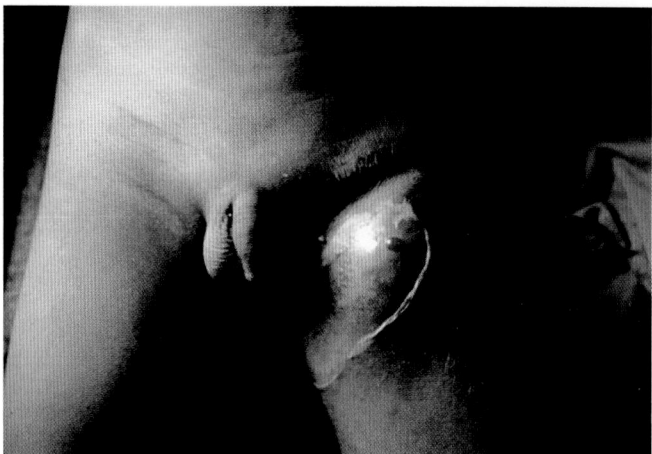

Figure 126-3 Left inguinal and femoral buboes, demonstrating surrounding edema and overlying desquamation.

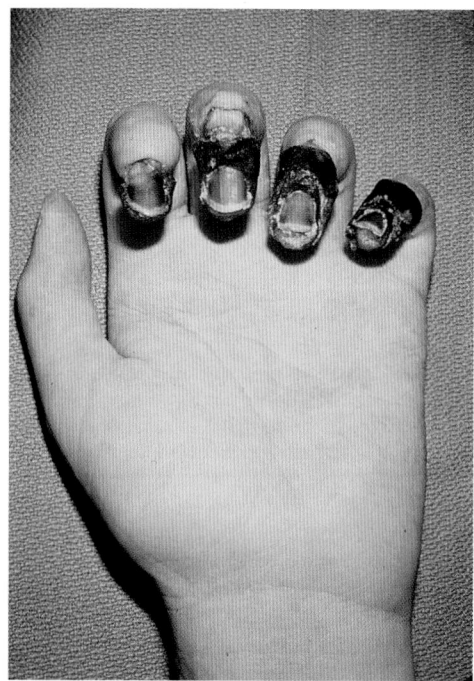

Figure 126-4 Septic plague patient who demonstrated disseminated intravascular coagulation, bleeding into the skin and acral gangrene as a late manifestation.

pressure near the bubo and guards against palpation. Tissues surrounding the bubo often become edematous and overlying skin may be reddened (Figure 126-3). Rarely, inspection of the skin around the bubo or distal to it may reveal a flea bite marked by a small scab, papule, pustule or ulcer. Larger furuncular lesions, sometimes with tularemia-like eschars, also occur rarely. Plague buboes differ from lymphadenitis of most other causes by their rapid onset, extreme tenderness, surrounding edema, accompanying signs of toxemia and absence of cellulitis or readily apparent ascending lymphangitis.

When treated soon after illness onset with an appropriate antimicrobial agent, bubonic patients usually experience defervescence and improvement of other systemic manifestations over a 2- to 3-day period.[1] Buboes frequently remain enlarged and tender for a week or more after initiation of treatment and rarely become fluctuant. Without antimicrobial treatment, bubonic patients typically exhibit an increasingly toxic state of fever, tachycardia, lethargy followed by prostration, agitation, confusion and, in severe cases, convulsions and delirium. Differential diagnostic options include staphylococcal or streptococcal adenitis, tularemia, cat-scratch disease, mycobacterial infection, acute filarial lymphadenitis, chancroid and strangulated inguinal hernia.

SEPTIC PLAGUE

Septic (septicemic) plague presents as a rapidly progressive, overwhelming endotoxemia that is usually fatal unless treated promptly.[1] Primary sepsis occurs in the absence of regional lymphadenitis, and a diagnosis of plague is likely to go unsuspected until results are available from blood cultures. Primary septic plague patients often present with gastrointestinal symptoms, including nausea, vomiting, diarrhea and abdominal pain, further complicating diagnosis. Petechiae, ecchymoses, bleeding from wounds or orifices, and ischemia of acral parts are manifestations of DIC (Figure 126-4). Pre-terminal signs can include refractory hypotension, renal shutdown, obtundation and other signs of shock. ARDS associated with septic plague may be confused with other conditions, including hantavirus pulmonary syndrome.

Differential diagnostic possibilities include sepsis caused by other bacterial infections, such as the agents of meningococcemia, bacterial endocarditis, tularemia or other gram-negative bacterial infections.

PNEUMONIC PLAGUE

Pneumonic plague is the most rapidly developing and life-threatening form of plague.[1,6] The incubation period for primary pneumonic plague is usually 2–5 days (range 1–6 days). Illness onset is most often sudden, with chills, fever, body pains, headache, weakness, dizziness and chest discomfort. Cough, sputum production, increasing chest pain, tachypnea and dyspnea typically predominate on the second day of illness; hemoptysis, increasing respiratory distress, cardiopulmo-

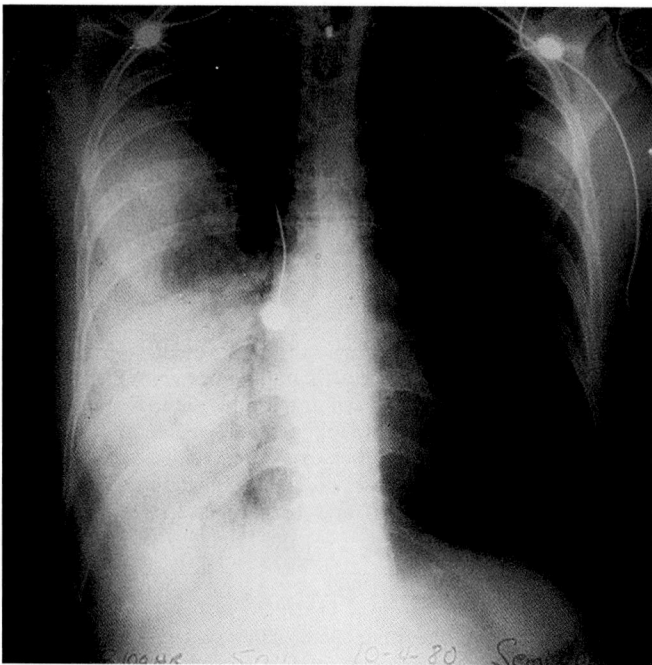

Figure 126-5 Chest radiograph of a patient who has primary plague pneumonia, showing extensive infiltrates in the right middle and lower lung fields.

nary insufficiency and circulatory collapse can also occur. The sputum of primary plague pneumonia patients is typically watery or mucoid, frothy and blood tinged, and can be bloody. Initially, chest signs may indicate localized pulmonary involvement and a rapidly developing segmental consolidation can appear before bronchopneumonia occurs elsewhere in both lungs (Figure 126-5). Liquefaction necrosis and cavitation can develop at sites of consolidation and result in residual scarring.

Secondary pneumonic plague resulting from metastatic spread typically manifests as a diffuse interstitial pneumonitis with sputum production that is scant and more likely to appear tenacious and inspissated than the sputum of primary pneumonic plague patients.

Differential diagnostic possibilities include other bacterial conditions such as tularemia, mycoplasma pneumonia or other community-acquired bacterial pneumonias, Legionnaires' disease, Q fever and staphylococcal or streptococcal pneumonia. Viral pneumonias requiring differentiation include influenzal pneumonitis, hantaviral pulmonary syndrome and those caused by respiratory syncitial virus or cytomegalovirus infection.

OTHER MANIFESTATIONS

Plague meningitis is unusual and typically arises as a complication among the treated survivors of bubonic plague.[1] Plague occasionally presents as pharyngitis accompanied by fever, sore throat and cervical lymphadenitis, and can be confused with other more common causes of pharyngitis. Primary plague pharyngitis can result from respiratory exposures or ingestion of infected undercooked meat and is usually associated with marked cervical glandular enlargement. Oculoglandular plague can arise from inoculation of Y. pestis through the conjunctiva.

Diagnosis

Except in outbreak situations, making a timely diagnosis of plague requires a high index of clinical suspicion, careful case history and physical examination. Treatment delays or misdiagnoses increase the likelihood of fatalities,[1,2,7] and infected travelers who seek medical care after returning from endemic areas are especially at risk. Laboratory tests for plague are highly reliable when conducted by experienced persons.

When plague is suspected, clinical specimens should be obtained promptly for microbiologic assays, chest radiographs taken and specific antimicrobial therapy initiated. Blood, bubo aspirates, sputum, tracheal washes, swabs of skin lesions or pharyngeal mucosa, and cerebrospinal fluid should be collected when appropriate and inoculated onto suitable media (e.g. brain–heart infusion broth, sheep blood agar, chocolate agar or MacConkey agar).[19] Bubo aspirates typically yield only small amounts of fluid and 1–2 mL of saline may need to be injected first to obtain adequate material. Smears of each specimen should be stained with Gram, Wayson or Giemsa stain. An acute-phase serum specimen should be collected for Y. pestis antibody testing, followed 3–4 weeks later by a convalescent-phase specimen. For fatal cases, samples from buboes, liver, spleen, lungs and bone marrow should be collected at autopsy for culture, fluorescent antibody,

immunohistochemical staining and histologic studies. Infected tissues can be transported in Cary-Blair medium. Presumptive identification of Y. pestis can be made by direct immunofluorescence assay, polymerase chain reaction or antigen capture enzyme-linked immunosorbent assay. A rapid immunogold dipstick assay that detects Y. pestis antigens in patient samples also appears promising and could be used in remote village clinics.[2]

Plague can be laboratory confirmed by isolation of Y. pestis from body fluids or tissues.[19] Plague bacteria are readily distinguished from other gram-negative bacteria by polychromatic and immunofluorescence staining properties, growth characteristics, biochemical profiles and lysis by Y. pestis-specific bacteriophage. Susceptible laboratory mice can be inoculated subcutaneously to make isolations from contaminated materials. Alternatively, confirmation can be provided by demonstration of a fourfold change in serum antibodies to Y. pestis.[19] Less than 5% of patients fail to seroconvert and some will develop detectable antibodies within 5 days of illness onset, although most seroconvert 1–2 weeks later and a few require more than 3 weeks to seroconvert. Early antibiotic therapy may delay seroconversion by several weeks. Positive serologic titers decrease gradually over time but can be present for months to years. Passive hemagglutination assay (PHA) is used for serodiagnosis; however, enzyme-linked immunosorbent assays that detect IgM and IgG antibodies to Y. pestis can identify antibodies characteristic of early infection and differentiate these from antibodies resulting from previous vaccination.

White blood cell counts for patients typically range from 10 to 25 x10^9/L and contain predominately early-stage polymorphonuclear leukocytes.[1] In some instances leukemoid reactions occur, with white cell counts in excess of 50 x10^9/L.

Management

Untreated, plague is fatal in over 50% of patients who have bubonic plague and in nearly all patients who have septic or pneumonic plague. Mortality rates in the USA were reportedly 14%, 22% and 57% for cases of bubonic, septic and pneumonic plague, respectively.[7] Fatalities are almost always due to delays in seeking treatment or misdiagnosis (Table 126-2).[1,7]

Streptomycin was considered the drug of choice for treating plague, but at present another aminoglycoside (gentamicin) is more commonly used because of its availability, ease of administration and efficacy as demonstrated by a treatment trial in Tanzania and a separate retrospective population-based study of 75 human plague cases in New Mexico.[1,7,8] Tetracyclines or chloramphenicol are also considered effective, and chloramphenicol is indicated for conditions that require high tissue penetration, such as plague meningitis, pleuritis,

TABLE 126-2	Treatment Guidelines for Plague		
Drug	**Patient**	**Dosage**	**Route of Administration**
Streptomycin	Adults	1 g q12h	im
	Children	15 mg/kg q12h*	im
Gentamicin	Adults	1–1.5 mg/kg q8h[†]	im or iv
	Children	2.0–2.5 mg/kg q8h	im or iv
	Infants/neonates	2.5 mg/kg BID	iv
Tetracycline	Adults	0.5 g q6h	po
	Children >8 years old	6.25–12.5 mg/kg q6h	po
Doxycycline	Adults	100 mg q12h	po or iv
	Children >8 years old and >45 kg	100 mg q12h	po or iv
	Children <8 years old and <45 kg	2.2 mg/kg q12h	po or iv
Chloramphenicol	Adults	12.5 mg/kg q6h[‡]	po or iv
	Children >1 year old	12.5 mg/kg q6h[‡]	po or iv

im, intramuscular; iv, intravascular; po, per os.
*Not to exceed 2 g/day.
[†]Daily dose should be reduced to 3 mg/kg as soon as clinically indicated.
[‡]Up to 100 mg/kg per day initially. Dosage should be adjusted to maintain plasma concentrations at 5–20 mg/ml. Hematologic values should be monitored closely.
See www.cdc.gov/plague/healthcare/clinicians.html.

endophthalmitis or myocarditis. The efficacy of doxycycline was demonstrated in the same Tanzanian treatment trial and retrospective New Mexico studies mentioned above. Trimethoprim–sulfamethoxazole (co-trimoxazole) has been used successfully to treat bubonic plague, but it is considered a secondary choice. Although fluoroquinolones have yet to be directly evaluated for treating human plague, animal experiments suggest these agents would be effective[9] and the FDA recently used its Animal Efficacy Rule to approve levofloxacin, ciprofloxacin and moxifloxacin for human plague treatment. Penicillins, macrolides and cephalosporins have a suboptimal effect and should not be used to treat plague. In general, antimicrobial treatment should be continued for either 7–10 days or for at least 3 days after the patient has become afebrile. Improvement is usually evident 2–3 days from the start of treatment, although fever may persist for several more days.

Complications of delayed treatment include DIC, ARDS and other consequences of bacterial sepsis; such patients require intensive monitoring and close physiologic support. Buboes may require surgical drainage and abscessed nodes can be a cause of recurrent fever. Viable *Y. pestis* have been isolated from buboes 1–2 weeks after clinical recovery. Although isolated reports exist of *Y. pestis* strains resistant to streptomycin or tetracycline, the few antibiotic-resistant *Y. pestis* strains isolated from humans have not been associated with treatment failure and typically have exhibited only partial resistance to a single agent. However, a multidrug-resistant strain of *Y. pestis* isolated from a plague patient in Madagascar appeared to be highly resistant to the antibiotics typically recommended for treatment (tetracycline, streptomycin and chloramphenicol).[2,20] Resistance was plasmid-mediated and could be transferred to other strains of *Y. pestis* and to *Escherichia coli*. Surveillance for multidrug-resistant *Y. pestis* in Madagascar and elsewhere has not provided evidence for the spread of similar strains. Postexposure treatment for 7 days with a tetracycline, chloramphenicol or trimethoprim–sulfamethoxazole is recommended for persons who have had close contact with pneumonic plague patients in the previous 7 days.[9]

In addition to fever watch, antimicrobial prophylaxis is sometimes recommended for persons who have handled an infected animal or for household members of bubonic plague patients because of likely flea exposures.[1,7] Antimicrobial prophylaxis also might be recommended following a bioterrorism attack.[9] Isolation and respiratory droplet precautions are recommended for patients with pneumonic plague, including the use of masks for persons caring for these patients while they are infectious. The use of masks may interrupt person-to-person transmission during pneumonic plague outbreaks. Pneumonic plague patients are considered to be noncontagious following 48 hours of antibiotic treatment.

References available online at expertconsult.com.

KEY REFERENCES

Boulanger L.L., Ettestad P., Fogarty J.D., et al.: Gentamicin and tetracyclines for the treatment of human plague: review of 75 cases in New Mexico, 1985–1999. *Clin Infect Dis* 2004; 38:663-669.

Butler T.: Plague into the 21st century. *Clin Infect Dis* 2009; 49:736-742.

Butler T.: Plague gives surprises in the first decade of the 21st century in the United States and worldwide. *Am J Trop Med Hyg* 2013; 89:788-793.

Chu M.C.: *Laboratory manual of plague diagnostic tests.* Atlanta, GA: Centers for Disease Control and Prevention/ Geneva: World Health Organization; 2000:1-129.

Dennis D., Meier F.: Plague. In: Horsburgh C.R., Nelson A.M., eds. *Pathology of emerging infections.* Washington, DC: ASM Press; 1997:21-47.

Eisen R.J., Gage K.L.: Transmission of flea-borne zoonotic agents. *Annu Rev Entomol* 2012; 57:61-82.

Gage K.L., Dennis D.T., Orloski K.A., et al.: Cases of cat-associated plague in the western US, 1977–1998. *Clin Infect Dis* 2000; 30:893-900.

Inglesby T.V., Dennis D.T., Henderson D.A. for the Working Group on Civilian Biodefense, et al.: Plague as a biological weapon: medical and public health management. *JAMA* 2000; 283:2281-2290.

Kool J.L.: Risk of person-to-person transmission of pneumonic plague. *Clin Infect Dis* 2005; 40:1166-1172.

MMWR: Summary of notifiable diseases – United States, 2006. *Morb Mortal Wkly Rep* 2008; 55(53):1-92.

Morelli G., Song Y., Mazzoni C.J., et al.: *Yersinia pestis* genome sequencing identifies patterns of global phylogenetic diversity. *Nat Genet* 2010; 42:1140-1143.

Mwenge W., Butler T., Mgema S., et al.: Treatment of plague with gentamicin or doxycycline in a randomized clinical trial in Tanzania. *Clin Infect Dis* 2006; 42:614-621.

Perry R.D., Fetherston J.D.: *Yersinia pestis* – etiologic agent of plague. *Clin Microbiol Rev* 1997; 10:35-66.

Willamson E.D., Oyston P.C.: The natural history and incidence of *Yersinia pestis* and prospects for vaccination. *J Med Microbiol* 2012; 61(Pt 7):911-918.

World Health Organization: Human plague: review of regional morbidity and mortality, 2004–2009. *Weekly Epidemiol Record* 2010; 85:40-45.

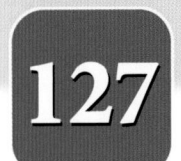

SECTION 6 International Medicine: Major Tropical Syndromes: Systemic Infections

127

Tularemia

JEANNINE M. PETERSEN | DAVID T. DENNIS | C. BEN BEARD

KEY CONCEPTS

- Tularemia is a potentially severe bacterial zoonosis caused by *Francisella tularensis*.

- In nature, the bacterium is associated with wild mammalian hosts and arthropod vectors.

- Transmission of *F. tularensis* to humans occurs by several modes, including bites by infective arthropods, direct inoculation of *F. tularensis* through skin or mucous membranes from handling infectious animal tissues, ingestion of contaminated water or food, or by inhalation of contaminated aerosols or dusts.

- The agent of tularemia is widely distributed throughout the northern hemisphere.

- Human infection results in differing clinical presentations of varying severity depending on the route of inoculation and the dose and virulence of the infecting strain. The most common clinical manifestations are fever, an ulcer at a cutaneous site of inoculation, and afferent lymphadenitis (ulceroglandular tularemia).

- Tularemia can be treated with aminoglycosides, tetracyclines, chloramphenicol and fluoroquinolones.

- Tularemia is considered to be an important potential weapon of bioterrorism.

Epidemiology

AGENT

Francisella tularensis is a small, facultatively intracellular, gram-negative coccobacillus. Within the species *F. tularensis*, there are three subspecies: *F. t. tularensis* (type A), *F. t. holarctica* (type B) and *F. t. mediasiatica*. Whereas type A strains occur only in North America, type B strains are distributed more broadly throughout the northern hemisphere, including North America.[1] Subspecies *mediasiatica* is limited in its distribution to central Asia.

Francisella tularensis is considered to be a potential agent of bioterrorism because its intentional misuse could result in large numbers of casualties and because it requires special actions for medical and public health preparedness.[2] The bacterium was previously weaponized for aerosol delivery by biowarfare programs during and after the Second World War, and it is assumed that this would be the most likely mode of delivery in a potential terrorism attack.

LIFE CYCLE

Francisella tularensis is widespread in nature and has been recovered from more than 100 species of wild mammals, at least nine species of domestic animals (including cats and dogs), birds, some amphibians and fish, and more than 50 species of arthropods.[3] The bacterium is most often associated with wild mammalian hosts, such as lagomorphs (wild hares and rabbits), terrestrial rodents (especially voles and meadow mice) and aquatic rodents (water rats, muskrats, beaver). Transmission among animals is accomplished by the bites of blood-feeding arthropods or by direct exposure to contaminated materials in the environment (Figure 127-1).[3]

Humans are incidental hosts and become infected:
- when they are bitten by ticks or by blood-feeding flies or mosquitoes
- by handling or ingesting infectious animal tissues or fluids
- by ingestion of contaminated water or food
- by inhalation of infective aerosols or dusts.

Cases also occur following infective bites or scratches by cats[4] with contaminated mouths or claws.

Person-to-person transmission has not been documented.

GEOGRAPHIC DISTRIBUTION

Tularemia is endemic throughout much of the region between latitudes 30°N and 71°N. This includes all of North America from the Arctic Circle to northern Mexico, and much of Eurasia.[1] In North America, the highest incidence of tularemia in humans occurs in the south-central region of the USA (Figure 127-2),[5] but cases have been reported throughout the continental USA, across Canada and in

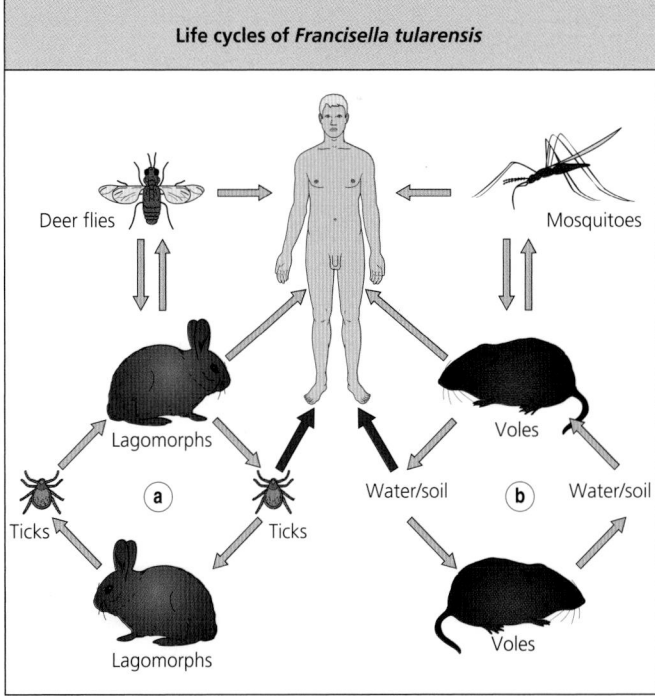

Figure 127-1 Life cycles of *Francisella tularensis*. The two major life cycles in nature are shown. In cycle (a), which is dominant in North America, *F. tularensis* is maintained predominantly among lagomorphs and hard ticks. In cycle (b), which is dominant in Eurasia, *F. tularensis* is principally maintained among cricetine rodents, especially field voles and mice, water voles and other aquatic rodents. Humans are incidental hosts that are infected by tick vectors and by the bites of flies or mosquitoes that have contaminated mouthparts, by direct contact with infected animal carcasses or other contaminated materials, by ingestion of contaminated matter or by inhalation of infectious aerosols or dusts.

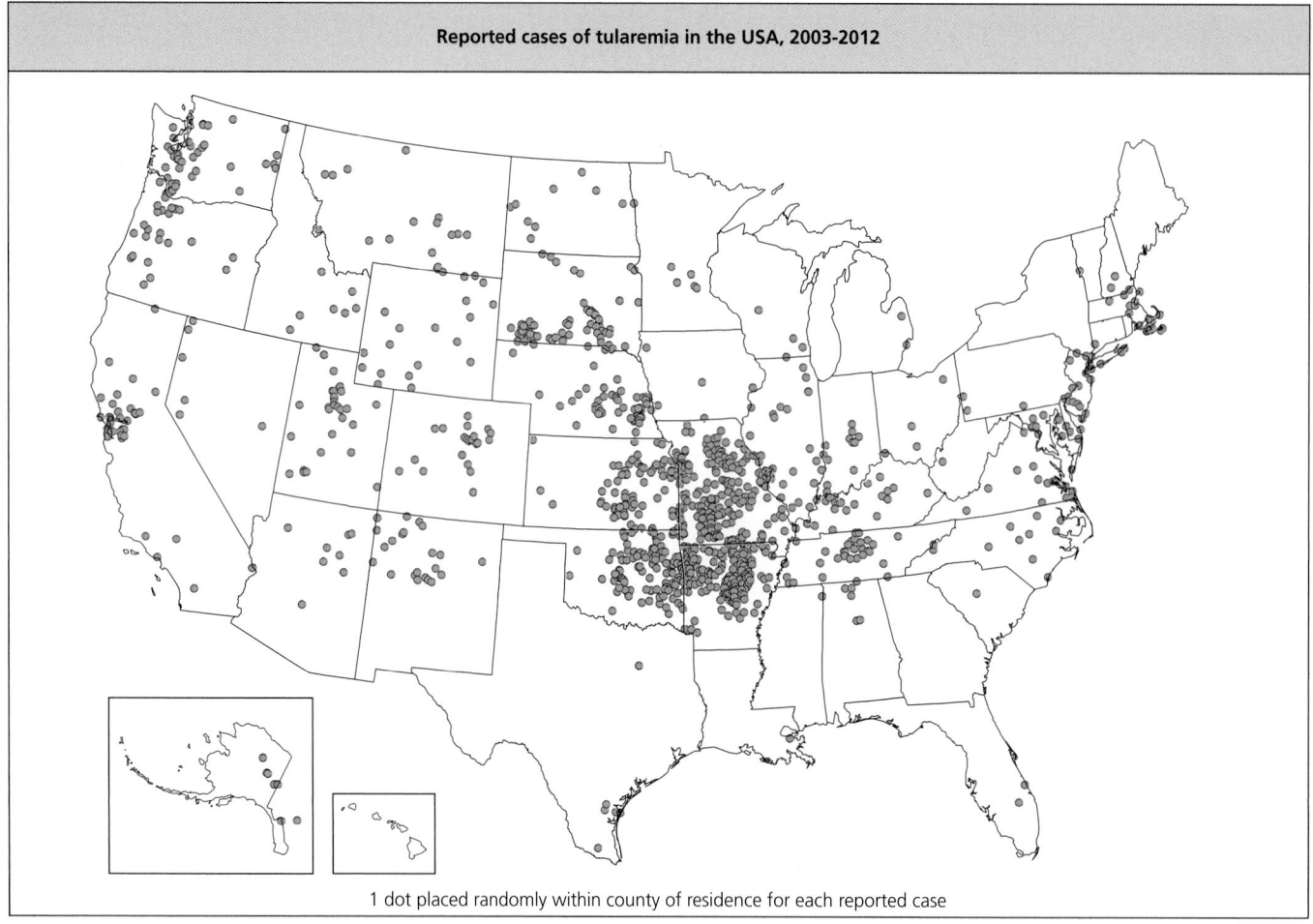

Reported cases of tularemia in the USA, 2003-2012

1 dot placed randomly within county of residence for each reported case

Figure 127-2 Reported cases of tularemia in the USA, 2003–2012.

Mexico as far south as Guadalajara. Tularemia also occurs throughout most of Europe and Russia, in some areas of the Near East and Middle East, in Central Asia and in Mongolia. It has not been documented in Central or South America, or Africa outside the Mediterranean littoral.

INCIDENCE

Global incidence figures are not available. In Eurasia, outbreaks involving hundreds of cases each have been reported from Sweden,[6] Kosovo,[7] Spain[8] and Turkey.[9] Tularemia incidence is relatively stable in the USA, where the disease has been in steady decline since the mid-1900s (Figure 127-3).[10] During 2001–2010, a total of 1208 cases were reported from 47 states, averaging 126.5 cases (range 90–154) per year.[5] Four states accounted for 49% of all reported cases: Missouri (19%), Arkansas (13%), Oklahoma (9%) and Massachusetts (7%).

SOURCES OF HUMAN INFECTION
Eurasia

Cricetine rodents (especially meadow voles, lemmings, water voles and muskrats), water and soil contaminated by these animals, hares (*Lepus* spp.) and bites by contaminated mosquitoes (especially *Aedes cinereus*) are the principal sources of human tularemia in Eurasia.[3,11,12] Sporadic cases also result in Eurasia from bites by infected ticks and by blood-feeding flies. Outbreaks of tularemia among farmers have been described in Europe following respiratory exposure to dusts from contaminated stored and fresh-mown hay.[12,13] Ingestion of water and food contaminated by infected rodents or hares has also resulted in outbreaks in the region, such as reported from Kosovo and Turkey.[7,9]

North America

The principal animal sources of infection in North America are the cottontail rabbit (*Sylvilagus* spp.), wild hares and rodents (muskrats, beaver, voles, ground squirrels).[3,14] The agent is vectored by certain species of hard ticks, especially the dog tick, *Dermacentor variabilis* (Figure 127-4a), the lone star tick, *Amblyomma americanum*, and the Rocky Mountain wood tick, *Dermacentor andersoni*.[15] Biting tabanid flies, especially deer flies (*Chrysops* spp.) (Figure 127-4b), mechanically transmit the infection.[15] Occasional cases arise as a result of the inhalation of dusts or aerosols. An outbreak of pneumonic tularemia associated with landscaping activities occurred on Martha's Vineyard in 2000, and since that time, Martha's Vineyard has recorded yearly cases.[16] The epidemiology of tularemia in North America has changed significantly since the 1930s and 1940s, when the disease most commonly called 'rabbit fever' had a much higher incidence and was more commonly due to direct exposures linked to the hunting, dressing and butchering of wild rabbits for meat and fur than to arthropod bites.[10]

SEASONALITY

Mosquito-borne transmission in Eurasia peaks in the summer months. In North America, cases occur year round, with a peak of tularemia cases in the spring and summer months attributed to bites by ticks and blood-feeding flies.[5,10] Cases in fall and winter primarily occur in hunters and trappers.

Pathogenesis and Pathology

The principal pathologic changes in localized disease occur at the cutaneous site of inoculation and in the regional lymph nodes draining

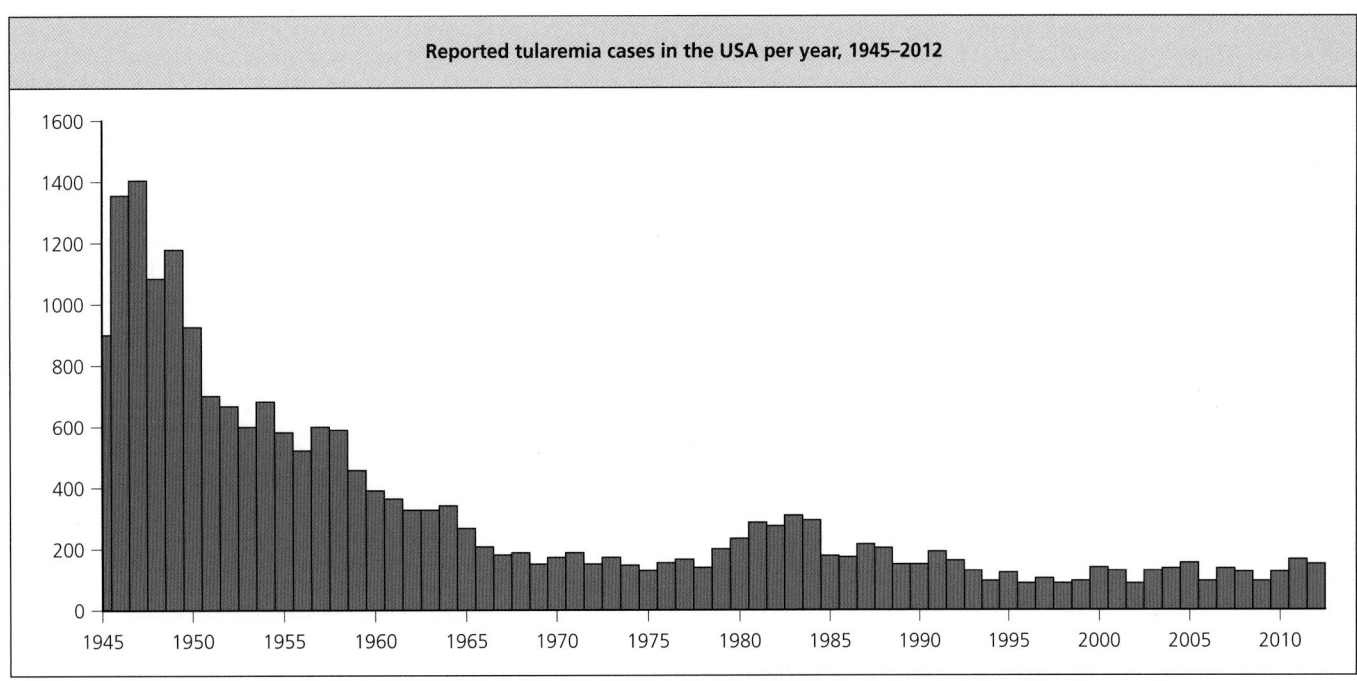

Figure 127-3 Reported tularemia cases in the USA per year, 1945–2012.

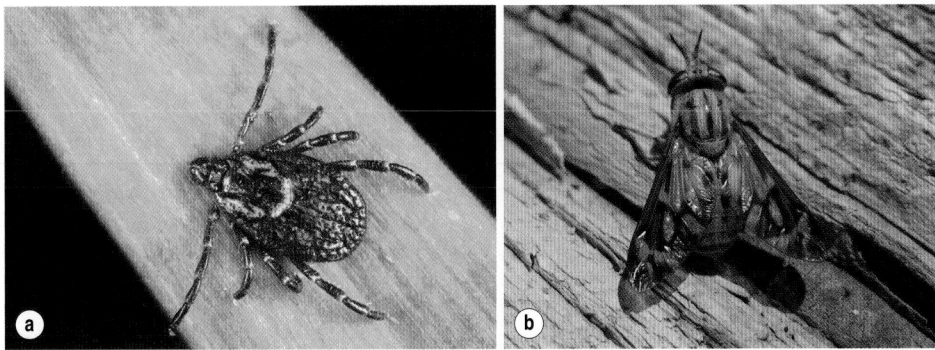

Figure 127-4 (a) The dog tick, *Dermacentor variabilis*, an important vector of tularemia in eastern and central USA. (b) The deer fly, *Chrysops discalis*, a primary vector of tularemia in western USA.

the site; when the disease is disseminated, the lungs, spleen, lymph nodes, liver and skin are most often involved.[17–19] The primary skin lesion begins as a papule several days following inoculation. The papule rapidly progresses to a vesicle that erodes and develops into an ulcer, which is typically 2–3 cm in diameter with an irregular, slightly raised and erythematous border. The base is necrotic, and frequently covered with a thick dark scab that can mimic the eschar of cutaneous anthrax. Secondary skin lesions have also been described in tularemia, including papular and papulovesicular lesions, erythema nodosum and erythema multiforme.

Francisella tularensis is an obligate intracellular organism within the vertebrate host, and replicates within macrophages, neutrophils, dendritic as well as other host cells.[12] Uncontrolled growth causes host cell damage and cell death. Histologically, infection with *F. tularensis* causes follicular hyperplasia in lymph nodes followed by focal necrosis and ultimately granuloma formation. The central area of necrosis is at first composed primarily of polymorphonuclear leukocytes and macrophages, which may be replaced by epithelioid cells in more advanced lesions. A wall of fibroblasts may surround the acute inflammatory reaction. A frequent finding on pathologic examination of affected lungs is small (3–12 mm), yellowish, necrotic subpleural nodules. The lungs in pneumonic tularemia show abundant fibrinous necrosis accompanied by various amounts of mixed inflammatory infiltrate;

bronchopneumonia is found in about 30% of pneumonic cases and lobar pneumonia with consolidation of an entire lobe, in about 15%. Lung abscesses occasionally occur. Hilar lymph nodes may be inflamed and enlarged.

PREVENTION

Persons exposed in endemic areas to ticks, biting flies or mosquitoes should, when feasible, wear protective clothing and apply repellents containing 20–30% DEET (*N,N*-diethyl-*m*-toluamide) to skin and clothing as directed by the manufacturer. Permethrin-based products will kill ticks, mosquitoes and biting flies and are recommended only for use on clothing and shoes – never on skin. When in tick-infested areas, frequent examinations should be made to identify and remove ticks on clothing and skin. Persons should always avoid direct contact with sick or dead animals, and hunters, trappers, dressers and butchers should wear impervious gloves when skinning and handling wild animal carcasses. Game meat should be cooked thoroughly before eating and surface water treated prior to ingestion. The use of fine particle masks while engaged in landscaping activities has been suggested as a possible means of reducing infective inhalation exposures, such as those which can result when using power tools that generate environmental dusts.

Currently, no tularemia vaccine is licensed for general use; this is, however, an important area of active research.[20] Persons exposed to a laboratory accident possibly resulting in aerosolization or inoculation of *F. tularensis* should be considered for prophylactic antibiotic administration or placed on fever watch and closely monitored for early signs of illness.

Clinical Features

POPULATIONS AFFECTED

Tularemia is a rural disease. It affects persons of all ages and both sexes. The highest incidence among five-year age groups was in 5–9-year-olds and 65–69-year-olds. Males accounted for 69% of reported cases during this period.[5] Groups at highest risk include:[14,21,22]

* hunters and trappers, wildlife specialists, animal skinners and dressers, and others who handle potentially infective animal carcasses
* farmers and landscapers who are exposed to water, soils, and dusts contaminated by infected wild animals or aerosols generated from infective materials (e.g. carcasses)
* persons exposed in enzootic areas to bites by certain hard ticks, tabanid flies or mosquitoes.

CLINICAL PRESENTATIONS

Clinical manifestations of *F. tularensis* infection range from subclinical to life-threatening and are determined by the route of exposure, the infecting dose and the infecting strain. Although the agent is highly infectious, requiring only 10–50 organisms to cause experimental infections of humans, person-to-person transmission has not been documented. The primary forms of tularemia include:[1,18,19]

* ulceroglandular tularemia (45–85% of cases)
* glandular tularemia (10–25% of cases)
* oculoglandular tularemia (<5% of cases)
* oropharyngeal tularemia (<5% of cases)
* pneumonic (inhalation) tularemia (<5% of cases).

The incubation period is usually 2–5 days (range 1–14 days). Onset is sudden; typically, the patient has fever of 38–40 °C (100–104 °F) and a constellation of nonspecific manifestations including chills, headache, generalized body aches (often prominent in the lumbosacral region), nausea, weakness, cough and chest pain. Without treatment, nonspecific symptoms usually persist for several weeks. Sweats, chills, progressive weakness and weight loss characterize the continuing illness. Any of the principal forms of tularemia may be complicated by bacteremic spread that may lead to secondary sepsis, pneumonia, or meningitis.

Clinical severity differs between the two subspecies causing human tularemia. Type A strains are associated with higher mortality rates in humans as compared to type B strains.[1] Before antibiotics became

available, the overall mortality rate from infections with type A strains was in the range of 5–10%; however, a considerably higher fatality rate was reported for septic and pneumonic forms of disease. A recent molecular epidemiologic study of 316 isolates obtained from human tularemia cases reported to the US Centers for Disease Control from 1964 to 2004 demonstrated genetic and virulence differences are also evidenced among type A strains from around the USA. Significantly higher case-fatality rates were observed for patients infected with type A strains from the eastern USA (A1b; 24%) as compared to those patients infected with type A strains from the western USA (A2; 0%).[4] A description of human infection due to *F. tularensis* subspecies *mediasiatica* is lacking in the published literature.

ULCEROGLANDULAR TULAREMIA

A local papule appears at the site of inoculation at the time of, or shortly after, the onset of fever and other generalized symptoms. This becomes vesiculated and pustular, and then ulcerates within a few days of its first appearance. Typically, the ulcer is tender, has an indolent character and may be covered by a scab (Figure 127-5a). By the time of ulceration, painful lymphadenitis occurs in one or more adjacent nodes in the afferent pathway. In persons infected by handling contaminated materials, the epitrochlear nodes (8%) and the axillary nodes (65%) are the most commonly affected. In persons infected by arthropod bites, the femoral–inguinal nodes (64%), the axillary nodes (24%) and the cervical nodes (6%) are commonly involved.[18] When treatment is delayed for 2 weeks or more there is risk that an abscessed node will suppurate, create a sinus tract and discharge purulent material to the outside.

GLANDULAR TULAREMIA

Glandular tularemia differs from the ulceroglandular type only in not having the local cutaneous ulceration. It is more likely to follow arthropod-borne inoculation than direct percutaneous inoculation of the hands and fingers of persons handling infected animal tissues.

OCULOGLANDULAR TULAREMIA

Oculoglandular tularemia (Parinaud's syndrome) follows contamination of the conjunctival sac. Ulceration may occur on the conjunctiva, which becomes severely inflamed, with marked edema and vasculitis. Characteristically, there is painful swelling of nodes draining the periorbital tissues, such as the preauricular, submandibular and cervical chain nodes.

OROPHARYNGEAL TULAREMIA

Oropharyngeal tularemia is acquired by ingesting inadequately cooked game, or contaminated water or food. The patient may develop a

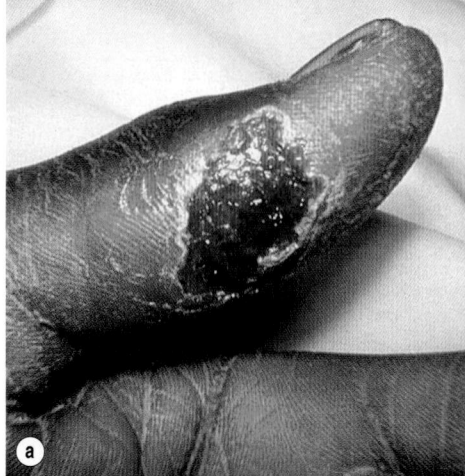
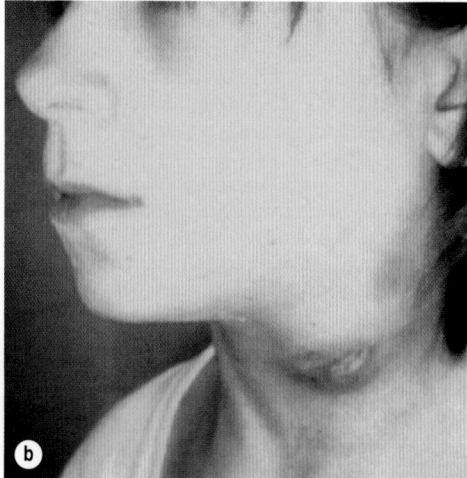

Figure 127-5   (a) Tularemic ulcer after percutaneous inoculation of *Francisella tularensis*. (b) Cervical lymphadenopathy after oral ingestion of *F. tularensis*.

painful exudative pharyngitis or tonsillitis, or a stomatitis, sometimes with ulceration, and tender cervical lymphadenopathy (Figure 127-5b). Suppuration, fistula formation and drainage of cervical nodes may occur.[9]

TYPHOIDAL TULAREMIA

Typhoidal tularemia was originally used to designate patients without skin lesions, lymphadenopathy or other localizing signs of infection.[1] With a better understanding of the routes of infection which, like inhalation and ingestion, may not be obvious and the potential for systemic spread, the term typhoidal tularemia is outdated.

PNEUMONIC TULAREMIA

Primary pneumonia can be severe and arises from inhalation of an infective aerosol or dust. Pneumonic tularemia is a common secondary complication of other forms of tularemia. In addition to fever, chills, fatigue and other generalized symptoms of infection, pneumonic manifestations include cough (usually with minimal sputum production), chest discomfort, sometimes with pleuritic pain, dyspnea, tachypnea and occasionally mild hemoptysis. Radiographic findings have included lobar and multilobar infiltrates, lung abscess and hilar adenopathy. Pleural effusions have been reported in 20–30% of cases.

Diagnosis

A clinical diagnosis of tularemia is made by medical examination combined with information on potentially infective exposures. Differential diagnostic possibilities are many, as follows:

- in persons who have glandular or ulceroglandular disease they include bubonic plague, cutaneous anthrax, sporotrichosis, cat-scratch fever, lymphogranuloma venereum, streptococcal or staphylococcal lymphadenitis, toxoplasmosis, mycobacterial infection, chancre and chancroid;
- in persons who have oropharyngeal tularemia, other bacterial and viral causes of stomatitis, pharyngitis and cervical adenitis must be considered, such as streptococcal infection, infectious mononucleosis, mycobacterial infection, adenoviral infection and diphtheria;
- in persons who have pneumonia, they include mycoplasmal pneumonia, chlamydial pneumonia, Legionnaires' disease, staphylococcal or streptococcal pneumonitis, *Haemophilus influenzae* pneumonia, plague, histoplasmosis and tuberculosis; and
- in persons without localizing signs of tularemia, they include bacterial endocarditis, disseminated mycobacterial or fungal infection, typhoid fever, brucellosis, listeriosis, leptospirosis, Q fever, plague and other causes of sepsis.

The clinical diagnosis of tularemia is confirmed by culture recovery of *F. tularensis*.[1] The organism is slow-growing and fastidious, therefore prolonged incubation times of 5–7 days at 35–37°C on cysteine-supplemented agar are often necessary for recovery from clinical specimens. *Francisella tularensis* may be present in human lesion exudates, respiratory secretions (bronchial/tracheal washes or aspirates, sputum, transthoracic lung aspirates and pleural fluid), blood and lymph node aspirates as well as biopsy and autopsy tissues. For blood culture, the BACTEC system or an equivalent system is recommended. Direct fluorescent antibody staining, using a FITC-labeled antibody against *F. tularensis*, is a rapid assay used for identification of *F. tularensis* recovered in culture and in primary clinical specimens.[1] Commercially available lateral flow assays have recently shown promise for identification of recovered cultures, but require validation for routine diagnostic use.[23] Polymerase chain reaction (PCR) for molecular detection of *F. tularensis* is particularly useful for rapid diagnosis in primary clinical specimens and when organisms are noncultivable. Real-time PCR has been applied to detect *F. tularensis* DNA in a variety of clinical specimens including ulcers, aspirates, pharyngeal swabs, lymph node specimens, bronchial washes and pleural fluid.[24–27] For additional details of the clinical microbiology see Chapter 183.

Acute and convalescent serum specimens that differ in titer by fourfold, with at least one serum-positive, are also considered confirmatory for the diagnosis of tularemia.[1] A first specimen should be collected as early in the course of infection as possible, followed by a second specimen taken in the convalescent period (at least 14 days apart and preferably 3–4 weeks after onset of symptoms). The agglutination reaction for combined IgM and IgG immunoglobulins is the serologic procedure used in many laboratories. Antibody titers usually do not rise before 10 days or more of illness onset.

Personnel handling diagnostic cultures of *F. tularensis* are at considerable risk for infection, due to the low infectious dose for *F. tularensis*. Tularemia has been one of the most commonly reported laboratory-associated bacterial infections.[28] Aerosol inhalation during manipulation of cultures presents the greatest risk to laboratory workers, due to the high concentration of organisms. BSL-3 practices, containment equipment and facilities are recommended for all manipulations of suspect cultures.[29] In the USA, *F. tularensis* is classified as a select agent. Laboratories identifying *F. tularensis* in culture are required to report this finding immediately. Report forms, contact information, laboratory registration information and pertinent citations of the US Federal Code may be found at www.selectagents.gov.

Management

Patients are best managed under hospital care until a full diagnostic evaluation and satisfactory treatment response has occurred. Presently, aminoglycosides, tetracyclines and chloramphenicol have been approved for treatment of tularemia by the US Food and Drug Administration (FDA). Streptomycin, which is bactericidal, has been the traditional drug of choice based on experience and efficacy.[2,30] It is given intramuscularly to adults in a dosage of 1 g and to children at 15 mg/kg (not to exceed 2 g/day), twice daily for 10 days. Gentamicin is given parenterally in an adult dosage of 5 mg/kg and to children at 2.5 mg/kg, per day for 10 days. A tetracycline (most commonly doxycycline) or chloramphenicol may be used in place of an aminoglycoside, especially in less severely ill patients, but use of these bacteriostatic agents occasionally results in primary treatment failures, and dosage schedules of at least 14 days are recommended to prevent relapses.

Although not yet FDA approved, oral or parenterally administered ciprofloxacin has been used to treat adults and children with good success in standard doses for 10 days.[31,32] Patients begun on parenterally administered antimicrobials can switch to oral administration upon clearing of symptoms and the ability to take medication orally.

F. tularensis strains produce β-lactamase and are resistant to β-lactam antibiotics and azithromycin. Penicillins and cephalosporins are therefore ineffective for treatment of tularemia.[33] Macrolides are also not recommended for treatment of tularemia, as type B strains from Central and Eastern Europe and Asia are naturally resistant to erythromycin and other macrolides. *F. tularensis* strains are uniformly susceptible to aminoglycosides, tetracyclines, chloramphenicol and quinolones.[34,35] No natural resistance to these antimicrobials has been observed.

Typically, fever and general symptoms of acute infection begin to regress within 24–48 hours of initiation of appropriate antibiotic administration. Factors associated with a poor outcome include delays in seeking medical care, or delays in diagnosis and treatment, and underlying medical disorders, such as diabetes or alcoholism.[36] Lymph node suppuration, refractive to all classes of antibiotics, can develop in patients who delay seeking treatment. Considerably longer recovery times are observed in these cases and can be >70 days.[37] Standard (universal) precautions only are required for purposes of hospital infection control.[2] Post-exposure prophylactic antibiotic treatment of close contacts is not recommended because human-to-human transmission is not known to occur.

References available online at expertconsult.com.

KEY REFERENCES

Centers for Disease Control and Prevention: Tularemia – United States, 2000–2010. *MMWR Morb Mortal Wkly Rep* 2013; 62:963-966.

Dennis D.T., Inglesby T.V., Henderson D.A., et al.: Tularemia as a biological weapon: medical and public health management. *JAMA* 2001; 285:2763-2773.

Eliasson H., Lindbäck J., Nuorti J.P., et al.: The 2000 tularemia outbreak: a case–control study of risk factors in disease-endemic and emergent areas, Sweden. *Emerg Infect Dis* 2002; 8:956-960.

Georgi E., Schacht E., Scholz H.C., et al.: Standardized broth microdilution antimicrobial susceptibility testing of *Francisella tularensis* subsp. *holarctica* strains from Europe and rare *Francisella* species. *J Antimicrob Chemother* 2012; 67:2429-2433.

Kugeler K.J., Mead P.S., Janusz A.M., et al.: Molecular epidemiology of *Francisella tularensis* in the United States. *Clin Infect Dis* 2009; 48:863-870.

Rossow H., Ollgren J., Klemets P., et al.: Risk factors for pneumonic and ulceroglandular tularaemia in Finland: a population-based case–control study. *Epidemiol Infect* 2013; 2:1-10.

Sjöstedt A.: Tularemia: history, epidemiology, pathogen physiology, and clinical manifestations. *Ann NY Acad Sci* 2007; 1105:1-29.

Tärnvik A., ed. *World Health Organization Guidelines on tularaemia*. Geneva: WHO Press; 2007:1-115.

Urich S.K., Petersen J.M.: In vitro susceptibility of isolates of *Francisella tularensis* types A and B from North America. *Antimicrob Agents Chemother* 2008; 52: 2276-2278.

Weber I.B., Turabelidze G., Patrick S., et al.: Clinical recognition and management of tularemia in Missouri: a retrospective records review of 121 cases. *Clin Infect Dis* 2012; 55:1283-1290.

128

Scrub Typhus and Other Tropical Rickettsioses

NICHOLAS P.J. DAY | PAUL N. NEWTON

KEY CONCEPTS

- Rickettsial pathogens are zoonotic intracellular bacteria transmitted by arthropods, such as ticks, mites, lice and fleas. Humans and other mammals are usually incidentally infected.

- They are clearly important pathogens but due to lack of awareness and problems with accessible and accurate laboratory diagnosis there are no evidence-based estimates of disease burden.

- Currently divided into four groups: scrub typhus (O. tsutsugamushi), the typhus group (Rickettsia typhi and R. prowazeckii), the spotted fever group (e.g. R. conorii indica and R. africae) and the transitional group (e.g. R. australis, R. akari and R. felis).

- Human incidence reflects the interaction of humans with the vectors, other mammals and their environment but there is little such ecologic understanding for these pathogens. An important exception is R. prowazeckii for which humans appear to be the reservoir.

- Serologic diagnostic tests for rickettsial diseases have low sensitivity and specificity and are rarely available and standardized. Polymerase chain reaction assays for rickettsial pathogens are available but low bacterial blood loads result in low sensitivity.

- The mainstay of management is doxycycline therapy with tetracycline and chloramphenicol as alternatives. Azithromycin may be appropriate for scrub typhus but fluoroquinolones are not. Given wide distributions and genotypic diversity it is unlikely that one treatment regimen will be appropriate everywhere.

- There is increasing realization that these pathogens cause severe diseases, especially of the central nervous system, and may be associated with poor maternal and pregnancy outcome.

- Coxiella burnetii is a related global pathogen in the order Legionellales, most commonly contracted via ingestion and inhalation from cattle, sheep and goats. It can cause acute fever, with hepatitis and pneumonia and a chronic endocarditis.

- There are no vaccines available for any of these pathogens except for C. burnetii.

Epidemiology

Tropical rickettsioses are a diverse group of zoonotic infectious diseases caused by obligate intracellular bacteria grouped in the family Rickettsiaceae of α-proteobacteria. These organisms are non-flagellate, small coccobacilli occurring within the host cytoplasm or nucleus and are not bounded in a vacuole. Transmitted to humans by arthropods, in which they may be maintained by transovarial and transstadial transmission, those responsible for human disease in the tropics include:

- *Orientia tsutsugamushi*, the causative organism of scrub typhus or tsutsugamushi disease transmitted by chigger mites.

- The typhus group (TG) of the genus *Rickettsia*, containing *R. prowazeckii*, the agent of epidemic (louse-borne) typhus, and *R. typhi*, which causes murine or endemic (flea-borne) typhus.

- The spotted fever group (SFG) *Rickettsia*, containing a large and ever-increasing number of species. These are mostly transmitted from mammals by ticks and include *R. conorii indica* (Indian tick typhus) and *R. africae* (African tick bite fever).

- The recently proposed transitional group includes *R. australis* (tick-borne), *R. akari* (mite-borne) and *R. felis* (flea-borne plus probably other vectors). For the purposes of this review we have included these in the SFG discussion.

Q fever has in the past been considered a rickettsiosis and will be covered in this chapter, though its causative agent *Coxiella burnetii* has been transferred to the α-proteobacteria order Legionellales.

The agents of rickettsioses are associated with mammals and crucially with arthropods, including ticks, mites, fleas and lice, which may act as vectors, reservoirs and/or amplifiers. Hence environmental determinants of the geographic distribution of vectors and probably mammals are the foundations for the risk to humans in different communities, interlinked with their relationships with vectors. Although some rickettsioses are distributed worldwide (Q fever, murine typhus), distribution is very heterogeneous through time and space. Table 128-1 summarizes the rickettsioses occurring in tropical areas of Africa, Asia, America and Australia.

Scrub typhus, caused by *Orientia tsutsugamushi*, is an important and widespread cause of fever in rural Asia and northern Australia (Figure 128-1).[1-3] It is contracted via the bite of larvae of several species of *Leptotrombidium* trombiculid mites ('chiggers'), which live in a wide range of vegetation types from scrub and primary forest to gardens and beaches; hence the term 'scrub' is misleading. At least in some habitats infected mites are characteristically found in discrete foci called mite islands, where the risk of contracting scrub typhus is high. The bacteria are maintained transovarially in the mite population, infecting rodents on which the mite larval stage feeds. As mites are thought to bite only once, humans and other mammals are incidentally infected and have little impact on O. tsutsugamushi ecology and selection apart from amplifying mite density (Figure 128-2) – though it is possible that mammals harbouring multiple infected mites provide an opportunity for bacterial recombination. That the *Orientia* genus may be a human pathogen outside Asia/Australia has been supported by the detection of *Orientia* DNA in rodents from Europe and West Africa, the description of a patient from the United Arab Emirates who contracted a new species, *O. chuto*, and case reports from Chile and Africa.[4-7] Their vectors are unknown.

Epidemic typhus, caused by *R. prowazeckii*, is one of the most dangerous of the arthropod-borne diseases.[8] It is transmitted by the human body louse (*Pediculus humanus corporis*), which lives in human clothing and thrives in conditions such as poverty and war. The bacteria are not transmitted vertically in lice and unlike all other rickettsial diseases humans are the major reservoir. Sporadic cases have been reported through contact with the flying squirrel *Glaucomys volans* in the USA.[9] R. prowazeckii is transmitted to people by infected louse feces (in which R. prowazeckii survives for weeks), through aerosols (thought to be the main route of infection for healthcare workers attending patients) or by skin autoinoculation, following scratching. Outbreaks

TABLE 128-1 Tropical Rickettsioses Throughout the World

Location by Continent	Vectors	Disease	Agent	Specific Areas	Risk of Exposure
AFRICA/MIDDLE EAST	**Ticks**				
	Rhipicephalus sanguineus	Mediterranean spotted fever	Rickettsia conorii	Mediterranean area, sub-Saharan Africa	Urban (2/3) and rural (1/3)
	Amblyomma spp., Hyalomma marginatum, Rhipicephalus spp.	African tick bite fever	R. africae	Sub-Saharan Africa, Israel*	Rural area; safari
	Hyalomma marginatum and other Hyalomma spp., Boophilus annulatum, Haemaphysalis sulcata	Unnamed	R. aeschlimannii	North Africa and sub-Saharan Africa	Infected ticks found on camels, domestic animals, and migratory birds
	Dermacentor marginatus	Tick-borne lymphadenopathy (TIBOLA)	R. slovaca	Morocco*	
	Dermacentor marginatus	Unnamed	R. raoultii	Morocco*	
	Rhipicephalus sanguineus and other Rhipicephalus spp., Haemaphysalis erinacei	Unnamed	R. massiliae	North Africa and sub-Saharan Africa	
	Hyalomma truncatum	Unnamed	R. sibirica mongolotimonae	North Africa and sub-Saharan Africa	
	Ixodes ricinus	Unnamed	R. monacensis	North Africa	
	Ixodes ricinus	Unnamed	R. helvetica	Algeria*	
	Fleas				
	Xenopsylla cheopis, Xenopsylla brasiliensis	Murine typhus	R. typhi	Ubiquitous. High prevalence in coastal areas	Contact with rats and rat fleas
	Ctenocephalides felis, Ct. canis, Ct. calceatus, Leptopsylla aethiopica, Pulex irritans (human flea)	Flea-borne spotted fever	R. felis	Mediterranean area sub-Saharan Africa	
	Lice				
	Pediculus humanus corporis	Epidemic typhus	R. prowazekii	North Africa and sub-Saharan Africa	Civil war, prisons refugee camps
	?Mites	Unnamed	Orientia chuto	Dubai	
AMERICAS	**Ticks**				
	Dermacentor andersoni, D. variabilis, Amblyomma spp. and Haemaphysalis leporispalustris	Rocky Mountain spotted fever	R. rickettsii	North and Central America	Rural areas
	Amblyomma triste	Unnamed	R. parkeri and rickettsial sp. Atlantic Rainforest strain (Brazil)	Brazil, Uruguay, Argentina	Rural areas
	Amblyomma spp.	African tick bite fever	R. africae	West Indies	Rural areas
	Unknown	Unnamed	R. massiliae	Argentina	
	Fleas				
	Xenopsylla cheopis	Murine typhus	R. typhi	Ubiquitous	Contact with rats and rat fleas
	Ctenocephalides felis, Ct. canis, Pulex irritans	Flea-borne spotted fever	R. felis	Central and South America	
	Lice				
	Pediculus humanus corporis	Epidemic typhus	R. prowazekii	Peru and Andes	Lack of hygiene in mountainous area
	Mites				
	Liponyssoides sanguineus	Rickettsialpox	R. akari	USA and Mexico	

TABLE 128-1 | **Tropical Rickettsioses Throughout the World** (Continued)

Location by Continent	Vectors	Disease	Agent	Specific Areas	Risk of Exposure
ASIA	**Ticks**				
	Rhipicephalus sanguineus	Indian tick typhus	*R. conorii indica*	India. Suspected in Thailand, Korea, Laos and Sri Lanka	
	Ixodes granulatus	Flinders Island spotted fever	*R. honei* (TT118)	Thailand	
	Ixodes ovatus, Haemaphysalis longicornis, Haemaphysalis flava, Dermacentor taiwanensis	Oriental or Japanese spotted fever	*R. japonica*	Japan†, China*	Agricultural activities, bamboo cutting
	Ixodes spp.	Unnamed	*R. helvetica*	Japan.† Suspected in Thailand, Laos	
	Hyalomma asiaticum	Lymphangitis-associated rickettsiosis	*R. sibirica mongolotimonae*	China† (Inner Mongolia)*	
	Dermacentor nuttalli, D. marginatus, Haemaphysalis concinna	North-Asian tick typhus	*R. sibirica sibirica*	Northern China, Central Asian Republics, Russia, Pakistan	
	Dermacentor silvarum	Far-Eastern tick-borne rickettsiosis	*R. heilongjiangii*	North-eastern China	
	Dermacentor silvarum	Tick-borne lymphadenopathy	*R. raoultii*	China–Russia border	
	Dermacentor silvarum	Tick-borne lymphadenopathy	*R. slovaca*	China*	
	Ixodes spp.	Unnamed	*R. monacensis*	Korea*	
	Amblyomma testudinarium	Unnamed	*R. tamurae*	Japan	
	Fleas				
	Xenopsylla cheopis	Murine typhus	*R. typhi*	Ubiquitous	
	Ctenocephalides felis, Ct. orientis, Xenopsylla cheopis	Flea-borne spotted fever	*R. felis*	Thailand, Laos, Taiwan, Korea, Malaysia*, Indonesia*, Afghanistan*	
	Mites				
	Leptotrombidium spp.	Scrub typhus	*Orientia tsutsugamushi*	Asia–Pacific Region	Rural activities, agricultural activities and soldiers
	Lice				
	Pediculus humanus corporis	Epidemic typhus	*R. prowazekii*	China, India (Kashmir)	Civil war, refugee camps
	House Mouse Mite				
	Liponyssoides sanguineus	Rickettsialpox	*R. akari*	Korea†	
AUSTRALIA	**Ticks**				
	Unknown	Flinders Island spotted fever	*R. honei*		
	Ixodes holocyclus	Queensland tick typhus	*R. australis*	North-eastern Australia	
	Fleas				
	Xenopsylla cheopis	Murine typhus	*R. typhi*	Ubiquitous	Contact with rats and rat fleas
	Ctenocephalides felis, Ct. canis	Flea-borne spotted fever	*R. felis*	Western Australia, Northern Territories*, Queensland*	
	Mites				
	Leptotrombidium spp.	Scrub typhus	*Orientia tsutsugamushi*	Northern Territory and Western Australia, Queensland	Rural activities, agricultural activities, soldiers

Note: Q fever caused by *C. burnetii* is distributed worldwide (except in New Zealand).
*Suspected by detection of the pathogen in the relevant arthropod.
†Isolated from voles (*Microtus fortis pelliceus*).

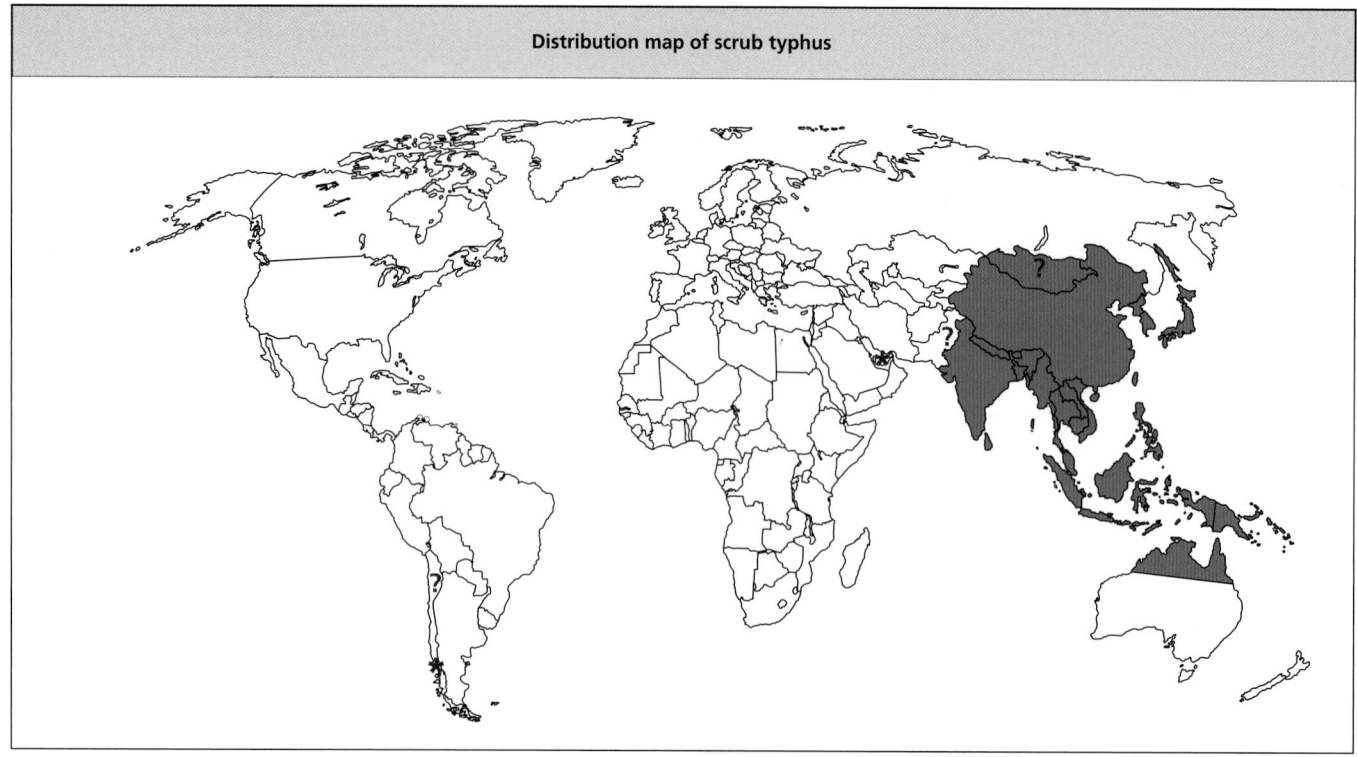

Figure 128-1 Distribution map of scrub typhus. Scrub typhus or tsutsugamushi disease (from a Japanese word meaning 'noxious bug') is caused by infection with *Orientia tsutsugamushi* and is transmitted by larval trombiculid mites of the genus *Leptotrombidium*. The disease occurs in the Indian subcontinent, South East Asia, the Far East and islands of the southwest Pacific, including the Republic of Palau. It seems likely that the *Orientia* genus has a wider distribution as a human pathogen, with reports from UAE and Chile (red stars). *(Adapted from Magill, et al., Hunter's tropical medicine and emerging infectious disease, 9th ed. Elsevier Inc., Copyright © 2012. Figure 63.1.)*

of epidemic typhus have recently occurred in Burundi. Sporadic patients have been reported in North Africa and France, and the homeless are at risk. Epidemic typhus is therefore a potential major health risk in tropical countries, particularly in environments such as refugee camps in cooler highlands.

Murine typhus, also known as endemic typhus, is a flea-borne rickettsiosis caused by *R. typhi*.[10] The rat flea *Xenopsylla cheopis* is the principal vector; rodents, mainly *Rattus norvegicus* and *R. rattus*, act as reservoirs. In suburban areas of the USA the cat flea, *Ctenocephalides felis*, has been identified as the principal vector. People become infected when flea feces containing *R. typhi* contaminate disrupted skin or are inhaled into the respiratory tract. Exposure to rat fleas is linked to exposure to rats, and high endemicity tends to occur in areas with large rat populations. Murine typhus has a worldwide distribution, occurring in urban as well as rural settings, though it probably has a higher incidence in warmer countries. Despite the name it has been given, it may also cause outbreaks, such as described in refugee camps and detoxification centres.

The spotted fevers are caused by a large and expanding number of rickettsial species, all of which are transmitted by ticks.[11] Ticks are not only vectors but also reservoirs of most of the currently known spotted fever group rickettsiae. Ecologic characteristics of the tick are keys to the epidemiology of tick-borne diseases. *R. felis*, of the related transitional group, is transmitted by fleas and probably other arthropods and recent data suggest that it is widespread.

Due to lack of awareness and problems in laboratory diagnosis there are no evidence-based burden of disease estimates for any tropical rickettsioses.

Q fever is a global zoonotic infection caused by *Coxiella burnetii*, usually acquired occupationally by the ingestion or inhalation of virulent organisms from infected mammals, mostly goats, sheep and cattle, and their products. *Coxiella burnetii* has been found to infect more than 40 species of ticks throughout the world, but the role of ticks in

human infections is not confirmed. It has caused large documented recent epidemics in the Netherlands and in Cayenne, French Guiana (associated with goats and three-toed sloths respectively), and there is growing realization of its global importance, especially in Africa.[12–14]

There are no known host predisposing factors, apart from human behavior, for rickettsial diseases but heart valve lesions predispose to chronic *C. burnetii* endocarditis. Neither human immunodeficiency virus (HIV) infection nor diabetes appears to predispose to rickettsial disease but scrub typhus infection appears to reduce HIV replication *in vitro* and *in vivo*.

Pathogenesis and Pathology

The rickettsial pathogens lead to a vasculitis-like syndrome in humans with proliferation in endothelial cells of small blood vessels (especially *Rickettsia* spp.).[15] Coagulation is disturbed but disseminated intravascular coagulation (DIC) is very rare.[16] In contrast to the typhus group bacteria that lack ability to directionally polymerize actin, SFG bacteria polymerize actin allowing spread from cell to cell. Cell-mediated immunity is thought to be vital in controlling the infection. In contrast, *O. tsutsugamushi* appears, at least early in the infection, to target dendritic cells, neutrophils, leucocytes and macrophages rather than endothelial cells, with cell invasion mediated by fibronectin.[17]

C. burnetii is more complicated, replicating intracellularly as two forms – a more frequent large cell variant (LCV) that replicates and a small cell variant (SCV) that does not.[18] The LCV is probably adapted to the host and the SCV to the environment. Acute Q fever may be characterized by granulomas (e.g. in the liver) but chronic Q fever (e.g. heart valves) is not.

Prevention

There are no vaccines available against any tropical rickettsioses. Prevention is based on avoiding arthropod bites, which is especially

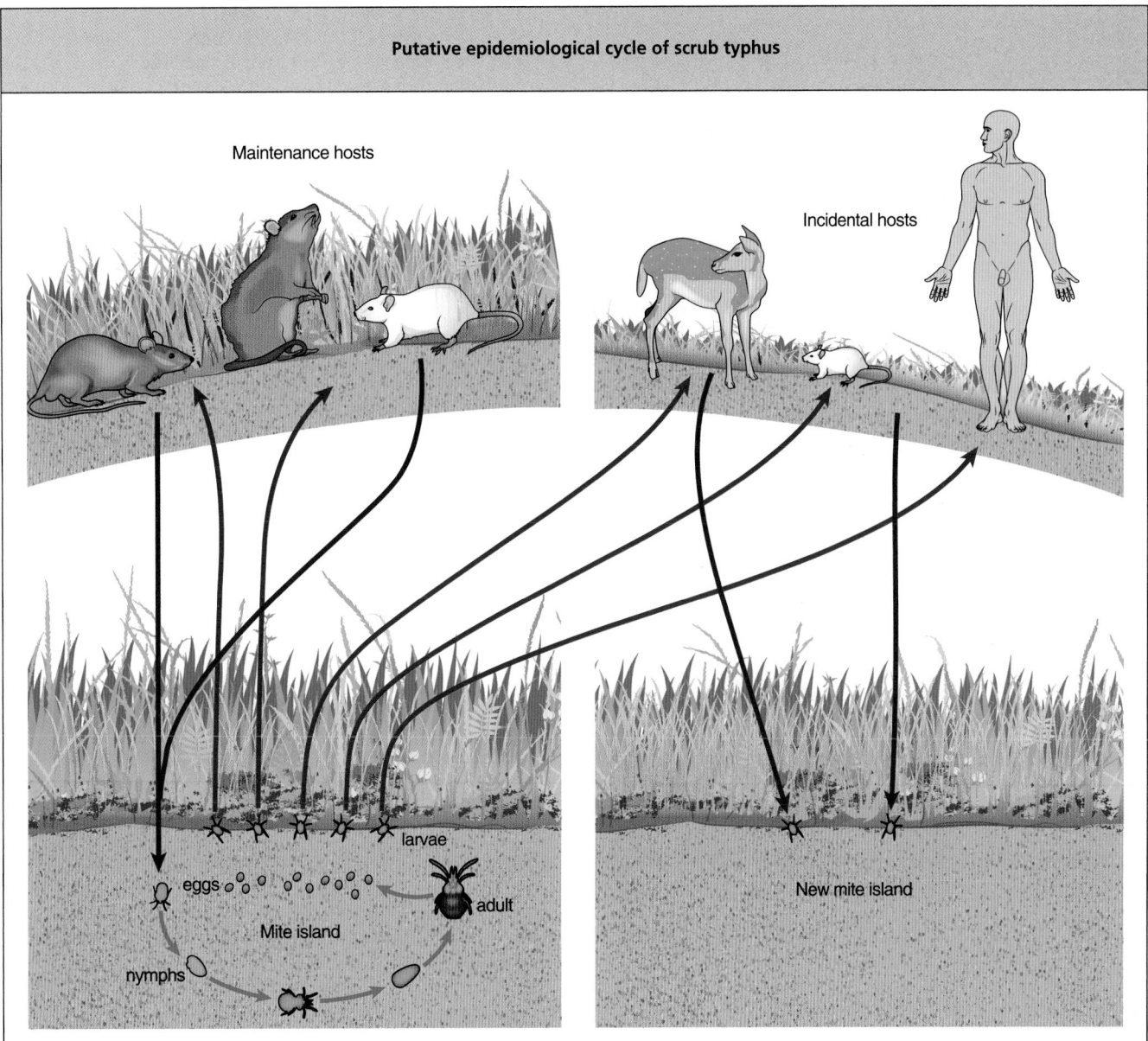

Figure 128-2 Putative epidemiological cycle of scrub typhus. *Orientia tsutsugamushi* is present in trombiculid-infested rodents. The mites occur in leaf litter in colonies known as 'mite islands' that are associated with the nests of the rodents on which they normally feed. They pass through a cycle that includes a parasitic, blood-feeding, six-legged larva followed by eight-legged, nonparasitic nymphal and adult stages. Vertical transmission occurs so that the reservoir of infection is the mite. Other mammals, humans and occasionally birds may be bitten by larvae. Thus, scrub typhus, although a zoonosis, can occur in small outbreaks if groups of people (e.g. farmers or soldiers) rest in the vicinity of a mite island. Whether this ecology and mite islands occur in all habitats is not known. *(Adapted from Audy JR. Red mites and typhus. London: Athlone Press; 1968.)*

difficult for those in rural communities. The best method to avoid tick, flea and chigger bites is to use topical DEET (*N,N*-diethyl-*m*-toluamide) repellent applied to exposed skin, and treat clothing with permethrin, which kills arthropods on contact. Bites may also be limited by wearing long trousers, tucked into boots. People staying in infested areas should be advised to check their bodies routinely for the presence of arthropods. Any tick found attached should be removed immediately using blunt, rounded forceps. Prevention of Q fever is assisted by milk pasteurization. A vaccine is available although further studies are needed to optimize safety and efficacy.[19]

Clinical Features

Symptoms of scrub typhus usually occur 6–10 days after the mite bite. The presenting features are typically fever, severe headache and myalgia with or without generalized or regional lymphadenopathy, and a macular or maculopapular rash (Figure 128-3) and eschar. Nausea and vomiting, diarrhea, constipation, conjunctival suffusion and reversible sensorineural deafness also occur.[20] A painless papule may occur at the bite site that later ulcerates, forming a black crust or 'eschar' (Figure 128-4) in a variable proportion of patients – this variability probably reflects, at least in part, the extent of the physical examination. However, the eschar and rash may be absent or unnoticed.

Complications include jaundice, meningoencephalitis, myocarditis, interstitial pneumonia leading on to adult respiratory distress syndrome (ARDS), and renal failure. Central nervous system *O. tsutsugamushi* infection usually presents with mildly raised cerebrospinal fluid white counts (neutrophils > lymphocytes), at a lower density than in patients with conventional bacterial meningitis. It has a high mortality and is not susceptible to conventional antibiotic therapy for

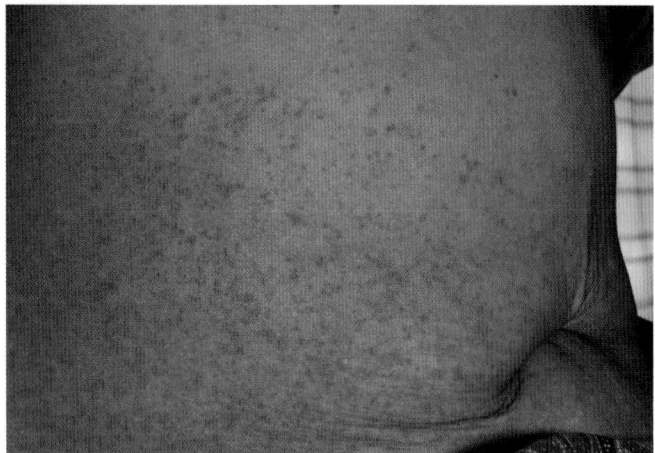

Figure 128-3   Macular rash in a patient with scrub typhus.

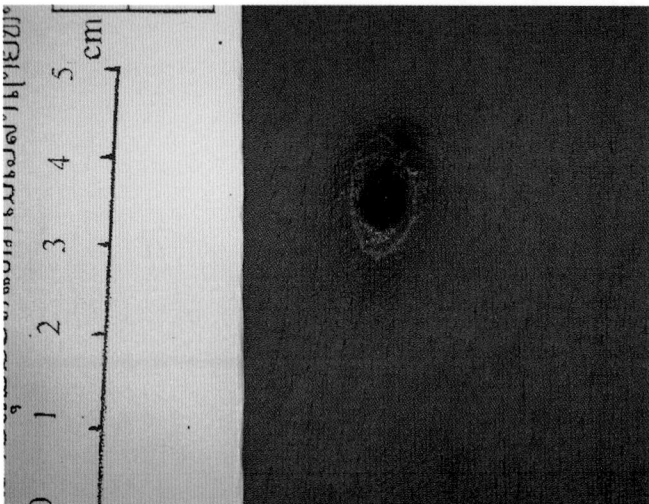

Figure 128-4   Eschar at the bite site, a hallmark of rickettsial diseases. They are not pathognomonic of scrub typhus as they also may occur in SFG infection.

meningitis, such as cephalosporins. Case series of scrub typhus in pregnancy suggest that *O. tsutsugamushi* infection may be associated with poor maternal and neonatal outcomes. Animal experiments indicate that disease severity may vary widely with the strain of bacteria. In the pre-antibiotic era high mortality rates were reported, and the disease still carries a significant risk of death in rural areas where effective treatment is unavailable or delayed, and everywhere if the diagnosis is not considered.

The incubation period of epidemic typhus is ~10–14 days with malaise and vague symptoms before the abrupt onset of fever (100%), headache (100%) and myalgia (70–100%).[21] Other common signs include nausea, vomiting, coughing and epistaxis. Meningoencephalitis is a common complication in severe cases, with meningism, tinnitus, deafness and altered consciousness, ranging from mild confusion through agitated delirium and coma. Diarrhea, pulmonary involvement, myocarditis, splenomegaly and conjunctivitis may also occur. Many patients (20–80%) develop a skin rash, classically centrifugal, that may be macular, maculopapular or petechial and difficult to detect on darker skin. The overall mortality is ~20%, rising to 60% in the malnourished and aged, though with appropriate antibiotic treatment mortality may be <4%. Recrudescence of epidemic typhus, unrelated to louse infestation, or Brill–Zinsser disease can appear many years after the acute disease and has milder symptoms.

Murine typhus usually presents with fever, severe headache and myalgia and, in a minority, a rash.[10] Dry cough is common. The incubation period is ~7–14 days. Nausea, vomiting, abdominal pain, diarrhea, jaundice, confusion, seizures and renal failure have been reported. Peripheral lymphadenopathy is significantly less frequent in murine typhus than in scrub typhus, and eschars do not occur – useful distinguishing clinical features in areas of Asia where the two diseases coexist. Mortality is probably low: around 1% with antibiotic treatment. However, severe disease can occur, especially of the central nervous system and in pregnant women.

The clinical symptoms of spotted fever group rickettsioses begin 6–10 days after the arthropod bite and typically include fever, headache, muscle pain, rash, local lymphadenopathy and a characteristic inoculation eschar ('tache noire') at the bite site. Despite the name 'spotted fever' many patients confusingly have no rash –'unspotted spotted fever'. The main clinical signs vary depending on the rickettsial species involved. For example, African tick bite fever is characterized by the occurrence of multiple inoculation eschars and cases occurring among groups of people, as numerous highly infected *Amblyomma* may attack and bite many people in several places at the same time. In contrast, in Mediterranean spotted fever due to *R. conorii*, a single eschar is usual because of the low likelihood of the tick biting people and a low rate of infection of the ticks. Details of each pathogen and clinical pictures are presented elsewhere (see Chapter 187).

Spotted fever group rickettsioses may result in mild to severe and fatal disease. For example, to date no mortalities or severe complications have been reported in patients with African tick-bite fever, whereas the mortality rate from Mediterranean spotted fever may be as high as 2.5%.

Acute Q fever is usually mild, with asymptomatic seroconversion occurring in 50–60% of infected individuals with an incubation period of 9–40 days. A self-limited fever occurs most frequently in symptomatic patients, but hepatitis, pneumonitis and prolonged fever may develop (see Chapter 187). Chronic Q fever may present as endocarditis in patients with underlying heart valve lesions or, more rarely, as vascular aneurysms, graft infections, chronic bone infections or pseudotumors of the lung.[22]

The differential diagnosis for these diverse pathogens is broad and dependent on geography. For *Orientia* and *Rickettsia* spp. sympatric diseases (i.e. diseases occurring in the same geographic region) such as malaria, leptospirosis, typhoid, causes of meningoencephalitis and diverse viruses, including dengue, are important. For acute *C. burnetii* hepatitis and pneumonia and for chronic *C. burnetii* other causes of endocarditis are key.

Diagnosis

The traditional gold standard diagnostic tests for rickettsial pathogens are the indirect immunoperoxidase and immunofluorescent assays (IFA), based on cell-culture-derived antigens, applied to paired admission and convalescent samples. Conventionally, a four-fold rise is regarded as significant and there are woefully few data to inform locally appropriate single-titer cut-offs.[23] These tests are not standardized across laboratories, are subjective, rarely available and cannot influence acute patient management.[24] Epidemic typhus can be diagnosed serologically by IFA, although Western blot combined with cross-adsorption tests is required for differentiation from murine typhus. The old Weil–Felix test (based on detection of antibodies cross-reactive to antigens of strains of *Proteus mirabilis*) has low sensitivity and specificity for all rickettsial groups. Mixed infections of other pathogens with rickettsioses have commonly been described, but care with over-interpretation of serologic tests is required.

Polymerase chain reaction (PCR) methods for detection of the 47 kDa, 56 kDa and GroEL protein genes of *O. tsutsugamushi* have been developed but are not standardized or in widespread use.[25–27] A quantitative real-time PCR assay targeting the *glt*A gene specific for *R. prowazekii* has been developed. PCR-based molecular methods have also been devised for detecting *R. typhi* but careful distinction from congeners in the SFG is needed. As rickettsial bacterial blood density is low, PCR sensitivity is also low. Such issues with serology and PCR suggest that they should be used in combination and that specific antigens should be sought. *O. tsutsugamushi* and *Rickettsia* spp. blood culture takes several weeks, and requires tissue culture techniques in biosafety level 3 facilities. Anti-*O. tsutsugamushi* IgM- and IgG-based rapid diagnostic tests have been developed and show some promise. A dot-blot semi-rapid test has been developed for murine typhus but there are no validated rapid diagnostic tests available. PCR for *O. tsutsugamushi* in swabs of eschars is a promising new technique for the molecular diagnosis of scrub typhus, in those with eschars.

Investigations using a spectrum of new molecular, immunologic and serologic tools have led to the recent dramatic expansion in the number of spotted fever rickettsial species now known to cause human disease.[28] In specialist centers a panel of antigens is used for testing for a range of possible SFG pathogens. Cross-reactivity within the SFG, between the SFG and the typhus group, and with other unrelated pathogens is a problem, so cross-adsorption assays and PCR-based techniques are often required to identify to the species level. A real-time PCR has been developed based on 47 kDa, *glt*A and *omp*B gene targets which will distinguish scrub typhus, typhus group and SFG on admission blood samples.[29]

The diagnosis of Q fever relies mainly on serology.[22] *Coxiella burnetii* exhibits phase variation, and in acute Q fever antibodies to phase II antigens predominate and their titer is higher than the phase I antibody titer. In chronic disease, however, elevated anti-phase I antibodies are uniformly detected. A phase I IgG titer of 800 or greater is one of the major modified Duke criteria for endocarditis. Q fever can also be diagnosed by PCR, though this test is not widely available and has low sensitivity using blood, as with rickettsial disease bacterial blood density is low, but is useful for diagnosis from resected cardiac valves.

Management

Doxycycline remains the mainstay of rickettsial disease management and should be given empirically if the diagnosis is suspected.[30] Unless contraindicated, doxycycline is the standard treatment (usual adult oral dose is 100 mg q12h for 7 days, following a 200 mg loading dose). Tetracycline 500 mg q6h for 7 days may also be used. Given the paucity of clinical trials, *in vitro* susceptibility data, the widespread distribution of these pathogens and the enormous genetic diversity of especially *O. tsutsugamushi*, it is unlikely that one treatment regimen will be appropriate in all communities.

For scrub typhus, trials of shorter courses are underway and azithromycin (500–1000 mg on the first day followed by 250–500 mg daily for 2 days) is an alternative that has been shown to be efficacious in a single dose.[31,32] Azithromycin may be particularly useful if doxy-cyclines are contraindicated, such as in pregnancy. Chloramphenicol is another alternative (500 mg q6h in adults or 50–75 mg/kg/day in children for 7 days).[33] Roxithromycin, telithromycin and rifampin have also been used successfully.[34–36] *O. tsutsugamushi* is intrinsically resistant to fluoroquinolones, and in 1996 doxycycline- and chloramphenicol-resistant scrub typhus was described from northern Thailand.[37,38] There has been a dearth of investigation of this potentially important problem since then.

Patients with suspected *R. prowazeckii* should be given antibiotics immediately. Doxycycline for 3 days or chloramphenicol for 7 days are considered efficacious.[39] In outbreaks a single 200 mg dose of doxycycline appears to be effective.[40] Louse eradication (e.g. in refugee camps or prisons) is the most important preventive measure and is essential in the control of outbreaks. Since body lice live only in clothing, the simplest method of delousing is to remove and destroy, or wash and boil, all clothing. Dusting of all clothing with 10% DDT, 1% malathion or 1% permethrin is also a rapid and effective method of killing body lice and reduces the risk of re-infestation.

The recommended treatment regimen for murine typhus is usually 7 days of doxycycline, but shorter courses may well be as effective – there are no published clinical trials of murine typhus treatment. Chloramphenicol can be used as an alternative and may be useful in pregnancy. Whether azithromycin is an efficacious alternative is currently unknown.

The treatment of choice for spotted fever rickettsioses is doxycycline for 1–7 days depending on the severity of the disease.[41] In children and pregnant women, macrolides including josamycin (50 mg/kg/day in children or 3 g/day in adults), roxithromycin, clarithromycin and azithromycin have all been used successfully for the treatment of Mediterranean spotted fever, as has chloramphenicol. However, there are very few data to inform therapy of this diverse group of pathogens.

There are also very few data to guide antibiotic therapy of severe typhus of any species, but intravenous or nasogastric doxycycline, chloramphenicol or azithromycin are likely to be efficacious. The key intervention is to include these neglected pathogens in the differential diagnosis of severe disease in endemic areas and in returning travelers and to actively consider whether an anti-rickettsial antibiotic should be added.

The treatment of choice for acute Q fever is doxycycline 100 mg 12 hourly for 14 days, though fluoroquinolones may also be used. The treatment of chronic disease is complex, involving long courses of doxycycline and hydroxychloroquine, with surgery if indicated.[42,43]

References available online at expertconsult.com.

KEY REFERENCES

Anderson A., Bijlmer H., Fournier P.E., et al.: Diagnosis and management of Q fever – United States, 2013: recommendations from CDC and the Q Fever Working Group. *MMWR Recomm Rep* 2013; 62(RR–03): 1-30.

Aung A.K., Spelman D.W., Murray R.J., et al.: Rickettsial infections in Southeast Asia: implications for local populace and febrile returned travelers. *Am J Trop Med Hyg* 2014; 91(3):451-460.

Bechah Y., Capo C., Mege J.L., et al.: Epidemic typhus. *Lancet Infect Dis* 2008; 8(7):417-426.

Blacksell S.D., Bryant N.J., Paris D.H., et al.: Scrub typhus serologic testing with the indirect immunofluorescence method as a diagnostic gold standard: a lack of consensus leads to a lot of confusion. *Clin Infect Dis* 2007; 44(3):391-401.

Botelho-Nevers E., Socolovschi C., Raoult D., et al.: Treatment of *Rickettsia* spp. infections: a review. *Expert Rev Anti Infect Ther* 2012; 10(12):1425-1437.

Civen R., Ngo V.: Murine typhus: an unrecognized suburban vectorborne disease. *Clin Infect Dis* 2008; 46(6): 913-918.

Kelly D.J., Fuerst P.A., Ching W.M., et al.: Scrub typhus: the geographic distribution of phenotypic and genotypic variants of *Orientia tsutsugamushi*. *Clin Infect Dis* 2009; 48(Suppl. 3):S203-S230.

Merhej V., Angelakis E., Socolovschi C., et al.: Genotyping, evolution and epidemiological findings of *Rickettsia* species. *Infect Genet Evol* 2014; 25:122-137.

Million M., Raoult D.: Recent advances in the study of Q fever epidemiology, diagnosis and management. *J Infect* 2015; 71(Suppl.1):S2-S9.

Paris D.H., Phetsouvanh R., Tanganuchitcharnchai A., et al.: *Orientia tsutsugamushi* in human scrub typhus eschars shows tropism for dendritic cells and monocytes rather than endothelium. *PLoS Negl Trop Dis* 2012; 6(1):e1466.

Parola P., Paddock C.D., Socolovschi C., et al.: Update on tick-borne rickettsioses around the world: a geographic approach. *Clin Microbiol Rev* 2013; 26(4):657-702.

Vanderburg S., Rubach M.P., Halliday J.E., et al.: Epidemiology of *Coxiella burnetii* infection in Africa: a OneHealth systematic review. *PLoS Negl Trop Dis* 2014; 8(4):e2787.

Watt G., Chouriyagune C., Ruangweerayud R., et al.: Scrub typhus infections poorly responsive to antibiotics in northern Thailand. *Lancet* 1996; 348(9020):86-89.

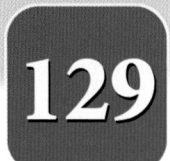

Brucellosis

NICK J. BEECHING | HAKAN ERDEM

Epidemiology

Brucellosis, also known as undulant fever or Malta fever, is a common zoonosis caused by gram-negative bacteria of the genus *Brucella*. The disease exists worldwide, with the highest prevalence in the Mediterranean countries, Asia, Africa and Central and South America. It is increasingly recognized in India, Pakistan and some Pacific countries. Around 500 000 new cases are reported annually worldwide but brucellosis is clearly underreported.[1–3]

Brucellosis is transmitted to humans by direct contact with infected animals, by ingestion of unpasteurized milk or milk products, through cuts and abrasions or by inhalation of aerosols. It is rarely acquired by eating uncooked liver of infected animals, blood transfusion or organ donation. It is common though infrequently diagnosed in pastoral rural populations in Africa and the Middle East. Most cases in Northern Europe or North America are acquired overseas or by consumption of imported unpasteurized cheeses. Otherwise it is mainly an occupational disease in farmers, abattoir workers and butchers. Veterinary surgeons may become infected by accidental inoculation of live attenuated *Brucella* vaccine. Person-to-person transmission (including sexual or perinatal) is extremely rare.

Four *Brucella* spp. can cause infection in humans:

- *B. melitensis*, which is found in goats, sheep and camels, is the most widespread and is the most virulent;
- *B. abortus*, which is found in cattle and camels, is less virulent;
- *B. suis*, which is found in pigs, is also less virulent; and
- *B. canis*, which is found in dogs, is the least common.

In addition, rare cases of human infections with *B. pinnipediae* or *B. cetaceae* have been acquired from marine mammals.

Wildlife such as elk and bison in the USA or feral pigs in Australia may provide a reservoir for brucellosis to infect domesticated animals, hampering eradication programmes.[1]

Pathogenesis

Brucellae are facultative intracellular coccobacilli that are able to survive and multiply within mononuclear phagocytes. The mechanism includes the suppression of degranulation of myeloperoxidase-containing granules, suppression of phagosome–lysosome fusion and production of protective enzymes.

The host reaction to brucellae is the formation of granulomas. *B. melitensis* and *B. suis* cause the most severe disease with caseating granulomas. Granulomas eventually heal with fibrosis and calcification.

Humoral antibodies play some role in protection against re-infection, but immunity is not solid and re-infections can occur. Control of the infection ultimately depends on cell-mediated immunity, but HIV infection does not increase susceptibility to infection or greatly alter clinical manifestations.

Prevention

The prevention of human brucellosis is dependent on the elimination of brucellosis in domestic animals. The use of live veterinary vaccines for *B. abortus* and *B. melitensis* together with pasteurization of milk has resulted in a dramatic decrease in the incidence of human brucellosis. There is no effective vaccine available for *B. suis*. People at high risk of infection, such as veterinary surgeons and abattoir workers, should wear protective clothing. Laboratory-acquired brucellosis can be prevented by adherence to biosafety level 3 precautions. No effective vaccine is available for human use. Travelers to high endemic areas should be advised not to drink unpasteurized milk.

Clinical Features

Brucellosis is a systemic infection that can involve any organ or organ system. The incubation period is normally between 2 and 4 weeks, but it may be months. The onset of clinical disease can be acute or insidious. Subclinical infection has been observed. Brucellosis is characterized by numerous somatic complaints in contrast to the few abnormal physical findings, and is further suggested by the presence of musculoskeletal symptoms in almost half of patients. Hepatosplenomegaly is present in around 25%, depending on the species of *Brucella*, and mild lymphadenopathy is present in 10–20% (more common in children). The nonspecific symptoms (e.g. fever, sweats, anorexia, fatigue, myalgia, malaise, headache and depression) are common and may mimic diseases such as malaria, tuberculosis, toxoplasmosis, mononucleosis, hepatitis, HIV seroconversion, systemic lupus erythematosus, enteric fever and many others.

When symptoms related to a single organ or organ system are dominant, it is often referred to as localized disease.[4,5] The most common complications are listed in Table 129-1. The term 'chronic brucellosis' should be reserved for patients who have complaints of ill health for more than 12 months.[2] This includes patients who have relapsing illness or persisting focal infection and patients complaining of weakness, fatigue and depression, but with no objective signs of infection and no elevation of IgG antibody titer, similar to other chronic fatigue syndromes (see Chapter 70).

TABLE 129-1	Common Complications of Brucellosis	
Organ System		**Patients (%)**
Cardiovascular		1–2
Endocarditis		0–2
Cutaneous		5–10
Gastrointestinal		50–70
Genitourinary		1–5
Orchitis		5–10
Neurologic		2–4
Osteoarticular		20–40
Sacroiliitis		10–15
Spondylitis		8–10
Pulmonary		5–10

COMPLICATIONS

Osteoarticular Complications

Osteoarticular complications affect 20–40% of patients. Sacroiliitis is the most common reported complication, especially when *B. melitensis* predominates.[4,5] The characteristic radiographic findings are blurring of articular margins and widening of the sacroiliac space (Figure 129-1). The clinical presentation is with systemic symptoms and pain.

Spondylitis is most often seen in the lumbosacral region in elderly men, probably reflecting pre-existing anomalies in the spine, and may be complicated by paraspinal abscesses. The main symptoms are fever and vertebral pain. The typical radiographic findings are epiphysitis of vertebrae and narrowing of the intervertebral disc (Figure 129-2). Bone scans and computed tomography (CT) scans detect infection earlier than radiography.

Differential diagnosis includes tuberculosis, fungal and pyogenic osteomyelitis, multiple myeloma and metastatic carcinoma.

Arthritis especially involves the hips, knees and ankles.

Gastrointestinal Complications

Up to 70% of patients have intestinal complaints such as anorexia, nausea, vomiting, abdominal pain, diarrhea or constipation.[4] The liver is probably always involved, but liver function tests are usually only mildly abnormal. Cirrhosis does not seem to follow *Brucella* infection.

Pulmonary Complications

Respiratory symptoms are reported by 15–25% of patients but radiological changes are seen in less than 10%.[6] They range from flu-like symptoms to bronchitis, lobar pneumonia, interstitial pneumonitis, lung abscesses, hilar lymphadenopathy and lung effusions.

Genitourinary Complications

Complications from the genitourinary tract are rare. Acute orchitis or epididymo-orchitis with signs of systemic infection do occur and pyelonephritis resembling tuberculosis has been described, particularly in females. Brucellosis during pregnancy is rare but it can result in abortion like any other systemic infection.

Neurologic Complications

Depression is a common complaint, but invasion of the central nervous system occurs in only 2–4% of cases. It usually presents as acute or chronic meningitis. Encephalitis, polyradiculopathy, psychosis and meningovascular complications have also been described, as well as rarer complex abscesses.[7] Analysis of cerebrospinal fluid reveals elevated protein, lymphocytic pleocytosis, low to normal glucose and most often intrathecally produced specific antibodies. Brucellae are isolated from cerebrospinal fluid in less than 30% of patients.

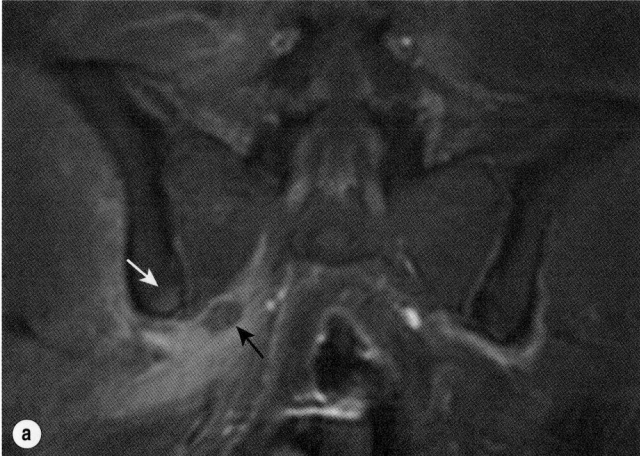
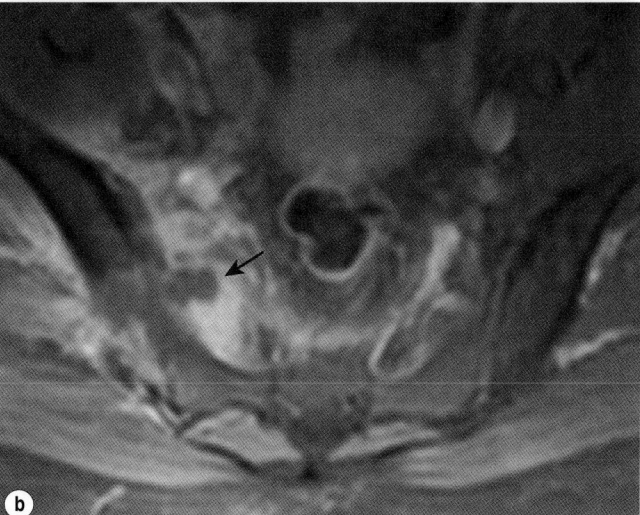

Figure 129-1 MRI showing sacroiliitis: (a) coronal; (b) axial. T1 fat-saturated images obtained after intravenous gadolinium contrast. There is osseous enhancement at the inferior part of the joint (white arrow) and huge soft tissue enhancement surrounding a non-enhancing abscess (black arrow).

Cardiovascular Complications

Endocarditis, although rare, is the main cause of death related to brucellosis.[1,4,5] The aortic valve is involved more often than the mitral valve. Other complications include mycotic aneurysms, myocarditis and pericarditis.

Cutaneous Involvement

Cutaneous manifestations of brucellosis consist mainly of transient nonspecific lesions including erythema nodosum, petechiae, vasculitis, papules and rashes.

Diagnosis

Because the symptoms of brucellosis are nonspecific, it is crucial that the attending physician anticipates the probability of the disease. A certain diagnosis of brucellosis is made when brucellae are isolated from blood, bone marrow or other body fluids or tissues. Traditional blood cultures rarely become positive before 7 days and need to be maintained for up to 42 days to isolate *Brucella* spp. successfully. Modern signaling blood culture systems (e.g. BACTEC) are usually positive within a few days but should not be discarded before 3 weeks. The laboratory must always be warned about possible brucellosis, both so that appropriate safety precautions are taken and also so that any gram-negative coccobacilli isolated are correctly identified, and serologic tests are performed correctly with adequate dilutions (see below). Bone marrow cultures are more sensitive than blood cultures in acute brucellosis and tend to remain positive later in the course of the infection, even during antimicrobial treatment.[8,9] There is limited experience with MALDI-TOF (matrix-assisted laser desorption/ionization time-of-flight mass spectrometry) to identify isolates to species level.[10]

Serologic tests are more sensitive than culture. The serum agglutination test (SAT) remains the best standardized and most widely used serologic test.[8] It measures both IgG and IgM antibodies; antibodies to *Vibrio cholerae*, *Francisella tularensis* and *Yersinia enterocolitica* can give false-positive reactions. False-negative reactions due to blocking IgA antibodies (prozone effect) are seen and dilutions of up to 1:640 should be made. A titer of 1:160 is normally considered positive, as is a fourfold or greater rise in titer. Most patients who have acute infection develop IgM and IgG antibodies. The IgG antibodies persist as long as the infection is active and they increase with relapse and decrease with cure. However, this is not reliable enough to be used to follow up success of treatment or to predict or detect relapse. The enzyme-linked immunosorbent assay (ELISA) is rapid and easy to perform and can be automated, and is preferred in some centres. Rose

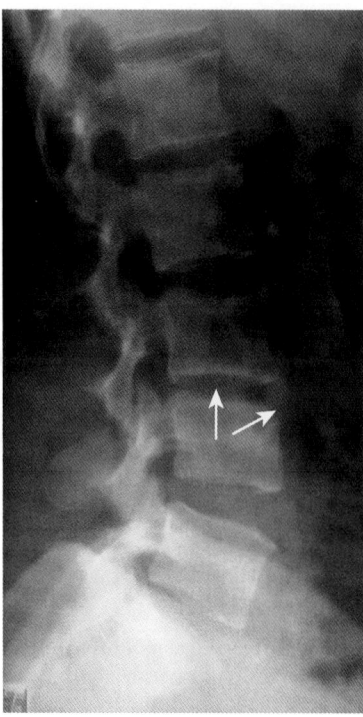

Figure 129-2   Radiograph of the lumbar spine in a patient who has discitis and spondylitis of L3–4 caused by brucellosis. Note the reduced disc space and the destruction of the upper articular margins of L4 (arrows). This contrasts with the severe bone and disc space destruction often seen in tuberculosis. Deformity and/or spinal cord compression are rare in brucellosis.

Bengal serologic tests are used in some centers instead of SAT for screening.[11,12] Polymerase chain reaction (PCR) using several different targets is sensitive and specific in reference laboratories, and should be very useful clinically for initial diagnosis, post-treatment follow-up and early detection of relapses. Unfortunately there is no international standardization of PCR tests and there has been controversy about the significance of continued PCR positivity in chronic infections.[8,11]

Management

Despite several recent meta analyses, there is still variation in treatment approaches.[13-17] As single drug treatment results in a high relapse rate (5–40%), combination therapy is usually recommended. Duration of treatment is normally 6 weeks for uncomplicated, nonfocal infections, extending to 3 months for most other cases. Most relapses are due to poor treatment adherence and/or too-short periods of treatment, rather than antimicrobial resistance.

Doxycycline forms the backbone for all combinations (replaced by trimethoprim–sulfamethoxazole in children). Addition of an aminoglycoside is more effective than addition of rifampin, particularly for prevention of relapse (roughly 5–10% vs 15–20% of cases respectively[13-17]). Gentamicin is often used instead of streptomycin as it has a better safety profile, is more readily available and familiar, and has better bactericidal activity. Fourteen days of streptomycin or gentamicin should be added to 6 weeks or more of doxycycline. There is no evidence that 21 days is superior to 14 days of streptomycin, and limited evidence that more than 7 days of gentamicin is needed if given as an alternative to streptomycin.[13-17] Fluoroquinolones have been disappointing and are usually kept as additional drugs for complex cases. Suggested regimens are summarized in Table 129-2. For post-exposure prophylaxis (e.g. after laboratory exposure), the combination of rifampin and doxycycline for 3 weeks is poorly tolerated and there is no evidence that this is superior to doxycycline alone.[18]

COMPLICATIONS

Complications of brucellosis such as meningitis and endocarditis require prolonged individualized courses of therapy, directed by the response.[19,20] A combination of at least three agents is usually recommended for 3–6 months; there are no prospective trials to demonstrate the shortest effective treatment period. Ceftriaxone is added to doxycycline/rifampin in central nervous system disease, while an aminoglycoside should be added to prolonged doxycycline/rifampin for 2–4 weeks, perhaps together with ceftriaxone or another fourth agent for endocarditis. Endocarditis often requires additional surgical intervention.

With chemotherapy the overall mortality rate is less than 1%.

ACKNOWLEDGMENT

This chapter is an updated version of chapters in previous editions by Finn T. Black.

References available online at expertconsult.com.

TABLE 129-2	Suggested Treatment Regimens for Brucellosis and Its Complications				
	Primary Choices	**Duration***	**Alternative Choices†**	**Duration***
Uncomplicated Brucellosis	Doxycycline 100 mg po twice daily	6 wks	Doxycycline 100 mg po twice daily	6 wks
	plus gentamicin 5 mg/kg iv/im daily	2 wks	*plus* rifampin 600–900 mg (15 mg/kg) once daily	6 wks
	or streptomycin 1 g im daily	2 wks		
Osteoarticular Involvement	Doxycycline 100 mg po twice daily	6–24 wks		
	plus rifampin 600–900 mg (15 mg/kg) po once daily	6–24 wks		
	plus gentamicin 5 mg/kg iv/im daily	2 wks		
	or streptomycin 1 g im daily	2 wks		

TABLE 129-2	**Suggested Treatment Regimens for Brucellosis and Its Complications** (Continued)				
	Primary Choices	**Duration***	**Alternative Choices†**	**Duration***
CNS Brucellosis	Doxycycline 100 mg po twice daily	16–24 wks	Doxycycline 100 mg po twice daily	16–24 wks
	plus rifampin 600–900 mg (15 mg/kg) po once daily	16–24 wks	*plus* rifampin 600–900 mg (15 mg/kg) po once daily	16–24 wks
	plus ceftriaxone 2 g iv twice daily	At least 4 wks	*plus* TMP–SMX 160/800 po twice daily	16–24 wks
Infective Endocarditis	Doxycycline 100 mg po twice daily	16–24 wks	*Consider* 1 mth of antibiotics after surgery	
	plus rifampin 600–900 mg (15 mg/kg) po once daily	16-24 wks		
	plus gentamicin 5 mg/kg iv/im daily	2–4 wks		
	or streptomycin 1 g im daily	2–4 wks		
	Consider adding ‡ceftriaxone 2 g iv daily	4–12 wks		
Genitourinary Involvement	As in the uncomplicated form of the disease			
Pulmonary Involvement	As in the uncomplicated form of the disease			
Hepatitis	As in the uncomplicated form of the disease			
Pregnancy	Rifampin 600–900 mg (15 mg/kg) po once daily	6 wks	Rifampin 600–900 mg (15 mg/kg) po once daily	6 wks
			plus TMP–SMX§ 160/800 mg po twice daily	6 wks
Post-exposure Prophylaxis	Doxycycline 100 mg po twice daily	3wks		
	Consider adding	3 wks		
	Rifampin 600–900 mg (15 mg/kg)			

CNS, central nervous system; TMP–SMX, trimethoprim–sulfamethoxazole.
*The duration should be individualized and can be extended according to clinical assessment.
†TMP–SMX should be used instead of doxycycline in children.
‡TMP–SMX or a fluoroquinolone might be added as fourth or fifth agents.
§>13th week and <36th week of gestation to prevent teratogenicity and kernicterus.

KEY REFERENCES

Dean A.S., Crump L., Greter H., et al.: Clinical manifestations of human brucellosis: a systematic review and meta-analysis. *PLoS Negl Trop Dis* 2012; 6:e1929.

Dean A.S., Crump L., Greter H., et al.: Global burden of human brucellosis: a systematic review of disease frequency. *PLoS Negl Trop Dis* 2012; 6:e1865.

Koruk S.T., Erdem H., Koruk I., et al.: Management of *Brucella* endocarditis: results of the Gulhane study. *Int J Antimicrob Agents* 2012; 40:145-150.

Solís García del Pozo J., Solera J.: Systematic review and meta-analysis of randomized clinical trials in the treatment of human brucellosis. *PLoS ONE* 2012; 7:e32090.

World Health Organization. Brucellosis in humans and animals. Available: www.who.int/csr/resources/publications/Brucellosis.pdf.

Yousefi-Nooraie R., Mortaz-Hejri S., Mehrani M., et al.: Antibiotics for treating human brucellosis. *Cochrane Database Syst Rev* 2012; (10):CD007179.

130

Leptospirosis

NICHOLAS P.J. DAY

KEY CONCEPTS

- Leptospirosis is the most geographically widespread zoonosis, occurring in both tropical and temperate climes, and in urban and rural settings.

- Infection is through exposure to pathogenic spirochetes of the genus *Leptospira* through contact with infected water, soil, or the reservoir mammals.

- Common settings for infection include exposure to infected floodwater, occupational exposure (farmers, abattoir workers, soldiers), and recreational exposure (canoeing, swimming).

- The clinical manifestations of leptospirosis are protean. Most cases are mild or subclinical, but severe and potentially fatal complications include renal failure, pulmonary hemorrhage and myocarditis.

- Reliable laboratory diagnosis is currently difficult and effectively retrospective, so timely management relies on empirical treatment of clinically suspected cases.

- All cases of suspected leptospirosis should be treated with antimicrobials with the aim of reducing the duration of illness and the risk of progression to severe disease.

Epidemiology

Leptospirosis is a geographically widespread zoonotic disease caused by pathogenic spirochetes of the genus *Leptospira*. A variety of wild and domestic mammals, particularly rodents, cattle, pigs, sheep, horses and goats, are the natural hosts. Humans are infected incidentally following exposure to animal urine, contaminated water or soil, or infected animal parts, and, rarely, through ingestion of infected material. Exposure can result from contact with contaminated floodwater (particularly in urban rodent-infested slums), occupational exposure (farmers, abattoir and tannery workers, soldiers, sewerage plant workers, pet traders and laboratory workers), and increasingly through exposure during recreational activities such as triathlons. Leptospirosis is an under-reported disease, and its true global incidence is unknown, though it is thought to be approximately 10 times more common in the tropics than in temperate regions.[1] Modeling conducted by the WHO estimated in 2013 that there are 873 000 cases worldwide annually, with 48 600 deaths.[2]

In most settings members of the rodent family are the most important reservoirs for maintaining transmission. Infection usually occurs during infancy, and infected animals may shed the organism in their urine intermittently or continuously throughout life, resulting in contamination of the environment, particularly water. Most animal infection is asymptomatic, but clinical disease also occurs and may be fatal.

Pathogenesis and Pathology

Leptospires are highly motile, obligate aerobic spirochetal bacteria, about $0.25 \times 6{-}25\ \mu m$ in size (Figure 130-1).[3] They can survive for days or weeks in warm, damp, slightly alkaline conditions, especially in still or slowly moving fresh water in the temperate summer, and in damp soil and water in the tropics, particularly in the rainy season.

On the basis of DNA–DNA hybridization studies the genus *Leptospira* is recognized as containing 21 species. Nine of these are regarded as pathogenic (*Leptospira interrogans, L. kirschneri, L. noguchii, L. alexanderi, L. weilii, L. alstonii, L. borgpetersenii, L. santarosai* and *L. kmetyi*), 5 are of intermediate or unclear pathogenicity (*L. inadai, L. fainei, L. broomii, L. licerasiae* and *L. wolffii*), and the remaining seven are nonpathogenic free-living saprophytic species that do not infect animal hosts (*L. biflexa, L. meyeri, L. wolbachii, L. vanthielii, L. terpstrae, L. yanagawae* and *L. idonii*). An older parallel classification system based on serology identifies more than 200 pathogenic and 60 nonpathogenic saprophytic serovars of *Leptospira*. Some serovars are strongly associated with a particular animal host, such as serovar Hardjo and cattle, and as some serovars are found in more than one species of *Leptospira*, by convention isolates are identified by both species and serovar.

Leptospirosis is a systemic infection with leptospires gaining access to the circulation through abraded skin, or via intact mucous membranes, including the oral cavity and conjunctivae. Transplacental infection can also occur, resulting in fetal death or neonatal infection.[4] Leptospires make their way into the bloodstream without producing any focal lesion at the inoculation site, leading to a bacteremia of as high as 10^6/mL of blood (similar to that seen in the spirochetemia of relapsing fever), and subsequent hematogenous spread to target organs including the liver, lung and kidney.

Histopathological findings include evidence of a systemic vasculitis with endothelial cell injury, with damaged endothelial cells showing varying degrees of swelling, denudation and necrosis. Leptospires are seen in large- and medium-sized blood vessels and in the capillaries and interstitial spaces of various organs. The major affected organs are:

- the kidneys, with a diffuse acute tubular necrosis and interstitial nephritis;

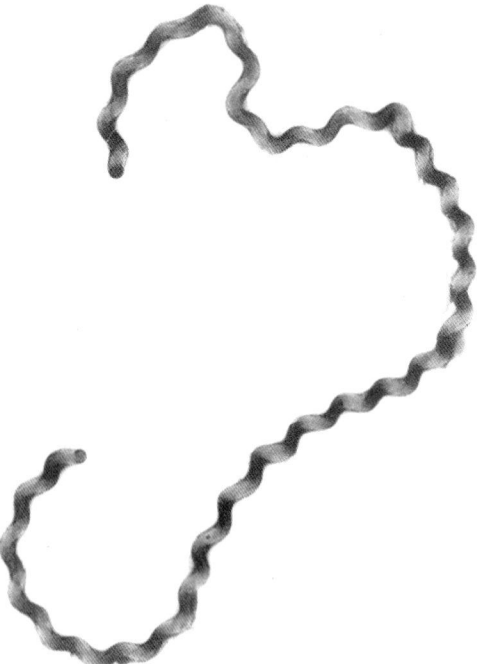

Figure 130-1 Electron micrograph of a leptospire.

- the lungs, usually congested, with focal or massive hemorrhage occurring in both the alveolar septa and intra-alveolar spaces; and
- the liver, which shows cholestasis associated with mild degenerative changes in hepatocytes and leptospiral infiltration of Disse's space and invasion of the perijunctional region between hepatocytes.

Other systems may also be affected, with myocarditis, meningoencephalitis and uveitis all occurring in severe disease. The pathological consequences of infection are probably mediated by a combination of a direct toxic effect of the leptospires and the resulting immune response. Pathogenic leptospires adhere directly to host cells and to the extracellular matrix, and pathogen-associated molecular patterns (PAMPs) including *Leptospira* outer membrane proteins (OMPs) and lipopolysaccharides activate the innate immune response through Toll-like receptor (TLR)2-dependent and TLR4-dependent pathways. In severe leptospirosis levels of pro-inflammatory cytokines are very high, and there is evidence of vigorous inflammasome activation leading to tissue damage, particularly in the kidneys and lungs. Thrombocytopenia and abnormalities of the coagulation system are also commonly seen. During recovery, leptospires continue to be excreted in the urine for some days.

Recent whole genome sequencing of both pathogenic and non-pathogenic *Leptospira* species and serovars have identified a series of genes possibly related to adhesion, invasion and the hematological changes that characterize leptospirosis, allowing in-depth studies of virulence and pathogenesis.

Prevention

Prevention measures are based on local knowledge of the epidemiology of the disease, and include avoidance of potential sources of infection such as animal farm water runoff and stagnant water, control of rodent populations, animal vaccination and antimicrobial prophylaxis with doxycycline 200 mg weekly for individuals at high risk of exposure.[5,6] No human vaccine is currently available.

Clinical Features

The clinical manifestations of leptospirosis are highly variable. Most cases are mild and self-limiting or subclinical, while some are severe and potentially fatal. Leptospirosis is classically described as a biphasic illness, with an acute bacteremic phase followed by an 'immune' phase characterized by leptospiruria, a rise in IgM antibodies, and the onset of severe complications such as jaundice, renal failure and pulmonary hemorrhage. Clinically, however, the two phases usually merge, particularly in severe disease. Following an incubation period of 2–26 days (usually 7–12 days), the acute phase of the illness generally presents with an abrupt onset of fever, rigors, headache and myalgias. Nausea, vomiting, diarrhea, abdominal pain, arthralgia and nonproductive cough may also occur. Conjunctival suffusion is common, and useful diagnostically when differentiating leptospirosis from other common causes of fever. Other clinical signs include muscle tenderness (particularly of the calves, abdomen and paraspinal region), splenomegaly, lymphadenopathy, pharyngitis, hepatomegaly, muscle rigidity, abnormal respiratory auscultation and skin rash.

In mild disease defervescence occurs after 3–9 days. In more severe disease the second or 'immune' phase begins either immediately or 2–3 days later, with fever recrudescence and signs of meningitis in 50–85% of cases. Optic neuritis, peripheral neuropathy and prolonged uveitis can also occur. Severe, potentially fatal illness characterized by jaundice and renal failure ('Weil's disease') occurs in a minority of patients, and a coagulopathy may develop with pulmonary hemorrhage as a potential complication.[7] Uveitis, acute respiratory distress syndrome, myocarditis and rhabdomyolysis may also occur.

Renal failure complicating leptospirosis is associated with hypokalemia and is often non-oliguric. Supportive renal replacement therapy may be required, though if the patient survives, renal recovery is generally complete.[8] The liver failure of leptospirosis is generally reversible and not a cause of death. Vasculitic necrosis of extremities is occasionally seen in severe cases.

Mortality rates in hospitalized patients range from 4 to 52%. Predictors of death include pulmonary involvement and central nervous system disease.[9]

Diagnosis

Leptospirosis may be difficult to distinguish from other infectious causes of fever, and a high index of suspicion is required based on the local epidemiology. Clinical and laboratory features may be nonspecific, and specific laboratory tests either take several weeks or are unavailable. Depending on the setting, the differential diagnosis includes malaria, dengue, scrub typhus and other rickettsial illnesses, ehrlichiosis and acute viral infections such as influenza. Conjunctival suffusion is rare in these conditions and is therefore one of the few diagnostically useful clinical signs. Hantavirus infection can mimic severe leptospirosis, causing hepatorenal syndrome and pulmonary hemorrhage.

Routine blood tests are usually nonspecific, with hyponatremia, mild to moderately increased transaminases, mildly raised white blood cell count, and thrombocytopenia all common. An elevated creatine kinase may be suggestive of leptospirosis, occurring in around 50% of patients. Urinalysis often shows proteinuria, pyuria and granular casts, and occasionally microscopic hematuria.

There is no adequate gold standard test for the diagnosis of leptospirosis, with the microagglutination test (MAT) and bacterial culture both imperfect in terms of sensitivity, even when combined.[10] The MAT is the most commonly used diagnostic test, and when applied to paired acute and convalescent samples is considered the reference standard; but it is complex to perform, serovar-dependent and restricted to reference centers. Recently developed serology-based rapid diagnostic tests perform variably in the field, particularly in endemic areas.[11] PCR-based molecular tests show considerable promise for rapid, accurate diagnosis but are not yet widely available. Pathogenic *Leptospira* spp. can be grown *in vitro* from clinical specimens including blood, urine and cerebrospinal fluid (CSF), though special media are required. Growth is usually observed in 1–2 weeks, but may take up to 3 months. A method of growing leptospires on solid agar (LVW media) has been developed recently, which facilitates more rapid growth, isolation of single colonies, and simplified antimicrobial sensitivity testing.[12]

In summary, timely diagnosis of leptospirosis remains problematic, and the emphasis should be on early empirical treatment of clinically suspected cases.

Management

Most cases of leptospirosis are self-limiting, and whether antimicrobials have a beneficial effect in mild disease has been the subject of controversy. However, the evidence increasingly supports the antimicrobial treatment of all patients suspected of having leptospirosis, both to reduce the duration of illness and to prevent progression to severe disease.[13,14]

For mild leptospirosis, doxycycline (200 mg initially then 100 mg twice a day for 7 days) and azithromycin (2 g then 1 g once a day for 2 further days) have been shown to be equally effective, though the latter was better tolerated. Both have the advantage of being effective against scrub typhus and other rickettsial diseases and therefore useful as empirical treatment in areas where both leptospirosis and rickettsioses are common causes of undifferentiated fever. For children under 8 years old and pregnant women azithromycin (or amoxicillin) is preferable and doxycycline should not be used.

For suspected severe leptospirosis 7 days' treatment with parenteral penicillin (1.5 million units four times a day), ceftriaxone (1 g once a day), cefotaxime (1 g four times a day) or doxycycline (200 mg initially then 100 mg twice a day) have all been shown to be equally effective.[13,15,16]

In severe cases, supportive care with renal replacement therapy (hemofiltration, hemodiafiltration or hemodialysis), ventilatory support and transfusion of blood products may also be required. Given the vasculitic nature of the disease adjunctive therapy with corticosteroids has been suggested, but there is currently insufficient evidence to recommend this routinely.

References available online at expertconsult.com.

KEY REFERENCES

Abela-Ridder B., Bertherat E., Durski K., on behalf of the World Health Organization Leptospirosis Epidemiology Reference Group: *Global burden of human leptospirosis and cross-sectoral interventions for its prevention and control.* Bangkok, Thailand: Prince Mahidol Award Conference; 2013.

Brett-Major D.M., Coldren R.: Antibiotics for leptospirosis. *Cochrane Database Syst Rev* 2012; (2):CD008264.

Hartskeerl R.A., Collares-Pereira M., Ellis W.A.: Emergence, control and re-emerging leptospirosis: dynamics of infection in the changing world. *Clin Microbiol Infect* 2011; 17:494-501.

Limmathurotsakul D., Turner E.L., Wuthiekanun V., et al.: Fool's gold: why imperfect reference tests are undermining the evaluation of novel diagnostics: a reevaluation of 5 diagnostic tests for leptospirosis. *Clin Infect Dis* 2012; 55:322-331.

McClain J.B., Ballou W.R., Harrison S.M., et al.: Doxycycline therapy for leptospirosis. *Ann Intern Med* 1984; 100:696-698.

Panaphut T., Domrongkitchaiporn S., Vibhagool A., et al.: Ceftriaxone compared with sodium penicillin G for treatment of severe leptospirosis. *Clin Infect Dis* 2003; 36:1507-1513.

Sehgal S.C., Sugunan A.P., Murhekar M.V., et al.: Randomized controlled trial of doxycycline prophylaxis against leptospirosis in an endemic area. *Int J Antimicrob Agents* 2000; 13:249-255.

Takafuji E.T., Kirkpatrick J.W., Miller R.N., et al.: An efficacy trial of doxycycline chemoprophylaxis against leptospirosis. *N Engl J Med* 1984; 310:497-500.

Tubiana S., Mikulski M., Becam J., et al.: Risk factors and predictors of severe leptospirosis in New Caledonia. *PLoS Negl Trop Dis* 2013; 7:e1991.

Wuthiekanun V., Amornchai P., Paris D.H., et al.: Rapid isolation and susceptibility testing of *Leptospira* spp. using a new solid medium, LVW agar. *Antimicrob Agents Chemother* 2013; 57:297-302.

Relapsing Fevers

DAVID A. WARRELL

- Relapsing fever group *Borrelia* spirochetes are genetically distinct from Lyme disease group *Borrelia*. They are widely distributed across Europe, Africa, Asia and the Americas and are the most frequent cause of bacterial infection in Africa.

- Clinically, the defining characteristic is repeated abrupt episodes of fever lasting 1–3 days, separated by afebrile periods of 3–10 days.

- Each febrile episode is associated with spirochetemia with an antigenically distinct population of the *Borrelia* species that is eliminated within a few days by specific IgM antibodies.

- Relapse strains are generated by rearrangements of the genes encoding the dominant outer surface variable major protein antigens, leading to evasion of the antibody response and relapse of symptoms.

- *Borrelia recurrentis* causes louse-borne relapsing fever, transmitted by human body lice. It has been responsible for several devastating historical pandemics.

- Tick-borne relapsing fever is caused by more than 20 *Borrelia* species, most of which are zoonotic infections, usually transmitted by soft (argasid) ticks that may also be reservoirs.

- Major pathophysiologic effects include high fever, coagulopathy with severe hemorrhagic diathesis, hepatic dysfunction, neurologic effects and transient immune-compromise that allows secondary infections by *Salmonella* and other pathogens.

- Essential antibiotic treatment is frequently complicated by severe Jarisch–Herxheimer reactions.

Epidemiology

TICK-BORNE RELAPSING FEVER

David Livingstone described fatal tick-borne fever in Angola in 1857, whose cause, tick-borne relapsing fever, is now known to be endemic in most temperate and tropical countries except in South and Far East Asia, Australasia, the Pacific, Arctic and Antarctic regions. Relapsing fever is the most frequent bacterial infection in Africa, and in the West African savanna region, *B. crocidurae* is the most prevalent bacterial infection, creating a medical problem second only to malaria.[1] It has increased during the recent drought. In parts of East Africa, *B. duttonii* is an important cause of abortion and perinatal mortality.[2] In North and West Africa, *Borrelia crocidurae*, *B. hispanica* and *B. merionesi* spirochetes responsible for relapsing fever in humans are prevalent in at least nine species of *Ornithodoros* ticks, and in small rodents and insectivores. South of latitude 13°N, longitude 01°E, these ticks are absent and small mammals are not infected.[1]

Borrelia–Tick Complexes

Spirochetes have been identified in a larval *Amblyomma* tick in fossilized amber from the Dominican Republic, dated at 15–20 million years old. Different species of *Borrelia* spirochetes are transmitted by particular species of soft ticks of the genus *Ornithodoros* (Argasidae) in

different parts of the world (Table 131-1). These ticks are found in dry savanna areas and scrub, particularly near rodent burrows, caves, piles of timber and dead trees, or in cracks and crevices in walls, roof spaces and beneath the floors of log cabins, anywhere inhabited by small rodents. Unlike louse-borne relapsing fever, tick-borne relapsing fevers are zoonoses with the exception of *B. duttonii* infection. Vertebrate reservoir species are rodents such as rats, gerbils, mice, squirrels and chipmunks, and also dogs and birds. Ticks ingest spirochetes while sucking blood from infected animals or humans. They attack at night, remaining attached for less than 30 minutes before returning to their hiding places. Infection is either by a bite, through infected saliva, or by contaminating mucosal membranes with infected coxal fluid. Borreliae are not excreted in tick feces. Ticks remain infected for life, even while starved of blood for as long as 7 years. Spirochetes can be transmitted transstadially, through successive stages of development of the tick; venereally from male to female ticks; and transovarially, by females to their progeny (except, perhaps, ticks of the *O. moubata* complex).

Borrelia miyamotoi was first described in Japan in 1995. Recently it was recognized as a human pathogen in the relapsing fever group of *Borrelia*. It is prevalent in hard ticks (Ixodidae), such as *Ixodes persulcatus* in Russia, *I. ricinus* in Western Europe and *I. scapularis* and *I. pacificus* in the USA. These ticks are also vectors of Lyme disease group *Borrelia*.[3]

TABLE 131-1	Geographic Distribution of some Important *Borrelia* and *Ornithodoros* spp.	
Borrelia spp.	**Ornithodoros spp.**	**Geographic Distribution**
NEW WORLD TICK-BORNE RELAPSING FEVER BORRELIAE		
B. hermsii	O. hermsi	Canada, Central and Western United States, Mexico
B. turicatae	O. turicata	Southwestern United States, Mexico
B. parkeri	O. parkeri	Western United States, Baja California
B. mazzotti	O. talaje	Mexico, Central America
B. venezuelensis	O. (venezuelensis) rudis	Colombia, Venezuela, Argentina, Bolivia, Paraguay
OLD WORLD TICK-BORNE RELAPSING FEVER BORRELIAE		
B. duttonii	O. moubata	Sub-Saharan Africa
B. crocidurae	O. (erraticus) sonrai	West, North, East Africa, Middle East
B. persica	O. tholozani	Middle East, Central Asia from Uzbekistan to western China
B. hispanica	O. erraticus	Iberian peninsula, Greece, Cyprus, North Africa
B. latyschewi	O. tartakowskyi	Eastern Europe, Iran, Iraq, Afghanistan
B. caucasia	O. asperus	Iraq, Eastern Europe

LOUSE-BORNE RELAPSING FEVER

Obermeier saw spirochetes in the blood of febrile patients in Berlin in 1866, now recognized to be *Borrelia recurrentis*, the cause of louse-borne relapsing fever. The incidence of this classic epidemic disease of armies, refugees and migrants has fallen in the last decade, but it remains endemic and seasonally epidemic in the highlands of Ethiopia and adjacent areas of Sudan and Somalia, hilly areas of Yemen and perhaps some parts of the Peruvian and Bolivian Andes.[4] In 2015, louse-borne relapsing fever was diagnosed in Germany, the Netherlands and Sicily in refugees from the Horn of Africa.[5] The human body louse, *Pediculus humanus humanus*, is an obligate blood-sucking human ectoparasite that ingests borreliae while feeding, but the role of head lice (*P. h. capitis*) remains controversial.[6] Infection follows scratching, which crushes lice so that their celomic fluid or feces are inoculated through broken skin or intact mucous membranes such as the conjunctiva. Unlike ticks, lice cannot infect their progeny. Humans are the only reservoirs of this infection.

Louse-borne relapsing fever thrives in the highlands of Ethiopia during the rainy season when impoverished people, encouraged to wear clothes by the cold wet climate, are crowded together and become heavily infested with lice. More than 20 000 lice were recovered from the clothes of one infected person.

OTHER MODES OF INFECTION

As well as transmission by arthropods, *Borrelia* may also be transmitted by needlestick, blood transfusion and transplacentally.

Pathogenesis and Pathology

In mouse models, *B. hermsii* infection induces expansion of a population of B1b cells that persists for extended periods after clearance of spirochetemia, and is responsible for resistance to reinfection.[7] Relapsing fever spirochetes in the blood are lysed by specific bactericidal IgM antibodies, independent of complement and T cells. However, some spirochetes persist extracellularly in various organs: spleen, liver, kidneys, eye and especially in the brain and cerebrospinal fluid. Relapse of spirochetemia and symptoms is explained by antigenic variation, which has been investigated mainly in *B. hermsii*.[8] Transposition of silent gene sequences from an archive stored in extrachromosomal plasmids and their recombination and expression on a linear plasmid results in the synthesis of a new major outer membrane lipoprotein. The spirochete possesses virulence and protective factors. *B. hermsii* surface protein CRASP-1 binds factor H (FH), FHR-1 and plasminogen. FH protects against opsonophagocytosis by inhibiting C3b. Plasminogen is bound and activated to plasmin, stimulating fibrinolysis that promotes spread. Erythrocyte rosetting shields spirochetes physically from host antibody.[9] Fibronectin-binding proteins, such as BHA007, are immunogenic and may interact with the complement system. Antigenic variation generates isogenic serotypes with properties such as enhanced invasiveness for cerebral vascular endothelium.

Prevention

TICK-BORNE RELAPSING FEVER

Tick infestation of dwellings can be reduced by improved house construction (e.g. rodent-proofing of cabins on the North Rim of the Grand Canyon), control of peridomestic rodent hosts and use of residual insecticides (pyrethroids, benzene hexachloride, lambda-cyhalothrin, malathion or dichlorodiphenyltrichloroethane – DDT). Travelers should avoid sleeping in places where ticks and rodents are abundant, such as poorly maintained log cabins, and should apply repellents to their skin (*N,N*-diethyl-*m*-toluamide – DEET). Postexposure prophylaxis with doxycycline (200 mg followed by 100 mg on the next 4 days) has proved effective against *B. persica* in Israel.[10]

LOUSE-BORNE RELAPSING FEVER

Infested clothing should be de-loused using heat (>60 °C), chlorine bleach or insecticide (10% DDT, 1% malathion, 2% temephos, 1% propoxur or 0.5% permethrin) and patients should be bathed with soap and 1% cresol (Lysol). Lice are abundant in hair, which should be washed or shaved off. Breaking transmission from lice to the susceptible population is essential for the control of an epidemic.

Clinical Features

TICK-BORNE RELAPSING FEVER

Ticks bite painlessly and detach after only a short feed and infection produces no eschar, unless there is a rickettsial coinfection, so exposure usually passes unnoticed.[11] After an incubation period of 3–18 days, the illness starts with sudden fever, chills, headache, muscle and joint pains, extreme fatigue, prostration and drenching sweats.[4] Epistaxis, abdominal pain, diarrhea, cough and erythematous or petechial rashes may follow. Up to 80% of patients may develop neurologic disturbances reminiscent of those in Lyme disease. These are most common with *B. duttonii* and *B. turicatae* and least common with *B. persica*, *B. hispanica*, and *B. hermsii* infections. Paresthesiae, visual symptoms, lymphocytic meningitis, cranial nerve palsies (especially VII), encephalitis, radiculomyelitis, delirium, hallucinations and nightmares are described. Ocular complications include iritis, cyclitis, choroiditis and optic neuritis.[12] Several cases of adult respiratory distress syndrome (ARDS) have been described in the USA.

The density of spirochetemia determines clinical severity. Symptoms abate after a few days, only to recur about 7–15 days later. As many as eight relapses may follow, becoming sequentially less severe. Abortion and perinatal mortality is common. In one study in Tabora, Tanzania, parturition was precipitated in 58% of infected pregnant women. Perinatal mortality was 436/1000 births; its risk related to low birth-weight and gestational age. The total loss of pregnancies including abortions was 475/1000. Spirochetemia was higher in pregnant than nonpregnant women.[2]

BORRELIA MIYAMOTOI INFECTION

Forty-six patients confirmed by polymerase chain reaction (PCR) in Yekaterinburg in the Russian Urals, were compared with local (*B. garinii*) and USA (*B. burgdorferi*) cases of Lyme disease.[13] Incubation period (12–16 days from tick bite) was longer for *B. miyamotoi* and systemic symptoms were more common. Maximum temperature (39.5 °C) was higher, headache and chills more common, but erythema migrans (9%) (none multiple) was far less frequent than with *B. garinii* or *B. burgdorferi* infections and arthralgia was less common than with *B. burgdorferi*. Relapsing fevers were detected in 11%. Other features included fatigue, myalgia, nausea, vomiting, neck stiffness, proteinuria, elevated hepatic transferases, leukopenia and thrombocytopenia. Tick-borne encephalitis virus, *B. garinii* and *B. afzelii* were found in the same *I. persulcatus* and *I. ricinus* ticks, creating the possibility of co-infections. Three cases of *B. miyamotoi* infection have been detected in the northeastern USA, an area endemic for other *I. scapularis*-borne infections: Lyme disease, babesiosis and human granulocytic anaplasmosis (ehrlichiosis). Two of the patients had clinical features similar to those reported from Russia[14] but the third, an elderly immunocompromised woman developed meningoencephalitis with deteriorating consciousness. Spirochetes were visible in her CSF.[15] Another elderly immunocompromised patient with meningoencephalitis was diagnosed in the Netherlands.[16] All these patients recovered completely after appropriate antibiotic treatment. Antibody against *B. miyamotoi* GlpQ protein was found in a number of patients in the same area, who had been screened for tick-borne infections including Lyme disease.[17]

LOUSE-BORNE RELAPSING FEVER[4]

After an incubation period of 4–17 (average 7) days, the first symptoms are fever, chills, headache, muscle and body aches, fatigue, dizziness, anorexia and nightmares. At least 50% of patients develop bleeding: epistaxis, subconjunctival hemorrhage (Figure 131-1) or petechial hemorrhages, especially on the trunk (Figure 131-2). An enlarged and tender liver, often with an enlarged spleen (Figure 131-3), is palpable in as many as 50% of cases in some outbreaks, and about half of these

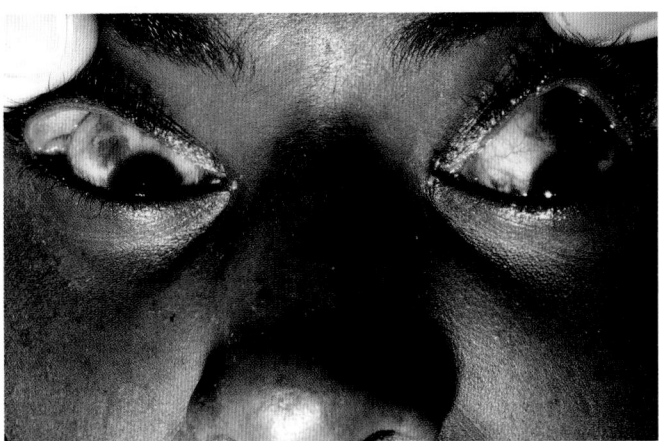

Figure 131-1 Subconjunctival hemorrhages and jaundice in an Ethiopian patient with louse-borne relapsing fever. *(Copyright D.A. Warrell.)*

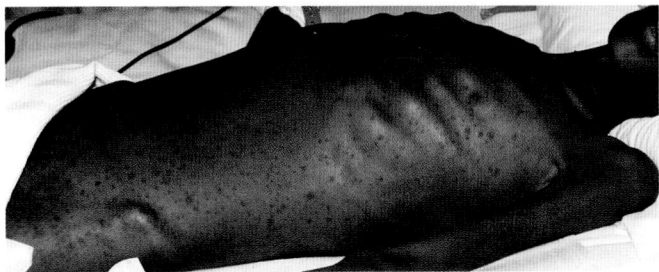

Figure 131-2 Petechial hemorrhages in an Ethiopian patient suffering from louse-borne relapsing fever complicated by typhoid. *(Copyright D.A. Warrell.)*

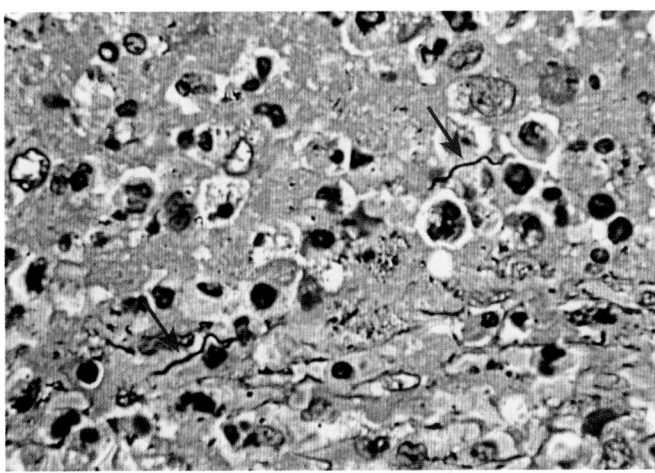

Figure 131-3 Spirochetes demonstrated in spleen in a fatal case of louse-borne relapsing fever in Ethiopia. *(Courtesy of Dr Ken Fleming.)*

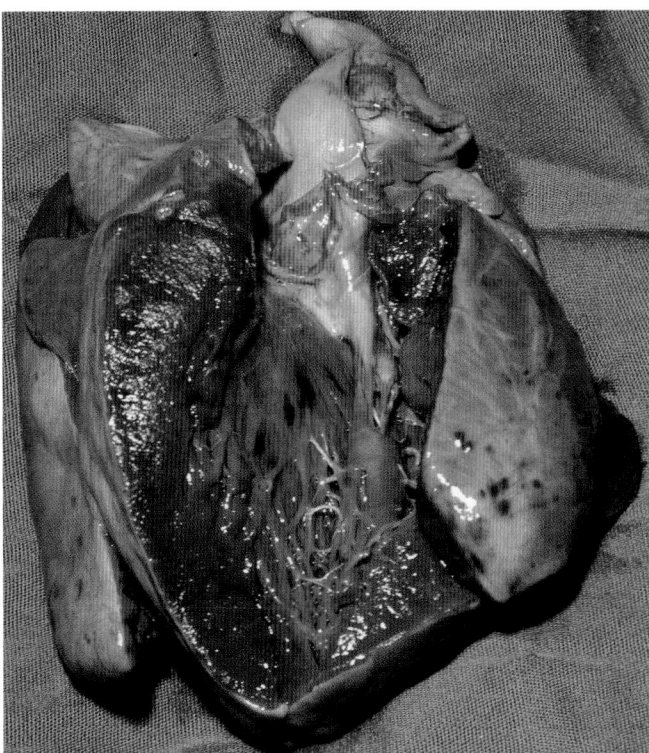

Figure 131-4 Epicardial and endocardial petechiae in a fatal case of louse-borne relapsing fever in Ethiopia. *(Copyright D.A. Warrell.)*

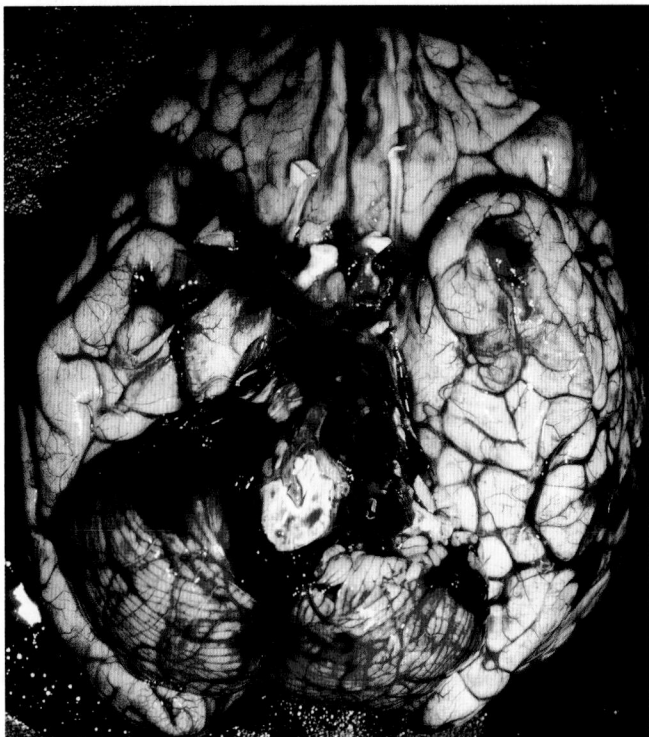

Figure 131-5 Fatal cerebral hemorrhage in louse-borne relapsing fever. *(Copyright D.A. Warrell.)*

are jaundiced. The respiratory system is affected in about 15% of cases. Cough may indicate pneumonia or acute pulmonary edema. Myocardial damage (Figure 131-4) may lead to acute left ventricular failure with pulmonary edema. Neurologic signs are less common than in tick-borne relapsing fever. Confusion or coma suggests circulatory failure, cerebral hemorrhage (Figure 131-5) or hepatic failure. Fetal loss is very common in pregnant women.

SPONTANEOUS CRISIS AND JARISCH–HERXHEIMER REACTION[18]

The clinical course of relapsing fever, especially louse-borne, usually ends either with a 'spontaneous crisis' on about day 5 of the untreated illness, associated with immune clearance of spirochetemia, or by a Jarisch–Herxheimer reaction (J-HR) that resembles a triphasic endotoxin reaction. About 1–3 hours after antibiotic treatment, the patient becomes restless. Violent rigors signal the chill phase associated with rapid increases in temperature, respiratory rate, pulse rate and blood

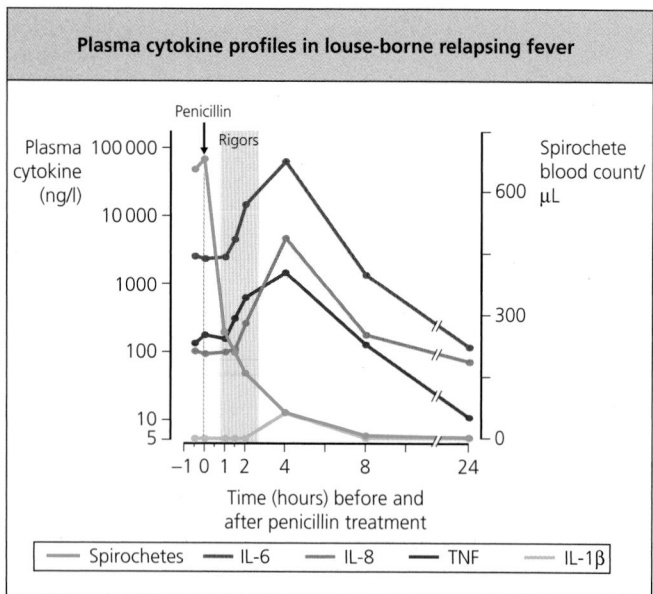

Figure 131-6 Plasma cytokine profiles in a patient with louse-borne relapsing fever during the Jarisch–Herxheimer reaction to penicillin treatment. *(Copyright D.A. Warrell.)*

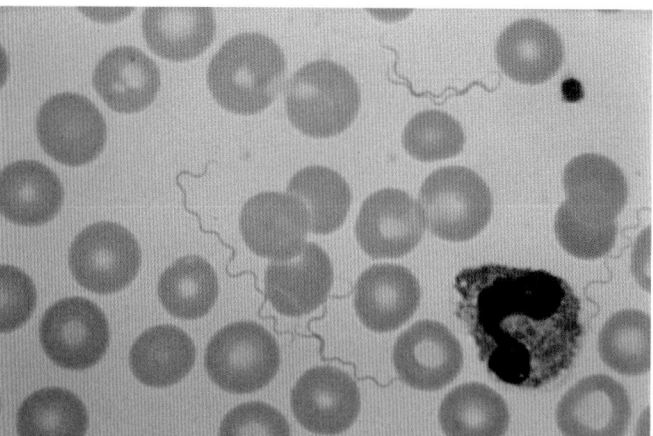

Figure 131-7 Spirochetes of *Borrelia recurrentis* in a thin blood film. *(Copyright D.A. Warrell.)*

pressure. There may be associated vomiting, diarrhea, coughing, musculoskeletal pains and delirium. Some patients die of hyperpyrexia at the height of the fever. During flush phase, there is profuse sweating, intense vasodilation and a fall in mean arterial pressure, and a slow decline in temperature over the next 6–12 hours during the recovery phase. Fatalities during this phase are due to hypovolemic shock or acute pulmonary edema resulting from myocarditis, sometimes precipitated by the patient getting out of bed and standing up. The incidence of Jarisch–Herxheimer reactions varies from 30% to almost 100% in different published reports of patients who were carefully observed.

A borrelial pyrogen, an outer membrane variable major lipoprotein[19] released by the action of antimicrobial agents, stimulates an explosive release of cytokines from macrophages through nuclear factor kappa B (NF-κB), principally tumor necrosis factor (TNF), interleukin (IL)-6, IL-8 and IL-1β, just before the start of the clinical manifestations of the Jarisch–Herxheimer reaction (Figure 131-6).[20] The reaction is unaffected by corticosteroids, but is delayed by the opiate agonist–antagonist meptazinol and can be prevented by a polyclonal antibody against TNF if this is given just before antibiotic treatment.

Laboratory Findings

There is a peripheral neutrophil leukocytosis but, during the Jarisch–Herxheimer reaction or spontaneous crisis, leukocytes almost disappear transiently from the peripheral blood. Thrombocytopenia is common and there is a coagulopathy attributable partly to hepatic dysfunction and partly to disseminated intravascular coagulation with increased fibrinolytic activity. Biochemical evidence of hepatocellular damage is found in most patients.[21] A few patients show transient, mild renal impairment. In tick-borne relapsing fever patients with meningism, a mild mononuclear cell pleocytosis has been described with associated mild increase in protein concentration.

Diagnosis

In patients with acute fevers who have been traveling in tropical countries it is essential to examine thick and thin blood films for malarial parasites. This may reveal relapsing fever spirochetes. Misidentification of microgametes of *Plasmodium vivax* has led to the diagnosis of 'pseudo-borreliosis'. Spirochetes are best demonstrated with Giemsa or Wright's stain, counterstained with 1% crystal violet (Figure 131-7).

Thick films have a 20-fold higher sensitivity than thin films. In louse-borne relapsing fever, spirochete density in peripheral blood may exceed 500 000/μL. In tick-borne relapsing fever, spirochetes may be difficult or impossible to find, even at the height of a relapse and, increasingly, PCR[22] and serology are being used. In Senegal, only 15% of patients positive for *Borrelia* by reverse transcription (RT)-PCR were detected by microscopy of thick films in hospital clinics and only 56% by expert microscopists.[23] ELISA, using the GlpQ gene product, can distinguish relapsing fever from Lyme disease.[24] In louse-borne relapsing fever, the higher and more persistent spirochetemia is more easily detected.

In vitro culture of borreliae, including *B. recurrentis*, *B. duttonii* and *B. crocidurae*, is now possible, using Barbour–Stoenner–Kelly medium.[25]

DIFFERENTIAL DIAGNOSIS

In a febrile patient with jaundice, petechial rash, spontaneous systemic bleeding and hepatosplenomegaly, the following differential diagnoses should be considered, depending on the geographic location: falciparum malaria, yellow fever and other viral hemorrhagic fevers (such as Rift Valley fever in the Horn of Africa), viral hepatitis, rickettsial infections (especially louse-borne typhus which has the same epidemiologic predispositions as louse-borne relapsing fever) and leptospirosis. Secondary infections, known to complicate louse-borne relapsing fever, include bacillary dysentery, salmonellosis, typhoid, typhus, malaria and tuberculosis. In Europe and Asia, differential diagnoses include other tick-borne infections such as Lyme disease, rickettsioses, babesiosis and tick-borne viral encephalitides. In North America, in addition, human anaplasmoses and ehrlichioses should also be considered, together with Colorado tick fever in the northwest.

In the differential diagnosis of travelers at risk, two less common causes of episodic recurrent fever are trench fever (caused by *Bartonella quintana*) if there was possible contact with lice, or rat-bite fever (caused by *Spirillum minus*).

Prognosis

Reported case fatalities during *B. recurrentis* epidemics have exceeded 40% but this can be reduced to less than 5% with antimicrobial treatment, provided that appropriate ancillary treatment is given during the life-threatening Jarisch–Herxheimer reaction. Tick-borne relapsing fever is less dangerous. Deaths during relapses are most unusual but have been reported in tick-borne relapsing fever.

Management

The principles of treatment are:

- to eliminate spirochetemia and prevent relapses, using antibiotics;

- to monitor the patient very carefully through the Jarisch–Herxheimer reaction; and
- to restore and maintain circulating volume during the 24 hours after starting antibiotic treatment.

ANTIBIOTIC AGENTS

The choice of agents is based on clinical experience.[26]

Tick-Borne Relapsing Fever

Doxycycline 100 mg per day for 10 days is recommended for adults. For pregnant women and young children, erythromycin can be used.

Borrelia miyamotoi Infection

Oral doxycycline 100 mg twice daily for 2 weeks or ceftriaxone 2 g daily intravenously for 2 weeks has proved effective.

Louse-Borne Relapsing Fever

A single 500 mg oral dose of tetracycline or erythromycin stearate is effective. In severely ill patients who are likely to vomit, effective parenteral treatment consists of either a single intravenous dose of tetracycline hydrochloride (250 mg)[27] or, for pregnant women and children, a single intravenous dose of erythromycin lactobionate (300 mg for adults, 10 mg/kg for children). In mixed epidemics of louse-borne relapsing fever and louse-borne typhus, a single oral dose of doxycycline 100 mg has proved effective.[28] Penicillins and chloramphenicol are also effective.[26,27] Some experienced clinicians prefer to use a low dose of penicillin (adult dose, 100 000–400 000 units by intramuscular injection) in severe cases and pregnant women because they believe that the incidence and severity of the Jarisch–Herxheimer reaction will be less although the risk of relapse is greater.

SUPPORTIVE TREATMENT

Postural hypotension and cardiac arrhythmias are prevented by nursing the patient flat in bed for 24 hours after antibiotic treatment. Hyperpyrexia and hypovolemia must be prevented. Acute heart failure with pulmonary edema responds to intravenous furosemide and digoxin. Bleeding and clotting problems are treated with vitamin K, platelets and clotting factor concentrates. Complicating infections, notably typhoid, salmonellosis, bacillary dysentery, tuberculosis, malaria and typhus in some endemic situations, must be treated appropriately.

References available online at expertconsult.com.

KEY REFERENCES

Barbour A.G., Dai Q., Restrepo B.I., et al.: Pathogen escape from host immunity by a genome program for antigenic variation. *Proc Natl Acad Sci USA* 2006; 103(48):18290-18295.

Bryceson A.D.M., Parry E.H.O., Perine P.L., et al.: Louse-borne relapsing fever: a clinical and laboratory study of 62 cases in Ethiopia and a reconsideration of the literature. *Q J Med* 1970; 39:129-170.

Fekade D., Knox K., Hussein K., et al.: Prevention of Jarisch–Herxheimer reactions by treatment with antibodies against tumor necrosis factor α. *N Engl J Med* 1996; 335:311-315.

Negussie Y., Remick D.G., De Forge L.E., et al.: Detection of plasma tumor necrosis factor, interleukin 6 and 8 during the Jarisch–Herxheimer reaction of relapsing fever. *J Exp Med* 1992; 175:1207-1212.

Perine P.L., Teklu B.: Antibiotic treatment of louse-borne relapsing fever in Ethiopia: a report of 377 cases. *Am J Trop Med Hyg* 1983; 32:1096-1100.

Platonov A.E., Karan L.S., Kolyasnikova N.M., et al.: Humans infected with relapsing fever spirochete *Borrelia miyamotoi*, Russia. *Emerg Infect Dis* 2011; 17:1816-1823.

Trape J.F., Diatta G., Arnathau C., et al.: The epidemiology and geographic distribution of relapsing fever borreliosis in west and north Africa, with a review of the *Ornithodoros erraticus* complex (Acari: Ixodida). *PLoS ONE* 2013; 8:e78473.

Vidal V., Scragg I.G., Cutler S.J., et al.: Variable major lipoprotein is a principal TNF-inducing factor of louse-borne relapsing fever. *Nat Med* 1998; 4:1416-1420.

Vuyyuru R., Liu H., Manser T., et al.: Characteristics of *Borrelia hermsii* infection in human hematopoietic stem cell-engrafted mice mirror those of human relapsing fever. *Proc Natl Acad Sci USA* 2011; 108:20707-20712.

Warrell D.A., Perine P.L., Krause D.W., et al.: Pathophysiology and immunology of the Jarisch–Herxheimer-like reaction in louse-borne relapsing fever: comparison of tetracycline and slow-release penicillin. *J Infect Dis* 1983; 147:898-909.

Warrell D.A., Pope H.M., Parry E.H.O., et al.: Cardiorespiratory disturbance associated with infective fever in man: studies of Ethiopian louse-borne relapsing fever. *Clin Sci* 1970; 39:123-145.

Viral Hemorrhagic Fevers

AMANDA ROJEK | GAIL CARSON | YASUYUKI KATO | PETER W. HORBY | HAKAN LEBLEBICIOGLU

> ## KEY CONCEPTS
>
> - Viral hemorrhagic fever (VHF) is a syndrome of acute febrile illness with hemorrhagic potential, and an often severe clinical course. VHFs are caused by viruses from one of four taxonomic families.
>
> - VHFs are an important public health problem. They can have an extremely high case fatality rate and some transmit through human-to-human contact, with epidemic potential.
>
> - The pathophysiology of VHFs is not well understood. However, increased microvascular permeability, platelet damage and impaired hemostasis occur. These explain, to some extent, hemorrhagic and shock complications. Early case detection and reporting is critical to mounting an effective public health response aimed at preventing an epidemic. The identification of index cases relies on the astute clinician.
>
> - Strict adherence to infection control procedures by healthcare workers is paramount in reducing personal risk and preventing further transmission of cases in healthcare facilities.

Introduction

The term viral hemorrhagic fever (VHF) is used to describe a group of viral infections in which a subset of patients develop a clinical syndrome of severe febrile illness with hemorrhagic signs. VHFs are of public health importance due to the high case fatality rate of some VHFs and the possibility of human-to-human transmission. VHFs are difficult to diagnose and treat. The history of VHFs is characterized by some notable outbreaks. In particular, the 2014–15 Ebola virus outbreak in West Africa, which resulted in loss of 1000s of lives and severely damaged the healthcare systems and economic development of the affected ountreis. This catastrophic outbreak has refocussed attention on the need for global leadership and coordination of outbreak preparedness and response. This chapter will aim to provide a clinically relevant overview of the most significant viruses (in terms of mortality and the risk of human-to-human transmission). It will discuss general measures for clinical management and public health containment that should be useful for known viruses, and adaptable to future novel VHF pathogens.

Virology

All known VHFs are caused by single-stranded enveloped RNA viruses, including arenaviruses, bunyaviruses, filoviruses and flaviviruses. There is no precise definition with which to classify VHFs, and dengue fever and henipavirus infections (Nipah and Hendra virus) are sometimes categorized as VHFs, although bleeding is rare in these infections.

Arenaviruses are classified into two categories: Old World and New World, based on geographic location in Africa and the Americas, respectively. Lujo and Lassa virus are the two Old World arenaviruses known to cause human disease. Of the New World arenaviruses, Junin virus, Machupo virus, Guanarito virus and Sabia virus are the etiologic agents of Argentine HF, Bolivian HF, Venezuelan HF and Brazilian HF, respectively.

In the Bunyaviridae family, Crimean–Congo hemorrhagic fever virus (CCHF), hantaviruses – particularly Andes virus, Hantaan virus and Sin Nombre virus – and Rift Valley fever virus cause VHFs in humans. Diseases caused by hantaviruses generally manifest as either hemorrhagic fever with renal syndrome (HFRS) or hantavirus pulmonary syndrome (HPS). SFTS virus (genus *Phlebovirus*, family Bunyaviridae) is one of the most recently discovered pathogens. It causes severe fever with thrombocytopenia syndrome (SFTS) in East Asia.

The Filoviridae (Ebola and Marburg viruses) are responsible for some of the most lethal VHFs. Figure 132-1 shows the areas in Africa at risk of four VHFs based on available data on the occurrence of these viruses in animals and humans, and the assumed ecologic niche for the known animal reservoirs. These maps are useful for targeting surveillance and preparedness activities but their accuracy is dependent on the current state of knowledge and the availability of data. As such the maps are guides only and cannot be assumed to be definitive. The *Ebolavirus* genus is comprised of four distinct species responsible for human disease (Zaire ebolavirus, Sudan ebolavirus, Bundibugyo ebolavirus and Tai Forest ebolavirus), each having different mortality rates. Marburg virus is a single species (Marburg marburgvirus).

Flaviviridae that cause HF include yellow fever virus (see Chapter 175) and dengue virus (see Chapter 133), both of which will not be discussed in depth here. Other flaviviruses can cause hemorrhagic fever, including Kyasanur Forest disease virus, Omsk hemorrhagic fever virus and Alkhumra virus, but transmission of these viruses is geographically restricted and they are not discussed further.

Epidemiology

The geographical extent of transmission, and transmission characteristics for different VHFs, are described in Table 132-1 and Figure 132-1. With the exception of dengue fever, humans are not the natural host for VHFs. Because the viruses rely on animal reservoirs for maintenance and transmission, index infections are geographically restricted to areas where the reservoir and vector reside. Consequently VHFs occur primarily in rural areas where there is substantial contact with rodents, ticks, bush meat, bats or mosquitoes. However, the 2014–15 Ebola outbreak in West Africa demonstrated how easily a VHF can spread into urban areas. Additionally, with increasing international travel, and in particular the return of international healthcare workers to their home countries, cases may present anywhere in the world. Figure 132-2 shows areas in Africa at risk of four VHFs based on available data on the occurrence of these viruses in animals and humans, and the assumed ecological niche for the known animal reservoirs. These maps are useful for targeting surveillance and preparedness activities but their accuarcy is dependent on the current state of knowledge and the availability of data. As such the maps are guides alone and cannot be assumed to be definitive.

Some VHFs are endemic (such as HFRS in China) or have predictable seasonal epidemiology (such as CCHF in Turkey). However, VHF epidemiology is notable for epidemics, ranging from small, well-contained outbreaks to complex humanitarian emergencies with thousands of fatalities. For various reasons, the overall incidence of VHFs is likely under-reported. The few seroprevalence studies that have been undertaken demonstrate a hidden burden of subclinical or mild infections or a broader geographical area of transmission. In addition, many isolated VHF cases likely go undiagnosed or unreported to public health authorities, particularly when they occur in an unusual region or present as mild, self-limiting disease. Furthermore, during epidemics, healthcare systems may become overwhelmed and case confirmation and reporting may be inadequate.

For viruses that demonstrate human-to-human transmission, infection can occur through exposure of mucosal membranes or skin

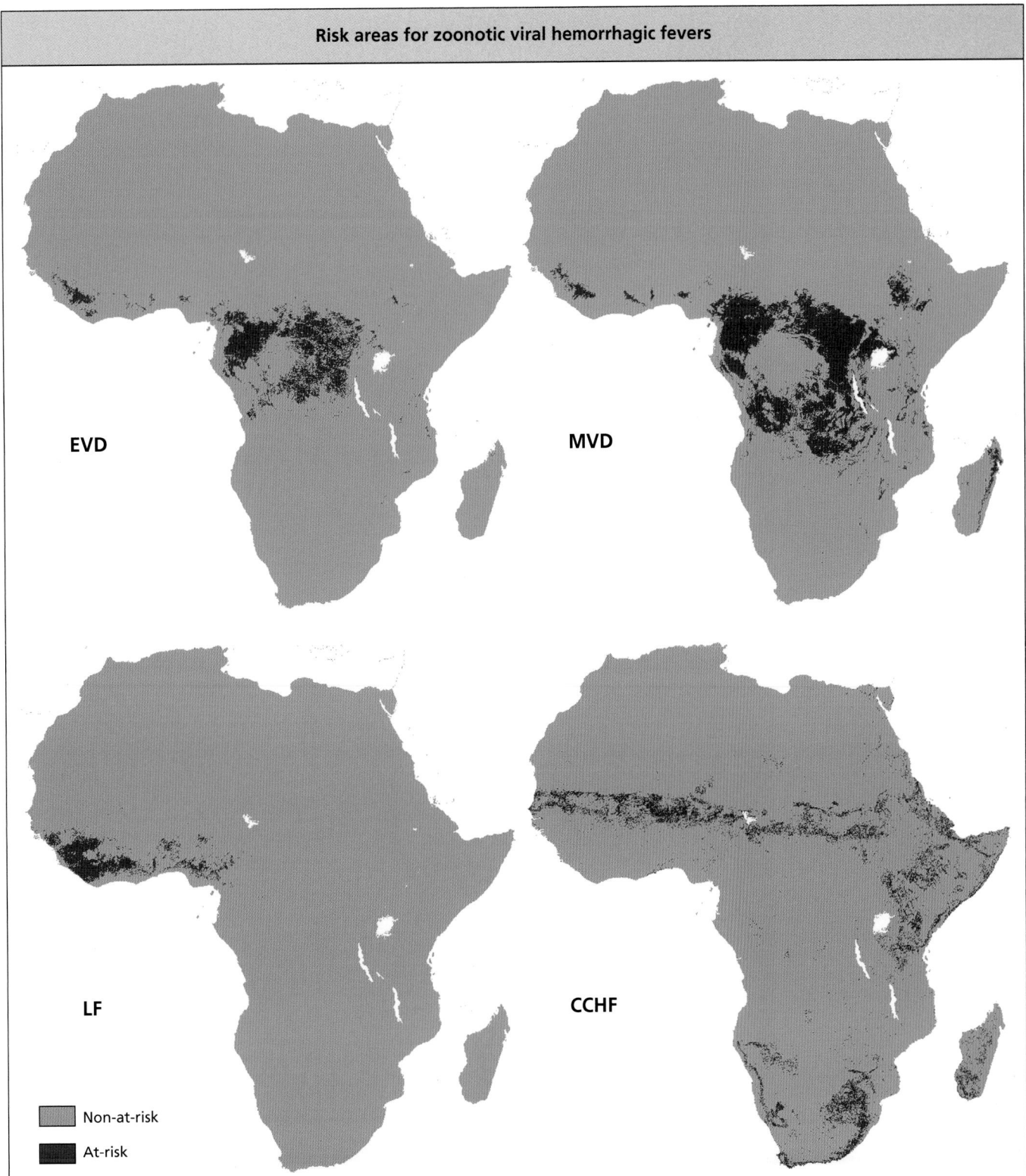

Risk areas for zoonotic viral hemorrhagic fevers

EVD

MVD

LF

CCHF

Non-at-risk

At-risk

Figure 132-1   Risk areas for zoonotic viral hemorrhagic fevers. Areas in red are regions predicted to be environmentally suitable for zoonotic spillover events to occur. The panels show (from top right, clockwise) predicted zoonotic niches for Ebola virus disease (EVD), Marburg virus disease (MVD), Crimean–Congo hemorrhagic fever (CCHF) and Lassa fever (LF). (Adapted from multiple sources. Messina JP, Pigott DM, Golding N, et al.: The global distribution of Crimean–Congo hemorrhagic fever. Trans R Soc Trop Med Hyg 2015;109:1–11; Mylne AQN, Pigott DM, Longbottom J, et al.: Mapping the zoonotic niche of Lassa fever in Africa. Trans R Soc Trop Med Hyg 2015;109(8):483-492. Pigott DM, Golding N, Mylne A, et al.: Mapping the zoonotic niche of Marburg virus disease in Africa. Trans R Soc Trop Med Hyg 2015;109(6):366–378. Pigott DM, Golding N, Mylne A, et al. Mapping the zoonotic niche of Ebola virus disease in Africa. 2014; eLife 3: e04395 doi:10.7554/eLife.04395.)

TABLE 132-1   Epidemiologic Characteristics of Common VHFs

	Arenaviruses			Filoviruses		Bunyaviruses				Flaviviruses
	Old World		New World							
	Lujo Virus	Lassa Virus	Junin, Machupo, Guanarito, Sabia	Ebola	Marburg	Hantavirus	Crimean–Congo	Rift Valley Fever	SFTS	Yellow Fever
Geography	Zambia	West Africa	South America, North America	Central and West Africa	East and Central Africa	Worldwide Old World (HFRS): eastern Asia New World (HPS): Americas	South Eastern Europe, Asia, Africa	Africa, Middle East	East Asia	South America, Africa
Primary reservoir	Unknown, likely rodent	Rodent (Mastomys natalensis)	Rodent (Calomys, Zygodontomys sp.)	Unknown, possibly fruit bat (Pteropodidae)	Fruit bat (Rousettus aegypti)	Rodents; species depends on location	Tick-borne	Mosquito	Tick-borne	Mosquito-borne (Aedes and Hemogogus spp.). Human reservoir in outbreaks
Transmission	Animal reservoir to human Nosocomial	Rodent to human, via direct contact or inhalation of excrement, or preparation of excrement Human to human Nosocomial	Rodent to human, via contact with excrement Human to human and nosocomial (for Machupo virus)	Fruit bat to human, via contact with saliva or excrement Possibly through other animals (chimpanzees, gorillas, duiker) prepared for consumption Human to human, including nosocomial		Rodent to human via contact with excrement Human to human for Andes virus	Tick bite to human Livestock to human via contact with blood or excrement Human to human Nosocomial	Animal to human via direct contact with infected body fluids or tissue Mosquito bite to human	Tick bite to human Nosocomial Human to human	Mosquito bite to human

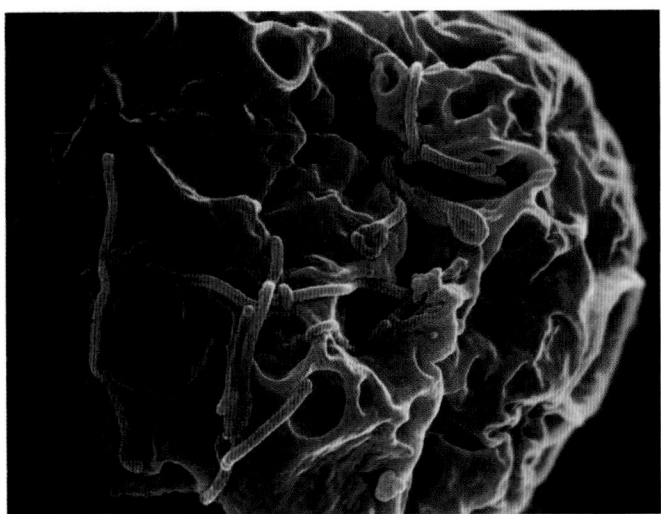

Figure 132-2 Scanning electron micrograph of Ebola virus budding from the surface of a Vero cell (monkey epithelial cell line) demonstrating characteristic filamentous shape. *(Image: NIAID.)*

breaks to infectious body fluids via mucosal memeranes or skin breaks. Secual transmission ocurs for Ebola. Notably, semen (along with other immune privileged fluids such as aqueous humour and CSF) can continue to harbour Ebolavirus following resolution of viraemia and sympoms. Sexual transmission probably also occuse for CCHF, LAssd, Marbury and Junin. There are reports of suspected airborne transmission of Lassa fever during an epidemic in a Nigerian hospital in 1970, and this is not thought to be a likely route of tansmission. Viral persistence on surfaces changes with aterial and environmental conditions the risk of transmission via fomites consequently is unclear and varies.[1] Nosocomial transmissions of CCHF and SFTS possibly associated with aerosol-inducing procedures have been reported. The risk of nosocomial infection and disease amplification in healthcare settings is especially important for Filoviridae, as exemplified by the high number of healthcare workers (HCWs) infected during the 2014–15 Ebola epidemic.

Pathogenesis

Following viral exposure, most initial viral replication occurs mostly in local tissues, monocytes, macrophages and/or dendritic cells, before migration to the lymphoreticular system.[2–5] The viruses causing VHFs have broad tissue tropism and subsequent dissemination occurs to the lymphatic system, blood (monocytes and macrophages) and a variety of solid organ targets, depending on the virus. The liver and spleen are commonly affected. High viral loads are common whilst the immune response is often poor, and may be worsened by viral-induced immunosuppression.[5–7] High viral loads are predictive of mortality, for some VHFs, such as Ebola and CCHF.[8,9]

Knowledge of the pathophysiology of VHF in humans is incomplete due to the geographic isolation of most outbreaks, reliance on historical data and the difficulty in safely collecting and managing biologic samples. While the pathogenesis differs between viruses, and the host–virus relationship is complex, there are common characteristics that contribute to the manifestations of shock and multiple organ failure.[10]

1. Excessive microvascular permeability occurs due to direct endothelial cell injury by the virus or via mediators such as pro-inflammatory cytokines/chemokines.[11]
2. Thrombocytopenia is common, as is inhibition of platelet function, leading to impaired platelet aggregation.[11,12]
3. To a varying extent for each of the VHFs, coagulopathy may be due to alterations to the fibrinolytic system, or consumption or activation of coagulation factors.[13] Together, these deficits may contribute to disseminated intravascular coagulopathy.

Volume depletion from vomiting and diarrhea and 'third spacing' due to vascular leakage frequently results in hypovoleamic shock in EVD patients. A substantial roportion of EVD patients in the 2014–15 outbreak had evidence of acute kidney injury on admission., although the mechanism for this may be partially independent of pre-renal failure caused by hypovolaemia.

Diagnosis and Clinical Features

The range of severity of VHFs, and the wide differential diagnosis for many of the symptoms, makes diagnosis difficult. Vigilance for clusters of cases (particularly if the cluster involves an HCW or exposure to a known VHF risk factor) may lead to early identification of a potential outbreak. The diagnosis of a VHF is based on three components: (a) a history of exposure, (b) clinical suspicion and (c) laboratory findings.[14]

A thorough case history must include the following information for the duration of the incubation period:
- All recent travel, particularly to endemic areas.
- Membership of an occupational risk group (e.g. HCW, veterinarian, abattoir worker).
- Contact with known or suspected cases of VHF (dead or alive), or severely ill febrile persons.
- Contact with deceased persons, who may have been infected with a VHF (usually during funeral practices).
- Contact with body fluids from a possible case of VHF or cadaver (e.g. laboratory workers).
- Contact with items contaminated by body fluids (bed sheets, medical instruments).
- Being breast-fed by a woman with a possible VHF.
- Sexual contact with a possible VHF case (including during convalescence).
- Contact with potential vectors.
- Contact with animals, animal droppings or animal products (cooking or consumption of bush meat, contact with bat droppings, etc.).
- Any entry into environments where a reservoir may have been present (e.g. caves housing bat populations or houses with rodent infestations).

The clinical manifestations of VHFs are heterogeneous. Typical symptoms for each virus are outlined in Table 132-2.[15,16] Importantly, although hemorrhage is eponymous, it is usually present in a minority of cases. After an incubation period of variable duration, there is usually a prodrome of a generalized febrile illness. Symptoms may include malaise, prostration, myalgia, headache and pharyngitis. At this early stage, the infection may resemble many other endemic diseases, and there is a broad differential diagnosis (Table 132-3). Clinical experience from the 2014–15 West African Ebola epidemic has provided useful experience of the range of clinical symptomatology and also the differential diagnosis.[17–20] It is important to note that not all patients are febrile on contact with the heatlhcare system.

As the disease progresses, specific organ involvement becomes more evident and pathognomonic features narrow the differential diagnosis. Gastrointestinal symptoms (commonly nausea, vomiting and diarrhea) can be severe and lead to significant volume depletion. Conjunctival injection, petechial rask, or hemorrhage is common. The likelihood of progression to life-threatening disease varies between viruses. When present, hemorrhagic symptoms include petechial rash, purpura, haematocchezia, melena, uterine or vaginal bleeding, oozing from intravenous sites, or epistaxis (Figure 132-3). These may be complicated by coagulopathy, notably, disseminated intravascular coagulopathy (DIC). Endothelium disruption manifests as pulmonary edema and peripheral edema. Neurologic disturbances include encephalopathy, seizures and coma. Hypovolemia and electrolyte disturbances may be common, and renal failure is predominant in some diseases (e.g. HFRS). Death may be due to septic shock or hypovolemic shock. It is suspected that the sudden death of some patients may be due to cardiac arrhythmias caused by electrolyte imbalances.

TABLE 132-2 Common Clinical Manifestations of Patients Infected with VHF*

	Arenaviruses			Filoviruses		Bunyaviruses				Flaviviruses
	Old World		New World							
	Lujo Virus[15]	Lassa Virus	Junin, Machupo, Guanarito, Sabia	Ebola[16]	Marburg	Hantavirus	Crimean–Congo	Rift Valley Fever	SFTS	Yellow Fever
Incubation period	9–13 days	1–3 weeks	10–14 days	2–21 days		HFRS:1–8 weeks HPS: 1–5 weeks	1–13 days. Faster onset of symptoms if infection acquired through tick bite than secretions	2–6 days	6–14 days	3–6 days
Range of disease	Severe. Mortality up to 80%	Asymptomatic or mild infections common (approx. 80%) in endemic areas. Ranges through to fatal disease 1% case fatality overall, up to 50% during epidemics Mortality high in third trimester women and fetuses	Case fatality 15–30%	Severe. Case fatality up to 90%. Differs between subtypes Mortality high in third trimester pregnant women and fetuses, the elderly, and those under age of 5		HFRS: case fatality is 1–15% HPS: case fatality is 38%	Ranges from mild through to fatal disease Case fatality rate in outbreaks is 9–50%	Often asymptomatic or mild disease Case fatality is 1%	Severe cases almost exclusively elderly people Case fatality is 10–30%	Often asymptomatic or mild disease Among those who develop severe disease, 20–50% case fatality
Early presentation	Rapid onset fever, malaise, headache and myalgia	Indolent onset of fever, malaise, weakness and headache. Additional common symptoms include exudative pharyngitis and productive cough, gastrointestinal symptoms, anemia and hypotension	Indolent onset of fever, malaise, weakness. At this stage similar to Old World fevers, but more likely to progress	Very similar for both viruses. Rapid onset of fever. Other common symptoms of weakness, malaise, myalgia, arthralgia, headache, dizziness and anorexia Nausea, vomiting and diarrhea common		HFRS: Sudden onset fevers, chills, nausea, back and abdominal pain, blurred vision, flushing of the face, red eyes, rash HPS: Fever, fatigue, myalgia, headache, gastrointestinal symptoms and dizziness	Rapid onset of fever, headache, myalgia, arthralgia, abdominal pain, vomiting, photophobia, red eyes, flushed face, petechial rash on palate, jaundice or changes in mood or sensory perception	Fever, weakness, backpain and dizziness	Fever, headache, weakness, myalgia, abdominal pain Nausea, vomiting and diarrhea common	Rapid onset of fever, chills, severe headache, back pain, myalgia, nausea, vomiting, fatigue, weakness

	C1	C2	C3	C4	C5	C6	C7	C8	C9
Disease progression in more severe cases	Pharyngitis, chest pain, gastrointestinal symptoms, rash, minor hemorrhage, subconjunctival injection, facial and neck edema Progresses to shock, DIC and multiorgan dysfunction. No frank hemorrhage	Occurs after 7 days. Includes facial or neck edema (about 10% of cases), mucosal or internal bleeding, encephalopathy and seizures, progressing to coma	Neurologic symptoms are more common than for Lassa fever (encephalopathy, irritability, seizure) Hemorrhage can be pronounced. Edema is common Disease progresses to shock	Hemorrhage may not be present. Severity ranges from mild to frank hemorrhage from orifices and venepuncture sites Gastrointestinal symptoms can be severe and may include 'cholera-like' diarrhea Neurologic manifestations include confusion and seizures Disease progresses to shock Miscarriage and IUFD are common in pregnant women	HFRS: hypotension, shock, acute kidney failure and fluid overload HPS: Occurs after 4–10 days. Coughing, dyspnea are predominant symptoms Renal and cardiopulmonary involvement can occur in either condition	Occurs after 3–5 days Agitation replaced with fatigue and depression Abdominal pain localizes and hepatomegaly may be present Hemorrhage is common and often severe Manifests as ecchymosis, severe epistaxis, bleeding from iv sites	At 2–4 days, jaundice and signs of liver impairment, hemorrhage (hematemesis, hematochezia, mucosal bleeding) At 1–4 weeks, encephalitis, causing headaches, seizures or coma	Occurs after 3–5 days Gastrointestinal symptoms and renal complication common Neurologic manifestations include confusion and seizures Hemophagocytic syndrome often seen	Biphasic. Period of improvement, then approx. 15% develop worsening symptoms that include high fever, jaundice, hemorrhage, multiorgan dysfunction, and shock
Convalescence	Recovery is slow and symptoms of prostration, weight loss and amnesia may last for months. Visual disturbances, including uveitis occurs for Ebola. Viable virus can persist in immune privileged body fluids Antibodies to Ebola may last for 10 years. Actual immunity and cross-reactivity is unknown	May include profound malaise. Temporary or permanent sensorineural deafness may occur in up to 30% of cases	Unknown in general. Junin fever appears to rapidly improve following period of diuresis	Unknown	HFRS: can take weeks to months	Unknown	Recovery after 2–7 days. Retinitis common, affects 1–10% of patients	Recovery after 7–10 days	Weakness and fatigue may be prolonged Lifelong immunity conferred

*Data are extracted from CDC reference material, unless otherwise referenced.

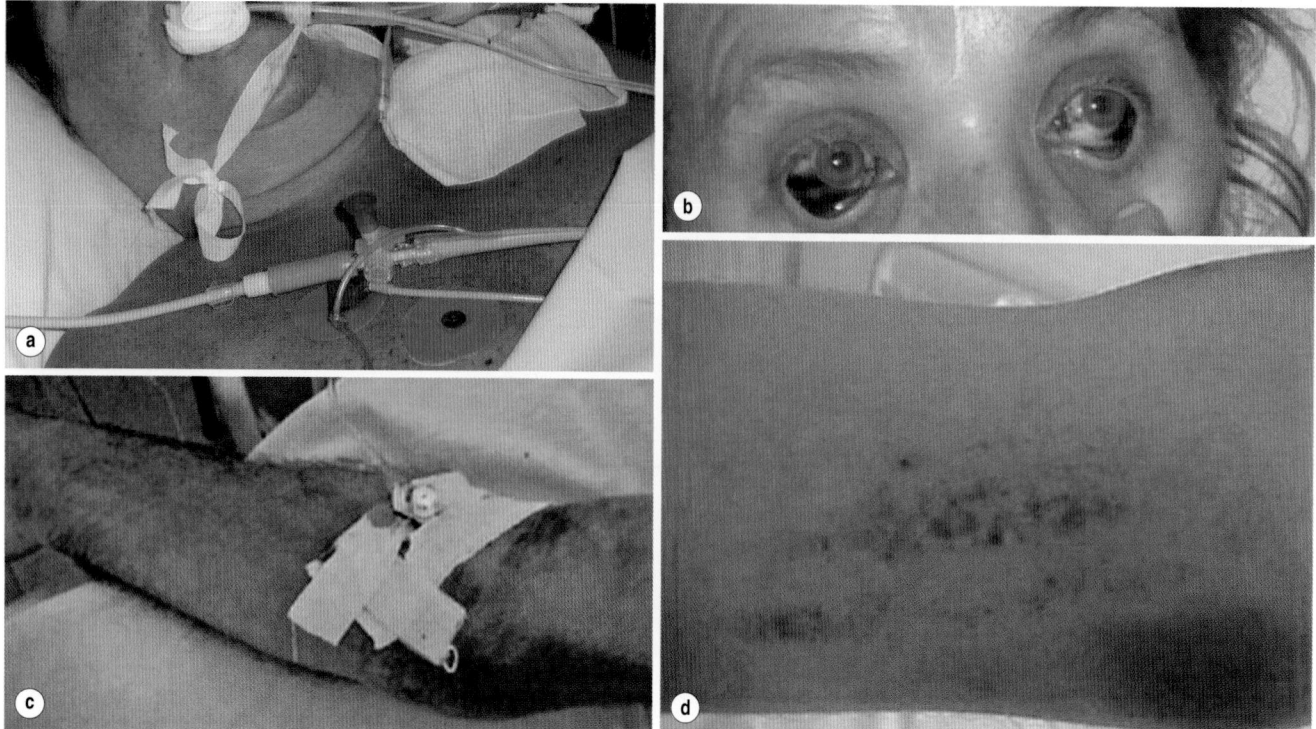

Figure 132-3   Characteristic clinical manifestations of severe VHF infection. Facial and neck swelling (a) and subconjunctival hemorrhage (b) in Lujo HF and ecchymosis (c) and petechial rash (d) in Crimean–Congo HF. *(Reprinted from (a,b) Sewall NH, Richards G, Duse A, et al.: Clinical features and patient management of Lujo hemorrhagic fever. PLoS Negl Trop Dis 2014;8(11):e3233 with permission of Nivesh Sewall; and (c,d) courtesy of Salih Ahmeti, in: Cook et al., Manson's tropical diseases, 22nd ed. Elsevier Ltd. Copyright © 2009.)*

TABLE 132-3	Differential Diagnosis for Viral Hemorrhagic Fever	
Viral	Other VHF Influenza	
Bacterial	Bacterial meningitis Bacillary dysentery Leptospirosis Typhoid fever Cholera *Yersina pestis*	
Other infectious causes	Malaria Rickettsial disease Hemolytic uremic syndrome	
Noninfectious causes	Thrombotic or idiopathic thrombocytopenic purpura Acute leukemia	

Please note, the above list is not exhaustive and the differential diagnosis will vary on presentation symptoms, severity and patient location.

For those who survive, weakness, fatigue and prostration are common in the post-infectious phase. Inflammatory complications have been reported and include uveitis, arthropathy, epidydimo-orchitis, hepatitis, pericarditis, meningitis, and transverse myelitis. There are a number of follow-up activities for the West African Ebola survivors which should further define these complications and, therefore, help manage them. For Ebola, localised disease, such as uveitis and meningtis, may arise dring convalescense as a result of persistence of the virus. Sensironeural deafness is a not uncommon complication for Lassa fever, and may be permanent. Stigmatization of persons returning to their communities may be severe and contribute to the psychological complications already experienced by this cohort.

INVESTIGATION FINDINGS

Great care must be taken in collecting, handling and transporting specimens. Potentially infectious specimens must be labeled as hazardous. Additional testing of patient samples should be minimized. Laboratories should be notified in advance that samples from a patient with suspected VHF will be transported to them. The samples must be packaged, labeled and transported according to national and international (i.e. IATA) guidance on the transport of infectious substances. Testing should be undertaken only by reference laboratories with adequate bio-containment facilities. Filoviruses, CCHF and most arenaviruses require BSL-4 handling. During an outbreak field laboratories capable of handling these dangerous pathogens can be established.

Laboratory diagnosis is usually based on blood or serum samples. Test methods include: RT-PCR, virus-specific IgM or IgG testing, detection of viral antigens using ELISA, virus isolation, visualizing using electron microscopy, or demonstrating a fourfold rise in antibody titre. Point-of-care rapid diagnostic tests for some VHFs are likely to be available in the near future.[21] Diagnosis may be possible from other body fluids, or from post-mortem tissue samples under some circumstances.

As safely acquiring and testing laboratory samples safely is difficult during an epidemic, the characteristic laboratory results for all viruses have not been fully elucidated. Hemoglobin may fall with hemorrhage, although hematocrit may rise due to hemoconcentration. Peripheral white blood cell counts are often low early in disease, but may increase later.[22] Thrombocytopenia is common for some conditions and platelet function is often impaired, even in the presence of low-normal platelet counts. Coagulation studies may demonstrate DIC.

Liver function is often abnormal. Aspartate aminotransferase (AST) is usually raised and virtually all VHFs distinguish themselves from viral hepatitis by the disproportionately high AST levels compared with alanine aminotransferase (ALT). Patients are rarely jaundiced (except in yellow fever) and the bilirubin is usually normal. Electrolyte disturbances commonly include sodium and potassium abnormalities. Renal failure is especially common in hantavirus infection in the Eurasia region (HFRS) and Ebola.

Management

For many of the VHFs, virus- or host-directed specific treatments are not available. However good supportive care likely improves outcomes and should be universally implemented.[23] The extent of clinical intervention available also differs between high- and low-income countries. Here, we focus on clinical management in low-income countries.

Healthcare workers must wear suitable personal protective equipment. Treatment of a patient as a suspected case of VHF should not be delayed to rule out other diagnoses, or while waiting for laboratory confirmation. A general approach to the clinical management of a suspected case (with presumed human-to-human transmission risk) is shown in Table 132-4.[14,24] Due to an evolving evidence base,

TABLE 132-4	Management Pathway for Patient with Suspected Viral Hemorrhagic Fever
1. Contain suspected and confirmed cases	1. Notify alert, cooperative patients of the requirement and process of isolation 2. Immediately isolate the suspected case 3. Implement appropriate infection control measures[24] 4. Urgently notify the appropriate public health authorities, such as the district health officer 5. If safe to do so, take blood samples and notify receiving laboratory of clinical suspicion 6. Perform malaria rapid diagnostic testing of all patients in endemic regions
2. Provide supportive management to all patients[14]	1. Treat for other co-morbidities 2. Treat empirically for suspected coinfections with broad spectrum antibiotics 3. Institute regular observation of vital signs (pulse, respiratory rate, blood pressure) 4. Manage fever with paracetamol 5. Provide supplemental oxygen for hypoxia 6. Provide oral rehydration solution in all patients and iv fluid resuscitation* for dehydration or hypovolemia 7. Monitor and correct electrolyte imbalances 8. Monitor and correct hypoglycemia 9. Provide simple analgesia† and opioid analgesia where required 10. Provide psychological support for anxiety 11. Provide environmental management for confusion and use sedation if required 12. Use antiemetics for gastrointestinal symptoms 13. Manage shock according to local practice or WHO guidelines for septic shock 14. Administer blood,* platelets or FFP if required, and available 15. Manage seizures
3. Consider further treatment options following confirmed diagnosis, ideally in the setting of a clinical trial	1. Consider anti-virals if available. 2. Consider other clinical trial agents 3. Consider convalescent blood/plasma
4. Provide additional intensive care interventions when they can be done safely	Consider ICU admission, when able. If indicated: 1. Provide mechanical ventilation 2. Administer vasopressors 3. Consider dialysis

*Careful fluid balance monitoring is required in these patients. Although fluid deficits may be severe and rapid infusion required, patients remain at increased risk of pulmonary edema.
†Avoid NSAIDs due to gastrointestinal bleeding and platelet complications.

management of the patient beyond the provision of symptom-based interventions, fluid replacement and electrolyte management must often be made on a case-by-case basis.

Pregnant women with a VHF have a high incidence of miscarriage, intrauterine fetal death and pregnancy-related hemorrhage. Pregnant women may present in an atypical manner, including with afebrile illness. Mortality is high in this population for both the mother and the child.

For patients responding poorly to supportive care, there are several additional treatment options to consider. The antiviral drug ribavirin is indicated for the treatment of Lassa fever,[25] and HFRS due to hantavirus infection.[26] While several small studies have been undertaken, there remains no strong evidence for the use of ribavirin in treating CCHF or SFTS. However, when available, it is often used for treatment of patients. It should not be used in treating filovirus infections. When used, the drug should be given early in the clinical course and in intravenous form. Anemia is a common complication of ribavirin treatment, and regular hemoglobin monitoring should be performed. Use of immune plasma is a beneficial treatment for Argentine Hemorrhagic Fever,[27] but there is insufficient evidence to support its routine use for other VHFs.

The following treatment strategies have insufficient clinical trial data in humans and should be used only as part of a clinical trial. Intravenous immunoglobulin has been used in human trials for CCHF, with no mortality benefit shown. Interferons have been used in animal model studies of arenavirus and filovirus infection but data on use in humans is not available to date. During the ongoing Ebola epidemic in West Africa, the WHO prioritized use of different experimental vaccines and therapeutics (including monoclonal antibodies, polymerase inhibitors, small interfering RNAs, and convalescent plasma), and vaccines.[28,29] While these efforts are ongoing at the time of writing, a coordinated approach to clinical research to improve the evidence base is a necessary component of the response to any VHF outbreak. For the future preparedness should conitinue around how clinical research can be better integrated rapidly into public health responses.

Prevention

Prevention of VHF index cases relies largely on avoidance of the reservoir species or vector, although this is difficult for viruses where the transmission cycle is incompletely understood. Vaccines exist for Argentine HF and HFRS in some countries in Asia, although these are not widely available. An experimental Vesicular Stomatitis Virus-Ebola Virus Vaccine (VSV-EBOV) has demonstrated excellent efficacy and adequate safety in an interim analysis of a ring vaccination cluster-randomised study.[30–33]

Prevention of secondary cases relies on a rapid, coordinated public health response, consisting of four elements – case detection, case isolation, contact tracing and safe burial. Screening for suspected VHF should be undertaken on entry to the healthcare system. Patients with suspected or confirmed VHF should be isolated, ideally in a dedicated isolation room with separate amenities, although during outbreaks use of shared facilities may be necessary. Healthcare workers designated to treating these patients require personal protective equipment, and training for its correct use. Equipment should be assigned to these patients exclusively and non-consumables decontaminated after use. Handling of deceased persons should be undertaken by trained staff and restricted to that necessary for safe and dignified disposal of the body. As the virus concentration is likely to be high at the time of death, the importance of infection control when handling a deceased patient cannot be understated. Healthcare workers who have experienced unprotected exposure to body fluids should immediately stop clinical tasks, decontaminate the area and notify the designated team physician for evaluation (as post-exposure prophylaxis and management differs between viruses). For Ebola, viable virus may persist in immune privileged body fluids (semen, aqueous humor) for a number of months following acute infection. Clinicians undertaking invasive procedures on people surviving Ebola should manage infection control according to the most current evidence.

Broader public health management relies on early notification of potential cases and activation of early warning systems to generate prompt intervention. Subsequent contact tracing of direct contacts (in viruses with human-to-human transmission) assists in controlling onward transmission.

Community perceptions of the meaning of the disease and mechanism of spread influence how an outbreak can be controlled. Cultural practices regarding social greetings and contact, care of unwell family members and burial practices can facilitate person-to-person transmission. At a time of extraordinary personal and social upheaval, community fears can be further exacerbated by an influx of foreign medical staff. Consequently, local leadership is a critical asset in control.

References and additional text available online at expertconsult.com.

KEY REFERENCES

Bah E.I., Lamah M.C., Fletcher T., et al.: Clinical presentation of patients with Ebola virus disease in Conakry, Guinea. *N Engl J Med* 2014; 372:40-47.

Blumberg L., Enria D., Bausch D.: Viral haemorrhagic fevers. In: Farrar J., Hotez P., Junghanns T., et al., eds. *Manson's tropical diseases.* 23rd ed. Philadelphia: Saunders/Elsevier; 2014.

Chertow D.S., Kleine C., Edwards J.K., et al.: Ebola virus disease in West Africa – clinical manifestations and management. *N Engl J Med* 2014; 371(22):2054-2057.

Kortepeter M.G., Bausch D.G., Bray M.: Basic clinical and laboratory features of filoviral hemorrhagic fever. *J Infect Dis* 2011; 204(Suppl. 3):S810-S816.

Paessler S., Walker D.H.: Pathogenesis of the viral hemorrhagic fevers. *Annu Rev Pathol* 2013; 8:411-440.

Schieffelin J.S., Shaffer J.G., Goba A., et al.: Clinical illness and outcomes in patients with Ebola in Sierra Leone. *N Engl J Med* 2014; 371(22):2092-2100.

Sewall N.H., Richards G., Duse A., et al.: Clinical features and patient management of Lujo hemorrhagic fever. *PLoS Negl Trop Dis* 2014; 8(11):e3233.

World Health Organization: Clinical management of patients with viral hemorrhagic fever: a pocket guide for the front-line health worker. Available: www.who .int/csr/resources/publications/clinical-management -patients/en/.

World Health Organization: Interim infection prevention and control guidance for care of patients with suspected or confirmed filovirus haemorrhagic fever in health care settings, with focus on Ebola. Available: www.who.int/ csr/resources/publications/ebola/filovirus_infection_ control/en/.

133

Dengue and Chikungunya

CAMERON P. SIMMONS | JAMES WHITEHORN | KATHERINE ANDERS | VINH CHAU VAN NGUYEN

KEY CONCEPTS

- Dengue and chikungunya are viral diseases transmitted by *Aedes* mosquitoes.

- Over 3 billion people are at risk of dengue.

- Explosive outbreaks of chikungunya occur in the Indian Ocean region and infection is spreading rapidly across the Caribbean region.

- The pathogenesis of both viruses is complex and incompletely understood – it involves an interplay between virus and host factors.

- Dengue treatment is currently limited to supportive care (fluid replacement and careful monitoring of fluid balance).

- No vaccines are currently available for either virus.

- Novel approaches to vector control may assist dengue control efforts (e.g. release of *Wolbachia*-infected *Aedes aegypti*).

Epidemiology

DENGUE

Dengue is a vector-borne, systemic viral infection and a globally important public health problem.[1] Dengue is transmitted predominantly by the mosquito *Aedes aegypti*, which bites in the daytime, is adapted to human habitats and has a preference for human blood meals. Mosquitoes become infected after feeding on the blood of a viremic human. More than 3 billion people living in over 100 countries throughout the tropics and sub-tropics are at risk of dengue (Figure 133-1). Recent probabilistic mapping studies suggest there are approximately 100 million clinically apparent cases of dengue each year, of which an estimated 2–5% are severe.[2] The global scale of the public health risk posed by dengue is in part due to the geographic expansion of *A. aegypti* into new territories. In endemic areas peak dengue transmission dynamics are influenced by factors such as mosquito density, human population density, co-circulation of dengue virus (DENV) serotypes, rainfall and humidity.

CHIKUNGUNYA

Chikungunya virus (CHIKV) is an alphavirus within the Togaviridae family, transmitted by *Aedes* mosquitoes.[3] CHIKV was first isolated in Tanzania in 1952. *Chikungunya* is the Makonde (an African dialect spoken in parts of Tanzania) for 'that which bends up'– the description eludes to the severe joint pain that can be seen in those infected. Typically major epidemics of the disease occur cyclically with long inter-epidemic periods.[4] CHIKV disease has been reported from Africa, Asia and Australasia; it has recently re-emerged resulting in millions of infections in the Indian Ocean and Caribbean regions.[5] Imported cases to Europe have resulted in autochthonous outbreaks in Italy. There is concern that a recent envelope mutation will result in increased infectivity to *Aedes albopictus* and a further spread of chikungunya's geographic footprint.[6]

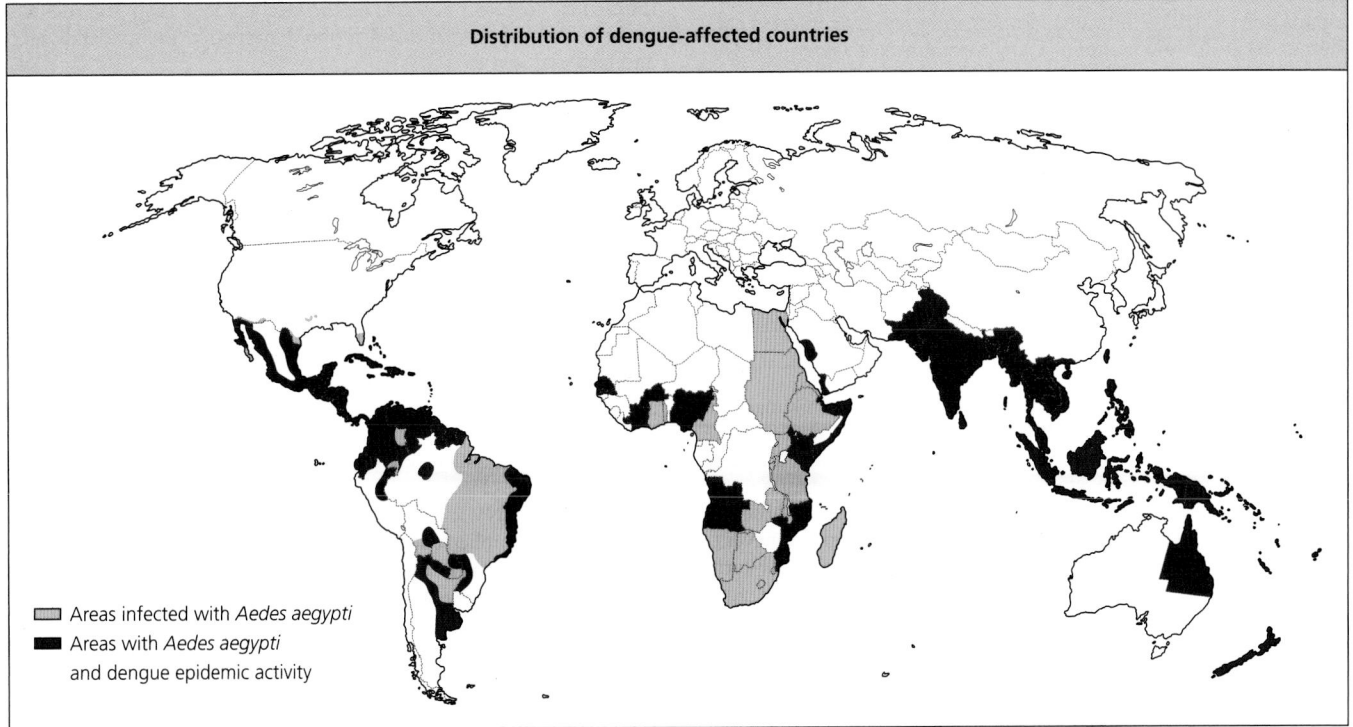

Distribution of dengue-affected countries

Areas infected with *Aedes aegypti*

Areas with *Aedes aegypti* and dengue epidemic activity

Figure 133-1 Distribution of dengue-affected countries.

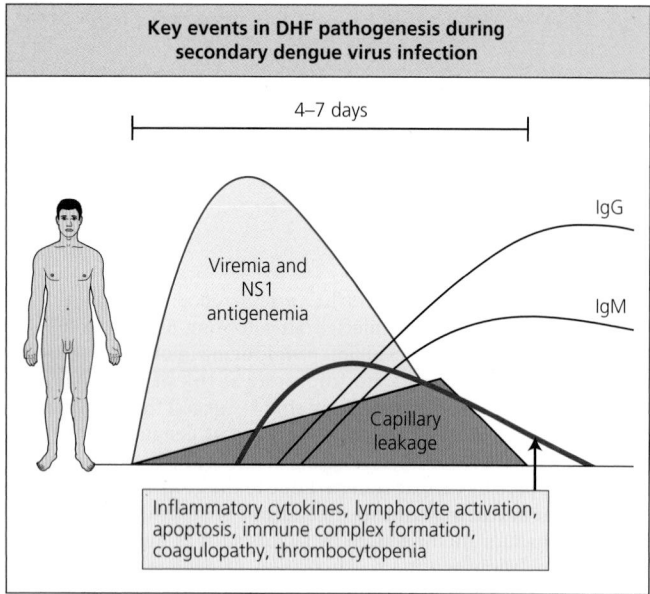

Figure 133-2   Key events in dengue pathogenesis during secondary dengue virus infection.

Dengue Pathogenesis and Pathology

The dengue viruses (DENV serotypes 1, 2, 3 and 4) are enveloped, single-stranded RNA viruses of the Flaviviridae family. Infection with any of the four serotypes of dengue virus can be clinically inapparent or, following an incubation period of 4–10 days, a systemic illness may develop that is characterized by fever, rash, headache, muscle and joint ache. Occasionally, more severe manifestations such as shock and hemorrhage occur, which are largely due to a transient increase in vascular permeability. Severe dengue is strongly associated with secondary, heterotypic infections (two sequential infections caused by different serotypes) (Figure 133-2).[7] Severe dengue also occurs during primary DENV infection of infants born to DENV-immune mothers.[8] Infants born to DENV-immune mothers and previously infected children or adults have in common a single immune risk factor – DENV-reactive IgG antibodies.[9] The capacity of subneutralizing concentrations of DENV-reactive IgG antibodies to enhance DENV infections in Fc receptor-bearing cells, a phenomenon called antibody-dependent enhancement (ADE), might explain the increased risk of severe dengue in secondary infections and in infants with primary infections.[10] Nonetheless, most secondary infections do not result in severe disease, suggesting there are other important factors involved. Young age, female gender, virus strain and genetic variants of the human major histocompatibility complex class I-related sequence B and phospholipase C epsilon 1 genes are also risk factors for severe dengue.[11,12]

Prevention

There are currently no licensed vaccines for dengue or chikungunya. Large phase III trials of a live-attenuated tetravalent dengue vaccine (ChimeriVax-DEN) indicated this vaccine was safe and well tolerated but delivered only partial efficacy (55–65%) against symptomatic dengue (any severity) during the 25-month period of study observation. Promisingly ChimeriVax-DEN was more efficacious in preventing dengue hospitalizations.[13,14] More recent results from longer-term follow-up suggest a sustained benefit in vaccine recipients aged between 9 and 16 years, but intriguingly showed higher rates of hospitalization in vaccine recipients aged under 9 in the third year after vaccination.[15] There remain many questions about the potential place of this vaccine in dengue control and the results suggest that partial, waning immunity could be a problem in the development of an efficacious dengue vaccine.

An alternative approach to dengue and chikungunya prevention is through the replacement of wild-type *A. aegypti* with *A. aegypti* infected with the intracellular bacterium *Wolbachia*.[16] *Wolbachia*-infected *A. aegypti* are resistant to DENV infection and these modified mosquitoes can be successfully established in the field.[16] Alternative approaches to mosquito control include the release of genetically modified mosquitoes that can suppress target populations – field trials of this approach are underway.[17] It is possible that combining these novel approaches with a partially efficacious vaccine may be a successful approach to dengue control.

Reduction of mosquito populations currently remains the best method of preventing transmission of dengue and chikungunya. Nevertheless, the relentless increase in the geographic footprint of dengue and the recent explosive outbreaks of chikungunya, indicates most vector control strategies in endemic areas are inadequate, not sustainable and/or poorly targeted. For travelers to tropical countries, the only practical method of prevention is to avoid bites from mosquitoes by wearing protective clothing and using appropriate *N,N*-Diethyl-*m*-toluamide (DEET)-based repellents.

Clinical Features

DENGUE

DENV infection causes a range of manifestations from asymptomatic infection through to fulminant shock and hemorrhage.[18] The previously used classification system categorized dengue infection into 'dengue fever' and 'dengue hemorrhagic fever (DHF)'. DHF was further subdivided into four severity grades, and grades III and IV were classified as dengue shock syndrome (DSS). Studies have shown that this rigid classification system had a low sensitivity for severe disease and that some cases resulting in shock and death did not meet the WHO case definitions for DHF/DSS.[19] The current WHO guidelines recognize that dengue is a clinical continuum from uncomplicated to severe disease.[18] This system places more emphasis on the early recognition of warning signs suggestive of severe disease, appreciating patients may move along the disease continuum during the course of their illness. These warning signs include abdominal pain, vomiting, liver enlargement, lethargy and restlessness.[18] In the early stages of illness the differential diagnosis of DENV infection is broad.[20] The differential diagnosis depends on the local epidemiology and includes malaria, chikungunya, measles, typhoid, influenza, Rickettsial diseases and bacterial sepsis.

In 'classic' dengue there is typically an abrupt onset of fever after a 4–7 day incubation period. This is often accompanied by headache, myalgia and severe retro-orbital pain.[21] Other clinical features seen are sore throat, diarrhea, vomiting, anorexia, conjunctival and pharyngeal injection.[18] Early in the illness the skin typically appears flushed, with petechiae appearing in the 'critical' phase and a macular rash developing in convalescence (Figure 133-3 and Figure 133-4). Severe arthralgia and myalgia can be a feature of the illness and perhaps explains the use of the descriptive term 'break-bone fever'.[22] The early febrile phase lasts for 2–7 days. Straddling the time of defervescence is a 24–72 hour 'critical' phase when an increase in capillary permeability with an associated rise in hematocrit can be observed. The degree of plasma leakage is variable – some patients will develop a detectable pleural effusion or ascites (Figure 133-5). When a critical volume of plasma is lost patients will develop hypovolemic shock, called dengue shock syndrome (Figure 133-6). Thrombocytopenia is almost universally seen in DENV infection and minor mucosal bleeding can be a feature of uncomplicated infection. In addition, in many cases elevation of the PT and APTT with associated reduced fibrinogen levels is observed. However, there is not the degree of FDP elevation that would be consistent with disseminated intravascular coagulation.[23] Severe gastrointestinal hemorrhage can occur and this is well described in patients with a history of peptic ulcer disease.[24] Less commonly, intracerebral and pulmonary hemorrhage can occur.[25] Other organs can be affected in dengue, and it is possible that these 'atypical' presentations are under-appreciated.[18] These 'atypical presentations'

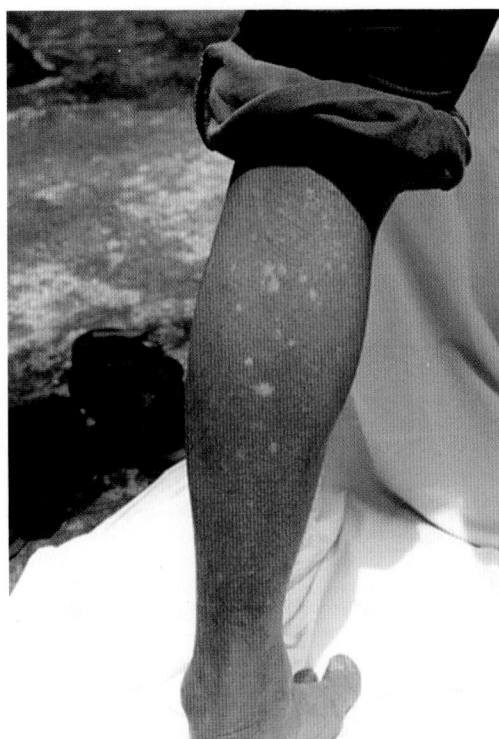

Figure 133-3 Diffuse macular recovery rash in an adult patient with dengue. The rash may appear between 3 and 6 days after fever onset. Note the 'islands' of normal skin surrounded by erythematous skin.

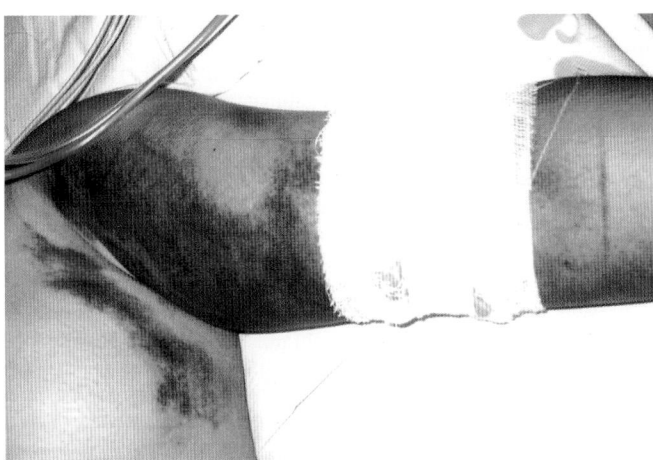

Figure 133-4 Hematoma in a patient with severe dengue. The combination of increased vascular fragility, platelet dysfunction/thrombocytopenia and coagulation disorders is believed to explain hemorrhagic manifestations in dengue. Frank hemorrhage, as pictured here, is relatively uncommon given the overall disease burden.

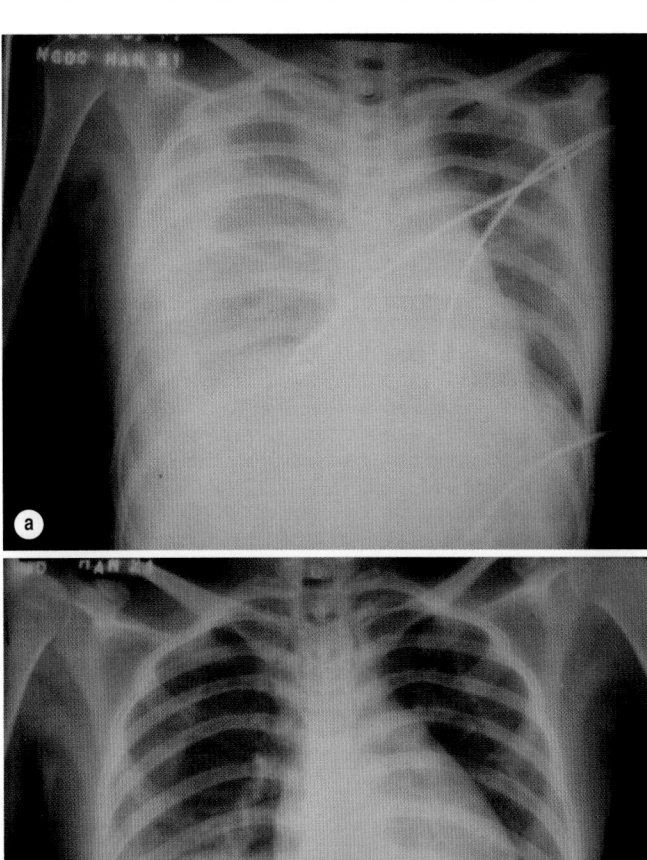

Figure 133-5 (a) Anteroposterior chest radiograph showing a large pleural effusion on the right side in an adult patient with dengue shock syndrome. (b) The same patient at hospital discharge. Such severe radiologic findings occur in dengue patients with capillary leakage and who have received an excessive volume of intravenous fluid.

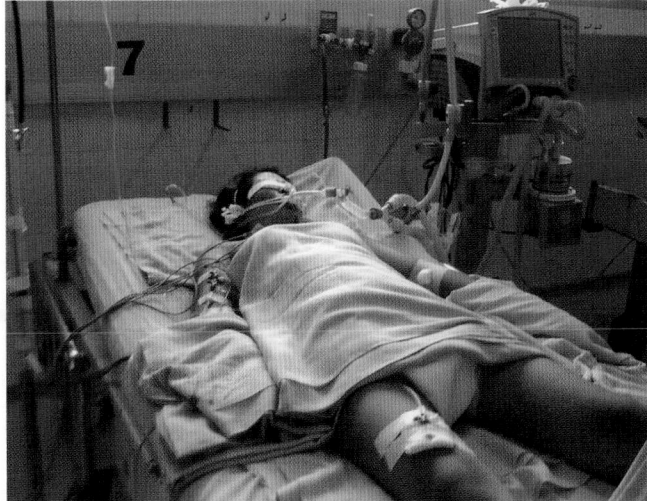

Figure 133-6 A patient with dengue shock syndrome. As shown in this image, patients with severe dengue require fluids (or blood products in cases with severe bleeding) to maintain hemodynamic stability. Respiratory support can be required in cases with severe pleural effusion and respiratory compromise.

include encephalitis, myocarditis, hepatitis, pancreatitis, retinitis and ARDS.[26]

CHIKUNGUNYA

After infection with CHIKV there is an incubation period of 2–4 days.[27] The onset of symptoms is abrupt with high fever, headache, myalgia and arthralgia. The symptoms resemble those seen with DENV infection. The skin is commonly involved, with maculopapular rashes being observed frequently – a bullous rash has been described in children.[28] The striking feature of CHIKV infection is severe arthralgia that can become chronic.[4] Less common features are eye involvement, minor bleeding, myocarditis and hepatitis.[29] The shock characteristic of severe dengue is not seen and severe hemorrhage is very rare. The laboratory features of CHIKV infection are distinct from those observed in DENV – lymphopenia and hypocalcemia are common.[30] Mild elevations of liver enzymes are observed but severe thrombocytopenia is rare.

Diagnosis

DENGUE

Virological confirmation of DENV infection can be obtained by detection of the virus-expressed NS1 protein in serum samples via enzyme-linked immunosorbent assays (ELISA) or rapid test. This method has high specificity but variable sensitivity. Real time reverse transcription (RT)-PCR can also be used to detect DENV nucleic acid and allow differentiation between serotypes, but this method is generally only used in research settings because of cost. Detection of NS1 and DENV nucleic acid is most sensitive in the febrile phase of illness.

A presumptive diagnosis of dengue can be obtained by detection of IgM antibodies in the acute phase. There are several commercially available ELISA and rapid tests for detection of DENV-reactive IgM, and some of these rapid tests combine IgM and NS1 tests in the same assay.

CHIKUNGUNYA

Diagnosis of CHIKV is often made on clinical and epidemiological grounds alone. Molecular assays are useful in the early stages of illness. RT-PCR assays are available that target the envelope or nonstructural protein genes.[31] Serological diagnosis via ELISA is an option – IgM is detectable after 2–3 days of illness and can persist for 3 months (in some cases years).[4] Rapid tests are also available but their reliability is uncertain.[3]

Management

DENGUE

Supportive care is the mainstay of dengue case management. Uncomplicated infections can be managed in the outpatient setting with access to further clinical reviews to assess for the development of any complications.[18] It is important that patients managed in the outpatient setting are able to tolerate oral fluids, and are encouraged to maintain a good oral intake.[18] Paracetamol is the recommended antipyretic as nonsteroidal anti-inflammatory drugs (NSAIDs) are associated with an increased risk of hemorrhage and gastritis, and aspirin has an association with the development of Reye's syndrome.[18]

Patients with warning signs suggestive of severe disease should be admitted. In addition, patients with co-morbidities and those who cannot practically be managed as outpatients should also be admitted.[18] Patients who have warning signs should have a baseline hematocrit measured and then should be started on parenteral isotonic fluids commencing at 5–7 ml/kg/hour for 1–2 hours – this infusion rate should be reduced according to the clinical response.[18] Parenteral fluids are generally needed for only 24–48 hours – the 'critical' phase.

Continuing parenteral fluids for longer than this carries a significant risk of fluid overloading the patient.

In severe cases the administration of parenteral fluid is life-saving.[18,32] Patients with shock require more intensive management with an initial 20 ml/kg fluid bolus. Further fluid administration is guided by the patient's clinical response. The use of isotonic fluids in the resuscitation of children with shock is supported by clinical evidence, and colloid solutions have been suggested for use in more severe cases.[32] In cases of hemorrhage the transfusion of blood products is often indicated. However cases involving mucosal bleeding without hemodynamic compromise require careful observation as opposed to transfusion.[18] Platelet transfusions are advocated in some settings as prophylaxis against hemorrhage. However this practice lacks an evidence base, has the potential to cause harm and is not recommended.[33]

Trials of both immunomodulatory and antiviral agents have been conducted but no intervention has demonstrated efficacy.[34]

CHIKUNGUNYA

There is currently no specific antiviral agent for CHIKV – management is predominantly supportive with analgesia and antipyretics. There is some evidence that those who have joint symptoms persisting for more than 2 weeks after the febrile illness may benefit from ribavirin.[35]

Zika

Zika virus is a flavivirus that was first described in Uganda in 1947 and until recently was a relatively mild and obscure infection confined to central Africa. Since 2010, in a manner very analogous to the spread of Chikungunya infection, it has crossed the world.[36] It has appeared in the Americas – initially in Brazil but then speading northwards to much of South America, Central America and the Caribbean. Additionally it has become endemic in South East Asia and Polynesia. Sporadic cases in returning travelers have been seen elsewhere. The virus is transmitted by aedes mosquitoes, especially *A. aegypti*. In most cases, infection has been asymptomatic or mild with fever, muscle aches, conjunctivitis and a maculopapular rash. Severe dengue-like infection has not been described. The most recent outbreaks have highlighted potential associations with severe neurological consequences. An outbreak in French Polynesia was associated with a parallel increase in Guillain-Barre syndrome. Of greatest concern is the potential link between infection in pregnant women and subsequent microcephaly in their infants. This was first noted in Brazil, but has been reported elsewhere. A cause and effect relationship remains unproven, but public health authorities in many countries are now advising additional precautions for women of child-bearing age including avoidance of pregnancy or travel to affected countries.[37] There is no specific treatment for Zika other than supportive care. Prevention efforts are similar to other arthropod-associated flaviviruses and center on vector avoidance and control.

References available online at expertconsult.com.

KEY REFERENCES

Anders K.L., Nguyet N.M., Chau N.V., et al.: Epidemiological factors associated with dengue shock syndrome and mortality in hospitalized dengue patients in Ho Chi Minh City, Vietnam. *Am J Trop Med Hyg* 2011; 84(1):127-134.

Bhatt S., Gething P.W., Brady O.J., et al.: The global distribution and burden of dengue. *Nature* 2013; 496(7446):504-507.

Capeding M.R., Tran N.H., Hadinegoro S.R., et al.: Clinical efficacy and safety of a novel tetravalent dengue vaccine in healthy children in Asia: a phase 3, randomised, observer-masked, placebo-controlled trial. *Lancet* 2014; 384(9951):1358-1365.

Dejnirattisai W., Jumnainsong A., Onsirisakul N., et al.: Cross-reacting antibodies enhance dengue virus infection in humans. *Science* 2010; 328(5979):745-748.

Khor C.C., Chau T.N., Pang J., et al.: Genome-wide association study identifies susceptibility loci for dengue shock syndrome at MICB and PLCE1. *Nat Genet* 2011; 43(11):1139-1141.

Moreira L.A., Iturbe-Ormaetxe I., Jeffery J.A., et al.: A *Wolbachia* symbiont in *Aedes aegypti* limits infection with dengue, chikungunya, and *Plasmodium*. *Cell* 2009; 139(7):1268-1278.

Simmons C.P., Farrar J.J., Nguyen v V., et al.: Dengue. *N Engl J Med* 2012; 366(15):1423-1432.

Villar L., Dayan G.H., Arredondo-Garcia J.L., et al.: Efficacy of a tetravalent dengue vaccine in children in Latin America. *N Engl J Med* 2015; 372(2):113-123.

Whitehorn J., Yacoub S., Anders K.L., et al.: Dengue therapeutics, chemoprophylaxis, and allied tools: state of the art and future directions. *PLoS Negl Trop Dis* 2014; 8(8):e3025.

134

Anthrax

MEHMET DOGANAY

- Anthrax is a zoonotic disease of herbivores.

- The source of infection in nature is contaminated soil.

- The etiological agent is *Bacillus anthracis* which is an aerobic or facultatively anaerobic, endospore-forming, rod-shaped bacterium. The bacteria produce capsules within the mammalian host.

- *B. anthracis* has two plasmid-mediated virulence factors: pOX1 and pOX2.

- Infection occurs within the agricultural or industrial environment. The spores of *B. anthracis* are a potential agent of bioterrorism.

- Humans are infected through contact with infected animal carcasses or contaminated animal products (meat, skin, hair etc.).

- The main clinical forms are cutaneous, ingestional and inhalation anthrax. Sepsis and meningitis can also be seen.

- Anthrax resulting from injecting drug use (heroin) is a newly described form.

- Diagnosis is based on the exposed history, demonstration of bacilli from lesions and culture.

- Penicillin G and amoxicillin are the first choice antibiotics; ciprofloxacin and doxycycline are the best alternatives in naturally occurring anthrax.

- An acellular vaccine is available and is used in the military setting.

Introduction

Anthrax is primarily a disease of herbivores which can be transmitted to humans and was one of the first zoonoses described. Currently, anthrax has assumed greater importance as a result of the potential use of *Bacillus anthracis* spores as an agent of bioterrorism and biological warfare.

Epidemiology

Anthrax occurs worldwide. It remains endemic or hyperendemic in both animals and humans in parts of the Middle East, West Africa, Central Asia, South America and Haiti, and the reservoir is contaminated soil. Figure 134-1 illustrates the cycle of infection in nature. Human anthrax is most common in enzootic areas in low- and middle-income countries, among people who work with livestock, eat undercooked meat from infected animals, or work in establishments where wool, goatskins and pelts are stored or processed.[1,2] The disease occurs only occasionally among humans in higher-income countries. Recently, a new clinical form of anthrax, 'injectional anthrax', has been described, which is transmitted by subcutaneous, intramuscular or intravenous injection of contaminated drugs in heroin users in European countries.[3–4]

The main route of transmission is contact with or inhalation of *B. anthracis* spores or consumption of contaminated food or water. Human cases may occur in both agricultural and industrial environments. Agricultural cases have occurred in individuals who came into contact with sick or dead animals in rural areas. In impoverished communities, livestock owners are driven by economic factors to slaughter animals at the first sign of infection in order to salvage the meat, hair and hides. Products made from contaminated hair (e.g. shaving brushes, wool coats), skins (e.g. drums, drumheads made of animal skin) and bone meal (e.g. fertilizer) can remain sources of infection for many years because of the hardy nature of the spores (Table 134-1).[1,2,5,6]

Insect vectors, such as horseflies, have been reported to transmit *B. anthracis* from an infected animal to a second animal. It is not well documented for human transmission.[1,2]

Industrial anthrax occurs as a result of the inhalation of spore-laden dust or other aerosols, or direct contact with spores. Spores in dust clouds can be created from the handling of dry hides, skins, sheep wool, goat hair and bone meal, and are either inhaled or spread through contact with the skin of workers. In industrialized countries most cases are associated with exposure to animal products, particularly goat hair imported from countries in which anthrax is endemic.[1,2]

Records of person-to-person spread exist but are very rare. All cases were cutaneous anthrax; there are no reports of inhalation or ingestion anthrax. Occasionally, laboratory-acquired infections have occurred.[1,2,5]

Pathogenesis and Pathology

Bacillus anthracis, the causative agent of anthrax, is a gram-positive, aerobic or facultatively anaerobic, endospore-forming, rod-shaped bacterium. Spores that lodge in a cut, abrasion or insect bite in the skin undergo germination and the emergent vegetative bacilli spread to the regional lymph nodes. Ingestion anthrax results if spores lodge in the gastrointestinal tract or achieve access to Peyer's patches. Inhaled spores may, on occasion, lead to infection of nasal-associated lymphoid tissues; those reaching the lungs do not germinate in the alveoli but remain dormant until carried by macrophages to the tracheobronchial lymph nodes. The spores germinate inside the macrophages and the emergent vegetative forms are released to multiply in the lymphatic system and enter the bloodstream, causing toxemia and sepsis.[2,7,8]

Bacillus anthracis has two principal virulence factors: the toxin complex and the polypeptide capsule. Both are plasmid mediated. The genes for the toxin components and virulence gene regulators AtxA and PagR are located on a large (182 kb) plasmid designated pX01 and the genes for capsule synthesis and their regulators AcpA and AcpB are

TABLE 134-1	Risk Factors for Anthrax	
General	**Occupational Risks**
• Workers involved in animal husbandry in endemic area	• Herdsman
• Consumers of traditional raw meat dishes in endemic area	• Slaughterhouse workers
• Drug users	• Butchers
• Laboratory workers	• Dairy workers
	• Veterinarians
	• Skinners
	• Tanners
	• Leather gift makers
	• Furriers
	• Shoemakers
	• Drum makers
	• Carpet weavers
	• Wool spinners
	• Bone meal processers
	• Wool textile factory workers

Adapted from references 2, 3, 4, 5, 6.

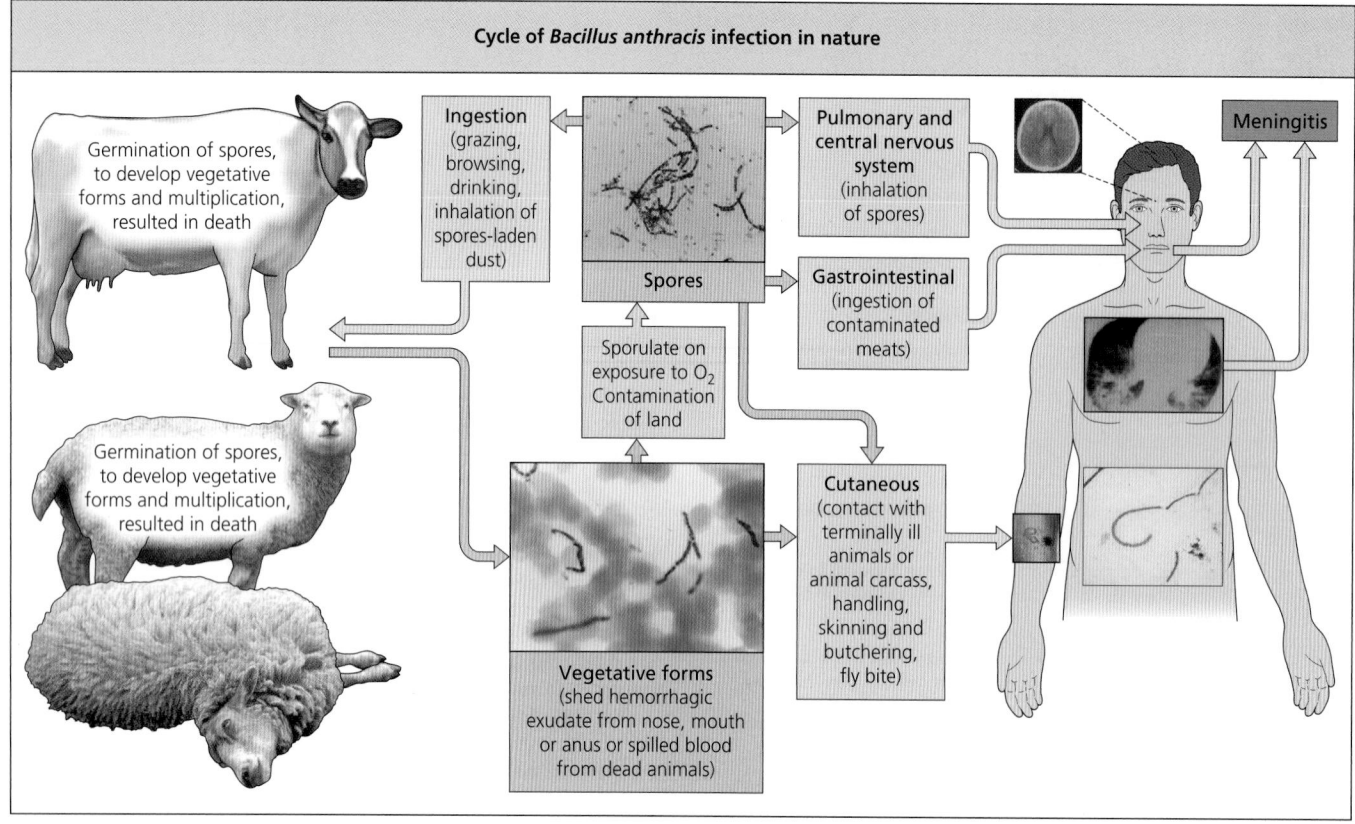

Figure 134-1 Cycle of *Bacillus anthracis* and anthrax infection in nature.

located on a smaller (95 kb) plasmid, pX02. Loss of either plasmid results in considerable reduction in virulence.[2,7,8,]

The toxin complex consists of three synergistically acting proteins: protective antigen (PA, 83 kDa), lethal factor (LF, 90 kDa) and edema factor (EF, 89 kDa). LF in combination with PA (lethal toxin, LeTx) and EF in combination with PA (edema toxin, EdTx) are secreted during multiplication of the vegetative cells and are accepted as responsible for the characteristic signs and symptoms of anthrax. EdTx is a calmodulin-dependent adenylate cyclase that increases intracellular levels of cyclic AMP (cAMP) on entry into most types of cell, leading to impaired maintenance of water homeostasis and characteristic edema. EdTx also inhibits macrophage activity by altering their cytokine production, decreases the circulating lymphocyte population and diminishes neutrophil function. LF is a zinc-dependent metalloprotease that cleaves the amino termini from mitogen-activated protein kinase kinases (MAPKKs), thereby disrupting signaling pathways with a range of resulting pathologic effects. LeTx kills or disrupts production and function of macrophages, dendritic cells, neutrophils and some epithelial and endothelial cells, downregulates cytokine production (preventing induction of chemokines integral to responses to viral or bacterial infection), inhibits B-cell proliferation and reduces B-cell production of immunoglobulin. Inflammatory mediators released in response to LeTx may also contribute to the sudden death characteristic of systemic anthrax and its lethal effect on microvascular endothelial cells is presumed to be responsible for the characteristic terminal hemorrhages.[2,7,8,9] Subsequently, the main pathologic changes seen in anthrax are edema, hemorrhage and necrosis with bacilli and limited leukocytic infiltration in involved organs.[2,7,8,10]

Prevention

The prevention of anthrax in humans is based on:

- control of infection in animals;
- prevention of contact with infected animals or contaminated animal products;
- environmental and personal hygiene;
- medical care of cutaneous anthrax;
- disinfection of fur and wool;
- education regarding the consumption of high-risk dishes made of raw meat in countries where anthrax is endemic, including Georgia, Turkey, Azerbaijan, Iran, Kyrgyzstan, Kazakhstan, African and Latin American countries.

The various strategies have recently been helpfully reviewed.[11]

Occupational groups at risk may be vaccinated. An acellular vaccine is available in the USA and the UK, and is used mostly in occupational and military settings. This vaccine is not recommended for normal travelers unless there is likely to be occupational exposure. A live spore vaccine has been produced and used in China and Russia.[1,2,12,13]

Clinical Features

The disease occurs primarily in three forms: cutaneous, gastrointestinal and respiratory. Sepsis and meningitis can rarely develop after the lymphohematogenous spread of *B. anthracis* from a primary lesion.

CUTANEOUS ANTHRAX

Cutaneous anthrax accounts for 95% of human cases.[5] The incubation period ranges from 1 to 19 days, usually 2–7 days. The lesion begins as a pruritic papule. The papule enlarges and a ring of vesicles develops around the papule at day 2–4 of the disease. Vesicular fluid may be a hemorrhagic exudate. This area is surrounded by a small ring of erythema and marked edema develops. Unless there is secondary infection, there is no pus and the lesion is not painful, although painful lymphadenitis may occur in the regional lymph nodes. Eventually, the vesicle or vesicular ring ruptures, discharging a clear fluid, and a central depressed black necrotic lesion known as an eschar is formed. Edema extends some distance from the lesion. The eschar begins to resolve about 10 days after the appearance of the initial papule. Resolution is slow (2–6 weeks), regardless of treatment.[2,6,7]

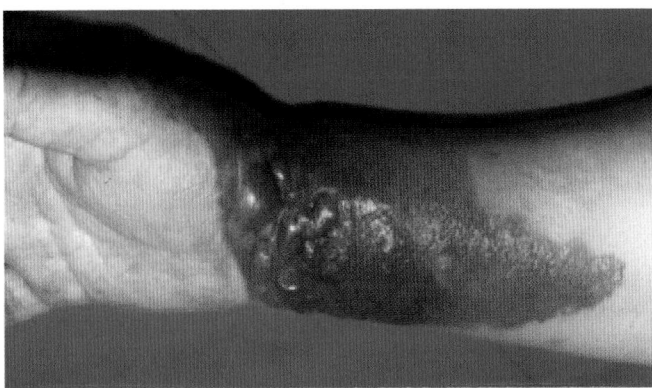

Figure 134-2 Typical appearance of mild cutaneous anthrax, characterized by a central depression, surrounded by vesicles filled with hemorrhagic fluid and erythema on the arm. *(Reproduced from Doganay M, Metan G, Alp E.: A review of cutaneous anthrax and its outcome. J Infect Public Health 2010;3:98-105.)*

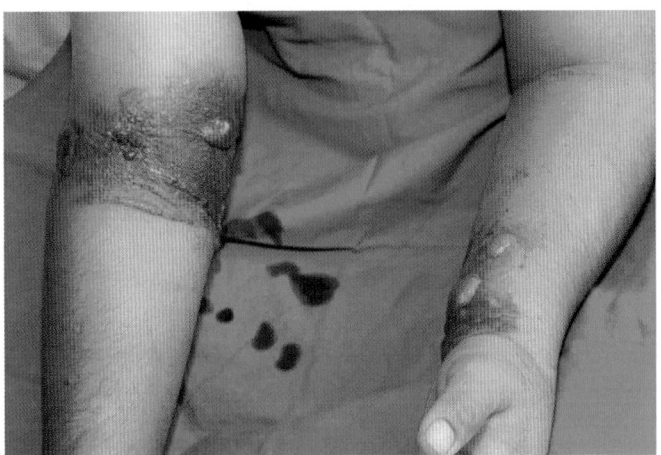

Figure 134-3 Typical appearance of severe cutaneous anthrax lesions. The patient had handled cattle and 6 days later lesions had appeared on the right and left arms. Extensive edema and hemorrhagic bullae in both arms. *(Reproduced from Doganay M, Metan G, Alp E.: A review of cutaneous anthrax and its outcome. J Infect Public Health 2010;3:98-105.)*

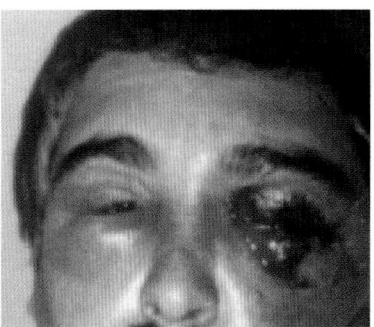

Figure 134-4 An anthrax lesion of the eyelids surrounded by erythema and massive edema extending from the left eye to the right and down to and beyond the neck. Such extensive edema is characteristic of anthrax lesions localized on the face. This lesion healed with antibacterial therapy and left a deep scar. *(Courtesy Professor Mehmet Doganay.)*

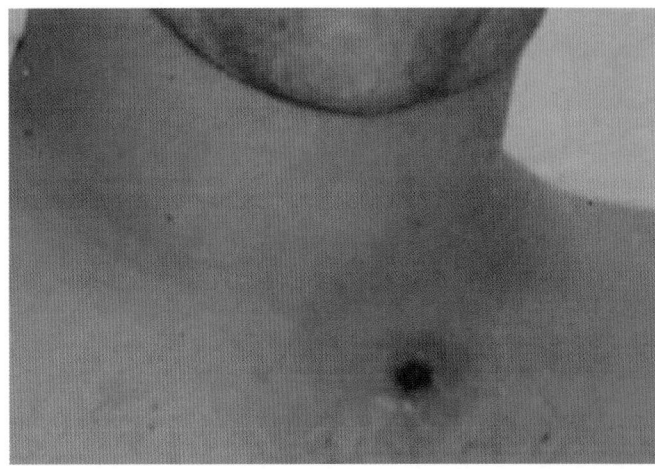

Figure 134-5 Typical appearance of cutaneous anthrax lesion but in an atypical localization on the anterior chest wall, characterized by a central depression, surrounding vesicles and erythema, and extensive edema. The patient gave a history of working with no clothes on the upper part of his body while building a new house for his family in their village during the summer. *(Courtesy Professor Mehmet Doganay.)*

The lesion is usually 1–3 cm diameter and remains round and regular (Figure 134-2). Rarely, a lesion may be larger and irregularly shaped. Systemic symptoms, including low-grade fever, malaise and headache, may be present. The cutaneous reaction may be severe in some patients and is characterized by significant local and spreading edema associated with blebs, bullae, induration, chills and fever (Figure 134-3). Clinical symptoms may be more severe if the lesion is located in the face, neck or chest. In these more severe forms, clinical findings are high fever, toxemia, regional painful lymphadenopathy and extensive edema; shock and death may ensue (Figure 134-4).[2,5–7]

More than 90% of lesions occur in exposed areas such as the face, neck, arms or hand.[2,5] The site of infection often reflects the occupation of the patient. Workers who carry hides or carcasses on their shoulders are prone to infection on the back of the neck. Handlers of contaminated animal products tend to be infected on the arms, wrists and hands. The patients generally have a single cutaneous lesion but sometimes they have two or more (Figure 134-3). Atypical localization can also be seen (Figure 134-5).[2,5–7]

A new clinical form of anthrax, injectional anthrax in drug users, has been described, firstly in Norway in 2000 and then in the UK in 2009. The clinical picture is characterized by severe soft tissue infection at the injection site, but without pain and abscess formation, and systemic symptoms of sepsis, organ dysfunction and shock. The bacterium is cultured from blood in most cases. Histological examination reveals capillary bleeding, superficial necrosis, extensive edema and necrosis along the needle tracks (Table 134-2). Mortality is very high (over 30%).[3,4,14,15]

GASTROINTESTINAL ANTHRAX

Ingestion of *B. anthracis* in contaminated food or drink can cause gastrointestinal anthrax. The incubation period is commonly 3–7 days. Two clinical forms are described: oropharyngeal and intestinal.[2,5,7,16,17]

Oropharyngeal Anthrax

The lesion is generally localized in the oral cavity, especially on the buccal mucosa or tongue, or the tonsils, and the posterior wall of the pharynx. In some cases, the lesion may be present in two or more places in the gastrointestinal system. The oral lesion is generally 2–3 cm in diameter and covered with a gray pseudomembrane surrounded by extensive edema. The main clinical features are sore throat, dysphagia, fever and painful regional lymphadenopathy in the neck. The illness progresses rapidly and edema develops around the lymph node and may extend to the upper anterior chest wall. Bacteremia may develop. The infection leads to toxemia and acute respiratory distress syndrome. Shock and coma ensue. In some cases, toxemia leads to sudden death. Despite intensive medical therapy, the mortality is about 50%.[2,7,16]

Intestinal Anthrax

The symptoms are initially nonspecific and include nausea, vomiting, anorexia and fever. With progression of the illness, abdominal pain,

TABLE 134-2	Comparison of Naturally Occurring Cutaneous Anthrax and Injectional Anthrax	
	Naturally Occurring Cutaneous Anthrax	**Injectional Anthrax**
Occurrence	Endemic areas, low- and middle-income countries	Drug users, industrialized countries
Incubation period	1–19 (2–7) days	1–10 days
Lesion site	Exposure site, mostly superficial	Injection site, deeper lesion, necrotizing soft tissue infection
Severity of infection	Mild to severe, rarely complicated	Severe and complicated (severe toxemia, sepsis, meningitis etc.)
Diagnosis	History, clinical examination, laboratory investigations	History, clinical examination, laboratory investigations
Treatment	Antibiotics, supportive therapy in severe and complicated cases	Supportive therapy, combination of antibiotics
Duration of antibiotic therapy	3–5 (may be 3–7) days	10–14 days. If snorting, up to 60 days?
Surgical intervention	Rarely	Multiple surgical debridement and reconstructive surgery
Mortality	<1%	>30%

Adapted from references 2, 3, 4, 5, 6, 7, 14.

hematemesis, bloody diarrhea and massive ascites occur, and signs suggestive of acute abdomen appear. Toxemia and shock then develop, followed by death. The lesions occur most commonly on the wall of the terminal ileum or cecum. The stomach, duodenum, upper ileum and large bowel are occasionally affected.[2,17]

INHALATION ANTHRAX

This form of anthrax was previously almost always caused by industrial exposure to spores; however, the most serious outbreaks of anthrax, in 1979 in Sverdlovsk in the former USSR and in October 2001 in the USA, have been accepted as bio-terrorism-related anthrax.[12,18]

Inhalation anthrax shows a biphasic clinical pattern with a mild initial phase followed by an acute and severe second phase. After an incubation period of 1–6 days (up to 43 days in the event at Sverdlovsk), the illness begins with mild fever, fatigue, malaise, myalgia, nonproductive cough and some chest or abdominal pain. The disease progresses to the second phase within 2–3 days. This is characterized by high fever, toxemia, dyspnea and cyanosis. Hypothermia and shock develop, resulting in death. In up to half of patients, meningitis develops as a complication.[2,12,18]

ANTHRAX MENINGITIS

Meningitis may be a complication of any of the three forms of primary anthrax and the mortality rate is over 90%. The most common portal of entry is skin (52%) followed by the lungs (22.9%). The organisms can spread to the central nervous system by hematogenous or lymphatic routes. However, the primary focus of infection cannot be determined in about 10% of cases and in these cases it is called primary anthrax meningitis. Blood cultures are positive for *B. anthracis* in 70% of patients who have meningitis.[2,5,19]

The clinical presentation includes sudden onset of fever, fatigue, myalgia, headache, nausea, vomiting, agitation, seizures, delirium and meningeal symptoms. The initial signs are followed by rapid neurologic deterioration and death. The cerebrospinal fluid is often bloody and contains many gram-positive bacilli.[2,5,19]

ANTHRAX SEPSIS

Sepsis may occur by spreading of *B. anthracis* via the lymphohematogenous route from a primary lesion. It is more commonly seen in patients with inhalation or gastrointestinal anthrax. Clinical features include fever, respiratory distress and changing mental status. Severe toxemia and shock may lead to death in a short time.[2,5]

Diagnosis

A history of exposure to contaminated animal materials, occupational exposure and living in an endemic area are all important clues for the suspicion of anthrax. Among laboratory findings, the leukocyte count

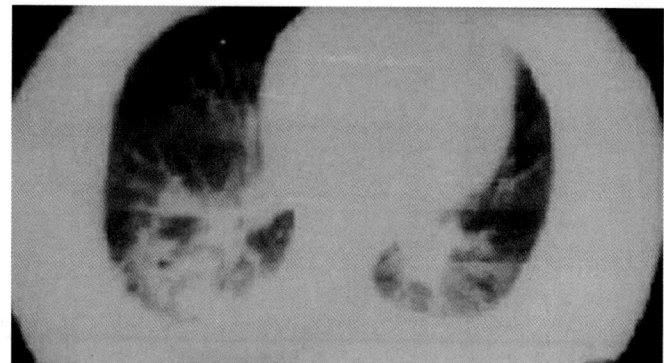

Figure 134-6 A 64-year-old male wool trader, diagnosed with inhalation anthrax complicated by hemorrhagic meningitis. A computerized tomograph of the chest revealed enlargement of the mediastinal lymph nodes, pulmonary infiltrations and small bilateral pleural effusions. *(Reproduced from Yorgancigil B, et al.: Turk J Med Sci 1998; 28:457-459.)*

is generally below 10×10^9/L in cases with mild cutaneous anthrax. Leukocytosis with neutrophilia, hemoconcentration, hypoalbuminemia, hyponatremia and an increase in AST and ALT levels may be seen in complicated cutaneous anthrax, toxemic shock and systemic anthrax. Severe sepsis due to anthrax may lead to leukopenia, thrombocytopenia and disseminated intravascular coagulation (DIC).[6,7]

In cutaneous lesions, swabs are used to sample vesicular exudates for microscopy and bacterial culture. In a well-formed eschar, in which vesicular exudate is absent, the edge of the eschar can be lifted with forceps and fluid obtained using a capillary tube. A smear is made from the material, stained with polychrome methylene blue and examined microscopically for the presence of the pink-staining encapsulated bacilli (McFadyean reaction). The samples are also inoculated on blood agar.[2,7]

For patients who have suspected gastrointestinal anthrax, swabs from oropharyngeal lesions and samples of vomit, feces, blood and ascites should be obtained. Specimens likely to be contaminated with commensal flora should be cultured on polymyxin-lysozyme-EDTA-thallous acetate (PLET) agar, which is a selective medium for *B. anthracis*.[2]

Radiographic examination of the chest usually reveals widening of the mediastinum in inhalation anthrax. Parenchymal infiltration and pleural effusion can also be seen (Figure 134-6). Direct examination of a smear of pleural fluid or blood, stained with polychrome methylene blue or Gram stain, may show encapsulated bacilli. *B. anthracis* can be isolated from the cultures of these specimens.[2,7]

Blood or cerebrospinal fluid smear stained with polychrome methylene blue should be examined for the encapsulated bacilli, which can be a useful rapid diagnostic test provided the patient has not received antibiotics. Blood and/or cerebrospinal fluid cultures should be taken for isolation of *B. anthracis* in cases of sepsis or meningitis. Blood culture is also positive in many cases with systemic anthrax.[2,5,7]

Serologic tests, immunohistochemical staining of clinical specimens and *B. anthracis*-specific polymerase chain reaction (PCR) are also useful for diagnosis of anthrax.[2,7]

Management

Antibiotic choice and administration route are based on the severity of infection. In cutaneous anthrax the patients may be divided into three groups according to severity: *mild cutaneous anthrax* (presence of a cutaneous lesion measuring <4 cm in diameter, surrounded by a narrow zone of erythema, and no systemic symptoms), or *severe cutaneous anthrax* (a cutaneous lesion measuring ≥4 cm in diameter, with a bullous reaction and/or extensive edema, and systemic symptoms including fever, tachycardia and tachypnea, or a small cutaneous lesion with extensive edema and systemic symptoms). *Complicated cutaneous anthrax* is defined as presence of septic shock or bacteremia and/or any organ involvement with a cutaneous lesion. An oral antibiotic may be given to patients with mild cutaneous anthrax in the outpatient clinic. In severe and complicated cutaneous anthrax, patients should be hospitalized and antibiotics should be given intravenously.[6,20]

In vitro human clinical isolates of *B. anthracis* are sensitive to many antibiotics: penicillins, aminoglycosides, macrolides, quinolones, carbapenems, tetracyclines, vancomycin, clindamycin, rifampin (rifampicin), cefazolin and linezolid.[2,21] Penicillin G is still the drug of choice in the therapy of naturally occurring anthrax. In mild uncomplicated cutaneous anthrax, intramuscular procaine penicillin (800 000 to 1 million units q12–24h) or amoxicillin (500 mg orally q6–8h) is suggested for 3–5 days. *B. anthracis* cannot be isolated from cutaneous lesions 24–48 hours after antibiotic administration. Early treatment will limit the size of the lesion but will not alter the evolutionary stages (Table 134-3).[2,21]

In patients showing signs of systemic involvement, such as inhalation anthrax or gastrointestinal anthrax, meningoencephalitis and sepsis, antibiotics should be given intravenously. Penicillin G is the first choice, given at a dose of 4 million units q4–6h (total daily dose should be 20–24 million units) until the patient's symptoms resolve and fever returns to normal. At this point, the intravenous antibiotic can be switched to intramuscular penicillin G or to an oral antibiotic. In the treatment of systemic anthrax, penicillin should be combined with one or two other antibiotics to which *B. anthracis* is susceptible. Penicillin G may be combined with clindamycin, clarithromycin or ciprofloxacin in treating inhalation anthrax or with an aminoglycoside (streptomycin is suggested) in gastrointestinal anthrax.[2,7,20]

Anthrax meningoencephalitis is a life-threatening infection. Currently, a combination of penicillin G and rifampin is the first choice of treatment. Other possible regimens would be penicillin G in combination with vancomycin, or vancomycin and rifampin or vancomycin and meropenem.[2,19]

In the event of allergy to penicillin, either doxycycline or ciprofloxacin is accepted as best alternative. Tetracyclines and erythromycin are also effective alternatives in mild cutaneous anthrax in low- and middle-income countries. In uncomplicated cutaneous anthrax, doxycycline or ciprofloxacin is given orally. In systemic anthrax, doxycycline or ciprofloxacin should be given intravenously and may be combined with another suitable antibiotic, such as penicillin.[2,5–7] Duration of antibiotic treatment in uncomplicated cutaneous anthrax is suggested as 3–5 days (may be 3–7 days). Therapy in cases of systemic and injectional anthrax should be continued for at least 10–14 days.[2,6,20]

In addition to antibiotic therapy, specific antitoxin serum for anthrax may be beneficial in systemic and injectional anthrax. Raxibacumab, an IgG1 monoclonal antibody that binds the protective antigen (PA) of *Bacillus anthracis*, has shown benefit in an animal model.[22] Supportive treatment for shock, intubation, tracheotomy or ventilatory support in respiratory problems and steroid administration or other anti-brain edema therapies for anthrax meningoencephalitis are life-saving in some cases.[2,7,19] In cutaneous anthrax, surgical intervention is not generally suggested. Surgical debridement or fasciotomies are rarely required in cutaneous anthrax. Large crusts should be removed and deep scars due to anthrax lesions may be reconstructed surgically. On the other hand, in injectional anthrax, surgical debridement removes the nidus of infection, provides diagnostic materials (Gram stain, culture and PCR) and may be life-saving. It is also noted that surgical resection of intestinal lesions along with medical treatment has shown a beneficial effect.[2–5,7,19]

References available online at expertconsult.com.

TABLE 134-3	Suggested Antibiotic Therapy for Anthrax in Adults		
Category	**Antibiotic**		**Duration**
Naturally occurring anthrax	*First choice** Procaine penicillin G 0.6–1.2 mU im q12–24h Penicillin G, sodium or potassium 4 mU iv q4–6h Amoxicillin 500 mg po q6–8h *Alternative** Doxycycline 100 mg iv/po q12h or Ciprofloxacin 200–400 mg iv q12h, followed as 500–750 mg po q12h		Uncomplicated cutaneous anthrax: 3–5 days (may be 3–7 days) Systemic anthrax†: 10–14 days
Injectional anthrax	Antibiotic combination with surgical debridement and later reconstructive surgery if required		10–14 days. If snorting, up to 60 days?
Biological weapon or bioterrorism-related anthrax	Ciprofloxacin 200–400 mg iv q12h, followed as 500–750 mg po q12h or Doxycycline 100 mg iv/po q12h		Up to 60 days

*Antibiotic therapy may be given orally in mild cutaneous anthrax. In cases of severe cutaneous anthrax or systemic anthrax, initial antibiotic therapy should be given intravenously; when fever has subsided to normal, antibiotic therapy may be switched to oral.
†In systemic anthrax, initial antibiotic choice should be combined with one or two of the following antibiotics: penicillin, ampicillin, ciprofloxacin, imipenem, meropenem, vancomycin, rifampin (rifampicin), clindamycin, linezolid, streptomycin or other aminoglycoside. Two or more antibiotics combination should be given in meningitis.
In anthrax meningitis, initial antibiotics should have good CSF penetration.
Additional to antibiotics, specific antitoxic serum for anthrax may also be given if available.
Adapted from references 2, 4, 6, 7, 12, 14, 19, 20.

KEY REFERENCES

Booth M.G., Hood J., Brooks T.J.G., et al.: Anthrax infection in drug users. *Lancet* 2010; 375:1345-1346.

Dixon T., Meselson M., Guillemin J., et al.: Anthrax. *N Engl J Med* 1999; 341:815-886.

Doganay M., Metan G.: Human anthrax in Turkey from 1990 to 2007. *Vector Borne Zoonotic Dis* 2009; 9(2):131-140.

Doganay M., Metan G., Alp E.: A review of cutaneous anthrax and its outcome. *J Infect Public Health* 2010; 3:98-105.

Grunow R., Werbek L., Jacob D., et al.: Injection anthrax – a new outbreak in heroin users. *Dtsch Arztebl Int* 2012; 109(49):843-848.

Inglesby T.V., O'Toole T., Henderson D.A., et al.: Anthrax as a biologic weapon, 2002. Updated recommendations for management. *JAMA* 2002; 287:2236-2252.

Kanafani Z.A., Ghossain A., Sharara A.I., et al.: Endemic gastrointestinal anthrax in 1960s Lebanon: clinical manifestations and surgical findings. *Emerg Infect Dis* 2003; 9:520-525.

Kayabas U., Karahocagil M.K., Ozkurt Z., et al.: Naturally occurring cutaneous anthrax: antibiotic treatment and outcome. *Chemotherapy* 2012; 58:34-43.

Sejvar J.J., Tenover F.C., Stephens D.S.: Management of anthrax meningitis. *Lancet Infect Dis* 2005; 5:287-295.

Turnbull P., WHO Anthrax Working Group: *Anthrax in humans and animals.* 4th ed. Geneva: World Health Organization; 2008.

135

The Patient Returning from the Tropics with Fever

CHRISTOPHER J.M. WHITTY

KEY CONCEPTS

- The commonest serious cause of fever from the tropics is malaria – this should always be excluded by testing.

- Prevalence of human immunodeficiency virus (HIV) is high in many tropical countries; have a low threshold for testing.

- A detailed travel history and then matching that against local epidemiology is the key to diagnosing most other serious tropical causes of fever.

- The differential diagnosis for patients whose symptoms start more than 21 days from tropical exposure is much shorter, with parasitic diseases and TB the main groups.

- Rash and jaundice are useful signs.

Introduction

In patients having recently arrived from tropical or low-resource environments, a history of undifferentiated fever or one with additional signs and symptoms such as headaches, rash or jaundice, is a common presentation. Case series suggest around a third of travellers presenting to healthcare have a fever syndrome. The differential diagnosis of infections that are potentially serious or treatable is significantly wider than for patients who have not traveled outside their home country. Which infections are commonly imported into countries depends on local travel patterns, often influenced by historical ties, so, for example, infections from Latin America are more commonly imported into the USA than Europe, but West African infections are more commonly seen in the UK and France. The area a traveler has come from determines the likely causes. This chapter will consider a systematic approach to excluding important tropical or parasitic causes of fever, but travelers may well have an infection which they could just as easily have caught without any travel, such as upper respiratory tract and urinary tract infections, or a noninfectious cause of fever. The chapter is aimed particularly at infectious disease physicians who have less recent experience of diagnosing tropical infections; treatment is covered in relevant chapters. Guidelines exist with more detailed national advice.[1]

The general history and examination of patients from the tropics is very similar to any other infectious disease, with one exception. A really detailed travel history, including exact timings of travel and onset of symptoms and specific questions about exactly what people did in the countries they have returned from, is the key to identifying the great majority of treatable tropical causes of fever. Most febrile patients returned from the tropics who do not have self-limiting viral illness have a relatively limited range of infections, and by excluding these the great majority of people who need treating with specific antimicrobials rather than just supportive care will rapidly be identified. There are several questions the physician will want to ask the patient and themselves to avoid missing an important imported infection.

Seven Questions to Ask

(1) Could the patient have malaria or HIV? If either of these is a possibility testing needs to be done at an early stage. Malaria remains the commonest serious cause of febrile illness in returning travelers from most of sub-Saharan Africa, and a significant risk for many parts of Asia and Latin America. Nothing in the history or examination will either prove or exclude it, so a malaria test will be needed if the traveler has been to anywhere where malaria transmission occurs.[2] Around half of travelers who present with malaria will not have a fever at the time of presentation so a recent history of fever is sufficient. In a typical series in London, around 20% of those returned from sub-Saharan Africa with a history of fever had malaria, with much lower but appreciable rates among those returning from other tropical areas.[3] HIV needs to be identified early because whilst relatively rarer than malaria it completely changes the differential diagnosis. Whilst a sexual history is useful in very short-term travelers such as holidaymakers, in those who have lived for extended periods in countries where a significant proportion of the general population has HIV it is usually better simply to exclude by testing.

(2) Has the patient been out of the last tropical country they were in for more than 21 days prior to development of symptoms? A very high proportion of the tropical infections, including the arboviruses such as dengue, and for practical purposes bacterial enteric fevers such as typhoid, are excluded if so. Thus the list of possible causes is much shorter if people present after this time, with parasitic causes such as malaria or amebic liver abscess, and tuberculosis relatively more likely if the fever is related to their tropical travel. Table 135-1 shows some of the most common tropical infections that can present after 21 days.

(3) Exactly where has the patient traveled, and was it to rural or exclusively urban environments? Whilst some of the important tropical infections such as malaria or dengue are very widespread, even in countries where they are common there is generally significant regional variation. This may depend also on the time of year. For example, malaria is unlikely if the patient has only been in Lagos, but more common if the patient has been in the less urbanized areas of southern Nigeria. Many tropical infections are extremely geographically defined.

TABLE 135-1	Pointers to Narrow the Differential Diagnosis in Imported Fevers	
Common Causes of Fever that Can First Present >21 Days After Last Tropical Exposure	Fever and Rash	Fever and Jaundice
Malaria	HIV seroconversion	Malaria
Tuberculosis	African tick typhus	Leptospirosis
HIV-associated	Katayama syndrome	Ascending cholangitis
Amebic abscess	Dengue and other arboviruses	Rarely
Katayama syndrome (4–8 weeks)	Measles and rubella	HIV-associated non-typhi salmonella
Visceral leishmaniasis	Secondary syphilis	Amebic liver abscess
Brucellosis	Meningococcal infection	

Melioidosis is a common cause of fever in certain parts of northern Thailand but rare elsewhere in the country, whilst over the border in Laos mite-borne typhus is common. Leishmaniasis concentrates in certain parts of Sudan and South Sudan, human African trypanosomiasis in others. Knowing which country people have gone to is therefore not sufficient; where they have been exactly will help narrow down the possibilities. Those who are not primarily trained in tropical medicine can use this information either to have an informed discussion with 'tropical specialists, or look up common diseases in particular geographical areas if they do not have access to tropical medicine expertise.

(4) Has the patient undertaken high-risk activities from the perspective of acquiring infections? Specific ones to ask about in addition to sexual history and risks for blood-borne viruses such as injections or tattoos are:

- Exposure to game parks in Africa. This significantly increases the risk of African tick typhus, and much more rarely, acute human African trypanosomiasis.
- Jungle exposure in Asia. In particular this is associated with leptospirosis and mite-borne typhus.
- Fresh water exposure such as swimming in lakes or rivers. Fever developing 4–8 weeks after this raises the possibility of Katayama syndrome in Africa. It is also a risk for leptospirosis globally.
- Visiting hospitals, sick friends or relatives, or traditional funerals. This has a number of increased risks but the one that concerns people most, although normally very rare, is viral hemorrhagic fever, especially Lassa from West Africa and Ebola in West and Central Africa. Both are excluded if the patient has been back more than 21 days since the last contact. If hemorrhagic fevers are within the differential diagnoses, there are clear national guidelines on the safe investigation and management of these patients, which must be followed.[4]
- Exposure in caves, where histoplasmosis in particular is more likely.

(5) Does the patient have any specific symptom or sign which might help narrow the differential diagnosis? Important ones for infectious diseases are jaundice (most common tropical causes in acutely febrile patients are severe malaria and leptospirosis) and rash (e.g. typhus, dengue, Katayama syndrome, HIV seroconversion). A longer list of potential causes of these syndromes is shown in Table 135-1.

(6) Is there a clue from the basic blood tests and chest radiograph? Important ones where the implications are sometimes missed include:

- Low platelet count (common in malaria, HIV seroconversion and several viral illnesses).
- A raised right hemidiaphragm on chest radiograph in the presence of raised neutrophils or inflammatory markers which is often associated with amebic liver abscess. This should trigger liver ultrasound or CT and serology.
- A significantly raised eosinophil count, which is associated with Katayama syndrome.
- It is easy to overdo testing for tropical diseases. Many tests, especially serological ones, have a specificity well short of 100% and with low pre-test probabilities for many of the diseases the chance of a false-positive is high.[5] For most patients malaria films, full blood count, blood culture, liver function tests, inflammatory markers and chest radiograph are sufficient, with a saved serum in case it is needed later.

(7) Is there a local outbreak or epidemic, and is there a risk of viral hemorrhagic fever? Some imported infections, such as dengue, can vary considerably by year depending on outbreaks.[6] There are several excellent free resources for providing latest news of these, including CDC, the WHO, Eurosurveillance and Health Protection England, but the most widely used resource is probably Promed (www.promedmail.org). In patients with rural exposure in West or Central Africa within 21 days consider viral hemorrhagic fever (VHF). In most countries there is a protocol for assessing and managing these patients; if in doubt isolate the patients and follow the protocol: (www.gov.uk/government/publications/viral-haemorrhagic-fever-algorithm-and-guidance-on-management-of-patients) or (www.cdc.gov/vhf/ebola/pdf/ebola-algorithm.pdf).

Some Common Infections by Region

Whilst there are significant local variations, some broad generalizations by region are reasonable as a guide to important infections causing fever, which should be considered when patients first present.

SUB-SAHARAN AFRICA ABOVE SOUTH AFRICA

Unless patients have been exclusively in highly urban areas or have HIV, falciparum malaria remains the most important thing to exclude. After that, relatively common identifiable causes of imported fever include amebic liver abscess and African tick typhus. Typhoid is substantially overdiagnosed within Africa due to overreliance on the Widal test – case series suggest it is actually rare except in urban slum areas. Fever and rash raise the possibility of Katayama syndrome, one of the many arboviruses (mosquito-borne), HIV or syphilis, and in unvaccinated travelers' measles. Physicians should remember that the meningococcus belt runs across West Africa and epidemics can make it a common disease at particular times although it is relatively rarely imported.

SOUTH AND SOUTH EAST ASIA

Whilst malaria should always be excluded, enteric fever (typhoid and paratyphoid) is commoner from most areas. Leptospirosis and dengue are both relatively commonly seen in travelers from this region. In addition, from the area around the Indian Ocean, Chikungunya is currently relatively frequently seen.

MIDDLE EAST AND NORTH AFRICA

Brucellosis is the main disease to be aware of that is significantly more common than from other areas. Malaria is rare except from Yemen.

LATIN AMERICA

Dengue is well established in parts of Latin America. Malaria is now rare except in restricted areas – it should be excluded but is unlikely.

Spotting Danger Signs, and Outcomes

As important as identifying the organism is identifying those patients who are at increased risk of doing badly, are likely to need admission to hospital, and in some cases high-intensity supportive care. The standard list of danger signs in malaria is a good screening tool for severe illness in most tropical infections. Reduced level of consciousness or neurological signs, shock or oliguria and rapid breathing are important but obvious signs of severity. Evidence of bleeding, or purpura, is a bad sign with any infection, and should additionally raise the possibility of viral hemorrhagic fevers or meningococcus. Jaundice in patients with fever from the tropics is always a worrying sign as it is most likely to be malaria with severe hemolysis, or leptospirosis, with a large amebic liver abscess and ascending cholangitis also possible. Of note in most cases of acute viral hepatitis the fever has resolved by the time jaundice appears. Two groups – pregnant women and elderly patients – are at particular risk of poor outcomes with imported tropical causes of fever such as malaria[7] and physicians should have a low threshold for admitting them.

The wide range of imported infections seen in returning travelers present a diagnostic challenge for physicians, but almost all of them are either self-limiting or easily treatable if diagnosed early. Unfortunately, every year a few patients die from severe malaria in Europe, the USA and other high-resource settings, but most have presented late and *in extremis*: it is important to stress to travelers the need to seek diagnosis and treatment early. In settings with good diagnostic and treatment facilities very few immunocompetent patients die or have significant long-term morbidity from imported febrile infections.

References available online at expertconsult.com.

KEY REFERENCES

Checkley A.M., Smith A., Smith V., et al.: Risk factors for mortality from imported *falciparum* malaria in the United Kingdom over 20 years: an observational study. *BMJ* 2012; 344:e2116.

Inojosa W.O., Augusto I., Bisoffi Z., et al.: Diagnosing human African trypanosomiasis in Angola using a card agglutination test: observational study of active and passive case finding strategies. *BMJ* 2006; 332:1479.

Johnston V., Stockley J.M., Dockrell D., et al.: British Infection Society and the Hospital for Tropical Diseases. Fever in returned travellers presenting in the United Kingdom: recommendations for investigation and initial management. *J Infect* 2009; 59:1-18.

La Ruche G., Dejour-Salamanca D., Bernillon P., et al.: Capture–recapture method for estimating annual incidence of imported dengue, France, 2007–2010. *Emerg Infect Dis* 2013; 19(11):1740-1748.

Nic Fhogartaigh C., Hughes H., Armstrong M., et al.: *Falciparum* malaria as a cause of fever in adult travellers returning to the United Kingdom: observational study of risk by geographical area. *QJM* 2008; 101:649-656.

Taylor S.M., Molyneux M.E., Simel D.L., et al.: Does this patient have malaria? *JAMA* 2010; 304:2048-2056.

UK Advisory Committee on Dangerous Pathogens: *Management of Hazard Group 4 viral haemorrhagic fevers and similar human infectious diseases of high consequence.* London: HPA; 2012.

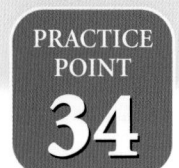

PRACTICE POINT

34

Respiratory Tract Infection in a Traveler Returning from the Hajj

SHRUTI SRIDHAR | JEAN-CHRISTOPHE LAGIER | PHILIPPE GAUTRET

Case Report

A 71-year-old woman returned from Saudi Arabia complaining of cough and fever for 10 days. The complaints started during the Hajj pilgrimage in Mecca. The initial episode started abruptly with dry cough, fatigue and subjective fever which were followed by diarrhea a few days later. Many pilgrims from her group presented with similar symptoms. On her arrival from Saudi Arabia, she immediately presented to the emergency ward and was subsequently transferred to the infectious disease ward in biologic safety level 3 (BSL3) conditions. She complained of fatigue, cough, dyspnea, diarrhea (five stools per day) and nausea.

She had a history of hypertension, chronic hypertensive heart disease, atrial fibrillation, hypothyroidism, gastritis, depression and allergy to penicillin. On admission, she was treated with furosemide, bisoprolol, ramipril, eplerone, rivaroxaban, L-thyroxine, esomeprazole and fluoxetine. She was vaccinated against meningitis before the pilgrimage but was not vaccinated against influenza in that year and never against invasive pneumococcal disease. She used face masks from time to time during the pilgrimage and practiced hand hygiene more often than usual. Physical examination in the emergency room revealed a body temperature of 39°C, dry cough, respiratory rate of 30 breaths per minute, bilateral diffused rhonchi and sibilants, without crepitant rales or decreased breathing sounds, blood pressure 130/70 mmHg, heart rate of 74 beats per minute (irregular). Oxygen saturation was 95% on ambient air. Chest radiography showed increased interstitial bilateral diffuse markings and moderate cardiomegaly. The laboratory results on admission were: white blood cell count 4.34×10^9/L (59% neutrophils, 34% lymphocytes); C-reactive protein 24 mg/L; serum sodium 141 mmol/L; serum phosphorus 85 IU/L; serum creatinine 11.5 mg/L; serum glutamate pyruvate transaminase 22 IU/L; serum oxaloacetate transaminase 41 IU/L; gamma glutamyl transferase 36 IU/L. Nasal swab polymerase chain reaction (PCR) detection of influenza H1N1 virus was positive. Nasal swab PCR detection of influenza A3N2, influenza B, parainfluenza viruses 1, 2, 3 and 4, rhinovirus, human metapneumovirus, human respiratory syncytial virus and Middle East Respiratory Syndrome coronavirus (MERS-CoV), E229 coronavirus, HKU1 coronavirus, NL63 coronavirus and OC 43 coronavirus were negative. *Legionella* antigens were negative in urine samples. Sputum bacterial cultures were negative. Blood cultures were negative. Atrial fibrillation was confirmed by the electrocardiogram. Oral levofloxacin and oseltamivir were administered. She was apyrexial on the second day and was discharged on day 6.

Discussion

The pilgrimage to Mecca, also known as the Hajj, is the fifth pillar of Islam and is mandatory for all adult Muslims who are physically and financially capable to undertake at least once during their lifetime. Therefore, about 2–3 million Muslims from more than 180 countries gather each year in the Kingdom of Saudi Arabia to perform the Hajj pilgrimage. As a result of overcrowding during the stay, acute respiratory infections are very common among pilgrims. Incidence rate of respiratory symptoms may be up to 90%, as observed in a French cohort survey during the 2012 Hajj season, with cough as the most frequently reported complaint (83% of respondents) followed by sore throat (78%) and rhinorrhea (69%). Respiratory diseases are by far the main reason for consultation at primary healthcare centers during the Hajj and major causes of hospitalization in tertiary care hospitals among pilgrims during their stay in Saudi Arabia. Recent studies demonstrated a rapid acquisition of respiratory viruses and bacteria nasal carriage among pilgrims during their stay in Saudi Arabia, most notably coronaviruses, rhinovirus, influenza virus and *Streptococcus pneumoniae*. According to a survey in 2012, out of the pilgrims who presented with fever and cough or sore throat (influenza-like illness), 7% were associated with *Strep. pneumoniae* nasal carriage and 37.5% with virus carriage. The majority of viral cases were associated with human rhinovirus, followed by influenza H3N2 virus. The differentiation between bacterial and viral infection is imperative in deciding the course of treatment. Also, this implies that antibiotics would be rendered ineffective in almost 40% of cases presenting with fever and cough.

According to the World Health Organization, there has also been an ongoing outbreak of MERS-CoV in Saudi Arabia since April 2012 with over 1060 laboratory confirmed cases as of August 2015 and a case fatality rate of approximately 38%. The majority of human cases of MERS-CoV infections are secondary cases and attributable to human-to-human transmission, primarily among healthcare workers. Cases have been acquired or reported in Saudi Arabia (>85%), Qatar, Jordan, Oman, Kuwait, United Arab Emirates and Yemen. Some cases have been exported from the Arabian Peninsula in Europe, the USA, North Africa, Asia and the Middle East. In addition, there has been a significant cluster of 186 cases in South Korea, associated with 36 deaths. This was traced to a traveler returning from the Middle East. There is evidence suggesting that camels may act as a reservoir. In the case presented here, we considered that the patient may have been infected by MERS-CoV and she was managed in a BSL3 environment until a diagnosis of influenza H1N1 was made. It is not always possible to identify patients with MERS-CoV early because some have mild or unusual symptoms. For this reason, it is important that healthcare workers apply standard precautions consistently with all patients, regardless of their diagnosis, in all work practices all the time. Droplet precautions should be added to the standard precautions when providing care to any patient with symptoms of acute respiratory infection. Contact precautions and eye protection should be added when caring for probable or confirmed cases of MERS-CoV infection. Airborne precautions should be applied when performing aerosol-generating procedures.

Preventive Measures Against Respiratory-Transmited Diseases at the Hajj

Hajj pilgrims should be up to date with routine immunizations and must have had the tetravalent meningococcal vaccine ≤3 years and ≥10 days before arriving in Saudi Arabia. Seasonal influenza vaccine is recommended for all pilgrims and pneumococcal vaccine for pilgrims aged ≥65 years and for younger pilgrims with co-morbidities. Behavioral interventions such as hand hygiene, wearing a face mask, cough etiquette, social distancing and contact avoidance can be effective at mitigating respiratory illness among Hajj pilgrims. Additionally, pilgrims should take precautions when visiting farms and markets where camels are present. These precautions include: avoiding contact with camels; not drinking raw camel milk or camel urine; and not eating meat that has not been thoroughly cooked.

Further reading available online at expertconsult.com.

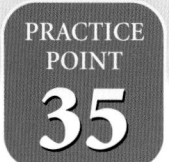

PRACTICE POINT 35

Jaundice in the Traveler Returning from Nepal

JUSTIN BEARDSLEY

Introduction

Jaundice is a symptom of many disease states, and in the case of a traveler who has returned from Nepal a working knowledge of the prevalence of particular infectious diseases in that country can help to narrow the differential diagnosis. Exposure is not only affected by the environment, but also by the traveler's behavior. It has been consistently demonstrated that travelers underestimate risks when overseas, resulting in behaviors such as drug-taking, casual sex and the consumption of excessive alcohol and potentially unsafe foods.

Background

Nepal is a popular destination for travelers, attracting more than 800 000 visitors each year. It is also a poor country with underdeveloped infrastructure, and the government hopes that increasing income from tourism will help to address this. Although traditional water spouts (Figure PP35-1) remain popular, access to improved drinking water has improved. UNICEF's report 'Progress on Drinking Water and Sanitation 2014' states that 23% of the population gained access to improved water between 2000 and 2012. However, even this improved supply may not be potable, due to contamination with arsenic and human waste. Beyond Kathmandu the mountainous terrain is a major obstacle to civil engineering projects, and waterborne disease is an important cause of illness. Malaria is endemic in lower-lying southern parts of the country but, apart from Chitwan National Park, these areas are off the main tourist trail. Reports of malaria in travelers, even those visiting Chitwan National Park, are rare. Selected comparative country health indicators are illustrated in Table PP35-1.

Potential Noninfectious Causes of Jaundice in a Traveler Returning from Nepal

Although the focus of this Practice Point is infectious causes of jaundice, noninfectious causes remain which must be excluded. In a tropical traveler, these include drug-induced hepatitis from antimalaria chemoprophylaxis (described with mefloquine, amodiaquine and atovaquone–proguanil) or self-treatment of travelers' diarrhea (described with macrolides and rarely with fluoroquinolones). Over-the-counter pharmaceuticals and traditional herbal remedies are readily available, so opportunities for self medication are greatly increased.

Potential Infectious Causes of Jaundice in a Traveler Returning from Nepal

A nonexhaustive list of infectious causes of jaundice is found in Table PP35-2. The outlook for most infectious diseases is improved by early diagnosis and treatment. Treatable potentially fatal diseases such as enteric fever and malaria should always be considered and excluded in patients returning from the tropics.

TABLE PP35-1 Selected Comparative Health Indicators			
Indicator	Nepal	WHO South East Asia Region Average	Global Average
Population living in urban areas (%)	17	34	52
Access to improved drinking water (%)	88	–	89
Access to improved sanitation (%)	35	–	63
Gross national income per person (USD)	1260	3747	11 536
Life expectancy at birth	68	67	70
Prevalence of TB (per 100 000)	243	271	170
Prevalence of HIV (per 100 000)	161	189	499
Incidence of malaria (per 100 000)	64	1773	4082
Distribution of years of life lost by cause (communicable/non-communicable %)	60/40	49/51	–

From WHO Health Statistics, 2014 and UNICEF Nepal, 2011.

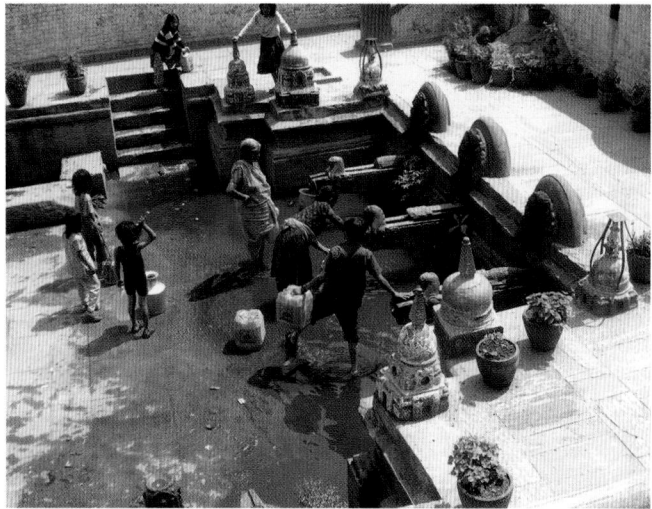

Figure PP35-1   Collecting water from traditional water spouts in Patan, Nepal.

TABLE PP35-2	Potential Infectious Causes of Jaundice in a Traveler Returning from Nepal	
	Pathogen	**Comment**
VIRAL	Hepatitis A virus Hepatitis B virus Hepatitis C virus Hepatitis D virus Hepatitis E virus Epstein–Barr virus Cytomegalovirus Human immunodeficiency virus	Requires coinfection with hepatitis B virus
BACTERIAL	*Listeria monocytogenes* *Neisseria* spp. Pneumococcus	As part of disseminated disease, i.e. severe sepsis
	Coxiella burnetti *Rickettsia conori*	Cause granulomatous hepatitis but jaundice is rare. No reported *Coxiella* infections from Nepal
	Treponema pallidum	In secondary syphilis. Primary disease may be asymptomatic depending upon the site of the lesion
	Chlamydia spp.	Fitz-Hugh–Curtis syndrome
	Brucella spp. *Leptospira* spp.	
	Salmonella enterica	Serovars Typhi and Paratyphi A
	Mycobacterium tuberculae	The commonest cause of granulomatous hepatitis worldwide
PARASITIC	*Entamoeba histolytica*	If there is compression of bile ducts by abscess
	Falciparum spp	The presence of jaundice defines severe malaria
	Leishmania spp.	Can cause granulomatous hepatitis, jaundice is rare
	Fasciola hepatica/gigantica	Abnormal liver enzymes common in acute disease, jaundice can be a feature of established infection

HEPATITIS E

Hepatitis E virus (HEV) is endemic in the developing world and is the commonest viral cause of acute hepatitis in Nepal. Disease is often asymptomatic but can be severe, particularly in pregnant women, with mortality up to 25%, and there is no specific treatment. There have been large-scale outbreaks reported from several countries, including Nepal, but the vast majority of disease burden is accounted for by sporadic cases. The route of infection is most commonly feco-oral, and the incidence is higher in the rainy season, possibly related to fecal contamination of drinking water. Some reports have attributed up to 90% of Nepali cases of acute infectious jaundice to HEV, but the incidence varies from year to year. There are four genotypes of HEV described but only one serotype, which aided the development of a vaccine, licensed and released in China in 2012, but not yet available globally.

With the exception of the high mortality in pregnancy, the presentation and clinical course of hepatitis E is similar to that of hepatitis A. It cannot be distinguished clinically from other causes of acute hepatitis, and definitive diagnosis relies on serologic testing. The period of viremia can be prolonged but resolution of biochemical hepatitis seems to correlate strongly with clearance of virus from stool.

HEPATITIS A

Hepatitis A virus (HAV) is endemic in Nepal with one survey showing 3–8% of acute hepatitis resulting from HAV. This is a vaccine-preventable disease for travelers and an immunization history is critical. Spread is feco-oral, and the incubation period is 2–6 weeks. Most infected adults (70%) become jaundiced, although children under 2 years are usually asymptomatic. Fulminant hepatic failure is rare (0.2%).

HEPATITIS B

Hepatitis B vaccination is increasingly offered to travelers. The relevant risk factors for HBV infection in travelers include sex and contaminated medical equipment/blood products – a careful history is essential as sex tourism is common in South and South East Asia. Diagnosis is by serologic testing. The incubation period is 2–6 months. HBV accounts for between 2 and 15% of cases of acute infectious hepatitis in Nepalese patients, though their risk factors include vertical transmission and childhood horizontal spread, so these rates may not be generalizable to travelers.

HEPATITIS C

Hepatitis C virus (HCV) accounts for 3–5% of acute infectious hepatitis cases in Nepal. Data are limited, but most infections are due to genotypes 1 or 3. HCV has a low risk of sexual transmission and is predominantly transmitted via blood, blood products and intravenous drug use. Both HBC and HCV viruses can be transmitted through tattooing, and this risk is often not recognized by travellers. The incubation period is between 2 weeks and 6 months. Most infections with HCV lead to chronic disease (80%) and are initially asymptomatic. Less than 25% of patients are acutely jaundiced. Early diagnosis and treatment of HCV may result in increased cure rates, and the diagnosis should be excluded in any jaundiced patient, or any asymptomatic patient with a significant exposure history.

ENTERIC FEVER

Up to 18% of patients with enteric fever are jaundiced, and it is the commonest identifiable cause of fever in patients presenting to Patan Hospital, Kathmandu. Between 2008 and 2011, 34.7% of ambulatory febrile patients at this hospital had culture-confirmed enteric fever. The incubation period is 1–4 weeks. Over the past 10 years *Salmonella enterica* serovar Paratyphi A has emerged as an important cause of enteric fever, and rates of drug resistance for this organism are increasing. Bone marrow culture is the most sensitive diagnostic test for enteric fever. The sensitivity of standard blood culture is improved with a large, 15 mL draw, as there often are very few organisms in the bloodstream.

LEPTOSPIROSIS

Leptospirosis is widely distributed in tropical countries and has been associated with popular recreational activities such as white water rafting, canoeing and triathlons. One survey of blood donors and army recruits in eastern Nepal found 12% of the population to be seropositive. Jaundice occurs in a subset of patients, although many infections are sub-clinical. Serologically confirmed leptospirosis accounted for 4% of all cases of fever in adults at Patan Hospital. The incubation period is between 5 and 14 days. Headache and fever are the most frequent symptoms; other manifestations include cough, pharyngitis, myalgia, abdominal pain, hepatosplenomegaly and conjunctival suffusion. The clinical features are similar to enteric fever, although jaundice is more common. Diagnosis is made through paired sera – isolation of the organism from blood culture is difficult. Nucleic acid amplification techniques, including real time polymerase chain reaction, have been developed as diagnostic tests, but are not widely available. Doxycycline or benzylpenicillin are commonly used for treatment.

MALARIA

Jaundice is a manifestation of severe malaria. There are around 3500 cases of malaria each year in Nepal. Most of these (75%) are *Plasmodium vivax*; *P. falciparum* accounts for the rest. Transmission is limited to elevations of less than 1500 m, and is commonest in the rainy season. The Terai region has the highest transmission rates whilst the Kathmandu valley and Himalayan districts, most popular with tourists, appear malaria-free. However, exclusion of malaria is cheap and simple and failure to diagnose malaria results in potentially fatal treatment delays, so it should be excluded in all unwell travelers returning from endemic countries. If there is doubt about the infecting species, the patient should receive artemisinin combination therapy. The SEAQUAMAT and AQUAMAT trials have demonstrated the superiority of artesunate over quinine for the treatment of severe malaria.

TYPHUS

Rickettsial diseases are a common cause of fever in Nepal, with previous surveys showing 16%, 17% and 46% of undifferentiated febrile illnesses were caused by either scrub (*Orientia tsutsugamushi*) or murine (*Rickettsia typhi*) typhus. Scrub typhus is acquired from the bite of a mite in rural areas, whereas murine typhus is associated with rat fleas and is likely to be commoner in urban areas. Although these conditions are caused by different organisms, and have different vectors, they are clinically indistinguishable. Patients usually present with fever, headache and a rash. Although the classically described eschar is not commonly identified in Nepalese patients, it can be diagnostically useful when seen. Derangement of liver function tests and jaundice are common, occurring in up to 35% of septic patients.

Summary

The most likely infectious cause of acute jaundice in Nepal is hepatitis E virus. Potentially life-threatening infections which may be rare in travelers, such as malaria and enteric fever, must be excluded. Meticulous history-taking with particular attention to environmental and behavioral risks is key in developing a coherent differential diagnosis and instituting timely treatment.

Further reading available online at expertconsult.com.

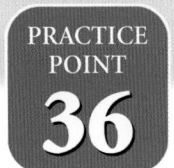
PRACTICE POINT
36

Sexually Transmitted Infection in a Traveler Returning from South Africa

A. WILLEM STURM

Case Study

A 38-year-old man seeks medical assistance because of the development of a single lesion on his penis. Four weeks ago he returned from a business trip to South Africa where he visited Johannesburg and Durban. He noticed the lesion about a week ago. He describes himself as bisexual and says he had unprotected sex in both cities with men whom he met in bars. The lesion is sore when in contact with clothes or when touched, it bleeds easily and the edges are partly undermined (Figure PP36-1). Your differential diagnosis is chancroid or genital herpes. You collect a specimen from the ulcer base and send this to the diagnostic laboratory for polymerase chain reaction (PCR) together with a blood specimen for syphilis and human immunodeficiency virus (HIV) serology. The results of the laboratory tests are shown in Table PP36-1.

Background Information

Although several other parts of sub-Saharan Africa do show considerable economic growth, South Africa is still the major economic hub on the African continent. Johannesburg, Cape Town and Durban are the cities in which most business activity takes place. In addition, Durban has the largest harbor of Africa while Cape Town is a major international tourist destination. South Africa has an incidence of HIV of 12.2% (2012) – the highest HIV incidence globally. The province of KwaZulu–Natal has the highest HIV prevalence (16.9%) and the Western Cape the lowest (5%). These provinces have Durban and Cape Town as their major centers respectively. Although no epidemiologic information is available for all parts of South Africa with respect to the other sexually transmitted infections (STIs), high prevalences of all of these infections have been reported where studies have been performed.

It is generally considered that STIs circulate within a limited number of individuals in a population. However, the existence of such a core group among the heterosexual population of South Africa is challenged by the presence of non-ulcerative STIs in a high percentage of first-time antenatal clinic attendees who perceive themselves to be asymptomatic (in KwaZulu–Natal 35% and 32% respectively in 2001 and in 2013). These figures show that STIs are widespread among the heterosexual population and are not restricted to individuals who seek medical care for such a disease. The STI prevalence among men who have sex with men (MSM) will be at least as high.

Studies on the prevalence of the different organisms that cause the different syndromes in patients attending STI clinics in KwaZulu–Natal are shown in Table PP36-2. Although these relative percentages change over time, it shows that all known causative agents of STIs are present in South Africa and Table PP36-2 shows the most recent available data. Unfortunately, the latest studies on the etiology of genital disease are from 2010, but although the percentages may differ one should assume that all causative agents are still present. In all syndromes, multiple infections are seen in approximately 10% of patients.

Susceptibility testing of *Neisseria gonorrhoeae* in patients from KwaZulu–Natal reveals high levels of resistance to penicillins, tetracyclines and fluoroquinolones and borderline resistance to spectinomycin. The minimum inhibitory concentrations (MICs) for third-generation cephalosporins are rising. This is a major concern but so far true resistance has been reported only in isolates from MSM.

General Approach

Since STIs are so prevalent in South Africa, any traveler to this country who has been sexually active with a South African partner during this visit can become infected with one or more pathogens. This is not restricted to patients who had contact with a commercial sex worker.

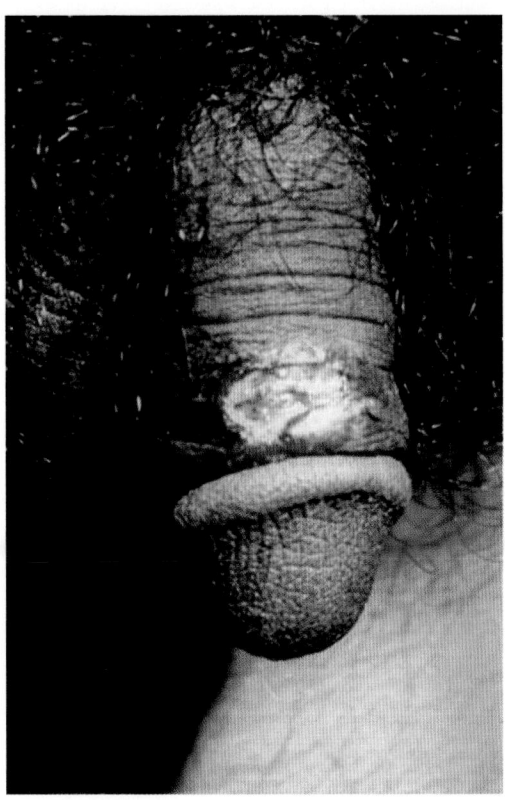
Figure PP36-1 Ulcerative lesion on the penis.

TABLE PP36-1	Results of Laboratory Tests in the Case Study Patient	
PCR	*Haemophilus ducreyi*	Negative
	Treponema pallidum	Positive
	Herpes simplex virus 2	Negative
	Chlamydia trachomatis, biovar LGV	Negative
Serology	HIV	Negative
	Fluorescent treponemal antibody absorption test (FTA-ABS)	Positive
	Rapid plasma reagin (RPR) test	1:4

TABLE PP36-2 Etiology of the Three Main STI Syndromes in KwaZulu–Natal, South Africa			
	PREVALENCE (%) IN PATIENTS WITH:		
	Male Urethritis Syndrome	Vaginal Discharge Syndrome	Genital Ulcer Syndrome
Neisseria gonorrhoeae	6		
Chlamydia trachomatis, biovar OG	16		
Mycoplasma genitalium			
Trichomonas vaginalis		22	
Bacterial vaginosis		52	
Chlamydia trachomatis, biovar LGV			6
Treponema pallidum			4
Haemophilus ducreyi			0
Herpes simplex virus 2			34
Klebsiella (Calymmatobacterium) granulomatis			6

TABLE PP36-3 Differential Diagnosis for Nonhealing Genital Ulcers	
Sexually Transmitted Infection	Other Causes
Noncompliance to treatment	Malignancy
Inadequate duration of treatment	Tuberculosis
Resistant STI microbes	Hydradenitis in the groin
Herpes simplex virus in an immunocompromised patient	Pyodermas
Secondary bacterial infection	Behçet's disease

When symptomatic, the infections present as one or more of three major clinical syndromes: male urethritis (MUS), vaginal discharge (VDS) and genital ulcer syndrome (GUS). MUS and VDS are caused by the same group of microbes while GUS has a different spectrum of pathogens. Each of these infections have their 'textbook' clinical presentation, but it has been well established that the clinical presentation is a poor predictor of the etiology for all three syndromes. Apart from atypical presentations, pathogens causing MUS and VDS also cause asymptomatic infections in a significant percentage of patients. Therefore, in a male patient presenting with GUS, the presence of MUS pathogens cannot be excluded and should be tested for.

An etiologic diagnosis is dependent on the laboratory diagnosis. Since microscopy and culture has a low sensitivity or is not available, nucleic acid amplification tests need to be performed. This technology is available for MUS and VDS pathogens in most laboratories in higher-income countries, but for GUS pathogens this is restricted mainly to specialized laboratories.

Principles of Management of Sexually Transmitted Infections

Laboratory test results indicate that the patient in this case study has primary syphilis. The polymerase chain reaction for *Treponema pallidum* is highly sensitive and specific. Of the serologic tests for syphilis, the fluorescent treponemal antibody test (FTA-ABS) becomes positive first while in early primary syphilis the rapid plasma reagin (RPR) test is often low or still negative. Negative PCRs for the other pathogens make a mixed infection with GUS pathogens unlikely, but other organisms should be considered if there is no response to the treatment with a single dose of benzathine–penicillin. Repeat serology in patients who do respond is not indicated. Patients should be followed-up weekly until the lesion has epithelized.

If there is no response to treatment after one week, a mixed infection should be considered and repeat PCRs should be performed. If these are still negative for herpes simplex virus, *Chlamydia trachomatis* (LGV) and *Haemophilus ducreyi*, infection with *Klebsiella* (*Calymmatobacterium*) *granulomatis* as well as the conditions listed in Table PP36-3 should be considered. The PCR for *T. pallidum* will remain positive for some time even after that component of the mixed infection has responded to the penicillin treatment.

The diagnosis of granuloma inguinale, caused by *Klebsiella* (*Calymmatobacterium*) *granulomatis*, is made by microscopy on Giemsa-stained impression smears. The presence of the typical Donovan bodies is diagnostic. As all microscopy, the test has a low sensitivity and should be repeated at least three times with multiple impression smears made on each occasion.

Further reading available online at expertconsult.com.

PRACTICE POINT

37

Lymphadenopathy, Splenomegaly and Anemia in a Traveler Returning from Sudan

TOM DOHERTY

A 31-year-old Caucasian woman had been working in Sudan as a logistician with an international aid agency for the previous 6 months. Apart from some menorrhagia that she had had since she was a teenager, she had no significant past medical history. She was fully compliant with appropriate antimalarial chemoprophylaxis (Malarone – atovaquone–proguanil daily) but was taking no other regular medication. For the last 3 months of her stay she had been in a relationship with a new male partner but they always used barrier protection.

Six weeks previously she developed a febrile illness associated with a nonproductive cough, myalgia, arthralgia and she had noticed that the glands in her neck were tender and swollen. She was seen at a health center in Sudan and diagnosed as having falciparum malaria on the basis of a positive rapid diagnostic test (RDT). At that time there were no abnormal findings and her vital signs were all within the normal range. She was prescribed a 3-day course of co-artemether, advised to drink adequate fluids and told to rest at home for several days. Three days later she had not improved and returned to the health center. On this occasion, an RDT for malaria was negative but she was diagnosed as having typhoid fever on the basis of a positive WIDAL test. On the second presentation, the attending physician noted minimal splenomegaly. She was prescribed a 10-day course of oral ciprofloxacin 400 mg BD. There were no facilities to perform blood cultures or other laboratory investigations.

Three days later she returned to the health center, having experienced no improvement. She had a fever of 38.0 °C and her spleen was noted to be still enlarged. A third RDT was negative for malaria and, because of the lack of diagnostic investigations, she was advised to return to the UK.

Twenty-four hours later she presented to hospital in London. Her cough and myalgia persisted but there were no other localizing symptoms to suggest a source for her infection. She was clinically pale, tired and drawn, but not acutely unwell and she was afebrile. On examination, she had palpable lymphadenopathy in both anterior cervical chains. Her throat looked red but there was no frank tonsillitis. Other than this, examination of her respiratory and cardiovascular systems was normal. Her spleen was easily palpable two fingers' breadth below the left costal margin but there was no hepatomegaly. She was fully conscious and alert with no signs of meningitis or encephalitis.

Preliminary investigations with both thick and thin blood films looking for malaria parasites were negative, but the parasitologist noted some abnormal lymphocytes on the thin film. Urine dipstick testing and a chest radiograph were both unremarkable. Her full blood count showed a normochromic, normocytic anemia at 9.8 g/dL with a normal total white cell count, no increase in her eosinophil count but she had a lymphocytosis at 4.9×10^9/L. Her platelet count was normal. Her liver function tests revealed raised transaminases (ALT 350 IU/L) with a normal bilirubin. She was admitted to hospital and

serological tests were sent urgently for blood-borne virus infections, Epstein–Barr virus (EBV) and cytomegalovirus infection and toxoplasmosis. Within 24 hours of admission, tests for human immunodeficiency virus (HIV), EBV and hepatitis C were all reported as negative, tests for hepatitis A and B were both consistent with previous vaccination, but her CMV serology was positive. A few days later, the reference laboratory confirmed she had a positive test for CMV IgM, confirming a diagnosis of acute CMV infection. She made a full recovery and at follow-up 2 weeks after discharge her abnormal liver function tests, splenomegaly and lymphadenopathy had all completely resolved. Her anemia persisted but this was attributed to her menorrhagia.

Discussion

The combination of anemia, lymphadenopathy and splenomegaly always raises the possibility of a lymphoproliferative disorder, particularly in the context of an unexplained febrile illness or one that has not responded to appropriate anti-infective treatment, but in this case, happily, the diagnosis was acute CMV infection, probably acquired from her recent new partner – who remained completely asymptomatic throughout. CMV, like EBV, is often contracted through close personal contact but there is also risk associated with exposure to urine – often through changing the nappies of small children. In immunecompetent individuals, the infection is almost invariably self-limiting but with HIV coinfection both colitis and retinitis are serious sequelae. Latent infection can re-activate, for example, following solid organ transplantation. The natural history of CMV disease is very similar to EBV; infected people are often completely asymptomatic but others can suffer from a quite prolonged debilitating fatigue.

CMV is a ubiquitous infection and the fact that this patient acquired her infection while in Sudan was probably a matter of chance. Other more exotic 'tropical' infections, particularly malaria, needed to be excluded. Even the most effective antimalarial prophylactics do not confer complete protection and may in fact increase the risk of a low-grade persistent infection which may lead to anemia and splenomegaly. Malaria seldom, if ever, causes lymphadenopathy. Enteric fever is usually acquired in the Indian subcontinent but is not uncommon in sub-Saharan Africa. Again, vaccination is only about 60% effective and ciprofloxacin has now been recognized to be far less effective than 10 years ago. Brucellosis is endemic throughout the Middle East and the Horn of Africa, commonly causes splenomegaly and anemia, rarely generalized lymphadenopathy but is much more common among the indigenous population than among travelers. Acute schistosomiasis or Katayama fever is usually acquired in sub-Saharan Africa and not uncommonly presents with splenomegaly but an eosinophilia is a characteristic finding. African tick typhus is not uncommon among travelers but is associated more with the savanna of East and Southern Africa than with countries like Sudan. Rift Valley fever, Crimean-Congo

---

BOX PP37-1 MAIN CAUSES OF SPENOMEGALY

MILD SPLENOMEGALY

- Malaria
- Epstein–Barr virus
- Cytomegalovirus
- Enteric fever
- Dengue/chikungunya fever
- Human immunodeficiency virus
- Katayama fever (schistosomiasis)
- Disseminated tuberculosis
- Toxoplasmosis
- Leptospirosis
- Brucellosis
- Trypanosomiasis
- Histoplasmosis
- Generalized sepsis
- Systemic lupus erythematosus
- Rheumatoid arthritis
- Still's disease
- Sarcoidosis

MODERATE SPLENOMEGALY

All of the above plus:
- Lymphoproliferative disorder
- Infective endocarditis
- Splenic abscess
- Portal hypertension

MARKED SPLENOMEGALY

- Visceral leishmaniasis
- Hyper-reactive malarial splenomegaly
- Myelofibrosis
- Chronic myeloid leukemia
- Glycogen storage disease

BOX PP37-2 CAUSES OF LYMPHADENOPATHY

COMMON

- Local sepsis, such as tonsillitis
- Epstein–Barr virus/cytomegalovirus
- Nonspecific viral infection

LESS COMMON, BUT IMPORTANT

- Human immunodeficiency virus
- Tuberculosis
- Lymphoproliferative disorder/neoplasia
- Toxoplasmosis
- Secondary syphilis
- Sarcoidosis
- African trypanosomiasis
- Typhus
- Chancroid
- Leishmaniasis – cutaneous and visceral
- Leptospirosis

UNCOMMON

- Lymphatic filariasis
- Parvovirus
- Q fever
- Lymphogranuloma venereum
- Castleman's disease
- Rheumatoid vasculitis/systemic lupus erythematosus
- Still's disease
- Cat-scratch disease
- Lepromatous leprosy/erythema nodosum leprosum (ENL)

---

hemorrhagic fever, other viral infections such as dengue, chikungunya, Ebola and Marburg, are all possible diagnoses – but very rare. HIV infection always needs to be excluded – however low the degree of perceived risk. Visceral leishmaniasis is endemic in Sudan and surrounding countries but usually presents with a pancytopenia rather than anemia alone.

Box PP37-1 gives a list of the causes of splenomegaly that is not exhaustive. Box PP37-2 provides a list of those conditions that commonly or very rarely cause lymphadenopathy.

Further reading available online at expertconsult.com.

PRACTICE POINT 38

What are the Treatment Options for a Pregnant Patient with Malaria?

ROSE MCGREADY | FRANÇOIS NOSTEN

Definition of the Problem

Malaria is the most important parasitic infection in humans, and in pregnancy is detrimental to the mother and fetus. In pregnancy the adverse effects of malaria infection result from:

- systemic infection, comparable to the effects of any severe febrile illness in pregnancy, i.e. maternal/fetal mortality, abortion, still-birth and premature delivery; and
- parasitization, i.e. birth-weight reduction, maternal/fetal anemia, interaction with human immunodeficiency virus (HIV) and susceptibility of the infant to malaria.

The hallmark of malaria in pregnancy is parasites sequestered in the placenta. Sequestered parasites evade host defense mechanisms including splenic processing and filtration. Sequestration is not known to occur in the benign malarias due to *Plasmodium vivax*, *P. ovale* and *P. malariae*. *P. falciparum* causes greater morbidity (principally low birth-weight and anemia) and mortality than non-*falciparum* infections. The clinical manifestations in pregnancy depend on premunition, that is, the degree of natural immunity to malaria: for example, in early pregnancy miscarriage is increased in symptomatic (4-fold) and asymptomatic (2.7-fold) malaria infections and the odds are similar for *P. falciparum* and *P. vivax* (Table PP38-1).

Premunition appears slowly following continuous and numerous re-infections by malaria parasites to prevent it waning. Premunition acquired in childhood is impaired during the first pregnancy but recovers during subsequent gestations. *P. falciparum* is unique in its ability to sequester in large numbers in the placenta and placental parasites have been shown to bind preferentially to chondroitin sulfate A. During the course of pregnancy or over successive pregnancies women develop variant specific immunity to chondroitin sulfate A binding infected red blood cells (IRBC). Thus, in areas of high transmission (conferring high premunition), severe anemia is common and is associated with mortality, predominantly affecting primigravidae; on the other hand, in areas of low transmission or in epidemics, pregnant women of any gravida are at risk of severe and cerebral malaria and death.

Ideally, malaria infection during pregnancy should be prevented. Failing this (an increasing problem due to drug resistance) prompt diagnosis and effective treatment will prevent fatal outcomes and help reduce morbidity in both mother and baby. Clinicians who assess and manage pregnant women with malaria in non-endemic countries will be unfamiliar with the condition. Delay and misdiagnosis, with subsequent failure to provide prompt effective treatment, are the main recurring themes in death from malaria. *P. vivax* relapse rates in pregnancy are high and commonly appear in the postpartum period. Genotyping of these relapses suggest they result from reactivation of the liver stage hypnozoites. Primaquine treatment, contraindicated in pregnancy, would be beneficial in the postpartum period, however the safety of primaquine and transfer into breast-milk is unknown.

Clinical Cases

CASE 1 – SEVERE MALARIA

A 37-year-old West African woman presented for the first time in pregnancy to a London maternity department at 29 weeks' gestation in her first pregnancy, with a 5-day history of fever. She had recently returned to her home in London (resident two years) after a 1-month visit to West Africa to take care of her mother (no prophylaxis). On admission her temperature was 39.5 °C (103.1 °F), pulse rate 130 beats/min (bpm) and blood pressure 108/56 mmHg. She was conscious and responsive. Her urine contained protein on ward testing and was sent for culture (subsequently negative). Her uterus was soft and fetal size was appropriate for 29 weeks. There was a fetal tachycardia (180 bpm) with a suspicious cardiac rhythm: a flat trace with reduced short-term variability (<5 bpm). Her initial investigation results were as follows: hemoglobin (Hb) 8.2 g/dL, white blood cell count 18.3×10⁹/L and platelets 50×10⁹/L. Apart from her thrombocytopenia, her coagulation screen was normal. Two hours after admission her malaria film was reported to be positive with 10% *P. falciparum* IRBC, including schizonts and malaria pigment. Her blood sugar was 2.6 mmol/L.

The patient was transferred to the intensive care unit and commenced on an infusion of 10% dextrose after a bolus of 50 mL of 50% dextrose. She received a loading dose of intravenous quinine 20 mg/kg over 4 hours and clindamycin 5 mg/kg. In view of the hyperparasitemia, she was transferred to a tertiary referral unit for consideration of exchange transfusion. During the transfer she became unconscious and her blood sugar was 1.4 mmol/L. She regained consciousness with 0.5 g/kg glucose. She had repeated episodes of hypoglycemia over the next few days. She required 2 units of blood for severe symptomatic anemia. After an initial rise in parasitemia (6-hourly blood smear) in the first 24 hours her parasitemia was down to 1% by the third day of treatment. On the fourth day she developed acute respiratory distress syndrome

TABLE PP38-1	Main Consequences of Malaria in Pregnancy in Different Transmission Situations		
	Non-Immune*	Low Premunition	High Premunition
Susceptibility	++++	+++	++
Risk of illness	++++	+++	+
Severe anemia	?	+++	+++
Severe/cerebral malaria	++++	+++	-
Maternal/fetal mortality	++++	+++	+
Birth-weight reduction	?	++	++
Fetal wastage	++++	++++†	+
Gravida at risk	All	All	Primigravidae
Placental parasitemia	?	+	+++

*Includes women never exposed to malaria and women who come from malaria-endemic areas but who have lived for a prolonged period outside an endemic area.

+, Level of severity.

?, No data available. (There are actually no collective data on the effects of malaria in nonimmune women, but the severity of the infections caused by *Plasmodium falciparum* in this group would probably mask the effect on maternal anemia and birth-weight.)

†See McGready R., Lee S.J., Wiladphaingern J., et al.: Adverse effects of *falciparum* and *vivax* malaria and the safety of antimalarial treatment in early pregnancy: a population-based study. Lancet Infect Dis 2012; 12(5):388–396.

and despite ventilation died the next day. Fetal heart beat was not detectable before she died.

CASE 2 – UNCOMPLICATED MALARIA

A 26-year-old Burmese woman in her third pregnancy presented at 24 weeks' gestation for antenatal booking. She had arrived in the UK 1 week previously, as part of the resettlement of Karen refugees from the Thai–Burmese border. She reported having had fever in the last 24 hours with headache, muscle and joint pain for 2 days. Much to the chagrin of the physician on duty she requested a malaria smear. This was agreed to and was positive for *P. falciparum*, 1.2% IRBC, and *P. vivax*, 0.2% IRBC. Routine booking investigations were carried out. All results were unremarkable apart from the hemoglobin (9.5 g/dL with iron-deficient indices). The patient was diagnosed as having uncomplicated malaria and was treated with coartemether 4 tablets with 200 mL of milk. She vomited all the tablets 15 minutes after treatment initiation and said it was because of the milk. The physician ordered metoclopramide and repeated the dose with soya milk and without further vomiting. The patient was admitted to the ward, spiked a fever that evening of 40.0 °C (104 °F), treated with paracetamol and oral fluids. There were no further febrile episodes, the remaining doses of coartemether were well tolerated and the patient was blood smear-negative on the second day of treatment. Ultrasound assessment revealed an appropriately grown fetus with normal amniotic fluid volume. There was bilateral notching of the uterine artery Doppler waveforms with raised resistance indices, suggesting a degree of placental dysfunction. The umbilical artery and fetal arterial Doppler studies were normal. By the next antenatal visit the uterine artery Doppler waveforms had normalized.

Six weeks later the woman complained again of headache, muscle and joint pain, no fever and again requested a malaria smear. *P. vivax* trophozoites 0.5% IRBC, schizonts and gametocytes were all reported. The physician on duty diagnosed *P. vivax* and treated the woman with chloroquine 10, 10 and 5 mg/kg once daily on days 0, 1 and 2, respectively. At 32 weeks' gestation the fundal height was 27 cm. By 37 weeks' gestation fundal height measurement and serial scans for growth demonstrated intrauterine growth retardation (IUGR), despite normal Dopplers. The woman had spontaneous onset of labor at 37.2 weeks' gestation and a normal vaginal delivery of a term 2.3 kg normal infant. At 18 hours postpartum the midwife on the labor ward recorded the temperature of the patient as 38 °C (100.4 °F). As everyone was aware of the woman's history of malaria a blood smear was ordered for the mother and baby (normal vital signs) and both were positive for *P. falciparum*. Attempts to salvage the placenta to do a malaria smear were made too late and were not done. The mother and the baby were successfully treated with 3 days of atovaquone–proguanil (Malarone).

Diagnosis

Failure to consider malaria as a possible diagnosis can result in death. The diagnosis of malaria in pregnancy, as in nonpregnant patients, relies on microscopic (the current gold standard) examination of thick and thin blood films for parasites, or the use of rapid diagnostic tests that detect specific parasite antigen (see Chapter 117). Microscopic diagnosis allows species identification and estimation of parasitemia, so that appropriate antimalarials can be prescribed. Always consider malaria in the febrile patient and never forget to ask for a history of travel. Thrombocytopenia, metabolic acidosis and elevated lactate levels are also highly suggestive of severe malaria. The investigation of a patient with suspected falciparum malaria in pregnancy should be treated with great urgency. Blood and urine should be cultured to exclude other infections. In the comatose patient, lumbar puncture should be considered to exclude meningitis and encephalitis, providing there is no evidence of raised intracranial pressure.

In a woman from a malaria-endemic country with severe anemia and suspected asymptomatic disease, presumptive treatment should be given even if a blood smear is negative.

Management

Prompt treatment is vital in pregnancy as the disease is more severe and mortality risk is 2–10 times higher than in nonpregnant patients. The disease in pregnancy is associated with higher parasitemia and is dangerous for both mother and fetus. The aim of treatment of uncomplicated malaria is to cure the patient and in severe malaria to save the mother's life. Severity of malaria is determined by the symptoms and microscopic findings (Table PP38-2).

Management of malaria in pregnancy depends on the infecting species, severity of the disease, the stage of pregnancy (first trimester or other), prophylaxis or intermittent preventive therapy and drug availability. The fast expansion of resistant isolates has compromised many of the standard antimalarials, including chloroquine, sulfadoxine–pyrimethamine and quinine monotherapy and more recently the artemisinin derivatives in South East Asia (Chapter 117). Patients may deteriorate under treatment, at which point management should be upgraded to account for severity. Drugs for treatment are summarized in Table PP38-3. Specific points related to treatment of malaria in pregnant women have been summarized in Table PP38-4.

TABLE PP38-2	Classification of Severity of Malaria in Pregnancy		
Grade of Malaria	**Microscopic Findings**	**Symptoms**	**Case Fatality Rate**
Uncomplicated	Positive blood smear with parasite count <4% IRBC or parasitemia of 150 000/μL	First symptoms are usually nonspecific and similar to a minor systemic viral illness Headache, lassitude, fatigue, abdominal discomfort, dizziness and muscle and joint aches, followed by fever, chills, sweating, anorexia, vomiting and worsening malaise are the typical features of uncomplicated malaria No signs of severity* or organ dysfunction	Low: ~0.1% for *P. falciparum* infections Non-*falciparum* spp. are rarely fatal
Uncomplicated hyperparasitemia	*P. falciparum* asexual parasitemia with ≥4% IRBC 2% should be used in nonimmune patients from nonendemic countries	As for uncomplicated	As for uncomplicated if treated adequately
Severe (rare reports with *P. vivax* monoinfection)	*P. falciparum* asexual parasitemia (or positive rapid diagnostic test)	No other obvious cause of symptoms and with signs of severity* and/or organ dysfunction	High: 15–20% in nonpregnant patients compared with 50% in pregnancy Untreated severe malaria is always fatal

IRBC, infected red blood cells.
*Signs of severity: *Clinical manifestations*: prostration, impaired consciousness, respiratory distress (acidotic breathing), multiple convulsions, circulatory collapse, pulmonary edema (radiologic), abnormal bleeding, jaundice, hemoglobinuria; *Laboratory tests*: severe anemia, hypoglycemia, acidosis, renal impairment, hyperlactatemia, hyperparasitemia, HRP-2 as a marker of sequestration (see cross-ref).
Adapted from World Health Organization: WHO guidelines for the treatment of malaria. Report No. WHO/HTM/MAL 2006/1108. Geneva: WHO; 2006

TABLE PP38-3   Drugs for Treatment of Malaria in Pregnancy

Species and Trimester	Severity	Treatment
P. vivax, P. ovale and *P. malariae*, regardless of trimester	Not usually severe If severe, see *P. falciparum* (severe)	Chloroquine phosphate (1 tablet contains 250 mg salt equivalent to 155.3 mg base) Dose: 10 mg/kg base q24h on days 1 and 2, followed by 5 mg/kg base on day 3 For chloroquine-resistant *P. vivax*, amodiaquine, quinine or artemisinin derivatives can be used
First trimester: *P. falciparum* or mixed species, i.e. *P. falciparum* and non-*falciparum* (usually *P. vivax*) coinfection	Uncomplicated	1st episode: quinine 10 mg/kg q8h for 7 days, preferably with clindamycin* 5 mg/kg q8h for 7 days Subsequent episodes: repeat treatment with quinine and clindamycin* as above ACT that is locally effective or artesunate 2 mg/kg q24h for 7 days with clindamycin* as above
Second and third trimesters	Uncomplicated	1st episode: ACT that is locally effective such as artemether–lumefantrine[§] or artesunate plus clindamycin* as above Malarone (atovaquone–proguanil)[†] alone can be used for treatment in pregnancy but it is highly recommended to use it with artesunate to maximize fever and parasite clearance times and ensure cure Subsequent episodes: artesunate plus clindamycin* as above Artesunate–atovaquone–proguanil and dihydroartemisinin–piperaquine[§] can be used for *P. falciparum* recurrence in the same pregnancy
Regardless of trimester	Uncomplicated hyperparasitemia	Artesunate: 4 mg/kg po loading dose then 2 mg/kg q24h for 7 days with clindamycin* as above, or quinine iv (see below)
Regardless of trimester	Severe[I]	Artesunate[‡]: 2.4 mg/kg iv at 0, 12 and 24h, then q24h until the patient can tolerate oral artesunate 2 mg/kg q24h for a total of 7 days, and clindamycin* 5 mg/kg q8h for 7 days, or quinine: 20 mg/kg iv loading dose given over 4h, then 10 mg/kg 8h after the loading dose was started, followed by 10 mg/kg q8h for 7 days. Once the patient has recovered sufficiently to tolerate oral medication both quinine 10 mg/kg and clindamycin 5 mg/kg q8h should be continued for/until 7 days

ACT, artemisin-based combination therapy. Dosages for pregnant women are likely to be revised when all the pharmacokinetic antimalarial pregnancy data become available.
*When clindamycin is not available, give artesunate monotherapy.
[†]Malarone use in pregnancy.
[‡]Intravenous artesunate is the best treatment but unfortunately is not available routinely in the UK. Some hospitals may have their own supply.
[§]Prescribe artemether–lumefantrine with fat.
[I]The two drugs (quinine and artesunate) should be combined in areas of resistance to artemisinin.
Adapted from World Health Organization: WHO guidelines for the treatment of malaria. Report No. WHO/HTM/MAL 2006/1108. Geneva: WHO; 2006
WHO guidelines for the treatment of malaria – 3rd edition. NLM classification WC 770 http://www.who.int/malaria/publications/atoz/9789241549127/en/

TABLE PP38-4   Problems Pertinent to Treatment of Malaria in Pregnant Women

Adjunctive Treatment	Relationship to Pregnancy	Details of Treatment
Antiemetics	There are no trials specifically in pregnancy but pregnant women have a higher tendency to vomit than nonpregnant women	If vomiting occurs within 30 min, the full dose should be repeated. If vomiting occurs from >30 to 60 min, repeat half the dose. An antiemetic (metoclopramide) can be given im or iv; wait 20 min before repeating the dose Antiemetics are widely used for treatment in malaria although there have been no studies of their efficacy. There is no evidence to indicate harm. If a patient vomits twice they will need parenteral treatment. Oral medication can be recommended when oral fluids are well tolerated. Although these patients may show no signs of severity, the treatment regimen should be switched to that used for severe cases
Antipyretics	Fever is a cardinal feature of malaria. In pregnant women it has been associated with premature labor	Paracetamol 1 g q4–6h (maximum 4 g q24h) is safe and effective
Intravenous infusions	Due to greater circulating volume in pregnancy and increased losses, hydration is essential Quinine is still widely used in pregnancy but can be a particularly offensive drug to take due to cinchonism (tinnitus, hearing loss, nausea, uneasiness, restlessness and blurring of vision)	Febrile pregnant women with nausea and vomiting may be dehydrated and oral fluids need to be encouraged and adequate urine output confirmed. Intravenous fluids may be required, particularly on quinine
Glucose	Pregnancy can predispose to hypoglycemia and the nausea associated with malaria prevents some women from taking an adequate oral intake, thus promoting hypoglycemia Hypoglycemia in pregnancy may be profound and recurrent, particularly on quinine	Hypoglycemia may manifest as fetal brady- or tachycardia. In the most severely ill patients it is associated with lactic acidosis and high mortality In patients who have been given quinine, abnormal behavior, sweating and sudden loss of consciousness are the usual manifestations
Tocolytic therapy	Pre-term labor appears to be associated with the fever from malaria	Usual pre-term labor protocols apply Monitor uterine contractions
Fetal distress	Exclude maternal hypoglycemia, particularly if the patient is being treated with quinine and hyperthermia is the cause	Normal labor protocols should be implemented but fetal heart rate must be monitored. This may reveal fetal tachycardia, bradycardia or late decelerations in relation to uterine contractions, indicating fetal distress

Continued on following page

TABLE PP38-4	Problems Pertinent to Treatment of Malaria in Pregnant Women (Continued)	
Adjunctive Treatment	**Relationship to Pregnancy**	**Details of Treatment**
Antibiotics	Secondary bacterial infection, principally gram-negative sepsis, has been reported in pregnancy	The patient is collapsed with a systolic blood pressure <80 mmHg in the supine position Blood cultures should be taken if the patient shows signs of shock or fever returns after apparent fever clearance Hypovolemia should be corrected and broad-spectrum antibiotics started immediately (e.g. ceftriaxone). Once the results of blood culture and sensitivity testing are available, give the appropriate antibiotic
Assisted ventilation	Pulmonary edema is a grave complication of severe malaria, with a high mortality rate in pregnancy (over 50%). Note: also associated with *P. vivax* infection (see cross ref).	May be present on admission or develop suddenly and unexpectedly, or develop immediately after childbirth The first indication of impending pulmonary edema is an increase in the respiratory rate which precedes the development of other chest signs Hypoxia may cause convulsions and deterioration in the level of consciousness and the patient may die within a few hours Ensure the pulmonary edema has not resulted from iatrogenic fluid overload
Blood transfusion	Severe anemia is associated with perinatal mortality, maternal morbidity and an increased risk of postpartum hemorrhage	Women who go into labor when severely anemic or fluid overloaded may develop acute pulmonary edema after separation of the placenta Transfuse pregnant women slowly, preferably with packed red blood cells, and furosemide 20 mg iv; alternatively exchange transfusion may be given

Conclusion

There is a paucity of data on antimalarials used for treatment and prevention in pregnancy. Most of what we know about chloroquine in pregnancy comes from research on autoimmune disease in pregnancy and for quinine from its historical use. Sulfadoxine–pyrimethamine has been widely advocated as a preventive antimalarial in pregnancy without clear evidence of the efficacy or pharmacokinetic properties in pregnant women. There have only been 10 randomized controlled trials (RCTs) specifically involving treatment for pregnant women with acute uncomplicated falciparum malaria involving a total of 1914 patients. Much larger numbers of women must be treated and followed prospectively until the data on efficacy, outcome and drug safety in pregnancy (including developmental assessment of the infant) are robust, and clear guidelines can be issued.

For first trimester antimalarials, there is not a single RCT published. Given the impact of malaria in pregnancy and the huge number of women affected, this is a major deficiency. The collective data on epidemiology, prevention and treatment of malaria in pregnancy clearly demonstrate how dangerous malaria in pregnancy is to both the mother and the baby. Malaria in pregnancy is a medical emergency. It can be prevented and treated with reasonable confidence using the guidelines outlined in Tables PP38-3 and PP38-4.

Further reading available online at expertconsult.com.

136

Principles of Anti-infective Therapy and Surgical Prophylaxis

EVELINA TACCONELLI | FEDERICO FOSCHI | CHRISTINA FORSTNER |
ROGER G. FINCH | MATHIAS W. PLETZ

KEY CONCEPTS

- Antimicrobial prescribing should be based on clear microbiological evidence of infection or sound clinical criteria, narrow spectrum if possible, and de-escalated as soon as the microbiological results are available.

- Knowledge of local epidemiological data of antimicrobial resistance in clinical samples is mandatory to increase the rate of appropriate empiric antibiotic therapy and improve clinical outcomes.

- Pharmacodynamic and pharmacokinetic properties of drugs are today essential in order to provide personalized therapy, reduce adverse events and improve effectiveness.

- Surveillance system for surgical site infections is indicated to monitor trends in healthcare-associated infections and rapidly detect new resistance patterns. Homogeneity on case definition needs to be achieved.

- Surgical prophylaxis has been proved to reduce post-surgical infections in different types of surgery. Although heterogeneity exists with respect to the type of antibiotic, timing, dosing, and type of procedure, a generalized benefit almost always is detected regardless of the degree of surgical contamination. Decolonization for methicillin-resistant *Staphylococcus aureus* is an important component in cardiothoracic and orthopedic surgery.

Introduction

In the last 70 years, major improvements in the early recognition and treatment of infectious diseases have resulted in an extraordinary reduction in the morbidity and mortality associated with these illnesses.[1] As more antibiotics were discovered, they had truly become the 'panacea' of medicine and were being widely misused and overused. Indeed, in many countries, antimicrobial drugs can be purchased by the public without prescription, leading to so-called 'over-the-counter' selling, which is largely unregulated and poorly defined in terms of impact on patient safety and public health. This inappropriate antibiotic use leads to preventable complications of treatment such as anaphylaxis, renal failure and, most importantly, development of antimicrobial resistance.[2] All these threats to patient safety are associated with increased mortality, length of hospital stay, readmission rates and treatment costs.[3,4] The selection of drug-resistant bacteria has also significant consequence not only at individual level (i.e. increased risk of infection in a colonized patient) but also at institutional level (i.e. increased risk of cross-transmission among hospitalized patients, environmental contamination, and spread of resistance in the community). Moreover, once the pipeline of antibiotics, in particular drugs for gram-negative, multidrug-resistant bacteria, drained dry over the last 20 years, other strategies needed to be developed to fight the spread of antibiotic resistance and to increase treatment effectiveness.[5] Thus, adequacy of therapy, for not microbiologically (empiric level in patients at hospital admission) and microbiologically confirmed infections (for severe bacterial infections), is a major challenge when addressing the problem of antimicrobial resistance and optimized treatment outcome in hospitalized patients. The overall adequacy of antimicrobial therapy depends on multiple parameters such as site of infection, the minimum inhibitory concentration of the causative pathogen, the pharmacodynamic/pharmacokinetic (PK/PD) indicators of the administered drug, host characteristics, co-morbidities and concomitant treatments. Therefore, more efforts and clinical guidance are urgently needed to tailor antimicrobial prescribing to the individual needs of different patients and specific clinical scenarios.

General Principles of Prescribing

Anti-infective drugs are generally classified according to their major microbial targets rather than by target disease or infection.[6,7] Pharmacopoeias and formularies categorize these as antibacterial, antiviral, antifungal and antiparasitic (antiprotozoal or anthelmintic) agents. Within these categories some specific indications can be found such as antiviral drugs used in the treatment of herpesvirus infections, chronic hepatitis C or HIV (Tables 136-1 and 136-2). Major antifungal and antiparasitic drugs are listed in Tables 136-3 and 136-4. Among anti-infective drugs the largest proportion is for the treatment of bacterial infections.

Antimicrobial prescribing should be based on clear evidence of infection established by either laboratory investigation or sound clinical criteria. In general, laboratory confirmation of infection, although desirable, is only possible in a minority of treated infections and is largely confined to hospitalized patients where access to laboratory investigation is readily available.

The results of microbiologic sampling may confirm the nature of an infection and support the continued use of initial empiric treatment or indicate alternative therapy. However, most prescribing is empiric, particularly in community practice, which accounts for about 80–90% of antimicrobial prescribing.

CHOICE OF AGENT OR AGENTS

Fundamental to the treatment of infectious diseases is the evidence-based selection of an antimicrobial regimen with established efficacy against the target infection and supported by widespread clinical use. The antimicrobial spectrum of activity should be based on local susceptibility data.[8] The National Committee for Clinical and Laboratory Standards Institute (CLSI) and the European Committee on Antimicrobial Susceptibility Testing (EUCAST) set 'breakpoints' for the minimum inhibitory concentration (MIC) based on the integration of MICs with achievable antibiotic levels in serum and tissues, clinical pharmacology and data from *in vitro* and animal models.

Broad-Spectrum Versus Narrow-Spectrum Antimicrobial Agents

The terms 'broad-spectrum' and 'narrow-spectrum' are widely used to distinguish between agents that target a limited range of pathogens in contrast to broad-spectrum agents to which many pathogens are susceptible. Historically, the terms have been applied to developments in the penicillin class of drugs. Penicillin G (benzylpenicillin) targeted a limited number of pathogens – for example, *Streptococcus pneumoniae*, hemolytic streptococci and *Neisseria* spp. (meningococci and gonococci). With the development of the aminopenicillins

TABLE 136-1	Antiviral Drugs: Non-HIV			
Agent	**Mechanism of Action**	**Antiviral Activity**	**Mechanisms of Resistance**	**Toxicity/Side Effects**
Aciclovir	Inhibits DNA polymerase, chain terminator. Requires viral thymidine kinase and cellular enzymes	**HSV-1/2**>VZV >EBV (*in vitro, in vivo* limited activity)>CMV	Mutations in thymidine kinase (more common) and mutations in DNA polymerase	Confusion, delirium, lethargy, tremors, nausea, vomiting, light-headedness, diaphoresis, rash Intravenous: phlebitis, crystalline nephropathy
Adefovir	Nucleotide analog	**HBV** >HIV, CMV	Mutational resistance	Renal impairment at >30 mg q24h
Amantadine	Inhibits transmembrane protein M2, reduced uncoating of viral genome	**Influenza A**	Point mutation in gene encoding transmembrane domain M2 protein	Nervousness, anxiety, light-headedness, confusion, insomnia
Boceprevir	NS3/4A protease inhibitor of HCV	**HCV**	Mutations in the protease gene (155K/T, and V36A/M substitutions, A156V/T mutation)	Fatigue, anemia, nausea, headache, dysgeusia
Cidofovir	Acyclic nucleoside phosphonate (does not require a virus-specific thymidine kinase)	**HSV-1, HSV-2, VZV, EBV, CMV**, adenovirus, HPV, polyomavirus	Mutations in DNA polymerase	Severe nephrotoxicity, neutropenia, ocular hypotony, metabolic acidosis. Carcinogenic, teratogenic
Daclatasvir	Inhibits the HCV nonstructural protein NS5A	HCV	Mutational resistance	Headache, nausea, fatigue, pruritus, diarrhea, anemia
Entecavir	Nucleoside reverse transcriptase inhibitor	**HBV**	Mutational resistance	Hepatotoxicity, headache, hyperglycemia, raised lipase
Famciclovir	Prodrug to penciclovir, incorporated into DNA molecule	**HSV-1, HSV-2, VZV** >EBV, CMV, HBV (*in vitro*)	Mutations in thymidine kinase and mutations in DNA polymerase	Headache, nausea, diarrhea, vomiting, pruritus, LFT abnormalities
Foscarnet	Noncompetitive inhibitor of viral DNA polymerase (does not require thymidine kinase)	**CMV**, HSV-1, HSV-2, VZV, HBV, HHV-6, EBV, HIV	In CMV, single mutation in conserved region of DNA polymerase	Renal impairment, electrolyte disturbances, seizures, anemia, neutropenia, fever, nausea, vomiting, diarrhea, headache
Ganciclovir	Inhibitor of DNA polymerase, also competitive inhibitor of deoxyguanosine triphosphate (monophosphorylation by infection-induced kinases in HSV and VZV, and viral-encoded phosphotransferase in CMV-infected cells)	**CMV**, HSV-1/2>VZV> EBV, HHV-6	One or more point mutations in UL97, mutations in CMV DNA polymerase	Bone marrow suppression, fever, rash, increased LFTs, nausea, vomiting, eosinophilia, seizures, confusion, encephalopathy
Interferon-α (including pegylated interferon)	Induces changes in infected/exposed cells to promote resistance to infecting virus. Produces proteins that inhibit RNA synthesis, cleaves cellular and viral DNA, inhibits messenger RNA, alters cell membranes, inhibits release of replicated virions	**HCV** (pegylated), HPV, HBV, HDV, HIV	Mutation of viral proteins such as C, E2, NS3/NS4, and NS5A; interaction with signal transducer and activator of transcription 1 (STAT-1) inhibits interferon signal transduction pathways	Fever, headache, chills, arthralgias, myalgias, fatigue, dizziness, neutropenia, thrombocytopenia, somnolence, depression, cognitive changes, suicidal ideation, increased LFTs, altered thyroid function, nausea, vomiting, diarrhea
Lamivudine	Competitively inhibits viral reverse transcriptase, terminates proviral DNA chain extension	HBV, HIV	Mutations at YMDD locus (conserved domain reverse transcriptase)	Low dose: equivalent to placebo. High dose: headache, fatigue, insomnia, myalgias, arthralgias, diarrhea, rash, lactic acidosis, hepatomegaly
Ledipasvir	Inhibits the HCV nonstructural protein NS5A	HCV	Mutational resistance	Fatigue, headache
Oseltamivir	Neuraminidase inhibitor	Influenza A, influenza B	Mutations in viral neuraminidase and viral hemagglutinin	Nausea, vomiting
Ribavirin	Guanosine analog, three possible mechanisms: competitive inhibition of host enzymes, inhibition of viral RNA polymerase complex, inhibition of messenger RNA formation	RSV, HCV; but also influenza A, influenza B, mumps, measles, parainfluenza, herpesviruses, togavirus, bunyavirus, adenovirus, coxsackievirus, hemorrhagic fever virus, HAV, HBV, Lassa fever virus, hantavirus	Mutations leading to resistance of HCV (NS5B mutation)	Anemia, hyperbilirubinemia, elevated uric acid, nausea, headache, lethargy. Teratogenic, mutagenic, embryotoxic, gonadotoxic

TABLE 136-1	Antiviral Drugs: Non-HIV (Continued)			
Agent	**Mechanism of Action**	**Antiviral Activity**	**Mechanisms of Resistance**	**Toxicity/Side Effects**
Rimantadine	Inhibits transmembrane protein M2, reduced uncoating of viral genome	Influenza A	Point mutation in gene encoding transmembrane domain M2 protein	Nervousness, anxiety, light-headedness, confusion, insomnia
Simeprevir	NS3/4A protease inhibitor of HCV	**HCV**	Mutations at the NS3 protease positions (F43, Q80, S122, R155, A156 D168)	Rash, pruritus, nausea, photosensitization
Sofosbuvir	Nucleotide polymerase inhibitor of the HCV nonstructural protein NS5B RNA-dependent RNA polymerase	**HCV**	High barrier to resistance compared to other anti-HCV agents (NS5B resistance-associated mutations, S282T)	Fatigue, headache, insomnia, pruritus, skin rash, nausea, anemia, fever
Telaprevir	NS3/A4 protease inhibitor of HCV	**HCV**	Mutations in the HCV protease gene (155K/T and V36A/M substitutions, A156V/T mutation)	Rash, serious skin reaction (some fatal in combination with peginterferon alfa and ribavirin); anemia, leukopenia, thrombopenia
Valaciclovir	Valine ester of aciclovir	See aciclovir	See aciclovir	Headache, nausea, abdominal pain
Valganciclovir	Valine ester of ganciclovir	See ganciclovir	See ganciclovir	Bone marrow suppression, fever, nausea, headache, vomiting, insomnia, abdominal pain, peripheral neuropathy, paresthesias, potential carcinogen
Zanamivir (aerosolized/intranasal)	Neuraminidase inhibitor	Influenza A, influenza B	Mutations in viral neuraminidase and viral hemagglutinin	Nasal, throat discomfort, bronchospasm in asthmatics

CMV, cytomegalovirus; EBV, Epstein-Barr virus; HAV, hepatitis A virus; HBV, hepatitis B virus; HCV, hepatitis C virus; HDV, hepatitis D virus; HHV, human herpesvirus; HPV, human papillomavirus; HSV, herpes simplex virus; LFT, liver function test; RSV, respiratory syncytial virus; VZV, varicella-zoster virus.

(e.g. amoxicillin), the spectrum increased to also include *Enterococcus faecalis, Listeria* spp., *H. influenzae,* and *E. coli* and were thus considered as broad-spectrum agents; however, as stated above, with time the latter two pathogens have become resistant as a result of β-lactamase production.

The antimicrobial spectrum of an antibiotic has important practical implications. Narrow-spectrum agents have a more limited range of indications and in general require greater diagnostic precision to ensure they are used appropriately. They also require greater emphasis on documenting the microbiologic nature of an infection. In contrast, broad-spectrum agents usually capture a greater range of micro-organisms and indications. They are also widely used as initial empiric therapy of respiratory tract and intra-abdominal infections.

One of the consequences of broad-spectrum agents is their impact on the normal flora, particularly that of the gastrointestinal tract. As a consequence, microbial overgrowth by organisms such as *Candida* spp. and *C. difficile* may occur and give rise to superinfection or *C. difficile*-associated diarrhea, respectively. A recent study on the structure and function of human gut microbiota revealed that the effect of antibiotics relates to the interaction and the properties of the antimicrobial agent and the structure, function and resistance genes among the microbial community.[9]

Bactericidal Versus Bacteriostatic Activity

Antibacterial drugs act by either killing or inhibiting the growth of micro-organisms. These bactericidal or bacteriostatic effects are determined by the mode of action of a drug against a particular target organism. Table 136-5 identifies the usual mode of action of commonly prescribed agents.

Cell wall active agents, such as the penicillins, cephalosporins and glycopeptides, are largely bactericidal, whereas most agents that interfere with protein synthesis are bacteriostatic. Examples of the latter include the tetracyclines, lincosamides and macrolides. Metabolic inhibitors of folic acid synthesis, namely the sulfonamides and trimethoprim, are also bacteriostatic but the combination of both (co-trimoxazole) is bactericidal. Cidality can be affected by drug concentration and *in vitro* conditions of testing and may also vary by target pathogen. Nonetheless, it is a useful distinguishing feature with clinical implications in selected circumstances.

In general, bactericidal and bacteriostatic agents are equally effective in the management of many mild to moderate infections. However, bacteriostatic agents are dependent upon an effective host immune response, notably the ability to phagocytose drug-exposed bacteria. There are a number of clinical conditions in which host immunity is either deficient or suppressed and where bacteriostatic agents should be avoided in favor of bactericidal agents. Other circumstances where bactericidal agents are recommended are in the management of infective endocarditis.[10] The infected vegetations are impermeable to phagocytic cells and require high plasma concentrations of bactericidal drugs to sterilize them.

DOSE SELECTIONS AND FREQUENCY OF ADMINISTRATION

The selection of antimicrobial chemotherapy is supported by a matrix of information that includes *in vitro* evaluation of antimicrobial activity, animal models of infections, pharmacokinetic studies of the drug in health and disease, and clinical trial data developed to support the approved indications. Table 136-6 identifies some common bacterial infections affecting adults and the agents used in their treatment.

PHARMACOKINETICS

The bioavailability of a drug indicates the degree of absorption from the gastrointestinal tract. Parenterally administered agents achieve 100% bioavailability. The bioavailability of orally administered antimicrobials ranges from only 15% to 30% for aciclovir to >90% for antimicrobials with a high degree of bioavailability such as

TABLE 136-2 Antiviral Drugs: HIV

Agent	Mechanism of Action	Toxicity/Side Effects
Abacavir	Nucleoside reverse transcriptase inhibitor	Hypersensitivity syndrome in 5% of patients include anaphylaxis, fever, rash, fatigue, nausea, vomiting, diarrhea, abdominal pain → abacavir has to be stopped immediately. Other side effects: elevated LFTs, depression, hypertriglyceridemia
Atazanavir	Protease inhibitor	Increased unconjugated bilirubin, gastrointestinal symptoms, rash
Darunavir	Protease inhibitor	Hepatotoxicity, rash, nausea, diarrhea, erythema multiforme, lipodystrophy
Delavirdine	Non-nucleoside reverse transcriptase inhibitor	Rash, headache, Stevens–Johnson syndrome, nausea, depression
Didanosine	Nucleoside reverse transcriptase inhibitor	Nausea, vomiting, diarrhea, abdominal pain, peripheral neuropathy, pancreatitis
Dolutegravir	Integrase inhibitor	Insomnia, headache, allergic reactions, abnormal liver functions
Efavirenz	Non-nucleoside reverse transcriptase inhibitor	Vivid dreams, dizziness, difficulty concentrating, nausea, vomiting, diarrhea, rash, flu-like symptoms
Elvitegravir	Integrase inhibitor	Diarrhea, nausea, headache
Emtricitabine	Nucleoside reverse transcriptase inhibitor	Nausea, diarrhea, headache
Enfuvirtide	Fusion inhibitor	Injection site inflammation
Etravirine	Non-nucleoside reverse transcriptase inhibitor	Rash, hypersensitivity reaction, nausea
Fosamprenavir	Protease inhibitor	Rash, hyperlipidemia, diarrhea, lipodystrophy, headache
Indinavir	Protease inhibitor	Nephrolithiasis, nausea, dysgeusia, benign hyperbilirubinemia
Lamivudine	Nucleoside reverse transcriptase inhibitor	Peripheral neuropathy, pancreatitis
Lopinavir	Protease inhibitor	Nausea, asthenia, diarrhea
Maraviroc	CCR5 co-receptor blocker	Hepatotoxicity, fever, rash, abdominal pain
Nelfinavir	Protease inhibitor	Diarrhea
Nevirapine	Non-nucleoside reverse transcriptase inhibitor	Dizziness, rash, difficulty concentrating, nausea, vomiting, diarrhea, flu-like symptoms
Raltegravir	Integrase inhibitor	Rash, hyperlipidemia,
Ritonavir	Protease inhibitor	Dysgeusia, nausea, vomiting, diarrhea, circumoral paresthesias, increased triglycerides, LFTs, CPK and uric acid
Saquinavir	Protease inhibitor	Nausea, vomiting, diarrhea, headache
Stavudine	Nucleoside reverse transcriptase inhibitor	Peripheral neuropathy, lipoatrophy
Tenofovir	Nucleoside reverse transcriptase inhibitor	Nausea, vomiting, diarrhea, headache, elevated LFTs and CPK
Tipranavir	Protease inhibitor	Nausea, vomiting, diarrhea, headache, abdominal pain, rash, hepatitis, hyperglycemia and diabetes, hyperlipidemia
Zidovudine	Nucleoside reverse transcriptase inhibitor	Anemia, neutropenia, nausea, vomiting, myositis, neuropathy

CPK, creatine phosphokinase; LFTs, liver function tests.

cephalexin, levofloxacin, moxifloxacin, doxycycline, clindamycin, linezolid, trimethoprim-sulfamethoxazole, voriconazole and metronidazole. As a rule, replacing an intravenous antimicrobial agent with an oral drug is unwise for oral agents with less than 50% bioavailability.

Drugs once absorbed or injected diffuse from the intravascular fluid space to extravascular fluid spaces and this distribution is best described by the drug's volume of distribution.[11] The volume of distribution (V_D), also known as apparent volume of distribution, is a pharmacological, theoretical volume that is calculated as follows: V_D = total amount of drug in the body/drug blood plasma concentration. V_D has nothing to do with the actual volume of the body or its fluid compartments but rather involves the distribution of the drug within the body. For a drug that is highly tissue-bound, very little drug remains in the circulation; thus, plasma concentration is low and V_D is high. Drugs that remain in the circulation tend to have a low V_D. V_D provides a reference for the plasma concentration expected for a given dose but provides little information about the specific pattern of distribution.

Drugs that distribute widely through the body tend to have large volumes of distribution and low serum concentrations. Drugs that remain only in the blood volume typically have small volumes of distribution and high serum concentrations. Anti-infective drugs are generally distributed in the blood and tissues bound to plasma proteins, most notably albumin. The degree of protein binding varies from drug to drug. It has to be emphasized that only the free concentration of an anti-infective drug exhibits antimicrobial activity. Therefore, despite apparently adequate total plasma levels of highly protein-bound drugs, the concentration of free (i.e. active) drug might be less than the MIC of the pathogen. As most sites of infection are extravascular, treatment of infections in these sites depends on movement of the antimicrobial agent out of the bloodstream and into interstitial and sometimes intracellular fluid. In general, hydrophilic agents (such as β-lactams) tend to reach higher concentrations in body fluids and the interstitium, whereas lipophilic agents (such as fluoroquinolones) are able to cross biologic membranes and achieve effective intracellular concentrations. Therefore, even within one organ, such as lung or brain, antibiotic concentrations can vary between anatomic or histological structures. For example, antibiotic concentrations in the epithelial lining fluid differ from concentrations within the bronchial epithelial cells or the interstitium of the lung. When the drug ultimately reaches the site of infection, local factors may play a role in the effectiveness of its antimicrobial activity such as pH, anaerobic

TABLE 136-3	Major Antifungal Drugs		
Agent	**Mechanism of Action**	**Specific Activity**	**Toxicity/Side effects**
Amphotericin B	Polyene, binds with ergosterol in the fungal cell membrane and leads to pore formation	*Candida* species (except *C. lusitaniae*), *Cryptococcus* species, *Aspergillus* species (except *A. terreus*), Mucorales, dermatophytes, endemic (dimorphic) fungi, *Leishmania* species; some activity against *Fusarium* spp. *Pseudallescheria boydii/Scedosporium apiospermum* and phaeohyphomycosis-associated fungi	Acute reaction after infusion (fever, shaking chills, headache, hypotension, nausea), nephrotoxicity (reduced with lipid-associated forms of amphotericin B), electrolyte imbalances; hepatotoxicity, anemia, leukopenia, thrombocytopenia, arrhythmias, skin reactions
Anidulafungin	Echinocandin, inhibition of (1,3) β-D-glucan synthase, an enzyme important to synthesis of the fungal cell wall	*Candida* species (limited activity against *C. parapsilosis* and *C. guilliermondii*), *Aspergillus* species, some activity against endemic (dimorphic) fungi, *Pseudallescheria boydii/Scedosporium apiospermum* (combination therapy) and *Pneumocystis jirovecii* (last line treatment)	Diarrhea, nausea, vomiting, flushing, convulsions, headache, exanthema, pruritus, coagulation disorders, thrombocytopenia, electrolyte imbalances
Caspofungin	Echinocandin, see anidulafungin	See anidulafungin	Fever, shivering, phlebitis, abdominal pain, nausea, vomiting, exanthema, pruritus, anemia, headache, hypokalemia, tachycardia, increased liver enzymes, increased plasma creatinine
Fluconazole	Triazole, inhibits fungal cytochrome P450 enzyme lanosterol 14 α-demethylase preventing conversion of lanosterol to ergosterol, an essential component of the fungal cytoplasmic membrane	*Candida* species (except *C. glabrata*, *C. krusei*), *Cryptococcus* species, some endemic dimorphic fungi, some dermatophytes	Rash, headache, nausea, vomiting, abdominal pain, diarrhea, elevated liver enzymes (in rare cases serious hepatotoxicity including liver failure), anorexia, fatigue, constipation, thrombocytopenia, electrolyte imbalances, prolonged QT interval
Flucytosine	Pyrimidine analog, by conversion it interacts with RNA biosynthesis and fungal DNA synthesis	*Candida* species (reduced activity against *C. krusei*), *Cryptococcus* species (as part of combination treatment)	Bone marrow depression, GI toxicity, hepatotoxicity, nephrotoxicity (crystalluria), adverse central nervous system effects, skin reactions, anaphylaxis, increased toxicity in combination with amphotericin B
Itraconazole	Triazole, see fluconazole	*Candida* species (reduced activity against *C. glabrata* and *C. krusei*), *Cryptococcus* species, *Aspergillus* species, dermatophytes, endemic dimorphic fungi, phaeohyphomycosis-associated fungi	Elevated liver enzymes, sometimes fatal liver failure, congestive heart failure. Cyclodextrin used to make syrup preparation can cause: nausea, vomiting, abdominal pain, fatigue, loss of appetite, jaundice, itching, dark urine, pale stool, headache
Micafungin	Echinocandin, see anidulafungin	See anidulafungin	Leukopenia, anemia, electrolyte imbalances, headache, phlebitis, nausea, vomiting, diarrhea, abdominal pain, increased liver enzymes (risk of liver tumors in rats), exanthema, fever
Posaconazole	Triazole, see fluconazole	*Candida* spp. (reduced activity against *C. glabrata* and *C. krusei*), *Cryptococcus* species, *Aspergillus* spp., Mucorales, endemic dimorphic fungi, phaeohyphomycosis, *Fusarium* species, *Pseudallescheria boydii/Scedosporium apiospermum*	Fever, diarrhea, nausea, vomiting, headache, anemia, thrombocytopenia, electrolyte imbalance, rash, hepatotoxicity, prolonged QT interval
Voriconazole	Triazole, see fluconazole	*Candida* spp., *Cryptococcus* spp., *Aspergillus* spp., endemic dimorphic fungi, phaeohyphomycosis, *Fusarium* species, *Pseudallescheria boydii/Scedosporium apiospermum*	Transient visual disturbances, fever, rash, vomiting, nausea, diarrhea, headache, peripheral edema abdominal pain, respiratory disorder, hepatotoxicity, increased risk of squamous cell carcinoma of the skin, prolonged QT interval
Co-trimoxazole (trimethoprim–sulfamethoxazole)	Antifolate, inhibits folate biosynthesis and metabolism	*Pneumocystis jirovecii* (first line treatment), paracoccidioidomycosis, broad antibacterial spectrum including multiresistant bacteria such as MRSA or *Stenotrophomonas maltophilia*	Fever, nausea, vomiting, diarrhea, rash, hyperkalemia, thrombocytopenia, headache, hepatotoxicity, peripheral neuritis, anemia, crystalluria, interstitial nephritis, myelosuppression, Stevens-Johnson syndrome, toxic epidermal necrolysis

TABLE 136-4	Major Antiparasitic Drugs		
Agent	**Mechanism of Action**	**Antiparasitic Activity**	**Toxicity/Side Effects**
Albendazole	Benzimidazole anthelmintic, inhibits the polymerization of the parasite tubulin into microtubules. The loss of the cytoplasmic microtubules leads to impaired uptake of glucose by the larval and adult stages of the parasites	Echinococcosis, cysticercosis, fasciolosis, enterobiasis, trichuriasis, toxocariasis, ascariasis, hookworm, cutaneous larva migrans, filariasis, myiasis, oxyuriasis, strongyloidiasis	Nausea, abdominal pain, headache, bone marrow suppression, hepatotoxicity
Artesunate	Artemisinin derivate, a prodrug which is converted to dihydroartemisinin (DHA). DHA is a blood schizonticide, potently inhibits the essential *Plasmodium falciparum* exported protein 1 (EXP1), a membrane glutathione S-transferase	*Plasmodium* species (indicated for severe forms of malaria), some effect against *Schistosoma haematobium*	Delayed hemolysis (two weeks after treatment), lower reticulocyte counts
Artemether + lumefantrine	Artemisinin-based combination, both substances are blood schizonticides. Artemether is rapidly metabolized into DHA (see above). Available data suggest lumefantrine inhibits the formation of ß-hematin by forming a complex with hemin	*Plasmodium* species (indicated for uncomplicated malaria)	Mild forms of headache, dizziness and anorexia; tinnitus, tremor, gastrointestinal disorders, anaphylactic reactions
Atovaquone + proguanil	Antimalaria combination treatment, atovaquone selectively inhibits the parasitic electron transport chain. Proguanil, via its metabolite cycloguanil, functions as a dihydrofolate reductase inhibitor, halting parasitic deoxythymidylate synthesis	*Plasmodium* species (malaria treatment and prophylaxis)	Headache, abdominal pain, stomach pain, nausea, vomiting, diarrhea, dizziness
Chloroquine	4-aminoquinoline drug with antimalarial activity, inhibits heme polymerase activity, in the lysosome chloroquine interferes with pigment formation and the Fe(II)-protoporphyrin IX-chloroquine complex is highly toxic to the parasite	*Plasmodium vivax, Plasmodium ovale, Plasmodium malariae* (malaria treatment and prophylaxis), no activity against most strains of *Plasmodium falciparum*	Gastrointestinal problems, stomach ache, itching, headache, hypotension, nightmares, blurred vision, retinopathy, cardiac toxicity
Diloxanide furoate	Dichloroacetamide derivative, luminal amebicide, the mechanism of action is unknown	*Entamoeba histolytica* (for mild intestinal amebiasis and to eradicate cysts)	No relevant toxicity
Ivermectin	Avermectin derivative anthelmintic, binds to glutamate-gated chloride ion channels in invertebrate muscle and nerve cells of the microfilaria. This leads to increased permeability of the cell membranes to chloride ions and results in hyperpolarization of the cell and death of the parasite	Onchocerciasis, strongyloidiasis, ascariasis, toxocariasis, trichuriasis, filariasis, enterobiasis, cutaneous larva migrans, scabies, lice	Neurotoxicity, fever, pruritus, headache, edema, abdominal pain, diarrhea, nausea
Liposomal amphotericin B	Polyene (see amphotericin B, Table 136-3)	Leishmaniasis, broad antifungal spectrum (see amphotericin B, Table 136-3)	(See amphotericin B, Table 136-3)
Mefloquine	Analog of quinine, produces swelling of the *Plasmodium falciparum* food vacuoles. It may act by forming toxic complexes with free heme that damage membranes and interact with other plasmodial components	*Plasmodium* species (malaria treatment and prophylaxis)	Psychotropic potential, gastrointestinal problems
Metronidazole	Nitroimidazole antibiotic with additional antiprotozoal activity, inhibits nucleic acid synthesis by disrupting the DNA of microbial cells	Anaerobic bacteria (e.g. *Clostridium difficile*, bacterial vaginosis), extra-intestinal amebicide (e.g. to treat amebic liver abscess), giardiasis, trichomoniasis	Nausea, diarrhea, abdominal pain, vomiting, headache, dizziness, metallic taste, hypersensitivity reactions, leukopenia, central nervous toxicity, interaction with alcohol
Miltefosine	Alkylphosphocholine derivative against leishmaniasis, interferes with cellular membranes and modulates membrane permeability and fluidity, membrane lipid composition, metabolism of phospholipids and proliferation signal transduction	*Leishmania* species, *Schistosoma mansoni*	Nausea, vomiting, diarrhea, weakness, leukopenia, anemia
Praziquantel	Isocholine derivative anthelmintic, mode of action is not exactly known, causes severe spasms and paralysis of the worms' muscles	Schistosomiasis, cysticercosis, taeniasis, toxocariasis, clonorchiasis, filariasis	Dizziness, headache, somnolence, fatigue, vertigo, gastrointestinal problems, transient increased liver enzymes, sensitivity reactions, arrhythmia, hypotension
Primaquine	8-aminoquinoline derivative, clearing malarial hypnozoites, mode of action is not exactly known, may be acting by generating reactive oxygen species or by interfering with the electron transport in the parasite	*Plasmodium vivax* and *ovale* (against dormant liver forms), *Pneumocystis jiroveci* (with clindamycin)	Hemolysis in patients with glucose-6-phosphate dehydrogenase deficiency; methemoglobinemia, nausea, vomiting, stomach pain, headache, visual disturbances, intense itching
Quinine	Crystalline alkaloid with antimalarial activity, interferes with the parasite's ability to digest hemoglobin. Inhibits the spontaneous formation of ß-hematin (hemozoin or malaria pigment) which is a toxic product of the digestion of hemoglobin by parasites	*Plasmodium* species (indicated for severe malaria)	Cinchonism, fever, hypotension, hypoglycemia, electrolyte imbalances, arrhythmia, nausea, vomiting

TABLE 136-5	Examples of Bactericidal and Bacteriostatic Antibacterial Agents	
Antibacterial Agent or Class	Target	Action
β-lactams	Peptidoglycan synthesis	Cidal
Glycopeptides	Transpeptidases	Cidal
Daptomycin	D-alanyl-D-alanine ligase	Cidal
	Dephosphorylation of lipids	
Isoniazid, ethionamide, ethambutol	Mycolic acid synthesis	Cidal
Aminoglycosides	Protein synthesis	Cidal
Tetracyclines, tigecycline	Ribosomal 30S subunit	Static
Macrolides, lincosamides, oxazolidinones	Ribosomal 50S subunit	Static
	tRNA dephosphorylation	
Mupirocin	synthetase	Cidal
Fusidic acid	Elongation factor G	Cidal
Metronidazole, nitrofurantoin	Nucleic acid synthesis	Cidal
Quinolones	DNA disruption	Cidal
Rifampin (rifampicin)	DNA gyrase A and topoisomerase IV	Cidal
	DNA-dependent RNA	
Trimethoprim, para-aminosalicylic acid	Folic acid metabolism	Static
	Dihydrofolate reductase	
Sulfonamides, diaminodiphenyl sulfone	Dihydropteroate synthase	Static
	Dihydrofolate reductase +	
Co-trimoxazole	synthase	Cidal

Pharmacokinetic and pharmacodynamic parameters and the resulting three different PK/PD indices

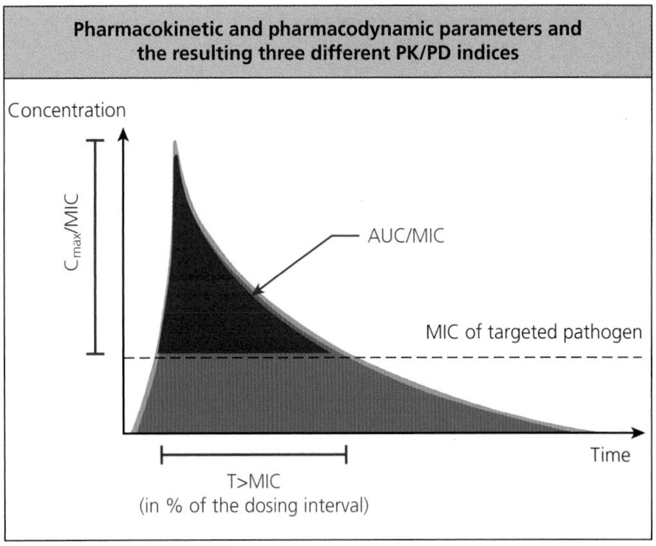

Figure 136-1   Pharmacokinetic (maximal concentration – C_{max} and area under the curve – AUC) and pharmacodynamic (relationship to minimal inhibitory concentration – MIC) parameters and the resulting three different PK/PD indices (red). *Reproduced with permission from M.W., Lipman J.: Intensive Care Med 2013; 39(7):1322-1324.*

environment or the presence of β-lactamases and other deactivating enzymes.

After a peak plasma level is attained, the plasma level declines as a consequence of drug distribution and elimination, usually by the kidneys, liver or both. The term 'clearance' describes a theoretic volume of plasma cleared of the drug within a period of time. Drugs may be excreted unchanged but in general undergo metabolism, especially in the liver for subsequent excretion in the bile. Typical metabolites are the result of glucuronidation, conjugation and acetylation. Drugs metabolized by the cytochrome P450 system may interact with other drugs which share this route. Drug–drug interactions involving antibiotics are mainly caused by inhibition of their metabolism or by additive toxic effects and can be responsible for severe complications. Conversely, enzyme induction may lead to subtherapeutic drug levels.

In those with impaired liver function, drugs excreted through the liver should be used with caution or avoided. Dose adjustment may be appropriate following careful assessment of liver function tests.

Drug excretion is also largely the result of renal excretion. The latter may be either a metabolically active or passive process, and involve the glomeruli or renal tubules or both. Impairment of renal function often leads to a prolonged drug half-life for renally excreted drugs. Dose modification may be required to avoid drug accumulation and drug toxicity.

A clear understanding of the elimination half-life ($t_{1/2elim}$) and excretion of antibiotics also influences dosage selection. Drugs with a short half-life, such as many β-lactams, are rapidly eliminated and need more frequent administration to produce satisfactory antibiotic concentrations at the site of infection. Drugs with a longer half-life, such as moxifloxacin, azithromycin, ceftriaxone or ertapenem, allow once-daily dosing. Recently, the US Food and Drug Administration (FDA) approved a novel lipoglycopeptide antibiotic for gram-positive skin and soft-tissue infections called dalbavancin with unusually long elimination half-life, ranging from 149 to 250 hours. This long half-life is the result of extensive, reversible binding of dalbavancin to plasma proteins and allows even once-weekly dosing.

PHARMACOKINETIC AND PHARMACODYNAMIC PARAMETERS

The success of antimicrobial therapy is determined by complex interactions among an administered drug, a host and an infecting agent. In the past, dose and drug selection was mostly based on MIC and on the drug's serum concentration. However, a pharmacodynamic effect *in vivo* is rather the result of a dynamic exposure of the infective agent to the unbound antibiotic drug fraction at the relevant effect site. To elucidate this dynamic relationship, PK/PD models have to be considered.[12,13] The most useful PK/PD variables are summarized in Table 136-7.

The efficacy of an antimicrobial agent can depend on the maximal concentration, on the exposure time and on the total exposure that the drug remains on its target sites. The integration of how high (concentration) and how long (time) an antibiotic's level remains above a zero concentration over a dosing interval is referred to as the area under the concentration-time curve (AUC). The different classes of antibiotics differ in their relevant PK/PD target parameters. For time-dependent antibiotics such as β-lactams or vancomycin, the duration of time during a dosing interval that the antibiotic's concentration remains above the MIC for a particular organism (time above MIC, t>MIC) is the best predictor of clinical outcome.[7,13] To prolong the duration of a β-lactam concentration above its MIC in severe infections, the drug has to be given in larger and more frequent doses or administered by a 24-hour constant infusion. For concentration-dependent agents such as aminoglycosides, fluoroquinolones, metronidazole, amphotericin B or daptomycin, the single dose is pivotal, whereas the dosage interval can be extended. Thus, for these agents, the pharmacodynamic parameter ratio of AUC/MIC can be simplified to the ratio of peak concentration to MIC (C_{max}/MIC). For a number of bacteriostatic antimicrobial agents such as azithromycin, clindamycin and tigecycline, the antimicrobial efficacy of the drug can be correlated best with the 24-hours AUC/MIC ratio.[14,15]

Data based on PK/PD parameters and timed plasma samples from volunteers and patients may be employed in mathematical models using approaches such as Monte Carlo simulations. Using this basic pharmacokinetic data and *in vitro* susceptibility profiles of microorganisms, the relationship between PK and PD variables can be characterized graphically.[16] Figure 136-1 illustrates these key parameters in relation to the MIC of a target pathogen.[17]

Such PK/PD data have supported single daily dosage regimens for the aminoglycosides[18] and dosage revisions for ciprofloxacin and levofloxacin.[19] Continuous or prolonged infusion of β-lactams is conducted with increasing frequency in intensive care units (ICU) and has

TABLE 136-6	Common Clinical Sites for Bacterial Infections in Adults, Frequently Encountered Organisms and Appropriate Antibiotics*

Infection Site	Common Bacterial Etiology	Appropriate Antibiotics[†]
Oropharynx, tonsil	Streptococcus pyogenes	Penicillin V × 10 days, macrolides, first-generation cephalosporin, clindamycin
Acute bacterial sinusitis	Streptococcus pneumoniae, Haemophilus influenzae, Moraxella catarrhalis, group A streptococcus	Amoxicillin, amoxicillin–clavulanate, first- or second-generation cephalosporin
Acute exacerbation of chronic bronchitis (AE-COPD) AE-COPD in patients with bronchiectasis and/or known P. aeruginosa colonization	Strep. pneumoniae, H. influenzae, M. catarrhalis Strep. pneumoniae, H. influenzae, M. catarrhalis, P. aeruginosa	Mild: oral – amoxicillin, clarithromycin, doxycycline Moderate to severe: ampicillin–sulbactam iv, cefuroxime iv, levofloxacin, moxifloxacin Piperacillin/tazobactam, carbapenem, levofloxacin, ciprofloxacin + antipneumococcal agent, ceftazidime + antipneumococcal agent The majority of mild to moderate AE-COPD is not caused by bacterial infection and does therefore not require antibiotic treatment. The cornerstone of all AE-COPD are inhaled bronchodilators and systemic steroids
Pneumonia, community-acquired Outpatient treatment possible	Strep. pneumoniae, H. influenzae, M. pneumoniae, respiratory viruses + Enterobacteriaceae, Staph. aureus	Without co-morbidities: amoxicillin, clarithromycin With co-morbidities: amoxicillin-clavulanate, fluoroquinolone (third or fourth generation)
Pneumonia, community-acquired, requires admission to a normal ward	Strep. pneumoniae, H. influenzae, M. pneumoniae, respiratory viruses, Enterobacteriaceae, Staph. aureus, Legionella spp.	Ampicillin–sulbactam plus clarithromycin, cefuroxime plus clarithromycin, fluoroquinolone (third or fourth generation)
Pneumonia, community-acquired, requires admission to ICU	Strep. pneumoniae, H. influenzae, M. pneumoniae, respiratory viruses, Enterobacteriaceae, Staph. aureus, Legionella spp., Pseudomonas aeruginosa	Piperacillin/tazobactam or extended-spectrum cephalosporin + clarithromycin, or fluoroquinolone
Urinary tract infection, uncomplicated cystitis	Enterobacteriaceae	Nitrofurantoin, pivmecillinam, fosfomycin, trimethoprim–sulfamethoxazole, trimethoprim, fluoroquinolone
Pyelonephritis	Enterobacteriaceae, Enterococcus spp.	Fluoroquinolone, ampicillin–sulbactam iv, third-generation cephalosporin, piperacillin–tazobactam
Urethritis, gonococcal	Neisseria gonorrhoeae	Ceftriaxone
Urethritis, nongonococcal	Chlamydia spp., Mycoplasma hominis, Ureaplasma spp.	Doxycycline, azithromycin
Pelvic inflammatory disease	N. gonorrhoeae, Chlamydia spp., Bacteroides spp., Enterobacteriaceae, Streptococcus spp.	Levofloxacin plus metronidazole, ceftriaxone plus doxycycline, ampicillin–sulbactam plus doxycycline
Prostatitis, <35 years old	N. gonorrhoeae, Chlamydia spp.	Ceftriaxone plus doxycycline
Prostatitis, >35 years old	Enterobacteriaceae	Fluoroquinolone, trimethoprim–sulfamethoxazole, aminoglycoside
Gastroenteritis	Shigella spp., Salmonella typhi/paratyphi Campylobacter spp., Salmonella enteritidis, Escherichia coli O157 H7	Fluoroquinolone, third-generation cephalosporin, ampicillin–sulbactam No antimicrobial treatment recommended
Cholecystitis	Enterobacteriaceae, enterococci, anaerobes	Ampicillin–sulbactam, ceftriaxone plus metronidazole, piperacillin/tazobactam, imipenem, meropenem
Diverticulitis	Enterobacteriaceae, anaerobes, enterococci	Ampicillin–sulbactam, piperacillin/tazobactam, imipenem, meropenem, metronidazole plus fluoroquinolone
Spontaneous bacterial peritonitis	Enterobacteriaceae, Bacteroides spp., enterococci	Ampicillin–sulbactam, ceftriaxone plus metronidazole, piperacillin/tazobactam
Erysipelas	β-hemolytic Group A streptococcus	Penicillin, cefazolin, clindamycin
Cellulitis	β-hemolytic Group A streptococcus, Staph. aureus	First-generation cephalosporin, dicloxacillin/flucloxacillin, ampicillin–clavulanate
Osteomyelitis	Staph. aureus	Dicloxacillin/flucloxacillin, first-generation cephalosporin, vancomycin (methicillin-resistant pathogen)
Meningitis	Strep. pneumoniae, N. meningitides Listeria monocytogenes	Ceftriaxone ± ampicillin
Endocarditis, native valve	Viridans streptococcus, staphylococci, other streptococcal species, enterococci	Penicillin (for streptococci), ampicillin (for enterococci), dicloxacillin/flucloxacillin (for methicillin-susceptible staphylococci), vancomycin or daptomycin (for MRSA, MRSE) plus gentamicin
Endocarditis, prosthetic valve	Staph. epidermidis, Staph. aureus	Vancomycin or daptomycin plus gentamicin ± rifampin (rifampicin)

*This table is not intended to be all-inclusive. Specific infections are considered in detail in other chapters. Note that some agents have restricted geographic availability.

[†]This is a general overview; the choice of antibiotics must consider the resistance pattern in any given geographic area (e.g. penicillin and macrolide resistance in Strep. pneumoniae; ampicillin and trimethoprim–sulfamethoxazole resistance among E. coli), as well as adjustments based on the identified etiologic agent and susceptibility testing.

TABLE 136-7	**Pharmacokinetic and Pharmacodynamic Parameters That Affect Antibiotic Therapy**	
Parameters		**Details**
Pharmacokinetic	F	Bioavailability, fraction of the administered dose absorbed intact; intravenous drugs have 100% bioavailability; oral drugs vary with absorption and are usually less bioavailable than intravenous forms
	C_{max}	Peak serum concentration after single or multiple doses
	t_{max}	Time after drug administration to reach C_{max}
	$t_{1/2elim}$	Elimination half-life; time to reduce peak serum concentration by 50%
	AUC	Area under the concentration–time curve (relates to total drug exposure following a dose)
Pharmacodynamic	C_{max}/MIC	Ratio of the peak serum concentration to the MIC (predicts activity of concentration-dependent bactericidal antibiotics)
	AUC/MIC	Ratio of the area under the concentration–time curve to the MIC (predicts best activity of some bacteriostatic antibiotics)
	t>MIC	Time above the MIC; the duration of time during a dosing interval that antibiotic concentration remains above the MIC (predicts activity of time-dependent bactericidal antibiotics)

recently been included as an option to increase antibiotic efficacy in the German guideline for the treatment of nosocomial pneumonia.[20] To date, evidence from RCTs showing that continuous infusion of β-lactams improves clinical outcome is increasing.[21,22]

DRUG SAFETY

Adverse reactions range from drug hypersensitivity to dose-related side effects and unpredictable or idiosyncratic phenomena. With regard to antibiotics, the penicillins and cephalosporins share the β-lactam ring structure and in turn have many adverse effects in common. These include hypersensitivity rashes and other reactions and toxicity to hematopoietic cells. However, there are differences between these two classes. Hypersensitivity reactions occur less commonly to the cephalosporins. This applies to anaphylaxis which is the most severe and feared hypersensitivity reaction. Any severe hypersensitivity reaction to a β-lactam is a bar to its future use and of the β-lactam agents in general. However, milder forms of hypersensitivity, such as rash or skin eruption to a penicillin, do not necessarily preclude the use of a cephalosporin. Usual alternatives to β-lactams in patients with severe allergies are vancomycin and clindamycin.

Many adverse drug events can be minimized in persons with known excretory organ malfunction by adjusting the dose. The aminoglycosides, such as gentamicin, have been extensively studied and dosage schedules developed which are adjusted for age, weight, gender and renal function.

THERAPEUTIC DRUG MONITORING

Therapeutic drug monitoring (TDM) aims to ensure safe and effective prescribing for drugs with a narrow therapeutic index. The latter reflects the limited margin between the therapeutic and toxic concentrations of a particular drug. In contrast, drugs such as penicillins have a wide therapeutic index and even when given in high concentration are generally safe.

In practice much TDM is directed at ensuring therapeutic nontoxic concentrations of the aminoglycosides or ensuring sufficient but nontoxic concentration of the glycopeptides. Other examples include TDM for antifungals such as itraconazole and voriconazole[23] in the treatment of severe fungal infections as well as, in some circumstances, antiretroviral agents such as the protease inhibitors and non-nucleoside reverse transcriptase inhibitors.[24]

There is increasing evidence that TDM is not only required to avoid toxic concentrations but also to achieve sufficient concentrations, particularly in septic patients with unpredictable and highly variable pharmacokinetics. Roberts *et al.* prospectively evaluated TDM in ICU patients and reported that β-lactam dose adjustment was necessary for 74% of patients; 50% of the total patients required a dose increment after the first measurement.[25] Recently, in a randomized controlled trial in 41 patients receiving piperacillin/tazobactam or meropenem, with and without therapeutic drug monitoring-based dose optimization, De Waele *et al.* showed that among critically ill patients with normal kidney function, a strategy of dose adaptation based on daily TDM led to an increase in PK/PD target attainment compared to conventional dosis (58% versus 16%).[26]

COMBINED DRUG REGIMENS

In general and whenever possible it is preferable to manage an infection with a single drug. However, there are an increasing number of diseases and circumstances where a combination of drugs is appropriate or necessary to control the infection. Examples include tuberculosis,[27] HIV infection[24] and, more recently, malaria[28] and gonorrhoea. In practice, drugs are frequently combined where there is uncertainty about the microbiologic nature of a diagnosis or where the spectrum of a single agent is inadequate, particularly in situations such as intraabdominal sepsis where the etiology is often polymicrobial. Combining an extended-spectrum cephalosporin, such as cefuroxime or cefotaxime, with metronidazole provides an appropriate 'broadspectrum' regimen. Another example is in the treatment of severe community-acquired pneumonia when both atypical and conventional pathogens need to be 'covered'.[29]

Another important reason for combined drug regimens is to prevent resistant organisms emerging on therapy. This was first demonstrated in the treatment of tuberculosis where minority populations of organisms can become resistant to the most active tuberculostatic drugs, isoniazid or rifampin (rifampicin) when applied as monotherapy. Therefore, the standard regimen for treating pulmonary tuberculosis includes isoniazid and rifampin combined with a third (pyrazinamide) and fourth (ethambutol) agent for the first 2 months, by which time the results of susceptibility testing are generally available. It is then usually safe to continue with a two-drug regimen of isoniazid and rifampin for the remaining 4 months of treatment (see Chapter 148).[27]

Similar principles are increasingly being applied to the treatment of severe malaria, particularly in regions of the world where chloroquine-resistant malaria is widespread. Examples include combinations of artemisinin with tetracycline or mefloquine.[28]

Other circumstances where combined regimens have become the norm are in the management of HIV[24] and chronic hepatitis C.[30] In both diseases clinical trials have shown greater efficacy with combined regimens. In the case of HIV, viral load is more rapidly controlled and sustained with faster immune reconstitution and decreased clinical progression. By selecting two or more agents from different classes of antiretrovirals, drug resistance is delayed in addition to providing a more efficacious regimen.

In the case of hepatitis C, recently new combination regimens have been developed including not only pegylated interferon and ribavirin, but also new nucleotide polymerase inhibitors (e.g. sofosbuvir) ± new protease inhibitors (e.g. simeprevir) enabling prompt and sustained viral response with high cure rates (see Chapter 155).[30,31]

Another rationale for combined drug regimens is to achieve synergistic inhibition of a target pathogen. The combining of a penicillin (for susceptible strains) with an aminoglycoside to treat enterococcal endocarditis is now standard therapy since *in vitro* and *in vivo* the combination is more effective than a penicillin alone.[10]

FAILURE OF ANTIMICROBIAL THERAPY

Failure to respond to antimicrobial treatment may have several explanations. These include the accuracy of the primary diagnosis, the choice of initial therapy, the selection of dose and route of administration, the duration of treatment and, in the case of trauma or implant surgery, an assessment of the possible presence of deep-seated infection. Surgical drainage of pus with abscess formation is often overlooked and needs emphasis.

Failure to make a correct diagnosis may be the result of an inaccurate clinical assessment and, in turn, presumptive microbiologic assessment to guide initial empiric therapy – for example, the incorrect diagnosis of superficial cellulitis instead of more deep-seated necrotizing fasciitis. Here the selection of oxacillin, dicloxacillin or flucloxacillin alone will be ineffective, particularly against methicillin-resistant *Staphylococcus aureus* (MRSA) or anaerobic pathogens.[32] The dose and route of medication are also of importance. For example, pneumococcal pneumonia can be effectively managed in the community with oral agents for patients with mild to moderate infection.

Most mild to moderate infections respond to 5–10 days of antibiotic therapy.[33,34] However, selected infections require more protracted therapy to avoid treatment failure and relapse. Severe *Legionella pneumophila* pneumonia may require up to 3 weeks of treatment,[29] as does meningitis caused by *Listeria monocytogenes*. Infection as a complication of the presence of foreign materials, notably vascular and articular prosthetic devices, is increasing. Infection is often caused by skin micro-organisms, notably coagulase-negative staphylococci. These are not only of variable sensitivity to many commonly used agents but also adhere to the foreign material as biofilms in which they are protected against host defenses and are less responsive to treatment. The so-called minimal biofilm eradicating concentration (MBEC) of a certain bacterial strain can exceed its MIC, which is measured in the planktonic phase, by more than 1000-fold. Prolonged therapy or surgical revision, sometimes with removal of the infected device, may be necessary to eliminate the infection.

Surgical Prophylaxis

Surgical site infection (SSI) is the most common postoperative complication and is associated with significant morbidity, and mortality.[35,36] Depending on the type of surgery, 2–20% of patients develop SSIs, with risk being highest for orthopedic, cardiac and intra-abdominal surgeries.[37,38] Length of stay can increase by 4–32 days compared to patients without complications after surgery.[39,40] Up to 25% of patients with SSI progress to severe sepsis/shock and are admitted to the ICU.[36] The US National Surgical Quality Improvement Program (NSQIP) has shown that postoperative complications can increase hospital costs by US$ 25 534 (for infectious complications) and mortality by 69%.[41,42] Moreover, an increasing proportion of SSIs are now being caused by multidrug-resistant (MDR) organisms such as MRSA and MDR gram-negative and fungi such as *Candida albicans*.[43–46]

Consequently, the selection of appropriate antimicrobial prophylaxis is becoming an increasingly complex issue.

Pathogenesis

SSI develop due to microbial contamination of the surgical wound, most commonly from patients' endogenous flora or from an exogenous source, such as personnel in the operating room or the environment. The role of wound contamination during the postoperative period, from direct inoculation or from hematogenous seeding, is less clear but is thought to be involved in late infections of prosthetic devices.

The risk of SSI is due to a combination of factors as follows:[47,48]

$$\frac{\text{Dose of bacterial contamination} \times \text{virulence}}{\text{Resistance of the host patient}} = \text{Risk of surgical site infection}$$

Preoperative antisepsis and antimicrobial prophylaxis are performed to decrease the bacterial load in the wound; however, it is not possible to completely sterilize it, as up to 20% of skin flora resides beneath the surface in sebaceous glands and hair follicles. Regarding the bacterial 'dose', studies demonstrate that a concentration of $>10^5$ organisms per gram of tissue is the critical threshold above which risk of SSI increases significantly.[49] As shown in the above equation, however, this dose could be lower if the virulence of the organism is high, host immunity is low or prosthetic material (including suture material) is in place.

Since the microbiology of SSIs is usually a function of the patient's skin flora, the causative organisms are most often staphylococci: *Staph. aureus* and coagulase-negative staphylococci. However, some patients can also be colonized with a variety of other organisms including gram-negative bacilli and *Candida* species which can then lead to infection of the wound. Finally, in intra-abdominal surgeries, gastrointestinal flora, such as enteric bacteria and anaerobes, can contaminate the wound and cause infection.

SSI Risk Classification Systems and SSI Risk Factors (Table 136-8)

Since 1964, surgical wounds have been categorized by the traditional wound classification system, which stratifies wounds into four categories based on the expected bacterial dose that would contaminate the wound: clean, clean–contaminated, contaminated, and dirty–infected. Data show that these wound categories have different associated infection rates, ranging from 5% for clean surgeries and up to 22% for the contaminated category, if antimicrobial prophylaxis is not administered (decreased to 0.8% and 10% respectively if antibiotics are administered).[50]

The surveillance system that is most widely used at present is the National Nosocomial Infection Surveillance (NNIS), which counts the numbers of risk factors present among the following:
- an American Society of Anesthesiologists (ASA) preoperative assessment score of 3, 4 or 5;
- an operation classified as either contaminated or dirty–infected; and
- an operation with duration of >T hours, where T depends on the type of operative procedure.

Surveillance for SSI

In the USA, the Centers for Disease Control and Prevention (CDC) developed the NNIS system as early as the 1970s as a voluntary reporting system. This system has since been renamed the National Healthcare Safety Network (NHSN) and enables confidential data exchange and analysis within its information technology architecture. In the 1990s, a number of European countries established national or regional healthcare-associated infections (HAI) surveillance systems, largely modeled on the NNIS system as the Hospitals in Europe Link for Infection Control through Surveillance (HELICS) and The European Surveillance System (TESSy).[51,52]

One key component of efficient SSI surveillance is having a case definition that is applied accurately and consistently. A recent study [53] assessed agreement in diagnosing SSIs. Twelve case vignettes based on SSI were submitted to 100 infection-control physicians (ICPS) and 86 surgeons in 10 European countries. Each participant scored eight randomly-assigned case vignettes using a 7-point Likert scale. The study showed an imperfect agreement among intra- and interspecialties in each country as well as across the countries.[53]

Indications for Antibiotic Prophylaxis

In most instances, antibiotic prophylaxis is administered to prevent an SSI by decreasing the microbial burden at the surgical site. While there is fairly good agreement between consensus statements regarding which surgery types require prophylaxis, the increase in less invasive

TABLE 136-8	Surgical Site Infection Risk Classification Systems	

Wound Classification System

I. Clean	An uninfected operative wound in which no inflammation is encountered and the respiratory, alimentary, genital or uninfected urinary tract is not entered. In addition, clean wounds are primarily closed and, if necessary, drained with closed drainage. Operative incisional wounds that follow nonpenetrating (blunt) trauma should be included in this category if they meet the criteria
II. Clean–contaminated	An operative wound in which the respiratory, alimentary, genital or urinary tract is entered under controlled conditions and without unusual contamination. Specifically, operations involving the biliary tract, appendix, vagina and oropharynx are included in this category, provided no evidence of infection or major break in technique is encountered
III. Contaminated	Open, fresh, accidental wounds. In addition, operations with major breaks in sterile technique (e.g. open cardiac massage) or gross spillage from the gastrointestinal tract, and incisions in which acute nonpurulent inflammation is encountered are included in this category
IV. Dirty–infected	Old traumatic wounds with retained devitalized tissue and those that involve existing clinical infection or perforated viscera. This definition suggests that the organisms causing postoperative infection were present in the operative field before the operation

SENIC (STUDY ON THE EFFICACY OF NOSOCOMIAL INFECTION CONTROL) INDEX

1 point	Operative time >2h
1 point	Abdominal procedure
1 point	Contaminated or dirty procedure
1 point	≥Three discharge diagnoses

NNIS (NATIONAL NOSOCOMIAL INFECTION SURVEILLANCE) RISK INDEX

1 point	ASA score of 3, 4 or 5
1 point	Contaminated or dirty procedure
1 point	Length of procedure >T hours (75th percentile duration of specific procedure)
Minus 1 point	Use of laparoscope

ASA, American Society of Anesthesiologists.
Reproduced from Gaynes R.P.: Surgical site infection (SSI) rates in the United States, 1992–1998: the National Nosocomial Infections Surveillance System basic SSI risk index. Clin Infect Dis 2001; 33(Suppl.2):S69-77.

procedures, including laparoscopic procedures and procedures performed by interventional radiology, has led to some controversy regarding the necessity of prophylaxis. In some instances, antibiotic prophylaxis is administered not to prevent an SSI, but rather to prevent endocarditis from procedure-induced transient bacteremia in patients with underlying cardiac disease.

A meta-analysis of meta-analyses including 250 clinical trials and 4809 patients has provided an estimation of the relative benefit of systematic prophylactic antibiotics to reduce infection for 23 different types of surgery.[54] Although the study showed heterogeneity as for the type of antibiotic, timing, dosing and type of procedure, the relative risk of developing infection for all types of operations comparing prophylactic systemic antibiotics versus no prophylaxis varied slightly from 0.19 to 0.82 relative risk (RR), suggesting a generalized benefit regardless of the degree of surgical contamination.[54]

General Principles of Antibiotic Prophylaxis

CHOICE

The choice of antibiotic should ideally be one which is safe, inexpensive, and bactericidal with an *in vitro* spectrum that covers the most probable intraoperative contaminants for the operation.[48] Thus the antibiotic choice varies depending on the type of procedure. Cephalosporins fit the criteria listed above; they have long duration of action and comparatively low cost. First-generation cephalosporins, such as cefazolin, are therefore frequently used for clean procedures (and some clean–contaminated procedures) due to their adequate coverage of gram-positive organisms, as well as some gram-negative organisms. For surgeries involving the distal intestinal tract, second-generation cephalosporins, such as cefoxitin, are used for their additional anti-anaerobic spectrum of activity.[47]

DOSE

It is crucial to achieve and maintain levels of the antibiotic in the serum and at the surgical site that exceed the MIC for likely pathogens, from the time of incision until the incision is closed. Therefore, both the dose and timing of administration of the antibiotic are important. To ensure that adequate serum and tissue concentrations of antimicrobial agents for prophylaxis of SSIs are achieved, antimicrobial-specific pharmacokinetic and pharmacodynamic properties and patient factors must be also considered when defining the dosage. The dose may need to be individualized based on a given patient's weight. For example, it is currently recommended to increase the cefazolin dose from 1 g to 2 g for patients weighing >80 kg and to 3 g for patients weighing >120 kg (2 g of cephalosporin should be used for repeat doses after the initial 3 g dose[55]) to increase the likelihood of serum and adipose tissue concentration above the MIC of likely organisms.[56] Moreover, cefazolin concentrations in patients undergoing gastric bypass surgery after a 2 g preoperative dose were found to be insufficient and decreased as patient body mass index increased.[57] Re-dosing of the antibiotic is key if the procedure extends beyond 4 hours and/or major blood loss occurs. The goal is to re-dose every 1–2 half-lives of the drug being used; assuming normal renal function, this is approximately every 4 hours for most cephalosporins (Table 136-7).

TIMING

The antimicrobial agent should be administered at such a time to provide serum and tissue concentrations exceeding the MIC for the probable organisms associated with the procedure, at the time of incision and for the duration of the procedure. In order to allow the antibiotic adequate time to distribute to the site of action and to maintain adequate levels throughout the procedure, guidelines recommend that most intravenous antibiotics should begin infusing within 1 hour of surgical incision time and complete before the incision. The exceptions to this recommendation are vancomycin and fluoroquinolones, which should begin infusing within 2 hours prior to surgical incision to minimize the potential for adverse reactions associated with rapid infusion and to ensure adequate tissue levels. However, a more precise or optimal time within this 1-hour window remains somewhat controversial.[47] Guidelines, including the US National Surgical Infection Prevention Project, recommend administering antibiotics 'as near to the incision time as possible to achieve low SSI rates'.[58]

Hawn et al. [59] reviewed 32 459 operations in which prophylactic antibiotics were administered at a median of 28 minutes prior to surgical incision. The amount of patients who developed an SSI was 4.6%. Higher SSI rates were observed for timing more than 60 minutes prior to incision but not after incision. The authors conclude that SSI risk varies by patient and procedure factors as well as antibiotic properties but is not significantly associated with prophylactic antibiotic timing.[59] Further studies are needed to clarify this issue.

DURATION

Antibiotic prophylaxis continued for more than 24–48 hours after surgery does not further decrease SSI rates but rather increases the emergence of antibiotic-resistant bacteria.[48,60,61] The exception is cardiac surgery, where most guidelines recommend prophylaxis for 48 hours, although it is very possible that 24 hours would be just as effective in preventing SSIs.[62,63]

MRSA

Staph. aureus is the most common pathogen causing SSIs, accounting for 30% of SSIs in the USA. Colonization with Staph. aureus, primarily in the nares, occurs in roughly one in four persons and increases the risk of SSI by 2- to 14-fold.[47,64,65] In recent years, given the increase in methicillin resistance among Staph. aureus at both the healthcare and community level, the issue of MRSA coverage for surgical prophylaxis has arisen, particularly in the cardiac and orthopedic surgery population. Risk factors for MRSA carriage include advanced age, recent healthcare contacts, dialysis, the presence of chronic open wounds, and previous antibiotic use.[66–68]

For patients known to be colonized with MRSA, in case decolonization is not achieved, consideration should be given towards using vancomycin for prophylaxis as opposed to a β-lactam such as cefazolin. In the last update of the CDC's SSI prevention guidelines,[69] the use of vancomycin for surgical antibiotic prophylaxis is recommended only in case of operative procedures in which prosthetic materials are placed and in case of patients undergoing median sternotomy or craniotomy. Several studies compared the efficacy of vancomycin versus a β-lactam in preventing SSI.[70–72] Finkelstein et al. conducted a study in an Israeli hospital with a 'high' prevalence of MRSA infections (rate was not specified) in which patients were randomly assigned to receive vancomycin or cefazolin prior to cardiac surgery.[70] They found that overall SSI rates were similar in the two groups and that infections due to methicillin-susceptible staphylococci were more common in the vancomycin group.

Recently a meta-analysis from Schweizer et al.[73] evaluated 39 studies that assessed nasal decolonization or glycopeptide prophylaxis, or both, for prevention of SSI due to gram-positive bacteria. Pooled effects of 15 prophylaxis studies showed that glycopeptide prophylaxis reduced significantly MRSA SSI compared with prophylaxis using β-lactam antibiotics (RR, 0.40) but not MSSA (RR, 1.47).

NONSYSTEMIC AGENTS

Chlorhexidine Gluconate

Chlorhexidine gluconate is an antiseptic agent that has been shown to decrease microbial flora on the skin and prevent infection risk in various settings, including as a skin preparatory agent for surgical procedures and for insertion of vascular access devices, as a surgical hand scrub, and for oral hygiene.[74,75] A Cochrane Collaboration review which evaluated data from six randomized controlled trials with a total of >10 000 participants did not show any significant decrease in SSI rates with antiseptic bathing or showering.[76]

Currently there is interest in the use of chlorhexidine-impregnated wipes as an alternative to bathing or showering with chlorhexidine soap. Although the wipes only contain 2% chlorhexidine, they have been shown to achieve higher chlorhexidine concentrations on the skin than the 4% chlorhexidine soap,[74] and may represent an attractive alternative for patients who are unable to shower or bathe thoroughly. Preoperative chlorhexidine bathing may be considered if other measures have been instituted and SSI rates remain high.

Mupirocin

Mupirocin is a topical antibiotic that can be administered intranasally in an attempt to eradicate a significant reservoir for Staph. aureus. The use of prophylactic intranasal mupirocin has been widely adopted for preoperative patients and is recommended by the Society of Thoracic Surgeons' practice guidelines for all patients undergoing cardiac surgery 'in the absence of a documented negative test for staphylococcal colonization'.[63]

Perl et al., in 2002, enrolled and decolonized more than 4000 preoperative patients in a randomized, placebo-controlled trial. Intranasal mupirocin did not significantly reduce the rate of Staph. aureus SSIs overall although there was a significant reduction in Staph. aureus SSIs among Staph. aureus carriers.[77] More recently a randomized, double-blind, placebo-controlled, multicenter trial, from Bode et al.,[78] assessed whether rapid identification of Staph. aureus nasal carriers, followed by treatment with mupirocin nasal ointment and chlorhexidine soap, reduces the risk of hospital-associated Staph. aureus infection. Their results show that the cumulative incidence of healthcare-associated Staph. aureus infection in surgical patients was significantly lower in the mupirocin–chlorhexidine group than in the placebo group.

Recommendations for Specific Procedures (Tables 136-9 and 136-10)

CARDIOTHORACIC SURGERY

Antimicrobial prophylaxis should be administered for all cardiac procedures with median sternotomy. The incidence of deep sternal wound infections is reported to be between 0.25% and 4% of surgeries with mortality ranging between 7 % and 9%.[79]

Prophylaxis should target staphylococcal species, namely Staph. aureus and coagulase-negative staphylococci. As mentioned above, the increasing prevalence of MRSA complicates antimicrobial choices and some guidelines have recommended the use of vancomycin in institutions with a 'high rate' of infection due to MRSA, but the threshold for a 'high rate' has not been established. Similarly, the Society of Thoracic Surgeons recommends consideration for the use of vancomycin combined with a β-lactam for patients with either presumed or known staphylococcal colonization, institutions with a 'high incidence' of MRSA, patients susceptible to colonization (hospitalized >3 days, transfer from another inpatient facility, already receiving antibiotics) or a procedure involving insertion of a prosthetic valve or vascular graft.[80]

Duration of prophylactic antibiotics beyond 48 hours does not decrease the potential for SSIs. Continuation of antimicrobial prophylaxis until chest tubes or other indwelling catheters are removed is not warranted.[80]

GASTROINTESTINAL SURGERY

Prophylaxis is recommended for most gastrointestinal procedures. The biliary tract is considered a sterile site, and the stomach contains few bacteria due to the highly acidic environment. However, the density of bacteria progressively increases from the small bowel to the colon, as does the proportion of anaerobic to aerobic bacteria. Prophylaxis is recommended for all procedures that enter the small bowel and colon. The intrinsic risk of infection associated with entry into other areas of the gastrointestinal tract is considered low and does not support routine antibiotic prophylaxis except in high-risk patients. In

TABLE 136-9   Antibiotic Prophylaxis Recommendations for Selected Surgical Procedures

Type of Surgery	Recommended Drugs	Alternative Drugs	Duration
Cardiothoracic	Cefazolin*†‡ or cefuroxime†† or ampicillin–sulbactam* or vancomycin (if high risk for MRSA) †‡	β-Lactam allergy: vancomycin †‡ ± cefazolin or gentamicin* or clindamycin†	Single dose‡ ≤48h† ≤72h*
Gastrointestinal			
Gastroduodenal	Cefazolin* (high risk only‡)	β-Lactam allergy: Clindamycin or vancomycin + gentamicin‡ or ciprofloxacin‡ or levofloxacin‡ or aztreonam‡	Single dose*‡
Biliary Open procedures	Cefazolin, cefoxitin, cefotetan, ceftriaxone, ampicillin–sulbactam*	β-Lactam allergy: Clindamycin or vancomycin + gentamicin or ciprofloxacin or levofloxacin or aztreonam	Single dose*
Laparoscopic procedures	Cefazolin (high risk only) cefoxitin, cefotetan, ceftriaxone, ampicillin–sulbactam*‡	β-Lactam allergy: Clindamycin or vancomycin + gentamicin‡ or ciprofloxacin‡ or levofloxacin‡ or aztreonam‡	Single dose‡
Appendectomy for uncomplicated appendicitis	Cefoxitin*‡ or cefotetan* or cefmetazole* or cefazolin + metronidazole‡ or ampicillin–sulbactam‡	β-Lactam allergy: Clindamycin + gentamicin‡ or ciprofloxacin‡ or levofloxacin‡ or aztreonam‡ or gentamicin + metronidazole*	Single dose*‡
Colorectal	Oral: Neomycin + erythromycin base*†‡ or neomycin + metronidazole†‡ Parenteral: Cefotetan*† or cefoxitin*†‡ or ceftriaxone* or cefazolin + metronidazole†‡ or ampicillin–sulbactam†‡ or ertapenem*	β-Lactam allergy: Clindamycin + gentamicin†‡ or fluoroquinolone†‡ or aztreonam†‡ or metronidazole + gentamicin† or fluoroquinolone†	Parenteral: Single dose (≤24 h)*†‡
Head and Neck			
Clean with prosthesis placement Incisions through oral or pharyngeal mucosa	Cefazolin or cefuroxime* Cefazolin or cefuroxime with metronidazole, ampicillin–sulbactam*‡ or clindamycin†	Clindamycin Clindamycin* or clindamycin + gentamicin‡	Single dose Single dose*‡
Neurosurgery			
Elective craniotomy or cerebrospinal fluid shunting	Cefazolin*‡ or vancomycin*‡ (if high risk for MRSA or β-lactam allergy)	Clindamycin or vancomycin*	Single dose*‡
Obstetrics/Gynecology			
Cesarean delivery	Cefazolin*‡	β-Lactam allergy: Clindamycin + gentamicin‡ or ciprofloxacin‡ or levofloxacin‡ or aztreonam‡	Single dose*‡
Hysterectomy	Cefotetan*† or cefazolin*†‡§ or cefoxitin††§ or ampicillin–sulbactam†‡ or metronidazole§ or tinidazole§	β-Lactam allergy: Clindamycin + gentamicin or fluoroquinolone or aztreonam or metronidazole + gentamicin or fluoroquinolone or clindamycin monotherapy	Single dose (≤24 h)*†‡§
Ophthalmic	Topical gentamicin*‡ or tobramycin*‡ or ciprofloxacin‡ or gatifloxacin‡ or levofloxacin‡ or moxifloxacin‡ or ofloxacin‡ or neomycin–gramicidin–polymyxin B*‡ or cefazolin by subconjunctival injection‡	Addition of tobramycin by subconjunctival injection*	Prior to procedure* 2–24 h‡
Orthopedic			
Hip fracture repair	Cefazolin*	Clindamycin or vancomycin*	24 h*
Implantation of internal fixation devices	Cefazolin*	Clindamycin or vancomycin*	24 h*
Total joint replacement	Cefazolin*†‡ or cefuroxime†‡ or vancomycin*†‡ (if high risk for MRSA)	β-Lactam allergy: Vancomycin*†‡ or clindamycin†	Single dose (≤24 h)*†‡
Urologic (high risk patients only)	Oral: Trimethoprim–sulfamethoxazole* or ciprofloxacin‡ Parenteral: Cefazolin ± aminoglycoside or aztreonam or metronidazole* or ciprofloxacin‡	Oral or parenteral: Levofloxacin	Single dose*‡
Vascular	Cefazolin*†‡ or cefuroxime†‡ or vancomycin (if high risk for MRSA)†‡	Vancomycin ± gentamicin* β-Lactam allergy: Vancomycin†‡ or clindamycin†	Single dose (≤24 h)*†‡

Continued on following page

TABLE 136-9	Antibiotic Prophylaxis Recommendations for Selected Surgical Procedures (Continued)			
Type of Surgery	Recommended Drugs		Alternative Drugs	Duration
Transplantation				
Heart	Cefazolin*		β-Lactam allergy:	48–72 h*
Lung and heart–lung	Cefazolin*		Clindamycin or vancomycin	48–72 h*
Liver	Piperacillin-tazobactam or cefotaxime + ampicillin*		Clindamycin or vancomycin	48 h*
Pancreas and pancreas–kidney	Cefazolin*		Clindamycin or vancomycin + gentamicin or ciprofloxacin or levofloxacin or aztreonam	Single dose*
Kidney	Cefazolin*		β-Lactam allergy: Clindamycin + gentamicin or ciprofloxacin or levofloxacin or aztreonam	Single dose*
			β-Lactam allergy: Clindamycin + gentamicin or ciprofloxacin or levofloxacin or aztreonam	

MRSA, methicillin-resistant *Staphylococcus aureus*.
*As recommended by the American Society of Health-System Pharmacists (ASHP) Therapeutic Guidelines on Antimicrobial Prophylaxis in Surgery.[47]
†As recommended by the National Surgical Infection Prevention Project.[58]
‡As recommended by The Medical Letter.[92]
§As recommended by the American College of Obstetrics and Gynecology.[82]

TABLE 136-10	Recommended Initial Dose, Half-Life and Time to Re-dosing Intraoperatively			
Antimicrobial	Usual Half-Life with Normal Renal Function (Hours)	Infusion Time (Min)	Usual Intravenous Dose (Weight-Based Dosing)	Re-dosing Interval (Hours)
Ampicillin	1–1.8	10–30	1–2 g (50 mg/kg/dose)	4
Ampicillin–sulbactam	1–1.8	10–30	1.5–3 g (50 mg/kg/dose ampicillin component)	4
Aztreonam	1.5–2	3–5 (slow iv push) 15–60 (intermittent infusion)	1–2 g (30 mg/kg/dose)	3–5
Cefamandole	0.5–2.1	3–5 (slow iv push) 15–60 (intermittent infusion)	1 g (20–40 mg/kg/dose)	3–4
Cefazolin	1.2–2.5	3–5 (slow iv push) 15–60 (intermittent infusion)	1–2 grams (20–30 mg/kg/dose)	2–5
Cefotaxime	1.5–6	3–5 (slow iv push) 15–60 (intermittent infusion)	1–2 g (50 mg/kg/dose)	4
Cefuroxime	1–2	3–5 (slow iv push) 15–60 (intermittent infusion)	1.5 g (50 mg/kg/dose)	3–4
Clindamycin	2–5.1	10–60 (do not exceed 30 mg/min)	600–900 mg (3–6 mg/kg/dose)	3–6
Ciprofloxacin	3.5–5	60	400 mg (10–15 mg/kg/dose)	4–10
Gentamicin	2–3	30–60	1.5 mg/kg/dose*	3–6
Levofloxacin	6–8	60	500 mg (10 mg/kg/dose)	12–18
Metronidazole	6–14	30–60	500 mg–1 g (15 mg/kg/dose)	6–8
Nafcillin	0.5–1.9	30–60	1–2 g (12–50 mg/kg/dose)	2–4
Oxacillin	0.5–1.8	10–30	1–2 g (12–50 mg/kg/dose)	2–4
Vancomycin	4–6	60 (≥60 min if >1 g)	1 g (10–15 mg/kg/dose)	6–12

*If the patient's body weight is >30% higher than their ideal body weight (IBW), the dosing weight (DW) can be determined as follows: DW‗IBW+[0.4 + (total body weight – IBW)

Reproduced from Bratzler D.W., Houck P.M.: Antimicrobial prophylaxis for surgery: an advisory statement from the National Surgical Infection Prevention Project. Clin Infect Dis 2004; 38:1706-1715.

gastroduodenal surgeries, patients at a higher risk of infection include those with achlorhydria, decreased gastric motility, gastric outlet obstruction, morbid obesity, gastric bleeding or cancer.[81] For biliary procedures, high-risk patients include the elderly, those with recent symptoms of inflammation, common duct stones, jaundice or those with a history of previous biliary surgery. Colorectal procedures have a high risk of infection and warrant routine antibiotic prophylaxis in all patients.

In gastroduodenal procedures, first- and second-generation cephalosporins have demonstrated effectiveness and are the most widely used, but the number of studies is limited compared to other types of surgery. The need to cover anaerobic bacteria increases in distal areas of the gastrointestinal tract, and antibiotics for prophylaxis of colonic procedures should be directed at both gram-negative aerobes and anaerobic bacteria.

HEAD/NECK SURGERY

Antimicrobial prophylaxis is recommended for all head and neck procedures that involve entry into the oropharynx (clean–contaminated procedures). Antimicrobial prophylaxis is not warranted for patients undergoing clean procedures of the head and neck.[47] Antimicrobial choice should target the normal flora of the mouth and oropharynx, especially streptococci and oropharyngeal anaerobes, as postoperative wound infections are frequently polymicrobial.

NEUROSURGERY

Clean neurosurgical procedures are associated with a relatively low risk of SSI, usually less than 5%. Nonetheless, antimicrobial prophylaxis is recommended for clean procedures, which include craniotomies, laminectomies and ventricular fluid-shunt placements. SSIs in this population are primarily associated with gram-positive bacteria, especially Staph. aureus and coagulase-negative staphylococci.

OBSTETRIC/GYNECOLOGIC SURGERY

Antimicrobial prophylaxis is recommended for hysterectomies (vaginal, abdominal) and Cesarean deliveries. For most SSIs following gynecologic procedures, the bacterial source is the skin or the vagina. Aerobic gram-positive cocci (e.g. staphylococci) predominate from the skin, but the potential for exposure to gram-negative aerobes and anaerobic bacteria can be expected when the vagina is opened or incisions are made near the perineum or groin.[82] Postoperative infections associated with hysterectomies are often polymicrobial. Cephalosporins have been the most widely studied in these procedures and studies comparing different cephalosporins have not shown differences in rates of infection.

For Cesarean sections, a first-generation cephalosporin is the drug of choice. Unlike in other surgical procedures, current guidelines recommend that the timing of antimicrobial administration for Cesarean deliveries should be delayed until after cord clamping to avoid effects on the child's normal bacterial flora. However, a joint publication by the American College of Obstetricians and Gynecologists and the American Academy of Pediatrics stated that administering antibiotics pre-incision appears to be more effective in preventing SSIs than post-cord clamping.[82]

ORTHOPEDIC SURGERY

Clean orthopedic procedures not involving implantation of foreign materials do not require routine antimicrobial prophylaxis as the risk of an SSI is low, while the usage of prophylaxis is suggested for the insertion of a prosthetic joint, ankle fusion, revision of a prosthetic joint, reduction of hip fractures, reduction of high-energy closed fractures and of open fractures.

Skin organisms account for most SSIs in orthopedic surgery, with Staph. epidermidis and Staph. aureus accounting for >70% of infections following total joint replacements. First-generation cephalosporins are the most widely studied antimicrobials for prophylaxis in this population. While second-generation cephalosporins offer no clear advantage, either cefazolin or cefuroxime is recommended as the preferred antimicrobial for prophylaxis in patients undergoing hip or knee arthroplasty without a β-lactam allergy. Similar to cardiac procedures, vancomycin is an alternative to consider in institutions with a 'high rate' of MRSA.

The duration of antimicrobial prophylaxis following orthopedic procedures has been debated. There is no evidence that extension of antimicrobial prophylaxis duration beyond 24 hours or until drains or catheters are removed is beneficial in reducing infections.[47]

UROLOGIC SURGERY

Most urologic procedures do not require prophylaxis in patients with sterile urine. The notable exceptions are in patients undergoing transurethral prostatectomy, transrectal prostatic biopsies and insertion of urologic prostheses.[83,47]

A wide range of antimicrobials has been studied as prophylaxis in urologic procedures. Current recommendations include the use of trimethoprim–sulfamethoxazole, cefazolin or a fluoroquinolone as the preferred antimicrobials in high-risk patients only (i.e. positive or unavailable urine culture, preoperative urinary catheter, transrectal prostatic biopsy or insertion of prosthetic material) and in patients undergoing a transurethral prostatic biopsy. Escherichia coli is the most common organism complicating these procedures, but other gram-negative bacilli and enterococci also cause infection. The choice of agent for urologic procedures must be dictated by patient-specific and local susceptibility data, given that significant increases in trimethoprim–sulfamethoxazole and fluoroquinolone resistance in E. coli have been noted.

VASCULAR SURGERY

Antimicrobial prophylaxis is indicated for abdominal and lower extremity vascular procedures including aneurysm repair, thromboendarterectomy and vein bypass.[47] The most common organisms associated with infections following vascular procedures include Staph. aureus, Staph. epidermidis and enteric gram-negative bacilli. Cefazolin and cefuroxime remain the drugs of choice, with the option to use vancomycin in institutions with a 'high rate' of infections caused by MRSA.[47]

Less Invasive Procedures

As technology advances, the ability to perform procedures in a minimally invasive way is progressively increasing. Many procedures that previously could only be performed openly in an operating room setting can now be performed laparoscopically or by a nonsurgical interventionalist. These procedures are associated with their own, usually lower, risk of infection. Because most of these procedures involve newer technology, there is a smaller body of literature associated with their infection risk and antibiotic prophylaxis. Here we discuss what is available for selected procedure types.

PREVENTION OF INFECTIVE ENDOCARDITIS IN DENTAL AND OTHER PROCEDURES

In 2006 the British Society for Antimicrobial Chemotherapy issued guidelines recommending prophylaxis only for patients with a history of previous infective endocarditis (IE) or who have had cardiac valve replacement or surgically constructed pulmonary shunts or conduits.[11] Similarly, in 2007 the American Heart Association (AHA) released revised and simplified guidelines which have greatly narrowed the settings in which antibiotic prophylaxis is recommended for infective endocarditis prevention[10] (see Table 136-11 and Box 136-1 for specific recommendations). Prophylaxis is indicated for all dental procedures that involve manipulation of gingival tissue or the periapical region of teeth or perforation of the oral mucosa (including standard dental cleanings) in patients at risk. Viridans group streptococci are the most common cause of endocarditis following these procedures. Prophylaxis is not recommended, however, for routine anesthetic injections through noninfected tissue, taking dental radiographs, placement of removable prosthodontic or orthodontic appliances, placement of orthodontic brackets, bleeding from trauma to the lips or oral mucosa, orthodontic appliance adjustment or shedding of deciduous teeth.[10]

BOX 136-1   CARDIAC CONDITIONS FOR WHICH PROPHYLAXIS IS REASONABLE WITH DENTAL PROCEDURES

- Prosthetic cardiac valve or prosthetic material used for valve repair
- Previous infective endocarditis
- Congenital heart disease (CHD). Only patients with the following conditions are candidates for prophylaxis:
  - Unrepaired cyanotic CHD, including palliative shunts and conduits
  - Completely repaired congenital heart defect with prosthetic material or device, whether placed by surgery or by catheter intervention, during the first 6 months after the procedure. After 6 months, prophylaxis is not recommended because endothelialization of prosthetic material occurs within this time
  - Repaired CHD with residual defects at the site or adjacent to the site of a prosthetic patch or prosthetic device (which inhibit endothelialization)
- Cardiac transplantation recipients who develop cardiac valvulopathy.

Reproduced from Allen U.: *Can J Infect Dis Med Microbiol* 2010; 21:74–77.

TABLE 136-11	Prophylactic Regimens for Dental, Oral, Respiratory Tract or Esophageal Procedures			
		DOSING REGIMEN: SINGLE DOSE 30–60 MIN BEFORE PROCEDURE		
Situation	Agent	Adults	Children	
ORAL PROPHYLAXIS				
Standard	Amoxicillin	2 g	50 mg/kg (max 2 g)	
Penicillin allergy	Clindamycin or Cephalexin*† or Azithromycin or clarithromycin	600 mg 2 g 500 mg	20 mg/kg (max 600 mg) 50 mg/kg (max 2 g) 15 mg/kg (max 500 mg)	
PARENTERAL PROPHYLAXIS				
Standard	Ampicillin	2 g iv or im	50 mg/kg (max 2 g) iv or im	
Penicillin allergy	Clindamycin or Cefazolin† Ceftriaxone†	600 mg iv 1 g iv or im 1 g iv or im	20 mg/kg (max 600 mg) iv 50 mg/kg (max 1 g) iv or im 50 mg/kg (max 1 g) iv or im	

*Or other first- or second- generation oral cephalosporin in appropriate equivalent dosage.
†Cephalosporins should not be used in individuals with immediate-type hypersensitivity reaction (urticaria, angioedema or anaphylaxis) to penicillins.
Adapted from Wilson, Kathryn A. Taubert, Michael Gewitz et al. *Prevention of Infective Endocarditis: Guidelines From the American Heart Association: A Guideline From the American Heart Association Rheumatic Fever, Endocarditis, and Kawasaki Disease Committee, Council on Cardiovascular Disease in the Young, and the Council on Clinical Cardiology, Council on Cardiovascular Surgery and Anesthesia, and the Quality of Care and Outcomes Research Interdisciplinary Working Group.* Circulation 2007; 116:1736-1754.

PACEMAKER/CARDIOVERTER-DEFIBRILLATOR IMPLANTATION

The estimated rate of infection after implantation of permanent endocardial leads is 1–2%, although published rates vary.[84] A large prospective survey (the PEOPLE study) in patients with implantation of pacemakers and cardioverter-defibrillators reported that antibiotic prophylaxis appeared to have a protective effect (adjusted odds ratio 0.4) against the development of a cardiac device-related infection.[84] Nonetheless, there was variability in type and duration of antibiotic prophylaxis (antibiotics were administered according to local guidelines). Hence, while it remains unclear as to the optimal duration and choice of antibiotics, there does appear to be a body of literature suggesting that antibiotic prophylaxis is beneficial in preventing cardiac device-related infections. A single dose of a β-lactam antibiotic, such as cefazolin, is probably appropriate to cover skin flora.

A meta-analysis evaluated 15[85] prospective randomized trials in which intravenous antibiotic was compared with no antibiotic, placebo, an alternative antibiotic, antibiotic delivered via another route of administration (e.g. oral), local antibiotic, or an alternative antibiotic regimen (e.g. different timing or duration). The analysis showed that perioperative systemic antibiotics plus antiseptics delivered 1 hour before the procedure significantly reduced the incidence of SSI compared with no antibiotics. Furthermore, perioperative systemic prophylaxis plus antiseptics significantly reduced the incidence of postoperative infection compared to antibiotics delivered postoperatively.

GASTROINTESTINAL ENDOSCOPY

Antibiotic prophylaxis has been used in the setting of gastrointestinal endoscopy for two purposes: to prevent endocarditis from bacteremia; and to prevent gastrointestinal or intra-abdominal infections from local seeding. It is no longer recommended for the prevention of infective endocarditis.

Endoscopic Retrograde Cholangiopancreatography

Cholangitis and pancreatitis can occur as a result of endoscopic retrograde cholangiopancreatography (ERCP), particularly when biliary drainage is incomplete.[86] Antibiotic prophylaxis is a common practice for some of these patients, but practices and guidelines vary widely as to which specific subsets of patients should receive antibiotics. Most randomized controlled trials investigating this issue are relatively small, and since infection rates are low it is probable that they were not adequately powered to detect a difference in infection rates. A

meta-analysis by Harris et al. summarized the results of five randomized controlled trials and found no significant difference in infection rates between the group that received prophylaxis and the group that did not.[93] A recent retrospective review followed outcomes over an 11-year period during which the use of prophylaxis was sequentially scaled back. Initially all patients with biliary or pancreatic obstruction, those likely to need therapeutic intervention and those with immunosuppression received prophylaxis. By the end of the study period, the only patients who received prophylaxis were those in whom drainage was suspected to be incomplete, or were considered immunosuppressed. The authors found no significant difference in infection outcomes during this time.[86] A meta-analysis by Brand et al. examined the evidence for antibiotic prophylaxis in ERCP and stated that prophylaxis for all patients was beneficial in preventing cholangitis, sepsis, bacteremia and pancreatitis. However, they suggested that the effect on patients with non-complicated ERCP may be less evident.[87]

The American Society for Gastrointestinal Endoscopy (ASGE),[88] the British Society of Gastroenterology Endoscopy Committee[89] and the European Society of Gastrointestinal Endoscopy all recommend antibiotic prophylaxis when ERCP is performed for pancreatic pseudocyst drainage or biliary obstruction. The antibiotic chosen should cover biliary organisms, including enterococci and enteric gram-negative bacteria. Fluoroquinolones or β-lactam/β-lactamase inhibitor combinations, such as ampicillin–sulbactam, are sometimes used.

Endoscopic Ultrasound-Fine Needle Aspiration

With regard to endoscopic ultrasound-fine needle aspiration (EUS-FNA) procedures, antibiotic prophylaxis is often administered when FNA of cystic lesions along the gastrointestinal tract is performed so as to prevent cyst infection; however, these infections are rare and there are no randomized studies evaluating the efficacy of antibiotic prophylaxis in these patients, despite the fact that expert opinion frequently recommends it.

Percutaneous Endoscopic Gastrostomy

Antibiotic prophylaxis is recommended for percutaneous endoscopic gastrostomy (PEG) tube placements, typically with single-dose cefazolin. A recent Cochrane Review did find a significant decrease in peristomal infections with antibiotic prophylaxis.[90]

INTERVENTIONAL RADIOLOGY

There are no randomized controlled trials in the interventional radiology arena proving the efficacy of antibiotic prophylaxis. Ryan et al. recommend antibiotic prophylaxis for specific IR procedures such as embolization procedures (uterine fibroid, hepatic chemoembolization, splenic, renal) and tube placements (cholecystostomy, gastrostomy, nephrostomy) although only a few studies support these recommendations.[94] When prophylaxis is given, a single-dose antibiotic covering the local organisms is sufficient (frequently used options include cefazolin for skin flora and ampicillin–sulbactam or ceftriaxone for gastrointestinal or genitourinary organisms).

LAPAROSCOPIC CHOLECYSTECTOMY

Most randomized controlled trials looking at the utility of antibiotic prophylaxis for laparoscopic cholecystectomy have included only a small number of patients. However, a meta-analysis combining results from five studies with a total of 899 patients found no significant difference in wound infection rates between those that received antibiotic prophylaxis and those that did not.[91] Hence, most experts do not recommend routine prophylaxis for laparoscopic cholecystectomy.

References available online at expertconsult.com.

KEY REFERENCES

Bowater R.J., Stirling S.A., Lilford R.J.: Is antibiotic prophylaxis in surgery a generally effective intervention? Testing a generic hypothesis over a set of meta-analyses. *Ann Surg* 2009; 49:551-556.

Bratzler D.W., Dellinger E.P., Olsen K.M., et al.; American Society of Health-System Pharmacists (ASHP); Infectious Diseases Society of America (IDSA); Surgical Infection Society (SIS); Society for Healthcare Epidemiology of America (SHEA): Clinical practice guidelines for antimicrobial prophylaxis in surgery. *Am J Health Syst Pharm* 2013; 70:195-283.

Center for Diseases Prevention and Control (CDC): Antibiotic resistance threat in the United States, 2013. Available: http://www.cdc.gov/drugresistance/threat -report-2013/pdf/ar-threats-2013-508.pdf.

Dulhunty J.M., Roberts J.A., Davis J.S., et al.: Continuous infusion of beta-lactam antibiotics in severe sepsis: a multicenter double-blind, randomized controlled trial. *Clin Infect Dis* 2013; 56(2):236-244.

Hawn M.T., Richman J.S., Vick C.C., et al.: Timing of surgical antibiotic prophylaxis and the risk of surgical site infection. *JAMA Surg* 2013; 148:649-657.

Korol E., Johnston K., Waser N., et al.: A systematic review of risk factors associated with surgical site infections among surgical patients. *PLoS ONE* 2013; 8(12):e83743.

Perez-Cobas A.E., Artacho A., Knecht H., et al.: Differential effects of antibiotic therapy on the structure and function of human gut microbiota. *PLoS ONE* 2013; 8:e80201.

Roberts J.A., Ulldemolins M., Roberts M.S., et al.: Therapeutic drug monitoring of beta-lactams in critically ill patients: proof of concept. *Int J Antimicrob Agents* 2010; 36(4):332-339.

Schweizer M., Perencevich E., McDanel J., et al.: Effectiveness of a bundled intervention of decolonization and prophylaxis to decrease Gram positive surgical site infections after cardiac or orthopedic surgery: systematic review and meta-analysis. *BMJ* 2013; 346:f2743.

World Health Organization: Global report on surveillance. WHO Library Cataloguing-in-Publication Data. Available: www.who.int.

137

Mechanisms of Action

FRANÇOISE VAN BAMBEKE | MARIE-PAULE MINGEOT-LECLERCQ |
YOURI GLUPCZYNSKI | PAUL M. TULKENS

KEY CONCEPTS

- Antibiotics should act on targets that are sufficiently different from those found in eukaryotic cells to avoid toxicity related to their pharmacological activity.

- Targets of current antibiotics include cell wall synthesis, protein synthesis, nucleic acids, metabolic pathways and membrane.

- Bactericidal drugs principally act by destabilizing the bacterial membrane or causing the synthesis of abnormal proteins.

- Resistance inexorably develops after a few years of clinical use, whatever the target, by highly variable, although often very specific, mechanisms.

- Over the last 10 years, new molecules have been obtained for most of the previously existing classes with increased affinity for their target(s) and/or activity on strains resistant to their parent compound. Molecules with truly novel modes of action and/or directed against so far unexploited targets, remain, however, scarce.

Antibiotics that Act on the Cell Wall

The bacterial cell wall is primarily made of peptidoglycan, a large and reticulated polymer containing alternating residues of *N*-acetyl-glucosamine and muramic acid in β-1→4 linkage. The carboxyl groups of muramyl residues are substituted by short peptides terminated by a D-Asp-D-Ala-D-Ala sequence. Cell-wall active antibiotics act by inhibiting the activity of enzymes involved in the synthesis of the precursors or in the reticulation of peptidoglycan.

β-LACTAMS

The β-lactam nucleus is the basic building block of an exceptionally large class of antibiotics that all share a common mode of action but have quite distinct properties in terms of spectrum, pharmacokinetics and, to some extent, activity against resistant strains.

Chemical Structure

All antibiotics in this class contain a four-membered cyclic amide (β-lactam). With the exception of the monobactams, this cycle is fused with a five- or six-membered cycle. According to the nature of these cycles and/or of the presence of a heteroatom, the following main classes have been described (Figure 137-1):[1-5]

- penams – β-lactams with a five-membered ring containing a sulfur atom (penicillins);
- clavams – β-lactams with a five-membered ring with an oxygen (or sulfur) atom and mostly used as β-lactamase inhibitors (e.g. clavulanic acid);
- carbapenems – β-lactams with a five-membered ring without heteroatom and with a double bond (e.g. imipenem or meropenem). Penems have also a double bond but no heteroatom (e.g. faropenem [not approved in USA or EU but commercialized in other countries]);
- cephems – β-lactams with a six-membered unsaturated ring with a sulfur atom (cephalosporins);
- oxacephems – oxygen analogs of cephems (latamoxef);

- monobactams – β-lactams without additional fused ring (four-membered ring [azetidine] only with a methylcarboxylate function in the case of nocardicins and a sulfonate in the case of the other monobactams e.g. aztreonam).

Other β-lactams include thiacephems, dethiacephems, dethiacephams, heterocephems and cephams, as well as diverse bicyclic systems but none has been approved for clinical use.

Mode of Action

β-lactams act primarily as inhibitors of transpeptidases (specialized acyl serine transferases), thereby impairing the synthesis of the cell wall (Figure 137-2).[1] β-lactams mimic the D-Ala-D-Ala sequence in that the distance between the carboxylate or the sulfonate (monobactams) and the cyclic amide is similar, and act as a false substrate for D-alanyl-D-alanine transpeptidases. The serine residue of the transpeptidases (also called penicillin-binding proteins, PBPs) reacts with the carbonyl

Diversity of β-lactam antibiotics		
Structure	Group	Examples
	Penam	Penicillins
	Clavam	β-Lactamase inhibitors (e.g. clavulanic acid)
	Carbapenem	(e.g. imipenem, meropenem)
	Cephem	Cephalosporins
	Oxacephem	(e.g. latamoxef)
	Monobactam	(e.g. aztreonam)

Figure 137-1 Diversity of β-lactam antibiotics: main ring structure names and representative antibiotics. The figure highlights the fact that all drugs share a common four-piece β-lactam ring and a carboxylate (or sulfonate) function at an appropriate, similar distance. (Clavams are weak antibiotics but efficient β-lactamase inhibitors.)

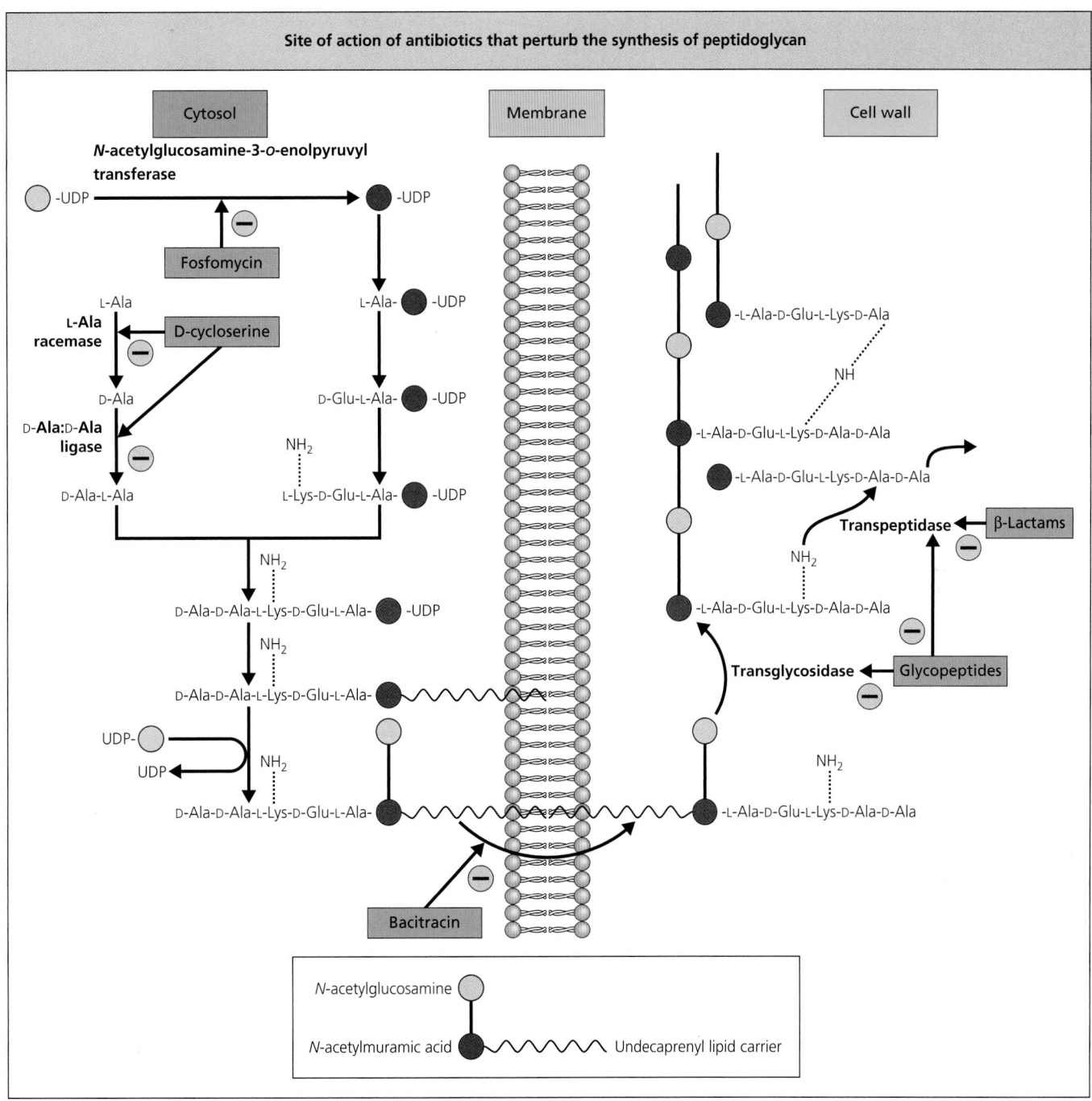

Figure 137-2 Site of action of antibiotics that perturb the synthesis of peptidoglycan. The peptidoglycan unit is formed in the cytosol of bacteria by binding to uridine diphosphate (UDP) *N*-acetylmuramic acid of a short peptide (the nature of which differs between bacteria). This precursor is then attached to a lipid carrier and added to *N*-acetylglucosamine before crossing the bacterial membrane. At the cell surface peptidoglycan units are reticulated by the action of transglycosylases (catalyzing the polymerization between sugars) and of transpeptidases (catalyzing the polymerization between peptidic chains). The antibiotics act as follows: fosfomycin is an analog of phosphoenolpyruvate, the substrate of the *N*-acetylglucosamine-3-O-enolpyruvyl transferase synthesizing *N*-acetylmuramic acid from N-acetylglucosamine and phosphoenolpyruvate; cycloserine is an analog of D-Ala and blocks the action of D-Ala racemase and D-Ala: D-Ala ligase; bacitracin inhibits the transmembrane transport of the precursor; vancomycin binds to D-Ala-D-Ala termini and thus inhibits the action of transglycosylases and transpeptidases; and β-lactams are analogs of D-Ala-D-Ala and suicide substrates for transpeptidases.

β-lactam ring to give inactive acyl enzymes ('suicide inhibition' by formation of a covalent bond; Figure 137-3).[2] Transpeptidases, located in the periplasmic space, are directly accessible in gram-positive bacteria but protected by the outer membrane in gram-negative bacteria, which β-lactams must cross (mainly via porin channels).

By inhibiting cell wall synthesis, β-lactams are usually active against rapidly dividing bacteria only. Their bactericidal effect results from indirect mechanisms (mostly the activation of autolytic enzymes).

Resistance

Resistance to β-lactams occurs by three main different mechanisms:
- Decrease of the accumulation of the antibiotics in gram-negative bacteria by alteration of porins (reducing the access of water-soluble β-lactams) or by overexpression of efflux transporters (mostly affecting lipophilic β-lactams).
- Production of hydrolyzing enzymes called β-lactamases,[5] encoded by genes carried either on chromosomes or on

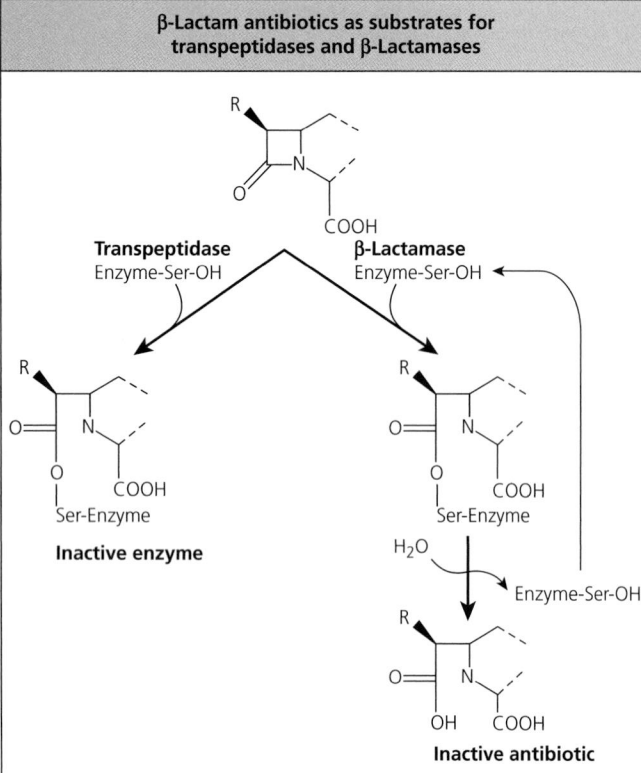

β-Lactam antibiotics as substrates for transpeptidases and β-Lactamases

Figure 137-3 β-Lactam antibiotics as substrates for transpeptidases and β-lactamases. The left part of the illustration shows how a β-lactam covalently binds to transpeptidases. Hydrolysis of this acylated enzyme is very slow (1 β-lactam per hour), making the enzyme inactive. The right part of the illustration shows that the same reaction occurs in the case of serine β-lactamases (in this example; there are non-serine β-lactamases). Hydrolysis of the acylated enzyme is, however, very rapid (1000 β-lactams per second), making the antibiotic inactive and regenerating the enzyme for a new cycle of hydrolysis.

plasmids. β-lactamases are serine or zinc (Zn^{2+}) proteases having a high affinity for β-lactams and cleaving the amide bond. X-ray data and genetic studies of β-lactamases and PBPs show a high level of structural homology, suggesting that both derive from a common ancestor. Although most β-lactamases open the β-lactam ring in the same way as transpeptidases, the hydrolysis rate of the acyl-enzyme is far quicker than in PBPs (see Figure 137-3), resulting in the regeneration of the enzyme and the production of an irreversibly inactivated antibiotic, and their turnover is much more rapid (1000 times per second vs once per hour for PBPs).

• Modification of PBPs, in particular PBP2 which is essential for the 'shaping' of bacteria. The most typical example is found in methicillin-resistant *Staphylococcus aureus* (MRSA) that produces an altered protein (called PBP2' or PBP2a) with a very low affinity for all conventional β-lactams. In other organisms (e.g. streptococci) PBPs show decreased affinity to some β-lactams only, leading to decreased susceptibility.

A number of β-lactams have been made to resist β-lactamases by appropriate steric hindrance or change in conformation (Figure 137-4a), giving rise to the so-called β-lactamase-resistant penicillins and cephalosporins. β-Lactamases, however, have an extraordinary plasticity and inevitably develop activity against all new derivatives at a rapid pace (Table 137-1). Thanks to their specific structure, clavams (Figure 137-4b) are poor antibiotics but bind tightly to β-lactamases and inactivate them. Given in combination with β-lactams, they provide protection unless the bacteria overproduce β-lactamases. Yet, they can be hydrolyzed by some β-lactamases. Avibactam is a novel β-lactamase inhibitor with a structure quite different from clavams and is active against a larger panel of β-lactamases (including some

class D enzymes such as OXA-48).[6] It is approved in combination with ceftazidime.

Ceftaroline and ceftobiprole are two recently approved cephalosporins that possess a bulky hydrophobic substituent near the carboxylate (see Figure 137-4c) and are active against MRSA. This results from the triggering of an allosteric conformational change of PBP2a, allowing for the opening of the enzymatic cavity and its acylation by the antibiotic.[3] Ceftolozane, showing enhanced activity against *P. aeruginosa*, has also been recently approved in combination with tazobactam to provide some protection against extended spectrum β-lactamases.

Pharmacodynamics

β-Lactams are relatively slow-acting antibiotics that must be present at a concentration above the minimum inhibitory concentration (MIC) for as long as possible. Conversely, concentrations above four to five times the MIC provide little gain in activity, so that frequent dosing is more appropriate than infrequent administration of large doses. Administration of β-lactams by continuous infusion is increasingly popular[7] but can be applied only for molecules remaining stable at room temperature for prolonged periods of time. Carbapenems are unstable and thus should not be given by continuous infusion; a 'prolonged' infusion time of 3–4 hours has been proposed for doripenem as part of the drug labeling. In general, β-lactams show only a moderate postantibiotic effect.

GLYCOPEPTIDES AND LIPOGLYCOPEPTIDES
Chemical Structure

Glycopeptide antibiotics (vancomycin, teicoplanin) contain two sugars and an aglycone moiety made of a relatively highly conserved heptapeptide core, bearing two chloride substituents. The aglycone fraction is responsible for the pharmacologic activity of the molecule, whereas the sugars modulate its hydrophilicity and its propensity to form dimers (see below). As a result of their large size, glycopeptides are unable to cross the outer membrane of gram-negative bacteria (against which they are, therefore, inactive). Lipoglycopeptides are semisynthetic derivatives characterized by the addition of a hydrophobic moiety, which confers additional properties to the drugs.

Mode of Action

Glycopeptides inhibit the late stages of cell wall peptidoglycan synthesis (see Figure 137-2) by binding to D-Ala-D-Ala termini of the pentapeptide-ending precursors localized at the outer surface of the cytoplasmic membrane. At the molecular level, glycopeptides form a high affinity complex with D-Ala-D-Ala by establishing hydrogen binding via their aglycone moiety.[8] The strength of this binding is greatly enhanced when forming dimers (via sugar moieties; vancomycin) or anchoring in the membrane (via a fatty acyl chain substituent; teicoplanin). The subsequent steric hindrance around the pentapeptide termini blocks the reticulation of peptidoglycan by inhibiting the activity of transglycosylases and transpeptidases.

Lipoglycopeptides (telavancin, oritavancin) show stronger inhibition of transglycosidase and also membrane-destabilization effects (causing rapid bacterial death), due to their membrane-anchoring properties and to dimerization of molecules (Figure 137-5) and, for oritavancin and enterococci, the possibility to bind an additional site in the peptidoglycan which is associated with an inhibition of transpeptidase activity.[8] Dalbavancin also has a lipophilic side chain but does not appear to destabilize bacterial membranes.

Resistance

Resistance to glycopeptides results from substituting a D-lactic acid or a D-serine in place of terminal D-Ala of the pentapeptide, reducing the affinity of the antibiotic to its target.[8] This mode of resistance is most prevalent in enterococci, but rare in *Staph. aureus*. In the latter, resistance is more commonly acquired as a result of thickening of the cell wall associated with an increased abundance of free D-Ala-D-Ala termini. This causes increase in MICs, producing the so-called vancomycin- or glycopeptide-intermediate phenotype (VISA and GISA

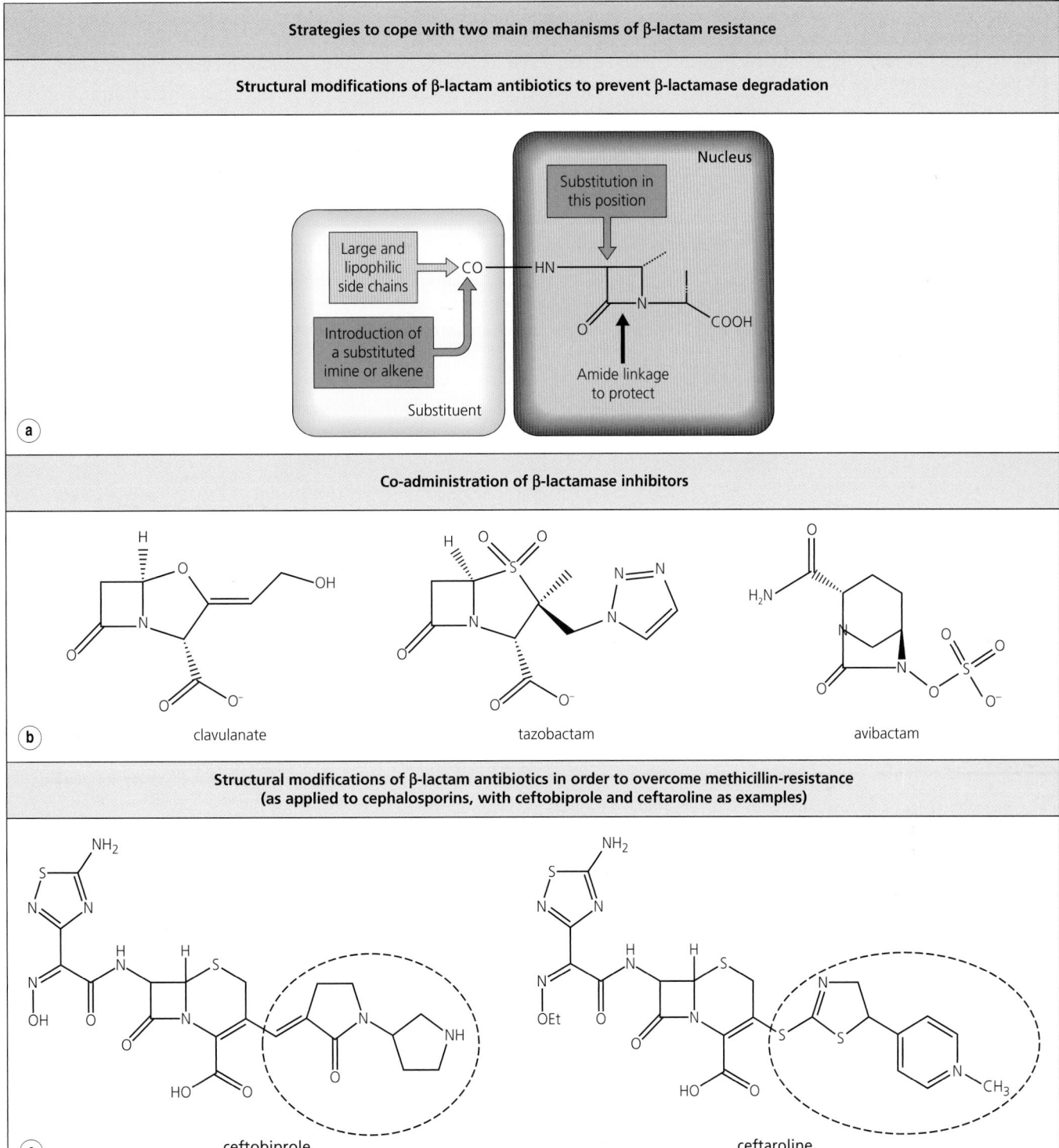

Figure 137-4   Strategies to cope with two main mechanisms of β-lactam resistance. (a) Structural modifications of β-lactam antibiotics that overcome β-lactamase degradation. A first strategy, applied in penicillins, cephalosporins, oxacephems and monobactams consists of the introduction of a large side chain on the nucleus, possibly containing a substituted imine or alkene. A second strategy, applied in oxacephems and cefoxitin as well as in temocillin, consists of the introduction of a methoxy group on the β-lactam ring. (b) Chemical structure of the main inhibitors of β-lactamases. Clavulanate and tazobactam both contain a β-lactam ring in their structure. They are active on class A enzymes. They react with the β-lactamase enzyme to form a covalent acyl-enzyme intermediate. Avibactam does not contain a β-lactam ring but keeps an acidic function and a cyclic amide function. It is a slowly reversible inhibitor of β-lactamase targets including class A, C (ESBLs and AmpC) and some class D enzymes, such as OXA-48. (c) Structural modifications of β-lactam antibiotics in order to overcome methicillin resistance, as applied to cephalosporins (with ceftobiprole and ceftaroline as examples). The bulky hydrophobic moieties (dotted-lined ellipse) added to the molecules forces a conformational change in PBP2a resulting in the opening of the active site and allowing acylation (inactivation) by the antibiotic. Although activity is largely restored towards methicillin-resistant organisms, MICs remain still typically one to four dilutions higher than for susceptible ones. The increase in lipophilicity also makes it necessary to administer the molecules as prodrugs – medocaril for ceftobiprole and fosamyl for ceftaroline (not shown).

TABLE 137-1 **Functional Classification of β-Lactamases**

(See regularly updated data on www.lahey.org/studies; note that as from July 1st 2016, updates must be directed and wil be found at http://www.ncbi.nlm.nih.gov/projects/pathogens/submit_beta_lactamase).

Group	Molecular Class	Preferred Substrates	Active β-Lactams	Typical Examples
Group 1: serine cephalosporinases not inhibited by clavulanic acid	C	Cephalosporins I, II and III (≫ cephalosporins IV, monobactams, penicillins)	Carbapenems Temocillin (cephalosporins III and IV; variable upon level of expression)	AmpC from gram-negatives; variable upon the species
GROUP 2: SERINE β-LACTAMASES				
2a: penicillinases inhibited by clavulanic acid	A	Penicillins (penicillin, ampicillin ≫ carbenicillin ≫ oxacillins)	Amoxicillin + clavulanic acid Cephalosporins Carbapenems	Penicillinases from gram-positives
2b: broad-spectrum β-lactamases inhibited by clavulanic acid	A	Penicillins (penicillin, ampicillin ≫ carbenicillin ≫ oxacillins) Cephalosporins I and II	Cephalosporins III and IV Monobactams* Carbapenems Amoxicillin + clavulanic acid	TEM-1,TEM-2, SHV-1 from Enterobacteriaceae, Haemophilus spp., Neisseria gonorrhoeae
2be: extended spectrum β-lactamases (ESBL) inhibited by clavulanic acid	A	Penicillins Cephalosporins I, II, III (IV) Monobactams	Carbapenems Temocillin	TEM-3 to -29, 42, 43, 46–49, 52, 53, 56, 60, 61, 63, 66, 71, 72, 75, 85-88, 91-94, 101, 102 in Enterobacteriaceae SHV-2 to -9, 12–13, 15-18, 24, 27, 30, 31, 38-42 in Klebsiella spp. CTX-M-1 to CTX-M-165 (five phylogenetic groups) in Enterobacteriaceae K1-OXY from Klebsiella oxytoca
2br: broad-spectrum β-lactamases with reduced binding to clavulanic acid	A	Penicillins	Most cephalosporins Monobactams* Carbapenems	TEM-30 to -40 (= IRT-1 to IRT-12), 44, 45, 50, 51, 54, 58 59, 65, 67, 73, 74, 76–84 from Escherichia coli SHV-10 from Klebsiella spp.
2c: carbenicillin-hydrolyzing β-lactamases inhibited by clavulanic acid	A	Penicillins Carbenicillin (Cephalosporins I and II)	Piperacillin + tazobactam Cephalosporins III and IV Monobactams* Carbapenems	CARB-1 to -16 from Pseudomonas aeruginosa
2d: cloxacillin-hydrolyzing β-lactamases generally inhibited by clavulanic acid	D	Penicillins Cloxacillin Cephalosporins I and II	Carbapenems Cephalosporin III Monobactams* Piperacillin† tazobactam	OXA-1 to OXA-4 in Enterobacteriaceae OXA-2, OXA-10 (PSE-2) in Pseudomonas aeruginosa (penicillins, cefpirome, cefepime ≫ cephalosporins III) OXA-11, OXA-14 to -19, 28, 32, 45 are ESBLs in P. aeruginosa (R to cephalosporins III and IV and aztreonam) OXA-48 and carbapenemase variants (OXA-162, OXA-181, OXA-204, OXA-244, OXA-245; low activity against carbapenems but hydrolyse penicillins [even with beta-lactamse inhbibitors] but not cephalosporins) OXA-23, -24, -58, -143 are carbapenemases in Acinetobacter baumannii
2e: cephalosporinases inhibited by clavulanic acid	A	Cephalosporins I and II	Cephalosporins III and IV Monobactams* Penems	FPM-1 from Proteus vulgaris Cep-A from Bacteroides fragilis
2f: carbapenem-hydrolyzing-nonmetallo-β-lactamases	B	Most β-lactams, including carbapenems (low or high resistance level depending on enzyme, species and genetic environment)	Carbapenems Monobactams and β-lactam inhibitors (variable activity depending on type of enzyme, bacterial host and genetic environment)	SME-1 to -5 from Serratia spp. IMI-1/2 and NMC-A from Enterobacter cloacae KPC-2 to -19 from Klebsiella spp., other Enterobacteriaceae and Pseudomonas GES-1 to -25 in Enterobacteriaceae, P. aeruginosa and A. baumannii
Group 3: metallo-β-lactamases inhibited by EDTA	B	Most β-lactams, including carbapenems	Monobactams*‡	L-1, XM-A from Stenotrophomonas maltophilia CcrA from B. fragilis A2h, CphA from Aeromonas hydrophila IMP-1 to -45, VIM-1 to -41, in Pseudomonas, other gram-negative non-fermenters and Enterobacteriaceae NDM-1 to -15 in Enterobacteriaceae, Acinetobacter baumannii and P. aeruginosa SPM-1, GIM-1, SIM-1, DIN-1 in P. aeruginosa and A. baumannii
Group 4: penicillinases not inhibited by clavulanic acid		Penicillins, including carbenicillin and oxacillins	Monobactams*‡ and generally carbapenems	SAR-2 from B. cepacia

*Monobactams are not active against gram-positive bacteria.
†Penems are the only molecules active in this case.
‡Remain active for most of the rare published studies.
EDTA, ethylenediaminetetraacetic acid.
Compiled from reference 5 and from www.lahey.org/studies (last accessed: 28 Feb 2015). The number of enzymes is continuously increasing and their spectrum also continuously evolving.

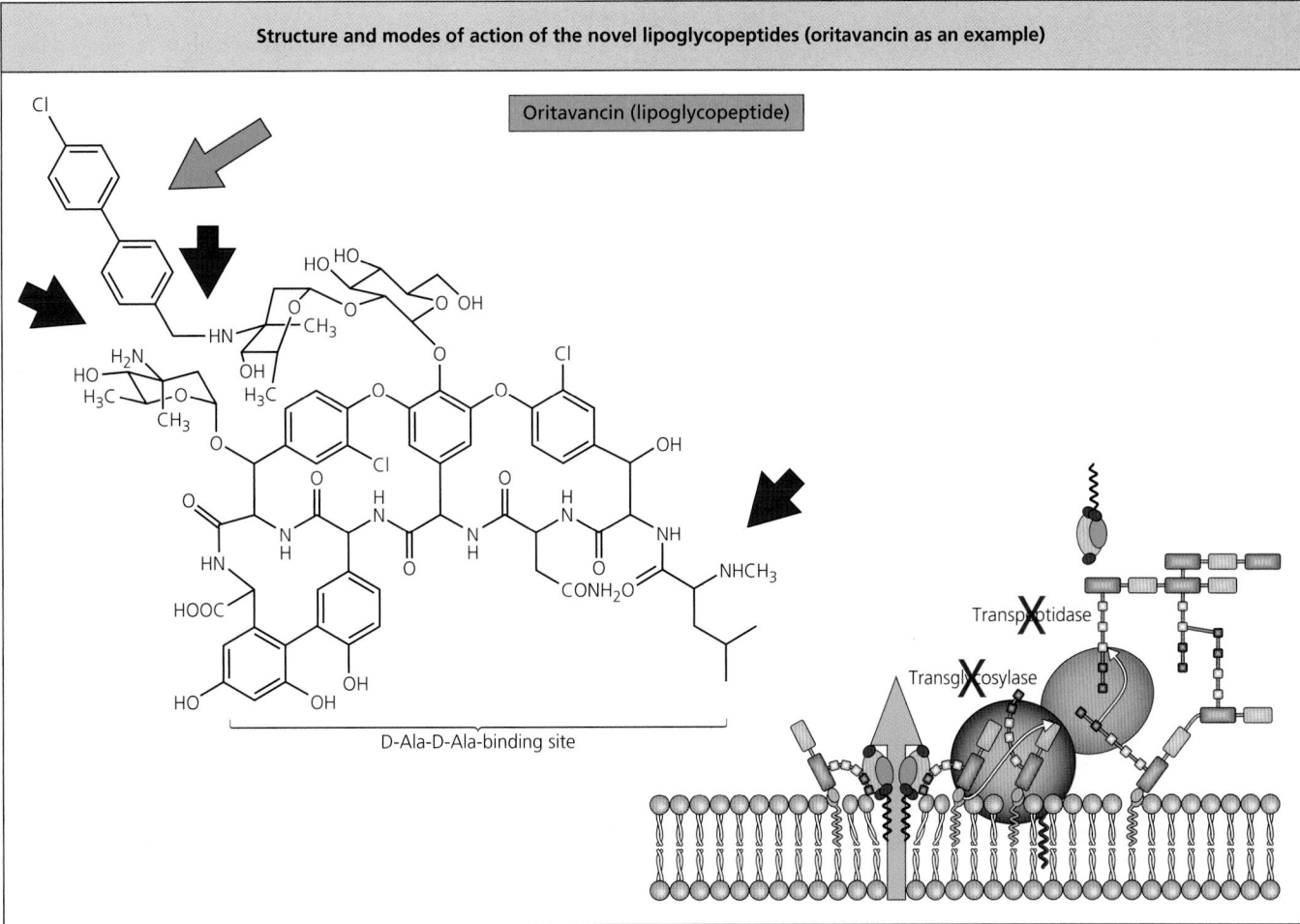

Figure 137-5   Structure and proposed modes of action of the novel lipoglycopeptides (oritavancin as an example). Left: The drugs are characterized by the presence of a bulky hydrophobic moiety (chlorodiphenyl in this example; dark green arrow) and either additional amino groups (red arrows) or other polar groups (phosphonate for telavancin; not shown), resulting in a global amphiphilic character for the whole molecule. Note that the D-Ala-D-Ala binding site of the molecule remains unchanged. Right: The molecule interacts with the D-Ala-D-Ala termini of the pentapeptide (closed squares) as vancomycin, inhibiting both the transpeptidase and the transglycosidase activities, but also inserts itself into the membrane through its lipophilic side chain (this is favored, in the case of oritavancin, by its strong capacity to dimerize). As a result, lipoglycopeptides induce membrane leakage and thereby display a marked, concentration-dependent bactericidal effect. This second mode of action is exerted even if bacteria display a D-Ala-D-Lac or D-Ala-D-Ser in place of the D-Ala-D-Ala moiety, as in vancomycin-resistant organisms. Specificity towards bacterial membranes probably stems from the fact that membrane anchoring is enhanced by the presence of acidic phospholipids (phosphatidylglycerol, cardiolipin) abundant in bacterial but not in eukaryotic pericellular cell membranes. (Adapted from Van Bambeke et al. Trends Pharmacol Sci 2008; 29(3):124-134.)

[these strains should actually be reported as resistant, based on current EUCAST breakpoints, and their presence is associated with clinical failures]). A further difficulty is the fact that the expression of this resistance is variable and may only affect a small proportion of a given inoculum, giving rise to a heteroresistant phenotype that makes detection by automated systems unreliable.[9] Telavancin and oritavancin are less affected by both resistance mechanisms thanks to their dual mode of action.

Pharmacodynamics

Conventional glycopeptide antibiotics exhibit slow bactericidal activity, which is largely concentration dependent. Because of their half-life however (about 8 hours for vancomycin and much longer for teicoplanin), their overall activity, depends rather on the 24-hour area under the serum concentration–time curve/MIC (AUC_{24h}/MIC) than on time above MIC or on concentration only.[10] Accordingly, they can be administered by discontinuous or continuous infusion the latter will make monitoring easier. For lipoglycopeptides, C_{max}/MIC ratios drive activity. Oritavancin accumulates greatly in macrophages and is therefore highly active on phagocytosed *Staph. aureus*. Due to their very prolonged half-life, dalbavancin and oritavancin allow for once-a-week or even single-dose treatment.

OTHER AGENTS ACTING ON CELL WALL SYNTHESIS

D-Cycloserine is a broad-spectrum antibiotic which has structural similarities to D-Ala (see Figures 137-2 and 137-6) and inhibits the conversion of L-Ala into D-Ala (catalyzed by a racemase) and the dimerization of D-Ala (catalyzed by the D-Ala:D-Ala ligase).[11]

Fosfomycin, which bears structural similarities to phospho-*enol*-pyruvate, inhibits very early stage synthesis of peptidoglycan by impairing the formation of uridine diphosphate (UDP)-*N*-acetylglucosamine-*enol*-pyruvate, a precursor of UDP-*N*-acetylmuramic acid (see Figures 137-2 and 137-6).[12]

Bacitracin is a polypeptide of complex structure that inhibits peptidoglycan synthesis at the level of translocation of the precursor across the bacterial membrane (see Figure 137-2).[13]

Antibiotics that Act on Protein Synthesis

Bacterial ribosomes comprise a 30S subunit that binds mRNA and initiates protein synthesis; and a 50S subunit that binds aminoacyl tRNA, catalyzes peptide bond formation and controls the elongation process.

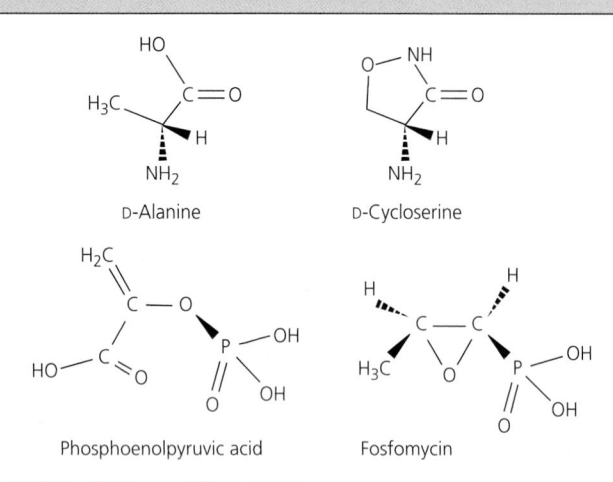

Figure 137-6 Analogy of structure between cycloserine and fosfomycin and their corresponding physiologic substrates involved in peptidoglycan synthesis.

The main sites identified in the 50S unit are the donor peptidyl site (P-site), where the growing peptide chain is fixed, and the acceptor aminoacyl site (A-site), where peptide bond formation occurs.

AMINOGLYCOSIDES
Chemical Structure

Streptomycin, discovered in 1944, has a limited spectrum of activity. Natural and semisynthetic derivatives with broader spectrum were discovered over time. Aminoglycosides comprise a dibasic cyclitol[14] (2-deoxystreptamine in most clinically used aminoglycosides) linked to cyclic sugars at positions 4 and 5 or 4 and 6 (Figure 137-7). All compounds are polycationic at physiologic pH.

Bacterial Targeting

Aminoglycosides selectively inhibit bacterial protein synthesis by binding to the prokaryotic 30S ribosomal subunit. Molecules displaying a hydroxyl function in C6' in place of an amino function (G-418, also known as geneticin) can also bind to eukaryotic ribosomes.

Mode of Action

Due to their polar nature, aminoglycosides cannot diffuse through membranes. They cross the outer membrane of gram-negative bacteria through a non-energy-dependent process involving drug-induced disruption of magnesium (Mg^{2+}) bridges between adjacent lipopolysaccharide molecules while their transport across the cytoplasmic membrane of both gram-positive and gram-negative bacteria is dependent upon electron transport (energy-dependent phase I; EDP-I). This transport is impaired in anaerobic environments, at low external pH or in high osmolality culture media, making aminoglycosides poorly active in these conditions.

Aminoglycosides bind largely to the aminoacyl site of the 30S subunit of ribosomes and, to a lesser extent, to specific sites of the 50S subunit, again through an energy-dependent process (energy-dependent phase II, EDP-II), disturbing the elongation of the nascent peptide. Their mechanism of action is complex, involving inhibition of the transfer of peptidyl tRNA from the A-site to the P-site and impairment of the proofreading process that controls translational accuracy. The aberrant proteins may compromise bacterial physiology, explaining the highly bactericidal, concentration-dependent activity of aminoglycosides.

Resistance

Resistance occurs mainly from the production of aminoglycoside-modifying enzymes (Figure 137-8). The semisynthetic derivatives (e.g. netilmicin, amikacin, isepamicin, and more recently plazomicin [in phase III clinical development]) were specifically designed to protect against the principal enzymes. However, multienzyme-producing bacteria have become increasingly common, causing multidrug resistance.[14]

A second mechanism of resistance causes membrane impermeabilization, the underlying mechanism of which is mainly active drug efflux, with at least five distinct systems described in bacteria such as *Escherichia coli* and *Pseudomonas aeruginosa*.[15]

A third mechanism involves post-transcriptional methylation of 16S rRNA occurring in Enterobacteriaceae and non-fermenters (Arm/Rmt mechanism). This affects all currently used 2-deoxystreptamine-containing aminoglycosides, with at least six distinct genes reported worldwide.[16,17]

Pharmacodynamics

Aminoglycosides demonstrate rapid, concentration-dependent killing as well as an important postantibiotic effect, probably due to their irreversible binding to the ribosomes. Simultaneously, toxicity (renal and auditory) is delayed as uptake of the drug into the target tissues is saturable.[18] As a result, once-a-day regimens provide the optimal mode of administration. Once-daily dosing has been instituted worldwide since the late 1990s to improve efficacy while reducing the toxicity of aminoglycosides.

Aminoglycosides are synergistic with antibiotics acting on cell wall synthesis by facilitating bacterial penetration of the aminoglycoside. In contrast, their activity is antagonized by bacteriostatic agents such as chloramphenicol and tetracyclines, probably by inhibition of their energy-dependent uptake and interference with the movement of the ribosome along mRNA.

TETRACYCLINES AND ALKYLAMINOCYCLINES
Chemical Structure

The early tetracyclines were derived from *Streptomyces* spp. (tetracycline, oxytetracycline), in contrast to more recent semisynthetic compounds (doxycycline, minocycline). All are characterized by four hydrophobic fused rings diversely substituted (principally by hydroxylated hydrophilic groups). Alkylaminocyclines possess an additional substituent with a bulky hydrophobic moiety and an ionizable amino function (Figure 137-9). Among them, tigecycline is often referred to as a glycylcycline based on the presence of a glycyl moiety as a spacer between the main part of the molecule and the ter-butyl-amino group.

Bacterial Targeting

Tetracyclines penetrate the outer membrane of gram-negative organisms through porins. Intrabacterial accumulation probably occurs via a bacterial transmembrane proton-driven carrier, which would explain their selectivity of action towards bacteria as opposed to eukariotic cells (Figure 137-10).

Mode of Action

Tetracyclines interfere with the initiation step of protein synthesis (Figure 137-10) by inhibiting the binding of aminoacyl tRNA to the A-site of the ribosome.[19] The 7S protein and the 16S RNA show the greatest affinity for tetracyclines and are therefore the main targets. This binding inhibits the fixation of a new aminoacyl tRNA on the ribosome. In addition, tetracyclines bind, or at least protrude, in the P-site by alteration in ribosome conformation in the post-translocational state, and may modify the ribosome conformation at the level of the head of the 30S subunit and the interface side of the 50S subunit.

Resistance

Resistance to tetracyclines is widespread. Some 29 genes on mobile elements have been identified in the so-called 'tetracycline' (tet) family

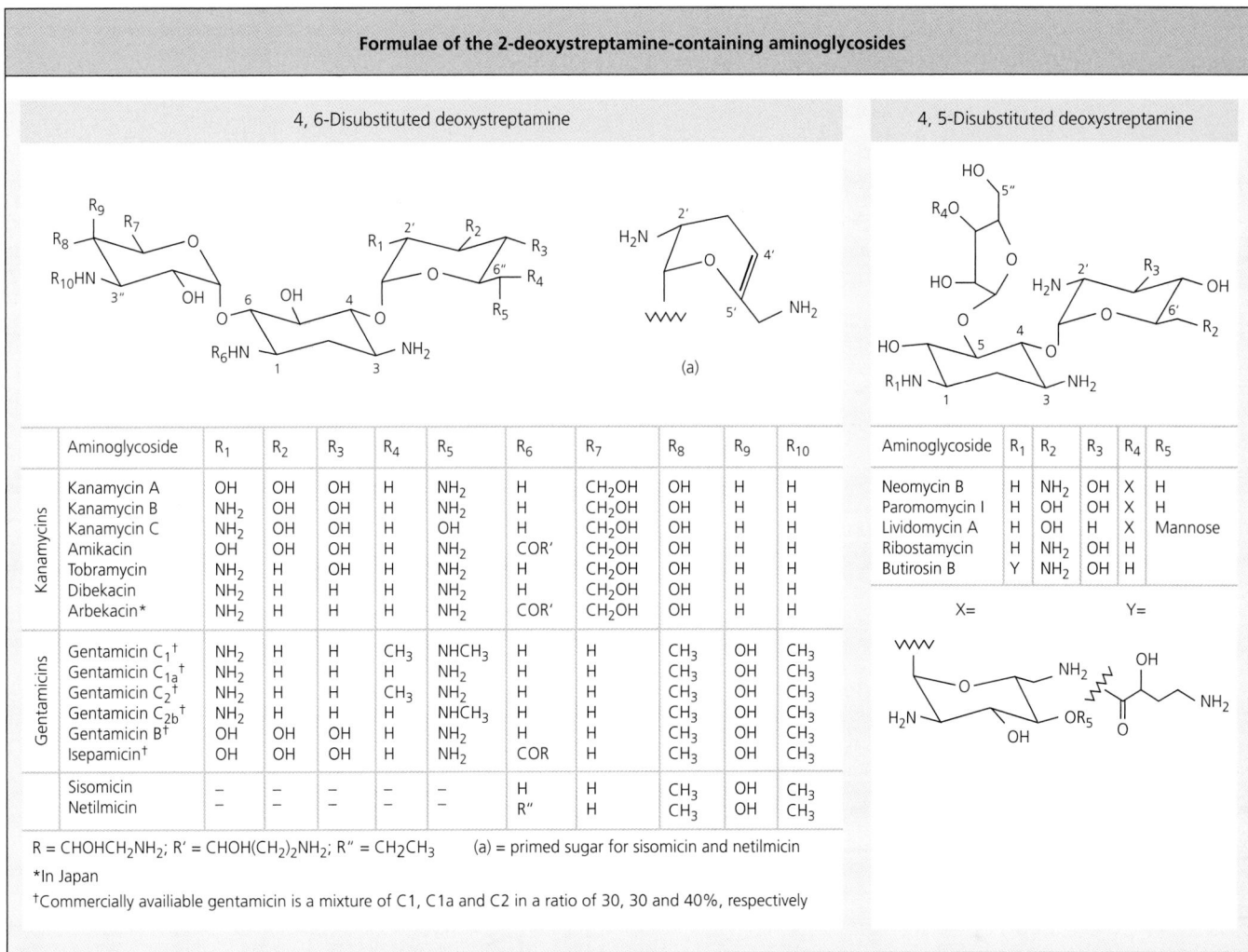

Aminoglycoside	R_1	R_2	R_3	R_4	R_5	R_6	R_7	R_8	R_9	R_{10}
Kanamycins										
Kanamycin A	OH	OH	OH	H	NH_2	H	CH_2OH	OH	H	H
Kanamycin B	NH_2	OH	OH	H	NH_2	H	CH_2OH	OH	H	H
Kanamycin C	NH_2	OH	OH	H	OH	H	CH_2OH	OH	H	H
Amikacin	OH	OH	OH	H	NH_2	COR'	CH_2OH	OH	H	H
Tobramycin	NH_2	H	OH	H	NH_2	H	CH_2OH	OH	H	H
Dibekacin	NH_2	H	H	H	NH_2	H	CH_2OH	OH	H	H
Arbekacin*	NH_2	H	H	H	NH_2	COR'	CH_2OH	OH	H	H
Gentamicins										
Gentamicin C_1[†]	NH_2	H	H	CH_3	$NHCH_3$	H	H	CH_3	OH	CH_3
Gentamicin C_{1a}[†]	NH_2	H	H	H	NH_2	H	H	CH_3	OH	CH_3
Gentamicin C_2[†]	NH_2	H	H	CH_3	NH_2	H	H	CH_3	OH	CH_3
Gentamicin C_{2b}[†]	NH_2	H	H	H	$NHCH_3$	H	H	CH_3	OH	CH_3
Gentamicin B[†]	OH	OH	OH	H	NH_2	H	H	CH_3	OH	CH_3
Isepamicin[†]	OH	OH	OH	H	NH_2	COR	H	CH_3	OH	CH_3
Sisomicin	–	–	–	–	–	H	H	CH_3	OH	CH_3
Netilmicin	–	–	–	–	–	R"	H	CH_3	OH	CH_3

Aminoglycoside	R_1	R_2	R_3	R_4	R_5
Neomycin B	H	NH_2	OH	X	H
Paromomycin I	H	OH	OH	X	H
Lividomycin A	H	OH	H	X	Mannose
Ribostamycin	H	NH_2	OH	H	
Butirosin B	Y	NH_2	OH	H	

R = CHOHCH₂NH₂; R' = CHOH(CH₂)₂NH₂; R" = CH₂CH₃   (a) = primed sugar for sisomicin and netilmicin

*In Japan

[†]Commercially availiable gentamicin is a mixture of C1, C1a and C2 in a ratio of 30, 30 and 40%, respectively

Figure 137-7   Formulae of the 2-deoxystreptamine-containing aminoglycosides. The numbering of the atoms shown is as in Mingeot-Leclercq *et al.*[18] with the primed numbers (') being ascribed to the sugar attached to C4 of the 2-deoxystreptamine (as this C is of the R configuration) and the doubly primed numbers (") being ascribed to the sugar attached to either the C6 (S configuration) for the 4,6-disubstituted 2-deoxystreptamine or the C5 (R configuration) for the 4,5-disubstituted 2-deoxystreptamine.

and three in the 'oxytetracycline resistance' gene family (otr). Two main mechanisms have been described, namely efflux and ribosomal protection. Resistance by enzymatic inactivation has been described but remains uncommon. Low levels of resistance can also result from mutations or decreased expression of porins.

As tigecycline increases the number of bonds to the target 16S RNA, the drug is unaffected by the ribosome protection mechanism.[20] Together with the vicinal hydrophobic moiety, it makes the molecule less susceptible to efflux, with the noticeable exception of resistance nodulation cell division (RND)-type efflux pumps constitutively expressed by *P. aeruginosa* and Proteae, against which it is inactive.[21] Moreover, mutants (related to efflux) have already been reported in *Acinetobacter* spp.

Pharmacodynamics

Tetracyclines are essentially bacteriostatic and need to be administered at intervals determined by the drug half-life in order to maintain their serum level above the MIC of the infecting organism for as long as possible. Because of their prolonged half-life, however, AUC_{24h}/MIC emerges as the main parameter driving the activity of tetracyclines (including tigecycline) *in vivo*. In contrast to conventional tetracyclines, tigecycline must be given by the intravenous route.

FUSIDIC ACID

Chemical Structure

Fusidic acid is a steroid-like structure, belonging to the fusidane class.

Mode of Action and Resistance

Fusidic acid prevents the dissociation of the complex formed between guanosine diphosphate, elongation factor 2 and the ribosome, thereby inhibiting the translocation step of the peptidyl tRNA from the P-site to the A-site of the ribosome.[22] Because of a lack of cross-resistance with other antistaphylococcal agents, fusidic acid is revived in several countries for the treatment of multiresistant *Staph. aureus*. More specifically, it is re-developed in the USA in view of the mounting epidemic of community-acquired MRSA. Fusidic acid is always used in combination because of the high rate of emergence of resistance when used as monotherapy. The latter seems to result from the acquisition of the *fusB* gene, which protects ribosomal protein synthesis inhibition from fusidic acid in a dose-dependent fashion.[23]

Pharmacodynamics

Fusidic acid is bacteriostatic but may be bactericidal at high concentrations.

Major aminoglycoside-modifying enzymes that act on kanamycin B

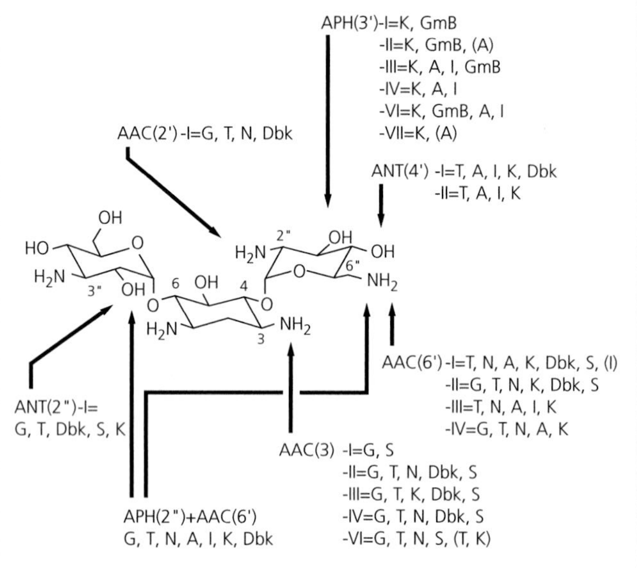

Figure 137-8 Major aminoglycoside-modifying enzymes that act on kanamycin B. This aminoglycoside is susceptible to the largest number of enzymes. The *N*-acetyltransferases (AACs) affect amino functions and the o-nucleotidyltransferases affect hydroxyl functions. Each group of enzymes inactivates specific sites, but each of these sites can be acted upon by distinct isoenzymes (Roman numerals) with different substrate specificities (phenotypic classification). At least one enzyme is bifunctional and affects both positions 2'; (o-phosphorylation) and 6' (*N*-acetylation). The main aminoglycosides used clinically on which these enzymes act are amikacin (A), dibekacin (Dbk), commercial gentamicin (G), gentamicin B (GmB), kanamycin A (K), isepamicin (I), netilmicin (N), sisomicin (S) and tobramycin (T). The drug abbreviations that appear in parentheses are those for which resistance was detectable *in vitro* although clinical resistance was not conferred. *(Adapted from Mingeot-Leclercq* et al.[18]*)*

Chemical structures of tetracyclines (tetracycline, doxycycline, minocycline) and alkylaminocyclines (tigecycline)

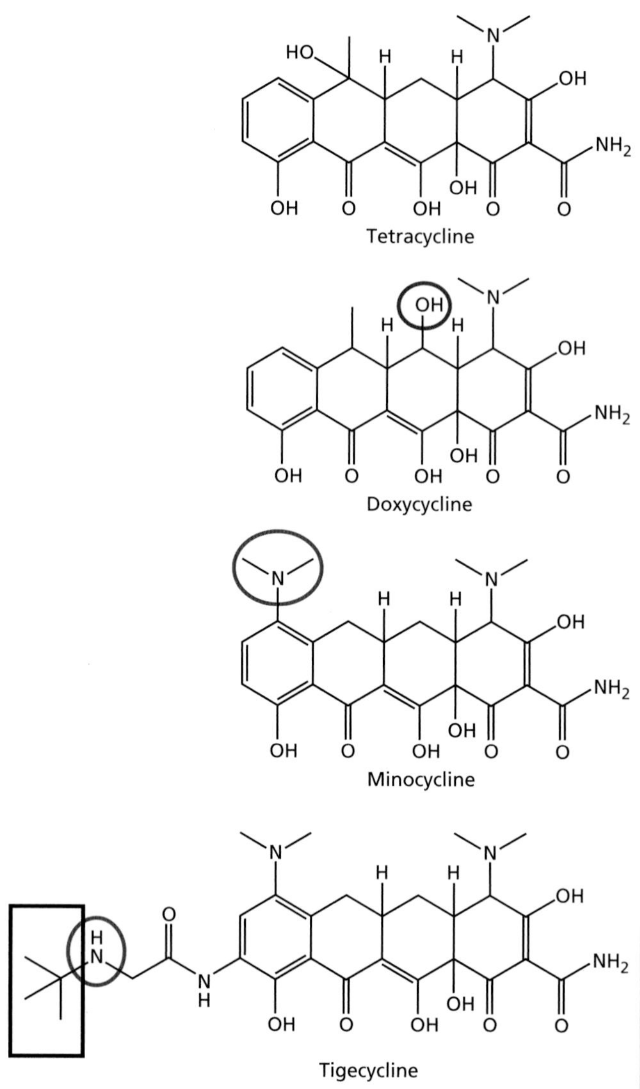

Figure 137-9 Chemical structures of tetracyclines (tetracycline, doxycycline, minocycline) and alkylaminocyclines (tigecycline). The figure highlights the displacement of a hydroxyl group (circled in blue) between tetracycline and doxycycline, and the additional ionizable amino function in minocycline (circled in red) which confer a more prolonged half-life and improved activity (minocycline). Tigecycline is the first of a new group of derivatives with a bulky hydrophobic moiety (black box; *ter*-butyl in the case of tigecycline) and an additional amino group (circled in red) that make the molecule less susceptible to efflux by tetracycline-specific transporters as well as to ribosomal protection, the two main mechanisms of bacterial resistance towards all other tetracyclines.

MUPIROCIN

Chemical Structure

Mupirocin contains a short fatty acid side chain (9-hydroxynonanoic acid) linked to monic acid by an ester linkage. Mupirocin is also called pseudomonic acid because its major metabolite (pseudomonic acid A; responsible for most of the activity) is derived from submerged fermentation of *Pseudomonas fluorescens*. Three other minor metabolites (pseudomonic acids B, C and D) share a similar chemical structure and antimicrobial spectrum.

Mode of Action and Resistance

Mupirocin inhibits bacterial RNA and protein synthesis by binding to bacterial isoleucyl tRNA synthetase, which catalyzes the formation of isoleucyl tRNA from isoleucine and tRNA.[24] This prevents incorporation of isoleucine into protein chains, leading to arrest of protein synthesis. Resistance to mupirocin develops through the production of a modified target enzyme. Because of its unique mechanism of action, there is no cross-resistance between mupirocin and other antimicrobial agents.

Pharmacodynamics

Mupirocin is bacteriostatic at low concentration but becomes bactericidal at concentrations achieved locally by topical administration. The *in vitro* antibacterial activity is greatest at acidic pH, which is advantageous in the treatment of cutaneous infections because of the low pH of the skin.

RETAPAMULIN

Retapamulin is a semisynthetic derivative of pleuromutilin, a naturally occurring tricyclic antibiotic, diterpene, discovered in the early 1950s, and out of which only veterinary antibiotics had been developed until now. Retapamulin inhibits bacterial protein synthesis by binding to domain V of 23S rRNA, thereby blocking peptide formation directly by interfering with substrate binding. Resistance occurs through mutations in the genes encoding 23S rRNA, but is not crossed with other antibiotics as the binding site in the ribosome is different from that of other antibiotics.[25] Retapamulin has been developed as a topical antibiotic for the management of impetigo and uncomplicated secondarily infected traumatic skin lesions. Other derivatives of pleuromutilins are in development for systemic use. Isolates of *Staph. aureus* with *cfr* mechanism of resistance to linezolid are also resistant to pleuromutilins (see oxazolidinones).

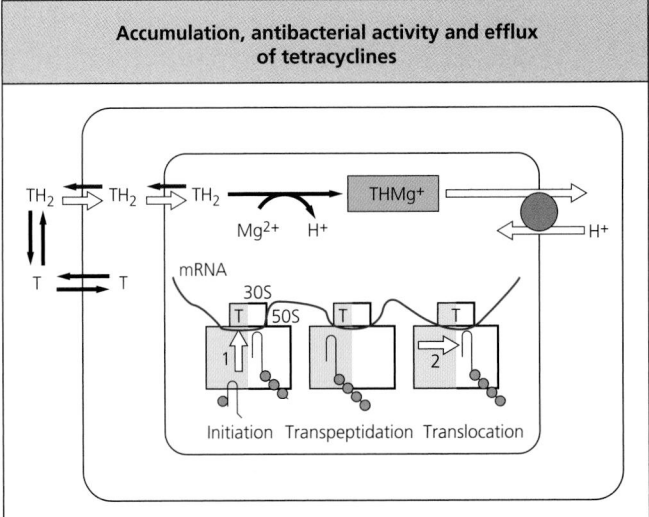

Accumulation, antibacterial activity and efflux of tetracyclines

Figure 137-10 Accumulation, antibacterial activity and efflux of tetracyclines. Tetracyclines freely diffuse through the extracellular membrane of gram-negative organisms. Penetration inside bacteria is an energy-dependent process, depending on the pH and Mg^{2+} gradient between the extracellular medium of gram-positive organisms or the periplasmic medium of gram-negative organisms and the intracellular medium. Only the protonated (uncharged) form is highly diffusible, so that accumulation is favored by a lowering of the extracellular pH. Once inside the cytosol, the tetracycline molecule forms a nondiffusible complex with Mg^{2+}. This type of complex with a bivalent cation is also the substrate of the efflux pumps present in the membrane of resistant bacteria and acting as H^+ antiports (purple circle). The antibacterial action of the tetracyclines (T) is due to their binding to the 30S subunit of the ribosomes. In the pretranslocational state, tetracyclines inhibit the binding of aminoacyl tRNA (arrow 1) to the A-site (yellow part of the ribosome). In the post-translocational state, tetracyclines protrude in the P-site (white part of the ribosome) and inhibit the binding of the peptidyl tRNA (arrow 2).

MACROLIDES
Chemical Structure
The main active macrolides are 14-, 15- or 16-membered lactone rings, substituted by two sugars, one of which bears an aminated function. In 15-membered macrolides (azithromycin), an additional aminated function is inserted in the lactone ring, conferring to this subclass of molecule the name of 'azalides'. Ketolides are 14-membered macrolides in which the cladinose is replaced by a keto function and which possess in their macrocycle a carbamate linked to an alkyl-aryl extension, represented by telithromycin as the only registered antibiotic so far (Figure 137-11).[26]

Erythromycin, the first clinically developed macrolide, is a natural product. Most of the more recent molecules are semisynthetic derivatives designed to be stable in acidic milieu, and are therefore characterized by an improved oral bioavailability. Both 16-membered macrolides and ketolides are intrinsically acid stable.

Bacterial Targeting
Macrolides specifically bind to the 50S subunit of the ribosomes (more precisely, to the 23S rRNA), which does not exist in eukaryotic cells.

Mode of Action
Macrolides reversibly bind to the peptidyl transferase center, located at the 50S surface, causing multiple alterations of the 50S subunit functions. While macrolides only bind to domain V of the 23S rRNA, ketolides also bind to domain II of 23S rRNA as a result of their carbamate extension, and thus are double anchored to their target (Figure 137-12).[27] Macrolides are classically thought to block the peptide bond formation or the peptidyl tRNA translocation from the A-site to the P-site. However, additional consequences of their binding to ribosomes have been reported. It has been proposed that they could also favor the premature dissociation of peptidyl tRNA from the ribosome during the elongation process, leading to the synthesis of incomplete peptides.[28] It has also been suggested that erythromycin prevents the assembly of the 50S subunit, a property not generalizable to other macrolides.

Resistance
Clinically meaningful resistance occurs by modification of the bacterial target and therefore affects all macrolides as well as by efflux.[29] Target modification also affects lincosamides and streptogramins because of the common binding site for these three classes of antibiotic and also explains why these classes have antagonist activity. Resistance to macrolides may be inducible or constitutive; however, it will not affect streptogramins and lincosamides if inducible since these are not inducers. Ketolides (due to their lack of cladinose) and 16-membered macrolides are not inducers and therefore show activity on a subset of resistant strains. Moreover, the double ribosomal anchoring of ketolides (through the presence of an additional side chain) confers a higher affinity not only for wild-type ribosomes, but also for ribosomes of strains resistant by methylation of domain V, with consequent improved activity against resistant strains.[26,30] However, telithromycin, the first approved ketolide, has been severely restricted due to concerns about toxicity (mainly liver).[31] Solithromycin (a fluoroketolide presently in phase III of clinical development) may have a better safety profile due to a different side chain.

Efflux mechanisms are being reported mainly in North America. 16-membered macrolides are again spared against this effect. The frequency of strains susceptible to 16-membered macrolides and resistant to 14- and 15-membered macrolides remains low, however. Isolates of *Staph. aureus* with *cfr* mechanism of resistance to linezolid are also resistant to 16-membered macrolides (see oxazolidinones).

Pharmacodynamics
Macrolides are essentially bacteriostatic antibiotics, except at high concentrations. Their concentration at the infected site therefore needs to be durably maintained above the MIC of the pathogen. Because of their prolonged half-life, the activity of clarithromycin, azithromycin and telithromycin have been shown to primarily depend upon AUC_{24h}/MIC parameter *in vivo*.[26]

LINCOSAMIDES
Chemical Structure
Lincomycin and its 7-chloro-7-deoxy derivative, clindamycin, comprise a propylhygrinic acid linked to an aminosugar.

Mode of Action
Lincosamides bind to the 50S ribosomal subunit and have a mode of action similar to that of macrolides.

Resistance
The main mechanism of resistance to lincosamides is similar to that of macrolides and streptogramins and consists of an alteration of the 50S subunit. Rare cases of enzymatic inactivation of the antibiotic have also been described for clindamycin. Resistance dissociation is, however, observed for those strains for which macrolide resistance is inducible, as clindamycin is not an inducer. Likewise, efflux-mediated resistance to macrolides does not affect lincosamides.[29] Isolates of *Staph. aureus* with *cfr* mechanism of resistance to linezolid are also resistant to clindamycin (see oxazolidinones).

Pharmacodynamics
Lincosamides are bacteriostatic and are antagonists of macrolides and streptogramins, which bind at the same site on the ribosomes.

STREPTOGRAMINS
Chemical Structure
Streptogramins are antibiotics that comprise a pair of synergistic constituents, namely a depsipeptide (group I) and a lactonic macrocycle (group II). Quinupristin–dalfopristin is the only combination used in the clinic.

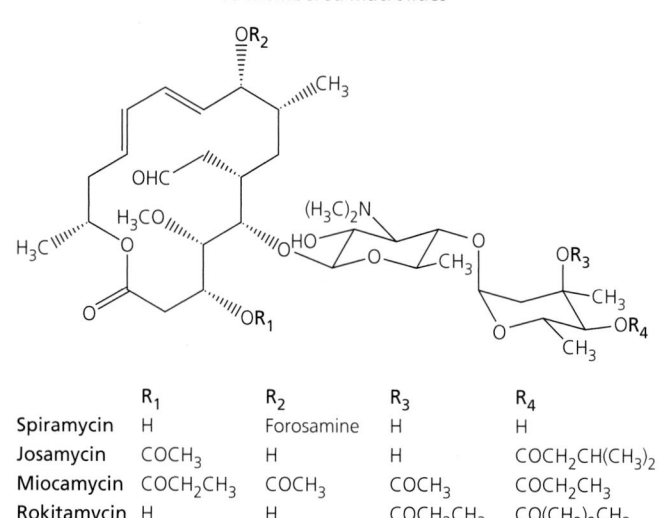

Figure 137-11 Chemical structure of the macrolides. The upper panel shows the degradation of erythromycin in the gastric milieu (substituents responsible for the instability of the molecule are shown in purple). 16-membered macrolides and ketolides are intrinsically stable. The structural modifications conferring stability in acidic milieu to 14- and 15-membered macrolides are highlighted in pink in the middle panel.

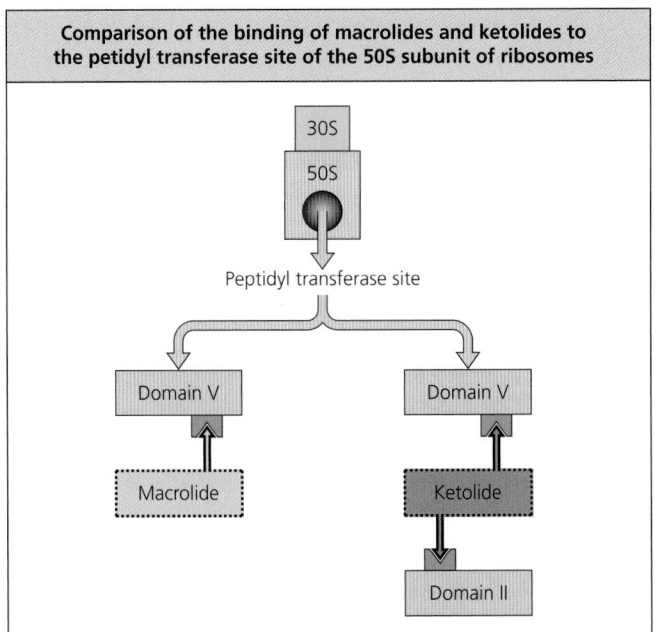

Comparison of the binding of macrolides and ketolides to the petidyl transferase site of the 50S subunit of ribosomes

Figure 137-12 Comparison of the binding of macrolides and ketolides to the peptidyl transferase site of the 50S subunit of ribosomes. Macrolides are characterized by a single anchoring point and ketolides by a double anchoring point, which increases the affinity of ketolides for wild type and methylated ribosomes.

Mode of Action

Streptogramins bind to the 50S subunit of the bacterial ribosome. They interfere with protein synthesis by a double mechanism, involving inhibition of the incorporation of aminoacyl tRNA in the ribosome and the translation of mRNA. The synergistic effects of the two components could be due to a modification of the conformation of the ribosome caused by binding of the group I component, which exposes a site of fixation for the group II component.[28]

Resistance

Resistance is by mutation of the ribosomal target and results in cross-resistance with macrolides and lincosamides. Because of the presence of two components, however, synergistins remain active against many macrolide and lincosamide-resistant isolates. Resistance to streptogramins alone is rare and occurs by enzymatic inactivation (hydrolase and acetylase). Isolates of *Staph. aureus* with *cfr* mechanism of resistance to linezolid are also resistant to streptogramins (see oxazolidinones).

Pharmacodynamics

Streptogramin constituents are highly synergistic; they exhibit dose-dependent bactericidal activity in combination and prolonged postantibiotic effect. In addition, they also increase the antibiotic activity of aminoglycosides and rifamycins.

CHLORAMPHENICOL AND THIAMPHENICOL

Chemical Structure

These antibiotics are constructed on a dichloroacetamide bearing a diversely substituted phenyl group.

Bacterial Targeting

Chloramphenicol acts principally by binding to the 50S subunit of the bacterial ribosomes. However, it can also interact with mitochondrial ribosomes of eukaryotic cells, which results in its toxicity.

Mode of Action

Chloramphenicol enters the bacteria by an energy-dependent process. Its antibiotic activity is due to competitive inhibition for the binding of aminoacyl tRNA to the peptidyltransferase domain of the 50S

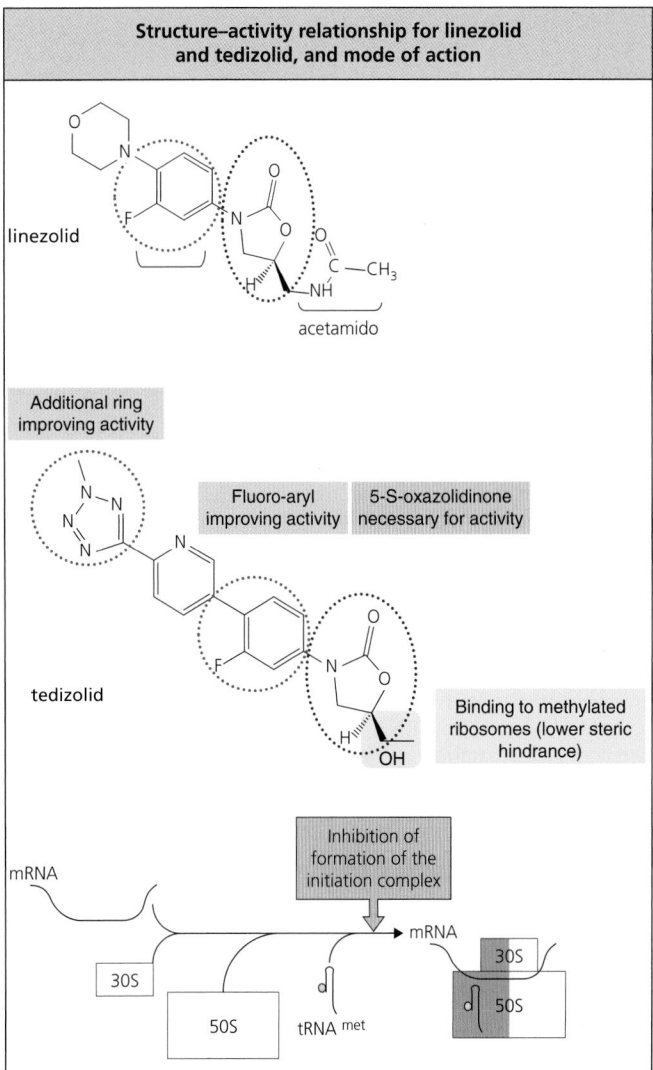

Structure–activity relationship for linezolid and tedizolid, and mode of action

Figure 137-13 Structure–activity relationship for linezolid and tedizolid, and mode of action. The drug prevents the formation of the ternary complex between mRNA, ribosome subunits and tRNA[met] necessary for protein synthesis.

subunit. This induces conformational change in the ribosome, which slows or even inhibits the incorporation of the aminoacyl tRNA and in turn the transpeptidation reaction.[32]

Resistance

Resistance to chloramphenicol is mainly due to the production of a specific inactivating chloramphenicol acetyltransferase (CAT). The CAT gene is widely disseminated on plasmids that also confer resistance to other antibiotic classes. Isolates of *Staph. aureus* with *cfr* mechanism of resistance to linezolid are also resistant to chloramphenicol.

Pharmacodynamics

Chloramphenicol is bacteriostatic. It competes in binding to the ribosomes with macrolides and lincosamides, making its combination with these drugs useless.

OXAZOLIDINONES

Chemical Structure

Oxazolidinones are synthetic molecules. The first derivatives were described in the 1970s, leading to linezolid that was brought on the market in the late 1990s (Figure 137-13). The 5-(S)-configuration of the oxazolidinone ring is essential for activity, which is further improved by its substitution by an *N*-fluorinated aryl group and a C5 acetamido group.[33]

Mode of Action

Oxazolidinones inhibit protein synthesis at an earlier step than other antibiotics acting on the ribosome (Figure 137-13). Their binding site is located in the vicinity of the peptidyl transferase with the A-site of the bacterial ribosome where they seem to interfere with the placement of the aminoacyl tRNA.[34] This interaction prevents the formation of the initiation ternary complex which associates tRNA[met], mRNA and the 50S subunit of the ribosome, and therefore the binding to the ribosome as well as the synthesis of peptide bonds, and the translocation of tRNA[met] into the P-site. They can compete for binding to the 50S subunit with other antibiotics (e.g. lincosamides, chloramphenicol) without being antagonistic.

Oxazolidinones show useful activity only against gram-positive cocci, due to active efflux in most gram-negative bacteria.[35]

Oxazolidinones also interact with mitochondrial ribosomes to inhibit protein synthesis (reversible upon drug elimination), which is probably the basis for their undesirable myelosuppressive, neurotoxic and metabolic effects (lactic acidosis).[36]

Resistance

Because of the unique mode of action of oxazolidinones, there was hope of absence of cross-resistance with other antibiotics acting on protein synthesis. Resistance, however, has developed following point mutations of the 23S rRNA (*cfr* mechanism),[34] which also affect phenicols, lincosamides, pleuromutilins, streptogramins and 16-membered macrolides. Another mechanism consists in base-pair deletions in the gene encoding riboprotein L4.[37] Tedizolid (Figure 137-13) is more potent that linezolid on susceptible strains (because of the presence of an additional ring permitting additional interactions with the ribosome) and keeps activity on strains carrying the *cfr* mechanism of resistance (because of the replacement of the acetamido by a less sterically-hindered hydroxymethyl group, allowing for binding to methylated ribosomes).[38] Although more inhibitory towards mitochondrial protein synthesis than linezolid on a molar basis, tedizolid does not cause more toxicity in humans because of a more favorable pharmacokinetic profile allowing a once-daily schedule, which leaves longer recovery periods than linezolid.

Pharmacodynamics

Oxazolidinones are essentially bacteriostatic against enterococci and staphylococci with a short postantibiotic effect, but is bactericidal against some streptococcal species. Because of their prolonged half-life, activity is primarily dependent on the AUC_{24h}/MIC parameter *in vivo*.[10]

Drugs That Affect Nucleic Acids (DNA/RNA)

FLUOROQUINOLONES

Chemical Structure

Fluoroquinolones are totally synthetic products originally derived from nalidixic acid. All current compounds have a dual ring structure, with a nitrogen atom at position 1, a free carboxylate at position 3 and a carbonyl at position 4. A fluor substituent at position 6 usually greatly enhances activity, whereas the substituents at positions 7, 8 and N1 modulate the spectrum, the pharmacokinetics and the side effects of the drugs (Figure 137-14).[39] More recent molecules like moxifloxacin have been designed to better cover gram-positive organisms, while retaining activity against gram-negative organisms and possibly also acting on anaerobes; they present a small hydrophobic substituent at N1 and a diaminated small-sized ring substituent at position 7.

Bacterial Targeting

Fluoroquinolones cross the outer membrane of gram-negative bacteria via porins. Their affinity for their bacterial target is 1000 times greater than for the corresponding eukaryotic enzyme, which ensures their specificity.

Mode of Action

Fluoroquinolones inhibit the activity of topoisomerases. These enzymes are responsible for the supercoiling of DNA (DNA gyrase) and the relaxation of supercoiled DNA (topoisomerase IV). Both enzymes have a similar mode of action, implying the binding of DNA to the enzyme; the cleavage of the DNA; the passage of the DNA segment through the DNA gate; and the resealing of the DNA break and release from the enzyme.

Gyrase and topoisomerase IV are tetramers composed of two types of subunit, namely two GyrA or ParC catalyzing the DNA cutting and resealing, and two GyrB or ParE responsible for the transduction and binding of ATP. The main target of fluoroquinolones is DNA gyrase in gram-negative bacteria and topoisomerase IV in gram-positive bacteria.

Fluoroquinolones form a ternary complex with DNA and the enzyme (Figure 137-15).[40] This binding site for fluoroquinolones is formed during the gate-opening step of the double-stranded DNA. Co-operatively, four fluoroquinolone molecules are fixed to single-stranded DNA. Their stacking is favored by the presence of the co-planar aromatic rings in their structure and by the tail-to-tail interactions between the substituents at N1. Interaction with DNA occurs by hydrogen bonds or via Mg^{2+} bridges established with the carbonyl and carboxylate groups. Interaction with the enzyme is mediated by fluoride at position 6 and the substituents at position 7. The binding of the fluoroquinolones stabilizes the cleavable complex (formed by the cut DNA and the enzyme) and leads to the dissociation of the enzyme subunits. The latter action is, however, observed only for potent molecules or at high concentrations for the others.

Fluoroquinolones are highly bactericidal, suggesting the formation of abnormal proteins as a consequence of DNA cleavage. Quinolones also induce an SOS (DNA repair) response, which involves three proteins (RecA, LexA and RecBCD). Induced RecA cleaves the repressor of the SOS regulon (LexA), stimulating repair of damage caused by fluoroquinolones to DNA. Induced RecBCD binds at the double-strand break created by the ternary complex of topoisomerase–DNA–quinolone, leading to mutagenesis as well as increased cell survival in the presence of quinolones. This system protects against the antibacterial activity of fluoroquinolones and could be a basis for emergence of resistance.[41]

Resistance

Resistance was long considered to be only chromosomally mediated from mutation of the topoisomerases, porin impermeabilization (for gram-negative bacteria) or efflux.[39] A methoxy substituent at position 8 (see Figure 137-14) lowers the ratio of the MIC in gyrase mutant strains to the corresponding MIC in the wild type, thereby reducing the risk of selecting resistant mutants during therapy. Plasmid-mediated resistance, however, is now increasingly observed,[42] related to the production of Qnr proteins capable of protecting DNA gyrase from quinolones or of AAC(6')-Ib-cr, a variant aminoglycoside acetyl-transferase capable of acetylating ciprofloxacin.

Pharmacodynamics

The activity of fluoroquinolones is largely both concentration dependent (which drives the bactericidal effect) and proportional to the amount of drug administered (which drives the global efficacy *in vivo*), making these drugs C_{max}/MIC and AUC_{24h}/MIC dependent for their activity. For fluoroquinolones with short half-life (e.g. ciprofloxacin), this imposes the use of repeated doses per day (to reduce the risk of C_{max}-related toxic reactions). For fluoroquinolones with more prolonged half-lives (levofloxacin, moxifloxacin), once-daily administration is possible, with the aim of obtaining both C_{max}/MIC (>8) and AUC_{24h}/MIC (from 30 to 125 or more) ratios. This pharmacodynamic property offers optimal efficacy while minimizing the selection of resistant subpopulations.[39] Novel fluoroquinolones (finafloxacin,

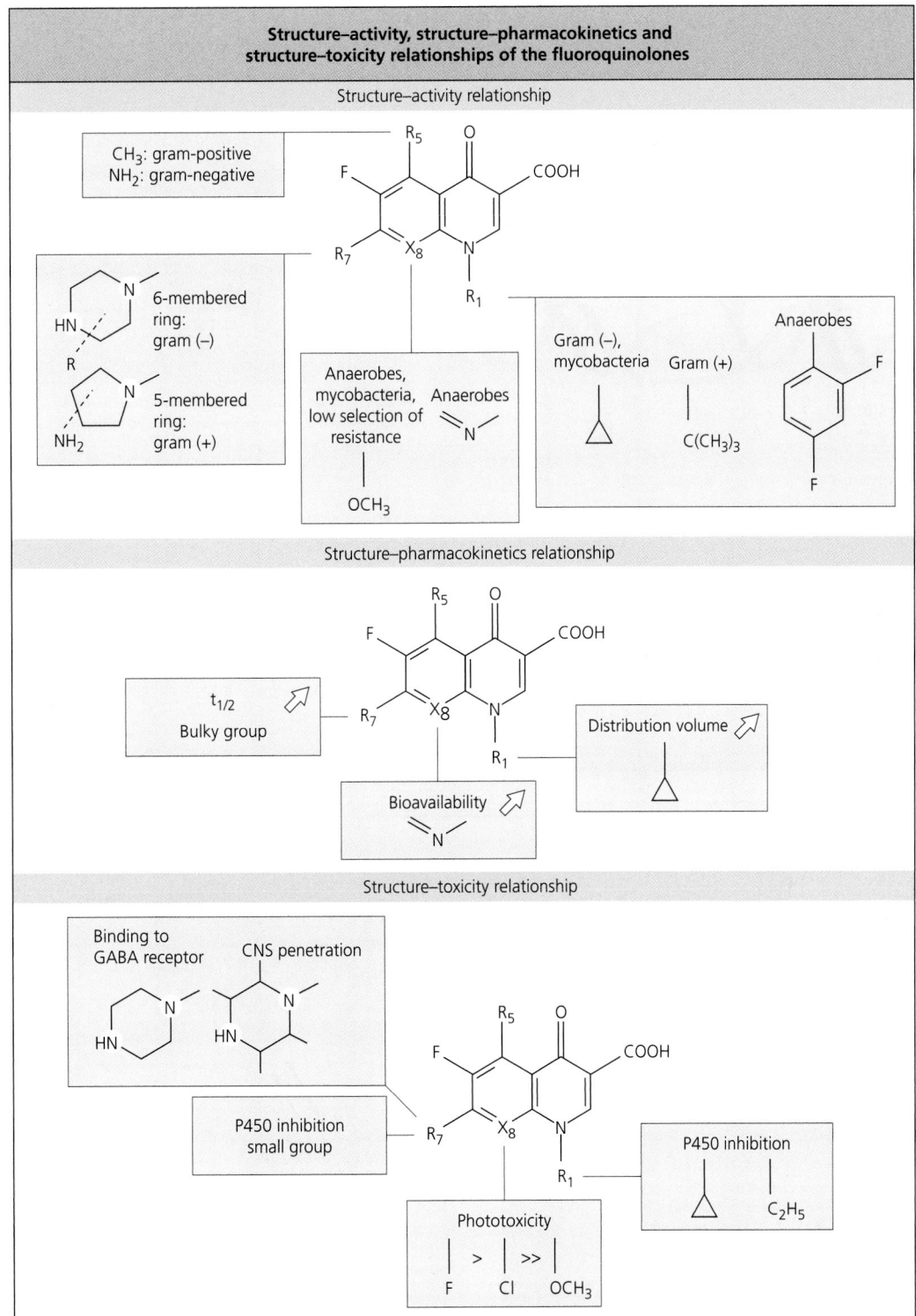

Figure 137-14 Structure–activity, structure–pharmacokinetics and structure–toxicity relationships of the fluoroquinolones. These considerations form the basis of the rational development of the new molecules of this class, which have a very extended spectrum (including gram-positive bacteria and anaerobes), a long half-life and minimal phototoxicity and metabolic interactions.

delafloxacin) show a markedly improved activity at acid pH, which could be of interest for activity against intracellular bacteria known to develop in phagolysosomes and related vacuoles where pH is acidic.

NITROIMIDAZOLES AND NITROFURANS
Chemical Structure
The nitroheterocyclic drugs include nitrofuran and nitroimidazole compounds (Figure 137-16).

Mode and Spectrum of Action
The activity of the nitroheterocyclic drugs requires activation of the nitro group attached to the imidazole or furan ring, which must undergo single- or two-electron enzymatic reduction in the bacteria.[43] Although the nitro radicals generated by reduction of the parent drugs are similar for the nitroimidazoles and the nitrofurans, these drugs differ by their reduction potential, and therefore their spectrum of activity. Thus nitroimidazoles must be fully reduced to generate the

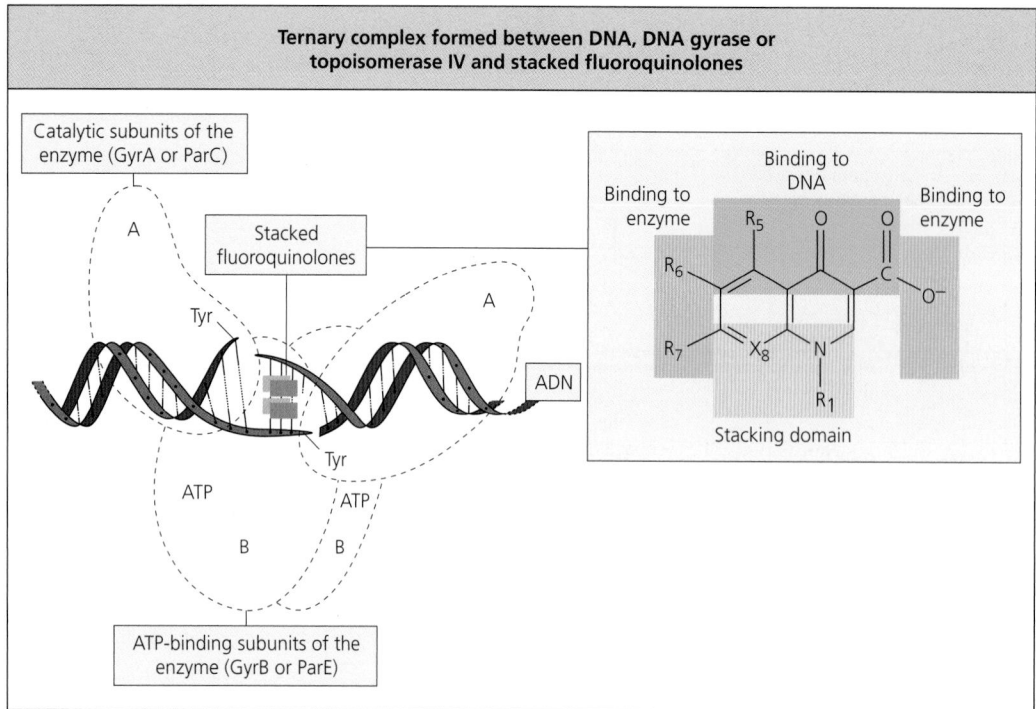

Figure 137-15 Ternary complex formed between DNA, DNA gyrase or topoisomerase IV, and stacked fluoroquinolones. Subunits A form covalent bonds via Tyr122 with the 5' end of the DNA chain. The binding site for fluoroquinolones is located in the bubble formed during the local opening of the DNA molecule. The right panel shows the parts of the antibiotic molecules interacting with DNA, with the enzyme, or favoring the stacking of the fluoroquinolone molecules. (*Adapted from Shen* et al. *Biochemistry 1989; 28(9):3886-3894.*)

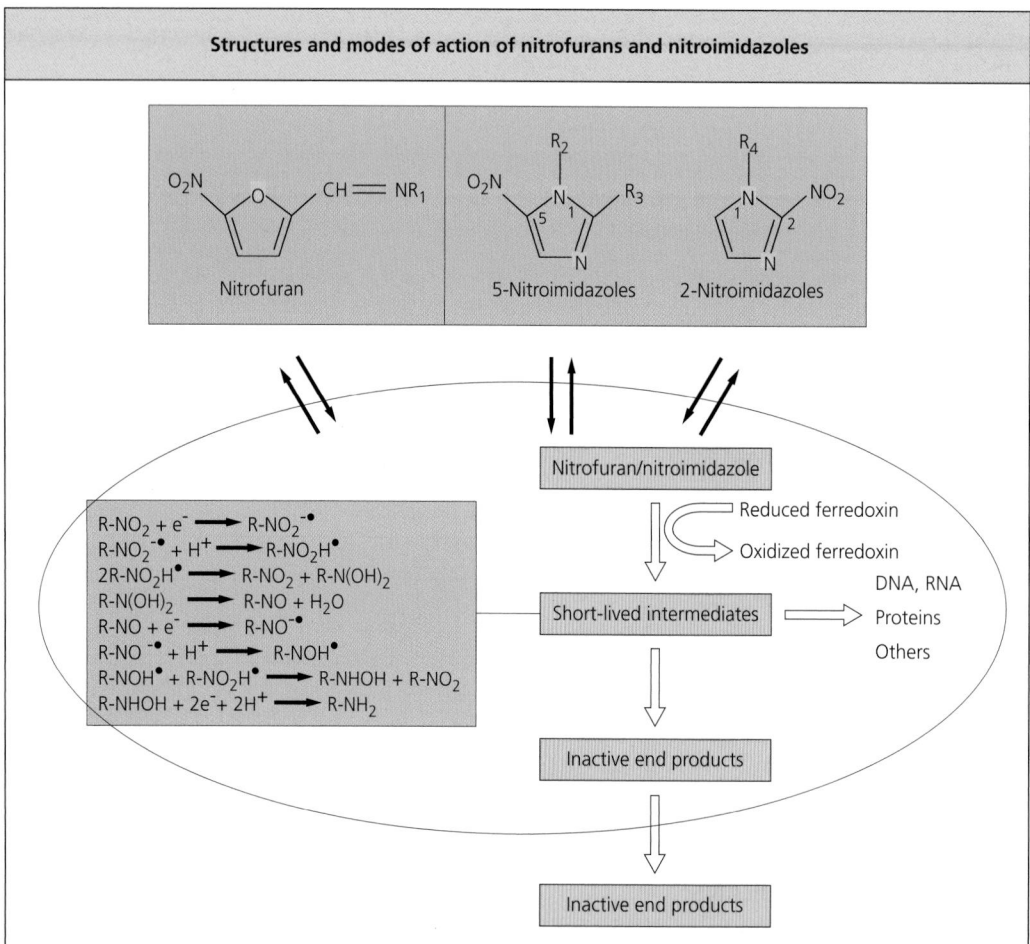

Figure 137-16 Structures and modes of action of nitrofurans and nitroimidazoles. The molecules must be reduced to form highly reactive products that interact with intracellular targets.

highly reactive species, whereas singly reduced nitrofurans may directly inhibit the activity of enzymes involved in the degradation of glucose and pyruvate and covalently bind to proteins and DNA by an alkylation reaction. Nitroimidazoles will, therefore, express activity only towards truly anaerobic and microaerophilic bacteria, and towards other parasitic organisms such as *Trichomonas vaginalis*, whereas nitrofurans are equally active against anaerobic and aerobic bacteria.

Resistance

Resistance to nitroimidazoles in true anaerobic bacteria is rare, but has been described in *Bacteroides fragilis* (combination of decreased antibiotic uptake, reduced nitroreductase and pyruvate:ferredoxin oxidoreductase activity and increased lactate dehydrogenase activity).[44] It has become significant in *Helicobacter pylori* (null mutations in *rdxA* encoding an oxygen-insensitive nitroreductase that normally prevents reoxidization of metronidazole in the microaerophilic environment of this bacterium).[45]

Pharmacodynamics

Nitroimidazoles show concentration-dependent killing, which is consistent with the current clinical pattern of dispensing a large dose in a single administration (although more frequent administration of lower dose is also recommended). Clinical failures of metronidazole (commonly observed in aspiration pneumonia or *C. difficile* colitis) may be due to reoxygenation of the infectious foci following initial decrease of bacterial load, with ensuing loss of activity of these compounds that only act in a strictly anaerobic milieu.

ANSAMYCINS AND LIPIARMYCINS
Chemical Structure

Ansamycins are lipophilic macrocyclic antibiotics that easily diffuse through membranes. They comprise two aromatic rings (containing a quinone), connected by a long chain (or 'ansa'– hence the name given to this class of antibiotics), which confers a rigid character to the whole molecule. The first clinically developed and major antibiotic in this class was rifampin (rifampicin). Successful successors have been rifapentin, rifamixin and rifabutin. Among lipiarmycins, fidaxomicin is a high molecular weight macrocyclic antibiotic which is virtually not absorbed by oral route. It is quickly metabolized by esterases in OT-1118 which keeps antibacterial activity.[46]

Mode of Action

Both types of drugs act on the RNA polymerase (Figure 137-17), an enzyme made of five subunits ($\alpha_2\beta\beta'\sigma$), namely: two α subunits establish contact with transcription factors; the β' subunit is a basic polypeptide that binds DNA; the β subunit is an acidic polypeptide and is part of the active site; and the σ initiates transcription and then leaves the polymerase nucleus. The core polymerase ($\alpha_2\beta\beta'$) retains the capacity to synthesize RNA but is defective in its ability to bind and initiate DNA transcription.

Ansamycins inhibit the initiation of the transcription of DNA in mRNA and therefore subsequent protein synthesis, by binding to the β subunit of the RNA polymerase or, to a lesser extent, of the DNA–RNA complex.[47] This binding is mediated by hydrophobic interactions between the aliphatic ansa chain and the β subunit. The precise site of binding has been identified only partly, by studying mutants in RNA polymerase that has acquired resistance to rifampin. All the mutations affecting drug binding belong to three clusters of amino acids in the central domain of the β subunit. Specificity of action depends on the fact that ansamycins alter mammalian cell metabolism only at concentrations 10 000 times those necessary to cause bacterial cell death.

Lipiarmycins act at an earlier stage, by binding to the DNA template–RNA polymerase complex prior to the formation of the open complex initiating transcription.[48]

Pharmacodynamics

Rifamycins are bactericidal. This effect could be due to either the high stability of the complex formed between rifampin and the enzyme or

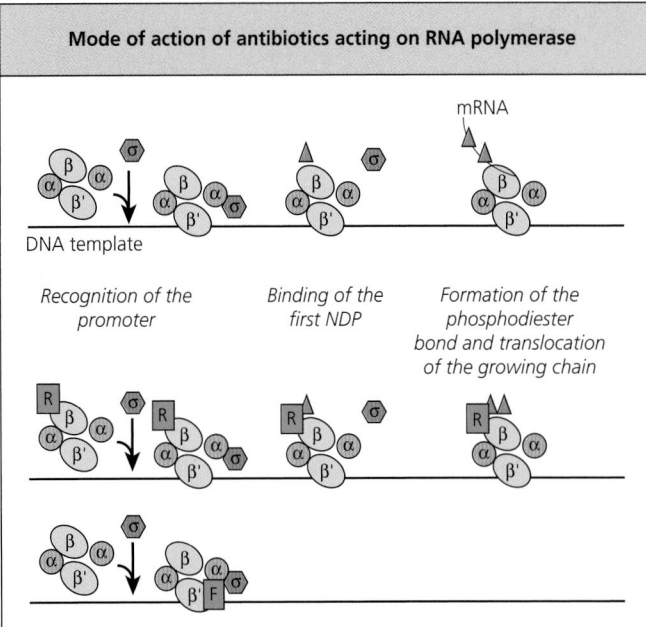

Figure 137-17 Mode of action of antibiotics acting on RNA polymerase. Synthesis of mRNA by RNA polymerase is shown in the upper panel and inhibition by rifamycins (R in the green squares) and by fidaxomicin (F in the green square) is shown in the lower panels. The RNA polymerase core is made up of four subunits, of which the β' subunit binds to the DNA template and the β subunit binds the ribonucleotide diphosphate (NDP; triangle). The σ factor only participates to the initiation step by allowing for the recognition by the enzyme core of promoter sequences on the DNA template. Rifamycins bind to the β subunit. They do not interfere with the binding of the nucleotide diphosphate, but rather inhibit the transcription initiation either by impairing the formation of the first phosphodiester bond or the translocation reaction of the newly synthesized dinucleotide. Fidaxomicin probably binds to the β' subunit and the σ factor, which inhibits transcription by blocking the formation of the transcriptionally competent complex.

the formation of superoxide ions of the quinone ring of the antibiotic molecule. Rifamycins show a long postantibiotic effect because of the irreversible character of their binding. The excellent penetration of rifamycins in eukaryotic cells has often been a major argument for supporting their use against intracellular organisms, including mycobacteria (exposure to critical concentrations of rifampin may be sufficient to kill intermittently metabolizing mycobacterial populations).[49]

Fidaxomicin shows excellent activity against *Clostridia*. Due to its null absorption, it shows high concentrations in the intestine, making it a drug of choice for the treatment of recurrent pseudomembranous colitis.[46]

Antimetabolites
SULFONAMIDES AND DIAMINOPYRIMIDINES

Prontosil (sulfamidochrysoidine, found by Domagk in 1932) was a prodrug which led to the development of the sulfonamides. With diaminopyrimidines, they inhibit the folate pathway in bacteria. Diaminopyrimidines are used in combination with sulfonamides except for specific indications (parasitic diseases) or for the treatment of uncomplicated cystitis.

Chemical Structure

Sulfonamides such as sulfamethoxazole (Figure 137-18a) are derived from *p*-amino-benzene-sulfonamide, which is a structural analog of *p*-aminobenzoic acid, a factor required by bacteria for folic acid synthesis. A free amino group at position 4 and a sulfonamide group at position 1 are required for antibacterial activity. Heterocyclic or

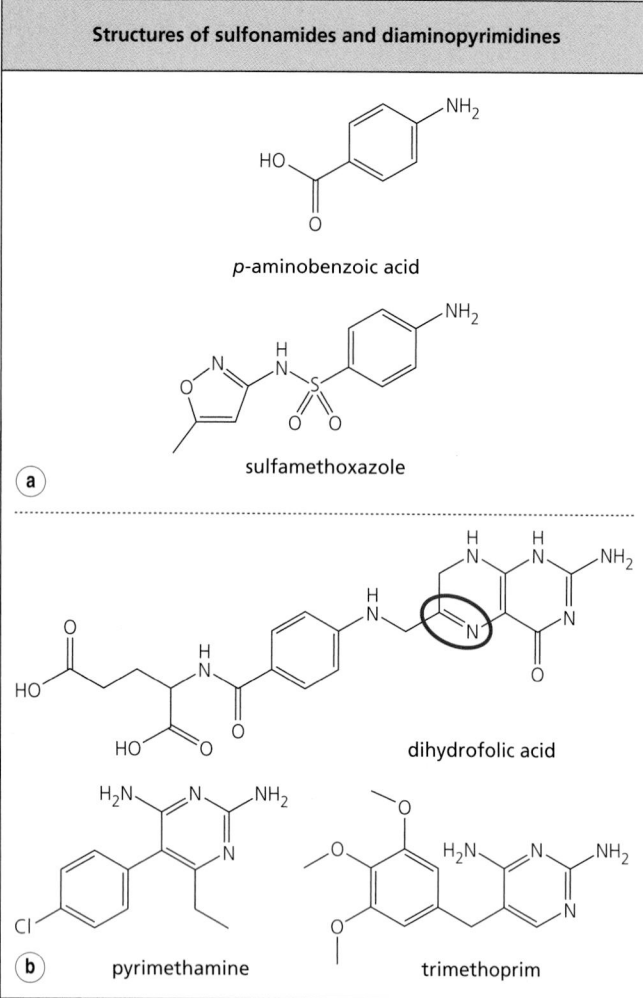

Structures of sulfonamides and diaminopyrimidines

p-aminobenzoic acid

sulfamethoxazole

(a)

dihydrofolic acid

pyrimethamine

trimethoprim

(b)

Figure 137-18 Structures of sulfonamides (a) and diaminopyrimidines (b). The figure highlights the similarity between these molecules and the substrates of the reactions with which they interfere, namely *p*-aminobenzoic acid (a) and dihydrofolic acid (b); in dihydrofolic acid, the red circle outlines the unsaturated positions that are reduced for conversion into tetrahydrofolic acid.

aromatic rings substituting the sulfonamide enhance this activity by modifying absorption and gastrointestinal tolerance.

Diaminopyrimidines such as trimethoprim and pyrimethamine (Figure 137-18b) are pyrimidines substituted at position 5 by an aromatic group (pyrimethamine has an additional ethyl substituent at position 6).

Mode of Action

Sulfonamides inhibit tetrahydrofolic acid synthesis, acting at the level of dihydropteroate synthetase as analogs of *p*-aminobenzoic acid (Figure 137-18a), and as alternative substrates to become incorporated into a product with pteridine.[50,51]

Diaminopyrimidines, which mimic the pteridine part of dihydrofolic acid (Figure 137-18b) are competitive inhibitors of bacterial dihydrofolate reductase.[50,51] Selectivity of action towards prokaryotes results from more binding interactions with the bacterial than with the corresponding eukaryotic enzymes.

Resistance

For sulfonamides, resistance mainly occurs from hyperproduction of *p*-aminobenzoic acid or a reduced affinity of dihydrofolate reductase for the antibiotic, causing resistance to the whole class. For

diaminopyrimidines, resistance mostly occurs via enzyme mutations which prevent binding and inhibition to the drug.[52]

Pharmacodynamics

Sulfonamides are bacteriostatic; however, in combination with diaminopyrimidines they are bactericidal.

Antibiotics Acting on the Membrane
LIPOPEPTIDES
Chemical Structure

Daptomycin is a cyclic peptide flanked by an oxodecyl side chain conferring a strong amphiphilic character to the molecule.

Mode of Action

Daptomycin binds to Ca^{2+} to form micelle-like oligomeric assemblies delivering daptomycin to the bacterial membrane in a 'detergent-like' form, causing leakage of cytosolic contents and a rapid bactericidal effect (Figure 137-19).[53] Daptomycin is only active against gram-positive bacteria since it cannot cross the outer membrane of gram-negative organisms. It is used against vancomycin-resistant enterococci and staphylococcal infections. Daptomycin shows preferential interaction with phosphatidylglycerol, a phospholipid abundant in prokaryotic cell membranes and largely absent from eukaryotic cell membranes, except in lung surfactant where it forms aggregates, thereby explaining the failure of daptomycin in treating pulmonary infections.

Resistance

Resistance to daptomycin results from mutations in genes encoding enzymes involved in the synthesis of phosphatidylglycerol. *Staph. aureus* with a VISA phenotype (see glycopeptides section) are less susceptible to daptomycin due to impaired access through the thickened cell wall.[9]

Pharmacodynamics

Daptomycin activity is concentration dependent, whereas its toxicity (mainly for skeletal muscle) is more related to the frequency of exposure. As a result, daptomycin should be administered once daily.

CYCLIC POLYPEPTIDES (POLYMYXINS/COLISTINS)
Chemical Structure

These are a collection of cyclic, branched polypeptides (molecular masses about 1000 Da) containing both cationic and hydrophobic amino acids. Some of these are of the D configuration or are non-DNA coded, which confers resistance to mammalian peptide-degrading enzymes. Polymyxins are obtained from *Bacillus polymyxa* and colistins from *Aerobacillus colistinus*. Only polymyxin B and colistin (identical to polymyxin E) are used in clinical practice. Commercial colistin contains at least two components (E1 and E2, also called colistin A and colistin B) differing by the length of the fatty acid chain.

Mode of Action

Because of their amphipathic character, polymyxins and colistins act as detergents and alter the permeability of the cytoplasmic membrane.[54] They therefore act at all stages of bacterial development. However, they cannot diffuse easily through the thick peptidoglycan layer of gram-positive bacteria. In contrast, they bind easily to the outer membrane of gram-negative bacteria (interacting with the lipopolysaccharide (LPS), displacing divalent cations that stabilize LPS and triggering a 'self-promoted uptake' process). The insertion of the hydrophobic moiety of the molecule in the membrane weakens the packing of fatty acyl chains and triggers the fusion of the inner leaflets of the outer membrane and the outer leaflet of the cytoplasmic membrane, causing osmotic imbalance and driving the antibiotic into the cytoplasmic membrane through polar and nonpolar channels (Figure 137-19). These properties explain their strong and fast bactericidal activity through disruption of membranes and their essentially gram-negative spectrum.

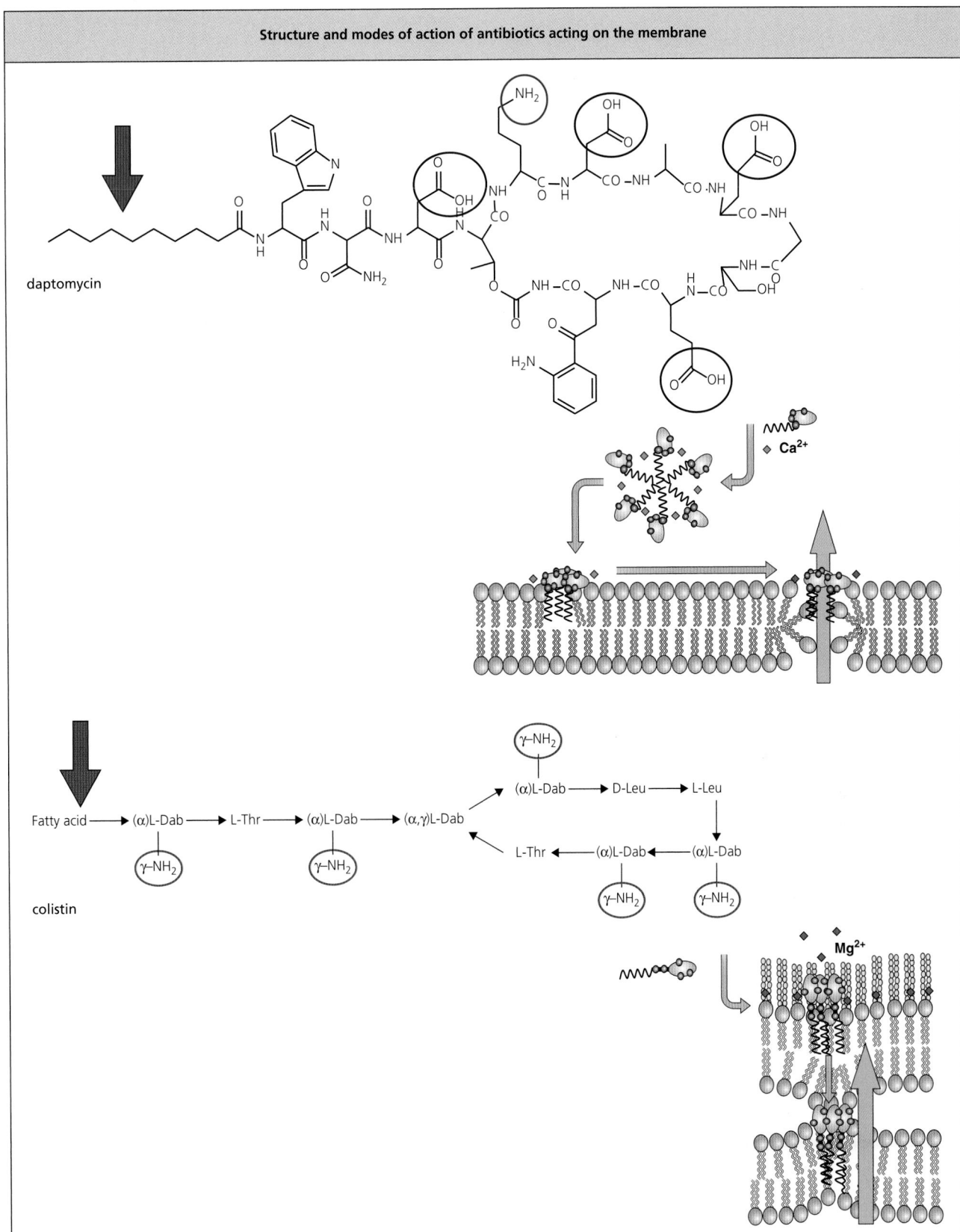

Figure 137-19   Structure and modes of action of antibiotics acting on the membrane. Daptomycin is a cyclic, polar depsipeptide (the ionizable residues are circled) flanked with a lipophilic oxodecyl side chain (purple arrow) conferring to the molecule a marked amphiphilic character. In the presence of Ca²⁺, daptomycin forms loose micelles that serve as a delivery system to the bacterial membrane where the drug lipophilic side chain can then interact with the fatty acid chains of the phospholipids causing permeabilization and rapid bacterial death. As for lipoglycopeptides, specificity towards bacterial membranes stems from the fact that daptomycin–membrane interactions are favored by the presence of phosphatidylglycerol, an acidic phospholipid abundant in bacterial but not in eukaryotic cell membranes (it is, however, present in lung surfactant, causing daptomycin inactivation in this environment and explaining clinical failures in pulmonary infections). Colistin is a cyclic polycationic peptide (the ionizable residues are circled) substituted by an alkyl chain (purple arrow) (the ionizable residues are circled). Colistin interacts with LPS at the outer leaflet of the outer membrane from which it displaces Mg²⁺ ions. The insertion of the hydrophobic chain in the membrane weakens the packing of fatty acyl chains causing expansion of the outer membrane monolayer favouring its fusion with the outer leaflet of the cytoplasmic membrane. Colistin then transits to the outer leaflet of the inner membrane by a self-promoted uptake mechanism and disrupts membrane integrity. *(Modified from Van Bambeke et al.[30])*

Resistance

Acquired resistance to polymyxins and colistins is chromosomal (but plasmid-mediated resistance has been recently observed in animal isolates in China) and globally results from decreased permeability of the outer membrane secondary to changes in its biochemical composition.[54] Bacteria with decreased sensitivity are characterized by a decreased phospholipid/lipid ratio and a higher content of divalent cations (Ca^{2+}, Mg^{2+}). Protein H1 from *P. aeruginosa* (OprH) prevents binding of polymyxins and colistins to lipopolysaccharide, and its overproduction correlates with reduced sensitivity. However, this change is not sufficient *per se* and must be combined with other modifications of the membrane; two genes downstream to OprH (PhoP and PhoQ) co-regulate OprH and polymyxin B resistance. Other mechanisms have been described like a loss of LPS production or a decrease of its anionic character, changes in the expression of outer membrane proteins, and active efflux. Resistance to polymyxins and colistins was previously uncommon but is now increasingly described in strains exhibiting multiple resistance to β-lactams and aminoglycosides. A puzzling observation is that the regrowth is easily observed *in vitro*, suggesting the occurrence of a so-called 'adaptive resistance', the mechanism of which is still uncertain.

Pharmacodynamics

Colistin A and polymyxin B show concentration-dependent activity and little or no postantibiotic effect, justifying the administration of repeated daily doses. It is proposed that the pharmacodynamic parameter governing the activity of colistin is the free AUC/MIC ratio.[55] Yet, exposure is still suboptimal in many patients if using the currently recommended doses.

Non-antibiotic Pharmacologic and Toxicologic Properties Related to Chemical Structure

As membrane-disrupting and lipid-binding agents, polymyxins and colistins display a number of non-antibiotic effects. Some of them are potentially useful, such as inactivation of endotoxins and synergy with serum bactericidal activities.[56] Others, however, are highly detrimental to the host and include activation of the alternate complement pathway, mastocyte degranulation with histamine release, decreased production of cytokines (but increased tumor necrosis factor release), increased membrane conductance in epithelia, and apoptosis.

Antibiotics Acting on ATP Synthase

Diarylquinolines are inhibitors of mycobacterial ATP synthase (a mechanism not exploited so far in Mycobacteriaceae) and show activity even on dormant organisms.[57] Bedaquiline is the first in this series to have been approved to treat multidrug-resistant tuberculosis.

References available online at expertconsult.com.

KEY REFERENCES

Artsimovitch I., Seddon J., Sears P.: Fidaxomicin is an inhibitor of the initiation of bacterial RNA synthesis. *Clin Infect Dis* 2012; 55(Suppl. 2):S127-S131.

Bozdogan B., Appelbaum P.C.: Oxazolidinones: activity, mode of action, and mechanism of resistance. *Int J Antimicrob Agents* 2004; 23(2):113-119.

Bush K., Jacoby G.A., Medeiros A.A.: A functional classification scheme for beta-lactamases and its correlation with molecular structure. *Antimicrob Agents Chemother* 1995; 39(6):1211-1233.

Chopra I., Roberts M.: Tetracycline antibiotics: mode of action, applications, molecular biology, and epidemiology of bacterial resistance. *Microbiol Mol Biol Rev* 2001; 65(2):232-260.

Fishovitz J., Rojas-Altuve A., Otero L.H., et al.: Disruption of allosteric response as an unprecedented mechanism of resistance to antibiotics. *J Am Chem Soc* 2014; 136(28):9814-9817.

Locke J.B., Finn J., Hilgers M., et al.: Structure-activity relationships of diverse oxazolidinones for linezolid-resistant *Staphylococcus aureus* strains possessing the *cfr* methyltransferase gene or ribosomal mutations. *Antimicrob Agents Chemother* 2010; 54(12):5337-5343.

Mingeot-Leclercq M.P., Glupczynski Y., Tulkens P.M.: Aminoglycosides: activity and resistance. *Antimicrob Agents Chemother* 1999; 43(4):727-737.

Van Bambeke F., Harms J.M., Van Laethem Y., et al.: Ketolides: pharmacological profile and rational positioning in the treatment of respiratory tract infections. *Expert Opin Pharmacother* 2008; 9(2):267-283.

Van Bambeke F., Michot J.M., Van Eldere J., et al.: Quinolones in 2005: an update. *Clin Microbiol Infect* 2005; 11(4):256-280.

Van Bambeke F., Van Laethem Y., Courvalin P., et al.: Glycopeptide antibiotics: from conventional molecules to new derivatives. *Drugs* 2004; 64(9):913-936.

Velkov T., Roberts K.D., Nation R.L., et al.: Pharmacology of polymyxins: new insights into an 'old' class of antibiotics. *Future Microbiol* 2013; 8(6):711-724.

138

Mechanisms of Antibacterial Resistance

GIAN MARIA ROSSOLINI | FABIO ARENA | TOMMASO GIANI

KEY CONCEPTS

- Unlike other drugs, antibiotics tend to lose their efficacy over time due to the emergence of microbial drug resistance.

- No antibiotic has escaped resistance, which has often emerged soon after the introduction of the antibiotic in clinical practice.

- Several biochemical mechanisms can be responsible for antibiotic resistance, including drug inactivation, target modification or by-pass, and reduced drug uptake.

- Resistance can be a feature typical of a bacterial species (intrinsic resistance) or acquired by individual strains of a species that are naturally susceptible (acquired resistance).

- Acquired resistance can emerge due to chromosomal mutations or acquisition of resistance genes by horizontal gene transfer mechanisms.

- Resistance to multiple antibiotics can be acquired by individual strains, resulting in multidrug-resistant (MDR) phenotypes.

- The acquisition of multiple resistance determinants can eventually result in strains that remain susceptible to only a few antibiotics, designated as extremely drug-resistant (XDR) strains.

Introduction

The activity of antibiotics against bacterial pathogens is a prerequisite for clinical efficacy. To this purpose, the activity of antibiotics against bacterial pathogens is normally measured by standardized laboratory methods for determining susceptibility and resistance. Infections caused by bacterial strains that are categorized as susceptible to an antibiotic can be treated with that drug with a high likelihood of clinical success (although additional factors can contribute to determine the eventual outcome). On the other hand, infections caused by bacterial strains that are categorized as resistant to an antibiotic are likely not to respond to treatment with that drug, which should not be used for treatment.[1] Categorization of bacterial strains as susceptible or resistant following susceptibility testing is based on comparison of results with reference values of minimal inhibitory concentrations (or of zone inhibition diameters) indicated as clinical breakpoints.

The biochemical mechanisms by which bacteria resist the inhibitory action of antibiotics include:
- the presence of an enzyme that inactivates the antibiotic;
- modification of the antibiotic target by mutation or by posttranslational mechanisms which reduce binding of the antibiotic to the target;
- by-pass of the function dependent on the antibiotic target by an alternative enzyme that is not inhibited by the antibiotic; and
- reduced uptake of the antibiotic inside the cell, due to reduced permeability of the cell envelopes or to active efflux.

When a resistance mechanism is present and functional in most or all strains of a bacterial species, the species is categorized as intrinsically resistant to the antibiotic(s) affected by that mechanism and resistance can be directly predicted from bacterial identification (Table 138-1). On the other hand, acquired resistance occurs when strains of a susceptible species acquire one or more resistance mechanisms. Acquired resistance is not predictable from species identification, and the purpose of *in vitro* susceptibility testing in the laboratory is to identify acquired resistance among infecting pathogens isolated from clinical specimens, to guide the choice of definitive antimicrobial therapy.

Acquired resistance can be due to mutations of chromosomal genes or to the acquisition of resistance determinants by horizontal gene transfer mechanisms. Transferable resistance genes are usually carried by plasmids or other types of mobile genetic elements (MGEs), and play a relevant contribution to the evolution of microbial drug resistance.

There is a strong correlation between the presence of some resistance determinants and the outcome of antimicrobial therapy. For instance, the presence of the *mecA* gene in *Staphylococcus aureus* is highly predictive of methicillin resistance and, therefore, resistance to all conventional β-lactam antibiotics. However, the presence of a resistance gene is not equivalent to treatment failure: the gene also must be expressed in sufficient amounts to lead to phenotypic resistance.

Resistance to β-Lactam Antibiotics

β-Lactam antibiotics interfere with peptidoglycan synthesis by inhibition of enzymes, called penicillin-binding proteins (PBPs), that are responsible for the formation of the peptide bonds which cross-link the peptidoglycan chains. Penicillin is the oldest β-lactam antibiotic, and the active β-lactam ring has been exploited to obtain a broad array of β-lactam antibiotics, including penicillins, cephalosporins, monobactams and carbapenems, characterized by different antimicrobial spectra and pharmacokinetic properties. Overall, β-lactams are among the most prescribed antibiotics in clinical practice due to their efficacy, safety and versatility.

Resistance to β-lactams can be caused by different mechanisms including: 1) the production of β-lactamases, which destroy the β-lactam ring; 2) the presence of altered PBPs, which have lower affinity for β-lactams; and 3) a reduced permeability of the outer membrane or active efflux of the drug from the periplasmic space, which impair the access of β-lactams to their PBP targets (in gram-negative bacteria).

β-LACTAMASE-MEDIATED RESISTANCE

Production of β-lactamase activity is a common mechanism of intrinsic and acquired resistance to β-lactams in gram-positive and gram-negative pathogens and, in the latter, is overall the most important mechanism of β-lactam resistance.

The number of β-lactamases detected in pathogenic bacteria has risen steadily since the introduction of penicillin. β-Lactamases have been classified according to their functional properties, considering the substrate preference and the behavior towards some inhibitors (Table 138-2).[2] From the clinical standpoint, the most challenging enzymes are: 1) the extended-spectrum β-lactamases (ESBLs), which are able to hydrolyze penicillins, cephalosporins (both narrow- and expanded-spectrum) and monobactams; 2) the carbapenemases, which are able to hydrolyze carbapenems and usually most other β-lactams.

β-lactamases have also been classified according to the amino acid sequence similarity and mechanistic features into four molecular

TABLE 138-1 **Examples of Intrinsic Resistances of Some Gram-Positive and Gram-Negative Pathogens**

Gram-positives[a]	Fusidic Acid	Ceftazidime	Cephalosporins (Except Ceftazidime)	Erythromycin	Clindamycin	Quinupristin–dalfopristin	Vancomycin	Teicoplanin
Staphylococcus aureus		R						
Streptococcus spp.	R							
Enterococcus faecalis	R	R	R	R	R	R		
Enterococcus faecium	R	R	R	R				
Listeria monocytogenes		R	R					
Leuconostoc spp., Pediococcus spp.							R	R

Gram-negatives[b]	Ampicillin	Amoxicillin–clavulanate	Piperacillin	Cefotaxime	Cefoxitin	Tetracyclines/ Tigecycline	Polymyxins	Ertapenem	Meropenem	Trimethoprim–sulfamethoxazole
Citrobacter freundii	R	R			R					
Enterobacter cloacae	R	R			R					
Klebsiella spp.	R									
Proteus mirabilis						R	R			
Serratia marcescens		R					R			
Pseudomonas aeruginosa	R	R		R	R	R		R		R
Acinetobacter baumannii	R	R		R	R			R		
Stenotrophomonas maltophilia	R	R	R	R	R			R	R	

[a]Gram-positive bacteria are also intrinsically resistant to aztreonam, temocillin, polymyxins and nalidixic acid.
[b]Gram-negative bacteria are also intrinsically resistant to glycopeptides, lincosamides, daptomycin and linezolid.
Modified from EUCAST expert rules in antimicrobial susceptibility testing, version 2 (www.eucast.org).

TABLE 138-2	Classification of β-Lactamases Based on Relevant Functional Properties and Molecular Class					
	RELEVANT FUNCTIONAL CHARACTERISTICS					
			Behavior With Inhibitors*			
Functional Group (Bush–Jacoby)	**Substrate Preference**		**SBLI**	**EDTA**	**Molecular Class**	**Representative Enzymes**
1	Cephalosporins (including cephamycins)		R	R	C	AmpC of *Pseudomonas aeruginosa*, ACT-1, CMY-1, FOX-1
1e	Same as group 1, but increased hydrolysis of oxyiminocephalosporins		R	R	C	GC1 of *Enterobacter cloacae* CMY-19, CMY-37
2a	Penicillins		S	R	A	PC1
2b	Penicillins, narrow-spectrum cephalosporins (broad-spectrum)		S	R	A	TEM-1, TEM-2, SHV-1
2be	Same as group 2b, but including expanded-spectrum cephalosporins and monobactams (extended-spectrum)		S	R	A	TEM-3, SHV-12, CTX-M-15, PER-1, VEB-1
2br	Same as group 2b but resistant to SBLI		R	R	A	TEM-30, SHV-10
2ber	Same as group 2be but resistant to SBLI		R	R	A	TEM-50
2c	Carbenicillin		S	R	A	PSE-1, CARB-3
2ce	Same as group 2c, but including oxyiminocephalosporins		S	R	A	RTG-4
2d	Penicillins (including cloxacillin)		V	R	D	OXA-1, OXA-2, OXA-10
2de	Same as group 2d, but including oxyiminocephalosporins (extended-spectrum)		V	R	D	OXA-11, OXA-15
2df	Penicillins, carbapenems		V	R	D	OXA-23, OXA-24, OXA-48
2e	Cephalosporins (excluding cephamycins)		S	R	A	CepA of *Bacteroides fragilis*
2f	Broad-spectrum including carbapenems		V	R	A	KPC-2, IMI-1, SME-1
3a	Broad-spectrum including carbapenems (not active on monobactams)		R	S	B (B1, B3)	IMP-1, VIM-1, NDM-1 L1 of *Stenotrophomonas maltophilia*
3b	Carbapenems (not active on monobactams)		R	S	B (B2)	CphA of *Aeromonas hydrophila*

*SBLI, mechanism-based serine β-lactamase inhibitors including clavulanate, sulbactam, tazobactam and avibactam; R, resistant; S, susceptible; V, variable susceptibility.
Adapted from Bush K., Jacoby G.A. Antimicrob Agents Chemother 2010; 54(3):969–76.

classes. Enzymes of classes A, C and D have a serine residue at their active site, whereas those of class B require a zinc co-factor for activity (metallo-β-lactamases, MBLs). The relationships between structure and function are complex: members of the same molecular class exhibit some conserved functional properties (dependent on the structural features and catalytic mechanism defining the class), but can also exhibit significant functional diversity, while functional similarities can exist among enzymes of different classes (Table 138-2).[2]

Class A β-lactamases are found as resident chromosomally-encoded enzymes in some species (e.g. *Klebsiella pneumoniae*, *Citrobacter koseri*, *Proteus vulgaris*, *Bacteroides fragilis*) and are among the most prevalent acquired plasmid-encoded β-lactamases encountered in the clinical setting. They include, for instance, the plasmid-encoded broad-spectrum TEM-1, TEM-2 and SHV-1 enzymes that have emerged and broadly disseminated in Enterobacteriaceae since the 1970s and have contributed the most common mechanism of acquired resistance to amino-penicillins in enterobacterial species such as *Escherichia coli*, *Proteus mirabilis* and *Salmonella enterica*. Their activity is usually inhibited by clavulanic acid, sulbactam, tazobactam and avibactam, thereby rendering penicillin derivatives active again. The broad-spectrum TEM and SHV β-lactamases are not active against the expanded-spectrum cephalosporins (e.g. cefotaxime, ceftriaxone and ceftazidime). However, under the selective pressure generated by the use of the latter compounds, the TEM and SHV enzymes have shown the ability to evolve an expanded spectrum of activity through mutations at specific positions, which may lead to resistance against the

expanded-spectrum cephalosporins and monobactams.[3] These TEM- and SHV-type ESBL derivatives, of which a large number of variants have been described (http://www.lahey.org/studies/), have played an important role in the evolution of resistance to expanded-spectrum cephalosporins among Enterobacteriaceae since the mid-1980s.

On the other hand, the TEM and SHV enzymes have also shown the ability to evolve mutations that confer resistance to β-lactamase inhibitors.[4] More recently, plasmid-encoded class A ESBLs other than TEM and SHV derivatives have also emerged in Enterobacteriaceae. Of these, the CTX-M-type enzymes have been the most successful. In fact, they have largely replaced the TEM- and SHV-type ESBLs in many clinical settings, and are currently the most prevalent ESBLs in Enterobacteriaceae from several regions.[5] The class A β-lactamases also include some enzymes with carbapenemase activity: the most important are the KPC-type (after *Klebsiella pneumoniae carbapenemase*) enzymes, which emerged in the late 1990s and have thenceforth disseminated worldwide providing a major contribution as a carbapenem resistance mechanism in carbapenem-resistant Enterobacteriaceae (CRE).[6]

Class C β-lactamases (also called AmpC-type enzymes) are found as resident chromosomally-encoded β-lactamases in several gram-negative bacilli including *Pseudomonas aeruginosa*, *Acinetobacter baumannii*, and some members of the family Enterobacteriaceae (e.g. *Citrobacter freundii*, *Enterobacter cloacae*, *Serratia marcescens* and *Morganella morganii*). Production of these enzymes is normally regulated and contributes to intrinsic resistance to those β-lactams that act as inducers and are hydrolyzed by the enzyme (e.g. ampicillin and narrow-spectrum cephalosporins). *Escherichia coli* is also provided with a chromosomally-encoded class C β-lactamase, but normally the gene is expressed only at negligible levels and is not inducible, which explains why most *Escherichia coli* strains remain susceptible to ampicillin and narrow-spectrum cephalosporins.[7] Some genes encoding AmpC-type enzymes have been mobilized to plasmids and can disseminate by horizontal transfer. These plasmid-encoded AmpC-type β-lactamases are usually produced constitutively, and their prevalence among Enterobacteriaceae is increasing.[4] Class C β-lactamases are active against penicillins and many cephalosporins (including cephamycins and some expanded-spectrum cephalosporins, but usually not cefepime), are not inhibited by clavulanic acid, sulbactam or tazobactam, but are inhibited by cloxacillin and avibactam.[7]

Class D β-lactamases (also called OXA-type enzymes after their efficient hydrolysis of oxacillin) are found as resident chromosomally-encoded enzymes in several bacterial species, and also as plasmid-encoded enzymes. They were originally considered to be less important due to their overall lower diffusion and narrow substrate profile (including penicillins and some narrow-spectrum cephalosporins). However, the recent emergence of plasmid-encoded class D enzymes endowed with carbapenemase activity, which are spreading among major gram-negative pathogens including *Acinetobacter* spp. (e.g. OXA-23, OXA-24 and OXA-58) and members of the family Enterobacteriaceae (e.g. OXA-48) and which are responsible for acquired carbapenem resistance in those species,[4] has remarkably increased the clinical relevance of these enzymes. Class D enzymes are usually resistant to clavulanate, sulbactam and tazobactam and, when co-produced with class A β-lactamases, can be responsible for an inhibitor-resistant phenotype.

Class B β-lactamases are zinc-dependent enzymes whose catalytic mechanism is completely different from that of the serine-β-lactamases. MBLs are resistant to serine-β-lactamase inhibitors including the diazabicyclooctane derivatives such as avibactam, and unlike serine-β-lactamases, are inhibited by EDTA. The clinical importance of MBLs is largely related with their constant and efficient carbapenemase activity, and their spectrum often extends to most other β-lactams. MBLs are found as resident chromosomally-encoded enzymes in some environmental species of low pathogenic potential (e.g. *Stenotrophomonas maltophilia, Aeromonas hydrophila, Elizabethkingia meningoseptica, Chryseobacterium indologenes*), but since the mid-1990s several plasmid-encoded MBLs have emerged as acquired carbapenemases in isolates of gram-negative non-fermenters and of Enterobacteriaceae. The VIM, NDM and IMP-type enzymes are currently the most prevalent and widespread acquired MBLs encountered among clinical isolates.[8]

β-LACTAM RESISTANCE MEDIATED BY ALTERED PBPS

Altered PBPs are also a major cause of resistance against β-lactam antibiotics, especially among gram-positive cocci. Acquisition of a novel PBP, which takes over the functions of the resident PBPs and is not inhibited by conventional β-lactams, is responsible for methicillin resistance in staphylococci. Both methicillin-resistant *Staph. aureus* (MRSA) and methicillin-resistant coagulase-negative staphylococci are important causes of difficult-to-treat nosocomial infections. Moreover, community-associated and livestock-associated MRSA strains have emerged, compounding the epidemiology of MRSA infections.[9,10] The modified PBP associated with methicillin resistance (PBP2a) is encoded by the *mecA* gene. Regulation of methicillin resistance is complex. Expression can be heterogeneous, whereby only a few cells express the phenotype. The *mecA* determinant apparently originated from some coagulase-negative staphylococci, and is associated with a peculiar type of MGE, named staphylococcal chromosome cassette *mec* (SCC*mec*), which is able to integrate at a specific locus (*orfX* gene) of the staphylococcal chromosome. Several types of SCC*mec* elements have been described, based on the type of *ccr* recombinase genes (involved in the mobilization of SCC elements) and on the structure

of the genetic context of the *mecA* gene.[9] Recently, *mecA*-negative MRSA strains carrying a second type of *mec* gene, named *mecC*, have been detected from animal and human infections. The *mecC* gene is about 30% divergent from *mecA* and is not detected by molecular probes targeting *mecA*.[11]

Resistance to penicillin in *Streptococcus pneumoniae* is due to the presence of altered PBPs, encoded by genes that have undergone recombination with PBP genes from other species, to yield mosaic PBPs.[12] On the other hand, in *Enterococcus faecium* mutations in PBP5 can be responsible for resistance to ampicillin, which is frequently detected in this species.[13] β-Lactam resistance by altered PBP targets can also be encountered in some gram-negative pathogens including *Neisseria gonorrhoeae, Neisseria meningitidis* and *Haemophilus influenzae*.[14]

β-LACTAM RESISTANCE MEDIATED BY IMPERMEABILITY OR EFFLUX

Reduced drug uptake is the third major mechanism responsible for β-lactam resistance in gram-negative bacteria, where β-lactams need to enter the periplasmic space to bind the PBP targets located in the cytoplasmic membrane. In fact, in gram-negative bacteria, the activity of β-lactams against the bacterial cell depends on the complex interplay of a number of factors (Figure 138-1), including:
- the concentration of the antibiotic in the environment;
- the rate of antibiotic entry through the outer membrane;
- the amount of β-lactamase produced;
- the catalytic efficiency of the β-lactamase for the antibiotic; and
- the affinity of the PBPs for the antibiotic.

Reduced drug uptake can be due either to a reduction or alteration in the porin channels used by β-lactams to cross the outer membrane, or to the presence of efflux pumps that can actively extrude β-lactams from the periplasmic space.

Reduced uptake is often encountered as a β-lactam resistance mechanism in *Pseudomonas aeruginosa*, but also in *Acinetobacter baumannii* and Enterobacteriaceae. In *Pseudomonas aeruginosa*, mutational loss or alterations of the OprD2 porin, which is the entry channel for carbapenems, is one of the most common mechanisms of acquired resistance to these drugs, while upregulation of the resident RND-type MexAB multidrug efflux pump can contribute to acquired resistance to several β-lactams which are effluxed by the pump from the periplasmic space, including meropenem, and anti-pseudomonas cephalosporins and penicillins.[15]

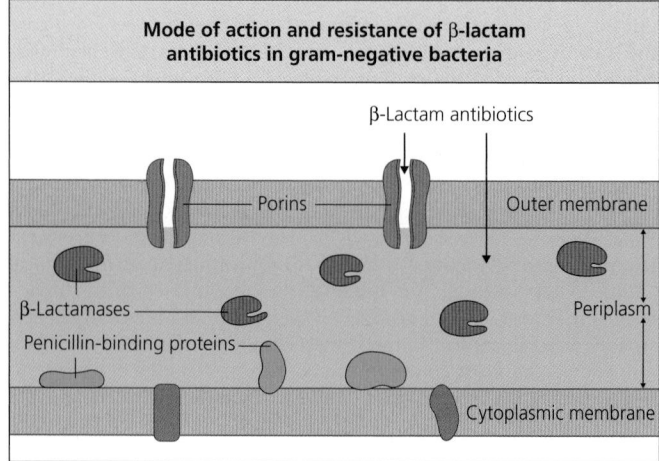

Figure 138-1 Mode of action and resistance of β-lactam antibiotics in gram-negative bacteria. In gram-negative bacteria, β-lactam activity depends on the complex interplay among several factors, including the concentration of the drug in the environment, the rate of entry through the outer membrane (usually across porins), the amount of β-lactamase produced and present in the periplasmic space, the catalytic efficiency of the β-lactamase for the antibiotic, and the affinity of the antibiotic for the penicillin-binding protein (PBP) targets, located in the cytoplasmic membrane.

TABLE 138-3	Characteristics of a Selected Set of Aminoglycoside-Modifying Enzymes				
				DISTRIBUTION	
Resistance Mechanism	Name	Resistance Phenotype*	Gram-negative		Gram-positive
N-acetyltransferases (AAC)	AAC(3)-I	Gm	Enterobacteriaceae, *Acinetobacter baumannii*, *Pseudomonas aeruginosa*		
	AAC(3)-II	Gm,Tm	Enterobacteriaceae		
	AAC(3)-III	Gm,Tm	*Pseudomonas* spp.		
	AAC(3)-IV	Gm,Tm	Enterobacteriaceae		
	AAC(3)-VI	Gm	Enterobacteriaceae		
	AAC(6′)-I	Ak, Tm	Enterobacteriaceae, *Acinetobacter* spp., *Pseudomonas aeruginosa*		*Enterococcus* spp.
	AAC(6′)-II	Gm, Tm	Enterobacteriaceae, *Pseudomonas* spp.		
	AAC(6′)-Ib-cr	Ak, Tm†	Enterobacteriaceae		
	AAC(6′)-APH(2″)	Ak, Gm, Tm, Sm			*Enterococcus* spp., *Staphylococcus* spp.
O-nucleotydyltransferases (ANT)	ANT(2″)-I	Gm, Tm	Enterobacteriaceae, *Pseudomonas aeruginosa*, *Acinetobacter baumannii*		
	ANT(3″)-I	Sm	Enterobacteriaceae, *Pseudomonas aeruginosa*, *Acinetobacter baumannii*		
	ANT(4′)-I	Ak, Tm			*Enterococcus* spp., *Staphylococcus* spp.
	ANT(4′)-II	Ak, Tm	Enterobacteriaceae, *Pseudomonas aeruginosa*, *Acinetobacter baumannii*		
	ANT(6)-I	Sm			*Enterococcus* spp., *Staphylococcus* spp., *Streptococcus* spp.
	ANT(9)-I	Sm			*Enterococcus* spp., *Staphylococcus* spp.
O-phosphotransferases (APH)	APH(3′)-III	Ak			*Staphylococcus aureus*, *Enterococcus* spp.
	APH(3′)-VI	Ak	Enterobacteriaceae, *Acinetobacter baumannii*		
	APH(6)-I	Sm	Enterobacteriaceae, *Pseudomonas aeruginosa*		

*Only the clinically relevant antibiotics are listed: Ak, amikacin; Gm, gentamicin; Tm, tobramycin; Sm, streptomycin.
†Also confers decreased susceptibility to some quinolones.
Data from Vakulenko S.B., Mobashery S. Clin Microbiol Rev 2003; 16(3):430–50 and Ramirez M.S., Tolmasky M.E. Drug Resist Updat 2010; 13(6):151–71.

In Enterobacteriaceae, reduced uptake by mutational loss or alteration of some porins, in combination with the overproduction of ESBLs or AmpC-type β-lactamases, can be responsible for a low-level carbapenem resistance phenotype that can be selected during carbapenem treatment.[16]

Resistance to Aminoglycosides

The first clinically effective aminoglycoside introduced in clinical practice was streptomycin, in the 1940s. Numerous aminoglycosides have since been isolated and synthetic derivatives were also produced. The most important aminoglycoside antibiotics for clinical practice are gentamicin, tobramycin, amikacin and streptomycin. They have an overall broad antimicrobial spectrum but are not active against anaerobes.

Aminoglycosides bind to the bacterial ribosome (30S subunit) and interfere with protein synthesis exerting a bactericidal action. To reach the ribosomal target, aminoglycosides enter the cytoplasmic membrane via an energy-dependent transport mechanism which is not active in anaerobes. In gram-negative bacteria, aminoglycosides first bind to anionic sites on the cell envelope. This binding displaces magnesium ions and allows entry of the aminoglycosides across the outer membrane.

Inactivation of aminoglycosides by aminoglycoside-modifying enzymes (AMEs) is the most common mechanism of acquired resistance against these antibiotics. Other resistance mechanisms include ribosomal target modification and reduced drug uptake. Aminoglycoside resistance genes encoding AMEs or rRNA methylases that modify the ribosomal target are believed to originate from genes present in aminoglycoside-producing species (e.g. *Streptomyces griseus*).

AMEs belong to three major classes, depending on the type of modification that causes inactivation: phosphotransferases (APH), acetyltransferases (AAC) and nucleotidyltransferases (ANT). Each class includes several enzymes that may differ by the site of modification on the substrate and by the substrate specificity (Table 138-3).[17,18] Often AMEs are able to modify several structurally related aminoglycosides, and the spectrum of resistance conferred by each enzyme depends on the substrate specificity. Some AMEs are bifunctional enzymes that can modify aminoglycosides by two different mechanisms. One such enzyme is the bifunctional AAC(6′)-APH(2″) enzyme, which is encoded by transposon Tn*4001* found in *Staph. aureus* and in *Enterococcus faecalis* isolates, that apparently arose through the fusion of two genes, each encoding one of the partners. The AMEs must inactivate their targets before they reach the ribosomes and are either located inside the cell or associated with the cytoplasmic membrane.

AMEs can be found as acquired resistance determinants in gram-positive and gram-negative bacterial pathogens. In staphylococci, aminoglycoside resistance mediated by AMEs is well documented. In enterococci, the acquisition of AMEs such as the bifunctional enzyme AAC(6′)-Ie-APH(2″)-Ia, is of clinical relevance since it is responsible for high-level aminoglycoside resistance and the loss of synergistic action with β-lactams.[17] In gram-negative bacilli, a large number of acquired AMEs has been detected, which can variably contribute to resistance to the various aminoglycosides. Some species have resident chromosomal AMEs that may contribute to the intrinsic resistance of that species versus some aminoglycosides (e.g. *Serratia marcescens*, which produces a chromosomally-encoded AAC(6′)-Ic enzyme that affects the activity of all aminoglycosides except streptomycin and gentamicin).[18]

Modification of the ribosomal binding site is another resistance mechanism to aminoglycosides. Modification can consist in methylation of the rRNA or in mutation of some ribosomal proteins. Methylation of rRNA can confer a high-level broad-spectrum aminoglycoside resistance including gentamicin, tobramycin and amikacin. Several types of plasmid-encoded 16S rRNA methylases have been discovered, spreading among gram-negative pathogens including Enterobacteriaceae and gram-negative non-fermenters. The most widespread 16S rRNA methylases are the ArmA and RmtB enzymes that have been detected worldwide in isolates from both human and animal origin and are often co-expressed with other clinically-relevant resistance determinants.[19]

Mutation of the S12 protein in the small ribosomal subunit can be associated with resistance to streptomycin.

Reduced uptake has also been reported as a mechanism of aminoglycoside resistance. In *Pseudomonas aeruginosa*, in particular, mutational upregulation of the resident RND-type MexXY efflux system can be responsible for acquired resistance to multiple aminoglycosides.[20]

Resistance to Quinolones

Quinolone antibiotics exert their antibacterial effects by inhibition of certain bacterial topoisomerase enzymes, namely DNA gyrase and topoisomerase IV. These bacterial enzymes regulate the topology of the bacterial chromosome (which is maintained in a supercoiled state) and their function is essential in chromosomal replication, segregation, transcription, recombination and repair. DNA gyrase and topoisomerase IV are heterotetrameric proteins composed of two subunits, designated A and B. The genes encoding the A and B subunits are referred to as *gyrA* and *gyrB* (DNA gyrase) or *parC* and *parE* (DNA topoisomerase IV; *grlA* and *grlB* in *Staph. aureus*). Quinolones bind to the quinolone-binding pocket of DNA topoisomerases while they are working on DNA by forming a ternary complex (enzyme–DNA–quinolone). This interaction blocks the enzyme activity and eventually results in DNA fragmentation and rapid killing of the bacterial cell.

The affinity of quinolones for their dual topoisomerase targets can be different depending on the quinolone and on the bacterial species. In gram-negatives, DNA gyrase is the primary target for most quinolones, whereas topoisomerase IV appears to be the primary target in *Staph. aureus* and *Strep. pneumoniae*. However, different quinolones can have different primary targets in the same bacterial species and the primary target can be dependent on the bacterial species as well as on the quinolone structure. For instance, in *Strep. pneumoniae* topoisomerase IV is the primary target for ciprofloxacin while DNA gyrase is the primary target for sparfloxacin.

Resistance to quinolones can be due to several different mechanisms including: 1) topoisomerase target modification by mutation; 2) reduced drug uptake by reduced permeability or active efflux; 3) topoisomerase target protection by specific proteins; and 4) drug inactivation. These mechanisms can variably cooperate among each other to increase stepwise the resistance level to quinolones.

QUINOLONE RESISTANCE BY TARGET MODIFICATION

Alterations of the target topoisomerases by mutations that reduce the affinity for quinolones without compromising the enzyme function are overall the most common mechanism of acquired resistance to quinolones and have been reported in many bacterial species.[21] The mutations associated with resistance are clustered in discrete regions of the enzyme subunits, which are called quinolone resistance determining regions (QRDRs). In most cases, the amino acid substitutions within the QRDR involve the replacement of a hydroxyl group with a bulky hydrophobic residue that alters the geometry of the quinolone-binding pocket present in the enzyme and impedes binding of the quinolone molecule.[22]

In *Escherichia coli* and other gram-negatives, DNA gyrase is usually the primary target and the first-step mutations leading to quinolone resistance usually occur in the QRDR of GyrA and also GyrB. Although quinolones are thought to interact primarily with the A subunit of DNA gyrase, there are mutations in the B subunit that also confer quinolone resistance in some species. However, the frequency of GyrB mutations has been shown to be lower compared with the frequency of GyrA mutations. No GyrB mutations have been reported as resulting in cross-resistance between quinolones and the B subunit inhibitors coumermycin and novobiocin. This is consistent with the fact that the GyrB protein comprises two distinct domains: an N-terminal domain containing the sites for hydrolysis of adenosine triphosphate and binding of novobiocin and coumermycin, and a C-terminal domain containing the QRDR. Topoisomerase IV is usually a secondary target for quinolones in *Escherichia coli* and other gram-negatives. Thus, mutations in the QRDR of ParC are typically selected for in GyrA mutants (second-step mutations) and result in further decreased susceptibility. Second-step mutations that result in decreased quinolone susceptibility have also been reported in ParE, but they are overall less common in clinical isolates. In *Staph. aureus* and *Strep. pneumoniae* topoisomerase IV is usually the primary target of quinolones, and first-step mutations leading to quinolone resistance are usually found in ParC and ParE, while second-step mutations leading to further increased quinolone resistance are found in the gyrase subunits.[21] In general, the nature of the primary target of each quinolone in a bacterial species can be deduced by the location of the first-step target mutations that are selected upon quinolone exposure.

Combinations of multiple mutations within individual targets can also increase the resistance level. For instance, combinations of multiple mutations in the GyrA proteins were shown to be associated with higher minimum inhibitory concentration (MIC) values for ciprofloxacin than single point mutations. Similarly, combinations of single point mutations within GrlA were shown associated with higher ciprofloxacin MIC values than single mutations in *Staph. aureus*.[23]

QUINOLONE RESISTANCE BY DECREASED UPTAKE/ACTIVE EFFLUX

DNA gyrase and topoisomerase IV are located in the cytoplasm of the bacterial cell. In order to reach their targets, quinolone antibiotics must enter the cell envelope. In gram-negative bacteria the fluoroquinolones must first cross the outer membrane. Changes in the outer membrane proteins of gram-negative bacteria have been associated with increased resistance to quinolones by decreased drug uptake.[21,24]

Active efflux as a mechanism of fluoroquinolone resistance has been reported in several bacterial species. In *Staph. aureus* the resident chromosomally-encoded NorA efflux pump is responsible for a low basal level of quinolone efflux, with a preference for hydrophilic fluoroquinolones, and can be responsible for increased resistance following mutations that cause overexpression of the *norA* gene.[25] In *P. aeruginosa*, resistance to fluoroquinolones as well as to a number of other antimicrobial agents is often associated with mutational upregulation of resident RND-type multidrug efflux pumps, such as MexAB, MexCD, MexEF and MexXY, that can efflux fluoroquinolones.[26] *Escherichia coli* has also been shown to possess resident efflux systems for quinolones, including EmrAB and AcrAB, that can decrease quinolone susceptibility upon mutational upregulation.[26]

Recently, plasmid-encoded quinolone efflux systems have also been reported in Enterobacteriaceae, namely QepA and OqxAB. QepA is a an efflux pump that belongs in the major facilitator superfamily (MFS) of transporters, and that can efflux some quinolones including nalidixic acid, ciprofloxacin and norfloxacin increasing the MICs up 2- to 64-fold.[27] The *qepA* gene is often associated with other resistance determinants (e.g. the *rmtB* gene encoding a 16S ribosomal methylase conferring protection to aminoglycosides) in transferable resistance plasmids, and has been detected at high rates in China, but occasionally also in other countries.[28] OqxAB is an RND-type efflux pump that was originally identified in animal isolates of *Escherichia coli* resistant to olaquindox, a quinoxaline derivative used in agriculture and as a growth promoter. OqxAB is a multidrug efflux pump that can extrude also chloramphenicol and some quinolones including nalidixic acid and ciprofloxacin, causing a moderate MIC increase

(8- to 16-fold) for these agents.[29] Plasmids encoding OqxAB have mostly been detected in animal isolates, but also in clinical isolates of Enterobacteriaceae including *Salmonella enterica* and *Escherichia coli*. The *oqxAB* genes are also present in the chromosome of *Klebsiella pneumoniae*.[30]

QUINOLONE RESISTANCE BY TARGET PROTECTION

Acquired quinolone resistance by protection of the topoisomerase target was discovered in the late 1990s and was the first example of plasmid-encoded transferable mechanism of quinolone resistance. Target protection is conferred by a family of small pentapeptide-repeat proteins, named Qnr proteins, that bind to the topoisomerase targets and protect them from the interaction with quinolones.[30] A similar mechanism has evolved in bacteria to protect topoisomerases from microcins, which are proteins of the pentapeptide-repeat family that are produced by some bacteria as a mechanism of biological competition and can kill susceptible bacteria by inhibiting their topoisomerases.

Qnr production leads to a 10- to 100-fold increase in the MIC for quinolones. Because MIC values for quinolones are often extremely low, the production of Qnr may be insufficient for MIC to reach the breakpoint for resistance (or even an intermediate level of susceptibility). Nevertheless, the MIC increase may significantly affect the mutant-prevention concentration (MPC) favoring the selection of QRDR mutants with higher levels of resistance.[30]

Several types of plasmid-encoded Qnr proteins, indicated by letters (e.g. QnrA, QnrB, QnrC, QnrD, QnrS) have been described, including multiple variants for some of these types, indicated by numbers (e.g. QnrA1, QnrA2 etc.).[31] Acquired *qnr* genes have been reported worldwide, mostly in strains of Enterobacteriaceae, and this resistance mechanism is now considered of growing importance.[28,30]

QUINOLONE RESISTANCE BY DRUG INACTIVATION

Inactivation by drug modification was the most recently described resistance mechanism to quinolones. Modification is due to acetylation, and is carried out by a plasmid-encoded AAC enzyme variant (named AAC(6')-Ib-cr) that, in addition to aminoglycosides, has evolved (by mutations) the ability to acetylate also some quinolone molecules that have unsubstituted piperazinyl secondary amines, such as ciprofloxacin and norfloxacin (other quinolones lacking unsubstituted piperazinyl secondary amines are not affected). In presence of this mechanism, the MICs of quinolones are increased by two- to fourfold and usually remain lower than the breakpoint for susceptibility. However, as observed with Qnr proteins, the MIC increase may significantly affect the MPC and favor the selection of QRDR mutants with higher levels of resistance. Following its discovery, plasmid-encoded AAC(6')-Ib-cr has been detected worldwide, mostly in *E. coli* but also in other enterobacterial species.[30]

Resistance to Macrolides, Lincosamides and Streptogramins

Macrolide, lincosamines and streptogramin (MLS) antibiotics are chemically distinct inhibitors of the protein synthesis acting by binding to the 50S subunit of the bacterial ribosome and usually resulting in a bacteriostatic effect.

Macrolides are hydrophobic molecules having a central 12- to 16-membered-ring lactone attached to amino or neutral sugars. The macrolides of human importance are natural or semisynthetic 14-, 15- and 16-membered-ring molecules. Lincosamines are alkyl-derivatives of proline and are devoid of a lactone ring. Clindamycin is a semisynthetic derivative of 7-chloro-7-deoxy lincomycin, the first-discovered member of the family, and represents the only member of lincosamines currently used in the clinical practice. Streptogramins are composed of a mixture of two types of molecules: group A streptogramins and group B streptogramins. The two molecules act via a

synergistic interaction in the binding of the two antibiotics to the ribosome. Dalfopristin–quinupristin, a hydrosoluble derivative of pristinamycin, is the unique member of this class used in clinical practice.

Although azithromycin has been used in the treatment of infections caused by some gram-negative bacilli such as *Salmonella typhi* and *Shigella* spp., Enterobacteriaceae and gram-negative non-fermenters are considered naturally resistant to MLS antibiotics due to resident efflux systems associated with a certain degree of impermeability of the outer membrane. Some clinically relevant enterococcal species, including *Enterococcus faecalis*, *Enterococcus avium*, *Enterococcus gallinarum* and *Enterococcus casseliflavus* are intrinsically resistant to lincosamides and streptogramins. Resistance in these species is mediated by the presence of a resident *lsa* gene encoding an efflux pump. For some species, notably *Haemophilus influenzae*, the correlation between susceptibility testing and clinical outcome is weak and wild-type isolates are currently categorized as intermediate (see EUCAST clinical breakpoint v 6.0, http://www.eucast.org/clinical_breakpoints/).

Acquisition of resistance to macrolides by naturally susceptible species was documented only one year after market introduction of erythromycin. In 1953, in fact, clinical isolates of macrolide-resistant staphylococci were described in reports from France, England, Japan and the USA.[32] After these first cases, resistance to MLS antibiotics has become of clinical relevance in several cases. Resistance to macrolides can impair the efficacy of macrolide-including empirical regimens for the treatment of community-acquired pneumonia since, in some epidemiological settings the concurrent presence of macrolide resistance and reduced susceptibility to β-lactams is not uncommon in *Strep. pneumoniae*.[33] Similarly, clindamycin resistance can impact on the treatment of skin, soft tissue and bone infections sustained by *Staph. aureus* and *Streptococcus pyogenes*.[34] Resistance to macrolide in *Strep. pyogenes* can represent also a limitation in the treatment of pharyngitis in penicillin-allergic patients.[35] Furthermore, from an epidemiological point of view, acquisition of resistance to MLS antibiotics by hyperepidemic clones has probably played a relevant role in the abrupt worldwide diffusion of strains of *Clostridium difficile*.[36]

Three main types of mechanisms can be responsible for acquired resistance to MLS antibiotics, including target modification, active efflux and drug inactivation by enzymatic modification.[37] Table 138-4 summarizes the most clinically relevant mechanisms of acquired resistance together with the resulting phenotypes and their distribution.

RESISTANCE BY TARGET MODIFICATION

Modification of the ribosomal target causing reduction of affinity for their binding site can cause resistance to MLS antibiotics.

The most frequently encountered mechanism consists in a post-transcriptional modification of the 23S rRNA by methylases, usually named Erm (erythromycin resistance methylase), which add one or two methyl groups to a single adenine residue (A2058 in *Escherichia coli*) in the 23S rRNA moiety. Since adenine 2058 is a common binding site for macrolides, lincosamides and streptogramin B, this modification confers cross-resistance to all these drugs and the phenotype is called MLS$_B$. After the first description in 1956, the number of Erm-type enzymes have grown and the nomenclature for these genes has varied. The nomenclature currently used, proposed by Roberts and colleagues in 1999,[37] assigns two genes of ≥80% amino acid identity to the same class and same letter designation, while two genes that show ≤79% amino acid identity are given a different letter designation. An updated database of genes encoding transferable mechanisms of resistance to MLS antibiotics is available at the website http://faculty.washington.edu/marilynr.

rRNA methylase genes have been reported from a large number of gram-positive and gram-negative bacterial genera including intracellular and anaerobic species. However their clinical relevance is mostly linked to the spread in *Staphylococcus* spp. and *Streptococcus* spp. *erm*(A) and *erm*(C) genes predominate in staphylococcal species while *erm*(B) and *erm*(TR) are prevalent in streptococcal isolates (Table 138-4). Dissemination of these genes is attributed to the fact that these determinants can be transported by transposons and plasmids.

| TABLE 138-4 | The Most Relevant Acquired Resistance Mechanisms to MLS Antibiotics and Resulting Resistance Phenotypes |

			DISTRIBUTION	
Resistance Mechanism	Gene	Phenotype	Gram-positive	Gram-negative
TARGET MODIFICATION				
rRNA methylases	erm(A)*	Inducible or constitutive MLS$_B$	Staphylococcus, Enterococcus, Streptococcus	Haemophilus, Bacteroides
	erm(B)	Inducible or constitutive MLS$_B$	Staphylococcus, Enterococcus, Streptococcus, Clostridium, Corynebacterium	Campylobacter, Escherichia, Haemophilus, Neisseria
	erm(C)	Inducible or constitutive MLS$_B$	Staphylococcus, Enterococcus, Streptococcus, Clostridium, Corynebacterium	Bacteroides, Escherichia, Haemophilus, Neisseria
	erm(D)	Inducible or constitutive MLS$_B$		Salmonella
	erm(E)	Inducible or constitutive MLS$_B$		Bacteroides, Shigella
	erm(F)	Inducible or constitutive MLS$_B$	Staphylococcus, Enterococcus, Streptococcus, Clostridium, Corynebacterium	Bacteroides, Haemophilus, Neisseria
	erm(G)	Inducible or constitutive MLS$_B$	Staphylococcus	Bacteroides
	erm(Q)	Inducible or constitutive MLS$_B$	Staphylococcus, Streptococcus, Clostridium	Bacteroides
	erm(T)	Inducible or constitutive MLS$_B$	Staphylococcus, Enterococcus, Streptococcus	
	erm(X)	Inducible or constitutive MLS$_B$	Corynebacterium	
	erm(Y)	Inducible or constitutive MLS$_B$	Staphylococcus	
	erm(33)	Inducible or constitutive MLS$_B$	Staphylococcus	
	erm(35)	Inducible or constitutive MLS$_B$		Bacteroides
	erm(37)	Inducible or constitutive MLS$_B$	Mycobacterium spp.[†]	
	erm(38)	Inducible or constitutive MLS$_B$	Mycobacterium spp.[†]	
	erm(39)	Inducible or constitutive MLS$_B$	Mycobacterium spp.[†]	
	erm(40)	Inducible or constitutive MLS$_B$	Mycobacterium spp.[†]	
	erm(41)	Inducible or constitutive MLS$_B$	Mycobacterium spp.[†]	
	erm(43)	Inducible or constitutive MLS$_B$	Staphylococcus	
rRNA methyltransferase	cfr	PhLOPS$_A$	Staphylococcus, Enterococcus	Escherichia
EFFLUX				
Major Facilitator Superfamily	mef(A)[‡]	M	Staphylococcus, Enterococcus, Streptococcus, Clostridium, Corynebacterium	Bacteroides, Haemophilus, Neisseria, Escherichia, Salmonella
	mef(B)	M		Escherichia
ATP-binding transporter	msr(A)	Inducible MS$_B$	Staphylococcus, Enterococcus, Streptococcus, Corynebacterium	
	msr(C)	Inducible MS$_B$	Enterococcus	
	msr(D)	Inducible MS$_B$	Staphylococcus, Enterococcus, Streptococcus, Corynebacterium, Clostridium	Escherichia, Neisseria, Bacteroides
	lsa(B)	LS$_A$Ph	Staphylococcus	
	lsa(C)	LS$_A$Ph	Streptococcus	
	lsa(E)	LS$_A$Ph	Staphylococcus, Enterococcus	
	vga(A)	LS$_A$Ph	Staphylococcus	
	vga(B)	LS$_A$Ph	Enterococcus, Staphylococcus	
	vga(C)	LS$_A$Ph	Staphylococcus	
	vga(D)	LS$_A$Ph	Enterococcus	
	vga(E)	LS$_A$Ph	Staphylococcus	
	eat(A)	LS$_A$Ph	Enterococcus	
	sal(A)	LS$_A$Ph	Staphylococcus	
INACTIVATING ENZYMES				
Esterases	ere(A)	M		Escherichia, Salmonella
	ere(B)	M	Staphylococcus	Escherichia
Lyases	vgb(A)	S$_B$	Enterococcus, Staphylococcus	
	vgb(B)	S$_B$	Staphylococcus	
Transferases	lnu(A)	L	Staphylococcus	Clostridium
	lnu(B)	L	Enterococcus, Staphylococcus, Streptococcus	Clostridium
	lnu(C)	L	Streptococcus	Haemophilus
	lnu(D)	L	Streptococcus	
	lnu(E)	L	Streptococcus	
	vat(A)	S$_A$	Staphylococcus	
	vat(B)	S$_A$	Enterococcus, Staphylococcus	
	vat(C)	S$_A$	Staphylococcus	
	vat(D)	S$_A$	Enterococcus	
	vat(E)	S$_A$	Enterococcus	
	vat(H)	S$_A$	Enterococcus	
Phosphorylases	mph(A)	M		Shigella, Escherichia
	mph(B)	M		Escherichia
	mph(C)	M	Staphylococcus	Escherichia
	mph(D)	M		Escherichia
	mph(E)	M		Escherichia

M, macrolides; L, lincosamides; S$_A$: streptogramins A; S$_B$: streptogramins B; O: oxazolidinones; Ph: phenicols; P: pleuromutilins.
*Includes also erm(TR).
[†]Acid-fast bacteria, nontuberculous mycobacteria.
[‡]Includes also mef(E).
Data from Roberts M.C., Sutcliffe J., et al. Antimicrob Agents Chemother 1999; 43(12):2823–30.

The expression of *erm* genes can be inducible or constitutive resulting in different phenotypes. When the expression is constitutive the resulting strain is resistant to all macrolides, lincosamides and streptogramin B. The synergy between streptogramin A and B is conserved, but in *Staphylococcus* spp. the bactericidal activity of the streptogramin combination is lost. In the inducible phenotype, the enzyme is only expressed in presence of 14- and 15-membered macrolides and the strain remains susceptible to 16-membered macrolides, lincosamides and streptogramins. The inducible expression depends on the sequence of the regulatory region upstream from the structural gene for the methylase. Regulation occurs by a translational attenuation mechanism in which the mRNA secondary structure normally prevents translation, which is released in the presence of inducing macrolides. Single nucleotide changes, deletions or duplications in the regulatory region can also convert inducibly resistant strains to constitutively resistant ones that are cross-resistant to MLS$_B$ antibiotics.[32] Since selection of resistant mutants is not unusual during clindamycin therapy, a conservative approach should be suggested in the treatment of infection caused by inducible strains and the use of clindamycin should be discouraged when other therapeutic options are available.

A new methyltransferase called Cfr, has recently been described in staphylococcal isolates. The target of this enzyme, differing by previously described Erm enzymes, is represented by the adenosine at position 2503 in 23S rRNA in the large ribosomal subunit. This modification does not confer resistance to macrolides but impairs the efficacy of lincosamides, streptogramin A, oxazolidinones, pleuromutilins and phenicols.[38]

RESISTANCE BY EFFLUX

Active efflux is another mechanism of resistance to MLS antibiotics, by pumping the antibiotic out of the cytoplasmic membrane, keeping intracellular concentrations low and avoiding the binding to the ribosomal target.

Two classes of efflux pumps of the ATP-binding cassette (ABC) transporter superfamily or of the MFS have been increasingly detected in gram-positive pathogens. ABC transporters are composed of a channel with two cytoplasmic domains and two ATP-binding domains situated on the internal surface of the membrane. ABC transporters use ATP as the energy source, while MFS efflux pumps derive energy from the proton-motive force.

The *msr*A gene, encoding a member of the ABC transporter superfamily, is a common cause of reduced susceptibility to 14- and 15-membered macrolides in staphylococcal isolates. Expression is inducible by macrolides. This determinant also confers resistance to streptogramin B, but only after induction by macrolides. However, the synergism between streptogramins A and B is conserved. Acquisition of two members of the MFS, *mef*(A) and *mef*(E) is clinically relevant in *Strep. pyogenes* and *Strep. pneumoniae* respectively. Due to the high degree of homology between the two genes they have been assigned to the same class (*mef*(A)). The resistance phenotype is characterized by reduced susceptibility to 14- and 15-membered macrolides. Clindamycin and 16-membered macrolide activity is preserved.

RESISTANCE BY ENZYMATIC MODIFICATION

Several enzymes can act in modifying specific antibiotics. These proteins usually confer resistance to only one of the three classes (M, L, or S) or one component such as streptogramin A, but not streptogramin B.

Enzymes which hydrolyze streptogramin B (encoded by *vgb*(A) and *vgb*(B) genes) or modify the antibiotic by adding an acetyl group (acetyltransferases) to streptogramin A (encoded by *vat*(A), *vat*(B) and *vat*(C) genes) have been described alone or in association in *Enterococcus* spp. and *Staphylococcus* spp. When present simultaneously, they confer resistance to dalfopristin–quinupristin. Nucleotidyltransferases of the *lnu*(A) class, encoding 3-lincomycin- and 4-clindamycin *O*-nucleotidyltransferases, have been identified as a cause of isolated lincosamides resistance in staphylococcal strains. Similarly *lnu*(B) and *lnu*(C) genes can be responsible of resistance to lincosamides in

Streptococcus agalactiae isolates. Although mainly reported in enterobacteria, the phosphotransferase MphC and the esterase EreA can be responsible for erythromycin inactivation in *Staph. aureus* isolates.[37]

Resistance to Tetracyclines

Tetracyclines are broad-spectrum bacteriostatic antibiotics that inhibit bacterial protein synthesis by binding the 30S ribosomal subunit and preventing the attachment of the aminoacyl-tRNA and eventually the elongation phase of protein synthesis.

Resistance to tetracyclines can be due to several different mechanisms. From the clinical point of view the principal mechanisms of tetracycline resistance are represented by active efflux and ribosomal target protection.

RESISTANCE TO TETRACYCLINE BY RIBOSOMAL PROTECTION

Acquired tetracycline resistance can result from production of elongation-factor G (EF-G)-like ribosomal protection proteins that interact with the ribosome so that protein synthesis is unaffected by the presence of the antibiotic. Several different *tet* determinants that confer tetracycline resistance by this mechanism have been identified (Table 138-5).[39]

The most studied determinants of ribosomal protection have been those encoded by the *tet*(M) and *tet*(O) genes. The ribosomal protection proteins encoded by the other classes have an amino acid sequence identity of at least 40% to Tet(M), and the mechanism of action is presumed to be similar for all ribosomal protection proteins. The Tet(M) ribosomal protection protein has amino acid sequence similarity to EF-G (which translocates the peptidyl transfer RNA during protein synthesis) and EF-Tu, has a ribosome-dependent guanosine triphosphatase activity, and seems to confer resistance by reversible binding to the ribosome. Ribosomal protection proteins interact with the ribosome at the level of the protein h34 causing the release of the tetracycline molecules. The ribosome returns to its standard conformational state and protein synthesis proceeds.[39]

Tet ribosomal protection proteins are encoded by different types of MGEs and are a common cause of acquired tetracycline resistance both in gram-positive and gram-negative bacteria (Table 138-5). This mechanism can confer resistance to both tetracycline and minocycline, but not to tigecycline, a new glycylcycline derivative of minocycline whose modified structure allows escaping most tetracycline resistance mechanisms including ribosomal protection and active efflux.

TETRACYCLINE EFFLUX SYSTEMS

Acquired tetracycline efflux systems encoded by plasmid-encoded *tet* genes have been described both in gram-positive and gram-negative bacteria. These efflux pumps, generally, are membrane proteins with 12–14 transmembrane domains, member of the MFS of efflux systems, that are able to actively pump tetracyclines out of the cell preventing intracellular accumulation and consequently ribosome binding.[39] The energy for the efflux is derived from the proton-motive force.

Several different classes of Tet efflux pumps have been described, encoded by different types of MGEs and found as a common cause of acquired tetracycline resistance in bacteria (Table 138-5). Tet efflux pumps generally confer resistance to tetracycline but, with the exception of Tet(B), not to minocycline. Tigecycline is not affected by Tet efflux pumps.

Expression of Tet efflux systems is often regulated by the presence of the antibiotic. In some cases (e.g. with Tet(A), Tet(B), Tet(C), Tet(D), Tet(E), Tet(G) and Tet(H)) expression is regulated by a repressor (TetR) which, in the absence of tetracycline, binds to the operator region upstream of the *tet* gene and represses the expression of the efflux pump.[39] When tetracycline enters the cell, it binds the TetR repressor promoting a conformational change that results in a decreased ability to bind the operator region, thus allowing expression of the efflux pump. In other cases (e.g. with Tet(K) and Tet(L)), expression is regulated by mRNA attenuation in a similar way to that

TABLE 138-5	The Most Relevant Acquired Resistance Mechanisms to Tetracycline Antibiotics and Resulting Resistance Phenotypes		
		DISTRIBUTION	
Resistance Mechanism	**Gene**	**Gram-positive**	**Gram-negative**
RIBOSOMAL PROTECTION	tet(M)	Enteroccoccus, Staphylococcus, Streptococcus, Mycobacterium spp.[†]	Enterobacteriaceae, Haemophilus, Stenotrophomonas
	tet(O)	Enteroccoccus, Staphylococcus, Streptococcus, Mycobacterium spp.[†]	Campylobacter, Enterobacteriaceae, Stenotrophomonas
	tet(Q)	Streptococcus	
	tet(S)	Enteroccoccus, Staphylococcus, Streptococcus	Enterobacteriaceae
	tet(T)	Enteroccoccus, Streptococcus	Stenotrophomonas
	tet(W)	Staphylococcus, Streptococcus	Enterobacteriaceae
	tet(32)	Streptococcus	
	tet(44)		Campylobacter
	otr(A)	Mycobacterium spp.[†]	
EFFLUX	tet(A)		Enterobacteriaceae
	tet(B)		Enterobacteriaceae, Haemophilus
	tet(C)		Enterobacteriaceae
	tet(D)		Enterobacteriaceae
	tet(E)		Enterobacteriaceae
	tet(G)		Enterobacteriaceae
	tet(H)		Enterobacteriaceae
	tet(J)		Enterobacteriaceae
	tet(K)	Enteroccoccus, Staphylococcus, Streptococcus, Mycobacterium spp.[†]	Haemophilus
	tet(L)	Enteroccoccus, Staphylococcus, Streptococcus, Mycobacterium spp.[†]	Enterobacteriaceae
	tet(V)	Mycobacterium spp.[†]	
	tet(Y)		Enterobacteriaceae
	tet(35)		Stenotrophomonas
	tet(39)		Enterobacteriaceae, Stenotrophomonas
	tet(38)	Staphylococcus	
	tet(40)	Staphylococcus, Streptococcus	
	tetAB(46)	Streptococcus	
	otr(B)	Mycobacterium spp.[†]	
ENZYMATIC INACTIVATION	tet(X)		Enterobacteriaceae
UNKNOWN	tet(U)	Enteroccoccus, Staphylococcus, Streptococcus	

[†]Acid-fast bacteria, nontuberculous mycobacteria.
Data from Roberts M.C. FEMS Microbiol Lett 2005; 245(2):195–203.

described for gram-positive *erm* genes encoding rRNA methylase (see above) and *cat* genes encoding chloramphenicol acetyltransferases.[40]

Tetracyclines can also be effluxed by some resident MDR efflux systems of gram-negative bacteria. In some species (e.g. *Proteus mirabilis, Pseudomonas aeruginosa*), the basal-level efflux confers intrinsic resistance to tetracyclines. In other species, the basal-level efflux is not sufficient to confer intrinsic resistance, but mutations upregulating the resident efflux systems can be responsible of acquired tetracycline resistance. One of the best known examples is represented by mutations of the *mar* locus in *E. coli*, which lead to an overexpression of the transcriptional activator MarA, that in turn causes the overexpression of the resident multidrug efflux pump AcrAB causing tetracycline resistance.[41] Efflux mediated by upregulation of some resident efflux systems has also been involved with acquired resistance to tigecycline in Enterobacteriaceae and *Acinetobacter baumannii*. In *Escherichia coli* and other enterobacteria, mutations of the regulatory genes *ramA, marA, rarA* and *soxS*, leading to overexpression of the resident AcrAB efflux system, have been associated with acquired tigecycline resistance.[42] In *Acinetobacter*, decreased tigecycline susceptibility was found associated with mutations upregulating the resident AdeABC efflux system.[43] In addition to point mutations, also insertion sequences can upregulate the expression of resident efflux systems.

Resistance to Chloramphenicol

Chloramphenicol is a bacteriostatic antibiotic that binds to the 50S ribosomal subunit and inhibits the peptidyltransferase step in protein synthesis. Resistance to chloramphenicol is mostly due to inactivation of the antibiotic by chloramphenicol acetyltransferase (CAT) enzymes that acetylate the antibiotic. In certain gram-negative bacteria, reduced drug uptake can also be responsible for resistance to chloramphenicol.

RESISTANCE BY DRUG INACTIVATION

Chloramphenicol contains two hydroxyl groups that are acetylated in a reaction catalyzed by CAT enzymes. Monoacetylated and diacetylated derivatives are unable to bind to the 50S ribosomal subunit and to inhibit the prokaryotic peptidyltransferase. The *cat* genes are usually associated with MGEs and often carried on plasmids that mediate their diffusion among bacterial pathogens.[44]

Expression of the *cat* genes in gram-positive pathogens (*Staph. aureus, Strep. pneumoniae* and *E. faecalis*) is often inducible, and appears to be regulated by translational attenuation in a similar manner to the *erm* genes conferring resistance to macrolides (see above). In these cases the *cat* gene is preceded by a nine amino acid leader peptide, and the leader mRNA can form a stable stem-loop structure which masks the ribosome binding site of the *cat* gene. Chloramphenicol appears to cause the ribosome to stall on the leader sequence, opening the stem-loop structure, thereby exposing the cat ribosome binding site and allowing *cat* gene expression. In gram-negative bacteria, resistance to chloramphenicol is usually mediated by plasmid-mediated *cat* genes that are expressed constitutively.[44]

RESISTANCE BY DECREASED DRUG UPTAKE

In gram-negative bacteria, resistance to chloramphenicol may also be due to reduced drug uptake mediated by chromosomal mutations or by acquired resistance genes. In *E. coli*, for instance, chromosomal mutations of the *mar* locus can result in resistance to chloramphenicol and structurally unrelated antibiotics as part of the MAR phenotype, mediated by a reduced drug uptake mechanism (see below). Moreover, the *cmlA1* gene carried on a mobile gene cassette associated with some integrons encodes a chloramphenicol efflux system that can contribute to acquired resistance to chloramphenicol in gram-negative bacteria.[44]

Resistance to Glycopeptides

The glycopeptide antibiotics vancomycin and teicoplanin inhibit peptidoglycan synthesis in gram-positive bacteria by binding with high affinity to the terminal D-alanyl-D-alanine (D-Ala-D-Ala) group of the pentapeptide side chains of peptidoglycan precursors and blocking the transglycosylation and transpeptidation reactions required for polymerization of peptidoglycan. Gram-negative bacteria are intrinsically resistant to glycopeptides since these relatively large molecules cannot cross the outer membrane and reach their peptidoglycan target.

Acquired resistance to glycopeptides is a major problem in enterococci, and has also been reported in staphylococci.

GLYCOPEPTIDE RESISTANCE IN ENTEROCOCCI

Acquired resistance to glycopeptides can be relatively common, especially in *Enterococcus faecium*. Infections caused by glycopeptide-resistant enterococci (usually named vancomycin-resistant enterococci, VRE) are difficult to treat since only few treatment options remain available.[45]

Resistance to glycopeptides is due to the production of low-affinity pentapeptide precursors, ending either with D-lactate (D-Lac) or D-serine (D-Ser) residues, which can be incorporated in the peptidoglycan. Production of these precursors is dependent on new biosynthetic pathways which include a new D-amino acid ligase and also enzymes that degrade the normal peptidoglycan precursors. Genes encoding these pathways (named *van* genes), together with regulatory genes, are usually found clustered on MGEs that, upon transfer, can confer glycopeptide resistance to the bacterial host.

Several different clusters of *van* genes have been described, indicated by letters, that can be associated with different resistance phenotypes (Table 138-6).[45]

vanA-type Resistance

The *vanA* gene cluster is one of the most frequent glycopeptide resistance determinants encountered in enterococci and, therefore, among the most clinically relevant. It confers high-level resistance to vancomycin and teicoplanin, since its expression can be induced by both drugs.

The *vanA* gene cluster is carried within a transposon (usually Tn*1546*) and is composed by genes involved in glycopeptide resistance (*vanHAXYZ*) and by regulatory genes (*vanRS*). VanA is the ligase that catalyzes the formation of D-Ala-D-Lac precursors. The *vanH* gene apparently encodes an enzyme that catalyzes the conversion of pyruvate, common in nature, to D-lactic acid, rarely found in nature. The VanA ligase uses this as a substrate to form the depsipeptide D-Ala-D-Lac, which is then incorporated into an alternative, vancomycin-resistant peptidoglycan precursor (Figure 138-2). The VanX protein cleaves the D-Ala-D-Ala dipeptide, decreasing the amount of substrate that is available for the formation of the normal pentapeptide. This step is important since resistance would not be expressed in the presence of wild-type precursors which allow binding of glycopeptides. The VanY protein is a carboxypeptidase that may reduce the levels of the normal precursor already present so that the alternative precursor predominates. The genes *vanR* and *vanS* encode a two-component signal transducing regulatory system that sense the presence of glycopeptides by the VanS sensor and responds by activating the VanR transcriptional activator that, in turn, activates the transcription of the other *van* genes. The environmental stimulus that triggers the initial phosphorylation of VanS has not been identified, but it is probably

TABLE 138-6	*van* Gene Clusters Mediating Resistance to Glycopeptides in Gram-positive Cocci		
Type of Target Modification	*van* Gene Cluster	Phenotype	Distribution
D-Ala–D-Lac	*vanA*	Inducible V,T	*Enterococcus* spp., *Staphylococcus aureus*
	vanB	Inducible V	*Enterococcus faecium*, *Enterococcus faecalis*
	vanD	Constitutive V, T	*Enterococcus faecium*, *Enterococcus faecalis*
	vanM	V,T	*Enterococcus faecium*
D-Ala–D-Ser	*vanC*	Inducible/constitutive V	*Enterococcus gallinarum*, *Enterococcus casseliflavus*
	vanE	Inducible/constitutive V	*Enterococcus faecalis*
	vanG	Inducible V	*Enterococcus faecalis*
	vanL	Inducible V	*Enterococcus faecalis*
	vanN	Constitutive V	*Enterococcus faecium*

V, vancomycin; T, teicoplanin.
Adapted from Cattoir V., Leclercq R. J Antimicrob Chemother 2013; 68(4):731–42.

related to the presence of the glycopeptide and its interaction with the D-Ala-D-Ala target site, which inhibits transglycosylation and transpeptidation.

Other van-type resistances

Other *van* gene clusters that are found as acquired resistance genes in enterococci are *vanB*, *vanD*, *vanE*, *vanG*, *vanL*, *vanM* and *vanN*, while the *vanC* gene cluster is intrinsic in *Enterococcus gallinarum* and *Enterococcus casseliflavus* (Table 138-6). Among them, *vanB* is the most widespread and clinically relevant. VanB-positive strains display various levels of inducible resistance to vancomycin but remain susceptible to teicoplanin that it is not an inducer. However, the emergence of mutants that express *vanB* constitutively and are also resistant to teicoplanin has been described.[46] Resistance mediated by *vanB* may also be transferable. The other acquired *van* genes are overall less common. In some cases the genes are located chromosomally and are constitutively expressed. In some cases (e.g. *vanD* and *vanM*), transfer by conjugation has been demonstrated.

The *vanC* resistance determinants are present on the chromosome in *Enterococcus casseliflavus* and *Enterococcus gallinarum* and are intrinsic characteristics of these species. VanC-harboring enterococci have low-level resistance to vancomycin and remain susceptible to teicoplanin. The pentapeptide that results from the action of the VanC ligase terminates in D-Ala-D-Ser.[47] This substitution probably reduces vancomycin binding, albeit not to the same degree as the depsipeptide found in VanA and VanB enterococci. VanC-harboring strains with high-level resistance to glycopeptides as a result of the acquisition of the *vanA* gene cluster have also been isolated.

GLYCOPEPTIDE RESISTANCE IN STAPHYLOCOCCI

The glycopeptides are front-line drugs for MRSA infections. Despite their abundant use, resistance to glycopeptides in *Staph. aureus* has remained overall uncommon and is phenotypically diverse, depending on the mechanism of resistance.[48]

High-level glycopeptide resistance is observed with strains that have acquired a VanA-type resistance mechanism identical to that

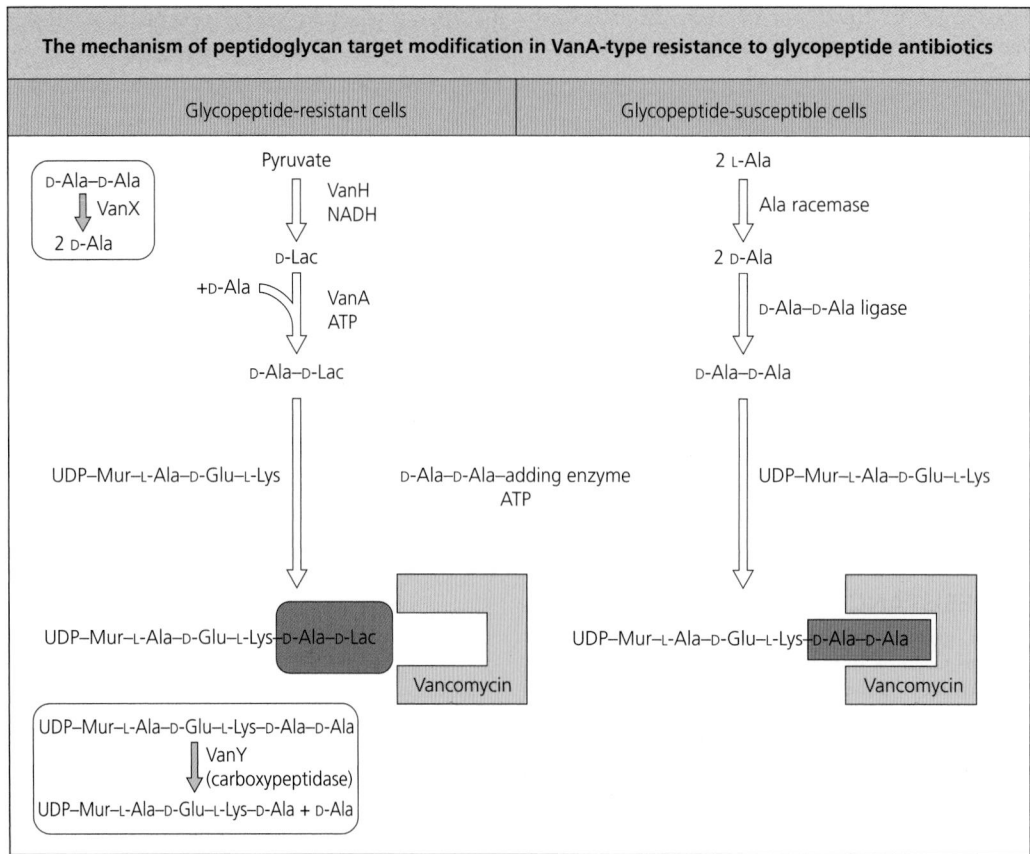

Figure 138-2   The mechanism of peptidoglycan target modification in VanA-type resistance to glycopeptide antibiotics. The various products of the *vanA* gene cluster are responsible for the synthesis of a modified peptidoglycan precursor and removal of the native precursors. ATP, adenosine triphosphate; Lac, lactate; UDP, uridine diphosphate. *Adapted from Cattoir V., Leclercq R. J Antimicrob Chemother 2013; 68(4):731–42.*

described for enterococci. These strains, indicated as vancomycin- or glycopeptide-resistant *Staph. aureus* (VRSA or GRSA), have been described since the early 2000s but thus far have remained unusual and do not exhibit a tendency to disseminate, possibly due to a remarkable fitness cost associated with the resistance mechanism.[49]

Lower level glycopeptide resistance is observed with strains that have acquired some chromosomal mutations. These mutants are also indicated as vancomycin- or glycopeptide-intermediate *Staph. aureus* (VISA or GISA). In some cases, named heteroresistant glycopeptide-intermediate *Staph. aureus* (hVISA or hGISA) resistance is expressed only in a minority of the bacterial population. These strains are susceptible to vancomycin (MICs ≤2 mg/L) but with minority populations (typically 1 organism on 10^5 to 10^6 colony forming units) with higher vancomycin MIC, and their detection needs a population analysis profile. The GISA and hGISA strains exhibit a thicker cell wall which limits the access of glycopeptides to the D-Ala-D-Ala target in the peptidoglycan precursors. Furthermore, most of these strains show reduced peptidoglycan cross-linking when compared with isogenic revertants. The genetic mechanism for this cell-wall thickening is not fully understood, but seems to be related to mutation of many genes involved in the regulation of peptidoglycan metabolism.[50] Several mutations associated with the GISA phenotypes have been characterized,[50] and it has also been documented how stepwise mutations involving certain loci (e.g. *graRS* and *vraSR* and *walKR*) can lead first to a hGISA and then to a homogeneous GISA phenotype.[51]

Resistance to Trimethoprim and Sulfonamides

Trimethoprim and sulfonamides are synthetic agents that affect the biosynthesis of tetrahydrofolic acid, an essential metabolite used in amino acid and nucleotide synthesis. Sulfonamides are analogs of *para*-aminobenzoic acid. They competitively inhibit the enzyme dihydropteroate synthase (DHPS), which catalyzes the condensation of dihydropteridine with *p*-aminobenzoic acid at an early step of the folate synthesis pathway. Trimethoprim is an analog of dihydrofolic acid which competitively inhibits the enzyme dihydrofolate reductase (DHFR). DHFR catalyzes the reduction of dihydrofolic acid to tetrahydrofolic acid, the final step in tetrahydrofolic acid synthesis. Trimethoprim–sulfamethoxazole (co-trimoxazole) is a formulation of trimethoprim with a sulfonamide, which has a synergistic effect showing a broader spectrum of activity and a bactericidal action.

A number of different resistance mechanisms to sulfonamides and trimethoprim have been described, including reduced drug uptake, target modification and target by-pass by resistant enzymes.

INTRINSIC RESISTANCE TO TRIMETHOPRIM AND SULFONAMIDES

Reduced drug uptake is responsible for intrinsic resistance to trimethoprim of *Pseudomonas aeruginosa*. Intrinsic resistance to trimethoprim in a number of other species (e. g. *Acinetobacter baumannii* and *Stenotrophomonas maltophilia*) is due to host DHFR enzymes with low affinity for the drug. Enterococci, which unlike other species are able to use exogenous preformed folates, exhibit reduced susceptibilities to sulfonamides and trimethoprim.

ACQUIRED RESISTANCE TO TRIMETHOPRIM

Both high- and low-level resistance has been reported in several species.

In some cases, acquired trimethoprim resistance may be due to chromosomal mutations leading to: 1) overproduction of the host DHFR caused by promoter mutation, thus requiring more trimethoprim concentration for the inhibition (described in Enterobacteriaceae); 2) mutations in the DHFR structural gene (described in streptococci, staphylococci). These two mechanisms are often associated in Enterobacteriaceae and in *Haemophilus influenzae* resulting in high-level resistance.[52]

High-level resistance to trimethoprim in enterobacteria is mostly caused by the acquisition of exogenous genes that encode a trimethoprim-resistant DHFR with an altered active site. Several different trimethoprim-resistant DHFRs have been characterized in gram-negative organisms, belonging in at least two groups, encoded by the *dfrA* and *dfrB* genes. In Enterobacteriaceae these genes are usually carried on mobile gene cassettes associated with integrons.[53]

The acquisition of the trimethoprim-resistant DHFR genes, *dfrA*, and the mutation of the chromosomal DHFR gene (*dfrB*) are currently considered to be key determinants of trimethoprim resistance in *Staph. aureus* of human origin.[54]

ACQUIRED RESISTANCE TO SULFONAMIDES

Chromosomally-encoded sulfonamide resistance has been described and resistance seems to be due to an increased production of *para*-aminobenzoic acid and to alterations of DHPS that lower the enzyme affinity for sulfonamides. Acquired sulfonamide resistance can also result from the acquisition of plasmids harboring genes that encode a drug-resistant DHPS. This mechanism is typical for gram-negative bacilli and there are at least three genes involved, named *sul1*, *sul2* and *sul3*. These genes code for a DHPS with low affinity for sulfonamide and confer high resistance levels.[52]

Resistance to Other Antibiotics

Linezolid has been the first licensed oxazolidinone agent, and is mostly used to treat infections caused by vancomycin-resistant enterococci and MRSA. Linezolid is a protein synthesis inhibitor that targets the large subunit of the bacterial ribosome. Acquired resistance to linezolid remains uncommon but has been reported both in enterococci and in staphylococci, either sporadically or even in small outbreaks.[55] Resistance can be due to mutations of the ribosomal target (nucleotide substitutions of 23S rRNA, such as G2505A or G2576U, or mutations of the L3 and L4 ribosomal proteins) or to target modification by methylation at specific positions of the 23S rRNA, that impede linezolid binding to the target.[56] Resistance mediated by ribosomal target mutations is usually selected after a long exposure to the drug and, in the case of rRNA target mutations, resistance can be expressed at variable levels depending on the number of rDNA genes that carry the mutation. Ribosomal rRNA methylation, on the other hand, is mediated by the plasmid-encoded Cfr methyltransferase, which modifies the 23S rRNA at residue A2503. The latter mechanism, which is of remarkable concern due to the transferable nature, is responsible for cross-resistance to linezolid and other anti-ribosomal drugs including phenicols, lincosamides, pleuromutilins and streptogramin A (the so-called PhLOPS$_A$ phenotype), and its dissemination has likely been promoted by the use of florphenicol in veterinary medicine.

Fusidic acid binds elongation-factor G (EF-G) preventing its release from the ribosome and blocking bacterial protein synthesis. In staphylococci, which are the main clinical target for fusidic acid, acquired resistance can be due either to mutations in the *fusA* gene, which encodes EF-G, or to the acquisition of resistance genes (*fusB* and *fusC*) that encode proteins able to bind the ribosome and protect it from fusidic acid.[57] Reduced uptake and enzymatic inactivation have also been occasionally reported as resistance mechanisms to fusidic acid.

Mupirocin inhibits bacterial protein synthesis by inhibition of isoleucyl tRNA synthetase (IleRS) and is used as a topical antibiotic for nasal decolonization of *Staph. aureus* (both MSSA and MRSA). Low-level resistance is caused by mutations in the chromosomal gene encoding the IleRS enzyme, which are not associated with high fitness cost. Acquisition of a novel mupirocin-resistant isoleucyl tRNA synthetase, encoded by the *mupA* gene can confer high-level resistance.

Plasmids carrying *mupA* have been detected in all major circulating MRSA clones. Recently a new plasmid-mediated mechanism for high-level mupirocin resistance, *mupB*, was detected, but the prevalence of this mechanism remains to be determined.[58]

Metronidazole resistance in *Helicobacter pylori* usually results from mutational inactivation of the *rdxA* gene that encodes NADPH nitroreductase. This enzyme converts metronidazole into a metabolite that is toxic for the bacterial cell. Inactivation of other reductase-encoding genes could also be involved in metronidazole resistance.[59]

Polymyxins are last-resort drugs for multiresistant gram-negative pathogens. They exert bactericidal action by damaging the bacterial membrane after binding to the lipid A moiety of the bacterial lipopolysaccharide (LPS) present in the outer membrane of gram-negative bacteria. The interest for these drugs was recently increased by the dissemination of extremely drug-resistant (XDR) gram-negative pathogens for which polymyxins are among the few drugs that retain activity. Resistance to polymyxins generally arises following modification of the LPS target by decoration of lipid A with amino-arabinose or phosphoethanolamine residues, thereby reducing the negative charge of lipid A and the binding of polymyxins. A similar resistance mechanism has been detected in polymyxin-resistant clinical isolates of Enterobacteriaceae, *Pseudomonas aeruginosa* and *Acinetobacter*, and can be due to different chromosomal mutations.[60] In *Acinetobacter*, acquired polymyxin resistance has also been associated with mutations causing a loss of the LPS target.

Fosfomycin is a peptidoglycan synthesis inhibitor that acts by blocking the MurA enzyme, involved in the first steps of the peptidoglycan biosynthetic pathway. Its interest was largely confined to treatment of uncomplicated urinary tract infections, but recently it has also been reconsidered as a salvage option for infections caused by some XDR gram-negative bacteria. Resistance to fosfomycin can be due to several mechanisms including: 1) chromosomal mutations that alter the expression of the transport systems (for 1-α-glycero-3 phosphate and for hexose monophosphates) that fosfomycin uses to enter the cytoplasmic membrane; 2) chromosomal mutations altering the affinity of MurA enzyme for fosfomycin; 3) chromosomal mutations causing overexpression of the MurA enzyme; and 4) inactivation of fosfomycin by modifying enzymes.[61] Several plasmid-encoded inactivating enzymes, such as FosA, FosB, FosC, FosD, FosK, FomX, FomA, and FomB have been described. FosA, the first characterized, is a glutathione S-transferase, which catalyzes the addition of glutathione to fosfomycin.

Resistance in *Mycobacterium tuberculosis*

Despite the global fall in incidence and mortality related to tuberculosis (TB), MDR and extensively drug-resistant (XDR) TB represents an emerging challenge. The World Health Organization (WHO) estimated there were 210 000 drug-resistant TB-related deaths in 2013 worldwide.[62]

Since isoniazid and rifampin represent the backbone agents of combination therapy commonly used in the treatment of TB, the emergence of resistance to these agents poses a serious clinical challenge.

Resistance to isoniazid was reported soon after its introduction in 1952. Isoniazid inhibits the synthesis of mycolic acid of the cell wall and triggers the production of toxic free radicals. Modification of numerous genes has been involved in the development of isoniazid resistance. The most common mechanism of resistance involves the *katG* gene that encodes for a catalase-peroxidase enzyme essential for the conversion of isoniazid to the active form. Mutations in this gene, causing enzyme conformational changes, usually lead to a high level of resistance. The most frequently observed mutation occurs at codon 315. Also mutations in the *inhA* gene, which encodes for an NADH-dependent enoyl-ACP reductase, and/or in its promoter cause low-level isoniazid resistance associated with ethionamide cross-resistance.

Rifampin and related antibiotics (rifabutin and rifapentine) block transcription initiation by binding to the β subunit of the bacterial RNA polymerase. Resistance is caused by mutation in the *rpoB* gene that encodes this subunit. Most often these mutations are located at codons between nucleotide 507 and 533 (numbered according to *rpoB* coding sequence of *Escherichia coli*).

From a clinical standpoint resistance to pyrazinamide and ethambutol also are relevant. Resistance to pyrazinamide is most commonly caused by mutations in the *pncA* gene, or its upstream region. The *pncA* product is required to convert pyrazinamide into its active form. The target of ethambutol is the arabinosyltransferase enzyme involved in mycolic acid synthesis. Acquired resistance is frequently caused by mutations in the *embB* gene encoding for this enzyme.[63]

Multidrug Resistance

Bacteria are often resistant to more than one antimicrobial agent. Multidrug resistance can be conferred by three mechanisms: 1) reduced permeability affecting more than one drug; 2) active efflux affecting more than one drug; 3) presence of multiple resistance genes.

Reduced permeability is generally caused by mutational alterations affecting the structure of the outer membrane of gram-negative bacteria, mostly consisting of the reduced expression of porins that are the main entry channel for several antibiotics. One of the best known examples is the reduction of the outer membrane protein OmpF in *Escherichia coli*, leading to a decreased uptake of antibiotics.[26]

Active efflux of antibiotics is a common resistance mechanism. Some efflux pumps are only able to pump out a single antibiotic and its close structural homologues (e.g. pumps dedicated to tetracycline efflux). However, more general-purpose efflux systems also exist. These pumps can handle a wide variety of different compounds, including many antibiotics, and thus contribute multidrug resistance phenotypes. Efflux systems may belong to a number of different families:[26]

- ATP-binding cassette (ABC);
- major facilitator superfamily (MFS);
- resistance-nodulation-division (RND);
- small multidrug resistance (SMR);
- multidrug and toxic compound extrusion (MATE).

Efflux systems can be composed of either a single polypeptide or multiple polypeptide components, depending on the family (Figure 138-3). Multicomponent efflux systems are typical of gram-negative bacteria, where the compounds must be transported across both the cytoplasmic and outer membrane. The ABC transporters are dependent on ATP as an energy source for their activity, whereas the proton-motive force is used by other transporters.

Many of these efflux systems are encoded by resident chromosomal genes and provide a contribution to the basal level of resistance to various antibiotics expressed by the corresponding bacterial species. In this case, mutations can be responsible for upregulation of the efflux system resulting in increased resistance to multiple antibiotics (depending on the spectrum of the substrates recognized by the system). Well known examples of similar systems are the AcrAB pump of *Escherichia coli* and the MexAB pump of *Pseudomonas aeruginosa*, which belong to the RND family. The latter pump is responsible for efflux of several different compounds under basal conditions, and can be upregulated by mutations. Mutational upregulation can contribute to acquired multidrug resistance to several anti-pseudomonas agents including fluoroquinolones, anti-pseudomonas penicillins and cephalosporins, and meropenem, but not imipenem or aminoglycosides.

Resistance to disinfectants is usually also mediated by efflux pumps.[26]

Genetic Bases of Acquired Antibiotic Resistance

Acquired antibiotic resistance can arise by mutations of chromosomal genes or by acquisition of exogenous resistance genes following events of horizontal gene transfer between bacteria.

Mutations leading to resistance can affect a single antibiotic or class of antibiotics, or can even be responsible for the emergence of MDR phenotypes. The latter occurs when mutations upregulate multidrug efflux pumps or affects regulatory systems that activate multiple resistance mechanisms. The MAR (**m**ultiple **a**ntibiotic **r**esistance) system in *Escherichia coli* is one of the best studied regulatory systems that controls resistance to multiple antibiotics by different mechanisms.[26] The system includes a three-gene operon containing *marRAB*. The MarR product acts as a negative regulator for the *mar* operon. The MarA product is required for resistance and acts by downregulating the expression of OmpF protein and upregulating the expression of the AcrAB efflux pump (Figure 138-4). Mutations in *marR* or in the promoter region of the *mar* operon can activate expression of *marA* leading to decreased susceptibility to multiple antibiotics (e.g. tetracycline, chloramphenicol, rifampin, nalidixic acid) that can be effluxed by the AcrAB pump and/or enter the cell via OmpF. Homologues of the *mar* locus exist in other members of the family Enterobacteriaceae as well as in other bacteria.

Acquisition of resistance genes by horizontal gene transfer is an important mechanism of evolution of microbial drug resistance. Acquired resistance genes are typically associated with MGEs, such as

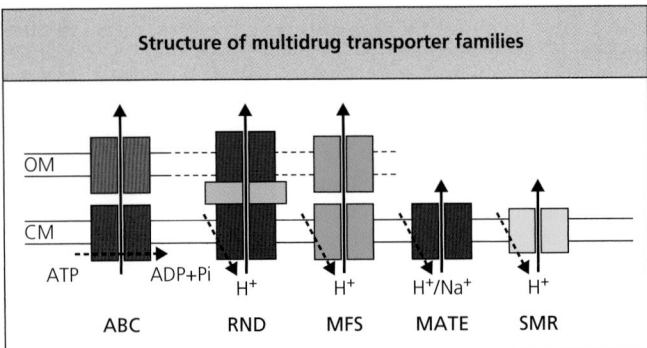

Figure 138-3 Structure of different multidrug transporter families. Different subunits are indicated by different colors. Efflux direction is indicated by a solid arrow. The energy source for efflux is indicated by a broken arrow. The cellular membrane (CM) is present in all cells, but gram-positive bacteria lack an outer membrane (OM). Some multidrug transporter families are present in both gram-positive and gram-negative bacteria as indicated by dotted lines for the OM (see text for details.)

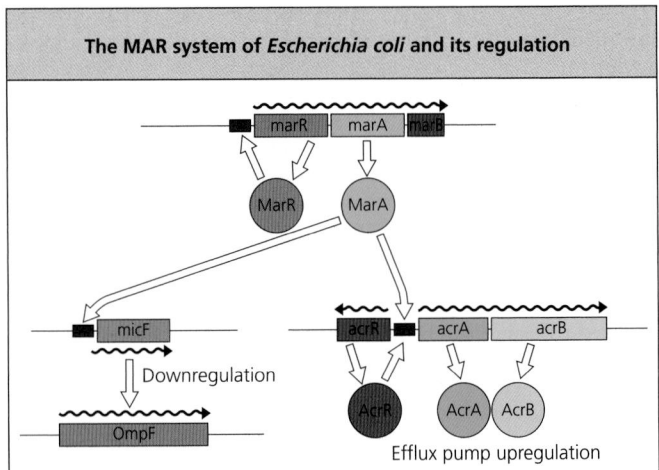

Figure 138-4 The MAR system of *Escherichia coli* and its regulation. The MarR product acts as a negative regulator for the *mar* operon. The MarA product acts by downregulating the expression of OmpF protein (via upregulation of *micF* antisense RNA) and upregulating the expression of the AcrAB efflux pump. Production of MarA is normally repressed. Mutations in *marR* or in the promoter region of the *mar* operon can activate expression of *marA* leading to decreased susceptibility to multiple antibiotics that can be effluxed by the AcrAB pump and/or enter the cell via OmpF.

plasmids or integrative and conjugative elements (ICEs, formerly named conjugative transposons), that can be transferred between different bacterial cells by conjugation.[53,64] Plasmids and ICEs can carry multiple resistance genes and, upon transfer, confer an MDR phenotype to the new host. Conjugative plasmids are circular DNA molecules that contain an origin of replication, a locus for partitioning, genes encoding plasmid maintenance and transfer functions, and accessory genes that often include one or more resistance determinants (Figure 138-5). Some plasmids are lacking transfer functions, but can be transferred if these functions are provided in *trans* by a conjugative plasmid simultaneously present in the cell.

Transposons and integrons can be responsible for the capture of resistance genes on plasmids and ICEs and for their dissemination among these elements. Transposons are MGEs that range in size from a few to more than 150 kilobases and can move from one site to another of the same or of another replicon by a mechanism named transposition (Figure 138-6). Several different transposons have been described, and many of them carry one or more antibiotic-resistance determinants.[64]

Integrons are a peculiar group of genetic elements consisting of an integrase gene and a nearby recombination site at which mobile gene cassettes can be directionally inserted or excised by a site-specific recombination mechanism catalyzed by the integron integrase. The mobile gene cassettes are small units usually containing a single gene and a recombination site, which is recognized by the integron integrase (Figure 138-7). There are two groups of integrons: resistance integrons and superintegrons. Superintegrons are found in many gram-negative species and are located on the chromosome. These integrons may contain tens to hundreds of gene cassettes, which encode a large variety of different functions. Resistance integrons contain a lower number of gene cassettes which usually carry resistance determinants to antibiotics or disinfectants. The most common resistance integrons belong to

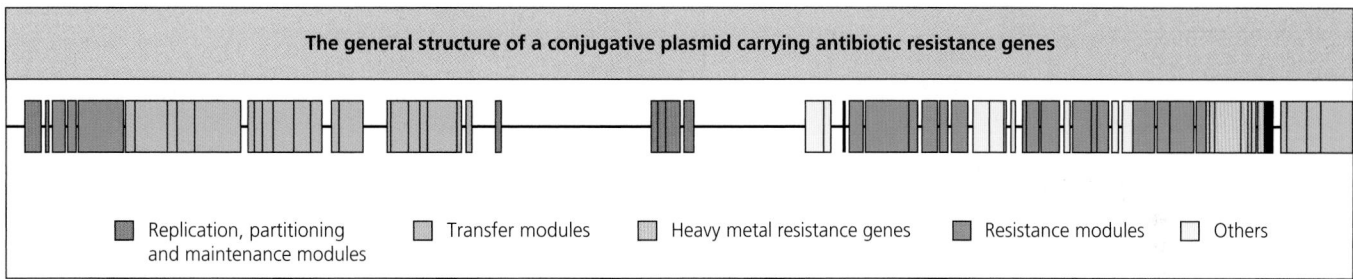

Figure 138-5 The general structure of a conjugative plasmid carrying antibiotic resistance genes. The plasmid is a circular DNA molecule (the map is shown linearized to facilitate readability). The plasmid has a modular structure including modules for plasmid replication, partitioning and stable maintenance, and for the plasmid transfer apparatus; in addition it carries resistance genes for antibiotics and heavy metals, which are associated with transposons.

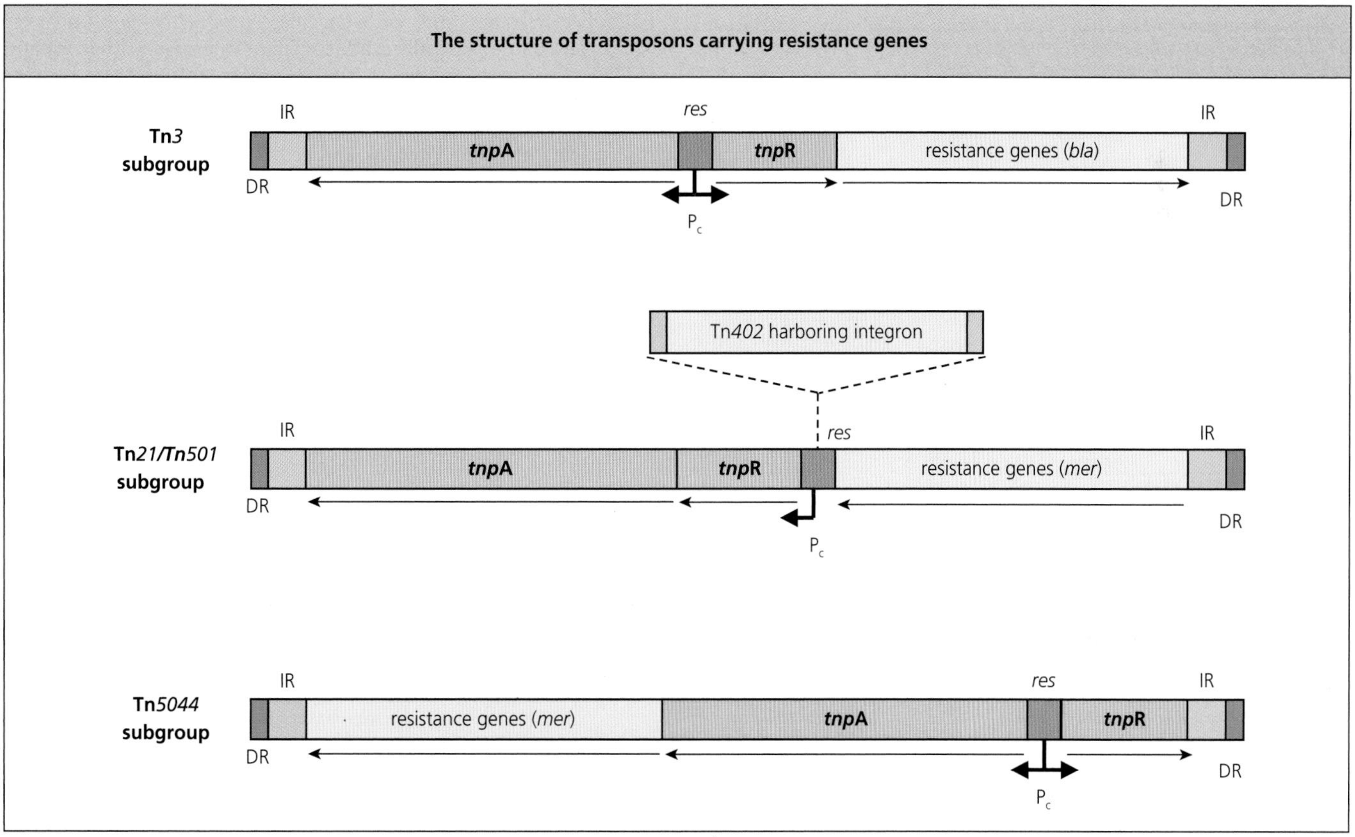

Figure 138-6 The structure of transposons carrying resistance genes. Transposons carry genes (*tnp*) encoding the enzymes (transposases and resolvases) responsible for the transposition process. The transposons are delimited by inverted repeats (IR) which are recognized by the transposases, and usually flanked by direct repeats (DR) that are generated following the transposition process. Resistance genes (to antibiotics, heavy metals, disinfectants) can be found at different positions and are mobilized together with the transposon.

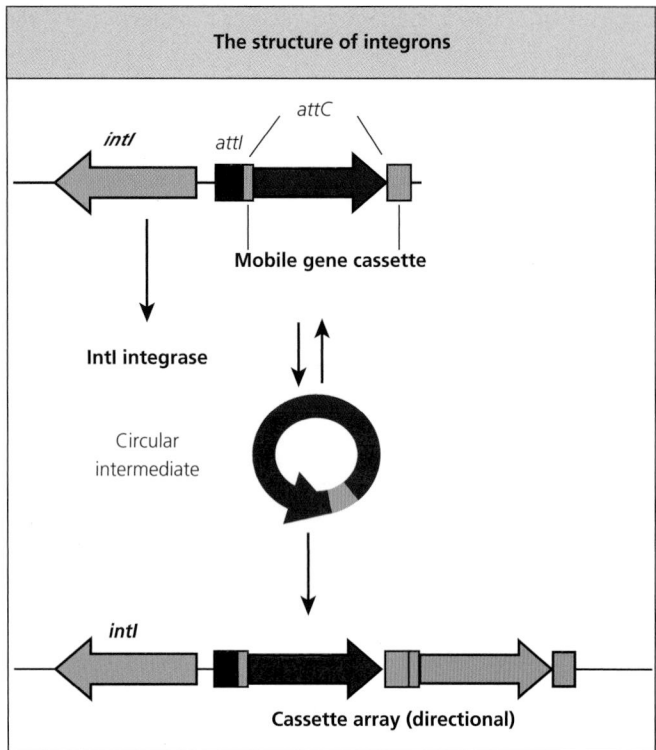

The structure of integrons

Mobile gene cassette

Intl integrase

Circular intermediate

Cassette array (directional)

Figure 138-7 The structure of integrons. The integron consists of an *intl* gene, encoding a DNA integrase, and a recombination site (*attl*), which is located upstream from the integrase gene. The integron integrase can insert and excise mobile gene cassettes at the *attl* recombination site via a site-specific recombination mechanism between *attl* and a recombination site (*attC*) that is present in the gene cassette. The gene cassettes are small mobile genetic units that normally contain a single gene (indicated by the red and blue arrows) and the *attC* recombination site. In resistance integrons most gene cassettes carry resistance genes to antibiotics and disinfectants (see text for details).

TABLE 138-7	Resistance and Mechanism of Resistance for Gene Cassettes
Antimicrobial Agents	**Resistance Determinants (Examples)**
β-Lactams	Class A β-lactamases (*bla*GES; *bla*PSE; *bla*CARB) Class B β-lactamases (*bla*IMP-type; *bla*VIM-type) Class D β-lactamases (*bla*OXA-10; *bla*OXA-9)
Aminoglycosides	Aminoglycoside adenylyltransferases (*ant(3′)-1a*) Aminoglycoside acetyltransferases (*aac(6′)-Ia*) Aminoglycoside phosphotransferases (*aphA15*)
Chloramphenicol	Chloramphenicol acetyltransferases (*catB2*) Chloramphenicol exporter (*cmlA, cmlB*)
Trimethoprim	Class A dihydrofolate reductases (*dfrA1*) Class B dihydrofolate reductases (*dfrB1*)
Erythromycin	Erythromycin esterases (*eraA1*)
Lincosamides	Lincomycin nucleotidyltransferases (*linF*)
Rifampin (rifampicin)	ADP ribosylation (*arr2*)
Fosfomycin	Fosfomycin inactivating enzyme (*fosA*)
Antiseptics and disinfectants	SMR-type efflux pumps (*smr1, qacE*)

Adapted from Partridge S.R., et al. FEMS Microbiol Rev 2009; 33(4):757–84.

class 1, but other classes are known as well. A large number of gene cassettes have been described, including resistance genes for β-lactams, aminoglycosides, trimethoprim, chloramphenicol and antiseptics and disinfectants (Table 138-7). Generally the cassettes do not have promoters, but transcription occurs from one of two promoter sequences present upstream from the integron recombination site. Integrons are widespread in Enterobacteriaceae and also in gram-negative nonfermenters. ISCRs are another type of MGEs that can capture resistance genes, and that are often found associated with integron platforms.[53,64]

Conclusions

Antibiotic resistance is ubiquitous and increasing. The most challenging resistant pathogens from the clinical and epidemiological standpoint are currently represented by MRSA, VRE, ESBL-producing Enterobacteriaceae, and carbapenemase-producing gram-negative bacilli. These strains usually exhibit MDR or extensively drug-resistant (XDR) phenotypes for which the treatment options may be very limited. Examples of XDR pathogens are represented by carbapenem-resistant *Acinetobacter baumannii* (CRAb), which usually remain susceptible only to polymyxins, and by CRE, which often remain susceptible only to polymyxins, tigecycline and some aminoglycosides.[65]

Selection and dissemination of resistant strains following the use of antimicrobial agents is unavoidable. However, the phenomenon can be minimized by the prudent use of antibiotics and a strict implementation of infection control and prevention measures. The misuse and overuse of antibiotics and the presence of poor hygienic conditions facilitate the cross-transmission of resistant strains in healthcare settings and also in the community.

References available online at expertconsult.com.

KEY REFERENCES

Almeida Da Silva P.E.A., Palomino J.C.: Molecular basis and mechanisms of drug resistance in *Mycobacterium tuberculosis*: classical and new drugs. *J Antimicrob Chemother* 2011; 66(7):1417-1430.

Bush K., Jacoby G.A.: Updated functional classification of beta-lactamases. *Antimicrob Agents Chemother* 2010; 54(3):969-976.

Cattoir V., Leclercq R.: Twenty-five years of shared life with vancomycin-resistant enterococci: is it time to divorce? *J Antimicrob Chemother* 2013; 68(4):731-742.

Chambers H.F., Deleo F.R.: Waves of resistance: Staphylococcus aureus in the antibiotic era. *Nat Rev Microbiol* 2009; 7(9):629-641.

Jacoby G.A.: Mechanisms of resistance to quinolones. *Clin Infect Dis* 2005; 41(Suppl. 2):S120-S126.

Macgowan A.P., BSAC Working Parties on Resistance Surveillance: Clinical implications of antimicrobial resistance for therapy. *J Antimicrob Chemother* 2008; 62(Suppl. 2):ii105-ii114.

Munoz-Price L.S., Poirel L., Bonomo R.A., et al.: Clinical epidemiology of the global expansion of Klebsiella pneumoniae carbapenemases. *Lancet Infect Dis* 2013; 13(9):785-796.

Poole K.: Efflux-mediated antimicrobial resistance. *J Antimicrob Chemother* 2005; 56(1):20-51.

Ramirez M.S., Tolmasky M.E.: Aminoglycoside modifying enzymes. *Drug Resist Updat* 2010; 13(6):151-171.

Roberts M.C.: Update on acquired tetracycline resistance genes. *FEMS Microbiol Lett* 2005; 245(2):195-203.

Roberts M.C., Sutcliffe J., Courvalin P., et al.: Nomenclature for macrolide and macrolide-lincosamide-streptogramin B resistance determinants. *Antimicrob Agents Chemother* 1999; 43(12):2823-2830.

Toleman M.A., Walsh T.R.: Combinatorial events of insertion sequences and ICE in Gram-negative bacteria. *FEMS Microbiol Rev* 2011; 35(5):912-935.

139

Optimizing the Use of Antimicrobial Agents: Antimicrobial Stewardship and Outpatient Parenteral Antimicrobial Therapy (OPAT)

MATTHEW S. SIMON | DAVID P. CALFEE

KEY CONCEPTS

- Antimicrobial agents are often used inappropriately and this inappropriate use is associated with adverse patient outcomes and development of antimicrobial resistance.

- Antimicrobial stewardship is a term that refers to coordinated interventions intended to optimize the use of antimicrobial agents.

- The introduction of antimicrobial stewardship activities has been associated with reductions in inappropriate antimicrobial use, improved patient outcomes, reductions in rates of antimicrobial resistance, and decreased healthcare costs in a variety of healthcare settings.

- With proper patient selection and adequate monitoring, outpatient parenteral antimicrobial therapy (OPAT) can provide excellent patient outcomes, reduce the risk of healthcare-associated infections, and improve the quality of life for patients requiring long-term parenteral antimicrobial therapy.

- Critical aspects of successful OPAT include identification of patients for whom OPAT is appropriate, selection of an appropriate antimicrobial regimen, education of the patient and the patient's caregivers, appropriate safety monitoring, and effective communication between members of the OPAT team (patient, visiting nurse, pharmacy, social worker or case manager and prescribing clinician).

Antimicrobial Stewardship

Since their introduction into clinical medicine in the early 20th century, antibiotics have saved millions of lives and prevented or minimized morbidity in countless others. Like any other medication or medical intervention, antimicrobial use is also associated with risks. These risks include complications that are the result of exposure to the drug (e.g. allergic reactions, drug-related toxicity), administration of the drug (e.g. central line-associated bloodstream infection), and alteration of the recipient's normal flora (e.g. *Clostridium difficile* infection (CDI)). Other risks include development or selection of antimicrobial-resistant organisms. In addition to the untoward effects that may be experienced by the recipient, antimicrobial use in one person can have an impact on the larger population due to ecologic changes in antimicrobial resistance resulting from antimicrobial selection pressure that occurs at the societal level. While the benefits of antimicrobial therapy outweigh the potential risks when antibiotics are used appropriately, inappropriate use of these agents alters the risk-benefit ratio and in some cases the potential risks exceed the potential for benefit. There are many ways in which antimicrobial agents can be misused (Table 139-1) and the reasons for misuse are numerous and complex.

Prevalence and Characteristics of Antimicrobial Use and Misuse

A large proportion of hospital patients receive antimicrobial therapy during their hospital stay. Data from 70 academic medical centers in the USA showed that 63.7% of adult patients were treated with antimicrobial agents.[1] While an understanding of the prevalence of antimicrobial use is important, it is even more important to consider the appropriateness of antimicrobial use. Several studies have demonstrated that nearly 50% of antimicrobial use in hospitals and 25–75% of systemic antibiotic use in long-term care facilities (LTCF) is inappropriate. Using data from nationally representative surveys of adult ambulatory visits in the USA, investigators found that antibacterial therapy was prescribed during 51% of outpatient visits for acute respiratory tract infections for which antibiotics are rarely indicated (e.g. bronchitis and laryngitis).[2] In outpatient hemodialysis units, a 3-year study found that the rate of parenteral antibacterial use was 32.9 doses per 100 patient-months and that nearly 30% of doses were inappropriate.[3]

Antimicrobial Stewardship Concepts and Strategies

Antimicrobial stewardship has been defined as 'coordinated interventions designed to improve and measure the appropriate use of antimicrobial agents by promoting the selection of the optimal antimicrobial drug regimen including dosing, duration of therapy, and route of administration.'[4] The purpose of these interventions is to optimize clinical outcomes, minimize antimicrobial-related toxicities and adverse events, and avoid unnecessary antibiotic selection pressure to limit the emergence and propagation of antimicrobial resistance. Multidisciplinary antimicrobial stewardship programs have been associated with a variety of beneficial outcomes, including improved appropriateness of antimicrobial prescribing and significant reductions in broad-spectrum antimicrobial use, adverse outcomes associated with antibiotic use, rates of antimicrobial resistance among healthcare-associated pathogens, mortality and hospital expenditures for antimicrobial agents. The Institute for Healthcare Improvement and the USA Centers for Disease Control and Prevention have developed an antimicrobial stewardship driver diagram and change package.[5] This document identifies four primary drivers of timely and appropriate antibiotic utilization in the acute care setting: 1) timely and appropriate initiation of antibiotics; 2) appropriate administration and de-escalation; 3) data monitoring, transparency, and stewardship infrastructure; and 4) availability of expertise at the point of care. Attention to each of the four primary drivers should increase the likelihood that the antimicrobial stewardship program will effectively achieve its goal.

There are a number of strategies that have been used to improve antimicrobial prescribing practices. These strategies can be described

TABLE 139-1	Inappropriate Antimicrobial Use	
Category of Inappropriate Use	Example(s)	Potential Adverse Outcomes Associated with Misuse
Use of antibacterial agents for treatment of syndromes that are not caused by bacteria	Common cold, viral upper respiratory tract infection, most sore throats	No potential for benefit; risk of toxicity, complications (e.g. *C. difficile* infection), development of antimicrobial resistance; unnecessary expense
Treatment for culture results that reflect colonization or contamination rather than infection	Asymptomatic bacteriuria, blood culture contaminants	No potential for benefit; risk of toxicity, complications, development of antimicrobial resistance; unnecessary expense
Administration of an antibacterial regimen with a broader than necessary spectrum of activity	Overly broad empiric therapy; failure to narrow the antibacterial spectrum of an empiric regimen based on culture results and other clinical data	Alteration of normal flora leading to increased risk of complications (e.g. *C. difficile* infection); antimicrobial selection pressure favoring antimicrobial-resistant organisms
Prescription of courses of antibacterial therapy for treatment or prophylaxis that are longer than necessary	Administration of surgical antimicrobial prophylaxis for >24 hours after the procedure	Risk of toxicity, complications (e.g. *C. difficile* infection), development of antimicrobial resistance; unnecessary expense
Prescription of antibacterial agents at inappropriate doses or dosing intervals	Lack of appropriate dose adjustment for abnormal renal function or body weight	Inappropriately high doses or inappropriately short dosing intervals: increased risk of toxicity, unnecessary expense Inappropriately low doses or inappropriately long dosing intervals: increased risk of treatment failure, increased risk of development of antimicrobial resistance
Treatment of an infectious process with agents that do not provide activity against the causative agent(s)	Failure to appropriately adjust antimicrobial regimen when antimicrobial susceptibility testing demonstrates that pathogen is resistant to empiric treatment regimen	Increased risk of treatment failure
Redundant spectra of antimicrobial activity among agents in a multidrug antimicrobial regimen	Simultaneous administration of two drugs with activity against anaerobic organisms	Increased risk of toxicity, complications; unnecessary expense

as restrictive, persuasive or structural.[6] Restrictive interventions are those that restrict the ability of prescribers to use certain antimicrobial agents. Examples of restrictive strategies include formulary restriction, requirement for approval prior to use of selected antimicrobial agents, and the requirement to use antimicrobial order forms or other processes to document an appropriate indication for use of the prescribed antimicrobial agent. Persuasive strategies, such as education, reminders and audit and feedback interventions, are intended to change behavior among clinicians who prescribe antimicrobial agents. Finally, structural strategies are changes in the healthcare delivery system that may contribute to optimization of antimicrobial prescribing. These changes are often technology-based (e.g. computerized decision support systems and rapid laboratory diagnostic testing modalities). Many stewardship programs use a combination of these three types of strategies. Guidelines published by the Infectious Diseases Society of America (IDSA) and the Society for Healthcare Epidemiology of America (SHEA) provide recommendations for developing antimicrobial stewardship programs in acute care hospitals.[7] There has been less experience with implementation of antimicrobial stewardship in other healthcare settings, such as LTCF and outpatient settings, but many of the interventions described for acute care hospitals would also be appropriate for use in these settings. Some of the more common and well-established strategies are described and illustrative examples are provided in the following paragraphs.

FORMULARY RESTRICTION AND PREAUTHORIZATION

Although technically two different strategies, formulary restriction and preauthorization are included together as one of two core strategies in the IDSA-SHEA guidelines.[7] These strategies limit the ability of individual clinicians to prescribe certain antimicrobial agents in an effort to reduce overall antimicrobial use and/or the use of specific antimicrobials or classes of antimicrobial agents. Formulary restriction refers to limiting the number of antimicrobial agents contained in the hospital's formulary. Preauthorization strategies may require the prescribing clinician to obtain approval from a member of the stewardship team before the pharmacy will dispense the requested antimicrobial

agent or require that certain pre-specified criteria for the drug's use are met and documented when the order for the antimicrobial agent is placed. One hospital that implemented a number of restrictive strategies reported a substantial reduction in the use of selected antimicrobial agents with an associated 25% reduction in antimicrobial expenditures and stabilization or improvement in antimicrobial resistance patterns for several pathogens, including *Staph. aureus* and *Pseudomonas aeruginosa*.[8]

Preauthorization programs should be designed to ensure that the approval process does not result in inappropriate delays in the administration of appropriate antimicrobial therapy. The use of strategies that involve specific drug class restrictions or favor the use of one specific agent may potentiate the development and propagation of antimicrobial resistance to that agent. Because of this, many authorities highlight the importance of maintaining some degree of diversity or heterogeneity in the use of antimicrobial drug classes in order to limit antibiotic selection pressure that may lead to emergence of resistance to a favored class of drugs. Other unintended consequences observed as a result of restrictive strategies have included an increase in prescriptions for nonrestricted drugs in an attempt to bypass the approval procedure and shifts in antimicrobial ordering practices so that restricted drugs are ordered at an increased frequency during periods (e.g. overnight) when the approval process is suspended.[9] Another potential pitfall of preauthorization programs is reliance on the requesting prescriber to provide correct and complete information. In a retrospective cohort study, investigators found that miscommunication of microbiologic data resulted in approval of antimicrobial therapy that was not indicated.[10]

PROSPECTIVE AUDIT WITH INTERVENTION AND FEEDBACK

The second of the two core strategies identified in the IDSA-SHEA guidelines is prospective audit with intervention and feedback, also known as post-prescription review. This strategy involves review by the antimicrobial stewardship team of the appropriateness of prescribed antimicrobial therapy with provision of recommendations for optimizing therapy, if such opportunities are identified, to the prescriber.

In one hospital, introduction of prospective audit and feedback in intensive care units (ICU) was associated with an immediate and sustained reduction in the use of the targeted broad-spectrum antimicrobial agents, a significant increase in meropenem susceptibility among gram-negative bacteria, and a 31% reduction (p=0.04) in nosocomial CDI in the participating ICUs.[11] A subsequent trial of the introduction of this same audit and feedback program on non-ICU wards detected a 21% reduction in use of the targeted antimicrobial agents among patients who met criteria for review. However, there was no change in the overall use of targeted antimicrobials, overall costs or microbiologic outcomes.

In a randomized, controlled study, patients receiving broad-spectrum antimicrobial therapy for at least 3 days who underwent post-prescription review and feedback were more likely to receive early antibiotic interventions, including discontinuation of therapy, shortened duration of therapy and streamlining of the antimicrobial regimen.[12] In addition, fewer patients in the intervention group required subsequent readmission for relapsed infection (3.4% vs 7.9%, p = 0.01). Reductions in the use of targeted antimicrobials have not, however, been observed in all hospitals that have introduced this type of intervention. In a before–after study in five academic hospitals, significant reductions in the use of targeted antibiotics were observed in two hospitals while increases were observed in two others and no change was observed in the fifth hospital.[13] Of note, the hospitals in which reductions were observed had well-established antimicrobial stewardship programs prior to the intervention. This suggests that factors such as program acceptance by prescribing clinicians and the antibiotic stewardship team's comfort with assessing antimicrobial use and making interventions may have contributed to the inconsistent findings among participating hospitals.

EDUCATION

Education for prescribing clinicians can be a useful persuasive component of an antimicrobial stewardship program, but it is most likely to be effective in changing antimicrobial prescribing practices when combined with an active intervention (e.g. preauthorization, prospective audit and feedback). Education topics should target the audience and address the priority antimicrobial use and resistance issues identified within the facility. Common topics addressed in these educational programs include general principles of antimicrobial therapy, interpretation of antibiotic susceptibility reports and hospital antibiograms, and facility-specific diagnostic and treatment guidelines.

GUIDELINES AND CLINICAL PATHWAYS

The development and distribution of guidelines and clinical pathways is a commonly used strategy to optimize antimicrobial use. Guidelines and clinical pathways typically provide recommendations for empiric antimicrobial therapy for specific infection syndromes (e.g. healthcare-associated pneumonia) based on national guidelines, hospital formulary, local antimicrobial resistance patterns, cost and other institutional considerations. Guidelines may also contain recommendations for selection of a definitive antimicrobial regimen based on pathogen identification, recommendations for duration of therapy based on site of infection and other considerations, and dosing recommendations for specific antibiotics. In addition to antimicrobial recommendations, guidelines and clinical pathways may also include recommendations for diagnostic testing and other aspects of clinical care to further optimize healthcare utilization and patient outcomes. The results of one randomized controlled trial suggest that direct interaction with an antimicrobial stewardship team is more effective in optimizing antimicrobial use than the availability of guidelines alone.[14]

STREAMLINING OR DE-ESCALATION OF THERAPY

Empiric antimicrobial regimens are often broad in spectrum in order to maximize the chance of providing activity against the infecting organism. Streamlining or de-escalation refers to changes made to a previously prescribed antimicrobial regimen based on available culture results and other laboratory data, imaging studies or clinical data. These changes can include adjustment of an empiric antibiotic regimen to a narrower spectrum of antimicrobial activity, discontinuation of unnecessary duplicative therapy, addition of a different antimicrobial agent to provide coverage for an organism for which coverage had not previously been provided, or complete discontinuation of antimicrobial therapy if the additional information reveals no evidence of an infectious process. De-escalation limits exposure to broad-spectrum antimicrobial therapy and thus may reduce the risk of toxicity and complications and the cost of antimicrobial therapy. Streamlining can be accomplished via a variety of approaches including reminders, automatic stop orders, and audit and feedback interventions.

DOSE OPTIMIZATION

Dose optimization includes strategies to ensure that characteristics of the drug, infectious agent, patient and site of infection are appropriately considered. Such strategies may improve rates of cure, minimize toxicity and reduce the risk of development of antimicrobial resistance. Examples include dose adjustments for patients with renal dysfunction who are receiving antimicrobials that are eliminated by renal mechanisms; weight-based dosing of certain antimicrobials; once-daily dosing of aminoglycosides in appropriate circumstances; and extended or continuous infusions of some β-lactam antibiotics. Extended or continuous infusion has been used to increase the percentage of the dosing interval during which the free antibiotic concentration exceeds the minimum inhibitory concentration (fT>MIC) of the infecting organism. Conventional dosing regimens may not provide the required fT>MIC for organisms with higher MICs,[15] an increasingly common occurrence in the era of multidrug-resistant gram-negative pathogens. For some drugs, such as vancomycin and aminoglycosides, dose optimization includes therapeutic drug monitoring to increase the likelihood of achieving the desired clinical outcome and/or to minimize the risk of toxicity. Hospitals with stewardship programs have demonstrated significantly lower rates of nephrotoxicity and ototoxicity associated with the use of vancomycin and aminoglycosides.[16]

PARENTERAL TO ORAL CONVERSION

Intravenous (iv) antimicrobial agents are often administered in situations where orally-administered (po) antimicrobial therapy would be sufficient.[17,18] Unnecessary use of intravenous antimicrobial therapy can result in prolonged hospital stay, an unnecessary risk of complications from the vascular access device required for administration of iv therapy, and unnecessary antimicrobial expenditures. Parenteral to oral conversion strategies may most easily be accomplished for antimicrobial agents for which similar concentrations are achieved whether the drug is administered intravenously or enterally, such as fluoroquinolones, azoles, metronidazole, clindamycin and oxazolidinones. However, iv to po conversion initiatives can also target inappropriate intravenous administration of other antimicrobial agents. Conversion from iv to po therapy requires that the patient is able to reliably take enterally-administered medications and is not suspected or known to be unable to absorb the orally-administered antibiotic. In some situations where the oral regimen will not achieve the same blood or tissues concentrations as iv therapy, evidence of clinical improvement may also be desirable prior to conversion. While iv to po switch recommendations should be included in facility-specific antimicrobial use guidelines, several studies have found that this approach alone is often insufficient. Additional strategies that may improve rates of appropriate conversion from iv to po therapy include pharmacist-driven initiatives, reminders and checklists, and computer-assisted decision support tools.

CLINICAL DECISION SUPPORT SYSTEMS (CDSS)

Clinical decision support systems (CDSS) have been used to assist clinicians in making wise antimicrobial treatment decisions and to assist the antimicrobial stewardship program with identification of patients for potential intervention. These systems may use medication administration or ordering data, microbiology data, estimates of creatinine clearance, drug allergy information, drug cost information and other information to guide clinician prescribing or to identify patients who may be receiving suboptimal antimicrobial therapy. CDSS have been shown to select appropriate empiric antimicrobial regimens significantly more frequently than physicians.[19] In a cluster-randomized trial of one such CDSS, the rate of appropriate empiric antimicrobial therapy was higher on wards assigned to the CDSS intervention but the difference failed to reach statistical significance after adjustment for location and clustering by ward. In a before-after study, introduction of a real-time CDSS was associated with a significant decrease in consumption of broad-spectrum antibacterial agents in the ICU and with statistically significant increases in antimicrobial susceptibility among *Pseudomonas, Acinetobacter* spp., and Enterobacteriaceae isolates.[20] The rapid expansion of the use of electronic medical record and automated surveillance systems provides an opportunity for the use of CDSS in antimicrobial stewardship programs; however, the capabilities of currently available systems are quite variable.

Antimicrobial Stewardship in Settings Other than the Acute Care Hospital

Although most studies of and the vast majority of experience with antimicrobial stewardship programs are in the acute care hospital setting, there is an increasing body of literature that suggests that antimicrobial stewardship interventions are feasible in other healthcare settings. Differences in resources, infrastructure, the population served and clinical practice within these other settings as compared to acute care hospitals, however, may require modifications in the way in which stewardship activities are implemented and carried out.

OUTPATIENT MEDICAL PRACTICES

Audit and feedback strategies have been used successfully in the outpatient setting. In a cluster-randomized trial conducted in 18 primary care pediatric practices, participation in a 1-hour education session and receipt of quarterly audit and feedback reports of physician-specific prescribing data for acute respiratory tract infections was associated with statistically significant reductions in broad-spectrum antibiotic prescribing and off-guideline prescribing for children with pneumonia.[21] CDSS have also been used successfully in outpatient settings. In a controlled, observational study, introduction of a CDSS that deployed guideline-based recommendations during order entry was associated with a significant reduction in inappropriate antimicrobial treatment for acute respiratory tract infections for which antimicrobial therapy was not warranted.[22]

LONG-TERM ACUTE CARE HOSPITALS

A prospective audit and feedback intervention that was staffed by a non-ID trained clinical pharmacist and an ID physician was introduced into a long-term acute care hospital.[23] This was associated with a 21% reduction in mean monthly antimicrobial use (p = 0.003) and a 28% reduction in mean monthly cost per patient (p = 0.004) with no observed changes in mortality or transfers to short-term acute care hospitals.

LONG-TERM CARE FACILITIES

A cluster-randomized study of a nurse-driven antimicrobial stewardship tool conducted in 30 LTCFs demonstrated a 4.9% reduction (p = 0.02) in total systemic antibiotic consumption relative to baseline in the intervention group, compared to a 5.1% increase (p = 0.04) in the control group, and a significant increase in the appropriateness of therapy.[24] In another LTCF, a 30% reduction in systemic antibiotic administration and a significant reduction in the rate of positive *C. difficile* tests were observed following the introduction of an infectious disease consultation service in which an ID physician and nurse practitioner visited the facility once per week and were available by telephone at other times.[25]

Implementation and Monitoring of an Antimicrobial Stewardship Program

Despite a growing body of evidence that antimicrobial stewardship programs can improve patient outcomes and provide additional ecologic and financial benefits, many hospitals do not have such programs in place.[26] Even among those facilities with a stewardship program, stewardship activities vary greatly and it is likely that there remain substantial opportunities to improve antimicrobial stewardship. Organized antimicrobial stewardship activities are even less common in non-acute care facilities, such as LTCF and ambulatory care settings. Lack of funding and personnel are the most commonly reported barriers to establishment of a functional and effective antimicrobial stewardship program.[26] Another commonly reported barrier is physician resistance to restriction of their autonomy in antimicrobial prescribing. Thus, obtaining the financial and philosophical support of the facility's administration and medical leadership is critical to the success of the antimicrobial stewardship program.[27] SHEA, IDSA and the Pediatric Infectious Diseases Society have outlined minimum requirements for antimicrobial stewardship programs in acute care hospitals, LTCF, long-term acute care facilities, ambulatory surgery centers and dialysis facilities.[4] These requirements include: a physician-led multidisciplinary team; a restricted antimicrobial formulary; guidelines for the management of common infection syndromes; additional interventions to improve the use of antimicrobials within the facility; processes to measure and monitor antimicrobial use; and periodic distribution of a facility-specific antibiogram. As with any quality improvement program, it is important to assess the antimicrobial stewardship program's activities and the clinical and microbiologic outcomes associated with those activities. An international expert panel developed a list of indicators that can be used to evaluate the structure and activities of antimicrobial stewardship programs in acute care hospitals.[28]

Outpatient Parenteral Antimicrobial Therapy

Since initially described in the 1970s, the use of outpatient parenteral antimicrobial therapy (OPAT) has expanded dramatically. In the 1990s, it was estimated that approximately 250 000 patients per year receive OPAT in the USA.[29] OPAT's acceptance has been driven by studies demonstrating safety and efficacy coupled with decreased hospital length of stay and reduced healthcare costs.[30] Additional benefits include avoidance of nosocomial complications and improved quality of life as patients receive treatment at home or return to work.[31] Conversely, OPAT has the potential to result in harm due to vascular access-related complications and medication-related adverse events. As OPAT utilization has increased over the past decade, there has been recognition of the importance of antimicrobial stewardship interventions to optimize antimicrobial prescribing as patients transition from the inpatient to outpatient setting.[32] This section will summarize the key components of a safe and effective OPAT program.

Development of an OPAT Team

Because of the medical, social and economic complexities of OPAT, a multidisciplinary team approach is recommended to enable effective and safe delivery.[33,34] An OPAT team typically consists of the patient and the patient's caregivers, a physician, an infusion nurse, a pharmacist and a case manager or social worker. Team members may vary depending on the setting in which OPAT is administered. OPAT settings include: 1) self-administration at home, usually in coordination with a home infusion company; 2) visiting nurse service; 3) a dedicated infusion center; or 4) a skilled nursing facility. Despite recommendations for a dedicated OPAT team, data suggest low rates of implementation in practice. In a survey of North American infectious disease physicians, lack of dedicated personnel was the most commonly identified barrier to providing safe OPAT care.[35] Mechanisms for reliable communication between team members should be established prior to the initiation of OPAT and maintained throughout treatment. A process map of a typical OPAT course identified 217 potential failures that could result in error or harm with the majority (57%) due to communication issues.[36]

Patient Selection

Prior to initiation of OPAT, it is crucial to ensure clinical stability and the presence of adequate social support at home. Key questions in selecting patients for OPAT include:[33]

- Is parenteral antimicrobial therapy needed?
- Do the patient's medical care needs exceed resources available in the community?
- Is the home environment safe and adequate to support care?
- Are the patient and caregiver willing and able to safely, effectively, and reliably deliver parenteral antimicrobial therapy?
- Are rapid and reliable communication mechanisms in place for monitoring of problems or complications?
- Do the patient and caregiver understand the benefits, risks and financial costs of OPAT?

Special populations who may require OPAT include the elderly and patients with substance abuse. Compared with patients younger than age 60, older OPAT patients have comparable outcomes but may be at increased risk for nephrotoxicity and require more urgent care visits.[37] Active substance abuse has often been considered a contraindication to OPAT because of concerns related to abuse of vascular access; however, it may be considered for carefully selected patients.[38]

Vascular Access and Drug Delivery Systems

Peripherally inserted central catheters (PICCs) are frequently used for the administration of OPAT because of their durability and ease of insertion and removal. Antibiotics that require dilution in large volume solution (e.g. vancomycin) may be administered via gravity drip. Battery-operated, computerized infusion pumps can be used and programmed to deliver an antibiotic via bolus or continuous infusion (e.g. nafcillin). Patients can wear these automated devices around their waist and often resume daily functioning while receiving therapy.

OPAT Indications, Prescribing and Monitoring

The most common indications for OPAT are bone and joint infections, endocarditis, skin and soft tissue infections (SSTIs) and bacteremia.[29] Additional infections for which OPAT is used include pyelonephritis, intra-abdominal, prosthetic device-related, and central nervous system infections. The decision to initiate treatment in the hospital or outpatient setting depends on infection severity, signs of systemic toxicity, need for surgical debridement and patient co-morbidities. ID consultation is recommended by US and UK practice guidelines.[33,34] ID consultation has been associated with cost-savings and, even more importantly, improved antimicrobial utilization and enhanced safety. In one study, ID consultation prior to hospital discharge determined that OPAT was not necessary in 27% of cases.[39]

Antimicrobial selection must balance tolerability, feasibility of administration, and cost while considering the site of infection and microbiologic data. Agents with once-daily dosing intervals, such as ceftriaxone, ertapenem and daptomycin, are well-suited for OPAT. New antimicrobials, such as dalbavancin and oritavancin, possessing long half-lives that allow for weekly administration, may dramatically alter the approach to OPAT for some infections. The most commonly reported complications include catheter occlusion, rash, gastrointestinal side effects, nephrotoxicity and cytopenias.[33,35] Premature discontinuation due to medication-related adverse events may occur in 3–10% of OPAT courses. Hospital readmission rates have ranged from 6–50%.[33,40] Few randomized studies have directly compared the safety

TABLE 139-2	Proposed Outpatient Parenteral Antibiotic Therapy Bundle	
Main Bundle Components	**Key Aspects**	
Patient identification/ selection	Fully aware of risks/benefits Appropriate home environment with adequate support No clinical contraindications to hospital discharge Feasibility and willingness to comply with follow-up Insurance/copayment issues resolved	
ID consultation	Prior to intravenous access Prior to discharge home	
Patient/family education	Vascular access education/teach back Emergency contact numbers for patients Physician responsible until patient seen in clinic Medication side effects Potential complications	
Care transition	ID appointment scheduled prior to discharge Clear communication between inpatient and outpatient providers OPAT plan documented in discharge summary Safety labs included as part of discharge plan	
Outpatient monitoring	Safety labs: identifying missing labs, addressing lab abnormalities, adjusting medication doses as indicated PICC line care, maintenance and removal at completion of OPAT course Change in management: communication between ID physician and infusion company/rehabilitation facility Monitoring of clinical and microbiologic response/cure	
OPAT program measures	Patient satisfaction Clinical outcomes Complications/Readmissions Program improvements	

Adapted from: Muldoon EG, Snydman DR, Penland EC, Allison GM. Are we ready for an outpatient parenteral antimicrobial therapy bundle? A critical appraisal of the evidence. Clin Infect Dis 2013; 57:(3)419-24

and efficacy of antimicrobial regimens used in OPAT. A retrospective cohort study of outpatients receiving vancomycin or daptomycin for antimicrobial-resistant gram-positive infections found daptomycin to have comparable efficacy and 60% fewer antimicrobial adverse events compared with propensity score-matched patients receiving vancomycin.[41]

Weekly clinical and laboratory monitoring for patients receiving OPAT is typically recommended but less frequent office visits may be appropriate for patients without significant co-morbidities and good social support.[33] Laboratory monitoring varies depending on the specific antimicrobial agent but typically involves at least weekly assessment of complete blood count, renal and liver function tests. For instance, daptomycin requires weekly monitoring of creatine kinase whereas aminoglycoside therapy necessitates twice weekly monitoring of renal function and instructing patients to monitor for changes in hearing and vestibular symptoms. A survey of North American infectious disease physicians suggested considerable variation in OPAT monitoring in clinical practice.[42] 29% of respondents did not see patients weekly, but greater than 90% reported weekly laboratory monitoring. In one retrospective study, non-availability of recommended labs was independently associated with hospital readmission.[40] Reliable systems to ensure appropriate monitoring and follow-up are essential for OPAT safety. To this end, an evidence-based bundle comprised of six core elements has been proposed to promote standardized, high-quality care for OPAT patients (Table 139-2).[43]

References available online at expertconsult.com.

KEY REFERENCES

Camins B.C., King M.D., Wells J.B., et al.: Impact of an antimicrobial utilization program on antimicrobial use at a large teaching hospital: a randomized controlled trial. *Infect Control Hosp Epidemiol* 2009; 30(10):931-938.

Chapman A.L., Seaton R.A., Cooper M.A., et al.: Good practice recommendations for outpatient parenteral antimicrobial therapy (OPAT) in adults in the UK: a consensus statement. *J Antimicrob Chemother* 2012; 67(5): 1053-1062.

Dellit T.H., Owens R.C., McGowan J.E., et al.: Infectious Diseases Society of America and the Society for Healthcare Epidemiology of America guidelines for developing an institutional program to enhance antimicrobial stewardship. *Clin Infect Dis* 2007; 44(2):159-177.

Gerber J.S., Prasad P.A., Fiks A.G., et al.: Effect of an outpatient antimicrobial stewardship intervention on broad-spectrum antibiotic prescribing by primary care pediatricians: a randomized trial. *JAMA* 2013; 309(22): 2345-2352.

Institute for Healthcare Improvement: Antibiotic Stewardship Driver Diagram and Change Package Atlanta GA:

Centers for Disease Control and Prevention. Available: http://www.cdc.gov/getsmart/healthcare/pdfs/Antibiotic_Stewardship_Change_Package.pdf.

Johannsson B., Beekmann S.E., Srinivasan A., et al.: Improving antimicrobial stewardship: the evolution of programmatic strategies and barriers. *Infect Control Hosp Epidemiol* 2011; 32(4):367-374.

Lane M.A., Marschall J., Beekmann S.E., et al.: Outpatient parenteral antimicrobial therapy practices among adult infectious disease physicians. *Infect Control Hosp Epidemiol* 2014; 35(7):839-844.

Lesprit P., Landelle C., Brun-Buisson C.: Clinical impact of unsolicited post-prescription antibiotic review in surgical and medical wards: a randomized controlled trial. *Clin Microbiol Infect* 2013; 19(2):E91-E97.

Muldoon E.G., Snydman D.R., Penland E.C., et al.: Are we ready for an outpatient parenteral antimicrobial therapy bundle? A critical appraisal of the evidence. *Clin Infect Dis* 2013; 57(3):419-424.

Paladino J.A., Poretz D.: Outpatient parenteral antimicrobial therapy today. *Clin Infect Dis* 2010; 51(Suppl.2): S198-S208.

Shrestha N.K., Bhaskaran A., Scalera N.M., et al.: Contribution of infectious disease consultation toward the care of inpatients being considered for community-based parenteral anti-infective therapy. *J Hosp Med* 2012; 7(5): 365-369.

Society for Healthcare Epidemiology of America: Infectious Diseases Society of America, Pediatric Infectious Diseases Society. Policy statement on antimicrobial stewardship by the Society for Healthcare Epidemiology of America (SHEA), the Infectious Diseases Society of America (IDSA), and the Pediatric Infectious Diseases Society (PIDS). *Infect Control Hosp Epidemiol* 2012; 33(4): 322-327.

Stevenson K.B., Balada-Llasat J.M., Bauer K., et al.: The economics of antimicrobial stewardship: the current state of the art and applying the business case model. *Infect Control Hosp Epidemiol* 2012; 33(4):389-397.

Tice A.D., Rehm S.J., Dalovisio J.R., et al.: Practice guidelines for outpatient parenteral antimicrobial therapy. IDSA guidelines. *Clin Infect Dis* 2004; 38(12):1651-1672.

140

β-Lactam Antibiotics

RICHARD R. WATKINS | ROBERT A. BONOMO

KEY CONCEPTS

• β-Lactam antibiotics have a broad range of clinical indications.

• The most important mechanism for bacterial resistance to β-lactams is the production of β-lactamases.

• Resistance to β-lactams continues to evolve especially among *Streptococcus pneumoniae* and certain gram-negative bacilli (e.g. *Pseudomonas aeruginosa*).

• Recommendations for antibiotic prophylaxis have been recently updated and there are now fewer indications.

• Continuous infusions may have advantages over conventional intermittent bolus dosing.

• β-Lactam antibiotics are generally safe and well tolerated compared to other classes, although toxicities are not uncommon in clinical practice.

Introduction

Despite Alexander Fleming's observation that a *Penicillium* mold inhibited the growth of bacteria in culture in 1928, it was not until 1941 that Florey, Chain and Abraham used penicillin for the first time to treat patients.[1] More than 70 years later, the β-lactam antibiotics remain a pillar of therapy for a variety of bacterial infections (Table 140-1) and currently include:

• penicillins
• cephalosporins
• monobactams
• carbapenems
• β-lactamase inhibitor combinations.

Penicillins

The natural penicillins, such as penicillin G, are used primarily for the treatment of selected gram-positive and gram-negative infections. The penicillinase-resistant penicillins, including nafcillin and oxacillin, had been used for the treatment of infections due to staphylococci prior to the emergence of widespread resistance among staphylococci from the acquisition of low-affinity penicillin-binding proteins. These agents are active against other gram-positive organisms and continue to remain agents of choice in treating methicillin-susceptible staphylococci (MSSA). The aminopenicillins, such as ampicillin and amoxicillin, have a similar spectrum of activity as the natural penicillins but have additional activity against gram-negative organisms including many Enterobacteriaceae. When used together with β-lactamase inhibitors, they have good activity against aerobic gram-positive, gram-negative and anaerobic organisms that produce β-lactamases, enzymes which can hydrolyze these agents. The carboxypenicillins (ticarcillin) and ureidopenicillins (piperacillin) have activity against aminopenicillin-resistant gram-negative bacilli, especially *Pseudomonas aeruginosa*, and can also be used in conjunction with β-lactamase inhibitors for extended activity against β-lactamase-producing organisms.

CEPHALOSPORINS

Cephalosporins are frequently designated as belonging to a generation, first through fifth, to suggest a general spectrum of activity of the agents. In this classification, first-generation cephalosporins have activity against gram-positive cocci, but have limited activity against gram-negative pathogens. The second-generation cephalosporins have improved gram-negative activity compared to the first-generation cephalosporins. Selected second-generation cephalosporins (i.e. cefoxitin and cefotetan) also have activity against anaerobes. Third-generation cephalosporins have further improved gram-negative activity, but their activity against gram-positive bacteria is variable (e.g. cefotaxime, ceftazidime and ceftriaxone). Cefepime (primarily USA) and cefpirome (Europe) are fourth-generation cephalosporins with demonstrated efficacy against most clinically important gram-positive and gram-negative bacteria. Ceftaroline is a fifth-generation cephalosporin with enhanced activity against methicillin-resistant *Staphylococcus aureus* (MRSA). Ceftazidime/avibactam has improved activity against KPC-producing gram-negative bacteria.

Another useful categorization of cephalosporins is based on chemical structure[2,3] and could become more widely accepted with the emergence of new agents having a unique microbiologic spectrum. As cephalosporin resistance increases due to extended-spectrum β-lactamases and carbapenemases, the antimicrobial spectrum of agents categorized within these generations will need to be redefined, especially for gram-negative bacteria.

MONOBACTAMS

Monobactams, with aztreonam as the only commercially available agent, are effective against aerobic gram-negative organisms and have no activity against gram-positive organisms or anaerobes.

CARBAPENEMS

The carbapenems (imipenem, meropenem, ertapenem and doripenem) have the broadest bacterial coverage of the β-lactam antibiotics.

TABLE 140-1	Clinical Use of β-Lactam Antibiotics by Site of Infection	
Infection Site	**β-Lactam Used**
Skin/soft tissue infections	Cephalosporins, penicillins, carbapenem (ertapenem)
Head and neck infections	
Dental infections	Penicillins
Pharyngitis	Cephalosporins, penicillins
Sinusitis	Penicillins, cephalosporins
Meningitis	Cephalosporins (third- and fourth-generation agents), carbapenem (meropenem)
Lower respiratory tract infections	Penicillins, cephalosporins, carbapenems (especially for hospital-acquired infections)
Urinary tract infections	Penicillins, cephalosporins, monobactams, carbapenems (especially for infections due to multidrug-resistant gram-negative bacilli)
Intra-abdominal infections	Cephalosporins (in combination with agents with anaerobic activity), carbapenems, ureidopenicillin with β-lactamase inhibitor
Bone and joint infections	Penicillins, cephalosporins
Infective endocarditis	Penicillins, cephalosporins

These agents are used to treat patients with infections caused by gram-positive, gram-negative and anaerobic bacteria.

MECHANISM OF ACTION (see also Chapter 137)

β-Lactam antibiotics inhibit bacterial cell wall synthesis, a bactericidal mechanism of action. These agents bind tightly to penicillin-binding proteins (PBPs) on the inner surface of the bacterial cell membrane, thereby interrupting the terminal transpeptidation process in bacterial cell wall biosynthesis. Ultimately, loss of viability and, in some bacteria, lysis, occurs as the result of the activation of autolytic enzymes.

BACTERIAL RESISTANCE (see also Chapter 138)

The main mechanisms leading to bacterial resistance to β-lactam antibiotics include:

- failure of the antibiotic to penetrate the bacterial cell membrane;
- modification to porins that do not allow passage of the antibiotic into the periplasmic space;
- efflux of the antibiotic from the periplasmic space by specific pumping mechanisms;
- alterations in PBPs that reduce the binding affinities of the β-lactams (intrinsic resistance);[4] and
- bacterial production of β-lactamases, which are enzymes that hydrolyze and inactivate the β-lactam ring. This is the most important and common cause of resistance, especially in gram-negative bacteria.[5]

Pharmacokinetics and Distribution

ABSORPTION

The β-lactams have variable absorption from the gastrointestinal tract. Some agents, such as the anti-pseudomonal penicillins and methicillin, are acid-labile and cannot be taken orally. The absorption characteristics and pharmacokinetics of the β-lactams are shown in Table 140-2.

DISTRIBUTION

Following absorption, β-lactams are variably and reversibly bound to serum proteins, mostly albumin. Protein-bound drug does not exert antimicrobial activity. Excretion of the β-lactams is primarily renal (glomerular filtration and tubular secretion) and, in general, the serum half-life of these drugs is short, often 1 hour or less.

Procaine penicillin G and benzathine penicillin G are intramuscular preparations that are absorbed slowly, allowing for longer dosing intervals. Nafcillin, the ureidopenicillins (20–30%), cefoperazone (20%), ceftriaxone (10–65%) and cefotetan (13%) have significant excretion in bile.[13]

Imipenem, a carbapenem, is inactivated by dehydropeptidase I, an enzyme present on the renal brush border and other tissues. Cilastatin, a dehydropeptidase inhibitor and nephroprotectant is administered along with imipenem to prevent subtherapeutic levels of the antibiotic. Cilastatin is not microbiologically active nor does it alter the pharmacokinetics of other drugs.[20]

The β-lactam antibiotics achieve therapeutic concentrations in most tissues including lung, kidney, bone, muscle and liver, and in secretions such as synovial fluid, pleural fluid, pericardial fluid, peritoneal fluid and bile. The microenvironment that may be found in an abscess, including a low pH, the presence of neutrophils and associated proteins, and low oxygen tension, does not inhibit the function of β-lactam antibiotics. In general, β-lactams are considered to be unable to penetrate host cells and are therefore relatively ineffective against intracellular organisms (*Listeria* and *Salmonella* spp. are important exceptions). Low concentrations of β-lactams are found in prostatic secretions, brain tissue, intraocular fluid and cerebrospinal fluid (CSF; Figure 140-1). In the presence of inflammation, however, concentrations in the CSF are much higher, accounting for the efficacy of some β-lactams in the treatment of meningitis.[21] The penicillins and cephalosporins can penetrate the aqueous humor of the eye, but do not reach therapeutic levels in the posterior chamber.

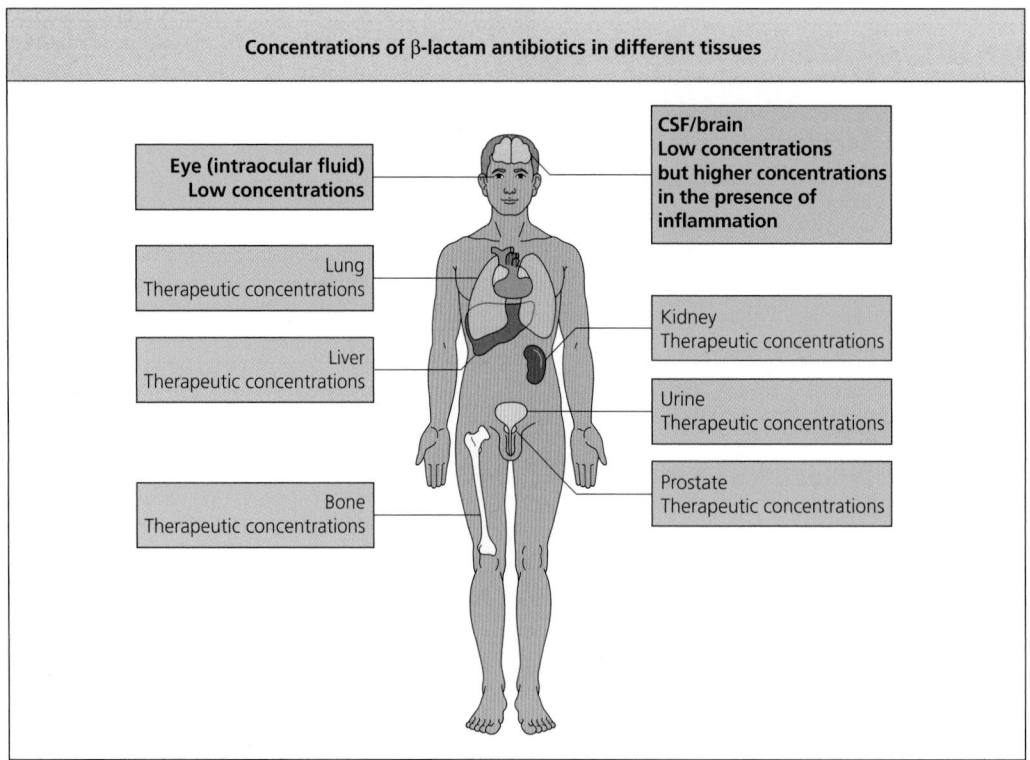

Concentrations of β-lactam antibiotics in different tissues

Eye (intraocular fluid) Low concentrations

CSF/brain Low concentrations but higher concentrations in the presence of inflammation

Lung Therapeutic concentrations

Liver Therapeutic concentrations

Kidney Therapeutic concentrations

Urine Therapeutic concentrations

Prostate Therapeutic concentrations

Bone Therapeutic concentrations

Figure 140-1 Concentration of β-lactam antibiotics in different tissues.

TABLE 140-2	Pharmacokinetics of Selected β-Lactam Antibiotics				
Generic Name	Oral Absorption (%)	Effect of Food on Absorption	Protein Binding (%)	Serum Half-Life (H)	Biliary Excretion (% of Dose)
PENICILLINS					
Amoxicillin–clavulanate	75/–	Minimal/increases	20/30	1.3/1.0	2–3/<1
Ampicillin–sulbactam	40/–	Decreases/–	28/38	1.1/1.0	3/0.24
Azlocillin	NA	30	0.8–1.5	5.3	
Bacampicillin	87–95	None	28	1.1	0.1
Carbenicillin (indanyl)	30–40	50–60	1.0	Minimal	
Cloxacillin	50	Decreases	90–98	0.5	2–10
Dicloxacillin	35–76	Decreases	95–97	0.7	Some penetration into bile
Flucloxacillin	50-70	Decreases	95	0.75-1	
Methicillin	NA	17–45	0.5–1.0	2–3	
Mezlocillin	NA	16–42	1.1	2.5	
Nafcillin	10–20	Decreases	90	0.5	8
Oxacillin	30	Decreases	94	0.5	2–10
Penicillin G	15	Decreases	65	0.5	5
Penicillin V	60	Lowers and delays peak	80	0.5	
Piperacillin–tazobactam	NA	26–33/31–32	1.0/0.7–0.9	20	
Ticarcillin–clavulanate	NA	45/30	1.2/1.0	4/<1	
CEPHALOSPORINS					
Cefaclor	52–95	Lowers and delays peak	22–25	0.6–0.9	Some penetration into bile
Cefadroxil	90	None	20	1.5	High conc. in bile
Cefazolin	NA	73–87	1.4–2.0	0.03	
Cefdinir	16–25	Reduced after a fatty meal	60–70	1.7	
Cefditoren (pivoxil)	14–16	Increased with fatty meal	88	1.6	Some penetration into bile
Cefepime	NA	20	2.0	Some penetration into bile	
Cefixime	40–50	65	3–4	5	
Cefoperazone	NA	82–93	1.9	20–30	
Cefotaxime	NA	30–51	1.0–1.5	0.1	
Cefotetan	NA	78–91	3–4.6	13	
Cefoxitin	NA	65–79	0.7–1.1	High conc. in bile	
Cefpodoxime (proxetil)	46–50	Increases	18–40	2.1–2.8	Some penetration into bile
Cefprozil	95	None	35–45	1.3–1.8	
Ceftaroline	NA	None	20	2.7	
Ceftazidime	NA	10–20	1.5–1.8	0.21	
Ceftibuten	>90	Lowers peak	65–77	2–2.4	
Ceftizoxime	NA	30	1.3–1.9	0.2–7.8	
Ceftobiprole (medocaril)	NA	16	3.0	<1%	
Ceftolozane–tazobactam	NA	None	16-20/30	3/1	
Ceftriaxone	NA	85–95	5–11	10–65	
Cefuroxime (axetil)	52	Increases	33–50	1.5	0.13
Cephalexin	90	Lowers and delays peak	5–15	0.7–1.1	0.29
Cephalothin	NA	65–80	0.5–1.0	High conc. in bile	
Loracarbef	~90	Decreases	25	1.2	
MONOBACTAM					
Aztreonam	NA	56	1.7–2.9	<1	
CARBAPENEMS					
Doripenem	NA	5–15	1.0	<1%	
Ertapenem	NA	85–95	4	Some penetration into bile	
Imipenem–cilastatin	NA	15–25	1.0	<0.3	
Meropenem	NA	2	1.0–1.5	Some penetration into bile	

Pharmacokinetic data as per references 6–19.
NA, not applicable because agent is administered by parenteral route only. Absence of information is due to lack of published data.

Route of Administration and Dosage

β-Lactams are available for oral, intravenous and intramuscular use. Generic names, routes of administration and standard dosages for adult and pediatric patients with normal renal function are listed in Table 140-3. In dosing the β-lactam antibiotics, it is important to remember that:

- food can have an effect on oral absorption; and
- absorption of both cefuroxime and cefpodoxime are decreased by H_2 blockers or nonabsorbable antacids.[22]

Dosing of β-lactams is based on achieving plasma drug concentrations above the minimum inhibitory concentration (MIC) of the infecting bacteria for substantial periods of the dosing interval; this is the critical pharmacodynamic relationship to consider in choosing a dose regimen. Many of these agents have short half-lives after intravenous dosing and therefore could be more optimally dosed if infused over several hours. Compared to intermittent boluses, prolonged infusions have been associated with reduced mortality.[23]

Indications

The β-lactam antibiotics are routinely used in the treatment of sinusitis, otitis, pharyngitis, epiglottitis, dental infections, bronchitis, pneumonia, meningitis, infective endocarditis, infections of the genitourinary tract, peritonitis, biliary and gastrointestinal infections, skin and soft tissue infections, osteomyelitis, septic arthritis and infection of prosthetic devices including venous access catheters (Table 140-1). The choice of antibiotic and recommended duration of therapy for these infections is discussed in the chapters on the specific diseases. The remainder of this section focuses on the use of the β-lactam antibiotics in special circumstances. Table 140-4 summarizes the relative susceptibilities of various microbes to the β-lactam antibiotics.

PROPHYLAXIS

Antimicrobial Prophylaxis in Surgery
(see also Chapter 136)

β-Lactam antibiotics are commonly prescribed to decrease the incidence of infection for selected surgical procedures.[26] A single dose of cefazolin had been shown to decrease the incidence of wound infection for selected 'clean' procedures. This approach is used commonly for cardiac, noncardiac thoracic, vascular, orthopedic, ophthalmic and neurosurgical procedures. With the emergence of MRSA, concern has been raised about the effectiveness of using β-lactams with no activity against MRSA, especially in centers where MRSA prevalence is high.

For 'clean–contaminated' procedures in which colonized mucosa is violated, such as head and neck surgery, abdominal surgery and gynecologic surgery, antibiotic prophylaxis may also be used. Cefazolin can be used before head and neck surgery. Similarly, patients undergoing biliary tract surgery who are at high risk of infection due to advanced age, acute cholecystitis, a nonfunctioning gallbladder, obstructive jaundice, or choledocholithiasis may benefit from preoperative cefazolin. In the setting of acute appendicitis, cefoxitin or ampicillin–sulbactam has been recommended. Women undergoing vaginal or abdominal hysterectomy, emergency Cesarean section or first trimester abortion may be candidates for antibiotic prophylaxis with cefazolin. Antibiotics should be used not only as prophylaxis but also as treatment for 'dirty' surgical procedures in which the surgical site is obviously contaminated by bacteria (e.g. a perforated viscus).

Endocarditis Prophylaxis

Patients who have underlying cardiac or congenital valvular abnormalities are candidates for antibiotic prophylaxis when they undergo procedures that can cause transient bacteremia. Cardiac conditions that place a patient at increased risk of endocarditis include prosthetic valves, a previous history of endocarditis, most congenital cardiac abnormalities (except an isolated secundum atrial septal defect), rheumatic and other acquired valvular dysfunction, hypertrophic cardiomyopathy, and mitral valve prolapse when accompanied by regurgitation.

Procedures that can cause transient bacteremia and may place a patient at risk of endocarditis include:

- dental procedures (including professional cleaning);
- tonsillectomy and/or adenoidectomy;
- surgical procedures involving intestinal or respiratory mucosa;
- rigid bronchoscopy;
- sclerotherapy for esophageal varices;
- esophageal dilatation;
- gallbladder surgery;
- cystoscopy;
- urethral dilatation;
- urethral catheterization and/or urinary tract surgery if there is infection;
- prostatic surgery; and
- incision and drainage of infected tissue.

Recommendations for using β-lactams for prophylaxis for patients at risk for infective endocarditis have recently been updated by an American College of Cardiology/American Heart Association Task Force on Practice Guidelines.[27] Prophylaxis is not recommended for patients undergoing non-dental procedures and is no longer recommended for many patients that had been considered candidates for prophylaxis in the past.

TABLE 140-3	β-Lactam Antibiotics – Spectrum Of Activity, Generic Names, Routes Of Administration And Dosages Used In Patients With Normal Renal Function			
Agent	Antimicrobial Spectrum	Generic Name	Route	Adult Dose (Pediatric Dose)
PENICILLINS				
Natural penicillins	Gram-positives, anaerobes and some gram-negatives	Penicillin V	po	250–500 mg q6–12h (6.25–12.5 mg/kg q8h)
		Penicillin G (benzathine)	im	1.2 million U every 3–4 weeks (25 000–50 000 U/kg every 3–4 weeks; or if <27 kg, 300 000–600 000 U and if >27 kg, 900 000 U)
		Penicillin G (procaine)	im	300 000–600 000 U q12h (25 000–50 000 U/kg q24h or 12 500–25 000 U/kg q12h)
		Penicillin G, sodium or potassium	iv	1–4 million U q4–6h (6250–100 000 U/kg q6h or 4166.6–66 666 U/kg q4h)
Penicillinase-resistant penicillins	Penicillin-resistant, methicillin-susceptible staphylococci (MSSA) and some streptococci	Cloxacillin	po	250–500 mg q6h
		Dicloxacillin	po	125–500 mg q8h
		Flucloxacillin	po/iv/im	250–500 mg q6h
		Methicillin	im/iv	1–2 g q6h
		Nafcillin	im/iv	1–2 g q4h (12.5–25 mg/kg q6h or 8.3–33.3 mg/kg q4h)
		Oxacillin	iv	1–2 g q4h (12.5–25 mg/kg q6h or 8.3–33.3 mg/kg q4h)

TABLE 140-3	β-Lactam Antibiotics – Spectrum Of Activity, Generic Names, Routes Of Administration And Dosages Used In Patients With Normal Renal Function (Continued)			
Agent	**Antimicrobial Spectrum**	**Generic Name**	**Route**	**Adult Dose (Pediatric Dose)**
PENICILLINS				
Aminopenicillins	Same as penicillin G plus β-lactamase-negative gram-negative bacilli and some Enterobacteriaceae	Amoxicillin	po	250–500 mg q8h or 875 mg q12h (12.5–25 mg/kg q8h or 7–13 mg/kg q8h)
		Ampicillin	im/iv po	500 mg–2 g q4–6h (25–50 mg/kg q6h) 250–500 mg q6h
		Bacampicillin	po	400–800 mg q12h (12.5 mg/kg q12h)
with a β-lactamase inhibitor	Expanded activity against β-lactamase-producing bacteria	Amoxicillin–clavulanic acid	po	250–500 mg q8h or 875 mg q12h (if >40 kg, dose as adult)
		Ampicillin–sulbactam	im/iv	1.5–3 g q6h (25–50 mg/kg q6h)
Carboxypenicillins	Some ampicillin-resistant gram-negatives including *Pseudomonas aeruginosa* (at highest dose regimens)	Ticarcillin	im/iv	3 g q4–6h (if <60 kg, 50 mg/kg q4–6h)
with a β-lactamase inhibitor	Expands activity against β-lactamase-producing bacteria	Ticarcillin–clavulanic acid	iv	3.1 g q4–6h (if <60 kg, 50 mg/kg [based on ticarcillin component] q4–6h)
Ureidopenicillins	Similar to carboxypenicillins	Mezlocillin	im/iv	3–4 g q4–6h (50 mg/kg q4h)
		Piperacillin	im/iv	3 g q4–6h (50–75 mg/kg q6h or 33.3–50 mg/kg q4h)
with a β-lacatamase inhibitor	Expands activity against β-lactamase-producing bacteria	Piperacillin–tazobactam	iv	3.375 g q4–6h (80 mg/kg q8h) 4.5 g q6h (for nosocomial pneumonia)
CEPHALOSPORINS				
Referred to as 'first generation'	Methicillin-susceptible staphylococci, streptococci and some gram-negative bacilli	Cefadroxil	po	500 mg–1 g q12h (15 mg/kg q12h)
		Cefazolin	im/iv	1–2 g q8h (16.6–33.3 mg/kg q8h)
		Cephalexin	po	250–500 mg q6h (6.25–12.5 mg/kg q6h or 8.0–16 mg/kg q8h)
		Cephalothin	im/iv	500 mg–2 g q4–6h (25 mg/kg q6h or 16.6 mg/kg q4h)
Referred to as 'second generation'	Greater activity than earlier agents against gram-negative bacilli. Some anaerobes for specific agents (especially cefotetan, cefoxitin)	Cefaclor	po	250–500 mg q8h (10–20 mg/kg q12h or 6.6–13.3 mg/kg q8h)
		Cefotetan	im/iv	1–3 g q12h (20–40 mg/kg q12h)
		Cefoxitin	im/iv	1 g q8h to 2 g q24h (27–33 mg/kg q8h)
		Cefprozil	po	250 mg q4h or 500 mg q12–24h (15 mg/kg q12h)
		Cefuroxime (axetil)	po	125–500 mg q12h (10–15 mg/kg q12h)
		Cefuroxime	im/iv	750 mg–1.5 g q6–8h (25–50 mg/kg q8h)
		Loracarbef	po	200–400 mg q12h (7.5–15 mg/kg q12h)
Referred to as 'third generation'	Many β-lactamase-positive gram-negatives, some *P. aeruginosa* (especially cefoperazone, ceftazidime) Gram-positives including MSSA, many gram-negatives including *P. aeruginosa*, and *Bacteroides fragilis*	Cefditoren (pivoxil)	po	200–400 mg q12h
		Cefdinir	po	300 mg q12h or 600 mg q24h (7 mg/kg q12h or 14 mg/kg q24h)
		Cefixime	po	200 mg q12h or 400 mg q24h (8 mg/kg q24h or 4 mg/kg q12h)
		Cefoperazone	im/iv	1 g q12h to 2 g q4h (25–100 mg/kg q12h)
		Cefotaxime	im/iv	1 g q12h to 2 g q4h (8.3–33.3 mg/kg q4h or 16.6–66.6 mg/kg q6h)
		Cefpodoxime (proxetil)	im/iv	100–400 mg q12h (5 mg/kg q12h)
		Ceftazidime	iv	1 g q12h to 2 g q8h (25–50 mg/kg q8h)
		Ceftibuten	im/iv	400 mg q24h (9 mg/kg q24h)
		Ceftizoxime	po	500 mg q12h to 4 g q8h (50 mg/kg q6–8h)
		Ceftriaxone	im/iv	1–2 g q24h
		Ceftolozane/tazobactam	im/iv	1.5 g IV q8h
		Ceftazidime/avibactam	iv	2.5 g IV q8h
Referred to as 'fourth generation'	Similar to above Gram-positives including MSSA, and many β-lactamase-positive gram-negatives, some *P. aeruginosa*	Cefepime	im/iv	1–2 g q8–12h (50 mg/kg q8–12h)
		Ceftobiprole (medocaril)	iv	500 mg q8h
Referred to as 'fifth generation'	Gram-positives including MRSA, many gram-negatives not including *P. aeruginosa*	Ceftaroline	iv	600 mg q12h for adults, safety and efficacy not established <18 years of age
MONOBACTAM				
	Gram-negatives	Aztreonam	im/iv	1–2 g q6–12h (30–40 mg/kg q6–8h)
CARBAPENEMS				
	Gram-positives (except MRSA), many gram-negatives (including ESBL-producers) and many *P. aeruginosa* (except ertapenem)	Doripenem	iv	500 mg q8h
		Ertapenem	im/iv	1 g q24h
		Imipenem–cilastatin	im/iv	500 mg–1 g q6h (15–25 mg/kg q6h)
		Meropenem	iv	1 g q8h (20–40 mg/kg q8h)

Dosing guidance as per references 9–12, 18, 19.

TABLE 140-4 Susceptibilities of Selected Bacteria to β-Lactam Antibiotics

Generic Name	Streptococci*	Oxacillin-Susceptible, Penicillinase-Producing *Staphylococcus aureus*†	Enterococci	Enteric Gram-Negative Bacilli‡	*Pseudomonas aeruginosa*	Anaerobes
PENICILLINS						
Amoxicillin	++	0	++	0	0	0
Amoxicillin–clavulanate	++	++	++	++	0	++
Ampicillin	++	0	++	0	0	0
Ampicillin–sulbactam	++	++	++	++	0	++
Carbenicillin	+	0	0	0	+	0
Cloxacillin	+	++	0	0	0	0
Dicloxacillin	+	++	0	0	0	0
Flucloxacillin	+	++	0	0	0	0
Methicillin	+	++	0	0	0	0
Mezlocillin	+	0	+	+	+	+
Nafcillin	+	++	0	0	0	0
Oxacillin	+	++	0	0	0	0
Penicillin	++	0	++	0	0	0
Piperacillin	++	0	+	+	++	+
Piperacillin–tazobactam	++	++	+	++	++	++
Ticarcillin	++	0	0	+	+	+
Ticarcillin–clavulanate	++	++	0	++	+	++
CEPHALOSPORINS						
Cefaclor	+	+	0	+	0	+
Cefadroxil	+	+	0	0	0	0
Cefazolin	++	++	0	0	0	0
Cefdinir	++	+	0	+	0	0
Cefditoren	++	+	0	+	0	0
Cefepime	++	+	0	++	++	0
Cefixime	++	0	0	++	0	0
Cefoperazone	++	+	0	+	+	+
Cefotaxime	++	+	0	++	0	0
Cefotetan	+	0	0	+	0	+
Cefoxitin	+	0	0	+	0	++
Cefpodoxime	++	++	0	+	0	0
Cefprozil	++	+	0	+	0	0
Ceftaroline	++	++	+	++	0	+
Ceftazidime	+	0	0	++	++	0
Ceftibuten	+	0	0	+	0	0
Ceftizoxime	++	+	0	+	0	+
Ceftobiprole	++	++	++	++	+	0
Ceftolozane–tazobactam	++	++	0	++	++	+
Ceftriaxone	++	+	0	++	0	0
Cefuroxime	++	+	0	+	0	+
Cephalexin	++	+	0	+	0	+
Cephalothin	++	++	0	+	0	+
Loracarbef	+	+	0	+	0	+

TABLE 140-4 Susceptibilities of Selected Bacteria to β-Lactam Antibiotics (Continued)						
Generic Name	Streptococci*	Oxacillin-Susceptible, Penicillinase-Producing Staphylococcus aureus†	Enterococci	Enteric Gram-Negative Bacilli‡	Pseudomonas aeruginosa	Anaerobes
MONOBACTAM						
Aztreonam	0	0	0	++	+	0
CARBAPENEMS						
Doripenem	++	++	+	++	++	++
Ertapenem	++	++	0	++	0	++
Imipenem	++	++	++	++	++	++
Meropenem	++	++	+	++	++	++

Interpretations: 0, not active, 90% of the minimum inhibitory concentrations (MICs) are greater than resistance breakpoint; +, intermediate activity, approximately 90% of the MICs are greater than susceptible, but less than the resistant breakpoint; ++, clinically useful activity, generally with 90% of the MICs within the susceptible range, using interpretive criteria as defined by the Clinical and Laboratory Standards Institute (CLSI) or the Food and Drug Administration (FDA). Susceptibility data based on references 17, 24, 25.

*Non-meningitis isolates.

†Methicillin-susceptible Staph. aureus and Staph. epidermidis. All methicillin-resistant Staph. aureus and Staph. epidermidis are resistant to all β-lactams, with the exception of ceftobiprole and ceftaroline.

‡Primarily Escherichia coli, Klebsiella pneumoniae and Proteus mirabilis.

This recommendation was made because evidence has shown the risks of prophylactic antibiotics outweigh the benefits for most patients. For at-risk patients undergoing dental procedures, the antibiotic of choice has remained constant for over two decades and is a single dose of amoxicillin 2 g (50 mg/kg for children) taken orally 30–60 minutes before the procedure. Alternatives exist for patients who are allergic to penicillins.[27] Guidelines posted by the National Institute for Health and Clinical Excellence (NICE)[28] and published by the British Society for Antimicrobial Chemotherapy[29] emphasize that past practices of using antibiotic prophylaxis in patients at risk for infective endocarditis need to be reconsidered. The current list of indications during dental procedures include patients with: 1) prosthetic heart valves; 2) cardiac transplant recipients; 3) complex, surgically corrected or unrepaired congenital heart disease; or 4) a previous episode of endocarditis (see Chapter 136 for detailed discussion on antimicrobial prophylaxis).

Rheumatic Fever Prophylaxis

Because patients who have had acute rheumatic fever are at risk of recurrent attacks if they have group A streptococcal infections, the American Heart Association (AHA) recommends prophylaxis with penicillin for these patients. The dose is either a single injection of benzathine penicillin G 1.2 million U intramuscularly every 4 weeks or penicillin V 250 mg orally q12h. Prophylaxis can be safely discontinued in patients with a history of carditis after 10 years or at age 25. In patients without a history of carditis, prophylaxis can be stopped after 5 years or at age 18. The decision to stop prophylaxis, however, must be individualized because a patient who is at continued risk of streptococcal infection (e.g. teacher or pediatrician) may benefit from continued antibiotic prophylaxis (see also Chapter 52).[30]

Intrapartum Prophylaxis

Penicillin G is the agent of choice for use in intrapartum prophylaxis for early onset group B streptococcal disease in newborns. Ampicillin is an acceptable alternative agent. These agents should be given to women in labor as soon as risk for intrapartum transmission of group B streptococcus is identified. Initial intravenous doses (5 million U penicillin G or 2 g ampicillin) should be followed with half doses every 4 hours until the newborn is delivered.

PNEUMOCOCCAL INFECTIONS

Penicillin and amoxicillin are the antibiotics of choice for infections (such as community-acquired pneumonia, bacteremia or meningitis) caused by penicillin-susceptible strains of Streptococcus pneumoniae.

However, an increasing proportion of isolates of this pathogen are not susceptible to penicillin. For meningitic isolates and epidemiologic purposes, an interpretation of intermediate is defined as a strain with a penicillin MIC of 0.1–1 µg/mL and resistance is defined by a penicillin MIC of ≥2 µg/mL. However, recent revisions to the interpretive criteria define penicillin MICs >2 µg/mL for non-meningitis-related Strep. pneumoniae isolates as nonsusceptible. Although only about 5% of pneumococcal clinical isolates in the USA were not susceptible to penicillin in the early 1990s, by 2007 25.4% were intermediate and 11.1% were resistant to penicillin.[31] Because of the emergence of resistance, some suggest that suspected cases of pneumococcal pneumonia and meningitis should be treated with vancomycin and/or a third-generation cephalosporin or meropenem until susceptibilities are known. There have been reports of failure of third-generation cephalosporins such as cefotaxime or ceftriaxone in the treatment of penicillin-resistant pneumococcal meningitis, again suggesting that vancomycin or meropenem should be included until susceptibilities are known.[32]

STAPHYLOCOCCAL INFECTIONS

Soon after the introduction of penicillin for the treatment of staphylococcal infections, penicillinase-producing strains rapidly emerged. Penicillinase-resistant penicillins (nafcillin, oxacillin, methicillin, dicloxacillin, cloxacillin, flucloxacillin) are often agents of choice for methicillin-susceptible strains of Staph. aureus (MSSA). Other β-lactam antibiotics that are effective in the treatment of susceptible staphylococcal infections are:

- the aminopenicillins in combination with a β-lactamase inhibitor (ampicillin–sulbactam or amoxicillin–clavulanate);
- the anti-pseudomonal penicillins in combination with a β-lactamase inhibitor (ticarcillin–clavulanate, piperacillin–tazobactam); and
- the carbapenems (doripenem, ertapenem, imipenem and meropenem).

The first-generation cephalosporins, which are as effective as the penicillinase-resistant penicillins in the treatment of staphylococcal infections, require less frequent dosing and may be used in patients with a history of mild penicillin allergy.

Isolates of Staph. aureus or Staphylococcus epidermidis that are resistant to methicillin should be considered to be resistant to all other β-lactams,[33] with the exception of ceftobiprole.[34] Ceftobiprole has received regulatory approval in Canada and some European countries for treating patients with complicated skin and skin-structure infections, including those caused by MRSA.[35,36]

GRAM-POSITIVE BACILLI

Penicillin G is the treatment of choice for:

- infections (oral–cervicofacial, thoracic, abdominal) due to actinomycosis;
- elimination of the carrier state of diphtheria;
- infections (pulmonary, cutaneous, gastrointestinal) due to anthrax, except for β-lactamase-producing strains;
- gas gangrene caused by species of *Clostridium* spp.;
- erysipeloid caused by *Erysipelothrix rhusiopathiae*; and
- syphilis.

Either penicillin G or ampicillin may be used for infections caused by *Listeria monocytogenes*. No currently available cephalosporin has useful activity against *L. monocytogenes*.

INFECTIONS CAUSED BY GRAM-NEGATIVE ORGANISMS INCLUDING *PSEUDOMONAS AERUGINOSA*

β-Lactam antibiotics with *in vitro* activity against *P. aeruginosa* are ticarcillin, carbenicillin, piperacillin, ceftazidime, cefoperazone, cefepime, ceftobiprole, ceftolozane–tazobactam, aztreonam, imipenem, meropenem and doripenem. Of these agents, the carbapenems–doripenem, imipenem and meropenem – have the most consistent activity against pseudomonads. Because resistance to carbapenems (most evident with imipenem) has emerged in many areas, it is important to be aware of *P. aeruginosa* resistance patterns for a particular healthcare facility. During treatment of pseudomonal infections, resistance to all β-lactam agents used as sole therapy has been observed.[24] For this reason, in serious infections a suitable β-lactam antibiotic is often used in conjunction with a second agent, such as a fluoroquinolone or an aminoglycoside.

The anti-pseudomonal penicillins piperacillin and ticarcillin are often used in conjunction with a β-lactamase inhibitor. However, the inhibitor does not confer improved activity against many β-lactam-resistant *Pseudomonas* spp., because the mechanism of resistance is typically not due to β-lactamase production.[25]

The development of drug-resistant isolates of *P. aeruginosa* and other gram-negative bacilli has emerged as a clinically important challenge, especially in considering treatment of patients with nosocomial infections. Many gram-negative bacteria, especially *Escherichia coli* and *Klebsiella* spp., may acquire extra DNA (e.g. a plasmid) that encodes for other types of β-lactamase, such as extended-spectrum β-lactamases (ESBLs). These bacteria may develop resistance to most β-lactams during therapy if they acquire an ESBL or hyperproduce chromosomal β-lactamases.[37] Older recommendations of concurrent use of an aminoglycoside in conjunction with a cephalosporin for the treatment of infections caused by these bacteria to prevent therapeutic failures have been challenged due to the realization that cross-resistance in ESBL-producing bacteria can occur due to the co-acquisition of modifying enzymes for both antibiotic classes.[38]

Among β-lactams, carbapenems have the broadest spectrum of activity against gram-negative organisms resistant to other antibiotics. Given the emergence of resistance, especially resistance due to ESBL-producing bacteria, carbapenems have been used more frequently as empiric therapy in seriously ill patients, especially those at risk for gram-negative infections. Although imipenem resistance in *P. aeruginosa* has risen in some centers to 10–15%, some of these isolates continue to be susceptible to meropenem and doripenem, carbapenems with more potent *in vitro* activity against most gram-negative bacteria.[39] Resistance to carbapenems is increasing in some centers due to the production of acquired carbapenem-hydrolyzing β-lactamases, including enzymes that require metal ions for hydrolysis. The metallo-β-lactamases confer resistance to all β-lactams except aztreonam, in contrast to other carbapenemases that generally are associated with resistance to all β-lactams.[40]

Among the cephalosporins, cefepime is effective in the treatment of severe infections due to a broad spectrum of pathogens that involve the lower respiratory and urinary tracts, the skin and soft tissue, and the female reproductive tract. It has been shown to be more effective than ceftazidime in the treatment of pneumonia in patients with cystic fibrosis where *P. aeruginosa* is a common pathogen.[41] In addition to having activity against strains of *P. aeruginosa* resistant to ceftazidime, cefepime has also shown activity against many Enterobacteriaceae, including *Enterobacter* spp., that are resistant to other cephalosporins.[42] However, cefepime is inactivated by many ESBLs. Although a meta-analysis suggested that a subset of seriously ill patients had higher mortality rates after treatment with cefepime compared with alternative agents,[43] a 2009 Food and Drug Administration (FDA) analysis did not show a statistically significant increase in mortality in cefepime-treated patients.

ANAEROBIC INFECTIONS

Anaerobic bacteria often have significant roles in abscess formation along with bone and soft tissue infections. Although β-lactam antibiotics are used extensively for treating anaerobic infections, there is a trend for increased resistance of anaerobes to some β-lactam antibiotics due to production of β-lactamases.[44]

Most *Clostridium* strains, with the exception of some strains of *C. ramosum*, *C. clostridioforme* and *C. innocuum*, remain susceptible to penicillin. Penicillin resistance is increasingly seen in the genus *Fusobacterium*, most commonly in *F. varium* and *F. mortiferum*, and although generally still sensitive to penicillin, the MICs for *F. nucleatum* have increased. Penicillin resistance is a major problem encountered in the treatment of infections caused by β-lactamase-producing *B. fragilis* and other *Bacteroides* spp.[44]

Penicillin is slightly more active than nafcillin against anaerobes, although neither is considered to be a potent anti-anaerobic agent. Ticarcillin, mezlocillin and piperacillin also have excellent activity against anaerobes, although there has been an increase in *B. fragilis* strains resistant to ticarcillin. Of the β-lactamase-stable cephalosporins, cefoxitin, cefotetan and ceftizoxime all show activity against anaerobes. Cefoxitin remains the most active cephalosporin against *B. fragilis*. Resistance to these cephalosporins is seen with some species of *Clostridium*, *Fusobacterium* and nonspore-forming gram-positive bacilli. Cephalosporins such as ceftazidime and the first-generation agents cefazolin and cephalothin have poor activity against gram-negative anaerobes whereas the broader spectrum cephalosporins cefotaxime, cefoperazone and ceftriaxone have modest activity (resistance seen in 30–60% of strains) and are therefore not the agents of choice for the empiric treatment of anaerobic infections.

β-Lactamases in anaerobes include the typical cephalosporinases in the *B. fragilis* group and the penicillinases in *Clostridium* spp. and *F. nucleatum*. Nearly all *B. fragilis* isolates produce β-lactamases, including a subset of isolates that produce a broad-spectrum metallo-β-lactamase. β-Lactamase production has not been reported in strains of *Clostridium perfringens*.[45]

The addition of a β-lactamase inhibitor increases the activity of some penicillins against β-lactamase producing anaerobes, in particular *Bacteroides* spp., resulting in efficacy for the combinations of ticarcillin–clavulanate, piperacillin–tazobactam, amoxicillin–clavulanate and ampicillin–sulbactam. The most active β-lactam agents against anaerobic isolates in the USA are the carbapenems, imipenem, meropenem, ertapenem and doripenem. Aztreonam has no activity against anaerobes and must be used with other agents when treating mixed aerobic and anaerobic infections.[46]

CENTRAL NERVOUS SYSTEM INFECTIONS (MENINGITIS) (see Chapter 19)

Certain β-lactam antibiotics are able to penetrate inflamed meninges and are commonly used to treat meningitis (e.g. penicillin G, ampicillin, nafcillin, oxacillin, cefotaxime, ceftizoxime, ceftriaxone, ceftazidime and meropenem). The most common pathogens in a series of adult patients with meningitis were *Strep. pneumoniae*, and *Neisseria meningitidis*.[47] With the widespread use of conjugate *Haemophilus influenzae* and *Strep. pneumoniae* vaccines, *N. meningitidis* has become the most important cause of bacterial meningitis in children in the

USA. These bacteria have remained consistently susceptible to β-lactam antibiotics.

Because of the severity of infections in the central nervous system there is a need to start effective therapy before the identity and susceptibility of the bacteria causing infection is known. The activity of β-lactams against the leading causes of these infections makes them appropriate choices for initial therapy. Although penicillin G at a dose of 20–24 million U/day intravenously q4h is a treatment of choice for susceptible strains of *Strep. pneumoniae* and for nearly all *N. meningitidis*, due to the possibility of infection by penicillin-resistant pneumococci, β-lactamase-producing *H. influenzae* and the rare β-lactamase-producing *N. meningitidis*, the use of ceftriaxone with vancomycin is generally considered the most appropriate β-lactam-containing regimen for use as empiric therapy for bacterial meningitis. β-Lactams are not sufficient to eliminate the carrier state of *N. meningitidis* that often occurs in patients recovering from bacterial meningitis. Thus, rifampin should be given at the completion of therapy. The agent of choice for the treatment of meningitis due to *L. monocytogenes* is ampicillin or penicillin alone or in combination with gentamicin.

In children, the preferred agents for the treatment of *H. influenzae* meningitis are the third-generation cephalosporins cefotaxime or ceftriaxone.[48] Cefuroxime is not considered an appropriate alternative to these newer agents because of failures of treatment as well as the development of meningitis during cefuroxime treatment. A randomized trial found that ceftriaxone resulted in less hearing impairment and sterilized the CSF earlier than cefuroxime when used as treatment for meningitis in children.[49]

Patients with staphylococcal meningitis (which is usually seen after trauma or neurosurgical procedures) are best treated with high doses of nafcillin or oxacillin if the organism is susceptible. *Pseudomonas aeruginosa* meningitis has been effectively managed with ceftazidime, although meropenem may be an alternative.[50]

Clinical trial experience has shown that early adjunctive therapy with dexamethasone can improve the outcome of bacterial meningitis.[51]

BILIARY SYSTEM INFECTIONS (CHOLANGITIS)

Infection of the biliary tract generally occurs if there is an abnormality such as gallstones, strictures or a stent. Infection rarely complicates malignant obstruction of the biliary tree. In the obstructed biliary tract, there is very little excretion of any antibiotic. The β-lactams that achieve significantly higher biliary than serum levels are nafcillin, mezlocillin, piperacillin, cefoperazone and ceftriaxone. Ampicillin achieves concentrations in the bile equal to or greater than those in serum. Biliary concentrations of ticarcillin, cefazolin, cefotaxime, ceftazidime and cefuroxime are all less than serum concentrations.[52]

Ureidopenicillins mezlocillin and piperacillin have been used in biliary tract infections as has cefoperazone. Cefoxitin, cefuroxime and ceftriaxone are also commonly used in conjunction with an aminoglycoside in patients with cholangitis. In patients undergoing biliary surgery, adequate serum levels of antibiotic have been shown to be more important than biliary levels when the goal is to reduce postoperative infection.

INTRA-ABDOMINAL INFECTIONS
(see also Chapter 41)

Intra-abdominal infections, such as acute appendicitis, diverticulitis, penetrating abdominal trauma and bowel perforation, are generally polymicrobial in nature and caused by a combination of aerobic, anaerobic and facultative anaerobic organisms. Clinical trials have confirmed the efficacy of β-lactam antibiotics alone or in combination with other agents for various intra-abdominal infections.[53] Cefotetan, cefoxitin, imipenem, piperacillin–tazobactam and ticarcillin–clavulanic acid have all been shown to be effective in treating intra-abdominal infections when used as monotherapy, while ceftolozane–tazobactam must be used in combination with metroni-

dazole. Meropenem has been shown to have efficacy similar to that of imipenem for the treatment of intra-abdominal sepsis.[54] Ertapenem has similar efficacy in treating intra-abdominal infections as piperacillin–tazobactam.[55] Doripenem has been shown to have similar efficacy to meropenem in treating patients with complicated intra-abdominal infections.[56] The combination of clindamycin with either ceftazidime or aztreonam has been successful in the treatment of intra-abdominal infections. Failures of ampicillin–sulbactam have occurred when pseudomonal infections occur.

Enterococci are commonly isolated from intra-abdominal infections (14–33%), although the necessity to treat these organisms routinely in the initial antibiotic regimen for this indication remains unclear. 'Breakthrough' enterococcal infections occur in patients who have been hospitalized for long periods of time with persistent or recurrent intra-abdominal sepsis or who are immunosuppressed.[57]

SPONTANEOUS BACTERIAL PERITONITIS

Few studies have evaluated the efficacies of different antibiotics in the treatment of spontaneous bacterial peritonitis (SBP). The organisms that typically cause SBP are the gram-negative bacilli (especially *E. coli* and *Klebsiella* spp.). However, gram-positive cocci (including pneumococci, other streptococci, enterococci and staphylococci) and anaerobes are occasionally isolated in SBP. Cefotaxime is often used in patients with cirrhosis and SBP, while amoxicillin/clavulanic acid is an effective oral option. Aztreonam monotherapy has been associated with gram-positive superinfection. Therefore, if aztreonam is to be used for SBP, then an additional antibiotic providing gram-positive coverage is needed.[58]

PANCREATITIS AND ITS COMPLICATIONS
(see also Chapter 41)

The prophylactic use of antibiotics in uncomplicated acute pancreatitis is controversial. Patients with acute necrotizing pancreatitis treated with imipenem for 14 days had a lower incidence of pancreatic sepsis than those not treated; however, a trend toward a decreased mortality rate was not statistically significant.[59] A study that used cefuroxime in patients with acute necrotizing pancreatitis found that rates of bacteremia and mortality were both lower than those of controls.[60]

It is clear that β-lactam antibiotics have a role in the management of infectious complications of pancreatitis such as abscess or infected pseudocyst. The agents commonly used in addition to cefuroxime and imipenem include ampicillin–sulbactam, meropenem, piperacillin–tazobactam and ticarcillin–clavulanic acid.

ENDOVASCULAR INFECTIONS (ENDOCARDITIS)
(see also Chapter 51)

Updated statements regarding the treatment of endocarditis were published by the AHA in 2005[61] and the British Society for Antimicrobial Chemotherapy (BSAC) in 2004.[62] The drug of choice for the treatment of endocarditis caused by viridans streptococci is penicillin G. Depending upon the drug susceptibility of the organism, gentamicin can be added for part or all of a 2–6 week course. A 2-week course of combination ceftriaxone with an aminoglycoside may be sufficient as therapy for patients with uncomplicated endocarditis due to viridans streptococci. Alternatively, a 4-week course of ceftriaxone can be used.[63] Enterococcal endocarditis is best treated with ampicillin or penicillin in combination with an aminoglycoside for 4–6 weeks. A recent study found ampicillin plus ceftriaxone to be as effective as ampicillin plus gentamicin in treating *Enterococcus faecalis* endocarditis but with far fewer adverse events, including new renal failure.[64]

The treatment of choice for native-valve endocarditis caused by methicillin-susceptible *Staph. aureus* is nafcillin, flucloxacillin or oxacillin for 6 weeks. Gentamicin has been used for the first 3–5 days to decrease the number of days of bacteremia, but has not been shown to change outcomes.[65]

Intravenous drug users with right-sided staphylococcal endocarditis have been successfully treated with 2 weeks of nafcillin and tobramycin.[66] Prosthetic valve endocarditis with methicillin-susceptible *Staph. aureus* (MSSA) is optimally treated with nafcillin or oxacillin (if the organism is sensitive) in combination with rifampin and gentamicin (for the first 2 weeks) for at least 6 weeks.

Endocarditis caused by the slow-growing fastidious gram-negative organisms *Haemophilus parainfluenzae, H. aphrophilus, Actinobacillus actinomycetemcomitans, Cardiobacterium hominis, Eikenella corrodens* and *Kingella kingae* (the HACEK group) can be treated with ampicillin and gentamicin for 4 weeks or ceftriaxone alone for 4 weeks.

NEUTROPENIC FEVER

β-Lactam antibiotics have been used for many years in managing febrile patients with cancer and treatment-induced neutropenia. Because life-threatening infections can occur due to gram-negative bacteria, especially *P. aeruginosa*, and resistance to β-lactams has continued to become more prevalent among gram-negative enteric pathogens, using these agents as monotherapy may not be as effective as has been previously reported.[67] Combining a β-lactam with a second agent that has activity against a broad-spectrum of gram-negative bacteria, typically an aminoglycoside, has been recommended in patients who present with high risk for rapidly progressing disease.[68] Most recently, the emergence of MRSA as an important cause of disease in this patient population has further complicated using β-lactams to provide reliable activity against gram-positive bacteria (see also Chapter 79).

LYME DISEASE

Early infection caused by *Borrelia burgdorferi* can be managed with either amoxicillin or doxycycline. Since co-infection with *Ehrlichia* or *Anaplasma* spp. occurs in several areas, many clinicians now prefer to use doxycycline. For later manifestations of Lyme disease, however, β-lactams are the agents of choice. Lyme carditis can be successfully treated with a 2-week course of ceftriaxone or intravenous penicillin G. Lyme meningitis and Lyme arthritis can also be treated with ceftriaxone or penicillin G, but for 2–4 weeks. A 30-day treatment course of amoxicillin and probenecid has been used for the treatment of Lyme arthritis. In pregnant women, doxycycline cannot be used so amoxicillin is given in early Lyme disease and intravenous penicillin G is used for disseminated early Lyme disease or any manifestation of late disease (see Chapter 46).[69]

SYPHILIS

Parenteral penicillin G is the preferred agent for treating all stages of syphilis and is the only therapy that has proved effective for neurosyphilis, syphilis in pregnancy and congenital syphilis.[70] Primary and secondary syphilis can be treated with a single dose of benzathine penicillin G. Late latent syphilis is treated with benzathine penicillin G 2.4 million units intramuscularly every week for 3 weeks. Procaine penicillin can be used where benzathine penicillin is unavailable, and there are alternatives for patients who are allergic to penicillin (see Chapter 61).

Patients being treated for any of the spirochete diseases – syphilis, Lyme disease or borreliosis – may develop a Jarisch–Herxheimer reaction, which may produce fever, tachycardia, chills, headaches, sore throat, malaise, myalgias, arthralgias, rash and, rarely, hypotension. This reaction has been observed in approximately 50% of patients treated for primary syphilis and 75% of patients with secondary syphilis.[71] Generally it occurs a few hours after the first dose of penicillin, lasts for only a few hours and does not occur with subsequent doses of the antibiotic. Pre-treatment of patients with hydrocortisone or acetaminophen does not prevent the Jarisch–Herxheimer reaction.[72] It is important to distinguish the reaction from penicillin allergy so that appropriate treatment is not discontinued.

Dosage in Special Circumstances
RENAL IMPAIRMENT

The majority of the β-lactam antibiotics are excreted almost entirely by the renal route, and so dose adjustments are necessary in the presence of kidney disease. Failure to reduce the dose of penicillin in uremic patients can result in toxicity, most notably encephalopathy.[73] In patients with high glomerular filtration rates, rapid clearance of renally excreted antibiotics may result in a need to increase dosages in order to achieve therapeutic exposures.[74] As biliary secretion plays a major role in the excretion of ceftriaxone, cefoperazone, nafcillin and oxacillin, the doses of these antibiotics do not need to be adjusted in renal failure. Because biliary secretion plays a lesser, although significant, role in the excretion of the ureidopenicillins, the dosages of these drugs do not have to be reduced as much as for the other penicillins. Specific dose adjustments are needed for patients with renal impairment and for patients on hemodialysis or peritoneal dialysis (Table 140-5).

HEPATIC IMPAIRMENT

The dosages of some β-lactams must be adjusted in patients with severe hepatic disease. As a result of reduced deacetylation in patients with liver disease, the half-life of cefotaxime may increase slightly, but the half-life of cefoperazone may increase significantly and dosage reductions are required. No dose adjustment is needed in patients with liver disease receiving ceftriaxone.

EXTREMES OF AGE

Dose reductions of the β-lactam antibiotics should be made in the elderly in the presence of renal dysfunction (see Table 140-5). Otherwise, elderly patients tolerate standard doses of the β-lactam antibiotics.

Because neonates do not have fully developed renal function, special modifications in dosage are necessary. In addition, because children have a high risk of cholestatic complications with ceftriaxone, another agent should be used when possible. Ceftriaxone should not be used in neonates with hyperbilirubinemia.

β-LACTAMS IN PREGNANCY

The penicillins, the β-lactamase inhibitors and the cephalosporins, aztreonam, meropenem, ertapenem and doripenem, are considered category B in pregnancy. When indicated, these antibiotics are commonly used in clinical practice in pregnant women. Imipenem–cilastatin is pregnancy category C. However, the benefit of using it may exceed the risk of not treating a serious infection in a pregnant woman when no alternatives exist.[79] Meropenem or doripenem may be a suitable alternative to imipenem for infections with resistant gram-negative aerobic organisms.

β-Lactam antibiotics that are not protein bound are transported across the placenta and reach the drug levels that are present in maternal serum. β-Lactams that are highly protein-bound reach only low concentrations in amniotic fluid and the fetus.[79]

As a general principle, the β-lactam antibiotics have accelerated elimination and lowered plasma concentrations in pregnant women as compared with nonpregnant women. As a result, the dose or frequency of administration should be increased in pregnant women.[80]

Adverse Reactions and Interactions

Adverse reactions that occur with the β-lactam antibiotics are summarized in Table 140-6.

ALLERGIC REACTIONS

The most common adverse event associated with the use of β-lactam antibiotics is an allergic reaction. The reported frequency of allergic reaction to penicillin varies from 0.7% to 10%. Anaphylaxis historically was documented to occur in 0.004–0.015% of patients.[81] A maculopapular rash occurs late in the treatment course of 2–3% of patients receiving a course of penicillin. Ampicillin and amoxicillin induce rashes in a higher percentage of patients (5.2–9.5%) than other β-lactams and almost invariably cause a rash when given during acute infectious mononucleosis (Epstein–Barr virus).

TABLE 140-5 Drug Dosages in Patients with Renal Failure

Generic Name	Dose in Normal Renal Function	Max. Daily Dose with Normal Renal Function	Adjustment in Dose (D) or Interval (I)	GFR (mL/min) >50	GFR (mL/min) = 10–50	GFR (mL/min) <10	Supplement after HD	Supplement with PD	CVVHD
PENICILLINS									
Amoxicillin	250–500 mg q8h	2–3 g/q24h	I	q8h	q8–12h	q24h	Yes, 250–500 mg	250 mg q12h	500 mg q8–12h
Amoxicillin–clavulanate	250–500 mg q8h		I	q8h	q8–12h	q24h	Yes, 250–500 mg q24h	Usual regimen	Usual regimen
Ampicillin	250 mg–2 g q6h	2–4 g/q24h	I	q6h	q6–12h	q12–24h	Yes	250 mg q 12h	1–2 g q6–12h
Ampicillin–sulbactam (AM–SB)	1–2 g AM–500 mg–1 g SB q6–8h	8 g AM–4 g SB/q24h	D	q6h	q8–12h	q24h	Yes	2 g AM–1 g SB/24h	3 g q8h
Dicloxacillin	125–500 mg q8h	2 g/q24h	I	100%	100%	100%	No	No	
Flucloxacillin	250–500 mg q6h	2 g/q24h	I	100%	100%	100%	No	No	
Mezlocillin	1.5–4.0 g q4–6h	24 g/q24h	D	q4–6h	q6–8h	q8h	No	No	
Nafcillin	1–2 g q4–6h	12 g/q24h	D	100%	100%	100%	No	No	2 g q4–6h
Oxacillin	1–2 g q4–6h	12 g/q24h	D	100%	100%	100%	No	No	2 g q4–6h
Penicillin G	0.5–4 million U q4–6h	24 million U	D	100%	75%	20–50%	Yes	Dose for GFR <10	0.5–3 million U q6h
Penicillin V	250–500 mg q6h	3 g/q24h	I	100%	100%	100%	Yes	Dose for GFR <10	300 mg q6h
Piperacillin	3–4 g q4–6h	24 g/q24h	I	q4–6h	q6–8h	q8h	Yes	Dose for GFR <10	
Piperacillin–tazobactam	3.375 g q6h	13.5 g/q24h	D&I	3.375 g q6h	2.25 g q6h	2.25 g q8h	Dose for GFR <10 + 0.75 g	Dose for GFR <10	2.25–3.375 g q6h
Ticarcillin	3 g q4h	24 g/q24h	D&I	1–2 g q4h	1–2 g q8h	1–2 g q12h	Yes, extra 3 g	Dose for GFR <10	
Ticarcillin–clavulanate	3.1 g q4h	24 g/q24h	D&I	3.1 g q4h	3.1 g q8–12h	2 g q12h	Yes, extra 3.1 g	3.1 g q12h	3.1 g q6h
CEPHALOSPORINS									
Cefaclor	250–500 mg q8h	1.5 g/q24h	D	100%	50–100%	50%	Yes	Usual regimen	
Cefadroxil	500 mg–1 g q12h	2 g/q24h	I	q12h	q12–24h	q36h	Yes, extra 500 mg–1 g	Usual regimen	
Cefazolin	1–2 g q8h	12 g/q24h	I	q8h	q12h	q24–48h	Yes, extra 500 mg–1 g	500 mg q12h	2 g q12h
Cefdinir	300 mg q12h	600 mg/q24h	I	q12h	q24h	q48h	Yes	Dose for GFR <10	
Cefditoren (pivoxil)	200–400 mg q12h	800 mg/q24h	D&I	100%	200 mg q12h	200 mg q24h	Dose for GFR <10	No data	
Cefepime	250 mg–2 g q8–12h	6 g/q24h	D&I	100%	50–100% q24h	25–50% q24h	Yes, dose for GFR <10	Dose for GFR <10	2 g q12h
Cefixime	200 mg q12h or 400 mg q24h	400 mg/q24h	D	100%	75%	50%	Yes	Usual dose	
Cefoperazone	1–2 g q12h	12 g/q24h	D	100%	100%	100%	Yes, extra 1 g	No	1 g q12h
Cefotaxime	1–2 g q6–12h	12 g/q24h	I	q6h	q6–12h	q24h or 50%	Yes, extra 500 mg–2 g	1 g q24h	2 g q12h
Cefotetan	1–2 g q12h	6 g/q24h	I	100%	q24h	q48h	Yes, extra 1 g	1 g q24h	

Continued on following page

TABLE 140-5 Drug Dosages in Patients with Renal Failure (Continued)

Generic Name	Dose in Normal Renal Function	Max. Daily Dose with Normal Renal Function	Adjustment in Dose (D) or Interval (I)	GFR (mL/min) >50	GFR (mL/min) = 10–50	GFR (mL/min) <10	Supplement after HD	Supplement with PD	CVVHD
CEPHALOSPORINS									
Cefoxitin	1–2 g q6–8h	12 g/q24h	I	q6–8h	q8–12h	q24–48h	Yes, extra 1 g	1 g q24h	
Cefpodoxime (proxetil)	100–400 mg q12h	800 mg/q24h	I	q12h	q24h	q24h	Yes	Dose for GFR <10	
Cefprozil	250–500 mg q12h	1 g/q24h	D	100%	50%	50%	Yes, extra 250 mg	Dose for GFR <10	
Ceftaroline	600 mg q12	1.2 g/q24h	D	100%	400 mg q12 (31–50 mL/min)	300 mg q12 (15–30mL/min) 200 mg q12 on HD	Yes, give dose after HD	No data	No data
Ceftazidime	1–2 g q8h	8 g/q24h	I	q8–12h	q12–24h	q24–48h	Yes, extra 1 g	500 mg q24h	2 g q12h
Ceftibuten	400 mg q24h	400 mg	D	100%	25–50%	25–50%	Yes, extra 400 mg	100–200 mg q24h	
Ceftizoxime	1–2 g q8–12h	12 g/q24h	I	q8–12h	q12–24h	q24h	Yes, extra 1 g	500 mg–1 g q24h	
Ceftobiprole (medocaril)	500 mg q8h	1.5 g/q24h	D&I	100%	500 mg q12h (30–50 mL/min)	250 mg q12h (<30 mL/min)	No data	No data	
Ceftolozane–tazobactam	1.5 g q8h	4.5 g/q24h	D	100%	375–750 mg q8h	750 mg × 1 then 150 mg q8h on HD	Yes, give dose after HD	No data	No data
Ceftriaxone	1–2 g q24h	4 g/q24h	D	100%	100%	100%	No	Usual regimen	2 g q12–24h
Cefuroxime (axetil)	250–500 mg q12h	1 g/q24h	D	100%	100%	100%	Yes	Dose for GFR <10	250–500 mg q12h
Cefuroxime	750 mg–1.5 g q8h	6 g/q24h	I	q8h	q8–12h	q24h	Yes	Dose for GFR <10	
Cephalexin	250–500 mg q6h	4 g/q24h	I	q6–8h	q8–12h	q12–24h	Yes	Dose for GFR <10	250–500 mg q12h
Loracarbef	200–400 mg q12h	800 mg/q24h	I	q12h	q24h	q3–5d	Yes	Dose for GFR <10	
MONOBACTAM									
Aztreonam	500 mg–2 g q8–12h	8 g/q24h	D	100%	50%	25%	Yes, extra 500 mg	Dose for GFR <10	2 g q12h
CARBAPENEMS									
Doripenem	500 mg q8h	1.5 g/q24h	D&I	100%	250 mg q8h (30–50 mL/min)	250 mg q12h (<30 mL/min)	No data	No data	250 mg q12h
Ertapenem	1 g q24h	1 g/q24h	D	100%	100%	50%	Yes, extra 150 mg if dose given within 6 h of HD	Dose for GFR <10	50%
Imipenem–cilastatin	250 mg–1 g q6h	4 g/q24h	D	100%	50%	25%	Yes	Dose for GFR <10	250 mg q6h, 500 mg q8h or 500 mg q6h
Meropenem	1 g q8h	4 g/q24h	D&I	100%	50% q12h	50% q24h	Yes	Dose for GFR <10	1 g q12h

Dosing guidance as per references 9, 10, 18, 75–78.
CVVHD, continuous veno-venous hemodialysis; GFR, glomerular filtration rate; HD, hemodialysis; PD, peritoneal dialysis.
Absence of information is due to lack of published data.

TABLE 140-6	Adverse Reactions Associated with β-Lactam Antibiotics	
Reaction Site/System	**Examples**
Local	Pain, induration, tenderness at site of intramuscular injection; burning during intravenous administration; phlebitis
Hypersensitivity	Rash, pruritus, urticaria, fever, chills, Stevens–Johnson syndrome, anaphylaxis
Gastrointestinal	Diarrhea, nausea, vomiting, abdominal pain, Clostridium difficile-associated diarrhea
Hematologic	Eosinophilia, leukopenia, anemia, positive Coombs' test, hemolytic anemia, neutropenia, lymphopenia, thrombocytosis, thrombocytopenia, elevated prothrombin time, bleeding, abnormal clotting time, abnormal platelet aggregation
Hepatic	Elevated serum transaminases (aspartate transaminase, alanine transaminase), hepatitis, elevated alkaline phosphatase, elevated bilirubin
Renal	Elevated blood urea nitrogen and creatinine, casts in urine
Central nervous system	Headache, dizziness, somnolence, confusion, tremor, myoclonus, seizures, encephalopathy
Genitourinary	Vaginitis
Superinfection	Thrush, vaginal candidiasis, infection with resistant bacteria

Reactions to penicillins are characterized according to the time of onset following administration of the drug:

- immediate reactions occur in the first hour;
- accelerated reactions occur 1–72 hours after drug administration; and
- late reactions occur 72 hours or more after starting a course of the antibiotic.

Previous exposure to penicillin does not seem to be a major risk factor for penicillin allergy. However, it is clear that people who have had allergic reactions to penicillin have a higher risk of allergic reactions than people who have tolerated therapy in the past. It is estimated that patients with a previous reaction to penicillin have a four- to sixfold increased risk for developing a subsequent reaction when rechallenged compared with those without a prior reaction.

Skin testing is a useful technique in the evaluation of patients with a history of penicillin allergy, but is not useful as a screening test for the general population because many skin test-positive patients without a history of penicillin allergy can tolerate penicillin therapy. Although fatalities have occurred as a result of the skin test itself, the procedure is generally regarded as safe. A wide range in the incidence of positive skin tests in patients with a previous history of penicillin allergy has been noted (8.75–63%), and therefore a significant proportion of patients who give a history of penicillin allergy can tolerate the drug.[82] In one large study, penicillin skin testing allowed the safe use of penicillin in 90% of patients who gave a history of penicillin allergy.[83] Skin test reactivity declines with time in patients with a history of penicillin allergy. People with dermatitis and allergic rhinitis do not have an increased risk of penicillin allergy, but the risk may be increased for atopic individuals.[84]

Patients with a history of penicillin allergy are four times more likely to have a reaction to first-generation cephalosporins than patients without a history of allergy (8.1 vs 1.9%). Second- and third-generation cephalosporins have an incidence of skin reaction (rash) ranging from 1% to 3%, similar to the incidence of rash with penicillin. Anaphylaxis, however, is uncommon with cephalosporins. Patients with allergy to penicillins were previously thought to be considered allergic to the carbapenems, but subsequent clinical experience indicates that carbapenems can be given to such patients. There seems to be no cross-reactivity with aztreonam. No major allergic reactions to aztreonam have been reported, but rarely patients will develop a rash. Allergic cross-reactivity between cephalosporin derivatives is greater than cross-reactivity between cephalosporins and penicillins.[85]

Occasionally it may be necessary to administer penicillin to patients with a previous severe reaction to the drug (e.g. a pregnant woman with syphilis). Effective methods of desensitization have been described,[86] but adverse reactions are common and the procedure should be done in an intensive care unit with close monitoring.

HEMATOLOGIC EFFECTS

Hematologic toxicity is rare, but leukopenia (occurring in 0.2% of patients on mezlocillin in one study) has been observed when the penicillins or cephalosporins are used at high doses,[87] and also rarely occurs with imipenem. Counts return when the drug is discontinued, and lower dosages can often be tolerated without neutropenia. Isolated eosinophilia can occur in patients on cephalosporins (1–7%). A Coombs positive hemolytic anemia is rarely observed with the penicillins and cephalosporins.[88] It is somewhat more common with ceftaroline and any patient who develops anemia while on the drug should be evaluated by a Coombs' test.

Dose-dependent defects of platelet aggregation and a prolongation of the bleeding time can be seen with carbenicillin and ticarcillin and can occur with all of the penicillins at high doses. Clinically significant bleeding can occur but is uncommon.[89]

Hypoprothrombinemia occurred frequently with cephalosporins that are no longer widely used. These agents all had a methylthiotetrazole (MTT) group (i.e. cefoperazone, cefotetan, cefmenoxime), which may interfere with the activation of factors II, VII, IX and X, and may also prevent the activation of vitamin K.[90] Isolated thrombocytopenia rarely complicates the use of the β-lactam antibiotics. An immune mechanism has been documented. Thrombocytopenia can occur as soon as 5 days after the initiation of the antibiotic and generally resolves when the agent is withdrawn.[91]

RENAL EFFECTS

Interstitial nephritis and occasionally acute kidney injury can be seen with the penicillins.[92] Cephalothin can cause renal damage that histopathologically resembles that of nafcillin.[93] The concurrent use of aminoglycosides may add to the nephrotoxicity of cephalosporins such as cephalothin. About 1% of patients on ceftazidime have elevated blood urea nitrogen or creatinine, but these are generally not clinically significant.[93] The sodium load of some penicillins can be high, most notably with ticarcillin (4.7 mEq/g), but also with ampicillin, methicillin, penicillin G, azlocillin, mezlocillin and piperacillin thereby posing a problem for patients with congestive heart failure.

NEUROLOGIC EFFECTS

Many of the β-lactams can cause neurotoxicity and, in particular, seizures. Notably, benzylpenicillin, cefazolin and imipenem have the highest neurotoxic potential of the β-lactam antibiotics. Seizures occur in 0.4–1.5% of patients taking imipenem.

Risk factors for neurotoxicity include:

- high drug doses;
- renal failure;
- disruption of the blood–brain barrier;
- pre-existing central nervous system (CNS) disease;
- advanced age;
- concurrent administration of nephrotoxic drugs;
- concurrent drugs that may reduce the seizure threshold; and
- concurrent administration of other β-lactam antibiotics.[94]

Neurotoxicity of penicillins is clearly related to elevated CSF antibiotic levels, such as may occur when high doses are being used in patients with impaired renal function. Penicillin levels in CSF should not exceed 5 mg/L.

GASTROINTESTINAL EFFECTS

Gastrointestinal upset and diarrhea are common side-effects of the β-lactams. Enterocolitis caused by *Clostridium difficile* may result from use of any of the β-lactams.

Hepatitis is a rare side-effect of certain penicillins like mezlocillin and nafcillin and resolves after discontinuation of therapy. Hepatitis from intravenous oxacillin is thought to result from a hypersensitivity reaction, is not dose related and is reversible on discontinuation of the drug.[95] Mild elevations in transaminases and alkaline phosphatase also occur with the cephalosporins and carbapenems, but the drug can usually be continued.[96] Serum transaminases become elevated in 2–4% of patients receiving aztreonam.

Gallbladder sludge formation[97] and cholelithiasis[98] have occurred in patients on ceftriaxone. Children, patients receiving prolonged or high doses, and patients on total parenteral nutrition appear to be at risk of this complication.

A disulfiram-like reaction has been associated with the cephalosporins with an MTT group.[99] Patients taking these agents and then ingesting alcohol have developed flushing, tachycardia, diaphoresis, headache, nausea, vomiting and dizziness.

OTHER REACTIONS

At the intramuscular injection site, patients may experience pain, tenderness and edema. Thrombophlebitis can occur in up to 5% of patients receiving parenteral therapy with some agents. Other reactions to penicillin are less common. Serum sickness can occur and, rarely, exfoliative dermatitis, the Stevens–Johnson syndrome and allergic vasculitis. Late-onset morbilliform rashes can develop as a result of penicillin therapy and may disappear, even if the penicillin is continued, but desquamation can occur.

DRUG INTERACTIONS

The most clinically important drug interaction with the β-lactams occurs with probenecid, which causes a two- to fourfold increase in the peak serum concentration of the antibiotics. Probenecid is used most often with penicillin (e.g. for treatment of gonococcal infections) but can also be used with ampicillin, methicillin, oxacillin, cloxacillin and nafcillin. The mechanism of action involves not only inhibition of renal tubular secretion of the β-lactams, but also a decrease in the apparent volume of distribution of the drug.[100] Probenecid has little effect on the serum drug levels of imipenem and aztreonam and none on ceftazidime. Adverse reactions, including anaphylaxis, can occur with probenecid and the clinician must also be aware that toxicity can result from supratherapeutic levels of the β-lactam antibiotics when used with probenecid.

Synergistic activity against various bacteria occurs when the penicillins, cephalosporins, carbapenems and monobactams are used in conjunction with aminoglycosides.[101] However, using two β-lactam antibiotics together may result in either synergy or antagonism.

The bactericidal effect of ampicillin may be reduced when other antibiotics (chloramphenicol, erythromycin, sulfa drugs and tetracycline) are used simultaneously. The clinical significance of this is unclear. When ampicillin is used in patients who are taking oral contraceptive agents, breakthrough bleeding may occur and the contraceptive may be less effective.

Piperacillin and ticarcillin must be used cautiously in any patient on vecuronium because the neuromuscular blockade can be further prolonged. Piperacillin can also lower serum levels of tobramycin if the drugs are used together but does not significantly affect tobramycin pharmacokinetics.

Fatal reactions associated with the appearance of precipitates of calcium and ceftriaxone have occurred in neonates; it is therefore recommended not to administer ceftriaxone within 48 hours of giving intravenous calcium-containing solutions.

References available online at expertconsult.com.

KEY REFERENCES

Baddour L.M., Wilson W.R., Bayer A.S., et al.: Infective endocarditis: diagnosis, antimicrobial therapy, and management of complications. A statement for healthcare professionals from the Committee on Rheumatic Fever, Endocarditis, and Kawasaki Disease, Council on Cardiovascular Disease in the Young, and the Councils on Clinical Cardiology, Stroke, and Cardiovascular Surgery and Anesthesia, American Heart Association-Executive Summary. *Circulation* 2005; 111:3167-3184.

de Gans J., van de Beek D.: Dexamethasone in adults with bacterial meningitis. *N Engl J Med* 2002; 347:1549-1556.

Fernandez-Hildaldo N., Almirante B., Gavalda J., et al.: Ampicillin plus ceftriaxone is as effective as ampicillin plus gentamicin in treating *Enterococcus faecalis* infective endocarditis. *Clin Infect Dis* 2013; 56:1261-1268.

Gilbert D.N., Moellering R.C. Jr, Eliopoulos G.M., et al.: eds. *The Sanford Guide to antimicrobial therapy*, 44th ed. Sperryville, VA: Antimicrobial Therapy; 2014.

Graham D.R., Lucasti C., Malafaia O., et al.: Ertapenem once daily versus piperacillin-tazobactam four times per day for treatment of complicated skin and skin-structure infections in adults: results of a prospective, randomized, double blind multicenter study. *Clin Infect Dis* 2002; 34:1460-1467.

Livermore D.M.: Beta-lactamases in laboratory and clinical resistance. *Clin Microbiol Rev* 1995; 8:557-584.

Mandell L.A., Wunderink R.G., Anzueto A., et al.: Infectious Diseases Society of America/American Thoracic Society consensus guidelines on the management of community-acquired pneumonia in adults. *Clin Infect Dis* 2007; 44:S27-S72.

Munar M.Y., Singh H.: Drug dosing adjustments in patients with chronic kidney disease. *Am Fam Physician* 2007; 75:1487-1496.

Norrby S.R.: Side effects of cephalosporins. *Drugs* 1987; 34(Suppl. 2):105-120.

Physicians' desk reference. 68th ed. Montvale, NJ: Medical Economics; 2014.

Queenan A.M., Bush K.: Carbapenemases: the versatile β-lactamases. *Clin Microbiol Rev* 2007; 20:440-458.

Teo J., Liew Y., Lee W., et al.: Prolonged infusion versus intermittent boluses of β-lactam antibiotics for treatment of acute infections: a meta-analysis. *Int J Antimicrob Agents* 2014; 43:403-411.

Trotman R.L., Williamson J.C., Shoemaker D.M., et al.: Antibiotic dosing in critically ill adult patients receiving continuous renal replacement therapy. *Clin Infect Dis* 2005; 41:1159-1166.

141

Macrolides, Ketolides, Lincosamides and Streptogramins

JENNIE H. KWON*

Macrolides and Ketolides

Introduction

Soon after the beginning of the antimicrobial era, it became apparent that bacteria could rapidly evolve resistance to antibacterial agents. In a search for new antibacterial compounds, researchers at Eli Lilly discovered the erythromycin complex in 1952.[1]

Erythromycin A, the most active component of the erythromycin complex, was initially intended to provide an alternative therapy to penicillinase-producing strains of *Staphylococcus aureus*. The later discoveries of vancomycin and the semisynthetic penicillins and cephalosporins led to a decline in the use of erythromycin A.

In the 1980s, the recognition of the pathogenic potential of *Chlamydia trachomatis* and the outbreak of 'Legionnaires' disease' led to a revival of interest in macrolides (the second wave of macrolides – azithromycin, clarithromycin, dirithromycin, flurithromycin, roxithromycin).[2] Macrolides have excellent activity against the intracellular pathogen *Legionella pneumophila*, in contrast to β-lactams, which do not accumulate in phagocytic cells.[3]

The third wave of macrolides (the ketolides – cethromycin, modithromycin, solithromycin, telithromycin) was in response to the emergence of erythromycin A-resistant strains among gram-positive cocci, *Campylobacter* spp., *Helicobacter pylori*, *Mycobacterium avium* complex, etc. Solithromycin and cethromycin are currently in clinical development.[4,5]

Definitions

The macrolides are hydrophobic molecules with a central 14- to 16-membered-ring lactone with few or no double bonds and no nitrogen atom. Several amino or neutral sugars may be attached to the lactone nucleus.

The azalides, such as azithromycin or tulathromycin, are not included as they have an endolactone nitrogen atom. Nevertheless, they are semisynthetic derivatives of erythromycin A and due to their antibacterial spectrum, belong to the macrolide family. Semisynthetic ketolides were obtained by the removal of the neutral sugar. The 3-OH group obtained was oxidized yielding a 3-carbonyl group, which characterizes the ketolides.[5]

Classification

There are several classifications of macrolides: a chemical and a simplified classification that considers the lactone structure and the natural or semisynthetic origin of the molecule. The natural macrolides of importance in human therapeutics are 14- or 16-membered-ring macrolides, the semisynthetic derivatives and the 15-membered-ring macrolides (azalides).

The 14-membered-ring macrolides are divided into two groups: those of natural origin such as erythromycin A (Figure 141-1) and oleandomycin, and the semisynthetic derivatives of erythromycin A. The latter may be separated into three subgroups:

- those with a modified substituent of the lactone nucleus, such as roxithromycin, clarithromycin, dirithromycin, flurithromycin and davercin (group II_A);
- those with a modified lactone nucleus, involving two subgroups, azalides (azithromycin, tulathromycin, gamithromycin) and oxolides (group II_{B1} and II_{B2}); and
- those with a modified neutral sugar – ketolides (3-keto group) and acylide derivatives (alkyl or alkyl aryl 3-substituent) (group II_C) (Figure 141-2).

Groups III and IV comprise, respectively, the 16-membered-ring natural molecules, such as josamycin, spiramycin and midecamycin, and the synthetic molecules such as miocamycin or rokitamycin.[5]

Physicochemical Characteristics

The main physicochemical properties of macrolides and ketolides are presented in Table 141-1.

STABILITY IN ACIDIC MEDIUM

Erythromycin A, spiramycin and josamycin are unstable in an acidic medium. Erythromycin A is degraded by the formation of a hemiketal or a spiroketal form of erythronolide A (Figure 141-3).

Josamycin (leucomycin A_3) may be converted in an acidic medium to isojosamycin, which has a hydroxyl group at C-13 because of the rearrangement of the dienole system.

*The editors would like acknowledge Dr. Andre Bryskier contribution to the previous edition.

Erythromycin A

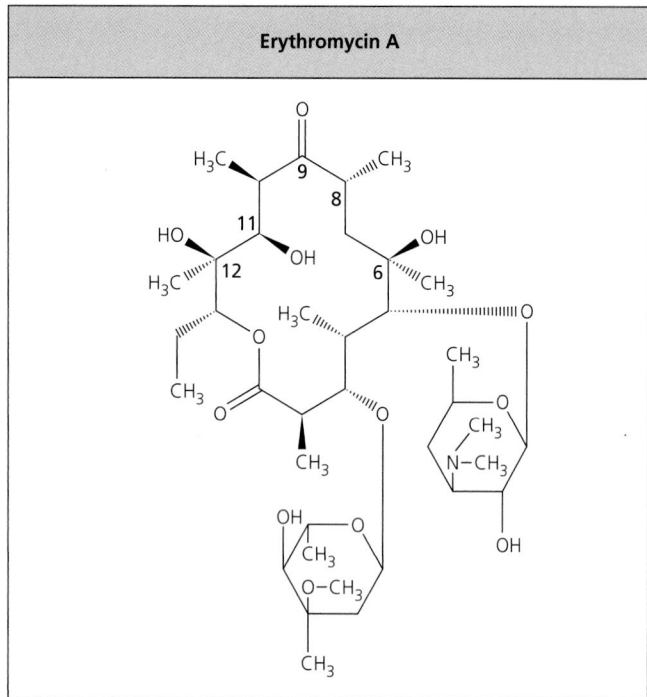

Figure 141-1   Erythromycin A.

| TABLE 141-1 | **Main Characteristics of Macrolides and Ketolides** |

Drug	pK	Molecular Weight
Azithromycin	8.9–9.1	748.9
Clarithromycin	8.3	747.96
Dirithromycin	9.2	835
Erythromycin A	8.6	733.94
Erythromycylamine	8.9	734
Flurithromycin	–	751.95
Josamycin	7.1	828.02
Midecamycin	6.9	813.99
Miocamycin	6.5	898.05
Oleandomycin	8.5	687.89
Rokitamycin	6.3	828
Roxithromycin	9.2	837.04
Spiramycin I	7.7	843.06
Telithromycin	8.7	812

Spiramycin is a complex formed by three major components (I–III), which differ in the substituent at position 3 of the lactone nucleus. The spiramycins are more stable than erythromycin A in an acidic medium.

Roxithromycin is highly stable at pH 4.2 (Figure 141-4). Clarithromycin is 6-O-methylerythromycin A, and the hydroxyl at position 11 remains free. A degradation product (pseudoclarithromycin) devoid of antibacterial activity occurs under conditions of extreme acidity (Figure 141-5).

Azithromycin and roxithromycin are hydrolyzed at the β-O-glycoside bond at position 3 in a highly acidic medium (pH 1.2). The resultant descladinose degradation product has a 3-hydroxyl group on

Classification of macrolides

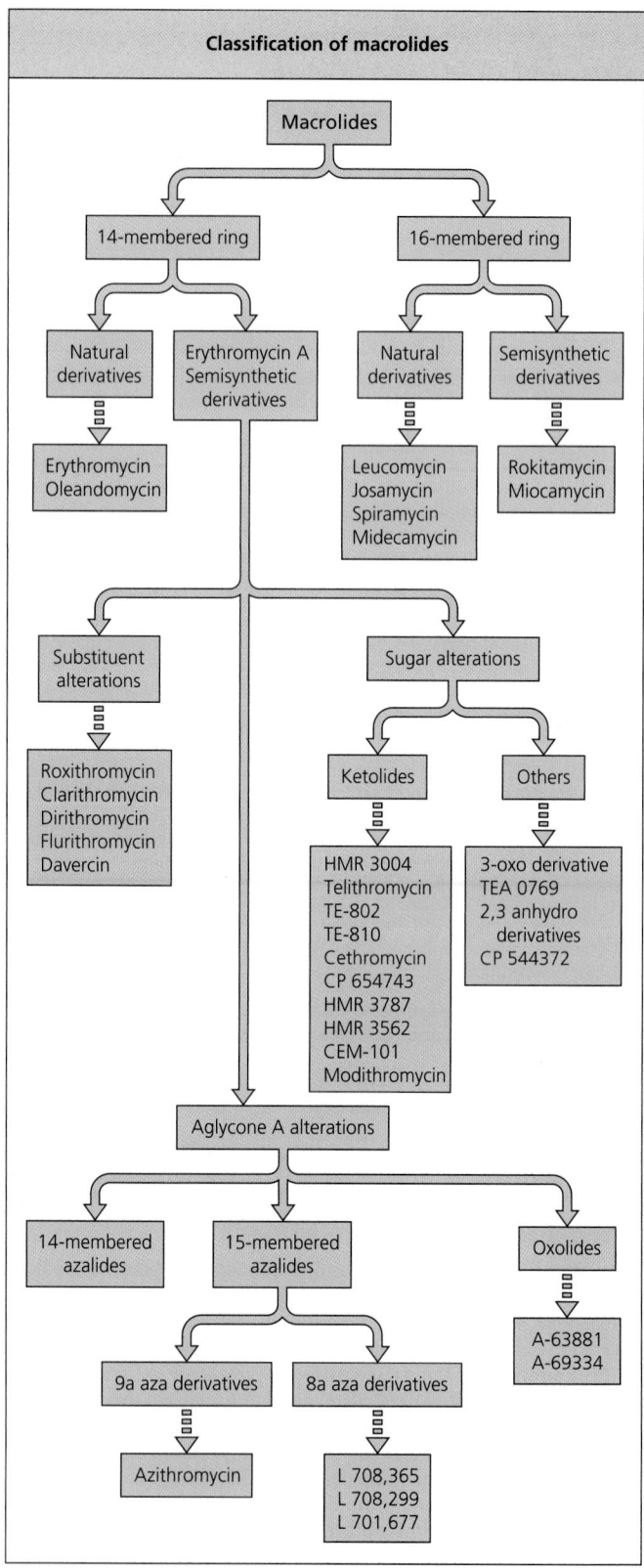

Figure 141-2   Classification of macrolides.

the lactone nucleus. These compounds are highly stable in an acidic medium (Figure 141-6).

Different ketolides are very stable in an acidic medium depending on the substituent fixed on aglycone. Ketolides are not destroyed at pH 1.2 after >6 hours of exposure.

Degradation of erythromycin A in an acidic medium

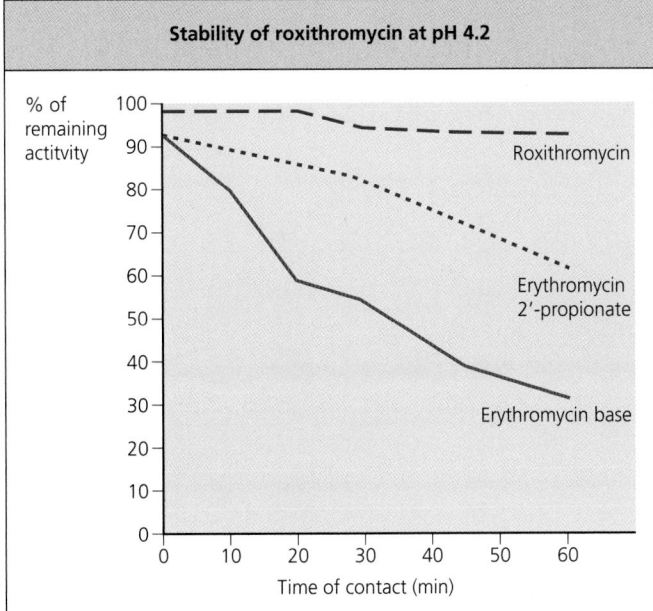

Figure 141-3   Degradation of erythromycin A in an acidic medium.

Stability of roxithromycin at pH 4.2

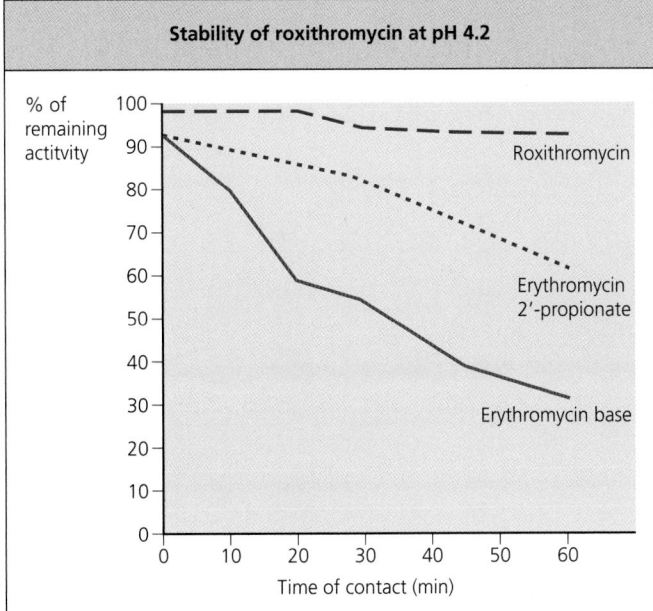

Figure 141-4   Stability of roxithromycin at pH 4.2.

Azithromycin: degradation in an acidic medium

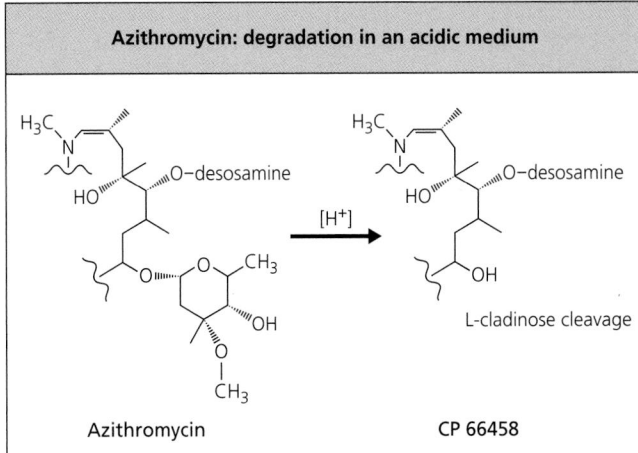

Figure 141-6   Azithromycin: degradation in an acidic medium.

Pseudoclarithromycin

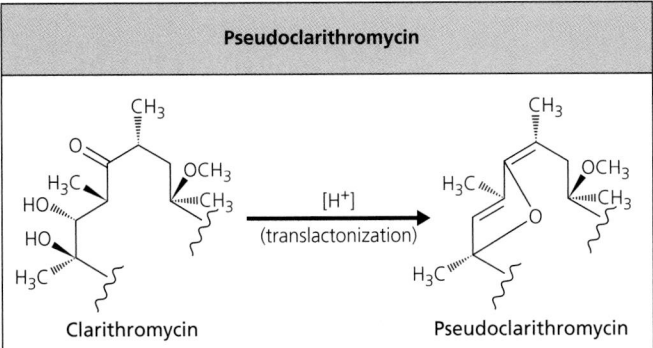

Figure 141-5   Pseudoclarithromycin.

In Vitro Activity (Table 141-2)

The antibacterial spectrum of the macrolides includes gram-positive bacteria[6] (e.g. *Staphylococcus* spp., *Streptococcus* spp., *Listeria* spp., *Erysipelothrix insidiosa*, *Corynebacterium* spp., *Lactobacilli* spp., *Leuconostoc* spp., *Pediococcus* spp.) and gram-negative cocci along with fastidious

gram-negative bacilli (e.g. *Haemophilus influenzae*, *Moraxella catarrhalis*, *Pasteurella* spp. and *Bordetella* spp.).[7,8] Some anaerobic bacteria, intracellular bacteria, atypical bacteria such as mycoplasmas, and related species are also susceptible to the macrolides. Some atypical mycobacteria, spirochetes, bacteria responsible for gastrointestinal infections (*Vibrio cholerae* and other *Vibrio* spp., *Campylobacter* spp. and *H. pylori*) and *Treponema pallidum* remain susceptible to macrolides.[9,10] They also display activity against *Leptospira*, *Borrelia* and *Bartonella* spp. However, these molecules are weakly active against enterococci and only have moderate activity against the viridans group of streptococci.

Erythromycin A overall is less active than clarithromycin but more active than azithromycin, roxithromycin and dirithromycin. Erythromycin A is 10 times more active than oleandomycin, 2–10 times more active than josamycin, 2–12 times more active than spiramycin and up to 10 times more active than midecamycin. The antibacterial spectrum of telithromycin, cethromycin and others encompasses that of the macrolides.[11]

Telithromycin is more active *in vitro* than clarithromycin against gram-positive and gram-negative cocci, and also against erythromycin A-susceptible strains of gram-positive bacilli. Telithromycin, like erythromycin A, is very active against β-hemolytic streptococci of Lancefield groups A, B, C and G when the strains are susceptible to erythromycin A. Telithromycin displays a good activity against viridans group streptococci, irrespective of the resistance phenotype (erythromycin A-resistant, penicillin G-resistant).[11]

Ketolides remain highly susceptible against isolates of *S. pneumoniae* whatever their phenotype of resistance to erythromycin A.

TABLE 141-2	*In Vitro* Activity of Macrolides and Ketolides				
	MIC$_{50}$ (mg/L)				
Organism	ERY	CLA	AZI	ROX	TEL
Bartonella spp.	0.06	0.03	0.03	–	0.006
Bordetella pertussis	0.06	0.015	0.03	0.12	0.01
Borrelia spp.	0.015–0.03	0.0006–0.0025	0.002–0.008	0.0025–0.006	–
Campylobacter jejuni	1.0	1.0	0.12	4.0	0.5–1.0
Chlamydophila pneumoniae	0.03	0.125	0.125	0.125	0.125
Corynebacterium diphtheriae	0.008	0.004	0.015	0.008	0.004
Corynebacterium jeikeium	>128	>128	>128	>128	0.06
Corynebacterium urealyticum	>64	>64	>64	>64	≥0.015
Enterococcus faecalis	4.0	4.0	8	8	0.12
Enterococcus faecium	>64	>64	>64	>64	2.0
Erysipelothrix rhusiopathiae	0.03	0.06	0.5	0.06	≥0.015
Gardnerella vaginalis	0.06	0.06	0.06	0.03	≥0.002
Haemophilus ducreyi	0.06	0.008	0.015	0.03	0.004
Haemophilus influenzae	4.0	4.0	1.0	8.0	1.0
Helicobacter pylori	0.25	0.015	0.25	0.12	0.25
Lactobacillus spp.	0.06	0.015	0.06	0.06	≥0.03
Legionella pneumophila	0.25	0.03	0.12	0.12	0.03
Leuconostoc spp.	0.06	0.03	0.125	0.125	0.25
Listeria monocytogenes	0.25	0.06	0.5	0.25	0.03
Moraxella catarrhalis	0.12	0.06	0.03	0.12	0.06
Mycoplasma pneumoniae	0.0039	0.019	0.0024	0.0039	0.00097
Neisseria gonorrhoeae	0.25	0.25	0.12	0.5	0.12
Neisseria meningitidis	0.12	0.015	0.015	0.06	0.0015–0.12
Nocardia spp.	16	16	>128	64	–
Pasteurella multocida	4.0	2.0	1.0	4.0	1.0
Pediococcus spp.	0.125	0.06	0.125	0.06	0.008
Rhodococcus equi	0.5	0.06	1.0	0.25	0.25
Staphylococcus aureus (methicillin sensitive)	0.25	0.25	1.0	0.5	0.06
Streptococcus agalactiae	0.06	0.015	0.06	0.12	0.008–0.12
Streptococcus groups C and G	0.06	0.03	0.12	0.12	≥0.008
Streptococcus pneumoniae	0.06	0.015	0.06	0.06	0.015
Streptococcus pyogenes	0.06	0.015	0.06	0.12	≥0.008
Viridans streptococci	2.0	1.0	4.0	4.0	≥0.03–0.25

ERY, erythromycin A; CLA, clarithromycin; AZI, azithromycin; ROX, roxithromycin; TEL, telithromycin.

Diphtheria antibiotic treatment is based on penicillin G or erythromycin A. Rare erythromycin A-resistant strains have been described. Telithromycin is active against toxigenic and nontoxigenic *Corynebacterium diphtheriae*.

The *in vitro* activity of macrolides and ketolides against *Listeria monocytogenes* and *Erysipelothrix rhusiopathiae* is good, and some reports have shown *in vitro* activity against *Bacillus anthracis*.

Macrolides are inactive against *Corynebacterium jeikeium* and *Corynebacterium urealyticum*; in contrast, telithromycin is very active against the majority of corynebacteria. Telithromycin activity against *C. jeikeium* is distributed in a bimodal population. There are discrepancies among authors with respect to the activity against *C. urealyticum*.[11]

Neisseria meningitidis strains with reduced susceptibility to penicillin G have been described and rifampin-resistant strains are increasingly common. Some erythromycin A or spiramycin-resistant strains have been observed which harbor an efflux mechanism of resistance mediated by Mtr (encoded by the *mtr* gene).[12]

Macrolides and ketolides are inactive against Enterobacteriaceae with few minor exceptions. Macrolides are weakly active or inactive against enterococci. Azithromycin exhibits a certain *in vitro* activity against *Salmonella*, *Shigella* spp. and *Escherichia coli*.

Macrolides and ketolides are highly active against *Leptospira inter-rogans* (minimum inhibitory concentrations (MICs) range from 0.01 to 0.04 mg/L) and *Bartonella* spp. (MICs 0.03–0.125 mg/L).

Lyme disease, caused by *Borrelia burgdorferi*, is divided into at least three subspecies associated with different syndromes: rheumatic (*B. burgdorferi sensu lato*), neurologic (*B. garinii*) and dermatologic (*B. afzelii*). Activity of macrolides/ketolides is species-dependent.

BACTERIA RESPONSIBLE FOR LOWER RESPIRATORY TRACT INFECTIONS

Lower respiratory tract infections are due to respiratory pathogens or to intracellular or atypical bacteria. Common pathogens are *Strep. pneumoniae, H. influenzae, Staph. aureus* and *Moraxella catarrhalis.*

The determination of the *in vitro* activity of antibiotics against *H. influenzae* is poorly standardized. Telithromycin has *in vitro* activity similar to that of azithromycin and greater than that of clarithromycin and roxithromycin, which are poorly active. Macrolides remain the first line treatment against *Bordetella pertussis*. Erythromycin A-resistant strains are of rare occurrence.[5,11]

Mycoplasma pneumoniae, a common cause of atypical pneumonia, is susceptible to macrolides and ketolides. Pneumonia due to *Chlamydophila pneumoniae* and *L. pneumophila* is highly susceptible to macrolides/ketolides.[2,3,10]

Parachlamydia and Simkania

Trophozoites of *Acanthamoeba* hosting *Chlamydia*-like bacteria have been isolated from patients with fever associated with humidifier use in Vermont (Hall's coccus strain) and from the nasal mucosa (strain Bn9). The use of antibiotics directed against *Parachlamydia* for community-acquired pneumonia has been reported.[12]

Tropheryma whipplei

The growth of *T. whipplei* (the organism responsible for Whipple's disease) in MRC5 cells is inhibited by macrolides/ketolides according to the method of quantification of the copies of DNA.

BACTERIA INVOLVED IN SEXUALLY TRANSMITTED DISEASES

There have been multiple reports of *Neisseria gonorrhoeae* with resistance to azithromycin.[13]

Strains of *Treponema pallidum* resistant to erythromycin A and azithromycin have been reported.

Chancroid is caused by *Haemophilus ducreyi*. Macrolides represent a standard treatment for this infection.

Chlamydia trachomatis is the causative agent of trachoma in endemic regions, nongonococcal urethritis and pelvic inflammatory disease. The activity of macrolides/ketolides is good, with MICs ranging from 0.008 mg/L to 0.06 mg/L.

The *in vitro* activity of macrolides/ketolides against *Ureaplasma urealyticum* is good, with MICs of 0.06 μg/mL.

Fourteen- and 15-membered-ring macrolides are inactive against *Mycoplasma hominis*, but 16-membered-ring macrolides exert good *in vitro* activity; activity of ketolides is structure dependent.[10]

ANAEROBIC BACTERIA

Macrolides exhibit variable activity against gram-positive anaerobes and are poorly active against gram-negative anaerobic bacilli. Telithromycin possesses excellent *in vitro* activity against gram-positive bacteria, moderate activity against gram-negative bacilli of the *Bacteroides* group, good activity against *Porphyromonas* and *Prevotella* spp. and variable activity against *Fusobacterium* spp.[11,14]

Mechanism of Action (see also Chapter 137)

The macrolides/ketolides inhibit protein synthesis by binding to the 50S subunit of the bacterial ribosome and by blocking the translation of messenger RNA. In the presence of macrolides/ketolides, peptidyl tRNA accumulates in the bacterial cell, causing depletion of the free transfer tRNA needed for α-amino acid activation. The presence of erythromycin A causes the release of a basic amino acid-rich peptide chain by transient inhibition of transpeptidation. It appears that erythromycin A modifies the interaction between peptidyl tRNA and the peptidyltransferase donor site.[5]

INTRA-BACTERIAL PENETRATION

Before reaching ribosomes, the molecule has to cross one (gram-positive) or two (gram-negative) barriers. Erythromycin A and its derivatives penetrate gram-positive bacteria and *H. influenzae* passively. The affinity for ribosomes is higher for ketolides than for erythromycin A.[11]

EXIT TUNNEL

The exit tunnel passes through the 50S ribosomal subunit and is paved mainly by the RNA loop. The nascent polypeptide being translated into the final protein product escapes the ribosome via this exit tunnel. The tunnel accommodates a peptide of 25–40 amino acids and is formed with proteins L22 and L4. The binding site of macrolides, lincosamide and streptogramin B (MLSB) antibacterials is located in the entrance of the exit tunnel before the ribosomal proteins L4 and L22 constrict it, causing destabilization of peptidyl tRNA during translocation and inducing dissociation of peptidyl tRNA from the ribosomes during protein synthesis.[5,15–20]

Fourteen- and 15-membered-ring macrolides reduce the diameter of the tunnel entrance blocking the progression of the nascent peptide by steric hindrance. Lincosamides and 16-membered-ring macrolides inhibit the peptidyltransferase enzymatic activity. However, 14- and 15-membered-ring macrolides as well as streptogramin B analogs block the entrance of the exit channel of the 50S ribosomal subunit.

The translation reaction contains a peptidyl-tRNA hydrolase, which hydrolyzes peptidyl tRNAs that dissociate from the ribosome by drop off, but not those remaining bound to the ribosome. The length of the drop off nascent peptide is compound-dependent.

PEPTIDYLTRANSFERASE CENTER

The peptidyltransferase center consists of domains II and V, forming a pocket with 5S rRNA.[5] Macrolides and ketolides are fixed on domain V; ketolides are also fixed on domain II.

Cethromycin and telithromycin interact like erythromycin A with domain V through desosamine sugar and aglycone.

Ketolides are composed of two additional parts: C11–C12 carbamate residue and a long side chain either on the carbamate moiety for telithromycin or through the 6-hydroxyl group for cethromycin.

Intracellular Concentrations in Host Cells

Macrolides penetrate and accumulate in phagocytic cells, thereby allowing the treatment of infections due to intracellular bacteria. The mean ratios of cell concentrations to those present in the extracellular medium are presented in Table 141-3.[5,21,22]

Like azithromycin, telithromycin gradually accumulates in polymorphonuclear neutrophils, particularly in the granules (60%), and is eliminated progressively from the cell (efflux). Telithromycin uses a transport system to penetrate the phagocytic cell.[11]

Mechanism of Resistance
EPIDEMIOLOGY

Since the first report in the mid-1970s of *Strep. pneumoniae* multidrug-resistant strains, the prevalence rate of erythromycin A resistance (along with *Strep. pyogenes* and other gram-positive cocci) has increased worldwide.[4,17] Surveillance programs such as Protek include detection of phenotypes and genotypes of resistance. For 2004–2005, the prevalence rate of erythromycin A resistance worldwide was 35%. The main resistance mechanism was methylation (*erm B* gene) and represented 66% of the resistant isolates. In the USA, the main resistance mechanism was efflux (*mef A* gene) and represented 80% of the

TABLE 141-3	Accumulation Ratio of the Main Macrolides (*In Vitro*)	
Drug	**Cells**	**C/E**
Azithromycin	PMN	80–300
Clarithromycin	PMN	9–16
Dirithromycin	PMN, MA	7–60668
Erythromycin A	PMN, MA	4.4–1818–38
Josamycin	PMN	16
Rokitamycin	PMN	30
Roxithromycin	PMN, MA	14–10061
Spiramycin	MA	20–35
Telithromycin	PMN	250–300

C/E, cellular to extracellular accumulation ratio; MA, alveolar macrophages; PMN, polymorphonuclear neutrophils.

resistant isolates. In Europe, the highest rate of *Strep. pneumoniae* resistance was in France (52.5%), Spain (32.2%) and Italy (33.5%).[23]

MOLECULAR MECHANISMS OF RESISTANCE

There are currently four recognized mechanisms of resistance to erythromycin A:

- modifications in the ribosomal target;
- inactivation of the molecule;
- efflux;
- mutations in the 23S ribosomal RNA and ribosomal proteins L4 and L22.

These resistance mechanisms are described in detail in Chapter 138.

Pharmacodynamic Properties

Thigh-infection models in neutropenic and normal mice have shown that macrolides/ketolides can be separated in two subgroups: those that are time dependent (T>MIC) such as erythromycin, roxithromycin, clarithromycin, and those that are concentration dependent such as azithromycin and dirithromycin.[5,16,24]

The pharmacodynamics of telithromycin data indicates that there is a good correlation between efficacy and concentration, particularly the area under the curve (AUC).

Pharmacokinetic Properties

ADULT VOLUNTEERS

Absorption and bioavailability vary according to the molecule.[25–28] Absorption can be rapid, with a lag time of 0.25 hours (roxithromycin, clarithromycin). The average peak serum concentration ranges from 0.4 mg/L (azithromycin 500 mg) to 11 mg/L (roxithromycin 300 mg). It is reached after a period of between 0.6 hour (rokitamycin) and 4.0 hours (dirithromycin) and is dose dependent. The relative bioavailability (AUC/F) ranges from 3.7 mg.h/L (rokitamycin) to 132 mg.h/L (roxithromycin 300 mg) and is dose dependent, but is not proportional to the dose for certain molecules with nonlinear pharmacokinetics. The elimination half-life ranges from 0.1 hour (miocamycin) to 44 hours (dirithromycin). The absolute bioavailability ranges from 10% (dirithromycin) to about 50–60% for roxithromycin and clarithromycin. It is in the order of 37% for azithromycin and 14-hydroxyclarithromycin (clarithromycin metabolite).

Plasma protein binding is mainly to the α_1-glycoproteins for macrolides, ranging from 15% (josamycin) to more than 90% (roxithromycin).

For telithromycin and cethromycin, peak plasma concentrations varied from 1.9 mg/L (telithromycin 800 mg) to 0.14–1.7 mg/L (cethromycin 100 mg and 1200 mg, respectively) and were reached 1.0

hour after administration, and the apparent elimination half-life ranged from 3.5–6.6 hours (cethromycin) to 7.16 hours (telithromycin 800 mg) (see Table 141-4).

ELDERLY PATIENTS

In elderly patients with no liver abnormalities the pharmacokinetic profiles were similar to those of adults (Table 141-5).

Renal Insufficiency

Clarithromycin requires a dose adjustment for renal insufficiency, whereas azithromycin does not. There is no established dose adjustment for telithromycin for severe renal insufficiency.

Clinical Studies

High concentrations in the respiratory tract and serum can be detected following single or multiple doses of macrolides (Table 141-6). Telithromycin concentrations in different parts of the lung tissue after a single dose of 800 mg are summarized in Table 141-7.

Adverse Reactions and Interactions

Common side effects of macrolides/ketolides are diarrhea, nausea and vomiting. Telithromycin has been associated with potentially fatal hepatotoxicity, and should be avoided in patients with hepatic dysfunction.[11] Patients on telithromycin should be monitored for signs and symptoms of liver dysfunction. Due to reports of potentially fatal exacerbations of myasthenia gravis associated with telithromycin, the US Food and Drug Administration (FDA) announced a black box warning stating that telithromycin should not be used in patients with myasthenia gravis. Additionally, the FDA recommends that telithromycin should not be used to treat acute sinusitis or bronchitis. If telithromycin is used for community-acquired pneumonia, the FDA recommends that it should be a secondary alternative.[29]

Azithromycin is contraindicated in patients with cholestatic jaundice or prior liver dysfunction related to azithromycin administration. QT prolongation has been described with macrolides, therefore the risk of cardiac complications should be considered when prescribing a macrolide. Macrolides have the capacity to interfere with the metabolism and pharmacokinetics of other drugs (Table 141-8) and may produce adverse events when administered with other drugs such as theophylline, carbamazepine, cyclosporine A, methotrexate, midazolam and terfenadine.[5,20,30,31]

Macrolides/Ketolides Versus Other Antibacterials: Advantages

Macrolides are mainly used as an alternative to β-lactam antibiotics, particularly in the outpatient setting. However, some primary indications remain for macrolides such as diphtheria, chancroid, *Helicobacter pylori* and *Mycobacterium avium*.

One of the major uses for macrolides is atypical and intracellular pathogenic infections such as *Chlamydia* and *Legionella* spp. in parenchymal lower respiratory tract infections or nongonococcal urethritis.[5,32]

Other major advantages of macrolides compared to other compounds is their safety in β-lactam-allergic patients, oral bioavailability, tolerability when used during pregnancy, and in the pediatric setting as well as in adult and elderly patients.

Lincosamides

Introduction

Lincomycin was isolated in 1962 from fermentation of *Streptomyces lincolnensis* subsp. *lincolnensis*. Numerous analogs have been prepared from lincomycin by semisynthesis to enlarge the antibacterial spectrum and enhance antibacterial activity. A series of derivatives have been synthesized, yielding clindamycin and lincomycin.

TABLE 141-4	Pharmacokinetics of Macrolides and Ketolides					
Drug	Dose (mg)	Compound or Metabolite	C_{max} (µg/mL)	T_{max} (h)	AUC/F (µg/h/mL)	$T\frac{1}{2}$ β (h)
Azithromycin	500	–	0.35 ± 0.1	0.9 ± 0.9	3.58 ± 1.2	–
	500	–	0.59 ± 0.2	2.2 ± 0.02	3.35 ± 0.4	41.2 ± 4.3
Clarithromycin	100	C	0.35	1.46	1.67	2.27
	200	C	0.6	1.56	2.99	2.3
	–	OH-C	0.41	2.29	3.4	3.37
	400	C	0.13	1.86	8.55	3.6
	–	OH-C	0.78	2.11	7.52	3.89
	600	C	2.03	1.83	15.44	3.64
	–	OH-C	1.06	2.45	9.95	3.84
	800	C	2.63	2.67	24.73	4.25
	–	OH-C	1.02	2.72	10.72	5.09
	1200	C	3.97	2.2	44.6	5.98
	–	OH	1.54	2.61	23.9	9.19
	250	C	0.7–0.8	1.7 ± 1.9	4–4.2	2.6–2.8
	–	OH	0.6–0.7	2.2–2.3	4.6–4.9	3.9–5.1
	500	C	1.77–1.89	2.3	11.1–11.7	3.3–3.5
	–	OH	0.7–0.8	2.3–2.8	6.1–6.9	6.4–6.6
Dirithromycin	250	–	ND	–	–	–
	500	–	0.29 ± 0.2	4	0.86 ± 0.6	32.5
	750	–	0.64 ± 0.4	4	1.84 ± 1.2	30.6
	1000	–	0.41 ± 0.2	4	1.61 ± 1.1	31.9
Flurithromycin	500	–	1 ± 0.7	0.92	0.4	3.54
	750	–	1.58 ± 0.3	0.72	3.52	2.8
	375	–	1.41 ± 0.5	1	4.41	3.94
Josamycin	1000	–	2.74	0.75	4.2	1.5
Josamycin	400	–	0.33	0.77	0.91	1.51
	1000	–	2.41	0.75	4.9	2
Midecamycin	400	–	0.25	0.5	0.34	1
Midecamycin	600	–	0.8	1	–	–
	1200	–	1.9	2	–	–
Miocamycin	600	–	3.01	2	3	1
	400	Mb12	0.6	0.48	0.73	1.24
	–	Mb6	0.17	0.6	0.28	1.47
	–	Mb9a	0.16	0.73	0.27	1.45
	800	Mb12	1.37	0.52	1.72	1.32
	–	Mb6	0.44	0.65	0.76	1.71
	–	Mb9a	0.4	0.83	1.46	2.34
	800	Mb12	1.73	0.79	2.59	1.31
	–	Mb6	0.66	0.83	1.46	2.34
	–	Mb9a	0.57	1.06	1.33	2.09
Oleandomycin	1000	–	2.8	2.6	10.8	3.4
Oleandomycin	1000	–	4	1	14	4.2
Rokitamycin	600	–	1.9	0.6	3.7	2
Roxithromycin	150	–	7.9 ± 0.6	1.9	81 ± 10	10.5 ± 1.4
	300	–	10.8 ± 0.6	1.5	132 ± 17	11.9 ± 0.5
	450	–	12.2 ± 0.7	1.3	170 ± 20	13.8 ± 0.9
Spiramycin	1000	–	0.96	3	5.43	5.37
	1500	–	1.53	3	9.8	5.52
	2000	–	1.65	4	11.26	6.23
	500	–	2.14	–	6.19	4.51
Telithromycin	800	–	1.90	1.0	8.25	7.16

C, parent compound; Mb, metabolite; OH-hydroxyl metabolite; AUC, area under the curve; F, bioavailability.

Chemical Structures

The lincosamides consist of three components: an amino acid, a sugar and an amide bond connecting these two moieties to one another. The amino acid residue is a substituted L-proline. The sugar is lincosamine.

Clindamycin is the 7(S)-chlorodeoxylincomycin derivative. Pirlimycin is the 4-cis-ethyl-L-pipecolic derivative of clindamycin. For oral use, a palmitate salt of clindamycin hydrochlorine is available; for injection, clindamycin phosphate is available.[33]

A number of compounds have shown drug incompatibility with lincomycin, including β-lactams (penicillin G, cloxacillin, methicillin, ampicillin, ticarcillin, cephalothin), novobiocin, hydrocortisone, streptomycin, vitamin B and potassium canrenoate. Drug incompatibility has been reported with clindamycin phosphate and: ampicillin, calcium gluconate, magnesium sulfate, phenytoin, group B vitamins

TABLE 141-5	Pharmacokinetics of Macrolides in Elderly Patients						
Drug	Young/Elderly	Dose (mg)	Route	C_{max} (µg/mL)	T_{max} (h)	$AUC_{0-\infty}$; (µg/h/mL)	$T\frac{1}{2}$ (h)
Azithromycin	Young	500	po	0.41	2.5	2.5	
	Elderly	500	po	0.38	3.8	3.0	
14-OH clarithromycin	Young	500	po	0.66			7.2
	Elderly	500	po	1.33			14.0
Clarithromycin	Young	500	po	2.41		18.9	4.9
	Elderly	500	po	3.28		30.8	7.7
Dirithromycin	Young	500	po	0.34	3.90	0.91	
	Elderly	500	po	0.52	4.80	2.42	
Josamycin	Young	1000	po			6.25	1.69
	Elderly	1000	po			6.25	3.4
Miocamycin (Mb12)	Young	800	po	1.34	0.67	1.92	1.24
	Elderly	800	po	1.15	0.58	2.52	2.36
Roxithromycin	Young	300	po	9.7	1.6	122.6	11.2
	Elderly	300	po	10.8	2.06	197.3	15.5
Spiramycin adipate	Young	500	iv	2.14		6.7	4.5
	Elderly	500	iv	2.51		16.7	9.8
Telithromycin	Young	800	po	3.0	0.5	11.56	11.46
	Elderly	800	po	1.9	1.0	7.25	10.64

TABLE 141-6	Tissue Distribution of Macrolides (Peak Concentrations mg/kg and µg/mL)					
				RESPIRATORY TRACT		
Drug	Dose (mg)	Serum (µg/mL)	Bronchial Mucosa	Bronchial Secretions	Sinus	
Azithromycin	500*		3.89	0.23	1.34	
Dirithromycin	500**	0.22	1.9	1.3		
Erythromycin	500**	3.08	7.20	1.05	0.9–1.8	
Josamycin	1000**	2.3		1.60	2.8	
Miocamycin	600**			5.16		
Oleandomycin	200*	6.26		3.77	2.68	
Roxithromycin	150**	2.51		3.10	4.15	
	500**	2.4			2.18	
Spiramycin	2000**	0.39	13–36	7.3	2–8.8	

*Single dose.
**Multiple doses.

TABLE 141-7	Telithromycin Concentration in Lung Tissues				
			CONCENTRATION OF TELITHROMYCIN		
Sampling Time (h)	Number of patients/ sample size	Plasma Concentration (mg/L)	Bronchial Mucosa (mg/kg)	ELF (mg/L)	Alveolar Macrophages (mg/L)
1–3	5	1.07	0.68	5.4	65
6–8	6	0.61	2.2	4.2	100
24	6	0.07	3.5	1.17	41
48	6	ND	ND	ND	2.15

ELF, epithelial lining fluid; ND, not detectable.

and barbiturates. Solutions containing tobramycin sulfate and clindamycin phosphate are unstable.

Antibacterial Activity

The antibacterial spectrum of lincosamides includes gram-positive cocci, anaerobic bacteria and certain atypical bacteria. Enterobacteriaceae, *Pseudomonas* spp. and *Acinetobacter* spp. are not susceptible to the lincosamides.

Lincosamides possess good antistaphylococcal activity. They are active against methicillin-susceptible *Staph. aureus* strains but not against methicillin-resistant strains (MIC >64 mg/L). They are active against coagulase-negative staphylococci, with the exception of *Staph. cohnii*, *Staph. sciuri* and *Staph. xylosus*, which have low-level resistance

TABLE 141-8	**A Selection of Drugs Whose Metabolism May Interfere With That of Macrolides**

Alfentanil, sufentanil	Felodipine
Antipyrine	Glibenclamide
Astemizole	Levodopa, carbidopa
Bromocriptine	Lovastatin
Carbamazepine	Methylprednisolone
Ciclosporin A	Phenytoin
Cimetidine	Rifampin (rifampicin), rifabutin
Cisapride	Sodium valproate
Clozapine	Theophylline
Diltiazem	Triazolam, midazolam
Digoxin	Verapamil
Dysopyramide	Warfarin
Ergotamine	Zidovudine
Ethylestradiol	

TABLE 141-9   *In Vitro* Activity of Clindamycin

Micro-organism(s)	MIC (mg/L) 50%	90%	Range
Actinomyces spp.			0.03–0.25
Bordetella pertussis			0.25–>8
Bordetella bronchiseptica			≥32
Campylobacter jejuni	0.4	0.8	0.1–>50
Chlamydia trachomatis			1.0
Coagulase-negative staphylococci	0.25	>16	
Corynebacterium diphtheriae			≥0.2
Enterococcus spp.	>16	>16	
Gardnerella vaginalis	0.003	0.06	0.2–2.0
Haemophilus influenzae			8.0
Helicobacter pylori	0.5	2.0	0.25–2.0
Legionella pneumophila			12.5
Mycoplasma hominis			0.03
Mycoplasma pneumoniae			1.0
Neisseria gonorrhoeae			2.0
Neisseria meningitidis			>5
Nocardia spp.			0.78–0.25
Staphylococcus aureus Met^s	0.12	0.125	
Staphylococcus aureus Met^r	1.0	>16	
Streptococcus agalactiae	0.06	0.5	
Streptococcus pneumoniae Pen^r	1.0	16	
Streptococcus pneumoniae Pen^s	0.125	0.25	
Streptococcus pyogenes	0.03	0.06	
Ureaplasma urealyticum			2.0
Viridans group streptococci	0.5	0.5	

Met^r, methicillin resistant; Met^s, methicillin sensitive; Pen^r, penicillin resistant; Pen^s, penicillin sensitive.

to lincomycin and to streptogramin B. The MICs of lincomycin are 4–8 mg/L, as opposed to 0.5–1 mg/L for susceptible strains. They are inactive against enterococci. They possess good activity against group A and B streptococci, viridans group streptococci and *Strep. pneumoniae*. These strains appear to be inhibited by concentrations of 0.4 mg/L. The lincosamides are active against *Corynebacterium diphtheriae*, *Nocardia* spp. and *Bacillus anthracis* but are inactive against *Listeria monocytogenes*.

Clindamycin is active against *Erysipelothrix rhusiopathiae*. They are inactive or weakly active against *Neisseria meningitidis* and *Neisseria gonorrhoeae*, *H. influenzae*, *Moraxella catarrhalis* and *Pasteurella* spp. Clindamycin is active against *Bordetella pertussis*, but inactive against *Bordetella bronchiseptica*. Clindamycin possesses good activity (MIC$_{50}$ 0.4 mg/L), against *Campylobacter jejuni*, whereas lincomycin is inactive. The activity of clindamycin against *Helicobacter pylori* is good (MIC 1 mg/L).

The lincosamides are inactive against *Legionella pneumophila*. Clindamycin has activity against *Chlamydia trachomatis* (MIC 1.0 mg/L), whereas lincomycin is inactive. Clindamycin is active against *Mycoplasma hominis* but is weakly active against *Mycoplasma pneumoniae* and *Ureaplasma urealyticum*. Clindamycin is active against *Gardnerella vaginalis*. Lincomycin is active against *Leptospira* spp. Clindamycin has good activity against anaerobes.

Among gram-positive anaerobes, clindamycin exhibits good activity against *Clostridium perfringens*, *Clostridium tetani* and *Clostridium difficile*. Its activity against *Bifidobacterium*, *Propionibacterium* spp. and gram-positive cocci is moderate. It exhibits good activity against *Eubacterium* spp.

Among gram-negative anaerobes, clindamycin displays good activity against the *Bacteroides fragilis* group, with the exception of *Bacteroides thetaiotaomicron*, *Porphyromonas* spp. and *Prevotella* spp. Activity against *Veillonella* spp. is good (MIC >0.05 mg/L) (Table 141-9).

Mode of Action and Resistance

Lincosamides act on the 50S ribosomal subunit of the bacterial ribosome. The binding sites are similar to those for erythromycin A. The lincosamides prevent transpeptidation during the formation of the nascent peptide chain by inhibiting peptidyltransferase.[5]

The intrinsic resistance of Enterobacteriaceae, *Pseudomonas* spp. and *Acinetobacter* spp. is due to the relative impermeability of the bacterial outer membrane. In gram-positive cocci, penetration is a passive phenomenon. The enterococci are resistant to the lincosamides. Acquired resistance to lincosamides may be due to modification of the bacterial target, modification of the antibiotics and reduced permeability.

In the constitutive form of resistance in *Staph. aureus*, all macrolides, lincosamides and streptogramin B are also resistant (*erm* gene); conversely, when it is an inducible resistance, there is dissociation between the three families and the lincosamides remain active, even if the activity is reduced. In streptococci, in contrast to *Staph. aureus*, the lincosamides can induce resistance. Inducible resistance may be highlighted by the D-test in *Staph. aureus* (see Chapter 138).

A plasmid-mediated 3-lincomycin or 4-clindamycin-O-nucleotidyltransferase has been detected in *Staph. aureus*. There is high-level resistance to lincomycin and a reduction in susceptibility to clindamycin has been noted. In coagulase-negative staphylococci, the main mechanism of resistance is adenine methylation (MLS$_B$ type), identical to that of *Staph. aureus*. These species possess more specific resistance mechanisms, such as a reduction in permeability to 14-membered-ring macrolides as has been described for *Staph. epidermidis*. The 14-membered-ring macrolides may also be inactivated enzymatically; this resistance phenotype has been described for *Staph. hominis*, *Staph. haemolyticus* and *Staph. saprophyticus*.

Like *Staph. aureus*, certain species may inactivate lincomycin or clindamycin by a plasmid-mediated enzyme.

Strains of *B. fragilis* are divided into three groups, those which are very susceptible to clindamycin (MIC ≤ 0.25 mg/l), moderately susceptible (MIC 0.25–8 mg/l), and resistant (MIC >16 mg/L).

Strains of *Strep. pneumoniae* and *Strep. pyogenes* susceptible to clindamycin and resistant to erythromycin A derivatives have been described.

ANTIPARASITIC ACTIVITY

In 1967, it was shown that clindamycin and its derivatives possessed antiplasmodial activity. Several clinical studies have been conducted with clindamycin administered at a dose of 450 mg every 6 hours for 14 days to four patients to treat a *Plasmodium vivax* infection. A relapse occurred between 41 and 51 days after the end of treatment.

In nonimmune patients, clindamycin (450 mg q6h for 3 days) was combined with quinine in the treatment of chloroquine-susceptible or chloroquine-resistant *P. falciparum* infections. A curative effect was obtained with the combination, but major gastrointestinal disorders were noted. Other studies have also been undertaken with various results obtained.

If clindamycin is used, it is recommended that a fast-acting schizonticide, such as quinine or amodiaquine, is administered first, followed by clindamycin, to avoid problems of gastrointestinal intolerance.

ACTIVITY AGAINST *TOXOPLASMA GONDII*

Clindamycin has been proposed as alternative therapy in the treatment of encephalic toxoplasmosis in patients intolerant to sulfonamides.[33,34]

There are contradictory studies on the *in vitro* activity of clindamycin. Clindamycin starts to exert an inhibitory effect at <1 mg/L, but the 90% inhibitory concentration is 100 mg/L. The discrepancy in the results between the different studies is probably due to slow inhibition of the growth of the parasite, which occurs after 24 hours. It has been shown that clindamycin alone or in combination with pyrimethamine possesses curative activity in acute murine toxoplasmosis. Clindamycin exhibits protective activity against murine cerebral toxoplasmosis. Multicenter studies have shown beneficial effects of clindamycin combined with pyrimethamine in the treatment of acute cerebral toxoplasmosis.[33,34] Clindamycin has also been proposed as treatment for toxoplasmic chorioretinitis.

Pharmacokinetics

LINCOMYCIN

Lincomycin has oral, intravenous, intramuscular, and rectal forms.

Oral Form

After administration of 500 mg and 1000 mg, peak serum concentrations are reached in 2–4 hours and are 1.8–5.3 mg/L and 2.5–6.7 mg/L, respectively. Food consumption affects oral bioavailability. Plasma concentrations are detectable for 12 hours. Absorption of lincomycin represents 20–35% of the administered dose. Fecal elimination is 30–40% of the administered dose over a 72-hour period.

Intravenous Form

After a 1-hour infusion, concentrations obtained range from 9.1 mg/L (300 mg) to 36.2 mg/L (500 mg). The AUCs are proportional to the administered doses (300–1500 mg). The mean apparent elimination half-life is 5 hours and 40% of the administered dose is eliminated in the urine.

Plasma protein binding albumin is dose dependent and ranges from 28–86% (average 75%), depending on the dose and the method of determination.

Plasma clearance is dose dependent because of protein saturation and is 13.32 L/h. The clearance of the free fraction is between 28.6 L/h for 2400 mg intravenously and 36.4 L/h for 1200 mg intravenously. Renal clearance is weak – 43 mL/min (2.6 L/h). Urinary elimination ranged between 30% and 40%. After an intravenous dose of 500 mg, fecal elimination of lincomycin is about 14% over 96 hours.

Intramuscular Form

After a single intramuscular administration of 600 mg, the peak concentration in serum is between 7.2 and 18.5 mg/L and is reached after between 0.5 and 5 hours. After repeated doses of 600 mg, the residual concentration (8 hours) is 6.4 mg/L. After a daily dose of 500 mg, the residual concentration at 24 hours is 1.1 mg/L. The apparent elimination half-life range is 4–5 hours. The plasma clearance is dose dependent and is between 0.098 and 0.139 L/kg. Urinary elimination is between 10% and 47%, depending on the study. Fecal elimination after a dose of 500 mg is 4–6% over a period of 48–72 hours. The bioavailability after intramuscular administration appears to be absolute.

Rectal Form

After administration of a 500 mg suppository of lincomycin, a peak concentration in serum of 1.1 mg/L is reached in 1.5 hours, with an AUC of 8.9 mg.h/L, compared to a peak of 2.8 mg/L and an AUC of 25.7 mg.h/L after administration of a rectal solution of lincomycin.

Safety

Lincomycin has been associated with severe *Clostridium difficile* infection, therefore it is recommended to be used only for serious bacterial infections for which alternate agents are not available. Lincomycin should be avoided in patients with hypersensitivities to lincosamides.

Specific Underlying Diseases

Renal Impaired Patients. After intramuscular administration of 600 mg of lincomycin, the apparent elimination half-life, the peak concentration in serum and the AUC are increased. Lincomycin is not dialyzable.

Hepatic Impaired Patients. After a single dose of 600 mg intramuscularly to patients with hepatic insufficiency, the apparent elimination half-life is increased (8.90 vs 4.85 hours) and the peak concentration in serum is decreased (9.2 vs 12.8 mg/L).

Metabolism

A small amount of lincomycin is inactivated in the liver. The metabolites have not been fully characterized and are devoid of antibacterial activity. Biliary elimination is extensive, ranging from 30% to 40% of the administered dose.

CLINDAMYCIN

Clindamycin is presented in the form of clindamycin phosphate for parenteral use and clindamycin hydrochloride for oral use.

Intravenous Form

Clindamycin phosphate is soluble in water. This solubility is pH dependent: at pH 7 the solubility is between 200 and 300 mg/mL, whereas at pH 4 it is 25 mg/mL. Clindamycin phosphate infusion is administered over 10–45 minutes, depending on the dose. Clindamycin phosphate is slowly hydrolyzed to clindamycin, with a hydrolysis half-life of between 3 minutes (1200 mg) and 1 minute (300← mg). 10% of the drug is present in the serum after 8 hours in the form of clindamycin phosphate. The peak concentration in serum of clindamycin appears about 3 hours after the end of the infusion and is between 5.4 mg/L (300 mg) and 15.87 mg/L (1200 mg). The elimination half-life of clindamycin is 2–3 hours, whereas that of clindamycin phosphate is 0.04–0.16 hour. Plasma clearance is of the order of 0.18 L/h/kg for clindamycin and 0.40 L/h/kg for clindamycin phosphate. Clindamycin binding to α_1-glycoprotein ranges from 92% to 93%.

Clindamycin is mainly eliminated in the hepatobiliary system. Metabolites of clindamycin are found in the urine and stool, but about 28% of the parent compound is found in the urine.

Intramuscular Form

After administration of single doses of clindamycin phosphate 300, 450 or 600 mg, peak concentrations in serum are between 3.17 and 6.56 mg/L and are reached in 1.5–3 hours. Clindamycin is detectable in the serum after 20 minutes. About 75% reaches the plasma in the form of clindamycin.

Oral Form

After absorption, clindamycin palmitate is rapidly hydrolyzed in the intestinal lumen before being absorbed in the form of the hydrochloride and the palmitate is undetectable in the serum. The bioavailability is of the order of 80%. The degrees of absorption are identical after single and repeated doses. Food consumption does not appear to alter the bioavailability of clindamycin, although absorption is delayed.

Clindamycin hydrochloride is poorly soluble in water and the solubility is pH dependent: when the pH <6, the solubility is greater than 160 mg/mL, whereas between 7 and 8 the solubility is weak, of the order of 2.7 ± 1.0 mg/L.

After administration of a single dose of 150, 300 or 450 mg of clindamycin hydrochloride, the peak concentrations in serum are between 2.56 and 5.58 mg/L and within 1 hour.

The dose eliminated in the urine ranges from 8%-26%. A number of metabolites are eliminated in the urine. Traces of clindamycin hydrochloride are in urine, in contrast to clindamycin phosphate, for which 1–2% of the administered dose is eliminated in this form.

Radiolabeled clindamycin hydrochloride (300 mg) was administered and the radioactivity was 61% and 28% over a period of 168 hours in feces and urine, respectively.

Metabolism

The free form of clindamycin is hydrolyzed in the liver. Fecal and urinary elimination of the metabolites differ.

After a single dose of 300 mg of clindamycin hydrochloride, the compounds eliminated in the urine are distributed as follows: clindamycin 27%, clindamycin sulfoxide 37%, N-demethyl clindamycin 6% and clindamycin-N-demethyl sulfoxide 2%. A hydroxyl derivative and a carboxyl derivative have been detected, and each accounts for 15% of the compounds eliminated in the urine.

Patients with Renal Impairment

Clindamycin is not significantly eliminated after hemodialysis or peritoneal dialysis.

It is recommended that when the creatinine clearance is <10 mL/min, the daily dosage be reduced by a half, as the apparent elimination half-life increases, with major interindividual variability (mean half-life of 5.28 hours compared to 2 hours).

In peritoneal fluid, about 3% of the dose of clindamycin phosphate is hydrolyzed to clindamycin in 2–4 hours. Peritoneal dialysis fluid must contain a concentration of 167 μg of clindamycin phosphate/mL to be certain of therapeutic activity.

Elderly Patients

After a single dose of 300 mg orally and intravenously the fractions absorbed were similar in young and elderly patients (0.92 vs. 0.85). The elimination half-life and plasma clearance after intravenous administration did not differ significantly (2.46 vs 2.79 hours, 0.71 vs 0.75 L/kg, 3.36 vs 3.11 mL/min/kg, respectively). No dosage modifications are indicated in elderly patients.

Patients with Hepatic Impairment

In patients with hepatic insufficiency, the apparent elimination half-life is prolonged from 5–15 hours compared to 2.5–3.6 hours in healthy volunteers. A reduction in the plasma clearance in cirrhotic patients has been demonstrated, with a reduction in protein binding to 79% (versus 93%).

Pregnancy

Clindamycin rapidly crosses the fetoplacental barrier. High concentrations have been detected in the liver, kidney and lungs, and low levels in cerebral tissue, bone or muscles of fetuses from spontaneous abortions occurring between the 10th and 22nd weeks of gestation.

Intraphagocytic Concentration. The intracellular:extracellular concentration ratio in neutrophils is between 11 and 15, while in macrophages and monocytes it is 23. Inside the cell, clindamycin is localized in the cytoplasm and granules.

Safety

The main adverse outcome related to clindamycin is pseudomembranous colitis due to *Clostridium difficile*. Hypotension and cardiorespi-

ratory arrest have been reported at high intravenous doses of lincomycin, particularly after rapid administration. Skin rashes and drug fever have been observed with clindamycin.

Streptogramins

Introduction

The streptogramins form a complex group of unique antibacterial agents.[35-38] Pristinamycin (oral natural form) has limited clinical introduction, mainly in French-speaking countries. For the injectable form (dalfopristin–quinupristin) the clinical introduction is wide, including the USA. A new oral streptogramin, linopristin–flopristin (NXL 103, XRP 2868), is currently under investigation.[39-41]

Properties of Natural Streptogramins

Streptogramins are composed of a mixture of two components: group A and group B.[5,42] These two components act synergistically at the microbiologic level. The two components are macrocyclic lactones and peptides, respectively.

Only two derivatives have been introduced in clinical practice: pristinamycin (Pyostacine) and virginiamycin (Staphylomycine). One injectable semisynthetic derivative has also been introduced in clinical practice, dalfopristin–quinupristin (Synercid), and one oral semisynthetic derivative is under development, linopristin–flopristin.[43-45]

The ratios between the two groups of components are 30–40% for component I (group B) and 60–70% for component II (group A).

ANTIBACTERIAL ACTIVITIES

These molecules exhibit different antibacterial activities, but their antibacterial spectra include gram-positive cocci and bacilli, gram-negative cocci and fastidious gram-negative bacilli such as *Haemophilus*, *Moraxella*, *Bordetella* and certain intracellular bacteria (*Chlamydia* and *Rickettsia*).

Pristinamycin is active against gram-positive cocci. It has good activity against methicillin-resistant or -susceptible strains and constitutive or inducible erythromycin A-resistant strains of *Staph. aureus* and against methicillin-resistant or -susceptible strains of *Staph. epidermidis*. Activities against common pathogens are given in Table 141-10. However, it is inactive against *Treponema pallidum* and *Brucella* spp.[45,46]

SYNERGY BETWEEN COMPONENTS A AND B

The combination of the two components is synergistic in terms of activity against erythromycin A-susceptible or -resistant strains of *Staph. aureus*. This synergy is independent of the respective percentages of the two components within a large range of (20–80%) for each factor. However, *in vivo*, a higher quantity of pristinamycin II than pristinamycin I must be administered for this synergy to manifest itself in experimental *Staph. aureus* infections in the mouse because of the poor absorption of pristinamycin II_A.

BREAKPOINTS

The French Antibiotic Sensitivity Test Committee has adopted a breakpoint of 2 mg/L for pristinamycin and virginiamycin. This corresponds to a diameter of ≥19 mm for a 15 μg disk.[45]

ANTIBIOTIC COMBINATIONS

The combinations of streptogramins plus aminoglycosides, rifampin or β-lactams are synergistic or additive. For staphylococci, pristinamycin combined with rifampin was bactericidal against 69% of the 16 tested strains responsible for sepsis; combination with an aminoglycoside induced bactericidal activity against 50% of the same strains.

Combination with fusidic acid or co-trimoxazole is synergistic, while the combination of pristinamycin and chloramphenicol is antagonistic.

TABLE 141-10	Antibacterial Activity of Streptogramins						

		MIC (mg/L)					
		LINOPRISTIN–FLOPRISTIN		PRISTINAMYCIN		DALFOPRISTIN–QUINUPRISTIN	
Organism(s)	Sample size (n), # isolates	50	90	50	90	50	90
Corynebacterium jeikeium	10	≥0.03	0.25	0.12	0.5	0.25	0.5
Enterococcus avium	10	0.5	1.0	0.5	2.0	2.0	4.0
Enterococcus casseliflavus	15	0.5	0.5	1.0	1.0	2.0	4.0
Enterococcus faecalis	21	1.0	2.0	2.0	8.0	8.0	16
Enterococcus faecalis Van^r	16	1.0	2.0	4.0	8.0	8.0	32
Enterococcus faecium	11	≥0.06	0.5	0.25	0.5	0.5	2.0
Enterococcus faecium Lin^r	12	0.12	0.25	0.25	0.5	1.0	–
Enterococcus faecium Q/D^r	3	1.0	2.0	4.0	–	–	–
Enterococcus faecium VanA	12	0.12	0.25	0.25	0.5	0.5	1.0
Enterococcus gallinarum	15	0.25	0.5	0.5	0.5	2.0	2.0
Enterococcus raffinosus	3	0.5	1.0	2.0	–	–	–
Haemophilus influenzae/β⁻	50	0.25	0.5	1.0	2.0	2.0	4.0
Haemophilus influenzae/β⁺	79	0.25	1.0	1.0	2.0	4.0	4.0
Haemophilus influenzae^{BLNAR}	21	0.25	0.5	1.0	1.0	2.0	4.0
Group C and G streptococci	15	0.12	0.25	0.25	0.25	1.0	1.0
Glycopeptide intermediate-resistant Staphylococcus aureus	3	0.12	–	0.25	–	0.12	–
Methicillin-resistant Staphylococcus aureus	25	0.12	0.25	0.25	1.0	0.25	0.50
Methicillin-sensitive Staphylococcus aureus	16	0.12	0.12	0.25	0.50	0.25	0.50
Staphylococcus aureus Lin^r	1	0.25	–	0.5	–	0.25	–
Streptococcus agalactiae	15	0.06	0.06	0.25	0.25	1.0	1.0
Streptococcus epidermidis	14	0.06	0.5	0.12	1.0	0.12	0.25
Streptococcus pneumoniae Ery^r	120	0.25	0.5	0.25	0.5	0.5	1.0
Streptococcus pneumoniae Ery^s	141	0.12	0.25	0.25	0.25	0.5	0.5
Streptococcus pyogenes	27	≥0.06	≥0.06	0.12	0.12	0.25	0.25
Viridans group streptococci	20	0.12	0.25	0.5	0.5	1.0	1.0

β⁻, non-β-lactamase producing; β⁺, β-lactamase producing; BLNAR, non-β-lactamase-producing strains; Ery^r, erythromycin resistant; Ery^s, erythromycin sensitive; Lin^r, lincomycin resistant; Q/D^r, quinupristin–dalfopristin resistant; VanA, vancomycin A phenotype; Van^r, vancomycin resistant.

Pristinamycin

MECHANISM OF ACTION

Streptogramins inhibit bacterial protein synthesis by binding sequentially to the 50S ribosomal subunit. Pristinamycin II binds irreversibly, thus releasing a receptor site for pristinamycin I. Both streptogramins cross the bacterial cell wall by passive diffusion.

Pristinamycin II acts on the early stage of protein synthesis, especially on the elongation phase of translation. Pristinamycin I exerts inhibitory activity at the end of the process during extension of the peptide chain, causing premature detachment of the nascent peptide.[37,45]

RESISTANCE

Epidemiology

In 1975, the first strain of Staph. aureus with plasmid-mediated pristinamycin I_A and II_A resistance was isolated in France.[47] Outbreaks associated with this plasmid have been reported in many hospitals, with a prevalence of 4–5% of strains isolated. However, the level of resistance has remained low and affects about 1% of methicillin-susceptible strains of Staph. aureus (MSSA) and 10% of methicillin-resistant strains (MRSA).

In the Protek study from 2000 to 2001, 0.02% of Strep. pneumoniae strains were resistant to dalfopristin–quinupristin. For Staph. aureus resistant to linezolid (MIC >128 mg/L), the MIC of dalfopristin–quinupristin is ≥0.25 mg/L. For Enterococcus faecium resistant to linezolid, the MIC at which 50% and 90% of isolates are inhibited ($MIC_{50/90}$) for dalfopristin–quinupristin is ≥0.5/1 mg/L.[23]

Mechanisms of Resistance

The antibacterial spectrum of the streptogramins does not include gram-negative bacilli such as Enterobacteriaceae, Pseudomonas spp. and other non-fermentative gram-negative bacilli.[1,5] Their intrinsic resistance is due to their outer membrane impermeability. Acquired resistance to this drug class is due to four mechanisms: modification of the antibiotic target, inactivation of the antibiotics, reduction of outer membrane permeability and efflux. Many genes encode streptogramin resistance, a complex phenomenon, which may be specific for each component.

Macrolide, lincosamide and streptogramin B (MLS$_B$) resistance in streptococci may be constitutive or inducible. Enterococci, *Strep. pneumoniae* and most viridans group streptococci have constitutive MLS$_B$ resistance. Inducible expression occurs above all in group A, C, G and B streptococci and in certain viridans group streptococcal strains.

Enzymatic inactivation of pristinamycin or virginiamycin has been described. Through a plasmid-mediated *O*-acetyltransferase, some strains of *Staph. aureus* are capable of acetylating the hydroxyl group at position 13, leading to a loss of ribosomal affinity and inactivating pristinamycin II. The macrolactone ring of pristinamycin I could be opened by a hydrolase which is carried by the same plasmid. The majority of these *Staph. aureus* strains have reduced susceptibility to lincosamides.

PHARMACOKINETICS

There are no published pharmacokinetic data for children, elderly patients or patients with renal or hepatic insufficiency. In adults, pristinamycin and virginiamycin are not inactivated by gastric fluid. About 15–18% of pristinamycin II$_A$ and virginiamycin M is absorbed in the ileojejunal section. There is also weak absorption of the I$_A$ fraction.[24,48,49]

After administration of 500 mg of pristinamycin or virginiamycin, the plasma concentration is 1 mg/L at 2 hours, and minimal or non-existent from 4 to 6 hours.

The apparent elimination half-lives are 4–5 hours for pristinamycin I and virginiamycin M and 2.8–8 hours for pristinamycin II and virginiamycin S. After administration of 2 g orally, the peak plasma concentrations of drug for pristinamycins I and II are, respectively, 0.8 and 0.6 mg/L and are reached in about 3 hours. The apparent elimination half-lives are, respectively, 4 and 2.8 hours. The lag time is about 20 minutes. The AUCs are 2.2 and 1.2 mg.h/L. The global peak concentration in serum (pristinamycins I and II) is 1.34 ± 0.7 mg/L (mean ± standard deviation) and is reached in 3 hours.[50] Plasma protein binding is 40–50% for pristinamycin I and 80–90% for pristinamycin II. Streptogramins are metabolized in the liver but this process has not been studied. Elimination occurs mainly in the bile and urinary elimination is weak (10% for pristinamycin I and 2% for pristinamycin II).

DRUG–DRUG INTERACTIONS

Pristinamycin does not interfere with cytochrome P450.[51] There is the possibility of a metabolic interaction between pristinamycin and cyclosporine, which may be responsible for acute nephrotoxicity.[30] Pristinamycin interferes with the metabolism of methotrexate.

Dalfopristin–Quinupristin

Due to the poor water solubility of pristinamycin, derivatives were synthesized with the same antibacterial activity but with greater hydrosolubility. One compound has been introduced in clinical practice, dalfopristin–quinupristin.[19]

Semisynthesis from the isolated I$_A$ and II$_A$ components has yielded hydrosoluble derivatives. The semisynthetic derivative of pristinamycin I$_A$ was obtained by introduction of an amino function at the 5δ position (5δ-thiomethylquinuclidine); the semisynthetic derivatives of pristinamycin II$_A$ with an amino substituent at position 26 (diethylaminoethylsulfonyl) are soluble in water.

ANTIBACTERIAL ACTIVITY

Dalfopristin–quinupristin possesses the same antibacterial spectrum as pristinamycin and similar *in vitro* activity. The approved National Committee on Clinical Laboratory Standards (NCCLS) breakpoint is ≥1 μg/mL (diameter of zone of inhibition ≥18 mm) for a disk load at 7.5 μg (ratio 30 : 70).[45] Dalfopristin–quinupristin MICs ranged between 0.5 and 1.0 mg/L for glycopeptide-intermediate *Staph. aureus* (GISA) strains.

PHARMACOKINETICS

After repeated administrations to 10 young male volunteers of dalfopristin–quinupristin 7.5 mg/kg for 5 days (q12h) and 4 days (q8h), there was no significant accumulation of either component (accumulation ratio range 1.16–1.43).

After an infusion over 1 hour, peak concentrations of dalfopristin–quinupristin were between 0.95 ± 0.22 mg/L (dose 1.4 mg/kg) and 24.20 ± 8.82 mg/L (dose 29.4 mg/kg). Quinupristin was rapidly converted to its active metabolite RP-12536. The activity of dalfopristin–quinupristin was detectable 6 hours after the end of the infusion.

Six volunteers received an infusion of a single dose of dalfopristin–quinupristin 12 mg/kg (ratio 30 : 70) for 60 minutes. Peak concentrations in serum and suction blisters were, respectively, 8.65 ± 0.92 and 2.41 ± 0.75 mg/L. The AUCs were, respectively, 11.2 ± 1.45 mg.h/mL and 9.19 ± 2.02 mg.h/L. The elimination half-life of dalfopristin–quinupristin was 1.48 ± 0.64 hours. The interindividual variabilities are 20–29% and 25–32% for quinupristin and dalfopristin, respectively.

Hepatic clearance and fecal elimination are 74.7% and 77.5% for quinupristin and dalfopristin, respectively. Protein binding rates are 55–78% and 11–26% for quinupristin and dalfopristin, respectively.

References available online at expertconsult.com.

KEY REFERENCES

Barrière J.C., Bouanchaud D.H., Desnottes J.F., et al.: Streptogramin analogues. *Expert Opin Investig Drugs* 1994; 3:115-131.

Barrière J.C., Bouanchaud D.H., Paris J.H., et al.: Antimicrobial activity against *Staphylococcus aureus* of semisynthetic injectable streptogramins, RP 59500 and related compounds. *J Antimicrob Chemother* 1992; 30(Suppl. A): 1-8.

Benazet F., Bourat G.: Etude radiographique de la répartition du constituant IA de la pristinamycine (7293 RP). *C R Acad Sci* 1965; 260:2522-2525.

Etienne S.D., Montay G., Le Liboux A., et al.: A phase 1, double-blind, placebo-controlled study of the tolerance and pharmacokinetic behaviour of RP 59500. *J Antimicrob Chemother* 1992; 30(Suppl.1):123-131.

Latorest H., Fourgesud M., Richet H., et al.: Comparative in vitro activities of pristinamycin, its components, and other antimicrobial agents against anaerobic bacteria. *Antimicrob Agents Chemother* 1988; 32:1094-1096.

Leclercq R., Nantas L., Soussy C.J., et al.: Activity of RP 59500, a new parenteral semisynthetic streptogramin, against staphylococci with various mechanisms of resistance to macrolide–lincosamide–streptogramin antibiotics. *J Antimicrob Chemother* 1992; 30(Suppl. A):67-76.

Le Goffic F.: Structure activity relationship in lincosamide and streptogramin antibiotics. *J Antimicrob Chemother* 1985; 16(Suppl.1):13-21.

Soreth J., Cox E., Kweder S., et al.: Ketek – the FDA perspective. *N Engl J Med* 2007; 356(16):1675-1676.

Vaquez D.: The streptogramin family of antibiotics. In: Corcoran J.N., Hahn P.E., eds. *Antibiotics*, vol. 3. Berlin: Springer-Verlag; 1975:521-534.

142

Oxazolidinones

FRANKLIN D. LOWY

Introduction

The oxazolidinones are bacteriostatic antimicrobials that are protein synthesis inhibitors. Because they work at the early stage of protein synthesis involving formation of the 70S initiation complex, there does not appear to be cross-resistance with other protein synthesis inhibitors. There are two FDA-approved oxazolidinones, linezolid (released in 2000) and tedizolid (released in 2014). A number of comprehensive reviews of oxazolidinones and linezolid, in particular, have been published.[1-5]

Pharmacokinetics and Distribution

Linezolid has similar pharmacokinetics whether administered parenterally or orally. It is completely absorbed following oral administration, achieving 100% bioavailability. Food causes a slight decrease in the rate of absorption but not in the overall amount absorbed. In normal volunteer studies, peak plasma concentrations were achieved in 1–2 hours. Steady state concentrations were approximately 12 μg/mL and 18 μg/mL following oral doses of 375 mg and 625 mg twice daily, respectively. Following intravenous administration of 625 mg twice daily for 7.5 days, the steady state level was 3.8 μg/mL. The half-lives of oral and intravenously administered linezolid are 5.4 and 4.8 hours, respectively. The drug is excreted by both renal and non-renal routes; 90% of linezolid is not metabolized, but there are two inactive metabolites that are the result of oxidation of the morpholine ring.

Linezolid is 31% bound to plasma proteins. It has a relatively large volume of distribution of 40–50 L. Studies suggest reasonable penetration of bone, fat and muscle. Mean ratios of linezolid in tissue fluid/plasma were 0.55, 1.2 and 0.71 for sweat, saliva and cerebrospinal fluid, respectively.

Route and Dosage

Both linezolid and tedizolid can be administered orally or intravenously. Adjustment of linezolid dosage is not necessary when switching from one route to the other. The recommended linezolid dosage for serious infections such as nosocomial pneumonia or complicated skin and soft tissue infections is 600 mg q12h. For uncomplicated infections, including community-acquired pneumonias or uncomplicated cutaneous infections, linezolid 400 mg q12h or tedizolid 200 mg once daily is adequate.

In patients with mild-to-moderate renal impairment (creatinine clearance 10–79 mL/min), dosage adjustment is not necessary. However, with more severe forms of renal disease dosage adjustment may be necessary. Renal excretion of tedizolid is limited so that dose adjustment even in the presence of significant renal dysfunction is unnecessary.

The pharmacokinetics of linezolid appears unaffected by age. Dosage adjustment for the elderly is unnecessary. The clearance of linezolid is more rapid in children than in adults. As a result, the dose recommended for infants and children is 10 mg/kg q8–12h.

Indications

The oxazolidinones are primarily used to treat bacterial infections caused by gram-positive bacteria including staphylococci, streptococci and pneumococci, although their spectrum of antibacterial activity extends beyond these species. Linezolid has excellent *in vitro* activity against methicillin-susceptible and -resistant staphylococci with little difference in the average minimal inhibitory concentrations (MICs). Linezolid is also active against *Staphylococcus aureus* isolates that are intermediate in susceptibility to glycopeptides.

Linezolid is active against all enterococci, including *Enterococcus faecalis* and *E. faecium*, as well as vancomycin-resistant enterococci. It is also active against penicillin-susceptible and penicillin-resistant *Streptococcus pneumoniae*, again with comparable MIC values (Table 142-1). Tedizolid is generally 4–16-fold more active than linezolid *in vitro* against staphylococci, enterococci and streptococci.

In addition to the common gram-positive pathogens, linezolid has activity (MIC = 4 μg/mL) against some of the less frequently encountered gram-positive organisms such as *Corynebacterium* spp., *Bacillus* spp., *Listeria monocytogenes*, *Erysipelothrix rhusiopathiae* and *Rhodococcus equi*.

Linezolid is moderately active against some anaerobes including *Clostridium* spp., *Peptostreptococcus* spp., *Bacteroides fragilis*, *Fusobacterium nucleatum* and *F. meningosepticum*. It has limited activity against some gram-negative bacteria such as *Moraxella*, *Bordetella* and *Haemophilus* spp. and has no activity against Enterobacteriaceae or *Pseudomonas* spp. Linezolid also has activity against *Mycobacterium tuberculosis* and *M. avium* complex. It is increasingly used for the treatment of multidrug-resistant tuberculosis.

TABLE 142-1	*In Vitro* Antimicrobial Susceptibility for Linezolid against Common Gram-Positive Pathogens			
Organism	MIC (μg/mL) 50%*	MIC (μg/mL) 90%	Overall (μg/mL)	
Staph. aureus (n = 52 256)				
Oxacillin susceptible	1–4	1–4	0.5–8	
Oxacillin resistant	1–4	1–4	0.5–8	
Coagulase-negative staphylococci (n = 548)				
Oxacillin susceptible	0.5–2	1–4	0.25–4	
Oxacillin resistant	0.5–2	1–2	0.5–4	
β-hemolytic streptococci (n = 547)	1–2	2–4	1–4	
Strep. pneumoniae (n = 5454)				
Penicillin susceptible	0.5	1	<0.016–1	
Penicillin resistant	0.5–1	1	0.06–4	
Enterococcus spp. (n = 5980)				
Vancomycin susceptible	1–4	1–4	0.5–4	
Vancomycin resistant	2–4	2–4	1–4	

*Minimum concentration at which 50% of strains are inhibited.
Adapted from multiple sources.

TABLE 142-2	Clinical Indications for the Use of Linezolid	
FDA-Approved Indications		
Nature of Infection		Potential Pathogens
Skin and soft tissue (complicated)		MSSA, MRSA, *Streptococcus pyogenes*, *Strep. agalactiae*
Skin and soft tissue (uncomplicated)		MSSA, *Strep. pyogenes*
Infection with bacteremia		Vancomycin-resistant *Enterococcus faecium*
Nosocomial pneumonia		MRSA, MSSA, *Strep. pneumoniae* (including multidrug-resistant strains)
Community-acquired pneumonia		*Strep. pneumoniae* (including multidrug-resistant strains), MSSA

NON-FDA-APPROVED (OFF-LABEL) INDICATIONS

Serious MRSA, VISA and VRSA infections or infections that are poorly responsive to vancomycin therapy
Infection with bacteremia caused by *Enterococcus faecalis* (including vancomycin-resistant strains)
Complicated infections requiring long-term oral therapy with an anti-staphylococcal or enterococcal agent where β-lactams cannot be used (e.g. chronic osteomyelitis)*
Treatment of infections (e.g. nosocomial pneumonia, endocarditis, meningitis) caused by highly resistant (but linezolid-susceptible) gram-positive bacteria where alternative agents are not available or are contraindicated
Combination therapy for anti-mycobacterial infections where first- and second-line agents cannot be used

*Close monitoring for toxicity is required with prolonged linezolid therapy.
MRSA, methicillin-resistant *Staphylococcus aureus*; MSSA, methicillin-susceptible *Staph. aureus*; VISA, *Staph. aureus* with intermediate susceptibility to vancomycin; VRSA, vancomycin-resistant *Staph. aureus*.

Linezolid is approved for the treatment of infections caused by a number of gram-positive organisms[6] (Table 142-2). Stevens *et al.*[7] reported that linezolid was comparable to vancomycin for the treatment of methicillin-resistant *Staph. aureus* (MRSA) infections primarily involving skin and soft tissue infections. A meta-analysis of randomized clinical trials compared linezolid with glycopeptides and β-lactams in the treatment of gram-positive infections and found that, overall, linezolid was more effective in clearing skin and soft tissue infections and bacteremia than the comparator antibiotics, but there was no overall difference in mortality.[3] A randomized controlled study comparing linezolid with vancomycin in the treatment of nosocomial MRSA pneumonia found linezolid to be superior in clinical outcome at the end of the study but again there was no effect on mortality.[8]

Tedizolid has FDA approval for the treatment of acute skin and skin structure infections. In a phase III study, oral tedizolid, once daily (200 mg) for 6 days was compared with linezolid (600 mg) twice daily for 10 days. Tedizolid was noninferior to linezolid for the treatment of acute bacterial skin and skin structure infections with fewer adverse events.[9] Its spectrum of activity is similar to linezolid although there is less clinical experience with its use.

There is additional clinical and experimental experience with linezolid suggesting that it may have a broader therapeutic role, although these other indications have not been FDA approved (Table 142-2). These reports, while limited, include the successful treatment of enterococcal endocarditis and meningitis; MRSA prosthetic hip infections, osteomyelitis, endocarditis and meningitis; and central nervous system infections caused by *Nocardia* spp., *Capnocytophaga* spp. and *C. jeikeium*.[10-12] There is also increasing evidence that linezolid may have utility in mycobacterial infections, most notably in the treatment of multidrug-resistant tuberculosis and *M. avium* complex.[13] It is still not clear how effective linezolid is in the treatment of infections that require bactericidal activity, such as endocarditis, but it may be a useful alternative in subjects who cannot tolerate vancomycin.[11]

Resistance to linezolid is uncommon but has been reported in enterococci and staphylococci (see also Chapter 138). It results from a chromosomal mutation in domain V of the 23S rRNA coding region. Enterococci and staphylococci carry multiple copies of this gene and the degree of resistance appears to correlate with the number of mutant copies. *In vitro* studies have shown that the appearance of resistance is strongly dependent upon the exposure dose and duration. A second form of resistance involves a plasmid-born gene, *cfr*, a ribosomal

methyl transferase. Because this gene can be horizontally transferred and does not appear to carry a fitness cost it is more likely to disseminate than the chromosomally-mediated resistance. An outbreak in an intensive care unit (ICU) setting with this latter form of resistance has been reported.[14]

Linezolid is an alternative agent for the treatment of resistant gram-positive infections (see Table 142-2). It has an antibacterial spectrum that is similar to vancomycin with advantageous pharmacokinetics. The availability of an oral preparation allows completion of therapy with the same therapeutic agent and therefore may help reduce the duration of hospital stays.

DOSAGE IN SPECIAL CIRCUMSTANCES

As noted above, adjustment of dosage for moderate degrees of renal failure is not necessary. Because linezolid, as well as the linezolid metabolites, are cleared during hemodialysis, it is recommended that patients receive a supplemental dose following dialysis. For moderate degrees of hepatic disease, dosage adjustment is not necessary.

Adverse Reactions and Interactions

Linezolid is generally well tolerated. The most common adverse events in the comparator-controlled trials were diarrhea (2.8–11%), nausea (3.4–9.6%) and headaches (0.5–11.3%).

Potentially the most serious adverse event, thrombocytopenia, was seen in 2.4% of patients. It was seen most often during prolonged therapy (longer than 2 weeks) and resolved upon completion of therapy. Others have reported a higher incidence of thrombocytopenia,[15] and there are reports of both anemia and leukopenia associated with linezolid therapy. As a result, hematologic monitoring of these parameters is recommended during prolonged therapy, especially for subjects who are already immunocompromised.

Several rare but important toxicities have emerged, including an irreversible peripheral neuropathy, a partially reversible optic neuropathy and severe lactic acidosis. Both the peripheral and optic neuropathies appear to occur after prolonged therapy (median 4 months and 10 months, respectively), whereas lactic acidosis has been reported after as little as 1 week of therapy.[16]

Linezolid is a relatively weak monoamine oxidase (MAO) inhibitor; there are now more than a dozen reports of serotonin syndrome in patients treated with linezolid while also taking selective serotonin reuptake inhibitors (SSRIs). Recommendations on the co-administration of linezolid with SSRIs vary, with some authors advocating a full washout of the SSRI before starting linezolid and other authors simply advising close clinical follow-up. Data on combination antibiotic therapy with linezolid are limited. There is limited clinical information on the adverse effects associated with tedizolid, though one comparative study suggested fewer events than linezolid.[9]

References available online at expertconsult.com.

KEY REFERENCES

Das D., Tulkens P.M., Mehra P., et al.: Tedizolid phosphate for the management of acute bacterial skin and skin structure infections: safety summary. *Clin Infect Dis* 2014; 58(Suppl.1):S51-S57.

Diekema D.J., Jones R.N.: Oxazolidinone antibiotics. *Lancet* 2001; 358(9297):1975-1982.

Falagas M.E., Siempos I.I., Vardakas K.Z.: Linezolid versus glycopeptide or beta-lactam for treatment of Gram-positive bacterial infections: meta-analysis of randomized controlled trials. *Lancet Infect Dis* 2008; 8(1):53-66.

Kuter D.J., Tillotson G.S.: Hematologic effects of antimicrobials: focus on the oxazolidinone linezolid. *Pharmacotherapy* 2001; 21(8):1010-1013.

Moellering R.C.: Linezolid: the first oxazolidinone antimicrobial. *Ann Intern Med* 2003; 138(2):135-142.

Moellering R.C. Jr: Tedizolid: a novel oxazolidinone for Gram-positive infections. *Clin Infect Dis* 2014; 58(Suppl.1):S1-S3.

Narita M., Tsuji B.T., Yu V.L.: Linezolid-associated peripheral and optic neuropathy, lactic acidosis, and serotonin syndrome. *Pharmacotherapy* 2007; 27(8):1189-1197.

Ntziora F., Falagas M.E.: Linezolid for the treatment of patients with mycobacterial infections: a systematic review. *Int J Tuberc Lung Dis* 2007; 11(6):606-611.

Prokocimer P., De Anda C., Fang E., et al.: Tedizolid phosphate vs linezolid for treatment of acute bacterial skin and skin structure infections: the ESTABLISH-1 randomized trial. *JAMA* 2013; 309:559-569.

Stevens D.L., Herr D., Lampiris H., et al.: Linezolid versus vancomycin for the treatment of methicillin-resistant *Staphylococcus aureus* infections. *Clin Infect Dis* 2002; 34(11):1481-1490.

Stevens D.L., Smith L.G., Bruss J.B., et al.: Randomized comparison of linezolid (PNU-100766) versus oxacillin–dicloxacillin for treatment of complicated skin and soft tissue infections. *Antimicrob Agents Chemother* 2000; 44(12):3408-3413.

143

Aminoglycosides

JAMES E. LEGGETT

KEY CONCEPTS

- The usual adult dose for aminoglycosides is 7 mg/kg every 24 hours (gentamicin, netilmicin, tobramycin) given intravenously (iv) or 20 mg/kg iv every 24 hours (for amikacin).

- The usual dose for synergy against gram-positive infections is 3 mg/kg/day gentamicin divided every 8, 12 or 24 hours.

- If impaired kidney function exists dose reduction is necessary depending on degree of impairment and is guided by therapeutic drug monitoring.

- Therapeutic drug monitoring is not always necessary for brief administration (<3d); trough concentrations following once-daily administration should be unmeasurable. Cerebrospinal fluid (CSF) penetration is relatively low and might require intrathecal administration in selected patients when relying upon aminoglycoside therapy for meningitis.

- Common adverse effects include nephrotoxicity, ototoxicity and occasional neurotoxicity.

- The major indications include atypical mycobacterial infections, brucellosis, cholangitis, cystic fibrosis, diverticulitis, endocarditis, endophthalmitis, meningitis, pelvic inflammatory disease, plague, healthcare-associated pneumonia, synergy for gram-positive infections, tularemia and urinary tract infections.

Introduction

Aminoglycoside antibiotics have been an important component of our antibacterial drug arsenal since the 1940s, especially for serious gram-negative infections. All aminoglycosides share similar physical, chemical and pharmacologic properties.[1] There are currently at least 10 available aminoglycosides for clinical use available worldwide with five major agents in widespread use (streptomycin, gentamicin, netilmicin, tobramycin and amikacin). They demonstrate concentration-dependent killing and prolonged postantibiotic effects against susceptible bacteria, and several have maintained predictable activity against most aerobic gram-negative bacilli.[2] Aminoglycoside antimicrobial activity may be additive to or synergistic with that of β-lactams against both gram-negative and gram-positive infections. The prevalence of aminoglycoside resistance has remained low, and emergence of bacterial resistance during therapy has been unusual. All aminoglycosides share the potential for nephrotoxicity, ototoxicity and, rarely, neuromuscular blockade. Allergic reactions are rare. The cost of many aminoglycosides is low compared to other agents. Despite the decline in aminoglycoside use over the past 10–20 years, recent reviews have reported that use is again increasing due to the emergence of gram-negative resistance to other available drugs.[3]

Microbiologic Activity

All aminoglycosides have an essential six-membered ring with amino group substituents and glycosidic bonds. Members of this group ending in -mycin are natural products derived from *Streptomyces* species (e.g. kanamycin, neomycin, paromomycin, streptomycin, tobramycin). Those with names ending in -micin are natural products derived from *Micromonospora* species (e.g. gentamicin). Amikacin is a semisynthetic aminoglycoside derived from kanamycin.[1] At neutral pH, aminoglycosides have a very high positive charge and are cationic. They are highly soluble in water, with limited ability to cross lipid-containing cellular membranes. They have a molecular size ranging from 445–600 daltons. Their positive charge contributes to both their antimicrobial activity and their toxicity. They bind to negatively charged RNA, lipopolysaccharide and cell membrane phospholipids. They may also interact chemically with β-lactam antibiotics. Patients with renal failure administered an aminoglycoside and an antipseudomonal penicillin concomitantly may experience a 10–20% reduction in serum aminoglycoside concentration compared to levels obtained when each drug is administered alone.[4]

MECHANISM OF ACTION (see also Chapter 137)

Aminoglycosides reversibly bind to the bacterial 30s ribosomal subunit, derailing translation and leading to misreading of the genetic code and accumulation of truncated or non-functional proteins in bacteria.[5] Moreover, aminoglycosides result in a rearrangement of the gram-negative bacterial outer membrane, leading to formation of transient holes in the cell wall and disruption of its normal permeability function.[6] The exact mechanisms of bactericidal activity remain unknown. Decreased activity in an acidic pH or an anaerobic environment significantly reduces activity of aminoglycosides *in vitro*, which may be clinically relevant in empyema or abscesses. However, their rapid bactericidal effect, whose rate increases with increasing drug concentration, is not significantly diminished with a high bacterial inoculum, unlike β-lactams.

Aminoglycosides bind to the bacterial ribosome, inhibiting protein synthesis, and thus exhibiting a postantibiotic effect, defined as the continued suppression of bacterial growth following transient antimicrobial exposure.[7] The postantibiotic effect correlates with duration of ribosomal impairment, lasting several hours *in vivo* (and several days clinically against mycobacteria). Both the extent of bactericidal activity and the duration of the postantibiotic effect are enhanced by increasing aminoglycoside concentrations, contributing to the biologically and pharmacokinetically plausible current clinical use of high doses and extended intervals. Clinical pharmacodynamic parameters best describing aminoglycoside activity include peak concentration/mean inhibitory concentration (MIC) and area under the curve (AUC)/MIC values, emphasizing the concentration-dependent activity of these drugs; high peak levels and increased doses correlate with antibacterial efficacy.[8]

SPECTRUM OF ACTIVITY

Although marked regional differences exist for *in vitro* susceptibility patterns, the majority of aerobic and facultative gram-negative bacilli remain susceptible. Aminoglycosides show no activity against *Burkholderia cepacia* or *Stenotrophomonas maltophilia*. Although >95% of coagulase-negative staphylococci and methicillin-susceptible *Staphylococcus aureus* isolates are inhibited by aminoglycosides (especially gentamicin and netilmicin), resistant small colony variants may appear within 24 hours unless another active antistaphylococcal β-lactam or vancomycin is co-administered. Some clonal strains of community-associated methicillin-resistant *Staph. aureus* isolates and all streptococci, including *Streptococcus pneumoniae*, are resistant. Since aminoglycosides require aerobic metabolism to exert an antibacterial effect, all anaerobic bacteria and facultative anaerobic bacteria growing in anaerobic environments are intrinsically resistant.

Although aminoglycosides alone are ineffective against streptococci, they have been used in combination therapy with β-lactams for serious infections such as endocarditis. However, recent reports have noted increasing resistance to gentamicin in enterococci, and a double β-lactam combination is more often being substituted for the traditional β-lactam + gentamicin combination in the treatment of enterococcal endocarditis.[9]

Current clinical use of aminoglycosides is mainly directed towards nosocomial gram-negative pathogens, including *Pseudomonas aeruginosa*. Minor differences in the relative *in vitro* potency, without significant differences in clinical activity, have been documented. For instance, while tobramycin demonstrates two-fold superior *in vitro* activity compared to gentamicin against *P. aeruginosa*, gentamicin has similarly enhanced potency against *Serratia* species, and amikacin demonstrates the broadest range of activity against otherwise aminoglycoside-resistant pathogens.[4] Activity against multidrug-resistant organisms producing extended-spectrum β-lactamases or carbapenemases is unpredictable. Among mycobacterial species, streptomycin is particularly active against *Mycobacterium tuberculosis*, while amikacin is generally the most active against atypical strains. Gentamicin or streptomycin are typically used against uncommon infections due to *Brucella abortus*, *Francisella tularensis* or *Yersinia pestis*, and all of the common aminoglycosides have been employed in *Vibrio vulnificus* sepsis.

RESISTANCE (see also Chapter 138)

Aminoglycoside resistance results from the combination of: 1) reduction of intracellular aminoglycoside accumulation due to reduced uptake and/or efflux systems; 2) decreased aminoglycoside binding to the ribosomal RNA binding site; and 3) most commonly, enzymatic deactivation (involving acetylation, adenylation or phosphorylation).[1] Since aminoglycosides require an active electron transport chain to enter a bacterium, anaerobic bacteria are intrinsically resistant. Reduced uptake (such as seen with small colony variants or multidrug efflux pumps) usually leads to low-level aminoglycoside resistance, and may explain adaptive resistance, a transiently resistant refractory state. This latter property has been used to theoretically support extended interval dosing. Ribosomal target mutation/methylation is uncommon, and most commonly noted among mycobacteria. The most common cause of aminoglycoside resistance is deactivation by specific enzymes, typically spread by plasmids or transposons. Enzymatic cross-resistance is generally incomplete. Emergence of resistance during therapy of an initially susceptible gram-negative pathogen is uncommon. All enterococci possess intrinsic resistance to aminoglycosides, although concomitant exposure to a cell wall active drug facilitates access of aminoglycosides to the ribosomal target and subsequent synergistic bactericidal activity.

Clinical Pharmacology

Aminoglycosides are generally administered intravenously over a 30–60-minute period, although slow-push infusion over 3–5 minutes has been safely administered in more than 5000 patients.[10] Aminoglycosides may be given intramuscularly with complete absorption; gastrointestinal tract absorption is minimal. Although aminoglycosides instilled into the pleural space or peritoneal cavity are absorbed rapidly, they have been administered as a bladder irrigant, as an aerosol and by direct instillation into the cerebrospinal fluid (CSF) without appreciable systemic absorption.

Given their low level of protein binding (approximately 10%) and high solubility in water, aminoglycosides are distributed freely in the vascular and interstitial spaces, albeit with significant interpatient variability, exhibiting a volume of distribution typically mirroring the extracellular fluid compartment of 0.2–0.3 L/kg (see Table 143-1). Due to their size, polycationic charge and lipid insolubility, aminoglycosides cross biologic membranes poorly except for renal tubular cells and perhaps inner ear cells that appear to have an inherent transport mechanism. Adequate aminoglycoside concentrations are achieved in most

TABLE 143-1	Typical Pharmacokinetic Parameters for Amikacin, Gentamicin, Netilmicin and Tobramycin
Parameter	**Mean (± SED) or Range**
Creatinine clearance (CrCl) (mL/min/kg) ≤1.5	1.33 (0.61)
Creatinine >1.5	0.53 (0.35)
CrCl ≥100 (mL/min)	1.51 (0.63)
VOLUME OF DISTRIBUTION (L/kg)	
Dehydration	0.07–0.15
Euvolemic	0.15–0.25
Expanded extracellular fluid (ECF)	0.35–0.70
HALF-LIFE (HR)	
Creatinine <1.5	0.15–15
CrCl ≥100	0.5–7.6
Age <30 yr	0.5–3
Age >30 yr	1.5–15
Urinary excretion	85–95%

Adapted from Schentag J.J., Meagher A.K., Jelliffe R.W. Aminoglycosides. In: Burton, M.E., et al., ed. Applied pharmacokinetics and pharmacodynamics: principles of therapeutic drug monitoring. Philadelphia; Lippincott Williams & Wilkins, 2006: Chapter 14.

body fluids although penetration into epithelial lining fluid ranges from 32–54% of serum concentrations, much below that which can be achieved by aerosol administration. Aminoglycosides traverse the blood–CSF and blood–brain barriers poorly, including tissues of the eye. On the other hand, since aminoglycosides are primarily eliminated unchanged by the kidney via glomerular filtration, urine concentrations exceed peak plasma levels 25–100-fold within 1 hour following drug administration. They remain above therapeutic levels for days following a typical multidose regimen, due to prolonged release from renal proximal tubules back into the urine, with a terminal half-life of 48–200 hours. Aminoglycosides can be removed by dialysis. Although no dosing adjustment is necessary for hepatic insufficiency, serum levels should be monitored in patients with severe hepatic disease, due to possible changes in volume of distribution.[3,6]

The pharmacokinetics of aminoglycosides in clinical use are similar, although interpatient variability is broad and associated with body weight and composition as well as renal function. Peak serum concentrations (typically obtained after the distributive phase, 1 hour after the start of drug administration) of gentamicin, netilmicin and tobramycin after a 7 mg/kg dose infused over 30 minutes range from 15–20 μg/mL and yield an AUC of 7200 mg/hr/L. Amikacin similarly infused at 15 mg/kg produces peak levels of 41–49 μg/mL and an AUC of 110–45 mg/hr/L.[2] Peak concentrations are higher and AUCs are larger in patients with renal impairment. Various dialysis modalities clear differing amounts of aminoglycosides, roughly one-half of the amount of circulating aminoglycoside per hemodialysis. Continuous hemofiltration usually results in a creatinine clearance (CrCl) equivalent of 10–50 mL/min. Because of interpatient variability, serum levels should be measured. Dosing for the morbidly obese appears to be best predicted by the chronic kidney disease-epidemiology equation (CKD-EPI) using lean body weight.[2] Although it remains debatable whether every patient administered an aminoglycoside requires an individual pharmacokinetic evaluation, individualized dosing is essential in critically ill patients with altered volumes of distribution and unstable renal function as well as those patients on prolonged courses of aminoglycosides.

Suggested initial dosing regimens for typical aminoglycosides in clinical use are listed in Table 143-2. Extended interval dosing is the

TABLE 143-2	Suggested Dosing Regimens for Adults		
Estimated Creatinine Clearance (mL/min)	DOSE (mg/kg)		Dosing Interval (hr)
	Gentamicin, Netilmicin, Tobramycin	Amikacin	
100	7	20	24
90	7	20	24
80	7	20	24
70	5	15	24
60	5	15	24
50	4	12	24
40	4	12	24
30	5	15	48
20	4	12	48
10	3	10	48
<10	2.5	7.5	48

Adapted from Gilbert D.N., Bennett W.M. Use of antimicrobial agents in renal failure. Infectious Diseases Clinics of North America 1989; 3:517-531.

TABLE 143-3	Estimated Frequency of Serious Clinical Adverse Reactions after Administration of Aminoglycoside Antibiotics	
Adverse Reaction	Estimated Usual Frequency (%)	
Nephrotoxicity	5–15	
Ototoxicity		
Cochlear	2–10	
Vestibular	3–14	
Neuromuscular blockade	Exceedingly rare	

Adapted from Gilbert D.N., et al. In: Mandell G.L., Bennett J.E., Dolin R., ed. Principles and practices of infectious diseases. Philadelphia: Churchill Livingstone; 2010:359-384.

norm, used in 75% of all acute care hospitals in the USA,[10] since traditional 8-hourly dosing frequently fails to provide optimal peak serum levels for many pathogens.[11] More than 55 clinical trials and nine meta-analyses comparing 24-hour with traditional 8- or 12-hour aminoglycoside administration have shown equivalency or superiority of extended interval dosing.[12,13] More than 6500 adults (including febrile neutropenic and critically ill patients, variable degrees of renal impairment and the elderly) have received aminoglycosides for 7–14 days, with comparable efficacy and toxicity for a broad range of serious infections (including gram-negative sepsis, pneumonia, intra-abdominal infections, febrile neutropenia, pelvic inflammatory disease and urinary tract infections). Five meta-analyses have shown statistically significantly improved clinical outcomes, and three have shown significantly lower nephrotoxicity with extended intervals between aminoglycoside doses.[12,13] Among trials identifying a time to onset of toxicity, use of extended interval dosing lessened the incidence of nephrotoxicity until total aminoglycoside duration approached 10–14 days.[14]

For routine anticipated aminoglycoside treatment lasting less than 3–6 days in hospitalized but not critically ill patients (with minimal anticipated renal fluctuation or aminoglycoside toxicity), obtaining a serum concentration may not be necessary. If obtained, a single random serum concentration 6–14 hours following the initial dose is often used with a nomogram to guide subsequent dosing intervals. For treatment regimens lasting longer than 5 or 6 days, individualized dosing overall results in greater efficacy and less toxicity when compared with the nomogram approach.[15] Following an initial dose (each dose being essentially a loading dose), typically two concentrations in the post-distribution phase (>1 hr after administration, separated by >1.5 half-lives) are used to individualize therapy (and to estimate AUC). Monitoring early peak concentration may assist in optimizing aminoglycoside efficacy, especially if an altered volume of distribution is expected. Monitoring renal function once- or twice-weekly may be used for prolonged therapy if renal function is stable. Lower aminoglycoside doses (typically 3 mg/kg/d) are employed in combination therapy against gram-positive pathogens.

SPECIAL POPULATIONS

Dosing of aminoglycosides in neonates and children is based upon age, varying from 4–5 mg/kg per day in neonates between 0 and 7 days, and 5–7.5 mg/kg per day in infants and children. Extended interval dosing has become the norm, as with adults. The volume of distribution in children under 1 year of age is slightly higher than that of an adult, whereas children over 1 year of age are similar to adults. Therefore, children under 1 year of age may require a higher dose than those over 1 year of age. Studies have shown that amikacin 20 mg/kg once daily in children undergoing bone marrow transplantation or with serious gram-negative bacillary sepsis are equivalent to standard intermittent dosing.[2] Pregnancy-induced physiologic changes include a possible larger volume of distribution and more rapid elimination.

For patients on hemodialysis, a traditional 1.7 mg/kg dose is given every 48–72 hours and an additional one-half of the full dose after dialysis in order to replace drug that was removed, or simply dosed after dialysis.[3] Serum levels should be monitored due to variability, depending upon the characteristics of the dialysis membrane, duration of dialysis, blood pressure during dialysis, and other factors. Continuous hemofiltration results in a CrCl equivalent of 10–50 mL/min. For patients undergoing continuous ambulatory peritoneal dialysis who have a systemic infection for which they are receiving 1.7 mg/kg intravenously every 48 to 72 hours, a small daily intravenous supplement to replace dialyzed drug may be given based upon serum concentrations.

Dosing for the morbidly obese has been traditionally based on excess body weight multiplied by 0.4 plus ideal body weight, but recent studies indicate that lean body weight permits simplified dosing across all weight strata, with clearance best predicted by CKD-EPI. On the other hand, the traditional Cockcroft–Gault-based model remains the best clinical descriptor of renal function for pharmacokinetic dosing in geriatric patients.[2]

Cystic fibrosis patients demonstrate increased volume of distribution and enhanced aminoglycoside elimination, requiring much larger doses of drug to achieve therapeutic serum levels, typically 7–10 mg/kg/day. Nebulized aminoglycoside therapy is frequently administered in these patients.[16]

TOXICITY

Aminoglycosides generally share the potential for causing injury to the renal proximal convoluted tubules, damage to the cochlea or vestibular apparatus or both, and neuromuscular blockade (see Table 143-3). The inherent toxicity and relative toxic potential of aminoglycosides correlate with their positive electrical charge at physiologic pH. Other untoward effects are encountered rarely – hypersensitivity reactions are uncommon and phlebitis is rare. Instillation into the pleural space, abdominal cavity or CSF causes no irritation, and incorporation of an aminoglycoside into methylmethacrylate prosthetic joint cement is well tolerated over protracted periods. They are not hepatotoxic, do not induce photosensitivity and have no adverse effect on hematopoiesis or the coagulation cascade. Aminoglycosides cross the placenta and produce detectable serum levels in the fetus. Nephrotoxicity has been rarely described following first trimester exposure; ototoxicity has been documented with streptomycin, and all aminoglycosides are classified as pregnancy category D.

Aminoglycosides accumulate in the kidney, accounting for 40% of the total drug in the body, and nearly 85% of this is located in the renal cortex.[17] Uptake into the proximal tubular cell is saturable so that the magnitude of toxicity is greatest when the dose is divided into multiple small increments and least when it is given as a single daily dose. Minimal clinical differences in toxicity among aminoglycosides were seen in a survey of approximately 10 000 patients in clinical trials between 1975 and 1982, averaging 14% for gentamicin, 15% for tobramycin, and 9% for amikacin and netilmicin. The reported incidence of significant nephrotoxicity in prospective randomized trials varies between 5% and 10%, with most other reports in the 5–15% range.[17]

In general, aminoglycoside-induced decrement in glomerular filtration rate is small with rare progression to dialysis-dependent oliguric renal failure. Clinical trial data support the concept that several days of therapy are needed to cause nephrotoxicity of clinical consequence, typically occurring after 6 or more days of extended interval administration.[18] Clinical risk factors for aminoglycoside nephrotoxicity include older age, pre-existing renal or hepatic disease, shock, larger volume of distribution, ICU stay, pneumonia, leukemia, duration of therapy, and concomitant vancomycin or other nephrotoxin (e.g. amphotericin B, foscarnet, furosemide, intravenous radiocontrast agents).[19]

Aminoglycoside antibiotics may cause cochlear and vestibular damage,[20] noted in 2–10% of patients in early clinical experience, with the predominant lesion usually being vestibular. Ototoxicity is of particular concern, since it is usually irreversible and can appear after the end of treatment; cumulative risk increases with repeated exposure.[21] It is unusual to see both nephrotoxicity and ototoxicity in the same patient.

Although few recipients of aminoglycoside complain of hearing loss, up to two-thirds have evidence of high frequency audiographic impairment (above normal speech perception). Overall, the incidence of cochlear toxicity ranges from 3% to 14%; controlled data show a three-fold increase in audiometric toxicity in aminoglycoside compared to β-lactam treated patients, and an initial onset after 9 days in subjects administered aminoglycosides for at least 4 days. Ototoxicity appears to be related to cumulative AUC, regardless of the frequency of dosing. The risk of ototoxicity varies negligibly among commonly used aminoglycosides, and is less than some chemotherapeutic agents. Prolonged therapy beyond 10 days, renal or hepatic impairment, and prior aminoglycoside exposure are major risk factors; aspirin use may mitigate the risk of ototoxicity.[22] The greatest potential risk for cochlear toxicity is genetic predisposition, due to mutations in the mitochondrial 12S rRNA gene, resulting in early, severe impairment in family members of multiple pedigrees.[23] No genetic predisposition to either vestibular or renal toxicity has yet been identified.

The true incidence of vestibular toxicity is difficult to determine since the injury is bilateral and initially symmetrical, compensated by visual and proprioceptive cues, enabling patients to suffer considerable damage before the onset of symptoms or clinical findings. Complaints of nausea, vomiting and imbalance should raise suspicion, and nystagmus may be evident. Functional recovery may occur in up to one-half of patients after cessation of drug exposure. Vestibular hair cells are purposely damaged by instillation of gentamicin into the middle ear as therapy for Ménière's disease that has not responded to conservative measures.[21]

Neuromuscular blockade following aminoglycoside administration is rare but potentially lethal, usually occurring in clinical situations in which a disease state or concomitant drug interferes with neuromuscular transmission. It has been reported anecdotally with all aminoglycosides, involving varied routes of administration.

Clinical Indications

Aminoglycosides are effective in the empiric therapy of most aerobic gram-negative bacillary infections, including Enterobacteriaceae, *P. aeruginosa*, *Acinetobacter* species and other non-fermentative gram-negative pathogens. Despite possessing *in vitro* activity, they are seldom used for *Salmonella* species, *Shigella* species, *Neisseria gonorrhoeae*, *Haemophilus influenzae* or *Legionella* species, due to safer alternatives. Despite their seemingly minimal *in vitro* activity in intracellular environments and their low concentration in acidic lysosomal compartments, aminoglycosides are used successfully in the treatment of intracellular infections such as brucellosis, tuberculosis, tularemia and yersiniosis. In contrast, they display minimal *in vitro* activity against *Burkholderia cepacia* and *Stenotrophomonas maltophilia*. Although they have *in vitro* activity against *Staph. aureus*, clinical failure occurs unless combination therapy with a cell wall active agent is administered. Likewise, activity against enterococci requires a concomitant cell wall active agent.

Aminoglycosides are often used in combination to enhance the spectrum of activity or to achieve an additive or synergistic effect with a β-lactam, vancomycin or anaerobically active drug. Observational studies have shown that between 25 and 50% of patients with bacteremia, surgical site infection or pneumonia, and over 50% of patients with shock in the intensive care unit, are administered combination antibiotic therapy. Despite *in vitro* synergy, clinical evidence to support these data are sparse and conflicting.[24] Meta-analyses of observational studies have tended to show benefit of combination therapy, while those including randomized, controlled trials have not.[24-30] Moreover, a meta-analysis of eight randomized, controlled trials comparing β-lactam monotherapy with aminoglycoside combination therapy showed that combination therapy neither prevented the emergence of resistance nor prevented superinfection;[27] many of the trials studied failed to employ optimal dosing strategies of aminoglycosides.

In febrile neutropenic patients, aminoglycosides may be administered in combination with a β-lactam, although newer guidelines suggest avoidance if possible, using empiric monotherapy with a broad-spectrum β-lactam instead.[31]

Several reviews have demonstrated inferior clinical efficacy of aminoglycoside monotherapy in severe gram-negative infections compared to therapy with β-lactams or fluoroquinolones, presumably related to the relatively low cut-off values for optimal peak MIC and AUC/MIC pharmacodynamic properties of aminoglyocosides.[25] In fact, traditional doses of gentamicin, netilmicin and tobramycin are optimal only with organisms whose MICs are 0.5 µg/mL or less (2 µg/mL for amikacin) and MICs of 1.0 µg/mL with 7 mg/kg extended interval dosing.[3] Although aminoglycosides have been used to enhance early killing in combination with β-lactams and fluoroquinolones, most older studies have failed to demonstrate improved outcomes with combinations compared to monotherapy.[24]

BACTEREMIA

In contrast to most older studies, many recent studies demonstrate improved outcome in patients with septic shock and gram-negative bacillary bacteremia treated with combination aminoglycoside plus β-lactam.[26-31] This is presumably due to a greater degree of initial appropriate therapy than β-lactam monotherapy, broader coverage than provided by fluoroquinolones, and improved outcomes even in neutropenic patients. In one recent international, propensity-adjusted trial involving over 4500 patients with septic shock whose pathogens were susceptible to all antibiotic classes employed, significant reduction in 28-day mortality as well as other parameters was seen with combination therapy, and greatest benefit with earlier combination.[28]

Reduced endotoxin release seen with aminoglycoside therapy may contribute to the diminished early mortality observed with combination therapy in patients with septic shock. The use of combination therapy in selected cases is endorsed in recent international guidelines for management of severe sepsis, such as neutropenic patients and patients with difficult-to-treat, multidrug-resistant bacterial pathogens such as *Acinetobacter* or *Pseudomonas*.[32]

Aminoglycoside use in combination with a β-lactam or vancomycin may benefit patients with streptococcal or enterococcal endocarditis.[33] Although the traditional dosage to achieve synergy is 1 mg/kg iv q8h, newer regimens have used 12–24- hour intervals with equal efficacy.[33] Although aminoglycoside combinations remain the standard of care for enterococcal endocarditis, dual β-lactam regimens are increasingly used as alternative therapy.[9] On the other hand, the formerly prevalent practice of administering combination gentamicin 1 mg/kg every 8 hours with β-lactams for staphylococcal bacteremia and endocarditis has recently been challenged due to its lack of improved efficacy and added nephrotoxicity. Others have instead emphasized the suboptimal dosing strategy used in these studies, or the earlier defervescence (2 days versus 4 days).

PNEUMONIA

Aminoglycoside use in pneumonia is typically employed with hospital-acquired or hospital-associated gram-negative bacillary infections, including those seen in patients on ventilators or with cystic fibrosis. β-lactam monotherapy for Enterobacteriaceae has been shown to be equivalent to combination therapy with an aminoglycoside and superior to aminoglycoside monotherapy. The role of combination therapy for *P. aeruginosa* pneumonia is still unclear, with one meta-analysis suggesting significant mortality benefit[28] and two additional large studies showing no additional benefit as long as the isolate was susceptible to more than one agent.[31,34]

While aerosolized aminoglycosides were initially used to treat cystic fibrosis exacerbations, they have recently been used more often in chronic bronchiectasis and ventilator-associated pneumonias, with inhaled aminoglycoside employed in conjunction with a systemic β-lactam. Aerosolized aminoglycosides in these studies were associated with improved clinical and microbiologic cure rates with less nephrotoxicity, and a large randomized placebo-controlled trial is underway. Tobramycin 300 mg once or twice daily is the usual regimen in this setting.

INTRA-ABDOMINAL INFECTIONS

Current guidelines on empiric therapy for intra-abdominal infections do not recommend the combination of an aminoglycoside with metronidazole, based on the toxic potential of aminoglycosides and availability of equally effective regimens.[35] Recent meta-analyses of more than 5000 patients demonstrated clinical inferiority of clindamycin + aminoglycoside therapy to its β-lactam comparator.[34] Alternative first-choice regimens include β-lactam-β-lactamase inhibitor combination plus a fluoroquinolone or monotherapy with a carbapenem.

URINARY TRACT INFECTIONS

A recent systemic review and meta-analysis in nearly 2500 patients showed that aminoglycoside monotherapy was equally effective to comparators, although few trials enrolled patients with sepsis, and a higher rate of bacteriologic failure and nephrotoxicity was observed with aminoglycosides.[36] Recent Infectious Diseases Society of America guidelines suggesting 7 days of therapy for pyelonephritis suggest that such a course of aminoglycoside therapy should easily provide equivalent clinical efficacy to previously recommended longer courses, given the presence of therapeutic aminoglycoside levels for most pathogens in the urine for 72 hours or longer after a single dose. Intravesicular gentamicin has been investigated anecdotally for recurrent urinary tract infections in intermittently catheterized patients.

CYSTIC FIBROSIS

Cystic fibrosis patients demonstrate altered aminoglycoside pharmacokinetics, requiring much larger doses of the drug to achieve therapeutic serum levels. The frequency of nephrotoxicity in such patients is less than that in non-CF patients, although the prevalence of hearing loss after aminoglycoside therapy in adult cystic fibrosis patients is approximately the same as the rate in non-CF patients.[21] Aerosolized therapy has long been used in cystic fibrosis patients showing an increase in forced expiratory volume in 1 second and reduced odds ratio of hospitalization in those receiving nebulized aminoglycosides.[15] Neither nephrotoxicity nor ototoxicity has been observed with aerosolized therapy, and sputum concentrations diminish rapidly within hours following an inhaled dose with minimal absorption into serum[15] (see also Chapter 34).

MYCOBACTERIAL INFECTIONS

Streptomycin has long been used in therapy against *M. tuberculosis*, although increasing streptomycin resistance and recognized toxicity have made it a second-line agent. Both streptomycin and amikacin, active against some streptomycin-resistant isolates, may be administered intermittently, to take advantage of a very prolonged postantibiotic effect against mycobacteria. Aminoglycosides, especially amikacin, are also often used in the initial course of therapy for atypical mycobacterial infections including *M. abscessus, M. fortuitum, M. chelonae,* and *M. kansasii.*

PROPHYLAXIS

Clinical practice guidelines for antimicrobial prophylaxis in surgery have recently been updated.[37] Gentamicin or tobramycin 5 mg/kg iv as a single dose is recommended as an alternative agent in patients with a β-lactam allergy in genitourinary and gastrointestinal procedures. Studies have shown that the risk of infection following elective colorectal procedures was significantly reduced by mechanical cleansing of the bowel plus oral administration of an aminoglycoside (usually neomycin together with erythromycin or metronidazole) in addition to standard iv antibiotic prophylaxis in recent controlled trials.[37] Other trials have shown that an oral selective digestive decontamination protocol containing gentamicin effectively eradicated carbapenem-resistant *Klebsiella pneumoniae* gastrointestinal carriage and may be used in nosocomial outbreaks. On the other hand, trials of topical gentamicin to prevent deep sternal wound infection in cardiac surgery have not shown unequivocal efficacy. Many tunneled catheter antibiotic lock trials have demonstrated the reduction in catheter-related infections, but emergence of resistance remains a concern.[37]

ANTIBIOTIC-IMPREGNATED CEMENT

Antibiotic-impregnated cement is increasingly used in primary hip and knee arthroplasties as well as revision procedures of infected total joint arthroplasties. Persistence of bacterial growth as adherent biofilms remains a potential problem and nephrotoxicity has been reported even with such local use.[37] A recent multicenter evaluation failed to show significant reduction in the risk of infection compared with traditional prophylaxis. Prospective trials of aminoglycoside-containing beads for established osteomyelitis and prosthetic joint-associated infections are needed.

References available online at expertconsult.com.

KEY REFERENCES

Craig W.A.: Pharmacokinetic/pharmacodynamic parameters: Rationale for antibacterial dosing of mice and men. *Clin Infect Dis* 1998; 26:1-10.

Drusano G.L., Amborse P.G., Bhavnani S.M., et al.: Back to the future: Using aminoglycosides again and how to dose them optimally. *Clin Infect Dis* 2007; 45:753-760.

Fernandez-Hidalgo N., Almirante B., Gavalda J., et al.: Ampicillin plus ceftriaxone is as effective as ampicillin plus gentamicin for treating *Enterocccus faecalis* infective endocarditis. *Clin Infect Dis* 2013; 56:1261-1268.

Hatala R., Dinh T., Cook D.J.: Once-daily aminoglycoside dosing in immunocompetent adults: A meta-analysis. *Ann Intern Med* 1996; 124:717-725.

Kumar A., Zarychanski R., Light B., et al.: Early combination antibiotic therapy yields improved survival compared with monotherapy in septic shock: a prospensity-matched analysis. *Crit Care Med* 2010; 38:1773-1785.

Martinez J.A., Cobos-Triqueros N., Soriano A., et al.: Influence of empiric therapy with a beta-lactam alone or combined with an aminoglycoside on prognosis of bacteremia

due to gram-negative microorganisms. *Antimicrob Agents Chemother* 2010; 54:3590-3596.

Micek S.T., Welch E.C., Kha J., et al.: Empiric combination antibiotic therapy is associated with improved outcome against sepsis due to gram-negative bacteria: A retrospective analysis. *Antimicrob Agents Chemother* 2010; 54: 1742-1748.

Paul M., Silbiger I., Grozinsky S., et al.: Beta-lactam antibiotic monotherapy versus beta-lactam-aminoglycoside antibiotic combination therapy for sepsis. *Cochrane Database Syst Rev* 2006; (1):CD003344.

144

Quinolones

ETHAN RUBINSTEIN[†] | PHILIPPE LAGACÉ-WIENS

KEY CONCEPTS

• Fluoroquinolones are a well-studied class of antimicrobial compounds with a wide variety of indications.

• Fluoroquinolones are most commonly prescribed for treatment of urinary tract infections and lower respiratory tract infections.

• Newer indications for fluoroquinolones include treatment of leprosy, prevention and treatment of BK virus infection in immunocompromised patients and treatment of multidrug-resistant tuberculosis.

• Fluoroquinolones available in the North American and European markets have favorable safety profiles with rare severe side effects that include cardiotoxicity, central nervous system irritability and tendinopathy.

• Resistance to fluoroquinolones, particularly in Enterobacteriaceae continues to increase and will reduce the utility of these agents in the future.

• Recent studies support that use of fluoroquinolones is safe in pediatric populations and that they may be viable treatment options when other treatments are not possible.

• Fluoroquinolones inhibit the activity of the P450 cytochrome system and dose adjustments may be required for other drugs with a low therapeutic index that are metabolized via this system.

Introduction

The quinolones are a heterogeneous group of synthetic antimicrobial agents. Originally derived from 1,8-naphthyridine compounds (e.g. nalidixic acid), modern quinolones have evolved to give compounds initially with improved activity against gram-negative bacteria (e.g. ciprofloxacin, ofloxacin) and more recently with greater activity against gram-positive bacteria (e.g. gatifloxacin, moxifloxacin) (Figure 144-1). A number of broader spectrum agents have been developed (e.g. clinafloxacin, trovafloxacin) but later were withdrawn due to toxicity. The notable market withdrawals of fluoroquinolones and their major toxicity issues are presented in Table 144-1.

As quinolones have excellent tissue and tissue fluid penetration, they are suitable for infections in a wide range of organ systems. Adverse reactions are uncommon in marketed agents and relate mainly to the skin, the gastrointestinal system and central nervous system (CNS), and rarely warrant cessation of therapy. However, there are a number of potentially more serious adverse effects such as arthropathy, cardiotoxicity and phototoxicity. These occur as a class effect (although to different extents with different compounds) and have been a problem in drug development.

Modern fluoroquinolones are available in both intravenous and oral formulations and have high to very high bioavailability. One of their major advantages has proved to be the ability to treat many serious infections with oral or intravenous-oral switch regimens, for example in the management of enteric fever, gram-negative bacterial pyelonephritis, osteomyelitis, nosocomial pneumonia and severe exacerbations of both chronic bronchitis and cystic fibrosis. Many of these diseases previously demanded lengthy therapy with intravenous β-lactams, aminoglycosides or their combinations.

The activity of fluoroquinolones, such as ciprofloxacin and ofloxacin in gram-positive infections, notably those caused by pneumococci, has been disputed. Newer compounds, such as moxifloxacin, have markedly improved activity against gram-positive pathogens and have found a place in the management of infections caused, for example, by penicillin-resistant pneumococci.

Antibacterial Spectrum and Potency

The antibacterial spectrum of quinolones is shown in Table 144-2. Quinolones are notable for the considerable knowledge that has been gained regarding structure-activity relationships.[1] The activity of the original naphthyridine and quinolone compounds (e.g. nalidixic acid) was limited to gram-negative pathogens, primarily the Enterobacteriaceae, including *Shigella* and *Salmonella* spp. A major step forward in the development of the class was the addition of a fluorine at position 6, giving rise to the fluoroquinolones (Figure 144-1). These agents are 10–100 times more active than their precursors against gram-negative pathogens, including *Pseudomonas aeruginosa*, and have gained activity against the organisms causing atypical pneumonia. Potency, spectrum of activity and adverse effects/drug interactions are largely determined by substitutions at positions 1, 5, 7 and 8:

• substitutions at position 1 (e.g. trovafloxacin) can alter potency (particularly against anaerobes) but may also affect interactions with theophyllines;

• substitutions at position 5 (e.g. grepafloxacin) can increase potency but may cause increased cardiotoxicity;

• substitutions at position 7 (e.g. moxifloxacin, gemifloxacin, garenoxacin) can increase activity against gram-positive organisms and increase the plasma half-life; and

TABLE 144-1	List of Fluoroquinolone Antibiotics Withdrawn from the Market Due to Adverse Events
Fluoroquinolone Antibiotic	**Reason/Adverse Event**
Clinafloxacin	Phototoxicity, dysglycemia
Enoxacin	Phototoxicity
Fleroxacin	Phototoxicity
Perfloxacin	Phototoxicity
Grepafloxacin	Cardiotoxicity
Sparfloxacin	Cardiotoxicity, phototoxicity
Temafloxacin	Hemolytic-uremic syndrome
Gatifloxacin	Dysglycemia
Trovafloxacin	Hepatotoxicity
Lomefloxacin	Phototoxicity, central nervous system toxicity
Tosufloxacin	Nephritis, thrombocytopenia

Reprinted from Rubinstein E. History of quinolones and their side effects. Chemotherapy 2001; 47 (Suppl 3):3-8; discussion 44-8.

[†]Deceased

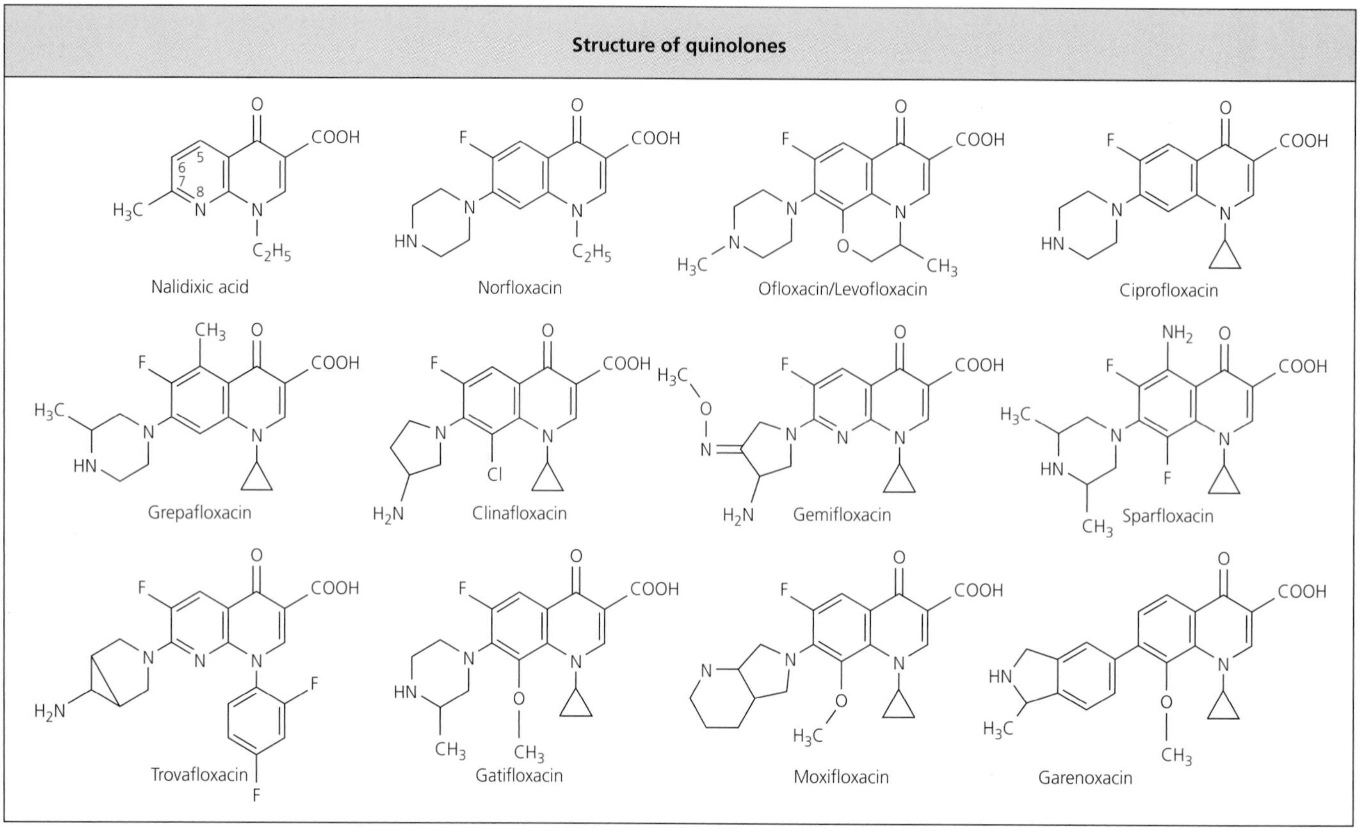

Structure of quinolones

Figure 144-1 Structure of quinolones.

- substitutions at position 8 (moxifloxacin, garenoxacin) can increase potency and reduce the rate of selection of resistant mutants but can be associated with increased phototoxicity (sparfloxacin).

Early representatives, such as ciprofloxacin, only have borderline activity against gram-positive pathogens. However, developments such as the addition of a five-membered ring (gemifloxacin) or an azabicyclo group (moxifloxacin, garenoxacin) at position 7 have brought increased gram-positive activity. Unfortunately, this has been partly at the expense of some activity against *P. aeruginosa*. Agents with good activity against both gram-positive and gram-negative bacteria have been developed (e.g. clinafloxacin) but have been withdrawn due to toxicity problems.

Fluoroquinolones have good activity *in vitro* against many intracellular pathogens such as *Legionella* spp., *Mycoplasma* spp., *Ureaplasma urealyticum*, *Chlamydia* spp., *Brucella* spp., *Salmonella enterica* including serovar Typhi and *Coxiella burnetii*. This may be enhanced by the concentrations of fluoroquinolones within cells (see below). As shown in Table 144-2, *Mycobacterium tuberculosis* is susceptible to most of the fluoroquinolones with greater activity displayed by most of the newer agents (e.g. gatifloxacin and moxifloxacin). Fluoroquinolones should be used with caution in the treatment of pneumonia if there is a suspicion of tuberculosis, in order to avoid inadvertent monotherapy and the attendant risks of reduced diagnostic yield and selection of quinolone resistance. Of the other mycobacteria, *M. kansasii*, *M. marinum* and *M. fortuitum* tend to be fluoroquinolone-susceptible, whereas *M. avium* complex, *M. chelonae* and *M. scrofulaceum* are more resistant.[2]

The quinolones are rapidly bactericidal against most susceptible species in a concentration-dependent manner and have a post-antibiotic effect (PAE) of 2–4 hours. The pharmacodynamic determinants of efficacy are C_{max}/MIC (ratio of the maximum plasma concentration to minimum inhibitory concentration) and AUC_{0-24}/MIC (ratio of the area under the 24-hour drug concentration curve to MIC). Various groups have attempted to define the AUC_{0-24}/MIC ratio

that would predict a successful outcome. It appears that the optimal ratio varies for different organisms so that a ratio of >125 has been proposed for infection caused by gram-negative enteric pathogens and *P. aeruginosa*, but a much lower ratio of >34 is proposed for pneumococcal lower respiratory tract infections.[3,4] In addition to clinical efficacy, recent studies have focused on therapeutic strategies which may reduce the risk of fluoroquinolone resistance. The concept of the 'mutant selection window' has emerged, in which the survival of resistant organisms may be selectively encouraged by agents that only narrowly exceed the MIC of the organism. In accordance with this hypothesis, the use of the most potent agents at high initial doses may help to limit the risk of development of resistance by reducing the mutant selection window.[5]

Mode of Action (see also Chapter 137)

Quinolones act by the rapid inhibition of bacterial DNA synthesis, leading to cell death. The primary targets are DNA gyrase and topoisomerase IV which are involved in the maintenance of the superhelical structure of DNA. Both enzymes are composed of two subunits that are homologous: DNA gyrase subunits encoded by *gyrA* and *gyrB*; topoisomerase IV encoded by *parC* (*grlA* in *Staphylococcus aureus*) and *parE* (*grlB* in *Staph. aureus*). The relative affinity of a quinolone antibiotic to either the topoisomerase or the gyrase depends both on the structure of fluoroquinolone and the organism in question and may vary from one agent to the next even within a single species. Some organisms (e.g. *Mycobacterium* spp. and *Campylobacter* spp.) do not have topoisomerase IV, such that the only target to quinolones is DNA gyrase in these organisms.[6,7]

Bacterial Resistance

The major mechanism for acquired resistance to quinolones is by mutational modification of the antimicrobial target site. Mutations around the active site of *gyrA* have been identified in many strains of

TABLE 144-2   Activity of Quinolones Against Common Pathogenic Bacteria: MIC$_{90}$ (mg/L)

Pathogen	Nalidixic Acid	Norfloxacin	Ciprofloxacin	Levofloxacin	Gemifloxacin	Moxifloxacin	Prulifloxacin[a]	Sitafloxacin[b]	Avarofloxacin[c]
Streptococcus pneumoniae	>64	2–16	1–4	2	0.06	0.12	4	0.06	0.12
Staphylococcus aureus	>64	2	0.5–2	0.25	0.03	0.06	.05–>4	0.03–0.5	0.25
Enterococcus spp.	>64	8–16	1–8	2–8	0.25–>16	0.5–4	2–4	N/A	0.5–4
β-hemolytic streptococci	>64	4–8	2	1	0.03	0.25	0.25–1	N/A	0.015
Listeria spp.	N/A	N/A	1	1	0.125	0.5	N/A	N/A	N/A
Haemophilus influenza	1	0.25	0.03	0.03	0.015	0.06	0.015	0.008	0.015
Moraxella catarrhalis	4	0.25	0.06–0.25	0.06	0.03	0.12	0.06	0.008	0.015
Neisseria spp.	0.5	0.03	0.03	0.015	0.008	0.03	N/A	0.008	N/A
Escherichia coli	4–8	0.12–2	0.06–0.25	0.06–0.25	0.015	0.016	0.015	0.5	0.25–16
Klebsiella spp.	8–16	025–1	0.12–0.25	0.06–0.5	0.25	0.12–0.5	0.12	0.12	0.25
Enterobacter spp.	8–16	0.12–0.5	0.12–0.5	0.12–2	0.25–1	0.25	0.12	0.25	0.12–0.25
Salmonella spp.	2–4	0.25	0.12	0.25	0.06	0.25	0.03	N/A	N/A
Shigella spp.	8	0.25	0.12	0.03	0.008	0.06	0.015	0.015	N/A
Campylobacter spp.	8	0.25	0.12	0.12	N/A	0.06	0.5	1[d]	N/A
Pseudomonas aeruginosa	>64	0.5–2	0.5–2	4	8	8	1	4	2
Acinetobacter spp.	>64	>16	1–2	0.25–8	0.5–>16	0.25–16	N/A	2	N/A
Stenotrophomonas maltophilia	>64	N/A	8	2–8	4	1	N/A	0.25	N/A
Bacteroides fragilis group	>64	16–32	4–16	2	1	0.5	N/A	1	N/A
Mycoplasma spp.	N/A	4–16	1–2	0.5	0.12	0.12	N/A	N/A	N/A
Chlamydia spp.	N/A	4–16	1–4	0.5	0.25	0.06	N/A	N/A	N/A
Legionella pneumophila	1	2	0.06	0.03	0.015	0.06	1	N/A	N/A
Mycobacterium tuberculosis	N/A	2–8	1–4	1	>4	0.12	N/A	0.12	N/A

N/A, not available.
[a]Prats G., Rossi V., Salvatori E., et al. Prulifloxacin: a new antibacterial fluoroquinolone. *Expert Rev Anti Infect Ther* 2006; 4(1):27-41.
[b]Zhanel G.G., Ennis K., Vercaigne L., et al. Critical review of the fluoroquinolones: focus on respiratory infections. *Drugs* 2002; 62(1):13-59
[c]Morrow B.J., He W., Amsler K.M., et al. In vitro antibacterial activities of JNJ-Q2, a new broad-spectrum fluoroquinolone. *Antimicrob Agents Chemother* 2010; 54(5):1955-64.
[d]Lehtopolku M., Hakanen A.J., Siitonen A. et al. In vitro activities of 11 fluoroquinolones against 226 Campylobacter jejuni strains isolated from Finnish patients, with special reference to ciprofloxacin resistance. *J Antimicrob Chemother* 56 (6): 1134-1138.

Escherichia coli and many other gram-negative bacilli, giving rise to greater resistance to nalidixic acid than the fluoroquinolones. Alterations in *gyrB* are less common and cause lower levels of resistance.[8] The main site for resistance mutations in gram-positive bacteria such as *Staph. aureus* and *Streptococcus pneumoniae* is the *parC* gene although mutations in *parE* have been described. In both gram-negative and gram-positive pathogens resistance develops in a stepwise fashion as mutations arise in one and then both targets. Following an initial mutation, the susceptibility to a quinolone will depend on the specificity of the agent for the alternative target. For example, in clinical practice it has been shown that an isolated *gyrA* mutation in *E. coli* will confer high-level resistance to nalidixic acid but only reduced susceptibility to ciprofloxacin. The acquisition of an additional *parC* mutation confers high-level resistance to ciprofloxacin.[9] For bacteria such as *P. aeruginosa* that inherently have less susceptibility to fluoroquinolones, a single mutation can give rise to clinically significant resistance.

Resistance to quinolones can also be achieved by active efflux of the drug from the bacterial cell. This has been best described in *P. aeruginosa* in which quinolone resistance has been associated with increased expression of the MexAB-OprM, MexCD-oprJ or MexEF-oprN efflux pumps.[10] In *E. coli* the pump is the acrAB-tolC system. Among gram-positive pathogens, the *norA* pump has been described in *Staphylococcus aureus* and the PmrA pump in *Strep. pneumoniae*.[11,12] On their own, efflux pumps will generally only cause low-level resistance and therefore may not be clinically important in inherently highly susceptible pathogens such as *E. coli*. However, the overexpression of efflux pumps becomes more significant in less susceptible organisms such as *P. aeruginosa*. The presence of efflux pumps may explain the reduced susceptibility of *Mycobacterium avium* when compared to other nontuberculous mycobacteria with similar susceptibility to gyrase inhibition.[13]

More recently, the spread of reduced susceptibility in Enterobacteriaceae by plasmid-mediated mechanisms such as Qnr proteins has been described. First discovered in the late 1990s, Qnr proteins protect gyrase and topoisomerase IV from quinolone inhibition. Qnr proteins confer low-level resistance which enhances the selection of resistant mutants *in vitro*, and may contribute to clinically significant levels of resistance by acting additively with other resistance mechanisms. The aminoglycoside acetyltransferase, AAC(6')-Ib-cr, is another recently discovered mechanism for transferring low-level resistance to both aminoglycosides and fluoroquinolones on mobile elements. AAC(6')-Ib-cr appears to act on piperazinyl-substituted quinolones such as ciprofloxacin.[14]

Resistance rates to quinolones continue to rise. A study spanning 2004–2007 across Europe revealed that 24.9% of *E. coli* were nonsusceptible to levofloxacin.[15] A similar study in the USA revealed that 23.9% of *E. coli* were nonsusceptible to levofloxacin.[16] In the UK, 2006 data from the Health Protection Agency reported that ciprofloxacin resistance among *E. coli* bacteremia isolates was 26%.[17] Among a global collection of Enterobacteriaceae, 29% were resistant to levofloxacin in 2010.[18] Resistance among other members of the Enterobacteriaceae is less common, with susceptibility rated generally over 90%.[15,16] Although methicillin-sensitive *Staph. aureus* is usually sensitive to fluoroquinolones, most studies report that methicillin-resistant strains are likely to be resistant to fluoroquinolones.[15,16] Resistance among pneumococci remains uncommon, with most countries, including the USA, Western Europe and Latin America, reporting rates of resistance to levofloxacin between 1 and 2%,[19] although in some areas there is evidence that resistance is more common among penicillin-resistant pneumococci.[20]

Cross-resistance between the older fluoroquinolones is almost complete and minor differences in activity are not usually clinically exploitable. The mechanisms of resistance to antimicrobial agents are discussed in detail in Chapter 138.

Pharmacokinetics and Distribution

The quinolones are generally well absorbed and are widely distributed in body tissues and fluids, including the intracellular environment. They are excreted either by glomerular filtration or hepatic biotransformation, or a combination of these routes, and by biliary or transintestinal elimination. Bioavailability is high and protein binding usually low to intermediate. Fluoroquinolone kinetics are summarized in Table 144-3.

ABSORPTION

Fluoroquinolones are well and rapidly absorbed after oral administration and exhibit linear absorption kinetics so that doubling the dose produces twice the plasma level.[13] Peak plasma concentrations are usually present 1–2 hours after an oral dose. Absorption may be delayed by food and is impaired by co-administration of antacids and ferrous iron, and possibly by zinc in multivitamin preparations.

DISTRIBUTION

The fluoroquinolones are extensively distributed to the tissues with most sites outside the CNS having concentration near-to-well-over serum levels. Apparent volumes of distribution are usually 2–3 L/kg,

TABLE 144-3	Basic Pharmacokinetic Parameters of Quinolones							
Agent	Dose (g)		C_{max} (mg/L)	AUC_{0-24} (mg*h/L)	$T_{1/2}$ (h)	Protein Binding %	% Dosage Excreted Unchanged in Urine	Route
Nalidixic acid	1	QDS	V	V	1.5	90	<1	po
Norfloxacin	0.4	BD	2	12.5	3	15	25–40	po
Ciprofloxacin	0.75	BD	3	30	4	40	30–50	po/iv
Levofloxacin	0.5	OD	6.4	54	7	40	85–90	po/iv
Gemifloxacin	0.32	OD	1.8	9	7	65	30	po
Moxifloxacin	0.4	OD	4.5	44	13	50	20	po/iv
Prulfloxacin[a]	0.6	OD	1.6	6.2	10.6	41–59	17–23	po
Sitafloxacin[b]	0.1	OD	1.0	5.6	4.7	50	72	po
Avarofloxacin[c]	0.25	BD	2.18	26.2	14.4	65	9.24	po/iv

V, variable.
[a]Picollo R., Brion N., Gualano V., *et al.* Pharmacokinetics and tolerability of prulifloxacin after single oral administration. *Arzneimittelforschung* 2003; 53(3):201-5.
[b]Zhanel G.G., Ennis K., Vercaigne L., *et al.* A critical review of the fluoroquinolones: focus on respiratory infections. *Drugs* 2002; 62(1):13-59.
[c]Davenport, J. M., Covington P., Gotfried M., *et al.* Summary of pharmacokinetics and tissue distribution of a broad-spectrum fluoroquinolone, JNJ-Q2. *Clin Pharmacol Drug Dev* 2012; 1(4): 121–130.
QDS, four times per day; BD, twice per day; OD, once per day.

although values for precursor compounds are lower (e.g. 0.5 L/kg). Protein binding varies from 15% to 40% with norfloxacin, ofloxacin and ciprofloxacin,[21] to 65% for gemifloxacin and higher still for garenoxacin and trovafloxacin (>80%).

Fluoroquinolones are concentrated approximately 10 times in neutrophils. Although it has been suggested that this may increase their *in vivo* efficacy against intracellular pathogens, there is evidence that the intracellular activity of different fluoroquinolones is variable, possibly related to where they are concentrated within the cell.[22] An additional result of the intracellular concentration of fluoroquinolones is that they may be transported by neutrophils to a site of infection and then released.[23]

ELIMINATION

Elimination half-lives vary from 1–2 hours for nalidixic acid to 3–5 hours for ciprofloxacin and 7–14 hours for newer agents.

Excretion of fluoroquinolones is primarily by renal glomerular filtration, hepatic metabolism and transintestinal elimination. The relative importance of glomerular filtration varies between agents and some compounds, such as ofloxacin, levofloxacin and gatifloxacin, exhibit minimal metabolism and are excreted largely unchanged in the urine. For these agents, renal clearance almost equals total clearance and dose modification is required in renal impairment.[21,24] Others, such as ciprofloxacin, moxifloxacin, prulifloxacin and avarofloxacin, have moderately extensive hepatic biotransformation (to oxo-, desethyl- and sulfo- derivatives, subsequently partly eliminated as inactive glucuronides in the bile). For these compounds, renal clearance is half of the total clearance and dosage modification may not be required in renal impairment as long as other routes of elimination are intact.[25]

In hepatic impairment, the dosage of agents primarily cleared by the kidney (ciprofloxacin, ofloxacin and levofloxacin) rarely requires modification.

Fluoroquinolones that are not primarily eliminated by the kidney are present in significant quantities in the stool, partly by biliary excretion and, notably with ciprofloxacin, by transintestinal elimination. The majority is bound to ligands in the stool.

Route of Administration and Dosage

Most agents are available in both oral and intravenous formulations. The high oral bioavailability of fluoroquinolones means that oral administration is adequate in most situations unless this route is unavailable. The manufacturers' dosage recommendations for quinolones are given in Table 144-4.

Indications

Early quinolones, such as nalidixic acid, were largely used for gram-negative urinary tract infection (UTI) and shigellosis. The development and evolution of fluoroquinolones have led to a number of agents with differences in spectrum of activity and therefore indications. Some, such as norfloxacin, are used almost exclusively for UTI. Agents such as ciprofloxacin and ofloxacin have been used for a broad range of infective syndromes. Newer compounds, such as levofloxacin, moxifloxacin and gemifloxacin, have improved activity against gram-positive pathogens and are more appropriate for respiratory tract infections.

GENITOURINARY TRACT INFECTIONS

Uncomplicated Lower Urinary Tract Infection

Oral fluoroquinolone therapy is highly effective – to limit selection pressure for resistance it should be used only when bacterial resistance precludes the use of other agents. Fluoroquinolones eradicate bowel reservoirs of uropathogenic *E. coli* and may reduce the incidence of early recurrence. Long-term suppression with low-dose norfloxacin or ciprofloxacin has been shown to be effective in preventing recurrent UTI in selected patients.[26,27]

Complicated Ascending Urinary Tract Infection

Fluoroquinolones given for 1–2 weeks are the recommended agents for the treatment of ascending or complicated UTI.[28] Oral ciprofloxacin has proved as efficacious as an intravenous regimen for initial empiric therapy.[29]

Prostatitis

Fluoroquinolones are concentrated in prostatic tissue and are recommended therapy for both acute and chronic bacterial prostatitis.[30] Ciprofloxacin for 28 days can give a clinical response of 98% in chronic bacterial prostatitis although relapse may occur in up to 40% of patients.[31]

Gonorrhea

The global prevalence of fluoroquinolone resistance continues to rise. In England and Wales the prevalence of ciprofloxacin resistance was 26.5% in 2006.[32] In the USA, the Centers for Disease Control and Prevention (CDC) treatment guidelines were updated in 2007 to recommend that fluoroquinolones should no longer be used to treat gonococcal infections in any patient group.[33] The new agents gemifloxacin and delafloxacin show promise for the treatment of fluoroquinolone-resistant gonorrhea.[34]

Nongonococcal Urethritis/Cervicitis

The antichlamydial activity of fluoroquinolones varies and ofloxacin is the most potent of the established agents. A 7-day course of ofloxacin is as effective as doxycycline therapy.[35] Newer compounds such as moxifloxacin have excellent *in vitro* activity and may have a role in therapy.

Chancroid

A single dose or 3-day course of ciprofloxacin is a recommended treatment for chancroid. Despite reports of isolates with reduced susceptibility to quinolones, a study in Nairobi showed a 92% cure rate for single-dose ciprofloxacin, comparable to a 7-day course of erythromycin.[36]

Pelvic Inflammatory Disease

The ideal antimicrobial treatment for acute pelvic inflammatory disease has not been established by randomized clinical trial. In view of the high rates of resistance of *Neisseria gonorrhoeae*, fluoroquinolones are no longer included in recommended treatment regimens.[33]

RESPIRATORY TRACT INFECTIONS

The fluoroquinolones, ciprofloxacin and ofloxacin, have been used extensively for upper and lower respiratory tract infections. However, there have been concerns regarding their activity against *Strep. pneumoniae*. Newer agents, such as gemifloxacin, moxifloxacin and garenoxacin, have improved activity against pneumococci, including macrolide- and penicillin-resistant strains, and are often termed 'respiratory quinolones'.

Sinusitis

Oral fluoroquinolones have comparable efficacy to macrolides or cephalosporins and give cure rates of >85% in acute sinusitis.[37–39]

Ear Infections

Topical preparations of ofloxacin or ciprofloxacin are effective for the treatment of acute otitis media in children with tympanostomy tubes and for chronic suppurative otitis media.[40] Clinical cure rates of >85% for otitis externa can be obtained with the topical preparations. Malignant otitis externa, which is usually caused by *P. aeruginosa*, can be treated with oral ciprofloxacin. A prolonged course is required (3 months) and gives cure rates in excess of 90%.[41]

Acute Exacerbations of Chronic Bronchitis

Fluoroquinolones are among the agents of choice for the management of moderate to severe exacerbations of chronic bronchitis. They have

TABLE 144-4 Dosing Recommendations for Quinolones (From Manufacturers' Data Sheets)

Indication	Norfloxacin po	Ofloxacin po/iv	Ciprofloxacin po	Ciprofloxacin iv	Levofloxacin po/iv	Gemifloxacin po	Prulifloxacin po	Moxifloxacin po/iv
Urinary tract infection	400 mg q12h (3–21 days)	200 mg q12h (3–10 days)	100–500 mg q12 (3–14 days)	200–400 mg q12h (7–14 days)	250 mg q24h (3–10 days)		600 mg q24h (1–10 days)	
Chronic bacterial prostatitis	400 mg q12h (28 days)	300 mg q12h (6 weeks)	500 mg q12h (28 days)	400 mg q12h (28 days)				
Acute sinusitis			500 mg q12h (10 days)	400 mg q12h (10 days)	500 mg q24 (7 days)			400 mg q24h (10 days)
Acute bacterial exacerbation of chronic bronchitis		400 mg q12h (10 days)	500–750 mg q12h (7–14 days)	400 mg q8-12h (7–14 days)	500 mg q24h (7 days)	320 mg q24h (5 days)	600 mg q24h (5–10 days)	400 mg q24h (5 days)
Community-acquired pneumonia		400 mg q12h (10 days)			500 mg q24h (7–14 days)			400 mg q24h (7 days)
Skin and skin structure infection		400 mg q12h (10 days)	500–750 mg q12h (7–14 days)	400 mg q8-12h (7–14 days)	500–750 mg q24h (7–14 days)			400 mg q24h (7 days)
Bone and joint infection			500–750 mg q12h (≥4–6 weeks)	400 mg q8-12h (≥4–6 weeks)				
Intra-abdominal infection			500 mg q12h (7–14 days)	400 mg q12h (7–14 days)				
Infectious diarrhea			500 mg q12h (5–10 days)					
Uncomplicated urethral and cervical gonorrhea	800 mg single dose	400 mg single dose	250 mg single dose					
Nongonococcal cervicitis/urethritis		300 mg q12h (7 days)						
Pelvic inflammatory disease		400 mg q12h (10–14 days)						
Inhalational anthrax (postexposure)			500 mg q12h (60 days)	400 mg q12h (60 days)				

equivalent efficacy to macrolides or β-lactam/β-lactamase inhibitor combinations and achieve cure rates of >90%.[42,43]

Community-Acquired Pneumonia

Older quinolones are not indicated for pneumococcal pneumonia when alternative antibiotics are available. However, results with ciprofloxacin and ofloxacin suggest clinical response and bacterial eradication rates of 90% or greater and, with levofloxacin, equivalence or superiority to ceftriaxone.[44] However, concerns have been raised regarding the efficacy of ciprofloxacin in severe pneumococcal pneumonia following reports of clinical failures.[45] Failures with levofloxacin have also been reported and in Europe it is suggested that it should be given at an increased dose of 500 mg twice daily or in combination with benzyl penicillin in cases of severe pneumonia.[46,47] Recent meta-analyses have suggested the superiority of quinolone therapy over macrolide therapy for community-acquired pneumonia, but the quality of these studies is hampered by the lack of resistance data, varied regimens studied and concerns with the use of macrolide monotherapy, which is not recommended for hospitalized CAP.[48]

Newer agents, such as gemifloxacin and moxifloxacin, which have improved activity against pneumococci and atypical pathogens, show promising results in clinical trials, with clinical cure rates in excess of 90%.[49] Additionally, *in vitro* tests suggest that the use of the most potent agents, or agents of intermediate potency with altered dose administration regimens, may reduce the emergence of resistance.

While high-level penicillin resistance was found to be associated with resistance to older quinolones, such as ciprofloxacin, the newer agents have comparable MIC values for both penicillin-sensitive and penicillin-resistant pneumococci.[50]

Legionellosis can be successfully treated with quinolones such as ciprofloxacin, ofloxacin or levofloxacin. There are few clinical data to show whether or not they are superior to macrolides and often they are given in combination with a macrolide or rifampin (rifampicin)[51] (see also Chapter 28).

Nosocomial Pneumonia

A large-scale study of ciprofloxacin showed equivalence with imipenem in moderately to severely ill patients, most of whom required ventilation and treatment in an intensive care unit.[52] In the 20–25% with infection caused by *P. aeruginosa*, the results with both regimens were less satisfactory, suggesting there are factors other than antimicrobial therapy at play in the outcomes of patients with *P. aeruginosa* pneumonia. Newer fluoroquinolones such as gemifloxacin and moxifloxacin have reduced *in vitro* potency against *P. aeruginosa* and will probably not have a role in the management of hospital-acquired pneumonia where *Pseudomonas* is the likely etiologic agent. A meta-analysis of efficacy in nosocomial pneumonia concluded that quinolones are an acceptable therapy and perform comparably to other standard regimes; the authors noted the importance of considering national and local antibiotic resistance trends when using fluoroquinolones (see Chapter 29).[53]

Cystic Fibrosis

Oral ciprofloxacin is effective for exacerbations caused by *P. aeruginosa*, producing results equivalent to those of standard β-lactam and aminoglycoside therapy. In the UK a 3-week course of ciprofloxacin combined with colistin is recommended for the treatment of early pseudomonal infection[54] (see Chapter 34).

MYCOBACTERIAL INFECTIONS

Older fluoroquinolones have only moderate activity against *Mycobacterium tuberculosis* and current evidence does not support the use of these agents in the treatment of drug-sensitive or resistant tuberculosis. Their role in therapy is currently limited to use in combination regimens for the treatment of multiple drug-resistant *M. tuberculosis* infection.[55] Newer agents such as moxifloxacin have enhanced antimycobacterial activity and its use is now established in the treatment of tuberculosis (see Chapter 31).[56]

As noted above, the susceptibility of nontuberculous mycobacteria to fluoroquinolones is variable. *Mycobacterium avium* complex is relatively resistant to quinolones and these agents are not recommended for first-line treatment of either pulmonary or disseminated infections. The addition of ciprofloxacin to standard therapeutic combinations has been shown to be of benefit in HIV patients with disseminated disease in one study.[57] Nonetheless, there is considerably more experience with alternate agents, such as macrolides, rifampin and ethambutol in combination, and they remain the first-line therapy.[57,58]

Leprosy

Fluoroquinolones in initial clinical trials have been shown highly effective in the treatment of the various forms of leprosy allowing for drastic shortening of the prolonged treatment duration.[58]

SKIN AND SOFT TISSUE INFECTIONS

The fluoroquinolones give excellent results when compared with cephalosporins for the treatment of both uncomplicated and complicated skin and soft tissue infections.[59,60] However, more effective agents are routinely available for gram-positive infections and usefulness in methicillin-resistant *Staph. aureus* (MRSA) infections is limited by high rates of quinolone resistance.

SKELETAL INFECTIONS

Oral fluoroquinolones are highly effective for gram-negative mixed acute (or chronic) contiguous osteomyelitis. They are also effective for postsurgical cases, *Salmonella* osteitis and in some cases of chronic *P. aeruginosa* osteomyelitis (ciprofloxacin), although resistance may emerge causing a failure of treatment or relapse.[61] In patients with orthopedic prostheses infected with staphylococci, ciprofloxacin or ofloxacin in combination with rifampin have been successfully used for conservative management (i.e. preserving the prosthesis).[62,63] The optimal duration of treatment for osteomyelitis has not been systematically studied and much controversy exists, particularly in the management of diabetic foot osteomyelitis. Guidelines suggest that good treatment outcomes are common in patients with acute osteomyelitis with shorter treatments while chronic osteomyelitis in the diabetic foot generally requires longer courses of therapy (>3 months), often in conjunction with surgical management.[64]

GASTROINTESTINAL INFECTIONS

Typhoid and Paratyphoid Fevers

Although fluoroquinolones are widely regarded as the agents of choice for typhoid and paratyphoid fevers,[65,66] a Cochrane systematic review in 2011 concluded there may be some advantage to the use of fluoroquinolones over first-line antibiotics in some settings, but that resistance trends and small studies made it difficult to make firm recommendations. It is therefore paramount for clinicians to be aware of local resistance patterns when managing these infections.[67] One potential advantage of fluoroquinolone therapy is that convalescent excretion states and long-term fecal carriage are rare after fluoroquinolone therapy, thereby reducing the human reservoir and possibly leading to a fall in incidence. Carriage states persisting after other antibiotic therapy may also respond to fluoroquinolones.

Decreased quinolone susceptibility has emerged in Asia over the last 10 years. Strains are typically resistant to nalidixic acid and have raised MICs of ciprofloxacin of 0.5–1 mg/L. These strains are ciprofloxacin susceptible by Clinical and Laboratory Standards Institute (CLSI) or British Society for Antimicrobial Chemotherapy (BSAC) criteria but the clinical response to fluoroquinolones in those infected by these strains is significantly worse than with nalidixic acid-sensitive strains, and longer courses or alternative agents are recommended.[65]

Salmonellosis

A 5- to 7-day course of oral fluoroquinolone is effective in reducing the duration and severity of severe salmonellosis.

Cholera

Three-day courses of oral fluoroquinolones are equal to standard trimethoprim-sulfamethoxazole or tetracycline regimens. A cure rate of >90% can be achieved with a single 1 g dose of ciprofloxacin.[68] Reports have emerged of strains of *Vibrio cholera* 01 with reduced susceptibility to ciprofloxacin, resulting in clinical and bacteriologic treatment failure.[69]

Shigellosis

Fluoroquinolones are the drugs of choice for invasive shigellosis. A single oral dose (ciprofloxacin 1 g) is effective in adults. Rising levels of resistance to nalidixic acid have led to the abandonment of this agent as a first-line treatment for acute shigellosis in some countries.[70]

Campylobacter

Fluoroquinolones have been used for gastrointestinal *Campylobacter* infections. However, resistance levels are increasing and travel-acquired campylobacteriosis appears to be associated with fluoroquinolone resistance in over 60% of cases.[71]

Travelers' Diarrhea

Single-dose fluoroquinolone (e.g. ciprofloxacin 750–1000 mg) in combination with loperamide has been shown to be as effective as longer treatments for travelers' diarrhea. However, the emergence of resistance to fluoroquinolones in many parts of the world has reduced the overall effectiveness of fluoroquinolones for this indication.[72]

OTHER TREATMENT INDICATIONS

Ocular Infections

Topical fluoroquinolones are effective for treatment of bacterial conjunctivitis and keratitis. Penetration of systemic quinolones into the vitreous is relatively good but may not exceed the MICs of all likely pathogens. Intravitreal ciprofloxacin has been used in the treatment of endophthalmitis.[73]

INFECTIONS ASSOCIATED WITH CHRONIC AMBULATORY PERITONEAL DIALYSIS

Ciprofloxacin and ofloxacin have been used with success both orally and intraperitoneally. However, the emergence of resistant staphylococcal infection has limited their usefulness as monotherapy.

Q Fever

Fluoroquinolones are active against *Coxiella burnetii in vitro* and a combination of a fluoroquinolone (ofloxacin) with doxycycline has been suggested for Q fever endocarditis.[74]

Anthrax

A 60-day course of ciprofloxacin is recommended for postexposure prophylaxis against anthrax.[75] In patients with inhalational anthrax a combination of ciprofloxacin plus another active agent (e.g. doxycycline) is recommended.[76]

Meningitis

Fluoroquinolones have been successfully used for gram-negative meningitis.[77] Newer agents such as moxifloxacin show promising results in animal models of pneumococcal meningitis.[78] Trovafloxacin had comparable efficacy to ceftriaxone in a trial of pediatric meningitis.[79]

BK VIRUS INFECTION AND PREVENTION

Several studies have demonstrated modest benefits of ciprofloxacin for the prevention and the treatment of BK virus viremia and viral hemorrhagic cystitis in immunocompromised patients.[80-82] The mechanism appears to be the inhibition of the virus-encoded DNA gyrase of polyomaviruses. Despite the apparent benefit for the prevention of BK-virus infections in immunocompromised hosts, the long-term benefit of prophylaxis has not yet been proven.[83]

CHEMOPROPHYLAXIS

Meningococcal Infection

Single-dose (500 mg) ciprofloxacin is effective in eradicating nasopharyngeal carriage in over 95% of subjects.[84]

Neutropenic Patients

Norfloxacin, ofloxacin and ciprofloxacin have been widely used in the prophylaxis of opportunistic infections among neutropenic patients. Although prophylaxis has been shown to prevent febrile episodes of an infectious nature, current recommendations do not suggest their use due to concerns regarding the emergence and spread of antimicrobial resistance.[85]

Surgical Infections

Fluoroquinolones have been used effectively for the prevention of infection following transurethral prostatectomy and biliary surgery.

PEDIATRIC USE OF FLUOROQUINOLONES

Pediatric use of fluoroquinolones has been limited by concerns regarding arthropathy observed in weight-bearing diarthrodial joints in juvenile dogs after prolonged high-dose administration. In the USA the only current licensed indications for fluoroquinolone use in patients under 18 years of age are complicated UTI, pyelonephritis and postexposure treatment for inhalational anthrax. Nevertheless, accumulated experience has established other situations in which the benefits of fluoroquinolones outweigh potential risks. These include typhoid fever, cholera and shigellosis, complicated UTI due to multiresistant pathogens, chronic suppurative otitis media caused by *P. aeruginosa*, multiresistant gram-negative sepsis (including osteomyelitis), prophylaxis of meningococcemia (single dose) and infection in neutropenia.

Treatment of pseudomonal infections in patients with cystic fibrosis is one of the commonest indications for the use of fluoroquinolones in children. Prolonged courses are often given but there has been little evidence of related arthropathy and fluoroquinolones continue to be widely used.

Dosage in Special Circumstances

RENAL IMPAIRMENT

The extent to which the dosage requires modification is dependent on the degree of renal elimination. Table 144-5 shows the manufacturers' recommendations for selected quinolones.

HEPATIC IMPAIRMENT

Apart for extensively metabolized quinolones, such as pefloxacin, dose modification is not necessary in patients with hepatic impairment. However, experience with newer agents such as moxifloxacin in patients with severe liver failure (Child–Pugh Class C) is limited.

ELDERLY PATIENTS

No specific adjustments in dosage are required for the elderly.

PEDIATRICS

Optimal pediatric doses have not been established. Suggested doses of ciprofloxacin are 7.5–40 mg/kg/day (oral) or 5–10 mg/kg/day (intravenous), administered on an 8–12-hourly basis.

PREGNANCY AND LACTATION

Quinolones are not approved for use in pregnancy or during lactation.

Adverse Reactions and Interactions

ADVERSE DRUG REACTIONS

Fluoroquinolones are generally well tolerated although there are a number of potentially serious adverse effects that have been seen in some agents.[86] When adverse effects are reported, they are usually

TABLE 144-5	Manufacturers' Dosage Recommendations for Patients with Renal Impairment		
	RENAL IMPAIRMENT		Hemodialysis/CAPD
	Mild	Moderate/Severe	
Ciprofloxacin iv		200–400 mg 18–24-hourly (CC = 5–29 mL/min)	
Ciprofloxacin po	250–500 mg q12h (CC = 30–50 mL/min)	250–500 mg 18-hourly (CC = 5–29 mL/min)	250–500 mg q24h after dialysis
Ofloxacin	400 mg q24h (CC = 20–50 mL/min)	200 mg q24h (CC <20 mL/min)	
Levofloxacin	250 mg q24h* (CC = 20–50 mL/min)	250 mg 48-hourly* (CC = 10–19 mL/min)	250 mg 48-hourly* (CC = 10–19 mL/min)
Norfloxacin		400 mg q24h (CC <30 mL/min)	
Gemifloxacin	120 mg q24h (CC <40 mL/min)	120 mg q24h (CC <40 mL/min)	120 mg q24h
Moxifloxacin	No adjustment required		

CC, creatinine clearance.
*Initial loading dose of 500 mg.

gastrointestinal (2–20%), dermatologic (0.5–3%) and CNS (0.5–2%) reactions which rarely necessitate withdrawal of therapy (1–3%). In most cases, there are no specific age, gender or racial predisposing factors.

Most fluoroquinolone adverse drug reactions are class effects, but incidence varies between compounds and can often be related to the specific structure of different agents. Certain group members have specific effects or more serious class effects that have led to restrictions on use or withdrawal. For example, the phototoxicity of sparfloxacin has restricted licensing by some registration authorities (e.g. US FDA), and temafloxacin, which caused hemolytic-uremic syndrome and hypoglycemia, was withdrawn in 1992.

GASTROINTESTINAL REACTIONS

The usual reported symptoms are nausea, anorexia and dyspepsia. While diarrhea, abdominal pain and vomiting are less frequent, they are more likely to result in discontinuation of treatment. Antibiotic-associated diarrhea caused by *Clostridium difficile* is associated with fluoroquinolone use, and all of the available fluoroquinolones have been implicated in *C. difficile* outbreaks.[87] Liver enzyme abnormalities occur in 2–3% of patients receiving fluoroquinolones and are usually mild and reversible. However, more severe liver abnormalities have been seen with some agents which led to the withdrawal of trovafloxacin from the market.

DERMATOLOGIC REACTIONS

Although nonspecific skin rashes, pruritus and urticaria have been reported, it is phototoxicity that has received most attention. This is a class effect and is thought to be related to the photodegradation of the fluoroquinolone and its ability to induce free radicals. The incidence and severity of phototoxicity differ between agents. Structurally, a fluorine moiety at position 8 causes more phototoxicity; sparfloxacin, which has this moiety, has caused a higher rate of phototoxicity. Phototoxic reactions are rare with ciprofloxacin, ofloxacin and levofloxacin. Gemifloxacin can cause a nonphototoxic rash which is seen particularly in female patients between the ages of 20 and 40 years, and postmenopausal women taking hormone replacement therapy; increased risk of rash was also associated with more than 7 days of therapy.[88]

CENTRAL NERVOUS SYSTEM REACTIONS

These occur in less than 2% of patients with most fluoroquinolones and usually manifest as headache, dizziness, mild tremor or drowsiness. Convulsions occur rarely both as a primary effect and as a result of interactions with theophylline or nonsteroidal anti-inflammatory drugs (NSAIDs). Although the mechanism of quinolone toxicity has not been fully elucidated, it is believed to be due to inhibition of $GABA_A$ receptors.

MUSCULOSKELETAL EFFECTS

Fluoroquinolones as a class produce destructive arthropathy in weight-bearing, diarthrodial joints of juvenile animals, notably dogs, by production of cartilage erosions after prolonged high dosage. Some agents, notably precursors such as nalidixic acid, are considerably more likely to induce arthropathy. This effect has never been observed in human children. MRI follow-up and autopsy studies in children receiving both nalidixic acid and modern fluoroquinolones have revealed no evidence of joint damange.[89] Experience with ciprofloxacin in 1500 children noted reversible arthralgia in 3.2% of patients treated for pulmonary exacerbations of cystic fibrosis.[90] In a retrospective study of more 6000 fluoroquinolone-treated children, the incidence of tendon or joint disorders was <1% and comparable to the reference group of azithromycin-treated children.[91]

Tendinitis occurs rarely as a class effect although it may be more common with concomitant corticosteroid therapy. The Achilles tendon is most commonly affected and patients are usually >50 years of age. Discontinuation is recommended at the first sign of tendon pain or inflammation.[92]

CARDIOTOXICITY

Cardiotoxicity is manifest as prolongation of the QT interval with the potential to cause ventricular arrhythmias. The significance of this effect varies between agents and appears to be affected by substitutions at position 5 (see Figure 144-1).[93] Of the currently available fluoroquinolones, the risk of QT interval prolongation appears to be greatest with moxifloxacin and lowest with ciprofloxacin; grepafloxacin was withdrawn voluntarily following reports of seven cardiac-related fatalities. Although adverse events due to cardiotoxicity are rare, the risk can be minimized by avoiding the use of multiple drugs that prolong the QT interval in high-risk patients, for example those with pre-existing cardiac disease or electrolyte disturbances.[94]

DYSGLYCEMIA

Two recent studies found gatifloxacin to be associated with an increased risk of both hypo- and hyperglycemia, probably due to the competing effects of the drug on both the beta cells and islet cells of the pancreas.[95] Gatifloxacin was removed from the market in 2006. In these studies levofloxacin therapy was found to be associated with a slightly increased risk of hypoglycemia, but no dysglycemic risk was noted with moxifloxacin or ciprofloxacin.

RETINAL DETACHMENT

An association between retinal detachment of the rhegmatogenous type and oral fluoroquinolones was established in two cohorts[96,97] with a hazard risk ratio of 2.07 (Cl 1.45–2.96). Retinal detachment occurred 35.5 days from start of treatment. A third study, however, could not support these findings.[98]

OTHER (RARE) EFFECTS

Hypersensitivity occurs at a frequency rate of ~1%. Crystalluria and secondary interstitial nephritis are rare and relate to pH-associated solubility of fluoroquinolones in urine.

INTERACTIONS WITH OTHER DRUGS

Interactions largely occur as a result of interference with fluoroquinolone absorption or by inhibition of biotransformation of unrelated drugs by the hepatic cytochrome P450 isoenzyme system. CNS interactions due to gamma-aminobutyric acid (GABA) receptor inhibition occur with NSAIDs, notably fenbufen, and convulsions may follow, as reported with enoxacin.

INTERACTIONS AFFECTING ABSORPTION OF FLUOROQUINOLONES

The absorption of fluoroquinolones is reduced by up to 80% by co-administration of aluminum- and magnesium-containing antacids, probably by the formation of insoluble complexes and, to a lesser extent, by calcium antacids, sucralfate and ferrous iron preparations. H_2 antagonists have no effect.

INTERACTIONS AFFECTING DRUG METABOLISM

Fluoroquinolones reduce the hepatic clearance of xanthines via the P450 cytochrome system. The effect is most marked with enoxacin and grepafloxacin, but ciprofloxacin and pefloxacin also reduce clearance of theophylline by 30% and co-administration may result in theophylline toxicity, usually nausea but possibly convulsions. Dosage of theophylline should be interrupted or reduced and serum levels monitored if enoxacin, pefloxacin or ciprofloxacin is to be administered.

A similar effect, induced by the same fluoroquinolones, is responsible for inhibition of caffeine metabolism and resultant insomnia. Metabolism of warfarin, cimetidine and ciclosporin is affected much less by P450 cytochrome inhibition and interaction may not be clinically significant.

References available online at expertconsult.com.

KEY REFERENCES

Centers for Disease Control and Prevention (CDC): Update to CDC's sexually transmitted diseases treatment guidelines, 2006: Fluoroquinolones no longer recommended for treatment of gonococcal infections. *MMWR Morb Mortal Wkly Rep* 2007; 56(14):332-336.

Fabrega A., Madurga S., Giralt E., et al.: Mechanism of action of and resistance to quinolones. *Microb Biotechnol* 2009; 2:40-61.

Fillastre J.P., Leroy A., Moulin B., et al.: Pharmacokinetics of quinolones in renal insufficiency. *J Antimicrob Chemother* 1990; 26(Suppl. B):51-60.

Kubin R.: Safety and efficacy of ciprofloxacin in paediatric patients - review. *Infection* 1993; 21:413-421.

Lipsky B.A., Baker C.A.: Fluoroquinolone toxicity profiles: a review focusing on newer agents. *Clin Infect Dis* 1999; 28:352-364.

Lode H., Hoflken G., Boeckk M., et al.: Quinolone pharmacokinetics and metabolism. *J Antimicrob Chemother* 1990; 26(Suppl. B):41-49.

Niederman M.S., Mandell L.A., Anzueto A., et al.: Guidelines for the management of adults with community-acquired pneumonia. Diagnosis, assessment of severity, antimicrobial therapy, and prevention. *Am J Respir Crit Care Med* 2001; 163:1730-1754.

Rubinstein E., Keynan Y.: Quinolones for mycobacterial infections. *Int J Antimicrob Agents* 2013; 42(1):1-4.

Van Bambeke F., Michot J.M., Van Eldere J., et al.: Quinolones in 2005: an update. *Clin Microbiol Infect* 2005; 11:256-280.

Van der Linden P.D., Sturkenboom M.C., Herings R.M., et al.: Increased risk of Achilles tendon rupture with quinolone antibacterial use, especially in the elderly patients taking oral corticosteroids. *Arch Intern Med* 2003; 163:1801-1807.

Warren J.W., Abrutyn E., Hebel J.R., et al.: Guidelines for antimicrobial treatment of uncomplicated acute bacterial cystitis and acute pyelonephritis in women. Infectious Diseases Society of America (IDSA). *Clin Infect Dis* 1999; 29:745-758.

145

Glycopeptides

DIANE M. PARENTE | KERRY L. LAPLANTE

Vancomycin

Vancomycin, a glycopeptide antibiotic that has been available clinically for half a century serves as the primary therapy for gram-positive infections due to methicillin-resistant *Staphylococcus aureus* (MRSA), other methicillin-resistant staphylococci, and ampicillin-resistant *Enterococcus* spp. The spectrum of activity of vancomycin also includes gram-positive anaerobes, diphtheroids and *Clostridium* spp., including *C. difficile*. Isolated from *Amycolatopsis orientalis*, vancomycin binds with high affinity to the D-alanyl-D-alanine (D-Ala-D-Ala) C-terminus of late peptidoglycan precursors and prevents reactions of cell wall synthesis (see Chapter 137).[1]

Its use today is greater than any other point in its history, with the surge in the past two decades of infections caused by β-lactam-resistant staphylococci and enterococci. As a result of increased vancomycin use, vancomycin-resistant enterococci (VRE), vancomycin-intermediate *Staph. aureus* (VISA), and vancomycin-resistant *Staph. aureus* (VRSA) have emerged (see Chapter 138). Recent studies demonstrate increased clinical failure of vancomycin therapy in MRSA infections where the isolates have increased minimum inhibitory concentrations (MICs) that are still within the susceptible range.[2-4] Further, isolates within the susceptible range have also been found to have heteroresistant subpopulations. We refer to these strains as heteroresistant-VISA (hVISA). As a result of these findings the Clinical and Laboratory Standards Institute (CLSI) have adjusted their susceptibility breakpoints (Table 145-1).

Pharmacokinetics and Distribution

Vancomycin is administered orally, intravenously, intraperitoneally and, based on limited data, via the intraventricular, intrathecal and intravitreal routes. The oral formulation is minimally absorbed into the systemic circulation with an oral bioavailability of <10%. However, therapeutic or potentially toxic concentrations of vancomycin have been documented in patients with impaired renal function who were administered oral vancomycin to treat *Clostridium difficile* infection (CDI).[5] Intraperitoneal vancomycin administration is used to treat peritonitis in patients receiving peritoneal dialysis (PD). Peritonitis causes inflammation of the peritoneal membrane, which facilitates absorption of vancomycin from the peritoneal to plasma side of the peritoneum.[6] Systemic absorption of vancomycin following intraperitoneal administration is 54–65% of a given dose in 6 hours and results in adequate serum concentrations.[6] Accumulation to appreciable serum concentrations is highly unlikely when administering vancomycin via intrathecal, intraventricular or intravitreal routes due to the small doses administered.

Data concerning the penetration of vancomycin into various body fluids and body compartments are summarized in Table 145-2.

Depending on the route of administration vancomycin can be excreted through the kidneys, feces, and minimally via the bile. After oral administration vancomycin is extensively concentrated in the feces with a fecal concentration greater than 100 mg/kg following multi-dose administration of 25 mg every 8 hours. Urinary concentration after oral vancomycin is less than 1%. The majority (70–90%) of an intravenous vancomycin dose is excreted unchanged in the urine of adults with normal to moderately impaired renal function through glomerular filtration. Disease states and conditions that affect a patient's renal function will influence vancomycin elimination.

The clearance rate for systemic vancomycin increases in proportion to creatinine clearance (CrCl). Patients with acute renal failure appear to eliminate vancomycin differently from patients with chronic renal failure. In patients with acute oliguric renal failure, substantial non-renal clearance (approximately 16 mL/min; range 3.8–23.3 mL/min)

TABLE 145-1	Vancomycin Susceptibility for *Staphylococcus Aureus*	
Vancomycin Susceptibility	**Abbreviation**	**MIC (µg/mL)**
Susceptible	VSSA	≤2
Heteroresistant	hVISA	1–2*
Intermediate	VISA	4–8
Resistant	VRSA	≥16†

hVISA, heteroresistant vancomycin-intermediate *Staph. aureus*; VISA, vancomycin-intermediate *Staph. aureus*; VRSA, vancomycin-resistant *Staph. aureus*; VSSA, vancomycin-susceptible *Staph. aureus*.
*Consist of subpopulations (≤10⁻⁶) that may grow in media containing >2 µg/mL vancomycin.
†Requires back-up primary testing with 6 µg/mL vancomycin overnight plate.
Data from Clinical Laboratory Standards Institute. Performance standards for antimicrobial disc susceptibility tests; 16th informational supplement. Report M100-S16. Wayne, PA: National Committee for Clinical Laboratory Standards; 2006.

TABLE 145-2	Vancomycin Penetration into Various Human Body Fluids and Tissues Following Intravenous Administration					
Body Fluid Or Tissue	Patient Description	N	Tissue Or Fluid Concentration Range (Mean), mg/L	Concomitant Serum Concentration Range (Mean), mg/L	% Tissue Or Fluid Penetration
Cerebrospinal fluid[7]	Adults receiving ventriculoperitoneal shunts for hydrocephalus	25	0.1–1.5 (0.9)	9.1–38.7 (22.3)	4.6
Cerebrospinal fluid[8]	Hemodialysis adults with proved or suspected central nervous system infection	3*	<0.5–1.54 (0.92)	8.8–24.0 (15.8)	5.9
Cerebrospinal fluid[9]	Premature infants	3	2.2–5.6	–	26–68
Heart valve[10]	Adults undergoing open heart surgery	33	0–2h post-dose: 4.2 5–6h post-dose: 2.3	28.9 4.4	14.5 52.3
Pleural fluid[11]	Critically ill, ventilated patients	14	0.4–8.1 (4.5)	9–37.4 (24)	~18.8
Lung tissue[12]	Adults with normal kidney and liver function undergoing thoracotomy	26	6.9–40.6	2.4–9.6	24–41
Mammary tissue[13] Capsular tissue Pericapsular tissue	Adult women undergoing reconstructive surgery	24	2.0–7.7 (4.6) 2.3–18.1 (6.4)	3.1–38.8 (14.0)	58 74
Peritoneal dialysis fluid[14]	Adults with peritonitis and on chronic intermittent peritoneal dialysis	6	Undetectable to 22.5	–	0–96 (mean, 27)

% Penetration = fluid or tissue vancomycin concentration/serum vancomycin concentration × 100.
*Two cerebrospinal fluid (CSF) and two serum samples obtained during each episode of meningitis.

of vancomycin appears to occur initially. Then, as the duration of renal failure increases, the nonrenal clearance decreases, and eventually approaches the total clearance observed in patients with chronic renal failure (4–6 mL/min).

The elimination half-life of vancomycin is significantly longer in elderly persons aged >65 years (12.1 hours) compared to younger subjects (7.2 hours).[15,16] Vancomycin dosing adjustments may be necessary in the elderly, even those with normal serum creatinine concentrations, due to the longer half-life of vancomycin in this patient population.

An important element that needs to be taken into consideration in patients undergoing hemodialysis is the elimination of vancomycin in different types of membrane and with different dialysis techniques (intermittent and continuous). Although vancomycin is not significantly dialyzable when hemodialysis is performed using a low-flux membrane, significant amounts of vancomycin are cleared in the dialysate with high-flux or high-efficiency hemodialysis using membranes such as polysulfone, polyacrylonitrile and polymethylmethacrylate.[17] Studies estimate that up to 40–50% of vancomycin is removed during high-flux hemodialysis. It is important to note that high-flux membranes have largely replaced traditional low-flux membranes in hemodialysis and dosing of vancomycin needs to reflect this transition in order to maintain adequate vancomycin concentrations in these patients.

In patients undergoing continuous ambulatory peritoneal dialysis (CAPD), the small but continuous drug loss is significant. Vancomycin is often administered intravenously approximately every 3–5 days or administered directly into the peritoneal space to maintain desired plasma concentrations.[18]

Pharmacodynamics

Data correlating pharmacodynamic indices with clinical response to vancomycin are summarized in Table 145-3. Studies suggest that vancomycin has concentration-independent cidal activity over gram-positive organisms, although some investigators propose the need to achieve certain trough concentrations for optimal activity.[19,20] The area under the serum drug concentration-versus time curve and the minimum inhibitory concentration ratio (AUC/MIC) is the preferred

pharmacodynamic parameter for predicting clinical effectiveness. Several studies suggest an AUC/MIC ratio of ≥400 to attain clinical effectiveness.[27] However, measuring multiple vancomycin concentrations to determine AUC/MIC can be difficult in the clinical setting. Therefore, trough serum concentrations, a surrogate marker for AUC, are recommended to monitor vancomycin effectiveness.

In invasive infections such as bacteremia, pneumonia, endocarditis, osteomyelitis and meningitis caused by MRSA the recommended optimal target trough concentration is 15–20 µg/mL and can be achieved by using standard vancomycin doses (15–20 mg/kg every 8–12 hours).[28] Target serum trough concentrations in that range should achieve an AUC/MIC of ≥ 400 in micro-organisms with an MIC of ≤ 1 µg/mL. In micro-organisms with MICs >1 µg/mL, larger doses may be required to achieve target concentrations. However, higher doses may increase a patient's risk of nephrotoxicity.[28]

Route of Administration and Dosage

Vancomycin administration via the oral route is primarily used for the treatment of gastrointestinal infections; primarily caused by *Clostridium difficile* with or without pseudomembranous colitis. Oral preparations of vancomycin are formulated in capsules and solution, and can be administered either by mouth, via nasogastric tube, rectal tube or ileostomy. The standard oral dose in adults ranges from 125 mg or 500 mg every 6 hours.

Intravenous administration of vancomycin is primarily used to treat systemic infections. The recommended dose in adults with normal renal function is 15 to 20 mg/kg every 8–12 hours. Doses should be based on actual body weight and should not exceed 2 g per dose. To prevent infusion-related reactions, vancomycin should be administered at a rate not to exceed 1 g per hour.[29]

Vancomycin may also be administered via intrathecal or intraventricular routes in patients with ventriculitis or shunt infections.

Dosing nomograms for vancomycin are available, but due to the pharmacokinetic variability of vancomycin arising from nonrenal factors, it seems impractical to rely exclusively on nomograms that are based on renal function alone. In addition, studies have shown that the published nomograms may significantly underpredict vancomycin steady-state peak and/or trough concentrations.

TABLE 145-3	Vancomycin Pharmacokinetic and Pharmacodynamic (PD) Data from Select *In Vitro*, Animal and Human Studies Predictive of Success		
Investigators	Organism	Model/Patients	PD Index Parameter
Larsson et al.[19]	Staphylococcus aureus	In vitro PD model	T >MIC ~100%
Duffull et al.[20]	Staphylococcus aureus	In vitro PD model	T >MBC ~100%
Ackerman et al.[21]	Staphylococcus aureus CONS	In vitro model	No relationship between VAN concentration and killing curves
Knudsen et al.[22]	Staphylococcus aureus Streptococcus pneumoniae	Murine peritonitis	T >MIC, C_{max}:MIC, AUC_{24h}:MIC
Ahmed et al.[23]	Streptococcus pneumoniae	Rabbit meningitis model	CSF C_{max}:MBC ≥4
Lisby-Sutch and Nahata[24]	Staphylococcus aureus CONS Enterococcus, group D	Infants with a variety of infections	C_{max} 25–35 mg/L (SBT ≥1:8) C_{min} 5–10 mg/L (SBT 1:2 to 1:8)
Schaad et al.[15]	Staphylococcus aureus Staphylococcus epidermidis	Children with a variety of infections	C_{max}>25 mg/L (SBT ~ 1:16) C_{min}<12 mg/L (SBT~1:4)
Iwamoto et al.[25]	MRSA	Patients with pneumonia or bacteremia	C_{max}>25 mg/L C_{min} 10–15 mg/L
Moise et al.[26]	MRSA	Adults with lower respiratory tract infections	Clinical success: AUC_{24h}:MIC >345 Bacterial eradication: AUC_{24h}:MIC >428

CONS, coagulase-negative staphylococci; CSF, cerebrospinal fluid; MBC, minimum bactericidal concentration; MIC, minimum inhibitory concentration; MRSA, methicillin-resistant *Staph. aureus*; SBT, serum bactericidal titers; AUC, area under the curve; VAN, vancomycin.

Monitoring

At this time, there appears to be no benefit in monitoring peak vancomycin serum concentrations. Trough concentrations are monitored and drawn 30–60 minutes before the fourth dose in patients whose CrCl is in steady state, and then weekly for patients on vancomycin therapy for more than 2 weeks. Ideally, a baseline serum creatinine concentration and complete blood count are obtained before vancomycin therapy is initiated and then weekly thereafter. If the CrCl is not in steady state or if the patient is receiving other nephrotoxic agents, such as aminoglycosides or amphotericin B, serum creatinine and vancomycin serum troughs may need more frequent monitoring (two or three times per week). If serum creatinine concentrations increase by more than 0.5 mg/dL over the baseline value (or more than 25–30% over baseline for serum creatinine values >2 mg/dL), and other causes of decrease in renal function are ruled out, alternatives for vancomycin may be warranted.

Indications

SKIN AND SOFT TISSUE AND OSTEOMYELITIS

While several antibiotics are FDA-approved for the treatment of severe acute bacterial skin and skin structure infections (ABSSSI) caused by MRSA in adult patients, none have demonstrated superiority over vancomycin. Using standard vancomycin intravenous dosing recommendations, MRSA ABSSSI infections can be treated with vancomycin typically for 7–14 days but should be individualized to the patient's clinical response. Vancomycin is also the primary treatment option for MRSA osteomyelitis and may be used in combination with rifampin to improve response rates. The recommended duration of treatment for MRSA osteomyelitis is at least 8 weeks.

PNEUMONIA

In patients with confirmed MRSA pneumonia, high vancomycin failure rates have been reported. These high failure rates may be due to vancomycin underdosing or poor penetration into pulmonary tissue.[30] Alternative antibiotics such as linezolid achieve higher concentrations in pulmonary tissue and in two clinical trials had comparable cure rates to that of vancomycin.[31,32] Another multicenter randomized control trial demonstrated significantly higher cure rates with linezolid in comparison to vancomycin for the treatment of MRSA nosocomial

pneumonia (57.6% vs 46.6%; p = 0.042) but no difference in 60-day mortality.[33] A majority of patients in the vancomycin arm had subtherapeutic vancomycin trough concentrations, concomitant bacteremia and kidney disease.

BACTEREMIA AND ENDOCARDITIS

Vancomycin is currently the standard therapy for the treatment of MRSA bacteremia and endocarditis at standard recommended doses. When the causative organism is MSSA, β-lactams are preferred over intravenous vancomycin because poorer outcomes have been demonstrated with vancomycin.[34] The recommended duration of treatment with vancomycin is 2–6 weeks and at least 6 weeks for MRSA bacteremia and endocarditis, respectively.[35] Enterococcal endocarditis can be treated with vancomycin in combination with an aminoglycoside when the infected organism is resistant to ampicillin.[35]

CLOSTRIDIUM DIFFICILE COLITIS

Oral vancomycin is one of three antibiotics available for the treatment of Clostridium difficile infection (CDI). In patients with severe uncomplicated CDI the recommended dose is 125 mg by mouth four times a day. In patients with severe complicated CDI, intravenous metronidazole should be added and the vancomycin dose increased to 500 mg administered either orally or via nasogastric tube. Further, adding a rectal instillation of vancomycin 500 mg every 4–12 hours may be considered in patients with a complete ileus. In mild CDI cases, studies have shown no differences in outcome and, in the effort to reduce the emergence of VRE, vancomycin should only be used when patients are not responding or are intolerant to metronidazole, or pregnant. The recommended duration of vancomycin therapy for CDI is 10–14 days (see Chapter 40).[36]

Dosage in Special Circumstances

As described above, vancomycin dose or frequency adjustments may be necessary in patients with advanced age, obesity or burns. Actual body weight is used to determine the initial dose (15–20 mg/kg) and adjustments are made based on serum trough concentrations. In obese and burn patients intravenous vancomycin may require more frequent dosing due to higher volumes of distribution and/or CrCl.

In patients with renal impairment vancomycin doses are typically that of standard doses (15–20 mg/kg) but the dosing interval is typically extended with CrCl <49 mL/min. Determining vancomycin dosing regimens for patients on hemodialysis is challenging and requires consideration of the following factors: body weight, timing of vancomycin administration and type of dialysis membranes. Vancomycin hemodialysis protocols vary between institutions. A recent hemodialysis vancomycin dosing protocol factoring a patient's weight was derived from a Monte Carlo simulation. Based on this validated protocol patients who weigh <70 kg should receive a loading dose (LD) of 1 g and a maintenance dose (MD) of 500 mg infused over the last 30 minutes of dialysis; 70–100 kg patients should receive a LD of 1.25 g and then a MD of 750 mg infused over the last hour of dialysis; > 100 kg patients should receive a LD of 1.5 g followed by a MD of 1 g infused over the last 90 minutes of dialysis.[37] Vancomycin trough levels should be obtained before each dialysis session to guide therapy.

Adverse Reactions and Interactions

Ototoxicity (<2%) and nephrotoxicity (5–43%) are well-recognized adverse events associated with vancomycin therapy and may be concentration related.[25,21] While many studies suggest that the current preparations of vancomycin may have less potential for nephrotoxicity than earlier preparations, increasing reports of vancomycin-induced nephrotoxicity have been reported when targeting 15–20 mg/L trough concentrations. In a meta-analysis comparing trough concentrations, the overall rates of vancomycin-induced nephrotoxicity ranged from 5–43%.[38] The highest rates of nephrotoxicity occurred in patients with other risk factors for nephrotoxicity. These data suggest that while vancomycin may not be solely responsible for nephrotoxicity, a vancomycin trough >15 mg/L was still independently associated with higher odds of nephrotoxicity. When vancomycin was administered concomitantly with an aminoglycoside to adults, the incidence of nephrotoxicity is higher in some of the studies (range 22–35%).[39-42] A higher incidence of acute kidney injury has also been reported with combination vancomycin and piperacillin-tazobactam (range 16.3–36.4%).[43-45] Other risk factors that may also increase the risk of developing nephrotoxicity include patients with neutropenia, peritonitis, increased age, male gender, liver disease, and receipt of contrast dye, concurrent amphotericin B, loop diuretic, nonsteroidal anti-inflammatory (NSAID), angiotensin-converting enzyme inhibitor (ACEI), or vasopressor therapy.

Investigations on vancomycin-induced ototoxicity (hearing loss or tinnitus) have raised the possibility that ototoxicity may be related to excessively high serum concentrations (>80 mg/L), with recommendations to avoid serum vancomycin concentrations >50 mg/L.[39,46] A comparison of once- versus twice-daily vancomycin found no statistically different rates in ototoxicity rates.[47]

Nonconcentration-related toxicities have also been reported with vancomycin. Rapid intravenous infusion of vancomycin, >500 mg per 30 minutes in normal adults, may result in a non-IgE-mediated histamine reaction characterized by flushing, local pruritus, erythema of the neck and upper torso, tachycardia and/or hypotension.[48,49] This reaction, often referred to as 'red man syndrome', may occur at any point in the infusion and may occur for the first time after several doses or with slow infusion.[49] The effects of this reaction can be relieved by antihistamines.[50,51] The incidence of red man syndrome varies between 3.7% and 47% in infected patients.[52] Use of concomitant opiates for analgesia can potentiate mast cell destabilization of vancomycin and may increase the risk for red man syndrome.[53] Eosinophilia, neutropenia, rashes (including exfoliative dermatitis), Stevens–Johnson syndrome (infrequent), immune-mediated thrombocytopenia and drug fever also have been reported with vancomycin.

Telavancin

In 2009 the US Food and Drug Administration (FDA) approved the first antimicrobial of the lipoglycopeptide class, telavancin, a semisynthetic derivative of vancomycin. In comparison to the chemical structure of vancomycin, telavancin contains an additional lipophilic side chain attached to the heptapeptide core and a negatively charged hydrophilic group.[54] These structural alterations improve binding affinity, and increase antibacterial activity, distribution, and clearance.

Unlike vancomycin, telavancin causes depolarization of the gram-positive bacterial membrane, thereby disrupting membrane potential and alterations in cellular permeability in both a time- and dose-dependent manner. This mechanism of action allows telavancin to be rapidly bactericidal.[54] Telavancin also shows bactericidal activity against MRSA and MSSA in their non-growing phase.[55]

Telavancin exhibits concentration-dependent, bactericidal activity against gram-positive micro-organisms (MRSA, MSSA, *Streptococcus pyogenes*, *Strep. agalactiae*, *Strep. anginosus* spp., vancomycin-susceptible *Enterococcus faecalis*) and no activity against gram-negative micro-organisms.

Pharmacokinetics and Distribution

Telavancin is approximately 93% protein-bound, primarily to serum albumin. Protein binding is not disturbed by renal or hepatic dysfunction. Telavancin does not undergo extensive metabolism and is excreted primarily in the kidneys (approximately 76% of the administered dose recovered in urine). The terminal elimination half-life of telavancin is approximately 8 hours. As with vancomycin, renal impairment increases the exposure to telavancin.

Administration and Dosage

Telavancin is administered once daily as a 1-hour intravenous infusion. A dose of 10 mg/kg/day (actual body weight) is recommended for the treatment of complicated skin and skin structure infections (CSSSIs) and nosocomial pneumonia (hospital-acquired and ventilator-associated) in adults with a CrCl >50 mL/min.

Indications

Telavancin is FDA-approved for the treatment of adults with complicated skin and soft tissue infections (cSSSI) caused by susceptible gram-positive micro-organisms, and hospital-acquired pneumonia (HAP) and ventilator-associated pneumonia (VAP) caused by MRSA and MSSA. Based on pooled clinical cure rates, telavancin demonstrated noninferiority to vancomycin for the treatment of cSSSIs caused by gram-positive pathogens.[56]

Dosage in Special Circumstances

In patients with renal impairment, dose adjustments are required. Renal dose adjustments are as follows: in patients with a CrCl (estimated using Cockcroft and Gault) between 30 and 50 mL/min, a dose of 7.5 mg/kg every 24 hours is recommended and those with a CrCl 10–29 mL/min the dose is 10 mg/kg every 48 hours. Dosage recommendations are not known for patients with a CrCl <10 mL/min or in those undergoing hemodialysis. Telavancin contains hydroxypropyl-beta-cyclodextrin, an ingredient to increase solubility, which is excreted in urine. In patients with renal impairment, accumulation may occur. The clinical significance of this accumulation is unknown. In patients with moderate hepatic impairment (Child-Pugh Class B) dose adjustments are not needed. Caution should be taken when administering telavancin in patients with severe hepatic impairment.

Adverse Reactions and Interactions

The highest concern of telavancin use is in regards to the safety profile. Telavancin has been associated with higher nephrotoxicity in comparison to vancomycin, particularly in patients with pre-existing renal impairment (CrCl <50 mL/min) or receiving concomitant nephrotoxic agents despite renal dose adjustment.[56,57]

In addition, patients with a CrCl <50 mL/min randomized to telavancin in two HAP/ VAP clinical trials had lower survival rates than those who received vancomycin (CrCl <50 mL/min, 59% vs 70%; CrCl <30 mL/min, 47% vs 61%; respectively).[58] Further investigation is warranted to clarify whether this finding is an issue of efficacy or safety.

Due to the increased risk of nephrotoxicity and mortality, telavancin should only be considered when alternative agents have been exhausted in renally impaired patients.

The most common adverse reactions reported in ≥5% phase III randomized clinical trials included metallic or soapy taste disturbance, nausea, vomiting and foamy urine and were described as mild to moderate in intensity and reversible.[56,57] Similar to vancomycin, symptoms associated with red man syndrome may occur with rapid infusion of telavancin.

Telavancin does not appear to be associated with any clinically relevant drug–drug interactions. Telavancin may falsely increase the values of coagulation tests when drawn up to 18 hours after the infusion. Therefore coagulation tests should be collected prior to telavancin administration.

Dalbavancin

Dalbavancin is a concentration-dependent bactericidal, semisynthetic lipoglycopeptide that inhibits cell wall synthesis. The use of dalbavancin in the USA was approved by the FDA in 2014. Dalbavancin is derived from a teicoplanin-like antibiotic produced naturally by actinomycete *Nonomuraea* spp. The chemical structure of dalbavancin includes a basic amide to improve activity against staphylococci, and a long lipophilic side chain which provides a prolonged half-life and enhances affinity for the terminal D-Ala-D-Ala. Similar to telavancin, dalbavancin has a spectrum of activity only against gram-positive micro-organisms including, MSSA, MRSA, *Strep. epidermidis, Strep. pneumoniae* (including penicillin-resistant) and enterococci with the exception of VanA-type enterococci.

Due to dalbavancin's long half-life, fewer antimicrobial administrations can potentially reduce healthcare costs while improving adherence and convenience. Dalbavancin appears to be a safe, effective therapeutic option, particularly in patients who are candidates for outpatient therapy.

Pharmacokinetics and Distribution

Dalbavancin exhibits linear, dose-proportional pharmacokinetics when administered in healthy patients. Reversible plasma protein binding of dalbavancin is 93–98% resulting in a long half-life of approximately 6–11 days. In comparison to telavancin and oritavancin, dalbavancin achieves the highest concentration in blister fluid (40% and 19% vs 60%, respectively).[59] Dalbavancin is not a substrate or inducer of CYP450 isoenzymes. The clearance of dalbavancin occurs through renal (45%) and fecal routes (20%) over 42 and 70 days, respectively, after a single 1 g intravenous dose.

ROUTE OF ADMINISTRATION AND DOSAGE

Dalbavancin is only available in intravenous formulation due to its poor absorption when administered orally. The standard administration of dalbavancin is a two-dose regimen of 1000 mg followed by a 500 mg dose 1 week later infused over 30 minutes.

Indications

Currently dalbavancin is only FDA-approved for the treatment of ABSSSI caused by susceptible gram-positive bacteria including MRSA. In phase III clinical trials dalbavancin was noninferior to vancomycin, linezolid and cefazolin.[60-63] In two phase III randomized double-blind double-dummy clinical trials, intravenous dalbavancin (1000 mg followed 1 week later by 500 mg) was compared with intravenous vancomycin (1000 mg or 15 mg/kg every 12 hours) with the option to switch to oral linezolid after 3 days for the treatment of ABSSSIs.[63] The primary endpoint clinical response at 48–72 hours after initiation of therapy in the first phase III trial was 83.3% and 81.8% in the dalbavancin and vancomycin/linezolid groups, respectively. In the second phase III trial the clinical response rates at 48–72 hours were 76.8% and 78.3%, respectively.

Dosage in Special Circumstances

Renal dose adjustments are not necessary in patients with an estimated CrCl of greater 30 mL/min or receiving hemodialysis three times a week (<6% of an administered dose is removed during a 3-hour hemodialysis session). However, dose adjustments are required in patients with a CrCl less than 30 mL/min or when hemodialysis is not regularly scheduled whereby the two-dose regimen is reduced to 750 mg then 375 mg 1 week later. In patients with mild hepatic impairment (Child-Pugh Class A) the standard dose can be administered. The use of dalbavancin should be used cautiously in patients with moderate to severe hepatic impairment (Child-Pugh Class B or C) until data regarding appropriate dosing are available. Factors such as gender, age, race, and serum albumin do not alter the pharmacokinetics of dalbavancin and therefore do not require any dose adjustments based on these factors alone.

Adverse Reactions and Interactions

Dalbavancin appears to be generally well tolerated and reported adverse drug events in clinical trials were similar to linezolid, cefazolin, cephalexin and vancomycin. The most common adverse events reported in phase II and III clinical trials (1778 total patients) included nausea (5.5%), headache (4.7%), and diarrhea (4.4%). A concern in an agent with a long half-life such as dalbavancin are late-onset events; however, the rate of such events were comparable with vancomycin and linezolid.[63] At the time of writing, no drug–drug interactions were identified in the published literature with the concomitant use of dalbavancin.

Oritavancin

Oritavancin is a concentration-dependent, bactericidal, intravenous, semisynthetic glycopeptide derived from naturally occurring chloroeremomycin. Oritavancin exhibits three mechanisms of action, inhibition of cell wall synthesis during transglycosylation (polymerization) and transpeptidation (crosslinking) steps as well as disruption of cell wall membrane function. Oritavancin may have clinical implications in the treatment of slow-growing or biofilm-producing micro-organisms because it is able to dissipate membrane potential in both stationary and exponential growth phases. While the spectrum of activity of oritavancin is similar to that of other glycopeptides, compared to dalbavancin and telavancin, oritavancin maintains activity against VanA VRE.

Oritavancin has the longest half-life (>10 days) of the glycopeptide class. However, the long half-life of oritavancin has also raised concerns with respect to delayed hypersensitivity reactions or other potential toxicities. Clinically, oritavancin provides another option for patients who cannot receive standard therapies or in patients who are candidates for outpatient therapy where compliance may be problematic. Of the currently available glycopeptides, oritavancin is the only agent with activity against VanA and VanB enterococci. Pending further study, oritavancin may potentially have a role in the treatment of VRE infections.

Pharmacokinetics and Distribution

Due to poor absorption from the gastrointestinal tract, oritavancin is administered intravenously to achieve therapeutic systemic concentrations. Oritavancin displays linear pharmacokinetics at doses up to 1200 mg. Protein binding of oritavancin is approximately 85% with extensive distribution into tissue. Oritavancin is slowly excreted unchanged in the urine with less than 5% recovered in urine and less than 1% in feces after 2 weeks.

Route of Administration and Dosage

In adults, oritavancin is administered as a single 1200 mg dose infused intravenously over 3 hours.

TABLE 145-4	Administration Route, Recommended Standard Dose and Dose Adjustments in Special Circumstances of Glycopeptides and Lipoglycopeptides		
Drug	**Administration Route**	**Recommended Dose**	**Dose Adjustments in Special Circumstances**
Vancomycin	Intravenous Oral	15–20 mg every 8–12 hours 125–500 mg every 6 hours	Renal impairment (CrCl < 49 mL/min), hemodialysis, advanced age, obesity, burn patients
Telavancin	Intravenous	10 mg/kg/day	Renal impairment (CrCl < 50 mL/min)
Dalbavancin	Intravenous	1000 mg followed by 500 mg 1 week later	Renal impairment (CrCl <30 mL/min) or hemodialysis not regularly scheduled
Oritavancin	Intravenous	One dose of 1500 mg	None
Teicoplanin	Intravenous Oral	Loading dose: 6–2 mg/kg every 12 hours for 3 doses Maintenance dose: 6–12 mg/kg/day 100–400 mg every 12 hours	Maintenance dose: renal impairment (CrCl 40–60 mL/min)

Indications

In 2014, oritavancin was FDA-approved for adults with ABSSSI caused by susceptible gram-positive pathogens. One phase II and two phase III trials were conducted using oritavancin in patients with ABSSSI.[64-66] The two phase III trials were identically designed, double-blind, multicenter, randomized, controlled trials (n = 1959). Patients were randomly assigned to receive either a single intravenous 1200 mg dose of oritavancin or intravenous vancomycin (1 g or 15 mg/kg every 12 hours) for 7–10 days. The efficacy primary endpoint in both trials was early clinical response (defined as cessation of spread or reduction in size of baseline lesion, absence of fever and no rescue antibacterial drug at 40–72 hours after initiation of therapy). In the first phase III trial, early clinical response rates were 82.3% and 78.9% in the oritavancin and vancomycin groups, respectively. Similar results were observed in the second phase III trial with rates of 80.1% and 82.9%. The use of oritavancin is currently limited to ABSSSI.

Dosage in Special Circumstances

Population pharmacokinetics analyses of oritavancin were conducted in phase III ABSSSI trials in patients with normal renal function (CrCl ≥ 80 mL/min), mild renal impairment (CrCl 50–79 mL/min) and moderate renal impairment (30–49 mL/min). Based on the analysis, dose adjustments are not needed in patients with mild to moderate renal insufficiency.[65,66] Dosing in patients with severe renal impairment or in hemodialysis have not yet been evaluated. In normal and moderate (Child–Pugh Class B) hepatic dysfunction, no dose adjustments of oritavancin are necessary. Whether the dose should be adjusted in patients with severe hepatic insufficiency is currently unknown.

Adverse Reactions and Interactions

In a pooled analysis of phase III ABSSSI clinical trials, adverse events that were drug-related (22.2% vs 28.4%), severe (5.2% vs 4.9%), or led to the discontinuation of the agent (3.7% vs 4.2%) were similar among patients who received oritavancin (n = 976) or vancomycin (n = 983), respectively.[65,66] The most commonly reported side effects in patients receiving oritavancin were nausea (9.9%), headache (7.1%), vomiting (4.6%), limb and subcutaneous abscess (3.8%), and diarrhea (3.7%).[65,66]

More cases of osteomyelitis in phase III ABSSSI clinical trials were reported in the oritavancin group (n = 6) than in the vancomycin group (n = 1). This led to a warning in the package insert. Although oritavancin did not exhibit a higher adverse event rate over 60 days compared with vancomycin in clinical trials, clinicians should be cautious in patients with a history of adverse effects to antimicrobials due to oritavancin's long half-life.

Oritavancin is a weak inducer of CYP3A4 and CYP2D6 as well as a weak inhibitor of CYP2C19 and CYP2C9. Caution and close monitoring should be used when administering oritavancin with drugs that are affected by these CYP450 enzymes, as oritavancin can decrease (CYP3A4 and CYP2D6 substrates) or increase (CYP2C10 and CYP2C9 substrates) the concentrations of these drugs.

The co-administration of oritavancin and warfarin may result in higher warfarin exposure leading to an increase risk in bleed. Oritavancin has been shown to falsely prolong activated partial thromboplastin time (aPTT) for 48 hours, and the prothrombin time (PT) and international normalized ratio (INR) for 24 hours. Therefore, monitoring the anticoagulation effect of warfarin may be unreliable in the first 24 hours after an oritavancin dose.

Other Therapies in the Glycopeptide Class

Teicoplanin

Teicoplanin is currently not approved by the FDA for use in the USA but is widely used in Europe, Asia and South America. Formerly called teichomycin A, teicoplanin is structurally similar to vancomycin and it is produced from the actinomycete *Actinoplanes teichomyceticus*. Teicoplanin binds to the terminal D-Ala-D-Ala sequence of peptides that form the bacterial cell wall.

Teicoplanin is similar but not identical to vancomycin in its spectrum of activity. The MICs for most gram-positive bacteria and anaerobes are comparable, but teicoplanin is less active against some strains of *Staph. haemolyticus* (MIC 16–64 mg/L compared to ≤4 mg/L for vancomycin). Both VanA-type VRE and VISA isolates are also resistant to teicoplanin.

Similar to vancomycin, teicoplanin's oral formulation is primarily used to treat CDI. The oral dose recommendation for teicoplanin is 100–400 mg by mouth every 12 hours for 10 days.[67] The recommended dosing regimen for intravenous teicoplanin in adults with normal renal function includes a LD ranging between 6 mg/kg and 12 mg/kg given every 12 hours for three doses, followed by a MD ranging from 6 mg/kg/day to 12 mg/kg/day.[68] Monitoring serum trough concentrations are not typically required unless the patient is receiving high doses (12 mg/kg), receiving treatment for a serious infection (endocarditis), has unstable renal function or is not responding to therapy. Target trough levels should be between 10–20 μg/mL. All patients regardless of renal function should receive LDs. For patients with a CrCl between 40 and 60 mL/min, the frequency of MDs should be increased to every 48–72 hours.

Teicoplanin has shown to be effective in the treatment of skin and soft tissue infections, pneumonia, febrile neutropenia, catheter-related infections and CDI caused by susceptible pathogens.

In both open and comparative clinical trials, teicoplanin has been well tolerated, and adverse reactions have rarely prompted discontinuation of treatment.[68,69] In comparison to vancomycin, nephrotoxicity caused by teicoplanin is uncommon, even when it is used concomitantly with aminoglycosides.

A summary of administration routes, recommended standard doses and dose adjustments in glycopeptides and lipoglycopeptides can be found in Table 145-4.

References available online at expertconsult.com.

KEY REFERENCES

Ackerman B.H., Vannier A.M., Eudy E.B.: Analysis of vancomycin time-kill studies with *Staphylococcus* species by using a curve stripping program to describe the relationship between concentration and pharmacodynamic response. *Antimicrob Agents Chemother* 1992; 36(8): 1766-1769.

Alwakeel J., Najjar T.A., al-Yamani M.J., et al.: Comparison of the effects of three haemodialysis membranes on vancomycin disposition. *Int Urol Nephrol* 1994; 26(2): 223-228.

De Lalla F., Nicolin R., Rinaldi E., et al.: Prospective study of oral teicoplanin versus oral vancomycin for therapy of pseudomembranous colitis and *Clostridium difficile*-associated diarrhea. *Antimicrob Agents Chemother* 1992; 36:2192-2196.

Hidayat L.K., Hsu D.I., Quist R., et al.: High-dose vancomycin therapy for methicillin-resistant *Staphylococcus aureus* infections: efficacy and toxicity. *Arch Intern Med* 2006; 166(19):2138-2144.

Matzke G.R., McGory R.W., Halstenson C.E., et al.: Pharmacokinetics of vancomycin in patients with various degrees of renal function. *Antimicrob Agents Chemother* 1984; 25(4):433-437.

Paton T.W., Cornish W.R., Manuel M.A., et al.: Drug therapy in patients undergoing peritoneal dialysis. Clinical pharmacokinetic considerations. *Clin Pharmacokinet* 1985; 10(5):404-425.

Rubinstein E., Lalani T., Corey G.R., et al.: Telavancin versus vancomycin for hospital-acquired pneumonia due to gram-positive pathogens. *Clin Infect Dis* 2011; 52(1): 31-40.

Rybak M.J., Lomaestro B., Rotschafer J.C., et al.: Therapeutic monitoring of vancomycin in adult patients: a consensus review of the American Society of Health-System Pharmacists, the Infectious Diseases Society of America, and the Society of Infectious Diseases Pharmacists. *Am J Health Syst Pharm* 2009; 66(1): 82-98.

Soriano A., Marco F., Martinez J.A., et al.: Influence of vancomycin minimum inhibitory concentration on the treatment of methicillin-resistant *Staphylococcus aureus* bacteremia. *Clin Infect Dis* 2008; 46(2):193-200.

Stryjewski M.E., Graham D.R., Wilson S.E., et al.: Telavancin versus vancomycin for the treatment of complicated skin and skin-structure infections caused by Gram-positive organisms. *Clin Infect Dis* 2008; 46(11): 1683-1693.

Tenover F.C., Moellering R.C. Jr: The rationale for revising the Clinical and Laboratory Standards Institute vancomycin minimal inhibitory concentration interpretive criteria for *Staphylococcus aureus*. *Clin Infect Dis* 2007; 44(9):1208-1215.

Van Hal S.J., Paterson D.L., Lodise T.P.: Systematic review and meta-analysis of vancomycin-induced nephrotoxicity associated with dosing schedules that maintain troughs between 15 and 20 milligrams per liter. *Antimicrob Agents Chemother* 2013; 57(2):734-744.

146

Tetracyclines and Chloramphenicol

JASON M. POGUE | MICHAEL N. DUDLEY | AMBIKA ERANKI |
KEITH S. KAYE

KEY POINTS

- The tetracyclines are broad-spectrum bacteriostatic antibiotics, with a wide range of clinical indications.

- The second-generation tetracyclines, doxycycline and minocycline, have essentially replaced tetracycline in clinical practice due to enhanced spectrum of activity and improved pharmacokinetics allowing less frequent dosing.

- The tetracyclines are highly bioavailable and oral doses of doxycycline and minocycline give similar concentrations to intravenous formulations.

- The tetracyclines are widely distributed in the body and thus a potential treatment option for a wide array of infections.

- Doxycycline remains the drug of choice in many instances for the treatment of Lyme disease.

- Tigecycline and, to a lesser degree, minocycline have an emerging role in the treatment of multidrug-resistant organisms, notably carbapenem-resistant gram-negative bacilli.

- Resistance to tetracyclines is mediated via ribosomal protection proteins and multidrug efflux pumps. Tigecycline avoids most tetracycline resistance mechanisms.

- Tetracyclines should be avoided in children <8 years old due to the risk of enamel hypoplasia. Use should also be avoided in pregnant patients.

- Tetracyclines can chelate with divalent cations in the gastrointestinal tract which can block absorption. They should be separated from supplements and multivitamins containing divalent cations (e.g. calcium, iron, magnesium).

Tetracyclines

Introduction

In 1948, Benjamin Duggar at the Lederle Laboratories isolated an antibiotic from a fungus producing a golden pigment called *Streptomyces aureofaciens* and the first tetracycline, chlortetracycline was identified. In 1953 tetracycline was produced semisynthetically from chlortetracycline; longer-acting tetracyclines, doxycycline and minocycline, were synthesized in 1966 and 1972, respectively.

In response to the increasing incidence of bacterial resistance to tetracyclines, a research program was initiated at Lederle Laboratories in the 1990s to seek new third-generation tetracyclines that would circumvent existing mechanisms of resistance. This led to the discovery of the glycylcyclines and the development of 9-(t-butylglycylamido)-minocycline (tigecycline) as a new therapeutic agent.

Chemically, the tetracyclines have a hydronaphthacene nucleus containing four fused rings. Specific analogs are obtained by substitutions at the fifth, sixth, seventh or ninth positions (Figure 146-1).

Tetracyclines are considered bacteriostatic agents in that they bind to the 30S subunits of the ribosomes in susceptible micro-organisms, inhibiting protein synthesis. However, there may be bactericidal effects against some pathogens. They have a weak association with the eukaryote 80S ribosomal subunit, which explains the general lack of toxic effects that can be associated with this action. However, they do inhibit mitochondrial protein synthesis in parasitic eukaryotes at the 70S subunit, which partially explains the antiparasitic activity of these agents (see also Chapter 137).

Second-generation tetracyclines (doxycycline and minocycline) are primarily used due to improved potency and more favorable pharmacokinetics and tolerability compared to tetracycline, allowing use for a broader spectrum of indications, and less frequent dosing. Tigecycline, available only intravenously, is FDA-approved for the treatment of complicated skin and skin-structure and intra-abdominal infections. In addition, the second-generation tetracyclines and tigecycline are increasingly used for treatment of drug-resistant organisms, notably carbapenem-resistant gram-negative bacilli.

Antimicrobial Spectrum

The tetracyclines have broad-spectrum activity against a variety of gram-positive and gram-negative bacteria, obligate intracellular bacteria (notably *Chlamydia*, *Legionella* and *Rickettsia* spp.) and importantly, potent activity against *Borrelia burgdorferi* (Table 146-1). The development of resistance has limited the activity of tetracycline against multiple organisms, including *Streptococcus pneumoniae*, *Staphylococcus aureus*, *Enterococcus* spp., *Acinetobacter* spp. and some Enterobacteriaceae. Doxycycline and minocycline often exhibit improved *in vitro* activity compared to tetracycline[1,2] against these organisms, but resistance is common in *Strep. pneumoniae*, many enterococci and Enterobacteriaceae. Importantly, minocycline and, to a lesser extent, doxycycline often retains excellent activity against drug-resistant organisms including methicillin-resistant *Staphylococcus aureus* (MRSA) and multidrug-resistant (MDR) *A. baumannii*. Tigecycline has expanded activity that includes potent coverage against vancomycin-resistant enterococci (VRE), MRSA and, often, carbapenem-resistant Enterobacteriaceae (CRE).[3,4] Tigecycline is active against many organisms displaying resistance to earlier tetracyclines.[5] *Proteus* spp. and *Pseudomonas* spp. are intrinsically resistant through expression of chromosomally encoded multidrug efflux pumps from the resistance–nodulation–division (RND) family.[6,7] Tetracyclines also retain activity against *Helicobacter pylori*, and can be used as second-line therapy.

Resistance (see Chapter 138)

Extensive use of tetracyclines in humans and in the veterinary field as growth promoters led to widespread selection and dissemination among bacteria of genetic determinants encoding ribosomal protection proteins (RPP) and major facilitator superfamily (MFS) drug efflux pump-mediated resistance mechanisms.[5] Most of these acquired tetracycline resistance genes reside on transposons, conjugative transposons and/or integrons which permit horizontal resistance transfer from one species to another and between unrelated genera.[5] Resistance to first- and second-generation tetracyclines is now relatively common among bacteria causing respiratory tract infections such as pneumococci. Obligatory intracellular pathogens such as *Chlamydia* and *Rickettsia* spp. have not yet acquired tetracycline resistance.

While RPPs, which release tetracyclines from the target site allowing protein synthesis to occur, confer resistance to both first- and second-generation tetracyclines, most efflux pumps efficiently remove only

Molecular structure of some tetracyclines

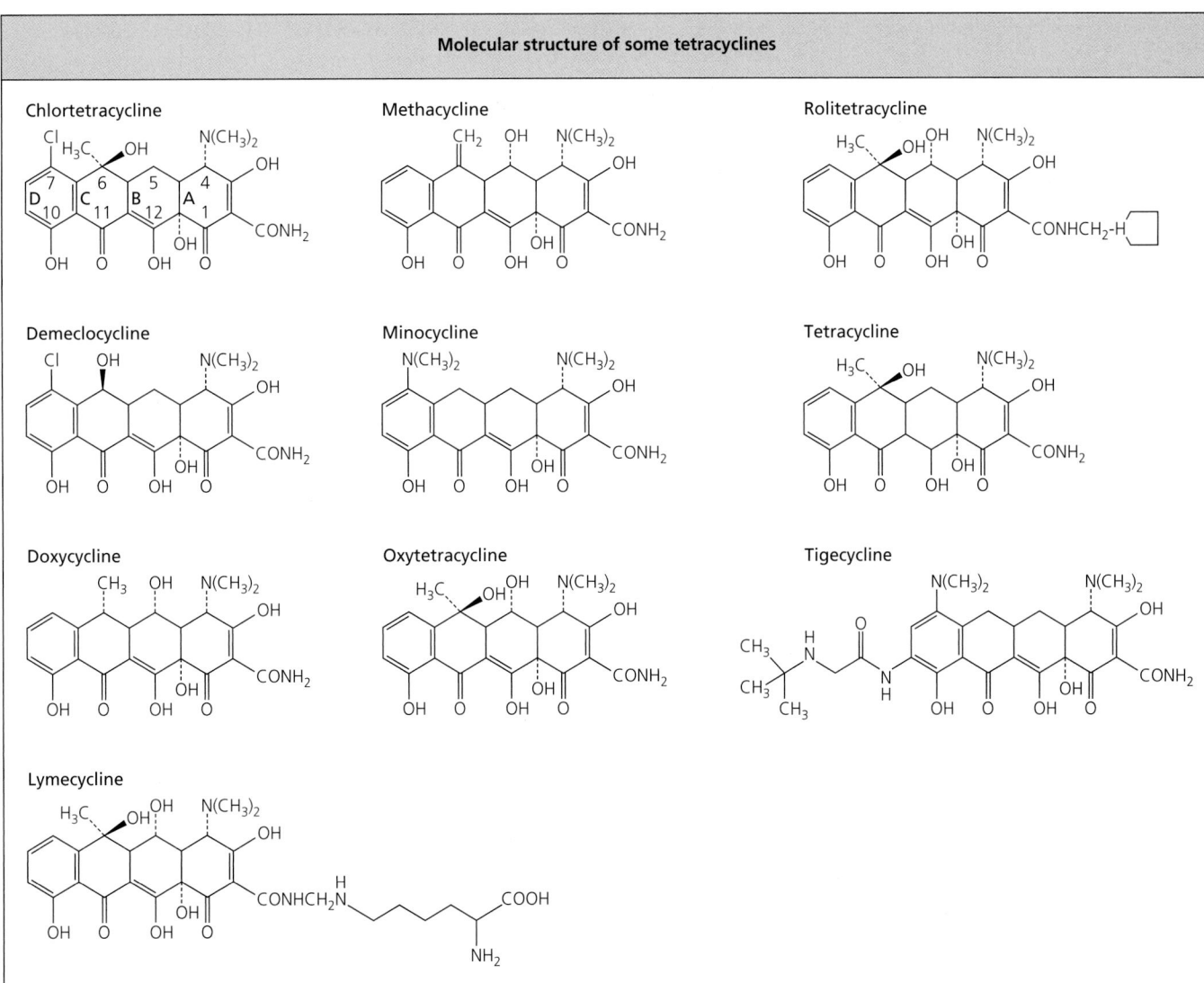

Figure 146-1 Molecular structure of some tetracyclines.

first-generation tetracyclines, allowing doxycycline and minocycline to retain activity. Since efflux pumps are the primary mechanism of resistance in many clinically relevant gram-negative bacilli (e.g. *Escherichia coli*, *Klebsiella*, *Citrobacter*, *Serratia*, etc.) the second-generation tetracyclines retain activity against many tetracycline-resistant gram-negative bacilli.

Tigecycline avoids most tetracycline resistance mechanisms. It has been suggested that tigecycline's tighter binding to the ribosome does not allow displacement by the RPPs. Importantly, however, in *Acinetobacter baumannii*, the AdeABC efflux pump, a well-characterized multidrug efflux pump, readily removes tigecycline from the intracellular space. Resistance to tigecycline in *A. baumannii* has been increasing over the past 5 years, and can develop during therapy. [8]

Pharmacokinetics and Distribution

ABSORPTION

After oral administration, tetracyclines are absorbed from the stomach and the small intestine. Absorption is usually highest in the fasting state, but doxycycline and minocycline are also well absorbed with food. The degree of absorption and other pharmacokinetic parameters for clinically relevant tetracyclines are shown in Table 146-2. [9] The nearly complete absorption of doxycycline salts is reduced if the gastric pH is increased, as occurs with atrophic gastritis or by acid-reducing

drugs. Tetracyclines chelate with divalent cations and this complex can impede absorption from the gastrointestinal tract.

DISTRIBUTION

Tetracyclines have relatively high volumes of distribution, and penetrate adequately into many infection sites. Provided that tetracycline-susceptible organisms are responsible for infection, doxycycline concentrations will be sufficient for treatment in the respiratory tract and lung tissue, the bile and the genital tract of both sexes. [10,11] Levels achieved in the central nervous system (CNS) are increased in chronic meningeal inflammation, [12] enabling treatment of neuroborreliosis. [13,14] Tigecycline has a large and variable volume of distribution. [3,15] It is concentrated in the colon, gallbladder, and lung. [16] Tetracyclines, including tigecycline, cross the placenta and bind to metal ions in fetal bone and teeth. First- and second-generation tetracyclines are also known to be excreted in human breast milk, however they form an insoluble complex with calcium and concentrations are undetectable in infant serum. It is not known whether tigecycline is excreted in human breast milk; however, studies of radiolabeled drugs in rats indicate that tigecycline is readily excreted via the milk of lactating rats. [17]

ELIMINATION

Tetracycline is metabolized in the liver in small amounts; this occurs more with doxycycline and minocycline. There is biliary excretion of the tetracyclines, particularly for minocycline and tigecycline.[18] The glomerular filtration of tetracyclines varies and is highest for tetracycline (>50%), followed by doxycycline and, to a lesser degree, minocycline and tigecycline. Concentrations achieved in the urine are considered efficient for both tetracycline and doxycycline for treating cystitis. Roughly 75% of doxycycline is removed via the feces.

Route of Administration and Dosage

Peak serum levels after an oral dose of 500 mg tetracycline or 200 mg of doxycycline or minocycline are usually 3–5 mg/L after 2 hours. Half-life in serum is longer for doxycycline and minocycline than tetracycline (Table 146-2), and they can be given orally less frequently. A loading dose is recommended for these drugs in order to achieve a steady-state level as soon as possible.

Doxycycline and minocycline are also available for intravenous infusion but there is little difference in serum levels compared with oral administration. Tigecycline is only available for intravenous infusion as a loading dose of 100 mg followed by 50 mg every 12 hours. The peak serum level of tigecycline after a 30-minute infusion of 100 mg is approximately 0.7 mg/L. Tigecycline efficacy in respiratory and bloodstream infections due to gram-negative infections appears to be limited due to poor pharmacokinetic/pharmacodynamic properties.[19]

Dosages of clinically relevant tetracyclines for adults are given in Table 146-3.

Dosage in Special Circumstances

Tetracycline is the only one of these compounds that requires dose adjustment in renal dysfunction. Additionally, use of tetracycline in end-stage renal disease might lead to accumulation and hepatotoxicity, and is not recommended. Doxycycline and minocycline have low renal clearance and thus no dosage adjustments are recommended in renal insufficiency. However, product labeling for minocycline recommends not giving more than 200 mg/day in renally-insufficient patients due to risk for accumulation and toxicity. Doxycycline may be given in normal doses to patients who have renal insufficiency and to those undergoing hemodialysis as the reduced renal excretion is compensated for by intestinal excretion of bound substance.[20] No dosage

TABLE 146-1	Susceptibility to First-, Second- and Third-Generation (Tigecycline) Tetracyclines	
	1st and 2nd Generation	**Tigecycline**
Generally susceptible species	Mycoplasma pneumoniae	Mycoplasma pneumoniae
	Ureaplasma urealyticum	Ureaplasma urealyticum
	Chlamydia spp.	Chlamydia spp.
	Rickettsia spp.	Rickettsia spp.
	Brucella spp.	Brucella spp.
	Francisella tularensis	Francisella tularensis
	Propionibacterium acnes	Propionibacterium acnes
	Borrelia burgdorferi	Borrelia burgdorferi
	Yersinia spp.	Yersinia spp.
		Streptococci
		Enterococci
		Staphylococci
		Enterobacteriaceae
		Haemophilus influenzae
		Meningococci
		Gonococci
		Serratia spp.
Resistance common	Streptococci	
	Staphylococci	
	Enterobacteriaceae	
	Haemophilus influenzae	
	Meningococci	
	Gonococci	
	Legionella pneumophila	
Resistance usually found	Enterococci	Proteus spp.
	Proteus spp.	Pseudomonas spp.
	Pseudomonas spp.	
	Serratia spp.	
	Bacteroides spp.	

TABLE 146-2	Pharmacokinetics of Some Tetracyclines in Humans			
	Tetracycline	**Doxycycline**	**Minocycline**	**Tigecycline**
Bioavailability	77–88%	95%	95–100%	NA
C_{max} (μg/mL)	3–5	1.7–5.9	3.1–4.1	<1
Half-life (hours)	6–12	18–22	12–21	36
Volume of distribution (L/kg)	1.3	0.7	1.2	2.5–7
Protein binding	55–64	82–93	76	73–79

NA, not applicable.
Reproduced from Agwuh K.N., MacGowan A. Pharmacokinetics and pharmacodynamics of the tetracyclines including glycylcyclines. Journal of Antimicrobial Chemotherapy 2006; 58, 256–265.

TABLE 146-3	Usual Adult Dosages for Clinically Relevant Tetracyclines				
Agent	**Loading Dose**	**Common Dosage***	**Renal Dosing**		
Tetracycline	NA	500 mg q6h	Clcr 50–80 mL/min 500 mg q8-12h	Clcr 10–50 mL/min 500 mg q12-24 h	Clcr <10 mL/min 500 mg q24h
Doxycycline	200 mg	100 mg q12h	No adjustment necessary		
Minocycline	200 mg	100 mg q12h	Do not exceed 200 mg in renal insufficiency		
Tigecycline	100 mg	50 mg q12h	No adjustment necessary		

Clcr = creatinine clearance.
*Doxycycline and minocycline may be given intravenously in the same doses. Higher doses of doxycycline are often used for sexually transmitted diseases and Lyme disease. Tigecycline is only available as an intravenous formulation.

adjustment of tigecycline is required in patients with renal impairment, or in patients undergoing hemodialysis.[18] Dosage adjustments are not required in patients with mild to moderate hepatic impairment, but patients with severe hepatic impairment should be treated cautiously and monitored for signs of worsening liver function as well as other side effects due to accumulation. Hepatotoxicity within the class has been observed, mostly in scenarios where older tetracyclines were used at high doses or given during pregnancy. In patients with severe hepatic impairment, the initial dose of tigecycline should be 100 mg followed by a reduced dose of 25 mg q12 hours.[17]

Tetracyclines use in pregnancy should be avoided because of the depressive effect on the skeleton of the child. In lactating patients, small amounts of older tetracyclines are excreted in breast milk, but may not be absorbed. Tetracyclines should be avoided in children <8 years of age.

In elderly patients with reduced renal function the daily dose of a tetracycline should be reduced unless doxycycline or tigecycline is used.

Indications

RESPIRATORY INFECTIONS

Tetracyclines were first used for respiratory tract infections. Because of increasing resistance in pneumococci and *H. influenzae*, they were replaced by other antibiotic classes, mainly β-lactams.

Doxycycline remains a first-line therapy for the treatment of chronic obstructive pulmonary disease (COPD) exacerbations. Doxycycline is distributed to sinuses and can be used as a second-line drug in sinusitis with β-lactam allergy or treatment failure.[21]

Tetracyclines have good activity in pneumonia caused by *Mycoplasma pneumoniae, C. pneumoniae, C. psittaci* and *Coxiella burnetii.* Tetracyclines have *in vitro* activity against *Legionella pneumophilia* as well, but clinical experience is lacking. Because of resistance in 'typical' pathogens associated with community-acquired pneumonia (CAP), doxycycline remains an alternative therapy only in clinically stable patients or in areas where pneumococcal resistance is low. These agents can be combined with antipneumococcal β-lactams for treatment of some hospitalized patients.

Tigecycline is also indicated for the treatment of CAP; however, due to its broad spectrum of activity, it should not be considered for this indication unless other, narrower spectrum therapies are not an option. Tigecycline was found to be inferior to imipenem-cilastatin in the treatment of hospital-acquired and ventilator-associated pneumonia[22] and should be reserved for treatment of these indications only if other options are not available (e.g. multidrug-resistant organisms).

SEXUALLY TRANSMITTED DISEASES

Older tetracyclines are effective therapy for nongonococcal urethritis caused by *Chlamydia trachomatis* or *Ureaplasma urealyticum*. The Centers of Disease Control recommends doxycycline for 7 days in patients who cannot tolerate a one-time dose of azithromycin for the treatment of *C. trachomatis.*[23]

First- and second-generation tetracyclines are usually effective for the treatment of lymphogranuloma venereum and granuloma inguinale. Additionally, although not recommended by guidelines, doxycycline remains a potential alternative for patients with syphilis and in patients who have immediate type hypersensitivity to penicillin and are not candidates for penicillin desensitization.[23]

LYME DISEASE AND EHRLICHIOSIS

Doxycycline (200 mg daily for 10 days) can be used in penicillin-allergic patients to treat erythema migrans and is as effective as penicillin. In erythema migrans with signs of dissemination, such as multiple erythema migrans lesions and fever, doxycycline is often recommended as the primary drug. Treatment of neuroborreliosis with doxycycline 200 mg daily for 2 weeks gave similar results to penicillin G (see Chapter 46).[24]

Doxycycline is also the preferred drug for infections due to *Ehrlichia* (see Chapter 187).[25]

OTHER INDICATIONS

First- and second-generation tetracyclines are effective drugs for rickettsial infections (see Chapter 187). Doxycycline has been used for single-dose treatment of louse-borne typhus, but for other infections 7–10 days of treatment is usually needed.

Doxycycline is also effective in a single dose for infections with *Borrelia recurrentis*. Tetracyclines are usually used in combination with other antibiotics such as streptomycin or rifampin for brucellosis and tularemia.

For cholera in adults, tetracycline 500 mg q6h for 5 days or a single dose of 300 mg doxycycline have been recommended.[26]

Doxycycline may also be used for malaria prophylaxis in areas where *Plasmodium falciparum* is resistant to other antimalarial drugs.[27]

Emerging Role in the Treatment of Multidrug-Resistant Organisms

Doxycycline, minocycline and tigecycline retain *in vitro* activity against a wide array of multidrug-resistant bacteria, including against MRSA, and VRE. Because enterococci will in some instances have RPPs, tigecycline is more active. Both minocycline and tigecycline have shown >70% activity against carbapenem-resistant *A. baumannii*, with tigecycline usually showing greater activity.[8,19,28]

Adverse Reactions and Interactions

ADVERSE DRUG REACTIONS

All oral preparations of tetracyclines can cause nausea and epigastric discomfort. Doxycycline and minocycline can be taken with food without decreasing absorption, to alleviate gastrointestinal symptoms. Diarrhea is less common but may occur, especially when tetracyclines with low absorption are used. Tigecycline is associated with a high rate of nausea and vomiting, the dose-limiting side effect of the drug.

Hypersensitivity reactions have been reported with the tetracyclines, although the incidence is relatively rare. Photosensitivity reactions can occur with all tetracyclines, and patients should avoid prolonged sun exposure while taking these drugs.

Tetracyclines should not be used in children younger than 8 years or during pregnancy because of the risk of enamel hypoplasia and tooth discoloration. Tetracycline should not be used in patients with end-stage renal disease, and caution should be exercised when using minocycline in this setting.

Vertigo and dizziness are CNS symptoms that occur with minocycline. It is reversible upon discontinuation of the agent, but can be severe.

Hepatotoxicity has been reported primarily after parenteral tetracycline therapy – often with high doses – and also when used during pregnancy.

DRUG–DRUG INTERACTIONS

Tetracyclines form chelate complexes with many drugs containing metal ions and form nonabsorbable complexes (Table 146-4). Tetracyclines should be administered separately from supplements with calcium, magnesium, iron, and others. Tetracycline and doxycycline are inhibitors and substrates of CYP 3A4 and metabolism based interactions are possible.

TABLE 146-4	Drug Interactions with Tetracyclines	
Interacting Drug	**Effect**
Antacids with metal ions, calcium and iron supplements, magnesium salicylates, magnesium-containing laxatives, multivitamins	Chelate formation and impaired absorption
Rifampin (rifampicin), phenobarbital, phenytoin, carbamazepine	Half-life of doxycycline shortened

Chloramphenicol

Introduction

Chloramphenicol was first isolated in 1947 from a sample of soil from Venezuela and the actinomycete was called *Streptomyces venezuelae*. Due to the association between chloramphenicol and aplastic anemia, as well as the availability of other less toxic agents, chloramphenicol use is rare in high-income countries.

Mode of Action and Spectrum

Chloramphenicol inhibits protein synthesis by binding to the 50S subunit of the bacterial 70S ribosome. It considered a bacteriostatic agent; however, bactericidal activity on some bacteria, such as *H. influenzae*, *Streptococcus pneumoniae* and *Neisseria meningitidis*, has been reported. This bactericidal activity enabled its use in the treatment of meningitis due to these pathogens (see Chapter 137).

Chloramphenicol has a broad spectrum, including aerobic and anaerobic bacteria, spirochetes, *Rickettsia*, *Chlamydia* and *Mycoplasma* spp. It is active against most anaerobic bacteria, including *Bacteroides fragilis*.

Chloramphenicol resistance occurs and is mediated by a bacterial enzyme, chloramphenicol acetyltransferase (CAT), which inactivates the drug. The gene that codes for CAT is carried on transmissible plasmids, and epidemics of chloramphenicol-resistant typhoid fever and *Shigella* infections have occurred. Other mechanisms, including reduced uptake into the cell, efflux and target site mutation, have also been described (see Chapter 138).

Pharmacokinetics and Distribution

Chloramphenicol undergoes 90% absorption after an oral dose. It is a small lipophilic molecule and is well distributed in the body. The serum protein binding is about 44%. It penetrates into the CNS better than most antibiotics and its concentration in the cerebrospinal fluid is often 30–50% of the serum concentration.

Chloramphenicol is conjugated with glucuronic acid and is then excreted in active form by the kidneys. The metabolites are not toxic and dose reduction is not needed in renal insufficiency.

Route of Administration and Dosage

Oral formulations are not available for use in the USA. Oral chloramphenicol 1 g gives a serum concentration of 10 mg/L and the half-life is 3–4 hours. It may also be given intravenously as a succinate ester, but intramuscular injections should be avoided as absorption is unreliable. Interestingly, the intravenous formulation results in slightly lower serum concentrations, due to incomplete hydrolysis of the succinate ester to the active form.

Indications

Chloramphenicol is toxic and should therefore be used only when alternatives are lacking. It can be used instead of tetracyclines for the treatment of rickettsial infections (particularly in pregnancy) and for bacterial meningitis in the few patients who have an allergy to β-lactam drugs and where other options such as the fluoroquinolones are not an option due to allergy or resistance.

Topical administration of chloramphenicol in drops or ointments is widely used for superficial bacterial infections of the eyes.[29,30]

Adverse Reactions and Interactions

ADVERSE DRUG REACTIONS

Neonates have a diminished ability to conjugate chloramphenicol and to excrete the active form in the urine. A dose of 25 mg/kg/day should not be exceeded[31] otherwise the 'gray baby syndrome' may develop, with severe cyanosis and circulatory collapse.

Dose-related reversible bone marrow depression can occur in adults given high doses of more than 4 g/day. Dose-related bone marrow suppression appears to be due to reduced utilization of iron, with elevation in serum iron concentrations observed in patients with reduced red blood cells and hematocrit. The daily dose should not exceed 3 g, and when the accumulated dose exceeds 25 g, reticulocytes should be monitored regularly (e.g. twice weekly).

A very severe reaction is aplastic anemia, which occurs with a frequency of 1/25 000–40 000 treatment courses.[32] The exact mechanism for the idiosyncratic reaction is not known but has been speculated to include metabolism to toxic metabolites. No clear correlation to dose or duration of treatment has been observed and no route of administration is exempt from causing this catastrophic complication.

DRUG–DRUG INTERACTIONS

Chloramphenicol is almost completely metabolized in the liver by cytochrome P450 enzymes, and there is a risk of drug–drug interactions. Chloramphenicol decreases the rate of metabolism of tolbutamide, phenytoin, cyclophosphamide and warfarin. Rifampin may lower chloramphenicol concentrations by induced metabolism.

References available online at expertconsult.com.

KEY REFERENCES

Agwuh K.N., MacGowan A.: Pharmacokinetics and pharmacodynamics of the tetracyclines including glycylcyclines. *J Antimicrob Chemother* 2006; 58:256-265.

Bhavnani S., Rubino C.M., Hammel J.P., et al.: Pharmacological and patient-specific response determinants in patients with hospital-acquired pneumonia treated with tigecycline. *Antimicrob Agents Chemother* 2012; 56:1065-1072.

Brogden R.N., Speight T.M., Avery G.S.: Minocycline: a review of its antibacterial and pharmacokinetic properties and therapeutic use. *Drugs* 1975; 9:251-291.

Burns L.E., Hodgman J.E., Cass A.B.: Fatal circulatory collapse in premature infants receiving chloramphenicol. *N Engl J Med* 1959; 261:1318-1321.

Chopra I., Roberts M.: Tetracycline antibiotics: mode of action, applications, molecular biology and epidemiology of bacterial resistance. *Microbiol Mol Biol Rev* 2001; 65:232-260.

Freire A.T., et al.: Comparison of tigecycline with imipenem/cilastatin for the treatment of hospital acquired pneumonia. *Diagn Microbiol Infect Dis* 2010; 68:140-151.

Pankey G.A.: Tigecycline. *J Antimicrob Chemother* 2005; 56:470-480.

Peleg A.Y., Potoski B.A., Rea R., et al.: *Acinetobacter baumannii* bloodstream infection while receiving tigecycline: a cautionary report. *J Antimicrob Chemother* 2007; 59:128-131.

Steigbigel N.H., Reed C.W., Finland M.: Susceptibility of common pathogenic bacteria to seven tetracycline antibiotics in vitro. *Am J Med Sci* 1968; 255:179-195.

Wallerstein R.O., Condit P.K., Kasper C.K., et al.: Statewide study of chloramphenicol therapy and fatal aplastic anemia. *JAMA* 1969; 208:2045-2050.

Zhanel G.G., Homenuik K., Nichol K., et al.: The glycylcyclines, a comparative review with the tetracyclines. *Drugs* 2004; 64:63-88.

147

Nitroimidazoles, Metronidazole, Ornidazole and Tinidazole; and Fidaxomicin

MARK H. WILCOX

KEY CONCEPTS

- Nitroimidazoles are widely used for infections caused by anaerobes, some vaginal infections and *Helicobacter pylori* gastritis.

- Aerobic bacteria are intrinsically resistant to nitroimidazoles.

- Nitroimidazoles are highly active against protozoa and are the first-line treatment options for giardiasis, amebiasis and trichomonal vaginitis.

- Resistance to nitroimidazoles is uncommon among target pathogens, except for *H. pylori* where high rates occur, especially in low- and middle-income countries.

- Increasing evidence highlights that metronidazole is inferior to vancomycin (and fidaxomicin) for the treatment of *Clostridium difficile* infection.

Introduction and Mode of Action

The nitroimidazoles, which include metronidazole, tinidazole and ornidazole, were initially introduced for the treatment of trichomonal vaginitis. They were subsequently recognized to be active against other protozoa, facultative anaerobes (*Helicobacter pylori* and *Gardnerella vaginalis*) and anaerobic bacteria, and so are very widely prescribed.

Once they have entered the cell by diffusion, the antimicrobial toxicity of the nitroimidazoles is dependent on reduction of the nitro moiety to the nitro anion radical and other highly active compounds, including nitroso and hydroxylamine derivatives.[1,2] These reduction products are damaging to macromolecules, and have been shown to cause DNA degradation and strand breakage.[1] The nitroimidazoles are selectively toxic for micro-organisms in which the redox potential of components of the electron transport chain are sufficiently negative to reduce the nitro group of metronidazole (see also Chapter 137). Aerobic bacteria are therefore intrinsically resistant to these antibiotics since they are unable to attain the low intracellular redox environment required for drug activation. In susceptible organisms, the ongoing reduction of metronidazole maintains a favorable transmembrane metronidazole concentration gradient, facilitating further diffusion into the cell. In general, micro-organisms develop resistance to the nitroimidazoles by reducing or abolishing the activity of elements of the electron transport reactions, with appropriate compensatory modifications of the normal fermentative pathway.[2–5] Resistance to metronidazole in *Bacteroides* spp. has been shown to be associated with specific nitroimidazole (*nim*) resistance genes that encode a 5-nitroimidazole reductase, which prevents the formation of the free radicals responsible for bactericidal activity.[6] There is evidence of the emergence of reduced susceptibility to metronidazole in some *Clostridium difficile* isolates with evidence for clonal spread, although the clinical relevance of such strains remains unclear.[7]

Route of Administration and Dosage

The two most frequently used nitroimidazoles – metronidazole and tinidazole – have parenteral and oral formulations and are also available as suppositories, as a gel for periodontitis and for vaginal administration. Dosing regimens of metronidazole are given in Table 147-1. The doses of tinidazole and ornidazole are similar but, because their

TABLE 147-1	Dosages of Metronidazole				
Type of Infection	Adult Dose	Pediatric Dose*	Duration of Treatment	Notes	
Trichomoniasis	2 g	Not applicable	Single dose	Or 400 mg q12h for 5–7 days (250–500 mg q8h)[†]	
Giardiasis	400 mg q8h (250 mg q12h or q8h)	15←mg/kg q12h	5–7 days	Or 2 g q24h for 3 days	
Amebic dysentery	800 mg q8h (500–750 mg q8h)	20 mg/kg q12h	5–10 days		
Amebic abscess	800 mg q8h	(500–750 mg q8h)	10 days	20 mg/kg q12h	
Bacterial vaginosis	400 mg q12h (500 mg q12h)	Not applicable	5–7 days	Or 2 g as a single dose	
Helicobacter pylori	400 mg q8h (250 mg q8h)	Not applicable	7–14 days		
Clostridium difficile	800 mg then 400 mg q8h (250 mg q6h or 500 mg q8h)	7.5 mg/kg q12h	10–14 days		
Anaerobic infection (treatment)	800 mg then 400 mg q8h (500 mg q12h–q6h)	7.5 mg/kg q8h	7–10 days		
Anaerobic infection (prophylaxis)	400 mg (15 mg/kg then 7.5 mg/kg 6 and 12 h after initial dose)	7.5 mg/kg	Single dose	Repeat every 3 h for prolonged procedures	

*Pediatric dose is for children aged 8 weeks or more.
[†]US dosages in parentheses.

half-lives are longer, these drugs can be administered less frequently.[8] Recommendations in the USA for certain infections are for shorter dose intervals, although it is recognized that the half-life of the nitroimidazoles means that dose intervals shorter than 8 hours should not be needed and in most cases 12-hour regimens should be adequate.

Pharmacokinetics

Following oral administration, all nitroimidazoles are almost completely absorbed.[9] After rectal administration of metronidazole, the bioavailability is approximately 60%, with considerable variability between individuals. When given vaginally the systemic bioavailability of metronidazole is 20% or less. Following a 400 mg oral dose of metronidazole or tinidazole, peak plasma concentrations of about 10 mg/L are achieved after 3–5 hours. Dose proportional kinetics have been seen for doses up to 2 g. The concentrations after normal oral doses are well above the minimum inhibitory concentrations (MICs) for anaerobes but are borderline for *G. vaginalis*. The nitroimidazoles are well distributed to peripheral compartments, including brain tissue and cerebrospinal fluid,[9] but concentrations in subcutaneous fat are low (15% or less of concurrent serum levels).[10] Nitroimidazoles are metabolized mainly by the liver, by both glucuronidation and oxidation to multiple metabolites, and are excreted in the urine. After oral administration, gut concentrations of metronidazole (of relevance to the treatment of *C. difficile* infection) peak at ~9 mg/L when diarrhea and an inflamed colonic mucosa are present, falling to zero as symptoms resolve.[11] The plasma half-life is about 8 hours for metronidazole and 12–13 hours for tinidazole. Metronidazole is partly metabolized to hydroxymetronidazole, which has a half-life of 10–13 hours. Metronidazole elimination is prolonged in premature newborns and in patients with impaired liver function, and dose reduction is necessary in these groups. Although dose adjustment is not normally required in patients with renal impairment, the hydroxymetronidazole metabolite may accumulate in patients with end-stage disease and dose reduction may be necessary. Hemodialysis increases the clearance of metronidazole, shortening the half-life to 2–3 hours.[12,13]

Indications

BACTERIAL INFECTIONS

Nitroimidazoles are the most active antibiotics for the treatment and prevention of infections caused by anaerobic bacteria (Table 147-2) and resistance in these organisms is rare.[14] Nitroimidazoles are therefore important in the treatment of intra-abdominal and gynecologic sepsis, abscesses and tetanus. They are also an important component of prophylactic regimens for surgical procedures where contamination with anaerobic flora is likely. Nitroimidazoles are used to treat bacterial

TABLE 147-2	Activity of Metronidazole Against Anaerobic Bacteria		
Organism	Metronidazole MIC (mg/L) for 90% Isolates	Percent Sensitive (NCCLS)	
Bacteroides fragilis	1–4	100	
Prevotella spp.	4	100	
Fusobacterium nucleatum	0.25–2	100	
Fusobacterium spp.	0.25–4	100	
Peptostreptococcus spp.	0.5–4	100	
Propionibacterium acnes	>1.0	0	
Clostridium difficile	0.5–4	100	
Clostridium spp.	2–16	95	

NCCLS, National Committee for Clinical Laboratory Standards.
Data from Wexler et al.[12] and Spangler et al.[13]

vaginosis (frequently associated with *G. vaginalis*) and dental infections, including acute necrotizing ulcerative gingivitis (Vincent's angina). Nitroimidazoles are also a component of modern triple eradication regimens for *H. pylori*, although resistance may affect 10–50% of strains isolated in high-income countries and virtually all strains from low- and middle-income countries (LMIC), likely reflecting prior exposure to these antibiotics.[15]

Metronidazole continues to be first-line treatment for mild/moderate *C. difficile* infection but is inferior to vancomycin in patients with severe, recurrent, complicated or fulminant disease (see also Chapter 40).[16] When the results of two recent, identically designed, phase 3 clinical trials were analyzed together, overall vancomycin was found to be superior to metronidazole, with clinical cure rates of 81.1% versus 72.7%, respectively; recurrence of infection occurred in 20.6% versus 23% of cases, respectively (no significant difference).[17] This finding questions the continued position of metronidazole as a first-line choice in mild/moderate *C. difficile* infection.

PROTOZOAL INFECTIONS

The nitroimidazoles are highly active against protozoa and provide the first-line treatment for giardiasis, amebiasis and trichomonal vaginitis. Although resistant strains of *Entamoeba histolytica* and *Trichomonas vaginalis* are rarely encountered, up to 20% of *Giardia lamblia* isolates may be resistant in general clinical practice.

OTHER

Topical metronidazole is used to reduce the odor produced by anaerobic bacteria in fungating cutaneous lesions and has also been used in the management of acne rosacea. Metronidazole may be beneficial for the treatment of diarrhea and perianal involvement in patients with active Crohn's disease.

Adverse Reactions and Interactions

The most common side effects of the nitroimidazoles are gastrointestinal (including nausea and diarrhea) and a metallic taste, especially when high doses are used. A reversible peripheral neuropathy may occur in patients receiving high doses for prolonged periods.

Severe central nervous system effects have also been reported and the drug should be discontinued if any abnormal neurologic symptoms are reported. If combined with alcohol, metronidazole may cause a disulfiram-like reaction, with nausea, vomiting, flushing of the skin, tachycardia, hypotension and palpitations. Although nitroimidazoles have been found to be mutagenic and carcinogenic in animal studies, there is a lack of evidence that they are carcinogenic to humans.[18] Although theoretical concerns of teratogenicity have not been confirmed,[19,20] it seems prudent that metronidazole should only be used in pregnancy when the benefits outweigh the risks and should be avoided altogether in the first trimester. Because the concentrations of metronidazole in breast milk are similar to those in serum, a risk assessment should be performed before using this drug in lactating mothers.

Fidaxomicin

Fidaxomicin is a novel, narrow-spectrum, macrocyclic antibiotic that has been recently marketed for the treatment of *C. difficile* infection. It inhibits RNA polymerase, but by a mechanism that is distinct from that of rifamycins, and thus there is no cross-resistance to the latter antibiotics. *In vitro* resistance to fidaxomicin has been described in a single clinical *C. difficile* isolate, recovered as part of a clinical trial. As *C. difficile* is not routinely cultured in most laboratories, the true potential for resistance emergence remains to be determined. However, typical gut concentrations of this orally administered, minimally absorbed antibiotic are typically >1000-fold higher than the MIC for *C. difficile*.

Fidaxomicin is dosed orally at 200 mg 12-hourly; tablets can be crushed for administration via a nasogastric tube if required. Fidaxomicin is similar to vancomycin in terms of initial clinical cure of *C.*

difficile infection, but is superior when recurrence rates are considered. This superiority was maintained in patients with severe infection and in those receiving concomitant antibiotic therapy, but not in cases caused by the epidemic NAP1 (ribotype 027) strain.[21-23]

There have been a few reports of hypersensitivity to fidaxomicin and may be associated in some cases with a history of macrolide allergy.

The true frequency of such reactions is unknown but appears to be very uncommon; it is unclear whether hypersensitivity reactions are associated with systemic exposure to fidaxomicin, noting that the drug is minimally absorbed.[24]

References available online at expertconsult.com.

KEY REFERENCES

Bagdasarian N., Rao K., Malani P.N.: Diagnosis and treatment of *Clostridium difficile* in adults: a systematic review. *JAMA* 2015; 313:398-408.

Bendesky A., Ménendez D., Ostrosky-Wegman P.: Is metronidazole carcinogenic? *Mutat Res* 2002; 511:133-144.

Caro-Paton T., Carvajal A., Martin de Diego I., et al.: Is metronidazole teratogenic? A meta-analysis. *Br J Clin Pharmacol* 1997; 44:179-182.

Cornely O.A., Crook D.W., Esposito R., et al.: OPT-80-004 Clinical Study Group. Fidaxomicin versus vancomycin for infection with *Clostridium difficile* in Europe, Canada, and the USA: a double-blind, non-inferiority, randomised controlled trial. *Lancet Infect Dis* 2012; 12:281-289.

Edwards D.I.: Nitroimidazole drugs – action and resistance mechanisms. II. Mechanisms of resistance. *J Antimicrob Chemother* 1993; 31:201-210.

Johnson S., Louie T.J., Gerding D.N., et al.: Polymer Alternative for CDI Treatment (PACT) investigators. Vancomycin, metronidazole, or tolevamer for *Clostridium difficile* infection: results from two multinational, randomized, controlled trials. *Clin Infect Dis* 2014; 59:345-354.

Lindmark D.G., Muller M.: Antitrichomonad action, mutagenicity, and reduction of metronidazole and other nitroimidazoles. *Antimicrob Agents Chemother* 1976; 10: 476-482.

Mégraud F.: Epidemiology and mechanism of antibiotic resistance in *Helicobacter pylori*. *Gastroenterology* 1998; 115:1278-1282.

Moreno S.N., Mason R.P., Muniz R.P., et al.: Generation of free radicals from metronidazole and other nitroimidazoles by *Trichomonas foetus*. *J Biol Chem* 1983; 258:4051-4054.

Viitanen J., Auvinen O., Tunturi T., et al.: Concentrations of metronidazole and tinidazole in abdominal tissues after a single intravenous infusion and repetitive oral administration. *Chemotherapy* 1984; 30:211-215.

Wilcox M.H.: Progress with a difficult infection. *Lancet Infect Dis* 2012; 12:256-257.

148

Antituberculosis Agents

GIOVANNI BATTISTA MIGLIORI | ALIMUDDIN ZUMLA

KEY CONCEPTS

- Treatment of drug-sensitive tuberculosis (TB) is of at least 6 months duration and involves two phases, 2 months of the four TB drugs – isoniazid (INH), rifampin (RIF), pyrazinamide (PZA) and ethambutol (EMB) – in the intensive phase and 4 months of two in the continuation stage.

- Anti-TB drugs can be classified into those that are synthetic molecules and those that are antibiotics or semisynthetic antibiotic derivatives.

- First-line drugs form the basis of the modern short-course regimens advocated by the World Health Organization (WHO) and second-line drugs are used in cases of drug resistance and when toxic reactions prevent the use of one or more first-line drugs.

- The targets of streptomycin and other aminoglycosides, rifamycins and fluoroquinolones are the same in mycobacteria as in other bacterial genera, and resistance is due to single amino acid substitutions in the target proteins.

- The targets of many important antituberculosis agents, notably isoniazid, pyrazinamide, ethambutol, ethionamide and prothionamide, are components of the complex and lipid-rich mycobacterial cell wall.

- Isoniazid (INH) has particularly high early bactericidal activity.

- After decades of inactivity in TB drug development, the past 10 years has seen a promising TB drug pipeline.

- The most rapid progress has been made by repurposing or re-dosing of known TB drugs such as high-dose rifampin and rifapentine (rifamycins), moxifloxacin and gatifloxacin (fluoroquinolones) and clofazimine (riminophenazine). These have all entered advanced phase III clinical trials.

- Historic advances include approval of two new drugs, delamanid and bedaquiline.

- Challenges with current therapy include: drug quality; directly observed therapy (DOT); drug intolerance and toxicities; pharmacokinetic interactions, particularly with antiretroviral (ART) drugs in TB patients coinfected with HIV; and patient adherence to treatment issues due to the lengthy treatment period.

- A number of new therapeutic agents are concurrently under investigation and new treatment regimens are in clinical trials.

Introduction

The discovery of the tubercle bacillus *Mycobacterium tuberculosis* by Robert Koch in 1882 raised hopes that an effective remedy for tuberculosis would soon be found. The discovery of streptomycin in 1944 by Albert Schatz and Selman Waksman in the USA opened the door to effective therapy. However, patients treated with streptomycin often made an initial improvement but soon relapsed because their tubercle bacilli became resistant to this agent. Fortunately, other active antituberculosis agents were discovered and, as a result of extensive trials initiated by Sir John Crofton in the UK, multidrug regimens that cured patients and prevented the emergence of drug resistance were developed.[1]

Therapy of tuberculosis with these early drug regimens, usually consisting of streptomycin, isoniazid and *para*-aminosalicylic acid, was beset with problems. Streptomycin had to be given by injection and *para*-aminosalicylic acid caused such severe gastrointestinal effects that patients often failed to comply with therapy. In addition, it was necessary to treat patients for 18–24 months in order to achieve a cure.

The second therapeutic revolution came in the early 1970s when regimens containing rifampin (rifampicin) were developed. The introduction of this drug had three major effects on the treatment of tuberculosis. First, the duration of therapy could be reduced to only 6 months. Secondly, regimens could be entirely oral and thirdly, hospitalization was often unnecessary.

Modern short-course therapy,[2] properly used, can achieve a cure in around 98% of patients and is among the most effective and cost-effective of all therapeutic interventions for a chronic disease.[3-5] However, tuberculosis remains one of the most prevalent causes of mortality and morbidity worldwide. It is responsible for one in seven deaths among young adults. The problem is currently exacerbated by the HIV pandemic, the increasing prevalence of multidrug-resistant tuberculosis (MDR-TB), defined as resistance to at least rifampin and isoniazid among the first-line drugs, and the more recent emergence of extensively drug-resistant tuberculosis (XDR-TB). After more than 40 years of the 'status-quo' of no new TB drugs, several new compounds have entered the drug development pipelines.[6-8]

Three new drugs have now been developed (delamanid, bedaquiline, PA-824) and are being evaluated in phase II and III trials to determine their optimal usefulness.[5,6,9]

Classification

Antituberculous agents can be classified in several ways (Table 148-1). They can be divided into:
- those that are synthetic molecules and those that are antibiotics or semisynthetic antibiotic derivatives;
- agents with a broad spectrum of activity and those only active against mycobacteria or, specifically, members of the *Mycobacterium tuberculosis* complex;
- first-line drugs that form the basis of the modern short-course regimens and second-line drugs that are used in cases of drug resistance and when toxic reactions prevent the use of first-line drug(s); and
- bacteriostatic and bactericidal agents, with a clinically important distinction of the latter between those that are bactericidal *in vitro* and those that are able to sterilize lesions of tubercle bacilli *in vivo* (Table 148-2).

Mode of Action and Pharmacokinetics

The sequencing of the genome of *M. tuberculosis*[10] has led to considerable advances in our understanding of the genetic basis of action of the drugs used for treating mycobacterial disease as well as the delineation of metabolic pathways that could serve as targets for novel drugs.

The targets of streptomycin and other aminoglycosides, rifamycins and fluoroquinolones are the same in mycobacteria as in other bacterial genera, and resistance is due to single amino acid substitutions in the target proteins. The targets of many important antituberculosis agents, notably isoniazid, pyrazinamide, ethambutol, ethionamide and prothionamide, are components of the complex and lipid-rich mycobacterial cell wall. The mode of action and target genes are discussed under the individual drug headings below and are summarized in Table 148-3; the targets are shown in Figure 148-1. Most of

TABLE 148-1	The World Health Organization's Recommended Classification of Antituberculosis Drugs		
Group Name		**Anti-TB agent**	**Abbreviation**
Group 1. First-line oral agents		Isoniazid	H or INH
		Rifampin	R or RIF
		Ethambutol	EMB or E
		Pyrazinamide	PZA or P
		Rifabutin[a]	Rfb
		Rifapentine[a]	Rpt
Group 2. Injectable anti-TB drugs (injectable agents or parenteral agents)		Streptomycin[b]	S
		Kanamycin	Km
		Amikacin	Am
		Capreomycin	Cm
Group 3. Fluoroquinolones (FQs)[d]		Levofloxacin	Lfx
		Moxifloxacin	Mfx
		Gatifloxacin[c]	Gfx
Group 4. Oral bacteriostatic second-line anti-TB drugs		Ethionamide	Eto
		Prothionamide	Pto
		Cycloserine	Cs
		Terizidone[e]	Trd
		Para-aminosalicylic acid	PAS
		Para-aminosalicylate sodium	PAS-Na
Group 5. Anti-TB drugs with limited data on efficacy and/or long-term safety in the treatment of MDR-TB. (This group includes new anti-TB agents)		Bedaquiline	Bdq
		Delamanid	Dlm
		Linezolid	Lzd
		Clofazimine	Cfz
		Amoxicillin/clavulanate	Amx/Clv
		Imipenem/cilastatin[f]	Ipm/Cln
		Meropenem[f]	Mpm
		High-dose isoniazid	High-dose H
		Thioacetazone[g]	T
		Clarithromycin[g]	Clr

MDR-TB: multidrug-resistant TB.

[a]Rifabutin and rifapentine have similar microbiologic activity as rifampin. Rifabutin is not on the *WHO Model List of Essential Medicines*; however, it has been added here as it is used routinely in patients on protease inhibitors in many settings. Rifapentine is part of a latent TB infection and active TB treatment in some countries but to date is not part of any WHO-endorsed treatment regimens.

[b]There are high rates of streptomycin resistance in strains of MDR-TB; therefore, streptomycin is not considered a second-line anti-TB injectable agent.

[c]Gatifloxacin can have 'life-threatening' side effects including serious diabetes (dysglycemia). The drug has been removed from the formula of a number of countries.

[d]Ofloxacin is considered a weaker agent with less activity against TB than other fluoroquinolones and has been removed as a choice in Group 3 drugs.

[e]Terizidone has limited programme data and effectiveness data as compared to cycloserine.

[f]Clavulanate (Clv) is recommended as an adjunctive agent to imipenem/cilastatin and meropenem.

[g]Limited data on the role of thioacetazone and clarithromycin in MDR-TB treatment has resulted in many experts not including these drugs as options for Group 5.

TABLE 148-2	Efficacy of First-Line Antituberculosis Agents*		
Agent	**Early Bactericidal Activity**	**Sterilizing Activity**	**Prevention of Emergence of Drug Resistance**
Ethambutol	Fair	Poor	Fair
Isoniazid	Good	Fair	Good
Pyrazinamide	Poor	Good	Poor
Rifampin (rifampicin)	Fair	Good	Good
Streptomycin	Poor	Poor	Fair

*In sterilizing lesions, reducing viable bacterial population rapidly and preventing the emergence of drug resistance.

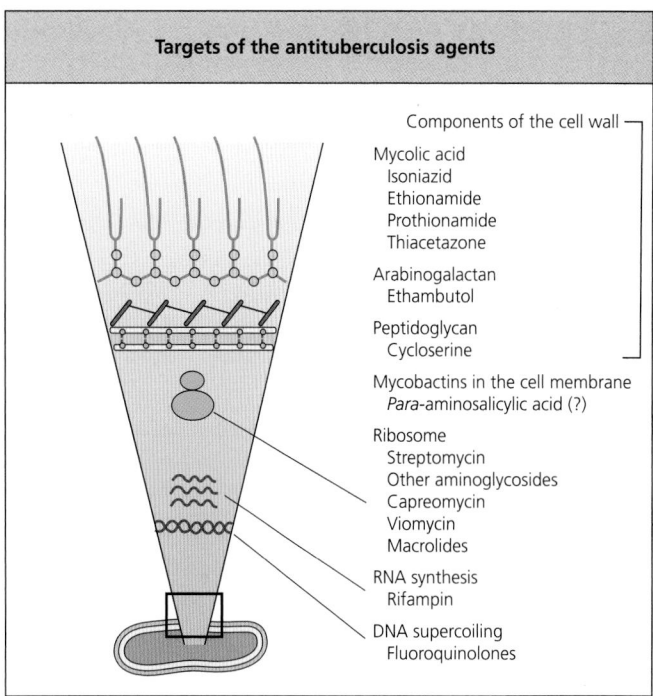

Figure 148-1 Targets of the antituberculosis agents.

the antituberculosis agents are readily absorbed from the gastrointestinal tract. Exceptions are streptomycin and other aminoglycosides, capreomycin and viomycin, which must be given parenterally. Binding to serum proteins varies, as does entry into the cerebrospinal fluid (CSF). Agents that enter into the CSF poorly in health often pass the inflamed meninges so that therapeutically useful levels are achieved. The pharmacokinetics of the conventional antimycobacterial drugs, their principal metabolites and routes of excretion are summarized in Tables 148-4 and 148-5.

Drug Toxicity

The major side effects are hepatotoxicity, peripheral neuropathy, mental disturbances, skin reactions (Figures 148-2 to 148-4) and fevers. Side effects are particularly likely to occur in HIV-positive patients and, of these, skin reactions due to thiacetazone are particularly serious and may be fatal.

The principal drugs used in modern short-course regimens – isoniazid, rifampin, pyrazinamide and ethambutol – are all potentially hepatotoxic. Some physicians advocate regular liver function tests during therapy.[11] The adverse effects of the various drugs are discussed under the individual headings below and are summarized in Table 148-6.

First-Line Drugs
ISONIAZID (ISONICOTINIC ACID HYDRAZIDE)

This is included in all modern regimens and is also used as preventive monotherapy for infected (tuberculin-positive, without clinical disease; also known as latent tuberculosis) persons.

It has a powerful bactericidal action against actively replicating tubercle bacilli and thus rapidly reduces infectiousness by reducing the number of viable bacilli in cavities. It has little or no activity against slowly replicating bacilli but is included in the continuation phase of modern short-course therapy to kill any rifampin-resistant mutants that commence replication. It inhibits the synthesis of mycolic acids – long-chain fatty acids that form an important part of the mycobacterial cell wall. Although mycolic acids are common to all mycobacteria, and similar molecules occur in the genera *Nocardia* and

Antituberculosis Agents: Targets and Genes for Resistance

Agent	Target	Gene(s) Encoding Target(s) or Those in Which Mutations Conferring Resistance Occur
FIRST-LINE DRUGS		
Isoniazid	Mycolic acid synthesis	*inhA, katG, KasA, oxyR-ahpC*
Rifampin (rifampicin)	DNA-dependent RNA polymerase	*rpoB*
Pyrazinamide	Fatty acid synthetase-1	*pncA*
Ethambutol	Arabinosyl transferase, involved in cell wall arabinogalactan synthesis	*embA, embB* and *embC*
Streptomycin	30S ribosomal subunit	*rspL* (encodes for ribosomal protein S12)
SECOND-LINE DRUGS		
Other aminoglycosides	30S ribosomal subunit	Genes encoding 16S-rRNA (and possibly *aac(2')* encoding aminoglycoside acetyltransferase)
Thiacetazone	Mycolic acid synthesis	Unknown
Para-aminosalicylic acid	Mycobactin synthesis (?)	Unknown
Ethionamide and prothionamide	Mycolic acid synthesis	*inhA*
Fluoroquinolones	Inhibition of bacterial DNA gyrase topoisomerase IV	*gyrA* and *gyrB* (gyrase) *parC* and *parD* (topoisomerase IV)
Capreomycin and viomycin	50S or 30S ribosomal subunit	*vicA* (50S) or *vicB* (30S)
Clofazimine	Unknown; possibly RNA polymerase	–
Cycloserine	Peptidoglycan	*alrA*

TABLE 148-4

Pharmacokinetics of the Antituberculosis Agents

Agent	Binding to Serum Proteins	Absorption From Gastrointestinal Tract (Time to Reach Peak Serum Level)	Entry into CSF (With Uninflamed Meninges)
FIRST-LINE DRUGS			
Isoniazid	Very low	Very rapid (30–60 minutes)	Good
Rifampin (rifampicin)	High (up to 95%)	Rapid (2 hours)	Poor
Pyrazinamide	Very low	Rapid (1–2 hours)	Good
Ethambutol	Binds to erythrocytes	Rapid (2 hours); 80% of dose absorbed	Poor
Streptomycin	Moderate (30–35%)	Not absorbed	Poor
SECOND-LINE DRUGS			
Thiacetazone	Not bound	Rapid (2 hours)	Limited data
Para-aminosalicylic acid	High (60–65%)	Very rapid	Poor
Ethionamide and prothionamide	Limited data	Very rapid (30 minutes)	Good
Capreomycin	Limited data	Not absorbed	Poor
Viomycin	Limited data	Not absorbed	Poor
Clofazimine	Limited data	Slow (8–12 hours)	Limited data
Cycloserine	Not bound	Rapid (3 hours)	Good
Ofloxacin	Low	Rapid (1–1.5 hours)	Moderate

Corynebacterium spp., susceptibility to isoniazid is essentially restricted to the *M. tuberculosis* complex and some strains of *M. xenopi* and *M. kansasii*. Isoniazid is a prodrug requiring oxidative activation by the mycobacterial catalase-peroxidase enzyme KatG. The commonest causes of isoniazid resistance are point mutations in, or deletion of, the *katG* gene that encodes this enzyme. Less frequent resistance-determining mutations are in the *inhA* locus (or in its promoter region) which codes for an NADH-dependent enoyl-acyl carrier protein reductase involved in mycolic acid synthesis and the *oxyR–ahpC* locus which, like the *katG* locus, is involved in protection against oxidative stress.[12] The predominant mutations conferring resistance to isoniazid differ between the various lineages of *M. tuberculosis* and therefore show geographic variations in their distribution.[13]

Isoniazid is readily absorbed from the gastrointestinal tract and is converted to inactive metabolites, principally by acetylation, the rate of which is genetically determined. Thus, patients can be divided into rapid acetylators and slow acetylators, in whom the elimination half-lives of the drug are 0.5–1.5 hours and 2–4 hours, respectively. About half of Caucasian and black patients but over 80% of Chinese and Japanese patients are rapid acetylators. If administered regularly, response to therapy is unaffected by acetylator status.

Owing to its widespread use since the 1950s, resistance to isoniazid is common and many strains that are resistant to other antituberculosis drugs, particularly to rifampin, are also resistant to isoniazid.

Adverse events are usually mild and are more likely to occur in slow acetylators. They include several neurologic effects, including

TABLE 148-5	Principal Metabolic Products and Excretion of the Antituberculosis Agents	
Agent	**Principal Metabolic Products**	**Excretion**
FIRST-LINE DRUGS		
Isoniazid	Acetyl derivatives: rate of acetylation is genetically controlled	Unchanged and as acetyl derivatives in urine (ratio depends on rate of acetylation)
Rifampin (rifampicin)	Desacetyl derivative	As desacetylrifampin in bile
Pyrazinamide	Pyrazinoic acid	Mostly as pyrazinoic acid in urine
Ethambutol	Oxidation products and aldehydes	Mostly unchanged in urine; about 15% as metabolites
Streptomycin	None	Unchanged in urine
SECOND-LINE DRUGS		
Other aminoglycosides	None	Unchanged in urine
Thiacetazone	Unknown	20% eliminated in urine, fate of remainder unknown
Para-aminosalicylic acid	Acetylation products and glycine conjugates	About 80% in the urine, mostly in the acetylated form
Ethionamide and prothionamide	Sulfoxide (biologically active) and methyl derivatives	Less than 1% unchanged in urine
Capreomycin	None	Unchanged in urine
Viomycin	None	Unchanged in urine
Clofazimine	Very small amounts of unidentified metabolites	Unchanged in urine and feces
Cycloserine	Up to 35% converted to unidentified metabolites	Varying amounts unchanged in urine
Ofloxacin	5% metabolized to oxides and dimethyl derivatives	70–95% unchanged in urine, small amounts in bile

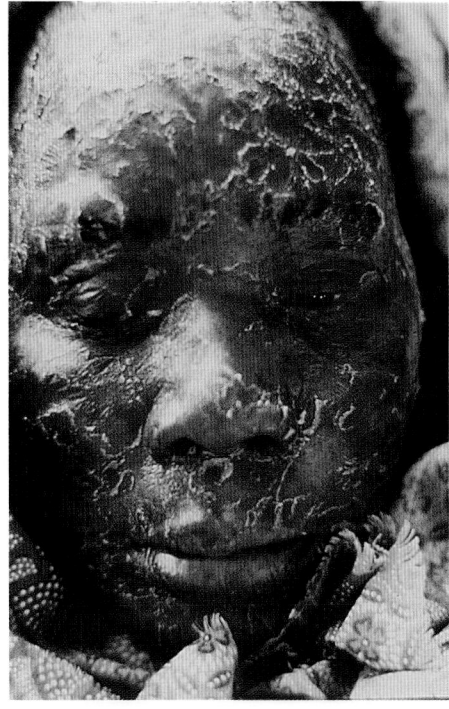

Figure 148-2 Severe dermal reaction to isoniazid. *Courtesy of Dr P. Mwaba, Zambia.*

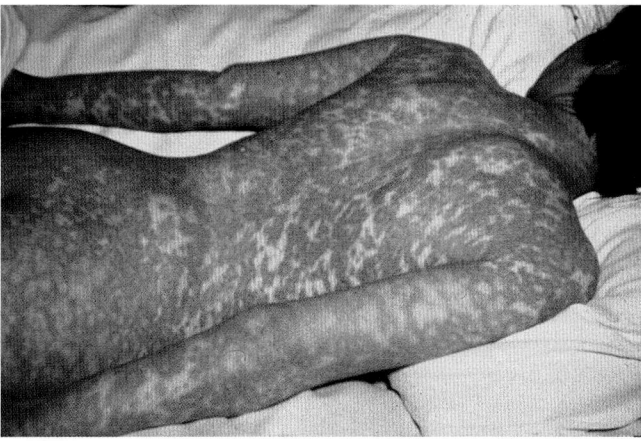

Figure 148-3 Erythema multiforme reaction to rifampin. *Courtesy of Dr P. Mwaba, Zambia.*

insomnia, restlessness, peripheral neuropathy, optic neuritis and mild psychiatric disturbances. More serious, but less common, neurologic effects include severe psychiatric disturbance and encephalopathy. The latter is particularly likely to occur in renal dialysis patients.[14]

Other adverse effects include hepatitis, particularly in patients aged over 35 years, arthralgia, fever and skin rashes. Very rare complications include hyperglycemia and agranulocytosis.

Adverse effects, particularly neurologic ones, are usually preventable by administration of pyridoxine (vitamin B6) 10 mg daily. Ideally all patients receiving isoniazid should be supplemented with pyridoxine. Accidental or intentional overdose of isoniazid can lead to refractory seizures and profound metabolic acidosis; treatment is with pyridoxine, given at a milligram to milligram dose equivalent to the amount of ingested isoniazid. Encephalopathy in renal dialysis patients may not respond to pyridoxine but usually resolves when isoniazid is withdrawn.[14]

RIFAMPIN (RIFAMPICIN) AND RIFAMYCINS

This is one of the rifamycins, semisynthetic derivatives of rifamycin S, a metabolite of *Amycolatopsis* (*Streptomyces*) *mediterranei*. Rifampin inhibits protein synthesis by a very specific inhibition of bacterial DNA-dependent RNA polymerase, thereby blocking the synthesis of mRNA. The corresponding mammalian enzyme is inhibited only by very high concentrations of rifampin. Resistance is due to single amino acid mutational changes in the *rpoB* gene, which encodes for the β subunit of the polymerase. Rifampin is a particularly effective drug because it kills both rapidly dividing bacilli and those that exhibit only occasional short bursts of metabolism. Ideally, therefore, it is given throughout the course of therapy. It is also used in the treatment of leprosy and for some other mycobacterial diseases.

TABLE 148-6	Adverse Reactions to the Antituberculosis Agents
Agent	**Adverse Reactions Reported By Drug, and – for Each Drug – Listed from More Common to Less Common**
ISONIAZID	
Uncommon reactions	Hepatitis, cutaneous hypersensitivity reactions including erythema multiforme, peripheral neuropathy
Rare reactions	Vertigo; convulsions; optic neuritis and atrophy; psychiatric disturbance; hemolytic anemia; aplastic anemia; dermal reactions including pellagra, purpura and lupoid syndrome; gynecomastia, hyperglycemia, arthralgia
RIFAMPIN (RIFAMPICIN)	
Uncommon reactions	Hepatitis, flushing, itching with or without a rash, gastrointestinal upsets, 'flu-like syndrome', headache
Rare reactions (usually associated with intermittent therapy)	Dyspnea, hypotension with or without shock, Addisonian crisis, hemolytic anemia, acute renal failure, thrombocytopenia with or without purpura, transient leukopenia or eosinophilia, menstrual disturbances, muscular weakness, pseudomembranous colitis
PYRAZINAMIDE	
Common reactions	Anorexia
Uncommon reactions	Hepatitis, nausea and vomiting, urticaria, nausea, arthralgia
Rare reactions	Sideroblastic anemia, photosensitization, gout, dysuria, aggravation of peptic ulcer
ETHAMBUTOL	
Uncommon reactions	Optic neuritis, arthralgia
Rare reactions	Hepatitis, cutaneous hypersensitivity including pruritus and urticaria, photosensitive lichenoid eruptions, paresthesia of the extremities, interstitial nephritis
STREPTOMYCIN	
Uncommon reactions	Vertigo, ataxia, deafness, tinnitus, cutaneous hypersensitivity
Rare reactions	Renal damage, aplastic anemia, agranulocytosis, peripheral neuropathy, optic neuritis with scotoma, severe bleeding due to antagonism of factor V, neuromuscular blockade in patients receiving muscle relaxants and in those with myasthenia gravis
OTHER AMINOGLYCOSIDES	
Common reactions	Vertigo, deafness, nephrotoxicity
Uncommon reactions	Neuromuscular blockade, particularly in high doses and in patients with myasthenia gravis or other neuromuscular disorders
Rare reactions	Agranulocytosis
PARA-AMINOSALICYLIC ACID	
Common reactions	Gastrointestinal upsets
Uncommon reactions	Cutaneous hypersensitivity, hepatitis, hypokalemia
Rare reactions	Acute renal failure, hemolytic anemia, thrombocytopenia, hypothyroidism
ETHIONAMIDE AND PROTHIONAMIDE	
Common reactions	Gastrointestinal upsets, salivation, metallic taste
Uncommon reactions	Cutaneous hypersensitivity, hepatitis
Rare reactions	Alopecia, convulsions, deafness, diplopia, gynecomastia, hypotension, impotence, psychiatric disturbance, menstrual irregularity, hypoglycemia, peripheral neuropathy
CAPREOMYCIN AND VIOMYCIN	
Common reactions	Eosinophilia (with capreomycin), pain and induration at injection site
Uncommon reactions	Loss of hearing, vertigo, tinnitus, electrolyte disturbances including hypokalemia, leukopenia or leukocytosis
Rare reactions	Renal impairment, hepatitis, thrombocytopenia
CLOFAZIMINE	
Common reactions	Discoloration of skin and body fluids, nausea, vomiting, abdominal pain, diarrhea
Uncommon reactions	Dryness of skin, ichthyosis, photosensitivity
Rare reactions	Intestinal obstruction
CYCLOSERINE	
Common reactions (especially with daily doses exceeding 500 mg)	Convulsions, drowsiness, sleep disturbance, headache, tremor, vertigo, confusion, irritability, aggression and other personality changes, psychosis (sometimes with suicidal tendencies)
Uncommon reactions	Cutaneous hypersensitivity, hepatitis, megaloblastic anemia
Rare reactions	Congestive heart failure

TABLE 148-6	Adverse Reactions to the Antituberculosis Agents (Continued)
Agent	**Adverse Reactions Reported By Drug, and – for Each Drug – Listed from More Common to Less Common**
FLUOROQUINOLONES	
Uncommon reactions	Gastrointestinal upsets, headache, dizziness, insomnia, cutaneous hypersensitivity reactions
Rare reactions	Restlessness; convulsions; psychiatric disturbances including psychotic reactions and hallucinations; edema of face, tongue and epiglottis; disturbance of taste and smell; anaphylactoid reactions; arthralgia, tendonitis, tendon rupture
LINEZOLID	
Described reactions	Thrombocytopenia, neutropenia and neuropathy which might require blood transfusion; metallic taste Adverse events have been lower with a dosage of 300 mg/day vs higher dosages (600 or 1200 mg/day)

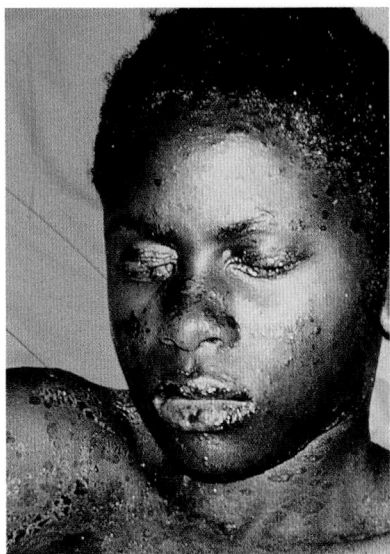

Figure 148-4   Stevens–Johnson syndrome induced by thiacetazone. *Courtesy of Dr P. Mwaba, Zambia.*

Rifampin is rapidly absorbed from the gastrointestinal tract, although absorption is delayed if it is given with food, and it is widely distributed. Only small amounts enter the CSF normally but much more enters when the meninges are inflamed. Rifampin enters cells and is therefore active against intracellular mycobacteria. It is metabolized by hepatic microsomal enzymes to the desacetyl derivative, which is excreted in the bile. As this enzymatic activity is inducible, the rate of plasma clearance of rifampin increases as treatment proceeds. Although principally excreted in the bile, some rifampin and the desacetyl derivative enter the urine and impart an orange-red color to it. It also enters saliva and lachrymal secretions and may cause pink staining of soft contact lenses. The induction of microsomal enzymes may have clinically significant effects on the metabolism of many other drugs (see below).

Rifampin may cause an influenza-like syndrome, which, paradoxically, occurs less often if the drug is given daily rather than intermittently. It causes transient abnormalities in liver function and, occasionally, clinically evident cholestatic hepatitis, although this is usually mild. Other adverse effects include gastrointestinal disturbances, skin rashes and antibody-mediated thrombocytopenia. Rifampin produces a deep orange pigment in the urine and other body fluids and the patient should be advised about this benign side effect.

Acute renal failure is a rare complication, although in some regions it is more frequent; in one center in India it accounted for 11 of 607 (1.8%) admissions for acute renal failure.[15] The renal prognosis is usually favorable. It typically occurs after re-introduction of rifampin and intermittent therapy is a risk factor.

Although the evidence that rifampin is teratogenic is very limited, it is best avoided if possible during the first 3 months of pregnancy. For the same reason, women receiving rifampin should avoid becoming pregnant. In this respect it is important to note that this drug interferes with the action of oral contraceptives, and women of childbearing age should be advised to use another form of birth control while receiving rifampin.

Rifabutin and rifapentine are closely related to rifampin, being semisynthetic derivatives of rifamycin S. Although rifabutin is considerably more active than rifampin *in vitro*, its *in vivo* action against *M. tuberculosis* is similar to that of rifampin. Cross-resistance between the rifamycins is usual, so the place for rifabutin in the treatment of MDR-TB is limited. Rifamycins induce cytochrome P450 enzymes in the liver leading to drug–drug interactions with antiretroviral agents, particularly HIV protease inhibitors, and other TB drug candidates such as bedaquiline.

PYRAZINAMIDE (PYRAZINOIC ACID AMIDE)

This is regularly included in the initial intensive phase of short-course chemotherapy because it has the important property of killing intracellular tubercle bacilli and, possibly, extracellular bacilli in anoxic, acidic inflamed lesions. It is inactive in neutral or alkaline microenvironments. The mode of action of pyrazinoic acid is poorly understood but the available evidence suggests that it disrupts bacterial membrane function. There is also evidence that it inhibits the mycobacterial fatty acid synthase (FAS)-1 enzyme.[16] Pyrazinamide requires conversion to pyrazinoic acid by mycobacterial pyrazinamidase enzymes encoded for by the 600 base-pair *pncA* gene. Resistance is usually associated with a wide range of point mutations in this gene, which are detectable by various techniques including microarrays.[17] Pyrazinamidase activity is not detectable in most pyrazinamide-resistant mutants of *M. tuberculosis* or in strains of *M. bovis*, which are naturally resistant to this agent. A few pyrazinamide-resistant strains, however, lack mutations in the *pncA* gene, suggesting alternative mechanisms for resistance to this agent, including defects in transportation of the agent into the bacterial cell.[18]

Pyrazinamide is readily absorbed from the gastrointestinal tract and freely enters the CSF, in which levels similar to those in plasma are found. It is metabolized in the liver; the metabolites, mostly pyrazinoic acid, are excreted in the urine.

Adverse effects are uncommon. It causes raised serum transaminase levels but overt hepatotoxicity is uncommon. It should be used with caution in alcoholics and in patients who have pre-existing hepatic disease, who should have regular liver function tests. Other adverse effects include anorexia, nausea, photosensitization of the skin,[19] arthralgia and gout caused by the inhibition of the excretion of uric acid by pyrazinoic acid.

ETHAMBUTOL

Ethambutol (*S,S'*-2,2'-(ethylenediimino)di-1-butanol) is included in the initial 2-month intensive phase of short-course antituberculosis regimens and also in some regimens for disease caused by other slowly growing mycobacteria, particularly members of the *M. avium* complex

(MAC), *M. kansasii*, *M. xenopi* and *M. malmoense*. By inhibiting the enzyme arabinosyl transferase, ethambutol blocks the synthesis of the polysaccharide arabinogalactan, a macromolecule essential for the structural integrity of the mycobacterial cell wall. Resistance is associated with mutations in the *embA*, *embB* and *embC* cluster of genes (principally *embB*), which code for this enzyme.[20]

There is conflicting evidence on its effect on resistance to other antituberculosis agents. Thus there is evidence that it may enhance the activity of some of the other drugs by affecting cell-wall permeability, particularly with MAC but possibly also in multidrug-resistant strains of *M. tuberculosis*.[21] There is also evidence that, in addition to determining resistance to ethambutol, a mutation in codon 306 of the *embB* gene predisposes *M. tuberculosis* to the development of resistance to a range of antituberculosis agents and transmission of such mutants has resulted in clusters of cases of drug-resistant tuberculosis.[22]

About 80% of the dose of ethambutol is absorbed from the gastrointestinal tract. Absorption is inhibited by antacids containing aluminum hydroxide. It does not cross the uninflamed meninges but up to 40% of the plasma level is found in the CSF in cases of tuberculous meningitis. It is mostly excreted unchanged in the urine but up to 15% is excreted as metabolites.

The principal side effect is optic neuritis which may have an irreversible effect on vision, but this is rare if the drug is given for no longer than 2 months at a daily dose of 25 mg/kg, or for longer at a dose not exceeding 15 mg/kg. Recommended dose and duration of therapy should never be exceeded, and the patient should be informed of the risk of visual impairment and advised to discontinue the drug if such impairment occurs. Loss of color discrimination is the first sign of visual toxicity. Where facilities are available, visual acuity should be assessed before therapy and at intervals during it.

Most guidelines recommend that the drug should not be given to children under the age of 5 years because their visual acuity cannot be readily assessed, even though ocular complications in such young children are extensively rare.

Other side effects of ethambutol include skin rashes, arthralgia, peripheral neuritis, hyperuricemia and, rarely, jaundice and thrombocytopenia.

STREPTOMYCIN

This was the first of the antituberculosis drugs to be discovered and it still has an important role in the treatment of tuberculosis. It inhibits protein synthesis by binding to the 30S subunit of the bacterial ribosome. It is active in neutral or alkaline environments such as the cavity wall but not in the more acidic environment of the closed, inflammatory foci and is therefore not a good sterilizing drug. It is very poorly absorbed from the gastrointestinal tract and must be given parenterally.

Streptomycin is toxic for the eighth cranial nerve (vestibular > cochlear), including that of the fetus, and its use should therefore be avoided in pregnancy. Other adverse reactions include impairment of renal function (uncommon) and hypersensitivity reactions – usually mild skin rashes or fever but occasionally anaphylactic reactions or exfoliative dermatitis.

Second-Line Drugs

There are, in addition to some agents used on anecdotal evidence of efficacy, six main classes of second-line antituberculosis agents; namely, aminoglycosides, polypeptides, thioamides, fluoroquinolones, cycloserine and *para*-aminosalicylic acid (Table 148-1).

AMINOGLYCOSIDES

In addition to streptomycin, the aminoglycosides kanamycin, amikacin and aminosidine (paromomycin) have activity against *M. tuberculosis*. Cross-resistance with streptomycin is usual. Kanamycin or amikacin is included in some regimens for the treatment of MDR-TB and amikacin in some regimens for the treatment of disease due to the MAC, particularly in HIV-positive patients. In common with streptomycin, these aminoglycosides are not absorbed from the gas-

trointestinal tract and must therefore be given parenterally. Nephrotoxicity and ototoxicity are the major toxicities.

POLYPEPTIDES: CAPREOMYCIN AND VIOMYCIN

In common with the aminoglycosides, these structurally closely related, cyclic polypeptides inhibit protein synthesis by blocking ribosomal function and must be given by intramuscular injection. They are completely cross-resistant and highly resistant mutants are cross-resistant to the aminoglycosides. They do not readily enter cells or the CSF and are mostly excreted unchanged in the urine. Adverse effects include ototoxicity, nephrotoxicity and pain, bleeding and induration at the injection site. There is some evidence that capreomycin is active against dormant or nonreplicating cells of *M. tuberculosis*.[23] Viomycin is rarely used and is seldom available.

THIOAMIDES: ETHIONAMIDE AND PROTHIONAMIDE

Ethionamide (ethylthioisonicotinamide) and prothionamide (propylthioisonicotinamide) are closely related drugs that are structurally similar to isoniazid; in common with isoniazid they inhibit the synthesis of mycobacterial mycolic acids by targeting the same molecule – enoyl-acyl carrier protein reductase encoded by the *inhA* gene.[24] Thus, in common with isoniazid, resistance is often associated with mutations in the *inhA* gene but, surprisingly, complete cross-resistance to isoniazid does not develop and partial cross-resistance is uncommon. Also in common with isoniazid, these agents are prodrugs that require activation by an enzyme encoded by the *ethA* locus but less than half the mutations conferring resistance to this agent occur in this locus.[25]

These two agents are degraded into several metabolites in the liver and less than 1% is excreted unchanged in the urine. The common occurrence of gastrointestinal irritation with these agents, even when they are given as enteric-coated tablets, limits their use. Prothionamide is slightly better tolerated and is used in some regimens for leprosy. Other adverse effects include skin reactions, hepatitis, impotence and gynecomastia in male patients, menstrual irregularities and various neurologic complications such as convulsions, mental disturbance and peripheral neuropathy.

FLUOROQUINOLONES

These agents inhibit the enzyme DNA gyrase encoded by the *gyrA* and *gyrB* genes, and DNA topoisomerase IV encoded by the *parC* and *parD* genes involved in the regulation of DNA supercoiling. Several fluoroquinolones have early bactericidal activities approaching those of isoniazid, and although results of clinical trials have been rather variable,[26] there is evidence that the addition of ofloxacin to the standard regimen of isoniazid, rifampin and pyrazinamide enables the duration of therapy to be reduced by 1–2 months.[27]

The role of second-generation fluoroquinolones (moxifloxacin in particular) has gained recent attention as they might be still active in the presence of resistance to first-generation drugs, and included in potential new regimens (together with pyrazinamide and PA-824) might have the potentiality of reducing the treatment duration to four months. Fluoroquinolones are readily absorbed from the gastrointestinal tract and enter tissues and fluids, including the CSF. Although metabolized to some extent by the liver, they are largely excreted unchanged in the urine. Doses therefore require modification in patients who have renal failure. Adverse effects include nausea and abdominal pain and various neurologic abnormalities including headache, vertigo, insomnia, restlessness, epileptiform attacks and psychiatric disturbances. They should be used with care in epileptic patients.

CYCLOSERINE

This D-alanine analog, a cyclic derivative of serine hydroxamic acid, inhibits synthesis of peptidoglycan. A related agent, terizidone, is a condensation product containing two cycloserine molecules. Cycloserine is bacteriostatic and thus of limited efficacy, although it is used in some cases of MDR-TB. Psychiatric symptoms, including acute psychotic episodes, occur commonly and further limit the usefulness of this drug, although the risk may to some extent be reduced by giving pyridoxine. Allergic skin rashes are rare.

PARA-AMINOSALICYLIC ACID

The mode of action of this bacteriostatic drug is poorly understood although there is some evidence that it inhibits the salicylate-dependent synthesis of the mycobactins – a class of iron-chelating lipids unique to the mycobacteria. It is readily absorbed from the intestine and rapidly acetylated in the liver. About 80% is excreted in the urine, mostly in the acetylated form.

It is rarely used as adverse effects are common. Gastrointestinal effects, including nausea, abdominal pain and diarrhea, occur in up to 30% of patients. Other adverse effects include thyroid dysfunction, crystalluria, blood dyscrasias and, rarely, Loffler's syndrome and encephalitis.

WHO CATEGORY 5 AND EXPERIMENTAL DRUGS

In common with isoniazid, thiacetazone (acetylaminobenzaldehyde thiosemicarbazone) inhibits the synthesis of mycolic acid, but by a poorly understood mechanism. Due to its very high incidence of severe, sometimes fatal, skin reactions – exfoliative dermatitis and Stevens–Johnson syndrome – thiacetazone should no longer be used.

Macrolides are broad-spectrum antibiotics that inhibit protein synthesis by binding to the ribosomal 50S subunit. The newer macrolides – clarithromycin, azithromycin and roxithromycin – are included in regimens used to treat disease due to MAC and other slowly growing mycobacteria including M. kansasii and M. xenopi. They have only partial in vitro activity against M. tuberculosis and evidence for their clinical usefulness is limited. They are well absorbed from the gastrointestinal tract and are excreted in urine. Adverse effects include gastrointestinal upset with occasional cases of pseudomembranous colitis and various psychiatric disorders, including rare episodes of acute mania.

Oxazolidinones are a new class of drugs that inhibit protein synthesis by binding to the 23S rRNA in the 50S ribosomal subunit. Linezolid (an oxazolidinone drug approved to treat drug-resistant, gram-positive bacteria) can substantially improve the outcome in patients with M/XDR-TB although cost and toxicity (thrombocytopenia and leukopenia) are major concerns.[28] The use of therapeutic drug monitoring (TDM) may minimize adverse events.[29]

Sutezolid, another oxazolidinone drug inhibiting protein synthesis, provides, as linezolid, a high barrier to resistance. It proved in mice to be more potent than linezolid with efficacy similar to that of isoniazid and rifampin, and a has synergistic effect with other first-line drugs, its toxicity being potentially lower.[30] In phase I trials in humans sutezolid appeared to be safe and well tolerated.[31,32] Recently, phase II clinical trials assessing safety and efficacy of sutezolid using early bactericidal activity (EBA) and whole-blood bactericidal activity were completed.[33]

A combination of amoxicillin and clavulanic acid has in vitro activity against M. tuberculosis and there is anecdotal evidence of a beneficial effect against MDR-TB.[34]

Meropenem-clavulanate added to a linezolid-containing regimen proved to be safe and effective in increasing the proportion of cases achieving bacteriological conversion.[35]

New TB Drug Development Pipeline

Figure 148-5 depicts the new TB drug development pipeline.[36,37]

Bedaquiline, a diarylquinoline, previously called TMC207 or R207910, specifically inhibits the c subunit of adenosine triphosphate (ATP) synthase thereby decreasing intracellular ATP levels. The drug was discovered using phenotypic screening and its target identified using whole genome sequencing of spontaneous bedaquiline-resistant mutants. In mice its bactericidal activity proved to be comparable to that of rifampin, isoniazid and pyrazinamide and its sterilizing activity comparable to that of rifampin. It has no cross-resistance with first antimycobacterial drugs, aminoglycosides, or fluoroquinolones. It has a long half-life (24 hours) and accumulates in tissues. Bedaquiline is given orally and is well absorbed and is metabolized by hepatic CYP450 enzymes to less active metabolite N-desmethyl M2.

Delamanid (OPC-67683), a nitro-dihydro-imidazooxazole derivative, is a new antituberculosis drug that inhibits mycolic acid synthesis and has shown potent in vitro and in vivo activity against drug-resistant strains of Mycobacterium tuberculosis. Delamanid[38] was recently pre-approved by EU authorities for inclusion in treatment regimens for MDR-TB.

PA-824, a nitroimidazole-oxazine drug, is active in vitro and in mouse models and shows cross-resistance with delamanid. The high

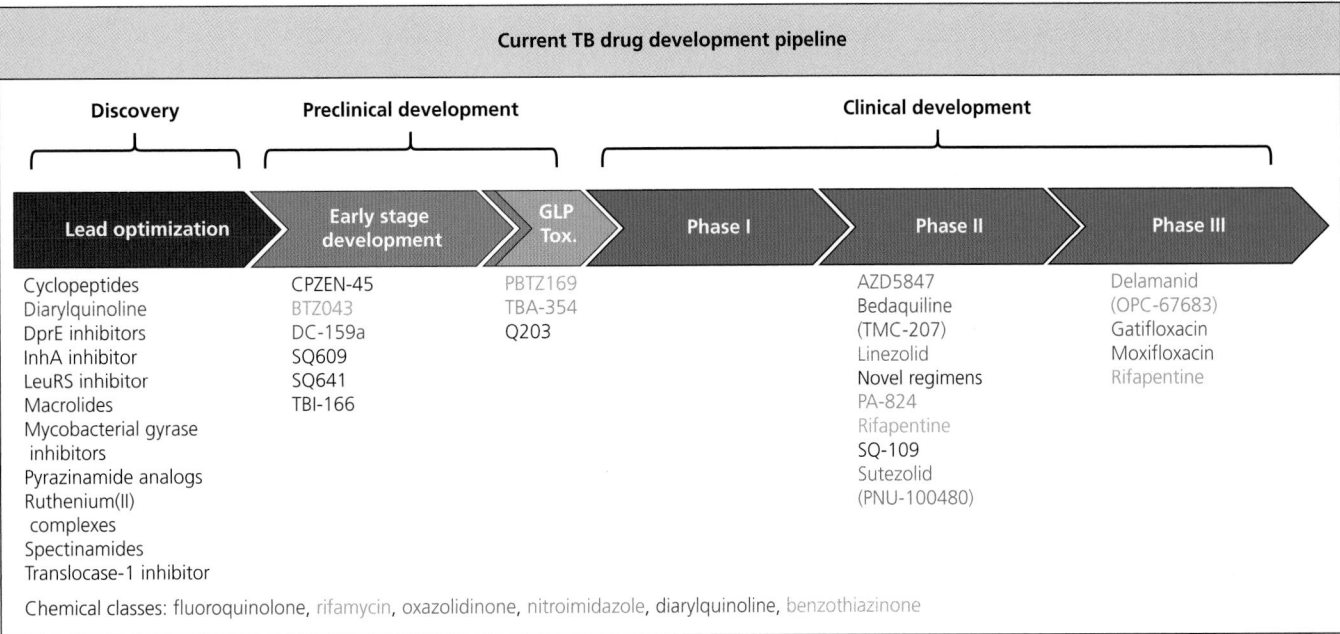

Figure 148-5 Current TB drug development pipeline. *Reprinted from Stop TB Partnership Working Group on New Drugs (www.newtbdrugs.org). Used with permission.*

protein binding may render PA-824 less accessible in cavities of pulmonary TB, being useful in combination regimens due to its synergistic action with other drugs (moxifloxacin and pyrazinamide in particular).

In addition, attempts to treat tuberculosis by enhancing or modifying immune defense mechanisms have been made with reported success.[39,40] Further clinical studies are required.

The Basis and Design of Therapeutic Regimens (see also Chapter 31)

The aims of modern chemotherapeutic regimens are:
- to cure the patient;
- to reduce infectivity as rapidly as possible; and
- to prevent the emergence of drug resistance.

In order to cure patients, it is necessary to destroy all the tubercle bacilli in the tissues; if even a few survive there is a high chance of relapse. Drugs that are bactericidal *in vitro* may not effectively sterilize the tissues *in vivo*.[41] This difference occurs because tubercle bacilli *in vivo* are in a number of different physiologic states or 'compartments':
- freely dividing extracellular bacilli, found mainly in the cavity walls;
- slowly dividing bacilli, found within macrophages and in acidic, inflammatory lesions; and
- dormant and near-dormant bacilli, within cells and in firm caseous material.

The antituberculosis drugs vary in their ability to destroy bacilli in these compartments and in preventing the emergence of resistance to a second drug.

During chemotherapy with modern short-course regimens, freely-replicating bacilli in the walls of the cavities are rapidly killed; this is termed the early bactericidal effect. Subsequently, the slowly replicating and near-dormant bacilli are destroyed, but at a much slower rate.

Isoniazid plays a key role in achieving the early bactericidal effect because it is particularly effective in destroying the freely-multiplying extracellular bacilli, particularly those in the walls of cavities. It has little or no effect on near-dormant bacilli and is therefore not a good sterilizing drug. Rifampin also contributes to the early bactericidal effect.

Ethambutol has bactericidal activity in the early stage of therapy but is not a sterilizing drug. Streptomycin is bactericidal in the slightly alkaline cavity walls but is likewise not a sterilizing agent because it is ineffective in the acidic environment within cells and caseous lesions. By contrast, pyrazinamide is effective within macrophages and acidic, anoxic inflammatory lesions, but not in the neutral or alkaline environment.

Thus, modern regimens commence with an intensive phase of therapy, usually lasting for 2 months, to optimize the early bactericidal effect, thereby eliminating most of the bacilli and rendering the patient noninfectious.[42] The principal drugs used are:
- isoniazid (active against bacilli in the cavity walls);
- pyrazinamide (active against bacilli in acidic closed lesions);
- rifampin (active against both); and
- ethambutol (active in the early stage of therapy and included as a fourth drug as drug resistance is increasingly prevalent).

The daily drug doses and the intermittent doses are listed in Table 148-7.

The intensive phase is followed by a continuation phase, usually lasting 4 months, in which any remaining dormant or near-dormant bacilli are destroyed. For this purpose, rifampin is the most powerful sterilizing drug. Although isoniazid is not a sterilizing drug, it is, by its potent activity against replicating bacilli, very effective at preventing the emergence of rifampin-resistant mutants. It is thus given together with rifampin throughout the regimen.

Accordingly, the most effective and widely used modern short-course regimens are based on a 2-month phase of rifampin, isoniazid, pyrazinamide and ethambutol, followed by a 4-month phase of rifampin and isoniazid (Table 148-8).[42]

TABLE 148-7	Doses of the Antituberculosis Agents				
FIRST-LINE DRUGS		**DAILY DOSE**		**THREE TIMES WEEKLY INTERMITTENT THERAPY**	
Agents	Adults	Children		Dose (Adults and Children) (mg/kg)	Maximum Dose
Rifampin (rifampicin)	450 mg if body weight <50 kg 600 mg if body weight ≥50 kg	10 mg/kg to maximum of 600 mg		15	600 mg
Isoniazid	200–300 mg	5 mg/kg		15	750 mg
Pyrazinamide	1.5 g if body weight <50 kg 2.0 g if body weight ≥50 kg	25 mg/kg		50	2.0 g if body weight <50 kg 2.5 g if body weight ≥50 kg
Ethambutol	15 mg/kg			30	1.8 g
Streptomycin	750 mg if body weight <50 kg 1 g if body weight ≥50 kg 750 mg if age ≥40 years 500 mg if age ≥60 years	15 mg/kg to maximum of 0.75 g		15–30	750 mg if body weight <50 kg 1 g if body weight ≥50 kg
SECOND-LINE DRUGS					
Agents	Adults		Children		
Thiacetazone	150 mg		50 mg		
Para-aminosalicylic acid	10–12 g		300 mg/kg		
Ethionamide and prothionamide	500 mg if body weight <50 kg 750 mg if body weight ≥50 kg		15–20 mg/kg		
Capreomycin	1 g		Avoid		
Viomycin	1 g		Avoid		
Cycloserine	500 mg if body weight <50 kg 750 mg if body weight ≥50 kg		Avoid		
Ofloxacin	800 mg		Avoid		

TABLE 148-8	Principal Antituberculosis Regimens for New TB Cases Recommended by the World Health Organization		
TB TREATMENT REGIMENS			
Intensive phase	**Continuation phase**	**Notes**	
2HRZE	4 HR	Standard regimen	
2HRZE	4 HRE	Level of H resistance among new TB cases is high and H susceptibility testing result is not available before the continuation phase.	

Notes: E has to be prescribed during the intensive phase in individuals with noncavitary, smear-negative pulmonary TB or with extrapulmonary TB and who are HIV-negative. In TB meningitis, it should be replaced by S.
H, isoniazid; R, rifampin; Z, pyrazinamide; E, ethambutol; S, streptomycin.

In most regimens, drugs are given daily but, provided that therapy is closely supervised so that all doses are taken, they may be given three times per week during the continuation phase or, in some regimens, throughout.

Some physicians continue therapy for up to 12 months as a precautionary measure for some extrapulmonary forms of tuberculosis; particularly TB meningitis or spinal TB, in which a relapse would be particularly devastating.

Drug-Resistant Tuberculosis

Resistance to any given anti-infective agent occurs by mutation at a low but constant rate, so that treatment with a single drug, however powerful, will inevitably lead to selection of resistant mutants. This is largely, but not entirely, avoided by the use of multidrug regimens. Under ideal conditions and in the absence of drug resistance, relapses after completion of a modern short-course chemotherapeutic regimen are uncommon and are mostly due to drug-susceptible bacilli. Deficiencies in the use of multidrug regimens has led to the increasing emergence of strains resistant to one or more drugs.[43]

Although resistance to isoniazid is common, patients whose disease is caused by such resistant strains usually respond to short-course chemotherapy. Resistance to rifampin is much more serious in view of the unique ability of this drug to eliminate near-dormant persisting bacilli. Many strains resistant to rifampin are also resistant to isoniazid. The term multidrug resistance has been adopted by the WHO to refer to strains that are resistant to these two drugs, with or without resistance to additional drugs.[44]

A combined initiative by the WHO and the International Union Against Tuberculosis and Lung Disease was launched in 1994 to perform a global survey of resistance to first-line antituberculosis drugs and now allows reliable monitoring of the prevalence of drug resistance globally.[45]

MDR-TB is presently a global phenomenon (although former Soviet Union countries represent the hot spot), potentially able to hamper the tuberculosis control efforts at the global level.[4,46] The 'world record' has been described in Belarus, with 35.3% among new cases and 76.5% among retreatment cases.[40]

EXTENSIVELY DRUG-RESISTANT TUBERCULOSIS (XDR-TB)

Tuberculosis resistant to many of the second-line, as well as first-line drugs, has been described in many countries and has been termed extensively drug-resistant tuberculosis (XDR-TB), defined as resistance to at least rifampin and isoniazid among the first-line agents, to any fluoroquinolone and to at least one of the injectable second-line agents (amikacin, kanamycin and capreomycin).[47-50]

The serious threat posed by XDR-TB became obvious during an outbreak in the Kwazulu-Natal province of South Africa. Despite

BOX 148-1	**FACTORS LEADING TO SUBOPTIMAL THERAPY AND THE EMERGENCE OF DRUG AND MULTIDRUG RESISTANCE**

Suboptimal Drug Regimens and Poor Adherence
During the continuation phase, a patient harboring an isoniazid-resistant strain is treated under rifampin monotherapy leading to rifampin resistance. Social determinants including interruptions interact to drive poor adherence and further acquired drug resistance.

Subtherapeutic Drug Levels (Below MICs)
- Efflux pump induction.
- Variability in drug metabolic rates driving subtherapeutic serum levels.
- Variability in drug absorption rates lead to subtherapeutic peak concentrations.
- Exposure of mycobacteria to suboptimal drug concentrations in fibro-cavitary lesions.

Enhanced Transmission of Drug-Resistant *M. tuberculosis*
- High bacterial burden.
- Strain genotype.
- Metabolic status of organisms in aerosolized sputum.
- Frequency and intensity of cough and sputum viscosity.
- Cavitary disease; number, dimension and location of cavities.
- Degree of ventilation, length of exposure, humidity and other factors enhancing transmission.

Effect of Genotype and Compensatory Mutations
- Epistatic interactions may modulate fitness (increased, decreased or unchanged).
- Compensatory mutations impact structural and physiological pathways because of changes in the proteome.
- Strain and types of mutations are associated with different cell wall characteristics, thickness and budding characteristics.
- Change in structure and the bacterial proteome by drug-resistant isolates impact host response.

antituberculosis and antiretroviral therapy, all patients except one with XDR-TB died, and the median survival was only 16 days after diagnosis.[51]

XDR-TB cases has been identified in 93 countries. In 2012 WHO estimated that 9.6% of the existing (estimated) 450 000 MDR-TB cases harbor XDR-TB strains.[4]

In the largest study available the probability of cure was significantly lower in those with XDR-TB and resistance to all second-line drugs (19% vs 43%), while the likelihood of failure and death was higher in XDR-TB patients with additional resistance ($\geq$48% vs 35%). These data suggest that patients with additional resistance beyond XDR-TB achieved poorer outcomes compared with those with MDR- and XDR-TB alone.

CAUSES OF ANTITUBERCULOSIS DRUG RESISTANCE

Two forms of drug resistance are encountered – acquired and primary (or initial):
- acquired resistance is the result of suboptimal therapy that encourages selective growth of mutants resistant to one or more drugs; and
- primary resistance is due to infection from a source case who has drug-resistant disease.

The development of drug resistance is due to many avoidable failures in the management of the disease (Box 148-1).

THERAPY OF MULTIDRUG-RESISTANT TUBERCULOSIS

Tuberculosis due to bacilli resistant to isoniazid alone usually responds to short-course drug regimens based on four drugs during the intensive phase but, by contrast, resistance to both isoniazid and rifampin (i.e. multidrug resistance) requires prolonged treatment with drugs that are much more costly, less effective and more toxic. The cost of such therapy is high; in the USA it can exceed US$250 000, compared with the cost of US$2000 for treating a patient who has drug-susceptible disease, while in Germany the cost (drugs only) of treating drug-susceptible TB is €7848, versus treating MDR-TB (€54 779) and XDR-TB (€168 310), respectively.[52] The prognosis for patients who have MDR-TB has improved considerably and, provided that the patient is diagnosed before severe lung damage has occurred and that the best supervised therapy and laboratory support is available, the outlook is good in the majority of cases. Under these optimal conditions, cure rates of 96% have been achieved.

Ideally regimens should be designed for each patient on the basis of *in vitro* susceptibility. Various regimens have been used and there have been few comparisons between them. Currently used regimens are usually based on a fluoroquinolone with at least two other drugs to which the strain is susceptible, such as kanamycin and ethionamide (or prothionamide).[53,54] Other agents include rifabutin, amikacin, capreomycin, clofazimine, cycloserine and *para*-aminosalicylic acid. Great care and dedication are required for the successful management of MDR-TB (Box 148-2).

Bedaquiline and Delamanid

These two new TB drugs are now available, under compassionate-use programs, to treat difficult cases, whenever the third or fourth active drugs are not available, and the disease is life-threatening.

According to the WHO recommendations, bedaquiline may be added to a WHO-recommended backbone regimen in adult MDR-TB patients under the following conditions:

- When an effective treatment regimen containing four second-line drugs in addition to pyrazinamide, cannot be designed.
- When there is documented resistance to any fluoroquinolone or injectables in addition to MDR.
- In adults older than 18 years of age under carefully monitored conditions.
- Per os at the dose of 400 mg daily for 2 weeks, then 200 mg three time a week, for a total duration of 24 weeks.

The EU regulatory (EMA) indications for delamanid recommend its use as part of an appropriate combination regimen for pulmonary MDR-TB in adult patients when an effective treatment regimen cannot otherwise be composed for reasons of resistance or tolerability.

THERAPY OF EXTENSIVELY DRUG-RESISTANT TUBERCULOSIS

When designing a regimen for an XDR-TB case the following principles need to be followed:

- Regimens should be constructed based on prevailing drug susceptibility testing (DST) patterns.
- One injectable is chosen from category 2, any drug that the isolate is susceptible to from category 1, and any remaining available drugs from category 3 or 4.

- Given the high background rates of TB and MDR-TB in several countries, regimens are often constructed around a backbone of capreomycin and PAS.
- Patients should be carefully monitored for adverse drug reactions, particularly for capreomycin (renal failure, hypokalemia and hypomagnesemia), which are common.
- Patients on capreomycin should have weekly urea and electrolytes monitored for the first 8 weeks and then monthly thereafter. Attention should be paid to correcting risk factors for renal failure (dehydration, nausea, vomiting and diarrhea), avoidance of other nephrotoxic drugs (co-trimoxazole and nevirapine) and early identification of underlying renal disease (diabetes and HIV-associated nephropathy).

Treatment of Patients in Special Circumstances

PATIENTS WHO HAVE RENAL OR HEPATIC DISEASE

Modification of drug regimens and dosages may be required when there is substantial renal impairment or liver disease. The first-line drugs (rifampin, isoniazid, pyrazinamide), and also ethionamide and prothionamide, are either completely metabolized or eliminated in the bile. They may therefore be used safely at normal doses in patients who have renal impairment. Isoniazid occasionally causes encephalopathy in patients who have renal failure and in those on dialysis but the risk is reduced, although not eliminated, by administering pyridoxine.[14] Although ethambutol is mainly eliminated by the kidney it can be used in reduced doses in patients who have impaired renal function. Streptomycin and other aminoglycosides are eliminated entirely by the kidney; as they are potentially nephrotoxic, special care must be taken.

In severe renal failure the dose of isoniazid should be reduced to 200 mg once daily (ensuring that pyridoxine is given to prevent peripheral neuropathy). Streptomycin and ethambutol are excreted by the kidney and adjustment to doses is necessary in renal failure. Streptomycin levels must be monitored and doses and spacing adjusted to achieve a peak level of 40 µg/mL and a trough level of <5 µg/mL to avoid toxicity. For patients on dialysis, a supplemental streptomycin dose should be given at approximately 5 mg/kg after hemodialysis.

Ethambutol dosages are dependent on creatinine clearances. For patients who have creatinine clearances between 50 mL/min and 100 mL/min, the dose is 25 mg/kg three times weekly; at 30–50 mL/min, the dose is 25 mg/kg twice a week; and at 10–25 mL/min the dose is 15 mg/kg at 2-day intervals. Patients on hemodialysis may be given 25 mg/kg ethambutol 6 hours before the procedure.

There is no clear evidence that the potentially hepatotoxic drugs rifampin and pyrazinamide are any more toxic in patients who have impaired hepatic function. Nevertheless, if they are used, hepatic function should be carefully and regularly monitored during therapy. Some physicians avoid them and treat such patients with isoniazid and ethambutol for 1 year, with the addition of streptomycin for the first 2–3 months. An alternative is to use a fluoroquinolone such as ofloxacin instead of rifampin.[55]

If rifampin is used, it should be used with caution; doses should be reduced in patients who have bilirubin concentrations exceeding 50 mmol/L (2.92 mg/dL). Liver function should be regularly monitored, where possible, in alcoholics, the elderly, malnourished children and children under 2 years of age.

If jaundice develops during antituberculosis therapy, treatment should be stopped until the jaundice resolves. In many cases resumption of treatment does not cause a recurrence of the jaundice. If the patient is seriously ill with tuberculosis, he or she may be treated with streptomycin and ethambutol even in the presence of jaundice.

HIV-POSITIVE PATIENTS WHO HAVE TUBERCULOSIS

The treatment of tuberculosis in HIV-positive patients (see also Chapter 96) follows the same well-established principles used in the treatment of non-HIV-infected patients.[56]

PREGNANCY AND THE POSTPARTUM PERIOD

There is general agreement that the management of tuberculosis in pregnancy and in the postpartum period should be similar to that in other patients, although some advocate avoiding pyrazinamide. Short-course regimens seem to have a minimal risk of causing fetal abnormalities, and side effects in the pregnant woman are no higher than in those who are not pregnant.[57] Opinions concerning the safety of pyrazinamide differ because there are limited experimental data on its effect on the fetus. Nonetheless, it is often used, particularly in regions where drug resistance is common. Streptomycin is avoided owing to its ototoxic properties. The treatment of drug-resistant tuberculosis, especially MDR-TB, during pregnancy and the management of the neonate requires careful consideration, and experience is very limited.[58] Expert clinical and laboratory guidance, if available, is required.

An increased incidence of isoniazid-related epileptiform attacks and other neurologic symptoms has been reported in pregnant women but these are preventable by the prescription of pyridoxine 10 mg daily. Mothers taking antituberculosis drugs at the time of birth can care for their infants with little risk, unless the mother's disease is drug resistant or not responding to therapy. Likewise, although some of the drugs enter the milk in small concentrations, breast-feeding has no adverse effects on the infant.[59]

Drug Interactions

Clinically significant interactions between the first-line antituberculosis drugs themselves have been described but are uncommon;[60] however, such reactions could well occur when more complex regimens are used to treat MDR-TB and XDR-TB. Antituberculosis drugs may interact with drugs used to treat unrelated conditions (Box 148-3). Rifampin is the most important in this respect because it is a potent inducer of cytochrome isoenzymes involved in the metabolism of many drugs. The increased metabolism and clearance of these drugs may lead to therapeutic failure unless levels are adjusted and then readjusted when rifampin therapy ceases. Patients on oral contraceptives should be advised to use alternative forms of birth control.

Rifampin reduces the plasma concentrations and half-lives of the imidazole and triazole antifungals and these agents reduce plasma levels of rifampin. Because some patients, notably those who are HIV-positive, may also require antifungal therapy, these interactions, which may lead to treatment failure, are of increasing importance. Patients who are HIV-positive may also be receiving trimethoprim–sulfamethoxazole for prevention or treatment of *Pneumocystis jirovecii* (formerly *P. carinii*) infection. This agent significantly increases the serum levels and half-life of rifampin, leading to an increased incidence of adverse effects, including hepatotoxicity.[61]

The catabolism of immunosuppressive agents administered to renal transplant patients, including azathioprine, corticosteroids, ciclosporin, sirolimus and tacrolimus, is increased by rifampin and dose adjustments may be required.[62] Streptomycin should be avoided in transplant patients as it increases the available level of ciclosporin, resulting in nephrotoxicity.

Drug interactions with isoniazid are more pronounced in slow acetylators. The effects of isoniazid are potentiated by insulin and opposed by prednisone (prednisolone); its absorption from the intestine, and that of ethambutol and the quinolones, is inhibited by antacids containing aluminum hydroxide. The effects of carbamazepine and phenytoin are potentiated by isoniazid and those of enflurane are opposed.

DRUG INTERACTIONS WITH ANTIRETROVIRAL AGENTS

Many antiretroviral agents interact with rifampin, but this is most marked with HIV non-nucleoside reverse transcriptase, protease and integrase inhibitors.[63] Rifampin accelerates the metabolism of HIV protease inhibitors (through induction of hepatic P450 cytochrome) and integrase inhibitors through inducing glucuronidation, resulting in subtherapeutic levels of these agents and thereby increasing the risk of the development of viral resistance. In addition, protease inhibitors

---

Drug Metabolism Induced by Rifampin (Decreased Therapeutic Effect)

Some antiretroviral agents (HIV integrase inhibitors, HIV protease inhibitors)
Azathioprine
Corticosteroids
Ciclosporin
Diazepam
Digoxin
Haloperidol
Imidazoles
Opioids
Oral contraceptives
Phenytoin
Propranolol
Quinidine
Theophylline
Tolbutamide
Warfarin

Potentiates the Effects of Rifampin (Rifampicin)

Trimethoprim–sulfamethoxazole

Effects Potentiated by Isoniazid

Phenytoin
Carbamazepine

Potentiates the Effects of Isoniazid

Insulin

Drug Metabolism Induced by Isoniazid (Decreased Therapeutic Effect)

Enflurane

Opposes the Effects of Isoniazid

Prednisone
Antacids (inhibit absorption)

Effects Potentiated by Streptomycin

Neuromuscular blocking agents

Effects Potentiated by Quinolones

Aminophylline and theophylline

Potentiates the Effects of Quinolones

Cimetidine

Interferes with the Absorption of Quinolones

Antacids, iron preparations, sucralfate, didanosine (all inhibit absorption)

---

retard the metabolism of rifampin, resulting in increased serum levels and the likelihood of increased drug toxicity (see Chapter 96).

Regimens not containing a rifamycin are much less effective than those that are rifamycin-based for treatment of HIV-infected patients. Thus, except in cases of resistance or intolerance to these agents, regimens containing a rifamycin throughout should be used and any interactions between these and the antiretroviral agents should be managed appropriately. Whenever possible, rifampin should be replaced by rifabutin, a much less powerful inducer of cytochrome enzymes, and to commence or continue with the antiretroviral drugs.[64] The clinical experience of antiretroviral regimens based on a non-nucleoside reverse transcriptase inhibitor such as efavirenz plus two nucleoside analogs with rifampin-based antituberculosis treatment regimens in terms of tolerance and impact on both tuberculosis and HIV disease has been favorable.[65,66]

The availability of new drugs (bedaquiline, delamanid, PA-824), which will hopefully include shorter, effective regimens not including rifampin and the ability to treat simultaneously drug-susceptible and MDR-TB cases, opens new scenarios in the treatment of TB/HIV coinfected patients.

Drug-Susceptibility Testing

The purpose of drug-susceptibility testing is not to detect small numbers of drug-resistant mutants, which will inevitably be present in

TABLE 148-9	Techniques Used To Determine Susceptibility to Antituberculosis Agents *In Vitro*	
Technique	**Where Technique is Used**	**Description of Technique**
Proportion method	USA and some European countries	Drug-free and drug-containing media are inoculated with test strains and the colony counts are compared; strains are reported as resistant if the colony count on the drug-containing medium is over 1% of that on the drug-free medium
Absolute concentration method	Some parts of Europe	Based on growth on media containing doubling dilutions of a known concentration of drug, so that the minimal bactericidal concentrations of drugs may be determined
Resistance ratio method	UK and those countries influenced by British bacteriologists	Similar to the absolute concentration method except that results are expressed as the ratio of the drug concentration inhibiting the test and drug-susceptible control strains, rather than as the actual inhibiting concentration
Disk diffusion method	Rarely used	Similar to absolute concentration method and resistance ratio method but technically simpler, as disks containing the drugs are placed on the solid media, thereby avoiding the need to prepare batches of media containing the various drugs

every patient who has tuberculosis and in every culture, but rather to determine whether the great majority of the bacilli are susceptible to levels of the drugs that are achieved clinically. In industrialized nations with the requisite facilities, and particularly where MDR-TB is common, susceptibility testing of all clinical isolates is definitely indicated. In most low and middle-income countries, facilities for conducting drug-susceptibility tests are limited. For this reason WHO has promoted the use of rapid tests (e.g. Xpert MTB/RIF, see below).

Global surveys on drug resistance have been compromised by the variety of methods used for surveillance and for drug-susceptibility testing and the lack of standardization of the methods. The WHO has therefore prepared guidelines for standardized surveillance techniques and has established a network of supranational reference laboratories to coordinate surveillance and to provide technical guidance and assistance.[67]

METHODS OF DRUG-SUSCEPTIBILITY TESTING

Methods for drug-susceptibility testing can be divided into those that:
- are based on inhibition of bacterial growth on drug-containing standard media;
- detect growth inhibition by automated systems;
- use biologic indicators of bacterial viability, such as enzyme activity and bacteriophage replication; and
- use nucleic-acid-based technology to detect mutations in genes determining susceptibility to drugs.

Methods for drug-susceptibility testing based on growth on conventional media are well established but have the great disadvantage that there is a long delay before results are available. Four methods are currently in use (Table 148-9).

In an (unpublished) investigation carried out by members of the European Society of Mycobacteriology, there were only minor discrepancies between results obtained by different workers using the first three of the methods listed in Table 148-9. All these methods may be used either for direct susceptibility tests on smear-positive sputum or for indirect susceptibility tests on cultures. The relative merits and usefulness of these methods in differing circumstances have been reviewed.[68]

Conventional tests for susceptibility to pyrazinamide pose particular problems because the drug acts only in acidic environments in which bacterial growth is poor. Thus, the tests require careful standardization and interpretation.

Automated techniques are widely used in high-income countries. They are more costly than the conventional methods but the rapidity of the results justifies the extra cost, especially where multidrug resistance is common. Susceptibility to all antituberculosis drugs, including pyrazinamide, can be determined by these methods. Although radiometric systems were used originally,[69] these have been largely replaced by nonradiometric systems, principally based on the unquenching of a fluorescent dye when oxygen is consumed by mycobacterial metabolism or on color changes in dyes when carbon dioxide is liberated from nutrients in the medium.[70]

Several rapid methods for the detection of mutations in the *rpoB* gene conferring resistance to rifampin have been described; Xpert MTB/RIF assay is a semi-nested quantitative real time polymerase chain reaction (PCR) assay that simultaneously detects TB and rifampin resistance.[71] It is validated for use with sputum, although evidence is emerging for its use on extrapulmonary samples. Xpert/RIF, which works also at primary care facility level, dramatically increases the number of TB cases detected and improves times to treatment initiation, as within less than 2 hours provides the crucial information the clinician needs: is it tuberculosis? Is there resistance to rifampin (considered a proxy of MDR-TB)?

Increased and earlier detection of rifampin resistance will hopefully facilitate earlier initiation of appropriate therapy and reduce transmission.

Alternative diagnostics are line probe assays, such as the MTB-DR*plus* assay which offers similar performance to Xpert MTB/RIF for TB detection directly from patient specimens and has excellent performance for the detection of MDR-TB. More recently, the MTBDR*sl* assay has been introduced which interrogates for drug resistance to second-line injectable drugs (SLID; mutations on the *rrs* gene), fluoroquinolones (*gyr A* gene) and ethambutol (*embB* gene). However, this has lower accuracy in smear-negative specimens.[72]

Bacteriophages have been used to detect bacterial viability in the presence of antituberculosis agents.[73]

References available online at expertconsult.com.

KEY REFERENCES

Centers for Disease Control and Prevention: Provisional CDC guidelines for the use and safety monitoring of bedaquiline fumarate (Sirturo) for the treatment of multidrug-resistant tuberculosis. *MMWR Recomm Rep* 2013; 62(RR–09):1-12. Erratum in: MMWR Recomm Rep 2013; 62(45):906.

Lechartier B., Rybniker J., Zumla A., et al.: Tuberculosis drug discovery in the post-post-genomic era. *EMBO Mol Med* 2014; 6(2):158-168.

Wallis R.S.: Sustainable tuberculosis drug development. *Clin Infect Dis* 2013; 56(1):106-113.

Wallis R.S., Maeurer M., Mwaba P., et al.: Tuberculosis-advances in development of new drugs, treatment regimens, host-directed therapies, and biomarkers. *Lancet Infect Dis* 2016; 16(4):e34-e46.

World Health Organization: *Treatment of tuberculosis guidelines*. 4th ed. Geneva: WHO; 2010. Available: http://whqlibdoc.who.int/publications/2010/9789241547833_eng.pdf.

Zumla A., Nahid P., Cole S.T.: Advances in the development of new tuberculosis drugs and treatment regimens. *Nat Rev Drug Discov* 2013; 12(5):388-404.

Zumla A.I., Gillespie S.H., Hoelscher M., et al.: New antituberculosis drugs, regimens, and adjunct therapies: needs, advances, and future prospects. *Lancet Infect Dis* 2014; 14(4):327-340.

Miscellaneous Agents: Fusidic Acid, Nitrofurantoin and Fosfomycin

ANGELA HUTTNER | STEPHAN HARBARTH

KEY CONCEPTS

- Fusidic acid is mainly used as an antistaphylococcal agent but has to be used in combination with other antibiotics to prevent the emergence of resistance during systemic treatment.

- Nitrofurantoin is currently recommended as first-line therapy for uncomplicated lower urinary tract infections. Its clinical efficacy is comparable to that of other antibacterial agents.

- Nitrofurantoin rarely causes side effects when given short-term (≤7 days).

- Oral fosfomycin is also recommended for uncomplicated lower urinary tract infections; while its single-dose administration is convenient, its clinical efficacy at this dose relative to other antibacterial agents is currently under investigation.

- Intravenous fosfomycin is available in some countries and is mostly used for staphylococcal infections; it should be used in combination with another antistaphylococcal agent to prevent the emergence of resistance.

Introduction

This chapter deals with three antibiotics that are chemically different and have varying antibacterial spectra and clinical uses.

Fusidic Acid

Fusidic acid has a steroidal chemical structure.

Mechanism of Action

It inhibits protein synthesis by binding to the ribosome elongation factor G complex (see Chapter 137).

Spectrum of Activity

Fusidic acid has a narrow spectrum of activity. It exhibits good activity against staphylococci including both methicillin-sensitive and methicillin-resistant strains of *Staphylococcus aureus* (MSSA and MRSA), as well as coagulase-negative staphylococci, but activity against other gram-positive cocci is poor. In addition, fusidic acid has anaerobic activity (including *Clostridium difficile*), has been found to be active against some mycobacteria and has limited activity against *Legionella pneumophila*.[1]

Mechanisms of Resistance

High-level resistance in *Staph. aureus* is conferred through mutations in the gene encoding elongation factor G. Several transferable mechanisms of resistance result in low-level resistance (see Chapter 138).[2]

Pharmacokinetics, Route of Administration and Dosage

Fusidic acid is available for intravenous (IV), oral or topical administration. The bioavailability after oral administration is 75–90% with

tablets but only about 23% in children given a suspension.[3] It has high inter-patient variability in pharmacokinetics, is almost entirely nonrenally eliminated by biliary excretion and is highly protein-bound (97%).

Conventional dosages are as follow:
- adults: 500 mg (as sodium fusidate tablets) q8h orally or intravenously;
- neonates: 50 mg/kg (as fusidic acid suspension) in three divided doses;
- children 1 month–1 year old: 15 mg/kg q8h;
- children 1–5 years old: 250 mg q8h;
- children 6–12 years old: 500 mg q8h.

Due to slow attainment of steady state, the use of loading doses (≥1200 mg twice daily on day 1 followed by ≥600 mg q12 h) was recently proposed to increase activity and prevent emergence of resistance.[4]

Doses should be reduced in patients who have hepatic and/or biliary disease. Full doses can be given to patients who have renal insufficiency and to the elderly. Because of its high protein binding, fusidic acid should be avoided in women in the third trimester of pregnancy and newborns to decrease the risk of kernicterus.

Indications

Fusidic acid is mainly used as an antistaphylococcal agent but has to be used in combination with other antibiotics to prevent the emergence of resistance during systemic treatment. Resistance has also emerged as a problem clinically when it has been used as a single agent topically for skin infections.[5]

Both *in vivo* and *in vitro* studies have shown that the antibacterial activity of the combination of fusidic acid with other antibiotics is unpredictable so that synergistic, antagonist, additive or indifferent effects have all been described.[6,7] For instance, in an experimental model of *Staph. aureus* meningitis, antagonism between methicillin and fusidic acid was observed.[8]

Fusidic acid is widely used for the treatment of bone and joint infections due to *Staph. aureus* as high bactericidal levels are achieved in infected joints and bone, including sequestra. It is usually combined with a penicillinase-stable penicillin (e.g. dicloxacillin or flucloxacillin) to prevent the emergence of resistance, although data from clinical trials are not available.

Fusidic acid is one of the few oral agents available for the treatment of methicillin-resistant staphylococci. Ideally it should be used in combination with another antibiotic to prevent the emergence of resistance. Oral rifampin (rifampicin) and fusidic acid have been used successfully together for MRSA decolonization and follow-up oral treatment of prosthetic joint infections, but monitoring of liver function is advisable as hepatic failure has been described with this combination.[9]

Adverse Reactions and Interactions

Fusidic acid has a good safety profile. Table 149-1 lists the most important adverse reactions to fusidic acid. Most common adverse reactions are minor (diarrhea, abdominal discomfort). Intravenous fusidic acid may cause thrombophlebitis, but this risk has decreased with newer

TABLE 149-1	Serious Adverse Reactions to Fusidic Acid, Nitrofurantoin and Fosfomycin	
Adverse Reaction	**Risk Factor**	
FUSIDIC ACID		
Thrombophlebitis	Use of intravenous preparation for more than 24 h	
Jaundice, liver impairment	Intravenous preparation, abnormal liver function	
NITROFURANTOIN		
Eosinophilic lung infiltrates, fever	Prolonged treatment time, high doses	
Pulmonary fibrosis	Elderly female patients, high doses prolonged therapy	
Polyneuropathy	High dose relative to renal function	
Hepatitis	Prolonged treatment time	
Hemolytic anemia	Hereditary glucose-6-phosphate dehydrogenase deficiency	
FOSFOMYCIN		
Angioedema	Renal insufficiency	
Aplastic anemia	Renal insufficiency	
Hepatic necrosis	Renal insufficiency	

intravenous formulations. Additionally, intravenous use appears to increase the risk of jaundice and liver impairment. In newborns, fusidic acid may cause kernicterus. Fusidic acid may interact with coumarin derivatives and oral contraceptives, reducing the bioavailability of these drugs.

Nitrofurantoin

Approved in 1953 for the treatment of lower urinary tract infections (UTIs), nitrofurantoin has the structure 1-{[(5-nitro-2-furanyl)methylene]amino}-2,4-imidazolidinedione and is the only compound of the nitrofuran class that has been used widely; the active component is the 5-nitro structure.

Mechanism of Action

Nitrofurantoin possesses several mechanisms of action, none of which is fully understood. It is known that intracellular nitroreductases produce the active form of the drug via reduction of the nitro group; resultant intermediate metabolites are highly active, binding to bacterial ribosomes as well as inhibiting several bacterial enzymes involved in the synthesis of DNA, RNA, and other metabolic enzymes.[10]

Spectrum of Activity

Nitrofurantoin has broad-spectrum activity against gram-negative and gram-positive bacteria, including enterococci but excluding *Pseudomonas aeruginosa* and the Proteae (e.g. *Proteus*, *Morganella* and *Providencia* spp.) and some limited activity against *Bacteroides* spp.[10] Resistance is still rare in *Escherichia coli* and other extended-spectrum β-lactamase (ESBL)-producing Enterobacteriaceae, but may increase with nitrofurantoin's recent reintroduction in many countries as first-line therapy for uncomplicated UTI.[11]

Mechanisms of Resistance

Acquisition of resistance to nitrofurantoin is infrequent, probably as a result of its multiple sites of action. When it does occur, resistance is thought to be due to loss of intracellular nitroreductase activity via sequential mutations in the DNA regions encoding these enzymes.[12]

Pharmacokinetics, Route of Administration and Dosage

Nitrofurantoin was initially produced in microcrystalline form (nitrofurantoin monohydrate); a macrocrystalline formulation with a slower absorption rate and thus improved gastrointestinal tolerance was later introduced. Currently most formulations are either purely macrocrystalline or mixed (25% macrocrystalline/75% microcrystalline).

Bioavailability is 80%, with roughly 25% of nitrofurantoin excreted in the urine unchanged. Except in patients with severe renal failure, serum concentrations are almost undetectable, with peak levels of 1 µg/mL. This is because of destruction of nitrofurantoin in the tissues and, in particular, a very rapid renal elimination by glomerular filtration (20%) and tubular secretion, resulting in a serum half-life of only 20 minutes in patients with normal renal function. Excretion is complete within 6 hours after intake and urine concentrations of 200–400 µg/mL are achieved after a dose of 100 mg q8h. Nitrofurantoin achieves therapeutically active concentrations only in the lower urinary tract; it does not penetrate other body sites in therapeutic concentrations.[13] Nitrofurantoin's use in most stages of pregnancy appears to be safe. However, some authorities advise avoidance in pregnant women at term (38–42 weeks' gestation) due to the possible risk of hemolytic anemia in the newborn.[14]

Therapeutic doses of nitrofurantoin are 100 mg q8h or q12h, or 50 mg q6h, for adults and 3 mg/kg/day q12h or q8h for children, for a duration of 5–7 days. To decrease gastrointestinal side effects, nitrofurantoin should be taken with food. Dosages are not affected by liver function.

Indications

Because of its pharmacologic site-specificity, nitrofurantoin is indicated only in the treatment and prophylaxis of lower UTI. In recent years nitrofurantoin has resumed its role in international guidelines as first-line therapy given the increase in fluoroquinolone and trimethoprim–sulfamethoxazole (TMP-SMX) resistance and uropathogens producing extended-spectrum β-lactamases (ESBL).[11] Several randomized trials in women with acute UTI have demonstrated clinical efficacy comparable to that of ciprofloxacin, TMP-SMX, and various β-lactam antibiotics.[15–17] It should be given for a minimum of 5 days, however; in a study comparing 3-day regimens of TMP-SMX, cefadroxil, amoxicillin and nitrofurantoin, significantly better results were obtained with TMP-SMX than with the other three regimens, which did not differ from each other.[18]

The use of a single dose (50–100 mg) of nitrofurantoin at night to prevent cystitis has been shown to be well tolerated with little emergence of nitrofurantoin-resistant organisms in the fecal flora.[19]

Adverse Reactions

Upper gastrointestinal adverse reactions (nausea, vomiting, anorexia) occur rarely and seem to be more common with the historical microcrystalline formulation than with the macrocrystalline and mixed formulations now in use. Table 149-1 lists severe adverse reactions to nitrofurantoin. They occur at low frequencies and their risk can be markedly reduced by:
- avoiding long-term (>7 days) treatment, especially in the elderly;
- avoiding daily doses higher than 300 mg in adults;
- reducing the dosage for patients with renal impairment.

Nitrofurantoin should be avoided in patients with renal failure (creatinine clearance <30 mL/min) primarily because urinary concentrations of the drug are subtherapeutic.[20]

Fosfomycin

Isolated in 1968 from strains of *Streptomyces*, fosfomycin is a phosphonic acid derivative (cis-1,2-epoxypropyl phosphonic acid).

Mechanism of Action

Fosfomycin is bactericidal; it inhibits bacterial cell wall synthesis by binding to uridine diphosphate-GlcNAc enol pyruvyl-transferase, also known as MurA.

Spectrum of Activity

Fosfomycin has broad-spectrum activity against gram-positive and gram-negative bacteria: *Staph. aureus*, *Staph. epidermidis*, *Strep. pneumoniae* and *Enterococcus faecalis* show *in vitro* susceptibility, as do *E. coli*, *Proteus* species, *Klebsiella pneumoniae*, *Enterobacter* species, and *Salmonella typhi*. Both carbapenemase- and ESBL-producing Enterobacteriaceae appear to be susceptible to fosfomycin. *Pseudomonas aeruginosa* is often resistant to fosfomycin, however, as are *Listeria monocytogenes*, *Acinetobacter baumanni*, and *Bacteroides fragilis*.[21]

Mechanisms of Resistance

Resistance to fosfomycin occurs through multiple mechanisms. The earliest reported were impairments in the L-alpha-glycerophosphate and hexose phosphate uptake systems that leave the drug unable to enter the bacterial cell. Fosfomycin resistance enzymes have also been described (see Chapter 138).[22]

The mounting use of oral fosfomycin in the community appears to be leading to increased resistance among *E. coli* strains, with resistance rates moving from roughly 3% to 11% in some countries.[23] Although some resistance mechanisms are plasmid-encoded, there is as yet little evidence of phenotypic cross-resistance between fosfomycin and agents from other antibacterial classes.[22]

Pharmacokinetics, Route of Administration and Dosage

Fosfomycin tromethamine, a synthetically prepared soluble salt with improved bioavailability, is the most commonly used oral form. Oral fosfomycin calcium is available in some countries, but appears to have decreased intestinal absorption. The intravenous formulation, available in some European countries, is fosfomycin disodium. Fosfomycin tromethamine has 34–41% bioavailability, a mean elimination half-life of roughly 5.7 hours, negligible protein binding and is primarily excreted unchanged in the urine. It distributes well into the tissues, achieving clinically relevant concentrations in serum, soft tissues, lung, bone, cerebrospinal fluid, heart valves and the prostate.[24,25] Fosfomycin crosses the placental barrier but appears safe for use in pregnancy; no teratogenicity in animals or adverse fetal effects in humans have been observed.[14]

Fosfomycin tromethamine is given as a single oral dose of 3 g for UTIs. The drug is not recommended in children weighing less than 50 kg. Intake with food leads to decreased serum concentrations, as does co-administration with metoclopramide. Intravenous fosfomycin disodium is given as a total daily dose of 100–200 mg/kg; it is typically administered every 8–12 hours in extended infusions of 4 g lasting 4–8 hours.

Indications

Oral fosfomycin is approved only for the treatment of lower UTIs. Like nitrofurantoin, it is now recommended in several countries' guidelines as first-line therapy for uncomplicated infections given increases in fluoroquinolone and TMP-SMX resistance and ESBL-producing uropathogens.[11] But, while fosfomycin's single-dose administration would appear advantageous, there are doubts concerning its overall clinical and bacteriologic efficacy when compared to other agents; these are the subject of ongoing randomized trials.[11,26]

Intravenous fosfomycin is approved in some countries for the treatment of meningitis caused by MRSA, but controlled clinical studies are lacking. It should be used in conjunction with another antistaphylococcal agent to avoid emergence of resistance; its activity in combination with β-lactams, vancomycin or aminoglycosides appears either additive or synergistic; antagonistic effects have not been observed.

Adverse Reactions

The most frequently observed side effects are diarrhea, headache and vaginitis. Serious adverse reactions are extremely rare and are listed in Table 149-1.

References available online at expertconsult.com.

KEY REFERENCES

Cunha B.A.: Nitrofurantoin – current concepts. *Urology* 1988; 32:67-71.

Drugeon H.B., Caillon J., Juvin M.E.: In-vitro antibacterial activity of fusidic acid alone and in combination with other antibiotics against methicillin-sensitive and -resistant *Staphylococcus aureus*. *J Antimicrob Chemother* 1994; 34:899-907.

Gupta K., Hooton T.M., Naber K.G., et al.: International clinical practice guidelines for the treatment of acute uncomplicated cystitis and pyelonephritis in women: A 2010 update by the Infectious Diseases Society of America and the European Society for Microbiology and Infectious Diseases. *Clin Infect Dis* 2011; 52:e103-e120.

Hooton T.M., Winter C., Tiu F., et al.: Randomized comparative trial and cost analysis of 3-day antimicrobial regimens for treatment of acute cystitis in women. *JAMA* 1995; 273:41-45.

Raz R.: Fosfomycin: an old–new antibiotic. *Clin Microbiol Infect* 2012; 18:4-7.

Sachs J., Geer T., Noell P., et al.: Effect of renal function on urinary recovery of orally administered nitrofurantoin. *N Engl J Med* 1968; 278:1032-1035.

Suarez J.E., Mendoza M.C.: Plasmid-encoded fosfomycin resistance. *Antimicrob Agents Chemother* 1991; 35:791-795.

Tsuji B.T., Okusanya O.O., Bulitta J.B., et al.: Application of pharmacokinetic-pharmacodynamic modeling and the justification of a novel fusidic acid dosing regimen: raising Lazarus from the dead. *Clin Infect Dis* 2011; 52(Suppl. 7):S513-S519.

150

Folate Inhibitors

EIRINI CHRISTAKI

KEY CONCEPTS

• Folate inhibitors antagonize the synthesis of folic acid and are used for treating bacterial, fungal and protozoal infections.

• This antimicrobial drug class includes sulfonamides, dihydrofolate reductase inhibitors and combinations of these two subclasses.

• Major indications for the use of folate inhibitor combinations are urinary tract infections, enteric infections caused by susceptible strains of gram-negative bacteria, specific respiratory infections and toxoplasmosis.

• Resistance rates of pathogens causing urinary tract infections and enteric infections to trimethoprim–sulfamethoxazole are increasing worldwide.

• Dose adjustment is necessary in case of renal impairment.

• Skin reactions are the most common adverse events of sulfonamides; however, serious reactions like toxic epidermal necrolysis are rare.

Pharmacokinetics and Distribution

Sulfonamides are competitive inhibitors of *para*-aminobenzoic acid (PABA), which is essential for folic acid synthesis in most bacteria, some protozoa and *Pneumocystis jirovecii* (formerly *P. carinii*).[1] The eukaryotic cell does not use PABA and sulfonamides do not interfere with human folic acid synthesis (see Chapter 137).

Trimethoprim is a diaminopyrimidine that competitively inhibits dihydrofolate reductase.[1,2] Pyrimethamine is also a competitive dihydrofolate reductase inhibitor, with a high affinity for the protozoal enzyme.

Combinations of sulfonamides and trimethoprim or pyrimethamine interfere with two consecutive steps in the same metabolic chain in the micro-organism. This may lead to synergistic antimicrobial activity. The rationale for a fixed combination of trimethoprim and sulfamethoxazole is that, although both antibiotics alone are bacteriostatic, the combination may be bactericidal. The optimal trimethoprim–sulfamethoxazole (TMP–SMX) ratio for synergism inside a bacterium is 1:20. Based upon the differential pharmacokinetics of the two agents, this ratio is obtained systemically with a 1:5 dosage combination.[3]

PHARMACOKINETICS

The sulfonamides are classically subdivided on the basis of their elimination time into short-acting (plasma half-life, $t_{1/2} < 8h$), medium-acting ($t_{1/2} = 8–16\,h$), long-acting ($t_{1/2} = 17–48\,h$) and ultra-long-acting ($t_{1/2} > 48\,h$). Sulfonamides used as single agents today are short- or medium-acting.

Plasma Kinetics

Currently used sulfonamides, as well as trimethoprim and pyrimethamine, are well absorbed after oral administration and have high bioavailability. Following an oral dose of 160 mg of trimethoprim and 800 mg of sulfamethoxazole, maximal plasma concentrations of 1.6–1.9 mg/L and 26–41 mg/L, respectively, are achieved.[4] After intravenous administration of 240 mg trimethoprim and 1200 mg

sulfamethoxazole q12h, peak plasma concentrations in the steady state are about 6 mg/L for trimethoprim and 180 mg/L for sulfamethoxazole.[5] The protein binding of the sulfonamides varies from less than 50% for sulfadiazine to more than 90% for sulfadoxine. Importantly, sulfonamides bind firmly to albumin and may displace other compounds (e.g. bilirubin). In newborns this may lead to toxic levels of unbound bilirubin with a subsequent risk of 'kernicterus' (see 'Central nervous system reactions' below).

Distribution

Trimethoprim is lipid soluble at physiologic pH and has a large volume of distribution (100–120 L), whereas sulfamethoxazole is a weak acid with poor lipid solubility at pH values above 7, leading to a volume of distribution corresponding to that of the extracellular space (i.e. 12–18 L). In tissues, concentrations similar to or higher than those in plasma are achieved with trimethoprim, whereas considerably lower levels of sulfamethoxazole reach peripheral compartments. Concentrations above the minimum inhibitory concentrations (MICs) of trimethoprim-susceptible strains are achieved in most tissues and tissue fluids. With sulfamethoxazole, the peripheral concentrations are sometimes so low that it should be questioned whether therapeutic levels are reached. All of the sulfonamides as well as trimethoprim achieve high urinary concentrations.

Elimination

The main routes of elimination of sulfonamides, trimethoprim and pyrimethamine are via liver metabolism and renal excretion.[6] In patients who have normal renal function, half-life varies from less than 6 hours for sulfisoxazole and sulfamethizole to 11–17 hours for sulfamethoxazole and sulfadiazine and more than 200 hours for sulfadoxine. Trimethoprim has a half-life of about 15 hours and pyrimethamine is eliminated slowly, with a half-life of about 100 hours.

Kinetics in Children

The kinetics of both sulfamethoxazole and trimethoprim differ between children and adults (Table 150-1). Elimination is faster in children, who must be given relatively higher doses than adults.

Route of Administration and Dosage

Most sulfonamides, trimethoprim and pyrimethamine are available for oral use. Trimethoprim, sulfamethoxazole and sulfadiazine are also used intravenously; intravenous use of TMP–SMX is recommended when patients are unable to take the drug orally. Dosages for some of the sulfonamides and for combinations of sulfonamides and dihydrofolic acid inhibitors are given in Table 150-2.

TABLE 150-1	Comparative Kinetics of Trimethoprim (T) and Sulfamethoxazole (S) in Children and Adults			
Parameter	**Age (Years)**			
	<1	1–9	10–19	20–63
T volume of distribution (L/kg)	2.0	1.6	1.5	1.4
S volume of distribution (L/kg)	0.5	0.5	0.4	0.4
T plasma half-life (h)	11	5.6	10	16
S plasma half-life (h)	7.5	9.8	10	15

TABLE 150-2	Adult Dosages of Some Folate Inhibitors*	
Drug	**Indication and Recommended Dose for Adults**

Pyrimethamine	Malaria prophylaxis (with sulfadoxine) 25 mg once weekly
	Malaria therapy (with sulfadoxine; Fansidar) 50–75 mg as single dose
	Toxoplasmosis encephalitis therapy (with sulfadiazine and calcium folinate) 75–200 mg loading dose,
	  followed by 25–100 mg q24h for 3–6 weeks, followed by 25–50 mg q24h (maintenance therapy in AIDS)
	Ocular toxoplasmosis (with sulfadiazine and calcium folinate) 100 mg loading dose q24h for 1–2 days
	  followed by maintenance doses of 25–50 mg q24h

Sulfadiazine	Toxoplasmosis encephalitis therapy (with pyrimethamine and calcium folinate) 0.5–1.5 g q6h Ocular toxoplasmosis (with pyrimethamine and calcium folinate) 0.5–1 g q6h
Sulfadoxine	Malaria prophylaxis 500 mg once weekly (with pyrimethamine; Fansidar); malaria therapy 1–1.5 g (with pyrimethamine; Fansidar) as single dose
Co-trimoxazole (trimethoprim with sulfamethoxazole ratio 1 part to 5 parts)	UTI 1.92 g single dose or 480–960 mg q12h; systemic bacterial infections 960 mg q12h *Pneumocystis* pneumonia treatment 1.92 g q8h or 15 mg of trimethoprim component/kg/day divided q6-8h *Pneumocystis* pneumonia prophylaxis 960 mg (ds tablet) thrice weekly or daily *Staphylococcus aureus* cellulitis 960-1920 mg q12h
Trimethoprim	UTI 100–200 mg q12h
Dapsone	*Mycobacterium leprae* infections 100 mg *Pneumocystis jirovecii* pneumonia prophylaxis 100 mg

*For pediatric doses, see the manufacturers' recommendations.

TABLE 150-3	Clinical Use of Trimethoprim–Sulfamethoxazole	
Type of Infection	**Limitations**
Uncomplicated UTI	None for short-term therapy (single dose or 3 days)
Other types of UTI	Resistance, safety
Shigellosis	Resistance
Salmonellosis	Resistance
Enteric fever	Resistance
Travelers' diarrhea	Resistance, safety
Otitis media	Resistance
Community-acquired pneumonia	Resistance, safety
Melioidosis	Resistance, efficacy
Prophylaxis in immunocompromised patients	Resistance, safety, efficacy
Pneumocystis jirovecii pneumonia	None

Indications

Folate inhibitor combinations are used for treating bacterial as well as fungal and protozoal infections. Emphasis will be put on combinations of sulfonamides and trimethoprim, especially the most widely used, namely TMP–SMX and pyrimethamine–sulfadoxine.

USE OF TRIMETHOPRIM–SULFAMETHOXAZOLE

TMP–SMX has lost some of its usefulness for the treatment of urinary, respiratory and gastrointestinal infections through the emergence of resistance and increased awareness of the risk of adverse reactions, which may be serious or life-threatening.

Urogenital Infections

Urogenital infections are the most common indications for TMP–SMX (Table 150-3); however, in some countries this has been replaced by the use of trimethoprim alone (see below). Urinary isolates of *Escherichia coli* show marked variation in susceptibility to TMP–SMX, not only between but also within countries. However, resistance is increasing and in many countries more than 12% up to 24% of urinary *E. coli* isolates are resistant to trimethoprim and TMP–SMX.[7,8]

Importantly, the use of TMP–SMX is well documented for single-dose or short-term treatment of uncomplicated cystitis in women. It is equally effective if given for 3 days compared with treatment for 5–10 days, and a single dose is only slightly less effective than 3-day treatment. For other types of urinary tract infections (UTI), longer treatment times are required. In countries where resistant uropathogens are uncommon, single-dose or short-term TMP–SMX is an inexpensive and effective treatment of cystitis in women, though if resistance prevalence is more than 20%, the empiric use of TMP–SMX should be avoided.[9]

Prostatitis is commonly treated with TMP–SMX and the few studies evaluating its use for this infection indicate a high degree of efficacy.[10]

The activity of TMP–SMX against enterococci is controversial. There are reports in the literature of enterococcal bacteremia during treatment with TMP–SMX despite full *in vitro* sensitivity pre-therapy, and of high failure rates and rapid emergence of resistance in enterococcal UTIs. Enterococci have the ability to incorporate exogenous folates and a large increase in MIC can been seen when *in vitro* susceptibility is determined in the presence of urine.[11]

For *Haemophilus ducreyi* infections, 160 mg of trimethoprim plus 800 mg sulfamethoxazole q12h for 3 days has resulted in high cure rates, whereas shorter treatment times seem ineffective.[12]

Infections caused by *Chlamydia trachomatis* respond poorly to TMP–SMX.[12]

Enteric Infections

These have been extensively treated with TMP–SMX because of its activity against *Salmonella* spp. (including *Salmonella typhi*), *Shigella* spp., *Vibrio cholerae* and enterotoxigenic *E. coli*; however, increasing resistance rates have limited its use in the treatment and prevention of enteric infections. In a well-controlled trial in patients who had enteritis of verified etiology, the causative pathogens were eliminated on treatment day 2 in 41% of patients treated with TMP–SMX compared with 23% of those receiving placebo and 91% of patients on norfloxacin.[13] A loading dose of TMP–SMX followed by standard dosing for 3 days was able to control symptoms in 12 hours in two-thirds of patients with travelers' diarrhea.[14]

Several studies have indicated a relatively high frequency of selection of resistance to TMP–SMX in Enterobacteriaceae when the antibiotic is used therapeutically or, in particular, prophylactically.[15]

Shigella and *Salmonella* spp. show varying sensitivity to TMP–SMX, with frequencies of resistance ranging from less than 5% to over 50%.

In most countries, due to the worldwide spread of resistant strains of *Shigella* species, TMP–SMX is no longer considered an appropriate treatment for shigellosis.

TMP–SMX had been widely used for the treatment of enteric fever caused by *S. typhi* and *S. paratyphi*. However, the emergence of multidrug-resistant strains has limited its usefulness and other agents are now preferred.[16] In salmonellosis TMP–SMX is effective for treatment of invasive infections caused by sensitive strains, but, like other antibiotics, it seems less effective in eliminating the carrier state of *Salmonella* spp.[17]

Treatment of cholera should be aimed mainly at rehydration of the patients. However, antibiotics may reduce symptoms and shorten the duration of the carrier state of *V. cholerae*, thereby reducing the risk of transmission. TMP–SMX has proved effective in patients who have cholera and one study showed that it was better than tetracycline or sulfamethoxazole alone.[18]

In several older studies, TMP–SMX has been shown to be effective in preventing travelers' diarrhea.[19] However, it has also been found to select for resistance which, along with serious adverse reactions, makes this type of prophylaxis of doubtful value.[20]

Respiratory Tract Infections

Reduced susceptibility or resistance to penicillin G by *Streptococcus pneumoniae* seems to be coupled to resistance to TMP–SMX in a very high percentage of strains studied.[21] Overall, resistance to TMP–SMX in pneumococci is a rapidly increasing problem.[22] Due to adverse drug reactions and the emergence of resistance in *Strep. pneumoniae* and *Haemophilus influenzae*, TMP–SMX is no longer considered first line for the treatment of lower and upper respiratory tract infections.[22]

In pneumonia caused by *Burkholderia pseudomallei*, melioidosis, TMP–SMX remains a choice for oral long-term treatment after standard treatment with ceftazidime, although some doubt exists about its effectiveness.[23] Trimethoprim–sulfamethoxazole is the drug of choice for the treatment and prevention of *P. jirovecii* pneumonia in the immunosuppressed (see Chapter 94).[24,25]

Other Infections

Both trimethoprim and sulfamethoxazole penetrate the blood–cerebrospinal fluid barrier and the combination has been found to be effective in experimental bacterial meningitis.[26] Trimethoprim–sulfamethoxazole has therefore been used as an alternative drug for the treatment of bacterial meningitis. Favorable clinical results have been reported in the treatment of meningitis caused by *Listeria monocytogenes* as well as other types of meningitis.[27]

TMP–SMX has activity against methicillin-resistant *Staphylococcus aureus* (MRSA) and is recommended for the outpatient empirical coverage of community-acquired MRSA in patients with skin and soft tissue infections.[28]

Several studies have shown excellent clinical results with TMP–SMX, alone or in combination with aminoglycosides, in the treatment of actinomycosis or nocardiosis.[29,30]

Trimethoprim–sulfamethoxazole is considered a first-line drug in the treatment of healthcare-associated infections due to *Stenotrophomonas maltophila*. This relatively avirulent gram-negative bacillus can cause infection in immunocompromised patients and is often a multidrug-resistant pathogen.

A controversial field for the use of TMP–SMX is prophylaxis in neutropenic patients. Early studies showed significant protection against bacterial infections but its role has generally been superseded by other classes (e.g. fluoroquinolones).

TMP–SMX is also used as a second-line agent for donovanosis caused by *Klebsiella granulomatis*.[31]

In patients who have brucellosis TMP–SMX can be considered a second-line drug.

TMP–SMX 160/800 mg twice daily for 6 weeks may be considered an alternative in the treatment of ocular toxoplasmosis.[32]

USE OF PYRIMETHAMINE–SULFADIAZINE AND PYRIMETHAMINE–SULFADOXINE

Pyrimethamine–sulfadiazine remains the first-line drug combination for the treatment of toxoplasmosis.[33]

Pyrimethamine–sulfadoxine is an alternative for the treatment of *Plasmodium falciparum* malaria in areas with chloroquine resistance.[34] However, resistance to pyrimethamine–sulfadoxine is not uncommon and safety concerns reduce its usefulness for prophylaxis.

USE OF FOLATE INHIBITORS ALONE

Because of the emergence of bacterial resistance and risks for adverse reactions, the sulfonamides have lost most of their usefulness as single agents.

USE OF TRIMETHOPRIM ALONE

In many European countries, trimethoprim is available as a single agent. Due to its better adverse reaction profile and avoidance of hypersensitivity reactions to sulfonamides, it is favored over TMP–SMX for some infections. Whilst resistance can sometimes be a problem, trimethoprim is the first-line drug for the treatment of uncomplicated UTI in many European countries[35] at a dose of 200 mg orally twice daily for 3 days. Also, trimethoprim has been shown comparable to TMP–SMX and doxycycline for the treatment of lower respiratory tract infections, although its first-line use is often hampered by emerging *Strep. pneumoniae* resistance.[36]

Dosage in Special Circumstances

Renal impairment results in prolonged elimination times. Table 150-4 gives dosages of sulfamethoxazole and trimethoprim in patients who had decreased renal function. There are no recommendations for reduced dosage of folate inhibitors in patients who have hepatic disease. Patients of advanced age often have renal impairment and therefore glomerular filtration rate based dosage adjustment is necessary. As pointed out, the above doses used in children should be higher than those in adults because of different kinetic profiles (see Table 150-1). All sulfonamides should be avoided in patients aged less than 6 weeks because of the risk of cerebral accumulation of free bilirubin (kernicterus). Most of the folate inhibitors pass to breast milk but at concentrations that make any toxic effects on the child unlikely. During pregnancy, particularly in the first trimester, trimethoprim and pyrimethamine should be avoided because of the possible risk of altered folate metabolism in the fetus. Sulfonamides should not be given during the last trimester of the pregnancy because of the risk of kernicterus.

TABLE 150-4	Effect of Renal Function on Dosage of TMP–SMX and Trimethoprim[37]	
Creatinine clearance	**Co-trimoxazole (TMP–SMX)**	**Trimethoprim**
>30–50 mL/min	Dose as in normal renal function	Dose as in normal renal function
15–30 mL/min	Normal dose for 3 days then use 50% of the normal dose at the normal frequency	Normal dose for 3 days then use 50% of the normal dose q18h
<15 mL/min	Normal dose for 3 days then use 50% of the normal dose at the normal frequency *Note:* High-dose treatment (60 mg/kg q12h) should only be given if hemodialysis facilities are available	Give 50% of the normal dose q24h

Body System	Sulfonamides	Trimethoprim–Pyrimethamine
Central nervous system	'Kernicterus' in newborns	Aseptic meningitis, especially in patients who have collagen diseases
Liver	Toxic hepatitis	Probably none
Skin	Hypersensitivity reaction, drug eruption, erythema multiforme (Stevens–Johnson)	Hypersensitivity reaction
Kidney	Crystalluria	Increased serum creatinine (inhibition of creatinine excretion); increased potassium
Hematologic	Hemolytic anemia (especially in G6PD deficiency)	Folate deficiency, megaloblastic anemia and pancytopenia

TABLE 150-5 Adverse Actions of Folate Inhibitors in Humans

Adverse Reactions and Interactions

A summary of the potential adverse effects of folate inhibitors is given in Table 150-5.

GENERAL SAFETY PROFILE

Since several studies have shown a correlation between the treatment time and the risk of adverse reactions to TMP–SMX when used for uncomplicated UTIs, short-course therapy (3 days) is encouraged.[38]

HEMATOLOGIC REACTIONS

The mode of action of trimethoprim has caused concerns over possible bone marrow toxicity. Studies in patients treated for 1 month or more with TMP–SMX have shown moderate folate deficiency.[39] The possibility of immune reactions causing hematologic adverse effects has been proposed.[40]

Serious and even fatal hematologic adverse reactions (usually cytopenias) to TMP–SMX have been reported. In a Swedish study of about 50 million daily doses an approximate frequency of fatal reactions to TMP–SMX was calculated to be 3.7/million treatments (data from SWEDIS, Medical Products Agency, Uppsala, Sweden). It was noteworthy that the mean age of the patients who died was 78 years (range 41–96 years) and that only three of 18 patients were below the age of 70. Taking into consideration the effect of aging on renal function, the doses of TMP–SMX were high. In addition, the treatment time was long (range 3–73 days, mean 17 days, median 12 days).

Pyrimethamine hematologic toxicity is less well described. Many use folinic acid to avoid folic acid deficiency. Support is lacking and hematologic reactions may very well be due to other mechanisms.

SKIN, MUCOCUTANEOUS AND ALLERGIC REACTIONS

Skin reactions (maculopapular rash, urticaria, diffuse erythema, erythema multiforme, morbilliform lesions, photosensitivity) are common; however, serious reactions like Stevens–Johnson syndrome or toxic epidermal necrolysis are rare.[41] Such reactions seem to be related to the sulfonamide component rather than to trimethoprim.

It is worth noting that, in most reports on the safety of TMP–SMX or sulfonamides, skin reactions are only rarely reported in children. Possible explanations for this are the reduced risk for overdosing in children due to efficient elimination and less risk of sensitization to trimethoprim or sulfamethoxazole from previous exposures.

High numbers of serious cutaneous reactions have been reported following treatment with pyrimethamine–sulfadoxine.[42] Between 1974 and 1989, 126 cases of mucocutaneous syndromes were reported, giving an estimated risk of about 1.1/million treatments. This risk, which is most probably related to the sulfadoxine component, is considered to be high enough to discourage routine use of the combination for malaria prophylaxis.

Patients who have AIDS and *P. jirovecii* pneumonia and are treated with high doses of TMP–SMX have high frequencies of cutaneous reactions as well as other adverse reactions.[43,44] These reactions seem to be related to dose and treatment time, and many patients who have AIDS who have developed skin reactions later tolerate low-dose TMP–SMX prophylaxis against *P. jirovecii*.

HEPATIC SIDE EFFECTS

Cases of hepatic necrosis associated with TMP–SMX use have been reported and are most likely to be caused by the sulfonamide component.[45]

GASTROINTESTINAL ADVERSE REACTIONS

Like many other orally administered antibiotics, TMP–SMX causes upper gastrointestinal adverse effects in some patients. Because of its low activity on the intestinal anaerobic flora it causes diarrhea only infrequently.

RENAL SAFETY

Sulfonamides with poor solubility can cause crystalluria. With sulfamethoxazole this does not seem to be a problem but, with sulfadiazine in high doses, crystalluria has been reported in AIDS patients who had toxoplasmal encephalitis.[46]

Hyperkalemia and increased serum creatinine have been reported in patients treated with TMP–SMX; elevated serum levels of creatinine seems to be related to competitive inhibition of the renal excretion of creatinine by trimethoprim.[47]

CENTRAL NERVOUS SYSTEM REACTIONS

Rarely, aseptic meningitis is related to trimethoprim therapy. Several cases have been reported in the literature with some over-representation of patients who have collagen vascular diseases (e.g. Sjögren's syndrome).[48] The pathogenesis remains obscure but seems to be of an allergic nature, with rapid onset and relapses after provocation.

Sulfonamides can cause central nervous system toxicity in newborns (kernicterus) because of displacement of bilirubin from albumin, resulting in toxic bilirubin concentrations in the brain.

DRUG–DRUG INTERACTIONS

The sulfonamides cause variable inhibition of the cytochrome P450 enzyme CYP2C9. Trimethoprim is a possible inhibitor of CYP2C8 and CYP2C9. Many of the resultant interactions (Table 150-6) are minor, with concurrent usage often only requiring increased monitoring. The major exception is with methotrexate where concurrent usage, especially of high-dosage regimens, has led to major morbidity.

Dapsone

Dapsone (diaminodiphenyl sulfone) inhibits bacterial dihydropteroate synthase, similarly to sulfonamides. It is well absorbed orally, has a long half-life of 12–44 hours and good tissue concentrations. Dapsone is mainly used in combination with rifampin and clofazimine in the treatment of leprosy.[49] Also, it is used for *P. jirovecii* pneumonia prophylaxis in patients with HIV and CD4 cell counts <200 cell/μL who cannot take trimethoprim–sulfamethoxazole.[50] Adverse events include hemolytic anemia, especially in those individuals with glucose-6-phosphate dehydrogenase deficiency, rash, gastrointestinal symptoms, methemoglobinemia and sulfone syndrome (fever, jaundice, lymphadenopathy).

References available online at expertconsult.com.

TABLE 150-6	Interactions between Trimethoprim (TMP), TMP–SMX and Sulfonamides with Other Drugs		
Drug	**Folate Inhibitor**	**Interaction**	**Suggested Management**
Angiotensin-converting enzyme (ACE) inhibitors	TMP (and TMP–SMX)	Serious hyperkalemia in older patients or those with concurrent renal impairment	Monitor potassium levels
Azathioprine	TMP (and TMP–SMX)	Increased risk of hematologic toxicity	If combination necessary, monitor for leucopenia
Ciclosporin A	TMP, TMP–SMX, many other sulfonamides	Not fully defined. Reversible decrease of renal function (TMP, TMP–SMX); risk of accumulation if function deteriorates. Possible reduction in ciclosporin levels with some sulfonamide	Monitor levels if sulfonamides are added to ciclosporin
Dapsone	TMP (and TMP–SMX)	Reduced clearance of both dapsone and trimethoprim	Monitor patient; increased dapsone toxicity has occurred
Digoxin	TMP (and TMP–SMX)	Reduced tubular secretion of digoxin	Monitor for toxicity
Folate inhibitors	TMP–SMX, sulfonamides, pyrimethamine	Concurrent use of pyrimethamine with sulfonamides has led to folate deficiency, megaloblastic anemia and pancytopenia	Supplementation with folinic acid (leucovorin) reduces the risk of folate deficiency
Lithium	TMP (and TMP–SMX)	Possible increased lithium levels	If combination necessary, monitor levels
Methotrexate	TMP, TMP–SMX	Potential severe bone marrow depression and pancytopenia	Combination of low-dose methotrexate with low-dose prophylactic TMP–SMX is commonly used in well-monitored patients without problems. Higher doses of either drug are likely to be more problematic and have led to major morbidity. Use only if absolutely necessary with close monitoring
Nucleoside reverse transcriptase inhibitors	TMP–SMX, TMP	Reduced urinary clearance of lamivudine, emtricitabine and zidovudine. Possible interaction between TMP and stavudine	Close monitoring advised if combinations used
Phenytoin	TMP (and TMP–SMX), sulfadiazine, sulfamethizole	Reduced metabolism of phenytoin	If combination necessary, monitor phenytoin levels
Procainamide	TMP (and TMP–SMX)	Reduced clearance of procainamide	Increased risk of toxicity; lower procainamide dose may be required
Repaglinide	TMP (and TMP–SMX)	Increased repaglinide levels likely to result in hypoglycemia	Avoid if possible; monitor closely if not
Sulfonylureas	TMP, some sulfonamides, TMP–SMX	Possible increased risk of hypoglycemia	Advise patients of risk
Warfarin	TMP–SMX, some other sulfonamides	Reduced metabolism of warfarin	Monitor international normalized ratio (INR) closely when initiating and stopping TMP–SMX

KEY REFERENCES

Basnyat B., Maskey A.P., Zimmerman M.D., et al.: Enteric (typhoid) fever in travelers. *Clin Infect Dis* 2005; 41:1467-1472.

Georgiev V.S.: Management of toxoplasmosis. *Drugs* 1994; 48:179-188.

Goldberg E., Bishara J.: Contemporary unconventional clinical use of co-trimoxazole. *Clin Microbiol Infect* 2012; 18(1):8-17.

Gupta K., Hooton T.M., Naber K.G., et al.: International clinical practice guidelines for the treatment of acute uncomplicated cystitis and pyelonephritis in women: A 2010 update by the Infectious Diseases Society of America and the European Society for Microbiology and Infectious Diseases. *Clin Infect Dis* 2011; 52(5):e103-e120.

Kovacs J.A., Gill V.J., Meshnick S., et al.: New insights into transmission, diagnosis, and drug treatment of Pneumocystis carinii pneumonia. *JAMA* 2001; 286:2450-2460.

Lawson D.H., Paice B.J.: Adverse reactions to trimethoprim–sulfamethoxazole. *Rev Infect Dis* 1982; 4:429-433.

Liu C., Bayer A., Cosgrove S.E., et al.: Clinical practice guidelines by the Infectious Diseases Society of America for the treatment of methicillin-resistant *Staphylococcus aureus* infections in adults and children: executive summary. *Clin Infect Dis* 2011; 52(3):285-292.

Murray B.E., Rensimer E.R., DuPont H.L.: Emergence of high-level trimethoprim resistance in fecal *Escherichia coli* during oral administration of trimethoprim or trimethoprim – sulfamethoxazole. *N Engl J Med* 1982; 306:130-135.

Norrby S.R.: Short-term treatment of uncomplicated urinary tract infections in women. *Rev Infect Dis* 1990; 12:458-467.

Sandberg T., Trollfors B.: Effect of trimethoprim on serum creatinine in patients with acute cystitis. *J Antimicrob Chemother* 1986; 17:123-124.

Sanchez G.V., Master R.N., Karlowsky J.A., et al.: In vitro antimicrobial resistance of urinary *Escherichia coli* isolates among U.S. outpatients from 2000 to 2010. *Antimicrob Agents Chemother* 2012; 56(4):2181-2183.

Spicehandler J., Pollock A.A., Simberkoff M.S., et al.: Intravenous pharmacokinetics and in vitro bactericidal activity of co-trimoxazole. *Rev Infect Dis* 1982; 4:562-565.

Thornsberry C., Sahm D.F., Kelly L.J., et al.: Regional trends in antimicrobial resistance among clinical isolates of *Streptococcus pneumoniae*, *Haemophilus influenzae* and *Moraxella catarrhalis* in the United States. Results from the TRUST surveillance program 1999–2000. *Clin Infect Dis* 2002; 34(Suppl.1):S4-S16.

151

Polymyxins

MICHAEL J. SATLIN | STEPHEN G. JENKINS

KEY CONCEPTS

- Polymyxins (colistin and polymyxin B) fell out of favor for clinical use because of concern for nephrotoxicity, but are now re-emerging as important last-line agents for the treatment of infections caused by gram-negative bacteria that are resistant to nearly all other antimicrobial classes.

- Although the exact mechanisms are unknown, polymyxins appear to exert their activity by binding to phosphate groups on lipids of gram-negative cell membranes, leading to membrane disruption and leakage of intracellular contents.

- Polymyxins are active in vitro against a broad range of gram-negative aerobic bacilli, with the notable exceptions of Burkholderia spp., Serratia marcescens, Proteus spp., and Morganella morganii.

- Their large size, positive charge, poor ability to diffuse in agar, and adherence to plastic and glass surfaces lead to challenges in performing in vitro susceptibility testing with the polymyxins.

- Colistin is administered intravenously as a prodrug, colistimethate sodium (CMS), whereas, polymyxin B is administered as the active drug, polymyxin B sulfate.

- Loading doses and higher daily dosages than previously recommended may be necessary to reach optimal plasma concentrations when using CMS or polymyxin B for the treatment of serious infections due to multidrug-resistant (MDR) gram-negative bacteria.

- CMS requires dosage adjustments for renal insufficiency, whereas polymyxin B does not.

- The combination of CMS and carbapenems frequently demonstrates in vitro synergy and has demonstrated clinical benefit compared to CMS alone in nonrandomized studies for the treatment of bacteremia caused by carbapenem-resistant Enterobacteriaceae.

- Given the poor penetration of intravenous CMS into pulmonary epithelial lining and cerebrospinal fluid, aerosolized or intrathecal CMS may be considered as adjunctive therapies (in combination with intravenous CMS) for ventilator-associated pneumonia and meningitis due to MDR gram-negative pathogens.

- Nephrotoxicity is the most common side effect of the polymyxins, is dose-dependent, and may occur more frequently with CMS than with polymyxin B. Neurotoxicity and hypersensitivity reactions are less common but serious side effects.

Introduction

Polymyxins are fermentation products of the bacteria *Bacillus polymyxa* and were first recognized to have antimicrobial activity in the 1940s.[1] Of the five polymyxins that were initially recovered (polymyxins A–E), only polymyxin B and polymyxin E (colistin) were put into clinical use, as these were shown to be the least nephrotoxic.[2] However, once newer gram-negative antibacterial agents became available that were perceived to be less toxic, polymyxins fell out of favor for clinical use. Unfortunately, with the emergence of gram-negative bacteria

resistant to nearly all other classes of antimicrobial agents, polymyxins have increasingly been relied upon as agents of last resort.[3]

Chemical Structure

The polymyxins are large, positively charged, cyclic polypeptides. Polymyxin B differs from polymyxin E (colistin) by a single amino acid.[3] Colistin is primarily composed of two polypeptides, colistin A and colistin B, and polymyxin B is primarily composed of polymyxin B_1 and polymyxin B_2.[4,5] Importantly, colistin is administered parenterally as a prodrug, colistimethate sodium (CMS), because it is thought to be less toxic than the parent drug, colistin sulfate. In contrast, polymyxin B is administered as the active compound, polymyxin B sulfate.[3]

Mechanism(s) of Activity

Polymyxins are surface-active amphipathic molecules harboring both lipophobic and lipophilic moieties. The exact mechanism(s) by which polymyxins result in bacterial cell death are unclear. The most frequently described mechanism is competitive displacement of divalent cations (Mg^{2+} and Ca^{2+}) from the phosphate groups of membrane lipids, leading to outer and cytoplasmic cell membrane disruption, leakage of intracellular contents and bacterial death.[6] This is evidenced by electron microscopic studies demonstrating that the bacterial cytoplasmic membrane is partially damaged upon polymyxin exposure and that components of the cytoplasmic membrane are released in fibrous forms through crevices.[7] By binding to the lipid A component of bacterial cell wall lipopolysaccharide (LPS, or endotoxin), polymyxins also may interfere with the biologic function of LPS.[8] Other findings suggest that polymyxins exert their effect through hydroxyl radical production, in addition to or instead of disruption of bacterial cell membranes.[9] Regardless of which of these mechanisms are most important, polymyxins have been shown to be rapidly bactericidal and demonstrate a significant postantibiotic effect (PAE) against *Pseudomonas aeruginosa*, with a lack, or only a modest PAE against *Acinetobacter baumannii* and *Klebsiella pneumoniae*.[10–12]

Spectrum of Activity

The polymyxins demonstrate activity against a broad range of gram-negative aerobic bacilli. The notable exceptions are listed in Table 151-1. Modifications in lipid A are associated with the innate resistance seen in intrinsically resistant organisms, such as *Proteus mirabilis* and *Burkholderia cepacia*.[13,14] The polymyxins usually retain activity against multidrug-resistant (MDR) gram-negative bacilli, including MDR strains of *K. pneumoniae*, *P. aeruginosa*, and *A. baumannii*, although heteroresistance is common among *A. baumannii* isolates.[15] Although minor differences in minimum inhibitory concentrations (MICs) between colistin and polymyxin B may be observed *in vitro*, cross-resistance is generally considered to be complete.

The mechanisms of acquired resistance to the polymyxins are still being elucidated. The most common mechanism is LPS modification, which interferes with the initial interaction between the negatively charged LPS and the positively charged peptides of the polymyxins.[16,17] In *A. baumannii*, mutations in the PmrAB two-component system have been shown to be responsible for modifications of lipid A and some colistin-resistant isolates have demonstrated a complete loss of LPS.[18,19] Other mechanisms of acquired resistance have also been identified. In *K. pneumoniae*, the capsule may contribute to polymyxin resistance.[20] In *P. aeruginosa*, polymyxin resistance may be due to increased production of the outer membrane protein OprH, a small, slightly basic protein that is structurally related to a porin and contributes to membrane stability by occupying Mg^{2+} binding sites in the outer membrane.[21] Additionally, multidrug efflux systems can also result in resistance to the polymyxins by *P. aeruginosa*.[22] A complete understanding of which of these mechanisms are most important for clinical resistance remains in evolution.

In Vitro Susceptibility Testing

A number of unique challenges exist when performing *in vitro* susceptibility testing with the polymyxins. First, the presence of excess calcium ions in the test system inhibits the activity of the polymyxins. Thus, divalent cation concentrations in the test media must be tightly controlled. Second, the polymyxins are large molecules that diffuse slowly in agar based assays. Resultantly, zones of inhibition are small, and very minor differences in zone sizes may result in interpretive errors. In fact, partly as a function of excessive error rates, Clinical and Laboratory Standards Institute (CLSI) disk zone size interpretive criteria do not exist for *Acinetobacter* spp. or the Enterobacteriaceae. Thirdly, the polymyxins have been shown to adhere to plastic and glass surfaces, potentially impacting MIC determinations. Currently, CLSI MIC interpretive criteria exist for *P. aeruginosa* and several other non-Enterobacteriaceae (Susceptible ≤2 µg/mL; Intermediate 4 µg/mL; Resistant ≥8 µg/mL), and *Acinetobacter* spp. (Susceptible ≤2 µg/mL; Resistant ≥4 µg/mL), but not the Enterobacteriaceae.[23] A joint European Committee on Antimicrobial Susceptibility Testing (EUCAST)/CLSI working group is in the process of developing breakpoints for the Enterobacteriaceae based upon recent pharmacokinetic/

pharmacodynamic advances, evaluations of testing methodologies, population distributions of MIC values, and animal model findings.

Available Preparations

Coly-Mycin M and Colomycin are the two colistimethate (CMS) prodrug formulations available for parenteral use. Coly-Mycin M is available in the USA and is distributed in vials containing 360 mg of CMS, corresponding to 150 mg of colistin base activity (CBA). Colomycin is produced in Europe and is dosed in international units (IU) instead of milligrams. One million IUs is approximately equal to 30 mg of CBA.[24] Polymyxin B is administered as the active drug, polymyxin B sulfate, and each mg of polymyxin B is equivalent to 10 000 IU.

Colistin sulfate and polymyxin B formulations are also available for topical use, where they are typically combined with other agents for expanded gram-negative activity. Colistin sulfate is also available as an oral formulation that is not absorbed systemically and has been used with limited efficacy to eradicate intestinal carriage of MDR Enterobacteriaceae.[25] Finally, CMS can be inhaled via a nebulizer to treat MDR gram-negative ventilator-associated pneumonia (VAP) or administered intrathecally for MDR gram-negative meningitis.[26,27]

Pharmacokinetics and Distribution

Given that the clinical use of polymyxins predated the availability of sophisticated pharmacokinetic and pharmacodynamic analyses, these properties have only recently been elucidated (Table 151-2). Colistin is administered as an inactive prodrug, CMS, and the percentage of CMS that is converted to colistin is highly variable, leading to marked variability in steady-state plasma colistin concentrations.[28,29] The fraction of CMS that is converted to colistin is particularly low in patients with intact renal function because CMS undergoes renal clearance more efficiently than the rate of hydrolysis to colistin. Furthermore, the inefficient conversion of CMS to colistin often results in a 4–6 hour delay until therapeutic plasma concentrations of colistin are achieved, even with the use of a loading dose.[30]

Colistin has a volume of distribution of approximately 0.76 L/kg in critically ill patients.[28] Distribution to the pleural space, bone, and joint fluid is poor and colistin concentrations in cerebrospinal and bronchoalveolar lavage fluid in patients receiving intravenous CMS are suboptimal.[3,31,32] Although colistin is not excreted by renal mechanisms, significant concentrations of colistin are recovered in urine because CMS, which undergoes renal excretion, converts to colistin in the urinary tract.[33] Colistin plasma protein binding is substantial (59–74%).[30] Similar to plasma colistin concentrations, the half-lives of CMS and colistin are inversely related to renal function (intact renal function: 4.6 and 11 hours, respectively; severely impaired renal function: 9.1 and 13 hours, respectively).[28]

In contrast to CMS/colistin, the administration of polymyxin B as the active drug leads to less variability in its pharmacokinetics and achievement of therapeutic plasma concentrations within 1–2 hours

TABLE 151-1	Bacteria Against Which the Polymyxins Either Lack or Exhibit Poor *In Vitro* Activity	
Innately Resistant		**Poor Activity**
Brucella spp.		*Aeromonas* spp.
Burkholderia spp.		*Edwardsiella tarda*
Chromobacterium violaceum		*Legionella* spp.
Helicobacter pylori		*Vibrio* spp.
Moraxella catarrhalis		Anaerobes
Morganella morganii		Gram-negative cocci
Neisseria (pathogenic spp.)		Gram-positive species
Proteus spp.		
Providencia spp.		
Serratia marcescens		

TABLE 151-2	Differences Between Colistin/Colistimethate (CMS) and Polymyxin B and Clinical Implications		
Characteristic	**Colistin/CMS**	**Polymyxin B**	**Clinical Implications**
Dosing form	Prodrug (CMS must be converted to colistin)	Active drug	Plasma concentrations of colistin are more variable than those of polymyxin B Longer time to achieve therapeutic concentrations of colistin after intravenous dosing
Dosing conversions	2.7 mg CMS = 1 mg colistin base activity (CBA) 1 million IU = 30 mg (CBA)	10 000 IU = 1 mg	The variations in reporting of dosages, particularly for CMS, is a source of confusion
Drug clearance	CMS undergoes renal clearance	Does not undergo renal clearance	CMS dosing, unlike polymyxin B dosing, must be adjusted for renal dysfunction
Urinary tract concentrations	High (CMS converts to colistin in the urinary tract)	Low	CMS may be a preferred option compared to polymyxin B for the treatment of urinary tract infections

IU, international units.

after intravenous dosing.[28,34] Also, unlike CMS, polymyxin B is predominantly cleared by non-renal mechanisms, and thus its plasma concentrations are not correlated with renal function. Thus, polymyxin B does not require dosing adjustment for renal insufficiency and achieves low urinary tract concentrations.[34] There are no substantial differences between the volume of distribution or degree of protein binding between colistin and polymyxin B.[28,30,34] The half-life of polymyxin B is 13–14 hours.[35]

Clinical Use

INTRAVENOUS FORMULATIONS

Given their high rates of toxicity and status as last-line agents, the use of parenteral polymyxins should be reserved for infections caused by gram-negative bacteria that are resistant to most other classes of antimicrobial agents. They are most commonly used for infections caused by carbapenem-resistant Enterobacteriaceae (CRE) and extensively drug-resistant isolates of *A. baumannii* and *P. aeruginosa*. Although CMS and polymyxin B can be administered intramuscularly, intravenous administration is preferred because intramuscular injections are very painful.[6] CMS can be administered intravenously over 3–5 minutes, whereas polymyxin B should be administered over 60–90 minutes. The recommend dosage of CMS for patients in the USA with normal renal function is 2.5–5 mg/kg/day (as determined by CBA), with an upper limit of 300 mg/day.[36] In Europe, where Colomycin is available, the recommended dosage is 3–6 million IU/day (90–180 mg of CBA/day). The recommended dosage of polymyxin B is 1.5–2.5 mg (15 000–25 000 IU)/kg/day.[36] Unlike polymyxin B, the dosage of CMS should be adjusted for renal insufficiency (Table 151-3).

Recent data suggest that current dosing recommendations of CMS (particularly when dosed using a maximum of 6 million IU/day) may be insufficient to achieve suggested plasma colistin concentrations in patients with normal renal function.[28] Observational clinical data also support the use of higher doses of CMS. In a single-center study of 258 patients who received CMS for MDR gram-negative bacterial infections, in-hospital mortality decreased from 39% to 28% to 20% when the median daily dosage of colistin was increased from 3 million IU to 6 million IU to 9 million IU, respectively.[37] Another study demonstrated that a higher colistin dosage was independently associated with microbiologic success.[38] Improved clinical outcomes have also been demonstrated for polymyxin B when dosages of ≥200 mg/day were used.[39]

The delay in achieving therapeutic concentrations of colistin and results from a pharmacokinetic study of 105 critically ill patients support consideration of a loading dose of CMS.[28,30] This study outlines suggested loading and maintenance doses based on the target colistin steady-state concentration, creatinine clearance and body weight. The clinical effectiveness of a loading dose of 9 million IU (270 mg CBA) of CMS was assessed in the treatment of 28 episodes of bacteremia or VAP due to MDR gram-negative bacteria.[40] The loading dose was followed by 4.5 million IU (135 mg CBA) every 12 hours, with adjustments for renal insufficiency. The clinical cure rate was 82%

with this dosing strategy, a result that compares favorably to those of other studies of critically ill patients who received CMS. Further studies are needed to better evaluate the role of a loading dose of CMS.

Given that polymyxin B achieves therapeutic plasma concentrations more rapidly than colistin, the rationale for a loading dose of polymyxin B is less clear. However, as with CMS, Monte Carlo simulations suggest a potential advantage to using a loading dose of polymyxin B of 2.5 mg/kg, followed by maintenance doses of 1.5 mg/kg every 12 hours, for patients with severe infections or harboring pathogens for which the polymyxin B MIC is ≥2 μg/mL.[34] Clinical data to support the use of a loading dose of polymyxin B are not available.

COMBINATION THERAPY

The suboptimal pharmacokinetic/pharmacodynamic parameters of polymyxins and the potential for emergence of resistance on therapy have led some experts to recommend combining polymyxins with an additional antimicrobial agent for the treatment of serious infections.[28] Among potential options for combination therapy, studies have most consistently demonstrated *in vitro* synergy between polymyxins and rifampin and polymyxins and carbapenems against MDR gram-negative pathogens.[41–43] Furthermore, the addition of rifampin and carbapenems to polymyxins has been shown to prevent the *in vitro* emergence of polymyxin resistance.[41,44]

Whether these *in vitro* advantages of combination therapy translate into improved clinical outcomes is unclear, as clinical data are conflicting and mostly observational. In the largest clinical trial to assess the benefits of polymyxin-based combination therapy, 210 patients with serious infections due to MDR *A. baumannii* were randomized to receive CMS alone or CMS plus rifampin.[45] There was no significant difference in 30-day mortality rates between treatment groups, although patients who received rifampin had improved microbiologic eradication rates. Four observational studies have demonstrated a mortality benefit to combining CMS with additional agents (primarily carbapenems, tigecycline and aminoglycosides) for the treatment of CRE bacteremia.[46–49] However, these studies were not randomized and did not evaluate polymyxin B. Furthermore, other observational studies have not demonstrated a benefit to combination therapy.[50] Well-designed randomized clinical trials of specific patient populations, therapies, and MDR pathogens are needed to clarify this issue.

URINARY TRACT INFECTIONS

The different pharmacokinetics of colistin and polymyxin B influence their role in the treatment of urinary tract infections (UTIs). Therapeutic urinary tract concentrations of colistin are attained because CMS is converted to colistin in the urinary tract.[29] Observational studies have generally shown high rates of clinical success when using intravenous CMS to treat MDR gram-negative UTIs, although the largest number of episodes evaluated in these studies was 12.[51] In order to avoid systemic toxicity caused by CMS, colistin has also been delivered directly into the bladder by instilling 3 mg (100 000 IU) CMS in 50 mL of saline through a urinary catheter three times daily.[52]

Unlike colistin, polymyxin B achieves low urinary tract concentrations and thus may not be as effective against UTIs.[29] In one study, the microbiologic clearance rate was significantly lower for episodes of carbapenem-resistant *K. pneumoniae* bacteriuria treated with polymyxin B (64%) compared to that of those treated with aminoglycosides (88%).[53] In another report of 17 UTIs treated with polymyxin B, clinical and microbiologic success rates were 82% and 53%, respectively.[54] Further clinical studies are needed to better evaluate the role of polymyxins in the treatment of UTIs caused by MDR gram-negative bacteria.

INHALED AND INTRATHECAL ADMINISTRATION

Inhalation therapy with aerosolized CMS has been used both as adjunctive therapy to intravenous antibiotics for MDR VAP and in the management of patients with cystic fibrosis. The rationale for using inhaled CMS is that intravenous CMS achieves suboptimal concentrations in lung epithelial lining fluid (ELF), whereas inhaled CMS

TABLE 151-3	Maintenance Dosing Adjustments for Intravenous Colistimethate (CMS) in Patients with Renal Insufficiency	
Creatinine Clearance (mL/min)	**Daily Dosage of Colistin Base Activity (Max: 300 Mg/Day)**
>80	5 mg/kg (divided into 2 doses per day)
50–79	2.5–3.8 mg/kg (divided into 2 doses per day)
30–49	2.5 mg/kg daily (once daily or divided into 2 doses)
10–29	1.5 mg/kg every 36 hours

Dosing should be based on ideal body weight.

achieves high lung ELF concentrations with minimal systemic absorption.[32,55] Clinical benefits of adding inhaled CMS to intravenous CMS in observational studies have been modest, with the largest study demonstrating a higher rate of clinical cure and fewer days requiring mechanical ventilation, but no mortality benefit.[26] The largest randomized clinical trial addressing this issue failed to find a significant difference in clinical cure rates or a mortality benefit with the addition of inhaled CMS, but found an improved microbiologic clearance rate.[56] Importantly, this trial also found an increased rate of bronchospasm (8% vs 2%) in patients randomized to inhaled CMS. There are no formal recommendations on dosing of inhaled CMS, but dosages between 30 and 75 mg (1–2.5 million IU) CBA every 12 hours have been most commonly reported.[56,57] Inhaled CMS should not be premixed until immediately before use.[58] Aerosolized polymyxin B has also been used to treat MDR gram-negative pneumonia, but its use has been limited because of an increased risk of bronchospasm compared to aerosolized CMS.[59]

In addition to being administered through a nebulizer, CMS has been administered through the intraventricular and intrathecal route, primarily to treat MDR *A. baumannii* meningitis.[27] The reason for considering the use of intraventricular or intrathecal colistin is that cerebrospinal fluid (CSF) concentrations of colistin in patients with meningitis receiving intravenous CMS range between 0.1 and 0.3 μg/mL, concentrations that are below the colistin MICs for most organisms.[60] However, the addition of 3.75 mg CBA (10 mg total; 125 000 IU) daily of intraventricular CMS achieves colistin CSF concentrations of 0.6–1.5 μg/mL. A recent review identified 83 reported episodes of MDR *A. baumannii* meningitis treated with intraventricular or intrathecal CMS.[27] In all cases, meningitis was secondary to neurosurgical procedures, and the majority of cases involved an external ventricular drain. The median dose of local CMS was 3.75 mg CBA and intravenous therapy was concurrently administered in the majority of cases. A successful outcome was achieved in 89% of cases. The primary toxicity related to treatment was a reversible chemical meningitis/ventriculitis that occurred in 11% of cases.

SPECIAL CIRCUMSTANCES

CMS dosing in the setting of renal impairment is outlined in Table 151-3. Dosage adjustments for hepatic insufficiency are unnecessary for either agent. The recommended dosages (in mg/kg) of CMS and polymyxin B also apply to children, although data to support recommendations in the pediatric population are sparse.[61] The manufacturer recommends dosing CMS based on ideal body weight. This is an important consideration in obese patients, as high rates of nephrotoxicity have been noted in this population when dosing was administered based on actual body weight.[62] Although polymyxin B has also traditionally been dosed based on ideal body weight, a recent pharmacokinetic study of 24 critically ill patients suggests that drug clearance is best correlated with total body weight.[34] Given that few obese patients were in this study, and the potential for increased toxicity using higher polymyxin B doses, further research is needed to clarify the optimal dosing strategy in obese patients. There is insufficient data to assess the safety of the polymyxins in pregnancy. According to the manufacturer, CMS is transferred across the placenta, and it is designated pregnancy Category C by the U.S. Food and Drug Administration.

Adverse Reactions

The most important and common side effect of intravenous polymyxins is nephrotoxicity, which typically manifests as acute kidney injury. In the two largest studies to evaluate the risk of nephrotoxicity using RIFLE criteria[63] in hospitalized patients receiving intravenous CMS, nephrotoxicity occurred in 40% and 43% of patients, respectively.[64,65] In the majority of cases, nephrotoxicity developed within the first week of therapy and was reversible after discontinuation of therapy. Modifiable independent risk factors for CMS-related nephrotoxicity include a daily dose of ≥5 mg CBA per kg of ideal body weight, duration of CMS therapy, and use of concomitant nephrotoxic medications.[64,66] This dose-dependent nephrotoxicity limits the amount of CMS that can be administered intravenously.

Intravenous polymyxin B was previously thought to be more nephrotoxic than intravenous CMS. However, this belief has been refuted by two studies of critically ill patients that reported a lower rate of nephrotoxicity with polymyxin B than with CMS.[67,68]

Neurotoxicity, particularly paresthesias (often perioral) and ataxia, are well known side effects of intravenous polymyxins.[3] In rare cases, polymyxins have caused respiratory paralysis,[69] and thus they should be avoided, if possible, in patients receiving neuromuscular blocking agents. Recent studies of polymyxin have identified a lower incidence of neurologic side effects than previously reported.[70,71] However, these studies may have underappreciated the risk of neurotoxicity because they were primarily retrospective and focused on nephrotoxicity. Older reports suggest that 2% of patients will develop allergic manifestations to polymyxins, but reports of hypersensitivity reactions in recent studies have been rare.[3]

Drug–Drug Interactions

Although there are no specific drug interactions related to the metabolism of the polymyxins, their use with other nephrotoxic or neuromuscular blocking agents increases the risk of these adverse effects.

References available online at expertconsult.com.

KEY REFERENCES

Akajagbor D.S., Wilson S.L., Shere-Wolfe K.D., et al.: Higher incidence of acute kidney injury with intravenous colistimethate sodium compared with polymyxin B in critically ill patients at a tertiary care medical center. *Clin Infect Dis* 2013; 57:1300-1303.

Durante-Mangoni E., Signoriello G., Andini R., et al.: Colistin and rifampicin compared with colistin alone for the treatment of serious infections due to extensively drug-resistant *Acinetobacter baumannii*: a multicenter, randomized clinical trial. *Clin Infect Dis* 2013; 57:349-358.

Falagas M.E., Kasiakou S.K.: Colistin: the revival of polymyxins for the management of multi-drug resistant Gram-negative bacterial infections. *Clin Infect Dis* 2005; 40:1333-1341.

Garonzik S.M., Li J., Thamlikitkul V., et al.: Population pharmacokinetics of colistin methanesulfonate and formed colistin in critically ill patients from a multicenter study provide dosing suggestions for various categories of patients. *Antimicrob Agents Chemother* 2011; 55: 3284-3294.

Karaiskos I., Galani L., Baziaka F., et al.: Intraventricular and intrathecal colistin as the last therapeutic resort for the treatment of multidrug-resistant and extensively drug-resistant *Acinetobacter baumannii* ventriculitis and meningitis: a literature review. *Int J Antimicrob Agents* 2013; 41:499-508.

Li J., Rayner C.R., Nation R.L., et al.: Heteroresistance to colistin in multidrug-resistant *Acinetobacter baumannii*. *Antimicrob Agents Chemother* 2006; 50:2946-2950.

Nation R.L., Velkov T., Li J.: Colistin and polymyxin B: Peas in a pod, or chalk and cheese? *Clin Infect Dis* 2014; 59:88-94.

Plachouras D., Giamarellos-Bourboulis E.J., Kentepozidis N., et al.: *In vitro* postantibiotic effect of colistin on multidrug-resistant *Acinetobacter baumannii*. *Diagn Microbiol Infect Dis* 2007; 57:419-422.

Poudyal A., Howden B.P., Bell J.M., et al.: *In vitro* pharmacodynamics of colistin against multidrug-resistant *Klebsiella pneumoniae*. *J Antimicrob Chemother* 2008; 62:1311-1318.

Rattanaumpawan P., Lorsutthitham J., Ungprasert P., et al.: Randomized controlled trial of nebulized colistimethate sodium as adjunctive therapy of ventilator-associated pneumonia caused by Gram-negative bacteria. *J Antimicrob Chemother* 2010; 65:2645-2649.

Sampson T.R., Liu X., Schroeder M.R., et al.: Rapid killing of *Acinetobacter baumannii* by polymyxins is mediated by a hydroxyl radical death pathway. *Antimicrob Agents Chemother* 2012; 56:5642-5649.

Sandri A.M., Landersdorfer C.B., Jacob J., et al.: Population pharmacokinetics of intravenous polymyxin B in critically ill patients: implications for selection of dosage regimens. *Clin Infect Dis* 2013; 57:524-531.

Tumbarello M., Viale P., Viscoli C., et al.: Predictors of mortality in bloodstream infections caused by *Klebsiella pneumoniae* carbapenemase-producing *K. pneumoniae*: importance of combination therapy. *Clin Infect Dis* 2012; 55:943-950.

PRACTICE POINT 39

Management Strategies for Drug-Resistant Infections

GEORGE L. DAIKOS | MARIA SOULI | ANASTASIA ANTONIADOU

Multidrug-Resistant Gram-Negative Bacteria

Examples of clinically important multidrug-resistant (MDR) gram-negative bacteria (GNB) are: *Acinetobacter baumannii*, *Pseudomonas aeruginosa*, and Enterobacteriaceae, primarily *Klebsiella pneumoniae* and *Escherichia coli*. Strategies for the management of MDR gram-negative infections are based on the following fundamental concepts: timely initiation of empiric therapy, selection of agents with high probability of activity and sufficient penetration to the site of infection, adequate dosing to attain optimal drug exposure, and prompt removal or drainage of infected source.

MDR-GNB-PRODUCING EXTENDED-SPECTRUM β-LACTAMASES (ESBLS)

Empirical treatment for infections that are potentially caused by ESBL-producing GNB should include: imipenem or meropenem; also consider using ertapenem against ESBL-producing Enterobacteriaceae in the absence of severe sepsis or septic shock. Once the susceptibility results are available and the patient's condition is stable, de-escalation to a carbapenem-sparing regimen should be considered. Cefepime in high doses (2g q 8–12h) can be used for isolates with minimum inhibitory concentration (MIC) ≤2 mg/L. Piperacillin–tazobactam (3.375–4.5 g q 6h) may be effective in patients with urosepsis caused by ESBL-producing *E. coli* with MIC ≤16 mg/L. The recent addition of avibactam as a novel beta-lactamase inhibitor and new combination formulations like ceftolozane/tazobactam (1.5-3 g q8h) are helpful against some ESBL-producing pathogens. Quinolones, aminoglycosides or trimethoprim/sulfamethoxazole (TMP-SMX) could be considered for urinary tract infections, but the frequent association of ESBL production with resistance to these agents precludes their use in most patients. In uncomplicated lower urinary tract infections, nitrofurantoin, fosfomycin and pivmecillinam may be considered as alternative agents.

Carbapenem-Resistant GNB

If the prevalence of carbapenem-resistant (CR) GNB is high, the empiric therapy should include a combination of two agents, one of which has high probability of activity against the infecting organism (e.g. a carbapenem with colistin or an aminoglycoside). The empiric regimen can be modified once susceptibility results are available. As CR GNB exhibit significant resistance, treatment options are usually limited to the following (see Table PP39-1):
- for Enterobacteriaceae: polymyxins, tigecycline, aminoglycosides, fosfomycin ceftazidime-avibactam and, in certain circumstances, aztreonam or carbapenems;
- for *Pseudomonas* spp.: polymyxins, aminoglycosides, fosfomycin; and
- for *Acinetobacter* spp.: polymyxins, aminoglycosides, tigecycline and, in certain circumstances, sulbactam.

Monotherapy with any of these agents results in unacceptably high mortality rates. Ceftazidime/avibactam has activity against Enterobacteriaceae producing KPC or OXA-48 types of carbapenemase but clinical experience is currently lacking. Despite the limitations in current evidence to guide treatment strategies against CR GNB infections, combination therapy appears to hold promise, particularly for severe infections in critically ill patients. For Enterobacteriaceae, carbapenems may be one of the core agents in combination treatment, provided that: 1) the MIC of meropenem is ≤ 8 mg/L and 2) a high-dose/prolonged infusion regimen is administered to attain acceptable drug exposure (Figure PP39-1). When the infecting organism is a metallo-β-lactamase (MβL)-producer and remains susceptible to aztreonam, combination of aztreonam with an aminoglycoside or colistin is reasonable. When no β-lactam agent can be used, a combination of two agents with *in vitro* activity against the infecting organism is recommended (e.g. colistin or aminoglycoside ± tigecycline or fosfomycin). In one study the triple drug combination of meropenem plus colistin plus tigecycline was an independent predictor of survival in patients with CR *Klebsiella pneumoniae* bloodstream infections. The sulbactam component of ampicillin–sulbactam may retain activity against CR *Acinetobacter* (MIC ≤8 mg/L); high-dose ampicillin–sulbactam (18–24 g/day), alone or in combination with colistin, can be administered. Rifampin or vancomycin have been proposed as part of combination therapy with colistin against CR *Acinetobacter*. In a randomized controlled trial, however, adding rifampin to colistin did not improve survival in serious infections due to extensively drug-resistant (XDR) *A. baumannii*. Finally, several studies support intrathecal administration of colistin for meningitis caused by CR GNB and the use of aerosolized colistin in the management of ventilator-associated pneumonia as an adjunct to intravenous colistin.

Multidrug-Resistant Gram-Positive Bacteria

The two major MDR gram-positive pathogens are *Staphylococcus aureus* and *Enterococcus* spp.

STAPHYLOCOCCUS AUREUS

Methicillin-resistant *Staphylococcus aureus* (MRSA, oxacillin MIC >2 mg/L) remains one of the principal pathogens, whereas vancomycin-intermediate or vancomycin-resistant *Staph. aureus* (vancomycin MIC 4–8 mg/L and ≥16 mg/L, respectively) are rare. In seriously ill patients with suspected or proven MRSA infection, a loading dose of vancomycin (25–30 mg/kg) may be considered followed by 15–20 mg/kg of actual body weight every 8–12h (not to exceed 2 g per dose). The available treatment options according to the site of infection are shown in Figure PP39-2.
- Skin and soft tissue infections (SSTIs): abscesses require incision and drainage, which may be sufficient for lesions smaller than 5 cm. Antimicrobial therapy is recommended in patients with extensive tissue involvement, rapid progression, systemic signs of infection, comorbid conditions, extremes of age and with failure of prior incision and drainage. The duration of therapy is usually 5–14 days.
- Osteoarticular infections: surgical debridement is the mainstay of therapy. Oral or initial parenteral followed by oral treatment is usually recommended for a total of 8–12 weeks. For septic arthritis, a 3–4-week course should be administered. For

TABLE PP39-1	Antimicrobial Agents Used Against Infections Caused by Carbapenem-Resistant Gram-Negative Bacilli (CR GNB)			
Drug	**Loading Dose**	**Daily Dose For Normal Renal Function**	**Comments**
Meropenem	Not required	2 g q 8 h iv infused over 3 h	Meropenem should be used in combination with another active agent; the probability of response is higher when meropenem MIC ≤8 mg/L is correct
Ceftazidime-avibactam	Not required	2.5 g q 8 h iv infused over 2 h	Approved for complicated urinary tract and intra-abdominal infections, active in vitro against Enterobacteriaceae producing ESBLs, AmpC as well as KPC and OXA-48 carbapenemases but clinical experience is currently lacking
Colistin	9 million IU infused over 1 h	4.5 million IU q 12h iv. First maintenance dose should be given within 24 h after loading dose Intrathecal/intraventricular: 125.000–250.000 IU q 24 Inhaled: 1–3 million IU q 8 h	For infections caused by organisms with MIC >0.5 mg/L, it is advisable to use colistin as part of combination therapy. For dosage adjustment in patients with renal failure refer to *Antimicrob Agents Chemother* 2011; 55: 3284
Polymyxin B (available in USA, Brazil, Malaysia and Singapore)	Not required	7500–12500 IU/Kg q 12 h iv Intrathecal/intraventricular: 50000 IU q 24 h	No dose adjustment for renal failure
Aztreonam	Not required	2 g q 6–8 h iv infused over 3 h	Aztreonam may be effective in infections caused by organisms producing metallo-β-lactamases and not co-producing an ESBL; use this agent in combination with an aminoglycoside or colistin
Sulbactam	Not required	6–8 g of sulbactam (18–24 g of ampicillin-sulbactam) iv in 4 divided dosages infused over 3 h	Only for *Acinetobacter* when ampicillin/sulbactam MIC ≤ 8 mg/L, preferably in combination with another active agent
Tigecycline	100 mg	50 mg q 12 h iv	For bloodstream infections or pneumonia or when tigecycline MIC >0.5 mg/L, higher doses are recommended (loading dose, 200 mg followed by 100 mg q 12 h), preferably in combination with another agent. Not to be used in urinary tract infections, no concentrations in urine Adjust doses according to Hartford nomogram (*Antimicrob Agents Chemother* 1995; 39: 650)
Gentamicin	Not required when administered in pulse dosing schemes	5–7 mg/kg iv infused over 1 h	Pulse dosing is preferable to multiple daily doses; desired peak serum levels are about 10 times the MIC of the organism Adjust doses according to Hartford nomogram (*Antimicrob Agents Chemother* 1995; 39: 650)
Amikacin	Not required when administered in pulse dosing schemes	15–20 mg/kg iv infused over 1 h	Adjust doses according to Hartford nomogram (*Antimicrob Agents Chemother* 1995; 39: 650)
Fosfomycin	Not required	18–24 g iv in 3–4 doses	The potential of fosfomycin to select resistant mutants precludes its use as a single agent

a. 1 mg of colistin base activity (CBA) is contained in 2.4 mg of colistimethate (CMS), which is equivalent to 30000 IU.
b. 1 mg of polymyxin B is equivalent to 10000 IU.

device-related infections, device removal is recommended using a 2-stage procedure. Retention is possible for early-onset (<2 months after surgery) or acute hematogenous infections involving a stable implant with short duration (<3 weeks) of symptoms.

- Bloodstream infections: a thorough clinical assessment and imaging including transesophageal echocardiography is recommended to identify and remove or drain the source of infection. A change of initial vancomycin to high-dose daptomycin (10 mg/kg) is recommended in cases of vancomycin failure. Daptomycin may be preferred for initial therapy in patients with serious infections when the vancomycin MIC is ≥2 mg/L. For cases refractory to both, consider: daptomycin in combination with another agent (β-lactam, linezolid, rifampin, gentamicin or trimethoprim/sulfamethoxazole), quinupristin/dalfopristin, linezolid, telavancin or ceftaroline. The duration of treatment is at least 2 weeks for uncomplicated bacteremia and 4–6 weeks for complicated bacteremia or endocarditis. Addition of gentamicin for 14 days and rifampin for 6 weeks to vancomycin is recommended for prosthetic valve MRSA endocarditis.
- Pneumonia: for hospitalized patients with severe pneumonia, empiric therapy for MRSA is recommended. If cultures do not grow MRSA, anti-MRSA treatment should be discontinued. In cases of confirmed MRSA infection, treatment with linezolid, vancomycin or telavancin is administered for up to 21 days.
- Central nervous system infections: for shunt infections, shunt removal is required and replaced only when cerebrospinal fluid cultures are repeatedly negative. Vancomycin is the treatment of choice; 2 weeks for meningitis and 4–6 weeks for brain abscess or empyema. Some experts recommend adding rifampin to vancomycin. Alternative agents are linezolid and TMP–SMX.

ENTEROCOCCI

Life-threatening infections due to enterococci should be treated with a cell-wall active agent in combination with an active aminoglycoside (gentamicin or streptomycin). Monotherapy is only used for less

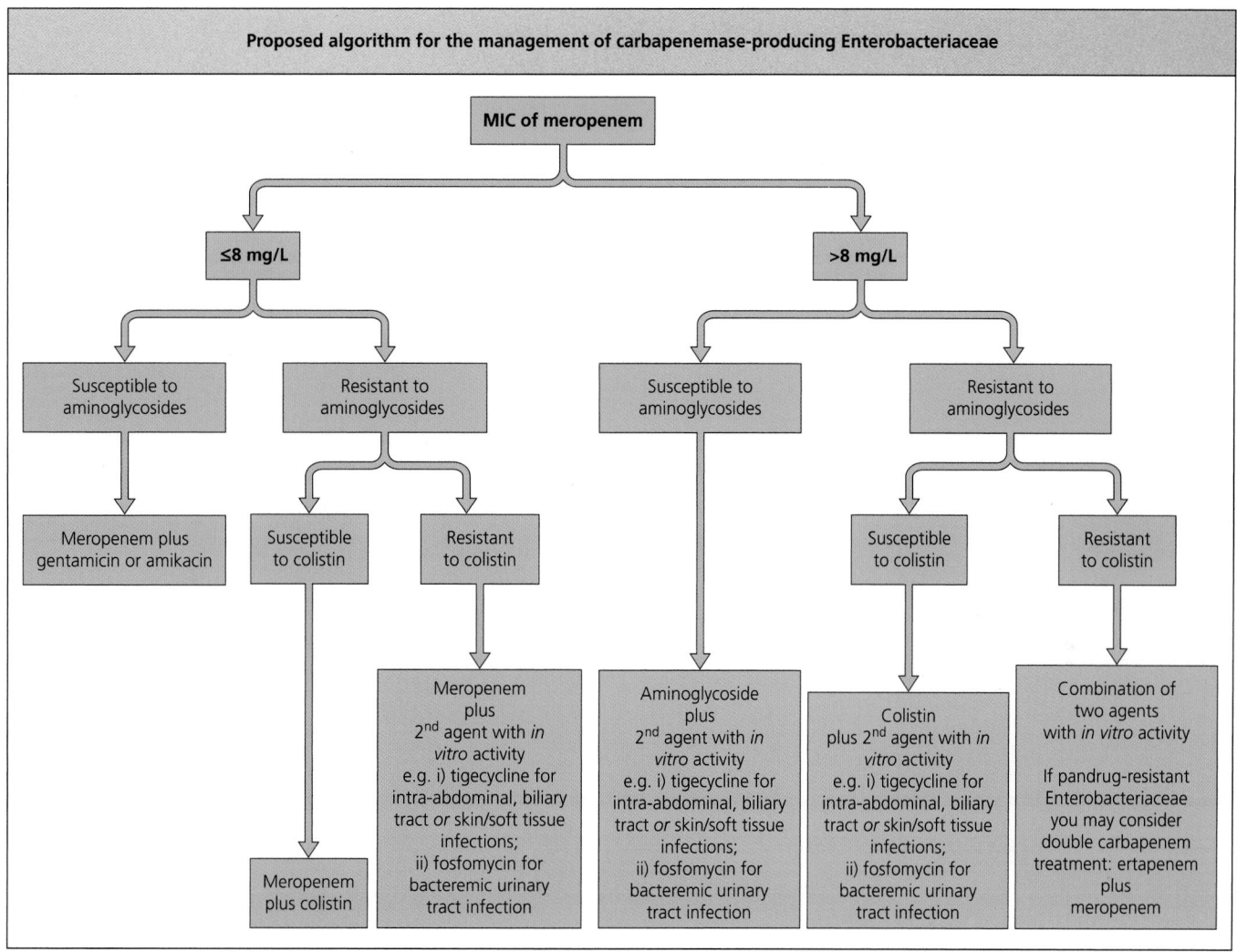

Figure PP39-1 Proposed algorithm for the management of carbapenemase-producing Enterobacteriaceae.

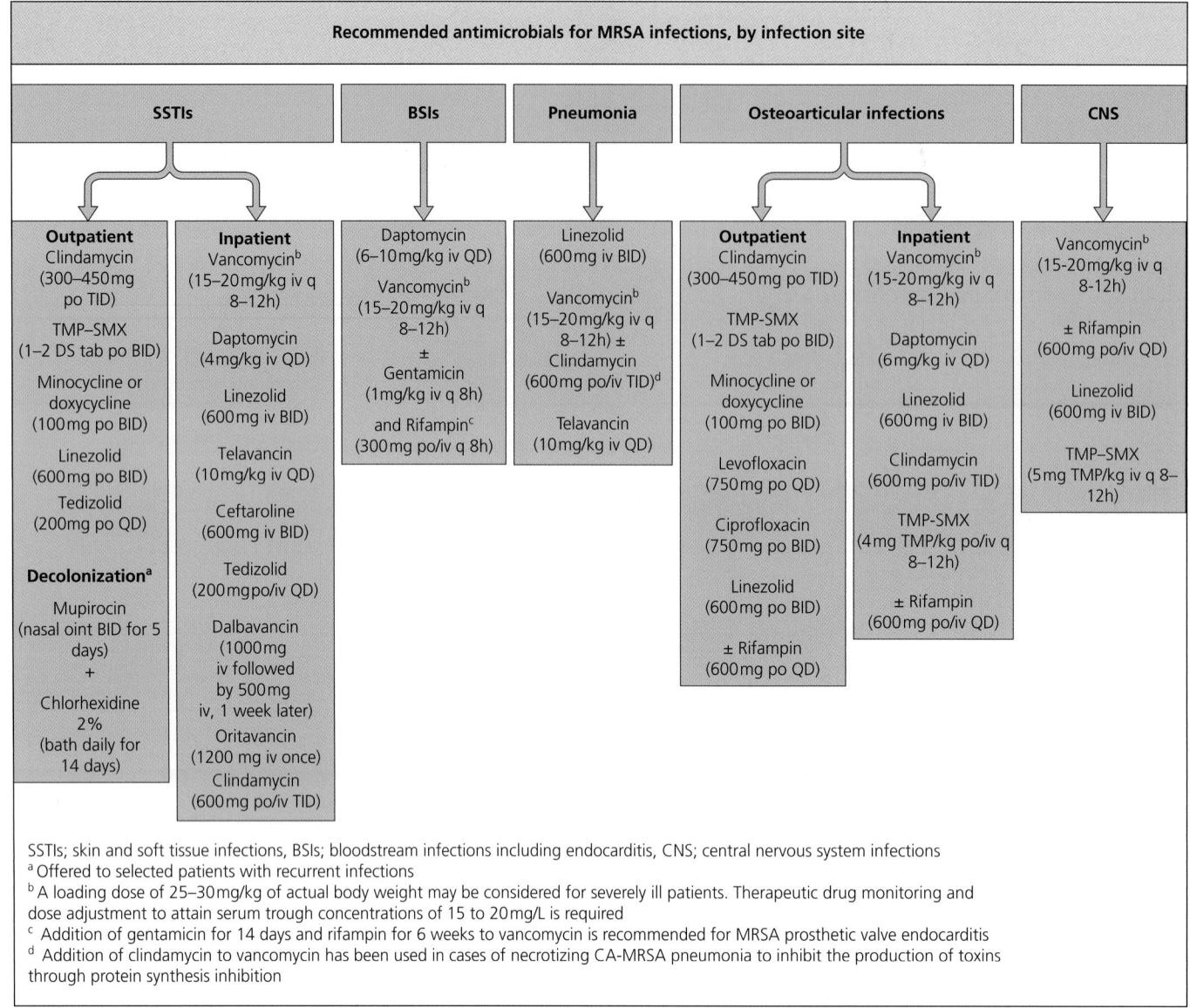

Recommended antimicrobials for MRSA infections, by infection site

SSTIs		BSIs	Pneumonia	Osteoarticular infections		CNS
Outpatient Clindamycin (300–450mg po TID) TMP–SMX (1–2 DS tab po BID) Minocycline or doxycycline (100mg po BID) Linezolid (600mg po BID) Tedizolid (200mg po QD) **Decolonization**[a] Mupirocin (nasal oint BID for 5 days) + Chlorhexidine 2% (bath daily for 14 days)	**Inpatient** Vancomycin[b] (15–20mg/kg iv q 8–12h) Daptomycin (4mg/kg iv QD) Linezolid (600mg iv BID) Telavancin (10mg/kg iv QD) Ceftaroline (600mg iv BID) Tedizolid (200mgpo/iv QD) Dalbavancin (1000mg iv followed by 500mg iv, 1 week later) Oritavancin (1200 mg iv once) Clindamycin (600mg po/iv TID)	Daptomycin (6–10mg/kg iv QD) Vancomycin[b] (15–20mg/kg iv q 8–12h) ± Gentamicin (1mg/kg iv q 8h) and Rifampin[c] (300mg po/iv q 8h)	Linezolid (600mg iv BID) Vancomycin[b] (15–20mg/kg iv q 8–12h) ± Clindamycin (600mg po/iv TID)[d] Telavancin (10mg/kg iv QD)	**Outpatient** Clindamycin (300–450mg po TID) TMP–SMX (1–2 DS tab po BID) Minocycline or doxycycline (100mg po BID) Levofloxacin (750mg po QD) Ciprofloxacin (750mg po BID) Linezolid (600mg po BID) ± Rifampin (600mg po QD)	**Inpatient** Vancomycin[b] (15–20mg/kg iv q 8–12h) Daptomycin (6mg/kg iv QD) Linezolid (600mg iv BID) Clindamycin (600mg po/iv TID) TMP-SMX (4mg TMP/kg po/iv q 8–12h) ± Rifampin (600mg po/iv QD)	Vancomycin[b] (15-20mg/kg iv q 8-12h) ± Rifampin (600mg po/iv QD) Linezolid (600mg iv BID) TMP–SMX (5mg TMP/kg iv q 8–12h)

SSTIs; skin and soft tissue infections, BSIs; bloodstream infections including endocarditis, CNS; central nervous system infections
[a] Offered to selected patients with recurrent infections
[b] A loading dose of 25–30mg/kg of actual body weight may be considered for severely ill patients. Therapeutic drug monitoring and dose adjustment to attain serum trough concentrations of 15 to 20mg/L is required
[c] Addition of gentamicin for 14 days and rifampin for 6 weeks to vancomycin is recommended for MRSA prosthetic valve endocarditis
[d] Addition of clindamycin to vancomycin has been used in cases of necrotizing CA-MRSA pneumonia to inhibit the production of toxins through protein synthesis inhibition

Figure PP39-2   Recommended antimicrobials for MRSA infections, by infection site.

serious infections such as uncomplicated bacteremia or urinary tract infections. The major categories of resistant enterococci include those with:

- β-lactam resistance (ampicillin MIC >8 mg/L): vancomycin is the agent of choice, in combination with an active aminoglycoside for serious infections. Daptomycin and tigecycline are approved for use in complicated SSTIs and tigecycline for complicated intra-abdominal infections caused by *E. faecalis*. Infections due to β-lactamase-producing enterococci can be treated with ampicillin–sulbactam. High-dose ampicillin (18–30 g/day) could be used for isolates with ampicillin MIC of 16–64 mg/L with or without an active aminoglycoside.
- High-level aminoglycoside resistance (HLAR, gentamicin MIC >128 mg/L, streptomycin MIC >512 mg/L): a double β-lactam

therapy (ampicillin plus ceftriaxone) is recommended for severe infections such as endocarditis.
- Vancomycin resistance (VRE, vancomycin MIC >4 mg/L): for *E. faecalis*, the standard combination of ampicillin with an aminoglycoside can be used, if susceptible. For MDR enterococci, linezolid, quinupristin/dalfopristin (only for *E. faecium*), high-dose daptomycin and tigecycline could be used. None of these agents has proven activity for the treatment of endocarditis. Daptomycin and tigecycline, although not approved for VRE, have been used successfully. For lower urinary tract infections requiring oral therapy, nitrofurantoin or fosfomycin or amoxicillin ± clavulanate can be used, depending on susceptibility.

Further reading available online at expertconsult.com.

152

Drugs for HIV Infection

BENJAMIN J. ECKHARDT | ROY M. GULICK

KEY CONCEPTS

- Currently 29 antiretroviral drugs, in six mechanistic classes, are approved for the treatment of human immunodeficiency virus (HIV).

- Antiretroviral drugs target critical steps in HIV replication including viral entry, reverse transcription, integration, and proteolytic processing.

- Antiretroviral therapy results in virologic suppression and CD4+ cell recovery, and consequently is associated with a dramatic reduction in HIV-related morbidity and mortality.

- Current antiretroviral drug regimens are potent, tolerable and as convenient as one pill once-a-day.

- Antiretroviral therapy is becoming increasingly available worldwide with an estimated over 15 million HIV-infected individuals currently receiving treatment.

- Life expectancy of HIV-infected individuals treated with effective antiretroviral therapy now approaches that of the general population.

- Antiretroviral therapy also is effective in preventing HIV transmission from pregnant mother to child, through sexual contact and through injection drug use.

- The development of effective treatment for HIV infection is among the greatest achievements in modern medicine.

Introduction

HIV/AIDS is a global pandemic with an estimated over 70 million people infected, over half of whom have died. The first cases of AIDS were reported in 1981 and the etiologic agent, the human immunodeficiency virus (HIV) was discovered in 1983–1984 and candidate compounds that interfered with steps of the viral life cycle were identified and tested (Figure 152-1). The first antiretroviral drug, AZT (later re-named zidovudine), a nucleoside analog reverse transcriptase inhibitor, was approved in 1987 on the basis of a short-term mortality benefit.[1] Two-drug therapy became the standard of care in the early-1990s, but also demonstrated only short-term benefits. Three-drug therapy led to potent virologic suppression and this translated into a dramatic reduction in morbidity and mortality in the late-1990s. Since 2000, antiretroviral therapy is increasingly available worldwide with an estimated over 15 million people currently treated. Antiretroviral therapy evolved to become more potent, less toxic, and more convenient allowing current therapy with one-pill, once-daily regimens. Currently, there are 29 drugs approved for the treatment of HIV infection (Table 152-1; Figure 152-2) and an HIV-infected person who takes antiretroviral therapy can expect a life expectancy similar to that of the general population. Clearly, the development of effective therapy for HIV/AIDS stands among the greatest achievements in modern medicine (see also Chapters 99 and 100).

Nucleoside Analog Reverse Transcriptase Inhibitors (NRTI)

Nucleoside analog reverse transcriptase inhibitors block the RNA-dependent DNA polymerase, reverse transcriptase, from synthesizing cDNA from viral RNA. After intracellular phosphorylation to the triphosphate forms, NRTIs compete with the natural substrate nucleoside triphosphate (Figure 152-3) and bind to the extending cDNA causing chain termination (Figures 152-1 and 152-4).

ZIDOVUDINE

Description

Zidovudine (ZDV; AZT; Retrovir; azidothymidine) is a thymidine analog reverse transcriptase inhibitor and was the first antiretroviral drug approved in 1987.[1] Zidovudine is considered an alternative initial therapy in the World Health Organization (WHO) Guidelines but is no longer recommended in US guidelines because of toxicity (Table 152-2).

Pharmacokinetics and Distribution

Zidovudine is rapidly absorbed following oral administration, and reaches peak serum concentrations within 0.5–1.5 hours. Oral bioavailability is 64% and plasma protein binding is <38%. Zidovudine is primarily eliminated by hepatic glucuronidation; urinary recovery of zidovudine is 14% (unchanged) and 74% (metabolites).

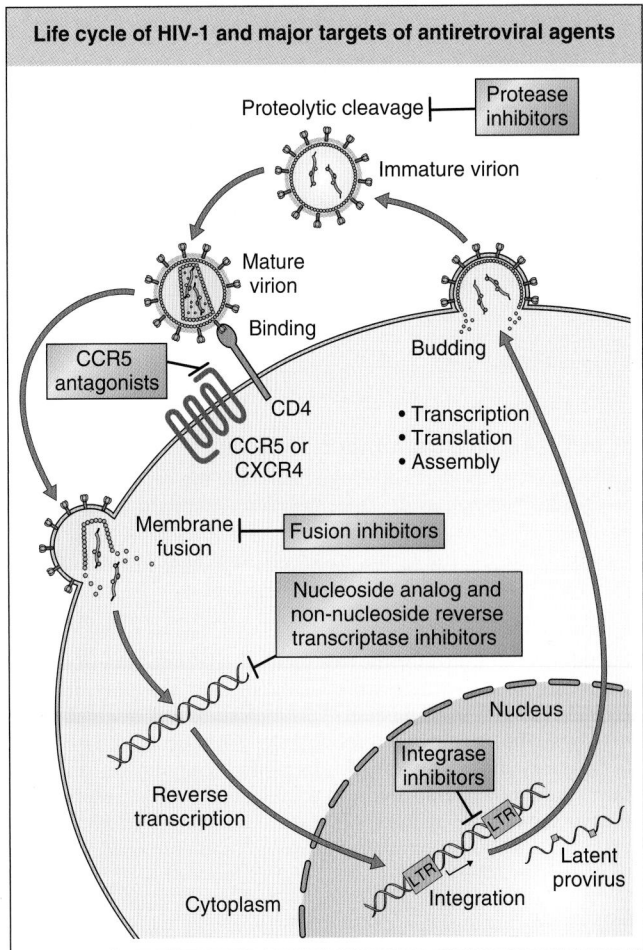

Figure 152-1 Life cycle of HIV-1 and major targets of antiretroviral agents.

TABLE 152-1	List of Approved Antiretroviral Agents and Combinations			
LIST OF ANTIRETROVIRAL DRUGS, IN ORDER OF US FDA APPROVAL				
Nucleoside/Nucleotide Reverse Transcriptase Inhibitors (NRTI)	Non-nucleoside Reverse Transcriptase Inhibitors (NNRTI)	Protease Inhibitors (PI)	Entry Inhibitors (EI)	Integrase Inhibitors (II)
Zidovudine (Retrovir) AZT	Nevirapine (Viramune) NVP	Saquinavir (Invirase) SQV	Enfuvirtide (Fuzeon) ENF	Raltegravir (Isentress) RAL
Didanosine (Videx, Videx EC) ddl	Delavirdine (Rescriptor) DLV	Ritonavir (Norvir) RTV	Maraviroc (Selzentry, Celsentri) MVC	Elvitegravir (Vitekta) EVG
Zalcitabine (Hivid) ddC*	Efavirenz (Sustiva, Stocrin) EFV	Indinavir (Crixivan) IDV		Dolutegravir (Tivicay) DTG
Stavudine (Zerit) d4T	Etravirine (Intelence) ETV	Nelfinavir (Viracept) NFV		
Lamivudine (Epivir) 3TC	Rilpivirine (Edurant) RPV	Amprenavir (Agenerase) APV†		
Abacavir (Ziagen) ABC		Lopinavir/ritonavir (Kaletra, Aluvia) LPV		
Emtricitabine (Emtriva) FTC		Fosamprenavir (Lexiva, Telzir) FPV		
Tenofovir disoproxil fumarate (Viread) TDF		Atazanavir (Reyataz) ATV		
Tenofovir alafenamide TAF		Tipranavir (Aptivus) TPV		
		Darunavir (Prezista) DRV		

List of FDA-Approved Fixed-Dose Combinations	Other Generic Fixed-Dose Combinations Found in Resource-Limited Settings (US PEPFAR-Approved)
Lamivudine/zidovudine (Combivir)	Atazanavir/ritonavir
Abacavir/lamivudine/zidovudine (Trizivir)	Lamivudine/tenofovir disoproxil fumarate/efavirenz
Abacavir/lamivudine (Epzicom, Kivexa)	Lamivudine/tenofovir disoproxil fumarate/nevirapine
Emtricitabine/tenofovir disoproxil fumarate (Truvada)	Lamivudine/zidovudine/nevirapine
Emtricitabine/tenofovir disoproxil fumarate/efavirenz (Atripla)	Lamivudine/stavudine/nevirapine
Emtricitabine/tenofovir disoproxil fumarate/rilpivirine (Complera)	Lamivudine/tenofovir disoproxil fumarate
Emtricitabine/tenofovir disoproxil fumarate/elvitegravir/cobicistat (Stribild)	Abacavir/lamivudine
Abacavir/lamivudine/dolutegravir (Triumeq)	Lamivudine/stavudine
Atazanavir/cobicistat (Evotaz)	
Darunavir/cobicistat (Prezcobix, Rezolsta)	
Emtricitabine/tenofovir alafenamide/elvitegravir/cobicistat (Genvoya)	

*Withdrawn in 2005.
†Withdrawn in 2004.

Route of Administration and Dosage

Zidovudine is available as 300 mg tablets, 100 mg capsules, or syrup (50 mg/5 mL) as well as in co-formulations. Standard adult dose of zidovudine is 600 mg/day in divided doses (e.g. 300 mg twice a day) with other antiretroviral agents, with or without food. Pediatric dosing is based on weight or body surface area.

Indications

Zidovudine is indicated for the treatment of HIV infection in combination with other antiretroviral agents and for the prevention of maternal-fetal HIV transmission. This indication was originally supported by studies of zidovudine monotherapy in patients with advanced HIV disease[1] and asymptomatic or mildly symptomatic disease.[6,7] A later study showed zidovudine in combination with lamivudine and indinavir significantly reduced AIDS and death compared with 2-drug therapy.[8] Zidovudine monotherapy reduced mother to child transmission of HIV by 69%.[9]

Resistance

Four or more substitutions in the HIV reverse transcriptase gene confer drug resistance to zidovudine; the thymidine analog-associated mutations (TAMs) are M41L, D67N, K70R, L210W, T215Y or F, and K219Q.[10] Cross-resistance to all other nucleoside/nucleotide analogs can occur. Zidovudine retains activity against viral strains with the K65R substitution (see Chapter 174).

Dosage in Special Circumstances

Zidovudine clearance is reduced with renal impairment; dose adjustment is necessary for patients with estimated creatinine clearance of <15 mL/minute (Table 152-3). There are insufficient data to recommend dose adjustment of zidovudine in patients with impaired hepatic function or liver cirrhosis. Zidovudine pharmacokinetics in pregnant or pediatric patients greater than 3 months of age is similar to those in adult non-pregnant patients. Zidovudine is pregnancy category C.

Adverse Reactions and Drug Interactions

The most commonly reported adverse reactions in adult HIV clinical studies were headache, malaise, nausea, anorexia, and vomiting. Hematologic toxicity including neutropenia and severe anemia occur commonly. Symptomatic myopathy and myositis associated with prolonged use (e.g. >1 year) of zidovudine occurs. Zidovudine also is associated with lipoatrophy (Table 152-4).

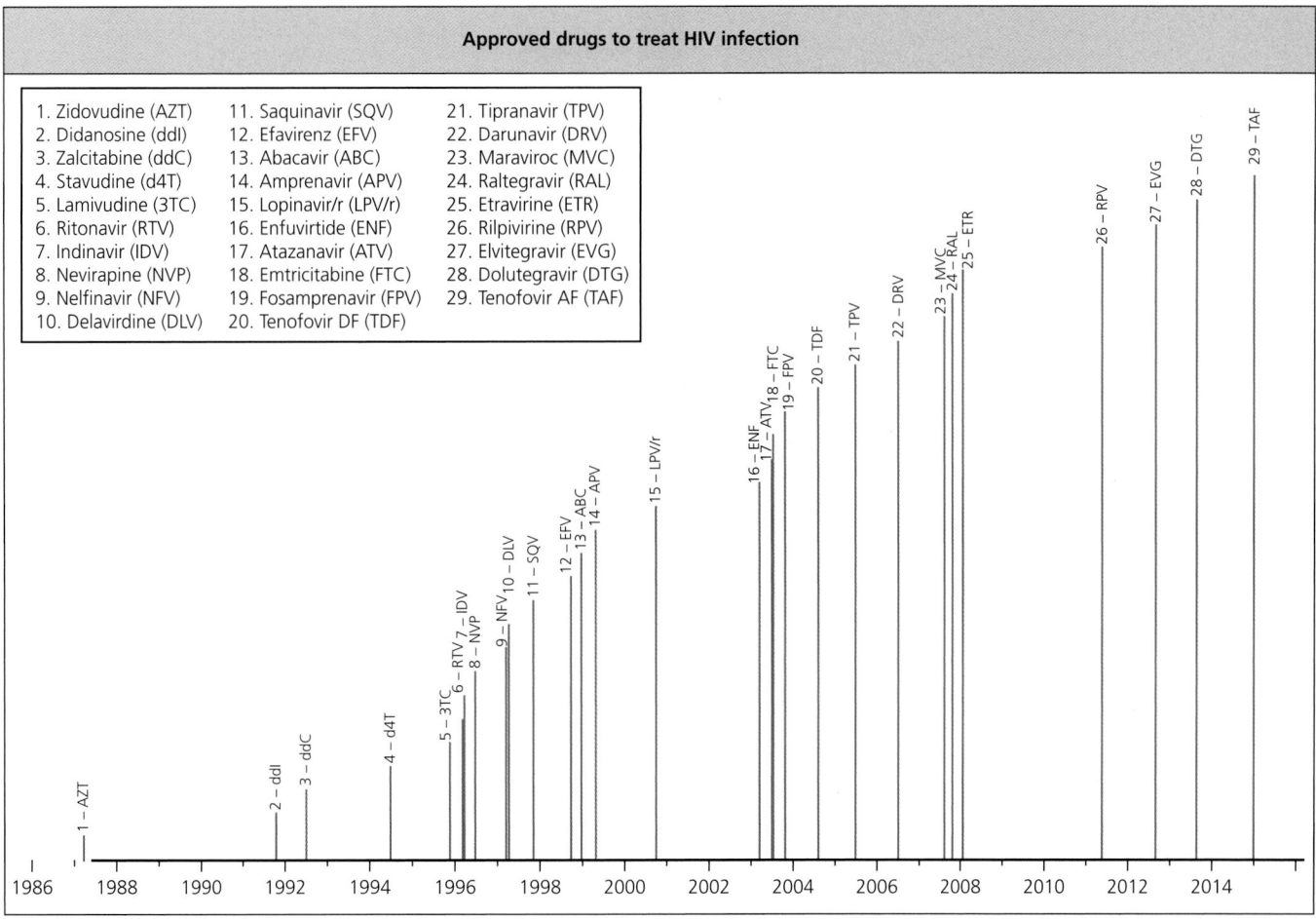

Figure 152-2   Approved drugs to treat HIV infection. (Antiretroviral agents listed by date of FDA approval. Agents in gray have been since removed from the market.)

Ribavirin reduces phosphorylation of zidovudine and antagonizes the antiviral activity; co-administration is not advised. Stavudine and doxorubicin each antagonize zidovudine; concomitant use should be avoided. Co-administration of ganciclovir, alfa interferon, ribavirin, and other bone marrow suppressants and cytotoxic agents may increase the hematologic toxicity of zidovudine.

DIDANOSINE

Description
Didanosine (ddl; Videx) is a nucleoside analog of adenosine that was approved in 1991 as the second antiretroviral drug (Figure 152-2). Didanosine is not in common use today and is no longer recommended in US treatment guidelines because of toxicities, including peripheral neuropathy and pancreatitis, and the need to administer when fasting.

Pharmacokinetics and Distribution
Didanosine is rapidly absorbed orally, with peak concentrations achieved by 0.25–1.5 hours. Oral bioavailability is 42%. Didanosine has an elimination half-life of 1.5 hours and 18% is excreted unchanged in the urine.

Route of Administration and Dosage
Didanosine delayed-release capsule with enteric-coated beadlets (EC) is available in 125 mg, 200 mg, 250 mg and 400 mg capsules. The recommended dose of didanosine enteric-coated formulation (EC) is 400 mg once daily for patients weighing at least 60 kg; 250 mg once daily for those weighing 25 kg to <60 kg; and 200 mg once daily for those weighing 20 kg to <25 kg. Since food reduces didanosine

absorption by nearly 50%, didanosine EC should be taken on an empty stomach. There also is a pediatric powder for oral solution available (2 g/4 ounces; 4 g/8 ounces).

Indications
Didanosine is indicated for use in combination with other antiretroviral agents for the treatment of HIV-1 infection. The original indication was based on clinical studies using monotherapy, where changing to didanosine decreased clinical progression in patients taking zidovudine[11] and a study in pediatric patients where didanosine or zidovudine and didanosine was superior with decreased clinical progression compared to zidovudine alone.[12] Didanosine EC was approved on the basis of a study showing comparability of a regimen of didanosine EC and stavudine versus zidovudine and lamivudine, each in combination with nelfinavir.[13] Later studies would demonstrate didanosine and stavudine was inferior virologically and associated with more toxicity than zidovudine and lamivudine each combined with a third drug[14] and this combination is no longer recommended.

Resistance
Resistance to didanosine is associated with amino acid substitutions in the HIV reverse transcriptase gene at positions K65R, L74V, and M184V. The L74V substitution was most frequently observed from resistant clinical isolates.[10]

Dosage in Special Circumstances
Renal impairment leads to decreased clearance of didanosine and daily dosing needs to be adjusted (Table 152-3).

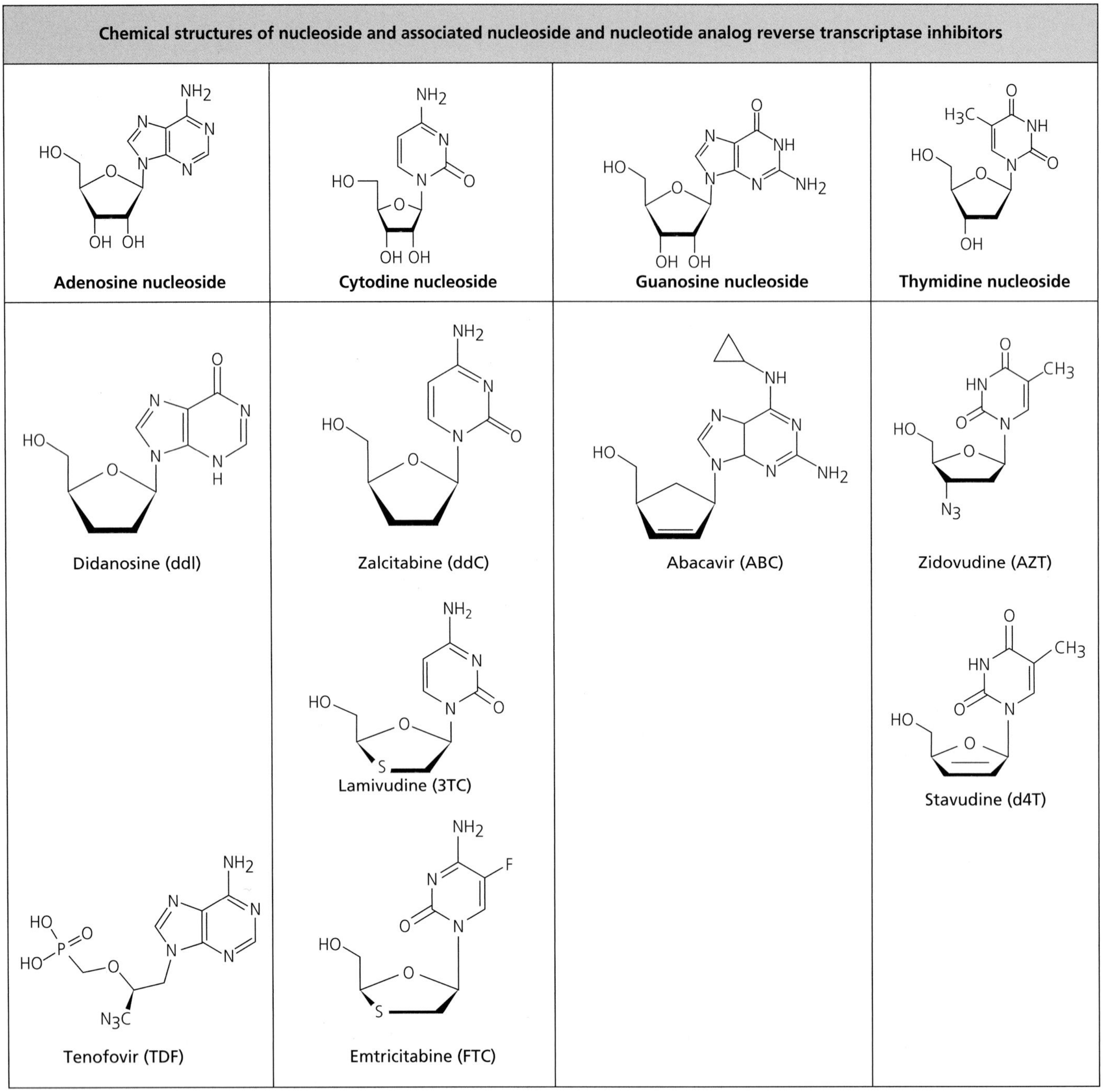

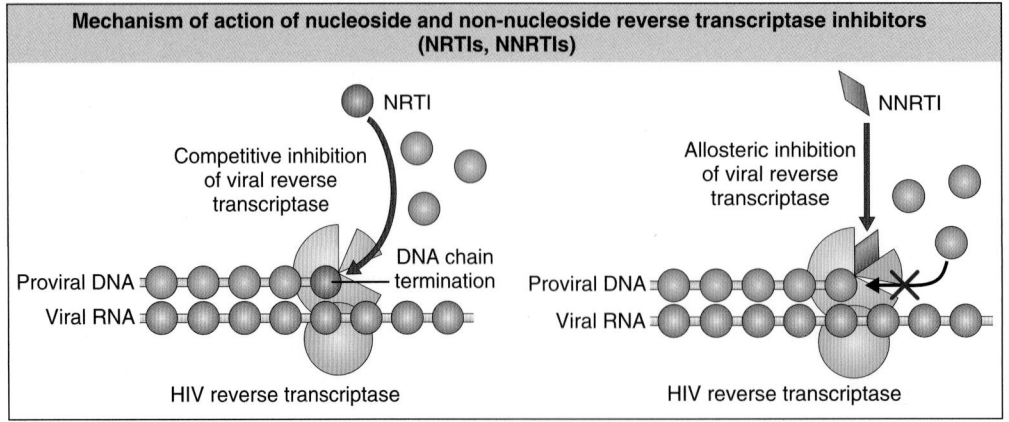

Chemical structures of nucleoside and associated nucleoside and nucleotide analog reverse transcriptase inhibitors

Adenosine nucleoside

Cytodine nucleoside

Guanosine nucleoside

Thymidine nucleoside

Didanosine (ddI)

Zalcitabine (ddC)

Abacavir (ABC)

Zidovudine (AZT)

Lamivudine (3TC)

Stavudine (d4T)

Tenofovir (TDF)

Emtricitabine (FTC)

Figure 152-3 Chemical structures of nucleoside and nucleotide analog reverse transcriptase inhibitors.

Mechanism of action of nucleoside and non-nucleoside reverse transcriptase inhibitors (NRTIs, NNRTIs)

NRTI

Competitive inhibition of viral reverse transcriptase

DNA chain termination

Proviral DNA

Viral RNA

HIV reverse transcriptase

NNRTI

Allosteric inhibition of viral reverse transcriptase

Proviral DNA

Viral RNA

HIV reverse transcriptase

Figure 152-4 Mechanism of action of nucleoside and non-nucleoside reverse transcriptase inhibitors.

TABLE 152-2	Recommended Initial Antiretroviral Regimens

RECOMMENDED INITIAL ANTIRETROVIRAL REGIMENS

	NNRTI-Based Regimens	PI-Based Regimens	INSTI-Based Regimens
US Department of Health and Human Service (DHHS) 2015[2]	–	DRV/r plus TDF/FTC	DTG/ABC/3TC DTG plus TDF/FTC EVG/cobi/(TDF or TAF)/FTC RAL plus TDF/FTC
European AIDS Clinical Society (EACS) 2014[3]	EFV plus ABC/3TC EFV/TDF/FTC RPV plus ABC/3TC* RPV/TDF/FTC*	ATV/r plus ABC/3TC ATV/r plus TDF/FTC DRV/r plus ABC/3TC DRV/r plus TDF/FTC	DTG/ABC/3TC DTG plus TDF/FTC EVG/cobi/TDF/FTC RAL plus ABC/3TC RAL plus TDF/FTC
International Antiviral Society (IAS)-USA 2014[4]	EFV/TDF/FTC EFV plus ABC/3TC RPV/TDF/FTC[†]	ATV/r plus ABC/3TC ATV/r plus TDF/FTC DRV/r plus TDF/FTC	DTG plus ABC/3TC DTG plus TDF/FTC EVG/cobi/TDF/FTC RAL plus TDF/FTC
WHO 2014[5]	EFV/TDF/3TC (or FTC)	–	–

ALTERNATIVE INITIAL ANTIRETROVIRAL REGIMENS

	NNRTI-Based Regimens	PI-Based Regimens	INSTI-Based Regimens	Other Regimens
US Department of Health and Human Service (DHHS) 2015[2]	EFV/TDF/FTC RPV/TDF/FTC*	ATV/cobi plus TDF/FTC ATV/r plus TDF/FTC DRV/cobi plus TDF/FTC DRV/(cobi or r) plus ABC/3TC	–	–
European AIDS Clinical Society (EACS) 2014[3]	NVP plus two NRTIs[‡]	LPV/r plus two NRTIs	–	AZT/3TC + 3rd drug DRV/r + RAL LPV/r + 3TC MVC + two NRTIs[§]
International Antiviral Society (IAS)-USA 2014[4]	NVP plus two NRTIs[‡] RPV/ABC/3TC*	ATV/cobi plus two NRTIs DRV/cobi plus two NRTIs DRV/r plus ABC/3TC LPV/r plus two NRTIs	RAL plus ABC/3TC	DRV/r plus RAL[¶] LPV/r plus 3TC LPV/r plus RAL
WHO 2014[5]	EFV/AZT/3TC NVP/AZT/3TC NVP/TDF/3TC (or FTC)	–	–	–

ABC, abacavir; ATZ, atazanavir; ATV, zidovudine; cobi, cobicistat; DRV, darunavir; DTG, dolutegravir; EFV, efavirenz; EVG, elvitegravir; FTC, emtricitabine; LPV, lopinavir; MVC, maraviroc; NVP, nevirapine; RAL, raltegravir; RPV, rilpivirine; r, ritonavir; TDF, tenofovir; 3TC, lamivudine.
*Recommended only if CD4 count > 200 cells/μL and HIV-VL < 100,000 copies/mL.
[†]Not recommended in patients with baseline HIV RNA levels >100000 copies/mL.
[‡]Severe hepatotoxicity may occur in initial therapy when CD4 cell count is >250 cells/μL in women and >400 cells/μL in men.
[§]For CCR5-tropic HIV only.
[¶]Less effective at CD4 cell counts of <200 cells/μL and possibly HIV-1 RNA levels >100000 copies/mL.

TABLE 152-3	Nucleoside and Nucleotide Reverse Transcriptase Inhibitors Dosage Modifications in Patients with Renal Dysfunction

Drug	Standard Adult Dosing (CrCl >50 mL/min)	RENAL IMPAIRMENT CrCl (mL/min)			
		30–49	10–29	<10	Hemodialysis
Zidovudine	300 mg q12h			100 mg q6-8h	
Didanosine	400 mg daily (> 60 kg)	200 mg daily	150 mg daily	100 mg daily	
Stavudine	40 mg q12h	20 mg q12h	20 mg q24h	20 mg q24h	
Lamivudine	150 mg q12h or 300 mg q24h	150 mg daily	150 mg first dose, then 100 mg daily	150 mg first dose, then 50 mg daily	50 mg first dose, then 25 mg daily
Abacavir	300 mg q12h or 600 mg daily	No dose adjustment required			
Emtricitabine	200 mg daily	200 mg q48h	200 mg q72h	200 mg q96h	
Tenofovir	300 mg daily	300 mg q48h	300 mg q72–96h	300 mg q7 days	

TABLE 152-4 Antiretroviral Class-Specific Toxicities		
Nucleoside/Nucleotide Reverse Transcriptase Inhibitors	Non-nucleoside Reverse Transcriptase Inhibitors	Protease Inhibitors
Lactic acidosis	Hepatotoxicity	Gastrointestinal intolerance
Lipoatrophy	Rash	Hepatotoxicity
Mitochondrial toxicity		Hyperglycemia
		Hyperlipidemia

No dose adjustment is required in patients with hepatic impairment, although the safety and efficacy of didanosine is not established in patients with significant underlying liver disease. Didanosine is pregnancy category B.

Adverse Reactions and Drug Interactions

In adults, the most common reported adverse reactions in clinical trials were diarrhea, peripheral neurologic symptoms/neuropathy, nausea, headache, rash and vomiting. Retinal changes and optic neuritis have also was reported. Didanosine also is associated with serious side effects linked to fatalities including pancreatitis, hepatotoxicity, and non-cirrhotic portal hypertension. In addition, like other nucleoside analogs, lactic acidosis and severe hepatomegaly (with fatal cases) have occurred with didanosine with or without stavudine.

Significant drug interactions occur with didanosine and tenofovir, increasing didanosine concentrations and the risk of toxicity and necessitating dose-reduction of didanosine (250 mg daily for ≥60 kg and 200 mg for <60 kg). Ganciclovir also increases didanosine concentrations. Drugs that cause pancreatitis or neurotoxicity should be used with caution with didanosine due to the potential for exacerbated toxicities.

ZALCITABINE

Zalcitabine (2',3'-deoxycytidine; ddC; Hivid), a cytosine nucleoside analog, was removed from the market in 2005 because of suboptimal virologic effect and association with significant peripheral neuropathy.

STAVUDINE

Description

Stavudine (d4T; Zerit) is a nucleoside analog of thymidine. Previously used widely, stavudine is no longer recommended in treatment guidelines because of toxicities, including peripheral neuropathy, lipoatrophy, and lactic acidosis.

Pharmacokinetics and Distribution

Stavudine is orally bioavailable and rapidly absorbed following oral dosing with a peak plasma concentration within 1 hour. The mean terminal elimination half-life is approximately 2.3 hours following a single oral dose. Stavudine undergoes negligible metabolism and is excreted 95% in urine, by glomerular filtration and active tubular secretion, and 3% in feces.

Route of Administration and Dosage

Stavudine is available in 15, 20, 30, and 40 mg capsules and in a 1 mg/mL oral solution. The standard adult dose is stavudine 40 mg every 12 hours orally for patients ≥60 kg and 30 mg every 12 hours for patients <60 kg, with or without food. The standard dose for children at least 2 weeks old and weighing under 30 kg is 1 mg/kg every 12 hours.

Indication

Stavudine is indicated for use in combination with other antiretroviral agents for the treatment of HIV-1 infection. This indication is based on the results of several studies, including a study in zidovudine-experienced patients of monotherapy with stavudine versus zidovudine that showed stavudine significantly delayed clinical progression;[15] a study of stavudine versus zidovudine, each in combination with lamivudine and indinavir demonstrating comparable virologic efficacy;[16] and a study of stavudine and didanosine versus zidovudine and lamivudine, each in combination with indinavir, demonstrating comparable or superior virologic efficacy.[17] Subsequent studies and clinical experience revealed the toxicity of stavudine and the combination of stavudine and didanosine and these are used uncommonly today.

Resistance

Four or more substitutions in HIV reverse transcriptase confer drug resistance to stavudine (and other nucleoside analogs); the thymidine analog-associated mutations or TAMs are M41L, D67N, K70R, L210W, T215Y/F and K219Q/E.[10]

Dosage in Special Circumstances

Stavudine dosing should be adjusted for renal insufficiency (Table 152-3). Since stavudine is not metabolized hepatically, no dose adjustment is necessary with hepatic insufficiency, although there are no data for use in patients with significant hepatic impairment. Stavudine is pregnancy category C.

Adverse Reactions and Drug Interactions

The most common side effects associated with stavudine are headache, diarrhea, neuropathy, rash, nausea and vomiting. Stavudine is associated with dose-related peripheral neuropathy, which is reversible upon discontinuation of the drug. Paradoxical increase in symptoms may occur following drug discontinuation. Stavudine is also associated with lactic acidosis and hepatic steatosis, and fatalities have been reported. The combination of stavudine and didanosine was associated with fatal pancreatitis and, in pregnant women, fatal lactic acidosis. Motor weakness, mimicking Guillain–Barré syndrome, also has been described in the setting of lactic acidosis. Stavudine also is associated with lipoatrophy (loss of fat in the face and extremities).

Stavudine should not be used in combination with hydroxyurea or didanosine because of liver and pancreatic toxicity. Stavudine should not be used in combination with zidovudine because, as another thymidine analog, zidovudine competitively inhibits the intracellular phosphorylation of stavudine and, clinically, decreases in CD4 cell counts occur.

Stavudine should not be used in combination with ribavirin, because ribavirin can reduce the phosphorylation of pyrimidine nucleoside analogs, such as stavudine, and hepatic decompensation in patients with HIV/HCV co-infection has been described.

LAMIVUDINE

Description

Lamivudine (3TC; Epivir) is the negative enantiomer of cytidine. Lamivudine has activity against HIV and hepatitis B virus. Lamivudine is a recommended first-line antiretroviral drug in treatment guidelines (Table 152-2).

Pharmacokinetics and Distribution

Lamivudine is rapidly absorbed after oral administration, reaching peak concentrations at 1.5 hours. Lamivudine is 86% orally bioavailable and protein binding is low (<36%). The elimination half-life is 5–7 hours. Lamivudine is eliminated primarily unchanged in the urine.

Route of Administration and Dosage

Lamivudine is available in 150 mg and 300 mg tablets and as an oral solution (10 mg/mL). Lamivudine is also available in several co-formulations (Table 152-1). Standard dose is 300 mg daily administered as either 150 mg twice-daily or 300 mg once-daily with or without food.

Indications

Lamivudine is indicated for the treatment of HIV infection in combination with other antiretroviral agents. This indication is based on the results of several studies: a large clinical endpoint study enrolled patients taking zidovudine-containing regimens and randomized them to add lamivudine (with or without an investigational non-nucleoside analog) or placebo and found that adding lamivudine significantly decreased disease progression and improved survival.[18] In patients with little or no zidovudine experience, a dual nucleoside regimen of zidovudine and lamivudine outperformed monotherapy with either drug both virologically and immunologically.[19] In zidovudine-experienced patients, zidovudine and lamivudine outperformed zidovudine and zalcitabine immunologically.[20] In a large study of treatment-naïve patients who received zidovudine and efavirenz, once-daily lamivudine demonstrated equivalence to twice-daily lamivudine.[21]

Resistance

Complete resistance to lamivudine is conferred by a single substitution in HIV reverse transcriptase at position 184 (M184V or I); this also confers complete cross-resistance to emtricitabine (see Chapter 174).[10]

Dosage in Special Circumstances

The dose of lamivudine should be modified in patients with renal impairment (Table 152-3). Lamivudine is not hepatically metabolized, so no dose adjustment is necessary in patients with hepatic impairment, although the safety and efficacy have not been established in patients with decompensated liver disease. Lamivudine is pregnancy category C.

Adverse Reactions and Drug Interactions

Lamivudine is well-tolerated; the most common adverse events in large clinical studies were nausea, dizziness, fatigue, malaise, headache, dreams, insomnia and skin rash. Laboratory abnormalities are uncommon with lamivudine. Pancreatitis, sometimes fatal, was observed rarely in some pediatric studies. Emergence of hepatitis B mutant viral strains during treatment, associated with reduced drug susceptibility and treatment response has been seen. Also, exacerbation of hepatitis B can occur following discontinuation of lamivudine. Drug interactions with lamivudine are uncommon.

ABACAVIR

Description

Abacavir (ABC; Ziagen; 1592U89) is a synthetic carbocyclic nucleoside analog of guanosine. Abacavir is a recommended or alternative first-line drug in treatment guidelines (Table 152-2).

Pharmacokinetics and Distribution

Abacavir is rapidly absorbed after oral administration; the oral bioavailability is 83%. Binding to plasma proteins is about 50%. The half-life of abacavir is about 1.5 hours. The primary routes of elimination of abacavir are metabolism by alcohol dehydrogenase and glucuronyl transferase. Abacavir is excreted in the urine as the parent compound (1%) and as metabolites (81%) with 16% eliminated in the feces.

Route of Administration and Dosage

Abacavir is available as 300 mg tablets or as an oral solution (20 mg/mL). The standard dose in adults is 600 mg daily or 300 mg twice daily, taken with or without food. The standard dose in pediatrics (aged 3 months–16 years) is weight based.

Indications

Abacavir is indicated in combination with other antiretroviral agents for the treatment of HIV infection. This indication is based on several large clinical studies: treatment-naïve patients received lamivudine and efavirenz and were randomized to receive either abacavir or zidovudine; the abacavir regimen was noninferior virologically to the zidovudine regimen and demonstrated improved CD4 cell counts.[22] In another study, treatment-naïve patients received zidovudine and lamivudine and were randomized to receive abacavir (triple nucleoside regimen) versus indinavir; in this study, the regimens were found equivalent.[23] However, a head-to-head comparative study in

treatment-naïve patients of zidovudine, lamivudine and abacavir versus zidovudine, lamivudine and efavirenz found the triple nucleoside regimen was virologically inferior.[24] Treatment-naïve patients received lamivudine and efavirenz with both once- or twice-daily abacavir, and once-daily dosing was found noninferior to twice-daily dosing.[25] Another study found that abacavir and lamivudine was virologically inferior with more toxicity compared to tenofovir and emtricitabine each when combined with either efavirenz or atazanavir/ritonavir in treatment-naïve patients with baseline HIV RNA levels greater than 100 000 copies/mL.[26] A more recent head-to-head comparative study found abacavir/lamivudine and dolutegravir superior virologically and better tolerated than tenofovir/lamivudine/efavirenz.[27]

Resistance

Abacavir resistance is associated with amino acid substitutions K65R, L74V, Y115F, and M184V/I in HIV reverse transcriptase.[10] An increasing number of thymidine analog mutations (TAMs: M41L, D67N, K70R, L210W, T215Y/F, K219E/R/H/Q/N) is associated with a progressive reduction in abacavir susceptibility (see Chapter 174).

Dosage in Special Circumstances

The pharmacokinetics of abacavir have not been determined in patients with renal insufficiency. Abacavir concentrations are increased in patients with mild hepatic insufficiency and dose adjustment to 200 mg twice daily is required; abacavir has not been studied in patients with more severe hepatic insufficiency and consequently, abacavir is contraindicated in these patients. Abacavir is pregnancy category C.

Adverse Reactions and Drug Interactions

The most important side effect of abacavir is a hypersensitivity reaction characterized by fever, rash, and constitutional, gastrointestinal, and/or pulmonary symptoms; re-challenge following a hypersensitivity reaction has led to fatalities and thus should be avoided. The hypersensitivity reaction is linked to a genetic marker, HLA-B*5701 and screening and avoiding abacavir administration in patients with the marker greatly reduces the risk.[28]

Other side effects are uncommon, although headache, malaise and fatigue, nausea and vomiting, and dreams/sleep disorders were reported in clinical trials. Abacavir has been associated with cardiovascular events in some clinical series, but not others.

Abacavir increases clearance of methadone and some patients may require an increase in methadone dose; other clinically significant drug interactions are uncommon.

EMTRICITABINE

Description

Emtricitabine (FTC; Emtriva; BW524W91; Coviracil) is a cytosine nucleoside analog HIV reverse transcriptase inhibitor. Emtricitabine also has activity against hepatitis B virus.

Emtricitabine is a recommended first-line drug in treatment guidelines (Table 152-2), and also in combination with tenofovir for pre-exposure prophylaxis (PrEP).

Pharmacokinetics and Distribution

Following oral administration, emtricitabine is rapidly absorbed with peak plasma concentrations occurring at 1–2 hours post-dose. Less than 4% of emtricitabine binds to human plasma proteins. Following a single oral dose, the plasma emtricitabine half-life is approximately 10 hours. Emtricitabine is renally metabolized by a combination of glomerular filtration and active tubular secretion and excreted; approximately 86% is recovered in the urine and 13% is recovered as metabolites.

Route of Administration and Dosage

Emtricitabine is available as 200 mg capsules and as an oral solution (10 mg/mL). Emtricitabine is available in several co-formulated preparations (Table 152-1). Standard dose of emtricitabine for adults (at least 18 years old and for children weighing at least 33 kg) is 200 mg once daily, with or without food.

Indications

Emtricitabine is indicated in combination with other antiretroviral agents for the treatment of HIV-1 infection. This indication is based on the results of several clinical studies: a large clinical study of treatment-naïve patients randomized to receive efavirenz with either tenofovir and emtricitabine or zidovudine and lamivudine found the tenofovir and emtricitabine regimen fulfilled noninferiority criteria but also was superior in terms of virologic response and CD4 cell count increases with fewer treatment-related discontinuations.[29] A second large study of treatment-naïve patients who received didanosine and efavirenz and were randomized to either emtricitabine or stavudine found emtricitabine was associated with significantly better and more durable virologic responses with fewer adverse events.[30]

Resistance

The signature emtricitabine substitution is M184V/I in the HIV reverse transcriptase, which confers complete resistance to emtricitabine as well as cross-resistance to lamivudine.[10]

Dosage in Special Circumstances

Emtricitabine is renally metabolized and dose interval adjustment is required for patients with renal insufficiency (Table 152-3). Emtricitabine is not significantly metabolized by the liver; no dose adjustments are required in patients with hepatic insufficiency. Emtricitabine is pregnancy category B.

Adverse Reactions and Drug Interactions

Emtricitabine is well-tolerated. In large clinical studies of adults, headache, diarrhea, nausea, fatigue, dizziness, depression, insomnia, abnormal dreams, rash, abdominal pain, asthenia, increased cough, and rhinitis were reported most commonly. Skin hyperpigmentation was common (≥10%) in pediatric patients. Drug interactions are uncommon with emtricitabine.

TENOFOVIR
Description

Tenofovir disoproxil fumarate (TDF; Viread; PMPA) is a prodrug acyclic nucleoside analog of adenosine monophosphate that is hydrolyzed in the blood to tenofovir. Tenofovir also demonstrates activity against hepatitis B virus. TDF is a recommended first-line drug in treatment guidelines (Table 152-2), and is also recommended in combination with emtricitabine for PrEP. An recently approved prodrug formulation, tenofovir alafenamide (TAF), with comparable virologic activity and less toxicity is now available.[31]

Pharmacokinetics and Distribution

Following oral administration of TDF, maximum tenofovir serum concentrations are achieved in 1 hour. Following a single oral dose of TDF, the terminal elimination half-life of tenofovir is approximately 17 hours. Tenofovir is renally metabolized by a combination of glomerular filtration and active tubular secretion and excreted and 70–80% is recovered as unchanged drug in the urine.

Route of Administration and Dosage

TDF is available as tablets of 150 mg, 200 mg, 250 mg, 300 mg and oral powder. The standard dose of TDF in adults and pediatric patients (12 years or older, 35 kg or greater) is 300 mg once daily with or without food. TDF is co-formulated with other antiretrovirals (Table 152-1).

Indications

TDF is indicated in combination with other antiretroviral agents for the treatment of HIV-1 infection in adults and pediatric patients 2 years of age and older. This indication was on the basis of a study in treatment-naïve patients where TDF, lamivudine, and efavirenz was highly effective and comparable to stavudine, lamivudine, and efavirenz, with better lipid profiles and less lipodystrophy[32] as well as a study in treatment-experienced patients in which TDF was associated with a significantly better virologic response than placebo.[33] In treatment-naïve patients, TDF, emtricitabine and efavirenz demonstrated noninferiority to zidovudine, lamivudine and efavirenz, with better virologic suppression, CD4 recovery and adverse event profile.[34] TDF co-formulated with emtricitabine (TDF/FTC, Truvada) also is indicated in combination with safer sex practices for PrEP to reduce the risk of sexually acquired or injection drug-acquired HIV in adults at high risk on the basis of randomized studies.[35-37]

Resistance

The signature tenofovir substitution is K65R in the reverse transcriptase enzyme.[10] Three or more nucleoside analog-associated substitutions among M41L, D67N, K70R, L210W, T215Y/F or K219Q/E/N also confer decreased susceptibility to tenofovir. Viral strains with the multinucleoside resistant substitution, Q151M retain susceptibility to tenofovir (see Chapter 174).

Dosage in Special Circumstances

Tenofovir is eliminated primarily by the kidney and dose adjustment of TDF is required for renal insufficiency (Table 152-3). For PrEP, TDF/FTC should not be used if the estimated creatinine clearance is <60 mL/min. Tenofovir is not significantly metabolized by the liver; no dose adjustments of TDF are required in patients with hepatic insufficiency. TDF is pregnancy category B.

Adverse Reactions and Drug Interactions

In HIV-infected patients, the most common reported side effects with TDF were diarrhea, nausea, fatigue, headache, dizziness, depression, insomnia, abnormal dreams, and rash. TDF causes renal insufficiency and Fanconi's syndrome (proximal renal tubular dysfunction), characterized by hypophosphatemia, glycosuria, proteinuria and, ultimately, renal insufficiency. TDF decreases bone mineral density and increases markers of bone metabolism, although this appears to stabilize after a year of treatment. The newer prodrug tenofovir alafenamide (TAF), when compared to TDF at 48 weeks, resulted in a smaller decrease in glomerular filtration rate, lower levels of proteinuria, and less reduction in bone mineral density.[31]

Discontinuing tenofovir in a patient with hepatitis B co-infection can result in acute exacerbations of hepatitis B.

Tenofovir increases didanosine concentrations that can lead to toxicity such as pancreatitis and peripheral neuropathy; co-administration also was associated with decreases in CD4 cell counts. Co-administration of TDF and atazanavir increases tenofovir concentrations and decreases atazanavir concentrations, necessitating the use of ritonavir boosting of atazanavir. Co-administration of TDF with ritonavir-boosted atazanavir, darunavir or lopinavir also increases tenofovir concentrations. TDF should be avoided with concurrent or recent use of nephrotoxic medications.

Non-nucleoside Reverse Transcriptase Inhibitors (NNRTI)

Non-nucleoside reverse transcriptase inhibitors bind to a different part of the enzyme and thereby block the RNA-dependent DNA polymerase, reverse transcriptase, from synthesizing cDNA from viral RNA. These agents are non-competitive inhibitors that cause a conformational change in the reverse transcriptase enzyme and render it inactive (Figures 152-1 and 152-4).

NEVIRAPINE
Description

Nevirapine (NVP; Viramune; BI-RG-587) was approved in 1996 as the first-in-class HIV NNRTI. Some current guidelines consider nevirapine as an alternative first-line drug; others no longer recommend nevirapine because of toxicity (Table 152-2).

Pharmacokinetics and Distribution

Nevirapine reaches peak serum concentrations 4 hours after oral administration. Additionally, nevirapine crosses the placenta and enters breast milk. Nevirapine undergoes oxidative metabolism by the hepatic CYP3A and CYP2B6 isozymes. With a terminal half-life of 25–30 hours following multiple doses, 10% of drug is eliminated in feces and 83% in urine (primarily as metabolites).

Route of Administration and Dosage

The drug is available as 200 mg immediate-release tablet, 400 mg extended-release (XR) tablet, and 50 mg/5 mL oral suspension. For nevirapine, a 14-day lead-in period of 200 mg once-daily (with monitoring for adverse reactions) is recommended before increasing to standard adult dosing of 200 mg twice-daily or extended-release 400 mg daily, with or without food. The newer extended-release formulation of 400 mg once daily demonstrated noninferiority to standard nevirapine 200 mg twice daily.[38] Body surface area-based pediatric dosing is available for children 15 days of age and older. In resource-limited settings, generic co-formulations are available (Table 152-1).

Indications

Nevirapine is indicated in combination with other antiretrovirals for treatment of HIV infection in adults and pediatric patients 15 days of age and older. Initiation is not recommended for females whose CD4$^+$ cell count >250 cells/µL or males with CD4$^+$ cell count >400 cells/µL due to increased risk for severe hepatotoxicity. Nevirapine was approved on the basis of clinical trials demonstrating higher rates of virologic suppression in patients receiving nevirapine, lamivudine and background therapy when compared with placebo, lamivudine and background therapy. Studies demonstrated similar rates of virologic suppression in treatment-naïve patients when compared with efavirenz (although nevirapine was associated with higher rates of adverse events)[39] and atazanavir/ritonavir-based regimens.[40]

Resistance

Single amino acid substitutions in the reverse transcriptase gene are associated with high-level resistance to nevirapine and the signature mutation is Y181C/I. Other common mutations leading to high-level nevirapine resistance include K103N, L100I, Y188C/L/H or G190A (see Chapter 174).[10]

Dosage in Special Circumstances

No dose adjustment is required for renal impairment. Patients on hemodialysis should receive an additional 200 mg dose of nevirapine after dialysis. Patients with mild hepatic impairment should be monitored for toxicity; nevirapine is contraindicated in patients with moderate and severe hepatic impairment. Nevirapine is pregnancy category B.

Adverse Reactions and Drug Interactions

The most common systemic side effects during clinical trials were rash, nausea and headache. Rash was seen in about 17% of patients, with 7% of all patients requiring discontinuation of the drug; severe rash was more common in patients with CD4$^+$ count >200 cells/µL. The 14-day lead-in dosing decreases the incidence of rash. Severe life-threatening hepatotoxicity is seen with nevirapine treatment especially in the first 18 weeks of treatment, often associated with rash. Women and individuals with higher CD4$^+$ counts have increased risk of toxicity.

Nevirapine is an inducer of hepatic CYP3A enzymes and may decrease concentrations of other drugs metabolized by CYP3A (Table 152-5).

DELAVIRDINE

Delavirdine (DLV; Rescriptor; U-90152S) is an HIV NNRTI. Clinical use of delavirdine is rare due to suboptimal potency, high pill burden and three-times daily dosing.

EFAVIRENZ

Description

Efavirenz, (EFV; Stocrin; Sustiva; DMP-266) is an HIV NNRTI. Treatment guidelines recommend efavirenz as first-line or alternative therapy (Table 152-2).

Pharmacokinetics and Distribution

Efavirenz reaches peak serum concentration 5 hours after oral administration. Food increases the systemic exposure to efavirenz; however, higher exposure results in higher rates of adverse events and efavirenz should be taken when fasting. Efavirenz is principally metabolized by the hepatic CYP3A and CYP2B6 enzymes. Efavirenz demonstrates prolonged serum concentrations with a terminal half-life of 40–55 hours; 16–61% of drug is eliminated in feces (primarily as parent drug) and 14–34% in urine (primarily as metabolites).

Route of Administration and Dosage

Efavirenz is available as 600 mg tablets and 50 mg or 100 mg capsules. Standard adult dosage of efavirenz is 600 mg once daily taken when fasting, preferably at bedtime. Pediatric dosing for children 3 months of age and older is weight based. Co-formulations are available, including generics (Table 152-1).

Indications

Efavirenz is indicated in combination with other antiretrovirals for the treatment of HIV infection in adults and children at least 3 months old and weighing at least 3.5 kg. Efavirenz was first approved for treatment of HIV after an efavirenz-based regimen demonstrated superior rates of virologic suppression compared with the protease inhibitor (PI) indinavir in patients with no prior exposure to NNRTIs, PIs, or lamivudine.[41] In antiretroviral-naïve patients, an efavirenz-based regimen proved superior virologically to a lopinavir/ritonavir-based regimen at 96 weeks.[42] Efavirenz has been extensively studied in treatment-naïve patients and has consistently shown similar rates of virologic suppression to other agents, specifically when compared to other

TABLE 152-5	Common Cytochrome P450 CYP3A4 Substrates, Inhibitors and Inducers		
		Inhibitors	**Inducers**
Substrates		**Concomitant use may increase side effects or toxicity of substrate drugs**	**Concomitant use may decrease therapeutic benefit of substrate drugs**
Benzodiazepines (alprazolam, midazolam and triazolam)		Amiodarone	Carbamazepine
Calcium channel blockers (amlodipine, diltiazem, verapamil and others)		Clarithromycin	**Efavirenz**
Hypnotics (zolpidem and eszopiclone)		Cyclosporine	**Etravirine**
Miscellaneous (buspirone, trazadone, estradiol, progesterone, ziprasidone, cyclosporine, and warfarin)		Erythromycin	**Nevirapine**
		Fluconazole	Rilpivirine
Opioids (methadone, oxycodone, and buprenorphine)		Grapefruit juice	Phenytoin
PDE5 inhibitors (sildenafil, tadalafil and vardenafil)		Itraconazole	Pioglitazone
Protease inhibitors (HIV & HCV)		Ketoconazole	Rifabutin
Statins (lovastatin, simvastatin and atorvastatin)		**Ritonavir**	Rifampin
		Verapamil	St John's wort

commonly used first-line agents including atazanavir,[43,44] raltegravir,[45] and elvitegravir.[46] Recently approved dolutegravir in combination with abacavir/lamivudine had unprecedented significantly higher rates of virologic suppression when compared with efavirenz/tenofovir/emtricitabine at 48 weeks (88% versus 81%),[47] although rates of virologic failure were similar.

Resistance

Single amino acid substitutions in the reverse transcriptase gene are associated with high-level resistance to efavirenz.[10] The signature substitution for efavirenz resistance is K103N, which confers cross-resistance to nevirapine and delavirdine. Newer diarylpyrimidine NNRTIs (etravirine and rilpivirine) retain susceptibility to viral strains with K103N. Single substitutions at codons 100, 106, 108, 181, 188, 190, or 225 also confer resistance (see Chapter 174).

Dosage in Special Circumstances

No dose adjustment is required for patients with renal impairment. Standard dosing should be used with caution in patients with mild hepatic impairment; efavirenz is not recommended in patients with moderate-to-severe hepatic impairment. Efavirenz is pregnancy category D; first trimester exposure to efavirenz was associated with case reports of neural tube defects.

Adverse Reactions and Interactions

Neuropsychiatric side effects (dizziness, headache, insomnia, impaired concentration, abnormal dreams) are the most common adverse reactions seen with efavirenz occurring in up to 50% of individuals, though many resolve within weeks. Rash is seen in 10% of patients; however these were typically mild and resolved with time, with only 2% severe enough to require treatment discontinuation. Serious psychiatric adverse experiences have been associated with efavirenz use including depression, anxiety, and rarely suicidality.

Efavirenz induces hepatic CYP3A enzymes and may decrease concentrations of drugs metabolized through this pathway (Table 152-5). An efavirenz dose increase to 800 mg should be considered when co-administered with rifampin.

ETRAVIRINE

Description

Etravirine (ETV; Intelence; TMC125) is a diarylpyrimidine (DAPY) NNRTI, with activity against some viral strains resistant to first-generation NNRTIs and is recommended only for treatment-experienced patients.

Pharmacokinetics and Distribution

Etravirine reaches peak serum concentrations within 2.5–5 hours after oral administration. Fasting state decreases systemic exposure by about 50%, and etravirine should be taken with food. Etravirine is principally metabolized by the CYP3A, CYP2C9, and CYP2C19 hepatic enzymes. With a terminal half-life of 41 hours, 94% of drug is eliminated through feces (primarily as parent drug).

Route of Administration and Dosage

Etravirine is available in oral tablets of 200 mg, 100 mg and 25 mg. Standard dosage of etravirine for adults and children weighing >30 kg is 200 mg twice-daily with food. Although labeled for twice-daily dosing, pharmacokinetic studies support once-daily dosing.[48] Dosing for children 6 years of age and older is weight based.

Indications

Etravirine is indicated for the treatment of HIV in combination with other antiretroviral agents for treatment-experienced patients aged 6 years and older, who have evidence of HIV resistance. Etravirine was initially granted accelerated approval based on 24 week data of two phase 3 studies in NNRTI- and PI-experienced patients.[49,50] Patients received an optimized darunavir-containing regimen with or without etravirine; in both studies, significantly more patients in the etravirine arm achieved suppressed viremia.

Resistance

Second-generation NNRTI compounds (etravirine and rilpivirine) tolerate substitutions in amino acids surrounding the active site of reverse transcriptase, allowing antiretroviral activity against viral strains resistant to first-generation NNRTIs.[51] Etravirine is active against many strains resistant to efavirenz or nevirapine. Combinations of mutations confer high-level resistance including Y181C and V179F/I (see Chapter 174).

Dosage in Special Circumstances

No dose adjustment is required for patients with renal impairment. As etravirine is highly protein bound, it is unlikely to be removed during dialysis. No dose adjustment is required in patients with mild or moderate hepatic impairment although higher etravirine levels have been demonstrated; safety in severe hepatic impairment has not been studied. Safety and efficacy has been demonstrated in children 6 years of age or older. Etravirine is pregnancy category B.

Adverse Reactions and Drug Interactions

The most common moderate-to-severe side effects seen in clinical trials included rash (10%) and peripheral neuropathy (4%). Rash was the most common side effect leading to treatment discontinuation (2%), and severe rash including Stevens–Johnson syndrome was seen. Hepatotoxicity (AST or ALT $\geq$2.5 times upper limit of normal) was seen in >7% of patients, with toxicity 3–4 times more common in hepatitis B or C co-infected patients.

Etravirine is an inducer of hepatic CYP3A, CYP2C9, and CYP2C19 enzymes (Table 152-5). Etravirine should not be co-administered with other NNRTIs, atazanavir, tipranavir, fosamprenavir, carbamazepine, phenytoin, rifampin, rifapentine, or St John's wort.

RILPIVIRINE

Description

Rilpivirine, (RPV; Edurant; TMC278) is an HIV NNRTI, with activity against many viral strains resistant to first-generation NNRTIs. Industrialized world treatment guidelines recommend rilpivirine as initial or alternative therapy in patients whose baseline HIV RNA is <100 000 copies/mL (Table 152-2).

Pharmacokinetics and Distribution

Rilpivirine reaches peak concentrations 4–5 hours after oral administration. Food increases systemic exposure of rilpivirine; fasting and taking with only protein-rich nutritional drinks decreased exposure significantly. Rilpivirine undergoes oxidative metabolism by the hepatic CYP3A enzyme system. With a terminal half-life of 50 hours, 85% of drug is eliminated in feces (25% as unchanged rilpivirine) and 6.1% in urine (almost exclusively as metabolites).

Route of Administration and Dosage

Standard adult dosage of rilpivirine is 25 mg once daily taken orally with a meal. The drug is available alone as a 25 mg tablet, and in a combination tablet (Table 152-1). An investigational long-acting parenteral formulation using a nanoparticle solution allowing once-monthly dosing with sustained-release of rilpivirine is in clinical trials.

Indications

Rilpivirine is indicated in combination with other antiretrovirals for treatment-naïve adult patients for the treatment of HIV; rilpivirine is approved only for patients with a baseline HIV RNA level of less than or equal to 100 000 copies/mL. In antiretroviral-naïve patients, a rilpivirine-based regimen demonstrated noninferiority to an efavirenz-based regimen.[52,53] Although the overall rates of virologic failure were similar, in the subset of patients whose baseline viral load was >100 000 copies/mL more patients on rilpivirine developed virologic failure compared to efavirenz.[54] Independent of baseline viral load, in patients whose baseline CD4+ count was less than 200 cells/μL, significantly more patients experienced virologic failure with rilpivirine than efavirenz.

Resistance

Susceptibility to rilpivirine was not affected by the presence of single common NNRTI drug resistance-associated substitutions, such as at codons 103, 106, 179 and 190.[10] In patients who developed virologic failure on rilpivirine, 63% developed NNRTI resistance-associated substitutions and E138K was most common (see Chapter 174).[55]

Dosage in Special Circumstances

No dose adjustment is required for patients with renal failure; however, those with end-stage renal failure should be monitored closely for increased adverse effects.[56] As rilpivirine is highly protein bound, it is unlikely to be removed during dialysis. No dose adjustment is required in patients with mild or moderate hepatic impairment although higher rilpivirine levels have been demonstrated; the safety in severe hepatic impairment has not been studied. Effectiveness and safety of rilpivirine has not been established for the pediatric population, although trials are ongoing. Rilpivirine is pregnancy category B.

Adverse Reactions and Drug Interactions

The most common moderate-to-severe systemic side effects associated with rilpivirine in clinical trials included dizziness, abnormal dreams/ nightmares and rash; the rash was typically mild and self-limited.[56] Although the incidence of depression was similar to that seen with efavirenz, rates of neurologic adverse events were lower.[57] Rilpivirine has little effect on serum lipids. A dose-dependent prolongation of the QTc interval was seen, and caution should be used when co-administered with drugs known to prolong the QTc interval.

Rilpivirine is metabolized by the hepatic CYP3A enzyme system (Table 152-5). Drugs that decrease gastric pH may decrease rilpivirine plasma concentrations. Proton pump inhibitors are contraindicated, and H_2-receptor antagonists should be administered at least 12 hours before and at least 4 hours after rilpivirine.

Protease Inhibitors (PIs)

The protease enzyme of HIV is responsible for cleavage of the gag and gag-pol polyprotein into their essential structural components. PIs block this enzyme, preventing development of mature HIV virus (Figure 152-1).

SAQUINAVIR

Saquinavir (SQV; Invirase [hard gel]; Ro 31-8959) was approved in 1995 as the first HIV PI. Saquinavir requires pharmacokinetic boosting by co-administration with ritonavir for optimal effect. Approval for ritonavir-boosted saquinavir was based on a clinical study in a heterogeneous group of HIV-infected patients who were treatment naïve, HIV PI-experienced, or had failed a prior HIV PI who were randomized to receive a saquinavir/ritonavir- or indinavir/ritonavir-based regimen.[58] However, due to side effects, the need for twice-daily dosing, and the lack of comparative data with contemporary HIV PIs, saquinavir/ritonavir is not recommended in current treatment guidelines (Table 152-2).

RITONAVIR

Ritonavir (RTV; Norvir; formerly ABT-538) was approved in 1996 as the second HIV PI at a dose of 600 mg twice daily on the basis of a demonstrated survival benefit;[59] today the drug is used exclusively as a pharmacokinetic booster at lower doses (100 mg once or twice daily). Ritonavir is one of the most potent inhibitors of CYP3A4 ever described and consequently, increases the concentrations of a number of other HIV PIs allowing lower doses and less frequent dosing intervals, and has numerous important drug-drug interactions (Table 152-5).

INDINAVIR

Indinavir (IDV; Crixivan; formerly MK 735,524) was approved in 1996 as the third HIV PI. Indinavir was a key component of early three-drug HIV therapy studies that first established the potency of highly active antiretroviral therapy,[8,60] however, because of side effects, particularly gastrointestinal and nephrolithiasis, and the need for three-times daily dosing or ritonavir boosting, this drug is rarely used today.

NELFINAVIR

Nelfinavir (NFV; Viracept; AG1343) is an HIV PI that was approved in 1997.[61] Although widely used in the late 1990s and the only HIV PI not requiring ritonavir boosting, this drug is rarely used today because of side effects, particularly diarrhea in at least 15–20% of patients.

LOPINAVIR/RITONAVIR

Description

Lopinavir (LPV; Kaletra; ABT 378) is part of a fixed-dose combination of two HIV PIs: lopinavir has an antiviral effect, and low-dose ritonavir acts as a potent CYP3A4 inhibitor, thereby increasing lopinavir concentrations. The drug was the first fixed-dose combination of HIV PI. Lopinavir/ritonavir is considered second-line therapy in the WHO guidelines and alternative therapy in industrialized world guidelines due to toxicity (Table 152-2).

Pharmacokinetics and Distribution

Peak plasma concentrations of lopinavir occur 4 hours after dosing and steady-state concentrations occur within 10–16 days. At steady state, 98% of lopinavir is bound to plasma proteins. Administration of lopinavir/ritonavir 400/100 mg twice-daily yields mean steady-state lopinavir plasma concentrations 15- to 20-fold higher than those of lopinavir monotherapy in HIV-infected patients. Lopinavir is metabolized primarily by oxidative hepatic metabolism resulting in at least 13 metabolites. At steady state, most lopinavir is eliminated in feces, with less than 3% eliminated in urine.

Route of Administration and Dosage

Lopinavir/ritonavir is available in three dosage forms: lopinavir 200 mg/ritonavir 50 mg co-formulated tablets; lopinavir 100 mg/ ritonavir 25 mg co-formulated tablets; and lopinavir 400 mg/ritonavir 100 mg per 10 mL oral solution. Lopinavir/ritonavir tablets may be taken with or without food; the oral solution must be taken with food. Adult dosage is lopinavir/ritonavir 400 mg/100 mg twice daily or lopinavir/ritonavir 800 mg/200 mg once daily. Twice-daily lopinavir/ ritonavir dosing should be used with three or more baseline lopinavir-associated drug resistance substitutions or when used with efavirenz, nevirapine, nelfinavir, carbamazepine, phenobarbital, or phenytoin. Pediatric dosing is weight based.

Indication

Lopinavir/ritonavir is an HIV PI indicated in combination with other antiretroviral agents for the treatment of HIV infection in adults and pediatric patients (14 days and older). Approval was based on large studies, including a head-to-head comparison in treatment-naïve individuals of two nucleosides with either lopinavir/ritonavir or nelfinavir where lopinavir proved virologically superior and well tolerated[62] and a study in treatment-experienced patients where lopinavir/ ritonavir outperformed an investigator-selected PI. In combination with two nucleosides, once-daily lopinavir/ritonavir was noninferior virologically to standard twice-daily dosing.[63] A three-drug combination of two nucleosides and lopinavir/ritonavir provided durable efficacy through 7 years, the longest published study of combination antiretroviral therapy.[64] More recent comparative studies find newer ritonavir-boosted PI (atazanavir, darunavir) to be better tolerated than lopinavir/ritonavir.[65,66]

Resistance

Lopinavir/ritonavir has a high barrier to resistance and multiple substitutions in HIV protease are required to confer drug resistance; specifically, three or more of the following substitutions in HIV protease:

L10F/I/R/V, K20M/N/R, L24I, L33F, M36I, I47V, G48V, I54L/T/V, V82A/C/F/S/T, and I84V.[10] Lopinavir/ritonavir demonstrates virologic activity in patients experiencing virologic failure on older PI-based regimens (see Chapter 174).

Dosage in Special Circumstances

Renal clearance of lopinavir/ritonavir is minimal; no dose adjustment is required for renal insufficiency. Because lopinavir/ritonavir is principally metabolized by the liver, a 20–30% increase in lopinavir concentrations in patients with mild-moderate hepatic impairment and decreased plasma protein binding occurs. Lopinavir/ritonavir has not been studied in patients with severe hepatic impairment. Lopinavir/ritonavir is pregnancy category C.

Adverse Reactions and Drug Interactions

The most common side effects associated with lopinavir/ritonavir are gastrointestinal. Diarrhea occurs in up to 50% of patients taking once-daily lopinavir/ritonavir, and about 20% have moderate or higher grade symptoms. Lopinavir/ritonavir also is associated with nausea, with about 10% experiencing moderate or greater grade symptoms and vomiting with about 7% experiencing moderate or greater grade symptoms, particularly initially after starting therapy. Lopinavir/ritonavir also associated with hypertriglyceridemia and hypercholesterolemia. Life-threatening hepatotoxicity has occurred, particularly in patients with underlying liver disease.

Lopinavir/ritonavir is contraindicated with drugs that are potent inducers of, or depend upon CYP3A for clearance (Table 152-5). Concomitant lopinavir/ritonavir and glucocorticoids can reduce lopinavir and increase glucocorticoid levels, including inhaled or intranasal steroids (e.g. fluticasone), resulting in clinical Cushing's syndrome.

AMPRENAVIR AND FOSAMPRENAVIR

Fosamprenavir (FPV; Telzir; Lexiva; GW433908) is a PI that is a prodrug of the previously approved HIV PI, amprenavir. Amprenavir was withdrawn from the market in 2004. Current treatment guidelines no longer recommend fosamprenavir due to high pill count (Table 152-2).

ATAZANAVIR

Description

Atazanavir (ATV; Reyataz; BMS-232632) is an azapeptide HIV PI with favorable pharmacokinetics allowing for once-daily dosing. Current industrialized world guidelines recommend atazanavir as first-line or alternative therapy (Table 152-2).

Pharmacokinetics and Distribution

Atazanavir reaches peak serum concentration 2.5 hours after oral administration. Food enhances systemic exposure to atazanavir, and administration is recommended with food. Atazanavir undergoes metabolism by the hepatic CYP3A enzymes and has a terminal half-life of 7 hours when administered alone, or 12 hours when co-administered with ritonavir. The drug is eliminated in feces (79% – primarily as metabolites) and in urine (13% – primarily as metabolites).

Route of Administration and Dosage

Atazanavir is available in capsules of 150 mg, 200 mg, and 300 mg, and is co-formulated with cobicistat. Standard adult dosage of atazanavir is 300 mg with ritonavir 100 mg once daily with food. In treatment-naïve patients unboosted atazanavir 400 mg once daily with food is an uncommonly used alternative. Dosing for children 6 years of age and older is weight based.

Indications

Atazanavir is indicated in combination for the treatment of HIV in adults and children 6 years of age or older. Initial studies of atazanavir-based regimens in treatment-naïve patients demonstrated noninferiority to nelfinavir-[67] and efavirenz-based[68] regimens. In an open-labeled,

randomized trial, an atazanavir/ritonavir-based regimen was noninferior to a lopinavir/ritonavir-based regimen, with fewer gastrointestinal side effects, although higher rates of elevated total bilirubin were seen with atazanavir. A large randomized study demonstrated similar virologic outcomes for treatment-naïve patients started on atazanavir/ritonavir-based regimens compared to efavirenz-based regimens. Most recently a large comparative study demonstrated comparable week 96 virologic responses with atazanavir-, darunavir-, and raltegravir-based regimens; however atazanavir had higher rates of treatment discontinuation largely due to hyperbilirubinemia and gastrointestinal intolerance.[69]

Resistance

Protease substitutions are uncommonly selected with virologic failure to atazanavir-based regimens. Accumulation of protease substitutions is typically required to lead to high-level resistance to atazanavir.[70] The three major protease substitutions contributing to resistance to atazanavir are I50L, I84V and N88S.[10] I50L is a signature mutation for unboosted atazanavir and does not confer cross-resistance to other PIs (see Chapter 174).

Dosage in Special Circumstances

No dose adjustment is required in patients with renal impairment. Lower serum concentrations were seen with patients on hemodialysis; treatment-naïve patients with end-stage renal disease on hemodialysis should receive standard-dose atazanavir and ritonavir, while atazanavir should be avoided in treatment-experienced patients on hemodialysis. Combined atazanavir/ritonavir is not recommended in patients with hepatic impairment, and unboosted atazanavir should be avoided in severe liver impairment. Atazanavir is safe and effective in children 6 years of age and older. Atazanavir is pregnancy class B.

Adverse Reactions and Drug Interactions

Elevation of total bilirubin (≥2.6 × normal) was seen in 34% of patients, with associated jaundice in 4%. This elevation in indirect bilirubin is related to the inhibition of UGT1A1 and is not associated with other hepatic abnormalities. The most common moderate-to-severe systemic side effects seen in clinical trials included headache and diarrhea.[71] Fewer metabolic complications were seen with atazanavir especially when compared to lopinavir, while nephrolithiasis has been reported.

Atazanavir is contraindicated with drugs that are potent inducers of, or depend upon, CYP3A for clearance (Table 152-5).

TIPRANAVIR

Tipranavir (TPV; Aptivus; PNU-140690) is a nonpeptidic HIV PI with activity against viral strains with resistance to older HIV PIs. Tipranavir is only recommended for treatment-experienced patients with resistance to one or more HIV PI. Tipranavir is used rarely because of gastrointestinal intolerance, hepatic toxicity in up to 20% of patients and the requirement for administration with food.

DARUNAVIR

Description

Darunavir (DRV; Prezista; TMC114) is a potent nonpeptidic PI with activity against PI-resistant viral strains. Darunavir/ritonavir-based regimens are recommended as first-line treatment in many industrialized world guidelines (Table 152-2).

Pharmacokinetics and Distribution

Darunavir reaches peak serum concentrations 2.5–4 hours after oral administration. Food increases systemic exposure to darunavir by 40%, and darunavir should be taken with food. Darunavir primarily undergoes oxidative metabolism by the hepatic CYP3A enzyme system. With a half-life of 15 hours when co-administered with ritonavir, 80% of drug is eliminated in feces (41% as unchanged darunavir) and 14% in urine (mostly as metabolites).

Route of Administration and Dosage

Darunavir oral solution (100 mg/mL), tablets of 75 mg, 150 mg, 400 mg, 600 mg, or 800 mg, and a co-formulation with cobicistat are available. Standard adult dosage of darunavir for treatment-naïve and treatment-experienced patients with no darunavir resistance-associated mutations is 800 mg with ritonavir 100 mg once daily with food. For treatment-experienced patients with at least one darunavir resistance-associated mutation, 600 mg with ritonavir 100 mg, both twice daily with food. Pediatric dosing is weight based, taken with ritonavir and food, for children of at least 3 years of age.

Indications

Darunavir, co-administered with ritonavir, is indicated in combination with other antiretrovirals for the treatment of HIV infection. In an open-label, randomized trial in treatment-naïve patients, a darunavir/ritonavir-regimen was noninferior virologically to lopinavir/ritonavir and better tolerated.[72] More patients with baseline HIV RNA levels >100 000 suppressed viremia in the darunavir/ritonavir arm than the lopinavir/ritonavir arm. In treatment-experienced patients receiving optimized therapy, darunavir/ritonavir demonstrated significantly higher rates of virologic suppression versus an investigator-selected PI.[73]

Resistance

No single PI mutation leads to complete loss of darunavir activity, and multiple cumulative mutations are needed to convey resistance. The most common protease enzyme substitutions are L33F, V32I and I54L, while others that result in reduced activity include V11I, I47V, I50V, I54M, T74P, L76V, I84V and L89V (see Chapter 174).[10]

Dosage in Special Circumstances

No dose adjustment is required for patients with mild-to-moderate renal failure; however, safety in severe renal failure has not been studied. As darunavir is highly protein bound, it is unlikely to be removed during dialysis. No dose adjustment is required in patients with mild or moderate hepatic impairment; darunavir is not recommended for patients with severe hepatic impairment. Darunavir is pregnancy category C.

Adverse Reactions and Drug Interactions

The most common moderate-to-severe adverse events seen in clinical trials were diarrhea, rash and nausea. Patients with underlying liver dysfunction, hepatitis B or C infection have an increased risk of liver function abnormalities. Severe rashes including Stevens–Johnson syndrome have been reported but occurred in <0.1%.[74]

Darunavir is contraindicated with drugs that are potent inducers of, or depend upon CYP3A for clearance (Table 152-5).

Entry Inhibitors (EI)

For HIV entry into a cell, the virus external membrane glycoprotein (gp120) attaches to the cellular CD4+ receptor causing a conformational change to the gp120 allowing it to bind to second cellular co-receptor (CCR5 or CXCR4). The CD4+ cell is then penetrated by a viral internal membrane glycoprotein, gp41, followed by membrane fusion as the heptad repeat regions of the gp41 fold over on themselves bringing together the cellular and viral membranes and allowing for the entry of the viral core into the cell. Enfuvirtide and maraviroc interrupt viral entry through distinct mechanisms (Figure 152-1).

ENFUVIRTIDE

Description

Enfuvirtide (ENF; Fuzeon; T-20) is a 36-amino-acid synthetic peptide that mimics the heptad repeat region-2 (HR2) of the HIV-1 envelope glycoprotein 41 (gp41), interfering with HR1-HR2 association, and preventing fusion of the viral and cellular membranes. As a twice-daily parenteral drug, enfuvirtide is used uncommonly.

Pharmacokinetics and Distribution

Enfuvirtide reaches peak serum concentration 8 hours after subcutaneous injection. With a half-life of approximately 4 hours, enfuvirtide, as a peptide, undergoes catabolism to its component amino acids.

Route of Administration and Dosage

Enfuvirtide is formulated as a lyophilized powder with 108 mg per single-dose vial to constitute a solution for injection, with no oral formulation available. Standard adult dosage of enfuvirtide is 90 mg every 12 hours by subcutaneous injection to the upper arm, anterior thigh, or abdomen with each injection given at a different site from the preceding injection. Pediatric dosing is weight based for children 6 years of age or older.

Indications

Enfuvirtide is indicated in combination with other antiretroviral agents for treatment-experienced HIV-infected patients with persistent viremia. This indication is based on two phase 3 randomized, controlled, open-label trials of optimized-background regimen with or without enfuvirtide in treatment-experienced patients where enfuvirtide was associated with improved virologic suppression rates.[75,76]

Resistance

Treatment-experienced patients who have continued viremia on enfuvirtide commonly develop mutations in the HR1 region of the gp41 gene at codons 36, 37, 38, 39, 40, 42, or 43, conferring high-level resistance.[10] Given its unique mechanism of action, enfuvirtide shares no cross-resistance with other classes of antiretrovirals.

Dosage in Special Circumstances

No dose adjustment is required in patients with renal or hepatic impairment. Safety and efficacy has been established in children 6 years of age and older. Enfuvirtide is pregnancy category B.

Adverse Reactions and Drug Interactions

The most common adverse reactions are injection site reactions (including pain, induration, erythema and subcutaneous nodules) that are seen in 98% of patients. Hypersensitivity reaction has also been reported. Initial clinical trial data demonstrated a significant increased frequency of bacterial pneumonia in patients receiving enfuvirtide compared to control for unclear reasons; a retrospective cohort trial did not confirm this association.[77] Enfuvirtide has no significant drug interactions.

MARAVIROC

Description

Maraviroc (MVC; Selzentry; Celsentri; UK-427,527) is the first-in-class CCR5 antagonist antiretroviral and the only approved antiretroviral drug that targets the host (CCR5 cellular receptor), rather than HIV itself. Maraviroc is active only against R5 virus. Current US treatment guidelines do not recommend maraviroc as initial therapy (Table 152-2) and it is used uncommonly.

Pharmacokinetics and Distribution

Maraviroc is rapidly absorbed following oral administration, reaches peak concentrations 1.6 hours after dosing, and achieves steady state by 7 days. Maraviroc does not affect cell surface levels of CCR5 or intracellular signaling. The drug is 76% protein bound and the terminal half-life is 14–18 hours. Maraviroc is metabolized by oxidation and N-dealkylation. Maraviroc and its metabolites are eliminated 76% in feces, 20% in urine.

Route of Administration and Dosage

Maraviroc is available as 150 and 300 mg tablets. The standard dose of maraviroc is 300 mg twice daily by mouth with or without food. This dose needs to be adjusted when maraviroc is co-administered with drugs that potently induce CYP3A4 (increased to 600 mg twice daily) or drugs that potently inhibit CYP3A4 (decreased to 150 mg twice daily).

Indications

Maraviroc, in combination with other antiretroviral agents, is indicated for adult patients infected with only CCR5-tropic (R5) HIV. Patients who are candidates for maraviroc must have their cellular tropism determined (R5 versus X4 versus dual/mixed R5/X4) with a tropism assay (phenotypic or genotypic). The drug is indicated for the treatment of HIV infection on the basis of results from two large phase 3 studies demonstrating improved virologic outcomes of HIV-infected, treatment-experienced patients who were randomized to receive an optimized-background antiretroviral drug regimen with or without maraviroc.[78] Maraviroc had no effect in patients infected with X4 or dual/mixed R5/X4 HIV.[79] A study in treatment-naïve patients found that a twice-daily maraviroc-based regimen was noninferior to an efavirenz-based regimen although maraviroc patients experienced more virologic failure and drug resistance; a once-daily maraviroc arm was discontinued early, but subsequent analyses demonstrated that 15% of the enrolled patients had R5/X4 virus and would not have been expected to respond.[80]

Resistance

Resistance to maraviroc most frequently occurs as a result of incomplete virologic suppression with emergence of pre-existing X4 virus.[81] Drug-resistant virus acquires the ability to bind to the CCR5-maraviroc complex to gain entry into the cell.[82] Discontinuing maraviroc most often results in the re-emergence of R5 virus.

Dosage in Special Circumstances

No dose adjustment is required for patients with mild-to-moderate renal impairment. Maraviroc should not be used in patients with severe renal impairment (CrCl <30 mL/min) who are taking potent CYP3A4 inducers or inhibitors. Maraviroc should be used with caution in patients with hepatic impairment or hepatitis B or C co-infection. No dose adjustment is required for patients with mild-to-moderate hepatic impairment; maraviroc should not be used in patients with severe hepatic impairment. Use of maraviroc in pediatric patients is limited; clinical trials are in progress. Maraviroc is pregnancy category B.

Adverse Reactions and Drug Interactions

Maraviroc prescribing information includes a boxed warning for hepatotoxicity, although a review of clinical trials data failed to associate maraviroc with a risk of hepatotoxicity.[83] Postural hypotension can occur with higher doses of maraviroc (600 mg twice daily and above) and in some patients with severe renal impairment taking CYP3A4 inhibitors or inducers with higher maraviroc concentrations.

Maraviroc is a substrate for CYP3A4 and the efflux transporter P-glycoprotein. Potent CYP3A4 inhibitors, including HIV PIs (with the exception of ritonavir-boosted tipranavir) and ketoconazole, increase maraviroc concentrations. Maraviroc concentrations were significantly reduced by CYP3A4 inducers such as rifampin (by 70%) and efavirenz (by 50%); increasing the maraviroc dose compensates for this reduction. A regimen with maraviroc, a ritonavir-boosted PI, and efavirenz reduced the magnitude of PI-mediated increase in maraviroc exposure by 50%; the overall effect was CYP3A4 inhibition.

Integrase Strand Transfer Inhibitors (INSTI)

HIV integrase catalyzes the random integration of cDNA into the host cellular genome. INSTIs block the integration of viral DNA into host DNA and subsequently inhibit viral replication (Figure 152-1).

RALTEGRAVIR

Description

Raltegravir (RAL; Isentress; MK-0518) is the first-in-class integrase strand transfer inhibitor (INSTI) with *in vitro* activity against HIV-1, approved in 2007. Raltegravir is a recommended first-line drug in industrialized world treatment guidelines (Table 152-2).

Pharmacokinetics and Distribution

Raltegravir reaches peak serum concentrations 3 hours after oral administration. Chewable tablets and oral solution formulations of raltegravir have higher oral bioavailability than film-coated tablets in adults. Raltegravir is predominately metabolized though uridine diphosphate-glucuronosyltransferase (UGT)-mediated glucuronidation in the liver, and is not a substrate for the cytochrome P450 system. With a terminal half-life of 9 hours, 51% of drug is eliminated in feces (mostly parent drug) and 32% in urine.

Route of Administration and Dosage

Raltegravir is available in 400 mg film-coated tablets, 100 mg or 25 mg chewable tablets, and an oral suspension (100 mg/5 mL). Standard dosage of raltegravir for adults and children weighing >25 kg is 400 mg twice-daily taken with or without food. Once-daily dosing of raltegravir was shown to be inferior to twice-daily dosing.[84] Pediatric dosing for children aged 4 weeks and >3 kg is weight based. Dosage recommendations for chewable tablets differ from film-coated tablets, and dose adjustment is required when switching between these two formulations.

Indications

Raltegravir is indicated in combination with other antiretroviral agents in the treatment of HIV in adults and children >4 weeks of age. In antiretroviral-naïve patients, a raltegravir-based regimen demonstrated noninferiority virologically to an efavirenz-based regimen and was better tolerated.[85] Five-year follow-up showed a significantly higher proportion with virologic suppression in the raltegravir arm than the efavirenz arm.[86] In treatment-experienced patients, raltegravir demonstrated superiority to placebo when combined with optimized-background therapy in patients with detectable viremia and documented resistance to at least one drug in each of three classes of antiretroviral agents (NRTI, NNRTI and PI). In a head-to-head comparative study in treatment-naïve participants, a raltegravir-based regimen was superior to either an atazanavir- or darunavir-based regimen.[69]

Resistance

Single mutations in the integrase gene are sufficient to confer high-level resistance to raltegravir; typically more than one mutation is present at the time of virologic failure. Three primary genetic pathway mutations lead to virologic failure, N155H, Q148H/K/R, and Y143C/H/R.[10] Substitution at either Q148 or N155 confer high-level resistance to elvitegravir, while Q148R/H substitutions confer high level resistance to elvitegravir and dolutegravir (see Chapter 174).

Dosage in Special Circumstances

No dose adjustment is required for patients with renal impairment. No dose adjustment is required in patients with mild or moderate hepatic impairment; safety in severe hepatic impairment has not been studied. Safety and efficacy has been established for children 4 weeks of age and older. Raltegravir is pregnancy category C.

Adverse Reactions and Drug Interactions

Side effects to raltegravir are uncommon. Rarely, severe, potentially life-threatening rashes (including Stevens–Johnson syndrome and toxic epidermal necrolysis), have been reported. Phase 2 studies demonstrated 6% of patients with grade 3–4 elevations of CPK,[87] and cases of rhabdomyolysis have been reported.

Raltegravir has few drug interactions. Rifampin decreases raltegravir levels, and dose increase of raltegravir to 800 mg twice daily is recommended.

ELVITEGRAVIR

Description

Elvitegravir (EVG; GS-9137; JTK-303) is an INSTI. In combination with cobicistat (a CYP3A4 inhibitor), it was the first approved once-daily INSTI. The co-formulation, elvitegravir/cobicistat/emtricitabine/tenofovir, is a recommended first-line regimen in industrialized world guidelines (Table 152-2).

Pharmacokinetics and Distribution

Pharmacokinetics of elvitegravir are enhanced when co-administered with inhibitors of CYP3A4. Studies demonstrated ritonavir 100 mg and cobicistat 150 mg similarly enhanced elvitegravir concentrations.[88] Boosted elvitegravir reaches peak serum concentrations approximately 4 hours after oral administration. Food increases systemic exposure, and elvitegravir should be taken with food. Elvitegravir is primarily metabolized by CYP3A enzymes in addition to undergoing glucuronidation via UGT1A1/3 enzymes. Elvitegravir has a terminal half-life of 13 hours when co-administered with cobicistat; elimination is primarily in feces.

Route of Administration and Dosage

Elvitegravir is available alone as 85 mg and 150 mg tablets and co-formulated as the once-daily combination tablet of 300 mg of TDF, 200 mg of emtricitabine, 150 mg of elvitegravir and 150 mg of cobicistat. Standard adult dosing of elvitegravir is one co-formulated pill, once daily.

Indications

Elvitegravir in a fixed-dose combination with cobicistat, emtricitabine, and TDF is indicated for the treatment of HIV-1 infection in antiretroviral-naïve adults. In a phase 3 trial elvitegravir was found noninferior virologically to efavirenz in antiretroviral-naïve patients.[46] A second phase 3 trial comparing an elvitegravir-based regimen to an atazanavir-based regimen in antiretroviral-naïve patients demonstrated similar rates of virologic suppression.[89] In treatment-experienced patients with resistance to at least two antiretroviral classes, elvitegravir was comparable to raltegravir.

Resistance

Single mutations in the integrase gene are sufficient to confer high-level resistance, although typically mutations are seen in combination. Reduced susceptibility to elvitegravir was associated with T66A/I, E92G/Q, S147G, or Q148R.[10] Mutations at codons T66, E92 and S147 do not confer resistance to other integrase inhibitors; however, Q148 confers cross-resistance to raltegravir and dolutegravir and N155 to raltegravir (see Chapter 174).

Dosage in Special Circumstances

Elvitegravir-cobicistat administered to healthy subjects with severe renal impairment showed no clinically significant difference in pharmacokinetics of either drug. However, the fixed-dose combination of elvitegravir/cobicistat/emtricitabine/tenofovir should not be started in patients whose baseline creatinine clearance is <70 mL/min, and should be discontinued if creatinine clearance falls below 50 mL/min while on treatment, due to the co-formulated nucleoside analogs. No dose adjustment is required in patients with mild-to-moderate hepatic impairment, while the safety in severe hepatic impairment has not been studied. Effectiveness and safety of elvitegravir has not been established for the pediatric population, although studies are ongoing. Elvitegravir is pregnancy category B.

Adverse Reactions and Interactions

The most common moderate-to-severe side effects seen in clinical trials in patients receiving co-formulated tenofovir/emtricitabine/elvitegravir/cobicistat were nausea, diarrhea and abnormal dreams.

Elvitegravir is dependent on CYP 3A4 for clearance, and drugs that induce, inhibit, or are metabolized by this system may affect plasma concentrations (Table 152-5).

DOLUTEGRAVIR

Description

Dolutegravir (DTG; Tivicay; Shionogi/GSK 572] is an INSTI with activity against HIV, and the first approved with once-daily dosing without pharmacologic boosting. Current treatment guidelines recommend dolutegravir-based regimens for initial therapy (Table 152-2).

PHARMACOKINETICS AND DISTRIBUTION

Dolutegravir reaches peak serum concentration 2–3 hours after oral administration.

Dolutegravir is primarily metabolized via glucuronidation by UGT1A1 in addition to CYP3A. With a terminal half-life of 14 hours, 53% of drug is eliminated in feces (primarily as parent drug), with 31% in urine (primarily as metabolites).

Route of Administration and Dosage

Dolutegravir is available alone as a 50 mg tablet and as part of a co-formulated tablet with abacavir/lamivudine (Table 152-1). For treatment-naïve adults and children >12 years of age, the standard dosage of dolutegravir is 50 mg once-daily taken orally with or without food. Higher doses (50 mg twice-daily) are recommended when co-administered with potent UGT1A/CYP3A inducers: efavirenz, fosamprenavir/ritonavir, tipranavir/ritonavir, or rifampin or with INSTI resistance.

Indications

Dolutegravir is indicated in combination with other antiretroviral agents for the treatment of HIV in adults and children 12 years and older weighing at least 40 kg. In antiretroviral-naïve patients, dolutegravir with two nucleosides was shown to have significantly higher rates of virologic suppression, compared to efavirenz/tenofovir/emtricitabine,[27] due to higher rates of treatment discontinuation in the efavirenz arm. Other phase 3 trials found dolutegravir was noninferior to raltegravir,[90] and superior to once-daily darunavir plus ritonavir.[91]

In treatment-experienced patients without prior integrase inhibitor resistance, dolutegravir resulted in higher rates of virologic suppression compared with raltegravir.[92] Dolutegravir also demonstrated effectiveness in suppressing viremia in patients with underlying raltegravir resistance.[93]

Resistance

Structural analysis suggests that dolutegravir establishes closer contact with viral DNA than raltegravir or elvitegravir, and has the ability to slightly adjust its position in response to active site changes conferred by raltegravir or elvitegravir resistance. This flexibility is thought to contribute to a higher barrier for dolutegravir resistance compared to raltegravir and elvitegravir. In treatment-experienced patients, mutations seen in dolutegravir-resistant virus were L74I/M, E92E/Q, Q95L/Q/R, T97A, G140A/S, Y143C/R, Q148H/R, V151I/V, N155H, E157E/Q, G163G/R, and R263K.[10] Dolutegravir remains active against raltegravir- or elvitegravir-resistant N155H and Y143C/K virus; however, dolutegravir has decreased activity against Q148 virus, especially when this mutation is seen in the setting of additional mutations (specifically at codons E138, G140, E92, or T97) (see Chapter 174).

Dosage in Special Circumstances

No dose adjustment is required for patients with renal insufficiency; however, those with severe renal failure have decreased dolutegravir concentrations and should be monitored closely. No dose adjustment is required for patients with mild or moderate hepatic impairment; dolutegravir has not been studied in patients with severe liver disease. Dolutegravir is pregnancy category B.

Adverse Reactions and Drug Interactions

Side effects to dolutegravir are uncommon. Dolutegravir inhibits renal tubular secretion through the OCT2 transporter, which is responsible for creatinine excretion. At 48 weeks dolutegravir resulted in a significant creatinine increase of 0.11 mg/dL (occurring mostly in the first 4 weeks),[27] without affecting glomerular function. Drugs whose primarily route of elimination are through the OCT2 transporter system may have increased plasma concentrations when co-administered with dolutegravir, specifically the antiarrhythmic dofetilide is contraindicated. Strong inducers of CYP3A4 results in decreased concentrations of dolutegravir; dolutegravir should be taken at least 2 hours before or at least 6 hours after taking cation-containing antacids or laxatives, sucralfate, oral iron supplements, oral calcium supplements, or buffered medications.

References available online at expertconsult.com.

KEY REFERENCES

Cameron D.W., Heath-Chiozzi M., Danner S., et al.: Randomised placebo-controlled trial of ritonavir in advanced HIV-1 disease. *Lancet* 1998; 351:543-549.

Connor E.M., Sperling R.S., Gelber R., et al.: Reduction of maternal-infant transmission of human immunodeficiency virus type 1 with zidovudine treatment. *N Engl J Med* 1994; 331:1173-1180.

Fischl M.A., Richman D.D., Grieco M.H., et al.: The efficacy of azidothymidine (AZT) in the treatment of patients with AIDS and AIDS-related complex; a double-blind placebo controlled trial. *N Engl J Med* 1987; 317:185-191.

Gallant J.E., DeJesus E., Arribas J.R., et al.: Tenofovir DF, emtricitabine, and efavirenz vs. zidovudine, lamivudine, and efavirenz for HIV. *N Engl J Med* 2006; 354:251-260.

Gulick R.M., Mellors J.W., Havlir D., et al.: Treatment with indinavir, zidovudine, and lamivudine in adults with human immunodeficiency virus infection and prior antiretroviral therapy. *N Engl J Med* 1997; 337:734-739.

Hammer S.M., Katzenstein D.A., Hughes M.D., et al.: A Trial Comparing Nucleoside Monotherapy with Combination Therapy in HIV-Infected Adults with CD4 Cell Counts from 200 to 500 Cubic Millimeter. *N Engl J Med* 1996; 335:1081-1090.

Hammer S.M., Squires K.E., Hughes M.D., et al.: A controlled trial of two nucleoside analogues plus indinavir in persons with human immunodeficiency virus infection and CD4 cell counts of 200 per cubic millimeter or less. *N Engl J Med* 1997; 337:725-733.

Hirsch M.S., Günthard H.F., Schapiro J.M., et al.: Antiretroviral drug resistance testing in adult HIV-1 infection: 2008 recommendations of an International AIDS Society-USA panel. *Clin Infect Dis* 2008; 47:266-285.

Lennox J.L., Landovitz R.J., Ribaudo H.J., et al.: Efficacy and tolerability of 3 nonnucleoside reverse transcriptase inhibitor-sparing antiretroviral regimens for treatment-naive volunteers infected with HIV-1: a randomized, controlled equivalence trial. *Ann Intern Med* 2014; 161:461-471.

Staszewski S., Morales-Ramirez J., Tashima K., et al.: Efavirenz plus zidovudine and lamivudine, efavirenz plus indinavir, and indinavir plus zidovudine and lamivudine in the treatment of HIV-1 infection in adults. *N Engl J Med* 1999; 341:1865-1873.

Walmsley S., Antela A., Clumeck N., et al.: Dolutegravir plus Abacavir-Lamivudine for the Treatment of HIV-1 Infection. *N Engl J Med* 2013; 369:1907-1918.

153

Drugs for Herpesvirus Infections

MICHELLE R. SALVAGGIO | JOHN W. GNANN, JR.

Drugs for Treatment of HSV and VZV Infections

ACICLOVIR AND VALACICLOVIR

Mechanism of Action and In Vitro Activity

Aciclovir, an acyclic analog of guanosine, is a selective inhibitor of the replication of herpes simplex virus (HSV) types 1 and 2 and varicella-zoster virus (VZV).[1] Valaciclovir is an orally-administered prodrug of aciclovir with improved pharmacokinetic properties. Aciclovir is converted to its monophosphate derivative by virus-encoded thymidine kinase (TK), a reaction that does not occur to any significant extent in uninfected cells (Figure 153-1). Subsequent diphosphorylation and triphosphorylation steps are catalyzed by cellular kinases, producing high concentrations of aciclovir triphosphate within HSV- or VZV-infected cells. Aciclovir triphosphate inhibits viral DNA synthesis by competing with deoxyguanosine triphosphate as a substrate for viral DNA polymerase. As aciclovir triphosphate lacks the 3'-hydroxyl group required for further DNA chain elongation, incorporation into viral DNA results in obligate chain termination. Viral DNA polymerase has much higher affinity for aciclovir triphosphate than does cellular DNA polymerase, resulting in little incorporation of aciclovir into cellular DNA. Aciclovir exhibits good *in vitro* activity against HSV-1, HSV-2 and VZV, with median inhibitory concentrations (IC_{50}) of 0.04, 0.10 and 0.50 μg/mL, respectively. Human cytomegalovirus (CMV) is not inhibited by aciclovir at clinically achievable concentrations.

Pharmacokinetics and Distribution

Following oral administration, aciclovir is slowly and incompletely absorbed, with bioavailability of about 15–30%. After oral doses of 200 mg or 800 mg of aciclovir, mean plasma peak concentrations (C_{max}) at steady state are about 0.66 μg/mL and 1.6 μg/mL, respectively. Steady-state peak plasma aciclovir concentrations after intravenous doses of 5 mg/kg or 10 mg/kg of body weight administered every

8 hours are about 10 μg/mL and 20 μg/mL, respectively. Plasma protein binding is less than 20%. Aciclovir penetrates well into most tissues, including the central nervous system. The cerebrospinal fluid (CSF) aciclovir area under the concentration–time curve (AUC) is about 20% of the serum AUC. In noninflamed eyes, the mean vitreous-to-serum concentration ratio for aciclovir is about 24%. Significant concentrations of aciclovir (up to 300% of the serum concentration) can be found in breast milk. Aciclovir is minimally metabolized and about 85% of an administered dose is excreted unchanged in the urine via glomerular filtration and renal tubular secretion. The terminal plasma half-life of aciclovir is 2–3 hours in adults and 3–4 hours in neonates with normal renal function, but is extended to about 20 hours in anuric subjects.

Valaciclovir is an orally-administered prodrug of aciclovir designed to overcome the problem of poor oral bioavailability.[2] Valaciclovir, the L-valine ester of aciclovir, is well absorbed from the gastrointestinal tract via a stereospecific transporter and undergoes essentially complete first-pass conversion in the gut and liver to yield aciclovir and L-valine. This prodrug improves bioavailability to about 54%, yielding peak plasma aciclovir levels that are three- to fivefold higher than those achieved with oral aciclovir. Oral doses of 500 mg or 1000 mg of valaciclovir produce peak plasma aciclovir concentrations of 3.3 μg/mL and 5–6 μg/mL, respectively. After administration of valaciclovir at a dose of 2 g orally four times daily, plasma aciclovir AUC values approximate those produced by aciclovir given intravenously at a dose of 10 mg/kg every 8 hours. Following enzymatic conversion of valaciclovir to aciclovir, the antiviral spectrum of activity, pharmacokinetic properties and excretion are the same as those described above.

Route of Administration and Dosage

Aciclovir is available in topical, oral and intravenous formulations. Outside of the USA, aciclovir is also available as a 3% preparation for topical ophthalmologic use. The dermatologic preparations consist of

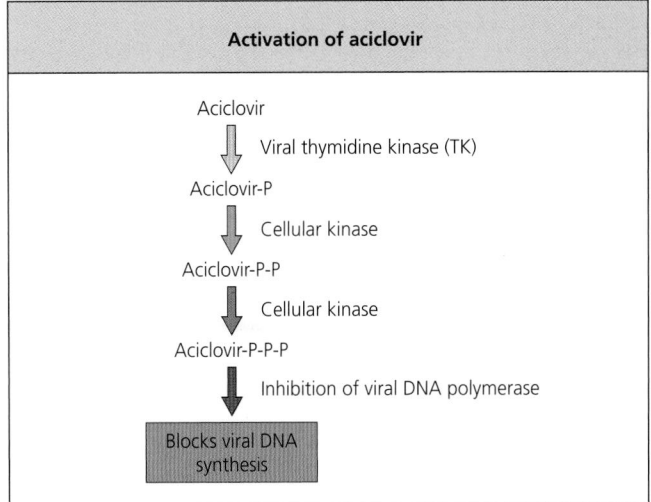

Figure 153-1 Activation of aciclovir is dependent on monophosphorylation via viral thymidine kinase (TK). Aciclovir triphosphate inhibits the activity of viral DNA polymerase, thus blocking viral replication. Penciclovir and ganciclovir are activated by similar mechanisms.

5% aciclovir in a polyethylene glycol ointment or propylene glycol cream base. Oral aciclovir products include a 200 mg capsule, 400 mg and 800 mg tablets, and a liquid suspension (200 mg/5 mL). Aciclovir sodium for intravenous infusion is reconstituted and diluted to a concentration of 50 mg/mL. A variety of sustained-release formulations (intravaginal rings, buccal tablets, *in situ* gels, aciclovir-loaded nanoparticles, etc.) are being evaluated.

The recommended dose of aciclovir varies with the specific indication (Table 153-1). Because of the greater intrinsic resistance of VZV to aciclovir, the doses required for treating VZV infections are higher than those used for HSV infections. In adults with normal renal function, oral aciclovir is given at a dose of 200 mg (for HSV) to 800 mg (for VZV) five times daily. The recommended dose of intravenous aciclovir is 5 mg/kg every 8 hours for HSV infections and 10 mg/kg every 8 hours for VZV infections, although higher doses (12–15 mg/kg every 8 hours) are sometimes used for life-threatening infections, especially in immunocompromised patients.

Valaciclovir recommended doses are 500 mg every 12 hours for episodic treatment of recurrent genital HSV infections and 1000 mg every 8 hours for treatment of herpes zoster.

Indications

HSV Infections. Aciclovir and valaciclovir are effective for treatment of initial and recurrent episodes of genital herpes as well as for suppressive therapy (see Table 153-2).[3,4] There is no evidence of cumulative toxicity or emergence of drug-resistant HSV in immunocompetent patients even after years of suppressive therapy. Suppression with aciclovir or valaciclovir will also significantly reduce (but not eliminate) the frequency of asymptomatic viral shedding and reduce the risk of transmission of genital herpes to an uninfected partner.[5]

Antiviral prophylaxis with aciclovir or valaciclovir can significantly reduce the necessity for Cesarean section due to active genital HSV lesions present at the onset of labor.[6] Intravenous aciclovir therapy can significantly reduce both morbidity and mortality in babies who develop neonatal herpes.

Valaciclovir (2 g every 12 hours for 1 day) has been shown to reduce the duration of an episode of recurrent herpes labialis by 1.1 days. Suppressive therapy with valaciclovir (1 g daily) can reduce the frequency of clinical recurrences of cold sores by about 50%.[7] Combination therapy with an antiviral drug (such as aciclovir or valaciclovir) plus corticosteroids is widely used for treatment of Bell's palsy, but the demonstrated benefit from the antiviral therapy has varied among clinical trials.[8] Oral aciclovir and valaciclovir have both been used successfully for treatment and prophylaxis of herpetic keratitis.

Aciclovir or valaciclovir prophylaxis of HSV infections is highly effective in severely immunocompromised patients, particularly those undergoing induction chemotherapy or organ transplantation. Clinical experience suggests that intravenous aciclovir (10 mg/kg every 8 hours) is the treatment of choice for disseminated or visceral HSV infection (e.g. pneumonitis, hepatitis, esophagitis, etc.) in immunocompromised patients, although data from controlled clinical trials are lacking. Aciclovir is the drug of choice for HSV encephalitis and should be given intravenously at a dose of 10–15 mg/kg every 8 hours for 14–21 days.

VZV Infections. Oral aciclovir therapy (20 mg/kg, up to a maximum of 800 mg, every 6 hours) is effective for immunocompetent children with chickenpox; however, the benefits are modest and many pediatricians consider antiviral treatment of chickenpox to be optional. Adolescents and adults are at greater risk for varicella complications; aciclovir therapy (800 mg orally five times daily for 7 days) is recommended for those who present within 24–48 hours of disease onset. Valaciclovir is also likely to be effective in this setting, but data from controlled clinical trials are unavailable. Immunocompromised patients with chickenpox should receive intravenous aciclovir (10 mg/kg or 500 mg/m^2 every 8 hours for 7–10 days). Clinical experience suggests that intravenous aciclovir is the treatment of choice for patients with VZV infections complicated by visceral involvement (e.g. pneumonitis, encephalitis, etc.).

TABLE 153-1	Indications for Aciclovir Therapy
Infection	**Route and Dosage***
Genital HSV	
Initial episode	400 mg po TID × 7–10 days
Initial episode with complications	5 mg/kg iv q8h × 5–7 days
Recurrent episodes	400 mg po TID × 5 days
Suppression	400 mg po BID daily
Mucocutaneous HSV in immunocompromised patient	400 mg po 5 times/d × 10–14 days, or 5 mg/kg iv q8h × 10 days
Disseminated or visceral HSV (including encephalitis)	10–15 mg/kg iv q8h × 14–21 days
Neonatal HSV	10–15 mg/kg iv q8h × 14–21 days
Varicella (chickenpox)	
Normal host	20 mg/kg (max. 800 mg) po 4–5 times/d × 5 days
Immunocompromised patient	10–15 mg/kg iv q8h × ≥7 days
Herpes zoster (shingles)	
Normal host	800 mg po 5 times/d × 7–10 days
Immunocompromised patient (disseminated or visceral VZV)	10–15 mg/kg iv q8h × ≥7 days

*Given doses are indicated for patients with normal renal function.
BID, twice daily; TID, three times daily; iv, intravenous; po, by mouth.

TABLE 153-2	Oral Antiviral Therapy for Genital Herpes*			
Drugs	**Initial Episode**	**Episodic Therapy**	**Suppressive Therapy**
Aciclovir	400 mg TID × 7–10 days *Alternative dose:* 200 mg 5 times daily × 7–10 days	400 mg TID × 5 days *Alternative doses:* 800 mg BID × 5 days 800 mg TID × 2 days	400 mg BID daily *Alternative dose (HIV positive):* 400-800 mg BID or TID daily
Famciclovir	250 mg TID × 7–10 days	125 mg BID × 5 days *Alternative dose:* 1000 mg BID × 1 day 500 mg × 1 dose, then 250 mg BID × 2 days	250 mg BID daily *Alternative dose (HIV positive):* 500 mg BID daily
Valaciclovir	1000 mg BID × 7–10 days	500 mg BID × 3 days *Alternative dose:* 1000 mg daily × 5 days	500 mg once daily *Alternative doses:* 1000 mg once daily *(HIV positive)* 500 mg BID daily

*Recommended doses for immunocompetent adults with normal renal function. (Workowski K.A., Berman S. Centers for Disease Control and Prevention (CDC). Sexually transmitted diseases treatment guidelines, 2010. MMWR Recomm Rep 2010; 59(RR-12):1-110.)
BID, twice daily; TID, three times daily.

Both aciclovir and valaciclovir are effective for treatment of localized herpes zoster in immunocompetent patients if therapy is initiated within 48–72 hours of rash onset. Valaciclovir has the advantage of a simpler dosing regimen. Severely immunocompromised patients (e.g. bone marrow transplant, cancer chemotherapy, etc.) with herpes zoster are at high risk for disseminated VZV infection and should be treated with intravenous aciclovir (10 mg/kg every 8 hours). Antiviral prophylaxis given to prevent HSV disease in this population also effectively suppresses VZV reactivation (Box 153-1).[9]

Other Viral Infections. While aciclovir is ineffective for established CMV infections, high-dose oral aciclovir or valaciclovir may have value for CMV prophylaxis in high-risk populations such as organ transplant recipients.[10–12] Aciclovir or valaciclovir can induce regression of Epstein–Barr virus (EBV)-associated oral hairy leukoplakia in HIV-infected patients. Aciclovir is considered the drug of choice for therapy of rare human infections caused by cercopithecine herpesvirus-1 (B virus). Aciclovir is not directly active against HIV; however, studies of HIV/HSV-2 co-infected persons have shown significant reductions in HIV plasma levels in those patients receiving aciclovir or valaciclovir.[13]

Dosage in Special Circumstances

Aciclovir is cleared primarily by renal mechanisms and dosage modification of aciclovir and valaciclovir is required for patients with significant renal dysfunction (Table 153-3). The mean elimination half-life of aciclovir after a single 1 g dose of valaciclovir is about 14 hours in patients with end-stage renal disease. No specific dosage modification is required for patients with hepatic impairment. Aciclovir and valaciclovir are not approved for use in pregnancy, but have been widely used to treat HSV and VZV infections in pregnant women without evidence of maternal or fetal toxicity.[14] Population pharmacokinetic studies suggest that higher-than-standard aciclovir doses may be required in infants and small children (<10 kg).[15] Experience with valaciclovir in very young children is limited as no commercial liquid preparation is commercially available. However, extemporaneous liquid valaciclovir for oral administration can be prepared by a compounding pharmacist by crushing 500 mg valaciclovir tablets and formulating a suspension at 25 or 50 mg/mL using suspension-structured vehicle (SSV) and flavoring. Aciclovir AUC values after oral valaciclovir dosing are slightly higher in elderly individuals when compared with younger control groups due to age-related decline in renal function.

Adverse Reactions

Aciclovir and valaciclovir are extremely well-tolerated drugs with few significant adverse effects. Allergic reactions to aciclovir or valaciclovir have been reported, but are very uncommon. With intravenous aciclovir therapy, inflammation and phlebitis may occur following localized drug extravasation.

Renal dysfunction (including cases of acute renal failure) resulting from accumulation of aciclovir crystals in the kidneys has been observed following administration of large doses of aciclovir by rapid intravenous infusion, but is uncommon and usually reversible. Formation of aciclovir aldehyde may also contribute to tubular toxicity.[16] The risk of nephrotoxicity can be minimized by administering aciclovir by slow infusion (over 1 hour) and ensuring adequate hydration. Risk factors for aciclovir-induced nephropathy include pre-existing renal dysfunction and concomitant use of other nephrotoxic drugs. Rarely, nephrotoxicity has been observed following oral dosing of aciclovir or valaciclovir.

Reports have linked administration of aciclovir (and less commonly valaciclovir) with central nervous system (CNS) disturbances, including agitation, hallucination, disorientation, tremors, clonus and seizures. Neurotoxicity has most often been recognized in elderly patients with underlying CNS abnormalities and renal insufficiency. Aciclovir-induced neurologic toxicity has been successfully treated by emergent hemodialysis.[17]

Patients receiving oral aciclovir or valaciclovir therapy occasionally complain of nausea, diarrhea, rash or headache, but at rates that do not differ from placebo recipients. The safety of oral aciclovir and valaciclovir for long-term administration has been confirmed in patients receiving the drug for over 5 years for suppression of recurrent genital herpes.

Significant interactions between aciclovir and other drugs are extremely uncommon. Probenecid decreases the renal clearance of aciclovir and can prolong the plasma excretion half-life. Additive aciclovir-induced nephrotoxicity in patients receiving concomitant cyclosporine therapy has been suggested. Concomitant administration of cimetidine and probenecid reduces the rate of valaciclovir conversion to aciclovir, but the effect is not clinically significant.

Resistance

HSV resistance to aciclovir can develop through mutation of the viral genes encoding TK or DNA polymerase.[18] Most aciclovir-resistant clinical HSV isolates are TK-deficient and are therefore unable to phosphorylate aciclovir. Consequently, these isolates will also be resistant to valaciclovir, penciclovir, famciclovir and ganciclovir, all of which have the same mechanism of action and require viral TK for activation.

Disease caused by aciclovir-resistant HSV isolates occurs almost exclusively in immunocompromised patients. The most common clinical presentation of infection caused by aciclovir-resistant HSV is chronic, progressive mucocutaneous ulcerations. Approximately 5–6% of HSV isolates recovered from HIV-seropositive patients are aciclovir-resistant (IC_{50}> 2.0 µg/mL). Aciclovir-resistant VZV isolates (which are less frequently encountered than resistant HSV isolates) are occasionally recovered from severely immunocompromised patients. Clinical disease caused by aciclovir-resistant VZV has usually been

---

BOX 153-1   ORAL ANTIVIRAL THERAPY FOR HERPES ZOSTER*

TREATMENT OPTIONS
- Aciclovir 800 mg 5 times daily for 7–10 days
- Famciclovir 500 mg TID for 7 days
- Valaciclovir 1000 g TID for 7 days
- Brivudin 125 mg once daily for 7 days

*Recommended doses for immunocompetent adults with normal renal function.

TABLE 153-3   Aciclovir Dosage Modification for Renal Impairment

Normal Dosage Regimen	CrCl (mL/min/1.73 m²)	Dose	Dosing Interval (Hr)
Aciclovir 200 mg po q4h	>10	200 mg	4 (5 times/day)
	0–10	200 mg	12
Aciclovir 400 mg po q12h	>10	400 mg	12
	0–10	200 mg	12
Aciclovir 800 mg po q4h	>25	800 mg	4 (5 times/day)
	10–25	800 mg	8
	0–10	800 mg	12
Aciclovir 5 mg/kg iv q8h	>50	5 mg/kg	8
	25–50	5 mg/kg	12
	10–25	5 mg/kg	24
	0–10	2.5 mg/kg	24
Aciclovir 10 mg/kg iv q8h	>50	10 mg/kg	8
	25–50	10 mg/kg	12
	10–25	10 mg/kg	24
	0–10	5 mg/kg	24

CrCl = creatinine clearance.

limited to cutaneous involvement, often characterized by atypical lesions. Antiviral options for systemic treatment of aciclovir-resistant HSV or VZV disease are foscarnet and cidofovir.

PENCICLOVIR AND FAMCICLOVIR

Mechanism of Action and In Vitro Activity

Penciclovir is an acyclic guanine derivative similar to aciclovir in structure, mechanism of action and spectrum of antiviral activity. In HSV- or VZV-infected cells, penciclovir is first monophosphorylated by virally-encoded TK and then further phosphorylated to the triphosphate moiety by cellular enzymes. Penciclovir triphosphate blocks viral DNA synthesis through competitive inhibition of viral DNA polymerase. Unlike aciclovir triphosphate, penciclovir triphosphate is not an obligate chain terminator and can be incorporated into the extending DNA chain. Compared with aciclovir triphosphate, intracellular concentrations of penciclovir triphosphate are much higher. For example, the half-life values for penciclovir triphosphate and aciclovir triphosphate in HSV-1-infected cells are 10 hours and 0.7 hour, respectively. However, this potential advantage is offset by a much lower affinity of penciclovir triphosphate for viral DNA polymerase. The *in vitro* activities of penciclovir against HSV-1, HSV-2 and VZV are similar to those of aciclovir, with median IC_{50} values of 0.4, 1.5 and 4.0 μg/mL, respectively, in MRC-5 cells.

As valaciclovir is a prodrug of aciclovir, famciclovir is a prodrug of penciclovir. Because penciclovir is very poorly absorbed, famciclovir (the diacetyl ester of 6-deoxy-penciclovir) was developed as the oral formulation. The first acetyl side chain of famciclovir is cleaved by esterases found in the intestinal wall. On first pass through the liver, the second acetyl group is removed and oxidation catalyzed by aldehyde oxidase occurs at the 6 position, yielding penciclovir, which is the active antiviral compound.

Pharmacokinetics and Distribution

Intravenous infusion of penciclovir at 10 mg/kg over 1 hour yields a peak plasma concentration of 12.1 μg/mL. Plasma protein binding of penciclovir is <20%. The drug is cleared by renal tubular secretion and passive filtration. The plasma elimination half-life of penciclovir is about 2 hours and approximately 70% is recovered unchanged in the urine.

When administered as the famciclovir prodrug, the bioavailability of penciclovir is about 77%. Following a single oral dose of 250 mg or 500 mg of famciclovir, peak plasma penciclovir concentrations of 1.9 μg/mL and 3.5 μg/mL, respectively, are achieved at 1 hour. The pharmacokinetics of penciclovir are linear and dose independent over a famciclovir dosing range of 125–750 mg. Food slows famciclovir absorption and lowers the peak plasma penciclovir concentration, but does not alter the AUC value.

Route of Administration and Dosage

Famciclovir is available as 125 mg, 250 mg and 500 mg tablets. Recommended dosages vary with indication. The usual dose of famciclovir is 125 mg every 12 hours for episodic therapy of recurrent genital herpes and 500 mg every 8 hours for herpes zoster. The intravenous preparation of penciclovir is not commercially available. A topical preparation of penciclovir is available as a 1% cream for treatment of HSV labialis.

Indications

Genital HSV Infections. Famciclovir is effective for initial and recurrent genital herpes and also provides effective suppressive therapy (see Table 153-3). Famciclovir suppressive therapy reduces mucosal viral shedding from HSV-2 infected persons,[19] but its effect on virus transmission has not been studied. Famciclovir is also effective for suppression and treatment of recurrent mucocutaneous (orolabial and anogenital) infections in HIV-infected patients.

Three drugs (aciclovir, valaciclovir and famciclovir) with proven efficacy for long-term suppression of recurrent genital herpes are

currently available.[20] For these drugs, a dose–response relationship exists, meaning that higher total daily doses generally produce more complete suppression. Dose titration of the selected drug may be necessary to identify optimal treatment for an individual patient (see Table 153-2).

Herpes Labialis. Topical 1% penciclovir cream (applied every 2 hours while awake) and oral famciclovir (1500 mg) have demonstrated efficacy for treatment of herpes labialis.[21]

Herpes Zoster. Famciclovir was shown to accelerate cutaneous healing and reduce the duration of viral shedding and postherpetic neuralgia in immunocompetent patients with dermatomal herpes zoster.[21] Famciclovir was proven effective for herpes zoster therapy in bone marrow transplant, cancer and HIV-seropositive patients. In the USA, the recommended dose of famciclovir for uncomplicated herpes zoster is 500 mg three times daily. Doses of 250 mg three times daily and 750 mg once daily are approved in Europe and the UK.

In a large randomized clinical trial, valaciclovir and famciclovir were shown to be therapeutically equivalent for treatment of herpes zoster.[22] Because of their improved pharmacokinetic profiles and simpler dosing regimens, valaciclovir and famciclovir are preferred over aciclovir for this indication.[23]

Other Viral Infections. Famciclovir suppresses hepatitis B virus (HBV) replication by targeting the viral polymerase, but treatment of hepatitis B using famciclovir monotherapy resulted in rapid emergence of HBV resistance.[24] Case reports have suggested that famciclovir is effective for treatment of EBV-induced oral hairy leukoplakia in HIV-infected patients.

Dosage in Special Circumstances

Penciclovir is cleared predominantly by renal mechanisms, so adjustments of famciclovir dosing are required in patients with advanced renal insufficiency. In patients with hepatic insufficiency, the rate of conversion of famciclovir to penciclovir is decreased, but the plasma AUC value for penciclovir is not significantly changed; no famciclovir dosage modification is necessary. Plasma penciclovir concentrations are slightly higher in elderly patients treated with famciclovir due to age-related reduction in glomerular filtration rates, but dosage modifications are not required. No liquid preparation of famciclovir is commercially available, thus data regarding use in children less than 12 years of age are limited. Famciclovir has not been approved for any indication during pregnancy.

Adverse Reactions

Safety data collected from over 3000 patients given famciclovir have shown the drug to be very safe and well tolerated. The most frequently reported adverse experiences have included occasional headache, nausea and diarrhea.[24]

No clinically significant drug interactions have been noted with famciclovir. Co-administration of famciclovir with cimetidine or theophylline will increase the penciclovir AUC by about 20%. Co-administration of famciclovir and digoxin results in a 19% increase in the peak digoxin concentration, but no change in the AUC.

Resistance

The majority of clinically encountered aciclovir-resistant HSV and VZV isolates are TK-deficient and thus will be resistant to penciclovir and famciclovir, which also require viral TK for activation. However, some HSV strains that are aciclovir-resistant by virtue of altered TK or DNA polymerase mutations may retain susceptibility to penciclovir.

BRIVUDIN

Brivudin is a highly potent antiviral agent selectively active against VZV and HSV-1 with therapeutic equivalence to aciclovir.[25–27] Because of concerns about potential toxicity, commercial development of brivudin has halted in some countries (including the USA), but the drug is widely available in Europe and other countries.

Mechanism of Action and In Vitro Activity

Brivudin (bromovinyl deoxyuridine; BDVU) is sequentially phophorylated by viral TK and cellular kinases to form BVDU triphosphate, a competitive inhibitor of viral DNA polymerase and alternate substrate for incorporation into viral DNA. The intracellular half-life in virus-infected cells is about 10 hours. The drug is highly active against VZV, with IC$_{50}$ values 28–1100-fold lower than those of aciclovir. Brivudin is active against HSV-1, but not against HSV-2. Thus, the clinical development of the drug has focused on its role for herpes zoster therapy.

Pharmacokinetics and Distribution

Brivudin is well absorbed after oral administration and absorption is not affected by food. There is high first-pass metabolism in the liver to bromovinyluracil, which lacks antiviral activity. At steady state (brivudin 125 mg daily for 5 days), the C_{max} and C_{min} are 1.7 μg/mL (at 1 hour) and 0.06 μg/mL, respectively. The plasma terminal elimination half-life is approximately 16 hours; metabolites are excreted in urine (65%) and plasma (21%). Brivudin is highly protein-bound (>95%).[28]

Route of Administration and Dosage

Brivudin is available as a 125 mg tablet and as a 0.1% ointment for ophthalmologic use. The standard dose for herpes zoster is 125 mg orally once daily for 7 days.

Indications

In randomized clinical trials, brivudin has been compared with aciclovir and famciclovir in immunocompetent patients with herpes zoster and was equivalent to the comparator drugs for end points of zoster lesion healing and pain resolution.[29] With its once-daily dosing, brivudin offers a potential advantage of convenience and improved patient adherence.

Dosage in Special Circumstances

The pharmacokinetic properties of brivudin in elderly patients or in patients with renal or hepatic failure are not significantly changed from those seen in healthy volunteers.

Adverse Reactions

In clinical trials with brivudin, the most commonly observed adverse effects were nausea (2.1%), abdominal pain (0.8%), vomiting (0.5%) and headache (1%) and did not differ significantly from adverse effects reported with aciclovir or famciclovir. Rare cases of brivudin-associated acute hepatitis and delirium have been reported.

Brivudin has a critically important drug interaction that has been an obstacle to its regulatory approval in some countries. Bromovinyluracil (the primary metabolite of brivudin) irreversibly inhibits dihydropyrimidine dehydrogenase (DPD), an enzyme that regulates nucleoside metabolism. Co-administration of brivudin with 5-fluorouracil (5-FU, a cancer chemotherapeutic agent) results in a 15-fold increase in systemic exposure to 5-FU, causing potentially lethal bone marrow suppression and gastrointestinal toxicity. Full recovery of DPD activity requires at least 18 days after brivudin dosing. Potential interactions with brivudin may also occur with other fluoro-pyrimidines such as flucytosine (5-FC), tegafur, floxuridine and capecitabine. Brivudin should be used with extreme caution in cancer patients to avoid concomitant dosing with 5-FU.

OTHER DRUGS

Trifluridine

Trifluridine, a fluorinated pyrimidine nucleoside with good in vitro activity against HSV, is a competitive inhibitor of HSV DNA polymerase. Trifluridine is widely used as a 1% ophthalmic solution for topical therapy of HSV keratitis. Topical trifluridine has also been used with moderate success for topical treatment of aciclovir-resistant mucocutaneous HSV infections.

n-Docosanol

n-Docosanol, a 22-carbon fatty alcohol with in vitro activity against HSV, acts by interfering with viral entry into target cells. n-Docosanol is available over-the-counter in a 2 g tube of 10% cream and is modestly effective for treatment of recurrent herpes labialis.

Drugs for Treatment of Cytomegalovirus Infections

GANCICLOVIR AND VALGANCICLOVIR

Mechanism of Action and In Vitro Activity

Ganciclovir is a nucleoside analog structurally similar to aciclovir, but has a hydroxymethyl group at the 3′ position of the acyclic side chain. This relatively minor structural modification accounts for enhanced activity of ganciclovir against human CMV as well as greater toxicity. Ganciclovir triphosphate is a potent inhibitor of herpesvirus DNA replication, acting as both an inhibitor of and a substrate for viral DNA polymerase.[30]

In HSV- or VZV-infected cells, monophosphorylation of ganciclovir is induced by viral TK, as also occurs with aciclovir. In CMV-infected cells, ganciclovir monophosphorylation is carried out by a protein kinase encoded by the UL97 gene. The di- and tri-phosphorylation steps are mediated by cellular kinases. On a molar basis, aciclovir triphosphate is actually a more potent inhibitor of CMV than is ganciclovir triphosphate. However, aciclovir is a poor substrate for phosphorylation by the UL97 gene product; consequently, the concentration of ganciclovir triphosphate in CMV-infected cells is 10-fold higher than that of aciclovir triphosphate. Furthermore, the half-life of ganciclovir triphosphate in CMV-infected cells is 16.5 hours, compared with 2.5 hours for aciclovir triphosphate. Ganciclovir triphosphate does not function as a chain terminator, and can be incorporated into elongating viral DNA (and, to a much lesser extent, human DNA) where it functions to slow DNA chain extension.

Ganciclovir and aciclovir have similar in vitro activity against HSV-1, HSV-2 and VZV. However, ganciclovir is much more active against CMV, with IC$_{50}$ values of 0.1–1.8 μg/mL against clinical isolates.

Pharmacokinetics and Distribution

Intravenous infusion of ganciclovir at a dose of 5 mg/kg yields peak and trough plasma levels of approximately 8 μg/mL and 1 μg/mL, respectively. Plasma protein binding is 1–2%. Reported plasma-to-CSF ratios for ganciclovir have ranged from 24% to 70%. Ganciclovir is not metabolized and is cleared by renal mechanisms, with an elimination half-life of about 3 hours. Ganciclovir is poorly absorbed after oral administration, with bioavailability of only 5–9%.

To overcome the limited oral bioavailability of ganciclovir, the prodrug valganciclovir was developed.[31] Valganciclovir, the L-valyl ester of ganciclovir, is rapidly and almost completely hydrolyzed to ganciclovir in the liver and intestinal wall. Bioavailability of ganciclovir from the prodrug formulation is about 60% and is significantly increased with food administration. Maximum plasma ganciclovir concentrations are four- to fivefold higher than those achieved after oral dosing with the parent drug. Oral valganciclovir doses of 450 mg and 875 mg once daily for 3 days produced peak plasma ganciclovir concentrations of 3.3 μg/mL and 6.1 μg/mL, respectively. The AUC of ganciclovir after administration of 900 mg valganciclovir is about 26 μg/mL/h, which is comparable to the AUC following administration of ganciclovir dosed at 5 mg/kg intravenously.

Route of Administration and Dosage

Ganciclovir is available as an intravenous formulation. Recommended doses vary with the indication. For treatment of acute CMV disease, the usual dose of intravenous ganciclovir is 5 mg/kg every 12 hours. An oral ganciclovir capsule and a delayed-release intraocular implant device previously available in the USA have been discontinued.

TABLE 153-4 **Systemic Antiviral Therapy for CMV Retinitis**

Drugs	Induction Therapy*	Maintenance Therapy[†]
Ganciclovir	5 mg/kg iv q12h × 4–21 days	5 mg/kg iv daily
Valganciclovir	900 mg po q12h × 14–21 days	900 mg po daily
Foscarnet	90 mg/kg iv q12h (or 60 mg/kg iv q8h) × 14–21 days	90–120 mg/kg iv daily
Cidofovir	5 mg/kg iv weekly × 2–3 weeks	5 mg/kg iv every other week

*Recommended doses for adults with normal renal function.
[†]Another therapeutic option includes intravitreal drug injections.

TABLE 153-5 **Ganciclovir and Valganciclovir Dosage Modification for Renal Impairment**

Normal Dosage Regimen	CrCl (mL/min)	Dose	Dosing Interval (Hr)
Ganciclovir 5 mg/kg iv q12h	≥70	5 mg/kg	12
	50–69	2.5 mg/kg	12
	25–49	2.5 mg/kg	24
	10–24	1.25 mg/kg	24
Ganciclovir 5 mg/kg iv q24h	≥70	5 mg/kg	24
	50–69	2.5 mg/kg	24
	25–49	1.25 mg/kg	24
	10–24	0.625 mg/kg	24
	HD	0.625 mg/kg	Post-HD (TIW)
Valganciclovir 900 mg po q12h	>60	900 mg	12
	40–59	450 mg	12
	25–39	450 mg	24
	10–24	450 mg	48
	Solution	225 mg	24
	HD	NR	–
	Solution	200 mg	Post-HD (TIW)
Valganciclovir 900 mg po q24h	>60	900 mg	24
	40–59	450 mg	24
	25–39	450 mg	48
	Solution	225 mg	24
	10–24	450 mg	Twice weekly
	Solution	125 mg	24
	HD	NR	–
	Solution	100 mg	Post-HD (TIW)

CrCl, creatinine clearance; HD, hemodialysis; NR, not recommended; post-HD, after each dialysis; TIW, three times weekly.

Valganciclovir is available as a 450 mg tablet as well as a 50 mg/mL solution. The recommended dose for induction therapy of acute CMV retinitis is 900 mg orally every 12 hours for a total of 21 days, followed by maintenance therapy of 900 mg orally once daily.[32] The dosage recommended for prophylaxis of CMV disease following solid organ transplantation is 900 mg orally once daily.[33] All doses should be administered with food.

Indications

Treatment of CMV Disease. Intravenous ganciclovir is used for therapy of serious CMV infections in immunocompromised patients, including CMV retinitis, pneumonitis, encephalitis and gastrointestinal disease. The usual dose of ganciclovir for induction therapy is 5 mg/kg given intravenously every 12 hours for 14–21 days, followed by a maintenance regimen (5 mg/kg once daily). Intravitreal injections of ganciclovir were formerly used for treatment of CMV retinitis, but systemic treatment of CMV in the setting of retinitis is associated with longer survival.[34]

Ganciclovir, valganciclovir, foscarnet and cidofovir are all effective for initial and maintenance therapy of CMV retinitis in HIV-seropositive patients (Table 153-4). All of these drugs are associated with significant toxicity; drug selection in an individual patient hinges, to some extent, on which adverse effects would be most tolerable. Ganciclovir is primarily myelosuppressive, while foscarnet and cidofovir are nephrotoxic. Despite the survival benefits shown for foscarnet therapy in some studies, most clinicians use ganciclovir or valganciclovir for initial therapy on the basis of more predictable adverse effects.

Prophylaxis of CMV Disease. Benefits of prophylaxis of CMV infection in solid organ transplant recipients have varied with the transplant type, immunosuppressive regimen and CMV serologic status of the donor and recipient. Prophylaxis with intravenous ganciclovir or oral valganciclovir significantly reduces the incidence of CMV disease in high-risk immunocompromised patients, but is often complicated by drug-induced neutropenia. An alternative scheme is to withhold ganciclovir until there is early laboratory evidence (by polymerase chain reaction) of CMV activation. This pre-emptive therapy approach permits initiation of antiviral treatment before CMV disease becomes symptomatic, while avoiding the risk of neutropenia associated with long-term ganciclovir administration.[35–42]

Dosage in Special Circumstances

Because ganciclovir is cleared by renal mechanisms, dosage reduction is necessary in patients with creatinine clearance of <70 mL/min (Table 153-5). About 50% of an administered dose is removed during 4 hours of hemodialysis; dosing after dialysis is recommended. Valganciclovir dosage adjustment is required for patients with creatinine clearance <60 mL/min; the solution should be used to provide doses less than 450 mg. No dosage adjustment for hepatic impairment is necessary.

Ganciclovir is mutagenic, carcinogenic and causes reproductive toxicity in animal models. Use of ganciclovir or valganciclovir in pregnant or nursing women is not recommended without careful consideration of the risk–benefit ratio. A retrospective study conducted among pediatric kidney transplantation recipients showed valganciclovir prophylaxis was more effective in preventing CMV reactivation than aciclovir plus CMV-specific immunoglobulin. However, data on valganciclovir use in children remains limited.[43,44]

Adverse Reactions

The most important adverse effects of ganciclovir noted in HIV-seropositive patients being treated for CMV retinitis were neutropenia and thrombocytopenia. About 40% developed granulocytopenia (absolute neutrophil count < 1.0×10^6/L) and 15% had thrombocytopenia (platelet count < 5×10^7/L).[45] Hematologic toxicity is also observed, although less commonly, in organ transplant recipients. Neutropenia and thrombocytopenia are usually reversible when ganciclovir therapy is discontinued. In many patients requiring ganciclovir therapy, neutropenia can be prevented or treated by co-administration of granulocyte colony-stimulating factor. Renal dysfunction has been reported in up to 20% of transplant recipients receiving ganciclovir prophylaxis, although this may be related to co-administration of other nephrotoxic drugs. In animal models, ganciclovir produces significant reproductive toxicity, especially azoospermia.

Valganciclovir appears to have hematologic toxicity similar to intravenous ganciclovir. In a study of valganciclovir 450 mg twice daily in kidney transplant recipients to prevent CMV disease, 5.7% (four patients) developed agranulocytosis (neutrophil count < 5×10^5/L) an average of 74 days after transplantation. Onset was abrupt and asymptomatic; all patients recovered after discontinuation of valganciclovir.[46]

Ganciclovir should be used with caution in combination with other myelosuppressive drugs such as zidovudine because of the risk of additive hematologic toxicity. When co-administered with didanosine, ganciclovir increases the AUC of didanosine from 50% to 114%; thus patients should be monitored for didanosine toxicity when these two drugs are administered together. Probenecid can reduce renal clearance of ganciclovir, resulting in clinically significant increases in ganciclovir AUC. Seizures have been reported in patients receiving concomitant therapy with ganciclovir and imipenem.

Resistance

HSV and VZV isolates that are TK deficient and aciclovir resistant will also be cross-resistant to ganciclovir. Ganciclovir resistance *in vitro* is defined as an $IC_{50} > 6\ \mu M$ (1.5 $\mu g/mL$). In a study of 72 HIV-seropositive patients treated with ganciclovir, five of 13 culture-positive patients treated for >3 months excreted resistant virus. Ganciclovir-resistant CMV has been identified as a cause of retinitis, encephalitis and polyradiculopathy in HIV-seropositive patients and enteritis and of viremia among solid organ transplant patients. Among solid organ transplant recipients, resistance rates of 1.5–14% have been reported.[47, 48] CMV resistance to ganciclovir is usually secondary to mutations in the UL97 gene, although alterations in the DNA polymerase gene have also been described. UL97 mutants remain susceptible to foscarnet, although polymerase mutants cross-resistant to ganciclovir, cidofovir, and foscarnet have been identified.[49] Foscarnet and cidofovir are therapeutic alternatives for treatment of disease caused by ganciclovir-resistant CMV.

FOSCARNET

Mechanism of Action and In Vitro Activity

Foscarnet is an analog of inorganic pyrophosphate that functions as a noncompetitive inhibitor of herpesvirus DNA polymerase.[50] Foscarnet blocks the pyrophosphate binding site, preventing cleavage of pyrophosphate from deoxynucleotide triphosphates. Viral DNA polymerase is inhibited at foscarnet concentrations 100-fold lower than those required to inhibit cellular DNA polymerase. Foscarnet is not a nucleoside analog, does not require intracellular activation by viral kinase, and is not incorporated into the viral DNA chain. Therefore, TK-deficient HSV and VZV isolates that are resistant to aciclovir will remain susceptible to foscarnet. Foscarnet has *in vitro* activity against HSV, VZV, CMV, EBV and human herpesvirus 6 (HHV-6). The IC_{50} for most clinical isolates of CMV is in the range of 100–300 μM, but varies considerably with the experimental conditions. Foscarnet can also inhibit viral reverse transcriptase and has *in vitro* activity against HBV and HIV.

Pharmacokinetics and Distribution

Foscarnet has low oral bioavailability (approximately 17%) and is administered intravenously. Peak plasma concentrations after steady-state dosing at 60 mg/kg every 8 hours or 90 mg/kg every 12 hours are about 500 μM and 700 μM, respectively. Plasma protein binding is about 15%. CSF foscarnet levels demonstrate wide interpatient variability, but average about 66% of plasma levels at steady state. Foscarnet is not metabolized and about 80% of an administered dose is excreted unchanged in the urine by glomerular filtration and tubular secretion within 36 hours. About 20% of the foscarnet dose is retained in bone, presumably due to the drug's structural similarity to inorganic phosphate. This results in a complex pattern of drug disposition, in which the initial elimination half-life is about 4.5 hours, followed by a prolonged terminal half-life of about 88 hours as drug is released from bone. Plasma foscarnet levels are reduced by about 50% following hemodialysis; dosing after dialysis is recommended.

Route of Administration and Dosage

Foscarnet is available only as an intravenous formulation. The usual dose for induction therapy of CMV retinitis is 90 mg/kg every 12 hours, with a maintenance dose of 90–120 mg/kg every 24 hours. For aciclovir-resistant HSV, the usual dose of foscarnet is 40 mg/kg every 8–12 hours. When given via a central venous catheter, the drug can be diluted to 24 mg/mL; for infusion through peripheral vein catheters, foscarnet must be diluted to 12 mg/mL to avoid local phlebitis. The foscarnet dose must be administered over at least 1 hour using an intravenous infusion pump; bolus infusion can result in severe toxicity. Intravitreal injections of foscarnet have been used for management of VZV retinitis.

Indications

Intravenous foscarnet is used primarily to treat diseases caused by drug-resistant strains of HSV, VZV or CMV, or to treat patients who are intolerant of first-line antiviral therapy. Use of foscarnet for prophylaxis is limited by toxicity.[51,52]

Dosage in Special Circumstances

Foscarnet is excreted by renal mechanisms and dosage adjustment is required even for minor degrees of renal insufficiency. Serum creatinine should be monitored at least every other day during foscarnet therapy to assess the need for further dose adjustment. Dosage modification in hepatic impairment is not required. The safety of foscarnet during pregnancy has not been adequately evaluated and use is not recommended unless no other alternative therapy is available. Little information has been published regarding foscarnet safety and tolerance in pediatric populations.

Adverse Reactions

The most serious adverse effect of foscarnet is nephrotoxicity. Dose-limiting renal toxicity occurs in at least 15–20% of patients treated with foscarnet for CMV retinitis. The primary mechanism of renal toxicity appears to be acute tubular necrosis, although interstitial nephritis and crystalline nephropathy have also been described. Loading the patient with intravenous saline prior to foscarnet infusion can help reduce the risk of nephrotoxicity. In most cases, the renal dysfunction is reversible and serum creatinine will return to normal within 2–4 weeks after foscarnet therapy is discontinued. However, irreversible renal failure may occur in patients who are volume depleted or who receive concomitant therapy with other nephrotoxic medications.

Foscarnet can induce a variety of electrolyte and metabolic abnormalities, most notably hypocalcemia. Hypercalcemia, hypomagnesemia, hypokalemia and hypo- and hyperphosphatemia have also been reported. The acute decline in ionized serum calcium that can occur with foscarnet infusion may be due to formation of a complex between foscarnet and free calcium. Further depletion of total serum calcium seen with long-term drug administration may be caused by renal calcium wasting, abnormal bone metabolism, concurrent hypomagnesemia, or some combination of these factors. Foscarnet-induced electrolyte disturbances can predispose the patient to cardiac arrhythmias, tetany, altered mental status or seizures. It is mandatory that serum creatinine and electrolyte levels be closely monitored during foscarnet therapy.

Foscarnet is much less myelosuppressive than ganciclovir, but anemia was reported in 10–50% of HIV-seropositive patients receiving foscarnet.[53] Patients, especially uncircumcised males, may develop genital ulcerations due to local toxicity from high foscarnet concentrations in urine. Nausea and vomiting have been reported by 20–30% of patients receiving foscarnet. Other infrequent adverse effects include headache, diarrhea and abnormal liver function tests. When possible, foscarnet should be administered through a central venous line with an infusion pump to avoid the risk of acute hypocalcemia and peripheral thrombophlebitis.

Specific drug interactions with foscarnet have not been described, although there is significant potential for additive toxicity. Concurrent therapy with foscarnet and intravenous pentamidine can result in severe and potentially lethal hypocalcemia. Concomitant administration of foscarnet with other nephrotoxic drugs (such as amphotericin B or aminoglycosides) can compound the risk of serious renal injury. Foscarnet can be safely administered to patients receiving zidovudine, although there may be an increased risk of anemia. Due to the chelating properties of foscarnet, a number of drugs may precipitate when administered through the same intravenous catheter. Thus, review of the package insert is recommended for dosing recommendations and drug incompatibilities prior to administration.

Resistance

Although uncommon, foscarnet-resistant isolates of CMV, VZV and HSV have been encountered in HIV-seropositive patients receiving foscarnet therapy.[54–56] Resistance is due to a mutation in the DNA polymerase gene, thus, in some circumstances, the foscarnet-resistant isolate may remain susceptible to aciclovir or ganciclovir. However, CMV isolates cross-resistant to both ganciclovir and foscarnet (containing both polymerase and UL97 mutations) have been recovered. Cidofovir may be an effective alternative drug in this setting, but *in vitro* antiviral susceptibility testing is necessary to guide drug selection.

CIDOFOVIR

Mechanism of Action and In Vitro Activity

Cidofovir is a nucleotide analog of cytosine monophosphate with potent broad-spectrum antiviral activity.[57] Unlike aciclovir and other nucleoside analogs, which require monophosphorylation by viral kinases for activation, cidofovir already carries a phosphonate group and does not require viral enzymes for conversion to cidofovir diphosphate, the active antiviral compound. Cidofovir diphosphate competitively inhibits the DNA polymerases of herpesviruses, thereby blocking DNA synthesis and viral replication. Cidofovir diphosphate inhibits viral DNA polymerases at concentrations much lower than those required to inhibit cellular DNA polymerases, accounting for its selectivity of action.

Cidofovir has potent *in vitro* activity against human CMV, with IC_{50} values in the range of 0.1–0.9 µg/mL. Cidofovir retains activity against most CMV clinical isolates that are resistant to ganciclovir. Cidofovir also demonstrates *in vitro* activity against HSV and VZV (including TK-deficient, aciclovir-resistant isolates), adenovirus, poxviruses (including smallpox virus) and human papillomaviruses.

Pharmacokinetics and Distribution

Serum cidofovir concentrations are dose proportional over a dosing range of 1.0–10.0 mg/kg. Intravenous infusion of cidofovir at a dosage of 5 mg/kg produces peak plasma concentrations of about 11 µg/mL. The terminal half-life is 2.6 hours. Approximately 90% of the intravenous cidofovir dose is excreted by the kidneys within 24 hours, with clearance involving both glomerular filtration and tubular secretion. At cidofovir doses higher than 3 mg/kg, concomitant administration of probenecid can block tubular secretion of cidofovir and reduce its renal clearance. Cidofovir diphosphate and its metabolites have prolonged intracellular half-lives, which permit cidofovir to be effectively administered at extended dosing intervals. An orally-administered prodrug formulation of cidofovir (brincidofovir; CMX001) with a long lipid side chain resulting in improved pharmacokinetic properties and reduced nephrotoxicity is undergoing clinical trials.

Route of Administration and Dosage

Cidofovir for intravenous administration is supplied as 375 mg of an aqueous solution (75 mg/mL). The selected dose is diluted in 100 mL of normal saline prior to administration. For induction therapy, the usual dose of cidofovir is 5 mg/kg infused over 1 hour once weekly for 2 weeks. The dose for maintenance therapy for CMV disease is 5 mg/kg administered once every 2 weeks. To minimize nephrotoxicity, patients should receive 1 liter of normal saline intravenously over 1–2 hours immediately prior to cidofovir dose and an additional 1 liter of normal saline immediately following the cidofovir dose. Probenecid is given at a dose of 2 g orally 3 hours before the cidofovir dose, then 1 g

doses at 2 hours and 8 hours after completion of the cidofovir infusion.

Indications

Cidofovir is used primarily to treat diseases caused by drug-resistant strains of HSV, VZV or CMV, or to treat patients who are intolerant of first-line antiviral therapy. Use of cidofovir for prophylaxis or pre-emptive therapy is limited by toxicity.

Dosage in Special Circumstances

Because intravenous cidofovir can cause significant nephrotoxicity, initiation of therapy in patients with pre-existing renal dysfunction (serum creatinine >1.5 mg/dL, calculated creatinine clearance <55 mL/min or proteinuria >100 mg/dL [>2+]) is not recommended. Declining renal function during cidofovir therapy mandates dosage adjustment. If the serum creatinine increases by 0.3–0.4 mg/dL above baseline, the cidofovir dose should be reduced from 5 mg/kg to 3 mg/kg. If the serum creatinine increases >0.5 mg/dL above baseline or if proteinuria >3+ develops, cidofovir therapy should be discontinued. Dosage adjustment in patients with hepatic impairment is not required. Cidofovir is embryotoxic in animals and the drug should not be used during pregnancy unless there are no other therapeutic options. In small studies of pediatric patients, cidofovir toxicity was similar to that seen in adults.[58]

Adverse Reactions

The most serious safety concern with cidofovir therapy is nephrotoxicity, specifically proximal renal tubule dysfunction, characterized by proteinuria, glycosuria, hypophosphatemia and renal insufficiency. Pretreatment with intravenous hydration and probenecid reduces the incidence of nephrotoxicity. In a clinical trial using cidofovir 5 mg/kg plus probenecid, proteinuria occurred in five of 41 patients (12%) and elevated serum creatinine levels in two of 41 patients (5%). Neutropenia (ANC $< 7.5 \times 10^5$/L) was observed in 15% of cidofovir recipients. Anemia, thrombocytopenia and hepatotoxicity have not been observed with cidofovir therapy. Ocular complications (including iritis, anterior uveitis and hypotony) have been described following intravenous or intravitreal cidofovir administration. Intravitreal injection is not recommended.

Cidofovir administration causes embryotoxicity and impaired spermatogenesis in animals; male and female patients are advised to use adequate birth control during and for 3 months after completion of cidofovir therapy.

No specific drug interactions with cidofovir have been described, although concomitant therapy with other nephrotoxic drugs may result in additive toxicity. Probenecid is known to alter the renal excretion of a wide variety of drugs.

Resistance

Instances of clinical failure of cidofovir therapy due to drug resistance have been reported. CMV resistance to cidofovir results from a mutation in the viral polymerase gene and resistant isolates may exhibit cross-resistance to ganciclovir and/or foscarnet. *In vitro* susceptibility testing is necessary in this circumstance to guide appropriate drug selection.

References available online at expertconsult.com.

KEY REFERENCES

Balfour H.H. Jr, Chace B.A., Stapleton J.T., et al.: A randomized, placebo-controlled trial of oral acyclovir for the prevention of cytomegalovirus disease in recipients of renal allografts. *N Engl J Med* 1989; 320: 1381-1387.

Chawla J.S., Ghobadi A., Mosely J. 3rd, et al.: Oral valganciclovir versus ganciclovir as delayed pre-emptive therapy for patients after allogeneic hematopoietic stem cell transplant: a pilot trial (04-0274) and review of the literature. *Transpl Infect Dis* 2012; 14:259-267.

Corey L., Wald A., Patel R., et al.: Once-daily valacyclovir to reduce the risk of transmission of genital herpes. *N Engl J Med* 2004; 350:11-20.

Drew W.F.: Cytomegalovirus resistance testing: pitfalls and problems for the clinician. *Clin Infect Dis* 2010; 50:733-736.

Hantz S., Garnier-Geoffroy F., Mazeron M.C., et al.: Drug-resistant cytomegalovirus in transplant recipients: a French cohort study. *J Antimicrob Chemother* 2010; 65:2628-2640.

Goral S., Ynares C., Dummer S., et al.: Acyclovir prophylaxis for cytomegalovirus disease in high-risk renal transplant recipients: is it effective? *Kidney Int Suppl* 1996; 57:S62-S65.

Jabs D.A., Ahuja A., Van Natta M., et al.: Comparison of treatment regimens for cytomegalovirus retinitis in patients with AIDS in the era of highly active antiretroviral therapy. *Ophthalmol* 2013; 120:1262-1270.

Jongsma H., Bouts A.H., Cornelissen E.A.M., et al.: Cytomegalovirus prophylaxis in pediatric kidney transplantation: The Dutch experience. *Pediatr Transplantation* 2013; 17:510-517.

Martin D.F., Sierra-Madero J., Walmsley S., et al.: A controlled trial of valganciclovir as induction therapy for cytomegalovirus retinitis. *N Engl J Med* 2002; 346: 1119-1126.

McDonald E.M., de Kock J., Ram F.S.: Antivirals for management of herpes zoster including ophthalmicus: a systematic review of high-quality randomized controlled trials. *Antivir Ther* 2012; 17:255-264.

Meyers J.D., Reed E.C., Shepp D.H., et al.: Acyclovir for prevention of cytomegalovirus infection and disease after allogeneic marrow transplantation. *N Engl J Med* 1988; 318:70-75.

Pasternak B., Hviid A.: Use of acyclovir, valacyclovir, and famciclovir in the first trimester of pregnancy and the risk of birth defects. *JAMA* 2010; 304:859-866.

Pescovitz M.D.: Valganciclovir: Recent Progress. *Am J Transplant* 2010; 10:1359-1364.

Piret J., Boivin G.: Resistance of herpes simplex viruses to nucleoside analogues: mechanisms, prevalence, and management. *Antimicrob Agents Chemother* 2011; 55: 459-472.

Long-term outcomes of pre-emptive valganciclovir compared with valacyclovir prophylaxis for prevention of cytomegalovirus in renal transplantation. *J Am Soc Nephrol* 2012; 23:1588-1597.

Truong Q., Veltri L., Kanate A.S., et al.: Impact of the duration of antiviral prophylaxis on rates of varicella-zoster virus reactivation disease in autologous hematopoietic cell transplantation recipients. *Ann Hematol* 2014; 93:677-682.

Wassilew S.: Brivudin compared with famciclovir in the treatment of herpes zoster: effects in acute disease and chronic pain in immunocompetent patients. A randomized, double-blind, multinational study. *J Eur Acad Dermatol Venereol* 2005; 19:47-55.

Workowski K.A., Berman S., Centers for Disease Control and Prevention (CDC): Sexually transmitted diseases treatment guidelines, 2010. *MMWR Recomm Rep* 2010; 59(RR-12):1-110.

154

Antiviral Agents Against Respiratory Viruses

MICHAEL G. ISON | FREDERICK G. HAYDEN

KEY CONCEPTS

- Most circulating strains of influenza are resistant to amantadine and rimantadine.

- There are four approved neuraminidase inhibitors: laninamivir, oseltamivir, peramivir and zanamivir.

- All of the neuraminidase inhibitors have the greatest clinical impact if started within 24–48 hours of symptom onset.

- For hospitalized adults and children, anti-influenza therapy should be initiated as soon as influenza is considered and should not be delayed for confirmatory testing.

- Neuraminidase inhibitors appear to reduce morbidity and mortality among hospitalized adults and children when started up to 5 days, and possibly longer, after symptom onset.

- Aerosol ribavirin is approved for the treatment of respiratory syncytial virus (RSV) but has very limited clinical indications; oral ribavirin is part of a triple drug regimen for influenza undergoing testing.

- Several new antivirals are in advanced development for the treatment of respiratory viral infections including RSV, rhinovirus and adenovirus.

- Neutralizing antibodies in the form of convalescent plasma or monoclonals appear to be promising for treatment in novel influenza and coronavirus infections.

Introduction

Few antiviral drugs are currently approved for treating respiratory virus infections and most of these are specific inhibitors of influenza viruses (Table 154-1). However, considerable progress is being made in the development of new therapeutics for other respiratory viruses.[1] The emergence of new pathogens such as Middle East respiratory syndrome coronavirus (MERS-CoV) has also led to screening efforts to identify new therapeutics.[2,3] Clinical studies to examine novel targets (Table 154-1), combinations designed to increase potency and reduce resistance emergence, therapeutic antibodies, and immunomodulatory agents selected to mitigate immunopathologic host responses, particularly for influenza, are in progress.[4] Neutralizing antibodies have been proven effective for prevention of respiratory syncytial virus (RSV) disease, although not for treatment,[5] but specific neutralizing antibodies (convalescent plasma, monoclonals) appear to be promising for treating novel influenza and coronavirus infections. This chapter reviews the properties and clinical applications of currently approved antiviral agents.

M2 Inhibitors

Amantadine (Symmetrel) and rimantadine (Flumadine) are symmetric tricyclic amines that specifically inhibit the replication of influenza A viruses at low concentrations (<1.0 μg/mL) by blocking the action of the M2 protein (Figure 154-1).[7–9] Unfortunately, widespread resistance to all M2 inhibitors has been documented in circulating influenza A strains, and this class of agents is not currently recommended for the prevention or treatment of influenza.[6]

PHARMACOKINETICS AND DISTRIBUTION

Both drugs achieve peak levels 3-5 hours after ingestion (see detailed pharmacokinetic data in Table 154-2).[10–12] Amantadine is excreted unchanged by the kidney while rimantadine undergoes extensive metabolism by the liver before being excreted by the kidney; as a result, dose adjustment with renal dysfunction is required (Table 154-2).

ROUTE OF ADMINISTRATION AND DOSAGE

Amantadine and rimantadine come as 100 mg tablets and a syrup formulation (50 mg/5 mL). In adults, the usual dose for treatment or prevention of influenza A infection is 100 mg q12h for both drugs (see Table 154-2).

INDICATIONS

The current recommendations of the Centers for Disease Control and Prevention (CDC) and the World Health Organization (WHO) should be consulted before using this class clinically, including in infections by novel strains of influenza-like avian H5N1. A triple drug regimen (amantadine, ribavirin, oseltamivir) is currently under study for influenza A infections, including those due to adamantane-resistant strains.[6] When used against susceptible strains, both agents are 70–90% effective in preventing infection and reduce duration of fever and symptoms when used for treatment.[15–17] Dosage in special circumstances is summarized in Table 154-1.

ADVERSE REACTIONS AND INTERACTIONS

The most common side-effects of the M2 inhibitors are minor central nervous system (CNS) complaints (anxiety, difficulty concentrating, insomnia, dizziness, headache and jitteriness) and gastrointestinal upset, which are particularly prominent in the elderly and those with renal failure.[11] Patients who receive amantadine may develop antimuscarinic effects, orthostatic hypotension and congestive heart failure. Rates of adverse effects are lower for rimantadine than amantadine.[11,18] Given drug–drug interactions, care should be used when co-administering either agent with antihistamines or anticholinergic drugs, trimethoprim–sulfamethoxazole, triamterene–hydrochlorothiazide, quinine, quinidine, monoamine oxidase inhibitors, antidepressants and minor tranquilizers.[19]

RESISTANCE

Cross-resistance to both agents occurs as the result of single amino acid substitutions in the transmembrane portion of the M2 protein.[9] The resistant virus appears to retain wild-type pathogenicity and causes an influenza illness indistinguishable from susceptible strains. Resistance has emerged within 2–4 days after the start of therapy in up to 30% of patients infected with initially susceptible strains.[11] Emergence of resistant variants may be associated with protracted illness and shedding in immunocompromised hosts[20]; spread to contacts causes failures of antiviral prophylaxis in nursing homes and households.[11]

TABLE 154-1	Agents Used to Prevent and Treat Influenza[6]				
Class	**Drug**	**USUAL ADULT DOSAGE***		**Dose Adjustment State**	**Suggested Dosage**
		Prophylaxis	Treatment		
M2 inhibitor	Amantadine	100 mg q12h	100 mg q12h	Age 1–9 years (yr) CrCl 30–50 mL/min CrCl 15–30 mL/min CrCl 10–15 mL/min CrCl 10 mL/min Age ≥65 yr	5 mg/kg to max of 150 mg in two divided doses 100 mg q24h 100 mg q24h 100 mg q week 100 mg q week 100 mg q24h
	Rimantadine	100 mg q12h	100 mg q12h	Age 1–9 yr* CrCl <10 mL/min Severe hepatic dysfunction Age ≥65 yr	5 mg/kg to max of 150 mg in two divided doses 100 mg q24h 100 mg q24h 100 mg q24h
Neuraminidase inhibitor	Laninamivir	20 mg QD × 2 days	40 mg once	Age <10 yr	20 mg once
	Oseltamivir[†]	75 mg q24h	75 mg q12h	CrCl <30 mL/min[‡] ≤15 kg[§] 15–23 kg[§] 23–40 kg[§] >40 kg[§] Any weight, 2 weeks to <1 yr	Treatment: 75 mg q24h Prophylaxis: 75 mg every other day 30 mg q12h (5 mL[¶]) 45 mg q12h (7.5 mL[¶]) 60 mg q12h (10 mL[¶]) 75 mg q12h (12.5 mL[¶]) 3 mg/kg q12hr (0.5 mL/kg[¶])
	Peramivir	NA	300 mg once	For patients with severe infection Children 6–17 yr Children 180 days– 5 yr CrCl 31–49 mL/min[§] CrCl 10-30 mL/min[§] CrCl <10 mL/min Intermittent hemodialysis (HD) (dose on HD days only)	600 mg QD as a single or multi-dose regimen 10 mg/kg QD for 5 days (max of 600 mg QD) 12 mg/kg QD Adult: 150 mg QD Age 6–17 yr: 2.5 mg/kg QD[§] Age 180 days–5 yr: 3 mg/kg QD Adult: 100 mg QD Age 6–17 yr: 1.6 mg/kg QD[§] Age 180 days–5 yr: 1.9 mg/kg QD Adult: 100 mg on day 1 then 15 mg QD Age 6–17 yr: 1.6 mg/kg on day 1 then 0.25 mg/ kg QD Age 180 days–5 yr: 1.9 mg/kg on day 1 then 0.3 mg/kg ≥18 yr: 100 mg on day 1 then 100 mg 2 hours after HD Age 6–17 yr: 1.6 mg/kg on day 1 then 1.6 mg/kg 2 hours after HD Age 180 days–6 yr: 1.9 mg/kg on day 1 then 1.9 mg/kg 2 hours after HD
	Inhaled zanamivir[‖]	2 puffs (10 mg) twice a day for 5 days	2 puffs (10 mg) twice a day for 5 days	No dose adjustment needed	
	iv zanamivir	NA	600 mg q12h	Renal insufficiency	Loading dose (all patients): 600 mg Maintenance dosing based on CL$_{cr}$/CL$_{CRRT}$ values: 80–50 mL/min: 400 mg 30–50 mL/min: 250 mg 15–30 mL/min: 150 mg <15 mL/min: 60 mg The interval between the initial dose and the start of maintenance dosing by CL$_{cr}$/CL$_{CRRT}$: 15–30 mL/min: 24 hrs <15 mL/min: 48 hrs

Recommendations based on those provided by the Advisory Committee on Immunization Practices.[4]
*Duration of treatment is usually 5 days. Duration of prophylaxis depends on clinical setting.
[†]Oseltamivir is indicated for prophylaxis in children ≥1 year old and for treatment in children in ≥2 weeks of age.
[‡]No treatment or prophylaxis dosing recommendations are available for patients undergoing renal dialysis.
[§]Initial loading dose of 600 mg or age adjusted equivalent; maximum dose 600 mg QD.
[¶]Volume of suspension.
[‖]Zanamivir is indicated for prophylaxis in children ≥5 years old and for treatment in children ≥7 years old.
CL$_{cr}$/CL$_{CRRT}$: Ratio of creatinine clearance to continuous renal replacement therapy clearance.

Neuraminidase Inhibitors

Influenza A and B viruses possess a surface glycoprotein with neuraminidase activity whereas influenza C viruses do not (Figure 154-1). This enzyme cleaves terminal sialic acid residues from various glycoconjugates and destroys the receptors recognized by viral hemagglutinin. This activity is essential for release of virus from infected cells, for prevention of viral aggregates, and for viral spread within the respiratory tract.[21] Oseltamivir (Tamiflu®, a prodrug of the active carboxylate), laninamivir (Inavir®), peramivir (Rapiacta®, Peramiflu®)

TABLE 154-2	Pharmacokinetic Properties of Antivirals with Activity Against Influenza[11–14]							
Drug	Dose	Route	C_{max} (µg/L)	T_{max} (h)	$AUC_{0-12 h}$ (mg/mL•h)	$T_{1/2}$ (h)	Bioavailability (Oral, %)	Protein Binding (%)
Amantadine[5,6]*	200 mg 200 mg	Oral (young) Oral (elderly)	510 (140) 800 (200)	2.1 (1) 2.2 (2.1)	10.2 (3.4) 17.6 (6.5)	14.4 (6) 19 (9.1)	62–93 54–100	67
Rimantadine[5,6]*	200 mg 200 mg	Oral (young) Oral (elderly)	240 (70) 250 (50)	4.6 (2.1) 4.0 (2.4)	9.8 (4.5) 11.5 (3.0)	36.5 (17.3) 36.5 (14.5)	75–93 NA	40
Laninamivir	40 mg	Inhaled	NA	NA	NA	3	~15	NA
Oseltamivir[8]*	100 mg q12h 100 mg q12h	Oral (18–55 years) Oral (≥65 years)	439 (40.8) 575 (83.8)	3.5 (1) 3.5 (1.4)	3.85 (0.6) 4.94 (1.0)	6–10 –	79 –	42
Peramivir	600 mg	Intravenous	46.8	NA	102.7	20	NA	<30
Zanamivir[7]†	16 mg 16 mg	Inhaled Inhaled	29 (23–69) 54 (34–96)	0.75 (0.08–2) 0.75 (0.25–1)	0.03 (0.02–0.06) 0.16 (0.02–0.32)	3.6 (2.2–9.4) –	4–17 4–17	10

C_{max}, maximum serum drug concentration; T_{max}, time to C_{max}; $T_{1/2}$, serum elimination half-life; AUC, area under the curve for serum drug concentration versus time for the dose interval; bioavailability, percentage of intravenous C_{max}.
*Values are mean (SD).
†Values are median (range).

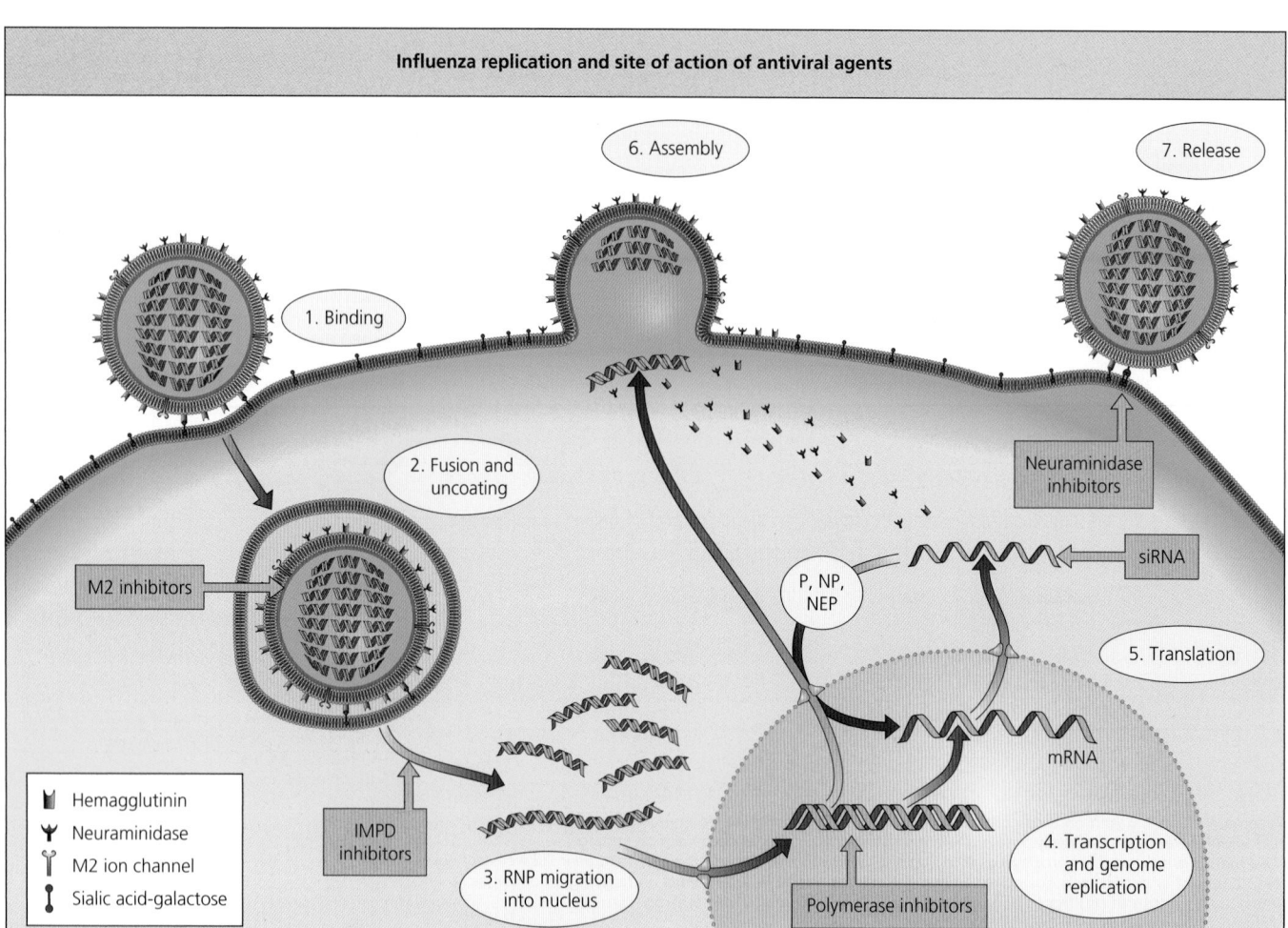

Figure 154-1 Influenza replication and site of action of antiviral agents. IMPD, inosine monophosphate dehydrogenase; NEP, nuclear export protein; NP, nucleoprotein; P, polymerase; RNP, ribonuclear protein; siRNA, small inhibitory ribonucleic acid. (*Reprinted from Beigel J, Bray M. Current and future antiviral therapy of severe seasonal and avian influenza. Antiviral Res 2008; 78:91–102.*)

and zanamivir (Relenza®) are sialic acid analogs that potently and specifically inhibit influenza A and B neuraminidases by competitively and reversibly interacting with the active enzyme site.[22,23] These drugs are active against all nine influenza neuraminidase subtypes in nature. Oseltamivir and zanamivir are globally available, while laninamivir is approved in Japan and peramivir is approved in China, Japan, South Korea and the USA.

Laninamivir
PHARMACOKINETICS AND DISTRIBUTION
Laninamivir octanoate (CS-8958) is a prodrug that is converted in the airway to laninamivir (R-125489), the active neuraminidase inhibitor and is retained at concentrations that exceed the IC_{50} for most influenza neuraminidases for at least 240 hours (10 days) after a single inhalation of 40 mg.[24] Only 15% of the drug is systemically absorbed after inhalation. Laninamivir has excellent *in vitro* activity against wild-type influenza A and B viruses currently circulating, including those H1N1 viruses containing H275Y mutations in the neuraminidase.

ROUTE OF ADMINISTRATION AND DOSAGE
Laninamivir octanoate (CS-8958) is currently only approved in Japan and is available as a 20 mg dry powder inhaler. It is undergoing clinical investigation outside of Japan at present.

INDICATIONS
Prophylaxis
Laninamivir is approved for the prevention of influenza in adults and children ≥ 10 years of age; a single inhalation of 20 mg daily for 2 days is recommended for this indication. Among household contacts of an index patient with influenza, 2 and 3 days of laninamivir 20 mg daily was associated with a 77% and 78% protective efficacy, respectively, compared with placebo.[25]

Treatment
Laninamivir is approved for the treatment and prevention of influenza A and B infection in Japan. For treatment, laninamivir is approved as a single inhalation of 40 mg for individuals ≥10 years of age and 20 mg for children less than 10 years of age. Laninamivir was associated with more rapid time to alleviation of influenza illness due to infections by seasonal H1N1 virus with the H275Y substitution in children compared to a standard 5-day oseltamivir regimen, while studies in adults demonstrated noninferiority versus oseltamivir in such patients.[26,27] Laninamivir demonstrates a similar duration of fever in ambulatory children when compared to patients treated with zanamivir.[28,29]

Dosage in Special Circumstances
No dose adjustment is currently indicated in any patient population.

Adverse Reactions and Interactions
Clinical studies in Asia found similar rates of nausea in laninamivir octanoate- and oseltamivir- treated patients, lower rates of vomiting in the laninamivir octanoate arm, and similar to slightly higher rates of diarrhea in laninamivir octanoate arms.[26,27] Dizziness was seen in 0.9–1.8% of laninamivir octanoate-treated patients but not oseltamivir-treated patients.[26] Laninamivir was not associated with significant bronchospasm or other respiratory adverse effects in patients with chronic respiratory disease.[30]

Oseltamivir
PHARMACOKINETICS AND DISTRIBUTION
Oral oseltamivir ethyl ester is well absorbed and rapidly cleaved by esterases in the gastrointestinal tract, liver or blood. The bioavailability of the active metabolite, oseltamivir carboxylate, is estimated to be ~80% in previously healthy persons (see Table 154-3).[13] The plasma elimination half-life is 6–10 hours but is more prolonged in the elderly, although dose adjustments are not generally necessary. Administration with food appears to decrease the risk of gastrointestinal upset without

decreasing bioavailability. Both the prodrug and parent are eliminated primarily unchanged through the kidney by glomerular filtration and anionic tubular secretion. The dose should be reduced by half for patients with a creatinine clearance less than 30 mL/min, and further reductions when clearance is below 10 mL/min.[31] Distribution is not well characterized in humans, but peak bronchoalveolar lavage, middle ear fluid and sinus fluid levels are similar to plasma levels.[13] Recent data suggest that significant relationships exist between oseltamivir carboxylate AUC_{0-24} and area under the curve (AUC) of symptom scores, time to alleviation of composite symptom scores, and time to cessation of viral shedding in experimentally infected volunteers.[32]

ROUTE OF ADMINISTRATION AND DOSAGE
Oseltamivir is available for oral delivery only. Oseltamivir comes as 30, 45, and 75 mg tablets and as a white tutti-frutti-flavored suspension (360 mg oseltamivir base for a final concentration of 6 mg/mL). The approved adult dose for treatment is 75 mg twice daily for 5 days and for prophylaxis is 75 mg once daily. Pediatric dosing is based on weight and is outlined in Table 154-2.

INDICATIONS
Prophylaxis
Oseltamivir is indicated for the prevention of influenza infection in patients ≥1 year, with dosing once a day. The efficacy of once-daily oseltamivir 75 mg for 6 weeks in preventing influenza illness in healthy, nonimmunized adults was 84% and in preventing influenza infection irrespective of symptoms was 50%.[13] In immunized nursing home residents, the efficacy of prophylaxis was 92% against illness compared to placebo.[23] Somewhat lower efficacy was seen in a household-contact prophylaxis study, and protection against influenza has been shown in children.[33] Seasonal prophylaxis of high-risk immunocompromised patients was documented to provide ~80% protective efficacy against RT-PCR-confirmed influenza illness.[34] Caution should be used when prescribing oseltamivir for prophylaxis in patients exposed to an index case as prophylaxis has been associated with emergence of resistant mutants;[35] empiric therapy or monitoring is generally recommended in these cases as a result.

Postexposure prophylaxis in nursing home influenza outbreaks is advised for 14 days or for at least 7 days after the last culture-confirmed illness in the ward or building is effective; this regimen should be given with concomitant influenza vaccination for those not previously provided. Seasonal prophylaxis, during the 4–8 weeks of peak influenza virus circulation within the community, can be used for protection of high-risk patients who cannot tolerate immunization, who do not develop an adequate immune response to vaccine, or when the strain circulating in the community does not match the vaccine strain.

Treatment
Oseltamivir 75 mg twice daily for 5 days when started within the first 2 days of symptoms was associated with a shorter time to alleviation of uncomplicated influenza illness (29–35 hours shorter) and with reductions in severity of illness, duration of fever, time to return to normal activity, quantity of viral shedding, duration of impaired activity, and complications leading to antibiotic use, particularly bronchitis, compared to placebo in previously healthy adults.[6,16,36] One recent study in Bangladesh suggests that oseltamivir may have efficacy up to 72 hours after symptom onset in children.[37] Pediatric studies enrolling children as young as 2 weeks of age demonstrated that oseltamivir is safe and is associated with significantly reduced illness duration and severity, time to resumption of full activities, and the occurrence of complications leading to antibiotic use, particularly acute otitis media.[38–42] Most existing literature on the safety and efficacy of oseltamivir in elderly or high-risk persons, including those with underlying cardiopulmonary conditions or immunodeficiency comes from observational studies[43–46] and suggests that among such high risk and hospitalized individuals, there is a benefit to starting antiviral therapy through at least 5 days after symptom onset with the greatest benefit in patients started within 48 hours after symptom onset.[47]

TABLE 154-3	Summary of Antiviral Agents in Advanced Clinical Development for Respiratory Viruses					
Drug	Spectrum	Target of Antiviral Action	Antiviral Resistance in Clinical Isolates	Route of Dosing	Pharmacokinetic Properties	Principal Adverse Effects	Clinical Effectiveness
Zanamivir	Influenza A + B	Enzymatic action of viral NA	Rare	iv	Renal excretion with plasma elimination half-life of ~2 hrs; dose adjustment required for renal insufficiency	iv delivery avoids bronchospasm risk with aerosol treatment	Significant antiviral effects in severely ill A(H1N1)pdm09-infected patients not responding to oseltamivir.
Favipiravir/ T-705	Influenza A, B, C and other RNA viruses	Influenza RNA polymerase; lethal mutagenesis	Not reported to date	Oral	Intracellular ribosylation and phosphorylation to its active triphosphate form. Good oral bioavailability; parent compound metabolized to inactive moiety by and also inhibitor of aldehyde oxidase >65% renally excreted as metabolite by 48 hrs	Dose-related hyperuricemia; teratogenic in preclinical testing – restricted use in pregnancy	BID dosing regimen more effective than TID regimen. Approved in Japan for use in novel or drug-resistant influenza infections. No data from severe influenza
DAS181	Influenza A + B, PIV	Host cell receptor for viral HA. Sialidase removes both the human-like a2,6- and avian-like a2,3-linked sialic acids from cellular receptors	Not reported to date	Inhaled	In ex vivo human airway epithelium and human bronchial tissue, the inhibitory effect of DAS181 treatment lasts ≥2 days. Tracheobronchial delivery and degree of systemic absorption dependent on particle size	Elevated alkaline phosphatase due to reduced clearance, no associated increases in transaminases	Reduced pharyngeal influenza virus detection but little clinical benefit in treating uncomplicated influenza; unstudied in serious influenza. Case reports of antiviral effectiveness and clinical improvement in serious PIV illness in transplant recipients; RCT in progress
Nitazoxanide	A + B and other RNA viruses	Influenza HA maturation; possible immune-modulatory and other antiviral mechanism of action	Not reported to date	Oral	Metabolized by plasma esterases to its active desacetyl derivative tizoxanide, which undergoes glucuronidation and urinary elimination with elimination half-life of ~7 hrs. Tizoxanide is highly bound by (>99%) plasma proteins. Need for dose adjustments uncertain	GI; respiratory distress	Shorter duration of viral replication and illness compared to placebo in phase 2 RCT in uncomplicated influenza; evidence for clinical benefit in influenza-like illness without detectable virus by RT-PCR
VX-787	Influenza A	Influenza RNA polymerase	Common	Oral		Not reported	Antiviral efficacy and associated reduction in illness measures in experimentally infected volunteers; no studies in natural influenza reported to date
AVI-7100	Influenza A	M1 (matrix) and M2 (ion channel) genes	Not reported	iv	Phosphorodiamidate morpholino oligomer with three modified linkages; active after topical or iv dosing in ferrets	Not reported	Phase 1 study of iv formulation in progress

Agent	Virus	Target	Route	Resistance	Class/comments	Adverse effects	Clinical status
Brincidofovir (CMX-001)	Adenovirus, other DNA viruses	Viral DNA polymerase	Oral	Infrequent	Infrequent dosing (weekly or bi-weekly) possible due to high intracellular concentration and long intracellular half-life (up to 4-6.5 days) of the active antiviral cidofovir-diphosphate	Diarrhea, other GI symptoms; transaminase elevations	Antiviral effects in case series of transplant recipients intolerant of or failing cidofovir for serious adenovirus infection and with bi-weekly dosing in RCT for pre-emptive treatment of adenoviremia; follow-up RCT in progress
GS-5806	RSV	F protein-fusion	Oral	Not reported but common in preclinical studies with other fusion inhibitors	Fusion inhibitor	Limited clinical data	Protective effects in experimentally infected volunteers; placebo-controlled RCTs in progress for treating elderly hospitalized with RSV and for transplant recipients with upper or lower respiratory illness due to RSV
ALS-8176	RSV	Polymerase	Oral	Not reported	Nucleoside analog	Not reported	Phase 1 studies in healthy adults completed; phase 2 in progress
MDT-637 (formerly VP-14637)	RSV	F protein-fusion	Inhaled	Not reported but common in preclinical studies with other fusion inhibitors	Fusion inhibitor	Not reported	Phase 1 studies up to 10 days dosing in healthy adults completed
ALN-RSV01	RSV	Nucleocapsid gene	Inhaled	Not reported	Small interfering RNA	Generally well-tolerated in studies to date	Protective against RSV infection in experimental human RSV challenge. Two placebo-controlled phase 2 RCTs in RSV-infected lung transplant patients found reduced incidence of new or progressive BOS

Note: this table summarizes small molecular weight inhibitors in active clinical development and does not include combinations, biologics like therapeutic antibodies, or immunomodulators.
Abbreviations: BOS, bronchiolitis obliterans syndrome; CNS, central nervous system; GI, gastrointestinal; HA, hemagglutinin; NA, neuraminidase; NAI, neuraminidase inhibitor; PIV, parainfluenza virus; RCT, randomized, controlled trial.

All of the studies in hospitalized adults suggest that early therapy is associated with reduced incidence of lower respiratory tract complications, requirement for ICU-level care, duration of illness, duration of shedding and mortality.[6,16,45,46,48]

DOSAGE IN SPECIAL CIRCUMSTANCES

The usual oseltamivir dose should be reduced to 75 mg once a day for treatment and 75 mg every other day or 30 mg of suspension daily for prophylaxis when a patient has a creatinine clearance of <30 mL/min. Doses of oseltamivir should be given after hemodialysis; detailed dosing for renal insufficiency and renal replacement therapy is available in Table 154-3. The safety and pharmacokinetics in patients with hepatic impairment have not been evaluated. Several studies in pregnancy suggest that oseltamivir is likely safe and provides clear therapeutic benefit to pregnant women infected with influenza.[49–51] There are conflicting data about optimal dosing of oseltamivir in pregnant women, with some studies suggesting need for higher doses (75 mg TID), while others suggest no dose adjustment is needed.[52–54] Current guidelines recommend treating pregnant women with influenza infection with one of the approved neuraminidase inhibitors. The recommended pediatric dosage is listed in Table 154-2.

Doubling the treatment dose of oseltamivir in hospitalized influenza patients does not appear to increase virologic efficacy, except perhaps for influenza B infections, or clinical effectiveness, although one ICU-based RCT reported that tripling the standard dose was associated with acceleration of viral RNA clearance from the respiratory tract.[55–57]

ADVERSE REACTIONS AND INTERACTIONS

Oral oseltamivir is generally well tolerated and no serious end-organ toxicity has been found in controlled clinical trials. Oseltamivir is associated with nausea, abdominal discomfort and, less often, emesis in a minority of treated patients. Nausea and vomiting occur at approximately 10–15% excess frequency in oseltamivir recipients. Gastrointestinal complaints are typically mild-to-moderate in intensity, usually resolve despite continued dosing, and are ameliorated by administration with food. Clinical studies comparing 75 mg and 150 mg twice daily found similar frequencies of adverse events with the two doses. Other infrequent possible adverse events include insomnia, vertigo and fever. Postmarketing reports suggest that oseltamivir may be associated rarely with skin rash, hepatic dysfunction or thrombocytopenia. Additionally, there have been reports of abnormal neurologic and behavioral symptoms which have rarely resulted in deaths among mostly children; most of these reports have come from Japan. Existing data suggest that these events are more likely secondary to influenza infections than oseltamivir therapy.[58,59] It is currently recommended that patients be monitored closely for behavioral abnormalities.

No clinically significant drug interactions have been recognized to date, including studies with amoxicillin, aspirin and acetaminophen. No interactions with the cytochrome P450 enzymes occur *in vitro* and oseltamivir does not affect steady-state pharmacokinetics of commonly used immunosuppressive agents.[60] However, probenecid blocks tubular secretion and doubles the half-life of oseltamivir. Protein binding is below 10%. Oseltamivir does not affect the immunogenicity of concomitant inactivated virus vaccine but might impair the immunogenicity of concurrent live-attenuated intranasal influenza vaccine.

Peramivir
PHARMACOKINETICS AND DISTRIBUTION

Peramivir has low oral bioavailability and is therefore delivered intravenously. Peramivir achieves exceptionally high maximum concentrations (~45 000 ng/mL after 600 mg intravenous dose) with excellent concentrations of drug in the nasal and pharyngeal secretions.[61] Peramivir is predominately eliminated unchanged by renal excretion with a plasma terminal elimination half-life of 12–25 hours.[41,62] Peramivir

has comparable or lower activity *in vitro* against influenza A and B viruses than oseltamivir carboxylate and zanamivir.[63]

ROUTE OF ADMINISTRATION AND DOSAGE

Peramivir is available in 150 mg and 300 mg solutions for intravenous use.

INDICATIONS

Peramivir randomized clinical trials have been conducted in previously healthy adults and children infected with uncomplicated influenza. When compared to placebo, a single 300–600 mg infusion of peramivir was associated with a significantly shorter time to alleviation of symptoms, significantly shorter time to resumption of their usual activities, and more rapid clearance of virus.[64] Another study found that a single 300–600 mg infusion of peramivir was noninferior to 5 days of oral oseltamivir 75 mg BID in a season when many of the viruses were resistant to oseltamivir as the result of the H275Y mutation; these data question the efficacy of peramivir in the management of viruses with the H275Y mutation.[65] In a study comparing 5 days of 200 mg or 400 mg QD of peramivir with oral oseltamivir 75 mg BID in hospitalized adults, there was a trend toward more rapid resumption of usual activities in peramivir-treated patients and greater reductions of influenza B viral titers in the nasopharynx than oseltamivir over the first 48 h.

DOSAGE IN SPECIAL CIRCUMSTANCES

Since peramivir is renally cleared, dosing must be adjusted based on renal function (see Table 154-3). There are limited data to guide dosing of peramivir in children, particularly among neonates.[66] Available data and models suggest that patients receiving intermittent hemodialysis need dose adjustment (see Table 154-3).[66] Dosing of patients on continuous renal replacement therapy (CRRT) should be based on CRRT clearance.[67] There is limited dosing information for patients on extracorporeal membrane oxygenation (ECMO). Based on modeling data and predicted drug concentrations, it is recommended that children ≥181 days and ≤ 5 years receive 12 mg/kg daily (daily maximum of 600 mg/dose), infants 91–180 days receive 10 mg/kg daily, infants 31–90 days receive 8 mg/kg daily, and neonates ≤30 days receive 6 mg/kg daily. No dose adjustments are needed for hepatic impairment.

ADVERSE REACTIONS AND INTERACTIONS

Recognized adverse events associated with the administration of peramivir are diarrhea, nausea, vomiting, and neutrophil count decreased; other less common adverse events observed in studies to date include dizziness, headache, somnolence, nervousness, insomnia, feeling agitated, depression, nightmares, hyperglycemia, hyperbilirubinemia, elevated blood pressure, cystitis, ECG abnormalities, anorexia, and proteinuria.[68]

Zanamivir
PHARMACOKINETICS AND DISTRIBUTION

The oral bioavailability of zanamivir is low (<5%), and most clinical trials have used intranasal or dry powder inhalation delivery. Following inhalation of the dry powder, approximately 7–21% is deposited in the lower respiratory tract and the remainder in the oropharynx.[14,69] Median zanamivir concentrations are above 1000 ng/mL in induced sputum 6 hours after inhalation and remain detectable up to 24 hours later. The peak plasma concentration averages 46 µg/L after a single 16 mg inhalation of zanamivir. The proprietary inhaler device for delivering zanamivir is breath-actuated and requires a cooperative patient.[70]

Intravenous zanamivir displays linear dosing kinetics and the volume of distribution is approximately equivalent to that of extracellular water (16L).[14] Intravenous zanamivir provides high peak plasma concentrations (~35 000 ng/mL after 600 mg dose in adults).[71] 90% of the drug is excreted unchanged in the urine with an elimination half-life of approximately 2 hours. Intravenous zanamivir clearance is highly correlated with renal function (CL ≅ 7.08 + 0.826 · CLCR).[72]

ROUTE OF ADMINISTRATION AND DOSAGE

Zanamivir is delivered by inhalation with a proprietary breath-activated device (Diskhaler®). The usual adult treatment dose is two inhalations (10 mg) twice a day for 5 days. Intravenous zanamivir is currently in advanced clinical development and available by compassionate use.

INDICATIONS

Prophylaxis

Zanamivir is indicated as once-daily inhalations for the prevention of influenza in patients >5 years old. Once-daily inhaled zanamivir for 4 weeks was 84% efficacious in preventing laboratory-confirmed illness with fever and 31% effective in preventing influenza infections, irrespective of symptoms.[69] When used for postexposure prophylaxis, inhaled zanamivir for 10 days reduced the risk of secondary influenza illness by 79% in households.[69] In nursing homes experiencing influenza outbreaks, inhaled zanamivir was more effective for prevention of influenza A illness than oral rimantadine, in part because of frequent resistance emergence to the M2 inhibitor.[69]

Treatment

In the USA, zanamivir is indicated for the treatment of uncomplicated acute illness due to influenza A and B viruses in adults and pediatric patients 7 years and older who have been symptomatic for no more than 2 days.[9] Inhaled zanamivir in adults has consistently shown at least 1 fewer day of disabling influenza symptoms, and most studies have found a reduction in the number of nights of disturbed sleep, in time to resumption of normal activities, and in the use of symptom relief medications.[6,16] Similar therapeutic benefits have also been shown in children aged 5–12 years old.[73] Zanamivir has also been associated with a 40% reduction in lower respiratory tract complications of influenza leading to antibiotics, particularly bronchitis and pneumonia.[74] Zanamivir appears generally well tolerated and effective in treating influenza in patients with mild-to-moderate asthma or, less often, chronic obstructive pulmonary disease.[74,75]

Intravenous zanamivir is in advanced clinical development and has been used in seriously ill influenza patients, especially those with suspected oseltamivir-resistant variants. Most of the emergency IND (eIND) use of intravenous zanamivir were in patients who were clinically failing other antiviral therapy with at least 25% of patients having proven or clinically suspected resistance to oseltamivir.[76] Available data from patients who were treated under eIND demonstrated that among those with reported outcomes, 10.5% died despite therapy.[76] A phase 2 study in critically ill pandemic 2009 H1N1 patients found that treatment was associated with significant antiviral effects, even though therapy was initiated a median of 4.5 days after symptom onset. In patients with influenza detected on initial sample, 2 days of therapy was associated with a median 1.42 $\log_{10}$ copies/mL decline in viral load.[71] There were no drug-related trends in safety parameters identified. The 14- and 28-day all-cause mortality rates were 13% and 17%, respectively.[71] A phase 3 study comparing iv zanamivir and oral oseltamivir in hospitalized adults is currently in progress.

DOSAGE IN SPECIAL CIRCUMSTANCES

Although the plasma elimination half-life increases with creatinine clearance ≤70 mL/min, drug accumulation is negligible after inhalation and dose adjustment is not necessary for renal or hepatic dysfunction. Certain populations, particularly very young, frail or cognitively impaired patients, may have difficulty using the drug delivery system.[70]

Intravenous zanamivir requires dose adjustment for renal insufficiency. All patients should receive an initial 600 mg loading dose. The maintenance dose and dosing interval are reduced with worsening renal function (see Table 154-2).[71,72]

ADVERSE REACTIONS AND INTERACTIONS

Topically applied zanamivir is generally well tolerated in controlled studies, including those involving patients with asthma and chronic obstructive pulmonary disease.[75] Postmarketing reports indicate that bronchospasm may be an uncommon but potentially severe problem, particularly in patients with acute influenza and underlying reactive airway disease.[6] Anecdotal reports of hospitalization and fatality indicate that inhaled zanamivir should be used cautiously in such patients.[6]

Low bioavailability is associated with low exposure to circulating zanamivir, and no clinically significant drug interactions have been recognized. In vitro studies suggest that zanamivir does not inhibit or induce cytochrome P450 enzymes. The drug does not affect the immunogenicity of concomitant immunization with inactivated virus vaccines but effects on intranasal, live-attenuated vaccine have not been studied. One randomized control trial in ambulatory adults found that the combination of inhaled zanamivir and oral oseltamivir was less effective than oseltamivir monotherapy.[77] Zanamivir is not associated with teratogenic effects in preclinical studies (FDA pregnancy category C) and should be considered as an option in pregnant women with proven influenza.[78]

NEURAMINIDASE INHIBITOR RESISTANCE

Neuraminidase inhibitor resistance in vitro results from mutations in the viral hemagglutinin and/or neuraminidase.[79,80] In the hemagglutinin variants, mutations in or near the receptor binding site make the virus less dependent on neuraminidase action, whereas neuraminidase mutations directly affect interaction with the inhibitors. The altered neuraminidases typically show reduced activity or stability, and the mutated viruses usually have decreased infectivity in animals.[79,80] The particular neuraminidase mutation determines the degree of resistance and cross-resistance (i.e. H275Y cause high-level resistance to oseltamivir but not zanamivir; R292K results in reduced susceptibility to both oseltamivir and zanamivir).[79,80] Oseltamivir-resistant variants have been recovered from <1% of treated adults and about 4% of treated children.[22] Assessment for resistance can be assessed by sequencing of the HA or NA gene or phenotypic testing.[79,80]

Ribavirin

Ribavirin (Virazole®, Rebetol®) is a guanosine analog with a wide range of antiviral activity including influenza viruses, RSV and parainfluenza viruses. Ribavirin is rapidly phosphorylated by intracellular enzymes and the triphosphate inhibits influenza virus RNA polymerase activity and competitively inhibits the guanosine triphosphate-dependent 5′-capping of influenza viral messenger RNA. In addition, ribavirin depletes cellular guanine pools[81,82] and may inhibit virus replication by lethal mutagenesis.

PHARMACOKINETICS AND DISTRIBUTION

Oral ribavirin has a bioavailability of 33–45% in adults and children and achieves peak plasma concentration of 0.6 µg/mL 1–2 hours after ingestion of a 400 mg dose in adults. Ribavirin has a short initial (0.3–0.7 hour) and a long terminal (18–36 hours) phase half-life and is eliminated by hepatic metabolism and renal clearance.[83] After aerosol administration, plasma levels increase with exposure and range from 0.2 to 1 µg/mL. Respiratory secretions have levels up to 1000 µg/mL, which decline with a half-life of 1.4–2.5 hours.

ROUTE OF ADMINISTRATION AND DOSAGE

Ribavirin comes in three formulations: oral (approved for combined use in hepatitis C), intravenous (investigational in USA) and aerosol. Ribavirin for aerosolization is available as a 6 g/100 mL solution which is diluted to a final concentration of 20 mg/mL and delivered by small particle aerosol for 12–18 hours with a proprietary device (SPAG-2 nebulizer). A higher concentration of aerosol solution (60 mg/mL) has been given over 2 hours three times daily in some studies and appears well tolerated.[84] Ribavirin also comes in 200 mg tablets and sterile solution for injection.

INDICATIONS

Ribavirin aerosol is currently indicated for the treatment of severe RSV in children. Trials of aerosolized ribavirin for the treatment of severe RSV infection in infants have shown no consistent effect on duration of hospitalization time, mortality or on pulmonary functions.[85] Current guidelines recommend that aerosolized ribavirin be considered in the treatment of high-risk infants and young children, as defined by congenital heart disease, chronic lung disease, immunodeficiency states, prematurity and age <6 weeks, as well as for those hospitalized with severe illness.[85] Aerosolized ribavirin has shown minimal efficacy in treating influenza in hospitalized children.[86]

Ribavirin has also been studied for the treatment of RSV and parainfluenza virus infections in immunocompromised patients. Intravenous ribavirin appears to be ineffective in reducing RSV-associated mortality in hematopoietic stem cell transplant (HSCT) patients with RSV pneumonia; there may be benefit among lung transplant recipients.[87] Aerosolized ribavirin may provide benefit in selected patient groups with less severe RSV disease. Survival was improved when treatment was started before respiratory failure or when infection was limited to the upper respiratory tract.[88] Observational studies suggest that combination therapy with antibodies (either intravenous immunoglobulin, RespiGam or palivizumab) appears more effective, particularly when started before severe respiratory distress.[88] Oral ribavirin has been tried in the management of RSV with variable success.[89] In the management of parainfluenza virus in bone marrow transplant recipients, two case series found that aerosolized ribavirin failed to improve 30-day mortality or reduce the duration of viral replication relative to no treatment.[90]

DOSAGE IN SPECIAL CIRCUMSTANCES

Systemic ribavirin is contraindicated in patients with creatinine clearance <50 mL/min and the dose should be reduced by one-third for patients under 10 years of age. Dose adjustment is needed if there is a substantial decline in hematocrit and the drug should be discontinued if the hemoglobin drops below 8.5 g/dL. There is a fixed combination of oseltamivir, amantadine and ribavirin that is active *in vitro* against susceptible and resistant strains and shows promise in clinical management of influenza infections.[91,92]

ADVERSE REACTIONS AND INTERACTIONS

Systemic ribavirin can cause a dose-related extravascular hemolytic anemia and, at higher doses, suppression of bone marrow release of erythroid elements. Aerosolized ribavirin can cause bronchospasm, mild conjunctival irritation, rash, psychological distress if administered in an oxygen tent and, rarely, acute water intoxication. Bolus intravenous administration may cause rigors. Antagonism of both drugs may occur when ribavirin is combined with zidovudine. Ribavirin is contraindicated in pregnant women and in male partners of women who are pregnant because of teratogenicity of the drug. Pregnancy should be avoided during therapy and for 6 months after completion of therapy in both female patients and in female partners of male patients taking ribavirin (pregnancy category X).

References available online at expertconsult.com.

KEY REFERENCES

Aoki F.Y., Sitar D.S.: Clinical pharmacokinetics of amantadine hydrochloride. *Clin Pharmacokinet* 1988; 14:35-51.

Duval X., van der Werf S., Blanchon T., et al.: Efficacy of oseltamivir-zanamivir combination compared to each monotherapy for seasonal influenza: a randomized placebo-controlled trial. *PLoS Med* 2010; 7:e1000362.

Fiore A.E., Fry A., Shay D., et al.: Antiviral agents for the treatment and chemoprophylaxis of influenza – recommendations of the Advisory Committee on Immunization Practices (ACIP). *MMWR Recomm Rep/CDC* 2011; 60:1-24.

Hayden F.G.: Advances in antivirals for non-influenza respiratory virus infections. *Influenza Other Respir Viruses* 2013; 7(Suppl. 3):36-43.

Ison M.G., Szakaly P., Shapira M.Y., et al.: Efficacy and safety of oral oseltamivir for influenza prophylaxis in transplant recipients. *Antivir Ther* 2012; 17:955-964.

Kaiser L., Keene O.N., Hammond J.M., et al.: Impact of zanamivir on antibiotic use for respiratory events following acute influenza in adolescents and adults. *Arch Intern Med* 2000; 160:3234-3240.

Keyser L.A., Karl M., Nafziger A.N., et al.: Comparison of central nervous system adverse effects of amantadine and rimantadine used as sequential prophylaxis of influenza A in elderly nursing home patients. *Arch Intern Med* 2000; 160:1485-1488.

Kimberlin D.W., Acosta E.P., Prichard M.N., et al.: Oseltamivir pharmacokinetics, dosing, and resistance among children aged <2 years with influenza. *J Infect Dis* 2013; 207:709-720.

Lee N., Ison M.G.: Editorial commentary. 'Late' treatment with neuraminidase inhibitors for severely ill patients with influenza: better late than never? *Clin Infect Dis* 2012; 55:1205-1208.

Louie J.K., Yang S., Acosta M., et al.: Treatment with neuraminidase inhibitors for critically ill patients with influenza A (H1N1)pdm09. *Clin Infect Dis* 2012; 55:1198-1204.

Marty F.M., Man C.Y., van der Horst C., et al.: Safety and pharmacokinetics of intravenous zanamivir treatment in hospitalized adults with influenza: an open-label, multi-center, single-arm, phase II study. *J Infect Dis* 2014; 209:542-550.

Nguyen H.T., Fry A.M., Gubareva L.V.: Neuraminidase inhibitor resistance in influenza viruses and laboratory testing methods. *Antivir Ther* 2012; 17:159-173.

Nguyen J.T., Smee D.F., Barnard D.L., et al.: Efficacy of combined therapy with amantadine, oseltamivir, and ribavirin in vivo against susceptible and amantadine-resistant influenza A viruses. *PLoS ONE* 2012; 7:e31006.

Shah J.N., Chemaly R.F.: Management of RSV infections in adult recipients of hematopoietic stem cell transplantation. *Blood* 2011; 117:2755-2763.

South East Asia Infectious Disease Clinical Research N: Effect of double dose oseltamivir on clinical and virological outcomes in children and adults admitted to hospital with severe influenza: double blind randomised controlled trial. *BMJ* 2013; 346:f3039.

Yamashita M.: Laninamivir and its prodrug, CS-8958: long-acting neuraminidase inhibitors for the treatment of influenza. *Antivir Chem Chemoth* 2010; 21:71-84.

155

Drugs to Treat Viral Hepatitis

LEAH A. BURKE | KRISTEN M. MARKS

KEY CONCEPTS

- Nucleoside and nucleotide analogs, which inhibit the hepatitis B virus (HBV) DNA polymerase, are the mainstays of chronic HBV therapy.

- Monotherapy with a single antiviral agent is unlikely to be sufficient for the eradication of HBV infection in the majority of patients who are chronically infected. However, studies of combinations of current HBV monotherapies have not consistently demonstrated an advantage over monotherapy.

- Oral direct-acting antiviral agents (DAAs), which inhibit various stages of the hepatitis C virus (HCV) life cycle, have become standard of care for the treatment of hepatitis C.

- Treatment with DAAs has greater efficacy than the combination of interferon and ribavirin and results in cure of HCV infection for the majority of patients.

- Interferon has fallen out of favor for the treatment of both hepatitis B (HBV) and hepatitis C (HCV) virus infections due to its potential for adverse effects, route of administration and efficacy profile.

Introduction

Tremendous progress in the treatment of viral hepatitis has been made over the past two decades, and the next several years hold similar promise. This chapter describes the mechanism of action, pharmacokinetics, indications and safety of drugs used for the treatment of chronic hepatitis B and C infections (in chronological order of approval by the United States Food and Drug Administration). Diagnosis, management, vaccination, and prevention strategies are discussed elsewhere (see Chapters 42 and 165, and Practice Points 31 and 32).

Oral nucleoside or nucleotide analog therapies now represent standard initial treatment for chronic hepatitis B infection, while interferon is used less commonly. Chronic hepatitis C infection is now treated with direct-acting antivirals (DAAs) that target the steps of the viral life cycle. In certain scenarios, DAAs may still be combined with ribavirin and/or pegylated (Peg)-interferon. As no targeted treatments exist for hepatitis A or E infections, they will not be discussed.

Chronic Hepatitis B Virus (HBV) Infection

Interferons

Interferons (IFNs) are naturally occurring proteins produced by eukaryotic cells that function as cytokines in an early response to viral infection. Interferons do not have direct antiviral activity, but instead induce an antiviral state and activate other immune functions. There are type I (IFN-α and -β) and type II (IFN-γ) interferons. The pharmaceuticals are termed 'IFN-alfa'. IFN-alfa can effectively inhibit HCV subgenomic RNA replication and suppress viral nonstructural protein synthesis via intracellular gene activation. Two pegylated varieties of IFN are available for subcutaneous (sc) injection, and their usage has, for the most part, replaced standard interferon. Peg-IFN alfa-2b by sc

injection has a half-life ($t\frac{1}{2}$) of 40 hours. Peg-IFN alfa-2a has a $t\frac{1}{2}$ of 80 hours. Dosages vary according to the specific preparation and indication (Table 155-1).

IFN-alfa-2a and Peg-IFN alfa-2b are approved for the treatment of chronic HBV infection. A response to IFN therapy is judged by a loss of HBV DNA and hepatitis B e antigen (HBeAg) from the plasma (in eAg-positive patients), along with biochemical and histologic improvements. A meta-analysis of 16 randomized trials comparing standard IFN versus control in HBeAg-positive patients found that loss of HBeAg and clearance of HBV DNA occurred in 21% and 20% more patients, respectively, who were receiving IFN.[1] While IFN or Peg-IFN treatment in HBeAg-negative patients results in high rates of HBV viral suppression, the response is generally not durable after treatment discontinuation.[2]

Patients receiving IFN may experience an 'influenza-like' syndrome characterized by fever, chills, headache, myalgia, and arthralgia. These symptoms appear a few hours after the IFN injection and usually resolve within 12 hours. The most frequent dose-limiting adverse effects are leukopenia and thrombocytopenia. IFNs are also associated with psychiatric disturbances including depression with suicidal ideation, paranoid psychoses or confusional states. Thus, caution is warranted when using IFNs and Peg-IFNs in patients with any history of depression or a psychiatric disorder.

Guidelines for adjusting IFN dosage in patients who have renal insufficiency are poorly defined. IFN may be poorly tolerated in patients with decompensated liver disease and its use is generally not advised. IFN has abortifacient effects in monkeys and should not be used in pregnant women, unless the potential benefits outweigh the risks to the fetus.

Recent years have seen a variety of effective oral medications for the treatment of HBV infection with improved rates of HBV DNA suppression and more favorable side effect profiles compared to IFN. As a result of these oral therapies, IFN monotherapy is no longer first-line treatment for HBV infection (see also Chapter 42).

HBV Polymerase Inhibitors: Nucleos(t)ide Analogs

Nucleoside and nucleotide analogs (NUCs) are oral agents that have been developed for use in the treatment of several viral pathogens and function either as nucleic acid chain terminators or as inhibitors of polymerase enzymes. Nucleoside analogs for HBV include lamivudine, emtricitabine, entecavir, and telbivudine, while nucleotide analogs include adefovir and tenofovir. Resistance to NUCs can be caused by mutations in the active site of the DNA polymerase enzyme.[3]

NUC therapy is generally indicated for patients with hepatitis B who have evidence of active viral replication and either persistent elevations in transaminases or histologically active disease (see Chapter 42). Based on the need for long-term treatment and their higher barrier to resistance, entecavir and tenofovir are the preferred first-line monotherapy choices.

LAMIVUDINE (3TC)

Lamivudine was the first nucleoside analog approved for HBV infection. It is also used for the treatment of HIV infection. Detailed pharmacokinetic and distribution data are provided in Chapter 152. The dose used for HBV (100 mg q24h) is lower than that used for HIV. Lamivudine therapy is associated with a significant improvement in

TABLE 155-1	**Medication Dosage Regimens for Adults**			
Disease	**Therapy**	**Route**	**Dose**	**Duration**
Chronic hepatitis B	IFN-alfa-2b*	sc	5×10^6 IU/day or 10×10^6 IU three times/week	HBeAg-positive: 16–32 weeks[†]
	Peg-IFN alfa-2a	sc	180 µg/week	HBeAg-negative: 12+ months[†]
	Peg-IFN alfa-2b (not available in the USA)			48 weeks[†]
	lamivudine (3TC)	po	100 mg q24h	Optimal duration unknown
	adefovir dipivoxil (ADV)	po	10 mg q24h	Optimal duration unknown
	entecavir (ETV)	po	0.5 mg q24h (lamivudine-inexperienced) or 1.0 mg (lamivudine-experienced)	Optimal duration unknown
	telbivudine (LdT)	po	600 mg q24h	Optimal duration unknown
	tenofovir[‡] (TDF)	po	300 mg q24h (also available in FDC with emtricitabine and other ARVs)	Optimal duration unknown
	emtricitabine[§] (FTC)	po	200 mg q24h (also available in FDC with tenofovir and other ARVs)	Optimal duration unknown
Chronic hepatitis C	IFN-alfa-2a*	sc	3×10^6 IU three times/week	24–48 weeks[¶]
	IFN-alfa-2b*	sc	3×10^6 IU three times/week	24–48 weeks[¶,#]
	IFN alfacon*	sc	9 µg three times/week	24–48 weeks[¶]
	Peg-IFN alfa-2a	sc	180 µg/week	12–48 weeks**
	Peg-IFN alfa-2b (not available in the USA)	sc		
	ribavirin (RBV)	po	800–1400 mg/day divided in two doses[§§]	Always part of combination therapy[§§]
Chronic hepatitis C: direct-acting antivirals				
Protease inhibitors	telaprevir (withdrawn from market)	po	750 mg 3 times daily or 1125 mg twice daily with high fat food	12 weeks telaprevir with 24–48 wks Peg-IFN+RBV[##]
	boceprevir (withdrawn from market)	po	800 mg 3 times daily	20–44 weeks boceprevir with 28–48 wks of Peg-IFN+RBV[##]
	simeprevir (SMV)	po	150 mg once daily with food	12–24 weeks when used with sofosbuvir** 12 weeks simeprevir with 24–48 wks of Peg-IFN+RBV[##]
	paritaprevir	po	150 mg once daily (always given with ritonavir boosting as part of FDC, see below)	
	grazoprevir	po	100 mg once daily (available only as a FDC, see below)	
Nucleos(t)ide analog RNA polymerase inhibitors	sofosbuvir (SOF)	po	400 mg once daily with or without food (also available in FDC with ledipasvir)	12–24 weeks when given with RBV, SMV, DAC, or Peg-IFN+RBV**
Non-nucleoside RNA polymerase inhibitors	dasabuvir	po	250 mg twice daily	12–24 weeks when given with paritaprevir/ritonavir/ombitasvir FDC**
NS5A inhibitors	daclatasvir (DCV)	po	60 mg once daily (adjust dose with certain ARVS[††])	12–24 weeks when given with sofosbuvir ±RBV**
	ledipasvir (LDV)	po	90 mg once daily (available only as a FDC, see below)	
	ombitasvir	po	25 mg once daily (available only as a FDC, see below)	
	elbasvir	po	50 mg once daily (available only as a FDC, see below)	
FDC	sofosbuvir /ledipasvir (SOF/LDV)(400mg/90mg)	po	1 tab daily with or without food	8–24 weeks**
	paritaprevir/ritonavir/ombitasvir (75 mg/50 mg/12.5 mg)	po	2 tabs daily every morning with food	12 weeks when given with RBV for genotype 4; 12–24 wks when given + dasabuvir ±RBV for genotype 1**
	grazoprevir/elbasvir (100 mg/50 mg)	po	1 tab daily with or without food	12 weeks-pending final regulatory approval**

Abbreviations: ARVs, antiretrovirals; FDC, fixed dose combination.

*The use of standard interferon has been replaced for the most part by the use of pegylated interferon for reasons of efficacy and convenience. Standard interferon may be used in certain situations (e.g. prior to liver transplant) when a shorter half-life is preferred.

[†]Optimal dosing and duration of interferons is unclear for HBV. Whether lower dose or shorter treatment of Peg-IFN may suffice for HBeAg-positive and whether longer treatment will improve response for HBeAg-negative patients is not known.

[‡]First-line therapy for HIV-infected patients who also require HBV treatment, usually in combination with lamivudine or emtricitabine as part of a combination antiretroviral regimen.

[§]FDA-approved for treatment of HIV infection but not HBV monoinfection.

[¶]Optimal duration of IFN therapy with these agents is based on genotype and what has become standard of care may vary from the package inserts.

[#]Dosing of 15 µg sc three times/week is recommended for patients with nonresponse or relapse to prior treatment. Daily dosing has also been studied and may be appropriate in certain circumstances.

**Duration depends on HCV genotype, the presence of cirrhosis, and co-administered HCV medications (see package insert and treatment guidelines[37]).

[§§]Optimal dose and duration of ribavirin varies with the co-administration of IFN as well as patient weight and HCV genotype. Refer to specific package inserts and treatment guidelines.[37]

[##]Duration depends on indication and response (see package insert).

[††]Decrease DCV dose to 30 mg QD with ritonavir-boosted atazanavir, nelfinavir, indinavir, or saquinavir; increase DCV dose to 90 mg QD with efavirenz and etravirine.

hepatic histology, normalization of hepatic enzymes and suppression of plasma HBV DNA.[4] However, in most patients, values return to baseline levels when lamivudine is discontinued. Furthermore, the emergence of drug-resistant HBV limits the value of lamivudine for long-term therapy.[5] Lamivudine is also available as a co-formulation with other drugs used in the treatment of HIV.

ADEFOVIR (ADV)

Adefovir is an approved nucleotide analog for the treatment of HBV infection. Unaffected by food, it achieves 60% oral bioavailability. Its half-life is 12–30 hours and it undergoes renal excretion without significant metabolites. It does not substantially affect the cytochrome P450 system. Dose adjustment is recommended for patients with creatinine clearances (CrCl) <50 mL/min. The most common adverse reactions are headache, gastrointestinal upset and elevated transaminases. The drug does not exhibit cross-resistance with lamivudine and is effective in the treatment of lamivudine-resistant HBV. As mutations associated with adefovir resistance emerge in 15% of patients by 96 weeks,[6] its use as first-line therapy has been supplanted by entecavir and tenofovir.

ENTECAVIR (ETV)

Entecavir is a guanosine nucleoside analog that functionally inhibits all three activities of the HBV DNA polymerase: base priming, reverse transcription of the negative strand and synthesis of the positive strand. Entecavir's active phosphorylated form has a half-life of 15 hours. Entecavir is cleared by the kidneys primarily, and dose adjustment is recommended for patients with CrCl <50 mL/min.

In studies of HBeAg-positive subjects comparing entecavir and lamivudine, entecavir was associated with superior rates of virologic suppression at 48 weeks compared to lamivudine (67% vs. 36% <300 copies/mL); however, rates of eAg loss were similar.[7] In lamivudine-naïve HBeAg-negative patients, entecavir was also shown to achieve superior rates of virologic suppression at 48 weeks.[8] Longer term treatment shows continued high rates of suppression for 4–5 years.

Resistance mutations associated with lamivudine and telbivudine predispose to the development of entecavir resistance, and its efficacy is reduced in the setting of prior lamivudine failure. For example, cumulative development of resistance was 43% in lamivudine-refractory subjects, compared to 1.2% in lamivudine-naïve subjects, at 4 years.[9] An increased dose is recommended for patients with probable or known lamivudine resistance. However, use of alternative drugs without cross-resistance may be preferable.

The dose is 0.5 mg once daily except for patients with probable or known lamivudine resistance, for whom the recommended dose is 1.0 mg daily. As its absorption is decreased by food, it is recommended that entecavir be administered at least 2 hours before or after a meal. In studies, safety was similar between entecavir and lamivudine or entecavir and placebo. The most commonly observed adverse events that were possibly related to entecavir included headache, fatigue, dizziness and nausea.

TELBIVUDINE (LDT)

Telbivudine is a thymidine nucleoside analog with activity against HBV. Telbivudine is excreted primarily by the kidneys and dose adjustments are recommended for CrCl <50 mL/min. There are no significant known drug interactions.

Telbivudine showed superior rates of HBV DNA viral suppression when compared with lamivudine for both HBeAg-positive and HBeAg-negative patients.[10] However, at 2 years, the development of genotypic resistance occurred in 21.6% and 8.6%, respectively.[11] The most commonly observed resistance mutation during treatment with telbivudine (M204I) confers cross-resistance to lamivudine. For these reasons, telbivudine monotherapy should generally be avoided.

Telbivudine was tolerated similarly to lamivudine in studies comparing the two drugs except that grade 3–4 creatine kinase elevations were observed more frequently with telbivudine (9% vs 3%). Myopathy with associated muscle weakness was rare (<1%).[10]

TENOFOVIR DISOPROXIL FUMARATE (TDF) AND TENOFOVIR ALAFENAMIDE (TAF)

TDF is a nucleotide analog approved for treatment of HIV and chronic hepatitis B. Detailed pharmacokinetic and safety data are given in Chapter 152. TDF exhibits potent viral suppression, with 85% and 73% of HBeAg-negative and HBeAg-positive patients having HBV DNA <400 copies/mL at 5 years of treatment.[12] No patients in these studies exhibited genotypic resistance, and only case reports of drug resistance have been described.

TDF has activity against lamivudine- and adefovir-resistant HBV isolates, and its efficacy has been shown in clinical trials of lamivudine- and adefovir-experienced patients.[13] TDF (usually in combination with lamivudine or emtricitabine) is the HBV treatment of choice for patients who require concomitant treatment of HIV infection. It is available with emtricitabine in several co-formulations used for treatment of HIV (see Chapter 152.)

TAF is a prodrug of tenofovir that is being studied in phase 3 trials, in comparison to TDF, for chronic hepatitis B infection. In studies of patients with HIV-1 monoinfection, compared with TDF, TAF demonstrated more potent antiviral activity, higher mononuclear cell intracellular tenofovir diphosphate levels, and lower plasma tenofovir (TFV) exposures, at approximately one-tenth of the dose.[14] The reduction in plasma exposures of TFV with TAF may result in decreased renal and bone toxicity.

EMTRICITABINE (FTC)

Emtricitabine is a cytosine nucleoside analog approved for treatment of HIV infection with efficacy against HBV. Because of its structural similarity to lamivudine, it shares a common resistance profile. Detailed pharmacokinetic and safety data are given in Chapter 152. In a study of both HBeAg-positive and HBeAg-negative patients, 200 mg of emtricitabine was associated with viral suppression in 54% compared to 2% of placebo-treated patients at 48 weeks.[15] As with lamivudine, resistance with monotherapy is unacceptably high, with emtricitabine resistance mutations detected in 13% of patients in this study. It is available with tenofovir in several co-formulations used for treatment of HIV.

Combination Therapies for Hepatitis B (see also Chapter 42)

Several studies have looked at combination HBV therapy involving nucleoside or nucleotide analogs with Peg-IFN but the results have been inconsistent.[16–18] A randomized open-label study of 740 patients with chronic HBV showed that 7.3% of patients treated with 48 weeks of tenofovir plus Peg-IFN experienced loss of HBsAg. Response rates were lower for patients treated with 16-week tenofovir plus Peg-IFN followed by tenofovir monotherapy for 48 weeks, and interferon monotherapy for 48 weeks. No subjects taking continuous tenofovir monotherapy experienced HBsAg loss. A majority of people in all the tenofovir-containing arms had undetectable HBV DNA at 48 weeks. However, viral load rebound or elevation of liver function tests occurred in >50% of all subjects who stopped treatment at 48 weeks.[19]

Studies comparing two antiviral agents of lamivudine and adefovir or lamivudine and telbivudine to a single antiviral agent suggest that the rate of virological response (HBV DNA suppression or HBeAg seroconversion) is not increased, but drug resistance is reduced.[20,21] One trial of adefovir plus emtricitabine showed a higher rate of alanine aminotransferase (ALT) normalization and reduction in HBV DNA without a difference in HBeAg seroconversion in comparison to adefovir monotherapy, but an emtricitabine monotherapy arm was not included.[22] A trial comparing the combination of tenofovir disoproxil plus entecavir to entecavir monotherapy in treatment-naïve patients found that overall responses were similar, but combination therapy resulted in more rapid viral suppression in HBeAg-positive patients with high baseline HBV DNA (>10^8 IU/mL). Whether this difference is clinically relevant is not clear.[23]

While combination therapy for HBV could theoretically offer the potential for long-term virologic suppression while avoiding drug resistance, no studies to date have convincingly demonstrated a significant advantage over available potent monotherapies. This may be due to the fact that all nucleoside(tide) analogs for HBV have the same viral target. For HIV/HBV co-infected patients who require combination therapy for the treatment of HIV, the use of the combination of tenofovir plus emtricitabine (available as a co-formulation) or tenofovir plus lamivudine is recommended as part of the regimen.

Chronic Hepatitis C Virus (HVC) Infection

Treatment of chronic HCV infection is recommended in all patients with detectable HCV RNA levels unless life expectancy is severely limited due to non-HCV co-morbidities. The goal of HCV treatment is to eliminate the virus to prevent further damage from HCV infection. The terminology used to describe treatment success or 'cure' is a sustained virologic response (SVR) to treatment, defined as a serum or plasma HCV RNA assay below the limit of assay quantification at 12 or 24 weeks after completion of therapy.

Interferons

The availability of direct-acting antivirals (DAAs) has made IFN-based therapy a less attractive option for HCV due to the unfavorable side effect profile. Pegylated IFN is no longer part of the recommended initial regimens for most genotypes, however, it may still play a role in treatment in select situations. It has been established that adding a DAA to pegylated IFN plus ribavirin (Peg-IFN+RBV) achieves SVR rates superior to Peg-IFN+RBV dual therapy for chronic HCV genotype 1 infection.[24–26] Thus, if Peg-IFN+RBV is to be used for chronic HCV, it should be used with a DAA.

Ribavirin (RBV)

Ribavirin is a guanosine analog with broad-spectrum antiviral activity that is used only in combination with DAAs and/or IFN for HCV

treatment. Proposed mechanisms of action include depletion of intracellular triphosphate pools, directly inhibiting viral mRNA and RNA polymerase, and mutagenesis, as well as effects on cytokines and interferon.[27] Oral bioavailability ranges from 33% to 69%. About 40% of the drug is eliminated via the kidneys. It can be used cautiously with dose adjustment in the setting of renal insufficiency. The recommended dose of ribavirin varies by weight and is divided into twice daily dosing to improve gastrointestinal tolerability (see Table 155-1) (see also Chapter 154).

The major side effect of ribavirin is hemolytic anemia, which may necessitate dose reduction. Ribavirin is teratogenic, so contraception is required if the drug is used by women of child-bearing age or their partners. In HIV-infected individuals, ribavirin should not be co-administered with didanosine because of excess toxicity, and co-administration with zidovudine should be avoided due to potentiation of anemia.

Direct-Acting Antivirals (DAAs)

HCV is a single-stranded RNA virus of about 9600 nucleotide bases in length. It is translated into a single polypeptide precursor, which is cleaved into several functional gene products.[28] DAAs that are approved or in pre-clinical or clinical development target key components of the viral life cycle, including inhibitors of viral entry, RNA polymerase activity (e.g. nucleoside and non-nucleoside inhibitors), RNA replication (e.g. NS5A inhibitors), protein translation, polyprotein processing (e.g. serine protease inhibitors) and viral assembly and release (see Figure 155-1). These drugs will be discussed in the order of their approval by drug class and dosing recommendations can be found in Table 155-1.

PROTEASE INHIBITORS

HCV protease inhibitors (PIs) inhibit the serine protease NS3/4A's cleavage of the HCV polypeptide. Monotherapy with PIs results in unacceptable rates of resistance, so the first use of PIs involved co-administration with Peg-IFN and ribavirin for treatment of HCV genotype 1. As drug classes targeting additional points of the life cycle

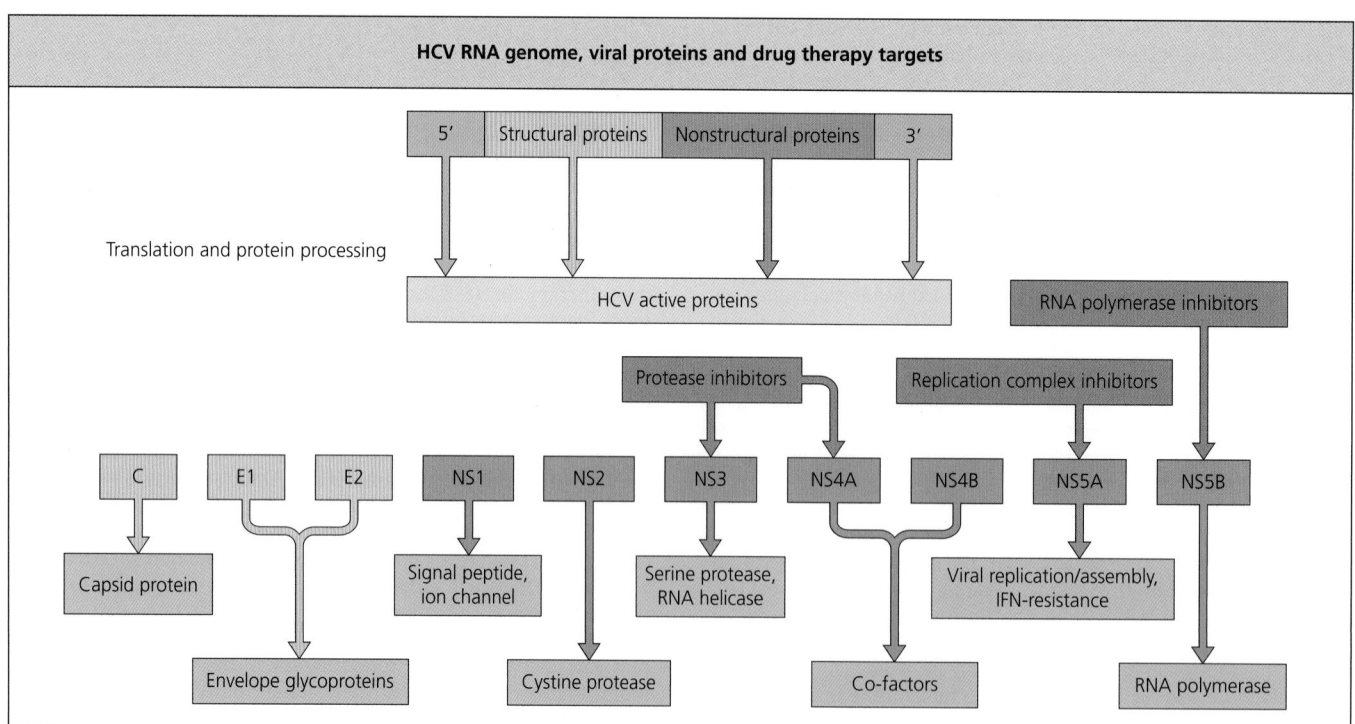

Figure 155-1 Hepatitis C genome, viral proteins and drug therapy targets. The protein targets of various classes of HCV direct-acting antiviral agents are shown in blue.

have been developed, later generations of PIs, some of which have activity against multiple genotypes, are being used as part of all-oral DAA combination therapy.

TELAPREVIR (TVR)

In 2011, telaprevir became the first approved DAA for use with Peg-IFN+RBV for treatment of HCV genotype 1 in treatment-naïve and IFN-experienced patients. This combination offered improved efficacy (69–75% SVR for initial treatment) and a shorter treatment duration (when patients met criteria for response-guided therapy) over Peg-IFN+RBV alone.[28] Issues with three times daily dosing, rash, drug interactions and resistance make it less preferable than DAAs in use today. Telaprevir has now been withdrawn from the market in the USA and Canada.

BOCEPREVIR (BCV)

Boceprevir was approved in 2011 for use in combination with Peg-IFN+RBV given its improved efficacy (42–53% and 67–68% SVR for initial treatment in black and non-black cohorts, respectively) for HCV genotype 1 over Peg-IFN+RBV for treatment-naïve as well as IFN-experienced patients.[29] Boceprevir is administered as four pills three times daily, started after a 4-week lead-in of Peg-IFN+RBV. The duration of treatment is determined by IFN-experience, on-treatment response and cirrhosis status. The main toxicities attributed to boceprevir include anemia and dysgeusia, while other on-treatment side effects of Peg-IFN and RBV remain. Drug interactions are common given boceprevir is both an inducer and substrate of CYP3A4 and P-glycoprotein (Pgp). It has not been studied with other DAAs and should not be used as part of DAA combination therapy. Given its limitations, newer PIs have supplanted the use of boceprevir and there are plans to withdraw it from the US market.

SIMEPREVIR (SMV)

Simeprevir was the first once-daily, oral, macrocyclic PI approved in 2013 for treatment of HCV genotype 1 in the USA and genotypes 1 and 4 in the European Union. Simeprevir should be administered with food to increase the oral bioavailability. It is metabolized in the liver primarily by the CYP3A system and eliminated by biliary excretion. Drug interactions remain common owing to metabolism by CYP3A, with drugs that induce or inhibit this pathway affecting SMV levels greatly. SMV accumulates in the setting of hepatic impairment and is not recommended in Child class B or C cirrhosis. Simeprevir was first FDA-approved for use with Peg-IFN+RBV, but subsequently approved as DAA combination therapy with sofosbuvir (a nucleotide analog, see below) ± RBV resulting in SVR rates from 79–100% with 12–24 weeks of treatment.[30] The combination of simeprevir and sofosbuvir represented the first available all-oral, IFN-free combination for treatment of HCV genotype 1. Adverse reactions are less common with simeprevir than first-generation PIs, the most frequent being a rash (photosensitivity) that often resembles a sunburn, hyperbilirubinemia, pruritus and nausea. The combination of simeprevir with Peg-IFN and RBV is not recommended for HCV genotype 1a harboring a Q80K polymorphism, since this mutation in the NS3 gene predicts a poorer response. At this time, this is the only FDA-approved regimen for which testing for resistance-associated mutations is recommended prior to treatment.

PARITAPREVIR

Paritaprevir was approved in 2014 for HCV genotype 1 and in 2015 for genotype 4 treatment. It exists only as a fixed dose combination (FDC) co-formulated with ritonavir and ombitasvir (an NS5A inhibitor, see below). The FDC is approved for used in combination with dasabuvir (a non-nucleoside polymerase inhibitor, see below) ± RBV for genotypes 1a and 1b, but also has been approved recently with RBV (without dasabuvir) for genotype 4. The combination does not require dose adjustment for patients with renal impairment, but is contraindicated in patients with severe hepatic impairment due to the risk of potential toxicity. Oral absorption of the FDC paritaprevir/ritonavir/

ombitasvir plus dasabuvir (will be referred to as PrOD) is increased in the presence of moderate/high fat meals and should always be administered with food. Paritaprevir is predominantly metabolized by CYP3A4, and to a lesser extent, by CYP3A5. Approximately 88% of the drug is eliminated in the feces, with the remainder eliminated in the urine. Owing to the presence of ritonavir for CYP3A4 inhibition in the combination regimen, drug interactions are common. When given for genotype 1a, RBV should be added to the PrOD regimen regardless of the stage of liver fibrosis; whereas genotype 1b only requires RBV for patients with cirrhosis. Side effects of paritaprevir/ritonavir/ombitasvir PrOD ± ribavirin are uncommon but include fatigue, nausea, pruritus, other skin reactions, insomnia and asthenia. A decrease in hemoglobin can also occur as a result of the RBV. In phase 3 trials of paritaprevir/ritonavir/ombitasvir PrOD ± ribavirin, less than 1% of subjects discontinued treatment as a result of side effects.[31]

GRAZOPREVIR

Grazoprevir is an investigational protease inhibitor with good activity against a range of HCV genotype variants, and is active against most variants that confer resistance to first-generation PIs. Grazoprevir is a substrate of CYP3A4, P-glycoprotein (Pgp) and the organic anion-transporting polypeptide (OATP1B). It is a weak inhibitor of CYP2C8, 3A4, and UDP glucuronosyltransferase 1 family, polypeptide A1 (UGT1A1). Dose modifications are not required for patients with renal insufficiency or mild-moderate hepatic impairment. In initial clinical trials with this drug, grazoprevir was well tolerated. Side effects reported include fatigue, headache, nausea and diarrhea; these were usually of mild intensity and temporary. The US Food and Drug Administration (FDA) has accepted for review the New Drug Application for grazoprevir/elbasvir (100 mg/50 mg), an investigational, once-daily, single-tablet combination therapy for the treatment of adult patients infected with chronic HCV genotypes 1, 4, or 6.

Nucleos(t)ide Analog Polymerase Inhibitors

Nucleos(t)ide analog polymerase inhibitors (NUCs) bind a highly conserved, active site of the NS5B RNA-dependent RNA polymerase and cause premature chain termination to inhibit HCV replication. NUCs represent an important class for treatment of HCV, as they are pangenotypic (active against HCV genotypes 1-6) with a high barrier to the development of resistance.

SOFOSBUVIR (SOF)

Sofosbuvir is the only FDA-approved (2013) NUC. Sofosbuvir can be administered with or without food. After absorption, sofosbuvir undergoes first-pass hepatic extraction and is metabolized in the liver to its active nucleoside triphosphate form and subsequently an inactive metabolite, GS-331007. Given that this metabolite is predominantly cleared renally, sofosbuvir is not recommended for use when GFR<30 mL/min, although studies are ongoing in patients with renal disease. Drug interactions are uncommon. However, drugs that are potent intestinal Pgp inducers (e.g. St John's wort, tipranavir, phenytoin) may lower sofosbuvir's concentration and should not be co-administered. No dose adjustments are required in the setting of hepatic impairment. Sofosbuvir was first approved for use in combination with ribavirin (IFN-free regimen) for genotype 2 (12 weeks), genotype 3 (24 weeks), genotype 1 (24 weeks) and as combination therapy with Peg-IFN+RBV (12 weeks) for genotype 1, as these regimens were proven to have superior response rates and fewer side effects than Peg-IFN+RBV. However for genotype 1, it should be used in co-formulation with ledipasvir (an NS5A inhibitor, see below) for genotype 1 and 4, given high SVR rates of 97–99% with initial treatment without the use of Peg-IFN or RBV.[31,32] Similarly for genotype 3, combination with daclatasvir ± RBV appears more effective than with RBV alone. Adverse reactions are infrequent with sofosbuvir but include fatigue, headache, and insomnia.

Non-Nucleos(t)ide Polymerase Inhibitors

Non-NUCs bind outside the active site of NS5B RNA polymerase and cause allosteric hindrance of the enzyme. They typically have a lower barrier to resistance than nucleos(t)ide polymerase inhibitors.

DASABUVIR

Dasabuvir was approved in 2014 as the first non-NUC approved for HCV genotype 1 infection. It must be administered with the FDC of paritaprevir/ritonavir/ombitasvir ± RBV. Dasabuvir achieves 70% oral bioavailability and is predominantly metabolized by CYP2C8, and to a lesser extent by CYP3A. Approximately 94% of the drug is excreted in the feces, with the remainder excreted in the urine. Side effects of FDC paritaprevir/ritonavir/ombitasvir plus dasabuvir ± RBV are detailed in the 'paritaprevir' section above.

NS5A Inhibitors

NS5A inhibitors target the NS5A protein, which is essential for HCV RNA replication and viral assembly. Those discussed below have activity against genotype 1 but vary in activity against other genotypes. Combining a pangenotypic NS5A inhibitor with a pangenotypic NUC may be a future strategy for decreasing treatment complexity due to genotype differences.

LEDIPASVIR (LDV)

Ledipasvir, the first NS5A inhibitor approved (2014) for HCV genotype 1 treatment, is available only as a FDC with sofosbuvir. *In vitro*, it is also active against genotypes 4, 5, and 6 and was subsequently approved for these indications. High pH inhibits ledipasvir absorption, thus recommendations exist for avoiding antacids with ledipasvir. Ledipasvir is an inhibitor and substrate of the drug transporters Pgp and breast cancer resistance protein (BCRP), so drug interactions are more common than with sofosbuvir alone. Ledipasvir is excreted in feces largely unmetabolized. Sofosbuvir/ledipasvir FDC is administered for 12 weeks in treatment-naïve, IFN-experienced and PI-experienced patients without cirrhosis and 24 weeks for patients with cirrhosis based on its high SVR rates in these populations.[33,34] Side effects are uncommon but include low-severity fatigue and headache. Less than 1% of subjects discontinued treatment as a result of side effects in phase 3 studies.

DACLATASVIR (DCV)

Daclatasvir, a pangenotypic NS5A inhibitor, is approved in the European Union (2014) for use as part of HCV combination therapy and in the USA (2015) for use specifically with sofosbuvir for treatment of HCV genotype 3. Daclatasvir is a substrate of CYP3A4 as well as a substrate and inducer of Pgp. Dose adjustment is recommended when used with medications that significantly affect these enzymes such as certain antiretrovirals (see Table 155-1). No dose adjustment is required in patients with renal or liver impairment. It has been studied in combination with Peg-IFN+RBV, sofosbuvir, and some investigational DAAs. The most common side effects include fatigue, nausea and headache.

OMBITASVIR

Ombitasvir was approved in 2014 for HCV genotype 1 and in 2015 for HCV genotype 4 as part of the FDC paritaprevir/ritonavir/ombitasvir. Ombitasvir is predominantly metabolized by amide hydrolysis followed by oxidative metabolism. Approximately 90% of the drug is excreted in the feces, with the remainder excreted in the urine. Side effects are detailed in the paritaprevir section above.

ELBASVIR

Elbasvir is an investigational NS5A replication complex inhibitor with broad genotypic activity. It is a substrate of CYP3A4, Pgp, and organic anion-transporting polypeptide (OATP). Dose modifications are not required for patients with renal insufficiency or mild-moderate hepatic impairment. Side effects are similar to those reported for grazoprevir. As stated above, this drug is being considered for FDA approval as part of a fixed-drug combination tablet with grazoprevir.

Combination Therapy for HCV Infection (see also Chapter 42)

INTERFERON-BASED COMBINATION THERAPY

Peg-IFN+RBV was the first combination therapy to be approved for treatment of HCV. However, treatment durations were long with significant side effects and suboptimal response rates, particularly in the setting of HCV genotype 1, cirrhosis, or HIV.[35,36] The addition of a PI to Peg-IFN+RBV improved response rates for genotype 1, but at the expense of treatment complexity.[24,25] Subsequently, sofosbuvir was approved for use with Peg-IFN+RBV for treatment of HCV genotype 1 as it led to high response rates (including in cirrhotics), further shortened treatment duration, and improved tolerability.[26]

DAA COMBINATION THERAPY (IFN-FREE) WITH OR WITHOUT RBV

IFN-free DAA combinations represent the current standard of HCV treatment, since they have accomplished the goal of making therapy more effective, safer, and more tolerable, as well as less complex to prescribe and monitor. It is difficult to predict which combinations may be used successfully together. Thus, only studied combinations are recommended for use. Several drug combinations have been studied as described above and many more are in clinical development. However, few have been compared head to head at this point. For the most up-to-date recommendations on DAA combination therapy for HCV, check treatment guidelines (e.g. www.hcvguidelines.org[37]) or package inserts.

References available online at expertconsult.com.

KEY REFERENCES

Afdhal N., Reddy K.R., Nelson D.R., et al.: Ledipasvir and sofosbuvir for previously treated HCV genotype 1 infection. *N Engl J Med* 2014; 370(16):1483-1493.

Afdhal N., Zeuzem S., Kwo P., et al.: Ledipasvir and sofosbuvir for untreated HCV genotype 1 infection. *N Engl J Med* 2014; 370(20):1889-1898.

Allen M.I., Deslauriers M., Andrews C.W., et al.: Identification and characterization of mutations in hepatitis B virus resistant to lamivudine. Lamivudine Clinical Investigation Group. *Hepatology* 1998; 27(6):1670-1677.

Chang T.T., Gish R.G., de Man R., et al.: A comparison of entecavir and lamivudine for HBeAg-positive chronic hepatitis B. *N Engl J Med* 2006; 354(10):1001-1010.

Ferenci P., Bernstein D., Lalezari J., et al.: ABT-450/r-ombitasvir and dasabuvir with or without ribavirin for HCV. *N Engl J Med* 2014; 370(21):1983-1992.

Lawitz E., Mangia A., Wyles D., et al.: Sofosbuvir for previously untreated chronic hepatitis C infection. *N Engl J Med* 2013; 368(20):1878-1887.

Lawitz E., Sulkowski M.S., Ghalib R., et al.: Simeprevir plus sofosbuvir, with or without ribavirin, to treat chronic infection with hepatitis C virus genotype 1 in non-responders to pegylated interferon and ribavirin and treatment-naive patients: the COSMOS randomised study. *Lancet* 2014; 384(9956):1756-1765.

Lim S.G., Ng T.M., Kung N., et al.: A double-blind placebo-controlled study of emtricitabine in chronic hepatitis B. *Arch Intern Med* 2006; 166(1):49-56.

Lok A.S., Trinh H., Carosi G., et al.: Efficacy of entecavir with or without tenofovir disoproxil fumarate for nucleos(t)ide-naïve patients with chronic hepatitis B. *Gastroenterology* 2012; 143(3):619-628, e1.

Marcellin P., Ahn S.-H., Ma X., et al. HBsAg loss with tenofovir disoproxil fumarate plus peginterferon alfa-2a in chronic hepatitis B: results of a global randomized controlled trial. American Association for the Study of Liver Diseases (AASLD) Liver Meeting. Boston, November 7–12, 2014. Abstract 193.

Poordad F., Hezode C., Trinh R., et al.: ABT-450/r-ombitasvir and dasabuvir with ribavirin for hepatitis C with cirrhosis. *N Engl J Med* 2014; 370(21):1973-1982.

Scheel T.K., Rice C.M.: Understanding the hepatitis C virus life cycle paves the way for highly effective therapies. *Nat Med* 2013; 19(7):837-849.

Wong D.K., Cheung A.M., O'Rourke K., et al.: Effect of alpha-interferon treatment in patients with hepatitis B e antigen-positive chronic hepatitis B. A meta-analysis. *Ann Intern Med* 1993; 119(4):312-323.

156

Systemic Antifungal Agents

SHMUEL SHOHAM | ANDREAS H. GROLL |
VIDMANTAS PETRAITIS | THOMAS J. WALSH

KEY CONCEPTS

• Invasive fungal infections have emerged as important causes of morbidity and mortality in immunocompromised and critically ill patients.

• For more than three decades, treatment had been limited to amphotericin B deoxycholate with or without flucytosine.

• Additional therapeutic options emerged with the clinical development of fluconazole and itraconazole in the late 1980s.

• The past two decades have witnessed a major expansion in our antifungal armamentarium through the introduction of less toxic formulations of amphotericin B, the development of improved antifungal triazoles and the advent of the echinocandin lipopeptides, a new class of antifungal agents that target the fungal cell wall.

• Accurate dosing of antifungal agents, which is essential for optimal outcome, requires careful consideration of renal and hepatic function, age (pediatric versus adult), potential drug interactions, and extremes of body mass.

Polyene Antifungal Agents

AMPHOTERICIN B DEOXYCHOLATE AND LIPID FORMULATIONS

Overview

Amphotericin B (AmB) is a natural polyene macrolide antibiotic that consists of seven conjugated double bonds, an internal ester, a free carboxyl group and a glycoside side chain with a primary amino group (Figure 156-1). It is amphoteric, virtually insoluble in water, and not orally or intramuscularly absorbed. For parenteral use, AmB has been solubilized with deoxycholate as a micellar suspension; this formulation has now been available for more than 50 years.

Three lipid formulations of AmB have been approved in the USA and most of Europe:
• a small unilamellar vesicle (SUV) liposomal formulation (L-AmB)
• AmB lipid complex (ABLC); and
• AmB colloidal dispersion (ABCD).

Because of their reduced nephrotoxicity in comparison to AmB deoxycholate, these compounds allow for the delivery of higher dosages of AmB. However, data from animal models also suggest that these higher dosages are required for equivalent antifungal efficacy.

Mechanism of Action

AmB primarily acts by binding to ergosterol, the principal sterol in the cell membrane of most fungi, leading to the formation of ion channels and concentration-dependent cell death (Figure 156-2).[1,2] With less avidity, the compound also binds to cholesterol, the main sterol of mammalian cell membranes, which is believed to account for most of its adverse effects. AmB may also induce cell damage through a cascade of oxidative reactions with formation of free radicals and an increase in membrane permeability.[3-5]

Pharmacokinetics and Distribution

After intravenous administration of AmB deoxycholate, AmB dissociates from its vehicle and becomes highly protein-bound before distributing predominantly into liver, spleen, bone marrow, kidney and lung. A unique property of AmB is that protein binding in plasma is enhanced with increasing drug concentration.[6] Clearance from plasma is slow with a terminal half-life of 5 days and longer.[7] Concentrations in body fluids other than plasma may vary greatly between patients and are substantially lower than serum drug levels.[8,9] The clinical relevance of this is unclear and despite mostly undetectable concentrations in the cerebrospinal fluid (CSF), AmB is effective in central nervous system (CNS) fungal infections. AmB is mostly excreted in urine and feces as unchanged drug and no metabolites have been identified.[7]

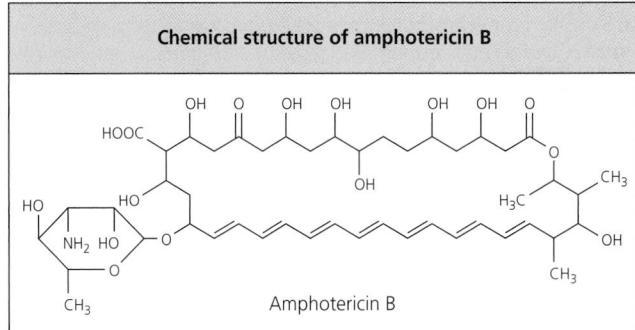

Figure 156-1 Chemical structure of amphotericin B.

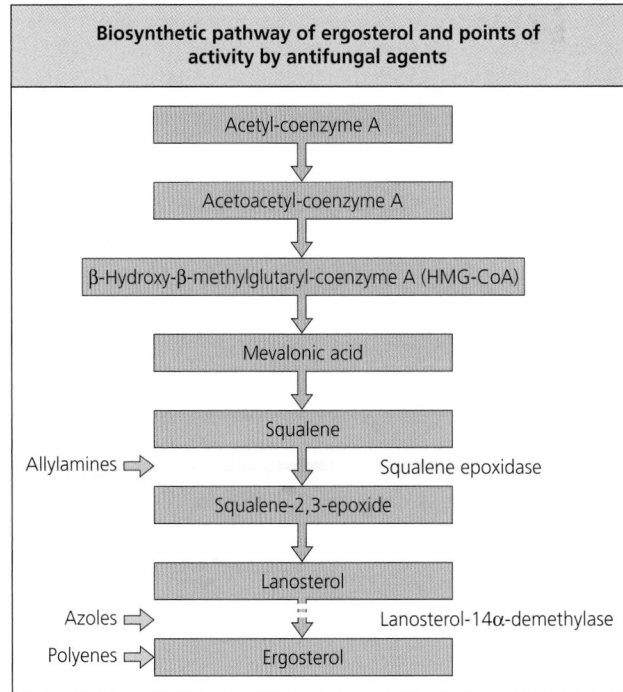

Figure 156-2 Biosynthetic pathway of ergosterol and points of activity by antifungal agents.

Each of the lipid formulations confers distinct plasma pharmacokinetic properties to AmB. All three formulations preferentially distribute to organs of the mononuclear phagocytic system (MPS) and functionally spare the kidney. L-AmB, the only truly liposomal AmB, is composed of small spherical unilamellar lipid vesicles averaging 60–70 nm in size. This preparation has a prolonged circulation time in plasma, achieves high peak plasma concentrations and area under the concentration-time curve (AUC) values and is only slowly taken up by the MPS. However, most of the AmB in plasma remains liposome-associated and free unbound drug concentrations are low.[6,7] ABLC is composed of ribbon-like lipid aggregates. It is efficiently bound by plasma proteins and rapidly taken up by the MPS to achieve high concentrations in cellular components of blood, liver, lung and spleen. ABLC exists as a depot in these tissues from which free AmB is slowly released. Fungal and inflammatory cell lipases at the site of infection act to release AmB from the lipid carrier.[10] ABCD, a colloidal dispersion of microscopic disc-shaped particles, also preferentially collects in tissues of the MPS and free drug is slowly released over time. Drug levels in the plasma and kidney are low and terminal elimination half-life is long. Comparisons of the different formulations of AmB against defined infections suggest potentially important differences in efficacy depending on agent, dose, type and site of infection.[11]

Pharmacodynamics

AmB displays concentration-dependent fungicidal activity against susceptible *Candida albicans*, *Cryptococcus (Cr.) neoformans* and *Aspergillus fumigatus* in time-kill assays and exhibits a postantifungal effect of up to 12 hours' duration against *C. albicans* and *Cr. neoformans in vitro*.[12-14] In neutropenic pharmacokinetic/pharmacodynamic mouse models of disseminated candidiasis and pulmonary aspergillosis, peak plasma concentration (C_{max})/minimal inhibitory concentration (MIC) is the parameter that provides the best correlation with outcome as measured by the residual organismal burden in tissue.[15,16] AmB may have immune stimulatory properties that enhance phagocytic responses to *Aspergillus* and *Fusarium* species.[15,16]

Route of Administration and Dosage

Despite its toxicity profile, AmB deoxycholate remains an important option for initial treatment of life-threatening fungal infections, particularly in resource poor circumstances and in infants, where nephrotoxicity is less apparent and reversible. Depending on the type of infection and the host, recommended daily dosages range from 0.5 mg/kg/day to 1.5 mg/kg/day administered over 2–4 hours as tolerated; the standard dosage for empiric therapy in persistently febrile neutropenic patients is 0.5–0.6 mg/kg/day.[17] Continuous infusion of AmB deoxycholate is counterintuitive to the concentration-dependent pharmacodynamics of AmB and is strongly discouraged. Treatment should be started at the full target dosage with careful bedside monitoring during the first infusion to allow for prompt intervention for infusion-related reactions.

The optimal dosages of each formulation for the various types and sites of invasive fungal infection largely remain to be defined. Based on animal data and the few randomized studies that have used AmB deoxycholate as comparator,[18] the authors and most other experts in the field consider a dose of 3–5 mg/kg/day of ABCD, ABLC and L-AmB equivalent to a dosage of 1 mg/kg/day of AmB deoxycholate. Accordingly, an initial dosage of 3–5 mg/kg/d of ABCD, ABLC or L-AmB is recommended for suspected or documented life-threatening infections, and 3 mg/kg/day when L-AmB is selected for empirical antifungal therapy in persistently febrile neutropenic patients; 3 mg/kg/day has been shown to be effective in aspergillosis, histoplasmosis and in patients with invasive candidiasis.[19,20] Some clinicians have successfully used L-AmB at 10 mg/kg/day and 15 mg/kg/day in patients with recalcitrant invasive fungal infections. However, such doses may provide no additional efficacy and more nephrotoxicity in aspergillosis.[21]

Nebulized AmB is increasingly used as anti-mold prophylaxis in lung transplant and neutropenic patients. All four AmB formulations can be aerosolized. This approach has shown promise in animal studies and in a randomized clinical trial.[22,23] Aerosol size and uniformity vary with AmB formulation and nebulizer technique.[24] Furthermore, among patients with compromised ventilation, the delivered dose may be suboptimal in some lung segments.[18] Common side effects are cough, adverse taste and nausea.[25,26] Tolerability remains a major drawback in fragile patients in whom cough and inability to use an aerosol delivery system are common limitations.[22]

Indications

AmB has broad-spectrum antifungal activity that includes most pathogenic fungi. Primary resistance has been associated with qualitative or quantitative variations in membrane sterols, but may also be related to increased catalase activity with decreased susceptibility to oxidative damage. Isolates of *Candida lusitaniae* and *C. guilliermondii* may be resistant to AmB, and this resistance can develop during treatment.[27] *Aspergillus* spp. and other opportunistic molds, but not the dimorphic molds, tend to have more variable susceptibility. *Aspergillus terreus*, *A. flavus*, *Fusarium* spp., *Scedosporium apiospermum*, *Scedosporium boydii*, *Scedosporium prolificans*, certain other dematiaceous fungi and *Trichosporon* spp. can be resistant to AmB at concentrations safely achievable in patients.[27-29]

Antifungal activity in biofilms has gained increasing attention. Biofilm-associated candidiasis typically occurs with infection of biomedical devices. Compared to planktonic yeast cells, biofilm-associated sessile cells show decreased susceptibility to AmB deoxycholate.[30]

The lipid formulations are indicated for the treatment of patients with AmB-susceptible invasive mycoses and, limited to L-AmB, for empirical therapy of persistently febrile neutropenic patients. The efficacy of the lipid formulations have been demonstrated in phase II and III studies in immunocompromised patients with a wide spectrum of underlying disorders.[17,20,31] The overall response rates in these trials ranged from 53% to 84% for invasive candidiasis and 34% to 59%, respectively, in probable or documented invasive aspergillosis. Clinical and microbiologic responses were observed even when lipid formulations were used after failure of conventional AmB deoxycholate. Several randomized controlled trials have compared lipid formulations with AmB deoxycholate. These studies have consistently shown at least equivalent efficacy and reduced nephrotoxicity in comparison to AmB deoxycholate. A meta-analysis of 1156 neutropenic patients from three trials found that prophylactic or empirical use of L-AmB tended to be more effective than AmB deoxycholate in preventing breakthrough fungal infections, was associated with less nephrotoxicity but did not alter survival.[32]

Lipid formulations of AmB are active against *Candida* biofilms including against sessile yeast population.[33] Animal models suggest a role for AmB lipid formulations as antibiotic lock therapy in catheter-associated candidiasis.[34]

Dosage in Special Circumstances

Dose adjustment of AmB is not necessary in patients with unrelated renal or hepatic dysfunction. Because of its high protein binding, hemodialysis usually does not affect plasma concentrations. Whether the enhanced plasma clearance of AmB deoxycholate reported in infants and young children has implications for dosing remains unknown. The available pediatric pharmacokinetic and safety data indicate no fundamental differences of AmB formulations in comparison to adults. Consequently, dosage recommendations for all pediatric age groups do not differ from those in adults.

Adverse Effects and Drug Interactions

Infusion-related reactions and nephrotoxicity are the major toxicities of AmB deoxycholate. Infusion-related reactions (fever, rigors, chills, myalgias, arthralgias, nausea, vomiting, headaches, hypotension, hypertension, and flushing) are mediated by cytokine release from monocytes. Infusion-related events can be noted in up to 73% of patients during the first dose, but may improve during continued therapy.[17] Slowing the infusion rate or premedication with acetaminophen (10–15 mg/kg), hydrocortisone (0.5–1.0 mg/kg) or meperidine (0.2–0.5 mg/kg) can blunt these reactions. Cardiac arrhythmias and cardiac arrest due to acute potassium release may occur with rapid infusion (<60 min), especially if there is pre-existing hyperkalemia and/or renal impairment. A randomized trial suggests that true allergic reactions to AmB are rare.[35]

AmB-induced nephrotoxicity is related to dose and duration of therapy, concomitant use of nephrotoxic agents, and pre-existing renal dysfunction.[5] AmB-associated nephrotoxicity occurs due to several mechanisms, including increased tubular glomerular feedback and alterations of membrane permeability in renal tubular cells and vascular smooth muscle cells. Tubular defects are responsible for potassium and magnesium wasting, renal tubular acidosis, and impaired urinary concentrating ability.[5] Hypokalemia can be refractory to replacement until hypomagnesemia is corrected. Azotemia is common and is mechanistically due to glomerular vasoconstriction. In a large prospective clinical trial of empirical antifungal therapy, baseline serum creatinine doubled in over one-third of patients receiving AmB.[17] AmB has the potential to lead to renal failure and dialysis.[36] Often, however, azotemia stabilizes on therapy and may be reversible after discontinuation of the drug. Avoiding concomitant nephrotoxic agents, and normal saline loading (10–15 mL 0.9% NaCl/kg/24hrs or 3mEq Na+/kg/24hrs) may ameliorate azotemia.

Hypokalemia may be aggravated by corticosteroids, and hypomagnesemia may become especially profound in cancer patients with platinum-associated nephropathy. AmB may enhance plasma levels and toxicity of renally cleared drugs, including aminoglycosides, vancomycin, flucytosine and cyclosporine. Nephrotoxic agents, such as aminoglycosides, calcineurin inhibitors and foscarnet, may enhance AmB-induced nephrotoxicity. Drug interactions due to shared metabolic pathways have not been described for AmB in humans. Simultaneous infusion of granulocytes has been associated with acute pulmonary reactions and should be used with extreme caution.

Amphotericin B may also cause a normochromic, normocytic anemia after chronic administration. As AmB deoxycholate is topically irritating, a central line should be used for infusion. Local instillation of AmB deoxycholate, including intrathecal administration, can cause focal areas of necrosis within the spinal cord with ensuing myelopathy.[37]

Relative to AmB deoxycholate, infusion-related side effects are less frequent with L-AmB but are increased with ABCD.[17,38,39] A distinctive severe acute infusion-related reaction of substernal chest discomfort, respiratory distress and sharp flank pain has been noted during infusion of L-AmB. Hypoxic episodes associated with fever and chills are more frequent with ABCD than with AmB deoxycholate.[35] Mild increases in serum bilirubin and alkaline phosphatases have been observed with lipid formulations and mild increases in pancreatic enzymes also have been observed with L-AmB.

FLUCYTOSINE
Overview
Flucytosine (5-fluorocytosine; 5-FC) is a low molecular weight water-soluble synthetic fluorinated analog of cytosine (Figure 156-3). The compound is taken up by the fungus-specific enzyme cytosine permease and converted in the cytoplasm by cytosine deaminase to 5-fluorouracil, which causes RNA miscoding and inhibits DNA synthesis via thymidylate synthase.[40,41]

Pharmacokinetics and Distribution
Oral 5-FC is readily absorbed from the gastrointestinal tract, has negligible protein binding and distributes evenly into tissues and body fluids, including the CSF and the eye. At usual dosages, the drug undergoes little hepatic metabolism and is eliminated predominantly in active form by glomerular filtration into the urine with a half-life in plasma of 3–6 hours. Individual dosage adjustment is necessary in patients with impaired renal function and those undergoing hemofiltration or dialysis.[41] Impaired liver function does not appear to alter 5-FC disposition.[42]

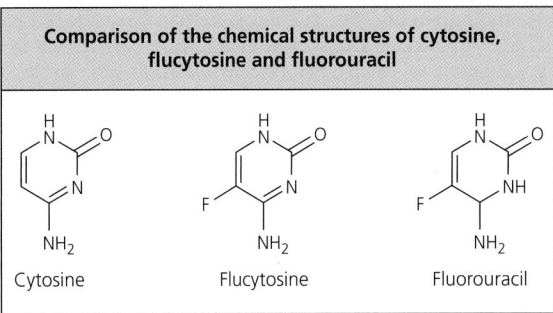

Figure 156-3 Comparison of the chemical structures of cytosine, flucytosine and fluorouracil.

Pharmacodynamics
Flucytosine has demonstrated predominantly concentration-independent antifungal activity against *Candida* spp. and *Cr. neoformans* in time-kill assays, and prolonged concentration- and exposure-dependent postantifungal effects of up to 10 hours.[43,44] Pharmacodynamic studies in mice with disseminated candidiasis indicate that time above the MIC and AUC/MIC are the most important parameters in predicting efficacy. Maximum efficacy was observed when levels exceeded the MIC for only 20–25% of the 24-hour dosing interval.[45] Thus, lower dosages or less frequent dosing may yield identical efficacy while reducing the mostly dose-dependent toxicities.

Route of Administration and Dosage
A starting dosage of 100 mg/kg daily divided in three or four doses is currently recommended in adults and children with normal renal function.

Monitoring of plasma concentrations and adjustment of dosage to changing renal function are essential to avoiding 5-FC toxicity.[46] Following oral administration, near-peak levels 2 hours post dosing overlap with trough levels as patients reach steady state and are thus sufficient for therapeutic monitoring. Peak plasma levels between 40 μg/mL and 60 μg/mL correlate with antifungal efficacy and are seldom associated with hematologic adverse effects.[40,47]

Indications
The antifungal spectrum of 5-FC *in vitro* encompasses *Candida* spp., *Cr. neoformans* and selected dematiaceous molds.[40] 5-FC is thought to have no or weak *in vitro* activity against *Aspergillus* spp. and other hyaline molds; however, more recent studies have shown that this lack of activity *in vitro* may be pH-dependent and that it does not correlate with the documented efficacy in animal models.[48,49] Synergistic or additive effects in combination with AmB have been observed against *Candida* spp. and in combination with AmB and fluconazole or posaconazole against *Cr. neoformans*.[50,51] Primary resistance to 5-FC is uncommon in *Cr. neoformans*. With the exception of *Candida krusei*, primary resistance occurs rarely in *Candida* spp. However, when used as a single agent, secondary resistance by selection of resistant clones can evolve rapidly and appears to result from a single point mutation. In *Cr. neoformans* resistance has been observed in 30–40% of isolates from patients with meningitis who relapsed following monotherapy.[41] As a consequence, 5-FC is rarely given alone but in combination with AmB or, more recently, fluconazole.

On the basis of randomized clinical trials, the combination of amphotericin B and flucytosine has become the standard for induction therapy of cryptococcal meningoencephalitis.[52,53] The pivotal role of 5-FC during initial treatment for cryptococcal meningoencephalitis has found strong support by several clinical trials conducted in the past decade[46,52,54] and, taken together, a large body of clinical evidence points to the benefits of 5-FC in induction treatment of cryptococcal meningoencephalitis with amphotericin B regardless of the patient's HIV serostatus.[53]

The combination of 5-FC with amphotericin B can also be recommended for complicated deep tissue candidiasis, particularly in critically ill patients and when non-*albicans Candida* spp. are involved. This includes meningitis, endophthalmitis, endocarditis, vasculitis and peritonitis, as well as osteoarticular, renal and chronic disseminated candidiasis.[42] Flucytosine with fluconazole may be used for cryptococcal meningitis, when treatment with AmB is not feasible. This combination may also be useful as second-line therapy for individual patients with invasive *Candida* infections involving aqueous body compartments. Due to the propensity for secondary resistance, 5-FC should not be administered alone. The one exception for monotherapy of 5-FC may be treatment of triazole-resistant *C. glabrata* lower urinary tract infection.

Dosage in Special Circumstances

Dose adjustment of 5-FC is critically important in patients with kidney dysfunction as 5-FC is excreted by glomerular filtration and toxic blood levels will occur if dosing is not modified according to kidney function. The adult oral dose is based on ideal body weight and is 25 mg/kg every 6 hr for glomerular filtration rate (GFR)>50 mL/min. The dose should be reduced to 25 mg/kg every 12–24 hr for GFR between 10–50 mL/min and 25 mg/kg every 48 hr for GFR<10 mL/min. 5-FC is readily dialyzable and the dose for hemodialysis patients should 25 mg/kg every 48 hours, administered post-dialysis on dialysis days. The dose for patients undergoing continuous veno-venal hemoperfusion/dialysis (CVVHD) is not well characterized. A starting dose of 25 mg/kg every 12 hours is reasonable with careful therapeutic drug monitoring (TDM) along with serial complete blood counts (CBCs).

TDM and follow up CBCs are strongly recommended with 5-FC treatment, especially in patients with pre-existing kidney disease, those receiving potentially nephrotoxic drugs, or in hemodynamically unstable patients with variable kidney function. The target blood level 2 hours after oral dosing of 5-FC after 3–5 days of starting therapy should be 50±20 µg/mL. Higher blood levels increase the risk of potentially severe bone marrow toxicity. No dose reduction for 5-FC is needed for hepatic dysfunction.

Adverse Effects and Drug Interactions

Common adverse effects of 5-FC include gastrointestinal intolerance, myelosuppression and elevations of hepatic transaminases and alkaline phosphatase. Myelosuppression, which may include neutropenia, thrombocytopenia or pancytopenia, is concentration dependent. Hematologic adverse effects are less frequent if plasma levels do not exceed 100 µg/mL.[42] Less common adverse reactions include rashes, eosinophilia, crystalluria, ulcerative colitis, and bowel perforation.[42] Among 202 AIDS patients receiving combination therapy with AmB and 5-FC for cryptococcal meningitis, the drug toxicity withdrawal rate of 3% was similar to those receiving AmB monotherapy.[53] Some adverse effects may be due to conversion of 5-FC to 5-fluorouracil by gastrointestinal bacteria and toxic effects of endogenous metabolites.[41]

Orally administered, non-resorbable antibiotics and aluminum/magnesium hydroxide-based antacids may delay oral 5-FC absorption.[42] Flucytosine is not known to interfere with the CYP450 enzyme system. However, drugs causing reduction in the GFR may increase 5-FC serum levels. Cytosine arabinoside competitively inhibits 5-FC and the drugs should not be given concomitantly.

ANTIFUNGAL TRIAZOLES
Overview

As a class, the triazoles are the most important group of antifungal agents for systemic use. These agents are now key components of prevention and treatment strategies for invasive fungal infections.

The antifungal triazoles target ergosterol biosynthesis by inhibiting the fungal cytochrome P450-dependent enzyme lanosterol 14-α-demethylase. Inhibition of lanosterol 14-α-demethylase interrupts the conversion of lanosterol to ergosterol, which leads to accumulation of aberrant 14-α-methylsterols and depletion of ergosterol in the fungal cell membrane (see Figure 156-2). This alters cell membrane physiology and, depending on organism and compound, may lead to cell death or inhibition of cell growth and replication. The various triazoles have different binding affinities to this enzymatic target. Tighter binding in the later generation agents (e.g. itraconazole, voriconazole and posaconazole) may account for their expanded spectrum of activity. The triazoles also inhibit cytochrome P450-dependent enzymes of the fungal respiration chain, further contributing to their antifungal activity.

Fluconazole and itraconazole are principally active against dermatophytes, *Candida* spp., *Cryptococcus neoformans*, *Trichosporon* spp. and some other uncommon yeast-like organisms, and against the dimorphic fungi *Histoplasma capsulatum*, *Coccidioides* spp., *Blastomyces dermatitidis*, *Paracoccidioides brasiliensis* and *Sporothrix schenckii*. These triazoles have less activity against *Candida glabrata* and almost none against *C. krusei*.[55] Itraconazole is active against *Aspergillus* spp. and dematiaceous molds. None of these are active against *Fusarium* spp. and the Mucorales. Voriconazole and posaconazole are active against *C. albicans* and *C. krusei*, *Aspergillus* spp. and some *Fusarium* spp. Posaconazole and isavuconazole are also active against the Mucorales.[56]

Selection and nosocomial spread of triazole-resistant *Candida* spp. is a matter of increasing concern. Resistance in *Candida* is encountered most commonly in the form of a primarily resistant species or through selection of resistant subclones during exposure to triazoles. Several mechanisms have been identified, including alterations at the target binding site, increased target expression and induction of cellular efflux pumps. *Candida* spp. in biofilm is significantly less susceptible to triazoles.[30] This effect is at least partly mediated by expression of efflux pumps and alteration in sterol composition.[57]

Reduced susceptibility or resistance to triazoles is seen in several settings: 1) oropharyngeal and esophageal candidiasis in patients with advanced HIV who have been extensively exposed to triazole antifungals;[58] 2) invasive candidiasis in patients with hematological malignancies and/or hematopoietic stem cell transplantation; and 3) breakthrough infections due to yeast or filamentous fungi in patients who are receiving an azole agent for prophylaxis. The latter group is increasingly important with the growing use of antifungal prophylaxis strategies for a range of at-risk patients. Because cross-resistance of *Candida* spp. to antifungal triazoles is common, a different class of antifungal agent should be used when resistance is suspected. However, some patients with fluconazole-resistant mucosal candidiasis may respond to other triazoles.

Acquired triazole resistance has been documented in patients with *Cr. neoformans* meningitis receiving maintenance therapy. Triazole-resistant *A. fumigatus* has emerged in the past decade and up to 6% of clinical isolates may have decreased susceptibility to newer triazoles.[59]

TDM to ensure appropriate serum levels is an important aspect of treatment with itraconazole, voriconazole and posaconazole. Serum drug concentrations can vary widely with these agents. Even with recommended dosing guidelines, many patients have subtherapeutic serum levels, which in turn are associated with reduced clinical efficacy.[60] Minimum trough levels of ≥0.5 µg/mL for itraconazole ≥1.0 (ideally ≥2) for voriconazole and ≥0.7 (ideally ≥1.25) for posaconazole are recommended.[61,62] Additionally, voriconazole toxicity is more common when levels exceed 5.5, making TDM particularly important.

There are many important interactions between antifungal triazoles and drugs metabolized through isoenzymes of the CYP450 system. Particular caution is advised when these agents are co-administered with CYP450 substrates that have the potential to prolong the QTc interval and when co-administered with HMG-CoA reductase inhibitors that have the potential to cause rhabdomyolysis. The concurrent use of terfenadine, astemizole, cisapride, pimozide, halofantrine, dofetilide, quinidine and vincristine is contraindicated.

Chemical structures of fluconazole, itraconazole, voriconazole, posaconazole and isavuconazole

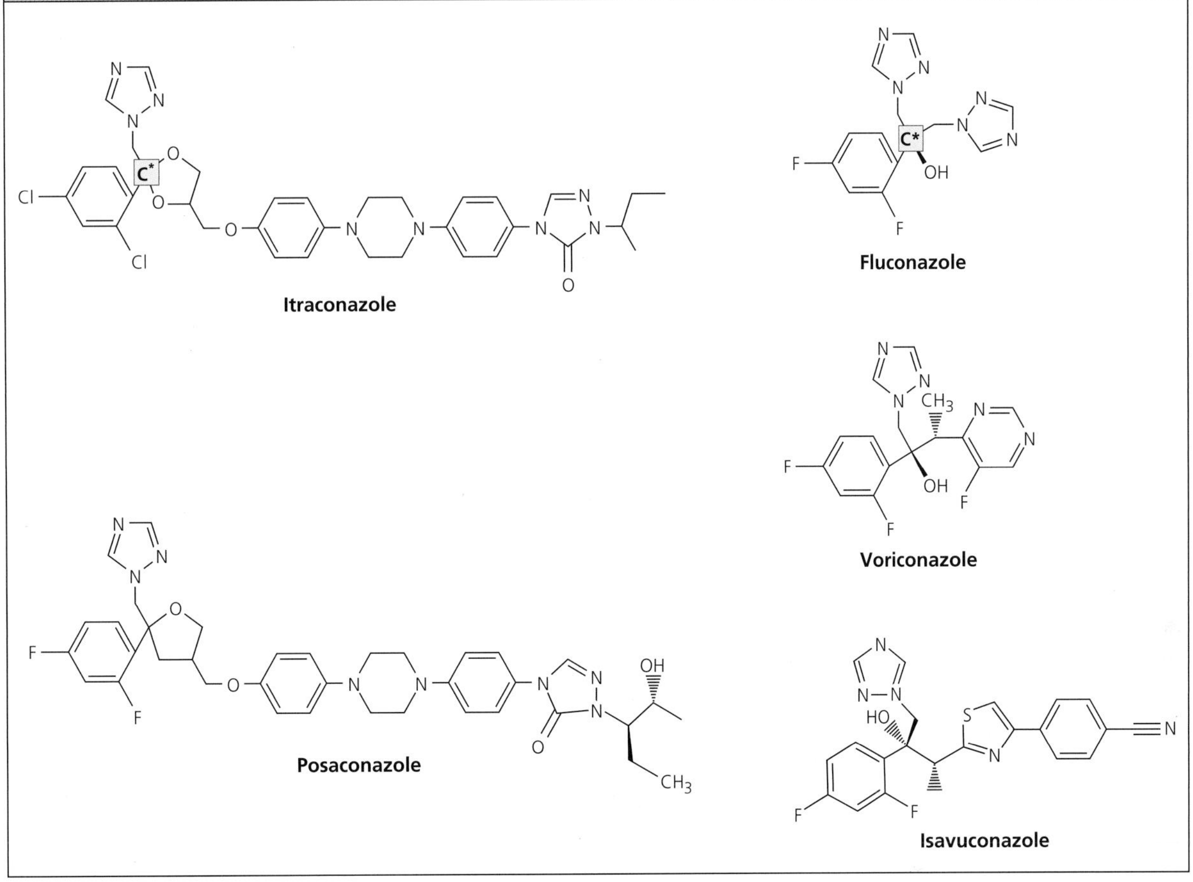

Figure 156-4 Chemical structures of fluconazole, itraconazole, voriconazole, posaconazole and isavuconazole.

FLUCONAZOLE (Figure 156-4)

Pharmacokinetics and Distribution

Fluconazole is available for oral and parenteral use, and exhibits linear plasma pharmacokinetics that are independent of route and formulation. Steady state concentrations are generally reached within 4–7 days following once-daily dosing, but can be rapidly achieved by doubling the dose on the first day. Protein binding is low, and the drug distributes evenly into virtually all tissue sites and body fluids, including the CSF, brain tissue and the eye. More than 90% of a dose is renally excreted, with approximately 80% recovered as unchanged active drug and 11% recovered as inactive metabolites. In patients with a creatinine clearance of ≤50 mL/min, a 50% reduction in dosage is required, and below 20 mL/min, a 75% reduction is needed. The initial loading dose need not be adjusted. Fluconazole is dialyzable; in patients undergoing hemodialysis, 100% of the target dose is given after each dialysis session. In continuous hemofiltration, clearance may be faster, requiring therapy at higher than usual dosages (e.g. 800 mg/day); in patients undergoing peritoneal dialysis, fluconazole can be administered either systemically or intraperitoneally.

Pharmacodynamics

Conventional time-kill assays performed over incubation periods of 24–48 hours in susceptible *Candida* spp. and *Cr. neoformans* show fungistatic activity of fluconazole with variable concentration-related growth effects. However, with extended incubation of up to 14 days and under nonproliferating growth conditions, fungicidal activity has been observed against *C. albicans*.[63,64] In serum-free growth media, fluconazole displays no measurable postantifungal effect (PAFE)

against *C. albicans* and *Cr. neoformans*, but concentration-dependent PAFEs of 1–3.6 hours were observed in the presence of fresh serum.[14] Clinical data and pharmacodynamic studies in murine models of disseminated *C. albicans* infection collectively suggest that the AUC/MIC ratio is the most predictive pharmacodynamic parameter of fluconazole.[65,66] Overall, the dose-independent pharmacokinetics and the available experimental and clinical data support once-daily dosing regimens of this triazole.

Route of Administration and Dosage

In adults, the recommended dosage range for treatment of invasive infections is 400–800 mg/day and for prevention, 200–400 mg/day.

Indications

Fluconazole is effective for treatment of superficial and invasive candidiasis, including infections in neutropenic patients.[67] However, echinocandins are replacing fluconazole as first line therapy of candidemia. For recipients of triazole prophylaxis, an alternative class is indicated for treatment of candidemia. Other indications for fluconazole include consolidation therapy for chronic disseminated candidiasis, cryptococcal meningitis and infections by *Trichosporon* spp. Fluconazole is the drug of choice for treatment of coccidioidal meningitis and has effectiveness in non-meningeal coccidioidal infections.[68,69] Against paracoccidioidomycosis, blastomycosis, histoplasmosis and sporotrichosis, fluconazole is less active than itraconazole.[70-73] In the prophylactic setting, fluconazole has proven efficacy for primary prevention of invasive candidiasis in high-risk patients with acute leukemia, bone marrow and liver transplantation,[74-77] for primary prevention of cryptococcosis in AIDS, and for secondary prevention of cryptococcosis and coccidioidomycosis in AIDS. Fluconazole is not active against filamentous fungi and should not be used for prevention or empiric therapy if there is a high-risk invasive infection.

Dosage in Special Circumstances

In children, the recommended dosage is 12 mg/kg/day to be comparable to the plasma exposure conferred by 400 mg/day in adults.[78] Given the extreme variability in extravascular water content and renal function, particularly in very low birth weight preterm infants, predictably effective and safe treatment with fluconazole may not be possible during the first days of life.[79] Hepatic insufficiency does not require dose adjustments, but careful monitoring of additional hepatic toxicity is warranted. The pharmacokinetics in children reflect developmental changes characteristic for a water-soluble drug with minor metabolism and predominantly renal elimination. Except for premature neonates, where clearance is initially decreased, children tend to have an increased weight-normalized clearance rate from plasma that leads to a shorter half-life in comparison to adults. As serum levels in neonates depend upon both gestational age at birth and postnatal age,[79] dosages at the high end of the recommended dosage range are necessary for the treatment of invasive mycoses in children.

Adverse Effects and Drug Interactions

In adults, fluconazole has been safely administered over prolonged periods of time at dosages of up to 1600 mg/day.[80] Compiled data from adults who received dosages of 100–400 mg/day indicate an incidence of significant adverse effects or laboratory abnormalities leading to drug discontinuation of 2.8%. Gastrointestinal symptoms are seen in <5%, rashes and headaches in <2% and are usually reversible, and asymptomatic transaminase elevations in up to 7% of adult patients. QT segment prolongation and ventricular tachycardia have been described with fluconazole.[81] In children, fluconazole is generally well tolerated.[82] Alopecia can be seen with higher doses (400 mg/day) given for 2 months or longer and is reversible with reduced dosage or drug discontinuation.[83]

Fluconazole undergoes minimal CYP-mediated metabolism, but inhibits intestinal and hepatic CYP3A4 and several other CYP isoforms in vitro. Fluconazole interacts with enzymes involved in glucuronidation and is a substrate of the drug transporter P-glycoprotein, leading to a number of significant drug interactions. Interactions with other CYP3A4 substrates, including calcineurin inhibitors, may be more pronounced with oral fluconazole.[84] On the other hand, drugs that induce hepatic enzymes – for example, rifampin (rifampicin) – may decrease fluconazole levels. Altogether, the number of relevant drug interactions is lower than with that of itraconazole and posaconazole.

ITRACONAZOLE

Pharmacokinetics and Distribution

Itraconazole is a high-molecular weight, highly lipophilic bis-triazole. It is available as capsules and as an oral solution in hydroxypropyl-β-cyclodextrin (HP-β-CD). Absorption from the capsule form is dependent on a low intragastric pH and is compromised in the fasting state, and thus is unpredictable in granulocytopenic cancer patients and in patients with hypochlorhydria. Absorption is improved when the capsules are taken with food or an acidic cola beverage. Itraconazole oral solution in HP-β-CD provides better oral bioavailability that is further enhanced in the fasting state.[85]

Following oral administration, peak plasma concentrations occur within 1–4 hours; systemic absorption of the cyclodextrin carrier is negligible. With once-daily dosing, steady state is achieved after 7–14 days, but can be reached more rapidly by doubling the dose over the first 2–3 days. Itraconazole is highly protein-bound and is extensively distributed throughout the body. Although concentrations in non-proteinaceous body fluids are negligible, tissue concentrations in many organs, including the brain, exceed corresponding plasma levels by 2–10 times.[85]

Itraconazole is extensively metabolized in the liver and excreted in metabolized form into bile and urine. The major metabolite, hydroxy-itraconazole, possesses antifungal activity similar to itraconazole. The elimination of itraconazole from plasma follows a biphasic pattern; in comparison to single dosing, the elimination half-life at steady state is about twice as long, reflecting saturable excretion mechanisms.

Pharmacodynamics

Itraconazole exerts species- and strain-dependent fungistatic or fungicidal pharmacodynamics in vitro. Time-kill experiments have demonstrated concentration-independent, fungistatic activity of itraconazole against Candida spp. and Cr. neoformans.[14] Against Aspergillus spp., however, itraconazole displayed time- and concentration-dependent fungicidal activity with >87% to >97% killing within 24 hours of drug exposure.[86] Persistent effects have not been reported thus far, and it remains to be determined which pharmacodynamic parameter best predicts antifungal efficacy in vivo.[14]

Route of Administration and Dosage

The recommended dosage range of oral itraconazole in adults is 100–400 mg/day (capsules) and 2.5 mg/kg q12h (HP-β-CD solution). For life-threatening infections, a loading dose of 600–800 mg/day for 3–5 days, followed by a maintenance dose of 400–600 mg/day, and monitoring of serum levels is recommended. Itraconazole is not approved for patients <18 years of age; based on the available pharmacokinetic data, a starting dosage of 2.5 mg/kg q12h of oral HP-β-CD itraconazole can be advocated. The recommended dosage range for the capsule formulation is 5–8 mg/kg/day with a loading dose of 4 mg/kg q8h for the first 3 days.

Indications

Itraconazole is effective against a range of fungal infections, but its current use is generally limited to chronic pulmonary aspergillosis, allergic bronchopulmonary aspergillosis, and certain endemic mycoses (e.g. nonsevere presentations of histoplasmosis and blastomycosis).[87,88]

Itraconazole also is effective for dermatophytic infections, pityriasis versicolor and cutaneous and mucosal candidiasis. Itraconazole has been successful for consolidation and maintenance treatment of cryptococcosis in the setting of HIV infection.[89] Itraconazole may be useful for certain dematiaceous molds, but is inactive against mucormycosis and fusariosis. Itraconazole is the current treatment of choice for lymphocutaneous sporotrichosis and non-life-threatening, non-meningeal paracoccidioidomycosis, blastomycosis and histoplasmosis. In progressive non-meningeal coccidioidomycosis, AmB remains the treatment of choice for most immunocompromised patients and for life-threatening infections.

Itraconazole has been successful as antifungal prophylaxis in patients undergoing stem cell transplantation or intensive chemotherapy. HP-β-CD itraconazole may reduce the incidence of proven or suspected invasive fungal infections in neutropenic patients with hematologic malignancies.[90] Itraconazole was at least as effective as conventional AmB and less toxic as empirical therapy in persistently febrile, neutropenic patients,[91] and is FDA-approved for this indication.

Dosage in Special Circumstances

The dosage of oral itraconazole does not need to be adjusted with renal insufficiency or dialysis. In patients with severe hepatic insufficiency, the elimination half-life of itraconazole can be prolonged and additional hepatic toxicity or possible drug interactions should be carefully monitored.[85] The pharmacokinetics of oral HP-β-CD itraconazole in pediatric patients beyond the neonatal period appear similar to that of adults.[92-94]

Adverse Effects and Drug Interactions

Itraconazole is usually well tolerated, with a similar spectrum and frequency of adverse effects as fluconazole. Adverse events leading to the discontinuation of itraconazole occur in approximately 4% of patients at dosages of up to 400 mg/day. Most observed reactions are transient, and include nausea and vomiting (<10%), hypertriglyceridemia (9%), hypokalemia (6%), elevated hepatic transaminases (5%), rash and/or pruritus (2%), headaches or dizziness (<2%) and pedal edema (1%).[95] Gastrointestinal intolerance is frequent with oral HP-β-CD itraconazole at dosages exceeding 400 mg/day. Severe hepatic injury is rare. Itraconazole can have negative inotropic effects and should not be administered to patients with ventricular dysfunction.[96] Oral HP-β-CD itraconazole was safe and relatively well tolerated in pharmacokinetic studies in pediatric patients with vomiting (12%), abnormal liver function tests (5%) and abdominal pain (3%) being the most common adverse effects.[97]

Drug–drug interactions are more common with itraconazole than with fluconazole. Itraconazole is a substrate of CYP3A4, but also interacts with the heme moiety of CYP3A, resulting in noncompetitive inhibition of oxidative metabolism of many CYP3A substrates and increased and potentially toxic concentrations of co-administered drugs. The adverse competitive interaction between vincristine and itraconazole, as well as other anti-mold triazoles, is one that is especially important in managing patients with lymphoid malignancies.[98] Increased metabolism of itraconazole resulting in decreased plasma levels can result from co-administration of inducers of hepatic enzymes, such as rifampin. Finally, the systemic availability of oral itraconazole depends in part on the activity of intestinal CYP3A4 and P-glycoprotein, which contributes to its variable bioavailability.

Second-Generation Antifungal Triazoles

Further improvements in the structure–activity relationship of antifungal triazoles have led to a new group of synthetic compounds that are collectively known as second-generation triazoles, comprising voriconazole, posaconazole, and isavuconazole. The second-generation triazoles possess enhanced target activity and specificity. They are active against a wide spectrum of clinically important fungi, including *Candida* spp., *Trichosporon* spp., *Cr. neoformans*, *Aspergillus* spp., *Fusarium* spp. and other hyaline molds, and dematiaceous and dimorphic molds. Similar to itraconazole, these novel triazoles exert fungistatic activity against susceptible yeast-like organisms and strain-dependent fungicidal activity against susceptible filamentous fungi. Isavuconazole and posaconazole appear to have the best activity against the Mucorales.

VORICONAZOLE

Pharmacokinetics and Distribution

Voriconazole is available as a tablet and parenteral solution that uses sulfobutyl ether-β-cyclodextrin (SE-β-CD) as a solubilizer. In tablet form, voriconazole is rapidly absorbed from the gastrointestinal tract. Although bioavailability is near 100%, steady-state plasma concentrations are achieved more rapidly with an intravenous loading dose. Multiple enzymes of the cytochrome P450 system including CYP2C19, which exhibits genetic polymorphism in certain racial groups, metabolize voriconazole. Drug levels in poor metabolizers, which may include up to 20% of Asian populations, can be significantly elevated. One such polymorphism is CYP2C19*2 and patients homozygous for this gene can have higher serum voriconazole levels.[99] Conversely, plasma levels in extensive or ultra-rapid metabolizers may be much lower.

In adults, voriconazole exhibits non-linear pharmacokinetics between 3 and 4 mg/kg, possibly due to saturable metabolism and systemic clearance.[100] In contrast, elimination of voriconazole in children is linear between 3 and 4 mg/kg and higher relative dosages may be required to achieve exposures consistent with those in adults.[101] TDM is increasingly used and may improve outcomes.[102]

CSF concentrations vary greatly, but are generally approximately half the serum concentration and have a linear relationship to dose.[103] Concentrations in the vitreous and aqueous fluids are 38% and 53% of serum levels, respectively.[104] The addition of a 1% topical voriconazole solution can further increase vitreous and aqueous levels and therapeutic concentrations against many pathogenic fungi

may be achieved with topical therapy alone.[105,106] Voriconazole may be applied to the cornea and directly injected into the anterior chamber and the vitreous in cases of invasive fungal keratitis and endophthalmitis.

Following its metabolism in the liver, the drug is mostly excreted in urine. The pharmacokinetics are unaffected by renal function. Current laboratory and clinical studies do not support the suggestions that the intravenous carrier solution, SE-β-CD, leads to renal dysfunction.[107,108]

Pharmacodynamics

In *Candida* spp. and *Cr. neoformans* voriconazole exhibits non-concentration-dependent pharmacodynamics. Near-maximal fungistatic activity is achieved at a drug concentration of approximately three times the MIC.[109] A postantifungal effect of up to 4 hours has been observed with *C. albicans*.[110] Voriconazole also has immunomodulatory properties that may enhance the immune response to *A. fumigatus*.[111]

Route of Administration and Dosage

For treatment of invasive fungal infections in adults, an intravenous loading dose of 6 mg/kg q12h on day 1 followed by 4 mg/kg q12h thereafter is employed. The oral dosage in adults consists of a loading dose of 450 mg q12h on day 1 followed by 300 mg q12h thereafter.

Indications

Voriconazole is indicated for primary treatment of aspergillosis and candidemia, as well as for salvage therapy for fusariosis and scedosporiosis. In a randomized, open-label trial of patients with invasive aspergillosis, initial therapy with voriconazole led to a significantly greater response rate, improved survival and less toxicity than the standard approach of initial therapy with AmB deoxycholate.[112] Voriconazole also has been used successfully in the treatment of invasive fungal infections including aspergillosis in children who were refractory to, or intolerant of, conventional antifungal therapy.[113] It is also effective in oropharyngeal and esophageal candidiasis in immunocompromised patients and as primary therapy for candidemia in non-neutropenic patients.[114,115] A large, randomized, multicenter trial compared 12-hourly administration of voriconazole (3 mg/kg intravenously or 200 mg orally) with liposomal AmB (3 mg/kg intravenously) for empiric antifungal therapy and showed comparable composite success rates, with fewer breakthrough infections, and less toxicity with voriconazole, although these patients had significantly more frequent episodes of transient visual disturbances and hallucinations.[116]

Dosage in Special Circumstances

For children, a dosage of 8 mg/kg intravenously q12h is initially used. Voriconazole by the oral route is administered at 200 mg q12h in adults. As SE-β-CD clearance is related to GFR, oral voriconazole should be used, when feasible, in patients whose creatinine clearance is <50 ml/min. In patients with mild to moderate hepatic cirrhosis, the standard loading dose is recommended, but the maintenance dose should be halved.

Adverse Affects and Drug Interactions

Mild and reversible visual disturbances of photopsia occur in approximately 30% of patients. This may manifest as altered color perception, photophobia or blurred vision. The mechanism is unknown, but is thought to be retinal. Other common adverse reactions include visual hallucinations, rashes, phototoxicity, gastrointestinal disturbances and hepatic abnormalities. Visual disturbances and/or hallucinations occur in up to 16.6% of patients, may be related to higher serum drug levels and are particularly associated with intravenously administered voriconazole.[117] Long-term voriconazole use has also been associated with elevated fluoride levels and painful periostitis that typically resolve with discontinuation of the drug.

In addition to undergoing metabolism by the P450 system, voriconazole inhibits several CYP enzymes, leading to extensive potential for drug–drug interactions. Extreme care must be taken when co-administering voriconazole with agents metabolized through the P450 system, particularly with drugs having narrow therapeutic windows such as vincristine, calcineurin inhibitors, and sirolimus.

POSACONAZOLE

Pharmacokinetics and Distribution

Three formulations of posaconazole are currently available; oral suspension, delayed-release tablets and intravenous injection. Most clinical experience is with the oral suspension, where optimal exposure is achieved when administered in two to four divided doses given with food or a nutritional supplement. Following repeat dosing, steady state is achieved after 7–10 days with a six- to eight-fold accumulation of plasma concentrations.[118] Posaconazole has a large volume of distribution on the order of 5 L/kg and a prolonged elimination half-life of approximately 20 hours. It is not significantly metabolized through the cytochrome P450 enzyme system but primarily excreted unchanged in the feces. Approximately 10% of the compound is metabolized through glucuronidation.

Route of Administration and Dosage

Recommended posaconazole dosage for prophylaxis of invasive fungal infections with the oral solution is 200 mg thrice daily, whereas delayed-release tablets and intravenous formulations are given with loading dose of 300 mg every 12 hours on the first day followed by 300 mg daily thereafter. The dosage of posaconazole solution for primary treatment of oropharyngeal candidiasis is 100 mg/day (day 1: 100 mg q12h) and 400 mg q12h for refractory disease. When using posaconazole for salvage treatment, the recommended daily dosage is 400 mg q12h of the solution given with food; for patients not tolerating solid food, a dosage of 200 mg q6h is recommended, preferentially together with a nutritional supplement.

Indications

Posaconazole is indicated for treatment of aspergillosis, fusariosis, chromoblastomycosis and coccidioidomycosis in patients who are refractory to, or intolerant of, standard therapies. It is also indicated for prophylaxis of invasive *Candida* and *Aspergillus* infections in high-risk patients ≥13 years of age with allogeneic hematopoietic stem cell transplantation and graft-versus-host disease or those with hematologic malignancies and prolonged neutropenia. In a large phase II study including 330 patients with invasive fungal infections mostly refractory to standard therapies, the rates of successful outcome were 42% for aspergillosis (107 patients),[62] 39% for fusariosis (18 patients), 69% (16 patients) for coccidioidomycosis and 81% for chromoblastomycosis (11 patients).[119,120] Efficacy has also been found against other invasive fungal infections, including mucormycosis, candidiasis, cryptococcosis and refractory oropharyngeal candidiasis.[121-126] Two studies demonstrated the preventive efficacy of posaconazole, in particular against invasive *Aspergillus* infections in high-risk patients, including a statistically significant survival benefit in patients with acute myeloid leukemia/myelodysplastic syndrome undergoing remission induction chemotherapy.[127,128]

Dosage in Special Circumstances

The pharmacokinetics of posaconazole in pediatric patients (<18 years of age) have not been adequately studied.[129]

Adverse Effects and Drug Interactions

The safety profile of posaconazole appears to be comparable to that of fluconazole or itraconazole.[127,128] In more than 400 patients with invasive fungal infections from two open-label clinical trials who received posaconazole suspension (800 mg/day in divided doses),[130,131] treatment-related adverse events occurred in 38% of patients; the most common were nausea (8%), vomiting (6%), headache (5%), abdominal pain (4%) and diarrhea (4%). Treatment-related abnormal liver function test results were observed in up to 3% of patients. The most common severe adverse events were altered drug levels, increased hepatic enzymes, nausea, rash, and vomiting (1% each).

Posaconazole is not significantly metabolized through the cytochrome P450 enzyme system, but inhibits cytochrome P3A4; it has no effect on 1A2, 2C8, 2C9, 2D6 and 2E1 isoenzymes.[132-135] As such, monitoring of cyclosporine, tacrolimus and sirolimus blood concentrations is mandatory, and dose adjustments should be made accordingly.

ISAVUCONAZOLE

Pharmacokinetics and Distribution

Isavuconazole is delivered in the form of a water-soluble prodrug, known as isavuconazonium. Isavuconazonium is administered orally or as an intravenous formulation. Isavuconazonium consists of an [N-(3-acetoxypropyl)-N-methylamino]-carboxymethyl group attached to isavuconazole via an ester linkage that is hydrolyzed in the presence of plasma esterases. In contrast to the intravenous formulations of other triazoles, isavuconazonium does not require cyclodextrin for solubility.

In healthy adult volunteers, isavuconazole has a relatively large volume of distribution (470-542 L), AUC_{0-24} following 200 mg load and 100 mg/day of 33.6–41.5 mg·h/mL, long terminal plasma half-life of approximately 56-104 h, clearance of 3 – 4 L/h, and steady state trough concentrations at 100 mg/d of approximately 1 μg/mL.

Route of Administration and Dosage

The following dosage regimen is used as either the parenteral or oral formulations: loading dose of 200 mg q8h intravenously or by mouth for the first 2 days followed by 200 mg/day intravenously or by mouth.[136]

Indications

Isavuconazole has broad-spectrum antifungal activity against *Candida* spp., *Aspergillus* spp., *Fusarium* spp. and several species of the Mucorales.[136-139] Isavuconazole is approved for primary treatment of invasive aspergillosis and mucormycosis in adult patients. Isavuconazole was studied in a randomized trial against voriconazole for the primary treatment of invasive aspergillosis that demonstrated that isavuconazole was noninferior to voriconazole and had a more favorable safety profile with significantly less visual toxicity, CNS adverse events, and cutaneous reactions. Results of the candidemia trial are pending.[139]

Isavuconazole is active against experimental murine disseminated mucormycosis by *Rhizopus oryzae*. Isavuconazole was as effective as liposomal amphotericin B in improving survival and decreasing residual fungal burden in cyclophosphamide/cortisone acetate immunosuppressed mice.[140] This activity of isavuconazole against mucormycosis was predictive of the favorable outcome of isavuconazole in a nonrandomized clinical trial for primary treatment of mucormycosis in immunocompromised patients.[141] Combination therapy with isavuconazole and micafungin is synergistic *in vitro* against *Aspergillus* spp., raising the hypothesis that this triazole-echinocandin combination may be active *in vivo*.

Dosage in Special Circumstances

Clearance in patients with liver impairment is significantly lower (estimates ranging from 2.73 to 1.43 L/h) in comparison to that of healthy volunteers with a near doubling of the elimination plasma half-life from a mean of 123 h in healthy volunteers to 302 h in patients with moderate hepatic impairment, indicating the need for dosage reduction in patients with liver dysfunction.

Adverse Effects and Drug Interactions

Among the minimal adverse effects observed in healthy adult volunteers receiving isavuconazole were nasopharyngitis, rhinitis and headaches. Elevations of serum serum hepatic transaminases could occur in some recipients of isavuconazole.

Because of its clearance through the CYP3A4 pathway, isavuconazole has been found to antagonize the metabolism of tacrolimus. Studies of other drug–drug interactions of isavuconazole are underway.

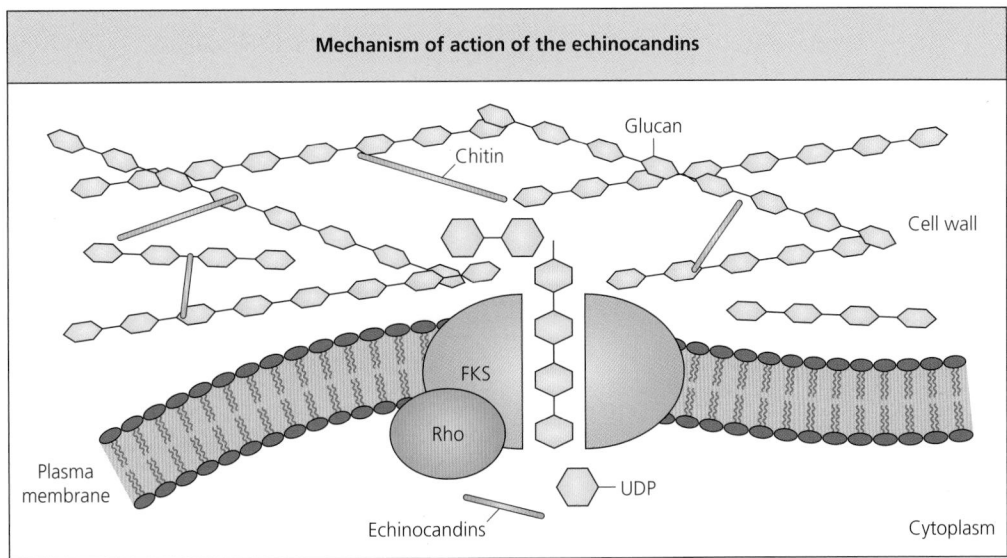

Figure 156-5 Mechanism of action of the echinocandins.

Echinocandin Lipopeptides
ANIDULAFUNGIN, CASPOFUNGIN, MICAFUNGIN
Mechanism of Action

The echinocandins are a novel class of semisynthetic amphiphilic lipopeptides composed of a cyclic hexapeptide core linked to a variably configured N-acyl-lipid side chain.[142-144] The echinocandins act by noncompetitive inhibition of the synthesis of $(1\rightarrow3)\beta$-D-glucan, a polysaccharide in the cell wall of many pathogenic fungi (Figure 156-5). Together with chitin, the rope-like glucan fibrils are responsible for the cell wall's strength and shape. They are important in maintaining the osmotic integrity of the fungal cell and play a key role in cell division and cell growth.[145,146] The structures of caspofungin, anidulafungin and micafungin are shown in Figure 156-6. The N-acyl aliphatic substitution with or without aryl mixed functional groups extends the antifungal spectrum of the cyclic hexapeptide to include *Candida* spp. and *Aspergillus* spp. and affects the pharmacokinetics of the molecules.

The echinocandins demonstrate a species-dependent mode of antifungal activity.[147] They have fungicidal activity against most *Candida* spp. but not against *Aspergillus* spp. In the latter, microscopic examination of exposed hyphae demonstrates a dose-dependent formation of microcolonies with progressively truncated, swollen hyphal elements that appear to be cell-wall deficient, but that can regain their cell walls upon subculture in the absence of drug. As exemplified by caspofungin, echinocandins preferentially kill cells at active centers of wall synthesis at the branch points and advancing tips of *A. fumigatus* hyphae.[148]

The echinocandins may have a role in biofilm-associated candidiasis. Therapeutic concentrations of echinocandins display potent *in vitro* activity against *C. albicans* in biofilms.[149] When used as catheter lock solutions echinocandins may effectively reduce or control fungal biofilms *in vitro* and in animal model systems.[30,150] Clinical studies are needed to define the role of the echinocandins in biofilms.

The mechanism of echinocandins includes immunomodulation and upregulation of innate host defenses. Data have emerged regarding interactions between echinocandins and phagocytic cells. Echinocandins alone do not completely inhibit *in vitro* growth of *Aspergillus fumigatus*, but a powerful antifungal effect is seen in combination with phagocytes. Echinocandins enhance neutrophil activity against *Aspergillus* and non-*Aspergillus* hyphae by unmasking β-glucans and activating host antifungal pathways via the dectin-1 receptor.[151,152]

Pharmacokinetics and Distribution

All current echinocandins are only available intravenously. They exhibit dose-proportional plasma pharmacokinetics with a plasma half-life of 10–15 hours that allows for once-daily dosing. Echinocandins are >95% protein bound and distribute into all major organ sites including the brain; however, concentrations in uninfected CSF are low. Caspofungin is transported into the liver and hepatically excreted largely unchanged. Micafungin is metabolized by arylsulfatase and catechol-O-methyl transferase followed by hepatic excretion. Anidulafungin is thermally and non-enzymatically degraded in serum with subsequent hepatic excretion. Only small fractions are excreted into urine in unchanged form.[153] The pharmacokinetic parameters are generally lower in children than in adults for caspofungin but not for anidulafungin. Drug levels are especially low in smaller, younger children and neonates for micafungin.[154]

Pharmacodynamics

In vitro pharmacodynamic studies in *Candida* spp. have shown predominantly concentration-dependent ($\geq 99.9\%$ reduction in CFU) fungicidal activity and *in vivo* concentration-dependent pharmacodynamics and prolonged postantifungal effects of up to 12 hours duration.[155]

Dosing and Administration

The recommended daily doses in adults with systemic infections are 100 mg for micafungin and anidulafungin, and 50 mg for caspofungin. A loading dose of 200 mg for anidulafungin and 70 mg for caspofungin is required on the first day.

Indications

Laboratory studies *in vitro* and in animals demonstrate synergy with the combination of an echinocandin and an anti-mold triazole in treatment of invasive aspergillosis.[156,157]

Although the current echinocandins differ in pharmacokinetic properties, all three have similar, potent, broad spectrum, and fungicidal *in vitro* activity against *Candida* species and inhibitory activity against *Aspergillus* spp. The median MICs for echinocandins against *C. albicans* are typically 0.03-0.06 μg/mL. The minimal effective concentration (MEC) against *Aspergillus fumigatus* also is typically low at 0.06–0.125 μg/mL. While still generally susceptible, *C. parapsilosis* isolates generally show elevated MICs for the echinocandins compared to most other wild type isolates of *Candida* spp. Wild type isolates of *C.*

Structures of echinocandins currently used in clinical practice or in clinical trials

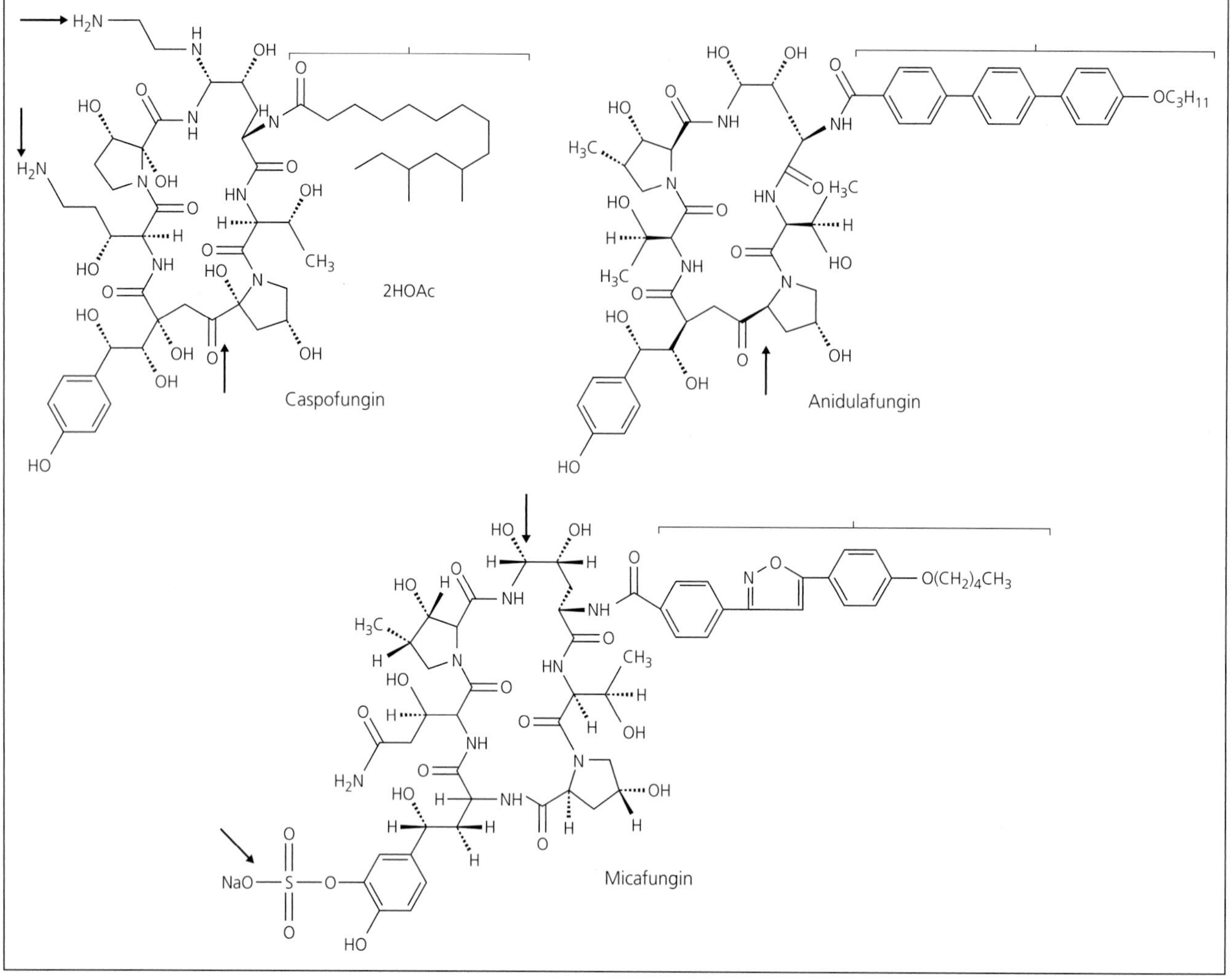

Figure 156-6 Structures of echinocandins currently used in clinical practice or in clinical trials.

parapsilosis demonstrate a proline to alanine polymorphism on the hot spot one region of the *FKS1* gene, which confers a higher MIC of approximately 1.0 µg/mL. The current echinocandins have variable *in vitro* activity against dematiaceous and endemic molds, and are inactive against most hyalohyphomycetes, *C. neoformans* and *Trichosporon* spp.[137,158] Echinocandins also have minimal *in vitro* activity against the Mucorales, but animal models of disseminated mucormycosis and clinical experience suggest a role for echinocandins, when combined with AmB.[159,160]

Primary resistance to echinocandins in otherwise susceptible fungal yeast species is uncommon and resistance-induction studies have demonstrated a low potential for secondary resistance in *Candida* spp. However, emergence of resistance to echinocandins has been observed increasingly in isolates of *Candida glabrata* in the setting of patients who have received 3–4 week courses of treatment.[161,162] This resistance coincides clinically with therapeutic failure and mechanistically with mutations within the hot spot regions of the FKS1p gene. Although the MICs of echinocandins against *C. parapsilosis* are elevated, most infections caused by this species can be successfully treated. The frequency of primary echinocandin resistance among clinical isolates of *Aspergillus* spp. is unknown, but induction of secondary resistance has been achieved *in vitro*.[163] The antifungal activity of echinocandins against *Candida* spp. and *Aspergillus fumigatus in vivo* has been demonstrated in several animal models, including those of oropharyngeal/esophageal candidiasis, disseminated candidiasis, and pulmonary aspergillosis.

A randomized comparative study of voriconazole plus anidulafungin versus voriconazole alone demonstrated significantly greater survival in a *post hoc* analysis in patients with hematological malignancies and probable invasive aspergillosis defined by galactomannan, suggesting the benefit of combination therapy in early infection.[164]

The clinical efficacy of anidulafungin, caspofungin and micafungin against *Candida* spp. was demonstrated in phase II or III studies of esophageal candidiasis.[165] Echinocandins are also effective for treatment of triazole-refractory esophageal and oropharyngeal candidiasis. Phase III studies of echinocandins for initial therapy of candidemia indicate that these agents are as effective, but less toxic than AmB, and superior to fluconazole in improving outcome and survival.[166-168]

Caspofungin as empirical therapy in patients with persistent fever and neutropenia was as effective and better tolerated than liposomal amphotericin B.[169] Micafungin was superior in overall efficacy to fluconazole in prevention of invasive fungal infections during neutropenia in patients undergoing hematopoietic stem cell transplantation.[170] The role of echinocandins in established invasive aspergillosis is less clear. In a salvage trial using caspofungin monotherapy, a complete or partial response was observed in 45% of patients.[171] As monotherapy, voriconazole, isavuconazole, or liposomal amphotericin B are preferred.

Dosage in Special Circumstances

In children caspofungin at 50 mg/m²/day, anidulafungin at 1.5 mg/kg/day provides comparable exposures to that of adults treated with standard dosing.[154,172-175]

Adverse Effects and Drug Interactions

Echinocandins are well tolerated. Only a small fraction of patients enrolled on the clinical trials (<5%) discontinued therapy due to drug-related adverse events. The most frequently reported adverse effects include increased hepatic transaminases, gastrointestinal upset and headaches. Like other basic polypeptides, the echinocandins have the potential to cause histamine release; however, histamine-mediated symptoms have been observed rarely. The current echinocandins appear to have no significant potential for drug interactions mediated by the CYP450 enzyme system. Caspofungin reduces the AUC of tacrolimus by approximately 20% but has no effect on cyclosporine levels. However, cyclosporine increased the AUC of caspofungin by approximately 35%; because of transient elevations of hepatic transaminases in single-dose interaction studies, concomitant use of both drugs is not recommended. Finally, inducers of drug clearance and/or mixed inducer/inhibitors, namely efavirenz, nelfinavir, nevirapine, phenytoin, rifampin, dexamethasone and carbamazepine may reduce caspofungin concentrations.

TERBINAFINE

Mechanism of Action

Terbinafine is a highly lipophilic and keratinophilic allylamine inhibitor of ergosterol biosynthesis. It is a potent noncompetitive inhibitor of fungal squalene epoxidase and prevents squalene epoxidation, an important early step in the synthesis of ergosterol. Cell death is associated with the accumulation of intracellular squalene, which interferes with fungal membrane function and cell wall synthesis. In addition to its antifungal properties, terbinafine is also anti-inflammatory and can act as a free radical scavenger.

Pharmacokinetics and Distribution

Oral terbinafine is rapidly absorbed, with peak concentration occurring at 60–90 minutes post dose.[176] It is quickly converted to multiple metabolites, which co-exist in plasma with the parent compound. Drug is delivered to peripheral tissues via sebum and by direct diffusion through the dermal layers. It is detected in sebum and hair within the first week of administration and by week 3 in stratum corneum and nail samples. The terminal half-life is approximately 3 weeks and fungicidal concentrations persist in peripheral tissues for weeks to months after administration of the last dose. Increasing age and concomitant hypertension are associated with higher plasma concentrations and smokers have lower levels than do nonsmokers.

Route of Administration and Dosage

Oral terbinafine at doses of 250 mg/day in adults and 62.5–250 mg/day in children is effective and generally safe.

Indications

Terbinafine is active *in vitro* against a wide range of pathogenic fungi, including dermatophytes, molds, dimorphic fungi, *Cr. neoformans* and some but not all *Candida* and *Aspergillus* spp.[177] Cross-resistance in *Candida* spp. following treatment with fluconazole can occur due to upregulation of target enzymes. Multidrug efflux pumps may also reduce susceptibility.[178]

Terbinafine is indicated for cutaneous dermatophytoses and onychomycoses that warrant systemic therapy. Recommended durations of treatment for tinea capitis, tinea corporis, tinea pedis and onychomycosis in adults are 4, 2, 6, and 12 weeks, respectively. Terbinafine cannot be recommended for the treatment of deeply invasive mycoses.

Adverse Effects and Drug Interactions

The drug is generally well tolerated, but gastrointestinal disturbances, skin rashes and headaches occur occasionally. Rare adverse reactions include induction and exacerbation of lupus, agranulocytosis, severe skin reactions, and hepatobiliary dysfunction including acute liver failure.

Multiple cytochrome P450 enzymes metabolize terbinafine, and agents that affect this system may alter drug concentrations.[179] Terbinafine competitively inhibits CYP2D6 and elevated levels of desipramine have been observed when the drugs are co-administered. Terbinafine may reduce the level of cyclosporin. Most of the drug and drug metabolites are eliminated in the urine.

GRISEOFULVIN

Mechanism of Action

Griseofulvin, a metabolic product of *Penicillium*, was the first oral agent available for treatment of dermatomycoses. This compound inhibits fungal cell mitosis and nucleic acid synthesis and disrupts spindle and cytoplasmic microtubule function.[180]

Pharmacokinetics and Distribution

Griseofulvin has extremely low water solubility and moderate lipid solubility. Absorption from the gastrointestinal tract is variable and enhanced by a fatty meal. The bioavailability of the ultra-microsize formulation is higher compared to the microsize formulation. The drug is highly protein-bound. Griseofulvin is detected in the outer layer of the stratum corneum soon after it is ingested and is diffused from the extracellular fluid and sweat. Deposition of drug in growing cells may account for entry into hair and nails. Concentration in plasma peaks at 3–4 hours and in skin blister fluid at 6 hours. The terminal half-life in plasma and in skin blisters is approximately 9–10 hours and during chronic administration, levels equilibrate. Griseofulvin is largely metabolized in the liver and degradation metabolites are excreted in the urine. Griseofulvin is also effective in several inflammatory skin conditions, possibly due to anti-inflammatory properties mediated by modulation of the expression of cell adhesion molecules on leukocytes and vascular endothelial cells.[181]

Route of Administration and Dosage

Doses of 500–1000 mg/day in adults have been used successfully. Length of treatment depends on the site and type of infection.

Indications

Griseofulvin is active against many, but not all, dermatophytes. High-level resistance can develop following drug exposure and a multiple-layered thick cell wall, which may limit griseofulvin entry, has been observed in resistant isolates. A meta-analysis of terbinafine and griseofulvin in treatment of tinea capitis demonstrated superiority of terbinafine in *Microsporum* infections and of griseofulvin in *Trichophyton* infections.[182]

For onychomycosis, griseofulvin has been largely supplanted by newer antifungal agents. Currently, its main indication is for the treatment of tinea capitis and other cutaneous mycoses.

Dosage in Special Circumstances

The dosage of griseofulvin in children is 15–20 mg/kg/day.

Adverse Effects and Drug Interactions

Adverse effects include gastrointestinal disturbances, headaches, hepatitis and rashes. Liver and thyroid neoplasia, abnormal germ cell maturation, teratogenicity and embryotoxicity have been observed in animal studies. The reproductive toxicity as well as the induction of chromosome aberrations in somatic cells may result from disturbance of microtubule formation. Griseofulvin also induces accumulation of porphyrins and formation of Mallory bodies in hepatocytes. These may represent additional carcinogenic mechanisms. Less common adverse events include exacerbation of lupus, porphyrias and blood dyscrasias. Drug interactions are related to induction of hepatic enzymes and include phenobarbital, oral anticoagulants and oral contraceptives.

References available online at expertconsult.com.

KEY REFERENCES

Andes D.R., Safdar N., Baddley J.W., et al.: Impact of treatment strategy on outcomes in patients with candidemia and other forms of invasive candidiasis: a patient-level quantitative review of randomized trials. *Clin Infect Dis* 2012; 54:1110-1122.

Cornely O.A., Maertens J., Bresnik M., et al.: Liposomal amphotericin B as initial therapy for invasive mold infection: a randomized trial comparing a high-loading dose regimen with standard dosing (AmBiLoad trial). *Clin Infect Dis* 2007; 44:1289-1297.

Cornely O.A., Maertens J., Winston D.J., et al.: Posaconazole versus fluconazole or itraconazole prophylaxis in patients with neutropenia. *N Engl J Med* 2007; 356(4):348-359.

Galgiani J.N., Catanzaro A., Cloud G.A., et al.: Fluconazole therapy for coccidioidal meningitis. The National Institute of Allergy and Infectious Diseases Mycoses Study Group. *Ann Intern Med* 1993; 119:28-35.

Herbrecht R., Denning D.W., Patterson T.F., et al.: Voriconazole versus amphotericin B for primary therapy of invasive aspergillosis. *N Engl J Med* 2002; 347:408-415.

Miceli M.H., Kauffman C.A.: Isavuconazole: A New Broad-Spectrum Triazole Antifungal Agent. *Clin Infect Dis* 2015; 61(10):1558-1565.

Mora-Duarte J., Betts R., Rotstein C., et al.: Comparison of caspofungin and amphotericin B for invasive candidiasis. *N Engl J Med* 2002; 347:2020-2029.

Reboli A.C., Rotstein C., Pappas P.G., et al.: Anidulafungin versus fluconazole for invasive candidiasis. *N Engl J Med* 2007; 356:2472-2482.

Rex J.H., Bennett J.E., Sugar A.M., et al.: A randomized trial comparing fluconazole with amphotericin B for the treatment of candidemia in patients without neutropenia. Candidemia Study Group and the National Institute. *N Engl J Med* 1994; 331:1325-1330.

Rotstein C., Bow E.J., Laverdiere M., et al.: Randomized placebo-controlled trial of fluconazole prophylaxis for neutropenic cancer patients: benefit based on purpose and intensity of cytotoxic therapy. The Canadian Fluconazole Prophylaxis Study Group. *Clin Infect Dis* 1999; 28:331-340.

Stevens D.A., Schwartz H.J., Lee J.Y., et al.: A randomized trial of itraconazole in allergic bronchopulmonary aspergillosis. *N Engl J Med* 2000; 342(11):756-762.

Ullman A.J., Lipton J.H., Vesole D.H., et al.: Posaconazole or fluconazole for prophylaxis in severe graft versus host disease. *N Engl J Med* 2007; 356(4):335-347.

van Burik J.H., Ratanatharathorn V., Stepan D.E., et al.: Micafungin versus fluconazole for prophylaxis of invasive fungal infections during neutropenia in patients undergoing hematopoietic stem cell transplantation. *Clin Infect Dis* 2004; 39:1407-1416.

Walsh T.J., Finberg R.W., Arndt C., et al.: Liposomal amphotericin B for empirical therapy in patients with persistent fever and neutropenia. National Institute of Allergy and Infectious Diseases Mycoses Study Group. *N Engl J Med* 1999; 340:764-771.

Walsh T.J., Teppler H., Donowitz G.R., et al.: Caspofungin versus liposomal amphotericin B for empirical antifungal therapy in patients with persistent fever and neutropenia. *N Engl J Med* 2004; 351:1391-1402.

157

Antiparasitic Agents

F. MATTHEW KUHLMANN | JAMES M. FLECKENSTEIN

KEY POINTS

- Many antiparasitic agents were developed years ago, treat rare infections and, as such, are understudied with few new agents in development.

- Treatment regimens for different infections vary despite using the same agent.

- The use of antiparasitics in pregnancy must weigh the potential risks to the fetus relative to the infection in the mother.

- Drug interactions are not well studied with many antiparasitics; use with caution in patients on multiple medications.

- The use of many agents in renal or hepatic impairment is understudied and many inferences are made based on pharmacokinetics. These agents should be used with caution.

Introduction

Antiparasitic agents are used to treat infestations caused by a diverse and complex group of organisms encompassing the unicellular protozoa, which have intricate life cycles often involving more than one host, as well as the helminths, which have highly developed organ systems. Many antiparasitic agents are old drugs that have never been subjected to the rigorous testing of efficacy and safety currently required by agencies in various countries, such as the US Food and Drug Administration. Given their rarity of use in low- and middle-income countries (LMIC), they are unlikely to undergo such testing in the future.

This chapter is divided in two classes of drugs, those to treat protozoa and those to treat helminths. The treatment options by organism or disease entity, along with the recommended adult and pediatric dosages, are listed in Table 157-1. Pharmacological information, dosage adjustments, pregnancy risk, adverse events, drug interactions and availability are provided in Table 157-2. The text also provides of list of adverse events, loosely ordered from common to uncommon. The decision to use of any of these agents in a pregnant patient must be made on an individual basis, weighing the severity of the illness and the benefit of treatment to the mother against the potential toxicity to the fetus.

Text continued on p. 1364

TABLE 157-1	**Antiparasitic Agents and Dosages** (Organism or Disease Entity is Listed Alphabetically)		
Infection and Comments	**Drug**	**Adult Dosage (po Unless Otherwise Indicated)**	**Pediatric Dosage (po Unless Otherwise Indicated)**
Acanthamoeba (keratitis)			
0.1% propamidine isethionate plus chlorhexidine (0.02%) or polyhexamethylene biguanide 0.02% (topical)			
Amebiasis (Entamoeba histolytica)			
Asymptomatic or following metronidazole or tinidazole therapy	Iodoquinol OR	650 mg q8h for 20 days	30–40 mg/kg/day (maximum 2 g) in three doses for 20 days
Alternatives	Paromomycin OR	25–35 mg/kg/day in three doses for 7 days	25–35 mg/kg/day in three doses for 7 days
	Diloxanide furoate	500 mg q8h for 10 days	20 mg/kg/day in three doses for 10 days
Mild-to-moderate intestinal disease			
	Metronidazole OR	500–750 mg q8h for 5–10 days	35–50 mg/kg/day in three doses for 10 days
	Tinidazole	2 g/day for 3 days	≥3 years: 50 mg/kg (maximum 2 g) per day for 3 days
Severe intestinal disease and extraintestinal disease			
	Metronidazole OR	750 mg q8h for 7–10 days	35–50 mg/kg/day in three doses for 10 days
	Tinidazole	2 g/day for 5 days	≥3 years: 50 mg/kg or 60 mg/kg (maximum 2 g) per day for 5 days

Durations and treatments of choice are provided if referenced elsewhere, otherwise clinical judgement should be used in deciding treatment options and duration.

Continued on following page

TABLE 157-1	**Antiparasitic Agents and Dosages** (Organism or Disease Entity is Listed Alphabetically) (Continued)		
Infection and Comments	**Drug**	**Adult Dosage (po Unless Otherwise Indicated)**	**Pediatric Dosage (po Unless Otherwise Indicated)**
Amebic meningoencephalitis (primary or granulomatous amebic encephalitis)[2] Exact treatment durations and combinations are unknown. Seek expert advice such as through the Centers for Disease Control (404) 718-4745 or www.cdc.gov to tailor treatment combinations and duration			
Naegleria spp.	Amphotericin B	1.5 mg/kg/day iv, uncertain duration	1 mg/kg/day iv, uncertain duration
	Rifampin	10 mg/kg iv daily (max 600 mg)	Same as adult
	Fluconazole	12 mg/kg iv daily	Same as adult
	Azithromycin	500 mg iv daily	20 mg/kg iv daily (max 500 mg)
Acanthamoeba spp.	Pentamidine	4 mg/kg iv daily	Same as adult
	Sulfadiazine	1.5 g q6h	200 mg/kg/day in 4-6 doses (max 6g/day)
	Flucytosine	37.5 mg/kg q6h (max 150 mg/kg/day)	Same as adult
	Fluconazole	12 mg/kg iv daily	Same as adult
	Miltefosine	< 45 kg: 100 mg/day po in 2 doses >45 kg: 150 mg/day in 3 doses	2.5 mg/kg/day in 2 doses (max 100 mg/day)
Balamuthia mandrillaris	Azithromycin	500 mg iv daily	20 mg/kg iv daily (max 500 mg)
	Clarithromycin	14 mg/kg/day in 2 doses (max 2 g/day)	Same as adult
	Pentamidine	4 mg/kg iv daily	Same as adult
	Sulfadiazine	1.5 g q6h	200 mg/kg/day in 4-6 doses (max 6g/day)
	Flucytosine	37.5 mg/kg q6h (max 150 mg/kg/day)	Same as adult
	Fluconazole	12 mg/kg iv daily	Same as adult
	Miltefosine	< 45 kg: 100 mg/day in 2 doses >45 kg: 150 mg/day in 3 doses	2.5 mg/kg/day in 2 doses (max 100 mg/day)
Sappinia diploidea	Azithromycin	250 mg q24h	
	Pentamidine	300 mg iv q24h	
	Itraconazole	200 mg q12h	
	Flucytosine	2.75 g q6h	
Ancylostoma caninum (eosinophilic enterocolitis)	Mebendazole OR	100 mg q12h for 3 days	100 mg q12h for 3 days
	Albendazole	400 mg, single dose	400 mg, single dose
Angiostrongyliasis			
Angiostrongylus cantonensis (Note: treatment may not be indicated)	Mebendazole	100 mg q12h for 5 days	100 mg q12h for 5 days
Angiostrongylus costaricensis Drug of choice	Mebendazole	200–400 mg q8h for 10 days	200–400 mg q8h for 10 days
Alternative	Thiabendazole	75 mg/kg/day in three doses for 3 days (maximum 3 g/day)	75 mg/kg/day in three doses for 3 days (maximum 3 g/day)
Anisakiasis (*Anisakis* spp.) Treatment of choice		Surgical or endoscopic removal	
Ascariasis (*Ascaris lumbricoides*, roundworm)	Mebendazole OR	100 mg q12h for 3 days or 500 mg, single dose	100 mg q12h for 3 days or 500 mg, single dose
	Albendazole OR	400 mg, single dose	400 mg, single dose
	Ivermectin	150–200 µg/kg once	Same as adult
Babesiosis (*Babesia* spp.) The recommendations below are for normal hosts. Immunocompromised individuals may require more prolonged (6 weeks or more) courses of therapy to achieve cure (see Krause et al., *Clin Infect Dis* 2008; 46:370–6)			
	Clindamycin PLUS	1.2 g q12h iv or 600 mg q8h po for 7 days	20–40 mg/kg/day po in three doses for 7 days
	Quinine OR	650 mg q8h for 7 days	25 mg/kg/day in three doses for 7 days
	Atovaquone PLUS	750 mg q12h for 7–10 days	20 mg/kg q12h for 7–10 days
	Azithromycin	600 mg q24h for 7–10 days	12 mg/kg q24h for 7–10 days
Balantidiasis (*Balantidium coli*) Drug of choice	Tetracycline	500 mg q6h for 10 days	40 mg/kg/day (maximum 2 g) in four doses for 10 days
Alternatives	Iodoquinol	650 mg q8h for 20 days	40 mg/kg/day in three doses for 20 days
	Metronidazole	750 mg q8h for 5 days	35–50 mg/kg/day in three doses for 5 days
Baylisascariasis (*Baylisascaris procyonis*) No drug proven effective – albendazole 3 mg/kg/day po with steroids has been used			
Blastocystis hominis (clinical significance controversial)	Metronidazole OR	750 mg q8h for 5–10 days	
	Iodoquinol	650 mg q8h for 20 days	
Capillariasis (*Capillaria philippinensis*) Drug of choice	Mebendazole	200 mg q12h for 20 days	200 mg q12h for 20 days
Alternative	Albendazole	400 mg/day for 10 days	400 mg/day for 10 days

Durations and treatments of choice are provided if referenced elsewhere, otherwise clinical judgement should be used in deciding treatment options and duration.

TABLE 157-1	Antiparasitic Agents and Dosages (Organism or Disease Entity is Listed Alphabetically) (Continued)		
Infection and Comments	**Drug**	**Adult Dosage (po Unless Otherwise Indicated)**	**Pediatric Dosage (po Unless Otherwise Indicated)**
Cryptosporidiosis (*Cryptosporidium parvum*) No agent has proven to be effective in immunocompromised patients. Nitazoxanide, in the doses listed below, showed efficacy in clearing infection from immunocompetent individuals	Nitazoxanide	500 mg q12h for 3 days	1–3 years: 100 mg q12h for 3 days 4–11 years: 200 mg q12h for 3 days
Cutaneous larva migrans (creeping eruption, dog and cat hookworm)	Albendazole OR Ivermectin	400 mg/day for 3 days 150–200 µg/kg, single dose	400 mg/day for 3 days 150–200 µg/kg, single dose
Cyclosporiasis (*Cyclospora cayetanensis*)	TMP–SMX	TMP 160 mg, SMX 800 mg q12h for 7–10 days	TMP 5 mg/kg, SMX 25 mg/kg q12h for 7–10 days
Cystoisosporiasis (formerly *Isospora belli*)	TMP—SMX	160 mg TMP, 800 mg SMX q6h for 10 days, then q12h for 3 weeks	TMP 5 mg/kg, SMX 25 mg/kg twice daily for 10 days
Dientamoeba fragilis	Iodoquinol OR Paromomycin	650 mg q8h for 20 days 25–30 g/kg/day in three doses for 7 days	40 mg/kg/day (maximum 2 g) in three doses for 20 days 25–30 mg/kg/day in three doses for 7 days
Dracunculiasis (*Dracunculus medinensis*, guinea worm)		Physical removal of worm	
Enterobiasis (*Enterobius vermicularis*, pinworm)	Pyrantel pamoate OR Mebendazole OR Albendazole	11 mg/kg, single dose (maximum 1 g); repeat in 2 weeks 100 mg, single dose; repeat in 2 weeks 400 mg, single dose; repeat in 2 weeks	11 mg/kg, single dose (maximum 1 g); repeat in 2 weeks 100 mg, single dose; repeat in 2 weeks 400 mg, single dose; repeat in 2 weeks
Filariasis			
Wuchereria bancrofti, Brugia malayi (alternative dosing regimens, including single dose regimens may be considered)	Diethylcarbamazine	Day 1: 50 mg after food Day 2: 50 mg q8h Day 3: 100 mg q8h Days 4–14: 6 mg/kg/day in three doses	Day 1: 1 mg/kg after food Day 2: 1 mg/kg q8h Day 3: 1–2 mg/kg q8h Days 4–14: 6 mg/kg/day in three doses
Loa loa	Diethylcarbamazine	Day 1: 50 mg after food Day 2: 50 mg q8h Day 3: 100 mg q8h Days 4–21: 9 mg/kg/day in three doses	Day 1: 1 mg/kg after food Day 2: 1 mg/kg q8h Day 3: 1–2 mg/kg q8h Days 4–21: 9 mg/kg/day in three doses
Mansonella ozzardi	Ivermectin	200 µg/kg single dose	
Mansonella perstans	Doxycycline	200 mg po daily for 6 weeks	
Mansonella streptocerca	Ivermectin OR Diethylcarbamazine	150 µg/kg, single dose 6 mg/kg/day for 14 days	
Tropical pulmonary eosinophilia	Diethylcarbamazine	6 mg/kg/day in three doses for 14 days	6 mg/kg/day in three doses for 14 days
Onchocerca volvulus (river blindness)	Ivermectin	150 µg/kg, single dose, repeated every 6–12 months	150 µg/kg, single dose, repeated every 6–12 months
Flukes (hermaphroditic) infection			
Clonorchis sinensis (Chinese liver fluke)	Praziquantel OR Albendazole	75 mg/kg/day in three doses for 1 day 10 mg/kg for 7 days	75 mg/kg/day in three doses for 1 day 10 mg/kg for 7 days
Fasciola hepatica (sheep liver fluke) Drug of choice Alternative	Triclabendazole Bithionol	10 mg/kg, single dose 30–50 mg/kg on alternate days for 10–15 doses	30–50 mg/kg on alternate days for 10–15 doses
Fasciolopsis buski, Heterophyes heterophyes, Metagonimus yokogawai (intestinal flukes)	Praziquantel	75 mg/kg/day in three doses for 1 day	75 mg/kg/day in three doses for 1 day 75 mg/kg/day in three doses for 1 day
Nanophyetus salmincola	Praziquantel	60 mg/kg/day in three doses for 1 day	60 mg/kg/day in three doses for 1 day
Opisthorchis viverrini (South East Asian liver fluke)	Praziquantel	75 mg/kg/day in three doses for 1 day	75 mg/kg/day in three doses for 1 day
Paragonimus westermani (lung fluke) Drug of choice Alternative	Praziquantel Bithionol	75 mg/kg/day in three doses for 2 days 30–50 mg/kg on alternate days for 10–15 doses	75 mg/kg/day in three doses for 2 days 30–50 mg/kg on alternate days for 10–15 doses

Durations and treatments of choice are provided if referenced elsewhere, otherwise clinical judgement should be used in deciding treatment options and duration.

Continued on following page

TABLE 157-1	Antiparasitic Agents and Dosages (Organism or Disease Entity is Listed Alphabetically) (Continued)		
Infection and Comments	**Drug**	**Adult Dosage (po Unless Otherwise Indicated)**	**Pediatric Dosage (po Unless Otherwise Indicated)**
Giardiasis (Giardia lamblia)			
Drugs of choice	Metronidazole OR	250 mg q8h for 5 days	15 mg/kg/day in three doses for 5 days
	Tinidazole	2 g, single dose	50 mg/kg, single dose (maximum 2 g)
Alternatives	Nitazoxanide OR	500 mg q12h for 3 days	1–3 years: 100 mg q12h for 3 days 4–11 years: 200 mg q12h for 3 days
	Furazolidone OR	100 mg q6h for 7–10 days	6 mg/kg/day q6h for 7–10 days
	Paromomycin OR	25–35 mg/kg/day in three doses for 7 days	25–35 mg/kg/day in three doses for 7 days
	Quinacrine	100 mg q8h for 5 days (maximum 300 g/day)	2 mg/kg q8h for 5 days (maximum 300 mg/day)
Gnathostomiasis (Gnathostoma spinigerum)			
Treatment of choice	Surgical removal OR Ivermectin OR	200 µg/kg/day for 2 days	200 µg/kg/day for 2 days
	Albendazole	400 mg q12h for 21 days	400 mg q12h for 21 days
Hookworm infection (Ancylostoma duodenale, Necator americanus)			
	Mebendazole OR	100 mg q12h for 2 days or 500 mg, single dose	100 mg q12h for 2 days or 500 mg, single dose
	Pyrantel pamoate OR	11 mg/kg (maximum 1 g) for 3 days	11 mg/kg (maximum 1 g) for 3 days
	Albendazole	400 mg, single dose	400 mg, single dose
Leishmaniasis (Leishmania mexicana, Leismania tropica, Leishmania major, Leishmania braziliensis, Leishmania donovani (kala-azar), Leishmania infantum). Treatment dependent on geography and infective species, of note, topical azole anti-fungals may be of benefit in cutaneous disease			
Visceral disease			
Drug of choice	Liposomal amphotericin B	15–20 mg/kg (total dose over 5 days or longer depending on species)	15–20 mg/kg (total dose over 5 days or longer)
Alternatives	Sodium stibogluconate OR	20 mg antimony (Sb)/kg/day iv or im for 20–28 days	20 mg Sb/kg/day iv or im for 20–28 days
	Meglumine antimonite OR	20 mg Sb/kg/day for 20–28 days	20 mg Sb/kg/day for 20–28 days
	Miltefosine OR	2.5 mg/kg/day (maximum 150 mg per day) for 28 days	2.5 mg/kg/day (maximum 150 mg per day) for 28 days
	Amphotericin B OR	0.5–1 mg/kg by slow infusion daily or every 2 days for up to 8 weeks	0.5–1 mg/kg by slow infusion daily or every 2 days for up to 8 weeks
	Paromomycin	15 mg/kg/day for 21 days	15 mg/kg/day for 21 days
Cutaneous disease			
Drugs of choice	Sodium stibogluconate OR	20 mg Sb/kg/day iv or im for 20–28 days	20 mg Sb/kg/day iv or im for 20–28 days
	Meglumine antimonite OR	20 mg Sb/kg/day iv or im for 20–28 days	20 mg Sb/kg/day iv or im for 20–28 days
	Miltefosine	2.5 mg/kg/day (maximum 150 mg per day) for 28 days	2.5 mg/kg/day (maximum 150 mg per day) for 28 days
Alternatives	Paromomycin OR	Topically q12h for 10–20 days	Topically q12h for 10–20 days
	Pentamidine	2–3 mg/kg iv or im q24h or q24 to 48 hours for 4–7 doses	2–3 mg/kg iv or im q24h or q24 to 48 hours for 4–7 doses
Mucosal disease			
Drugs of choice	Sodium stibogluconate OR	20 mg Sb/kg/day iv or im for 20–28 days	20 mg Sb/kg/day iv or im for 20–28 days
	Meglumine antimonite OR	20 mg Sb/kg/day iv or im for 20–28 days	20 mg Sb/kg/day iv or im for 20–28 days
	Amphotericin B OR	0.5–1 mg/kg by slow infusion daily or every 2 days for up to 8 weeks	0.5–1 mg/kg by slow infusion daily or every 2 days for up to 8 weeks
	Miltefosine	2.5 mg/kg/day (maximum 150 mg per day) for 28 days	2.5 mg/kg/day (maximum 150 mg per day) for 28 days
Malaria treatment (Plasmodium falciparum, Plasmodium ovale, Plasmodium vivax, Plasmodium malariae). See http://www.cdc.gov/malaria/resources/pdf/treatmenttable.pdf, accessed 19 February 2016 for more information			
Uncomplicated chloroqine-resistant Plasmodium falciparum (oral regimens)			
	Artemether/ lumefantrine OR	Four tablets/dose administered at 0, 8, 24, 36, 48 and 60 hours	<15 kg: one tablet/dose at same intervals as adults 15–25 kg: two tablets/dose at same intervals 25–35 kg: three tablets/dose at same intervals >35 kg: same as adult dosage

Durations and treatments of choice are provided if referenced elsewhere, otherwise clinical judgement should be used in deciding treatment options and duration.

TABLE 157-1	Antiparasitic Agents and Dosages (Organism or Disease Entity is Listed Alphabetically) (Continued)		
Infection and Comments	Drug	Adult Dosage (po Unless Otherwise Indicated)	Pediatric Dosage (po Unless Otherwise Indicated)
	Atovaquone/proguanil OR	Two adult tablets (250 mg atovaquone/100 mg proguanil) q12h for 3 days or four adult tablets q24h for 3 days	5–8 kg: two peds tablets/day (62.5 mg atovaquone/25 mg proguanil) for 3 days 9–10 kg: three peds tablets/day for 3 days 11–20 kg: one adult tablet/day for 3 days 21–30 kg: two adult tablets/day for 3 days 30–40 kg: 3 adult tablets/day for 3 days >40 kg: adult dose
	Quinine sulfate PLUS	650 mg q8h for 3–7 days	25 mg/kg/day q8h for 3–7 days
	Doxycycline OR PLUS	100 mg q12h for 7 days	2 mg/kg/day for 7 days
	Clindamycin	900 mg q8h for 5 days	20–40 mg/kg/day q8h for 5 days
Alternative	Mefloquine	750 mg followed by 500 mg 12h later	15 mg/kg, single dose (if body weight <45 kg), followed by 10 mg/kg 12h later
Uncomplicated chloroquine-sensitive *P. falciparum*			
	Chloroquine phosphate	600 mg base po then 300 mg base po at 6, 24, and 48 hours	10 mg base/kg then 5 mg base/kg at 6, 24, and 48 hours
Chloroquine-resistant *Plasmodium vivax* or *P. ovale* (if chloroquine-sensitive, treatment as above plus primaquine)			
	Atovaquone/proguanil OR	Two adult tablets (250 mg atovaquone/100 mg proguanil) q12h for 3 days or four adult tablets/day for 3 days	5–8 kg: two peds tablets/day (62.5 mg atovaquone/25 mg proguanil) for 3 days 9–10 kg: three peds tablets/day for 3 days 11–20 kg: one adult tablet/day for 3 days 21–30 kg: two adult tablets/day for 3 days 30–40 kg: three adult tablets/day for 3 days >40 kg: adult dose
	Mefloquine	750 mg followed by 500 mg 12h later	15 mg/kg, single dose (if body weight <45 kg), followed by 10 mg/kg 12h later
Alternative	Quinine sulfate PLUS	650 mg q8h for 3–7 days	25 mg/kg/day in three doses for 3–7 days
	Doxycycline	100 mg q12h for 7 days	2 mg/kg/day for 7 days
All *P. vivax* and *P. ovale* regimens followed by:			
	Primaquine phosphate	30 mg base/day for 14 days or 45 mg base/week for 8 weeks if borderline G6PD deficient (10–60% of normal enzyme function, WHO class II definition)	0.5 mg base/kg/day for 14 days
Severe Malaria, all species (parenteral regimens must be given with doxycycline, tetracycline, or clindamycin)			
	Quinidine gluconate OR	10 mg/kg iv loading dose (maximum 600 mg) in normal saline slowly over 1–2h, followed by continuous infusion of 0.02 mg/kg/min until oral therapy can be started	10 mg/kg iv loading dose (maximum 600 mg) in normal saline slowly over 1–2h, followed by continuous infusion of 0.02 mg/kg/min until oral therapy can be started
	Quinine dihydrochloride OR	20 mg/kg iv loading dose in 5% dextrose over 4h, followed by 10 mg/kg over 2–4h, q8h (maximum 1800 mg/day) until oral therapy can be started	20 mg/kg iv loading dose in 5% dextrose over 4h, followed by 10 mg/kg over 2–4h, q8h (maximum 1800 mg/day) until oral therapy can be started
	Artesunate (must be combined with another agent)	2.4 mg/kg/dose iv for 3 days with doses at 0, 12, 24, 48 and 72 hours	2.4 mg/kg/dose iv for 3 days with doses at 0, 12, 24, 48 and 72 hours
Prevention of relapses (*Plasmodium vivax* and *Plasmodium ovale* only)			
	Primaquine phosphate	26.3 mg (15 mg base)/day for 14 days or 79 mg (45 mg base)/week for 8 weeks	0.3 mg base/kg/day for 14 days
Malaria prevention **Chloroquine-sensitive areas**			
	Chloroquine phosphate	500 mg (300 mg base) once per week	5 mg/kg base once per week, up to adult dose of 300 mg base
Chloroquine-resistant area			
	Atovaquone/proguanil OR	One adult tablet/day starting 1–2 days before travel and continuing for 1 week after return	5–8 kg: ½ ped tablet/day 9–10 kg: ¾ ped tablet/day 11–20 kg: one ped tablet/day 21–30 kg: two ped tablets/day 31–40 kg: three ped tablets/day >40 kg: adult dose
	Mefloquine OR	250 mg once per week starting 1 week prior to travel and continuing for 4 weeks after return	Weight <5 kg, no data; weight 5–9 kg, ⅛ tablet; weight 10–19 kg, ¼ tablet; weight 20–30 kg, ½ tablet; weight 31–45 kg ¾ tablet; weight >45 kg, one tablet
	Doxycycline	100 mg/day starting 1–2 days prior to travel and continuing for 4 weeks after return	2 mg/kg/day, up to 100 mg/day
Alternative	Primaquine	30 mg base po daily starting 1 day prior to travel and continuing for 5 days after return	0.5 mg/kg base/day

Durations and treatments of choice are provided if referenced elsewhere, otherwise clinical judgement should be used in deciding treatment options and duration.

Continued on following page

TABLE 157-1	Antiparasitic Agents and Dosages (Organism or Disease Entity is Listed Alphabetically) (Continued)		
Infection and Comments	**Drug**	**Adult Dosage (po Unless Otherwise Indicated)**	**Pediatric Dosage (po Unless Otherwise Indicated)**
Microsporidiosis			
Ocular microsporidiosis (*Encephalitozoon hellem, Encephalitozoon cuniculi, Vittaforma corneae (Nosema corneum)*			
	Albendazole PLUS Fumagillin eye drops	400 mg q12h	15 mg/kg/day in 2 doses (max 400 mg)
Intestinal microsporidiosis (*Enterocytozoon bieneusi, Encephalitozoon (Septata) intestinalis*)			
	Albendazole (*E. intestinalis*) OR	400 mg q12h	15 mg/kg/day in 2 doses (max 400 mg)
	Fumagillin (*E. bieneusi*)	60 mg q24h for 14 days	
Disseminated microsporidiosis (*Enterocytozoon hellem, Enterocytozoon cuniculi, Enterocytozoon intestinalis, Pleistophora* ssp.)			
	Albendazole	400 mg q12h	15 mg/kg/day in 2 doses (max 400 mg)
Moniliformis moniliformis			
	Pyrantel pamoate	11 mg/kg, single dose, repeat twice 2 weeks apart	11 mg/kg, single dose, repeat twice 2 weeks apart
Oesophagostomum bifurcum			
	Albendazole (may also use pyrantel pamoate at standard dosing)	400 mg once	15 mg/kg/day once (max 400 mg)
Schistosomiasis (bilharziasis)			
Schistosoma haematobium			
	Praziquantel	40 mg/kg/day in two doses for 1 day	40 mg/kg/day in two doses for 1 day
Schistosoma japonicum			
	Praziquantel	60 mg/kg/day in three doses for 1 day	60 mg/kg/day in three doses for 1 day
Schistosoma mansoni			
Drug of choice	Praziquantel	40 mg/kg/day in two doses for 1 day	40 mg/kg/day in two doses for 1 day
Alternative	Oxamniquine	15 mg/kg, single dose	20 mg/kg/day in two doses for 1 day
Schistosoma mekongi			
	Praziquantel	60 mg/kg/day in three doses for 1 day	60 mg/kg/day in three doses for 1 day
Strongyloidiasis (*Strongyloides stercoralis*, threadworm)			
Drug of choice	Ivermectin	20 µg/kg/day for 1–2 days	200 µg/kg/day for 1–2 days
Alternative	Albendazole	400 mg twice daily for 7 days	400 mg twice daily for 7 days
Tapeworm infection (adult (intestinal stage))			
Diphyllobothrium latum (fish), *Taenia saginata* (beef), *Taenia solium* (pork), *Dipylidium caninum* (dog)			
Drug of choice	Praziquantel	5–10 mg/kg, single dose	5–10 /kg, single dose
Alternative	Niclosamide	2 g single dose	50 mg/kg, single dose
Hymenolepis nana (dwarf tapeworm)			
	Praziquantel	20 mg/kg, single dose	25 mg/kg, single dose
Tapeworm infection (larval (tissue stage))			
Echinococcus granulosus (hydatid cyst)			
	Albendazole	400 mg q12h for 28 days, repeated as necessary	15 mg/kg/day for 28 days, repeated as necessary
Echinococcus multilocularis			
Treatment of choice	Surgical excision	Surgical excision	
Alternative (refractory to surgery)	Albendazole	15 mg/kg/d po in 2 doses (max 800 mg)	
Taenia solium (cysticercosis, larval stage of *T. solium*). Treatment may not be necessary, steroids and antiepileptics are a frequent adjunct, surgery may be necessary for hydrocephalus			
	Albendazole OR	400 mg q12h for 8–30 days, repeated as necessary	15 mg/kg/day (maximum 800 mg) in two doses for 8–30 days, repeated as necessary
	Praziquantel	50 mg/kg/day in three doses for 15 days	50 mg/kg/day in three doses for 15 days
Toxoplasmosis (*Toxoplasma gondii*)			
Drugs of choice	Pyrimethamine PLUS	25–100 mg/day for 3–4 weeks	2 mg/kg/day for 3 days, then 1 mg/kg/day (maximum 25 mg/day) for 4 weeks
	Sulfadiazine	1–1.5 g q6h for 3–4 weeks	100–200 mg/kg/day for 3–4 weeks
Alternative	Spiramycin	3–4 g/day	50–100 mg/kg/day for 3–4 weeks

Durations and treatments of choice are provided if referenced elsewhere, otherwise clinical judgement should be used in deciding treatment options and duration.

TABLE 157-1	Antiparasitic Agents and Dosages (Organism or Disease Entity is Listed Alphabetically) (Continued)		
Infection and Comments	**Drug**	**Adult Dosage (po Unless Otherwise Indicated)**	**Pediatric Dosage (po Unless Otherwise Indicated)**
Trichinosis (*Trichinella spiralis*) Corticosteroids for severe symptoms			
Drug of choice	Albendazole	400 mg po BID for 1-2 weeks	400 mg po BID for 1-2 weeks
Alternative	Mebendazole	200–400 mg q8h for 3 days, then 400–500 mg q8h for 10 days	200–400 mg q8h for 3 days, then 400–500 mg q8h for 10 days
Trichomoniasis (*Trichomonas vaginalis*)			
	Metronidazole OR	2 g, single dose or 500 mg q12h for 7 days	15 mg/kg/day in three doses for 7 days
	Tinidazole	2 g, single dose	50 mg/kg, single dose (maximum 2 g)
Trichostrongyliasis (*Trichostrongylus* spp.)			
Drug of choice	Pyrantel pamoate	11 mg/kg, single dose (maximum 1 g)	11 mg/kg, single dose (maximum 1 g)
Alternatives	Mebendazole OR	100 mg q12h for 3 days	100 mg q12h for 3 days
	Albendazole	400 mg, single dose	400 mg, single dose
Trichuriasis (*Trichuris trichiura*, whipworm)			
Drug of choice	Albendazole	400 mg, single dose	400 mg, single dose
Alternatives	Mebendazole OR	100 mg q12h for 3 days or 500 mg, single dose	100 mg q12h for 3 days or 500 mg, single dose
	Ivermectin	200 µg/kg/d for 3 days	Same as adult
Trypanosomiasis			
***Trypanosoma cruzi* (American trypanosomiasis, Chagas disease)**			
	Benznidazole OR	5–7 mg/kg/day for 30–90 days	≤12 years: 10 mg/kg/day in two doses for 30–90 days
	Nifurtimox	8–10 mg/kg/day in three or four doses for 90 days	1–10 years: 15–20 mg/kg/day in four doses for 90 days 11–16 years: 12.5–15 mg/kg/day in four doses for 90 days
***Trypanosoma brucei gambiense* (West African trypanosomiasis) – hemolymphatic stage**			
Drug of choice	Pentamidine isethionate	4 mg/kg/day im for 7 days	4 mg/kg/day im for 7 days
Alternative	Suramin	100–200 mg (test dose) iv, then 1 g on days 1, 3, 7, 14 and 21	20 mg/kg iv on days 1, 3, 7, 14 and 21
***Trypanosoma brucei gambiense* (West African trypanosomiasis) – late stage**			
Drugs of Choice	Eflornithine (DFMO) OR	400 mg/kg/day iv in 4 doses for 14 days	Same as adult
	Eflornithine (DFMO) PLUS	400 mg/kg/day iv in 4 doses for 7 days	
	Nifurtimox	15 mg/kg/day po in 3 doses for 10 days	
Alternative	Melarsoprol	2.2 mg/kg/day iv for 10 days	2.2 mg/kg/day iv for 10 days
***Trypanosoma brucei rhodesiense* (East African trypanosomiasis) – hemolymphatic stage**			
	Suramin	100–200 mg (test dose) iv, then 1 g on days 1, 3, 7, 14 and 21	20 mg/kg iv on days 1, 3, 7, 14 and 21
***Trypanosoma brucei rhodesiense* (East African trypanosomiasis) – late stage**			
	Melarsoprol	2.2 mg/kg/day iv for 10 days	2.2 mg/kg/day iv for 10 days
Visceral larva migrans (toxocariasis)			
	Albendazole OR	400 mg q12h for 3–5 days	400 mg q12h for 3–5 days
	Mebendazole	100–200 mg q12h for 5 days	100–200 mg q12h for 5 days

Durations and treatments of choice are provided if referenced elsewhere, otherwise clinical judgement should be used in deciding treatment options and duration.
Sb, antimony; SMX, sulfamethoxazole; TMP, trimethoprim.
Data modified from Med Lett 2013; (11 Suppl):e1-31.

| TABLE 157-2 | **Dosing, Pharmacokinetics, Adverse Events, Drug Interactions and Availability of Select Agents** | | | |

Drug	Pharmacokinetics	Indication	DOSING Adult Dosage	DOSING Pediatric Dosage
ANTIPROTOZOALS				
Amodiaquine	Metabolized by liver, excreted by kidneys, 50% protein bound, $t_{\frac{1}{2}elim}$ = 12–16 hours	Used in combinations with artesunate for malaria	Artesunate 4 mg/kg and amodiaquine 10 mg/kg for 3 days	Do not use in children weighing < 5 kg
Amphotericin B	Detailed in Chapter 156	Cutaneous and visceral leishmaniasis, *Naegleria* meningoencephalitis	Detailed in Chapter 156, see also Table 157-1	
ANTIFOLATES				
Proguanil	Orally absorbed, metabolized by liver, excreted by kidneys, 75% protein bound, $t_{\frac{1}{2}elim}$ = 12–21 hours	Used with atovaquone against malaria	Used in fixed combinations with atovaquone (see below or Table 157-1)	Used in fixed combinations with atovaquone (see below or Table 157-1)
Pyrimethamine	Metabolized by liver, 20-30% excreted in the urine, 85% protein bound, $t_{\frac{1}{2}elim}$ = 4–6 days	As combination therapy for malaria or toxoplasmosis, and *Cystoisospora belli*	See below or Table 157-1	See below or Table 157-1
Trimethoprim	Metabolized by liver, excreted by kidneys, 50% protein bound, $t_{\frac{1}{2}elim}$ = 9–11 hours	Used with sulfamethoxazole for *C. belli* and *C. cayetanensis*	TMP–SMX 160/800 (double strength) every 6 hours for 10 days then every 12 hours for 3 weeks (*C. belli*) and 1 DS tablet every 12 hours for 7–14 days (cyclosporiasis)	Children ≥2 months: 4–6 mg/kg/day TMP in divided doses every 12 hours
Trimetrexate	Lipid-soluble intravenous medication, renally excreted, ~90% protein bound, $t_{\frac{1}{2}elim}$ = biphasic, first phase is 1 hour, second phase up to 18 hours	*T. gondii* infections	< 50 kg use 1.5 mg/kg/day, 50–80 kg use 1.2 mg/kg/day, >80 kg use 1 mg/kg/day	Not established, use adult dosing guide with caution
Sulfonamides – group of related antifolates				
Sulfadiazine	Penetrates central nervous system (CNS), metabolized by liver, excreted by kidneys, 45–55% protein bound, $t_{\frac{1}{2}elim}$ = 12 hours	Used with pyrimethamine for *T. gondii*	2-4 g/day in 3–6 divided doses	> 2 months, 75 mg/kg initial dose then 150 mg/kg/day in 4–6 divided doses
Sulfadoxine	Not metabolized, $t_{\frac{1}{2}elim}$ = 7–9 days	Used with pyrimethamine for malaria	Treatment: 3 tablets po	Treatment: 2–11 months (5–10 kg), ¼ tablet; 1–3 years (11 to 20 kg), ½ tablet; 21 to 30 kg, ¾ tablet; 4–8 years (31 to 45 kg), 1 tablet; 9–14 years, 2 tablets
Sulfamethoxazole	Metabolized by liver, excreted by kidneys, 50–70% protein bound, $t_{\frac{1}{2}elim}$ = 7–12 hours	See Table 157-1	TMP–SMX 80/400 (SS) or 160/800 (DS) every 12 to 24 hours	Based on TMP component 8 mg/kg/day TMP in 2–3 divided doses

Renal Impairment	Hepatic Impairment	FDA Pregnancy Category/Risk	Adverse Reactions	Drug Interactions	Availability in USA
	Contraindicated	Not established	Agranulocytosis, hepatitis		Not available
				Detailed in Chapter 156	Readily available
CrCl > 60 = 200 mg daily, CrCl 20–59 = 100 mg daily, CrCl 10-19 = 50 mg every other day, CrCl <10 50 mg weekly	No dosage adjustment	Presumed safe, no data available	Nausea, vomiting, and abdominal pain, rarely oral ulcerations, hair loss, scaling of palms and soles, and urticaria occur	Monitor interactions with warfarin	Readily available in combination with atovaquone
No dosage adjustment	No dosage adjustment	FDA Category C, contraindicated in the first trimester	Blood dyscrasias, rash	Avoid with artemether and lumefantrine	Readily available
Reduce dose for CrCl 15–30, avoid if CrCl < 15	No dosage adjustment	FDA Category C	Rash, pruritus, nausea, transaminitis, vomiting, cytopenias, fever, aseptic meningitis, renal failure	Avoid with dofetilide and leucovorin, several other interactions require monitoring therapy	Readily available
Not well studied, monitor renal function and stop if creatinine increases above 2.5 g/dl	Monitor therapy	FDA Category D, avoid in pregnancy	Rash, leukopenia (administer with leucovorin), transaminitis, peripheral neuropathy	Avoid with zidovudine and natalizumab	Production discontinued in 2007 in the USA
CrCL 25–50, decrease interval to every 24 hours, CrCl 10–25, decrease to every 24 hours, CrCl < 10, avoid	No dosage adjustment, use with caution	FDA Category C, contraindicated in the third trimester		Avoid with methenamine, potassium p-aminobenzoate, and procaine, several other interactions require monitoring therapy	Readily available
No adjustment, use with caution	No dosage adjustment, use with caution	FDA Category C, contraindicated in the third trimester		Avoid with artemether, lumefantrine, methenamine, potassium p-aminobenzoate, and procaine	Available in combination with pyrimethamine
CrCL 15–30 use 50% of dose, CrCl <15 not recommended	Use with caution in severe impairment	FDA Category C, contraindicated in the third trimester	Hypersensitivity reactions including rash, fever, and transaminitis, agranulocytosis, hemolytic anemia, crystalluria occurs with sulfadiazine; sulfadoxine/ pyrimethamine has a US boxed warning for Stevens–Johnson syndrome	Avoid TMP–SMX combination with dofetilide, leucovorin, methenamine, potassium p-aminobenzoate, and procaine	Available in combinations with trimethoprim

Continued on following page

TABLE 157-2	Dosing, Pharmacokinetics, Adverse Events, Drug Interactions and Availability of Select Agents (Continued)			
			DOSING	
Drug	**Pharmacokinetics**	**Indication**	**Adult Dosage**	**Pediatric Dosage**
ARTEMISININS				
Artemisinin	$t_{\frac{1}{2}elim}$ = 2–4 hours	Used in combination therapy against malaria, see Table 157-1	Oral and suppository, 25 mg/kg initial dose followed by 12.5 mg/kg dose at 24 and 48 hours, use in combination therapy	Same as adult
Artesunate	Water soluble, metabolized by the liver to dihydroartemisinin which is 50-75% protein bound, $t_{\frac{1}{2}elim}$ = 3–30 minutes		Oral, intravenous, and intramuscular iv: 2.4 mg/kg/dose initially, then 2.4 mg/kg/dose at 12 hours, 24 hours, and 48 hours after the initial dose	iv: same as adult dosing
Artemether	Oil soluble, metabolized by the liver to dihydroartemisinin, 95% protein bound, $t_{\frac{1}{2}elim}$ = 3–11 hours		Oral and intramuscular, combination tablet (20 mg artemether and 120 mg lumefantrine) 4 tablets on day 1 at 0 and 8 hours, then 4 tablets every 12 hours on days 2 and 3, 3 tablets if <35 kg	5-15 kg, 1 tablet per adult schedule; 16 to 25 kg, 2 tablets per adult dosing schedule
Dihydroartemisinin (DHA)	Active metabolite, $t_{\frac{1}{2}elim}$ = 30 minutes to 12 hours based on route		Oral, regimens vary, DHA-piperaquine fixed combination 1.6/12.8 mg/kg dose at 0, 8, 24, and 48 hours, tablets contain 40 mg of DHA	
Atovaquone	Absorption increased with dietary fat, metabolized by liver, excreted in stool, 99% protein bound, $t_{\frac{1}{2}elim}$ = 2–3 days in adults	Used with proguanil for malaria, azithromycin for *Babesia*, and has activity against *T. gondii*	See Table 157-1	See Table 157-1
Atovaquone/proguanil	See individual drugs	Malaria prophylaxis and treatment, see Table 157-1 for treatment doses	Atovaquone/proguanil 250/100 mg; for prophylaxis, 1 tablet daily starting 1–2 days prior to travel and continuing for 1 week after return	Atovaquone/proguanil: 11–20 kg: 62.5 mg/25 mg 21–30 kg: 125 mg/50 mg 31–40 kg: 187.5 mg/75 mg >40 kg: adult dosing
Benznidazole	60–70% renally excreted, 44% protein bound, $t_{\frac{1}{2}elim}$ = 12 hours	*T. cruzi* infections	5–7 mg/kg divided in two doses given every 12 hours for 60 days	Same as adult dosing for children >7 months of age
Chloroquine	Metabolized by liver, excreted by kidneys, 50% protein bound, $t_{\frac{1}{2}elim}$ = 4-6 days	Malaria treatment and prophylaxis in chloroquine-sensitive areas	Prophylaxis: 50 mg (300 mg base) weekly begin 1–2 weeks prior to exposure; continue until 4 weeks after leaving Treatment: 1 g (600 mg base) on day 1, then 500 mg (300 mg base) 6, 24, and 48 hours after first dose	Prophylaxis: 8.3 mg/kg base weekly for same duration as adults Treatment: 10 mg/kg initial dose followed by 8.3 mg/kg on same schedule as adults
Clindamycin	See Chapter 141 Metabolized by liver, excreted by kidneys, 90% protein bound, $t_{\frac{1}{2}elim}$ = 2.5–3 hours	*P. falciparum*, *T. gondii*, and *Babesia* spp.	See Table 157-1 for specific dosing	See Table 157-1 for specific dosing
Difluoromethylornithine (DFMO, eflornithine)	Excreted in the kidneys, $t_{\frac{1}{2}elim}$ = 3 hours	*T. brucei* infections	100 mg/kg every 6 hours for 2 weeks, or 200 mg/kg every 12 hours for 10 days combined with nifurtimox	Not well established, some use 100–150 mg/kg/dose based on adult schedules

Renal Impairment	Hepatic Impairment	FDA Pregnancy Category/Risk	Adverse Reactions	Drug Interactions	Availability in USA
	No adjustment	Understudied, must weigh risks and benefits of severe malaria in pregnant women	Diarrhea, abdominal pain, transient first degree heart block	No significant drug interactions known	Not currently available
No adjustment	No adjustment	Teratogenicity observed in animal models, must weigh risks and benefits of severe malaria in pregnant women	QT prolongation, neurological toxicity (ataxia, slurred speech)	No significant drug interactions known	Available through the CDC Drug Service
No adjustment	No adjustment	FDA Category C	Possible QT prolongation, some neurological toxicity	No significant drug interactions known for artemether, other antimalarials may enhance effects of lumefantrine; CYP3A4 inducers increase metabolism of artemether and should be avoided; avoid with ivabradine, mifepristone, QT prolonging agents, St John's wort and thioridazine	Available in combination with lumefantrine
No adjustment	No adjustment	FDA Category C	Possible QT prolongation, no severe effects noted	No significant drug interactions known	Not readily available; available in combination with piperaquine
No dosage adjustment, not studied	No dosage adjustment, not studied, use with caution	FDA Category C	Rash, nausea, and diarrhea are common	Avoid with efavirenz, rifamycins, and ritonavir	Readily available
Contraindicated for prophylaxis if CrCl <30	No dosage adjustment	FDA Category C	Rash, nausea, vomiting, diarrhea, headache, fever, anemia, transaminitis, hyponatremia and hyperglycemia	Avoid with artemether, efavirenz, lumefantrine, rifamycins, ritonavir	Readily available
Contraindicated in severe disease	Contraindicated in severe disease	Teratogenic in animals, avoid	Dermatitis, nausea, neuropathy, cytopenias	Avoid alcohol	Available through the CDC Drug Service
No adjustment	Use with caution	FDA Category C, considered safe	Bitter taste, headache, GI disturbances, blurred vision, dizziness, fatigue, pruritus, leukopenia, hair depigmentation, eczematous eruptions, psychosis (rarely)	Avoid with agalsidase, artemether, conivaptan, fusidic acid, ivabradine, lumefantrine, mefloquine, mifepristone, and thioridazine	
No adjustment needed	No adjustment needed	FDA Category B	Diarrhea, nausea, vomiting, abdominal pain, rash, hepatotoxicity, cytopenias	Avoid with erythromycin	Readily available
No clear recommendations, use with caution as renally excreted	Use with caution, no guidelines available	FDA Category C	Cytopenias, arrhythmias, abdominal pain, arthralgia, seizures, hearing loss, and alopecia	No significant interactions known	Available through the CDC Drug Service

Continued on following page

TABLE
157-2 **Dosing, Pharmacokinetics, Adverse Events, Drug Interactions and Availability of Select Agents** (Continued)

Drug	Pharmacokinetics	Indication	DOSING	
			Adult Dosage	**Pediatric Dosage**
Diloxanide furoate	Poorly absorbed and activated by intestinal esterases, metabolized by liver, excreted by kidneys, $t_{\frac{1}{2}elim}$ = 6 hours	*E. histolytica* cysts	500 mg three times daily	20 mg/kg/day divided in 3 equal doses
Fumagillin	No information available	Microsporidial infections	20 mg every 8 hours for 14 days, ocular formulations at 70 µg/mL	Used at 20 mg/day in one case report
Furazolidone	Orally absorbed, excreted in the urine and feces	Alternative therapy for Giardiasis, trichomoniasis, *C. belli*	100 mg po every 6 hours	1.25 mg/kg every 6 hours
Melarsoprol	Excreted in the urine, $t_{\frac{1}{2}elim}$ = 35 hours	Late-stage *T. brucei* infections	3.8 mg/kg/day for 3 days, maximum dose of 180–200 mg	1.8 mg/kg day vs 15-25 mg/kg total dose given in increasing doses over 1 month
Miltefosine	Orally absorbed, near-complete protein binding, metabolized by liver, $t_{\frac{1}{2}elim}$ = 6 days	*Leishmania* spp., free living amebae	<45 kg, 50 mg po twice daily; >45 kg, 50 mg po three times daily for 4 weeks	Same as adult
Nifurtimox	Orally absorbed, metabolized by the liver, limited renal excretion, $t_{\frac{1}{2}elim}$ = 3 hours	*T. cruzi* and *T.b. gambiense* infections	*T. cruzi*: 8–10 mg/kg/day in 3 divided doses for 90 days	*T. cruzi*: 15-20 mg/kg/day in 3 divided doses for 90 days
Nitazoxanide	Metabolized by liver, excreted in urine and bile, 99% protein bound	Giardiasis, amebiasis, and cryptosporidial infections	500 mg po every 12 hours for 3 days	Children 1–3 y.o. 100 mg po twice daily for 3 days; 4–11 y.o. 200 mg po twice daily
NITROIMIDAZOLES				
Metronidazole	Minimal protein binding, metabolized by the liver, excreted by the kidneys, $t_{\frac{1}{2}elim}$ = 6–11 hours	*Entamoeba* infections, giardiasis, trichomoniasis, *B. hominis*, *B. coli*, eases removal of guinea worms	500 mg po three times daily for 5–8 days depending on organism	15–30 mg/kg/day in three divided doses
Ornidazole	Metabolized by the liver, excreted by the kidneys, $t_{\frac{1}{2}elim}$ = 12–13 hours	Amebiasis, giardiasis, trichomoniasis	500 mg twice daily for 5 days	10-40 mg/kg/day in two divided doses depending on the type of infection
Tinidazole	10% protein bound, metabolized by the liver, excreted by the kidneys and feces, $t_{\frac{1}{2}elim}$ = 14 hours	Amebic liver abscess, metronidazole-resistant trichomoniasis	2 g daily, duration dependent on organism	50 mg/kg/day in children >3 y.o.
Paromomycin	Nonabsorbable, excreted in the feces	*E. histolytica, D. fragilis, T. saginata, T. solium, D. latum, D. caninum*, and *H. nana* infections, used topically for cutaneous leishmaniasis	25–35 mg/kg/day divided in 3 doses for 7 days total	Same as adult

Renal Impairment	Hepatic Impairment	FDA Pregnancy Category/Risk	Adverse Reactions	Drug Interactions	Availability in USA
No information available	No information available	No information available, avoid in first trimester	Flatulence, abdominal pain, and urticaria	No information available	Not readily available
No information available	No information available	No information available, considered unsafe	Neutropenia, thrombocytopenia	No information available	Not readily available
No information, use with caution	No information, use with caution	Avoid at term, consider alternatives	Diarrhea, fever, nausea, vomiting, hemolysis with G6PD deficiency	Monoamine oxidase inhibitor	Not readily available
Use with caution, renally excreted	Not studied	FDA Category C, defer treatment	Fever, fatal encephalopathy, arthralgia, rash, hypertension, proteinuria, transaminitis, exacerbation of erythema nodosum leprosum, and hemolysis in G6PD deficiency	Caution with G6PD deficiency	Available through the CDC Drug Service
No adjustment needed though not studied	No adjustment needed though not studied	Teratogenic, avoid	Abdominal pain, transaminits, renal insufficiency	No known drug interactions	Available through the CDC by IND for treatment of free-living ameba infections, recently FDA-approved for leishmaniasis
No adjustment needed though not well studied	Use with caution in severe disease	Avoid in the first trimester, preferably until after delivery	Abdominal pain, polyneuritis, neuropathy, rash, neutropenia	No significant interactions, follow tacrolimus levels	Available through the CDC Drug Service
No adjustment needed though not studied	No adjustment needed though not studied	FDA Category B	Headache and abdominal pain	No significant interactions known	Readily available
No adjustment needed, consider additional doses after dialysis	Do not use extended release tablets with liver failure	FDA Category B	Headache, metallic taste, abdominal pain, urticarial, pruritus, neutropenia, candidiasis, peripheral neuropathy, pancreatitis, US boxed warning regarding carcinogenic potential	Disulfiram-like reaction with alcohol and drugs using alcohol in their preparations, avoid with disulfiram and pimozide	Readily available
No adjustment needed, consider additional doses after dialysis	Increase interval with hepatic impairment	Not well studied but presumed safe	Headache, dizziness, and anorexia	Disulfiram-like reaction with alcohol	Not readily available in the USA
No adjustment needed, administer half the total dose after dialysis if first dose taken prior to dialysis	No adjustment needed	FDA Category C	Headache, dizziness, metallic taste, and anorexia	Disulfiram-like reaction with alcohol	Readily available
No adjustment needed though not studied	No adjustment needed though not studied	FDA Category C, not studied but considered safe due to lack of absorption, consider avoiding in the first trimester	Abdominal pain, headache, rash, and vertigo	No known interactions	Readily available

Continued on following page

TABLE 157-2	Dosing, Pharmacokinetics, Adverse Events, Drug Interactions and Availability of Select Agents (Continued)			

Drug	Pharmacokinetics	Indication	DOSING Adult Dosage	Pediatric Dosage
Pentamidine isethionate	No oral absorption, limited renal excretion, $t_{\frac{1}{2}elim}$ = 6–8 hours	Early stages of *T. brucei* infections, leishmaniasis, *Acanthamoeba* infections, and babesiosis	See Table 157-1 for various indications, usually given 3–4 mg/kg iv daily	Same as adult
PENTAVALENT ANTIMONIALS				
Meglumine antimonite	Poorly absorbed, excreted by the kidneys, $t_{\frac{1}{2}elim}$ = 2 hours in the first phase and 33 to 76 hours in the second phase	Cutaneous and visceral leishmaniasis	Intravenous or intramuscular, 20 mg/kg/day	Follow adult dosing
Sodium stibogluconate	Excreted by the kidneys, $t_{\frac{1}{2}elim}$ = 2 hours in the first phase and 33–76 hours in the second phase	Cutaneous and visceral leishmaniasis	Intravenous or intramuscular, 20 mg/kg/day for 20–28 days	Follow adult dosing
Piperaquine	Slow oral absorption, metabolized by the liver, excreted by the kidneys, $t_{\frac{1}{2}elim}$ = 22 days	Malaria	Available in tablets 320 mg piperaquine/40 mg dihydroartemisinin: 36–75 kg, 3 tablets; 75–100 kg, 4 tablets; >100 kg no data	Available in tablets 160 mg piperaquine/20 mg dihydroartemisinin: 5–7 kg, ½ tablet; 7–13 kg, 1 tablet; 13–24 kg, 1 adult tablet; 25–35 kg, 2 adult tablets
Primaquine	Orally absorbed, metabolized by the liver, excreted by the kidneys, $t_{\frac{1}{2}elim}$ = 6–7 hours	*P. vivax* and *P. ovale* malaria treatment and prophylaxis	Prophylaxis: 30 mg po daily for 2 days prior to departure and 7 days after return; Treatment: 30 mg daily for 14 days	0.5 mg/kg, same schedule as adults
Quinacrine	Orally absorbed, excreted in feces, 80–90% protein bound, $t_{\frac{1}{2}elim}$ = 5–14 days	Giardiasis with metronidazole, malaria prophylaxis	100 mg every 8 hours for 5–7 days in giardiasis	2 mg/kg every 8 hours for 5–7 days
Quinidine	Metabolized by the liver, excreted by the kidneys, 80–90% protein bound, $t_{\frac{1}{2}elim}$ = 6–8 hours. 267 mg of quinidine gluconate = 200 mg of quinidine sulfate	Severe malaria	Quinidine gluconate 10 mg/kg iv over 2 hours then 0.02 mg/kg/minute continuous infusion for ≥24 hours; alternative dosing 24 mg/kg loading dose over 4 hours, then 12 mg/kg over 4 hours every 8 hours	Same as adult

Renal Impairment	Hepatic Impairment	FDA Pregnancy Category/Risk	Adverse Reactions	Drug Interactions	Availability in USA
CrCl 10–30, increase interval to 36 hours in children, CrCl <10, increase interval to 36 hours in adults or 48 hours in children	No adjustment needed though not studied	FDA Category C	Hypotension, dyspnea, tachycardia, headache, vomiting, hypoglycemia, pancreatitis, hyperglycemia, renal insufficiency, arrhythmias, hypocalcemia, confusion, cytopenias, transaminitis	Avoid with agents prolonging the QT interval, ivabradine, mifepristone, and pimozide	Readily available
Not well studied, contraindicated in severe failure	Not well studied, use with caution in severe disease	Unknown risk, use with caution	Similar to sodium stibogluconate	Not well studied, no known interactions	Not readily available in the USA
Not well studied, contraindicated in severe failure	Not well studied, use with caution in severe disease	Unknown risk, use with caution	Abdominal pain, headache, arthralgia, myalgias, fever, rash, transaminitis, nephrotoxicity, pancreatitis, and QT prolongation. Arrhythmias and sudden death have occurred	Not well studied, no known interactions	Available through the CDC Drug Service
Not well studied, use with caution	Not well studied, use with caution	Not well studied, teratogenic in animals, avoid if able	Headache, anemia, and QT prolongation	Metabolized and inhibits CYP3A4; use with caution with QT-prolonging agents, HIV protease inhibitors, and cyclosporine	Available in Europe combined with dihydroartemisinin
No adjustment needed	No adjustment needed	FDA Category C, avoid in pregnancy	Hemolysis in G6PD deficiency, must test for G6PD deficiency prior to use; headache, nausea, vomiting, abdominal pain, cytopenias. Neurotoxicity, arrhythmias, hypertension and agranulocytosis rarely occur	Avoid with agomelatine, artemether, lumefantrine, mefloquine, pimozide, pirfenidone, pomalidomide, and tasimelteon	Readily available
Not well studied, use with caution	Not well studied, use with caution	Not well studied, avoid during pregnancy	Bitter taste, nausea, vomiting, dizziness, yellow skin discoloration, psychosis, cytopenias, dermatitis	Disulfiram-like effect with alcohol, increases primaquine concentrations	Not readily available
Decrease dose by 25% for CrCl <10	No adjustment needed	FDA Category C	QT prolongation (requires telemetry) and hypotension, contraindicated in myasthenia gravis, cinchonism (see quinine)	Avoid with amiodarone, anti-fungal azoles, bosutinib, conivaptan, crizotinib, enzalutamide, fingolimod, fusidic acid, ivabradine, macrolides, mefloquine, mifepristone, pazopanib, pimozide, propafenone, HIV protease inhibitors, silodosin, tamoxifen, thioridazine, topotecan and vincristine	Available but not routinely carried by pharmacies

Continued on following page

TABLE 157-2	Dosing, Pharmacokinetics, Adverse Events, Drug Interactions and Availability of Select Agents (Continued)			
			DOSING	
Drug	**Pharmacokinetics**	**Indication**	**Adult Dosage**	**Pediatric Dosage**
Quinine	Orally absorbed, metabolized by the liver, excreted by the kidneys, 90% protein bound, $t_{1/2elim}$ = 11 hours	Malaria, *Babesia*	650 mg salt every 8 hours for 3-7 days	30 mg/kg/day in three divided doses every 8 hours
Suramin	Excreted by the kidneys, 99% protein bound, persists for months, does not penetrate the CNS	Early stage *T. brucei* infections, active against *O. volvulus*	100–200 mg iv test dose, then 1 g on days 1, 3, 7, 14, and 21	20 mg/kg on adult schedule
TETRACYCLINES				
Doxycycline	Orally absorbed, metabolized in the GI tract, excreted in the feces and urine, 90% protein bound, $t_{1/2elim}$ = 18–21 hours	Malaria prophylaxis and treatment	Prophylaxis: 100 mg po daily starting 2 days before travel and 4 weeks after returning; Treatment: 100 mg iv/po twice daily for 7 days	2–5 mg/kg/day in two divided doses, contraindicated if less than 8 years old
Tetracycline	Orally absorbed, 65% protein bound, excreted by the kidneys, $t_{1/2elim}$ = 8–11 hours	Malaria treatment	250 mg four times daily for up to 7 days	25 mg/kg/day in 4 divided doses, avoid in children <8
ANTHELMINTICS				
Albendazole	Poorly absorbed, metabolized by the liver, excreted in bile, $t_{1/2elim}$ = 9–15 hours	*A. lumbricoides, E. vermicularis, A. duodenale, N. americanus, S. stercoralis, Echinococcus* spp., and *T. solium*. Activity against *A. caninum, C. philippinensis*, cutaneous and visceral larva migrans, *C. sinensis, G. spinigerum, O. bifurcum, Trichostrongylus* spp., microsporidia, giardiasis, used in combination therapy against filariasis	400 mg one time dose for many infections, see Table 157-1 for more details	400 mg one time dose, see Table 157-1 for more details, use with caution in children under 2 years of age
Bithionol	Bithionol is an older drug with limited data available, its use has largely been supplanted	*Fasciola hepatica* and *Paragonimus* spp.	30–50 mg/kg every other day for 10–15 days	Same as adult dosing
Diethylcarbamazine (DEC)	Metabolized by the liver, excreted by the kidneys, $t_{1/2elim}$ = 10 hours	Filariasis	6 mg/kg/day in 3 divided doses for 3 weeks	Same as adult dosing

Renal Impairment	Hepatic Impairment	FDA Pregnancy Category/Risk	Adverse Reactions	Drug Interactions	Availability in USA
CrCl 10–50: dose every 8 to 12 hours; CrCl <10: dose every 24 hours	Avoid use in severe impairment	FDA Category C	Cinchonism (tinnitus, hearing loss, headache, abdominal pain, and visual disturbances), hypoglycemia, rash, respirator depression in myasthenia gravis, hemolysis with G6PD deficiency	Avoid with antacids, artemether, bosutinib, conivaptan, fusidic acid, halofantrine, ivabradine, lopinavir, lumefantrine, macrolides, mefloquine, mifepristone, neuromuscular blocking agents, pazopanib, pimozide, rifampin, ritonavir, silodosin, thioridazine, topotecan, and vincristine	Readily available
Avoid in severe impairment	Avoid in severe impairment	Potentially teratogenic	Malaise, abdominal pain, fatigue, fever, shock, rash, stomatitis, dermatitis, lacrimation, photophobia, headache, hyperesthesia, renal dysfunction, transaminitis, diarrhea, cytopenias	No known interactions	Available through the CDC Drug Service
No dose adjustment	No dose adjustment	FDA Category D, avoid in pregnancy	Abdominal pain, photosensitivity, candidiasis	Avoid with pimozide, retinoic acid derivatives (except adapalene), and strontium ranelate	Readily available
CrCl 50–80: decrease to every 8–12 hours; CrCl 10–50: decrease to 12–24 hours; CrCl <10: every 24 hours	No dose adjustment	FDA Category D, avoid during pregnancy	Pericarditis, photosensitivity, rash, abdominal pain, and transaminitis, rarely associated with pseudotumor cerebri	Avoid with bosutinib, ibrutinib, ivabradine, lomitapide, pimozide, retinoic acid derivatives (except adapalene), simeprevir, strontium ranelate, and tolvaptan	Readily available
Not well studied, unlikely to be affected	Not well studied, use with caution	FDA Category C, avoid in pregnancy if able	Abdominal pain, transaminitis, alopecia, cytopenias	No significant interactions known, especially with single dose treatment	Readily available
Dose reduction advised	Not well studied	FDA Category C, not recommended	Anorexia, abdominal pain, headache, dizziness, diarrhea, urticaria, and proteinuria. Rarely used due to severe photosensitivity reactions	Not well studied	Previously available through the CDC, no longer provided
Avoid with severe impairment	Not well studied, use with caution in severe impairment	Avoid in pregnancy	Headache, malaise, arthralgia, anorexia, nausea, Mazzotti reaction (pruritus, edema, rash, arthralgia, lymphadenopathy, fever, hypotension, proteinuria, splenomegaly and eosinophilia in response to O. volvulus antigen release), encephalopathy with Loa loa infections	No known interactions	Available through the CDC Drug Service

Continued on following page

TABLE 157-2	Dosing, Pharmacokinetics, Adverse Events, Drug Interactions and Availability of Select Agents (Continued)			
			DOSING	
Drug	**Pharmacokinetics**	**Indication**	**Adult Dosage**	**Pediatric Dosage**
Flubendazole	Fluoride analog of mebendazole, poorly absorbed, limited information availability in humans	*Enterobius vermicularis* and other intestinal helminths	100 mg po twice daily for three days	Same as adult
Ivermectin	Well absorbed, 90% protein bound, metabolized by the liver, excreted in feces, $t_{\frac{1}{2}elim}$ = 18 hours	Onchocerciasis and other filarial infections, strongyloidiasis, *E. vermicularis, A. lumbricoides,* and *T. trichiura*	See Table 157-1 for specific treatment	In children > 15 kg, follow adult dosing, see Table 157-1
Mebendazole	Metabolized by the liver, excreted in feces, 95% protein bound, $t_{\frac{1}{2}elim}$ = 3–6 hours	*A. lumbricoides, E. vermicularis, T. trichiura, A. duodenale, N. americanus, S. stercoralis, C. philippinensis, A. cantonensis, A. costaricensis, T. canis, Trichostrongylus* spp., *T. spiralis,* some filariasis, dracunculiasis, *T. saginata, T. solium, H. nana,* and activity against *Echinococcus* spp.	In general, 100 mg twice daily for 3 days, see Table 157-1 for specific indications	Children > 2 y.o., same as adult, no information in children < 2 y.o.
Metrifonate	Minimal information available, orally available, $t_{\frac{1}{2}elim}$ = 2–3 hours	*S. haematobium*	7.5–10 mg/kg orally every 2 weeks for three doses	Same as adult
Niclosamide	Poorly absorbed	*D. latum, D. caninum, H. nana, T. saginata, T. solium, Echinostoma* spp., *F. buski,* and *H. heterophyes*	2 gram single dose except for *H. nana* infections	> 6 y.o., adult dosing; 2-6 y.o., 1 gram dose; < 2 y.o., ½ tablet
Oxamniquine	Orally absorbed, metabolized by the liver, excreted by the kidneys, $t_{\frac{1}{2}elim}$ = 2 hours	*S. mansoni*	15 mg/kg every 12 hours for 1-3 days	Same as adult dosing
Piperazine	Some hepatic metabolism, mostly excreted by kidneys	*A. lumbricoides, E. vermicularis*	75 mg/kg (max 4 grams) on 2 consecutive days	2–12 years old, 75 mg/kg on 2 consecutive days, max 2.5 grams/dose; > 12 y.o. see adult
Praziquantel	Orally absorbed, metabolized by the liver, excreted by the kidneys, 80% protein bound $t_{\frac{1}{2}elim}$ = 1.5 hours	*Schistosoma* spp., *C. sinensis, D. dendriticum, Echinostoma* spp., *F. buski, H. heterophyes, M. yokogawai, M. conunctus, N. salmincola, O. viverrini, Paragonimus* spp., *D. latum, H. diminuta, T. saginata,* and *T. solium*	See Table 157-1	See Table 157-1
Pyrantel pamoate	Poorly absorbed and excreted in the feces	*E. vermicularis, A. lumbricoides, A. caninum,* hookworm, *M. moniliformis, Trichostrongylus* spp.	Solution or 180 mg tablets: dose at 11 mg/kg	Same as adult
Thiabendazole	Orally absorbed, metabolized by the liver, excreted by the kidneys, $t_{\frac{1}{2}elim}$ = 1 hour	*Strongyloides* spp., *A. costaricensis, C. philippinensis, D. medinensis, Trichostrongylus* spp., *T. spiralis,* cutaneous and visceral larva migrans, *A. lumbricoides, E. vermicularis, T. trichiura,* and hookworm	13.5-23 kg, 250 mg; 23 kg to 34 kg, 500 mg; 34 kg to 45 kg, 750 mg; 45 kg to 57 kg, 1 g; 57 kg–68 kg, 1.25 g; over 68 kg, 1.5 g	Same as adult
Triclabendazole	Excreted in the feces, $t_{\frac{1}{2}elim}$ = 6–7 hours	*F. hepatica, Paragonimus* spp.	10 mg/kg	Same as adult, not well studied

When available, FDA pregnancy categories were described:
Category A, safe based on well-controlled studies in humans; B, presumed safe, animal studies fail to show risk; C, some risk, animal studies show harm;
  D, evidence of risk in human populations; and X, clear evidence of harm and risk outweighs benefit.

Renal Impairment	Hepatic Impairment	FDA Pregnancy Category/Risk	Adverse Reactions	Drug Interactions	Availability in USA
Not well studied, use with caution	Not well studied, use with caution	Contraindicated	Similar to mebendazole	Avoid with phenytoin, carbemazepine, and cimetidine	Not readily available
No adjustment needed	No adjustment needed	FDA Category C	Headache, fever, pruritus, lymphadenopathy, myalgias, arthralgia, and orthostatic hypotension	No significant risks known	Readily available
No adjustment needed	Not well studied, use with caution	FDA Category C	Abdominal pain, diarrhea, cytopenias, neutropenia, alopecia, allergic skin reactions, hepatitis, vertigo	No significant interactions, use with caution when combined with metronidazole	Readily available
Not well studied, appears safe, use with caution	Not well studied, use with caution	Not well studied, avoid if able	Nausea, vomiting, vertigo, lethargy	Neuromuscular blocking agents and insecticides	Not readily available
No dosage adjustment needed	No dosage adjustment needed	FDA Category B, consider avoiding in first trimester	Abdominal pain, dizziness, and rash	No known interactions	Not readily available
No adjustment needed	No adjustment needed	Avoid	Drowsiness, dizziness, orange/red urine discoloration, seizures	Not well studied, no significant drug interactions known	Not readily available
Avoid using in severe impairment	Avoid using in severe impairment	FDA Category B	Gastrointestinal disturbances, headache, dizziness, urticaria, and seizures. Contraindicated in patients with seizures	Avoid with pyrantel pamoate	Not readily available
No adjustment needed	No adjustment needed, use with caution in severe impairment	FDA Category B	Headache, dizziness, nausea, abdominal pain, rare events include fever and rash	Avoid with conivaptan and fusidic acid	Readily available
No adjustment needed	No adjustment needed, use with caution in severe impairment	FDA Category C, considered safe due to minimal absorption	Headache, dizziness, insomnia, nausea, anorexia, and abdominal pain	Avoid with piperazine	Readily available
No dosage adjustment, use with caution	No dosage adjustment, use with caution	FDA Category C, avoid if able	Nausea, vomiting, anorexia, dizziness, pruritus, abdominal pain, headache, drowsiness, diarrhea, tinnitus, hallucinations, numbness, seizures, altered perception and olfaction, hypotension, bradycardia, crystalluria, cytopenias, transaminitis, fever, angioneurotic edema, erythema multiform, and Stevens–Johnson syndrome	Theophylline	Not readily available
Limited information available	Limited information available	Risk not established	Well tolerated with abdominal pain reported, no significant adverse events have been reported	Limited information available	Not readily available

Antiprotozoal Agents

Amodiaquine

Amodiaquine is a 4-aminoquinoline with antimalarial activity and a mechanism of action similar to that of chloroquine.[1,2] The side effect profile is also similar to that of chloroquine but agranulocytosis and severe hepatitis have been reported with long-term use (as chemoprophylaxis). The activity of amodiaquine against some chloroquine-resistant strains of *Plasmodium falciparum* has led to a revival in its use, particularly as part of combination therapy with artesunate.[3] While resistance to amodiaquine in certain parts of Africa may limit the usefulness of this combination in those regions, the artesunate–amodiaquine combination has proved very effective in areas where responses to amodiaquine alone exceed 80%.[4]

Amphotericin B

Amphotericin B, a polyene antifungal agent, is the drug of choice for primary amebic meningoencephalitis caused by *Naegleria* spp.[5] (see Chapter 193), and is used for the treatment of visceral leishmaniasis (see Chapter 123).[6,7] Its pharmacokinetics and side effects are detailed in Chapter 156. Lipid-associated formulations of amphotericin B are effective in the treatment of visceral leishmaniasis, and in one study in India single-dose therapy with liposomal amphotericin B gave cure rates of more than 92% with minimal toxicity.[6]

Antifolate Agents

Antifolate agents act at various steps in the folic acid cycle. For *Plasmodium* spp., *Toxoplasma* spp. and other sensitive parasites, reduced folic acid derivatives are essential for *de novo* pyrimidine synthesis. Unlike mammalian cells, these parasites cannot use preformed pyrimidines. Antifolate agents are most commonly used in combination to block sequential steps in the folic acid metabolic pathway (see Chapter 150).

PROGUANIL

Proguanil is a biguanide that inhibits plasmodial dihydrofolate reductase.[1,2] Although it is seldom used for monotherapy because of its slow action, in combination with atovaquone it is effective in the prevention and treatment of *P. falciparum* malaria (see below, under atovaquone).[8,9]

Proguanil is metabolized to the active triazine metabolite, cycloguanil, and is excreted in urine (40–60%) and feces (10%).

PYRIMETHAMINE

Pyrimethamine is a diaminopyrimidine that inhibits plasmodial dihydrofolate reductase at a concentration that is 1000 times less than that required to inhibit the mammalian enzyme.[1,2] It is effective against the erythrocytic stages of all *Plasmodium* spp. that are pathogenic for humans, but resistance has significantly limited its usefulness as a single agent.[10] In combination with sulfadiazine, clindamycin or atovaquone, it is used for the treatment of *Toxoplasma gondii*.[11,12] Pyrimethamine also has activity against *Cystoisospora belli*.[13]

Although pyrimethamine is available as 25 mg tablets, it is almost exclusively used in combination with a sulfonamide (sulfadiazine, sulfadoxine) or a sulfone (dapsone; see below). The dosage for toxoplasmosis is listed in Table 157-1. Some clinicians give an initial pyrimethamine loading dose of 200 mg. In patients who cannot tolerate sulfonamides, clindamycin (1.8–2.4 g/day in divided doses) or atovaquone (1.5 g q12h) may be substituted. Side effects of pyrimethamine include blood dyscrasias, rash and, very rarely, seizures or shock. At high doses, pyrimethamine causes bone marrow suppression, which can be prevented by concurrent administration of folinic acid (leucovorin). Sulfadoxine–pyrimethamine as 25 mg pyrimethamine and 500 mg sulfadoxine is used in combination with artesunate for the treatment of *P. falciparum* malaria in areas where susceptibility to sulfadoxine and pyrimethamine remains high (South America, the Middle East, South Asia).[4]

TRIMETHOPRIM

Trimethoprim (TMP) is another diaminopyrimidine that inhibits microbial dihydrofolate reductase. It has activity against:

- a variety of bacteria (see Chapter 150);
- *Pneumocystis jirovecii* (see Chapter 94); and
- the parasites *Cystoisospora belli* and *Cyclospora cayetanensis* (see Chapter 191).[13]

For parasitic infections, TMP is used in fixed combination with sulfamethoxazole (SMX; see below). TMP inhibits the secretion of creatinine into the renal tubule, elevating its levels without changing the creatinine clearance.[14] Side effects include rashes, pruritus, nausea, vomiting, glossitis, elevated liver enzymes, cytopenias, megaloblastic anemia, fever, aseptic meningitis and impaired renal function.

SULFONAMIDES

Sulfonamides, which are derivatives of sulfanilamide, interfere with microbial folic acid synthesis by competitively inhibiting the enzyme dihydropteroate synthase.[1,2] This enzyme is involved in the step in folic acid synthesis that precedes the step blocked by pyrimethamine and TMP. Sulfonamides are separated into four groups:

- short- and intermediate-acting agents;
- long-acting agents;
- agents that are limited to the bowel lumen; and
- topical agents.

Only agents from the first two of these categories are used to treat parasitic diseases; these are generally combined with either pyrimethamine or TMP.

Sulfamethoxazole

Sulfamethoxazole is an intermediate-acting sulfonamide available in a fixed combination with TMP (see below) for numerous indications.

Sulfadiazine

Sulfadiazine, another intermediate-acting sulfonamide, is used with pyrimethamine in the treatment of toxoplasmosis, as detailed above.

Sulfadoxine

Sulfadoxine, a long-acting sulfonamide, is available in a fixed combination with pyrimethamine for the treatment of malaria (see pyrimethamine above).

Side Effects of Sulfonamides

Side effects of sulfonamides are numerous. Nausea, vomiting and anorexia occur in 1–2% of patients. Hypersensitivity reactions include:

- drug eruptions (ranging from morbilliform rash to severe exfoliation);
- fever;
- serum sickness; and
- hepatocellular dysfunction and necrosis.

Acute hemolytic anemia, agranulocytosis and aplastic anemia are rare. Reversible bone marrow suppression is not uncommon in immunocompromised patients, particularly those who have AIDS. Crystalluria can occur with sulfadiazine and can be avoided by increasing fluid intake, following sulfa levels, or alkalinizing the urine.

TRIMETHOPRIM–SULFAMETHOXAZOLE

Trimethoprim–sulfamethoxazole (TMP–SMX) is a combination used to treat bacterial infections, *P. jirovecii* and the parasites *C. belli* and *C. cayetanensis*.[13] This combination also has some efficacy against *P. falciparum*, but resistance to the TMP component limits its use.[15] It is available as single-strength tablets (80 mg TMP and 400 mg SMX) and as double-strength tablets (160 mg TMP and 800 mg SMX). An oral suspension (40 mg TMP and 200 mg SMX per 5 mL) and an intravenous formulation (80 mg TMP and 400 mg SMX per 5 mL vial) are available as well.

The dose for cystoisosporiasis is one double-strength tablet orally q6h for 10 days, followed by one double-strength tablet q12h for 3 weeks. Immunocompromised patients usually require maintenance therapy of one double-strength tablet daily or three times weekly. For cyclosporiasis, one double-strength tablet q12h for 7–10 days is generally used, but some clinicians extend treatment to 14 days. Immunocompromised patients sometimes require four tablets per day and usually need maintenance therapy as well.

Side effects of TMP–SMX include those listed for each of the two component drugs, as detailed above. Dermatologic reactions (3–4%) and gastrointestinal disturbances (3–4%) are the most common side effects in non-immunocompromised patients. For unclear reasons, patients who have AIDS have a much higher rate of complications, ranging in different series from 45% to 90%.

TRIMETREXATE
Trimetrexate is a lipid-soluble dihydrofolate reductase inhibitor that was originally developed as a myelosuppressive agent but was found to have antiparasitic activity against *P. jirovecii* and *T. gondii*.[11] It is available for intravenous injection only. Adverse effects include rash, leukopenia, elevated liver enzymes and a reversible peripheral neuropathy. Folinic acid is administered concurrently to diminish the incidence of bone marrow suppression.

Artemisinin and Its Derivatives
A major change in malaria therapy over the past 6 years has been the growing use of combination therapy for chloroquine-resistant *Plasmodium falciparum* infections. Artemisinin-based combination treatments (ACTs) have become a foundation of this effort.[4] Artemisinin, or qinghaosu, is a sesquiterpene lactone derived from the leaves of the sweet wormwood *Artemisia annua*.[2,4] It has been used for centuries in traditional Chinese medicine and is now known to be active against intraerythrocytic forms of *P. falciparum* and *P. vivax*, *Schistosoma mansoni*, *Schistosoma japonicum*, *Clonorchis sinensis* and *Naegleria fowleri*. Its main clinical use is the treatment of drug-resistant *P. falciparum* infections.

ROUTE OF ADMINISTRATION AND DOSAGE
Artemisinin and its derivatives, the water-soluble hemisuccinate artesunate, the oil-soluble derivatives artemether and artemotil, and the active metabolite dihydroartemisinin are the most rapidly acting antimalarials known and appear to be quite safe. These compounds can be given by several routes:
- artemisinin is available in oral and suppository forms;
- artesunate is available in oral, intravenous and intramuscular forms;
- artemether is available in oral and intramuscular forms;
- artemotil is available for intramuscular injection; and
- dihydroartemisinin is available in oral form.

They are rapidly absorbed and eliminated, with half-lives ranging from minutes (artesunate) to hours (artemether). The parent drug and derivatives are hepatically hydrolyzed to the active metabolite, dihydroartemisinin. These compounds are believed to act by disrupting parasite protein synthesis via the production of oxygen free radicals. While delayed parasite clearance has been noted as a harbinger of resistance, the mechanisms underlying this phenomenon are just beginning to be understood.[16]

Artemisinin and its derivatives must be administered in conjunction with a longer-acting antimalarial (e.g. mefloquine, lumefantrine, amodiaquine, sulfadoxine–pyrimethamine) to decrease the emergence of resistance and enhance efficacy. Recrudescence is a significant problem when artemisinin compounds are used as single agents. Artesunate (4 mg/kg orally) is usually given q24h for 3 days and is followed by a course of mefloquine. A fixed combination of artesunate (200 mg) and mefloquine (400 mg) base dosed at mefloquine 8 mg/kg/day for 3 days has been used with good success and, as noted above, the combination of artesunate and amodiaquine has been effective in certain regions.[4,17] Artemether can be given at a dose of 3.2 mg/kg intramus-

cularly initially, followed by 1.6 mg/kg q24h. It is available orally in combination with lumefantrine (artemether 80 mg/lumefantrine 480 mg) as a six-dose regimen. This has been used effectively and is well tolerated, but requires twice daily dosing and co-administration of fat for optimal absorption.[4] The fixed dose combination of dihydroartemisinin (40 mg) and piperaquine (a 4-aminoquinolone related to chloroquine) (320 mg) has been used successfully to treat *P. falciparum* infections in Asia and Africa.[4,18]

ADVERSE REACTIONS
Adverse events from artemisinin and its derivatives include diarrhea, abdominal pain, transient first-degree heart block and reversible mild decreases in reticulocyte and neutrophil counts. Neurotoxicity has been described in animals but not with clinical use in humans. In the USA the only artemisinin derivative currently available is the intravenous form of artesunate, which must be obtained from the US Centers for Disease Control and Prevention (http://www.cdc.gov/malaria/index.html, call the Malaria Hotline: 770-488-7788 or 770-488-7100) and is currently released only for patients that cannot receive or tolerate quinidine.[8]

Atovaquone and Atovaquone–Proguanil
Atovaquone, a synthetic hydroxynaphthoquinone derivative, has activity against *P. jirovecii*, *P. falciparum*, *T. gondii* and *Babesia microti*.[8,9,12,19] It interferes with pyrimidine synthesis by uncoupling mitochondrial electron transport. Because of its erratic absorption it is usually administered with a fatty meal. Atovaquone is an alternative oral agent for the treatment of mild-to-moderate *P. jirovecii* pneumonia in those who are intolerant of TMP–SMX, and experimental data indicate that it is synergistic with pyrimethamine or sulfadiazine for *T. gondii* infection. Atovaquone has also been used with azithromycin in the treatment of babesiosis.

The combination of atovaquone and proguanil has become a treatment of choice for *P. falciparum* malaria contracted in areas where chloroquine resistance is present (most of the malarious world with the exception of Central America west of the Panama Canal, Mexico, Hispaniola, parts of China and the Middle East)[8] and the combination pill containing atovaquone 250 mg and proguanil 100 mg has rapidly become a leading drug for malaria prophylaxis in travelers.[8,9,20] A randomized controlled trial comparing mefloquine and atovaquone–proguanil for malaria prophylaxis in nonimmune travelers found equivalent efficacy for the two agents, with a similar number of adverse events, but fewer adverse effects of moderate or severe intensity were reported in the atovaquone–proguanil group.[20] The adult dosage for prophylaxis is one tablet q24h (250 mg atovaquone/100 mg proguanil), beginning 1–2 days prior to arrival in the malarious area and continuing for 1 week after return. Side effects include rash, nausea, vomiting, diarrhea, headache, fever, anemia, elevated liver function tests, hyponatremia and hyperglycemia. *P. falciparum* strains resistant to atovaquone–proguanil resulting in treatment failures have now been identified, with most strains showing mutations in the parasite cytochrome b gene.[21] Combination therapy of artesunate with atovaquone–proguanil has been tested and found to be well tolerated and highly effective in limited clinical trials.[22]

Benznidazole
Benznidazole is a nitroimidazole derivative that is active against both the trypomastigote and amastigote forms of *Trypanosoma cruzi*.[1,2,23] It is dosed at 2.5–3.5 mg/kg given every 12 hours for 60 days. Efficacy in indeterminate-phase disease has been established in retrospective studies. Recently, a dose of 150 mg twice daily was shown to be effective in clearing latent parasitemia.[24]

Chloroquine
Chloroquine, a 4-aminoquinoline that was first synthesized in 1934 but did not become popular until the end of the Second World War,

has been the agent most widely used for treating the erythrocytic stage of uncomplicated malaria caused by *P. vivax, P. ovale, P. malariae* and chloroquine-sensitive *P. falciparum*.[1,2,8,9] Its precise mechanism of action has not been delineated, but chloroquine and other antimalarial quinolones, such as mefloquine, appear to inhibit the ability of the parasite to polymerize the heme moiety of hemoglobin, resulting in toxic levels of free heme.[25]

PHARMACOKINETICS AND DISTRIBUTION

Absorption after oral ingestion is excellent (90%), and the volume of distribution is large owing to its extensive tissue sequestration, particularly in the liver, spleen, kidneys and erythrocytes. Chloroquine is metabolized by the liver to the active metabolite desethylchloroquine, but 50% is cleared by the kidneys unchanged. Thus, dosing need not be altered for abnormal renal function, but caution must be exercised in patients who have hepatic, gastrointestinal, neurologic or hematologic disorders.

ROUTE OF ADMINISTRATION AND DOSAGE

The drug is formulated as a phosphate, sulfate or hydrochloride salt and is dosed by base content. It can be administered orally or rectally or by intravenous, intramuscular or subcutaneous injection. In the USA, chloroquine is available in 500 mg salt tablets (equal to 300 mg base). The dosage for the treatment and prophylaxis of malaria is given in Table 157-1. If chloroquine hydrochloride is given intravenously, it must be administered by slow, constant infusion to avoid respiratory depression, hypotension, heart block, cardiac arrest and seizures that may occur with transient toxic levels. A dose of 300 mg base q8–12h may be given by intramuscular injection.

ADVERSE REACTIONS

Reversible side effects include headache, gastrointestinal disturbances, blurred vision, dizziness, fatigue and pruritus. Rarer side effects include hair depigmentation, weight loss, myalgias, leukopenia and eczematous eruptions. Very rarely, acute psychosis may occur. Permanent retinal damage has been observed with long-term (longer than 5 years) prophylactic use. The drug is contraindicated in patients who have retinal disease, psoriasis and porphyria. An oral dose of 5 g is fatal without immediate mechanical ventilation, adrenaline (epinephrine) and diazepam.

RESISTANCE OF *PLASMODIUM FALCIPARUM* TO CHLOROQUINE

Resistance of *P. falciparum* to chloroquine is ubiquitous in regions where malarial transmission occurs with the exception of the Caribbean, and much of Central America and the Middle East (although there are reports of resistance from Yemen, Oman and Iran).[8] There is a report that withdrawal of chloroquine as preferred treatment from a region can, after an 8-year period, result in the re-emergence of chloroquine-sensitive *P. falciparum*.[26] Resistance to chloroquine among *P. vivax* isolates has been reported in Brazil, Colombia, India, Myanmar, Papua New Guinea and Indonesia.[8,27,28] A single oral dose of mefloquine (15 mg base/kg) has been used successfully in such cases.

Clindamycin

Clindamycin, a lincosamide antibiotic, is active against bacteria, *P. falciparum, T. gondii* and *Babesia* spp.[15,29,30]

Dosages for malaria and babesiosis are listed in Table 157-1. For cerebral toxoplasmosis in the case of sulfonamide hypersensitivity, 1.8–2.4 g divided into three daily doses is combined with a course of pyrimethamine. Clindamycin has been used in combination with quinine for short-course (3-day) treatment of travelers who have *P. falciparum* malaria, with excellent results.[31] Side effects include rash, diarrhea, nausea, vomiting, abdominal pain, pseudomembranous colitis, hepatotoxicity and cytopenias.

Difluoromethylornithine (DMFO, Eflornithine)

Difluoromethylornithine, also referred to as DMFO or eflornithine, is effective in the treatment of both early and late sleeping sickness caused by *Trypanosoma brucei gambiense*.[7,32] It has minimal efficacy against *T. brucei rhodesiense* because many strains are resistant. Difluoromethylornithine inhibits ornithine decarboxylase, an enzyme involved in the first step in polyamine synthesis. It is available as the hydrochloride salt for both oral and intravenous administration.

Side effects of DMFO include anemia, thrombocytopenia, leukopenia, abdominal pain, nausea, vomiting, weight loss, arthralgias, seizures, hearing loss and alopecia. The usual dose of DMFO is 400 mg/kg intravenously every 6 hours for 14 days, which is logistically challenging. DMFO (400 mg/kg every 12 hours) has recently been combined with nifurtimox (15 mg/kg per os every 8 hours) as first-line therapy for late-stage *T.b. gambiense* infections.[33]

Diloxanide Furoate

Diloxanide furoate is a dichloroacetamide derivative that is a luminally active agent used to eradicate cysts of *E. histolytica* in asymptomatic carriers and in those who have mild, noninvasive disease, as well as after treatment with metronidazole in those who have invasive amebiasis.[6,34] It is not useful in extraintestinal disease. After oral administration, diloxanide furoate is hydrolyzed by intestinal esterases, thus releasing diloxanide, the absorbable component, and the ester furoic acid, which is not well absorbed and thus attains higher intraluminal concentrations in the colon. Both compounds are amebicidal, but the mechanism of action is not known.

Fumagillin

Fumagillin, a water-insoluble antibiotic derived from *Aspergillus fumigatus*, was discovered in 1949 and originally used in humans as an amebicide. Fumagillin is an inhibitor of parasite RNA synthesis, but may also act by inhibiting a key proteinase, type 2 methionine aminopeptidase.[35] Topical fumagillin has been used to treat microsporidial keratoconjunctivitis caused by *Encephalitozoon hellem, Encephalitozoon cuniculi, Encephalitozoon (Septata) intestinalis* and, with less success, *Vittaforma corneae (Nosema corneum)* in AIDS patients.[36] Oral fumagillin has been used successfully for *Encephalitozoon beineusi* infections inherently resistant to albendazole.[37]

Furazolidone

Furazolidone is a nitrofuran derivative that is commonly used to treat giardiasis in children because of its availability in a liquid form for oral use.[1,38] Furazolidone also has activity against *C. belli* and *Trichomonas vaginalis* as well as many enteropathogenic bacteria, and is also used for treatment of *Helicobacter pylori* infections. The mechanism of action involves damage to DNA.

Adverse reactions include diarrhea, fever, nausea and vomiting. Urticaria, serum sickness, hypoglycemia and orthostatic hypotension occur rarely. Furazolidone has disulfiram-like properties and patients should therefore be warned to avoid alcohol. Furazolidone has monoamine oxidase inhibitor activity, but hypertensive crises have not been reported in association with this agent. Furazolidone may cause hemolysis in patients who have glucose-6-phosphate dehydrogenase (G6PD) deficiency.

Halofantrine

Halofantrine is an oral synthetic 9-phenanthrene methanol with activity against the intraerythrocytic stages of chloroquine-sensitive and chloroquine-resistant *P. falciparum* and *P. vivax*.[1,2,9,39] It is more active and generally better tolerated than mefloquine. Its mechanism of action is poorly understood.

There is some evidence of cross-resistance with mefloquine; therefore halofantrine may not be useful for those patients in areas with mefloquine resistance. Its side effects include prolongation of the PR and QT_c intervals on the electrocardiogram, diarrhea, abdominal pain, pruritus and rash. Because of reports of sudden death associated with halofantrine therapy, it is absolutely contraindicated in individuals with a history of congenital QT prolongation, other conduction defects or anyone taking medications known to prolong the QT interval.

Iodoquinol and Iodochlorhydroxyquin

Iodoquinol, a halogenated hydroxyquinoline, is a luminal amebicide used to eradicate cysts in patients who have asymptomatic *E. histolytica* infection.[1,34] It is also given after metronidazole therapy to eradicate cysts in patients who have invasive disease. Iodoquinol is the drug of choice for *Dientamoeba fragilis* infection and is an alternative for *Balantidium coli*.[40] It has also been used to treat *Blastocystis hominis*. Iodoquinol also has activity against *Giardia lamblia* and *T. vaginalis*, but other agents are typically employed. The mechanism of action of iodoquinol is uncertain. It is available in oral form, but is poorly absorbed and should be given with meals. Side effects include nausea, vomiting, diarrhea, abdominal pain, headache, fever, seizures and encephalopathy.

Iodochlorhydroxyquin, a related compound, is better absorbed than iodoquinol, but is rarely used because of the high incidence of subacute myelo-optic neuropathy described with its use in Japan in the early 1970s. Because iodoquinol may rarely cause this syndrome when given at high dose or for prolonged periods, treatment recommendations should not be exceeded. For this reason many clinicians prefer alternative agents such as paromomycin or diloxanide furoate for these indications.

Lumefantrine

Lumefantrine is an aryl amino alcohol compound that is structurally related to mefloquine and halofantrine. It is active against all *Plasmodium* spp. that infect humans.[4] As noted above, a fixed tablet combination of lumefantrine and artemether has proven to be highly effective in the treatment of multidrug-resistant *P. falciparum* infection.[4]

Macrolide Antibiotics

SPIRAMYCIN

Spiramycin is used to prevent the transmission of *T. gondii* from mother to fetus.[11] The drug is concentrated in the placenta and has been shown to reduce transmission by 60%. It is given at a dose of 1 g orally q8h on an empty stomach. If fetal infection has not occurred (as assessed by amniotic fluid polymerase chain reaction testing for *T. gondii*), spiramycin is continued until delivery. Because spiramycin does not cross the placenta well, it cannot be used to treat fetal toxoplasmosis; pyrimethamine and sulfadiazine are recommended in this situation. Oral spiramycin is generally well tolerated; gastrointestinal distress is the main side effect.

AZITHROMYCIN

Azithromycin (see Chapter 141), both alone and in combination with pyrimethamine, has been shown to be effective in cerebral toxoplasmosis in AIDS patients.[11] It is considered relatively safe in pregnancy, but has not been extensively studied in preventing the vertical transmission of *T. gondii*. Azithromycin has also been used with both quinine and atovaquone for babesiosis.[29] Azithromycin has activity against *Plasmodium* spp., and is being evaluated as a component of combination therapy for *P. falciparum* paired with pyrimethamine–sulfadoxine, artesunate or quinine.[41]

Mefloquine

Mefloquine is a fluorinated 4-quinoline methanol derivative of quinine. It is an oral formulation that was developed as part of a search for new antimalarials.[1,2,8,9] It is a blood schizonticide effective against all *Plasmodium* spp. that infect humans, including *P. falciparum* isolates that are resistant to chloroquine and pyrimethamine–sulfadoxine. It is ineffective against exoerythrocytic forms and gametocytes. The mechanism of action is unknown, but mefloquine may interfere with the function of *Plasmodium* food vacuoles or inhibit the polymerization of heme.

Common side effects at therapeutic doses include nausea, vomiting, dizziness, weakness and dysphoria.[22,42] Neuropsychiatric reactions, including acute psychosis, sleep disturbances and seizures, have been documented in approximately 0.5% of patients taking therapeutic doses and in less than 0.5% of those taking prophylactic doses. The US FDA issued a boxed warning for those who have a history of seizures or psychiatric disorders. Judicious use is suggested for those whose occupations require spatial discrimination and fine motor coordination. Cardiac rhythm and conduction abnormalities and at least one instance of nonfatal cardiac arrest have occurred in patients on β-adrenergic blockers who took mefloquine; caution should be exercised in any patient who has cardiac disease. Mefloquine may also decrease the response to the live *Salmonella typhi* oral vaccine, and thus the vaccine series should be completed at least 3 days before beginning mefloquine prophylaxis.

Mefloquine resistance in *P. falciparum* isolates has been increasing along the Thailand–Myanmar and Thailand–Cambodia borders, in western Africa and in the Amazon region. In these areas, doxycycline at a dose of 100 mg/day or atovaquone–proguanil may be used for prophylaxis. Even the combination of mefloquine and artesunate may no longer be effective for treatment of acute falciparum malaria in those regions.[17,43] Treatment options include:

- quinine plus tetracycline or doxycycline for 7 days;[44]
- lumefantrine and artemether;[4]
- doxycycline plus artesunate;[45]
- atovaquone–proguanil and artesunate;[22]
- quinine plus clindamycin;[30] and
- dihydroartemisinin and piperaquine.[4]

Melarsoprol

Melarsoprol is a trivalent arsenical compound introduced in 1949 and used for the treatment of late-stage African trypanosomiasis caused by either *T. brucei gambiense* or *T. brucei rhodesiense*.[1,2] Its use in late-stage *T. brucei gambiense* has been supplanted by NECT (nifurtimox–eflornithine combination therapy). It is also effective in treating the early or hemolymphatic stage of infection, but its toxicity prohibits routine use for this stage and it should be used only in patients who have failed to respond to suramin and pentamidine.

Melarsoprol acts by interacting with protein sulfhydryl groups and subsequently inactivating enzymes, a nonspecific action that is also responsible for the toxicity of the drug. Melarsoprol, formulated as a 3.6% weight per volume solution in propylene glycol, is given intravenously. A small, but adequate amount of the drug penetrates the cerebrospinal fluid, where it is taken up and concentrated by susceptible trypanosomes. Resistant organisms appear to concentrate the drug poorly.

Melarsoprol is highly toxic. It is irritating to tissues and a fine gauged needle must be used to prevent extravasation. Fever is commonly seen. Reactive encephalopathy occurs in up to 18% of patients and may be fatal; it usually occurs during the first 3–4 days of therapy.[46] It is manifested by headache, confusion, dizziness, mental slowing and ataxia, with seizures and a progressive decline in mental status, and it is felt to be an immunologic reaction to parasite antigens released during therapy. Corticosteroids have been used to treat the encephalopathy with some success. Very rarely, a hemorrhagic encephalopathy, which is almost always fatal, may occur. Abdominal pain and vomiting may be minimized by slow administration of the drug to a patient who is supine and fasting. Erythema nodosum leprosum may be precipitated in patients who have leprosy. Hemolysis may be seen in G6PD-deficient patients.

Miltefosine

Miltefosine, an alkyl phospholipid compound, was developed as an anticancer agent, but had dose-limiting gastrointestinal toxicity that outweighed its clinical benefits. However, it was discovered to have excellent antileishmanial activity and became the first oral drug in the treatment of visceral leishmaniasis.[47] Its mechanism of action remains unknown, but parasite death appears to occur via apoptosis.[47] A 28-day course of miltefosine has proven safe and effective in the treatment of adults with visceral leishmaniasis in India.[47] It has also been studied in the treatment of cutaneous leishmaniasis in the Americas where it showed variable efficacy depending on the region and parasite strain.[48] Gastrointestinal side effects including nausea, vomiting and diarrhea are frequent, occurring in roughly one-third of subjects. Elevations in transaminases may be seen in 15% of recipients, and increases in serum creatinine in 10%; both tend to normalize during treatment. Recently, miltefosine has been used in combination therapy for treatment of amebic encephalitis due to *Balamuthia* or *Acanthamoeba*.[49]

Nifurtimox

Nifurtimox, an oral nitrofuran, is used to treat acute Chagas disease (American trypanosomiasis), although benznidazole is a first-line agent in some regions with endemic Chagas disease (see Chapter 124).[1,2,23] Nifurtimox has also been used in late-stage *T. brucei gambiense*.[32] It acts by inhibiting nucleic acid synthesis by oxygen free radical formation. There is considerable geographic variation in responsiveness to nifurtimox; better results are obtained in Argentina and Chile than in Brazil and other countries. Effectiveness in indeterminate-phase and chronic-phase infection is variable and organ damage is not reversible.

Gastrointestinal side effects, including nausea, vomiting, anorexia and abdominal pain, and weight loss may occur. Neurologic side effects include headache, restlessness, insomnia, disorientation, paresthesias, polyneuritis, weakness and seizures. Rash, decreased sperm counts and neutropenia have also been described. Adherence to a full 3 months of therapy is often poor.

Nitazoxanide

Nitazoxanide is a nitrothiazole benzamide derivative with *in vitro* activity against a wide variety of bacterial, protozoal and helminthic pathogens. In randomized, double-blind, placebo-controlled clinical trials it showed efficacy comparable to metronidazole in the treatment of giardiasis and amebiasis, and was very successful in eradicating helminths from individuals in Egypt and Mexico.[50] Healthy adults treated with nitazoxanide cleared cryptosporidia from their stool more rapidly than did placebo controls, but nitazoxanide lacks efficacy in AIDS patients.[52]

Nitroimidazole Derivatives

METRONIDAZOLE

Metronidazole (see Chapter 147) has activity against many anaerobic parasites. It is the drug of choice for the treatment of:

- invasive enterocolitis and liver abscess caused by *E. histolytica* and the rarely reported *Entamoeba polecki*;[1,2,34]
- vaginitis caused by *T. vaginalis*;[51] and
- enteritis caused by *G. lamblia*.[38]

It has been used to treat *Blastocystis hominis* in the stool (although its efficacy remains unproven) and is considered an alternative agent for *Balantidium coli* infection. Metronidazole is also used in the treatment of infections with the guinea worm, *Dracunculus medinensis*; it decreases inflammation and facilitates worm removal, but has no direct toxic effect on the worm itself.

Metronidazole acts as an electron sink under anaerobic or microaerophilic conditions, depriving the parasite of necessary reducing equivalents, such as nicotinamide adenine dinucleotide phosphate (NADPH). Reduced metronidazole (i.e. drug molecules that have gained electrons) causes a loss of the helical structure of DNA and strand breakage.

The most common side effects are headache, metallic taste, dry mouth and nausea. Less frequent are urticaria, pruritus, urethral burning, reversible neutropenia, and vaginal and oral candidiasis. Rarely, patients may experience central nervous system toxicity, including dizziness, vertigo, ataxia, encephalopathy and seizures, as well as peripheral neuropathy. Acute pancreatitis has been reported. Patients should be advised to avoid consuming alcohol because of the disulfiram-like effects of metronidazole, including headache, flushing, abdominal pain, and vomiting. Some patients may experience a red–brown discoloration of the urine owing to the presence of metabolites of metronidazole.

TINIDAZOLE AND ORNIDAZOLE

Tinidazole and ornidazole are two other nitroimidazole derivatives (see Chapter 147). Their antimicrobial spectrum is similar to that of metronidazole,[1,2,34] and tinidazole has been used successfully for single-dose therapy of amebic liver abscess.[52] Tinidazole has also been used to treat metronidazole-resistant *Trichomonas* spp. and may show greater efficacy in the treatment of bacterial and trichomonal vaginitis.[51] These compounds are well absorbed orally and are widely distributed. Generally, these drugs are better tolerated than metronidazole; the main side effects are headache, dizziness and anorexia.

Paromomycin

Paromomycin (also known as aminosidine) is a nonabsorbable aminoglycoside antibiotic (see Chapter 143) that is concentrated in the lumen of the colon. It is active against *E. histolytica*, *D. fragilis* and *G. lamblia* as well as the cestodes *Taenia saginata*, *Taenia solium*, *Diphyllobothrium latum*, *Dipylidium caninum* and *Hymenolepis nana*.[1,34,38,40] Paromomycin with methylbenzethonium chloride or gentamicin has been used topically in the treatment of cutaneous leishmaniasis and systemically for visceral leishmaniasis.[53,54] Paromomycin is available as the sulfate salt for oral administration.

The dose is 25–35 mg/kg/day in three divided doses for 7 days. Side effects include cramps, nausea, vomiting, diarrhea, rash, headache and vertigo. Burning may occur with topical preparations.

Pentamidine Isethionate

Pentamidine isethionate, an aromatic diamidine derivative, is effective in the treatment of the early or hemolymphatic stages of sleeping sickness caused by *T. brucei gambiense*, some forms of leishmaniasis and *P. jirovecii* pneumonia.[1,2,32] It is less effective against *T. brucei rhodesiense*. It has also been used in the treatment of disseminated *Acanthamoeba* spp. infections and babesiosis.[55,56] The mechanism of action of pentamidine is unclear, but it may involve the binding of DNA and the interruption of DNA replication. The drug is available for parenteral and inhalational use; the latter mode is used only in the prophylaxis *P. jirovecii* pneumonia because little of the inhaled drug is absorbed systemically. Parenterally administered pentamidine isethionate penetrates extensively and is excreted slowly from tissues such as liver, spleen, kidneys and adrenal glands. Very little crosses the blood–brain barrier, accounting for the lack of utility of pentamidine in late-stage trypanosomiasis.

ROUTE OF ADMINISTRATION AND DOSAGE

There are different recommendations for dosing pentamidine isethionate. For early *T. brucei gambiense* infection, the Centers for Disease Control and Prevention (CDC) recommends 4 mg/kg/day for 10 days. The World Health Organization (WHO) recommends 3–4 mg/kg/day or every other day for 7–10 doses. Because of the rapidity with which *T. brucei rhodesiense* invades the central nervous system, this drug is generally not used for this organism. Pentamidine has also been used for prophylaxis against infection with *T. brucei gambiense* at a dose of 4 mg/kg (to a maximum of 300 mg) given every 3–6 months.

For leishmaniasis, the CDC recommends 2–4 mg/kg/day or every other day for 12–15 doses; a second course is sometimes given after an interval of 1–2 weeks. Alternatively, the WHO recommends 4 mg/kg three times a week for 5–25 weeks or longer. The dosage regimen varies slightly depending on the species of *Leishmania* and the region of the body affected. A study of 315 patients in Surinam found good results in the treatment of cutaneous leishmaniasis with a single dose weekly for 3 weeks.[57]

ADVERSE REACTIONS

Pentamidine isethionate may cause toxicity in 50% of patients. Precipitous hypotension with dizziness, dyspnea, tachycardia, headache, vomiting and syncope can occur with rapid intravenous infusion. Intramuscular administration may result in sterile abscesses. Hypoglycemia, which may be life-threatening, pancreatitis, hyperglycemia and diabetes mellitus probably result from a direct toxic effect of pentamidine on pancreatic β cells. Reversible renal failure occurs in up to 25% of patients. Other side effects include fever, arrhythmias (particularly torsades de pointes), hypocalcemia, confusion, hallucinations, leukopenia, thrombocytopenia and elevated transaminases.

Pentavalent Antimonial Compounds

The pentavalent antimonial compounds remain a mainstay of therapy for leishmaniasis and are less toxic than the older trivalent compounds.[1,2,58] Sodium stibogluconate has been the most extensively studied and is the only pentavalent antimonial available in the USA. Meglumine antimoniate is used largely in French-speaking countries and parts of Latin America. These compounds appear to inhibit bioenergetic pathways such as glycolysis and fatty acid oxidation in *Leishmania* amastigotes. Antimonial resistance in visceral leishmaniasis is common leading to the development of new therapies.[6,47]

These compounds are available as aqueous solutions for intravenous or intramuscular use only. Each milliliter of sodium stibogluconate contains the equivalent of 100 mg of pentavalent antimony, whereas each milliliter of meglumine antimoniate contains 85 mg. They are rapidly absorbed and are eliminated in two phases. The first has a half-life of 2 hours, but the second is longer, with a half-life of between 33 hours (after intravenous administration) and 76 hours (after intramuscular administration). This slow terminal elimination may result from a conversion to trivalent antimony, which thus may be responsible for the toxicity seen with long-term therapy. Excretion is primarily renal.

Piperaquine

Piperaquine phosphate is a bisquinolone antimalarial drug that is structurally related to chloroquine and has activity against *P. vivax* and *P. falciparum*. Piperaquine is used in combination with dihydroartemisinin for the treatment of chloroquine-resistant *P. falciparum*. The drug is generally well tolerated, with relatively few adverse events noted to date.[59]

Primaquine

Primaquine, an 8-aminoquinoline active against hypnozoites of *P. vivax* and *P. ovale* in the liver, is the only agent with the potential for yielding complete resolution of malaria caused by these organisms.[1,2,8,9] Primaquine combined with clindamycin is also effective in the treatment of *P. jirovecii* pneumonia. Recently, primaquine in a dose of 30 mg base/day (52.6 mg salt/day) showed efficacy as prophylaxis against *P. falciparum* (88% protection) and *P. vivax* (92% protection) malaria.[60] Primaquine acts by interfering with plasmodial mitochondrial function, possibly through its effects on the electron transport chain and pyrimidine biosynthesis. Primaquine phosphate, which is available only in oral form, is rapidly absorbed (bioavailability 96%), widely distributed and hepatically converted to three metabolites. It is unclear whether the parent compound or the metabolites possess the antimalarial activity.

Primaquine phosphate is formulated in tablets containing 26.3 mg of the salt, equivalent to 15 mg of the base. Dosages are given in Table 157-1. Relapse of *P. vivax* after conventional primaquine treatment has been described in up to 30% of cases in Papua New Guinea, the Solomon Islands, Thailand and other parts of South East Asia.[61]

Therefore, for cases acquired in South East Asia or Oceania, the dose should be increased to 22.5 mg base per day.

The principal toxicity of primaquine is hemolysis in patients who are G6PD-deficient, and thus G6PD levels should be measured before therapy is begun. Alternative dosing regimens of primaquine are required in G6PD-deficient patients. Headache, nausea, vomiting and abdominal cramps have been reported. At higher doses, mild anemia, cyanosis (due to methemoglobinemia) and leukopenia may occur. Rarely, neurotoxicity, arrhythmias, hypertension and agranulocytosis occur.

Quinacrine

Quinacrine is an acridine dye derivative that is effective against *G. lamblia*.[1,38] It has been used as combination therapy with metronidazole for individuals who failed therapy with metronidazole alone.[62] It also has activity against adult cestodes, but for this indication it has been supplanted by less toxic alternatives. In the Second World War, quinacrine was used for malaria prophylaxis and treatment. The mechanism of antiparasitic action is unclear, but the drug has been shown to intercalate with DNA and inhibit nucleic acid synthesis.

The dosage in giardiasis is 100 mg q8h for 5–7 days. A second treatment course may be given 2 weeks later. The drug has a bitter taste and may induce nausea and vomiting. Dizziness and headache are also common. Reversible yellow skin discoloration (with spared sclerae) is seen in 4–5% of those treated with quinacrine for giardiasis. Under Wood's light, a bright yellow–green fluorescence distinguishes this side effect from hyperbilirubinemia. Toxic psychosis may occur in 0.1–1.5% of patients. Other rare side effects include blood dyscrasias, ocular toxicity and urticaria. Patients who have psoriasis may experience exfoliative dermatitis.

Quinidine

Quinidine is the dextrostereoisomer of quinine. It is a blood schizonticide and is the parenteral therapy of choice for chloroquine-resistant *P. falciparum* as a result of its wide availability as an antiarrhythmic.[1,2,8,9]

During treatment, continuous electrocardiographic and blood-pressure monitoring are recommended. Widening of the QRS complex and prolongation of the QT_c interval may be seen, and hypotension may ensue if the drug is infused rapidly. Other side effects are similar to those of quinine.

Quinine

Quinine is an alkaloid derived from the bark of the South American cinchona tree. It has been used as an antimalarial for over 350 years.[1,2,8,9] It is effective against the asexual blood stages of all four *Plasmodium* spp. that cause malaria in humans, and is used for chloroquine-resistant *P. falciparum* infections. Quinine is also used with clindamycin in the treatment of *Babesia microti* infection.[29] The basis for the antimalarial activity of quinine is unclear, but three mechanisms have been proposed:

- intercalation with parasite DNA, interrupting replication and transcription;
- interaction with erythrocyte fatty acids, promoting hemolysis and preventing schizont maturation; and
- alkalinization of parasite digestive vacuoles, interfering with hemoglobin degradation.

PHARMACOKINETICS AND DISTRIBUTION

Quinine is available as the sulfate, bisulfate, hydrochloride, dihydrochloride, hydrobromide and ethylcarbonate salts for oral administration and as the dihydrochloride salt for parenteral use. The therapeutic range in plasma is 8–15 mg/L, which is achieved within 1–3 hours after a single oral dose. In cases of severe illness, the volume of distribution decreases, clearance is reduced and the half-life is prolonged. Thus, on a given dosage schedule, plasma quinine concentrations are elevated with acute illness and decrease as the patient improves. Monitoring blood levels is recommended in those who have renal or hepatic dysfunction; dosage reduction is needed with severe renal failure.

ROUTE OF ADMINISTRATION AND DOSAGE

The oral dose of quinine sulfate (unlike other antimalarial agents, it is dosed by weight of salt) is 650 mg salt q8h for 3–7 days. A longer course is preferred for those in areas where *P. falciparum* is less sensitive to quinine, including South East Asia and western Africa.[63]

Intravenous quinine dihydrochloride may be used for severe infections. A 20 mg salt/kg loading dose in 5% dextrose is given over 4 hours, followed by 10 mg salt/kg over 2–4 hours q8h (maximum 1800 mg salt/day) until oral therapy can be given. The loading dose should be omitted in those who have received oral quinine, quinidine or mefloquine during the previous 24 hours. Intravenous quinidine gluconate has become the parenteral therapy of choice worldwide but its use may be supplanted by artesunate.

ADVERSE REACTIONS

The term cinchonism refers to a cluster of dose-related and reversible side effects of quinine, including tinnitus, decreased hearing, headache, nausea, vomiting, dysphoria and visual disturbances. Hypoglycemia can occur secondary to quinine stimulation of insulin release in conjunction with parasite consumption of glucose. Skin rashes (urticaria, flushing), pruritus, hepatitis, thrombocytopenia, agranulocytosis and massive hemolysis with hemoglobinuria (with resultant bilirubinuria, termed blackwater fever) occur rarely. Quinine can cause respiratory depression in patients who have myasthenia gravis and hemolysis in those who have G6PD deficiency. Myocardial depression, vasodilatation and shock may result from rapid intravenous infusion. Overdose can result in delirium, seizures, coma, respiratory depression, cortical blindness, shock and death. An oral quinine dose of 2–8 g may be fatal for adults.

Suramin

Suramin is a sulfated naphthylamine introduced in 1920 and is used in the treatment of the early or hemolymphatic stage of African trypanosomiasis.[1,2,32] It is more effective against *T. brucei rhodesiense* than against *T. brucei gambiense*, for which pentamidine is often used for early disease. Suramin has also been used for prophylaxis in those who have intense exposure. Additionally, suramin is active against the adult forms of *Onchocerca volvulus*, but is rarely used for this infection because of its toxicity.

The mechanism of action of suramin is unclear; it is a polyanion that inhibits many cellular enzymes. Notably, its antitrypanosomal activity correlates with inhibition of glycerol-3-phosphate oxidase and dehydrogenase, enzymes involved in energy metabolism.

ROUTE OF ADMINISTRATION AND ADVERSE REACTIONS

Suramin is available only for intravenous use. The dosage for trypanosomiasis is given in Table 157-1. Suramin has a variety of side effects, which are generally more severe in malnourished patients. Immediate reactions include malaise, nausea, vomiting, fatigue, fever, urticaria, shock, loss of consciousness and, rarely, death. Late reactions include fever, rash, stomatitis, exfoliative dermatitis, lacrimation, photophobia, headache and hyperesthesia. Renal dysfunction (hematuria, proteinuria, casts and elevated creatinine), hepatic dysfunction (elevated transaminases and bilirubin), diarrhea, thrombocytopenia and agranulocytosis may occur. Additional side effects during treatment for onchocerciasis include pruritus, dermal edema, papular eruptions, palmoplantar paresthesias and iridocyclitis.

Tetracyclines

Tetracycline (see Chapter 146) is used in combination with quinine in the treatment of drug-resistant *P. falciparum* in South East Asia, where resistance to chloroquine, sulfadoxine/pyrimethamine and quinine is common.[1,2,8,9,44] Doxycycline, a longer-acting derivative, is used for malaria prophylaxis in this area, and worldwide in individuals unable to tolerate mefloquine, although atovaquone–proguanil is now preferred for this indication.[8,9] Tetracycline is also the drug of choice for infection with the ciliate, *Balantidium coli*.

Tetracyclines are well absorbed after oral administration and are probably active against parasite protein synthesis. Side effects include gastrointestinal distress, photosensitivity and vaginal candidiasis.

Anthelmintic Agents

Albendazole

Albendazole is a benzimidazole carbamate that has a broad spectrum of anthelmintic activity, including against *Ascaris lumbricoides*, *Enterobius vermicularis*, *Ancylostoma duodenale*, *Necator americanus*, *Strongyloides stercoralis*, *Echinococcus* spp. and *T. solium* cysticerci.[1,2,64–67] The drug has also been used to treat eosinophilic enterocolitis caused by *Ancylostoma caninum*, *Capillaria philippinensis*, cutaneous and visceral larva migrans, *C. sinensis*, *Gnathostoma spinigerum*, *Oesophagostomum bifurcum* and *Trichostrongylus* spp. It is also used in combination with diethylcarbamazine or ivermectin for mass treatment of lymphatic filariasis (*Brugia malayi* and *Wuchereria bancrofti*).[68] Additionally, it has variable efficacy in the treatment of microsporidiosis caused by *Encephalitozoon hellem*, *E. cuniculi*, *E. intestinalis*, *E. bieneusi* and *Vittaforma corneae*.[69] Albendazole has some activity against *G. lamblia*.[38]

The mechanism of action is similar to that of mebendazole with blockade of parasite microtubule assembly. Albendazole is poorly soluble in water and should be taken with a fatty meal to enhance absorption.

Single doses of albendazole are generally well tolerated; abdominal discomfort, diarrhea or migration of *Ascaris* into the mouth and nose occur infrequently. Prolonged, high-dose treatment can be associated with reversible aminotransferase elevations, bone marrow suppression and alopecia.

Bithionol

Bithionol is a chlorinated bisphenol that is used for infections with *Fasciola hepatica*, but has been supplanted by triclabendazole. Bithionol is also an alternative agent against *Paragonimus* spp.[1,2] It has activity against many other flukes, but has been replaced by praziquantel. Its mechanism of action is poorly understood.

Side effects include anorexia, abdominal pain, nausea, vomiting, headache, dizziness, diarrhea, urticaria and proteinuria, some of which may be allergic responses to liberated fluke antigens.

Diethylcarbamazine

Diethylcarbamazine is a piperazine derivative used in the treatment of filariasis. It is microfilaricidal for *W. bancrofti*, *B. malayi* and *B. timori*.[1,2,64,70] It appears to be macrofilaricidal for these species as well (i.e. it kills adult worms) and is considered to be the drug of choice for these three infections. Diethylcarbamazine is a key component of mass chemotherapy approaches for the eradication of lymphatic filariasis.[68] It has been used as a sole agent for single-dose therapy, administered long term as diethylcarbamazine-fortified dietary salt, and as a component of combination single-dose regimens with ivermectin or albendazole. Diethylcarbamazine is also the mainstay of therapy against *Loa loa* and *Mansonella streptocerca*. It has been used to treat tropical pulmonary eosinophilia, supporting the contention that the pulmonary infiltrates in this disorder are due to migrating microfilariae. It has also been used for visceral larva migrans.

Diethylcarbamazine is effective in eliminating microfilariae of *O. volvulus* in the skin and eye, but the resulting inflammation can cause permanent ocular damage, including uveitis, punctate keratitis and retinal pigment epithelium atrophy. Adult *Onchocerca* worms are not killed, however, and the infection may return once treatment has stopped. Ivermectin has largely replaced diethylcarbamazine for ocular onchocerciasis. Diethylcarbamazine also has activity against *A. lumbricoides*.

The mechanism of action of diethylcarbamazine involves two processes:

- first, filarial muscular activity decreases, probably secondary to hyperpolarization of membranes by the piperazine moiety of diethylcarbamazine; and
- second, microfilarial surface membranes are altered by making them more susceptible to host defenses.

Toxicity can result from the destruction of organisms and release of antigens which provoke an inflammatory response. This reaction is most severe in patients who are heavily infected with *O. volvulus*. This is termed the Mazzotti reaction and consists of severe pruritus, edema, rash, arthralgias, lymphadenopathy, fever, hypotension, increased eosinophilia, proteinuria and splenomegaly. These symptoms persist for 3–7 days. Nodular swellings along lymphatics and lymphadenitis may occur with *W. bancrofti* and *B. malayi* infections. Patients heavily infected with *L. loa* may experience encephalopathy and other neurologic complications.[71] Pre-treatment with corticosteroids may lessen the severity of these inflammatory responses.

Flubendazole

Flubendazole is a fluorine analog of mebendazole and the two drugs have similar spectra of activity.[1,2] Flubendazole is poorly absorbed after oral administration. It has been used against many of the common intestinal helminths and, with limited success, in the treatment of neurocysticercosis.

Ivermectin

Ivermectin is a derivative of avermectin B1, a type of macrocyclic lactone that was discovered in the 1970s as a product of the actinomycete *Streptomyces avermitilis*.[1,2,65,72] Ivermectin is used as a broad-spectrum veterinary agent for infections with helminths and arthropods. Since the 1980s, it has become the drug of choice for onchocerciasis because it kills microfilariae in the skin and the eye while provoking much less inflammation than diethylcarbamazine. The response to ivermectin is rapid and can last for 6–12 months. Adult worms appear to be unaffected by ivermectin, but the drug seems to prevent developing larvae from leaving the uterus. The drug also has activity against *W. bancrofti*, *B. malayi*, *B. timori*, *L. loa*, *Mansonella ozzardi* and *Mansonella streptocerca*, and is being used as a component of mass chemotherapy for lymphatic filariasis.[66] Ivermectin is effective against *S. stercoralis* and is active against *E. vermicularis*, *A. lumbricoides* and *Trichuris trichiura*. Ivermectin causes tonic paralysis of the helminth musculature, but the mechanism of action is poorly understood, although it is known to include γ-aminobutyric acid (GABA) blockade.

Mebendazole

Mebendazole is a benzimidazole carbamate with a broad range of anthelmintic activity.[1,2,64,65] It is active against the larvae and adults of *E. vermicularis*, *A. lumbricoides*, *T. trichiura*, *N. americanus* and *A. duodenale*. It is ovicidal for *Ascaris* and *Trichuris* spp. It is less effective than thiabendazole against *S. stercoralis*. Mebendazole has been used at high doses and for long periods in the treatment of *C. philippinensis*. It can also be used for infections caused by *Angiostrongylus cantonensis*, *Angiostrongylus costaricensis*, *Toxocara canis* and *Trichostrongylus* spp. The drug has activity against adult *Trichinella spiralis*, with some activity against larval forms, and it is currently recommended in the treatment of trichinosis.

Mebendazole is also effective in the treatment of certain types of filariasis; it is considered the drug of choice against *Mansonella perstans* (diethylcarbamazine is ineffective) and has been shown to have efficacy against *L. loa*, *O. volvulus* and *Dracunculus medinensis* infections. The drug has activity against *T. saginata*, *T. solium* and *Hymenolepis nana*, although praziquantel is more effective. Although mebendazole does not eradicate echinococcal infection, the drug prevents progression of existing cysts and the development of new cysts when administered in high dose for a prolonged period. Mebendazole has largely been replaced by albendazole for echinococcosis.

Mebendazole acts by binding parasite tubulin, thus blocking microtubule assembly and interfering with glucose absorption. Susceptible helminths become paralyzed and depleted of energy stores, but death and clearance of the worms from the gastrointestinal tract can take days. Mebendazole, formulated as 100 mg tablets, has low water solubility and is poorly absorbed. It is 95% protein-bound in plasma and undergoes rapid and extensive first-pass metabolism in the liver. Thus, systemic bioavailability is low, accounting not only for its poor tissue levels and relative lack of usefulness in extraintestinal infections, but also for its low rate of side effects.

Abdominal pain and diarrhea may occur after mebendazole administration. The drug also has been reported to prompt the migration of adult *Ascaris* spp. into the mouth and nose. At high doses, reversible bone marrow suppression with neutropenia, alopecia, allergic skin reactions, hepatitis, vertigo and oligospermia occur rarely.

Metrifonate

Metrifonate is an organophosphate inhibitor of acetylcholinesterase that was originally developed as an insecticide. It has activity against *Schistosoma haematobium*[1,2,73] but has largely been replaced by praziquantel as primary therapy.

The dosage is 7.5–10 mg/kg orally once every 2 weeks for three cycles. Side effects include nausea, vomiting, vertigo and lethargy. Patients receiving metrifonate should neither be exposed to other insecticides nor receive neuromuscular blocking agents in the 2 days before or after taking metrifonate.

Niclosamide

Niclosamide is a salicylamide derivative that is active against the cestodes *Diphyllobothrium latum*, *D. caninum*, *H. nana*, *T. saginata* and *T. solium*, as well as the trematodes *Echinostoma* spp., *Fasciolopsis buski* and *Heterophyes heterophyes*.[1] It acts by interfering with oxidative phosphorylation and production of adenosine triphosphate. Treatment failures of *Taenia* spp. with niclosamide have been reported, and praziquantel has been used successfully in these cases.[74]

Oxamniquine

Oxamniquine is a tetrahydroquinoline that is effective in *S. mansoni* infections.[1,2,73] Its mechanism of action is unclear, but it causes adult worms to become paralyzed and dislodged from the veins they inhabit, resulting in subsequent killing by host defenses. The drug should be given cautiously to patients who have a history of seizures.

Piperazine

Piperazine has activity against *A. lumbricoides* and *E. vermicularis*.[1,2] In many parts of the world it has been replaced by less toxic agents such as mebendazole. However, because of its lower cost, piperazine is still frequently used. Piperazine blocks the helminth muscle response to acetylcholine by altering membrane ion permeability and causing hyperpolarization and decreased action potentials. Flaccid paralysis ensues and the worms are eliminated in the stool.

Praziquantel

Praziquantel, a pyrazinoisoquinoline derivative developed in the early 1970s, has broad activity against trematodes and cestodes but not nematodes.[1,2,64,73] All *Schistosoma* spp. that infect humans are susceptible. The drug also has activity against the trematodes *C. sinensis*, *Dicrocoelium dendriticum*, *Echinostoma* spp., *F. buski*, *H. heterophyes*, *Metagonimus yokogawai*, *Metorchis conjunctus*, *Nanophyetus salmincola*, *Opisthorchis viverrini* and *Paragonimus westermani* and other *Paragonimus* spp. *Fasciola hepatica* does not appear to be adequately treated with praziquantel. Praziquantel is effective in treating adult cestodes, including *D. latum* and other *Diphyllobothrium* spp., *D. caninum*, *H. nana*, *Hymenolepis diminuta*, *T. saginata* and *T. solium*. It has been used successfully to treat neurocysticercosis (larval *T. solium*) but it is not useful in echinococcosis. The drug has several actions, including promoting calcium influx and parasite muscle contraction and causing vacuolization and bleb formation in the helminth tegument, thereby activating host defenses.

Pyrantel Pamoate

Pyrantel pamoate, a tetrahydropyrimidine that was originally developed as a veterinary anthelmintic, has a broad range of activity in humans.[1,2,64,65] It is considered by many to be the treatment of choice for *E. vermicularis*. It is also effective for *A. lumbricoides*, eosinophilic enterocolitis caused by *Ancylostoma caninum*, hookworm, the acanthocephalan *Moniliformis moniliformis* and *Trichostrongylus* spp. It does not have activity against *T. trichiura*. Oxantel pamoate, an *m*-oxyphenol derivative, can be given in a single dose for *Trichuris* spp. Pyrantel pamoate and its analogs act by causing depolarizing neuromuscular blockade and by blocking acetylcholinesterase, which result in spastic paralysis and muscle contracture, respectively, and allow expulsion of the worms.

Pyrantel pamoate, which causes depolarization and increased spike frequency in worm muscle cells, should not be given with piperazine, which causes hyperpolarization and a reduction in spike frequency.

Thiabendazole

Thiabendazole is a substituted benzimidazole compound that has better activity against *S. stercoralis* and *Strongyloides fuelleborni* than mebendazole.[1,2,64,65,73] It is active against *A. costaricensis*, *C. philippinensis*, *D. medinensis*, *Trichostrongylus* spp. and *T. spiralis*. In trichinosis, however, larval stages are often resistant to thiabendazole. The drug is also used in the treatment of both cutaneous and visceral larva migrans. Thiabendazole has some activity against *A. lumbricoides*, hookworm, *E. vermicularis* and *T. trichiura*, but mebendazole is less toxic and is thus preferred. The drug acts by inhibiting parasite fumarate reductase, and it may bind tubulin as well.

Triclabendazole

Triclabendazole, a benzimidazole derivative used as a veterinary fasciolicide, has been used safely and successfully in cases of human chronic hepatic fascioliasis.[75] Resistance to triclabendazole has been described in the Netherlands.[76] It is now considered the drug of choice for human hepatic fascioliasis, but in the USA it is available only through compounding pharmacies.

ACKNOWLEDGMENTS

The authors thank Dr Samuel L. Stanley Jr., author of the chapter, Antiparasitic agents, in previous editions of Cohen *et al.*, *Infectious Diseases*, for his significant contributions.

References available online at expertconsult.com.

KEY REFERENCES

Bern C., Montgomery S.P., Herwaldt B.L., et al.: Evaluation and treatment of Chagas disease in the United States. A systematic review. *JAMA* 2007; 298:2171-2181.

Campbell W.C., Rew R.S.: eds. *Chemotherapy of parasitic diseases*. New York: Plenum Press; 1986.

De Silva N., Guyatt H., Bundy D.: Anthelmintics: a comparative review of their clinical pharmacology. *Drugs* 1997; 53:769-788.

Frayha G.J., Smyth J.D., Gobert J.G., et al.: The mechanisms of action of antiprotozoal and antihelminthic drugs in man. *Gen Pharmacol* 1997; 28:273-299.

Fung H.B., Kirschenbaum H.L.: Treatment regimens for patients with toxoplasmic encephalitis. *Clin Ther* 1996; 18:1037-1056.

Griffith K.S., Lewis L.S., Mali S., et al.: Treatment of malaria in the United States. *JAMA* 2007; 297:2264-2277.

Keiser J., Utzinger J.: Efficacy of current drugs against soil transmitted helminthic infections: systematic review and meta-analysis. *JAMA* 2008; 299:1937-1948.

Stanley S.L. Jr: Amoebiasis. *Lancet* 2003; 361:1025-1034.

Winstanley P., Ward S.: Malaria chemotherapy. *Adv Parasitol* 2006; 61:47-76.

SECTION 7 Anti-infective Therapy

158

Probiotics

JASMIN ISLAM

KEY CONCEPTS

- The microbiota is the collective name for the micro-organisms that reside in the human body and helps prevent infection by a process known as colonization resistance.

- Antibiotics can disrupt the host microbiota and leave individuals susceptible to pathogen adherence and colonization.

- Probiotics are live micro-organisms that ameliorate the harmful effects of antibiotics by re-establishing an equilibrium.

- All probiotic effects are strain and site specific.

- Probiotics have a good safety profile and have been successfully used in necrotizing enterocolitis and bacterial vaginosis.

- Recommending routine clinical use of probiotics for infection is limited by a lack of large randomized controlled trials.

Introduction

The microbiome is a community of micro-organisms that inhabit the body with a highly diverse and complex structure that has co-evolved with humans and serves a mutually beneficial role, out-competing pathogens for nutrients and receptor binding sites by a process known as colonization resistance.[1] Antibiotics can disrupt the microbiome, leading to complications.[1] In an era of increasing antimicrobial use there is a growing need for alternative therapies to prevent infection and limit antimicrobial side effects such as antibiotic-associated diarrhea (AAD).

Probiotics are live micro-organisms that ameliorate the harmful effects of antibiotics by helping re-establish the resting equilibrium. Probiotics are named based on the genus, species and a specific strain identifying name (e.g. *Lactobacillus rhamnosus GG*) and exist in a variety of different formulations that include yogurt drinks, capsules and dietary supplements (Table 158-1).

Guidelines exist outlining criteria that must be met before an organism can be classified as a probiotic (Figure 158-1). Probiotics can be categorized into three separate groups based on their efficacy in health and disease.[2] The first group contains organisms with no health claims. The second group contains strains used as food supplements that state specific health claims and should be supported by efficacy data from clinical trials and meta-analyses. The final group are probiotic strains classed as drugs and must meet stringent safety and regulatory standards outlined by national bodies, which include the Food and Drug Administration and Medicines and Healthcare Regulatory Agency.

Gastrointestinal Disease

Probiotics exert their effects in the gastrointestinal tract through different mechanisms (Figure 158-2). It is important to note that any observed effects are site and strain specific. This may be explained by structural differences in the micro-organism-associated molecular patterns found on bacterial cell surfaces, which are recognized by epithelial cell receptors.[4]

Pathogen inhibition occurs by direct competitive exclusion of surface receptors and indirectly through secretion of enzymes and bactericidal products. For example, the yeast, *Saccharomyces boulardii*

produces a serine protease, which can hydrolyse and inhibit the binding of *Clostridium difficile* toxin A to its glycoprotein receptor.[5] Bacteriocins are antimicrobial peptides synthesized by bacteria that enable the producers to compete within their own ecological niche. *Lactobacillus salivarius* was able to prevent *Listeria monocytogenes* infection in mice using the bacteriocin Abp118.[6]

A more subtle mechanism involves preservation of an existing host defense, such as the intestinal barrier, through direct strengthening of epithelial tight junctions or up-regulation of mucus production through signaling pathways. The probiotic *E. coli* Nissle 1917 conferred protection against colitis in a murine model of disease through induction and up-regulation of specific scaffolding proteins (zonula occludens 1 and 2), which led to a reduction in mucosal permeability and strengthening of epithelial tight junctions.[7] Mucins are proteins, encoded by MUC genes, which play an important role in host defense by thickening the intestinal mucus layer resulting in the reduced translocation of bacteria across the intestinal lumen. An increase in MUC2 gene expression was observed in Wisteria rats treated with a multi-species probiotic, accompanied by an accumulation of mucin in the colonic lumen.[8]

Immune system modulation occurs through secreted factors and metabolites that affect the growth and function of intestinal epithelial and immune cells. Following incubation of intestinal epithelial cells with the pathogen *Salmonella typhimurium*, the probiotics *L. salivarius* UC118 and *Bifidobacterium infantis* 35624 caused attenuated secretion of the pro-inflammatory cytokine IL-8 and increased the production of the anti-inflammatory cytokine IL-10, which resulted in an overall reduction in inflammation.[9]

The best evidence for clinical efficacy of probiotics exists for the prevention of necrotizing enterocolitis (NEC) in preterm infants. Preterm infants often receive courses of broad-spectrum antibiotics, undergo protracted lengths of stay in hospital and exhibit different patterns of intestinal colonization that all contribute to the pathogenesis of NEC. A Cochrane review recommended probiotics for the prevention of NEC, although not all strains were of equivalent efficacy.[10] *Helicobacter pylori* infection is a common cause of duodenal and gastric ulcers and causes gastric adenocarcinoma. The addition of different probiotic strains of *Lactobacillus* spp., *Bifidobacteria* spp. and *S. boulardii* to standard *H. pylori* triple therapy (two antibiotics and a proton pump inhibitor) has demonstrated a reduction in bloating, nausea and taste disturbance associated with treatment. Therefore, by improving tolerability, probiotics may increase compliance and eradication rates.[11]

Several studies have investigated the role of probiotics for the prevention and treatment of antibiotic-associated diarrhea (AAD). A meta-analysis of 63 randomized controlled trials (RCT) and 11 811 patients concluded that there was a statistically significant pooled relative risk (RR) in favor of probiotic reduction of AAD (RR 0.58, 95% confidence interval (CI) 0.50–0.68, p < 0.001, number needed to treat).[12,13] However, variations in probiotic strain, patient age and antibiotic class introduce heterogeneity, which make it difficult to generalize such findings. The largest RCT to date (n = 2981), evaluated a multi-strain preparation containing two *Lactobacillus* spp. and two *Bifidobacterium* spp. for AAD prevention in hospitalized patients aged over 65 years.[14] No significant difference in AAD occurred between the probiotic group (10.8%) and placebo (10.4%) groups (RR 1.04; 95% CI 0.84–1.28, p = 0.71) and provides the most compelling evidence to date that probiotics may not be beneficial for preventing AAD.

1373

TABLE 158-1 Probiotics Used to Treat Infection

Infection	Probiotic Strain	Formulation
Respiratory	*Lactobacillus casei* DN114001 *Lactobacillus acidophilus* + *Bifidobacterium bifidum* *Lactobacillus rhamnosus* GG	Fermented yogurt drink Capsules Yogurt, capsules
Bacterial vaginosis	*L. rhamnosus* Lcr35	Vaginal capsules
Wound infection	Kefir	Fermented milk
GASTROINTESTINAL		
Necrotizing enterocolitis	*L. rhamnosus* GG (LGG) *L. casei* and *Bifidobacterium breve* *Saccharomyces boulardii* Mixture of *Lactobacillus bifidus*, *S. thermophillus* and *Bifidobactrium infantis* *L. acidophilus* and *B. infantis* *Clostridium butyricum* 588	Added to infant milk, breast milk or enteral feeds
Helicobacter pylori	*L. casei* subsp. *shirota* *Lactobacillus johnsonii* La1 *S. boulardii* CNCM 1-745 (lyo) *Lactobacillus helveticus* R0052 (CNCM I-1722) + *L. rhamnosus* R0011 (CNCM I-1720) *L. casei* DN114001	Tablets, drink Fermented milk Milk Capsules Capsules, sachets
Antibiotic-associated diarrhea	*C. butyricum* 588 *L. rhamnosus* GG (ATCC 53013) *L. acidophilus* CL 1285 + *L. casei* Lb80r + *L. rhamnosus* CLR2 *S. boulardii* CNCM 1-745 (lyo) *L. helveticus* R0052 (CNCM I-1722) + *L. rhamnosus* R0011 (CNCM I-1720) *L. acidophilus* subsp. *gasseri* + *B. infantis*	Fermented yogurt drink Tablets, drink Yogurt, capsules Fermented drink, capsules Capsules Capsules, sachets
Clostridium difficile	*S. boulardii* CNCM 1-745 (lyo) *L. acidophilus* CL 1285 + *L. casei* Lb80r + *L. rhamnosus* CLR2	Fermented drink, capsules Capsules

Adapted from McFarland L.V. Meta-analysis of probiotics for the prevention of antibiotic associated diarrhea and the treatment of Clostridium difficile disease. Am J Gastroenterol 2006; 101(4):812.

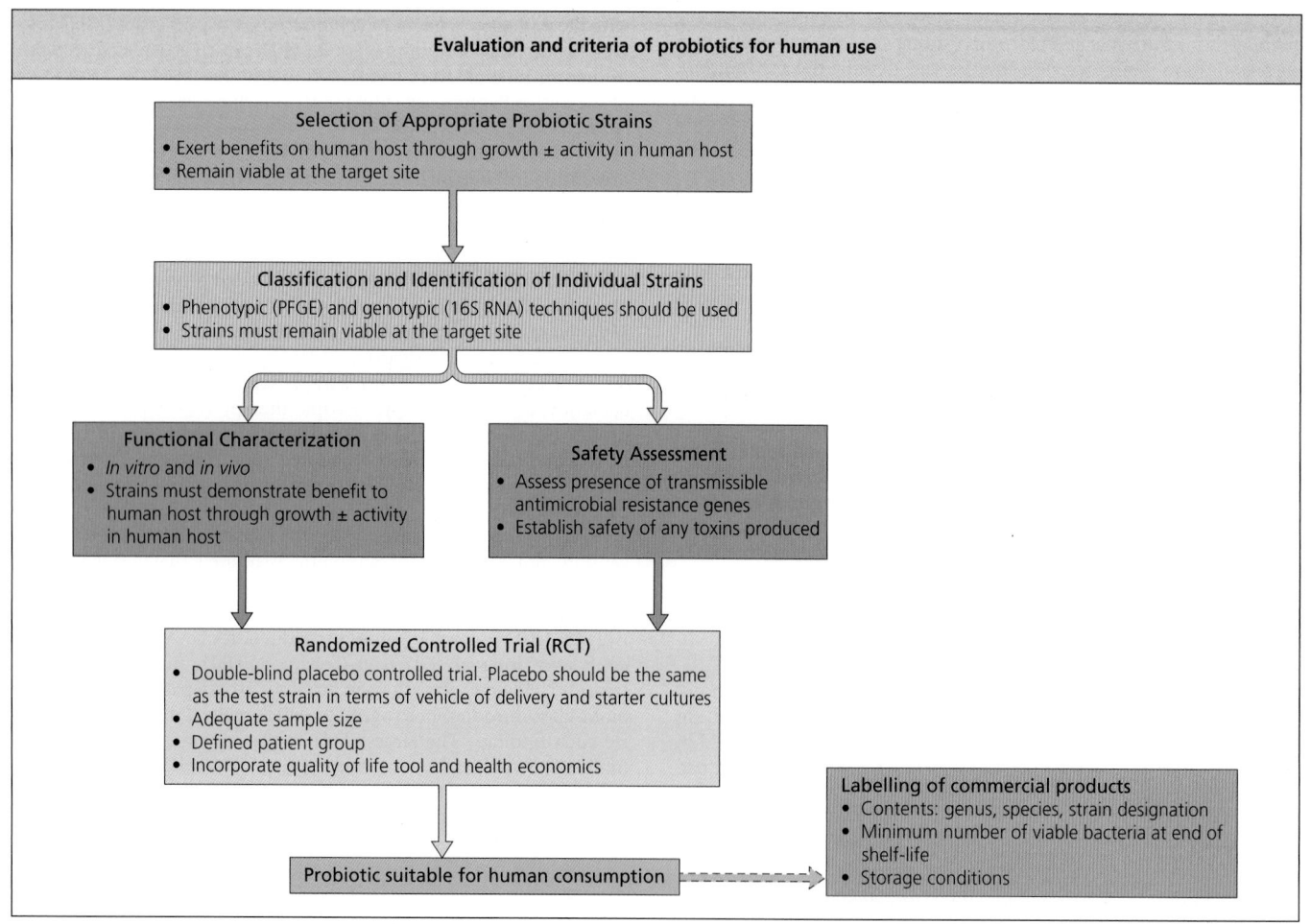

Figure 158-1 Evaluation and criteria of probiotics for human use. *(Adapted from joint guidelines released by the Food and Agricultural Organization and World Health Organization.[3])*

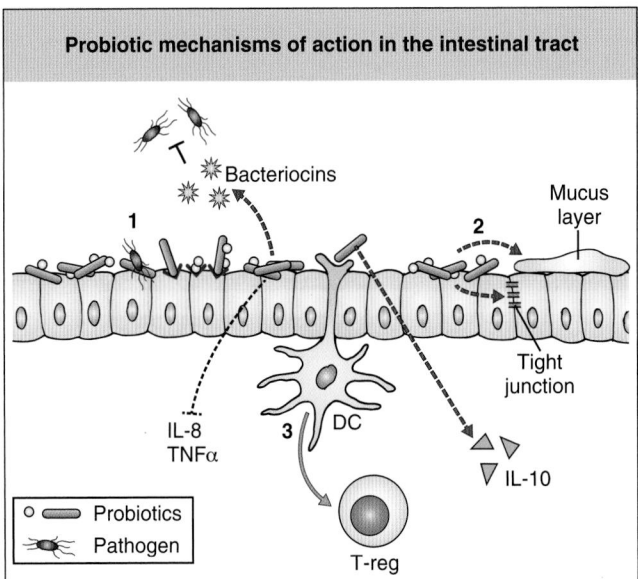

Probiotic mechanisms of action in the intestinal tract

Figure 158-2   Probiotic mechanisms of action in the intestinal tract. The three main mechanisms of action are 1) competitive inhibition of pathogens; 2) reinforcement of the epithelial barrier and tight junctions; 3) immunomodulation. DC, dendritic cell; T-reg, T regulatory cell. (*Adapted from O'Toole P.W., Cooney J.C. Probiotic bacteria influence the composition and function of the intestinal microbiota. Interdiscip Perspect Infect Dis 2008;2008:175285. doi: 10.1155/2008/175285.*)

Nevertheless, as effects are strain specific, alternative combinations of bacterial strains may still prove effective and further RCTs are needed to definitively address this question.

Fewer studies have addressed the effect of probiotics on *C. difficile* infection (CDI), which is usually measured as a secondary outcome in AAD studies. Currently there is insufficient evidence to support the use of probiotics for the treatment of CDI.[14] However, *S. boulardii* used in combination with standard treatment did reduce recurrence of CDI (RR 0.43, 95% CI 0.2–0.97) in a small clinical study.[15]

Respiratory Infections

Ventilator associated pneumonia (VAP) occurs due to abnormal colonization and translocation of pathogens during intubation and mechanical ventilation in intensive care, complicated by on-going micro-aspiration of oropharyngeal secretions around the endotracheal cuff. The prophylactic use of *L. rhamnosus GG* has resulted in a reduction in VAP; however, the effects have not been replicated in other studies and routine probiotic use is not recommended.[16,17] In the context of upper respiratory tract infections, *L. helveticus* MIMLh5 and *Streptococcus salivarius* ST3 have demonstrated pharyngeal mucosa adherence and can directly antagonize *Streptococcus pyogenes*, which causes Group A streptococcal throat infection.[18] Contradictory evidence exists for probiotic use in upper respiratory tract infection (URTI) in children and further studies are needed.[19]

Urogenital Tract Infections

Bacterial vaginosis (BV) is a condition characterized by vaginal discomfort that occurs in one-third of females. The condition is characterized by a rapid shift in the vaginal microbiota from one dominated by lactobacilli to a predominance of anaerobic bacteria. Affected individuals are at increased risk of acquiring sexually transmitted diseases and in pregnancy, BV has been linked to preterm labor.[20] Spontaneous resolution occurs in one-third of cases, but for symptomatic individuals metronidazole is the treatment of choice. Probiotics can help accelerate the natural recovery of the host vaginal microbiota. In a study of 40 female patients, those treated with intra-vaginal capsules of *L. rhamnosus* GR-1 and *L. reuteri* RC-14 experienced a significantly higher cure rate at 6 days, than patients treated with intra-vaginal metronidazole gel (p = 0.016).[21]

Soft Tissue Infections

Compared to intact skin, chronic wounds demonstrate reduced bacterial diversity that leaves the skin susceptible to opportunistic pathogens. Kefir, a fermented milk product containing probiotic bacteria and yeasts, demonstrated improved epithelialization and collagen formation when applied as a gel to *Pseudomonas aeruginosa*-infected burns in rats.[22] This suggests a potential role for stabilizing the microbiota that may be adopted in clinical practice to treat chronic conditions such as diabetic ulcers.

Safety

Probiotics have demonstrated a good safety profile with no cases of systemic bacteremia or fungemia reported in otherwise healthy adults, including trials involving older people.[23] However, in patients with chronic co-morbidity, such as diabetes or cardiac valve disease, at least two cases of infective endocarditis and one case of liver abscess have been observed.[24–26]

At least 24 cases of fungemia have been reported in the literature, following consumption of *S. boulardii*. However, all occurred in patients with underlying chronic disease and included critically ill patients with central venous catheters *in situ*.[27]

Concern remains regarding probiotic use in the immunocompromised. A review of 756 oncology patients revealed five cases of systemic infection following probiotic consumption (three following *S. boulardii*, two following *L. acidophilus* and one following *Bacillus subtilis*). However, four cases were effectively treated with antibiotics with no recurrence of infection.[28] The fifth case involved a patient with chronic lymphocytic leukemia (CLL), who had persistent positive blood cultures for *B. subtilis* despite recurrent courses of antibiotics and who subsequently died during the same admission.[29] Of note, the cause of death was attributed to progressive CLL with central nervous system involvement and the *B. subtilis* bacteremia was not listed as a contributing factor. Furthermore, probiotics have been used in HIV patients with no reported adverse events.[30] Therefore, although probiotics appear safe in certain groups of immunocompromised patients, they should be used with caution until more robust clinical trial data are available.

Concern regarding the potential deleterious metabolic effects of probiotics was raised following the PROPATRIA trial, which involved patients with severe acute pancreatitis in a critical care setting.[31] The study reported higher rates of intestinal ischemia and mortality in patients treated with a multispecies probiotic preparation (Ecologic 641) compared to those receiving placebo. However, the results might be explained by the compromise of a metabolically unstable environment, in the setting of severe pancreatitis, caused by the introduction of billions of live probiotic organisms. Reassuringly, subsequent probiotic studies in critically ill patients have not been associated with increased mortality.[32]

Additional theoretical risks posed by probiotics include potential excessive immune stimulation in susceptible individuals and plasmid-mediated transfer of antibiotic resistance genes to the host microbiota.[3] However, neither have been observed in clinical practice.

Conclusion

Current evidence suggests probiotics work best as prophylactic agents or adjuncts, rather than as sole treatments for infection. Despite promising *in vitro* work, the role of probiotics in infection remains controversial and existing evidence is weakened by a lack of RCTs. Although further research is needed to translate the *in vitro* effects to the human host, the field of probiotics offers considerable optimism due to recent advances in molecular sequencing, which have allowed identification of previously undetected micro-organisms using metagenomics. Universal efforts are underway to define the functions of micro-organisms that predominate in the skin, vaginal tract and intestinal tract and may reveal the probiotics of the future.

References available online at expertconsult.com.

KEY REFERENCES

AlFaleh K., Anabrees J.: Probiotics for prevention of necrotizing enterocolitis in preterm infants. *Cochrane Database Syst Rev* 2014; (4):CD005496.

Agency for Healthcare Research and Quality. Safety of probiotics used to reduce risk and prevent or treat disease. Available: http://www.ahrq.gov/downloads/pub/evidence/pdf/probiotics/probiotics.pdf.

Allen S.J., Wareham K., Wang D., et al.: Lactobacilli and bifidobacteria in the prevention of antibiotic-associated diarrhoea and *Clostridium difficile* diarrhoea in older inpatients (PLACIDE): a randomised, double-blind, placebo-controlled, multicentre trial. *Lancet* 2013; 382(9900):1249-1257.

Besselink M.G., van Santvoort H.C., Buskens E., et al.: Probiotic prophylaxis in predicted severe acute pancreatitis: a randomised, double-blind, placebo-controlled trial. *Lancet* 2008; 371(9613):651-659.

Esposito S., Rigante D., Principi N.: Do children's upper respiratory tract infections benefit from probiotics? *BMC Infect Dis* 2014; 14(1):194.

Hempel S., Newberry S.J., Maher A.R., et al.: Probiotics for the prevention and treatment of antibiotic-associated diarrhea: a systematic review and meta-analysis. *JAMA J Am Med Assoc* 2012; 307(18):1959-1969.

Medeiros J.A., Pereira M.-I.: The use of probiotics in *Helicobacter pylori* eradication therapy. *J Clin Gastroenterol* 2013; 47(1):1-5.

Pillai A., Nelson R.L.: Probiotics for treatment of *Clostridium difficile*-associated colitis in adults. In: The Cochrane Collaboration, Pillai A., eds. *Cochrane Database of Systematic Reviews*; 2008. Available: http://www2.cochrane.org/reviews/en/ab004611.html.

Report of a joint FAO/WHO working group on drafting guidelines for the evaluation of probiotics in food. Available: http://www.who.int/foodsafety/fs_management/en/probiotic_guidelines.pdf.

Van der Waaij D., Vries J.M.B., der Wees J.E.C.L.: Colonization resistance of the digestive tract in conventional and antibiotic-treated mice. *J Hyg (Lond)* 1971; 69(3):405-411.

Wang J., Liu K., Ariani F., et al.: Probiotics for preventing ventilator-associated pneumonia: a systematic review and meta-analysis of high-quality randomized controlled trials. *PLoS ONE* 2013; 8(12):e83934.

159

Infections Associated with Biologics

RUSSELL J. McCULLOH

Introduction

Biological immunomodulating agents are widely used in several medical disciplines, including organ transplantation, autoimmune diseases, and various inflammatory diseases affecting many organ systems. These agents have revolutionized the treatment of many illnesses that would otherwise result in severe disability, pain, or (in the case of organ transplantation) death from loss of vital organ functional capacity. Definitions of immunomodulatory biological agents differ by discipline, but these agents generally comprise five categories: 1) glucocorticoids; 2) systemic compounds with immunomodulatory activity ; 3) cytotoxic agents and antimetabolites; 4) monoclonal antibodies and receptor antagonists that block the action of pro-inflammatory

cytokines; and 5) immunoglobulins used as modulators of the immune response. These biologic agents primarily exert their therapeutic effect by decreasing systemic, organ-specific and/or local inflammation through down-regulation of deleterious immune responses. These agents can thus help reduce end-organ damage, chronic degeneration of osteoarticular tissue, and preserve the functional capacity of transplanted organs.

The use of biological agents carries the price of increased risk of infection due to altered host immune responses (Table 159-1).[1] These infections arise from three general sources: 1) opportunistic infections affecting immune-compromised hosts; 2) reactivation of latent infections acquired prior to immune suppression/modulation; and 3) development of severe disease from common infectious pathogens that would otherwise cause mild infection in immune-competent hosts. Consequently specialists treating patients with conditions that necessitate the use of biologic immunomodulating agents and infectious disease experts must be aware of the potential infectious complication risks associated with the use of specific agents.[2] Clinicians can then utilize appropriate risk-mitigation, diagnostic and treatment strategies based upon the knowledge of infectious complication risk that is specific to the use of any given biologic.

This chapter will provide clinicians with a brief overview of some of the most commonly-used biologic agents, their mechanism of action, and the infectious complications associated with each agent's use. Immunobiologics (i.e. the monoclonal antibodies and receptor agonists) are discussed in more detail in Chapter 88 and will be referenced only briefly here. Recommendations for screening for the presence of latent infections prior to initiation of biologic agents, vaccination of the patient receiving biologic agents, and surveillance and treatment strategies for selected infectious agents, are discussed in more detail in Chapters 80 to 88.

Glucocorticoids

Glucocorticoids remain the mainstay for anti-inflammatory therapy, and have demonstrated efficacy over the past 75 years of clinical use. Glucocorticoids diffuse across cell membranes and bind to their specific receptors.[3] These glucocorticoid receptors dissociate from Heat Shock Protein 90 upon glucocorticoid entry into the cell. The receptor-glucocorticoid complex then dimerizes and translocates to the nucleus, resulting in significant changes in transcriptional activity. These changes include up-regulation of IκB-α, which inhibits nuclear

TABLE 159-1	Biologic Agent Categories and Associated Infection Risk	
Agent Category	**Example Medications**	**Infection Risk**
Glucocorticoids	Prednisone, hydrocortisone	Fungal infection, MTB, PCP, *Strongyloides stercoralis*
Systemic immunomodulators	Cyclosporine, tacrolimus, sirolimus, mycophenolate mofetil, thalidomide	EBV, CMV, HSV, VZV, BK virus disseminated infection/reactivation, bacterial infections
Cytotoxic agents/antimetabolites	Azathioprine, cyclophosphamide, leflunomide, methotrexate, cisplatin	Invasive bacterial, fungal infections
Monoclonal antibodies/receptor antagonists	Anakinra, alemtuzumab, infliximab, rituximab, others	Varies by agent, but can include MTB, EBV, CMV, HSV, VZV, PCP, invasive fungal disease
Immunoglobulins	Immune globulin (pooled IgG)	No significant risk; must delay live virus vaccine administration

MTB, *Mycobacterium tuberculosis*; EBV, Epstein-Barr virus; CMV, cytomegalovirus; HSV, herpes simplex virus; VZV, varicella-zoster virus; PCP, *Pneumocystis jirovecii* pneumonia.

factor-κB (NFκB) translocation across the nuclear membrane, thus reducing pro-inflammatory gene activation.[4] Glucocorticoids also block transcription of inflammatory gene programs at the level of the essential co-activator complex of the transcriptional machinery of the cell. Steroids also block the actions of other transcriptional activators including several mitogen-activated protein kinases and activator protein 1. Glucocorticoids impair mRNA stability by limiting mRNA translation into protein products, including pro-inflammatory cytokines, chemokines and enzymes necessary for prostaglandin generation and other inflammatory mediators.

Glucocorticoid-related side effect risk is both dose- and time-dependent.[5,6] Risks include metabolic and infectious complications, although significant side effects are relatively rare within the first 14–21 days of therapy. Similarly, administering low doses of glucocorticoids (<10 mg daily prednisone or equivalent agents) can be tolerated with minimal infection risk for years of continuous therapy. However, glucocorticoid use affects both the innate and adaptive immune systems which accounts for the increased risk of infection from steroids. Neutrophilia with initial use is common and results from decreased egress from the circulation and increased release from bone marrow stores. Conversely, glucocorticoid use results in T lymphocyte, NK cell and eosinophil redistribution to extravascular sites. Steroid use also reduces the surface expression of Fc receptors, complement receptors (CR3 receptor) and expression of class II major histocompatibility complex (MHC) molecules and co-stimulatory signals by macrophages, eosinophils and monocytes. Corticosteroids reduce monocyte chemotaxis, intracellular killing, and cytokine and chemokine signaling, resulting in poor microbial clearance and excess infection risk.

Within 2 weeks of glucocorticoid exposure, lymphocyte populations, particularly T cells (both CD4 and CD8 lymphocytes), develop reduced proliferative capacity and cytokine generation.[7] Steroid use reduces IL-2 generation, resulting in impaired T cell proliferative capacity to respond to intracellular pathogens. Conversely, anamnestic antibody responses remain well preserved due to the relatively mild effect of high-dose corticosteroids on B cell and plasma cell populations. NK cell function is well preserved even after long-term glucocorticoid exposure. It is important for clinicians to remember that therapeutic doses of steroids impair fever generation via up-regulation of lipocortins that block phospholipase A₂, resulting in reduced arachidonic acid availability to produce prostaglandin E2 alpha (PGE2). PGE2 is critical to induce fever within the thermoregulatory center of the hypothalamus. Steroid-induced blockade of fever generation not only removes this cardinal sign of inflammation, but it also likely impairs the capacity to clear pathogens.

Several opportunistic pathogens and routine pathogens remain a constant concern with long-term glucocorticoid use. Isoniazid preventive therapy is indicated in steroid-treated patients with evidence of latent *Mycobacterium tuberculosis* (MTB) infection.[8] Opportunistic fungi and endemic mycoses are an important consideration in specific geographic regions where coccidioidomycosis and histoplasmosis are prevalent in the environment. Hyper-infection syndromes with strongyloidiasis is a real risk in steroid-treated patients and should be screened for in endemic regions of the world before beginning immunosuppressive doses of corticosteroids.[9]

Calcineurin Inhibitors and mTOR Inhibitors

CYCLOSPORINE

Cyclosporine (cyclosporin A; CSA) is used in a variety of circumstances, including organ transplantation, treating graft-versus-host disease (GVHD) after hematopoietic stem cell transplantation (HSCT), and for treating autoimmune disorders including rheumatoid arthritis (RA), psoriasis and uveitis. It is a peptide antibiotic that blocks T cell activation during antigen receptor-mediated induction of differentiation by binding to cyclophilin, an intracellular protein belonging to the immunophilin protein class. Cyclosporine forms a complex with cyclophilin that inhibits calcineurin, a cytoplasmic phosphatase crucial to activating nuclear factor of activated T cells (NF-AT). This transcription factor is necessary for synthesis of several interleukins, including IL-2, IL-3 and IFN-gamma, by activated T cells. However, cyclosporine does not block the effects of these cytokines on primed T cells or interaction with antigen. Cyclosporine is metabolized by the CYP450 3A isoenzymes, which means it has multiple drug–drug interactions and requires monitoring of drug levels. Infection risks associated with cyclosporine are related to suppression of cell-mediated immunity and are mediated by dosing and duration of treatment. Invasive fungal infections, infection from environmentally-acquired bacteria, such as *Nocardia* species, and reactivation of latent viral infections such as those caused by cytomegalovirus (CMV) can occur.[10] Epstein-Barr-virus (EBV) can reactivate in patients treated with cyclosporine, particularly transplant recipients receiving higher-dose therapy, resulting in the long-term risk of post-transplant lymphoproliferative disorder (PTLD) and progression to lymphoma.

TACROLIMUS

Tacrolimus (FK 506) is a macrolide antibiotic produced by *Streptomyces tsukubaensis*. It suppresses T cell transcription of NF-AT by binding to the immunophilin FK-binding protein (FKBP). Its immunosuppressive activity is similar to the calcineurin inhibitor (CNI) cyclosporine. Tacrolimus is used in solid organ transplant, hematopoietic stem cell transplant HSCT, and treatment or prevention of GVHD. It is used topically to treat various dermatologic conditions including atopic dermatitis and psoriasis. Tacrolimus is metabolized via the CYP450 pathway with similar drug interaction concerns as cyclosporine. Trough levels should be monitored in patients. Infectious complications of tacrolimus are similar to cyclosporine, although relative risk appears to be lower among patients taking tacrolimus compared to cyclosporine, likely due in part to lower doses of glucocorticoids used in tacrolimus-containing immunosuppressive regimens.[11]

SIROLIMUS

Sirolimus (rapamycin) is the prototype immunosuppressive macrolide antibiotic that inhibits the kinase activity of mammalian (or mechanistic) target of rapamycin (mTOR). Other 'rapalogs' in this group include everolimus and temsirolimus. Inhibition of the mTOR pathway has pleiotropic effects on various cellular processes including angiogenesis, metabolism and cellular proliferation such as interleukin-mediated T-cell activation and proliferation. Sirolimus and the other rapalogs have potential applications in both targeted oncologic therapies as well as immunosuppression. Sirolimus is used in preventing solid organ allograft rejection, prevention and treatment of GVHD, and in topical preparations for dermatologic disorders. Sirolimus is metabolized by CYP450 3A and P-glycoprotein, with similar concerns for drug–drug interactions as the CNIs. Its half-life is 60 hours, resulting in prolonged toxicity even after drug cessation. Use of the mTOR inhibitors has been associated with myelosuppression, and infection risks can include increased susceptibility to bacterial infection, poor wound healing, and similar opportunistic viral and fungal infection risks as those of the CNIs. Although initially thought to have antifungal properties, sirolimus has not been found to have an associated decreased risk of invasive fungal infections in randomized trials.[12] Sirolimus has been used in combination with reduced-dose CNIs therapy, which may be associated with lower overall risk of opportunistic infection, however.

MYCOPHENOLATE MOFETIL

Mycophenolate mofetil (MMF) inhibits several T- and B-lymphocyte actions, including mitogen and mixed lymphocyte responses, most likely via inhibition of purine synthesis. A semisynthetic derivative of mycophenolic acid, MMF can be given orally or intravenously. Unlike sirolimus and the CNIs, MMF is not metabolized via the CYP450 3A system. Mycophenolate mofetil is used in combination with prednisone as an alternative to CNI therapy in patients intolerant to these medications. It also is used in refractory solid organ rejection and GVHD. Outside of transplant medicine, MMF is used to treat lupus nephritis, RA, inflammatory bowel disease and severe atopic dermatitis. Reversible myelosuppression is a common side effect of MMF. Infectious complications associated with MMF include increased risk of BK-virus-associated nephropathy, particularly in renal transplants, as well as increased risk of cytomegalovirus (CMV) and varicella-zoster virus (VZV) reactivation/disease and bacterial infections.[13]

Thalidomide and Derivatives

THALIDOMIDE

Historically known as a sedative drug withdrawn from the market due to its severe teratogenic effects when used in pregnant women, thalidomide is being tested and/or used in a variety of clinical applications due to its anti-inflammatory, immunomodulatory, and anti-angiogenic effects.[14] It inhibits tumor necrosis factor alpha (TNF-α), decreases neutrophil phagocytic activity, increases IL-10 production, alters adhesion molecule function, and enhances cell-mediated immunity through interaction with T cells. Current approved applications include treatment of multiple myeloma, erythema nodosum leprosum, and dermatologic disease due to systemic lupus erythematosus (SLE). Currently thalidomide may only be prescribed through a restricted distribution program, administered by the drug manufacturer. The severe side effect profile has prompted the development and study of alternative agents known as immunomodulatory derivatives of thalidomide or IMiDs.

LENALIDOMIDE

The first IMiD approved for treating patients with myelodysplastic syndrome and multiple myeloma, lenalidomide has fewer side effects than thalidomide, although concomitant use of anticoagulant therapy, close monitoring of renal function and monitoring for neutropenia and thrombocytopenia remain important.[15] Reported infectious complications include increased risk of bacterial infections (e.g. pneumonia and bacteremia) and herpes simplex virus (HSV) reactivation.

Cytotoxic Agents and Antimetabolites

AZATHIOPRINE

Azathioprine is a prototypic immunosuppressive antimetabolite. It is a prodrug of mercaptopurine that is well-absorbed from the gastrointestinal (GI) tract. Azathioprine is cleaved by xanthine oxidase to 6-thiouric acid. Once metabolized, azathioprine inhibits purine nucleic acid metabolism resulting in destruction of stimulated lymphoid cells, causing cell-mediated and humoral immune suppression. Azathioprine and mercaptopurine are used in renal allograft maintenance, lupus nephritis, Crohn's disease, RA, multiple sclerosis, and steroid-resistant idiopathic thrombocytopenic purpura and autoimmune hemolytic anemias. Infection risks are similarly broad-based but are predominantly related to the risk of invasive bacterial and fungal infections.[16] Concomitant glucocorticoid use increases this risk.[17]

CYCLOPHOSPHAMIDE

Cyclophosphamide is an alkylating agent that is highly toxic to proliferating lymphoid cells and has some effect against resting cells. High doses may induce tolerance to a new antigen if the drug is administered with or immediately after the antigen, which can help improve rates of successful engraftment after HSCT. It is also used to prevent or treat GVHD. In addition to its use in oncology, it is used in low doses for SLE, antibody-mediated factor XIII deficiency, pure red cell aplasia and Wegener's granulomatosis. Cyclophosphamide poses similar infection risks as azathioprine.[17]

LEFLUNOMIDE

Leflunomide is an orally-active prodrug of a pyrimidine synthesis inhibitor. It has a half-life of several weeks, and is currently used for treatment of RA. Owing to its relative lack of hepatic cytochrome P450 enzyme interactions and antiviral activity against cytomegalovirus, leflunomide is being studied in a wide array of transplant-associated and rheumatologic conditions. Leflunomide can be associated with increased risk of bacterial infection and *Pneumocystis jirovecii* pneumonia (PJP), but this may be due to its concomitant use with other immunosuppressants, particularly prednisone and methotrexate.[18]

METHOTREXATE

An inhibitor of dihydrofolate reductase, methotrexate is used both in chemotherapy and in the treatment of various malignancies as well as in RA and psoriasis. It is a substrate of P-glycoprotein and has multiple drug–drug interactions. Due to its potential to cause myelosuppression, methotrexate use is associated with increased risk of bacterial infections and sepsis. Methotrexate is also associated with an increased risk of HSV reactivation and PJP.[19]

Alkylating Agents and Platinum Coordination Complexes

These agents, which include nitrogen mustards, ethyleneamines, alkyl sulfonates, nitrosoureas, triazines, and DNA-methylating drugs, are primarily used in the treatment of neoplastic diseases. Their mechanisms of action all involve the alkylation of reactive amines, oxygens or phosphates on DNA, resulting in cytotoxic effects. They are most effective in rapidly-proliferating tissues, which accounts in part for their immunosuppressive effects. This can result in suppression of all bone marrow-derived cell lines. For some agents, their effects can also be seen on resting-phase immune cells such as mature lymphocytes. Immunosuppression and infectious complications can be quite broad, and depend in part on the duration of immune suppression and co-administration of other potentially immunosuppressive drugs.[16,20] Immune suppression in the treatment of malignancy is discussed in more detail in Chapter 79.

Monoclonal Antibodies and Receptor Antagonists

Immune-modulating antibodies are the fastest-growing set of biological agents and are used in a diverse array of autoimmune and inflammatory diseases.[21-25] Monoclonal antibodies are also used in pre-transplant conditioning regimens to reduce the likelihood of graft rejection or the development of GVHD. These agents are composed of hybrid antibodies consisting of murine- or human-derived constant regions paired with specific active regions that target cell receptors and cytokines. Humanized murine monoclonal antibodies and fully human monoclonal antibodies are both in clinical use. Monoclonal antibodies directly target cell-surface receptors, circulating chemokines, or facilitate apoptosis of immune cells. The level of immune suppression depends upon the antibody target. Table 159-2 lists the common biologic agents currently in use for a variety of indications with immunosuppressive or immunomodulatory effects and major infection risks. Some of the agents are markedly immunosuppressive (e.g. rituximab, tumor necrosis factor (TNF) inhibitors, alemtuzumab) and place the patient at major risk for opportunistic infections, while others are well tolerated or increase infection risk for a specific set of pathogens. Infections arising from the use of immunobiologics are discussed in more detail in Chapter 88.

Other Immunosuppressive Drugs

Additional selected agents with immunosuppressive properties are listed in Table 159-3.

References available online at expertconsult.com.

TABLE 159-2	**Common Biologic Agents and Their Principal Immunologic Effects and Infection Risks**		
Biologic Agent or Antibody [Generic (trade) names]	**Molecular Target**	**Indication(s)**	**Major Infection Risk**
ANTICYTOKINES			
Anakinra (Kineret)	IL-1 receptor antagonist targets IL-1 beta	RA	Upper respiratory infection, pneumonia (viral or bacterial)
Basiliximab (Simulect)	mAb blocks IL-2R (CD25) on T cells	Transplant rejection	CMV reactivation
Brodalumab (AMG 827)	Blocks IL-17AR	Psoriasis	Increased pharyngitis, URI
Daclizumab (Zenapax)	Humanized mAb blocks IL-2R (CD25) on T cells	Transplant rejection	CMV, other OIs (viral and bacterial)
Tocilizumab (Actemra)	Blocks IL-6R on T and B cells	Autoimmune disease, neoplastic disease	URI, might increase risk of other infections (uncertain risk)
ANTILYMPHOCYTE ANTIBODIES			
Polyclonal antithymocyte or antilymphocyte antibodies	T lymphocytes	Organ transplant rejection	Impaired cell-mediated immunity increases risk of numerous OI (viral, bacterial, fungal)
ANTILYMPHOCYTE RECEPTOR/COMPONENT ANTIBODIES			
Alemtuzumab (Campath)	Blocks CD52 on T and B cells, NK cells, myeloid cells	Transplant rejection, CLL, neoplastic disease	Neutropenia; multiple OI with bacterial, viral, fungal pathogens, PJP, PTLD
Belatacept	Blocks co-receptor CD28 on T cells	Kidney transplantation	EBV-associated PTLD, ?PML, UTI, CMV infection
Natalizumab (Tysabri)	Blocks alpha4 integrin and trafficking of lymphocytes	MS, Crohn's disease	PML, especially if JC virus antibody+ and prolonged immune suppression
Rituximab (Rituxan)	Blocks CD20 on B cells	RA, SLE, B cell neoplastic disease	Bacterial infections, CMV, VZV, HBV, PML
ANTI-TNF AGENTS			
Adalimumab (Humira)	Humanized anti-TNF mAb targets sTNF, tmTNF	RA, psoriasis, AS, Crohn's disease	MTB, viral, bacterial, and fungal OIs
Certolizumab pegol (Cimzia)	Pegylated humanized anti-TNF Fab fragment	Crohn's disease, RA	Limited data, likely similar to other TNF inhibitors
Etanercept (Enbrel)	Type 2 TNFr:Fc IgG blocks sTNF and lymphotoxin	RA, psoriasis, AS, JRA	MTB, viral, bacterial, fungal OIs, geographic fungi
Golimumab (Simponi)	Human anti-TNF mAB targets sTNF and tmTNF	RA, psoriasis, AS	MTB, viral, bacterial OIs
Infliximab (Remicade)	Chimeric murine-human mAb blocks TNF and tmTNF	RA, psoriasis, AS, ulcerative colitis, Crohn's disease	MTB, HSV, viral, bacterial, fungal OIs, geographic fungi

AS, ankylosing spondylitis; CLL, chronic lymphocytic leukemia; CMV, cytomegalovirus; cocci, coccidioidomycosis; EBV, Epstein-Barr virus; Geographic fungi: *Coccidioides immitis*, *Histoplasma capsulatum*, *Blastomyces dermatitidis*; HBV, hepatitis B virus; histo, histoplasmosis; IL, interleukin; JRA, juvenile rheumatoid arthritis; mAb, monoclonal antibody; MS, multiple sclerosis; OI, opportunistic infections; PJP, *Pneumocystis jirovecii* pneumonia; PML, progressive multifocal leukoencephalopathy; PTLD, post-transplant lymphoproliferative disorder; R, receptor; RA, rheumatoid arthritis; SLE, systemic lupus erythematosus; TNF, tumor necrosis factor; URI, upper respiratory infection; UTI, urinary tract infection; VZV, varicella-zoster virus.

TABLE 159-3	**Other Immunosuppressive Drugs**		
	Mechanism of Action	**Indication(s)**	**Potential Infectious Complications**
ANTIMETABOLITES			
Fluorouracil (5-FU)	Blocks DNA methylation during DNA synthesis	Chemotherapy for various solid-organ cancers	Bacterial, viral reactivation, MTB
Cytarabine	Pyrimidine synthesis inhibitor	Acute leukemias	Bacterial infections, HSV, MTB
CYTOTOXIC AGENTS			
Dapsone	Inhibits neutrophil migration, adherence	Leprosy, dermatitis herpetiformis	Bacterial infection
Vincristine	Inhibits mast cell degranulation	Leukemia, lymphoma, and/or solid tumor tx	Bacterial, fungal infections, HSV
Bleomycin	Causes DNA strand breaks	Squamous cell carcinoma, Hodgkin's lymphoma	Bacterial infection, HSV, VZV
Pentostatin	Adenosine deaminase inhibitor	Hairy cell leukemia	Bacterial infections
Fingolimod	Decreases lymphocyte recirculation	Multiple sclerosis	Bacterial, invasive fungal infections
Hydroxychloroquine	Suppression of MHC class II antigen processing	Systemic lupus erythematosus, rheumatoid arthritis	Bacterial infections (rare)

MTB, *Mycobacterium tuberculosis*; HSV, herpes simplex virus; VZV, varicella-zoster virus.

KEY REFERENCES

Askling J., Fored C.M., Brandt L., et al.: Time-dependent increase in risk of hospitalization with infection among Swedish RA patients treated with TNF antagonists. *Ann Rheum Dis* 2007; 66:1339-1344.

Avivi I., Stroopinsky D., Katz T.: Anti-CD20 monoclonal antibodies: beyond B-cells. *Blood Rev* 2013; 27(5):217-223.

Gea-Banacloche J.C., Opal S.M., Jorgensen J., et al.: Sepsis associated with immunosuppressive medications: An evidence-based review. *Crit Care Med* 2004; 32(11):S578-S590.

Kusne S., Fung J., Alessiani M., et al.: Infections during a randomized trial comparing cyclosporine to FK 506 immunosuppression in liver transplantation. *Transplant Proc* 1992; 24(1):429-430.

Lacaille D., Guh D.P., Abrahamowicz M., et al.: Use of non-biologic disease-modifying antirheumatic drugs and risk of infection in patients with rheumatoid arthritis. *Arthritis Rheum* 2008; 59(8):1074-1081.

Mehrabi A., Fonouni H., Kashfi A., et al.: The role and value of sirolimus administration in kidney and liver transplantation. *Clin Transplant* 2006; 20(Suppl. 17):30-43.

Moynagh P.N.: Toll-like signaling pathways as key targets for mediating the anti-inflammatory and immunosuppressive effects of glucocorticoids. *J Endocrin* 2003; 179: 139-144.

Segal B.H., Sneller M.C.: Infectious complications of immunosuppressive therapy in patients with rheumatic diseases. *Rheum Dis Clin North Am* 1997; 23:219-237.

Stebbins W.G., Lebwohl M.G.: Biologics in combination with nonbiologics: efficacy and safety. *Dermatol Ther* 2004; 17(5):432-440.

Ritter M.L., Pirofski L.: Mycophenolate mofetil: effects on cellular immune subsets, infectious complications, and antimicrobial activity. *Transpl Infect Dis* 2009; 11(4):290-297.

160

Antibacterial Drugs: Looking Ahead From the Past

DAVID M. SHLAES

KEY CONCEPTS

- New, rapid and feasible regulatory pathways for the development and approval of antibiotics targeting resistant pathogens are needed.

- These could involve the use of externally or historically controlled superiority trials.

- Controls could come from pharmacometric data from contemporary trials or from prospective observational studies.

- New financial incentives will also be necessary to entice large pharmaceutical companies back into the business of antibiotic discovery and development.

- These can be justified by the value of new drugs active against highly resistant bacterial pathogens.

Introduction

The great fear among public health officials and scientists around the world is that we are approaching a postantibiotic era where common pathogens are resistant to available antibiotics. In this apocalyptic view, routine surgery becomes extraordinarily risky and toxic chemotherapy is out of the question. There is a small but finite risk that this scenario will come to pass. Even if the postantibiotic era has not yet arrived, the state of affairs of bacterial resistance is of increasing concern.[1] While there are many factors contributing to progressive loss of antibiotic effectiveness, a constant pipeline of new antibiotics active against increasingly resistant pathogens needs to be maintained. To assure that this need will be fulfilled, we must accomplish two tasks: 1) establish regulatory pathways such that these antibiotics can be developed rapidly and without the enormous expense; 2) create an antibiotic marketplace attractive to large and small pharmaceutical companies.

The Regulatory Environment for Antibiotics

The history of antibiotics and the history of the US Food and Drug Administration (FDA) are intimately intertwined.[2] Antibiotics were some of the first drugs approved by the FDA in the 1930s and 1940s (sulfonamides and penicillin). During those years, small numbers of patients were studied and were compared to either patients receiving placebo or to historical controls who had not been treated with the antibiotic. The antibiotic effect was dramatic and obvious to all. Since then, for the most part, it has become unethical to conduct placebo-controlled, antibiotic trials in patients with potentially serious bacterial infections. Since it is statistically impossible to show that two treatments are equivalent, a noninferiority design has been instituted. In this design, two treatment groups are compared and a statistical margin is used to define an acceptable level of statistical difference to define the noninferiority of the test drug to a previously approved control drug. The noninferiority margin was not chosen on the basis of scientific or statistical principles, but to make the trials more rapid and feasible. The more difficult a trial was to enroll, for example hospital-acquired pneumonia, where enrollment rates are notoriously low, the greater the margin allowed, such that the total number of patients required was smaller.

However, statisticians have begun to question the scientific basis for the different margins being used for different infectious disease indications such as otitis media, complicated skin and skin structure infections and nosocomial pneumonia. Moreover, a noninferiority study is only valid to approve a new drug if the control drug has a therapeutic effect beyond placebo. Statisticians began to question whether any antibiotic developed after the 1940s actually worked to treat infections. They worried about a so-called 'biocreep'. In biocreep, the antibiotic effect from serial noninferiority trials could diminish with each new antibiotic approved until the latest antibiotic approved is no better than placebo. This led the FDA at first to tighten the noninferiority margins that they required for antibiotic trials. So, for example, in complicated skin and skin structure infections, where the margins defined for such trials in the 1980s were around 15%, they suddenly became 10%. This change more than doubled the numbers of patients required for the trial and therefore more than doubled the cost of each trial. This expense discourages industry from continuing to discover and develop antibiotics. Between 1999 and 2006, most large companies halted their antibiotic research.

In 2006, the Ketek scandal occurred.[2,3] Ketek or telithromycin is a ketolide antibiotic (related to the macrolides) that is active against a number of macrolide-resistant pathogens, especially *Streptococcus pneumoniae* and *Strep. pyogenes*. The drug was developed for the treatment of sinusitis, acute bacterial exacerbations of chronic bronchitis and community-acquired pneumonia. The FDA review of telithromycin was complicated by safety concerns around the potential for cardiac toxicity (prolongation of the QT interval). To respond to those concerns, the drug sponsor undertook a 24 000 patient safety trial where intensive EKG monitoring was employed. The trial was highly controversial. The investigator contributing the greatest number of patients was later convicted of fraud. The FDA announced that it would be unable to use the trial data to approve the drug, but the FDA then took the unprecedented step of using voluntary reporting of adverse events associated with telithromycin's use in Europe. The drug had been marketed for over a year where over a million courses of therapy had been dispensed. Finding nothing untoward, they approved the drug. Several FDA staffers disagreed with this approach and leaked internal FDA emails to the press. Shortly afterwards, there were three reported cases of serious liver toxicity associated with telithromycin therapy. The US Congress became involved and threatened public hearings on the way telithromycin was approved. They also attacked the use of noninferiority trials for antibiotic approvals in general. The FDA responded with a new series of guidance documents after they voided all previous guidance on the development of antibiotics. They insisted on 'justification' for the proposed noninferiority trials for any infection studied. Drugs having completed trials based on prior agreements with FDA were not approved. Companies went bankrupt. Additional companies abandoned antibiotic research.[3]

Following this scandal, the FDA began to issue series of guidance statements calling for trial designs that were simply not feasible. The only exception to this was a guidance for trials in so-called acute bacterial skin and skin structure infections (ABSSSI) that called for a feasible design but recommended a peculiar end point of halting of the spread of the skin lesion (cellulitis or erysipelas) within 24–48 hours. The clinically relevant end point for this indication remains cure (no need for further antibiotic treatment).[4]

After years of uncertainty, the FDA began a 'reboot' process in 2012. That has led to new guidances for trials that are more streamlined and that are, most importantly, feasible. The most important features of the 'new' FDA policy are shown in Table 160-1. The new approach still requires controversial end points that may be of limited clinical relevance – most being early end points rather than cure. One exception to this is the end point for hospital-acquired pneumonia (HAP), which is mortality at day 14–30.[5] This end point is problematic as a number of studies[6] have shown that about half the mortality occurring in this group at day 30 is related to underlying co-morbidities rather than the infection being treated.[6]

In Europe, the other key regulatory agency, the European Medicines Agency or EMA, has steadfastly stuck to feasible designs and test of cure endpoints. They have been the most open to novel trial designs and have generally made the development of new antibiotics active against resistant bacteria a priority. This means that all trials to be submitted globally will have a primary endpoint in Europe of cure while the primary endpoint in the US will be the early endpoints (except HAP). The end result is the need to create a separate statistical plan for each trial for the two agencies.

In their reboot, the FDA and the EMA have followed the recommendations of Rex *et al.*[7] (Figure 160-1). The figure proposes a middle road between the two major existing strategies for antibiotic development – Tiers A and D. In Tier A, two noninferiority trials are required to establish efficacy of a new antibiotic for any given infection (urinary tract, skin, etc.). In Tier D, the animal rule is used to approve therapies for bioterror infections. Efficacy, pharmacokinetics and pharmacodynamics are studied in animals and safety and pharmacokinetic studies are carried out in humans. A pharmacodynamic argument supplants the need for clinical trials in humans showing efficacy since these are not possible with biohazardous pathogens. To support trial designs in the middle tier strategies, Tier B and C, strong pharmacodynamics data from preclinical models are absolutely required as are solid *in vitro* antibacterial data. Based on this, in Tier B, a single noninferiority trial could be paired with, for example, an open label trial of the new antibiotic demonstrating efficacy in infections that would not have been expected to respond to standard therapy – such as those caused by essentially pan-resistant pathogens. The antibiotic would then be approved for the infection studied in the noninferiority trial and for use when other options are not thought to be available. In Tier C, the only trials might be those where the antibiotic is targeting highly resistant infections. In this case, the trials might be pathogen-specific, such as drugs that only treat infections caused by *Pseudomonas aeruginosa*. Patients might have different infections such as pneumonia or urinary tract infection. This means that antibiotics targeting resistant pathogens could be developed. The FDA, in their recently released guidance[8] on antibacterial drugs for unmet needs, lists possible approaches to new drug development. All approaches would require strong supporting nonclinical data.

The approaches listed include statistically powered, active control, superiority trials in either one indication or patients with varying sites of infection. Noninferiority trials with a nested superiority component are possible along with externally-controlled or historically-controlled trials.

The premarket safety database could be as small as 300 patients for these antibiotics. Guidance from FDA is remarkably similar to that from EMA where the EMA preceded the FDA by roughly 1 year.

One looming question for developers is, how could one design a superiority trial for a new antibiotic targeting resistance?[9,10] There are several possible meanings of the idea of a 'superiority trial':

1. Head-to-head: a head-to-head prospective comparison of the new drug vs an existing drug.
2. Subanalysis: a superiority subanalysis (or analyses) embedded in a noninferiority trial.
3. External (historical) control: an indirect comparison of a new drug with data from patients treated (inadvertently) with ineffective therapy for resistant pathogens.

The first definition (head-to-head) seems logical but is practically unrealistic except under rare circumstances. In such a design, one group of patients would be randomized to standard of care whereas the second group would receive the new drug (perhaps alone or in a combination). In the case of antibiotics the standard of care patients are assumed to be getting therapy that might actually work. Indeed, the trial cannot be designed to deliberately seek superiority in a way that puts patients at risk: it is a requirement of the trial that a patient can NOT be enrolled if they are infected with a resistant organism.

The only possible loophole is that if the only available regimen is highly toxic (e.g. colistin-based), then a demonstration of superiority based on safety might be possible. However, the success of even one drug here would then create a new tool for future trials that would make it next to impossible to study the next new drug via a head-to-head superiority trial.

TABLE 160-1	The Evolution of FDA Policy	
FDA Pre-2012	**FDA Post-2012 Reboot**
In general, two independent NI trials	Single NI trial in ABSSSI plus a single NI trial in CABP – allows for approval in both indications
Required for each indication	Single NI trial in cUTI plus single NI trial in cIAI – allows for approval in both indications
Exception – 2 trials in CABP + 1 in HABP	Small, pathogen-specific trials may be allowed. Controls and other parameters for such trials
NI margins generally 10%	Margins remain to be established for individual products
Exception – HABP – 15–20%	
AOM, ABS, ABECOPD – placebo controls required	Placebo controls no longer required for AOM

ABECOPD, acute bacterial exacerbations of chronic obstructive pulmonary disease; ABS, acute bacterial sinusitis; ABSSSI, acute bacterial skin and skin structure infection; AOM, acute otitis media; CABP, community-acquired bacterial pneumonia; cIAI, complicated intra-abdominal infection; cUTI, complicated urinary tract infection; HABP, hospital-acquired bacterial pneumonia; NI, noninferiority.

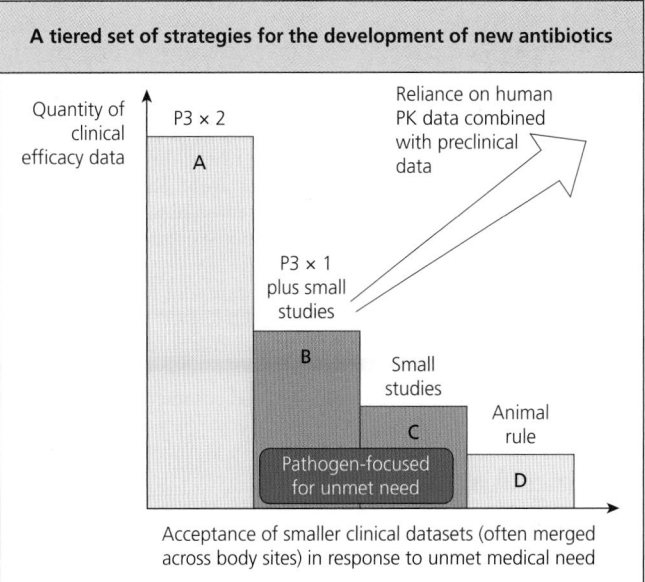

A tiered set of strategies for the development of new antibiotics

Figure 160-1 A tiered set of strategies for the development of new antibiotics. *(Courtesy of J. Rex)*

What are the alternative feasible superiority designs for antibiotics? There are three possibilities.

1. Embed a superiority trial within the context of a standard non-inferiority trial. In this design the new drug must not be inferior to some gold standard treatment. If you achieve superiority in a noninferiority trial – that is, your new drug is not only not inferior but is actually superior (the lower bound of the 95% confidence interval does not cross 0) to the gold standard – you can make that claim and get approved on that basis. But if you are noninferior in the large population, you can carry out a pre-designed analysis on a subpopulation (patients where the activity of the gold standard drug might be equivocal, for example) and show superiority there. If the new drug is not superior, approval might still be possible based upon noninferiority to a gold standard antibiotic. If the new drug cannot show noninferiority, then it is not approved.

2. Historically or externally controlled superiority trials might be a desirable study design depending on the definition of 'historical'.

   (a) The first such design would use a historical control based on pharmacokinetic analysis of previous but contemporary trial data. The best example of this is Paul Ambrose's analysis of the tigecycline trial in ventilator-associated pneumonia.[11] In that analysis, patients who do not achieve therapeutic drug levels are more likely to fail. The results in inadequately treated patients show what happens when you treat resistant infections with antibiotics that are unlikely to work because you cannot achieve high enough levels of drug to kill the infecting bacteria. If the new drug is superior in effect to this inadequate therapy, you should be able to achieve approval. The major criticism here is that the controls are still historical and therefore the patient populations under study might be different.

   (b) A second approach would be to carry out a prospective observational study of patients with highly resistant infections being treated with so-called standard of care (like colistin or tigecycline or others). This treatment would have some result in these patients. You then carry out a trial where patients receive the new drug, either in combination with 'standard of care' or with some gold standard antibiotic. Only those with infections resistant to the standard therapy would be evaluable to show that the new drug was better than standard of care. The patients are compared to the standard therapy patients enrolled in this prospective observational study. Similar inclusion and exclusion criteria are required for both the observational study and the prospective trial. This would then validate a superior result from the trial portion of the study.

3. Finally, there is the option to carry out an uncontrolled trial to demonstrate efficacy in a situation where there would be no reason to expect efficacy of any other agent. Such might be the case in the rescue therapy of patients infected with pan-resistant pathogens who have already failed prior standard of care or even 'salvage' therapy.

All of these approaches could involve exposing fewer patients to the test product and could be run in an accelerated time frame. The final label would, of course, reflect the higher risk posed by such agents and would attempt to limit use to patients for whom there might be little other choice. This would limit the final commercial value of the product.

Making Antibiotics Financially Attractive

Which business models work and how would this effect taxpayers and governments? First – we all must realize that there is no free lunch. Either we spend money on antibiotics that can cure resistant infection, or we pay the price in longer hospital stays, more time on ventilators and in lives lost.

1. Financial support for research and development – especially late stage clinical trials – will positively impact the net present value of the antibiotic by reducing upfront costs. This is a so-called 'push incentive'.

2. The traditional pricing model. New directly acting drugs for hepatitis C infection is a good example. In this scenario, small numbers of patients with demonstrated infection with a resistant pathogen would receive an antibiotic active against the resistant strain and pay up to $30 000 for a course of therapy. The cost would be covered by private or publicly supported health insurance or governmental health services.

3. Guaranteed government purchases. Here, governments would guarantee a certain upfront purchase of the antibiotic at the time of approval by the regulatory agencies. The price charged per course of therapy in each country would depend partly on the amount of its advance purchase. This serves to de-link the drug to some extent from the need for the company to spend money on marketing. Marketing costs about 25–30% of total sales of any antibiotic. Also, the guaranteed purchase increases the overall value of the antibiotic by decreasing its associated costs. Such a purchase is all the more powerful since an immediate revenue stream provides the greatest impact on the overall net present value of a product by eliminating the downstream correction for inflation in the value calculation.

4. The wild card patent exclusivity. In this formulation, a drug company that brought forward a new antibiotic would be allowed to have 6 months–2 years of additional patent exclusivity on another drug of their choice. For example, a drug company would be able to have additional time to sell its branded, highly profitable, trade name drugs, making new antibiotic development more appealing.

To justify these approaches, a number of studies have already been published. The London School of Economics and the Office of Health Economics have both focused on the costs of resistant infections – mainly in Europe, and both have proposed economic solutions.[12,13] A net cost study by Spellberg and Rex[14] showed that in a traditional pricing model, up to $50 000 per course of therapy for a drug active against highly resistant *Acinetobacter baumannii* could be justified based on cost savings in the therapy of such infections.

Current Late Stage Antibacterial Pipeline

At the time of writing, there are approximately 14 antibacterial compounds in late stage trials according to clinicaltrials.gov (Table 160-2). Almost half are being studied in gram-positive infections while the rest are directed towards gram-negative infection. Some (plazomicin and RPX-7009) are following the FDA's unmet needs guideline. None will work for all of our highly resistant infections.

Conclusions

By adapting regulatory policies to urgent medical needs for new antibiotics and by paying for these antibiotics in an appropriate way, we can bring pharmaceutical companies back into antibiotics research and development. Such a step will be required if we are ever to return to the days of the robust antibiotic pipelines we enjoyed during the 1970s and 1980s. And we need novel antibiotics to keep pace and continue to stay ahead of continually emerging bacterial resistance to the new therapies that are brought to the marketplace.

References available online at expertconsult.com.

TABLE
160-2 **The Late Stage Antibiotic Pipeline**

Antibiotic	Phase (II or III)	Indication(s)	Class
Plazomycin	II	cUTI	Aminoglycoside
Ceftaroline–avibactam	II (approved in USA)	cUTI	Cephalosporin plus DABCO β-lactamase inhibitor
Ceftazidime–avibactam	III (approved in USA)	cIAI, cUTI, HABP, resistant infections	Cephalosporin plus DABCO β-lactamase inhibitor
Ceftolozane–tazobactam	III (approved in USA)	cUTI, cIAI, VABP	Cephalosporin plus sulfone β-lactamase inhibitor
RPX-7009	III	cUTI, and in CRE infections	Novel boron β-lactamase inhibitor with biapenem meropenem
MK-7655	II	cUTI, cIAI	DABCO β-lactamase inhibitor combined with imipenem–cilastatin
Finafloxacin	II	cUTI	Fluoroquinolone
Delafloxacin	III	ABSSSI	Fluoroquinolone
Solithromycin	III	CABP	Ketolide
GSK1322322	II	ABSSSI	Novel peptide deformylase inhibitor
AFN-12520000	II	ABSSSI	Novel – specific for staphylococci
Lefamulin	II	ABSSSI	Pleuromutilin
Eravacycline	III	cUTI, cIAI	Tetracycline
Omadacycline	II	ABSSSI	Tetracycline

This pipeline is based on information available via clinicaltrials.gov.
Only pre-approval compounds in phases II or III of clinical development are included.
ABSSSI, acute bacterial skin and skin structure infection; CABP, community-acquired bacterial pneumonia; cIAI, complicated intra-abdominal infection; CRE, carbapenem-resistant Enterobacteriaceae; cUTI, complicated urinary tract infection; DABCO, diazabicyclooctane; HABP, hospital-associated bacterial pneumonia; VABP, ventilator-associated bacterial pneumonia.

KEY REFERENCES

Ambrose P.G., Hammel J.P., Bhavnani S.M., et al.: Frequentist and Bayesian pharmacometric-based approaches to facilitate critically needed new antibiotic development: overcoming lies, damn lies, and statistics. *Antimicrob Agents Chemother* 2012; 56(3):1466-1470.

Guidance for industry acute bacterial skin and skin structure infections: developing drugs for treatment. Available: http://www.fda.gov/downloads/Drugs/Guidance ComplianceRegulatoryInformation/Guidances/ UCM071185.pdf.

Guidance for industry antibacterial therapies for patients with unmet medical need for the treatment of serious bacterial diseases. Available: http://www.fda.gov/downloads/Drugs/GuidanceComplianceRegulatory Information/Guidances/UCM359184.pdf.

Guidance for industry hospital-acquired bacterial pneumonia and ventilator-associated bacterial pneumonia: developing drugs for treatment. Available: http://www.fda.gov/downloads/Drugs/GuidanceComplianceRegulatory Information/Guidances/UCM234907.pdf.

Infectious Diseases Society of America: White paper: recommendations on the conduct of superiority and organism-specific clinical trials of antibacterial agents for the treatment of infections caused by drug-resistant bacterial pathogens. *Clin Infect Dis* 2012; 55:1031-1046.

Melsen W.G., Rovers M.M., Groenwold R.H., et al.: Attributable mortality of ventilator-associated pneumonia: a meta-analysis of individual patient data from randomised prevention studies. *Lancet Infect Dis* 2013; 13(8):665-671.

Mossialos E., Morel C., Edwards S., et al. Policies and incentives for promoting innovation in antibiotic research. Available: http://www.lse.ac.uk/intranet/ LSEServices/ERD/pressAndInformationOffice/PDF/ Policiesandincentivesforpromotinginnovationinanti biotic.pdf.

Rex J.H., Eisenstein B.I., Alder J., et al.: A comprehensive regulatory framework to address the unmet need for new antibacterial treatments. *Lancet Infect Dis* 2013; 13(3): 269-275.

Shlaes D.M.: *Antibiotics: the perfect storm.* New York: Springer-Verlag; 2010.

Shlaes D.M. Superiority trials for antibiotics. Available: http://antibiotics-theperfectstorm.blogspot.com/2014/ 04/superiority-trails-for-antibiotics.html.

Shlaes D.M., Moellering R.C.: Telithromycin and the FDA: implications for the future. *Lancet Infect Dis* 2008; 8:83-85.

Shlaes D.M., Sahm D., Opiela C., et al.: The FDA reboot of antibiotic development. *Antimicrob Agents Chemother* 2013; 57(10):4605-4607.

Sharma P., Towse A. New drugs to tackle antimicrobial resistance: analysis of EU Policy options. 2011. Office of Health Economics. Available: https://www.ohe.org/ publications/new-drugs-tackle-antimicrobial-resistance -analysis-eu-policy-options.

Spellberg B., Rex J.H.: The value of single-pathogen antibacterial agents. *Nat Rev Drug Discov* 2013; 12(12):963.

161

Advances in Diagnostic Microbiology

GRÉGORY DUBOURG | PIERRE-EDOUARD FOURNIER

KEY CONCEPTS

- Clinical microbiology laboratories play a central role in optimizing the management of infectious diseases.

- Syndrome-based sampling and molecular testing, as well as extended automation, are major improvements in the clinical microbiology workflow.

- Mass spectrometry enables a rapid and cost-effective identification of bacterial and fungal pathogens, cultivated on agar or within blood culture vials.

- Real-time genomics has reached a stage when it may impact infectious disease outbreaks.

- Point-of-care assays and laboratories reduce the time to diagnosis and allow better patient management.

Introduction

The identification of bacterial, viral, fungal and parasitic agents that cause human diseases is crucial to enable adequate clinical management of patients as well as prevent infectious disease transmission.[1] Although culture remains a milestone of routine clinical microbiology, new tools, including improved sampling and culture strategies, molecular methods (polymerase chain reaction (PCR), high-throughput genome sequencing)[2] and matrix-assisted laser desorption/ionization time-of-flight-mass spectrometry (MALDI-TOF-MS) have been developed recently. These technological advances have revealed a much larger microbial world than was believed a few years ago and questioned our knowledge inherited from Pasteur and Koch, notably the fact that a given disease is caused by a given micro-organism.[3] Herein, we review the main advances that have recently influenced the diagnosis of infectious diseases in clinical microbiology laboratories (CMLs), notably in the fields of syndrome- and disease-based sampling kits, new culture approaches, direct pathogen detection, point-of-care testing and clinical isolate identification. We also propose our view of the CML of the future.

Syndrome-Based Sampling

The fact that the number of known pathogens in a given clinical situation has increased dramatically since the introduction of molecular methods has prompted the use of standardized kits that enable optimized sampling and testing of panels of the most likely micro-organisms, and which significantly reduce the time between sampling and final diagnosis, avoiding the need to re-sample or re-test. The design of these test panels is based on the prevalence of the pathogens involved in each syndrome and the use of the most efficient techniques for their identification (Figure 161-1). In addition, multi-site sampling enables both direct detection of pathogens by culture, molecular assays or pathological examination, and indirect detection, mainly represented by serological testing. To date, syndrome-driven kits are available for endocarditis, pericarditis, diarrhea, osteomyelitis, meningitis, encephalitis, uveitis and keratitis.[4-7] Syndrome-based sampling and testing may be cost-effective, despite misleading evidence, when considering the possibility of early appropriate antimicrobial therapy and shorter hospital stay, as well as suppression of unjustified treatments in cases of viral infections.[8]

The Renewal of Culture

Over recent years, innovative culture strategies have permitted an improved isolation of fastidious bacteria from both environmental and clinical samples.[9-11] These included the empirical change of culture conditions, starting with the culture medium. As an example, the growth of *Mycobacterium tuberculosis*, known to be slow on usual media for mycobacteria, has progressively been accelerated using blood-enriched media[12] and then ascorbic acid-enriched media.[13] The 'culturomics' strategy, based on the systematic diversification of all culture conditions (medium, temperature, incubation time and atmosphere), enabled the isolation of more than 100 novel bacterial species using up to 212 distinct culture conditions.[14]

In addition, in a recent study, antioxidant-supplemented agar was used (ascorbic acid, glutathione and uric acid) to cultivate aerobically 100% of anaerobic bacteria tested (Raoult *et al.*, unpublished data), allowing the avoidance of anaerobic conditions routinely used in clinical microbiology, and enabling a workflow improvement currently required in CML.

Identification of Micro-organisms

The usual identification methods for bacterial and fungal isolates using phenotypic characteristics and biochemical properties, although automated, are time- and money-consuming, and have progressively been replaced over the past decade, initially in Europe, by MALDI-TOF-MS.[15] MALDI-TOF-MS is a robust and cost-effective technology that enables a rapid and accurate identification of micro-organisms from culture despite the potential spectral variation introduced by different culture conditions, protein extraction methods and different laboratory processes (Figure 161-2). The rapidity of identification (6–10 minutes) has the greatest potential impact on the clinical management of patients allowing earlier decision-making regarding the tailoring of antimicrobial treatment. It is a sensitive technique able to generate mass spectra from samples of $<10^4$ micro-organisms and has the added benefit of not requiring a predefined target (in contrast with PCR-based methods of identification). However, a culture of the micro-organism is currently still required and it is unable to deal with mixed cultures. Additionally, the quality and taxonomic breadth of the reference database is critical, as an accurate identification is only possible if the micro-organism in question is in the database. There is also difficulty in distinguishing between some organisms that are closely genetically related, for example, *Streptococcus pneumoniae* and some of the viridans group streptococci, and further testing to confirm identification may be required. However, despite these drawbacks, MALDI-TOF-MS has been adopted by many large CMLs worldwide, allowing cost reduction and improved workflow.[16] In addition, it may also enable strain comparison for subtyping, as was demonstrated for *Corynebacterium striatum* or *Klebsiella pneumoniae*.[17-19] Regular database updates now also allow a correct identification of rare pathogenic[20] or fastidious bacteria.[21]

Over the last decade, Raman spectrometry has been described as a powerful identification tool for micro-organisms, exhibiting a high discriminatory power with a short delay. In this technique, a spectrum generated from light scattering from an illuminated colony is compared with a spectrum database. This method is inexpensive, due to the absence of the need for reagents, is as rapid as MALDI-TOF-MS and can be applied to bacterial species.[22,23] However, Raman spectrometry has not been widely deployed in CMLs, due in part to the initial

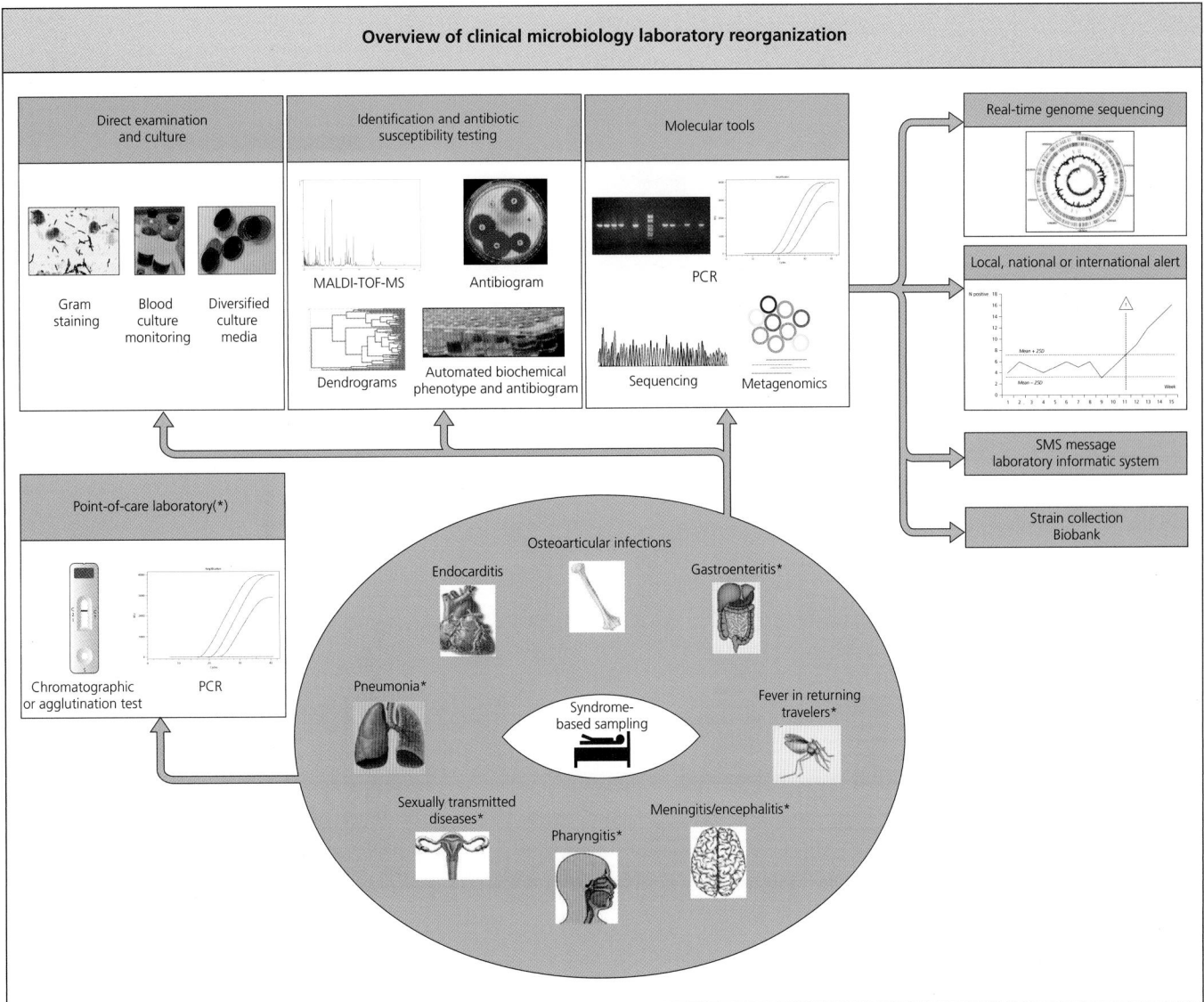

Figure 161-1 Overview of clinical microbiology laboratory reorganization. Specimens are collected and labeled using syndrome-based sampling kits. Those that can be tested by point-of-care assays are indicated with an asterisk. Culture, identification and antibiotic susceptibility testing are performed in the core laboratory, together with direct molecular detection applied to the sample in parallel. Unknown or unusual pathogens are further characterized by genome sequencing, and preserved in a strain collection. *(Adapted from Fournier, P.E., et al. Nature Reviews Microbiology 2013; 11(8):574-585.)*

instrument cost, and to the technical pitfalls inherent to the technique.

Detection of Antibiotic Resistance

Classical *in vitro* antimicrobial susceptibility tests are time-consuming as they require bacterial growth and interpretation. When bacterial growth is slow, as is the case for *M. tuberculosis*,[24] these assays may not be compatible with the urgency required in some situations.

In contrast, the use of real-time PCR (RT-PCR) enabled rapid detection of the most common antibiotic resistance genes of clinical relevance such as OXA-48[25] or MecA[26] (which code carbapenem resistance in Enterobacteriaceae and methicillin-resistance in *Staph. aureus*, respectively). In addition, single nucleotide polymorphisms (SNPs) or other gene mutations associated with resistance to antituberculous agents can be detected by pyrosequencing[27] or nonfluorescent microarrays.[28] In parallel, recent studies have shown that MALDI-TOF-MS can also be used routinely to detect antibiotic resistance, in particular in the case of β-lactamase activity where imipenem hydrolysis can be identified[29] as for *Acinetobacter baumannii* or those belonging to the family Enterobacteriaceae, with a high specificity and sensitivity in only 1–4 hours.[30-32] This technique has the advantage that it may detect the activity of unknown enzymes, and by extension allow the discovery of new antibiotic resistance genes.

In Situ Detection and Identification of Pathogens

MASS SPECTROMETRY

In addition to identifying bacteria from colonies, MALDI-TOF-MS has been demonstrated to be able to identify efficiently microorganisms directly within clinical samples. The first study, conducted on bacteria grown from blood collected in culture bottles, showed that MALDI-TOF-MS was able to identify blood-borne bacteria in less than 2 hours with a success rate of 97.5%.[33] The method was optimized using commercially-available extraction kits[34] and a minimum bacterial load of approximately 10^6–10^8 colony forming units per mL (CFU/mL).[35] This method was later adapted to the identification of bacteria in urine specimens with a success rate of identification of 91.8% but for lower concentrations of 10^3 CFU/mL.[36]

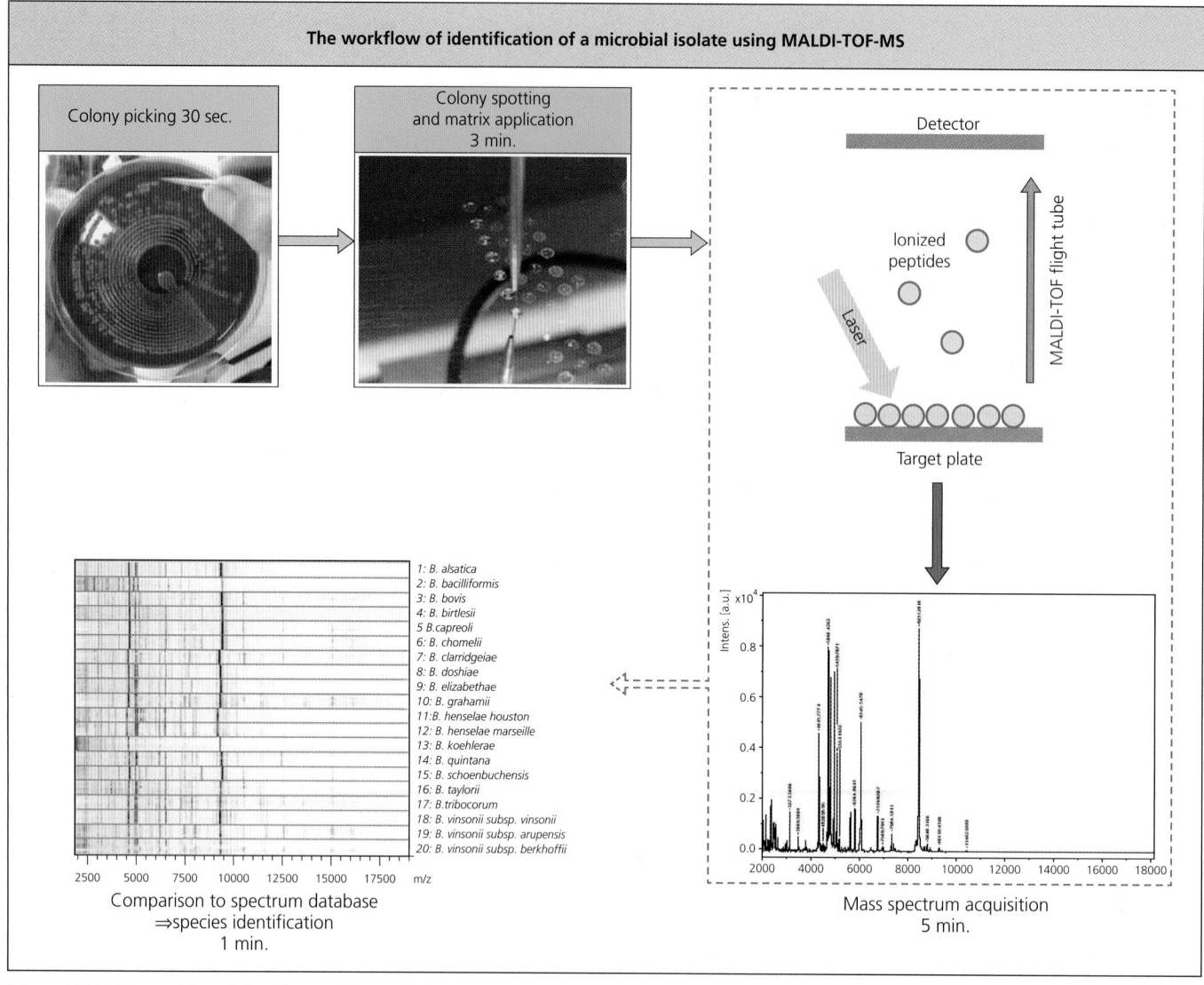

Figure 161-2   The workflow of identification of a microbial isolate using MALDI-TOF-MS. The example of *Bartonella alsatica* was taken. The time lapse of each step is indicated.

MOLECULAR DETECTION

In the past decade, RT-PCR constituted another significant step forward in terms of sensitivity and speed of diagnosis. By identifying the concentration of micro-organisms, it provides a way to evaluate infection severity or treatment efficiency.[37,38] The combination in multiplexed RT-PCR assays enabled the rapid and concomitant detection, using automated systems, of several pathogens responsible for a given disease. Several multiplexed RT-PCR systems are currently commercially available. As an example, the MagicPlex™ sepsis system (Seegene, Korea) enables an automated identification of 90 pathogens from blood specimens, 25 of which are at the species level, and three antibiotic resistance genes. However, despite a good analytic sensitivity, these systems can complement, but not replace, blood cultures due to an inadequate correlation rate.[39,40] Similar multiplexed assays dedicated to specific syndromes have been developed including meningitis, community-acquired pneumonia,[41] sexually transmitted diseases[42] or urogenital infections.[43]

Recently, Abbot introduced a micro-organism detection and identification system combining PCR and electron spray ionization MS (ESI-MS®) (Abbot Molecular, Carlsbad, CA, USA). This system can detect >1000 distinct pathogens on the basis of multiple broad-range PCR assays using 16 pairs of primers generating amplicons thereafter identified by ESI-MS in 1 minute, which constitutes a significant gain of time when compared to Sanger sequencing.[44,45]

Genotyping

Many clinical situations require a better understanding of the source and spread of micro-organisms, including outbreaks, endemic infections and emergence of novel pathogens or circulation of hypervirulent strains. Multi-locus sequence typing (MLST), commonly used to characterize strains using a combination of housekeeping genes,[46] has been recently extended to the genome level (genome-sequence-designed MLST) to discriminate micro-organisms with high variability such as *Escherichia coli*, *Neisseria meningitidis* or *Staphylococcus aureus*.[47-49] Finally, the affordability of whole-genome sequencing (WGS), facilitated by a better access to sequencing platforms, makes this approach very promising, offering the best discriminatory tool, as was demonstrated for a cholera outbreak[50,51] or the worldwide spread of methicillin-resistant *Staph. aureus*.[52]

Advances in Genomics and Metagenomics

Resolution of complex microbial communities is a major challenge of the 21st century. If high-throughput sequencing methods have permitted significant advances in this domain, the precision in characterizing these ecosystems is continuously increasing, as shown, for example, by the introduction of Illumina®-sequenced environmental metagenomes (mi-tags) that allow a better estimation of richness and evenness of microbial communities when compared with traditional 454 tags.[53] However, sequences obtained are compared to genome reference databases and thus only allow the identification of previously known organisms. Nevertheless, recent innovative methods such as co-abundance gene binning,[54] enabled the discovery of new bacteria and viruses in complex ecosystems, and may be a starting point of the high-resolution metagenomics era.

Despite these substantial advances, cultivation of an organism is a necessary condition to obtain highly informative genomic data. Recently, single-cell genome sequencing that does not require prior cultivation enabled sequencing of uncultivated bacteria and thus the study of virulence factors or the acquisition of antibiotic resistance genes.[55]

Finally, the study of gene function in complex ecosystems is now made possible by metatranscriptomics and metaproteomics by recovering mRNA and protein from diverse environments. Despite technical pitfalls, these tools have shown promising results.[56]

Point-of-Care Laboratories (POCLs)

Working around the clock, POCLs considerably reduce the turn-around time (TAT), performing mostly agglutination or immuno-chromatographic assays, for which the results are available in less than 1 hour, as well as RT-PCR assays that make possible the rapid molecular detection of many pathogens in emergency circumstances such as meningitis. POC assays are selected to provide an answer, having a clear impact on patient management: hospitalization; isolation of contagious individuals; or onset of specific anti-infective therapy. A large variety of agents can be tested, including bacteria, parasites or viruses.[8] Finally, POCLs are easily implementable in any environment and may thus be established in remote areas, as was the case in rural Senegal[57] or on a commercial ship.[58]

Conclusions and Perspectives

Medical microbiology is facing a sudden evolution, through the development of high-throughput approaches, represented by the 'omics' technologies and the centralization of biomedical analyses that enable a significant workflow improvement. Thus, reducing the time to diagnosis has become a major challenge for CMLs, making them a major actor in early patient management and thus helping reduce hospitalization costs.[59] In addition, recent technologies allowing rapid and more discriminatory identification of strains mean that CMLs can play a key role in detecting emerging infections, in syndromic surveillance or in outbreak detection and warning medical authorities, as was the case for the *Clostridium difficile* O27 outbreak in France,[60] for which management coupled with the use of new therapeutic tools, such as fecal transplantation, enabled resolution of the outbreak. In addition, with specialized staff and an expertise in advanced technologies, CMLs have to play an educational role in training and updating the current knowledge in microbiology. Finally, the involvement of CMLs in scientific discoveries has a significant impact on scientific literature. If balanced with cost, these developments can improve the workflow and output of CMLs and, by identifying and characterizing emerging microbial pathogens, provide significant breakthroughs in human medicine.

References available online at expertconsult.com.

KEY REFERENCES

Ashton L., Lau K., Winder C.L., et al.: Raman spectroscopy: lighting up the future of microbial identification. *Future Microbiol* 2011; 6(9):991-997.

Chin C.S., Sorenson J., Harris J.B., et al.: The origin of the Haitian cholera outbreak strain. *N Engl J Med* 2011; 364:33-42.

Cohen-Bacrie S., Ninove L., Nougairede A., et al.: Revolutionizing clinical microbiology laboratory organization in hospitals with in situ point-of-care. *PLoS ONE* 2011; 6(7):e22403.

Didelot X., Bowden R., Wilson D.J., et al.: Transforming clinical microbiology with bacterial genome sequencing. *Nat Rev Genet* 2012; 13(9):601-612.

Fournier P.E., Drancourt M., Raoult D.: Bacterial genome sequencing and its use in infectious diseases. *Lancet Infect Dis* 2007; 7:711-723.

Fournier P.E., Thuny F., Richet H., et al.: Comprehensive diagnostic strategy for blood culture-negative endocarditis: a prospective study of 819 new cases. *Clin Infect Dis* 2010; 51(2):131-140.

Lagier J.C., Hugon P., Khelaifia S., et al.: The rebirth of culture in microbiology through the example of culturomics to study human gut microbiota. *Clin Microbiol Rev* 2015; 28(1):237-264.

Maiden M.C., Bygraves J.A., Feil E., et al.: Multilocus sequence typing: a portable approach to the identification of clones within populations of pathogenic microorganisms. *Proc Natl Acad Sci USA* 1998; 95:3140-3145.

Nielsen H.B., Almeida M., Juncker A.S., et al.: Identification and assembly of genomes and genetic elements in complex metagenomic samples without using reference genomes. *Nat Biotechnol* 2014; 32(8):822-828.

Seng P., Rolain J.M., Fournier P.E., et al.: MALDI-TOF-mass spectrometry applications in clinical microbiology. *Future Microbiol* 2010; 5:1733-1754.

162

Acute Gastroenteritis Viruses

ARTURO S. GASTAÑADUY | RODOLFO E. BÉGUÉ

KEY CONCEPTS

- Acute diarrhea is the leading cause of morbidity and second commonest cause of mortality in children <5 years old worldwide.

- Most acute diarrheal illnesses are caused by viruses.

- Noroviruses are the commonest cause of diarrhea in all age groups combined, and rotaviruses are still the leading cause of diarrhea for children <5 years old.

- Transmission is mainly by the fecal–oral route through person-to-person contact, contaminated food and water.

- Most cases of viral diarrhea are mild and self-limiting, but severe cases occur, leading to dehydration and death. Repeated episodes lead to malnutrition.

- Most cases can be managed at home with oral rehydration solutions and feeding a regular diet.

- Vaccines will be the best preventive measure. Only rotavirus vaccines are available.

- Breast-feeding, vitamin A supplementation and zinc significantly reduce the frequency and/or severity of diarrhea.

Introduction

Acute diarrhea is the leading cause of morbidity and second commonest cause of mortality in children aged 0–5 years old. Worldwide estimates for this age group in 2010 were: 1.731 billion cases, with 36 million severe episodes, and 700000 deaths.[1] For older children, adolescents and adults, the estimate is 2.8 billion cases of diarrhea per year.[2] Viruses account for most of acute diarrhea illness,[3] mainly caliciviruses in all age groups and rotaviruses in children. Morphological, epidemiological and clinical characteristics of the main gastroenteritis viruses are presented in Tables 162.1 to 162.3.

Rotaviruses

Described in 1973 by Bishop et al.[4] human rotaviruses (RVs) represent the main agent of acute gastroenteritis in infants and young children worldwide.

Nature

Rotaviruses (RVs) belong to the family Reoviridae.[5] Intact 75 nm particles have a triple-layered structure with a core, and the inner and outer capsid layers. The core encloses the viral genome, consisting of 11 segments of double-stranded RNA. Each segment encodes for one protein, except segment 11 that encodes for two (Figure 162-1, Table 162-4). Six proteins (VP1–VP4, VP6–VP7) form the virion structure. The core is made of VP1, VP2 (its major constituent) and VP3; VP6 is the sole component of the inner capsid; and the outer capsid is composed of VP7 (90%) and VP4. VP4 forms the capsomers, spike-like structures that radiate from the inner to the outer capsid giving the virus its characteristic wheel-like appearance (rota = wheel). In addition, six nonstructural proteins (NSP1–NSP6) are expressed in the infected cell and participate in the replicative cycle.[6,7]

VP6 defines eight antigenic groups (A–H)[8] with group A RVs causing most human infections. The outer capsid proteins VP7 and VP4 elicit neutralization antibodies and determine serotypes, respectively designated as G (for glycoprotein), and P (for protease-sensitive protein). Nowadays, serotyping has been largely replaced by genotyping. Rotaviruses are designated with a dual system of G and P letters followed by a number to notate the serotype and a second number in brackets after P for the genotype, or – more frequently now – a genotype-only designation. For example, the human RV strain Wa is designated G1P1A[8] or G1P[8]. There are at least 27 G and 37 P genotypes.[9]

Epidemiology

Transmission of RVs is mainly from person-to-person by the fecal–oral route.[10] Spread is favored by the large number of virions excreted in feces ($\sim 1 \times 10^{12}$ per mL) and the low infective dose ($\sim 1 \times 10^4$ RV particles).[11] Asymptomatic shedding is frequently detected, especially among young children.[12] Fecal excretion starts immediately before the onset of symptoms and lasts for 5–7 days;[13] longer as detected by polymerase chain reaction (PCR).[14] Outbreaks have been described in nursing homes, hospitals and military bases, with food or water contamination implicated in some outbreaks.[7] Since RVs can survive for 60 days on environmental surfaces,[15] fomites may play a role in settings such as daycare centers and nurseries. RVs have been detected in 20% of cases of travelers' diarrhea.[16] The role of respiratory transmissions is controversial and likely of limited importance.[17]

RVs are the most commonly identified viral enteropathogens of infants and young children worldwide[18] – especially for severe diarrhea. In the USA, before vaccination, RVs caused 3.5 million cases, 55000 hospitalizations, 20–40 deaths and costs of $1 billion annually.[19] Worldwide, the annual estimates were 111 million episodes, 2 million hospitalizations and 600000 deaths.[20] Most affected are children under 5 years of age, with incidence rates peaking at 6–24 months old. Neonates are affected infrequently, and exposed adults become infected frequently (11–70%) but rarely develop clinical disease.[21,22] RVs present as characteristic winter epidemics in North America, marching from the southwest to the northeast.[23] In tropical climates, RVs are endemic throughout the year, with some clustering in the cooler, drier months.

Globally, group A types G1–G4 and G9, in conjunction with P[8] or P[4], constitute most human infections, the most common combination being G1P[8]. However, there is much geographic and temporal variability.[6,24] Multiple types can co-circulate during a specific year.

Pathogenicity

The replication cycle of RV has been reviewed elsewhere.[7] RVs preferentially infect the mature enterocytes of the small intestine. VP4 attaches to sialic acid residues or oligosaccharides of the histo-blood group family on the host cell. Individuals lacking a functional *FUT2* gene (about 20% of the white population) appear resistant to RV infection.[25] VP4 is cleaved into VP5* and VP8* by host proteases initiating the infection. The virus enters enterocytes either by direct membrane penetration or by receptor-mediated endocytosis.[26] Intracellular Ca^{2+} levels trigger virus uncoating and RNA synthesis proceeds in the core of the virion, mediated by VP1.[27,28] RV proteins are synthesized utilizing the host cell translational machinery. The initial steps of virus replication occur in cytoplasmic inclusions. The viral subparticles bud through the membrane of the endoplasmic reticulum and become

TABLE 162-1   Structure and Morphological Characteristics of Gastroenteritis Viruses

Characteristics	Norovirus	Sapovirus	Rotavirus	Astrovirus	Enteric Adenovirus
Family	Caliciviridae	Caliciviridae	Reoviridae	Astroviridae	Adenoviridae
Virion size (nm)	27–35	27–40	70–75	41	70–80
Envelope	Non-enveloped	Non-enveloped	Non-enveloped	Non-enveloped	Non-enveloped
Capsid	Icosahedral	Icosahedral	Triple shelled	Icosahedral	Icosahedral
Genome type	Positive-sense ssRNA	Positive-sense ssRNA	Segmented dsRNA	Positive-sense ssRNA	dsDNA
Morphology on electron microscopy	Round surface, cup-shaped indentations	Round surface, cup-shaped indentations	Wheel-like capsid with radiating spokes	Round, 28–30 nm, 5–6-pointed star shape	Fiber-like projections from vertices
Electron micrograph					

ds, double-stranded; ss, single-stranded.
Norovirus and sapovirus electron micrographs courtesy of C. Humphrey, (CDC). Rotavirus, astrovirus and enteric adenovirus electron micrographs, courtesy of S. Spangenberger.

TABLE 162-2   Epidemiological Characteristics of Gastroenteritis Viruses

Characteristic	Norovirus	Sapovirus	Rotavirus	Astrovirus	Enteric Adenovirus
Age group	All ages	Children	6–24 months	<7 years, elderly	<4 years
Seasonality	Winter	No	Winter	Winter	Summer
Disease pattern	Outbreaks, endemic	Endemic, outbreaks	Endemic, annual epidemics	Endemic, nosocomial outbreaks	Endemic
Transmission	Person-to-person, water, food, shellfish	Person-to-person, water, cold foods, shellfish	Person-to-person, food, water	Person-to-person, food, water	Person-to-person
Fecal excretion (days)	13–56 Median: 28	–	10	–	Persistent, months
Outpatient prevalence (%)	Endemic: 10–25 Outbreaks: 90	1–10	5–10	7–8	4–8
Inpatient prevalence (%)	Frequent	3–5	35–40	3–5	5–20

TABLE 162-3   Usual Clinical Characteristics of Gastroenteritis Virus Infections

Signs and Symptoms	Norovirus	Sapovirus	Rotavirus	Astrovirus	Enteric Adenovirus
Prodrome (days)	1–2	1–3	1–3	3–4	8–10
Diarrhea: watery	66–95% 4–8/day Adults >children	88–95% mild	96–100% 10–20/day	72–100% 2–4/day	97% 1/3 >14 days
Vomitus	57–95% Children >adults	44–65%	80–90% Early	20–50% 1/day	79% Early
Fever	24–48% Low grade	18–34%	60–65% Moderate	20% Low grade	Occasionally Low grade
Abdominal pain	11–91% cramps	–	Colicky	50%	–
Dehydration	~1%	Infrequent	Frequent in young children	Infrequent	Infrequent
Other symptoms	Myalgia 26%, headache 22%	Respiratory 22%, myalgia, headache	Respiratory 22–52%	Malaise, respiratory	Respiratory occasionally
Duration of illness (days)	0.5–2.5	4	3–8	2–3	5–12

mature particles. NSP4 plays a key role in the assembly process of these particles, which is Ca^{2+} dependent. Lastly, mature viruses are released by cell lysis or by vesicular transport.[7]

Infected intestinal cells change from columnar to cuboidal, with fewer and shorter microvilli; the cells are sloughed off resulting in shorter villi. Changes occur within 24 hours of infection, start proximally and progress caudally.[4,29] Diarrhea results from a mixture of causes: decreased absorption of salt and water secondary to enterocyte damage and replacement of absorptive intestinal cells by secreting cells from the crypts; loss of disaccharides at the damaged brush border

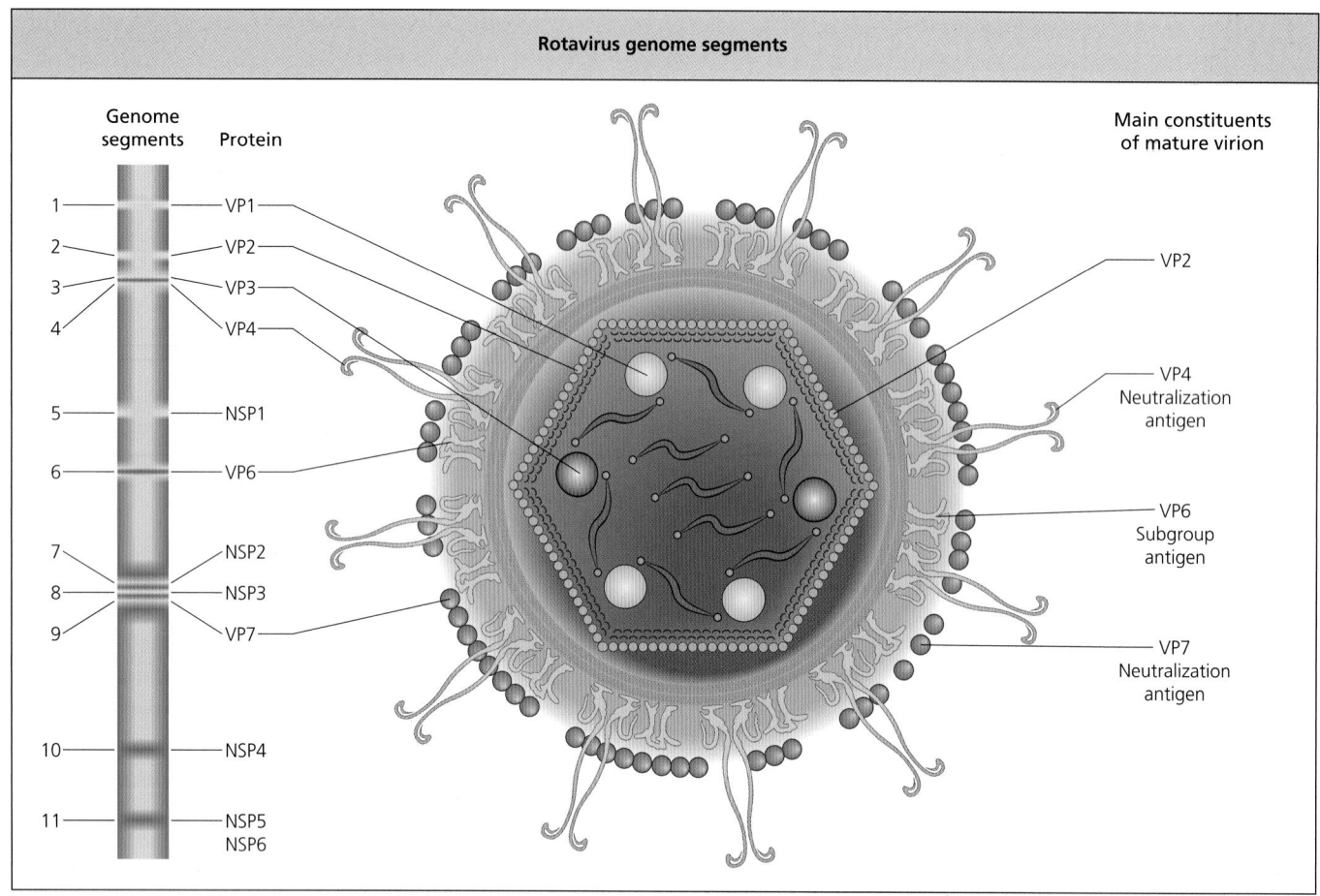

Figure 162-1   Rotavirus genome segments, protein products and their location in the viral particle. (*Adapted with permission from Gentsch J.R., Laird A.R., Bielfelt B., Griffin D.D., Banyai K., Ramachandran M., et al. Serotype diversity and reassortment between human and animal rotavirus strains: implications for rotavirus vaccine programs. J Infect Dis 2005; 192 (Suppl 1):S146-59.*)

TABLE 162-4	Rotavirus Genome Segments and Their Corresponding Viral Proteins			
Genome Segment (Size, Bp)	**Protein Product (MW, Kda)**	**Location in Virus Particles**	**Function**	
1 (3302)	VP1 (125)	Core capsid	RNA-dependent RNA polymerase, complex with VP3	
2 (2729)	VP2 (94)	Core capsid	Main constituent of core, RNA binding	
3 (2591)	VP3 (88)	Core capsid	Complex with VP1, guanylyl and methyl transferase, synthesis of capped mRNA transcripts	
4 (2359)	VP4 (86.7)	Outer capsid	Hemagglutinin, cell attachment, neutralization antigen, determines P serotypes, cleaved by trypsin into VP5*(52.9) and VP8*(24.7) virulence	
5 (1566)	NSP1 (58.6)	Nonstructural	Basic protein, RNA binding	
6 (1356)	VP6 (44.8)	Inner capsid	Main constituent of inner capsid, determines group specificity, protection, required for transcription	
7 (1074)	NSP3 (34.6)	Nonstructural	Acidic protein, RNA binding, inhibits host cell translation	
8 (1059)	NSP2 (36.7)	Nonstructural	Basic protein, RNA binding, forms viroplasms with NSP5	
9 (1062)	VP7 (37.4)	Outer capsid	Glycoprotein, major constituent of outer capsid, determines G serotypes	
10 (750)	NSP4 (20.2)	Nonstructural	Role in morphogenesis, interacts with viroplasms, modulates intracellular Ca^{2+} and RNA replication, enterotoxin, virulence	
11 (664)	NSP5 (21.7)	Nonstructural	Role in morphogenesis, forms viroplasms with NSP2, interacts with VP2 and NSP6	
11 (664)	NSP6 (12)	Nonstructural	Interacts with NSP5, present in viroplasms	

Bp, base pairs; MW, molecular weight.
Adapted with permission from Estes M.K., Kapikian A.Z. Visualization by immune electron microscopy of a 27 nm particle associated with acute infectious nonbacterial gastroenteritis. J Virol 1972; 10:1075-81.

resulting in carbohydrate malabsorption and osmotic diarrhea; and the effect of NSP4, a viral enterotoxin that increases plasma membrane chloride permeability leading to secretory diarrhea.[30] RV RNA and replicating viruses are frequently detected in blood and cerebrospinal fluid,[31] showing that RV represents a systemic infection with increase of pro-inflammatory cytokines.[32]

Immunity against RVs is likely multifactorial; involving local (mucosal) and systemic (serum) antibodies as well as innate and cellular immunity.[33,34] VP7 and VP4 induce serum-neutralizing antibodies against the infecting serotype (homotypic) that appear within 2 weeks of infection and correlate with protection.[21] Heterotypic antibodies (those against different serotypes) also occur, but mainly among adults and are dependent on the infecting strain. Homotypic protection lasts longer than heterotypic protection but is incomplete and short lived.[21] Anti-RV antibody levels are high at birth (transplacentally acquired), decline by 3–6 months, rise to a peak at 2–3 years and remain elevated throughout life (probably because of repeated, mostly asymptomatic infections).[35] Serum antibodies do not always prevent infection, pointing to the potential role of mucosal immunity. For example, IgA deficient mice shed RV for a prolonged time and are not protected against reinfection.[31] Furthermore, mucosal immunity, passively acquired by breast-feeding[36] or by orally administered immune globulins[37] ameliorates RV symptoms. Mucosal immunity develops 4 weeks after infection and persists for several months, eventually decreasing with advancing age.[38] Experimental and clinical data suggest a role for non-neutralizing anti-VP6[39-41] and other antibodies[42] in protection against RV disease. Cell-mediated immunity also seems important. In mice, RV-specific cytotoxic T cells appear in the intestinal mucosa soon after infection, and mice with severe combined immunodeficiency are able to clear RV infection when reconstituted with CD8 T cells, despite their lack of antibodies against the virus.[43] Lastly, the role of innate immunity is being explored.[44]

Clinical Manifestations

The clinical spectrum of RV infections ranges from asymptomatic to severe disease with dehydration and death; severity may be associated with antigenemia.[45] The usual clinical picture is presented in Table 162-3; in addition, transaminase elevation occurs in about 15% of cases[46] and neurological manifestations are increasingly recognized.[47] The disease is self-limiting and chronic infection has not been described in the normal host.[35] Neonatal RV infections are symptomatic in only 10–20% of cases and usually mild,[48] but severe infections may occur among premature infants and those in special care units.[49] Immunodeficient individuals can present a chronic or serious course with associated mortality.[50] Children with human immunodeficiency virus (HIV) infection, and not receiving antiretroviral therapy, may have a twofold risk of RV symptomatic infection and more prolonged virus shedding, but the severity of the illness itself may be similar to that seen in HIV-uninfected children.[51,52]

Diagnostic Microbiology

Antigen detection kits based on enzyme immunoassays (EIAs) and latex agglutination are the tests of choice for most clinical circumstances with high sensitivity and specificity (70–100%). Samples should be obtained during the symptomatic period. If samples are not to be processed immediately, they can be stored at 39.2°F (4°C) or frozen. A semi-nested reverse transcription polymerase chain reaction (RT-PCR) test allows for G and P genotyping.[53] In special situations, other tests can be considered: electron microscopy (EM), gel electrophoresis of viral RNA, hybridization of radiolabeled nucleic acid probes and viral culture. Serologic tests are rarely used. Neutralizing antibodies can be detected by plaque reduction or cytopathic effect inhibition.

Caliciviruses: *Norovirus, Sapovirus*

In 1972, Kapikian *et al.*, investigating a gastroenteritis outbreak in Norwalk, Ohio, visualized 27 nm particles in a stool filtrate and noted

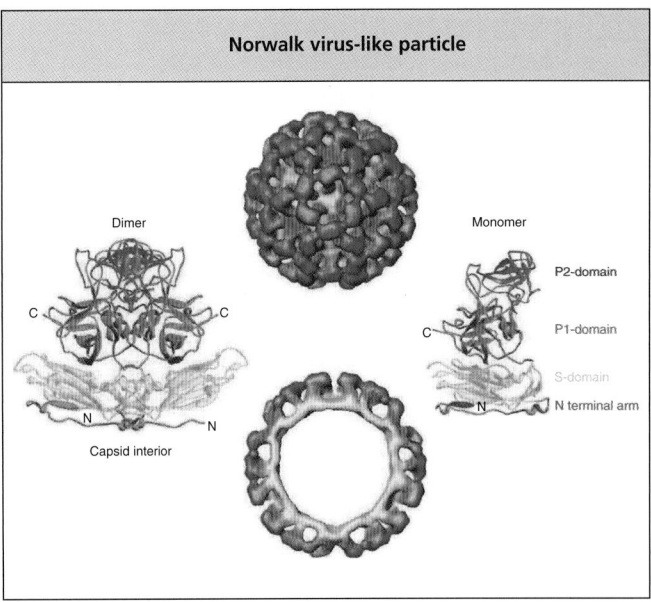

Figure 162-2   Norwalk virus-like particle. (*Adapted from Hutson* et al. Trends Microbiol 2004; 12:279–87, with permission.)

that infected individuals developed specific antibody response against the particles. The particles were named Norwalk virus (NV). This was the first confirmation of a virus as an etiological agent of gastroenteritis.[54] Similar viruses were named by the location where they were first identified (Hawaii, Sapporo, etc.) and, as a group, were known as Norwalk-like viruses or small round structured viruses (SRSVs). Cloning of the NV genome led to the classification of these viruses within the Caliciviridae family.[55]

Nature

Caliciviruses (CV) are small (27–40 nm), non-enveloped viruses with a single-stranded positive-sense RNA genome. They have an icosahedral capsid with cup-like depressions on the viral surface (*calici* is derived from the Latin word *calyx* = cup) (Figure 162-2).

Five genera have been identified in the Caliciviridae family: *Lagovirus, Nebovirus, Vesivirus, Norovirus* (NoV) and *Sapovirus* (SaV). *Lagovirus, Nebovirus* and *Vesivirus* only infect animals. NoV and SaV have human and animal strains and are further classified into genogroups, genotypes (genetic clusters) and subgenotypes or variants (Table 162-5).[5,56] Both NoV and SaV produce diarrheal illness in humans and NoV is the leading cause of acute gastroenteritis worldwide.

The CV genomes are about 7.3–8.5 kilobases in length and organized in two or three open reading frames (ORFs). In the genera with three ORFs (NoV and *Vesivirus*) the first ORF (ORF1) encodes for a large protein that by proteolytic cleavage produces the NSPs. The ORF2 encodes for the single major structural protein (VP1), and the ORF3 encodes for a minor structural protein (VP2). The *Nebovirus* and *Lagovirus* have only 2 ORFs. In these viruses, VP1 and VP2 are encoded in ORF1 and ORF2, respectively.[56]

A typical CV (Norwalk virus) capsid is formed by 90 VP1 dimers with 90 arch-like protruding capsomers arranged in such a way as to leave 32 calices on the viral surface. The VP1 has two major domains: the shell (S) domain and the protruding (P) domain. The S domain forms the inner part of the capsid. It has 225 amino acids (aa), including aa 10-49 corresponding to the N terminal region of the protein (N subdomain), which faces the interior of the capsid. The P domain includes amino acids 226–520 and is subdivided into subdomains P1 and P2. The P1 subdomain (aa 226–278 and 406–520) form the sides of the capsomers whereas the P2 subdomain (aa 279–405) form the most protruding part of the capsomers' arch (Figure 162-2). Each virion has only one or two copies of the VP2 (~22–29 kDa). The VP2

TABLE 162-5	Taxonomy of the Caliciviridae Family			
Genus	**Genogroups**	**Genetic Clusters**	**Representative Species**	**Representative Strain***
Norovirus (NoV)	I	1–8	Norwalk virus	Hu/NoV/GI.1/Norwalk/1968/US
	II	1–19	Hawaii norovirus	Hu/Nov/GII.1/Hawaii/1971/US
	III	1–2	Bovine norovirus	Bo/NoV/GIII.1/Jena/1980/DE
	IV	1	Alphatron virus	Hu/Nov/GIV.1/Alphatron98-2/1998/NL
	V	1	Murine norovirus	M/NoV/GV.1/MNV-1/2003/US
Sapovirus (SaV)	I	1–3	Sapporo virus	Hu/SaV/G1.1/Sapporo/1982/JP
	II	1–3	London sapovirus	Hu/SaV/GII.1/London/1992/UK
	III	1	Swine sapovirus	Sw/SaV/GIII.1/PEC-Cowden/1980/US
	IV	1	Houston sapovirus	Hu/SaV/GIV.1/Hou7-1181/1990/US
	V	1	Argentina sapovirus	Hu/Sav/GV.1/Argentina 39/AR
Lagovirus (LaV)			Rabbit hemorrhagic disease virus	Ra/LaV/RHDV/GH/1988/DE
			European brown hare syndrome virus	Ha/LaV/EBHSV/GD/1989/FR
Vesivirus (VeV)			Vesicular exanthema of swine virus	SW/VeV/VESV/A48/1948/US
			Feline calicivirus	Fe/VeV/FCV/F9/1958/US
Nebovirus (NeV)			Newbury 1 virus	Bo/BV/Newbury-1/1976/UK

Host species abbreviations: Bo, bovine; Fe, feline; Ha, hare; Hu, human; M, murine; Ra, rabbit; Sw, swine.
Country abbreviations: AR, Argentina; DE, Germany; FR, France; JP, Japan; NL, Netherlands; UK, United Kingdom; US, United States.
*Host species/genus/species or genogroup/strain name/year of occurrence/country of origin.
Adapted with permission from Green et al. J Infect Dis 2000; 181:S322-S330.

function is not completely understood; it appears to interact with the genome RNA during virus replication.[57] VP1 and VP2 self assemble into virus-like particles (VLPs) without RNA participation. VP2 is not needed for VLPs assembly but is essential for infections in feline calicivirus. The VLPs are morphologically and antigenically similar to natural virions.[58] The NoV has six nonstructural proteins with different functions: NSP 1/2 (p48), replication complex formation; NSP3 (NTPase), nucleoside triphosphatase/RNA helicase; NSP4 (p22), replication complex formation; NSP5 (VPg), genome linked protein involved in translation and replication; NSP6 (3CL, Pro), protease; and NSP7 (Pol, RdRp), RNA-dependent RNA polymerase. They play a role in the replication process of the genome RNA.[57,59]

Epidemiology

Human caliciviruses (HuCV) have worldwide distribution, and NoV infects persons of all ages, both in high-income and low- and middle-income countries (LMIC).[60] They are the most common cause of gastroenteritis outbreaks, and they are also recognized as the most common cause of endemic gastroenteritis.[61] In the USA, NoV produces 400 000 emergency department visits and 1.7 million office visits per year;[62] it also accounts for 19–21 million illnesses, 56 000–71 000 hospitalizations and 570–800 deaths.[63] Norovirus is the most commonly detected pathogen (26%) in adults with gastroenteritis.[64,65] In a 2009–2010 study of children under 5 years of age with acute gastroenteritis, RV and NoV were detected in 12 and 21 of the cases, respectively. The study conclusion is that 'norovirus has become the leading cause of medically attended gastroenteritis in US children' being responsible for approximately 1 million healthcare visits yearly.[66]

Norovirus infections occur mainly during the cold seasons. Almost 80% of cases and 71% of outbreaks occur from October to March in the northern hemisphere and from April to September in the southern hemisphere. The reasons for seasonality are not well understood but rainfall may play a role. Breaks in seasonality pattern have been observed with the emergence of new variant strains.[67]

Norovirus infections start early in life; a Finnish study found that the prevalence of GII-4 IgG antibodies was 47% in children aged 7–23 months and 91% after 5 years of age.[68] A birth cohort study in Peru followed 220 and 189 children for 1 and 2 years, respectively. By 1 year 80% of the children had at least one norovirus infection and by 2 years 71% had one or more episodes of norovirus-associated diarrhea.[69] Genogroups I and II strains produce the majority of infections. At a given time, most infections are caused by a major circulating strain. For example, after 2000, GII genogroup caused 96% of sporadic infections in children worldwide[70] and genogroup II.4 strains has caused more than 80% of US outbreaks since the 1990s.[71] Coinfections with different strains occur, giving the opportunity for the exchange of genetic material between strains and the generation of new virus variants.[72] Pandemic variants emerge every 2–4 years. Outbreaks occur mainly in daycare centers, schools, colleges, hospitals, nursing homes, military barracks, restaurants, vacation facilities and cruise ships. NoV also causes travelers' diarrhea. NoV can spread internationally through contaminated food or beverages.[73] A study of 8271 food-borne outbreaks of gastroenteritis showed a median of affected persons of 25 versus 10 for the bacterial outbreaks. Ten percent of the individuals required medical care and 1% were hospitalized.[74]

Sapovirus epidemiology is summarized in Table 162-2. Detection rates vary for different countries, and are much lower than those of NoV and illness is milder. Environment, eating habits and hygiene practices likely play a role in the different attack rates.[75]

Caliciviruses are ubiquitous and stable in the environment, providing a persistent source of infection. Noroviruses survive freezing, heating to 60°C (140°F) for 30 minutes and are stable in water chlorinated to 6.25 mg/L; most municipal water systems contain <5 mg/L of chlorine. The virus is also acid-resistant and ether-stable.[76,77] Caliciviruses are transmitted by the fecal–oral and vomit–oral routes. Sporadic and outbreak cases are spread mainly by person-to-person contact; the patients are more contagious during the first few days of illness. Contaminated food or water are important causes of outbreaks. Transmission through contaminated objects or surfaces in the environment is likely important and may last 2 weeks or longer.[78] Inhalation and swallowing of aerosols produced by vomiting or toilet flushing may also play a role in norovirus spread.[79]

Pathogenicity

The 50% human infectious dose is 1320 genome equivalents.[80] The median incubation period is 1.2 days, 5% of patients develop symptoms in 0.5 days and 95% of them will be symptomatic in 2.6 days.[81] Studies of NoV infections in volunteers described pathological changes in the proximal portions of the small intestine with broadening and blunting of the villi, crypt cell hyperplasia, cytoplasm vacuolization and mononuclear cell infiltration in the lamina propria. Brush border enzymes are decreased, producing malabsorption of carbohydrates and fat. The changes are transient and resolve within 2 weeks.[82,83] No histological lesions are seen in the gastric or rectal mucosa, and the secretion of hydrochloric acid, pepsin and intrinsic factor remain normal.[84] Gastric emptying is markedly delayed, which could explain the frequency of nausea and vomiting; however, the degree of delay does not correlate with the severity of vomiting.[85] Reduction of villous surface area, and sealing junctional proteins as well as increased active anion secretion, cytotoxic intraepithelial lymphocytes and apoptosis, have been observed suggesting that norovirus diarrhea is caused by a leak flux and secretory component.[86] Virus shedding in the stools begins during the prodrome stage, lasts 13–56 days (median 28 days)[87] and it can persist for several weeks after resolution of symptoms, especially in infants and for months to years in immunocompromised patients.[88,89]

Norovirus infection starts when the protruding domain (P) of the VP1 binds specific carbohydrate receptors on the cell membrane; thereafter NoV enters the cell by a process that requires a protein receptor. This is followed by virus uncoating and release of VPg-linked RNA genome to the cytoplasm. Genome replication starts with a negative-sense RNA intermediate. This process is performed by NSP7 (RdRp). The genome functions as an mRNA for the first viral RNA translation, and becomes a template for a double-stranded replication form (RF). Thereafter positive-sense RNA synthesis begins. During the replication process, full genome and subgenomic RNA are formed. Subgenomic RNA consists of the last 2.4 kb of the genome (ORF2+ORF3), and it is also attached to VPg. The ORF1 generates the polyprotein that after cleavage produces the NSPs. NS1/2 and NS4 recruit cellular membranes to form a replication complex. Both VP1 and VP2 capsid proteins are translated mainly by subgenomic RNA. VP1 self-assembles to form the capsid or VLP. Nevertheless VP2 is required for infectivity. The mechanisms of viral assembly and release of the virions are poorly understood; apoptosis has been proposed as an exit strategy. It is assumed that HuNoV replication occurs in the epithelial cells of the upper gastrointestinal tract; however, no viral particles have been observed by EM of the jejunum mucosa[59,90] (Figure 162-3).

Susceptibility to NV is peculiar. Some individuals have natural resistance to the infection. They lack virus receptors; repeated challenges with the virus fail to produce illness or antibody response. Norovirus receptors are the histo-blood group antigens (HBGAs). HBGAs are complex carbohydrates present on the surface of erythrocytes, enterocytes and other mucosal cells. HBGAs include the ABO, Lewis and secretor families. HBGAs production is genetically controlled. The *FUT2* gene controls the expression of fucosyltransferase 2 in saliva and mucosal secretions. Individuals who do not have the *FUT2* gene are called non-secretors. Twenty percent of Europeans are non-secretors and resistant to infection with the NV. Recognition of carbohydrate receptors is a common characteristic of calicivirus. Different CV have different carbohydrates receptors which determine host and tissue tropism.[91,92]

Norovirus immunity studies are difficult because there is no cell culture system or small animal model. Human volunteer and natural infections studies demonstrate virus-specific antibody response. Serum IgG, IgM and IgA as well as mucosal IgA antibodies are produced. Cell-mediated immunity has been induced by VLP. Serum IgG antibodies persist for months, IgM and IgA are short lived, mucosal IgA persistence is not known.[90,93] Antibody presence does not always correlate with protection; however, early (<5 days) mucosal IgA

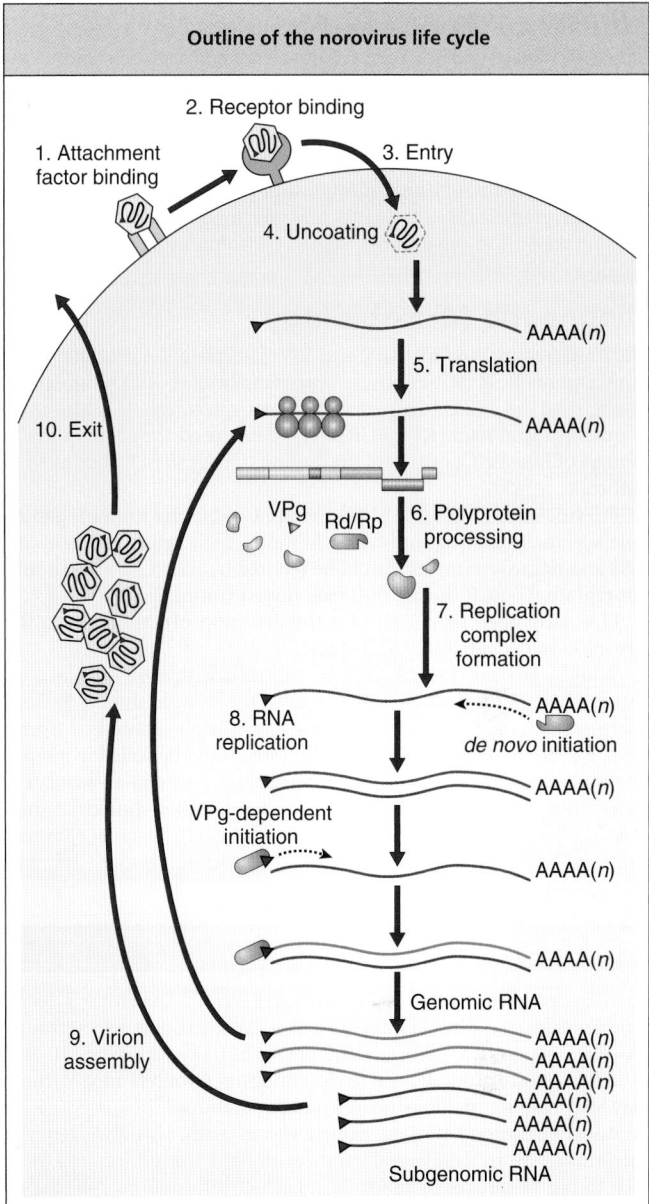

Figure 162-3   Outline of the norovirus life cycle. (1) HuNoV and MNoV are thought to attach to the cell surface using various carbohydrate attachment factors. This is not sufficient to mediate entry, and binding to an unidentified protein receptor is thought to be required (2). Entry (3) and uncoating (4) proceed through as-yet-undefined pathways. (5) The incoming viral genome is translated, through interactions with VPg at the 5' end of the genome (red triangle) and the cellular translation machinery. (6) The ORF1 polyprotein is co- and post-translationally cleaved by the viral protease NS6. (7) The replication complex is formed by recruitment of cellular membranes to the perinuclear region of the cell (not shown), through interactions in part with NS1/2 and NS4. (8) Genome replication occurs via a negative-strand intermediate, and genomic and subgenomic RNA are generated by the viral RdRp (NS7), using both *de novo* and VPg-dependent mechanisms of RNA synthesis. (9) The replicated genomes are translated (within the replication complex) or packaged into the capsid, VP1, for virion assembly and exit (10). *(Adapted from Thorne L.G., Goodfellow I.G. Norovirus gene expression and replication. J Gen Virol 2014; 95(Pt 2):278-91.)*

production protects against infection.[94] Earlier studies suggested that immunity is mostly short-term (6 months–2 years) and type-specific; however, several clinical and epidemiological observations were inconsistent with this notion. Mathematical models of community transmission of norovirus estimated immunity duration for gastroenteritis at 4.1– 8.7 years.[95]

Clinical Manifestations

The usual clinical characteristics of norovirus and sapovirus infections are presented in Table 162-3. Most of the time, infections are acute, short-lived or asymptomatic. Nevertheless, severe or prolonged illness and death may occur. Severe outcomes have been associated with the GII.4 NoV strains. Populations at risk include the elderly in healthcare facilities, young infants, and immunosuppressed individuals. Chronic debilitating conditions are usually present. Immediate causes of death include: aspiration pneumonia, sepsis, gastrointestinal bleeding, perforation or necrotizing enterocolitis.[96]

Diagnostic Microbiology

The preferred method for NoV and SaV detection is real-time reverse transcription-PCR (RT-PCR). It is very sensitive (10–100 virions) and can be used for clinical and environmental specimens. It is also used to quantify viral load (RT-qPCR). RT-PCR is used for genotyping by Centers of Disease Control and Prevention (CDC) surveillance of NoV outbreaks.

Enzyme immunoassays (EIAs) are rapid and useful for testing multiple specimens during outbreaks; however, their sensitivity is about 50% and negative samples should be retested by RT-PCR. EIAs should not replace RT-PCR during outbreak investigations.

EIAs have been very useful for the detection of antibodies to the viruses in sero-epidemiological studies.[97]

Whole diarrhea stools should be collected within 48–72 hours of illness. If testing is done within 3 weeks, the sample should be kept refrigerated at 39°F (4°C); for longer times, samples should be frozen at −4°F (−20°C). For shipping, each sample should be sealed in a separate plastic bag and kept on frozen refrigerant packs in an insulated, waterproof, polystyrene container. Vomitus samples should be processed in the same way as stools. Water and environmental samples, and food and shellfish samples, should be processed under CDC and FDA guidance respectively.[98]

Enteric Adenoviruses

Enteric adenoviruses were first described in 1975.[99] The family Adenoviridae includes 57 human adenoviruses classified into seven groups (A–G). Most are respiratory adenoviruses but two, serotypes 40 and 41 that belong to group F, are enteric pathogens. Group D adenoviruses may also be enteropathogenic in some populations.[100]

Adenoviruses are non-enveloped viruses with a dsDNA genome surrounded by an icosahedral capsid with fiber-like projections from each of the 12 vertices (Table 162-1). Each virion contains 240 hexons (the major surface protein) and 12 pentons. Each penton consists of a base and a fiber. Genus-specific antigens are located in the hexon. Type-specific antigens are located in the hexon and the fiber and elicit serum-neutralizing antibodies. The fiber protein of most adenoviruses binds to the coxsackie–adenovirus receptor (CAR) of epithelial cells. The penton base mediates internalization of the virus. Infected cells degenerate in a process dependent on the E3 virus protein.[101] The mechanism(s) by which serotypes 40 and 41 induce gastroenteritis remains unclear.

Enteric adenoviruses have worldwide distribution, mainly affecting young children, and are responsible for 4% of acute gastroenteritis episodes seen in outpatient clinics and 2–22% seen in hospitalized children.[102] Outbreaks lasting 7–44 days have occurred in hospitals and daycare centers with approximately 40% of children infected, half of them asymptomatically.[103] Transmission is person-to-person by the fecal–oral route. Infected persons develop group- and type-specific antibodies that confer long-term immunity. Stool excretion of adenoviruses lasts 10–14 days, from 2 days before to 5 days after end of diarrhea. Asymptomatic excretion may last months to years; thus, their isolation in diarrheic stools does not necessarily mean acute infection. Adenoviruses are less resistant than RVs and are rapidly inactivated at 133°F (56°C) and by exposure to ultraviolet light or formalin. Viral antigen detection in stool by immunoassay is the diagnostic test of choice, sensitivity and specificity are 98% when compared with EM. Real-time RT-PCR has proven superior to immunoassays and EM.[104] PCR amplification can be used for serotype determination. Serological tests are rarely used but specific antibodies can be detected by neutralization or hemagglutination inhibition assays. Enteric adenoviruses are difficult to grow in routine cell lines (e.g. Intestine 407, HEK293 and others), but isolation methods are improving.[105] The clinical manifestations of enteric adenoviruses are presented in Table 162-3. In general, the disease is milder but more prolonged than that with RV. Treatment is supportive. Cidofovir (or its oral lipid conjugate brincidofovir) alone or with ribavirin have been used for immunocompromised patients.

Astroviruses

Astroviruses belong to the family Astroviridae. They were first described in 1975 as small (28 nm) particles with a five- or six-pointed star appearance on EM.[106] Later studies showed an icosahedral, 41 nm morphology with well-defined spikes (Figure 162-4). Subjected to high pH, they transform to the previously described star.[106] The virus is non-enveloped, with a single-stranded, positive-sense RNA genome that contains three ORFs. ORF1a and ORF1b encode the viral protease and polymerase, respectively. ORF2 encodes a protein capsid precursor, which gives rise to VP32, VP29 and VP26 (structural capsid proteins). VP26 and VP29 appear to be responsible for antigenic variation.[107] Eight serotypes have been described (HAstV-1 to HAstV-8). Astroviruses infect mammals and birds and some transmission may be zoonotic.[108] Human astroviruses are responsible for 2–4% of endemic diarrhea in children worldwide; HAstV-1 is the most prevalent.[109,110] They have been associated with outbreaks in daycare centers, schools and pediatric wards. Infection confers protective antibodies, which increase with age (>80% of adults have antibodies). Immunocompromised subjects and the elderly may also be affected.[111]

Histopathologic studies show infection of mature epithelial cells of the small intestine,[112] without inflammatory response. The virus is inactivated by methanol 70–90% and heating at 140°F (60°C) for 10 minutes; however, it is resistant to chloroform and ethanol. Diagnosis can be made by commercial immunoassays with good sensitivity and specificity when compared with EM and RT-PCR.[110] Astroviruses can be grown in Caco-2 cells. The clinical characteristics of astrovirus infection are presented in Table 162-3. Symptoms are similar to those of RV infection but less severe. Management is supportive.

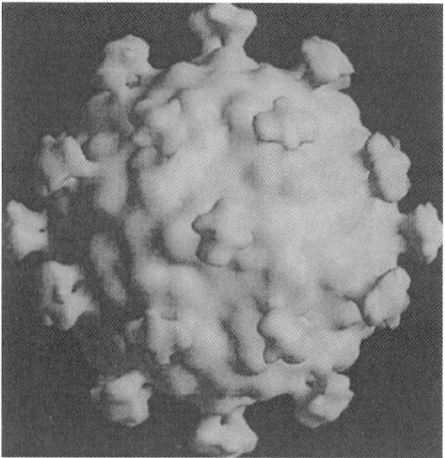

Figure 162-4 Three-dimensional reconstruction of cryoelectron microscopy image of human astrovirus. (*Reproduced with permission from Mendez E., Arias C. Astroviruses. In: Knipe D.M. et al., eds. Field's virology. 5th ed. Philadelphia: Lippincott Williams and Wilkins 2007: 981-1000.*)

Other Viruses

Cases of human gastroenteritis have been associated with parechoviruses, enteroviruses, cardioviruses, kuboviruses, coronaviruses, toroviruses, pestiviruses; parvoviruses, picobirnaviruses; and others, but their role as agents of gastroenteritis is under study.

Management

Most viral gastroenteritis cases are of mild to moderate severity and self-limited. Severe illness occurs mainly in young children, the elderly and immunocompromised patients. No specific antivirals exist for any of the gastroenteritis viruses.

Primary objectives of management are prevention and treatment of dehydration and malnutrition. Most patients can be treated at home with oral rehydration solutions (ORS) and feeding with their regular diet.[113] ORS may prevent 93% of diarrheal deaths.[114] Occasionally, hospitalization and intravenous fluids may be needed for severe illness.

Although lactose malabsorption develops frequently during acute gastroenteritis, most children can be fed lactose-containing formulas in small frequent feeds. Human milk, despite its high lactose content, reduces stool output and provides excellent nutrients and anti-infectious factors; therefore, breast-feeding should be continued. The protective effects of breast-feeding on diarrhea morbidity and mortality have been confirmed.[115]

A specially formulated ORS (ReSoMal) with less sodium, more potassium and glucose and the addition of magnesium, copper and zinc, as well as continuous feeding with calorie-dense foods, are recommended for malnourished patients.[116] The Ready-to-Use Therapeutic Foods have been proven successful.[117]

In LMIC, vitamin A supplementation reduces all-cause diarrhea mortality by 30% in children aged 6–59 months; and zinc, given for 10–14 days during and after a diarrheal episode, decreases diarrhea mortality by 23%.[118,119]

Antiemetics are usually unnecessary; single dose ondansetron can reduce vomiting, use of intravenous fluids and length of stay[120] but its routine use is not supported by the CDC.[121] Adsorbents (kaolin, pectin) and antimotility agents (opiates, loperamide) do not affect the diarrhea mechanisms and may have serious side effects such as paralytic ileus.

Nitazoxanide, bismuth subsalicylate, probiotics, bovine colostrum and human serum immunoglobulin have been tried in patients with severe illness with modest effect. Development of specific antivirals is still in a very early stage.[122]

Prevention

Hygienic measures decrease person-to-person spread; however, these measures are difficult to enforce in situations involving crowding, young children, nursing homes, etc. Some viruses may survive in the environment for weeks and are resistant to commonly used disinfectants, so transmission of the disease continues even in places with good sanitation. Outbreaks require furloughing ill personnel, thoroughly cooking food, disinfecting the environment and properly handling food, water and sanitation. Careful hand washing cannot be overemphasized, especially among food handlers and personnel from hospitals, schools and daycare centers. Hospitalized or other institutionalized patients should be placed under universal precautions with added contact isolation until 48–72 hours after symptoms resolution.[123]

Chemical disinfectants can interrupt virus spread from the environment. Special attention should be given to bathrooms, door knobs, hand rails and food preparation surfaces. Commonly used disinfectants are 70% ethanol, 6% hydrogen peroxide, 2500 ppm chlorine, povidone–iodine, ultraviolet radiation and heat. Since fecal matter inactivates the hypochlorites, it should be removed before application. Household laundry can be washed with detergent and bleach, followed by a drying cycle. Heat (176°F (80°C)) for at least 1 minute or high pressure processing have also been used.[124]

Breast-feeding may reduce the severity and duration of RV illness, but not the incidence,[36] and depending on the population being

TABLE 162-6	Comparison of Two Licensed Rotavirus Vaccines	
Name	**RotaTeq®**	**Rotarix®**
Producer	Merck & Co., Inc.	GlaxoSmithKline
Vaccine type	Live, bovine–human reassortant	Live-attenuated human RV strain (RIX4414)
Serotypes	Pentavalent: G1, G2, G3, G4, P1[8]	Monovalent: G1P[8]
Dose	>2 × 10⁶ infective doses, each	>1 × 10⁶ infective doses
Administration	Oral, three doses at 2, 4 and 6 months of age	Oral, two doses at 2 and 4 months of age
Intussusception risk*	~1/100 000	~5/100 000
Efficacy:†		
RV GE, any severity	74 (67–80)	73 (27–91)
RV GE, severe	98 (88–100)	85 (72–92)
All diarrhea hospitalization	59 (52–65)	42 (29–53)
Virus shedding	9%	50–80%

GE, gastroenteritis; RV, rotavirus.
*Odds ratio vaccine vs placebo (95% CI).
†Percent decrease vaccine vs placebo (95% CI).

studied,[125,126] artificial formulas supplemented with probiotics may reduce the incidence of diarrhea and shorten RV shedding.[127] The most practical and effective intervention to prevent gastroenteritis is vaccination. However, such vaccines are available only for rotavirus.

The first commercial RV vaccine, RotaShield® (Wyeth-Ayerst Laboratories), was licensed in the USA in 1998. The vaccine was 49% effective in preventing all RV diarrheas and 80% effective in preventing severe RV diarrhea,[128] but it was suspended due to an association with intussusception, estimated as one additional case/10 000 vaccinated infants.[129] A decade later, two new RV vaccines were licensed. RotaTeq® (or RV5), a live vaccine (Table 162-6) containing five bovine–human reassortant strains, four expressing human G1–G4 with bovine P7⁵ specificity, and one expressing bovine G6 with human P1[8]. Three doses administered at 2, 4 and 6 months of age demonstrated 74% efficacy to prevent any RV disease and 98% of severe disease.[130] A second RV vaccine, Rotarix® (or RV1) is a live monovalent vaccine (Table 162-6) derived of a human attenuated strain 89–12 of G1P[8] specificity. Two doses at 2 and 4 months proved effective in preventing any (73%) or severe (85%) RV disease.[131] The World Health Organization recommended inclusion of RV vaccines into national immunization programs in the Americas and Europe in 2007 and worldwide in 2009.[132]

In the USA, RV5 was introduced in 2006 and RV1 in 2008, resulting in >80% reduction in RV-related hospitalization, emergency department (ED) visits and outpatient visits. Concomitantly, there was ~50% decrease in all-cause gastroenteritis visits and hospitalizations. The benefit has been noted even with single dose of either vaccine and has included heterotypic protection.[133] Herd immunity is also present with either vaccine.[134] Countries that introduced RV vaccines have seen a virtual disappearance of the previously predominant G1P[8] strains and a proportional increase of other genotypes, especially G3P[8] (mainly seen in those using RV5) and G2P[4] (mainly in those using RV1).[135-137] Whether the change represents an effect of vaccine pressure or rather secular changes in circulating RV strains is unclear.

Studies in LMIC in Africa[138] and Asia[139] showed lower efficacy of RV5 and RV1 with prevention of severe disease varying between 39% and 77%.[140]

Post-licensure surveillance has detected risk of intussusception for RV5 and RV1, mainly after the first dose and estimated at 1–5 additional cases/100 000 infants vaccinated.[141,142] This risk is considered small and is outweighed by the benefits of vaccination.[143]

Some countries are pursuing their own RV vaccines but few have advanced through clinical testing. The Lanzhou Lamb RV (LLR) vaccine has been licensed in China since 2000 with reported effectiveness of 73% and 44% for RV-hospitalizations and all RV diarrhea respectively.[144,145] In India, a vaccine is being developed based on a natural human-bovine RV reassortant (116E) with 54% efficacy to prevent severe RV disease.[146] Few other candidate vaccines have entered early phase clinical trials.

No licensed vaccine exists against norovirus. Vaccine development has been complicated by several factors including: multiple virus types; antigenic variation; inability to culture the virus; no small animal model; partial understanding of immunity; and effect of previous infections. NoV VLPs given orally to mice and human volunteers are safe and induce IgG1 and IgA antibody responses[147] and a NoV VLP vaccine given intranasally to volunteers reduced the frequency of gastroenteritis and subclinical infections when the participants were given the Norwalk virus.[148]

References available online at expertconsult.com.

KEY REFERENCES

Desselberger U., Huppertz H.I.: Immune responses to rotavirus infection and vaccination and associated correlates of protection. *J Infect Dis* 2011; 203(2):188-195.

Franco M.A., Angel J., Greenberg H.B.: Immunity and correlates of protection for rotavirus vaccines. *Vaccine* 2006; 24(15):2718-2731.

Glass R.I., Parashar U.D.: Rotavirus vaccines – balancing intussusception risks and health benefits. *N Engl J Med* 2014; 370(6):568-570.

Hall A., Lopman B., Payne D., et al.: Norovirus disease in the United States. *Emerg Infect Dis* 2013; 19(8):1198-1205.

Hemming M., Huhti L., Rasanen S., et al.: Rotavirus antigenemia in children is associated with more severe clinical manifestations of acute gastroenteritis. *Pediatr Infect Dis J* 2014; 33(4):366-371.

Imdad A., Yakoob M., Sudfeld C., et al.: Impact of vitamin A supplementation on infant and childhood mortality. *BMC Public Health* 2011; 11(Suppl. 3):S20, :1-15.

Kotloff K.L., Nataro J.P., Blackwelder W.C., et al.: Burden and aetiology of diarrhoeal disease in infants and young children in developing countries (the Global Enteric Multicenter Study, GEMS): a prospective, case-control study. *Lancet* 2013; 382(9888):209-222.

Mukhopadhya I., Sarkar R., Menon V.K., et al.: Rotavirus shedding in symptomatic and asymptomatic children using reverse transcription-quantitative PCR. *J Med Virol* 2013; 85(9):1661-1668.

Munoz M., Walker C., Black R.: The effect of oral rehydration solution and recommended home fluids on diarrhoea mortality. *Int J Epidemiol* 2010; 39(Suppl.1):175-187.

Patel M., Widdowson M., Glass R., et al.: Systematic Literature Review of Role of Noroviruses in Sporadic Gastroenteritis. *Emerg Infect Dis* 2008; 14(8):1224-1231.

Santos N., Hoshino Y.: Global distribution of rotavirus serotypes/genotypes and its implication for the development and implementation of an effective rotavirus vaccine. *Rev Med Virol* 2005; 15(1):29-56.

Walker C., Rudan I., Liu L., et al.: Global burden of childhood pneumonia and diarrhea. *Lancet* 2013; 381(9875):1405-1416.

Yih W.K., Lieu T.A., Kulldorff M., et al.: Intussusception risk after rotavirus vaccination in U.S. infants. *N Engl J Med* 2014; 370(6):503-512.

Yu T.H., Tsai C.N., Lai M.W., et al.: Antigenemia and cytokine expression in rotavirus gastroenteritis in children. *J Microbiol Immunol Infect* 2012; 45(4):265-270.

163

Measles, Mumps and Rubella Viruses

SCOTT H. JAMES

KEY CONCEPTS

- Measles, mumps and rubella viruses are single-stranded RNA viruses with worldwide distributions.

- These viruses are of moderate to high communicability, with measles being the most contagious of the three.

- Clinically, measles and rubella infections are often marked by prodromal symptoms and distinctive exanthems, and can be associated with potentially serious complications and sequelae.

- Infection with mumps virus may consist of prodromal symptoms and a characteristic parotitis, with further complications being common but typically self-limiting.

- With sufficient vaccination coverage, endemic transmission of measles and rubella can be interrupted, whereas mumps outbreaks have been known to occur even in highly vaccinated populations.

- Measles and rubella have been targeted for elimination by collaborative global vaccination initiatives.

Introduction

The epidemiology of the viruses (measles, rubella and mumps) has changed dramatically since the successful introduction of live attenuated vaccines. With prevention, clinicians are less familiar with their clinical presentations and surveillance based solely on clinical recognition is not always sufficiently accurate. Laboratory confirmation of suspected cases is essential and should be complemented by genotyping of circulating viral strains for effective surveillance.[1]

Measles

Nature

Measles (rubeola) was first identified over 2000 years ago, although its infectious nature was not recognized until the mid-19th century when epidemics in island communities were described.

Measles virus is a member of the *Morbillivirus* genus of the Paramyxoviridae and was first isolated in cell culture in 1954; the first live attenuated vaccine became available in 1963. Pleomorphic, with a diameter of 150 nm, the single-stranded RNA is enclosed in a capsid of helical symmetry of 18 nm that is enclosed within an envelope, the surface of which expresses hemagglutinin and fusion proteins. Replication is mainly cytoplasmic; however, there is some nuclear involvement. Although there is only one measles virus serotype, 23 genotypes have been described, which are organized in eight clades (A–H).[2]

Epidemiology

Measles is endemic worldwide except in those countries in which immunization is routine (Figure 163-1). Childhood infection before the impact of immunization was almost 100%, confirming measles as one of the most infectious of microbial pathogens. Epidemics occur every 2–3 years, but are less well defined in the tropics.

The epidemiology of measles has been profoundly modified by immunization strategies, with a 78% reduction in measles deaths globally from 562 000 in 2000 to 122 000 in 2012, but measles remains common in many low- to middle-income countries (LMIC). The target set by the Global Vaccine Action Plan 2011–2020, a collaborative effort endorsed by the World Health Assembly, is to achieve elimination of endemic measles in at least 5 of 6 World Health Organization (WHO) global regions by 2020.[3]

Despite efforts to eradicate measles, outbreaks continue to occur in high-income countries; the number of measles cases reported to the Centers for Disease Control and Prevention (CDC) in the first half of 2014 was already more than double the highest year-to-date figure of the past decade.[4,5] Most measles cases were reported in unvaccinated children. Suboptimal vaccine uptake due to parental concerns and/or religious reasons remains a major obstacle to achieving and maintaining elimination of the disease.

Pathogenicity

Infection is spread by droplet from person to person. The incubation period to onset of rash is about 14 days, with prodromal symptoms starting 1–3 days earlier. Maximum infectivity is during the prodrome, although patients are considered to be infective from 4 days before to 4 days after onset of the rash.

After infection, initial replication occurs in the respiratory epithelium with local spread by lymphatics and a primary viremia 2–3 days after infection. A secondary viremia occurs 3–4 days later and lasts for up to 7 days. The peak viremia coincides with the prodromal symptoms. The rash results from the immunologic reaction between the virus antigens and host antibody with involvement of capillary walls. Intrauterine infection has not been convincingly reported.

Prevention

Live attenuated measles vaccine became available in 1963 based on the Edmonston strain, but those in current use, such as Schwarz and Moraten strains, are further attenuated. Measles vaccine is available in monovalent form, as well as in combination with mumps and rubella vaccine (MMR). Two doses of the vaccine are necessary to achieve high levels of immunity (>98% efficacy). They are included in the routine childhood immunization scheme at age 12–15 months and at school entry (4–6 years). Administration before 12 months can result in lower protection because of interference by residual maternal antibody. This is especially problematic for LMIC, where many cases of measles occur in infants under 12 months of age. For most LMIC, the WHO recommends immunization at 9 months of age.

In HIV-infected children the vaccine is less effective but protective antibody levels can be achieved for those on highly active retroviral therapy with immune recovery.[6] Measles vaccine is contraindicated in pregnancy and in those with impaired cell-mediated immunity. Previous concerns have been expressed as to whether there may be a link between MMR immunization and autism, but strong evidence demonstrates no association.[7,8]

Diagnostic Microbiology

Virus isolation may be attempted from throat swabs, conjunctival swabs, nasopharyngeal aspirates (NPAs) and urine, but is technically demanding and unreliable. The cell line used in global reference laboratories for virus isolation is a Vero/SLAM cell line – a Vero cell line transfected with a plasmid encoding human SLAM (signaling lymphocyte-activation molecule) which is a cellular receptor for the measles virus. Cytopathic effect can take up to 15 days after inoculation to develop.

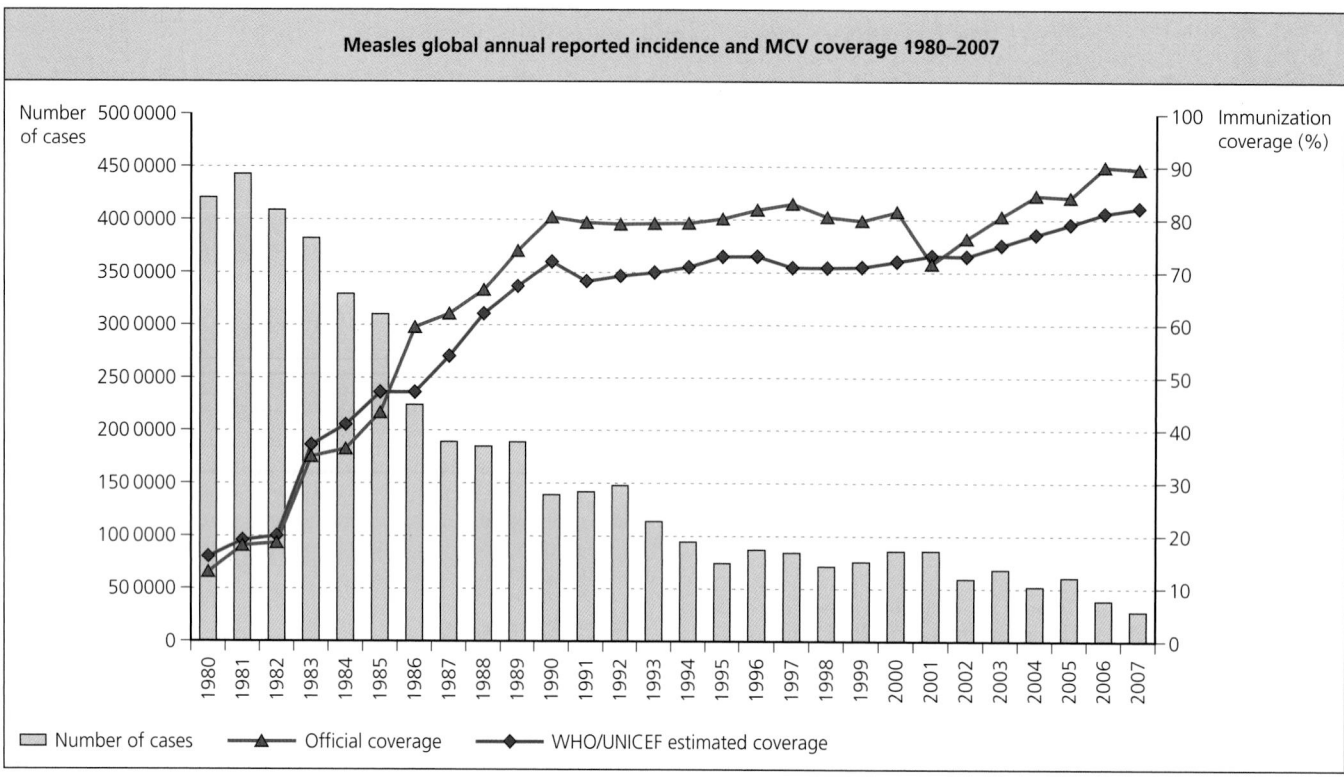

Figure 163-1 Measles global annual reported incidence and measles-containing vaccine coverage 1980–2007.

Immunofluorescent antigen detection in NPA cells may be performed and is particularly useful for diagnosing atypical cases or infection in the immunocompromised host. Measles virus genome, amplified from throat swabs or NPAs by RT-PCR is used for genetic characterization.[2]

As RT-PCR can detect the viral genome in the absence of viable virus, a diagnosis can be made up to several weeks after rash onset. Serologic diagnosis is dependent on demonstrating seroconversion or detecting specific IgM. Hemagglutination inhibition and complement fixation testing (CFT) were the established methods in the past, but are now replaced by immunoglobulin-specific enzyme immunoassays (EIAs). Serum-based IgM EIAs are currently recommended for the rapid laboratory detection of measles. False-negative IgM assays can occur if serum is collected within 3 days of rash onset.[9]

IgG assays require the collection of two serum specimens 10–30 days apart. A fourfold rise in the IgG titer is considered to be diagnostic. IgG assays are not routinely used for the diagnosis of acute measles virus infection but are used for the clarification of equivocal IgM results and in seroprevalence studies.[1] Simultaneous detection of IgM and viral RNA from dried blood specimens or oral fluid sampling are possible alternatives for diagnosis and surveillance of measles, especially in countries where specimen transport or refrigeration is challenging.

Subacute sclerosing panencephalitis (SSPE) may be diagnosed by detection of the genome or isolation of virus by co-cultivation from brain tissue. A more usual approach, however, is the detection of elevated concentrations of measles antibody in serum and concentrations indicating intrathecal synthesis in cerebrospinal fluid (CSF) by CFT.

Clinical Manifestations

Towards the end of the incubation period, prodromal symptoms of fever and malaise develop and persist for up to 4 days before the rash appears. Pyrexia may rise to 103–104°F (39.4–40°C) and is often accompanied by conjunctivitis, cough and coryza (the three 'C's of

measles). Koplik's spots are a pathognomonic feature of measles, and can be seen for up to 2 days before rash onset as punctate white spots on an erythematous background on the buccal mucosa (Figure 163-2).

The rash usually begins on the face and neck, and evolves to the body and limbs (Figure 163-3). Although lesions are usually discrete, they can coalesce and desquamate. The rash usually persists for 5–6 days. Generalized lymphadenopathy and diarrhea are common.

Complications are most common in younger and older patients (Table 163-1) and those with underlying malnutrition, particularly vitamin A deficiency. Pneumonia, either viral or, more usually, secondary bacterial, occurs in up to 4% of patients. Neurologic complications include convulsions, in up to 1% of cases, and encephalitis in 1/1000 cases, with a mortality rate of 15% and residual neurologic deficit rate of 25%. Overall, estimates of measles mortality are 1 per 1000 patients in high-income countries but higher in LMIC.

SSPE manifests months to years after the initial measles infection or immunization; the mean interval is 7 years after natural measles and 3.3 years after immunization. The risk is less after measles immunization (1 : 1 million) than after natural infection (1 : 100 000), and is three times more common in boys than in girls. Specific risk factors for the development of SSPE have not been identified. SSPE is a progressively fatal degenerative disease of the central nervous system, manifesting as a progressive intellectual impairment, which advances to convulsions, motor abnormalities and coma; death is inevitable after a gradual deterioration over months or years. Measles viruses associated with SSPE have phenotypic features that are distinct from those of wild-type measles virus, being more neuropathogenic in hamsters, mice and other rodents. Also, SSPE viruses produce few infectious virus particles, if any, and thus its spread from infected to uninfected cells is almost completely dependent on cell-to-cell infection. This phenotype is thought to be caused by mutations affecting the viral matrix (M) protein and the cytoplasmic tail of the fusion (F) glycoprotein. Accumulation of viral genetic mutations during viral persistence occurs over a long period of time, especially after the initial onset of SSPE symptoms.[11]

TABLE 163-1	Complications of Reported Measles Cases by Age Group, USA, 1987–2000					
		NO. (%) OF PERSONS WITH COMPLICATION, BY AGE GROUP				
Complication	Overall (67 032 Cases with Age Information)	<5 Years (n = 28 730)	5–9 Years (n = 6492)	10–19 Years (n = 18 580)	20–29 Years (n = 9161)	>30 Years (n = 4069)
Any	19 480 (29.1)	11 833 (41.4)	1173 (18.1)	2369 (12.8)	2656 (29.0)	1399 (34.4)
Death	177 (0.3)	97 (0.3)	9 (0.1)	18 (0.1)	26 (0.3)	27 (0.7)
Diarrhea	5482 (8.2)	3294 (11.5)	408 (6.3)	627 (3.4)	767 (8.4)	386 (9.5)
Encephalitis	97 (0.1)	43 (0.2)	9 (0.1)	13 (0.1)	21 (0.2)	11 (0.3)
Hospitalization	12 876 (19.2)	7470 (26.0)	612 (9.4)	1612 (8.7)	2075 (22.7)	1107 (27.2)
Otitis media	4879 (7.3)	4009 (14.0)	305 (4.7)	338 (1.8)	157 (1.7)	70 (1.7)
Pneumonia	3959 (5.9)	2480 (8.6)	183 (2.8)	363 (2.0)	554 (6.1)	379 (9.3)

Adapted from[10] Perry RT, Halsey NA. The clinical significance of measles: a review. J Infect Dis 2004;189 (Suppl 1):S4-16.

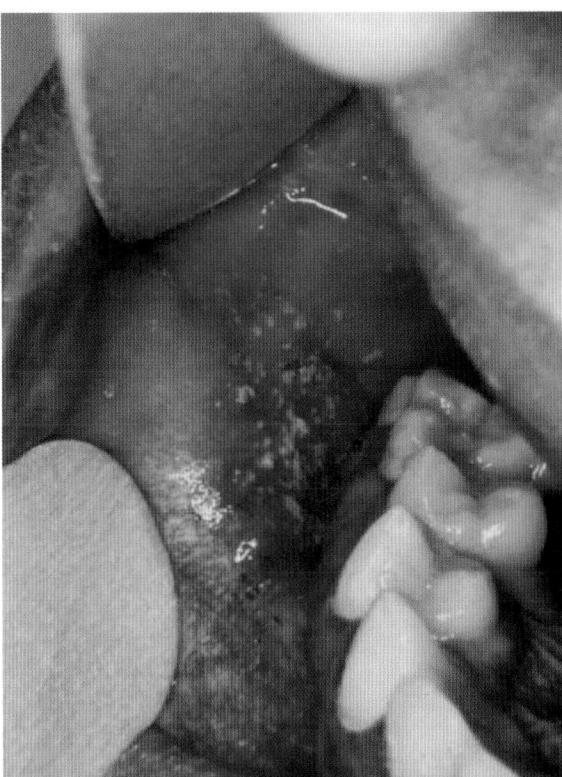

Figure 163-2   Koplik's spots: white lesions on the buccal mucosa characteristic of measles. (Reprinted from Goldman L. Schafer A.I., eds. Goldman's Cecil Medicine, 24th ed. Philadelphia: Elsevier Saunders; 2012: 2105-2107).

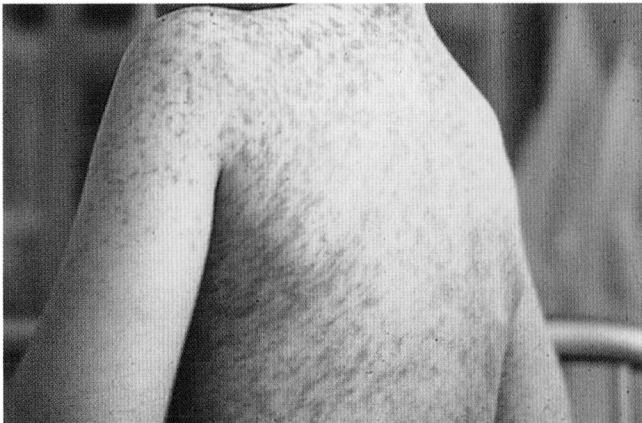

Figure 163-3   Measles. A disseminated erythematous rash can be seen over the trunk and arms.

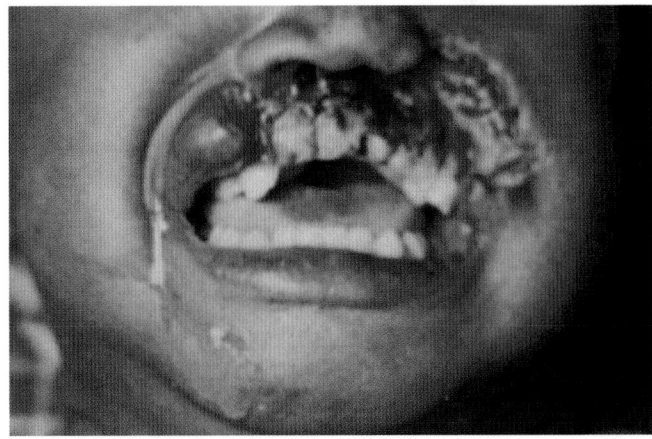

Figure 163-4   Cancrum oris. Necrosis of the upper lip.

Immunocompromised patients with T-cell deficiencies, such as those who have leukemia or HIV, are at particular risk for the development of complications. The typical rash is often missing and infection persists, manifesting as a giant cell pneumonitis or rapidly progressive encephalitis; the fatality rate is high.[12]

Measles in pregnancy seems to carry a higher risk of complications but has not been associated with congenital abnormalities, although there is an increased risk of intrauterine death or premature delivery.[13]

Measles presents special problems in LMIC, where case fatality rates of up to 25% have been described. The high mortality rate is associated with malnutrition and, in particular, vitamin A deficiency.[14] Death usually results from bacterial superinfection, such as pneumonia, or diarrheal illness, although cancrum oris, a progressive oral necrosis, is also seen (Figure 163-4).

Management

Postexposure prophylaxis with human immunoglobulin is indicated for those who are susceptible and at risk for complications, in particular immunocompromised children and pregnant women. In outbreak situations and in immunocompetent persons, administration of measles vaccine within 3 days of contact can provide protection.

Uncomplicated measles is managed symptomatically, with vitamin A supplementation for malnourished children. Antimicrobial therapy active against *Streptococcus pneumoniae* and *Haemophilus influenzae* is indicated for presumed bacterial superinfection. In those with major complications, such as pneumonitis in immunocompromised patients, specific antiviral treatment with ribavirin may be of limited benefit;[15] however, such treatment is of no value in SSPE.

Rubella

Nature

Although rubella had been recognized as a distinct clinical illness since the 18th century, it was not until 1941 that Sir Norman Gregg, an Australian ophthalmologist, made the association between rubella in early pregnancy and congenital abnormalities.[16] In 1962 the causative virus was isolated, leading to techniques for specific diagnosis and the development of attenuated live vaccines.

Rubella is a single-stranded RNA virus, with an icosahedral nucleocapsid surrounded by an envelope. Replication occurs in the cytoplasm. It is the sole member of the genus *Rubivirus* within the family Togaviridae. There are three major virus polypeptides: C, E_1 and E_2. Polypeptide E_1 is present in the envelope and has hemagglutinating properties. Only one serotype is recognized, but phylogenetic analysis of the coding region of E_1 revealed at least seven distinct genotypes grouped in two clades.[17] Humans are the only species known to be infected.

Epidemiology

Rubella is a mild disease presenting with fever and rash. Existing vaccines, single or in combination with measles and/or mumps, are highly efficacious. With the implementation of rubella-containing childhood immunization schedules, there has been an 82% global decrease in reported rubella cases, from 670 894 in 2000 to 121 344 in 2009.[18] Rubella elimination is one of the primary targets of the WHO since infection during the early months of pregnancy can lead to fetal death or serious congenital birth defects (congenital rubella syndrome; CRS). CRS cases are vastly underreported, but it is estimated that more than 100 000 infants are born with CRS each year, the majority occurring in countries without an effective rubella vaccination program.[19]

Pathogenicity

Infection is transmitted by the airborne route, by direct contact or indirectly through fomites. Patients are infectious from 1 week before to 1 week after the onset of rash. After replication in the upper respiratory tract and local lymph nodes, viremia infects target organs such as skin, joints and placenta. Similar to measles, the rash is immunologically mediated and marks the production of specific antibodies.

If the patient is pregnant, placental infection can occur; transmission to the fetus is possible but not inevitable.[20] Confirmed rubella during the first trimester of pregnancy results in damage to 50–90% of fetuses (see Box 163-1 and Chapter 56).[21]

Prevention

Passive prophylaxis with human IgG has not reduced the risk of rubella after contact, although it may attenuate the illness. Control of rubella has resided in using the live attenuated vaccines available since the early 1970s. The vaccine strain RA27/3 induces seroconversion in over 95% of susceptible vaccinees, and protection persists for at least 15–20 years.[22] A mild, transient rubelliform rash illness with arthralgia can occur 2–3 weeks after immunization. If vaccine virus is inadvertently administered to pregnant women fetal infection occurs in approximately 1% of cases, but extensive postvaccine surveillance has not detected any fetal damage.[23] Rubella immunization presents no significant risk to the individual who has HIV infection.

Control of rubella has focused on preventing infection in women of childbearing age by combining rubella vaccine with measles and mumps vaccines (MMR), and offering it to all children in the second year of life to eradicate rubella from the community. This policy is supplemented by identifying and immunizing susceptible women of childbearing age. If uptake rates of more than 90% can be obtained, control of endemic rubella is achievable (Figure 163-5). Elimination of congenital rubella syndrome has been accomplished in the USA and in other high-income countries although it is a problem in sub-Saharan Africa.[24]

Diagnostic Microbiology

With the clinical diagnosis of rubella being unreliable, laboratory confirmation of infection is required. In pregnancy it is imperative to

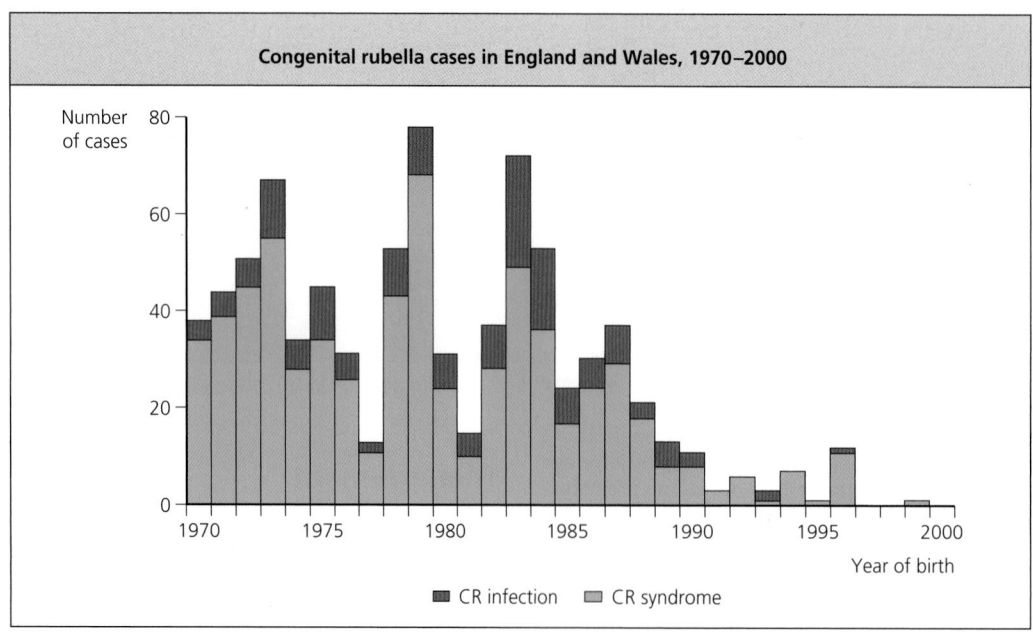

Figure 163-5 Congenital rubella cases in England and Wales, 1970–2000. The number of confirmed cases was substantially reduced by the introduction of MMR vaccine in 1988. (*Data from National Congenital Rubella Surveillance Programme and the PHLS Communicable Disease Surveillance Centre.*)

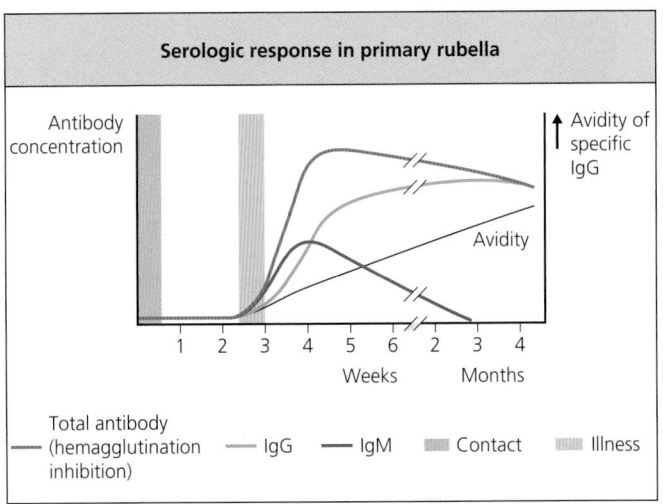

Figure 163-6 Serologic response in primary rubella. The development of specific IgG and IgM and the increasing avidity of specific IgG are illustrated.

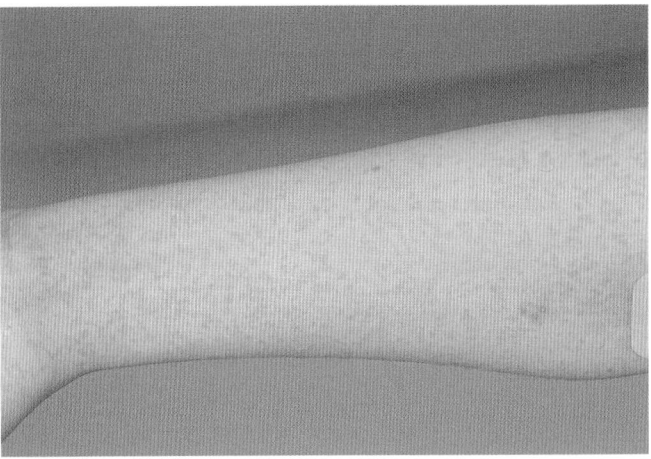

Figure 163-7 Rubella. A pink macular rash can be seen on the forearm.

investigate both a rash illness and contact with a rash illness because subclinical rubella may occur, and this has been proven to be a risk to the fetus.[25]

The diagnosis of postnatal rubella infection is made by serology, as detailed in Figure 163-6; tests for total rubella antibody (such as hemagglutination inhibition) have been progressively replaced with tests specific for IgG and IgM, particularly EIAs. Serum should be obtained as soon as possible after onset of illness or after contact. Detection of rubella-specific IgG, but failure to demonstrate specific IgM, indicates immunity to rubella and that the illness being investigated is not rubella. If neither rubella-specific IgG nor specific IgM are detected, repeat testing of a later serum is needed. The incubation period after contact may be up to 21 days, and it may take up to 10 days after onset of illness for rubella antibody to be detectable, therefore it may not be until about 4 weeks after contact that a subclinical illness can be excluded.

Detection of rubella-specific IgM indicates recent primary rubella infection, but care is needed in interpretation. Rubella-specific IgM reactivity persists for about 1–3 months and false-positive IgM results occur with other infections such as parvovirus B19 and Epstein–Barr virus. Rubella-specific IgM reactivity may also occur in rubella re-infection (see below). In the first 2 days after rash onset RT-PCR testing of oral fluid specimens can identify more cases than IgM testing.[26] Other serologic approaches, such as determining specific IgG avidity, are of value in confirming primary rubella,[27] with specific IgG early after infection being less tightly bound to antigen (low avidity) than the antibody found in the mature antibody response (high avidity; see Figure 163-6).

For the diagnosis of congenital rubella isolation of virus in cell culture is of value because infected infants can excrete high titers of virus in the throat and urine during the first year of life; congenitally infected infants can be highly infectious to susceptible contacts until approximately 6 months of age. Rubella isolation can be performed in many cell culture lines, but a cytopathic effect is only produced in a few of them, for example RK 13. Immunofluorescence is probably the best method for detecting virus growth.

Congenital rubella is routinely diagnosed by detecting specific IgM; all congenitally infected infants are positive for the first 3 months of life and most for the first 6 months. As passively transmitted maternal IgG antibodies have declined by 6 months of age, persistence of IgG antibodies beyond this time period indicates fetal infection as well.

Occasionally, intrauterine diagnosis of rubella may be considered. Approaches used, but of limited availability, have included virus isolation and genome detection from amniotic fluid or trophoblast, or detection of specific IgM in fetal blood; this latter method is unreliable before 24 weeks' gestation, however, because the infected fetus may not be capable of an IgM response until that age.

The majority of high-income countries have programs in place to identify susceptible women of childbearing age and offer immunization. Tests for specific IgG include EIAs and latex agglutination. An area of contention is the concentration of rubella-specific IgG taken to indicate protection (or, more correctly, as not necessitating immunization), with opinions varying from any confirmed antibody (possibly as low as 3–5 IU) up to 15 IU; 10 IU has been recommended in the USA.[28]

Clinical Manifestations

In childhood, primary rubella is subclinical in approximately 50% of patients, but in adolescence or adulthood it is usually (90% or more) clinically apparent. After an incubation period of up to 21 days (usually 15–17 days) a pinkish-red maculopapular rash develops, starting on the face and neck and rapidly spreading over body and limbs (Figure 163-7). Individual spots may coalesce but the rash usually clears in 3–4 days. Nonspecific symptoms such as fever, malaise and upper respiratory tract symptoms may precede and accompany the rash. In childhood the illness is usually benign and may have no systemic impact. Lymphadenopathy commonly occurs, the suboccipital nodes being frequently involved.

In adolescence and adulthood, rubella is often far more severe, not only because of complications but also because of a more severe systemic illness. Arthralgia is a frequent complication in adults, with women (30% or more) suffering more often than men. Joints frequently involved are those of the hands and wrists; resolution usually occurs in 2–4 weeks but can persist for some months or even years. Thrombocytopenia and postinfectious encephalitis are rare complications, occurring in less than 1/5000–10 000 patients, with fatal outcome virtually unknown. Even in patients with HIV infection or other immunocompromised states, rubella rarely carries any additional risk.[29]

Primary rubella infection in the first 16 weeks of pregnancy presents major risks to the fetus. Consequences include abortion, miscarriage or stillbirth or multiple birth defects (Box 163-1). The congenital rubella triad comprises cardiac, ophthalmic and auditory lesions, but purpura, intrauterine growth and neurologic problems are also frequent (see also Chapter 56).

The gestational age at which the mother suffers her rubella infection is critical for the outcome. Onset of rubella before conception carries little, if any, risk,[30] whereas from conception to the 12th week the risk is about 90%.[22] Between 12 and 16 weeks' gestation the risk falls to about 20%, with sensorineural hearing loss being the primary sequela. Beyond 16 weeks any risk is minimal, with only rare cases of sensorineural hearing loss.

BOX 163-1 FEATURES OF CONGENITAL RUBELLA

Cardiovascular defects
 Persistent ductus arteriosus
 Pulmonary artery stenosis
 Myocarditis
Ocular defects
 Cataracts (unilateral or bilateral)
 Pigmentary retinopathy
 Microphthalmus
 Glaucoma
 Iris hypoplasia
Auditory defects
 Sensorineural deafness (unilateral or bilateral)
Central nervous system
 Microcephaly
 Psychomotor retardation
 Meningoencephalitis
 Behavioral disorders
 Speech disorders
Intrauterine growth retardation
Hepatitis/hepatosplenomegaly
Thrombocytopenia, with purpura
Bone 'lesions'
Pneumonitis*
Diabetes mellitus*
Thyroid disorders*
Progressive rubella panencephalitis*

*These disorders become apparent in infancy or later.

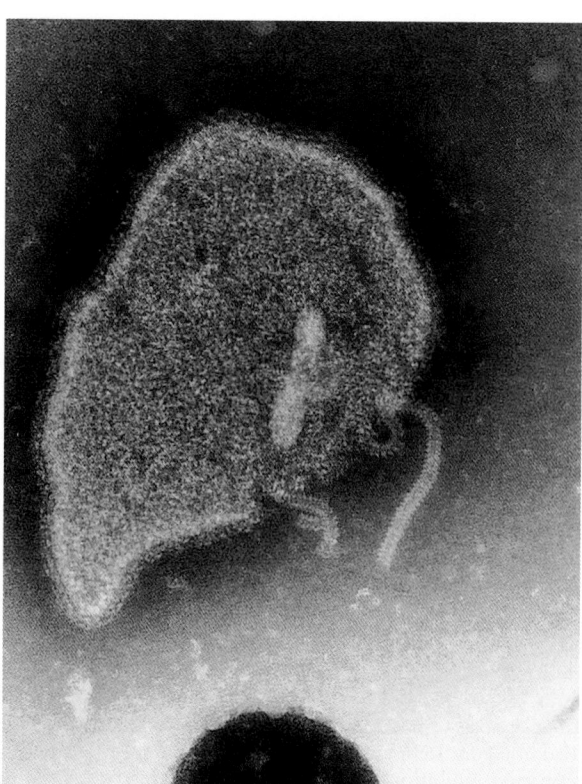

Figure 163-8 Electron micrograph of mumps virus. *(Courtesy of Dr A. Curry.)*

Re-infections can occur in those with a past history of natural rubella or successful immunization. Such re-infections are rarely clinically apparent and are usually identified by a serologic response after exposure. Fetal infection can occur after maternal re-infection but is rare, with the fetal risk probably being less than 5%.[31] Because of the difference in risk to the fetus, it is critical to distinguish between subclinical primary rubella and re-infection in early pregnancy. This may be difficult in the absence of past rubella-specific IgG test results because a specific IgM response can occur in both; IgG avidity testing will usually resolve the problem because re-infection would be characterized by the presence of high avidity IgG.

Management

Rubella is a self-limiting illness that usually runs a benign course. Supportive and symptom-relieving therapy is indicated for complications such as arthralgia, and the patient can be reassured that symptoms are unlikely to persist beyond a few months.

Management of rubella in pregnancy is first dependent on achieving a correct diagnosis. A serum sample must be taken as soon as possible after contact or onset of illness, and the testing laboratory given full details of past testing and/or vaccination. If primary rubella or re-infection in the first 16 weeks of pregnancy is diagnosed, it is likely that fetal health will be significantly impacted and further intervention will have to take into account social, legal and religious perspectives.

Mumps

Nature

Mumps was first identified as a distinct clinical illness by Hippocrates in the 5th century BCE, but has only attracted attention in the past two to three centuries. Natural infection is limited to humans and is endemic worldwide.

Mumps virus is a member of the *Paramyxovirus* genus of the Paramyxoviridae family. It was first isolated in chick embryos in 1945, with the first live attenuated vaccine being licensed in 1967. On electron microscopy it is pleomorphic (Figure 163-8) and varies in size from 80 to 350 nm, although it is usually approximately 200 nm. The envelope is studded with projections containing hemagglutinin/neuraminidase or fusion proteins. Within the envelope the nucleoprotein has helical symmetry with a diameter of 15–19 nm. The RNA is single stranded and of negative sense; the nucleocapsid contains an RNA-dependent RNA polymerase. This enzyme enables replication of the RNA in the cytoplasm once the cell has been penetrated.

Twelve mumps virus genotypes (A–L) with different geographic distribution have been described. There is only one serologic type although studies suggest that cross-neutralization between genotypes might not be complete.[32]

Epidemiology

Mumps is endemic worldwide, with epidemics occurring every 2–3 years in nonvaccinated populations. In the pre-vaccine era 50% of children aged 4–6 years and 90% aged 14–15 years were mumps seropositive.[33] With vaccine introduction the epidemiology of the disease shifted, but mumps outbreaks remain common even in countries with routine mumps vaccination. The Netherlands experienced a nationwide epidemic from 2009–2012 and the UK had a large-scale outbreak in 2004/2005.[34,35] Outbreaks in the USA led to over 6500 reported mumps cases in 2006, as well an additional 3000 cases in a 2009/2010 outbreak. During these outbreaks, the majority of infections were associated with university students or their contacts. When outbreaks occur in a predominantly vaccinated population, it is typically because suboptimal vaccine effectiveness and insufficient vaccine uptake allows ongoing transmission. Whereas natural infection results in lifelong immunity, immunity induced by vaccination can decrease.[36]

Pathogenicity

Infection is acquired by droplet, direct contact or contaminated fomites. Replication in the upper respiratory epithelium is followed by spread to local lymph nodes and subsequent primary viremia, with seeding of target organs such as parotid glands, central nervous system and genital organs. A secondary viremia occurs at the onset of symptoms. Intrauterine infection has been reported only rarely.

The incubation period is usually 16–18 days, with infectivity commencing 2 days before onset of symptoms and persisting for 5–7 days after onset. Patients with mumps should be isolated with droplet and contact precautions for a 5-day period after onset of parotitis.[37]

Prevention

Two live attenuated vaccine strains have been mainly used since 1967: Jeryl Lynn and Urabe strain vaccines. Both are produced in chick embryo cell culture and are available in monovalent form or combined as MMR. The vaccine is usually administered as MMR at 12–15 months of age, with second doses being given later in childhood. Protective efficacy is 75–85%, with clinically apparent mumps in immunized individuals being well documented. Minor complications of mumps vaccine include mild parotitis, fever and, very rarely, orchitis.

Mumps vaccine is contraindicated in pregnancy, although adverse implications for the fetus have not been reported, and immunocompromised patients, with the exception of children with HIV infection who do not have severe immunosuppression.[38]

Diagnostic Microbiology

Virus isolation may be achieved from throat swabs, saliva, CSF and possibly urine. Mumps virus is readily isolated in either Vero (African green monkey kidney) or Caco-2 (human colorectal adenocarcinoma epithelium) cell lines. Although cytopathic effect may be observed, isolation is usually confirmed by immunofluorescence staining. RT-PCR can be performed directly on the clinical specimen and sequencing of the amplified product allows identification of individual genotypes. RT-PCR was found to be more sensitive than culture methods in detecting virus in cerebrospinal and oral fluid.[39]

Serologic diagnosis is usually achieved by detection of virus-specific IgM antibody by direct or indirect enzyme-linked immunosorbent assay (ELISA). False-negative IgM results can occur for serum collected before day 4 of clinical presentation.[40] A fourfold rise of IgG titer between acute and convalescent serum is considered diagnostic. Serologic testing can be performed on CSF specimens in patients with mumps, meningitis or encephalitis. Saliva can be used for specific IgM detection and is valuable for surveillance of mumps-like illness in the community.[33]

Clinical Manifestations

Towards the end of the incubation period, prodromal symptoms such as pyrexia and malaise develop, followed by the characteristic tender swelling of the parotid glands; often accompanied by headache and earache. Recovery is usually complete within 4–5 days. Asymptomatic mumps is common and occurs in about one-third of infections. Parotitis is present in 95% of symptomatic infections and is unilateral in about one-quarter; other salivary glands are involved in about 10% of patients.

Complications are common; the risk is the same at all ages except for orchitis and oophoritis, which are typically limited to post puberty. Orchitis generally arises a few days after parotitis. The risk of orchitis in adolescent or adult males is about 35%, with bilateral involvement in one-third of these. There may be some persisting testicular atrophy, but sterility is remarkably uncommon. Oophoritis is only observed about 5% of the time in adult women and causes lower abdominal pain; it is uncertain whether there may be long-term consequences.

Meningeal involvement, with CSF pleocytosis, occurs in about 50% of patients, with signs of meningismus in about 1–10%. Up to 50% of meningitis cases occur without concomitant parotitis. Mumps virus may also cause encephalitis, presenting as impaired level of consciousness, seizures, or aphasia. Mumps meningitis is, in general, a benign disease; persistent sequelae are found in a small percentage of encephalitis cases, more commonly in adults.

The incidence of encephalitis is about 1/6000 patients, with a mortality rate of 1.4%. Transient hearing impairment as a result of a labyrinthitis is common, with persistent hearing loss occurring in about 1/20000 patients. Other possible complications include pancreatitis, arthritis, mastitis, thyroiditis and myocarditis. Investigation of renal function will often demonstrate kidney involvement, but there are usually no significant clinical consequences.

In general, mumps seems to carry no undue risk in immunocompromised patients, although it has been associated with graft failure after renal transplantation.[41]

First trimester infection can lead to spontaneous abortion, but infection later in pregnancy carries no increased risk, and congenital infection and damage have not been convincingly shown.

Management

Postexposure prophylaxis with human immunoglobulin is of no benefit, and specific mumps immunoglobulin is no longer available, although it may have reduced the risk of orchitis in adult men. Mumps vaccine administered as postexposure prophylaxis is of no benefit.

There is no specific antiviral treatment available; management of infection is symptomatic, with the patient being reassured that recovery occurs in a few days, even when complications are present.

References available online at expertconsult.com.

KEY REFERENCES

Centers for Disease Control and Prevention: Measles – United States, January 1-May 23, 2014. *MMWR* 2014; 63(22):496-499.

Galazka A.M., Robertson S.E., Kraigher A.: Mumps and mumps vaccine: a global review. *Bull World Health Organ* 1999; 77:3-14.

Helfand R.F., Heath J.L., Anderson L.J., et al.: Diagnosis of measles with an IgM capture EIA: the optimal timing of specimen collection after rash onset. *J Infect Dis* 1997; 175(1):195-199.

Hornig M., Briese T., Buie T., et al.: Lack of association between measles virus vaccine and autism with enteropathy: a case-control study. *PLoS ONE* 2008; 3(9): e3140.

McLean H.Q., Fiebelkorn A.P., Temte J.L., et al.: Prevention of measles, rubella, congenital rubella syndrome, and mumps, 2013: Summary recommendations of the Advisory Committee on Immunization Practices (ACIP). *MMWR Recomm Rep* 2013; 62(RR-04):1-34.

Perry R.T., Halsey N.A.: The clinical significance of measles: a review. *J Infect Dis* 2004; 189(Suppl.1):S4-S16.

Plotkin S.A.: The history of rubella and rubella vaccination leading to elimination. *Clin Infect Dis* 2006; 43: S164-S168.

Reef S.E., Strebel P., Dabbagh A., et al.: Progress toward control of rubella and prevention of congenital rubella syndrome – worldwide, 2009. *J Infect Dis* 2011; 204(Suppl.1):S24-S27.

Uchida K., Shinohara M., Shimada S., et al.: Rapid and sensitive detection of mumps virus RNA directly from clinical samples by real-time PCR. *J Med Virol* 2005; 75:470-474.

Vandermeulen C., Roelants M., Vermoere M., et al.: Outbreak of mumps in a vaccinated child population: a question of vaccine failure? *Vaccine* 2004; 22:2713-2716.

World Health Organization: *Global Vaccine Action Plan 2011-2020*. Geneva: WHO; 2013. Available: http://www.who.int/immunization/global_vaccine_action_plan/en/.

164

Human Enteroviruses

JOSÉ R. ROMERO

KEY CONCEPTS

- Enteroviruses are non-enveloped, positive sense, single-stranded viruses. Modern molecular techniques have allowed for a realignment of the serotypes that make up the original species into four new species: Enteroviruses A–D. These species encompass over 110 types. More will certainly be discovered in the near future.

- Enteroviruses are found worldwide. A higher prevalence of infection is seen during the summer months in temperate climates and during the rainy season in tropical regions.

- Transmission is most commonly by the fecal–oral route. The enteroviruses are responsible for diseases or clinical syndromes involving almost every organ system.

- A global initiative to eradicate polioviruses began in 1988 and has made great strides toward its goal. Polioviruses are currently endemic in only three countries: Afghanistan, Pakistan and Nigeria.

- Traditional cell culture methodologies for the detection and identification of the Enteroviruses have been replaced by more sensitive nucleic amplification assays.

- Currently only the polioviruses can be prevented by vaccines. Clinical trials are underway to develop a vaccine for the prevention of subgenotype C4 enterovirus A71 infections.

The Viruses

Discovering the Enteroviruses

HISTORY

The enteroviruses appear to have been human pathogens since antiquity. Depictions of poliomyelitis, the most recognizable of the enteroviral diseases, date to the ancient Egyptians. A stele from approximately 1300 BCE, on display at the Carlsberg Museum in Copenhagen, Denmark, depicts an Egyptian priest with an atrophic lower extremity and an equinus foot deformity characteristic of loss of lower motor neuron innervation observed with poliomyelitis.[1] The first known clinical description of poliomyelitis is attributed to Michael Underwood in 1789. In 1840 Jakob von Heine described the clinical symptoms of poliomyelitis, which were expanded by Karl Medin. The syndrome was named Heine–Medin disease.

In 1908 Karl Landsteiner and Erwin Popper successfully transmitted the etiologic agent of poliomyelitis to two Old World monkeys through intraperitoneal inoculation of a spinal cord suspension from a child who succumbed to poliomyelitis. The discovery of poliovirus and a model system with which to study it opened the way for the identification of other poliovirus serotypes and a better understanding of the disease, its pathology, immunology and epidemiology. The search for new poliovirus strains led to the identification, by suckling mouse inoculation, of two new species of enteroviruses: the group A and B coxsackieviruses by Gilbert Dalldorf and Joseph Melnick in 1948 and 1949.

Pivotal work by John Enders, Thomas Weller and Fredrick Robbins on refinement of tissue culture technique led not only to the development of the inactivated (Salk) and live oral (Sabin) polio vaccines, but also the identification of a fourth enterovirus species: echovirus. The development of reverse transcription-polymerase chain reaction (RT-PCR) methodologies for the detection of the enteroviruses, as well as computational methods for the analysis of viral genomes in the late 1980s and early 1990s, led to the discovery of nearly 50 novel types and a realignment of the taxonomy of the enteroviruses and rhinoviruses.

PHYSICAL AND CHEMICAL PROPERTIES

The pathology, transmission and general epidemiology of enteroviruses are all shaped by their biophysical properties (Table 164-1). Their structural stability in various environments are key factors in their transmission.

CLASSIFICATION

Members of the family Picornaviridae are small, positive sense, single-stranded RNA viruses. The family is subdivided into 26 genera of which *Enterovirus* is one (Table 164-2).[2-4] The genus *Enterovirus* comprises 12 species, seven of them pathogenic for humans and each with

TABLE 164-1	Physical and Chemical Properties of Enterovirus Particles	
Characteristic	**Properties**	
Sedimentation	Buoyant density in cesium chloride: 1.30–1.34 g/cm³	
Stability	Stable in weak acid, retain the infectivity for 1–3 hours at pH values up to 3.0 (allows replication in the alimentary tract) Environmental: stable at room temperature for days, 4°C for weeks, and years at freezing temperatures	
Structural stability	Insensitive to lipid solvents (ether and chloroform) Stable in many detergents at ambient temperature Resistant to laboratory disinfectants (70% ethanol, isopropanol, lysol, quaternary ammonium compounds)	
Inactivation	Chemical: formaldehyde, glutaraldehyde, strong acid, sodium hypochlorite, free residual chlorine Environmental: temperatures higher than 50°C (no inactivation in the presence of molar MgCl), ultraviolet light, drying on surfaces	

TABLE 164-2	Genera in the Family *Picornaviridae*[2-4]	
Aphthovirus	Gallivirus	Pasivirus
Aquamavirus	Hepatovirus	Passerivirus
Avihepatovirus	Hunnivirus	Rosavirus
Avisivirus	Kobuvirus	Salivirus
Cardiovirus	Megrivirus	Sapelovirus
Cosavirus	Mischivirus	Senecavirus
Dicipivirus	Mosavirus	Teschovirus
Enterovirus	Oscivirus	Tremovirus
Erbovirus	Parechovirus	

<table>
<tr><td colspan="2">TABLE 164-3   Classification of Enterovirus Species A–D and Serotypes</td></tr>
</table>

Species	Serotypes
Enterovirus A	CV-A2 to 8, CV-A10, CV-A12, CV-A14, CV-A16, EV-A71, EV-A76, EV-A89 to EV-A91, EV-A114, EV-A119 to EV-A121 (contains most of the old coxsackievirus A species members of the old nomenclature)
Enterovirus B	CV-A9 CV-B1 to B6 E-1 to E-7, E-9, E-11 to E-21, E-24 to E-27, E-29 to E-33 EV-B69, EV-B73 to EV75, EV-B77 to EV-B88, EV-B93, EV-B97, EV-B98, EV-B100, EV-B101, EV-B106, EV-B107, EV-B110, EV-B11 (contains all of the coxsackievirus B and echovirus species members of the old nomenclature)
Enterovirus C	PV-1 to 3 CV-A1, CV-A11, CV-A13, CV-A15, CV-A17 to CV-A22, CV-A24, EV-C95, EV-C 96, EV-C99, EV-C102, EV-C104, EV-C105, EV-C105, EV-C109, EV-C113, EV-C116 to EVC118 (contains the remainder of the members of coxsackievirus A species and all poliovirus species members of the old nomenclature)
Enterovirus D	EV-D68, EV-D70, EV-D94, EV-D111, EV-D120

<table>
<tr><td colspan="2">TABLE 164-4   Criteria for Species Classification of the Enteroviruses</td></tr>
</table>

Taxonomic Level	Criteria
Enterovirus species (ICTV)	Members of a species of the genus *Enterovirus*: • Share greater than 70% aa identity in the polyprotein • Share greater than 60% aa identity in P1 • Share greater than 70% aa identity in the nonstructural proteins 2C+3CD • Share a limited range of host cell receptors • Share a limited natural host range • Have a genome base composition (G+C) which varies by no more than 2.5% • Share a significant degree of compatibility in proteolytic processing, replication, encapsidation and genetic recombination

a variable number of serotypes. The species Enterovirus A–D will be discussed (Table 164-3).

The original classification of serotypes with in the enteroviral genus was based on physicochemical characteristics, host range and pathogenic potential. This classification defined serotypes into four species:

- polioviruses;
- coxsackie A viruses (CV-A);
- coxsackie B viruses (CV-B);
- echoviruses (E); and
- enteroviruses (EV). Since 1970, new enterovirus types have been assigned type numbers, starting with 68, forming the fifth species within the genus.

While originally useful, the scheme misclassified several enteroviruses and incorporated non-enteroviruses within the genus.[2] The advent of methods for amplification, rapid genomic sequencing and computation analysis of viral genomes has led to a classification scheme based on RNA homology within the VP1 capsid coding region. Under the new scheme, enteroviruses are subdivided into four species of Enterovirus, A to D.[2,3] New enteroviruses are phylogenetically assigned to their species[5–11] rather than being antigenically characterized. The International Committee on Taxonomy of Viruses (ICTV) has proposed criteria for inclusion of a new enterovirus within a species (Table 164-4).[2]

STRUCTURE AND GENOME ORGANIZATION

The enteroviral virion is non-enveloped, spherical, with icosahedral symmetry and approximately 30 nm in diameter. The capsid is composed of four structural proteins: VP1, VP2, VP3 and VP4. For all but VP4, the amino acid chains comprising the protein are arranged to form eight antiparallel β-sheet structures or 'β-barrels'.[12] The amino acids that connect β-strands and C-termini of the β-barrels are exposed on the virion's external surface and determine its topography and unique serotype antigenicity. A total of 60 structural proteins comprise the capsid. One copy of each of the four proteins form a capsid promoter. Five protomers assemble to form a pentamer and 12 pentamers form the virion. VP4 lacks external surface exposure but stabilizes the capsid through interactions of its conserved residues and the viral RNA.

The structure of multiple enteroviruses, including poliovirus, has been determined revealing conserved structural motifs.[12] At the five-fold axis of symmetry (i.e. pentameric apex) is a star-shaped plateau surrounded by a deep depression (canyon), which is the receptor-binding site for several of the enteroviruses. In the canyon floor is a hydrophobic 'pocket' that tunnels toward the fivefold axis.

The enteroviral genome is a single, positive-stranded RNA molecule. It has an average length of approximately 7.4 kb consisting of four regions: a 5' nontranslated region (NTR), a single open reading frame (ORF), a 3' NTR and a polyadenylated tail (Figure 164-1). A small protein, VPg, is covalently linked at the extreme 5' end of the genome.

Infection by Enterovirus

Pathogenicity

VIRAL CYCLE

Picornavirus replication occurs in the cell cytoplasm. The cycle of polioviruses has been the most studied and best characterized.

The replication stages can be divided into:

- attachment;
- entry and uncoating;
- translation of the viral genome and viral RNA synthesis; and
- assembly and release of the virus.

Attachment

Enterovirus attachment at the cell surface is determined by binding to cellular receptors. Enterovirus host range appears to be mainly determined by the specific recognition of the virus by receptors on the surface of susceptible cells (Table 164-5).[13] For some viruses of the species (i.e. poliovirus) viral binding to a cellular receptor is sufficient to initiate viral uncoating (infection).[14] For most, however, interaction with the receptor is insufficient for infection as they require a second molecule, a co-receptor, for viral entry.[15,16] The picture is further complicated in that some serotypes can use different receptors depending on cell type and different serotypes have different surface interactions with the same receptor.[17]

The poliovirus receptor (PVR, CD155) is a membrane protein composed of three extracellular immunoglobulin (Ig)-like domains: a membrane-distal V-type domain followed by two C2-type domains.[14] PVR is a member of the Ig supergene family. The first Ig-domain contains the poliovirus binding site and fits within the canyon. PVR transgenic mice are susceptible to poliovirus, but infection by the oral route is not possible unless the alpha/beta interferon receptor has been knocked out.[18] PVR transgenic mice have proved to be a valuable model for studying the pathogenesis of poliomyelitis.[19,20]

Some species C enteroviruses use another member of the Ig-superfamily, intercellular adhesion molecule-1 (ICAM-1, CD54), as their receptor or co-receptor. ICAM-1 is a type 1 membrane protein with five Ig-like domains. The viral binding occurs in the canyon and is located to the first Ig-like domain.

The receptor for all CV-Bs has two Ig-like extracellular domains, a transmembrane domain and a cytoplasmic domain that is also used as

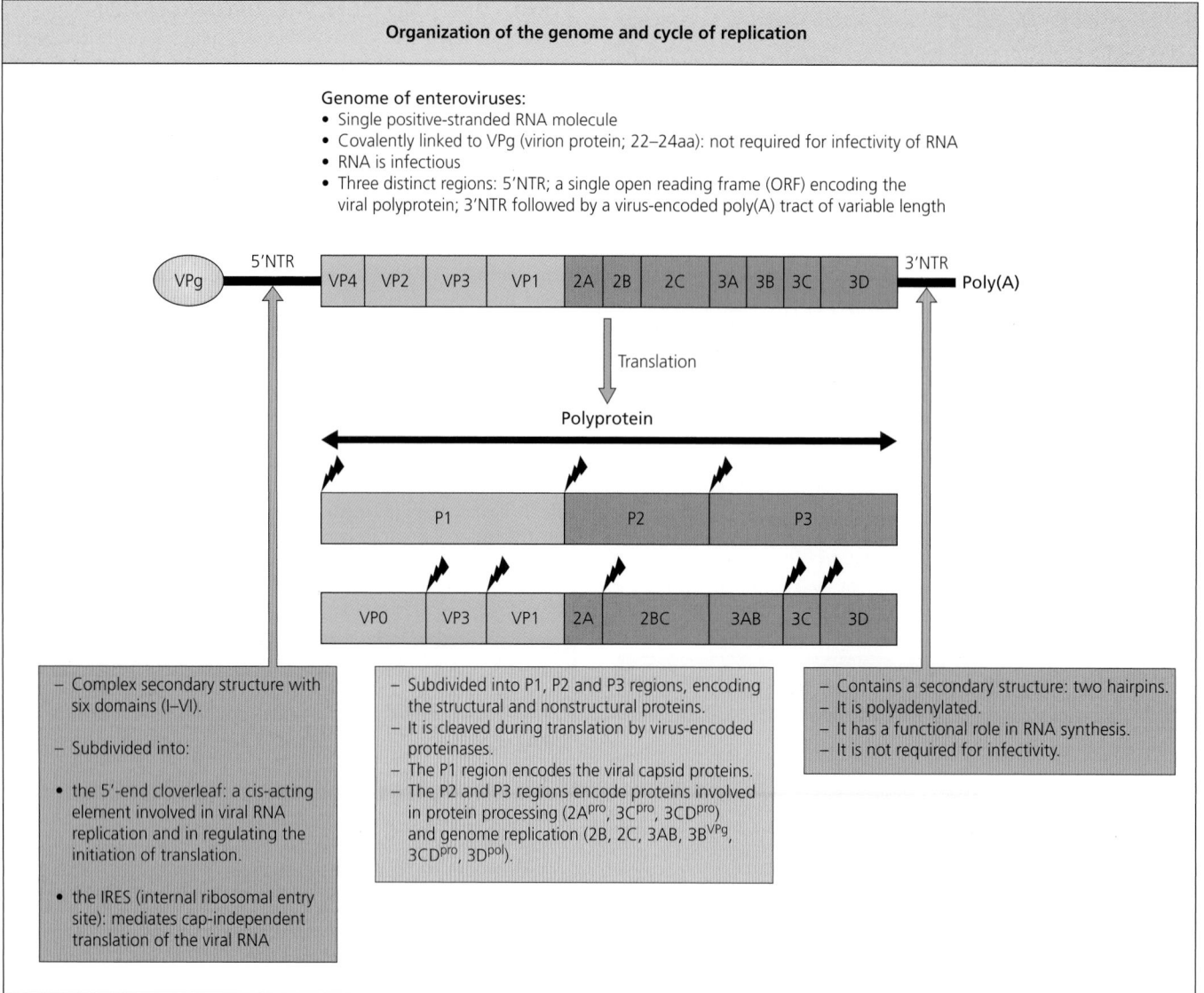

Organization of the genome and cycle of replication

Genome of enteroviruses:
- Single positive-stranded RNA molecule
- Covalently linked to VPg (virion protein; 22–24aa): not required for infectivity of RNA
- RNA is infectious
- Three distinct regions: 5'NTR; a single open reading frame (ORF) encoding the viral polyprotein; 3'NTR followed by a virus-encoded poly(A) tract of variable length

5'NTR | VP4 VP2 VP3 VP1 | 2A 2B 2C 3A 3B 3C 3D | 3'NTR Poly(A)
VPg

Translation

Polyprotein

P1 | P2 | P3

VP0 | VP3 | VP1 | 2A | 2BC | 3AB | 3C | 3D

- Complex secondary structure with six domains (I–VI).
- Subdivided into:
  - the 5'-end cloverleaf: a cis-acting element involved in viral RNA replication and in regulating the initiation of translation.
  - the IRES (internal ribosomal entry site): mediates cap-independent translation of the viral RNA

- Subdivided into P1, P2 and P3 regions, encoding the structural and nonstructural proteins.
- It is cleaved during translation by virus-encoded proteinases.
- The P1 region encodes the viral capsid proteins.
- The P2 and P3 regions encode proteins involved in protein processing ($2A^{pro}$, $3C^{pro}$, $3CD^{pro}$) and genome replication (2B, 2C, 3AB, $3B^{VPg}$, $3CD^{pro}$, $3D^{pol}$).

- Contains a secondary structure: two hairpins.
- It is polyadenylated.
- It has a functional role in RNA synthesis.
- It is not required for infectivity.

Figure 164-1 Organization of the viral genome and cycle of replication. NTR, nontranslated region.

a receptor by human adenoviruses 2 and 5; thus, it is named the coxsackievirus and adenovirus receptor (CAR). CAR functions in intracellular adhesion and is found at the tight junction. Viral binding to CAR occurs at the canyon.

Decay-accelerating factor (DAF, CD55), an extracellular protein of the complement system, comprises four short consensus repeat sequences and a glycosylphosphatidylinositol plasma membrane anchor. DAF has been shown to be the attachment receptor for various enteroviruses, although the sites of attachment on the viral surface differ (Table 164-5). DAF plays an important role in infection of polarized cells of the gastrointestinal and respiratory tracts by CV-B3. CAR is absent at the apical surface of these cells. Binding of CV-B3 to DAF triggers actin rearrangement that moves the DAF-CV-B3 complex to the tight junction where it can bind to CAR and cause infection.[21]

The superfamily of integrins contains enterovirus receptors: $\alpha_v\beta_6$, $\alpha_v\beta_3$ (vitronectin receptor) and $\alpha_2\beta_1$ (very late-activating antigen-2 [VLA-2]). CV-A9 binds to integrins using an Arg-Gly-Asp (RGD) sequence located in the C-terminus of VP1. E-2 does not require the RGD motif to bind $\alpha_2\beta_1$ in the canyon.

Entry and Uncoating

A series of conformational changes occur during virus entry. The interaction of poliovirus with PVR leads to expulsion of a lipid molecule

from the pocket and major structural changes in the virus. The N-terminus of the VP1 becomes exposed after release of the VP4, resulting in altered (or A) particles. In the most widely accepted hypothesis of poliovirus RNA entry, the N-terminal VP1 domain inserts into the cell membrane, forming a pore though which viral RNA enters the cytoplasm. VP4 may contribute to the formation of the pore.[22] Recently, a new model has been proposed in which an umbilicus, composed of the N-terminus of VP4 and VP1 is formed through which the viral RNA can pass.[23]

Translation of the Viral Genome and Viral RNA Synthesis

Following uncoating, the viral positive-stranded RNA serves as a template for protein and RNA synthesis. After release of VPg, viral protein synthesis takes place at the rough endoplasmic reticulum (ER). Enteroviral RNA lacks the m7G cap group required to bind the 40S ribosomal subunit. Instead, 40S ribosomal subunit binding and initiation of translation take place at the internal ribosome entry site (IRES) within the 5' NTR.

Translation of viral RNA produces a polyprotein that is cotranslationally processed to yield 11 mature viral proteins and several functional intermediates through cleavage by the viral proteinases. The

TABLE 164-5	Cell Receptors for Enterovirus Species A–D		
Virus	**Receptor**		**Co-receptor**
PV-1, PV-2, PV-3	PVR (CD-155)		
CV-A9	$\alpha_v\beta_3$, $\alpha_v\beta_6$		β2-microglobulin, GRP78, MHC-1
CV-A13, CV-A18, CV-A21	ICAM-1		
CV-A16	Scavenger receptor class B (SCARB2), P-selectin glycoprotein ligand-1 (PSGL-1)		
CV-A21	Decay-accelerating factor (DAF, CD55)		ICAM-1
CV-A24	Sialic acid		
CV-B1 to B6	Coxsackievirus–adenovirus receptor (CAR)		
CV-B1, CV-B3, CV-B5	Decay-accelerating factor (DAF, CD55)		αvβ6-integrin
E-1, E-8	$\alpha_2\beta_1$-integrin (VLA-2)		β2-microglobulin
E-3, E-6, E-7, E-11 to E-13, E-20, E-21, E-24, E-29, E-30, E-33	Decay-accelerating factor (DAF, CD55)		β2-microglobulin
E-5	Heparin sulfate		
E-9	$\alpha_v\beta_3$-integrin		
EV-D68	Sialic acid		
EV-D70	Decay-accelerating factor (DAF, CD55)		
EV-A71	Scavenger receptor class B (SCARB2), P-selectin glycoprotein ligand-1 (PSGL-1)		

2A protease catalyzes the first cleavage of the nascent polyprotein resulting in release of the P1 precursor. Subsequent cleavages of P1 into VP0, VP3 and VP1 are mediated by the 3CD protease. Cleavage of P2 and P3 precursors into stable end products is mediated by the 3C protease (3C[pro])/3CD protease (3CD[pro]).

The replication of viral RNA takes place on the cytoplasmic surface of double membraned vesicles. The viral proteins 3A and 2BC localize to the ER and promote vesicle formation. VPg, the protein primer for RNA synthesis, is anchored to the vesicle membrane by 3AB. 3AB also binds 3D[pol], the enterovirus RNA-dependent RNA polymerase, and 3CD[pro], recruiting them to the replication complex. 2C, also found on the membrane, could also anchor the viral RNA to the membrane via its RNA binding domain. The replication of viral RNA takes place using intermediate negative-stranded RNA copies of the viral genome. 3D[pol] regulates viral transcription by interaction with viral and cellular factors through secondary structural motifs in the NTRs of positive- and negative-stranded RNAs.

Assembly and Release of the Virus

Virus morphogenesis is characterized by intermediate assembly steps of the virus capsid via precursors and a procapsid. At the final stage, one molecule of positive-stranded RNA is encapsidated in the provirus and a final proteolytic cleavage of the precursor protein VP0 into VP2 and VP4 finalizes the virus maturation.

Cytopathic Effects

The replication cycle of poliovirus is 6–8 hours. Infected cells become rounded and contain cytoplasmic protrusions. The nucleus is pyknotic and the chromatin is condensed. During the early stage of the cycle, mitosis is enhanced; at later stages, mitosis is arrested at metaphase. Two hours after infection, poliovirus shuts down synthesis of cellular protein, RNA and DNA. Cellular protein synthesis inhibition is caused by proteolytic cleavage of eukaryotic initiation factor eIF-4G by 2A. Scanning electron microscopy reveals initial changes in the cell surface as early as 3 hours after infection. Eight hours after infection condensation of collapsed microvilli, formation of elongated filopodia and 'rounding up' of the cell is observed. At this time, up to 10 000 virus particles have been synthesized in a single cell.

Epidemiology

HOSTS

The natural host of enteroviruses is the human. Some animals are susceptible to natural and experimental infection with human enteroviruses: nonhuman primates and CD155 transgenic mice for poliovirus; mice and some species of monkeys for coxsackie A and B viruses and echovirus. CV-B5 is interesting in that it is antigenically and genetically (50% homology) related to the porcine enterovirus, swine vesicular disease (SVD) virus. Epidemiologic studies from SVD outbreaks suggest that CV-B5 was introduced into swine decades ago and led to establishment in this new host.[24]

The routes of enterovirus transmission are summarized in Table 164-6.

IMMUNE RESPONSE

Innate Immune System

The major factor affecting the outcome of an enteroviral infection is the efficacy of the immune response. The role of the innate immune system is important as an early determinant of pathogenesis. Studies of poliovirus in CD155 transgenic mice demonstrate that the interferon (INF) response is an important determinant of tissue tropism and pathogenicity.[25] Protection against poliovirus infection is mediated by IFN-alpha-induced 2',5'-oligoadenylate synthetases and ribonuclease L, and IFN-gamma-induced double-stranded RNA-dependent RNA-activated protein kinase in CV-B-infected pancreatic islet cells.[26] Nuclear factor kappa B, a regulator that activates INF-beta and initiates the cascade of proinflammatory cytokines, has been shown to be activated early after poliovirus infection. IFN-stimulated gene effects may be complex; reductions in inflammation have been associated with a slight increase in survival in animal transgenic models.[27] The role of innate lymphocytes and natural killer cells has been less studied. These cells may play a role, not only in protection, but also in mediating disease.

B-cell Response

The host humoral immune response is essential for protection from and elimination of enteroviral infections. Individuals with congenital or acquired humoral immunodeficiencies (e.g. agammaglobulinemia, severe combined immunodeficiency, rituximab therapy, etc.) are at risk for persistent or severe infections. Poliovirus neutralization sites are generally conformational antigenic sites that correspond to exposed loops of the capsid proteins, although some internally located regions of the virion can also function as neutralization sites. Studies to identify neutralization sites of nonpolio enteroviruses (nonPV-EV) are limited; however, results suggest similarities in the location of their antigenic sites to those of poliovirus.

CIRCULATION AND GEOGRAPHIC SPREAD

Enteroviruses have a worldwide distribution and are most prevalent during the summer in temperate climates and during the rainy season in the tropics. Within a given geographic locality, some serotypes may be endemic, with little or only gradual change in the serotypes isolated from year to year. Other serotypes, rarely encountered in the community, may be introduced periodically causing epidemics. Occasionally, enteroviruses have caused pandemics or outbreaks involving large geographic areas (e.g. EV-D70 and EV-A71).[28,29]

Clinical Manifestations

ASYMPTOMATIC INFECTIONS

Most enterovirus infections are subclinical, or mild. Since the cells of the gut epithelia normally have a high rate of turnover, it has been hypothesized that enterovirus passage through the gut may be the reason for the high incidence of subclinical infections.

CLINICAL SYNDROMES

Nonpolio Enteroviruses

NonPV-EVs are the causal agents in a wide variety of clinical syndromes involving multiple organ systems including the central nervous system (CNS) (aseptic meningitis, acute flaccid paralysis (AFP), encephalitis, transverse myelitis, Guillain–Barré syndrome), muscular (pleurodynia, acute inflammatory muscle disease), respiratory (upper respiratory tract infection, pneumonia), skin and mucous membranes (exanthema, herpangina, hand, foot and mouth disease (HFMD)), ocular (acute hemorrhagic conjunctivitis), cardiac (myocarditis and pericarditis) and neonatal sepsis-like infections (Table 164-7). Enterovirus D68 (EV-D68) is an emergent viral pathogen associated with severe respiratory illness, especially in children with asthma.[30]

TABLE 164-6 Routes of Transmission of Enterovirus Species A–D

Type	Route
Individual	Fecal–oral route (associated with poor sanitary conditions). Respiratory route (CV-A24, EV-D70, EV-D68) Other proven routes of transmission: • Environmental sources • Contaminated sources of water (swimming pools, ponds, salt water) • EV-D70 and CV-A24 (causing hemorrhagic conjunctivitis) can be isolated from eye secretions; those causing vesicular exanthema can be spread by direct and indirect vesicular fluid. In both cases, common routes for infection are hand contact with secretions, and autoinoculation of mouth, nose and eyes Possible routes of transmission: • Breast milk • Flies • EV have been isolated from mollusks and crustaceans
Groups	Enterovirus household transmission and familial outbreaks Schools Daycare centers Camps Sports teams Orphanages Nosocomial transmission Military installations Laboratory

---

TABLE 164-7 Clinical Manifestations of Enterovirus Species A–D Infections

Clinical Disorders	Enterovirus Serotypes	Characteristics
Paralysis	PV-1–3 (severe paralysis) CV-A4, A7, A9 E-4–6 EV-D70, A71	Transient mild paresis with aseptic meningitis may occur Younger children have milder disease
Aseptic meningitis	CV-A2, A4, A7, A9, A10, A12, A16 CV-B1–B6 PV-1 to 3 E-4, 6, 7, 9, 11, 30 EV-A71	Benign in infants and children May involve rash or encephalitis Virus isolated from the throat, stool or cerebrospinal fluid
Acute hemorrhagic conjunctivitis	EV-D70 CV-A24 variant	May produce subconjunctival hemorrhage and keratitis Pain, blurred vision, aversion to light, discharge from the eye Rarely accompanied by transient radiculomyelopathy or poliomyelitis-like paralysis
Hand, foot and mouth disease	CV-A10, A6, A16 , EV-A71 (less commonly CV-A4, A5, A9)	Vesicular exanthem, usually brief and benign, initially as a sore throat involving the tongue, followed by a rash on the hands and sometimes the feet The rash may form small blisters, which lead to ulcers Symptoms generally resolve within a week
Rash and exanthema with fever	CV-A2, A4 to A6, A9, A16 CV-B1, B3, B4, V5 E-2, 4, 9, 11, 14, 16, 19, 25	Nonpruritic, does not desquamate, on the face, neck, chest and extremities Maculopapular, morbilliform; occasionally hemorrhagic, petechial or vesicular Summer and fall rashes in children
Respiratory disease	E-4, 8, 9, 11, 20 CV-A2, A10, A21, A24 CV-B1–B6 EV-D68	Fever, coryza, pharyngitis; in some patients vomiting and diarrhea Bronchitis and interstitial pneumonia are seen occasionally
Herpangina	CV-A1–A6, A8– A10, A16, A21, A22	Palatal and pharyngeal lesions particularly severe, multiple ulcers in the throat Swallowing becomes very painful; symptoms can persist for several weeks
Myocarditis	CV-B1–B6 CV-A4, A16 E-9	Newborns infected after birth or rarely *in utero* can present with sepsis with fever, lethargy, disseminated intravascular coagulation, bleeding and multiple organ failure; death may occur from circulatory collapse or hepatic failure Older children or adults may make a complete recovery

TABLE 164-8	Characteristics of Poliovirus Vaccines	
Properties	**Inactivated Poliovirus Vaccine**	**Oral Poliovirus Vaccine**
Antigen	Three wild reference strains: PV1 Mahoney; PV2 MEF-1 and PV3 Sauckett	Three attenuated
Administration	Injection	Orally
Induces	Circulating antibodies	Circulating antibodies and local immune response in intestinal lining
Protection	Protects individual against spread of the virus to CNS	Protects individual against infection and passive immunization of close contacts (risk for revertants and AFP)
Local immunity	Very low levels of local immunity (in the gut)	Induces intestinal local immunity
Viral circulation	Cannot interrupt wild type poliovirus circulation	Interrupts wild type poliovirus transmission

In the postpolio era, the more important syndromes caused by the enteroviruses are those of the CNS. Meningitis can be caused by most enteroviruses. Constitutional symptoms include fever, malaise, headache, nausea, emesis and abdominal pain. CNS signs include nuchal rigidity, Brudzinski's and Kernig's signs, photo- or phonophobia, irritability, or lethargy. A nonspecific rash may be present. Rarely, seizures or a mild, transient paresis may occur. Enteroviruses are the most common cause of aseptic meningitis in children and adults in higher-income countries.

Encephalitis, and, less commonly, transverse myelitis, cerebellar ataxia and Guillain–Barré syndrome have been associated with enterovirus infections. Encephalitis is manifested by an altered state of consciousness, focal neurologic signs or seizures. If accompanied by meningitis it is termed meningoencephalitis. Depending on the country, enteroviruses may be responsible for up to 15% of encephalitis cases.[31] EV-A71 HFMD may be complicated by rhombencephalitis (brainstem encephalitis), meningitis and AFP.[32] EV-A71 has caused epidemics of severe neurologic disease in Australia, Europe, and Asia. Fatal cases of rhombencephalitis have occurred during large HFMD outbreaks in countries of the Asia-Pacific rim.[29]

Acute Flaccid Paralysis

Poliovirus and some nonPV-EV can cause AFP. The pathogenesis of polioviruses is the best studied. Following ingestion, poliovirus replicates in the submucosal lymphatic tissue at implantation sites (e.g. tonsils, ileal Peyer's patches and the mesenteric lymph nodes) and spreads to the regional lymph nodes. Replication at these sites results in a 'minor viremia' which disseminates virus throughout the body, leading to infection of reticuloendothelial tissues and multiple organs. Additional replication in these organs leads to a 'major viremia' that ceases once type-specific antibodies are produced. The method of poliovirus access to the CNS is yet unknown but evidence exists for either a bloodstream or retrograde axonal transport route.

The overwhelming majority of poliovirus infections are asymptomatic. In 4–8%, infection results in abortive poliomyelitis, characterized by 2–3 days of fever, headache, sore throat, anorexia, vomiting or abdominal pain. The neurologic examination is normal. Nonparalytic poliomyelitis differs by the presence of signs of meningeal irritation (see above) and is identical to meningitis caused by other enteroviruses. AFP occurs in < 1% of poliovirus infections in susceptible individuals. The onset of paralysis is preceded by 1–3 days of minor illness and, at times, by a symptom-free interval, followed by fever, meningismus, severe myalgias and the acute onset of flaccid paralysis. Paralysis is usually asymmetric and may affect skeletal muscles (spinal poliomyelitis), respiratory systems (bulbar poliomyelitis), or both (bulbospinal poliomyelitis). The loss of motor neurons is permanent and the denervated muscles atrophy.

A small number of infected individuals developed recrudescence of paralysis and muscle atrophy several decades after paralytic poliomyelitis. This postpolio syndrome results from the additive effects of physiologic aging and the prolonged loss of neuromuscular function from the earlier infection.

TABLE 164-9	Objective and Milestones of the WHO Polio Eradication and Endgame Strategic Plan 2013–2018	
Major Objectives	**Milestones**	
Poliovirus detection and interruption of transmission	Stop all poliovirus transmission by the end of 2014	
Strengthen routine immunization programs and withdrawal of the oral polio vaccine	Withdraw the Sabin type 2 component of the oral polio vaccine in all immunization programs by middle of 2016	
Containment and certification	Certification of all six WHO regions as having eradicated wild type poliovirus by the end of 2018	
Legacy planning	Have a legacy planning strategy in place by the end of 2015	

Reprinted from World Health Organization. Poliomyelitis: intensification of the global eradication initiative. Report by the Secretariat.

Control of Infection

VACCINES

Two different vaccines have been developed for the prevention of poliovirus: the Salk inactivated poliovirus vaccine (IPV) and Sabin's attenuated oral poliovirus vaccine (OPV) (Table 164-8).[33] Both contain strains of each of the three poliovirus serotypes and have played important roles in poliovirus elimination. Both are effective, each with particular advantages and disadvantages.[34] In approximately one in every 2.5 million vaccine doses the live attenuated vaccine viruses in OPV can cause paralysis, either in the vaccinated child or in a close contact. Immune deficiency of the recipient may be among the possible causes.

ERADICATION OF POLIOMYELITIS AND THE ENDGAME OF POLIOVIRUS VACCINATION

The global effort to eradicate poliomyelitis has been a massive public health initiative. Recently, the WHO has intensified the global eradication initiative in an effort to achieve polio eradication by 2018 (Table 164-9).[35] Since the launch of the Global Polio Eradication Initiative, the number of cases of polio has fallen by >99%, from >350 000 cases in 1988 to 416 cases in 2013.[36] Four of the six WHO regions have been declared polio-free: the Americas (1994) the Western Pacific Region (2000), the European Region (2002) and the South East Asia Regions (2014). While these successes are heartening, polio remains endemic to Afghanistan, Nigeria and Pakistan and introductions into previously polio-free countries (Somalia, Cameroon, Equatorial Guinea, Iraq, Syria, Ethiopia, Kenya) continue to occur. The impact of the global initiative can also be monitored by the declining genetic diversity of wild poliovirus genotypes. Wild poliovirus type 2 has been eradicated.[37] Wild poliovirus type 3 has not been detected since November 2012.[35]

Recombination between the Sabin OPV strains and species C enteroviruses has resulted in circulating vaccine-derived polioviruses (cVDPVs). Outbreaks of AFP secondary to cVDPVs have been reported in underimmunized populations.[38,39]

In high-income countries without incidence of wild type poliovirus (wtPV)-associated paralytic poliomyelitis, use of OPV is avoided in favor of the safer IPV. IPV is ineffective at producing gut immunity. As a result, it provides individual protection against polio but, unlike OPV, is less effective in preventing the spread of wtPV. Current WHO recommendations call for use of OPV alone for immunization in all polio-endemic countries, countries at high risk for polio importation, and countries with moderate or high potential for wtPV transmission.[40] Due to the international spread of polio the WHO declared an international public health emergency in May 2014 and issued vaccine recommendations for travelers from countries with active wtPV transmission.[41]

TREATMENT AND PREVENTION

With the exception of EV-A71, infections caused by nonPN-EVs cannot be prevented by vaccination. Recent successful vaccine trials show promise for a vaccine effective against EV-A71 subgenotype C4.[42-45] Pooled immunoglobulin has been used with limited success in enterovirus CNS infections in immunocompromised patients and neonates.[46] WIN-type compounds such as pleconaril (VP63843, licensed to Schering-Plough) showed broad *in vitro* inhibitory activity against nonPN-EVs tested.[47] It was not licensed due to adverse effects.

Diagnosis

Key to understanding the epidemiology of the enteroviruses, their diversity and clinical spectrum is their identification and characterization. Effective diagnostic virology depends on appropriate timing, collection and transport of appropriate clinical specimens.

SPECIMENS FOR DIAGNOSIS

For viral diagnosis, the specimens of choice will depend on the organ system involved and diagnostic assay available (classic or molecular), usually stool, rectal or throat swabs, blood and cerebrospinal fluid (CSF) samples. Stool has the highest yield of enteroviral detection, since it contains high virus concentrations (see Figure 164-3). However, the detection of enteroviruses in stool or throat swabs can be misleading in terms of causality of the disease due to asymptomatic viral

shedding. Generally, etiologic association of enterovirus with disease requires virus isolation from fluids or tissues manifesting lesions. Stool and rectal swabs are the specimens of choice for poliovirus diagnosis and AFP surveillance, CSF for neurologic syndromes and throat swabs for respiratory illness, vesicular fluid for vesicular rashes, ocular secretions for hemorrhagic conjunctivitis, and tissue from heart, muscle or brain for myocarditis, myositis or encephalitis, respectively.

CLASSIC TECHNIQUES

These involve direct detection, virus isolation, seroneutralization and serology.

Nonmolecular Direct Detection

Direct detection of the enteroviruses by immunofluorescence (IF), agglutination or enzyme-linked immunosorbent assay (ELISA) are not useful due to low viral burden in most specimens and antigenic diversity. Electron microscopy was used to visualize virus directly (Figure 164-2).

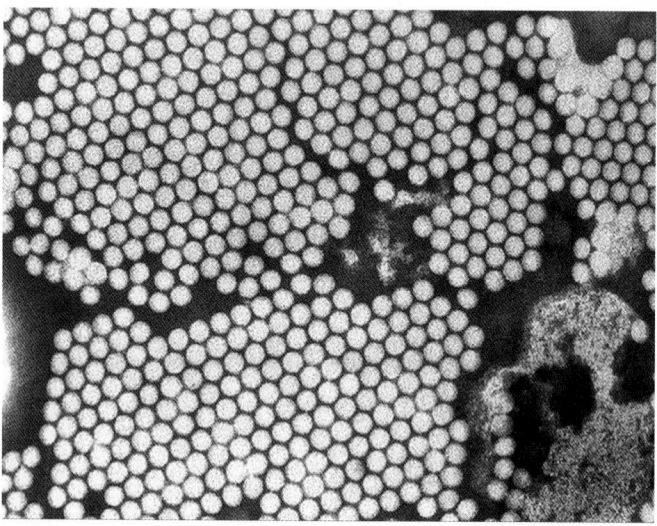

Figure 164-2 Electron micrograph showing poliovirus particles negatively stained with 2% phosphotungstic acid.

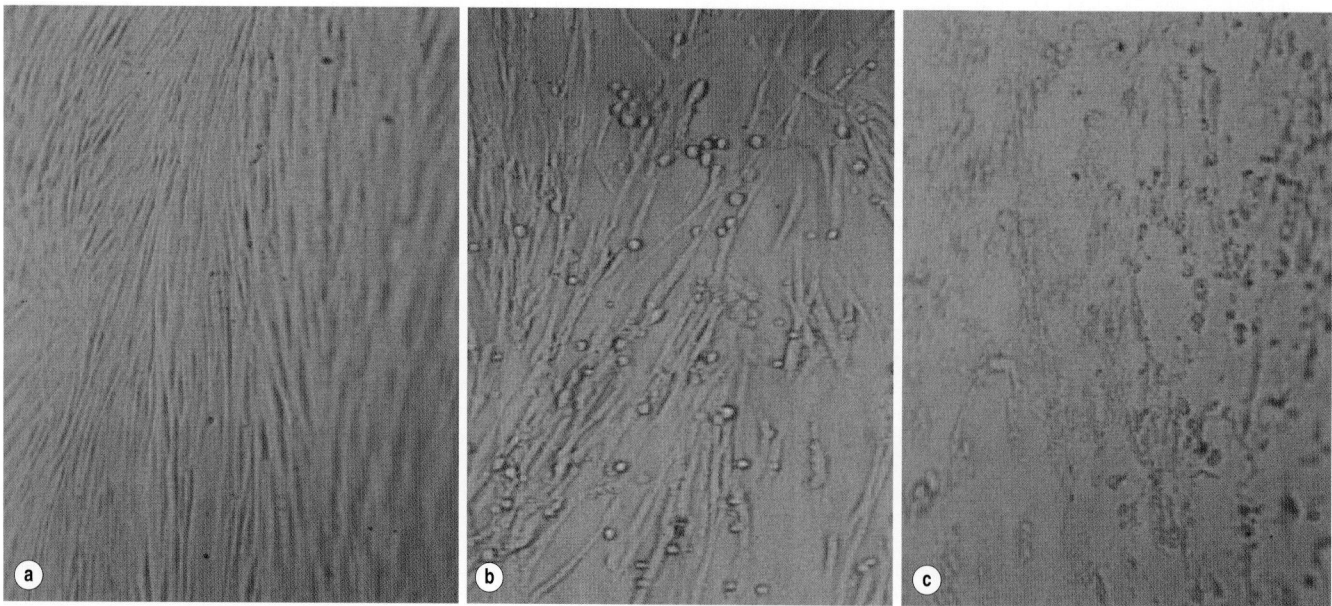

A.FP: uninoculated　　　**B.FP: CPE=1+**　　　**C.FP: CPE= 3+**

Figure 164-3 Enterovirus (EV) cytopathic effect (CPE). Lung fibroblasts (FP) in culture: normal and EV-infected, neither fixed nor stained. (a) Uninoculated FP monolayer. (b) FP showing typical early stage CPE by EV (25% CPE), especially rounding, indicating virus multiplication (1+). (c) FP illustrating more advanced CPE (3+); almost 100% of the cells are affected. Most of the cell sheet has come loose from the culture tube wall.

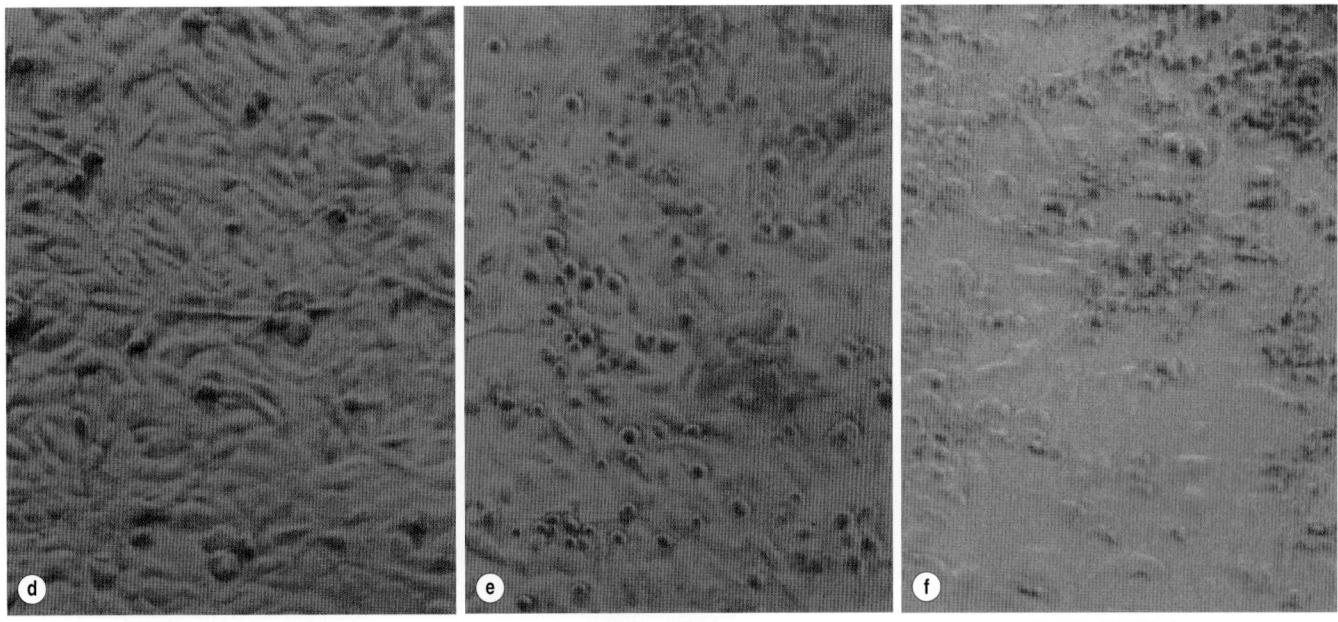

D.RD: uninoculated   **E.RD: CPE=1+**   **F.RD:CPE=3+**

Figure 164-3 Cont'd   Enterovirus (EV) cytopathic effect (CPE). Rhabdomyosarcoma (RD) cells in culture: normal and EV-infected, neither fixed nor stained. (d) Uninoculated RD monolayer. (e) RD showing typical early stage CPE by EV (25% CPE), especially rounding, indicating virus multiplication (1+). (f) RD illustrating more advanced CPE (3+); almost 100% of the cells are affected. Most of the cell sheet has come loose from the culture tube wall.

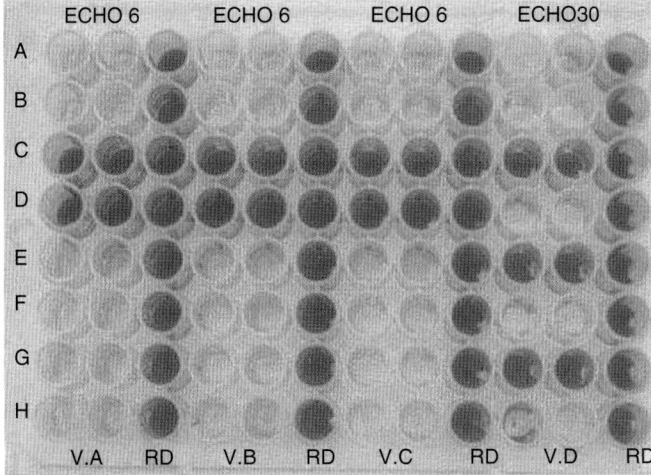

Figure 164-4   Typing of enterovirus by seroneutralization. Rhabdomyosarcoma-stained microplate showing neutralization patterns of A, B, C and D virus with Lim Benyesh-Melnick antiserum pools (A–H). Viruses A, B and C are considered E6 as a result of neutralization with C and D pools containing specific antisera. Virus D is neutralized by C, E and G pools; thus, it is considered an E30.

Enterovirus Isolation

Most enteroviruses will show a characteristic cytopathic effect (CPE) in cell culture – rounded and refractile, with cell detachment (Figure 164-3). To increase the sensitivity of cell culture several cell lines must be used. Isolation is usually attempted using Buffalo green monkey kidney (BGM), human cell lines: rhabdomyosarcoma (RD), lung carcinoma (A-549) and embryonic fibroblasts (HEF). The WHO recommends inoculation into L20B (a genetically engineered mouse cell line expressing PVR) and RD cells for specimens suspected to contain polioviruses.[48] If CPE is detected, identification of enterovirus using neutralization, IF or by molecular techniques is performed.

Serotyping of Enterovirus Isolates

Traditional typing of the nonPV-EVs relies on neutralization with specific antisera. Standardized hyperimmune equine antiserum developed by Lim and Benyesh-Melnick (LBM) is used to identify 42 common enterovirus serotypes.[49] The method employs a panel of eight combined pools (A–H). Isolates are identified by their neutralization pattern against these pools (Figure 164-4). A second panel of antisera was prepared by the National Institute of Public Health and the Environment (RIVM, Bilthoven, the Netherlands) to identify 19 coxsackievirus A serotypes.[50] After identification with these pools, further confirmation is needed by neutralization with the serotype specific antiserum. However, since such broad collections of specific reagents are rarely available in diagnostic and reference laboratories, this last step is normally ignored.

Polioviruses can be serotyped by IF with a panel of monoclonal antibodies (Chemicon, USA) or by neutralization with polyclonal antisera (RIVM). Differentiation between wtPV and vaccine-derived poliovirus (VDPV) strains (intratypic differentiation) is made by ELISA using cross-adsorbed antisera, probe hybridization, RT-PCR, neutralization with monoclonal antibodies or PCR-RFLP.[48] Recently, a dual-stage real-time RT-PCR has been developed which permits sensitive identification of OPV-related viruses.[51]

Despite the use of these techniques, some enteroviral isolates will remain unidentified because of:
- representing an novel serotype;
- representing a mixture of two or more viruses;
- problems with virus aggregation;
- extreme antigenic drift;
- microbial contamination of clinical samples; and
- low concentration of virus in the specimen.

Because of these issues, many diagnostic laboratories around the world have switched to molecular methods for the detection of the enteroviruses in clinical specimens and their identification.

Serologic Analysis

Several methods such as complement fixation, ELISA and immunoblotting are used to screen and detect enterovirus group-specific antibodies. However, the use of serologic techniques for primary diagnosis of suspected enteroviral illness is impractical due to virus diversity. These methods are useful to confirm poliovirus infection and immunization. Serologic diagnosis is performed by comparing titers in paired acute and convalescent serum specimens, in order to detect a significant fourfold antibody titer increase.

Many studies have examined the prevalence of antibodies to enteroviruses in specific populations.[52–54] The number of persons who show neutralizing antibody to any given enterovirus is large, indicating a high incidence of past infection. A high incidence of recent infection is suggested by immunoglobulin M (IgM). Infections with one serotype of enterovirus can boost the antibody titers to other serotypes. The pattern of the heterotypic response varies by serotype and among individuals, and the pattern of serotype antibody prevalence varies by geographic location, by time and by age. Thus prevalence data from different years and locations are not directly comparable. These general

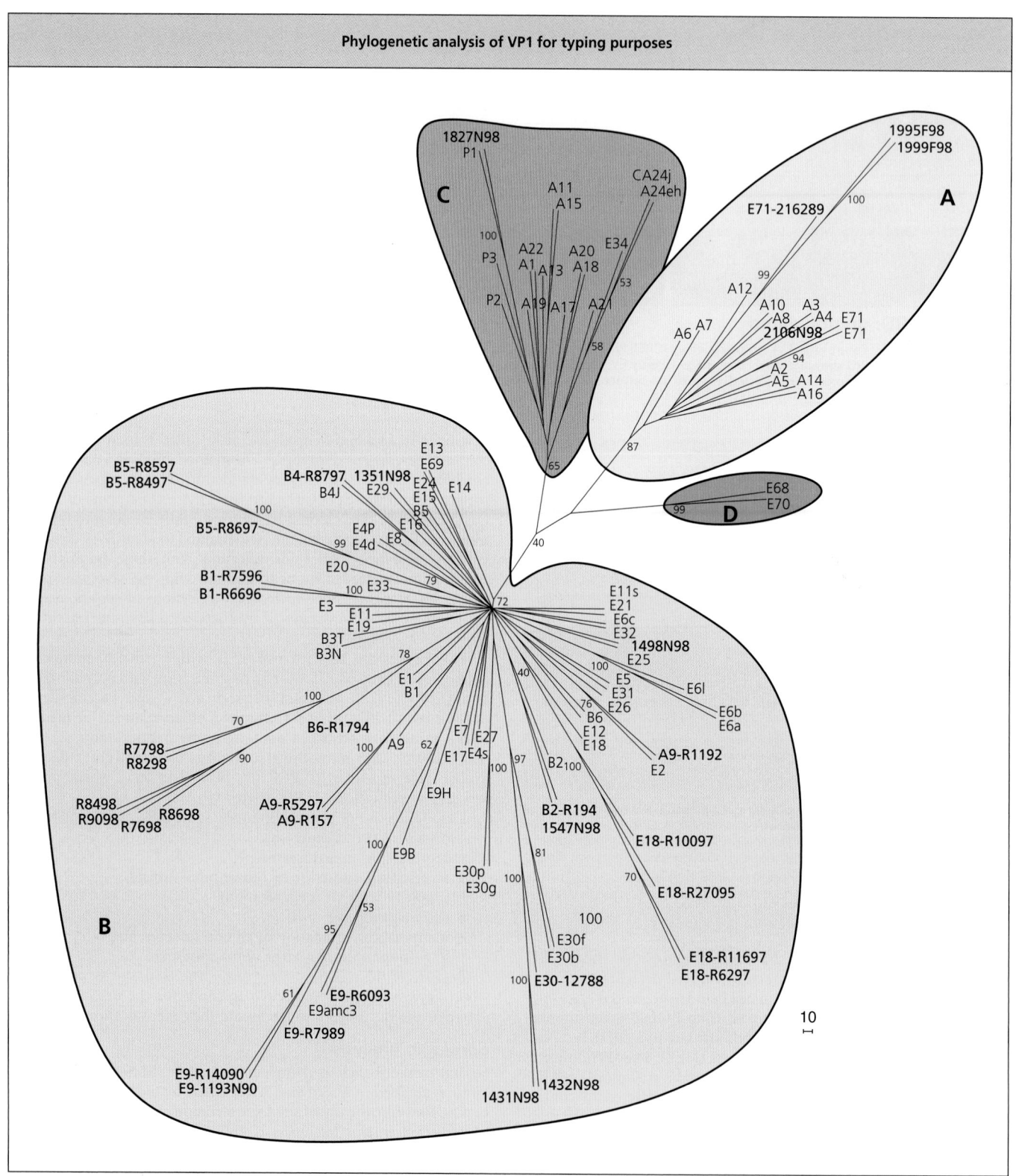

Figure 164-5 Phylogenetic analysis of VP1 for typing purposes.

Molecular epidemiology of EV through the phylogenetic analysis of VP1 sequences

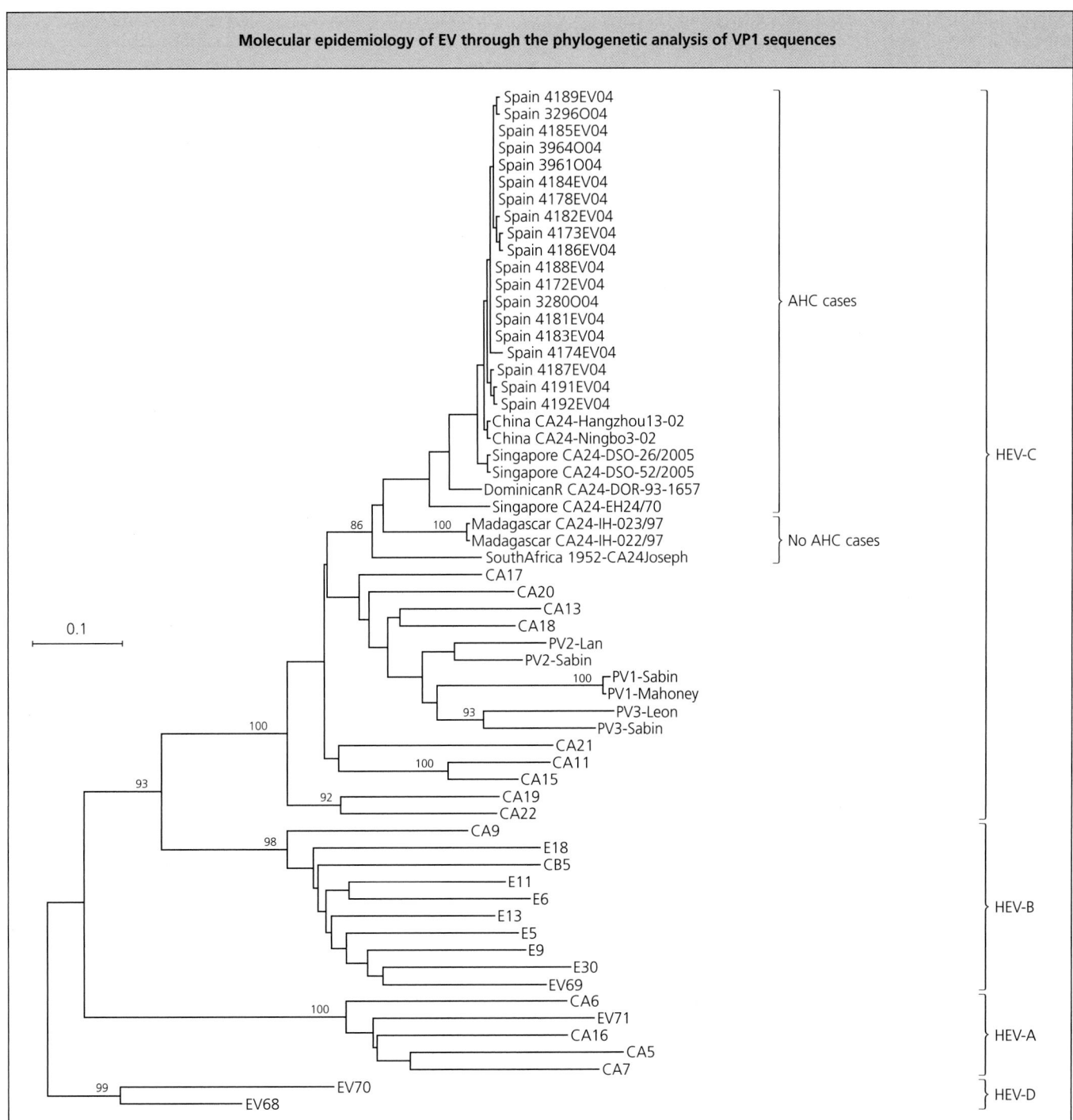

Figure 164-6 Molecular epidemiology of enterovirus though the phylogenetic analysis of VP1 sequences. Phylogenetic tree with 28 CV-A24 sequences and other reference strains of species EV-A to D based on 415 nucleotides within the 3′-VP1 region. EV-D was used to root the dendrogram. The dendrograms were constructed by the neighbor-joining method, with 1000 bootstrap pseudoreplicates. Only bootstrap values >70% are shown at nodes. Genetic distances were calculated with Tamura-Nei's evolution model, and the horizontal branch lengths are drawn to scale.

characteristics must be considered when interpreting the findings of serologic studies of associations between enterovirus infection and disease.

MOLECULAR TECHNIQUES
Detection and Molecular Typing

Application of molecular biology techniques to clinical virology has introduced significant changes in enteroviral diagnosis. Sensitivity and specificity has increased significantly.[54] In addition, molecular techniques provide short detection times, detection of isolates that do not readily grow in cell culture, and allow typing of enteroviruses that are difficult to identify by traditional techniques.[7,56]

Nucleic acid probe hybridization tests were used to detect enteroviruses, but have been replaced by RT-PCR assays. In general, diagnostic assays for enterovirus are targeted to amplify regions of the 5' NTR.[55]

The availability of sequence data for all members of the genus has enabled differentiation of viruses based on the nucleic acid sequence encoding VP1.[56] Molecular identification can be performed using sequences of RT-PCR products obtained directly from clinical specimens[57,58] or virus isolates.[59,60] Although other regions have been used for molecular typing they fail to provide reliable identification. Only VP1 capsid sequence correlates with serotype, due to the high frequency of interspecies recombination among co-circulating enteroviruses (e.g. within HEV-B).[9,61,62] Multiple new enteroviruses have been detected and characterized using molecular typing and sequencing (Figure 164-5).[5,6,8,9] Phylogenetic studies of clinical isolates are useful in examining enteroviral evolution and to characterize enterovirus molecular epidemiology[63-65] (Figure 164-6).

References available online at expertconsult.com.

KEY REFERENCES

Hogle J.M., Chow M., Filman D.J.: Three-dimensional structure of poliovirus at 2.9 Å resolution. *Science* 1985; 229:1358-1365.

Huang C.C., Liu C.C., Chang Y.C., et al.: Neurologic complications in children with enterovirus 71 infection. *N Engl J Med* 1999; 341:936.

Kew O.M., Sutter R.W., de Gourville E.M., et al.: Vaccine-derived polioviruses and the endgame strategy for global polio eradication. *Annu Rev Microbiol* 2005; 59:587-635.

Lukashev A.N.: Recombination among picornaviruses. *Rev Med Virol* 2010; 20:327-337.

Mendelsohn C.L., Wimmer E., Racaniello V.R.: Cellular receptor for poliovirus: molecular cloning, nucleotide sequence and expression of a new member of the immunoglobulin superfamily. *Cell* 1989; 56:855-865.

Nix A.W., Oberste S.M., Pallansch M.A.: Sensitive, semi-nested PCR amplification of VP1 sequences for direct identification of all enterovirus serotypes from original clinical specimens. *J Clin Microbiol* 2006; 44:2698-2704.

Racaniello V.R.: One hundred years of poliovirus pathogenesis. *Virology* 2006; 344:9-16.

Romero J.R., Modlin J.F.: Poliovirus. In: Bennette J.E., Dolin R., Blaser M.J., eds. *Mandell, Douglas, and Bennett's Principles and Practice of Infectious Diseases.* 8th ed. Sanders; 2015; 2073-2079.

Solomon T., Lewthwaite P., Wong S.C., et al.: Virology, epidemiology, pathogenesis, and control of enterovirus 71. *Lancet Infect Dis* 2010; 10:778-790.

Strauss M., Levy H.C., Bostina M., et al.: RNA transfer from poliovirus 135S particles across membranes is mediated by long umbilical connectors. *J Virol* 2013; 87:3903-3914.

World Health Organization: *Polio laboratory manual.* 4th ed. Geneva, Switzerland: Publications of the World Health Organization; 2004:1-157.

World Health Organization: Poliomyelitis: intensification of the global eradication initiative. Report by the Secretariat. Available: http://apps.who.int/gb/ebwha/pdf_files/WHA66/A66_18-en.pdf.

World Health Organization: Polio vaccines and polio immunization in the pre-eradication era: WHO position paper. *Wkly Epidemiol Rec* 2010; 85:213-228.

Romero J.R.: Reverse-transcription polymerase chain reaction detection of the enteroviruses. *Arch Pathol Lab Med* 1999; 123:1161-1169.

Zhu F., Xu W., Xia J., et al.: Efficacy, safety, and immunogenicity of an enterovirus 71 vaccine in China. *N Engl J Med* 2014; 370:818-828.

Hepatitis Viruses

STÉPHANE CHEVALIEZ | JEAN-MICHEL PAWLOTSKY

KEY CONCEPTS

- Hepatitis A virus infection remains endemic in many low- to middle-income countries posing risks for travelers from high-income countries where infection is uncommon.

- While hepatitis E virus infection is usually benign, chronic infection with cirrhosis occurs in immunocompromised hosts, especially transplant recipients and HIV-infected individuals.

- Hepatitis B virus infection remains a leading cause of death globally, resulting in nearly one million deaths annually from cirrhosis and hepatocellular carcinoma.

- Approximately 5% of chronic hepatitis B virus carriers are co-infected with hepatitis D virus and therefore at greater risk for progression to cirrhosis. However the incidence is decreasing with greater deployment of the hepatitis B vaccine.

- New hepatitis C virus infections continue to occur in higher-income societies.

- Hepatitis C virus infection remains a leading cause of liver transplantation.

Introduction

Viral hepatitis is a major public health problem throughout the world that affects several hundreds of millions of people worldwide. Viral hepatitis is a cause of considerable morbidity and mortality, both from acute infection and, mostly, from chronic infection. Chronic viral hepatitis is the leading cause of cirrhosis and hepatocellular carcinoma worldwide, and accounts for more than 1 million deaths per year.[1]

There are five recognized viruses responsible for viral hepatitis, which share the common property of replicating in the main liver cells, hepatocytes: hepatitis A virus (HAV); hepatitis B virus (HBV); hepatitis C virus (HCV); hepatitis D or delta virus (HDV), which is a defective viroid using the hepatitis B surface antigen (HBsAg); and hepatitis E virus (HEV) (Table 165-1). All these viruses can cause chronic hepatitis, except HAV. HEV generally does not cause chronic hepatitis, except in immunosuppressed patients. Other viruses may also cause inflammatory liver disease, including members of the Herpesviridae family, such as human cytomegalovirus, Epstein-Barr virus, or herpes simplex virus. It is unclear to what extent other viruses, such as parvovirus B19 or human herpesvirus 6, can also cause hepatitis.

Hepatitis A Virus

Infection with HAV is the commonest viral cause of acute liver disease and represents an important public health problem worldwide. The World Health Organization (WHO) estimates that about 1.5 million of clinical HAV cases occur yearly, with up to 20% requiring hospitalization. HAV transmission is principally fecal–oral, resulting from consumption of contaminated water or food. The incidence of hepatitis A varies greatly from country to country and is associated with socioeconomic factors that impact on the quality of sanitation and access to potable water. Primary infection confers lifetime protection elicited by antibodies generated during infection. An HAV vaccine exists. It is not recommended in highly endemic countries, where infection occurs early in life in the vast majority of individuals and confers lifelong protection. In contrast, it is desirable in countries of intermediate to low endemicity to prevent infection in exposed individuals, especially if they are likely to acquire it at an age when hepatitis is likely to be severe.

Virology of Hepatitis A Virus

HAV is a member of the Picornaviridae family, genus *Hepatovirus*. The hepatitis A viral particle is a 27 nm non-enveloped icosahedral capsid that is composed of multiple copies of the structural proteins and contains a single-stranded positive RNA genome of 7.5 kilobases (kb). Although the genomic organization and expression pattern of HAV are close to those of picornaviruses, differences exist. Recent crystallographic studies suggested that the HAV capsid is intermediate in structure between that of primitive insect dicistroviruses and mammalian picornaviruses, such as poliovirus.[2] A recent study suggested that HAV is released from infected hepatocytes cloaked in host membranes and thereby hidden from neutralizing antibodies.[3] These membrane-wrapped virions are infectious and possess key attributes of conventional enveloped viruses, including loss of infectivity upon extraction with organic solvents. The membrane cloaking the virus is not decorated with glycoproteins, providing an important distinction and leading to the conclusion that HAV particles are quasi-enveloped.

HAV LIFE CYCLE

HAV particles reach the liver after systemic circulation and infect hepatocytes via an interaction with hepatitis A virus cellular receptor 1 (HAVCR1/TIM-1), a member of the TIM (T-cell membrane, immunoglobulin and mucin) gene family, which plays critical roles in regulating immune cell activity. The capsid is generally devoid of the

TABLE 165-1	Features of Hepatitis Viruses					
	HAV	**HBV**	**HCV**	**HDV**	**HEV**
Type of nucleic acids	RNA	DNA	RNA	RNA	RNA
Route of transmission	Fecal–oral	Blood, sexual, mother-to-child	Blood	Blood	Fecal–oral
Seriousness of acute hepatitis	+ 0.1%*	++ 1%	− 0%	++ 10–20%	++ 10%
Chronic infection	No	Yes	Yes	Yes	Yes
Vaccine	Yes	Yes	No	Yes (HBV)	Yes (some strains)

*Risk of fulminant hepatitis.

surface topology that provides binding sites for cellular receptors on other picornaviruses,[2] raising the question as to how HAV enters cells. The positive-strand RNA genome released by uncoating of the HAV virion acts as a messenger RNA for the synthesis of the large polyprotein. Protein translation is initiated in a 5' cap-independent fashion, under the control of an IRES (internal ribosome entry site). Maturation of the polyprotein occurs in a co- and post-translational manner to generate the structural and nonstructural viral proteins. The 3D^{pol} RNA-dependent RNA polymerase of HAV serves as the catalytic core of a large, membrane-bound macromolecular complex that acts as an RNA replicase. Within the replicase complex, the positive-strand viral RNA serves as a template for negative-strand RNA synthesis. This negative-strand intermediate then acts in turn as a template for synthesis of new positive-strand RNA molecules, than can either be translated into viral proteins or packaged into new virions. Substantial evidence suggests that the mechanisms of HAV particles assembly differ from those of the picornaviruses. Newly assembled HAV particles appear to be transported to the apical plasma membrane of the hepatocytes. After replication in the liver, the virus is released into the bile, and eventually shed in feces. In animal models, HAV antigens can be detected in the stomach and small and large intestine, suggesting that viral replication also occurs in the intestine.

HAV GENETIC DIVERSITY

Based on sequence analysis of the full-length VP1 nonstructural protein-coding region of the genome, 7 HAV genotypes (I–VII) have been described. Genotypes I, II and III are further divided into subtypes A and B. Genotypes I, II, III and VII have been associated with infections in humans, whereas genotypes IV, V and VI are of simian origin. Genotype I is the most prevalent genotype worldwide, with subtype IA being more frequent than subtype IB. It is currently unclear to what extent different genotypes are associated with distinct clinical courses of infection. However, a recent study suggested that acute infection with subtype IB was more severe than infection with other genotypes.[4]

Epidemiology

INCIDENCE AND PREVALENCE

HAV has a worldwide distribution. Infections can be sporadic or occur in epidemic outbreaks. Approximately 1.5 million clinical cases of HAV infection are reported to occur worldwide annually, but the rate of infection is probably as much as 10 times higher.

In 2010, the WHO published a systematic review of the global prevalence of, and susceptibility to, HAV infection. Worldwide geographic areas can be characterized with high, intermediate, low, or very low levels of endemicity for hepatitis A. The levels of endemicity are related to hygienic and sanitary conditions in each area. In low- and middle-income countries, such as those in Africa, parts of South America, the Middle East, and India, HAV infection is very common. Most infections are acquired during childhood. Infections that occur at an early age are often asymptomatic. In countries with intermediate endemicity, such as China, some Eastern European countries and some South East Asian countries, community-wide outbreaks may occur.

In industrialized countries, such as North America, Western Europe, Scandinavia, Australia, and Japan, HAV infection is less common. Infection rates in children are generally low, and disease tends to occur in adolescents and young adults. Infections in these countries with good hygiene conditions occur in specific settings and are mainly associated with travel to countries with higher endemicity. In high-income countries, there is a general lack of immunization against HAV, although it is considered as an important travel-associated infection. In the past, the risk of HAV infection in unvaccinated travelers was considered to be 3 per 1000 individuals per month of travel to a low- and middle-income country (LMIC) in good quality accommodations. Currently, with improvements in sanitary conditions, the risk of infection for nonimmune travelers who visit high- or medium-endemicity

areas has been reduced to 6 to 30 per 100 000 individuals per months traveled.[5]

ROUTES OF TRANSMISSION AND AT-RISK GROUPS

HAV is generally transmitted via the fecal–oral route, directly from person to person or through the ingestion of fecally contaminated food or water. Transmission by blood transfusion has been reported, and isolated cases of apparent perinatal transmission have been described. High-risk groups for acute hepatitis A include travelers to countries with high endemicity, children in daycare centers and their parents, men who have sex with men, injection drug users, hemophiliacs who receive plasma products, and persons in institutions.

Pathogenicity

Typically, the incubation period is 15–45 days. In most cases, acute infection takes a mild, and often unrecognized, course. The incidence of symptomatic, icteric cases increases with the age at infection. Acute hepatitis A in adults may require hospitalization in up to 13% of cases; prolonged courses of 6–9 months have been reported in 10% of adult patients with a diagnosis of acute hepatitis A. Acute hepatitis A infection generally resolves without complications in 3–4 weeks and never evolves to chronic infection. Prolonged elevations of serum aminotransferase levels have been reported. Relapses a few weeks after the acute case have also been observed. Prolonged courses may occur in children and immunosuppressed individuals. Hepatitis A is the most common cause of relapsing cholestatic hepatitis. However, cholestatic hepatitis A is unusual and has a good prognosis, with full recovery within a few weeks. Acute liver failure (ALF) is rare, occurring in less than 0.1% of cases, but its incidence and mortality increase with the patient's age at acquisition. In the USA, 2.2% of all cases of fulminant hepatitis are caused by HAV infection.[6] Overall, mortality of acute hepatitis A is 1.8% in patients older than 50 years. In patients with chronic hepatitis B, superinfection with HAV is associated with a 6- to 23-fold higher morbidity and mortality.

The molecular mechanisms responsible for the wide range of disease severity are not well understood, but probably involve cytotoxic CD8$^+$ T-cell activity. The considerable variability in clinical outcomes among individuals and populations was initially attributed to the genetic variability of the pathogens, but recent studies have demonstrated that host factors probably influence the course of infection and disease. HAV induces a minimal intrahepatic type I interferon (IFN) response in chimpanzees, much weaker than that observed in acute HCV infection.[7] Despite this, intrahepatic viral levels are 100- to 1000-fold higher in acute HAV than in HCV infection. HAV expresses a protease that cleaves MAVS and TRIF, key adaptor proteins in RIG-I-like receptor and Toll-like receptor 3 pathways. Plasmacytoid dendritic cells (pDC) produce substantial amounts of IFN alpha when co-cultured with HAV-infected cells.[8] In chimpanzees, numerous pDCs are present within the liver at the end of the first week of HAV infection. For unknown reasons, they disappear and can no longer be detected at the peak of virus replication and acute inflammation 2–3 weeks later. HAV-specific humoral and cellular immune responses typically appear 4–5 weeks after infection. Neutralizing antibodies recognize a small number of epitopes in the highly conserved VP1, VP3 and VP2 capsid proteins. HAV-specific cytotoxic CD8$^+$ T-cell responses were first described in the blood and liver of jaundiced patients with acute hepatitis A. This CD8$^+$ T-cell response, as well as the expansion of functional CD4$^+$ T cells, was correlated with the control of virus replication.

Diagnostic Virology

The diagnosis of acute hepatitis A is based on the detection of anti-HAV IgM in serum by means of enzyme immunoassay (Box 165-1). Serum anti-HAV IgM levels peak during the second month of infection. HAV RNA can be transiently detected in stool and other body fluids by polymerase chain reaction (PCR) 3–10 days before the onset of illness and for 1–2 weeks thereafter; however, HAV RNA testing is generally not necessary. When the infection resolves, anti-HAV IgM disappears after 4–12 months, whereas anti-HAV IgG persists for life and confers definitive protection against infection. Total (IgG) anti-HAV antibodies must be sought to determine whether a patient has been exposed or infected in the past, in epidemiological studies or to assess the patient's status before vaccination.

Hepatitis E Virus

Retrospective studies in India of large water-borne epidemics of hepatitis, originally attributed to HAV, suggested the existence of a new enteric infectious agent, which was later named HEV. Oral administration of pooled stool extracts from Soviet soldiers in Afghanistan who suffered from unexplained hepatitis to a volunteer caused acute hepatitis. Viral particles were detected in stool samples from this volunteer shortly before and during the clinical phase of hepatitis. The viral genome was subsequently cloned and sequenced using bile samples from experimentally infected macaques.

Human HEV infection has two distinct epidemiological patterns. In areas of poor sanitation, HEV is transmitted by the fecal–oral route, generally via contaminated water. In high-income countries with good hygiene conditions, consumption of HEV-contaminated undercooked meat is the main source for HEV infections.

HEV infection is usually an acute self-limiting disease but, in high-income countries it may cause chronic infection that rapidly progresses toward cirrhosis (within 1–2 years), principally in organ transplant recipients, patients with hematological malignancies that require chemotherapy, and immunosuppressed HIV-infected individuals, either from a latent virus reactivated by immunosuppression or from a virus transmitted at the time of transplantation.

Virology of Hepatitis E Virus

HEV is a member of the Hepeviridae family, genus *Hepevirus*. The HEV particle is a 27 to 34 nm non-enveloped icosahedral capsid that contains a single-stranded positive RNA genome of 7.2 kb.

HEV LIFE CYCLE

Until recently, there was no robust cell culture system for HEV, impairing detailed analysis of the basic biology of HEV. However, knowledge of the HEV life cycle has improved after the development of replicons and *in vitro* infection systems, such as the HEV-like particles expressed in *Escherichia coli*. The HEV particle first binds to heparin sulfate proteoglycans at the surface of the host cell membrane. The high-affinity cellular membrane receptor(s) remain(s) unknown. The following step is internalization through a dynamin-2-, clathrin- and membrane-cholesterol-dependent pathway.[9] The capped viral genome is released from the virion during the uncoating process and directly translated by the host cell ribosomal machinery. The nonstructural proteins allow the replication of the viral genome in the cytoplasm and the production of subgenomic RNA that is translated into the structural proteins from open reading frames (ORF) ORF2 and ORF3. Full-length RNA progeny is then assembled with the capsid protein into viral particles that are released from the cells in a nonlytic fashion.[10]

HEV GENETIC DIVERSITY

Based on complete genome sequences from human and animal strains, three groups of mammalian Hepeviridae have been identified. The first group includes viruses infecting humans, pigs, deer and rabbits. This group includes the four human HEV genotypes (genotypes 1–4) and their 24 subgenotypes isolated from infected patients. The second group includes viruses infecting rats and ferrets, whereas the third group includes bat viruses. There is no known animal reservoir for HEV genotypes 1 and 2. In contrast, genotype 3 can infect humans, but also other animal species, including pigs, deer, mongooses, shellfish and rodents.

Epidemiology

In LMIC, hepatitis E is a water-borne infection caused by genotype 1 or 2. Genotype 1 is responsible for most endemic and epidemic cases in Asia, whereas genotype 2 is prevalent in Central America. In these areas, anti-HEV IgG seroprevalence studies showed that most children under the age of 10 years have never been exposed to HEV. The seroprevalence dramatically increases between the age of 15 and 30 years, to reach a plateau around 30%. This is in contrast with the HAV seroprevalence, which shows nearly universal exposure to HAV by the age of 10 years. The seroprevalence varies between and within countries and may reflect the populations studied and the sensitivity of the assay used. The incidence of infection varies between and within countries and over time. Hepatitis E is particularly common in some South East Asian countries, and there have been numerous large outbreaks in African refugee camps in the last 20 years. Sporadic cases of hepatitis E caused by genotypes 1 and 2 occur in travelers or workers returning to their country of origin from areas of endemicity.

In industrialized countries, a number of studies showed that autochthonous hepatitis E is present in Europe, North America, New Zealand and Japan. In contrast to HEV in LMIC, autochthonous HEV infection in high-income areas is a zoonotic infection caused by HEV genotypes 3 and 4, and the principal route of transmission is the consumption of uncooked or poorly cooked pork or game meat. HEV seroprevalence in these regions is probably underestimated, because most of the studies used poorly sensitive anti-HEV assays. These studies showed a considerable geographic variation in seroprevalence and incidence. For instance, the seroprevalence of HEV in the south of France is substantially higher than that found in the North (16.6% versus 2.9%, respectively).[11, 12] In the USA, the estimated overall anti-HEV IgG prevalence declined by approximately 40% from 1988–1994 (10.2%) to 2009–2010 (6.0%). The reasons for this decrease remain unknown. In particular, no clear association was found with changes in food consumption.[13] A similar trend was also recently observed in southeastern Germany.[14] Few data on the incidence of hepatitis E in industrialized countries are available, but estimates are high: 0.2% in the UK and 0.7% in the USA per year.

Pathogenicity

ACUTE HEPATITIS E

The incubation period is roughly 4–6 weeks from infection to onset of symptoms. In most patients, hepatitis E causes a self-limiting illness, which lasts a few weeks, characterized by nonspecific symptoms including fever and nausea followed by abdominal pain, vomiting, anorexia, malaise and hepatomegaly. Viremia generally persists for less than a month following the onset of symptoms, and HEV RNA can be undetectable in serum or stool by the time patients come to clinical attention. Jaundice occurs in up to 40% of cases during large outbreaks in LMIC, but is rare in sporadic cases in high-income countries. A high mortality rate was observed in pregnant women and individuals suffering from chronic liver disease during large outbreaks with HEV genotypes 1 or 2 in LMIC, the mechanisms of which remain unknown. No such phenomenon has been reported in patients with sporadic acute hepatitis E in industrialized areas. Recovery occurs within 4–6 weeks. Approximately 5% of patients with acute HEV infection also present with neurological disorders, including Guillain–Barré syndrome or acute meningoencephalitis.

Both human and animal studies have suggested that the immune response, rather than the viral damage to hepatocytes, drives the clinical manifestations of hepatitis E, including both self-limiting acute viral hepatitis and ALF. Several studies suggested that natural killer cells play an important role in mediating the immune response to HEV infection. Indeed, an elevated level of IFN gamma was observed in HEV-infected patients that could have contributed to hepatocyte death. On the other hand, the activity of nuclear factor kappa B (NF-κB), a regulator of transcription during the response to infections, appears to be altered by HEV. Elevated antibody titers, proinflammatory cytokines and low-level viral RNA were found in patients with HEV-associated liver failure compared to less severe acute hepatitis E cases. However, discrepant results have been reported, such as higher HEV RNA levels in pregnant women with ALF than in those with mild hepatitis.

Serologic evidence and animal studies suggested that HEV infection confers cross-protection against other strains, even across genotypes, owing to the existence of a common serotype. However, studies in animals suggested that protective immunity is not always complete. Longitudinal follow-up studies in humans have provided inconsistent results. These findings must be interpreted with caution, because of the marked variability in the sensitivity and specificity of HEV assays used for antibody detection.

CHRONIC HEPATITIS E

Immunocompromised patients can develop chronic infection. Chronic HEV infection can rapidly evolve toward cirrhosis. Although the majority of chronic HEV infections are diagnosed in the transplant population, cases have also been reported in HIV-infected patients and in patients with hematological malignancies or patients treated with anticancer chemotherapy. All chronic HEV cases reported thus far were due to HEV genotype 3. The diagnosis of chronic hepatitis E is based on persisting HEV replication lasting for at least 6 months.

Diagnostic Virology

Patients with otherwise unexplained acute hepatitis should be tested for hepatitis E. The diagnosis of HEV infection is based on anti-HEV antibody detection in blood and/or HEV RNA detection in blood or in feces. Anti-HEV antibodies, including both IgM and IgG, can be sought by means of commercial enzyme immunoassays and rapid immunochromatographic kits based on ORF2/ORF3 peptides or recombinant antigens from HEV1.

The presence of anti-HEV IgM is a marker of acute infection, whereas the presence of anti-HEV IgG alone is a marker of past HEV infection (Box 165-1). Anti-HEV IgM persists at relatively high levels for 8 weeks and rapidly declines thereafter, falling below the cutoff level of the assays after 32 weeks in most patients. IgG antibodies reach their peak level approximately 4 weeks after the onset of symptoms and high levels persist for more than 1 year.

The performance of commercial anti-HEV IgM immunoassays is variable. The lower limit of detection of these assays ranges from 0.25 to 2.5 WHO unit/mL. Their sensitivity varies between 78% and 98%, whereas their specificity varies between 78% and 96%. Two IgM assays,

TABLE 165-2	Diagnosis of Chronic Viral Hepatitis	
Diagnosis	**Screening Tests**	**Confirmatory/Complementary Tests**
Chronic hepatitis B	HBsAg	HBV DNA, HBeAg, anti-HBe antibodies
Chronic hepatitis C	Anti-HCV antibodies	HCV RNA
Chronic hepatitis D	Anti-HDV antibodies	HDV RNA
Chronic hepatitis E	Anti-HEV antibodies	HEV RNA

commercialized by Adaltis and Wantai, respectively, were recently shown to have acceptable sensitivity in immunocompetent patients with acute HEV infection. The sensitivity of these assays for the detection of acute HEV infection was altered in immunocompromised patients.

In patients with acute HEV infection, HEV RNA becomes detectable in blood 3 weeks after the onset of symptoms but can be detected in feces for another 2 weeks. Serum HCV RNA levels in the acute phase range from 2 to 8 Log copies/mL in immunocompetent patients. HCV RNA detection and quantification is based on real-time PCR with primers and a probe targeting conserved regions among HEV genotypes. Most PCR assays target ORF3 of the virus.

Anti-HEV IgM assays can be used as first-line diagnostic assays in immunocompetent patients. In immunocompromised patients, HEV RNA testing should be considered as the first-line diagnostic assay. In addition, HEV RNA testing is useful for molecular characterization and is essential to diagnose chronic infection, defined by the persistence of HEV RNA in blood for more than 6 months (Table 165-2).

Hepatitis B Virus

HBV was the first human hepatitis virus from which the proteins and genome were identified and characterized. HBV infection was known to cause acute and chronic liver disease and, based on epidemiological findings, it was postulated as early as the 1970s that this virus might represent a cause of liver cancer. Approximately 2 billion people worldwide have been infected, 240 million are chronically infected, and nearly 1 million people die every year as a result of the complications of chronic HBV infection, including cirrhosis and hepatocellular carcinoma.

Virology of Hepatitis B Virus

HBV is a member of the *Hepadnaviridae* family, which comprises two genera, the Orthohepadnaviruses, that infect mammals, and the avihepadnaviruses, that infect birds. The infectious virion, the Dane particle, is a spherical lipid-containing structure of 42–47 nm in diameter. It possesses an icosahedral nucleocapsid or core that contains the partially double-stranded, circular DNA genome and an envelope made up from three forms of the viral envelope proteins, large (L), middle (M) and small (S), acquired together with host lipids during budding into the endoplasmic reticulum.

HBV LIFE CYCLE

The HBV genome is the smallest known human virus genome, with approximately 3000 nucleotides. The viral genome contains at least four overlapping open reading frames that encode a number of structural and nonstructural viral proteins. The pre-S/S gene encodes the three surface proteins (S, M and L) that express HBsAg. The pre-C/C gene encodes the core protein that expresses the hepatitis B core (HBc) antigen and the hepatitis B e (HBe) protein, a nonstructural protein that plays a role in immune tolerance to HBV replication. The P gene encodes the HBV polymerase, whose two motifs, a reverse transcriptase motif and an RNase H motif, code for two enzymes involved in HBV replication. Finally, the X gene encodes the X protein, a transactivator involved in HBV replication that bears oncogenic properties. The blood of infected patients contains not only infectious viruses but also a large excess of empty, noninfectious HBV envelopes.

The complex HBV life cycle involves multiple steps. The first step is its fixation to a receptor at the surface of hepatocytes. Sodium taurocholate cotransporting polypeptide (NTCP) has been recently identified as a receptor for HBV (and also for HDV that is infectious within empty HBV envelopes).[15] The next steps of the HBV life cycle are internalization, fusion and release of the nucleocapsid containing the HBV DNA genome and the associated HBV polymerase molecule in the cell cytoplasm. The nucleocapsid is then transported into the nucleus, where decapsidation occurs, releasing the DNA genome molecule. In the nucleus, the HBV genome is transformed by the viral polymerase into a covalently closed circular DNA (cccDNA), the episomal form responsible for persistence of the HBV genome in the nucleus of infected hepatocytes. Messenger RNAs are generated from cccDNA for the synthesis of the different viral proteins. In addition, a pregenomic RNA is generated and serves as a template for reverse transcription that generates, in turn, the long genomic DNA strand. The pregenomic RNA is then degraded by the ribonuclease (RNase) H activity of the viral polymerase, whereas the viral reverse transcriptase synthesizes the short complementary DNA strand within the newly formed viral nucleocapsids. Finally, the new HBV virions bud into the endoplasmic reticulum, are matured and exported. HBV infections also lead to the production of noninfectious subviral particles that represent the most abundant structures released into the blood from infected livers. Their exact role in the HBV life cycle is not known. One hypothesis is that, by adsorbing virus-neutralizing antibodies, they facilitate virus spread and maintenance in the host.

HBV GENETIC DIVERSITY

Ten HBV genotypes (A–J), which differ by approximately 8% of their genomic nucleotide sequence, have different geographic distributions and may be associated with different clinical outcomes. Genotype A predominates in northern and Western Europe, whereas genotype D is the most frequent genotype in the Mediterranean area and in Eastern Europe. In non-Asian populations in the USA, genotype A predominates in men who have sex with men, whereas genotype D is the most frequent in intravenous drug users. In Asia and in Asian immigrants living in high-income countries, genotypes B and C predominate. Genotype C has been associated with a higher incidence of severe liver disease and hepatocellular carcinoma compared with genotype B in Asia, perhaps because this genotype spread earlier than the others.

Epidemiology
INCIDENCE AND PREVALENCE

More than 240 million individuals have chronic HBV infection worldwide.[16] In the 2010 Global Burden of Disease study, HBV infection ranked in the top health priorities in the world, being the 10th leading cause of deaths (nearly a million deaths attributable to HBV infection each year).[17] Age-specific HBsAg seroprevalence varies markedly by geographic region. Indeed, HBV carrier rates vary from very low (0.1–2.0%) in the USA and Western Europe, to intermediate (2–8%) in Mediterranean countries and Japan, to high (8–20%) in sub-Saharan Africa and most parts of Asia. Overall, almost half of the global population lives in areas with high endemicity. The prevalence of hepatitis B e antigen (HBeAg)-negative disease has been increasing over the past decade, as a result of aging of the HBV-infected population. It accounts for the majority of cases in many regions, including Western Europe.

ROUTES OF TRANSMISSION AND AT-RISK GROUPS

HBV virions are produced and circulate in very high amounts in HBV-infected individuals, who are highly contagious. Four major modes of transmission are responsible for HBV infection.

The principal cause of HBV transmission in areas of high endemicity is perinatal, from infected mothers to neonates. HBV is not transmitted *in utero*, but transmission occurs at or soon after birth when the neonate comes into contact with the mother's blood or secretions. Infection at birth is associated with a very high (>90%) rate of chronic infection. In low endemicity areas, sexual transmission is predominant. The risk of infection is higher in people with a high number of sexual partners, in men who have sex with men, and in people with histories of other sexually transmitted infections. The third major source of infection is percutaneous transmission by blood and blood products, unsafe medical or surgical materials, or injection drug use. Although screening of blood products has substantially reduced transfusion-associated HBV infection, this route of transmission is still frequent in LMIC. Finally, horizontal transmission through nonsexual inter-individual contacts is frequent at a young age in Africa and associated with chronic evolution in approximately 15% of cases. Other possible accidental sources of HBV infection include nosocomial infection, needlestick injuries and organ, tissue or cell transplantation.

Pathogenicity
ACUTE HEPATITIS B

Typically, the incubation period is 30–150 days. Jaundice has been reported in up to one-third of adult patients with acute hepatitis B, but most cases are unrecognized. Among symptomatic patients, the manifestations are similar to those of other causes of acute viral hepatitis, including fever and nausea followed by abdominal pain, vomiting, anorexia, malaise and hepatomegaly.

The main cellular target of HBV is the hepatocyte. HBV infection, replication and virus shedding are not cytopathic to hepatocytes. A strong immune response that kills large numbers of hepatocytes is needed for clearance of the infection. More than 99% of immunocompetent adults are able to mount such a response and to clear acute infection spontaneously. In the remaining 1%, as well as in the majority of children infected at birth and in a proportion of children infected before the age of 10 years, HBV cannot be eliminated by the adaptive immune response and chronic infection develops. The cytotoxic T-cell response in chronic HBV infection has been described as weak and mono- or oligospecific, in comparison with the robust T-cell response that develops during resolution of acute self-limiting infection.

CHRONIC HEPATITIS B

Chronic hepatitis B is usually asymptomatic. The most common symptom is fatigue, but sleep disorders, difficulty concentrating and upper right quadrant pain are often observed. Chronic hepatitis B is characterized biologically by elevated aminotransferase levels, and alanine aminotransferase (ALT) levels can fluctuate substantially during the immune elimination phase. Moderate cholestasis, with mildly elevated alkaline phosphatase and γ-glutamyl transpeptidase levels, can also be present, especially in patients with cirrhosis.

Chronic hepatitis B infection is a heterogeneous disease with markedly variable levels of viral replication and liver disease activity. It is characterized by liver injury mediated by a T-cell immune response targeting hepatocytes that express viral antigens. Chronic HBsAg carriage typically evolves through three phases: immune tolerant; immune elimination; and inactive.

The immune tolerant phase is generally short if the infection occurred during adulthood, but it persists for years to decades in patients infected at birth or during early childhood. At the immune tolerant stage, the immune response of the host 'tolerates' HBV infection and does not cause liver inflammation or hepatocyte destruction. The immune tolerant phase is characterized by the presence of hepatitis B e antigen (HBeAg), very high levels of HBV DNA in blood, normal serum or plasma aminotransferase levels, and no or minimal inflammatory activity on liver biopsy.

The immune elimination phase is characterized by an active immune response that causes necroinflammatory lesions and triggers

TABLE 165-3	Virological Marker Profiles in Patients with Chronic Hepatitis B Virus Infection						
					ANTI-HBc Ab		
Chronic Hepatitis	HBsAg	Anti-HBs Ab	HBeAg	Anti-HBe Ab	IgM	Total	HBV DNA
HBeAg-positive	+	−	+	−	−*	+	>2 × 10⁴ IU/mL
HBeAg-negative	+	−	−	+	−*	+	>2 × 10³ IU/mL
Inactive carrier	+	−	−	+	−	+	<2 × 10³ IU/mL
Reactivation	+	−	+/−	+/−	+/−	+	>2 × 10³ IU/mL

*Anti-HBc IgM can be detected at low titers.
Ab, antibodies; Ag, antigen; HBc, hepatitis B core; HBe, hepatitis B e; HBs, hepatitis B surface; IgM, immunoglobulin M.

hepatic fibrogenesis and progressive fibrosis. ALT and aspartate aminotransferase (AST) levels are increased, but HBV DNA levels are lower than during the immune tolerant phase and frequently fluctuate. The immune elimination phase has a variable duration, ranging from a few weeks to several decades. HBeAg, when present, defines HBeAg-positive chronic hepatitis B. HBeAg can be cleared spontaneously and replaced by anti-HBe antibodies, defined as HBe seroconversion. The incidence of spontaneous HBe seroconversion among HBeAg-positive patients is 8–12% per year when they are in the immune elimination phase; HBe seroconversion often follows a transient ALT flare. Some of these patients evolve toward inactive HBsAg carriage, whereas others switch into an HBeAg-negative form of chronic hepatitis B, with elevated ALT levels and an HBV DNA level greater than 2000 IU/mL (Table 165-3).

Patients with HBeAg-positive chronic hepatitis B are infected with a wild-type virus and are able to secrete the HBe protein. Patients with HBeAg-negative chronic hepatitis B are infected with so-called precore mutant viruses, which cannot produce the HBe protein because they have a stop codon in the pre-C gene, and/or with core promoter mutant viruses, which produce considerably lower amounts of HBe protein. HBeAg-negative chronic hepatitis B is generally more severe than the HBeAg-positive variety. Because of the prevalence of the HBV genotype D in Euro-Mediterranean and African countries, HBeAg-negative/anti-HBe-positive chronic hepatitis B is 7–9 times more frequent than HBeAg-positive disease in those locations.

The inactive HBsAg carriage phase is the result of successful immune elimination leading to HBe seroconversion. ALT and AST levels are normal, HBV DNA is undetectable or at very low levels, and patients without pre-existing cirrhosis have normal liver histology. Inactive HBsAg carriers are exposed to reactivation when profoundly immunosuppressed.

COMPLICATIONS OF CHRONIC HEPATITIS B
The annual incidence of cirrhosis varies from 2% to 10% in patients with chronic HBV infection, with a cumulative incidence of approximately 20% at 5 years. The risk of cirrhosis is two- to fourfold higher in HBeAg-negative patients compared with HBeAg-positive ones, probably because they are older and have more severe disease at the time of diagnosis.

The annual incidence of hepatocellular carcinoma in patients with chronic hepatitis B varies from 1% in patients without cirrhosis to 2–8% in cirrhotic patients, with the higher rates occurring in older patients. More than 50% of hepatocellular carcinoma cases develop in the context of liver cirrhosis. There has been substantial progress in understanding the molecular mechanisms and risk factors of primary liver cancer. HBV usually persists as an episome (cccDNA), but HBV DNA sequences can integrate into host cellular DNA and drive hepatocellular carcinoma (HCC) development by promoting genetic alterations, although the small-size integrated genome portions cannot generate HBV replication. Insertions of HBV DNA into host cell DNA are found in 85–90% of HBV-related HCCs as single or multiple discrete integrations. They may lead to chromosomal deletions, translocations, the production of fusion transcripts and generalized genomic instability, which ultimately gives rise to the selection and clonal expansion of a pre-/neoplastic hepatocyte. The insertion of viral DNA sequences into the cellular genome also leads to cis-/transactivation, which results in modifications of cellular gene expression, possibly inducing malignant transformation. In human HBV-related HCC there seem to be no specific host genome regions or oncogenes where integration typically occurs. HBV DNA integration may play a particularly important role in patients with HBV-related HCC occurring in the context of a non-cirrhotic liver, in chronically infected children and young adults, or in the case of an occult infection in patients negative for HBsAg. Several studies have reported procarcinogenic properties of HBV proteins or of their randomly truncated transcripts after integration, including the HBx and envelope proteins.

Rarely, chronic HBV infection is associated with extrahepatic manifestations, including glomerulonephritis, most often in children, and polyarteritis nodosa, mostly in adults.

Diagnostic Virology
Four markers should be sought for the diagnosis of acute hepatitis B: HBsAg, total anti-HBc antibodies, anti-HBc IgM, and anti-HBs antibodies. Acute hepatitis B is characterized by the simultaneous presence of both HBsAg and anti-HBc IgM (Box 165-1). Total anti-HBc antibodies are also present, whereas anti-HBs antibodies are absent or present at very low levels. During the convalescence phase, patients lose HBsAg before the appearance of anti-HBs antibodies; they have isolated anti-HBc antibodies, and the diagnosis is based on the presence of anti-HBc IgM. Recovery is characterized by the appearance of anti-HBs antibodies. The presence of both total anti-HBc and anti-HBs antibodies characterizes recovery from acute hepatitis B. Anti-HBc IgG remains at high levels for the patient's lifetime, whereas anti-HBs antibody titers may fluctuate and become undetectable after several years. Quantitative HBsAg assessment may be useful during the course of acute hepatitis B, because if the HBsAg level does not rapidly decrease, the patient is at risk for chronic evolution.

Chronic HBV infection is defined by the persistence of HBsAg in the serum for more than 6 months after the acute episode (Table 165-2). The majority of subjects with isolated anti-HBc antibodies are not viremic. However, some individuals who test positive for anti-HBc antibodies, but not for HBsAg or anti-HBs antibodies, may be viremic; in these cases, amino acid substitutions in the HBsAg sequence are responsible for the lack of HBsAg detection with current enzyme immunoassays (although the most frequent mutants can now be detected with the new generations of assays). Other individuals have very low-level HBV replication in their liver with undetectable HBV DNA in blood: this condition is called 'occult HBV infection' (OBI).

Serum or plasma ALT and HBV DNA levels are markers of disease severity and prognosis. The assessment of severity, including the grade of necroinflammation and the stage of fibrosis, is typically based on the liver biopsy. However, noninvasive assessment using serologic markers, transient elastography, or acoustic radiation force impulse imaging can discriminate cirrhosis from mild hepatitis and fibrosis.

Although they are not accurate enough for intermediate stages, these methods will likely replace liver biopsy in the pretreatment assessment of the severity of chronic hepatitis B in the future.

Hepatitis D Virus

HDV is a small defective RNA virus that is related to plant viroids. It can propagate only in subjects who have coexistent HBsAg carriage. HDV infection has a worldwide but not uniform distribution. It is estimated that 5% of HBsAg carriers are also infected with HDV, which signifies that there might be between 10 and 15 million HDV-infected individuals. Studies have shown that most patients with HBV and HDV coinfection have more severe liver disease, more rapid progression to cirrhosis and increased hepatic decompensation and death than those with HBV infection alone. However, the mechanisms by which HDV causes more severe liver disease are not fully understood.

Virology of Hepatitis D Virus

Hepatitis D virus is a small, spherical particle of about 36 nm in diameter. The HDV particle is composed of an outer coat containing the three HBV envelope glycoproteins and host lipids surrounding an inner nucleocapsid consisting of a single-stranded circular RNA of approximately 1700 nucleotides, and about 200 molecules of hepatitis delta antigen (HDAg) per genome.

HDV LIFE CYCLE

The first step is its fixation to a receptor at the surface of hepatocytes. NTCP has been recently identified as a receptor for HBV, thus also for HDV.[15] The virus is uncoated after entering into hepatocytes and a signal in delta antigen (HDAg) translocates the nucleocapsid to the nucleus. The antigen has no RNA polymerase activity. To replicate its genome, the virus hijacks the cellular RNA polymerase, which considers the genome as a double-stranded DNA. Three forms of RNA are synthesized in the host during replication: circular genomic RNA, circular complementary antigenomic RNA, and a linear polyadenylated antigenomic RNA, which is the messenger RNA containing the open reading frame. Replication of the circular HDV RNA template occurs via a rolling mechanism that is unique to animal viruses, but analogous to that of plant viroids. HDV RNA is first synthesized as a linear molecule, potentially containing many copies of the genome. In the genomic and antigenomic RNAs, a sequence of 85 nucleotides acts as a ribozyme, which self-cleaves the linear HDV RNA into monomers. The monomers are then ligated to form circular RNAs. HDAg is the only protein encoded by the HDV genome. It consists of two isoforms: the large HDAg and the small HDAg. Post-translational modification of the large HDAg is required for its ability to bind HBsAg and assemble the viral particle. Other post-translational modifications occur including phosphorylation and sumoylation of the small HDAg.

HDV GENETIC DIVERSITY

The sequence of the HDV RNA genome is highly variable, and there is divergence of up to 16% within the same genotype, compared with 20–40% between different genotypes. HDV has evolved in eight major genotypes that differ in their global distribution. Genotype 1 has a worldwide distribution, whereas genotypes 2 and 4 are found in Asia, genotype 3 in the Amazon region and genotypes 5, 6, 7 and 8 in Africa. Several studies showed that genotypes 3 and 4 are associated with more severe liver disease, including fulminant hepatitis.[18]

Epidemiology

Of the 240 million chronic HBV carriers worldwide, more than 10 million have serological evidence of exposure to HDV. Traditionally, the regions with high rates of HDV carriage where the virus is endemic are central Africa, the Horn of Africa, the Amazon, eastern and Mediterranean Europe, the Middle East and parts of Asia. Rates of HDV infection are generally highest in regions where HBV is endemic, but there are some exceptions (e.g. Vietnam, Indonesia and China).

Longitudinal studies have shown a recent decrease in the HDV prevalence in some endemic areas, such as Italy, where infection in HBsAg carriers has fallen from 24% in 1990 to 8.5% in 2006, for unclear reasons.[19] In the past three decades, reductions in HDV prevalence have also been reported in Spain, Taiwan and Turkey. Vaccination programs for HBV have probably contributed substantially to the decline in HDV in these regions, but additional factors, including increased awareness of the virus and its mode of transmission, may also be involved.

Pathogenicity

Like HBV, HDV is transmitted via the parenteral route through exposure to infected blood or body fluids. Thus, transmission rates remain high in intravenous drug users. HDV is usually associated with a severe form of hepatitis, but the range of clinical manifestations is wide, going from asymptomatic cases to fulminant hepatitis.

HDV can be acquired at the same time as HBV (coinfection) or by a chronic HBsAg carrier (superinfection). Acute HBV-HDV coinfection is generally more severe than HBV monoinfection, but results in the clearance of both viruses in approximately 95% of adult patients. In contrast, HDV superinfection of a chronic HBV carrier results in chronic HDV infection in most cases. Patients with chronic hepatitis B and D have a high rate of progression to cirrhosis; however, not all studies showed an increased incidence of hepatocellular carcinoma, perhaps because of the suppression of HBV replication by HDV generally observed in carriers of both viruses.

The mechanisms that determine whether or not an individual clears HDV spontaneously and the processes that cause severe hepatitis and rapid progression to fibrosis remain unclear. Hepatitis delta antigen is not directly cytopathic in human hepatocytes. The level of HDV RNA is not associated with the severity of liver injury. The host immune response is thought to have an important role in both HDV clearance and liver injury. A recent study showed a marked impairment of NK cell function in patients with HDV infection, in spite of a relative increase in the number of NK cells compared to healthy controls. Similar alterations were observed in patients with HBV and HCV infections, suggesting a common mechanism depending on disease activity rather than a virus-specific phenomenon.[20] The adaptive immune response probably plays an important role in HDV infection, but this role remains elusive. Several studies have shown that HDV infection is associated with a dominant T-helper-2 (Th2) response, with a high frequency of T cells secreting interleukin-10.

Diagnostic Virology

There are four markers of HDV infection that can be sought in serum or plasma: the HD antigen, total anti-HDV antibodies, anti-HDV IgM, and HDV RNA that can be detected and quantified by real-time PCR (Table 165-2). All HBsAg-positive patients should be tested for the presence of HDV markers.

During acute HDV infection, the presence of HD antigen and anti-HDV IgM is transient and they are often missed. Both markers are absent at the chronic stage. Thus, total anti-HDV antibodies should be systematically sought in patients with detectable HBsAg. In the presence of antibodies, HDV infection is confirmed by the detection of HDV RNA. Serial HDV RNA level measurements are useful to assess the response to antiviral therapy. HDV genotyping is only available in specialized centers and does not have clinical utility. However, some clinical studies suggested that HDV genotype 1 patients are at higher risk of developing end-stage liver disease and have a lower response to treatment with pegylated interferon than patients with African genotypes.

In patients with an HBV-HDV coinfection, HD antigen, anti-HDV IgM and HDV RNA are only transiently present and they are often missed. Anti-HBc IgM indicates concomitant acute HBV infection. In HDV superinfection of a chronic HBsAg carrier, no anti-HBc IgM is present. Total anti-HDV antibodies are present. HDV RNA is found in serum or plasma before and during the acute episode, whereas both total anti-HDV antibodies and anti-HDV IgM are present during the acute phase. Both total anti-HDV antibodies and anti-HDV IgM remain at high levels in chronic HDV infection, and HDV RNA is present. Although all chronic HDV carriers also are chronic HBsAg carriers, chronic HDV carriers generally have low or undetectable HBV DNA levels because HDV inhibits HBV replication.

Hepatitis C Virus

HCV infection is a major cause of chronic liver disease, with an estimated 130–170 million people infected worldwide. Chronic hepatitis C is becoming the main cause of hepatocellular carcinoma in the industrialized world. The global mortality rate related to chronic HCV infection has been estimated to be at least 350 000 each year. Nearly half of HCV-infected individuals are not aware of their serological status, in spite of the existence of accurate tools to diagnose infection. In contrast to HBV, HCV infection is curable by therapy. Numerous therapeutic options, in particular the recently approved interferon-free regimens, are available for the treatment of chronic infection, with infection cure rates over 90% for most groups of infected patients.

Virology of Hepatitis C Virus

HCV is a member of the Flaviviridae family, genus *Hepacivirus*. The hepatitis C viral particle is made of a 50–80 nm enveloped icosahedral capsid that is composed of multiple copies of the core protein and contains a single-stranded positive RNA genome of approximately 9.6 kb. Several lines of evidence suggest that the HCV particles circulate in the bloodstream as hybrid lipoviroparticles (LVP). Indeed, the majority of viral RNA in human infected plasma co-elutes with very low-density lipoproteins (VLDLs).

HCV LIFE CYCLE

The HCV life cycle takes place in the cytoplasm of hepatocytes, in close relationship to the lipid metabolism. Several cell surface molecules mediate HCV binding and internalization, including glycosaminoglycans and the low-density lipoprotein (LDL) receptor, which could serve as the initial docking site for HCV attachment; the tetraspanin CD81, which could act as a post-attachment entry co-receptor; the scavenger receptor B1, an essential component of the cellular HCV receptor complex; claudin-1 and occludin, which appear to act late in the entry process. After attachment, HCV entry into cells is pH-dependent and related to clathrin-mediated endocytosis. Entry is followed by a fusion step within an acidic endosomal compartment. Decapsidation of viral nucleocapsids liberates free positive-strand genomic RNAs in the cell cytoplasm, where they serve, together with newly synthesized RNAs, as messenger RNAs for synthesis of the HCV polyprotein. The large precursor polyprotein generated by HCV genome translation is targeted to the endoplasmic reticulum membrane. The co- and post-translational processing of the HCV polyprotein results in the generation of at least 11 proteins, including three structural proteins (C or core, E1 and E2), a viroporin, p7, and 6 nonstructural (NS) proteins (NS2, NS3, NS4A, NS4B, NS5A and NS5B). The viral proteins remain associated with intracellular membranes after processing. Replication is catalyzed by the HCV RNA-dependent RNA polymerase in the 'membranous web' or replication complex that supports and compartmentalizes HCV replication. The replication complex associates viral proteins, cellular components and nascent RNA strands. The positive-strand genome RNA serves as a template for the synthesis of a negative-strand intermediate of replication. Then, negative-strand RNA serves as a template to produce numerous strands of positive polarity that will subsequently be used for polyprotein translation, synthesis of new intermediates of replication or packaging into new virus particles. Viral particle formation is probably initiated by the interaction of the core protein with genomic RNA. HCV uses the lipoprotein production pathway to generate mature viral particles and export them. Cytoplasmic lipid droplets serve as virus assembly platforms and the VLDL synthesis/secretion machinery appears to be involved in infectious HCV production. The mechanisms underlying exportation of mature virions in the pericellular space or their transfer to neighboring cells have yet to be understood.

HCV GENETIC DIVERSITY

Seven major HCV genotypes (1–7) and numerous subtypes within each genotype have been identified.[21] HCV genotypes 1, 2, 3 and 4 have a worldwide distribution, whereas genotypes 5 and 6 are found essentially in South Africa and South East Asia, respectively. Genotype 1 is the most prevalent genotype in Europe, the USA, Asia and Australia. A recent study suggested that the viral genotype could influence the outcome of acute HCV infection. Indeed, genotype 1 was associated with more frequent spontaneous clearance of acute infection, particularly in females.[22] In contrast, the severity of chronic liver disease or of extrahepatic manifestations associated with HCV infection does not appear to be influenced by the viral genotype. HCV genotype determination is mandatory before starting antiviral treatment because the choice of the drugs and treatment duration depend on it.

Epidemiology
INCIDENCE AND PREVALENCE

Hepatitis C virus is present in all continents, and a recent estimate suggested that between 130 and 170 million individuals have chronic HCV infection, corresponding to a global prevalence of 1.1% .[23] In high-income countries, the incidence of HCV infection has declined considerably, owing to blood screening and measures to prevent viral infections in intravenous drug users. However, approximately 2000 new cases of acute hepatitis C probably still occur annually in the USA according to the Centers for Disease Control in 2012. The HCV incidence and prevalence is higher in LMIC, where the main route of HCV infection is unsafe medical or surgical procedures; only about 50% of blood products are screened for anti-HCV antibodies in these countries, and about 40% of all injections are given via reused equipment. A high prevalence of chronic HCV infection has been reported in African and Eastern Mediterranean countries, the highest prevalence being 14.7% in the general population of Egypt (9% with replicating virus), whereas the HCV prevalence varies from 0.4–0.8% in Sweden, Germany, the Netherlands and France to over 1.6% in the USA, and over 5% in some communities in Italy.[24-26] Because chronic hepatitis C is often asymptomatic until advanced stages of liver disease develop, up to approximately 60% of infected patients are unaware of their infection and related liver disease.[27]

ROUTES OF TRANSMISSION AND AT-RISK GROUPS

HCV is transmitted almost exclusively by infected blood. Preventive screening with highly sensitive enzyme immunoassays and, more recently, nucleic acid testing has virtually eliminated the risk of post-transfusional HCV infection (theoretical risk: 1 in 2 million donations in the USA, 1 in 8 million donations in France). As a result, the principal route of HCV transmission in high-income countries is now intravenous drug use, which is responsible for 80% of new cases of HCV infection.[28, 29] The incidence of HCV infection in this high-risk group is as high as 39 per 100 person-years. In this context, imprisonment is an important risk factor for acquiring HCV infection in high-income countries.

Nosocomial transmission through the use of improperly decontaminated materials or the contaminated hands or gloves of healthcare workers is responsible for a substantial number of new infections worldwide. HCV can also be transmitted by tattooing, piercing, mesotherapy or acupuncture if standard precautions are not implemented. Although HCV can be acquired after accidental needlestick exposure, the risk of infection is low (<1%), and healthcare workers have only a slightly higher prevalence of HCV than the general population. HCV can be transmitted to household members who share instruments such as scissors, razors and combs. Sexual transmission is unusual, but outbreaks of acute hepatitis have been reported in HIV-positive communities of men who have sex with men. The risk of mother-to-infant transmission of HCV is less than 5% and is generally related to exposure to the mother's blood in the perinatal period. Cesarean sections are not advocated as a means of preventing infection, and breast-feeding is not contraindicated. The risk of perinatal transmission is higher when the mother is coinfected with HIV. Other factors possibly associated with high transmission rates include the level of HCV viremia and maternal intravenous drug abuse. In 10–30% of cases, no apparent risk factor for HCV infection is identifiable, suggesting other potential sources of 'community-acquired' hepatitis C.

Pathogenicity

HCV RNA becomes detectable in the serum 3–7 days after exposure. HCV RNA levels rise rapidly during the first weeks, followed by serum aminotransferase levels 2–8 weeks after exposure. Anti-HCV antibodies arise late in the course of acute hepatitis C and may not be present at the onset of symptoms and serum aminotransferase elevation. After an incubation period that ranges from 15 to 120 days, acute hepatitis C usually remains asymptomatic and is undiagnosed. Nonspecific symptoms such as fatigue, low-grade fever, myalgias, nausea, vomiting or itching may be present. Jaundice occurs in only 20–30% of patients, usually 2–12 weeks after infection. Serum aminotransferase levels commonly exceed 10 times the upper limit of normal in the acute stage, even in the absence of symptoms. Fulminant hepatitis C has been reported but appears to be exceptional in the absence of another chronic underlying liver disease.

Chronic HCV infection is the leading cause of end-stage liver disease, hepatocellular carcinoma and liver-related death in the Western world. It is generally a slowly progressive disease characterized by a persistent inflammation leading to the development of cirrhosis in approximately 10–20% of patients over 20–30 years. Once cirrhosis is established, the disease progression remains unpredictable: cirrhosis may remain indolent for many years in some patients, whereas it rapidly progresses in others toward HCC, hepatic decompensation and death. Overall, once cirrhosis has established there is a 1–5% annual risk of HCC and a 3–6% annual risk of hepatic decompensation. Following an episode of decompensation, the risk of death in the following year is between 15% and 20%. Although hepatitis C causes persistent hepatitis, the viral RNA genome does not integrate into the host genome and viral replication can be eradicated and a virological cure achieved by treatment. Spontaneous resolution of chronic hepatitis C is exceptional, but has been described. Fibrosis progression rates are extremely variable and can be influenced by host, viral and environmental factors. The rates of progression are not linear and may vary between fibrosis stages and accelerate with duration of infection or aging. The factors that may influence disease progression include age, age at acquisition, male gender, alcohol consumption of more than 50 g/day, obesity, insulin resistance, type 2 diabetes, coinfection with HBV or HIV, immunosuppressive therapy, and host genetic factors.

Chronic infection with hepatitis C is known to cause extrahepatic manifestations. Several diseases including sicca syndrome and lichen planus have been reported to be more frequent in HCV-infected patients. Overall, 15–35% of patients with chronic HCV have circulating cryoglobulins. Among them, between 5% and 25% will develop clinical manifestations of mixed cryoglobulinemia, including systemic vasculitis, peripheral neuropathy, Raynaud's phenomenon, and/or membranoproliferative glomerulonephritis. Non-Hodgkin's lymphomas are more frequent in patients with chronic hepatitis C. HCV is also recognized as influencing metabolic pathways, with increased rates of insulin resistance, type 2 diabetes and vascular disease.

Diagnostic Virology

The diagnosis of acute HCV infection is based on the detection of total anti-HCV antibodies by means of a third-generation enzyme immunoassay (EIA) and of HCV RNA by a sensitive molecular method with a limit of detection of the order of 10–15 IU/mL. Four marker profiles can be observed, based on the presence or absence of either marker (Table 165-4). The presence of HCV RNA in the absence of anti-HCV antibodies is strongly indicative of acute HCV infection, which will be confirmed by seroconversion (i.e., the appearance of anti-HCV antibodies) a few days to weeks later. Acutely infected patients can have both HCV RNA and anti-HCV antibodies at the time of diagnosis; in this case, it is difficult to distinguish acute hepatitis C from an acute exacerbation of chronic hepatitis C or acute hepatitis of another cause in a patient with chronic hepatitis C. Acute hepatitis C is very unlikely if both anti-HCV antibodies and HCV RNA are absent or if anti-HCV antibodies are present without HCV RNA. Patients in the latter group should be retested a few weeks later, because HCV RNA may be temporarily undetectable owing to transient, partial control of viral replication before the infection becomes chronic. Apart from such cases, the presence of anti-HCV antibodies in the absence of HCV RNA is generally seen in patients who have recovered from a past HCV infection. Nevertheless, this pattern cannot be differentiated from a false-positive enzyme immunoassay result, the exact prevalence of which is unknown.

Chronic HCV infection is defined as the persistence of HCV RNA over 6 months. Chronic hepatitis C is characterized by the presence of both total anti-HCV antibodies and HCV RNA in individuals with clinical and/or biological signs of chronic liver disease.

References available online at expertconsult.com.

TABLE 165-4	Patterns of Hepatitis C Virus Markers and Their Significance during Acute Hepatitis

Anti-HCV Antibodies	HCV RNA	Diagnosis
–	–	Not acute hepatitis C
–	+	Acute hepatitis C
+	–	Probably not acute hepatitis C (retest a few weeks later)
+	+	Difficult to differentiate acute from chronic hepatitis C

KEY REFERENCES

Denniston M.M., Klevens R.M., McQuillan G.M., et al.: Awareness of infection, knowledge of hepatitis C, and medical follow-up among individuals testing positive for hepatitis C: National Health and Nutrition Examination Survey 2001-2008. *Hepatology* 2012; 55:1652-1661.

Dalton H.R., Kamar N., Izopet J.: Hepatitis E in developed countries: current status and future perspectives. *Future Microbiol* 2014; 9:1361-1372.

Gower E., Estes C., Blach S., et al.: Global epidemiology and genotype distribution of the hepatitis C virus infection. *J Hepatol* 2014; 61:S45-S57.

Hajarizadeh B., Grebely J., Dore G.J.: Epidemiology and natural history of HCV infection. *Nat Rev Gastroenterol Hepatol* 2013; 10:553-562.

Ott J.J., Stevens G.A., Groeger J., et al.: Global epidemiology of hepatitis B virus infection: new estimates of age-specific HBsAg seroprevalence and endemicity. *Vaccine* 2012; 30:2212-2219.

Lozano R., Naghavi M., Foreman K., et al.: Global and regional mortality from 235 causes of death for 20 age groups in 1990 and 2010: a systematic analysis for the Global Burden of Disease Study 2010. *Lancet* 2012; 380:2095-2128.

Wang X., Ren J., Gao Q., et al.: Hepatitis A virus and the origins of picornaviruses. *Nature* 2015; 517:85-88.

Wenzel J.J., Sichler M., Schemmerer M., et al.: Decline in hepatitis E virus antibody prevalence in southeastern Germany, 1996-2011. *Hepatology* 2014; 60:1180-1186.

166

Herpesviruses

TYREL T. SMITH | RICHARD J. WHITLEY

KEY CONCEPTS

- Herpesviruses possess double-stranded, linear DNA contained in an icosahedral capsid surrounded by tegument proteins further encased in a lipid envelope dispersed with membrane-associated glycoproteins.

- The Herpesvirales order is split into three families. Human herpesviruses are representative of the Herpesviridae family, which is divided into three subfamilies: Alphaherpesvirinae, Betaherpesvirinae and Gammaherpesvirinae.

- Human herpesviruses are lytic by nature and production of viral progeny ultimately leads to cell death.

- The establishment of latency is central to the success of herpesviruses as a pathogen, allowing the virus to persist to cause lifelong infection in the presence of a fully developed immune response.

- The majority of efficacious antiherpetic drugs are nucleoside analogs that depend on the viral thymidine kinase to activate compounds that inhibit the viral DNA polymerase thus terminating viral DNA replication.

Nature

TAXONOMY

The herpesviruses are double-stranded DNA (dsDNA) viruses belonging to Herpesvirales order.[1] More than 150 individual viruses have been described that have been discovered in almost all species of vertebrates and invertebrates. Their widespread presence suggests that they first colonized animal species at an early stage of evolution, and this primordial colonization has led to adaptations to their natural host resulting in increased host specificity.[2] These adaptations are exemplified by their high rates of infection, the generally mild symptoms associated with infection, and their perpetuation in a population with a high level of immunity by establishing latent infections.

Genetic analysis divides the Herpesvirales order into three distinct families.[1] The family containing the human herpesviruses, Herpesviridae, is further divided into three subfamilies – Alphaherpesvirinae, Betaherpesvirinae and Gammaherpesvirinae based upon biologic properties (Table 166-1).

At present, eight herpesviruses are known to infect man (Table 166-2). Additionally, the primate herpesvirus belonging to the *Simplexvirus* genus of the Alphaherpesvirus subfamily, B virus (Macacine herpesvirus 1), can also cause severe and sometimes fatal infections in humans.[3] The virus is enzootic among Old World macaques and usually causes minimal or no morbidity in its natural host.

STRUCTURE

Herpesviruses are morphologically distinct from all other viruses.[4] The virion often has a pleomorphic appearance when visualized by transmission electron microscopy (Figure 166-1). Examination of herpes simplex virus type 1 (HSV-1) using cryo-electron tomography (Figure 166-2), which permits three-dimensional visualization of the virion, displays the lipid bilayer membrane with an average diameter of 186 nm. An array of spikes protruding from eleach virion extends the full diameter to approximately 225 nm.[5]

The tegument consists of proteins between the capsid and envelope that aid the virion in successful infection. Studies with HSV-1 suggest that the tegument contains at least 20 proteins that are believed to have important functions in the early stages of virus replication following penetration of the host cell.

GENOME

A linear molecule of dsDNA encodes the genetic information of the virus, and its size varies for different herpesviruses, from approximately 124–245 kbp (80 000–150 000 kDa). The G+C composition of human herpesvirus DNA ranges from 36% to 69%. The complete sequence of each of the human herpesviruses is known (Table 166-3), and the phylogenetic relationships of the human herpesviruses are shown in Figure 166-3.

Epidemiology

TRANSMISSION PATHWAYS

Herpesviruses are relatively fragile in that they require a lipid envelope to achieve attachment to, and penetration of, the host cell. Consequently, these viruses transmit most easily on contact of warm and moist mucosal layers. Two broad groupings of virus transmission can be distinguished:

TABLE 166-1	Biologic Properties of Herpesviridae
Common properties	Spherical enveloped virions, 150–200 nm in diameter
	Large, linear, dsDNA genome of 125–290 kbp contained within a T = 16 icosahedral capsid, which is surrounded by a proteinaceous matrix named the tegument and then by a lipid envelope containing membrane-associated proteins
	Synthesis of DNA and assembly of capsid within the nucleus, acquire envelope by budding through host cell membranes
	Specify a large array of enzymes involved in nucleic acid metabolism and synthesis
	Production of progeny virus results in destruction of the host cell
	Establish latency in their natural host
Alphaherpesvirinae	Variable host range
	Short reproductive cycle
	Rapid spread in cell culture
	Efficient destruction of infected cells
	Establish latency primarily but not exclusively in sensory ganglia
Betaherpesvirinae	Restricted host range (a nonexclusive property of this subfamily)
	Long reproductive cycle
	Infection progresses slowly in culture, frequently forming enlarged (cytomegalic) cells
	Latency in secretory glands, lymphoreticular cells, kidneys and other tissues
Gammaherpesvirinae	Experimental host range limited to family or order of natural host
	In vitro replication in lymphoblastoid cells
	In vivo replication and latency in either T or B cells

TABLE 166-2	**Human Herpesviruses**		
ICTV* Name	**Common Name†**	**Subfamily**	**Genus**
Human herpesvirus 1	Herpes simplex virus type 1	Alphaherpesvirinae	*Simplexvirus*
Human herpesvirus 2	Herpes simplex virus type 2	Alphaherpesvirinae	*Simplexvirus*
Human herpesvirus 3	Varicella-zoster virus	Alphaherpesvirinae	*Varicellovirus*
Human herpesvirus 4	Epstein–Barr virus	Gammaherpesvirinae	*Lymphocryptovirus*
Human herpesvirus 5	Human cytomegalovirus	Betaherpesvirinae	*Cytomegalovirus*
Human herpesvirus 6	Human herpesvirus 6	Betaherpesvirinae	*Roseolovirus*
Human herpesvirus 7	Human herpesvirus 7	Betaherpesvirinae	*Roseolovirus*
Human herpesvirus 8	Kaposi's sarcoma-associated herpesvirus	Gammaherpesvirinae	*Rhadinovirus*

Two variants, 'a' and 'b', of human herpesvirus 6 are known.
*The International Committee on Taxonomy of Viruses (ICTV) classification scheme names the herpesviruses according to the taxon of the host that (in its natural setting) harbors the virus.[1]
†As many viruses have acquired commonly used names – for example, human herpesvirus 1 is commonly known as herpes simplex virus (HSV) type 1 – the classification is not yet rigorously applied. However, newly discovered viruses are now named in accordance with this classification scheme, for example human herpesviruses 6, 7 and 8.

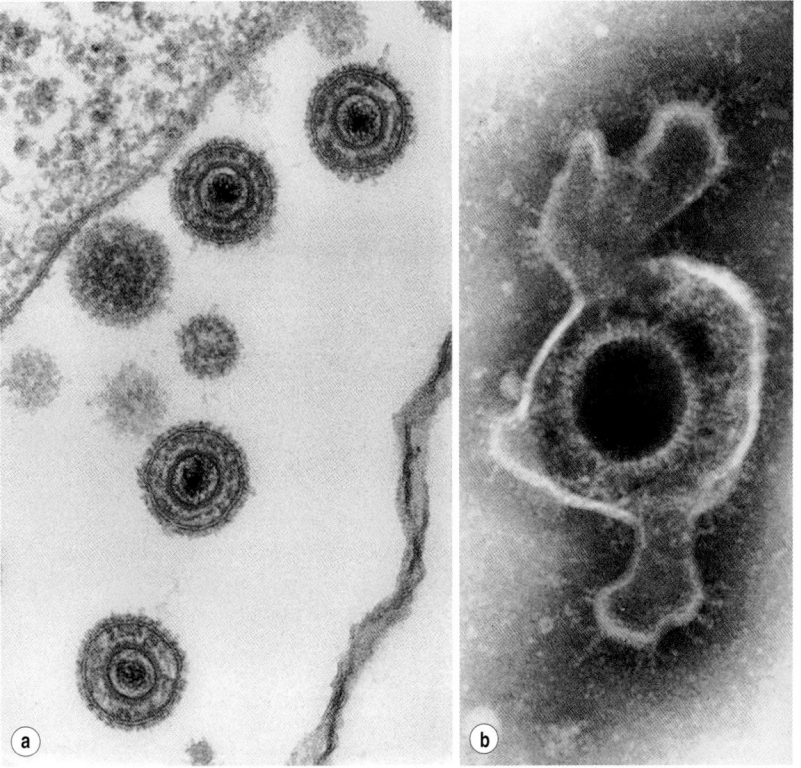

Figure 166-1   Enveloped virus particle. (a) Thin section. (b) Negative staining. These electron microscopic views show HSV. The DNA is surrounded by a nucleocapsid which comprises 162 individual protein subunits (150 hexavalent capsomers and 12 pentavalent capsomers) arranged in the form of an icosahedron. The nucleocapsid is in turn enclosed by the tegument and virus envelope bearing glycoprotein spikes. *(Courtesy of Hans Gelderblom.)*

- virus is transmitted most effectively by oral secretions and non-genital contact – HSV-1, varicella-zoster virus (VZV), Epstein–Barr virus (EBV), cytomegalovirus (CMV), human herpesvirus 6 (HHV-6) and HHV-7; and
- virus is transmitted most effectively by genital secretions – HSV-2 and Kaposi's sarcoma-associated herpesvirus (HHV-8).

These modes of transmission have a profound influence upon the epidemiology of the individual viruses. Also, it is important to note that EBV, CMV, HHV-6 and -7 can also be transmitted by blood transfusion.

PREVALENCE

Herpesviruses transmitted predominantly by oral secretion or non-genital contact have a peak incidence of infection in early childhood (Table 166-4), while the peak for genital transmission is in adolescence and young adults. The infection rates of viruses transmitted by genital route are generally not as high as viruses transmitted by nongenital routes. However, for both groups there is a further distinct relation between rates of acquisition, sexual preference and the socioeconomic status of the study population (i.e. low socioeconomic status equates with high seroprevalence). In addition, the seroprevalence of genital

TABLE 166-3	Properties of the Human Herpesviruses			
Virus	Site of Latency	G+C (%)	Genome (kb Pairs)	Sequence*
HHV-1	Sensory nerve ganglia	68	152	X14112
HHV-2	Sensory nerve ganglia	69	154	Z86099
HHV-3	Sensory nerve ganglia	46	125	X04370
HHV-4	Leukocytes, epithelial cells	60	172	V01555
HHV-5	B lymphocytes	57	229	X17403
HHV-6A	T lymphocytes (CD4+), epithelial cells	43	159	X83413
HHV-6B	T lymphocytes (CD4+), epithelial cells	43	162	AF157706
HHV-7	T lymphocytes (CD4+)	36	153	AF037218
HHV-8	B lymphocytes, epithelial cells	59	170	AF402655

*European Molecular Biology Laboratory Accession Numbers (http://www.embl-heidelberg.de).

TABLE 166-4	Features of Herpesvirus Infections				
	PEAK INCIDENCE OF PRIMARY INFECTION		Adult Seroprevalence (%)	Principal Route(s) of Transmission	Notes
Virus	Childhood	Adolescence			
HSV-1	+++	+	75–95+	Oral secretions, close contact	Overall seroprevalence predominantly determined by socioeconomic status
HSV-2	–	+++	4–95	Genital secretions, close contact	Lifetime number of sex partners is predominant influence on rates of seropositivity
VZV	+++	+	90–95	Aerosol, close contact	Epidemic spread in childhood, in tropics relatively more common in adults than children
CMV	++	++	40–95+	Oral secretions, genital secretions	Infection common in infancy, but a significant proportion of women of child-bearing age are susceptible; overall seroprevalence predominantly determined by socioeconomic status
EBV	++	++	70–95	Oral secretions	Second peak of incidence in early adolescence (glandular fever)
HHV-6	+++	–	>85	Oral secretions	Infection common in infancy – peak age of acquisition 2 years
HHV-7	+++	–	>85	Oral secretions	Infection common in infancy – peak age of acquisition 3 years
HHV-8	–	+++	10–25	Oral secretions, genital secretions	Men who have sex with men and have AIDS show highest seroprevalence

CMV, cytomegalovirus; EBV, Epstein–Barr virus; HHV, human herpesvirus; HSV, herpes simplex virus; VZV, varicella-zoster virus.

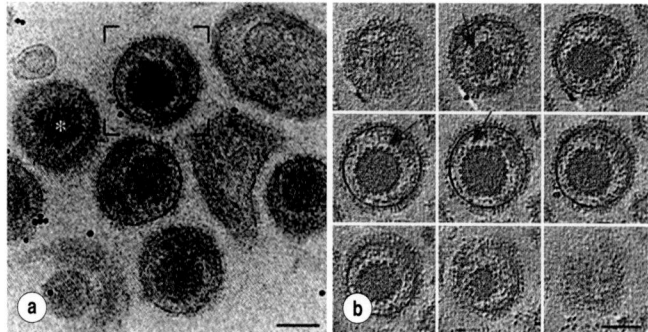

Figure 166-2   Herpes simplex virus type 1 cryo-electron tomography. Tomographic reconstruction of HSV-1 virions in vitreous ice. (a) Zero-tilt projection from a tilt series. Black dots are 10 nm gold particles used as fiducial markers. (b) Gallery of parallel slices, 15.5 nm apart and 5.2 nm thick, through the virion framed in (a). Each slice represents the average over seven planes. Red arrowheads mark filaments in the tegument. Scale bars, 100 nm. *(Reproduced with permission from Grünewald K., et al. Science 2003; 302:1396-14148.)*

HSV infection is skewing to more primary infection cases caused by HSV-1.[6]

GEOGRAPHIC ASPECTS

Herpesviruses are distributed worldwide and no animal reservoirs of infection are known for any of the human herpesviruses. There is evidence that varicella is less prevalent in childhood in tropical regions than in temperate climatic areas.[7] Possible explanations for this include the relative isolation of clusters of populations in rural areas, epidemiologic 'interference' through infections caused by other viruses, and perhaps decreased efficiency of transmission as a result of the lability of VZV in areas where there is a high ambient temperature. Other complications of herpesvirus infection, such as Burkitt's lymphoma, which is associated with EBV infection, are endemic only in tropical Africa.[8] Nasopharyngeal carcinoma is also associated with EBV infection and is endemic in Japan and Southern China.[9] A sporadic, nonimmunocompromised-associated Kaposi's sarcoma is found predominantly in countries bordering the Mediterranean and in Central Africa.[10]

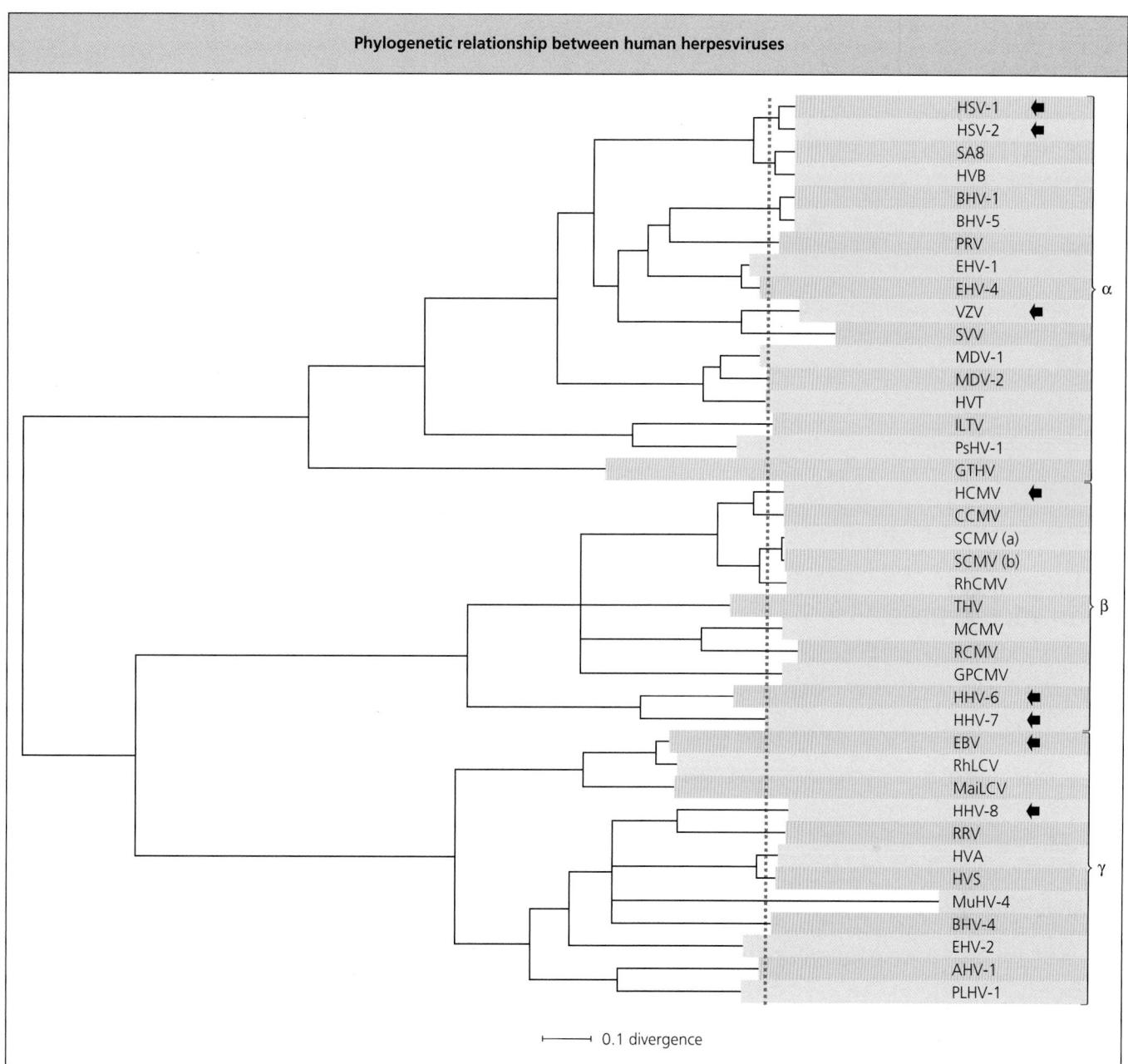

Figure 166-3 Phylogenetic relationship between the human herpesviruses. The tree was constructed based on an alignment of amino acid sequences for six genes of HSV-1: UL15, UL19, UL27, UL28, UL29 and UL30. *(Reproduced with permission from McGeoch D.J., et al., Virus Res 2006; 117:90-104.)*

PERIODICITY

The human herpesviruses are endemic in human populations as a result of establishing latent infections. Additionally, no seasonal variation in the efficiency of transmission exists due to their modes of transmission. For infections in which reactivation is infrequent (e.g. VZV infection) there may be 'outbreaks' of infection (mini-epidemics) when infection spreads rapidly through a nonimmune population. Outbreaks can also occur if large numbers of susceptible individuals are brought together (e.g. infectious mononucleosis among college students).[11]

DETERMINANTS OF INFECTION

Early acquisition of infection is common for all herpesviruses transmitted by the nongenital route (see Table 166-4). In a classic study of

HSV infection, Burnet and Williams showed that there was a clear relationship between the age of acquisition of the virus and socioeconomic status.[12] Populations associated with a low socioeconomic environment collectively showed earlier acquisition of HSV infection than more affluent populations, although in both groups, infection rates of 90–95% were observed by early adulthood. Primary HSV-1 infection was rare in those over 30 years of age. In recent years several seroepidemiologic studies have shown a general decrease in the overall prevalence of HSV-1 antibody in high-income countries.[13,14] However, even within individual countries there are variations in seroprevalence; for example, the seroprevalence rates are generally higher among inner city residents than among those from rural areas. Here, the major factor determining the seroprevalence is the frequency of direct person-to-person contact rather than the socioeconomic status of the individual populations.

If infection does not occur in infancy, transmission routes other than direct oral contact can constitute important risk factors. An example is found in the acquisition of CMV. Although most CMV infections occur in infancy, a significant proportion (40–50% in high-income countries) of women of child-bearing age is still susceptible to infection and may acquire the infection during pregnancy. Sexual transmission of infection then becomes an important mode of acquisition of infection for these women and can result in congenital CMV infection. In addition, contact with young children of less than 24 months of age is a further important risk factor.

Viruses such as HSV-2, for which the principal mode of transmission is sexual, are generally not acquired until the onset of sexual activity in adolescence and early adulthood. HSV-2 prevalence, overall and by age, varies markedly by country, region within country, population subgroup and in populations with higher risk sexual behavior.[15]

The seroprevalence of HHV-8 infection is low (<5%) in most northern, western and central European countries except for parts of Italy, Greece and, to a lesser extent, Spain. It is also low in the USA (0–5%). In many African countries, particularly sub-Saharan Africa, rates of 40–60% are found in adults and adolescents. In accordance with the high rates of Kaposi's sarcoma seen in HIV-infected men who have sex with men, HHV-8 antibodies are more common in these groups than in the general population of the same country.

Pathogenicity

VIRION POLYPEPTIDES

HSV-1 virions contain approximately 33 virus-specific proteins, but more than double this number are found within an infected cell. The transcription of mRNAs from the genome proceeds from both strands of the linear dsDNA, in either direction, with evidence of overlapping transcription and splicing of genes and gene products.[16] Three stages of transcription and translation are observed:

- α phase (resulting in the production of 'immediate-early proteins');
- β phase (proteins responsible mainly for DNA metabolism); and
- γ phase (principally structural proteins).

REPLICATION

The replicative cycle of the virus is illustrated in Figure 166-4. Attachment of herpesvirus to a host cell is mediated by glycoproteins projecting from the virus envelope interacting with receptors on the host cell.[17]

Initial low-affinity binding to glycosaminoglycans, namely heparan sulfate, concentrates virions on the cell surface, thus facilitating subsequent binding to entry receptors. The major pathway for virus entry is fusion of the envelope with the plasma membrane, introduction of tegument proteins and viral nucleocapsid into the cell cytoplasm, and transport of the released nucleocapsid to the nuclear pore. Alternate ancillary pathways have also been identified in cell culture, including fusion within an acidic or neutral endosome.[18]

The tegument proteins serve to both 'disable' the host cell and initiate viral replication. Soon after virus entry, host cell DNA synthesis is shut off, host cell protein synthesis declines rapidly and glycosylation of host cell proteins ceases to ensure that the metabolic machinery of the cell is fully available for virus replication. Simultaneously, the virion nucleocapsid is transported via microtubules of the cell cytoskeleton to a nuclear pore. The viral nucleocapsid breaks down at the nuclear pore, releasing its DNA into the cell nucleus where the linear DNA molecule immediately circularizes.

Transcription of viral DNA takes place within the host cell nucleus. The first sets of viral genes to be transcribed are the immediate-early or α genes; these produce checkpoint proteins that stimulate and regulate all the subsequent steps in the replication cycle. Their production is essential to stimulate the synthesis of β proteins involved in viral nucleic acid replication (e.g. DNA-dependent DNA polymerase).

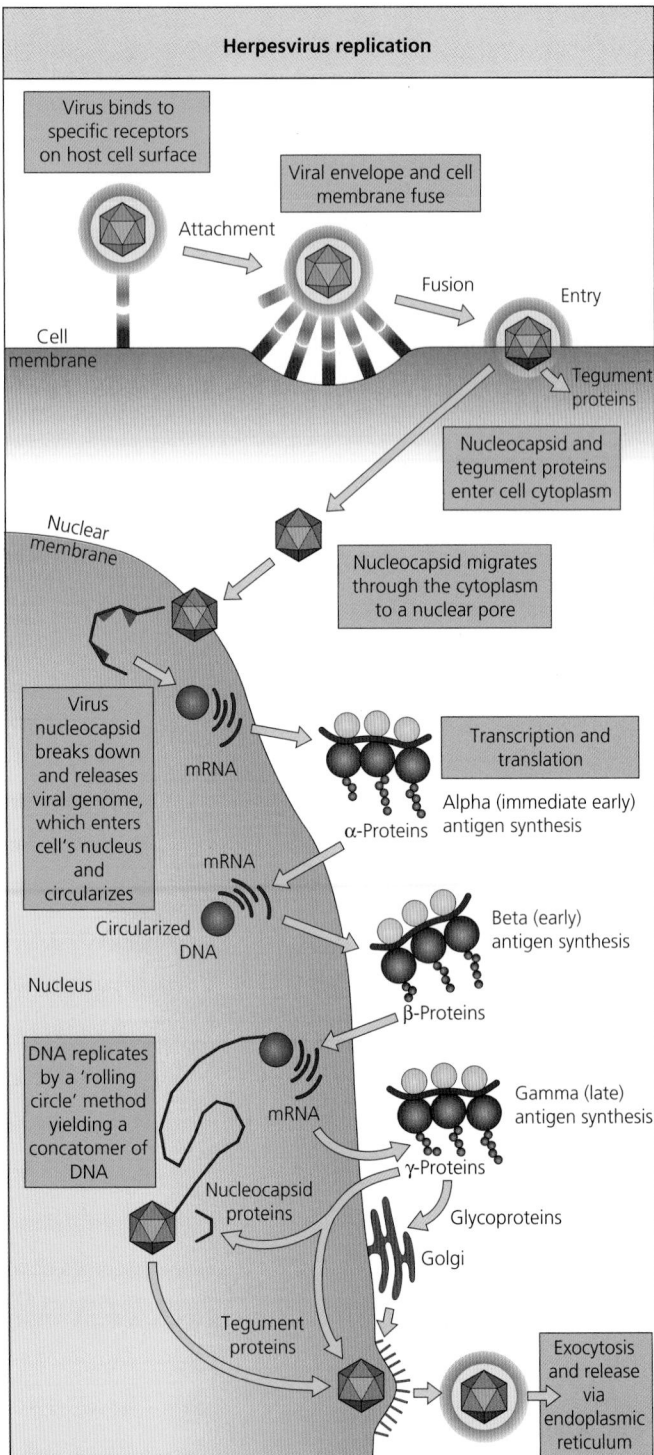

Figure 166-4 Herpesvirus replication. The tegument proteins affect the shutdown of host cell metabolism. On entry to the nucleus the DNA circularizes and binds a tegument protein and cellular factors to initiate transcription. Transcription and translation occur in three phases: immediate-early, early and late. Capsid proteins migrate into the nucleus and the viral DNA is encapsulated. The viral glycoproteins are extensively modified post-translationally by transit through the Golgi apparatus. The glycoproteins diffuse to the nuclear envelope. The nucleocapsids are enveloped at the inner nuclear membrane and are either transported within vesicles that fuse with the plasma membrane to release the enveloped capsids into the extracellular milieu, or undergo de-envelopment at the outer nuclear membrane and re-envelopment at cytoplasmic membranes. Alternatively, nuclear pores become enlarged sufficiently to allow egress of naked capsids and the capsids then become enveloped at cytoplasmic membranes.

TABLE 166-5	Principal Sites of Latency for Herpesviruses	
Virus	**Established (Most Probable) Sites of Latency**	**Other Possible Sites of Latency**
HSV-1	Neurons (trigeminal ganglia)	Other sensory nerve ganglia, brain, eye
HSV-2	Neurons (sacral ganglia)	Other sensory ganglia
VZV	Neurons (dorsal, thoracic and trigeminal ganglia)	Brain, other sensory ganglia
EBV	B cells (epithelial cells of nasopharynx and submandibular salivary glands)	–
CMV	Monocytes, lymphocytes, epithelial cells	Salivary glands, renal tubule cells
HHV-6, HHV-7	T cells	Bone marrow progenitors, monocytic/macrophage cells
HHV-8	Not firmly established	B cells

Gene products of α and β phases transactivate the γ genes, which produce the late or γ proteins, the virion structural proteins including the viral capsid and glycoproteins.

Nucleocapsids are assembled around viral scaffolding proteins in the nucleus. These proteins then interact with replicated viral DNA to allow encapsulation. The DNA-filled capsids proceed to associate with tegument (matrix) proteins near the nuclear membrane. Three different models for the release of mature nucleocapsids from cells have been proposed (see Figure 166-4). Whichever method the viruses use for their release, productive infection is fatal for the host cell because host cell chromosomes are degraded in the process of viral DNA replication.

LATENCY

During the course of a primary infection, a latent infection is established with the exact site(s) of latency varying for each subfamily of herpesvirus (Table 166-5). No virions can be detected within the latently infected cell. In the latent state, the virus is believed to exist as extrachromosomal circularized DNA (analogous to plasmids). The host immune response to infection rapidly eliminates virus and virus-infected cells from peripheral sites but does not recognize latently infected cells as harboring virus since no viral antigens are expressed on the cell surface.

This establishment of latency is central to the success of herpesviruses as a pathogen, allowing the virus to persist to cause lifelong infection in the presence of a fully developed immune response. Through periodic reactivation of latent virus, viral shedding occurs at intervals throughout life, allowing the virus to spread to new susceptible hosts. Such shedding is usually asymptomatic. In order to avoid eradication by the host immune system, each herpesvirus encodes multiple proteins that circumvent components of immune detection.[19–21] A key mechanism is to reduce or prevent expression of virus-specific peptide-MHC class I complexes at the cellular membrane, thus preventing recognition by cytotoxic T lymphocytes (CTLs) that would kill the infected cell.

MOLECULAR AND CELLULAR BASIS OF PATHOGENICITY

The combination of virion surface glycoproteins and the distribution of cellular receptors provide a partial explanation of the cell- and tissue-specific tropism of members of the human herpesviruses. After primary infection, herpesviruses persist in their host by a combination of lytic infectious processes (cellular persistence) and latency established in other sites. In response to various stimuli, latent virus can be reactivated to a lytic state that can cause disease and provide a source of virus for transmission to susceptible individuals.

Herpes Simplex Virus

In vitro, HSV can infect most types of human cells and even cells of other species, but *in vivo* it is host specific. It causes lytic infection of fibroblasts and epithelial cells, and establishes latent infection in neurons. The two biotypes of HSV, HSV-1 and HSV-2, show some predilection for infecting defined anatomic sites – oropharyngeal and genital, respectively. Both viruses are capable of infecting and producing latent infection at either site, but HSV-2 reactivation 'above the waist' and HSV-1 reactivation 'below the waist' is infrequent.[22]

Varicella-Zoster Virus

Primary VZV infection begins in the mucosa of the respiratory tract and progresses via the blood and lymphatic system to cells of the reticuloendothelial system. A secondary viremia at 11–13 days disseminates virus to the skin where the characteristic vesicular lesions of chickenpox are produced. The virus establishes latent infection in the cranial, dorsal root and autonomic nervous system ganglia during this viremic phase. The molecular basis of latency and reactivation is poorly understood. In contrast to studies in neurons latently infected with HSV-1 (where only the LAT transcript is found), neurons latently infected with VZV have four transcripts corresponding to VZV genes 21, 29, 62 and 63.[23]

Epstein–Barr Virus

During primary infection EBV establishes a productive infection in the epithelial cells of the oropharynx. Virus is shed in the saliva and gains access to B cells in lymphatic tissue and the blood.[8] A lytic infection leads to the production of EBV proteins, including the early antigens, viral capsid and membrane glycoproteins, and resulting virions (Figure 166-5). EBV is a B-cell mitogen, stimulating the growth and immortalization of B cells by preventing apoptosis. In EBV-immortalized cells, the genome is maintained as a circular episome which is replicated by cellular DNA polymerase and is equally distributed to daughter cells when EBV-infected cells divide. The resting cell contains nine latent proteins and several noncoding RNAs that are under the master control of Epstein–Barr nuclear antigen (EBNA) 2. These act jointly to drive the cell to resemble an antigen-activated lymphoblast. EBV-transformed proliferating lymphocytes are constantly held in check by the immune response.[19] By promoting cell growth and preventing apoptosis, the latency program of EBV is believed to assume the prime role in oncogenesis.

Cytomegalovirus

CMV is capable of producing lytic infection of epithelial, endothelial, smooth muscle, stromal, fibroblast and neuronal cells *in vivo*. However, viral latency only appears to occur in a restricted subpopulation of myeloid and dendritic progenitor cells.[24] Hematopoietic cell precursors (CD34+) are a common precursor of both lymphoid and myeloid cells. Cells of the monocyte/myeloid lineage have been shown to become latently infected by as yet undefined mechanisms.[25] In the latently infected cell there is absence of lytic gene transcription although transcripts of the major immediate-early gene (IE) region of the CMV genome can be detected with the exception of the major IE transcripts IE72 and IE86. Between 2 and 10 copies of the CMV genome are carried in an episomal form in mononuclear cells of healthy seropositive individuals. It is presently unknown how the viral genome is maintained in dividing progenitor cells.

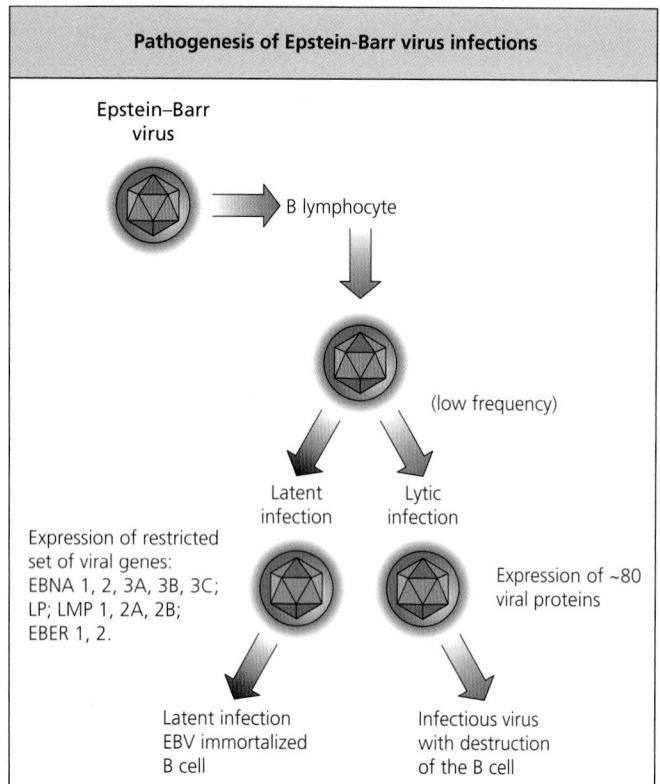

Pathogenesis of Epstein-Barr virus infections

Epstein–Barr virus

B lymphocyte

(low frequency)

Latent infection

Lytic infection

Expression of restricted set of viral genes: EBNA 1, 2, 3A, 3B, 3C; LP; LMP 1, 2A, 2B; EBER 1, 2.

Expression of ~80 viral proteins

Latent infection EBV immortalized B cell

Infectious virus with destruction of the B cell

Figure 166-5 Pathogenesis of Epstein–Barr virus (EBV) infections. Infection may result in lytic infection of the cell or cell immortalization, which can be distinguished by the production of virus and the expression of different viral proteins and antigens. T cells limit the outgrowth of EBV-infected cells. EBER, Epstein–Barr encoded small RNA; EBNA, Epstein–Barr nuclear antigen; LMP, latent membrane protein; LP, EBNA leader protein.

Human Herpesviruses 6 and 7

Human herpesvirus 6 was originally isolated from T cell cultures derived from the blood of patients who had AIDS, and HHV-7 was isolated from the $CD4^+$ T cells of a healthy individual. Both viruses infect and kill $CD4^+$ T cells, similar to HIV, yet the outcome of infection is markedly different.[26] In contrast to HIV infection, infection by HHV-6 or HHV-7 is rapidly controlled by the host immune response, and the virus establishes a state of latency. HHV-6 and HHV-7 establish chronic persistent infection with low-level replication in salivary, submandibular and parotid glands. Candidate sites for true latency are found in monocytes and early bone marrow progenitor cells. In HHV-6, the product of gene U94 has been shown to enable establishment and/or maintenance of latent infection in these cells.[27]

HHV-6 exists as two variants: HHV-6A and HHV-6B. Although closely related, consistent differences have been observed in their biologic, immunologic, epidemiologic and molecular properties. HHV-6B is the primary etiologic agent of exanthem subitum (also known as roseola or sixth disease; see Chapter 9), whereas no single disease has been definitively associated with HHV-6A. HHV-7 is responsible for a subset of exanthem subitum and other exanthema cases, but like HHV-6A, it also remains an 'orphan' virus with no firm disease association.[28]

Human Herpesvirus 8

Using representational difference analysis, HHV-8 was initially identified in 90% of AIDS-related Kaposi's sarcoma (KS) lesions and in 15% of non-KS tissues from people who had HIV infection.[29] Following these observations HHV-8 sequences were identified using polymerase chain reaction (PCR) in all forms of KS, including KS from different geographic locations in individuals with or without HIV infection.[10] Most KS spindle cells can be shown to be latently infected; only a small

proportion (1–3%) show lytic, replicative markers. Although HHV-8 can infect many cell types *in vitro*, only infection of primary epithelial cell cultures results in changes in morphology and growth. Once latency is established in these cells, dramatic elongation occurs to produce spindle-like cells. These changes can be traced to organization of the actin cytoskeleton and related to the expression of a single viral gene – v-FLIP.[10] The modifications are not, however, related to cell immortalization and this marks a clear difference between the latency program of HHV-8 and that of EBV. Six proteins are expressed in the latently infected KS cell; latency associated antigen (LANA), v-cyclin, v-FLIP and kaposin proteins A, B and C.

CELL TRANSFORMATION

Human herpesviruses can induce mutations in host cell DNA; however, greater oncogenic potential can be demonstrated for the human gammaherpesvirinae EBV and HHV-8.[8,10] EBV-infected human lymphocytes can be transformed into lymphoblast cell lines. All cells that carry the EBV genome express virus-specific nuclear antigens (EBNAs), regardless of virion shedding. There are also clear epidemiologic links to several types of tumor: Burkitt's lymphoma, infectious mononucleosis that progresses to fatal B-cell lymphoma in boys with an X-linked immunodeficiency, nasopharyngeal carcinoma and post-transplant lymphoproliferative disease in immunosuppressed solid organ transplant recipients.[8] HHV-8 similarly has strong epidemiologic links to KS and primary effusion lymphoma. HHV-8 DNA is found in all forms of KS and infection rates are higher in groups in which KS is frequent.[10]

Prevention

In a well-controlled environment, such as that of a hospital, prevention of host-to-host transmission for most human herpesviruses is achieved by simple hygiene as most disinfectants rapidly inactivate virus. In the home or other social situations, prevention of transmission by avoiding contact with a person who has evidence of recurrent infection is only partially effective. This is because infectious virus is often excreted before the appearance of overt symptoms of recurrent infection and 'silent' recurrent infections can also occur.

ACTIVE IMMUNIZATION

Except for VZV infection (for which a live attenuated vaccine is available) there are currently no licensed vaccines available to prevent herpesvirus infections. VZV infection causes particular problems in immunosuppressed children. Primary infection in immunosuppressed patients can result in a fulminant, generalized infection or severe respiratory disease. A live attenuated VZV vaccine has been licensed for use and is administered using the same schedule as the measles, mumps and rubella vaccine. The vaccine has an excellent safety record and although breakthrough infections can occur, they usually result in mild illness. In the USA the vaccine is recommended for use for all children over 12 months of age and susceptible healthy adolescents and adults. In other countries vaccination is only recommended for patients who are immunocompromised and who have never had chickenpox. A single dose is 80–85% effective in preventing disease of any severity and >95% effective in preventing severe varicella.[30] (See also Chapter 87.)

Studies of the Oka-derived strain of VZV vaccines showed that these could elicit a significant increase in VZV cell-mediated immunity (CMI) in immunocompetent older adults. This led to a study of immunization of older adults with live attenuated Oka VZV vaccine (at 14 times the minimum potency of the standard vaccine) to boost their waning VZV CMI. The vaccine significantly reduced the morbidity of herpes zoster (by 61.1%) and the incidence of postherpetic neuralgia, the most common debilitating complication of herpes zoster, by 66.5%.[31]

Research on the production of effective vaccines against HSV has been actively pursued since the 1920s. Two HSV-2 glycoprotein adjuvant vaccines (gB2 + gD2 and gD2) have reached phase III clinical evaluation. The overall protection rates were not significant. A gD2 vaccine formulated with an adjuvant alum and 3-deacetylated monophosphoryl lipid A showed a 73–74% protection from disease, but not infection, in women seronegative to HSV-1 and HSV-2. Gender differences and pre-existing HSV-1 serologic status influence vaccine efficacy in these trials.[32] Further, the changing epidemiology of genital infection, namely being caused by HSV-1 at increasing frequency, makes HSV-2 vaccines less appealing.[6]

Attempts to develop a prophylactic EBV vaccine have focused on the gp350 and EBNA3 antigens. Immunization with gp350 antigen has been shown to prevent infectious mononucleosis but not EBV infection in seronegative young adults.[33] Synthetic peptides based on the EBNA3 latent antigen have been the subject of small scale clinical trials. The latent antigen epitopes presented through common MHC class I can induce CD8+ T cell responses in the vaccinated. The value of this approach has been underscored by studies which show that autologous CD8+ cells against EBNA3 propagated in vivo and then given to immunosuppressed patients at risk of post-transplant lymphoproliferative disease (PTLD), can prevent PTLD and in some cases cause regression of PTLD.[34]

PASSIVE IMMUNIZATION

VZV hyperimmune globulin (VZVIG) is an effective prophylaxis for babies born to mothers who develop varicella (but not herpes zoster) in the 1-week period before or after delivery.[35] VZVIG is also recommended for VZ antibody-negative infants exposed to chickenpox or herpes zoster (other than in the mother) in the first 7 days after delivery. It is also given to VZ antibody-negative pregnant women exposed at any stage of pregnancy, providing VZVIG can be given within 10 days of contact. The rationale for the use of VZVIG prophylaxis in this situation is twofold: reduction in severity of maternal disease and reduction of risk of fetal infection for women contracting varicella in the first 20 weeks of pregnancy. The risk of fatal varicella is estimated to be about five times higher in pregnant than nonpregnant adults with fatal cases concentrated late in the second or early in the third trimester. VZVIG is also administered to immunocompromised and seronegative children at risk for severe disease.

Recently, adoptive cell therapy was reported as feasible treatment for ganciclovir-resistant CMV disease in a renal transplant recipient. CMV-specific CTLs from a healthy unrelated donor were partially matched at three of six major human leukocyte antigen (HLA) antigens. Infusion of third party cells resulted in significant reduction of CMV viremia and resolution of CMV-related kidney disease.[36] Additionally, neutralizing monoclonal antibodies have shown promise for protecting the fetus in a guinea pig model of congenital CMV infection by targeting glycoprotein H/glycoprotein L.[37]

ANTIVIRAL CHEMOTHERAPY

A number of specific antiviral compounds are available for the treatment of herpesvirus infection (Table 166-6) and prophylactic use of

antiviral chemotherapy to control infection is well established. Most antiherpetic drugs are nucleoside analogs that inhibit virus-specific DNA polymerases and terminate DNA chain elongation.

Aciclovir is the prototype of the current generation of antiviral drugs. Its high specificity and subsequent safety is based on its specific interaction with viral enzymes. It is an acyclic analog of guanosine that is activated by the viral and not the cellular thymidine kinase to serve as substrate for the viral DNA polymerase. Aciclovir is a safe, relatively nontoxic drug and is effective for therapeutic use as well as long-term suppressive treatment.

The oral bioavailability of aciclovir is relatively low and for this reason a prodrug – the L-valyl ester of aciclovir, valaciclovir – was developed. Valaciclovir hydrochloride is rapidly adsorbed from the gastrointestinal tract and almost completely converted to aciclovir and L-valine by first-pass intestinal and/or hepatic metabolism. The mode of action, safety profile and clinical spectrum of activity of valaciclovir are identical to that of aciclovir. However, because of improved pharmacokinetics and pharmacodynamics, it is preferred over aciclovir.

Penciclovir is another acyclic nucleoside analog whose mode of action and safety profile is essentially identical to that of aciclovir. The drugs differ in their rate of cellular uptake, phosphorylation rate, stability of the intracellular triphosphate and inhibitory concentration for viral DNA polymerase (100-fold higher for penciclovir triphosphate than for aciclovir triphosphate). The intracellular half-life of penciclovir triphosphate is substantially longer (7–20 hours) than that of aciclovir triphosphate (0.7–1 hour), which compensates for the slightly lower activity of the drug.

Famciclovir is the diacetyl 6-deoxy prodrug of penciclovir. Famciclovir achieves high levels of systemic bioavailability following oral administration. Following administration the drug is deacetylated and oxidized to form penciclovir. The mode of action and clinical spectrum of activity is thus identical to that of penciclovir.

The alternate antiherpetic drugs, ganciclovir (and its prodrug valganciclovir), foscarnet and cidofovir have similar mechanisms of action (i.e. inhibition of the viral DNA polymerase), but generally have a higher toxicity profile, including neutropenia and thrombocytopenia for ganciclovir, and nephrotoxicity for foscarnet and cidofovir. The recently studied antiviral maribavir directly inhibits UL97 kinase, an early gene involved in viral DNA elongation, DNA packaging and egress of viral capsids from the cell nucleus. Maribavir does not cause nephrotoxicity or hematologic toxicity and has activity against ganciclovir-resistant CMV. However, it failed in a phase III evaluation to prevent CMV infection in hematopoietic stem cell transplant recipients.[38]

Antiviral resistance has been described for all of the antiherpetic compounds mentioned, particularly when antivirals are administered to immunocompromised patients over extended periods of time. Studies in these patients have shown resistance to aciclovir in 5% and to ganciclovir in 7% of patients. Antiviral resistance is due to

TABLE 166-6	Currently Used Antiherpesvirus Drugs		
Antiviral Drug	**Chemical Class**	**Mechanisms of Action**	**Target Virus**
Aciclovir	Guanosine analog	Virus-activated DNA polymerase inhibitor	HSV-1, HSV-2, VZV
Valaciclovir	Guanosine analog	Virus-activated DNA polymerase inhibitor	HSV-1, HSV-2, VZV
Penciclovir	Guanosine analog	Virus-activated DNA polymerase inhibitor	HSV-1, HSV-2, VZV
Famciclovir	Guanosine analog	Virus-activated DNA polymerase inhibitor	HSV-1, HSV-2, VZV
Cidofovir	Cytidylic acid analog	DNA polymerase inhibitor	CMV, HSV-1, HSV-2
Foscarnet	Pyrophosphate analog	DNA polymerase inhibitor	CMV, HSV-1, HSV-2
Ganciclovir	Guanosine analog	Virus-activated DNA polymerase inhibitor	CMV, HSV-1, HSV-2
Maribavir	Benzimidazole riboside	Inhibits UL97 kinase	CMV, EBV

CMV, cytomegalovirus; EBV, Epstein–Barr virus; HSV, herpes simplex virus; VZV, varicella-zoster virus.

mutations in the viral thymidine kinase or in the DNA polymerase. Resistant viruses, however, appear to be less virulent. Significant circulation in the general population has not yet been found. Because of their similar mechanisms of action, cross-resistance frequently occurs (e.g. among aciclovir, famciclovir and valaciclovir).

Therapy is initiated early in infection, even before laboratory confirmation of the clinical diagnosis (Table 166-7).

EBV and HHV-6 have shown *in vitro* susceptibility to various antiherpetic drugs such as aciclovir, ganciclovir and cidofovir. However, apart from aciclovir treatment of oral hairy leukoplakia in patients who have AIDS, no significant clinical benefit has so far been demonstrated. Anecdotal use of ganciclovir or foscarnet for HHV-6, HHV-7 and HHV-8 infections has been reported. However, so far no data from well-designed clinical studies have been reported to show the effectiveness of these drugs in the treatment of these infections.

Further information on antiviral drugs is given in Chapter 153.

Diagnostic Virology

A key feature of the herpesviruses is their close adaptation to their host. In general, primary infection is usually asymptomatic or is accompanied by nonspecific mild signs and symptoms. Consequently, most primary infections and many recurrent infections are not recognized as herpesvirus infections. Where symptoms are observed, speed in using diagnostic procedures is important because the peak of virus replication and shedding is likely to precede the appearance of symptoms, which is why molecular biology techniques are commonly used. The diagnostic method chosen (Table 166-8) varies for different herpesviruses and also depends upon the type of infection (whether primary or recurrent), duration of symptoms and clinical manifestations.

TEST SPECIMENS

If visible lesions are present (HSV-1, HSV-2, VZV), the base of the lesion may be sampled with a dry cotton-tipped swab, which should be placed in virus transport medium and delivered to the laboratory as quickly as possible. If there are vesicles, vesicle fluid can be aspirated using a fine (intradermal) needle. The fluid should then be transported directly to the laboratory for virus detection by PCR testing, electron microscopy, direct immunofluorescent antibody staining or culture.

Viremia and viruria are common during both primary infection and recurrent infection with HSV, CMV, EBV, HHV-6, HHV-7 and HHV-8. Urine collected in urine transport medium is a useful specimen for detection of CMV. Blood collected in anticoagulant (EDTA)

TABLE 166-7   Indications for Antiherpesvirus Drug Treatment

Antiviral Drug	Target Virus	Infections	Possible Side Effects
Aciclovir, valaciclovir, famciclovir	HSV-1,2	Severe and/or frequent mucocutaneous HSV infection, including genital herpes; herpes encephalitis, herpes keratitis	Headache, nausea, diarrhea
	VZV	Severe cases of varicella, varicella in patients at risk for complications (immunocompromised, adolescents, adults) Severe cases of herpes zoster, including those at risk of developing postherpetic neuralgia, herpes zoster ophthalmicus, oticus	Headache, nausea, diarrhea
Cidofovir	CMV	CMV retinitis	Severe nephrotoxicity
Foscarnet	CMV, HSV-1, HSV-2, VZV; severe disease due to aciclovir-, valaciclovir- and famciclovir-resistant HSV or VZV strains	Severe CMV disease refractory to ganciclovir treatment	Nephrotoxicity, crystalluria
Ganciclovir	CMV	Severe CMV disease in immunocompromised host (e.g. retinitis, esophagitis, colitis, pneumonia, encephalitis)	Neutropenia, thrombocytopenia

CMV, cytomegalovirus; HSV, herpes simplex virus; VZV, varicella-zoster virus.

TABLE 166-8   Laboratory Diagnosis of Herpesvirus Infections

Virus	Disease Manifestation	Virus Culture	Serology	Antigen Detection	DNA Amplification
HSV-1	Skin lesions	++	+	+	+++
	CNS infection	–	++	–	+++
HSV-2	Genital lesions	++	+	+	+++
	CNS infection	–	+	–	+++
VZV	Skin lesions	+	++	++	+++
	CNS infection	–	+	–	+++
CMV	Mononucleosis-like illness	–	+++	–	–
	Neonatal disease	++	++	–	+++
	Systemic infection in immunocompromised	+	+	++	+++
	CNS disease	–	+	–	+++
EBV	Mononucleosis-like illness	–	+++	–	–
	Systemic infection in immunocompromised	–	+	+	+++
	CNS disease	–	+	–	+++
HHV-6	Exanthem subitum	+	+++	–	–
	CNS disease	–	++	–	+++
HHV-8	Kaposi's sarcoma	–	+	–	+++

CMV, cytomegalovirus; EBV, Epstein–Barr virus; HHV, human herpesvirus; HSV, herpes simplex virus; VZV, varicella–zoster virus.

can be used in direct detection of virus. In neurologic disease, cerebrospinal fluid (CSF) and a clotted peripheral blood specimen (for CSF and blood serology) are essential. Clotted blood specimens should be collected during the acute stages of illness and again after 10–14 days.

POLYMERASE CHAIN REACTION

Nucleic acid amplification, in particular PCR, is most widely applied to diagnose herpesvirus infections. A wide variety of PCR techniques have been used, including single, semi-nested and nested, with product detection via gel electrophoresis, Southern blotting, ELISA-like hybridization, microarray or bead-based arrays such as the Luminex® procedure. 'Real-time' PCR is now the most commonly used procedure; this offers testing of high sensitivity, reduced risk of intralaboratory cross-contamination of samples from amplicon release and reduces test turnaround times by combining the detection of amplification within the thermal amplification process. The test allows direct detection of the products of amplification in 'real time', is quantitative, and can allow, for example, typing of HSV-1 and HSV-2 within the same test. Multiplex PCR procedures are also available in both real-time and conventional PCR formats. Careful optimization of these test procedures is necessary to ensure that the sensitivity of detection of each of the individual target viruses within the test is maintained when targets are combined.

Many types of clinical samples contain substances that prove inhibitory to the PCR, which, if not efficiently removed, will result in the production of false-negative test results. The use of internal positive controls within PCR tests is used to monitor for test failure through test sample inhibition. Where internal molecules are not available, the same check may be performed by 'spiking' a sample with a known amount of virus or by checking for an alternate human gene always expected to be present within a clinical sample.

Nucleic acid amplification techniques are now considered essential for the diagnosis of herpesvirus infections, particularly for HSV infection of the central nervous system (CNS) or in the diagnosis of the acute retinal necrosis syndrome.[39,40] Determination of the viral load in blood is an indispensable tool for early detection, monitoring and medical management of CMV, EBV, HHV-6, and HHV-8 infections in hematopoietic stem cell transplantation (HSTC) and solid organ transplant (SOT) patients.[41] Rigorous quality control and attention to detail is of course essential for routine application of any PCR technique, but in the latter application of quantitative PCR, standardization of variables through parallel comparative and proficiency testing, development of standards and of uniform units for expressing results, have all become essential to allow clinical correlation with the results of these molecular assays.

GENOTYPIC ANALYSES

Sequencing of products of PCR is a useful method for the comparison of strains of virus detected. For example, sequencing of viruses obtained from different bodily sites or from different persons provides a more rapid method for epidemiologic and population diversity investigation than the technically demanding restriction-fragment polymorphic analyses previously applied in such studies.[42] The widespread use of ganciclovir to treat CMV infections in immunosuppressed patients has led to the development of drug resistance. Phenotypic assays for CMV drug resistance are presently too time-consuming to be therapeutically useful and this has led to the development of genotypic assays for ganciclovir resistance.[43] For other human herpesviruses the genomic mutations resulting in antiviral drug resistance have not all been identified. Phenotypic tests are easier to interpret and may detect resistance that genotypic analysis cannot yet discriminate. Maintenance of the capability of cell culture in diagnostic laboratories is thus important.

VIRUS CULTURE

While the use of virus culture has declined in many diagnostic virus laboratories, it remains an essential tool in reference laboratories when live virus is required for detailed analysis such as drug resistance. The fragility of the viral envelope presents a problem if virus is to be cultured. Collection of specimens into appropriate viral transport medium and rapid transportation of specimens to the diagnostic laboratory is essential for successful isolation in cell culture systems. Virus culture is only usually attempted for HSV-1, HSV-2, VZV and CMV.

VIRUS SEROLOGY

Complement fixation and indirect immunofluorescence tests are still used in many viral diagnostic laboratories; however, their use is declining in favor of more reproducible and sensitive enzyme-linked immunosorbent assay (ELISA) methodologies. Neutralizing antibody tests for herpesvirus antibodies are not routinely performed in diagnostic laboratories, and none of these viruses have hemagglutinating capability.

Immunoassays are available for the detection of IgM or IgG antibodies from HHV-1 to HHV-8. Although IgM antibody is produced during both acute (primary) infection and recurrent disease, quantitation of virus-specific IgG antibody in serial samples (10 or more days apart) often provides a more reliable diagnostic procedure. Determination of the avidity of IgG can provide valuable information when only a single, acute phase sample of blood is available. IgG antibody avidity matures with time after onset of infection, thus detection of IgG antibody of low avidity provides evidence of recent (primary) infection; detection of high avidity IgG antibody allows differentiation of recurrent infection from primary infection. Serology serves as a practical approach to differentiating between HSV-1 or HSV-2 infection when symptoms are mild or sporadic. Detection of glycoprotein G (gG) 1 or 2 serves as the key indicator for diagnosing HSV serotypes 1 or 2, respectively, because other immunogenic antigens are so similar between the two viruses and are likely to be cross-reactive.[44]

Clinical Manifestations

With the exception of VZV, primary herpesvirus infections in the immunocompetent host are usually asymptomatic or are associated with a minor illness with no specific symptoms. As a consequence, primary herpesvirus infections may not be recognized. When symptoms do occur, herpesvirus infections in the immunocompetent host are normally self-limiting and require only symptomatic treatment. Antiviral therapy is available for a number of herpesviruses, but is usually only indicated for those patients who have more severe disease manifestations or when it is appropriate to minimize the likelihood of complications. Herpesvirus infections in the immunocompromised host are frequently severe and sometimes life-threatening. Antiviral drug therapy is required for these patients to control the infection (see Table 166-6 and also Chapters 87 and 153).

HERPES SIMPLEX VIRUSES

Oropharyngeal Infection

Primary oropharyngeal HSV-1 infection is often asymptomatic. In symptomatic infections, acute gingivostomatitis is accompanied by fever and submandibular lymphadenopathy. The incubation period varies from 2 to 12 days (mean 4 days). The duration of clinical illness may extend from 2 to 3 weeks, with virus excretion from the oropharynx for an average of 7–10 days.

The severity and duration of clinical illness in recurrent infection is considerably less than in primary HSV infection. Recurrent orolabial lesions ('cold sores') are heralded by a prodrome of pain, burning, itching or tingling for several hours before the development of the characteristic vesicles. The vesicular stage persists for less than 48 hours and progresses to the ulcerative and crusting stage within 3–4 days. Pain resolves quickly during the same period, and healing is generally complete within 8–10 days. Systemic illness is usually absent in recurrent infection. Recurrence rates are highly variable and the precipitating factors involved are not well defined, but include the type of HSV (HSV-1 is more likely to recur than HSV-2), fever, stress, exposure to ultraviolet light and impaired CMI in the host.

Genital Infections

Primary genital herpes is, in the majority of cases (50–70%), asymptomatic or so mild that the infection is not recognized. Where lesions are observed the disease is characterized by the appearance of vesicular lesions – in males usually on the glans penis, on the penile shaft or in the perianal region, and in women involving the vulva, vagina, cervix and perineum. Extragenital lesions (on the buttocks and thighs) occur in 10–20% of patients.

The recurrence rate of genital HSV-2 infections is 10 times higher than that of genital HSV-1 infections. The signs and symptoms of recurrent genital herpes are usually restricted to the genital region and are relatively mild and of shorter duration than for primary disease. As for primary disease, recurrent lesions in women are more often painful and of longer duration than in men (60–90% vs 30–70%, and mean 5.9 vs 3.9 days, respectively).

Other Manifestations

A wide variety of other manifestations of infection are known (Figure 166-6) including herpes simplex virus encephalitis, neonatal herpes, herpes gladiatorium and keratoconjunctivitis.[15] Immunocompromised patients are at risk of developing a severe primary infection and more severe and frequent recurrent disease. Disease severity is directly related to the degree of immunosuppression or immunodeficiency.

VARICELLA-ZOSTER VIRUS

Varicella (chickenpox) and herpes zoster (shingles) are due to infection with the same virus, VZV. Varicella is the usual manifestation of primary infection, herpes zoster the most usual manifestation of recurrent infection.

Varicella

Varicella is a common childhood exanthematous disease, usually affecting children in their early school years. The incubation period is 14–15 days (range 10–20 days). The rash is characterized by maculo-papular lesions that vesiculate in about 3–4 days before crusting and scab formation. Scabs may remain *in situ* for up to 3 weeks. The exanthem is centripetal rather than centrifugal, with most lesions being present on the trunk and proximal extremities. Secondary bacterial infection of the lesions as a result of scratching is the most frequent complication. Occasionally cerebellar ataxia, transverse myelitis or Reye's syndrome may complicate the infection. Primary VZV infection occurring in adolescence and adult life is often associated with more severe disease including visceral complications such as pneumonitis, encephalitis and hepatitis.

Primary VZV infection may be more severe in pregnant women. This frequently includes visceral complications, notably pneumonitis. The fetus is at risk of infection and there is a low risk of severe fetal abnormalities ranging from long-lasting rash, limb or dermatomal scarring, to severe neurologic damage.[45] Severe neonatal varicella may occur when maternal varicella presents within 5 days of delivery.

Primary VZV infection of immunocompromised patients, such as children undergoing cancer chemotherapy or corticosteroid treatment, usually has a more severe protracted course with an increased rate of complications, particularly pneumonitis. With the advent of the VZV vaccine in childhood, chickenpox is becoming a rare disease in some countries of the world.

Herpes Zoster

Herpes zoster is typically a disease of the elderly. Usually there is a prodrome of pain followed within a few days by the development of a unilateral vesicular rash within the dermatome served by the sensory nerve from the affected ganglion. The sites most commonly affected by herpes zoster are the dermatomes T3–L3, often the same as those that were most affected during chickenpox. New lesions form over 2–5 days and the rash then pustulates and scabs over 2–3 weeks.

The most significant component of herpes zoster is pain, whether it is acute or chronic. Complications including motor weakness and visceral manifestations may occur, but are unusual. However, in up to

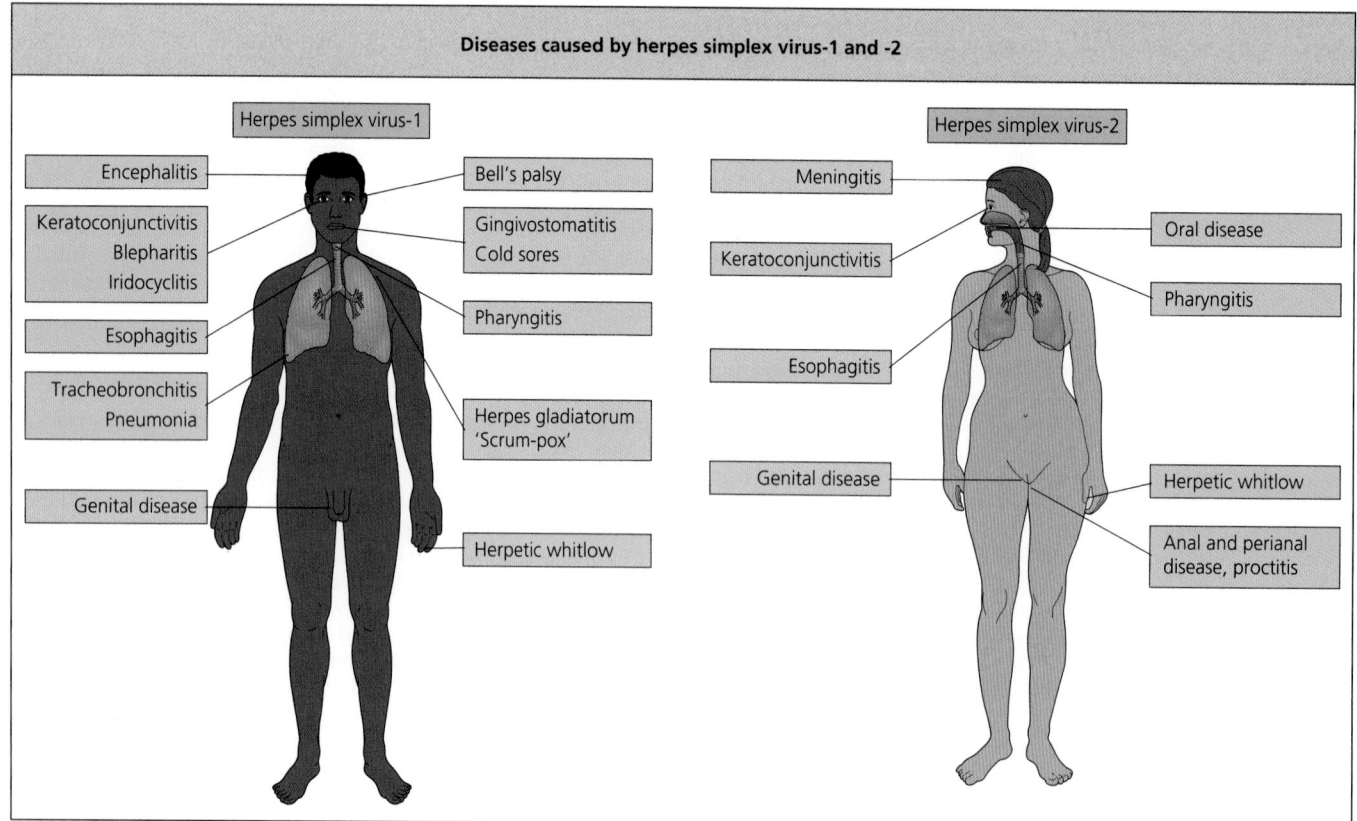

Figure 166-6   Diseases caused by herpes simplex virus-1 and herpes simplex virus-2.

50% of patients where herpes zoster involves the trigeminal nerve, ocular manifestations such as conjunctivitis, ulcerative keratitis, uveitis and iridocyclitis occur. Ocular complications are particularly common when the zosteriform lesions extend to the tip of the nose. Herpes zoster oticus, also called Ramsay Hunt syndrome, consists of lesions on the ear or within the auditory canal, which are sometimes barely visible, and can result in hearing loss and facial paralysis. Persisting pain, known as postherpetic neuralgia, is the most common complication of herpes zoster. It can be severe and last for several months. The rate, severity and duration of postherpetic neuralgia are directly related to age. It is uncommon in patients under 50 years of age, but occurs in over 40% of those over 60 years of age.

Herpes zoster is frequently observed in patients who are immunocompromised. Chronic cutaneous lesions and disseminated infections have been described, particularly in patients who have HIV infection. Meningoencephalitis, pneumonitis or hepatitis can also occur in immunocompromised patients, but are rare.

CYTOMEGALOVIRUS

CMV is an uncommon cause of disease in people who are immunocompetent. Primary infection may occasionally cause a glandular fever-type illness resembling EBV mononucleosis. In such patients, persistent fever, myalgia and asthenia accompanied by atypical lymphocytosis and elevated liver transaminases are common signs and symptoms. Occasionally hepatitis is the presenting symptom. The presence of fever and atypical lymphocytes distinguishes CMV mononucleosis with liver involvement from infections by the usual hepatitis viruses.

Congenital and Perinatal Infections

(see also Chapter 56)
CMV infections are the most common cause of congenital viral infection in high-income countries.[46] Both primary and recurrent infection in a pregnant woman can cause congenital and perinatal disease, but the frequency of severe disease is at least 10-fold higher after primary maternal infection. Overt clinical symptoms occur in 5–10% of cases of intrauterine CMV infection and include growth retardation, hepatosplenomegaly and thrombocytopenic purpura, and less frequently jaundice, microcephaly and chorioretinitis. The prognosis is poor for these infants. Another 10–15% of cases are neonates who are asymptomatic at birth and develop late sequelae, particularly mental retardation and sensorineural hearing loss.

Perinatal infections are nearly always asymptomatic, but neonates occasionally develop CMV pneumonitis, particularly when born prematurely. Severe disseminated disease may follow transfusion of CMV-infected blood products to premature neonates who have CMV-seronegative mothers.

Immunocompromised Patients

The pathogenesis and clinical spectrum of CMV disease in patients who are immunocompromised depend upon the cause and degree of immunosuppression. Persistent intermittent fever is often the presenting symptom of CMV infection in patients who have had a transplant. The infection may progress to cause pneumonitis, gastrointestinal disease, hepatitis and retinitis. In recipients of SOT, CMV disease most frequently occurs when the donor is CMV seropositive and the recipient is CMV seronegative. In bone marrow transplant patients, however, CMV disease most commonly results from reactivation of latent virus in the recipient, usually 20–90 days after the transplant. The most frequent manifestation is CMV pneumonitis. Unless treated very early, preferably before the appearance of respiratory symptoms, pneumonitis in these patients is often fatal.

Reactivation of latent CMV is usually the cause of CMV disease in patients who have HIV infection, frequently occurring in the later stages of the HIV infection when CD4$^+$ T cell counts are less than 50/μL. The most frequent manifestation is CMV retinitis presenting with blurred vision and decreased acuity.

Gastrointestinal disease, hepatitis, encephalitis and pneumonia also occur in patients who have HIV infection. Gastrointestinal disease includes esophagitis, gastritis, enteritis and colitis and is usually associated with fever and weight loss. Although CMV is often detected in respiratory specimens from patients with AIDS who have pneumonitis, the pulmonary process is usually caused by other pathogens, particularly *Pneumocystis jirovecii*.

EPSTEIN–BARR VIRUS

In most individuals EBV infection does not cause overt disease.[8] Primary infections in adolescents can, however, result in infectious mononucleosis. Immunocompromised hosts may develop severe manifestations during both primary and recurrent EBV infection.

Immunocompetent Host

Infectious mononucleosis (glandular fever) usually presents as fever, fatigue and malaise accompanied by a sore throat, cervical lymphadenopathy, hepatomegaly and splenomegaly. A rash may develop, particularly in those treated with ampicillin. Disease manifestations, especially fatigue and malaise, can persist for several weeks. Relapses and a chronic course have been described but the relationship to EBV infection is uncertain.

Immunocompromised Host

Immunocompromised patients are at risk of developing lymphoproliferative disorders following EBV infection. PTLD can result from EBV infection while patients are taking immunosuppressive drugs after organ transplant. Polyclonal B lymphocyte proliferation is often associated with fever, lymphadenopathy and hepatosplenomegaly and is frequently life-threatening in severely immunocompromised patients such as bone marrow transplant patients.

Patients who have AIDS may develop oral hairy leukoplakia, which is characterized by white plaques on the lateral margin of the tongue. EBV is associated with lymphocytic interstitial pneumonia (which is common in pediatric patients who have AIDS) and rapidly progressing, diffuse encephalitis.

EBV-associated hemophagocytic lymphohistiocytosis (HLH) is a rare syndrome predominantly characterized by macrophage phagocytosis of erythrocytes, leukocytes, platelets and their precursor cells. EBV-infected T cells are thought to play a role in HLH pathogenesis due to hyperproduction of immune-activating cytokines like interferon-gamma and tumor necrosis factor-alpha. Familial HLH may occur after acute infection of EBV in patients with autosomal recessive immunodeficiency, usually infants, with dismal prognosis.

HUMAN HERPESVIRUS 6

HHV-6, variant B, is the cause of exanthem subitum (roseola infantum) in young children. Symptomatic infection is characterized by a high fever, often associated with inflammation of tympanic membranes and sometimes associated with a mild respiratory illness and lymphadenopathy. This is followed by the appearance of a fine maculopapular rash spreading from the trunk to the extremities. Only a small proportion of these (<10%) develop exanthema subitum.[27] Recovery is usually rapid and uneventful, although a more protracted and severe course characterized by severe meningoencephalitis, fulminant hepatitis or fatal pancytopenia has been described. In adolescents and adults primary HHV-6 infection can cause a mononucleosis-like illness.

In severely immunocompromised patients, such as those who have AIDS or who have received a bone marrow transplant, reactivation of HHV-6 infection has an immunosuppressive effect, subsequent to which other pathogens may cause severe disease. In bone marrow transplant patients HHV-6 reactivation is associated with bone marrow suppression, probably as the result of viral replication in particular progenitor cells.[27] HHV-6 has also been associated with interstitial pneumonia and encephalitis in these patients.

HUMAN HERPESVIRUS 7

Although some cases of exanthem subitum appear to be due to HHV-7, a causal association between human disease and HHV-7 infection has not yet been established. HHV-7 has been associated with infant febrile illness as well as subsequent CNS complications. In renal transplant patients, evidence has been obtained that HHV-7 may be a co-factor in the development of CMV disease.

HUMAN HERPESVIRUS 8

No association has been recognized between primary HHV-8 infection and specific clinical disease, but it is now generally accepted that HHV-8 has a causal role in KS, primary effusion lymphoma and multicentric Castleman's disease.[10]

HERPES B VIRUS

Macacine herpesvirus 1 (herpes B virus) causes a benign latent infection in macaques that is analogous to HSV infection in humans. The infection is infrequently transmitted to humans. After an incubation period varying from 3 days to 3 weeks there may be localized pain, redness and vesicular skin lesions near the site of the viral inoculation, followed by localized neurologic symptoms. Encephalopathy is common and fatal in up to 70% of patients. The virus is susceptible to aciclovir and early treatment can be life-saving.

Management

As most herpesvirus infections in the immunocompetent host are self-limiting, patients usually only require supportive care. The type of supportive treatment required varies for different disease manifestations and may consist of rest, hydration, the appropriate use of antipyretics and analgesics, and treatment to soothe skin lesions and prevent secondary bacterial infection. Effective antiviral therapy is available for more severe cases of infection caused by HSV, VZV or CMV. It is stressed, however, that although antiviral drugs can help to control a herpesvirus infection they cannot eliminate the infection (see Table 166-7).

References available online at expertconsult.com.

KEY REFERENCES

Davison A.J., Eberle R., Ehlers B., et al.: The order Herpesvirales. *Arch Virol* Springer Vienna 2009; 154(1):171-177.

De Bolle L., Naesens L., De Clercq E.: Update on human herpesvirus 6 biology, clinical features and therapy. *Clin Microbiol Rev* 2005; 18:217-245.

Forgren M., Klapper P.E.: Herpes simplex virus type 1 and type 2. In: Banatvala J., et al., eds. *Principles and practice of clinical virology*, 6th ed. Chichester: Wiley; 2009:93-129.

Ganem D.: KSHV infection and the pathogenesis of Kaposi's sarcoma. *Ann Rev Pathol Mech Dis* 2006; 1:273-296.

Heldweina E.E., Krummenacher C.: Entry of herpesviruses into mammalian cells. *Cell Mol Life Sci* 2008; 65:1653-1668.

Kutok J.L., Wang F.: Spectrum of Epstein–Barr virus-associated disease. *Ann Rev Pathol Mech Dis* 2006; 1:375-404.

Kemble G., Spaete R.: Herpes simplex vaccines. In: Arvin A., Campadelli-Fiume G., Mocarski E., et al., eds. *Human herpesviruses*. Cambridge: Cambridge University Press; 2007:1253-1261.

Lafferty W.E., Downey L., Celum C., et al.: Herpes simplex virus type 1 as a cause of genital herpes: impact on surveillance and prevention. *J Infect Dis* 2000; 181(4):1454-1457.

LeGoff J., Péré H., Bélec L.: Diagnosis of genital herpes simplex virus infection in the clinical laboratory. *Virol J* 2014; 11(1):83.

McGeoch D.J., Rixon F.J., Davison A.J.: Topics in herpesvirus genomics and evolution. *Virus Res* 2006; 117:90-104.

Pellett P.E., Roizman B.: Herpesviridae. In: Knipe D.M., Howley P.M., eds. *Field's virology*, 6th ed. Philadelphia: Wolters Kluwer/Lippincott Williams & Wilkins; 2013:59-65.

Turner K.M., Lee H.C., Boppana S.B., et al.: Incidence and impact of CMV infection in very low birth weight infants. *Pediatrics* American Academy of Pediatrics 2014; 133(3):e609-e615.

Zuo J., Rowe M.: Herpesviruses placating the unwilling host: manipulation of the MHC class II antigen presentation pathway. *Viruses* 2012; 4(8):1335-1353.

167

Papillomaviruses

RAPHAEL P. VISCIDI | PATTI E. GRAVITT

KEY CONCEPTS

- Papillomaviruses are species specific and largely epitheliotropic. There are more than 100 different human papillomavirus (HPV) types which infect the cutaneous or the mucosal epithelium.

- HPV infection is very common in both men and women. Anogenital and oral HPV is largely transmitted by sexual activity and the vast majority of infections are self-limiting with no clinical consequences.

- Approximately 12–14 HPV types are carcinogenic to humans, causing cancers of the anogenital tract and oral cavity in both men and women. Carcinogenicity of HPV is highest in the female cervix.

- Prophylactic immunization with the quadrivalent HPV vaccine (Gardasil®) reduces incidence of genital warts and HPV6/11/6/18-associated neoplasia, and immunization with the bivalent HPV vaccine (Cervarix®) reduces the incidence of HPV 16/18-associated neoplasia. These vaccines are likely to reduce the burden of HPV-associated cancers.

- Early detection and treatment of cervical precancers reduce risk of incident cervical cancer. Screening based on cervical cytology, HPV nucleic acid testing, and visual inspection are all suitable methods for secondary prevention of cervical cancer.

Nature

Papillomaviruses are widely distributed in nature; among mammals they infect humans, cattle, dogs, rabbits, monkeys and other species. Human papillomaviruses (HPVs) are strictly epitheliotropic and infect the skin or the mucous membranes. Papillomaviruses cannot be propagated in cell culture. Therefore, rapid advances in the knowledge about papillomaviruses date from the 1970s, when molecular cloning of the viral genomes allowed comparisons between viruses from different species and from different sites of the same species.

The papillomavirus particle (Figure 167-1) is about 55 nm in diameter and has a double-stranded, covalently closed, circular genome of about 8000 bp. The genome is divided into an early region, a late region and a noncoding long control region, which contains regulatory elements for viral DNA replication and transcription. The late region encodes for the major L1 capsid protein, which accounts for most of the virion mass and mediates viral attachment. The L1 protein displays immunodominant type-specific neutralizing epitopes. The prophylactic HPV vaccines are based on the use of the L1 protein expressed by recombinant DNA technology and self-assembled as virus-like particles (VLPs). Experimental vaccines based on the minor L2 capsid protein, which displays a subdominant cross-neutralizing epitope, may provide cross protection against multiple HPV genotypes.[1] The early region genes E6 and E7 of high-risk HPVs code for the transforming proteins of the virus that mediate the oncogenic properties of the virus.

The molecular mechanisms of cellular transformation by E6 and E7 genes of high-risk HPVs are well understood. Briefly, the E6 protein complexes with tumor suppressor protein p53 and targets it for destruction (Figure 167-2). The E7 protein complexes with tumor suppressor protein Rb, which in turn induces expression of genes that activate the cell cycle. In the normal cell cycle, tumor suppressor proteins p53 and Rb inhibit cellular proliferation. In HPV infected cells, the HPV oncoproteins lead to continued cell proliferation without time for repair of DNA damage. This leads to genetic instability and accumulation of additional cellular mutations and chromosomal changes. Thus, infections with high-risk HPVs prepare the ground for the cellular genetic alterations that underlie cervical cancer.

Epidemiology

More than 100 individual HPV types have been described to date; they naturally fall into two groups, mucosal HPVs and cutaneous HPVs.[2]

MUCOSAL HUMAN PAPILLOMAVIRUSES

About 40 HPV types infect the genital tract. Genital HPV infections are the most prevalent sexually transmitted pathogens, infecting over 79.1 million individuals aged 14–59 years at any given time in the USA.[3] A history of multiple sexual partners, and having a male sexual partner who has many sexual partners, are the main risk factors for a woman for the acquisition of HPVs. Circumcision may decrease the risk of HPV acquisition in the male and his female partner.[4] Cervical HPV prevalence reaches its peak in young adults around the age of sexual debut. Cervical HPV prevalence at older ages differs significantly by region, declining in the USA and many western European countries, increasing at older ages in several central and south American countries, and remaining stable across age in many parts of Asia.[5] HPV infections are largely asymptomatic and of 1–2 years' duration. Infection probably confers partial immunity to re-infection with the same type. The course of HPV infection is altered profoundly by HIV-induced immunosuppression, which may reflect loss of immune-mediated control of latent HPV infection.[6,7]

HPV-6 and HPV-11 are the etiologic agents of genital warts (condylomas), which occur in sexually active individuals, and also of recurrent respiratory papillomatosis (RRP), which may have onset in childhood or in adult life. HPV-16, -18, -31, -45 and some other types account for nearly all cervical cancers, as described in later sections of this chapter.

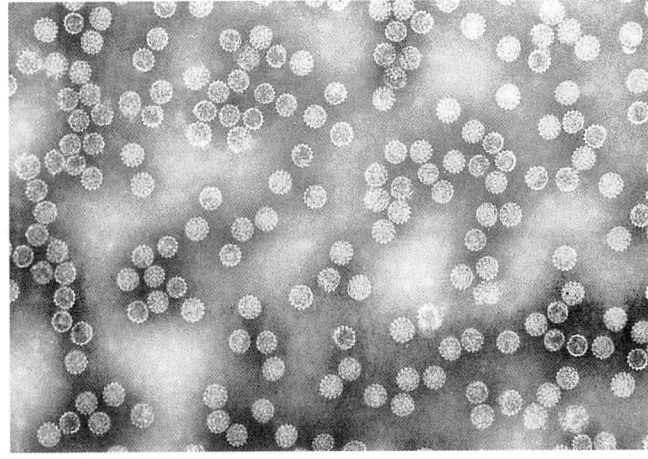

Figure 167-1 Human papillomavirus particles. The particles are non-enveloped, have icosahedral capsids and are 55 nm in diameter. *(Courtesy of Dr M. Reissig.)*

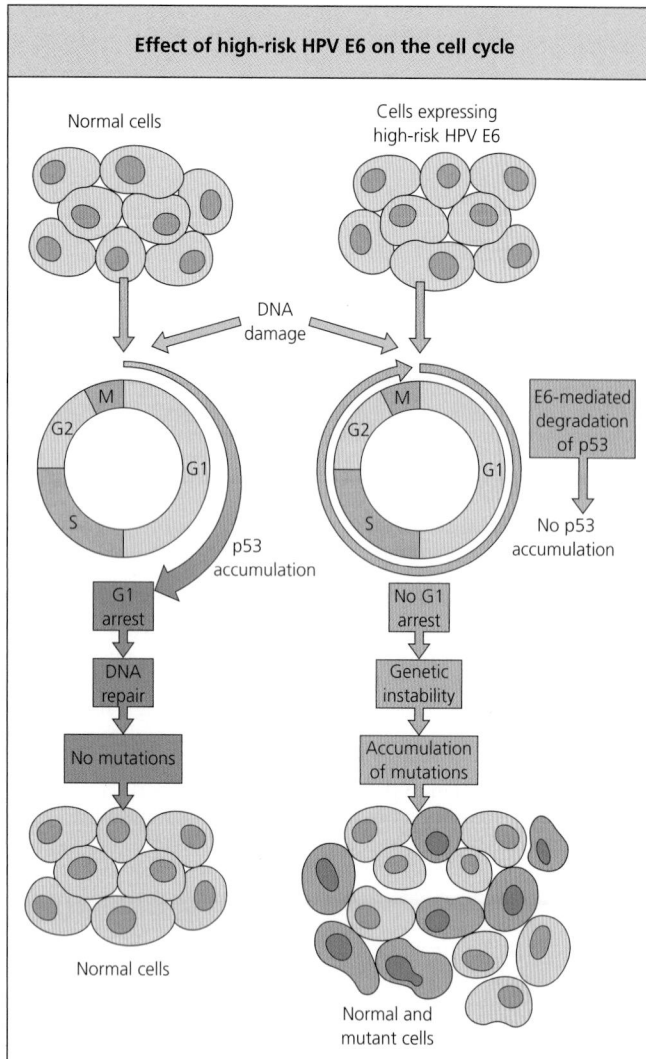

Figure 167-2 Effect of high-risk HPV E6 on the cell cycle. In normal cells (left), DNA damage results in increased p53 production, which leads to arrest of cell cycle in G1 phase, allowing the cell time to repair DNA damage. In cells infected with high-risk HPVs (right), the HPV E6 mediates degradation of p53, so there is no accumulation of p53, no cell-cycle arrest, and continued cell multiplication. This leads to genetic instability and accumulation of cellular mutations. (Courtesy of Dr T.D. Kessis.)

CUTANEOUS HUMAN PAPILLOMAVIRUSES

Skin warts are transmitted by direct contact with an infected tissue or indirectly by contact with virus-contaminated objects. There is some specificity between HPV type, and site and morphology of the warts; plantar warts are most often positive for HPV-1, common warts HPV-2 and flat warts HPV-3 and HPV-10. In addition to warts, the cutaneous types HPV-5 and HPV-8 can cause a rare condition, epidermodysplasia veruciformis (EV)[8] and these flat or reddish-brown macular plaques can undergo malignant transformation in about one-third of patients in association with sunlight exposure.[8,9] It is not clear if HPVs play a role in nonmelanoma skin cancer,[10] but this remains an active area of research.

Pathogenicity

Papillomaviruses have a high degree of species and tissue specificity. Genital HPVs are rarely detected on skin other than that of the anogenital tract, but they can infect other mucosal sites in the body such as the aerodigestive tract. Cutaneous HPVs are almost never encountered in the genital tract.

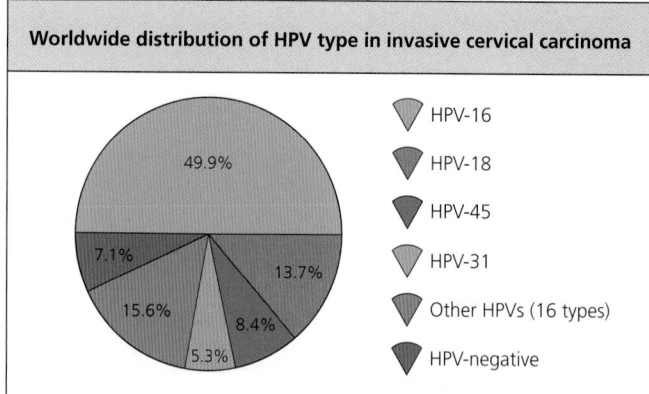

Figure 167-3 Worldwide distribution of HPV type in invasive cervical carcinoma. The data are based on tests of over 900 cancers from different countries. (Data from Bosch F.X., et al. J Natl Cancer Inst 1995; 87:796-802.)

Nearly all cervical cancers originate in the 'transformation zone', located at the lower end of the cervix, where the stratified squamous epithelium of the vagina forms a junction with the columnar cells of the endocervix. The cells in the transformation zone of the cervix must be highly susceptible to the oncogenic effects of HPVs, because cancers arise much less frequently at other sites in the genital tract (vulva, vagina, penis) that are infected with HPVs as frequently as the cervix but do not have an area similar to the transformation zone. A specific type of stem cell unique to the cervical squamocolumnar junction appears to have particular sensitivity to the transforming properties of HPV infections.[11]

Although almost all squamous cell abnormalities of the cervix including cervical cancer are the result of HPV infections, the probability of any one HPV infection progressing to cervical cancer is quite small (for review see reference 12). Most HPV infections produce only transient cytologic abnormalities and are resolved completely without a trace. Cytologic abnormalities are seen in only about 10% of women who are positive for HPV DNA in the genital tract, and range in severity from atypical squamous cells of undetermined significance (ASCUS), low-grade squamous intraepithelial lesions (LSILs) to high-grade squamous intraepithelial lesions (HSILs). The progression from initial HPV infection to invasive cancer may take 15–20 years.

A large majority of LSILs regress completely. In the USA, annually, there are tens of millions of HPV infections but only about 15 000 cases of invasive cancer. The relatively small number of cases is partly the result of treatment of LSILs and HSILs identified from Pap smear screening programs, but it is also, in a large measure, because most HPV infections do not result in significant cervical disease. In countries that have no effective Pap smear screening programs, the number of cases of cervical cancer is still a small fraction of the number of HPV infections in women.

HPVs are found in nearly all lesions spanning the entire spectrum of cytologic abnormalities from a LSIL to invasive cancer. The distribution of HPV types changes markedly with increasing severity of disease.[13] Almost all genital HPV types are represented in HPV DNA-positive cytologically normal specimens and in ASCUS and LSIL cases, but only about a dozen HPV types are found in invasive cervical cancer. HPV-16, -18, -45 and -31 account for nearly 80% of invasive cancers (Figure 167-3). The genital HPV types have therefore been categorized as high-risk, intermediate-risk or low-risk types (Table 167-1) on the basis of their prevalence in invasive cervical cancer.

Prevention

HPV-related diseases for which preventive strategies are being investigated are cervical and other lower genital tract cancers, tonsillar/oropharyngeal cancers, genital warts and recurrent respiratory papillomatosis (RRP).

TABLE 167-1	Major Clinical Associations of HPV Infections	
Disease	**HPV Types**	**Transmission**
Cervical cancer 　High risk 　Intermediate risk 　Low risk	 HPV-16, -18, -45, -31 HPV-33, -35, -39, -51, -52, -56, -59, -68, -73 HPV-6, -11, -26, -42, -43, -44, -53, -54, -55, -62, -66	Sexual
Cancer of vulva, vagina, anal canal, penis	HPV-16	Sexual
Oropharyngeal cancer	HPV-16	Sexual
Anogenital warts	HPV-6, -11	Sexual
Juvenile-onset RRP	HPV-6, -11	Mother–child, at birth
Adult-onset RRP	HPV-6, -11	Unclear
Cutaneous warts	HPV-1, -2, -3, -4, -10	Nonsexual contact
Epidermodysplasia verruciformis (EV)	HPV-5, -8, -9, -12, -14, -15, -17, -19, -25, -36, -38, -47, -50	Nonsexual contact
Nonmelanoma skin cancer	EV HPVs and novel HPVs	Unclear
Focal epithelial hyperplasia of the oral cavity	HPV-13, -32	Nonsexual contact

RRP, recurrent respiratory papillomatosis.

IMPROVED SCREENING FOR CERVICAL CANCER

Implementation of Pap smear screening and treatment of cervical cancer precursor lesions identified by follow-up investigation of abnormal Pap smears has resulted in a marked reduction in the incidence of cervical cancers in high-income countries but it has been difficult to establish effective Pap smear screening programs in low- and middle-income countries (LMIC). Primary cervical cancer screening by examination of cervical scrapes for DNAs of high-risk HPVs has been shown to have sensitivity greater than that of Pap smears for the detection of HSIL and cancer.[14] Primary screening with HPV testing or HPV cotesting with cytology is replacing cytology screening in many high-income countries. Some algorithms include triage of HPV positive test results using HPV16/18 genotyping, where HPV16/18 positive women are referred immediately to colposcopy and other high-risk HPV infections are followed with repeat testing at 1 year. These algorithms were developed in response to the high absolute risk of precancer in HPV16 positive women regardless of cytology, and the strong association of HPV18 with adenocarcinoma, which is more easily missed by cytology screening.

Because of the infrastructure required for the screening programs used in the industrialized world, the World Health Organization (WHO) has recommended that screening and treatment be performed at a single visit (i.e. 'screen-and-treat approach') using HPV tests where available and affordable or visual inspection with acetic acid, a low-cost test that has shown sensitivity comparable to Pap testing in pre-menopausal women.[15] In this strategy, treatment via cryotherapy is recommended for screen-positive women without further diagnostic verification.

Furthermore, adequate genital tract specimens for HPV testing can be self-collected by the women themselves, thus making it possible to avoid a pelvic examination. Self-sampling strategies are being employed to increase screening coverage in organized programs as well as rural and resource-limited populations lacking organizing screening.

PROPHYLACTIC VACCINES

VLPs that self-assemble from the L1 capsid protein when it is expressed by baculovirus or yeast recombinant DNA vectors have provided the immunogen for prophylactic vaccines. The VLPs are free of viral DNA and possess conformational epitopes of authentic virions. Gardasil® from Merck is a quadrivalent vaccine that has VLPs of high-risk HPV-16 and HPV-18 (which account for about 70% of invasive cervical cancers) and of low-risk HPV-6 and HPV-11 (which are

responsible for 90% of genital warts and 100% of recurrent respiratory papillomas). Cervarix® from GlaxoSmithKline is a bivalent vaccine with VLPs of HPV-16 and HPV-18. In clinical trials, both vaccines exhibited excellent safety and immunogenicity profiles.

The vaccines also demonstrated remarkably high and similar efficacy against the vaccine-targeted types for persistent infections and cervical precancerous lesions in women naïve to the corresponding type at the time of vaccination. However, protection from incident infection or disease from nonvaccine types was restricted, and the vaccines had no effect on prevalent infection or disease. In women, Gardasil® also demonstrated significant protection against genital warts and vulvar/vaginal neoplasia associated with the vaccine types. In other trials, Gardasil® protected middle-aged adult women from precancerous lesions caused by the vaccine types and protected men from genital warts and anal intraepithelial neoplasia caused by the vaccine types. Cervarix® protected against vaccine-targeted anal infections in one study. No clinical trials have been conducted of HPV vaccines for prevention of oropharyngeal cancers. Clinical trials of HPV vaccines have been reviewed recently.[16] Currently, the USA's Centers for Disease Control and Prevention (CDC) recommends that HPV vaccination is routinely targeted at girls and boys aged 11–12 years. Gardasil® is approved for use in boys and girls, whereas Cervarix® is only approved for use in girls. Catch-up vaccination is recommended up to age 26 years for young women and up to age 21 for young men. HPV vaccines are also recommended for gay and bisexual men, and men and women with compromised immune systems, including people living with HIV/AIDS, up to age 26 years. Similar schemes are in use elsewhere (for the UK see https://www.gov.uk/government/publications/the-complete-routine-immunisation-schedule).

The HPV vaccination rate for young women in the USA in 2012 was only 34% and rates were especially low among women with limited access to care.[17] The principal barriers to HPV vaccination in the USA are the high cost of the vaccines and parental attitudes and concerns with respect to risk of HPV infection, effects on sexual behavior, social influences and, for boys, perceived lack of direct benefit.[18] Major limitations of current vaccines are the high cost, incomplete coverage for all high-risk HPV types, need for intramuscular delivery and instability of the antigen at ambient temperatures. Second generation vaccines are being developed to address these limitations.[19] Merck has developed a nonavalent vaccine, which, in addition to the HPV types contained in Gardasil®, also contains VLPs for types 31, 33, 45, 52 and 58. Phase III trials of this vaccine are ongoing. Development is also underway for a pan-oncogenic vaccine based on the L2 minor capsid protein, which can elicit cross-neutralizing antibodies and thus holds promise for much broader protection. Capsomere vaccines, which can be produced less expensively in *Escherichia coli*, are also in development. Both the L2 and capsomere vaccines can potentially be delivered by noninjectable routes.

INTEGRATION OF HPV PROPHYLACTIC VACCINE AND SCREENING

As the prevalence of high-risk HPV infections and associated precancers decline in vaccinated populations, the positive predictive values from screening are anticipated to fall in parallel. Screening must continue even in women receiving current bivalent or quadrivalent vaccines, though implementation of more sensitive HPV-based screening tests with longer intervals between screens represents a more cost-effective integration of primary and secondary prevention. Even more efficient strategies will be needed to prevent the small numbers of cancers that will occur due to types not present in the next generation nonavalent vaccines (Figure 167-4).

THERAPEUTIC VACCINES

Several strategies are also being evaluated for therapeutic immunization, aimed at destroying established lesions of HSIL and invasive cancer.[20] For this purpose, the objective is to generate cytotoxic T cells directed against cells expressing the E6 and E7 proteins of high-risk HPVs. Chimeric vaccines which may have both prophylactic and therapeutic properties are also under investigation.

Diagnostic Microbiology
HPV NUCLEIC ACID DETECTION

The presence of HPV in a tissue is most often defined by the presence of HPV viral nucleic acid, using either DNA or RNA-based assays. A variety of HPV assays are commercially available.[21] In the USA, four commercial tests have received FDA approval for reflex testing of ASCUS positive cytology and cotesting with cytology in women over age 30 years:

- Hybrid Capture® 2 (hc2) HPV DNA test (QIAGEN Inc., Gaithersburg, MD)
- Cervista® HPV HR Test (Hologic, Madison, WI)
- APTIMA® HPV Test (Gen-Probe, Inc., San Diego, CA)
- cobas® 4800 HPV Test (Roche Molecular Systems Inc., Pleasanton, CA).

The Roche cobas® HPV test automatically separates positive results into HPV16/18 positive versus 'other' high-risk HPV. Cervista® also has a US FDA-approved test for HPV16/18 genotyping (Cervista® HPV 16/18 Test), though this must be performed separately from their general high-risk assay. In 2014, the US FDA also approved the cobas® 4800 HPV Test for use in primary screening of women aged 25–65, with immediate referral of HPV16/18 positive women to colposcopy, and triage of other HR-HPV positive women by cytology.

PROTEIN BIOMARKERS

The OncoE6 Test® by Arbor Vita Corporation (Fremont, CA) is a CE-marked lateral flow assay, which detects the presence of the HPVE6

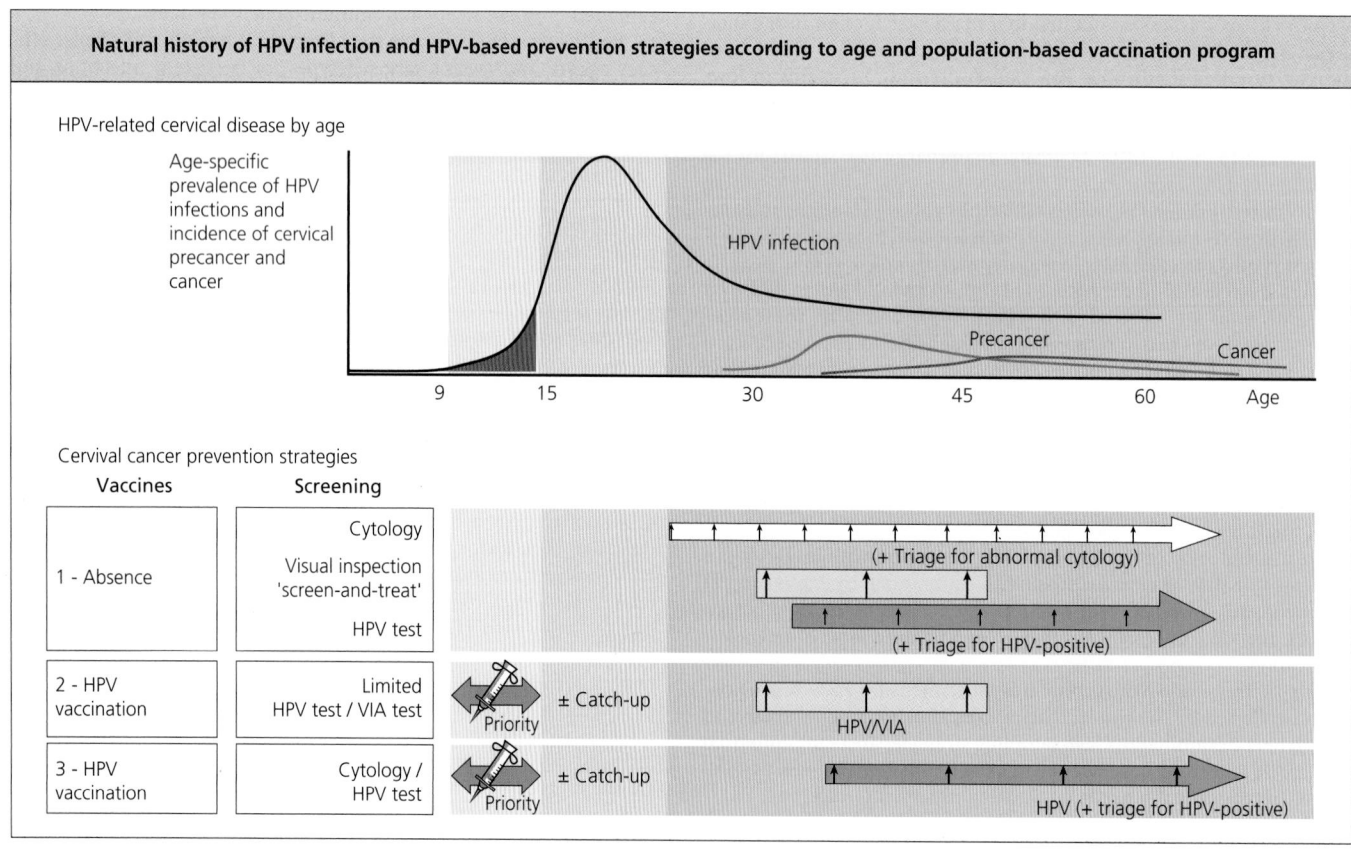

Figure 167-4   Natural history of HPV infection and HPV-based prevention strategies according to age and population-based vaccination program. Screening strategy 1 applies to settings where vaccination has not been introduced and conventional screening exists. Screening can be based on the Pap smear, can employ novel forms of automated reading of cytology or can use HPV nucleic acid detection technology (DNA and RNA tests). HPV-based screening has shown increases in sensitivity as compared with cytology with a moderate loss of specificity, allowing for increased screening intervals. For low- and middle-income countries (LMIC) where vaccination has not been introduced and established screening programs are not in place, a screen-and-treat strategy can be employed utilizing either visual inspection with acetic acid (VIA) or HPV DNA testing. Screening strategy 2 is likely to represent many LMIC without routine screening programs and where immunization appears as the primary component of the preventive strategy. Screening in these circumstances might develop slowly and few lifetime screening events may be offered. Novel low-cost HPV technologies paired with screen-and-treat protocols might be the model for large populations in the world. Screening strategy 3 is likely to be adopted by most high-income countries and some LMIC in which combinations of generalized immunization of adolescents and HPV screening of adult women will coexist until broad spectrum vaccines become established. *(Adapted from Bosch F.X., et al. Vaccine 2013; 31 (Suppl 5):F1-31.)*

oncoprotein in cervical cell lysates from HPV types 16 and 18. This presence of E6 protein has been shown to have superior specificity to nucleic acid-based HPV and morphology-based tests when used both as a primary screen or a triage test.[22] Detection of elevated levels of the p16(INK4a) host protein, which is upregulated by HPVE7 gene expression, has also been shown to have a higher specificity for detection of cervical precancer compared to HPV nucleic acid tests and cytology, with only minimal decreases in test sensitivity.[23] Because this test is genotype-agnostic, it may offer a reasonable solution for screening vaccinated populations.

IMMUNOLOGIC ASSAYS

Immunologic assays are rarely used for type-specific HPV diagnosis. In most HPV infections, viral particles and capsid proteins are present in very small amounts and so are difficult to detect with antiviral serum. Also, as cervical squamous intra-epithelial lesions (SILs) progress toward higher grade disease and cervical cancer, synthesis of capsid proteins and infectious particles is completely shut down. Type-specific antiserum is not available for any HPV type.

Antibody response to HPVs may be measured using enzyme-linked immunosorbent assay (ELISA) with VLPs. Antibody response to HPV infections is low-titered and detectable in only about 40–50% of infected individuals. The proportion of infected individuals who are antibody positive increases with the duration of infection and viral load in the genital tract specimens. Antibodies to E6 and E7 proteins are markers of HPV-associated invasive cancer. These antibodies may be detected by peptide-based ELISA or by radioimmunoprecipitation assays with *in vitro* synthesized full length E6 and E7 proteins. Elevated levels of E6 or E7 antibodies are found in about 70% of patients who have invasive cervical cancer but in less than 5% of controls.[24] Elevated E6 antibodies are also observed in patients with HPV-associated oropharyngeal cancer[25] and in about 35% of patients may be present more than 10 years before the clinical diagnosis is established.[26]

Clinical Manifestations

The major clinical associations of HPVs are listed in Table 167-1. Aspects not covered in the earlier sections of this chapter are discussed below. Clinical features of these infections are also discussed in Chapter 63.

CERVICAL CANCER

Cervical cancer is the most common female malignancy in LMIC. Approximately 500 000 cases of cervical cancer occur worldwide per year. The incidence of cervical cancer varies widely in different countries. Cervical cancer has long been known to have all the epidemiologic characteristics of a sexually transmitted disease. Observations from field, clinical and laboratory studies are mutually corroborative in building a compelling case for the HPV etiology of cervical cancer (Table 167-2), making it the first major human cancer with a single infectious etiology. The sexual behavior of the female, the sexual behavior of her male partners and the availability of an effective Pap smear screening program explain the wide differences in cervical cancer incidence in different countries. In many high-incidence areas, male sexual behavior is the key factor for the high cervical cancer rates among relatively monogamous women.

OTHER ANOGENITAL CANCERS

HPV infections are responsible for the basaloid or warty vulvar cancers that occur in younger women but are not related to the more common typical keratinizing squamous cell carcinomas that occur in older women. They are strongly associated with cancers of the anal canal, vagina and penis.

OROPHARYNGEAL/TONSILLAR CANCER

A subset of oropharyngeal/tonsillar cancer is etiologically linked to high-risk HPVs, especially HPV-16.[27] Virologically, these tumors have a transcriptionally active HPV genome localized to tumor cell nuclei.

TABLE 167-2	Evidence Linking HPVs with Invasive Cervical Cancer
Field	**Evidence**
Epidemiology	HPVs present in nearly 100% of cancers in low- and high-incidence areas HPV infection precedes cancer HPV epidemiology and cervical cancer screening practices account for differences in worldwide incidence of cervical cancer
Pathogenesis	HPV genome present in every cancer cell HPV associated with entire spectrum of cervical neoplasia, from low-grade cytologic abnormalities to invasive cancers HPV types most frequent in cancers are the most oncogenic in laboratory assays HPV oncogenes E6 and E7 invariably expressed in cancers HPV genome is episomal in preinvasive disease and integrates into cellular DNA in invasive cancers
Molecular mechanisms	E6 and E7 proteins of high-risk HPV types distort cell cycle and promote genetic instability by degradation of tumor suppressor protein p53 and inactivation of tumor suppressor protein Rb Integration of viral genome into cellular DNA enhances E6 and E7 expression

HPV-16 accounts for more than 90% of the HPV-associated cancers at this site. As compared with other patients with head and neck cancers, these patients are less likely to have a history of alcohol and tobacco exposure, more likely to have a history of multiple sexual partners and of oral sex, and a significantly better prognosis. A majority of the estimated 51 000 annual cases of oropharyngeal cancers worldwide are due to HPV infection and are very likely vaccine-preventable.

GENITAL WARTS

Although they are benign, genital warts (condylomas) are a significant problem in sexually active populations and especially in immunocompromised individuals. Vaccines which contain HPV-6 and HPV-11 VLPs have had a major impact on reductions of the incidence of genital warts in populations with high vaccine coverage (Figure 167-5).[28, 29]

RECURRENT RESPIRATORY PAPILLOMATOSIS (RRP)

This results from the transmission of HPV-6 and HPV-11 infections from the genital tract to the respiratory tract. For juvenile-onset disease, a large majority of the transmissions occur at birth, during passage of the fetus through an infected birth canal (for review of the clinical spectrum of juvenile-onset RRP, see reference 30). Some reports suggest occasional intrauterine transmission. About 25% of the cases occur in the first year of life and most of these in the second 6 months. There are progressively fewer cases in each year thereafter.

The most common site of the papilloma is in the larynx on the vocal cords. The tumors are benign but may threaten life if they grow and obstruct respiration. The tumors tend to recur after surgical removal, and in the worst cases operations may be required every few weeks. Rarely, the tumor may undergo malignant transformation. Cesarean delivery when there is an active infection of the maternal genital tract will reduce the risk of juvenile-onset disease in the child. Mothers who have been immunized with HPV vaccines that have HPV-6 and HPV-11 VLPs are probably protected against having a child with juvenile-onset RRP.

Management

The clinical conditions associated with HPV infections are very diverse. Regular screening and follow-up of women who have abnormalities

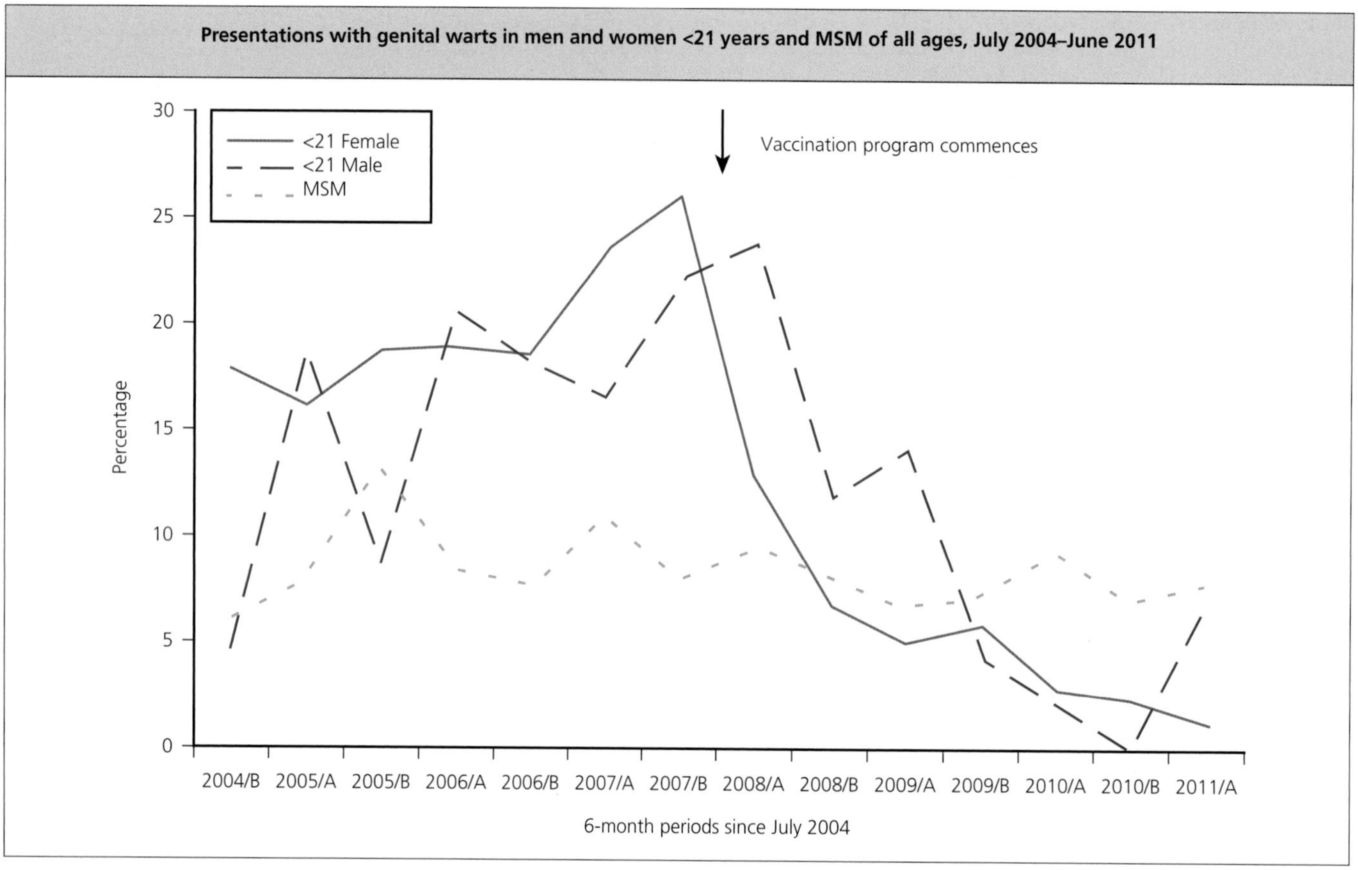

Presentations with genital warts in men and women <21 years and MSM of all ages, July 2004–June 2011

Figure 167-5   Presentations with genital warts in men and women <21 years and men who have sex with men (MSM) of all ages, during a 3-year period before and after introduction of mandatory HPV vaccination for girls in Australia. Proportion of male and female patients aged <21 years having genital warts in 6-month time intervals from 2004 until 2010, compared to the proportion of MSM having genital warts in the same time intervals. Males exclude MSM and nonresidents. Mandatory vaccination of young women was implemented in July 2007. Among females and heterosexual males the incidence of genital warts decreased dramatically after introduction of the HPV vaccine while no change was observed in MSM, as males were not routinely vaccinated at this time. *Adapted from Read, T.R., et al. Sex Transm Infect 2011; 87:544-547.*

greatly decreases the risk of cervical cancer. Newer strategies for screening include HPV testing and many have sufficiently high negative predictive value to allow less frequent screening, which increases efficiency of screening where programs exist and the feasibility of screening in lower resource settings. Preinvasive cervical disease is readily treated by excision (e.g. loop electroexcision procedure, or LEEP) or ablation (e.g. cryotherapy) with greater than 90% cure rates. Genital and skin warts may regress spontaneously or may be treated

with caustic agents (podophyllin), cryotherapy, and application of an immunomodulating agent (imiquimod) or by surgical removal. Intralesional or parenteral administration of interferon has been successful in the treatment of refractory genital warts (see Chapter 63 for additional information).

References available online at expertconsult.com.

KEY REFERENCES

Bosch F.X., Broker T.R., Forman D., et al.: Comprehensive control of human papillomavirus infections and related diseases. *Vaccine* 2013; 31(Suppl. 5):F1-F31.

Bruni L., Diaz M., Castellsague X., et al.: Cervical human papillomavirus prevalence in 5 continents: meta-analysis of 1 million women with normal cytological findings. *J Infect Dis* 2010; 202:1789-1799.

D'Souza G., Kreimer A.R., Viscidi R., et al.: Case-control study of human papillomavirus and oropharyngeal cancer. *N Engl J Med* 2007; 356:1944-1956.

Gravitt P.E.: The known unknowns of HPV natural history. *J Clin Invest* 2011; 121:4593-4599.

Kreimer A.R., Johansson M., Waterboer T., et al.: Evaluation of human papillomavirus antibodies and risk of subsequent head and neck cancer. *J Clin Oncol* 2013; 31:2708-2715.

Qiao Y.L., Jeronimo J., Zhao F.H., et al.: Lower cost strategies for triage of human papillomavirus DNA-positive women. *Int J Cancer* 2014; 134:2891-2901.

Read T.R., Hocking J.S., Chen M.Y., et al.: The near disappearance of genital warts in young women 4 years after commencing a national human papillomavirus HPV vaccination programme. *Sex Transm Infect* 2011; 87:544-547.

Schiffman M., Castle P.E., Jeronimo J., et al.: Human papillomavirus and cervical cancer. *Lancet* 2007; 370:890-907.

Schiller J.T., Castellsague X., Garland S.M.: A review of clinical trials of human papillomavirus prophylactic vaccines. *Vaccine* 2012; 30(Suppl. 5):F123-F138.

Schmidt S., Parsons H.M.: Vaccination interest and trends in human papillomavirus vaccine uptake in young adult women aged 18 to 26 years in the United States: an analysis using the 2008-2012 National Health Interview Survey. *Am J Public Health* 2014; 104:946-953.

168

Polyomaviruses

RAPHAEL P. VISCIDI | CHEN SABRINA TAN

KEY CONCEPTS

- Human polyomaviruses are ubiquitous in the general population and cause disease in immunocompromised individuals.

- JC polyomavirus (JCPyV) can be detected in the urine of one-third of healthy and immunosuppressed individuals alike.

- JCPyV causes the demyelinating central nervous system (CNS) disease – progressive multifocal leukoencephalopathy (PML) – in up to 5% of untreated AIDS patients, in patients with hematological malignancies, and in patients treated with monoclonal antibodies, especially in multiple sclerosis patients treated with natalizumab.

- The risk of PML in patients taking natalizumab is related to JCPyV antibody status, prior use of immunosuppressive drugs and the duration of natalizumab treatment.

- BK polyomavirus (BKPyV) is detected in the urine of 2–5% of healthy individuals.

- BKPyV reactivation causes nephropathy in graft kidney of transplant patients that can result in graft loss.

- BKPyV reactivation in patients after hematopoietic transplantation can result in hemorrhagic cystitis.

- Merkel cell polyomavirus (MCPyV) is closely linked to Merkel cell cancer, a rare neuroendocrine cancer of the skin.

- TSPyV causes trichodysplasia spinulosa, a follicular papular skin disease in patients with solid organ transplantation.

- There is no effective antiviral therapy against human polyomavirus; treatment and preventions are achieved through reduction of immunosuppression, such as treating human immunodeficiency virus (HIV) in AIDS patients.

Nature

Polyomaviruses are small, non-enveloped viruses, which are widespread in nature. They are highly adapted to grow in the species and the tissue they infect. The first human polyomaviruses were isolated in 1971 from immunocompromised patients. JC polyomavirus (JCPyV) was isolated from the brain of a patient with Hodgkin's disease, who died of progressive multifocal leukoencephalopathy (PML), a demyelinating disease of the central nervous system (CNS).[1] BK polyomavirus (BKPyV) was isolated from the urine of a renal transplant patient who developed ureteral stenosis.[2]

In 2007, genomes of two new human polyomaviruses, KIPyV virus and WUPyV virus, were independently detected in respiratory tract secretions of children by use of molecular techniques.[3,4] These two viruses share 65–70% amino acid similarity with each other, but only 15–50% similarity with JCPyV and BKPyV. In 2008, another new human polyomavirus, Merkel cell polyomavirus (MCPyV), was detected by employing mass sequencing of a messenger RNA library of tumor cells and bioinformatics analysis of the data to identify non-human sequences with homology to known infectious agents.[5] Since the discovery of WUPyV, KIPyV and MCPyV, seven more new

polyomaviruses have been discovered and named based on their geographic origins, MWPyV (Malawi) and STLPyV (St Louis), or on the diseases they cause, TSPyV (trichodysplasia spinulosa), or on the order of discovery, HPyV6, HPyV7, HPyV9, HPyV12 and HPyV13 (human polyomaviruses 6, 7, 9, 12 and 13).[6] So far, with the exception of TSPyV, no disease association has been found for any of these viruses (Table 168-1).

Epidemiology

Both BKPyV and JCPyV primary infections occur in childhood, but BKPyV occurs at an earlier age than JCPyV. BKPyV seropositivity increases rapidly with age and reaches 98% at 7–9 years of age. JCPyV seropositivity increases more slowly with increasing age, reaching 50% among children aged 9–11 years and 60–70% by adulthood.[7] The likely modes of transmission of BKPyV and JCPyV are the respiratory tract and the urine-oral route. Seroprevalence data for the newer polyomaviruses are more limited but the available data indicate that these viruses circulate widely in humans and exposure is most intense in childhood, although the observation that seroprevalence for some viruses rises with age suggests infection may occur throughout life, with some differences among the viruses in terms of age-specific seroprevalence.[8]

Pathogenicity

Primary BKPyV and JCPyV infections are either entirely asymptomatic or may be associated with nonspecific flu-like symptoms. After primary infection, the viruses remain latent in the kidney for an indefinite period of time. The viruses may activate periodically and be associated with asymptomatic shedding of virus in the urine. BKPyV DNA can be detected in the urine of ~2–5% of healthy persons and JCPyV DNA can be found in ~35% of healthy individuals, with a higher incidence of JCPyV shedding in older individuals.[9] After primary infection JCPyV also persists in the hematopoietic system, such as B lymphocytes and bone marrow, and has been reported to persist as a latent infection of the brain.[10] Nearly all significant illnesses due to BKPyV and JCPyV occur in immunocompromised hosts, mostly as a result of reactivation of latent virus but sometimes as a primary infection in an immunocompromised host. Conditions in which viruses are reactivated include pregnancy, diabetes, organ transplantation, anti-tumor therapy, treatment with monoclonal antibodies, particularly natalizumab, a monoclonal antibody to alpha-4 integrin that prevents entry of inflammatory cells into brain and other tissues, and AIDS and other immunodeficiency diseases.

Prevention

No attempt has been made to prevent primary BKPyV or JCPyV infection since infection is harmless in immunocompetent individuals and disease is uncommon even in immunocompromised individuals. However, PML occurs in up to 1.1% of multiple sclerosis (MS) patients treated for 24 consecutive months with natalizumab. To prevent or minimize the risk of PML in MS patients, JCPyV serology can be obtained prior to treatment and periodically during the treatment course.[11] Seropositivity or seroconversion is associated with an increased risk of PML, and has prompted clinicians to stop natalizumab treatment and monitor for signs and symptoms of PML.

TABLE 168-1	Human Polyomaviruses and Associated Disease, Site of Isolation and Seroprevalence in Adults			
Name	Abbreviation	Associated Disease	Site of Isolation	Adult Seroprevalence (%)
BK	BKPyV	Polyomavirus-associated nephropathy Hemorrhagic cystitis	Urine	98
JC	JCPyV	Progressive multifocal leukoencephalopathy	Brain Urine	55–65
Washington University	WUPyV	None known	Nasopharynx	70–90
Karolinska Institute	KIPyV	None known	Nasopharynx	55–90
Merkel cell	MCPyV	Merkel cell carcinoma	Carcinoma lesion, normal skin	60–65
Number 6	HPyV6	None known	Skin	70
Number 7	HPyV7	None known	Skin	35
Trichodysplasia spinulosa (TS)	TSPyV	Trichodysplasia spinulosa Pilomatrix dysplasia	TS spicules	70–80
Number 9	HPyV9	None known	Urine, blood, skin	25–50
Malawi	MWPyV (HPyV10)	None known	Stool, wart	42
Saint Louis	STLPyV	None known	Stool	Unknown
Number 12	HPyV12	None known	Liver from patient with colon cancer	30
New Jersey	NJPyV (HPyV13)	None known	Muscle endothelial cells form pancreatic transplant patient	Unknown

Additional risk factors are duration of natalizumab treatment and prior use of immunosuppressive drugs. Since human immunodeficiency virus (HIV)-associated PML occurs in the context of severe immunodeficiency, treatment of HIV with antiretroviral drugs and partial reversal of immune dysfunction will reduce the incidence and severity of PML.[12] Screening of renal transplant recipients for BKPyV viruria and viremia can identify patients at risk for BKPyV-associated disease and allow clinicians to change or reduce immunosuppressive regimens, which may reduce the risk of disease or allow patients with BKPyV-associated disease to recover more rapidly.[13]

Diagnostic Microbiology

BKPyV can be cultivated in several cell lines of human origin. JCPyV grows best in human fetal glial cultures. None of the more recently discovered polyomaviruses can be propagated in cell cultures. Cells and tissue infected with BKPyV and JCPyV can be identified by immunoperoxidase and immunofluorescence staining with antiviral antibodies. BKPyV and JCPyV DNA, as well as the DNA genomes of other polyomaviruses, can be readily identified by polymerase chain reaction (PCR) assays. PCR assays have been developed for JCPyV and BKPyV in academic centers and are used for clinical research; however, the only Food and Drug Administration (FDA)-approved polyomavirus PCR assays are those developed for BKPyV, the Focus Diagnostics Simplex® BKPyV assay and the QIAGEN Artus® BK virus RG PCR test.[14,15] The greatest limitation for the clinical application of BKPyV PCR assays is the uncertain clinical relevance of a positive test given the inherently high sensitivity of PCR assays and the potential to detect infections that are not clinically important. Serologic diagnosis of BKPyV and JCPyV infection can be made by hemagglutination-inhibition assays or by enzyme-linked immunosorbent assays (ELISA), which use virus-like particles formed by self-assembly of VP1 protein produced in eukaryotic expression systems. Because BKV and JCV infections occur early in life and are very common, serologic assays have limited utility for clinical diagnosis. A two-step ELISA assay for JCPyV serum antibodies (Focus Diagnostics STRATIFY JCV DxSelect®) has been used to risk-stratify MS patients on treatment with natalizumab.[16] The diagnosis of specific polyomavirus-associated diseases is discussed in greater detail below.

Clinical Manifestations
PROGRESSIVE MULTIFOCAL LEUKOENCEPHALOPATHY

PML is an often fatal, subacute demyelinating disease of the CNS that results from JCPyV infection of oligodendrocytes in the brain.[17] It occurs as a complication of conditions associated with T-cell deficiency, including lymphoproliferative disorders, primary immunodeficiency diseases, prolonged immunosuppressive therapy and secondary immunodeficiency disorders such as HIV infection. Until the advent of HIV/AIDS, PML was a rare disease with onset typically at middle age or later life. At present, HIV is estimated to be the underlying cause of immunosuppression in 55–85% of cases of PML, and PML is diagnosed in approximately 5% of AIDS cases.[18] In 2006, three patients with either MS or Crohn's disease developed PML in association with administration of natalizumab.[19] Approximately 400 cases of natalizumab-associated PML have been documented. PML has also been associated with other monoclonal antibodies, including rituximab for lymphoma or lupus, and efalizumab for psoriasis.

PML has an insidious onset. The neurological deficits correspond to the demyelinated white matter areas of the brain. Thus, symptoms can vary, including early signs of impairment of speech and vision and mental deterioration. Paralysis of limbs, cortical blindness and sensory impairment occur in later stages of the disease. Typically, the disease is progressive, often resulting in death within 3–6 months after onset. The introduction of combined antiretroviral therapy (cART) for HIV has had only a modest effect on the incidence of PML, but prognosis is improved from 10% of the HIV-infected patients with PML surviving past 1 year after diagnosis to 50% of this population.[20] At disease onset, factors associated with better survival include higher CD4 cell count, lower JCPyV viral load, presence of JCPyV-specific cellular immune responses, prior exposure to cART, elevated myoinositol in PML lesions on MRI and higher levels of macrophage chemoattractant protein (MCP)-1 in cerebrospinal fluid (CSF).

The definitive diagnosis of PML is established by pathologic examination of biopsy tissue. Demyelination is most frequently found in subcortical white matter. Microscopically, the presence of enlarged nuclei of oligodendrocytes is the pathognomonic lesion of PML. These altered nuclei contain abundant numbers of JCPyV viral particles. Brain biopsy has an operator-dependent sensitivity range from 64% to 96% and a specificity of 100%. Noninvasive techniques, particularly MRI of the brain, provide an effective means for diagnosis of PML.[21] The typical abnormalities are localized to subcortical white matter and are characterized by increased T2 signal and little contrast enhancement after gadolinium administration. CSF analysis typically shows minimal pleocytosis and modestly elevated protein. PCR of CSF for JCPyV DNA is the best noninvasive test for diagnosis of PML. Sensitivity of PCR is 80% and specificity is 100%.[22]

OTHER JCPyV ASSOCIATED SYNDROMES

PML-Immune Reconstitution Inflammatory Syndrome (IRIS)

Treatment of patients with HIV-associated PML with intensive antiretroviral drug therapy or of MS patients with plasma exchange to remove natalizumab can be paradoxically associated with clinical deterioration and pathological evidence of inflammation in the brain, a condition known as immune reconstitution syndrome (IRIS). Up to 57% of PML-IRIS lesions may display contrast enhancement on MRI. High doses of steroids have been used to treat the inflammation.

JCPyV Meningitis, JCPyV Encephalopathy and JCPyV Granule Cell Neuronopathy

JCPyV meningitis, JCPyV encephalopathy and JCPyV granule cell neuronopathy are other presentations of JCPyV infection in the brain. Multiple case reports have described these syndromes. Diagnosis of these syndromes is usually made by detection of JCPyV in CSF in patients with the associated clinical syndromes and after exclusion of other possible diagnoses.

BK VIRUS NEPHROPATHY IN KIDNEY TRANSPLANT RECIPIENTS

BK virus nephropathy (BKVN), also designated polyomavirus-associated nephropathy (PVAN), has been recognized as an important cause of graft dysfunction and graft loss in patients with renal allografts. The incidence of BKVN is 1–10% and graft loss occurs in from 10% to 80% of cases.[23] The majority of cases occur in the first year post transplantation (Figure 168-1). The variable incidence and outcome

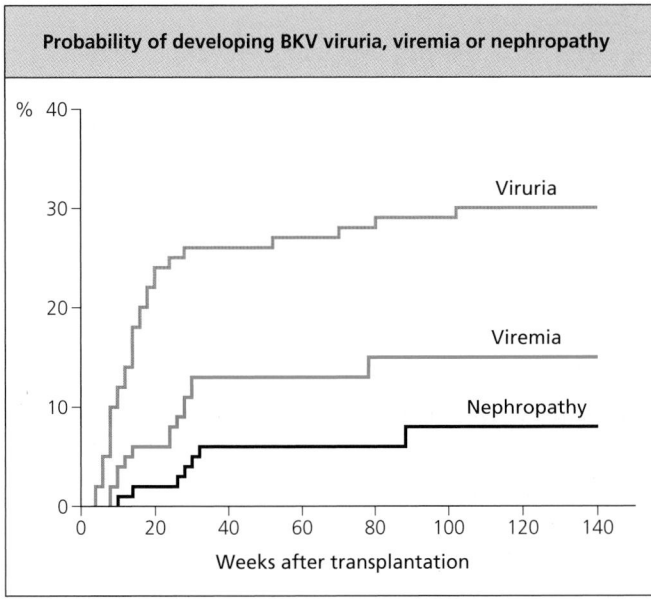

Figure 168-1 Probability of developing BKV viruria, viremia or nephropathy in the weeks following renal transplantation. (*Adapted from Hirsch H.H., et al. Prospective study of polyomavirus type BK replication and nephropathy in renal-transplant recipients. N Engl J Med 2002; 347:488–496*).

of BKVN most likely reflect differences across renal transplant centers in diagnostic criteria for BKVN, patient populations, immunosuppressive regimens and management strategies.

The definitive diagnosis of BKVN requires a renal biopsy showing polyomavirus-induced cytopathic changes in tubular or glomerular epithelial cells.[24] For early diagnosis, polyomavirus-bearing 'decoy cells' can be detected in urine with a Papanicolaou-stained cytology preparation. The positive predictive value for BKVN of the detection of decoy cells is 25–30%. BKPyV DNA can be detected in urine and plasma by PCR. Because of the high rate of excretion of BKPyV in urine of renal transplant recipients, the finding of BKPyV DNA by PCR in urine is of limited clinical value for diagnosis of BKVN. On the other hand, detection of BKPyV DNA in plasma by PCR has been shown to have a sensitivity of 100% and a specificity of 85% for biopsy-confirmed BKVN.[25]

HEMORRHAGIC CYSTITIS IN BONE MARROW TRANSPLANT RECIPIENTS

BK viruria occurs in 50% of patients after bone marrow transplantation (BMT). Hemorrhagic cystitis is the most prevalent and serious clinical manifestation of BKPyV infection in BMT recipients, with an incidence of 10–25%.[26] Less common clinical manifestations of BKPyV infection in BMT include ureteral stenosis and interstitial nephritis. Patients with hemorrhagic cystitis experience urgency, frequency of urination, dysuria, suprapubic pain and variable degrees of hematuria. BKPyV-associated hemorrhagic cystitis must be distinguished from cytomegalovirus- or adenovirus-caused hemorrhagic cystitis, as well as noninfectious hemorrhagic cystitis resulting from direct cytotoxic effects of antineoplastic treatment. BKPyV-associated hemorrhagic cystitis occurs after neutrophil engraftment; as early as 40 days after transplantation. Thus, cellular immune response to actively replicating BKPyV may be part of the pathogenesis. Potential risk factors for BKPyV-associated hemorrhagic cystitis include acute graft-versus-host disease, intensive immunosuppressive conditioning regimens, allogeneic transplant and magnitude of BKPyV urine viral load. BKPyV DNA can be detected by PCR in urine of patients with BKV-associated hemorrhagic cystitis; however, detection of BKPyV DNA does not have high specificity. A high urine viral load or viremia has greater specificity.

ROLE OF POLYOMAVIRUSES IN HUMAN MALIGNANCIES

Merkel cell cancer (MCC) is a rare aggressive neuroendocrine cancer of the skin. Exposure to sunlight and ultraviolet light, as well as immunosuppression, are risk factors for MCC. As mentioned above, a human polyomavirus, MCPyV, was identified in cancer cells in 2008. The evidence for an etiological role of the virus in oncogenesis is widely accepted in the scientific community.[27]

TRICHODYSPLASIA SPINULOSA

Trichodysplasia spinulosa (TS) is a rare skin disease which occurs in recipients of solid organs on immunosuppressive therapy and in patients with lymphocytic leukemia. The patients develop follicular papules and keratin spines on the face, often accompanied by alopecia of the eyebrows and eyelashes. The presence of TSPyV in high copy numbers in the lesions of TS suggests that the virus may be etiologically related to the disease.[28] However, the virus is widespread in human populations with a seroprevalence around 80%. Apart from immunosuppression other factors that lead to TS in infected patients are unknown.

Management

The majority of patients with BKPyV and JCPyV infections are asymptomatic and do not require treatment. There are no antiviral drugs with proven clinical efficacy against human polyomaviruses. The mainstay of treatment for BKPyV nephropathy is the reduction, change in drugs or discontinuation of immunosuppressive therapy.[29] While multiple small studies have shown benefits of treatment with fluoroquinolones, cidofovir or brincidofovir, randomized controlled studies are needed to determine efficacy. For ureteral stenosis, the treatment is surgical relief of the obstruction. Treatment of hemorrhagic cystitis is symptomatic and includes continuous bladder irrigations, analgesia, hyperhydration, forced diuresis, and transfusion.

Historically, the prognosis for PML was poor with death occurring within 3–4 months of diagnosis. However, for HIV patients, the introduction of cART has improved survival of patients with PML.

References available online at expertconsult.com.

KEY REFERENCES

Bloomgren G., Richman S., Hotermans C., et al.: Risk of natalizumab-associated progressive multifocal leukoencephalopathy. *N Engl J Med* 2012; 366:1870-1880.

Casado J.L., Corral I., Garcia J., et al.: Continued declining incidence and improved survival of progressive multifocal leukoencephalopathy in HIV/AIDS patients in the current era. *Eur J Clin Microbiol Infect Dis* 2014; 33:179-187.

DeCaprio J.A., Garcea R.L.: A cornucopia of human polyomaviruses. *Nat Rev Microbiol* 2013; 11:264-276.

Feng H., Shuda M., Chang Y., et al.: Clonal integration of a polyomavirus in human Merkel cell carcinoma. *Science* 2008; 319:1096-1100.

Ferenczy M.W., Marshall L.J., Nelson C.D., et al.: Molecular biology, epidemiology, and pathogenesis of progressive multifocal leukoencephalopathy, the JC virus-induced demyelinating disease of the human brain. *Clin Microbiol Rev* 2012; 25:471-506.

Hirsch H.H., Knowles W., Dickenmann M., et al.: Prospective study of polyomavirus type BK replication and nephropathy in renal-transplant recipients. *N Engl J Med* 2002; 347:488-496.

Randhawa P., Ho A., Shapiro R., et al.: Correlates of quantitative measurement of BK polyomavirus (BKV) DNA with clinical course of BKV infection in renal transplant patients. *J Clin Microbiol* 2004; 42:1176-1180.

Stolt A., Sasnauskas K., Koskela P., et al.: Seroepidemiology of the human polyomaviruses. *J Gen Virol* 2003; 84:1499-1504.

169

Parvoviruses

ALOYS C.M. KROES

KEY CONCEPTS

- Parvoviruses are among the smallest pathogenic viruses and their replication depends upon host cell DNA polymerase.

- Their genetic material is single-stranded DNA, which may persist in tissues, potentially causing diagnostic confusion.

- Human parvovirus B19 belongs to the genus *Erythroparvovirus*, typically replicating in erythroid precursor cells. This specific tissue tropism determines the pathogenesis of the most relevant clinical consequences of infection: fetal anemia with hydrops, aplastic crisis in patients with underlying disorders of erythropoiesis and chronic anemia in immunocompromised hosts.

- Additional frequent clinical manifestations are attributed to immunopathological antiviral host responses, including the common childhood exanthema erythema infectiosum or fifth disease and acute symmetric polyarthritis.

- Occasional and rare clinical manifestations include viral hepatitis, central and peripheral neurological syndromes, vasculitis and nephropathy.

- The role of parvovirus B19 in cardiac diseases including myocarditis is unclear, as passive persistence of viral DNA in myocardial tissue is well documented. Release of viral DNA may therefore suggest a relationship to cardiac disorders, which is not causal.

- A highly relevant intervention is possible in cases of fetal hydrops, consisting of intrauterine blood transfusion, which may be life saving for the fetus.

- Intravenous administration of immunoglobulins is an effective therapeutic option in cases of chronic anemia attributable to parvovirus B19 infection in immunocompromised hosts.

Nature

The family Parvoviridae consists of remarkably small (*parvus* in Latin), non-enveloped, single-stranded DNA viruses of animals, divided into the subfamilies Parvovirinae of vertebrates and Densovirinae of arthropods. The Parvovirinae subfamily is currently divided into eight genera.[1] Among these, the genus *Erythroparvovirus* contains the most relevant human parvovirus, B19 virus or primate erythroparvovirus 1. Further human viruses in the family include human bocavirus in the *Bocaparvovirus* genus (or primate bocaparvovirus 1 and 2), which is considered a respiratory pathogen (see Chapter 28) and the blood-borne virus human parvovirus 4 (PARV4, primate tetraparvovirus 1) that is classified in the genus *Tetraparvovirus* and is not associated with clinical disease.[2] Human infections with adeno-associated virus (AAV), belonging to the *Dependoparvovirus* genus, are not associated with disease but are currently being developed as vectors for gene therapy, as they can infect many cell types but do not replicate without the presence of helper viruses. Other parvoviruses include well-known canine and feline pathogens of veterinary relevance.

The name of the human parvovirus B19 (B19V) does not refer to any systematic nomenclature but was assigned by Yvonne Cossart who, in 1974, detected an immunoreactive antigen in human serum obtained from a donor referred to as B19. This antigen was subsequently determined to be part of a small icosahedral viral particle on electron

microscopy, with parvovirus-like features.[3] The corresponding antibodies were widely present in the human population and increased in prevalence with age but it took some time before several important disease associations were revealed. First, infection with this virus was associated with aplastic crisis among persons with sickle cell disease,[4] subsequently with the common childhood exanthema known as erythema infectiosum[5] and finally with a serious complication during pregnancy, hydrops fetalis.[6] These three clinical entities are still the most relevant consequences of infection by parvovirus B19, although a number of other clinical manifestations have been added since.[7]

The B19 virus appeared a typical member of the *Parvoviridae* family: a small (23 nm) viral particle, with a small (5.6 kb) genome consisting of single-stranded DNA (Figure 169-1). The DNA has palindromic hairpin structures at either end and encodes only three major viral proteins, the viral capsid proteins VP1 and VP2 and one nonstructural protein, NS1, in addition to two smaller products of unknown significance.[8] As a typical and unique property of the genus *Erythroparvovirus*, human parvovirus B19 requires erythroid precursor cells for productive infection. This is likely to be related to the presence of the cellular receptor, blood group P-antigen or globoside and to the necessary mitotic S phase activity of host cells to enable viral DNA synthesis. As the virus does not encode a polymerase, replication is dependent upon cellular DNA polymerase. Progeny virus is assembled in the nucleus and may be observed as intranuclear inclusions. Equal numbers of positive and negative sense DNA strands are encapsidated. The VP1 and VP2 proteins are overlapping, with the VP2 (58 kDa) fully contained in the VP1 (84 kDa) sequence. VP2 is the major constituent of the viral capsid (96%). NS1 has helicase activity and is involved in viral DNA transcription and replication. In addition, this protein has effects on the host cell, causing cell cycle arrest and apoptosis. Three distinct viral clades are known to circulate, indicated as genotypes 1, 2 and 3a/b, differing in nucleotide sequence by 10–15%.[8,9] Genotype distribution is geographically determined and also likely undergoing long-term shifts but presently genotype 1 is strongly

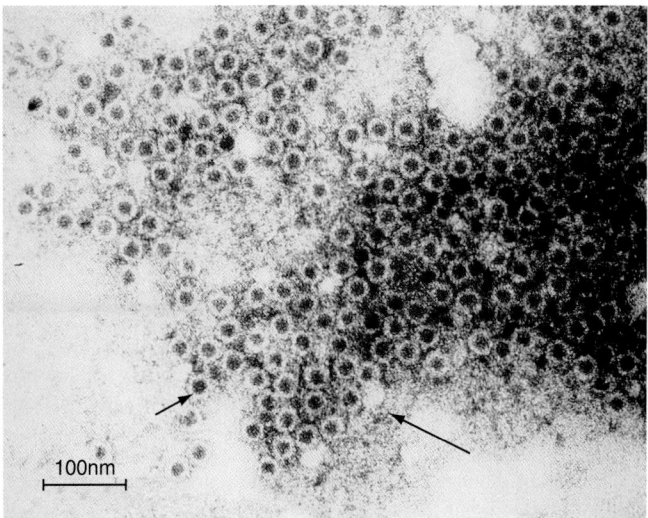

Figure 169-1 Electron micrograph of parvovirus B19 particles showing both full particles (short arrow) and empty capsids (long arrow). (*Courtesy of Stanley Naides, MD.*)

predominant. No clear correlations are present between the three genotypes and distinctive pathologic and clinical manifestations.

Epidemiology

Parvovirus B19 is found worldwide and infections occur in all seasons. In addition, two patterns can be recognized with regard to the occurrence of infections in time: a yearly peak in late winter and early spring in most moderate climates and a peak occurring at an approximate 4-yearly interval. This latter phenomenon of a cyclic pattern has been observed with other childhood exanthems, at least before vaccinations intervened, and is related to the proportion of susceptible hosts in the population. Transmission of B19 virus occurs via nasopharyngeal secretions and the infection spreads efficiently in households. Populations of children acquire B19 antibodies in an age-dependent fashion, beginning with entry into schools. Most surveys indicate that 50–70% of adults are anti-B19 virus IgG seropositive, indicating past infection and immunity. Clinical signs of infection occur after an incubation period of 7–18 days,[10] while infectivity is already present before this time. After infection B19 virus may be present in blood for some time[11,12] and may also resist current methods of blood decontamination. Therefore blood transfusion and pooled blood products may lead to transmission of infectious B19 virus, although this risk appears to be very small.

Pathogenicity

The particular tropism of parvovirus B19 for erythroid precursor cells plays a central role in the understanding of the pathogenesis of associated diseases. About 7–8 days after exposure to the virus, local replication in the bone marrow leads to a brisk viremia of 10^{11} or more viral particles/mL. In this same phase, the virus becomes detectable in respiratory secretions, leading to further spread. Viral replication causes maturation arrest at the giant pronormoblast stage of erythroid development, probably through viral induction of apoptosis.[13] Nonerythroid lineages may be affected as well, although these are less efficient in supporting B19 viral replication. Interestingly, in all infected individuals a temporary total disappearance of reticulocytes occurs reflecting an arrest of erythropoiesis, which is usually too short in duration to lead to any effect on hemoglobin levels. However, any underlying disorder affecting erythrocyte survival and the capacity to recruit additional erythroid progenitors will lead to prolonged and more severe effects on erythropoiesis, up to an aplastic crisis with severe anemia. Parvovirus B19 infection may also lead to an aplastic crisis in recipients of a recent hematopoietic stem cell transplant. Importantly, the same vulnerability applies to the expanding hematopoietic system of the fetus, explaining the observation of extreme fetal anemia with associated hydrops fetalis which may follow maternal infection during pregnancy. A few days after the peak of viremia antibodies appear and in this phase the clinical signs of erythema infectiosum may develop, characteristically consisting of a skin rash and arthralgia (see Chapter 9). This temporal association is a clear indication of the likely immunopathogenic origin of these signs.

Upon the development of immunity there is a strong decrease in viral titers in the blood, which does not always immediately lead to viral clearance. Virus may remain detectable in the blood at a low level for an extended period in some hosts, possibly reflecting a steady state level of viral clearance and replication.[11] Ultimately, in normal hosts the virus will be cleared from the blood but an impaired immune response may result in persistent or recurrent viremia and chronic or recurrent bone marrow suppression.[14] This sequence of events results in two clinical phases of illness (Figure 169-2), as observed in experimental infections.[10] In the first phase, mild fever, malaise and myalgia may occur during the viremia with associated areticulocytosis, leukopenia and thrombocytopenia. In the second phase, the appearance of antiviral antibodies is associated with a rash and arthralgia. In an infected pregnant woman, the virus may cross the placenta, most likely during the initial extreme peak of viremia.[15] This may lead to persistent arrest of the highly active erythropoiesis in the fetal liver, also because of the absence of an effective immune response in the fetus. The

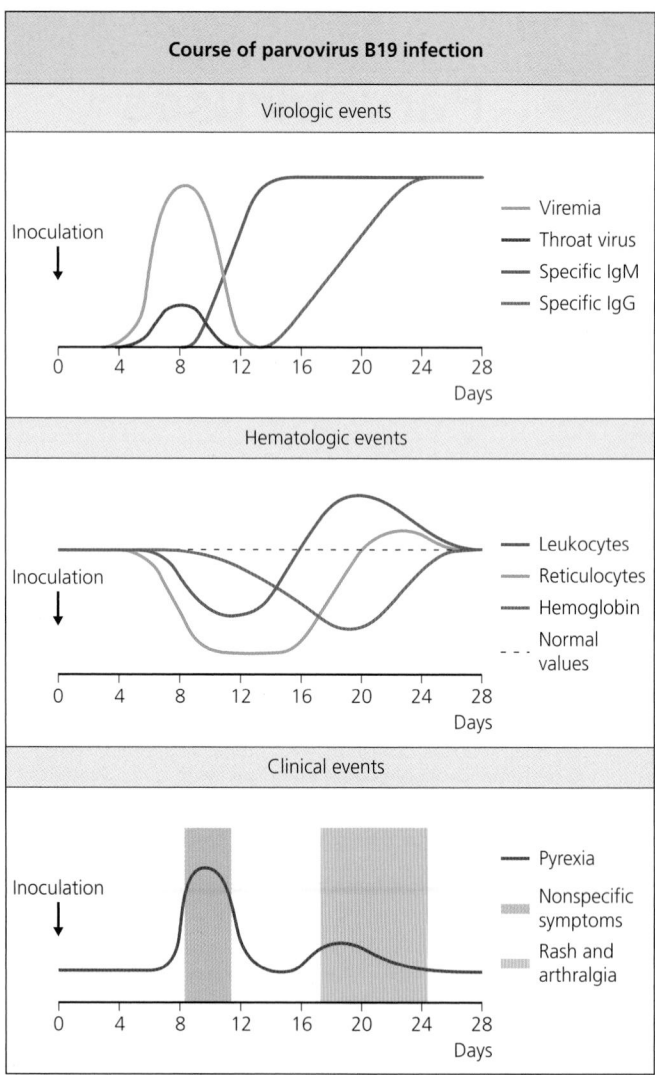

Figure 169-2 Course of parvovirus B19 infection. Volunteers were inoculated nasally with viremic serum and virologic, hematologic and clinical events observed. *(Courtesy of Stanley Naides, MD.)*

ensuing severe anemia results in high-output congestive heart failure, presenting as hydrops fetalis. Myocardial expression of the P-antigen in the fetus could imply an additional role of viral myocarditis as a cause of fetal cardiac failure but this has not been firmly established.

Prevention

Infected patients shed virus in nasopharyngeal secretions, following the viremic peak which occurs before the typical signs of erythema infectiosum are apparent. This severely limits the effects of measures based on clinical recognition of this disease. Hygiene regarding contact with secretions as well as precautions against the spread of infectious droplets are warranted if susceptible persons are involved. Patients should be considered infectious until 1 or 2 days after onset of rash.[16] Generally, attention is focused on pregnant women who have been in contact with (preferably proven) cases of erythema infectiosum. In these cases, it is important to determine potential susceptibility by testing for B19 virus-specific antibodies. Nonimmune exposed pregnant women should be offered further monitoring to enable a timely diagnosis of potential maternal and eventually fetal infection, which could necessitate an intrauterine blood transfusion.[17] The potential risk of viral transmission by blood transfusion could be relevant to recipients that are specifically vulnerable to this infection. Preventive strategies are an ongoing issue and include screening for the virus or selection of long-term seropositive donors for this purpose. A parvovirus B19 vaccine based on viral proteins VP1 and VP2, without the side effects associated with earlier candidates, has been described[18] but has not yet been clinically evaluated. There is no experience with the prophylactic administration of immunoglobulins.

Diagnostic Microbiology

The antibody response against the virus is very useful for diagnostic purposes. An acute infection can be confirmed by testing for IgM antibodies against B19 virus and immunity is demonstrated by the presence of IgG antibodies. Antibody determination employs recombinant capsid antigens (VP1, VP2), as the virus itself cannot be readily grown in tissue culture. The B19 virus can be demonstrated by testing for viral DNA by amplification techniques, although the extreme values during the initial peak in blood also allow detection by less sensitive hybridization techniques. This viral detection is particularly useful in cases of suspected fetal infections. Maternal serology alone is unable to confirm such infections, as maternal IgM does support the presence of this complication but may also notoriously be lacking in cases of established B19 virus-associated hydrops fetalis. Viral DNA can then be detected, often at extremely high levels, in amniotic fluid as well as umbilical cord blood samples obtained before intrauterine transfusion is started.[17] Quantitative viral DNA detection may provide useful additional information on the stage of the infection.[15,19–21] In such cases viral DNA is also present in maternal blood but levels are consistently much lower, suggesting a fetal origin of this viremia.

Detection of viral DNA is also important in the diagnosis of persisting infections in immunocompromised individuals, who may have chronic or recurrent viremia accompanied by poor IgM or IgG responses.[22] The extreme sensitivity of DNA-based techniques enables a diagnosis in outbreak settings if minute samples are used, as obtained by finger pricks.[23]

Unlike serological testing, viral DNA detection may encounter issues related to different viral genotypes, occasionally leading to false-negative results.[24]

Clinical Manifestations

The most frequently observed consequence of infection by parvovirus B19 is classic erythema infectiosum or 'fifth disease', characterized by a fairly typical exanthema described as 'slapped cheek' (Figure 169-3 and Chapter 9). It is clear that in persons with detectable B19-specific antibodies it is not always possible to recollect such a presentation and it is likely that only in a minority the full blown picture develops. The macular or maculopapular rash spreads to trunk and extremities and may be recurrently present for some time with conditions increasing skin perfusion. The rash as a clinical presentation is not highly specific and may be confused with several other conditions. Serologic confirmation is therefore advised to make a reliable diagnosis.

Accompanying joint symptoms are rare in children but may be severe in adults, more often in women. These consist of an acute, symmetric, rheumatoid-like polyarthritis which usually improves within 2 weeks but occasionally may persist for months. A more severe cutaneous disease, consisting of pruritic and painful acral erythema and edema is known as papular-purpuric gloves and socks syndrome. In addition to hands and feet, oral and genital mucosa may also be involved. Parvovirus B19 infection is most often associated with this condition.[25] In individuals with underlying disorders of erythropoiesis, such as sickle cell disease or hereditary spherocytosis, parvovirus B19 infection may lead to a transient aplastic crisis with severe anemia.[26] Although the erythroid precursors are most severely affected, in some cases thrombocytopenia or pancytopenia may occur, rarely even

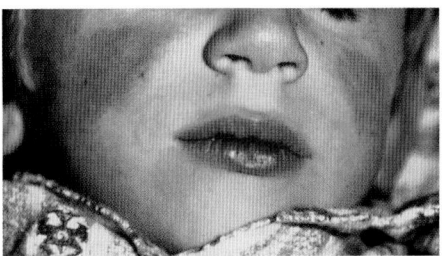

Figure 169-3 Classic 'slapped cheeks' of a child with erythema infectiosum, or fifth disease, caused by parvovirus B19. A lacy macular erythematous eruption is also present on the trunk but not shown. *(Courtesy of Dr K. Motton.)*

without an underlying hematologic disorder. Failure to clear parvovirus B19 effectively after infection in immunocompromised hosts may lead to a chronic suppression of erythropoiesis. Persistent B19 virus infection should be suspected in cases of transplant recipients[22] or untreated HIV infections,[27] presenting with chronic anemia. B19 virus can also complicate recovery after chemotherapy for leukemia.[28] As a consequence of infection during pregnancy, infection of the unborn child occurs in up to half of the cases. This may lead to the development of hydrops fetalis, again as a consequence of erythroid suppression. Affected fetuses present with extremely low hemoglobin values; if untreated, fetal death is often the consequence, although spontaneous recovery may occur (see also Chapter 56).

A number of other conditions have more rarely been associated with a concomitant parvovirus B19 infection, mainly based on case reports but with a consistent pattern emerging. These include viral hepatitis,[29] glomerulonephritis[30] and a variety of peripheral as well as central neurologic complications, notably brachial plexus neuritis and encephalitic syndromes.[31] A frequent association with cardiac disorders, including myocarditis, that was initially reported based on finding viral DNA in blood in affected patients, has been refuted by the clearly documented persistence of viral DNA in myocardial tissue in probably all seropositive persons.[32] The passive release of viral DNA upon any myocardial damage explains the finding of viral DNA without any further indications of infection. Since parvovirus DNA is indeed known to persist in several tissues after the initial high viremic peak,[33] any disease association based only on finding viral DNA should be approached with caution.

Management

No specific antiviral therapy is available to treat parvovirus B19 infection. Erythema infectiosum usually does not require treatment, though joint pain may benefit from anti-inflammatory drugs if it is severe. Transient aplastic crisis usually requires blood transfusion to reduce the consequences of severe anemia but will recover in a matter of weeks. In immunocompromised patients with persistent B19 virus infection and chronic anemia, intravenous immunoglobulin treatment is often effective, leading to clearance of the infection and resolution of bone marrow suppression.[22,27] B19 virus-associated fetal hydrops requires urgent intrauterine transfusion to correct the severe anemia present with this condition and to prevent fetal death.[17] Although B19 virus in general is not considered a cause of congenital anomalies, it appears that correction of the anemia does not prevent some neurodevelopmental delay in these children.[34]

References available online at expertconsult.com.

KEY REFERENCES

Barah F., Whiteside S., Batista S., et al.: Neurological aspects of human parvovirus B19 infection: a systematic review. *Rev Med Virol* 2014; 24:154-168.

Chisaka H., Morita E., Yaegashi N., et al.: Parvovirus B19 and the pathogenesis of anaemia. *Rev Med Virol* 2003; 13:347-359.

De Jong E.P., Walther F.J., Kroes A.C., et al.: Parvovirus B19 infection in pregnancy: new insights and management. *Prenat Diagn* 2011; 31:419-425.

Schenk T., Enders M., Pollak S., et al.: High prevalence of human parvovirus B19 DNA in myocardial autopsy samples from subjects without myocarditis or dilative cardiomyopathy. *J Clin Microbiol* 2009; 47:106-110.

Servant-Delmas A., Lefrère J.J., Morinet F., et al.: Advances in human B19 erythrovirus biology. *J Virol* 2010; 84:9658-9665.

Young N.S., Brown K.E.: Parvovirus B19. *N Engl J Med* 2004; 350:586-597.

170

Poxviruses

R. MARK L. BULLER

Nature

VIRION MORPHOLOGY, STRUCTURE AND BIOCHEMISTRY

Using negative-staining electron microscopy and/or cryo-electron microscopy, parapoxvirus virions appear ovoid with long and short axes of approximately 260 and 160 nm, respectively, whereas all other poxviruses are 'brick'-shaped, with dimensions of 350 × 250 nm on average (Figure 170-1).

Depending on the poxvirus, the genome can range from 130 kbp for the parapoxviruses to 300 kbp for the avipoxviruses. A schematic intracellular replication cycle based on the poxvirus vaccinia is presented in Figure 170-2 and described in more detail by Moss.[1] The poxvirus virion is notoriously stable in the environment, and this stability is increased by its association with the A-type inclusion bodies or scab material. Thus for poxviruses, fomites must be considered in disease transmission.

POXVIRUSES PATHOGENIC FOR HUMANS

Ten poxviruses infect humans (Table 170-1).[2] Except for the 'extinct' variola virus and molluscum contagiosum virus, the poxvirus diseases are zoonoses. With rare exception these zoonotic poxviruses fail to establish a human chain of transmission. Recently, outbreaks of human orthopoxvirus diseases have become more frequent due to the cessation in smallpox vaccination.[3] Most human poxvirus infections occur through minor abrasions in the skin. Orf, molluscum contagiosum and monkeypox viruses cause the most frequent poxvirus infections worldwide. Individuals with atopic dermatitis may be predisposed to poxvirus infections such as molluscum contagiosum, orf or cowpox.

Prevention

Because most poxvirus infections are rare zoonoses or cause only superficial 'nuisance' skin lesions in immunocompetent individuals, there are no recommended prevention strategies other than education of patients and various types of workers as to how the diseases are spread.

Molluscum Contagiosum Virus

Epidemiology

GEOGRAPHIC RANGE

Molluscum contagiosum virus has a worldwide distribution. Restriction endonuclease analysis of genomic DNA from molluscum contagiosum virus isolates has revealed the existence of at least four virus subtypes or strains, and one recent study suggests the distribution of subtypes can vary geographically.[4]

PREVALENCE AND INCIDENCE

For nonsexually-transmitted molluscum contagiosum, the disease appears more prevalent in the tropics than in Europe. For example, molluscum contagiosum was diagnosed in 1.2% of outpatients in Aberdeen, UK between 1956 and 1963, the mean age of infection was between 10 and 12 years and spread within households and schools was infrequent. On the other hand, in Fiji in 1966, 4.5% of an entire village had the disease, mean age of infection was between 2 and 3 years and 25% of households harbored more than one case.[5,6] Prevalence of infection in New Guinea was greater than 50% in many villages. A more recent study of 289 German adults and children found an overall seroprevalence of 14.8% with a low rate in children below the age of one (4.5%), a high rate in children between 2 and 10 years (25%) and an intermediate rate in subjects between ages 11 and 40 years (12.5%).[7] In England between 1971 and 1985 there was a 400% increase in cases of genital molluscum contagiosum; the majority of patients were aged 15–24 years, with affected women being younger than affected men. Molluscum contagiosum is a common and sometimes severely disfiguring opportunistic infection of patients with untreated HIV infection. Pre-existing atopic dermatitis may predispose children to infection as one study found 24% of molluscum contagiosum patients were also diagnosed with atopic dermatitis.[8]

Pathogenicity

TRANSMISSION

Molluscum contagiosum is observed in children and adults, with spread within this latter group governed in part by sexual practices. Nonsexual transmission is a consequence of infection by direct contact or through fomites. Case histories have suggested transmission from surgeons' fingers, swimming pools, bath towels in gymnasia, contact

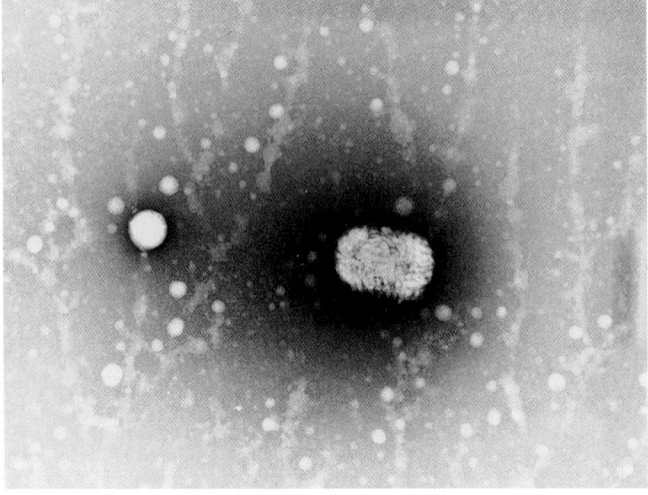

Figure 170-1 Negative-stained molluscum contagiosum virus from lesion material.

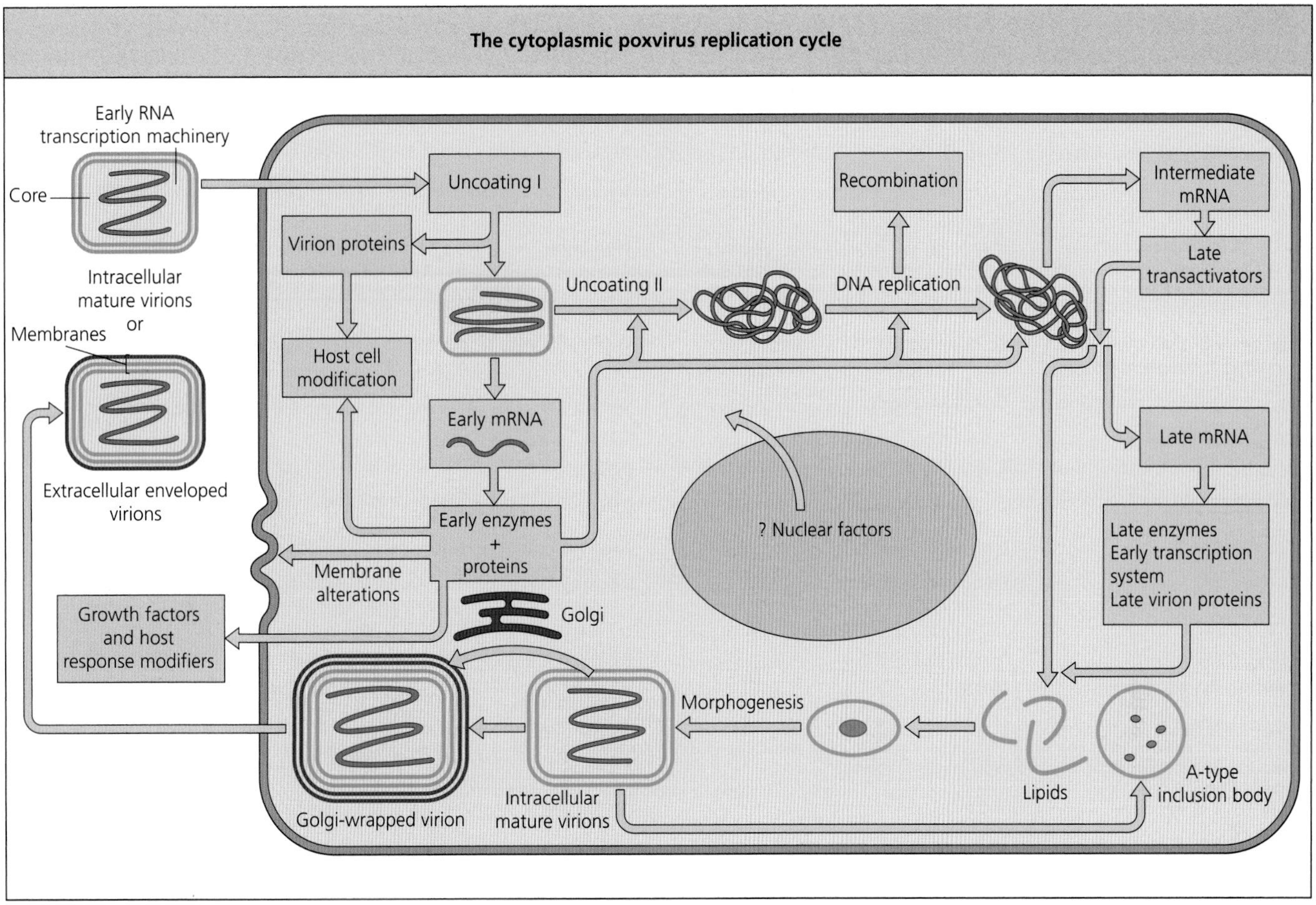

The cytoplasmic poxvirus replication cycle

Figure 170-2 The cytoplasmic poxvirus replication cycle. Poxvirus virions containing early RNA transcription machinery attach to, and fuse with, the plasma membrane (uncoating I). Early genes are expressed that code for a variety of functions that modify the host cell for optimal virus replication, attenuate the host response to infection and mediate virus synthetic processes. After further uncoating (II), the virus genome is replicated via concatemers, late transcription factors are expressed from interme-diate genes and late gene RNA is synthesized. Late genes encode the early transcription system, enzymes and structural proteins necessary for virion assembly, which commences with the formation of membrane structures in the intermediate compartment and the packaging of resolved unit length genomic DNA. The intracellular mature virion has one membrane derived from the intermediate compartment. It may remain in the cytoplasm or (in certain virus species) become occluded in an A-type inclusion body or become wrapped by a further two membranes in the Golgi and exported from the cell with the loss of one membrane (extracellular enveloped virions). The extracellular enveloped virions are thought to be most important in cell-to-cell spread and systemic disease. This replication scheme is based on the study of the prototypic poxvirus vaccinia.[1] Other poxvirus species probably vary from this model mainly in the types of growth factors and host response modifiers encoded by the virus and the amounts of extracellular enveloped virions produced. *(Adapted from Moss, B. In: Fields, B.N., et al. [eds]. Fields virology, 5th ed. Philadelphia: Lippincott Williams and Wilkins; 2007:2905-2945.)*

between wrestlers and as a result of tattooing.[5] Lesions can be commonly observed on opposing surfaces and the virus can be further spread on the person by autoinoculation.

LESION HISTOPATHOLOGY

Molluscum contagiosum virus has one of the narrowest cell tropisms of any virus, replicating only in the human keratinocyte of the epidermis. As the virus-infected cell approaches the surface of the skin, the accumulation of progeny virions in a granular matrix in the cytoplasm forces the cell organelles, including the nucleus, to the periphery of the cell. Under light microscopy these cells stain as hyaline acidophilic masses, are referred to as molluscum or Henderson–Patterson bodies and are pathognomonic for disease (Figure 170-3). Higher magnifications of molluscum bodies reveal them to be entirely filled with virions, partial virions and debris.

Clinical Manifestations

SIGNS, SYMPTOMS AND SEVERITY

Molluscum contagiosum manifests as small clusters of lesions in immunocompetent individuals. The lesions are generally painless; they appear on the trunk and limbs (rarely palms and soles) in the nonsexually-transmitted disease. In children, the virus can also be

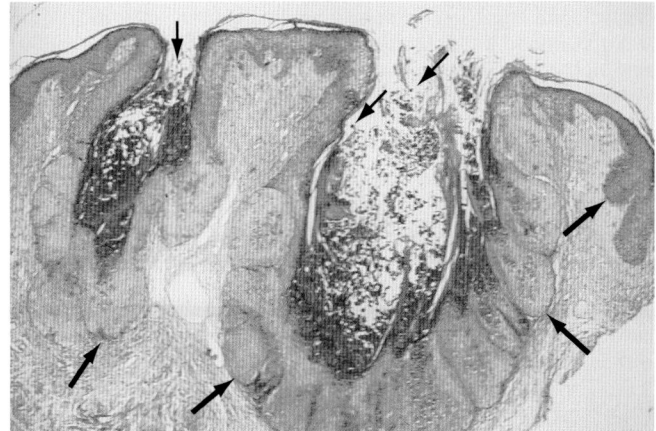

Figure 170-3 Molluscum contagiosum lesion. In this lesion a major and minor umbilicus has formed as a result of the hypertrophy of infected cells and hyperplasia of the basal cells, which caused a severe invagination of the epidermis but no loss of integrity of the basement membrane. The molluscum bodies stain as pink to purple acidophilic hyaline masses up to 37 × 27 µm in size. Small arrows: molluscum bodies. Large arrows: epidermis–dermis boundary. (H & E.)

TABLE 170-1	Poxviruses Pathogenic for Humans Presented by Genus in Order of Importance for Human Disease		
Genus/Species	**Hosts**	**Geographic Distribution**	**Disease**
MOLLUSCIPOXVIRUS			
Molluscum contagiosum virus	Humans*	Worldwide	Molluscum contagiosum, single or multiple skin nodules
PARAPOXVIRUS			
Orf virus (contagious pustular dermatitis virus or contagious ecthyma virus)	Sheep*, goats, dogs, bighorn sheep, thinhorn sheep, Rocky Mountain goat, chamois, reindeer, musk-ox, Himalayan tahr, steenbok, alpaca	Worldwide	Orf, localized skin lesions
Pseudocowpox virus (milkers' nodule or paravaccinia)	European cattle*	Worldwide	Milkers' nodule, localized skin lesions
Bovine papular stomatitis virus	European cattle*	Worldwide	Localized skin lesions
ORTHOPOXVIRUS			
Cowpox virus	Rodents*, cats, cows, zoo animals	Europe, western Asia	Cowpox, localized pustular lesions
Monkeypox virus	Squirrels*, monkeys	Western and central Africa	Monkeypox, rash, generalized disease
Vaccinia virus	Natural host unknown (buffalo† and cattle)	Asia, India, Brazil and laboratory	Buffalopox, localized pustular lesions
Variola virus	Eradicated from humans in 1977	Was worldwide	Smallpox, rash, generalized disease
YATAPOXVIRUS			
Tanapox virus	Monkeys?, rodents?	Eastern and central Africa	Tanapox, localized nodular skin lesions
Yaba monkey tumor poxvirus	Monkeys?	Western Africa	Localized nodular skin lesions

*Natural reservoir.
†During the smallpox eradication program, water buffalo in India and cattle in Brazil were infected with the local vaccine strain of vaccinia virus, which apparently persists in these animals and occasionally infects humans.
?Putative host

fairly common in the skin of the eyelids, with solitary or multiple lesions, and can be complicated by chronic follicular conjunctivitis and later by a superficial punctate keratitis. There may be an associated erythema 1–11 months after the appearance of the lesion, with no correlation to a history of allergy or eczema. Lesions can persist for as little as 2 weeks or as long as 2 years. Re-infections can be common. As a sexually transmitted disease in teenagers and adults, the lesions are mostly on the lower abdominal wall, pubis, inner thighs and genitalia. As yet there is no solid correlation of virion DNA type with specific pathology or location of lesions (i.e. genital versus nongenital).[9]

In immunocompromised individuals (especially those with untreated HIV infection), the infection is not self-limiting, with more frequent and larger lesions present especially on the face, neck, scalp and upper body. Multiple adjacent lesions sometimes become confluent. Molluscum contagiosum can be considered a cutaneous marker of severe immunodeficiency.

GROSS LESION PATHOLOGY

In immunocompetent patients, molluscum contagiosum virus lesions are epidermal, flesh-colored, raised nodules of 2–5 mm in diameter (Figure 170-4). Occasionally the gross lesions may have a hypopigmented or erythematous halo, which can precede resolution. Rarely they will present as a large lesion called giant molluscum (>5 mm in diameter). Both types of lesion usually have an umbilicated center and have been reported frequently in severely immunodeficient individuals with HIV infection.

Diagnosis and Differential Diagnosis

The diagnosis is usually made clinically, based on the gross appearance of the lesions and their chronic nature. Confirmation is easily obtained through the detection of molluscum bodies.

Molluscum contagiosum (especially giant molluscum) can be confused with a number of other disorders such as keratoacanthoma, warty dyskeratoma, syringomas, hidrocystomas, basal cell epithelioma,

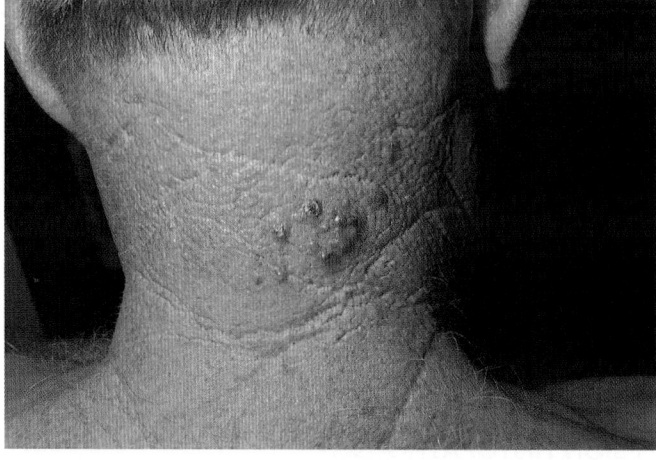

Figure 170-4 Molluscum contagiosum lesions. These are the more typical, but still large, lesions of molluscum contagiosum. (*Courtesy of J. Burnett.*)

trichoepithelioma, ectopic hyperplastic sebaceous glands or giant condylomata acuminata, chalazion, sebaceous cysts, verrucas, milia, lid abscess or granuloma on eyelids.[10] In immunodeficient patients, disseminated cutaneous cryptococcosis and cutaneous histoplasmosis can resemble typical molluscum contagiosum.[10] An inflamed molluscum lesion without the association of typical lesions can be mistaken for a bacterial infection.

Parapoxviruses

The parapoxviruses orf, bovine stomatitis and pseudocowpox collectively cause occupational infections known as the 'farmyard-pox' diseases, with orf infections being the most common.

Epidemiology

GEOGRAPHIC RANGE

Orf in sheep and goat populations has been reported in Canada, the USA, Europe, Japan, New Zealand and Africa. Pseudocowpox virus and bovine papular stomatitis virus are both maintained in European-derived dairy herds in all parts of the world.

PREVALENCE AND INCIDENCE

In a 1-year New Zealand study, 500 meat workers out of a population of 20 000 at risk were infected with orf; those involved in the initial stunning, killing and hanging of the sheep had the highest risk (4%) of infection.[11] Serologic surveys of orf-infected sheep and goat herds yielded orf antibody prevalence of up to 90%. The high seroprevalence of orf antibody in herds is likely attributable to the highly stable nature of the orf virion, which contaminates the pasture.

Pseudocowpox virus and bovine papular stomatitis are probably endemic in all European-derived dairy herds.

Pathogenicity

TRANSMISSION

Direct transmission of orf virus has been observed as a consequence of bottle-feeding lambs, from animal bites to the hand and contact with sheep and goat products during slaughter. Fomites such as splinters, barbed wire or farmyard surfaces, including soil, feeding troughs or barn beams, have been implicated as sources of virus. No human-to-human transmission of parapoxvirus infections has been reported.

Pseudocowpox virus from lesions on teats of cows is a major source of virus for milkers' nodule of the hand.

Bovine papular stomatitis virus infection of humans occurs generally from lesions confined to the mouth, tongue, lips or nares and occasionally from the teats of infected cattle.

LESION HISTOPATHOLOGY

Epidermis

The most striking change in the epidermis is hyperplasia in which strands of epidermal keratinocytes penetrate the dermis.[12] Generally, a mild to moderate degree of acanthosis is detected, and parakeratosis is a common feature. Cytoplasmic vacuolation, nuclear vacuolation and deeply eosinophilic, homogeneous cytoplasmic inclusion bodies often surrounded by a pale halo are also characteristic of the infection. An intense infiltrate of lymphocytes, polymorphs or eosinophils frequently involves the epidermis.

Dermis

A dense, predominantly lymphohistiocytic inflammatory cell infiltrate is present in all cases with marked edema. The most striking feature of the dermis is the massive capillary proliferation and dilatation.

Clinical Manifestations

SIGNS, SYMPTOMS AND SEVERITY

Clinical manifestations of orf usually occur 3–4 weeks after infection. The disease involves the appearance of single or multiple nodules (diameters of 6–27 mm),[12] which are sometimes painful, usually on the hands and, less frequently, on the head or neck (Figure 170-5). Orf illness can also be associated with a low-grade fever, swelling of the lymph nodes and/or erythema multiforme bullosum. Disease resolution occurs over 4–6 weeks, usually without complication; however, autoinoculation of the eye can lead to serious sequelae, and enlarged lesions can arise in humans suffering from immunosuppressive conditions, burns or atopic dermatitis.[13] Lesion healing can be complicated by bullous pemphigoid. Re-infections have been documented.

Pseudocowpox virus lesions usually appear on the hands and are relatively painless, but may itch. The draining lymph node may be enlarged. The nodules are gradually absorbed and disappear in 4–6 weeks.[14]

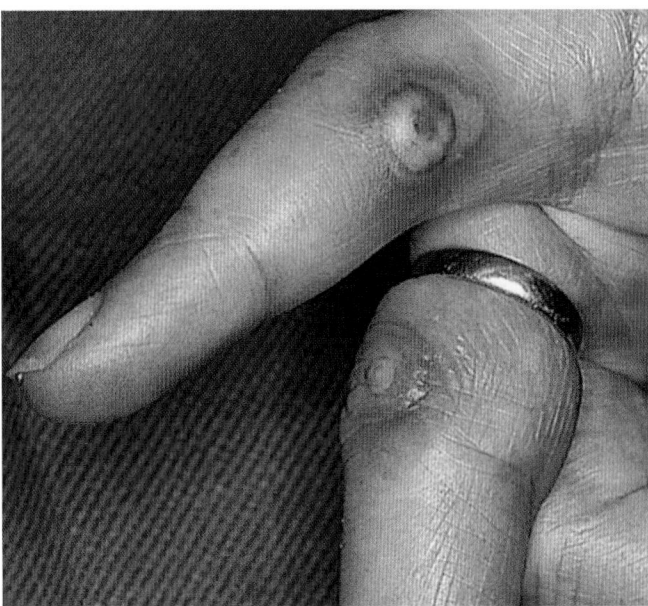

Figure 170-5   Typical lesions of orf on the hand. *(From Viral infections – warts and other viral infections. In: Gawkrodger, D.J., Arden-Jones, M.R., eds. Dermatology: an illustrated colour text. Edinburgh: Churchill Livingstone Elsevier; 2012: 52-53.)*

In bovine papular stomatitis, lesions occur on the hands, diminish after 14 days and are no longer evident 3–4 weeks after onset.[15]

GROSS LESION PATHOLOGY

The orf lesion characteristically evolves through a maculopapular target stage in which a red center is surrounded by a white ring of cells and a red halo of inflammation (approximately 1–2 weeks after infection); however, patients usually present later when the lesion is at the granulomatous or papillomatous stages.[13]

In pseudocowpox virus infection, milkers' nodules are first observed as round, cherry-red papules; these develop into purple, smooth nodules of up to 2 cm in diameter and may be umbilicated. The lesions rarely ulcerate.[14]

The lesions of bovine papular stomatitis appear as circumscribed wart-like nodules that gradually enlarge until they are 3–8 mm in diameter.[15]

Diagnosis and Differential Diagnosis

Parapoxvirus disease diagnosis is by clinical (lesion morphology), epidemiologic (recent contact with cattle or sheep) and laboratory findings (the presence in scab material of genomic DNA or ovoid-shaped virions with distinctive criss-cross filament patterns).[12] Orf should be included in the differential diagnosis of patients with clinically compatible skin lesions and a history of household meat processing or animal slaughter.[16]

Without knowing the animal source of the infection, orf cannot easily be differentiated from milkers' nodule on the basis of clinical finding, histology or electron microscopy (i.e. disease acquired from sheep is orf and from cattle is milkers' nodule or possibly bovine papular stomatitis).[12] Atypical giant orf lesions in patients who are immunocompromised or suffering from burns or atopic dermatitis may be confused with pyogenic granuloma.[13] Orf can also be misdiagnosed as inflammatory vascular neoplasms.

Orthopoxviruses

Although four orthopoxviruses have been shown to cause disease in humans, only two still cause significant human infections. With the global eradication of smallpox in 1977, the causative agent variola virus no longer circulates in human populations, but there is concern that it may be used as a biologic weapon by terrorist groups or rogue nations (see Chapter 75).[17]

In nature, vaccinia virus infections are limited to exposure to a vaccinia-like virus infecting milking buffalos and dairy cattle in Asia and Africa (called buffalopox) and cattle in Brazil (Cantagalo virus).[18] Vaccinia virus (smallpox vaccine) is used also in the immunization of personnel in the laboratory, but is not recommended at this time for the general population due to the occurrence of frequent and sometimes severe complications;[17] however, it may be used in a post-exposure capacity in the event of an outbreak of a highly transmissible human orthopoxvirus infection.[19] Currently only monkeypox virus causes significant human infections.

Epidemiology

GEOGRAPHIC RANGE

Traditionally monkeypox virus is found in the tropical rain forests of countries in western and central Africa, most notably the Democratic Republic of Congo, but its range may be expanding. In 2003 monkeypox virus was imported into the USA in a shipment of rodents destined for the pet trade, and in 2005 an outbreak was recorded in southern Sudan.[20] The reservoir of monkeypox virus in nature is most likely the African arboreal squirrels (*Funisciurus* and *Heliosciurus* spp.), other rodents and perhaps monkeys. Cowpox virus is extremely diverse genetically[21] and is endemic in Europe and some western states of the former Soviet Union. Rodents (voles, wood mice and rats) have been implicated as reservoirs of cowpox virus; cows, zoo animals and cats are incidental hosts.

PREVALENCE AND INCIDENCE

Intensive surveillance between 1981 and 1986 in Zaire by the World Health Organization confirmed 338 cases of human monkeypox, with the greatest risk of infection to inhabitants of small villages within 100 m of tropical rain forests.[22] In recent years there has been an increase in frequency of human monkeypox in Africa, perhaps due in part to cessation of vaccination for smallpox.[23]

Although humans have been infected by cows and rodents, the domestic cat is responsible for the majority of human cowpox infections. Between 1969 and 1993 there were approximately 45 human cowpox cases in the UK, three published case histories from Germany and two each from Belgium, Sweden and France.[24]

Pathogenicity

TRANSMISSION

The route of monkeypox virus infection of humans from animal sources has not been well-studied. Person-to-person transmission (like eradicated smallpox) is believed to be by the upper respiratory tract, with virus released in oropharyngeal secretions of patients who have a rash.[22] Unlike smallpox, monkeypox person-to-person transmission is very inefficient and rarely surpasses three generations.[22]

Cowpox virus is acquired usually by direct introduction of the virus from an animal source into minor abrasions in the skin; however, 30% of infections show no known risk factor.[24]

LESION HISTOPATHOLOGY

Orthopoxvirus lesions are characterized by epidermal hyperplasia, with infected cells becoming swollen, vacuolated and undergoing 'ballooning degeneration'.

Clinical Manifestations

SIGNS, SYMPTOMS AND SEVERITY

Approximately 12 days after infection with monkeypox virus, fever and headache occur. This is followed 1–3 days later by rash and generalized lymphadenopathy. The rash (the number of lesions is variable) appears first on the face and generally has a centrifugal distribution. The illness lasts 2–4 weeks, depending on its severity. The case fatality rate is approximately 12% when caused by strains from the Congo River Basin.[22]

With cowpox virus infection, a lesion, usually solitary, appears on the hands or face; this can be extremely painful, and the patient can present with systemic symptoms, including pyrexia, malaise, lethargy, sore throat and local lymphadenopathy. Complete recovery takes between 3 and 8 weeks. Person-to-person transmission has not been reported. Complications can include ocular or generalized infections; the latter occurs in patients who have atopic dermatitis, allergic asthma or atopic eczema and in one case was associated with death.[24]

GROSS LESION PATHOLOGY

The monkeypox virus skin lesions begin as macules but rapidly progress to pustules. About 8 or 9 days after the onset of rash the pustules become umbilicated and dry up; by 14–16 days after the onset of the rash a crust has formed. Most skin lesions are about 0.5 cm in diameter.[22]

The cowpox lesion appears as an inflamed macule, progresses through an increasingly hemorrhagic vesicle stage to a pustule that ulcerates and crusts over by the end of the second week to become a deep-seated, hard black eschar 1–3 cm in diameter.[24]

Diagnosis and Differential Diagnosis

The diagnosis of monkeypox infection requires clinical (rash), epidemiologic (equatorial Africa) and laboratory findings (the presence of genomic DNA or brick-shaped virions in scab material). Although the rash with associated lymphadenopathy is usually pathognomonic, the sporadic nature of the disease makes it difficult to arrive at an accurate diagnosis solely on clinical grounds.[22]

Diagnosis of cowpox virus infection is rarely made on clinical findings (lesion morphology and systemic illness) and usually requires laboratory results (the presence of genomic DNA or brick-shaped virion in scab material). Cowpox should be considered in patients who have had contact with cats and who present in July to October with a painful hemorrhagic vesicle or black eschar, with or without erythema, accompanied by lymphadenopathy and a systemic illness.[24]

Monkeypox can be confused with a number of other conditions that result in a rash:

- chickenpox, although its varicella-zoster lesions are more superficial, appear in crops and have a centripetal distribution;
- tanapox, except the tanapox lesions evolve slowly, are nodular and large, without pustulation; and
- syphilis, although the secondary rash of syphilis does not evolve past the papular stage.[22]

Generalized cowpox can be misdiagnosed as eczema herpeticum, whereas localized cowpox is most frequently misdiagnosed as:

- orf or milkers' nodules, although the parapoxvirus lesion is clinically distinct, and there are often no systemic disease symptoms;
- herpesvirus reactivation, even though herpes lesions are not usually hemorrhagic or erythematous and the scab is not so deep-seated and of lighter color; and
- anthrax, although the anthrax lesion is painless and rapidly progresses to the eschar stage (5–6 days).[24]

Diagnostic Microbiology

The appropriate biosafety level precautions must be taken for the handling, transport and processing of infected lesion material.

MOLLUSCUM CONTAGIOSUM VIRUS

For a squash preparation the keratotic dome-shaped molluscum lesion is placed on a regular slide and under a coverslip or second slide. The lesion is flattened and can be examined using light microscopy either directly or after staining with Wright's or methylene blue stains. Round to ovoid molluscum bodies up to 37 × 27 μm are diagnostic of molluscum contagiosum.[5]

For histopathologic analysis, a biopsy specimen is fixed in 10% formal saline and submitted for wax embedding, sectioning at 5 μm and staining with hematoxylin and eosin. Microscopic examination should provide a field of view similar to that shown in Figure 170-3.

PARAPOXVIRUS, ORTHOPOXVIRUS AND YATAPOXVIRUS

Orthopoxvirus (brick-shaped), parapoxvirus (ovoid) and tanapox virus (enveloped brick-shaped) virions can be differentiated from one another by an experienced electron microscopist. Polymerase chain reaction is rapidly becoming the assay of choice for laboratory diagnosis of poxvirus infections.[25,26]

Management

The management of parapoxvirus, orthopoxvirus and yatapoxvirus infections is mainly supportive in immunocompetent subjects.

MOLLUSCUM CONTAGIOSUM VIRUS

There is no FDA-approved therapy for molluscum contagiosum. Since infection of immunocompetent patients is generally self-limiting and resolves within 6 to 9 months, no therapeutic intervention is an effective and rational approach in certain situations with a small number of lesions. Curettage, cryotherapy, and cantharidin are considered the first-line treatment strategies, with cantharidin the most popular treatment of American dermatologists.[27,28] Immunocompromised patients can develop severe and persistent molluscum contagiosum infections that can be treated with intravenous cidofovir or topical 2% cidofovir ointment.[28]

PARAPOXVIRUS, ORTHOPOXVIRUS AND YATAPOXVIRUS

At this time there are no approved systemic or topical chemotherapeutic agents commercially available for the treatment of poxvirus infections. Vaccinia immune globulin (VIG) is available from Centers for Disease Control and Prevention (CDC) as an investigational new drug, but its efficacy has yet to be convincingly demonstrated for orthopoxvirus infections. Brincidofovir and tecovirimat are two promising therapies for poxviruses and orthopoxviruses, respectively.[29]

References available online at expertconsult.com.

KEY REFERENCES

Breman J.G., Henderson D.A.: Diagnosis and management of smallpox. *N Engl J Med* 2002; 346:1300-1308.

Damon I.K.: Poxviruses. In: Fields B.N., Knipe D.M., Howley P.M., eds. *Fields virology*, 5th ed. Philadelphia: Lippincott Williams and Wilkins; 2007:2947-2975.

Keckler M.S., Reynolds M.G., Damon I.K., et al.: The effects of post-exposure smallpox vaccination on clinical disease presentation: Addressing the data gaps between historical epidemiology and modern surrogate model data. *Vaccine* 2013; 31:5192-5201.

McCollum A.M. Damon I.K.: Human monkeypox. *Clin Infect Dis* 2014; 58:260-267.

Moye V.A., Cathcart S., Morrell D.S.: Safety of cantharidin: A retrospective review of cantharidin treatment in 405 children with molluscum contagiousum. *Ped Derm* 2014; 31:450-454.

Nguyen H.P. Tyring S.K.: An update on the clinical management of cutaneous molluscum contagiousm. *Skin Therapy Letter* 2014; 19:5-8.

Rimoin A.W., Mulembakani P.M., Johnston S.C., et al.: Major increase in human monkeypox incidence 30 years after smallpox vaccination campaigns cease in the Democratic Republic of Congo. *Proc Nat Acad Sci USA* 2010; 107:16262-16267.

Shchelkunov S.N.: An increasing danger of zoonotic orthopoxvirus infections. *PLOS Pathogens* 2013; 9(12): e1003756.

171

Rabies and Rabies-Related Viruses

MARY J. WARRELL | DAVID A. WARRELL

KEY CONCEPTS

- Rabies encephalitis due to canine rabies virus is 100% fatal in unvaccinated patients.

- No deaths have been reported in anyone who had had both pre-exposure vaccination and postexposure boosting.

- Pre-exposure immunization should be encouraged for residents of, and travelers to, dog rabies enzootic countries.

- Dog rabies is the source of 98% of human rabies deaths.

- Rabies virus types found in bats in the Americas appear to be less pathogenic in humans.

- There is not yet any specific treatment for rabies encephalitis.

- Intensive care therapy is only recommended for certain encephalitis patients, those previously immunized or if infected by an American bat rabies virus.

- Palliation is advised for the vast majority of symptomatic patients.

Nature

Rabies is a zoonosis of dogs and other mammals that is occasionally transmitted to humans, causing fatal encephalomyelitis. Dog rabies virus is universally fatal in unvaccinated humans causing more than 98% of human rabies deaths. However, prophylaxis can be 100% effective, so all human deaths represent failure of prevention.

Lyssaviruses are members of the large Rhabdoviridae family infecting animals and plants. The *Lyssavirus* classification and terminology have changed from genotypes to species. Rabies virus is the type species, species 1 of the genus, which also contains 11 rabies-related *Lyssavirus* species. They are divided into three phylogroups. All six species known to cause the typical fatal encephalitis in man are in phylogroup I. (See end of chapter.)

Structure

The bullet-shaped virions contain a nonsegmented negative strand of rabies RNA encoding five proteins. The RNA is coiled with a nucleoprotein, a phosphoprotein and an RNA-dependent RNA polymerase to form a helical ribonucleoprotein complex or nucleocapsid. This is covered by a matrix protein. An outer envelope studded with the virus-coded, glycoprotein-bearing, club-shaped projections is acquired by budding through a host cell lipid membrane. Rabies virus strains from different vector species and geographic areas are distinguished by nucleotide sequencing.

Epidemiology

ANIMAL RABIES

Rabies is enzootic in most parts of the world. Globally, the domestic dog is the most important reservoir species and is the dominant vector in Asia, Africa and some areas of Latin America[1] including Bolivia, Brazil, Haiti and the Dominican Republic. Separate reservoirs of enzootic infection occur in certain wild mammalian species (Table 171-1). Sylvatic rabies[2] predominates in North America, Europe, parts of southern Africa and the Caribbean. All mammals are potentially susceptible, and infection may be transmitted to other species, including domestic animals, especially cats, and to humans. Lyssaviruses have not been reported from a few areas including Iceland, Italy, Cyprus, some other Mediterranean islands, Singapore, Sabah, Sarawak, New Guinea, New Zealand, Antarctica, Oceania, Hong Kong islands, Japan and some Caribbean islands. Although these countries have no apparent current indigenous rabies, infected animals cross national boundaries and so infection may be imported. Rabies (species 1) infects terrestrial mammalian reservoir species and bats in the Americas. Western Europe and Australia are free of rabies in terrestrial mammals, but rabies-related lyssaviruses are found in bats (see end of chapter). As the epizootiology changes constantly, up-to-date local advice should be sought for detailed information.

HUMAN RABIES

Estimates of human rabies mortality are notoriously unreliable in tropical areas where about 99% of the deaths occur. The much quoted estimate of 55 000 deaths annually in Asia and Africa was deduced and extrapolated from data on the incidence of human dog bites. A well-designed Indian verbal autopsy survey discovered 12 700 furious encephalitic rabies deaths annually.[3] This estimate excluded paralytic cases. Other areas of high incidence include Bangladesh and Pakistan. There is very little surveillance in Africa.

In Europe over the last 10 years, the average annual mortality was nine deaths, predominantly in Russia and Ukraine.[4] Ten percent were imported, mainly from Asia or Africa. In the USA, an average of three cases are diagnosed annually. About 60% of cases are indigenous, of which 95% are caused by insectivorous bat rabies virus. Although fewer than 20 percent of such North American patients remember a bat bite, possible bat contact is more often reported.

Pathogenicity

TRANSMISSION

Human infection usually results from bites by rabid dogs or other mammals. Virus in saliva can enter via broken skin or intact mucous membranes, and so scratches or licks by a rabid animal may cause infection.

On two occasions, human rabies may have resulted from inhalation of virus in caves in Texas that were densely populated by insectivorous bats. Unnoticed skin contact was a more likely route of infection.[5] However, inhalation of virus aerosols has occurred in rare laboratory accidents. The saliva, respiratory secretions and tears of rabies patients contain virus,[6] which could infect another person but the only documented instances of human-to-human transmission have been through human tissue transplants from donors in whom rabies had not been suspected. At least 11 cases of infection by corneal graft have been reported. In the USA and Germany, three donors transmitted rabies to eight recipients of solid organ transplants (kidney, liver, lung, pancreas) and one patient received only a segment of artery.[7-9] Several women with rabies encephalitis have delivered healthy infants. Only one case of neonatal rabies has been reported, although vertical transmission is documented in animals.

PATHOGENESIS (Figure 171-1)

Rabies virus attaches to a variety of cellular receptors, but in a bite wound, competitive binding to acetylcholine receptors may concentrate virus at neuromuscular junctions where it is poised for entry into a peripheral nerve pre-synaptic axon terminal.[10] The virus or viral components then travel to the cell soma by retrograde axonal transport.[11] Experimentally, infection can be halted by sectioning the nerve

TABLE 171-1	**Distribution of Rabies Reservoir Species**	
Africa	Domestic dog (*Canis familiaris*)	Widespread dominant reservoir
	Black-backed jackals (*Canis mesomelas*)	Southern Africa
	Yellow mongoose (*Cynictis penicillata*)	Southern Africa
	Bat-eared fox (*Otocyon megalotis*)	Southern Africa
	Frugivorous and insectivorous bats – (bat lyssaviruses)	see Table 171-3
Asia	Domestic dog (*Canis familiaris*)	Widespread dominant reservoir
	Wolf (*Lupus lupus*)	Middle East
	Chinese ferret badgers (*Melogale moschata*)	China, Taiwan
Americas	Arctic fox (*Alopex lagopus*)	Alaska, northwest Canada
	Red fox (*Vulpes fulva*)	Western Canada and northeast USA
	Gray fox (*Urocyon cinereoargenteus*)	Texas, Arizona
	Striped skunk (*Mephitis* spp.)	Texas, central USA, California
	Raccoon (*Procyon lotor*)	Eastern USA, southeast Canada
	Insectivorous bats	Very widespread
	Vampire bat (*Desmodus* spp.)	Mexico, Trinidad and Tobago, Isla de Margarita, northern South America
	Frugivorous bats	South America
	Mongoose (*Herpestes* spp.)	Puerto Rico, Granada, Cuba, Dominican Republic
	Domestic dog (*Canis familiaris*)	Mexico, parts of central and South America eg. Haiti, Bolivia, Brazil, Dominican Republic
Australia	Flying foxes or fruit bats (*Pteropus* spp.)	Eastern coastal area
	Insectivorous bats – (Australian bat Lyssavirus see Table 171-3)	
Europe	Red fox (*Vulpes vulpes*)	Eastern Europe, Russian Federation
	Arctic fox (*Alopex lagopus*)	Northern Russian Federation
	Raccoon dog (*Nyctereutes procyonoides*)	Eastern Europe
	Wolf (*Lupus lupus*)	Eastern Europe, Russian Federation
	Domestic dog (*Canis familiaris*)	Turkey (act as vectors in Eastern Europe and Russian Federation)
	Insectivorous bats – (European bat lyssaviruses)	Widespread see Table 171-3

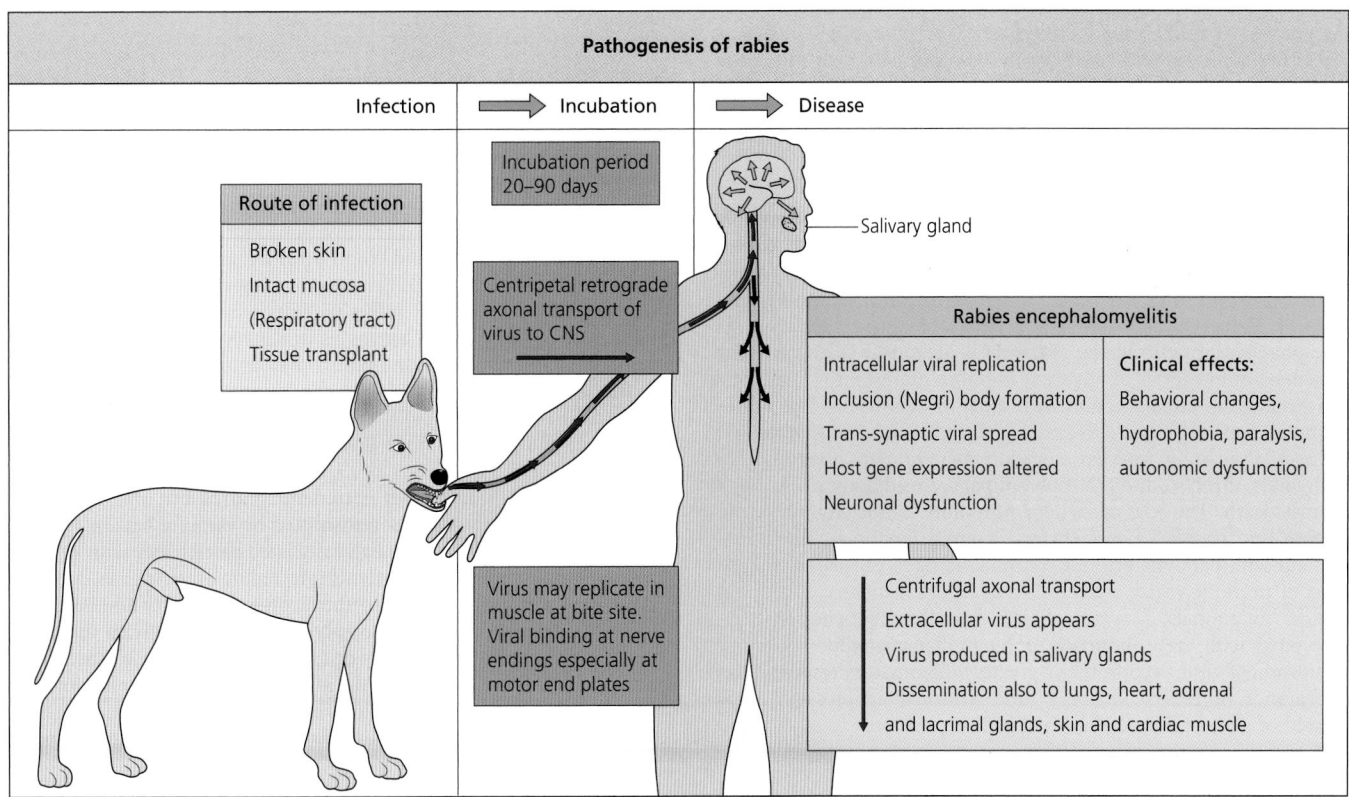

Figure 171-1   The pathogenesis of rabies.

or by poisoning microtubular function. The route of viral entry into the central nervous system (CNS) after superficial inoculation by bats is unknown.

Viral replication is intraneuronal. Accumulations of viral proteins form inclusions, such as classic Negri bodies (Figure 171-2). The virus spreads up the spinal cord towards the brain, passing intraneuronally by budding from synaptic membranes, during which it acquires its glycoprotein envelope. Rabies virus remains confined to neurons where it evades immune recognition throughout the incubation period.

Experimentally, neurophysiological disturbance is indicated by abnormal neurotransmitter activity, electroencephalograph patterns

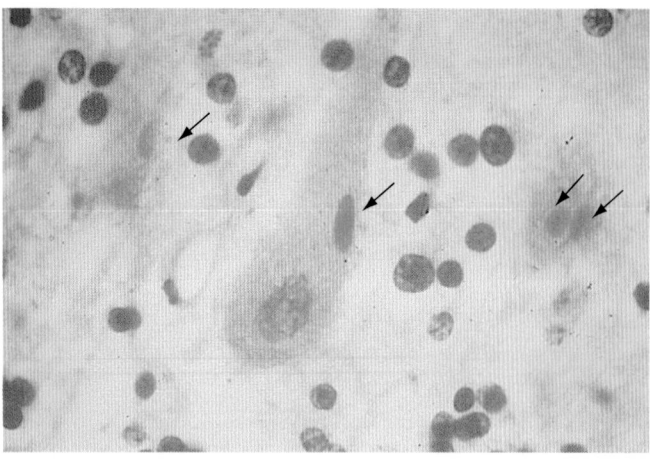

Figure 171-2 Negri bodies in cerebellar Purkinje cells in a human victim of rabies encephalitis. The intracytoplasmic, dark-staining Negri bodies are marked with arrows. (*Courtesy of Armed Forces Institute of Pathology, Bethesda, USA.*)

and ion-channel function. The demonstrated viral effects on host gene expression include upregulation of genes which could enhance viral spread and replication, and downregulation of genes related to cell protein synthesis. The latter will impair cell metabolism and innate immune responses and contributes to the widespread dysfunction of intact neurons.[12] Viral pathogenicity correlates with low levels of rabies glycoprotein expression, a minimal inflammatory response and little if any apoptosis. Pathological features of diffuse encephalomyelitis may be minimal or even absent in humans.

Rabies virus spreads centrifugally via peripheral and autonomic nerves to many tissues including the salivary and lacrimal glands where replication produces extracellular virus that may initiate an immune response (Figure 171-1).

IMMUNOLOGY

Following infection, rabies virus evades the immune system.[13] No immunological response can be detected in unvaccinated patients before signs of encephalitis develop. Rabies antibody does not appear until 1–2 weeks after the onset of symptoms, if at all, and later in the CSF. Rabies-specific IgM is not detectable any earlier than IgG. The presence of neutralizing antibody is diagnostic in unvaccinated patients, but low levels of apparent immunofluorescent (IF) antibody can result from cross-reaction with other viral antigens. The virus is immunosuppressive, as reflected by the minimal histopathological changes in the brain. Interferon production in humans is very low, and high levels of IFN-α and IFN-β in animal brains did not protect them against death. The role of cellular immunity is not clear in human disease, but specific T lymphocytes are found experimentally in rabid animals with paralytic but not encephalitic signs. Surprisingly, apoptosis of immune reactive CD3⁺ T cells has been observed in mouse brains.[13] In animals, clearance of virus from the brain and recovery is associated with early induction of neutralizing antibody, increased expression of viral glycoprotein, a greater inflammatory response, early appearance of IFN-γ and very little neuronal apoptosis. Neurons cleared of virus still have abnormal gene expression.

Control

The elimination of rabies virus from domestic dogs would prevent 98% of human rabies deaths, obviating the need for expensive prophylaxis. This has been achieved, for example, in Western Europe, North America, Japan, several urban areas of Latin America[1] and even in one study area in India.[14] Mass killing of reservoir species is ineffective, but campaigns of dog vaccination and population control can be successful, if accompanied by enthusiastic education and publicity supported by adequate funding. Although oral vaccination of dogs is possible, it remains impractical.

Appropriate rabies control strategies are based on surveillance to determine the principal domestic or wild reservoir species, with laboratory diagnosis to confirm the local prevalence of infection.

Sylvatic rabies has been eliminated in the red fox, *Vulpes vulpes*, in Western Europe by distributing oral vaccine in suitable baits around the countryside.[15] Repeated campaigns of oral vaccination are needed over many years, using live attenuated rabies, vaccinia or adenovirus recombinant vaccine expressing rabies glycoprotein. In North America, raccoons, foxes and skunks, and in southern Africa, jackals, have been similarly immunized. Control of vampire bat rabies, a cause of human and many cattle deaths in Latin America, is attempted by treating cattle with small doses of anticoagulant in order to poison the bats. Vaccination of cattle is possible but expensive. No active measures are taken to control rabies in insectivorous or fruit bats in the Americas, Europe, Africa or Australia, but the population is educated to avoid direct contact with these animals.

Clinical Features

The incubation period (bite to first symptom) ranges from 4 days to a documented 19 years, but in about 75% of cases it ranges 20–90 days. Of the many reported prodromal symptoms, only itching, pain or paresthesiae, radiating proximally from the site of the healed causative bite wound, suggest imminent encephalomyelitis. After 1–7 days of generally nonspecific symptoms, features of furious or paralytic rabies develop.

The pathognomonic symptom of furious rabies is hydrophobia[16] – jerky, violent inspiratory muscle spasms associated with an inexplicable terror provoked by water – or aerophobia – an identical response provoked by a draught of air on the skin. The hydrophobic response may be provoked by attempts to drink liquid or by the sight, sound or mere mention of water. An hydrophobic spasm may end in extreme opisthotonos, reminiscent of severe tetanus; in generalized convulsions; or in cardiorespiratory arrest. Other features of furious rabies include periods of excitement, sometimes with hallucinations or, rarely, with aggression; interspersed with lucid intervals during which victims can be aware of their terrible predicament; fever; tachycardia and other arrhythmias; hypersalivation; lacrimation; sweating; and fluctuating temperature and blood pressure; and priapism. These features suggest stimulation of the autonomic nervous system as in severe tetanus. Hypersexuality in rabies patients may be attributable to hippocampal or amygdaloid lesions as in Klüver–Bucy syndrome. Conventional neurological examination may prove surprisingly normal, unless hydrophobia is provoked, but meningism, cranial nerve lesions (especially III, VI, VII, IX–XII), upper motor neuron lesions, fasciculations, myoclonus and other involuntary muscular contractions are sometimes detected.

Paralytic or dumb rabies is underdiagnosed but was recognized during an epidemic of rabies transmitted by vampire bats in Trinidad in the 1920s and 1930s. Although associated particularly with vampire bat rabies, it is also seen in patients infected by other species. After the prodromal symptoms described above, often with fever and headache, local paresthesiae and flaccid paralysis develop, usually in the bitten limb, and ascend symmetrically or asymmetrically. There is accompanying pain and fasciculation in the affected muscles and mild objective sensory disturbances. Death follows paralysis of the muscles of deglutition and respiration; there is usually no evidence of hydrophobia or aerophobia.

Patients with rabies whose lives are prolonged by intensive care may develop a variety of respiratory, cardiovascular, neurological and gastrointestinal complications including fatal cardiac arrhythmias, pneumothorax, cerebral edema, diabetes insipidus, syndrome of inappropriate secretion of antidiuretic hormone (SIADH), hypo- or hyperpyrexia, diffuse axonal neuropathy and Mallory–Weiss hematemesis.

DIFFERENTIAL DIAGNOSIS

Severe and unusual neurological symptoms, whether encephalitic or paralytic, should suggest the possibility of rabies in any unimmunized person who has had contact with mammals in rabies-endemic areas. Children may not report animal contact and rabies patients infected by bats in the USA often deny exposure to bats.

Rabies in children has been misdiagnosed as cerebral malaria. Furious rabies can be mimicked by the pharyngeal form of cephalic tetanus ('hydrophobic tetanus'); however, severe tetanus usually has a shorter incubation period than rabies and there is sustained muscle rigidity, often associated with trismus. Delirium tremens and the excitatory effects of some plant toxins and recreational drugs[7] have been confused with rabies. Paralytic rabies is indistinguishable from other encephalitides, and the many causes of Landry-type ascending paralysis, including postvaccinal encephalomyelitis complicating the use of obsolete nervous tissue rabies vaccines, and Guillain–Barré syndrome.

No convincing or diagnostically useful differences have been proven between the clinical features of rabies encephalitis acquired from terrestrial mammals, classic (species 1) rabies compared to those from bats infected with rabies-related species (Table 171-3).

PROGNOSIS AND RECOVERY

Without intensive care, victims of furious rabies encephalitis usually die within a few days, but some patients with paralytic rabies have survived for as long as 1 month, even without this support.

During the virological era, only 10 documented cases of recovery or prolonged survival with neurological deficits after rabies encephalomyelitis have been reported. In two of them, rabies polymerase chain reaction (PCR) or antigen was detected and in eight, the diagnosis was based on detection of very high neutralizing antibody levels. Six had been infected by dogs and had received at least one dose of vaccine postexposure before the onset of symptoms.[17,18] A seventh, who inhaled an attenuated vaccine virus, had received pre-exposure nervous tissue vaccine. Six of these seven suffered debilitating residual neurological sequelae but one has recently recovered: a 17-year-old Turkish shepherd who was bitten on the forearm and shoulder by a proven rabid dog. Four days later he was given a single dose of Vero cell vaccine, but 20 days after that he developed typical symptoms of rabies including hydrophobia. PCR on saliva and IFA corneal smear tests were positive for rabies, with high serum-neutralizing antibody. Equine rabies immunoglobulin and vaccine were given, and he was discharged after 66 days, apparently fully recovered.[19]

Three of the survivors were bitten by bats. One was bitten by a vampire bat in Brazil. He received postexposure prophylaxis, was diagnosed by PCR and has neurological sequelae. Another was a 6-year-old boy bitten on the thumb by a big brown bat (*Eptesicus fuscus*) in 1970 in Ohio, USA.[20] He started having duck embryo rabies vaccine 4 days later but developed an encephalitic illness with

very high rabies neutralizing antibody in the serum and CSF. After intensive care but no specific treatment he recovered completely in 6 months. The most surprising case, the only unvaccinated person known to have survived, is a 15-year-old girl in Wisconsin, USA, bitten by a bat in 2004.[21] She developed paresthesiae of the bitten hand and features of paralytic rabies: progressive cranial nerve paralyses and leg weakness, with fever and hypersalivation. Rabies antibody had appeared by the sixth day after the onset of symptoms, but no virus or antigen was detected. Her intensive treatment included ketamine-induced coma and the antiviral agents ribavirin and amantadine. She made a slow recovery with only minor residual neurologic deficits, and she graduated from high school. This case has features similar to the boy in Ohio. It is likely that they both had rabies antibody present at, or soon after, the onset of symptoms. The American bat viruses are all rabies (species 1), which has a different pattern of infection from the dog rabies strains experimentally. It is slower to evolve and progress and there is relatively little neuronal apoptosis.

The Milwaukee treatment protocol that was apparently effective in the Wisconsin girl, has not proved effective in at least 30 other patients infected by bats or dogs. It is not recommended by the World Health Organization (WHO). There is no evidence that it is superior to normal intensive care unit (ICU) therapy.

Two patients initially reported to have recovered from rabies in the USA were diagnosed by finding low levels of IFT antibody. They are now considered to have been misdiagnoses due to a nonspecific serological cross-reaction.[18]

In summary, no unvaccinated patient is known to have survived rabies encephalitis if infected by a terrestrial mammal. Three people have recovered: two were vaccinated, after being bitten by a dog or bat, and a single unvaccinated patient recovered from a bat infection. All other survivors were left with severe neurological sequelae.

Diagnosis

Confirmation of the diagnosis of rabies encephalitis should be possible within a day, if optimal samples are supplied to a specialist laboratory (Table 171-2). Rapid identification of antigen can be followed by virus isolation and, in unvaccinated patients, by detecting neutralizing antibody.[22]

Skin, saliva, respiratory secretions, CSF, tears and brain are all suitable samples, but a full-thickness skin biopsy is the most likely to yield a rapid result. A punch biopsy is taken from a hairy area, usually at the nape of the neck. Frozen sections show the characteristic IF staining of rabies antigen visible in nerve fibers around the base of hair follicles.[23] With controls to ensure specificity and examination of many

TABLE 171-2	Rabies Diagnostic Methods	
Diagnostic Sample	**Aim**	**Method**
Full-thickness **skin*** punch biopsy	Antigen detection	IFA test on frozen section RT-PCR
Saliva Tears CSF	Virus isolation and antigen detection	Tissue culture Mouse inoculation test RT-PCR
Serum	Antibody test	Detectable antibody is diagnostic in unvaccinated patients Save sample for comparison later if vaccinated previously
CSF	Antibody test	Test in parallel with serum
REPEAT skin and saliva samples daily until a diagnosis is confirmed		
Brain post-mortem: needle biopsy† or autopsy sample brain stem and cerebellum	Virus isolation and antigen detection	Tissue culture Mouse inoculation test IFA test-impression smear RT-PCR

*__Bold__, most important, potentially helpful, samples.
†See text for details.

sections, sensitivity is 60–100%. False-positive results have not been reported, whereas the corneal impression test is insensitive and false-positive results do occur. RT-PCR can be performed on the samples mentioned. Skin and saliva are the most likely to be positive. Viral isolation in tissue culture is the ideal method. Genetic analysis will indicate the likely reservoir species and geographic origin of the virus. Tests should be repeated until the diagnosis of rabies is excluded.

In unvaccinated patients, diagnostic seroconversion may occur in the second week of illness or thereafter.[24] In vaccinated patients, high levels of antibody both in the serum and in the CSF have been considered diagnostic.[20]

To confirm the diagnosis post-mortem, brain samples should be cultured, but antigen can readily be detected by IF staining of impression smears, enzyme immunoassay or RT-PCR. Without a full autopsy, a needle necropsy sample of brain can be obtained by inserting a long biopsy needle percutaneously through the medial canthus of the eye and the superior orbital fissure, the foramen magnum, the nose and ethmoid sinus or, in young children, through an open fontanelle.

Management

No antiviral or ancillary treatments have proved effective in animal models and, in unvaccinated people, rabies of canine origin remains 100% fatal. Patients should be admitted to hospital so that their agonizing symptoms can be palliated with adequate doses of analgesic and sedative drugs.[25] Friends, family and medical staff in close contact with the patient should be vaccinated as reassurance, even though such person-to-person transmission has not been documented.

Intensive care should be considered for previously vaccinated patients, or those infected by an American bat virus. A better prognosis is associated with previous good health, early presentation and seroconversion. Novel approaches to rabies antiviral methods are needed, perhaps with immunological enhancement. Intrathecal injection of a live attenuated rabies virus is currently the most promising experimental method. Until a treatment has proved effective in animals, intensive care therapy is usually inappropriate, especially in low- to middle-income countries (LMIC).

Prevention

POSTEXPOSURE PROPHYLAXIS[26-28]

In rabies-endemic areas, the risk of infection, and hence the decision to give postexposure prophylaxis, depends on the species of animal, its behavior and the circumstances of contact. An unprovoked attack by a known local vector suggests a high risk of exposure to rabies, especially if the animal is unvaccinated, unusually excitable, partially paralyzed or if a wild animal is unusually tame. Vaccinated animals have, however, transmitted rabies. The virus gains access through any bite, scratch or contamination of broken skin or mucous membrane, but intact skin is an adequate barrier against infection. Bites or scratches by bats may pass unnoticed. The risk of infection is greatest from bites on the head, neck and hands, and multiple bites carry a higher risk than single bites. Before vaccines were available, the mortality from proven rabid dog bites in India was 35–57%.

The biting animal's brain should be tested for rabies. The routine IF test for antigen may give a false-negative rate of 1–2%. This test is unreliable for rabies-related lyssaviruses, and so viral culture and PCR are important in highly suspicious cases. Postexposure prophylaxis should not await laboratory results but must be started immediately, irrespective of the time that has elapsed since the bite.

Postexposure prophylaxis aims to inactivate rabies virus in the wound and to stimulate immunity to kill the virus before it enters the nervous system, where it is protected from immune attack. Postexposure therapy includes urgent wound treatment, active prophylaxis with vaccine and passive immunization with rabies immune globulin (RIG). The complete therapy is very effective, and failures of optimal treatment started on the day of exposure are very rare. However, many deaths occur because treatment is often delayed, unaffordable, inadequate or incomplete.

TREATMENT OF MAMMAL BITES, SCRATCHES OR LICKS

The treatment can be summarized as follows:

1. Scrub wounds vigorously with soap or detergent and water, reaching into the depth and removing foreign material. Local or even general anesthesia may be necessary, especially for children.
2. Swab with a virucidal agent: povidone iodine or 40–70% ethanol. (The virucidal effect of quaternary ammonium compounds is neutralized by soap, and so they are not recommended.)
3. Suturing of wounds should be avoided or delayed for fear of inoculating virus deeper into the wound.
4. Tetanus prophylaxis (tetanus immune globulin or toxoid booster plus metronidazole) must not be forgotten. Antibiotic prophylaxis against other potential wound pathogens is recommended in the case of bites on the hands.
5. If there is a risk of rabies, start specific postexposure prophylaxis immediately.

RABIES VACCINES

Vaccines of Nervous Tissue Origin

Human rabies vaccines contain killed virus. Vaccines produced from infected sheep, goat or suckling mouse brain (SMB) should no longer be used. However, Fermi vaccine is still produced in Ethiopia and SMB in Peru. These are weak antigens and neurological reactions still occur.

Purified Tissue Culture Vaccines

Tissue culture-grown vaccines are in general use. The original human diploid cell vaccine (HDCV) *Imovax*, Sanofi Pasteur has given way to vaccines of equivalent efficacy and safety, including German and Indian purified chick embryo cell vaccines (PCECV) *Rabipur*. *RabAvert* GSK, and a French purified Vero cell vaccine (PVRV), *Verorab*, Sanofi Pasteur which meet the WHO standards. Several other Indian and Chinese tissue culture vaccines are exported whereas Russian and Japanese vaccines are used locally.

Immunological Response to Vaccination

The presence of serum-neutralizing antibody is the best available indicator of protection against rabies. It appears 7–14 days after starting a primary course of a modern rabies vaccine. A level of 0.5 IU/mL is considered satisfactory, although the protective level cannot be determined in humans. Only the viral surface glycoprotein molecules induce neutralizing antibody. They also stimulate helper and cytotoxic T-lymphocyte responses.

The speed and size of the antibody response to vaccine vary, influenced by genetic factors. Relatively delayed, lower antibody levels are found in about 3% of vaccinees. Increasing age and immunosuppression, including by HIV infection also impair the response.

The induction of neutralizing antibody is related to the amount of antigen (within limits) and the route of inoculation. Intradermal (ID) injection delivers antigen into the dermis, rich in antigen-presenting dendritic cells which stimulate T lymphocytes to initiate antibody production, an advantage over intramuscular (IM) inoculation.

POSTEXPOSURE VACCINE REGIMENS

Intramuscular Vaccine Regimens

- The standard **five-dose intramuscular (Essen) regimen** is one dose of vaccine (1 mL or 0.5 mL, depending on the product) into the deltoid on days 0, 3, 7, 14 and 28. A recent change, to omit the final dose, has been sanctioned in the USA for otherwise healthy patients if RIG is also given.
- An alternative **2-2-1 (Zagreb) regimen** is two doses intramuscularly into deltoids on day 0 and one dose on days 7 and 21.

Intradermal Vaccine Regimens

The five-dose intramuscular regimen is unaffordable by the vast majority of patients in LMIC. Multiple-site ID vaccination is economical but only recommended using specified vaccines – PVRV, PCECV and HDCV. The manufacturers' instructions must be used for all other vaccines.

The **four-site ID 1-month regimen**[28,29] is the original eight-site regimen[30] adapted by halving the number of injection sites and doubling the intradermal (ID) dose per site. The regimen is:

- Day 0: four ID injections – the entire contents of the vial are divided between four sites: the deltoid and either the thigh or suprascapular areas. *The ID dose depends on the volume per vial: for 0.5 mL/vial PVRV vaccine the ID dose is 0.1 mL/site, and for less concentrated 1.0 mL/vial PCECV vaccine it is 0.2 mL/ site.*
- Day 7: two ID injections in deltoid areas [0.1/ 0.2 mL]
- Day 28: one ID injection in a deltoid area [0.1/ 0.2 mL].

If there is difficulty injecting 0.2 mL ID, the needle is withdrawn and the remainder injected nearby.

This four-site regimen meets the WHO criteria of immunogenicity and supersedes the eight-site regimen, recognized as highly immunogenic and recommended by WHO for many years. The regimen is as immunogenic as the five-dose IM Essen method. It requires three visits and is the most economical, both for the patient and the healthcare provider. It is practical in rural areas because on the first crucial day a whole vial of vaccine is used. Vaccine wastage can be minimized by asking the patient to bring relatives with them on day 7, in case there is any left-over vaccine available for pre-exposure immunization. The timing of the day 28 dose may be adjusted to enable sharing of vials.

- A **two-site ID regimen** is: on days 0, 3, 7 and 28, two 2 ID injections in deltoid areas [0.1 mL]. (Although originally 0.1 or 0.2 mL depending on the vaccine.)

This regimen has been used in thousands of patients in urban areas in Thailand, the Philippines and Sri Lanka, where RIG treatment is likely to be available.

PASSIVE IMMUNIZATION WITH RABIES IMMUNE GLOBULIN

Except in the case of trivial exposures, every primary postexposure vaccine course should be accompanied by RIG to cover the first 7–10 days before vaccine-induced immunity appears. RIG treatment is especially important after bites on the head, neck or hands, or multiple bites. A dose of 20 IU/kg of human RIG or 40 IU/kg of equine RIG is given, preferably with analgesia, at the same time as the first dose of vaccine. As much as possible is infiltrated into and around the wound, but care is needed when injecting into fingers or other tight tissue compartments. Any remaining vaccine is injected intramuscularly, avoiding the gluteal region. Increasing the dose of RIG may impair the response to vaccine, but if the volume is insufficient for infiltration, it can be diluted in saline two- or threefold in order to infiltrate all wounds. Skin testing with equine RIG does not predict early (anaphylactic) reactions and is no longer recommended.[26] Adrenaline (epinephrine) should always be ready in case of very rare anaphylaxis. Reactions occur in 1.8% of equine RIG recipients and serum sickness is seen in 0.7%, but not after human RIG therapy.[31]

Postexposure Boosting of Previously Vaccinated Patients

Treatment is always urgent. Provided that the patient has previously had a complete pre-exposure or postexposure course of tissue culture vaccine or if a neutralizing antibody level >0.5 IU/mL has been recorded anytime previously, only booster vaccination is needed without RIG.

- **Two-dose intramuscular regimen**: one dose on days 0 and 3.
- **Single day four-site ID regimen**: four ID injections in deltoid and thigh or suprascapular areas.[26]

SIDE EFFECTS OF TISSUE CULTURE VACCINES[32]

The incidence of minor symptoms is very variable. Local pain or erythema occurs in about 15% of people vaccinated and irritation is more common following intradermal injections. Generalized nonspecific symptoms are reported by about 7% of patients and transient maculopapular and urticarial rashes are occasionally seen. Neurologic symptoms, either Guillain–Barré-like or local limb weakness, are extremely rare, and the incidence following treatment is no greater than those following other routine vaccines. No complications have been observed in pregnancy.

PRE-EXPOSURE PROPHYLAXIS[26–28]

Pre-exposure vaccination is recommended for anyone at risk of exposure to rabies virus, particularly veterinary surgeons, animal handlers, zoologists, all bat handlers, laboratory staff working with rabies, wildlife officers and people living in or traveling[33] to rabies-endemic areas where dogs are the dominant reservoir species. A total of three doses of cell culture vaccine are needed on days 0, 7 and day 28. The last dose can be advanced towards day 21 if time is short. The dose can be intramuscular or 0.1 mL ID. Families or student groups who cannot afford intramuscular vaccine can share ampoules economically if inoculated the same day. If immunosuppression is suspected, or if taking chloroquine, give vaccine intramuscularly rather than ID. A single booster dose after 1 or 2 years prolongs the antibody response, which usually lasts 5–10 years.[34] Unnecessary boosters can be avoided if antibody is detected. Booster doses are not needed for travelers who will have access to vaccine if exposed. If not, boost after 5 years. Serologic testing is useful to determine the need for booster injections and is advised if immunosuppression is suspected.

Rabies-Related Viruses Infecting Humans

With one exception, these are viruses of bats. Five of the six are phylogroup I viruses, causing typical rabies-like encephalitis (Table 171-3). New unclassified lyssaviruses are emerging.

AFRICA[2]

Duvenhage virus, a bat virus, is fatal in humans[2,35,36] (Table 171-3). Its true prevalence is uncertain as the diagnosis of human rabies is normally made on clinical grounds and rabies-related viruses may give a weak or negative result with the routine diagnostic rabies IF test.

EUROPE

There are two species of European bat lyssaviruses[2] (EBLVs): EBLV type 1 is widely distributed in insectivorous bats across Europe and EBLV type 2, which is rare. There are four reports of EBLV fatal rabies-like encephalitis following bat bites in Europe (see Table 171-3).[2,37–39] Irkut virus caused a human death in Eastern Russia.[40]

AUSTRALIA

Australian bat Lyssavirus,[2] found in flying foxes or fruit bats (*Pteropus* spp.) and other bats, has caused three human deaths.[41]

CHINA AND ASIA

In China there is serological evidence of lyssaviruses in bats, but only a single isolate of Irkut virus from a bat which fatally infected a woman.[40] Rabies was diagnosed clinically in one other victim of a Chinese bat bite.

There is indirect evidence of bat lyssaviruses in India. A case of typical furious rabies followed a bat bite in Andhra Pradesh in 1954 and an untyped Lyssavirus was isolated from a bat in Chandigarh in 1978. In South East Asia, seropositive bats have been found in the Philippines, Thailand, Cambodia, Bangladesh and Vietnam.

References available online at expertconsult.com.

TABLE 171-3	Rabies and Rabies-Related Lyssaviruses Known to Infect Humans			
Lyssavirus Species*	Phylogroup	Virus Distribution§	Animal Reservoirs (Potential Vectors)	Disease in Humans
1 Rabies	I	Widespread	Dogs, some wild mammals and bats in the Americas	Tens of thousands annually
3 Mokola	II	South Africa, Nigeria, Cameroon, Ethiopia (rare)	Shrews, rodents (cat, dog)	Child febrile convulsion;[†] recovered[2] Child encephalitic signs;[‡] died[2] Vaccinated laboratory worker, mild illness; recovered
4 Duvenhage	I	South Africa, Zimbabwe, Kenya (very rarely identified)	Insectivorous/fruit bats (cats)	Man bitten by a bat, signs of typical furious rabies; died[2] Man scratched by a bat, signs of classic rabies encephalitis; died[35] Woman scratched by a bat, signs of rabies encephalitis; died[36]
5 European bat Lyssavirus EBLV type1a EBLV type 1b	I	Northern and Eastern Europe Western Europe	Insectivorous bats	Girl had bat bite, had acute ascending paralysis and encephalitis; died (clinical diagnosis only) Girl had bat bite, signs of furious rabies; died of EBLV 1a[37]
6 European bat Lyssavirus EBLV type 2a EBLV type 2b	I	Netherlands, UK, Germany, France Switzerland, Finland	Insectivorous bats (*Myotis* spp.)	Bat conservationist bitten by bats, typical signs of rabies encephalitis; died of EBLV 2a[38] Zoologist bitten by sick bat, signs of furious rabies; EBLV type 2b[39]
7 Australian bat Lyssavirus	I	Australia	Fruit bats (*Pteropus* spp.), insectivorous bats	Woman bat carer, scratched by bats, typical signs of rabies encephalitis; died Woman, bitten by a fruit bat, signs of paralytic rabies; died[39] Boy scratched by bat, developed typical rabies encephalitis; died[41]
10 Irkut	I	Eurasia, China	Insectivorous bats	Woman bitten on lip by bat, paralytic rabies-like encephalitis, died[40]

*Bat Lyssavirus species not found in humans.
In Africa, Phylogroup II: 2 Lagos bat virus; 12 Shimoni bat virus.
In Eurasia: Phylogroup I: 8 Aravan; 9 Khujand virus; Phylogroup III: West Caucasian bat virus.
§There is serologic evidence of lyssaviruses in bats in the Philippines, Cambodia, Thailand, Bangladesh and Vietnam.
†Doubtful diagnosis.
‡Alternative diagnosis possible.

KEY REFERENCES

Gautret P., Parola P.: Rabies in travelers. *Curr Infect Dis Rep* 2014; 16:394.
Helmick C.G., Tauxe R.V., Vernon A.A.: Is there a risk to contacts of patients with rabies? *Rev Infect Dis* 1987; 9:511-518.
Jackson A.C., Warrell M.J., Rupprecht C.E., et al.: Management of rabies in humans. *Clin Infect Dis* 2003; 36:60-63.
Nel L.H., Markotter W.: Lyssaviruses. *Crit Rev Microbiol* 2007; 33:301-324.

Noah D.L., Drenzek C.L., Smith J.S., et al.: Epidemiology of human rabies in the United States, 1980 to 1996. *Ann Intern Med* 1998; 128:922-930.
Schnell M.J., McGettigan J.P., Wirblich C., et al.: The cell biology of rabies virus: using stealth to reach the brain. *Nat Rev Microbiol* Jan 2010; 8:51-61.
Warrell D.A., Davidson N.M., Pope H.M., et al.: Pathophysiologic studies in human rabies. *Am J Med* 1976; 60:180-190.

Warrell M.J.: Current rabies vaccines and prophylaxis schedules: preventing rabies before and after exposure. *Travel Med Infect Dis* 2012; 10:1-15.
Warrell M.J., Riddell A., Yu L.-M., et al.: A simplified 4-site economical intradermal post-exposure rabies vaccine regimen: a randomised controlled comparison with standard methods. *PLoS Neglect Trop Dis* 2008; 2(4): e224.

172

Influenza Viruses

SCOTT H. JAMES | RICHARD J. WHITLEY

KEY CONCEPTS

- The A(H1N1)pdm09 pandemic strain of influenza remains in circulation and, therefore, remains a key constituent of global vaccines.

- Highly pathogenic avian influenza H5N1 remains a cause of localized disease around the world.

- Avian influenza has been detected in poultry populations around the world and most recently the USA.

- Vaccination with either an inactivated or live attenuated vaccine remains the method of prevention of choice.

- Vaccine efficacy varies significantly according to its match with circulating influenza strains.

- The deployment of neuraminidase inhibitors is of both therapeutic and prophylactic value for select populations.

- Antiviral resistance remains uncommon in adults but is higher in children.

Introduction

Influenza is a seasonal respiratory viral infection that results in some 250 000–500 000 deaths globally each year.[1] The illness is characterized by a sudden onset of high temperature and debilitating systemic symptoms. In healthy individuals, infection is typically self-limited; however, complications often occur in certain high-risk groups such as infants, the elderly and the immunocompromised host. Despite the availability of preventive vaccines and influenza therapeutics, seasonal influenza remains a major global health problem. In addition to the direct medical costs, the indirect social and economic costs remain significant.

While seasonal influenza epidemics occur annually in the autumn and winter, global pandemics also occur, albeit less frequently. In 2009, the world experienced the first influenza pandemic of the 21st century. The virus involved was a novel H1N1 virus of swine origin that originated in Mexico in the spring of 2009. Having spread globally, this pandemic strain now remains in circulation and continues to be a constituent of current vaccines. The emergence of this new pandemic serves to secure influenza's place in history as 'the last great uncontrolled plague of mankind'.[2]

Nature

VIRUS STRUCTURE

Influenza viruses are enveloped, single-stranded, negative-sense RNA viruses of the family Orthomyxoviridae. There are three major antigenic types, A, B and C. These can be differentiated not only on the basis of antigenic differences in their nucleocapsid and matrix proteins, but also with respect to the number of gene segments and viral proteins, host range and capacity to cause disease.[2]

Influenza viruses possess segmented genomes: influenza A and B contain eight RNA segments and influenza C seven. Influenza A, the predominant pathogen in seasonal influenza and the cause of pandemic influenza, provides the main focus for the remainder of this section. The influenza A genome encodes 11 viral proteins:

- hemagglutinin (HA), which is divided into two subunits (HA1 and HA2);
- neuraminidase (NA);
- two matrix proteins (M1 and M2);
- heterotrimeric RNA-dependent RNA polymerase, composed of one polymerase acidic (PA) and two polymerase basic (PB1 and PB2) subunits and the alternatively transcribed proapoptotic peptide, PB1-F2;
- nucleoprotein (NP);
- two nonstructural proteins (NS1 and NS2; NS2 is also known as NEP, or nuclear export protein).[2-4]

The virus particle (virion) has an irregular spherical shape with a lipid envelope, approximately 80–120 nm in diameter. The surface is covered with spike-like projections composed of the two primary viral glycoproteins, HA and NA, which are involved in host cell attachment and host cell egress, respectively. In addition, M2 (a transmembrane ion channel) is also present on the external surface of the virus. M1 is found within the lipid bilayer, which surrounds the virus core. The core is a ribonucleoprotein (RNP) complex, which consists of the viral RNA segments and the NP and the RNA polymerase (Figure 172-1). Influenza A is currently classified on the composition of the HA and NA proteins. At present, 16 different HA (H1–H16) and nine different NA (N1–N9) molecules are known to exist.[4]

VIRUS REPLICATION

At the initiation of human infection, the HA binds to receptors on the host cell surface that contain $\alpha2$, 6-linked sialic acid residues, and virion entry occurs via receptor-mediated endocytosis. In the host cell cytoplasm, the vesicle containing the virus undergoes an acidification process through fusion with intracellular endosomes. This triggers a conformational change in the HA, exposing a fusion peptide and permitting exit from the endosome; in addition, hydrogen ions are pumped from the endosome through the M2 ion channel into the virus particle. This allows the viral RNPs to be released, and they are then actively transported into the nucleus through the nuclear pore complex.[2] The M2 inhibitor class of antiviral agents, the adamantanes, inhibits this acidification process.

Transcription of the influenza viral genomic RNA (vRNA) into messenger RNA (mRNA) takes place in the nucleus. Following transcription, viral mRNA strands are exported to the cytoplasm where new viral proteins are synthesized. Newly synthesized viral RNAs are exported via a vRNP–M1–NEP protein complex. Packaging of progeny virions occurs at the host cell surface where the RNP–M1–NEP complex assembles at the cytoplasmic membrane under regions containing viral glycoproteins. As the new viruses bud and are released from the host cell, the NA is responsible for cleaving sialic acid residues that would cause the virus to remain bound to either the cell surface or other viral particles (Figure 172-2). The neuraminidase inhibitor class of antiviral agents prevents this cleavage process and thereby the release of virus and subsequent infection of new host cells.

Epidemiology

NATURAL RESERVOIRS OF INFLUENZA VIRUSES

Wild aquatic birds are the natural reservoir of all influenza A viruses.[5,6] Influenza A viruses in humans are maintained by human-to-human transmission during acute infection; however, other animals including primates, poultry, swine, ferrets, horses, seals, whales and mink can also become infected.

Structure of the influenza virion

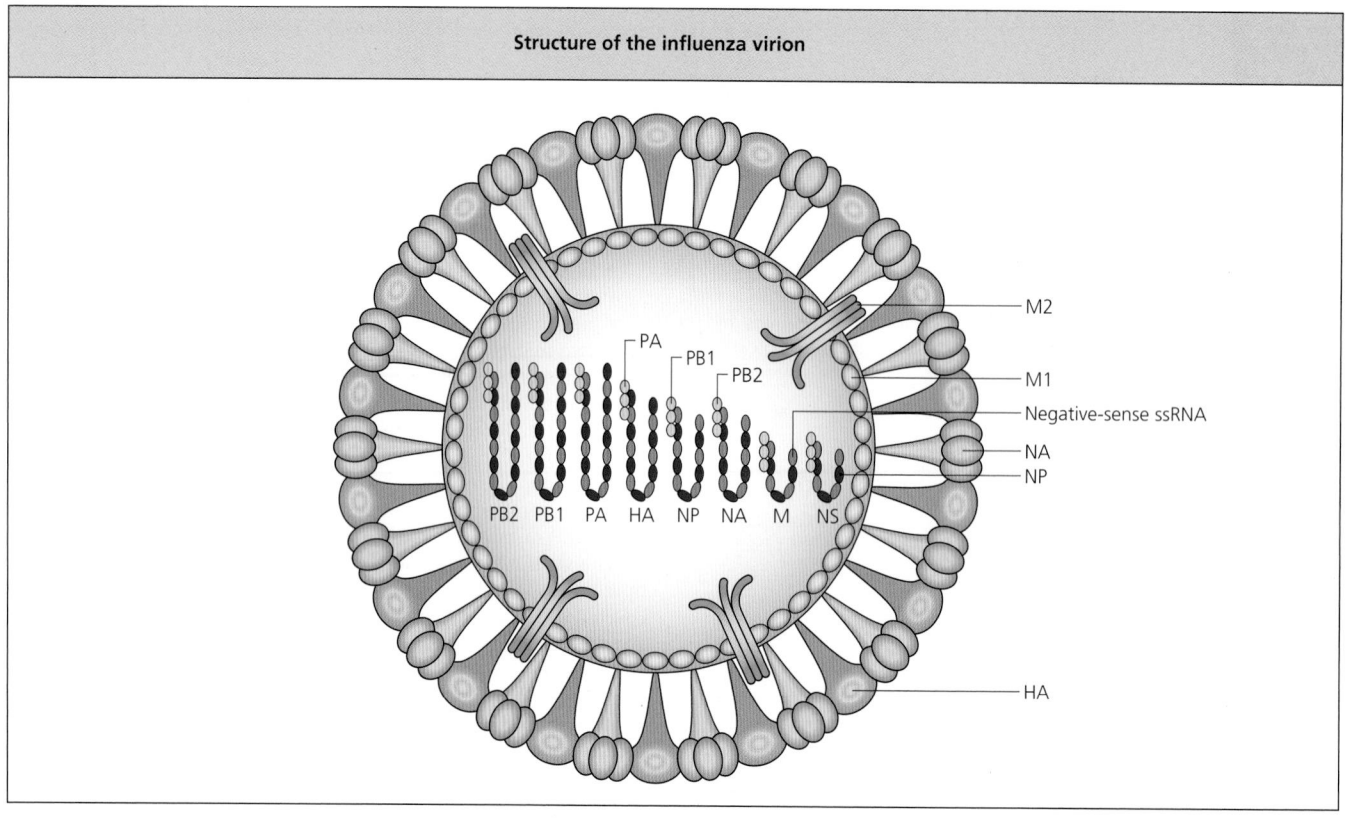

Figure 172-1   Structure of the influenza virion. The genome of the influenza A virus is composed of eight genomic segments and each segment contains a region that encodes one or two proteins. In all, the eight segments encode 11 proteins. Details of the proteins, their biologic functions and their roles in virus replication are summarized in the text. (*Reproduced with permission from Nelson M.I., Holmes E.C. Nature Reviews Genetics 2007; 8(3):196-205. Epub 2007/01/31.*)

ANTIGENIC VARIATION: ANTIGENIC DRIFT AND SHIFT

The influenza A viruses evolve rapidly, primarily because of the absence of a proofreading mechanism during the copying of the vRNA to mRNA. The antigenic variation in influenza viruses occurs as a result of small changes, *antigenic drifts*, over time within the RNA segments encoding the surface glycoproteins NA and, in particular, HA. Antigenic drift leads to positive selection of these escape mutants from neutralizing antibody responses elicited by previous exposure(s) to wild-type viruses.

Human influenza virus HA molecules preferentially bind α2,6-linked sialic acid expressed on respiratory epithelia, whereas the HA of avian viruses binds predominantly α2,3-linked sialic acid receptors. Reassortment of influenza vRNA segments can occur if different viruses simultaneously infect a single cell, allowing RNA exchange. This can result in the production of a novel progeny virus and is known as *antigenic shift*. Reassortment may occur in an intermediate host species such as swine (the mixing vessel hypothesis), which can be infected with both human and avian viruses as swine epithelia possess both α2,3- and α2,6-linked sialic acid receptors. Antigenic shift can lead to the introduction of a new influenza subtype into an immunologically naïve population, and has the potential for pandemic spread, as occurred with the 2009-H1N1 pandemic.

INFLUENZA PANDEMICS

During pandemics, virus spreads rapidly, resulting in significant morbidity and mortality. The 'Spanish influenza' pandemic of 1918–19 was caused by a highly virulent influenza A, subtype H1N1 virus that infected approximately one-third of the human population, leading to the deaths of more than 50 million people.[7,8] One striking feature of the 1918–19 pandemic was the disproportionately high numbers of healthy young individuals who succumbed to infection, which has

been attributed to an uncontrolled immune response with increased production of pro-inflammatory cytokines, the so-called 'cytokine storm'. In 1957–58, the 'Asian' influenza pandemic arose after genetic shift of the circulating H1N1 virus to an H2N2 subtype.

The H2N2 viruses were subsequently supplanted by the H3N2 'Hong Kong' influenza pandemic of 1968. Lindstrom and co-workers performed a whole genome phylogenetic analysis of human influenza H2N2 viruses isolated from 1957 to 1968 and human H3N2 viruses isolated from 1968 to 1972.[9] The data suggest that H2N2 viruses continued to circulate for some time after 1968 and that the subsequent establishment of human H3N2 was associated with multiple reassortment events that increased the genetic diversity. In 1977 an outbreak of H1N1 occurred by an unknown mechanism involving a virus which was identical to that circulating in humans in the 1950s. Since then, seasonal influenza outbreaks have involved two main subtypes, H1N1 and H3N2, and these viruses continue to undergo antigenic drift.

TRANSMISSION OF AVIAN INFLUENZA TO HUMANS

Until 1997, the difference in HA receptor-binding specificities was thought to provide a host range barrier such that direct infection of humans by an avian-origin virus seemed highly unlikely. However, in 1997 avian influenza A, subtype H5N1 virus was transmitted to humans from infected chickens in poultry markets in Hong Kong, resulting in the deaths of six of the 18 patients infected.[10] This and subsequent avian influenza viruses have become known as highly pathogenic avian influenza (HPAI) viruses. The high case fatality rate and the subsequent global spread of highly pathogenic H5N1 in birds raised the possibility of a significant future pandemic. The cumulative number of confirmed human cases from 2003 to the present has been reported as 826 with 440 deaths, a 53% case fatality rate.[11] In most cases, infected individuals have had close contact with infected poultry.

Life cycle of influenza virus

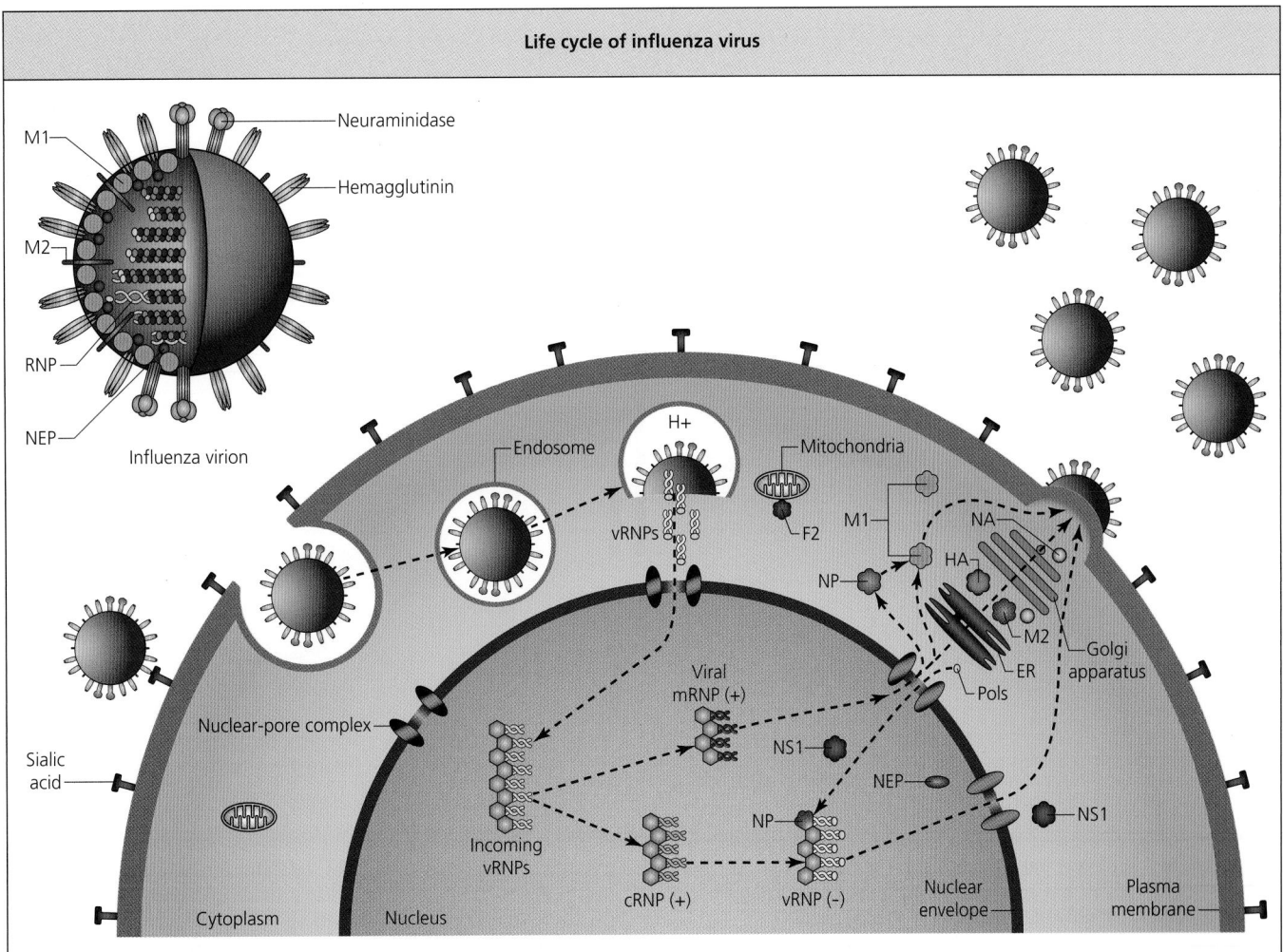

Figure 172-2   Life cycle of the influenza virus. Virus particles initially associate with the host cell by binding to sialic acid-containing receptors on the cell surface. The bound virus is endocytosed, with the eventual release of the uncoated viral ribonucleoprotein (vRNP) complex into the cytoplasm. The ribonucleoprotein complex is transported through the nuclear pore complex into the nucleus. The incoming viral RNA (vRNA) is transcribed into messenger RNA (mRNA). The viral proteins are expressed and processed and eventually assemble with vRNAs at budding sites within the host cell membrane. The viral protein complexes and ribonucleoproteins are assembled into viral particles that bud from the host cell. Further details are provided in the text. *(Reproduced with permission from http://www.reactome.org.)*

On rare occasions human-to-human transmission has been reported in Thailand, China, Vietnam, Indonesia and Azerbaijan; however, fortunately, there has been no evidence of sustained human-to-human transmission.[12-18] In March 1999, influenza A (H9N2) viruses infected two children in Hong Kong; however, these two cases were mild and self-limiting.[19] Subsequently, an outbreak of HPAI A H7N7 occurred in early 2003 in commercial poultry farms in the Netherlands, which resulted in 89 human infections of whom 83 developed conjunctivitis. Notably, one fatality occurred in a veterinarian who developed acute respiratory distress and fatal pneumonia.[20]

During 2015, H5N2 has been detected in poultry flocks in the Midwest of the US with several states declaring it an 'emergency'.[21] However, there has been no evidence of transmission to humans, in large part because of the rapid culling of infected flocks.

SWINE INFLUENZA (H1N1v) PANDEMIC 2009

In March 2009, public health authorities in Mexico City observed a large increase in the number of patients presenting with influenza-like illness. Subsequent testing in Canada and the USA confirmed that a previously undescribed influenza A virus was responsible. In April 2009, a novel swine-origin influenza A virus (also identified as 2009 H1N1 and per the World Health Organization (WHO) nomenclature A(H1N1)pdm09) infection was reported to the WHO by the Centers

for Disease Control and Prevention (CDC) in two children presenting with a febrile respiratory illness from neighboring counties in southern California.[22] These cases were not epidemiologically linked and neither child had exposure to swine. Phylogenetic characterization of the virus from the US index case (A/California/04/2009) showed that the virus had a unique gene constellation not previously seen in humans or other animal reservoirs. Six genes (PB2, PB1, PA, HA, NP and NS) were similar to viruses previously identified in triple-reassortment swine influenza viruses in North American pigs and the remaining two gene segments (NA and M) were derived from Eurasian swine influenza viruses (Figure 172-3).[23,24]

Globally the pandemic took on unique clinical and epidemiologic characteristics but did not lead to the devastating mortality of prior pandemics. Deaths predominantly occurred in individuals with underlying medical conditions, pregnant women, immunocompromised hosts, infants and the neurologically impaired but not, as would have been anticipated, in the elderly. In retrospect, the absence of morbidity and mortality in individuals >60 years has been attributed to exposure to a similar circulating strain decades ago.

After the original identification of A(H1N1)pdm09, sustained human-to-human transmission has occurred globally and on June 11 2009, the WHO declared the first pandemic of the 21st century. In addition to the rapid global spread, a major concern is the continued

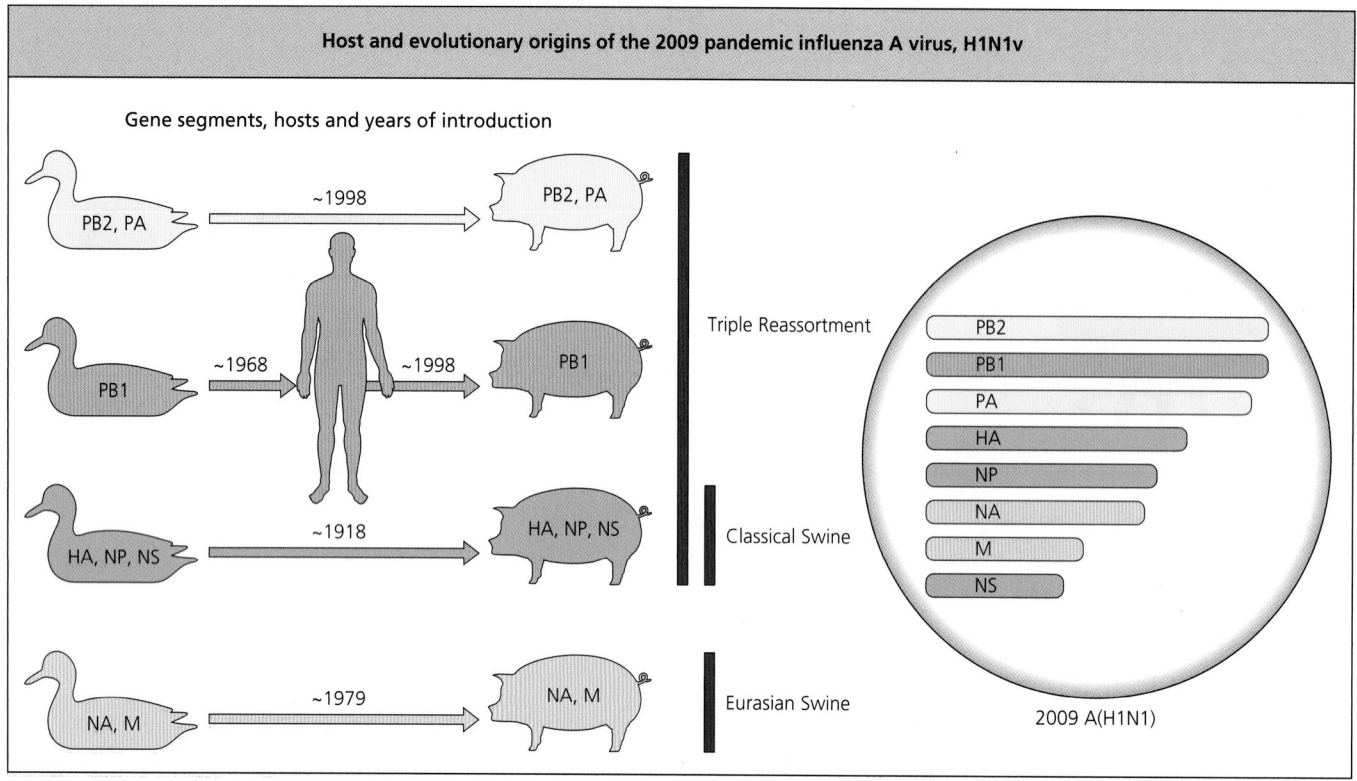

Figure 172-3   Host and evolutionary origins of the 2009 pandemic influenza A virus, H1N1v. Host and lineage origins for the gene segments of the 2009 A (H1N1) virus: PB2, polymerase basic 2; PB1, polymerase basic 1; PA, polymerase acidic; HA, hemagglutinin; NP, nucleoprotein; NA, neuraminidase; M, matrix gene; NS, nonstructural gene. Color of gene segment in circle indicates host. *(Reproduced with permission from Garten R.J. et al. Science 2009; 325 (5937):197-201. Epub 2009/05/26.)*

co-circulation – and potential reassortment – of the novel H1N1v with seasonal H1N1 (which has acquired oseltamivir resistance approaching 100%) and the highly pathogenic H5N1 avian virus.

Pathogenesis

Influenza virus is classically acquired by the inhalation of infectious droplets. However, transmission by airborne droplet nuclei, small-particle aerosols, or self-inoculation (via virus-contaminated hands or fomites) may also occur. Following inhalation, the virus attaches to specific $\alpha2$, 6-linked sialic acid receptors expressed on respiratory epithelial cells. Although these receptors are widespread, the virus attaches preferentially to tracheal and bronchial epithelium.[25] In contrast, human infection by avian influenza viruses preferentially involves the distal airways.[26]

In uncomplicated influenza, histologic examination reveals diffuse mucosal inflammation with edema of the upper airways: epithelial cells become vacuolated, edematous and lose their cilia, accompanied by hyperemia and infiltration with primarily lymphocytes and histiocytes. Virus replication peaks at about 48 hours and the level of viral shedding correlates directly with severity of symptoms.[2] In the more severe primary viral pneumonia, the pathologic process extends distally to the lung causing an interstitial pneumonitis. Damage to the alveoli with formation of hyaline membranes allows exudates and hemorrhage from alveolar capillaries into the alveolar lumina, resulting in impaired gas exchange and severe respiratory dysfunction.

The host immune response against influenza virus is complex. Following infection of the respiratory epithelial cells, pro-inflammatory cytokines – primarily interleukin (IL)-6 and interferon-alpha (IFN-α) – are produced by, and secreted from, infected cells. Cytokine production typically peaks by day 2 after infection, and corresponds with the peak of systemic symptoms.[27] In addition to cytokines, neutralizing antibodies (predominantly of the IgA subclass) are also produced at the site of infection. However, it is serum antibody levels (to HA and NA) that correlate with protection from illness and with restriction of infection. Serum antibodies (IgM, IgG and IgA) are present within 1 week of the onset of illness, and may provide immunity and protection against re-infection by homotypic viruses for many years, if not longer.[28] Cell-mediated immune responses are detectable before humoral responses and involve the activity of both CD8+ cytotoxic T cells and CD4+ helper T cells. Although these two classes of T cells closely interact, animal models have demonstrated that the response of either alone is capable of clearing infection.[3]

Prevention

VACCINATION

Vaccination remains the cornerstone of the prevention of seasonal influenza. Current recommendations in the USA by the Advisory Committee for Immunization Practices (ACIP) include annual vaccination for everyone 6 months and older, with rare exception.[29] Other countries have similar regimens; in the UK for example, there is a slightly more selective approach (https://www.gov.uk/government/collections/annual-flu-programme).

As a result of antigenic drift, the process of candidate vaccine selection is complex. The WHO in collaboration with the CDC is responsible for decisions as to which influenza strains should be included in the vaccine, and separate recommendations are made annually to regional health authorities in the Northern and Southern hemispheres. The WHO conducts global surveillance programs through a network of national and regional virology reference laboratories, which provide information on circulating viruses. In parallel, serologic surveys are performed on recipients of the previous year's vaccine to evaluate immune responses to the emerging strains of the current season.[30] Decisions regarding vaccine composition are made early in the calendar year and usually prior to the end of the current influenza season. Improvements are an ongoing enterprise.[31]

Since 1977, seasonal influenza has been caused by two co-circulating influenza A viruses (H1N1 and H3N2) and influenza B with a second

B strain contributing to disease more recently. Routinely, available seasonal vaccines contain three strains and, more recently, a quadrivalent vaccine has been developed that contains two influenza B strains. During influenza outbreaks where a close match exists between circulating virus strains and those in the vaccine, efficacy has been estimated at 80%. In seasons with a poor match, as occurred during the 2014–2015 influenza season, this can fall to as low as 50%, if not lower.[32]

Seasonal influenza vaccines may comprise either inactivated virus particles or live attenuated virus. Both vaccine formulations have been shown to be safe and efficacious in healthy children and adults, although the immune responses tend to be poorer among the elderly and young children. Live attenuated influenza virus vaccine (LAIV) is presently only licensed for use in healthy children aged 2 years and older, and in healthy nonpregnant adults through the age of 49 years. Trivalent inactivated influenza vaccine (TIV) is licensed for use in all persons aged 6 months and older and all high-risk groups. Studies have shown that both vaccine types have equivalent efficacy.[32] Of note, a high antigen content vaccine is available for individuals over the age of 65, although its enhanced efficacy is questioned.

Seasonal influenza vaccination is both clinically and cost-effective. It results in lower rates of laboratory-confirmed influenza cases, lower rates of clinical influenza-like illness, reduced numbers of physician visits, days of illness, days of work loss, hospitalization rates and mortality. The impact of vaccination on public health has been studied extensively by the US CDC. For example, during the 2013–2014 influenza season, vaccination decreased illness by over 2 million cases and hospitalization by 80 000. From a logistics perspective, LAIV has the advantage of intranasal administration, thus avoiding the need for injections. As patient surveys have indicated a preference for intranasal immunization over parenteral, more widespread use of the former would be expected to lead to an increased uptake of seasonal vaccine.[30]

Vaccination is generally well tolerated. Local reactions to TIV (discomfort, erythema and swelling) are typically mild. Systemic symptoms, which include fever, malaise and myalgia, may also occur. Despite widespread concern following an association between swine influenza vaccine and Guillain–Barré syndrome (GBS) in the USA in 1976, no definitive association between seasonal influenza vaccination and GBS has been demonstrated.[33]

CHEMOPROPHYLAXIS

According to the Infectious Diseases Society of America, 'influenza vaccination is the primary tool to prevent influenza and antiviral chemoprophylaxis is not a substitute for vaccination'.[34] However, antiviral chemoprophylaxis is effective and should be considered in the following groups:

- high-risk individuals within 2 weeks of influenza vaccination (before an adequate immune response develops);
- high-risk individuals for whom vaccination is contraindicated, unavailable or expected to have low effectiveness (significantly immunocompromised);
- high-risk individuals who have not yet been vaccinated (influenza vaccine should be also administered);
- those who are in close contact with people at high risk of developing influenza complications;
- all residents (vaccinated and unvaccinated) of institutions experiencing influenza outbreaks.

The deployment of antiviral drugs for treatment of influenza is detailed below. However, the same medications are used for chemoprophylaxis. The adamantane M2 inhibitors amantadine and rimantadine exhibit resistance to virtually all strains of influenza with the exception of some H3N2 strains and are therefore no longer routinely used for either therapy or prophylaxis when the circulating strain is known. As a consequence the neuraminidase inhibitors oseltamivir and zanamivir are recommended for the chemoprophylaxis of influenza A and influenza B virus infections.[34] Chemoprophylaxis is estimated to be 70–90% effective in preventing illness in healthy adults.[35] In hospital or residential institution settings, strategies for the prevention of nosocomial transmission of influenza should be implemented. These include staff and patient vaccination programs, chemoprophylaxis if appropriate, and compliance with droplet isolation precautions.

Diagnostic Microbiology

Laboratory diagnosis plays a crucial role in the management of influenza. The development of highly sensitive and specific methods for virus detection allows the laboratory to provide a rapid definitive diagnosis, enabling clinicians to initiate prompt and appropriate management.

VIRUS ISOLATION IN CULTURE

Influenza viruses can be isolated in culture from a range of specimens taken from the upper and lower respiratory tract; preferred specimen types are nasopharyngeal or nasal swabs and nasal washes or aspirates. Recently, the capital costs and longer turnaround times of culture compared with other more rapid detection systems have called into question the relevance of culture isolation methods.[36] However, it is clear that virus isolation remains essential for phenotypic antiviral susceptibility testing. In addition, the isolation process can be accelerated using centrifugation-enhanced ('shell vial') techniques.[37]

SEROLOGY

Serologic assays, such as hemagglutinin inhibition and complement fixation, require an acute-phase serum to be collected within 7 days of the onset of symptoms and compared with a convalescent serum specimen taken 14–21 days later to demonstrate a greater than fourfold rise in strain-specific, antibody titer. Because of the time required for host response, serology is of little use for the diagnosis of acute influenza; however, it remains important in basic research, epidemiologic investigations and the evaluation of antibody responses to vaccination.[38]

RAPID ANTIGEN TESTING

Rapid antigen or point-of-care (POC) testing has become increasingly important as timely results can lead to the prompt initiation of antiviral therapy, implementation of outbreak control measures and a reduction of inappropriate antibiotic usage.[39] The POC testing devices are simple to use and easily interpretable. However, while they have high specificities for virus detection, they have a lower sensitivity than 'gold standard' methods such as virus culture and reverse transcriptase polymerase chain reaction (RT-PCR), particularly in adult populations.[40-44] In general, the sensitivity of POC tests in adults is lower than in pediatric patient populations, attributable to the higher viral loads and antigen shedding in younger age groups.[45] Thus, a negative test may not definitively exclude a positive diagnosis.

IMMUNOFLUORESCENCE MICROSCOPY

The detection of influenza virus by direct fluorescent antibody (DFA) or immunofluorescence antibody (IFA) testing is extremely rapid and employs specific monoclonal antibodies to influenza virus antigens and visualization by fluorescence microscopy. The specificity and the sensitivity of this approach depend on sample collection and the presence of infected cells in the specimens. This is widely employed as an excellent first-line choice for clinicians requesting a laboratory confirmation of POC positives already identified in the clinical setting.

MOLECULAR DETECTION

Molecular diagnostic approaches are increasingly replacing virus isolation and to a lesser extent immunofluorescence and rapid antigen testing for the detection of influenza due to rapidity of performance, cost-effectiveness and standardization. Molecular detection of nucleic acids extracted from respiratory specimens, employing real-time RT-PCR, is the method of choice. In addition, multiplex PCRs have been developed for the identification of multiple viral and bacterial respiratory pathogens, and are being incorporated into diagnostic algorithms for the differential diagnosis of respiratory tract infections.[46-48] Rapid real-time influenza subtyping approaches have also been developed and these can be employed downstream of universal influenza molecular detection assays, allowing the differentiation of seasonal human influenza, H1N1 and H3N2, avian H5N1 subtypes and novel swine H1N1v.[49] Molecular methods have been developed to detect single nucleotide polymorphism underlying resistance.[50,51] More recently, pyrosequencing ('sequencing by synthesis') has also been applied for the detection of drug resistance.[52]

Clinical Manifestations

SEASONAL INFLUENZA

Influenza A and B cause an acute respiratory illness, with fever, cough, coryza, malaise, myalgia and headache. However, it is the associated systemic symptoms that distinguish influenza from other respiratory virus infections, such as rhinovirus or respiratory syncytial virus. The incubation period for influenza infection averages 2 days (range 1–4 days). The classic illness has an abrupt onset with headache, high-grade fever, chills, dry cough, myalgia and malaise. Rhinorrhea, nasal congestion and pharyngitis may also be present. Fever typically peaks within the first 24 hours of illness. It begins to decline on the second or third day and is usually resolved by day 6; however, fever may be continuous or intermittent. Systemic symptoms usually resolve within a similar timescale. Weakness and fatigue, which on occasions can be accompanied by cough, can persist for an additional 1–2 weeks. Influenza attack rates are higher in children compared with adults, with fever, cervical lymphadenopathy, nausea and vomiting being frequent manifestations; bronchiolitis and croup (laryngotracheitis) may also occur. Indeed, young children may present with primarily abdominal complaints initially rather than those involving the respiratory tract.

Subclinical or asymptomatic infection can also occur, particularly in individuals with pre-existing immunity to the circulating strains of virus. In contrast to influenza A and B, influenza C typically causes only a sporadic and usually afebrile upper respiratory tract illness.

Complications

Complications occur not infrequently. The most common complications are bronchitis in adults and otitis media in children; yet, exacerbations of pre-existing chronic medical conditions, such as asthma, chronic obstructive pulmonary disease and congestive heart failure, have been well described.

Pulmonary. Three distinct syndromes of severe pneumonia can occur after influenza infection in children or adults:

- primary viral pneumonia;
- combined viral–bacterial pneumonia; and
- secondary bacterial pneumonia.

Pneumonia complicates influenza predominantly in the elderly, patients with chronic cardiopulmonary disease, pregnant women and immunocompromised individuals.

Primary influenza virus pneumonia develops abruptly after the onset of symptoms and progresses within 24 hours to a clinical picture resembling severe acute respiratory distress syndrome (ARDS) associated with hypotension, hypoxia and cyanosis. Fatality rates are as high as 50%, with death typically occurring within 4 days.

Combined viral–bacterial pneumonia is more common than primary viral pneumonia, with *Streptococcus pneumoniae*, *Staphylococcus aureus* and *Haemophilus influenzae* being predominantly involved. The clinical syndrome is indistinguishable from primary viral pneumonia. However, the later onset and the detection of both virus and bacteria in clinical samples confirm the diagnosis. The case fatality rate for combined pneumonia is about 10%, although this is frequently higher in cases of *Staphylococcus aureus* coinfection.

Secondary bacterial pneumonia typically manifests after the patient has started to improve clinically from the original influenza illness. The onset of new respiratory symptoms is accompanied by localized clinical and radiologic findings. Bacteria may be isolated from clinical specimens, but usually virus is no longer detectable. The case fatality rate for this group of patients has been reported at around 7%.

Extrapulmonary. A variety of extrapulmonary manifestations have been described. Central nervous system (CNS) involvement, ranging from irritability and drowsiness to seizures and coma, has been reported, although the pathogenesis remains unclear. Influenza-associated acute encephalopathy (IAAE), which is associated histologically with diffuse cerebral congestion and edema, is a recognized, uncommon but potentially fatal neurologic syndrome generally occurring in children and adolescents and typically presenting during the early phase of infection.[53] A post-influenza encephalitis may also occur 2–3 weeks following recovery from the acute illness; fortunately, complete recovery occurs in the majority of cases. Reye's syndrome has also been reported following influenza (B more frequently than A) infection. Though the etiology is unknown, the risk of Reye's appears to be increased by the administration of therapeutic doses of salicylates and their use is now contraindicated in influenza infection.

Myocarditis has also been reported but the pathogenesis is poorly understood and is probably due to a combination of viral and host factors. Clinically, myocarditis may be associated with heart failure, pericardial effusion or conduction system disorders. Myositis or myopathy have also been described. While most cases recover, this may be so severe that acute renal failure secondary to myoglobinuria can occur. Toxic shock syndrome may also present in the context of influenza virus infection. It is believed that this is the consequence of bacterial exotoxin (TSST-1) secreted by colonizing or co-infecting *Staph. aureus* strains.

Infection in Specific Groups

In the immunocompromised host, influenza virus infection is associated with an increased risk of complications, hospitalizations and death. While the observed illness typically reflects that seen in the healthy individual, the clinical presentation may be atypical in the elderly (e.g. confusion, lethargy, low-grade fever) or in the transplant population (e.g. pneumonia, rejection). A prolonged disease course with viral shedding and the rapid emergence of antiviral resistance are also features of influenza in the immunocompromised.

Pregnant women in the second or third trimester have an increased risk of mortality from influenza. Although this is more commonly seen in the pandemic setting, it is also a feature of seasonal influenza, and the cause of death is usually overwhelming pulmonary disease. There are no clear explanations for the increased risk of pulmonary disease in pregnancy; however, it has been postulated that the increased pulmonary blood flow in pregnancy may predispose to pulmonary edema when alveoli are damaged.[54] While maternal influenza infection has been reported to be associated with an increased risk of congenital anomalies and fetal loss, no specific teratogenic effect has been attributed to influenza virus.

Infants, particularly those less than 1 year of age, have both increased morbidity and mortality. Mortality is now a reportable event in this population to the US CDC. However morbidity and mortality are greatest in the elderly. As a consequence, all efforts should be made to prevent disease in those over 75.

AVIAN INFLUENZA (H5N1)

H5N1 avian influenza, in contrast to seasonal influenza and A(H1N1) pdm09, is highly pathogenic in humans with high morbidity and mortality. Although a definitive explanation for the severity of H5N1 infection remains to be established, much is known.[55] The virus is capable of infecting pulmonary epithelial cells, thereby causing diffuse alveolar damage and hemorrhage (this process is not dissimilar to primary viral pneumonia as described above). In addition, H5N1 (unlike seasonal influenza) disseminates beyond the respiratory tract during infection. The virus also has the capacity to impair cytotoxic T-cell activity *in vitro*, thereby reducing the capacity of the host to clear infection. Studies indicate that aberrant production of pro-inflammatory cytokines may also contribute to the pathogenesis of H5N1 influenza.

TABLE 172-1	**Antiviral Drugs for Influenza**					
Drug (Trade Name)	**Virus**	**Administration**	**Treatment Indications**	**Chemoprophylaxis Indications**	**Adverse Effects**
Oseltamivir (Tamiflu®)	A and B	Oral	Birth or older	3 mo or older	Nausea, vomiting
Zanamivir (Relenza®)	A and B	Inhalation	7 y or older	5 y or older	Bronchospasm
Amantadine (Symmetrel®)	A	Oral	1 y or older	1 y or older	Central nervous system (CNS), anxiety, gastrointestinal
Rimantadine (Flumadine®)	A	Oral	13 y or older	1 y or older	CNS, anxiety, gastrointestinal
Peramivir	A	iv	13 y or older	13 y or older	NA

PANDEMIC INFLUENZA (A(H1N1)pdm09)

In general, the clinical presentation of pandemic influenza is similar to that described above, although some symptoms atypical for seasonal influenza may be more prominent. This is the case in the A(H1N1)pdm09 pandemic with diarrhea and/or vomiting being reported in some 38% of patients. This pandemic was characterized by the mildness of symptoms in the overwhelming majority of patients.[56] However, despite mild disease, the hospitalization rate is significant and reports from Australia indicated this may be in the region of 10% of 'laboratory-confirmed' cases.[57] Severe respiratory disease and death have been reported, both in previously healthy individuals and those with underlying chronic disease.[58] Pregnant women, those with a body mass index (BMI) of >40 and those with pre-existing pulmonary disease were particularly at risk of severe respiratory distress following A(H1N1)pdm09 infection.[59,60] As noted above, initial serologic studies suggest that a degree of pre-existing immunity to A(H1N1)pdm09 exists in adults >60 years.[61]

Management

The majority of individuals infected with influenza virus have a self-limited, uncomplicated illness. However, in those patients with severe illness, early treatment with antiviral therapy reduces the severity and duration of symptoms, the number of hospitalizations, the incidence of complications, the use of outpatient facilities and, in some cases, the inappropriate use of antibiotics.[34] Of note, the use of antivirals for the treatment of influenza has been controversial in some countries, particularly the UK;[62] however, recently published data have established the unequivocal value of treatment by public health officials of Europe and the USA. In an individual patient meta-analysis, oseltamivir therapy decreased mortality, hospitalization and lower respiratory tract infections in adults.[63]

Antiviral therapy for influenza has been covered in detail elsewhere in this text (see Chapter 154). However, in brief, there are two classes of agents with anti-influenza activity: the adamantane M2 inhibitors (amantadine and rimantadine) and the neuraminidase inhibitors (oseltamivir, zanamivir and peramivir [US and Japan]), as illustrated in Table 172-1. Additionally, laninamivir is licensed in Asia while favipiravir and Fludase® are under investigation in Europe and the USA. Because of global resistance, the use of the adamantines is now restricted to only the pre-2009 seasonal H1N1 strain. Of the three neuraminidase inhibitors, oseltamivir is administered orally; zanamivir is delivered by inhalation and peramivir is given intravenously. To be effective, antiviral therapy must be administered within 24–48 hours of the onset of symptoms. In general, both classes of agents are well tolerated, although zanamivir-induced severe bronchospasm has also been described, particularly in individuals with a history of asthma. The effectiveness of oseltamivir was best illustrated by an individual patient meta-analysis.[63]

In the years leading up to the 2009 pandemic, antiviral drug resistance had become prevalent for both classes of antivirals. Widespread resistance to the M2 inhibitors was documented in the H3N2 virus and the prevalence of oseltamivir resistance in seasonal H1N1 virus prior to 2009 increased to greater than 90%. Since the A(H1N1)pdm09 strain became the predominantly circulating seasonal strain of influenza A, rare, oseltamivir resistance (H275Y mutation in NA) has been reported. However, the virus remains sensitive to zanamivir. A recent multiyear prospective study designed to assess emerging resistance to oseltamivir has reported an approximate incidence of only 2%.[64] These resistant viruses were no more virulent in animal models than wild-type virus. In children, the incidence of resistance approaches 10%.[65]

The following groups should be considered for antiviral therapy if influenza virus infection is documented: unvaccinated infants aged 1–24 months and individuals with any of the following: chronic pulmonary disease; hemodynamically significant cardiac disease; HIV infection; sickle cell anemia or other hemoglobinopathies; disease requiring long-term aspirin therapy; chronic renal dysfunction; cancer; chronic metabolic conditions; neuromuscular disorders; and seizure disorders. In addition, all adults over 65 years of age and all residents of nursing homes (or other long-term care facilities) should be considered for treatment.[34] Key to successful therapy is the early introduction of treatment after the onset of symptoms, a time frame that is usually 48 hours.

References available online at expertconsult.com.

KEY REFERENCES

Dobson J., Whitley R.J., Pocock S., et al.: Oseltamivir treatment for influenza in adults: a meta-analysis of randomised controlled trials. *Lancet* 2015; 385(9979): 1729-1737.

Kimberlin D., Acosta E., Prichard M., et al.: Oseltamivir pharmacokinetics, dosing, and resistance in children from birth to two years of age with influenza. *J Infect Dis* 2012; 207(5):709-720.

Krammer F., Palese P.: Advances in the development of influenza virus vaccines. *Nat Rev Drug Discov* 2015; 14(3):167-182.

Harper S.A., Bradley J.S., Englund J.A., et al.: Seasonal influenza in adults and children – diagnosis, treatment, chemoprophylaxis, and institutional outbreak management: clinical practice guidelines of the Infectious Diseases Society of America. *Clin Infect Dis* 2009; 48(8):1003-1032.

Havers F., Flannery B., Clippard J.R., et al.: Use of influenza antiviral medications among outpatients at high risk for influenza-associated complications during the 2013-2014 influenza season. *Clin Infect Dis* 2015; 60(11): 1677-1680.

Hayden F., Palese P.: Influenza virus. In: Richmann D., Whitley R., Hayden F., eds. *Clinical virology*. 3rd ed. Washington: ASM Press; 2009:943-976.

Shaw M., Palese P.: Orthomyxoviridae. In: Knipe D., Howley P., eds. *Fields Virology*. 6th ed. Philadelphia: Lippincott, Williams and Wilkins; 2013:1151-1185.

Whitley R.J., Boucher C.A., Lina B., et al.: Global assessment of resistance to neuraminidase inhibitors, 2008-2011: the Influenza Resistance Information Study (IRIS). *Clin Infect Dis* 2013; 56(9):1197-1205.

World Health Organization: *Cumulative number of confirmed human cases of avian influenza A/(H5N1) reported to WHO 2003-2015*. Geneva: WHO; 2015. Available: http://www.who.int/influenza/human_animal_interface/EN_GIP_20150501CumulativeNumberH5N1cases.pdf?ua=1.

Wright P., Neumann G., Kawaoka Y.: Orthomyxoviruses. In: Knipe D., Howley P., eds. *Fields Virology*. 6th ed. Philadelphia: Lippincott, Williams and Wilkins; 2013: 1186-1243.

173

Noninfluenza Respiratory Viruses

MICHAEL G. ISON | NELSON LEE

KEY CONCEPTS

- Novel strains of adenovirus 11 and 14 have recently been identified as a cause of clinically significant, sometimes severe infection, in otherwise healthy adults and children.

- The novel coronavirus, MERS-CoV, has emerged to cause severe respiratory infections in the Arabian Peninsula.

- A short inhibitory RNA has shown promise in the management of respiratory syncytial virus (RSV) in lung transplant recipients but is not yet approved for the treatment of RSV.

- Human rhinoviruses are the most common cause of the common cold and are also common triggers of exacerbations of asthma and chronic obstructive pulmonary disease (COPD).

- Human metapneumovirus is a significant cause of disease in young children

- Human bocavirus 1 is a newly discovered respiratory pathogen although coinfection with other viruses is often documented.

Adenovirus

Nature

Human adenoviruses (hAdV) are members of the Adenoviridae family, which are enveloped, double-stranded DNA (dsDNA) viruses. hAdV are divided into 57 serotypes and seven species (A, B, C, D, E, F, and G; see Table 173-1) based on serum neutralizing and hemagglutination epitopes, genome sequence and function, oncogenic properties and pathology in humans.[1-3]

Epidemiology

Adenoviruses cause a range of infections from mild, self-limited respiratory viral infections, conjunctivitis and diarrhea to severe disseminated disease.[4] Adenoviruses have a worldwide distribution and infections occur throughout the year without significant seasonal variability. Most infections occur as sporadic events, although local or regional epidemics have been described.[5,6] Infection is more common in children (66.9%), generally less than 5 years of age.[7] About 4.4% of children with diarrhea are infected with adenovirus, typically with AdV 40 and 41.[8] Recently, several, often fatal, outbreaks of AdV 14 occurred starting in 2005 in the USA.[5,6] AdV 55, which is an AdV 11 and 14 recombinant virus, has been recognized to cause significant outbreaks of disease in China.[9,10] Adenovirus is the leading cause of respiratory viral infections among military recruits.[11,12]

Pathogenicity

Adenoviruses infect susceptible hosts by the mouth, nasopharynx or ocular conjunctiva. Key cellular receptors include CAR (coxsackie-adenovirus receptor), CD46, desmoglein 2 and GD1a glycan.[13] In addition, adenovirus hexon-factor X complexes can result in CAR-independent binding involving heparin sulfate glycosaminoglycans or αv integrins.[14]

Replication causes desquamation of epithelial cells, which induces changes in regional lymphatic tissue, including hypertrophy and active, proliferative germinal centers and can result in lymphadenopathy and intussusception, particularly in children.[15,16] The innate and adaptive immune responses are critical for the control of adenovirus replication.[17,18] CD4+ and CD8+ T lymphocytes play a particularly important role in the control and clearance of replicating adenovirus in humans with deficits associated with progressive dissemination in immunosuppressed patients.[4,19-21] Group- and type-specific neutralizing and non-neutralizing antibodies play a significant role, too, in limiting infection.[22]

Prevention

Vaccination and careful attention to infection control practices are the only existing preventative strategies.[11] To date, the vaccine is only available to members of the military in the USA who are 17–50 years old.[11] Contact and droplet precautions are recommended to prevent healthcare-associated and institutional outbreaks of adenovirus infections, including epidemic keratoconjunctivitis.[23] Likewise, careful attention to hand hygiene and standard sterilization of medical equipment that comes in contact with patients with proven or suspected adenovirus infection is essential.[24]

Diagnostic Microbiology

Diagnosis of adenovirus depends on the isolation of the virus from infected tissue and either histopathologic evidence of local replication or clinical symptoms consistent with infection. Confirmation of infection can be confused by latent infection in some tissues, such as the tonsils, and intermittent and sometimes prolonged shedding of virus from throat or in the stool for months to years after primary infection.[25,26] Direct detection of adenovirus from clinical isolates is generally achieved by culture, direct fluorescent antigen detection, or polymerase chain reaction (PCR).[2,27] Adenovirus can readily be grown in HEK and A549 cell lines (see Figure 173-1), with typical cytopathic effect or fluorescent antibodies used to confirm infection. Molecular

TABLE 173-1	Adenovirus Subgroup, Serotype and Major Site of Infection	
Subgroup	Serotype	Major Site of Infection
A	12, 18, 31	Respiratory, urinary, gastrointestinal (GI)
B1	3, 7, 16, 21, 50	Respiratory, eye, urinary, GI
B2	11, 14, 34, 35	
C	1, 2, 5, 6, 57	Respiratory, urinary, GI
D	8–10, 13, 15, 17, 19, 20, 22–30, 32, 33, 36–39, 42–49, 51, 53, 54, 56	Eye, GI
E	4	Eye, respiratory
F	40, 41	GI
G	52	GI

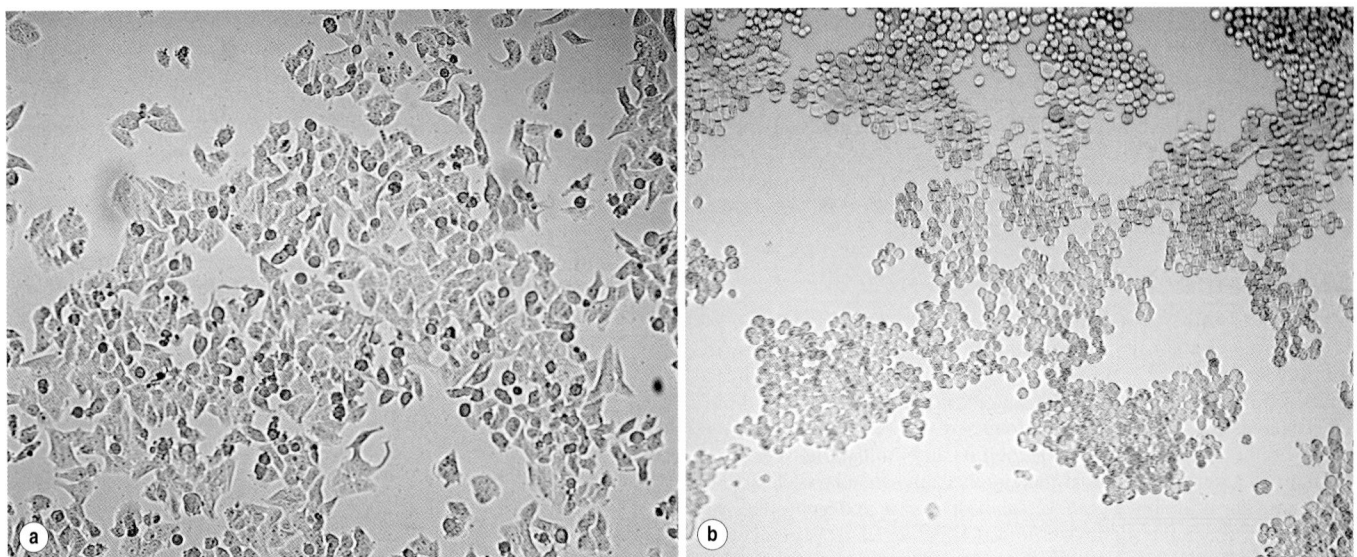

Figure 173-1 Cytopathic effect caused by adenovirus on Hep-2 cell line culture. (a) Uninoculated cell line. (b) Enlarged, refractile, rounded cells forming grape-like clusters.

techniques are used increasingly for the diagnosis of adenovirus and generally have the highest yield of the various diagnostic methods.[27,28] Unfortunately many respiratory virus multiplex panels have low yields for adenovirus in patients with clinical infection; this is especially true if respiratory samples are collected and the respiratory tract is not the primary site of infection.[29] Quantitative PCR assays can be used to predict progression to disseminated disease in pediatric and, to a lesser extent, adult stem cell transplant (HSCT) recipients and to assess response to antiviral therapy.[28,30–33]

Clinical Manifestations

Adenovirus infections are associated with a wide range of clinical manifestations, including respiratory tract, ocular, gastrointestinal tract, genitourinary tract, and central nervous system (CNS) infections, among others. Disseminated infection can also occur, typically in the immunosuppressed host.

RESPIRATORY TRACT INFECTIONS

Pharyngitis, laryngotracheitis, bronchitis and pneumonia have all been described. Typically, symptoms that include nasal congestion, coryza and cough are often accompanied by systemic manifestations, such as generalized malaise, fever, chills, myalgia and headache; abdominal pain, an exudative tonsillitis and cervical adenopathy are often frequently observed.[34,35] If conjunctivitis accompanies the above signs and symptoms, the disease is designated as pharyngoconjunctival fever.[7,36] Rarely a pertussis-like syndrome has been described, typically caused by AdV 5.[37,38] Pneumonia, usually with diffuse bilateral interstitial infiltrates, has been described and may be particularly severe with AdV 3, 7, 14 and 21.[5,39–44] The recent outbreak of severe AdV 14 resulted in significant morbidity and mortality in some patients.[5,44] Most individuals presented with fever and cough and most required hospitalization (76%), supplemental oxygen (61%), and critical care (47%), while a minority received vasopressors (24%) or died (18%).[5] Older age, chronic underlying condition, low absolute lymphocyte counts and elevated creatinine levels were associated with severe illness.

OCULAR INFECTIONS

The two most common manifestations of ocular adenovirus infection are pharyngoconjunctival fever and epidemic keratoconjunctivitis (EKC). Pharyngoconjunctival fever is typically a milder form of acute follicular conjunctivitis that accompanies febrile pharyngitis or cervical adenitis.[7,36] Symptoms typically resolve without sequelae and no treatment is indicated. Epidemic keratoconjunctivitis (EKC) is a more

serious disease with a much longer time to recovery. Following an 8–10 day incubation, a follicular conjunctivitis with edema of the eyelids, pain, lacrimation, photophobia, preauricular lymph node hypertrophy and, rarely, self-limited painful corneal opacities develop.[45,46] Epidemic keratoconjunctivitis, typically caused by adenovirus types 8, 19, and 37, was first seen in shipyard workers whose eyes had been slightly injured by chips of rust or paint. Although patients may experience significant pain and blurry vision, EKC typically resolves without permanent corneal damage over 4 weeks.[47,48]

GASTROINTESTINAL TRACT INFECTIONS

Up to 10% of pediatric cases of diarrhea are caused by the group F AdV 40 and 41. Higher rates of adenovirus-induced diarrhea have been described with seasonal outbreaks in low- and middle-income areas of the world.[2] Adenovirus-associated diarrhea is typically prolonged, lasting 8–12 days. Outbreaks in closed communities and clinical settings have been described.[49] Mesenteric adenitis is common and clinically mimics appendicitis or results in intussusception in young children.[16,50] Adenovirus infection may masquerade as rejection in small bowel transplant recipients and should be ruled out on all biopsies from such patients.[4,51]

GENITOURINARY TRACT INFECTIONS

Hemorrhagic cystitis typically presents as microscopic or macroscopic hematuria and pain and cramping of the bladder, and is associated with AdV 11 and 21.[52] Adenovirus tubulointerstitial nephritis occurs mostly commonly in kidney transplant recipients and presents as transient elevation of serum creatinine and hemorrhagic cystitis.[53–55]

OTHER MANIFESTATIONS OF ADENOVIRUS

Other rare manifestations include meningitis, encephalitis, myocarditis and dilated myocardiopathy.[56–58] Additionally, echogenic liver lesions with or without hydrops and neural defects in fetuses have also been described.[59]

ADENOVIRUS DISEASES IN IMMUNOCOMPROMISED PATIENTS

Adenovirus disease in immunocompromised adults and children ranges from asymptomatic shedding to progressive, often fatal disseminated disease.[28,60–63] Risk factors for adenoviral infection in the HSCT population includes allogeneic donor (8.5–30% vs 2–12% for autologous donor), pediatric age groups (20–47% vs 9–13.6% for adults), T cell-depleted grafts (45% vs 11%), use of alemtuzumab, cord blood donor and patients with acute graft-versus-host disease

(GVHD).[4,28,63–65] Although disseminated disease only effects 1–7% of HSCT recipients it is associated with a significant risk of mortality (8–26%).[4,28,63,66] Incidence among solid organ transplant recipient populations is highest in small bowel and liver transplant recipients, pediatric transplant recipients, patients who receive antilymphocyte antibodies, and patients with donor-positive/recipient-negative adenovirus status.[60] Asymptomatic adenovirus DNAemia is common among solid organ transplant recipients and generally is not associated with progression to symptomatic disease.[67,68]

Management

Although no antivirals are specifically approved for the treatment of adenovirus, several have *in vitro* and *in vivo* experimental data to support their use.[4,63,69–73] While no single agent has consistently been effective in all cases, existing data suggest that cidofovir and its lipid ester analogs (CMX001 or brincidofovir) are most effective in managing adenovirus infections.[4,63,74] Adenovirus- and multi-virus-specific T cells are an emerging potential therapy that can safely be used with a low frequency of de novo graft-versus-host disease and a complete or partial response in the adenovirus infection.[75,76] Serial measurement of quantitative viral load is predictive of response to any therapeutic intervention.

Coronavirus

Nature

Coronaviruses are large, lipid-enveloped, positive-sense, single-stranded RNA viruses. Human coronaviruses (e.g. hCoV 229E, OC43, NL63) commonly cause mild upper respiratory tract infections, although occasionally result in more severe disease in immunocompromised individuals.[77] However, two novel human coronaviruses, the severe acute respiratory syndrome-associated coronavirus (SARS-CoV), and a recently identified Middle East respiratory syndrome-associated coronavirus (MERS-CoV) may cause serious viral pneumonitis, leading to hospitalizations and deaths.[78,79,289] Viral genome analyses revealed that SARS-CoV belongs to Group B and MERS-CoV belongs to Group C betacoronavirus, respectively, and both are closely related to coronavirus strains found in bats.[78–80] Intermediate mammalian hosts, such as civet cats, have been implicated for SARS-CoV before its adaptation for human transmission, and emerging evidence (through virus or antibody detection) suggest that the dromedary camels are likely the host for MERS-CoV.[78,79,81,290] The surface spike glycoprotein (S-protein) of coronaviruses is a key virulence factor which attaches the virus to host cells, determining its host range and tissue tropism, and it is a target of the neutralizing antibodies. SARS-CoV uses human angiotensin-converting enzyme 2 (ACE-II) as the primary cellular receptor; the human cellular C-type lectin (DC/L-SIGN) may be the alternative.[82] MERS-CoV has been shown to bind to dipeptidyl peptidase 4, (DPP4; also called CD26), an interspecies-conserved protein found on the surface of several cell types, including the non-ciliated cells in human airways, which can explain its broadened host range and its ability to cause cross-species, zoonotic transmission.[83]

Epidemiology

HCoVs are ubiquitous among humans and are the major cause of respiratory disease, accounting for up to 30% of all common colds. Serologic studies have also suggested that one-half of the infections with coronaviruses are asymptomatic.[84] Two more newly-described coronaviruses, HKU1 and NL63, are also common causes of typically mild, self-limited colds.[85] More severe clinical disease has been described in young children, the elderly and in immunocompromised patients.[86]

SARS-CoV emerged in Southern China (Guangdong province) in late 2002; the first victims were those involved in live animal trade and food handlers at restaurants which serve exotic animal meat.[79] Through international air travel, the disease quickly spread to Hong Kong, Vietnam, Singapore, Taiwan and Canada in a matter of weeks; at the end of the 6-month epidemic, more than 30 countries were affected, resulting in 8096 confirmed infections, and 774 deaths (9.6%).[87] The primary mode of transmission was via respiratory droplets; the basic reproductive number (R0) of SARS was in the range of 2.2–3.7.[79,82,87] However, frequent nosocomial outbreaks and 'super-spreading events' had greatly exacerbated its transmission.[88] Notably, 21% of SARS victims were healthcare workers; and the disease attack rate in hospitals was between 10% and 60%.[78,82] Viral kinetics (peak at the time of clinical deterioration), application of aerosol-generating procedures and devices (e.g. intubation, resuscitation, oxygen or nebulizer therapy, bilevel positive airway pressure (BiPAP)), overcrowdedness and lack of proper isolation facilities in hospitals are some of the explanations.[88–90] A community 'super-spreading event' that occurred in a private housing estate in Hong Kong involved over 300 residents. Drying up of a 'U-shaped' bathroom floor drain and backflow of contaminated sewage (from a SARS patient with diarrhea), coupled with the toilet's exhaust fan, might have created infectious aerosols that rose with warm air along the building's air-shaft; these were then dispersed by wind flow, causing long-range transmission to nearby buildings.[90] This and other evidence suggested that SARS could be 'opportunistically' airborne.[78,89]

The first cases of MERS-CoV infections emerged in June 2012 in Saudi Arabia and Qatar. As of May 2015, a total of 1180 confirmed infections and 483 (41%) deaths had been reported.[78,91] The Middle Eastern countries of Saudi Arabia, Qatar, Jordan and United Arab Emirates were predominantly affected, but imported cases to UK, Netherlands, USA and Asia were reported.[91,291] The largest outbreak outside the Middle East occurred in South Korea in 2015, which involved multiple hospitals and 185 individuals, causing 36 (19.5%) deaths. Although zoonotic transmission is implicated, the majority of infected cases did not report a history of direct animal contact. Epidemiological investigations suggested sporadic transmission of disease with multiple introductions into the at-risk population. It was found that occupational exposure to camels (e.g. shepherds, slaughter-house works) was associated with 15–23 times higher risk of seroconversion (2.3–3.6%) than the general population (<0.2%). Also, a large number of younger (15–44 years) infected individuals, who develop no or mild symptoms might exist and serve as the source of infection for those without direct animal contact.[78,91,92,292] Secondary transmission in household is not uncommon, which occur in over 20% of case clusters. Transmission is typically highly efficient in the hospital settings via infectious droplets/aerosols, leading to frequent occurrence of nosocomial outbreaks, as in the case of SARS.[78,93–96,293,294]

Pathogenicity

The cellular receptor for HCoV-229E is aminopeptidase N (APN) or CD13; the cellular receptor for HCoV-OC43 is 9-O-acetylated sialic acid on the cell surface. Like SARS-CoV, HCoV-NL63 binds to ACE2.[85]

Humans have no pre-existing immunity to SARS-CoV or MERS-CoV. These novel viruses have the ability to evade innate host defenses (e.g. type I interferon responses and related mechanisms), and replicate efficiently in host tissues (respiratory and intestinal tract cells; kidney cells also for MERS-CoV).[78,80,82,83] In addition to lytic cell damage, uncontrolled replication of SARS-CoV leads to unabated inflammatory cytokine activation (commonly known as 'cytokine storms'), which is implicated in the development of progressive pneumonitis, diffuse alveolar damage and acute respiratory distress syndrome (ARDS), and hemophagocytic syndrome.[79,97] High viral load and slow viral clearance due to inefficient host responses are associated with progressive disease and fatal outcomes.[82,98,99] Pathogenesis data for MERS-CoV are limited; a macaque model has shown active viral replication in lung tissues causing localized-to-widespread lesions and clinical illness, which only abates after 1 week of illness. Infected marmosets can develop severe interstitial pneumonia similar to humans cases. Neutrophil and macrophage infiltration and alveolar oedema are noted.[78,100,101]

Prevention

There is no vaccine or chemoprophylaxis available for coronaviruses at present.[102] Droplet and contact precautions, including the use of face masks, are advisable to prevent transmission. As transmission could be opportunistically airborne, appropriate isolation precautions (in negative-pressure facilities if available) should be implemented in all hospitalized patients confirmed with novel coronavirus infections, particularly when respiratory procedures and devices are applied.[88–91]

Diagnostic Microbiology

A high index of suspicion, together with detailed clinical and epidemiological assessments (e.g. travel history to affected areas, case clustering), is required for the diagnosis of novel coronavirus infections.[88,103] RT-PCR is the diagnostic test of choice. A combination of upper respiratory (nasal, pharyngeal, nasopharyngeal), lower respiratory (higher yield due to higher viral levels, e.g. sputum, tracheal aspirate, bronchoalveolar lavage (BAL) whenever available), blood and fecal samples, and repeated sampling should be considered to maximize the chance of virus detection.[103–105] A single negative test from an upper respiratory sample may be insufficient to rule out the diagnosis. For SARS-CoV, plasma RT-PCR can detect viremia as early as day 2–3 after symptom onset, and its level may have prognostic value.[88,99] Virus culture (e.g. using Vero cells) is confirmatory, but the delay to a result prevents its use for clinical management; also biosafety level-3 facilities are required. Serological diagnosis is retrospective and largely used for epidemiological surveillance purposes.[103] Clinicians should refer to their local reference laboratories for coronavirus testing (e.g. pan-coronavirus RT-PCR, specific SARS-CoV and MERS-CoV RT-PCR).[87,91]

Clinical Manifestations

The incubation period of SARS is about 4–6 days (range 2–16 days). Patients initially develop fever, chills and rigor, which partially subside in a few days. These are then followed by resurgence of high fever, cough, shortness of breath and the development of pneumonia.[78,88] Chest radiographs first reveal patches of consolidation and ground-glass changes, which rapidly progress in the next few days to involve multiple lobes. CT scan of thorax may show features resembling bronchiolitis obliterans or organizing pneumonia, such as peripheral air-space consolidation.[78,79,88] Laboratory features include lymphopenia, thrombocytopenia, elevated transaminases, creatinine kinase and lactate dehydrogenase.[88] Around day 10–14, 15–25% of patients further deteriorate and develop refractory respiratory failure and ARDS.[106] About 20% of patients develop profuse diarrhea which contains highly infectious virus particles; renal failure is rare.[107] Other complications include ventilator-associated pneumonia (e.g. MRSA), pneumothorax and pneumomediastinum.[106] The overall death rate of SARS was 6–16%. The age-stratified case fatality rate was: <25 years: <1%; 25–44 years: 6%; 45–64 years: 15%; and >65 years: >50%.[78,87,106] Young children (e.g. <5 years) typically have mild disease; fatality is rare.

Available data indicate that the clinical features of MERS-CoV are similar to those of SARS. Patients develop high fever and chills, cough, shortness of breath and progressive pneumonia in about 1 week after symptom onset. Imaging findings include multiple, patchy consolidations and ground-glass changes. In addition to lymphopenia, thrombocytopenia and elevated liver enzymes, acute renal failure seems to be a common feature.[80,92,95,104,108] The majority of adult patients with severe infection are older (mean age 60 years), and had underlying conditions (e.g. diabetes mellitus, renal impairment) and required ICU care because of respiratory failure and ARDS; the associated fatality rate in such patients can be as high as 60–76% despite maximal medical support.[92,108,109] Notably, affected children usually have mild or no symptoms, as in the case of SARS.[78,79,110]

Management

At present, there is no established therapy for coronavirus infection. During the SARS outbreak in 2003, a range of agents had been used but their efficacies are questionable.[78,102,111] Ribavirin, though shown to be active *in vitro*, did not seem to provide any clinical benefit. An HIV protease-inhibitor (lopinavir-ritonavir) with *in vitro* activity against SARS-CoV was reported to cause viral load reduction and fewer ARDS and deaths in 41 patients; however, the study was uncontrolled.[112] Another study reported that 19 patients who received 'convalescent-plasma' from recovering individuals, which contained neutralizing antibodies, had better clinical outcomes (survival 100% vs 66%, discharge rates 78% vs 23%).[113] Subsequent *in vitro* and animal (ferrets, hamsters, macaques) studies have shown that monoclonal antibodies targeting the S-protein may provide neutralizing activity against SARS-CoV, resulting in viral load reduction and resolution of lung lesions.[114,115] *In vitro* and animal (mice, macaques) studies show that type I interferons, if given prophylactically or shortly after exposure, may protect against SARS.[116] In a small clinical study (n=9), interferon-alpha given within 5 days was associated with lower rates of intubation (11% vs 23%) and death (0% vs 8%).[117] Against MERS-CoV, available data have shown that type I and type III interferons are active *in vitro*; a combination of IFN-α 2b and ribavirin given hours after infection appears to reduce lung injury in a macaque model.[118] Clinical data are limited; among the few patients who received such treatment, no consistent result was observed. In one retrospective study, survival was 30% versus 17% at 28 days, but it did not reach statistical significance.[80,92,95,104,108–110,295] Animal models have suggested potential benefits of other antiviral agents or antibody-based therapies, but no clinical data have been published to date.[119,296,297]

Systemic corticosteroid treatment is highly controversial. While favorable clinical and radiological responses have been reported, controlled data are lacking.[102,106,111] In the only randomized, placebo-controlled study performed during the SARS outbreak, early corticosteroid treatment within the first few days delayed viral clearance.[98] A later systematic review has ded that corticosteroid is not associated with definite benefit, but is likely to be harmful (e.g. metabolic side effects, bacterial and fungal superinfections, avascular osteonecrosis, acute psychosis).[111] Currently, corticosteroid therapy is not recommended in SARS-CoV, MERS-CoV and avian influenza infections, perhaps except in cases with refractory septic shock and adrenal insufficiency, and should only be given at a low dose (e.g. hydrocortisone 50 mg Q8H).[78,91]

Respiratory Syncytial Virus

Nature and Pathogenicity

Respiratory syncytial virus (RSV) is an enveloped, single-stranded RNA paramyxovirus that includes two major groups, A and B, each of which consists of 5 to 6 genotypes. The RSV genome encodes two nonstructural (NS1 and NS2) and nine structural proteins, including the F (fusion) and G (attachment) glycoproteins on the viral envelope. Antibodies against the F and G proteins are neutralizing, and have been shown to confer protection against RSV infection in animal models. Immunity after primary infection (which generally occurs by 2 years of age) is partial and short-lived; thus, reinfections can occur throughout life.[120] Low serum neutralizing antibody levels in adults predicts infection risk and disease severity.[121] Immunologic mechanisms (e.g. cytokine responses) have been implicated in the pathogenesis of severe RSV diseases; however, emerging evidence suggests that uncontrolled viral replication, as indicated by high respiratory tract viral load, drives disease manifestations and is associated with severe clinical outcomes.[120,122–125] Such findings provide an important rationale for the approach to antiviral drug development against RSV.[122]

Epidemiology

RSV is known to be an important cause of lower respiratory tract infection in infants and young children (e.g. acute bronchiolitis, wheezy attacks), resulting in hospitalizations and deaths.[126] In adults, it has been estimated that RSV infects 3–10% of the population annually. Although most infections are mild, severe lower respiratory tract infections can occur, especially among older adults (e.g. >65 years) and those with underlying conditions (e.g. chronic lung diseases, chronic cardiovascular diseases).[120,127] RSV has been shown to account for 5–15% of community-acquired pneumonia, 9–10% of hospital admissions for acute cardiorespiratory diseases and excessive deaths among adults during seasonal peaks.[120,128,129] Outbreaks among nursing home residents are common, but under-recognized. The disease burden of RSV has been shown to approach that of seasonal influenza.[129–131] Patients who are profoundly immunosuppressed, such as hematopoietic stem cell transplant (HSCT) recipients, are at particularly high risk for severe RSV infection (2–17%), which can be rapidly fatal.[132]

Diagnostic Microbiology

RSV infection is clinically indistinguishable from other viral respiratory infections and diagnosis requires laboratory testing. Upper respiratory tract specimens (e.g. nasal, throat, nasopharyngeal) are commonly used, but lower respiratory samples (e.g. tracheal aspirate, BAL) should be considered whenever available. The gold standard for diagnosis is by RT-PCR; other tests such as antigen assays (e.g. enzyme immunoassays) and culture have much lower sensitivities (see Figure 173-2), especially among adults because of their lower viral loads.[120,131] A negative antigen assay result cannot be used to rule out RSV infection. Serology to detect RSV-specific IgG antibodies may also assist with the diagnosis and, if available, can be used in combination with RT-PCR to maximize the yield.[120]

Clinical Manifestations

RSV infections in infants and young children can lead to severe lower respiratory tract illnesses such as pneumonia and bronchiolitis.[126] The clinical manifestations of RSV infection in adults are diverse and often determined by the underlying conditions (e.g. chronic lung diseases) and degree of immunosuppression. In healthy young adults, RSV may cause self-limiting upper respiratory illnesses; in the profoundly immunosuppressed, progressive pneumonitis can occur (17–84%), resulting in high mortality (7–83%).[120,132] Older adults hospitalized for RSV infection may present with fever, cough, sputum production, wheezing and dyspnea. Although wheezing and dyspnea may be more common with RSV, and the magnitude of fever sometimes lower, such findings could not reliably differentiate it from influenza.[120,131] Radiographically, about 50–60% of cases show active pneumonic changes

such as consolidation and ground-glass opacities, which are typically small, patchy and unilateral.[97,120,131] The majority (>70%) of adults hospitalized with RSV develop severe lower respiratory complications, including pneumonia, acute bronchitis and exacerbations of COPD/asthma resulting in respiratory failure and hypoxemia, and 10–15% develop cardiovascular complications such as congestive heart failure or acute coronary syndrome.[127–129,131] Bacterial superinfection occurs in at least 12–17%.[120,127,131] Published data suggest that around 10–18% of patients required ventilatory support because of respiratory failure and the overall mortality was approximately 8–10%; the outcomes are generally comparable to that of seasonal influenza.[128,131]

Treatment and Prevention

At present, there is no established antiviral therapy or vaccine available for RSV. Ribavirin has *in vitro* activity against RSV and in animal models, palivizumab (an RSV-specific monoclonal antibody directed against the F glycoprotein) has been shown to reduce viral titers and replication in pulmonary tissues.[120,133] In randomized clinical trials, palivizumab given prophylactically to very young high-risk children was shown to reduce hospitalizations related to RSV infections.[134] In immunocompromised adults, ribavirin (aerosolized or systemic administration) and palivizumab have been used to treat RSV infection with the aim of reducing progression to lower respiratory disease and death, with variable results.[120,132,133,135] There is lack of controlled data, and it is not known whether these approaches can be applied to older, non-immunocompromised adults. New antiviral agents (e.g. fusion protein and polymerase inhibitors, siRNA) and newer generation antibody therapies are under active research.[120,136,137,298] Systemic corticosteroids are commonly used to treat wheezing and exacerbations of COPD/asthma in adults, including those triggered by viral infections. Randomized controlled trials of corticosteroid therapy in young children with RSV infections have revealed a lack of clinical benefit and inconsistent control of inflammatory cytokine responses.[138,139] A recent study of corticosteroids in adults reported that virus control seemed to be unaffected but humoral immunity against RSV was diminished.[140] It is suggested that the decision to treat RSV patients with corticosteroids should be weighed against the potential risks (e.g. bacterial superinfections) and be limited to a short course if used.[131,140] Because of the high rates of secondary infections, it is prudent to test and treat bacterial pathogens according to local resistance profiles. In addition to *Streptococcus pneumoniae* and *Haemophilus influenzae*, *Pseudomonas aeruginosa* and other gram-negative bacilli

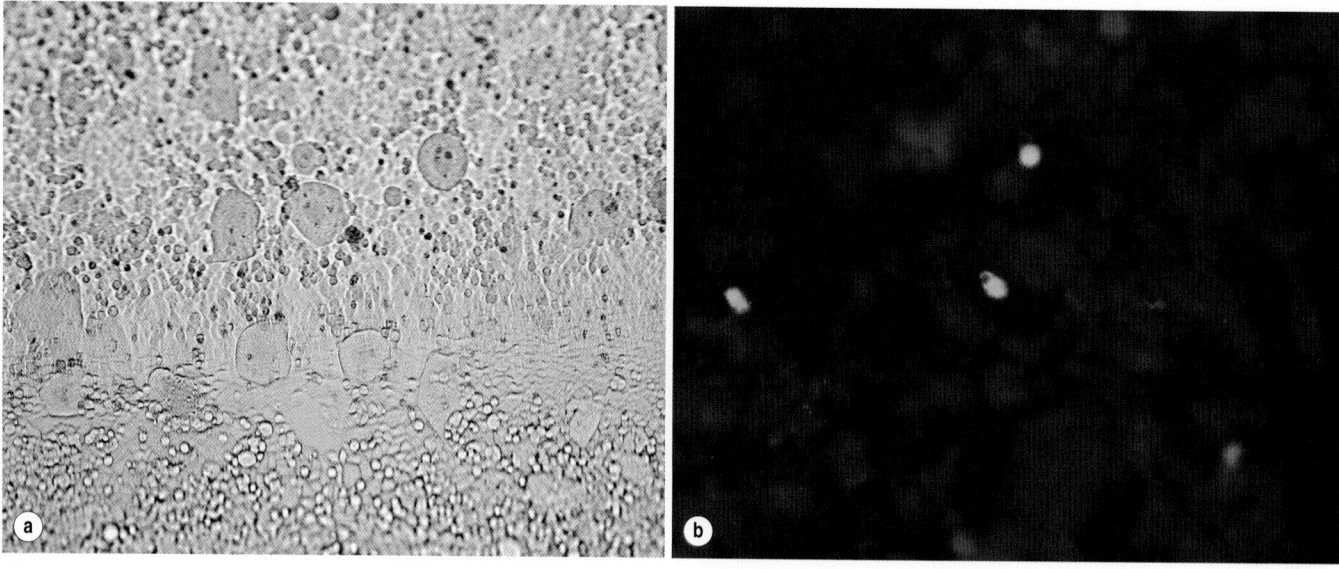

Figure 173-2 Cytopathic effect of RSV on Hep-2 cell line culture and identification of RSV antigen by means of IFA. (a) Syncytia formation in cell line culture. (b) Positive cells coloring green under IF microscope.

may need to be considered in patients with underlying chronic lung diseases.[127,131]

Rhinovirus

Nature

Human rhinoviruses (HRVs) are members of the family Picornaviridae and the genus *Enterovirus*. The HRVs are positive-sense, single-stranded-RNA viruses that encode a single protein that is cleaved by the virally mediated protease. The VP1-4 proteins make up the viral capsid.[141] There are well over 100 serotypes that are generally phylogenetically organized into three different species: HRV-A (74 serotypes), HRV-B (23 serotypes) and a more recently identified HRV-C (>50 serotypes have been identified to date).[142,143]

Epidemiology

HRV infections occur worldwide with peak incidence in the early fall and spring in temperate climates, although infection can occur year round. HRV-C has its peak incidence in the fall and winter in temperate regions and during the rainy season in tropical regions.[144,145] Infections occur in all age groups. HRVs are responsible for over half of all common colds and have been increasingly associated with more severe upper and lower respiratory tract infections in children, the elderly and the immunocompromised.[141] Young children are typically responsible for introducing the virus in household settings with a secondary attack rate of about 50%. With challenge studies, most (95%) develop infection while about 75% demonstrate clinical illness.[146]

Pathogenicity

HRVs are transmitted from person to person via contact (either direct or through a fomite) or aerosol (small or large particle).[147] HRVs can survive from a few hours to as long as 4 days on nonporous surfaces and for over 2 hours on human skin.[148] The majority of HRVs bind to intercellular adhesion molecule 1 (ICAM-1) whereas a minor group of HRVs adhere to the low-density lipoprotein receptor (LDLr).[141] Heparan sulfate has also been demonstrated as an additional receptor for some HRVs. Following infection of the respiratory epithelium, significant inflammatory cytokines, including IFN-β and IFN-γ and RANTES, IP-10, IL-6, IL-8, epithelial cell-derived neutrophil-activating peptide 78 (ENA-78), bradykinins, prostaglandins and histamine, are released locally.[141,149,150] This, in turn, results in vasodilation of nasal blood vessels, transudation of plasma and increased glandular secretions.[151] Together, these result in local congestion and trigger sneeze and cough reflexes. Immunity, which is type-specific and short-lived, results in eventual clearance of virus locally.

While the majority of replication was initially felt to be limited to the upper airway, a growing body of evidence suggests that HRVs can and frequently may replicate in the lower airways. This is likely to be more common among individuals with lower airway signs and symptoms and may contribute to pneumonia, which may occur rarely in immunocompromised adults and children. Further, this lower airway involvement may contribute to asthma and COPD exacerbations.[141,152]

Prevention

There are currently no available vaccines against HRV. The cornerstone against transmission is diligent hand hygiene. Symptomatic adults should be advised to wash hands frequently and use disposable tissues. Currently, droplet precautions are recommended to prevent nosocomial transmissions of rhinoviral infections.

Diagnostic Microbiology

While HRV can be grown in cell culture, molecular diagnostics are more sensitive and are currently widely available.[141,153] Typical cytopathic effects can be seen when HRV are grown on human embryonic kidney and human fibroblast cell lines, including WI-38, human foreskin fibroblasts (HFF), MRC-5 and HeLa (see Figure 173-3). HRV are acid labile which allows differentiation from other enteroviruses; they preferentially grow at pH 7.0 and not at 3.0.[148] Most molecular assays target the 5'UTR, a region highly conserved among all HRVs and enteroviruses; as a result, most molecular assays detect but do not differentiate between HRV and enteroviruses, although newer diagnostic platforms are circumventing this problem.[141,153]

Clinical Manifestations

The most common manifestations of HRV infections include the common cold and exacerbations of asthma and COPD, although more serious infections, including pneumonia, have been described, particularly in immunocompromised adults and children. Following a typically 2-day incubation period, patients with colds then develop watery rhinorrhea, nasal congestion, sneezing, cough, sore throat, headaches and sometimes fever that last 7–14 days.[154] Rhinoviral colds cannot be differentiated from those caused by other pathogens. Primary viral

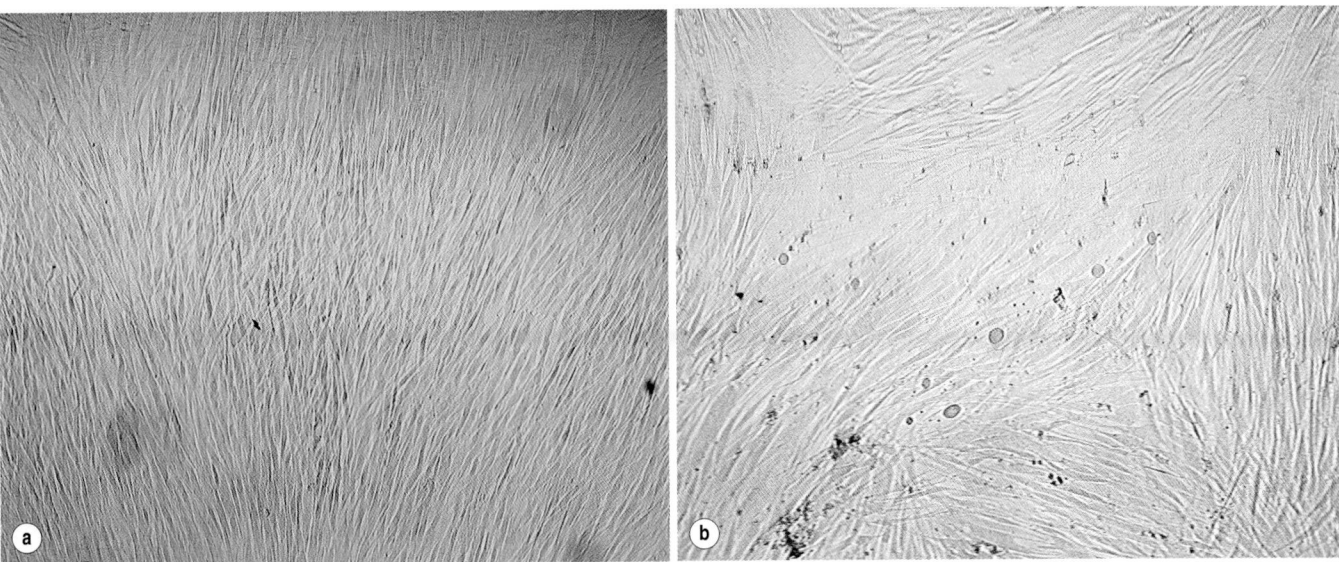

Figure 173-3 Cytopathic effect caused by rhinovirus on human foreskin fibroblasts (HFF) cell line culture. (a) Uninoculated cell line. (b) Formation of small teardrop- to oval-shaped highly refractile cells indicative of adenovirus-induced cytopathic effect.

otitis or rhinosinusitis may also occur with HRV and typically occurs earlier than bacterial superinfections that occur later in the course of colds. Lower airway infections, including croup, bronchiolitis and pneumonia have been described.[148,155,156] HRV are common triggers for exacerbation of asthma and COPD and may be caused by the direct infection of the lower airway or the stimulation of inflammatory, immunological, or neurogenic mechanisms.[157]

Management

While a number of small molecule antivirals (capsid-binding agents: pleconaril, vapendavir and pirodavir; 3C protease inhibitors: rupintrivir; soluble ICAM-1: tremacamra) and complementary medical interventions (echinacea, zinc) have been studied for the treatment of rhinoviral colds, none has been approved for use. Interferons have been shown to prevent HRV colds, but they have not been documented to have positive therapeutic effects. As a result, the mainstay of treatment of rhinoviral colds remains symptomatic treatment with analgesic agents, decongestants, antihistamines and antitussives.[141]

Parainfluenza Virus

Nature

Parainfluenza viruses (PIVs) are single-stranded, enveloped RNA viruses belonging to the genus *Paramyxovirus* in the Paramyxoviridae family.[158,159] The single strand of negative-sense RNA encodes at least six viral proteins: the nucleocapsid protein (NP), the phosphoprotein (P), the matrix protein (M), the fusion glycoprotein (F), the hemagglutinin-neuraminidase glycoprotein (HN), and the RNA polymerase (L).[160] There are four major serotypes of human PIV (PIV-1, 2, 3, 4) that are defined by complement fixation and hemagglutinating antigens.[161–163] PIV-1 and 3 are members of the genus *Respirovirus*, whereas PIV-2 and 4 are members of the genus *Rubulavirus*.

Epidemiology

Initial infection with parainfluenza typically occurs early in childhood, most commonly in children less than 5 years old. Serologic studies have demonstrated that PIV-3 affects up to 50% of children within the first year of life with PIV-1 and 2 causing initial infections later, generally between 3 and 5 years old.[164,165] Most adults have antibodies to PIV. PIV is responsible for 20–40% of lower respiratory tract infections and is the second most common viral cause of hospitalization in children.[166] With contemporary molecular diagnostics, PIV has also been demonstrated to be the second or third most commonly isolated virus in hospitalized adults, aged 16–64 years old.[167–169] In both adults and children, re-infection is common despite the presence of antibodies formed during prior infection.[170]

In tropical and subtropical regions, parainfluenza viruses do not show seasonal variations, while in temperate regions, such as the USA, PIV-1 and PIV-2 cause seasonal outbreaks in the fall (September–December) and PIV-3 causes epidemics during the spring (April–June).[171,172] In years when there is no PIV-1 circulating (typically even-numbered years), PIV-3 activity is generally greater.[172] PIV-4, which generally causes a milder degree of illness, is more common in the autumn and winter months.[173]

Parainfluenza is one of the more common causes of respiratory viral infections in patients with hematologic malignancies, hematopoietic stem cell transplantation, or solid organ transplantation and is associated with a high rate of progressive disease involving the lower airway and an increased mortality rate.[174,175]

Pathogenicity

Parainfluenza viruses are transmitted by direct person-to-person contact through large respiratory droplets and contact with fomites contaminated with respiratory secretions.[176] Clinical symptoms typically develop after a 2–6 day incubation period. After initial infection of upper airway ciliated epithelial cells,[177] infection spreads to the large and small airways.[178] Peak symptoms correlate with peak viral replication. Infection of the larynx and upper trachea is associated with croup whereas bronchiolitis and pneumonia are associated with infection of the distal airways.[179]

The host immune response appears to play a more important role in the pathogenesis of PIV infection than direct viral replication.[179,180] Specifically, the key host immune responses which contribute to viral clearance, including the innate immune responses, CD8+ and CD4+ T-cell responses, interferon production and local and system IgA, IgE and IgG responses, are also the key drivers of the clinical signs and symptoms of infection.[179] While both humoral and cellular immune responses are critical for clearance of infection, defects in cytotoxic T-cell response are associated with progressive disease, as is demonstrated by the increased risk of progressive and fatal disease in HSCT recipients.[174]

Prevention

There is currently no licensed vaccine against PIV, although several candidates that appear to produce neutralizing antibodies to the HN and F proteins are being investigated.[163] Most of the contemporary vaccine candidates have focused on reverse genetic technology applied to live, attenuated intranasal vaccines.[159] Further, some of the candidate vaccines afford protection against both PIV and RSV.[181] Nosocomial outbreaks of PIV infection have been documented, highlighting the importance of standard and contact precautions and use of private rooms whenever possible.[24] Respiratory precautions are not necessary, because the droplets are large and do not aerosolize.

Diagnostic Microbiology

PIV can be diagnosed by culture, antigen detection, or nucleic acid testing. PIV is stable in viral transport medium at 4°C for up to 5 days. Freezing to −20°C does decrease infectivity of the virus, but long-term storage can be achieved easily by adding sucrose or glycerol to the holding media and freezing to less than −70°C.[162] LLC-MK2 rhesus monkey kidney, Vero African green monkey kidney, and NCI-H292 human lung carcinoma cell lines using standard and shell vial techniques can be used to culture PIV;[163] fixed-mixed cell lines, such as R-Mix (Diagnostic Hybrids, Athens, OH), have a sensitivity that approaches that of standard cell culture lines for the detection of PIV.[162,182–184] Trypsin is required for the growth of PIV-1 and PIV-4 but not PIV-2 and PIV-3.[163] Hemadsorption-inhibition, hemagglutination inhibition or immunofluorescence is used to identify the PIV in cultures (see Figures 173-4 and 173-5).[162] There are currently no approved rapid antigen kits available for the detection of PIV although monoclonal antibodies can be used to detect the PIV serotypes in primary patient samples and from cell cultures.[162,185]

Polymerase chain reaction (PCR)-based tests, typically directed toward the hemagglutinin-neuraminidase (HN) gene, are now considered the gold standard for the diagnosis of PIV. Such assays typically have higher yield over cultures for the diagnosis of PIV.[186–189] Despite the advantages of highly multiplexed PCR-based systems in detecting a wide range of viruses, the diagnostic yield for PIV is not consistent for all available systems.[190–192]

Clinical Manifestations

Parainfluenza viruses cause a variety of upper and lower respiratory tract illnesses, ranging from mild cold-like syndromes to life-threatening pneumonias.

PEDIATRIC DISEASE

Most infections in children are limited to the upper respiratory tract with only about 15% involving the lower respiratory tract.[193] Upper tract disease may involve the entire airway, including the middle ear and sinuses.[193–195] PIV-1 and -2 are associated with croup or laryngotracheobronchitis in children, which is characterized by fever, rhinorrhea and pharyngitis and is typically followed by a barking cough.[161,196]

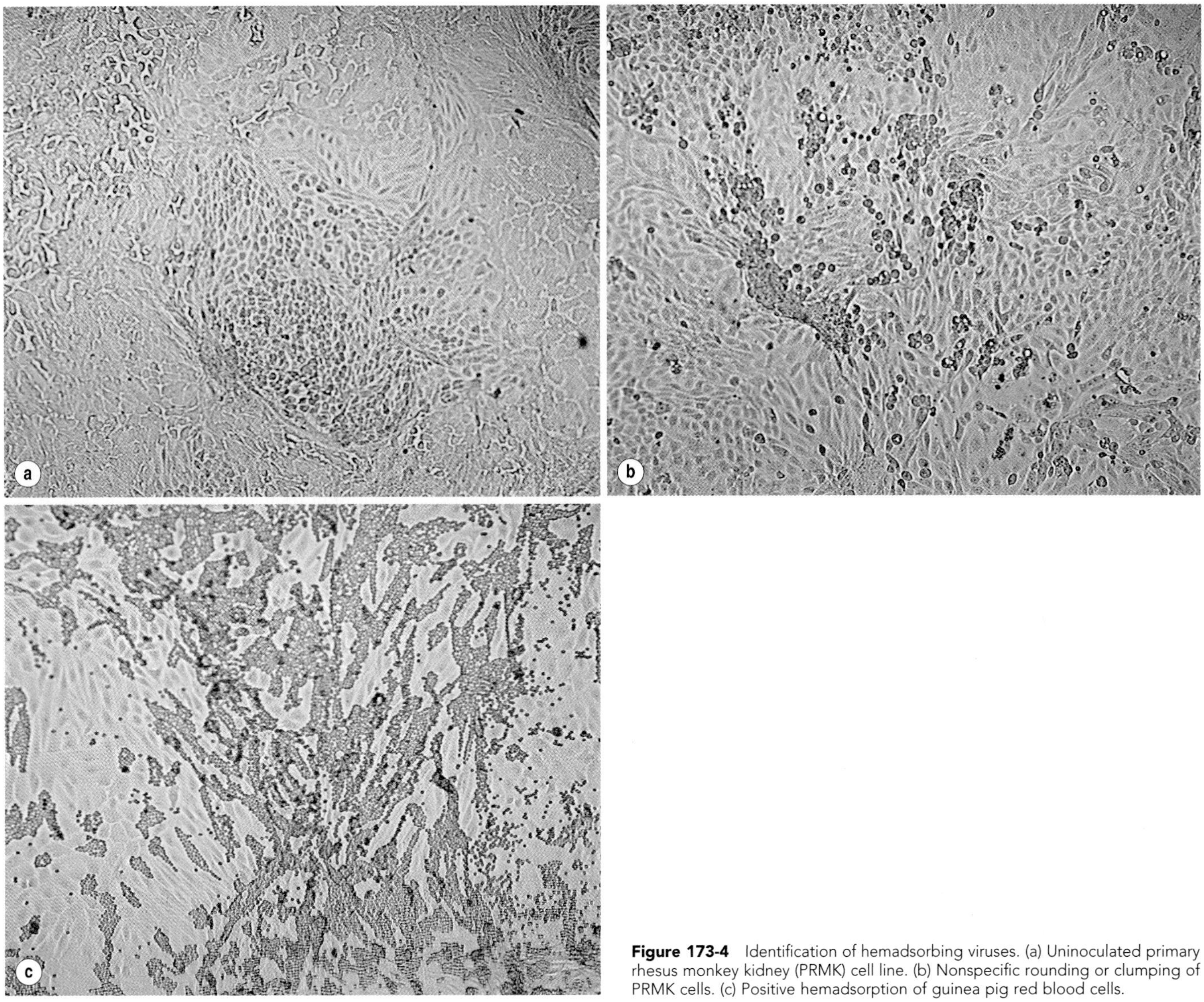

Figure 173-4 Identification of hemadsorbing viruses. (a) Uninoculated primary rhesus monkey kidney (PRMK) cell line. (b) Nonspecific rounding or clumping of PRMK cells. (c) Positive hemadsorption of guinea pig red blood cells.

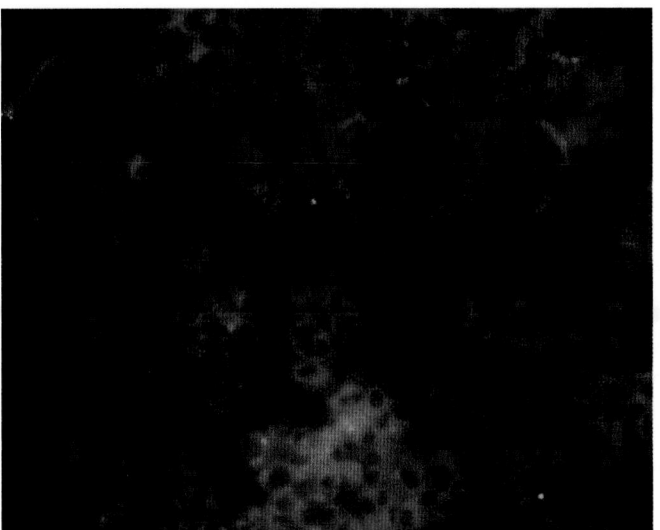

Figure 173-5 Differentiation of hemadsorbing viruses by means of IFA. Negative control.

PIV-3 is associated with more distal lung involvement, particularly in the first 6 months of life.[161,197] PIV-4 is generally associated with mild upper respiratory infections or asymptomatic infection, although more severe disease has been described in children with underlying cardiopulmonary disease or immune compromise.[161,198] Nonrespiratory complications of PIV include meningitis, myocarditis, pericarditis, and Guillain–Barré Syndrome.[199–202]

ADULT DISEASE

PIV is responsible for 1–15% of acute, typically mild respiratory illnesses in adults with higher rates and more significant morbidity in older adults.[203,204] Higher rates of pneumonia (11–14%) have been described in the elderly.[205,206] Wider use of more sensitive molecular assays have demonstrated that PIV is a significant cause of community-acquired pneumonia and exacerbations of asthma and chronic bronchitis.[207–213]

PARAINFLUENZA VIRUS IN IMMUNOCOMPROMISED PATIENTS

Parainfluenza virus causes significant direct and indirect morbidity and mortality among immunocompromised adults and children.[174] PIV can cause asymptomatic shedding, particularly among HSCT recipients, which may contribute to nosocomial spread.[214] Progression to the lower respiratory tract complicates 13–43% of cases and is associated with enhanced mortality.[175,214–219] Rarely, lower airway involvement will be characterized by small peribronchial nodules on CT radiography.[220] Steroids, in a dose dependent manner, are associated with increased risk of progression from upper to lower tract disease and mortality.[217,221,222] Other risk factors for progressive disease include onset early post-transplant, allogeneic (matched unrelated and matched related) donor, presence of lymphocytopenia, active graft-versus-host disease and pediatric age group.[174,175,221,223] Reduced intensity conditioning appears to be a risk factor for late onset (≥ 30 days) PIV infection.[223] PIV infection is associated with a 17.9 greater odds of developing severe airflow declines following infection.[224]

Parainfluenza has also been demonstrated to cause severe disease in patients undergoing chemotherapy, with enhanced risk of progression to severe lower respiratory infection in patients with severe lymphocytopenia.[225,226]

Parainfluenza virus infections among lung transplant recipients have been associated with significant short- and long-term pulmonary dysfunction.[71,227] In addition to local acute, direct virologic effects on the lung of transplant recipients, PIV, particularly with lower tract infection, is associated with development or progression of bronchiolitis obliterans or bronchiolitis obliterans syndrome (BOS).[71,227–230]

Management

There are currently no antivirals with proven efficacy approved for the treatment of PIV infections. For children with croup, glucocorticoids and nebulized epinephrine have been associated with improved clinical outcomes.[231,232] When approved antivirals such as ribavirin have been studied, typically in immunocompromised patients, treatment was not associated with reduction in viral shedding or mortality.[175,202,216–219,223,227,233–240] One investigational agent, DAS181, which acts by cleaving the sialic acid receptors from the surface of human respiratory epithelial cells, has been shown to improve symptoms, oxygenation, pulmonary function and nasopharyngeal viral loads in treated subjects with PIV infection.[241–244]

Human Metapneumovirus

Nature

Human metapneumovirus (hMPV) is a nonsegmented negative-sense RNA virus that is a member of the Pneumovirinae subfamily of the Paramyxoviridae. There are two subgroups each with two clades of hMPV (A1, A2, B1 and B2); although all four subtypes typically co-circulate, each season often has one subtype that predominates.[245,246] hMPV codes for similar genes to RSV except that the order is slightly different (3'-N-P-M-F-M2-SH-G-L-5') and there are no NS1 or NS2 genes.[247]

Epidemiology

hMPV results in typically self-limited upper and lower respiratory tract infections in all age groups with a global distribution.[248] Symptomatic disease appears to be more common among young children and the elderly.[249] Risk factors for hospitalization from hMPV infections in children include age <6 months and the presence of three or more children in the home, whereas female gender, prematurity and genotype B infection were risk factors for severe disease.[250] About 4–9% of children require hospitalization for severe respiratory symptoms or pneumonia.[248,250] hMPV is identified in 8.5% of adults hospitalized with acute cardiorespiratory illness.[251] Risk factors for hospitalization and severe disease in the elderly include a diagnosis of COPD, asthma, cancer or lung transplantation. The average rate of hospitalization for hMPV (9.8 per 10 000 residents) is similar to the rate for influenza (11.8 per 10 000 residents) in adults ≥ 50 years old.[252] Severe, sometimes fatal infections, including pneumonia, have

been described more frequently among immunocompromised patients and the elderly.[248,251,253]

Most children are infected by 5 years of age.[254] hMPV is the second most frequently isolated viral pathogen, after RSV, in children presenting with bronchiolitis.[248] Infections typically occur in the late winter and spring in temperate climates and in the spring and summer in subtropical regions.[254,255] Epidemic peaks typically occur 1–2 months later than RSV epidemics annually.[248]

Pathogenicity

hMPV is likely to be transmitted by direct or close contact with contaminated secretions; large particle aerosols, droplets and fomites may also result in transmission. There is typically a 5-day interval between onset of symptoms in an index case and the onset of symptoms in household exposed contacts.[256] hMPV G protein binds to the integrin α-V-β-1 receptors on respiratory epithelial cells.[248,257] Local replication in the airway is associated with upper respiratory tract signs and significant airway inflammation.[258] Viral replication also induces mucus hyperproduction and hyperplasia of the respiratory epithelium which may result in airway obstruction and hyperresponsiveness to methacholine challenge.[259] Replication results in an increase in IL-8, IL-12, tumor necrosis factor, IL-6, and IL-1β, although levels are lower than those observed with RSV infection.[260]

Prevention

There is currently no licensed vaccine against hMPV, although several are currently under investigation. Most of the candidate vaccines utilize chimeric viruses, live-attenuated viruses and subunits of the virus.[248] Nosocomial outbreaks have been described which highlight the importance of droplet and contact precautions to prevent transmission.

Diagnostic Microbiology

Although hMPV may be grown in tertiary monkey kidney cells, Vero cells, LLC-MK2-cells, BEAS-2B cells, A549 cells and HepG2 cells, yields are often low and require prolonged incubation.[248] Cytopathic effects typically can be observed after 10–21 days and range from syncytia formation to rounding of the cells.[254] Direct immunofluorescence assays (DFA) with virus-specific antibodies are available and allow detection of virus in direct patient specimens and cell culture. DFA is less sensitive than PCR but is often more widely available.[248] Molecular diagnostics, as either a singleplex or multiplex assay, are commercially available and have the highest yield in detecting hMPV. Most PCR assays detect all hMPV genotypes and rely on conserved and essential regions within the N, F or L gene.[248,261] The sensitivity varies by assay and is lower for most multiplex assays as compared to singleplex assays. Serologic diagnosis can be made by ELISA methods but is not widely available.[248]

Clinical Manifestations

hMPV is associated with respiratory tract infections in all age groups. Among children, the most common symptoms are rhinorrhea, cough or fever, although conjunctivitis, vomiting, diarrhea and rash have been reported infrequently.[262] Encephalitis is a rare manifestation of hMPV infection.[263,264] Although hMPV and RSV are generally indistinguishable, fever is more frequent in children with hMPV, while rhinorrhea is more commonly observed in RSV-infected individuals.[248,265] Children appear to be at higher risk of developing bronchiolitis, pneumonia, croup and possibly asthma exacerbation, particularly when younger than 2 years of age. Most hospitalizations are the result of bronchiolitis and pneumonia in children. Coinfection with hMPV and RSV results in more severe disease and an increased risk for admission to the ICU and a 10-fold increase in the need for mechanical ventilation.[266] The typical duration of symptoms is around a week with viral shedding typically for 1–2 weeks.[254,255] Repeat infection has clearly been documented although subsequent infections are typically limited to the upper airway. Severe, sometimes fatal infections, often involving the lower airway, have been described in adults and children with malignancy, hematopoietic stem cell and solid organ transplantation. The severity of illness is likely related to reduced cellular immune responses. Likewise, elderly adults, adults with severe cardiopulmonary disease, and residents of long-term care facilities have a higher incidence of hMPV infection with an increased risk of lower airway involvement, complications including bacterial superinfections, and death.[248] Although asymptomatic infection is common for otherwise healthy adults, such individuals may present with cold- and influenza-like illnesses.[267] Adults commonly present with cough, nasal congestion and rhinorrhea, but rarely have fever.[130] The role of hMPV in exacerbations of COPD is unclear as one large study demonstrated an association whereas another failed to identify hMPV in patients with COPD exacerbations.[268,269]

Management

Generally, patients can be safely managed with supportive care, including supplemental oxygen and intravenous hydration when indicated. Bronchodilators and corticosteroids are often used empirically although there are no controlled trials of these medications for hMPV.[248] Ribavirin shows equivalent activity against hMPV (mean EC50 74μM) and RSV (mean EC50 88 μM).[270] Likewise, standard IgIV has neutralizing antibodies against hMPV (10 $\log_2$/0.05mL) and RSV (11 $\log_2$/0.05mL), whereas RSV-specific monoclonal antibodies have no activity against hMPV.[270] Neither agent has been studied prospectively for the treatment of hMPV, although there are a number of case series demonstrating clinical response in some cases.[135,271–273]

Human Bocavirus

Nature

Human bocaviruses were first identified through molecular screening in 2005.[274] Bocaviruses are non-enveloped, linear, single-stranded DNA viruses that are members of the Parvoviridae family.[275] There are currently four species of human bocaviruses (HBoV1-4); HBoV2 can be further divided into two strains (A and B).[276] The viral genome encodes two forms of the nonstructural protein (NS1), nuclear phosphoprotein (NP1) and two major structural proteins (VP1 and VP2).[275,277]

Epidemiology

Human bocaviruses have been detected worldwide from respiratory and stool specimens. HBoV1 is predominantly a respiratory pathogen whereas HBoV2-4 have been mostly found in stool and are less clearly associated with respiratory tract infections. Although HBoV1 is most commonly detected in children 6–24 months old, it has been detected less frequently in other age groups.[275] Infection appears to occur year round with peaks of detection in the winter and spring. Although HBoV2-4 are felt to be predominantly gastrointestinal viruses, HBoV2 has been detected in nasopharyngeal specimens.[278,279] Most children have antibodies to HBoV1 by age 6 and most adults have detectable HBoV1 antibodies.[275]

Pathogenicity

A key challenge to understanding the pathogenesis and clinical implications of HBoV is the fact that up to 83% of HBoV DNA-positive respiratory samples have evidence of coinfection with other respiratory viruses. Further, the virus is often shed for at least 6 months after initial infection in immunocompetent individuals. In studies of wheezing children, 64% had serologic evidence of primary infection. Further, several studies that include asymptomatic control patients have documented an association between presence of HBoV and clinical symptoms. Additionally, these studies have documented a positive correlation between high copy numbers of HBoV1 DNA and HBoV1 monoinfection and respiratory symptoms.[275]

Although the exact route of transmission of human bocaviruses is unknown, transmission by inhalation or contact with infectious sputum, feces or urine is probable. The mechanism of cell entry and host range are not known. Although most HBoV1 is detected in the upper airway, clinical symptoms and positive BAL specimens suggest that HBoV1 is capable of infecting the lower airways down to at least the bronchioles.[275] HBoV1 DNA is detectable in the serum suggesting dissemination beyond the airway. Likewise, HBoV1 can rarely be detected in stool with and without gastrointestinal symptoms suggesting passive spread from the respiratory to the gastrointestinal tract.[275]

In vitro, HBoV1 induces IL-13, IFN-γ and IL-10 in CD4+ T cells. Children with HBoV1-associated bronchiolitis have increased levels of IFN-γ, IL-2 and IL-4 in nasopharyngeal aspirates. [280–282]

Prevention

There is no vaccine available for HBoV.[275] Specialist advice should be sought regarding appropriate isolation practice for patients with proven HBoV infections.

Diagnostic Microbiology

Diagnosis of HBoV depends on molecular and serologic methods. While HBoV can be cultured on differentiated human airway epithelial cells, these are not widely available in the clinical microbiology laboratory.[283] PCR is not an optimal diagnostic method because of prolonged shedding and the potential for persistent infection in some tissues. Presence of HBoV1 DNA in serum may provide enhanced specificity of active infection as it correlates with HBoV1-specific IgM 61% of the time.[284,285] Quantitative virology may also help improve the probability that HBoV detection is associated with the clinical presentation, as high viral loads (>2 × 10^8 genomes/mL) in nasopharyngeal aspirates appear to correlate with illness severity and fewer coinfections.[275,286] Serology, particularly IgG avidity EIA, may also increase the probability that detected HBoV is truly associated with clinical disease.[275] Given the limitations of diagnostic strategies, most would recommend using two diagnostic modalities to diagnose HBoV infection.

Clinical Manifestations

Because of the limitations outlined above, there remains controversy in the causal link between HBoV1 and respiratory disease. A number of studies have correlated HBoV1 detection and the common cold, asthma, acute wheezing, bronchiolitis, pneumonia, acute otitis media and plastic bronchitis. The strongest link in the available literature is that HBoV1 may be the cause of wheezing and pneumonia. One study found a link between HBoV1 DNA in serum, cerebrospinal fluid (CSF) or stool and Kawasaki disease,[287] although this study was not confirmed by two other groups.[278,288]

Management

No comparative studies of available antivirals have been conducted in patients with HBoV infection. Supportive measures are the only currently available therapy.[275]

References available online at expertconsult.com.

KEY REFERENCES

Advisory Committee on Healthcare Infection Control Practices, Centers for Disease Control and Prevention: Guidelines for preventing health-care-associated pneumonia, 2003 recommendations of the CDC and the Healthcare

Infection Control Practices Advisory Committee. *Respir Care* 2004; 49:926-939.
Centers for Disease Control and Prevention: Acute respiratory disease associated with adenovirus serotype 14 – four

states, 2006–2007. *MMWR Morb Mortal Wkly Rep* 2007; 56:1181-1184.
Chan J.F., Lau S.K., To K.K., et al.: Middle East respiratory syndrome coronavirus: another zoonotic

betacoronavirus causing SARS-like disease. *Clin Microbiol Rev* 2015; 28(2):465-522.

Chan J.F., Yao Y., Yeung M.L., et al.: Treatment With Lopinavir/Ritonavir or Interferon-β1b Improves Outcome of MERS-CoV Infection in a Nonhuman Primate Model of Common Marmoset. *J Infect Dis* 2015; 212(12):1904-1913.

Corti D., Zhao J., Pedotti M., et al.: Prophylactic and post-exposure efficacy of a potent human monoclonal antibody against MERS coronavirus. *Proc Natl Acad Sci USA* 2015; 112(33):10473-10478.

DeVincenzo J., Lambkin-Williams R., Wilkinson T., et al.: A randomized, double-blind, placebo-controlled study of an RNAi-based therapy directed against respiratory syncytial virus. *Proc Natl Acad Sci USA* 2010; 107: 8800-8805.

DeVincenzo J.P., Whitley R.J., Mackman R.L., et al.: Oral GS-5806 activity in a respiratory syncytial virus challenge study. *N Engl J Med* 2014; 371(8):711-722.

Drosten C., Meyer B., Müller M.A., et al.: Transmission of MERS-coronavirus in household contacts. *N Engl J Med* 2014; 371(9):828-835.

Garbino J., Gerbase M.W., Wunderli W., et al.: Respiratory viruses and severe lower respiratory tract complications in hospitalized patients. *Chest* 2004; 125: 1033-1039.

Gern J.E.: Rhinovirus and the initiation of asthma. *Curr Opin Allergy Clin Immunol* 2009; 9:73-78.

Hall C.B.: Respiratory syncytial virus and parainfluenza virus. *N Engl J Med* 2001; 344:1917-1928.

Hui D.S., Memish Z.A., Zumla A.: Severe acute respiratory syndrome vs. the Middle East respiratory syndrome. *Curr Opin Pulm Med* 2014; 20:233-241.

Jacobs S.E., Lamson D.M., St George K., et al.: Human rhinoviruses. *Clin Microbiol Rev* 2013; 26:135-162.

Khalafalla A.I., Lu X., Al-Mubarak A.I., et al.: MERS-CoV in Upper Respiratory Tract and Lungs of Dromedary Camels, Saudi Arabia, 2013-2014. *Emerg Infect Dis* 2015; 21(7):1153-1158.

Korea Centers for Disease Control and Prevention: Middle East Respiratory Syndrome Coronavirus Outbreak in the Republic of Korea, 2015. *Osong Public Health Res Perspect.* 2015; 6(4):269-278.

Louie J.K., Kajon A.E., Holodniy M., et al.: Severe pneumonia due to adenovirus serotype 14: a new respiratory threat? *Clin Infect Dis* 2008; 46:421-425.

Müller M.A., Meyer B., Corman V.M., et al.: Presence of Middle East respiratory syndrome coronavirus antibodies in Saudi Arabia: a nationwide, cross-sectional, serological study. *Lancet Infect Dis* 2015; 15(5):559-564.

Oboho I.K., Tomczyk S.M., Al-Asmari A.M., et al.: 2014 MERS-CoV outbreak in Jeddah – a link to health care facilities. *N Engl J Med* 2015; 372(9):846-854.

Omrani A.S., Saad M.M., Baig K., et al.: Ribavirin and interferon alfa-2a for severe Middle East respiratory syndrome coronavirus infection: a retrospective cohort study. *Lancet Infect Dis* 2014; 14(11):1090-1095.

Peiris J.S., Yuen K.Y., Osterhaus A.D., et al.: The severe acute respiratory syndrome. *N Engl J Med* 2003; 349: 2431-2441.

Raza K., Ismailjee S.B., Crespo M., et al.: Successful outcome of human metapneumovirus (hMPV) pneumonia in a lung transplant recipient treated with intravenous ribavirin. *J Heart Lung Transplant* 2007; 26:862-864.

Schildgen V., van den Hoogen B., Fouchier R., et al. Human Metapneumovirus: lessons learned over the first decade. *Clin Microbiol Rev* 2011;24:734-754.

Walsh E.E.: Respiratory syncytial virus infection in adults. *Semin Respir Crit Care Med* 2011; 32:423-432.

174

Retroviruses and Retroviral Infections

GEORGE B. KYEI | WILLIAM G. POWDERLY

KEY CONCEPTS

- Retroviruses are RNA viruses that require reverse transcription of their RNA to a DNA intermediate and integration into the host genome.

- The retroviruses of clinical importance are the human immunodeficiency viruses (HIVs) and the human T-lymphocyte leukemia virus-1(HTLV-1).

- Several steps of the HIV life cycle, including entry, reverse transcription, integration and maturation, have been successfully targeted for therapy.

- Modern diagnostic tools using viral RNA detection and fourth-generation serological assays have shortened the time from infection to diagnosis of HIV to less than 2 weeks.

- The most important obstacle to HIV cure is viral latency: its ability to remain as a provirus in resting T cells and other potential cellular reservoirs.

- Current attempts at cure include bone marrow transplant for special populations, gene therapy and latency reversing agents.

Introduction

The Retroviridae constitute a large family of viruses that predominantly infect both human and animal vertebrates. They are positive-stranded enveloped RNA viruses that reverse transcribe their RNA into a DNA intermediate during viral replication, hence the name 'retroviruses'.[1] Retroviral infections can cause a wide spectrum of diseases ranging from malignancies to immune deficiencies and neurologic disorders. However, most retroviral infections occur without any detectable deleterious effect to the host. Examples of retroviruses are the human immunodeficiency virus (HIV) and the human T-cell leukemia viruses (HTLVs). Several human retroviruses have been identified, of which only the HIVs and HTLV-1 are of clinical importance and are discussed in this chapter. Additionally, the human genome is replete with endogenous retroviruses (HERVs, also known as retrotransposons) that have entered the human germline at various times in the evolutionary past and now occupy 8.3% of the genome. They are mostly silent, although some HERVs have physiologic roles (see Chapter 69 for further details).

Nature

Various classifications exist for retroviruses. For our purposes, we will consider the following:

1. Endogenous or exogenous: retroviruses that occur as part of the human genome and can be inherited through the germ line are called human endogenous retroviruses (HERVs). Current estimates put them at about 8% of the human genome with over 100 000 HERV elements.[2,3] Despite the large number, their role in disease causation in humans is not established. Exogenous retroviruses are those that can be acquired, such as HIV or HTLV.

2. Lentiviruses are a genus of the Retroviridae family that cause disease after a long incubation period. They also have the unique ability to replicate in nondividing cells. Examples include

the HIV, feline immunodeficiency virus (FIV) and simian immunodeficiency virus (SIV).

3. Simple and complex retroviruses. The genome of retroviruses is approximately 10 000 base pairs (bp) in length. Each end of the genome consists of repeating nucleotide sequences of 4–6 bp, called the long terminal repeats (LTRs). The LTRs flank the three genomic regions that encode for sets of structural genes common to all retroviruses:
   - the group antigen (*gag*) region, which codes for the core antigens;
   - the polymerase (*pol*) region, which codes for the enzymes protease (PT), reverse transcriptase (RT) and integrase (IN); and
   - the envelope (*env*) region, which codes for glycoproteins of the envelope.

The structural genes always appear in the same order: *gag-pol-env* (Figure 174-1).[4] The genomes of so-called simple retroviruses only contain *gag, pol* and *env* genes. Retroviruses that encode additional regulatory genes are called complex retroviruses; examples of these are the HIVs and the HTLVs.

The electron microscopic view of retroviral particles shows spherical particles approximately 100 nm in diameter with an electron-dense core (Figure 174-2). Retroviruses are enveloped viruses (Figure 174-3). The envelope consists of a phospholipid double layer derived from the plasma membrane of the host cell. Viral-encoded transmembrane glycoproteins are inserted into the envelope, enabling the virus to attach to the host cell. The envelope surrounds the nucleocapsid core, which contains the viral genome: two identical RNA molecules with the same polarity as mRNA, with which an RNA-dependent DNA polymerase enzyme, RT, is closely associated. Also present in the core is the integrase enzyme.[5]

The Human Immunodeficiency Viruses

Nature

The human immunodeficiency viruses HIV-1 and HIV-2 are members of the family of lentiviruses. Although both viruses can cause the acquired immunodeficiency syndrome (AIDS), HIV-1 is by far the more pathogenic and is largely responsible for the AIDS pandemic. HIV-2 is localized mainly in portions of West Africa and parts of Europe and India, all with links to West Africa. A comparison of HIV-1 and HIV-2 is shown in Table 174-1.

Genome Organization and Life Cycle

HIV-1 genome has nine open reading frames and encodes a total of 15 proteins (Figure 174-4).[4] The proteins can be divided broadly into:

1. Structural proteins: these consist of Gag, Env and Pol proteins. The gag protein is translated as one entity (p55) and cleaved by HIV protease into capsid (CA;p24) which surrounds the viral RNA and enzymes, matrix (MA;p17) and nucleocapsid (NC;p7) which is at the core of the virus and bound to the RNA. Other products of Gag include p6 (important for viral budding), p1 and p2. The env glycoprotein (gp) is produced as the polyprotein gp160, which is cleaved by the cellular protease, furin, to form trimers of surface gp120 and transmembrane gp41.

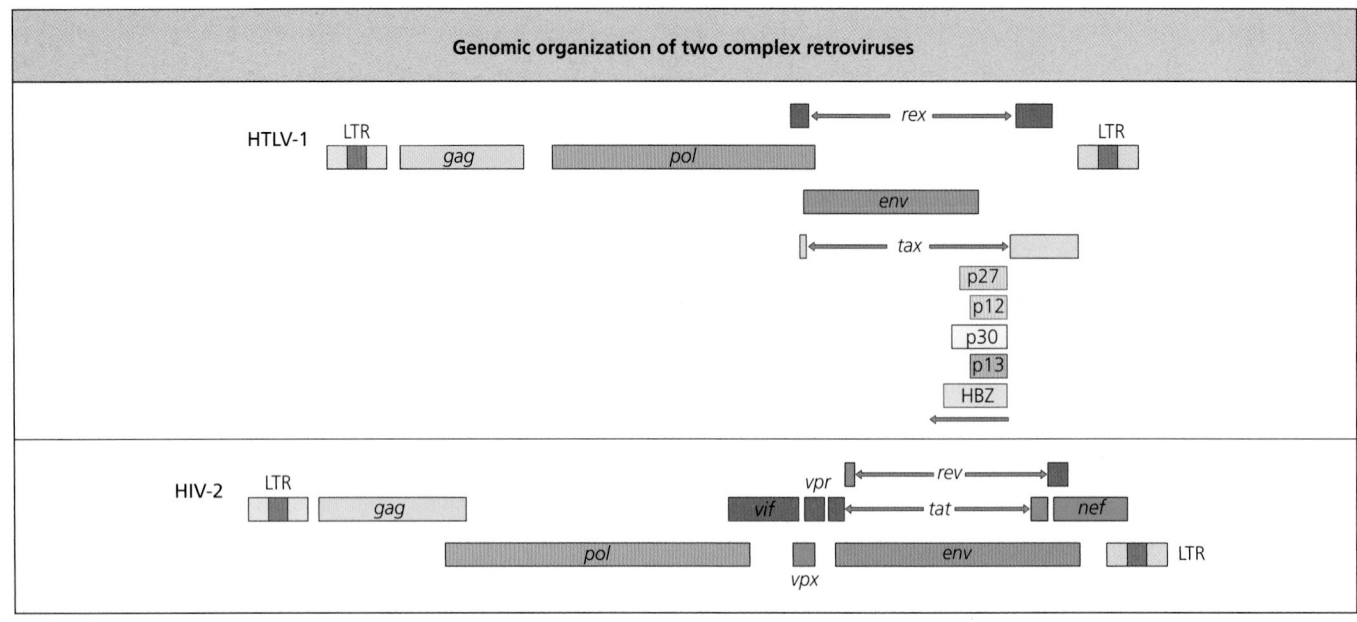

Figure 174-1   Genomic organization of two complex retroviruses. The diagram shows HTLV-1 and HIV-2. The components of the long terminal repeats are shaded. (*Adapted from Galasso G. J. et al., eds. Antiviral agents and human diseases, 4th ed. Philadelphia: Lippincott Raven; 1997.*)

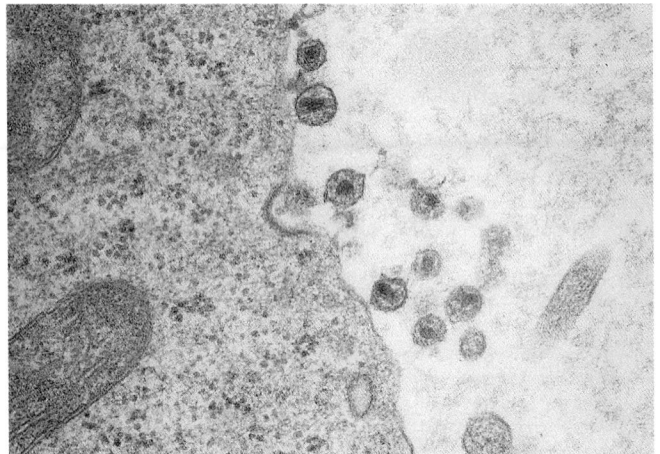

Figure 174-2   Typical electron microscopic view of retroviruses (HIV) showing an electron-dense core. (*Courtesy of Dr Piet Joling.*)

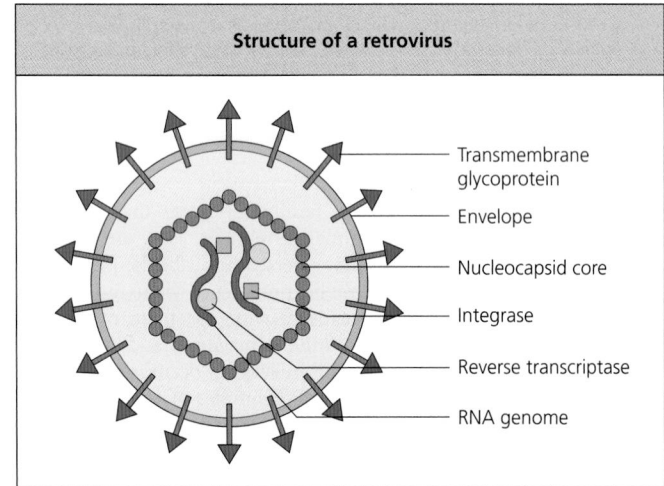

Figure 174-3   Structure of a retrovirus.

TABLE 174-1	Comparison of HIV-1 and HIV-2	
Characteristic	**HIV-1**	**HIV-2**
Molecular structure	Lacks the accessory protein *Vpx* Has *Vpu* important for efficient budding	Lacks *Vpu* Has *Vpx* which enables efficient infection of macrophages and resting T cells by targeting the restriction factor *SAMHD1* for degradation
Immune deficiency	Over 90% progress to AIDS High viral load, low CD4 count	Less than 20–30% progress to AIDS Low viral load, higher CD4 count
Epidemiology	Worldwide Prevalence increasing Average age at diagnosis 20–30 years	Localized to parts of West Africa and places with historical ties to West Africa Prevalence decreasing Age at diagnosis 40–50 years
Diagnosis	HIV1/2 ELISA WB detects gp40, gp160/140 and p24	HIV 1/2 ELISA WB detects gp36/gp105
Treatment	NRTI, NNRTI, PI, IN, co-receptor, fusion inhibitors	NRTI, PI, IN Intrinsically resistant to NNRTIs and fusion inhibitor enfuvirtide

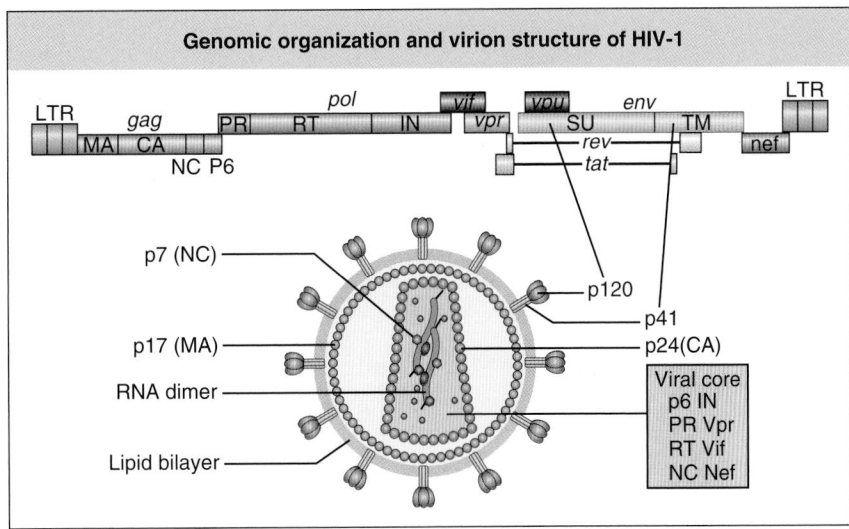

Figure 174-4 Genomic organization and virion structure of HIV-1. (*Adapted from Frankel A.D., Young J.A. Annu Rev Biochem 1998; 67: 1-25.*)

The pol protein is initially made as a gag-pol polyprotein. This is because the *gag* and *pol* open reading frames (ORFs) overlap. The *pol* ORF is positioned in the −1 frame relative to gag ORF. During translation of full-length mRNA, approximately 5–10% of the ribosomes slip back one nucleotide (frame shift) and gain access to the pol ORF, and translation continues resulting in a Gag-Pol polyprotein. The Pol protein is then cleaved by HIV protease to form the three active enzymes RT, PR and IN.

2. Regulatory proteins: these are also called accessory proteins and consist of Tat, Rev, Nef, Vpu, Vpr and Vif. Their functions as related to the life cycle are highlighted below and in Figure 174-5. HIV-2 lacks Vpu but has an extra accessory protein, Vpr, believed to be a duplication of *vpr* during evolution.

The viral life cycle can be artificially divided into the following steps (Figure 174-5):[6]

1. **Entry.** Infection starts with the binding of gp120 to the cellular surface CD4 molecule, which acts as a high-affinity receptor.[7, 8] This causes conformational change in gp120, enabling it to bind to a co-receptor. Two co-receptors can be used: CCR5 and CXCR4 (also known as fusin). These co-receptors are members of the 7-transmembrane G-protein coupled receptor family. All HIV strains tested to date can use either CCR5 (R5 viruses) or CXCR4 (X4 viruses), or both (dual tropic or R5X4 viruses). Binding of the co-receptor by gp120 initiates fusion of the HIV outer membrane and the target plasma membrane, a process mediated by gp41, finally leading to the delivery of the viral core, containing the viral genome, into the host cell cytoplasm.

   With rare exceptions, R5 or R5X4 (not X4) viruses are transmitted from person to person, making the CCR5 co-receptor critical for initiation of infection.[9] About 1% of the Caucasian population have a 32 nucleotide deletion in both alleles of CCR5 (*CCR5Δ32δΔ32*) resulting in a stop codon.[10] These individuals make a non-functional protein which cannot be expressed on the cell surface. People who are homozygous for this allele have profound resistance to HIV infection although infections with X4 viruses in these patients have been reported. Heterozygous individuals, when infected by HIV, have slower progression of disease.

   Maraviroc is an HIV entry inhibitor that inhibits binding of HIV to the CCR5 co-receptor. If this drug is to be used in clinical practice, patients should be tested to ensure that they have only R5 viruses prior to initiation of therapy. Enfuvirtide is an injectable peptide that inhibits HIV membrane fusion by preventing gp41 binding to its target. Several other entry inhibitors are currently under development (see Chapter 152).

2. **Reverse transcription and integration.** Once inside the cytoplasm, the RNA in the viral core is reverse transcribed into DNA by the viral RT enzyme using cellular nucleotides.[11] The backbone of current antiretroviral therapy is to block RT using nucleoside reverse transcriptase inhibitors (NRTI) and non-nucleoside reverse transcriptase inhibitors (NNRTI) (see Chapters 102 and 103). Synthesis of DNA results in the formation of a pre-integration complex (PIC) consisting of the newly made DNA, cellular proteins and viral proteins like the enzyme IN, matrix (MA) and Vpr protein. The PIC is transported into the nucleus through the nuclear pore and integrated into the host genome. Integration involves the covalent attachment of the viral LTR ends into the host DNA catalyzed by viral IN. The activity of IN is enhanced by its binding to the host protein LEDGF/p75 which tends to guide IN to favorable sites.[12-14] Integration occurs at transcriptionally active sites of the host genome, allowing for efficient viral transcription. The integrated virus is called the provirus. Raltegravir, elvitegravir and dolutegravir are HIV integrase inhibitors currently in clinical use (see Chapter 152).

3. **Transcription and nuclear export.** The integrated provirus is transcribed into mRNA by the host enzyme, RNA polymerase II. About half of the mRNA made is spliced into over 40 different alternatively spliced products, the respective ratios of which seem to be important for efficient viral replication. In general, there are three kinds of mRNA products made:

   a. 9 kb unspliced product which is full-length mRNA. From this product, the next viral RNA, full-length Gag and Gag-Pol are derived;

   b. 4 kb singly spliced product from which Env/Vpu (one mRNA), Vif, Vpr and some parts of Tat are made; and

   c. 1.8 kb multiply spliced product from which Tat, Rev and Nef are derived.[15] During the replication cycle, the first synthesized transcription products are the viral regulatory proteins Nef, Tat and Rev. The Tat protein will bind to the transactive response element region on the proviral DNA and, as a consequence, high-level expression of all viral genes occurs. The Nef protein is required for high-level viral replication *in vivo* and it decreases CD4 on the cell membrane. The Nef protein may also enhance the efficiency of reverse transcription and enhance HIV replication in multiple ways.[16]

   The Rev protein facilitates the nuclear transport of unspliced and singly spliced RNA transcripts that contain the *rev*-responsive element, located in the *env* gene. In addition it promotes

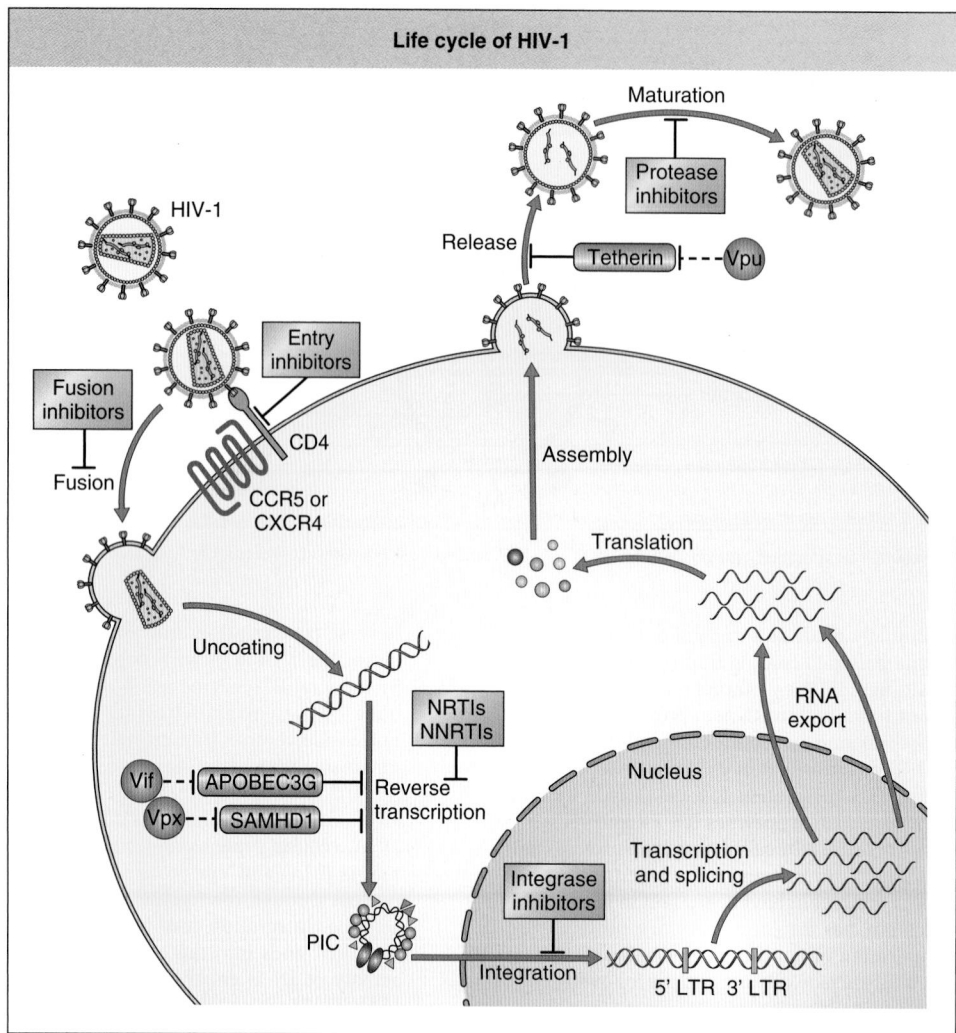

Figure 174-5 Life cycle of HIV-1. Accessory proteins and points of therapeutic intervention are highlighted. (*Modified from Barré-Sinoussi et al. Nat Rev Microbiol 2013; 11: 877-883.*)

translation of messages containing the *rev*-responsive element. Transport of the completely spliced (multiply spliced) RNA to the cytoplasm follow the normal cellular pathway and is rev-independent.

4. **Assembly and budding and maturation.** Once in the cytoplasm, translation of Gag, Gag-Pol and most of the accessory proteins occur on aggregates of cellular ribosomes while translation of Env/Vpu takes place on the rough endoplasmic reticulum. Since viral assembly occurs at the plasma membrane, all viral proteins must traffic to the membrane. Gag is the main structural protein and is targeted to the membrane through a post-translation lipidation (myristoylation) of the MA domain. The envelope glycoprotein is transported to the membrane independent of Gag though interaction of the TM domain of the envelope and the MA domain of Gag seem to be important for viral particle formation. Assembly takes place at cholesterol and sphingolipid-rich microdomains of the plasma membrane termed 'lipid rafts'. The full-length Gag protein begins the assembly into immature viral particles. Several copies of Vpr are incorporated into the virion through direct interaction with the p6 domain of gag. In addition few copies of Nef and Vif proteins are also incorporated. A dimer of full-length RNA is incorporated into the immature virion through interaction between the gag nucleocapsid (NC) and the RNA dimer. Vif plays a critical role in maintaining the integrity of the new viral genome. It

binds to and targets the host cytidine deaminase enzyme APO-BEC3G (apolipoprotein B mRNA-editing, enzyme-catalytic, polypeptide-like 3G) for proteasomal degradation. Without the activity of Vif, APOBEC3G will cause hypermutation of the viral genome and make reverse transcription in the next cell abortive.[17]

Viral budding occurs through interaction between the *gag* p6 domain and the cellular membrane sorting system called the ESCRT (endosomal sorting complexes required for transport) machinery.[18,19] The virus hijacks this conserved trafficking system to bud from the cell surface. The accessory protein Vpu plays a critical role in the budding process by inhibiting the cellular restriction factor Tetherin (also called bone marrow stromal antigen-2). HIV-1 with a *vpu* mutation gets sequestered at the cell surface due to the action of Tetherin. The viral membrane is a phospholipid bilayer derived from the host cell plasma membrane.

Viral maturation occurs during and immediately following budding and is essential for the infectivity of the viral particle. The budding process activates the viral aspartic protease which recognizes and cleaves gag at specific sites into its constituents: MA, CA, NC, p6 proteins along with the peptides sp1 and sp2. Several protease inhibitors (PIs) are in clinical use and they form a key component of current combination antiretroviral therapy. Maturation leads to the formation of an infectious particle ready to engage CD4 and co-receptors on the next cell surface to complete the life cycle.

Transmission (see Chapter 89)

The three major routes of transmission of HIV are by sexual contact, blood or blood products and vertically through maternal–fetal transmission. Infection can occur through the vaginal lining and even more readily through the endocervix or rectal mucosa, which are devoid of squamous epithelium. Infection begins with interaction of viral envelope with dendritic cells (DCs), Langerhans cells (LCs) and/or T cells expressing CD4/CCR5. The DCs and LCs express large amounts of mannose-binding C-type lectins, including one termed the DC-SIGN. DCs and LCs have long dendritic cytoplasmic processes that stretch across into the epithelium and may be available for high-affinity binding of their C-type lectins with viral gp120. Since DCs and LCs do not support productive infections, it is believed that these cells capture virus and transport it to mucosal T cells or macrophages through the process of transcytosis by way of the virological synapse. During episodes of inflammation, such as a sexually transmitted disease or trauma, T cells migrate in large numbers to the mucosa or breached epithelium and will be available for direct infection. Recent evidence suggests that CD4+CCR5+ mucosal memory T cells may be the principal cell type involved in early infection.[20,21] Infection is initially established by a single founder R5 virus that utilizes exclusively a CCR5 co-receptor. In about 50% of patients, co-receptor shift occurs from R5 to X4, usually late in disease[22] (see also Chapter 92).

Diagnosis of HIV

SEROLOGIC ASSAYS

Assays have been developed for detection of HIV antibodies in serum, whole blood, saliva, urine and dried blood collected on filter paper.

Enzyme Immunoassays

HIV diagnosis by enzyme-linked immunosorbent assays (ELISA) has undergone significant evolution since it was first introduced in 1985.[23] The first and second generation assays could only detect the serum IgG and took about 6–8 weeks post infection to be positive, giving a long window period for diagnosis. Significant advance was made when third generation assays were introduced that detect both serum IgM and IgG shortening the window period to about 3 weeks post infection. Currently, fourth-generation assays that detect HIV antigen p24, as well as IgM and IgG antibodies simultaneously, are recommended. They have significantly shortened the time to diagnosis to as early as 2 weeks post infection.[24]

Western Blot

The western blot (WB) method has traditionally been the most widely used method for confirmation of HIV diagnosis with a sensitivity and specificity over 99%. In a WB, viral proteins are separated by polyacrylamide gel electrophoresis and transferred by blotting onto a nitrocellulose strip. The strips are then reacted with the test serum to determine which, if any, viral proteins are recognized by patient antibodies. Figure 174-6 shows a typical WB positive for HIV-1, with the different reactive proteins. Serologic differentiation between HIV-1 and HIV-2 can be done using detection of specific antibodies against the HIV-2 transmembrane protein (gp36). WB assays are reported as positive, negative or indeterminate. A positive result means any two of p24, gp41 or gp120/160 bands are present. A negative result means there are no bands on the blot. An indeterminate result is anything in between, commonly an isolated p24 band. If a WB is reported as indeterminate, then additional testing such as a p24 antigen ELISA, or an approved HIV-1 RNA assay like the Gen-probe® APTIMA® viral load assay, should be considered to confirm HIV infection.

Testing Algorithm

The high sensitivity and specificity of the WB test is valid only if seroconversion has occurred because it detects serum IgG. Hence it can lag behind a fourth-generation ELISA by as much as 3 weeks. The current recommended algorithm does not require a WB and is more efficient at detecting early infections as well as HIV-2 (see Figure 174-7 and

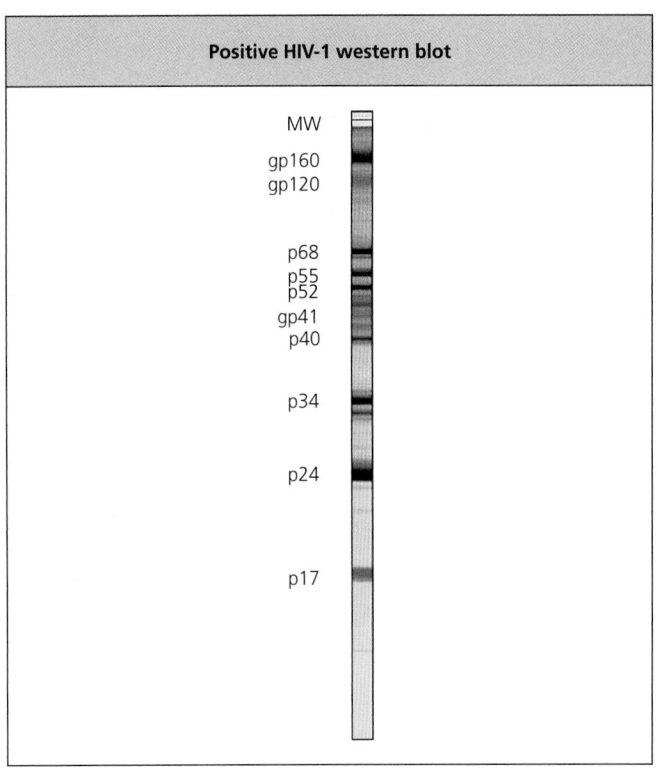

Figure 174-6 Positive HIV-1 western blot. The binding of the patient's antibodies to viral antigens coated on the strip is revealed by an enzyme-labeled antihuman globulin. gp160, gp120 and gp41 are *env* gene products; p55, p24 and p17 are *gag* gene products; p68, p52 and p34 are *pol* gene products. MW, molecular weight of the viral proteins.

Table 174-2). The recommendation is to use a fourth-generation antigen/antibody assay to screen for HIV.[25] Positive tests undergo a second generation ELISA for IgG to differentiate between HIV-1 and HIV-2, also serving as a second specimen to confirm the initial screening test. Confirmed reactivity will diagnose HIV. If the second generation IgG testing comes back as negative for both HIV-1 and HIV-2, then an HIV-1 polymerase chain reaction (PCR) assay is warranted. If the PCR test is positive, the patient likely has acute HIV infection. There is no approved RNA diagnostic assay for HIV-2 although this can be performed in some reference labs. Since most hospital laboratories still use third generation assays, and some resource-poor countries still use second generation tests, it is important for the provider to know which assay is being used to help interpret test results.

Rapid Tests

Diagnostic tests based on red cell or particle agglutination as well as dot-blot assays have been developed that permit rapid diagnosis of HIV-1 infection. In laboratory comparisons, sensitivity and specificity are similar to those of the ELISA, but performance is typically lower in the field.[26] The simplicity and wide operating temperature of these tests make them suitable for use in home testing in at-risk groups, resource-poor settings, for women during labor and delivery, and for source patients following an occupational needlestick injury. They typically consist of lateral flow or flow through cassettes and can detect anti-HIV IgM and/or IgG from a variety of samples including whole blood, plasma, serum and saliva. In this regard, they are equivalent to second or third generation ELISAs. Fourth-generation rapid assays are now available. The turnaround time for rapid tests is typically less than 30 minutes.

HIV Isolation and Resistance Testing

HIV can be isolated from blood, plasma, CSF, genital secretions or tissue by co-culture with lymphocytes from a seronegative donor that

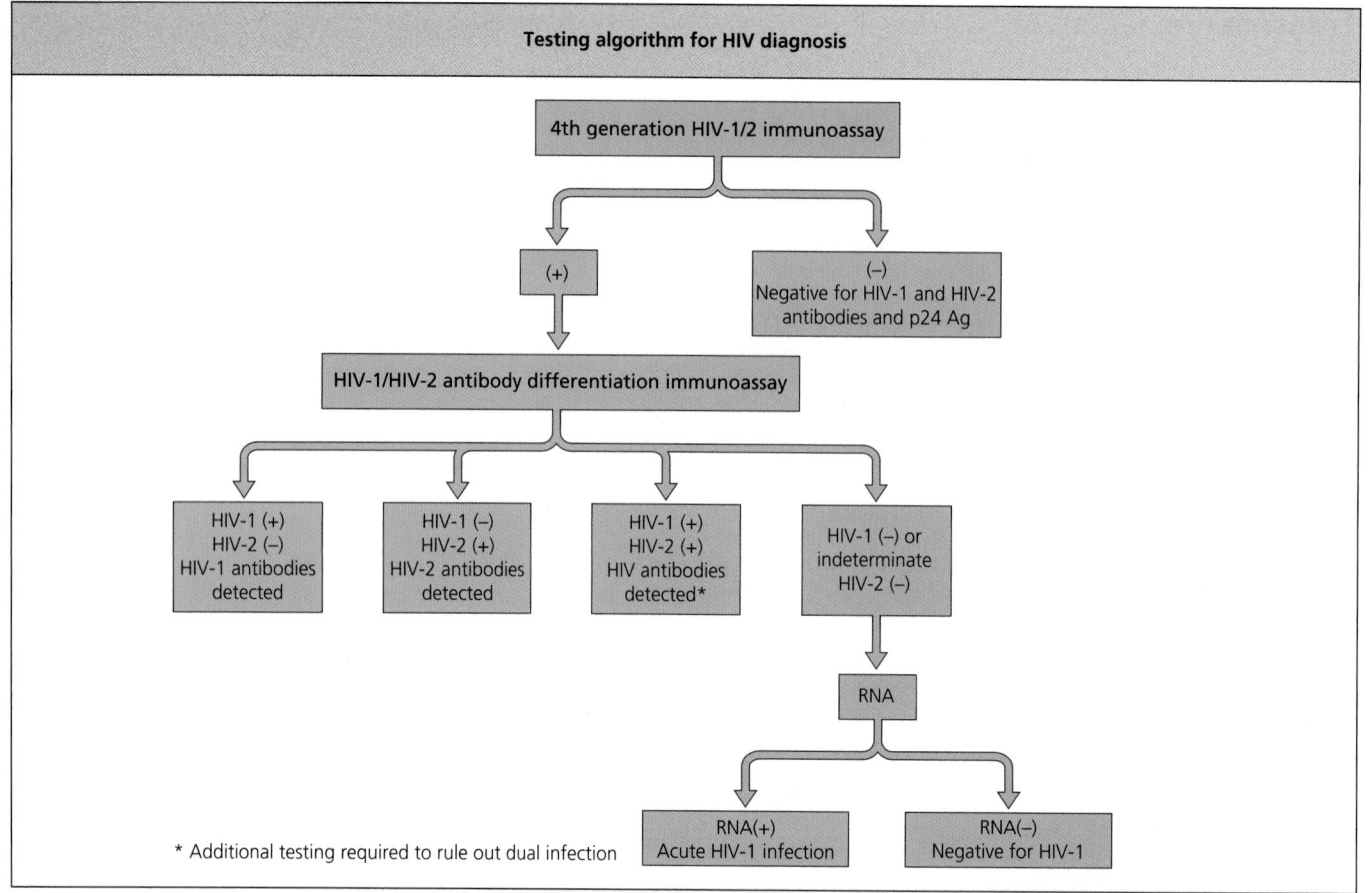

Figure 174-7 Testing algorithm for HIV diagnosis.

TABLE 174-2	HIV Diagnostic Tests and Their Limitations		
Test Type	**What It Detects**	**Limitations**	**First Positive**
4th generation ELISA	HIV antigen p24, plus specific antibodies IgM and IgG	May miss acute HIV infection prior to antigenemia Not available in all settings	14 days
3rd generation ELISA	HIV-specific antibodies IgM and IgG	May be negative even if viral Ag is present Requires WB for confirmation	21 days
2nd and 1st generation ELISA	HIV-specific IgG	Long window period Less sensitive and specific	4–6 weeks
Western blot	Panel of HIV antigens are detected with patient serum IgG	Technically complex Less sensitive than 3rd and 4th generation ELISAs Typically negative for acute HIV infections	4–6 weeks
Nucleic acid amplification tests (NAAT)	HIV DNA or RNA is amplified using specific primers	Not widely available for HIV-2 May not be available in resource-poor settings	1–3 weeks

have been stimulated with phytohemagglutinin and interleukin-2 before use. Virus isolation is successful in more than 95% of individuals infected with HIV-1, but sensitivity is lower in patients with higher CD4 cell counts.

HIV-1 DNA POLYMERASE CHAIN REACTION

HIV-1 DNA PCR assays are used almost exclusively for early diagnosis of infection in neonates. These tests have limited utility in adults, but occasionally may be useful in resolving cases in which results of serologic tests are ambiguous.

QUANTITATIVE HIV-1 RNA ASSAYS

Use of these assays is now standard in the management of HIV-1-infected patients in high-income countries. Several different assay formats have been developed for HIV-1 RNA quantification. In PCR-based assays HIV-1 RNA is converted into DNA by reverse transcription followed by PCR amplification of the DNA. The PCR product is detected by hybridization to an enzyme-conjugated probe specific for HIV-1, and quantified by reacting bound probe with a substrate that undergoes a color change. Branched DNA assay uses nonenzymatic means to amplify the signal from HIV RNA. In this assay, viral RNA is 'captured' by hybridization to complementary oligonucleotides that are bound to the wells of a microtiter plate. The captured viral RNA target is then hybridized to branched oligonucleotides (hence the name 'branched' DNA assay), which in turn are hybridized to enzyme-conjugated oligonucleotides that can be quantified as above. Performance characteristics of most commercially available assays are similar. Most assays have a lower limit of quantification of approximately

TABLE 174-3	HIV Resistance Mechanisms	
Drug Class	Mechanism of Action	Mechanism of Resistance
NRTIs	Act as nucleoside analogs but lack the 3' hydroxyl group leading to HIV DNA chain termination	1. Nucleoside/nucleotide associated mutations (NAMs) – prevent NRTI incorporation into the nascent DNA chain e.g. M184V 2. Thymidine analog mutations – ATP-dependent pyrophosphorolysis that removes the NRTI from the DNA chain thus reversing chain termination.
NNRTIs	Bind RT proximal to its active site. RT amino acids Y181 and K103 are critical for this inhibition	1. Amino acid substitutions such as K103N or Y181C prevent NNRTIs binding 2. HIV-2 and some HIV-1 group O isolates have Y181C as wild type making NNRTIs ineffective
Protease inhibitors	Bind to the active site of the HIV protease enzyme and prevents processing of gag and gag-pol	1. Mutations in the protease gene that prevent PI binding 2. Mutations in major cleavage sites in gag and gag-pol
Integrase inhibitors	Inhibit HIV strand transfer to the host genome. Bind specifically to the part of IN that interacts with the ends of the viral DNA and chelate essential Mg^{2+} at the enzyme active site	Primary mutations at the active site, accompanied by specific secondary mutations
CCR5 inhibitors	Bind to hydrophobic helices within the transmembrane regions of CCR5 inducing a conformational change	Emergence of X4 virus
Fusion inhibitor (Enfuvirtide)	A 36-amino acid peptide that binds to gp41 and prevents the conformational changes needed for viral-host membrane fusion	Mutations in the N-terminal heptad repeats 1 (HR1) domain of gp41 mediate resistance

20–40 copies/mL. Assay sensitivity can be extended by concentrating plasma virus from larger sample volumes.

Plasma HIV-1 RNA levels that appear to be lower than expected in a patient with advanced disease can be a clue to infection with a non-subtype B strain. Incorporation of alternative primer sets in the latest versions of the HIV-1 molecular quantitative assays has improved the ability of these assays to detect diverse HIV-1 subtypes.

HIV DRUG RESISTANCE
(SEE ALSO CHAPTER 103)

The HIV RT has no proofreading ability and is error prone. It is estimated that one mutation is introduced in the genome for every 1000–10 000 nucleotides synthesized resulting in about 1–10 mutations generated for every viral particle made. In the untreated individual, viral turnover is about 10^9 per day, and this gives opportunity for the emergence of many quasi-species of virus with variable fitness that may be resistant to one or more of the current antiretrovirals. Combination antiretroviral therapy keeps replication to a minimum and prevents the development of new mutations.

Mechanisms of resistance and common clinically relevant mutations are summarized in Tables 174-3 and 174-4.

DRUG RESISTANCE ASSAYS

The assessment of drug resistance has now become routine practice in Europe and the USA.[27] A variety of assays are available including: *genotypic* assays, in which nucleotide sequencing of viral genetic material is used to detect the presence or absence of critical drug resistance mutations; and *phenotypic* assays, in which the concentration of drug necessary to inhibit virus replication *in vitro* is estimated in a drug susceptibility assay.

Each method has potential advantages and disadvantages. An important limitation of both approaches is that they provide a measure of the characteristics of the predominant viral species but do not indicate the presence of minor species that may emerge as resistant variants during subsequent treatment.

GENOTYPIC TESTS OF HIV-1 DRUG RESISTANCE

Several approaches to genotyping are available, ranging from full-length sequencing of the target gene to point mutation assays, which focus only on a particular mutation of interest. The most commonly used genotypic assays rely on automated DNA sequencing. Using this technique, the nucleotide sequence of some or all of the gene of interest (e.g. protease, RT or integrase) is obtained, then translated into the predicted amino acid sequence in order to determine whether specific mutations are present or absent. Automated sequencing offers the most complete data on viral genotype, but generates more information than is needed for most clinical purposes. For example, HIV-1 RT has 550 amino acids, but mutations at only a small number of these positions are implicated in drug resistance. Therefore, interpretation of the genotype is needed in order to help distinguish which changes are merely polymorphisms and which might be significantly associated with drug resistance. The Stanford HIV resistance database is a useful resource for interpreting genotype results (http://hivdb.stanford.edu/).

In most commercially available genotypic tests, viral RNA is extracted from a sample of plasma and reverse transcribed into complementary DNA in the laboratory. The protease and RT or integrase coding regions of the cDNA are then amplified by PCR, and the nucleotide sequence of the PCR product is determined on an automated DNA sequencer. Some laboratories use specific diagnostic kits that provide standardized reagents needed for the RT-PCR and DNA sequencing steps. Generally, these kits are part of an HIV-genotyping system that includes equipment for running the sequencing assays and software for interpreting assay results.

The frequency of false-positive and false-negative results is 0.1% for genotypic assays when assessed using samples that carry predominantly mutant or predominantly wild-type virus populations. However, sensitivity for detecting presence of a mutation is variable when both wild-type and mutant viruses are present as a mixture. In general, mutant species must constitute 10–20% of the population to be detected by standard sequencing methods. Some mutations may go undetected unless they are present as the majority species.

PHENOTYPIC TESTS OF HIV-1 DRUG RESISTANCE

Drug susceptibility tests with HIV-1 are usually performed using a recombinant virus assay, in which the viral genes of interest (e.g. protease and RT) are introduced into a plasmid that carries all of the other viral genes needed for replication in cell culture (Figure 174-8). Modification of the assay allows introduction of the integrase (*in*) or envelope (*env*) genes in order to determine susceptibility to integrase inhibitors and entry inhibitors, respectively. Using these assays, small differences in susceptibility can be detected (approximately two- to

TABLE 174-4	Common HIV Drug Resistance Mutations
Mutation/HIV Gene	**Drug Resistance and Implications**
NRTI MUTATIONS	
M184V	3TC, FTC, DDI, ABC
K65R	All NRTIs except AZT
Q151M	All NRTIs affected, although tenofovir retains activity
TAMs: M41L, L210W, T215Y, D67Y, K70R, K219Q	4 or more TAMS induce resistance to all NRTIs
L74V	ABC and DDI; possibly increased susceptibility to TDF and AZT
T69S-XX insertion mutations	Resistant to all NRTIs
NNRTI MUTATIONS	
K103N	High-level resistance efavirenz (EFV) and nevirapine (NVP), etravirine (ETR) retains activity
Y181C	High-level resistance for EFV and NVP. Provides the foundation for ETR resistance though it may have activity
E138 A/G/K/Q/R	Rilpivirine
PIs/PROTEASE GENE	*Boosting with ritonavir reduces the likelihood of resistance; multiple mutations in the protease gene are usually required before resistance emerges with ritonavir-boosted PIs*
D30N	Nelfinavir with no cross-resistance
G48V	Saquinavir, no cross-resistance
L76V	When combined with other PI mutations (>3), decreases susceptibility to lopinavir/ritonavir and darunavir/ritonavir
L90M	Nelfinavir, saquinavir
INTEGRASE INHIBITORS/IN GENE	
Q148H/K/R	Raltegravir and elvitegravir resistance
N155H	Raltegravir and elvitegravir
Y143C	Raltegravir
T66I	Elvitegravir
Combination of Q148H, G140S and other integrase mutations	Decreased susceptibility to dolutegravir

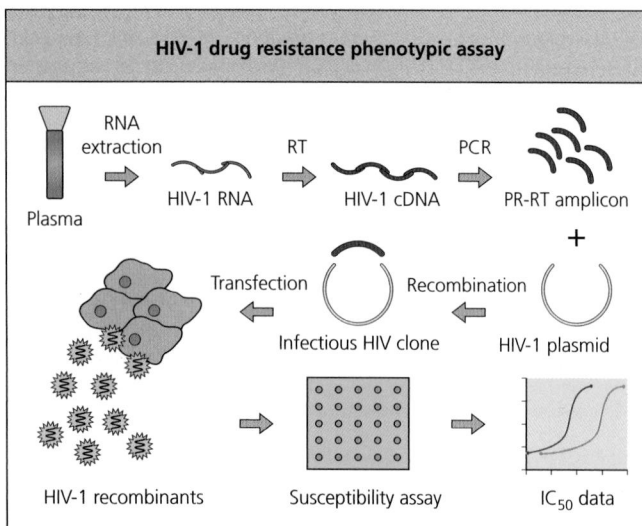

Figure 174-8 HIV-1 drug resistance phenotypic assay. RT, reverse transcription reaction; cDNA, complementary DNA; PR-RT, protease and reverse transcriptase gene; IC$_{50}$, 50% inhibitory concentration.

fourfold compared with control). Phenotypic assays are more complex and labor intensive than genotypic assays. Automation makes it possible to test many samples simultaneously, and allows for high throughput. However, the cost and complexity of the automation limit availability of these assays to a few reference laboratories.

HIV Latency and Prospects for Cure

(see Chapter 105)

The most important obstacle to HIV cure is the existence of proviral DNA in long-lived resting CD4 T cells forming a latent reservoir that is not affected by highly active antiretroviral therapy (HAART) or the immune system. These cells serve as the source of viral production once antiretrovirals are discontinued, thus necessitating lifelong therapy. Owing to the long half-life of resting T cells, some estimates suggest that it will take up to 70 years for the reservoir to fully decay with current HAART therapy.[28,29]

BONE MARROW TRANSPLANT

The apparent cure of the so-called 'Berlin patient' has renewed optimism that HIV cure is possible. Following a diagnosis of leukemia, this patient underwent double hematopoietic stem-cell transplant from a donor who was homozygous for the CCR5Δ32 allele. Since 2007, there is no trace of active HIV replication in this patient. Attempts to eradicate HIV using stem-cell transplant in other leukemia patients have not so far been successful.[10,30,31]

CO-RECEPTOR TARGETING

Since the homozygous CCR5Δ32 confers natural resistance to HIV infection, therapeutic approaches are being explored that will disable this co-receptor. The general approach is to obtain CD4 T cells from the infected patient and knock down the co-receptor gene using lentiviral or adenoviral vector-derived small hairpin RNA (shRNA) or zinc finger nucleases (ZFN). The CD4 T cells are then expanded and infused into the patient. A recent Phase I clinical trial using ZFN modified CCR5 CD4 T cells was shown to be safe. Attempts to target the CXCR4 receptor are ongoing.[32]

EXCISION OF PROVIRUSES FROM GENOME

Since HIV integrates into the genome, one approach using an engineered Tre recombinase enzyme to specifically excise the HIV provirus from the human genome is being pursued. This approach has been tried in humanized mice so far and found to have good antiviral activity.[33]

LATENCY REVERSING AGENTS (LRAs)

An approach that has received a lot of attention is to use pharmacological means to reactivate HIV from latency while patients are on HAART. The idea is that reactivation will cause viral replication in latently infected cells leading to cell death without opportunity to infect bystander cells. Histone deacetylase inhibitors (HDACi) are the primary candidates for this approach.[34,35] HDACs are enzymes that remove acetyl groups from the lysines of histones leading to tighter chromatin remodeling. The use of HDAC inhibitors (HDI) leads to more efficient transcription of latent genes. Several HDIs have been shown *in vitro* and in *ex vivo* models to induce HIV from latency. Of these, suberoylanilide hydroxamic acid (SAHA/vorinostat), already approved for cutaneous T-cell lymphoma, has been shown to induce HIV reactivation in a Phase I trial.[36] Other latency reversing agents being considered include protein kinase C modulators such as bryostatin-1, transcriptional regulators such as small molecule JQ1 and the zinc-chelating agent disulfiram. Despite this enthusiasm, recent research indicates that LRAs may need to be combined with some form of CD4 T-cell activation to be able to make a considerable dent in the HIV reservoir.[37,38]

Human T-Lymphocyte Leukemia Viruses

Nature

The human T-lymphocyte leukemia viruses are complex retroviruses. Of the four species identified so far (HTLV-1, -2, -3 and -4), only HTLV-1 has been associated with disease in humans and is the focus of this section. In addition to the standard genes encoded by all retroviruses (*gag, pol, env*), HTLV-1 also encodes several accessory proteins in its N- terminal (pX) region including *tax, rex*, p12, p13, p21, p30 and HBZ (Figure 174-1).[39]

The Rex protein is involved in splicing, processing, stabilization and transport of viral mRNA from nucleus to cytoplasm. The Tax protein is a transactivator protein; by acting on the LTR located 5' to the viral *gag* gene, Tax induces the transcription of viral mRNA. Current research implicates Tax and HBZ for initiation and maintenance of adult T-cell leukemia (ATL).

Epidemiology

Seroepidemiologic studies have shown that the highest incidence of anti-HTLV-1 antibodies is found in south-western Japan, ranging from 5% to 35% in endemic areas. Other areas with high incidence are the Caribbean islands, some regions of South and Central America, the south-west Pacific and Papua New Guinea. The general incidence in the USA and Europe is low (0.05%), although an increasing incidence has been reported among homosexuals and intravenous drug users.

Pathogenesis

HTLV-1 is transmitted by infected lymphocytes and not as free virus in cell-free body fluids. Three transmission routes for HTLV-1 have been described.
- transmission of HTLV-infected lymphocytes via the placenta, during birth or after birth through the mother's milk;
- transmission from male to female during sexual intercourse; and
- blood transfusion.

Human T-lymphocyte leukemia virus-1 is a lymphotropic virus that preferentially infects CD4+ T cells. Usually, the leukemic cells in ATL have the following phenotype: CD2+, CD3+, CD4+, CD5+, CD25+, CD29+, CD45RO+, CD52+, HLA-DR+, T-cell receptor αβ+ and variably CD30+, and lack CD7, CD8 and CD26 expression.

The molecular mechanisms by which HTLV-1 is able to induce cell transformation have not been unraveled. Human T-lymphocyte leukemia virus does not contain a typical oncogene. Several hypothetical mechanisms of HTLV-induced oncogenesis have been formulated including a role for Tax and HBZ. However, these hypotheses do not explain why it takes an average incubation time of 20–30 years to develop ATL or why only a small number of HTLV-1-infected people develop clinical manifestations of ATL.[40]

Diagnostic Microbiology

Infection with HTLV-1 and HTLV-2 can be diagnosed using serologic assays (ELISA and rapid tests) to detect antibodies against the virus. Confirmation and distinction between HTLV-1 and HTLV-2 can be done through PCR detection of proviral DNA in lymphocytes. HTLV PCR assays are only available in specialized laboratories.

Clinical Features

In addition to ATL, HTLV-1 is associated with uveitis, polymyositis, arthropathy, Sjögren's syndrome and myelopathy. Individuals infected with HTLV-1 are also at risk for infections such as disseminated strongyloidiasis, pneumocystis pneumonia, cryptococcal disease and toxoplasmosis.

ADULT T-LYMPHOCYTE LEUKEMIA

Several pieces of evidence established the causal relationship between HTLV-1 and ATL:
- ATL has an identical geographic distribution to that of HTLV-1, having a high incidence in south-western Japan, as was shown in seroepidemiologic studies.
- All ATL tumor cells contain one or more copies of the HTLV-1 provirus in their genomic DNA.
- *In vitro* infection of human T cells with HTLV-1 results in T-cell immortalization.
- HTLV-1 has been demonstrated to be oncogenic in animals.

The lifetime chance of an infected person developing ATL is very low (about 1%). The first clinical manifestations of ATL generally occur 20–30 years after infection with HTLV-1. The median age of ATL onset is 52.7 years.

TROPICAL SPASTIC PARESIS

Infections with HTLV-1 have also been associated with a neurologic syndrome affecting the pyramidal tract, called HTLV-1-associated myelopathy or tropical spastic paresis (HAM/TSP). This disorder is characterized by a slowly progressive symmetric myelopathy combined with high titers of antibodies to HTLV-1 in plasma and cerebrospinal fluid. The myelopathy primarily affects the pyramidal tract. The mechanism by which HTLV-1 infection causes HAM is unclear.

References available online at expertconsult.com.

KEY REFERENCES

Barre-Sinoussi F., Ross A.L., Delfraissy J.F.: Past, present and future: 30 years of HIV research. *Nat Rev Microbiol* 2013; 11:877-883.

Battistini A., Sgarbanti M.: HIV-1 Latency: an update of molecular mechanisms and therapeutic strategies. *Viruses* 2014; 6:1715-1758.

Centers for Disease Control and Prevention: Detection of acute HIV infection in two evaluations of a new HIV diagnostic testing algorithm – United States, 2011-2013. *MMWR Morb Mort Wkly Rep* 2013; 62(24):489-494.

Cook L.B., Elemans M., Rowan A.G., et al.: HTLV-1: persistence and pathogenesis. *Virology* 2013; 435:131-140.

Frankel A.D., Young J.A.: HIV-1: fifteen proteins and an RNA. *Annu Rev Biochem* 1998; 67:1-25.

Hirsch M.S., et al.: Antiretroviral drug resistance testing in adult HIV-1 infection: 2008 recommendations of an International AIDS Society-USA panel. *Top HIV Med* 2008; 16:266-285.

Hu W.S., Hughes S.H.: HIV-1 reverse transcription. *Cold Spring Harb Perspect Med* 2012; 22(10):pii: a006882.

Passaes C.P., Saez-Cirion A.: HIV cure research: Advances and prospects. *Virology* 2014; 454-455:340-352.

Stoltzfus C.M.: Chapter 1. Regulation of HIV-1 alternative RNA splicing and its role in virus replication. *Adv Virus Res* 2009; 74:1-40.

Sundquist W.I., Krausslich H.G.: HIV-1 assembly, budding, and maturation. *Cold Spring Harb Perspect Med* 2012; 2:a006924.

175

Zoonotic Viruses

LYLE R. PETERSEN | THOMAS G. KSIAZEK

KEY CONCEPTS

- Zoonotic infections are infections of animals that can naturally infect humans.

- More than 80 arthropod-borne viruses (arboviruses) can cause human disease.

- Arboviral infections produce three main clinical syndromes: febrile illness accompanied by rash and arthralgia, neuroinvasive disease and hemorrhagic fever.

- Flaviviruses are major causes of arboviral disease globally: dengue, West Nile, yellow fever, and tick-borne encephalitis.

- Arenaviruses are infections of rodents and can be acquired by contact with rodents and their excretions or by contact with secretions from infected patients.

- Arenavirus infection can be severe and cause meningoencephalitis and hemorrhagic fever.

- Hantaviruses are infections of rodents that can be acquired by humans by contact with rodents and their excretions.

- Hantaviruses are significant causes of illness in some parts of the world and are associated with two main clinical syndromes: hemorrhagic fever with renal disease and severe pulmonary disease.

- Marburg and Ebola viruses are filoviruses that derive from bats in Africa.

- Marburg and Ebola viruses cause hemorrhagic fever with high mortality and outbreaks occur from contact with secretions from infected patients.

- Nipah and Hendra viruses are infections of fruit bats. Humans can become infected by contact with infected animals or by contact with body fluids of infected patients.

Introduction

Zoonotic infections are infections of animals that can naturally infect humans. Of the approximately 213 viruses known to cause human disease, most have known (60%) or presumed (8%) nonhuman vertebrate hosts.[1] Humans can be infected directly from the host animal species, for example following the bite of a rabies-infected animal, through inhalation of rodent urine (hantavirus) or by direct contact with rodent urine (Lassa fever). However, most zoonotic infections are spread by arthropod vectors and are classified as arboviruses.[1]

Arboviruses

Approximately 83 viruses that cause human disease are classified as arboviruses.[1] These are distributed worldwide because of their close association with lower vertebrates and insects and their wide host range. All arbovirus infections of humans are caused by RNA viruses, most commonly by the alphaviruses (genus *Alphavirus*, family Togaviridae), flaviviruses (genus *Flavivirus*, family Flaviviridae), and bunyaviruses (genus *Orthobunyavirus*, *Nairovirus* and *Phlebovirus*).[1,2]

Many arboviruses that infect humans cause nonspecific symptoms such as acute fever. Three broad clinical patterns are recognized with arbovirus infection:

- fever, rash and arthritis or retinitis;
- encephalitis; and
- viral hemorrhagic fevers (VHFs).

Most arboviruses circulate in complex life cycles that involve non-human vertebrate hosts and blood-feeding arthropod vectors, most commonly mosquitoes, ticks, sand flies (*Phlebotomus* spp.) and midges (*Culicoides* spp.). Many arboviruses have several vertebrate hosts and many can be transmitted by several vectors. Because arboviruses typically have little or no clinical impact on their primary vertebrate hosts, these arboviral enzootic life cycles often only become evident when humans are bitten directly by the natural enzootic vectors, such as exposure to West Nile virus (WNV)-infected *Culex* mosquitoes, or when humans are exposed to a virus that has escaped the primary enzootic transmission cycle via a secondary vector or vertebrate host. An example of the latter is Eastern equine encephalitis, which circulates between *Culiseta melanura* mosquitoes and birds. Humans become infected when bitten by so-called bridge mosquito vectors that feed on infected birds as well as humans and other mammals.

In most instances, humans are considered dead-end hosts since they develop insufficient viremia to efficiently infect arthropods and thus do not contribute to arboviral transmission cycles (see Figure 175-1). However, the dengue, yellow fever, chikungunya and Zika viruses cause sufficient viremia in humans to allow transmission directly between humans and *Aedes* mosquitoes in urban settings (Figure 175-2). The key features of the clinically important arboviruses transmitted to humans by hematophagous arthropod vectors, such as mosquitoes, ticks and *Phlebotomus* flies (sand fly), are given in

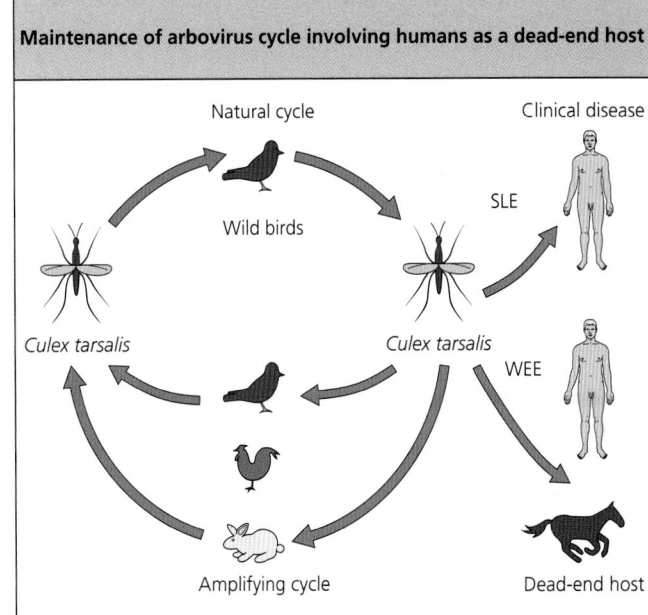

Figure 175-1 Maintenance of arbovirus cycle involving humans as a dead-end host (e.g. St Louis (SLE) and Western equine encephalitis (WEE) viruses).

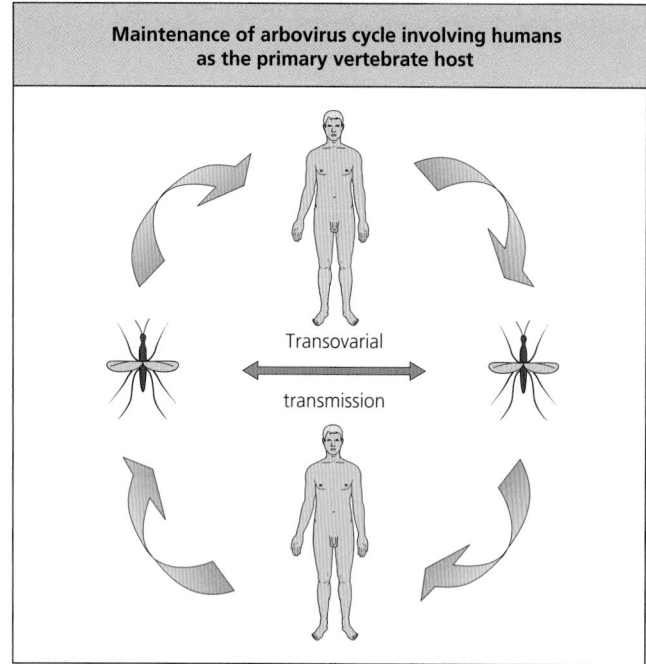

Figure 175-2 Maintenance of arbovirus cycle involving humans as the primary vertebrate host (e.g. dengue, chikungunya, Zika).

Table 175-1. Yellow fever and WNVs are examples of mosquito-borne zoonotic infections.

Yellow Fever

Nature

Yellow fever has historically been one of the great killers of humans. Regrettably, this mosquito-borne virus continues to exact a considerable toll on human populations living in endemic areas.

Epidemiology

Yellow fever occurs in sub-Saharan Africa and tropical South America, where it is endemic and intermittently epidemic. Since 1996, fewer than 300 cases in South America and fewer than 1200 in Africa have been reported annually to the World Health Organization (WHO). However, the potential for recurrence of large urban outbreaks was demonstrated in West Africa from 1986 to 1994 during which more than 20 000 cases and 4000 deaths were recorded (Figure 175-3).[3]

There are three transmission cycles of yellow fever (Figure 175-4). The jungle (sylvatic) transmission cycle consists of a natural reservoir of disease in nonhuman primates with transmission by forest-dwelling mosquitoes (mainly by *Haemagogus* sp. mosquitoes in South America and *Aedes africanus* in sub-Saharan Africa). The urban (or epidemic) cycle of yellow fever consists of a human-to-human transmission cycle vectored by the human-adapted mosquito *Aedes aegypti*. The intermediate (savanna) cycle in Africa involves viral transmission from mosquitoes to humans living or working in jungle border areas. In this cycle the virus can be transmitted from monkey to human or from human to human via mosquitoes.

All susceptible populations appear to be at equal risk for disease yet most cases occur in children or young men (particularly those involved in the logging industry or construction in heavily forested areas). Population expansion, economic development and ecotourism in rainforest areas and inadequate distribution of yellow fever vaccine in endemic regions of the world are of concern. From 1990 to 2011, nine yellow fever cases were reported in unvaccinated residents of the USA and Europe who traveled to West Africa (5 cases) or South America

(4 cases). Expanding commercial trade and international travel increases the risk of yellow fever outbreaks in non-endemic regions of the world in which the mosquito vector is found.[4]

Pathogenicity

Yellow fever is a prototypic mosquito-borne viral hemorrhagic fever. The virus is a 38 nm ssRNA virus with a genome of approximately 4 $\times$ 10^6 Da. The virus is injected into humans during the course of a mosquito bite. Local viral replication takes place in human skin and regional lymph nodes, followed by viremia and dissemination to multiple organs of the body.

Major pathologic findings are found in the liver, kidney, heart and gastrointestinal tract. The virus infects the liver and causes massive hepatic necrosis. The characteristic pathologic finding is that of midzone necrosis with sparing of hepatocytes around the central vein and portal triads. Another characteristic finding is that of Councilman bodies within degenerating hepatocytes. Councilman bodies are acidophilic cytoplasmic deposits and not viral inclusion bodies. Diffuse areas of petechial hemorrhage are found throughout the body with the most marked changes found in the brain, kidney and gastrointestinal tract.

Prevention

Control of *Aedes aegypti* mosquitoes responsible for urban yellow fever transmission has proven ineffective in most contemporary urban settings. Thus, prevention largely relies on vaccination programs with the live, attenuated 17-D yellow fever virus vaccine strain.[5] The vaccine is highly effective; 99% of healthy persons develop neutralizing antibody and more than 80% have neutralizing antibodies 30–35 years after vaccination. Adverse events following yellow fever vaccine are generally mild; however, two patterns of severe adverse reactions occur. Yellow fever vaccine-associated neurologic adverse disease includes several neurologic conditions beginning 3–28 days after vaccination, including meningoencephalitis, Guillain–Barré syndrome and acute disseminated encephalomyelitis. The risk is estimated to be 0.8 per 100 000 doses and is higher in recipients aged more than 60 years. Yellow fever vaccine-associated viscerotropic disease is a severe illness resembling wild-type disease occurring 0–8 days after vaccination. The estimated risk is 0.4 per 100 000 doses and is higher in recipients aged more than 60 years. Travelers to yellow fever endemic areas and residents within endemic areas should be considered for vaccination.[5,6]

Diagnostic Microbiology

The virus can be isolated from several cell lines including Vero cells and AP-61 cells. Virus isolation represents an extreme biohazard and should only be attempted in specialized laboratory facilities. Serodiagnosis is possible within 1 week of onset of infection, with IgM antibodies detectable using enzyme-linked immunosorbent assay (ELISA), microsphere-based immunoassay (MIA), hemagglutination inhibition or plaque-reduction neutralization tests. Virus detection can also be accomplished using reverse transcriptase semi-nested polymerase chain reactions (PCRs) from blood as well as tissue samples. Immunohistochemical staining of formalin-fixed material can detect yellow fever antigen on histopathologic specimens.

Clinical Manifestations

Human illness with yellow fever follows three discrete phases. The first phase of illness lasts approximately 72 hours and is initiated by fever, headache, malaise, weakness, nausea and vomiting. The virus is replicating rapidly and high titers of infectious virus are found in the body fluids of patients at this point. This initial period of infection is followed by a brief period of remission where fever and symptoms remit. After 24–48 hours, in about 15% of patients, symptoms recur and are dominated by acute hepatic and renal failure. Patients develop jaundice and very high fever (hence the name yellow fever) followed by a

TABLE 175-1   Important Arbovirus Infections That Cause Human Disease

Genus	Virus diseases	Afr.	Asia	Aust.	Eur.	N. Am.	C. Am.	S. Am.	Pac.	Main hosts	Clinical
MOSQUITO VECTOR											
Alphavirus	Western equine encephalitis	−	−	−	−	+	−	+ −	−	Rodents, birds, marsupials, equines	Encephalitis
	Eastern equine encephalitis	−	−	−	−	+	+	+	−	Wild birds, bats, rodents, equines, reptiles	Encephalitis
	Venezuelan equine encephalitis	−	−	−	−	+	+	+	−	Rodents, birds, marsupials, equines	Encephalitis
	Chikungunya	+	+	−	+	+	+	+	+	Primates	Fever, rash, myalgia, polyarthritis
	Ross River fever	−	−	+	−	−	−	−	+	Large mammals, marsupials	Fever, rash, myalgia, arthralgia, hemorrhagic fever
Flavivirus	Dengue	+	+	+	−	+	+	+	+	Humans	Encephalitis
	Japanese encephalitis	−	+	+	−	−	−	−	−	Birds, pigs	Encephalitis
	St Louis encephalitis	−	+	+	−	+	−	+	−	Birds	Encephalitis
	Murray Valley encephalitis	−	+	+	−	−	−	−	−	Birds	Encephalitis
	West Nile	+	+	+	+	+	+	+	−	Birds	Fever, rash, myalgia, polyarthritis, encephalitis
	Yellow fever	+	−	−	−	−	+	+	−	Primates	Hemorrhagic fever
	Zika	+	−	−	−	−	−	−	+	Primates	Fever, rash
Phlebovirus	Rift Valley fever	+	−	−	−	−	−	−	−	Wild mammals, domestic livestock	Hemorrhagic fever, retinitis, encephalitis
TICK VECTOR											
Flavivirus	Central European encephalitis	−	−	−	+	−	−	−	−	Rodents	Encephalitis
	Russian spring-summer encephalitis	−	−	−	+	−	−	−	−	Rodents	Encephalitis
	Omsk hemorrhagic fever	−	+	+	−	−	−	−	−	Water voles, muskrats	Encephalitis
	Powassan	−	−	+	−	+	−	−	−	Rodents	Encephalitis
Nairovirus	Crimean–Congo hemorrhagic fever	+	+	−	+	−	−	−	−	Wild and domestic mammals	Hemorrhagic fever
Coltivirus	Colorado tick fever virus	−	−	−	−	+	−	−	−	Wild and domestic mammals	Febrile illness
SAND FLY VECTOR											
	Sand fly fever Naples	+	+	−	+	−	−	−	−	Rodent	Febrile illness, myalgia, conjunctivitis
	Sand fly fever Sicilian	+	+	−	+	−	−	−	−	Rodent	Febrile illness, myalgia, conjunctivitis
	Toscana	−	−	−	+	−	−	−	−	Rodent	Febrile illness, myalgia, conjunctivitis

hemorrhagic diathesis with petechiae, mucosal hemorrhages and gastrointestinal bleeding. A characteristic physical finding is marked bradycardia in the face of high fever (Faget's sign). Patients develop delirium, seizures, coma, acute renal failure and death within 7–10 days of illness. Most persons with mild yellow fever illness recover completely. However, the case : fatality ratio is 20–50% among patients with severe disease.[7]

Management

The management of yellow fever remains primarily supportive. Intravenous fluids, blood products and management of hepatic and renal insufficiency are the mainstays of therapy. Ribavirin does not appear to be effective and no other antiviral agent has been shown to be useful. Transmission to healthcare workers, particularly after needlestick injuries, has been described. Patients should be isolated as their blood and body secretions contain infectious virus.

West Nile Virus

Nature

WNV is a prototypic example of an emerging arboviral disease, with anthropogenic and virologic factors contributing to widened geographic distribution and increased public health importance. Following its initial discovery from the blood of a febrile woman in the West Nile district of Uganda in 1937, WNV caused sporadic disease as well as outbreaks of mostly mild febrile illness in Africa and occasionally in Europe and Israel. The virus was first identified in the western hemisphere during an outbreak of human neuroinvasive disease and an epizootic in birds in 1999 in the New York City (NYC) area.[8] Repeated large outbreaks of severe neuroinvasive disease – meningitis, encephalitis, and acute flaccid paralysis – have occurred subsequently in the USA, Canada, Europe and Israel.

Epidemiology

WNV is a flavivirus most closely related to the Japanese encephalitis, Murray Valley encephalitis and St Louis encephalitis viruses. WNVs can be designated into at least five phylogenetic lineages, although only lineage 1 and 2 viruses have been associated with substantial human morbidity. The initial North American isolates (East Coast genotype) from 1999 in NYC were closely related to a lineage 1 WNV isolated from Israel in 1998, suggesting Middle Eastern origin.[9] However, subsequent genetic analysis suggested independent importation of both viruses from a common African ancestor.[10] The means of importation to NYC from Africa remains unknown, although air transport of an infected animal is a likely possibility. Although lineage 2 viruses were thought initially to be of low pathogenicity, they have caused outbreaks of human and animal disease in South Africa and Europe in recent years. Interestingly, the North American lineage 1 isolates and the lineage 1 and 2 isolates in Europe that have caused large human neuroinvasive disease outbreaks all contain a single genetic mutation in the NS3 helicase gene that confers high avian mortality.[11,12] Since

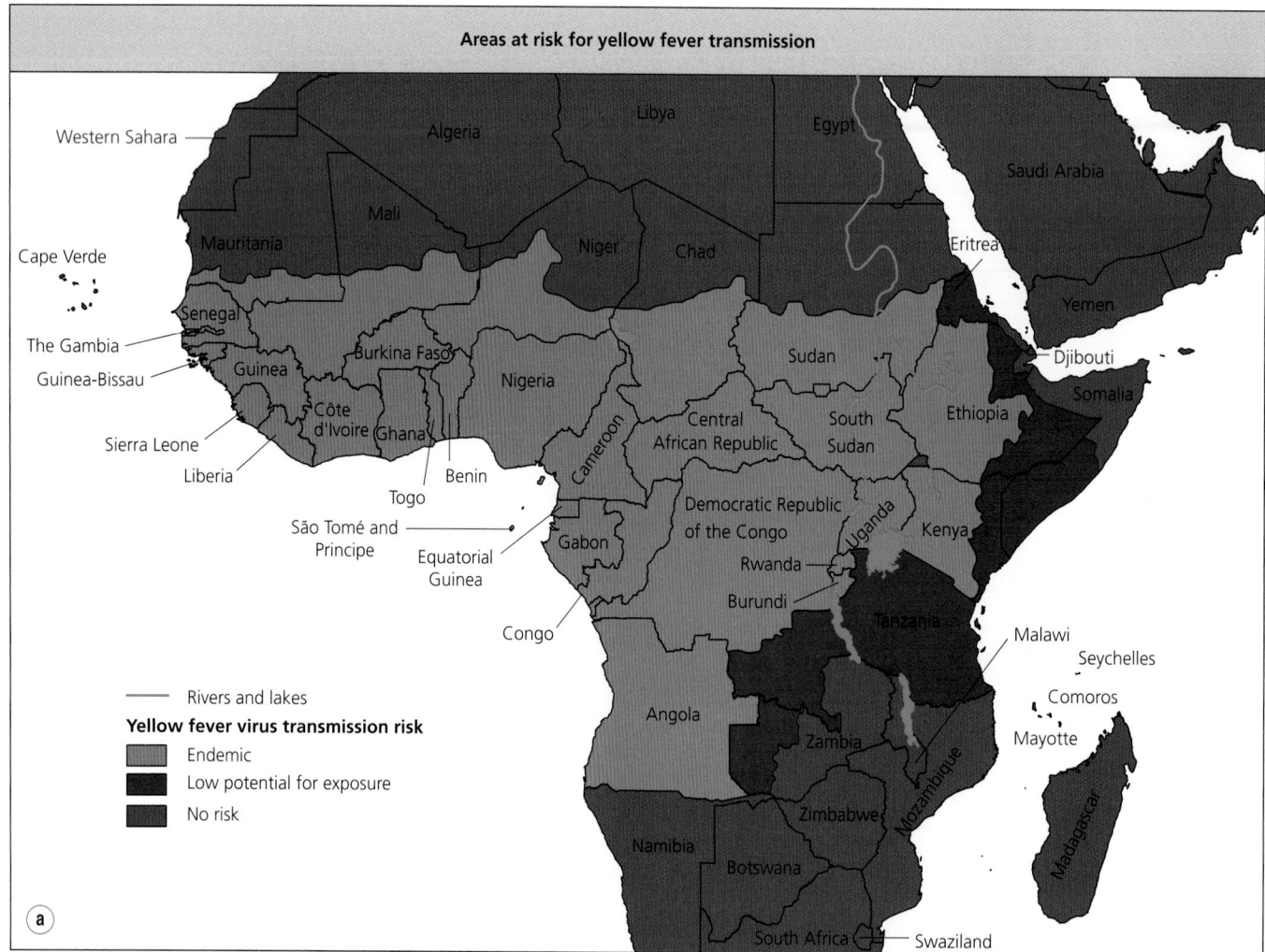

Figure 175-3 Areas at risk for yellow fever transmission. (a) Africa. (*Source: Lancet Infect Dis 2011; 11: 622-32.*)

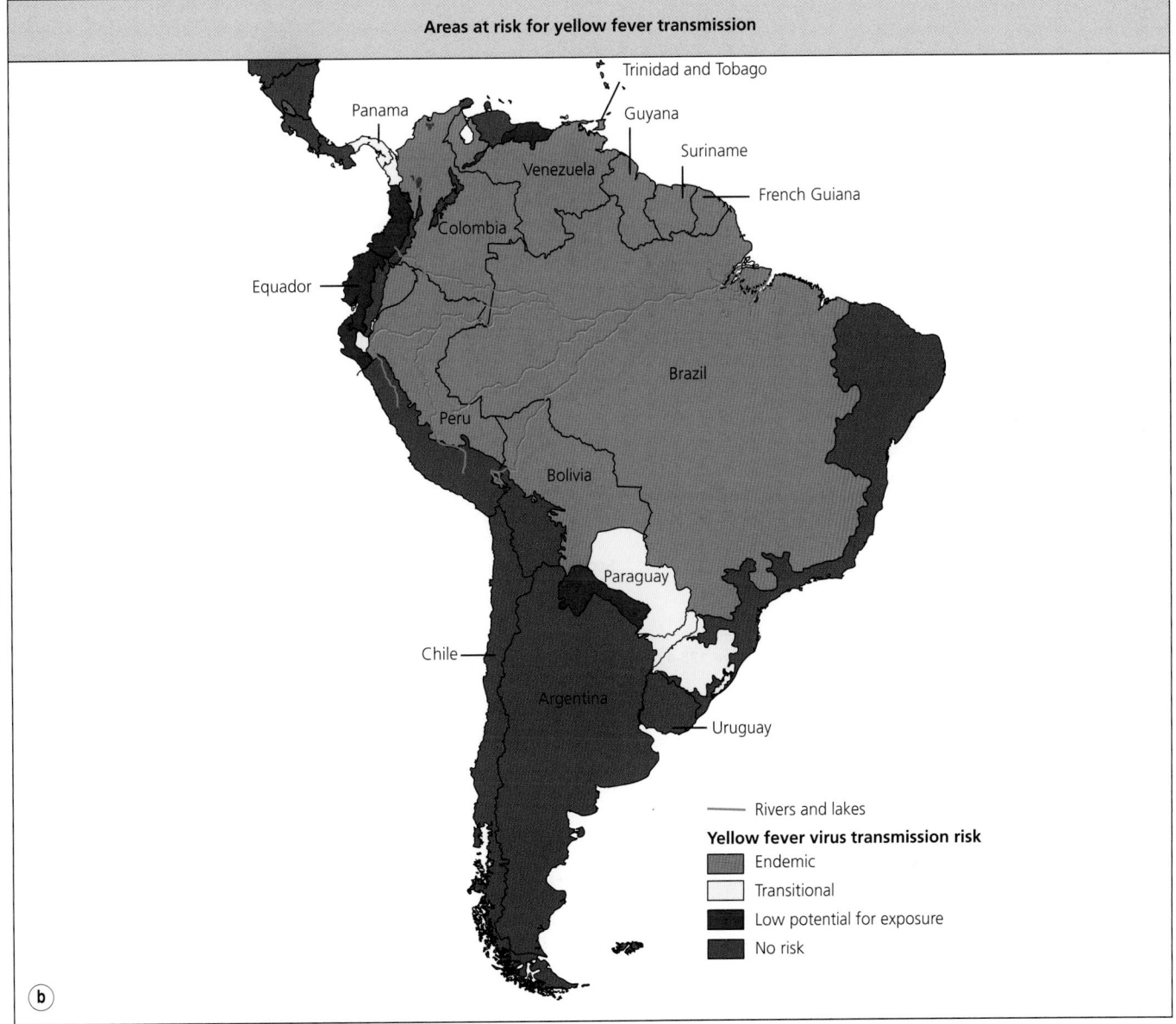

Figure 175-3, cont'd   Areas at risk for yellow fever transmission. (b) South America. *(Source: Lancet Infect Dis 2011; 11: 622-32.)*

approximately 2002, the East Coast genotype has largely been displaced by a new genotype (WN02 genotype) encompassing several conserved amino acid substitutions that may have increased the efficiency and rapidity of viral transmission in North American mosquito vectors.[13,14]

WNV circulates in a bird–mosquito–bird transmission cycle, predominately among *Culex* mosquitoes, which are most active around dawn and dusk. Many bird species are susceptible to infection, although morbidity and mortality varies greatly by species. Humans and horses are considered dead-end hosts since they do not develop sufficient viremia to efficiently infect mosquitoes. WNV has spread rapidly throughout the western hemisphere since 1999; however, large human disease outbreaks and avian mortality have only occurred in the USA and Canada.[15] Although the virus is now endemic throughout the USA, certain areas have a higher incidence of sporadic disease and outbreaks (Figure 175-5). While the vast majority of humans are infected via mosquito bite in late summer and early fall, infection can occur via blood transfusion, organ transplantation, breast milk, percutaneous exposure and transplacentally.[15]

Pathogenicity

The virus is injected into humans during the course of a mosquito bite. Local viral replication takes place in human skin and regional lymph nodes, followed by viremia and dissemination to multiple organs of the body. Postulated methods by which the virus gains entry into the central nervous system include direct viral crossing of the blood–brain barrier (BBB) due to cytokine-mediated vascular permeability, a Trojan horse mechanism in which infected tissue macrophages are trafficked across the BBB, direct infection and passage through the endothelium of the BBB and retrograde axonal transport of the virus to the central nervous system (CNS) via infection of olfactory or peripheral neurons.[16]

Many of the clinical features of WNV are attributed to the virus homing to certain areas of the CNS. For example, asymmetrical paralysis is associated with destruction of anterior horn cells and Parkinsonian symptoms with involvement of the basal ganglia. Histopathologic changes include microglial nodules composed of lymphocytes and histiocytes, perivascular inflammation consisting predominantly of

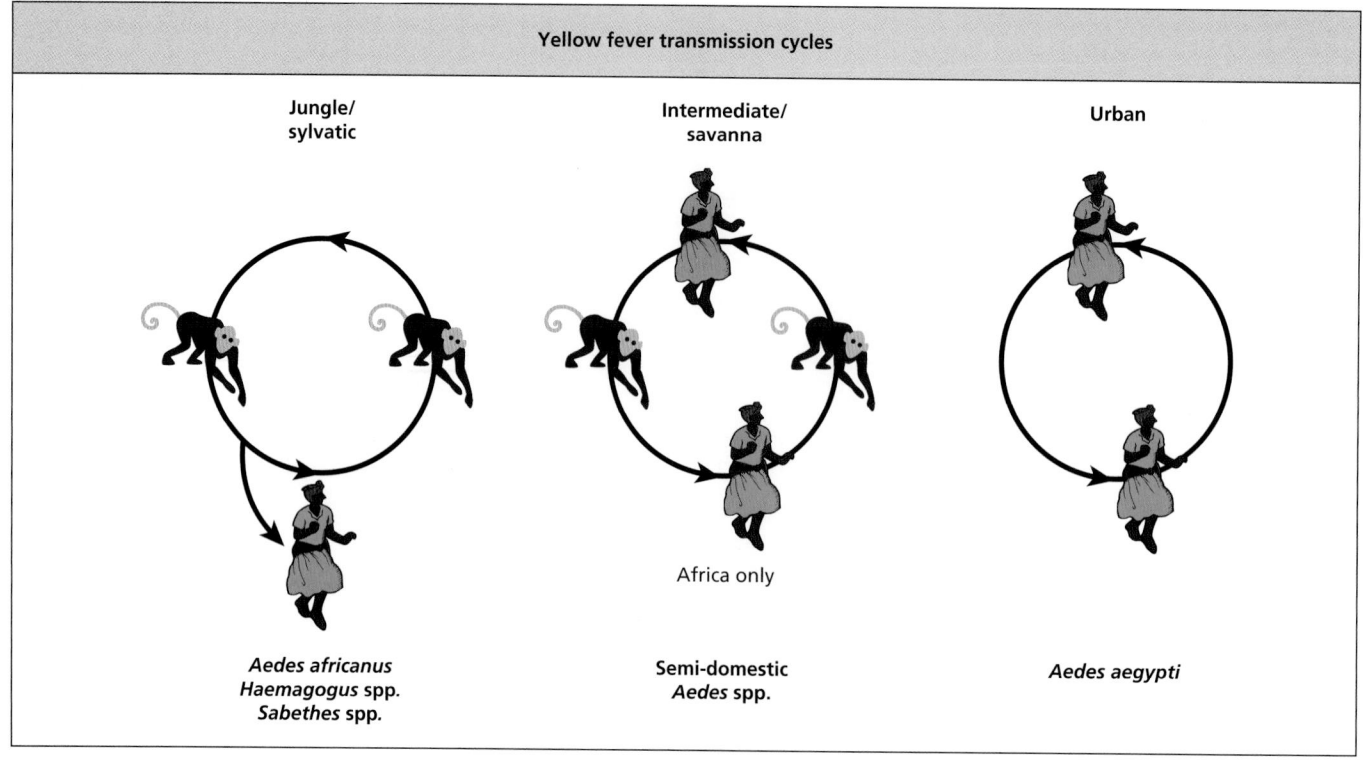

Figure 175-4 Yellow fever transmission cycles.

CD8 T-lymphocytes, and leptomeningeal mononuclear inflammatory infiltrates when meningitis is present.[17,18]

Prevention

WNV prevention relies in part on methods to reduce contact with infected mosquitoes, such as encouraging the use of repellents and reducing the numbers of WNV-infected mosquitoes. Human health risks associated with pesticide use to reduce adult mosquito populations appear negligible, largely because the timing of application and low volume of pesticide used result in minimal human exposure.[19,20] Routine screening of donated blood for West Nile viral nucleic acid has almost eliminated the risk of transfusion transmission. Several effective equine WNV vaccines are marketed.

Diagnostic Microbiology

Routine diagnosis is made by the detection of IgM antibody to WNV in serum or cerebrospinal fluid (CSF) using the IgM antibody capture ELISA (MAC-ELISA) or microsphere-based immunoassay (MIA). As IgM does not cross the blood–brain barrier, IgM antibody in the CSF strongly suggests CNS infection. At least 90% of patients with encephalitis or meningitis have demonstrable IgM antibody in CSF within 8 days of symptom onset. WNV-specific IgM antibody may not be detected initially in serum or plasma; one study showed that only 58% of patients with WNV fever had a positive MAC-ELISA result at clinical presentation.[21] Recent yellow fever or Japanese encephalitis vaccination or infection with a related flavivirus such as St Louis encephalitis or dengue may produce a positive WNV IgM antibody test result. The plaque-reduction neutralization test can help distinguish serologic cross-reactions among the flaviviruses. WNV IgM antibodies persist for at least 1 year after initial illness in about one-fifth of patients; thus, IgM antibodies may be unrelated to current illness.[22]

Nucleic acid amplification testing has utility in certain clinical settings as an adjunct to MAC-ELISA. Among patients presenting with West Nile fever, one study showed that cases were identified with

nucleic acid testing, serology, or a combined approach of these two methods in 45%, 58% and 94% of cases, respectively.[21] Nucleic acid amplification testing may prove useful in the immunocompromised when antibody development is delayed or absent.

Clinical Manifestations

Approximately 25% of humans infected with WNV become ill, with an incubation period of 2–14 days. Most of those who become ill develop West Nile fever, which is characterized by the sudden onset of symptoms such as headache, malaise, fever, myalgia, chills, vomiting, rash, eye pain, and later skin rash.[23] Fever may be low-grade or absent. While the initial illness may last for several days to a week, persistent fatigue, headaches and difficulty in concentrating lasting weeks or months are common.

Approximately one in 150–250 persons infected with WNV develop neuroinvasive disease.[24,25] Advancing age and the presence of immunocompromising conditions profoundly increases the risk of neuroinvasive disease. WNV meningitis is similar to that of other viral meningitides with abrupt onset of fever and headache with meningeal signs and photophobia. WNV encephalitis ranges in severity from a mild, self-limited confusional state to severe encephalopathy, coma and death. Extrapyramidal disorders are frequently observed. WNV paralysis is usually characterized by asymmetric weakness developing within 48 hours after symptom onset.[26] Respiratory failure may develop. Other causes of weakness associated with WNV infection such as Guillain–Barré syndrome may occur uncommonly.

Patients with uncomplicated West Nile fever or meningitis usually recover fully, although extreme fatigue may be prolonged. Patients with WNV encephalitis have a highly variable outcome that may not correlate with the severity of initial symptoms. Nevertheless, a high proportion is left with substantial long-term functional and cognitive impairments.[27] Among patients with acute flaccid paralysis, about one-third recover strength to near baseline, one-third have some improvement and one-third have little or no improvement.[28]

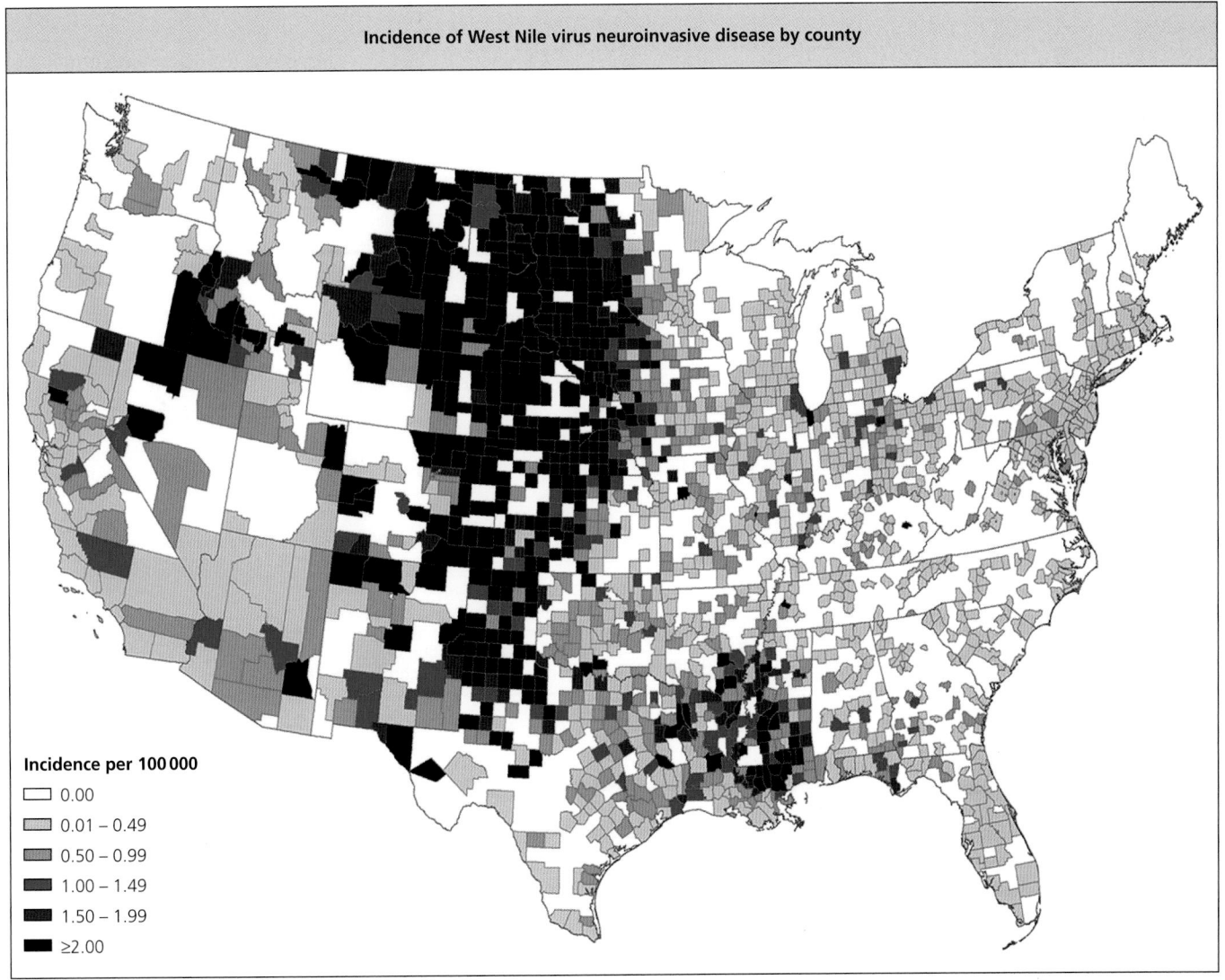

Figure 175-5 Incidence of West Nile virus neuroinvasive disease by county.

Management

Treatment of WNV infection is supportive. Several investigated therapeutic approaches include immune γ-globulin, WNV-specific neutralizing monoclonal antibodies, corticosteroids, ribavirin, interferon-α-2b and anti-sense oligomers.[27,29,30] No study has documented efficacy, in part due to difficulty in recruiting sufficient numbers of patients. Case reports or uncontrolled clinical series suggesting efficacy should be interpreted with extreme caution due to WNV's highly variable clinical course.

Arenaviridae

Nature

Members of the family Arenaviridae have been isolated from diverse species of rodents, which are their natural hosts, in a wide range of geographic locations. One arenavirus, Tacaribe, has been isolated from bats rather than rodents and a new member of the genus, California Academy of Science virus, was more recently identified in boid snakes with inclusion body disease.[31] Two arenavirus complexes are recognized – the complex of lymphocytic choriomeningitis virus and Lassa virus (LCMV-LASV), or Old World arenaviruses, and the Tacaribe

complex, or New World arenaviruses.[32] This broad antigenic classification is supported by more detailed phylogenetic comparisons. A wide range of arenaviruses have been described in their host species; several cause human infection, of which the most important human pathogens are listed in Table 175-2.

Arenavirus virions range from spherical to pleomorphic and have a mean diameter of 110–130 nm. Particles are characterized by a variable number of electron-dense ribosomes (diameter 20–25 nm) within the virus particles that are the source of the name of the genus as they appear sand-like in electron micrographs. They have a lipid membrane with glycoprotein spikes that project 8–10 nm from the surface.

The genome consists of two ssRNA molecules, L (large) and S (small). The L and S RNAs of arenaviruses have an ambisense coding arrangement; nucleocapsid (N) is encoded in the viral-complementary sequence corresponding to the 5′ half of segment S, whereas the viral glycoprotein precursor (GPC) is encoded in the viral-sense sequence corresponding to the 3′ half of S.[32]

The N protein, which is the most abundant polypeptide, is non-glycosylated and forms a ribonucleoprotein (RNP) complex with the genomic RNA. Two glycosylated proteins, GP-1 and GP-2, are derived by post-transitional cleavage from the GPC. The L segment codes for the L protein, which is an RNA polymerase, and the Z protein, a putative zinc binding protein. α-Dystroglycan has recently been identified

TABLE 175-2	Arenaviruses Known to Cause Human Disease		
Virus	**Host in Nature**	**Geographic Distribution**	**Main Features of Human Disease**
Lymphocytic choriomeningitis virus (LCMV)	*Mus domesticus, Mus musculus*	Europe, Americas, perhaps elsewhere	Isolated 1933; causes lymphocytic choriomeningitis, which usually presents as an aseptic meningitis with a mortality rate <1%
Lassa fever	*Mastomys* spp.	West Africa	Isolated 1969; causes Lassa fever, a severe systemic illness; severe cases suffer shock and hemorrhages; mortality rate between 2% and 16% among those hospitalized
Junin	*Calomys musculinus*	Argentina	Isolated 1958; causes Argentine hemorrhagic fever, which causes a similar illness to Lassa but hemorrhage and CNS disease more frequent; mortality up to 30%
Machupo	*Calomys callosus*	Beni region of Bolivia	Isolated 1963; causes Bolivian hemorrhagic fever; similar clinical picture to Argentine hemorrhagic fever; mortality rate 25%
Guanarito	*Zygodontomys brevicauda; Sigmodon alstoni*	Venezuela	Isolated 1989; similar to Argentine hemorrhagic fever; mortality rate 25%
Sabia	Unknown	Brazil	Isolated 1993; only three human cases described, one fatal; clinical picture probably similar to Argentine hemorrhagic fever
Lujo	Unknown	Zambia	Isolated 2008; only five human cases described, four fatal; similar clinical picture to Lassa fever

as a receptor for LCMV and Lassa fever virus.[33] This belongs to a highly conserved family of proteins found in epithelial, muscle and neurologic cells in humans.

Pathogenicity

In their natural rodent hosts, during the neonatal period arenavirus infections cause a chronic viremia that does not have major clinical sequelae for the infected rodent[32] while infections in adults is transient and self-limiting. In humans several arenavirus infections cause severe illness, including meningoencephalitis and hemorrhagic fever, with significant mortality. Microscopic changes found at autopsy reflect little direct tissue damage and do not account for the severity of illness. Modulation of the host innate immune response dampens the response to the virus and leads to cytokine and chemokine dysregulation in a manner that may account for much of the disease. Petechial hemorrhages of the skin occur, along with hemorrhages and focal necrosis of internal organs. Serous effusions and interstitial pneumonia have been described. Hemorrhages are more common with South American arenavirus infections. In contrast to modest pathologic lesions, physiologic changes are extensive. Shock characteristic of severe disease reflects an increase in vascular permeability. The mechanism involved is not fully understood, but may be an indirect effect of immune mediators on endothelial cells produced by infected macrophages and monocytes, rather than direct viral damage.

Epidemiology

The epidemiology of individual arenaviral disease in humans depends on the geographic distribution of infected rodents and their habits influencing their contact with humans (Figure 175-6).

Several distinct patterns are seen. In Lassa fever, which is a common human infection, the reservoir host is *Mastomys* spp., which is a peridomestic rodent found in sub-Saharan Africa. The rodents are persistently infected and contaminate the environment with the virus, which may generate infectious aerosols on drying. Other routes of transmission include direct contact with rodent excretions during the capture and killing of these animals for consumption. The host of Junin virus, the cause of Argentine hemorrhagic fever, is *Calomys musculinus*. The natural habitat of this rodent is the border areas of uncultivated/cultivated fields and transmission occurs at harvest time, presumably because of aerosol generation from infected rodents during mechanical harvesting.

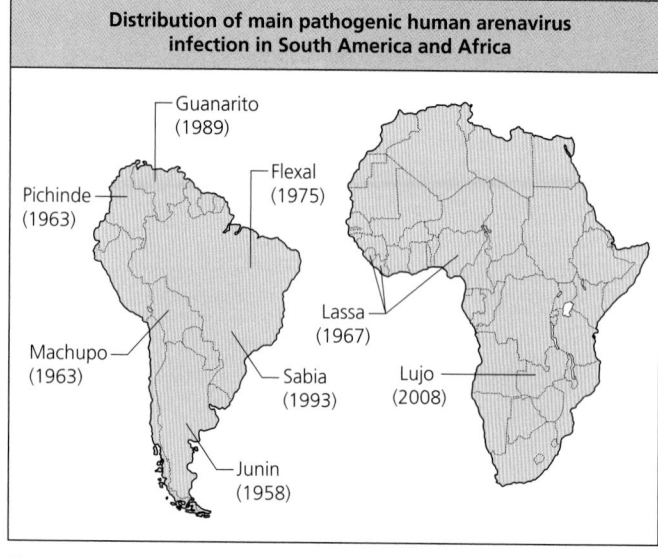

Distribution of main pathogenic human arenavirus infection in South America and Africa

Figure 175-6 Distribution of main pathogenic human arenavirus infection in South America and Africa, and year of first isolation of each virus.

Infection by LCMV is found worldwide, wherever its natural hosts *Mus musculus* are infected. The burden of disease is not well established, but LCMV infection is linked with up to 10% of CNS disease of suspected viral origin. Antibody studies show a prevalence of ~5% in urban populations in the USA,[34] 9% in urban populations in Germany and 2.2% in Argentina. The increased frequency of cases reported in the autumn may result from the reservoir host moving into homes for the winter. The potential for LCMV to cause human disease was recently highlighted by a group of cases linked to organ transplantation.[35, 36]

Lassa fever is a serious public health problem in West Africa, particularly in Sierra Leone, Guinea, Liberia and Nigeria. A case identified in Côte d'Ivoire suggests a wider distribution in West Africa.[37] Infections are seen throughout the year, but peak incidence is in the dry season. An estimated 400 000 human cases may occur annually, with an overall mortality of 2%.[38] More severe hospitalized cases have a mortality of 16%.[39]

Before the use of a live attenuated Junin virus vaccine, several hundred cases of Argentine hemorrhagic fever occurred annually and were associated with the harvest. Most cases occur in adult males.

Bolivian hemorrhagic fever was first identified in 1963–4, during an outbreak in San Joaquin involving 113 deaths.[40] However, the disease has since been uncommon, with only occasional cases reported in rural areas among those more likely to come into contact with the infected rodent host.

A new, previously unknown Old World arenavirus appeared in 2008. The virus, now known as Lujo (a contraction of Lusaka and Johannesburg), originated in Lusaka, Zambia in a resident who became ill and was air-evacuated to Johannesburg, Republic of South Africa. A subsequent chain of nosocomial transmissions eventually involved six healthcare workers, four of whom died.[41]

Prevention

Prevention strategies involve rodent control and vaccination. The local eradication of *Calomys callosus* was important in controlling Bolivian hemorrhagic fever outbreaks in small hamlets. The house mouse, *Mus domesticus*, can be effectively eliminated from homes, thus reducing exposure to LCMV. However, *Mastomys natalensis* is widespread and it has not proved practical to control rodent populations with living conditions found in West Africa. Both *C. callosus* and *C. musculinus* inhabit rural areas and control is not feasible.

A live, attenuated Junin virus vaccine (Candid–1®) has been developed and proven effective.[42] The vaccine is manufactured in Argentina and is used for occupationally at-risk workers.[43]

Lassa fever is the most important human arenavirus infection and vaccination seems to be the best hope for control. Several vaccine constructs have been developed and evaluated in animal models, and the most promising candidate vaccine is a vaccinia recombinant containing the Lassa virus glycoprotein gene. No human studies have been performed.

Diagnostic Microbiology

All arenavirus infections present similar diagnostic problems; the virus can be isolated early in the disease and this is followed by the later development of IgM and IgG antibody responses. Relatively little development of diagnostic assays for these agents has occurred since they are relatively rare and geographically localized.

Infection by LCMV is generally diagnosed by the detection of specific antibody usually by immunofluorescence, but ELISA tests for IgG and IgM have been described. For virus isolation, blood and CSF samples are the most useful. Mice and guinea pigs are the most sensitive culture system, but isolation in Vero cells is more practical.

Lassa fever and several of the South American hemorrhagic fevers cause severe infections and can be transmitted by aerosol. Consequently, they have been classified as BSL 4 viruses. Because ribavirin is an effective treatment for Lassa fever if started early in the disease course, laboratory confirmation of infection is important. Detection of Lassa-specific antibody can be achieved by immunofluorescence ELISA-based tests for LASV antigen and IgM and IgG antibodies.[44] RT-PCR is now the first line diagnostic test because it enables same-day diagnosis, and RNA extraction steps also inactivate the virus. This improves biosafety, and diagnosis in endemic areas. In one study all Lassa fever patients were diagnosed by RT-PCR within 3 days of admission.[45] Quantitative real-time PCR has now been applied to the diagnosis of Lassa fever and the issue of high variability of Lassa strains from different endemic areas overcome.[46] The ability to quantify and monitor viral load by PCR probably has prognostic value, as has been found with infectious virus quantification and amount of virus antigen.[44,47]

The South American arenaviruses can be cultured from acute blood samples in newborn mice and hamsters or Vero cells. The detection of virus-specific IgG and IgM by immunofluorescence was widely used, and more recently ELISA using baculovirus-expressed viral proteins to detect antibody and RT-PCR tests have been described.

Clinical Manifestations

Arenavirus infections are often mild or subclinical. Even in severe infections, early illness is characterized by nonspecific symptoms, such as fever and myalgia.

In LCMV infection headache, nausea or vomiting accompanies the febrile prodrome. In the second week of illness, CNS disease develops in a minority of cases and usually presents as aseptic meningitis. In severe cases encephalitis can develop. Full recovery is the most common outcome, but occasional deaths occur.

The incubation period of Lassa fever is about 10 days. Illness generally begins with a gradual onset of fever and malaise. As the disease progresses, abdominal pain, nausea and vomiting become more pronounced and an exudative pharyngitis and conjunctivitis are common signs. More pathognomonic signs and symptoms develop during the second week of illness, including facial edema, pleural edema, encephalopathy and shock. High viremic loads and LASV antigen loads have correlated with poor prognosis. In severe cases illness is progressive, with shock followed by death. In survivors, defervescence is followed by recovery in 2–3 weeks. Infection during pregnancy is associated with high mortality. Fetal loss is also common. Hemorrhagic complications are frequent in severe cases and generally present with epistaxis, bruising and conjunctival hemorrhage. Pericarditis has been described in the convalescent period. Unilateral or bilateral deafness is now recognized as a late complication. It is not related to the severity of disease and may be immune mediated.[48]

Argentine and Bolivian hemorrhagic fever present with a similar clinical picture. The progression of illness is more rapid than in Lassa fever, with severe prostration developing 3–4 days after onset. Unlike LASV infection, patients with the New World arenavirus infections have both low white cell and platelet counts. In more severe cases, mucous membrane hemorrhage and bruising at intravenous injection sites indicate a poor prognosis. In a few cases substantial neurologic involvement leads to convulsions. Recovery usually starts at the end of the second week of illness.

Management

Lassa fever has caused nosocomial infections in Africa and is a BSL 4 agent most commonly imported into non-endemic countries. Consequently, many countries have developed containment guidelines for the management of suspected Lassa fever cases to prevent secondary transmission.[49,50] Transmission is through direct contact with infected body fluids and little evidence suggests that airborne transmission is important in patient management. The guidelines include an initial patient risk assessment, which leads to different levels of investigation, containment and monitoring of close contacts, depending on risk (see also Chapter 132).

Ribavirin is effective *in vitro* against arenaviruses. Ribavirin dramatically reduces the mortality rate from severe Lassa fever provided it is given early in the illness.[51] Its use for prophylaxis of contacts with Lassa fever cases and for the treatment of other arenavirus infections has been proposed, but no reports have been published.

Treatment of Argentine hemorrhagic fever infections with convalescent human plasma is effective in reducing the mortality rate from 15–30% to less than 2% if given during the first 8 days of illness. Convalescent plasma could potentially play a role in Lassa fever treatment, but this has not been established in practice.

Hantaviruses

Nature

The genus *Hantavirus* in the family Bunyaviridae comprises a growing number of viruses, including those that cause hemorrhagic fever with renal syndrome (HFRS) and hantavirus pulmonary syndrome (HPS).[52,53] Many of the recently recognized viruses identified by molecular genetic analysis have not yet been isolated (Table 175-3).

TABLE 175-3	Characteristics of Some Known Hantaviruses Found in Europe, Asia, Russia and India				
Species	Human Illness	Pathology	Mortality Rate (%)	Reservoir	Geographic Virus Distribution
Hantaan (HTN)	Severe: HFRS, EHF, KHF	Renal	5–15	*Apodemus agrarius* (striped field mouse)	China, Russia, Korea
Dobrava/Belgrade (DOB)	Severe: HFRS	Renal	5–15	*Apodemus flavicollis* (yellow neck mouse)	Balkans
Seoul (SEO)	Moderate: HFRS	Renal	1	*Rattus norvegicus* (Norway rat)	Worldwide
Puumala (PUU)	Mild; NE	Renal	1	*Myodes glareolus* (bank vole)	Europe, Russia, Scandinavia
Khabarovsk (KHB)	?	?	?	*Microtus fortis* (reed mole)	Russia
Tula (TUL)	?	?	?	*Microtus arvalis* (European common vole)	Europe
Thailand (THAI)	?	?	?	*Bandicota indica* (bandicoot rat)	Thailand
Thottapalayam (TMP)	?	?	?	*Suncus murinus* (musk shrew)	India
Topografov (TOP)*	?	?	?	*Lemmus sibiricus* (Siberian lemming)	Siberia

EHF, epidemic hemorrhagic fever; HFRS, hemorrhagic fever with renal syndrome; KHF, Korean hemorrhagic fever; NE, nephropathia epidemica; ?, not yet documented.

*Virus not yet isolated/molecular analysis suggests they are probable hantavirus species.

Hantaviruses contain a tripartite, single-stranded, negative-sense RNA genome. The three segments are designated as small (S), medium (M) and large (L), and encode for the nucleocapsid (N) protein of 50–53 kDa, the two envelope proteins (G1 and G2) of 65 and 74 kDa, respectively, and an associated virus polymerase of 200 kDa.[54]

Epidemiology

The epidemiology of hantavirus disease in humans is dependent on the geographic distribution of persistently infected rodent hosts.[55] The hantaviruses linked with HFRS are associated with specific rodent hosts, each named for the region in which they were first isolated:

- *Apodemus agrarius* (the striped field mouse) for Hantaan virus;
- *Rattus norvegicus* (the Norway rat) and *Rattus rattus* (the black rat) both for Seoul virus; and
- *Apodemus flavicollis* (the yellow necked field mouse) for Dobrava virus.

The hantaviruses from Korea, Russia and China and the Dobrava virus (DOBV) from the Balkan countries of Europe (Bosnia and Herzegovina, Croatia, Yugoslavia, Albania, Slovenia, Greece, Bulgaria and Russia) are associated with the severe form of HFRS, with an estimated mortality of 5–15% (see Table 175-3).[56, 57] DOBV appears to be the most life-threatening hantavirus in Europe; a moderate form of HFRS is also caused by the Seoul virus, which (along with its hosts, *Rattus norvegicus* and *Rattus rattus*) is found worldwide. Seoul viruses and serologic evidence for infection with Seoul-like hantaviruses has been found in rodents in major cities within the USA with a few human cases recently described.[58,59]

A mild form of HFRS, caused by the Puumala virus (PUUV), is responsible for nephropathia epidemica (NE) in Scandinavia, the European regions of the former USSR and through much of Europe to France, Spain and Portugal.

The hantavirus associated with HPS, Sin Nombre virus (SNV), has been recognized throughout the USA since its discovery in 1993.[60] Subsequently, a substantial number of similar viruses also associated with HPS illness – Black Creek Canal (BCC), New York, Bayou (BAY) and Andes – have been discovered. This has extended the geographic range of these viruses from North America to Mexico and South America (Table 175-4). Two novel hantaviruses, with unknown pathogenic potential, were found in Africa[61-63] and a large number of hantaviruses have more recently been discovered among insectivorous small mammals (shrews and moles).[64] However, at present, little or no human disease has been linked to this grouping of viruses.

All rodent hosts are persistently infected with specific hantavirus strains that apparently cause no illness. In wild rodent populations, most infections occur through age-dependent horizontal routes, predominately in mature males. Horizontal transmission among cage mates was experimentally demonstrated via the aerosol route at median infectious doses of 1.0 plaque forming units (pfu) for each virus tested; however, their greater susceptibility by inoculation (median infectious doses 0.003–0.016 pfu) supports the concept of horizontal transmission by aggressive encounters (biting). Vertical transmission from dam to pup has proved negligible or absent, both in wild and experimental settings.

Hantavirus disease, irrespective of strain, is a seasonal disease associated with population dynamics of the rodent hosts and their interaction with humans. Rurally-acquired HFRS in Asia and Europe is linked to human rodent contact during the planting and harvesting of crops (late autumn and early winter). Similarly, in Scandinavia, PUUV causes most cases of NE during the same period. PUUV outbreaks in Scandinavia and the original HPS outbreak in America were associated with increases in the natural rodent population. Rodent species that naturally invade human habitation or are present in habitats that put them into contact with humans are most likely to be associated with human hantavirus disease. These cases point to higher risk among people such as forestry workers and shepherds. In China HFRS induced by Seoul virus appears to be most common in the spring.

The aerosol route of infection is regarded as the most common means of transmission to humans. Rodent bites cannot be excluded as a way of maintaining the disease among rodents or occasionally resulting in human infection. Epidemiologic investigations link virus exposure to farming activities, sleeping on the ground and military exercises. Indoor exposure has been linked to rodent infestation of homes and activities, such as cleaning, or entering heavily infested vacant buildings where aerosols may be created from the excreted and secreted virus from the resident rodents. Many hantavirus infections are identified among people who live in poor housing conditions, prone to rodent infestation, or in those who pursue recreational activities such as camping. Human-to-human transmission has been rare with Old World hantaviruses and consequently hantaviruses have not posed a risk to hospital workers. However, recent outbreaks of HPS caused by Andes virus in South America suggest that minimal exposure to body

TABLE 175-4	Some Known Hantaviruses Found In North and South America					
Species	**Human Illness**	**Pathology**	**Mortality Rate (%)**	**Reservoir**	**Geographic Virus Distribution**
Sin Nombre virus (SNV)	Severe: HPS	Pulmonary	50	*Peromyscus maniculatus* (deer mouse)	USA, Canada, Mexico
New York (NY)	HPS	Pulmonary	Not recorded	*Peromyscus leucopus* (white-footed mouse)	USA
Black Creek Canal (BCC)	HPS	Pulmonary	Not recorded	*Sigmodon hispidus* (cotton rat)	USA
El Moro Canyon (ELMC)	?	?	?	*Reithrodontomys megalotis* (Western harvest mouse)	USA, Mexico
Bayou (BAY)*	HPS	Pulmonary/renal	?	*Oryzomys palustris* (rice rat)	USA
Andes (AND)*	HPS	Pulmonary	50	*Oligoryzomys longicaudatus* (long tailed pygmy rice rat)	Argentina
Unnamed*	HPS	Pulmonary	?	*Calomys laucha* (vesper mouse)	Paraguay
Rio Segundo (RIOS)*	?	?	?	*Reithrodontomys mexicanus* (Mexican harvest mouse)	Costa Rica
Rio Mamoré (RIOM)*	?	?	?	*Oligoryzomys microtis* (small-eared pygmy rice rat)	Bolivia
Isla Vista (ISLA)*	?	?	?	*Microtus californicus* (California vole)	USA
Bloodland Lake (BLL)*	?	?	?	*Microtus ochrogaster* (prairie vole)	USA

HPS, hantavirus pulmonary syndrome.
?, not yet documented.
*Virus not yet isolated/molecular analysis suggests they are unique hantavirus strains.

fluids of infected patients resulted in apparent person-to-person spread.

The annual incidence of HFRS involving hospitalization throughout the world is estimated to be between 150 000 and 200 000 cases. More than half these cases predominate in the endemic center of epidemic hemorrhagic fever in the Chinese provinces of Hubei, Heilongjiang, Jiangxi, Jilin and Shanxi. Annual incidence rates range from 0.05 to 3.0/1000. Russia and Korea also report hundreds to thousands of cases of HFRS each year. Most of the remaining cases (a few hundred) are reported from Japan, Finland, Sweden, Belgium, The Netherlands, Greece, Hungary, France and the Balkan countries formerly constituting Yugoslavia. Mortality rates range from less than 0.1% for HFRS caused by PUUV to approximately 5–10% for HFRS caused by Hantaan virus.

Several hundred cases of HPS have been reported throughout North and South America (see Table 175-4).[65] Most of identified cases in the USA and Canada are caused by SNV, while cases of HPS in the southern USA and South America are caused by viruses that include BAY, BCC and Andes viruses.[66]

Several laboratory-associated outbreaks of HFRS have occurred, all of which were traced to persistently infected rodents obtained from breeders, wild-caught naturally infected rodents or experimentally infected rodents. No illness has been associated with laboratory workers using cell-culture adapted viruses, although asymptomatic infections have been documented serologically.

Pathogenicity

The process by which hantaviruses cause multisystem organ dysfunction syndrome is unclear. Thrombocytopenia, defects in platelet function, transient disseminated intravascular coagulation (DIC) and increased vascular fragility are all thought to play a key role in the early stages of the disease. Hantavirus disease is mainly microvascular in nature and endothelium is the predominant cell type involved. The presence of hantavirus antigen has been demonstrated by immunochemistry in vascular endothelial cells of fatal HFRS infections, experimentally-infected rodents and endothelium of lung capillaries in the highly lethal form of HPS.[67] Endothelial damage or dysfunction leads to capillary engorgement, leakage of erythrocytes and increased permeability.

Studies have implicated the disease process as immunologically based, with lymphocytes playing a key role, especially T cells. The CD4:CD8 ratio is greatly decreased, although abundant CD4+ and CD8+ lymphocytes have been reported in the lung interstitium of HPS patients.[67] Lymphocyte induction of migrating macrophages and other inflammatory cells results in the production of cytokines, such as tumor necrosis factor (TNF), interleukin (IL)-1 and IL-2, and interferon-gamma (IFN-γ), which in turn increases vascular permeability.

Prevention

Prevention of hantavirus infection relies on reducing contact between humans and infected rodents. However, many rodent control programs in known highly endemic areas, such as China, have been ineffective. Guidelines in the USA to control HPS infections have been aimed at reducing rodent access to homes, recommendations for clean-up of buildings with heavy rodent infestations, and precautions for workers with occupational exposure to rodents and for campers and hikers in areas with infected rodents.

Vaccines for hantaviruses have been licensed and used in China and Korea, where the disease burden is high and the need for vaccines is clear. Vaccine developmental efforts exist outside of these countries, but none have been licensed or used.[68]

Both wild-caught rodents introduced into laboratories and laboratory-bred colonies have caused several laboratory-based infections. Current recommendations directed at the manipulation of hantaviruses call for handling of clinical materials at biosafety containment level 2 and for work with the viruses associated with HPS BSL3. Work with infected laboratory rodents that may lead to the generation of infectious aerosols in urine or feces should be undertaken in facilities that utilize primary containment of animals (such as individual ventilated caging systems with HEPA filtration), have suitable room ventilation and high-efficiency particulate air (HEPA) filtration, cage changing and animal manipulation within laminar flow biosafety cabinets and personal protective equipment that offers a high level of personal protection, such as powered air purifying respirators. Precautions should ensure suitable decontamination of animal bedding, cages and animal waste.

It is prudent to introduce hantavirus screening of laboratory-bred and wild-caught rodents and cell lines that originate from rodent tissue before use. Such animals and cells should be segregated from other animals, with care being taken to prevent possible aerosolized spread of infectious virus. As for other rodent-borne viruses, control and exclusion of wild rodents from the facility is of great importance.

Diagnostic Microbiology

Diagnosis of hantavirus infection relies upon the recognition of characteristic clinical features, a history consistent with the epidemiology of the disease and serologic or RT-PCR confirmation. RT-PCR is best done on whole blood or buffy coat cells rather than upon serum.

The method of choice to diagnose acute hantavirus infection is an IgM antibody assay of high sensitivity and specificity.[69] Currently, two alternatives are available:

- M antibody capture IgM enzyme immunoassay (EIA) based on the use of cell-culture grown hantavirus antigen; and
- M antibody capture IgM EIA based on baculovirus or *Escherichia coli* expressed full-length nucleocapsid protein.[70]

As IgG antibodies persist for life in both humans and rodents, the presence of IgG antibody in acute diagnostic samples may not reflect a recent infection. Rising IgG antibody titers are of diagnostic value, but require the collection of a convalescent sample to be of any diagnostic value. The IgG ELISA or immunofluorescent antibody (IFA) test is well suited for epidemiologic studies; however, both assays offer little virus specificity and determination of the specific infecting virus is best achieved by neutralization tests, or more commonly by sequencing of an informative part of the virus genome using RT-PCR to amplify from clinical materials. Infected rodents bear viral RNA in their tissues (and in whole blood) long after initial infection and this can be exploited in conjunction with serology to determine the hantavirus present in rodent populations.

Clinical Manifestations

The HFRS complex comprises three distinct clinical diseases, each caused by a specific hantavirus.[55,56] The spectrum of disease ranges from inapparent infection to fulminant hemorrhagic fever with renal failure (sometimes having a fatal outcome). Fatality rates range from less than 1% for hemorrhagic fever with renal syndrome (HRFS) caused by PUUV to approximately 5–10% for HFRS caused by Hantaan virus (Table 175-5).

The clinical course of pathogenic hantavirus infection comprises an acute febrile illness characterized by variable degrees of hemorrhagic and renal dysfunction. More severe disease involves five overlapping stages – febrile, hypotensive, oliguric, diuretic and convalescent.

The onset of the disease is abrupt and characterized by high fever of 102.2–104°F (39–40°C), chills, intensive headache, malaise, myalgia, dizziness and anorexia. A petechial rash may also appear on the face, neck and trunk. The main laboratory findings include normal-to-elevated white blood count (WBC), decreasing platelets, rising hematocrit and rising proteinuria.

As the febrile phase ends, hypotension can abruptly develop and last for a few hours or days. Prominent features are tachycardia, falling arterial pressure and narrowing pulse pressure, and in severe cases, classic shock. Laboratory findings include leukocytosis with a left shift, thrombocytopenia and prolonged bleeding times. Urinalysis shows proteinuria, mild hematuria and hyposthenuria. About one-third of fatalities occur during this phase.

The oliguric phase lasts 3–7 days, during which blood pressure returns to normal or is slightly raised because of hypervolemia. Laboratory findings include normal WBC and platelet counts, initially normal and then depressed hematocrit, continual marked hematuria and elevated blood urea nitrogen and creatinine. Hyponatremia, hyperkalemia and hypocalcemia result from renal failure. Pulmonary edema may occur if fluid management is not handled with care. Almost half of the deaths occur during this phase, often from pulmonary edema or infection, electrolyte imbalance, late shock or hemorrhage into the brain.

Clinical recovery is signaled by a diuretic phase, with improved renal function and normal clotting. Diuresis over a few hours or days is evident, with an output of 3–6 liters. Fluid management must be maintained to prevent negative fluid balance that may lead to shock. The final (convalescent) phase can last weeks to months before recovery is complete.

Seoul virus infections (generally leading to mild HFRS) are less severe than those caused by Hantaan virus. Typically the phases are shorter and difficult to recognize or even absent. The disease is characterized by fever, anorexia, chills and nausea and vomiting. Palatal injection is common, although other hemorrhagic signs (epistaxis, melena, hematemesis) are observed in fewer than 30% of patients. Laboratory findings include lymphocytosis, thrombocytopenia, microscopic hematuria and proteinuria, and elevation of serum transaminase. Renal involvement is less severe and fatalities are uncommon.

PUUV infection, the cause of NE, is characterized by a sudden onset of fever accompanied by headache. Characteristically, by the fourth day of illness nausea, vomiting, petechiae in the throat and soft palate, and facial flush and petechial rash have occurred. A mild thrombocytopenia can be observed. Hypotension occurs, but evidence of shock is rare. Onset of oliguria or recognition of renal failure around the sixth day of disease is the main cause of hospital admission. Serum creatinine levels rise and dialysis may be required in 10% of cases. As with other hantavirus infections, the onset of polyuria indicates the recovery process.

First recognized as a severe, often fatal respiratory illness in adults in the Southwestern USA, HPS was characterized as a severe, systemic illness with a nonspecific onset, fever, myalgia, cough or dyspnea, gastrointestinal symptoms and headache that typically lasted 3–5 days.[71,72] Rapid and abrupt onset of noncardiogenic edema and hypotension (systolic blood pressure ≤80 mmHg) then follow, resulting in shock and death in over half of the early recognized cases (see Table 175-5). Laboratory findings indicate leukocytosis, an increase in

TABLE 175-5	**Main Characteristics of the Two Severe Forms of Hantavirus Disease**	
Characteristics	Hemorrhagic Fever With Renal Syndrome	Hantavirus Pulmonary Syndrome
Primary target organ	Kidney	Lung
Acute phase	Febrile	Febrile 'prodrome'
Later phases	Shock, hemorrhage	Shock, pulmonary edema
Disease progression	Hypotensive, oliguric, diuresis, convalescence	Diuresis, convalescence
Other clinical and laboratory features	Thrombocytopenia, leukocytosis, proteinuria, hematuria, creatinine >100 mmol/L, hemoconcentration, raised transaminases	Thrombocytopenia, leukocytosis, hemoconcentration, shortness of breath, abnormal respiratory rate, lung infiltrates
Mortality rate (%)	1–15	≥50

polymorphonuclear leukocytes, left shift, increased hematocrit, thrombocytopenia, prolonged prothrombin and partial thromboplastin time, elevated serum lactate dehydrogenase, decreased serum protein concentrations and proteinuria. Increases in hematocrit and thromboplastin time are considered to be predictors of death. Radiographic examinations show bilateral pulmonary infiltrates and evidence of pleural effusions in the majority of hospitalized patients. Histopathologic features seen in lung tissue reveal mild-to-moderate interstitial pneumonitis with variable degrees of congestion, edema and mononuclear infiltrates. Immunohistochemistry has identified virus antigen extensively within endothelial cells of the pulmonary microvasculature, spleen and lymph nodes.

Current understanding of the disease indicates little evidence of renal damage as a feature of the New World hantavirus infection. The extensive pulmonary endothelial involvement and severe pulmonary edema hinder clinical management.

Management

Effective management of HFRS and HPS requires early diagnosis, knowledge of disease course and prompt hospitalization. Aggressive clinical management is essential to improve survival. Care should be phase specific, with special attention given to fluid management. Ribavirin may be efficacious in the treatment of HFRS patients, but its treatment of HPS, probably because of the rapid progression of HPS relative to HFRS, has not been proven.

Filoviridae

Nature

The family Filoviridae consists of two distinctive genera, *Marburgvirus* and *Ebolavirus*, which cause severe and often fatal hemorrhagic disease in humans and monkeys (see Chapter 132). The viruses have a distinctive filamentous morphology under the electron microscope with a genome that consists of a nonsegmented, negative-stranded RNA approximately 19 kb in length. Several features of their molecular organization and structure have linked these viruses to members of the Paramyxoviridae and Rhabdoviridae under the taxonomic order Mononegavirales.[73] The virions are composed of a central core formed by an RNP complex, which is surrounded by a lipid envelope derived from the host cell plasma membrane. The RNP is composed of a genomic RNA molecule bound by the NP, virion structural protein 30 (VP30), VP35 and the L protein (RNA transcriptase polymerase). The three remaining structural proteins are membrane associated – GP, VP24 and VP40 are located on the inner side of the membrane.

Marburg and Ebola were first detected in 1967[74] and 1976,[75,76] respectively. The original Ebola outbreaks in Zaire and DRC have been followed in recent years by the discovery of three additional viruses, which have been afforded species status bringing the total number to five: *Zaire ebolavirus*, *Sudan ebolavirus*, *Reston ebolavirus*, *Taï Forest ebolavirus* (formerly *Côte d'Ivoire ebolavirus*) and *Bundibugyo ebolavirus*. Among the newly isolated Ebola viruses are differences in molecular structure, pathogenicity and virulence in humans.[77] Importation of Reston virus-infected monkeys into the USA (1989–1990, 1996) and Italy (1992) attracted extensive worldwide media coverage and raised public concerns about the potential public health threat of these pathogens through international travel and commerce.[78, 79] *Reston ebolavirus* has more recently been recognized in several commercial swine herds in the Philippines with some infection in humans, again without recognition of overt disease.[80] A virus related to Ebola and Marburg viruses has recently been described in sick and dead insectivorous bats in Spain, but no human disease has yet been associated with the virus.[81]

The natural history and reservoirs of the Ebola viruses remains to be established, but the potential role of bats has been highlighted and the role of the cave-dwelling fruit bat, *Rousettus aegyptiacus*, as a reservoir of Marburg virus has been well established.[82, 83]

Pathogenesis

The precise mechanisms by which filoviruses cause the most severe forms of VHF remain somewhat obscure. The viruses suppress the host's early innate immune response and stimulate untoward levels of certain cytokines and chemokines resulting in 'cytokine storms' that have severe clinical consequences. This results in marked hepatic involvement, DIC and shock, and multiorgan failure, producing extremely high fatality (ranging from 30–90% depending on the virus). In the early stages of infection, laboratory findings, such as high aspartate transaminase/alanine transaminase (AST/ALT) ratios and marked lymphopenia followed by a marked neutropenia with left shift, suggest other extrahepatic targets are also affected by the virus and or the host's response. As with other VHF infections (HFRS, Lassa, dengue) fluid imbalance and platelet abnormalities indicate endothelial cell and platelet damage or dysfunction. Human monocytes and/or macrophages, fibroblasts and endothelial cells support virus replication. Infected monocyte and/or macrophages have been shown in models *in vitro* to secrete the cytokines which have the ability to increase vascular endothelial cell damage.[84] The data currently available support mediator-induced vascular damage that leads to increased permeability and shock observed in severe cases.[85]

Epidemiology

In 1967, a fulminating hemorrhagic fever, Marburg disease, occurred in Marburg and Frankfurt, Germany, and Belgrade, Yugoslavia among laboratory workers handling blood and tissue from a shipment of African green monkeys (*Cercopithecus aethiops*, now known as *Chlorocebus pygerythrus*) soon after being imported from Uganda via London. Among the 31 human cases, 25 of which were primary infections, there were seven (23%) deaths.[74] None of the secondary cases died. Since then, sporadic cases and outbreaks have been reported from South Africa and Kenya, Democratic Republic of Congo, Angola and Uganda (Figure 175-7). An outbreak associated with a former commercial mine in Durba, Democratic Republic of Congo, was actually a series

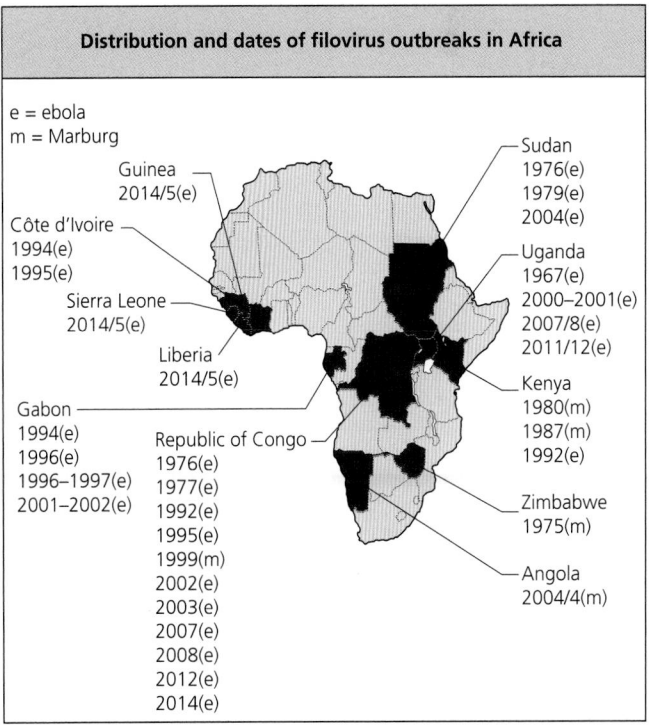

Figure 175-7 Distribution and dates of filovirus outbreaks in Africa.

of mini-outbreaks in which a miner was infected and transmitted the virus to those who cared for the primary case in each instance. This circumstance strongly implicated the mine and its associated fauna as the source of the virus. Subsequent investigation provided the strongest evidence for bats, particularly *Rousettus aegyptiacus*, as the principal reservoir of Marburg virus.[86-88] The known geographic distribution (and case fatality) widened with a major outbreak caused by Marburg virus in Uige Province, Angola during 2004–5 where 252 cases were identified with 227 deaths (case fatality rate 90%).

In 1976, the first known cases of Ebola hemorrhagic fever were identified in southern Sudan and in a simultaneous outbreak in northern Democratic Republic of Congo (Zaire at the time), with fatality rates of about 60% and 90%, respectively. Subsequently, multiple outbreaks have been noted in the Republic of Congo, Sudan, Ivory Coast, Gabon, and Uganda (see Figure 175-6). These outbreaks occasionally involved hundreds of persons with extremely high mortality rates.[76] In 2008, a newly discovered Ebola virus was found responsible for an outbreak in Bundibugyo District, Uganda.[83] A large outbreak in Guinea, Sierra Leone, and Liberia beginning in 2014 has dwarfed all previous outbreaks.[89,90] This outbreak, involving more than 20 000 cases and 8200 deaths as of January 2015, emphasizes the potential for significant public health events if an outbreak becomes urban and control efforts are not exercised with vigor.[91,92] In addition, more than 800 healthcare workers have become infected, emphasizing the hazards of exposure to infected bodily fluids.

Ebola virus has also appeared outside Africa among shipments of imported cynomolgus monkeys in Reston, Philadelphia and Texas, USA, in 1989, 1990 and 1996, respectively, and Sienna, Italy, in 1992.[93] The monkeys involved in each epizootic event were imported from the Philippines and traced to the same handling facility, where the presence of the virus was also documented. The epizootics indicate that monkeys acutely infected with filoviruses present a major veterinary emergency, which threatens a valuable biomedical resource. Current interest in this strain of Ebola virus has increased with the description of Ebola-Reston in samples originating from domestic pigs originating in the Philippines. Several healthcare workers infected during the care of patients in West Africa have received care in the USA and Europe. A Spanish nurse was infected during the care of a missionary who had become infected in West Africa and two nurses were infected in the USA during the care of a recent traveler from Liberia.[94]

Prevention

The imposition of ecologic controls to prevent outbreaks is impossible until the natural history of the viruses has been discovered. It is important that healthcare workers in areas where hemorrhagic fever exists are aware of the high risk of nosocomial spread if patients are not recognized early and placed in complete isolation.[95] In non-endemic areas an awareness of the changing epidemiology associated with viral re-emergence or emergence should always be considered, bearing in mind the threat and consequences of importation. High-risk patients are those who during the 3 weeks before illness had:

- traveled into areas where VHF occurred recently;
- been in contact with body fluids from a person with VHF; or
- worked in a laboratory environment handling the virus. (See also Chapter 132.)

Practical advice on triaging potential imported cases can be found on government websites, for example:

https://www.gov.uk/government/publications/viral-haemorrhagic-fever-algorithm-and-guidance-on-management-of-patients.

Importantly, filovirus illness is a rare event if patients do not meet any of these criteria.

As nonhuman primates are responsible for the introduction of Marburg into Europe, and of Ebola into the USA and Italy, the management of transportation, quarantine facilities and animal husbandry must ensure that personnel understand the hazards of handling nonhuman primates, and thus reduce the risks of future human outbreaks.

Diagnostic Microbiology

The clinical diagnosis of Ebola or Marburg should be considered in patients who show acute, febrile illness and have traveled in known epidemic or suspected endemic areas of rural sub-Saharan Africa and Asia, particularly when hemorrhagic signs are present. As the differential diagnosis in the early acute phase of illness is difficult, other causes (malaria, typhoid) should not be excluded and treatment delayed. Laboratory diagnosis carried out on patient specimens is undertaken by more than one procedure to guard against false-positives.

Care should be taken when drawing or handling blood specimens at the acute stage of illness as blood contains infectious virus with onset of fever; increasing amounts of infectious virus are present as the disease progresses. High virus loads indicate a poor prognosis. Although the virus is relatively stable, it is also quite susceptible to disinfection with commonly used medical disinfectants.

Although their morphologic appearance is similar by electron microscopy, Marburg and Ebola are immunologically distinct. The basic diagnostic tool for filovirus infection for the diagnosis of human filovirus disease is the detection of the virus RNA or virus antigen by RT-PCR or antigen detection ELISA. Detection of antibody is not of great value in acute diagnosis as many patients may die without developing detectable antibody levels. Indirect fluorescent antibody testing for antibody has largely been replaced by IgG and IgM ELISA tests, which have demonstrated improved specificity over the immunofluorescence assay. The presence of specific IgM antibodies or rising IgG titers is evidence of past infection and is useful in epidemic settings to identify surviving patients who were not sampled during the acute illness.

Filoviruses can be readily isolated from fresh or stored (−70°C) specimens of blood or serum collected during the acute phase of illness. Vero cells (clone E6) and MA104 have proved the most sensitive for the isolation and propagation of Marburg and Ebola viruses. As primary isolation using tissue culture may produce somewhat variable cytopathic effect, evidence of infection is confirmed by immunofluorescence staining using specific monoclonal or polyclonal reference antibodies or the use of proven RT-PCR assays with known reactivity with all filovirus strains. The isolation or propagation of filoviruses should not be attempted outside a biosafety containment level 4 laboratory.

More recently in outbreak settings, early detection of filovirus infections was considerably improved by the development of an antigen-capture ELISA and amplification of filovirus RNA by RT-PCR. However, several approaches, including virus isolation in appropriate labs, are considered best practice, particularly for early cases in outbreaks with suspected filovirus etiology. Use of a number of the above assays has proven useful in outbreak settings where the tests have been deployed by experienced teams to local facilities to support on-site diagnostic testing. Immunohistochemistry performed on tissue from expired patients has also proven useful for identification of Ebola and Marburg viruses in fatal cases; a technique of utilizing skin biopsies was shown to be of utility in the diagnosis of Ebola in patients who had died of the disease. Skin biopsies can be obtained with minimal risk and then fixed in formalin which can be safely transported to reference facilities for confirmation without the need for low temperature preservation.

Clinical Manifestations

The incubation period for Ebola ranges from 4 to 10 days and for Marburg from 3 to 9 days.[74] The shorter incubation periods have been associated with exposure to contaminated needles. Although aerosol infection can be demonstrated in the laboratory, epidemiological studies do not suggest that aerosols generated by patients play a large role in creating infections in outbreak settings. Filoviruses enter the host through close and unmanaged contact with contaminated body fluids; thus, extra care must be taken with contaminated body fluid, tissue, hospital material and waste.

Both Marburg and Ebola virus infections follow a similar pattern of illness. Initial symptoms following exposure include fever, severe frontal headache, malaise and myalgia. The initial diagnosis of a filovirus infection is very difficult as these symptoms are similar to those of many viral illnesses that originate locally and in tropical areas. Disease progression is characterized by pharyngitis, nausea, epigastric pain, and prostration.[96] A characteristic maculopapular rash occurs 7–10 days (range 1–21 days) after onset of the clinical disease. Overt bleeding is not a consistent finding, but it may occur in approximately 50% of patients and includes hemorrhages seen from under the skin, from venipuncture sites and from other orifices of the body. If fatal, death from shock and multiorgan failure occurs 6–9 days after onset of the clinical disease. Convalescence is slow, taking many weeks, and is marked by weight loss, prostration and amnesia of the acute phase of illness.

Clinical laboratory findings in the early acute phase include lymphopenia followed by neutrophilia, marked thrombocytopenia and abnormal platelet aggregation. Serum AST and ALT are elevated and characterized by an AST/ALT ratio of between 10 and 3:1.

Management

No specific treatment is available. Treatment is limited to the provision of intensive nursing and effective control of blood volume and electrolyte balance. Shock, renal failure, depletion of blood clotting factors, bleeding and oxygen depletion must be managed. Human interferon, human convalescent plasma, antivirals and monoclonal antibodies have been used to treat patients, but their efficacy is not proved.[97] Laboratory studies have confirmed that ribavirin has no therapeutic value.

Patient management is further complicated by the need to isolate the patient and protect medical and nursing staff.[98,99] In outbreak settings strict barrier nursing techniques have been key to stopping outbreaks. The latter can be supplemented using HEPA filter respirators for protection against aerosols if considered feasible. Particular emphasis should be placed on ensuring that high-risk procedures (such as handling blood, secretions, catheters and introducing intravenous lines) are undertaken under barrier nursing conditions. It is recommended that patients who die from the disease should be buried or cremated promptly and that measures to stop traditional contact with the body be directly supervised.

Nipah and Hendra Viruses

Nature

Both Hendra virus (HeV; briefly known as equine morbillivirus) and Nipah virus (NiV) have been recognized relatively recently. They are viruses belonging to a new genus, *Henipavirus*, within the family Paramyxoviridae. They are zoonotic in nature with fruit bat reservoirs. The distribution of the viruses is widening with the recognition of related viruses in bats belonging to the family Pteropodidae extending from Australia through South East Asia, South Asia and into Africa. Hendra and Nipah viruses seem to be limited to fruit bats (also known as flying foxes) belonging to the genus *Pteropus*.

Both NiV and HeV share a nonsegmented, negative-stranded RNA genome and similar genome organization, replication strategy and domain structure in the polymerase proteins to members of the Filoviridae, Paramyxoviridae, Rhabdoviridae and Bornaviridae. While being related to these families, they are closely related to the Paramyxoviridae and more specifically the morbilliviruses. Within the subfamily Paramyxovirinae, the extent of nucleotide homology in the N gene between different viruses in the same genus ranges from 56% to 78%, whereas the extent of nucleotide similarity between viruses from different genera is 39–78%. The N genes of HeV and NiV have 78% nucleotide homology, but the two viruses have no more than 49% similarity with any other members of the Paramyxovirinae.[100]

Phylogenetic analysis of the N gene sequences show that HeV and NiV form a distinct cluster within the subfamily Paramyxoviridae.

The genome organization of NiV and HeV is the same as for the rest of the Paramyxoviridae. There are a total of six transcription units encoding six structural proteins. These are the nucleocapsid protein (N), phosphoprotein (P), matrix protein (M), fusion protein (F), glycoprotein (G) or attachment protein, and large protein (L) or RNA polymerase. They are found on the genome in the order 39-N-P-M-F-G-L-59. Evidence suggests that NiV and HeV form a distinct group of viruses within the subfamily Paramyxovirinae and they have been afforded genus status as *Henipavirus*.[101]

Epidemiology

Two outbreaks of a new zoonotic disease affecting horses and animals in Australia occurred within 1 month of each other in Brisbane (southeast Queensland) and Mackay (central Queensland) in 1994. The Brisbane case was the first to attract attention when horses and two human cases occurred in a racing stable in the Brisbane suburb of Hendra. The Mackay incident was not associated with the virus until the single human case associated with the incident became ill and a post-mortem was conducted on a horse that had died. A third event involving a single fatal equine case occurred near Cairns (North Queensland) in 1999. To date, two humans and 16 horses with this disease have died from acute respiratory failure.[102-104]

Another member of the Paramyxoviridae (NiV) was responsible for an outbreak of severe febrile encephalitis in humans in Malaysia in 1998–9. The outbreak was associated with respiratory illness in pigs and was initially considered to be Japanese encephalitis. Of a total of 256 cases, 105 were fatal. In March 1999, a cluster of 11 cases (one fatality) was described in Singapore in abattoir workers who handled pigs imported from the outbreak regions in Malaysia.[105] Control measures, which involved finding and culling infected swine herds, resulted in the culling of over one million pigs (almost half the national pig herd) and had major domestic and international trade implications.

Nipah virus has also been a public health problem in South Asia beginning with a hospital-based outbreak in which person-to-person transmission occurred in Siliguri, West Bengal, India.[106] Outbreaks of NiV have continued to occur in Bangladesh after they were first noted in 2001.[107] Limited person-to-person transmission has been noted in Bangladesh, but unlike the outbreak in Malaysia, much of the initial infection appears to come from the fruit bat reservoir through indirect contact and food-borne (palm sap) transmission.[108]

The geographic distribution of both HeV and NiV is currently undefined, although Australia and South East Asia are considered endemic based on the known incidents reported in the literature. Fruit bats of the genus *Pteropus* are considered to be the reservoir hosts of HeV and NiV and are found in north, east and southeast areas of Australia, Indonesia, Malaysia, Philippines, the Indian subcontinent and some of the Pacific Islands.[101] Pigs were the apparent source of infection among most human cases in the Malaysian outbreak of NiV.[109]

Clinical Manifestations

The emergence of NiV and HeV has raised clinical concerns in the management of individuals returning from Australia and South East Asia presenting with pyrexia and other nonspecific signs and symptoms. The incubation period for NiV and HeV is generally from 4 to 18 days. Onset of disease is usually influenza-like with high fever and myalgia. Sore throat, dizziness and drowsiness and disorientation have been described. The case fatality rate for clinical cases is about 50% and subclinical infections may be common.[110]

Experimental studies have confirmed the possibility of transmission through close contact with infected body fluids and that aerosol transmission does not seem to be significant, probably because the amount of virus found in oropharyngeal secretions and urine are low.[111] Human-to-human transmission has been reported within the Bangladesh community.[112] The risk of transmission of Hendra virus from horse to human, primarily veterinarians or veterinary assistants, has occurred repeatedly in Australia and has precipitated the use of a vaccine in horses, primarily as a public health measure.[113]

Diagnostic Microbiology

Virus isolation has been an important primary diagnostic tool in early outbreaks. Both NiV and HeV grow well in Vero cells. A cytopathic effect (CPE) usually develops within 3 days but two 5-day passages are recommended before virus isolation is considered to be unsuccessful. However, isolation should only be attempted in a containment level 4 laboratory.

Virus neutralization tests are considered to be the reference standard in the serologic identification of NiV and HeV infection. This procedure needs to be carried out at a containment level 4 laboratory. Sera are added into the media covering virus-inoculated Vero monolayers in a 96-well plate format. Positive results are demonstrated by the inhibition of CPE production by sera.[114]

To reduce the dependence on high containment facilities (CL4), both the indirect IgG and capture IgM ELISA NiV and HeV systems can use irradiated viral antigens purified from cell culture. The level of sample processing involved to make the antigen safe to use outside Advisory Committee on Dangerous Pathogens (ACDP) 4 containment reduces the specificity and sensitivity of the assay.

NiV-specific primers that amplify a 228 bp segment of the N gene region of the virus will form the basis of the RT-PCR detection system that has proven of diagnostic value when used in conjunction with specimens (sera, tissue from humans and animals) implicated in HeV and NiV outbreaks. In addition, another published primer pair that amplifies a 200 bp region of the matrix (M) protein will form a proven alternative primer set for the RT-PCR detection of HeV originally designed by Halpin *et al.*[115]

Management

As there are neither a vaccine nor antivirals for treatment and because the viruses are potentially able to transmit by the aerosol route,[111] work with both HeV and NiV requires the use of BSL 4 laboratories. Therefore, with the increasing movement of horses and travelers to endemic areas, both clinicians and veterinarians have increasingly expressed a need to consider these infections as part of the current differential diagnosis. Care in the management of patients should be exercised as NiV has been isolated in the respiratory secretions and urine of patients identified as having Nipah virus encephalitis in Malaysia[111] and risk of person-to-person transmission recognized in Bangladesh and India.

References available online at expertconsult.com.

KEY REFERENCES

Barrett A.D., Higgs S.: Yellow fever: a disease that has yet to be conquered. *Annu Rev Entomol* 2007; 52: 209-229.

Barrette R.W., Metwally S.A., Rowland J.M., et al.: Discovery of swine as a host for the *Reston ebolavirus*. *Science* 2009; 325:204-206.

Bausch D.G., Rollin P.E., Demby A.H., et al.: Diagnosis and clinical virology of Lassa fever as evaluated by enzyme-linked immunosorbent assay, indirect fluorescent-antibody test, and virus isolation. *J Clin Microbiol* 2000; 38:2670-2677.

Cao W., Henry M.D., Borrow P., et al.: Identification of alpha-dystroglycan as a receptor for lymphocytic choriomeningitis virus and lassa fever virus. *Science* 1998; 282:2079-2081.

Centers for Disease Control and World Health Organization: Infection control for viral haemorrhagic fevers in the African health care setting. 1998; 1-198.

Duchin J.S., Koster F., Peters C.J., et al.: Hantavirus pulmonary syndrome: a clinical description of 17 patients with a newly recognized disease. *N Eng J Med* 1994; 330:949-955.

Groen J., van der Groen G., Hoofd G., et al.: Comparison of immunofluorescence and enzyme-linked immunosorbent assays for the serology of Hantaan virus infections. *J Virol Methods* 1989; 23:195-203.

Mostashari F., Bunning M.L., Kitsutani P.T., et al.: Epidemic West Nile encephalitis, New York, 1999: results of a household-based seroepidemiological survey. *Lancet* 2001; 358:261-264.

Mackenzie R.B.: Epidemiology of Machupo virus infection. I. Pattern of human infection, San Joaquin, Bolivia, 1962-1964. *Am J Trop Med Hyg* 1965; 14:808-813.

Olschlager S., Lelke M., Emmerich P., et al.: Improved detection of Lassa virus by reverse transcription-PCR targeting the 5' region of S RNA. *J Clin Microbiol* 2010; 48:2009-2013.

Riquelme R., Riquelme M., Torres A., et al.: Hantavirus pulmonary syndrome, southern Chile. *Emerg Infect Dis* 2003; 9:1438-1443.

Salvato M.S.: *The arenaviridae.* New York: Plenum Press; 1993.

176

Staphylococci and Micrococci

DAVID J. HETEM | SUZAN H.M. ROOIJAKKERS | MIQUEL B. EKKELENKAMP

KEY CONCEPTS

- *Staphylococcus aureus* is a major cause of infections and can cause a wide range of usually purulent infections, ranging from skin and soft tissue infections to endocarditis.

- *Staph. aureus* pathogenicity is mediated by various virulence factors.

- *Staph. aureus* virulence factors include adhesins, immune evasion molecules and cytolytic toxins.

- *Staph. aureus* carriers have an increased risk in developing nosocomial *Staph. aureus* infection; decolonization of *Staph. aureus* can reduce these risks.

- Even though the rise of methicillin-resistant *Staph. aureus* has stalled, MRSA is still a major source of infections in healthcare settings and the community in certain areas.

- Evidence of resistance against vancomycin, linezolid and daptomycin potentially threaten current treatment regimens for MRSA.

- Coagulase-negative staphylococci are important causative agents of foreign body-related infections, catheter-associated bloodstream infections and drain-associated meningitis.

- Coagulase-negative staphylococci are often resistant to multiple classes of antibiotics and treatment should be guided based on their antibiotic susceptibility profile.

- *Micrococcus* species are common human colonizers, rarely causing infections.

Nature

Staphylococci are gram-positive spherical bacteria about 1 micrometer in diameter, which divide in three dimensions and, due to incomplete cell separation, form a 'bunch of grapes' cluster that defines the genus.[1] The genus *Staphylococcus* has been classified together with genera including *Bacillus*, *Gemella*, *Listeria* and *Planococcus*, in the order of Bacillales and the family of Staphylococcaceae. Approximately 50 species have been described thus far (www.bacterio.cict.fr) (Figure 176-1), which are able to colonize or infect multiple animal species. For instance: *Staph. hyicus* is the main causative agent of infectious dermatitis and arthritis in swine, *Staph. aureus* causes bovine mastitis, and has also been reported in pigs, pigeons, cats and dogs, and *Staph. intermedius* causes infections in dogs, foxes, mink, pigeons and horses.

The genus *Micrococcus* currently contains 16 species, including *M. luteus*, *M. lylae* and *M. cohnii*, and resides in the family Micrococcaceae of the order of the Actinomycetales.[2,3] *Micrococcus* spp. colonize humans and are frequently found as contaminants of blood cultures. Rarely they cause disease, and then mostly in immunocompromised patients. The genera of *Rothia* and *Kuceria* can also be found in the family of Micrococcaceae.

Staphylococci

Epidemiology of *Staphylococcus aureus*

Staphylococci, in particular *Staphylococcus aureus*, are ubiquitous and frequent causes of infection in humans, and have been so throughout history. As the cause of post-influenza necrotizing pneumonias, *Staph. aureus* was considered responsible for at least a quarter of the deaths during the Spanish influenza pandemic of 1917–1918, and it is estimated that half of the casualties in the trenches of the First World War were due to septic wound infections with *Staph. aureus*.

In healthy humans, carriage (or colonization) of *Staph. aureus* may occur on multiple sites of the skin and mucosal surfaces (including the intestine and vagina), the main reservoir being the anterior nares (vestibulum nasi/nostrils). In the general population 20% are persistently colonized, 30% intermittently colonized and the remaining 50% are non-susceptible to colonization, but colonization rates can differ extensively among healthy subjects.[4] Person-to-person spread is believed to occur mainly by direct hand/skin contact; nosocomial spread is primarily mediated by healthcare workers. Furthermore, up to 10% of healthy *Staph. aureus* carriers disperse the bacterium into the air. Under normal circumstances, when airborne dispersers are at rest, they are surrounded by 0.01–0.1 colony-forming units (cfu)/m³ but up to 0.3 cfu/m³ in selected cases. However, the bacterial density may increase 40-fold with movement (due to release of bacteria from the clothing) and with respiratory tract infections. Multiple outbreaks have been attributed to single airborne spreaders. Although (methicillin-resistant) *Staph. aureus* has been reported to persist on inanimate surfaces for up to 7 months, the role of environmental contamination or airborne transmission is controversial. Although acquisition occurs primarily on the skin, *Staph. aureus* can only persist in the long term if the nares or perineum become colonized. Generally, the established flora of the nose prevents the acquisition of new strains.

Patients with type 1 diabetes, patients undergoing hemodialysis, surgical patients, intravenous drug users and HIV-infected patients have an increased risk of *Staph. aureus* colonization. Heavy antibiotic pressure may lower (detectable) colonization rates.[4]

Methicillin-susceptible *Staph. aureus* (MSSA) strains have a high genetic diversity across Europe and the USA.[5,6] In contrast, methicillin-resistant *Staph. aureus* (MRSA) shows a high degree of geographic clustering. Based upon multilocus sequence typing (MLST) the population structure of hospital-acquired MRSA (HA-MRSA) is characterized by five major clonal complexes (CCs) with pandemic clones: CC5, CC8, CC22, CC30 and CC45. Within these five clonal complexes different SCC*mec* types are found, indicating that MRSA clones emerged by multiple independent introductions of the *mecA* gene.[7]

NOSOCOMIAL *STAPHYLOCOCCUS AUREUS* INFECTIONS

Staph. aureus is the major cause of severe nosocomial infections, and empiric treatment of such infections will always need to include *Staph. aureus* coverage. Nosocomial transmission of resistant *Staph. aureus* strains, in particular MRSA and strains with reduced susceptibility against vancomycin, convey a risk to hospitalized patients:

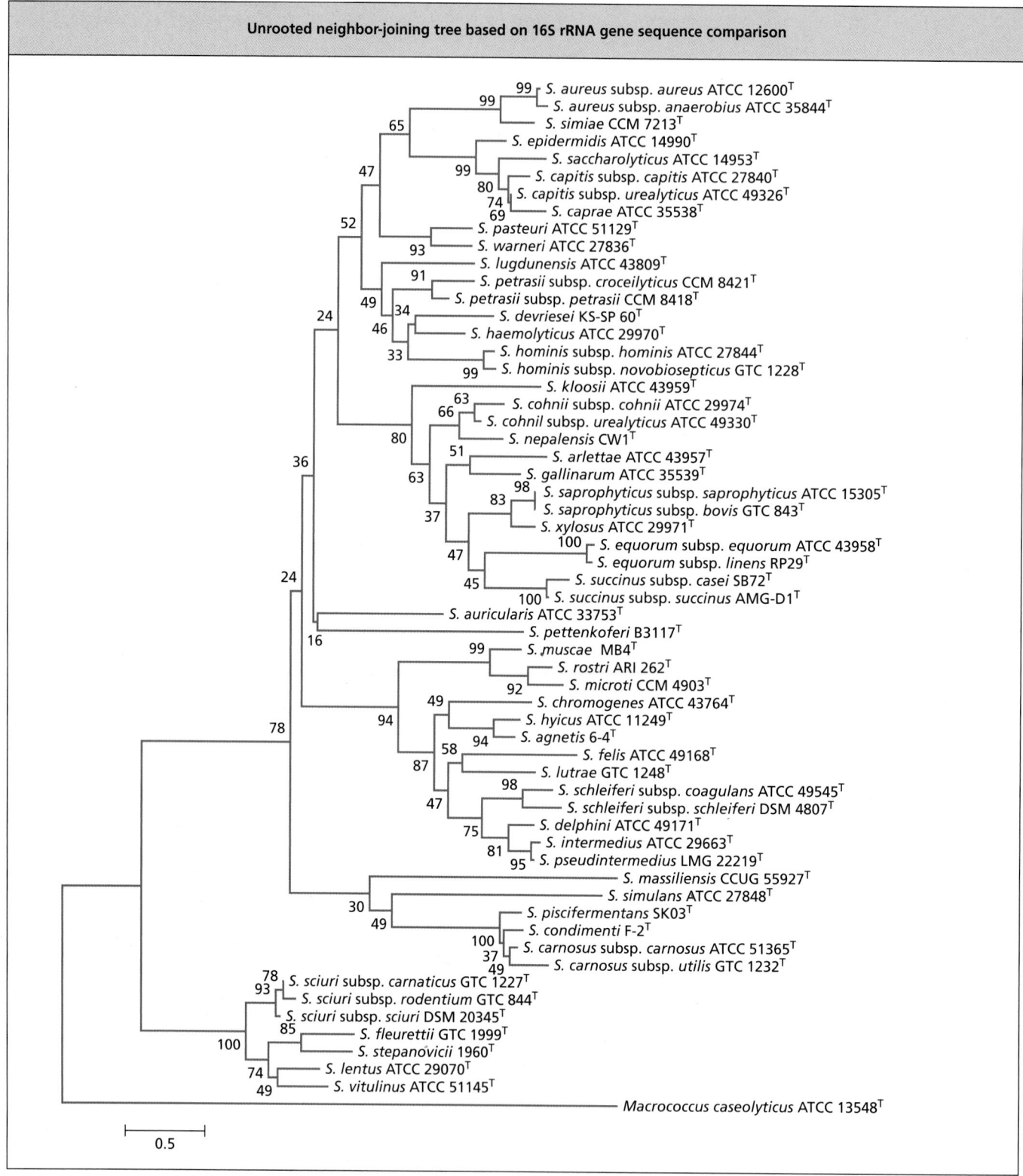

Unrooted neighbor-joining tree based on 16S rRNA gene sequence comparison

Figure 176-1 Unrooted neighbor-joining tree based on 16S rRNA gene sequence comparison, showing the phylogenetic relationships of Staphylococcal (S.) reference type strains of all species. *Macrococcus caseolyticus* ATCC 13548[T] sequence was used as an outgroup. Bootstrap probability values (percentages of 1000 tree replications) are indicated at branch points. The bar represents the number of base substitutions per 100 nucleotide positions. (*Adapted from Pantucek R, et al. Syst Appl Microbiol 2013;36(2):90-95.*)

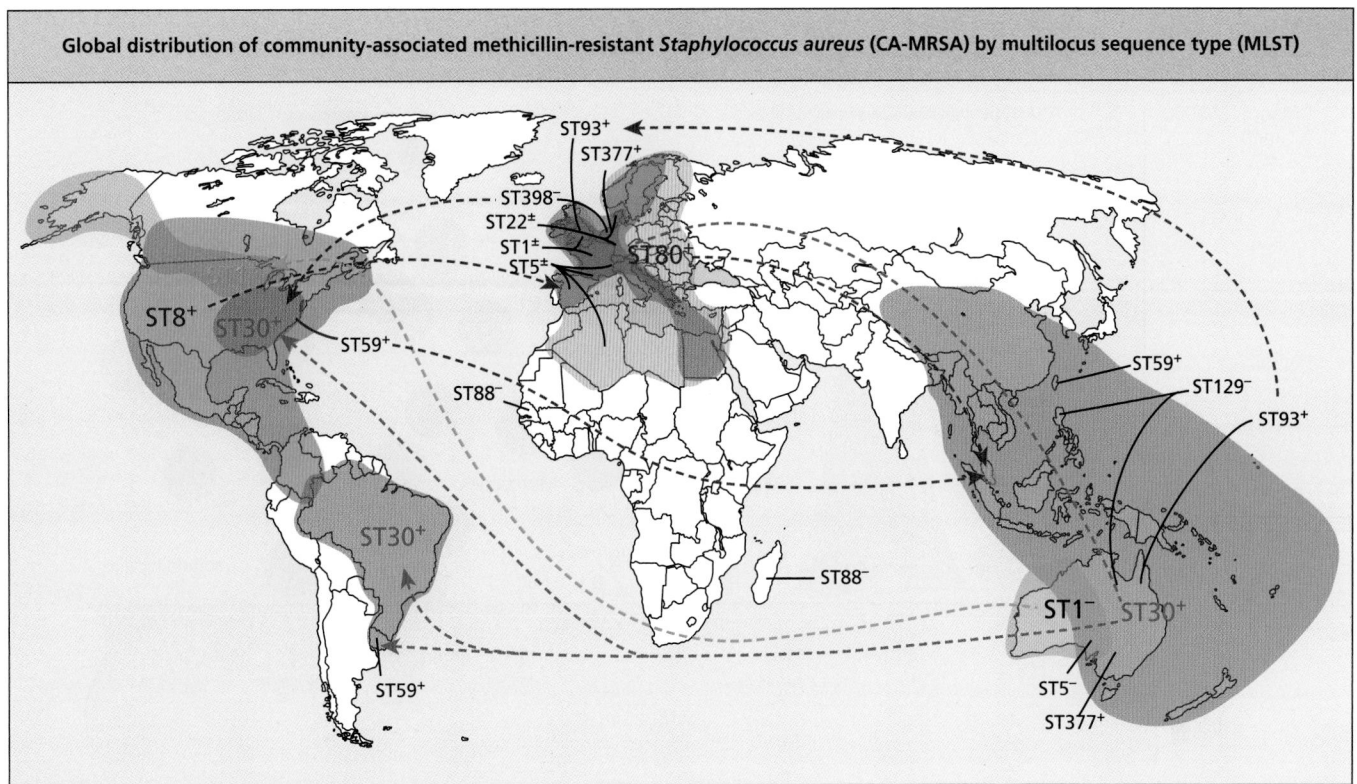

Figure 176-2 Global distribution of community-associated methicillin-resistant *Staphylococcus aureus* (CA-MRSA) by multilocus sequence type (MLST). Dotted lines indicate possible route of dissemination of the CA-MRSA strains. Estimates of the areas are shown in which infections with the main strains have been reported, i.e. ST1 (green), ST8 (red), ST30 (blue) and ST80 (purple). +, Panton–Valentine leukocidin (PVL)-positive strains; –, PVL-negative strains; ±, combination of PVL-positive and PVL-negative strains. *(Adapted from DeLeo FR, et al. Lancet 2010;375:1557–1568.)*

MRSA-transmission in hospitals has been demonstrated to lead to higher rates of invasive infection with *Staph. aureus*.[8]

Some countries, such as the Netherlands and the Scandinavian countries, have succeeded in containing the nosocomial spread of MRSA by adhering to extensive infection-control measures and restrictive antibiotic policies, but in general MRSA-colonization is widespread in hospitals. In the USA, for instance, the proportion of MRSA infections among patients with nosocomial *Staph. aureus* bacteremia increased from 2.4% in 1975 to 29% in 1991, and in American intensive care units the proportion of MRSA infections had risen to nearly 60% by 2003.[9] Interestingly, in recent years a decline in the percentage of nosocomial *Staph. aureus* infections due to MRSA has been observed in countries such as the UK and the USA.[10] Despite a variety of government-led interventions, it is still not entirely clear what has led to this decline.

Nasal carriage of *Staph. aureus* is a risk factor for subsequent infection in hospitalized patients. Colonized surgical patients had an absolute risk of wound infection of roughly 5–15%, which was two to eight times the risk of control patients.[11] Persistent urinary tract colonization with *Staph. aureus* carries a high risk for subsequent *Staph. aureus* infection and bacteremia. Intestinal carriage of *Staph. aureus* is associated with an increased risk of subsequent *Staph. aureus* infection when compared to nasal carriage alone.[12,13] A large observational study showed that nosocomial *Staph. aureus* bacteremia was three times more frequent in *Staph. aureus* carriers than in non-carriers and ~80% of the strains causing *Staph. aureus* bacteremia in carriers were from endogenous origin (i.e. they were colonized at admission).[14] However, mortality in *Staph. aureus* bacteremia was higher in patients who were not colonized at hospital admission.

COMMUNITY-ACQUIRED MRSA

For several decades, MRSA colonization and infection was largely confined to healthcare settings, but in the USA during the 1990s MRSA strains emerged which were able to sustain themselves and spread in the community. The major community-associated MRSA (CA-MRSA) clone is the USA300 strain (this number is based on pulsed-field gel electrophoresis analysis), a Panton-Valentine leukocidin (PVL)-positive *Staph. aureus*, of sequence type (ST) 8 by MLST. USA300 has a propensity to cause skin and soft tissue infections, and was at first found mostly in outbreaks, but currently this clone causes the majority of *Staph. aureus* infections in both hospitals and the community in the USA.[15] Several other CA-MRSA clones have emerged around the world, such as the European clone CC80 (*pvl*-positive, ST80) and the South-West Pacific clone (*pvl*-positive, ST30) (Figure 176-2).[16]

Although CA-MRSA is still uncommon as a cause of disease in Europe, in several European countries MRSA is widely spread among livestock, with subsequent transmission of MRSA to humans. Nosocomial transmission of livestock-associated MRSA (LA-MRSA) is low, however, and hospital outbreaks are therefore rare.[17] Phylogenetically, LA-MRSA is not related to any of the major MRSA CCs: in Europe most strains belong to CC398 (ST398), whereas in South East Asia CC9 is more common as LA-MRSA.

COAGULASE-NEGATIVE STAPHYLOCOCCI: EPIDEMIOLOGY AND INFECTIONS

Colonization with coagulase-negative staphylococci (CoNS) occurs shortly after birth, the normal habitats of these staphylococci being the skin and the mucous membranes. *Staph. epidermidis* is the predominant species; other frequent colonizers include *Staph. hominis, Staph. haemolyticus* and *Staph. warneri*. Although in general CoNS are non-pathogenic colonizers, their propensity to adhere to biomaterials and form biofilms makes them important causative agents of foreign body-related infections. CoNS are the main pathogens isolated in catheter-associated bloodstream infections (CR-BSI) and drain (shunt)-associated meningitis. They are amongst the foremost causes of prosthetic joint infections and prosthetic heart valve endocarditis,

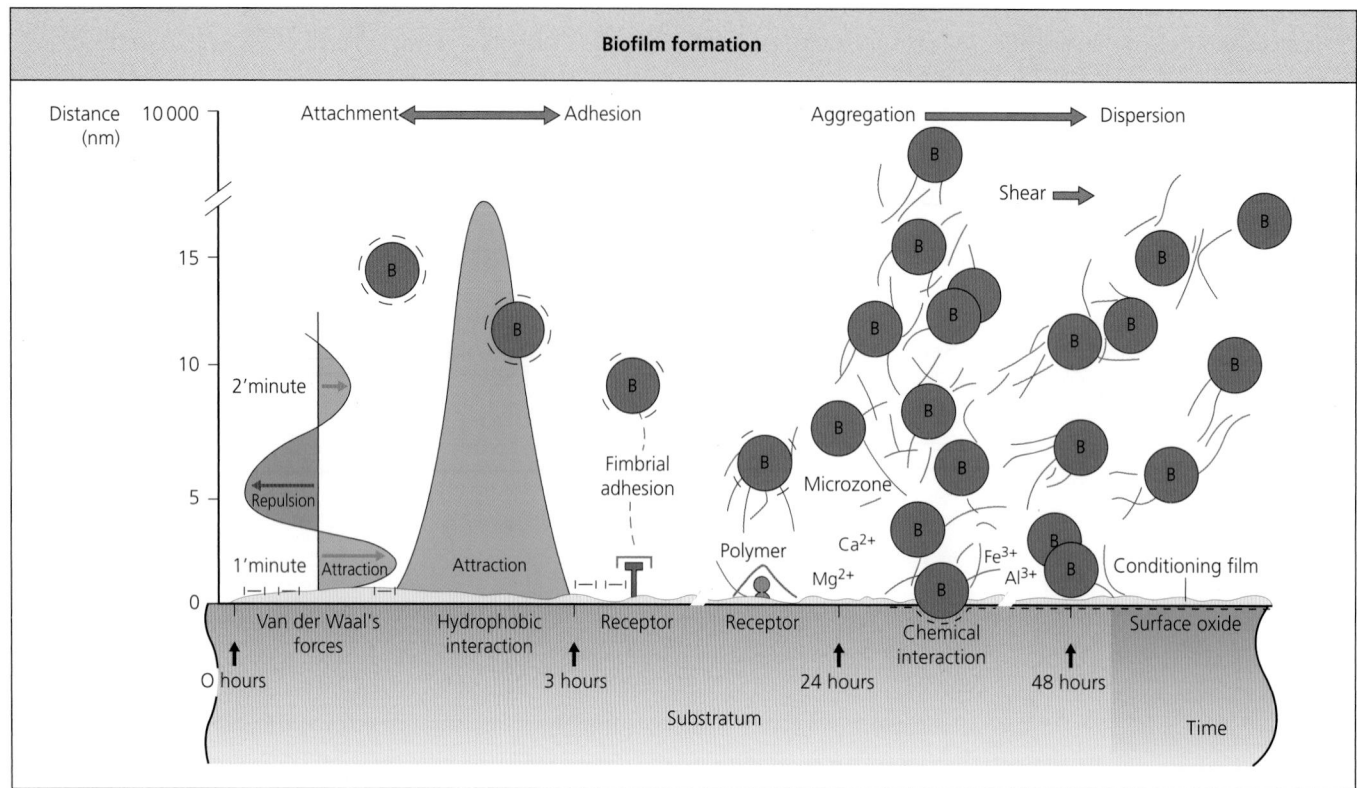

Figure 176-3 Biofilm formation. The events associated with bacterial (B) adherence to a biomaterial in relation to time and the molecular sequence in bacterial attachment, adhesion, aggregation and dispersion at substratum surface. A number of possible interactions may occur depending on the specificities of the bacteria or substratum system, the distance from the biomaterial and the stage of adherence. The attachment stage is mediated by nonspecific forces. Adhesion is driven by specific adhesin–receptor interactions. The final aggregative step results in a bacterial macrocolony on the biomaterial surface in which the bacteria are firmly adherent to the biomaterial and each other. Bacterial exopolysaccharide blankets the macrocolony and may serve to improve the nutritional microenvironment and protect the bacteria from host defenses. In the dispersion phase, bacteria disaggregate, break loose from the macrocolony and drift free into the bloodstream. (Adapted with permission from Gristina AG. Science 1987;237:1588. © 1987 American Association for the Advancement of Science.)

and they cause ~10% of all cases of native valve endocarditis.[18] *Staph. epidermidis* is primarily responsible for foreign body infections, and both prosthetic and native valve endocarditis. *Staph. saprophyticus* causes urinary tract infections (see Chapter 57) and *S. lugdunensis* and *S. schleiferi* may cause infections very similar to those of *Staph. aureus*, including abscesses, endocarditis and wound infections. Infections in humans with *Staph. intermedius* are rare and have been associated with exposure to animals, in particular dogs.

The colonizing CoNS flora may be influenced by antibiotic therapy. In hematology and neonatology wards with high antibiotic pressure, a population of more resistant and/or more virulent CoNS strains may be selected and become epidemic among patients and healthcare workers: multiple reports describe outbreaks of *Staph. epidermidis* clones causing intravascular CR-BSI.[19]

Pathogenicity of *Staphylococcus aureus*

The broad spectrum of diseases caused by *Staph. aureus* is due to its production of many surface-bound and extracellular virulence factors. These include molecules that adhere to host tissues, counteract the host defense or lyse cells (Table 176-1).

ADHERENCE TO HOST CELLS AND TISSUES

Staph. aureus expresses a number of adhesion molecules that facilitate interactions with host cells and extracellular matrix (ECM) components. These 'microbial surface components recognizing adhesive matrix molecules' (MSCRAMMs) are surface-anchored molecules that bind host molecules like collagen, laminin, fibronectin, elastin, vitronectin and fibrinogen.[20] MSCRAMMs are involved in colonization and sepsis, and also mediate the attachment of *Staph. aureus* and *Staph.*

epidermidis to foreign body materials and indwelling devices because coating of the biomaterials with host proteins and platelets results in biofilm formation (Figure 176-3).[21]

BLOCKING HOST DEFENSES

The immune response against *Staph. aureus* largely depends on the innate immune system: antimicrobial peptides, the complement system and phagocytes. The bacterium, in response, produces highly specific proteins that enable it to suppress the immune response.

Resistance to Antimicrobial Peptides

In response to infectious stimuli, skin keratinocytes, mucosal epithelial cells and neutrophils produce high levels of antimicrobial peptides (AMPs) known as cathelicidins (LL-37) and defensins. The *Staph. aureus* metalloproteinase aureolysin cleaves LL-37, while staphylokinase (SAK) inhibits the bactericidal effect of α-defensins.[22] Furthermore, modification of cell wall teichoic acids promotes *Staph. aureus* resistance to AMPs.[23]

Complement Evasion

The complement cascade serves three major functions in innate immunity:

- to opsonize bacteria (through C3b) (Figure 176-4)
- to attract phagocytes (through C3a and C5a)
- to perturb bacterial membranes of gram-negative bacteria (C5b–9, the membrane attack complex or MAC).[24,25]

Complement activation is initiated by three different pathways (classical, lectin or alternative) that all result in the formation of C3 convertase enzymes that cleave the central complement protein C3. The C3 cleavage product C3b covalently binds to the bacterial surface and is recognized by phagocytic cells expressing complement receptors.

TABLE 176-1   Virulence Factors of *Staphylococcus aureus*

Virulence Factor	Acronym or Gene	Activity
IMMUNE EVASION MECHANISMS		
Clumping factor	ClfA, ClfB	Binds fibrinogen, coating the bacterial cell and inhibiting phagocytosis
Chemotaxis inhibitory protein of *Staph. aureus*	CHIPS	Downregulates the C5a receptor and the formylated peptide receptor (FPR) on neutrophils; inhibits chemotaxis
Extracellular adherence protein	EAP	Binds to ICAM-1, fibrinogen, vitronectin. Blocks leukocyte adhesion, diapedesis and extravasation
Extracellular fibrinogen-binding protein/ extracellular complement binding protein	Efb/Ecb	Bind to C3 molecules, inhibit convertases. Efb creates an antiphagocytic fibrinogen shield
Staphylococcal complement inhibitor	SCIN/SCIN-B/SCIN-C	Inhibit C3 convertases, inhibiting C3b deposition and phagocytosis
Staphylokinase	SAK	Activates human plasminogen at the bacterial surface to cleave opsonins; inhibits bactericidal effect of α-defensins
Staphyloxantin (golden pigment)		Resist oxidant killing
Polysaccharide capsule		Antiphagocytic function
FLPR1 inhibitory proteins	FLIPr/FLIPr-like	Block Fc receptors, impair neutrophil responses to formylated peptide receptor-like-1 agonists
Polysaccharide intercellular adhesin	PIA	Holds multilayered cell complexes that form biofilms together; decreases susceptibility to defensins
Catalase		Inhibits bacterial killing by inactivating hydrogen peroxidase and free radicals formed by the myeloperoxidase system within phagocytic cells
Protein A	SpA	Binds Fc part of human IgG and prevents phagocytic uptake by Fc receptors; stimulates B lymphocytes
Coagulase/von Willebrand binding protein	coa/vwbp	Bind and activate prothrombin into thrombin
Staphylococcal superantigen-like 3	SSL3	Inhibits TLR2 activation
Staphylococcal superantigen-like 5	SSL5	Binds PSGL-1 and inhibits P-selectin-mediated neutrophil rolling
Staphylococcal superantigen-like 7	SSL7	Binds IgA and blocks FcαRI-mediated responses. Binds C5 and blocks C5 cleavage into C5a and C5b
Staphylococcal superantigen-like 10	SSL10	Binds IgG and inhibits FcR recognition and complement activation
Aureolysin	Aur	Metalloproteinase that cleaves LL-37 and complement C3
Staphylococcal immunoglobulin-binding protein	SBI	Binds IgG and C3. Blocks complement activity
Staphopain A	ScpA	Cleaves CXCR2 and blocks chemotaxis
INVASION MECHANISMS		
α-Hemolysin	hla	Lyses macrophages, lymphocytes and erythrocytes
β-Hemolysin	hlb	Sphingomyelinase; damages eukaryotic cell membranes containing sphingomyelin; causes lysis of sheep erythrocytes on blood agar
γ-Hemolysin	hlgA, hlgB	Consists of two proteins that assemble to form membrane-perforating complexes; toxic to PMNs, monocytes and macrophages, lytic for red blood cells
Panton–Valentine leukocidin	lukS (lukS-PV, lukF-PV)	Lyses human neutrophils after binding to the C5a receptor
Leukocidin E/D	LukED	Lytic to leukocytes
δ-Hemolysin	hld	Variety of attributed actions: multimerizes on eukaryotic membranes to form lytic pores; possible mediator of staphylococcal membranous enterocolitis; linked to atopic dermatitis by activating mast cells
Exfoliative toxins	eta, etb	Epidermolytic proteases that cleave desmoglein. Cause of staphylococcal scalded skin syndrome
Fibrinolysins		Break down fibrin clots
Hyaluronidase	hysA	Hydrolyzes intercellular matrix of mucopolysaccharides
DNAse/thermonuclease	nuc	Hydrolyzes RNA and DNA, frees nutrients
Lipase	geh	Facilitates spread in subcutaneous tissues; associated with furunculosis
Superantigens/pyrogenic exotoxins		Stimulate T cells nonspecifically to cytokine release
Enterotoxins A, B, C, D, E, G, H, K (and others)	sea, seb, sec, sed, see, seg, seh, sek	Cause staphylococcal food poisoning and half of the cases of nonmenstrual toxic shock syndrome (TSS)
Toxic shock syndrome toxin	TSST-1/tst	Responsible for about 75% of cases of TSS, including all cases of menstrual TSS

Continued on following page

TABLE 176-1	Virulence Factors of *Staphylococcus aureus*—cont'd	
Virulence Factor	**Acronym or Gene**	**Activity**
ATTACHMENT MECHANISMS (MSCRAMMS)		
Fibronectin-binding protein	*fnbpA, fnbpB*	Binds fibronectin, fibrinogen and elastin
Collagen-binding protein	*cna*	Binds collagen/cartilage
Clumping factor	*clfA, clfB*	Binds fibrinogen

ICAM-1, intercellular adhesion molecule 1; MSCRAMM, microbial surface components recognizing adhesive matrix molecules; PMNs, polymorphonuclear leukocytes; PSGL-1, P-selectin glycoprotein ligand-1.

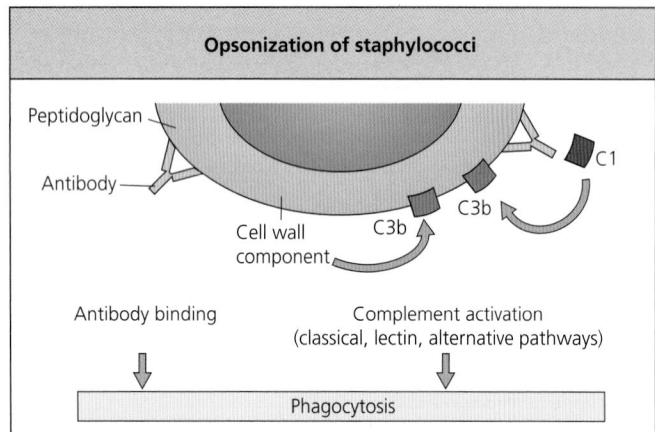

Figure 176-4 Opsonization of staphylococci with antibody molecules and complement activation products is essential for effective phagocytosis. Antibodies bind to the surface and are recognized by Fc receptors on phagocytic cells. Complement activation, either triggered by antibodies or cell wall components, results in labeling of bacteria with C3b and iC3b, which are recognized by complement receptors.

Furthermore, C3b associates with C3 convertases to form a C5 convertase that cleaves C5 into C5a (a potent chemoattractant) and C5b (part of the MAC). *Staph. aureus* produces a variety of molecules that interfere with multiple steps of the complement cascade (Table 176-1). For instance, the secreted staphylococcal complement inhibitor (SCIN) blocks C3 convertases to interfere with C3b deposition and phagocytosis,[26] while staphylococcal superantigen-like (SSL) protein 7 specifically binds to C5 to prevent cleavage by C5 convertases and formation of C5a.[27]

Mutagenesis studies have indicated that staphylococcal complement inhibitors contribute to the pathogenesis of *Staph. aureus in vivo*.[28]

Inhibition of Neutrophil Recruitment and Activation

Effective eradication of *Staph. aureus* depends on phagocytosis and intracellular killing by immune cells, mainly neutrophils.[29] This critical role is reflected by the increased risk for *Staph. aureus* infections in patients with defects in granulocyte function, both inherited (e.g. chronic granulomatous disease, myeloperoxidase deficiency, leukocyte adhesion deficiencies) and acquired (e.g. diabetes mellitus, rheumatoid arthritis, HIV). During an infection, neutrophils are rapidly recruited from the circulation to sites of microbial invasion by host stimuli (complement fragment C5a, interleukin 8, leukotriene B4) and pathogen-derived stimuli (fMLP, phenol-soluble modulins (PSMs)).[30] These chemotactic factors activate neutrophils, increase vascular permeability and induce expression of adhesion molecules on endothelial cells. Neutrophils express selectins and integrins that bind these adhesion molecules; the cells start to roll on the endothelial lining and firmly adhere to it.[31] Subsequently, the neutrophils migrate through the endothelial cell layer (diapedesis) and move towards the site of infection under a gradient of chemoattractant substances.

Staph. aureus secretes several molecules that specifically block phagocyte recruitment: the staphylococcal superantigen-like 5 (SSL5) inhibits neutrophil rolling by blocking the interaction between P-selectin on endothelial cells and P-selectin glycoprotein ligand-1 (PSGL-1) on neutrophils;[32] the chemotaxis inhibitory protein of *Staph. aureus* (CHIPS) prevents chemotaxis by blocking the formylated peptide receptor and the C5a receptor and the cysteine protease Staphopain A cleaves the chemokine receptor CXCR2.[33] *Staph. aureus* also prevents neutrophil activation by the staphylococcal superantigen-like protein 3 that binds Toll-like receptor 2.[34]

Resistance to Phagocytosis and Intracellular Killing

Staph. aureus is most efficiently phagocytosed after opsonization by both complement and antibodies. Upon bacterial uptake, the interaction of opsonic ligands with receptors triggers the release of oxygen radicals and granular contents (e.g. myeloperoxidase, proteases) into the phagosome that can destroy the ingested particle.[35] *Staph. aureus* resists phagocytosis by expression of complement inhibitory proteins that decrease surface deposition of C3b (Table 176-1). Furthermore, the extracellular fibrinogen binding protein (Efb) effectively inhibits phagocytosis by covering bacteria in an antiphagocytic shield of fibrinogen.[36] Some *Staph. aureus* strains surround themselves with a loose-fitting polysaccharide capsule (Figure 176-5) that hinders the binding of surface-bound complement factors to phagocyte receptors.[37] Alternatively, *Staph. aureus* specifically modulates Fc-dependent uptake by secretion of the formyl peptide receptor-like 1 inhibitor (FLIPr) protein family that potently bind and antagonize Fc receptors on neutrophils. The *Staph. aureus* surface protein A (SpA) also blocks antibody-dependent phagocytosis since this protein binds the Fc terminal of human IgG and covers the bacterial surface with outward-facing IgG molecules that cannot react with Fc receptors (Figure 176-5).

Once phagocytosed, staphylococci may inhibit killing and travel through the bloodstream within neutrophils. The golden pigment staphyloxanthin (for which *Staph. aureus* is named) is a carotenoid molecule with antioxidant properties that scavenges free oxygen radicals.[38] Furthermore, *Staph. aureus* can resist oxidative stress by two superoxide dismutase enzymes that remove superoxide.

CYTOLYTIC TOXINS AND PROTEASES

Staph. aureus secretes a variety of cytotoxins that lyse host cells by forming β-barrel pores in cytoplasmic membranes. These toxins are secreted as monomers but form multimeric pores in the membrane of target cells (Table 176-1). The five different bicomponent pore-forming leukocidins all 'recognize' their target cells via G-protein-coupled receptors. The best-known leukocidin, Panton–Valentine leukocidin (PVL), specifically binds the C5a receptors on human neutrophils to cause lysis before the bacteria are engulfed.[39] PVL is well known for its association with furunculosis and hemorrhagic pneumonia and is strongly associated with recent outbreaks by community-associated MRSA strains (CA-MRSA).[29] *Staph. aureus* can also lyse neutrophils after engulfment via PSMs.[40] Delta toxin, also part of the

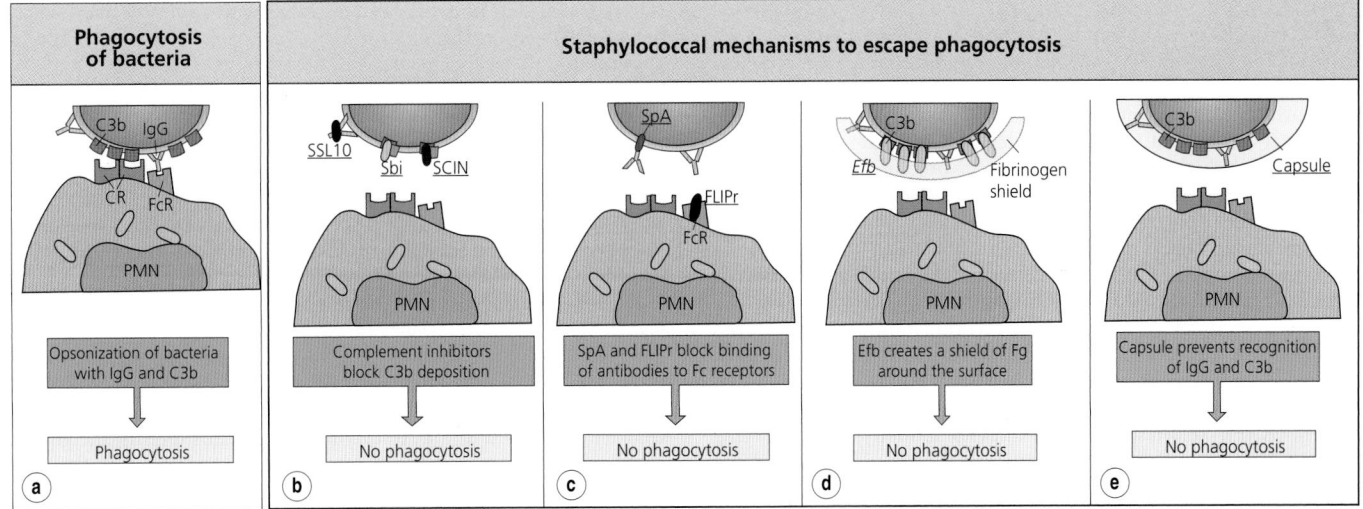

Figure 176-5 Phagocytosis of bacteria and staphylococcal mechanisms to escape phagocytosis. (a) Phagocytosis requires opsonization of bacteria with antibodies (IgG) and complement fragments (C3b). (b–e) *Staphylococcus aureus* uses different mechanisms to block phagocytosis: (b) complement inhibitors block the labeling of *Staph. aureus* with C3b; (c) surface-bound SpA binds Fc domains of IgG, thereby orienting the molecule in the wrong orientation and FLIPr/FLIPr-like proteins bind the Fc receptor; (d) Efb binds C3b and attracts fibrinogen that hides opsonins from phagocyte receptors; (e) the capsule prevents recognition of opsonins on the cell wall of *Staph. aureus* to complement and Fc receptors on PMNs.

PSM family, was recently identified as a potent mast cell degranulation factor causing allergic skin disease.[41]

IMMUNOSTIMULATORY MOLECULES

Superantigens (or pyrogenic exotoxins) are the agents responsible for toxic shock syndrome (TSS) (Figure 176-6). These extracellular proteins bind to the exterior surface of major histocompatibility complex (MHC) class II molecules on antigen-presenting cells (APCs), and link them to receptors on the surface of T-helper cells, activating them without the need for antigen presentation by the APCs.[29]

Toxic shock syndrome toxin 1 (TSST-1) causes most cases of TSS, including all cases of tampon-associated TSS; approximately one-fourth of the cases are caused by enterotoxins. Apart from their superantigenic activity, when ingested orally the heat-resistant enterotoxins may also cause *Staph. aureus* food poisoning, characterized by emesis with or without diarrhea. The target responsible for initiating the emetic reflex is located in the abdominal viscera, where putative (unidentified) cellular receptors for the enterotoxins exist.

INTERACTIONS WITH THE COAGULATION SYSTEM

Staph. aureus produces two extracellular coagulases (coagulase and von Willebrand binding protein) which bind and activate prothrombin into thrombin. The activated thrombin converts fibrinogen to fibrin, causing localized clotting and shielding the bacteria from host defenses.[42] In addition, most strains express a fibrinogen binding protein (clumping factor) which promotes attachment to blood clots and traumatized tissue.

GENETIC LOCATION AND REGULATION OF VIRULENCE FACTORS

Staph. aureus virulence factors can be chromosomally encoded and uniformly present, or located on mobile genetic elements such as bacteriophages, plasmids, transposons and pathogenicity islands. The genes for exfoliative toxins A and B are located on a bacteriophage and a plasmid respectively (0–2% of strains); PVL is located on a bacteriophage (2% of isolates). The pathogenicity island harboring TSST-1 is found in 14–24% of strains. The immune modulators CHIPS, SCIN, SAK and SEA are clustered on a bacteriophage present in 90% of clinical *Staph. aureus* isolates.[43]

The expression of virulence factors in *Staph. aureus* is controlled by a complex system of regulatory mechanisms. A well-studied

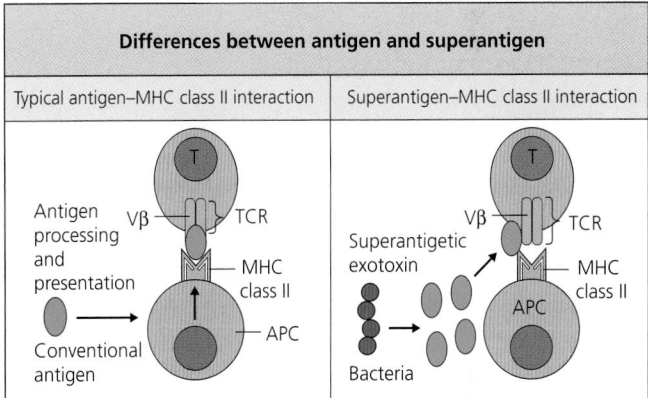

Differences between antigen and superantigen

Figure 176-6 Differences between antigen and superantigen. Staphylococcal enterotoxin and TSST-1 act as superantigens, binding directly to MHC class II and the Vβ chains of the T-cell receptor (TCR) without the need for normal antigen processing. *(Courtesy of Jan Verhoef, Ad C. Fluit and Franz-Josef Schmitz.)*

response regulator is the accessory gene regulator (*agr*), a two-component quorum sensing system that switches the preferential expression of surface adhesins during the exponential growth phase to the expression of secreted proteins during the postexponential and stationary growth phases.[44] This system is turned on at high bacterial densities and recent studies showed that *agr* is turned on when bacteria are inside the phagolysosomal vacuole of the neutrophil. There, *agr* drives expression of PSMs that subsequently lyse the neutrophil.[45] Another important regulator is the SaeRS system that drives expression of most immune evasion molecules.[46]

Pathogenicity of *Staphylococcus epidermidis*

Most of the pathogenicity studies in coagulase-negative staphylococci (CoNS) have focused on virulence factors involved in foreign-body infections by the most common and relevant species, *Staphylococcus epidermidis*. These infections are characterized by the formation of biofilms: first the bacteria adhere to the foreign body or indwelling device, followed by an accumulation phase in which the bacteria form multilayered cell clusters embedded in extracellular material.

Hydrophobic interactions, Van der Waal's forces and bacterial surface proteins play a role in initial bacterial adherence to the foreign material. On insertion or implantation, the material is rapidly coated with plasma proteins and extracellular matrix proteins (e.g. fibronectin, fibrinogen, vitronectin and von Willebrand factor), providing additional attachment sites. Molecules that mediate attachment to polymers include the staphylococcal surface proteins SSP-1 and SSP-2, the surface-associated autolysin AtlE, biofilm-associated protein (Bap) and the capsular polysaccharide/adhesin (PS/A). Molecules that bind to extracellular matrix proteins include fibrinogen-binding protein (Fbe, a protein with similarity to ClfA in *Staph. aureus*), cell-wall teichoic acid (attachment to fibronectin) and AtlE (binds to vitronectin). A number of factors involved in the accumulation phase have been identified: the polysaccharide intercellular adhesin (PIA), also known as slime-associated antigen (SAA); the capsular polysaccharide/adhesin (PS/A); biofilm-associated protein (Bap); and accumulation-associated protein (AAP).[47] Elastases, proteases, lipases and fatty-acid modifying enzymes have been identified in *Staph. epidermidis* and are considered possible virulence factors.[47]

Prevention

Staph. aureus is the main pathogen causing postoperative wound infections. Strict compliance with prophylactic antibiotic regimens for surgery (i.e. timely administration) and adaptation of these regimens to the local susceptibility patterns are essential to maximally reduce such infections.

PREVENTION OF MRSA/SPREAD

During the 1980s several countries implemented nationwide 'search-and-destroy policies' to limit the spread of MRSA within hospital settings. At that time carriage of MRSA among hospitalized patients was still extremely low. The cornerstone of the search-and-destroy policies is that colonized patients are treated in strict isolation; admitted patients with an increased risk of MRSA carriage are screened (see below) and isolated until culture results rule out MRSA carriage. Finally, contact patients and healthcare workers are screened for MRSA carriage in case of unexpected detection of MRSA in a hospitalized patient. In the United Kingdom multiple MRSA prevention initiatives were implemented to reduce the spread of MRSA in hospitals, and the effects were assessed via a mandatory MRSA bacteremia reporting scheme. Mandatory reporting of MRSA bacteremia showed a reduction in MRSA infections of more than 50% between 2003 and 2010.[48] Infection control is further discussed in Chapter 77.

PREVENTION OF HOSPITAL-ACQUIRED INFECTIONS BY DECOLONIZATION

Perioperative eradication of *Staph. aureus* carriage, using mupirocin nasal ointments and chlorhexidine body wash for 5 days, may reduce the number of nosocomial *Staph. aureus* infections by up to 60%.[49] Topical mupirocin is highly effective for short-term nasal eradication of *Staph. aureus*; 90% of patients remain negative after 1 week, and around 60% after a longer follow-up period.[50]

In smaller populations, such as CAPD patients, hemodialysis patients and patients with recurrent skin infections, mupirocin treatment was associated with significant reductions in *Staph. aureus* infections.[51]

Diagnostic Microbiology

The name 'staphylococcus' (derived from the Greek σταφύλή [staphyle], a bunch of grapes) was introduced by Alexander Ogston, a Scottish surgeon who, in 1881, described the presence of grape-like clusters of spherical micro-organisms in pus from abscesses.[52] The first to isolate and culture staphylococci was the German surgeon Friedrich Rosenbach. Rosenbach distinguished two different species of staphylococci based on colony color: a species with yellow/orange/golden colonies which he named *Staphylococcus aureus* (derived from the

word *aurum*, gold in Latin), and a species with white colonies which he called *Staphylococcus albus* that was later renamed *Staphylococcus epidermidis*.

Staphylococci are nonmotile, nonspore-forming bacteria with a genome size of between 2000 and 3000 kbp, and a 30–39% GC-content. Most staphylococcal species demonstrate catalase activity and are facultative anaerobes. Only *Staph. aureus* subsp. *anaerobius* and *Staph. saccharolyticus* require anaerobic conditions for growth. Further characteristics of the genus include susceptibility to furazolidone, resistance to bacitracin and production of acid from glucose under anaerobic conditions or in the presence of erythromycin.

The main constituents of the staphylococcal cell wall are peptidoglycan, which constitutes 50% of the dry cell mass, and teichoic acid (40% of the dry cell mass). The glycan chains of the peptidoglycan layer are built with approximately 10 alternating subunits of *N*-acetylmuramic acid and *N*-acetylglycosamine. Pentapeptide side chains are attached to the *N*-acetylmuramic acid subunits; the glycan chains are then cross-linked with peptide bridges between the side chains. The teichoic acids are macromolecules of phosphate containing polysaccharides. Teichoic acid is bound both to the peptidoglycan layer (wall teichoic acids, WTA) and to the cytoplasmic membrane (lipoteichoic acid, LTA). The polysaccharides are species-specific; *Staph. aureus* cell walls contain ribitol teichoic acids while *Staph. epidermidis* makes glycerol teichoic acids.

ISOLATION AND DETERMINATION

Most staphylococcal lesions contain numerous polymorphonuclear leukocytes (PMNLs) and large numbers of *Staph. aureus*, which may readily be demonstrated by a direct Gram smear of pus (Figure 176-7). Direct Gram smears of sputum samples may occasionally assist in rapid identification of staphylococcal pneumonia.

In general, staphylococci grow overnight on most conventional bacteriologic media. The preferential medium for isolation is (sheep) blood agar, on which they form colonies of 2 mm or more in diameter (Figure 176-8). Blood cultures from untreated bacteremia patients are usually positive after overnight incubation. Staphylococci may grow at a temperature range of 15–45°C and at NaCl concentrations as high as 15%. Differentiation from other gram-positive cocci may be aided by the determination of a couple of characteristics (Table 176-2). The fermentation of mannitol by *Staph. aureus* is used in mannitol salt agar to screen for this bacterium in clinical and environmental samples.[53]

Staph. aureus colonies on blood agar can be differentiated from other staphylococci by their yellowish (gold-colored) pigment. Confirmation tests include latex agglutination assays that detect protein A and clumping factor ('bound coagulase') on the cell surface of *Staph. aureus* (Figure 176-9), testing for free coagulase and for DNAse/thermostable endonuclease. However, non-optimal sensitivity of these

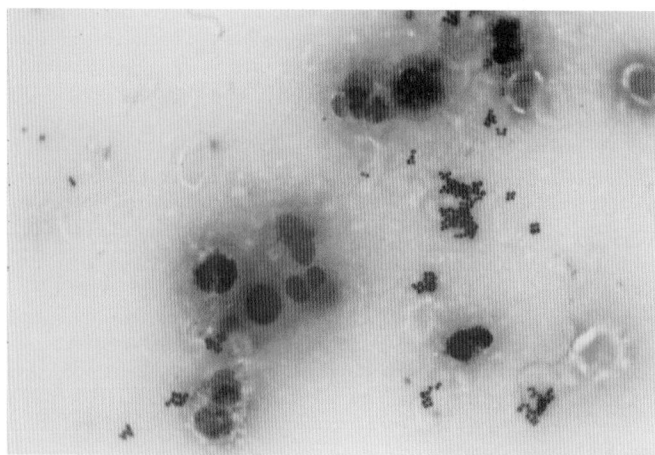

Figure 176-7 *Staphylococcus aureus in a Gram stain of pus. (Courtesy of Jan Verhoef, Ad C. Fluit and Franz-Josef Schmitz.)*

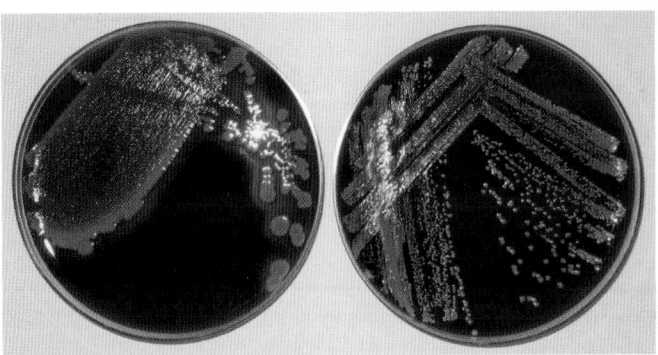

Figure 176-8 Growth of *Staphylococcus aureus* (left) and *Staphylococcus epidermidis* (right) on trypticase soy agar with sheep blood.

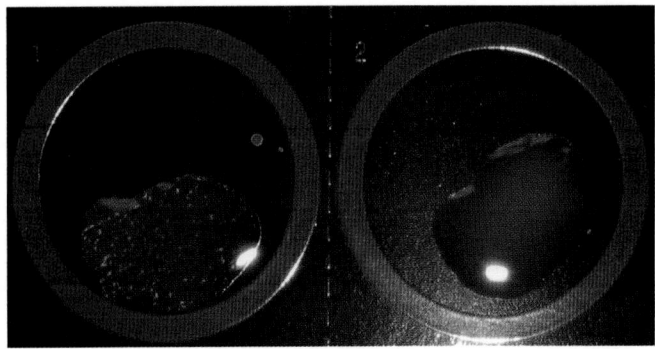

Figure 176-9 Slide coagulase test. Latex particles coated with fibrinogen and IgG agglutinate when a colony of *Staphylococcus aureus* is suspended in the solution (left), and negative control (right).

TABLE 176-2	Differentiation of *Staphylococcus aureus* and Coagulase-Negative Staphylococci from Other Gram-Positive Cocci				
	Staphylococcus aureus	**CoNS**	**Micrococcus spp.**	**Kocuria kristinae**	**Rothia mucilaginosa**
Gram stain	Gram-positive cocci, in clusters	Gram-positive cocci, in clusters	Gram-positive cocci, in clusters	Gram-positive cocci in tetrads	Gram-positive cocci in pairs or clusters with capsules
Color	Cream-colored to golden	White to cream	Cream-colored to canary yellow	Cream-colored to canary yellow	Clear to white
Mupirocin	Susceptible	Susceptible or resistant	Resistant	Resistant	–
Bacitracin	Resistant	Resistant	Susceptible	Susceptible	Susceptible
Growth in 6.5% NaCl	Yes	Yes	Yes	Yes	No
Oxidase	Negative	Negative	Positive	Positive	Negative
Catalase	Positive	Positive	Positive	Positive	Weakly positive or negative
Coagulase	Positive	Negative	Negative	Negative	Negative

CoNS, coagulase-negative staphylococci.

TABLE 176-3	Susceptibility Profiles of Different *Staphylococcus aureus* Strains*			
Antimicrobial Agent	**MSSA (Miko *et al.*)**		**MRSA (Diekema *et al.*)**	
	Outpatient (*n* = 298)	Inpatient (*n* = 410)	HA-MRSA USA100 (*n* = 368)	CA-MRSA USA300 (*n* = 2093)
Clindamycin	97	92	5	91
Erythromycin	67	70	2	8
Levofloxacin	90	87	3	47
TMP–SMX	100	99	98	99
Daptomycin	100	100	99	100
Linezolid	100	100	100	100
Vancomycin	100	100	100	100

*Data are percentages of isolates being susceptible. CLSI breakpoints were used.
CA-MRSA, community-associated methicillin-resistant *Staphylococcus aureus*; HA-MRSA, hospital-associated methicillin resistant *Staph. aureus*; MRSA, methicillin-resistant *Staph. aureus*; MSSA, methicillin-susceptible *Staph. aureus*; TMP–SMX, trimethoprim–sulfamethoxazole.

tests has been reported, especially in identifying MRSA. Most CoNS species can be determined with carbohydrate utilization tests and enzyme tests (e.g. phosphatase, urease, nitrate reduction). *S. saprophyticus* from urine samples may be identified by demonstrating novobiocin resistance.

The introduction of matrix-assisted laser desorption/ionization time-of-flight (MALDI-TOF) mass spectrometry in microbiology labs facilitated the identification and differentiation of staphylococcal species, as MALDI-TOF can rapidly and accurately identify staphylococci and discriminate between *Staph. aureus* and CoNS species.[54]

PHENOTYPIC SUSCEPTIBILITY TESTING

Staph. aureus susceptibility testing can be performed by disc diffusion or E-test on several standard bacteriologic media, and by microbroth or macrobroth dilution. Guidelines and breakpoints are available from the Clinical and Laboratory Standards Institute (CLSI), and the European Committee on Antimicrobial Susceptibility Testing (EUCAST). A number of automated systems are available for broth dilution susceptibility testing. These tests are adequate for most antibiotics, but certain special considerations apply (see below). Susceptibility profiles of different *Staph. aureus* strains can differ extensively (Table 176-3).

Clindamycin Susceptibility Testing

Methylation of the ribosomal target, usually encoded by *ermA* or *ermC*, is the main mechanism of resistance against clindamycin, and also results in cross-resistance to macrolides, lincosamide and streptogramin B (MLS$_B$) (Table 176-4).[55] Clindamycin does not induce expression of these methylase genes *in vitro* and tested strains may wrongly appear susceptible. An induction test with erythromycin (erythromycin and clindamycin disk placed 20–26 mm from each other) should, therefore, be performed on erythromycin-resistant *Staph. aureus* strains.

Isoxazolyl Penicillins (Oxacillin, Cloxacillin, Flucloxacillin, Nafcillin)

Methicillin resistance results from the production of an alternative penicillin-binding protein, PBP2A (or PBP2'), encoded by the *mecA* gene on the staphylococcal cassette chromosome *mec* (SCC*mec*), a mobile genetic element, supposedly acquired through horizontal gene transfer from CoNS (Table 176-4). Although the gold standard for identification of MRSA is in fact the detection of the *mecA* gene, recently a homolog to *mecA*, called *mecC*, has been detected in MRSA from human and bovine origin.[56,57] In heterogeneous MRSA populations, expression of PBP2a may be suppressed in most colony-forming units, hindering detection by disk diffusion or by automated (microbroth dilution) systems. A screening assay with 30 μg cefoxitin disks has the highest sensitivity for MRSA detection, with specificity being comparable to other susceptibility assays.[58] Screening for MRSA colonization can be performed on selective media (both liquid and solid) containing either oxacillin or cefoxitin. Several chromogenic MRSA detection media are available which contain an indicator agent to distinguish *Staph. aureus* from CoNS. Sensitivity and specificity of most of these tests are reported to be higher than 90–95%.[59]

In some cases, overexpression of penicillinases may lead to resistance against isoxazolyl penicillins. These strains do not harbor the *mecA*-gene and may have minimum inhibitory concentrations (MICs) in the susceptible range for β-lactam/β-lactamase-inhibitor combinations. They are not considered 'true' MRSA and have thus far not been associated with outbreaks.

Glycopeptides

To reliably determine the susceptibility of staphylococci for glycopeptides, MIC testing should be performed, as disk diffusion has insufficient sensitivity and specificity. Vancomycin-intermediately-susceptible *Staph. aureus* (VISA), defined by a MIC of >2 and ≤8 mg/L, is associated with thickening of the bacterial cell wall, thereby creating an

TABLE 176-4	Resistance Genes and Resistance Mechanisms for *Staphylococcus aureus*			
Antibiotic	**Resistance Gene(s)**	**Gene Product(s)**	**Mechanism(s) of Resistance**	**Location(s)**
β-Lactams	*blaZ*	β-Lactamase	Enzymatic hydrolysis of β-lactam nucleus	Plasmid: Transposon
	mecA	PBP2a	Reduced affinity for PBP	Chromosome: SCC*mec*
Glycopeptides	GISA: unknown	Altered peptidoglycan	Trapping of vancomycin in the cell wall	Chromosome
	VRSA: *vanA*	D-Ala-D-Lac	Synthesis of dipeptide with reduced affinity for vancomycin	Plasmid: Transposon
Quinolones	*parC*	ParC (or GrlA) component of topoisomerase IV	Mutations in the QRDR region, reducing affinity of enzyme-DNA complex for quinolones	Chromosome
	gyrA or *gyrB*	GyrA or GyrB components of gyrase		
Aminoglycosides (e.g., gentamicin)	Aminoglycoside-modifying enzymes (e.g., *aac*, *aph*)	Acetyltransferase, phosphotransferase	Acetylating and/or phosphorylating enzymes modify aminoglycosides	Plasmid, Plasmid: Transposon
TMP–SMX	Sulfonamide: *sulA*	Dihydropteroate synthase	Overproduction of p-aminobenzoic acid by enzyme	Chromosome
	TMP: *dfrB*	DHFR	Reduced affinity for DHFR	
Tetracyclines	Tetracycline, doxycycline and minocycline: *tetM*	Ribosome protection protein	Binding to the ribosome and chasing the drug from its binding site	Plasmid: Transposon
	Tetracycline: *tetK*	Efflux protein	Efflux pump	Plasmid
Erythromycin	*msrA*	Efflux protein	Efflux pump	Plasmid
	erm (A, C)	Ribosomal methylase (constitutive or inducible)	Alteration of 23S rRNA	Plasmid: Transposons
Clindamycin	*erm* (A, C)	Ribosomal methylase (constitutive or inducible)	Alteration of 23S rRNA	Plasmid: Transposons
Linezolid*	*cfr*	Ribosomal methyltransferase	Methylation of the 23S rRNA that interferes with ribosomal binding	Plasmid
Daptomycin†	*mprF*	Lysylphosphatidylglycerol synthetase (LPG) synthetase	Increasing: synthesis of total LPG, outer LPG translocation and positive net charges on cell membrane	Chromosomal
Mupirocin‡	*mupA*	Alternative isoleucyl-tRNA synthetase (IleRS-II)	Reduced affinity for mupirocin	Plasmid

DHFR, dihydrofolate reductase; GISA, glycopeptide-intermediate-susceptible *Staphylococcus aureus*; LPG, lysylphosphatidylglycerol; QRDR, quinolone resistance-determining region; TMP–SMX, trimethoprim–sulfamethoxazole; VRSA, vancomycin-resistant *Staph. aureus*.
*Other mechanisms for linezolid resistance involve mutations to the central loop of domain V of 23S rRNA or in the ribosomal proteins L3 and/or L4 of the peptide translocation center.
†Other mechanisms were also proposed, such as increased cell wall thickening, decreased membrane fluidity, and increased expression of *vraSR*.
‡High-level resistance is mediated by *mupA*, whereas low-level resistance results from a point mutation in the native chromosomal *IleRS*.
Adapted from Stryjewski ME, Corey GR. Methicillin resistant Staphylococcus aureus: an evolving pathogen. Clin Infect Dis 2014; 58(Suppl 1):S10–S19.

excess of binding sites to 'trap' vancomycin.[60,61] Vancomycin-susceptible strains producing subcolonies (at a frequency of ≥1/10[6] according to the population analysis profile) with MICs in the VISA range are called heterogeneous vancomycin-intermediately-resistant *Staph. aureus* (hVISA); these are difficult to detect using standard laboratory methods. VISA isolates can return to susceptible strains in the absence of antibiotic pressure of vancomycin.[62] Both VISA and hVISA phenotypes are associated with an impaired clinical response to vancomycin.[63,64]

High-level vancomycin-resistant *Staph. aureus* (VRSA) is extremely rare (MIC ≥16 mg/L) and results from acquisition of the enterococcal *vanA* resistance gene by *Staph. aureus*. Recently, a vancomycin-resistant CA-MRSA strain phylogenetically related to USA300 was reported from Brazil.[64] Worryingly, the strain carried a plasmid containing *vanA* cluster which was readily transmissible to other staphylococci. The European Committee on Antimicrobial Susceptibility Testing (EUCAST) considers that it is unclear whether increased doses of vancomycin improve clinical outcome in infections with VISA, and therefore does not differentiate between VISA and VRSA. EUCAST recommends reporting all *Staph. aureus* with an MIC>2 as VRSA.

Most vancomycin-resistant strains are also resistant against teicoplanin. Furthermore, resistance against vancomycin has also been associated with reduced susceptibility to daptomycin.[65]

Linezolid

Linezolid resistance in *Staph. aureus* and CoNS has been detected in patients previously treated with linezolid and has been reported in nosocomial outbreaks from several countries. Linezolid resistance is associated with mutations in the 23S rRNA or the presence of a transmissible cfr ribosomal methyltransferase.[66]

GENOTYPIC SUSCEPTIBILITY TESTING

On demand automated rapid cartridge-based amplification assays can identify *Staph. aureus* and MRSA carriers within 3–4 hours. These systems can also identify *Staph. aureus* and MRSA from cultured colonies, clinical samples taken from skin and soft tissue infections, and from positive blood culture vials containing gram-positive cocci. Polymerase chain reaction (PCR) targets are usually the *mecA* gene in combination with a specific *Staph. aureus* gene (e.g. the *spa* gene, the coagulase gene (*coa*) or the nuclease gene (*nuc*)). However, none of these techniques is 100% sensitive or specific. MRSA isolates containing the *mecC* gene can result in false-negative PCR results, depending on the platform used.

The main *Staph. aureus* genes involved in conferring resistance against antimicrobial agents are described in Table 176-4. Applying such resistance databases, considerable progress has been made with whole-genome sequencing (WGS) to predict a susceptibility profile of bacterial strains.[67]

TYPING METHODS

The epidemiology of (methicillin-resistant) *Staph. aureus* may be studied by typing the isolated strains. Numerous typing methods are available, differing in reproducibility, cost, ease, speed and discriminatory capacity.

Pulsed Field Gel Electrophoresis

Pulsed field gel electrophoresis (PGFE) is based on the digestion of bacterial DNA with restriction endonucleases (for MRSA usually *smaI*), generating large fragments of DNA (10–800 kb). PFGE has a high discriminatory power and the results are highly reproducible. However, there are limitations to its use, such as the long time interval until the final results are obtained, limited transferability, multiple nomenclatures and the cost of reagents and specialized equipment.

Multilocus Sequence Typing

Multilocus sequence typing (MLST) characterizes bacterial isolates by using the sequences of internal fragments of seven housekeeping genes.[68] Every polymorphism of a housekeeping gene is assigned a number, yielding a code consisting of seven numbers for each bacterial isolate; subsequently, each new code receives a sequence type (ST) number. Advantages of MLST include its unambiguous nomenclature, easy global exchange of typing data and the possibility for population structure and evolutionary analyses. On the downside, MLST is less discriminatory than PFGE and more expensive.

Multilocus Variable Number Tandem Repeat Analysis

Multiple locus variable number tandem repeat analysis (MLVA) uses the variability in the number of short tandem repeat sequences to create DNA profiles for epidemiologic studies. Multiple MLVA schemes have been designed and used for *Staph. aureus*. MLVA has lower costs than MLST, can be as discriminatory as PFGE, and has an improved resolution compared to *spa* typing.[69] Limitations include the absence of an international protocol for MLVA and the absence of universal nomenclature.

Spa Typing

Spa typing is a single-locus sequence typing technique for *Staph. aureus*, based on the polymorphic region X of the protein A gene.[70] *Spa* typing is highly reproducible and easy to interpret. It has less discriminatory power than PFGE and MLVA, but is less costly and easier to perform. A web-based reference database (www.spaserver.ridom.de), which uses a standardized spa-type nomenclature, permits global epidemiologic comparison of isolated MRSA strains.

Whole Genome Sequencing

Recent advances in technology have made whole-genome sequencing (WGS) of bacteria more accessible and affordable. The latest generation of sequencing platforms can produce a whole genome sequence of a bacterium within 24 hours. The increased resolution of WGS can disprove transmission events which were otherwise indicated by conventional methods and can also reveal otherwise unsuspected transmission events. The increased resolution is especially useful in countries and healthcare centers with a single dominant strain.[71] However, the lack of universal nomenclature still hampers the comparison between laboratories and with historical isolates. Currently, *Staph. aureus* core genome allele-based typing, based on a standardized analysis of whole-genome sequences, is being developed,[72] enabling comparisons between historical and current isolates by WGS. Next to providing insight into transmission events, WGS may provide comprehensive information about the presence of resistance genes and virulence factors.

Clinical Manifestations of *Staphylococcus aureus* Infections

Staph. aureus is an invasive micro-organism with a propensity for abscess formation. Community-acquired infections mostly involve skin and soft tissue infections such as cellulitis and furunculosis, but also pneumonia (typically post-influenza), osteomyelitis and acute endocarditis. *Staph. aureus* is the most common causative agent of infective endocarditis, accounting for 28% and 21% of native valve and prosthetic valve endocarditis cases, respectively.[18] Staphylococcal toxins are responsible for food poisoning, staphylococcal toxic shock syndrome (TSS) and staphylococcal scalded skin syndrome (SSSS).[73]

In nosocomial settings *Staph. aureus* is the main causative agent of postoperative wound infections, often leading to abscess formation. It is notorious for infecting prosthetic materials, such as prosthetic joints, prosthetic heart valves and internal pacemakers. Furthermore, it is one of the main causes of intravascular CR-BSI, causing 10% of all CR-BSI, second only to CoNS with 34% of the CR-BSI caused.[74] *Staph. aureus* is also a frequent cause of hospital-acquired pneumonia (HAP) and ventilator-associated pneumonia (VAP). *Staph. aureus* bacteremia (SAB) is often regarded as a specific clinical entity due to its associated mortality risk and high rate of relapses and complications.[75,76]

Infrequently, *Staph. aureus* causes urinary tract infections, predominantly in patients with recent urinary tract surgery or other manipulations, and in patients with urinary tract obstruction.[12]

Management of *Staphylococcus aureus* Infections

Management of *Staph. aureus* infections involves the combination of source control and antibiotic therapy. Uncomplicated wound or skin and soft tissue infections should be treated locally by drainage (after incision in case of abscess formation or necrotectomy in case of necrosis) or local antiseptics. Systemic antibiotics may be required if there is severe cellulitis or associated deep tissue infection. First choice for systemic therapy are the narrow-spectrum β-lactams such as the isoxazolyl penicillins or first-generation cephalosporins. Alternative (oral) regimens include trimethoprim–sulfamethoxazole (TMP–SMX), clindamycin (used especially in the treatment of abscesses, for its high tissue penetration) or linezolid; these agents are usually also active against CA-MRSA. The main characteristics of antimicrobial agents effective against *Staph. aureus* and MRSA are described in Table 176-5.

β-Lactam antibiotics are the agents of first choice in the treatment of (severe) systemic methicillin-sensitive *Staph. aureus* (MSSA) infections. Comparative studies between different β-lactam antibiotics are lacking, as are studies evaluating different durations of treatment. Isoxazolyl penicillins, penicillin/β-lactamase inhibitor combinations, first- and second-generation cephalosporins and carbapenems are considered equally effective in the treatment of MSSA infections. Clinical experience with the isoxazolyl penicillins and their narrow

spectrum of activity makes them the first choice of therapy. Vancomycin, a glycopeptide, has been the antibiotic of choice for (severe) systemic infections with MRSA and in patients with β-lactam allergy. The glycopeptides are significantly less active than the β-lactams,[77] and trough levels should be monitored to ensure adequate (high enough) dosing of vancomycin in patients with severe infections. Vancomycin-induced nephrotoxicity may occur after longer durations of administration.[78] In the majority of cases nephrotoxicity is reversible, and patients seldom require dialysis. Recent studies suggest daptomycin may be preferred to treat patients failing on vancomycin therapy and patients whose infections are caused by strains with vancomycin MICs greater than 2 mg/L.[65] However, daptomycin is inhibited by pulmonary surfactant, and should not be used to treat pneumonia.[79] Alternative agents for severe *Staph. aureus* infections include teicoplanin, tigecycline, quinupristin–dalfopristin and televancin. For MRSA infections the fifth-generation cephalosporins ceftaroline and ceftobiprole may also be considered.

Because of the severe complications of *Staph. aureus* bacteremia and its propensity to relapse,[75] treatment with systemic antibiotic therapy for a minimum of 2 weeks is recommended.[80] Follow-up bloodcultures should be taken after 48 hours of therapy. Positive follow-up bloodcultures or persistant fever for more than 72 hours should prompt the search for a deep abscess or intravascular focus of infection. Infections complicated by metastatic foci should be treated for 4–6 weeks; infections with non-removable intravascular foci

TABLE 176-5	Characteristics of Antimicrobial Agents Effective Against *Staphylococcus aureus*				
Agent	**Mechanism of Action**	**Bacterial Effect**	**Principal Adverse Events**	**Advantages**	**Caveats**
Isoxazolyl penicillins (oxacillin, cloxacillin, flucloxacillin, nafcillin)	Inhibiting cell wall synthesis	Bactericidal	Neurotoxicity and bone marrow suppression at high dosing, interstitial nephritis	Well tolerated, rapidly bactericidal against MSSA	Not active against MRSA, low bioavailability (~50%) in oral formulations
First-generation cephalosporin (cefazolin, cephalexin)	Inhibiting cell wall synthesis	Bactericidal	Hepatitis, renal impairment	Well tolerated, rapidly bactericidal against MSSA, formulations with high bioavailability available, broad spectrum	Not active against MRSA, poor CSF penetration
Rifampin	Inhibiting RNA synthesis	Bactericidal	Elevated liver enzymes, discoloration of bodily fluids	High bioavailability in oral formulation. Good penetration in biofilms	Inducible resistance, should not be given as monotherapy. Numerous drug interactions
Fusidic acid	Inhibiting protein synthesis	Bacteriostatic	GI side effects (nausea, diarrhea, discomfort). Elevated liver enzymes	High bioavailability in oral formulation, high concentrations in bones and joints	Not available in all countries, little experience with treating invasive infections
Vancomycin	Inhibiting cell wall assembly	Bactericidal	Nephrotoxicity; red man syndrome	Inexpensive, >50 years of clinical experience	MIC >2 mg/L associated with poor outcomes (VISA, hVISA, VRSA), nephrotoxicity may develop with longer durations of therapy
Linezolid	Inhibiting protein synthesis (23S RNA at 50S ribosomal subunit)	Bacteriostatic	Peripheral and optic neuropathy, thrombocytopenia and anemia, lactic acidosis	High bioavailability in oral formulation, good drug penetration into lung, recommended for treatment of pneumonia by MRSA	Bacteriostatic, not suitable for longer duration of therapy (maximum 28 days) due to serious adverse events with long-term use
Daptomycin	Membrane depolarization (Ca++ dependent)	Bactericidal	CK elevation, myopathy; peripheral neuropathy, rhabdomyolysis and eosinophilic pneumonia	Rapidly bactericidal, effective for MRSA bloodstream infections and right-side endocarditis	Not suitable for treatment of pneumonia, due to inactivation by pulmonary surfactant; elevated vancomycin MICs have been associated with daptomycin resistance

TABLE 176-5	Characteristics of Antimicrobial Agents Effective Against *Staphylococcus aureus*—cont'd				
Agent	**Mechanism of Action**	**Bacterial Effect**	**Principal Adverse Events**	**Advantages**	**Caveats**
Tigecycline	Inhibiting protein synthesis by binding to 30S ribosomal subunits	Bacteriostatic	GI side effects (nausea, vomiting)		Bacteriostatic, GI side effects are common. Higher risk of mortality than comparator agents. Low serum and ELF concentration
Telavancin	Inhibiting formation of cell wall and depolarizes membrane	Bactericidal	GI side effects, nephrotoxicity, QT prolongation	Rapidly bactericidal against MRSA, VISA and VRSA; active against MRSA strains resistant to vancomycin, linezolid and daptomycin	Nephrotoxicity, lower clinical outcomes in patients with reduced renal function, coagulation test interference
TMP–SMX	Sequential blockade in the synthesis of folic acid	Bactericidal	GI side effects, rash, hematologic suppression with longer use	Virtually no CA-MRSA resistance, oral formulation	No data to support treatment of invasive infections
Quinolones (moxifloxacin, levofloxacin)	Inhibiting DNA synthesis by inhibiting the DNA gyrase and topoisomerase	Bactericidal	GI side effects (nausea, diarrhea). Tendon inflammation/rupture, QT prolongation, irreversible peripheral neuropathy	High bioavailability oral formulation, broad spectrum	Resistance may be induced with limited number of mutations; limited clinical experience in severe infections. Very broad spectrum, especially against gram-negatives
Clindamycin	Inhibiting protein synthesis by binding to 50S ribosomal subunits	Bacteriostatic or bactericidal depending on drug concentration, infection site	GI side effects (diarrhea, CDAD, severe colitis)	Decreases toxin production, good bioavailability (90%) with oral formulation	Inducible resistance, inadequate penetration into the CSF
Ceftaroline	Inhibiting cell wall synthesis	Bactericidal	Well tolerated (<5% incidence of diarrhea, nausea, rash)	Bactericidal, well tolerated	Most clinical data on bacterial skin and soft tissue infections

CA-MRSA, community-associated methicillin-resistant *Staphylococcus aureus*; CDAD, *Clostridium difficile*-associated disease; CK, creatine kinase; CSF, cerebrospinal fluid; DNA, deoxyribonucleic acid; GI, gastrointestinal; hVISA, heterogeneous vancomycin-intermediate-resistant *Staph. aureus*; MIC, minimal inhibitory concentration; MRSA, methicillin-resistant *Staph. aureus*; MSSA, methicillin-susceptible *Staph. aureus*; RNA, ribonucleic acid; TMP–SMX, trimethoprim–sulfamethoxazole; VISA, vancomycin-intermediate-susceptible *Staph. aureus*; VRSA, vancomycin-resistant *Staph. aureus*.

(including infected thrombosis and endocarditis) should be treated with 6 weeks of intravenous, bactericidal therapy. ID consultation is associated with better adherence to quality measures (including echocardiography, repeat blood culture, removal of infectious foci and antibiotic therapy), reduced in-hospital mortality, and earlier discharge in patients with SAB.[81] *In vitro*, aminoglycosides act synergistically in *Staph. aureus* killing, and the addition of an aminoglycoside (most often gentamicin) may shorten the duration of fever and bacteremia, although improved outcome with this combined therapy has not been demonstrated.

Linezolid or vancomycin should be added for anti-staphylococcal coverage in patients with a severe community-acquired pneumonia suspected to be caused by CA-MRSA, and in patients developing HAP or VAP in institutions in which MRSA is a frequent nosocomial pathogen.

The optimal treatment for severe pneumonia caused by a PVL-producing *Staph. aureus* is still unclear. The UK Health Protection Agency (HPA) recommends starting treatment with an empiric combination of clindamycin, linezolid and rifampin for severe pneumonia suspected to be caused by a PVL-positive *Staph. aureus*, and discontinuing the linezolid if the cultured isolate is sensitive to clindamycin. The HPA also advises adding intravenous immunoglobulin (IVIG) for severe cases and explicitly dissuades the use of β-lactams.[82]

In treatment of prosthetic joint infections (with retention of the prosthesis) and prosthetic valve endocarditis, rifampin is part of the antibiotic combination regimen, because of high penetration of this antibiotic in biofilms and its activity on slowly dividing bacteria.[83] *Staph. aureus* requires only a single mutation to become resistant to rifampin and this may happen rapidly when the drug is used as monotherapy or with inadequate drug levels of the combination antibiotic. Therefore, it is recommended not to start rifampin therapy before adequate levels of the other antibiotic have been secured and bacterial load reduction has been achieved, for instance after a minimum of 2 days' therapy. Fusidic acid has been used as an alternative to rifampin in the treatment of prosthetic valve endocarditis. Fusidic acid in combination with a second antibiotic agent (e.g. rifampin) has been used as an oral step-down regimen in the treatment of bone infections, joint infections and prosthetic joint infections caused by methicillin-resistant staphylococci.[84] Fusidic acid is also used in some places (notably the UK) for furunculosis and other skin and soft tissue infections.

Management of Coagulase-Negative Staphylococcal Infections

Vancomycin is usually the agent of choice in the treatment of CoNS infections, but when thorough laboratory testing indicates that a CoNS is methicillin-susceptible, the isoxazolyl penicillins or first-generation cephalosporins are preferred. Other antibiotics that may be considered include clindamycin, teicoplanin, linezolid, daptomycin, TMP–SMX, quinupristin–dalfopristin, ceftabiprole and ceftaroline. Similar to the treatment of prosthetic joint infections caused by *Staph. aureus*, rifampin is an integral part in the treatment of prosthetic joint infections with CoNS. CoNS are often multiresistant, and therapy should be guided by the susceptibility test results.

Micrococci

Micrococci are human commensals that colonize the skin, mucosa and oropharynx. Micrococcal species may occasionally cause invasive disease, usually in immunocompromised patients, the majority caused by *M. luteus*. Micrococci have occasionally been reported as the cause of pneumonia, meningitis associated with ventricular shunts, septic arthritis, bacteremia, peritonitis, endophthalmitis, CR-BSI and endocarditis.

Diagnostic Microbiology

Micrococci are catalase-positive, oxidase-positive, strictly aerobic gram-positive cocci that grow in clusters. On sheep blood agar they form cream-colored to yellow colonies. Resistance to mupirocin and staphylolysin, and susceptibility to bacitracin and lysozyme differentiate them from the staphylococci. Micrococci isolated from clinical specimens usually represent contamination, either from the skin and mucous membranes or from the environment.

Management

For micrococcal species MICs at achievable concentrations can be obtained for most β-lactams, aminoglycosides, glycopeptides, clindamycin, daptomycin, linezolid and the most active drug *in vitro*, rifampin. Fosfomycin, erythromycin and fusidic acid should be considered inactive.[85] Clinical data on infections with micrococci are too scarce to formulate any clear therapeutic recommendations. In case of infections of prosthetic materials, combination therapy with rifampin should be considered.

References available online at expertconsult.com.

KEY REFERENCES

Ammerlaan H.S., Harbarth S., Buiting A.G., et al.: Secular trends in nosocomial bloodstream infections: antibiotic-resistant bacteria increase the total burden of infection. *Clin Infect Dis* 2013; 56(6):798-805.

Bode L.G., Kluytmans J.A., Wertheim H.F., et al.: Preventing surgical-site infections in nasal carriers of *Staphylococcus aureus*. *N Engl J Med* 2010; 362(1):9-17.

Deleo F.R., Otto M., Kreiswirth B.N., et al.: Community-associated meticillin-resistant *Staphylococcus aureus*. *Lancet* 2010; 375(9725):1557-1568.

Garcia-Alvarez L., Holden M.T., Lindsay H., et al.: Meticillin-resistant *Staphylococcus aureus* with a novel mecA homologue in human and bovine populations in the UK and Denmark: a descriptive study. *Lancet Infect Dis* 2011; 11(8):595-603.

Gu B., Kelesidis T., Tsiodras S., et al.: The emerging problem of linezolid-resistant *Staphylococcus*. *J Antimicrob Chemother* 2013; 68(1):4-11.

Holmes N.E., Turnidge J.D., Munckhof W.J., et al.: Antibiotic choice may not explain poorer outcomes in patients with *Staphylococcus aureus* bacteremia and high vancomycin minimum inhibitory concentrations. *J Infect Dis* 2011; 204(3):340-347.

Price J.R., Golubchik T., Cole K., et al.: Whole-genome sequencing shows that patient-to-patient transmission rarely accounts for acquisition of *Staphylococcus aureus* in an intensive care unit. *Clin Infect Dis* 2014; 58(5):609-618.

Spaan A.N., Surewaard B.G., Nijland R., et al.: Neutrophils versus *Staphylococcus aureus*: a biological tug of war. *Annu Rev Microbiol* 2013; 67:629-650.

Spaulding A.R., Salgado-Pabon W., Kohler P.L., et al.: Staphylococcal and streptococcal superantigen exotoxins. *Clin Microbiol Rev* 2013; 26(3):422-447.

Wertheim H.F., Melles D.C., Vos M.C., et al.: The role of nasal carriage in *Staphylococcus aureus* infections. *Lancet Infect Dis* 2005; 5(12):751-762.

177

Streptococci and Enterococci

ANDROULLA EFSTRATIOU | THERESA LAMAGNI | CLAIRE E. TURNER

KEY CONCEPTS

- The vast clinical and taxonomic diversity of the genus *Streptococcus*.
- The diverse range of clinical diseases from sore throat to serious invasive infections.
- The public health impact of novel genomics on streptococcal epidemiology and pathogenicity.
- Latest methods and guidance for prevention, control and management.

Introduction

The genus *Streptococcus* currently comprises 99 recognized species, many of which are associated with disease in humans and animals (www.bacterio.net/streptococcus.html).

The streptococci are gram-positive cocci that are usually arranged in chains of varying lengths and in some cases pairs. The detection of cytochrome enzymes with the catalase test distinguishes members of the catalase-positive family of Micrococcaceae (see Chapter 176) from the members of the family of Streptococcaceae, which are catalase negative. Most species in this genus grow well on conventional culture media but growth is almost always enhanced on culture media containing sterile blood (usually sheep or horse) and in an aerobic environment or an environment enhanced with CO_2. Most of these species will grow both aerobically and anaerobically and are referred to as 'facultative anaerobes'. Some species of streptococci are true obligate anaerobes.

The genus *Enterococcus* consists of gram-positive, catalase-negative, nonspore-forming, facultative anaerobic bacteria that can occur both as single cocci and in chains. Enterococci belong to a group of organisms known as lactic acid bacteria (LAB) that produce bacteriocins. They are able to survive a range of stresses and hostile environments, including those of extreme temperature (5–65°C), pH (4.5–10.0) and high NaCl concentration, enabling them to colonize a wide range of niches. The nosocomial pathogenicity of enterococci has emerged in recent years, as well as increasing resistance to glycopeptide antibiotics.

Taxonomy and Identification

The traditional division of streptococci into α-streptococci, β-streptococci and γ-streptococci on the basis of their capacity to hemolyze erythrocytes in the blood agar medium and coupled with the traditional Lancefield grouping (which subdivides the genus into 20 groups based on the cell wall polysaccharide) are still considered as first steps for classification of streptococci.[1] Since the mid-1970s the ease of performing the grouping of hemolytic streptococci has been radically simplified through the introduction of latex agglutination based typing reagents.

The identification of streptococci has long been recognized as unsatisfactory, with the result that significant proportions remain misidentified or unidentified by the diagnostic microbiology laboratory. However, the taxonomic classification (mainly for α and non-hemolytic streptococci) was substantially simplified by Facklam in 2002.[2] With the advent of genomics and molecular technologies (next

generation sequencing) the classification has now been revisited to allow for a greater understanding of the genera and their bacterial diversity.

A variety of molecular methods have been developed over the years for the identification of gram-positive cocci, in particular streptococci, enterococci and other related organisms. Bishop and colleagues[3] used multilocus sequence analysis (MLSA) of concatenated sequences of seven housekeeping genes to describe the phylogenetic relationship between the genus *Streptococcus* with special attention to the phylogenetically diverse 'other nonpyogenic group' commonly nicknamed as the 'viridans group' and other closely-related genera for example, *Enterococcus* (Figure 177-1). Recently several studies have determined that matrix-assisted laser desorption ionization-time of flight mass spectrometry (MALDI-TOF-MS) appears to be a reliable and rapid alternative for group-level identification of streptococci but it does not discriminate genetically related species of certain groups.[4]

Applications of chemotaxonomic approaches, DNA hybridization and 16S rRNA gene sequencing have resulted in the proposal of 'species groups' for streptococci. The main species groups have been named as, 'Pyogenic', 'Mitis', 'Anginosus', 'Bovis', 'Mutans' and 'Salivarius' respectively[5-7] (Figure 177-2) and encompass the majority of

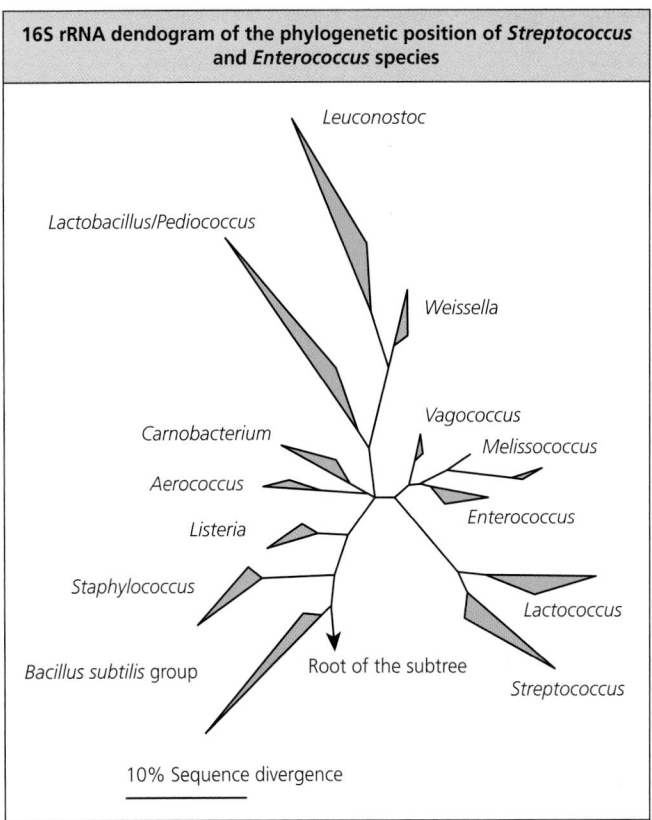

16S rRNA dendogram of the phylogenetic position of *Streptococcus* and *Enterococcus* species

Leuconostoc

Lactobacillus/Pediococcus

Weissella

Carnobacterium

Vagococcus

Melissococcus

Aerococcus

Enterococcus

Listeria

Staphylococcus

Lactococcus

Bacillus subtilis group

Root of the subtree

Streptococcus

10% Sequence divergence

Figure 177-1 16S rRNA dendogram of the phylogenetic position of *Streptococcus* and *Enterococcus* species (*Adapted from Klein, G.: Taxonomy, ecology and antibiotic resistance of enterococci from food and the gastro-intestinal tract. Int J Food Microbiol 2003; 88:123–131 and Fisher, K., Phillips, C. The ecology, epidemiology and virulence of Enterococcus. Microbiol 2009; 155:1749-1757*).

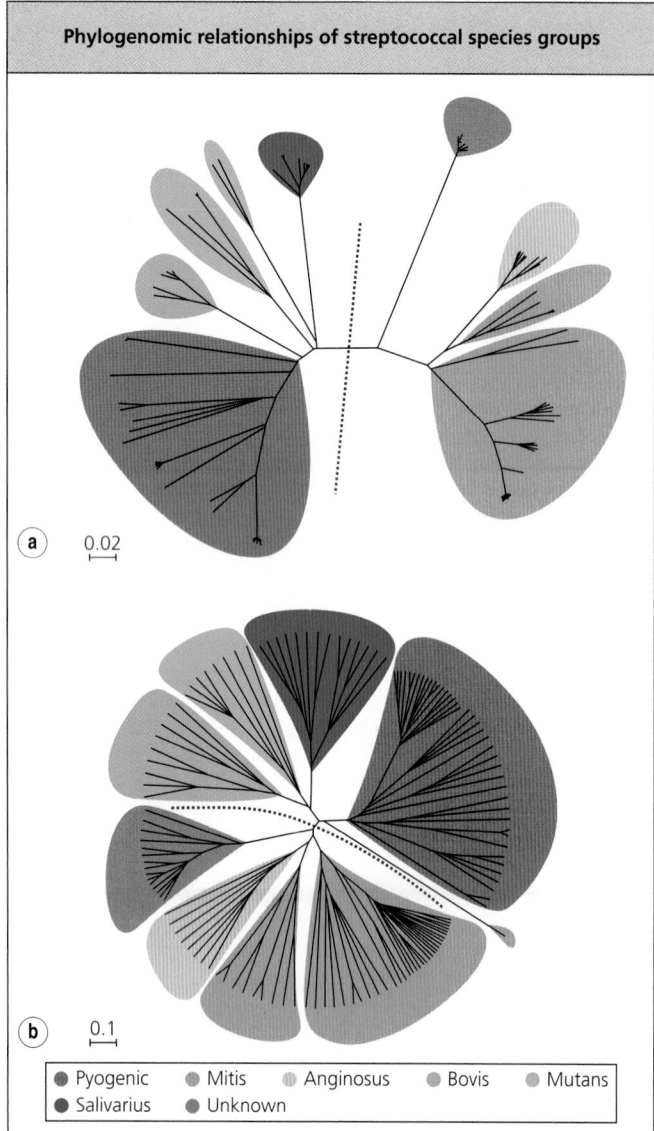

Phylogenomic relationships of streptococcal species groups

a   0.02

b   0.1

- ● Pyogenic
- ● Mitis
- ● Anginosus
- ● Bovis
- ● Mutans
- ● Salivarius
- ● Unknown

Figure 177-2 Phylogenomic relationships of streptococcal species groups. The clustering results of seven species groups were based on phylogenomic tree and gene content dendrograms. Each species group was painted with the assigned color as the above analysis. The supermatrix tree was constructed based on maximum likelihood (ML, bootstrap value indicated as numerator) and neighbor-joining (NJ, bootstrap value indicated as denominator) algorithms, using a concatenated alignment of 278 orthologous proteins. All the 138 *Streptococcus* strains analyzed were assigned to the corresponding species groups and were marked with related colored circles. Different color-coded branches denoted different species. *(Reprinted from PLoS One 2014; 9(6): e101229.)*

TABLE 177-1	**Typing of Streptococci**	
Serologic methods	M typing and T typing group A streptococci (GAS) R typing (GAS) OF typing (inhibition of the opacity reaction) (GAS) **Polysaccharide antigen typing: GBS** Lipoteichoic acid typing: Enterococci	
Molecular methods	DNA fingerprinting	**Pulsed-field gel electrophoresis** Amplified fragment length polymorphism Restriction fragment length polymorphism (RFLP) of specific genes
	Ribotyping DNA sequencing	**Multilocus sequence typing (MLST)** *emm* **gene sequencing**
	PCR-based	Multiple locus variable number of tandem repeat analysis (MLVA) Random amplification of polymorphic DNA (RAPD)
	Whole Genomes	**Whole Genome Sequencing (WGS)**
Rarely used	Multilocus enzyme electrophoresis (MEE) Whole cell protein analysis (WCPA) Bacteriophage typing Bacteriocin typing	

Bold: Key methods currently used for typing streptococci.

distinct from the other streptococci to be designated another genus, *Enterococcus*, which now includes 28 species.[8] The molecular data that were collected using 16S rRNA sequencing of *Streptococcus* enabled the construction of a 16S rRNA-dendrogram showing the relationship between *Streptococcus*, *Enterococcus* and *Lactococcus* species (Figure 177-1).[6] This method also allowed the grouping of *Enterococcus* species, with the key pathogens being *Enterococcus faecalis* species group and the *Enterococcus faecium* species group.[5] The discrimination of enterococci from streptococci is mainly established by Lancefield group D antigen, as only the 'Streptococcus bovis group', *Streptococcus alactolyticus* and *Streptococcus equinus* are serogroup D. These groups can be distinguished from *Enterococcus* species by the lack of growth in 6.5% (w/v) sodium chloride at 10°C. The use of fermentation patterns, enzyme activities such as pyroglutamyl aminopeptidase (PYRase),[9] growth at defined temperatures and physiological characteristics is essential in the identification of *Enterococcus* species.[9,10]

Various methods are used to type streptococci and enterococci (Table 177-1). Multilocus sequence typing (MLST) made it possible to unambiguously assign names or codes to genotypes, and has improved worldwide tracking of clinically relevant (i.e. particularly virulent or resistant) circulating clones. MLST also allowed construction of web-based international databases (see http://www.mlst.net, http://pubmlst.org/databases/). In addition, comparative whole genome analyses of a large number of streptococcal genomes have revealed diversities within both streptococci and enterococci, especially with respect to the virulence-related genes and metabolic pathways.

GROUP A STREPTOCOCCI (GAS)

The cell wall proteins of group A streptococci (GAS) that are used in strain typing include T protein and M protein. The M protein antigen, a potent virulence factor, was the basis for the further serologic and genetic identification of more than 100 M types. However, given the limitations with M typing this method has been largely replaced by the analysis of the *emm* gene encoding the M protein.[11] More than 223 *emm* types have thus far been reported globally, with considerable variation in *emm* type distribution both at country and regional level.[12] A new *emm*-cluster system was recently proposed[13] that classifies the

described species although several remain ungrouped. Comparative genomics using population structure, phylogenetic and phylogenomic analyses of 138 *Streptococcus* genomes offers insights into the evolution of species and species groups within this genus.[5] The population structure of streptococcal species groups suggests that there are two major evolutionary lineages within this genus.[8]

Molecular Characterization and Population Structure

Many attempts have been made to distinguish *Enterococcus* species from *Streptococcus* species. In 1984, through the use of DNA hybridization and 16S rRNA sequencing, it was established that the species *Streptococcus faecium* and *Streptococcus faecalis* were sufficiently many GAS *emm* types into 48 discrete *emm* clusters containing closely related M proteins that share binding and structural properties. Genomic studies are also proving to be pivotal in understanding the level of diversity that exists in the streptococcal population. The first M1 GAS genome was published in 2001[14] with genomes from other *emm* types following soon after.[15] A striking resurgence of severe infections caused by *emm*1 was reported in many countries from the late 1980s to the early 1990s.[16] Nasser and colleagues recently sequenced 3615 strains of *emm*1 and discovered that the contemporary epidemic clone emerged from a precursor cell that contained the phage encoding the SpeA2 variant of the streptococcal pyrogenic exotoxin A superantigen and had acquired, by homologous recombination, a locus with enhanced expression of the toxins NADase and streptolysin O (see Pathogenesis). A key finding was that the molecular evolutionary events transpiring in just one bacterial cell ultimately produced millions of severe infections globally.[16]

GROUP B STREPTOCOCCI (GBS)

MLST studies have shown that *Strep. agalactiae* (group B streptococcus, GBS) isolated from carriage and disease in different countries cluster into five major clonal complexes (CC) (CC1, 10, 17, 19 and 23).[17] CC17 strains are considered hypervirulent as they are responsible for the vast majority of meningitis cases among neonates, and for more than 80% of late onset cases in infants 7–90 days old.[18] However, whole genome sequencing (WGS) of GBS strains has concluded, thus far, that the classic serotyping scheme based upon the capsular polysaccharide does not reflect the genetic diversity. Strains that belong to different serotypes can be more closely related than strains of the same serotype. This information therefore, will impact upon vaccine development and a larger collection of strains from carriage and infected neonates need to be examined.

Streptococcus pneumoniae

Genome comparisons of completely sequenced *Strep. pneumoniae* strains have revealed extensive variation in gene content and confirmed that lateral gene transfer and recombination is the most important driving mechanism generating genetic diversity and mosaicism in the pneumococcal genome.[19] A remarkable feature of the *Strep. pneumoniae* genome is the presence of many insertion sequence (IS) elements and repeated sequences, which may have facilitated genome plasticity of this organism and the generation of pseudogenes. This extreme level of genetic diversity, most likely facilitated by genetic transformation, is also exemplified by the presence of over 90 distinct capsular serotypes. This, however, may not be true within all *Strep. pneumoniae* lineages since, despite its high potential of genetic variation, the genomes of strains R6 and D39 showed nearly 100% conserved gene synteny, suggesting that rearrangements and transpositions have not occurred frequently since R6 was separated from D36 several decades ago.[20] Comparative genomics has shown that *Strep. mitis* is the main external reservoir of genetic variability of *Strep. pneumoniae*, and that most events of horizontal gene transfer involve closely-related species that share a similar ecological niche.[21]

Enterococcus

Extensive genetic variation driven by recombination has also been reported for *E. faecalis* and *E. faecium*.[22-24] In contrast to *Strep. pneumoniae*, horizontal gene transfer in enterococci is most likely the result of conjugation, involving conjugative plasmids and/or conjugative transposons. Enterococci have become especially notorious for their unprecedented abilities to acquire and disseminate antibiotic-resistance genes. As for GAS and pneumococci, enterococcal intra- and interspecies genetic exchange facilitates rapid adaptation of enterococci to stringent and changing environmental conditions.

The first enterococcal genome sequence for *E. faecalis* V583 was published in 2002 and complete genome sequences of various enterococcal strains now number in the hundreds (http://www.ncbi.nlm.nih.gov/genome). The availability of the completely sequenced *Enterococcus* genome, *E. faecalis* V538,[25] underlined the enormous potential for genomic rearrangement, with more than 25% of the genome consisting of mobile or exogenously acquired genetic elements. Virulence and antibiotic-resistance genes are distributed among multiple genetic lineages, but in high-risk enterococcal clonal complexes (HiRECC), antibiotic-resistance and virulence genes converged, causing infections and outbreaks globally.[26,27]

Epidemiology

β-HEMOLYTIC STREPTOCOCCI OF GROUPS A, C AND G

Whilst the frequency of disease manifestations caused by groups A, C and G streptococci differ, they share commonalities with respect to colonization sites and disease presentations, a likely reflection of similarities in microbiological characteristics. All are known colonizers of the oropharynx, genital mucosa, rectum and skin, especially at the site of lesions. Person-to-person transmission occurs through inhalation of respiratory droplets or direct skin contact. Transmission through contaminated environmental reservoirs, ranging from personal objects to bathing facilities, has also been well documented. Transmission through consumption of inoculated food has become less common but still occurs.[28] In the absence of antibiotic therapy, colonized or infected individuals may remain infectious for several weeks (see Prevention).

Representative studies quantifying carriage rates in different sites are severely lacking, but for GAS, studies suggest low levels of colonization in healthy adults, less than 5% for throat and less than 1% for vaginal or rectal carriage.[29] Studies of pharyngeal GAS carriage in healthy children are rather more variable ranging from 2–17%.[30,31] Of the few recent studies that have assessed asymptomatic pharyngeal carriage of group C (GCS) or group G (GGS) streptococci, rates of <4% have been identified in adults.[30,32] In areas of high endemicity of rheumatic fever, carriage studies have pointed to higher rates for GGS than GAS in some but not all studies.[33-36] Vaginal carriage rates of GCS and GGS have been estimated at 5–6%.[37]

Of the more superficial conditions caused by these streptococci, pharyngitis and tonsillitis are likely to number among the most common in temperate climates. Streptococcal pharyngitis/tonsillitis and scarlet fever share a similar seasonal pattern, peaking in springtime in temperate countries. Widespread upsurges in scarlet fever incidence have been noted in recent years in Hong Kong and most recently in the UK.[38,39] Whilst all age groups succumb to scarlet fever, incidence is most common in children, peaking around 4 years.

Of the skin and soft-tissue infections caused by groups A, C and G streptococci, impetigo (pyoderma) is considered the most common. In tropical climates, the incidence of impetigo is strongly elevated with particularly high rates documented in native populations of Australia and South Pacific islands, with scabies a key risk factor in these populations.

Immunological sequelae of acute respiratory tract and GAS skin infections, notably rheumatic fever and glomerulonephritis, continue to be a source of substantial disease burden in low- and middle-income countries (LMIC). An extensive World Health Organization (WHO) review estimated 2.4 million children aged 5–14 years to be affected by rheumatic heart disease with prevalence highest within south and central Asia, sub-Saharan Africa and native populations of Australasia (Figure 177-3), ranging from 2 to 6 per 1000 children.[40]

Contemporary estimates suggest an approximate incidence of 2–4 per 100 000 population for invasive GAS infections in high-income countries with incidence highest in the elderly and to a lesser extent in children.[41]

Invasive GAS disease incidence follows a similar seasonal pattern to GAS pharyngitis/tonsillitis and scarlet fever with lowest rates in the autumn and highest rates in winter and spring. A characteristic feature of invasive GAS infections is their occurrence in individuals with no known risk or predisposing factors, with 15–30% of adult and close to 50% of pediatric infections occurring in such individuals.[42] Skin lesions, traumatic, surgical or chronic, are the most common risk

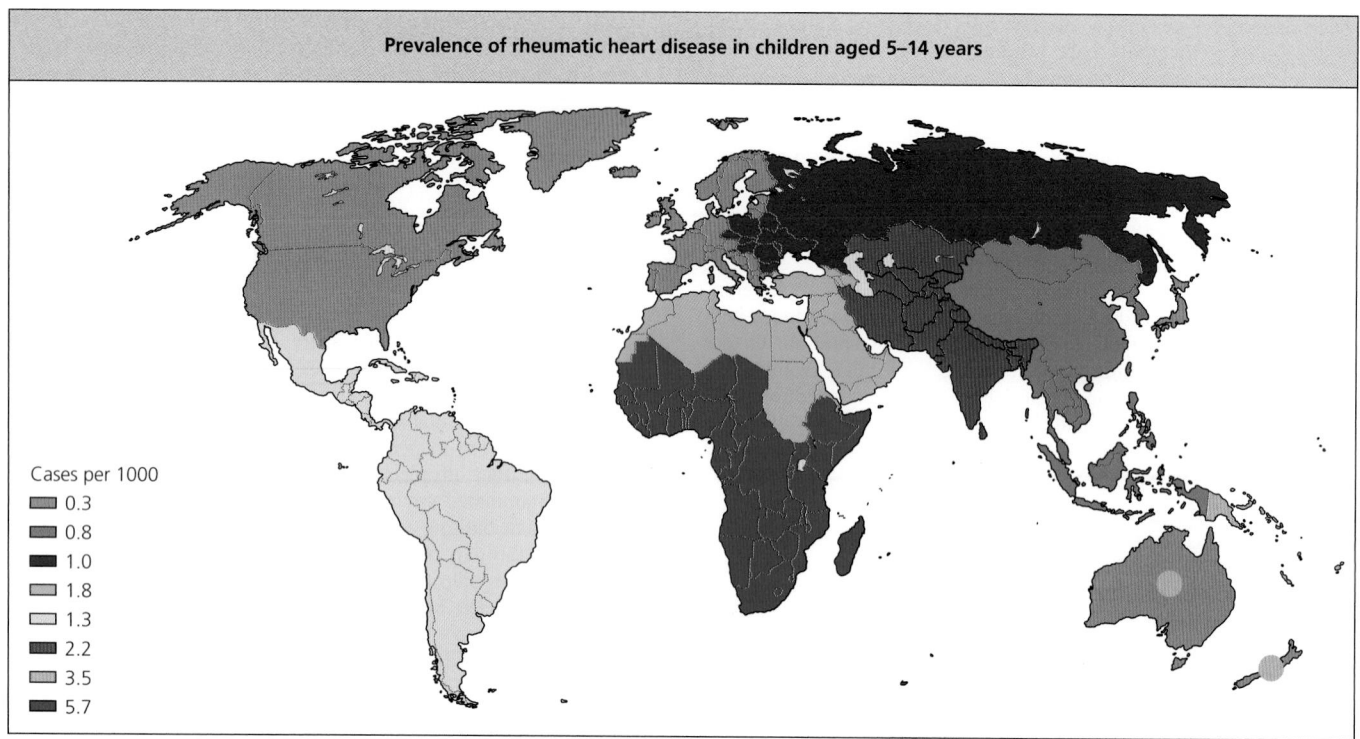

Figure 177-3   Prevalence of rheumatic heart disease in children aged 5–14 years. The circles within Australia and New Zealand represent indigenous populations. (*Adapted from*[40] *Carapetis, J.R.: Lancet Infect Dis 2005; 5:685-694*).

factors, providing a portal of entry for the organism. Among children, chickenpox is one of the more common risk factors, present in around 1 in 5 of cases, and particularly linked to development of severe soft-tissue infections such as necrotizing fasciitis. Acute viral respiratory infections, in particular influenza and herpes zoster[43,44] are well recognized factors predisposing to invasive GAS infection with secondary infections generally occurring within 1 week of influenza diagnosis.[43] Intrinsic risk factors are numerous and include a range of co-morbidities such as heart disease, diabetes and malignancy.[41] Between 2–4% of invasive GAS infections are associated with pregnancy and childbirth (see Clinical Manifestations).

Estimates of invasive GCS and GGS are less plentiful than for GAS. Bacteremia surveillance in European countries suggests a population incidence of approximately 2-4 per 100 000 for GGS and <2/100 000 for GCS.[45] Unlike GAS infection, invasive GCS and GGS infections are generally closely tied to individuals with predisposing factors, with disease incidence more highly concentrated in the elderly than for GAS infection.[45-50]

GROUP B STREPTOCOCCI (GBS)

The principal reservoir for group B streptococci (GBS) is the gut from which the genital or urinary tract may become infected or colonized. Rectal–vaginal carriage rates of 20–30% are typically identified in women of childbearing age and, although less studied, similar rates have been identified for anogenital carriage in young men and older adults.[51-53] Studies in the USA have identified higher carriage rates in non-white ethnic groups, which may in part explain the higher incidence of invasive disease in black Americans compared to white.[54] Pharyngeal GBS colonization is known to occur but less common at <10% in adults.[32,53,55]

Perinatal transmission of GBS results in colonization in around 9% of neonates.[56] Whilst the overriding majority of colonized neonates remain healthy, for a small proportion transmission results in preterm delivery, stillbirth or early-onset sepsis, defined as infection within the first week of life. Outbreaks of GBS infection in neonatal intensive care wards are uncommon but have been documented. Rates of early-onset invasive GBS disease vary markedly internationally, in part but not wholly reflecting differing approaches to prevention. Within European countries, rates of early-onset GBS disease vary from 0.4 to 0.75 per 1000 live births whereas in the USA, where programs of antenatal screening have been in place for some time, rates are currently estimated at 0.24/1000.[57] LMIC estimates are variable but suggest higher rates in African countries.[58,59]

Infections arising from day 7 to 90 are termed late onset with transmission routes for these infants far less well understood but likely to arise from direct maternal contact or from the wider environment. Prematurity is a key risk factor for late onset disease with increases in premature births potentially driving a rise in late onset disease reported in some regions. Estimates of late onset disease incidence are generally around 0.3/1000 live births.[57,59] Combined with early-onset disease, this gives overall infant rates generally between 0.5-0.8 in Europe and USA and 1–2 per 1000 live births in Africa (Figure 177-4).

Increases in invasive GBS infections in adults have been reported in several countries, potentially linked to a rise in diabetes mellitus.[60-63] Between 12% and 24% of adult cases are thought to be healthcare-associated, in particular linked to surgery. High rates of infection have also been noted in nursing home residents.[63-65] Other key risk factors for adult disease include pregnancy and childbirth. Population rates in over 65s in UK, Canada and USA range from 20 to 70 per 100 000 with incrementally higher rates according to age.[46,60,62]

ENTEROCOCCI

Enterococci are the most prevalent aerobic cocci in the bowel. Resistance against glycopeptides has been emerging since 1990, especially in *E. faecium* isolated in intensive care units and nursing homes in the USA. This emergence can be attributed to epidemic spread of a single clonal lineage, CC17 (see above). CC17 is characterized by high-level ampicillin and quinolone resistance.[66,67] Ampicillin resistance preceded

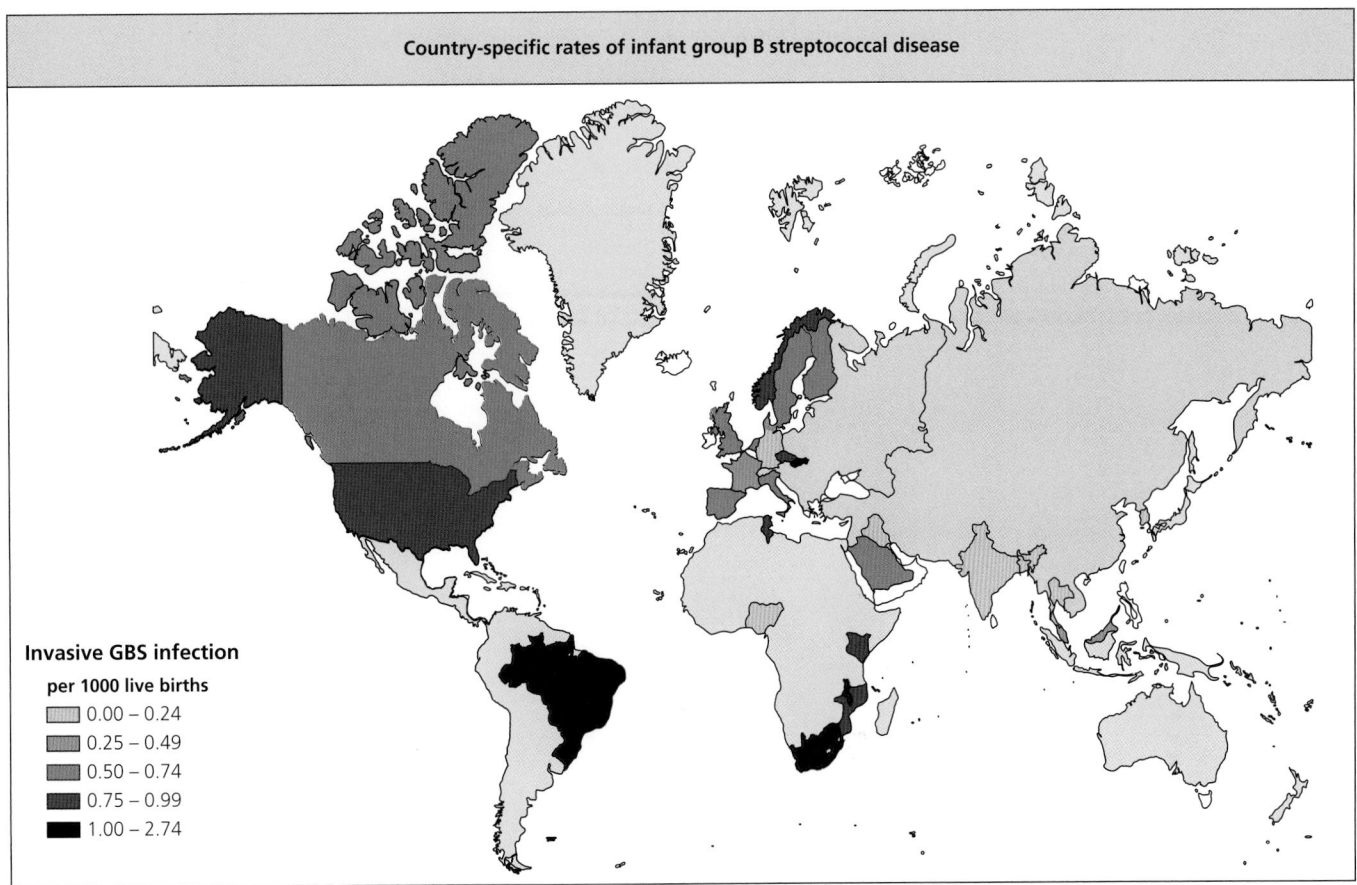

Figure 177-4 Country-specific rates of infant group B streptococcal disease. (*Adapted from*[58] *Edmond et al.: Lancet 2012; 379:547-556 and*[69] *Dagnew et al.: Clin Infect Dis 2012; 55:91-102.*)

and may have facilitated the emergence of glycopeptide-resistant *E. faecium* in the USA. In Europe, prevalence of vancomycin-resistant enterococci (VRE) started to increase after the turn of the century, with prevalence rates above 10% in countries such as Greece, Ireland, Israel, Italy, Portugal and the UK (Figure 177-5). In other countries, such as the Netherlands, the prevalence of VRE has remained low but the number of ampicillin-resistant *E. faecium* has increased explosively during the past 10 years.[68]

STREPTOCOCCUS PNEUMONIAE

Strep. pneumoniae is an obligate parasite in humans that colonizes the nasopharynx and is frequently carried and transmitted by children but less so among adults. The risk of developing invasive pneumococcal disease (IPD) is dependent upon both the host susceptibility and invasiveness of the pneumococcus which is largely determined by its polysaccharide capsule.[69] Pneumococci can be distinguished into >90 different serotypes based on specific antibody responses generated by their polysaccharide capsule. The capsular types 6a, 6b, 14, 19a, 19f and 23f are the dominant types found in pneumococcal infection during the first 2 years of life, whereas in adults these types and the types 1, 3, 4, 7f, 8, 9, 10a, 11a, 12f, 14, 15b, 17f, 18c, 20 and 22f seem to cause the greatest number of bacteremic infections recorded in the USA. Population rates of IPD show wide variation from <1 to over 10 per 100 000 population in Nordic countries.[70] Differences in clinical practices in terms of microbiological investigation, as well as surveillance methods, may account for some of these differences.

Despite the high frequency of horizontal sequence transfer in the pneumococcal population, the spread of multidrug-resistant (MDR)

pneumococci has primarily reflected the global dissemination of particular clones rather than the acquisition of resistance by resident, sensitive genotypes.[71] Since the 1980s, the prevalence of penicillin non-susceptible pneumococci has been constantly increasing worldwide with alarmingly high prevalence in countries bordering the Mediterranean (Figure 177-6). Continued global surveillance is important since serotype distributions and age-related incidences of IPD vary from country to country and the use of new vaccines is expected to have a further impact.

NONPYOGENIC/OTHER STREPTOCOCCI

The nonpyogenic/other streptococci encompass four phylogenetic clusters: Mitis, Mutans, Salivarius and Anginosus, which are part of the human microbiota, being isolated from the oral cavity, gastrointestinal and genitourinary tracts. The organisms are most abundant in the mouth, and one member of the group, *Strep. mutans*, is the etiologic agent of dental caries in most cases and populations. *Strep. sanguinis* is also another potential cause. Others may be involved in other mouth or gingival infections such as periodontitis. If they are introduced into the bloodstream, they have the potential of causing endocarditis, in particular in individuals with damaged heart valves, and are the most common causes of subacute bacterial endocarditis. Some of these streptococci (notably the mutans group) have the unique ability to synthesize dextrans from glucose, which allows them to adhere to fibrin-platelet aggregates at damaged heart valves. However, despite the substantial clinical effect of the other nonpyogenic streptococci, the epidemiology and pathogenesis of all these streptococci are minimally understood.[72]

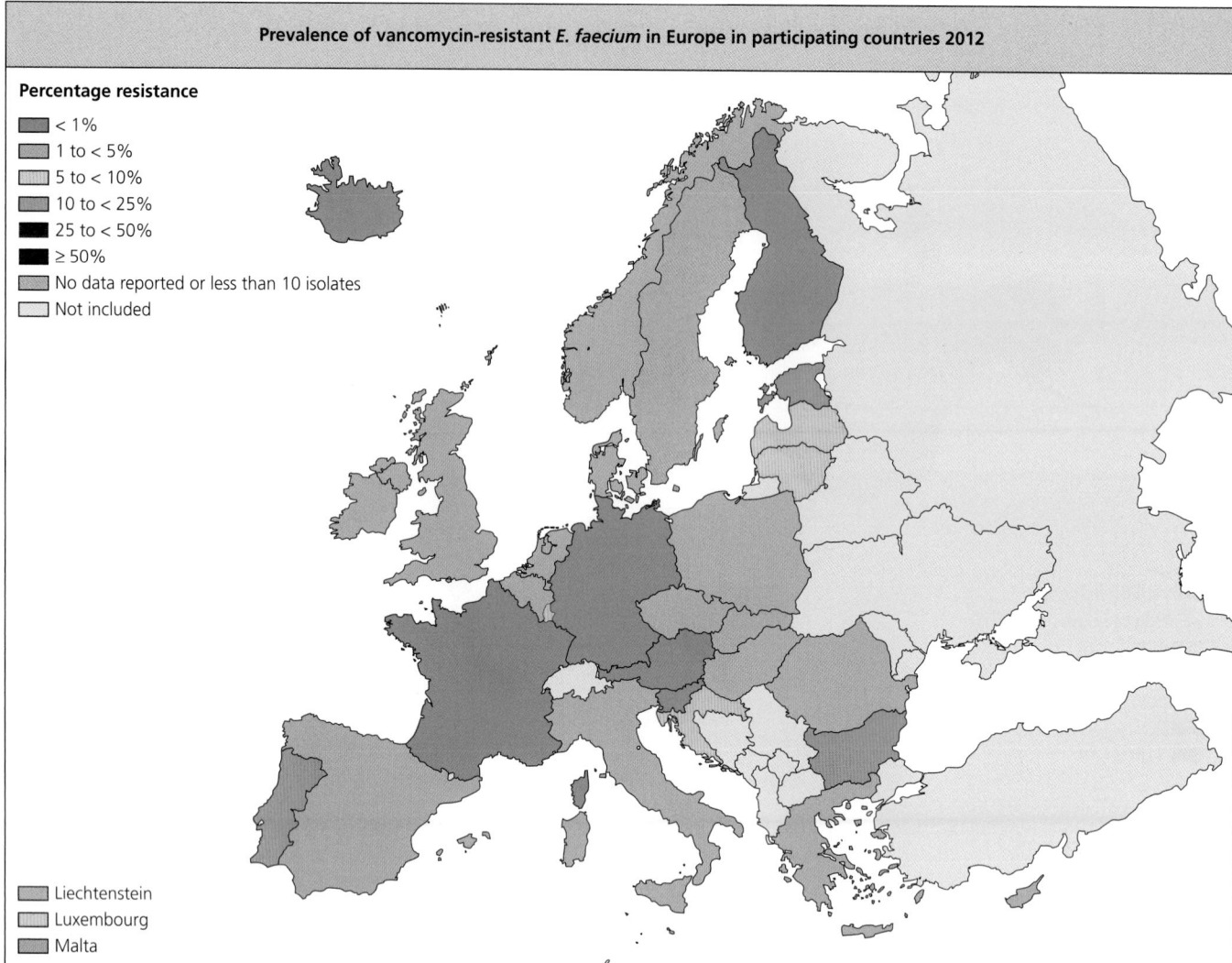

Figure 177-5 Prevalence of vancomycin-resistant *E. faecium* in Europe in participating countries 2012. (http://www.ecdc.europa.eu/en/healthtopics/antimicrobial_resistance/database/Pages/map_reports.aspx.)

Pathogenesis

GROUP A STREPTOCOCCI (GAS)

Group A streptococci can produce a variety of virulence factors that can be surface-associated or secreted (Figure 177-7), where each contribute in enabling the bacterium to evade the host immune system and to cause disease (Figure 177-8).

Surface Antigens and Hyaluronic Acid Capsule

The biggest threat to GAS survival within the host is the neutrophil response and opsonin-mediated phagocytosis. The coiled-coil surface M protein and M-like proteins play major roles in the prevention of opsonophagocytosis of the bacterium. Their anti-opsonic properties are derived from their ability to bind host complement regulators C4BP and Factor H or Factor H-like proteins that prevent complement activation and deposition of the opsonin C3b on the bacterial cell surface. M protein and M-like proteins can also bind fibrinogen and fibronectin that then act like a shield preventing the opsonin accessing the bacterial surface.[73,74] The hyaluronic acid capsule that is secreted by the bacterium to surround itself also protects against deposition of opsonins.[73] GAS are also susceptible to antimicrobial peptides released by many cell types, including epithelial cells and phagocytes. The GAS hyaluronic acid capsule can prevent the antimicrobial peptide LL-37 reaching the bacterial cell surface.[75] Cationic antimicrobial peptides are electrostatically attracted to the negatively charged bacterial surface where they then assemble to form pores in the bacterial membrane. To enhance their resistance to these peptides GAS can positively increase their surface charge by incorporating alanine residues into the cell wall teichoic acids.[74]

Proteases

To prevent neutrophil activation and migration to the site of infection, GAS produces two proteolytic enzymes. C5a peptidase (ScpA) inactivates the polymorphic leukocyte (including neutrophils) chemotactic C5a component of complement;[76] GBS also produce this enzyme. The *Strep. pyogenes* cell envelope proteinase (SpyCEP) specifically cleaves and inactivates chemokines required for neutrophil recruitment and activation, including interleukin-8. Active homologs of this protease have also been identified in group C streptococcal species *Strep. zooepidemicus* and *Strep. equi.*[77]

Group A streptococci make several DNA degrading enzymes (DNAses) whose contribution to pathogenesis is still not entirely clear. Previously they were regarded to be required for bacterial spread through purulent material; however in recent years a new role was identified with the discovery of neutrophil extracellular traps (NETs) released by neutrophils. The main component of

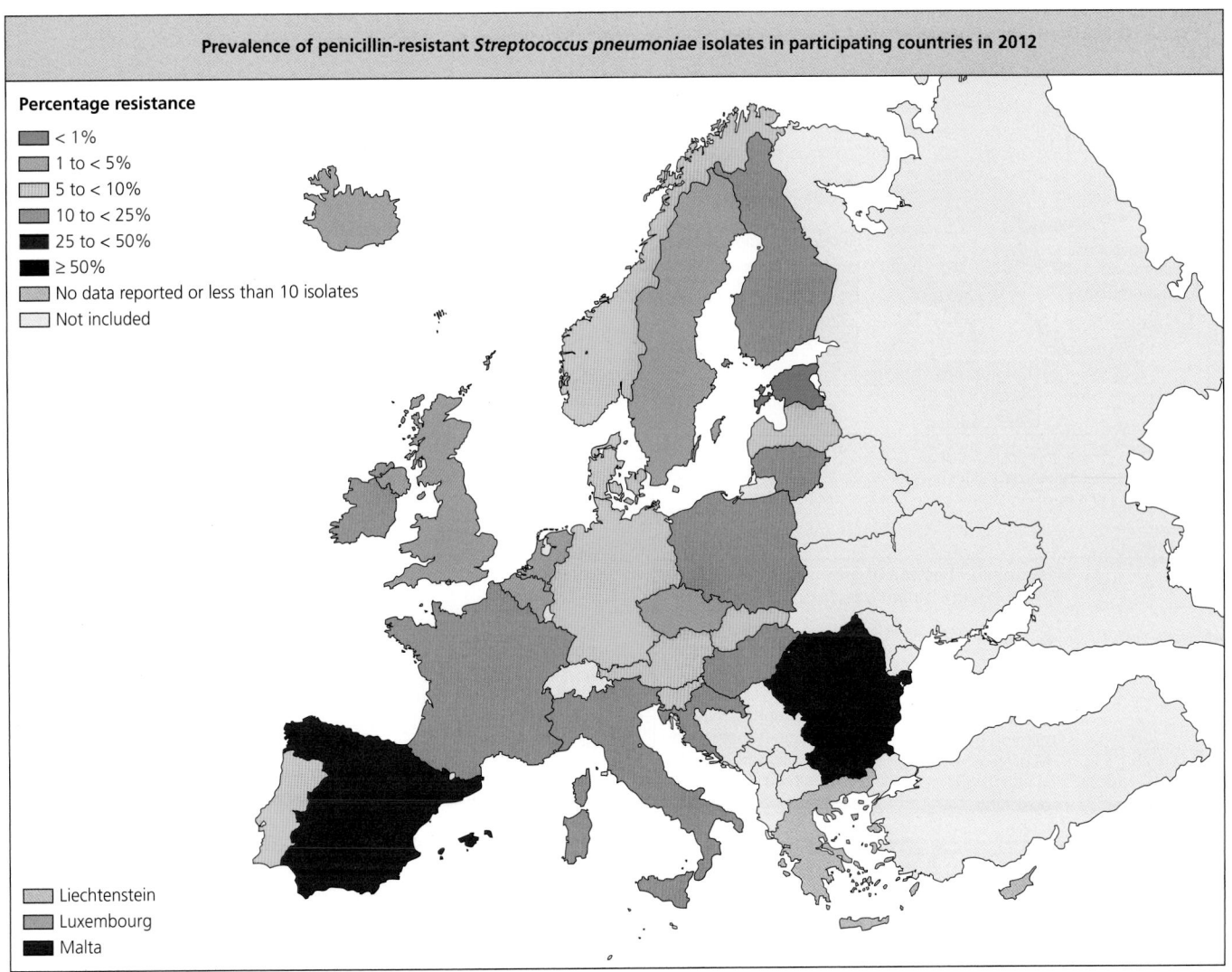

Prevalence of penicillin-resistant *Streptococcus pneumoniae* isolates in participating countries in 2012

Percentage resistance
- < 1%
- 1 to < 5%
- 5 to < 10%
- 10 to < 25%
- 25 to < 50%
- ≥ 50%
- No data reported or less than 10 isolates
- Not included

- Liechtenstein
- Luxembourg
- Malta

Figure 177-6 Prevalence of penicillin-resistant *Streptococcus pneumoniae* isolates in participating countries in 2012. (http://www.ecdc.europa.eu/en/healthtopics/antimicrobial_resistance/database/Pages/map_reports.aspx.)

NETs is DNA that is able to entrap bacteria and kill it with associated antimicrobial factors. DNAses expressed by GAS can degrade NETs and protect against this mechanism of neutrophil-mediated killing.[74]

Leukotoxins

GAS leukotoxin streptolysin O (SLO) is able to form pores in host cell membranes, including neutrophils, macrophages and epithelial cells, which will lead to host cell apoptosis. SLO is co-transcribed with the toxin NAD-glycohydrolase (NADase) which can enter through SLO-induced pores and further damage host cells by depleting energy stores. Another GAS leukotoxin streptolysin S (SLS) is lytic toward a broad range of target cells including epithelial cells, lymphocytes, erythrocytes and platelets and is responsible for the beta hemolytic phenotype of GAS.[78]

Secreted Toxins

The streptococcal pyrogenic toxins, (SPE)A, C, G-M, streptococcal superantigen SSA, and streptococcal mitogenic exotoxin SMEZ, all have superantigenic properties able to trigger massive nonspecific T-cell proliferation, resulting in inflammatory cytokine release (Figure 177-9). These toxins are thought to be responsible for scarlet fever and streptococcal toxic shock syndrome.[79] The advantage of these toxins to the bacterium is unclear but generation of a nonspecific response

may prevent the host immune system producing a bacterium-targeted response.

GROUPS C AND G STREPTOCOCCI

The group C/G streptococcus *Strep. dysgalactiae* subsp. *equisimilis* is able to cause a significant amount of human infection in a similar manner to group A streptococcus and they share several virulence factors.[80] These virulence factors include M protein, C5a peptidase, leukotoxins SLO and SLS, and DNAses.[81] *Strep. equisimilis* is also able to cause toxic shock syndrome, although no isolates have been found carrying superantigens other than SpeG, which was subsequently shown to be inactive.[80] Group C streptococcus *Strep. zooepidemicus*, which can cause zoonotic infection in humans, produces a hyaluronic acid capsule, a chemokine cleaving protease and superantigens.

GROUP B STREPTOCOCCI (GBS)

GBS produce a sialic acid-rich capsular polysaccharide which, like the hyaluronic acid capsule of GAS, provides a critical defense mechanism against opsonophagocytosis.[82,83] There are 10 different GBS capsule serotypes, designated Ia, Ib, II-VIII and the recently identified IX; each unique in their repeating monosaccharide structures.[83] Crucially, sialic acid is present in all capsule serotypes and this confers protection from immune recognition through molecular mimicry as it is also present

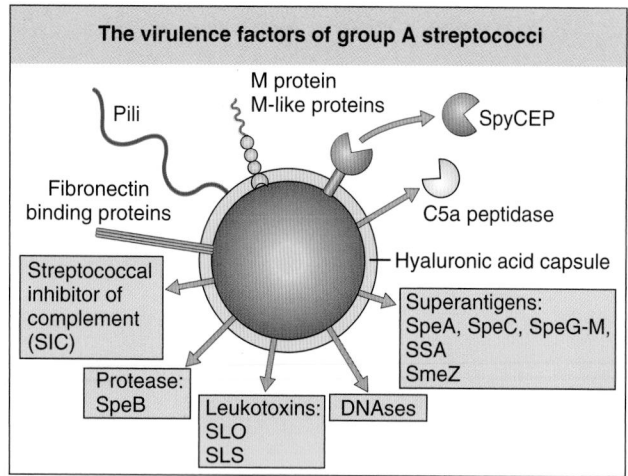

Figure 177-7 The virulence factors of group A streptococci. The hyaluronic acid capsule is secreted by the bacterium and surrounds it. SpyCEP is both cell wall anchored and secreted. SLO; streptolysin O, SLS; streptolysin S.

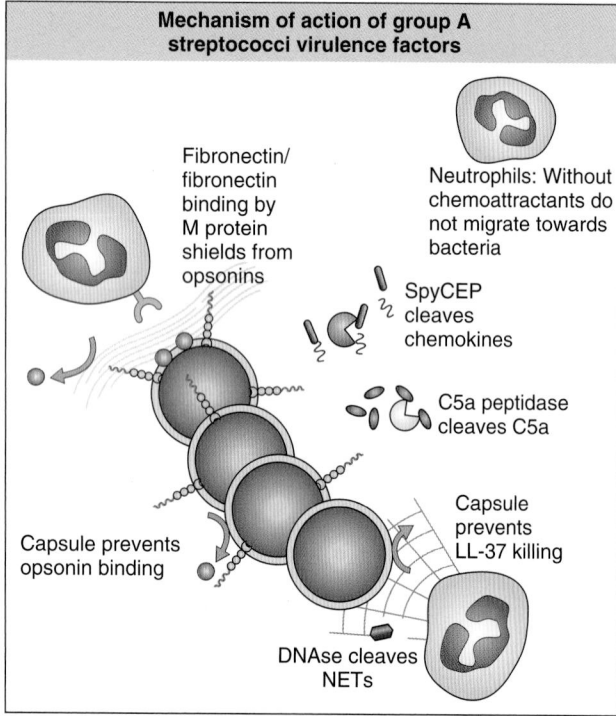

Figure 177-8 Mechanism of action of group A streptococci virulence factors. Neutrophil extracellular traps (NETs) are composed of DNA which can be degraded by streptococcal DNAses. Within NETs there are antimicrobial peptides, such as LL-37, which can be inhibited by the streptococcal inhibitor of complement (SIC) as well as the hyaluronic acid capsule. The M protein and M-like proteins can bind fibrinogen/fibronectin which, like the hyaluronic acid capsule, can prevent opsonins from binding and shield epitopes and any bound opsonins from the neutrophil receptors. SpyCEP and C5a peptidase cleave and inactivate chemokines and C5a, respectively, preventing neutrophil recruitment and activation.

on the surface of host cells. The capsule also prevents opsonizing C3b deposition on the bacterial cell surface and can limit the production of complement chemoattractant C5a.[82,83] Resistance to the complement system is also provided by C5a peptidase ScpB, which acts in the same manner as ScpA from GAS, and BibA which, in addition to a role in adherence, also binds complement regulator C4BP.[84]

Pore-forming toxins expressed by GBS include β-hemolysin/cytolysin (β-H/C) and CAMP, which can disrupt host cells including

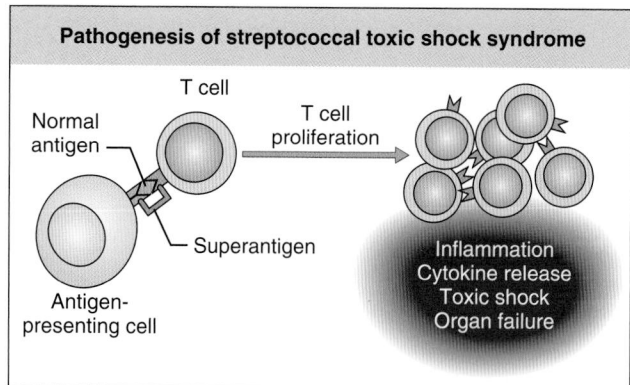

Figure 177-9 Pathogenesis of streptococcal toxic shock syndrome. Streptococcal superantigens lead to unregulated T-cell activation resulting in toxic shock syndrome and organ failure. A normal antigen is presented to a T cell from an antigen-presenting cell through the MHC class II receptor to the T-cell receptor. A streptococcal superantigen bypasses this system to cross-link the MHC class II receptor to the variable beta-chain of T-cell receptor. The Vβ specificity demonstrated by superantigens means that a given superantigen can activate up to 20% of circulating T cells. The result is uncontrolled cell expansion and cytokine release leading to inflammation, toxicity and multiple organ failure. (Adapted from[79] Reglinski, M., Sriskandan, S. The contribution of group A streptococcal virulence determinants to the pathogenesis of sepsis. Virulence 2014; 5:127-136.)

phagocytes and epithelial cells contributing to opsonophagocytosis resistance and bacterial pathogenesis and dissemination.[82,83]

Like GAS, GBS can alter their surface charge to enhance their resistance to antimicrobial peptides. In addition, the backbone component of pilus, PilB and the surface-anchored penicillin-binding protein PBP1a also enhances resistance to antimicrobial peptides.[82,83]

An important step in GBS disease is adherence to mucosal surfaces. Binding of fibrinogen by the bacterium can aid in adherence, biofilm formation, invasion of host epithelial cells and, as previously described, evasion of opsonophagocytosis. Three fibrinogen binding proteins have been described in GBS; FbsA, FbsB[83] and a recently identified FbsC.[85] FbsC (also known as BsaB) is able to bind fibronectin as well as fibrinogen, contributing significantly to host cell interactions.[85,86] Mutants lacking FbsA, the laminin-binding protein LmB or the pilus protein PilB had reduced adherence or invasion of brain microvascular endothelial cells, suggesting they are essential for the bacterium to cross the blood–brain barrier and go on to cause meningitis.

Many strains of GBS express the C antigen on their surface. The C antigen comprises either or both α protein and β protein. The family of α proteins, which include α, R28, Rib and Alp2, vary significantly in size due to the number of repeat regions. The function of these proteins is unclear but they may play a role in adherence. The β protein can bind the complement inhibitor, Factor H and the Fc region of immunoglobulin A.[83,87]

ENTEROCOCCI

Members of the genus *Enterococcus*, despite their ability to cause a range of disease, display relatively low virulence and do not produce pro-inflammatory toxins like many streptococci species.[88] Their pathogenic success seems to stem from their natural ability to maintain and exchange extra-chromosomal plasmids that can be associated with virulence factors or antibiotic-resistance mechanisms, allowing them to adapt to different environments. The ability of *Enterococcus* to adhere, aggregate and form biofilm contributes significantly to the nature of enterococcal disease, particularly endocarditis, but also allows the bacterium to survive for long periods on environmental surfaces.[88] A number of adhesins have been implicated in these processes including microbial surface components recognizing adhesive matrix molecules (MSCRAMMs) and the *E. faecalis* proteins Ace and Esp, or Acm and Esp of *E. faecium*.[88,89] Biofilm formation and adherence to host tissue may also be mediated by the plasmid-encoded enterococcal aggregation substance proteins and the enterococcal pili.

Capsular polysaccharides, encoded by the *epa* cluster, mediate resistance to phagocytic killing of both *E. faecalis* and *E. faecium*.[90] Extracellular toxins such as cytolysin, gelatinase and a serine protease also contribute to *E. faecalis* pathogenesis.[88]

STREPTOCOCCUS PNEUMONIAE

Like the other streptococci described, the ability of the pneumococcus to cause disease hinges on its ability to colonize successfully and to evade the complement system[91,92] (Figure 177-10). Pneumococcal infections often occur after a viral respiratory tract infection that has damaged the epithelium, aiding the pneumococci to establish themselves in the mucous membranes. Factors that disrupt the normal clearing process in the airways also predispose patients to pneumococcal lung infections. Defects in systemic host defenses (i.e. HIV infection, asplenia, immunoglobulin deficiency) may also contribute to pneumococcal infections and can lead to more invasive infections such as bacteremia, meningitis and endocarditis.

Expression of a polysaccharide capsule is important for survival in blood and is strongly associated with the ability of *Strep. pneumoniae* to cause invasive disease. Like other streptococcal capsules, the pneumococcal capsule presents a shield against complement and antibody binding. The pneumococcal capsule is structurally distinct for the 90 known serotypes. During mucosal colonization, the capsule prevents entrapment in mucus allowing the bacterium to reach the epithelial surface for attachment.[93] At the epithelium, however, capsule expression is switched off as it impedes interactions between bacterial adhesins and host ligands.[93]

Phosphorylcholine (*P*Cho), a component of pneumococcal cell wall-associated acids and lipoteichoic acids, mediates interactions with host factors through pneumococcal *P*Cho-binding proteins PspA and PspC (also known as CbpA or SpsA). PspA can protect the bacterium from the antimicrobial apolactoferrin (ALF) and can also limit C3b deposition.[91-93] PspC can bind polymeric immunoglobulin receptor (PIgR) providing a mechanism for host cell attachment. PspC also

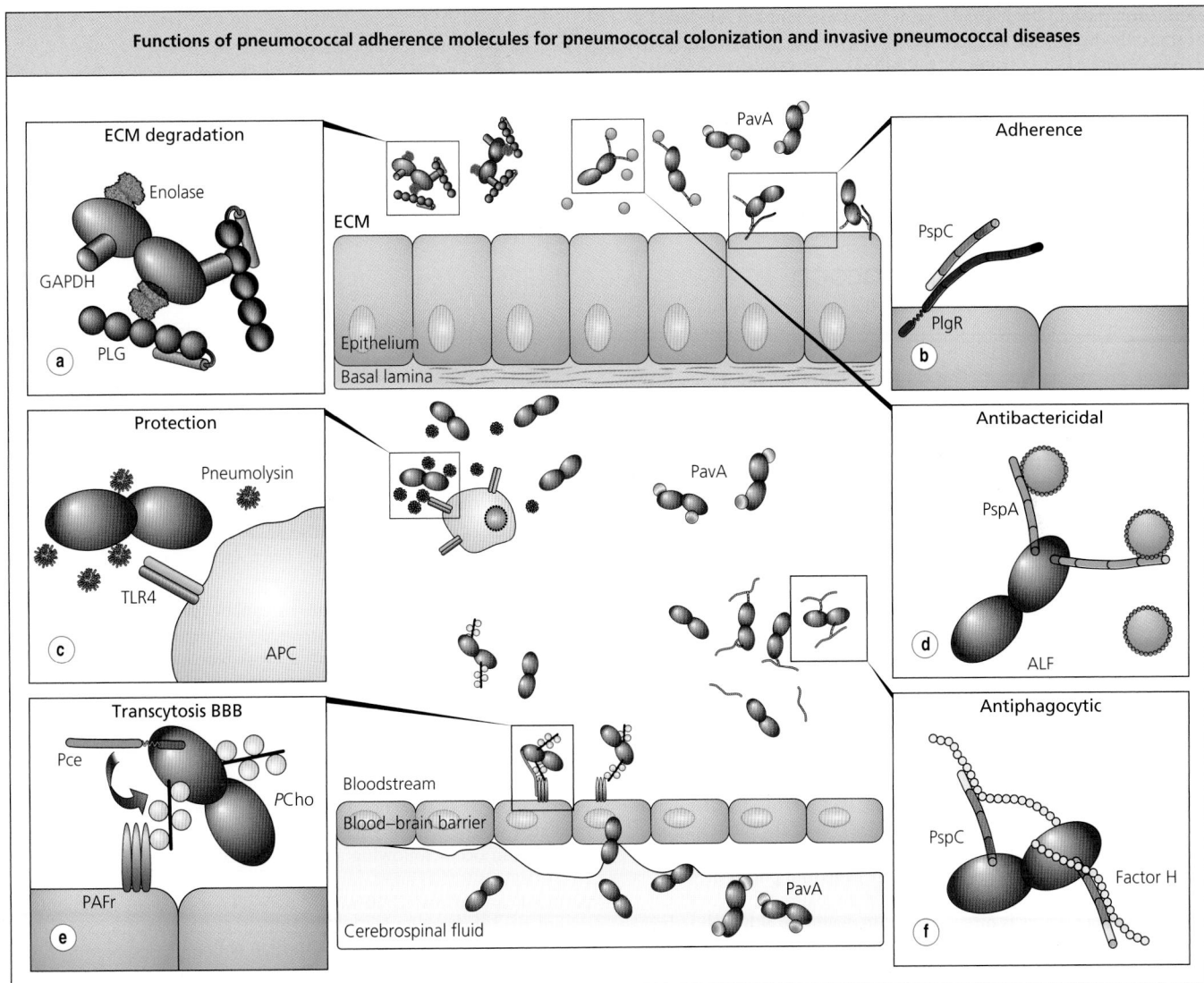

Figure 177-10 Functions of pneumococcal adherence molecules for pneumococcal colonization and invasive pneumococcal diseases. (a) The acquisition of plasmin(ogen) (PLG) by binding to surface-exposed GAPDH and enolase promotes degradation of the extracellular matrix (ECM). (b) The adhesin PspC mediates adherence of pneumococci to epithelial cells through binding to PIgR. (d) Binding of antimicrobial apolactoferrin (ALF) by PspA on mucosal surfaces protects against the bactericidal effect of ALF. (f) Within the blood, binding of complement regulator Factor H by PspC/Hic protects against complement-mediated phagocytosis and (c) pneumolysin functions as the pathogen-associated molecular pattern for Toll-like receptor 4 (TLR4) on antigen-presenting cells (APC). It is suggested that the pneumolysin–TLR4 interaction provides protection against the innate immune response of the host. (e) On stimulated cells, the PAFr is targeted by the *P*Cho of pneumococci. This interaction is involved in transcytosis of pneumococci through the blood–brain barrier (BBB). The amount of *P*Cho is modulated by another choline-binding protein, the Pce protein. PavA, a fibronectin-binding protein of pneumococci, has also been shown to have a crucial impact on pneumococcal adherence and invasive diseases including sepsis and meningitis. (*Adapted from*[92] *Hammerschmidt, S.: Curr Opin Microbiol 2006; 9:12-20.*)

provides protection against complement through binding of Factor H.[91-93] PCho can be involved directly in adherence by binding to the receptor for platelet activating factor (rPAF); binding also activates host cell signaling and can aid in transcytosis across the blood–brain barrier.[92] Other adhesins include PavA, PavB and PfbA, which can bind fibronectin, and enolase and PsrP, which can bind plasminogen and keratin respectively.[91-94] Pneumococcus can also express pili which may also contribute to adherence.[95]

OTHER/NONPYOGENIC STREPTOCOCCI

The streptococcal species generally considered to be commensals, particularly oral commensals, are also capable of causing endocarditis, bacteremia and abscesses. Of the oral streptococci, *Strep. mitis* is the leading cause of endocarditis and bacteremia and is closely related to the more pathogenic pneumococcus. Some known virulence factors of pneumococcus are also shared by *Strep. mitis*, including autolysins, PCho-binding proteins and adhesins. It does not produce a polysaccharide capsule, which may limit its pathogenicity, but does show tolerance to antimicrobial peptides. In addition *Strep. mitis* is able to produce an immunoglobulin A1 protease, which may aid resistance to clearance by the immune response.[96]

The *Streptococcus anginosus* group (SAG) rarely cause endocarditis but are often found in blood cultures and abscesses. Abscess formation suggests some ability to interact with neutrophils but this has not been fully elucidated. Some SAG strains do produce a capsule that is similar to the pneumococcal capsule. They are also able to produce an SLS homolog and DNAses.[97]

Clinical Manifestations

GROUPS A, C AND G STREPTOCOCCI

Group A streptococcus is considered the most pathogenic species of β-hemolytic streptococci. *Strep. dysgalactiae* subsp. *equisimilis* has also emerged as an important human pathogen able to cause a similar range of disease as GAS.[80] The clinical syndromes can range from uncomplicated superficial infections to severe and potentially lethal invasive infections, and can also include autoimmune sequelae.

Superficial Infections

Uncomplicated Throat Infections. See also Chapter 25.

Uncomplicated Skin Infections. Streptococci can cause skin infections of various forms and the clinical features are determined by which skin layers are infected:

- infections immediately below the stratum corneum result in impetigo;
- infections in the epidermis can give rise to ecthyma; and
- infections in the dermis give rise to erysipelas and cellulitis.

Clinical descriptions of these conditions can be found in Chapter 10.

Invasive Infections

GAS can cause severe invasive disease that can be lethal. Examples are bacteremia, puerperal sepsis, pneumonia, septic arthritis, meningitis and necrotizing fasciitis.[74] The skin often serves as the main portal of entry, in particular when damaged by varicella co-infection, penetrating injuries or burns, although in many cases the portal of entry is unknown and there can be a history of blunt trauma.[98]

Necrotizing fasciitis is often difficult to diagnose; although redness and bullae may be visible, edema is sometimes the only superficial sign. Discrepancy between the unimpressive clinical observations and the extremely severe pain indicated by the patient is then the only clue to the correct diagnosis. Subsequent surgery may reveal massive tissue necrosis along the fascial planes. Invasive disease may be complicated by clinically defined streptococcal toxic shock syndrome (Box 177-1),[99] which culminates in hypotension and multiple organ failure. Despite adequate antibiotic treatment and intensive care, STSS-associated infections are characterized by a high mortality rate of between 23% and 81%.[74]

BOX 177-1 DEFINITION FOR STREPTOCOCCAL TOXIC SHOCK-LIKE SYNDROME[99]

I. Isolation of GAS from:
  A. Normally sterile site (e.g. blood, cerebrospinal, pleural or peritoneal fluid, tissue biopsy, surgical wound, etc.)
  B. Nonsterile site (e.g. throat, sputum, vagina, superficial skin lesion, etc.)
II. Clinical signs of severity
  A. Hypotension: systolic blood pressure ≤90 mmHg in adults or <5th percentile for age in children
  and
  B. 2 or greater of the following signs:
  - Renal impairment: creatinine ≥177 µM for adults or ≥2 × the upper limit of normal for age. In patients with pre-existing renal disease, a ≥twofold elevation over the baseline level
  - Coagulopathy: platelets ≤100 × 10⁹/L or disseminated intravascular coagulation defined by prolonged clotting times, low fibrinogen level and the presence of fibrin degradation products
  - Liver involvement: alanine aminotransferase, aspartate aminotransferase or total bilirubin levels ≥2 × the upper limit of normal for age. In patients with pre-existing liver disease, a ≥twofold elevation over the baseline level.
  - Adult respiratory distress syndrome defined by acute onset of diffuse pulmonary infiltrates and hypoxemia in the absence of cardiac failure or evidence of diffuse capillary leak manifested by acute onset of generalized edema or pleural or peritoneal effusions with hypoalbuminemia
  - Generalized erythematous macular rash that may desquamate
  - Soft-tissue necrosis, including necrotizing fasciitis or myositis or gangrene.

An illness fulfilling criteria IA and II (A and B) is defined as a definite case; an illness fulfilling criteria IB and II (A and B) is defined as a probable case if no other etiology for the disease is identified.

Although considered a 'historical disease' there has been a recent and unexplained increase in severe maternal sepsis caused by GAS following child birth (post-partum sepsis). Symptoms can occur within 24–48 hours post-partum, but is defined as maternal infection within 30 days of giving birth. Disease can be wide ranging, including pneumonia, bacteremia, necrotizing fasciitis and STSS, meaning diagnosis and treatment can be delayed.[100]

Autoimmune Sequelae

In some cases, streptococcal disease is followed by autoimmune sequelae, either acute rheumatic fever (see Chapter 52) or acute glomerulonephritis.

Acute Rheumatic Fever. Acute rheumatic fever (ARF) is a delayed, nonsuppurative sequela of an untreated pharyngeal infection, thought to be caused by the development of cross-reacting antibodies. Symptoms of ARF can vary between patients and so clinical diagnosis of initial attacks of ARF are made based on the updated Jones criteria (Table 177-2).

Acute Glomerulonephritis. Acute poststreptococcal glomerulonephritis (APSGN) is an immune-complex mediated disease that can be triggered by streptococcal antigens and followed by complement-mediated injury. Unlike ARF which follows a pharyngeal infection, APSGN can occur following a skin infection, with a latent period of 14-21 days, as well as an upper respiratory tract infection, with a latent period of approximately 10 days.[101] APSGN occurs most commonly in school-aged children and in less high-income countries incidence rates have been estimated at 24.3 per 100 000 children compared to 6 per 100 000 in high-income countries.[40] Among Australian Aboriginal children living in remote communities, where scabies is common and streptococcal pyoderma is endemic, APSGN occurs in a sporadic and epidemic form with rates as high as 94.3 cases per 100 000 children.[102,103] In these remote communities, high levels of chronic kidney disease and end-stage renal failure occur in adults, likely due to repeat or prolonged APSGN during childhood.[103] Diagnosis is on the basis of the clinical presentation in combination with evidence of a recent infection (in the previous 1–6 weeks) with GAS. Patients typically present with

TABLE 177-2	Revised Jones Criteria for the Diagnosis of Poststreptococcal Rheumatic Fever		
Major Manifestations	**Minor Manifestations**		
Carditis	Clinical	Previous rheumatic fever or rheumatic heart disease	
Polyarthritis		Arthralgia	
Chorea		Fever	
Erythema marginatum	Laboratory	Acute phase reactants	
Subcutaneous nodules		Leukocytosis	
Positive throat culture		Elevated erythrocyte sedimentation rate	
Increased titer(s)		Elevated C-reactive protein	
Recent scarlet fever		Prolonged P–R interval on electrocardiogram	
		Supporting evidence of streptococcal infection (positive throat culture, positive rapid streptococcal antigen test, elevated or rising streptococcal antibody titer)	

The presence of two major criteria or of one major and two minor criteria is highly suggestive of rheumatic fever, if supported by evidence of preceding group A streptococcal infection.
Adapted from[121] Gerber et al. Circulation 2009; 119:1541-1551.

hematuria and proteinuria. Arterial hypertension and edema are common, due to water and salt retention. Proliferative glomerulonephritis with diffuse hypercelluarity can be observed by histopathology. C3 and IgG deposits can be observed by immunohistochemistry in early biopsies, while IgM, IgA and other complement components are rarely detected. Three patterns of immunohistochemistry have been identified. In the early stages of disease the 'starry sky' pattern is typically observed with subepithelial granular deposits scattered in the tuft and is associated with diffuse endocapillary proliferation. In approximately 25% of early biopsies a 'garland' pattern may be observed as large granular deposits form in the basal membrane which may also be associated with subendothelial and mesangial deposits. The third is a 'mesangial' pattern which occurs in later stages of disease and corresponds to mesangial proliferation with deposits of C3 in the mesangium. Large electron-dense deposits can be observed by electron microscopy as humps in the capillary walls located on the epithelial side of the basal membrane.[104]

For children the outcome is generally favorable, with the majority of cases being self-limiting with supportive care.[101] Infection in adults, however, can be more aggressive and 25% may require dialysis and a complete recovery is only seen in 40–50% of patients.[104] In contrast to ARF, recurrences with subsequent GAS infection are rare and therefore long-term antibiotic prophylaxis is not required.[101] During an outbreak situation there is evidence to suggest that community-wide administration of penicillin can halt continuing transmission, but treatment may not prevent the development of APSGN.[101,105]

Chorea and Other Neurologic Syndromes. Sydenham's chorea (St Vitus' dance) is characterized by rapid involuntary movements, sometimes associated with emotional lability and other neuropsychiatric features.[106] Approximately 10% of patients with ARF can present with Sydenham's chorea, in which case diagnosis is relatively easy. However, it may present many years later as a seemingly distinct clinical syndrome, making the association with past streptococcal infection in these cases very difficult.

Additionally, a syndrome termed 'poststreptococcal autoimmune neuropsychiatric disorder associated with streptococci' (PANDAS) has been described to encompass a range of neurologic conditions such as tics and obsessive compulsive disorder.[107] The precise relationship with streptococcal infection is unclear, but is currently being investigated under the auspices of a Pan-European study (http://www.emtics.eu).

GROUP B STREPTOCOCCI

Neonatal Disease

GBS are a leading cause of bacteremia and meningitis in neonates. Most early-onset (within first week of life) GBS infections are thought to be transmitted to the infant from the maternal genital tract during delivery (see Practice Point 17).

Approximately half of early-onset GBS infections occurs in infants born to mothers with recognized obstetric risk factors, namely premature onset of labor, prolonged rupture of membranes before delivery, maternal fever, anogenital colonization of the mother and having a previous child with infant GBS disease.[108] Clinical presentations of early-onset disease include sepsis, pneumonia and meningitis. Prematurity is a key risk factor for late onset (7–90 days of age) disease with these cases having a higher likelihood of developing meningitis, linked to higher frequency of capsular serotype III infection. Given a substantial proportion of children with GBS sepsis develop meningitis, lumbar punctures should be performed in all infants with suspected sepsis. Overall mortality rate for infant GBS is around 5–10% with close to half of meningitis survivors suffering long-term neurodevelopmental sequelae.[109,110] Death rates are generally lower for late than in early-onset disease.

Adult Disease

Epidemiological changes in invasive GBS infection are resulting in increasing incidence of adult disease. Two groups of adults are at increased risk of GBS infection: pregnant women and patients with serious underlying disease, in particular diabetes mellitus, malignancy, and cardiovascular disease. The spectrum of GBS disease in nonpregnant adults is very wide and includes bacteremia with or without sepsis, cellulitis and other soft-tissue infections, pneumonia, arthritis, meningitis, osteomyelitis, endocarditis and urinary tract infection. Case fatality rates are higher in nonpregnant adults with invasive GBS than infants, ranging from 12–25%.[62] Clinical presentations in pregnancy-associated infections include focal and non-focal bacteremia, genital tract sepsis, bacteremic chorioamnionitis, pneumonia and endocarditis. Pregnancy outcomes in such women are often poor with around half resulting illness including spontaneous abortions and stillbirths.[110]

ENTEROCOCCI

Initially thought of as merely harmless commensals because of their low intrinsic virulence compared with other organisms, such as GAS, enterococci have become the third most common nosocomial pathogen overall. This appears to have been caused by selection of these organisms by the widespread use of broad-spectrum antibiotics, such as the cephalosporins, which lack enterococcal activity, and acquisition of new mechanisms of antibiotic resistance.[111] Infections commonly caused by enterococci include urinary tract infection (UTIs), endocarditis, bacteremia, catheter-related infections, wound infections, and intra-abdominal and pelvic infections. Many infecting strains originate from the patient's intestinal flora. From here, they can spread and cause UTI, intra-abdominal infection and surgical wound infection. Bacteremia may result with subsequent seeding of more distant sites. Meningitis, pleural space infections, and skin and soft-tissue infections have also been reported. Individuals at risk for colonization include critically ill patients who have received lengthy courses of antibiotics (particularly those in long-term care facilities), solid organ transplant recipients and patients with hematologic malignancies, and healthcare workers. Unfortunately, spontaneous decolonization is uncommon, and antimicrobials are unlikely to eradicate VRE colonization. Identified risk factors for VRE bacteremia include prior intestinal colonization, prior long-term antibiotic use, increased severity of illness, hematologic malignancy, bone marrow transplant, mucositis, neutropenia, indwelling urinary catheters, corticosteroid treatment, chemotherapy and parenteral nutrition.

It has been reported that 60% of enterococcal infections are nosocomial, with half of them occurring in intensive care units. Originally,

E. faecalis was responsible for 80–90% of enterococcal infections and *E. faecium* for 10–20%.[66,106] This ratio, however, has changed during the last decade in favor of *E. faecium*.

STREPTOCOCCUS PNEUMONIAE

Streptococcus pneumoniae is an important agent of human disease at the extremities of age and in those who have underlying disease. Pneumococcal disease is most commonly associated with an antecedent viral respiratory infection, such as influenza, or with chronic conditions such as chronic obstructive pulmonary disease, diabetes mellitus, congestive heart failure, renal failure, smoking and alcoholism. Immunodeficiency such as that caused by splenic dysfunction or splenectomy is an additional risk factor for the development of severe pneumococcal disease because of decreased bacterial clearance and defective production of antibodies.

The pneumococcus can cause noninvasive or invasive disease and is a common cause of community-acquired pneumonia (CAP), meningitis and bacteremia in both children and adults.[112]

Pneumococcal pneumonia is discussed in Chapter 28; pneumococcal meningitis in Chapter 19.

NONPYOGENIC, OTHER STREPTOCOCCI

These streptococci are usually found as normal inhabitants of the oral cavity, the upper respiratory tract and the bowel. When these organisms gain access to the bloodstream, people who have damaged heart valves are at increased risk of endocarditis. Infection is usually endogenous and is preceded by disease, dental extraction or trauma to a mucosal surface. It is often associated with an immunocompromised condition. However, although blood cultures that are positive for α-hemolytic streptococci or non-hemolytic streptococci have no clinical relevance in many cases, it has been estimated that approximately 21% of blood cultures are clinically significant. If the same strain is isolated from more than one blood culture bottle or is isolated on repeated occasions, the assumption of clinical relevance is strengthened. A special population prone to develop infections with other streptococci is those with hematologic malignancies who are treated with cytotoxic drugs with high cytotoxicity for mucosal surfaces. The course of infection in these patients may vary from mild to highly severe, with shock, adult respiratory distress syndrome and death.

The 'Strep. anginosus group' are considered commensals of the human mouth, throat and gastrointestinal and genital tracts, but may cause opportunistic infections such as bacteremia, and serious purulent infections in sites of the oral, thoracic, abdominal and central nervous system.[108] In addition, studies have identified members of the anginosus group as etiologically important in pulmonary exacerbations in patients with cystic fibrosis.[108]

The main species within the 'Strep. bovis' group (SBG) are *Streptococcus gallolyticus* subsp. *gallolyticus* (formerly Strep. bovis biotype I), *Strep. gallolyticus* subsp. *pasteurianus* (biotype II/2), *Strep. infantarius* subsp. *infantarius* and *Streptococcus lutetiensis* (biotype II/1). *Strep. gallolyticus* subsp. *macedonicus* is also a member of the group, but is generally considered as nonpathogenic for humans.

Because there is a strong association between infections with the SBG, notably *Strep. gallolyticus* subsp. *gallolyticus* and colonic neoplasms and other lesions of the gastrointestinal tract, evaluation of the gastrointestinal tract with colonoscopy is important for patients with infections due to this organism.[114]

The other two 'groups' are mutans and salivarius. The 'mutans group' is most commonly isolated from the oral cavity and the main species are *Strep. mutans*, *Strep. sobrinus*, *Strep. cricetus* and *Strep. ratti*.

The mutans group comprises seven species, with *Strep. mutans* being the main causative organism of dental caries.[115] *Streptococcus mutans* resides in the mouth and can thrive in temperatures ranging from 18-40°C. It metabolizes different kinds of carbohydrates, creating an acidic environment in the mouth that causes the tooth decay, and *Strep. mutans* is considered to be the most cariogenic of all of the oral streptococci. They occasionally cause bacteremia, abscesses and infective endocarditis.[116]

The 'salivarius group' colonizes the mouth and upper respiratory tract of humans a few hours after birth, making further exposure to the bacteria harmless in most circumstances. The bacteria are considered opportunistic pathogens, rarely finding their way into the bloodstream, where they have been implicated in cases of sepsis in people with neutropenia. Some strains of *Strep. salivarius* are being trialed for their use as a probiotic in the prevention of oral infections.

Management

GROUPS A, C AND G STREPTOCOCCI

Penicillin is the traditional first-choice therapy for infections caused by groups A, C or G streptococci. *Strep. pyogenes* is still extremely sensitive to penicillin, and erythromycin is a good alternative in case of penicillin allergy. However, there has been an increase in the prevalence of erythromycin-resistant GAS strains over the past 20 years. Notable outbreaks of macrolide resistant strains have also occurred in some countries.[116] Generally, macrolide resistance exists in 5–10% of strains.[116]

Failure of GAS infection to respond to penicillin therapy may occur in some patients, leading to prolonged carriage or recurrent infection. The mechanism behind this is unclear but may be due to internalization of the bacterium into host cells or the formation of resistant biofilm.[74]

Rapid diagnosis and immediate treatment of severe and life-threatening necrotizing fasciitis and streptococcal toxic shock syndrome are essential.[99] Surgery (debridement of necrotic tissue or even amputation) is the key event in the treatment of necrotizing fasciitis. Treatment with penicillin in combination with a protein synthesis inhibitor such as clindamycin, to inhibit toxin production, is the therapy of choice.[118] The addition of pooled human intravenous immunoglobulin may also aid in treatment of severe infection,[118] although clinical trial data are lacking.

GROUP B STREPTOCOCCI

GBS remain susceptible to penicillin. However, the minimum inhibitory concentration (MIC) of penicillin G for GBS is considerably higher (average 0.04 µg/mL) than that observed for GAS with recent reports from the Far East and USA documenting clinical isolates with reduced susceptibility to penicillin. Resistance to erythromycin and clindamycin occurs in 15–20% of invasive isolates and tetracycline resistance is seen in 80–90% of isolates.

ENTEROCOCCI

The antibiotic resistance of *Enterococcus* is well documented and has been of concern for many years. Resistance rates (particularly to glycopeptides) have reached endemic or epidemic proportions in North America, with Europe having lower but increasing levels. Hence, antimicrobial therapy for enterococcal infections is complicated because most antibiotics are not bactericidal at clinically relevant concentrations. Combination therapy with a cell wall agent plus an aminoglycoside improves the outcome of enterococcal endocarditis and probably of enterococcal meningitis, but may not improve the outcome in bacteremia. High-level aminoglycoside resistance, vancomycin resistance and high-level ampicillin resistance are increasing in prevalence.

Enterococcus faecium is typically high-level penicillin- and ampicillin-resistant and this type of resistance has been reported as a significant predictor of lack of cure. Therapy of enterococcal infections caused by vancomycin-resistant *E. faecium* is very difficult because these organisms are usually resistant to alternative antibiotics currently available. The newly developed streptogramins (quinupristin and dalfopristin), oxazolidinones (linezolid), daptomycin and tigecycline appeared promising against VRE. Nitrofurantoin is active against many strains of VRE and should be useful for UTIs.

Streptococcus gallolyticus should be 'differentiated' from the enterococci because it is usually susceptible to penicillin alone, and both endocarditis and meningitis due to *Strep. gallolyticus* have a better prognosis.

STREPTOCOCCUS PNEUMONIAE

Penicillin used to be the first-choice therapy for pneumococcal disease, and in penicillin-sensitive strains it still is. For patients who have penicillin allergy, cephalosporins and erythromycin are valuable alternatives.

Resistance to penicillin is associated with a decreased affinity of the antibiotic for penicillin-binding proteins present in the bacterial cell wall. Following widespread reports of increased resistance during the 1990s, the introduction of the conjugated PCV7 vaccine into routine childhood immunization schedules had a substantial impact in reducing antimicrobial resistance in adults and children with further decreases expected following the introduction of PCV13. Current estimates of penicillin nonsusceptibility in the USA stand at around 6%. Use of different breakpoints hampers direct comparison but penicillin nonsusceptibility above 10% is reported in several European countries with recent trends indicating a rise in prevalence (Figure 177-6).[119] A worrying increase in the prevalence of multidrug-resistant strains, such as serotype 19A, has been documented, potentially due to serotype replacement and capsular switching following the introduction of PCV7.[119,120]

International surveillance studies demonstrate a high global prevalence of macrolide resistance of up to 30% among pneumococcal isolates obtained from patients with community-acquired respiratory tract infections. Low-level resistance to macrolides (usually <16 μg/mL) is due to the *mefA* gene encoding an efflux pump. High antibiotic concentrations might overcome the pump and exert an antibacterial effect. High-level resistance is due to the *ermB* gene that encodes methylation of the 23S rRNA. In this case increasing the dose will exert little effect.

Remarkably, the rate of resistance to erythromycin, tetracycline and trimethoprim–sulfamethoxazole is much greater in penicillin-resistant strains than in penicillin-sensitive strains.

OTHER NONPYOGENIC STREPTOCOCCI

The other or nonpyogenic streptococci were considered to be uniformly susceptible to β-lactams, macrolides, lincosamines, rifampin (rifampicin) and vancomycin. Occasionally, however, mostly under the pressure of long-term penicillin therapy, serious infections due to penicillin-resistant or penicillin-tolerant strains have been reported. In endocarditis, high-dose penicillin in combination with an aminoglycoside is recommended. In cases of penicillin allergy, vancomycin is a good alternative. Surgical drainage remains central to the management of abscesses (caused by anginosus group) and is often augmented by antibiotics.

Prevention

The potentially serious nature of infections caused by streptococci mean that clinical and public health guidelines to prevent infection, minimize risk of complications and control spread to others are warranted. Preventive measures include:

- improved hygiene;
- communication of elevated risk;
- exclusion from workplace or school;
- bacteriological screening;
- antibiotic prophylaxis and treatment; and
- vaccination.

GROUP A STREPTOCOCCI

Whilst the clinical presentation is generally not severe for patients with superficial GAS infection, the potential for complication makes antibiotic therapy essential as a means to lower this risk as well as reducing onward transmission. No vaccine is at present available for protection against GAS infections, although intensive research is ongoing.

Large numbers of pyogenic streptococci are shed in the immediate environment, where the bacteria may be cultivated from clothing as well as from sheets and mattresses belonging to the infected person.

Whilst GAS infections are thought to be exclusively human pathogens, reports suggesting pets may act as a source of infection have been published. GCS infections are more firmly established as potentially zoonotic pathogens through close contact with infected horses.[120]

Primary prevention of rheumatic fever is dependent on successful management of pharyngitis. Criteria have been established to guide treatment of pharyngitis by identifying patients more likely to have an infection of GAS etiology.[120]

Individuals diagnosed with ARF will require long-term treatment to minimize risk of permanent damage to the heart (secondary prevention) (see Chapter 52 for details).[121] In contrast to rheumatic fever, the beneficial effect of penicillin prophylaxis in cases of glomerulonephritis has never been demonstrated, with relapses of glomerulonephritis occurring at such low frequency that prophylaxis is not warranted.

As a primarily community-acquired infection, assessments of secondary household risk from contact with invasive manifestations of GAS infection have been undertaken in the USA, Canada, UK and Australia, all of which pointed to a considerable elevation in risk.[29] The period of excess risk appears to be confined to within 4 weeks of the index case, with many 'secondary' cases presenting near simultaneously with the primary case, therefore limiting opportunities for prevention.[118,123] Different strategies for managing this risk have been adopted by different countries but include antibiotic prophylaxis to all close contacts or in selected situations.[122,124] Given the rapid onset of invasive GAS infection, provision of advice on signs and symptoms to be aware of is an essential component of risk management.

GROUP B STREPTOCOCCI

Studies have clearly demonstrated that intrapartum administration of penicillin reduces transmission GBS from the mother to the infant, and as such offers an effective intervention for the prevention of early-onset GBS infection. Different prevention strategies have been designed and deployed to target intrapartum antibiotic prophylaxis. These have been based on vaginal–rectal carriage detected through universal screening programs and/or identification of infants at increased risk on the basis of obstetric risk factors.[58] The risks and benefits of each approach remain highly controversial for countries with low incidence of infant GBS disease.

STREPTOCOCCUS PNEUMONIAE

A number of multivalent vaccines have been developed to target disease burden caused by specific pneumococcal serotypes. Currently there are two types of vaccine available for prevention of pneumococcal infections, namely the polyvalent pneumococcal conjugate vaccines (PCV: PCV7, PCV10, PCV13) and the plain pneumococcal polysaccharide vaccines (PPV23). The most common vaccines are the PPV containing polysaccharides from 23 serotypes (PPV23) and the PCV containing polysaccharide from 13 serotypes (PCV13), conjugated to a carrier protein that is nontoxic and nearly identical to diphtheria toxin (CRM197). PPV23 is specifically for adults and elicits an immune response via a T-cell independent mechanism whereas PCV13 for children elicits a T-cell dependent immune response. Many countries have reported changes in the prevalence of nonvaccine-related serotypes, felt likely to be due to antibiotic and vaccine selection combined with natural serotype variation.[70]

PREVENTION OF ENDOCARDITIS

Recommendations for the routine use of antibiotics for the prevention of (mainly streptococcal) endocarditis have recently been the subject of substantial review and discussion. More recently, guidelines for the diagnosis and antibiotic treatment of endocarditis in adults were published by a British Society for Antimicrobial Chemotherapy (BSAC) working party[125,126] (Table 177-3). For a more detailed discussion see Chapter 51.

TABLE 177-3	Endocarditis Prophylaxis
Patients at the highest risk	Prophylaxis was recommended only in those settings associated with the highest risk of developing an adverse outcome if infective endocarditis (IE) were to occur. Patients with the following cardiac conditions were considered to meet this criterion: • prosthetic heart valves, including bioprosthetic and homograft valves • a prior history of IE • unrepaired cyanotic congenital heart disease, including palliative shunts and conduits • completely repaired congenital heart defects with prosthetic material or device, whether placed by surgery or by catheter intervention, during the first 6 months after the procedure • repaired congenital heart disease with residual defects at the site or adjacent to the site of the prosthetic device • cardiac 'valvulopathy' in a transplanted heart (valvulopathy is defined as documentation of substantial leaflet pathology and regurgitation) Similar limited criteria for prophylaxis were proposed in 2006 by the Working Party of the British Society for Antimicrobial Chemotherapy (BSAC) and also more recently guidelines for the diagnosis and antibiotic treatment of endocarditis in adults have been published by the working party of BSAC in 2012.[127] 'Valvulopathy' in a transplanted heart was not included, but these guidelines also included complex left ventricular outflow abnormalities including aortic stenosis and bicuspid aortic valves, or acquired valvulopathy or mitral valve prolapse with echocardiographic evidence of substantial leaflet pathology and regurgitation
No longer indicated	Common valvular lesions for which antimicrobial prophylaxis is no longer recommended in the 2007 American Heart Association guidelines include: bicuspid aortic valve; acquired aortic or mitral valve disease (including mitral valve prolapse with regurgitation and those who have undergone prior valve repair); and hypertrophic cardiomyopathy with latent or resting obstruction

Adapted from[128] Wilson et al. Circulation 2007; 116:1736-1754.

STREPTOCOCCAL VACCINES

Vaccines have a significant impact on public health, and vaccinology in the era of genomics is taking advantage of new technologies to tackle diseases for which vaccine development has so far been unsuccessful.

Active efforts are underway to develop vaccines, primarily against GAS and GBS.[127,128] Currently these are not available for routine clinical use.

References available online at expertconsult.com.

KEY REFERENCES

Carapetis J.R., Steer A.C., Mulholland E.K., et al.: The global burden of group A streptococcal diseases. *Lancet Infect Dis* 2005; 5:685-694.

Edmond K.M., Kortsalioudaki C., Scott S., et al.: Group B streptococcal disease in infants aged younger than 3 months: systematic review and meta-analysis. *Lancet* 2012; 379:547-556.

Facklam R.: What happened to the streptococci: overview of taxonomic and nomenclature changes. *Clin Microbiol Rev* 2002; 15:613-630.

Fisher K., Phillips C.: The ecology, epidemiology and virulence of *Enterococcus*. *Microbiol* 2009; 155:1749-1757.

Gerber M.A., Baltimore R.S., Eaton C.B., et al.: Prevention of rheumatic fever and diagnosis and treatment of acute Streptococcal pharyngitis: a scientific statement from the American Heart Association Rheumatic Fever, Endocarditis, and Kawasaki Disease Committee of the Council on Cardiovascular Disease in the Young, the Interdisciplinary Council on Functional Genomics and Translational Biology, and the Interdisciplinary Council on Quality of Care and Outcomes Research: endorsed by the American Academy of Pediatrics. *Circulation* 2009; 119:1541-1551.

Gould K.F., Denning D.W., Elliott T.S.J., et al.: Guidelines for the diagnosis and treatment of endocarditis in adults: a report of the Working Party of the British Society for Antimicrobial Chemotherapy. *JAC* 2012; 67:269-289.

McMillan D.J., Danderson-Smith M.L., Smeesters P.R., et al.: Molecular markers for the study of streptococcal epidemiology. *Curr Top Microbiol Immunol* 2013; 368:29-48.

Rantala S.: *Streptococcus dysgalactiae* subsp. *equisimilis* bacteremia: an emerging infection. *Eur J Clin Microbiol Infect Dis* 2014; 33:1303-1310.

Reglinski M., Sriskandan S.: The contribution of group A streptococcal virulence determinants to the pathogenesis of sepsis. *Virulence* 2014; 5:127-136.

Steer A.C., Law I., Matatolu L., et al.: Global emm type distribution of group A streptococci: a systematic review and implications for vaccine development. *Lancet Infect Dis* 2009; 10:611-616.

Vernatter J., Pirofski L.: Current concepts in host-microbe interaction leading to pneumococcal pneumonia. *Curr Opin Infect Dis* 2013; 26:277-283.

Walker M.J., Barnett T.C., McArthur J.D., et al.: Disease manifestations and pathogenic mechanisms of group A streptococcus. *Clin Microbiol Rev* 2014; 27:264-301.

178

Aerobic Gram-Positive Bacilli

GUY PROD'HOM | JACQUES BILLE

KEY CONCEPTS

- Some aerobic gram-positive bacilli cause severe diseases, thanks to many virulence factors, and toxins in particular.

- The recent implementation of MALDI-TOF mass spectrometry in diagnostic microbiology has contributed to quicker and more accurate identification of aerobic gram-positive bacilli than before.

- *Listeria monocytogenes* is a food-borne pathogen targeting at-risk populations at the two extremes of life as well as the growing immunocompromised population.

- Interest in *Bacillus anthracis* has exploded after its implication in bioterrorism, leading to a huge increase of new knowledge on its pathogenicity, microbiologic diagnosis, prevention and treatment.

- Due to the low incidence of diphtheria, clinicians should inform the laboratory when a clinical case is suspected, since the laboratory should include specific laboratory procedures for *C. diphtheriae* detection.

- Among aerobic actinomycetes, *Nocardia* spp. represent the most important pathogen. Prolonged microbiologic culture is mandatory to enhance the rate of positive culture. MALDI-TOF mass spectrometry and 16S rRNA gene sequencing are becoming common diagnostic tools for species identification.

Introduction

The past 20 years have seen an explosion of new bacterial species being described, and aerobic gram-positive bacilli are not an exception. Although most of the new species have been recovered only occasionally from human material, the key representative species have enjoyed renewed interest, for very different reasons.

Listeria monocytogenes, feared for its high associated morbidity and mortality, has extended its clinical presentations from the classic invasive food-borne pathogen to a sporadic or epidemic gastroenteritis. *Bacillus anthracis*, once an occasional agent of cutaneous anthrax in exposed persons, is now the most studied agent of bioterrorism. *Corynebacterium* spp. also enjoy renewed attention with their propensity to colonize and infect foreign materials. Finally, *Nocardia* spp. are still a rare but classic finding in the growing population of severely immunosuppressed patients.

Thus, this chapter will essentially focus on the few pathogenic species that play a major role in infectious diseases. Practical algorithms will be proposed to speed up their preliminary identification (Figure 178-1). The major emphasis is on the laboratory diagnosis of these bacteria; their associated clinical presentations are discussed elsewhere in this book.

If most of the aerobic gram-positive rods have an irregular shape, the most important (*Listeria, Bacillus, Erysipelothrix*) have a regular one. Almost all are non-pigmented, except *Oerskovia*. All are nonsporeforming except *Bacillus* spp. A few exhibit filamentous growth: *Nocardia, Gordonia, Rhodococcus, Tsukamurella* and *Streptomyces*.

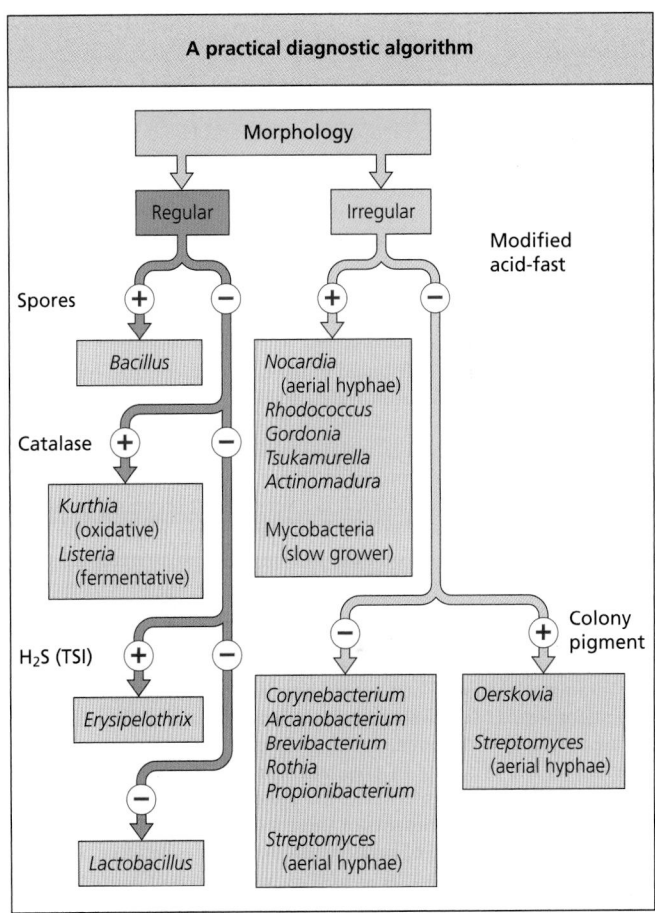

Figure 178-1 A practical diagnostic algorithm.

Commonly found aerobic gram-positive rods can be preliminarily differentiated by a few simple tests:

- *Listeria monocytogenes* is catalase-positive, motile and β-hemolytic on blood agar plates;
- *Bacillus* spp. display spores;
- *Erysipelothrix* is catalase-negative and produces H₂S in triple sugar iron (TSI) slants;
- *Corynebacterium* spp. are catalase-positive, club-shaped, non-branching rods.

Listeria monocytogenes

Nature

The genus *Listeria* comprises at least nine species, among them *L. monocytogenes, L. ivanovii, L. seeligeri, L. innocua, L. welshimeri* and *L.*

grayi. Only *L. monocytogenes* is regularly pathogenic for humans; *L. ivanovii* very rarely causes clinical disease but it is pathogenic for animals. The genus *Listeria* belongs to the *Clostridium* subdivision of gram-positive bacilli, where it forms a family with *Brochothrix* with a characteristic low G+C DNA content (<42%). The *Listeria* species are separated into two lineages, one comprising *L. monocytogenes*, *L. innocua* and *L. ivanovii*, and the other *L. welshimeri*, *L. seeligeri* and *L. grayi*.[1]

Morphologically, *Listeria* colonies appear as nonspore-forming, non-branching, regular short (0.5–2 × 0.4–0.5 µm) gram-positive rods occurring singly or in short chains. *Listeria* is motile at room temperature but not at 37°C (99°F). On blood agar plates, *Listeria* grows as smooth, gray, small colonies (1–2 mm in diameter after 1–2 days of incubation at 35°C (95°F)). Its growth is optimal at 35–37°C (95–99°F) in an aerobic atmosphere, but occurs also at lower temperatures (including refrigerator temperature), in an anaerobic atmosphere, at low pH (≥4.5) and in a high salt concentration (up to 10% NaCl).

Listeria spp. produce catalase but not oxidase, and characteristically hydrolyze esculin. Indole reaction is negative and H_2S is not produced. Acid production from various sugars allows a differentiation within species. In addition, *L. monocytogenes* is β-hemolytic on blood agar plates, and can be differentiated from another β-hemolytic species, *L. ivanovii*, by the CAMP reaction (enhancement of β-hemolysis in the vicinity of *Staphylococcus aureus* streak culture).[2]

Epidemiology

Listeria spp. are widely distributed in the environment, and have been regularly recovered from soil, water, sewage, vegetables and animal feed.

L. monocytogenes has been isolated from a wide variety of food or food products such as milk products, raw or transformed meat, smoked fish, seafood and raw vegetables. It is a very robust organism, resisting many adverse conditions in the food processing chain or during storage.[3] *L. monocytogenes* colonizes or causes disease in many animals, mainly in bovines, ovines and caprines, but also in fish, crustaceans and birds. In humans, it can be carried asymptomatically and transiently in feces in up to 5% of the healthy population.

L. monocytogenes infections are almost all caused by the ingestion of contaminated food. They occur as sporadic cases or as outbreaks. Two major forms of clinical presentation can occur: the classic invasive disease causing bacteremia, meningitis or meningoencephalitis or infection of the offspring in pregnant women, and the newly recognized, less severe gastroenteritis form.[4] Host factors and level of inoculum are the main determinants of these two presentations.

The annual incidence of invasive listeriosis varies between 3 and 15 cases per 10^6 population in countries with a surveillance system. Although much less common than *Salmonella* or *Campylobacter*, food-borne listeriosis is much more severe, with an associated hospitalization rate of more than 95%, and a mortality rate of 20–40%. At particular risk of developing an invasive disease are the populations at the two extremes of age, as well as some immunocompromised patients (transplant patients and those with HIV infection with a low CD4+ cell count). Other predisposing conditions are diabetes, untreated hemochromatosis, alcoholism, liver or renal insufficiency and a high gastric pH. During outbreaks, immunocompetent persons exposed to a high inoculum can develop invasive disease. Outbreaks of invasive cases have been ascribed to different food vehicles. Among them, milk products (in particular ripened cheese), raw or undercooked meat and smoked fish have been implicated. When known, the level of contamination has been as high as 10^5 to 10^6 cfu/g of food. In these outbreaks the proportion of the maternofetal versus nonpregnant adult cases has varied greatly, as well as the distribution between bacteremia, meningitis and meningoencephalitis cases.

Not all *L. monocytogenes* strains are able to cause an invasive disease or an outbreak. Whereas *L. monocytogenes* strains can be classified into three serogroups and 13 serotypes, only three usually cause invasive disease (serotypes 4b, 1/2a and 1/2b). Most of the outbreaks described were caused by *L. monocytogenes* serotype 4b and within this serotype by restricted clones defined by phage or various molecular typing methods. Recently it has been shown that only the isolates harboring an intact internalin sequence are associated with invasive disease.[5]

Outbreaks of gastroenteritis seem to be associated with different strains and particularly with a very high level of contamination (>10^6 cfu/g of food). Major vehicles have been milk-based beverages, various salads or cold prepared dishes served during hot weather.[6]

Small nosocomial outbreaks have occasionally occurred in neonatal wards.

Pathogenicity

The mechanisms of pathogenicity of *L. monocytogenes* from its ingestion to its multiplication in selected target organs are incompletely understood. The inoculum necessary to trigger an invasive infection is not known, but it probably varies according to the magnitude of defects in host defenses. Resistant to the pH of gastric fluid, *L. monocytogenes* cells first attach to epithelial cells of the intestinal mucosa. The initial event involves the bacterial surface protein internalin A (InIA), a potent virulence factor which attaches to E-cadherin, a transmembrane glycoprotein adhesin molecule at the surface of intestinal epithelial cells. E-cadherin interacts with actin which polymerizes. A second protein, internalin B (InIB), contributes to *Listeria* entry by a different mechanism.[7]

After entry into the cell, *Listeria* cells are able to escape from the internalization vacuole thanks to listeriolysin O (LLO), a pore-forming toxin. In the cytosol, *Listeria* replicates freely and moves by the recruitment and polymerization of actin at one pole of the bacterium, the surface protein ActA. Moving to the opposite surface of the cell, *Listeria* protrudes into the neighboring cell and, by cell-to-cell spread, is able to disseminate in tissues. Recent advances have been made in the understanding of the very peculiar tropism of *Listeria* for specialized tissues such as placenta or the central nervous system (CNS). Both have an E-cadherin at the surface of some specialized cells (syncytiotrophoblasts, choroid plexus epithelium), allowing attachment of the bacteria.[8]

Acquired immunity after infection is mediated by phagocytosis (by macrophages and monocytes), followed by binding of the bacterial peptides to major histocompatibility complex (MHC) class I molecules. This complex is then recognized by CD8+ cytotoxic T cells and by T-helper cells. Cytokines – interferon-gamma (IFNγ), macrophage colony-stimulating factor (M-CSF) and tumor necrosis factor (TNF) – are produced, which enhance host resistance. In the premature infant and the neonate, macrophage activation is delayed and the number of natural killer (NK) cells reduced, increasing the susceptibility to *Listeria*. Both antibodies against somatic (O) and flagellar (H) antigens are produced after infection, but their determination is too complex to be used for diagnosis. More recently, the detection of antibodies to listeriolysin O in the blood has been claimed to be both sensitive and specific, but has not yet been used extensively.

Diagnostic Microbiology
DIRECT EXAMINATION

Gram staining of clinical material should be attempted, particularly in normally sterile samples such as cerebrospinal fluid (CSF), amniotic fluid or placenta. Small gram-positive bacilli or coccobacilli are suggestive in an appropriate specimen.

Listeria may sometimes be confused with enterococci, streptococci or corynebacteria.

The sensitivity of Gram stain direct examination of CSF to detect *Listeria* is rather low (30–40%) due to the usual low number of organisms.[9] It is much higher in meconium or ear swabs of the infected neonate.

CULTURE

L. monocytogenes is easy to isolate from normally sterile clinical samples such as blood, CSF, placenta or amniotic fluid. These specimens can be plated onto blood agar plates and blood inoculated in standard blood culture bottles.

Normally contaminated samples such as stool, genital swabs, gastric fluid and ear swab require the addition of selective solid or liquid media.

Food samples require special handling, with selective enrichment steps and indicator media.

On solid media, *L. monocytogenes* will grow in 18–24 hours as small, grayish, smooth colonies with a discrete β-hemolysis underneath the colonies.

IDENTIFICATION

Key characteristics to identify *L. monocytogenes* from colonies on agar media are the Gram stain morphology, tumbling motility in a wet mount or in semisolid agar slant (Figure 178-2a), a positive catalase reaction and hydrolysis of esculin. A correct determination of hemolysis is essential to differentiate *L. monocytogenes* from other hemolytic or nonhemolytic *Listeria* spp. The CAMP test (for Christie, Atkins, Munch–Peterson) uses a strain of *Staph. aureus* producing a betalysin and a strain of *Rhodococcus hoagii* streaked in one direction on a sheep blood agar plate, and the *Listeria* spp. culture to test streaked at right-angles (Figure 178-2b).[1] *Staph. aureus* betalysin enhances the hemolysis of *L. monocytogenes* whereas *R. hoagii* enhances the hemolysis of *L. ivanovii*.

Commercial kits allow the identification of *Listeria* to the genus level or to the species level (API-Listeria test, Vitek 2). A DNA probe assay performed on colonies provides rapid confirmation of *L. monocytogenes*. MALDI-TOF (matrix-assisted laser desorption ionization time of flight) mass spectrometry allows the rapid identification of *Listeria* to the genus level, but not to the species level.[10]

Antimicrobial susceptibility testing is not mandatory for *L. monocytogenes*, the susceptibility pattern of which is rather predictable. Penicillin, aminoglycosides and trimethoprim–sulfamethoxazole (TMP–SMX) are bactericidal. Cephalosporins are inactive *in vitro*, and should not be used when *Listeria* is among the suspected agents of CNS infection.

There is no currently commercially available serologic test to be recommended.

Several typing systems have been developed primarily for the investigation of food-borne outbreaks. Serotyping is still the reference phenotypic method whereas pulsed field gel electrophoresis is the most widely used for molecular typing. More recent methods (multilocus sequence typing, polymerase chain reaction (PCR)-based methods) are increasingly used.[11]

Clinical Manifestations

Listeria monocytogenes causes invasive disease in two categories of populations: adults, often immunocompromised, and the pregnant woman and/or her offspring. In the nonpregnant adult population, *L. monocytogenes* causes two main types of disease: an invasive disease characterized by a bacteremic episode, with or without focal organ involvement (CNS, disseminated disease), and a febrile gastroenteritis.[4]

Invasive disease varies in presentation according to the age of the patient and the level of immunosuppression. Classically, one differentiates uncomplicated bacteremia without obvious organ involvement from bacteremia with CNS involvement. Several presentations of CNS disease can occur: meningitis, meningoencephalitis, rhombencephalitis and, rarely, brain abscesses.

Isolated bacteremia is the most frequent presentation of listeriosis, particularly among severely immunocompromised patients, representing about 40% of all cases of invasive diseases.

Associated clinical symptoms are rather nonspecific: fever, myalgia, nausea and diarrhea in a minority of patients. Focal infections following bacteremia are uncommon. The most frequently reported are liver abscess, cholecystitis, peritonitis, splenic abscess, joint infections and endophthalmitis. Endocarditis is rare and can occur both on native and prosthetic valves. *Listeria* endocarditis is a severe disease with a high rate of complications and a high mortality (>50%).

CENTRAL NERVOUS SYSTEM INFECTIONS

Listeria display a particular tropism for CNS tissue, which has been recently explained at the molecular level.[8] Following bacteremia, three main presentations may occur: meningitis, meningoencephalitis and brain abscess. A peculiar form of encephalitis involving the pons is classically described under the name of rhombencephalitis.

Meningitis due to *Listeria* ranks as number four or five in terms of frequency, but it has a disproportionately high case mortality rate (typically 15–30%, sometimes up to 60%), probably because of its predilection for patients with other risk factors such as advanced age or immunosuppression. In neonates and patients older than 60 years, *Listeria* represents 20% of all bacterial etiologies of meningitis. In patients with lymphoma, solid organ transplant or on steroid therapy, it ranks as number one. Almost all patients are either immunocompromised or older than 50 years, or both.

The clinical presentation is subacute to acute, nuchal rigidity is less common than with other etiologic agents, movement disorders can be seen in 15–20% of the cases, as well as seizures and fluctuation of

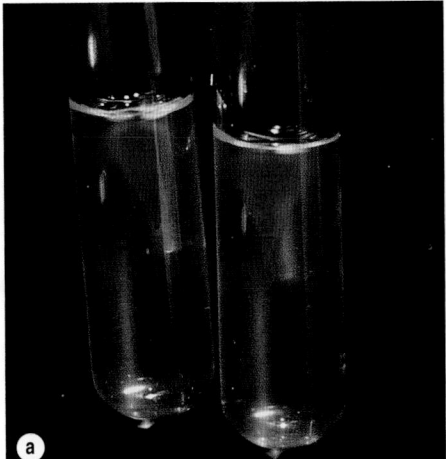
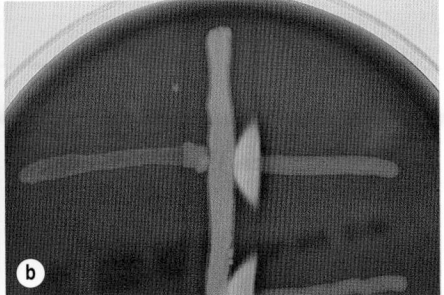

Figure 178-2 Tests for the identification of *Listeria monocytogenes*. (a) Demonstration of motility of *L. monocytogenes* grown in semisolid agar at room temperature. Note that the migration of the organism from the central stab is more pronounced at the surface of the soft agar, forming the typical umbrella-shaped pattern in both tubes. (b) CAMP test. Enhanced hemolysis patterns of *L. monocytogenes* (left) and *Streptococcus agalactiae* (right) colonies are shown; these are growing adjacent to a streak of *Staphylococcus aureus* colonies in the center. (*Courtesy of Robert Bortolussi and Timothy Mailman.*)

mental status. The triad of fever, neck stiffness and alterations of mental status is present in less than 50% of cases.[9]

The diagnosis is based on blood cultures (positive in up to 75% of the cases) and CSF culture (40% of the cases have a low glucose level and a positive direct Gram stain). There is usually a moderate CSF pleocytosis; despite its name, listerial meningitis can be characterized by neutrophils rather than monocytes.

Listeria encephalitis, also named rhombencephalitis due to its similarity to the circling disease described in sheep, is more frequent in previously healthy adults than the meningitic form. It classically occurs in two phases, starting with an episode of fever, headaches, nausea and vomiting, followed 3–5 days later by the development of cranial nerve deficits, cerebellar signs or hemiparesis.[12,13] Nuchal rigidity is seen in about 50% of the cases and respiratory failure in 40%. Mortality is very high, in part due to the often delayed diagnosis and treatment. The microbiologic diagnosis of *Listeria* rhombencephalitis is sometimes particularly difficult because blood cultures are positive in only 60% of the cases and CSF culture in no more than 40%. Magnetic resonance imaging is more helpful than computed tomography to document the lesions.

Brain abscess represents about 10% of CNS listerial infections, usually with a concomitant bacteremia, and in 25–40% of cases of concomitant meningitis. Typical locations are the thalamus, the pons and the medulla. Most occur as a single lesion. Associated mortality is high (40%), as well as the occurrence and severity of sequelae in surviving patients.[14]

In pregnant women, listeriosis presents classically in two phases. The first phase presents as an acute influenza-like illness with fever, chills, fatigue, myalgia and headaches, mostly in the second half of the pregnancy. When this episode is unnoticed and/or untreated, premature labor and delivery occur 2–14 days after the acute presentation. It is thus important to diagnose the first episode by blood culture. Early appropriate antibiotic treatment can prevent progression of the infection to the fetus. When the infection progresses (second phase), it can lead to death *in utero* or to the (premature) birth of an infected neonate. Neonatal mortality reaches 40–50%. The clinical manifestations of neonatal listeriosis differ greatly, as well as the mortality and the sensitivity of the diagnostic procedures according to the rapidity of disease onset at or after birth.[15]

Early-onset neonatal listeriosis is present at delivery or within the first 48 hours of life, and corresponds to an infection acquired *in utero*. The most common presentation is a pneumonia with or without sepsis (Table 178-1). The diagnosis is generally made by blood cultures or culture of meconium. Anemia and thrombocytopenia are common. The mortality of early-onset neonatal listeriosis is about 20%. Late-onset neonatal listeriosis develops generally after the first week of life and corresponds to the acquisition of this pathogen during birth or shortly thereafter from an infected mother or from the environment. The main presentation is meningitis.

Interestingly, the proportion of fetomaternal listeriosis has diminished considerably during the last two decades, most probably reflecting a higher awareness among pregnant women of at-risk food. On the whole, the incidence of invasive listeriosis has also decreased in many higher-income countries, reflecting the positive impact of various measures taken at many steps during food production and among consumers.

Listeria gastroenteritis is a rather recently described entity, undisputedly documented in several large outbreaks involving numerous previously healthy subjects exposed to a highly contaminated food product, as for example, chocolate milk, rice or corn salad. Major symptoms have been fever, vomiting, abdominal cramps and diarrhea, abating after 48 hours. Very few patients develop bacteremia.[6]

Treatment

Listeria monocytogenes is almost uniformly susceptible to penicillins, aminoglycosides and TMP–SMX. Based on animal studies showing synergism, the current recommendations for a severe infection is the combination of intravenous ampicillin (2 g q4h) and intravenous gentamicin (1.5–2 mg/kg q8h) for 2–4 weeks. Fewer cases have been successfully treated with intravenous TMP–SMX (20 mg/kg q24h trimethoprim part divided into two to four doses) for 2–3 weeks. Meropenem (2 g iv q8h) is an alternative. Bacteremia without distant focal infection can be treated by intravenous amoxicillin for 10–14 days. In the neonate, the combination of ampicillin (150 mg/kg q24h divided into three to four doses), amoxicillin (2 g intravenously q4h) and gentamicin (2–2.5 mg/kg q8h) is recommended.

Listeria gastroenteritis is usually not treated by antibiotics due to its benign and rapidly favorable course, and low risk of associated invasive disease. Oral ampicillin or TMP–SMX may be considered in patients at risk.[6] In pregnant women with positive blood cultures, intravenous ampicillin (2 g q6h) should be administered.

Prevention

The great majority of *Listeria* infections are food-borne, occurring more often sporadically (>90%) than as an outbreak.[16]

Several measures have been, or should be, taken at various levels in the food chain:

- pathogen elimination at production level of ready-to-eat at-risk food (especially meat or poultry); and
- in the consumer kitchen, wash raw vegetables, keep refrigerator temperature below 5°C, keep raw food products separate, wash hands and kitchen instruments after use, and cook raw meat properly.

Individuals at risk, such as pregnant women and the immunocompromised, should not eat at-risk food products such as cold meat, refrigerated patés or meat spreads, unwashed salad, various soft cheeses or smoked seafood.

Bacillus

Nature

The genus *Bacillus* comprises more than 200 species of which two, *B. anthracis* and *B. cereus*, are especially important as agents of disease in humans. *Bacillus* spp. are ubiquitous gram-positive bacilli. They are characterized by their production of resistant endospores in the presence of oxygen. They have a wide range of G+C content (from 32 to 69). Morphologically, *Bacillus* spp. cells appear as spore-forming, large (3–5 × 1 μm), gram-positive aerobic or facultative anaerobic mesophilic rods occurring singly or in pairs. Some *Bacillus* spp. are motile, others are not. On agar media, *Bacillus* spp. usually grow as large, irregular colonies easy to recognize. Most are saprophytes widely distributed in the environment.[17]

TABLE 178-1	**Neonatal Listeriosis**	
	Early Onset (1–2 days of life)	Late Onset (>7 days of life)
Pneumonia	62%	
Meningitis	21%	94%
Anemia	62%	
Thrombocytopenia	35%	
Positive blood culture	73%	
Positive meconium stain and culture	69%	17%
Mortality (live-born)	20%	

Bacillus anthracis

Epidemiology

Known since 1877 when Robert Koch first cultivated *Bacillus anthracis*, this agent received increased attention only after its use as a bioterrorism agent in 2001.[18]

  B. anthracis is ubiquitous and can be recovered worldwide as a saprophytic organism from soil, water and dust. It belongs to the normal intestinal flora of many mammals, including humans. As a sporulating bacterium, *B. anthracis* can survive for decades in soil before being ingested, usually by herbivore animals in which it can transform into a vegetative form or is eliminated in feces. In animals, *B. anthracis* causes severe gastrointestinal damage and high losses, particularly in nonimmunized herds in low- and middle-income countries. Major outbreaks involving thousands of bovines have been reported in Africa, whereas the incidence of animal anthrax is very low in the Western world, particularly for inhalation anthrax. In humans the most frequent presentation by far is cutaneous anthrax (>95% of the reported cases), with very few cases of inhalation anthrax or gastrointestinal anthrax, which is the most frequent form in ruminants. Accidental anthrax can occur in laboratory workers or in relation to a bioterrorism event, leading to pulmonary anthrax. Naturally acquired human infections occur by accident, when *B. anthracis* spores or cells enter the body, generally through an abrasion. It is mainly restricted to persons in contact with an infected animal (farmers or veterinarians) or with animal products (skin handlers).

  There are no documented cases of human-to-human transmission. The incubation time can vary widely, from a few days (1–7) to months when few spores have been inhaled. The lethal dose is probably small (2500–50 000 spores), as suggested by the tragic episode in Russia (Sverdlovsk) in 1979, when an explosion in an arms manufacturing plant caused at least 66 deaths, some of them up to 60 km from the epicenter.[19]

Pathogenicity

The virulence of *B. anthracis* is mediated by a complex interplay of three thermolabile proteins under the control of two plasmids. In addition, a large capsule made of poly-D-glutamic acid contributes to the virulence.[20]

  The three components of the toxins are a protective antigen (PA, 83 kDa), an edema factor (EF, 89 kDa) and a lethal factor (LF, 90 kDa). Individually, they have no harmful effect. PA binds to two cell surface receptors – the tumor endothelium marker 8 (TEM8) and the capillary morphogenesis protein 2 (CMG2) – and is subsequently cleaved by a cell protease.[21] The cleaved particle (PA 63) binds to the two other components and enters by endocytosis. EF activity depends on calcium; LF interferes with the protein kinase signal transduction pathway. When assembled, PA–EF and PA–LF kill macrophages by proteolysis and induce release of cytokines, particularly interleukin (IL)-1 and TNF, interfering with the coagulation system and causing edema (PA–EF). Lethal toxin and edema toxin induce host lethality by co-ordinately damaging two vital systems, cardiomyocytes and hepatocytes, respectively.[22]

  The large capsule observed mostly *in vivo* in clinical specimens is made of linear polymer of glutamic acid, and is antiphagocytic and very weakly immunogenic. These virulence factors are under the control of two large interconnected plasmids, pX01 (controlling for toxin production and carrying a pathogenicity island) and pX02 (controlling for capsule production). The toxins are mainly produced during the multiplication of the vegetative form in host tissues. External factors such as the temperature and the sodium bicarbonate concentration act on regulatory plasmid genes. In addition to the capsule, *B. anthracis* possesses another unique cell-wall structure named the S layer, which is made of glycoproteins and is responsible for the shape of the bacterium.

Diagnostic Microbiology

DIRECT EXAMINATION

Gram staining of appropriate clinical material (skin lesion or ulcer biopsy, blood, CSF, sputum, pleural fluid) shows large, encapsulated, box-shaped, gram-positive bacilli without spores. The sensitivity of direct examination in skin material from cutaneous anthrax is rather low (<30%). A direct fluorescent antibody (DFA) stain using an antibody against the capsular glutamic acid or a special stain (McFadyean methylene blue) can enhance detection of the capsule.

  Direct detection in clinical samples can also be attempted by *B. anthracis*-specific molecular amplification or by antigen detection.[23]

CULTURE

Bacillus anthracis grows rapidly on aerobic standard agar media as large, flat, spreading, nonhemolytic, white to gray sticky colonies, with a typical morphology called 'medusa-head'. Cells are catalase-positive, non-motile and produce endospores but no capsule on solid media.

IDENTIFICATION

Key characteristics to identify *B. anthracis* from appropriate clinical material are the Gram staining morphology, a positive catalase reaction, and the absence of motility and of frank hemolysis on blood agar. Confirmation of identification can be achieved with species-specific PCR and/or by lysis of colonies by a specific phage (γ phage) and recently by MALDI-TOF mass spectrometry.[24,25] Growth on agar medium enriched in sodium bicarbonate (at 0.8%) and incubated under 5% CO_2 will favor the formation of a large capsule. DFA assay and a rapid immunochromatographic test targeting the S layer to be used with colonies are also available.

  Antibiotic susceptibility testing is generally not attempted because *B. anthracis* wild strains are usually susceptible to penicillins, tetracyclines, quinolones, rifampin (rifampicin), vancomycin, daptomycin and clindamycin, and resistant to the cephalosporins and to TMP–SMX.

CLINICAL MANIFESTATIONS

There are three clinical presentations due to *B. anthracis* directly related to the mode of infection: a cutaneous form by direct transdermal inoculation of spores, a respiratory form following spore inhalation and a digestive form following ingestion of spores. By number of cases the most important is the cutaneous form and by severity the respiratory form. The digestive form, predominant in ruminants, is exceedingly rare in humans. (For further discussion, see Chapter 134.)

Bacillus cereus

Nature

Bacillus cereus is the second *Bacillus* species of interest in human diseases. It is ubiquitous in nature, and can easily contaminate various raw or processed foods or damaged human skin.

  B. cereus is a large gram-positive bacillus with four major properties, differentiating it from *B. anthracis*: motility, hemolysis, absence of capsule and resistance to penicillin.

Epidemiology

B. cereus represents a significant cause of food poisoning (variable incidence, usually 1–3%). It is widely present in various raw or processed food products such as rice, vegetables, turkey meat and spices. Spores usually naturally contaminate the food environment.

Pathogenicity

B. cereus carries two toxins, one responsible for a diarrheal syndrome (enterotoxin) and one for an emetic syndrome. The enterotoxin is a 38–57 kDa thermolabile protein, preformed or produced in the small intestine, acting on adenylcyclase. The emetic toxin is a 10 kDa peptide which is highly thermostable and resistant to proteolytic degradation. Its effect is classically observed when rice or pasta meals are consumed cold after cooking. In both cases, spores of *B. cereus* resist the heating process, and germinate and multiply during storage of the leftover food.[26]

Diagnostic Microbiology

In clinical material – particularly in tissue – *B. cereus* appears as a large bacillus with a central endospore. *B. cereus* can be cultured easily from blood or tissue biopsies, and appears on blood agar as large, flat, granular to ground-glass, β-hemolytic colonies of variable shape (circular to irregular) (Figure 178-3, lanes 6C and 6D). They can be easily taken up with a loop, as opposed to *B. anthracis* colonies, which are sticky. Its isolation from contaminated material such as feces, vomitus or food items requires selective media usually containing mannitol, egg yolk and antibiotics. *B. cereus* is a facultative anaerobe and gives a positive lecithinase reaction on egg yolk medium.[17]

Clinical Manifestations and Management

The diarrheal syndrome caused by the enterotoxin is characterized by an episode of profuse diarrhea with abdominal pain and cramps, occurring 8–16 hours after ingestion of the contaminated food. Fever and vomiting occur rarely.

The other clinical syndrome is food poisoning. For an extensive clinical discussion, see Chapters 37 and 38.

As well as the classic gastrointestinal diseases, *B. cereus* also occasionally causes an array of focal or invasive diseases:

- in immunocompromised hosts, bacteremia, meningitis, endocarditis, brain abscess, pneumonia;
- in surgical patients, wound infections, after traffic accidents or burns;
- in neonates, infection of the umbilical cord;
- in contact lens-wearing patients, keratitis or endophthalmitis.

It is important to consider the potential pathogenic role of *B. cereus* in these situations and not automatically disregard a positive culture for *Bacillus* considered as a simple contamination.

B. cereus is resistant to penicillins and cephalosporins (due to the presence of a β-lactamase) but is usually susceptible to aminoglycosides, glycopeptides, clindamycin, ciprofloxacin and erythromycin. The recommended therapy for severe infection is the combination of vancomycin and an aminoglycoside, and clindamycin with gentamicin for ophthalmic infections. Ciprofloxacin has been used successfully to treat wound infections and bacteremia.

Erysipelothrix

Nature

Erysipelothrix rhusiopathiae is a small gram-positive bacillus, widespread in nature, causing self-limited illnesses or systemic infections in various animals, swine in particular, and occasionally in humans. *E. rhusiopathiae* is a thin, elongated ($0.2–0.4 \times 0.8–2.5\,\mu m$) gram-positive to gram-labile, aerobic to facultative anaerobic bacillus, nonmotile, nonsporulated and non-encapsulated, belonging to the clade of gram-positive bacilli with a low G+C content (36–40%) (*Listeria, Lactobacillus, Kurthia, Brochothrix*).[27]

Epidemiology

E. rhusiopathiae is ubiquitous in nature, found on plants, in humid soil and used water, as well as in many animals as asymptomatic carriers. The major reservoir is the pig, where it is carried in the pharynx or digestive tract as a commensal. It can also cause a disease in pigs called swine erysipelas, presenting as skin infection, arthritis or sepsis.[28]

Humans usually develop a local infection, called erysipeloid, through direct contact with an infected animal or animal product. At particular risk are butchers and fishermen handling crabs, but also farmers, abattoir workers and veterinarians. There is no documented human-to-human transmission.

Pathogenicity

Several components of *E. rhusiopathiae* are thought to play a role in virulence: these include an antiphagocytic capsule, a surface protein (Spa A), the enzyme neuraminidase and the capacity to survive in macrophages. The exact mechanisms, however, are not firmly established.

Diagnostic Microbiology

For localized erysipeloid lesion(s), the best clinical specimen is a deep tissue biopsy or liquid when present in vesicles. Swabs of the skin surface are to be discouraged. Blood cultures are taken for systemic disease.

The microscopy of a tissue biopsy is occasionally positive for thin gram-positive bacilli. On blood agar, *E. rhusiopathiae* appears as punctiform colonies, α-hemolytic after 2 days, either as gray, translucent and regular S colonies (smooth variant) or as larger, opaque, irregular R colonies (rough variant). Growth is enhanced in 5–10% CO_2 at 33–37 °C (91–99 °F) and usually present in liquid media.

Preliminary identification relies on the pleomorphic Gram stain and cultural appearance of the colonies. *E. rhusiopathiae* is catalase-negative, nonmotile and non-β-hemolytic, but H_2S-positive in 24–48 hours on TSI or Kligler slant agar.[2] There is an indirect immunofluorescence test, as well as a mouse inoculation test used in reference laboratories. There is no serologic test currently available.

E. rhusiopathiae isolates can be typed in two serogroups (A and B) and 23 serovars for epidemiologic purposes. *E. rhusiopathiae* is susceptible *in vitro* to penicillins, cephalosporins, clindamycin and erythromycin, more or less susceptible to tetracyclines and chloramphenicol, and resistant to vancomycin, aminoglycosides, sulfonamides and TMP–SMX.[29]

Clinical Manifestations and Management

E. rhusiopathiae has three distinct clinical presentations, as follows.

- A cutaneous lesion called erysipeloid, localized to the upper extremities (generally the fingers) around an inoculation site, and characterized by a painful itching and burning erythematous, violaceous, well-demarcated lesion developing over 10 days after inoculation. Fever or arthralgias are uncommon, but localized lymphangitis (30%) and lymphadenopathy (30%) are frequent. In the absence of treatment, spontaneous healing generally occurs.
- A diffuse cutaneous disease with skin and soft tissue extension from the original inoculation site. This form is less frequent and is observed in some immunocompromised patients, in whom systemic manifestations (fever, arthralgia) are common.
- A disseminated disease, usually sepsis, often (up to 90%) complicated by an endocarditis on native valve. This form is usually a primary infection but can follow an erysipeloid lesion in about 40% of cases. The disease is often characterized by a long-lasting fever, with multiple cutaneous lesions on the trunk or the extremities. Classic underlying conditions are alcohol abuse and/ or chronic liver disease, as well as corticosteroid use or chemotherapy. The associated mortality is rather high (38%).[30]

The treatment of uncomplicated erysipeloid skin lesions (with oral penicillin, 500 mg q6h, for 1 week or another active drug, such as another β-lactam, fluoroquinolones or clindamycin) will accelerate natural healing. For severe cutaneous disease or disseminated disease the recommended therapy is intravenous benzylpenicillin (2–4 million units q4h), ceftriaxone (2 g q24h) or ciprofloxacin (400 mg q12h) for 2–4 weeks.[28] As there are no human vaccines, the only form of disease prevention is to limit occupational exposure to the organism.

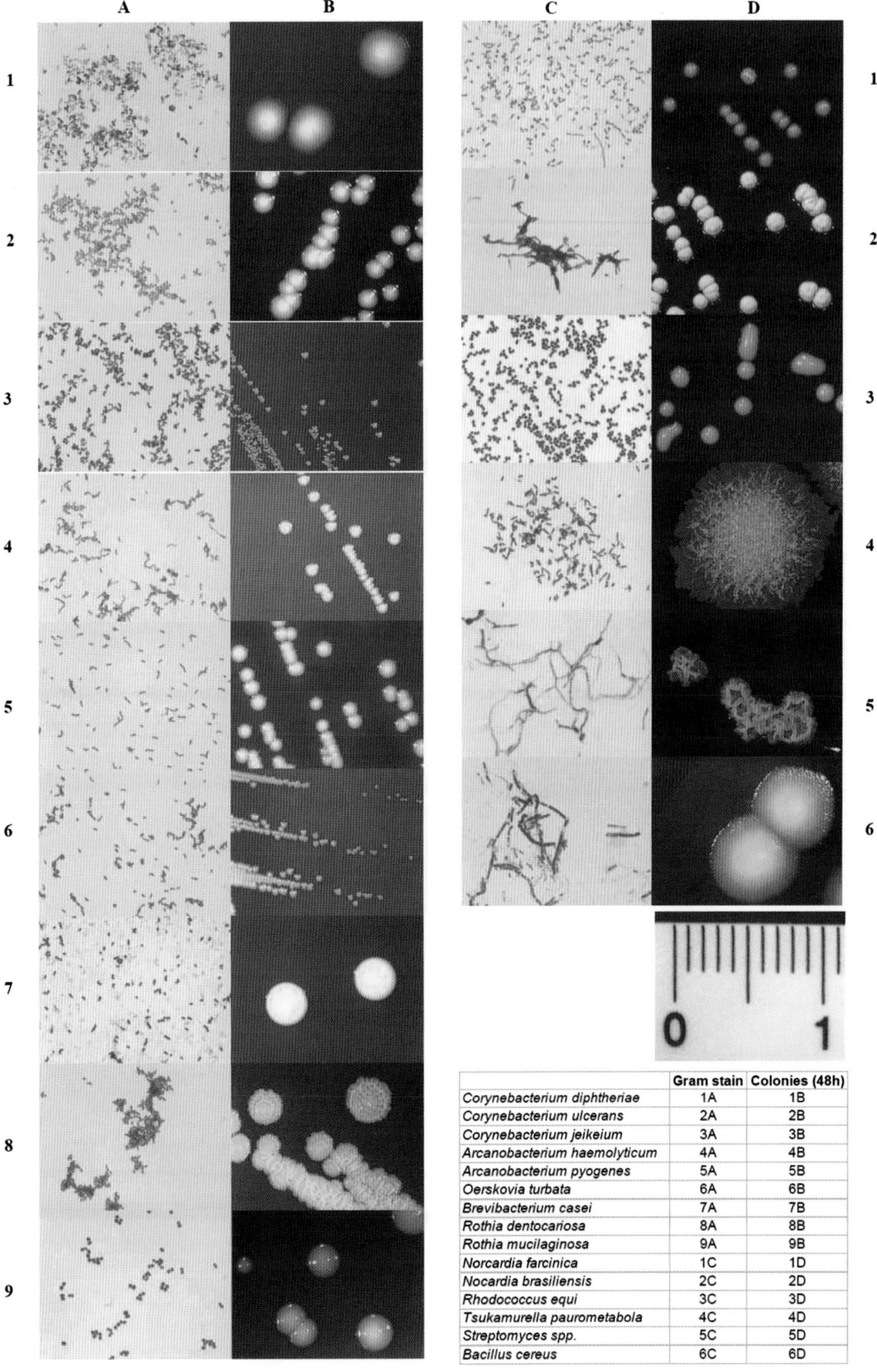

	Gram stain	Colonies (48h)
Corynebacterium diphtheriae	1A	1B
Corynebacterium ulcerans	2A	2B
Corynebacterium jeikeium	3A	3B
Arcanobacterium haemolyticum	4A	4B
Arcanobacterium pyogenes	5A	5B
Oerskovia turbata	6A	6B
Brevibacterium casei	7A	7B
Rothia dentocariosa	8A	8B
Rothia mucilaginosa	9A	9B
Norcardia farcinica	1C	1D
Nocardia brasiliensis	2C	2D
Rhodococcus equi	3C	3D
Tsukamurella paurometabola	4C	4D
Streptomyces spp.	5C	5D
Bacillus cereus	6C	6D

Figure 178-3   Gram stain and colonies (48-hour incubation) of different gram-positive bacilli.

Corynebacterium diphtheriae, C. ulcerans

Nature

Diphtheria is now a rare disease. This communicable infectious and vaccine-preventable disease may result in acute localized respiratory infection with typical 'croup' symptomatology due to the development of oropharyngeal adherent pseudomembranes. The mortality is due to airway obstruction or myocarditis caused by toxin production. *Corynebacterium diphtheriae* is a small, irregular, nonsporulated, gram-positive bacillus with enlarged extremities and a typical 'club-shaped' morphology. A 'palisade' or 'V' arrangement or clusters with a so-called Chinese-letter appearance are observed in liquid media (Figure 178-3, lanes 1A and 1B). *Corynebacterium* spp. belong to the broad class Actinobacteria. Phylogenetic studies show that *Corynebacterium* spp. are closely related to acid-fast bacilli such as *Mycobacterium*.

Corynebacterium ulcerans shares certain common features with *C. diphtheriae*. *C. ulcerans* causes a rare oropharyngeal diphtheria-like illness, as well as extrapharyngeal infections due to the presence of a toxin similar to diphtheria toxin. Taxonomic studies show that *C. ulcerans* is closely related to *C. diphtheriae*.[31-]

Epidemiology

Diphtheria remains endemic in numerous countries throughout the world – Eastern Europe, South East Asia, South America and the Indian subcontinent. In higher-income countries, diphtheria occurs sporadically and most cases are imported from areas of endemicity.[32]

During the 1990s, an important outbreak occurred in Russia and the newly independent states of the former Soviet Union, with more than 157 000 cases and 5000 deaths. Several factors may explain the re-emergence of epidemic diphtheria, notably the introduction of a toxigenic strain, insufficient coverage of vaccination of children and an increasing proportion of adults with waning vaccine-induced immunity. Contrary to the prevaccine era, where diphtheria was essentially a childhood disease, a shift in the age of patients was observed. The epidemic began in towns and in groups with close contacts (e.g. hospitals, military troops), before dissemination to socioeconomically disfavored groups (e.g. alcoholics).[33–35]

Achieving a high coverage (90–95%) of primary immunization is mandatory for diphtheria elimination and periodic booster doses for adults are necessary in regions at high risk of diphtheria. Control measures allow the control of epidemic diphtheria. In 1997, the World Health Organization (WHO) identified 10 countries with more than 10 cases for a total number of 15 839 cases reported, whereas in 2006 the number of reported cases decreased to 4000.

Humans represent the sole significant reservoir for *C. diphtheriae*. Acquisition occurs essentially through direct transmission (or via airborne droplet) with contaminated respiratory secretions or skin lesions.

In temperate climates, respiratory infections due to toxigenic strains predominate, while in the tropics, cutaneous diphtheria is more commonly caused by nontoxigenic strains. A peak incidence of respiratory infections is observed during the cold months.

In diphtheria-endemic areas with high prevalence of cutaneous diphtheria, respiratory diphtheria is rare due to the high rate of natural immunity attained through exposure to cutaneous diphtheria. In most cases, transmission of *C. diphtheriae* to susceptible individuals results in transient pharyngeal carriage rather than in disease. Cutaneous diphtheria appears to be more contagious than the respiratory form of diphtheria and persists longer than *C. diphtheriae* infections of the tonsils or nose in a carrier state.

C. ulcerans is a commensal of wild and domestic animals. Human *C. ulcerans* infection is considered a zoonosis, since human transmission occurs via manipulation of infected dairy animals or consumption of contaminated milk; however, these risk factors are absent in half of the cases. Global epidemiologic data on *C. ulcerans* infection are missing but *C. ulcerans* strains represent 58% of toxigenic *Corynebacterium* strains submitted to WHO reference laboratories.[35]

Pathogenicity

C. diphtheriae contains pili or fimbriae involved in initial adhesion of the bacteria to host-cell receptors; the pili also promote the aggregation of other bacteria to ensure colonization. These structures contain subunits of pilin proteins, a backbone protein component (SpaA; Spa for sortase-mediated pilus assembly) and two ancillary proteins (SpaB, SpaC). The pili are covalently linked to the peptidoglycan structure of the bacterial cell wall. Minor pilins, SpaB and SpaC, are required for pharyngeal cell adhesion, the specific receptor being currently unknown.[36] This type of pilus is encoded on a pathogenicity island, probably acquired by recent horizontal transfer. *C. diphtheriae* is responsible for a localized predominantly pharyngeal infection with the appearance of a so-called 'pseudomembrane' made of fibrin, neutrophilic inflammation and abundant colonies of *C. diphtheriae*. The major virulence factor is a 58 kDa exotoxin responsible for the systemic complications of diphtheria, notably for myocardial and neurologic toxicity.[37] This exotoxin is very effective, since one molecule introduced into a cell can kill it.

The exotoxin gene (*tox*) is present on a family of corynephages hosted by some *C. diphtheriae* strains. The expression of toxin is reliant on an iron-dependent regulatory element (*dtxR*). The presence of iron activates *dtxR* and blocks the transcription of *tox*. Under iron-limiting conditions, generally observed on the mucosal surface, *dtxR* is inactivated and diphtheria toxin is produced. The toxin is excreted through the bacterial cell and diffuses both locally and via the circulation to all organs, the myocardium and the peripheral nerves being the most affected. Diphtheria toxin has a complex activity, resulting in cytolysis through cell-protein inhibition.

Three distinct domains of diphtheria toxin have been described:
- the carboxyl-terminal R-domain (fragment B), which is responsible for binding to the heparin-binding epidermal-like growth factor, the specific receptor for the toxin;
- internalization into endocytic vesicles, which is mediated by the central part of the toxin;
- the amino-terminal C-domain (fragment A) which is delivered in the cytosol and is responsible for the inhibition of protein synthesis by inactivating the eukaryotic elongation factor 2 (eEF-2) through adenosine diphosphate (ADP) ribosylation of diphthamide residue[38] (Figure 178-4).

Histology of heart tissues shows necrosis associated with active inflammation in the interstitial space. Cardiac conduction tissue may also be affected. Diphtheria toxin may affect peripheral nerves, causing a demyelination localized around the nodes of Ranvier. In severe cases, axonal degeneration can occur.[39]

C. ulcerans also carries a corynephage coding for the diphtheria toxin, and the *C. ulcerans tox* gene has 95% homology with *C. diphtheriae tox* gene. Most differences are located in the B fragment of the toxin in the translocation (T) region and in the receptor-binding (R) domain.[40]

Diagnostic Microbiology

Due to the declining incidence of diphtheria, the policy for screening throat swabs varies in different countries. In endemic regions, routine screening for *C. diphtheriae* in throat swabs is recommended since milder infections or atypical infections may be misdiagnosed. When diphtheria is suspected, clinicians should inform the laboratory.

Cotton or polyester-tipped swabs are appropriate for sampling. When membranes are removed, they should be sent to the laboratory for culture and a swab from areas under the membranes should be obtained. Standard Amies transport media ensure adequate maintenance of viability during transport to the laboratory. When molecular testing is available, Dacron polyester swabs are preferred for sampling. Suspected cases should have specimens taken from both the nose and

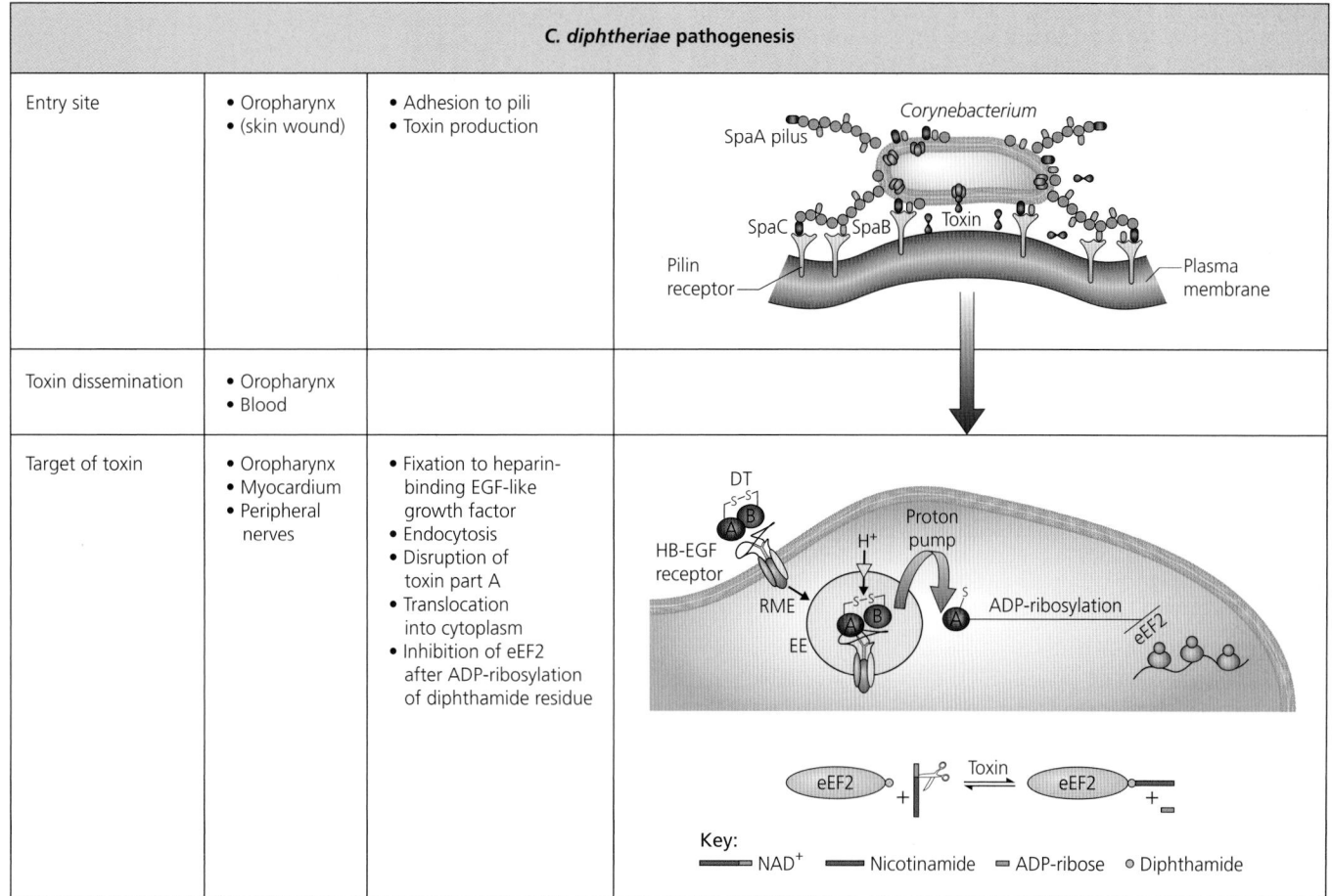

Figure 178-4 *C. diphtheriae* pathogenesis. *(Adapted from Mandlik et al., Mol Microbiol 2007;64(1):111–124, and Yates et al., Trends Biochem Sci 2006;31(2):123–133.)*

the throat. For wound infections, swabs or aspirates of inflamed lesions are recommended.

For culture, selective media such as cysteine–tellurite blood agar or Tinsdale medium and nonselective sheep blood agar are recommended.[41] When selective media are not available, multiple colonies from sheep blood agar are picked and biochemically identified to rule out *C. diphtheriae*. Commercial biochemical tests and MALDI-TOF mass spectrometry accurately identify *C. diphtheriae* strains. *C. diphtheriae* appear as small 0.5 mm up to 2 mm large colonies with a gray to white opaque surface (see Figure 178-3, lanes 1A and 1B). Some strains (biotype intermedius) appear dysgonic on standard media, their colonies being enlarged on lipid-enriched media (lipophilism). Based on colony morphology and biochemical reactions, *C. diphtheriae* can be divided into four biotypes: *gravis, mitis, belfanti* and *intermedius*. However, biotyping is of limited use and is generally carried out only in reference laboratories.

C. ulcerans grows on standard sheep blood agar media, but the use of selective media such as cysteine–tellurite blood agar or Tinsdale medium facilitates the isolation of pathogenic corynebacteria.

After 24 hours, 1 mm colonies are observed with a gray–white appearance (see Figure 178-3, lanes 2A and 2B) and slight hemolysis on sheep blood agar. Presence of urease and a positive reverse CAMP test (inhibition reaction) differentiate *C. ulcerans* from *C. diphtheriae*.[42]

The detection of toxin is the most important test; molecular tests based on the amplification of the *tox* gene constitute an alternative to the classic Elek immunoprecipitation test. Recently, the direct detection of the *tox* gene from clinical specimens has been described; the

amplification test can differentiate the *C. diphtheriae tox* gene from toxin-producing *C. ulcerans*.[43]

Some toxigenic *C. ulcerans* strains show atypical results in real-time PCR for toxin detection. Specific amplification of the *C. ulcerans tox* gene has been described based on the polymorphic region of the *tox* gene.[44]

Clinical Manifestations

RESPIRATORY TRACT DISEASE

C. diphtheriae is responsible for localized infection of the upper respiratory tract. The oropharynx and rhinopharynx are most frequently affected. Symptoms generally occur 2–5 days after transmission, the most common symptoms being a moderate fever and sore throat followed by weakness, painful swallowing and headaches. Classic adherent and gray pseudomembranes are not always present and their extent can vary from small patches on infected tonsils to an extensive involvement of the posterior oropharynx and larynx. A serous or serosanguinous discharge can be observed in nasal diphtheria, which is often milder and chronic. Signs of toxicity may be present with edema of the neck, hoarseness and stridor and a marked local lymphadenopathy. In adults, atypical presentations are observed with oral lesions.[40]

Respiratory infections due to *C. ulcerans* are similar to infection due to *C. diphtheriae*.

CUTANEOUS DISEASE

Cutaneous diphtheria appears usually as a chronic and nonspecific disease. In fact, *C. diphtheriae* may colonize any kind of primary cutaneous lesion. Superinfection with *C. diphtheriae* begins with vesicles or pustules evolving as skin ulcers, with edematous surrounding tissues. Dark pseudomembranes may be observed during the first 1–2 week(s). Their localization is predominantly on the legs and hands. Coinfection with other pathogens such as *Staph. aureus* and *Streptococcus pyogenes* is common. Systemic toxic manifestations of cutaneous diphtheria are rarely seen. Chronic cutaneous infections with gray membranes due to toxigenic *C. ulcerans* have been described.[45]

Infections due to *C. diphtheriae* and *C. ulcerans* are undoubtedly underreported since cutaneous manifestations may be mild and corynebacteria are often considered as contaminants.

MYOCARDIAL DISEASE

Myocardial toxicity occurs in 10–20% of patients with respiratory diphtheria and is associated with a mortality rate of 40%. Its frequency depends on the extension of the oropharyngeal infection and on the delay until antitoxin therapy is started. Cardiac manifestations appear during the second week of the disease with a dilated cardiomyopathy and depressed left ventricular function. Electrocardiography shows anomalies of conduction and dysrhythmia may be observed with atrioventricular block, bundle branch block and hemi block. Markers of poor prognosis and carditis in children are a high myoglobin level and an increased lactate dehydrogenase (LDH) isoenzyme level, with an LDH1/LDH2 ratio >1.[46]

NEUROLOGIC DISEASE

Neuronal toxicity appears generally in severe respiratory diphtheria. Distinct types of damage are observed due to the regional effect of the toxin, with paralysis of the soft palate, of the posterior pharyngeal wall with dysphonia, dysphagia and defects of ocular accommodation; a delayed complication consisting of a peripheral neuritis affecting the limbs and/or the diaphragm can also occur up to 3 months later. Recovery is slow and only 20% of patients with diphtherial peripheral neurotoxicity were completely healthy after 1 year.[47] The incidence of severe paralysis seems reduced when prompt antitoxin therapy is initiated within the first 2–3 days of infection.

SYSTEMIC DISEASE

Deep-seated infections due to *C. diphtheriae* (e.g. endocarditis, septic arthritis, osteomyelitis and splenic abscesses) have also been documented. Risk factors such as intravenous drug use, homelessness and alcoholism have been identified. The portal of entry is likely to be skin colonization or skin infections with *C. diphtheriae*. Strains belonging to different biotypes (*gravis*, *mitis*, *belfanti*) have been isolated and are generally nontoxigenic.[48] These strains may represent a potential reservoir for the emergence of toxigenic *C. diphtheriae* strains since they possess the functional regulation machinery represented by the 'diphtheria toxin repressor (*dtxR*) genes' and thus could become toxigenic by acquiring the *tox* gene.[49]

Management

The management of respiratory tract diphtheria includes specific and nonspecific measures. Specific measures include the administration of diphtheria antitoxin and antibiotic treatment for *C. diphtheriae* eradication, whereas nonspecific measures are the surveillance and support of respiratory and cardiac functions. Neutralization of circulating toxin through diphtheria antitoxin represents the mainstay of diphtheria therapy. Since diphtheria antitoxin is prepared with horse hyperimmune serum, the sensitivity of the patient to horse serum should be tested before administration. According to the extent and duration of the illness, a variable dose of antitoxin is administered (Table 178-2).[50] Penicillin or erythromycin constitutes the standard antibiotic treatment. *In vitro* resistance to penicillin has not yet been described but *in vitro* penicillin tolerance has been documented and could explain some eradication failures.[51] Erythromycin is generally highly active *in vitro* but inducible resistance has been described.[52]

Antibiotics are used to reduce the carrier state and are combined with antitoxin to treat the disease. Erythromycin 40–50 mg/kg/day

TABLE 178-2	Dosage of Antitoxin Recommended for Various Types of Diphtheria		
Type of Diphtheria	**Dosage (units)**	**Route**	
Nasal	10 000–20 000	Intramuscular	
Tonsillar	15 000–25 000	Intramuscular or intravenous	
Pharyngeal or laryngeal	20 000–40 000	Intramuscular or intravenous	
Combined types or delayed diagnosis	40 000–60 000	Intravenous	
Severe diphtheria: extensive membrane and/or severe edema (bull-neck diphtheria)	40 000–100 000	Intravenous or part intravenous and part intramuscular	

From Bonnet JM, Begg NT. Control of diphtheria: guidance for consultants in communicable disease control. World Health Organization. Commun Dis Public Health 1999;2(4):242–9.

intravenously for 7–14 days is the treatment of choice, but oral penicillin (benzylpenicillin G 50 000 IU/kg/day for 5 days followed by penicillin V 50 mg/kg/day for 5 days) has been shown to be superior in a randomized trial.[52]

Testing for *C. diphtheriae* eradication is recommended at the end of treatment. Continue treatment for 10 days if culture remains positive.[50]

Close contacts should receive a single dose of penicillin or a 7-day course of erythromycin.[50]

Prevention

The following measures to control diphtheria have been proposed by international experts:

- primary prevention of disease based on a childhood immunization program;
- secondary prevention through rapid investigation of close contacts of index cases to prevent emergence of secondary cases, with investigation of carriage rate, clinical surveillance, penicillin prophylaxis and administration of a booster dose of diphtheria toxoid-containing vaccine;
- tertiary prevention based on early diagnosis and proper management to prevent complications of suspected cases.[53]

Primary prevention with diphtheria toxoid obtained from formaldehyde-treated toxin is highly effective, providing high immunization rates. Recent epidemics have shown that more than 90% of children should be vaccinated to interrupt efficiently the transmission of epidemic clones.[54] The primary vaccination is based on a series of three doses started at 6 weeks of age and given at intervals of 4 weeks. Three doses induce the formation of protective toxin-neutralizing antibodies in 95.5% of children. This series is completed by at least one booster dose in the preschool period. The waning of adult immunity should be prevented with booster doses of diphtheria toxoid every 10 years throughout life. Recently, a new vaccine formulation called Tdap (for tetanus toxoid, reduced diphtheria toxoid and acellular pertussis vaccine) has been recommended for adults aged 19–64 years.[55] In endemic regions, booster doses are less necessary since natural boosting of immunity may occur through *C. diphtheriae* colonization.

Coryneforms

Nature

The genus *Corynebacterium* contains more than 70 species, half of them being considered as pathogenic for humans in case reports or small series of cases. Taxonomic studies have shown that the genus is quite homogeneous except for a distinct subgroup formed by *C. diphtheriae, C. kutscheri, C. pseudotuberculosis, C. vitarumen* and *C. ulcerans*.[31] Some *Corynebacterium* spp. have been reported as opportunist pathogens with some frequency, including *C. amycolatum, C. jeikeium* (formerly group JK) and *C. urealyticum*.

The so-called coryneforms represent a heterogeneous group of asporogenous, irregularly shaped, nonacid-fast, generally gram-positive rods. This group contains the following genera considered as human pathogens: *Arcanobacterium, Brevibacterium, Oerskovia* and *Rothia* (Tables 178-3 and 178-4).

Epidemiology

For most *Corynebacterium* spp. and coryneforms, the reservoir and ecology are unknown. *Corynebacterium* spp. may be isolated from normal skin and mucous membranes, whereas *C. jeikeium* has also been isolated from inanimate hospital environments. *Arcanobacterium* may colonize mucous membranes from humans and farm animals. *Brevibacterium* can be isolated from dairy products (e.g. cheese) and *Oerskovia* from the inanimate environment. *Rothia* are members of the oropharyngeal microflora. Possible human-to-human or animal-to-human transmission may occur with *Arcanobacterium*.

Pathogenicity

Except for *Arcanobacterium*, most coryneforms and *Corynebacterium* spp. are opportunistic human pathogens. The major risk factors are immunosuppressive diseases such as malignancy, organ transplantation, iatrogenic manipulation (e.g. urinary tract instrumentation for *C. urealyticum*), breaks in the skin barrier (e.g. medical devices for *C. jeikeium, Brevibacterium* spp., *Oerskovia* spp., *Rothia* spp.) and therapy with broad-spectrum antibiotics (*C. jeikeium, C. urealyticum, C. amycolatum*).

Diagnostic Microbiology

Several *Corynebacterium* spp. and coryneforms colonize the mucocutaneous epithelium and are part of the normal microflora. Their isolation from clinical specimens is difficult to interpret. Criteria have been proposed to help clinical microbiologists and clinicians to distinguish colonization from a possible role in infection (Box 178-1).

With few exceptions, *Corynebacterium* spp. and coryneforms grow in 24–48 hours in aerobic conditions in standard liquid media (blood culture) or on solid media (blood-containing media). *C. jeikeium* (see

Figure 178-3, lanes 3A and 3B) and *C. urealyticum* grow better in lipid-enriched media such as those containing Tween. Some morphologic or physiologic characteristics of colonies may help to differentiate them; for example (see Figure 178-3, lanes 4–9A and 4–9B):

- *C. amycolatum* produces dry colonies;
- β-hemolysis is observed around *Arcanobacterium* spp. colonies;
- *Brevibacterium* produces a cheese-like smell;
- *Oerskovia* colonies are pigmented in yellow to orange;
- white colonies with a 'spoked-wheel' aspect are observed in *Rothia dentocariosa*;
- *Rothia mucilaginosa* produces mucoid colonies which adhere on agar.

Antibiotic susceptibility testing is obtained generally by using E-test technology which allows the determination of the minimal inhibitory concentration on blood-containing agar. However, standardized interpretation criteria are lacking for these bacteria.

C. jeikeium, C. urealyticum and *C. amycolatum* exhibit high levels of resistance to several antibiotics (including resistance to penicillins, cephalosporins, macrolides and aminoglycosides) but are uniformly susceptible to glycopeptides. Resistance to glycopeptides attributed to the presence of the *vanA* gene has been described in *Oerskovia turbata* and *Arcanobacterium haemolyticum* strains.[56]

Clinical Manifestations and Management

Corynebacterium spp. and coryneform bacteria have a low index of pathogenicity and are considered as opportunistic. Clinical syndromes that have been reported include bacteremia, endocarditis, infections of prosthetic joints, infections of the urinary tract and pneumonia in immunocompromised hosts.

For detailed discussions, see specific chapters and Table 178-4.

Aerobic Actinomycetes

Nature

The term 'aerobic actinomycetes' helps clinical microbiologists to define noncoryneform gram-positive rods which grow better under aerobic conditions. Table 178-5 shows the different genera belonging to this heterogeneous group. Only the most frequently encountered species in human pathology will be discussed. Important pathogens

TABLE 178-3	Taxonomy of Medically Relevant Actinomycetales			
Suborders	**Families**	**Genera**	**Frequency**	**Practical Classification**
Actinomycineae	Actinomycetaceae	*Actinobaculum, Actinomyces, Arcanobacterium,* * *Mobiluncus*	+	Ac
Propionibacterineae	Propionibacteriaceae	*Propionibacterium*	+++	An
Micrococcineae	Micrococcaceae	*Arthrobacter, Micrococcus, Rothia**	+	Co
	Cellulomonadaceae	*Cellulomonas, Oerskovia,** *Tropheryma*[†]	+	Co
	Dermatophilaceae	*Dermatophilus*	+	Aa
	Brevibacteriaceae	*Brevibacterium**	+	Co
	Dermabacteraceae	*Dermabacter*	+	Co
	Microbacteriaceae	*Microbacterium*	+	Co
Corynebacterineae	Corynebacteriaceae	*Corynebacterium,** *Turicella*	+++	Co
	Mycobacteriaceae	*Mycobacterium*[†]	++	My
	Nocardiaceae	*Nocardia,** *Rhodococcus**	+	Aa
	Gordoniaceae	*Gordonia**	+	Aa
	Tsukamurellaceae	*Tsukamurella**	+	Aa
	Dietziaceae	*Dietzia*	+	Aa
Streptomycineae	Streptomycetaceae	*Streptomyces**	+	Aa
Streptosporangineae	Nocardiopsaceae	*Nocardiopsis*	+	Aa
	Thermomonosporaceae	*Actinomadura**	+	Aa

Aa, aerobic actinomycetes; Ac, actinomycetes; An, anaerobic gram-positive rods; Co, coryneforms; My, mycobacteria.
*Genera dealt with in this overview.
[†]Genera discussed in separate chapters.

TABLE 178-4 **Medically Relevant Corynebacterium Species and Coryneform Bacteria***

Genera	Predominant Species	Gram Stain	Natural Habitat	Site of Infection	Risk Factors, Transmission	Diagnostic Comments
Corynebacterium	C. diphtheriae	Club-shaped morphology, arrangement in liquid media: V forms, in palissades or in clusters with so-called Chinese letter appearance	Human	Upper respiratory tract, wound	No or insufficient vaccination, human-to-human transmission (close contact)	Four biotypes: gravis, mitis, belfanti and intermedius. C. diphtheriae biotype intermedius: lipophilism (growth enhanced in presence of Tween 80)
	C. ulcerans		Cattle, domestic cats and dogs	Upper respiratory tract, wound	Contact with animals, rural setting, ingestion of unpasteurized dairy products	Small β-hemolytic colonies; reverse CAMP test with S. aureus positive; positive urease test
	C. jeikeium		Human skin (axillary, inguinal and perineal areas), mucous membranes (urinary tract), inanimate hospital environment	Bacteremia, endocarditis, foreign body infections, wound infections	Immunosuppression, medical devices, prolonged hospital stay, therapy with broad-spectrum antibiotics	Lipophilism; multiresistance to antibiotics
	C. amycolatum		Human skin	Bacteremia, endocarditis, foreign body infections, wound infections	Immunosuppression, underlying heart disease (endocarditis)	—
	C. urealyticum		Urinary tract, skin (axilla and groin of hospitalized patients)	Bacteremia, urinary tract infections, alkali-encrusted cystitis (struvite stones), wound infections	Immunosuppression (kidney transplant), urologic procedures	Lipophilism; strong positive urease test; multiresistance to antibiotics
Arcanobacterium	A. haemolyticum	Gram-positive rod (to gram-variable, with branching bacilli)	Oropharyngeal microflora	Pharyngitis (20% with morbilliform rash), soft tissue infections, sepsis (immunosuppression), endocarditis	Possible human-to-human transmission (pharyngitis in teenagers and young adults), immunosuppression	Small β-hemolytic colonies; reverse CAMP test with S. aureus positive
Trueperella	Trueperella pyogenes (formerly Arcanobacterium pyogenes)	Gram-positive rod (to gram-variable, with branching bacilli)	Normal flora of farm ruminants and swine	Abdominal abscesses, soft tissue abscesses, bacteremia, endocarditis	Contacts with animals, rural setting	Small β-hemolytic colonies
Brevibacterium	B. casei (formerly CDC coryneform groups B-1 and B-3)	Small gram-positive rods (coccoid forms – old colonies)	Dairy products/skin flora	Bacteremia, endocarditis	Immunosuppression, medical devices (intravascular catheter)	Nonhemolytic colonies; typical cheese-like smell
Oerskovia	O. turbata	Branching bacilli, coccoid forms (breaking up of mycelia)	Inanimate environment (soil)	Bacteremia, endocarditis	Immunosuppression, medical devices (intravascular catheter)	Yellow-orange pigmented colonies
Rothia	R. dentocariosa	Gram-positive rods	Oropharyngeal microflora	Bacteremia, endocarditis, meningitis	Immunosuppression, medical devices, underlying heart disease (endocarditis)	First isolation from carious lesions; nonhemolytic white colonies with a 'spoked-wheel' aspect, charcoal-black pigmented variants
	R. mucilaginosa (formerly Stomatococcus mucilaginosa)	Coccoid forms, encapsulated	Oropharyngeal microflora	Bacteremia, endocarditis, meningitis, lower respiratory tract infections	Immunosuppression, indwelling foreign material	Nonhemolytic white to gray mucoid colonies; adherence of older colonies to the agar surface

*All acid-fast stain-negative.

such as *Mycobacterium* and *Tropheryma* are covered elsewhere (see Chapters 31, 39 and 185), and anaerobic actinomycetes (e.g. *Actinomyces israelii*) are discussed in Chapters 35 and 184.

Epidemiology

The prevalence of disease due to aerobic actinomycetes is not precisely established but remains rare. For nocardiosis, which represents the most frequently encountered disease in this group of micro-organisms, a frequency of about 2 per million cases annually has been proposed.[57,58] During the period prior to highly active antiretroviral therapy (HAART), the incidence of nocardiosis in AIDS patients with fewer than 100 CD4 cells/μL was estimated to vary from 0.3% to 1.8% according to geographic differences, and predominated in rural environments.[59] In organ transplant recipients, nocardiosis was diagnosed in 0.6% of the patients in a recent case–control study. Independent risk factors were high-dose steroids, history of cytomegalovirus disease and high levels of calcineurin inhibitors.[60]

Rhodococcus hoagii (formely *R. equi*), the second most frequent aerobic actinomycete, occurs in patients with the same predisposing factors. Rarely, infection may be observed in immunocompetent patients with a male-to-female ratio of 3:1 and a history of exposure to livestock.[61]

The reservoir of all aerobic actinomycetes is the soil environment where micro-organisms are implicated in decaying plant matter. *R. hoagii* is found in high proportion in dung from horses and foals. Aerobic actinomycetes are thought to be acquired essentially by inhalation from the soil. Colonization or infections may also be acquired through a traumatic lesion contaminated with soil, wound infections or catheter colonization.

Pathogenicity

Few studies have investigated the virulence mechanisms of aerobic actinomycetes. The complete genome sequence of *Nocardia farcinica* has revealed the presence of potent virulence determinants such as mammalian cell entry (Mce) proteins with homology with *Mycobacterium tuberculosis* Mce proteins,[62] allowing mycobacteria to multiply in a mammalian host. Similar Mce genes have also been identified in *R. hoagii*[63] and *Streptomyces coelicolor*.[64]

N. farcinica and *R. hoagii* also possess adherence factors with proteins belonging to fibronectin-binding protein families presenting a homology with antigen 85 of *M. tuberculosis*.[62,63]

Murine models have shown the importance of cell-mediated immunity in nocardiosis.[65] Studies with human monocytes show a resistance of *Nocardia* spp. to killing mechanisms of phagocytes by inhibition of phagosome–lysosome fusion and by bacterial detoxification enzymes (superoxide dismutase, catalase).[65] *In vitro* studies have also demonstrated the induction of apoptosis related to caspase activation during contact of cells with *N. asteroides*.[66] This may play a role in the progression of nocardiosis.

Abscess formation with polymorphonuclear cell infiltration and later cell necrosis represents the hallmark of histologic lesions of both *Nocardia* and *Rhodococcus*. Malakoplakia is a granulomatous inflammation in which large macrophages have basophilic inclusions known as Michaelis–Gutmann bodies. This entity is observed in *R. hoagii* infection in HIV-infected patients.[67] The origin of Michaelis–Gutmann bodies is attributed to an abnormal degradation of bacteria by phagocytes.

Diagnostic Microbiology

Microscopy and culture on appropriate media are critical for the precise clinical diagnosis of these infections, and contact with the laboratory is mandatory. Samples from the respiratory tract represent the majority of specimens, others being blood, cutaneous tissue, subcutaneous tissue biopsy and abscess collection from a large variety of organs. Multiple specimen examination is recommended, particularly from the respiratory tract.

Macroscopic examination of skin and soft tissue specimens is important to detect the presence of granules or concretions. These granules will be used selectively for microscopic examination since they represent masses of filaments embedded in necrotic tissue. Gram staining is preferred to modified acid-fast stain for visualization of this group of micro-organisms. However, determination of acid fastness is used as confirmatory staining. According to the species, the microscopic appearances may vary from coccoid and diphtheroid bacteria seen for *Rhodococcus* spp. and *Gordonia* spp. to branched and filamentous gram-positive bacilli for *Nocardia* spp. and *Streptomyces* spp. (see Table 178-5 and Figure 178-3, lanes 1–5C and 1–5D).

Routine media are generally used for recovery of aerobic actinomycetes; for specimens containing surface or mixed flora, selective media with antibiotic cocktails such as buffered charcoal yeast extract (BCYE) agar is recommended, particularly for *Nocardia* and for respiratory tract specimens. Media appropriate for mycobacteria such as Löwenstein may also be used. The incubation period for bacterial growth is prolonged, up to 2–3 weeks. Conventional blood cultures may be used for the detection of bacteremia due to *Rhodococcus* or *Gordonia*, but prolonged incubation is mandatory. In a review of *Nocardia* bacteremia, the detection time ranged from 2 to 14 days with a median of 4 days.[68]

A minimum of 48–72 hours is necessary before colonies become visible on routine media. Phenotypic aspects such as pigmentation or aerial hyphae appear later (see Table 178-5). Aerial hyphae give a powdery aspect to most *Nocardia* and *Streptomyces* isolates; sparse aerial hyphae can be observed with *Actinomadura* isolates or rarely for *Rhodococcus* strains. Mucoid colonies are typically seen for *R. hoagii* strains and *Actinomadura*. Only a small fraction of bacteria appear acid-fast using modified acid-fast stain, this property being enhanced in lipid-rich media such as Löwenstein.

Biochemical identification to species level is difficult since most commercial kits are not appropriate for aerobic actinomycete differentiation. MALDI-TOF mass spectrometry is a promising tool but improvement of the database is required for the diagnosis of actinomycetes.[69] Molecular techniques, notably sequencing of 16S rRNA, have now replaced biochemical identification.[70] Analysis of heat shock protein genes by PCR paired with restriction fragment length polymorphisms has also been described.[71]

The distinction of pattern of resistance to antimicrobial agents has been used to subtype *N. asteroides* complex into six different groups.[72] Species most frequently isolated in human specimens are *N. asteroides sensu stricto* type VI, *N. brasiliensis*, *N. farcinica* and *N. nova*, the proportion of each species varying according to the type of specimen and the geographic location.

TABLE 178-5	Medically Relevant Aerobic Actinomycetes						
Genera	Gram Stain	Acid-Fast Stain*	Predominant Species	Natural Habitat	Site of Infection	Risk Factors, Transmission	Diagnostic Comments
Nocardia	Branched filamentous gram-positive bacilli, short rods (breaking up of mycelia)	Positive	N. asteroides, N. nova, N. brasiliensis, N. farcinica	Inanimate environment (soil)	Soft tissue infection, nonmycetomic (mycetoma), respiratory and disseminated infection	Penetrating wound (occupational disease, male predominance, tropical and subtropical regions), immunosuppression (inhalation), underlying chronic lung disease	Presence of white to yellow intralesional grains (mycetoma); colonies white to red, superficially chalky appearance (powdery aerial hyphae); slow growth with aerial mycelium (3–7 days)
Rhodococcus	Coccoid forms to coccobacilli (may be dismissed as diphtheroids)	Weakly positive	R. hoagii	Inanimate environment (coprophilic soil – dung of horses)	Pulmonary (lung abscesses) and bacteremic infections, rare cutaneous infections (traumatic wounds)	Immunosuppression (AIDS, organ transplant recipients), contact with animals	Pink mucoid colonies (variant: yellow pigmentation, rough appearance)
Gordonia	Thin gram-positive coccobacilli (may be dismissed as diphtheroids)	Weakly positive	G. terrae	Inanimate environment (soil)	Bacteremia, endocarditis	Immunosuppression, indwelling foreign material, wound infections	Dry, wrinkled beige to orange colonies
Tsukamurella	Gram-positive rods	Positive	T. paurometabola	Inanimate environment (soil)	Bacteremia, endocarditis	Immunosuppression, indwelling foreign material	Psychrophilic micro-organism (grows best at cooler temperatures); slow growth
Actinomadura	Branched filamentous gram-positive bacilli with short chains of spores	Negative	A. madurae, A. pelletieri	Inanimate environment (soil)	Soft tissue infection (mycetoma), rare nonmycetomic disseminated infection, pneumonia (immunosuppression)	Penetrating wound (occupational disease, tropical and subtropical regions), inhalation (immunosuppression)	Colonies white to red, usually mucoid, 'molar tooth' appearance after a few days of growth; aerial hyphae if present are sparse and appear later during growth incubation
Streptomyces	Filamentous gram-positive bacilli	Negative	Streptomyces somaliensis	Inanimate environment (soil)	Soft tissue infection (mycetoma), perianal soft tissue infection	Penetrating wound (occupational disease, tropical and subtropical regions)	Presence of yellow to brown intralesional grains (mycetoma); smooth to rugous colonies, generally with powdery aerial hyphae

*Modified acid-fast staining with reduced acid decoloration.

Antibiotic susceptibility testing with broth microdilution is the recommended method.[73] The breakpoints for *Nocardia* and other aerobic actinomycetes are based on pharmacokinetic/pharmacodynamic (PK/PD) data. For clinical laboratories not performing these tests, collaboration with reference laboratories is important since these tests remain problematic due to the slow growth and the degradation of the antimicrobial agent.

Clinical Manifestations and Management

PULMONARY INFECTIONS AND DISSEMINATED INFECTIONS

Nocardiosis

Pulmonary infections and disseminated infections represent the most frequent form of nocardiosis. The patients are generally severely immunocompromised due to advanced HIV infections with low (<100) CD4 counts or are receiving chemotherapy with cytotoxic agents or immunosuppressive drugs. Pulmonary nocardiosis is also observed in patients with impaired local defenses due to chronic lung disease such as chronic obstructive pulmonary disease, bronchiectasis and chronic sarcoidosis.

Clinical presentation is subacute or chronic with cough, dyspnea, productive sputum, hemoptysis and systemic symptoms such as fever, weight loss and sweats. Lung infiltrates with and without abscess formation represent a frequent radiologic finding. Other findings are the presence of nodules, reticulonodular infiltrates, interstitial infiltrates and pleural effusions. Nocardial lesions are poorly localized and may extend to adjacent tissues with pleural effusion, pericarditis or mediastinitis. Misdiagnosis as malignancy or tuberculosis is frequent. In a recent observational study performed on adult patients diagnosed with pulmonary nocardiosis during a 13-year period, disseminated nocardiosis was observed in 30% of patients.[74] Any organ may be involved; however, a predilection for brain and cutaneous dissemination is frequently mentioned. In a review of 1050 cases in the literature, 44% of patients with systemic nocardiosis had cerebral infections, with pulmonary infection being the primary site.[65] Brain abscess may be an unapparent infection; in other cases seizures, headache or focal deficits predominate.

Pulmonary and disseminated nocardiosis treatment is based on antibiotic therapy. Standard treatment is TMP–SMX (co-trimoxazole) (15 mg/kg/day TMP component) in 2–4 divided doses for 3–6 months. Combination therapy with meropenem (2 g intravenously q8h) or imipenem (500 mg intravenously q6h) with or without amikacin is recommended for severely ill patients or for those with cerebral lesions.[75] There is, however, considerable debate over the extent to which *in vitro* antibiotic susceptibility testing is helpful in guiding the choice of therapy.

Clinical management of nocardial brain abscess has been reviewed.[76] If the nocardial infection is not documented elsewhere, aspiration or biopsy is recommended. When the nocardial infection is already documented, medical management is feasible for a brain abscess smaller than 2 cm. Surgical intervention and aspiration are needed if the clinical condition deteriorates, if the lesion does not shrink within 1 month or if the lesion is larger than 2.5 cm.

Mortality of pulmonary nocardiosis remains high in spite of adequate therapy. In one recent series, the mortality from pulmonary nocardiosis was 39%, 64% in case of disseminated nocardiosis and 100% in case of cerebral abscess.[74] In another series of organ recipients, 89% of patients were cured, including six of seven cases with disseminated disease.[60] The mortality rates may vary from series to series according to diagnostic procedure, optimization of treatment and the severity of the patient's immunosuppression.

Rhodococcus equi hoagii (formely R. equi)

The lung represents the primary site of infection due to *R. hoagii*. Inhalation is the portal of entry and severe immunosuppression is the major predisposing factor, in particular advanced HIV infection. In a large retrospective study in HIV patients, the lung was involved in more than 90% of cases.[77] The clinical presentation develops insidiously over days to weeks, with fever, nonproductive cough, dyspnea and pleuritic pain predominating. Lung infiltrates or nodules are observed on chest radiographs and pleural effusions may occur. Cavitation is seen in 63% of immunocompetent patients and in 41–77% of HIV-immunosuppressed patients.[61,78] Bacteremia is detected in more than 50% of cases and dissemination to the CNS, bone and soft tissue may occur.

Treatment of *R. hoagii* lung infection is based on antibiotic therapy. Surgical resection is considered for isolated lung abscesses and failure of medical treatment. *Rhodococcus hoagii* is usually susceptible *in vitro* to erythromycin, rifampin, fluoroquinolones, aminoglycosides, glycopeptides and imipenem. Several successful antibiotic regimens exist. A few principles guide the treatment:

- a combination regimen is necessary to avoid the appearance of resistance;
- prolonged therapy (2–6 months) is recommended to avoid frequently observed relapses;
- initial intravenous therapy with bactericidal agents such as imipenem and vancomycin is followed by oral therapy (e.g. macrolide plus quinolone);
- antibiotics able to kill intracellular micro-organisms are used;
- HAART is initiated in HIV patients to reduce mortality.[77]

Rhodococcus hoagii causes a serious disease with a high mortality rate. The outcome depends on predisposing factors. In the pre-HAART period, mortality was estimated to be greater than 50%. In an extensive series of *R. hoagii* infections in patients with HIV, HAART was the unique independent factor associated with reduced mortality.[77] In transplant recipients and immunocompetent patients, mortality is about 20%.[61,79]

CUTANEOUS AND SOFT TISSUE INFECTION

Nocardia spp., Actinomadura, Streptomyces

Cutaneous nocardiosis can be divided into two main groups: primary lesions observed generally in immunocompetent patients and secondary lesions observed following dissemination in immunosuppressed patients representing metastatic lesions due to a bacteremic episode. In primary cutaneous nocardiosis, infection results from inoculation of the micro-organism during skin trauma (outdoor activities) or following iatrogenic trauma such as surgery. Rarely, in immunosuppressed patients, primary cutaneous lesions may evolve in a disseminated disease.[80]

The clinical presentation of primary cutaneous lesions is as cellulitis or abscess, or as mycetoma. *Nocardia brasiliensis* is isolated in the majority of cases.[72] Mycetoma predominates in men living in rural and subtropical or tropical areas. Lesions are usually on the feet, legs, shoulders and back. Mycetoma is a general term for a chronic granulomatous infection of the subcutaneous tissue due to either aerobic actinomycetes (actinomycetoma) or filamentous fungi (eumycetoma) (see Chapter 190). In actinomycetoma the following etiologic agents predominate: *Nocardia*, *Streptomyces* and *Actinomadura*. Mycetoma begins as nodules that fistulate to the skin. Exudates contain granules corresponding to masses of bacteria embedded in necrotic tissue. The lesion is chronic, and pain or systemic manifestations are generally absent. In late-stage infection, deep soft tissue and bone are implicated. Superinfection with pyogenic bacteria is frequent. Identification of the etiologic agent is necessary to determine the appropriate antibiotic regimen. TMP–SMX prescribed for several months is the treatment of choice.[81] For treatment failure, amoxicillin–clavulanate is recommended.[82]

BACTEREMIA AND CATHETER-RELATED INFECTIONS

Nocardia

A positive blood culture for *Nocardia* is a rare event. In a large review, the incidence was estimated at 0.003%.[68] Secondary bacteremia associated with pulmonary infection and cutaneous infection predominates. In this series, less than 20% of *Nocardia*-positive blood culture was attributed to contamination. Catheter-related nocardial infections are also rare and catheter removal is recommended.

Rhodococcus hoagii (formely R. equi)

Bacteremia due to *R. hoagii* represents a secondary bacteremia during disseminated or lung infection. In HIV coinfected patients, up to 50% with *R. hoagii* lung disease have bacteremia.[77]

Gordonia

Gordonia is a rarely isolated human pathogen and only case reports or small series have been published. Several of these infections were bacteremias associated with an intravenous catheter.[83] The propensity of *Gordonia* spp. to biodegrade rubber may contribute to the pathogenesis of these infections.[84] Infections generally resolved with catheter removal and an antibiotic regimen containing vancomycin.[85] *In vitro,*

Gordonia strains are susceptible to imipenem and ciprofloxacin, frequently susceptible to gentamicin, vancomycin, azithromycin, ceftriaxone and ceftazidime (80–90% of isolates) and variably susceptible to doxycycline, TMP–SMX, erythromycin, penicillin, ampicillin and rifampin (30–70% of isolates).[85]

Tsukamurella

Tsukamurella have also been isolated in relation to central venous catheter-related infection.[86] In a review published in 2004, fewer than 20 cases of *Tsukamurella* infections were identified, the majority being catheter-related, generally in immunosuppressed patients.[87]

Management is based on medical device removal associated with an antibiotic regimen, generally with a β-lactam and an aminoglycoside.

References available online at expertconsult.com.

KEY REFERENCES

Brown-Elliott B.A., Brown J.M., Conville P.S., et al.: Clinical and laboratory features of the *Nocardia* spp. based on current molecular taxonomy. *Clin Microbiol Rev* 2006; 19(2):259-282.

Collier R.J., Young J.A.: Anthrax toxin. *Annu Rev Cell Dev Biol* 2003; 19:45-70.

Corti M.E., Villafane-Fioti M.F.: Nocardiosis: a review. *Int J Infect Dis* 2003; 7(4):243-250.

Cossart P., Sansonetti P.J.: Bacterial invasion: the paradigms of enteroinvasive pathogens. *Science* 2004; 304(5668):242-248.

Efstratiou A., Engler K.H., Mazurova I.K., et al.: Current approaches to the laboratory diagnosis of diphtheria. *J Infect Dis* 2000; 181(Suppl.1):S138-S145.

Funke G., Bernard K.: Coryneform gram-positive rods. In: Versalovic J., Carroll K.C., Funke G., et al., eds. *Manual of clinical microbiology: 1.* 10th ed. Washington, DC: ASM Press; 2011:413-443.

Hadfield T.L., McEvoy P., Polotsky Y., et al.: The pathology of diphtheria. *J Infect Dis* 2000; 181(Suppl.1):S116-S120.

Liu S., Zhang Y., Moayeri M., et al.: Key tissue targets responsible for anthrax-toxin-induced lethality. *Nature* 2013; 501(7465):63-68.

Logan N.A., Hoffmaster A., Shadomy S.V., et al.: *Bacillus* and other aerobic endospore-forming bacteria. In: James V., Carroll K.C., Funke G., et al., eds. *Manual of clinical microbiology: 1.* 10th ed. Washington, DC: ASM Press; 2011:381-402.

Ng L.S., Sim J.H., Eng L.C., et al.: Comparison of phenotypic methods and matrix-assisted laser desorption ionisation time-of-flight mass spectrometry for the identification of aero-tolerant *Actinomyces* spp. isolated from soft-tissue infections. *Eur J Clin Microbiol Infect Dis* 2012; 31(8):1749-1752.

Wellinghausen N.: *Listeria* and *Erysipelothrix.* In: Versalovic J., Carroll K.C., Funke G., et al., eds. *Manual of clinical microbiology: 1.* 10th ed. Washington, DC: ASM Press; 2011:403-412.

179

Neisseria

TONE TØNJUM | JOS VAN PUTTEN

Nature

The genus *Neisseria* was named after Albert Neisser who observed gonococci (*Neisseria gonorrhoeae*) in leukocytes in urethral exudates from patients with gonorrhea in 1879. Eight years later Weichselbaum isolated meningococci (*Neisseria meningitidis*) from six of eight cases of primary sporadic community-acquired meningitis. The gonococcus and the meningococcus are exclusively human pathogens and the most studied neisserial species.

Neisseria gonorrhoeae is an obligate pathogen that causes gonorrhea, a sexually transmitted disease. Gonorrhea was named by Galen in CE 130 after the Greek words *gonor* (seed) and *rhoia* (flow), suggesting that the disease was related to the flow of semen. In the 13th century, Maimonides recognized that the urethral discharge of male gonorrhea patients was not semen, but a sexually transmitted disease. In 1885 Bumm proved gonococci as the cause of gonorrhea by inoculating human volunteers.

Neisseria meningitidis is an opportunistic pathogen that can cause endemic and epidemic meningitis and/or sepsis worldwide. Epidemic meningococcal meningitis was first described by Vieusseaux in 1805 in Geneva. Throughout the 19th century periodic epidemics occurred, involving mainly young children and adolescents including military recruits. In 1896 Kiefer described the nasopharyngeal meningococcal carrier state among healthy people.

TAXONOMY

The family Neisseriaceae consists of the genus *Neisseria* as well as the heterogeneous genera (in order of decreasing relatedness to genus *Neisseria*) *Kingella, Eikenella, Alysiella, Simonsiella, Microvirgula, Lari-* *bacter, Vogesella, Vitreoscilla, Chromobacterium, Aquaspirillum, Prolinoborus, Formivibrio* and *Iodobacter* (Figure 179-1).[1] The taxonomy of the family has been extensively revised over the past decades, mainly based on 16S rRNA gene sequence analysis and whole genome sequencing, even though these methodologies do not reflect all the complex levels of relationships between these heterogeneous polyphyletic entities.

The members of the genus *Neisseria* are typically gram-negative cocci. The bacteria appear in pairs (diplococci). Diplococci have flattened opposing sides, imparting the characteristic kidney or coffee-bean appearance seen in stained smears. Some species are medium-to-large plump rods that sometimes occur in pairs or short chains (*N. elongata, N. weaveri, N. bacilliformis* and *N. shayeganii*). Several species possess capsules and are fimbriated (piliated). Endospores and exotoxins are not found and flagella are absent. Some *Neisseria* spp., including *N. gonorrhoeae* and *N. meningitidis*, may show surface-bound twitching motility due to pilus retraction. All species are aerobic.

N. gonorrhoeae and *N. meningitidis* are genetically very closely related human pathogens (Figure 179-1). The genus *Neisseria* is composed of 17 species that may be isolated from humans and six species that colonize various animals (Table 179-1).[2] *N. lactamica* and *N. cinerea* are most closely related to the pathogenic *Neisseria*, and frequently colonize the nasopharynx of children and adults. The saccharolytic *Neisseria* (*N. polysaccharea, N. subflava, N. sicca* and *N. mucosa*) are more distantly related to the other *Neisseria* and colonize humans less frequently. Commensal *Neisseria* species are widespread in animals and non-mammalian hosts and are even more distantly related to the human pathogens.[2]

TABLE 179-1	Members of the Genus *Neisseria*	
NEISSERIA SPECIES		
Humans		**Animal Hosts Only**
Urogenital Tract	**Oropharynx**	**Host/Species**
N. gonorrhoeae	N. meningitidis	Dogs/N. weaveri, N.
	N. lactamica	flavescens, N. animaloris,
	N. gonorrhoeae	N. mucosa, N. flavescens,
	N. animaloris	N. sicca, N. canis,
	N. bacilliformis	N. shayeganii, N.
	N. cinerea	zoodegmatis
	N. elongata	Guinea pigs/N. animalis,
	subsp. elongata	N. denitrificans
	subsp. glycolytica	Cow/N. dentiae
	subsp. nitroreducens	Cat, leopard, lion, tiger/N.
	N. flavescens	animaloris
	N. mucosa	Iguanas/N. iguanae
	var. mucosa	Dolphins/N. mucosa var.
	var. heidelbergensis	heidelbergensis
	N. polysaccharea	Monkeys/N. macacae
	N. sicca	Vulture/N. sicca
	N. subflava	Duck/N. mucosa
	bv. flava	Mosquito, fly, tick/
	bv. perflava	Neisseria spp.
	bv. subflava	Honey bee/N. meningitidis
	N. zoodegmatis	Louse/N. perflava, N.
	N. weaveri	mucosa, N. flavescens

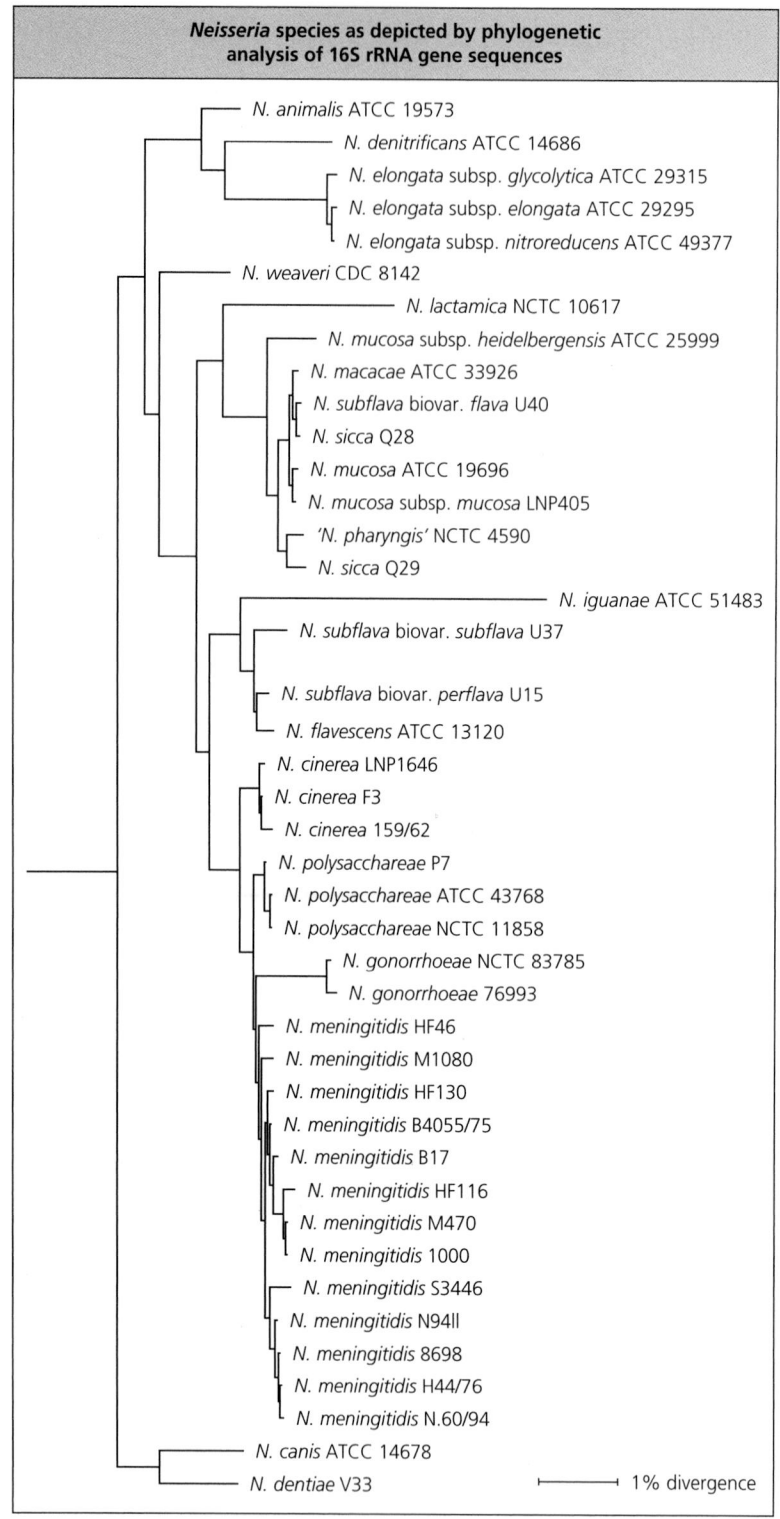

Figure 179-1   *Neisseria* species as depicted by phylogenetic analysis of 16S rRNA gene sequences. *(Redrawn from Tønjum.[1])*

GROWTH CHARACTERISTICS

Neisseria spp. grow best aerobically in an atmosphere containing 5–10% carbon dioxide at a temperature of 89.6–98.6°F (32–37°C) and a pH of 7–7.5. Cell size ranges from 0.6 to 1.5 mm depending upon the species source of the isolate and the age of the culture.

Neisseria spp. are fastidious. Blood agar and chocolate medium (blood heated at 176–194°F/80–90°C) are suitable growth media. Bacterial colonies usually appear after 24–48 hours of growth. Colonies of

N. gonorrhoeae are 0.5–1 mm in size. Colonies of *N. meningitidis* are usually larger (1–2 mm) and flatter. Colonies of the nonpathogenic *Neisseria* spp. are similar in size, appearance and consistency, except for the saccharolytic *Neisseria* spp. (*N. subflava, N. sicca* and *N. mucosa*) that are larger (1–3 mm), more convex and smooth (*N. mucosa*). Colonies of *N. subflava* and *N. sicca* are opaque and have varying consistency. *N. sicca* adhere to the agar surface and become wrinkled with prolonged incubation. Some nonpathogenic *Neisseria* spp. form a yellow pigment (*N. flavescens*) or a greenish-yellow pigment (*N. mucosa, N. subflava*).

Neisseria spp. are oxidase positive and catalase positive, except *N. elongata*, which is catalase negative. All species produce acid from a few carbohydrates by oxidation. The ability to produce polysaccharide from sucrose, to produce catalase and deoxyribonuclease, to reduce nitrate and nitrite, and to oxidize the tributyrin fatty acid can also be used to identify *Neisseria* spp.

GENOME DYNAMICS

The size of the *Neisseria* chromosome is approximately 2.2–2.3 Mb. The average G+C content is 48–56 mol%. *N. meningitidis* and *N. gonorrhoeae* share about 95% of their gene content.[1] The vast majority of genes are also present in nonpathogenic *N. lactamica*, but gene regulation may be different in pathogenic and commensal strains.[3] Due to genetic instability, the *Neisseria* spp. have hyperdynamic genomes.[4] The genome plasticity contributes to adaptation and immune evasion and thereby to the pathogenic potential of *N. meningitidis* and *N. gonorrhoeae* and the development of hypervirulent lineages. The most important sources of neisserial genome instability (Figure 179-2) are as follows:

- *Phase variation*, i.e. variable protein expression due to slipped-strand mispairing of nucleotide runs found within or close to the promoter region (affect transcription) or within open reading frames (affect translation). There are more than 100 phase-variable genes in the pathogenic *Neisseria* spp.[5]
- *Recombination*, i.e. the genetic exchange or rearrangement of DNA from external or internal sources. This may, for example, lead to the generation of millions of variants of pilin subunits.

- *Horizontal gene transfer*, i.e. the introduction of genes predominantly via natural transformation (mediated by the DNA uptake sequences, DUS) and integration into the chromosome by RecA-mediated homologous recombination. *Neisseria* spp. are naturally competent for transformation throughout their growth cycle.
- *Hypermutation*, i.e. increased global mutation rates often associated with DNA repair deficiencies, replication infidelity or overexpression of DNA translesion polymerases.

The pathogenic *Neisseria* spp. share several genomic regions, including up to nine prophage and eight genetic islands, that are absent from *N. lactamica*.[6] There are no classic pathogenicity islands as are present in many other bacterial species. *N. meningitidis*-specific DNA sequences include the *cps* locus encoding the polysaccharide capsule, genes that encode the RTX family of toxins and an ortholog of the filamentous hemagglutinin of *Bordetella pertussis*. Certain hypervirulent lineages contain the filamentous prophage Nf1.[7] About 80% of the gonococcal clinical isolates and *N. meningitidis* strains of serogroups W135, H and Z contain the 'gonococcal genetic island' (GGI, 57 kb).[6] This often chromosomally integrated conjugative plasmid encodes a type IV secretion system involved in DNA secretion. The genome of *Neisseria* spp. has a variable number of noncoding repeat arrays and insertion (IS) elements among which IS*1655* appears unique to *N. meningitidis*.

Most isolates of *N. gonorrhoeae* but not *N. meningitidis* carry plasmids.[8] Nearly all gonococcal strains carry a 4.2 kb cryptic plasmid of unknown function and many strains carry plasmids encoding β-lactamase causing resistance to penicillin.

Genome-based phylogenetic reconstruction indicates that some hundreds of years ago pathogenic *N. meningitidis* emerged from a

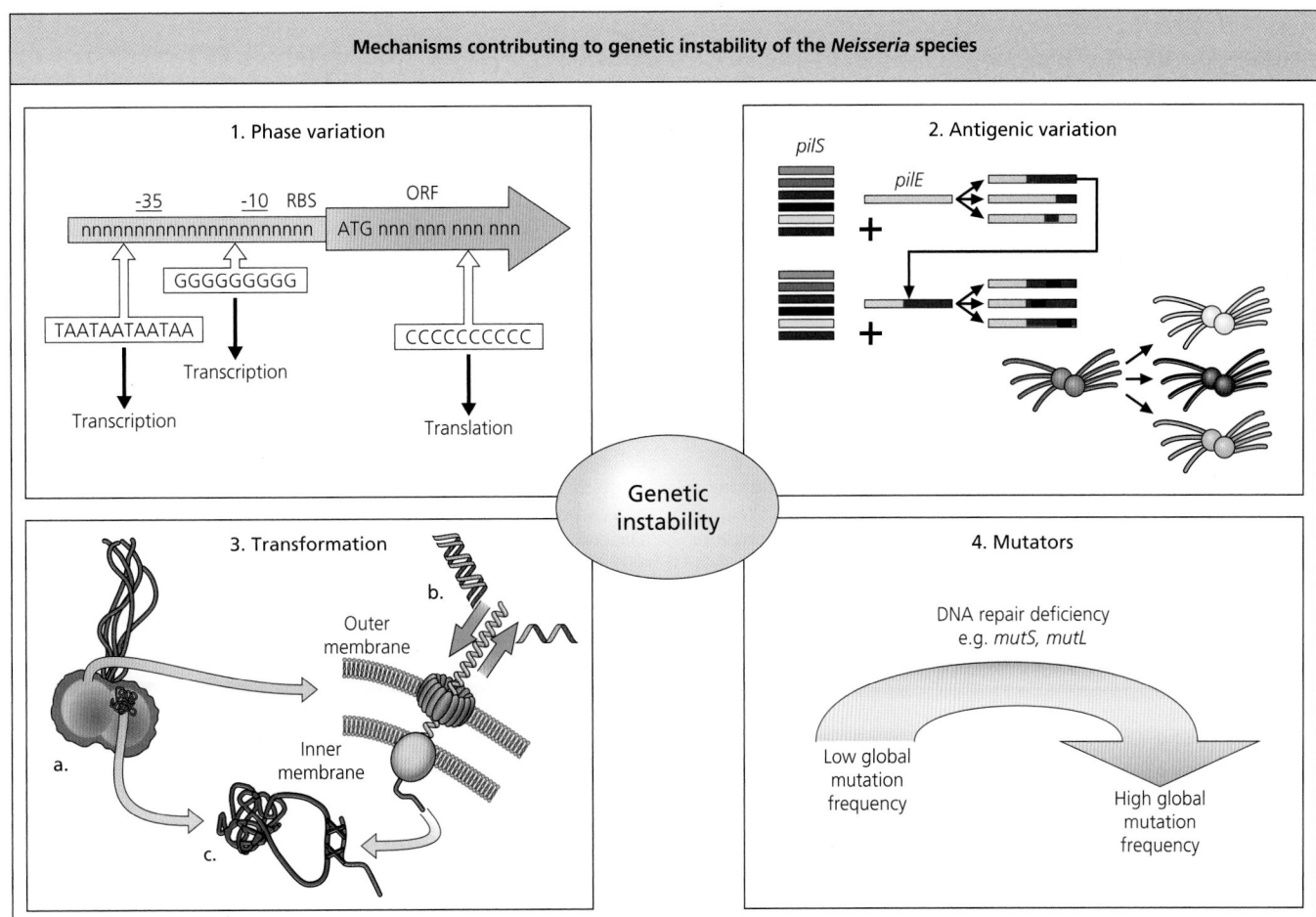

Figure 179-2 Mechanisms contributing to genetic instability of the *Neisseria* species. (*Redrawn from Davidsen et al.*[4])

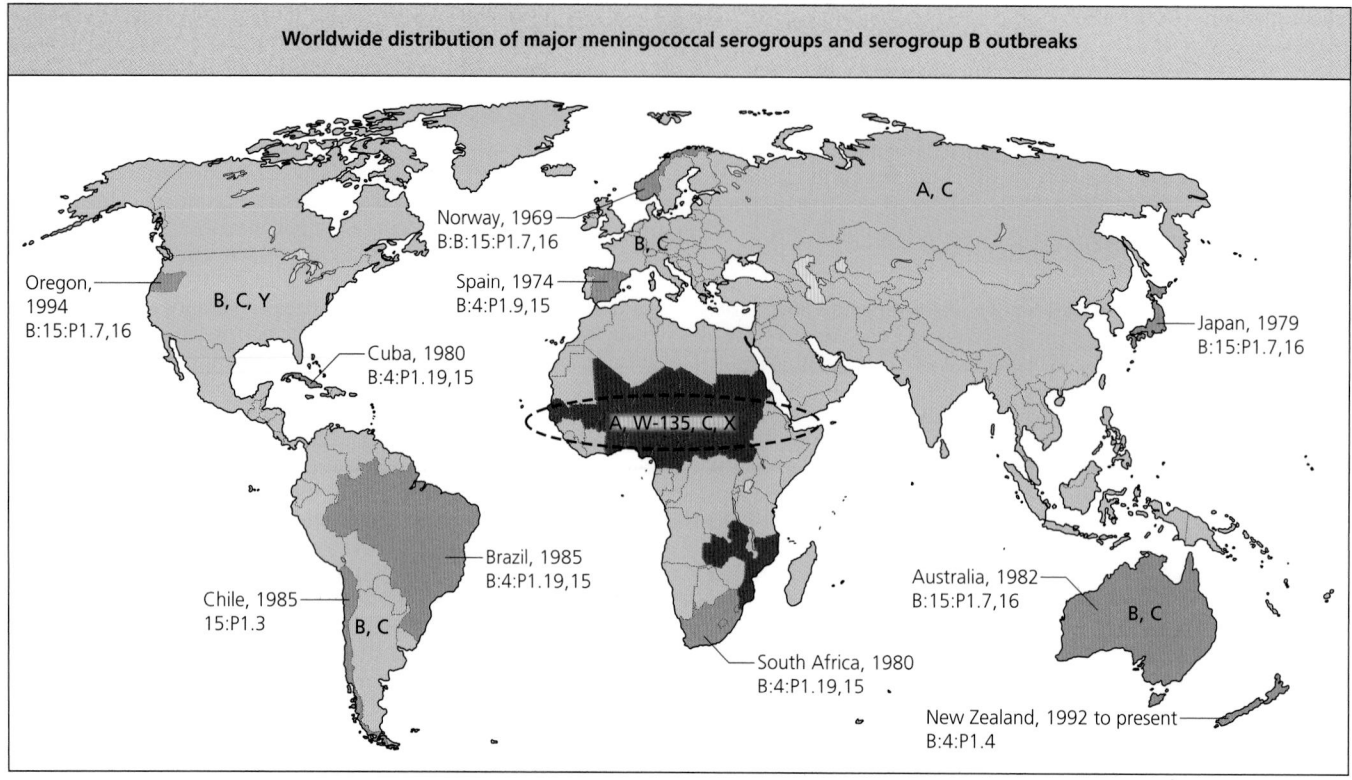

Worldwide distribution of major meningococcal serogroups and serogroup B outbreaks

Oregon, 1994
B:15:P1.7,16

B, C, Y

Norway, 1969
B:B:15:P1.7,16

Spain, 1974
B:4:P1.9,15

B, C

A, C

Japan, 1979
B:15:P1.7,16

Cuba, 1980
B:4:P1.19,15

A, W-135, C, X

Brazil, 1985
B:4:P1.19,15

Chile, 1985
15:P1.3

B, C

Australia, 1982
B:15:P1.7,16

B, C

South Africa, 1980
B:4:P1.19,15

New Zealand, 1992 to present
B:4:P1.4

Figure 179-3 Worldwide distribution of major meningococcal serogroups and serogroup B outbreaks (in purple). The meningitis belt (dotted line) of sub-Saharan Africa and other areas of substantial meningococcal disease in Africa are shown. *(Redrawn from Stephens et al.[12])*

common unencapsulated ancestor by acquisition of capsule genes, probably from members of the family Pasteurellaceae.[9]

Epidemiology
GONORRHEA

Gonorrhea is a common sexually transmitted disease worldwide. *N. gonorrhoeae* infection is the second most common notifiable disease in the USA, with 333 004 cases reported in 2013.[10] Incidences in Europe and in the developing world are 10–30 and 4000–10 000 per 100 000 population, respectively.[11] The actual disease burden is probably higher due to underdiagnosis and underreporting. The highest attack rates occur in 15–25-year-old men and women. In regions where collected statistics include sexual orientation, rates of gonococcal infection more than quadrupled from 1995 to 2013 among men who have sex with men (MSM).

Gonococci are exclusive human pathogens. The risk of acquiring a urethral infection for men is approximately 20% after a single vaginal exposure to an infected woman, rising to 60–80% after four or more exposures. The transmission rate from male to female is approximately 50% per contact, rising to 90% after three exposures. Gonococci are transmitted by orogenital contact or rectal intercourse. Perinatal transmission may also occur. Although gonococci can survive for brief periods outside the human reservoir, extracorporeal transmission is extremely rare.

The major reservoir for continued spread of gonorrhea is the asymptomatic patient. Among infected women, 30–50% are asymptomatic or show no symptoms associated with a sexually transmitted disease.[11] Among infected men, only 5–10% are asymptomatic. Asymptomatic women and men remain infectious for months. Maintenance and transmission of gonorrhea are also related to a social subset of 'core transmitters' who have unprotected intercourse with multiple new partners and either are asymptomatic or choose to ignore symptoms. The average incubation period for developing gonorrhea is 2–7 days but can vary between 1 and 14 days.

MENINGOCOCCAL DISEASE

Meningococcal disease is a global major health problem (Figure 179-3).[12] The annual number of invasive disease cases worldwide is estimated to be at least 1.2 million, with 135 000 deaths related to invasive meningococcal disease.[13] Disease patterns differ among populations and infecting strains and can be endemic, hyperendemic, epidemic and pandemic. The case fatality rate is 5–10% in industrialized countries, and 10–20% of survivors develop permanent sequelae. Transmission of meningococci occurs by respiratory aerosol droplets and hand-to-mouth contact in children, requiring close contact. Invasive disease occurs particularly when bactericidal antibodies against the invading strain are lacking.[14] Concurrent viral or mycoplasmal respiratory tract infections facilitate systemic invasion.

The major virulence factor of disease-associated meningococci is the polysaccharide capsule.[14] Most infections are caused by strains belonging to serogroups A, B, C, Y and W135 (see Figure 179-3).[11] In Western Europe and the Americas, meningococcal disease is endemic and caused mainly by serogroups B or C with incidences of 1–3/100 000. Periodically, local hyperendemic outbreaks occur when new lineages spread through the population. A serogroup B infection has spread worldwide, culminating in outbreaks in Australia and New Zealand in 2001–2006.[11] In China, the Middle East and parts of Africa, serogroups A and C predominate. Large epidemics are attributed predominantly to serogroup A strains. In the African 'meningitis belt', major periodic epidemics of serogroup A disease occur every 5–12 years, with attack rates of 500/100 000 population or higher.[15] The emergence and global importance of serogroups W135, X and Y has been recognized only in the last 10 years. Serogroup W135 was identified in 2002–2003 as a major threat and the main pathogen during outbreaks in Africa. An unprecedented incidence of serogroup X meningitis was observed in Niger in 2006.[16] Occasionally, particularly virulent strains arise that cause pandemic outbreaks across continents.[12] In the USA, Israel and Sweden, disease due to serogroup Y strains has increased.[17]

The occurrence of meningococcal disease varies with climate, age and social behavior. Serogroup A and C disease increases during the

TABLE 179-2	Neisserial Virulence Factors
Virulence Factor	**Function**
Lipopolysaccharide (LPS/LOS)	Lipo-oligosaccharide (LOS) has endotoxin activity and is released as bacterial outer membrane vesicles (blebs) or through cellular lysis. LOS is responsible for toxic damage to the human tissue, development of septic shock and disseminated intravascular coagulation (DIC) through interactions with Toll-like receptors (TLR4) and cytokine induction
Polysaccharide capsule (*N. meningitidis* only)	Polysaccharide surface component which works as a protective shell and blocks the insertion of the membrane attack complex of the complement system and protects the bacteria from phagocytosis. The capsule is the main component enabling bacterial survival in blood and resisting bactericidal antibodies. The serogroup B capsule can also mimic human antigens
Type IV pili	Major adhesins that mediate initial attachment to non-ciliated human cells. Also required for efficient transformation of DNA
Outer membrane proteins (OMP)	Dominant antigens. Porin proteins promote intracellular survival. Opacity proteins mediate firm attachment to eukaryotic cells. RmpM protein may protect other antigens from bactericidal interactions with antibodies. Frequent antigenic variation makes it difficult for the host immune system to recognize the porin and opacity protein antigens
Iron-binding proteins	Transferrin-, lactoferrin- and hemoglobin-binding proteins. Pathogenic *Neisseria* spp. are dependent on a constant iron supply for growth
IgA1 protease	Destroys mucosal IgA which is a part of the local immune system
β-Lactamase	An enzyme that hydrolyzes the β-lactam ring of penicillin. Important for antibiotic resistance development in *Neisseria* spp.

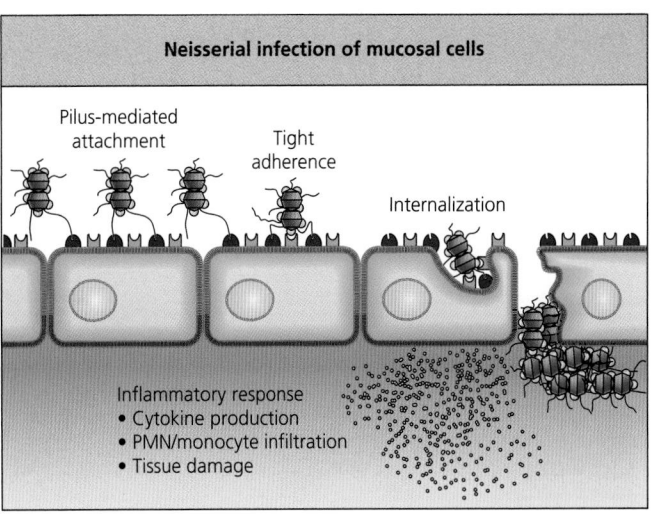

Figure 179-4   Neisserial infection of mucosal cells.

dry season in Africa. The number of serogroup B and C cases peaks during the winter months in higher-income countries.[11] In the meningitis belt, young school-aged children represent the peak age group. In higher-income countries, children aged between 1 and 4 years account for the majority of cases with a second peak among teenagers.[11] Young adult smokers who socialize frequently at discos and parties may be particularly at risk.[12] Passive smoking predisposes children to contract meningococcal disease.[12] The attack rate among family members of a clinical case is 1000-fold higher than in the general population. The acquisition of meningococcal disease requires a combination of a pathogenic organism, a susceptible host, and possibly coincidental mucosal damage by other infections, nutrition or low humidity. Hereditary factors such as late complement deficiencies and receptor polymorphisms may be additional predisposing factors.[12,18]

Pathogenicity
GONOCOCCAL PATHOGENESIS
At the cellular level, a large repertoire of often phase-variable adhesins and invasion-promoting surface factors enables gonococcal infection of different niches and with different cell tropism (Table 179-2).[19] The first step in gonococcal infection is the type IV pilus-mediated attachment to mucosal cells (Figure 179-4).[20] Once attached, PilT-mediated pilus retraction brings the bacteria into intimate contact with the cell surface and stimulates mechanosensitive host cell signaling pathways.[21] Shortly after initial attachment Opa proteins interact with carcinoem-

bryonic antigen-related cell adhesion molecules (CEACAM) and/or heparan sulfate proteoglycan (HSPG) receptors.[22] Different Opa proteins bind to distinct receptors types. *In vitro* Opa-receptor interactions result in efficient internalization of the gonococci by host cells (Figure 179-4).[19] PorB-IA expressing strains also efficiently invade cells in the absence of Opa proteins.[22,23] Bacteria carrying distinct lipo-oligosaccharide (LOS) variants may invade through binding of lectin receptors.[24] Bacteria with sialylated LOS variants are impaired in invasion but more resistant to killing by complement. Gonococci induce recruitment of and show intimate association with polymorphonuclear leukocytes (Figure 179-4). Type IV pili and distinct Opa proteins confer non-opsonophagocytosis.[19] Some of the gonococci ingested may resist killing by phagocytes.

The presence of *N. gonorrhoeae* is sensed by the host innate immune system. Neisserial LOS is recognized by the Toll-like receptor (TLR)4–MD2 complex. Porins interact with the TLR2 receptor complex. Peptidoglycan fragments activate the cytoplasmic Nod-1 receptors. These interactions induce the secretion of cytokines, chemokines and antimicrobial peptides.

Gonococcal infection elicits a strong humoral immune response. Dominant antigens are PorB, Opa proteins, RmpM, LOS and iron-regulated proteins. Nevertheless, the antibodies provide limited protection due to bacterial surface variation and bacterial immune evasion mechanisms (see Table 179-2). The extensive phenotype variation and immune escape mechanisms are major obstacles in the generation of a broadly protective gonococcal vaccine.

MENINGOCOCCAL PATHOGENESIS
Meningococcal colonization of the nasopharynx largely resembles the events following gonococcal infection (see above).[19] Type IV pili facilitate initial adherence, and opacity-associated proteins (Opa and Opc) and PorB trigger uptake of the bacteria into the cells largely via similar types of receptor (CEACAM, HSPG). Particular sets of Opa protein variants are found in hyperinvasive meningococcal lineages. Opa and Opc proteins that bind heparan sulfate and thus are able to recruit heparin-binding proteins such as vitronectin and fibronectin enter cells via integrin receptors. This is accompanied by a downregulation of pili and capsule, enabling optimal contact between bacterial adhesins and the host mucosa. Transferrin (TbpA, TbpB) and hemoglobin (Hbp) binding proteins recruit the iron sources required for growth.[25] Ciliated mucosal cells may be damaged by released peptidoglycan fragments and LOS. Meningococcal (and gonococcal) infection of the oropharynx is usually entirely asymptomatic, possibly because of the relatively high threshold for activation of an inflammatory response in the oropharynx compared to more sterile anatomic niches such as the urethra.

Steps in pathogenesis of *N. meningitidis* infection

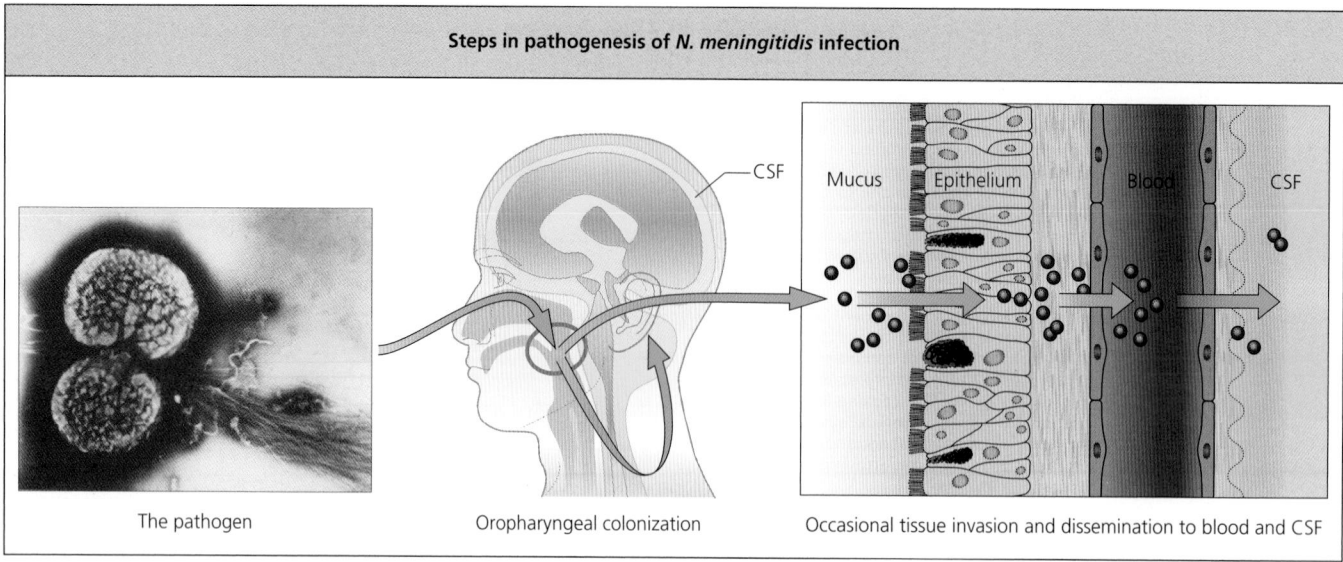

| The pathogen | Oropharyngeal colonization | Occasional tissue invasion and dissemination to blood and CSF |

Figure 179-5   Steps in pathogenesis of *N. meningitidis* infection. (*Redrawn from Davidsen et al.*[26])

The mechanism of meningococcal penetration and passage of the mucosa is only partially understood.[20] The major difference in pathogenesis between gonococci and meningococci is the ability of distinct meningococcal lineages to survive in the bloodstream and to access the cerebrospinal fluid (CSF) (Figure 179-5).[26] The few phylogenetic groups of *N. meningitidis* that cause meningococcal disease often carry a filamentous prophage in their genome that is released from the bacteria via the type IV pilus secretin.[7] The prophage may promote the development of new epidemic clones. Meningococci survive and multiply during epithelial cell traversal. The IgA1 protease and PorB may promote survival on mucosal surfaces and inside epithelial cells, respectively. Meningococci isolated from the bloodstream invariably produce polysaccharide capsule. The capsule protects the bacterium from phagocytosis and complement-mediated lysis by preventing insertion of the terminal complement attack complex. Invasive meningococci express sialylated LOS which influences binding of C4b, while the proteins PorA and GNA1870 recruit the negative regulators of complement activation C4BP and factor H.[18] Individuals with inherited deficiencies in the late complement components (C6–C9) have a high risk of developing meningococcal disease. Intriguingly, they acquire the infection at a much later age, have frequent recurrences, and the fatality rate is much lower than for normo-complementemic individuals.[18] This may be because the complement deficiency results in less effective cell lysis and therefore less endotoxin release.[27]

STRUCTURE AND VIRULENCE FACTORS

Neisseria spp., like other gram-negative bacteria, have a cell wall that consists of two membranes separated by a thin peptidoglycan layer (Figure 179-6). The inner cytoplasmic membrane consists of proteins embedded in a phospholipid bilayer that is impermeable for hydrophilic compounds. The outer membrane is an asymmetric bilayer composed of phospholipids in the inner leaflet and LOS in the outer leaflet. The LOS renders the outer membrane relatively resistant to detergents and is semipermeable due to the presence of protein channels, called porins. Other surface-exposed outer membrane proteins and extracellular appendages such as capsular structures and type IV pili particularly contribute to neisserial survival and virulence.[19] Neisserial outer membrane vesicles (OMVs, blebs) that contain nucleic acids, protein and high levels of LOS are continuously shed by the bacteria.

Capsules

N. meningitidis produces a polysaccharide capsule (see Figure 179-6). On the basis of structural differences in capsule, meningococci are

Architecture of the neisserial cell wall

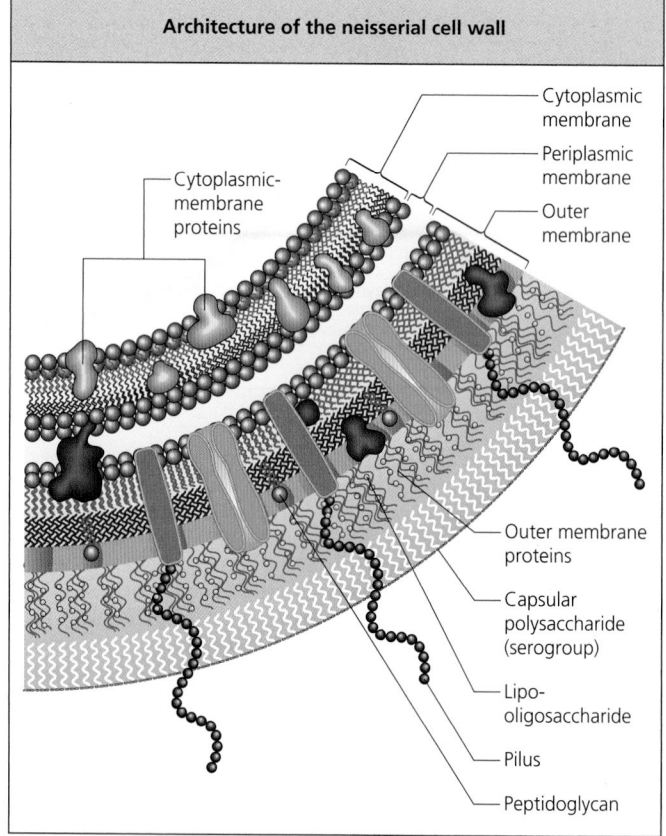

Cytoplasmic-membrane proteins

Cytoplasmic membrane

Periplasmic membrane

Outer membrane

Outer membrane proteins

Capsular polysaccharide (serogroup)

Lipo-oligosaccharide

Pilus

Peptidoglycan

Figure 179-6   Architecture of the neisserial cell wall. (*Redrawn from Stephens et al.*[12])

divided into at least 13 serogroups (A, B, C, D, 29E, H, I, K, L, W135, X, Y and Z). Serogroups A, B, C, Y and W135 cause more than 90% of meningococcal disease. Capsular types are normally stable but strains can acquire variant capsule gene alleles by transformation.[28] Serogroup B can thus switch to C or vice versa. The serogroup A capsule contains *N*-acetyl-mannosamine-1-phosphate. The capsules of the serogroups B, C, Y and W135 consist of polymers of

N-acetylneuraminic (sialic) acid. The B polysaccharide resembles structures present in human neural tissues, limiting its immunogenicity and vaccine potential. The carbohydrates can be variably *O*-acetylated. Isolates from healthy carriers are frequently unencapsulated due to reversible changes in capsule gene expression. A substantial proportion of meningococcal carrier isolates are incapable of capsule production due to deletions in or a lack of capsule genes. Isolates from the bloodstream or CSF are invariably encapsulated.

N. gonorrhoeae does not produce a polysaccharide capsule. However, both meningococci and gonococci are covered with a loosely adherent capsular-like structure containing high-molecular weight polyphosphate. This layer provides protection against environmental stress.

Pili

Pili are hair-like fibers consisting of thousands of protein subunits (pilin, 16–20 kDa).[20] Pathogenic *Neisseria* spp. have long pili (up to 4300 nm in length), termed type IV pili, that protrude from the bacterial surface (see Figure 179-6). Nonpathogenic *Neisseria* spp. may express both long and short pili (175–210 nm in length). Type IV pili confer bacterial cell-to-cell interactions and twitching motility – a form of locomotion that is powered by extension and retraction of the pilus filament.[19] Pili are essential for adhesion to epithelial and endothelial cells and impart tissue tropism.[19] Expression of type IV pili is also required for transformation of DNA.[4]

During infection pilins undergo rapid phase shifts and antigenic variation. The single *pilE* expression locus is changed by unidirectional donation of coding sequences from multiple silent partial *pilS* genes in a process similar to gene conversion (see Figure 179-2), producing an extensive repertoire of antigenic variants.[20] The frequency of antigenic pilus variation may be as high as 10^3. Pilin can be post-translationally modified with phosphorylcholine, phosphoethanolamine and variable acetylated O-linked glycans.[29,30]

N. gonorrhoeae produces one type of pili (class I). *N. meningitidis* can express class I or class II pili which are antigenically and structurally distinct, while commensals express only class II pili. Class II pili are encoded by a different *pilE* gene that has no silent cassette counterparts.

Surface Proteins

The repertoire of the meningococcal and gonococcal surface proteins is very similar.[19] Trimeric protein channels (porins) confer transport of low-molecular nutrients across the outer membrane. The principal gonococcal porin is PorB (formerly protein I). The gonococcal PorB porin is essential for bacterial survival. Gonococci express either of two PorB isotypes, termed PorB-IA and PorB-IB. The proteins are stably expressed and display interstrain variation due to amino acid differences in surface-exposed regions. The antigenic heterogeneity is the basis for gonococcal PorB-based serologic typing. PorB-IA strains are resistant to normal human serum and can cause disseminated gonococcal infection.

N. meningitidis can express two types of porins simultaneously: PorA and PorB. PorA (class 1 protein, 44–47 kDa) is variably expressed and PorA-negative variants can be isolated from patients.[11] Expression of at least one of the porin types is required for meningococcal survival. PorA antigenic differences serve as the basis for serologic subtyping of meningococci. Meningococcal PorB is equivalent to the gonococcal PorB protein and is present as either PorB-IA (class 2 protein) or PorB-IB (class 3 protein).[11] Serotyping of meningococci is also based on antigenic differences in PorB.

The neisserial RmpM protein (formerly protein III or class 4 protein) is complexed to and likely stabilizes outer membrane protein complexes including porins.[31] The protein is stably expressed by gonococci and meningococci. Its C-terminal periplasmic region resembles *Escherichia coli* OmpA domains and interacts with peptidoglycan. Rmp-specific antibodies may interfere with the bactericidal activity of antibodies directed to other surface antigens and increase the risk of infection.[31]

Both pathogenic *Neisseria* spp. can express different opacity (Opa) proteins (formerly protein II or class 5 proteins, 20–28 kDa).[19] Colonies of gonococci expressing Opa proteins often have a more opaque appearance. In meningococci colonial opacity is most evident at 88°F (31°C) when capsule production is low. The gonococcus contains up to 11 different *opa* genes. The meningococcal genome contains three to four *opa* genes. The expression of each Opa protein can independently be switched on and off, enabling expression of multiple proteins simultaneously.[19] This phase and antigenic variation limits their vaccine potential.

In addition, both pathogenic *Neisseria* spp. express more than 80 other outer membrane proteins, among which the pilus-related secretin complex PilQ is the most abundant.[4] Protein expression may vary, depending on the bacterial growth conditions. Iron-regulated proteins are essential for survival of gonococci and meningococci *in vivo*.[26] The transferrin-binding proteins (Tbp-1 and Tbp-2) and the lactoferrin-binding proteins (Lbp) are scavenger proteins that mediate internalization of iron into the bacterium. Conserved surface-exposed proteins such as NspA, NadA, GNA1870 (factor H binding protein) and GNA2132 (hypothetical lipoprotein) are recognized vaccine antigens.[32]

Lipo-Oligosaccharide

Approximately half of the neisserial surface comprises lipid-anchored oligosaccharides (LOS) (see Figure 179-6). Neisserial LOS is composed of hexa-acylated lipid A, two keto-deoxyoctulosonate, a carbohydrate (KDO) molecules, and one or more carbohydrate chains of 8–12 saccharide units, the core oligosaccharide. Lipid A anchors LOS in the outer membrane and is one of the most potent bacterial endotoxins.[24,33]

The core oligosaccharide of neisserial LOS is divided into an inner and an outer core region. The composition of the inner core is heterogeneous due to variable substitutions (phosphoethanolamine, glycine, glucose, *O*-acetyl groups).[24] This variation in glycoforms is partially regulated by environmental cues. The outer core is highly variable and undergoes high-frequency phase and antigenic variation due to frequent nucleotide mismatching during replication of LOS biosynthesis genes and horizontal gene transfer.[24] A single strain can simultaneously express up to six related LOS structures. The terminal structure of neisserial LOS is the target for sialylation by bacterial sialyltransferase. Gonococci utilize host sialic acid (CMP-NeuNAc) to modify their LOS. Meningococci produce their own CMP-NeuNAc. The terminal LOS of the pathogenic *Neisseria* spp. often shares epitopes with host glycolipids.[25] This molecular mimicry is exploited by the pathogens to interact with host cell lectin receptors and limits the vaccine potential of the LOS.

Peptidoglycan

Neisserial peptidoglycan consists of long chains of repeated disaccharide units cross linked via peptide bridges.[34] Peptidoglycan metabolism is a dynamic process involving coordinated activity of lytic and synthetic enzymes. The peptidoglycan is synthesized by up to four penicillin-binding proteins (PBPs). *O*-acetylation of peptidoglycan protects against autolysis by endogenous lytic transglycosylases and host lysozymes. Released peptidoglycan fragments activate the innate immune response and contribute to the inflammatory response.

Secreted Factors

Meningococcal and gonococcal genome analyses predict the presence of autotransporter-, two-partner-, type I and type II secretion mechanisms.[35] The pathogenic *Neisseria* spp. secrete immunoglobulin A1 (IgA1) protease. This serine protease directs its own transport across the outer membrane and secretion into the environment. The enzyme cleaves in the hinge of IgA1 separating the Fab and Fc regions, making IgA ineffective. IgA protease also cleaves other proteins such as endosomal Lamp1, which is important for intracellular vesicle trafficking. The function of the other secreted proteins including the filamentous hemagglutinin (FHA)-like protein TpsA and FrpA/C is largely unknown. A subset (≈80%) of gonococcal strains secrete DNA via a type IV secretion system.[36] *Neisseria* spp. lack a type III secretion mechanism which is present in many other pathogens.

Prevention

GONOCOCCAL INFECTION

Condoms provide a high degree of protection from acquisition of gonorrhea, as well as other sexually transmitted diseases (STDs). Other preventative measures are early diagnosis and treatment, partner notification and screening, and case finding. A new approach is the use of topical microbicides for intravaginal or intrarectal use.

Attempts to develop a gonococcal vaccine have been hampered by the multitude of gonococcal immune evasion strategies including a high degree of antigenic variability in pili, outer membrane proteins and LOS during the natural course of infection. Transfected animals expressing human proteins involved in *Neisseria* infection such as transferrin receptors, CR3, CD46, CEACAMs and Toll-like receptors may aid vaccine development.

MENINGOCOCCAL DISEASE

Prevention of meningococcal disease is based on chemoprophylaxis and vaccination.[33]

Chemoprophylaxis

The aim of chemoprophylaxis is to reduce secondary cases of meningococcal disease and to arrest outbreaks. The risk of a secondary case among close contacts in the household setting is 150–1000 times higher than that in the general population. Children are at greatest risk, but secondary disease can occur at all ages. Risk is maximal in the week following recognition of the index case but extends for several weeks.

Ceftriaxone as a single intramuscular dose is 97% effective in household contacts 1–2 weeks after infection. The advantage of ceftriaxone is that it can be used in pregnancy and in small children. Many antibiotics used for therapy do not effectively eradicate or prevent carriage of meningococci because of inadequate levels in oropharyngeal secretions. Rifampin, ceftriaxone, azithromycin and the quinolones are effective against meningococci in the naso- and oropharynx.[12] However, rifampin and quinolone resistance can develop rapidly in meningococci. Chemoprophylaxis is recommended only for close household contacts of cases and other intimate contacts.

Vaccines

Polysaccharide meningococcal vaccines against serogroups A, C, W135 and Y conjugated to tetanus toxoid are available and used successfully worldwide. The immunogenicity of polysaccharide vaccines is greatly improved by chemical conjugation to a protein carrier. These vaccines are safe and immunogenic, are anticipated to provide long-term protection (as they induce a T-cell-dependent response) and are also effective in young children.[37] Introduction of the C conjugate meningococcal vaccines in 2000 markedly reduced the incidence of serogroup C disease in the UK and other European countries with estimated vaccine efficacies of 88% in young children and 95% in young adolescents. Immunization also decreased nasopharyngeal carriage by 66% and transmission of the pathogen (herd immunity).[38] These conjugated vaccines are also used to contain outbreaks of meningococcal infections in MSM in Europe and the USA.

A polysaccharide vaccine against serogroup B meningococci is not available due to carbohydrate mimicry and poor immunogenicity. However, a universal vaccine that protects against *N. meningitidis* serogroup B, which causes most cases of disease in temperate countries, was released for use in 2014.[32] Relevant conserved candidate vaccine antigens were identified by the 'reverse vaccinology' approach.[39] In the current vaccine against serogroup B meningococcal disease recombinant NHBA (*Neisseria* heparin binding antigen), NadA (Neisserial adhesin A) and fHbp (factor H binding protein) in combination with OMV (with PorA P1.4 2) are included (Bexsero, GlaxoSmithKline).[39]

The absence of an efficient serogroup B vaccine until very recently has limited the effective control of meningococcal disease. Meningococcal vaccines are given to small children, young people at risk including military recruits and are used by travelers visiting countries with a high incidence of meningococcal disease. However, widespread use of monovalent serogroup conjugate vaccines may become ineffective when the capsule types switch due to genetic exchange or strains arise that show reduced capsule expression.

Capsule polysaccharide vaccines for the pathogenic meningococcal serogroups A, C, Y and W135 used before the era of conjugated vaccines reduced the incidence of infection among military recruits, reduced the progress of epidemics of serogroup A disease and protected susceptible complement factor-deficient individuals.[12] These vaccines are safe, with mild local adverse events, and have good efficacy (>85%) in older children and adults. However, due to lack of a T-helper response, nonconjugated capsule vaccines are poorly immunogenic below 2 years of age, fail to induce immunologic memory and provide protection for only 3–5 years.

Outer Membrane Vesicle

OMV vaccines with a low LOS composition show efficacies of 50–80% in clinical trials, but do not protect young children and are in general too strain-specific, i.e. the vaccines can be used against clonal disease outbreaks, but not for prevention of sporadic disease caused by diverse strains.[12] Multivalent vaccine strains based on common variants of PorA (a major inducer and target of bactericidal antibodies) may provide protection against multiple subtypes of *N. meningitidis*.

Diagnostic Microbiology

GONOCOCCAL INFECTION

Diagnosis of gonococcal infection is made at two levels: presumptive and confirmed. Antimicrobial treatment must be started based on the results of the presumptive tests, but additional tests must be performed to yield a confirmatory diagnosis.

Collection of specimens for diagnosis depends on the clinical manifestations and the sites exposed. Male urethral exudates and female cervical swabs should be taken from all cases of suspected gonococcal infection for direct examination and culture. Neutrophils containing gram-negative cocci in the Gram-stained smear are presumptive evidence of gonococcal infection (Figure 179-7). Gram stain is highly sensitive and specific for diagnosing genital gonorrhea in men. Gram-stained smears from endocervix specimens of symptomatic women have a sensitivity of only 40–60% relative to culture, but have a high predictive value. In asymptomatic women, Gram stain has a low predictive value and is not useful. Direct detection (i.e. with or without culture) of gonococci is performed by rapid and sensitive diagnostic nucleic acid amplification tests (NAATs) that simultaneously detect

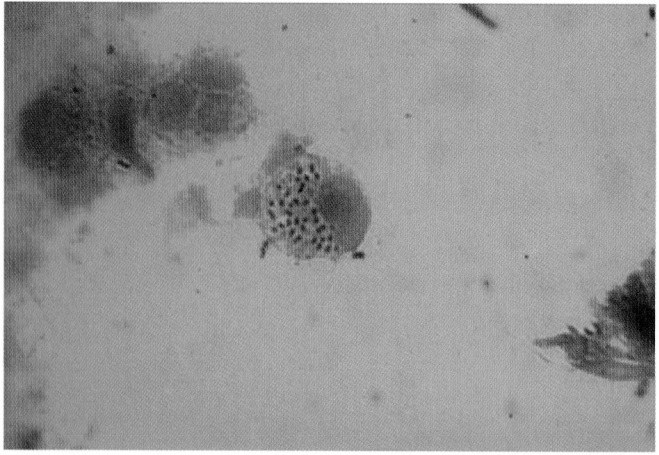

Figure 179-7 Gram stain of a urethral discharge from a male who has gonorrhea. Note the intracellular gram-negative diplococci with neutrophils.

TABLE 179-3	Specimens and Culture Media for the Isolation of *N. Gonorrhoeae* and *N. Meningitidis*		
Species	Disease	Specimen/Site	Media for Cultivation
N. gonorrhoeae	Cervicitis	Endocervix, urethra (Bartholin's glands, rectum, pharynx)	Selective
	Pelvic inflammatory disease (PID)	Endocervix, endometrium, fallopian tubes	Selective, nonselective
	Disseminated infection (DGI)	Endocervix, urethra, skin lesions Joint fluid Blood	Selective, nonselective Nonselective, selective Blood culture medium
	Ophthalmic	Conjunctiva	Nonselective, selective
N. meningitidis	Meningitis/sepsis	Cerebrospinal fluid	Nonselective, blood culture medium
		Blood	Blood culture medium
		Nasopharynx	Selective, nonselective
		Skin lesions	Nonselective

N. gonorrhoeae and *Chlamydia trachomatis*.[40] NAATs require only a freshly voided urine sample. Limitations are cost, risk of carryover contamination, inhibition and inability to provide antibiotic resistance data.[41] Frequent horizontal genetic exchange leading to commensal *Neisseria* spp. acquiring *N. gonorrhoeae* genes may give false-positive results. Furthermore, some *N. gonorrhoeae* subtypes may lack specific sequences targeted by a particular NAAT due to sequence variation in the dynamic gonococcal populations, leading to false-negative results.

Maximal culture recovery of gonococci by culture requires immediate plating of the collected specimen.[1,11] If this is not possible, swabs can be transported in commercially available charcoal-containing transport media. When appropriate, cultures should be obtained from blood and biopsies from skin lesions and joint fluid aspirates. Commonly used culture media are Thayer–Martin and Martin–Lewis. These media contain lysed or heated blood (chocolate agar) supplemented with growth factors and a variety of antimicrobials to suppress the growth of other bacteria and yeast. Specimens taken from sites that are normally sterile are cultured on antibiotic-free media to enable growth of occasional strains that are susceptible to the antibiotics added to the growth media. Growth is performed in an atmosphere with 5–10% carbon dioxide at 95–98.6°F (35–37°C) for 48 hours. Gram-negative diplococci with a positive oxidase and catalase test may be *N. gonorrhoeae*.

Confirmatory culture identification includes mass spectrometry (MALDI-TOF) analysis and carbohydrate utilization tests, which can be supplemented by monoclonal antibody testing (PorB), chromogenic detection of specific enzyme activities and DNA-based culture confirmation tests. Gonococci oxidize glucose, but not maltose, sucrose or lactose.

MENINGOCOCCAL INFECTION

CSF, blood, nasopharyngeal swabs and aspirates are the most relevant specimens for the diagnosis of meningococcal disease.[1,11] Additionally, skin biopsies, synovial fluid, sputum and conjunctival swabs may be cultured if clinically indicated. Because meningococci, like gonococci, are susceptible to desiccation and temperature extremes, specimens should be cultured as soon as possible.

For presumptive diagnosis, specimens are examined by Gram stain. Gram-stained smears are made directly from CSF, if the CSF is cloudy, or after centrifugation if the CSF is clear. The majority of the smears will show gram-negative diplococci inside and outside polymorphonuclear leukocytes (PMNs) when the CSF bacterial count is $>10^5$/mL. Smears from CSF containing $<10^3$ mL of bacteria will be positive in only 25%; on average 60–90% of culture-positive CSF specimens are positive in the Gram stain. Gram-stained smears from petechial skin lesions due to meningococcemia may detect meningococci in more than 70% of cases.

Direct detection of meningococci is performed by NAAT.[40,41] NAATs are also useful in confirming the diagnosis in patients who had antibiotic treatment prior to collection of CSF and whose CSF Gram stain, antigen test and culture are negative.

The proportion of PMNs in CSF from patients who have meningitis ranges from 49% to 98% (mean of 86%). Other CSF abnormalities include low glucose and an elevated protein concentration. In patients partially treated with antibiotics, the CSF leukocyte count, glucose and protein concentration, and the antigen tests remain abnormal for several days, whereas bacteria might not be evident on smear or by CSF culture. Blood cultures are positive in only 50% of patients with meningococcal disease. A nasopharyngeal swab from young children will provide valuable information in cases of suspected meningococcal disease.

For isolation of *N. meningitidis* by culture, the clinical specimen should be inoculated on selective and nonselective growth media (Table 179-3).[1] Appropriate nonselective media are 5% sheep blood agar (in contrast to gonococci, meningococci grow well on this medium) and chocolate agar.[11] Selective media used to culture nasopharyngeal specimens are the same as those mentioned for gonococci. Most blood-containing media support the growth of meningococci. Meningococci are grown on agar media in a 5–10% carbon dioxide-enriched atmosphere with rather high humidity at 95–98.6°F (35–37°C). After 18–24 hours, flat, gray-brown, translucent, smooth, 1–3 mm in diameter colonies of *N. meningitidis* are present, which can be analyzed by Gram stain.[1] The finding of oxidase- and catalase-positive gram-negative diplococci is sufficient to support a tentative diagnosis of meningococcal disease, to be confirmed by MALDI-TOF analysis. For conventional confirmatory identification, differentiation characteristics are the production of acid from glucose and maltose. Gonococci acidify only glucose and *N. lactamica* produces acid from glucose, maltose and lactose, although a number of commensal *Neisseria* spp. may be misidentified as *N. meningitidis* on the basis of carbohydrate oxidation. Isolation of *N. meningitidis* can also be confirmed by NAAT or 16S rRNA gene sequencing.[40]

MOLECULAR TYPING OF *N. GONORRHOEAE* AND *N. MENINGITIDIS*

The current methods for monitoring transmission of *N. gonorrhoeae* are multilocus sequence typing (MLST) and genome sequencing.[42] Gonococcal serotyping is based on a panel of monoclonal antibodies directed against variant epitopes on PorB-IA and PorB-IB. At least 55 serovars have been identified.

For larger studies on *N. meningitidis* genome evolution and surveillance, MLST shows that epidemics are often caused by specific complexes of related hypervirulent lineages.[42,43] Targeted and complete genome sequencing are the next generation of typing methods that are being applied, along with MALDI-TOF.[11]

Phenotypic classification of *N. meningitidis* is based on antigenic differences of the major surface antigens which provides information about the serogroup (capsule, e.g. B), serotype (PorB porin, e.g. 15),

TABLE 179-4 Characteristics of the Most Common Human *Neisseria* spp. That Can Be Used in Species Differentiation

Species	Colony morphology on chocolate agar	Glucose	Maltose	Lactose	Sucrose	Fructose	Reduction of Nitrate
		ACID FROM					
N. gonorrhoeae	Gray-brown, translucent, smooth (0.5–1 mm diameter)	+	−	−	−	−	−
N. meningitidis	Gray-brown, translucent, smooth (1–3 mm diameter)	+	+	−	−	−	−
N. lactamica	Gray-brown, translucent, smooth (1–2 mm diameter)	+	+	+	−	−	−

TABLE 179-5 Examples of Nonpathogenic Neisserial Species Rarely Isolated From Clinical Disease in Humans

Neisserial Species	Clinical Disease Observed When Isolated
N. lactamica	Meningitis or sepsis in adults and children
N. cinerea, N. polysaccharea, N. sicca, N. subflava	Native and prosthetic endocarditis, often in patients with heart abnormalities or intravenous drug use
N. sicca	Native and prosthetic valve endocarditis Meningitis cases Rarely pneumonia and osteomyelitis
N. subflava	Rarely endocarditis, meningitis and sepsis
N. flavescens	Once in an outbreak of meningitis Occasionally in sepsis resembling chronic meningococcemia
N. mucosa	Occasional endocarditis, meningitis, ocular infections, cellulitis, pneumonia and empyema
N. cinerea	Conjunctivitis in newborns (ophthalmia neonatorum) Proctitis and lymphadenitis Meningitis in patients with facial trauma Pneumonia in immunodeficient patients
N. elongata	Endocarditis or sepsis, wound infections, osteomyelitis after oral surgery
N. weaveri	Human wounds due to dog bites

TABLE 179-6 Clinical Disease Caused by the Pathogenic *Neisseria* spp.

Neisseria spp.	Clinical Diagnosis	Reference
N. gonorrhoeae	Most common manifestations Local urogenital: Urethritis Cervicitis Salpingitis/PID Proctitis	11, 44, 45, 47
	Less common manifestations Pharyngitis	44, 45
	Uncommon manifestations Acute conjunctivitis Acute keratitis	45, 46
	Systemic dissemination, uncommon Dermatitis–arthritis–tenosynovitis syndrome Monoarticular septic arthritis/perihepatitis Endocarditis Meningitis	44, 45
N. meningitidis	Most common manifestations Systemic infections: Meningoencephalitis/meningitis Sepsis with meningitis Sepsis without meningitis Meningococcemia without septic complications	11, 12, 13, 33, 48, 49
	Less common Persistent meningococcemia Low-grade fever, rash and arthritis: arthritis–dermatitis syndrome Pharyngitis Community-acquired pneumonia	11, 12

serosubtype (PorA porin, e.g. P1.7) and LOS immunotype (e.g. L3) of a particular strain. This results in the classification: B, 15, P1.7, L3. Multiple epitopes may be recognized depending upon the presence of phase or antigen variants in the bacterial population. Antigen-based typing, however, is relevant only for vaccine efficacy studies.

IDENTIFICATION OF NONPATHOGENIC *NEISSERIA* SPECIES

The commensal *Neisseria* spp. colonize the human nasopharynx and oropharynx.[1, 2] They can be isolated on nonselective rich media and identified by MALDI-TOF. Strains of *N. lactamica, N. gonorrhoeae and N. meningitidis* can be differentiated by their patterns of acid production (see Table 179-4).[1,2] *N. lactamica* produces acid from lactose and can thus be differentiated from meningococci. This and other nonpathogenic neisserial species are only occasionally associated with disease, although *N. lactamica* has been isolated from cases of meningitis or sepsis in both adults and children (Table 179-5).

In general, the commensal *Neisseria* spp. are susceptible to penicillin, ampicillin and tetracyclines. Only *N. mucosa* is penicillin-resistant and sensitive to chloramphenicol. Some strains of *N. lactamica* have an altered penicillin-binding protein 2 as found in relatively penicillin-resistant *N. meningitidis*. Rare strains of *N. sicca, N. flavescens* and *N. subflava* are penicillin-resistant because of production of β-lactamase. Such strains are a potential source of β-lactamase genes that are transferable to meningococci and gonococci.[1]

Clinical Manifestations

GONORRHEA

N. gonorrhoeae usually causes an infection of the urethra (urethritis) and cervix (cervicitis). Ascending gonococcal infection in infected women can result in pelvic inflammatory disease (PID) (Table 179-6) (see also Chapters 53 and 54). Other frequently infected anatomic niches are the rectum, oropharynx and conjunctiva.[44] All *N. gonorrhoeae* strains are considered to be pathogenic. The infective dose for the male urethra is as low as 250 gonococci; for the uterine cervix this ranges from 10^2 to more than 10^7 gonococci. Certain gonococcal strains may cause disseminated infection and/or arthritis.[45] Dissemination to more distant sites occurs in about 0.5–3% of gonococcal infection.[44]

Urogenital Gonococcal Infection

In men, acute anterior urethritis is the most common manifestation of gonorrhea. Symptoms are a purulent urethral discharge and dysuria.

Acute epididymitis is the most common local complication. In women, the endocervix is the primary site of infection. This infection is characterized by (muco)purulent discharge and intermenstrual bleeding, but is often asymptomatic. Urethral infection is present in 70–90% of women who have gonococcal cervicitis. Infection of the Bartholin's glands leads to abscess formation in about 35% of the patients. Gonococcal infection in women may ascend to cause endometritis, acute salpingitis or PID in 10–20% of the cases.[11]

In males infection usually manifests after development of inflammation caused by local induction of cytokines and influx of PMNs. Examination of male biopsies and exudates shows gonococci attached to and within the epithelial cells, development of (sub)mucosal microabscesses and exudation of pus with gonococci inside PMNs.[11]

In women gonococcal infection can ascend to the upper genital tract and selectively adhere to nonciliated cells of the fallopian tubes. Ciliated cells are lost through cytotoxic effects of released peptidoglycan fragments and LOS. Tissue invasion and the inflammatory responses generated may manifest as PID and can lead to infertility.

Gonorrhea in Children. Historically gonococcal infection in children included only ophthalmia neonatorum (acute gonococcal conjunctivitis).[46] However, children can acquire gonococcal infection by sexual contact with an infected person.[47] Such infection indicates sexual abuse.

Localized Gonococcal Infection Outside the Urogenital Tract

Proctitis. Anorectal gonorrhea is only present in up to 5% of women who have gonorrhea, while gonococci can be cultured from the anorectal region of 40% of women and homosexual men with gonorrhea.

Pharyngeal Gonorrhea. Pharyngeal infection occurs in 10–20% of women who have gonorrhea, in 10–25% of homosexual men who have the infection and in 3–7% of heterosexual men with gonorrhea. The infection is due to orogenital sexual exposure. Most cases are asymptomatic and resolve spontaneously.

Acute Conjunctivitis. Ophthalmia neonatorum is acquired during passage through an infected birth canal.[46] In adults ocular infection usually results from autoinoculation of the conjunctiva in a person who has the infection. Gonococcal conjunctivitis is usually severe, with an overt purulent exudate and corneal ulceration.

Disseminated Gonococcal Infection

Disseminated gonococcal infection is reported in 1–2% of patients who have gonococcal infection and can occur as dermatitis–arthritis–tenosynovitis syndrome, monoarticular septic arthritis, perihepatitis, endocarditis or meningitis.[44,45]

MENINGOCOCCAL INFECTION

The clinical spectrum of meningococcal disease includes meningoencephalitis, meningococcemia without meningitis, and bacteremia without septic complications.[12, 48] The disease usually begins abruptly with headache, meningeal signs including stiffness of the neck and fever (Figure 179-8a).[49] Mortality approaches 100% in untreated cases, but is around 10% when appropriate antibiotic therapy is instituted. The incidence of reported neurologic sequelae is low, with hearing deficits, epilepsy and arthritis most commonly noted.

Meningitis (see also Chapter 19)

The most frequent form of meningococcal infection is acute pyogenic meningitis due to inflammation of the meninges, with or without meningococcemia.[48] Among patients who have meningococcal disease, 75% have meningitis; 40% of them also have bacteremia.

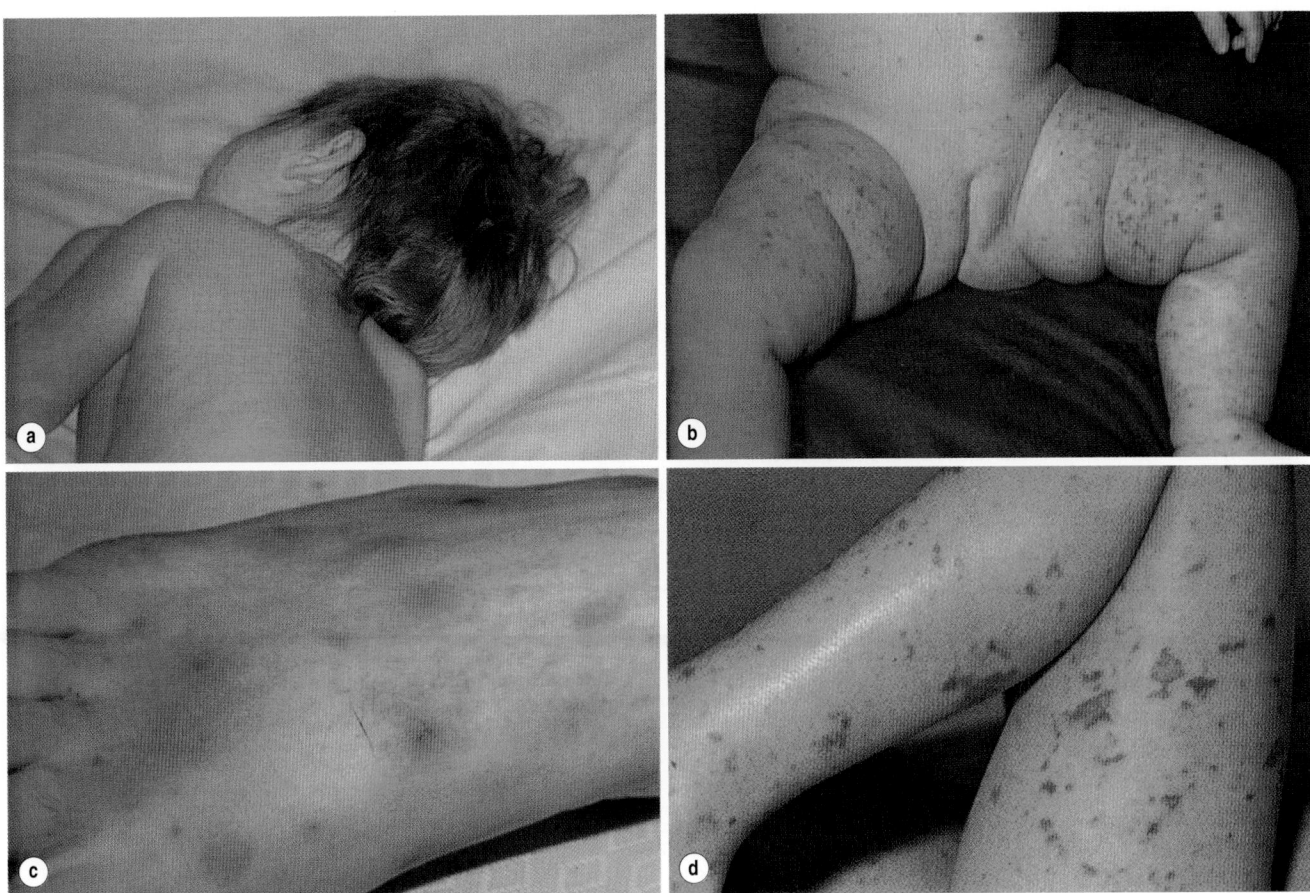

Figure 179-8 Typical symptoms of meningococcal infection. Stiffness of the neck may indicate meningitis. Fine erythematous macules, maculopapular petechial eruptions and purpuric/petechial or ecchymotic skin lesions that are hemorrhagic and necrotic may accompany meningococcal sepsis. *(From Brandtzæg et al.[49])*

Meningococcemia

Meningococcemia may be transient, occult or result in severe sepsis. Bacteremia without meningitis occurs in 7–10% of patients. Meningococcemia can manifest as pink maculopapular petechial eruptions (Figure 179-8b).[12,33] Rapidly progressive infections may result in purpuric petechial or ecchymotic skin lesions that are hemorrhagic and necrotic (Figure 179-8c,d). Fulminant shock may dominate the clinical picture of acute meningococcal sepsis.[12,33] Sepsis may progress to disseminated intravascular coagulation (DIC) characterized by increasing petechiae or purpura fulminans, resulting in extensive areas of tissue destruction secondary to coagulopathy, rapid onset of hypotension and adrenal hemorrhage (Waterhouse–Friderichsen syndrome).

In the blood *N. meningitidis* replicates to high levels and sheds OMVs. The OMVs may subvert the complement system and high levels of circulating LOS overactivate the innate immune system. Circulating levels of the proinflammatory mediators tumor necrosis factor (TNF), interleukin (IL)-1 and interferon-gamma (IFN-γ) strongly correlate with development of lethal septic shock.[33,48] In patients with complement deficiencies the clinical picture can be milder and they may only present with fever, while the blood culture is positive.

Encapsulated meningococci enter the CSF likely by the hematogenous route via the veins in the subarachnoidal space (the blood–CSF barrier) and the choroid plexi rather than through the brain parenchyma (blood–brain barrier).[33, 48] The absence of opsonophagocytosis in CSF enables uncontrolled bacterial growth and inflammation of the leptomeninges and subarachnoid space. Attracted PMNs aggravate the inflammatory response and release cytotoxic mediators.

Other Meningococcal Infections

Due to hematogenous spread meningococci may cause a plethora of infections (Table 179-6). Persistent meningococcal bacteremia is associated with low-grade fever, rash and arthritis (arthritis–dermatitis syndrome).[11,12] Meningococci are implicated as the etiologic agent in approximately 5–14% of patients who have community-acquired pneumonia. Pharyngitis is associated with recent contact with individuals who are colonized by meningococci and is often a symptom prior to serious meningococcal disease.

Meningococcal Carriage

Infection due to *N. meningitidis* commonly results from asymptomatic oronasopharyngeal mucosal carriage.[43] At any time about 10% of the general population is colonized with meningococci. In children under 4 years of age the carriage rate is less than 1%, but this progressively increases with age to peak at about 20–25% in late teenage and early adult life. During carriage, non-groupable meningococci are most often isolated. Immunohistochemistry has also demonstrated meningococci within the tonsillar tissues in 45% of patients undergoing tonsillectomy.[49]

Meningococcal carriage induces bactericidal antibodies within 1–2 weeks after colonization. Antibodies may last for several months after carriage. *N. lactamica* carriage elicits bactericidal antibodies that cross-react with various meningococcal serogroups and serotypes. Carriage of *N. lactamica* is approximately 4% by 3 months of age and peaks at 21% by 18–24 months of age.[43] *N. lactamica* may contribute to

TABLE 179-7	The Most Prevalent Neisserial Antibiotic Resistance Markers		
Antibiotic	Drug Resistance Gene	Gene Product	Reference
Penicillin/ β-lactams	PbpA,B	Penicillin-binding protein	51
	mtr	Efflux pump	11
	env	Accessory outer membrane protein	11
	penA	TEM-1 type β-lactamase, PPNG	8
Ciprofloxacin	gyrA parC	DNA gyrase Topoisomerase IV	11
Sulfonamide	sul1	Dihydrofolatesynthase	12
Tetracycline	tetM	Soluble ribosomal protein	11
Rifampin	rpoB	RNA polymerase subunit B	11

protection against meningococcal disease as development of invasive meningococcal disease correlates with the absence of bactericidal antibodies.[43]

Management

GONORRHEA

The treatment of gonorrhea is discussed in Chapter 65.

Drug resistance in gonococci is increasing, and the main drug resistance markers are depicted in Table 179-7. Since 1976, gonococcal isolates with a decreased sensitivity for penicillin (minimum inhibitory concentration (MIC) >0.1 mg/L) have been emerging. Fluoroquinolones (i.e. ciprofloxacin, ofloxacin or levofloxacin) are also no longer recommended for treatment of gonococcal infections due to the sharp increases in antibiotic resistance.[10]

Treatment of hospitalized PID cases takes into account the important role of both gonococci and *C. trachomatis* in addition to anaerobic cover in PID patients, and is described in Chapter 54.

MENINGOCOCCAL DISEASE

Patients with meningococcal disease are treated with benzylpenicillin when susceptible or a third-generation cephalosporin (e.g. cefotaxime or ceftriaxone).[33,49] When the etiology is not known at admission, ceftriaxone or cefotaxime is used for the first 24–48 hours to cover the possibility of other bacterial pathogens.[33,50] The management of meningitis is discussed in detail in Chapter 19. There are *N. meningitidis* strains that have decreased sensitivity to penicillin due to reduced affinity of penicillin to PBPs 2 and 3, resulting from a *penA* gene altered by transformation.[51] In addition, β-lactamase-producing strains have occasionally been recovered. Cefotaxime or ceftriaxone is used when relatively penicillin-resistant strains are isolated.

References available online at expertconsult.com.

KEY REFERENCES

Bowler L.D., Zhang Q.Y., Riou J.Y., et al.: Interspecies recombination between the penA genes of *Neisseria meningitidis* and commensal *Neisseria* species during the emergence of penicillin resistance in *N. meningitidis*: natural events and laboratory simulation. *J Bacteriol* 1994; 176:333-337.

Elias J., Frosch M., Vogel U.: Neisseria. In: Jorgensen J., Pfaller M., Carroll K., et al., eds. *Manual of clinical microbiology*. 11th ed. Washington DC: ASM Press; 2015: 635-651.

Giuliani M.M., Adu-Bobie J., Comanducci M., et al.: A universal vaccine for serogroup B meningococcus. *Proc Natl Acad Sci USA* 2006; 103:10834-10839.

Maiden M.C., Bygraves J.A., Feil E., et al.: Multilocus sequence typing: a portable approach to the identification of clones within populations of pathogenic microorganisms. *Proc Natl Acad Sci USA* 1998; 95:3140-3145.

Pizza M., Rappuoli R.: *Neisseria meningitidis*: pathogenesis and immunity. *Curr Opin Microbiol* 2015; 23:68-72.

Stephens D.S., Greenwood B., Brandtzaeg P.: Epidemic meningitis, meningococcaemia, and *Neisseria meningitidis*. *Lancet* 2007; 369:2196-2210.

van Deuren M., Brandtzaeg P., van der Meer J.W.: Update on meningococcal disease with emphasis on pathogenesis and clinical management. *Clin Microbiol Rev* 2000; 13:144-166.

Vogel U., Claus H., Frosch M.: Rapid serogroup switching in *Neisseria meningitidis*. *N Engl J Med* 2000; 342: 219-220.

Yazdankhah S.P., Caugant D.A.: Neisseria meningitidis: an overview of the carriage state. *J Med Microbiol* 2004; 53:821-832.

180

Enterobacteriaceae

CLAIRE JENKINS | ROB J. RENTENAAR | LUCE LANDRAUD |
SYLVAIN BRISSE

KEY CONCEPTS

- Impact of multilocus sequence typing and whole genome sequencing on informing the taxonomy of the Enterobacteriaceae family.

- Molecular approach to detection and typing of pathogenic Enterobacteriaceae species.

- Incidence and prevalence of disease.

- Modes of transmission.

- Clinical features and symptoms.

- Pathogenicity mechanisms.

- Laboratory procedures.

- Emerging resistance to the extended-spectrum cephalosporins and carbapenems.

Introduction

The family Enterobacteriaceae are ubiquitous and members are found worldwide in various ecological sources such as soil, water, vegetation and animals.[1–3] Some species are important pathogens of plants and have economic importance in crop production.[4] Certain species are part of the normal flora of animals including humans, although many are frequently associated with diarrheal disease and extraintestinal infections.[2,5] Some of the most important pathogens in human history, such as the agent of plague *Yersinia pestis*, belong to the Enterobacteriaceae family and other members currently represent a huge public health concern (e.g. *Salmonella enterica* serotype Typhi, *Shigella*, *Escherichia coli*).

Two main types of infectious disease are associated with Enterobacteriaceae: intestinal and extraintestinal diseases. The transmission route of intestinal infection is classically fecal–oral either by person-to-person, direct contact with animals or their environment, or by consumption of contaminated food or water. An endogenous pathway of infection is also possible (e.g. bacterial translocation from the gut to blood), resulting in extraintestinal disease, and is more often observed in immunocompromised hosts or persons with underlying conditions such as cirrhosis or those undergoing chemotherapy.

Members of the Enterobacteriaceae should not be confused with the term 'enteric bacteria', which refers specifically to species of the gut and includes all species found in that habitat. This chapter focuses on aspects of taxonomy, pathogenesis, clinical diagnosis and management of human Enterobacteriaceae infections.

Taxonomy, Phylogeny and Clonal Relationships

In the prokaryotic taxonomy, the Enterobacteriaceae represent the only family within the order Enterobacteriales, one of 15 orders within class Gammaproteobacteria, which belongs to phylum Proteobacteria. Based on 16S rRNA gene sequences, the closest phylogenetic relatives of Enterobacteriaceae are the Pasteurellaceae, the Vibrionaceae, and members of the orders Aeromonadales and Alteromonadales (Figure 180-1).

The family Enterobacteriaceae currently includes (as of June 2014) more than 210 species and 53 genera, and these numbers continue to increase. A history of taxonomic changes and synonyms of species is maintained at http://www.bacterio.cict.fr. Some recent taxonomic changes for taxa of medical relevance include the creation of the species *Escherichia albertii* for *eae*-positive diarrhea-causing strains that are closely related to *Shigella boydii* serotype 13,[6] the transfer of *Calymmatobacterium granulomatis*, the agent of granuloma inguinale (donovanosis), to the genus *Klebsiella*,[7] the definition of novel *Klebsiella* species closely related to *K. pneumoniae*[8] and an extensive revision of the genus *Enterobacter*.[9] The review by Janda[3] provides detailed information on some of the recent changes to Enterobacteriaceae taxa, including a review of the evidence for their medical significance.

A precise phylogeny of Enterobacteriaceae genera and species would be useful for taxonomic purposes and would allow understanding of the evolution of characteristics, such as biochemical capabilities,

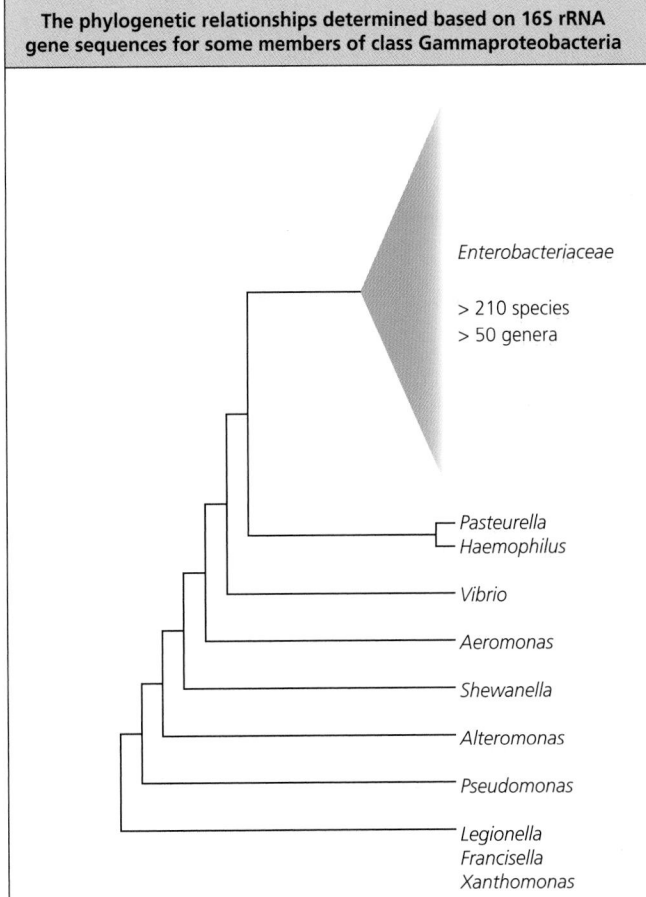

The phylogenetic relationships determined based on 16S rRNA gene sequences for some members of class Gammaproteobacteria

Enterobacteriaceae

> 210 species
> 50 genera

Pasteurella
Haemophilus

Vibrio

Aeromonas

Shewanella

Alteromonas

Pseudomonas

Legionella
Francisella
Xanthomonas

Figure 180-1 The phylogenetic relationships determined based on 16S rRNA gene sequences for some members of class Gammaproteobacteria. Bacterial groups most closely related to Enterobacteriaceae are families Pasteurellaceae and Vibrionaceae, order Aeromonadales, genus *Shewanella* and order Alteromonadales. (*Data from the Ribosomal Database Project, http://rdp.cme.msu.edu.*)

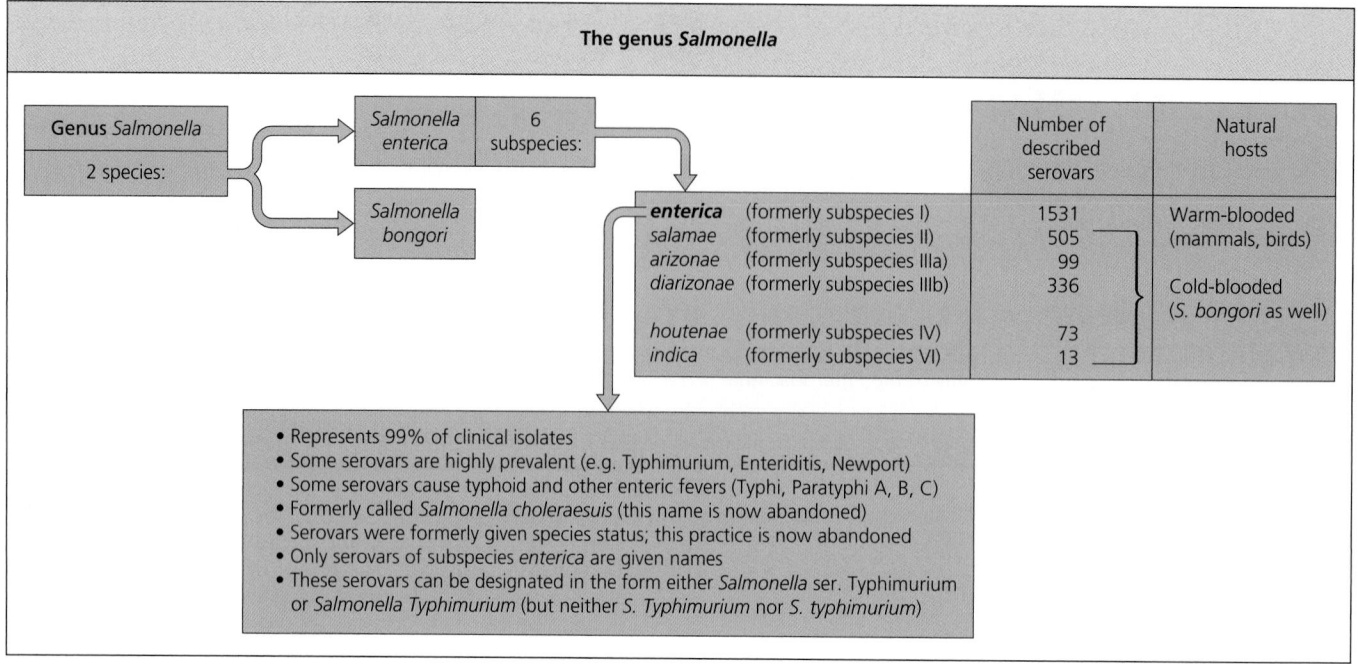

Figure 180-2 The genus *Salmonella* includes two species, *S. bongori* and *S. enterica* (formerly *S. choleraesuis*), with the latter including six subspecies. Nomenclature has evolved from a system where all serovars (the combination of O antigen and the two phases of the H antigen) were considered as species (e.g. *Salmonella typhi*) into the current system, which gives names to serovars of subspecies *S. enterica* subsp. *enterica* (e.g. *S. enterica* subsp. *enterica* serotype Enteritidis), but designates the serovars of other subspecies and of *S. bongori* simply by their antigenic formula. *(More details can be found at http://www.bacterio.cict.fr/s/salmonella.html.)*

host range, ecology and virulence. Although the 16S rRNA molecule is a good phylogenetic marker for most bacterial species, it is poorly informative within this family.[10] Analyses of whole genome sequences of a wide range of bacteria are currently being performed in academic, clinical and public health settings and data will be used to establish a robust phylogeny of Enterobacteriaceae species.[11,12]

All *Salmonella* strains are currently classified into two species: *S. enterica* and *S. bongori*. *Salmonella enterica* itself is subdivided into six subspecies: *enterica*, *arizonae*, *diarizonae*, *houtenae*, *indica* and *salamae*. *Salmonella enterica* subsp. *enterica* is by far the most important from a medical standpoint, representing 99% of clinical infections. For details of *Salmonella* nomenclature, including serovar naming, see Figure 180-2 and http://www.serotest-thailand.com/upload/news/download/9-8310-0.pdf.

The genus *Escherichia* currently includes the species *E. coli*, *E. fergusonii*, *E. albertii*, *E. hermanii*, *E. vulneris* and *E. blattae*. Clinically, *E. coli* is by far the most important species. Sequence comparisons indicate that *E. fergusonii* and *E. albertii* are closely related to *E. coli*, while the three remaining species may be evolutionarily more distant.

The clonal diversity of *E. coli* strains was initially described based on multilocus enzyme electrophoresis (MLEE) and large-scale multilocus sequence typing (MLST) studies.[13] These studies indicated that recombination events were a major influence on evolutionary relationships in *E. coli*.[14] Genome-wide sequence data of multiple strains has confirmed the important contribution of horizontal gene transfer, demonstrating that the core genome of *E. coli* comprises ~2200 genes but each strain has a large accessory genome that renders the total gene pool across the species effectively infinite.[14]

Shigella species were distinguished historically based on clinical and biochemical characteristics, but whole genome sequencing (WGS) has confirmed that *Shigella* strains are phylogenetically more closely related to some *E. coli* strains than some *E. coli* strains are among themselves.[15] In addition, the three taxonomic *Shigella* species *S. flexneri*, *S. dysenteriae* and *S. boydii* do not correspond to three phylogenetic clusters within the *E. coli* species and evolved in parallel on multiple occasions.[16] In contrast, both *S. sonnei* and *S. dysenteriae*

serotype 1 form unique and genetically homogeneous clusters. WGS has confirmed that other pathotypes of *E. coli*, such as enteropathogenic *E. coli*, enterotoxigenic *E. coli*, enteroinvasive *E. coli*, enteroaggregative *E. coli* and enterohemorrhagic *E. coli*, also show multiple independent origins and parallel evolution (see Figure 180-3).[12,15]

Diagnostic Microbiology

All Enterobacteriaceae are gram-negative, nonspore-forming bacilli. They are either motile by peritrichous flagella (except *Tatumella ptyseos*) or nonmotile. With a few exceptions (e.g. *Klebsiella granulomatis*), they grow rapidly on ordinary laboratory media, under either aerobic or anaerobic conditions. Growth is generally optimal at 99°F (37°C). Some specific properties are common: all species utilize glucose fermentatively (often with gas production), are oxidase-negative (with the exception of *Plesiomonas shigelloides*) and catalase-positive, and reduce nitrates to nitrites (except *Photorhabdus* and *Xenorhabdus*). Some useful features for identification of Enterobacteriaceae species that are common in clinical samples are given in Table 180-1; more details on identification methods can be found in other reference texts.[1,17]

In classic nonselective media, colonies are circular and convex, with a smooth surface and a diameter of 1–3 mm after 24 hours. Selective media are used to recover Enterobacteriaceae from fecal samples or other specimens containing complex flora. These media enhance the growth of specific Enterobacteriaceae species, while inhibiting nondesired species. Classically, these media (e.g. MacConkey lactose- or sorbitol-containing media) contain substrates selectively used by one or a few species and facilitate distinction between colonies. More precise distinction of genera and species is obtained by differences in biochemical activity (enzyme profiles, carbon source utilization, pH-based reactions). Several miniaturized tests are available commercially (e.g. Api 20E or Biotype-100 strips from BioMerieux). Typically, isolates are identified by comparison of their biochemical profile with a reference database that contains the percentages of positive results for each substrate/species pair. More automated identification systems based on the same approach are classically used in larger microbiology

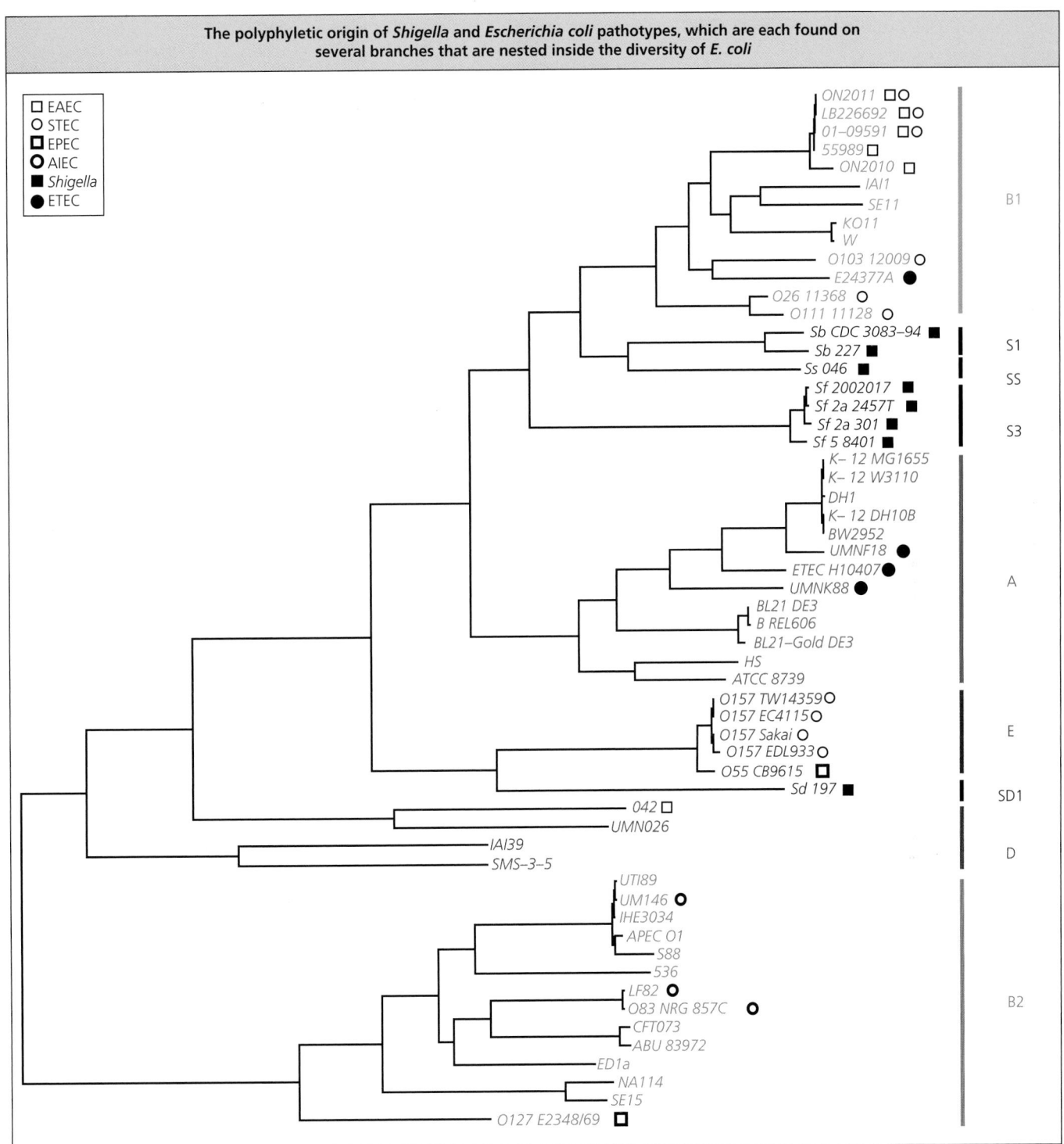

Figure 180-3   The polyphyletic origin of *Shigella* and *Escherichia coli* pathotypes, which are each found on several branches that are nested inside the diversity of *E. coli*. *Shigella* (black squares), enterotoxigenic *E. coli* (ETEC; black circles) and shiga toxin-producing *E. coli* (STEC; thin black circles) pathotypes have several independent origins from ancestral strains that have incorporated virulence genes by horizontal transfer. EAEC (enteroaggregative *E. coli*; thin open squares; EPEC-(enteropathogenic *E. coli*; bold open squares); AIEC-adherent invasive *E. coli*; thick open circles) hybrid EAEC and STEC stains denoted as open thin squares and open thin circles *(Reprinted from Croxen M.A., et al. Clin Microbiol Rev 2013; 26:822–80.)*

laboratories[18,19] although there are limitations to this approach. For example, isolates that are biochemically atypical or correspond to rare or novel species (thus not incorporated in the reference databases) cannot be identified or can even be misidentified. Furthermore, biochemically inactive or closely related bacteria may also be misidentified by certain automated systems. Automated methods can also test antimicrobial susceptibility, which is important with respect to the

increasing levels of antibiotic resistance detected in clinically important strains belonging to the Enterobacteriaceae family.

Matrix-assisted laser desorption/ionization time-of-flight mass spectrometry (MALDI-TOF-MS) is the first step in the identification of Enterobacteriaceae in many clinical microbiology laboratories (see also Chapter 161). Sample preparation can be fast and simple. A typical sample preparation method used in the identification of

TABLE 180-1	Major Properties Used to Identify the Most Common Enterobacteriaceae Implicated in Human Infections						
	BIOCHEMICAL TESTS						
Species	TDA	VP	ONPG	Indole Production	Citrate (Simmons)	Remarks	
Escherichia coli	(−)	(−)	(+)	(+)	(−)	Utilization of inositol (−)	
Citrobacter spp.	(−)	(−)	(+)	Variable	(+)	Urease variable, H₂S (−) except *C. freundii*	
Shigella spp.	(−)	(−)	(−) except *S. sonnei*	(+)*	(−)	Utilization of xylose (−)	
Salmonella enterica	(−)	(−)	(−) except *S. arizonae*	(−)	(+) except Typhi and Paratyphi A	H₂S (+)	
Yersinia spp.	(−)	(−)	Variable	Variable	(−)	H₂S (−), urease (+) except *Y. pestis*	
Enterobacter spp.	(−)	(+)	(+)	(−)	(+)	LDC (−) except *E. aerogenes* and *E. gergoviae*, ODC (+)	
Klebsiella spp.	(−)	(+)†,‡	(+)†	(−) except *K. oxytoca*	(+)†	ODC (−) except *K. ornithinolytica*	
Serratia spp.	(−)	(+)	(+)	(−)	(+)	Gelatin hydrolysis (+) except *S. fonticola*	
Proteus spp.	(+)	(−)	(−)	(−) except *P. vulgaris*	Variable	H₂S (+), urease (+)	
Morganella morganii	(+)	(−)	(−)	(+)	(−)	H₂S (−), urease (+)	
Providencia spp.	(+)	(−)	(−)	(+)	(+)	H₂S (−)	

*30–70% positive reaction for *S. dysenteriae* or *S. flexneri*, and negative for *S. sonnei*.
†Except *K. pneumoniae* subsp. *rhinoscleromatis*.
‡Except *K. pneumoniae* subsp. *ozaenae*.
(−), 70–100% negative reaction; (+), 70–100% positive reaction; variable, different reactions between different species or <70% positive/negative reaction for strains of the species. H₂S, hydrogen sulfide production; LDC, lysine decarboxylase; ODC, ornithine decarboxylase; ONPG, O-nitrophenyl-β-D-galactopyranoside; TDA, phenylalanine deaminase; VP, Voges–Proskauer.

Enterobacteriaceae is the 'direct transfer method': a thin film of biomass from a colony is smeared on a target plate and overlaid with a small volume of matrix solution. Fresh colonies from solid media are used, colonies from selective media are generally acceptable. Sample preparation from blood culture bottles is more complicated. However, in comparison with biochemical identification of Enterobacteriaceae, MALDI-TOF-MS is much faster. For many extraintestinal infections with Enterobacteriaceae, MALDI-TOF-MS may be sufficiently accurate to be used for final identification. Thereby, MALDI-TOF-MS-based identification of Enterobacteriaceae may lead to early instalment of appropriate antibiotic treatment.[20] In contrast, routine MALDI-TOF-MS analysis is insufficiently accurate for most species or serotype identifications of pathogenic Enterobacteriaceae from human intestinal infections. If MALDI-TOF-MS is employed in such infections, identification results typically require additional biochemical, nucleic acid amplification tests and/or serotyping. One exception may be the MALDI-TOF-MS identification of *Plesiomonas shigelloides*, which seems reliable in at least one of the commercial systems. In contrast, *Shigella* is identified as *E. coli* by commercial MALDI-TOF-MS systems. Therefore, a lactose-negative colony isolated from a fecal sample from a patient with diarrheal illness, identified as *E. coli* by MALDI-TOF-MS, requires additional biochemical and serological testing for definitive identification. Differentiation of *E. coli* pathotypes is currently not feasible in routine MALDI-TOF-MS analyses with commercial databases. MALDI-TOF-MS identification of *Salmonella* is highly reliable at the 'genus level', but incapable of serotype differentiation. Similarly, MALDI-TOF-MS identification of *Yersinia* genus is accurate, but species differentiation of pathogenic *Yersinia* spp. may be problematic and may at least require additional 'security relevant' databases of mass spectra. MALDI-TOF-MS-based detection and identification of Enterobacteriaceae directly from urine from patients with urinary tract infections, detection of β-lactam hydrolyzing enzymes in Enterobacteriaceae and/or typing of Enterobacteriaceae in outbreak settings may reveal relevant and relatively fast and accurate information. However, these techniques are not widely adopted in clinical microbiology laboratories.

In some species, serotyping remains the predominant means by which routine identification is performed beyond the species level.

Serotyping is important because of the high epidemiologic and medical significance of serotype characterization for strains of *Salmonella*, *Shigella* and *E. coli*. In fact, biochemical profiling is not sufficient for diagnosis of the serotypes causing typhoid or typhoid-like fevers (Typhi, Paratyphi A, B and C). Moreover, *Shigella* and *E. coli* are notoriously difficult to distinguish using biochemistry alone and serotyping is often essential to differentiate the two groups. Serotyping of Enterobacteriaceae is based on antigenic variation of the O (somatic, corresponding to the polysaccharide side chain of the lipopolysaccharide), H (flagellar) and K (capsular) surface antigens. In some species, most or all strains do not have a capsule (*E. coli*, *Salmonella*), whereas the capsule is the predominant and most discriminatory antigen of *Klebsiella*. Serotyping is typically performed by slide agglutination using sets of O, H and K antisera, and the resulting combination of antigens defines the serotype (also called serovar). The most familiar serotyping scheme is the Kauffman–White scheme used for *Salmonella*, which distinguishes more than 2540 serotypes.[21] A re-evaluation of serotypes in the light of multilocus sequence typing[22] has shown that many serotypes are actually polyphyletic, meaning that the same serotype can be found in isolates belonging to unrelated lineages of *S. enterica* subsp. *enterica*. In *E. coli*, serotyping is important for identification of particular pathovars, such as the enterohemorrhagic *E. coli* O157:H7 or O26:H11 strains associated with hemolytic–uremic syndrome, or for identification of *E. coli* strains that possess the K1 capsular type implicated in neonatal infections.

In the clinical microbiology laboratory, where the focus is on the detection of pathogenic members of the Enterobacteriaceae family, knowledge of the mechanisms of infection has facilitated the development of rapid molecular diagnostic methods targeting specific virulence genes, especially those associated with gastrointestinal bacterial pathogens.[23,24] In-house and commercial polymerase chain reaction (PCR) assays for the direct detection from fecal specimens of *Salmonella*, *Shigella* and the pathogenic strains of *E. coli* are routinely used in many clinical microbiology laboratories (e.g. http://www.iss.it/binary/vtec/cont/EU_RL_VTEC_Method_02_Rev_0.pdf). Target genes are typically associated with either invasion, toxin production or adherence to the host gut mucosa. These genotypic methods are important in differentiating between diarrheagenic *E. coli* and

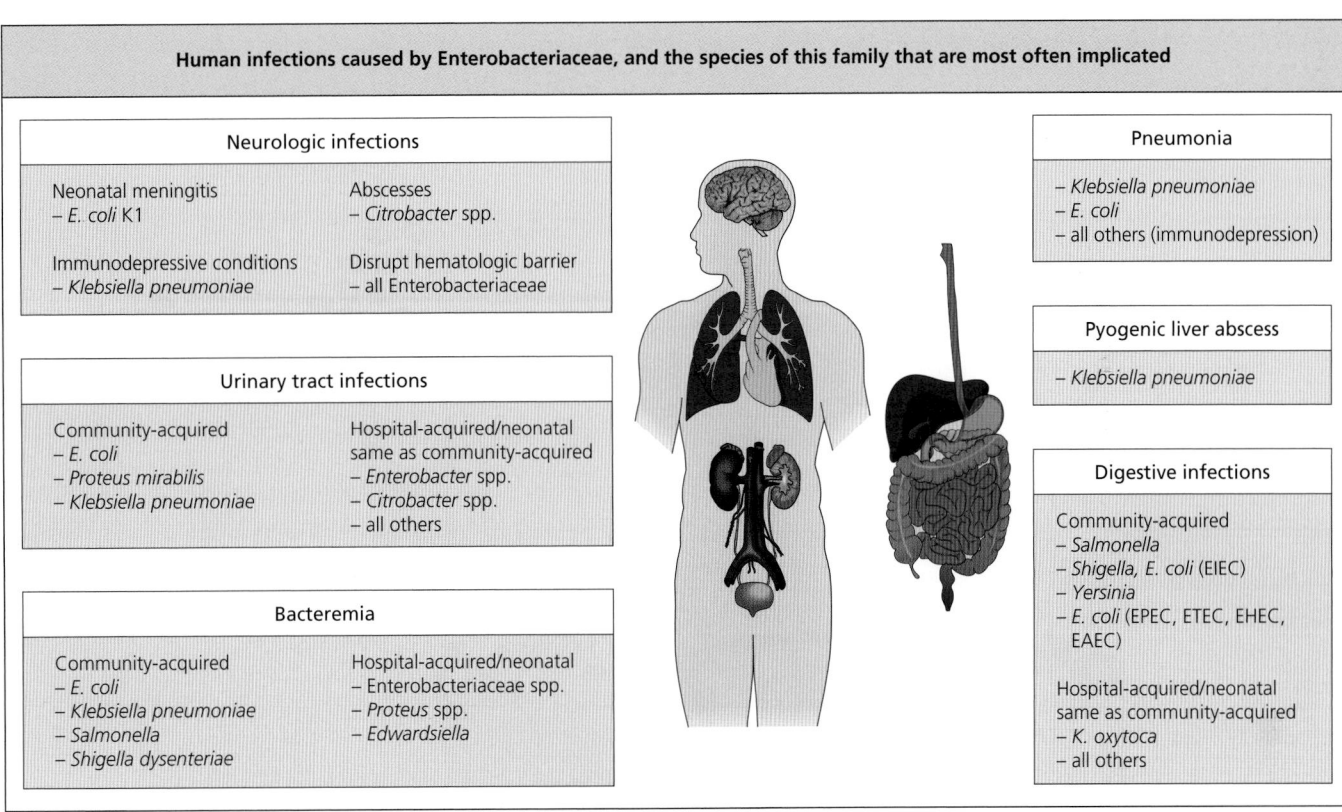

Human infections caused by Enterobacteriaceae, and the species of this family that are most often implicated

Neurologic infections	
Neonatal meningitis – *E. coli* K1	Abscesses – *Citrobacter* spp.
Immunodepressive conditions – *Klebsiella pneumoniae*	Disrupt hematologic barrier – all Enterobacteriaceae

Urinary tract infections	
Community-acquired – *E. coli* – *Proteus mirabilis* – *Klebsiella pneumoniae*	Hospital-acquired/neonatal same as community-acquired – *Enterobacter* spp. – *Citrobacter* spp. – all others

Bacteremia	
Community-acquired – *E. coli* – *Klebsiella pneumoniae* – *Salmonella* – *Shigella dysenteriae*	Hospital-acquired/neonatal – Enterobacteriaceae spp. – *Proteus* spp. – *Edwardsiella*

Pneumonia
– *Klebsiella pneumoniae* – *E. coli* – all others (immunodepression)

Pyogenic liver abscess
– *Klebsiella pneumoniae*

Digestive infections
Community-acquired – *Salmonella* – *Shigella*, *E. coli* (EIEC) – *Yersinia* – *E. coli* (EPEC, ETEC, EHEC, EAEC)
Hospital-acquired/neonatal same as community-acquired – *K. oxytoca* – all others

Figure 180-4 Human infections caused by Enterobacteriaceae and the species of this family that are most often implicated.

commensal strains or rapidly detecting strains associated with life-threatening disease, such as the enterohemorrahgic *E. coli* group, associated with hemolytic–uremic syndrome.

General Pathophysiologic Considerations

Enterobacteriaceae are associated with both gastrointestinal and extraintestinal infections including urinary tract infection, bacteremia, pneumonia, abdominal or pelvic infection, surgical site infections, meningitis and various abscesses including wound infections (Figure 180-4). The balance between host defenses and virulence factors of Enterobacteriaceae members is a key factor that determines commensalism or disease (Figure 180-5).[25,26]

Extraintestinal pathogenic *E. coli* (ExPEC) are facultative pathogens that belong to the normal gut flora of a certain fraction of the healthy population where they live as commensals.[5] Infections occur through microbial colonization of normally sterile sites. Each anatomic site presents specific molecular structures and defenses against infection, and bacteria must therefore express specific colonization factors to adhere to these structures and specific virulence factors to counter these defenses.

Commensal bacteria represent an important barrier against infection, as colonization by harmless commensals protects the host from invading pathogens. The host 'tolerates' the commensal gut flora and homeostasis is maintained by 1) the physical barrier of the mucus and antibacterial molecules that keeps commensal bacteria separate from the epithelial surface; 2) specific features of commensal species enabling them to escape or alter the inflammatory response; 3) particular characteristics of epithelial cells, such as the reduced expression of Toll-like receptor 4 (TLR4) at the gut surface epithelium that reduce the effects of bacterial stimuli, thus avoiding inflammation that would be detrimental for the host.[25] In contrast, enteric pathogens modulate inflammation leading to host responses that facilitate their survival and restrain other commensal flora.[25] Genomic approaches to the human

microbiota of the gut will further elucidate the interactions between commensal and pathogen.[24] The mechanisms by which the well-known gastrointestinal (GI) pathogens, *E. coli*, *S. enterica*, *Shigella* spp. and *Yersinia*, breach the intestinal barrier and cause disease are described below.

Many pathogenicity factors have been described in Enterobacteriaceae. These factors are often phage-encoded or clustered in chromosomal regions called pathogenicity islands (PAIs), which were first described in uropathogenic and diarrheagenic *E. coli*.[27,28] Most pathogenic Enterobacteriaceae are characterized by specific sets of PAIs (Table 180-2) whereas these PAIs are absent in nonpathogenic strains. PAIs are acquired by horizontal transfer and are typically associated with tRNA genes, flanked by repeated sequences, and may differ from the core genome in guanine and cytosine (G+C) content and in codon usage.

Clinical Manifestations
INTESTINAL INFECTIONS

The most important enteric pathogens are *S. enterica*, some strains of *E. coli*, *Shigella* and *Y. enterocolitica*. Although other Enterobacteriaceae are occasionally implicated in gastrointestinal infections, clinical significance is sometimes controversial (e.g. for *Plesiomonas shigelloides* or diarrhea-associated *K. pneumoniae*). Indeed, Enterobacteriaceae isolated from stool specimens during acute diarrhea could reflect the drastic change in stool flora, rather than being the cause of the symptoms.

Escherichia coli

Six distinct pathotypes of diarrheagenic *E. coli* are classically distinguished: enterotoxigenic, enteropathogenic, enterohemorrhagic, enteroinvasive, enteroaggregative and diffusely adherent *E. coli*. Identification of diarrheagenic *E. coli* strains requires their distinction from commensal *E. coli* strains, which is rendered possible by their specific sets of virulence factors, sometimes in combination with serotyping.[29]

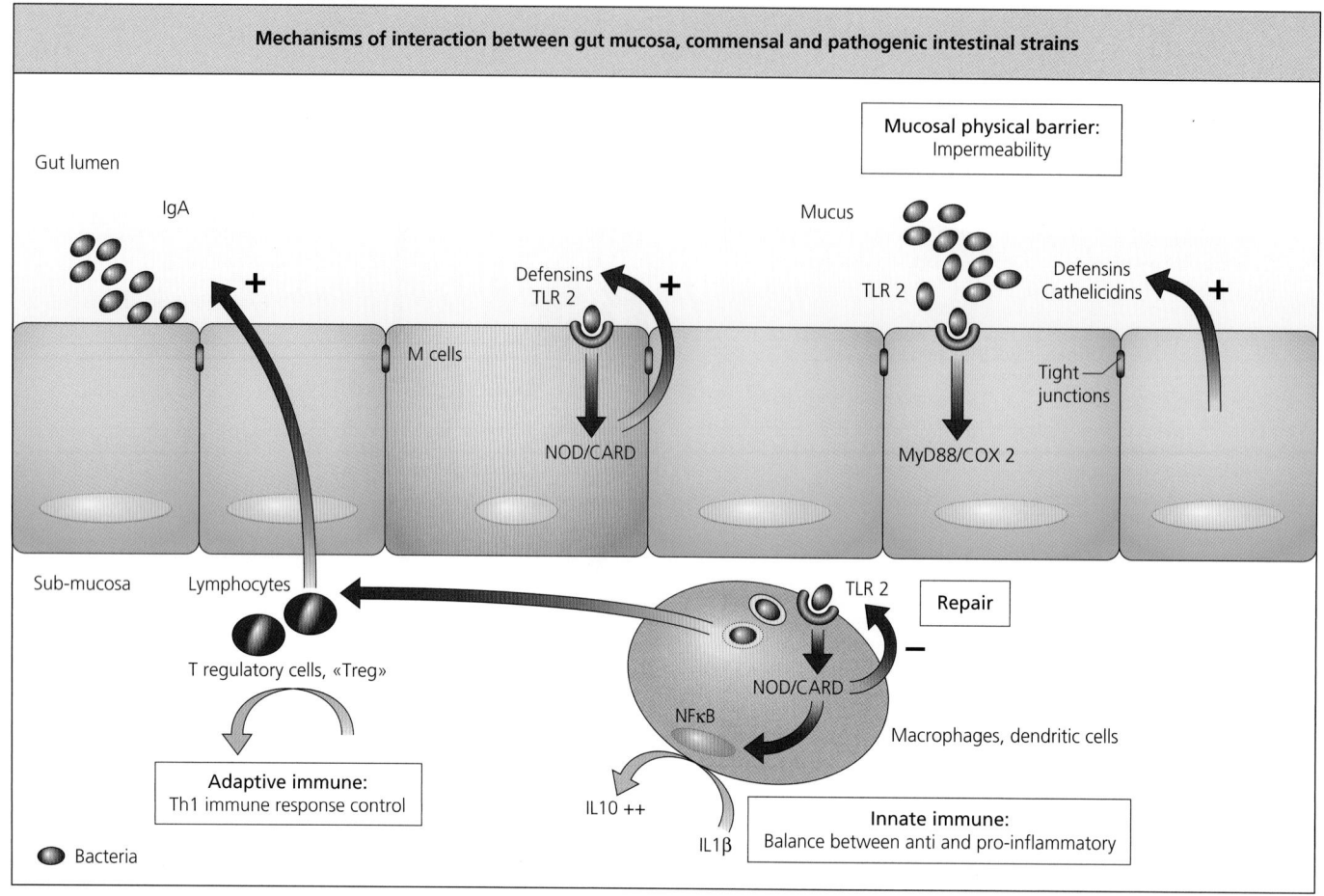

Figure 180-5 Mechanisms of interaction between gut mucosa, commensal and pathogenic intestinal strains. At the proximity of the intestinal mucosa, physical barriers exclude bacteria by the impermeability of the epithelium with tight junctions, and by production of factors excreted by epithelial cells themselves such as defensins or cathelicidins. The mucus is composed of mucin glycoproteins that interplay with bacteria, which are trapped and maintained at a distance from the epithelium. When the intestinal mucosa is exposed to bacteria (pathogens or commensal in hosts with underlying conditions), an effective immune activation is essentially based on three major regulated events. 1) Activation of TLR2/MyD88-dependent signaling is essential for effective intestinal repair in response to epithelial damage in the presence of commensal bacteria. 2) Innate immune mechanisms with activation of macrophages, dendritic cells or neutrophils are central in the control of local inflammation (NOD2/CARD15 pathway). A central role of the NOD/CARD system implicated in the controlled production of NF-κB is demonstrated. 3) Induction of regulatory T cells by commensal bacteria, with low induction of Th1 differentiation, is observed and explains at least in part the associated tolerance.

Table 180-3 summarizes clinical, epidemiologic and biologic features of the distinct pathotypes.

Enterotoxigenic *Escherichia coli* (ETEC). First described in Calcutta in 1956, ETEC is one of the top four etiologic agents of severe diarrhea in infants younger than 5 years of age in low- and middle-income countries (LMIC)[30] responsible for approximately 280 million cases in this age group and 840 million cases in total. ETEC are also a common cause of travelers' diarrhea associated with ~30% of cases in North American and European travelers.[31] The illness caused by ETEC has a short incubation period and symptoms of watery diarrhea, similar to *Vibrio cholerae* infection. ETEC is endemic all year round in many countries in Africa, Asia and Latin America but more common in warm and wet months. Outbreaks occur and are associated with food or water contaminated with human feces.

ETEC are defined by the presence of plasmid-encoded LT-I and LT-II heat-labile oligomeric toxins and STa and STb heat-stable monomeric toxins and the expression of fimbrial antigens, also plasmid encoded. The fimbrial antigens were known previously as colonization factor antigens (CFAs) but are now referred to as coli surface (CS) antigens suffixed with a number e.g. CS2.[32] CFA/I are still referred to as such. More than 25 different CS antigens are known. ETEC cause disease by adhering to the host gut mucosa via CS antigens (and possible other colonizing factors) and producing either one or both of the LT/ST enterotoxins.[33]

Serotyping has limited use in identifying strains of *E. coli* belonging to the ETEC group as there are a large number of associated serotypes (at least 78 O antigens and 34 H antigens) and common serotypes change over time. ETEC can be detected by PCR targeting the LT and ST genes in isolated colonies or directly from fecal specimens but are rarely sought in diagnostic laboratories. PCR methods are also available to detect ETEC colonization factors.

Enteropathogenic *Escherichia coli* (EPEC). EPEC was the first group of diarrheagenic *E. coli* to be identified and was associated with morbidity and mortality in infants with diarrhea in the 1940s and 50s in the UK and USA. EPEC is still a global cause of diarrhea in infants younger than 2 years today and is especially common in LMIC where mortality rates are high. It is more rarely associated with diarrhea in adults where symptoms are attributed to ingestion of large inocula and/or travel. Clinical manifestations include profuse, persistent diarrhea, vomiting and fever, all of which contribute to severe dehydration, which can be life-threatening in very young and/or malnourished children.

Initially strains of *E. coli* belonging to the EPEC group were defined by serotype and then by their localized adherence (LA) pattern on HEp-2 cells. Currently EPEC are defined as having the *intmin* or *eae* (for *E. coli* **a**ttaching and **e**ffacing) gene, encoding a 97 kDa bacterial outer-membrane protein. During infection, the bacterium intimately attaches to the host gut mucosa disrupting the apical cytoskeleton of

TABLE 180-2	Classification of Virulence Factors Described in Enterobacteriaceae Species		
	DESCRIPTION		
Type of Virulence Factor (VF)	**Bacterial Source**	**VF-Specific Nomenclature**	**Major Function**
Colonization factors, adhesins	*Escherichia coli*	P-fimbriae: type 1 common pili; sfa fimbriae: CFA/I, CS2-25 in ETEC; bundle-forming pilus (BFP) in EPEC; AAF/I-V in EAEC; Afa adhesins in DAEC	Adherence to target epithelial cells via specific receptors
	Shigella	–	
	Salmonella	Type1 fimbriae; Long polar fimbriae; Curli fimbriae	
	Yersinia	Invasin	
	Proteus	MR/P fimbriae; PMF (*P. mirabilis* fimbriae), ATF (ambient temperature fimbriae), NAF (nonagglutinating fimbriae)	
	Klebsiella	Type 1 common fimbriae, type 3 and type 6 fimbriae	
Component of secretion system	*Escherichia coli*	T3SS *sep/esp* locus in EPEC and EHEC	Molecular needle that permits export of secreted bacterial proteins across bacterial membranes and injection directly into target eukaryotic cells
	Salmonella	T3SS *inv/spa* locus	
	Shigella	T3SS *mxi/spa* locus (also described in EIEC)	
	Yersinia	T3SS *ysc* and *ysa* loci	
Flagella	Many members of Enterobacteriaceae except *Shigella*	–	Mobility, pro-inflammatory activity
Capsular polysaccharide	*Escherichia coli*	K1 antigen	Resistance to antimicrobial complement activity and prevention of antibacterial serum resistance
	Salmonella serotype Typhi	Vi antigen	
	Klebsiella	K capsular antigens: K1, K2, K4 and K57 emergent capsule	
	Yersinia	YadA, Ail (attachment invasion locus)	
Iron capture system	*Escherichia coli*	Aerobactin, chu protein, yersiniabactin in EAEC	Iron acquisition
	Shigella	*foc*, *fet*, *iuc* and *iut* loci	
	Yersinia	Yersiniabactin	
Toxins, cytotoxic effectors	*Shigella* spp.	SPATEs	Mucolytic activity; modification of 28S ribosomal subunit leading to apoptosis of target cells
	Shigella dysenteriae	Shiga toxin (Stx1) (ADP ribosyltransferase toxins)	
	Enterohemorrhagic *Escherichia coli*	Shiga-like toxins (Stx1 and Stx2)	
	Enterotoxigenic *Escherichia coli*	Thermolabile and thermostable enterotoxins (LT, ST)	Increase of intracellular cAMP causes modification of apical ion channel activity in target cells
	Enteroaggregative *Escherichia coli*	EAST-1, plasmid-encoded toxin (Pet), SPATEs	Unknown
	Uropathogenic *Escherichia coli*	Hemolysin alpha (RTX toxins), CNF1	Pro-inflammatory activity; modification of Rho GTPase (for CNF1)
T3SS EFFECTORS			
Effectors targeting or mimicking Rho GTPase family members	*Salmonella*	SopE2, SopE, SptP	Modification of cytoskeletal actin and macropinocytosis
	Shigella	IpaA, IpaC, IpgB1, IpgB2	
	Yersinia	YopT, YopE, YpkA/YopO	
Effectors targeting innate immune signaling pathways	*Salmonella*	SipB (SspB), AvrA, SspH1, SpvC	Apoptosis in macrophages and dendritic cells; inhibition of NF-κB signaling and IL-8 production
	Shigella	OspG, OspF, IpaB	
	Yersinia	YopJ	
Effectors targeting actin polymerization directly	Enteropathogenic *Escherichia coli*	Tir	Actin nucleation and pedestal formation
	Salmonella	SipA (SspA), SipC (SspC)	Induction of actin polymerization
	Shigella	IcsA (VirG), IcsP, VirA	Actin nucleation
	Yersinia	YopH	Antiphagocytic activity targeting a major focal adhesin
Effectors promoting intracellular survival	*Salmonella*	SseF, SseG, SseJ, SopD2, SifA, PipB2, SspH2, SptP	Contribution of Sif formation and microtubule formation
	Shigella	IcsB	Host cell survival and prevention of autophagic recognition of IcsA/VirG

cAMP, cyclic adenosine monophosphate; DAEC, diffusely adherent *E. coli*; EAEC, enteroaggregative *E. coli*; EHEC, enterohemorrhagic *E. coli*; EIEC, enteroinvasive *E. coli*; EPEC, enteropathogenic *E. coli*; ETEC, enterotoxigenic *E. coli*; IL, interleukin; NF-κB, nuclear factor kappa B; SPATEs, serine protease autotransporters of Enterobacteriaceae.

Escherichia coli and Intestinal Infections

Pathotype of E. coli	Clinical Manifestations	Histologic Effects	Specific Virulence Factors	Diagnostic Methods
Enterotoxigenic E. coli (ETEC)	Watery diarrhea; travelers' diarrhea; endemic cholera-like illness in children; low- and middle-income countries (LMIC)	LT-B subunit binding GM1 and LT-A subunit increase cyclic AMP production, leading to chloride and neutral sodium chloride secretion	LT (enterotoxin, heat labile) and ST (enterotoxin, heat stable); various colonization factors (CFs) including CS1, CS7, CFA/I and CFA/II	PCR targeting the LT and/or ST gene
Enteropathogenic E. coli (EPEC)	Watery diarrhea with vomiting and fever; infantile diarrhea in children <2 years old; LMIC	A/E adhesion; actin-rich pedestal	Outer-membrane intimin adhesin (eae gene); LEE pathogen (T3SS, esc genes, Esp effectors); EAF plasmid (bundle-forming pilus); intimin receptor Hp90 or Tir; EAST-1 (astA gene)	PCR targeting the eae gene encoded on the LEE PAI and/or bfp gene encoded on the EAF plasmid
Enterohemorrhagic E. coli (EHEC)	Bloody diarrhea, hemolytic–uremic syndrome triad (thrombocytopenia, hemolytic anemia, renal failure); children and young adults; industrialized countries	A/E adhesion; actin-rich pedestal (identical to EPEC)	Major virulence determinant – stx genes; intimin adhesin (eae gene); LEE pathogen (T3SS, esc genes, Esp effectors); pO157 plasmid encoding enterohemolysin gene (in O157:H7 strains); EAST-1 (astA gene)	PCR targeting the phage-encoded stx genes and the eae gene encoded on the LEE
Enteroinvasive E. coli (EIEC)	Classic watery diarrhea; occasionally dysentery syndrome	Shigella-like invasion of epithelium	Large virulence plasmid (220 kb, 100 genes); TTSA type secretion (mxi/spa locus); Ipa, Ipg and Osp effectors; Vir regulators; IcsA/VirG	PCR targeting the ipaH gene encoded in the pINV; guinea pig keratoconjunctivity or Sereny test for differentiation of EIEC from Shigella
Enteroaggregative E. coli (EAEC)	Watery diarrhea; travelers' diarrhea; children and adults; HIV patients; LMIC and industrialized world	Adherence to epithelial cells with typical 'stacked-brick' pattern; mucoid biofilm formation; toxic effects	Large plasmid pAA (typical strains); EAST-1; transcriptional activator gene; she patho-island; AAF/I-AAF/V	PCR targeting the aggR gene encoded in the pINV and the aaiC gene encoded on the chromosome
Diffusely adherent E. coli (DAEC)	Watery diarrhea persistent in young children; LMIC and industrialized world	–	Afa, dra operon	PCR targeting the daaC gene

A/E adhesion, 'attaching and effacing' adhesion; PCR, polymerase chain reaction.
From Croxen M.A., Law R.J., Scholz R., et al.: Recent advances in understanding enteric pathogenic Escherichia coli. *Clin Microbiol Rev 2013; 26:822-80.[29]*

the epithelial cells lining the gut mucosa, effacing the microvilli and forming pedestal-like structures.[34] The process is coordinated by a type III secretion system (T3SS) and multiple EPEC-secreted protein (Esp) effectors on a 35 kb chromosomal pathogenicity island called the locus of enterocyte effacement (LEE). One of the effectors, the translocated intimin receptor (Tir), acts as a receptor for intimin. Symptoms of diarrhea are not toxin-mediated and are likely to be caused by the cellular changes in the host's gut mucosa; for example, changes in the electrolyte balance within the epithelial cells and destruction of the microvilli, resulting in the reduction in the absorptive capacity of the intestinal epithelium.[34]

Certain strains of EPEC also carry an adherence factor (EAF) plasmid encoding a cluster of 14 genes coding for the expression and assembly of the bundle-forming pilus (BFP) and are known as typical (tEPEC) or classical EPEC. Like ETEC, transmission of tEPEC is human-to-human or from food or water contaminated by human feces. EPEC without the EAF plasmid are designated atypical EPEC (aEPEC) – although epidemiological studies show they are more common than tEPEC. aEPEC is associated with a varied animal reservoir, including domesticated and wild animals, and these animal isolates share many characteristics with strains known to cause diarrhea in humans.[35]

Historically, EPEC was identified at diagnostic laboratories by serotyping, as tEPEC comprised relatively few serotypes and subsequently confirmed at reference laboratories by the technically-demanding fluorescent actin staining (FAS) test. This approach has now been replaced by PCR targeting the intmin gene and bfp genes.

Enterohemorrhagic *Escherichia coli* (EHEC). First reported in 1983, EHEC strains are responsible for gastrointestinal illnesses including severe abdominal pain and grossly bloody diarrhea that can develop into hemolytic–uremic syndrome (HUS) between 4 and 15 days after the onset of diarrhea.[36] HUS is specifically associated with thrombocytopenia and hemolytic anemia, as well as acute renal failure and cases often require dialysis treatment. EHEC is the most common etiologic agent of infectious HUS in children and is an emerging pathogen in industrialized countries. The infectious dose is low (10–100 organisms) and transmission is via contaminated food or water, direct contact with animals, especially ruminants, indirect contact with a contaminated environment or person-to person.

The EHEC group is defined by the production of two phage-encoded Shiga toxins, Stx1 (identical to Stx1 of *S. dysenteriae* type 1) and Stx2. Both toxin types have a number of variants and Stx2, specifically the stx2a subtype, is most commonly associated with HUS.[37] Stx, circulating via the bloodstream, is thought to cause vascular damage in the colon and kidneys, specifically by adhering to cell surface globotriaosylceramide (gb3) and the induction of apoptosis.[29] Many EHEC associated with causing severe bloody diarrhea or HUS also have a LEE pathogenicity island, and adhere to the host gut mucosa in a similar way to EPEC. More recently, stx-positive, LEE-negative strains causing HUS were found to harbor the aggR and aai genes, previously associated with EAEC group (see below). EHEC negative for both the LEE and aggR/aai genes have also been associated with HUS and it is likely that other, as yet unknown, attachment mechanisms exist.[38]

Microbiological diagnosis is difficult as the onset of HUS often occurs several days after the diarrheal prodrome, when patients no longer have detectable levels of EHEC in their stools. The recommended diagnostic method is the detection of *stx* genes directly from fecal specimens using PCR and the subsequent culture and identification of *stx*-positive colonies using the same PCR. The most common EHEC serotype, EHEC O157:H7, does not ferment D-sorbitol (as opposed to most other *E. coli* strains), and can be clearly identified as colorless, sorbitol non-fermenting colonies on sorbitol MacConkey agar containing cefixime and tellurite (CT-SMAC). HUS can be caused by other serogroups of *stx*-producing *E. coli* (e.g. O26, O103, O111 and O145), that (unlike EHEC O157:H7) do not have specific biochemical characteristics that aid identification and this further complicates the bacterial diagnosis of HUS. Immunomagnetic separation techniques, involving magnetic beads coated in antibodies to the most commonly detected serogroups, may facilitate detection when EHEC is present in the fecal specimen at low levels.

Enteroinvasive *Escherichia coli* (EIEC). First described in 1971 as being capable of causing diarrhea in volunteers, EIEC has similar pathogenic, biochemical and genetic properties to *Shigella*. EIEC infections occur most commonly in LMIC and are associated with travelers recently returned from these regions. Like *Shigella*, EIEC is transmitted mainly through contaminated water and food or direct person-to-person spread.

The major virulence factor is a 220 kb plasmid, designated the invasion plasmid (pINV). The pathogenic mechanism of EIEC is virtually identical to that of *Shigella* (Figure 180-6). Although EIEC can be responsible for dysentery with fecal blood, mucus and leukocytes, this clinical presentation is less common than with *Shigella* infection and volunteer studies indicate that the infectious dose is higher. Watery diarrhea is common and indistinguishable from *Shigella* infections.

Differential diagnosis from *Shigella* is difficult even using the PCR approach as the *ipaH* gene, the target for detecting *Shigella* is on the pINV plasmid and is also carried by EIEC. EIEC and *Shigella* can only be clearly differentiated by the guinea pig keratoconjunctivity or Sereny test (now rarely used) or by extended biochemical tests and serology.

Enteroaggregative *Escherichia coli* (EAEC). Nataro *et al.*[39] first described the aggregative adherence (AA) or stacked-brick formation of bacteria attached to HEp-2 cells that characterizes the EAEC group. EAEC is the most common bacterial cause of diarrhea in studies in the USA and UK[40,41] and an emerging cause of travelers' diarrhea. It makes a significant contribution to morbidity in children younger than 2 years of age in LMIC and is also an important cause of diarrhea in HIV-infected patients. The typical illness is characterized by a persistent watery, mucoid, secretory diarrhea with low-grade fever and symptoms may continue for more than 10 days. Transmission of EAEC is thought to be similar to that of EIEC and *Shigella*, via food and water contaminated with human feces or person-to-person spread. EAEC strains have been reported in animals but there is, as yet, little evidence to suggest a significant animal reservoir.

Certain EAEC harbor a plasmid, designated pAA, encoding a number of putative virulence factors including AggR (involved in the regulation of many of the virulence genes involved in both the aggregation and toxin production stages of EAEC pathogenesis) and are known as typical EAEC. Atypical strains also adhere to HEp-2 cells in a stacked-brick formation but do not have the pAA plasmid. Although the exact mechanism of pathogenesis is not fully understood, a model in three stages has been proposed:[29]

1. Adherence to host gut mucosa by fimbrial and afimbrial adhesins. To date, five types of aggregative adherence fimbriae have been described (AAFI-V) all encoded on pAA and regulated by aggR.

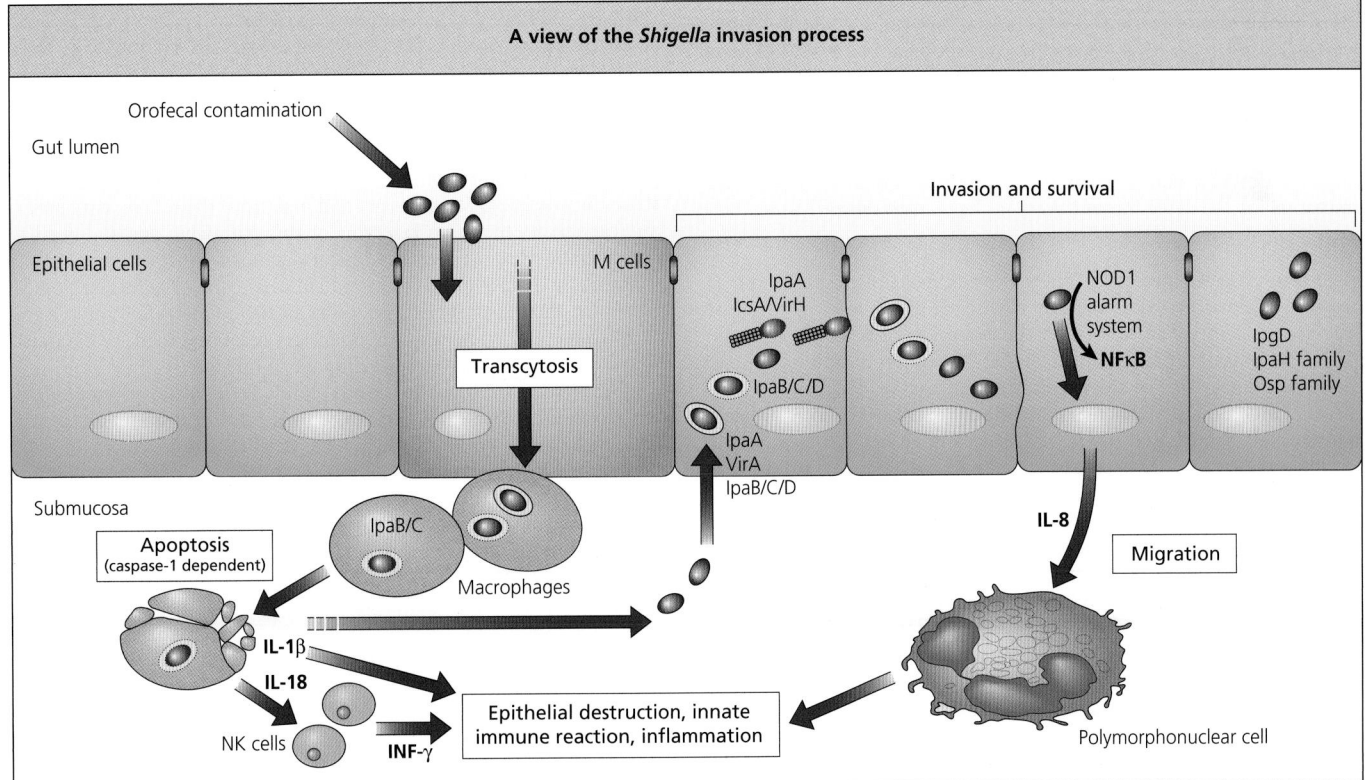

Figure 180-6 A view of the *Shigella* invasion process. *Shigella* transmitted by the fecal–oral route reach the large intestine, transcytose across the epithelial layer through M cells, and encounter resident macrophages. *Shigella flexneri* is capable of survival in macrophages, inducing apoptosis and release of proinflammatory cytokines such as IL-1β or IL-8. IL-8 induces a massive infiltration of neutrophils, which destroy the integrity of the epithelial layer. Once released from macrophages, bacteria invade the epithelial cells from the basolateral side, escape to phagosomal vesicles, and move in the intracellular cytoplasm by polymerization of actin, ultimately invading neighboring cells. (*Adapted from Schroeder & Hilbi Clin Microbiol Rev 2008; 21:134–156.*)

2. Production of enterotoxins and cytotoxins including a cytoskeleton-altering plasmid-encoded toxin (Pet), SHet, a toxin also produced by *Shigella flexneri*, heat-stable enterotoxin (EAST-1) and Pic, a mucinase, both encoded by many other pathogens.[42]

3. Mucosal inflammation induced by both the pathogen and the host's own immune system.

Recent studies suggest that the *aggR* gene also regulates chromosomally-encoded genes located on the Aai operon.[43]

EAEC strains are phenotypically and genetically diverse and, therefore, comprehensive diagnostic assays based on biochemical, serological or molecular approaches all have limitations. The gold standard method for the identification of EAEC is the HEp-2 adherence assay with the characteristic aggregative or 'stacked-brick' adherence pattern but this is technically demanding and unsuitable as a routine diagnostic tool. PCR targeting the *aggR* and *aaiC* genes is the most commonly used method.

In 2011, 4321 previously healthy people from 16 countries were associated with an outbreak of food-borne illness caused by an EAEC Shiga toxin-producing strain identified as *E. coli* O104:H4. Over 900 cases developed HUS and more than 50 people died.[44] This hybrid pathogen carried virulence genes found in both typical EAEC strains (*aggA, aggR, set1, pic,* and *aap*) and EHEC (*stx2*). Other examples of the acquisition of Shiga toxin genes by EAEC isolated from patients with HUS have been reported in Japan, France, Northern Ireland and Central African Republic.

Diffusely Adherent *Escherichia coli* (DAEC).

Diffusely adherent *E. coli* defined by a diffuse adherence (DA) pattern to HEp-2 or HeLa culture cells were originally described as being associated with watery diarrhea in children older than 1 year of age.[45] The adherence phenotype is due to the production of adhesins encoded by a family of operons related to *afa/dra/daa* genes encoding both afimbrial (such as Afa) or fimbrial (such as F1845 encoded by daaC or Dr) adhesins. Afa/Dr DAEC was reported initially in extraintestinal *E. coli* infection by a uropathogenic strain[29] and does not appear specific to strains associated with diarrheal diseases (DAEC). Moreover, these structures were also described among commensal *E. coli* from normal digestive flora. Although the interaction between Afa/Dr adhesins and receptors leads to cell signaling resulting in actin modification, the implication of Afa/Dr DAEC strains in diarrhea remains controversial. Epidemiological studies are hampered by the fact there are no universally agreed methods for the detection of DAEC in the clinical setting.

Shigella

The four *Shigella* species (*S. dysenteriae, S. flexneri, S. sonnei* and *S. boydii*), a genus first described by Kiyoshi Shiga in 1897, are part of the genomic species *E. coli* (with the exception of *S. boydii* serotype 13). The Shigellae can be divided into 49 serotypes and additional subtypes. Symptoms of shigellosis are mild watery diarrhea or more severe inflammatory bacillary dysentery, characterized by fever, abdominal cramps, and blood and mucus in stools. *S. dysenteriae* 1 produces Stx1 and has been associated with HUS similar to the syndrome caused by EHEC.[46] A large proportion of all diarrheal episodes worldwide are attributed to *Shigella*, with 1.1 million fatal cases annually; approximately 99% of cases occur in LMIC with the majority occurring in children under the age of 5 years.

Shigella dysenteriae and *S. boydii* are rare, the latter being largely restricted to the Indian subcontinent. *S. flexneri* is the most commonly isolated species, endemic in LMIC and isolated in industrialized countries, mainly in travelers returning from abroad. Recently, outbreaks of *S. flexneri* have been associated with transmission between men who have sex with men (MSM) in Europe, North America and Australia. *S. sonnei* are the most common species isolated in industrialized countries, often linked to outbreaks in nurseries and schools.

The Shigellae are facultative intracellular pathogens derived from *E. coli* by a combination of gene loss and acquisition. Acquisition genes are associated with bacterial invasion and intracellular survival (e.g. *virB* and *mxiE*), iron acquisition (e.g. *iuc* and *fuc*) and toxin

production (e.g. *set1A* and *set1B*) encoded on the invasion plasmid pINV and the chromosomally located *Shigella* PAIs (SHIs) SHI-1 and SHI-2, SHI-O, and SRL. The *Shigella* genome is also characterized by deletions associated with the loss of metabolic pathways (e.g. *cadA*) no longer required for an intracellular lifestyle and antivirulence factors (e.g. *nadA* and *nadB*) that would suppress pathogenicity.[14,29,47] In the large intestine, during the invasion process, the bacteria cross the epithelial layer through M-cells and are engulfed by macrophages on reaching the submucosa. They survive in the macrophage, eventually inducing apoptosis and the release of cytokines that destroy the integrity of the epithelial layer. On escaping from the macrophage, they invade the epithelial cells from the basolateral side and traverse the intracellular cytoplasm of the invaded cell and neighboring cells by formation of an actin tail on the bacterial surface that provides the propulsive force required for directed motility (Figure 180-6). Diarrhea results from the breakdown of the integrity of the epithelium and subsequent reduction in its capacity to resorb fluid.

Detection of *Shigella* from feces relies on the use of differential and selective media (e.g. deoxycholate agar (DCA)) and xylose-lysine deoxycholate (XLD). Biochemically, *Shigella* are unable to ferment lactose or utilize citrate, urea or produce lysine decarboxylase, are nonmotile and produce acid from glucose but no gas. The PCR targets to invasion plasmid antigen H (*ipaH*) gene. Strains are serotyped (*S. dysenteriae, S. boydii* and *S. flexneri*) or phage typed (*S. sonnei*) to facilitate outbreak investigations. Molecular typing methods include PFGE, MLST, MLVA and WGS.

Salmonella

There are two clinical manifestations of salmonellosis: gastroenteritis and typhoid (enteric) fever. *Salmonella enterica* serovars Typhi and Paratyphi A, B and C are responsible for typhoid and typhoid-like fevers. These pathogens only infect humans and are transmitted via the fecal–oral route by contaminated food or water, or by person-to-person spread. This systemic illness leads to an estimated 20 million cases and 200 000 deaths worldwide each year. Typhoid fever is characterized by a systemic infection where bacteria colonize the liver, spleen and bone marrow. Cases often report a short bout of nausea and diarrhea prior to malaise, headache, fever, myalgia and minor upper respiratory symptoms. Complications include persistent infection resulting in relapse or chronic carriage where the bacterium may persist in the gallbladder. WGS data has shed light in the population structure and evolution of Typhi and highlights the role of asymptomatic carriers as the main reservoir of this pathogen, and the need to identify and treat carriers.[48] Clinical diagnosis can be confirmed by isolating the bacterium from blood culture, urine or feces. Serological assays for the detection of antibodies to the *Salmonella* Typhi O and H antigens (e.g. Widal test) are no longer recommended for diagnosis as cross-reactions make results difficult to interpret.

The global burden of nontyphoid *Salmonella* gastroenteritis remains high at 93.8 million cases, with 155 000 deaths and an average incidence of 1.14 episodes/100 person-years each year. The incubation period is from 4 hours to 72 hours after the ingestion of contaminated food or water. Symptoms include fever and chills, nausea and vomiting, abdominal cramping and diarrhea. Gastroenteritis can be caused by a large number of serovars, most commonly Typhimurium and Enteritidis. Infection is localized to the intestine, without systemic diffusion in most cases. Some serovars cause disease in both humans and animals and have a wide host range (e.g. Typhimurium associated with humans, cattle, swine, horses, sheep, poultry, and wild rodents), whereas others are host restricted (e.g. *S. gallinarum* associated with poultry).[49]

Salmonella pathogenicity factors are encoded on five *Salmonella* PAIs, SPI1-SPI5. In the small bowel, salmonellae cross the intestinal mucus layer and adhere to intestinal epithelial cells using a variety of adhesins including type I fimbriae, curli fimbriae, Pef fimbriae, and Std fimbriae. The invasion of the host epithelial cells by *Salmonella* is mediated by T3SS1 effectors (SipA, SipC, SopB, SopE, SopE2) that trigger the rapid appearance of membrane ruffles on the surface of the host cell, and subsequent formation of spacious phagosomes or vacuoles.[50,51] Alternatively, at least two non-fimbrial outer-membrane proteins, Rck and PagN, can mediate invasion of nonphagocytic cells.[52] Following invasion, the bacteria remain within a modified phagosome known as the *Salmonella*-containing vacuole (SCV), where their survival and replication is controlled by the down regulation of T3SS1 and up-regulation of T3SS2 (SseF, SseG, SifA and SseJ).[53] The SCVs cross the basolateral membrane and release the bacteria into the submucosa, where they are internalized within phagocytes and disseminated through the lymph and the bloodstream.[51]

Like *Shigella*, detection of *Salmonella* from feces relies on the use of differential and selective media (e.g. deoxycholate agar (DCA) or XLD). There are exceptions but generally *Salmonella* are unable to ferment lactose or urea but do utilize citrate and hydrogen sulfide. They produce lysine decarboxylase and acid from glucose and gas and are motile. A variety of published PCR assays exist; generic assays targeting the *ttr* genes required for tetrathionate respiration and assays specific for subspecies 1 targeting in invasion genes such as *hilA*. Molecular typing methods include PFGE, MLST, MLVA and WGS. MLST correlates well with the traditional serotyping scheme.[22]

Yersinia

Of the 11 established *Yersinia* species, only *Y. enterocolitica, Y. pseudotuberculosis* and *Y. pestis* are clinically important. *Yersinia pestis*, the agent of plague, has species status in the nomenclature for obvious clinical and historic reasons[54] and is discussed in Chapter 126. *Yersinia enterocolitica* and *Y. pseudotuberculosis* can cause acute gastroenteritis with fever, abdominal pains and diarrhea, more commonly in children, and acute terminal ileitis and mesenteric lymphadenitis with abdominal pain mimicking appendicitis in adults, erythema nodosum, reactive polyarthritis, and, occasionally, bloodstream infections.[55] Yersiniosis represents the third most frequently reported food-borne gastroenteritis in Europe; the most important source of infection is believed to be contaminated porcine products.

Pathogenic *Y. enterocolitica* colonize the terminal ileum, invade Peyer's patches and disseminate to lymphoid tissues, including liver and spleen, where they replicate, suppress and reorient the immune system. Virulence factors are located on the chromosome and on a 70 kb plasmid. Key invasion proteins are encoded by *inv, yadA* and *ail*. Pathogenesis involves many effectors (named Yop for 'Yersinia outer proteins'), which translocate via a secretory mechanism designated Ysc T3SS (encoded by the virulence plasmid) directly into eukaryotic cells and inhibit phagocytosis and down-regulate the host immune response by hijacking the host's intracellular machinery. The most pathogenic *Y. enterocolitica* biotype 1B carries an additional recently described T3SS, Ysa T3SS.[56]

On *Yersinia* selective agar, CIN (cefsulodin, irgasan, novobiocin), *Yersinia enterocolitica* and *Y. pseudotuberculosis* appear as translucent, well-defined colonies with a deep red center (bull's eye colonies) due to mannitol fermentation. *Y. enterocolitica* is a heterogeneous group of strains classified into six biotypes, of which 1A is regarded as nonpathogenic and 1B and 2-5 are pathogenic. Strains belonging to serogroups O3 (biotype 4), O5, 27 (biotypes 2 and 3), O8 (biotype 1B) and O9 (biotype 2) are most frequently isolated worldwide. MLST and WGS have been used to investigate the population structure and evolution of the genus.[57]

EXTRAINTESTINAL INFECTIONS

Urinary Tract Infections

Urinary tract infections (UTIs) are among the most common bacterial infections in humans and account for significant morbidity and high medical costs (see Chapters 53, 55 and 56). UPEC infections account for roughly 80% of all UTIs, causing cystitis in the bladder and acute pyelonephritis in the kidneys.

The ability to cause UTI requires a combination of highly regulated virulence factors, including multiple pili, secreted toxins (for example Sat and vacuolating autotransporter toxin (Vat)), multiple iron acquisition systems and polysaccharide capsules, often encoded on PAIs.

Attachment is mediated by fimbrial adhesin H (FimH), which is found at the tip of the phase-variable type 1 pili and binds to proteins called uroplakins that coat the uroepithelium, a specialized stratified transitional epithelium composed of three cell layers. Uroplakin Ia is the receptor for one important adhesive appendage of UPEC, the type 1 pili. FimH also mediates UPEC invasion and once internalized, UPEC can rapidly replicate and certain strains produce hemolysin A (HlyA) toxin causing tissue damage and apoptosis. Adhesins include the fimbrial adhesins such as the type 1 pili, P-fimbriae and S-fimbriae, and the afimbrial adhesins such as AfaE. Crosstalk between P fimbriae, type 1 pili and other adhesion clusters prevents co-expression of multiple surface structures.[28,58,59]

Other common Enterobacteriaceae associated with UTIs are *Klebsiella pneumoniae* and *Proteus mirabilis*.[60] These species infect specific groups of patients, such as those with diabetes mellitus or dysfunctional bladders and urinary catheters. A common pathogen in both community and hospitalized UTIs, *K. pneumoniae* possesses a number of virulence determinants, including adhesins, urease activity, capsule and iron-scavenging systems.[61] *Proteus mirabilis* is an important agent of UTI, particularly in hospitalized patients and notably those who are catheterized. A hallmark of infection with this species is stone formation, resulting from active urease which hydrolyzes urea to ammonia, raising urinary pH and subsequently leading to precipitation of magnesium ammonium phosphate and calcium phosphate. Another specific characteristic of *Proteus* infections is the ability to colonize the surfaces of catheters forming biofilms.[62]

Respiratory Tract Infections

Enterobacteriaceae may cause community-acquired pneumonia in the elderly and are implicated in ventilator-associated pneumonia.[63] In particular, *K. pneumoniae* and *E. cloacae* are among the most frequent bacteria responsible for ventilator-associated pneumonia, after *Staphylococcus aureus* and *Pseudomonas aeruginosa*. *Klebsiella pneumoniae* was originally described as the agent of Friedländer's pneumonia, a severe lobar pneumonia, and remains an important cause of hospital- and community-acquired pneumonia, even though the incidence of community-acquired pneumonia has decreased in North America and Europe[61] (see 'Other infections and rare or emerging Enterobacteriaceae pathogens' below and Chapter 28).

Meningitis and Neurologic Infections

Certain types of *E. coli* can cause gram-negative-associated meningitis (neonatal meningitis *E. coli* or NMEC) in newborns. Fatality rates can approach 40%, and survivors are usually burdened with severe neurological sequelae.[64] Survival in the blood is facilitated by an antiphagocytic polysialic acid capsule and manipulation of the classical complement pathway by the bacterial outer-membrane protein A (OmpA).[65] Invasion of macrophages and monocytes prevents apoptosis and chemokine release, providing a niche for replication before dissemination back into the blood. A lambdoid phage that encodes O acetyltransferase acetylates the O antigen to provide phase variation and diversity to the capsule, hiding the bacteria from host defenses. Attachment to the endothelial cells of the blood–brain barrier is mediated by FimH of the type 1 pili binding to CD48 and by OmpA binding to its receptor, ECGP96. Invasion occurs through the actions of Ibe proteins, FimH, OmpA and cytotoxic necrotizing factor 1 (CNF1).[28] The K1 capsule – which is found in approximately 80% of NMEC isolates – also has a role in invasion by preventing lysosomal fusion and thus allowing delivery of live bacteria across the blood–brain barrier.[66] In the central nervous system the bacterium can induce edema, inflammation and neural damage.

Citrobacter koseri is another classic bacterium described in neonatal neurologic infections, in particular as a cause of devastating neonatal meningitis characterized by the formation of multiple brain abscesses.[67] There is some evidence that *C. koseri* is able to resist phagocytosis and the presence of a 32 kDa protein in the external membrane of the bacteria may be linked to meningeal tropism and abscess formation.

Bacteremia

Bacteremia is a major complication of infection by Enterobacteriaceae as it can lead to severe sepsis with acute organ failure and septic shock (see Chapter 47).

In recent years *E. coli* bacteremia has increased and in the UK the species now accounts for more than 30% of bacteremia in those aged over 75 years.[68] There have also been significant increases in bacteremia caused by other gram-negative pathogens. The primary source of bacteremia is UTIs. Other classic sources of blood infections include the digestive tract, implicating both specific intestinal pathogens and opportunistic enteric bacteria, which can translocate from the intestinal lumen to blood in hosts with underlying conditions (e.g. digestive solid tumor, cholecystitis or immunosuppressive treatment). *Salmonella* serovars that cause typhoid fever[69] and, more rarely, nontyphoidal *Salmonella* can cause sepsis.

OTHER INFECTIONS AND RARE OR EMERGING ENTEROBACTERIACEAE PATHOGENS

Many, if not most, Enterobacteriaceae can cause infection, even if rarely, and those species that are considered medically most important are described in Table 180-4. *Klebsiella* spp., principally *K. pneumoniae* and to a lesser extent *K. oxytoca*, are second only to *E. coli* as a nosocomial cause of urinary tract, respiratory tract or blood infections.[61] *K. pneumoniae* also cause serious community infections such as pneumonia, bacteremia and meningitis. *Klebsiella pneumoniae* owes its name to Friedländer's pneumonia, a severe form of lobar pneumonia that used to devastate chronic alcoholics. A recent population study by MLST[61] has defined a number of virulent clones of *K. pneumoniae*, one of which is associated with pyogenic liver abscess and two of which correspond to *K. pneumoniae* subsp. *rhinoscleromatis* and *K. pneumoniae* subsp. *ozaenae*, respectively. The latter two are regarded as a cause of chronic upper respiratory disease. *Klebsiella planticola* and *K. terrigena* are often misidentified as *K. pneumoniae* or *K. oxytoca*; as a result, knowledge of their clinical importance remains poor (note that the validity of genus *Raoultella*, which was proposed for the two former species, has been questioned). Cytotoxin-producing *K. oxytoca* were recently shown to be a cause of antibiotic-associated hemorrhagic colitis.[74]

Klebsiella (Calymmatobacterium) granulomatis is the causative agent of donovanosis (granuloma inguinale), a chronic genital ulceration (see Chapter 64). Specific diagnosis is possible by detection of large mononuclear cells with intracytoplasmic cysts filled with deeply stained gram-negative Donovan bodies in biopsy samples or PCR targeting two unique base changes in the *phoE* gene.[73] In fact, comparison of *phoE* sequences of *K. granulomatis* and *K. pneumoniae* suggests that the former may represent particular strains of *K. pneumoniae*.[61]

Serious infections by *Cronobacter* (formerly *Enterobacter*) *sakazakii* with fatal outcome have been described, particularly in children. This species has been associated with small outbreaks or sporadic cases of sepsis, meningitis and necrotizing enterocolitis reported in infants younger than 1 month, especially in premature babies and neonatal intensive care units (ICUs). High morbidity and mortality were associated with neurologic forms of this infection. Powdered infant formulas were incriminated as a source of *C. sakazakii* infections.[71]

Other species such as *Enterobacter cloacae* (itself a complex of several species), *Citrobacter freundii*, *Citrobacter koseri*, *Proteus mirabilis*, *Hafnia alvei*, *Morganella morganii*, *Serratia marcescens*[62,67,76,81] and others can cause disease in humans. These are generally considered as opportunistic pathogens, as they ordinarily occur as commensals in the gastrointestinal tract. The clinical significance of most unusual Enterobacteriaceae species remains unclear, given limited data and that specific virulence factors remain unknown in most.

Rare pathogenic species are more difficult to identify with classic methods than more frequent pathogens. Molecular methods, such as the sequencing of 16S rRNA or *rpoB* genes, are especially helpful in

these cases and may also lead to the discovery of novel species. For example, some strains that were misidentified as *Hafnia alvei* expressing the *eae* gene have now been reclassified as *Escherichia albertii*, leading to reconsideration of the implication of *H. alvei* in gastrointestinal disease.[6,70]

Prevention, Management and Control of Infections

SYMPTOMATIC TREATMENT

Rapid oral rehydration using intravenous fluids is the first recommended therapy in digestive Enterobacteriaceae infections, specifically during EPEC infection affecting very young children or ETEC-related diarrhea and shigellosis.[29] Symptomatic treatment of EHEC infections is critical for management of HUS, which requires dialysis in more than half of cases[36] (see Chapters 37 and 38 for a discussion on the management of these conditions).

ANTIMICROBIAL RESISTANCE AND EMERGENCE OF MULTIDRUG RESISTANCE

Resistance mechanisms to antimicrobial agents can be intrinsic and acquired. The latter mechanisms result from mutational events (especially for quinolone resistance) or, more often, acquisition of various mobile genetic elements such as transposons and plasmids.

First reported in the early 1980s in Germany and France, a major problem in the medical field in recent times is the increasing numbers of Enterobacteriaceae strains found to produce extended-spectrum β-lactamases (ESBLs).[82] ESBLs are defined as enzymes produced by certain bacteria that are able to hydrolyze extended-spectrum cephalosporins. The 'workhorse hospital antibiotics', such as ceftazidime, ceftriaxone and cefotaxime, are rendered ineffective against ESBL-producing bacteria. There are three important types of ESBLs: TEM, SHV and CTX-M.[82] The numbers of TEM and SHV type antibiotics each currently exceeds 100. The most common types are carried by *E. coli* and *K. pneumoniae*[83] but they are also found in *Enterobacter*, *Proteus*, *Morganella* and *Salmonella* species. TEM and SHV enzymes, widespread in *E. coli* and *Klebsiella*, have evolved by mutation of common plasmid-encoded penicillinases, whereas CTX-M enzymes represent examples of plasmid acquisition of beta-lactamase genes normally found on the chromosome in *Kluyvera* species. CTX-M family, first described in Japan in 1986, hydrolyze cefotaxime in preference to ceftazidime and are prevalent among community-acquired infections. In *E. coli*, one predominant CTX-M clone, CTX-M-15, represented two-thirds of all extended-spectrum β-lactamase (EBSLs) isolated in 2004 in the UK.[84] CTX-M is also a common ESBL identified in Enterobacteriaceae isolated in fecal flora.

A recent study showed that community ESBL fecal carriage, which was unknown before the turn of the millennium, has since increased significantly everywhere, with LMIC being the most affected. Intercontinental travel may have emphasized and globalized the issue and CTX-M enzymes, especially CTX-M-15, are the dominant type of ESBL. The authors of the study suggest that CTX-M carriage is evolving toward a global pandemic.[85]

Most outbreaks reported in ICUs, involve unrelated strains of the same species but may involve the dissemination of the ESBL plasmid to different species. Risk factors for infection by ESBL-producing Enterobacteriaceae included increased length of hospital stay, admission to the ICU or pre-existing co-morbidities and specifically prior use of third-generation cephalosporins.[81]

Developed in the 1980s, carbapenems (the most widely used is imipenem, followed by meropenem and ertapenem) are derivatives of thienamycin and have broad-spectrum activities and are used to treat infections caused by ESBL-producing strains. Three distinct mechanisms have been described for carbapenem resistance:[86]

- outer-membrane protein mutation causing decreased permeability;

TABLE 180-4	Unusual, Emerging or Recently Reclassified Enterobacteriaceae Species Causing Human Infections			
Species	**Human Infections**	**Properties**	**Risk Factors**	**Recent References**
Escherichia albertii	Diarrhea	Eae-positive strains, previously misidentified as *Hafnia alvei*; closely related to *Shigella boydii* serotype 13	–	Hyma et al.,[6] Nimri[70]
Enterobacter (Cronobacter) sakazakii	Bacteremia, meningitis and cerebrolysis, necrotizing enterocolitis	Described in 1980, phenotypically close to *E. cloacae* but sorbitol-negative, specific yellow pigment, α-lucosidase activity detected in specific agar medium	Neonatality, low birth weight	Holý & Forsythe[71]
Klebsiella pneumoniae subsp. *rhinoscleromatis*	Rhinoscleroma, a chronic granulomatous disease of upper airways	Related to *K. pneumoniae* but ONPG-negative; no acid production with lactose; urease-, LDC- and citrate-negative; K3 capsular type	Nutritional deficiency, tropical and subtropical areas	Brisse et al.[61] Botelho-Nevers et al.[72]
Klebsiella pneumoniae subsp. *ozaenae*	Ozena, a chronic rhinitis with atrophic nasal mucosa	Closely related to *K. pneumoniae* but always urease-negative; K4 or rarely K5	LMIC	Brisse et al.[61] Botelho-Nevers et al.[72]
Klebsiella granulomatis	Donovanosis (granuloma inguinale)	Previously named *Calymmatobacterium granulomatis*; uncultured in defined medium	Southern Africa or Asia, Papua New Guinea, northern and central Australia	O'Farrell et al.[73]
Enterobacter hormaechei	Intra-abdominal abscesses, urinary tract infections (UTIs), bacteremia	Often misidentified as *E. cloacae*; a frequent cause of nosocomial infections	–	Mezzatesta et al.[74]
Edwardsiella tarda	Gastrointestinal disease (controversial), bacteremia, wound infections with abscesses following trauma in aquatic environment	Described in 1965, resides in intestine of cold-blooded animals and water. LDC-, ODC-, H_2S- and indole reaction-positive; absence of fermentation of most sugars except glucose and maltose	Immunocompromised	Leung et al.[75]
Hafnia alvei	Bacteremia, respiratory tract infections associated with abscesses, gastroenteritis (controversial)	Voges–Proskauer reaction-positive, indole production-negative, absence of fermentation of lactose, motility at 22°C positive	Immunocompromised	Janda & Abbott[76]
Kluyvera ascorbata	UTIs, soft tissue infections, intra-abdominal abscesses	Described in 1936, including four species (*ascorbata, cryocrescens, cochleae, georgiana*) closely related to *E. coli* but esculin-negative, citrate- and malonate-positive, growth in KCN	Neutropenia, underlying malignancy	Isozaki et al.[77]
Leclercia adecarboxylata	Bacteremia, wound infections, pneumonia	Described in 1962, closely related to *E. coli* but lysine decarboxylase-negative, malonate-positive; acid production from arabitol and cellobiose but not from adonitol and sorbitol	Immunocompromised status, neutropenia, cirrhosis	Keren et al.[78]
Pantoea agglomerans	Bacteremia associated with venous catheter, bone or joint infections, soft tissue infections with abscesses	Includes strains originally named *Enterobacter agglomerans* or *Erwinia herbicola*; presents a characteristic LDC-, ADH- and ODC-negative profile	Blood products, intravenous fluids; wounds from thorns or knives	Cruz et al.[79]
Plesiomonas shigelloides	Water-borne gastrointestinal infections	Oxidase-positive	Consumption of seafood or untreated water; biliary tract diseases or acute cholangitis	Salerno et al.[80]

ADH, antidiuretic hormone; H_2S, hydrogen sulfide production; LDC, lysine decarboxylase; ODC, ornithine decarboxylase.

- production of carbapenemases (four classes encoded either on chromosomes or plasmids are known; classes A and B are mostly identified in Enterobacteriaceae); and
- altered affinity of the penicillin-binding proteins for carbapenems.

IMI-1 was the first acquired carbapenemase identified in *Serratia marcescens* isolated in Japan in 1991. KPC-1 was reported from a *K. pneumoniae* isolate from the USA in 2001. Both molecules are β-lactamase enzymes that hydrolyze β-lactams, conferring a high level of resistance even to carbapenems and thus compromising treatment.[87] Their dissemination has significantly increased over the last decade among various Enterobacteriaceae, as the corresponding genes are often located on transferable plasmids.

VACCINATION AND PREVENTION

Prevention of digestive infections depends on adequate treatment of drinking water and food contamination control, which remains very difficult in many places in the world.

Vaccination constitutes a major challenge for the control of frequent Enterobacteriaceae infections specifically against digestive illnesses affecting several millions of people globally.[29] The emergence and rapid dissemination of multidrug resistance and the challenges faced by the development of novel agents makes vaccination an attractive option. The key Enterobacteriaceae vaccination programs currently being developed include vaccines against *Salmonella* Typhi[88] and Shigellae,[89,90] the rCTB-CF ETEC vaccine consisting of a combination of recombinant cholera toxin B subunit and formalin-inactive ETEC bacteria,[91] and EHEC vaccines to prevent human disease as well as carriage of EHEC in animals.[92]

References available online at expertconsult.com.

KEY REFERENCES

Chaudhuri R.R., Henderson I.R.: The evolution of the *Escherichia coli* phylogeny. *Infect Genet Evol* 2012; 12:214-226.

Croxen M.A., Finlay B.B.: Molecular mechanisms of *Escherichia coli* pathogenicity. *Nat Rev Microbiol* 2010; 8:26-38.

Croxen M.A., Law R.J., Scholz R., et al.: Recent advances in understanding enteric pathogenic *Escherichia coli*. *Clin Microbiol Rev* 2013; 26:822-880.

Fàbrega A., Vila J.: *Salmonella enterica* serovar Typhimurium skills to succeed in the host: virulence and regulation. *Clin Microbiol Rev* 2013; 26:308-341.

Fleckenstein J.M., Munson G.M., Rasko D.A.: Enterotoxigenic *Escherichia coli*: orchestrated host engagement. *Gut Microbes* 2013; 4:392-396.

Grad Y.H., Lipsitch M., Feldgarden M., et al.: Genomic epidemiology of the *Escherichia coli* O104:H4 outbreaks in Europe, 2011. *Proc Natl Acad Sci USA* 2012; 109: 3065-3070.

Hazen T.H., Sahl J.W., Fraser C.M., et al.: Refining the pathovar paradigm via phylogenomics of the attaching and effacing *Escherichia coli*. *Proc Natl Acad Sci USA* 2013; 110:12810-12815.

Holt K.E., Parkhill J., Mazzoni C.J., et al.: High-throughput sequencing provides insights into genome variation and evolution in *Salmonella* Typhi. *Nat Genet* 2008; 40:987-993.

Karmali M.A.: Host and pathogen determinants of verocytotoxin-producing *Escherichia coli*-associated hemolytic uremic syndrome. *Kidney Int Suppl* 2009; 112:S4-S7.

Lai Y., Rosenshine I., Leong J.M., et al.: Intimate host attachment: enteropathogenic and enterohaemorrhagic *Escherichia coli*. *Cell Microbiol* 2013; 15:1796-1808.

Papp-Wallace K.M., Endimiani A., Taracila M.A., et al.: Carbapenems: past, present, and future. *Antimicrob Agents Chemother* 2011; 55:4943-4960.

Reuter S., Connor T.R., Barquist L., et al.: Parallel independent evolution of pathogenicity within the genus *Yersinia*. *Proc Natl Acad Sci USA* 2014; 111(18):6768-6773.

Schroeder G.N., Hilbi H.: Molecular pathogenesis of *Shigella* spp.: controlling host cell signaling, invasion, and death by type III secretion. *Clin Microbiol Rev* 2008; 21:134-156.

Steyert S.R., Sahl J.W., Fraser C.M., et al.: Comparative genomics and stx phage characterization of LEE-negative Shiga toxin-producing *Escherichia coli*. *Front Cell Infect Microbiol* 2012; 2:133.

Woerther P.L., Burdet C., Chachaty E., et al.: Trends in human fecal carriage of extended-spectrum β-lactamases in the community: toward the globalization of CTX-M. *Clin Microbiol Rev* 2013; 26:744-758.

Pseudomonas spp., Acinetobacter spp. and Miscellaneous Gram-Negative Bacilli

HILMAR WISPLINGHOFF

KEY CONCEPTS

- Nonfermenting gram-negative bacilli (NFGNB), such as *Pseudomonas aeruginosa*, *Acinetobacter baumannii*, and *Stenotrophomonas maltophilia*, are important nosocomial pathogens contributing significantly to morbidity and mortality, while others are being increasingly recognized as clinical pathogens.

- NFGNBs such as *A. baumannii* or *P. aeruginosa* have been implicated in nearly all kinds of infections, including bloodstream infections (BSI), pneumonia and meningitis.

- Clinical presentation of BSI due to *A. baumannii* or *P. aeruginosa* varies. It may range from benign transient bacteremia to fulminant septic shock with high mortality and is not different from other gram-negative bacteria.

- Most NFGNB have a high intrinsic resistance which makes them frequently resistant to the major classes of antimicrobial agents, often leaving few therapeutic options.

- Several NFGNB are highly resistant to environmental conditions favoring epidemic spread.

Introduction

Strictly aerobic gram-negative bacilli have become increasingly important as human pathogens over the past decades.[1-3] Molecular methods for identification have led to a number of changes in taxonomy, contributing insights into the clinical significance and epidemiology. While *Pseudomonas aeruginosa*[1] remains the clinically most prevalent species among the nonfermenting gram-negative bacilli (NFGNB), other species, mainly *Acinetobacter baumannii*, have emerged as important nosocomial pathogens.[2] *Stenotrophomonas maltophilia* and *Burkholderia cepacia* are commonly isolated from intensive care unit (ICU) patients and patients with cystic fibrosis (CF).[3,4] Species of *Acidovorax*, *Alcaligenes*, *Brevundimonas*, *Comamonas*, *Chryseobacterium* (*Flavobacterium*), *Pandoraea* and *Ralstonia* groups have been recognized as potential pathogens since the late 1980s.[4]

Epidemiology

Most of the NFGNB can survive or even replicate under adverse environmental conditions. *Pseudomonas* spp. and other NFGNBs, in particular *Acinetobacter* spp., may survive for extended periods of time in dry, cold or warm environments, and have been isolated from a variety of surfaces, medical products and foods such as dairy products, poultry and frozen foods. Most species are saprophytic organisms and can be recovered from water, soil, plants, vegetables, insects and various other sources due to their ability to use a wide variety of substrates as sole carbon and energy sources and to grow in environments providing only limited nutrients.[1-4] Combining intrinsic resistance to antimicrobial agents with the protective conditions of clie skin (such as dryness, low pH, the resident normal flora and toxic lipids), the mucous membranes (such as the presence of mucus, lactoferrin and lactoperoxidase) and to environmental conditions, these organisms may pose an important problem in the susceptible host and in healthcare facilities.

Pathogenic Role

Aerobic NFGNB can be part of the transient physiologic flora. Although most species are considered low-virulent, some like *P. aeruginosa* and *A. baumannii* are recognized as important human pathogens (Table 181-1).[1,2]

Antibiotic Therapy

Most aerobic NFGNB have a high intrinsic resistance to the major classes of antimicrobial agents, often leaving few therapeutic options.[1-4] Various mechanisms of both intrinsic and acquired

TABLE 181-1	Predominant Sites and Incidences of Nosocomial Infections due to *Acinetobacter baumannii*, *Burkholderia cepacia*, *Pseudomonas aeruginosa* and *Stenotrophomonas maltophilia*	
Organism	**Clinical Presentation**	**Incidence (% of Patients)**
Pseudomonas aeruginosa	Bloodstream infection	3–5
	Pneumonia (VAP)	21–24
	Urinary tract infection	11–15
	Wound infection	8–10
	Cystic fibrosis respiratory infection	70–90
	Burn wound infection	1–10
Stenotrophomonas maltophilia	Bloodstream infection	<1 to 6
	Pneumonia (VAP)	2
	Urinary tract infection	3–9
	Wound infection	8–17
	Cystic fibrosis respiratory infection	7
	Burn wound infection	–
Burkholderia cepacia	Bloodstream infection	<1
	Pneumonia (VAP)	<1
	Urinary tract infection	4
	Wound infection	–
	Cystic fibrosis respiratory infection	80
	Burn wound infection	–
*Acinetobacter baumannii**	Bloodstream infection	<1 to 14
	Pneumonia (VAP)	5–10
	Urinary tract infection	10–30
	Wound infection	2–32
	Cystic fibrosis respiratory infection	–
	Burn wound infection	–

*Includes *Acinetobacter* genomic species 2, 3 and 13TU.
–, no data available; VAP, ventilator-associated pneumonia.

resistance have been identified, their type and frequency varying widely among different species.

Antimicrobial therapy should be guided by *in vitro* susceptibility testing results; when possible, minimal inhibitory concentrations (MICs) of the respective antimicrobials should be determined.

Pseudomonas aeruginosa and Other *Pseudomonas* spp.

Nature and Taxonomy

The taxonomic classification of *Pseudomonas* spp. (historically, based on the utilization of various organic compounds as sole energy sources) has significantly changed since the proposition of the genus in 1894. Using rRNA–DNA hybridization, five different groups have been identified:[1]

- I: *Pseudomonas* spp.
- II: *Burkholderia* spp. and *Ralstonia* spp.
- III: *Comamonas* spp., *Acidovorax* spp., *Delftia* spp. and *Hydrogenophaga* spp.
- IV: *Brevundimonas* spp.
- V: *Xanthomonas* spp. and *Stenotrophomonas* spp.

The taxonomic status of *Pseudomonas* spp. (see Table 181-2) continues to evolve with the advances of polyphasic taxonomy. Some species display a high genetic diversity, such as *P. stutzeri* (at least 18 genovars, additional three proposed),[5] *P. fluorescens* (biotype A (I), B (II, reclassified as *P. marginalis*), C (III), D and E (IV, V, reclassified together as *P. chlororaphis*), F and G), and *P. putida* (at least biovars A and B). However, most have so far not been isolated from clinical specimens.[1]

Epidemiology

Currently, there are 160 *Pseudomonas* spp., most of which are ubiquitous organisms and are widely distributed in nature.[1] To date, at least 12 *Pseudomonas* spp., including *P. aeruginosa*, *P. alcaligines*, *P. fluorescens*, *P. luteola*, *P. mendocina*, *P. oryzihabitans*, *P. putida* and *P. stutzeri*,[1,6,7] have been implicated in human infections. *P. aeruginosa* remains the most prevalent aerobic NFGNB identified as the causative pathogen in a large variety of nosocomial infections.

Studies have shown the ability of *P. aeruginosa* strains to acquire or discard genomic segments, giving rise to strains that can survive in a wide range of environmental habitats and serve as reservoirs for the infecting organisms.[8] For example, *P. aeruginosa* has been isolated from surgical instruments, disinfectants (quaternary ammonium compounds) and contact lens cleaning solutions, ventilatory equipment in ICUs and surgical equipment such as ultrasonic aspirators used in neurosurgical procedures.[7,9] Surveys using molecular typing methods (exotoxin A typing) also linked *P. aeruginosa* isolates from sinks, wash basins and toilets to those isolated from the hands of staff and the urinary tracts of paraplegic patients. Transmission over a 6-month period in an ICU for newborns has also been related to a source implicating air valves in the ventilator tubes.[10] *Pseudomonas* spp. are not part of the normal flora and colonization of healthy individuals with *Pseudomonas* spp., particularly *P. aeruginosa*, is rare.[11] Recovery of these bacteria, especially mucoid variants, should prompt the search for infections.[1] In hospitalized patients intestinal colonization reaches 18% (up to 73% in patients recovering from gastrointestinal surgery). In neutropenic patients intestinal colonization has been identified as the source of subsequent *P. aeruginosa* bloodstream infection (BSI).

Pseudomonas spp., such as *P. fluorescens*, *P. stutzeri* and *Sphingomonas paucimobilis* (*P. paucimobilis*), are more frequently isolated from clinical specimens than other *P. non-aeruginosa* species and have been implicated in a variety of infections in adult and pediatric patients. There have also been individual reports of common source outbreaks due to these organisms.

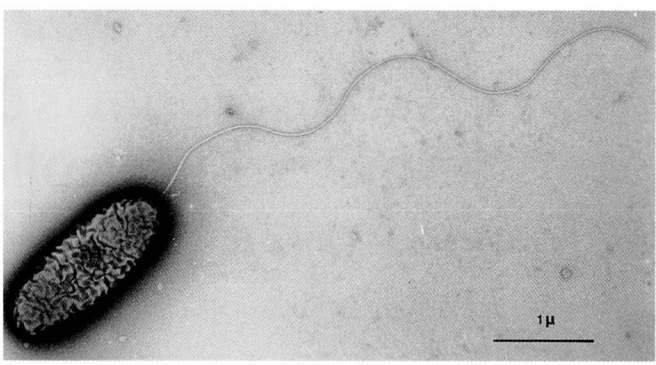

Figure 181-1 *Pseudomonas aeruginosa* monotrichous polar flagellum seen on electron microscopy. *(Courtesy of Professor A. Marty.)*

EPIDEMIOLOGIC MARKERS

A variety of typing methods (phenotypic and molecular) have been assessed for epidemiologic and clinical purposes.[12,13] A selection of methods is summarized in Table 181-3.

Diagnostic Microbiology
BACTERIOLOGY OF *PSEUDOMONAS* SPP.

Pseudomonas spp. are thin, rod-shaped, non spore-forming gram-negative bacilli with a guanine/cytosine content of 57–68 mol%. *Pseudomonas* spp. are motile due to one (e.g. *P. aeruginosa*, *P. stutzeri*, *P. oryzihabitans*; Figure 181-1) or more polar flagella (e.g. *P. fluorescens*, *P. putida*, *P. luteola*). *Pseudomonas* spp. are strictly aerobic, although in some cases anaerobic growth is possible if a nitrate source can be utilized. *P. aeruginosa* and other clinically relevant *Pseudomonas* spp. are oxidase-positive with the exception of *P. luteola* and *P. oryzihabitans*.[1,6] *Pseudomonas* spp. can be recovered from clinical and environmental specimens using standard collection, transport and storage techniques. It can also be cultured using standard broth or solid media including all nonselective (e.g. Columbia or tryptic-soy agar) as well as a number of selective media including MacConkey agar. While selective media containing inhibitors such as acetamide, nitrofurantoin or cetrimide may be helpful for the isolation of *Pseudomonas* spp., inhibition of some strains of *P. aeruginosa* (isolated from specimens from CF patients) by cetrimide and nalidixic acid has been reported.

Some *Pseudomonas* spp. (*P. fluorescens*, *P. putida*) have the ability to grow at temperatures as low as 4 °C (39 °F), but most grow between 28 and 42 °C (82 and 108 °F), achieving visible growth within 24–48 hours. *P. aeruginosa* colonies on solid media are usually flat, but small colony variants (SCV)[14] and mucoid forms have been described (Figure 181-2). Mucoid forms are particularly observed in patients suffering from CF and can pose problems for identification and susceptibility testing. Pyoverdin (fluorescein, yellow) is produced by all fluorescent *Pseudomonas* spp.; *P. aeruginosa* may also produce pyocyanin (blue), pyorubin (red) or pyomelanin (black). The distinct green color of *P. aeruginosa* colonies (Figure 181-2) usually results from a combination of pyoverdin and pyocyanin. *P. aeruginosa* can be separated from the other fluorescent *Pseudomonas* spp. (e.g. *P. fluorescens*, *P. putida*) by its ability to grow at 42 °C (108 °F).

Automated systems can usually identify *P. aeruginosa*; however, additional testing is often required for identification of *Pseudomonas* spp., including mucoid or other forms of *P. aeruginosa* from cystic fibrosis (CF) patients.

Other identification methods include conventional and real-time polymerase chain reaction (PCR), probes directed at or sequencing of species-specific 16S rRNA,[15] fluorescence in situ hybridization (FISH) and matrix-assisted laser desorption/ionization-time of flight (MALDI-TOF) mass spectrometry.[16]

TABLE 181-2	Current Nomenclature of Nonfermenting Gram-Negative Bacilli*	
Genus	**Current Name**	**Previous Name(s)**
Achromobacter	Achromobacter denitrificans Achromobacter piechaudii Achromobacter ruhlandii Achromobacter xylosoxidans	Alcaligenes xylosoxidans subsp. denitrificans, Alcaligenes denitrificans CDC group VD-3 Alcaligenes piechaudii Alcaligenes ruhlandii Alcaligenes xylosoxidans subsp. xylosoxidans, Alcaligenes denitrificans subsp. xylosoxidans, Achromobacter xylosoxidans CDC groups IIIa, IIIb
Acidovorax	Acidovorax delafieldii Acidovorax facilis Acidovorax temperans	Pseudomonas delafieldii Pseudomonas facilis Pseudomonas temperans
Acinetobacter	Acinetobacter baumannii Acinetobacter baylyi Acinetobacter bouvetii Acinetobacter calcoaceticus Acinetobacter gerneri Acinetobacter grimontii Acinetobacter haemolyticus Acinetobacter johnsonii Acinetobacter junii Acinetobacter lwoffii Acinetobacter nosocomialis Acinetobacter parvus Acinetobacter pittii Acinetobacter radioresistens Acinetobacter schindleri Acinetobacter tandoii Acinetobacter tjernbergiae Acinetobacter towneri Acinetobacter ursingii Acinetobacter venetianus	Acinetobacter anitratus, A. calcoaceticus, Diplococcus mucosus, Micrococcus calcoaceticus, Alcaligenes haemolysans, Mima polymorpha, Herellea vaginicola, Bacterium anitratum, Moraxella lwoffi var. glucidolytica, Neisseria winogradskyi, Achromobacter anitratus, Achromobacter mucosus Acinetobacter anitratus, Acinetobacter calcoaceticus subsp. anitratus Acinetobacter anitratus Acinetobacter anitratus, Moraxella lwoffi, Acinetobacter calcoaceticus subsp. lwoffi Acinetobacter genospecies 13 Acinetobacter genospecies 3
Agrobacterium	Agrobacterium tumefaciens	
Alcaligenes	Alcaligenes faecalis	Alcaligenes odorans, Pseudomonas odorans
Bergeyella	Bergeyella zoohelcum	Weeksella zoohelcum
Brevundimonas	Brevundimonas aurantiaca Brevundimonas diminuta Brevundimonas intermedia Brevundimonas subvibrioides Brevundimonas variabilis Brevundimonas vesicularis	Caulobacter henricii subsp. aurantiacus Pseudomonas diminuta Caulobacter intermedius Caulobacter subvibrioides Caulobacter variabilis Pseudomonas vesicularis
Burkholderia	Burkholderia ambifaria Burkholderia anthina Burkholderia arboris Burkholderia cenocepacia Burkholderia cepacia Burkholderia contaminans Burkholderia diffusa Burkholderia dolosa Burkholderia gladioli Burkholderia lata Burkholderia latens Burkholderia mallei Burkholderia metallidurans Burkholderia multivorans Burkholderia pseudomallei Burkholderia pyrocinia Burkholderia seminalis Burkholderia stabilis Burkholderia vietnamensis	 Burkholderia cepacia complex genomovar III Pseudomonas cepacia, Pseudomonas multivorans, Pseudomonas kingae CDC group EO-1 Pseudomonas gladioli, Pseudomonas marginata Pseudomonas mallei, Actinobacillus mallei Pseudomonas pseudomallei
Chryseobacterium	Chryseobacterium gleum Chryseobacterium indologenes Chryseomonas luteola	Flavobacterium gleum CDC group IIb Flavobacterium indologenes CDC group IIb Pseudomonas luteola CDC group Ve-1
Comamonas	Comamonas aquatica Comamonas kerstersii Comamonas terrigena Comamonas testosteroni	 Pseudomonas terrigena Pseudomonas testosteroni CDC group EF-19
Cupriavidus	Cupriavidus necator	Wautersia eutropha, Ralstonia eutropha, Pseudomonas/Alcaligenes eutrophus
Delftia	Delftia acidovorans	Comamonas acidovorans, Pseudomonas acidovorans

Continued on following page

TABLE 181-2	Current Nomenclature of Nonfermenting Gram-Negative Bacilli* (Continued)	
Genus	**Current Name**	**Previous Name(s)**
Elizabethkingia	Elizabethkingia meningoseptica	Chryseobacterium meningosepticum, Flavobacterium meningosepticum CDC group IIa, Flavobacterium meningosepticum
Kerstersia	Kerstersia gyiorum	Alacligines faecalis (some strains)
Myroides	Myroides odoratus	Chryseobacterium odoratum, Flavobacterium odoratum CDC group M-4f
Ochrobactrum	Ochrobactrum anthropi Ochrobactrum intermedium	Achromobacter Vd Ochrobactrum sp. nov.
Oligella	Oligella ureolytica Oligella urethralis	CDC group IVe Moraxella urethralis, CDC group M-4
Pandoraea	Pandoraea spp.	Burkholderia spp.
Pedobacter	Pedobacter heparinum Pedobacter piscium	Sphingobacterium heparinum Sphingobacterium piscium
Pseudomonas	Pseudomonas aeruginosa Pseudomonas alcaligenes Pseudomonas chlororaphis Pseudomonas delafieldii Pseudomonas fluorescens Pseudomonas kingii Pseudomonas mendocina Pseudomonas oryzihabitans Pseudomonas pertucinogena Pseudomonas pseudoalcaligenes Pseudomonas putida Pseudomonas sp. group 1 Pseudomonas stutzeri Pseudomonas stutzeri-like Pseudomonas-like group 2	 Pseudomonas fluorescens Biotype D Pseudomonas fluorescens Biotype E Pseudomonas aureofaciens CDC group Vb-2 Bordetella pertussis rough phase IV Pseudomonas alcaligenes biotype B Pseudomonas denitrificans CDC group Vb-1 CDC group Vb-3 CDC group IV-d
Psyrobacter	Psyrobacter faecali Psyrobacter pulmonis	Psyrobacter immobilis
Ralstonia	Ralstonia pickettii	Burkholderia pickettii, Pseudomonas pickettii, CDC groups Va-1, Va-2, Pseudomonas thomasii
Rhizobium	Rhizobium radiobacter Rhizobium rhizogenes Rhizobium rubi Rhizobium vitis	Agrobacterium radiobacter, Agrobacterium tumefaciens, Agrobacterium radiobacter CDC group Vd-3 Agrobacterium rhizogenes Agrobacterium rubi Agrobacterium vitis
Shewanella	Shewanella algae Shewanella hanedai Shewanella putrefaciens	 Alteromonas hanedai Pseudomonas/Alteromonas putrefaciens, CDC group Ib, Achromobacter putrefaciens
Sphingobacterium	Sphingobacterium antarcticum Sphingobacterium faecium Sphingobacterium mizutaii Sphingobacterium multivorum Sphingobacterium spiritivorum Sphingobacterium thalpophilum Sphingobacterium yabuuchiae	 Flavobacterium mizutaii Flavobacterium multivorum CDC group IIk-2 Flavobacterium spiritivorum, Sphingobacterium versatilis CDC group IIk-3 Flavobacterium thalpophilum Flavobacterium yabuuchiae
Sphingomonas	Sphingomonas paucimobilis	Pseudomonas paucimobilis CDC group IIk-11
Stenotrophomonas	Stenotrophomonas maltophilia	Xanthomonas maltophilia, Pseudomonas maltophilia
Weeksella	Weeksella virosa	Flavobacterium genitale CDC group II-f

*The list is limited to those potentially involved in human infections.[1,6,7]

Pathogenicity and Pathogenesis

P. aeruginosa expresses a variety of virulence factors some of which have been characterized in recent years (Table 181-4).

HOST-RELATED FACTORS

Host-related factors such as anatomic and physiologic barriers play an important role in the pathogenesis of *P. aeruginosa* infections. Several important *P. aeruginosa* infections such as burn wound infections or the colonization of the upper respiratory or gastrointestinal tract, largely depend on the impairment of the natural barriers provided by intact skin or mucous membranes. Animal studies showed that *P. aeruginosa* can cause lethal infections originating from as little as 10 colony forming units (cfu) inoculated into burned skin, while similar infections of the intact skin require five to six logs more organisms.

Disruption of the integrity of the corneal mucosa has been identified as the major factor in severe *P. aeruginosa* infections of the eye. Mucosal surfaces provide protection against *P. aeruginosa* colonization and infection by a variety of mechanisms such as mucus-containing antimicrobial factors including lysozyme, lactoferrin and defensins, the presence of physiologic flora, and mucociliary clearance. However, if impaired by underlying diseases such as CF or therapeutic

TABLE 181-3 Epidemiologic Markers for *Acinetobacter baumannii* and *Pseudomonas aeruginosa* Typing

Epidemiologic Markers		Species	Principles and Characteristics	Advantages	Drawbacks
Phenotypic	Biotyping	A. baumannii	Utilization of substrates, production of enzymes, biotyping schemes for identification, commonly carbon-source utilization test using levulinate, citraconate, L-phenylalanine, phenylacetate, 4-hydroxybenzoate and L-tartrate	Rapid, easy to perform, inexpensive, also useful for identification to species level	Unstable, variability of metabolic characters, limited discriminatory power
		P. aeruginosa	Utilization of substrates, production of enzymes, biotyping schemes for identification	Rapid, easy to perform, API 20NE panel or automated identification systems (Vitek, MicroScan, Phoenix), inexpensive	Unstable, variability of metabolic characters, poorly discriminating
	Resistance phenotype	A. baumannii, P. aeruginosa	Antimicrobial susceptibility pattern always obtained, multiple resistance markers	Rapid, easy to perform, standardized (national/international guidelines), automated systems (Vitek, MicroScan, Phoenix) can be used, early and often useful during outbreak	Unstable profiles, plasmid acquisition or loss during an outbreak, derepression of inducible enzymes, mutations, poorly discriminating, unreliable
	Serotyping	A. baumannii	O-antigenic polysaccharide of the lipopolysaccharide, 34 O-antisera	No advantages for A. baumannii	Not all strains typeable, low discriminatory power
		P. aeruginosa	Based on somatic O-specific antigen (LPS), polyclonal/monoclonal antibodies, 20 serotypes, 17 antisera (IATS)	Rapid, early results, easy to perform, inexpensive	50–70% of CF strains nontypeable, polyagglutination of some CF strains, reproducibility of anti-LPS monoclonal antibodies is 75%, only available in specialized laboratories
	Phage typing	A. baumannii	Two systems (21 and 14 phages, respectively)	Limited requirements, inexpensive	Lack of reproducibility, low discriminatory power, approx. 20% of strains nontypeable, only available in specialized laboratories
		P. aeruginosa	Colindale set of 21 phages, cell surface receptors (OM, LPS, slime)	Limited requirements, inexpensive	Lack of reproducibility, low discrimination, insensitivity of CF- and LPS-defective strains, only available in specialized laboratories
	Pyocin typing	P. aeruginosa	R, F, S pyocins, specific lytic activity, 105 types, 26 subtypes	Limited requirements, inexpensive	Poor discrimination, complexity of the system, time-consuming technique, only available in specialized laboratories
Genotypic	Plasmidotyping	A. baumannii	Plasmids present in many A. baumannii strains	No advantage for A. baumannii typing	Plasmids are easily transferable and may be gained or lost, cumbersome technique
		P. aeruginosa	Relatively rare plasmid in P. aeruginosa, plasmids of 1.2–60 MDa in 15% of strains	No advantage for P. aeruginosa typing	Low frequency, acquisition or loss during epidemics
	Genomic DNA, total DNA	P. aeruginosa	Polymorphism of DNA, REA endonucleases (EcoR1, HindII, SmaI), conventional agarose gel electrophoresis	Good discriminatory power	Large number of fragments making resolution of bands difficult to interpret
	DNA RFLP	P. aeruginosa	Detection of genes coding for exotoxin A (exoA), elastase (lasB), alginate (algD), two probes necessary	Good discriminatory power, good correlation with ribotyping	Laborious techniques, small numbers of isolates can be compared
	Ribotyping (ribosomal DNA)	A. baumannii	HindIII, HincII, EcoR1, ClaI	Results comparable to AFLP, automated systems available	Limited discriminatory power, labor intensive, PFGE and others provide more accurate results for A. baumannii
		P. aeruginosa	Three genes coding for rRNA, probes for 16S and 23S RNA, restriction enzymes (EcoR1, ClaI, SalI)	Universal, excellent reproducibility, stable ribotype patterns within outbreaks	Laborious techniques, sensitivity and specificity not established for P. aeruginosa

Continued on following page

TABLE 181-3	Epidemiologic Markers for *Acinetobacter baumannii* and *Pseudomonas aeruginosa* Typing (Continued)				
Epidemiologic Markers		**Species**	**Principles and Characteristics**	**Advantages**	**Drawbacks**
Genotypic	Pulsotyping (PFGE)	*A. baumannii*	Apal and/or Smal	Gold standard for *A. baumannii*, highest discriminatory power, interlaboratory reproducibility possible with standardized protocols	Labor intensive
		P. aeruginosa	DNA fingerprinting, restriction enzymes *DraI*, *SpeI*	The most specific discriminatory technique	Interpretation somewhat delicate, heavy workload
		S. maltophilia	DNA fingerprinting	The most specific discriminatory technique	Interpretation somewhat delicate, heavy workload
	ERIC-PCR	*S. maltophilia*	Amplification of DNA sequences using ERIC2 primer	Good discriminatory power	Inter- and intralaboratory reproducibility difficult to achieve
	RAPD-PCR	*A. baumannii*	Amplification of random DNA sequences	Fast, easy and low cost, relatively high discriminatory power	Inter- and intralaboratory reproducibility difficult to achieve, not suited for large-scale epidemiologic studies, discriminatory power inferior to PFGE
		P. aeruginosa	Amplification of random DNA sequences	Fast, easy and low cost, relatively high discriminatory power	Inter- and intralaboratory reproducibility difficult to achieve
		S. maltophilia	Amplification of random DNA sequences	Fast, easy and low cost, relatively high discriminatory power	Inter- and intralaboratory reproducibility difficult to achieve
	REP-PCR	*A. baumannii*	PCR-based typing method, amplification of highly conserved REP sequences using specific primers	Simple, rapid	Inter- and intralaboratory reproducibility remains to be determined, expensive
		S. maltophilia	PCR-based typing method, amplification of highly conserved REP sequences using specific primers	Simple, rapid	Inter- and intralaboratory reproducibility remains to be determined, expensive
	AFLP	*A. baumannii*	PCR-based typing method, amplification of restriction fragments (*HindIII* and *TaqI*) using specific primers	Can be used for typing and species identification, relatively robust method, high discriminatory power	*Acinetobacter* only, requires a high level of standardization and extensive experience, cumbersome and expensive, restricted to reference laboratories, not suited for routine epidemiologic analyses, data are not readily transportable
	MLST	*A. baumannii, Acinetobacter* genomic species 13TU, *P. aeruginosa*	Amplification and sequencing of several specific loci in different housekeeping genes: *A. baumannii* and *Acinetobacter* genomic species 13TU: *gltA*, *gyrB*, *gdhB*, *recA*, *cpn60*, *gpi*, *rpoD*; *P. aeruginosa*: *acsA*, *aroE*, *guaA*, *mutL*, *nuoD*, *ppsA*, *trpE*	Highly portable, highly reproducible	Time-consuming, very expensive
	PCR/ESI-MS	*A. baumannii*	Amplification of specific sequences of six housekeeping genes (*efp*, *trpE*, *adk*, *mutY*, *fumC*, *ppa*), detection by ESI-MS	Results similar to MLST, easy, high throughput, fastest method to date	Novel method, not suited for routine laboratories, expensive equipment, detailed evaluation warranted

AFLP, amplified fragment length polymorphism; CF, cystic fibrosis; ERIC-PCR, enterobacterial repetitive intergenic consensus polymerase chain reaction; ESI-MS, electrospray ionization mass spectrometry; IATS, International Antigenic Typing Scheme; LPS, lipopolysaccharide; MLST, multilocus sequence typing; OM, outer membrane; PCR, polymerase chain reaction; PFGE, pulsed-field gel electrophoresis; RAPD, random amplified polymorphic DNA; REA, restriction endonuclease analysis; REP-PCR, repetitive extragenic palindromic polymerase chain reaction; RFLP, restriction fragment length polymorphism.

interventions, such as antimicrobial or anticancer chemotherapy, *P. aeruginosa* has a high propensity for colonization and infection of the respective site.

A variety of soluble factors is involved in the pathogenesis of *P. aeruginosa* infections, such as complement, collectins, cytokines, chemokines and immunoglobulins, as well as cellular mediators. A detailed summary of their function can be found elsewhere.[1,17]

BACTERIAL FACTORS

Virtually all major classes of bacterial virulence systems (see Table 181-4) have been reported in *P. aeruginosa*, including endo- and exotoxins, pili, flagella, proteases, lipases, iron-binding proteins and exopolysaccharides. Adherence of *P. aeruginosa* to host tissue is in part promoted by pili (*pilA* gene, regulated by *rpoN*, *pilS* and *pilR*), flagella (*fliC* [flagella] and *fliD* [protein caps]) and other appendage-like

TABLE 181-4	*Acinetobacter baumannii* and *Pseudomonas aeruginosa* Virulence-Associated Factors		
Category	**Pathogen**	**Classes of Virulence Factors (examples)**	**Effects in Humans**
Enzyme	*A. baumannii*	Antibiotic-inactivating enzymes (β-lactamases) Proteases Protein S	Inactivation of antimicrobial agents Tissue damage Interference with phagocytosis
	P. aeruginosa	Adhesins (exoenzyme S) Antibiotic-inactivating enzymes (β-lactamases) Elastolytic activity (two enzymes Las A, Las B) Glycolipid-rhamnolipid (heat-stable) Hemolysins (phospholipase C) Neuraminidase Cytoplasmic lectins, *P. aeruginosa* lectin I (PA I), PA II Proteases (alkaline and neutral metalloproteinase)	Binding specificity for glycolipids (glycosphingolipid) Inactivation of antimicrobial agents Break down elastin of blood vessels, hemorrhages Disruption of phospholipids of cell membranes, hydrolysis of lung surfactant and ciliostatic action Enhances pilin-mediated adherence PA I specific for D-galactose, PA II specific for D-mannose Tissue damage (active on elastin, collagen, fibrin), digestion of protecting host defense proteins
Structural	*A. baumannii*	Aerobactin Fimbriae Iron-repressible outer membrane receptor proteins Iron-uptake components Lipopolysaccharide Lipopolysaccharide (hydrophobic sugars in the O side chain) Outer membrane proteins Pili Polysaccharide capsule	Increased virulence (mechanism to be determined) Adhesion to epithelial cells Increased virulence (mechanism to be determined) Survival in the bloodstream Proinflammatory response Adhesion to host cells Interference with cell permeability Adhesion to epithelial cells Interference with phagocytosis, survival in dry environment
	P. aeruginosa	Efflux pumps Lipopolysaccharide Mucopolysaccharide capsule (alginate) Pili (fimbriae) Siderophores (pyochelin and pyoverdin) Quorum sensing Type III secretion factors	Increase resistance to antimicrobial agents Cascade of inflammatory events Adhesion to epithelial cells, barrier to antibiotics, increased viscosity of bronchial secretions (cystic fibrosis) Adhesion to epithelial cells Help growth in iron-limited condition, generation of toxic oxygen-free radicals Biofilm formation, regulation of virulence factors Facilitate injection of type III effectors
Toxin	*A. baumannii*	Lipid A Outer membrane protein A (Omp 38)	Toxicity, pyrogenicity Cytotoxicity, apoptosis, cell death
	P. aeruginosa	Cytotoxins (leukocidin) Endotoxins Exotoxin A Type III secretion (ExoS, ExoT, ExoU, ExoY) Phenazine pigment (pyocyanin)	Cytopathic effects on leukocytes and alteration of phospholipids of cell membrane Septic shock Tissue damage, inhibition of phagocytes, inhibition of protein synthesis Cytotoxicity, cell death Ciliary disruption

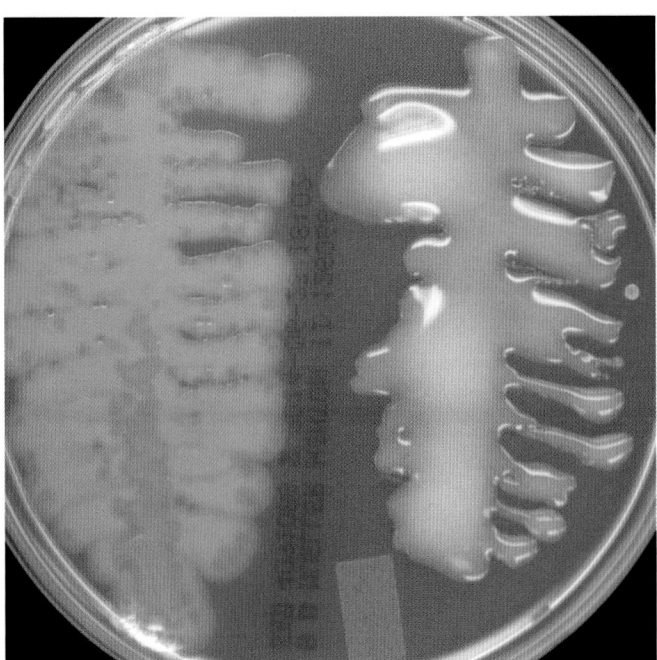

Figure 181-2 *Pseudomonas aeruginosa* mucoid (right side of plate) and non-mucoid colonies (left side of plate) on MH-agar. *(Courtesy of H. Wisplinghoff.)*

structures that have recently been identified in multidrug-resistant strains of *P. aeruginosa*. In addition, lipopolysaccharide may bind to the cystic fibrosis transmembrane conductance regulator (CFTR). Defective expression of the CFTR contributes to the hypersusceptibility of CF patients to *P. aeruginosa* infection. Recent studies have identified numerous CFTR-dependent factors that are recruited to the epithelial plasma membrane in response to infection and are needed for bacterial clearance. Several factors mediating resistance to host defenses have been identified in *P. aeruginosa* – including lipopolysaccharide O (LPS O) which prevents lysis by complement and proteases (e.g. protease IV, elastolytic proteases and alkaline protease) – that are involved in the evasion of innate immunity, degradation of cells and host proteins, and syndecan 1.

Manifestation of infection largely depends on the expression of a variety of substances that damage host cells, such as ferripyochelin (destroying endothelial cells) alone or in combination with hydrogen peroxide. *P. aeruginosa* toxins include exotoxin A (inhibition of protein biosynthesis by inactivating elongation factor 2), leukocidin, plcHR (a hemolytic phospholipase C), pyocyanin and rhamnolipids. Most toxins and hydrolytic enzymes involved in virulence are regulated by a complex system, components of which are influenced by environmental factors.

Intoxication of the host cells via type III secretion systems is another important factor in *P. aeruginosa* infections and the production of type III secretor proteins (PcrG, PcrV, PcrH, PopB, and PopD, encoded by the pcrGVH-popBD operon) has repeatedly been identified as an independent risk factor for poor outcome.[18]

In *P. aeruginosa* three major quorum-sensing systems have been identified to date, termed las, rhl and PQS. These interacting systems seem to play an important role in the regulation of biofilm formation and expression of virulence factors. Degradation of acyl-homoserine lactones, the signaling molecules of the quorum-sensing system, has been discussed as a treatment option. In addition, the GacS/GacA two-component system positively controls the transcription of two sRNAs (RsmY, RsmZ) that are crucial for the expression of virulence genes and regulate the response to oxidative stress in *P. fluorescens*. The spread of *P. aeruginosa* and invasion of the bloodstream requires a smooth LPS substituted with O side chains and is likely enhanced by bacterial factors stimulating the release of tumor necrosis factor (TNF) and quorum-sensing molecules.

MUCOID *PSEUDOMONAS AERUGINOSA*

In the early 1960s the importance of mucoid variants of *P. aeruginosa* was recognized. Mucoid strains are morphologic and functional variants characterized by the ability to produce copious amounts of alginate, an acetylated polymer of D-mannuronic and L-glucuronic acids regulated by ClpXP proteases, AlgB, Alg8 and Alg44 (Figures 181-3 and 181-4). Expression is regulated by the extracytoplasmatic sigma factor (σ(22), AlgU/T) and negatively impacted by the cognate anti-sigma factor MucA. Alginate has been implicated in the pathogenesis of respiratory tract infections due to *P. aeruginosa* as well as in chronic oropharyngeal colonization.[19,20]

In vivo, in areas with impaired local defenses, such as in the airways of CF patients, the organism grows in microcolonies surrounded by a thick polysaccharide matrix adherent to the walls of larger airways and in the alveoli. Mucoid *P. aeruginosa* is present in foci of active inflammation in small bronchioles but not in destroyed parenchymal areas. This is consistent with the simultaneous role of bacterial growth in the active inflammatory process and of toxins produced by *P. aeruginosa* diffusing away from microcolonies. Several studies have addressed the role of antibodies against alginate and their failure to confer protection against infection in CF patients, showing that the biofilm-like growth may interfere with the opsonizing capabilities of the alginate antibodies. An exopolysaccharide–alginate conjugate vaccine has been discussed as a therapeutic approach.

Clinical Manifestations

BACTEREMIA/BLOODSTREAM INFECTION

Assessment of the incidence of *P. aeruginosa* BSI is difficult. *P. aeruginosa* accounted for 20–35% of all BSI isolates in older series, but only for 4.4% in recent series. Among 24 179 nosocomial BSIs from 52 hospitals in the USA over a 7-year period, *P. aeruginosa* (incidence 2.1 per 10 000 admissions) accounted for 3.8% of all BSI isolates from non-ICU wards and 4.7% from ICUs, making it the seventh and fifth most commonly isolated pathogen, respectively.[21] Historically, crude mortality rates of 50–70% have been reported in patients with *P. aeruginosa* BSI, while more recent studies found crude mortality rates of 28% in non-ICU and 48% in ICU patients, respectively,[21] as well as an attributable mortality ranging from 15% to 44%.

Secondary *P. aeruginosa* BSI most often originates from the respiratory tract (Table 181-5) followed by the urinary tract or burn wounds. Colonization of the gastrointestinal tract, which may develop in the presence of risk factors such as hospitalization in an ICU, neutropenia or treatment with cytotoxic chemotherapy, has also been discussed as a source of *P. aeruginosa* BSI, particularly in neutropenic patients receiving chemotherapy. Approximately 50% of these patients develop intestinal carriage, compared to only 5–15% of the general population, and translocation has been implicated as the potential mechanism for invasion. In addition, contaminated medical equipment used for endoscopic retrograde cholangiopancreatography (ERCP), placement of left ventricular assist devices and other invasive procedures have been reported as sources of *P. aeruginosa* BSI.[22]

The clinical presentation of *P. aeruginosa* BSI does not differ from sepsis due to other gram-negative pathogens and may range from benign transient bacteremia to fulminant septic shock with high mortality. In neutropenic patients, typical skin lesions (e.g. ecthyma gangrenosum; see Chapter 13) may present. Even though these lesions may on rare occasions present in non-neutropenic patients or be associated with other pathogens, such as *Aspergillus* spp. or *Mucor* spp., ecthyma gangrenosum in a septic patient should prompt antimicrobial chemotherapy active against *P. aeruginosa*.[1]

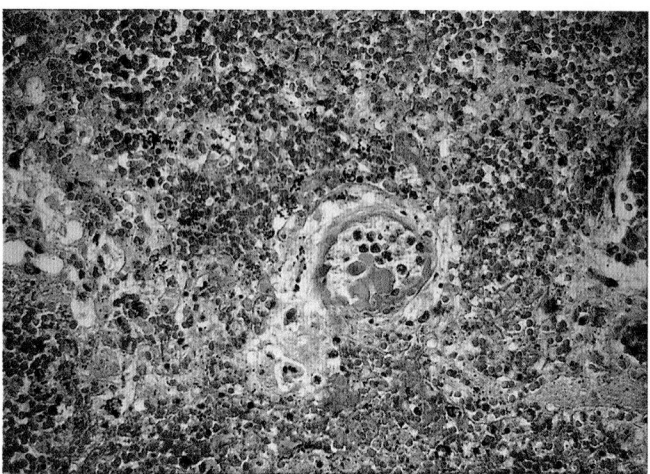

Figure 181-3 Anatomic pathology of *Pseudomonas aeruginosa* pneumonia showing acute inflammatory exudate, necrosis of alveolar membranes and fibrinous thrombosis in a venula. Hematoxylin–eosin stain. (*Courtesy of Professor Groussard.*)

ENDOCARDITIS (see also Chapter 51)

P. aeruginosa is the second most common cause of endocarditis due to non-HACEK GNB (after *Escherichia coli*), accounting for 22% (*n*=11) of all cases caused by non-HACEK GNB in a recent observational study from the International Collaboration on Endocarditis-Prospective Cohort Study (ICE-PCS) database, including 2761 cases of definite endocarditis from 61 hospitals in 28 countries.[23] *P. aeruginosa* is also the second most common cause of cardiac device-related endocarditis (CDE) in a retrospective survey of CDE-cases occurring between 1980 and 2011. In contrast to older studies that reported endocarditis due to *P. aeruginosa* predominantly in intravenous drug users,[22] the ICE-PCS study found that 57% of patients with non-HACEK GNB endocarditis had a healthcare-associated infection (IVDA in only 4%), and implanted endovascular devices and prosthetic heart valves were frequent risk factors.[23] The in-hospital mortality of patients with endocarditis due to *P. aeruginosa* reached 21% in recent studies despite high rates of cardiac surgery (55%).[23]

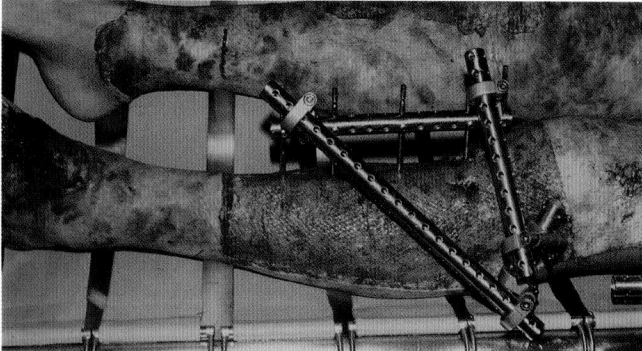

Figure 181-4 Burned leg superinfected with *Pseudomonas aeruginosa*. (*Courtesy of Professor H. Carsin.*)

TABLE 181-5   **Infections Due to *Acinetobacter baumannii* and *Pseudomonas aeruginosa***

Infection		Associated Factors
Respiratory tract infections	*A. baumannii* pneumonia, nosocomial, 60% mortality with BSI	Mechanical ventilation Endotracheal or tracheostomy tube Neurologic disease
	P. aeruginosa pneumonia (30–60% mortality rate)	Nasogastric tube Prolonged stay in intensive care unit Broad-spectrum antibiotics
	P. aeruginosa pneumonia, nosocomial, with BSI (80–100% mortality rate)	Neutropenia Underlying malignant neoplasm Cytotoxic chemotherapy Chronic bronchiectasis (terminal state) Diabetes mellitus Severe immunosuppression Severe burns
	A. baumannii pneumonia (community acquired, 60% mortality in bacteremic pneumonia)	Chronic obstructive pulmonary disease Smoking Alcoholism
	P. aeruginosa respiratory tract infection in people with cystic fibrosis (ultimately fatal unless a pulmonary transplant is carried out)	Presence of the lethal genetic disease cystic fibrosis Chronic colonization with *P. aeruginosa* Progressive lung deterioration Altered immune response to *P. aeruginosa*
Bloodstream infection (BSI)	*A. baumannii*	Prolonged stay in intensive care unit, mechanical ventilation, underlying immunosuppression, intravenous devices Leukemia, lymphoma Colonization with *A. baumannii* Various endoscopic instrumentation procedures
	P. aeruginosa	Prolonged stay in intensive care unit, broad-spectrum antibiotics, invasive procedures, underlying immunosuppression, intravenous devices Leukemia, lymphoma Mechanical ventilation Intravenous drug use Trauma Prematurity Ulceration of the gastrointestinal tract Solid organ or bone marrow transplant Various endoscopic instrumentation procedures
Skin and soft tissue infections	*P. aeruginosa*	Burn wound sepsis Wound infection Ecthyma gangrenosum Invasive procedures, surgery Dermatitis, pyoderma
UTI	*A. baumannii* *P. aeruginosa*	Invasive procedures, urinary catheters Acute (rare) Chronic (obstruction)
Endocarditis	*P. aeruginosa*	Intravenous drug use Prosthetic heart valves
Miscellaneous	*A. baumannii* *P. aeruginosa*	Meningitis (secondary) Brain abscesses, meningitis (secondary, following neurosurgical procedures) Bone and joint infections (chronic osteomyelitis) Ear infections (otitis externa, malignant external otitis) Eye infections (keratitis, endophthalmitis, contact lens keratitis)

LOWER RESPIRATORY TRACT INFECTIONS (see also Chapter 29)

P. aeruginosa is the most common gram-negative pathogen causing ventilator-associated pneumonia (VAP) and is consistently associated with a measurable attributable mortality.[24,25]

In a recent prospective multicenter study from Spain, *P. aeruginosa* (together with *L. pneumophila*) was the second most common bacterial pathogen (after *S. pneumoniae*) in patients with healthcare associated pneumonia accounting for 4.8% of cases.[26]

Since *P. aeruginosa* is also a frequent colonizer of endotracheal tubes and the nasopharynx of patients with mechanical ventilation receiving antimicrobial chemotherapy, the significance of a culture from the upper respiratory tract yielding *P. aeruginosa* in the absence of clinical and/or radiologic signs of pneumonia is less clear. The delay in eradication of *P. aeruginosa* in patients with VAP may be explained by an increased apoptosis in neutrophils.[24]

Typical pathologic features include necrosis of alveolar septa (see Figure 181-3) and arterial walls, with areas of focal hemorrhage and, in intact areas, infiltration with macrophages, mononuclear cells and polymorphonuclear leukocytes. A different lung pathology has been described in bacteremic pneumonia, which is rarely seen and mainly affects patients with severe underlying conditions. Risk factors are listed in Table 181-6. The clinical course is characterized by a rapid progression with a diffuse and often bilateral infiltration, usually in combination with pleural effusion. On cross-section, the lesions are nodular, hemorrhagic with necrotic foci or umbilicated nodules surrounded by dark hemorrhage. Intra-alveolar hemorrhage with patchy alveolar septal necrosis is seen on microscopy. Lesions contain many bacteria but lack infiltration with macrophages, mononuclear cells and polymorphonuclear leukocytes. Pulmonary edema and necrotizing bronchopneumonia are associated with a poor prognosis. The case fatality rate in patients with fulminant bacteremic pneumonia due to *P. aeruginosa* is extremely high (80–100%).

TABLE 181-6	Sources, Means of Transmission and Risk Factors for Nosocomial Infections Due to Aerobic Gram-Negative Bacilli		
Organisms	Settings*	Sources/Means of Transmission	Risk Factor/Comments
Achromobacter (Alcaligenes) xylosoxidans	ICU, hemodialysis units	Contaminated chlorhexidine solution, dialysis fluid, aerosols, respirators	Aqueous source, hemodialysis, severe underlying disease
Acinetobacter baumannii	ICU	Contaminated ventilators, intravascular catheters	Severely ill patients, cross-contamination, outbreaks
Burkholderia cepacia	ICU	Airborne transmission, contaminated skin preparations, ventilator, thermometer, antiseptic solutions	Cystic fibrosis patients, hand carriage, immunocompromised patients
Elizabethkingia (Chryseobacterium) meningosepticum	NICU	Contaminated water, ice, disinfectants, humidifiers	Wounds, mechanical ventilation
Pseudomonas aeruginosa	ICU, burns units	Contaminated equipment, solutions, antiseptics, endogenous	Cross-contamination, exposure to broad-spectrum antibiotics, severely ill patients, outbreaks in burn patients
Pseudomonas putida, Pseudomonas fluorescens	ICU	Contaminated blood and blood by-products, antiseptics	Large (burn) wounds, intravascular devices
Stenotrophomonas maltophilia	ICU, hematology/oncology units	Contaminated devices, disinfectants, catheters	Dialysis fluids, exploratory procedures, neutropenia, respiratory devices, tracheostomized patients, backflow from nonsterile tubes

*Most frequently reported occurrence.
ICU, intensive care unit; NICU, neonatal intensive care unit.

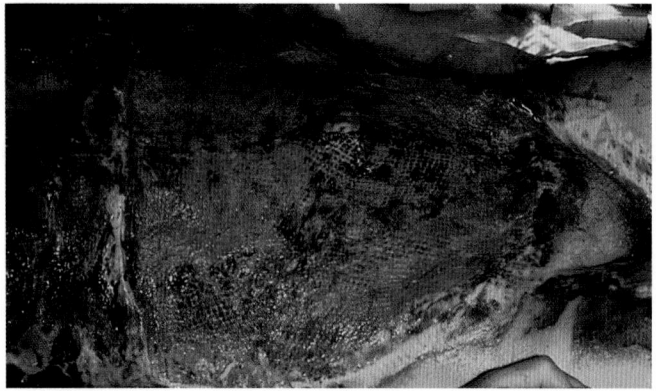

Figure 181-5 Burned abdominal wall superinfected with *Pseudomonas aeruginosa*. (Courtesy of Professor H. Carsin.)

Historically, community-acquired pneumonia due to *P. aeruginosa* was mainly seen in immunocompromised patients, such as human immunodeficiency virus/acquired immune deficiency syndrome (HIV/AIDS) patients with low CD4 counts or patients suffering from CF, but has also been reported in previously healthy non-immunocompromised patients, especially in patients with structural lung defects (e.g. COPD).

Inappropriate antibiotic therapy has been identified as a significant risk factor for adverse outcome.[24]

SKIN AND SOFT TISSUE INFECTIONS

Skin and soft tissue infections are usually dermatitis or superinfections of predisposing skin lesions. Folliculitis due to *P. aeruginosa* has been described and outbreaks have been linked to swimming pools, whirlpools, hot tubs and, recently, contamination of an industrial closed loop water recycling system.[27] See also Chapters 10, 11 and 13.

Burn Wound Sepsis

P. aeruginosa is the most common cause of burn wound sepsis, the predominant form of skin and soft tissue infection complicating thermal injury (see Figures 181-4 and 181-5). The mortality rate is high (50–78%) despite improvements in management and antibiotic therapy.[22] The incidence of *P. aeruginosa* BSI, however, has declined

considerably from 10% in older reports to about 1% in current studies.[28]

Colonization of the burned skin may result from the patient's own flora or from environmental sources. The bacteria penetrate into the subcutaneous tissues via hair follicles and break in the burned skin and may enter the bloodstream with the help of proteolytic enzymes. Other virulence factors (see Table 181-4) contribute significantly to the severity of the infection. Gr-1+/CD11b+ cells have been identified as an accelerator of sepsis originating from wound infection in thermally injured mice. Sepsis requires specific management in burn centers (Figures 181-4 and 181-5). Recent studies comparing BSI in burn patients due to *P. aeruginosa*, *A. baumannii*, *Klebsiella pneumoniae* and *S. aureus* showed that *K. pneumoniae* had the greatest impact on mortality relative to all other pathogens.

EYE INFECTIONS (see also Chapters 16 to 18)

P. aeruginosa is the most common gram-negative pathogen causing infections of the eye. Infections most commonly originate from an exogenous source and are related to (superficial) injuries. Ocular infections vary from mild (conjunctivitis) to extremely severe (orbital cellulitis).

Keratitis

Keratitis is the most frequent eye infection. Keratitis due to *P. aeruginosa* has been reported only secondary to an injury of the corneal surface. The predominant predisposing factors are contact lenses, congenital abnormalities, burns or trauma, altered host defenses (in particular HIV/AIDS) and prematurity. Contact lens-associated keratitis due to *P. aeruginosa* has mainly been observed in association with extended-wear contact lenses, inappropriate disinfecting regimens and poor hygiene. The bacteria may adhere to the lens, resulting in a coat of mucopolysaccharides forming a biofilm similar to other prosthetic devices. Viral keratitis may also be associated with secondary bacterial infection.

Exocellular products of *P. aeruginosa* and strong adhesion to the exposed basement membrane of the epithelium increase the corneal damage; exotoxins, proteases and phospholipases degrade the corneal stroma, resulting in extensive loss of collagen fibers from the stroma. Keratitis due to *P. aeruginosa* may progress rapidly, leading to endophthalmitis and loss of eyesight.

Endophthalmitis

Endophthalmitis most often results from an endogenous origin, occurring by hematogenous spread from other infected sites or after intraocular inoculation of *P. aeruginosa* by trauma, burns or ocular surgery. Endophthalmitis may present as an acute fulminant disease with severe pain, chemosis and decreased acuity, and can progress rapidly to panophthalmitis. The prognosis is poor without appropriate local and systemic management.

URINARY TRACT INFECTIONS (see also Chapter 57–60)

Urinary tract infections (UTI) due to *P. aeruginosa* are usually healthcare associated. Risk factors include the presence of a foreign body (e.g. long-term catheter or stent), surgery, obstruction of the urinary flow or persistent infection (e.g. chronic prostatitis). While *P. aeruginosa* UTI usually affect patients with prolonged hospitalization, antimicrobial therapy and/or other risk factors, infections in otherwise healthy children with no known risk factors have also been reported.

P. aeruginosa UTIs have no specific clinical presentation but tend to evolve with frequent recurrences, treatment failures and chronic evolution. A characteristic picture of ulcerative or necrotic lesions and multiple renal abscesses is seen in patients who have metastatic bacteremia with urinary tract invasion.[22]

EAR INFECTIONS

P. aeruginosa is frequently isolated from the external auditory canal, particularly in infants. Infections may range from benign transient colonization to severe infections with a prolonged clinical course that may be associated with permanent neurologic sequelae and adverse outcome. *P. aeruginosa* has been identified as the cause of a mild superficial infection of the external ear canal (e.g. swimmer's ear). Although this benign infection usually resolves without sequelae, it may proceed to invasion of the epithelium between cartilage and bone in the lateral portion of the auditory canal, penetrating soft tissue, cartilage and bone.

Malignant (Necrotizing) Otitis Externa

Malignant or necrotizing otitis externa is a severe invasive ear infection, clinically characterized by decreased hearing, otalgia, otorrhea, early facial nerve paralysis and a swollen erythematous external auditory canal. Adjacent soft tissue is often involved and the infection may progress to the middle ear, mastoid, temporal bone and cranial nerves. Clinical presentation may include visible extension with cellulitis, bone erosions and purulent discharge from the inner ear if the tympanic membrane is perforated.[22] *P. aeruginosa* may be isolated from superficial swabs of the external auditory canal and from surgical specimens. Most cases occur in elderly people with diabetes mellitus, but cases have also been reported from HIV/AIDS patients, elderly patients without immunosuppression or infants with severe underlying diseases.

Management requires prolonged antibiotic therapy, surgical debridement and drainage. The fatality rate is high (about 15–20%). Relapses are frequent and malignant external otitis requires prolonged follow-up.

MISCELLANEOUS

Central Nervous System Infections (see also

Chapters 19, 21 and 24)

Infections of the central nervous system are rarely due to *P. aeruginosa*. Meningitis, epidural or subdural empyema and brain abscesses have been reported in adults and children, usually as a result of either direct inoculation (head trauma, surgery), a contiguous infection (sinus, mastoid) or following BSI.

Bone and Joint Infections (see also Chapters 43 to 45)

Bone and joint infections are infrequently caused by *P. aeruginosa*. Direct inoculation (trauma, surgery), contiguous infection from surrounding tissue or hematogenous seeding following BSI are the most common routes of infection. Studies in war casualties found that *P. aeruginosa* was more frequently seen in primary osteomyelitis, whereas gram-positive pathogens were more likely to be isolated from recurrent episodes.

Infections predominantly occur in patients with predisposing factors such as diabetes mellitus, intravenous drug use and chronic debilitation. More frequently reported associations include:

- vertebral osteomyelitis and arthritis involving the sternoclavicular or sternochondral joints in intravenous drug users
- vertebral osteomyelitis in elderly patients following genitourinary instrumentation or surgery
- osteochondritis of the foot in children following puncture wounds or in patients with diabetic foot ulcers.

While *P. aeruginosa* seems to have a particular affinity for cartilaginous joints of the axial skeleton, infections at a distant site, such as pneumonia, rarely spread to the vertebral column or the axial skeleton. Following pelvic surgery or femoral catheterization, osteomyelitis of the pubic symphysis has been reported as well as rare cases of pelvic osteomyelitis in children.

Clinical presentation may be discrete; pain, swelling, fever and other systemic signs are variable.[22] The diagnosis may be difficult as blood cultures are frequently negative and imaging studies may also be normal in the earlier stages.

Pathogenicity and Clinical Manifestations of *Pseudomonas* spp. Other than *P. aeruginosa*

Some of the non-*aeruginosa Pseudomonas* spp. have been isolated from human clinical specimens (blood, urine, stools) and occasional cases of opportunistic infection as a result of transfusions, contamination of indwelling catheters, antiseptics or dialysis fluid and various other mechanisms of transmission have been reported. For example, *P. fluorescens* may grow at 4°C (39°F), which favors its presence in blood products and infusates such as heparin. Outbreaks of bacteremia, respiratory infections, wound infections and rare cases of community-acquired pneumonia have been reported. Other *Pseudomonas* spp., particularly *P. fluorescens*, *P. stutzeri* and *Sphingomonas paucimobilis* (*P. paucimobilis*), have also been implicated in rare cases of brain abscess, arthritis, endophthalmitis and keratitis while *P. alcaligenes* and *P. mendocina* have been isolated from patients with endocarditis. Most cases occur in patients with severely impaired host defenses such as immunocompromised patients in the ICU setting (Table 181-7).[22]

Antimicrobial Resistance and Therapy

Although *P. aeruginosa* is intrinsically resistant to many antimicrobials, several agents from different classes remain potentially active (Tables 181-8 and 181-9). However, the percentage of multi- or pandrug-resistant clinical *P. aeruginosa* strains has increased considerably in the past decade. Antimicrobial agents with potential antipseudomonal activity include semisynthetic penicillins such as carboxypenicillins (ticarcillin), ureidopenicillins (piperacillin), some third- (group IIIb), fourth-, and fifth generation cephalosporins (ceftazidime, cefpirome, cefepime, ceftaroline, ceftobiprole), carbapenems (imipenem, meropenem, doripenem), monobactams (aztreonam), aminoglycosides (gentamicin, tobramycin, amikacin), fluoroquinolones (ciprofloxacin, levofloxacin) and polymyxins (polymyxin B, polymyxin E). A summary of anti-pseudomonal treatment options in various indications is given in Table 181-10.

P. aeruginosa displays a wide array of resistance determinants, most of which are chromosomally located. The incidence of plasmids is relatively low. Mechanisms of resistance include altered outer membrane permeability (altered protein porins or lack of protein porin OprD), production of β-lactamases, aminoglycoside-inactivating enzymes and efflux pump systems actively removing different antibiotic classes from the bacterial cell (Table 181-11).

TABLE 181-7	Epidemiology and Pathogenicity of *Acinetobacter* spp. and *Pseudomonas* spp.	
Species	**Habitat and Epidemiology**	**Clinical Significance**
Acinetobacter non-*baumannii*, i.e. *A. johnsonii, A. junii, A. lwoffii, A. radioresistens, A. ursingii*	Ubiquitous, soil, water, sewage water, hospital environment, antiseptics, injectable solutions, more susceptible to antibiotics than other species	Outbreaks of pseudobacteremia involved in catheter-related bloodstream infection, isolation from wounds, urine, blood, cerebrospinal fluid
A. baumannii, A. pittii, A. nosocomialis (*Acinetobacter* genomic species 2, 3, 13TU)	Hospital environment, colonized patients, healthcare personnel	Opportunistic pathogen, severe infections mostly in immunocompromised patients
Pseudomonas alcaligenes, P. pseudoalcaligenes	Environment, water, plants, hospital environment, rare opportunistic pathogens	Occasional bacteremia (contaminated blood products, solutions)
P. putida, P. fluorescens, P. aeruginosa	Soil, water, plants, hospital sinks, floor, food spoilage (eggs, meat, fish, milk), opportunistic pathogens	Rarely isolated from clinical specimens, rare cases of colonization in patients with cystic fibrosis, bacteremia, urinary tract infection, wounds
P. stutzeri	Ubiquitous, soil, water, sewage water, hospital environment, antiseptics, injectable solutions, relatively more frequent than other non-*aeruginosa Pseudomonas* spp., opportunist, more susceptible to antibiotics than other species	Outbreaks of pseudobacteremia, isolation from pus, urine, blood, cerebrospinal fluid, contamination of bone marrow transplant
P. aeruginosa, P. fluorescens	Hospital environment, patients, healthcare personnel	Opportunistic pathogen, severe infections mostly in immunocompromised patients

TABLE 181-8	Antibiotic Susceptibility of *Acinetobacter baumannii* and *Pseudomonas aeruginosa*				
		A. baumannii		**P. aeruginosa**	
Antibiotic Class		MIC_{50} (mg/L)	MIC_{90} (mg/L)	MIC_{50} (mg/L)	MIC_{90} (mg/L)
β-Lactams	Ampicillin	64	>256	64	>256
	Ampicillin–sulbactam	1	16	32	256
	Amoxicillin	32	256	32	>256
	Amoxicillin–clavulanic acid	2	256	32	256
	Mezlocillin	16	512	16	128
	Piperacillin	8	512	8	512
	Piperacillin–tazobactam	4	128	4	128
	Ticarcillin	64	512	32	512
	Ticarcillin–clavulanic acid	32	256	16	512
	Cefazolin	256	512	128	512
	Cefuroxime	32	128	32	256
	Ceftriaxone	8	128	8	128
	Cefotaxime	16	128	16	64
	Ceftazidime	4	128	4	32
	Cefepime	4	16	4	16
	Imipenem	0.06	0.25	1	2
	Meropenem	0.25	1	0.5	2
	Aztreonam	16	64	4	16
Aminoglycosides	Amikacin	2	8	0.5	2
	Gentamicin	1	32	0.5	8
	Tobramycin	0.5	8	0.125	4
Quinolones	Ofloxacin	0.5	16	2	4
	Ciprofloxacin	0.5	64	0.06	0.25
	Levofloxacin	0.25	8	1	32
	Moxifloxacin	0.12	16	4	32
Miscellaneous	Trimethoprim–sulfamethoxazole	2	256	128	>128

From Zhanel et al. Diagn Microbiol Infect Dis 2008; 62:67–80 and Seifert et al. J Antimicrob Chemother 2006; 58:1099-1100.

β-Lactamases as well as IMP, GES and VIM metallocarbapenemases may be augmented by a number of efflux systems and decreased OprD expression which together confer multidrug resistance to β-lactam antibiotics. In clinical settings, these are often encountered in combination with other mechanisms conferring resistance to fluoroquinolones and aminoglycosides, thus considerably limiting the remaining therapeutic options.

Recent multicenter studies report rates of multidrug-resistant (MDR, i.e. resistance to three or more antimicrobial classes) *P. aeruginosa* ranging from 3% to 50%, with considerable variation between countries. In the USA, the prevalence of MDR-*P. aeruginosa* was approximately 15-fold higher than the prevalence of carbapemen-resistant *Enterobacteriaceae* in nationwide data from 2000 to 2009.[29,30]

The therapy of serious *Pseudomonas* infections should be based on the results of adequately performed antimicrobial susceptibility testing, including determination of MICs. Of note, in mucoid strains of *P. aeruginosa*, susceptibility testing with commercial systems may not be accurate, and the addition of agar dilution or gradient diffusion techniques (such as E-test) may be warranted. Data shown in Table 181-9

to colistin-only susceptible *P. aeruginosa,* aerosolized colistin may be a beneficial adjunct to intravenous colistin.[34] In CF patients, eradication of *Pseudomonas* spp. as well as other pathogens, such as *Burkholderia cepacia* or *Stenotrophomonas maltophilia,* from the airways occurs temporarily only, whatever strategy is used. A recent review did not find any conclusive evidence that oral anti-pseudomonal antibiotics are more or less effective than alternative treatments for either pulmonary exacerbations or long-term treatment.[35] Acute exacerbations of *Pseudomonas* lung infection in these patients usually require combination therapy and higher dosing. Fluoroquinolones have been successfully both in adult and pediatric CF patients, and a combination of ciprofloxacin with fosfomycin has demonstrated *in vitro* synergy. Repeated courses of aggressive antibiotic therapy every 3 months in combination with other measures such as mucolytics, antiproteases, topical (inhaled) antibiotic therapy and physiotherapy have increased the long-term survival of patients with CF. Treatment options have been extensively reviewed elsewhere. Inhalation therapy utilizing aminoglycosides and colistin is generally well tolerated, although some reduction of the maximum expired volume per second has occasionally been observed. Currently, tobramycin, polymyxin B and aztreonam are being used successfully in prevention and therapy of respiratory tract infections due to *P. aeruginosa* as well as *B. cepacia* in patients with CF.

Prevention

Prevention plays a major role in controlling *Pseudomonas* infections. Preventive measures can be based on the identification of sources and interruption of ways of transmission (see Table 181-3). Guidelines have been established in the USA and Europe, implementing isolation policies, administrative and regulatory measures and hospital epidemiology surveillance. Attempts to reduce the risk of colonization in high-risk patients have included:

- elimination of endogenous nosocomial *P. aeruginosa* and reduction of oropharyngeal, intestinal and skin colonization in ICU patients
- prevention of cross-contamination and monitoring of various sources of *P. aeruginosa*
- prevention of contamination in burn patients, in surgical wounds and in the oropharyngeal area in ventilated patients.

Active vaccination has been discussed and a variety of antigenic determinants are being evaluated as potential vaccine targets including outer membrane proteins, flagella and pili. In addition, vaccination with live attenuated strains has been shown to be efficacious in animal models. Current approaches to vaccines and immunotherapy against *P. aeruginosa* have recently been reviewed in detail.[36]

Acinetobacter spp.

Nature and Taxonomy

The genus *Acinetobacter* currently consists of 41 different species, nine of which have not been assigned names (see Table 181-2). While most *Acinetobacter* spp. (Figure 181-6) are considered to be of minor clinical importance, *A. baumannii* (see Figure 181-7), *A. pittii* and *A. nosocomialis* (together also referred to the *A. baumannii* group, ABG) have emerged as important clinical pathogens. Due to their phenotypic similarity, these three species have been grouped together with the environmental organism *A. calcoaceticus* in the so-called *A. calcoaceticus–A. baumannii* (Acb) complex. Overall, *A. baumannii* has emerged as one of the most significant nosocomial pathogens, especially in patients with impaired host defenses in the ICU, and has been implicated in a variety of infections including BSI, pneumonia and meningitis, with mortality rates as high as 64%. Major epidemiologic features of these organisms include their propensity for clonal spread and their involvement in hospital outbreaks as well as the ability to express or acquire resistance determinants, making it one of the most resistant organisms known to date.

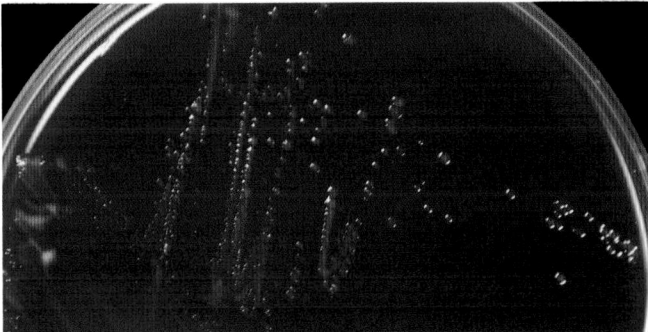

Figure 181-6 Example of *A. non-baumannii* spp. Colonies of *Acinetobacter lwoffii* on TSA-blood agar. *(Courtesy of H. Wisplinghoff.)*

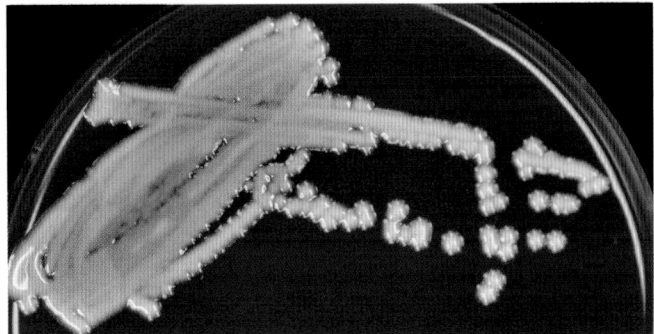

Figure 181-7 *Acinetobacter baumannii* on TSA-medium. *(Courtesy of H. Wisplinghoff.)*

Epidemiology

Acinetobacter spp. are widely distributed in nature, but not all *Acinetobacter* spp. are found in the environment (some, such as *A. schindleri* and *A. ursingii,* have until now been recovered only from human specimens) and the clinically important species (e.g. *A. baumannii*) are in fact not ubiquitous even though reservoirs outside the hospital have been described.[3,37] A variety of *Acinetobacter* spp. recovered from the axilla, groin and toe webs, the oral cavity, the respiratory tract and normal intestine have been identified as part of the commensal human flora. In contrast, some *Acinetobacter* spp., such as *A. baylyi, A. bouvetii, A. grimontii, A. tandoii, A. tjernbergiae* and *A. towneri,* have as yet never been observed in human specimens. Studies investigating the colonization of human skin and mucous membranes found *Acinetobacter* spp. in up to 44% of nonhospitalized and up to 75% of hospitalized individuals. The most frequently isolated species were *A. lwoffii* (58–61%), *A. johnsonii* (20%), *Acinetobacter* genomic species 15BJ (12%), *A. junii* (10%), *A. radioresistens* (8%) and *A. pittii* (5%), whereas *A. baumannii* was found only rarely on human skin (0.5–3%) and in human feces (0.8%).[38] Recent studies investigating potential skin contamination in healthy US soldiers did not report any *Acinetobacter* spp., but the lack of enrichment techniques and long transport time may have contributed to this finding. In addition, seasonal and geographic variations in skin colonization with *Acinetobacter* spp. have been reported from different geographic locations where *A. pittii* (36%), *A. nosocomialis* (15%), *Acinetobacter* genomic species 15TU (6%) and *A. baumannii* (4%) were the most frequently recovered species, whereas *A. lwoffii, A. johnsonii* and *A. junii* were only rarely found.[39,40]

MOLECULAR EPIDEMIOLOGY

After 1986, the taxonomy of the genus *Acinetobacter* was revised when molecular methods enabled identification of *Acinetobacter* at the species level, and studies of the epidemiology of the different members of this genus became possible. Methods include ribotyping, pulsed-field gel electrophoresis, random amplified polymorphic

DNA analysis, amplified fragment length polymorphism, multilocus sequence typing[41,42] and polymerase chain reaction/electrospray ionization mass spectrometry.[43]

Acinetobacter outbreaks published between 1977 and 2004 have been extensively reviewed.[44,45] Recent studies have increasingly reported outbreaks involving MDR *A. baumannii*. The persistence of endemic strains of *A. baumannii* over an extended period of time and the spread of single clones within a medical center have been documented in several institutions worldwide. Some outbreaks have been linked to a common source, such as computer keyboards, blood pressure cuffs, enteral nutrition or dust inside of mechanical ventilators or continuous venovenous hemofiltration dialysis machines, others do not seem to have a common source despite extensive environmental surveillance.

Several large studies failed to detect interinstitutional spread of *A. baumannii* while studies from New York, London and Johannesburg reported involvement of several different medical centers within a city, or even of healthcare facilities in several cities within one country. Following reports of the European clones I, II and III,[46] some authors suggested that few epidemic strains may be involved in outbreaks across countries; however, no epidemiologic link in time or space could be established. Studies investigating the population structure using MLST and REP-PCR show evidence of the distribution of several *A. baumannii*-clones designated as worldwide or international clones.[47,48]

Diagnostic Microbiology

Acinetobacter spp. are nonfermenting, nonmotile, oxidase-negative, aerobic gram-negative coccobacilli (Figure 181-8) and may be mistaken for gram-negative (or even gram-positive) cocci. Strictly aerobic, *Acinetobacter* spp. grow on most routinely used media at temperatures of 20–44 °C (68–111 °F). *Acinetobacter* spp. isolated from human specimens grow readily at 37 °C (99 °F). In contrast to the species of the Acb complex, other *Acinetobacter* spp. do not grow on MacConkey agar or may show hemolysis on sheep blood agar (*A. haemolyticus*, *Acinetobacter* genomic species 6, 13BJ, 14BK, 15BJ, 16 and 17).

Presumptive identification at genus level is possible using the above-mentioned criteria; unambiguous identification of *Acinetobacter* spp. is possible by transformation of the naturally transformable tryptophan auxotroph *A. baylyi* ADP1 by crude DNA of any *Acinetobacter* to wild-type phenotype.[49] Phenotypic identification of 11 of the 12 initially described (but not the novel) species is possible using a scheme proposed by Bouvet and Grimont.[50] A variety of molecular methods may be used for identification to species level.[41] While most

of these methods are not suitable for the routine laboratory, MALDI-TOF mass spectrometry can be used to identify at least the members of the *A. baumannii* group and may be an interesting option in the future for identification of all *Acinetobacter* spp.[51]

Species identification using current commercial systems such as API 20NE, Vitek 2, Phoenix and MicroScan WalkAway remains problematic, especially since *A. baumannii*, *A. pittii* and *A. nosocomialis* are uniformly identified as *A. baumannii* by the most widely used identification systems.[2]

Pathogenicity and Pathogenesis

Several factors may be responsible for the virulence of *Acinetobacter* spp., including a polysaccharide capsule formed of L-rhamnose, L-glucose, D-glucuronic acid and D-mannose, factors facilitating adhesion to human epithelial cells in the presence of fimbriae and/or mediated by the capsular polysaccharide; enzymes, such as butyrate esterase, caprylate esterase and leucine arylamidase, which are potentially involved in damaging tissue lipids; and the LPS component of the cell wall and the presence of lipid A, which are likely to participate in the pathogenicity of *Acinetobacter* spp.

Recent studies using whole genome sequencing identified a large number of antibiotic drug resistance determinants as well as several pathogenicity islands,[52] some of which likely originated in other species including *Pseudomonas* spp., *Salmonella* spp. and *E. coli*.[52] Relevant genes included those encoding the cell envelope, pilus biogenesis, iron uptake and metabolism, as well as sensor kinases. Several studies in *A. baumannii* have described siderophore-mediated iron acquisition systems, biofilm formation, adherence and outer membrane protein function and a specific lipopolysaccharide.

The LPS of *Acinetobacter* seems to be equally potent to *E. coli* LPS at similar concentrations. Humoral immune responses include antibodies targeted toward iron-repressible outer membrane proteins and the O-polysaccharide component of LPS that have bactericidal and opsonizing *in vitro* activity. While several potential host response mechanisms have been described in recent studies, the role of the host responses in the pathogenesis of *A. baumannii* infections remains to be determined.

CLINICAL MANIFESTATIONS

Acinetobacter spp. (mainly *A. baumannii*, *A. pittii* and *A. nosocomialis*) have been implicated as the causative pathogen in nearly all types of nosocomial infection, including BSI, pneumonia, urinary tract infection, wound infection and meningitis (see Table 181-5). Overall, clinical significance remains controversial. Some studies report high mortality in patients with pneumonia and BSI, others argue that these rates are associated rather with the underlying conditions. Crude mortality in patients with *A. baumannii* BSI ranges from 32% to 52%,[53] but mortality rates as high as 73% have been reported in patients with meningitis due to *A. baumannii*. *Acinetobacter* spp. other than the ABG, such as *A. johnsonii*, *A. junii*, *A. lwoffii*, *A. parvus*, *A. radioresistens*, *A. schindleri* or *A. ursingii*, have been isolated from clinical specimens, representing transient colonizers of the human skin rather than true pathogens.[54] Community-acquired infections – with the exception of *A. baumannii* pneumonia – are less common and usually less severe. In contrast to other pathogens, *A. baumannii* infections are frequently reported in association with natural disasters (Marmara earthquake, 1999; Indian Ocean tsunami, 2004) or military operations (Operation Enduring Freedom, from 2001).

Pneumonia

A. baumannii accounts for 5–10% of cases of ICU-acquired pneumonia in the USA and is usually observed in patients with a prolonged ICU stay. In a recent series analyzing almost 13 000 patients hospitalized with pneumonia in the USA and Europe, *Acinetobacter* spp. were the eighth (USA) and fifth (Europe) most common pathogens, accounting for 3.7 and 7.5% of isolates, respectively.[55] Predisposing factors include endotracheal intubation, surgery, prior antibiotic therapy and underlying pulmonary disease. The clinical presentation

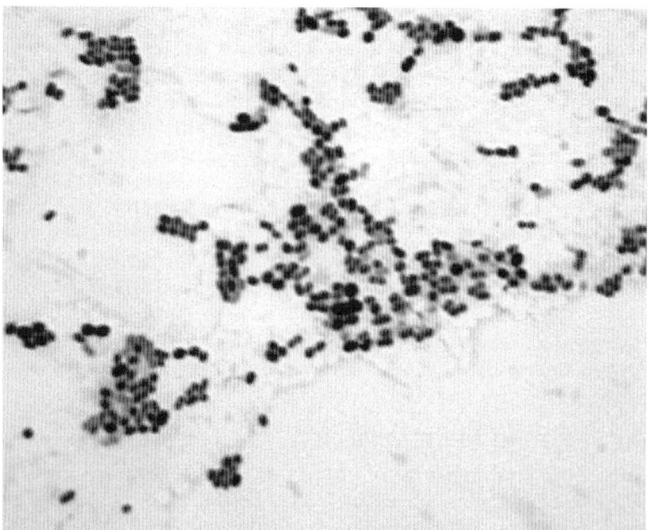

Figure 181-8 *Morphology of Acinetobacter baumannii on Gram stain. (Courtesy of H. Wisplinghoff.)*

may include multilobular involvement, pleural effusion and formation of a bronchopulmonary fistula. Mortality rates of up to 70% have been reported, but this may reflect the patients' underlying condition rather than the virulence of the organism. Community-acquired pneumonia due to *A. baumannii*, which is characterized by a fulminant clinical course, secondary BSI and high mortality of 40–60%, has mainly been reported from tropical regions of Australia and Asia, affecting patients with impaired host defenses (diabetes, renal failure, chronic alcohol abuse) or underlying pulmonary disease.

Bloodstream Infection

In a recent series analyzing almost 25 000 cases of nosocomial BSI, *A. baumannii* was the tenth most common pathogen, accounting for 1.3% of all monomicrobial BSIs (0.6 BSIs per 10 000 admissions), occurring late during hospitalization (mean, 26 days after admission).[21] Sources include intravascular catheters, pneumonia, urinary tract infection and wound infection. Crude mortality rates in patients with *A. baumannii* BSI ranged from 16.3% to 43.4% and was exceeded only by *P. aeruginosa* and *Candida* spp. Even though studies reported a significantly higher mortality in *A. baumannii* BSI, none of the studies formally adjusted for severity of illness or co-morbidities. *Acinetobacter* spp. other than the members of the ABG – in particular *A. johnsonii*, *A. lwoffii*, as well as *A. haemolyticus*, *A. junii*, *A. radioresistens* and *Acinetobacter* genomic species,[10] *A. ursingii* and *A. schindleri* – have been mainly associated with catheter-related BSIs.

Wound Infection

A. baumannii has been implicated in 2.1% of ICU-acquired skin/soft tissue infections, but has been isolated from up to 32.5% of wound infections in combat casualties sustained in Iraq or Afghanistan. Even though colonization is one of the major risk factors for BSI in these patients, the impact of *A. baumannii* infection on the outcome of burn patients or combat casualties remains to be determined. While a combination of early microbiologic diagnosis, adequate antimicrobial therapy, surgical debridement and early wound closure may be effective, there are no data on the impact of *A. baumannii* colonization on the wound healing process.[56]

Miscellaneous

A. baumannii is responsible for 1.6% of ICU-acquired UTI. Most cases of pyelonephritis and other UTIs have been associated with a urinary catheter or nephrolithiasis. Nosocomial, post-neurosurgical *A. baumannii* meningitis has increasingly been reported. Risk factors include neurosurgery and external ventricular drainage. Crude mortality rates of up to 73% have been reported. Other infections include endocarditis (commonly associated with prosthetic valves), endophthalmitis or keratitis, as well as osteomyelitis and arthritis.

Management and Resistance
ANTIBIOTIC RESISTANCE

Since 1980 successive surveys have shown increasing resistance in clinical isolates of *A. baumannii*. High proportions of strains are now resistant to the most commonly used antibacterial drugs, including aminopenicillins, ureidopenicillins, cephalosporins of the first (cephalothin) and second generation (cefamandole), cephamycins, such as cefoxitin, chloramphenicol and tetracyclines, and resistance to all known antibiotics (i.e. pandrug resistance) has been reported. In addition, with reports of resistance to polymyxins and tigecycline there is currently no antimicrobial agent to which *A. baumannii* can be considered uniformly susceptible.

Therapy of serious *A. baumannii* infections should be based on the results of adequately performed antimicrobial susceptibility testing, and empiric therapy should consider recent institutional level susceptibility data.[2] To date, carbapenems remain the agents of choice for serious *A. baumannii* infections, but increasing resistance (up to 70%) has been reported from several countries, including Portugal, Spain, France and the USA.[48] The increasing prevalence of carbapenem-resistant *A. baumannii* isolates (CRAB) is highly problematic since

there are few therapeutic options and studies have indicated that patients with CRAB infections may have a worse prognosis.

In the case of multi- or pandrug-resistant strains, combination therapy or the use of agents such as colistin may be considered. Even though polymyxins remain highly active in recent *in vitro* studies, there are increasing reports of resistant strains and clinical data suggest that combination therapy may be benficial.[57]

Tigecycline remains controversial, despite being active *in vitro* against most strains including CRAB, because several studies reported development of resistance or the emergence of *A. baumannii* infections despite tigecycline therapy as well as higher mortality associated with a tigecycline MIC of ≥ 2 mg/L.[58,59] Several recent studies summarize the currently available antimicrobial agents and their potential use in the therapy of *A. baumannii* infections, even though there are no data from prospective trials and most recommendations are based on *in vitro* data and small case series.

Burkholderia spp.

Nature and Taxonomy

Burkholderia spp. (as well as *Ralstonia* spp.) were transferred from rRNA group II of the former genus *Pseudomonas*. The genus *Burkholderia* currently consists of more than 60 species, most of which have been assigned species names. Some of the novel *Burkholderia* spp. have recently been reclassified as *Pandoraea* species. *Burkholderia* spp. are ubiquitous organisms, being widespread in water, soil and plants, and are present in the human environment.

The *B. cepacia* complex currently harbors nine genovars:
I: *B. cepacia*
II: *B. multivorans*, *B. gladioli*
III: genovar III, *B. cenocepacia*
IV: *B. stabilis*
V: *B. vietnamensis*
VI: genovar VI
VII: *B. ambifaria*
VIII: *B. anthina*
IX: *B. pyrrocinia*
and represents the most frequently isolated clinical pathogen among the *Burkholderia* spp., followed by *B. mallei* and *B. pseudomallei*. It has recently been proposed that five other species be added to the novel species within the *B. cepacia* complex: *Burkholderia latens* sp. nov., *Burkholderia diffusa* sp. nov., *Burkholderia arboris* sp. nov., *Burkholderia seminalis* sp. nov. and *Burkholderia metallica* sp. nov.[60]

Epidemiology

Burkholderia spp. can be isolated from a variety of environmental sources. *B. cepacia* has no specific nutritional requirements and may survive for months in water, sinks, antiseptic solutions (chlorhexidine, quaternary ammoniums, povidone–iodine) and pharmaceutical products. It may also survive on environmental surfaces[4] and has been found in nebulizers and other medical devices (see Table 181-6).

Person-to-person transmission has been reported for strains of the *B. cepacia* complex and *B. pseudomallei*, but so far there have been no reports for *B. mallei* and *B. gladioli*. Overall, about 3% of pediatric and 7% of adult CF patients are colonized or infected with strains of the *B. cepacia* complex, with a considerable geographic variation of species. *Ralstonia pickettii* (*B. pickettii*) and *B. gladioli* are ubiquitous organisms that can be found in water and soil and may play a role as nosocomial pathogens. Rare outbreaks of infection have been described and emergence of multidrug resistance is a potential problem.[4]

B. mallei and *B. pseudomallei* are predominantly found in Asia, Africa and South America. *B. pseudomallei*, the causative agent of melioidosis, can be isolated from environmental samples such as soil and water.

Transmission to humans usually occurs by percutaneous inoculation, ingestion or inhalation from the environment; however, person-to-person transmission, zoonotic disease and laboratory-acquired infections have been reported. *B. mallei* is the causative agent of glanders, a disease primarily affecting horses and donkeys. In contrast to *B. pseudomallei*, *B. mallei* does not survive in the environment, although laboratory infections have been reported.[61]

Diagnostic Microbiology

Commercial test systems such as API 20NE, Phoenix, MicroScan and Vitek 2 can identify bacteria of the *B. cepacia* complex. However, misidentification (*B. gladioli* as *B. cepacia*) is frequent and differentiation of species within the complex, as well as differentiation from other NFGNB such as *Achromobacter* spp. or *Ralstonia* spp., may require additional testing. *B. pseudomallei* and *B. mallei* cannot be distinguished by morphology or serologic tests and may be falsely identified as *B. cepacia*, *P. stutzeri* or other *Pseudomonas* spp., and molecular methods such as 16S rRNA gene sequencing or MALDI-TOF MS may be required for species identification.[62]

Pathogenicity and Pathogenesis

Although only weakly virulent with a limited invasive capacity in the normal host, *B. cepacia* has become an important nosocomial pathogen that has been isolated from a variety of nosocomial infections including BSI, UTI, arthritis, peritonitis, endophthalmitis and pneumonia,[22] most commonly in patients with impaired host defenses such as CF patients or patients in the ICU. The predominant site of infection is the respiratory tract (Table 181-1).

Virulence factors of *B. cepacia* include exoproducts (proteases, lipases, exopolysaccharides) that act in addition to the LPS-forming part of O-antigen and which are responsible for severe pneumonia and sepsis in CF patients. Cellular virulence factors have recently been reviewed in detail.[63]

Attachment to epithelial cells is mediated by pili, followed by penetration, biofilm formation and invasion, which is in part aided by flagella and LPS. In addition, intracellular survival of clinical *B. cepacia* has been demonstrated. As in *Pseudomonas* spp., quorum-sensing system(s) may be responsible for the regulation of virulence factors.

In *B. pseudomallei*, host-related factors such as diabetes, chronic renal disease or alcoholism seem to play a major role in the acquisition and clinical course of disease. Production of LPS and the ability of *B. pseudomallei* to survive intracellularly have been identified as important factors in the pathogenesis of melioidosis.

Clinical Manifestations

While several *Burkholderia* spp. such as *B. gladioli*, *B. thailandiensis* or *B. oklahomensis* have been isolated only occasionally from clinical specimens, the *B. cepacia* complex (including *B. cepacia*, *B. multivorans*, *B. cenocepacia*), *B. mallei* and *B. pseudomallei* are classified as human pathogens. *B. gladioli* has been reported to cause disease in patients with CF or chronic granulomatous disease and other immunocompromising conditions.

Respiratory tract infection and pneumonia are the most frequent manifestations of the *B. cepacia* complex, mainly affecting patients with CF. Most commonly isolated species are *B. cenocepacia*, *B. multivorans* and in some series *B. cepacia*, even though with the exception of *B. ubonensis* all species of the *B. cepacia* complex have been recovered from clinical specimens (see Table 181-1). In patients with CF, increased mortality and a higher rate of fatal complications following lung transplantation has been associated with *B. cepacia* colonization. While chronic colonization of the respiratory tract with little or no clinical symptoms is frequent, cases of fulminant necrotizing pneumonia and sepsis with a rapidly fatal outcome have been reported. In addition, *B. cepacia* has been associated with catheter-related BSI, ventilator-associated pneumonia, and skin and soft tissue infections following burns, surgery or invasive diagnostic procedures.

B. mallei and *B. pseudomallei* can cause glanders and melioidosis in humans. Clinical manifestations of melioidosis (*B. pseudomallei*, recently reviewed in detail[64]) in humans include pneumonia, genitourinary manifestations, osteomyelitis and skin or soft tissue abscesses,

commonly associated with BSI and sepsis (see Chapter 125). Clinical presentation of BSI may range from transient bacteremia to fulminant septic shock with mortality rates of up to 87%.

Management and Resistance

In vitro efficacy against *B. cepacia* has been demonstrated for ureidopenicillins, third-generation cephalosporins, carbapenems, fluoroquinolones, TMP–SMX, chloramphenicol and minocycline.[65] Among the novel antimicrobials, tigecycline has shown less activity compared to minocycline. Resistance to several classes of antimicrobial agents is often observed, especially in patients receiving multiple courses of antibiotics over a prolonged period of time. Therapy of *B. cepacia* infections should be based on the results of antimicrobial susceptibility testing. In cases of multi- or pandrug-resistant strains, combination therapy is recommended and the use of agents such as polymyxins may be considered. In addition, inhalation therapy in combination with intravenously administered antimicrobials can control pulmonary exacerbation by *B. cepacia* infection.[66] Management of *B. mallei* and *B. pseudomallei* infections is discussed elsewhere in this book (see Chapter 125) and has been recently reviewed.[64]

Stenotrophomonas maltophilia

Nature and Taxonomy

Stenotrophomonas maltophilia is a ubiquitous environmental bacterium that has also emerged as an important nosocomial pathogen contributing substantially to morbidity and mortality of immunocompromised patients, particularly in the ICU setting.[3]

Epidemiology

S. maltophilia is a water-borne organism that can be readily isolated from soil, plants, water and raw milk. It can also be recovered from the hospital environment where it has been isolated from a variety of sources such as ventilatory equipment, nebulizers, endoscopes, prosthetic devices, as well as dialysis fluids and antiseptic solutions (see Table 181-6). There is a high incidence of infections due to *S. maltophilia* in immunocompromised patients such as those with solid malignancies, leukemia or lymphoma.[67] In addition, *S. maltophilia* is increasingly implicated in pulmonary infections in CF patients (see Table 181-1). Recent surveys report a point prevalence of 11% of CF patients with transient colonization with *S. maltophilia*, even though the importance of *S. maltophilia* in patients with CF remains to be determined.[3]

Diagnostic Microbiology

S. maltophilia grows readily on most routinely used media and is characterized by the presence of a single or a small number of polar flagella (motile bacteria), frequently pigmented colonies (yellow or yellowish-orange) and a negative oxidase reaction, even though some isolates may be oxidase-positive.[3] *S. maltophilia* acidifies sugars (except for rhamnose and mannitol) and is generally proteolytic. Co-isolation of *S. maltophilia* with other NFGNB, such as *A. baumannii*, *Burkholderia* spp. and *P. aeruginosa*, from respiratory specimens can be challenging. Current automated biochemical panels usually identify *S. maltophilia* with high certainty as well as molecular methods or MALDI-TOF.[3]

Pathogenicity and Pathogenesis

S. maltophilia produces proteolytic enzymes and other pathogenic extracellular enzymes such as DNAse, RNAse, elastase, lipase, hyaluronidase, mucinase and hemolysin, which may contribute to the severity of *S. maltophilia* infection. In addition, cytotoxic activity has been reported from clinical isolates. Other pathogenicity factors include LPS, flagella and a diffusible signal factor system which may play a role in adherence to and invasion of bronchial epithelial cells, biofilm formation, chronic colonization and antimicrobial resistance.

Pathogenicity, including the role of *S. maltophilia* in the CF lung environment, has been recently reviewed in detail.[3]

Clinical Manifestations

S. maltophilia has been implicated in respiratory tract infections, endocarditis, bacteremia, meningitis and UTI. In addition, severe cutaneous infections (ecthyma gangrenosum similar to that due to *P. aeruginosa*), cellulitis and abscesses (wounds resulting from agricultural machinery) have been reported. Several studies listing *S. maltophilia* among the top 15 pathogens with recovery rates around 3% from hospitalized patients with pneumonia have been summarized in a recent review.[3] In a series analyzing almost 13 000 patients hospitalized with pneumonia in the USA and Europe, *S. maltophilia* was the sixth (USA) and eighth (Europe) most common pathogen, accounting for 4.4% and 3.2% of isolates, respectively. Crude mortality in patients with *S. maltophilia* BSI ranges from 14% to 69%, and attributable mortality as high as 37.5% has been reported.[3,55]

Management and Resistance

S. maltophilia displays intrinsic resistance to most classes of antimicrobial agents (see Table 181-8). Mechanisms of resistance include production of several β-lactamases, rendering it susceptible only to latamoxef and combinations of ticarcillin plus clavulanic acid or piperacillin plus tazobactam, as well as carbapenemase production conferring resistance to carbapenems.[3,68] Few strains are susceptible to gentamicin, neomycin and kanamycin, and susceptibility to doxycycline is reported in less than 50% of strains.

Currently, TMP–SMX remains the drug of choice for treatment of infections due to *S. maltophilia*, although *in vitro* studies and retrospective case series indicate that ticarcillin–clavulanic acid, minocycline, some of the new fluoroquinolones, colistin and tigecycline may be alternative agents in case of resistance or allergy.[68,69] Due to increasing rates of resistance, therapy should always be guided by susceptibility testing. Of note, susceptibility testing results may not correctly predict clinical treatment response. Severe infections may require combination therapy.

Miscellaneous Aerobic Nonfermenting Gram-Negative Bacteria

Many other NFGNB have been identified from clinical specimens, some of which are increasingly involved in human infection.[3,70] These genera and species have undergone many taxonomic changes; some have been identified recently and the wide use of analysis of ribosomal 16S RNA gene sequences has allowed a clearer taxonomic position to be established for most of these organisms. The following section includes a short description of the pathogenic role of NFGNB involved in human infections and of the management of these infections. For easy reading, the generic groups are described in alphabetical order. Details regarding conventional identification have been summarized elsewhere.[3,70]

Alcaligenes spp. (Including Achromobacter spp., Ochrobactrum spp., Kerstersia spp. and Advenella spp.)

The genera *Alcaligenes*, *Achromobacter* and *Ochrobactrum* have undergone confusing taxonomic changes in the past decade (see Table 181-2). Currently *Alcaligenes faecalis* remains the only *Alcaligenes* species of clinical importance, after several other *Alcaligenes* spp. have been transferred to the genus *Achromobacter*, including *A. denitrificans*, *A. xylosoxidans*, *A. ruhlandii* and *A. piechaudii*.

The genus *Kertersia* harbors *Alcaligines faecalis* strains that have been reclassified as *K. gyiorum*, while *Advenella* consists of *A. incenata* and several other currently unnamed species.

EPIDEMIOLOGY

The natural habitat of *Alcaligenes* spp. is the same as that of *Pseudomonas* spp. In the hospital environment, *A. faecalis* and *A. xylosoxidans* have been isolated from various environmental sources such as respirators, hemodialysis systems, intravenous solutions and disinfectants.[1]

DIAGNOSTIC MICROBIOLOGY

Achromobacter spp. and *Alcaligines* spp. are gram-negative, oxidase- and catalase-positive, indole-negative nonfermenting rods, strictly aerobic and motile, with one to eight peritrichous flagella. In contrast to *A. xylosoxidans*, *A. faecalis*, *A. piechaudii* and *A. denitrificans* are not saccharolytic. Biochemical identification to species level is not possible for all *Alcaligenes* spp. or *Achromobacter* spp.

PATHOGENESIS AND CLINICAL MANIFESTATIONS

Alcaligenes spp. and *Achromobacter* spp. have been isolated from various clinical sources such as blood, feces, sputum, urine, CSF, wounds, burns and swabs taken from throat, eyes and ear discharges. *Alcaligenes* strains do not seem to possess any specific virulence determinants. They are infrequent causes of hospital-acquired infections in patients who often have severe underlying disease. Rare cases of peritonitis, pneumonia, bacteremia, meningitis and UTI have been reported. In many instances the organism is considered to be a colonizer.[71] Nosocomial outbreaks are usually associated with an aqueous source. *Alcaligenes* spp. are predominantly isolated from respiratory tract specimens and recovery of these organisms from the sputum of CF patients has been associated with an exacerbation of pulmonary symptoms.

Alcaligenes xylosoxidans has been implicated in BSI (mostly catheter-related), pneumonia, endocarditis, meningitis, osteomyelitis, peritonitis and urinary tract infection, often in patients with underlying malignancy, HIV and CF.

MANAGEMENT

As with other NFGNB, available susceptibility data for *Alcaligenes* spp. and *Achromobacter* spp. are based on a limited number of isolates, and antimicrobial therapy should be guided by appropriate susceptibility testing. *Alcaligenes faecalis* is generally resistant to aminoglycosides, chloramphenicol and tetracyclines and usually susceptible to TMP–SMX and β-lactam antibiotics such as ureidopenicillins, ticarcillin–clavulanic acid, cephalosporins and carbapenems. *A. xylosoxidans* is usually susceptible to ureidopenicillins, imipenem and polymyxins and variably resistant to fluoroquinolones. In contrast to *A. faecalis*, *Achromobacter* spp. are often resistant to cephalosporins. There have been several reports of resistance to broad-spectrum penicillins in *A. xylosoxidans* due to constitutive β-lactamase production. *Kerstersia* spp. are usually susceptible to ciprofloxacin and cefotaxime.

Bergeyella spp. and Weeksella spp.

Bergeyella zoohelcum and *Weeksella virosa* (see Table 181-2) have been implicated in infections in humans. *W. virosa* has been recovered from urine and vaginal swabs, *B. zoohelcum* has been isolated from wound infections following animal bites, but individual cases of BSI and meningitis have also been reported.[72] Both grow as pigmented colonies (brown or yellow) and can be distinguished by urease (positive in *B. zoohelcum*) and susceptibility to polymyxin B (*B. zoohelcum* is resistant). Both organisms are usually susceptible to most antimicrobial agents, but susceptibility testing is nevertheless warranted in all cases.

Chryseobacterium spp., Elizabethkingia spp., Flavobacterium spp. and Myroides spp.

The clinically important *Chryseobacterium* spp. (*C. meningosepticum* and *C. indologenes*) have been reclassified from the genus *Flavobacterium* (see Table 181-2), while other *Flavobacterium* spp. such as *F.*

multivorum and *F. spiritivorum* have been moved to the genus *Sphingobacterium*. In addition, *F. odoratum* has been reclassified as *Myroides odoratus* and *M. odoratimimus*.

C. *meningosepticum* has been reclassified as *Elizabethkingia meningoseptica*.[73] *Chryseobacterium* spp. and *Elizabethkingia* spp. are ubiquitous organisms that can be found in soil and water and have also been recovered from foods and the hospital environment. Epidemiologic studies have traced the bacterial source to contaminated water, ice machines and humidifiers. Phenotypic markers used for the delineation of outbreaks of *E. meningoseptica* infections were serology based on the O-antigenic type; nine O-serovars have been identified (A–H and K).

MICROBIOLOGY

Chryseobacterium spp. usually grow between 5° and 30°C (41° and 86°F), but strains isolated from human specimens including *E. meningoseptica* readily grow at 37°C (99°F). On nutrient agar, colonies are 1–2 mm in diameter, and are frequently pigmented light yellow or yellowish-orange. The metabolism is strictly aerobic, except for *M. odoratus* and *Sphingobacterium multivorum* which do not acidify glucose. Indole-positive species (i.e. *E. meningoseptica*, *C. gleum*) are usually strongly proteolytic; esculin, citrate and urease tests are variably positive.

CLINICAL MANIFESTATIONS

E. meningoseptica and *C. indologenes* have been isolated from patients with sepsis, osteomyelitis, meningitis and endocarditis.[74] Meningitis due to *E. meningoseptica* has often been observed in neonates but has been reported infrequently in immunocompromised adult patients. BSIs due to *E. meningoseptica*, *E. miricola* and *C. indologenes* have been associated with intravascular catheters or contaminated infusates and often present as benign transient bacteremia. In otherwise healthy individuals *E. meningiseptica* has been implicated in cellulitis, arthritis and community-acquired pneumonia.[74]

MANAGEMENT

E. meningoseptica and *Chryseobacterium* spp. are intrinsically resistant to many commonly used antimicrobial agents, including aminoglycosides, third-generation cephalosporins, penicillins (mezlocillin, piperacillin, ticarcillin), aztreonam, imipenem and tetracycline. However, most of these species, including *E. meningoseptica*, are generally susceptible to agents that are usually active against gram-positive bacteria such as rifampin (rifampicin), clindamycin, erythromycin and vancomycin. Cases of neonatal sepsis have been treated with clindamycin combined with piperacillin. Recent studies have reported the highest *in vitro* activities in minocycline, rifampin, TMP–SMX and levofloxacin. One reported case of *E. miricola* BSI has been successfully treated with tigecycline and levofloxacin. *C. indologenes* is uniformly resistant to aztreonam, third-generation cephalosporins, aminoglycosides, erythromycin, clindamycin, vancomycin and teicoplanin. Therapy should be guided by antimicrobial susceptibility testing using MICs, since disk-diffusion results are unreliable in predicting susceptibility of *Chryseobacterium* spp.[70]

Comamonas spp., Delftia spp. and Acidovorax spp.

Previously designated as *Pseudomonas* rRNA homology group III, the family Comamonadaceae now includes the genera *Comamonas*, *Delftia* and *Acidovorax*. The genus *Comamonas* consists of four named species – *C. aquatica*, *C. kerstersii*, *C. terrigena* and *C. testosteronei* – that have been isolated from human specimens, as well as several other species that so far have been recovered from environmental samples only. The genus *Delftia* consists of *D. acidovorans*, formerly designated *Comamonas acidovorans*. Three clinically relevant species – *Acidovorax facilis*, *A. delafieldii* and *A. temperans* – currently belong to the genus *Acidovo-*

rax in addition to several environmental species that have recently been identified or reclassified from the genus *Pseudomonas*.

Members of these genera are aerobic, gram-negative, oxidase-positive rods that are commonly found in soil, water and on plants but are seldom implicated in human infections. Rare cases of catheter-related bacteremia (*C. testosteroni*, *D. acidovorans*, *Acidovorax* spp.), meningitis (*C. testosteroni*), endocarditis (*C. testosteroni*, *D. acidovorans*), conjunctivitis (*C. testosteroni*) and otitis media (*D. acidovorans*) have been reported.[75]

Ochrobactrum spp.

Derived from the genus *Achromobacter*, two species have been recognized as clinical pathogens: *Ochrobactrum anthropi* and *O. intermedium*. These nonfastidious bacteria grow readily on most conventional media and can be identified to genus level by classic biochemical tests; however, no biochemical reaction can separate the two species.

Ochrobactrum spp. are environmental organisms and are considered opportunistic pathogens of low virulence in humans. *O. anthropi* has been associated with catheter-related BSIs, and individual cases of meningitis, endocarditis and other infections have been published. In contrast, *O. intermedium* has been implicated only in one case of pyogenic liver infection; however, due to the biochemical indistinguishability, these data should be interpreted with caution.

Ochrobactrum spp. are usually resistant to most β-lactam antibiotics except carbapenems. Aminoglycosides (except tobramycin in *O. intermedium*), fluoroquinolones, tetracycline and TMP–SMX are usually active. In addition, *O. intermedium* is resistant to polymyxins.[70]

Oligella spp.

This genus was created in 1987 and includes *O. urethralis* (derived from *Moraxella urethralis* and CDC group M-4) and *O. ureolytica* (derived from CDC group IVe). These small rods, often occurring in pairs, grow slowly on blood agar and exhibit only limited metabolic activity. They are oxidase- and catalase-positive. *O. ureolytica* is motile, while *O. urethralis* is not. Both species have been implicated in bacteremia, arthritis and genitourinary infections including urosepsis, although the causative role could not be established in all cases.[76]

Both species are usually susceptible to most antimicrobial agents, with *O. ureolytica* being the more resistant species. Therapy should be guided by the results of antimicrobial susceptibility testing.

Pandoraea spp.

Pandoraea spp. are aerobic, gram-negative, nonspore-forming rods that are usually isolated from soil, water, plants, fruits and vegetables. *Pandoraea* spp. have been recovered from blood cultures and other specimens in patients with CF or other predisposing pulmonary conditions.[4]

Psyrobacter spp.

Most of the more than 30 species of the genus *Psyrobacter* have so far not been isolated from human specimens. Recent studies using 16S rRNA data suggest that *P. faecalis* and *P. pulmonis* (both coccoid gram-negative rods) are the only species isolated from clinical material, and infections attributed to *P. immobilis* in earlier reports may have been also due to one of the other *Psyrobacter* spp.[70]

Ralstonia spp. and Cupriavidus spp.

Ralstonia spp. were reclassified from *Pseudomonas* rRNA group II and originally consisted of *R. pickettii* (formerly *Burkholderia pickettii* or *Pseudomonas pickettii*) and *R. eutropha* (formerly *Alcaligenes eutrophus*). More recently, *R. eutropha* has been reclassified as *Cupriavidus necator*, after intermittently being named *Wautersia eutropha*.[77] *R. mannitolilytica* (formerly *R. pickettii* biovar 3) has been reported to account for the majority of infections due to *Ralstonia* spp. and has been implicated in nosocomial outbreaks. *C. pauculus* has been associated with BSI and peritonitis. While other species such as *R. pickettii*,

R.insidiosa, C. respiraculi and *C. metallidurans* have been recovered from CF patients, their role has not been entirely clarified.[2,77,78]

Rhizobium spp. (Formerly Agrobacterium spp.)

The genus *Rhizobium* currently consists of four species – *R. radiobacter, R. rhizogenes, R. rubi* and *R. vitis* – all of which were transferred from the genus *Agrobacterium* (see Table 181-2). *Rhizobium* spp. are phytopathogenic organisms, present in water, soil and environmental plants; they are strictly aerobic coccobacilli, motile with peritrichous flagella (one to six). They grow easily on conventional media, produce oxidase and catalase and can be identified by most commercially available systems.

Thus far, only *R. radiobacter* has been implicated in infections in humans, mostly device-related. Individual cases of endocarditis, catheter-related BSI, peritonitis and UTI have been published.[79]

Rhizobium spp. are generally susceptible to cephalosporins (second- and third-generation), ticarcillin, imipenem, tetracyclines, colistin, TMP–SMX and fluoroquinolones. In device-related infections, removal of the device may be necessary.[79]

Shewanella spp.

Shewanella putrefaciens, formerly CDC group Ib, *Alteromonas, Pseudomonas* and *Achromobacter putrefaciens*, currently belongs to the genus *Shewanella*, which also includes *Shewanella algae*. *Shewanella* spp. grow in media used for Enterobacteriaceae and produce H_2S, which may result in misidentification as *Salmonella* spp. or *Proteus* spp., even though *Shewanella* spp. are nonfermenting. *S. putrefaciens* is present in the environment and has occasionally been isolated from meningitis, otitis media, keratitis, intra-abdominal infections and bacteremia, most cases occurring in immunocompromised patients.[80] In contrast, *S. algae* accounts for the majority of clinical isolates and has been associated with a broad range of diseases, including BSI, peritonitis, osteomyelitis, skin and soft tissue infections and otitis media.[80]

Shewanella spp. are generally resistant to penicillins but susceptible to third-generation cephalosporins, imipenem, ciprofloxacin, aminoglycosides, TMP–SMX and tetracyclines.[80]

Sphingobacterium spp.

Two species of the genus *Sphingobacterium, S. multivorum* and *S. spiritivorum*, are derived from several *Flavobacterium* spp. and CDC groups IIk-2 and -3 (see Table 181-2). In addition, the genus also harbors *S. antarcticum, S. faecium, S. thalpophilum* and *Sphingobacterium* genospecies 1 and 2. *S. mizutaii* has been transferred to the genus *Flavobacterium*. Other species formerly included in the genus, *S. heparinum* and *S. piscium*, have been reclassified as *Pedobacter* spp., none of which has been implicated in clinical manifestations in humans. *Sphingobacterium* spp. are characterized by colonies that develop a yellow pigment after a few days at room temperature. *S. multivorum, S. spiritivorum* and *S. thalpophilum* have been isolated from a variety of infections, including BSIs, peritonitis, wound infections, UTI and abscesses.[81]

Sphingobacterium spp. *in vitro* are usually resistant to aminoglycosides and polymyxin B and susceptible to fluoroquinolones and TMP–SMX.

References available online at expertconsult.com.

KEY REFERENCES

Antunes L.C., Visca P., Towner K.J.: *Acinetobacter baumannii*: evolution of a global pathogen. *Pathog Dis* 2013; 71(3):292-301.

Brooke J.S.: *Stenotrophomonas maltophilia*: an emerging global opportunistic pathogen. *Clin Microbiol Rev* 2012; 25(1):2-41.

Eveillard M., Kempf M., Belmonte O., et al.: Reservoirs of *Acinetobacter baumannii* outside the hospital and potential involvement in emerging human community-acquired infections. *Int J Infect Dis* 2013; 17:e802-e805.

Higgins P.G., Dammhayn C., Hackel M., et al.: Global spread of carbapenem-resistant *Acinetobacter baumannii*. *J Antimicrob Chemother* 2010; 65:233-238.

Mathee K., Narasimhan G., Valdes C., et al.: Dynamics of *Pseudomonas aeruginosa* genome evolution. *Proc Natl Acad Sci USA* 2008; 105:3100-3105.

Peleg A.Y., Seifert H., Paterson D.L.: *Acinetobacter baumannii*: the emergence of a successful pathogen. *Clin Microbiol Rev* 2008; 21(3):538-582.

Polverino E., Torres A., Menendez R., et al.: Microbial aetiology of healthcare associated pneumonia in Spain: a prospective, multicentre, case–control study. *Thorax* 2013; 68:1007-1014.

Samonis G., Karageorgopoulos D.E., Maraki S., et al.: *Stenotrophomonas maltophilia* infections in a general hospital: patient characteristics, antimicrobial susceptibility, and treatment outcome. *PLoS ONE* 2012; 7:e37375.

Wiersinga W.J., Currie B.J., Peacock S.J.: Melioidosis. *N Engl J Med* 2012; 367:1035-1044.

Zilberberg M.D., Shorr A.F.: Prevalence of multidrug-resistant *Pseudomonas aeruginosa* and carbapenem-resistant Enterobacteriaceae among specimens from hospitalized patients with pneumonia and bloodstream infections in the United States from 2000 to 2009. *J Hosp Med* 2013; 8:559-563.

182

Curved and Spiral Bacilli

FRANCIS MÉGRAUD | DIDIER MUSSO | MICHEL DRANCOURT |
PHILIPPE LEHOURS

KEY CONCEPTS

- *Campylobacter jejuni* is the leading worldwide cause of bacterial enteritis. In a few cases severe complications can occur such as the Guillain–Barré syndrome. Campylobacters are part of the normal flora in birds, and poultry is the main source of human infection leading to cross-contamination in the kitchen.

- *Helicobacter pylori* is a chronic, lifelong infection of half of the world population. *H. pylori* transmission is person-to-person and occurs at a young age, essentially in the family. Gastritis is always present and may evolve towards peptic ulcer diseases and gastric cancers. The main pathogenic factors are a pathogenicity island called *cag* and a cytoxin, VacA.

- *Vibrio cholerae*, which belongs to either serogroup O1 or serogroup O139, has been associated with epidemic cholera. Cholera is an acute diarrheal disease in which fluid loss is the essential clinical manifestation of the disease. Vaccination should be considered as an adjunct for controlling epidemics and also for volunteer healthcare workers who provide services in low- and middle-income countries.

- Relapsing fevers caused by various species of soft tick-borne *Borrelia* are neglected infections in endemic regions in tropical Africa and Asia, the Middle East and American mountains. Clinical presentation is variable, but may result in miscarriage or death, depending on the causative species.

- Leptospirosis is a worldwide zoonosis. Its incidence is underestimated, especially in highly endemic areas (tropics and subtropics) due to the lack of point-of-care diagnostic tools. Clinical presentation is nonspecific and may mimic a number of other unrelated infections such as common viral infections (especially dengue in endemic areas) or bacterial infections such as typhoid fever. During the acute phase of leptospirosis, serodiagnosis is insensitive and diagnosis relies on molecular technologies.

Introduction

The curved and spiral bacilli are a heterogeneous group of gram-negative bacteria that share little morphology. Using nucleic acid sequence determination of 16S rRNA, the genera *Campylobacter* and *Helicobacter* have been classified (together with *Arcobacter*, *Sulfurospirillum* and *Wolinella*) as members of the superfamily VI of gram-negative bacilli now called Epsilonproteobacteria (Table 182-1).[1] Only Epsilonproteobacteria that are involved in human infections are discussed in this chapter.

Treponema, *Borrelia* and *Leptospira* are all members of Spirochaetales. These spirochetes are thin, helical, gram-negative bacteria. Syphilis is discussed in Chapter 61, and the endemic treponematoses in Chapter 109.

Campylobacter spp.

Microbiology

Campylobacter spp. are micro-aerophilic, gram-negative, curved rods which obtain their energy by using fatty acids and amino acids rather than carbohydrates, and are adapted to life in mucus of the digestive tract. With the genera *Arcobacter* and *Sulfurospirillum*, they form the family Campylobacteraceae. At least 24 species and 10 subspecies have been differentiated. New species have been described since publication of the last edition of the Bergey's manual.[1] Not all, however, cause disease in humans.[2] *Campylobacter jejuni* and *Campylobacter coli* are responsible for enteric infections and are the most common Campylobacters found in humans. *Campylobacter fetus* is the third most frequently isolated, but is mostly involved in systemic diseases. The other species, e.g. *Campylobacter lari*, *Campylobacter upsaliensis*, occur only anecdotally. They also lead to enteric infections.

Epidemiology

Campylobacter spp. infections can be considered as zoonoses. These bacteria are essentially present in the digestive tract of animals, especially birds, where they do not cause disease. Only *C. fetus* spp. *venerealis* causes septic abortion in cattle. Humans can become infected by ingesting contaminated food or water or through contact with infected animals, including pets. The majority of *Campylobacter* spp. infections are sporadic, although outbreaks mostly of limited size do occur. Large outbreaks involving water as a vehicle have also been described. *Campylobacter* enteritis is more common than *Salmonella* and *Shigella* enteritis and is a major cause of travelers' diarrhea. Infections can be caused by the ingestion of undercooked, contaminated poultry or contaminated milk as well as by cross-contamination of foods which will be consumed raw.[3] Taking acid suppression drugs, especially proton pump inhibitors, is a risk factor for *Campylobacter* infection.[4] It has been estimated that there are 1.4 million cases annually in the USA[3] and 9.25 million cases in the European Union.[5] In temperate countries there is a peak incidence in summer and early autumn, although infections occur throughout the year.[6] The highest incidence is found in young children, with a second peak in young adulthood. Infants can also be infected but the risk factors appear to be different. The incidence in low- and middle-income countries (LMIC), with less hygienic living conditions, is even higher than in high-income countries and direct transmission from poultry to humans seems to occur.

Pathogenesis

Campylobacter bacilli are acid sensitive and the gastric acid environment is the first barrier against the infection. Histologic examination of gut biopsies obtained from patients who have *Campylobacter* enteritis reveals inflammation and edema of the mucosa, with infiltration of neutrophils in the lamina propria. *Campylobacter* colonizes the small bowel but lesions are mainly restricted to the ileum and colon.

In vitro co-culture of epithelial cells with *C. jejuni* has shown that these bacteria can adhere and penetrate into cells. *C. jejuni* can adhere to epithelial cells via a number of different adhesins: a surface-exposed lipoprotein (JlpA) which binds to Hsp90α,[7] a fibronectin-binding protein (CadF)[8] and also an ABC binding protein (Peb1), and a putative autotransporter (CapA). *C. jejuni* is able to circumvent the induction of innate immunity, Toll-like receptors 5 and 9 not being efficiently stimulated. *C. jejuni* is also able to synthesize proteins, which may play a role in internalization and cytoskeletal rearrangement.[9] Cia proteins (for *Campylobacter* invasion antigens) are secreted through the flagella filament upon contact with a eukaryotic cell and appear to contribute to the invasion.[10] Another protein, HtrA, is also important in this

TABLE 182-1	Epsilonproteobacteria Species Described		
FAMILY CAMPYLOBACTERACEAE		**FAMILY HELICOBACTERACEAE**	
Genus Campylobacter	**Genus Arcobacter**	**Genus Helicobacter**	
Campylobacter avium	Arcobacter butzleri	Helicobacter acinonychis	
Campylobacter coli	Arcobacter cryaerophilus	Helicobacter anseris	
Campylobacter concisus	Arcobacter nitrofigilis	Helicobacter aurati	
Campylobacter cuniculorum	Arcobacter skirrowii	Helicobacter brantae	
Campylobacter curvus		Helicobacter canadensis	
Campylobacter fetus		Helicobacter canis	
Campylobacter gracilis		Helicobacter cetorum	
Campylobacter helveticus		Helicobacter cholecystus	
Campylobacter hominis		Helicobacter cinaedi	
Campylobacter hyoilei		Helicobacter cynogastricus	
Campylobacter hyointestinalis		Helicobacter equorum	
Campylobacter insulaenigrae		Helicobacter felis	
Campylobacter jejuni		Helicobacter fennelliae	
Campylobacter lanienae		Helicobacter ganmani	
Campylobacter lari		Helicobacter heilmannii	
Campylobacter mucosalis		Helicobacter hepaticus	
Campylobacter peloridis		Helicobacter muridarum	
Campylobacter rectus		Helicobacter nemestrinae	
Campylobacter sputorum		Helicobacter pametensis	
Campylobacter subantarcticus		Helicobacter pullorum	
Campylobacter upsaliensis		Helicobacter pylori	
Campylobacter ureolyticus		Helicobacter rodentium	
Campylobacter volucris		Helicobacter salomonis	
		Helicobacter suis	
		Helicobacter trogontum	
		Helicobacter typhonius	
		Helicobacter valdiviensis	
		'Candidatus Heliobacter bovis'	
		'Candidatus Heliobacter suis'	
		Related species:	
		'H. winghamensis'	
		'H. muricola'	
		CLO-3	
		'Gastrospirillum hominis'	

respect. Recent data emphasize the role of the intestinal microbiota to prevent the initial stage of colonization.[11] *C. jejuni*'s translocation may occur by a transcellular as well as a paracellular route. The disruption of tight junctions of epithelial cells leads to proinflammatory cytokine response and allows the bacterium to move to the basolateral side and reinvade epithelial cells or be taken up by macrophages. For recent detailed information see Backert *et al.*[12]

During this process the transcription factors NF-κB and MAP kinases are activated contributing to both inflammatory diarrhea and clearance of the infection. In addition, *C. jejuni* produces a cytolethal distending toxin (CDT) acting on the cell cycle and leading to apoptosis.[13] Nevertheless, the role of CDT in diarrheal disease caused by *C. jejuni* remains unclear.

The molecular mimicry of human ganglioside with the lipo-oligo-saccharide (LOS) molecules present in strains of *C. jejuni* expressing the O:19 antigen has been implicated in the association of *C. jejuni* infection with the Guillain–Barré syndrome.[14]

Immune persons in endemic areas, where infections are frequent, can become asymptomatic carriers. Infection can have a protracted course in the case of immune deficiencies, such as in patients suffering from hypogammaglobulinemia. In HIV-infected patients, opportunistic infections with *C. jejuni* and atypical *Campylobacter* spp. also suggest a role for cellular immunity.

The presence of *Campylobacter*-specific secretory IgA and serum IgA in breast milk correlates with protection against diarrhea. IgG also plays an important role against disease.[15]

Interestingly, almost all *C. fetus* strains express a surface protein that abrogates complement C3b binding. This prevents opsonization, thereby conferring resistance to killing by phagocytes and adds to the pathogenicity of the species.[16]

In summary, pathogenesis remained poorly understood because of the lack of an animal model that mimics human diarrheal disease, as well as because of the genetic variability resulting from genomic reorganization and phase variation.[17]

Prevention

Preventive measures for *Campylobacter* spp. infections include adequate heating of contaminated food and reinforcement of hygiene in the kitchen in order to avoid cross-contamination as well as adequate disinfection of drinking water supplies.[18] The habit of washing raw poultry in order to decrease the bacterial load is not recommended because it contributes to spreading Campylobacters in the kitchen. Eradication of the animal reservoir is extremely difficult and costly but adequate measures taken in poultry farms and abattoirs can at least decrease the level of contamination. Other measures currently being investigated are the use of phage cocktails and the development of vaccines.[19,20]

Diagnostic Microbiology

The curved motile rods can be observed in a fecal sample using Gram staining or dark-field microscopy. Culturing *Campylobacter* spp. necessitates special conditions. Cultures are commonly performed with an atmosphere comprising 5% oxygen, 10% carbon dioxide and 85% nitrogen. Some species, such as *Campylobacter rectus* and *Campylobacter hyointestinalis*, also require hydrogen in the atmosphere for growth. Selective culture media contain antibiotics such as cefoperazone to suppress the growth of normal gram-negative intestinal bacteria, vancomycin to suppress the growth of gram-positive bacteria, and an antifungal compound, as well as blood or charcoal to neutralize inhibiting factors such as oxygen-free radicals. Commonly used media are Skirrow's, Butzler's, or Karmali's agar and cefoperazone charcoal deoxycholate agar. An important disadvantage of selective media is that some *Campylobacter* species such as *C. hyointestinalis*, *C. fetus* and

C. upsaliensis, which are sensitive to antibiotics used in these selective media, can be missed. To circumvent this problem, membrane filtration of feces can be performed to eliminate contaminants followed by culturing on nonselective media. However, this filtration technique is less sensitive than direct plating.

Although the most important species (i.e. *C. jejuni* and *C. coli*) grow at 42°C, some species (e.g. *C. fetus*) grow best at 37°C and will be missed when cultures are only incubated at 42°C. Typically, *C. jejuni* and *C. coli* colonies with a gray color and growing flat and confluently are visible after 2–3 days of culture. To make a definite identification of suspicious colonies, the best method is MALDI-TOF mass spectrometry (MALDI-TOF-MS).[21]

Campylobacter jejuni is the only *Campylobacter* spp. that is capable of hydrolyzing hippurate, which is essential for its differentiation from other Campylobacters, especially *C. coli*, however, some *C. jejuni* strains may appear hippurate-negative. Growth at 25°C is essential for diagnosing *C. fetus*. Given the high level of resistance of Campylobacters to quinolones, the nalidixic acid susceptibility test is no longer a key test in *Campylobacter* identification. A strip (API®Campy, bioMérieux) containing the most important tests can be used for identification.

Molecular identification (PCR, sequencing) is being performed more frequently in this group of bacteria. Real-time PCR is now essentially used.[22]

Campylobacter spp. can also be detected using PCR or enzyme-linked immunosorbent assay (ELISA) directly on feces with a sensitivity higher than detection by culture.[23] In contrast, rapid immunochromatographic tests have a good sensitivity but specificity must be confirmed. At this stage they can only be recommended as screening methods.[24] Typing of isolates is important for epidemiologic studies. More than 60 serotypes of *C. jejuni* and *C. coli* have been identified with the Penner O typing system but molecular typing methods are now commonly used, including PCR-RFLP of the *fla* gene, macrorestriction of the genomes, amplified fragment length polymorphism and multilocus sequence typing (MLST).[25] The development of a MLST system has offered important insight into the population structure and the epidemiology of *C. jejuni* and *C. coli* infections.[26] Some clonal complexes (CC) are associated with the predisposition to infect particular animals. *C. jejuni* CC from poultry and *C. coli* CC from poultry and ruminants have been shown to be the major CC in humans indicating the role of these sources in contamination.[27] Serology can also be helpful in diagnosing a *Campylobacter* spp. infection because serum IgG and IgM levels start to rise in response to infection 5 days after infection and reach a peak 2–4 weeks later. This is the essential method to diagnose the Guillain–Barré syndrome due to *C. jejuni*.

Clinical Features

Most *Campylobacter* spp. infections manifest as acute enteritis. The ensuing diarrhea can vary from modest to voluminous stools that may be watery or bloody. The infection can also run a subclinical course, especially in hyperexposed populations. Disease will develop 1–3 days after ingestion of the bacilli and symptoms usually disappear after a week. Stool samples typically remain positive for *Campylobacter* spp. for several weeks. In most cases, *Campylobacter* enteritis is a self-limiting disease and it tends to be more severe in patients at the extreme ages of life. Fever, malaise and abdominal pain may precede diarrhea or may be the most predominant signs. Infection with *Campylobacter* spp. gives rise to inflammation of the gut mucosa. *Campylobacter jejuni* can grow in bile and can occasionally cause acute cholecystitis and pancreatitis.

Only a few patients who have a *C. jejuni* infection develop systemic disease. Bacteremia can occur, but generally in patients who have an underlying disease.[28]

As with other pathogenic bacteria, a postinfectious syndrome may occur after *C. jejuni* infection. One is reactive arthritis which is very similar to the complication seen after enteritis caused by *Salmonella* spp., *Shigella* spp. or *Yersinia* spp. and appears to be associated with the presence of the HLA-B27 antigen. It also appears that *C. jejuni* is the major cause of postinfectious irritable bowel syndrome.[29] *C. jejuni* has also been associated with a rare form of mucosa-associated lymphoid tissue (MALT) lymphoma called immunoproliferative small intestinal disease (IPSID).[30]

An important complication of *Campylobacter* enteritis is Guillain–Barré syndrome, and its variant Miller Fisher syndrome. Guillain–Barré syndrome is an acute demyelinating disease affecting the peripheral neurons and is characterized by an ascending paralysis.[14] *Campylobacter jejuni* enteritis is the infection most frequently observed before Guillain–Barré syndrome and occurs in 20–40% of cases. The risk of developing Guillain–Barré syndrome after *Campylobacter* spp. infection is estimated at 1 per 2000 infections. Major neurological sequelae exist in 20% of the cases. This disease is associated significantly with a particular sequence type (ST22) as defined by MLST.

Campylobacter coli infections are very similar to infections with *C. jejuni*, but they are found in slightly older patients, in patients having traveled abroad, and occur less often in summertime than *C. jejuni*.[31]

Infections with *C. fetus* tend to disseminate from the intestine, especially in patients who have conditions that cause impaired immunity, such as chronic alcoholism, diabetes mellitus, malignancies and HIV infection, and in the elderly. Systemic *C. fetus* infections can lead to endocarditis, thrombophlebitis, mycotic aneurysm, meningitis, bone and joint infections and septic abortion.

Campylobacter upsaliensis, *C. lari* and *C. hyointestinalis* can also cause enteritis. *Campylobacter concisus*, *C. gracilis*, *C. curvus*, *C. mucosalis*, *C. rectus*, *C. showae*, *C. sputorum* and *Campylobacter* (*Bacteroides*) *ureolyticus* can be associated with periodontal infections. *C. concisus* has also been associated with acute gastrointestinal infections and is considered as a putative agent in the pathogenesis of inflammatory bowel diseases.

Management

Disease management is primarily symptomatic. Depending on the severity of the diarrhea, fluid replacement can be performed with oral rehydration fluids. Antibiotic treatment is especially effective early in the disease and is of benefit in cases of prolonged illness, recurrent disease and secondary sepsis. The first-choice antibiotic is azithromycin 500 mg (10 mg/day for children) for 5 days or another macrolide, resistance being low for this class of antibiotics. Ciprofloxacin (500 mg q12h orally for 5 days) can also be used, but only after antimicrobial susceptibility testing because a high prevalence of resistance to quinolones exists. Indeed, the withdrawal of fluoroquinolones from use in poultry in some countries may reverse this tendency.[32] Other alternatives include amoxicillin–clavulanic acid and doxycycline. Gentamicin in association with imipenem or amoxicillin–clavulanic acid are the antibiotic of choice for systemic infection. Susceptibility testing can be performed according to the The European Committee on Antimicrobial Susceptibility Testing (EUCAST) protocol (www.eucast.org).

Helicobacter pylori

Helicobacter pylori was cultured for the first time in 1982, being isolated from the stomach which was previously thought to be a sterile site.[33] It is the first bacterium known to be involved in a cancer in humans.

Nature

Helicobacter spp. are spiral-shaped, flagellated gram-negative bacilli. They are microaerophilic and use amino acids and fatty acids rather than carbohydrates to obtain their energy. At present, about 35 species of *Helicobacter* have been identified, only eight of which cause disease in humans (Table 182-1).[1]

Epidemiology

The prevalence of *H. pylori* infection is strongly linked to the socioeconomic level of a community.[34] The infection rate decreases as the socioeconomic level increases. Infection usually occurs in childhood and the bacilli persist in the stomach for decades and possibly for life. The socioeconomic level of the family into which a child is born and raised is a more important risk factor than his or her socioeconomic status in adult life. The corresponding risk factors are poor sanitation, poor education and sharing a bed,[35] i.e. transmission occurs mainly within families. Given the substantial improvement in socioeconomic conditions in high-income countries during recent decades, there has been a gradual decrease in the acquisition of the infection. Because the infection is lifelong, a cohort effect is present: the oldest people in a population are infected more often than the youngest.[36]

The prevalence in young adults in Western countries does not exceed 10%. The incidence of *H. pylori* infection is low in adulthood (less than 0.5%), but higher in low- and medium-income countries (LMIC) than in the West. Although the source of the infection is known (i.e. the stomach of humans), the mode of transmission remains uncertain: it may be fecal–oral or oral–oral. Vomiting may play an important role. The fecal–oral route appears to be more important in LMIC than in high-income countries.

Pathogenesis

Helicobacter pylori is adapted to the acid milieu of the stomach: it produces urease, which breaks down the urea diffusing from the mucosa and buffers the pH around the bacterium. *Helicobacter pylori* moves into the mucus and produces different kinds of adhesins, BabA being the most important, that allow it to adhere very specifically to epithelial cells. *H. pylori* appears in the duodenum when metaplasia of these antral cells is present and disappears from the stomach when intestinal metaplasia is present.

H. pylori can persist by escaping host-defense mechanisms. For example, it synthesizes catalase and superoxide dismutase enzymes which destroy bactericidal products from inflammatory cells. Moreover, urease increases the pH of the phagolysosomal compartment, thereby disturbing phagocyte function. It has also been proposed that the large amount of released antigens could saturate local antibodies. In addition, *H. pylori* triggers a response from T helper (Th)l lymphocytes with IgG production and inflammation, whereas a Th2 lymphocyte response would be more appropriate.[37]

H. pylori strains do not all share the same virulence factors; the most important are the *cag* pathogenicity island and the vacuolating cytotoxin VacA. VacA may be responsible for the epithelial cell damage observed in *H. pylori* infection. The main action of VacA is on the mitochondria. Typing has been proposed: s1-ml, s1-m2 and s2-ml, corresponding to high, low and no production of toxin, respectively. Type s1 and i1 VacA alleles are found associated with gastric cancer.[38] The *cag* pathogenicity island is a 40kB fragment containing 27–31 open reading frames. Six of them have sequence similarities to genes coding for a type IV secretion system, i.e. a complex protein structure that allows the bacterium to inject compounds into eukaryotic cells. The CagA protein is phosphorylated by cellular kinases and interacts with a number of host cell signalling pathways in both tyrosine phosphorylation-dependent and -independent manners including a reorganization of the actin cytoskeleton. CagA can be considered as an oncoprotein and transgenic mice producing CagA in the stomach develop more gastric cancers than controls, independently of *H. pylori* infection.[39] Another effect associated with the *cag* pathogenicity island is an increased production of IL-8 via an NF-κB pathway.[40] The complex balance between *H. pylori* and host factors allows the majority of individuals to be asymptomatic during their entire life.

Prevention

Because the route of transmission is unclear, it is difficult to take preventive measures. The first vaccination attempts in humans used a recombinant urease vaccine as the only antigen and were not successful. Protective immunity can be obtained in animal models but no clear mechanism of protection has been delineated and no correlation of protection identified, hampering the development of a human vaccine.

Diagnostic Microbiology

Invasive methods for diagnosing *H. pylori* infection depend on endoscopy to obtain biopsies. These biopsies can then be processed for histological examination and stained with hematoxylin-eosin, Giemsa stain or silver stain. *H. pylori* is usually abundant and its typical morphology and the presence of polymorphs make diagnosis easy. However, previous treatment with proton pump inhibitors may render histological diagnosis more difficult. The use of immunoperoxidase staining can be considered when atypical bacilli are detected.

Because *H. pylori* is a fragile organism, transport conditions are extremely important for culture. It is recommended to transport gastric biopsies in transport medium maintained at 4°C before being ground with a homogenizer and plated on media enriched with 5–10% blood and supplemented with antibiotics to inhibit growth of contaminant bacteria. The plates must then be incubated for up to 10 days in a microaerobic atmosphere. Growth usually occurs within 3–4 days. *H. pylori* colonies are easily identified by their morphology and their urease, catalase and oxidase activities. Molecular tests must be added when they are grown from specimens other than the stomach. MALDI-TOF-MS is not a good method for identification because of the diversity of the species.

The urease test is specific for *H. pylori*. A color change is observed if *H. pylori* urease is present when the biopsy is introduced into a medium containing urea and a pH indicator. Tests using semisolid agars show an optimal sensitivity after 24 hours. In contrast, strip tests show a high sensitivity after just 2 hours.

Polymerase chain reaction for diagnosing *H. pylori* infection does not require specific transport conditions and can be performed with a urease test kit sent by mail. Several genes can be targeted. A real-time PCR targeting the 23S rRNA has been developed which allows detection of both *H. pylori* and its resistance to macrolides.[41]

Less invasive methods for obtaining material are aspiration of gastric juice or a capsulated string. Diagnosis can also be made using noninvasive tests. The urea breath test measures urease production by *H. pylori*. Samples of breath air are collected by having the patient blow into a tube before and 30 minutes after ingestion of ^{13}C-labeled urea. The tubes can be maintained for months and sent by mail to a laboratory equipped with a mass spectrometer in order to measure the ^{13}C : ^{12}C ratio.

Another good method is based on the detection of *H. pylori* antigens in stools using ELISA with monoclonal antibodies.

Antibodies are mainly detected by ELISA. There are numerous kits commercially available with different sensitivities and specificities.[42] Immunoblot methods can also be used. Detection of specific antibodies in urine has also been proposed but shows a lower sensitivity than in blood.

Rapid one-step immunoassays have been developed for detection either of *H. pylori* antigens in stools or *H. pylori* specific antibodies in blood or urine, but they do not reach a sufficient level of sensitivity to be recommended.

Since none of the tests are perfect in terms of sensitivity, a combination of tests is recommended.[43] All tests have a comparable sensitivity except for the smear examination, the agar-based urease and rapid serology tests which are inferior. The urea breath test is ideal for follow-up 4–6 weeks after eradication therapy. Serology cannot be used for this purpose because the antibody titer may be high for months after the disappearance of *H. pylori*.[44]

Clinical Features

The presence of *H. pylori* in the stomach is always accompanied by inflammation of the mucosa. However, this infection is not always symptomatic. Duodenal ulcer, gastric ulcer, gastric carcinoma, gastric lymphoma and some nonulcer dyspepsia syndromes can develop.

Symptoms of these diseases (e.g. epigastric pain and dyspepsia) are not specific.

DUODENAL ULCER

Duodenal ulcer occurs in subjects who are infected by *H. pylori* and who also have gastric metaplasia in the duodenal bulb, which will be colonized with *H. pylori*. Hyperproduction of acid following a decrease in somatostatin and an increase in gastrin production are observed. Antral gastritis is the usual pattern of histological lesions. Smoking and infection with *cag*-positive *H. pylori* strains are important risk factors. The incidence of duodenal ulcers is decreasing following the decrease in *H. pylori* prevalence.

GASTRIC ULCER

In contrast, gastric ulcer occurs in patients who have multifocal gastritis or pangastritis leading to a decreased acid production. Gastric ulcer in Western countries is about five times less frequent than duodenal ulcer and occurs in older people. Smoking, dietary factors (e.g. high salt intake) and infection with *cag*-positive *H. pylori* strains are important risk factors. In some instances, gastric ulcer may be a precursor of gastric carcinoma, motivating endoscopic follow-up.

GASTRIC CARCINOMA

The incidence of gastric carcinoma is currently decreasing in industrialized countries. This decrease has been attributed to a decrease in the rate of *H. pylori* infection. Indeed, gastric carcinoma is virtually absent when gastric mucosa is histologically normal.[45] Most gastric carcinomas are of the intestinal type and are thought to result from chronic gastritis followed by atrophy, intestinal metaplasia and dysplasia ultimately leading to carcinoma. These events occur over several decades. They can be reproduced in an animal model: the Mongolian gerbil infected with *H. pylori*.[46] A very early acquisition of the bacterium, infection with *cag*-positive strains and dietary factors (e.g. high salt consumption and low vitamin intake), are risk factors for this evolution. The diffuse type of gastric cancer does not follow the pattern described above, but it is associated with *H. pylori* infection.

A systematic review and meta-analysis of six randomized clinical trials aiming to eradicate *H. pylori* to prevent gastric cancer in healthy asymptomatic infected individuals showed the benefit of this intervention (RR:0.66, 95% CI 0.46–0.95) with no heterogeneity between studies.[47]

GASTRIC LYMPHOMA

Gastric lymphoma involves mucosa associated lymphoid tissue (MALT). The stomach is normally free of lymphoid follicles; they only occur when *H. pylori* is present. T cells stimulated by *H. pylori* antigens trigger a monoclonal B-cell proliferation, giving rise to lymphoid follicles. *H. pylori* infection is responsible for most gastric MALT lymphomas.

No specific *H. pylori* pathogenic factor has been associated with gastric MALT lymphoma development, nor host genetic or environmental factor.[48] *H. pylori* eradication is able to cure this cancer in most of the cases.

NONULCER DYSPEPSIA

Nonulcer dyspepsia occurs in dyspeptic patients in whom no organic lesion is found at endoscopy. *H. pylori* is found in almost 50% of the cases in Western countries. In most of these cases, however, the presence of *H. pylori* is probably incidental, with only about 10% of cases being the consequence of *H. pylori* infection.[49] The benefit of eradication must be looked at after 1 year.

OTHER DISEASES

H. pylori infection also causes immune thrombocytopenic purpura and iron deficiency anemia. In children it has been implicated in growth retardation and recurrent abdominal pain. It may be a risk factor for myocardial infarction, possibly because of the long-lasting chronic inflammation it induces.[50] *H. pylori* or enterohepatic Helicobacters may also play a role in liver diseases.[51]

Management

Eradication of *H. pylori* in duodenal ulcer and gastric ulcer avoids relapses, increases the healing process and normalizes the mucosa and gastric physiology. In low-grade gastric MALT lymphoma, eradication leads to a disappearance of the lesions. Nevertheless, follow-up is needed over several years. Eradication of *H. pylori* at an early stage can prevent gastric carcinoma while after the occurrence of intestinal metaplasia it can only decrease the risk.

The optimal regimen to eradicate *H. pylori* consists of two orally administered antibiotics for 14 days with a proton pump inhibitor. The combinations favored are:
- clarithromycin (500 mg q12h) and amoxicillin (1 g q12h), or
- clarithromycin (250 mg q12h) and metronidazole (500 mg q12h).

A double dose of proton pump inhibitors is also given. Follow-up is performed 4–6 weeks after the end of the treatment. Currently, resistance to amoxicillin is seldom found, whereas resistance to macrolides may occur in up to 30% of the strains.

In countries with clarithromycin resistance higher than 15%, the recommended treatment is quadruple therapy with metronidazole, tetracycline, bismuth salts and a proton pump inhibitor for 10 days, or the so-called sequential therapy of 5 days proton pump inhibitor and amoxicillin followed by 5 days of proton pump inhibitor, clarithromycin and metronidazole, which can eliminate clarithromycin-resistant *H. pylori*.[52] Another alternative is to test for clarithromycin resistance and give a tailored treatment. In the case of failure, the second treatment will depend on the initial treatment prescribed. An alternative for salvage therapy is to use a proton pump inhibitor with amoxicillin and a fluoroquinolone (levofloxacin) for 10 days.[53]

Vibrio cholerae

Microbiology

Vibrio cholerae is a gram-negative, comma-shaped rod belonging to the family Vibrionaceae. Its natural habitat consists of fresh-water and salt-water environments. Based on differences in the composition of the major cell wall antigen (O), 139 serotypes have been differentiated. *V. cholerae*, which belongs to either serogroup O1 or serogroup O139, has been associated with epidemic cholera. *V. cholerae* serogroup O1 can be subdivided into El Tor and classic biotypes as well as the Ogawa, Inaba and Hikojima serotypes. *V. cholerae* O1 strains can interconvert and switch between the Ogawa and Inaba serotypes. Other serogroups of *V. cholerae*, in addition to nontoxigenic *V. cholerae* O1 or O139, do not cause epidemic cholera; they may, however, cause individual cases of diarrhea.

Epidemiology

Cholera has raged in seven pandemics since 1817. It is possible that an eighth is superimposed on the seventh. The fifth and sixth pandemics have been explored and were caused by the classic biotype and originated in the Indian subcontinent. The seventh and current one was caused by the El Tor strain and began in 1961 in Indonesia. It has gradually affected most of Asia and Africa and is found incidentally in parts of Europe. In 1991, this pandemic reached South America and has since spread throughout Latin America. Persons who have blood group O are at higher risk of El Tor cholera than those with blood group A, B or AB. This is particularly important for Latin America, where 73% of the population carries the blood type O. In 1992, a novel *V. cholerae* variant O139 (synonym Bengal), which has the same origin as the El Tor strain, emerged in southern Asia. This 1992 epidemic was the first one caused by a serogroup other than O1, and it occurred in populations assumed to be largely immune to *V. cholerae* O1. The Bengal strain has the potential to spread pandemically. It has now affected areas throughout the Indian subcontinent, neighboring states and other parts of Asia. The distribution and sub-distribution of 632 reported outbreaks has been reviewed from the Program for Monitoring Emerging Diseases (ProMED) from 1995 to 2005. Of the reported outbreaks, 66% occurred in sub-Saharan Africa followed by South East Asia. In West and Southern Africa, the most commonly cited risk factor was heavy rainfall and flooding. The lack of infrastructure and economic development, and especially poor sanitation and the lack of clean water, has made many parts of Africa susceptible to cholera.

In 2010, only 10 months after an earthquake, Haiti experienced the most severe cholera epidemic observed during the past 100 years. During the epidemic period, diarrhea was associated with 33.7% of hospitalizations and 11.5 % in-hospital deaths in children ≤5 years old (mainly children ≤2 years old). Examination of the complete genome sequences of Haitian strains obtained from the outbreak, demonstrated that they were genetically identical, consistent with a clonal source for the outbreak. It was suggested that cholera was introduced into Haiti through human transmission from a distant geographic source, most probably from South Asia (i.e. Bangladesh, Nepal).[54,55] Despite the strong evidence supporting the human transmission hypothesis, the role of climate was also investigated to explain the emergence of cholera in Haiti.[56]

In fact, whatever the source of introduction of this bacterium, Haiti's catastrophic sanitation infrastructure meant that *V. cholerae* introduced from almost any source could have caused an epidemic. As a general rule, populations around the world that live without drinking water and proper management of human fecal waste remain vulnerable for cholera.

Cholera can also occur in high-income countries. In the USA, between 2001 and 2011, cholera was mostly associated with international travel, in particular to Asia, but also linked to the cholera epidemic in Haiti. For patients who acquired cholera domestically, the consumption of seafood, especially consumption of Gulf Coast seafood, was an important source.[57]

In Europe, cholera infections are found only rarely and, as in the USA, most patients have a history of travel from countries where the disease is endemic. However, *V. cholerae* belonging to the non-O1, non-O139 serogroups are present in some coastal waters or lakes where they can cause gastroenteritis and extra-intestinal infections. Non-O1, non-O139 strains from diarrheal patients possess the type III secretion system (TTSS) and/or repeats-in-toxin (RTX) toxins. One of the consequences of global climate warming is that continued surveillance of *V. cholerae* non-O1, non-O139 in Europe should be carried out in order to detect a putative increase in the prevalence of *Vibrio* spp.[58]

V. cholerae are relatively robust and can survive a range of environmental conditions.[59] There is a correlation between cholera incidence and elevated sea surface temperature. The extreme weather conditions of higher temperature, increased rainfall and consequent flooding associated with El Niño may explain the global increase in the number of reported outbreaks from 1997 to 1999. Finally, it should be noted that under-reporting of cholera is a notorious problem, and the estimation of 3 and 5 million cases and 120 000–200 000 deaths per year due to cholera annualy could represent a small proportion, perhaps only 10–20% of all cases.[60]

Pathogenesis

The infectious dose is high due to the acid sensitivity of the bacteria. Persons who have impaired gastric acidity or who take acid-suppressing medication have an increased risk of infection. The surviving bacteria adhere to and colonize the small intestine epithelial cells, producing the cholera toxin and causing acute watery diarrhea. In the intestine, *V. cholerae* is faced with growth inhibitory substances such as bile salts and defense factors, e.g. complement and defensins, against which it has developed survival strategies. In the course of cholera pathogenesis, *V. cholerae* expresses a transcriptional activator ToxT, which subsequently transactivates expression of two crucial virulence factors: toxin-coregulated pilus and cholera toxin.[61] The powerful enterotoxin then released is a 68kDa protein consisting of an active (A) subunit

and five binding (B) subunits. The cholera toxin is released from *V. cholerae* via an extracellular protein secretion machinery which excretes more than 90% of the toxin. The genes encoding the cholera toxin are part of a single-stranded DNA filamentous bacteriophage CTXΦ.[62] More precisely, the cholera toxin is composed of two types of subunit, a single toxic-active A subunit (CTA) and a circular B-subunit heptamer (CTB) responsible for toxin binding to cells. CTA is synthesized as a single polypeptide chain, which is post-translationally modified via the action of a *V. cholerae* protease which generates two fragments CTA1 and CTA2. CTA1 possesses an ADP-ribosylating activity whereas CTA2 inserts CTA into CTB. The CTB subunits attach to the GM1 ganglioside receptors on the apical membrane and undergo vesicular trafficking to endoplasmic reticulum, where they exploit endoplasmic reticulum-associated protein degradation systems to release a catalytic A1 subunit (CTA1) into the cytoplasm. CTA1, in turn, catalyzes ADP ribosylation of alpha subunits of stimulatory G proteins, leading to a persistent activation of adenylate cyclase and elevation of intracellular cAMP. Increased cAMP in human intestinal epthelial cells accounts for the pathogenesis of profuse diarrhea and severe fluid loss in cholera.

The A subunit triggers a cascade of reactions involving cyclic adenosine monophosphate, prostaglandins, 5-hydroxytryptamine and calmodulin. This results in an increased level of intracellular cAMP leading to an increase in intestinal chloride secretion and a decrease in sodium chloride absorption. The outcome is a passive watery excretion that leads to diarrhea. The volume typically exceeds 1 liter per hour in adults and 10 mL/kg/h in children. Since cholera results from a locally acting enterotoxin, it is not accompanied by systemic manifestations caused by a cytokine-induced acute-phase reaction.

The genome consists of two circular chromosomes of approximately 3 Mb and 1 Mb. Most of the genes that are essential for cell functions (such as DNA replication, transcription, translation and cell wall biosynthesis) and pathogenicity (for example, toxins, surface antigens and adhesins) are located on the large chromosome. In contrast, the small chromosome contains a larger fraction of hypothetical genes and may have originally been a megaplasmid that was captured by an ancestral *Vibrio* species.[63] To date, around 30 complete or draft genome sequences have been deposited in databases. A toxin-coregulated pilus (TCP) was identified as the most important colonization factor. The bacterium first colonizes the intestinal surface utilizing TCP and then may receive a signal that induces full cholera toxin and TCP expression and the onset of disease. The genes required for TCP synthesis (*tcp* operon) are located on a pathogenicity island (PI) named Vibrio PI (VPI). VPI contains a G+C content lower than the rest of the genome (35.6% versus 47.7%) suggesting an external origin.[64,65] VPI also encodes the regulator ToxT, which has been demonstrated to coordinate the expression of TCP and cholera toxin. ToxT is under the control of several regulatory systems that are known to respond to various environmental conditions (osmolarity, pH and nutriment composition) and to bacterial cell density.[66]

Motility, surface antigens (capsule, LPS, outer membrane proteins) and hemagglutination protease are additional important virulence factors. Finally, the role of extracellular capsular polysaccharides in the intestinal adherence, virulence and biofilm formation have also been characterized.

In *V. cholerae*, quorum-sensing regulation is considered as the key mechanism regulating the virulence gene expression to that of cell population density.[67] Once in the intestinal environment, quorum-sensing signals within the biofilm repress the expression of virulence factor genes such as those encoding for the cholera toxin and TCP. Then the bacterium detaches from the biofilm and colonizes the intestines where quorum-sensing signals are low and cholera toxin and TCP are expressed.[68]

Prevention

Cholera re-emerged as a major infectious disease in the recent past, with a global increase in its incidence. *V. cholerae* is difficult to eradicate from water and is likely to remain a serious threat to public health for some time. Measures to prevent cholera include separating sewage and drinking water systems, disinfection of drinking water and food, hygiene measures (e.g. handwashing with soap), active case finding and effective case management with the use of oral rehydration. Breast-feeding provides important protection to infants, not because of transmission of maternal antibodies but because of the lower exposure to contaminated food and water.

Vaccination should be considered as an adjunct for controlling the epidemics and also for volunteer healthcare workers who provide services to LMIC.[69] The currently licensed, parenteral, killed cholera vaccine is no longer recommended by the World Health Organization (WHO) because of its limited protective efficacy. To induce mucosal immunity, oral vaccines, both inactivated (whole-cell/cholera toxin B-subunit or WC-BS) and live (CVD103-HgR), have been developed. WC-BS is currently recommended by the WHO (Dukoral™, licensed by SBL Vaccine, Sweden) and consists of four batches of heat- or formalin-killed whole-cell *V. cholerae* O1, representing both serotypes (Inaba and Ogawa) and both biotypes (classic and El Tor), supplemented with purified recombinant cholera toxin B-subunit. Vaccines that include the B-subunit of the toxin provide cross-protection against heat-labile enterotoxigenic *Escherichia coli*, a result of the close relationship between the two toxins.[70] A variant of the Dukoral killed whole-cell vaccine containing no recombinant CTB-subunit has been produced and tested in Vietnam. It is administered in two doses 1 week apart and an efficacy of 66% against *V. cholerae* El Tor was obtained after 8 months in all age groups tested.

CVD103-HgR consists of a live attenuated genetically modified *V. cholerae* O1 Inaba strain which has been engineered to produce CTB but not the A subunit of CT and produces higher protection to the homologous classic strain than to the El Tor strain. Attenuation of El Tor has led to several new candidate vaccines that have proven safe and highly effective against El Tor cholera.[71] The vaccine (Orochol™, Berna Biotech, Switzerland) is given orally along with buffer to neutralize stomach acidity. The vaccine is available in two formulations, either a low dose formulation for non-endemic countries or a 10-fold higher dose formulation for cholera-endemic LMIC. The vaccine is currently licensed in several high-income countries. The safety and immunogenicity of a single dose of Orochol has been demonstrated.[72]

Because immunity against the O1 type is not protective against O139, *V. cholerae* O139 type vaccines have been developed. New attenuated strains of serogroup O139 for use as oral vaccines (CVD112 and Bengal 15) as well as new candidate vaccines have been developed.[73] A bivalent O1 and O139 whole-cell oral vaccine without CTB was also recently developed in Vietnam and shown to be safe and immunogenic in both adults and children, generating 90% anti-O1 and 68% anti-O139 vibriocidal responses after administration of a two-dose regimen. It elicits a robust immune response and can be produced at a low cost.[74] This vaccine provides 50% protection for at least 3 years after vaccination. For epidemic cholera, population-level immunity is relatively high, making control possible with relatively low vaccine coverage levels. This vaccine should be used in areas where cholera is endemic, particularly in those at risk of outbeaks, in conjunction with other prevention and control strategies.

T-cell memory responses are markedly diminished in children receiving oral cholera vaccine (OCV), especially young children, compared to responses following naturally-acquired cholera, and these differences affect subsequent development of memory B-cell responses. These findings may explain the lower efficacy and shorter duration of protection afforded by oral-killed cholera vaccines in young children. The impact of host factors such as malnutrition, genetics and coinfection with other pathogens also remains to be fully defined.[75]

Diagnostic Microbiology

For rapid diagnosis, dark-field examination of a fresh, unstained stool specimen is highly sensitive and specific: a characteristic finding is the 'shooting star' phenomenon caused by the motility of the single polar flagellum of the organism. The diagnosis of cholera is confirmed when *V. cholerae* is identified by stool culture on thiosulfate-citrate-bile salts-sucrose (TCBS) agar directly or after enrichment in alkaline peptone water, taking advantage of *V. cholerae* tolerance to alkaline conditions. Cary-Blair transport medium is recommended for specimen transport. Filter paper, which is mainly used during epidemics, can be replaced by rectal swab specimens. Suspicious, oxidase-catalase-positive isolates are serotyped in monovalent antisera.[76] Sucrose-postive, smooth, yellow colonies grown on TCBS agar are submitted to identification. The use of MALDI-TOF-MS analysis for species discrimination and identification of *Vibrio* spp. has recently been highlighted.[77] Isolation of *V. cholerae* 01 is necessary for cholera outbreak confirmation. Rapid diagnostic testing of fecal specimens, based on lipopolysaccharide detection of *V. cholerae* O1 or O130 may assist in early outbreak detection and surveillance. For the detection of *V. cholerae* O1 an immunochromatographic strip test may be the simplest, most rapid and most sensitive and specific test. Several rapid immunodiagnostic test kits are also available. In epidemic settings in LMIC, a bacteriological diagnosis is not indicated in all suspected cases because the management of dehydrating diarrhea is guided by the extent of fluid loss rather than by the nature of the infecting organism. In contrast, the diagnosis should be confirmed in individual cases of suspected cholera in high-income countries. PCR assays have the ability to detect the lowest amount of bacteria, however immunochromatographic assays achieve both low detection thresholds and high sensitivity and specificity.[78]

Molecular methods, when available, are more suitable for *Vibrio* spp. detection directly from environmental water samples, since they can detect dead bacteria and viable but nonculturable (VNC) bacteria. Several molecular techniques based on DNA amplification have been developed and could be useful in the detection of *V. cholerae* O1 directly from environmental water in cholera-endemic areas and in complementing the identification of toxigenic strains isolated by culture.[79,80]

Clinical Features

Cholera is an acute diarrheal disease in which the fluid loss is the essential clinical manifestation of the disease. Most cases are so mild that they may escape detection, but a small percentage are so serious that death can occur within a few hours of the onset of symptoms. *V. cholerae* needs to be considered among the possible diarrheal causes in children living in endemic areas.[60,81] In the past decade, cholera has caused devastating outbreaks in many parts of Africa, illustrated by the recent cholera epidemics in Zimbabwe and regions of central Africa.[82] A putative reservoir has been suggested in the Rift Valley lakes and the possible contribution of the lakes' fishing industry to the spread of cholera was highlighted.[83]

The fatality rates there also tend to be higher (about 10%).[84] Children are more likely to have only subclinical infection or mild diarrhea, whereas adults tend to develop more severe disease and require hospitalization. Cholera is in principle a self-limiting disease if dehydration is sufficiently corrected. Cholera gravis is a voluminous painless watery diarrhea that can lead to dehydration and even death within a few hours. The case fatality rate for untreated cholera gravis is 50%. Symptoms include nausea, vomiting (especially early in the illness) and muscle cramps, followed by signs of hypovolemic shock. With adequate treatment, mortality is reduced to 1% or less in all age groups. After an incubation period of between 18 hours and 5 days, symptoms are generally abrupt and include watery diarrhea and vomiting. The most distinctive feature of cholera is the painless purging of rice-water stools with a fishy odor. The incubation period does not differ between strains (except O1 El Tor Ogawa) and is estimated to be around 1–2 days. Only a small percentage of cholera cases develop symptoms within a day; most infected patients develop symptoms after 4.4 days of infection. The vomitus is generally a clear, watery, alkaline fluid. The rate of diarrhea may reach 500–1000 mL/h, in severe cases, leading to severe dehydration. Most patients have no urine output until the dehydration is corrected. Because *V. cholerae* does not invade the epithelial lining of the intestine, there is little inflammatory response and hence the stools contain few if any leukocytes, and patients don't have fever. Metabolic abnormalities may also occur, including hypokalemia as the result of potassium loss, acidosis from both bicarbonate loss and increased lactate production resulting from anaerobic glycolysis, and hypoglycemia due to deficient gluconeogenesis resulting in seizures and other neurologic abnormalities. Hyperventilation (Kussmaul breathing) may occur as a result of the metabolic acidosis. Shock from cholera can precipitate abortion in pregnant women, although this is less likely to occur if rehydration is prompt. WHO recommends the use of oral rehydration solutions (ORS) of reduced osmolarity for the treatment of acute noncholera diarrhea and the use of rice-based ORS for the management of cholera diarrhea.[85]

Management

The management of cholera patients consists of two components:
- rehydration, which is critical; and
- antimicrobial therapy, which is optional and intended to shorten the duration of the illness and prevent spread of the disease.

Antibiotic treatment shortens the illness and saves rehydration fluids. Incomplete courses have contributed to antibiotic resistance. Antibiotic therapy currently faces difficulties due to the rapid emergence and spread of multidrug-resistant *V. cholerae* strains, which include production of extended-spectrum β-lactamases, enhanced multidrug efflux pump activity, plasmid-mediated quinolone resistance and chromosomal mutations. Horizontal transfer of resistance determinants with mobile genetic elements like integrons and the integrating conjugative elements, SXTs, help in the dissemination of drug resistance.[86] Numerous multidrug-resistant strains of *V. cholerae* have been isolated from both clinical and environmental settings, indicating that antibiotic use has to be restricted and alternative methods for treating cholera have to be implemented.[87]

Therapy is guided by local sensitivity patterns. These include tetracycline (250 mg q12h for 7–10 days) or amoxicillin (250 mg q6h for 5 days). During epidemics, prophylactic antibiotics should be used for the immediate family only and should be limited to a single-dose therapy.

Apart from fluid replacement, novel and potentially useful strategies to reduce diarrhea in cholera have been developed. First, the inhibition of toxin binding is a particularly attractive approach because binding inhibitors can be administered prophylactically in high-risk areas or as therapy after the infection has begun, as well as administrated orally.[88] Second, enkephalin inhibitors, such as racecadotril, can be effective in *V. cholerae* and *E. coli*-related pediatric diarrhea.[89] Third, small-molecule thiazolidonone inhibitors of CFTR Cl-conductance have been shown to be effective in preventing Cl and fluid secretion in human intestinal cells and rodents.[90]

Other Pathogenic *Vibrio* spp.

Vibrio parahaemolyticus is a halophilic (salt-requiring) *Vibrio* sp. that has been related to food poisoning and ingestion of raw or inadequately cooked seafood. The epidemiology results from the ubiquitous presence of the organism in coastal waters. Preventive measures include the use of boiled water for cooking food. It is not known whether clinical disease confers immunity. There is no effective vaccine available. Stool culture on selective TCBS agar demonstrates distinct opaque green colonies; final identification is made using MALDI-TOF-MS[91] or standard biochemical tests. The clinical picture ranges from mild, watery diarrhea with low-grade fever to frank dysentery. Specific treatment is not required in most cases because the illness is self-limiting and no benefit has been established from antimicrobial agents.

Other less common halophilic *Vibrio* spp. include *Vibrio vulnificus*, *Vibrio alginolyticus*, *Vibrio fluvialis*, *Vibrio hollisae* and *Vibrio damselae*. Molecular methods, especially PCR, can be used for identification or detection of these species, including in the environment. In contrast to the *Vibrio* spp. discussed so far, *V. vulnificus* and *V. alginolyticus* are more frequently associated with soft tissue wound infection and sepsis than with diarrhea. *V. vulnificus* may be considered an emerging pathogen and its virulence is the strongest among the noncholera *Vibrio* spp. Infections generally occur in immunocompromised hosts and are also related to disease states that exhibit high serum iron levels, including liver disease (cirrhosis). Prevention involves avoidance of contaminated salt water. Immunocompromised patients should be warned against the ingestion of raw oysters and shellfish.

V. vulnificus infections are the cause of two main clinical syndromes:
- primary sepsis secondary to ingestion of raw oysters; and
- localized infection from wound exposure to salt water in which the organism lives.

Both syndromes demonstrate characteristic skin lesions (ecthyma gangrenosum) of the trunk and extremities. They are characterized by hemorrhagic bullae which progress to necrotic ulcerations. Necrotizing fasciitis of the foot associated with *V. vulnificus* can cause death within 48 hours and has an overall mortality rate of 50%, even with appropriate antibiotic and surgical treatment. Besides these two syndromes, *V. vulnificus* may also cause acute diarrhea in those on antacid therapy. Early suspicion is critical, because *V. vulnificus* is not always susceptible to aminoglycosides, and tetracycline is the first-choice treatment.

V. alginolyticus may cause bacteremia and death in immunocompromised hosts. Among immunocompetent hosts, it may cause cellulitis and otitis media in swimmers and fishermen.

Vibrio mimicus, a nonhalophilic *Vibrio*, produces a clinical spectrum that is indistinguishable from that of *V. parahaemolyticus*. The epidemiology of *V. mimicus* reflects a global distribution; outbreaks have been associated with heavy contamination of water sources. Prevention involves adequate purification of water sources and proper cooking practices. The diagnosis is confirmed by identifying the agent on TCBS agar and subsequent specific antiserum testing. Treatment is limited to fluid and electrolyte replacement.

V. alginolyticus represents a diagnostic obstacle, because it is often outnumbered by other *Vibrio* spp. in environmental and seafood samples. *V. parahaemolyticus* is the species responsible for most seafood-borne outbreaks worldwide[92] thus the differentiation of this species from other *Vibrio* spp. is of great importance. For this purpose Bauer *et al.* have recently developed a novel multiplex PCR for the identification of *V. parahaemolyticus*, *V. cholerae* and *V. vulnificus* which could be very useful for clinical laboratories.[93]

Vibrio fluvialis is a pathogen found in coastal environments. Following the recent increase in numbers of diarrheal outbreaks and sporadic extraintestinal diseases, this species has been considered as an emerging pathogen. Molecular tools are useful to detect *V. fluvialis* although identification can be a problem due to a close phenotypic resemblance either with *V. cholerae* or *Aeromonas* spp.[94]

Relapsing Fever Borreliae

Microbiology

In the genus *Borrelia*, genome sequence comparisons confirmed that relapsing fever borreliae form a phylogenetic group distinct from the Lyme disease group,[95,96] comprising 11 species (Figure 182-1). Taxonomy and nomenclature still rely on geography and main vector, but modern identification can be done by MALDI-TOF[97] and gene sequencing; two approaches allowing dual identification of the vector and the *Borrelia*.[97] Molecular typing techniques including multilocus sequence analysis[98] and multispacer sequence analysis[99] are also available.

Epidemiology and Prevention

The epidemiology of relapsing fever is driven by contacts with small mammal reservoirs and their tick ectoparasites acting as vectors. Ectoparasite *Ornithodoros* soft ticks transmit most relapsing fever borreliae

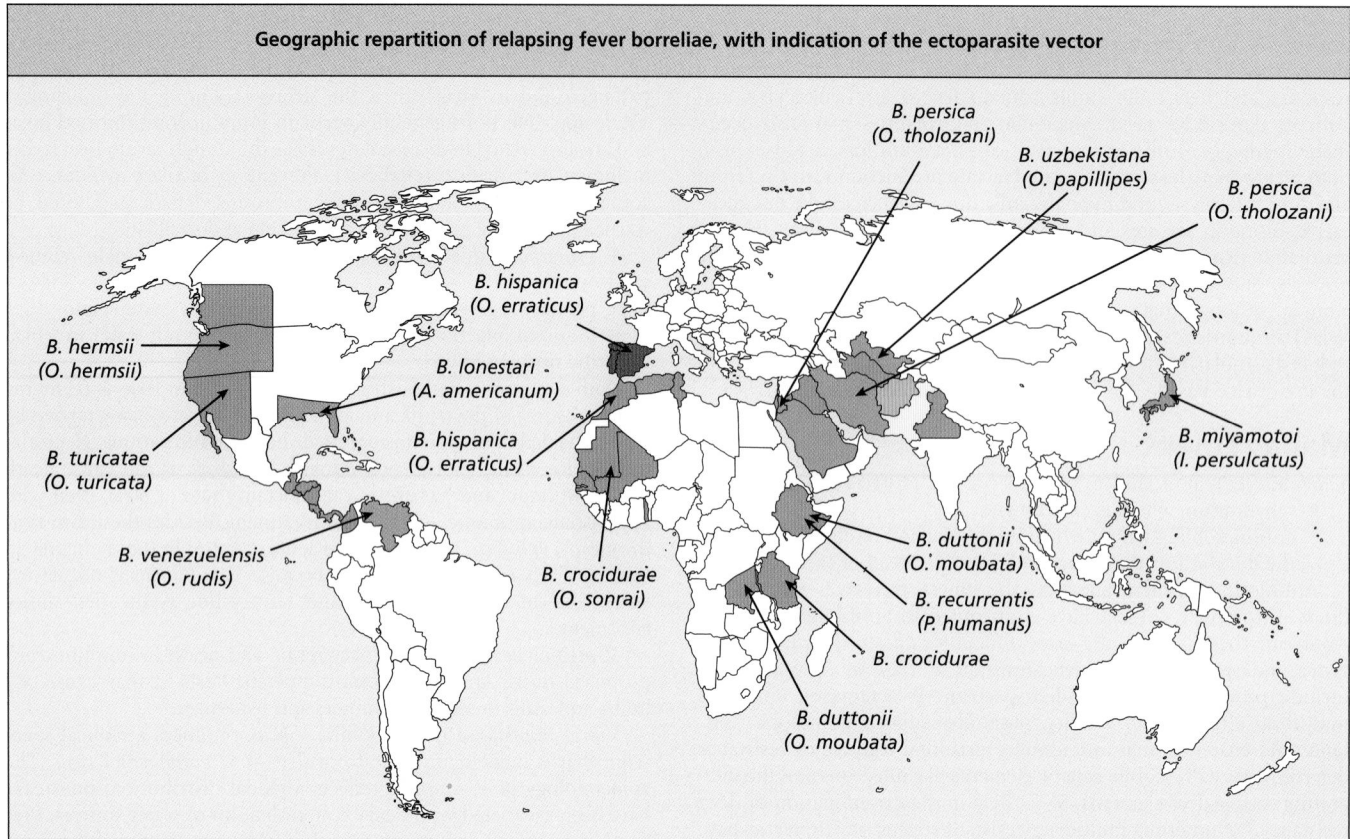

Figure 182-1 Geographic repartition of relapsing fever borreliae, with indication of the ectoparasite vector. O., *Ornithodoros*; A., *Amblyoma*; I., *Ixodes*; P., *Pediculus*.

by contaminating the biting site with infected salivary and coxal secretions, while *Borrelia miyamotoi* is uniquely transmitted by *Ixodes ricinus* (the same vector as for Lyme disease group *Borrelia* spp.) hard ticks, and *Borrelia recurrentis* by the human louse found in people with poor hygiene, such as in displaced and homeless populations.[100] Accordingly, transmission of *B. recurrentis* may occur by louse crushing and more efficiently by louse feces.[101] Typically, *Borrelia* species are transmitted through tick bites at night in cabins and rooms where small mammals enter. *Borrelia hermsii* is the main pathogen in western North America in persons exposed at high elevation in mountain cabins.[102,103] Companion dogs are also susceptible to the infection *Borrelia turicatae*[104] and, more recently, *B. miyamotoi* has been occasionally documented in the coastal north-east.[105] In Africa, *Borrelia hispanica* is prevalent in the North, *Borrelia crocidurae* in the West, *Borrelia duttonii* in the East and *B. recurrentis* in the Horn of Africa.[106,107] In Eurasia, *B. hispanica* is reported in Spain and Portugal,[108] and *Borrelia persica* in eastern Mediterranean countries and Central Asia. *B. miyamotoi* is reported in Japan.[109] Effective prevention relies on limiting contacts with mammal reservoirs[109] including avoiding sleeping in epidemic sites such as caves and mountain cabins. There is no recommended antibiotic prophylaxis and no vaccine.

Diagnosis and Management

The severity of relapsing fever mainly depends on the etiologic *Borrelia*, ranging from mild fever to malaria-like infection and death. Relapses within days are the hallmark of these infections but this has not been reported with *B. miyamotoi*. The clinical picture initially includes fever >39°C with chills and polyalgia. Abdominal signs may include vomiting, abdominal pain and diarrhea. Physical examination may find inconstant rash, splenomegaly and hepatomegaly. The fatality rate is estimated to be 2–5%, depending on the causative *Borrelia*, the highest mortality rate being observed with *B. recurrentis*.[106] More specifically, *B. duttonii* is responsible for miscarriage;[110] and all species may

provoke iritis, iridocyclitis, uveitis and central nervous system infection, the latter being the main clinical form reported for *B. miyamotoi*. Laboratory confirmation should no longer rely on poorly sensitive (70%) direct microscopic examination of blood smear. Quantitative stained buffy coat is more sensitive and specific, but PCR-based detection of specific sequences is the modern method for laboratory diagnosis. Relapsing fevers may cause false-positive syphilis serology. Point-of-care tests[111] may be soon available to help distinguish relapsing fevers and malaria, in areas where both infections are endemic.

Relapsing fevers are highly susceptible to many antibiotics, with penicillins and cyclins being well adapted to field prescription. Suspected and laboratory-confirmed cases should be promptly treated with doxycycline (200 mg per day; 1–2 mg/kg/day in children aged >8 years) with a single dose used to treat *B. recurrentis* and a 2–3-week course to prevent relapses in tick-borne infection.[112,113] Because of concern of teeth discoloration, children <8 years old and pregnant women should receive 1.5 g/day amoxicillin for 7–21 days. Patients with neurological involvement may be treated with 2 g ceftriaxone/day for 14 days. A Jarisch–Herxheimer reaction has been observed in almost all patients with *B. recurrentis* infection, in up to 59% in *B. duttonii* patients, and in up to 54% in *B. hermsii* patients but not in *B. crocidurae* patients, treated with β-lactams, tetracyclines, erythromycin, and ciprofloxacin.[114-116] Therefore, a short surveillance is mandatory in order to provide such patients with a supportive therapy after initiation of the antibiotic treatment.[115]

Leptospira spp.

Microbiology

Leptospires belong to the order Spirochaetales, family Leptospiraceae, genus *Leptospira*.[117] Before 1989, the genus *Leptospira* was divided into two species: *Leptospira interrogans* (pathogenic strains) and *Leptospira biflexa* (saprophytic strains).[118] The species were divided into serovars and the serovars were grouped into serogroups. More than 24 serogroups and 250 serovars of pathogenic leptospires have been described. The serologic classification has been replaced by a genotypic one. The genomospecies include all *L. interrogans* and *L. biflexa* serovars. The genus *Leptospira* is divided into 20 species classified into saprophytic, intermediate and pathogenic groups. There is no serovar-specific presentation of infection and any serovar may cause mild or severe disease in different hosts.

Epidemiology

Leptospirosis is the most widespread zoonosis in the world and is considered as an emerging global public health concern.[119,120] Numerous animals, primarily mammals including livestock and companion animals, are sources of human infections. Rodents are the most important and widely distributed reservoirs of leptospires. Infected animals may carry leptospires in their kidneys and shed them in the environment with their urine.[121]

Human infection results from direct or indirect exposure to the urine of infected animals.

Leptospirosis occurs worldwide with a higher incidence in warm than in temperate regions. Incidences range from 0.1–1 per 100 000 per year in temperate climates, 10–100 per 100 000 in the humid tropics and may reach over 100 per 100 000 during outbreaks and in high-exposure risk groups.

In countries with temperate climate, in addition to locally acquired leptospirosis, contamination due to recreational exposures is increasing, often in association with adventure tourism in tropical areas. In the tropics and subtropics the disease is often associated with climatic conditions (high rainfall, following natural disasters such as cyclones and floods) and local agriculture practice (such as rice farming), poor housing and waste disposal.

Diagnosis of leptospirosis requires specific laboratory tools that are often lacking in highly endemic countries, so leptospirosis is often overlooked and under-reported in these countries.

Pathogenesis

Leptospires penetrate through abrasions or cuts in the skin and probably through waterlogged skin. They can also enter via intact mucous membranes (nose, mouth, eyes). Human-to-human contamination by sexual intercourse and from mother to child transplacentally are described.

After infection, leptospires appear in the blood and can invade practically all tissues and organs.

Prevention

Transmission can be interrupted by avoiding contact with animal urine and by using protective clothing during at-risk occupational or recreational exposure. A human vaccine is available but with protection being serovar-specific, the vaccine cannot protect against all infective serovars. In some countries, vaccination is recommended for workers with high-risk occupations but it is not current practice. Immunization of animals by vaccines is of short duration and boosting at regular intervals is necessary to maintain protective antibody titers.

Control measures can target the reservoir species which is difficult because wild animals represent a reservoir from which domestic animals are continually infected.

The use of prophylactic doxycycline has been reported to give some protection against infection and disease.[122]

Diagnostic Microbiology

Laboratory diagnosis of leptospirosis is challenging.[123] Leptospires are not stained by conventional Gram staining, direct examination by dark-field microscopy is neither sensitive nor specific, and culture of leptospires requires specific culture media and can take many months. Serodiagnosis using the microscopic agglutination test (MAT) has been considered as the 'gold standard' but it is long and complex; it detects both class M and G antibodies so cannot differentiate between current, recent or past infections; the cut-off value on a single serum depends on the seroprevalence of the disease in the studied population, ranging from ≥100[124] to ≥1600 in very endemic areas. The Leptospirosis Burden Epidemiology Reference Group consider a single MAT ≥ 1 : 400 (or single MAT ≥1 : 100 in non-endemic regions) to be consistent with leptospirosis.[125] Commercial ELISA tests are now routinely used and allow detection of specific IgM but the cut-off point is determined on the same considerations as for the MAT. Commercial rapid diagnosis tests have been developed and are primarily IgM detection assays.[126,127]

Seroconversion usually occurs during the second week of the illness and detection of antibodies is variable: antibodies can be undetectable (especially if antibiotic treatment has been initiated), detectable for a short time or may persist for several years. In addition, as antibodies usually appear from the second week of the illness, serology is not accurate for diagnosis in the acute phase of the disease.[128]

Acute phase diagnosis now relies on molecular technologies.[129] Where it is available, PCR allows a rapid diagnosis in the acute phase of the disease before antibodies are detectable. PCR detects DNA in blood in the first 5–10 days after the onset of the disease and sometimes up to the 15th day.

Clinical Manifestations

The spectrum of the disease is wide and may mimic a number of other unrelated infections,[130] such as common viral infections and dengue in endemic area, or bacterial infections such as typhoid fever. Incubation is usually 1–2 weeks.

A substantial proportion of cases are subclinical and people do not seek medical attention. Common symptoms are fever of sudden onset, chills, intense myalgia, abdominal pain, headache, conjunctival suffusion, nausea, and vomiting. Confusion with dengue is common in the tropics.

The clinical presentation of leptospirosis is often reported as biphasic with complications occurring during the second week of the illness; however, in many severe cases, the distinction between the two phases is not apparent.

Complicated forms may include liver involvement (jaundice) with or without acute renal failure, and hemorrhage (Weil's disease), pulmonary involvement, cardiac involvement (myocarditis), ocular involvement (uveitis) and aseptic meningitis.

Pulmonary involvement can be a prominent manifestation and may occur in the absence of hepatic and renal failure.[131]

Nonspecific abnormalities can be detected on standard blood testing (leukocytosis, thrombocytopenia, elevated erythrocyte sedimentation rate, creatinine, urea, aminotransferase, bilirubin, alkaline phosphatases), on urine testing (proteinuria, microscopic hematuria), and cerebrospinal fluid testing (increase in polymorphs or lymphocytes, usually below 0.5 10^9/L).

For case definition, the 'Leptospirosis Burden Epidemiology Reference Group' definition is reported in Box 182-1.

Management

The WHO guidelines strongly promote the use of antibiotic therapy as soon as leptospirosis diagnosis is considered and, according to the common recommendations, antibiotic treatment should be initiated without waiting for the results of laboratory tests.

Severe cases of leptospirosis are usually treated with intravenous penicillin (1 million units [600 mg] q4-6h for 7 days). Less severe cases can be treated with oral antibiotics such as amoxicillin, ampicillin, doxycycline or erythromycin. Third-generation cephalosporins, such as ceftriaxone and cefotaxime, and quinolone antibiotics also appear to be effective. Despite its higher cost, interest in azithromycin for leptospirosis is increasing due to its broad activity against confounding pathogens.

In severe cases, hospitalization is necessary and aggressive supportive care with strict attention to fluid and electrolyte balance is essential. Hemodialysis is indicated in renal failure.

Nevertheless, the role of antibiotics in the treatment of leptospirosis remains controversial. Among survivors who were hospitalized for leptospirosis, use of antibiotics may have decreased the duration of clinical illness by 2–4 days, though this result was not statistically significant. Even if it is current practice, the benefit of antibiotic therapy in the treatment of leptospirosis remains unclear, particularly for severe diseases.[132,133]

References available online at expertconsult.com.

KEY REFERENCES

Bessede E., Delcamp A., Sifre E., et al.: New methods for detection of Campylobacters in stool samples in comparison to culture. *J Clin Microbiol* 2011; 49(3):941-944.

Bharti A.R., Nally J.E., Ricaldi J.N., et al.: Leptospirosis: a zoonotic disease of global importance. *Lancet Infect Dis* 2003; 3(12):757-771.

Cutler S.J., Abdissa A., Trape J.F.: New concepts for the old challenge of African relapsing fever borreliosis. *Clin Microbiol Infect* 2009; 15(5):400-406.

de Jong A.E., Verhoeff-Bakkenes L., Nauta M.J., et al.: Cross-contamination in the kitchen: effect of hygiene measures. *J Appl Microbiol* 2008; 105(2):615-624.

Havelaar A.H., Ivarsson S., Lofdahl M., et al.: Estimating the true incidence of campylobacteriosis and salmonellosis in the European Union, 2009. *Epidemiol Infect* 2013; 141(2):293-302.

Karaolis D.K., Somara S., Maneval D.R. Jr, et al.: A bacteriophage encoding a pathogenicity island, a type-IV pilus and a phage receptor in cholera bacteria. *Nature* 1999; 399(6734):375-379.

Krause P.J., Narasimhan S., Wormser G.P., et al.: Human *Borrelia miyamotoi* infection in the United States. *N Engl J Med* 2013; 368(3):291-293.

Lescot M., Audic S., Robert C., et al.: The genome of *Borrelia recurrentis*, the agent of deadly louse-borne relapsing fever, is a degraded subset of tick-borne *Borrelia duttonii*. *PLoS Genet* 2008; 4(9):e1000185.

Megraud F., Lehours P.: *Helicobacter pylori* detection and antimicrobial susceptibility testing. *Clin Microbiol Rev* 2007; 20(2):280-322.

Miller M.B., Skorupski K., Lenz D.H., et al.: Parallel quorum sensing systems converge to regulate virulence in *Vibrio cholerae*. *Cell* 2002; 110(3):303-314.

Oleastro M., Menard A., Santos A., et al.: Real-time PCR assay for rapid and accurate detection of point mutations conferring resistance to clarithromycin in *Helicobacter pylori*. *J Clin Microbiol* 2003; 41(1):397-402.

Vakil N., Megraud F.: Eradication therapy for *Helicobacter pylori*. *Gastroenterology* 2007; 133(3):985-1001.

Yuki N.: Infectious origins of, and molecular mimicry in, Guillain–Barré and Fisher syndromes. *Lancet Infect Dis* 2001; 1(1):29-37.

183

Gram-Negative Coccobacilli

FIONA J. COOKE | MARY P.E. SLACK

KEY CONCEPTS

The pathogens covered in the chapter exemplify a number of diverse aspects of the interaction between man and microbes, as exemplified by:

• Zoonotic and imported infections, such as *Brucella, Francisella, Pasteurella* and *Yersinia*.

• Mucosal infections, such as *Moraxella* and nontypeable *Haemophilus influenzae* (NTHi), which emphasize the importance of biofilms and microbial interactions in the pathogenesis of mucosal disease.

• Environmental infections such as *Legionella* sources. International alerting systems are critical in many outbreak investigations.

• Vaccine-preventable infections, notably pertussis and *Haemophilus influenzae* type b (Hib).

• Commensal bacteria, which can cause serious disease, such as the HACEK group causing endocarditis.

Introduction

The gram-negative coccobacilli (GNCB) that are important human pathogens include *Bordetella, Brucella, Francisella, Haemophilus, Legionella, Pasteurella, Moraxella* and *Yersinia* spp. Other GNCB including *Actinobacillus, Aggregatibacter, Cardiobacterium, Eikenella,* and *Kingella* spp. occasionally cause human disease. All of these genera except *Yersinia* are fastidious, requiring special nutrients and growth factors for isolation.

Other less common GNCB not discussed further in this chapter include *Oligella ureolytica, Psychrobacter phenylpyruvicus* (formally *Moraxella phenylpyruvica*) and *Psychrobacter immobilis*. *Actinobacillus ureae* is an occasional opportunist human pathogen, associated with pneumonia, lung abscess and invasive infections.

Bordetella spp.

Nature

Bordetella spp. are minute GNCB. All nine species in the genus are strict aerobes, except for *Bordetella petrii*, and grow optimally at 35–37°C. *Bordetella pertussis* and *B. parapertussis* are nonmotile. *B. pertussis* is the most fastidious and requires special media for isolation; *B. parapertussis* is slightly less exacting, while *B. bronchiseptica* grows on ordinary laboratory media. *B. pertussis* and *B. parapertussis* are human pathogens of the respiratory tract and cause pertussis or whooping cough. *Bordetella holmesii* causes both invasive infections and pertussis-like respiratory symptoms.[1] *B. bronchiseptica, B. hinzii, B. trematum, B. petrii, B. avium* and *B. ansorpii* infrequently cause infection in humans and tend to affect immunocompromised hosts. *B. bronchiseptica* and *B. avium* are primary respiratory tract pathogens of birds and mammals. Whole genome sequencing has confirmed the close genetic relatedness of the three 'classical' *Bordetella* species (*B. pertussis, B. parapertussis* and *B. bronchiseptica*) and genomic analysis suggests that *B. pertussis* and *B. parapertussis* are probably human-adapted subspecies of *B. bronchiseptica*.[2]

Epidemiology

Pertussis is the most prevalent vaccine-preventable disease in high-income countries and an important cause of death in malnourished children. In 2011 the World Health Organization (WHO) estimated there were at least 16 million cases and 200 000 deaths annually, mostly in low- and middle-income countries (LMIC). In most populations the disease is endemic, with epidemics occurring every 4 years in autumn and winter. There is no animal reservoir.

Pertussis is highly contagious, being transmitted via aerosolized droplets of respiratory secretions. In the prevaccine era nearly all children became infected between the ages of 1 and 5 years. Attack rates range from 50% for school contacts to 80–90% for close family contacts. Patients may disseminate organisms for weeks or months and are highly infectious in the nonspecific catarrhal and early paroxysmal stages of the infection. The infection can therefore be transmitted to susceptible individuals before the possibility of whooping cough is considered. There is little evidence of asymptomatic carriage.

Vaccination against pertussis has resulted in a decline in the incidence of the disease in children aged 3 months to 9 years (Figure 183-1). However, infants less than 3 months old remain susceptible to pertussis as they cannot be fully protected by immunization. Over the last decade, pertussis has emerged in adolescents and adults in many higher-income countries,[3] probably due to waning immunity after natural infection or vaccination. Other important factors include improved molecular diagnostic testing, increased awareness of the disease leading to increased reporting of cases, active surveillance, changes in disease susceptibility and characteristics of the vaccine.[3] Combination vaccines containing diphtheria toxoid, tetanus toxoid and an acellular pertussis component (DTaP) are less potent than vaccines containing whole-cell pertussis (DTP)[4] and vaccine-induced immunity may wane more rapidly when DTaP is used.[5] It has also been postulated that genetic changes in circulating strains of *B. pertussis* may be a factor in the recent resurgence[4] though this is not proven. Older patients who develop pertussis can act as a source of transmission to very young children.

Vaccination schedules vary between countries, but administration of boosters at different ages may reduce individual morbidity and onward transmission, and increase herd protection. Rates of infection in the 2011–2013 UK outbreak were greatest in infants less than three months old, who are at most risk of complications and death (Figure 183-1). A temporary program to offer pertussis vaccination to pregnant women from 28–32 weeks of gestation was introduced in the UK in 2013 and successfully reduced cases in very young infants.[6] Due to the success of the maternal immunization program in preventing pertussis in infants, the UK Joint Committee on Vaccines and Immunisation (JCVI) has decided to continue the temporary policy for at least 5 more years (https://www.gov.uk/government/publications/vaccine-update-issue-217-july-to-august-2014).

The three serotypes of *B. pertussis* pathogenic for humans contain agglutinins 1,2; 1,2,3; and 1,3. Strains may switch serotype both *in vitro* and *in vivo*. Various genotypic methods, such as multiple locus variable number tandem repeat analysis (MLVA), pulsed-field gel electrophoresis (PFGE), multiple antigen sequence typing (MAST) and more recently whole genome sequencing have been applied to the epidemiological typing and population analysis of *B. pertussis*.

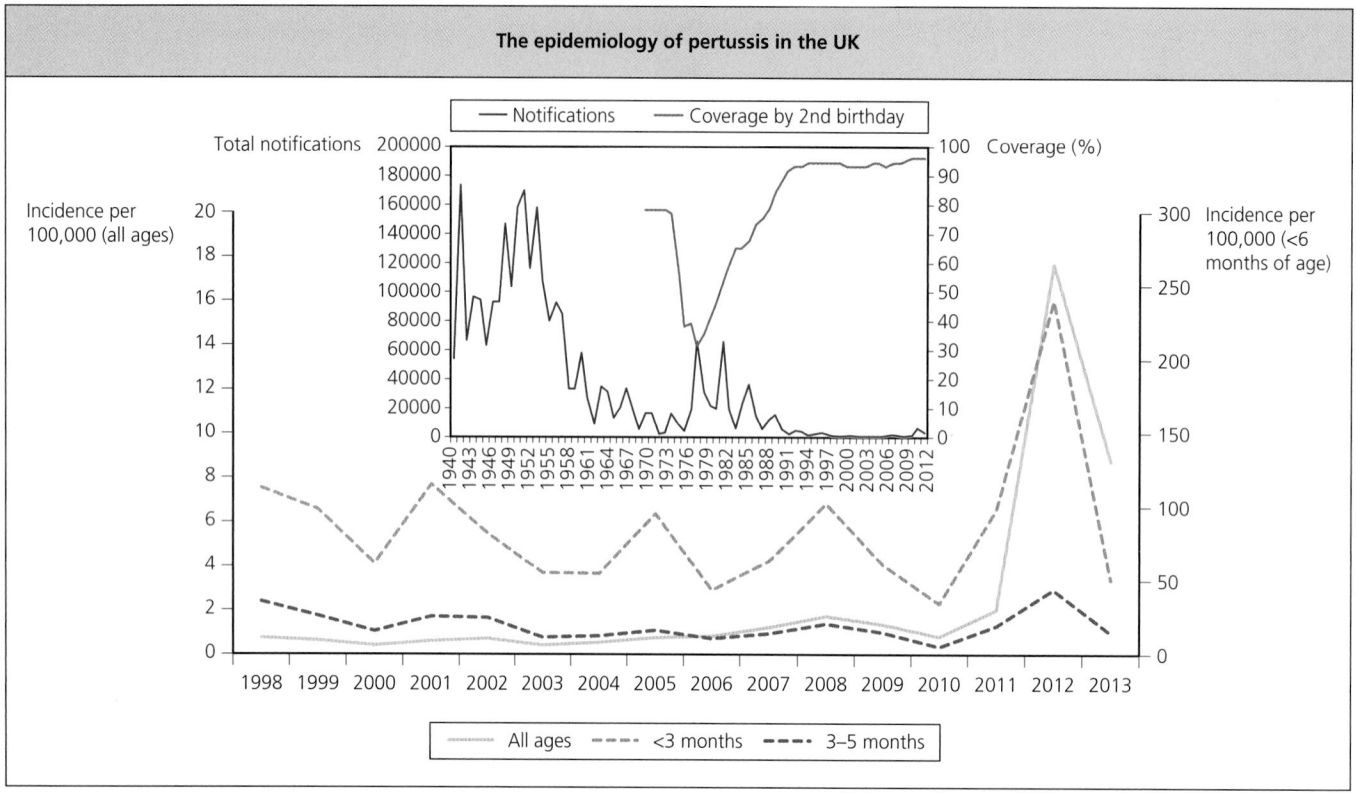

Figure 183-1 The epidemiology of pertussis in the UK. The main graph shows the incidence of confirmed pertussis in infants under 6 months old and at all ages, England only, 1998–2013. The insert graph shows vaccine coverage data by second birthday for England between 1940 and 2012, and the incidence of confirmed pertussis over this period. Data supplied by Public Health England.

Pathogenicity

Bordetella pertussis, *B. parapertussis* and *B. bronchiseptica* all possess a virulence control system regulated by BvgAS operon, which is a two-component phospho-relay system that responds to environmental conditions by switching between three phenotypic phases.[7] The Bvg+ phase occurs with respiratory tract colonization and is associated with the expression of a number of virulence factors. The Bvg[i] phase is associated with respiratory transmission and Bvg− is an avirulent phase that enables *B. bronchiseptica* to survive in the environment.[7] Some Bvg-regulated genes are expressed in all three subspecies. Others, although they are present, are differentially expressed. Importantly the *ptx-ptl* operon, which encodes pertussis toxin (PT), is present in *B. pertussis*, *B. parapertussis* and *B. bronchiseptica* but only expressed in the Bvg+ phase of *B. pertussis*.

Bordetella pertussis produces a number of adhesins and toxins, which are important in pathogenesis (Table 183-1).[8] Following inhalation, *B. pertussis* adheres to ciliated epithelium in the trachea and bronchi. Adhesion is mediated by filamentous hemagglutinin, pertactin and, possibly, PT. The bacteria then begin to multiply and produce various toxins: PT (disrupts cell function); tracheal cytotoxin (inhibits ciliary motion); adenylate cyclase toxin (interferes with phagocytosis) and dermonecrotic toxin (causes local necrosis). The organisms remain localized on the respiratory epithelium, and do not invade.

Prevention

Prevention of pertussis depends on immunization. Whole-cell pertussis vaccine, consisting of killed suspensions of whole bacterial cells adsorbed with the adjuvant aluminum hydroxide, was introduced in the UK during the 1950s and resulted in a steady decline in the size of pertussis epidemics until the mid-1970s. Concerns about the safety of whole-cell vaccines and fears of possible neurologic sequelae led to a dramatic fall in vaccine uptake in the UK, and three large epidemics

of pertussis occurred in the late 1970s (Figure 183-1). There is no strong evidence that whole-cell pertussis vaccine produces long-term adverse effects but it may trigger the appearance of pre-existing neurological problems.

A number of acellular pertussis vaccines, containing up to five *B. pertussis* antigens, including PT, filamentous hemagglutinin, pertactin and fimbrial antigens FIM2 and FIM3, have been developed. These have replaced whole-cell pertussis vaccines in routine infant immunization programs in many high-income countries, including the UK. They are generally less reactogenic than whole-cell preparations and may be used for booster immunization in older children and adults. There is no vaccine against *B. parapertussis*.

Continual review of vaccination strategies, together with the development of new immunogenic and efficacious vaccines, is critical to control the resurgence of this potentially fatal disease.

Diagnostic Microbiology

With careful sampling and culture techniques *B. pertussis* can be recovered during the catarrhal phase and the first 2–3 weeks of the paroxysmal phase of the illness. Nasopharyngeal aspirates, pernasal swabs or nasopharyngeal swabs are the specimens of choice, and are superior to 'cough plates'. Material collected for bacterial culture should be plated immediately onto appropriate agar, or placed in charcoal transport medium. Charcoal blood agar, containing cephalexin to enhance selectivity, has largely replaced the traditional Bordet–Gengou agar. Cultures should be incubated in a moist aerobic atmosphere at 98.6°F (37°C) for at least 7 days. After 3–5 days of incubation, typical 'bisected pearl' colonies appear (Figure 183-2). Suspect colonies should be Gram-stained and identified using slide agglutination with type-specific antisera. *B. pertussis*, *B. parapertussis* and *B. bronchiseptica* can be identified using a commercial test kit such as API 20NE. Matrix-assisted laser desorption/ionization time-of-flight (MALDI-TOF) mass spectrometry reliably identifies the classical *Bordetella* species.

TABLE 183-1	Virulence Factors of *Bordetella pertussis**			
Toxin	**Synonyms**	**Composition**	**Actions**	**Comments**
Filamentous hemagglutinin	FHA	Filamentous protein	Adhesin, binds to ciliated respiratory tract epithelium, and macrophage CR3 promoting phagocytosis	Highly immunogenic component of acellular pertussis vaccines
Pertactin	PRN	Outer membrane protein	Adhesin, important in colonization of ciliated respiratory tract epithelium	Enhances protective immunity
Pertussis toxin	PT	A-protomer (S1 subunit) and B-oligomer which consists of four subunits (S2 to S5)	Attachment to ciliated respiratory epithelium Activation of cAMP, HSF, IAP, LPF Impairs leukocyte function Hemolytic	Adjuvant component of acellular pertussis vaccines
Adenylate cyclase toxin	ACT	Protein	Activation of cAMP Antiphagocytic Anti-inflammatory Hemolytic	Calmodulin-activated RTX toxin
Dermonecrotic toxin	DNT	Polypeptide, heat-labile	Vascular smooth muscle contraction Dermal necrosis Activates host GTP binding protein Rho	
Tracheal cytotoxin	TCT	Glycopeptide	Ciliostasis Inhibits DNA synthesis	
Lipopolysaccharide	LPS	Lipopolysaccharide	Endotoxin	
Tracheal colonization factor	TCF-A	Proline-rich protein	Cytotoxin Adhesin predominantly in trachea Contributes to destruction of respiratory epithelium	
Serum resistance factor	BRK	Protein	Potential adhesin and serum resistance factor Complement resistance	
Fimbriae	FIM	Filamentous proteins composed of subunits	Facilitates persistent tracheal colonization	Component of some acellular pertussis vaccines

cAMP, cyclic adenosine monophosphate; HSF, histamine sensitizing factor; IAP, islet-activating protein; LPF, lymphocytosis promoting factor; RTX, repeats in toxin.
*With the exception of pertussis toxin, similar toxins are expressed in *B. parapertussis* and *B. bronchiseptica*.

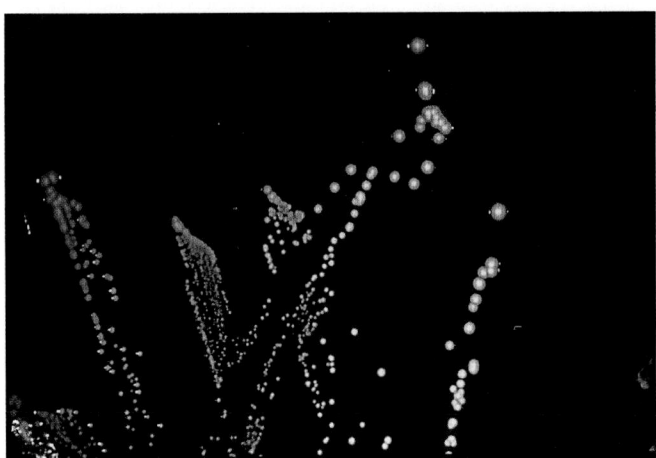

Figure 183-2 Colonies of *Bordetella pertussis* on charcoal blood agar.

Real-time polymerase chain reaction (PCR) is more sensitive than culture, especially for specimens collected more than 3–4 weeks after onset of the cough and following antibiotic treatment. A number of different primers have been used, including *IS481*, which detects *B. pertussis* and *B. holmesii*; *IS1001*, which detects *B. parapertussis* and *B. holmesii*; and *ptxA*, which is specific for *B. pertussis*. Serotyping of *B. pertussis* is based on the three major surface agglutinogens (1, 2 and 3). Type 1,3 is more common than serotypes 1,2 and 1,2,3, and accounts for 90% of isolates. Typing by MLVA facilitates comparison between laboratories.

Serological diagnosis of *B. pertussis* is based on enzyme-linked immunosorbent assay (ELISA) of IgG and IgA antibodies to PT. A rise in titer of IgG or IgA (twofold or greater) in acute and convalescent phase samples taken at least 2 weeks apart is considered significant. In adolescents and adults a single high titer of antipertussis toxin IgG has a good predictive value of acute pertussis infection, with reported sensitivity of 76% and specificity of 99%.[9] Serology is unreliable in young infants.

Clinical Manifestations

Bordetella pertussis is the cause of pertussis (whooping cough). Typically, following an incubation period of 7–14 days, the patient develops red eyes, a runny nose, mild cough and sneezing ('catarrhal stage'). Symptoms are clinically indistinguishable from many viral upper respiratory tract infections. After approximately 1 week the cough becomes more severe and the patient experiences paroxysmal bouts of a severe, hacking cough ('paroxysmal stage'). A paroxysm consists of repeated coughing followed by an inspiratory gasp as the patient finally inspires. This is the characteristic 'whoop'. Paroxysms may be triggered by a variety of stimuli, including cold air and loud noises. A child may become cyanosed during a paroxysm and can suffer fatal hypoxia. Often the child vomits at the end of a paroxysm and is left exhausted. This paroxysmal stage may last for 1–4 weeks, and is followed by a lengthy 'convalescent stage' as the paroxysms decline and the patient slowly recovers.

Common complications include pneumonia (which may be primary or secondary to a supervening infection with another pathogen) and otitis media. The child may suffer cerebral hypoxia during a paroxysm, which can lead to encephalopathy or fitting. Other possible complications include intraventricular hemorrhage, subconjunctival hemorrhages, umbilical or inguinal herniae, fractured ribs, ruptured diaphragm and rectal prolapse. Pertussis is most severe in very young infants and in this age group the presentation may be atypical with no characteristic paroxysmal whooping. Partially immunized children and adults may have an atypical form of pertussis.[10]

Bordetella parapertussis is a cause of acute bronchitis or pertussis-like infections in children. *Bordetella bronchiseptica* may rarely cause pneumonia, meningitis or whooping cough in highly immunocompromised patients.[10] *Bordetella holmesii* is associated with pertussis-like symptoms, but may also cause invasive infections, including meningitis, bacteremia, pneumonia, endocarditis and arthritis. While respiratory infections with *B. holmesii* tend to occur in healthy adults and adolescents, invasive infections generally affect patients with underlying co-morbidities, including asplenia, HIV infection or immunosuppression. Infection with *B. holmesii* may be misidentified as being due to *B. pertussis* because routine diagnostic tests are not species-specific.[1]

Management

Antimicrobial therapy for pertussis, when administered early in the illness, can decrease transmission to susceptible contacts and possibly ameliorate symptoms. Macrolides are the antibiotics of choice and appear to reduce the severity and duration of the disease. Co-trimoxazole or fluoroquinolones are alternatives. Corticosteroids may be indicated in infants who have life-threatening disease. Secondary bacterial infections should be treated with appropriate antibiotics. Antibiotic prophylaxis should be offered to all close contacts, regardless of their immunization status, where there is an unimmunized or partially immunized vulnerable close contact.[11] Immunization should be considered for those offered antibiotic prophylaxis.[11]

Brucella spp.

Nature

Brucella spp. are small, nonmotile, nonsporing, noncapsulate GNCB. They are aerobic, but some strains require 5–10% carbon dioxide for primary isolation. Growth *in vitro* is slow and primary isolation may require 4 weeks incubation. Growth may be improved by addition of serum or blood. *Brucella* spp. are catalase-positive and usually oxidase-positive.

Brucella is a monospecific genus (*Brucella melitensis*) with multiple biovars. In practice it is more useful to refer to separate species, which have different preferential host specificities. There are 10 'species' of *Brucella*: *B. melitensis* is the most virulent and is responsible for most human infections (Table 183-2). *B. melitensis*, *B. abortus* and *B. suis* cause considerable morbidity in countries where brucellosis persists in domestic animals. Human infections with *B. canis* and the marine species (*B. ceti*, *B. pinnipedialis*) are rare. Complete genome sequences

of at least 25 *Brucella* strains are available, and analysis has confirmed that members of the genus are genetically homogeneous. Investigating *Brucella* diversity helps our understanding of evolution and taxonomy, and also directs the development of new molecular typing tools.[12]

Epidemiology

Brucellosis is a true zoonosis, because humans acquire the infection directly or indirectly from infected animals. It is the commonest zoonotic infection worldwide, with more than 500 000 cases of human brucellosis reported annually, which is likely to be an underestimate. Brucellosis is prevalent in Mediterranean countries, the Middle East, the Indian subcontinent, Mongolia and Central and South America.[13] Some countries have eradicated brucellosis, including the UK, much of northern Europe, Australia, New Zealand and Canada.

In their natural hosts, *Brucella* spp. cause chronic infections which are mild or asymptomatic. The bacteria localize in the reproductive tissues of ruminants, which are rich in mesoerythritol. Erythritol stimulates the multiplication of *Brucella* spp. Thus the main symptoms of brucellosis in animals include sterility or abortion. *Brucella* organisms are shed in large numbers in the products of conception, urine and milk, and when infected animals are slaughtered. Humans are infected either by direct contact with infected animals or animal products or indirectly by ingesting infected milk or dairy produce.

In endemic areas, most cases occur in dairymen, herdsmen, abattoir workers, butchers and veterinary surgeons. Children may become infected in rural areas of LMIC if they live in close proximity to domestic animals. The general public is usually infected by ingesting unpasteurized milk and milk products such as fresh soft cheese. Case-to-case transmission in humans is very rare. Self-inoculation with live *Brucella* vaccine is a risk among veterinary surgeons, and laboratory workers are at risk if they handle as-yet unidentified gram-negative coccobacilli without adequate precautions. Brucellosis is considered a potential biologic weapon via airborne transmission.

Pathogenesis

Brucella spp. are facultative intracellular parasites, their survival and persistence within the body being dependent on their ability to survive and multiply within cells of the reticuloendothelial system.[14] The organisms enter the body by inhalation, ingestion or after penetration of intact skin, abrasions or the conjunctival mucosa. The lipopolysaccharide (endotoxin) of smooth strains (S-LPS) is a major virulence determinant. S-LPS is antiphagocytic, facilitates cell entry, inhibits the fusion of *Brucella*-containing vacuoles (BCV) with lysosomes and inhibits host cell apoptosis. A two-component regulatory system, BvrR/BvrS is important for invasion and intracellular survival, and acts by regulating the expression of outer membrane proteins, Omp3a

TABLE 183-2	*Brucella* species		
Species (Number Of Biovars)	Primary Host	Humans As Secondary Host	Notes Regarding Human Infections
B. abortus (6)	Cattle, camels, yaks, buffalo	++	Usually sporadic, in people who work with cattle
B. melitensis (3)	Goats	++++	Responsible for the majority of human infections. Primarily food-borne
B. suis (5)	Pigs	+	Usually sporadic, in people who work with pigs
B. canis	Dogs	+	Unusual
B. ceti	Whales	+	Very rare
B. pinnipediae	Seals	+	Very rare
B. neotomeae	Desert rats	–	–
B. ovis	Sheep	–	–
B. microti	Voles	–	–
B. inopinata	?	?	1 case report of human infection in breast implant

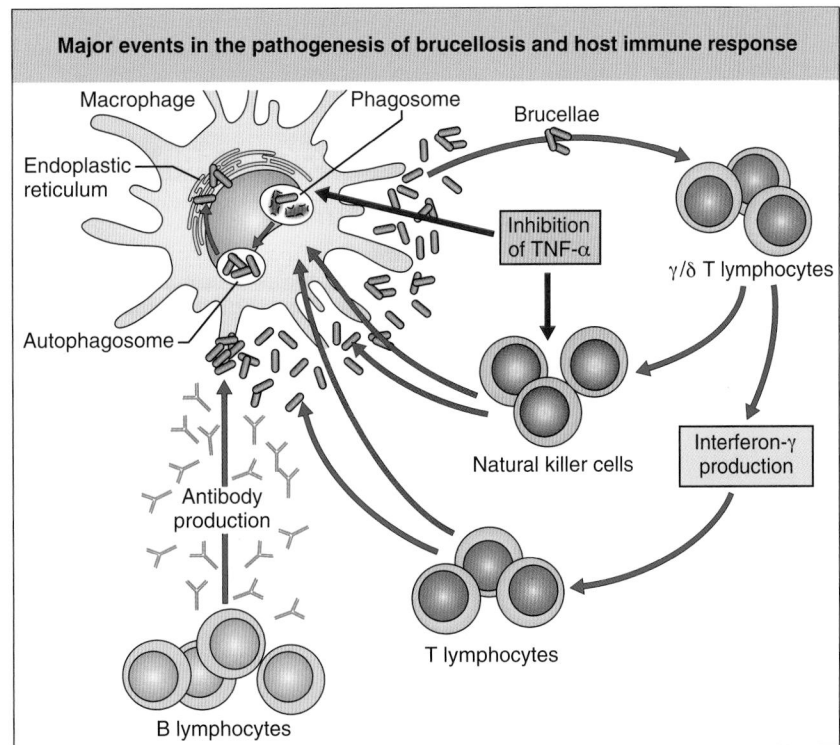

Figure 183-3   Major events in the pathogenesis of brucellosis and the host immune response. *(From Pappas G. et al. N Engl J Med 2005; 352:2325-2336.)*

(Omp25) and Omp3b (Omp22). The altered expression of surface proteins permits *Brucella* to bind to and penetrate host cells. The type IV secretion system (VirB) of *Brucella*, encoded by the *virB* operon, is also important for adherence, cell entry and bacterial survival and replication within macrophages.

After ingestion by phagocytic cells, the organisms proliferate in local lymph nodes. The infection spreads hematogenously to tissues rich in elements of the reticuloendothelial system, including the liver, bone marrow, lymph nodes and spleen. Organisms may also localize in other tissues, including the central nervous system, joints, heart and kidneys.

Endotoxin and hypersensitivity to *Brucella* antigens may explain some of the symptoms of brucellosis, including fever and weight loss. Antibodies against the *Brucella* LPS appear within a few days of onset of the acute phase of the disease and are important in preventing re-infection. However, cell-mediated immunity, particularly the production of activated mononuclear phagocytes, is more important in promoting recovery (see Figure 183-3).

Prevention

The ideal method of prevention of human brucellosis is elimination of the disease from domestic livestock. There are effective vaccines for cattle (S19) and goats (Rev-1). Where eradication has not been achieved, individuals with at-risk occupations should wear protective clothing, gloves, goggles and masks, especially when handling post-partum animals.

Previously, live attenuated animal vaccines have been given to workers at high risk of contracting brucellosis. However, these vaccines may produce infection in humans and are far from ideal. Candidate vaccines, including an LPS–protein conjugate vaccine and a subunit vaccine against the outer membrane vesicle are under development.[14]

Boiling or pasteurizing milk eliminates the risk of transmission via dairy products, as *Brucella* is killed by heating at 140°F (60°C) for 10 minutes. If laboratory workers are exposed to *Brucella*, postexposure antibiotic prophylaxis, for example with doxycycline or co-trimoxazole, should be considered.

Diagnostic Microbiology

Clinicians should inform laboratory staff if brucellosis is suspected (or when investigating febrile patients who have visited or resided in *Brucella*-endemic areas) to ensure samples are processed appropriately. Definitive diagnosis depends on isolating *Brucella* spp. from cultures of blood, bone marrow or tissue obtained early in the disease. Bone marrow cultures reportedly give a slightly higher yield than blood cultures. However, automated blood culture methods may produce positive results in approximately 80% of cases, so bone marrow cultures are rarely required. Cultures should be incubated at 98.6°F (37°C) for at least 6 weeks, but commercial systems may show growth in a few days. In LMIC where automated blood culture systems are not available, blood clot culture is more sensitive than whole blood culture and lysis centrifugation may increase yield.

Positive cultures should be subcultured onto serum dextrose agar or similar agar. Selective media may be required for contaminated material. After 48 hours of incubation at 98.6°F (37°C) in air plus 5–10% carbon dioxide, *Brucella* spp. produce small, smooth, translucent colonies. Commercial galley-test identification systems (API) may misidentify *Brucella* spp. as *Moraxella phenylpyruvica*. MALDI-TOF MS is a rapid and reliable method to identify *Brucella* spp.

The biovar of the strain is usually determined by reference laboratories, based on production of hydrogen sulfide, urease activity, tolerance to bacteriostatic dyes and agglutination. Tbilisi (Tb) phage typing may also be used. A number of PCR assays for diagnosing brucellosis in clinical samples have been described and may rapidly diagnose acute brucellosis and enable early detection of relapse.

Many serological tests have been described for brucellosis, including rose bengal test, serum agglutination, Coombs, competitive ELISA lateral flow immunochromatography for IgM and IgG detection and immunoprecipitation with *Brucella* proteins. Interpretation of results is often difficult since both IgG and IgM antibodies can persist for a long time.

The serum agglutination test (SAT) using *B. abortus* strain 119 is widely used, preferably on serum collected very early in the course of the disease. False-negative results may occur if serum samples are not diluted beyond 1:320, owing to a prozone phenomenon. False-positive reactions may occur due to cross-reactivity with *Escherichia coli*, *Vibrio cholerae*, *Yersinia enterocolitica* and *Francisella tularensis*. The SAT measures both IgM and IgG. The best indicators of acute infection are IgG and IgA antibodies. A rise in antibody titer is observed in more than 97% of patients who have acute brucellosis and positive blood cultures. An initial IgM antibody response is followed after 1–2 weeks by a rise in IgG. During recovery the IgG antibody titers slowly decline over a period of months but IgM antibodies may persist at a low level in the serum for several years. Sustained IgG antibody titers or a second rise in IgG antibody levels are seen in chronic infection or relapse. The SAT test does not detect *B. canis* as it lacks surface LPS, and specific serology for this organism should be requested.

Commercial ELISA tests based on antibodies to S-LPS are highly sensitive but appear to be less specific than the SAT. Again, because *B. canis* lacks surface LPS it provokes minimal anti-LPS-specific antibody response.

Rapid point-of-care tests, including fluorescent polarization immunoassay (FPA) and immunochromatographic *Brucella* IgM/IgG lateral flow assay (LFA) are highly sensitive and specific and have been used successfully to diagnose brucellosis in endemic areas. Ideally the diagnosis of brucellosis should be based on clinical suspicion, isolation of the organism and positive serology.

Clinical Manifestations (see also Chapter 129)

Brucellosis, also known as Malta fever or undulant fever, is a systemic infection that can affect any tissue of the body, and tends to present with nonspecific clinical symptoms.[15] The possibility of brucellosis should be considered in any fever of unknown origin, especially in patients who have occupational exposure or relevant travel history. See Chapter 68.

Management

Before the introduction of antibiotics, brucellosis was a chronic, relapsing illness. *In vitro* antibiotic activity does not always correlate with clinical efficacy, and agents that achieve adequate intracellular concentrations should be used. A prolonged course of treatment is recommended to reduce relapse. Most recommendations center on dual or triple therapy, usually involving an aminoglycoside. Examples include oral doxycycline plus rifampin (rifampicin) for at least 6 weeks, or oral doxycycline for 6 weeks supplemented by a parenteral aminoglycoside for the first 2–3 weeks (see also Chapter 129). In cases of accidental laboratory exposure, post-exposure prophylaxis should be offered as soon as possible. Possible regimens include oral doxycycline or co-trimoxazole. In all such cases the patient should

be monitored for 6 months for signs of infection, including the development of fever, headache, malaise, myalgia, arthralgia, anorexia or weight loss.

Francisella spp.

Nature

Francisella spp. are very small, faintly staining, pleomorphic, nonmotile and nonspore-forming GNCB, surrounded by a thin lipid-rich capsule. They are strictly aerobic, oxidase-negative and weakly catalase-positive. They attack carbohydrates slowly, producing acid but no gas. *Francisella tularensis* requires cysteine or cystine for growth and grows slowly at 98.6°F (37°C) on suitably enriched media.

F. tularensis causes tularemia in animals and humans. Within the species *F. tularensis* there are three subspecies, which differ in their geographical distribution and virulence in man (Table 183-3). Comparative genomics suggest that these subspecies are genetically distinct groups.[16]

Epidemiology

The majority of human infections with *F. tularensis* occur in the northern hemisphere between latitudes 30° and 71°. It is well recognized in North America, Scandinavia and Russia, and cases have been reported from central and southern Europe, including Czech Republic, Kosovo, Bulgaria, Germany, Spain and France. All cases in the UK are imported. The organism is found in more than 250 host animal species including wild and domestic animals, birds, fish, amphibians, protozoa and blood-sucking arthropods. In the USA the most important reservoirs of *F. tularensis* are cottontail rabbits, jackrabbits, hares and muskrats. In Scandinavia and Russia, hares and rabbits are important reservoirs. The modes of transmission to humans include tick or mosquito bites, contact with infected animal tissues, inhalation of infectious aerosols or ingestion of contaminated meat or water.

F. tularensis may survive in soil, water (possibly in association with free-living amebae) and animal carcasses for several weeks. In endemic areas, tularemia is seasonal with the majority of cases occurring during the late spring, summer and autumn. There are approximately 200 cases each year reported in the USA, with over 60% occurring in the southern and southern-central states of Missouri, Oklahoma, Arkansas, Texas and Kansas.

People who handle infected animals, including hunters, farmers and veterinary surgeons are at increased risk of infection. Laboratory workers are at high risk through handling infected laboratory animals or cultures of the organism. Person-to-person transmission of *Francisella tularensis* has not been documented.

TABLE 183-3 The Subspecies and Biovars of *Francisella tularensis*

Subspecies	Geographical Distribution	Virulence In Humans	Main Animal Hosts
F. tularensis (type A)			
Clade AI (sub-groups AIa and AIb)* Clade AII	Central USA (east of Rocky Mountains) Western USA	+++	Cottontail rabbits, jackrabbits, hares, ground squirrels
F. holarctica (type B)			
Biovar I Biovar II Biovar japonica	North America, Europe, Siberia, Eurasia, Japan	++	Beavers, voles, muskrats Hares Voles
F. mediasiatica	Central Asia	+	Rodents, rabbits
F. novicida†	North America, Australia, Thailand	+	?§

*Human infections with *F. tularensis* subspecies *tularensis* AIb run a fulminant course with a high mortality rate compared with infections due to AIa, AII or Type B strains.
†Less virulent. Infection mainly occurs in immunocompromised hosts.
§Infections associated with brackish water.

Pathogenicity

The infectious dose for humans depends on the subspecies and the route of entry. Inhalation of fewer than 10 organisms of *F. tularensis* subsp. *tularensis* can result in infection. The infecting dose rises to 10^8 when the organisms are ingested.

F. tularensis subsp. *tularensis* (type A) is more virulent to animals and humans than the other subspecies. The low infecting dose, aerosol transmission, high virulence and high mortality of consequent infection with *F. tularensis* subsp. *tularensis* mean that this organism is a potential bioweapon.[17]

The virulence of *F. tularensis* is based on its ability to survive and replicate within the cytosol of infected cells, including macrophages, hepatocytes and endothelial cells.[18] After entering the body, the organisms spread to the regional lymph nodes, from where they may disseminate via the lymphatic system or bloodstream to involve multiple organs. There is probably a transient bacteremia at this early stage. Intracellular survival is enabled by a number of virulence genes, including the 'macrophage growth locus' (mgl) A and B and the '*Francisella* pathogenicity island'. Organisms are protected from humoral antibodies, which are directed against carbohydrate antigens. Recovery from tularemia depends largely on cell-mediated immunity, which is directed against the protein antigens of the organism.

Prevention

Prevention of tularemia is best achieved by avoiding exposure to the organism. Gloves, masks and goggles should be worn when skinning or eviscerating animals. Animals that look sick should be left intact. Game meat should be thoroughly cooked and fresh water that is possibly contaminated should not be drunk. Ticks should be promptly removed and chemical insect repellants may be used.

There is no licensed vaccine available. To be effective a vaccine would need to elicit a T-cell memory response. The live attenuated vaccine (LVS) given to laboratory staff working with *F. tularensis* in the USA was withdrawn because of variable immunogenicity and risk of reversion to virulence. Killed and subunit vaccines have not been effective. A vaccine using an attenuated strain of Type A tularemia, SchuS4, appears to provide protection against parenteral and intranasal challenge with a fully virulent SchuS4 strain.[19]

Diagnostic Microbiology

F. tularensis is a Hazard Group 3 pathogen, so it is imperative that the laboratory is notified if tularemia is suspected so appropriate containment precautions can be taken. The detection of *F. tularensis* in a Gram-stained smear of aspirates or other samples is rarely successful.

Specialized culture media such as cysteine–glucose–blood agar or cysteine-enriched media, such as buffered charcoal yeast extract agar (BCYE), have been developed for *F. tularensis*. It also grows on chocolate blood agar supplemented with cysteine (e.g. IsoVitaleX™). Plates should be incubated at 98.6°F (37°F) with carbon dioxide-enriched air. *F. tularensis* grows slowly, taking 2–4 days to produce visible colonies, and incubation should be extended for 3 weeks. Colonies appear blue-gray, round, smooth and somewhat mucoid. They are β-hemolytic on blood-containing media. Identification can be confirmed by slide agglutination or fluorescent antibody staining. Alternatively, PCR targeting the *fopA* or *tul4* gene may be used.[20] Real-time PCR for *F. tularensis* is based on four target genes, *ISFtu2, 23kDA, tul4* and *fopA*[21] and real-time PCR has been used to differentiate subspecies *tularensis* and *holarctica*.

Antibody titers reach detectable levels 10–20 days post-infection. A fourfold rise in antibody titer or a single titer greater than 1:160 is considered diagnostic. ELISA is more sensitive than agglutination assays. IgG and IgM antibodies can persist for months or years and it may be difficult to distinguish past from current infection. Infections with *Brucella* spp. can give rise to antibodies that cross-react with *F. tularensis*.

Clinical Manifestations (see also Chapter 127)

The clinical manifestations of *F. tularensis* infection depend on the portal of entry, the virulence of the infecting strain, infecting dose and host immune status. Up to 30% of untreated infections can be lethal.

Management

Fluoroquinolones, such as ciprofloxacin, are effective treatment for uncomplicated tularemia. For the treatment of more severe cases, including pneumonic tularemia, aminoglycosides are indicated. A high rate of relapse has been associated with the use of tetracyclines. For postexposure prophylaxis, oral doxycycline or ciprofloxacin for 14 days should be considered.

Haemophilus spp.

Nature

Haemophilus spp. are small, pleomorphic, nonmotile, nonsporing gram-negative rods or GNCB. They are aerobic and facultatively anaerobic, and addition of 5–10% carbon dioxide to the incubation atmosphere may enhance growth. The oxidase and catalase reactions vary. The differential requirements for X and V factors are important criteria for defining species of *Haemophilus*. X factor can be provided by hemin, protoporphyrin IX or other iron-containing porphyrins. X-dependent *Haemophilus* spp. cannot synthesize protoporphyrin from δ-aminolevulinic acid, a process involving several enzyme-mediated steps, some or all of which may be defective. V factor is nicotinamide adenine dinucleotide (NAD) or NAD phosphate or certain unidentified precursors of these compounds. It is essential for the oxidation–reduction processes.

The species of *Haemophilus* associated with human infections are shown in Table 183-4. *Haemophilus influenzae* is the major human pathogen in the group. There are six distinct antigenic types of encapsulated *H. influenzae*, designated a–f. *H. influenzae* type b (Hib) has a polyribosyl-ribitol-phosphate (PRP) capsule and before the introduction of Hib conjugate vaccines, was associated with most invasive infections. There is considerable debate as to whether *H. aegyptius* (which is associated with purulent conjunctivitis) is a species distinct from *H. influenzae*. The syndrome of epidemic purpura fulminans and purulent conjunctivitis, known as Brazilian purpuric fever, was first described in Brazil in the 1980s and was caused by a single clone of *Haemophilus* (*H. influenzae* biogroup aegyptius).[22]

The name *Haemophilus quentini* has been proposed for variant strains of *H. influenzae* isolated from the genitourinary tract which may be associated with maternal-neonatal infections.[23] These strains are distinguishable from typical strains of nontypeable *Haemophilus influenzae* (NTHi) by multilocus enzyme electrophoresis, 16S rRNA gene sequence and DNA hybridization. Most of these strains were reported to be biotype IV and were described as a 'cryptic genospecies of *Haemophilus* biotype IV'. Subsequent studies, however, have reported more diverse *H. influenzae* biotypes causing such infections.

H. haemolyticus is a pharyngeal commensal of low pathogenicity, which can be hemolytic or nonhemolytic, and may be misidentified as *H. influenzae*.[24] V-factor requiring species of *Haemophilus* include *H. parainfluenzae, H. parahaemolyticus, H. paraphrohaemolyticus, H. pittmaniae* and *H. sputorum*.[23]

H. ducreyi, the cause of chancroid, is not closely related to the other *Haemophilus* spp.

H. aphrophilus and *H. paraphrophilus* have recently been combined as a single species and reassigned to the genus *Aggregatibacter* as *Aggregatibacter aphrophilus*.[23] This species forms part of the HACEK group (see below). *H. segnis* (*Aggregatibacter segnis*) is occasionally associated with acute appendicitis and bacteremia.

DNA sequencing is increasingly being used for identification and typing of *Haemophilus* spp. and MALDI-TOF is a valuable tool for

TABLE 183-4	Species of *Haemophilus* and *Aggregatibacter* Associated with Human Infection							
	REQUIREMENT FOR				**ACID FROM**			**IgA1 protease (probable virulence factor)**
Species	**X factor**	**V factor**	**CO_2**	**Hemolysis**	**Sucrose**	**Mannose**	**Lactose**	
H. influenzae	+	+	−	−	−	−	−	+
H. aegyptius	+	+	−	−	−	−	−	+
H. haemolyticus	+	+	−	+§	−	−	−	−
H. parainfluenzae	−	+	−	−	+	+	−	−
H. parahaemolyticus	−	+	−	+	+	−	−	+
H. paraphrohaemolyticus	−	+	−	+	+	−	−	−
H. sputorum	−	+	−	+	+	−	−	−
H. pittmaniae	−	+	−	+	+	+	−	−
H. ducreyi	+	−	−	v	−	−	−	−
*Aggregatibacter aphrophilus**	h	v	+	−	+	+	+	−
A. segnis†	+	−	−	−	w	w	−	−
A. actinomycetemcomitans	−	−	−	−	−	+	−	−

h, *A. aphrophilus* requires hemin for primary isolation; w, weak reaction; v, variable.
H. aphrophilus and *H. paraphrophilus* have been reassigned to the genus *Aggregatibacter* as *Aggregatibacter aphrophilus* sp. nov. comb.
†*H. segnis* has been reassigned to the genus *Aggregatibacter* as *Aggregatibacter segnis*.
§*H. haemolyticus* strains can be hemolytic or nonhemolytic.

identification in a clinical microbiology laboratory. Of note, the genome of *Haemophilus influenzae* strain Rd was the first bacterial genome to be fully sequenced.[25]

Epidemiology

Haemophilus influenzae is only found in humans and colonizes the throat and nasopharynx, and, to a lesser extent, the conjunctivae and genital tract. The respiratory tract is mainly colonized by *H. parainfluenzae* and nontypeable (noncapsulate) *H. influenzae* (NTHi). Carriage rates for Hib are low (3–5%).

The epidemiology of invasive infections caused by *H. influenzae* is distinct from noninvasive infections. NTHi is a major cause of mucosal infections such as otitis media, sinusitis, conjunctivitis and exacerbations of chronic obstructive pulmonary disease, associated with the formation of biofilms.[26]

Pathogenicity

H. influenzae is transmitted by aerosols of respiratory secretions or by direct contact with contaminated material. The primary event is colonization of the nasopharynx. Prior infection with respiratory viruses (e.g. influenza) predisposes to nasopharyngeal colonization by mechanisms including obstruction to the outflow of respiratory secretions, depression of local immunity and suppression of mucociliary clearance. Contiguous spread (usually of NTHi) may result in noninvasive mucosal infections including acute sinusitis and otitis media.

Colonization may be promoted by microbial factors such as fimbriae and other adhesins, lipo-oligosaccharide (LOS) and IgA1 protease.[26] LOS consists of two covalently linked moieties, lipid A (which mediates endotoxic effects) and core oligosaccharide. LOS is a ciliotoxin and is important for colonization, persistence and survival of the bacteria in the human host.

IgA1 protease inactivates secretory IgA, facilitating bacterial access to the mucosal surface. Fimbriae and the autotransporter proteins Hap, HMW1/HMW2 and Hia/Hsf are associated with binding to respiratory tract epithelium. Hap promotes bacterial entry into epithelial cells. HMW1/HMW2 proteins are expressed by the majority of NTHi but are not found in capsulate strains. Hia is found in nearly all NTHi. Its analog, Hif, is expressed in almost all capsulate strains. Possession of the outer membrane protein P2 is another important

virulence factor for NTHi. Lipoprotein D (LPD) impairs respiratory ciliary function.

In the pre-Hib vaccine era, invasive infections, notably meningitis and epiglottitis, were mainly caused by Hib and resulted from invasion of the bloodstream. The capsule of type b *H. influenzae* is the single most important virulence determinant for invasion because it protects the organism from phagocytosis and complement-mediated lysis. The rarity of infections in the first 2 months of life correlates with the presence of maternal antibodies to PRP, and the occurrence of infection in early infancy with the absence of antibodies having such specificity. As the mean level of PRP antibodies in the population rises, so Hib infections become less common. It is unclear whether natural antibody production is stimulated by exposure to Hib or to some other organism (e.g. *E. coli* K100) that possesses cross-reacting antigens.

With the widespread use of Hib conjugate vaccines, invasive Hib infections have become uncommon and the majority of invasive infections are caused by NTHi or other capsulated serotypes. Invasive NTHi infections mainly occur in very young infants and in the elderly. Pregnant women have an increased susceptibility to invasive NTHi disease, which is associated with miscarriage, premature labor and post-partum infection in the mother and the neonate.[27]

Prevention
VACCINATION

H. influenzae type b conjugate vaccines consist of the PRP covalently linked to a protein carrier, such as tetanus toxoid, diphtheria toxoid, a non-toxic mutant diphtheria and an outer membrane protein complex from *Neisseria meningitidis* group B. These vaccines produce a lasting anamnestic response, which is not age related. They can be given to infants as young as 2 months of age and are also effective in high-risk patients who have a poor response to polysaccharide vaccines. In the UK Hib vaccine is administered at 2, 3 and 4 months as a component of a pentavalent vaccine (diphtheria, tetanus, acellular pertussis, Hib and inactivated polio vaccine), with a booster dose (Hib combined with meningococcus C vaccine) at 12–13 months of age. Countries where Hib vaccine is routinely offered have witnessed a dramatic decline in the occurrence of Hib infections (Figure 183-4). Immunization of infants with conjugate Hib vaccine results in a reduction in the rate of nasopharyngeal colonization by Hib and a marked

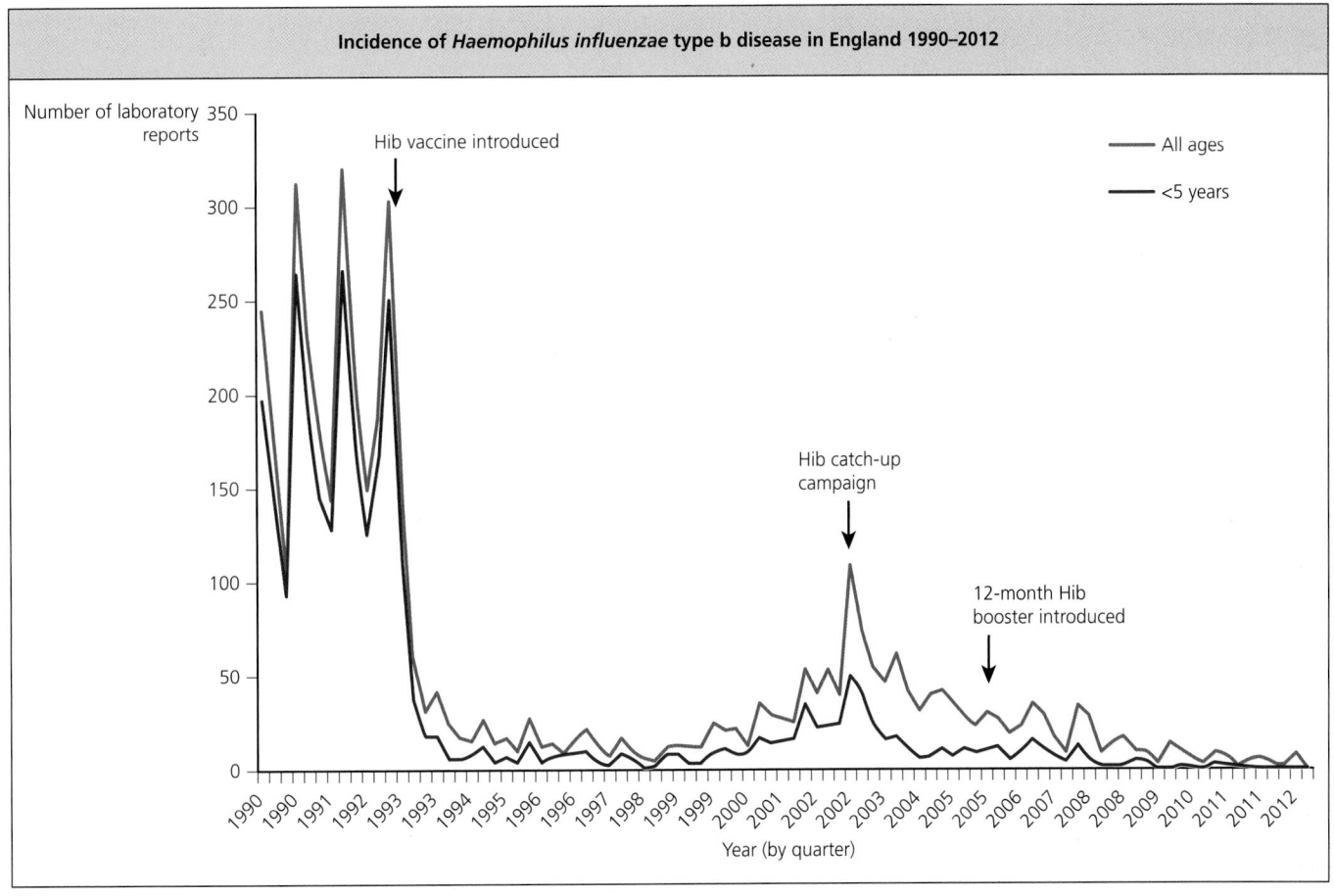

Incidence of *Haemophilus influenzae* type b disease in England 1990–2012

Number of laboratory reports

Hib vaccine introduced

All ages
<5 years

Hib catch-up campaign

12-month Hib booster introduced

Year (by quarter)

Figure 183-4   The incidence of *Haemophilus influenzae* type b disease in England, 1990–2012. Routine laboratory data combined with reference laboratory data. Data supplied by Public Health England.

herd immunity effect. Hib vaccine is recommended post splenectomy and for patients with functional asplenia, together with pneumococcal and meningococcal vaccines.

There is currently considerable interest in developing vaccines for NTHi.[28] A 10-valent pneumococcal conjugate vaccine, using *H. influenzae*-derived protein D as a carrier protein for the pneumococcal polysaccharide, showed protection against both pneumococcal and noncapsulate *H. influenzae* otitis media.[29] Outer membrane vesicles (OMVs) present a combination of multiple heterologous antigens to the immune system which may increase vaccine efficacy against heterologous strains.[30] Orally administered killed vaccines which aim to prevent acute exacerbations of chronic obstructive pulmonary disease are under investigation. Several other candidate antigens are being investigated (Table 183-5).[31]

CHEMOPROPHYLAXIS

Oral rifampin for 4 days is recommended for eradicating carriage of *H. influenzae* type b and has been used to prevent secondary infection in household and nursery contacts. Its effectiveness is unproven.

Diagnostic Microbiology

Gram-stained smears of clinical samples such as cerebrospinal fluid or pus may aid rapid diagnosis, although *H. influenzae* tends to stain poorly. Dilute carbol fuchsin is a better counterstain than neutral red or safranin. Rapid tests for Hib capsular antigens, such as latex agglutination or a PCR-based method, can be applied to clinical material. False-positive latex agglutination results have been reported in cerebrospinal fluid samples collected from children who had recently received Hib vaccine.

TABLE 183-5   Candidate Vaccine Antigens of Nontypeable *Haemophilus influenzae* (NThi)

Antigen	Protective In Animal Model	Comments
Lipo-oligosaccharide (LOS)	+	Common epitopes among NTHi strains
P6	+	Highly conserved lipoprotein
OMP26	+	Highly conserved
OMP P5	+	Highly conserved
Lipoprotein D (LPD)	+	Recombinant deacylated form (protein D) used as carrier protein for pneumococcal conjugate vaccine
OMP P2		>50% of total OMP of NTHi Heterogeneous and conserved regions
HtrA	±	
HMW1/HMW2	+	Found in >75% NTHi strains
P4 lipoprotein	+	Highly conserved
OMVs	+	Present a combination of multiple heterologous antigens

Chocolate agar is used most commonly to culture *Haemophilus* spp. The addition of bacitracin suppresses growth of other respiratory organisms, thus assisting the recovery of *H. influenzae* from respiratory samples. Cultures should be incubated at 98.6°F (37°C) in an aerobic atmosphere enriched with 5–10% carbon dioxide. After 24 hours of incubation, colonies of nontypeable *H. influenzae* (NTHi) are small, circular, smooth and pale gray. Capsulated strains produce somewhat larger, mucoid colonies, with a characteristic seminal odor. Phenotypic identification depends on growth factor requirement. To perform the 'disk test', the culture is plated onto nutrient agar with paper disks containing X factor alone, V factor alone, and both X and V factors. After overnight incubation, growth is observed around the disks supplying the required growth factor(s) (Figure 183-5). Besides *H. influ-*

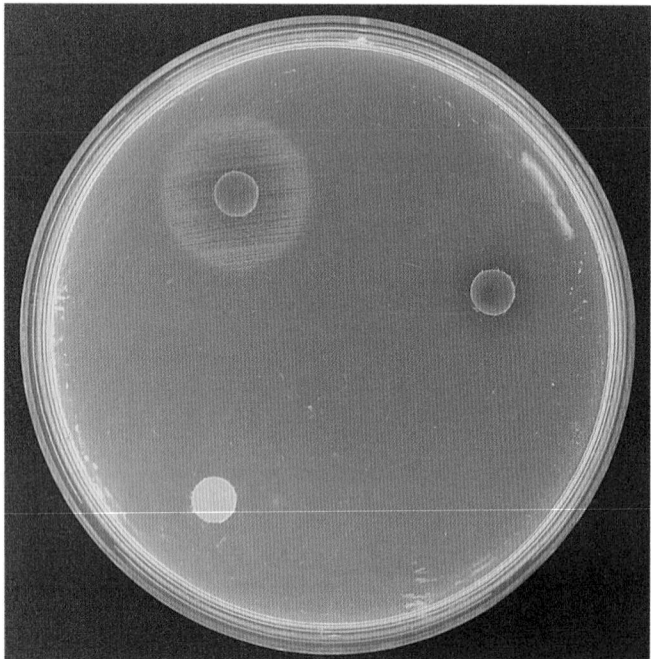

Figure 183-5   Growth factor requirement of *Haemophilus influenzae*. Strain of *H. influenzae* sown on Columbia agar plate. Filter paper disks containing X factor, V factor and both X and V factors were placed on the surface of the inoculated plate, but colonies of *H. influenzae* grow only around the disk with both X and V factors.

enzae, a second X- and V-factor dependent species, *H. haemolyticus*, is frequently found in the upper respiratory tract, and has long been regarded as a commensal. Until recently, microbiologists relied on the production of zones of β-hemolysis on horse blood agar to differentiate *H. haemolyticus* from NTHi. However, 10-40% of *H. haemolyticus* strains are nonhemolytic,[24] so a scheme including hpd- and iga-based PCR assays has been recommended to improve the identification of *H. haemolyticus*.[31]

The capsular serotype of *H. influenzae* is normally determined by slide agglutination using type-specific antisera. This method is prone to misinterpretation, with problems of autoagglutination, cross-reacting antisera and observer error. There are eight biotypes of *H. influenzae* (I-VIII) and eight biotypes of *H. parainfluenzae*, based on indole production, ornithine decarboxylase and urease activity. In clinical practice the designation of biotype is of little value. The definitive method of typing *H. influenzae* is capsular genotyping using a PCR-based method.

Clinical Manifestations

Haemophilus influenzae is associated with two distinct types of infection: invasive and noninvasive infections (Table 183-6).

INVASIVE INFECTIONS

Introduction of the Hib conjugate vaccine has resulted in a dramatic decline in the incidence of invasive *H. influenzae* infections. In countries with established Hib vaccination programmes, most invasive *H. influenzae* infections are caused by NTHi with a median age of onset of approximately 60 years. Disease in neonates is almost invariably due to NTHi. Epiglottitis is almost always caused by Hib, and has a peak incidence in children aged 2–3 years (see also Chapter 25). Most invasive NTHi cases in children (40–70%) and adults (60–80%) occur in individuals with underlying co-morbidities, particularly chronic respiratory disease and impaired immunity. *H. influenzae* type b (Hib) childhood meningitis and bacteremia remain common where the Hib vaccine is not used.

Other less common invasive *H. influenzae* infections include pneumonia, endocarditis, periorbital cellulitis, osteomyelitis, septic arthritis and a bacteremia with no obvious focus of infection. *H. influenzae* pneumonia is a major cause of mortality in young children in LMIC.

H. parainfluenzae is the most common cause of non-*H. influenzae* bacteremia and infective endocarditis. *Aggregatibacter aphrophilus* may cause infective endocarditis and cerebral abscesses, *Aggregatibacter actinomycetemcomitans* also causes infective endocarditis and is associated with periodontal disease. *Aggregatibacter segnis* is a rare cause of endocarditis, acute appendicitis and bacteremia.

TABLE 183-6	Spectrum of Infections Caused by *Haemophilus influenzae*		
Infection	**Age Group Affected**	**Details**	**Strains**
Invasive infections: Meningitis Epiglottitis Pneumonia Septic arthritis Osteomyelitis Cellulitis Bacteremia	90% children <4 years old* 10% older children and adults	Hib meningitis principally affects children aged 2 months–2 years. Epiglottitis occurs in slightly older children (peak incidence 2–3 years). Risk factors for invasive disease include overcrowding, attendance at daycare centers, chronic illness and poor access to healthcare facilities	~90% type b (Hib) ~10% NTHi 1% types e and f
Neonatal and maternal sepsis	Neonates Parturient mothers		>90% NTHi
Noninvasive respiratory infections: Otitis media Sinusitis Conjunctivitis Acute exacerbations of chronic bronchitis	Children and adults		>90% NTHi

Hib, *Haemophilus influenzae* type b.
NTHi, nontypeable (noncapsulated) *Haemophilus influenzae*.
*Figures reflect prevaccine incidence and age distribution.

NONINVASIVE INFECTIONS

Respiratory tract infections, acute exacerbations of chronic bronchitis, otitis media, sinusitis and conjunctivitis are usually caused by NTHi (see Chapter 27).

H. influenzae biogroup aegyptius is a distinct strain of nontypeable *H. influenzae*. For more than a century this organism was known to cause seasonal epidemics of acute purulent conjunctivitis, especially in warmer climates. In 1984, a virulent clone of *H. influenzae* biogroup aegyptius, emerged in Brazil as the cause of an acute febrile illness in children with a high mortality rate.[22] This infection, subsequently known as Brazilian purpuric fever, caused a series of outbreaks and sporadic cases almost exclusively in Brazil over the next decade but has virtually disappeared since then.

Unusual infections due to *H. influenzae* include urinary tract infections, cholecystitis, salpingitis and epididymo-orchitis. These may be associated with pre-existing damage, e.g. the presence of urinary stones or gallstones. *Haemophilus pittmaniae* is part of the normal oropharyngeal flora and may be isolated from various sites of infection, including blood and bile. It may cause respiratory tract infections in patients with chronic lung disease.

Management

Third-generation cephalosporins are the treatment of choice for *Haemophilus* meningitis. They are bactericidal for *H. influenzae*, achieve high concentrations in the meninges and cerebral tissues, and have proved highly effective in clinical practice. Ampicillin is also effective but resistance due to a β-lactamase is now high (for example, 13% of Hib strains in the UK are β-lactamase-producers). The β-lactamase is usually TEM-1 and, rarely, ROB-1. No TEM-type extended-spectrum β-lactamases (ESBLs) have yet been detected in *H. influenzae*. In addition to β-lactamase production, BLNAR (β-lactamase negative ampicillin resistant) strains occur, especially in Japan, South East Asia, Spain and France. BLNAR strains have mutations in the *fts*I gene, which encodes penicillin-binding protein 3 (PBP3) involved in septum formation of dividing cells. BLNAR are subdivided into genotypes I, II (low gBLNAR) and III (high gBLNAR) linked to different minimum inhibitory concentration (MIC) values: genotype I/II strains usually have ampicillin MIC values between 0.5–2 μg/mL and genotype III strains have MICs ranging between 1.0–16 μg/mL, often combined with reduced susceptibility to cephalosporins. There are also BLPACR, which are β-lactamase positive amoxicillin–clavulanic acid-resistant strains. These strains combine β-lactamase production with the presence of PBP3 mutations. Compared to BLNAR with the same PBP3 mutations but without a β-lactamase, these BLPACR strains have higher ampicillin MICs and similar amoxicillin–clavulanic acid and cephalosporin MICs. BLPACR can also be subdivided based on the specific *fts*I mutations.[26,32]

For the treatment of less serious respiratory infections, oral antibiotics including amoxicillin (if β-lactamase negative), amoxicillin–clavulanate, tetracycline or macrolides are usually effective.

Haemophilus ducreyi

Epidemiology

Haemophilus ducreyi (see Chapter 64) which causes chancroid, or soft sore, has declined in importance as a sexually transmitted pathogen in most countries where it was previously endemic (Central and Southern Africa, South East Asia, India, and the Caribbean). The epidemiology of chancroid is not well characterized because of syndromic management and inadequate diagnostic laboratories and surveillance systems. However, it still occurs sporadically in other countries, and is more common in non-white, uncircumcised males in low socioeconomic groups. Genital ulcers, including chancroid, are associated with increased transmission of HIV. Co-infection with *Treponema pallidum* or herpes simplex virus (HSV) is common. There have been recent reports of *H. ducreyi* causing chronic skin ulceration in Papua New Guinea.

Pathogenicity

The pathogenesis of chancroid is poorly understood. *Haemophilus ducreyi* gains access via a break in the epithelium and establishes infection in a focal area of mucosa or skin in the genital tract. Hemolysin is important in epithelial cell invasion and ulcer formation. Superoxide dismutase enzymes contribute to survival of the bacteria within the host. Potential virulence factors include fimbriae, pili, LPS, cytotoxins and outer membrane proteins (OMP).

Prevention

The use of condoms dramatically reduces the transmission of *H. ducreyi*. All sexual partners should be identified by contact tracing and treated. Education is vitally important. *H. ducreyi* hemolysin or hemoglobin receptor (HgbA) are possible candidates for vaccine development.

Diagnostic Microbiology

Gram-stained examination of material from ulcers or buboes may reveal pleomorphic GNCB or short rods. The organisms characteristically resemble 'shoals of fish'. However, microscopy is not recommended as a diagnostic test, as ulcer material is generally contaminated and direct Gram staining identifies only 10% of culture-positive cases.[33] Specimens collected from the base and margins of ulcers or by aspirating a bubo should be plated directly onto culture media and incubated in a humid atmosphere with 5% carbon dioxide at 91.4°F (33°C) for 2–3 days.

H. ducreyi is a fastidious organism that grows slowly on chocolate agar. Alternatives include GC agar supplemented with 1–2% bovine hemoglobin plus 5% fetal calf serum (or 0.2% activated charcoal) or Mueller–Hinton agar enriched with 5% chocolatized horse blood. Both of these media should be supplemented with 1% IsoVitaleX and 3 mg/L vancomycin to prevent overgrowth by gram-positive organisms.

The appearance of colonies of *H. ducreyi* varies with the medium used. Typically they are pinpoint, yellow-gray and translucent or semiopaque. Cultures often appear mixed, with a variety of colonial forms. The colonies are very cohesive and can be pushed across the agar surface with an inoculating loop.

H. ducreyi requires X factor but not V factor for growth. It can be identified using a number of rapid test systems (for example API-ZYM and RapIDNH) and MALDI-TOF (which can also identify strain-specific biomarkers from different patients). PCR is the most sensitive diagnostic technique and has been shown to be 95% sensitive compared to culture. Multiplex PCR tests that also amplify *Treponema pallidum* and HSV have been developed. PCR may be negative in some culture-positive cases due to the presence of Taq polymerase inhibitors in DNA extracts from genital ulcers. Antigen detection and serological methods have been described but are not in common use.

Sequencing of 16S rRNA and nucleic acid hybridization studies suggest *H. ducreyi* is a valid member of the family Pasteurellaceae, but is more similar to the *Actinobacillus* rather than the genus *Haemophilus*.

Clinical Manifestations

These are described in Chapter 64.

Management

The susceptibility of *H. ducreyi* to antimicrobial agents varies from one geographic area to another. Azithromycin, ceftriaxone or ciprofloxacin may be used, but strains with intermediate resistance to ciprofloxacin have been reported. HIV-infected patients require careful follow-up due to reports of treatment failure with single dose regimens. Buboes should be drained to prevent sinus formation.

HACEK Group

Nature

The HACEK group comprises the *Haemophilus* species, *Aggregatibacter actinomycetemcomitans* (formerly *Actinobacillus actinomycetemcomitans*), *Aggregatibacter aphrophilus* (formerly *Haemophilus aphrophilus* and *Haemophilus paraphrophilus*), *Aggregatibacter segnis* (formerly *H. segnis*), *Cardiobacterium hominis*, *Cardiobacterium valvarum*, *Eikenella corrodens* and *Kingella* species (*Kingella kingae*, *Kingella denitrificans* and *Kingella oralis*). This group of fastidious GNCB account for 1–3% of cases of infective endocarditis.[34]

All of the HACEK group are small, fastidious, pleomorphic GNCB and are commensals of the oropharyngeal/respiratory tract. They cause endocarditis and a range of other infections.[35-38] *K. kingae* has recently emerged as a major cause of septic arthritis in children less than 2 years of age[39] and has been associated with outbreaks of invasive infection in daycare facilities.[40] *K. kingae* has a polysaccharide capsule and virulence factors include type IV pili and an RTX toxin which is cytotoxic to synovial cells, respiratory epithelium, and macrophage-like cells.[41]

Diagnostic Microbiology

The slow growing HACEK group requires enriched culture media and an increased carbon dioxide tension. *Cardiobacterium hominis* and *Eikenella corrodens* usually require hemin (X factor) and carbon dioxide for primary isolation and may be misidentified as *Haemophilus* spp.; these requirements are lost on subculture. The colonies of *E. corrodens* have a characteristic 'bleach-like' odor and often 'pit' the surface of the agar. Older cultures of *E. corrodens* may appear yellow. Colonies of *K. kingae* produce slight β-hemolysis on blood agar and may be misidentified as pathogenic *Neisseria* species as they grow on *Neisseria* selective agar. *A. actinomycetemcomitans* colonies may be firm, adherent, star-shaped and difficult to remove from the agar surface. When *Aggregatibacter* spp. produce extracellular slime, cultures appear sticky on primary isolation. MALDI-TOF is a reliable tool for identification of HACEK organisms.[42]

Clinical Manifestations

These organisms cause infective endocarditis and a variety of other infections (see Chapter 51).

Prevention

Approximately 60% of cases of endocarditis caused by HACEK organisms are associated with poor oral hygiene, bad dentition or recent dental work.[43] Prevention of endocarditis should therefore be based on good dental and oral hygiene in patients at risk of endocarditis.

Management

The treatment of endocarditis caused by HACEK organisms should be based on antimicrobial susceptibility tests, including tests for β-lactamase activity. Currently, third-generation cephalosporins are the agents of choice. While *Eikenella corrodens* is generally susceptible to penicillin, broad-spectrum antibiotics are usually used to treat mixed infections, such as human bites.

Legionella spp.

Nature

Legionella spp. are slender, aerobic, noncapsulated, nonspore-forming, pleomorphic gram-negative coccobacilli. They may stain poorly in clinical material but can be filamentous in older cultures. Basic fuchsin may be a better counterstain. *Legionella* are motile with a single polar flagellum.

Legionella can grow in the temperature range 68–107.6°F (20–42°C). They are nutritionally fastidious and cannot be cultured on

TABLE 183-7	*Legionella* Species Associated With Human Disease	
Species	**Number of Serogroups**	
Legionella pneumophila	16	
Legionella anisa	1	
Legionella bozemanii	2	
Legionella cincinnatiensis	1	
Legionella dumoffii	1	
Legionella feeleii	2	
Legionella gormanii	1	
Legionella hackeliae	2	
Legionella jordanis	1	
Legionella longbeachae	2	
Legionella lansingensis	1	
*Legionella lytica**	1	
Legionella maceachernii	1	
Legionella micdadei	1	
Legionella oakridgensis	1	
Legionella parisiensis	1	
Legionella sainthelensi	2	
Legionella tucsonensis	1	
Legionella wadsworthii	1	

*Formerly called *Legionella*-like amebal pathogen (LLAP).

ordinary media. They generally grow well on BCYE supplemented with L-cysteine, α-ketoglutarate and ferric ions, adjusted to pH 6.9. Some species of *Legionella* grow poorly on BCYE but can be isolated by co-cultivation with amebae. Originally called *Legionella*-like amebal pathogens (LLAP), these have been renamed *L. lytica*, *L. drozanskii*, *L. falloni* and *L. rowbothamii*.[44]

There are more than 50 species of *Legionella* and human infections have been documented for 19 of these species (Table 183-7). Infections due to species other than *L. pneumophila* are rare and usually occur in immunocompromised hosts. The exception is *Legionella longbeachae* serogroup 1 which causes community-acquired pneumonia in Western Australia, possibly associated with handling compost and soil.[45]

Epidemiology

Legionella spp. are distributed worldwide, in fresh water streams, rivers, ponds, lakes and mud. The organisms can survive in moist environments for long periods and can withstand temperatures of 32–154°F (0–68°C) and chlorination. They proliferate in air-conditioning cooling towers, hot water systems, shower heads, taps, whirlpool spas and respiratory ventilators, and form biofilms which render them less susceptible to biocides and chlorine. The growth of *Legionella* spp. is aided by coexisting bacteria and algae, which provide nutrients, and protozoa, in which the *Legionella* spp. can live and multiply.

The exact incidence of *Legionella* infections is unknown. Exposure to *Legionella* spp. occurs fairly frequently and serological surveys suggest that asymptomatic infection and seroconversion are common. Large-scale surveys of pneumonia suggest that *Legionella* spp. cause 2–5% of community-acquired pneumonia and up to 30% of nosocomial pneumonia.

Cases may be sporadic or occur as part of an outbreak. The original description of Legionnaires' disease was of an outbreak of a febrile respiratory illness in delegates at an American Legion convention in Philadelphia in 1976. A total of 221 people developed pneumonia and 34 died.[46] Retrospective studies have revealed that the first proven case occurred in 1947 and the first known epidemic was in 1965 in Washington, DC.

Legionnaire's disease usually occurs in the middle-aged and elderly, especially in smokers, the immunocompromised and people with impaired respiratory and cardiac function. Cases have been documented in children. Person-to-person spread has not been demonstrated.

Legionella is a good example of an organism that has been present in the environment for a long time but has been brought into close contact with humans as a result of technical developments. Organisms are disseminated via contaminated water droplets from nebulizers and humidifiers and in aerosols from cooling towers, whirlpools and evaporative condensers. Infection arises from inhalation of contaminated aerosols, direct instillation during surgery or possibly by ingestion of contaminated water. Hospital equipment that has been rinsed in tap water prior to use may be a source of infection.

L. pneumophila contains 16 different serogroups. More than 80% of human infections are caused by *Legionella pneumophila* serogroup 1. This serogroup can be divided into subtypes, on the basis of monoclonal antibody typing or genotyping, which is important during outbreak investigation.

Pathogenicity

Legionella spp. are transmitted to humans via aerosols. Droplet nuclei of less than 5 μm reach the alveoli, where alveolar macrophages ingest the organisms. *Legionella* is a facultative intracellular parasite and multiplies freely within the macrophages. The bacteria bind to alveolar macrophages via complement receptors and are engulfed in phagosomes. The bacteria resides in a specialized 'Legionella-containing vacuole' (LCV), and phagolysosome fusion is inhibited. LCVs provide an intracellular niche for replication and help prevent release of bacterial components into the cytoplasm. The Dot/Icm type IVB secretion system effector SdhA maintains LCV integrity (see below). The bacteria respond to depletion of nutrients by expressing virulence proteins, which cause host cell lysis and release of bacteria. These bacteria are then taken up by other macrophages and the infection cycle is repeated.[47] This process produces chemotactic substances that attract polymorphonuclear leukocytes and monocytes, and the inflammatory response results in a destructive pneumonia.

There are two phases in the life cycle of *Legionella pneumophila* – an intracellular replicative phase (RP) and an infectious nonreplicating transmissive phase (TP). Bacteria in the RP are avirulent, nonflagellated and sodium resistant, whereas those in the TP are virulent, flagellated and motile. Complex regulatory systems govern the differentiation between these two phases.[48]

Multiple virulence factors are involved in initial attachment and early intracellular infection, including type IV pili, Hsp60, the pore-formation protein RtxA, the macrophage infectivity potentiator Mip and the macrophage-specific infectivity protein MilA. The *icm* (intracellular multiplication) and *dot* (defect in organelle trafficking) groups of genes form a type IV secretion system and enable bacterial survival and intracellular replication. Other effectors (including RalF LidA; LepA/B), regulators (RpoS; LetA), a type II protein secretion system, iron-uptake systems and iron-acquisition genes (*feoB*; *iraA*; *ccmC*) have been described.

Prevention

Prevention of legionellosis depends upon identifying the environmental source and reducing colonization. The simple preventive measure of keeping water from hot taps 'hot' and water from cold taps 'cold' should always be observed. Periodic superheating and flushing of water supplies may be useful during an outbreak. The continuous chlorination of hot and cold water service systems, after initial disinfection, is not recommended because chlorine has a limited ability to penetrate biofilms and inactivate sessile micro-organisms. Treatment using copper/silver ionization or chlorine dioxide can be used. Despite numerous costly measures it is often impossible to eliminate *Legionella* spp. from water supplies.[49]

New water systems should be designed to minimize the risk of heavy colonization with *Legionella* spp., avoiding 'dead spaces', stagnation, materials that support the growth of *Legionella* spp. and the build-up of sediment. Regular monitoring for *Legionella* spp. is advisable, particularly in high-risk areas.

Vaccination may be a future option for highly susceptible patients.

Diagnostic Microbiology

Legionella spp. can be cultured from sputum, endotracheal aspirates, bronchoalveolar lavages, lung biopsies and pleural fluid. Sputum samples should be diluted in distilled water because saline can inhibit some *Legionella* spp. Gram-stained smears may reveal poorly staining gram-negative rods or coccobacilli. Direct immunofluorescence using a monoclonal antibody to a major outer membrane protein common to all serogroups of *L. pneumophila* gives a rapid diagnosis, but is less sensitive than culture and only detects *L. pneumophila*.

Cultures should therefore also be carried out, using a selective and non-selective agar incubated at 98.6°F (37°C) in 2–5% carbon dioxide for up to 14 days. *Legionella* species will grow on *Legionella* agar base (BCYE) supplemented with L-cysteine. Those colonies that fail to grow on the BCYE without L-cysteine, are presumptive *Legionella*. Growth on both plates indicates it is not *Legionella*.

Colonies of *Legionella* may take 3–5 days to appear, and have a ground-glass appearance, which may be white, gray, pale blue or purple-tinged (Figure 183-6). Some species, other than *L. pneumophila*, fluoresce blue-white under long-wave UV light while others fluoresce dull yellow or brick red. *Legionella lytica* (and other LLAPs) can be isolated on BCYE if the plates are incubated at 86°F (30°C).

Colonies that grow on L-cysteine-containing BCYE, but not on BCYE lacking L-cysteine, which are catalase-positive, oxidase-negative and have characteristic Gram stain, should be regarded as presumptive *Legionella* spp. Biochemical tests contribute little to identification. Serologic typing using direct or indirect fluorescent antibody tests with polyclonal or monoclonal antibodies will confirm the identity. Sequence analysis of the *mip* gene can be used to differentiate most *Legionella* spp.[50] and real-time PCR-based on the *mip* gene can provide a rapid diagnosis.

Urine samples can be examined for *Legionella* soluble antigen using either an enzyme immunoassay or a radioimmunoassay kit, or commercially available immunochromatographic tests. These rapid tests are specific for *L. pneumophila* serogroup 1, which is most common,

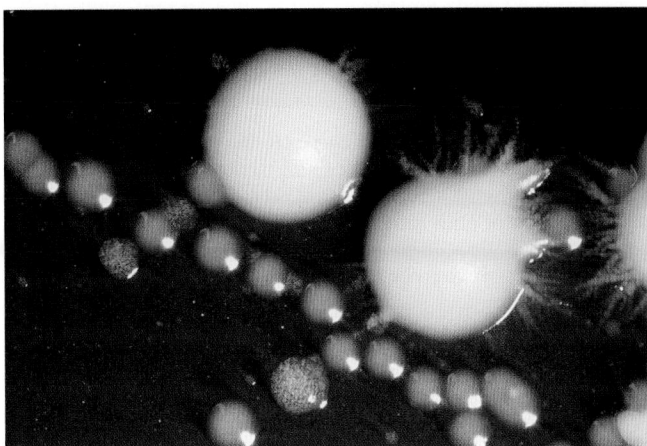

Figure 183-6 Colonies of *Legionella pneumophila* on BCYE agar, showing the typical ground-glass appearance. *(With permission from Harrison T.G., Taylor A.G., eds. A laboratory manual for Legionella. Chichester: John Wiley; 1998.)*

but will not detect other species. The antigen persists in urine for 1–2 weeks, and occasionally for months.

The most commonly used serological technique is an indirect fluorescent antibody test (IFAT), but ELISA or rapid microagglutination tests are also available. A fourfold or greater rise in antibody titer in a patient who has had clinical pneumonia indicates *Legionella* infection. Serology is useful in epidemiological studies, rather than diagnosis of acute diseases, as it may take weeks or months for the antibody titer to rise, and antibodies can persist for years. The only validated serologic test is for *L. pneumophila* serogroup 1, and patients with *Campylobacter* infections may have cross-reacting antibodies.

Clinical Manifestations

Asymptomatic *Legionella* infections are relatively common. Symptomatic *Legionella* infection can present as a severe pneumonia (Legionnaires' disease) or an acute influenza-like illness (Pontiac fever). See Chapter 28.

Management

For an acutely ill patient with Legionnaires' disease, quinolones are the treatment of choice; macrolides are an alternative. The co-administration of rifampin does not appear to give any additional benefit. Cases of Pontiac fever usually resolve spontaneously.

Moraxella spp.

Nature

Moraxella spp. are gram-negative short rods, coccobacilli or, in the case of *M. catarrhalis*, diplococci (GNDC) that phenotypically resemble *Neisseria* spp. diplococci (GNDC) that phenotypically resemble *Neisseria* spp. They are strictly aerobic, oxidase-positive, catalase-positive, DNAse-positive, non-encapsulated and asaccharolytic. *Moraxella catarrhalis* causes upper and lower respiratory tract infections in children and adults.

Moraxella lacunata is associated with conjunctivitis. *Moraxella nonliquefaciens* is an upper respiratory tract commensal which may be a secondary invader in respiratory infections. *Moraxella osloensis* is a genital tract commensal which may be misidentified as *Neisseria gonorrhoeae*. *M. osloensis* has also been reported in cases of septic arthritis, osteomyelitis and bacteremia. *Moraxella atlantae* can cause bacteremia in immunocompromised patients.

Epidemiology

Moraxella catarrhalis is exclusively found in humans. Up to 75% of children are colonized within the first year of life. Adults with chronic lung disease are more likely to be carriers than healthy adults. Nasopharyngeal carriage rates are significantly higher in autumn and winter.[51]

Pathogenicity

M. catarrhalis is a mucosal pathogen, causing infections of the upper respiratory tract in young children and the lower respiratory tract in adults with chronic lung disease. *M. catarrhalis* is the third most common cause of otitis media in children (after *Haemophilus influenzae* and *Streptococcus pneumoniae*). Binding of *M. catarrhalis* to host epithelial cells and extracellular matrix (ECM) is multifactorial. Adhesins include ubiquitous surface proteins (Usp) A1, A2 and A2H, *M. catarrhalis* IgD-binding protein hemagglutinin (MID/Hag), OMP CD and OMP M35, Mha B1 and B2 and C, OlpA, McaP and LOS.[52] Following colonization of the host epithelium and ECM, *M. catarrhalis* invade host cells, enabling evasion of both humoral and cellular immunity and antimicrobial therapy. The organisms persist within the cytoplasm in vacuoles. *M. catarrhalis* can form biofilms, which are important in the development of acute and chronic respiratory mucosal infections.

TABLE 183-8	Candidate Vaccine Antigens of *Moraxella catarrhalis*	
Antigen	**Action**	**Comments**
UspA1, A2 and A2H	Adhesin, interfere with complement-mediated killing	Highly immunogenic Contains both conserved and variable regions
MID/Hag	IgD binding Adhesin Hemagglutinin	Highly immunogenic Contains both conserved and variable regions
McaP	Adhesin, transporter	Highly conserved
OMP CD	Porin, mucin-binding	Highly conserved
OMP M35	? porin	Highly conserved
MhaB1, MhaB2, MhaC	Filamentous haemagglutinin, adhesion	–
OlpA	?	Highly conserved Immunogenic
TbpA, TbpB	Transferrin-binding proteins	Immunogenic
LbpA, LbpB	Lactoferrin-binding proteins	Immunogenic
OMP B2/CopB	Iron acquisition	Immunogenic
OMP E	? porin	Immunogenic
LOS A, LOS B, LOS C	Lipo-oligosaccharide,? adhesin	Immunogenic

Prevention

A number of vaccine candidates are under development or clinical testing. However the phase-variable expression of several important virulence factors (e.g. UspA1, UspA2, UspA2H, MID/Hag) and high genotypic heterogeneity of *M. catarrhalis* suggest that a multicomponent vaccine will be required to prevent colonization and pathogenesis (Table 183-8).[53]

Diagnostic Microbiology

M. catarrhalis grows well on blood and chocolate agar, producing small, nonhemolytic, grayish-white colonies that slide across the agar surface, like a hockey puck, when pushed with a bacteriologic loop. Gram-stained films reveal GNDC but *M. catarrhalis* often resists decolorization and thus may appear gram-positive. *M. catarrhalis* is DNAse positive, reduces nitrate and hydrolyses tributyrin (enabling differentiation from most *Neisseria* spp.). PCR (multiplexed with other respiratory pathogens, or bacteria causing middle ear infections) and MALDI-TOF are useful diagnostic tools.

Clinical Manifestations (see also Chapter 26)

M. catarrhalis causes upper respiratory tract infections, otitis media and sinusitis in children. In adults *M. catarrhalis* is associated with acute exacerbations of chronic bronchitis, pneumonia or invasive infections, including bacteremia, meningitis, septic arthritis and endocarditis.

Management

Most strains of *M. catarrhalis* are β-lactamase-positive. The β-lactamase enzymes (BRO-1 and BRO-2) are unique to this genus and are inducible; therefore ampicillin therapy should be avoided.[54] Many infections due to *M. catarrhalis* can be treated with oral antibiotics, such as amoxicillin–clavulanate. Other options include tetracyclines, macrolides and fluoroquinolones, although antibiotic resistance to these agents has been reported.

Pasteurella spp.

Nature

Pasteurella spp. are very small, nonmotile, nonspore-forming gram-negative bacteria that are coccoid, oval or rod-shaped. *Pasteurella* spp. grow on ordinary laboratory media at 98.6°F (37°C), and most species are catalase-positive and oxidase-positive. There are 15–20 species currently included in the genus *Pasteurella*, but some are more closely related genotypically to *Actinobacillus*. The type species is *P. multocida*, which is subdivided into four subspecies – *multocida, septica, gallicida* and *tigris*.

Epidemiology

Pasteurella spp. are distributed worldwide. They are commensals or parasitic organisms in the upper respiratory tract and gastrointestinal tracts of many domestic and wild animals and birds.

Many *Pasteurella* spp. are opportunistic pathogens that can cause endemic disease and are associated increasingly with epizootic outbreaks. *Pasteurella multocida* is found in the oropharynx of 50–90% of domestic cats, 50–70% of dogs and 50% of pigs. It causes hemorrhagic sepsis and bronchopneumonia in cattle and water buffalo, pneumonia in pigs and sheep, swine atrophic rhinitis, snuffles in rabbits and fowl, and fowl cholera in chickens, ducks and turkeys. It is generally carried asymptomatically by cats and dogs, and humans become infected through contact with infected animals.

Pasteurella multocida can remain viable in soil and water for up to 4 weeks and may survive in animal carcasses for up to 3 months. Most human infections are caused by *P. multocida* subsp. *multocida* and *P. multocida* subsp. *septica*. Occasionally, *Pasteurella canis, Pasteurella dagmatis* or *Pasteurella stomatis* may be implicated.

Pathogenicity

Pasteurella multocida is transmitted to humans by contact with infected animals, usually following bites or scratches from cats or dogs. Respiratory tract infections may occur through airborne transmission (see Chapter 73). Occasionally, an animal source of infection is not documented.

Virulence in *P. multocida* is associated with the degree of encapsulation, which prevents phagocytosis. There are five serogroups based on capsular antigens – A, B, D, E and F – and 16 serovars (1–16) based on lipopolysaccharide (LPS) antigens. Capsular types A and D produce a dermonecrotic toxin (PMT), encoded by the *toxA* gene, which modulates the immune response. Enhanced survival in the host environment also depends on membrane lipopolysaccharide that confers serum resistance, iron-acquisition mechanisms that enable growth, surface components such as fimbriae, which provide adherence properties, extracellular matrix-degrading enzymes, such as neuraminidases, hyaluronidases and proteases that facilitate colonization and/or dissemination.[55]

Prevention

The only way of effectively preventing *Pasteurella* infections is avoiding contact with domestic or wild animals. Prophylactic antibiotics may be indicated after cat and dog bites, particularly if the patient is immunocompromised or diabetic or the wound affects the hands or face. Vaccine research is focused on controlling animal disease, as the incidence of human infections is relatively low.

Diagnostic Microbiology

A clinical history of animal bites should alert the laboratory to the possibility of *Pasteurella* spp. After 24 hours of culture on blood agar plates at 98.6°F (37°C) *P. multocida* appear as small, gray, nonhemolytic colonies, with a strong odor of indole. *P. multocida* does not grow on MacConkey agar, but can grow poorly on some cystine lactose electrolyte deficient (CLED) agars. The organisms often show bipolar staining in methylene blue preparations. Identification can be confirmed by biochemical tests, serology or MALDI-TOF.

Clinical Manifestations

Pasteurella multocida causes opportunistic soft tissue infections in humans, especially the elderly and immunocompromised. Up to 75% of cat bites and 50% of dog bites are contaminated with *P. multocida*. The infection may spread rapidly along fascial planes. Patients with underlying respiratory disease or cirrhosis are more susceptible to respiratory infections and systemic infections respectively (see Chapter 73).

Management

Penicillin is the treatment of choice for *Pasteurella* infections. Other agents with good activity include ampicillin, amoxicillin–clavulanate, cefuroxime and ciprofloxacin. Broad-spectrum antibiotics are usually recommended for infected animal bites, which are often polymicrobial.

Yersinia spp.

Nature

Yersinia spp. are members of the Enterobacteriaceae. They are short, pleomorphic gram-negative rods or GNCB, which often exhibit bipolar staining. *Yersinia pestis* is nonmotile. Other species are nonmotile at 98.6°F (37°C) but motile at temperatures less than 86°F (30°C) by means of peritrichous flagella. They are nonlactose fermenters, oxidase-negative and catalase-positive. *Yersinia pestis* is urease-negative; *Y. enterocolitica* and *Y. pseudotuberculosis* are both urease-positive. *Yersinia* spp. grow on simple laboratory media and are tolerant of bile salts. The optimal temperature for growth is 82–86°F (27.8–30°C). They do not form spores or capsules, but *Y. pestis* produces a capsule-like envelope. They share antigens with other members of the Enterobacteriaceae.

In total, there are 11 species of *Yersinia*, three of which are important human pathogens associated with zoonotic infections – *Y. pestis* causes plague and *Y. pseudotuberculosis* and *Y. enterocolitica* give rise to yersiniosis. These two diseases are very different so are described separately below. Genomic studies suggest that *Y. pseudotuberculosis* (serotype O:1b) is the direct evolutionary ancestor of *Y. pestis*.[56] This occurred 15–20 000 years ago by lateral gene transfer and gene inactivation. The acquisition of the pFra plasmid by *Y. pestis*, plus the ability to express chromosomally-encoded proteins not expressed in *Y. pseudotuberculosis*, conferred transmissibility from one mammalian host to another via a vector flea.

Yersiniosis

The clinical features of yersiniosis range from gastroenteritis, enterocolitis, mesenteric adenitis, reactive arthritis to sepsis (see Chapters 43 and 47). Recipients of blood transfusions, or patients with iron overload, are at particular risk of infection with this siderophilic bacterium.

EPIDEMIOLOGY

Yersinia enterocolitica is harbored in the gastrointestinal tract of a range of mammals, including rodents, cattle, sheep, pigs, cats and dogs. Infected animals tend to become chronic carriers and excrete large numbers of bacteria, which may contaminate water and dairy products. Humans are infected by eating inadequately cooked meat (especially pork) or other contaminated food, or through contact with an infected domestic animal. In the USA, outbreaks associated with dairy products, chocolate and milk have been reported. The ability of *Y. enterocolitica* to grow at 39°F (4°C) means that refrigerated meat and meat products can become a potent source of infection. *Yersinia enterocolitica* sepsis has been reported following transfusion of blood stored for more than 3 weeks at 39°F (4°C).

Yersinia enterocolitica are classified phenotypically into six bio-groups, five of which (1B and 2–5) are regarded as pathogens. There are more than 57 'O' serogroups, based on the lipopolysaccharide surface antigen, only a few of which have been associated with human or animal disease. In Europe, serogroup O:3 is most important followed by O:9, whereas in the USA, where yersiniosis is less common, serogroup O:8 predominates.

Yersinia pseudotuberculosis infection is less common. The organism is harbored in the gastrointestinal tract of rodents, farm animals and birds. Human infections have been reported worldwide, but as with *Y. enterocolitica*, it is most common in northern Europe.

PATHOGENICITY

Yersinia enterocolitica and *Y. pseudotuberculosis* usually enter the body via the gastrointestinal tract. Organisms invade the ileal mucosa via specialized follicle-associated epithelial cells (M cells) involved in antigen uptake. Adherence and invasion of epithelial cells requires two chromosomally-encoded proteins, Invasin and Ail.[57] Following invasion the bacteria enter Peyer's patches and macrophages, and can survive intracellularly and multiply. In Peyer's patches the organisms express Yad A, which protects them against phagocytosis. Yad A and Ail facilitate dissemination of bacteria to regional lymph nodes. Yad A also helps adhesion to collagen, which is crucial in the development of reactive arthritis in *Y. pseudotuberculosis* infection.

Y. enterocolitica usually causes acute gastroenteritis, while *Y. pseudotuberculosis* infection causes mesenteric adenitis, which can mimic acute appendicitis. Systemic dissemination may cause sepsis and splenic/hepatic abscesses. A reactive polyarthritis can occur, particularly in HLA-B27 positive patients. Erythema nodosum is also a recognized post-infectious complication. A clone of *Y. pseudotuberculosis* which produces a superantigenic exotoxin mitogen (YPM) causes a toxic-shock like syndrome called Far East scarlet-like fever (or Izumi fever in Japan).[58]

PREVENTION

Prevention of yersiniosis depends on good animal husbandry and careful slaughtering techniques. Meat should not be consumed raw and should not be stored at 39°F (4°C) for prolonged periods before consumption. There is no effective vaccine.

DIAGNOSTIC MICROBIOLOGY

Material for culture includes stool, blood, lymph nodes, abscesses and food samples. Specimens should be cultured on blood and MacConkey agars at 80°F (26.7°C) for 24 hours. A selective medium, CIN (cefsulodin, irgasan, novobiocin), is available.

TABLE 183-9	Key Virulence Factors of *Yersinia* species					
	Location	*Y. pestis*	*Y. enterocolitica*	*Y. pseudotuberculosis*	Action	
Phospholipase D	pFra plasmid	+	–	–	Promotes survival of *Y. pestis* in flea vector	
F1 antigen	pFra plasmid	+	–	–	Fibrillar capsule inhibits macrophage activity	
Plasminogen activator (Pla)	pPCP1 plasmid	+	–	–	Activates mammalian plasminogen and anticomplementary serum resistance. Promotes dissemination from subcutaneous inoculation of *Y. pestis*	
Yersinia outer protein (YOPs) Yad A	Plasmid encoded	-	+	+	Invasion epithelial cells	
Lipopolysaccharide	Chromosomal	+	+	+	Endotoxin	
Yersiniabactin	Chromosomal	+	+	+	Siderophore-essential for full virulence of *Y. pestis* by subcutaneous inoculation	
YOPs	Chromosomal	+	+	+		
Yad BC		+	+	+	Adhesion	
YopH		+	+	+	Antiphagocytic	
YopE		+	+	+	Antiphagocytic	
YopT		+	+	+	Antiphagocytic	
YpKA/YopO					Antiphagocytic	
pH 6 antigen	Chromosomal	+	+	+	Fimbrial adhesin. Binds host lipoprotein. Antiphagocytic	
Invasin	Chromosomal	–	+	+	Invasion of epithelial cells	
Ail	Chromosomal	–	+	+	Host cell attachment and serum resistance	
HPI (high pathogenicity island)	Chromosomal	+ (*pgm* locus)*	Biotype 1B	Serotype O1	Iron uptake	

pgm locus includes (i) *hms* (hemin storage); (ii) *irp1* and *irp2* (iron-repressible high molecular weight proteins HNWP1 and HMWP2) and (iii) *fyuA* or *psn* gene (ferric yersiniabactin uptake or pesticin sensitivity).

Cold enrichment of heavily contaminated samples such as feces involves inoculation into phosphate-buffered saline and incubation at 39°F (4°C) for at least 3 weeks. To reduce contamination the broth can be treated with potassium hydroxide. The broth is subcultured at weekly intervals on to MacConkey or CIN agar. *Y. enterocolitica* colonies give a 'bulls-eye' appearance on CIN agar, while *Y. pseudotuberculosis* colonies are smaller on CIN, with a deep-red center and a sharp border surrounded by a translucent zone. Confirmation of identification is usually by biochemical or molecular tests or MALDI-TOF. The serotype of *Yersinia* can be determined using slide agglutination tests. A serologic diagnosis depends on demonstrating a significant rise of serotype-specific antibodies. *Yersinia pseudotuberculosis* is rarely isolated from feces.

CLINICAL MANIFESTATIONS

Yersiniosis encompasses a variety of clinical presentations including gastroenteritis, enterocolitis, mesenteric adenitis, and reactive arthritis.

MANAGEMENT

Yersinia enteritis and mesenteric adenitis do not generally require antimicrobial chemotherapy. Sepsis, extra-intestinal foci of infection and enteritis in immunocompromised patients should be treated with antimicrobials, such as aminoglycosides, quinolones, tetracyclines or third-generation cephalosporins. *Yersinia pseudotuberculosis* is usually sensitive to benzylpenicillin and ampicillin.

Plague

Plague is a zoonotic infection caused by *Y. pestis*, and has caused devastating pandemics such as the 'Plague of Justinian' in 541–3CE and the Black Death of the Middle Ages. Plague is still responsible for many thousands of human infections annually.[59] The clinical features, pathogenesis, epidemiology and management of plague are discussed in detail in Chapter 126.

Y. pestis possesses unique proteins associated with virulence, including Pla, Yad A, and Yad C (Table 183-9).[60,61] The key step in evolution of virulence appears to be the acquisition of the Fra plasmid, which together with the expression of chromosomal proteins not expressed in *Y. pseudotuberculosis* conferred the transmissibility from mammalian host to mammalian host via vector fleas.[56]

DIAGNOSTIC MICROBIOLOGY

Plague should be suspected in febrile patients exposed to flea bites or rodents in endemic areas. There is a considerable risk of laboratory-acquired infection, so high-risk samples must be handled in a containment level 3 laboratory by experienced trained personnel. Gram stain of smears taken from bubo aspirates, blood, sputum or cerebrospinal fluid may reveal pleomorphic GNCB with rounded ends. Wright–Giemsa or Wayson staining may demonstrate bipolar staining. *Yersinia pestis* appear light blue with dark blue polar bodies. Direct immunofluorescence of smears may be beneficial.

Culture of material on blood or MacConkey agars or in broth cultures, at 80°F (26.7°C), may reveal tiny, translucent, nonhemolytic colonies after 24 hours. After further incubation the colonies enlarge and become opaque. *Yersinia pestis* grows poorly on MacConkey agar and the colonies tend to autolyse after 2–3 days. In fluid culture *Y. pestis* tends to form chains.

Typically, *Y. pestis* is oxidase-negative, catalase-positive, urea-negative and indole-negative. Strains may be misidentified as *Y. pseudotuberculosis* or other Enterobacteriaceae. Definitive identification can be confirmed by immunofluorescence of F1 antigen or molecular techniques, such as real-time PCR for *Y. pestis pla* gene.[62] A serologic diagnosis can be made by a passive hemagglutination test using tanned sheep red cells to which F1 antigen has been adsorbed, or a complement fixation test. ELISA tests for antibodies to F1 antigen are useful in large-scale seroepidemiologic surveys.

References available online at expertconsult.com.

KEY REFERENCES

Achtman M., Zurth K., Morelli G., et al.: *Yersinia pestis*: the cause of plague is a recently emerged clone of *Yersinia pseudotuberculosis*. *Proc Natl Acad Sci USA* 1999; 96: 14043-14048.

Adalga A.A., Toner E., Inglesby T.V.: Clinical management of potential bioterrorism-related conditions. *N Engl J Med* 2015; 372:954-962.

Brouqui P., Raoult D.: Endocarditis due to rare and fastidious bacteria. *Clin Microbiol Rev* 2001; 14:177-207.

Butler T.: Review article: Plague gives surprises in the first decade of the 21st century in the United States and Worldwide. *Am J Trop Med Hyg* 2013; 89:788-793.

Chambers S.T.1., Murdoch D., Morris A., et al.: HACEK infective endocarditis: characteristics and outcomes from a large, multi-national cohort. *PLoS ONE* 2013; 8(5):e63181.

McCrea K.W., Xie J., LaCross N., et al.: Relationships of nontypeable *Haemophilus influenzae* strains to hemolytic

and nonhemolytic *Haemophilus haemolyticus* strains. *J Clin Microbiol* 2008; 46(2):406-416.

Mattoo S., Cherry J.D.: Molecular pathogenesis, epidemiology and clinical manifestations of respiratory infections due to *Bordetella pertussis* and other *Bordetella* subspecies. *Clin Microbiol Rev* 2005; 18:326-382.

Melvin J.A., Scheller E.V., Miller J.F., et al.: *Bordetella* pertussis pathogenesis: current and future challenges. *Nat Rev Microbiol* 2014; 12:274-288.

Muder R.R., Yu V.L.: Infection due to *Legionella species* other than *L. pneumophila*. *Clin Infect Dis* 2002; 35:990-1108.

Nørskov-Lauritsen N.: Classification, identification and clinical significance of *Haemophilus* and *Aggregatibacter* species with host specificity for humans. *Clin Microbiol Rev* 2014; 27:214-240.

Pappas G., Papadimitriou P., Akritidis N., et al.: The new global map of human brucellosis. *Lancet Infect Dis* 2006; 6:91-99.

Titball R.W., Petrosino J.F.: *Francisella tularensis* genomics and proteomics. *Ann N Y Acad Sci* 2007; 1105:98-121.

Tristram S., Jacobs M.R., Appelbaum P.C.: Antimicrobial resistance in *Haemophilus influenzae*. *Clin Microbiol Rev* 2007; 20:368-389.

Van Eldere J., Slack M.P.E., Ladhani S., et al.: Non-typeable *Haemophilus influenzae*, an under-recognised pathogen. A review of the literature. *Lancet Infect Dis* 2014; 14:1281-1292.

Verduin C.M., Hol C., Fleer A., et al.: *Moraxella catarrhalis*: from emerging to established pathogen. *Clin Microbiol Rev* 2002; 15(1):125-144.

184

Anaerobic Bacteria

ITZHAK BROOK

Introduction

Infections caused by anaerobic bacteria are common and may be serious and life-threatening. Anaerobes are the predominant components of the bacterial flora of normal human skin and mucous membranes,[1] and are therefore a common cause of bacterial infections of endogenous origin. Because of their fastidious nature, they are difficult to isolate and are often overlooked. Delay in appropriate therapy often leads to clinical failures. Their isolation requires proper methods of collection, transportation and cultivation of specimens.[2-5] Treatment is complicated by the slow growth of these organisms, by the infection's polymicrobial nature and by the organisms' growing antimicrobial resistance.

Epidemiology

Most infections are caused by normal flora anaerobes that contaminate a previously sterile body site or gain access to the body from an external source of normal flora such as a bite. They also occur when the local defenses are decreased. Some infections are caused by wound contamination by soil anaerobes (i.e. Clostridia). *Clostridium difficile* can lead to hospital epidemics when these bacteria are transmitted from patient to patient. Toxin-producing *Clostridium botulinum* causes food poisoning.[5]

Microbiology

Anaerobes do not grow in the presence of room air (0.05% carbon dioxide and 21% oxygen), whereas facultative anaerobes grow both in the presence and in the absence of air. Microaerophilic bacteria grow poorly or not at all aerobically, but grow better under 10% carbon dioxide or anaerobically. Anaerobes can be divided into strict anaerobes that are unable to grow in the presence of more than 0.5% oxygen and moderate anaerobes that are capable of growing in between 2% and 8% oxygen.[4] Anaerobes generally do not possess catalase, but some produce superoxide dismutase that can protect them from oxygen.

The clinically important anaerobes are:
- six genera of gram-negative rods (*Bacteroides, Prevotella, Porphyromonas, Fusobacterium, Bilophila* and *Sutterella* spp.);
- gram-positive cocci (primarily *Peptostreptococcus* spp.);
- gram-positive spore-forming (*Clostridium* spp.) and nonspore-forming bacilli (*Actinomyces, Propionibacterium, Eubacterium, Lactobacillus* and *Bifidobacterium* spp.); and
- gram-negative cocci (mainly *Veillonella* spp.) (Table 184-1).[3,4]

The frequency of recovery of anaerobes differs in various infectious sites (Table 184-2). Mixed infections caused by numerous aerobic and anaerobic organisms are observed commonly in clinical situations (Figure 184-1).[2]

Approximately 95% of the anaerobes isolated from clinical infections are members of these genera. The remaining isolates belong to species not yet described, that can be assigned to the appropriate genus.

TABLE 184-1	Predominant Anaerobic Bacteria
Gram-positive cocci	*Peptostreptococcus* spp.: P. magnus, P. asaccharolyticus, P. prevotii, P. intermedius, P. anaerobius, P. micros Microaerophilic streptococci (not true anaerobes)
Gram-positive nonspore-forming bacilli	*Propionibacterium* spp.: P. acnes, P. propionicum, P. granulosum *Eubacterium tentum* *Bifidobacterium* spp.: B. eriksonii, B. dentium *Actinomyces* spp.: A. israelii, A. naeslundii, A. viscosus, A. odontolyticus, A. meyeri
Gram-positive spore-forming bacilli	*Clostridium* spp.: C. perfringens, C. ramosum, C. septicum, C. novyi, C. histolytica, C. sporogenes, C. difficile, C. bifermentans, C. butyricum, C. innocuum, C. sordellii, C. botulinum, C. tetani
Gram-negative bacilli	*Bacteroides fragilis* group: B. fragilis, B. thetaiotaomicron, B. distasonis, B. vulgatus, B. ovatus, B. uniformis Other *Bacteroides* spp.: B. gracilis, B. ureolyticus, Bilophila wadsworthia, *Sutterella* spp., pigmented *Prevotella* spp.: P. melaninogenica, P. intermedia, P. denticola, P. loescheii, P. corporis, P. nigrescens, other *Prevotella* spp.: P. oris, P. buccae, P. oralis group (P. oralis, P. buccalis, P. veroralis), P. bivia, P. disiens, Porphyromonas spp.: P. asaccharolytica, P. gingivalis, P. endodontalis, Fusobacterium spp.: F. nucleatum, F. necrophorum, F. gonidiaformans, F. naviforme, F. mortiferum, F. varium

TABLE 184-2	Anaerobic Bacteria Most Frequently Encountered in Specific Infection Sites	
Organism		**Infection Site**
Gram-positive cocci	Peptostreptococcus spp. Microaerophilic streptococci (not obligate anaerobes)	Respiratory tract, intra-abdominal and soft-tissue infections, sinusitis, brain abscesses
Gram-positive bacilli	Nonspore-forming: Actinomyces spp.	Intracranial abscesses, chronic mastoiditis, aspiration pneumonia, head and neck infections
	Propionibacterium acnes	Shunt infections (cardiac, intracranial), infections associated with foreign body
	Bifidobacterium spp.	Chronic otitis media, cervical lymphadenitis, abdominal infections
	Spore-forming: Clostridium perfringens	Soft-tissue infection, sepsis, food poisoning
	Clostridium septicum	Sepsis, neutropenic enterocolitis
	Clostridium difficile	Colitis, antibiotic-associated diarrheal disease
	Clostridium botulinum	Botulism
	Clostridium tetani	Tetanus
	Clostridium ramosum	Soft-tissue infections
Gram-negative bacilli	Bacteroides fragilis group	Intra-abdominal and female genital tract infections, sepsis, neonatal infections
	Pigmented	Orofacial infections, aspiration pneumonia, periodontitis
	Prevotella and Porphyromonas spp.	Orofacial infections
	Prevotella oralis, Prevotella oris-buccae	Orofacial infections, intra-abdominal infections
	Prevotella bivia, Prevotella disiens	Female genital tract infections
	Fusobacterium nucleatum	Orofacial and respiratory tract infections, brain abscesses, bacteremia
	Fusobacterium necrophorum	Aspiration pneumonia, bacteremia

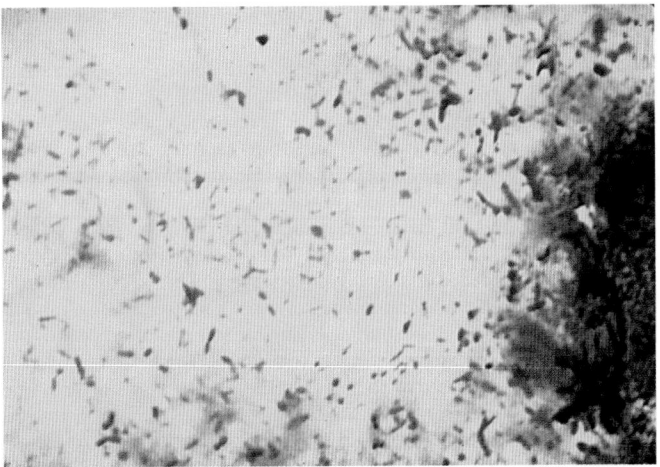

Figure 184-1 Gram stain of a perirectal abscess caused by polymicrobial aerobic and anaerobic flora.

The taxonomy of anaerobes has changed because of improved characterization methods using genetic studies.[3] The ability to differentiate between similar strains enables better characterization of type of infection and predicted antimicrobial susceptibility.[4]

GRAM-POSITIVE SPORE-FORMING BACILLI

Anaerobic spore-forming bacilli belong to the genus *Clostridium*. Morphologically, they are highly pleomorphic, ranging from short, thick bacilli to long filamentous forms, and are either ramrod straight or slightly curved. The clostridia found most frequently in clinical infections are *Clostridium perfringens*, *Clostridium septicum*, *Clostridium ramosum*, *Clostridium novyi*, *Clostridium sordellii*, *Clostridium histolyticum*, *Clostridium fallax*, *Clostridium bifermentans* and *Clostridium innocuum*.

Clostridium perfringens inhabits soil and the intestines of humans and animals. It is the most frequently encountered histotoxic clostridium and elaborates several necrotizing extracellular toxins.[6] It is a stout gram-variable rod of varying length, frequently surrounded by a capsule. It can cause devastating illness with a high mortality rate and bacteremia associated with extensive tissue necrosis, hemolytic anemia and renal failure.

Isolation of *C. septicum* can be associated with gastrointestinal malignancy. The intestinal tract is thought to be the source of the organism, and most of the isolates are recovered from blood and subcutaneous tissue.[7] *Clostridium sordellii* infections occur in women undergoing therapeutic abortion, during natural childbirth and in injection drug users.[8]

Although *C. botulinum* is usually associated with food poisoning, wound infections caused by this organism are being recognized with increasing frequency. Proteolytic strains of types A and B have been reported from food poisoning and wound infections. Infant botulism occurs with types A, B and F.[5] Disease caused by *C. botulinum* is usually an intoxication produced by ingestion of contaminated food (uncooked meat, poorly processed fish, improperly canned vegetables) containing a highly potent neurotoxin.[6] The polypeptide neurotoxin is relatively heat labile, and food containing this toxin may be rendered innocuous by exposure to 212°F (100°C) for 10 minutes. Infection of a wound with *C. botulinum* occurs rarely and can produce botulism.

Clostridium difficile causes antibiotic-associated and spontaneous diarrhea and colitis.[9] *Clostridium tetani* is found in soil and is rarely isolated from human feces. Infections result from wound contamination with soil containing *C. tetani* spores.[6] The spores will germinate in devitalized tissue and produce the neurotoxin that causes clinical findings.

Laboratory Diagnosis of C. difficile

Many options are available for testing *C. difficile*; each has inherent advantages and disadvantages. Most laboratories perform toxin testing using an enzyme immunoassay method.[10] Symptomatic patients with negative test should be tested by another more sensitive method. Until recently, cell culture cytotoxicity neutralization assays (CCNAs) were considered the gold standard in the USA. A two-step algorithm using an enzyme immunoassay (EIA) for glutamate dehydrogenase (GDH) detection followed by testing positives using CCNA offered an improved alternative until the availability of molecular assays. Recent comparisons of GDH to toxigenic culture and polymerase chain reaction (PCR) have shown >80% sensitivity.[10] Toxigenic culture became the new gold standard against which newer assays are compared.

Direct Stool Toxin Assays
Cell Culture Cytotoxicity Neutralization Assays (CCNAs). The test is performed by adding a prepared stool sample (diluted, buffered and filtered) to a monolayer of cultured cells.[11] If *C. difficile* toxins (A and/

or B) are present, they exert a cytopathic effect characterized by rounding of fibroblasts in tissue culture. If cytopathic effect is observed, a neutralization assay with specific antiserum is performed. Although toxin B is primarily detected in this assay, toxin A is also detected to some extent.

This method lacks the desired sensitivity to be the gold standard as their sensitivities ranging from 60% to 70% and specificities of 98%.[12,13] Most clinical laboratories do not perform this assay routinely given its relative inadequate sensitivity, high cost, long turnaround time (24–48 hours), and the requirement for expertise in maintenance of cell cultures and interpretation of results.

Enzyme Immunoassay. Enzyme immunoassays (EIA) use monoclonal or polyclonal antibodies against *C. difficile* toxins and allow direct detection of the toxin.[6,14] There are a number of commercially available EIAs for *C. difficile* toxins, including rapid immunochromatographic/lateral flow membrane immunoassays and microwell and solid-phase assays that can detect toxin A alone or both toxins A and B. EIA for both toxins can detect strains with toxin A mutation or strains that produce only toxin B.[15] The sensitivity and specificity of these assays vary from about 40% to 100%.[16,17]

Because EIA is relatively simple and results are available within 24 hours it is the preferred diagnostic assay. Despite good specificity (99%), EIA has only moderate and variable sensitivity (60–95%).[13] There is a relatively high false-negative rate since 100–1000 pg of toxin must be present for the test to be positive.[12] Up to three serial EIA tests may increase the diagnostic yield by as much as 10% if the initial test is negative. Supplementing negative EIA stool tests with tissue culture assay may also be useful.[14] Due to inadequate sensitivity, EIA is no longer recommended as a stand-alone test for diagnosing *C. difficile* infection.[18]

Organism Detection Assays. An inherent problem with detection of the organism rather than the toxin is that up to 30% of hospitalized patients are colonized without disease.[17] Some laboratories use one of these methods to screen stool samples, with subsequent cytotoxin testing for positive samples.

Anaerobic Culture

Anaerobic culture is used less frequently for diagnosis of *C. difficile*. Although the test is extremely sensitive, culture requires about 3 days. However, it remains an important tool for epidemiologic surveillance. Isolating the organism from fecal specimens and determining if it is a toxin-producing strain (toxigenic culture) is considered by many to be the gold standard for *C. difficile* detection in fecal specimens.[19] However, others argue that although toxigenic culture may result in more positive specimens, it might not be a superior test for the diagnosis of clinical disease compared to cytotoxic assays.[20]

Polymerase Chain Reaction. Real-time PCR using primers targeting a region of the toxin B gene is a useful diagnostic tool.[15] Several nucleic acid amplification assays are available to clinical laboratories. Because these assays detect a gene that encodes toxin and not the toxin itself, testing should be performed only in symptomatic patients. These molecular assays are superior to toxin EIAs, cell CCNAS and two-step algorithms, but not to toxigenic culture.[21]

Common Antigen Testing. Common antigen testing detects glutamate dehydrogenase (GDH) antigen, an essential enzyme produced constitutively by all *C. difficile* isolates. Some laboratories use this method to screen stool samples, with subsequent cytotoxin testing for positive samples.[22]

Endoscopy

Endoscopy can be a useful adjunctive tool for the diagnosis of *C. difficile* in the following settings:

- high clinical suspicion for *C. difficile* with negative laboratory assay(s);
- prompt *C. difficile* diagnosis needed before laboratory results can be obtained;

- failure of *C. difficile* infection to respond to antibiotic therapy; and
- atypical presentation with ileus or minimal diarrhea.[9]

Endoscopy is not warranted in patients with classic clinical findings and a positive stool toxin assay. In the setting of fulminant colitis, care should be taken to introduce minimal amounts of air given the risk of perforation.

GRAM-POSITIVE, NONSPORE-FORMING BACILLI

Anaerobic, gram-positive, nonspore-forming rods comprise part of the microflora of the gingival crevices, the gastrointestinal tract, the vagina and the skin. Several distinct genera are recognized: *Actinomyces, Arcanobacterium, Atopobium, Bifidobacterium, Eubacterium, Lactobacillus, Mobiluncus, Propionibacterium* and *Pseudoramibacter*. The most frequently recovered species are *Propionibacterium, Eubacterium, Bifidobacterium* and *Lactobacillus*.

The *Actinomyces, Arcanobacterium* and *Bifidobacterium* spp. are gram-positive, pleomorphic, anaerobic to microaerophilic bacilli.

Actinomyces israelii, Actinomyces naeslundii and *Propionibacterium propionicum* are normal inhabitants of the human mouth and throat and are the most frequent cause of actinomycosis. They have been recovered from intracranial abscesses, chronic mastoiditis, aspiration pneumonia and peritonitis.[2,4] Actinomycosis usually presents as an anatomically localized infection and can often be misdiagnosed as malignancy. Orocervicofacial actinomycosis is the most common presentation, characteristically occurring after trauma to the mouth or dental surgery. The usual presentation is a chronic soft-tissue swelling of the perimandibular region, with or without fever. The swelling can be painful or painless; sinus tracts can develop over time. If undiagnosed, infection can invade local muscle and bone. Thoracic actinomycosis usually results from aspiration of oropharyngeal secretions. The usual presentation is one of a chronic pneumonia, with fever, weight loss and hemoptysis, mimicking lung cancer. Invasion into the pleural space or mediastinum has been described. Abdominopelvic actinomycosis most often results from perforation of an abdominal viscus (classically, a ruptured appendix); presentation is nonspecific with abdominal pain, fever and weight loss and a mass (which may not be clinically apparent). Sinus tracts to the abdominal wall or perianal region can occur. Pelvic actinomycosis was classically associated with intrauterine devices, but has become rare in recent years. Diagnosis is usually made by demonstration of gram-positive filamentous organisms and sulfur granules on histopathology. Culture provides definitive identification but is often negative.

Management of actinomycosis requires long-term antibiotic therapy, usually in the form of 6–12 months of penicillin. Doxycycline, clindamycin and the macrolides appear suitable for patients allergic to penicillin. Surgical resection may also be required, especially in cases with extensive tissue destruction, sinus tracts or fistulas.[23]

Eubacterium and anaerobic lactobacilli are part of mixed flora in the oral, vaginal and gastrointestinal areas. They are associated with malignancy, previous surgery, immunodeficiency, diabetes mellitus, presence of a foreign body, dental extraction and broad-spectrum antibiotic therapy.[23,24]

Propionibacterium spp. are ordinarily nonpathogens but can cause infections of implanted cardiac prostheses or central nervous system (CNS) shunt infection and endocarditis in previously damaged heart valves. They have been recovered from parotid and dental infections, brain abscesses, conjunctivitis associated with contact lens, peritonitis and foreign body and pulmonary infections. The commonest species, *Propionibacterium acnes*, may be isolated from blood cultures but is associated only rarely with bacteremia or endocarditis. Because these organisms are part of the normal skin flora, they are common laboratory contaminants or may grow in blood cultures from skin contamination. *Prop. acnes* can cause bacteremia, especially in association with shunt infections,[25,26] and is believed to play a role in the pathogenesis of acne vulgaris.[27]

GRAM-NEGATIVE BACILLI

Bacteroides fragilis group are the most frequently recovered species of Bacteroidaceae in clinical specimens. *Bacteroides fragilis* group are resistant to penicillins, mostly through the production of β-lactamase. They include several members – the most commonly isolated ones are *B. fragilis* (the most commonly recovered member), *Bacteroides thetaiotaomicron*, *Bacteroides distasonis*, *Bacteroides ovatus* and *Bacteroides vulgatus*. They are part of the normal gastrointestinal flora[1] and predominate in intra-abdominal infections and other infections that originate from the gut flora (i.e. perirectal abscesses, decubitus ulcers).[2,4] *Bilophila wadsworthia* and *Centipeda periodontii* are new genera and species found in abdominal and endodontal infection, respectively.[28]

Pigmented *Prevotella* spp. (*Prevotella melaninogenica*, *Prevotella intermedia*), *Porphyromonas* spp. (*Porphyromonas asaccharolytica*) and nonpigmented *Prevotella* spp. (*Prevotella oralis*, *Prevotella oris*) are part of the normal oral and vaginal flora and are the predominant anaerobic gram-negative bacilli (AGNB) isolated from respiratory infections and their complications, aspiration pneumonia, lung abscess, chronic otitis media, chronic sinusitis, abscesses around the oral cavity, bite infections, paronychia, brain abscesses and osteomyelitis.[29] *Prevotella bivia* and *Prevotella disiens* are important isolates from obstetric and gynecologic infections.

FUSOBACTERIUM SPP.

Fusobacterium spp. are moderately long and thin organisms with tapered ends, and have typical fusiform morphology. The species of *Fusobacterium* seen most often in clinical infections are *Fusobacterium nucleatum*, *Fusobacterium necrophorum*, *Fusobacterium mortiferum* and *Fusobacterium varium*. *F. nucleatum* predominates in clinical specimens and is often associated with oral, pulmonary and intracranial infections.[30] *Fusobacterium* spp. are frequently isolated from abscesses, obstetric and gynecologic infections, blood and wounds.

A growing resistance of AGNB to penicillins has been noted in recent years.[31] Resistance was noted in pigmented *Prevotella* and *Porphyromonas*, *Prev. oralis*, *Prev. disiens*, *Prev. bivia* and *Fusobacterium* spp. The main mechanism of resistance is through the production of the enzyme β-lactamase.

The recovery rate of the different AGNB in infected sites is similar to their distribution in the normal flora.[2,4] *B. fragilis* group were more often isolated in sites proximal to the gastrointestinal tract (abdomen, bile), pigmented *Prevotella* spp. were more prevalent in infections proximal to the oral cavity (bones, sinuses, chest), and *Prev. bivia* and *Prev. disiens* were more often isolated in obstetric and gynecologic infections (Table 184-2). Knowledge of this mode of distribution allows for logical choice of antimicrobials that are adequate for the therapy of infections in or proximal to these sites.

GRAM-POSITIVE COCCI

The species most commonly isolated are *Peptostreptococcus magnus*, *Peptostreptococcus asaccharolyticus*, *Peptostreptococcus anaerobius*, *Peptostreptococcus prevotii* and *Peptostreptococcus micros*. Additional anaerobic cocci include *Coprococcus*, *Peptococcus*, *Ruminococcus sarcina* and *Staphylococcus saccharolyticus*. These organisms are part of the normal flora of the mouth, upper respiratory tract, intestinal tract, vagina and skin.

These organisms can be isolated in all types of anaerobic infection. They also predominate in all types of respiratory infection (including chronic sinusitis, mastoiditis, acute and chronic otitis media, aspiration pneumonia and lung abscess) and necrotizing, subcutaneous and soft-tissue infections.[32] They are generally recovered mixed with other aerobic or anaerobic organisms, but in many cases they are the only pathogens recovered. This may be of particular significance in cases of bacteremia. Microaerophilic streptococci are not true anaerobes as they can also become aerotolerant after subculture; however, they grow better anaerobically and are often grouped under anaerobes in many studies. These organisms include the *Streptococcus anginosus* group (previously called *Streptococcus milleri* group, which includes

Streptococcus constellatus and *Streptococcus intermedius*) and *Gemella morbillorum* (previously called *Streptococcus morbillorum*). Microaerophilic streptococci are common in chronic sinusitis and brain abscesses. They are also recovered from obstetric and gynecologic infections and abscesses.[33]

GRAM-NEGATIVE COCCI

There are three anaerobic gram-negative cocci genera: *Veillonella*, *Acidaminococcus* and *Megasphaera* spp. There are two described species of *Veillonella* and only one each of the other two genera. *Veillonella* spp. is the most common of the three genera and is part of the normal flora of the mouth, vagina and the small intestine. They are occasionally isolated from almost every type of anaerobic infection.[2,4]

Pathogenicity

ANAEROBES AS PART OF THE NORMAL FLORA

The human mucosal and epithelial surfaces are colonized with aerobic and anaerobic micro-organisms.[1] Differences in the environment, such as oxygen tension, pH and variations in bacterial adherence, account for changing patterns of colonization. The microflora also vary at different locations, as the organisms in the oral buccal folds vary in their concentration and strain types from those isolated from the tongue or gingival sulci. However, the organisms that prevail in one body system tend to belong to certain major bacterial species, and their presence in that system is predictable. The relative and total number of organisms can be affected by various factors, such as age, diet, anatomic variations, illness, hospitalization and antimicrobial therapy. However, the predictable patterns of bacterial flora remain stable throughout life, despite their subjection to perturbing factors. Anaerobes outnumber aerobic bacteria in all mucosal surfaces, and certain organisms predominate at different sites (Table 184-3).

Knowledge of the composition of the flora at certain site is useful for predicting which organisms may be involved in an infection adjacent to that site and can assist in the selection of empiric antimicrobial therapy. Recognition of the normal flora can also help the clinical microbiology laboratory identify appropriate culture media.[1]

The anaerobic microflora of the skin is largely made up of the genus *Propionibacterium* (mostly *Prop. acnes*) and, to a lesser extent, *Peptostreptococcus* spp. The perineum and lower extremity may harbor anaerobic members of the colonic and vaginal flora.

The microflora of the upper airways, including oral cavity, nasopharynx and oropharynx, is complex and contains many types of obligate anaerobes. The distribution of bacteria within the mouth seems to be a function of their ability to adhere to the oral surfaces. The differences in numbers of the anaerobic microflora probably occur because of considerable variations in the oxygen concentration in parts of the oral cavity. The ratio of anaerobic to aerobic bacteria in saliva is approximately 10:1. The total count of anaerobes in the saliva and elsewhere in the oral cavity reaches 10^7–10^8 bacteria/mL.[1,2] The predominant anaerobes in the upper airways include *Fusobacterium* spp. (especially *F. nucleatum*), pigmented *Prevotella* and *Porphyromonas* spp., *Prev. oralis* and *Peptostreptococcus* spp.

The gastrointestinal flora varies in bacterial concentration at different levels. The stomach acidity reduces the number of organisms swallowed from the oropharynx. The stomach, duodenum, jejunum and proximal ileum normally contain relatively few bacteria. However, the flora becomes more complex, and the number of different species increases in the distal gastrointestinal tract. Interruption in intestinal motility may result in an increase in the number of anaerobic and aerobic bacteria. The bacterial counts in the small intestine are relatively low, with total counts of 10^2–10^5 organisms/mL.[1,2] The organisms that predominate up to the ileocecal valve are gram-positive facultative bacteria, whereas below that structure *Bacteroides*, *Peptostreptococcus* and *Clostridium* spp. and coliform bacteria are the major isolates.[2] The mean number of bacteria in the colon exceeds 10^{11} bacteria/g fecal material; 99.9% are anaerobic (ratio of aerobes to

TABLE 184-3   **Normal Flora**

Site	No. of Organisms/g Fecal Material		Anaerobe/aerobe ratio	Predominant anaerobic bacteria
	Aerobes	Anaerobes		
Skin	–	–	–	Propionibacterium acnes Peptostreptococcus spp.
Mouth/upper respiratory tract	10^8–10^9	10^9–10^{11}	Nasal washings 3–5:1 Saliva 1:1 Tooth surface 1:1 Gingival crevice 1000:1	Pigmented Prevotella and Porphyromonas spp. Fusobacterium spp. Peptostreptococcus spp. Actinomyces spp.
Gastrointestinal tract: Upper Lower	 10^2–10^5 10^5–10^9	 10^3–10^7 10^{10}–10^{12}	Stomach 1:1 Small bowel 1:1 Ileum 1:1 Colon 1000:1	Bacteroides fragilis group Clostridium spp. Peptostreptococcus spp. Bifidobacterium spp. Eubacterium spp.
Female genital tract	10^8	10^9	Endocervix 1–5:1 Vagina 1–5:1	Peptostreptococcus spp. Prevotella bivia Prevotella disiens

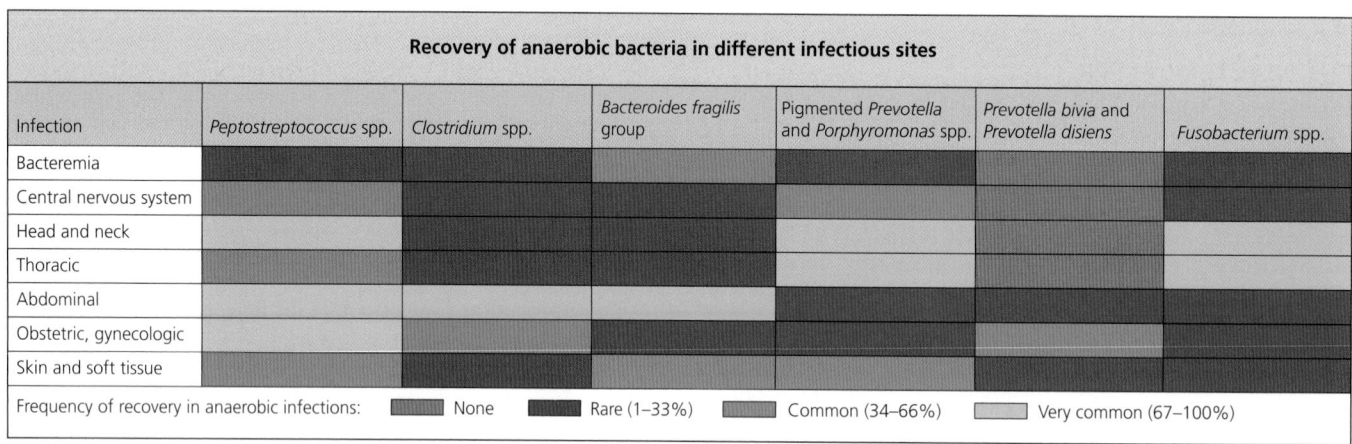

Figure 184-2   Recovery of anaerobic bacteria in different infectious sites.

anaerobes is 1:1000–10000).[34] In the colon 300–400 different species or types of bacteria can be found, many not yet identified.

The female genital flora is composed of mixed aerobic and anaerobic bacteria. However, the concentration and type of bacteria is less stable than that of the gastrointestinal flora and can be influenced by antimicrobial therapy, hormones, menstrual cycle, pregnancy and gynecologic surgery. A concentration of 10^8 organisms/mL is found during the reproductive years. Changes occur in the number of organisms at the various stages of the menstrual cycle.[35] The predominant aerobic organisms are aerobic lactobacilli, and the main anaerobic bacteria are anaerobic Lactobacillus, Peptostreptococcus, Prevotella, Bacteroides and Clostridium spp. Other anaerobes include Porphyromonas, Fusobacterium, Bilophilia, Bifidobacterium, Actinomyces, Eubacterium and Propionibacterium spp. Enterobacteriaceae can be found in postmenopausal flora. Bacterial vaginosis is associated with an increase in the number of anaerobic flora and a decrease in the concentration of lactobacilli.[35]

Most anaerobic infections originate from the endogenous mucosal membrane and skin flora. An exception is C. difficile, the major cause of antibiotic-associated colitis. Anaerobes belonging to the indigenous flora of the oral cavity can be recovered from various infections adjacent to that area, such as cervical lymphadenitis, subcutaneous abscesses and burns in proximity to the oral cavity, human and animal bites, paronychia, tonsillar and retropharyngeal abscesses, chronic sinusitis, chronic otitis media, periodontal abscess, thyroiditis, aspiration pneumonia and bacteremia associated with one of the above

infections.[2,4] The predominant anaerobes recovered in these infections are Prevotella, Porphyromonas, Fusobacterium and Peptostreptococcus spp., which are all part of the normal flora of the mucous surfaces of the oropharynx (Figure 184-2).

A similar correlation exists in infections associated with the gastrointestinal tract. Such infections include peritonitis after rupture of a viscus, liver and spleen abscess, abscesses and wounds near the anus, intra-abdominal abscess, and bacteremia associated with any of these infections.[2,4] The anaerobes that predominate in these infections are B. fragilis group, Clostridium spp. (including C. perfringens) and Peptostreptococcus spp.

Such a correlation also occurs in the genitourinary tract. The infections involved are amnionitis, septic abortion and other pelvic inflammations.[2,4] The anaerobes usually recovered are species of AGNB and Peptostreptococcus spp. Organisms belonging to the vaginal–cervical flora are also important pathogens of neonatal infections. They can be acquired by the newborn before delivery in the presence of amnionitis or during passage through the birth canal.

CONDITIONS PREDISPOSING TO ANAEROBIC INFECTION

Poor blood supply and tissue necrosis lower the oxidation and reduction potential and favor the growth of anaerobic bacteria. This can occur in the context of trauma, foreign body, malignancy, surgery, edema, shock, colitis and vascular disease. Other predisposing conditions include diabetes mellitus, splenectomy, immunosuppression, hypogammaglobinemia, neutropenia, leukemia, collagen vascular disease and cytotoxic drugs. Previous infection with aerobic or facultative organisms may make the local tissue conditions more favorable for the growth of anaerobic bacteria. Host defense mechanisms may also be impaired by anaerobic conditions and anaerobic bacteria. These include impairments in phagocytosis and intracellular killing (often caused by encapsulated anaerobes[36] and by succinic acid produced by *Bacteroides* spp.), inhibition of chemotaxis (by *Fusobacterium*, *Prevotella* and *Porphyromonas* spp.), degradation of serum proteins by proteases (by *Bacteroides* spp.) and production of leukotoxins (by *Fusobacterium* spp.).[37]

Suppuration, abscess formation, thrombophlebitis and gangrenous destruction of tissue associated with gas formation are the hallmarks of anaerobic infection (Box 184-1). Anaerobes are especially common in chronic infections, and are commonly seen after failure of therapy with antimicrobials that are not effective against them, such as aminoglycosides, trimethoprim–sulfamethoxazole (co-trimoxazole) and many quinolones.

Certain infections are very likely to involve anaerobes as important pathogens, and their presence should always be assumed. Such infections include brain abscess, oral and dental infections, human and animal bites, aspiration pneumonia and lung abscesses, peritonitis after perforation of viscus, amnionitis, endometritis, septic abortions, tubo-ovarian abscess, abscesses in and around the oral and rectal areas, pus-forming necrotizing infections of soft tissue or muscle and postsurgical infections following procedures on the oral or gastrointestinal tract or female pelvic area.[4] Certain solid malignant tumors, such as colon, uterine and bronchogenic carcinomas, and necrotic tumors of the head and neck, can become infected with anaerobes.[38] The anoxic conditions in the tumor and exposure to the endogenous adjacent mucous flora may predispose to these infections.

VIRULENCE FACTORS

Anaerobes possess a number of virulence factors including toxins, polysaccharide capsules and lipopolysaccharides.

Anaerobes possess several virulence factors that assist them to adhere to and invade epithelial surfaces. These factors include the presence of surface structures (such as capsule polysaccharide or lipopolysaccharide), production of superoxide dismutase and catalase, immunoglobulin proteases, coagulation promoting, spreading factors (such as hyaluronidase, collagenase and fibrinolysin) and the production of toxins.[37] Other factors that enhance the virulence of anaerobes include mucosal damage, oxidation–reduction potential drop and the presence of hemoglobin or blood in an infected site.

Toxins

These include the exotoxins produced by clostridial species including botulinum toxins, tetanus toxin, *C. difficile* toxin A and B,[39] and five toxins produced by *C. perfringens* (as well as many other clostridial species);[40] these are among the most virulent bacterial toxins in mouse

lethality assays. Alpha toxin is the major toxin produced by *C. perfringens*, but studies have shown a complex interaction between alpha and theta toxin in the production of experimental gas gangrene.[6] Both toxins appear to be involved in upregulation of intercellular adhesion molecule (ICAM)-1 and platelet aggregating factor (PAF), which contribute to vascular leukostasis and absence of a polymorphonuclear leukocyte (PMN) response to the infection.[4]

Clinical expression of histotoxic clostridial syndromes depends upon the site of toxin production and the physiologic effects of the toxin (see epidemiology, microbiology and pathophysiology of *Clostridium difficile* infection (Chapter 40), clostridial myonecrosis (Chapter 11) and botulism (Chapter 22)).

An enterotoxin has also been identified in *B. fragilis*, which is a metalloprotease.[41] Strains producing the toxin were recovered more often from patients with diarrhea as compared with healthy controls.[42]

Capsular Polysaccharides

B. fragilis is the most common anaerobe isolated from intra-abdominal infections and blood cultures even though it constitutes only 0.5% of normal colonic flora.[1,43]

Rat models showed that *B. fragilis* alone is capable of producing abscesses without a synergistic facultative organism and that heat-killed *B. fragilis* retained this capacity.[44] The polysaccharide capsule was also able to provoke abscesses in animal models. Further study of the capsular polysaccharide has led to an appreciation that it is actually a complex of polysaccharides with zwitterionic properties (containing alternating oppositely charged sugars).[45] Adherence of the capsular polysaccharide complex to mesothelial cells *in vitro* stimulates ICAM-1 and tumor necrosis factor (TNF); pre-treatment of mice with antibodies to ICAM-1 or TNF results in failure of the animals to develop intraperitoneal abscesses in a mouse model of intra-abdominal sepsis.[46]

Lipopolysaccharides

Anaerobic gram-negative bacteria possess lipopolysaccharide (LPS) that can be extracted from the envelope, but the biologic activity of this endotoxin is 100–1000 times less than that of LPS from Enterobacteriaceae.[47] The LPS of *B. fragilis* contains a lipid A moiety, but there are structural and chemical composition differences which render this LPS less potent than the LPS of *Escherichia coli*.[47]

Other gram-negative bacteria, such as fusobacteria, are thought to contain endotoxin with substantial biologic activity. The LPS from *F. nucleatum* had biologic activity equal to the LPS of Enterobacteriaceae that inhibits gingival fibroblasts.[48] Thus, LPS of fusobacteria may play a pathogenic role in periodontal disease and presumably accounts for the severity of illness with Lemierre's disease.[49]

Volatile Fatty Acids

The characteristic production of short chain volatile fatty acids by anaerobes is another virulence factor. These acids are used to identify anaerobes in the microbiology laboratory and may be responsible for the characteristic putrid drainage. These acids have been shown to inhibit phagocytic killing of bacteria.[50]

Ability to Tolerate Oxygen

A number of anaerobes, including *B. fragilis*, can tolerate exposure to oxygen. These organisms contain varying concentrations of superoxide dismutase, an enzyme present in aerobic bacteria which protects against oxygen's toxic effects.[51] The ability to survive exposure to oxygen facilitates the survival and thus pathogenicity of the organism.

Synergistic Capabilities

Anaerobes contribute to the severity of infection through their synergy with their aerobic counterparts and with each other.[52] Anaerobes generally take longer than aerobic bacteria to become virulent. This is because some of the major virulence factors of certain anaerobic bacteria (i.e. the production of a capsule) are expressed only after the infection has become chronic.[36]

BOX 184-2 PRINCIPAL β-LACTAMASE-PRODUCING ANAEROBES

Fusobacterium spp.: *F. nucleatum, F mortiferum, F. varium*
Pigmented *Prevotella* and *Porphyromonas* spp., *Prevotella oralis* group
Other *Prevotella* spp.: *P. oris, P. buccae, P. bivia, P. disiens*
Bacteroides fragilis group, *Bacteroides splanchnicus*
Bilophila wadsworthia
Clostridium spp.: *C. ramosum, C. clostridioforme* and *C. butyricum*

Production of β-Lactamase

An indirect pathogenic role of some anaerobes is their ability to produce the enzyme β-lactamase (Box 184-2). β-lactamase-producing bacteria (BLPB) can protect not only themselves but also other penicillin-susceptible organisms from the activity of penicillins. This can occur when the enzyme β-lactamase is secreted into the infected tissue or abscess fluid in sufficient quantities to degrade the β-lactam ring of penicillin before it can kill the susceptible bacteria.[53]

In vitro and *in vivo* studies have demonstrated protection of penicillin-susceptible bacteria from penicillin by aerobic and anaerobic BLPB.[53] The predominant anaerobic BLPB are pigmented *Prevotella* and *Porphyromonas, Bacteroides* and *Fusobacterium* spp.

Prevention

Early and aggressive treatment of acute infection can prevent it from becoming chronic.

Prevention and early therapy of conditions that may lead to anaerobic infection can reduce their rate. Preventing oral flora aspiration by improving neurologic status, suctioning oral secretions, improving oral hygiene, and maintaining lower stomach pH can reduce the risk of aspiration pneumonia and its complications. Irrigation and debridement of wounds and necrotic tissue, drainage of pus and improvement of the blood supply help prevent skin and soft-tissue infections.

Prophylactic antimicrobial therapy before surgery is generally administered when the operative field is expected to be contaminated by the mucosal membrane flora. Cefazolin is effective in surgical prophylaxis in sites distant from the oral or rectal areas, when anaerobic coverage is not required. Cefoxitin, cefotetan or ertapenem are used in procedures that involve the oral, rectal or vulvovaginal flora (i.e. abdominal surgery) because their spectrum includes the aerobic and anaerobic flora likely to be encountered.

Vaccination with tetanus toxin can prevent *C. tetani* infection.[54] Prevention of botulism depends mainly on adequate food preparation (see Chapter 22 for further details).

Collection, Transport and Diagnostic Microbiology

COLLECTION OF SPECIMENS FOR ANAEROBIC BACTERIA

Collection of specimens for anaerobic bacteria is important because documentation of an anaerobic infection is through isolation of organisms from the infected site. Appropriate documentation of anaerobic infection requires proper collection of appropriate specimens, expeditious transportation, and careful laboratory processing.[3] Inadequate techniques or media can lead to missing the presence of anaerobic bacteria or the assumption that only aerobic organisms are present in a mixed infection.

Because anaerobes are present on skin and mucous membranes, even minimal contamination with normal flora can be misleading. Unacceptable or inappropriate specimens can yield normal flora and can be misleading and have no or little diagnostic value. Appropriate materials should be obtained by using techniques that bypass the normal flora (Table 184-4).

Acceptable specimens (Table 184-5) include those obtained from normally sterile sites, such as blood or spinal, joint or peritoneal fluids,

---

TABLE 184-4 Methods for Collection of Specimens for Anaerobic Bacteria

Infection Site	Methods
Abscess or body cavity	Aspiration by syringe and needle Incised abscesses: syringe or swab (less desirable); specimen obtained during surgery after cleansing the skin
Tissue or bone	Surgical specimen using tissue biopsy or curette
Sinuses or mucuos surface abscesses	Aspiration after decontamination or surgical specimen
Ear	Aspiration after decontamination of ear canal and membrane; in perforation, cleanse ear canal and aspirate through perforation
Pulmonary	Transtracheal aspiration, lung puncture, bronchoscopic aspirate (using double-lumen catheter and quantitative culture)
Pleural	Thoracentesis
Urinary tract	Suprapubic bladder aspiration
Female genital tract	Culdocentesis after decontamination, surgical specimen Transabdominal needle aspirate of uterus Intrauterine brush (using double-lumen catheter and quantitative culture)

TABLE 184-5 Appropriate and Inappropriate Specimens for Anaerobic Culture

Appropriate	Inappropriate
Feces or rectal swabs Throat or nasopharyngeal swabs Sputum or bronchoscopic specimens Routine or catheterized urine Vaginal or cervical swabs Material from superficial wound or abscesses not collected properly to exclude surface contaminations Material from abdominal wounds obviously contaminated with feces (e.g. an open fistula)	All normally sterile body fluids other than urine (e.g. blood, pleural and joint fluids) Urine obtained by suprapubic bladder aspiration Percutaneous transtracheal aspiration or direct lung puncture Culdocentesis fluid obtained after decontamination of the vagina Material obtained from closed abscesses Material obtained from sinus tracts or draining wounds

---

or are collected after thorough skin decontamination. Two approaches are used to culture the maxillary sinus by aspiration following sterilization of the canine fossa or the nasal vestibule, via either the canine fossa or the inferior meatus. Urine is collected by percutaneous suprapubic bladder aspiration. Specimens can be collected from abscess contents, from deep aspirates of wounds, and via special techniques, such as transtracheal aspirates or direct lung puncture. Specimens of the lower respiratory tract are difficult to obtain without contamination with indigenous flora. Double-lumen catheter bronchial brushing and bronchoalveolar lavage, cultured quantitatively, can be useful.

Culdocentesis fluid obtained after decontamination of the vagina is acceptable.

Transportation of Specimens

Prompt delivery of specimens to the laboratory to allow for microbiologic processing is essential. Transportation of specimens should be prompt unless anaerobic transport devices are available. Transport devices generally contain oxygen-free environments provided by a mixture of carbon dioxide, hydrogen, and nitrogen, plus an aerobic condition indicator. Specimens should be placed into an anaerobic transporter as soon as possible.

BOX 184-3 BACTERIOLOGIC FINDINGS SUGGESTIVE OF ANAEROBIC INFECTION

Organisms seen on Gram stain that cannot be grown in aerobic cultures.
Typical morphology for anaerobes on Gram stain.
Anaerobic growth on proper media containing antibiotic-suppressing aerobes.
Growth in anaerobic zone of fluid or agar media.
Gas, foul-smelling odor in specimen or bacterial culture.
Characteristic colonies on anaerobic plates.
Colonies of pigmented *Prevotella* or *Porphyromonas* spp. may fluoresce red under ultraviolet light, and older colonies produce a typical dark pigment.

BOX 184-4 ANAEROBIC INFECTIONS FOR WHICH SUSCEPTIBILITY TESTING IS INDICATED

1. Serious or life-threatening infections (e.g. brain abscess, bacteremia or endocarditis).
2. Infections that failed to respond to empiric therapy.
3. Infections that relapsed after initially responding to empiric therapy.
4. Infections where an antimicrobial will have a special role in the patient's outcome.
5. When an empirical decision is difficult because of absence of precedent.
6. When there are few susceptibility data available on a bacterial species.
7. When the isolate(s) is often resistant to antimicrobials.
8. When the patient requires prolonged therapy (e.g. septic arthritis, osteomyelitis, undrained abscess, or infection of a graft or a prosthesis).

Liquid or tissue specimens are always preferred to swabs. Liquid specimens are inoculated into an anaerobic transport vial or collected in a syringe and a needle. All air bubbles are expelled from the syringe. Insertion of the needle tip into a sterile rubber stopper is no longer recommended. Because air gradually diffuses through the plastic syringe wall, specimens should be processed in less than 30 minutes.

Swabs are placed in sterilized tubes that contain carbon dioxide or pre-reduced anaerobically sterile Carey-Blair semisolid media. Tissue specimens can be transported in an anaerobic jar or in a sealed plastic bag rendered anaerobic.

Laboratory Diagnosis

For the laboratory diagnosis of *C. difficile*, see above.

Certain findings are suggestive of anaerobic infection (Box 184-3). Gram stain of a smear of the specimen provides important preliminary information regarding the types of organisms present, helps determine appropriate initial therapy and serves as a quality control.

Cultures should be immediately placed under anaerobic conditions and should be incubated for 48 hours or longer. An additional 36–48 hours is generally required for species- or genus-level identification by using biochemical tests. Kits that contain these tests are commercially available.[3]

A rapid enzymatic test enables identification after only 4 hours of aerobic incubation. Gas-liquid chromatography of metabolites can be used. Nucleic acid probes and PCR methods are also being developed for rapid identification.

Matrix-assisted laser desorption/ionization time-of-flight mass spectrometry (MALDI-TOF MS) Biotyper is a fast and reliable identification of the most clinically relevant anaerobic bacteria; it is less time-consuming, the cost for reagents is minimized and it does not require dedicated personnel.[55]

Detailed procedures of laboratory methods can be found in microbiology manuals.[3]

Identification of an anaerobe to a species level is often cumbersome, expensive and time-consuming, taking up to 72 hours. Identification is most helpful in selecting an antibiotic against a species that has predictable antibiotic susceptibility. The level of speciation adequate for identifying an anaerobe is often controversial.

Occasionally, species identification of an organism will provide the diagnosis, as with *C. difficile* in patients who have colitis or *C. botulinum* in infants with botulism. However, because most anaerobes are endogenous, there are rarely epidemiologic reasons to perform complete identification. Identifying *B. fragilis* group, which often cause bacteremia and septic complications, has significant prognostic value.

Antimicrobial Susceptibility Testing (Box 184-4)

The antimicrobial susceptibility of anaerobes has become unpredictable and multiresistant clinical isolates are appearing confounding the concept of foolproof anaerobic therapy.[56] Resistance to even the most active drugs such as imipenem, piperacillin–tazobactam, ampicillin–sulbactam and metronidazole is reported.[56]

Routine susceptibility testing of all anaerobic isolates is extremely time-consuming and in many cases unnecessary. The Clinical and Laboratory Standards Institute (CLSI) suggests testing isolates from blood, brain abscess, endocarditis, osteomyelitis and joint infection, infection of prosthetic devices and vascular grafts.[57] Also, any bacteria isolated from normally sterile body sites should be tested (as long as they are not likely to be contaminants). Isolates from patients likely to undergo long-term therapy should be tested so that any development of resistance can be recognized; any isolate from a therapy failure, or in a case in which the therapeutic decisions will be influenced by the results, should be tested.

Antibiotics tested should include penicillin, a broad-spectrum penicillin, a penicillin plus a β-lactamase inhibitor, clindamycin, a second-generation cephalosporin (e.g. cefoxitin), an extended-spectrum fluoroquinolone, tigecycline, metronidazole and a carbapenem (e.g. imipenem).

The method recommended by the CLSI, includes agar dilution testing, microbroth and macrobroth dilution.[57] Newer methods include the E-test and the spiral gradient end-point system. For *C. difficile* no resistance testing is needed because there are no data to substantiate a relation between outcome and resistance.

Clinical Manifestations

Anaerobes have been recovered in infections at all anatomic locations. However, their frequency of isolation and the types of bacterial isolate depend on the microbial flora at their source or the adjacent mucocutaneous sites.

Central Nervous System Infections

Anaerobes can cause a variety of intracranial infections. These include brain abscess, subdural empyema and infrequently cause epidural abscess and meningitis. The main source of brain abscess is an adjacent, generally chronic infection in the ears, mastoids, sinuses, oropharynx, teeth or lungs.[58] Ear or mastoid infection tends to spread to the temporal lobe or cerebellum, whereas facial sinusitis often causes abscess of the frontal lobe. Hematogenous spread often occurs after dental, oropharyngeal or pulmonary infection. Rarely, bacteremia of another origin or endocarditis can lead to such infection.

Meningitis is uncommon and can follow respiratory or cerebrospinal fluid shunt infection. Shunt infections are generally caused by skin flora such as *Prop. acnes*,[25] or in instances of ventriculoperitoneal shunts that perforate the gut, by anaerobes of enteric origin (i.e. *B. fragilis*).[59] *Clostridium perfringens* has been reported as a cause of brain abscesses and meningitis after head injuries or after intracranial surgery.[2]

The anaerobes generally recovered from brain abscesses that complicate respiratory and dental infections include *Prevotella*,

TABLE 184-6	Aerobic and Anaerobic Bacteria Isolated in Head and Neck and Upper Respiratory Tract Infections	
Type of Infection	Aerobic and Facultative Organisms	Anaerobic Organism
Otitis media and mastoiditis: Acute Chronic	Streptococcus pneumoniae Haemophilus influenzae* Moraxella catarrhalis* Staphylococcus aureus* Escherichia coli* Klebsiella pneumoniae* Pseudomonas aeruginosa*	Peptostreptococcus spp. Pigmented Prevotella and Porphyromonas spp.* Bacteroides spp.* Fusobacterium spp.* Peptostreptococcus spp.
Peritonsillar and retropharyngeal abscess	Streptococcus pyogenes Staphylococcus aureus*	Fusobacterium spp.* Pigmented Prevotella and Porphyromonas spp.*
Recurrent tonsillitis	Streptococcus pyogenes Haemophilus influenzae* Staphylococcus aureus*	Fusobacterium spp.*
Suppurative thyroiditis	Streptococcus pyogenes Staphylococcus aureus*	Pigmented Prevotella and Porphyromonas spp.* Peptostreptococcus spp.
Sinusitis: acute/chronic	Haemophilus influenzae* Streptococcus pneumoniae Moraxella catarrhalis* Staphylococcus aureus* Streptococcus pneumoniae Haemophilus influenzae*	Peptostreptococcus spp. Pigmented Prevotella and Porphyromonas spp.* Fusobacterium spp.* Bacteroides fragilis group*
Cervical lymphadenitis	Staphylococcus aureus* Mycobacterium spp.	Pigmented Prevotella and Porphyromonas spp.* Peptostreptococcus spp.
Postoperative infection disrupting oral mucosa	Staphylococcus spp.* Enterobacteriaceae* Streptococcus pyogenes	Fusobacterium spp.* Bacteroides spp.* Pigmented Prevotella and Porphyromonas spp.* Peptostreptococcus spp.
Deep neck abscesses and parotitis	Streptococcus spp. Staphylococcus spp.*	Bacteroides spp.* Fusobacterium spp.* Peptostreptococcus spp.*
Odontogenic complications	Streptococcus spp. Staphylococcus spp.*	Pigmented Prevotella and Porphyromonas spp.* Peptostreptococcus spp.
Oropharyngeal: Vincent's angina	Streptococcus spp. Staphylococcus spp.*	Fusobacterium necrophorum*

*Organisms that have the potential of producing β-lactamase.

Porphyromonas, Bacteroides, Fusobacterium and Peptostreptococcus spp. Microaerophilic and other streptococci are also often isolated. Actinomyces are less frequently encountered.

At the stage of encephalitis, antimicrobial therapy accompanied by measures to control the increase in intracranial pressure can prevent abscess formation. Once an abscess has formed, surgical excision or drainage may be needed, combined with a long course of antibiotics (4–8 weeks). Some neurosurgeons advocate complete evacuation of the abscess, whereas others recommend repeated aspirations.[60] In patients who have multiple abscesses or in those who have abscesses in essential brain areas, repeated aspirations are preferable. High-dose antibiotics for an extended period may represent an alternative approach in this group of patients and have often replaced surgical drainage.[61]

Because of the difficulty involved in the penetration of various antimicrobial agents through the blood–brain barrier, the choice of antibiotics is restricted. The antimicrobials advocated for these infections are metronidazole, penicillins, meropenem and chloramphenicol. However, the choice may vary according to the specific isolates and their susceptibilities. A significant improvement in the mortality rate has been associated with the introduction of computed tomography (CT) and use of metronidazole therapy.

Head and Neck and Upper Respiratory Tract Infections

Anaerobes can be recovered from a variety of head and neck and upper respiratory tract infections and predominate more in their chronic forms (Table 184-6). These include chronic otitis media, sinusitis and mastoiditis, tonsillar, peritonsillar and retropharyngeal abscesses, deep neck space infections, parotitis, sialadenitis, thyroiditis, odontogenic infections, and postsurgical and nonsurgical head and neck wounds and abscesses. The predominant organisms are of oropharyngeal flora origin and include Prevotella, Porphyromonas, Bacteroides, Fusobacterium and Peptostreptococcus spp. Other isolates include microaerophilic streptococci and Streptococcus salivarius.

Most dental infections involve anaerobes. These include endodontal (e.g. pulpitis) and periodontal (gingivitis, periodontitis and periimplantitis) infections, periapical and dental abscesses, perimandibular space infection, and postextraction infection.[61,62] Pulpitis may progress to an abscess and eventually involve the mandible and other neck spaces. In addition to the organisms mentioned above, microaerophilic streptococci and Streptococcus salivarius can also be involved. Vincent's angina (or trench mouth) is a distinct form of ulcerative gingivitis; the causative organisms include Fusobacterium spp. and anaerobic spirochetes.[2]

Ludwig angina and Lemierre's syndrome are life-threatening deep neck infections. Ludwig angina is a deep tissue infection of the floor of the mouth. Lemierre's syndrome is characterized by thrombosis and suppurative thrombophlebitis of the internal jugular vein that is associated with spread of septic emboli to the lungs and other sites (Figure 184-3).[30] Fusobacterium is the predominant genus and F. necrophorum is the most prevalent species.

Deep neck infections are usually polymicrobial. These include mediastinitis following perforation of the esophagus, extension of retropharyngeal abscess or cellulitis and dental abscess.[63]

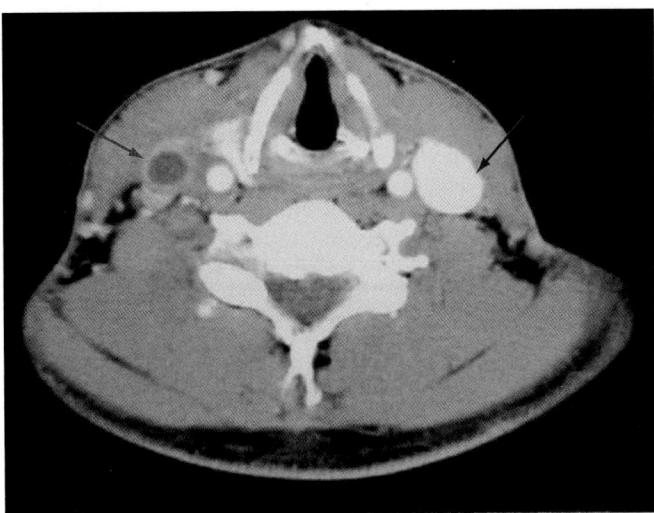

Figure 184-3 CT of a clotted jugular vein indicating Lemierre's syndrome (red arrow). A normal-appearing jugular vein is indicated by the blue arrow.

OTITIS MEDIA

Anaerobes were isolated in 5–15% of patients with acute otitis media[64] and 42% of culture-positive aspirates of patients who had serous otitis media.[65] The predominant isolates in acute otitis media were *Peptostreptococcus* spp. and *Prop. acnes*. These organisms, as well as AGNB, were recovered in serous otitis media.

Anaerobes were recovered in about 50% of the patients with chronic suppurative otitis media.[2,4,66,67] The infection is often polymicrobial and the predominant anaerobes are gram-negative bacilli and peptostreptococci. The predominant aerobes are *Pseudomonas aeruginosa* and *Staph. aureus*. Many of these organisms can produce β-lactamase and might have contributed to the high failure rate of β-lactam antibiotics. Anaerobes were isolated from 23 out of 24 (96%) specimens of chronic mastoiditis[68] and from most patients who have intracranial abscesses complicating chronic suppurative otitis media.[2,4,58]

Anaerobes were recovered from infected cholesteatomas.[69,70] The production of organic acids by anaerobes may promote bone destruction in cholesteatoma.[70] Because infected cholesteatoma contains bacteria similar to those recovered from chronically infected ears, it may serve as a nidus for chronic infection.

SINUSITIS

Sinus disease may develop when viral infection, allergy or anatomic obstruction prevents drainage. Earlier infection is caused by pathogens similar to those recovered in acute otitis media: *Streptococcus pneumoniae*, *Haemophilus influenzae* and *Moraxella catarrhalis*. Anaerobes become involved as the infection becomes chronic and tissue oxygen concentration declines. The bacterial flora transition from aerobic to anaerobic has been demonstrated.[71] An elevated serum antibody level to *Prevotella* and *Fusobacterium* spp. was demonstrated in patients with chronic sinusitis.[72] Although anaerobes are generally isolated from only about 7% of patients with acute sinusitis (generally in maxillary sinusitis secondary to periodontal infection), they can be isolated from up to 67% of those with chronic infection.[2,4,73] An average of three anaerobes per aspirate were recovered in chronic sinusitis.[74]

Sinus infection may spread via anastomosing veins or contiguously to the CNS. Complications include orbital cellulitis,[75] meningitis, cavernous sinus thrombosis, and epidural, subdural and brain abscesses.[2,4]

PAROTITIS

Viral parotitis can be caused by paramyxo- (mumps), Epstein–Barr, coxsackie, HIV, influenza A and parainfluenza viruses. Acute suppurative parotitis is generally caused by *Staph. aureus*, streptococci and,

rarely, aerobic gram-negative bacteria. Anaerobes, mostly *Peptostreptococcus*, *Bacteroides*, and pigmented *Prevotella* and *Porphyromonas* spp., have also been isolated.[76] Empiric antibiotic therapy should be directed against both aerobic and anaerobic bacteria. Surgical drainage may be indicated when pus has formed.

CERVICAL LYMPHADENITIS

The anterior cervical, submandibular and posterior cervical nodes are the most infection-prevalent sites. The commonest causes in children and young adults are viruses, particularly Epstein–Barr virus. The organisms causing acute unilateral infection associated with facial trauma or impetigo are *Staph. aureus* and *Streptococcus pyogenes*. *Bartonella henselae* and mycobacteria are important in chronic infections. Anaerobes (mostly *Fusobacterium* and *Peptostreptococcus* spp.) were isolated in about 25% of the infections, often in pure culture,[77] and were associated with dental, periodontal or tonsillar infection.

INFECTION AFTER HEAD AND NECK SURGERY

Infections after head and neck surgery are caused by the exposure of the surgical site to the oropharyngeal flora, and are enhanced by decreased blood supply and by the presence of necrotic tissue. They are common after surgery for tumors. Surgical wounds are generally infected by polymicrobial aerobic and anaerobic flora; the number of isolates varies from one to nine (average six).[78] The commonest isolates are peptostreptococci, *Staph. aureus*, AGNB (i.e. *Bacteroides* spp.), *Fusobacterium* spp. and Enterobacteriaceae. The presence of this flora warrants the use of antimicrobials effective against these organisms in the prophylaxis and therapy of this infection.[79]

TONSILLITIS

Clinical and laboratory evidence supports the role of anaerobes in acute and chronic tonsillitis. Anaerobes play a major role in complications of tonsillitis (i.e. bacteremia, abscesses).[73] The organisms recovered in these infections are *Fusobacterium* and *Peptostreptococcus* spp. and AGNB. Polymicrobial flora predominate in peritonsillar and retropharyngeal abscesses, where the number of isolates is one to 12.[3,5,80] Anaerobes were isolated from the cores of tonsils of children with recurrent group A β-hemolytic streptococci (GABHS)[55,74,81] and non-GABHS tonsillitis.[81] Anaerobes were isolated from 25% of suppurative cervical lymph nodes, dental and tonsillar infections,[78] and internal jugular vein thrombophlebitis causing postanginal sepsis.[2,4]

The pathogenic role of anaerobes in the acute inflammatory process in the tonsils is supported by these observations:

- recovery in tonsillar or retropharyngeal abscesses, often without any aerobic bacteria;[80]
- isolation from tonsils in Vincent's angina;[4]
- recovery of encapsulated pigmented *Prevotella* and *Porphyromonas* spp. in acutely inflamed tonsils and isolation from the core of recurrently inflamed non-GABHS tonsils;[81] and
- response to antibiotics in patients who have non-GABHS tonsillitis.[81]

Furthermore, an immune response against *Prev. intermedia* can be detected in patients with non-GABHS tonsillitis and against *Prev. intermedia* and *F. nucleatum* in patients who recovered from peritonsillar cellulitis or abscesses and infectious mononucleosis.[81]

Metronidazole therapy alleviated the symptoms of tonsillar hypertrophy and shortened the duration of fever in patients with infectious mononucleosis.[81] Because metronidazole has no antiviral or aerobic antibacterial efficacy, suppression of oral anaerobes may contribute to reduce the inflammation caused by the Epstein–Barr virus. This is supported by the increased recovery of *Prev. intermedia* and *F. nucleatum* during the acute phases of mononucleosis.[81]

Recurrent pharyngotonsillitis and failure to eradicate the GABHS with penicillin can be a serious clinical problem. One explanation for penicillin failure is that repeated administrations result in selection of BLPB.[53,82] β-lactamase-producing strains of pigmented *Prevotella* and *Porphyromonas* spp., *B. fragilis*, *Fusobacterium* spp., *H. influenzae* and *Staph. aureus* were isolated from the tonsils of more than 75% of children with recurrent GABHS tonsillitis[54,76,81] and from 40% of children with non-GABHS tonsillitis.[81] Similar organisms were found in adenoiditis and adenoid hypertrophy.[81]

The recovery of BLPB in >75% of patients with recurrent GABHS tonsillitis,[54,81] the ability to measure β-lactamase activity in the core of their tonsils[81] and the response of patients to antimicrobials effective against BLPB (i.e. clindamycin or amoxicillin/clavulanate)[81,82] support the role of aerobic and anaerobic BLPB in the inability of penicillin to eradicate GABHS tonsillitis.

Pleuropulmonary Infections

Aspiration of oropharyngeal secretions or gastric contents, and severe periodontal or gingival disease are the most prevalent risk factors for developing anaerobic pleuropulmonary infection. The infection can progress from pneumonitis to necrotizing pneumonia and pulmonary abscess, and empyema.[83] The lesions tend to develop in dependent pulmonary segments, in either of the superior segments of the lower lobes, or the posterior segments of the upper lobes. The infection is generally polymicrobial where the causative organisms of community-acquired infection (in 60–80% of cases) are aerobic and anaerobic members of oropharyngeal flora. The anaerobes isolated are *Prevotella*, *Porphyromonas*, *Fusobacterium* and *Peptostreptococcus* spp., and the aerobes are GABHS and microaerophilic streptococci (Table 184-7).[84] Anaerobes can also be recovered in about one-third of patients who have nosocomial-acquired aspiration pneumonia and pneumonia associated with tracheostomy with and without mechanical ventilation,[85] where they are generally recovered mixed with Enterobacteriaceae, *Pseudomonas* spp. and *Staph. aureus*.

Cultures should be obtained without contamination by oral flora using bronchoalveolar lavage, bronchoscopy via bronchial brush protected in a double-lumen plugged catheter (using quantitative cultures in the last two methods), percutaneous transtracheal aspiration, lung biopsy, or thoracentesis (of empyema fluid). Management includes drainage of empyema and antimicrobials effective against anticipated anaerobic and aerobic bacteria (see Chapter 29).

Intra-Abdominal Infections

Most visceral abscesses (e.g. hepatic, splenic); chronic cholecystitis; perforated and gangrenous appendicitis; perforations resulting from obstruction, inflammatory bowel disease, trauma, diverticulitis or infarction; and postoperative abdominal surgery wound infections and abscesses are polymicrobial caused by the gastrointestinal aerobic and anaerobic bacteria.[86]

The initial infection following perforation is peritonitis; a synergistic polymicrobial infection. Characteristically, the more types of bacteria involved, the graver the morbidity. The organisms involved are generally those of the gastrointestinal tract flora.[1] Of the more than 400 bacterial species that constitute the gut flora, only the virulent ones survive in the peritoneum to cause the infection. The more distal the perforation, the greater the types and number of organisms involved. An average of 11.6 organisms per specimen (8.5 anaerobes and 3.1 nonanaerobes) were recovered in a study of 71 patients with gangrenous and perforated appendicitis.[87] The predominant aerobic and facultative bacteria are *E. coli* and *Streptococcus* spp. (including *Enterococcus* spp.), and the anaerobes are the *B. fragilis* group, and *Peptostreptococcus*, *Clostridium*, *Fusobacterium* and *Eubacterium* spp. (Table 184-7).[2,4]

Intra-abdominal infections are characteristically biphasic: an initial generalized peritonitis primarily associated with *E. coli* sepsis, followed by abscess formation due to anaerobes (mainly *B. fragilis*).[88]

The clinical manifestations of secondary peritonitis reflect of the underlying disease process. Fever, diffuse abdominal pain, nausea and vomiting are characteristic. Physical examination reveals signs of peritoneal inflammation, including rebound tenderness, abdominal wall rigidity and decrease in bowel sounds. The early findings may be followed by shock associated with ruptured viscus, followed by toxemia, restlessness and irritability, fever, an increase in pulse rate, chills and convulsions.

Biliary tract infection is generally caused by *E. coli*, *Klebsiella* and *Enterococcus* spp. Anaerobes (mostly *B. fragilis* group and rarely *C. perfringens*) can be recovered in complicated infections associated with carcinoma, recurrent infection, obstruction, bile tract surgery or manipulation.[89]

Laboratory studies reveal leukocytosis (>12 000/mm³) with a predominance of polymorphonuclear forms. Radiographs of the abdomen may reveal free air in the peritoneal cavity, evidence of ileus or obstruction and obliteration of the psoas shadow. Diagnostic ultrasound, gallium and CT scanning[90] may be useful in detecting appendiceal or other intra-abdominal abscesses.

TABLE 184-7	Aerobic and Anaerobic Bacteria Isolated in Various Types of Infection	
Type of Infection	**Aerobic and Facultative Organisms**	**Anaerobic Organism**
Pleuropulmonary	*Staphylococcus aureus** Viridans streptococci *Pseudomonas aeruginosa** Enterobacteriaceae*	Pigmented *Prevotella* spp. (*P. denticola, P. melaninogenica, P. intermedia, P. nigrescens, P. loescheii*) Nonpigmented *Prevotella* spp. (*P. oris, P. buccae, P. oralis*) *Fusobacterium nucleatum* *Peptostreptococcus* spp. (*P. micros, P. anaerobius, P. magnus*) *Bacteroides fragilis* group, nonspore-forming gram-positive rods (*Actinomyces, Eubacterium, Lactobacillus* spp.)
Intra-abdominal	*Escherichia coli* *Enterococcus* spp. *Pseudomonas aeruginosa**	*Bacteroides fragilis* group *Bilophila wadsworthia* *Peptostreptococcus* spp. (especially *P. micros*) *Clostridium* spp.
Female genital tract	*Streptococcus* (groups A, B, others) *Escherichia coli* *Klebsiella pneumoniae, Neisseria gonorrhoeae* (in sexually active patients) *Chlamydia* spp. (in sexually active patients) *Mycoplasma hominis* (in postpartum patients)	*Peptostreptococcus* spp. *Prevotella* spp. (especially *P. bivia, P. disiens*) *Bacteroides fragilis* group *Clostridium* spp. (especially *C. perfringens*) *Actinomyces* *Eubacterium* spp. (in intrauterine contraceptive device-associated infections)
Skin and soft tissue	*Staphylococcus aureus* *Streptococcus* (*Strep. milleri* group, groups A and B, viridans group) *Enterococcus* spp. Enterobacteriaceae‡; *Pseudomonas aeruginosa**	*Peptostreptococcus* spp. (*P. magnus, P. micros, P. asaccharolyticus*) Pigmented *Prevotella* spp.†, *Actinomyces* spp. *Fusobacterium nucleatum*† *Bacteroides fragilis* group‡ *Clostridium* spp.‡

*Recovered in hospital-acquired infection.
†After exposure to oral flora.
‡After exposure to colonic flora.

Appropriate management of intra-abdominal infections requires administration of antimicrobials effective against both aerobic and anaerobic components of the infection,[2,4,91] as well as surgical correction and evacuation of pus.[91] Single and easily accessible abscesses can be drained percutaneously. The outcome of the infection depends on a variety of factors that include the general condition of the patient (as measured by the Apache score[92]), site of perforation, bacteriology and antimicrobials given.

Antimicrobials should cover Enterobacteriaceae and anaerobes (mainly *B. fragilis* group). This can be achieved by combination or single-agent therapy. For mild-to-moderate community-acquired infections in adults, the agents recommended for empiric regimens are: ticarcillin–clavulanate, cefoxitin, ertapenem, moxifloxacin, or tigecycline as single-agent therapy or combinations of metronidazole with cefazolin, cefuroxime, ceftriaxone, cefotaxime, levofloxacin, or ciprofloxacin. Agents no longer recommended are: cefotetan and clindamycin (because of *B. fragilis* group resistance), ampicillin–sulbactam (*E. coli* resistance) and aminoglycosides (toxicity).[93]

For high-risk community-acquired infections in adults, the agents recommended for empiric regimens are: meropenem, imipenem–cilastatin, doripenem, piperacillin–tazobactam, ciprofloxacin or levofloxacin in combination with metronidazole, or ceftazidime or cefepime in combination with metronidazole. Quinolones should not be used unless hospital surveys indicate >90% susceptibility of *E. coli* to quinolones.[56]

Empiric therapy against enterococci is recommended in high-risk patients, and agents effective against methicillin-resistant *Staph. aureus* (MRSA) or yeast is not recommended in the absence of evidence of infection caused by these organisms.

Antimicrobial prophylaxis for colonic surgery includes either oral preparation such as erythromycin plus neomycin or a parenteral antimicrobial such as cefoxitin or ertapenem. Use of prophylaxis has reduced the rate of postsurgical wound infection (see also Chapter 76).[94]

Female Genital Tract Infection

Female genital tract infections involving anaerobes are polymicrobial and include: soft-tissue, and perineal; bacterial vaginosis; vulvar and Bartholin gland abscesses; endometritis; pyometra; salpingitis; tubo-ovarian abscesses; adnexal abscess; pelvic inflammatory disease, which may include pelvic cellulitis and abscess; amnionitis; septic pelvic thrombophlebitis; intrauterine contraceptive device-associated infection; septic abortion; and postsurgical obstetric and gynecologic infections.[2,4,95] Obtaining proper cultures is often difficult, and avoiding specimen contamination by normal genital flora can be achieved by use of culdocentesis, laparoscopy or quantitative endometrial cultures of transcervical samples obtained with a telescoping catheter.

The predominant anaerobes include *Prev. bivia*, *Prev. disiens* and *Peptostreptococcus*, *Porphyromonas* and *Clostridium* spp. *Bacteroides fragilis* group is less often isolated in these infections than in intra-abdominal infection.[95] *Actinomyces* spp. and *Eubacterium nodatum* are commonly isolated in infections associated with intrauterine devices. *Mobiluncus* spp. may be involved with bacterial vaginosis.[2,4,95] The aerobes isolates include Enterobacteriaceae, *Streptococcus* spp. (including groups A and B), *Neisseria gonorrhoeae* and *Chlamydia* spp. (in sexually active females) and *Mycoplasma genitalium* (Table 184-7).

Clinical findings associated with the presence of anaerobes include gas in the tissues, abscess formation and foul-smelling discharge. Management of polymicrobial pelvic infection includes the treatment with antimicrobials effective against all potential aerobic, anaerobic and sexually transmissible pathogens. Outpatient regimens include cefoxitin, ceftriaxone or other parenteral third-generation cephalosporins plus doxycycline, with or without metronidazole. Regimens for in-patient therapy are: cefoxitin, cefotetan, or ampicillin–sulbactam plus doxycycline; and clindamycin or metronidazole plus doxycycline and gentamicin.[96]

Skin and Soft-Tissue Infections

Skin and soft-tissue infections involving anaerobes include superficial infections, such as infected cutaneous ulcers, cellulitis, pyoderma, paronychia, hidradenitis suppurativa and a variety of secondary-infected sites. These include secondary-infected diaper rash, gastrostomy or tracheostomy site, subcutaneous sebaceous or inclusion cysts, eczema, psoriasis, poison ivy, atopic dermatitis, eczema herpeticum, scabies, kerion infections and postsurgical wound.[2,4,97-100]

Subcutaneous tissue infections that may also include skin involvement include cutaneous and subcutaneous abscesses, breast abscess, decubitus ulcers, infected diabetic (vascular or trophic) ulcers (Figure 184-4), bite wound (Figure 184-5), anaerobic cellulitis, gas gangrene, bacterial synergistic gangrene, infected pilonidal cyst or sinus, Meleney's ulcer and burn wound infection.[98,100] Deeper soft-tissue infections include necrotizing fasciitis (see Figure 11-5), necrotizing synergistic cellulitis, gas gangrene and crepitus cellulitis.[100] These infections can involve the fascia and the muscle surrounded by the fascia, and can cause myositis (Figure 184-6) and myonecrosis.

The isolated organisms vary according to the type and circumstances leading to the infection, and often involve members of the normal flora of the region (Figure 184-7).

Aspirates from wounds and subcutaneous tissue infections and abscesses of the rectal area (i.e. decubitus ulcer, perirectal abscess) or those that originate from the gut flora (i.e. diabetic foot infection) tend to yield organisms found in the colonic flora.[2,4,98-100] These include *B. fragilis* group, *Clostridium* spp., Enterobacteriaceae and *Enterococcus* spp. In contrast, infections in and around the oropharynx, or those

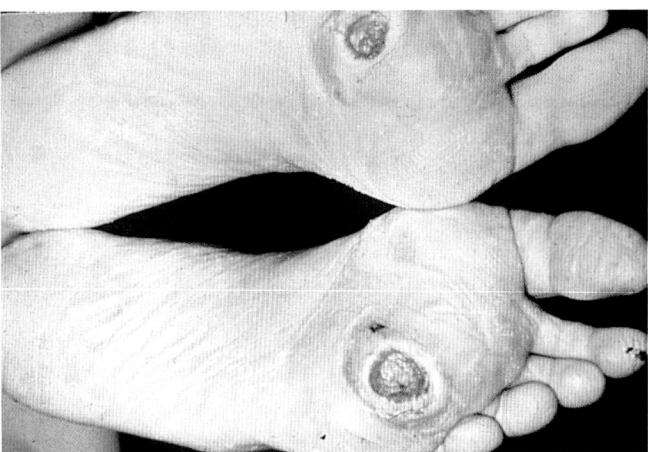

Figure 184-4 Infected diabetic ulcer.

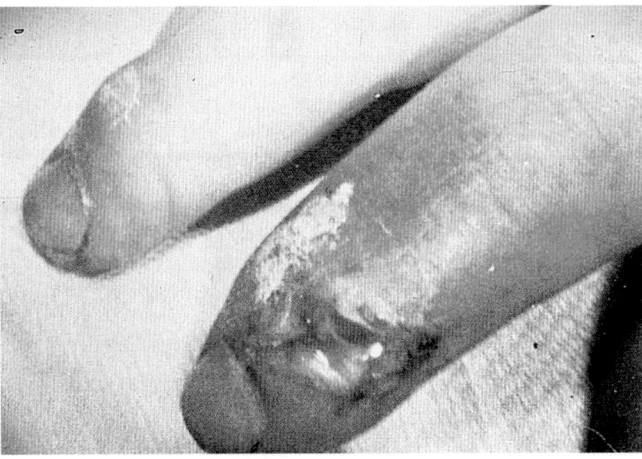

Figure 184-5 Human bite wound.

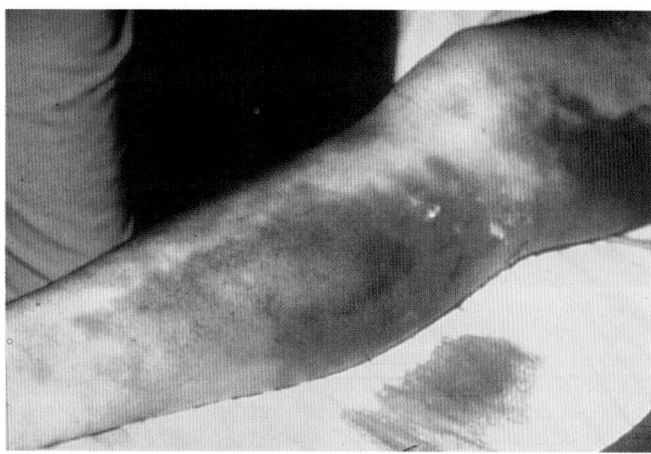

Figure 184-6 Anaerobic streptococcal myositis involving muscle and fascial planes.

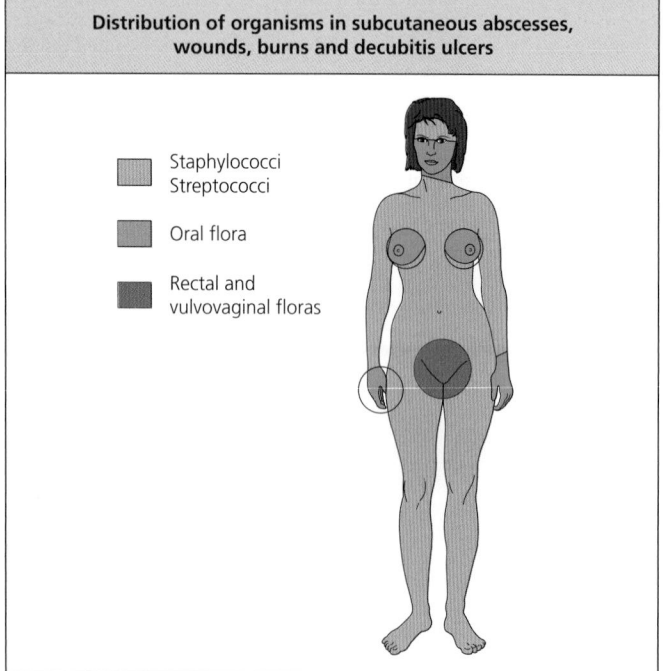

Figure 184-7 Distribution of organisms in subcutaneous abscesses, wounds, burns and decubitus ulcers.

that originate from that site (i.e. paronychia, bites, breast abscess), generally contain members of the oral flora. These include pigmented *Prevotella* and *Porphyromonas*, *Fusobacterium* and *Peptostreptococcus* spp. Skin flora organisms such as *Staph. aureus* and *Streptococcus* spp. and nosocomially acquired organisms can be isolated at all body sites (Table 184-7). In addition to oral flora, human bite infections often contain *Eikenella* spp. and animal bites harbor *Pasteurella multocida*.[101]

Infections involving anaerobes are generally polymicrobial, and in some (i.e. decubitus ulcers, diabetic foot ulcer) are often complicated by osteomyelitis or bacteremia.[43,102] Deep tissue infections such as necrotizing cellulitis, fasciitis and myositis often involve *Clostridium* spp., *Strep. pyogenes* or polymicrobic aerobic and anaerobic bacteria. They often contain free gas in the tissues, putrid-like pus with a gray thin quality, and are associated with a high rate of bacteremia and mortality.[43,100]

Management of deep-seated soft-tissue infection includes surgical debridement, drainage and vigorous surgical management. Improvement of oxygenation through enhancement of blood supply and administration of hyperbaric oxygen (HBO), especially in clostridial infection, may be helpful.[2,4]

Osteomyelitis and Septic Arthritis

Osteomyelitis caused by anaerobes is often indistinguishable from infection caused by aerobic bacteria. Anaerobes are especially notable in osteomyelitis of the cranial and facial bones and long bones after trauma and fracture; and osteomyelitis related to peripheral vascular disease, and decubitus ulcers.[102] Most of these infections are polymicrobial.

Anaerobic osteomyelitis of cranial and facial bones is generally caused by spread from a contiguous soft-tissue source or from sinus, ear or dental infection. The high number of anaerobes within the oral flora accounts for their importance in cranial osteomyelitis. The predominance of intestinal anaerobes in pelvic osteomyelitis has been related to their spread from decubitus ulcers.[4] The anaerobes in osteomyelitis associated with peripheral vascular disease access the involved bone from adjacent soft-tissue ulcers. Osteomyelitis of long bones is generally caused by hematogenic spread, trauma or the presence of a prosthetic device.

Anaerobic streptococci and *Bacteroides* spp. are the most common organisms at all sites, including osteomyelitis associated with bites and cranial infection. Pigmented *Prevotella* and *Porphyromonas* spp. are prevalent in skull and bite infections, *B. fragilis* group is associated with vascular disease and neuropathy. Fusobacteria are frequently isolated from bites and from cranial and facial infections. Clostridia are often found in long bones, especially in association with environmental wound contamination after trauma. Because clostridia colonize the lower gastrointestinal tract, they may contaminate compound fractures of the lower extremities.

Septic arthritis caused by anaerobes is uncommon, and is often associated with hematogenous and contiguous spread, trauma and prosthetic joints.[102] Most infections are monomicrobial and the predominant isolates are peptostreptococci and *Prop. acnes* (often in prosthetic joint infection), *B. fragilis* and fusobacteria (often in infections of hematogenic origin), and clostridia (associated with trauma).

Bacteremia

The incidence of anaerobes in bacteremia is 5–15%.[43] However, in the 1990s the incidence was lowered to approximately 4% (0.5–12%) of bacteremias, with variation by geographic location, hospital patient demographics and patient age.[103] Recent studies documented a resurgence in bacteremia due to anaerobes.[103] This increase is due to the higher incidence of anaerobic bacteremia in immunosuppressed patients and those with complex underlying disease.[103] The common isolates are *B. fragilis* group (>75% of anaerobic isolates), *Clostridium* (10–20%), *Peptostreptococcus* (10–15%), and *Fusobacterium* spp. (10–15%) and *Prop. acnes* (2–5%).

The specific organisms involved in bacteremia largely depend on the portal of entry and underlying disease. Recovery of *B. fragilis* group and clostridia is mostly associated with a gastrointestinal source, pigmented *Prevotella* and *Porphyromonas* spp. and fusobacteria with oropharynx and pulmonary sources, fusobacteria with the female genital tract, *Prop. acnes* with foreign body, and peptostreptococci with all sources, but especially with oropharyngeal, pulmonary and female genital tract. The predominance of these isolates in conjunction with the specific sources is related to the origin of the primary infection and the endogenous flora at the infection site.

Predisposing factors to anaerobic bacterial bacteremia include malignant neoplasms; hematologic disorders; organ transplant; recent gastrointestinal, obstetric, or gynecologic surgery; intestinal obstruction; decubitus ulcers; dental extraction; the newborn; sickle cell disease; diabetes mellitus; splenectomy; and the use of cytotoxic agents or corticosteroids.[2,4]

The clinical presentation of anaerobic bacteremia is often similar to the aerobic one, except for the signs of infection at the portal of entry of infection. It commonly includes fever, chills, hypotension, leukocytosis, shock, disseminated intravascular coagulation and anemia. Features typical of anaerobic infection include metastatic lesions, hyperbilirubinemia and suppurative thrombophlebitis. Mortality rate is 15–30% and it improves with early and appropriate antimicrobial therapy and resolution, when present, of the primary infection.

Management

The recovery from an anaerobic infection depends on prompt and proper management. The principles of managing anaerobic infections include neutralizing toxins produced by anaerobes, preventing the local proliferation of the organisms by changing the environment and hampering their spread into healthy tissues.

Toxin neutralization by specific antitoxins may be employed, especially in infections caused by *Clostridium* spp. (tetanus and botulism). Controlling the environment is achieved by debriding necrotic tissue, draining pus, improving circulation, alleviating obstructions and increasing tissue oxygenation. Certain types of adjunct therapy such as HBO may also be useful. The primary role of antimicrobials is in limiting the local and systemic spread of the organisms.

HYPERBARIC OXYGEN

There is controversy regarding whether HBO should be used in infection of gram-positive spore-forming anaerobic rods. There are several uncontrolled reports that demonstrated efficacy in individual cases.[2,4,104] However, because no well-controlled studies are available, the efficacy of HBO is unproved. Using HBO in conjunction with other therapeutic measures is not contraindicated, except when it may delay the execution of other essential procedures. Topical application of oxygen-releasing compounds may be useful as an adjunct to other procedures.

SURGICAL THERAPY

In many cases surgical therapy is the most important and sometimes the only form of treatment required, whereas in others surgical therapy is an important adjunct to a pharmacologic approach. Surgery is important in draining abscesses, debriding necrotic tissues, decompressing closed space infections and relieving obstructions. When surgical drainage is not used, the infection may persist and serious complications can develop.

ANTIMICROBIAL THERAPY

Appropriate management of mixed aerobic and anaerobic infections requires the administration of antimicrobials effective against both the aerobic and the anaerobic components. A number of factors should be considered when choosing appropriate antimicrobial agents. They should have efficacy against all target organisms, induce little or no resistance, achieve sufficient levels in the infected site, and have minimal toxicity and maximum stability.

Antimicrobials often fail to cure the infection. Among the reasons for this are the development of bacterial resistance, achievement of insufficient tissue levels, incompatible drug interaction and the development of an abscess. The environment of an abscess is detrimental to many antibiotics. The abscess capsule interferes with the penetration of drugs, and the low pH and the presence of binding proteins or inactivating enzymes (i.e. β-lactamase) may impair their activity. The low pH and the anaerobic environment within the abscess are especially unfavorable for the aminoglycosides and quinolones. However, an acidic pH, high osmolarity and an anaerobic environment can also develop in the absence of an abscess.

When choosing antimicrobials (Tables 184-8 and 184-9) for the therapy of mixed infections, their aerobic and anaerobic antibacterial spectrum (Figure 184-8) and their availability in oral or parenteral

TABLE 184-8	Antimicrobial Drugs Recommended for the Therapy* of Site-Specific Anaerobic Infections		
Infection Site	**Surgical Prophylaxis**	**Parenteral**	**Oral**
Intracranial	Penicillin Vancomycin	Metronidazole[b] Chloramphenicol	1. Metronidazole[b] 2. Chloramphenicol
Dental	Penicillin Erythromycin	Clindamycin Metronidazole[b] Ticarcillin + CA, ampicillin + SU[d]	Clindamycin, amoxicillin + CA Metronidazole[b]
Upper respiratory tract	Cefoxitin Clindamycin	Clindamycin Ticarcillin + CA, ampicillin + SU[d] Metronidazole[b]	Clindamycin, amoxicillin + CA Metronidazole[c]
Pulmonary	NA	Clindamycin[c] Ticarcillin + CA, ampicillin + SU,[d] imipenem or meropenem	Clindamycin[f] Metronidazole[c] Amoxicillin + CA
Abdominal	Cefoxitin 2. Clindamycin[c]	Metronidazole[a] Imipenem or meropenem ertapenem, piperacillin–tazobactam, tigecycline, Cefoxitin[c]	Metronidazole[f] Amoxicillin + CA
Pelvic	Cefoxitin Doxycycline	Cefoxitin,[d] clindamycin[a] Piperacillin–tazobactam,[d] ampicillin + SU,[d] metronidazole[d]	Clindamycin[d] Amoxicillin + CA,[d] metronidazole[d]
Skin and soft tissue	Cefazolin[e] Vancomycin	Clindamycin, cefoxitin Metronidazole + vancomycin Tigecycline	Clindamycin, amoxicillin + CA Metronidazole + linezolid
Bone and joint	Cefazolin[e] Vancomycin	Clindamycin, imipenem or meropenem Metronidazole + vancomycin, piperacillin–tazobactam	Clindamycin Metronidazole + linezolid
Bacteremia with BLPB	NA	Imipenem or meropenem, metronidazole Cefoxitin, ticarcillin + CA	Clindamycin, metronidazole Chloramphenicol, amoxicillin + CA
Bacteremia with non-BLPB	NA	Penicillin Clindamycin, metronidazole, cefoxitin	Penicillin Metronidazole, chloramphenicol, clindamycin

*Therapies are given as drug(s) of choice (alternative drugs). BLPB, β-lactamase-producing bacteria; CA, clavulanic acid; NA, not applicable; SU, sulbactam.
1., drug(s) of choice; 2., alternative drugs; a, plus aminoglycoside; b, plus a penicillin; c, plus a macrolide (i.e. erythromycin); d, plus doxycycline; e, in locations proximal to the rectal and oral areas use cefoxitin; f, plus a quinolone (only in adults).

TABLE 184-9 Antimicrobial Drugs of Choice for Anaerobic Bacteria		
Bacteria	**Drug of Choice**	**Alternative Drugs**
Peptostreptococcus spp.	Penicillin	Clindamycin, chloramphenicol, cephalosporins
Clostridium spp.	Penicillin	Metronidazole, chloramphenicol, cefoxitin, clindamycin
Clostridium difficile	Vancomycin	Metronidazole, bacitracin
Fusobacterium spp.	Penicillin	Metronidazole, clindamycin, chloramphenicol
Bacteroides (BL–)	Penicillin	Metronidazole, clindamycin, chloramphenicol
Bacteroides (BL+)	Metronidazole, a carbapenem, a penicillin and β-lactamase inhibitor, clindamycin	Cefoxitin, chloramphenicol, piperacillin, tigecycline

Gram-negative bacilli include *Bacteroides fragilis* group and *Prevotella, Porphyromonas* and *Fusobacterium* spp. BL, β-lactamase.

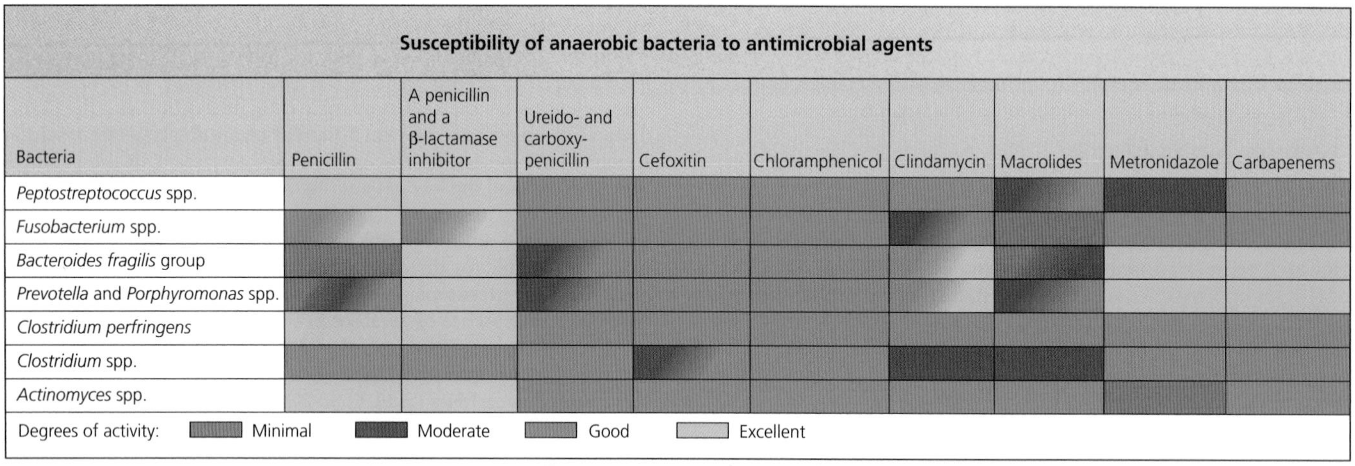

Bacteria	Penicillin	A penicillin and a β-lactamase inhibitor	Ureido- and carboxy-penicillin	Cefoxitin	Chloramphenicol	Clindamycin	Macrolides	Metronidazole	Carbapenems
Peptostreptococcus spp.									
Fusobacterium spp.									
Bacteroides fragilis group									
Prevotella and *Porphyromonas* spp.									
Clostridium perfringens									
Clostridium spp.									
Actinomyces spp.									

Degrees of activity: ▨ Minimal ▨ Moderate ▨ Good ▨ Excellent

Figure 184-8 Susceptibility of anaerobic bacteria to antimicrobial agents.

form should be considered.[56] Some antimicrobials have a limited range of activity. Metronidazole is active only against anaerobes and therefore cannot be administered as a single agent for the therapy of mixed infections. Others (i.e. carbapenems) have wide spectra of activity against Enterobacteriaceae and anaerobes.

The selection of antimicrobials is simplified when reliable culture results are available. However, this may be difficult to achieve in anaerobic infections because of inability to obtain appropriate specimens. For this reason, many patients are treated empirically on the basis of suspected, rather than established, pathogens. Fortunately, the types of organism involved in many anaerobic infections and their antimicrobial susceptibility patterns tend to be predictable. However, resistance patterns to antimicrobials may vary in a particular hospital; resistance to antimicrobials has consistently increased in the past three decades and may emerge while a patient is receiving therapy.

B. fragilis group's susceptibility to frequently used antimicrobials varies among different geographic regions and institutions, and some antimicrobials used in the past are no longer adequate for empiric therapy.[56,105] A significant increase in resistance of AGNB is to clindamycin, cefoxitin and cefotetan. Resistance to other agents varies, but *B. fragilis* group is almost uniformly susceptible to metronidazole, carbapenems, chloramphenicol and combinations of β-lactam/β-lactamase inhibitors.[56,105]

Recent reports of multiple drug-resistant *B. fragilis* group underscores the need for improved antibiotic stewardship.[57,106] Although *B. fragilis* has long been considered reliably susceptible to a number of broad-spectrum anti-anaerobic drugs, these reports suggest that clinicians should no longer rely on cumulative susceptibility data alone to direct treatment and should consider performing susceptibility testing when treating serious infections by *B. fragilis* group.

Aside from susceptibility patterns, other factors influencing the choice of antimicrobial therapy include the pharmacologic characteristics of the drugs, their toxicity and effect on the normal flora. Although identification of the infecting organisms and their antimicrobial susceptibility may be needed for selection of optimal therapy, the clinical setting and Gram-stain preparation of the specimen may suggest the types of anaerobe present as well as the nature of the infectious process.

ANTIMICROBIAL AGENTS

Some classes of agents have poor activity against anaerobic bacteria. These include the aminoglycosides, monobactams and older quinolones. Antimicrobials suitable for use in controlling anaerobic infections are discussed in detail below.[56]

Penicillins

Penicillin G can be used when the infecting strains are susceptible. These include anaerobic streptococci, most *Clostridium* spp. and non-sporulating anaerobic bacilli, and most non-β-lactamase-producing AGNB (i.e. *Bacteroides, Fusobacterium, Prevotella* and *Porphyromonas* spp.).[56,57] However, in addition to the *B. fragilis* group, which is known to resist the drug, many other anaerobic gram-negative bacteria show increased resistance. These include *Fusobacterium* spp., pigmented *Prevotella* and *Porphyromonas* spp. (prevalent in orofacial infections), *Prev. bivia* and *Prev. disiens* (common in obstetric and gynecologic infections), *Bilophila wadsworthia* and *Bacteroides splanchnicus*. Resistance to penicillin of some *Clostridium* spp. through production of β-lactamase has also been noted. These included *C. ramosum, C. clostridioforme* and *C. butyricum*.

Ampicillin and amoxicillin are equally active as penicillin G, but the semisynthetic penicillins are less active. Methicillin, nafcillin, and the isoxazolyl penicillins (oxacillin, cloxacillin, and dicloxacillin) are also not active against *B. fragilis* group and have unpredictable activity and frequently are inferior to penicillin G against anaerobes.[56]

Penicillin therapy against a susceptible pathogen might be rendered ineffective by the presence of BLPB.[53,82] The combinations of β-lactamase inhibitors (e.g. clavulanic acid, sulbactam, tazobactam) with a β-lactam antibiotic (ampicillin, amoxicillin, ticarcillin or piperacillin) can overcome this phenomenon in organisms that produce a β-lactamase that can be bound by the inhibitor. Other mechanisms of penicillin resistance include alteration in the porin canal and changes in the penicillin-binding protein.

In high concentrations, ticarcillin, piperacillin, and mezlocillin have good activity against Enterobacteriaceae and most anaerobes; however, up to 30% of B. fragilis group are resistant.[56]

Cephalosporins

The activity of first-generation cephalosporins against anaerobes is similar to penicillin G. B. fragilis group, Prevotella species and Porphyromonas species are resistant to first-generation cephalosporins by virtue of cephalosporinase production.[107] Cefoxitin is the most effective cephalosporin against the B. fragilis group, although 5–15% may be resistant. Cefoxitin is inactive against most clostridial organisms, except C. perfringens. Other second-generation cephalosporins, cefotetan and cefmetazole, have a longer half-life than cefoxitin but are as effective against B. fragilis; however, they are less efficacious against other members of the B. fragilis group.[56] Cefotetan is no longer recommended for treatment of intra-abdominal infections because of its poor B. fragilis group activity and resultant clinical failures.[56,93]

Carbapenems (Imipenem, Meropenem, Doripenem, Ertapenem)

Carbapenems have excellent activity against a broad spectrum of aerobic and anaerobic bacteria. Resistance of B. fragilis group is rare (<1%). They are usually employed in serious infections such as intra-abdominal, and skin and soft tissue. Two recent reports have noted the development of carbapenem resistance among anaerobes: (1.1–2.5%) in a multicenter survey[105] in the USA and a higher rate (7–12%) in a small study from Taiwan.[108] Ertapenem has similar efficacy but is not active against Pseudomonas spp. and Acinetobacter spp.[56]

Chloramphenicol

Chloramphenicol shows excellent in vitro activity against most anaerobes and resistance is rare.[56,57] Its unique lipid solubility permits its penetration across lipid barriers and achieving high concentrations in the CNS, even in the absence of inflammation. However, the experience of using this drug in intra-abdominal sepsis was disappointing. The toxicity of chloramphenicol, the rare but fatal aplastic anemia and the dose-dependent leukopenia, limit its use.

Clindamycin

This antimicrobial is effective against aerobic gram-positive cocci.[56] Although the patterns differ by region, B. fragilis resistance to clindamycin is increasing worldwide.[56] Resistance of the B. fragilis group in some centers has reached about 40%[57] and it is no longer recommended as empiric therapy for intra-abdominal infections.[93] Up to 10% resistance was noted for Prevotella, Fusobacterium, Porphyromonas, and Peptostreptococcus spp., with higher rates for some Clostridium spp. (especially C. difficile).[56] Antibiotic-associated colitis due to C. difficile, although associated with most antimicrobials, was first described following clindamycin therapy.

Metronidazole and Tinidazole

These nitroimidazoles have excellent activity against anaerobes; however, this efficacy is limited to anaerobes. Microaerophilic streptococci, Prop. acnes and Actinomyces spp. are often resistant, therefore adding an antimicrobial that is effective against these organisms (e.g. penicillin) is often necessary. Resistance to metronidazole among B. fragilis group is very rare.[56] Concern was raised about the carcinogenic and mutagenic effects of these drugs, however, these effects were shown only in one species of mice and were never substantiated in other animals or humans.[2,4]

Macrolides (Erythromycin, Azithromycin, Clarithromycin)

The macrolides have moderate to good in vitro activity against anaerobes other than B. fragilis group.[56] Macrolides are active against pigmented Prevotella and Porphyromonas spp. and microaerophilic streptococci, gram-positive nonspore-forming anaerobic bacilli and certain clostridia. They are less effective against Fusobacterium and Peptostreptococcus spp.[109] They show relatively good activity against C. perfringens and poor or inconsistent activity against AGNB. Clarithromycin is the most active of the macrolides against gram-positive oral cavity anaerobes, including Actinomyces, Propionibacterium, and Lactobacillus spp. and Bifidobacterium dentium. Emergence of erythromycin-resistant organisms during therapy has been documented.[110]

Glycopeptides (Vancomycin, Teicoplanin)

The glycopeptides are effective against gram-positive anaerobes (including C. difficile), but are inactive against AGNB.[56]

Tetracyclines

Tetracycline is of limited use because of the development of resistance by all types of anaerobe. Resistance to Prop. acnes has been related to previous use.[111] The newer tetracycline analogs doxycycline and minocycline are more active than the parent compound. Because there is significant resistance to these drugs, they can only be used if the organisms are susceptible or in less severe infections in which a therapeutic trial is feasible.

Tigecycline

This glycylcycline is active against aerobic gram-negative and gram-positive bacteria, anaerobes and certain drug-resistant pathogens.[112] It is active against Streptococcus anginosus group (includes Strep. anginosus, Strep. intermedius and Strep. constellatus), B. fragilis group, C. perfringens, C. difficile and Parvimonas micra (Peptostreptococcus micros).[56,112] Resistance of members of the B. fragilis group is 3.3–7.2%.[105]

Fluoroquinolones

Quinolones with low activity against anaerobes include ciprofloxacin, ofloxacin, levofloxacin, pefloxacin, and lomefloxacin. Compounds with intermediate anti-anaerobic activity include sparfloxacin and grepafloxacin. Gatifloxacin and moxifloxacin yield low minimum inhibitory concentrations (MICs) against most groups of anaerobes. Quinolones with the greatest in vitro activity against anaerobes include clinafloxacin and sitafloxacin.[113] Moxifloxacin has been used as monotherapy in intra-abdominal infections in adults. However, concern over increasing fluoroquinolone resistance in E. coli and B. fragilis group reduced its use.[108,113] The use of quinolones is restricted in growing children and during pregnancy because of their possible adverse effects on cartilage.

Other Agents

Bacitracin is active against pigmented Prevotella and Porphyromonas spp. but is inactive against B. fragilis and Fusobacterium nucleatum.[2] Quinupristin–dalfopristin shows antibacterial activity against C. perfringens, Lactobacillus and Peptostreptococcus spp.[56] Linezolid is active against Fusobacterium, Porphyromonas, Prevotella and Peptostreptococcus spp.[109] Little clinical experience has, however, been gained in the treatment of anaerobic bacteria using these agents.

CHOICE OF ANTIMICROBIAL AGENTS

The available parenteral antimicrobials for most infections (Tables 184-8 and 184-9) include the combination of metronidazole, a penicillin (i.e. ticarcillin, ampicillin, piperacillin) plus a β-lactamase inhibitor (i.e. clavulanic acid, sulbactam, tazobactam) or a carbapenem (e.g. imipenem, meropenem, doripenem, ertapenem).

An agent effective against gram-negative enteric bacilli (e.g. aminoglycoside, a fluoroquinolone) or an antipseudomonal cephalosporin (e.g. cefepime) are generally added to metronidazole, and occasionally to cefoxitin when treating intra-abdominal infection.

Penicillin can be added to metronidazole in the therapy of intracranial, pulmonary and dental infections to cover microaerophilic streptococci, *Actinomyces* and *Arachnia* spp. A macrolide is added to metronidazole in upper respiratory infections to treat *Staph. aureus* and aerobic streptococci. Penicillin is added to clindamycin to supplement its coverage against *Peptostreptococcus* spp. and other gram-positive anaerobic organisms.

Doxycycline is added to most regimens in the treatment of pelvic infections to provide therapy for *Chlamydia* and *Mycoplasma*. Penicillin is still the drug of choice for bacteremia caused by susceptible non-BLPB. However, other agents should be used for the therapy of bacteremia caused by BLPB.[2,4]

Because the duration of therapy for anaerobic infections, which are often chronic, is generally longer than for infections caused by aerobic and facultative anaerobes, oral therapy is often substituted for parenteral therapy. The agents available for oral therapy include amoxicillin plus clavulanic acid, clindamycin, chloramphenicol and metronidazole. The duration of therapy ranges between 2 and 4 weeks, but should be individualized depending on the response. In some cases, such as lung abscesses, treatment may be required for as long as 6–8 weeks, but can often be shortened with proper surgical drainage. Some infections (i.e., osteomyelitis) require longer treatment.

Clinical judgment, personal experience, safety and patient compliance should direct the physician in the choice of the appropriate antimicrobial agents.

References available online at expertconsult.com.

KEY REFERENCES

Bartlett J.G., Gorbach S.L., Finegold S.M.: The bacteriology of aspiration pneumonia. *Am J Med* 1974; 56:202-207.

Bratzler D.W., Dellinger E.P., Olsen K.M., et al.: Clinical practice guidelines for antimicrobial prophylaxis in surgery. *Surg Infect (Larchmt)* 2013; 14:73-156.

Brook I.: The role of beta-lactamase-producing bacteria in the persistence of streptococcal tonsillar infection. *Rev Infect Dis* 1984; 6:601-607.

Brook I.: *Pediatric anaerobic infection: diagnosis and management*, 3rd ed. New York: Marcel Dekker; 2002.

Brook I.: The role of anaerobic bacteria in tonsillitis. *Int J Pediatr Otorhinolaryngol* 2005; 69:9-1983.

Brook I.: Microbiology and antimicrobial treatment of orbital and intracranial complications of sinusitis in children and their management. *Int J Pediatr Otorhinolaryngol* 2009; 73:1183-1186.

Brook I., Frazier E.H.: Aerobic and anaerobic microbiology of empyema. A retrospective review in two military hospitals. *Chest* 1993; 103:1502-1507.

Brook I., Wexler H.M., Goldstein E.J.: Antianaerobic antimicrobials: spectrum and susceptibility testing. *Clin Microbiol Rev* 2013; 26:526-546.

Centers for Disease Control and Prevention (CDC): Updated recommendations for use of tetanus toxoid, reduced diphtheria toxoid, and acellular pertussis vaccine (Tdap) in pregnant women – Advisory Committee on Immunization Practices (ACIP), 2012. *MMWR Morb Mortal Wkly Rep* 2013; 62:131-135.

Clinical and Laboratory Standards Institute: *Methods for antimicrobial susceptibility testing of anaerobic bacteria*. Approved Standard-eighth edition. CLSI Document M11-A9. Wayne, PA: Clinical and Laboratory Standards; 2012.

Cohen S.H., Gerding D.N., Johnson S., et al.: Clinical practice guidelines for *Clostridium difficile* infection in adults: 2010 update by the Society for Healthcare Epidemiology of America (SHEA) and the Infectious Diseases Society of America (IDSA). *Infect Control Hosp Epidemiol* 2010; 31:431-455.

Nord C.E.: The role of anaerobic bacteria in recurrent episodes of sinusitis and tonsillitis. *Clin Infect Dis* 1995; 20:1512-1524.

Pieracci F.M., Barie P.S., Bartlett J.G.: Intra-abdominal infections. *Curr Opin Crit Care* 2007; 13:440-449.

Snydman D.R., Jacobus N.V., McDermott L.A., et al.: Update on resistance of *Bacteroides fragilis* group and related species with special attention to carbapenems 2006-2009. *Anaerobe* 2011; 17:147-151.

Solomkin J.S., Mazuski J.E., Bradley J.S., et al.: Diagnosis and management of complicated intra-abdominal infection in adults and children: guidelines by the Surgical Infection Society and the Infectious Diseases Society of America. *Clin Infect Dis* 2010; 50:133-164.

Walker C.K., Wiesenfeld H.C.: Antibiotic therapy for acute pelvic inflammatory disease: the 2006 Centers for Disease Control and Prevention sexually transmitted diseases treatment guidelines. *Clin Infect Dis* 2007; 44(Suppl. 3): S111-S122.

185

Mycobacteria

JAKKO VAN INGEN

Introduction

Mycobacterial diseases remain an important burden to man and a serious and frequent challenge to health systems. Tuberculosis, leprosy, Buruli ulcer disease and the infections caused by nontuberculous mycobacteria all provide specific challenges to physicians and microbiologists, in frequencies that differ strongly between geographical areas.

Mycobacterium tuberculosis and *M. leprae* were traditionally considered key players in global mycobacterial disease. During the past decade the Buruli ulcer disease (caused by *M. ulcerans*) and diseases caused by nontuberculous mycobacteria (NTM) have become subject of extensive investigations as well; for the former this is due to improved therapeutics, for the latter it is largely because of the increasing incidence of human disease and increasing awareness. As a consequence, accurate laboratory diagnosis of all mycobacterial species, is an important element for effective treatment and control of any mycobacterial disease.

General Characteristics of Mycobacterial Organisms

Lehmann and Neumann first introduced the genus *Mycobacterium* into the scientific literature in 1896. The subsequent history of the genus has been profoundly influenced by the fact that only very few of the more than over 150 currently recognized species have been a cause of human disease, above all *M. tuberculosis*. Thus, studies of microbial physiology, structure, genetics and diagnostic tools have mainly focused on *M. tuberculosis* and secondarily on *Mycobacterium leprae*.

The genus *Mycobacterium* is the only genus in the family of the Mycobacteriaceae and is related to other mycolic acid-containing genera. All mycobacteria are aerobic (though some species are able to grow under a reduced oxygen atmosphere), nonspore-forming, nonmotile, slightly curved or straight rods. The most prominent feature of mycobacteria that is uniformly present and distinctive to the genus

is the lipid-rich cell envelope.[1,2] Indeed, it is the complex cell envelope of mycobacteria that confers upon these bacteria the property of 'acid-fastness' (i.e. resistance to decolorization when stained with carbol-fuchsin and decolorized with dilute hydrochloric acid). Uniformly, they do not stain well with Gram stain and should be considered gram-neutral. Mycobacteria possess a cell wall polysaccharide that resembles that of gram-positive bacteria; however, the mycobacterial peptidoglycan contains lipids in place of proteins and polysaccharides.[1,2] Furthermore, the mycobacterial envelope contains a plasma membrane that is quite similar in structure and function to the plasma membrane of other bacteria, except for the presence of lipoarabinomannan (LAM), lipomannan and phosphatidylinositol mannosides (Figure 185-1). As a whole, the cell wall component of the envelope confers size, shape, protection against osmotic pressure and probably protects the plasma membrane from deleterious molecules in the environment of the cell. In summary, the peptidoglycan confers cell shape while the next layer of the envelope, arabinogalactan esterified to the mycolic acids, provides a hydrophobic permeability barrier. Other important fatty acids are waxes, phospholipids and mycoserosic and phthienoic acids, and tuberculostearic acid (10-R-methyl-octadecanoic), a unique cell component within the Actinomycetales, including the mycobacteria.[1,2]

In 1947, Middlebrook first described growth of tubercle bacilli in the shape of serpentine cords ('cording'). For many years cording was correlated with virulence and considered a distinctive feature of *M. tuberculosis* (Figure 185-2). However, it is now known that several mycobacterial species display cording and the correlation with virulence, if any, is unclear. Cord factor appears to be a mixture of

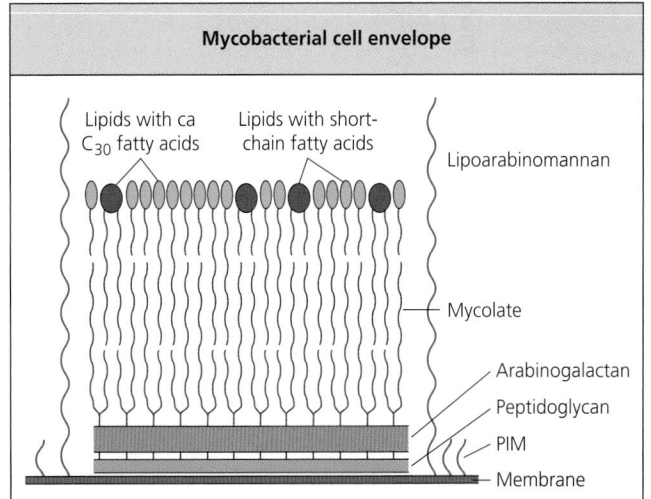

Figure 185-1 Mycobacterial cell envelope. This model displays the asymmetric array of the structural elements extending from the plasma membrane that surrounds the cytoplasm of the mycobacterial cell. The arabinogalactan is covalently linked to the peptidoglycan, which along with the lipoarabinomannan (LAM) and phosphatidylinositol mannosides (PIM) are associated with the plasma membrane. The cell wall lipids are shown in a possible arrangement with the mycolates linked to the arabinogalactan. Two classes of polar lipids with medium and short chain fatty acids complement the varying hydrocarbon chains of the mycolates to create an even cell envelope. There is evidence for a small number of porins within the hydrophobic bilayer. (*Adapted from Brennan & Draper. American Society for Microbiology; 1994:271-284.*)

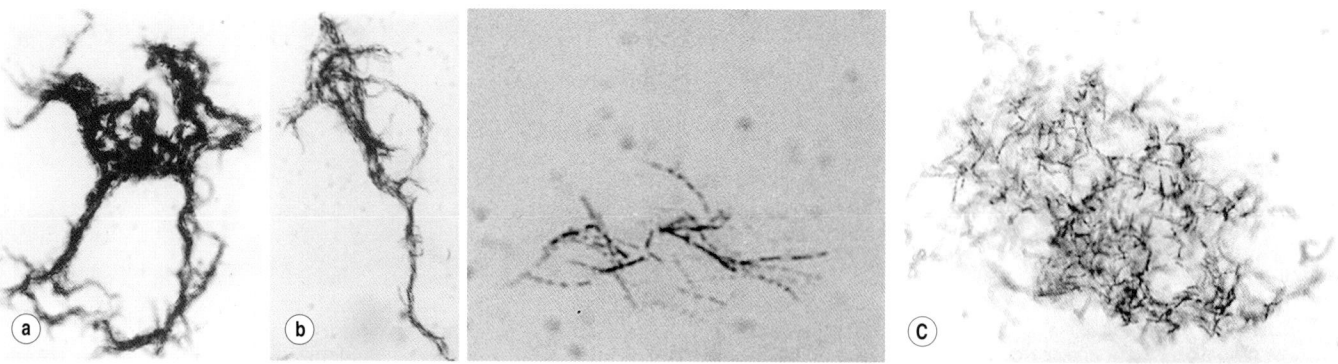

Figure 185-2 Microscopic clusters of three different species of mycobacteria. (a) Serpentine cording of *M. tuberculosis*. (b) Cross-banding of *M. kansasii*. (c) Loose clusters of *M. avium* complex. *(Photomicrographs taken from Attorri et al. J Clin Microbiol 2000; 38:1426-1429.)*

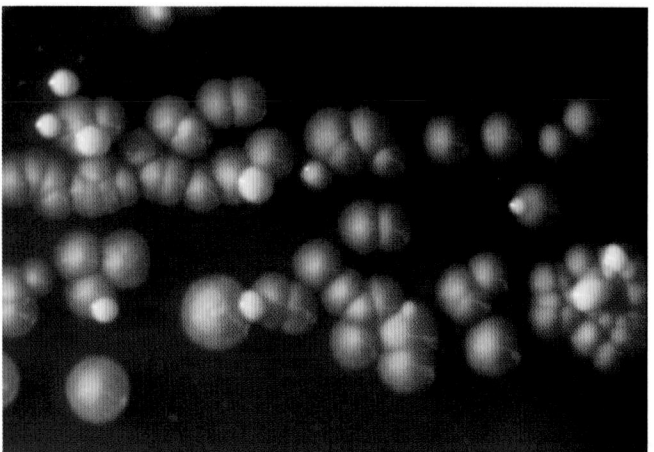

Figure 185-3 *Mycobacterium scrofulaceum*, a scotochromogenic mycobacterium, grown on Middlebrook 7H10 agar.

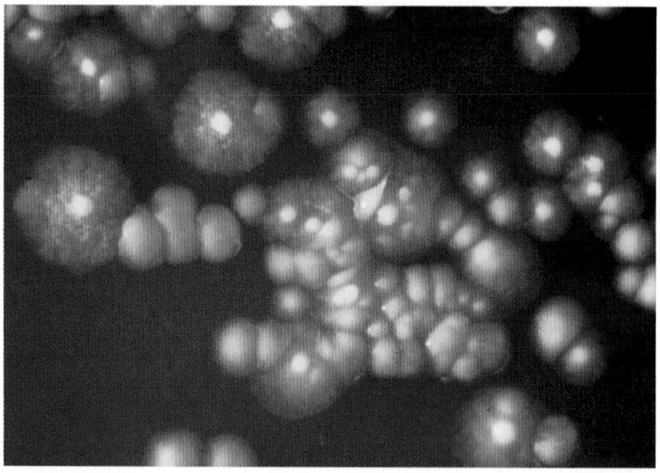

Figure 185-4 *Mycobacterium szulgai*, a scotochromogenic mycobacterium, grown on Middlebrook 7H10 agar.

mycolate-containing molecules including the original cord factor associated with *M. tuberculosis*, trehalose 6,6'-dimycolate.

Many species of mycobacteria are capable of producing carotenoids (carotene and xanthophylls) and this feature was part of classical biochemical identification schemes of mycobacteria. The production of carotenoids is strongly influenced by the composition of the media and growth conditions. Light has a significant effect on pigment production for some species. Scotochromogens, e.g. *M. scrofulaceum* (Figure 185-3) or *M. szulgai* (Figure 185-4) produce a yellow pigment in the absence of light, whereas photochromogens, e.g. *M. kansasii* (Figure 185-5), produce pigment when stimulated by light. Nonchromogens, e.g. *M. tuberculosis* or *M. avium*, do not produce carotenoids (Figure 185-6). The function of mycobacterial carotenoids is largely unknown, but some evidence suggests that carotenoids provide protection against phototoxic effects.

The genome of mycobacteria displays a typical bacterial chromosomal structure, i.e. a single large circular DNA molecule with a high G + C content of 60–70 mol% (except *M. leprae*; <57%). *M. tuberculosis* was among the first bacterial species to have its full (4.41 Mb) genome sequenced.[3] Many NTM species contain plasmids. The size and number of plasmids vary and they appear to be species-specific without evidence of transfer. Most contain genes involved in resistance to environmental hazard such as heavy metals. *M. tuberculosis* does not contain plasmids.

Analyses of whole genome sequence information have revealed differences within the *M. tuberculosis* complex. For example, comparisons of *M. tuberculosis* H37Rv (a human isolate that is also virulent in mice) with Bacille Calmette–Guérin (BCG) Pasteur led to the discovery of the so-called Region of Difference 1 (RD1), which encodes for two key secreted virulence factors (ESAT-6 and CFP-10) and their

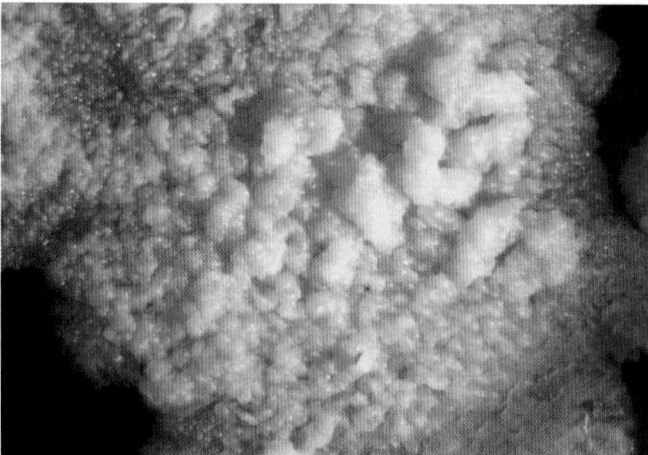

Figure 185-5 *Mycobacterium kansasii*, a photochromogenic mycobacterium, grown on Middlebrook 7H10 agar, after exposure to light.

secretion system, which is present and functional in *M. tuberculosis* but absent from the almost avirulent *M. bovis* BCG vaccine strains. Furthermore, the genome size of *M. bovis* is significantly smaller than that of *M. tuberculosis*. Given the role of reductive genomics in mycobacterial evolution, this indicates that, contrary to long-held belief, all members of the *M. tuberculosis* complex, i.e. *M. tuberculosis*, *M. bovis*, *M. bovis* BCG, *M. caprae*, *M. africanum*, *M. mungi*, *M. orygis*, *M. microti*, 'M. canettii' and *M. pinnipedii* (Table 185-1), gradually evolved from a common ancestor and 'M. canettii' segregated some 2.4–2.8 million years ago. M. tuberculosis, in its present form, is estimated to be only some 35 000 years old and was always a human pathogen.[4,5]

Epidemiology and Clinical Manifestations of the Most Important Mycobacterial Pathogens
TUBERCULOSIS

Tuberculosis is the second most common infectious cause of death in adults, and is ranked 10th of all causes of loss of healthy life

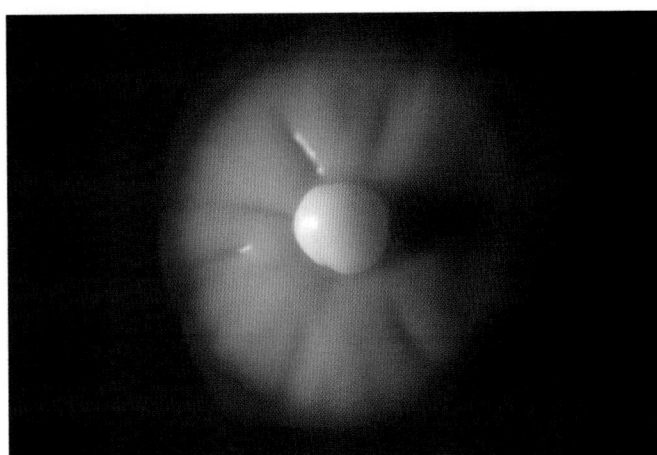

Figure 185-6 *Mycobacterium fortuitum*, a nonchromogenic rapid grower, grown on Middlebrook 7H10 agar.

worldwide. In 2013, an estimated 9.0 million people developed tuberculosis and 1.5 million died from the disease, 360 000 of whom were HIV-positive.[6] Before the development of effective chemotherapy, the mortality rate for tuberculosis was 50–60%. Following the discovery of isoniazid (INH) and rifampin (rifampicin; RMP), the majority of pulmonary and extrapulmonary tuberculosis became treatable with relatively short (6 months) treatment regimens. Nevertheless, treatment of tuberculosis remains problematic in many areas because of the lack of/or intermittent access to therapy, poor adherence to therapy, poor drug quality and, above all, the worldwide emergence of resistance.

Multidrug-resistant *M. tuberculosis* strains (i.e. resistant to INH and RMP at least) are responsible for 3.5% of new and 20.5% of previously treated tuberculosis cases in 2013. This translates into an estimated 480 000 people having developed MDR-TB in 2013. About 9% of the patients actually have XDR-TB (extensively drug-resistant tuberculosis).[6] Occurring worldwide, such XDR strains are resistant against INH and RMP as well as against the two most important second-line drug classes, a fluoroquinolone (e.g. moxifloxacin) and an injectable drug (e.g. amikacin) and pose a significant threat for humans and healthcare systems.

The most common form of tuberculosis is a chronic pulmonary disease classified as either primary or post-primary disease. Post-primary disease can be a consequence of either reactivation (endogenous infection) or re-infection (exogenous infection). By far the most common (95%) route of infection is inhalation of infectious droplet nuclei, but neither does exposure to *M. tuberculosis* bacilli always lead to infection, nor are all patients with disease infectious. The risk of infection is directly related to the number of tubercle bacilli in the inhaled air and the duration of exposure, emphasizing the importance of infectious droplet nuclei to airborne transmission. The appearance and extent of disease varies with only one-half of infected patients

TABLE 185-1	Major Characteristics of the *Mycobacterium tuberculosis* Complex		
Species	**Geographic Distribution**	**Remarks**	**Identifying Features**
M. tuberculosis	Widespread, humans are the definite host; disease also in elephants and other mammals	Based on genetic analyses, present day *M. tuberculosis* is relatively young (~35 000 years old)	Usually PZA-susceptible, nitrate reductase activity-positive, niacin-positive, aerobic
M. bovis	Widespread, broad host range including nonhuman primates, cattle, goats, cats, dogs, buffalo, badgers, possums, deer and bison. Humans are viewed as a 'spillover' host	Mainly extrapulmonary manifestation in humans	PZA-resistant, nitrate reductase activity-negative, niacin-negative, microaerophilic
M. bovis BCG	Nonvirulent vaccine strain	First reported in 1908 as a nonvirulent strain of *M. tuberculosis*; lacks the RD1 region/esat-6 and cfp-10 virulence genes	PZA-resistant, nitrate reductase activity-negative, niacin-negative, aerobic
M. caprae	Mainly in goats, few infections in humans		PZA-susceptible, nitrate reductase activity-negative, niacin-negative, microaerophilic
M. africanum	West Africa		Mostly PZA-susceptible, predominantly nitrate reductase activity-negative, niacin-variable, microaerophilic
M. microti	Initially considered strictly an animal pathogen (e.g. voles, llamas, cats), several human cases were reported in 1998[15]		'Croissant-like' cell morphology; does not grow well in culture; identification via molecular methods
'M. canettii'	East Africa, occurrence appears to be limited to the African continent	Based on genetic studies, ancestor of all members of the *M. tuberculosis* complex, ~2.4–2.8 million years old; 'living fossil'	Smooth colonies, distinct patterns upon DNA typing
M. pinnipedii	Pinnipeds as major hosts		
M. orygis	Africa, Saudi Arabia and South Asia. Antelopes, cows and monkeys as host, human cases reported		
M. mungi	Mongoose as host		

PZA, pyrazinamide.

developing disease within the first 2 years. Hematogenous spread of tubercle bacilli from the lung probably invariably occurs, but the bacteremia is usually occult and does not produce symptoms or disease. Nevertheless, hematogenous dissemination accounts for the occurrence of extrapulmonary involvement of lymph nodes, kidneys, reproductive organs, bones, and gastrointestinal tract (see Chapter 31).

Compared with the global incidence of tuberculosis, there is a small proportion of human disease caused by *M. africanum* and the other – mostly animal-adapted – members of the *M. tuberculosis* complex such as *M. bovis*, *M. caprae*, *M. microti*, *M. pinnipedii* and 'M. canettii'.

LEPROSY

Leprosy (Hansen's disease) is a chronic disease of the skin, nerves and mucous membranes. The immunologic response (e.g. hypersensitivity) becomes an important component of the pathogenesis of the disease. The clinical manifestations of leprosy have been separated into six categories (Ridley–Jopling classification scheme).[7] The system is both a clinical classification based on the nature and severity of symptoms and a histopathologic classification. The classification groups are: 1) polar tuberculoid; 2) borderline tuberculoid; 3) borderline; 4) borderline lepromatous; 5) lepromatous (subpolar); and 6) lepromatous polar.

Lepromatous leprosy is the most severe form of the disease with numerous skin lesions involving face and nose. Acid-fast bacilli (AFB) are numerous and present in immature macrophages, which contrasts to tuberculoid leprosy, where macrophages have matured into epithelioid cells (see also Chapter 108), and AFB are hard to detect.

Epidemiology of leprosy is difficult to assess because of the lack of a diagnostic skin test, inability to cultivate the organism *in vitro* and the nature of the geographic distribution of endemic disease. Even though the disease is of great antiquity, the source for *M. leprae* and the portal of entry are not clear to date. Human-to-human transmission occurs via droplets, from the nose and mouth, during close and frequent contacts with untreated cases. The worldwide implementation of the standardized multidrug therapy has dramatically decreased the number of registered leprosy patients. Official figures from 103 countries from five WHO regions show the global registered prevalence of leprosy to be at 180 618 at the end of 2013; during the same year, 215 656 new cases were reported, suggesting that therapy fails to prevent transmission.[7]

The vast majority of patients are in low- and middle-income countries, predominantly South East Asia and mostly in India.

BURULI ULCER/BAIRNSDALE ULCER

Mycobacterium ulcerans is the etiologic agent of Buruli ulcer in Africa and Bairnsdale ulcer in Australia, an emerging disease involving chronic and necrotizing skin ulcers. Occurring mostly in rural tropical regions it is the third most common mycobacterial disease in immunocompetent humans after tuberculosis and leprosy (Figure 185-7). Disease typically begins as a lump under the skin, followed by a shallow ulcer at the site of the lump. *M. ulcerans* produces mycolactone, a toxin that causes necrosis. The type of disease ranges from a localized nodule or ulcer to widespread ulcerative or nonulcerative disease including, for instance, osteomyelitis.[8]

Surgical removal of the affected tissue, often followed by skin grafting, was for long the mainstay of treatment. In the last decade, significant progress has been made in antibiotic treatment; 8-week regimens of rifampin and streptomycin (or 4 weeks rifampin–streptomycin and 4 weeks rifampin–clarithromycin) are effective in early nodular disease and regimens of rifampin and fluoroquinolones are currently under investigation.[9]

Adequate surveillance data are missing for most of the endemic areas, therefore the incidence and prevalence of Buruli ulcer are not precisely defined. Ghana, an exception, has reported an overall national prevalence rate of active lesions of 20.7 per 100 000, but the rate was as high as 150.8 per 100 000 in districts where the disease was more endemic.[8] Reservoirs and routes of transmission remain poorly

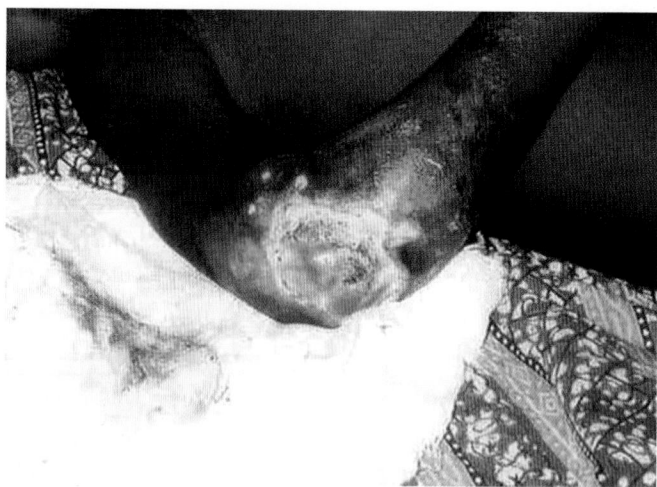

Figure 185-7   Buruli ulcer on the elbow of an African girl caused by *M. ulcerans*. *(Courtesy of F. Portaels.)*

TABLE 185-2	Clinically Important Nontuberculous Mycobacteria and Associated Diseases	
Growth Rate	**Species**	**Main Site of Infection**
Slow	M. avium complex (M. avium, M. intracellulare, minor species)	Pulmonary, lymph node, disseminated
	M. kansasii	Pulmonary, disseminated
	M. xenopi	Pulmonary
	M. malmoense (North-western Europe)	Pulmonary, lymph node
	M. simiae	Pulmonary, disseminated
	M. haemophilum	Skin, lymph node
	M. ulcerans (West Africa, Australia)	Skin
Intermediate	M. marinum	Skin (aquarium granuloma)
Rapid	M. abscessus	Pulmonary, skin, soft tissues
	M. chelonae	Skin, soft tissues, eye
	M. fortuitum	Skin, soft tissues, pulmonary

Note: all skin disease caused by rapid growers and *M. haemophilum* can be localized after traumatic inoculation or disseminated disease of the immunocompromised.

understood. *M. ulcerans* is a fastidious organism and has an unusually long generation time. Molecular tests have been developed which have accelerated diagnosis in select settings.[10]

Nontuberculous Mycobacterial Diseases

Over the past three decades it has been increasingly recognized that NTM are important opportunistic pathogens of humans, capable of causing a wide array of diseases. Diagnostic criteria, clinical presentation and treatment of diseases caused by more than 20 NTM have been meticulously reviewed and have improved diagnosis and treatment practices.[11] Subsequent reviews have focused on all laboratory diagnostic aspects of NTM including susceptibility testing.[11-14] Therefore, the following discussion only focuses on the most prominent NTM species causing disease in humans (Table 185-2).

MYCOBACTERIUM AVIUM COMPLEX

Mycobacterium avium complex (MAC) is common in soil, water and animals and can occur in pools and hot water tubs. Routes of infection are gastrointestinal and pulmonary by ingestion of contaminated water and food and inhalation of aerosols, as well as direct inoculation through trauma or existing wounds.[11]

MAC bacteria can cause a chronic pulmonary infection in patients with pre-existing pulmonary disease (e.g. COPD), cervical lymphadenitis in immunocompetent children, localized infections after traumatic inoculation and disseminated disease in the severely immunocompromised, e.g. HIV-infected, transplant recipients, patients with deficiency in interferon-gamma (IFN-γ) production or IFN-γ receptors.[11] The use of highly active antiretroviral therapy (HAART) has significantly decreased the incidence of MAC disease in people with HIV infection.

MAC pulmonary disease is seen worldwide but its incidence seems to vary between 1/100 000 persons per year in Eastern European countries with a high tuberculosis incidence to 6/100 000 persons per year in the USA and Canada. The incidence of pulmonary disease increases in many countries, particularly those where the tuberculosis incidence is in decline.[15] The traditionally recognized presentation of MAC pulmonary disease has been an apical fibrocavitary lung disease, sometimes showing large cavities, in males in their late 40s and early 50s who have a history of smoking and, sometimes, alcohol abuse.[11] This disease manifestation is very similar to tuberculosis in its clinical and radiological presentation, but its course is typically slower. In postmenopausal, nonsmoking, white females, a different manifestation of MAC pulmonary disease is seen, with nodular and interstitial nodular infiltrates and bronchiectasis, frequently involving the right middle lobe or lingula ('Lady Windermere Syndrome' or nodular-bronchiectatic disease).[11] The symptoms may vary and be nonspecific, including chronic productive cough, malaise, fatigue, dyspnea and sweats (see Chapter 32).

MAC cervical lymphadenitis is mostly a pediatric disease and primarily seen in children under 5 years of age. Lymphadenitis in immunocompetent children usually presents as an insidious, painless, unilateral process involving one or more lymph nodes. Mycobacteria isolated from infected lymph nodes are mostly (60–80%) MAC with the remainder being *M. haemophilum*, *M. malmoense* and *M. tuberculosis*; their relative frequencies differ strongly between various geographical areas (see Chapter 32). MAC lymph node infection of children over 12 years of age is rarely simple lymphadenitis and may indicate disseminated disease and immunodeficiency.

Disseminated MAC disease in people with HIV infection is a progressive illness characterized by intermittent fever, sweats, weakness, anorexia and weight loss. Patients may have nausea, diarrhea and vomiting along with abdominal pain. The microbiologic hallmark of MAC disease is a positive blood or bone marrow culture; however, liver biopsies may be diagnostic as well (Figure 185-8).

Treatment of all MAC diseases is by combination therapies of a rifamycin (rifampin or rifabutin), ethambutol and a macrolide (clarithromycin or azithromycin). Adjunctive amikacin may be added for severe cases and surgical resection of worst affected tissues should always be considered.[11]

MYCOBACTERIUM KANSASII

Mycobacterium kansasii is the second most frequent NTM isolate in many settings, but there are important geographical differences. The spectrum of disease equals that of MAC, although *M. kansasii* is less frequently associated with pediatric lymphadenitis.

RAPID GROWERS

Although the number of newly discovered rapidly growing mycobacteria is increasing constantly and the pathogenic potential of many of them is well recognized,[11] the vast majority (>90%) of disease in humans is caused by three species: *M. abscessus*, *M. chelonae* and *M. fortuitum* (see Figure 185-6). These species are important causes of pulmonary, cutaneous and postsurgical wound infections (skin, soft tissue, bone), especially following catheter placement, augmentation mammoplasty and cardiac bypass surgery. Disseminated disease is rare

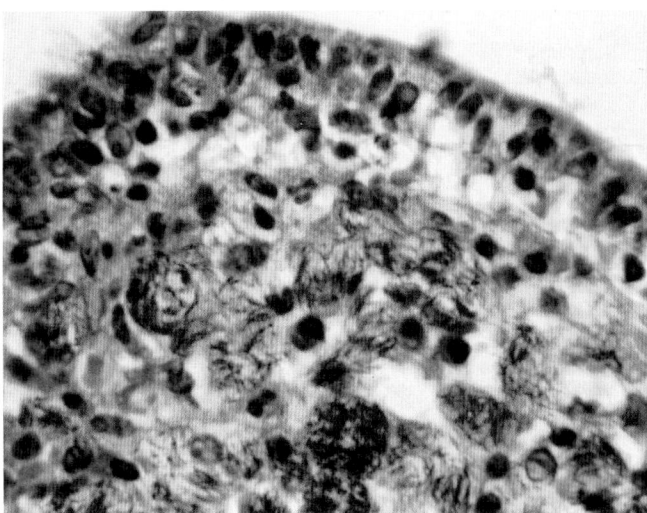

Figure 185-8 Acid-fast stain of a section of small intestine from a patient with HIV infection and disseminated *M. avium* disease. The photomicrograph shows many AFB within a villus tip of the intestinal tract biopsy. The cuboidal cells at the periphery of the tip are in disarray and appear abnormal with cell nuclei not evenly distributed at the base of the cells. There is no evidence of granuloma, but the overwhelming number of mycobacteria may be partially obscuring the host's cellular response. The histopathology is consistent with the symptoms of patients with MAC gastrointestinal tract infections, including abdominal pain, diarrhea and wasting. *(Courtesy of L.S. Young.)*

and almost invariably occurs in immunocompromised patients, but disease is not common in people with HIV infection.

The pulmonary disease caused by *M. abscessus* has received significant attention in recent years, owing to its emergence in specific risk groups (cystic fibrosis patients) and specific geographical areas (East Asia, pockets in the USA) and particularly because of the very poor outcomes of treatment. Owing to its natural resistance to most antibiotics, treatment is very complex with important roles for drugs that can only be given by the intravenous route (amikacin, cefoxitin, imipenem, tigecycline).[16]

Pathogenicity

The pathogenicity of mycobacterial infections in the immunocompetent host has as much to do with the immune response of the host as with destructive virulence properties of the mycobacterial pathogen. Thus, the principal virulence factor of mycobacteria is the ability to invade and persist or replicate within macrophages. The bacilli enter the macrophage by phagocytosis and once internalized the bacilli are surrounded by a membrane-bound vacuole to form a nascent phagosome. With the maturation of the phagolysosome, bacilli are exposed to a variety of antimicrobial factors including reactive oxygen intermediates, hydrolytic activities and a highly acidic pH. Virulent mycobacteria obstruct the maturation of phagosomes, inhibiting acidification, and can escape from the phagolysosome into the cytoplasm.[17]

The immunopathogenesis of mycobacterial infections primarily involves a cell-mediated immune response. This response includes the activation of macrophages to identify and inhibit or kill mycobacteria and the detection and lysis of phagocytes in which mycobacteria are in a state of growth and replication (Figure 185-9).

Mycobacterial antigens are presented by antigen-presenting cells (monocyte/macrophage lineage) resulting in secretion of interleukin (IL)-2 and clonal proliferation of CD4+ and CD8+ lymphocytes (α/β T cells). Mycobacterial antigens arising from the phagosome are presented by major histocompatibility complex (MHC) class II molecules while antigens arising from the cytoplasm are presented by MHC class I molecules. This difference determines, in part, the fate of the antigen-presenting cell, stimulation or destruction, because the presentation of antigen arising from the cytoplasm indicates that the cell has failed to

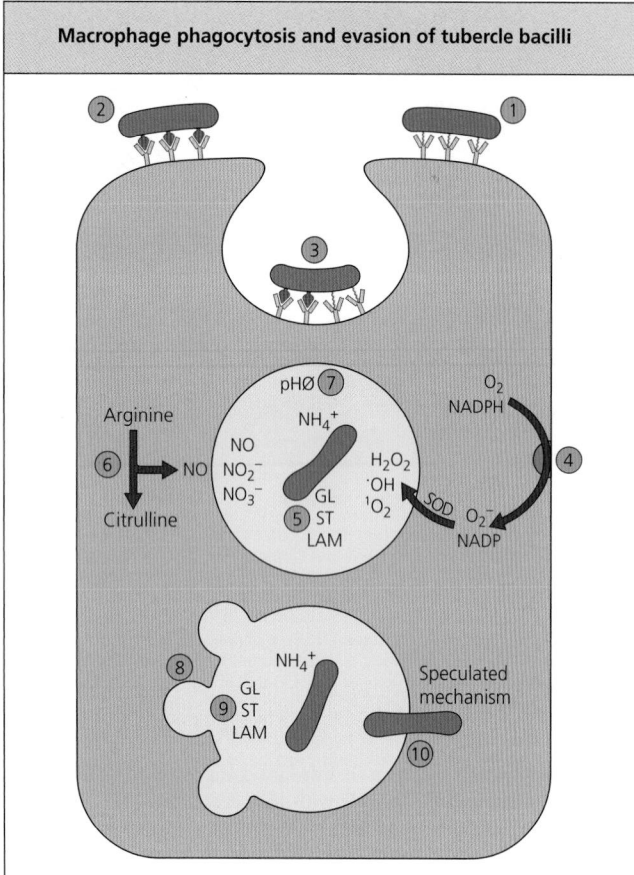

Figure 185-9 Macrophage phagocytosis and evasion of tubercle bacilli. The tubercle bacilli bind via lipoarabinomannan (LAM) (1) or complement receptors (2); phagocytosis occurs (3) with the activation of an oxidative burst (4); glycolipids (GL), sulfatides (ST) and LAM can downregulate the oxidative burst (5); reactive nitrogen intermediates may play a role in antimycobacterial activity (6), as does the acidic pH of the phagolysosome (7). Finally, the production of ammonia by tubercle bacilli may diminish the effect of reactive nitrogen intermediates (8) and contribute to the failure to form a phagolysosome fusion (9). Tubercle bacilli may evade the antimycobacterial activities of the phagolysosome by producing a hemolysin that releases the bacilli into the cytoplasm (10). NADP, nicotinamide adenine dinucleotide phosphate; NADPH, nicotinamide adenine dinucleotide phosphate, reduced form; SOD, superoxide dismutase. *(Adapted from Chan J., Kaufmann S.H.E.: Immune mechanisms of protection. In: Bloom B.R., ed. Tuberculosis: pathogenesis, protection and control, Washington DC: American Society for Microbiology; 1994:389-415.)*

control the mycobacteria. The release of IFN-γ by the clonally expanded CD4 cells, but also to a lesser extent by CD8 cells, natural killer (NK) cells and γδ cells, activates macrophages. This initiates a cascade of events including the hydrolysis of vitamin D that leads to further activation of macrophages and the release of tumor necrosis factor (TNF) by the activated macrophages. The sequence of cellular responses at the site of mycobacterial infection appears to be polymorphonuclear granulocytes (PMNs), NK cells, γδ cells and then α/β T cells; however, with time the α/β T cells become predominant in the cellular response. The sequence of recruitment is probably determined by the proximity of the cells to the site of infection; for example, γδ cells are likely to be one of the first cells recruited to the site of *M. tuberculosis* infection in the lung. The PMNs produce highly proteolytic enzymes that cause tissue liquefaction while each of the T-cell types possesses cytotoxic activity. Activated macrophages have an increased capacity for seeking out, engulfing and destroying mycobacteria, but the production of TNF by macrophages contributes to tissue necrosis and, therefore, to the immunopathology of the disease.[18]

Granulomas develop as a mycobacterial infection becomes more chronic. Granulomas are aggregates of activated macrophages that take on epithelial cell-like morphology (epithelioid cells) and, typically, lymphocytes are found at the periphery of the granuloma. Although the formation of a granuloma effectively contains the mycobacteria where they can be killed, bacilli can persist within giant cells (fused epithelioid cells) and the granuloma may never sterilize. With time a fibrotic wall (collagen) will encapsulate the granuloma and the center of the granuloma may become necrotic with a cheese-like appearance, which is the source of the descriptive word caseation.

Laboratory Diagnosis of Mycobacteria

GENERAL REMARKS

The detection and identification of mycobacteria in clinical specimens requires expertise and is associated with a considerable safety risk when specimens are handled improperly. Given the low infectious dose of *M. tuberculosis* for humans (50% infective dose, <10 AFB), specimens from known or suspected cases of tuberculosis must be considered potentially infectious and handled with appropriate precautions.[19,20] Aerosol-generating manipulations should be conducted in a biosafety cabinet class II. Level 3 facilities are required for laboratories performing high-risk procedures (processing specimens for culture, identification and susceptibility testing; extraction of DNA from culture).

The technologies available to assist in the laboratory diagnosis of mycobacterial infections have improved remarkably. Major achievements are:

- fully automated, nonradiometric culture systems for culture and drug susceptibility testing;
- nucleic acid amplification assays for the direct detection of *M. tuberculosis* complex in clinical specimens;
- identification at the species level by nucleic acid probes, line probe assays and gene sequencing;
- molecular assays for the rapid detection of antimicrobial resistance; and
- improved DNA typing methods to study transmission routes, distinguish reactivation from re-infection and to study genetic diversity of strain populations.

In discussing diagnostic mycobacteriology it is important to emphasize two general principles of laboratory medicine. First, the quality of any clinical test is highly dependent on the quality of the specimen, including the time of collection in the course of the disease, the appropriateness and sufficiency of the specimen, and the prompt and proper transport of the specimen to the laboratory. Second, the intended purpose of the test must be understood by the physician who orders the test. Was the test designed to screen for disease, to provide a definitive diagnosis based on a clinical index of suspicion, to confirm another test, to monitor therapy (test of cure), or to provide epidemiologic information? Use of a test for a purpose for which it was not designed and evaluated could be misleading. For example, nucleic acid amplification assays for the direct detection of *M. tuberculosis* complex in clinical specimens were evaluated as diagnostic assays for the detection of disease and explicitly not for monitoring response to therapy or cure.

COLLECTION OF SPECIMENS

The quality, quantity, timing, transport and appropriateness of the specimen have a greater impact on the outcome of a laboratory test than almost any other factor (Table 185-3).[20] It is important that physicians notify the laboratory if they suspect an uncommon or fastidious mycobacterial infection (such as *M. ulcerans*, *M. genavense* or *M. haemophilum*) because these and other species of mycobacteria have growth requirements that are significantly different from the majority of other species of mycobacteria isolated from clinical specimens.[14]

Respiratory Specimens

Expectorated sputum specimen should be collected early in the morning on at least two occasions for tuberculosis diagnostics and at least three for NTM pulmonary disease diagnostics. The

TABLE 185-3	Specimen Types and Requirements for the Diagnosis of Mycobacterial Infections		
Specimen Type	**Requirements**	**Collection**	**Note**
Abscess and fluid	10 mL*	Collect with syringe, submit in sterile container	Dry swab or swab submitted in transport medium unacceptable
Blood	8–10 mL (adult), 1–5 mL (child)	SPS tube, tube with heparin or citrate, Isolator tube	EDTA tube and coagulated blood unacceptable. Do not refrigerate
Bone	Bone chip	Sterile container, no fixative	Formalin-fixed unacceptable
Bone marrow	100 mg* or 1–3 mL aspirate	SPS tube, heparin or citrate tube, Isolator tube	Aspirate volumes >5 mL may be primarily peripheral blood. Do not refrigerate
Bronchoalveolar lavage or bronchial washing	≥5 mL	Sterile container	Avoid contamination of bronchoscope with tap water (possible false-positive results)
Cerebrospinal fluid	5–10 mL*	Sterile tube	
Fluids (pleural, pericardial, peritoneal, synovial, etc.)	10–15 mL*	Collect with syringe, submit in sterile container	Swabs unacceptable
Gastric lavage	5–10 mL	Sterile container, collecting in morning before arising and eating	Neutralize with 10% sodium carbonate if delayed processing
Lymph node	Whole node or part*, caseous part	Sterile container	Formalin-fixed unacceptable
Skin biopsy	Sterile container, aspirate	Biopsy at periphery or aspirate from under margin of lesion	Note if suspicion of *M. ulcerans, M. haemophilum* or *M. marinum* (need special culture conditions or extended incubation)
Sputum	5–10 mL	Early morning sputum in sterile plastic container	Use sterile hypertonic saline for induced sputum, avoid exposure to tap water. Do not pool sputum specimens
Stool	≥1 g	Sterile plastic container, no transport medium	Refrigerate, but do *not* freeze
Tissue biopsy	1 g*	Sterile container	Caseous portion, formalin-fixed unacceptable
Urine	50 mL*	First morning specimen, catheter urine in sterile container	24-hour urine and pooled urine specimens unacceptable. Refrigerate

SPS, sodium polyanetholsulfonate.
*As much as possible (up to or in excess of the weight/volume shown).
Adapted and modified from CLSI, Laboratory detection and identification of mycobacteria; approved standard M48-A, Villanova, PA, CLSI, 2008.

wide-mouthed, sterile, plastic container (wax free) with a tight fitting cap containing the sputum specimen should be immediately transported to the laboratory or held at 39.2°F (4°C) until processed. Prompt processing of sputum is required to minimize overgrowth of mycobacteria by the normal respiratory tract microflora. Alternative respiratory tract specimens are induced sputum, endotracheal aspiration, bronchial washings or aspirates taken during bronchoscopy, and gastric lavage. Bronchoscopes must be carefully cleaned and decontaminated after collecting specimens from patients.[14,20]

Gastric Lavage

Gastric lavage (for swallowed sputum) is useful for collecting specimens from patients who, for a variety of reasons, are unable to produce sputum by other means. Gastric lavage is the specimen of choice from infants and children (up to 12 years) suspected of having pulmonary tuberculosis. A gastric lavage must be sent to the laboratory promptly because it must be processed as soon as possible or neutralized with 10% sodium carbonate to avoid loss of mycobacteria due to gastric acidity. As with expectorated sputum specimens, gastric lavage specimens should be collected early in the morning, before eating, and on three separate occasions. Culturing NTM from these samples has little if any clinical significance.

Urine

Three early morning midstream urine specimens should be collected into a sterile plastic container with a leak-proof cap. Large volumes of urine can be concentrated by filtration, but 24-hour urine should not be used because of contamination and dilution of any mycobacteria present.

Blood and Bone Marrow

Blood, bone marrow aspirates or cores are ideal specimens for the diagnosis of disseminated mycobacterial infections, in particular of MAC infections. If blood has to be transported before inoculation of the medium, sodium polyanethol sulfonate (SPS), heparin or citrate may be used as an anticoagulant. Blood collected in EDTA and coagulated blood are not acceptable for culture; neither is direct inoculation of blood onto a solid medium. If the laboratory cannot process the specimen immediately, it should be stored at room temperature.

Other Fluids

Pleural, pericardial, synovial and ascitic fluids as well as pus and cerebrospinal fluid (CSF) may also be submitted for diagnostic analyses. *Mycobacterium tuberculosis* meningitis is a medical emergency and CSF specimens should be collected, transported and processed in a manner that reflects the urgent nature of such a diagnosis; polymerase chain reaction (PCR) is faster and – in most studies – more sensitive than culture from CSF.[21]

Tissues

Tissue should be submitted for both histology and mycobacteriology. As tissue is preferred over necrotic material or pus for culture, it is therefore important to have fresh tissue and not swabs submitted to the microbiology laboratory. Formalin-preserved tissue should be submitted for histologic studies. Although not suitable for culture, formalin-preserved and paraffin-embedded tissue may be submitted for PCR analysis, especially if AFB are observed on microscopic examination of the tissue sections.

Feces

Feces are not a particularly useful specimen for the diagnosis of tuberculosis or other mycobacterial infections, with the exception of suspected gastrointestinal tract infection with MAC or other NTM in the severely immunocompromised, including HIV-positive patients. However, the recovery of MAC from feces is poor (low sensitivity) even in HIV-positive patients. If *M. avium* is isolated from the feces the positive predictive value of the culture is high, meaning that the patient is likely to develop disseminated disease.[22] To avoid overgrowth of normal gastrointestinal tract microflora, feces must be rather harshly decontaminated, but this is likely to also decrease the yield of mycobacteria.[23]

PROCESSING

Contaminated Specimens

Most respiratory tract specimens will be contaminated with normal respiratory tract microflora. In addition, the mucin matrix both protects and traps micro-organisms and makes the specimens difficult to process. Therefore such specimens have to be decontaminated (to reduce or eliminate other micro-organisms that would be likely to overgrow the mycobacteria that might be present in the specimen) and liquefied. The most common agents used to pretreat respiratory specimens are *N*-acetyl-L-cysteine (NALC) and dithiothreitol (DTT or Sputolysin®). Both NALC and DTT are unstable in air and must be prepared fresh. A combination of NALC and sodium hydroxide is most commonly used for digesting and decontaminating sputum. Finally, the pretreated specimen is centrifuged to increase sensitivity of microscopy and the recovery of mycobacteria from culture.

There is no ideal method for digesting and decontaminating respiratory tract specimens. Invariably, mycobacteria are lost during decontamination. Detailed descriptions of the various procedures for digesting and decontaminating sputum and other contaminated specimens have been well described elsewhere.[12,14]

UNCONTAMINATED SPECIMENS

The primary concern about specimens from sterile body sites is the quantity of specimen submitted for smear and culture. Swabs usually contain insufficient material for culture, and 1 g of tissue or 10 mL of fluid are ideal. To improve recovery of mycobacteria, centrifugation should be used to concentrate large volumes of fluids. Aseptically collected tissues and fluids from normally sterile body sites usually do not require processing. These specimens can initially be inoculated on a chocolate agar plate to check for purity. If sterile, specimens are concentrated and inoculated into a liquid growth medium as well as on solid media without decontamination.

ACID-FAST STAIN AND SMEAR MICROSCOPY

An acid-fast stain remains the most rapid and least expensive method for directly detecting mycobacteria in clinical specimens, and is highly specific. Nevertheless, there are organisms other than mycobacteria with various degrees of acid-fastness such as *Rhodococcus* spp., *Nocardia* spp. and *Legionella micdadei*, as well as cysts from *Cryptosporidium*, *Isospora*, *Cyclospora* and *Microsporidium* spores. The presence of AFB in a specimen from a patient with signs and symptoms of tuberculosis or another mycobacterial infection is an important guide to effective treatment and the initiation of public health measures. Furthermore, an acid-fast stain can quickly assess patient infectiousness, and is also used to confirm that a cultured bacterium is acid fast. The detection limit of an acid-fast stain has been estimated to be 5000–10 000 bacilli/mL of sputum; overall sensitivity is between 22% and 78%.[24]

The three stains that are commonly used to detect AFB are Ziehl–Neelsen, Kinyoun and auramine–rhodamine fluorochrome stains. With each of these procedures, acid-fastness is defined as resistance to decolorizing with acid–alcohol (e.g. 3% hydrochloric acid in 95% ethanol). When mycobacteria are stained with Gram's crystal violet and safranin they often appear as beaded gram-positive bacilli or fail to stain at all (and are thus to be considered gram-neutral).

The preparation of the smear is the critical first step in performing an acid-fast stain. Using a glass slide cleaned with ethanol, make a smear of approximately 1×2 cm of a single specimen or isolate. For CSF specimens previously concentrated by centrifugation, three drops of the concentrate are placed on a clean glass slide, one drop at a time. The drop is allowed to air dry before the next drop is added. The slide is air dried or alternatively dried at 176°F (80°C) for 15 minutes in a biosafety cabinet class II – it is important to note that heat fixing may not kill all the mycobacteria on the slide. Mycobacteria appear brightly fluorescent against a dark background in the auramine–rhodamine stain and the increased sensitivity of the fluorescence stain compared with the other stains is used to rapidly screen slides at a lower (250–450×) magnification. However, fluorescent objects must be examined at 1000× magnification to confirm morphology. Positive fluorescent smears should be confirmed with either the Ziehl–Neelsen or Kinyoun stains. The Ziehl–Neelsen stain requires that the carbolfuchsin stain be heated for the stain to penetrate the mycobacterial cell. In contrast, heating is unnecessary with the Kinyoun stain because the concentration of basic fuchsin and phenol have been increased to ensure that the basic fuchsin penetrates the mycobacterial cell wall. Using a 100× oil immersion lens, 100–300 fields of a properly prepared smear and stain should be examined. It should be remembered that in examining even 100–300 fields, only 1–4% of a 1×2 cm smear would be examined. Mycobacteria usually appear as pink, slender rod-shaped bacilli; however, pleomorphic shapes are common and range from coccoid to long rods with curves or bends (Figure 185-10).

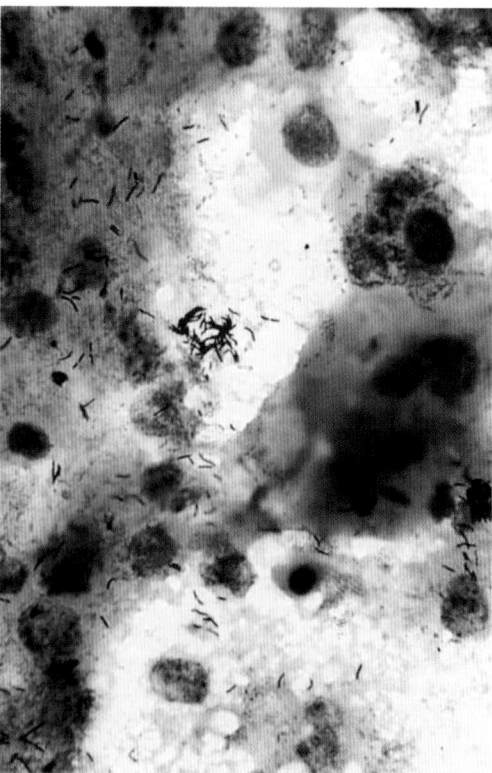

Figure 185-10 Ziehl–Neelsen acid-fast stain of sputum containing 4+ tubercle bacilli. (*Courtesy of S. Froman and A. Gaytan.*)

CULTURE

In detecting approximately 10^2 viable organisms/mL of specimen, culture is more sensitive than smear microscopy. Also, it is the only reliable means to monitor effectiveness of therapy in tuberculosis patients.[24] A variety of solid (e.g. Löwenstein–Jensen, Ogawa, Middlebrook agar) and liquid media (see below) are available for the culture of mycobacteria from clinical specimens. It is highly recommended to use a combination of solid and liquid media to ensure good recovery for subsequent species identification and susceptibility testing.[25] The macroscopic and microscopic characteristics, together with the rate of growth and pigmentation, are valuable in making a presumptive identification (see Figure 185-2).

Manual or automated liquid culture systems used for the detection of mycobacteria are the Mycobacteria Growth Indicator Tube (MGIT; Becton Dickinson) and – to a lesser degree – the BacT/ALERT® (bioMérieux) and VersaTrek® (Trek Diagnostic Systems, Cleveland, OH) systems. The MGIT contains a modified Middlebrook 7H9 broth in conjunction with a fluorescence quenching-based oxygen sensor (silicon rubber impregnated with a ruthenium pentahydrate). Growth is detected by exposing an inoculated MGIT to ultraviolet light and examining for fluorescence, which is an indication of growth and oxygen consumption. The performance of these manual systems is mostly equal and – in combination with conventional solid media – is satisfactory. Adding solid media to liquid media for primary isolation of mycobacteria increases sensitivity by 10%.[25]

For many years the Isolator System (Wampole, Cranbury, NJ) and the radiometric BACTEC 13A blood culture medium (Becton Dickinson) were the only reliable systems for mycobacterial blood cultures. The Isolator System is associated with a not negligible safety risk, but is still used in conjunction with liquid culture systems that do not have specific blood culture bottles for mycobacterial culture (BacT/ALERT and VersaTrek). A more widely used system for blood and bone marrow specimens are MYCO/F Lytic bottles (Becton Dickinson) in conjunction with conventional BacTec blood culture systems (Becton Dickinson).[26]

IDENTIFICATION

The first challenge for the clinical mycobacteriology laboratory is to distinguish between members of the *M. tuberculosis* complex (see Table 185-1) and NTM, a taxonomically imprecise, but clinically important distinction.

Growth of *M. tuberculosis* on Middlebrook 7H10 or 7H11 agar at 95°F (35°C) is usually detected in 2–3 weeks. The colonies are beige colored, rough, dry, corded, flat and with irregular borders (Figure 185-11). On egg media, such as Löwenstein–Jensen or Ogawa media, the colonies are frequently warty and granular and with time heap into a cauliflower shape (Figure 185-12). Although the growth of *M. tuberculosis* is quite distinct and it is not unreasonable for an experienced mycobacteriologist to make a presumptive report of *M. tuberculosis* based on the rate and appearance of growth, identification must always be confirmed by immunochromatographic or – preferably – molecular tests. Identification based on this morphology is no longer particularly relevant in the era of rapid liquid culture systems.

Three clinically significant species of mycobacteria have lower optimal growth temperatures (86°F/30°C): *M. ulcerans*, *M. marinum* and *M. haemophilum*. In addition, *M. haemophilum* requires hemin for growth and, therefore, specimens suspected to harbor this species should be inoculated onto chocolate agar, or on Middlebrook 7H10 agar or 7H9 broth supplemented with an iron source such as hemolysed blood, a hemin-containing paper strip or disk or ferric ammonium citrate/Fastidious Organisms Supplement (FOS; BD Bioscience).[11,12,14]

MAC organisms isolated from blood or sputum appear as either glossy, whitish colonies or smaller, translucent colonies on Middlebrook 7H10 or 7H11 agar after 10–14 days (Figure 185-13). The NTM vary widely in their colony morphology. *Mycobacterium abscessus* is

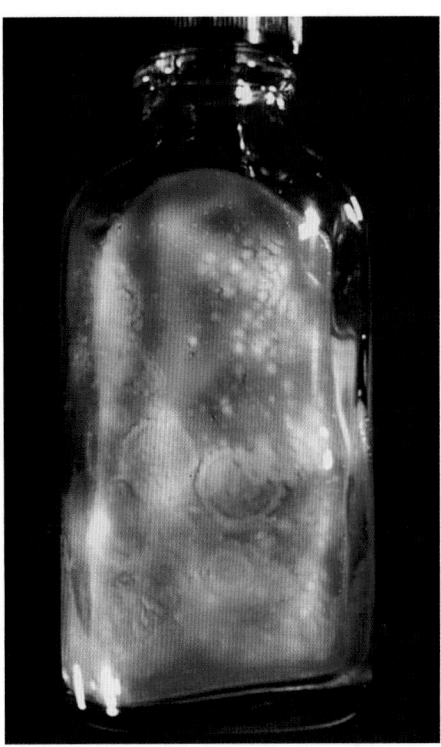

Figure 185-11   Primary isolate of *M. tuberculosis* grown from sputum on Löwenstein–Jensen medium displaying characteristic beige, rough and dry-appearing growth. *(Courtesy of S. Froman and A. Gaytan.)*

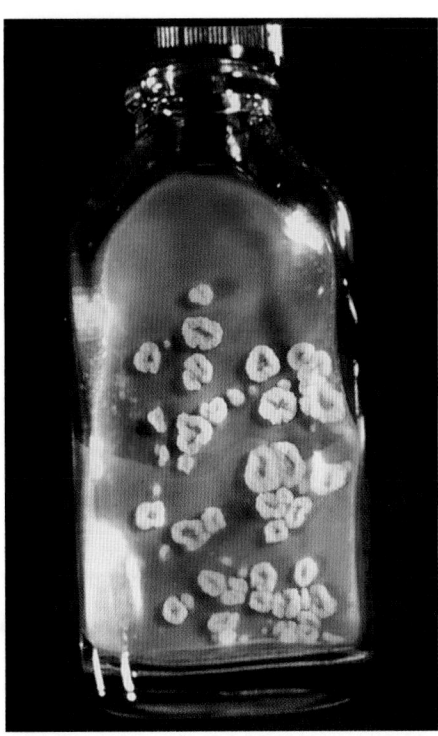

Figure 185-12   Primary isolate of *M. tuberculosis* grown from sputum on Löwenstein–Jensen medium displaying 'cauliflower' or verrucose colonies. These are also characteristic of other mycobacteria including MAC and rapid growers, especially as a culture ages. *(Courtesy of S. Froman and A. Gaytan.)*

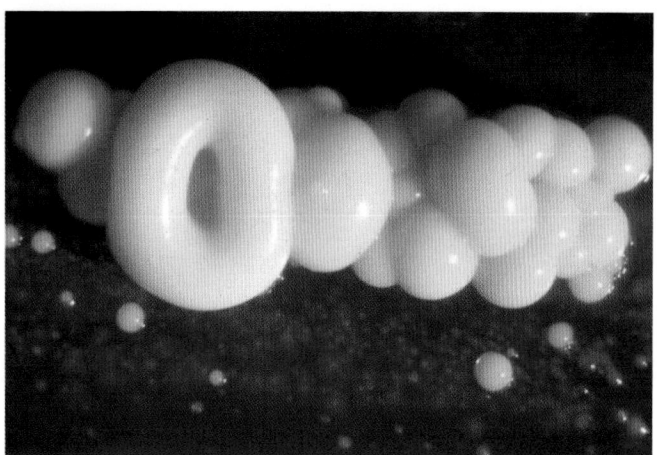

Figure 185-13 *M. avium* grown on Middlebrook 7H10 agar. The two most frequent morphologies are shown (beige opaque colonies and smaller translucent colonies).

well known to show both smooth and rough colonies; the latter are associated with invasive disease and are more difficult to grow and more resistant to antibiotics.

Conventional Biochemical Tests

Biochemical identification of mycobacteria is slow, labor-intensive and inaccurate owing to the limited discriminatory power and reproducibility. Biochemical testing (including HPLC of cell wall lipids) should no longer be used in clinical laboratories.

Immunochromatography Methods

With the advent and spread of liquid cultures systems, new rapid tools to distinguish *M. tuberculosis* complex bacteria from the NTM were sought. One very promising target was the MPT64 antigen, which is produced and secreted by virtually all *M. tuberculosis* complex organisms (of note: some *M. bovis* BCG strains do not produce MPT64). Several commercial immunochromatography tests are now available, with good diagnostic accuracy from both liquid and solid media.[27]

Molecular Methods

For some time nucleic acid probes (AccuProbe; Gen-Probe, San Diego, CA) have been commercially available for the identification of *M. tuberculosis* complex, *M. avium*, *M. intracellulare*, MAC, *M. gordonae* and *M. kansasii* from culture. The AccuProbe culture confirmation test is based on the use of acridinium ester labeled DNA probes that are complementary to species-specific rRNA, which is released from the mycobacteria after lysis. The AccuProbe test cannot be used for direct detection of mycobacteria in clinical specimens. In general, the Accu-Probe tests are highly reliable and simple to perform. Their use is largely restricted to the USA, where they are the only FDA-approved method for identification of mycobacteria.

Another widely used format is the line probe assay. In the INNO-LiPA multiplex probe assay (INNO-LiPA MYCOBACTERIA; Innogenetics, Ghent, Belgium), probes consist of the ~280 bp internal transcribed spacer (ITS) region in between the 16S and the 23S rRNAs. With this assay both *M. tuberculosis* complex as well as a number of NTM can easily be identified.[28] The GenoType kits of Hain Lifescience (Nehren, Germany) are based on similar technology but target the 23S rDNA gene and are able to identify 23 (GenoType CM) and 14 (Geno-Type AS) additional species, respectively. Concordant results have been obtained for 92.6% of previously sequenced mycobacterial strains with the CM assay and 89.9% with the AS assay.[29] There is a separate GenoType assay for (sub)species identification within the *M. tuberculosis* complex.

Another way to identify mycobacteria at the species level is via PCR and PCR-restriction enzyme analysis (PRA). Telenti *et al.*[30] established a method based on the *hsp65* gene encoding for the 65 kDa heat shock protein and developed an algorithm of species identification based on the restriction profiles generated by Hae*III* and BstE*II*. Although the method is widely used the major drawbacks of the technique are the facts that ambiguous profiles may occur and the database is very complex and does not feature all species (http://app.chuv.ch/prasite/index.html).

Gene sequencing for identification purposes remains the 'gold standard' for identification. Identification of species-specific signatures within variable regions of highly conserved genes such as the 16S rDNA gene or *hsp65* gene generated PCR protocols using genus-specific primers followed by direct sequencing of the PCR products.[11,12,14] In addition to these genes, the *rpoB* gene coding for the RNA polymerase or the ITS 16S–23S sequence may be used (for references, see reference 14). Even with the possibilities of gene sequencing the user has to be aware that each protocol has its limitations. For example, 16S rDNA sequencing has limited discriminatory power, particularly among rapidly growing mycobacteria, whereas *hsp65*, *rpoB* and ITS public databases are less complete and not quality controlled.

SERODIAGNOSIS, URINE-BASED DIAGNOSIS AND PLEURAL FLUID CHEMISTRY

Serodiagnostic techniques do not perform well enough for routine use, producing inconsistent and imprecise estimates of sensitivity and specificity.[31] Indeed WHO has actively discouraged their use. Assays to detect lipoarabinomannan (LAM) in urine samples may be of some use in HIV-infected adults and those with disseminated disease, either alone (sensitivity for culture positive disease in HIV-positive patients of approximately 50%, specificity >95%) or in combination with other diagnostic tests.[32] To detect tuberculous pleurisy, a paucibacillary disease in which culture and PCR have proven to have low sensitivity, chemical analyses of pleural fluid can be helpful. Detecting increased concentrations of interferon-gamma, adenosine deaminase (ADA) and lysozyme can be helpful. Of these three, detection of increased interferon-gamma concentrations has the highest sensitivity and specificity.[33]

DIRECT DETECTION OF M. TUBERCULOSIS COMPLEX BY NUCLEIC ACID AMPLIFICATION

A vast number of studies have concentrated on four nucleic acid amplification (NAA)-based kits designed to detect *M. tuberculosis* complex directly from clinical specimens:

- the Amplicor *M. tuberculosis* Test (Roche Molecular Systems, Inc., Branchburg, NJ);
- the Amplified *M. tuberculosis* Direct Test (MTD; Gen-Probe);
- the BDProbeTec Strand Displacement Amplification (SDA; Becton Dickinson); and
- GeneXpert MTB/RIF (Cepheid).

The Amplicor *M. tuberculosis* PCR and amplified *M. tuberculosis* direct (MTD) assays are based on amplification of a 16S rDNA gene fragment. The specificity for smear-positive specimens ranges from 90% to 100%. Sensitivity is significantly lower for smear-negative specimens, from 60% to 95%. The BDProbeTec SDA co-amplifies sequences of the IS*6110* (specific to *M. tuberculosis* complex) and the 16S rDNA gene (common to most mycobacterial species), but has similar sensitivity and specificity.

The most recent addition to the landscape of molecular detection of *M. tuberculosis* is the GeneXpert MTB/RIF assay. This semi-quantitative PCR-based system comes in a fully automated and closed cartridge-based platform; this allows for its use by untrained personnel in settings with very little infrastructure other than electricity. It generates a result within 2 hours after pipetting in the buffered sputum (or other) sample. In a recent meta-analysis, a pooled sensitivity of 89% (95% CI 85–92%) and pooled specificity of 99% (95% CI 98-99%) were calculated for detection of *M. tuberculosis*.[34] This assay also detects the major mutations responsible for rifampin resistance and thus predicts whether the strain infecting the patient is rifampin susceptible or not (see below).

DNA FINGERPRINTING

Molecular typing helps to differentiate relapses from exogenous re-infections in patients and to demonstrate false-positive cases due to contaminated bronchoscopes or laboratory cross-contamination of clinical specimens during workup. It also allows the definition of prevalent families of strains and elucidates the intraspecies genetic microevolution. Most importantly, it helps to identify transmission chains. Lastly, DNA typing methods are also useful in identifying members within the M. tuberculosis complex such as M. microti, M. caprae or M. canettii. For M. tuberculosis, a number of methods have been developed to carry out DNA typing with high discriminatory power, the most important ones are listed below. Molecular typing of NTM is still in its infancy and has not yet seen significant standardization.

IS6110 Restriction Fragment Length Polymorphism

The IS6110-based analysis of M. tuberculosis centers on differences in fragment length and copy number of this insertion element. There are 0–20 copies of the 1355 bp IS6110 in most strains of M. tuberculosis. The distribution of IS6110 within the genome appears to be stable over several months to years. Basically, the method involves extraction of genomic DNA, restriction of the DNA with an appropriate enzyme (e.g. PvuII) and electrophoretic separation of the restriction fragments (RFLP analysis). The IS6110 pattern is revealed by Southern hybridization using a labeled fragment of the IS6110 sequence.[35] A drawback of this method was the large amount of DNA (about 2 μg) that is required for analysis, requiring long subculture, as well as its technical complexity. Therefore, it has now been superseded by PCR-based typing methods of equal or better discriminatory power.

Multi-locus Variable Number of Tandem Repeats Analysis (MLVA/VNTR)

Genotyping based on a variable number of tandem repeats (VNTRs) of different classes of interspersed genetic elements, the mycobacterial interspersed repetitive units (MIRUs), is a fast and elegant alternative to the labor-intense classic IS6110-based DNA typing, and has a very similar discriminatory power.[36] It has become the gold standard for molecular typing for epidemiological or surveillance purposes. It relies on:

- PCR amplification of multiple loci using primers specific for the flanking regions of each repeat locus; and
- the determination of the sizes of the amplicons which reflect the numbers of the targeted MIRU-VNTR copies.

This method has been standardized several years ago.[37] Some suggestions for technical improvements have been published.[38]

Whole Genome Sequencing

Whole genome sequencing is currently being explored as a tool for molecular epidemiology studies and surveillance of M. tuberculosis. The very high discriminatory power can identify transmission chains and even allows inference of direction of transmission.[39] The cost per strain has come down dramatically, but data analysis still requires highly trained staff and is very time-consuming. These aspects still hamper its use as a tool for surveillance of tuberculosis in health systems.

Antimicrobial Resistance and Susceptibility Testing

RESISTANCE

During bacterial multiplication resistance to antimycobacterial drugs develops spontaneously and with a defined frequency. Genetic mutations resulting in resistance of M. tuberculosis to rifampin (rifampicin; RMP) lead to an estimated prevalence of 1 in 10^8 bacilli in drug-free environments. Antimicrobial resistance in mycobacteria is fundamentally a reflection of the large populations of mycobacteria present in infected tissues and fluids and the frequencies of individual gene mutations that result in a resistant phenotype. In pulmonary tuberculosis there are 10^7–10^9 bacilli in lung cavities, but only 10^2–10^4 bacilli in

caseous lesions. The likelihood of spontaneous mutations leading to an isoniazid (INH)- and RMP-resistant phenotype of M. tuberculosis (MDR-TB) is very low, i.e. in 10^{-14} ($10^{-6} \times 10^{-8}$) AFB.[40-42] Therefore, the worldwide emergence of resistant strains cannot be explained by the phenomenon of natural mutations only. More important is the man-made impact leading to the high rate of acquired resistance,[3,6] mainly because of the patients' nonadherence to therapy (see above).

Antimicrobial resistance in M. tuberculosis is classically defined as a significant difference in the activity of an antimycobacterial drug between a wild-type strain and another strain. A wild-type strain is defined as a strain isolated from a patient before treatment and less than 1% of a population of that strain is resistant to any antimycobacterial agent. Resistance emerges as a consequence of individual mutations in mycobacterial genes that lead to a structural or functional change such that an antimycobacterial agent is no longer active against that strain. In the recent past, several resistance mechanisms at the molecular level have been elucidated (for references, see reference 39). For example, resistance to INH results from a mutation or a combination of mutations in the katG, ahpC, inhA, ndh or the kasA genes of M. tuberculosis (Table 185-4). In M. tuberculosis, resistance to RMP is a result of a mutation within an 81 bp (27 amino acid) sequence of the core region of the rpoB gene (RNA polymerase β subunit); streptomycin resistance has been attributed to mutations in either the rrs gene (16S rRNA gene) or the rpsL gene (ribosomal protein S12). Fluoroquinolone resistance has been ascribed to mutations in the gyrA and gyrB genes and pyrazinamide resistance to mutations in the pncA gene that encodes pyrazinamidase/nicotinamidase activity.[39-42] The targets for the major classes or types of antimycobacterial agent are shown in Figure 185-14. Antibiotic resistance does not transfer between strains of mycobacteria by either plasmid exchange or resistance transfer factors. The M. tuberculosis MDR as well as the XDR phenotypes appear to be entirely the result of a stepwise accumulation of individual mutations.

Intrinsic resistance to antimicrobial agents is also common in both slowly and rapidly growing NTM. In most instances, this form of

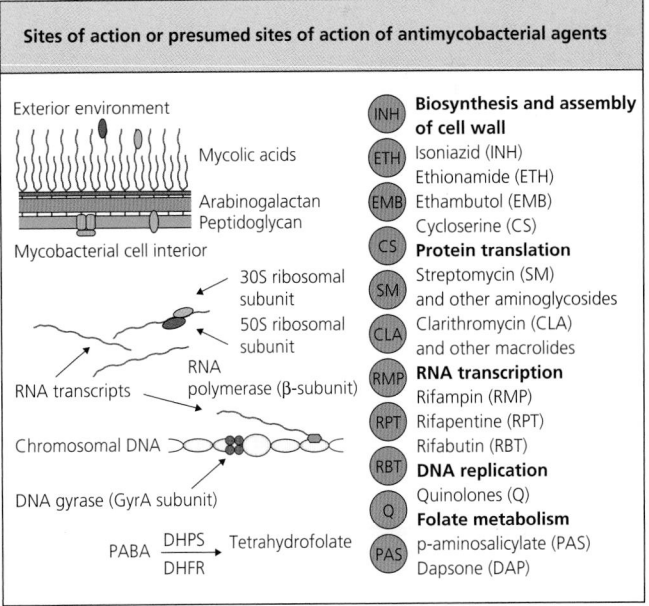

Figure 185-14 Sites of action or presumed sites of action of antimycobacterial agents. DHFR, dihydrofolate reductase; DHPS, dihydropteroate synthase; PABA, p-aminobenzoic acid; PAS, p-aminosalicylic acid. (Adapted from Parsons L.M., Driscoll J.R., Taber H.W., Salfinger M.: Drug resistance in tuberculosis. In: Tenover F.C., McGowan Jr J.E., ed. Infectious Diseases Clinics of North America: antimicrobial resistance, Philadelphia: WB Saunders; 1997:905-928 with additional data from Young D.B.: Strategies for new drug development. In: Bloom B.R., ed. Tuberculosis: pathogenesis, protection and control, Washington, DC: American Society for Microbiology; 1994:559-567.)

TABLE 185-4	Mycobacterial Genes with Mutations Associated with Antimicrobial Resistance			
Antimicrobial Agent	Species	Gene(s) Involved	Gene Function	Mechanisms of Action
Rifampin (rifampicin)	M. tuberculosis complex M. leprae	rpoB	β-subunit of RNA polymerase	Inhibition of transcription
Isoniazid	M. tuberculosis complex	katG inhA locus ndh ahpC acpM (kasA)	Catalase-peroxidase Enoyl ACP reductase NADH dehydrogenase II Alkyl hydroperoxidase β-ketoacyl ACP synthase	Inhibition of mycolic acid biosynthesis and multiple effects on DNA, lipids, carbohydrates, NAD metabolism
Ethambutol	M. tuberculosis complex	embCAB	Arabinosyltransferase	Inhibition of arabinogalactan synthesis
Streptomycin	M. tuberculosis complex M. smegmatis	rpsL rrs	S12 ribosomal protein 16S rRNA	Inhibition of protein synthesis
Pyrazinamide	M. tuberculosis complex	pncA	Nicotinamidase/pyrazinamidase	Acidification of cytoplasm and de-energized membrane
Fluoroquinolones	M. tuberculosis complex M. smegmatis	gyrA gyrB	DNA gyrase subunit A and subunit B	Inhibition of DNA gyrases
Azithromycin–clarithromycin	M. avium M. intracellulare M. chelonae M. abscessus	V domain 23S rRNA (rrl)	23S rRNA	
Amikacin–kanamycin	M. tuberculosis M. avium M. intracellulare M. abscessus	rrs	16S rDNA	Inhibition of protein synthesis
Ethionamide	M. tuberculosis	etaA/ethA inhA	Flavin mono-oxygenase	Inhibition of mycolic acid biosynthesis

Proportion of resistance represents the estimated percentage of resistance that can be accounted for by mutations in the respective genes. Mutations in katG, ahpC, inhA and/or kasA collectively probably account for 90% of isoniazid resistance.

resistance appears to be the result of the impermeability of the mycobacterial cell envelope and a broad repertoire of efflux pumps, chelating and lysing enzymes and target-blocking proteins. For example, most MAC isolates have very high minimum inhibitory concentrations (MICs) to RMP despite the fact that the isolate has a wild-type rpoB gene.

SUSCEPTIBILITY TESTING

The susceptibility testing of M. tuberculosis and the NTM has developed along very different lines and now involves very different methodologies. Extrapolation of methods and interpretive criteria of M. tuberculosis to NTM provides misleading and potentially harmful results.[13] Susceptibility testing of mycobacteria should be performed in laboratories with extensive experience, particularly for testing second-line drugs against M. tuberculosis and testing of NTM. Application of those results to the treatment of a patient with an uncommon or first line drug-resistant mycobacterial infection is likely to require the involvement of a physician with experience in the management of such infections.

Drug susceptibility testing is mandatory on initial isolates of M. tuberculosis complex species from all patients. If culture remains positive over an extended period of time, susceptibility testing should be repeated to monitor a possible development of drug resistance. The current guidelines of the Clinical Laboratory Standards Institute (CLSI) recommend repeating susceptibility testing at least every 3 months.[43]

There are three accepted methods for drug susceptibility testing of M. tuberculosis: the absolute concentration method, the resistance ratio method and the agar proportion method, the latter being used most widely in the Western hemisphere.

Agar Proportion Method

This method is based on the concept of 'critical concentrations' of antituberculosis agents and the percentage of resistant tubercle bacilli within a test population ('critical proportion'). Critical concentrations

for antituberculosis agents were established on an empiric clinical basis. Therapeutic success was unlikely if the proportion of drug-resistant mutants within a population of M. tuberculosis isolated from a patient exceeded a threshold of 1% at a concentration of the antituberculosis agent that was known to be therapeutically effective against a 'wild-type' or fully susceptible strain. The critical concentration may not be the same as the peak serum concentration of a drug and there might be an interest in applying the use of the MIC in the future. However, there are no standardized methods for MIC testing of mycobacteria and the testing of M. tuberculosis continues to follow the conventions of critical concentrations and the 1% growth inhibition threshold.

The proportion method can be applied as either a direct or an indirect test.[43] The basis of the agar proportion method is the inoculation of several dilutions of a standardized suspension of mycobacteria onto Middlebrook 7H10 agar plates. The number of colony forming units (cfu) that grow on the drug-containing plates or quadrants are compared with the number of cfu on a drug-free plate or quadrant. If the number of cfu that grow on drug-containing medium exceeds 1% of the total number of cfu on the drug-free medium, then the isolate is considered 'resistant' to that drug at that concentration. The agar proportion method is a standard[43] against which all newer developments of culture-based drug susceptibility testing have to be validated (see below).

Modified Proportion Testing By Nonradiometric Broth-Based Methods

The new, nonradiometric methods, such as the BACTEC MGIT 960, BacT/ALERT (Biomérieux) and VersaTrek (Trek Diagnostics), show excellent agreement with the agar proportion method and the now no longer available BACTEC 460 TB System for drug susceptibility testing.[44-46] However, to date, only the BACTEC MGIT 960 System offers pyrazinamide (PZA) and second-line drug testing.[47-49] For INH and RMP, the BACTEC MGIT 960 was in 99–100% agreement with the resistance ratio method, and showed a concordance for ethambutol (EMB) and PZA of 85% and 92%, respectively. Good correlation was also found for second-line drugs.[47-49] For the MGIT960 system, critical concentrations for second-line drugs for this system have been established in multicenter studies.[47-49] It should be noted that these critical concentrations stem from wild-type MIC distributions and not from pharmacokinetic studies or treatment outcome data from proper clinical trials. The labeling as 'susceptible' or 'resistance' thus might not accurately predict treatment outcomes in patients.

MAC, Mycobacterium kansasii and Other Slowly Growing NTM

The clinical significance of NTM has now been clearly established and this has created a need for drug susceptibility testing methods that can help to design treatment regimens and predict treatment outcomes in individual patients.

In general, the *in vitro* susceptibility testing of MAC has value particularly for the macrolides (clarithromycin is tested as the class representative) which have proven clinical and microbiologic efficacy in treatment of MAC pulmonary and disseminated disease,[11,50] with interpretive criteria based, at least in part, on treatment trials in humans. Although wild-type MAC is uniformly susceptible to macrolides, macrolide resistance develops quickly with monotherapy. An analysis of these resistant isolates showed that over 95% of clinically significant macrolide resistance in MAC is a consequence of mutations in the V domain of the 23S rRNA gene.[11,13,20]

Establishing baseline MIC values for a MAC isolate may prove valuable in interpreting susceptibility test results for a subsequent isolate from the same patient later on in case of treatment failure or relapse. Susceptibility to first line drugs including rifampin and ethambutol should not be determined since these drugs have an adjunctive role, in that they prevent the emergence of macrolide resistance. They should not be considered active components of MAC treatment regimens and should be given regardless of MICs *in vitro*.[11,13,20] For adjunctive amikacin or streptomycin, recommended for patients with severe cavitary MAC pulmonary disease, phenotypic susceptibility testing by broth microdilution was recently shown to correlate well with mutational resistance after previous exposure and thus has clinical significance. If resistance (MIC >64 mg/L) is detected, adjunctive aminoglycoside therapy is not warranted.[51]

Mycobacterium marinum is predictably susceptible to RMP and EMB; alternative agents are tetracyclines, clarithromycin and trimethoprim–sulfamethoxazole (co-trimoxazole). There are several suitable methods for susceptibility testing of *M. marinum* isolates.[43] Wild-type isolates of *M. haemophilum* are susceptible to fluoroquinolones, rifamycins and clarithromycin; the clinical significance of the elevated MICs to ethambutol is not known and treatment is usually similar to that of MAC disease.[11,43,52] The need for media supplementation means that susceptibility testing for *M. haemophilum* is far from standardized.[13] *Mycobacterium simiae* is highly resistant to antimycobacterial agents; however, there are exceedingly few cases of disease on which to base any firm conclusions about *in vitro–in vivo* correlations.[11,13,53] Clarithromycin in combination with EMB and moxifloxacin appears to be effective in some cases and the use of clofazimine and amikacin is under investigation.[11,53,54]

Rapid Growers

Although four methods have been described for measuring the *in vitro* susceptibility of rapidly growing mycobacteria, the CLSI now recommends only the microdilution method using cation-adjusted Mueller Hinton broth.[43] Broth microdilution provides a quantitative result and better supports the growth of *M. chelonae*. The broth microdilution method is essentially a modification of a standard method for nonmycobacteria that grow aerobically. Commercially prepared broth microdilution panels which can be used as specific plate formats for both slow and rapid growers are available. Alternatively, broth microdilution panels can be prepared in-house. Correlations with *in vivo*

outcome of treatment are strongest for macrolides, tetracyclines, co-trimoxazole, aminoglycosides and selected β-lactams (mainly cefoxitin). Testing rapidly growing mycobacteria should be restricted to laboratories with more extensive experience.

PRACTICAL VALUE OF MOLECULAR DETECTION OF RESISTANCE

Molecular detection of mutations associated with first line drug resistance in *M. tuberculosis* has moved from a research tool to clinical tests that have impacted on tuberculosis treatment worldwide. The most widely used assay is probably the GeneXpert MTB/RIF (Cepheid), which detects *M. tuberculosis* in clinical samples and predicts rifampin susceptibility based on probes targeting the 81bp hotspot region of the *rpoB* gene. A recent meta-analysis of is performance measured a pooled sensitivity of 95% and a pooled specificity of 98% for the detection of rifampin resistance.[34] The other widely used assay to detect resistance to first line antituberculosis drugs based on genomic mutations is the GenoType MTBDR*plus* assay (Hain Lifescience, Nehren, Germany). This assay can be performed on cultures as well as directly in clinical samples. In a recent meta-analysis, this assay showed a pooled sensitivity of 96% and a pooled specificity of 98% for detection of rifampin resistance.[55] Their sensitivity and specificity for detecting isoniazid resistance amount to 88% and 100% if *katG* and *inhA* data are combined.[56]

An important limitation of both these assays is that their positive predictive value is limited in settings with very low rates of resistance/MDR-TB (typically <5%).[55,56] Another limitation is that most were validated against crude phenotypic assays with a breakpoint concentration (particularly for rifampin) based entirely on wild-type MIC distribution, not on pharmacokinetic/pharmacodynamic science.

The latest addition to this widening array of diagnostic tests is the GenoType MTBDR*sl* which can detect mutations associated with resistance to aminoglycosides and fluoroquinolones (thus predict XDR-TB) as well as ethambutol.[57] As a test for fluoroquinolone resistance, the pooled sensitivity was 84% (95% confidence interval (CI) 78.7–86.7%) and the pooled specificity was 98% (95% CI 94.3-99.1%). The pooled sensitivity of MTBDR*sl* to detect second-line injectable drug (aminoglycosides and capreomycin) resistance was 77% and the pooled specificity was 99%; the low sensitivity was a result of poor correlation particularly with kanamycin and capreomycin resistance by phenotypic testing. As a test for XDR-TB, the pooled sensitivity and specificity were 71% and 99%.[57]

Ultimately, drug resistance and susceptibility may be predicted directly from whole genome sequences obtained straight from clinical samples; there is promising advance in this field.[58]

Immunodiagnostic Tests for Tuberculosis

Historically, the first immunodiagnostic test was the tuberculin skin test (TST). Shortcomings of this test include the inability to distinguish active disease from patient sensitization, unknown predictive values and cross-reaction with NTM. None of the numerous serologic tests has found wide clinical use, mainly because of the lack of sensitivity and specificity.

In contrast, the recently developed and commercially available whole-blood IFN-γ assays (interferon-gamma release assays, often called IGRAs) are promising candidates to improve the current level of diagnostic accuracy for tuberculosis infection, particularly if skin testing remains equivocal. The two test systems – the QuantiFERON®-TB Gold In-Tube (QFNG-IT; Cellestis, Victoria, Australia) and the T-SPOT.TB (Oxford Immunotec, Oxford, UK) – are not affected by BCG vaccination, do not cross-react with the majority of NTM and are less prone to variability and subjectivity associated with placing and reading of the TST (Table 185-5).

Although both tests measure T-cell INF-γ responses to similar *M. tuberculosis*-specific antigens over a 16- to 24-hour incubation period,

TABLE 185-5	Characteristics of the Commercially Available Tests for the Diagnosis of Tuberculosis Infection		
Variable	Tuberculin Skin Test	QuantiFERON-TB Gold/ QuantiFERON-TB Gold In-Tube	ELISPOT T-SPOT.TB
Administration	In vivo (intradermal)	Ex vivo, ELISA-based	Ex vivo, ELISPOT-based
Antigens	PPDS or RT-23	ESAT-6, CFP-10 and TB7.7	ESAT-6 and CFP-10
Standardized	Mostly	Yes	Yes
Reading prone to subjectivity	Yes	No	No
Units of measurement	Millimeters of induration	Units of IFN-γ	IFN-γ spot-forming cells
Definition of positive test results	5, 10 and 15 mm	Patient's IFN-γ ≥ 0.35 U/mL (after subtracting IFN-γ response in nil control)	≥ 6 spot-forming cells in the antigen wells, with 250 000 cells/well, and at least double-negative well
Indeterminate	If anergy (rarely tested)	Poor response to mitogen (<0.5 U/mL in positive control) or high background response (>8.0 U/mL in nil well)	Poor response to mitogen (<20 spot-forming cells in positive control well) or high background (>10 spot-forming cells in negative well)
Time to result	48–72 h	Same day (but longer if run in batches)	16–24 h (but longer if run in batches)
Consultation(s)	2	1	1
COST PER TEST (US DOLLARS)			
Materials		17.29	57.33
Labor/other		20.02	20.02
Total cost	11.58	37.31	77.35

Adapted from Menzies et al. Ann Intern Med 2007; 146:340-354.[59]

they are based on different technologies. The T-SPOT.TB assay is based on ELISPOT methodology and requires the isolation and incubation of peripheral blood mononuclear cells (PBMC) and the standardization of 250 000 PBMC in each of its test wells. The T-SPOT.TB assay requires, overall, two working days, and may be more laborious than the QFNG-IT. Nevertheless, the use of a standardized number of washed PBMC might contribute to the greater sensitivity reported in the literature. In contrast, the QFNG-IT has technical advantages over the T-SPOT.TB assay, since the stimulation of T-cell IFN-γ response in whole blood is performed in tubes precoated with the *M. tuberculosis* antigens. Also, the enzyme-linked immunosorbent assay (ELISA) is simple and rapid to perform. Since background noise may occur, a 'nil' control is required to adjust for this background, as well as for heterophile antibody effects and nonspecific IFN-γ in blood samples.

It is important to stress that neither of these tests distinguishes between latent and active infection. To date, there are a large number of publications available which focus on the performance characteristics of each test; however, there are only a few published head-to-head comparisons of the QFNG-IT and the T-SPOT.TB assays in different patient cohorts. In a systematic review of the literature Pai *et al.*[60] concluded that QFNG-IT has a specificity of 99% (T-SPOT.TB 96%) among non-BCG-vaccinated participants and a specificity of 96% (T-SPOT.TB 93%) among BCG-vaccinated participants, while the T-SPOT.TB appears to be more sensitive than QFNG-IT and TST. Diel *et al.*[61] compared both IFN-γ release assays in TST-positive persons recently exposed to pulmonary tuberculosis cases. In this study, factors independently influencing the risk of *M. tuberculosis* infection and their interactions with each other were evaluated by multivariate analysis. There were five variables which significantly predicted a positive IFN-γ release assay result, i.e. age, AFB-positivity of the source case, cough, cumulative exposure time and foreign origin of the patient. There was excellent agreement between the two assays (93.9%, kappa = 0.85), with QFNG-IT finding 30.2% of contacts positive and T-SPOT.TB finding 28.7% of them. Overall, the IFN-γ release assays were more accurate indicators of the presence of latent tuberculosis than TST.

In HIV-positive asymptomatic individuals (n=286) both QFNG-IT and T-SPOT.TB assay were more sensitive than TST (20.0% and 25.2%, respectively, compared with 12.8% [TST]), but seemed, as a whole, to be less sensitive than in immunocompetent patients.[62]

The performance of IFN-γ release assays in children is less understood, although their sensitivity and specificity compare well with the TST[63] and without the inconvenience and complications associated with TST. In latent tuberculosis the agreement between QFNG-IT and T-SPOT.TB assay was very good (92%) in children, with moderate agreement between TST and QFNG-IT (77%) and TST and T-SPOT.TB (75%), respectively.[64] For culture-confirmed active tuberculosis, however, the same authors stated that the sensitivity of the TST was 83%, compared to 80% for the QFNG-IT and 58% for the T-SPOT.TB.

The problem of indeterminate results occurs with both IFN-γ release assays. In HIV-infected individuals, T-SPOT.TB provided more indeterminate results than the QFNG-IT (8 vs 1/256, p<0.01),[61] similar to that confirmed by others (14% versus 1.8%).[65] Indeterminate results appear to be dependent on the number of CD4 cells inasmuch as patients with a CD4 count <200 cells/mL were significantly more likely to have an indeterminate result.[62,65] In children less than 4 years of age indeterminate results were more often seen using the QFNG-IT than the T-SPOT.TB.[66] In applying the T-SPOT.TB assay after indeterminate results have been obtained from the QFNG-IT test, 65% of the 40 patients yielded a valid result.[66]

Recently, large studies by the TB-NET network have shown that among various groups of immunocompromised patients, progression toward tuberculosis was highest in HIV-infected individuals and was poorly predicted by TST or IGRAs.[67] This predictive value needs further studies in other high-risk populations, including children.[68,69] A large meta-analysis has pointed out very clearly areas of uncertainty and recommendations for research.[60] Other problems concern the phenomena of conversions, reversions and nonspecific variations in serial testing[70] and altered performance characteristics of the assays in conjunction with ethnicity (e.g. Malay and Indian race versus Chinese race).[71]

From the present state of knowledge it is obvious that application of IFN-γ release assays for tuberculosis infection should be tailored to different high-risk groups. In addition, caution should be exercised in their current use in immunosuppressed patients.

For therapy of tuberculosis see Chapter 31.

References available online at expertconsult.com.

KEY REFERENCES

Beissner M., Herbinger K.H., Bretzel G.: Laboratory diagnosis of Buruli ulcer disease. *Future Microbiol* 2010; 5(3):363-370.

Bergamini B.M., Losi M., Vaienti F., et al.: Performance of commercial blood tests for the diagnosis of latent tuberculosis infection in children and adolescents. *Pediatrics* 2009; 123:e419-e424.

Chaidir L., Ganiem A.R., Van der Zanden A., et al.: Comparison of real time IS6110-PCR, microscopy, and culture for diagnosis of tuberculous meningitis in a cohort of adult patients in Indonesia. *PLoS ONE* 2012; 7(12):e52001.

de Beer J.L., van Ingen J., de Vries G., et al.: Comparative study of IS6110 restriction fragment length polymorphism and variable-number tandem-repeat typing of *Mycobacterium tuberculosis* isolates in the Netherlands, based on a 5-year nationwide survey. *J Clin Microbiol* 2013; 51:1193-1198.

Klimiuk J., Krenke R., Safianowska A., et al.: Diagnostic performance of different pleural fluid biomarkers in tuberculous pleurisy. *Adv Exp Med Biol* 2015; 852:21-30.

Lenaerts A., Barry C.E. 3rd, Dartois V.: Heterogeneity in tuberculosis pathology, microenvironments and therapeutic responses. *Immunol Rev* 2015; 264:288-307.

Menzies D., Pai M., Constock G.: Meta-analysis: New tests for the diagnosis of latent tuberculosis infection: areas of uncertainty and recommendations for research. *Ann Intern Med* 2007; 146:340-354.

Mugo D., Musyimi R., Mutiso A., et al.: Performance of the MGIT TBc identification test and meta-analysis of MPT64 assays for identification of the *Mycobacterium tuberculosis* complex in liquid culture. *J Clin Microbiol* 2011; 49:4343-4346.

Nessar R., Cambau E., Reyrat J.M., et al.: *Mycobacterium abscessus*: a new antibiotic nightmare. *J Antimicrob Chemother* 2012; 67:810-818.

Nienhuis W.A., Stienstra Y., Thompson W.A., et al.: Antimicrobial treatment for early, limited *Mycobacterium ulcerans* infection: a randomised controlled trial. *Lancet* 2010; 375(9715):664-672.

Sester M., van Leth F., Bruchfeld J., et al.: Risk assessment of tuberculosis in immunocompromised patients. A TBNET study. *Am J Respir Crit Care Med* 2014; 190:1168-1176.

Shah M., Ssengooba W., Armstrong D., et al.: Comparative performance of urinary lipoarabinomannan assays and Xpert MTB/RIF in HIV-infected individuals. *AIDS* 2014; 28(9):1307-1314.

Simons S.O., van der Laan T., de Zwaan R., et al.: Molecular drug susceptibility testing in the Netherlands: the performance of the MTBDRplus and MTBDRsl assay. *Int J Tuberc Lung Dis* 2015; 19:828-833.

Steingart K.R., Flores L.L., Dendukuri N., et al.: Commercial serological tests for the diagnosis of active pulmonary and extrapulmonary tuberculosis: an updated systematic review and meta-analysis. *PLoS Med* 2011; 8(8):e1001062.

Steingart K.R., Schiller I., Horne D.J., et al.: Xpert® MTB/RIF assay for pulmonary tuberculosis and rifampicin resistance in adults. *Cochrane Database Syst Rev* 2014; (1):CD009593.

Stephan C., Wolf T., Goetsch U., et al.: Comparing QuantiFERON-tuberculosis gold, T-SPOT tuberculosis and tuberculin skin test in HIV-infected individuals from a low prevalence tuberculosis country. *AIDS* 2009; 22:2471-2479.

Theron G., Peter J., Richardson M., et al.: The diagnostic accuracy of the GenoType(®) MTBDRsl assay for the detection of resistance to second-line anti-tuberculosis drugs. *Cochrane Database Syst Rev* 2014; (10):CD010705.

van Ingen J., Kuijper E.J.: Drug susceptibility testing of nontuberculous mycobacteria. *Future Microbiol* 2014; 9(9):1095-1110.

van Ingen J.: Diagnosis of nontuberculous mycobacterial disease. *Semin Respir Crit Care Med* 2013; 34(1):103-109.

van Ingen J.: Microbiological diagnosis of pulmonary disease caused by nontuberculous mycobacteria. *Clin Chest Med* 2015; 36(1):43-54.

Walker T.M., Ip C.L., Harrell R.H., et al.: Whole-genome sequencing to delineate *Mycobacterium tuberculosis* outbreaks: a retrospective observational study. *Lancet Infect Dis* 2013; 13:137-146.

Walker T.M., Kohl T.A., Omar S.V., et al.: Whole-genome sequencing for prediction of *Mycobacterium tuberculosis* drug susceptibility and resistance: a retrospective cohort study. *Lancet Infect Dis* 2015; 15(10):1193-1202.

186

Mycoplasma and Ureaplasma

JØRGEN SKOV JENSEN

Introduction

The class Mollicutes (meaning 'soft skin'), trivially known as mycoplasmas, comprise some of the smallest free-living micro-organisms. They lack the cell wall found in most other bacteria and, consequently, they are resistant to β-lactam antimicrobials. The small size of the mycoplasma genome limits the metabolic capabilities, making culture of some mycoplasmas difficult or impossible. Mycoplasmas isolated commonly from humans belong to the genera Mycoplasma and Ureaplasma within the order Mycoplasmatales. The genus Ureaplasma ('ureaplasmas') is unique in the ability to hydrolyze urea.

The Mollicutes are also economically important plant and animal pathogens. Although most species have strict host specificities, some of the animal mycoplasmas may occasionally cause infections in humans.

Currently, 14 Mycoplasma species and two Ureaplasma species are considered human mycoplasmas (summarized in Table 186-1). In this chapter, only the five species of clinical significance will be considered:

- Mycoplasma pneumoniae
- Mycoplasma genitalium
- Mycoplasma hominis
- Ureaplasma urealyticum
- Ureaplasma parvum

Mycoplasma pneumoniae

Nature

Mycoplasma pneumoniae is an important respiratory tract pathogen. It grows slowly in specialized bacteriological media, and infection is primarily diagnosed by nucleic acid amplification tests (NAAT), or indirectly by serology.

Epidemiology

M. pneumoniae causes mild upper respiratory tract symptoms more often than severe disease, and infections have been described from most parts of the world. In temperate climates, most infections are reported during late summer until mid-winter. However, the infection is endemic throughout the year with epidemic peaks about every 4–7 years.[1] The incubation period ranges from 2 to 4 weeks. Spread from person to person occurs slowly, usually where there is continual or repeated close contact, as within a family.[2,3]

M. pneumoniae is only responsible for a minority of all upper tract infections, where viral infection is the dominating cause, but it is a significant cause of lower respiratory tract infections being reported in 15–20% of all pneumonias in the USA.[4] In closed communities such as military camps and institutions, outbreaks with a high attack rate have been reported.[3]

Pathogenicity

Infection with *M. pneumoniae* probably happens in all age groups but the risk of developing pneumonia varies with age. Approximately 25% of children 5–15 years old with *M. pneumoniae* infection develop pneumonia, whereas this is the case in only about 7% of younger adults, although they often experience milder disease. Pneumonia is less frequent thereafter, but is more severe in older patients.[5]

A crucial step in *M. pneumoniae* infection is the adherence of the organisms to respiratory mucosal epithelial cells, which is mediated by a specialized terminal tip-structure carrying the P1 main adhesion protein and accessory proteins. After attachment to the ciliated epithelium, *M. pneumoniae* secretes hydrogen peroxide leading to ciliostasis, and subsequent necrosis of the epithelium.[6] The pneumonia is mainly caused by peribronchiolar and perivascular pulmonary infiltration with lymphocytes and is mainly an immune-pathological process since immunosuppression prevents pneumonia or diminishes its severity.[7]

Prevention

No vaccine against *M. pneumoniae* has been developed, and early attempts with vaccination resulted in more severe disease. Azithromycin treatment has been used successfully to prevent spread of epidemics in confined settings, but is not generally recommended.[8]

Diagnostic Microbiology

Diagnosis can be made by molecular methods such as NAAT, serology and culture. Traditionally, serology has been the primary diagnostic method, but this is increasingly being replaced by molecular methods. NAATs such as polymerase chain reaction (PCR) are capable of providing rapid diagnostic results in the acute phase of the disease, where it may direct antimicrobial treatment. Various gene targets have been used, but no standardization or general recommendations exist.[9] Recently, commercially available detection kits have received US Food and Drug Administration (FDA) approval.

Serology is generally less costly than NAATs, but since antibodies peak at 3–4 weeks after onset of disease, this method may have less relevance in the acute phase of the disease. Commercially available enzyme immunoassays specific for IgG and/or IgM are commonly used. IgM detection is much less reliable in re-infection, which is most often the case in adults. Cold agglutinins, detected by agglutination of O Rh-negative erythrocytes at 4 °C, correlate with specific IgM and are

TABLE 186-1	*Mycoplasma* and *Ureaplasma* Species Considered of Human Origin, Their Preferred Colonization and Disease Association					
	DETECTION RATE					
Species	**Respiratory Tract**	**Genitourinary Tract**	**Rectum**	**Blood**		**Cause of Disease**
M. amphoriforme	Rare	—*	—*	—*		Possibly
M. buccale	Rare	—	—	—		No
M. faucium	Rare	—	—	—		No
M. fermentans	Common	Rare	—	Very rare		Possibly
M. genitalium	Rare	Common	Rare	?		Yes
M. hominis	Rare	Common	Common	Rare		Yes
M. lipophilum	Rare	—	—	—		No
M. orale	Common	—	—	—		No
M. penetrans	—	Rare	Very rare	?		?
M. pirum	?	—	Rare	Very rare		?
M. pneumoniae	Rare†	Very rare	—	—		Yes
M. primatum	—	Rare	—	—		No
M. salivarium	Common	Rare	—	—		No
M. spermatophilum	—	Rare	—	?		?
U. parvum	Rare	Common	Common	Very rare		Yes
U. urealyticum	Rare	Common	Common	Very rare		Yes

*No reports of detection.
†Except in disease outbreaks.

suggestive of a recent *M. pneumoniae* infection, but have a low specificity and the test is rarely used.[10]

Complex culture media are needed for isolation of *M. pneumoniae*, and as culture may take up to 5 weeks, it is of no clinical value. It does, however, allow for antimicrobial susceptibility testing and is therefore important in surveillance and research.[11]

Clinical Manifestations

M. pneumoniae produces a range of clinical manifestations from asymptomatic infection and mild, afebrile, upper respiratory tract disease to severe pneumonia. The most typical clinical syndrome is tracheobronchitis, often accompanied by upper respiratory tract symptoms, such as acute pharyngitis. *M. pneumoniae* pneumonia cannot be distinguished from other etiologies without laboratory testing.[12] Illness often starts with a few days of malaise and headache before respiratory symptoms appear, and pneumonia is seen radiographically before physical signs, such as rales, are detectable. Usually, only one of the lower lobes is involved and the radiograph shows patchy opacities but approximately 20% of patients have bilateral pneumonia. Pleuritis and pleural effusions are unusual. Illness is often protracted, and symptoms may persist for several weeks, and may relapse. *M. pneumoniae* can persist in respiratory secretions for weeks despite antibiotic therapy and apparent clinical cure. Mortality is low, although patients with immunodeficiency or sickle cell anemia may experience severe infections. In children, illness may be prolonged with paroxysmal cough followed by vomiting, simulating whooping cough. *M. pneumoniae* has been implicated in bronchial asthma, but this is controversial.

EXTRAPULMONARY MANIFESTATIONS OF *M. PNEUMONIAE* INFECTION

Infections with *M. pneumoniae* are occasionally associated with various extrapulmonary symptoms which may occur simultaneously with the respiratory symptoms or after these have resolved.[13] Hemolytic crisis

can be precipitated by cold agglutinins, which are autoimmune antibodies against the I-antigen on erythrocytes. Cross-reacting autoantibodies may be responsible for neurological and other complications, although direct invasion of the central nervous system may explain a small proportion of cases. Skin manifestations such as an urticarial rash are quite common and may be misinterpreted as allergic reactions to the commonly prescribed macrolide treatment. Stevens–Johnson syndrome is often associated with *M. pneumoniae* infection (Table 186-2). *Mycoplasma* has been thought of as a cause of bullous myringitis but more recent studies suggest this is a false association.

Management

M. pneumoniae is generally susceptible to tetracyclines and macrolides. Ciprofloxacin and similar quinolones have only moderate activity, whereas the newer quinolones, such as moxifloxacin, are highly active *in vitro*. They should not be used as first-line therapy but may have a role in immunosuppressed patients, as they are bactericidal. High-level macrolide resistance in *M. pneumoniae* has become extremely common in some areas, with nearly 95% resistance reported among infected patient in parts of Asia.[14] However, only 1–10% resistant strains have been reported from Europe and the United States.[15]

Tetracyclines and macrolides significantly reduce the duration of fever, pulmonary infiltration and other signs and symptoms, and treatment with an active antimicrobial is recommended. In areas with low levels of macrolide resistance, azithromycin is commonly used, often as 500 mg once daily for 3 days.

Mycoplasma genitalium

Nature

Mycoplasma genitalium is an emerging sexually transmitted infection and the bacterium is very closely related to *M. pneumoniae*. Indeed, all

TABLE 186-2	Extrapulmonary Manifestations of *M. pneumoniae* Infections	
System	Manifestation	Estimated Frequency
Dermatological	Urticaria, erythema multiforme, Stevens–Johnson syndrome, other rashes	Some involvement in about 25%
Gastrointestinal	Anorexia, nausea, vomiting and transient diarrhea	14–44%
	Hepatitis	?
	Pancreatitis	?
Musculoskeletal	Myalgia, arthralgia, arthritis	14–45%
Genitourinary	Acute glomerulonephritis	Insignificant
Hematological	Cold agglutinin production	About 50%
	Hemolytic anemia	?
	Thrombocytopenia	?
	Intravascular coagulation	>50 reported cases
Neurological	Meningitis, meningoencephalitis, ascending paralysis, transient myelitis, cranial nerve palsy, poliomyelitis-like illness, Guillain–Barré syndrome	6–7% in a few studies based on serology
Cardiovascular	Myocarditis, pericarditis	<5%

M. genitalium genes present in the very small genome (580 kbp) can be found in the larger (816 kbp) *M. pneumoniae* genome.[16]

Epidemiology

M. genitalium is strongly associated with acute non-gonococcal urethritis (NGU) in both men and women. It is detected in approximately 25% of cases but in only 5–10% of asymptomatic sexually transmitted disease (STD) clinic attendees and in 1–3% of asymptomatic healthy controls.[17] In symptomatic men it has been detected almost independently of *Chlamydia trachomatis*.[18] In both men and women, the highest prevalence is found in individuals slightly older than those with *C. trachomatis*.[19]

Pathogenicity

Similar to *M. pneumoniae*, *M. genitalium* has a specialized terminal structure mediating cell-adherence.

Experimentally, *M. genitalium* causes urethritis in male chimpanzees,[20] and adheres to and enters epithelial cells.[21] Intracellular *M. genitalium* may be partially protected from antimicrobials, resulting in persistent or recurrent non-gonococcal urethritis.

Prevention

No vaccine against *M. genitalium* is available, but as with other sexually transmitted infections, consistent use of condoms provides good protection.

Diagnostic Microbiology

Culture of *M. genitalium* is extremely difficult and time-consuming and is not useful for diagnosis. Serology is severely hampered by cross-reactions with pre-existing *M. pneumoniae* antibodies, which are present in most adult patients. Consequently, NAATs are the only useful diagnostic methods, but at present, no commercially available FDA approved test exists. Test performance may vary significantly between laboratories due to the low amount of *M. genitalium* present

in many samples.[22,23] From men, the optimal diagnostic sample appears to be first-void-urine (FVU), whereas in women, a combination of FVU and cervical or vaginal swabs detects most infections.[24] As mentioned below, macrolide resistance is a major problem in some populations, and rapid NAAT-based detection of macrolide resistance mediating mutations has been introduced in a few laboratories to guide treatment.[25]

Clinical Manifestations
DISEASE IN MEN
Acute Non-gonococcal Urethritis
M. genitalium was isolated initially from men with acute NGU and more than 35 studies have shown *M. genitalium* to be strongly and almost uniformly associated with acute NGU.[17] Among STD clinic populations, about 90% of *M. genitalium*-infected men have microscopic evidence of urethritis and 70–80% report symptoms. The association between *M. genitalium* and urethritis is even stronger in acute non-chlamydial NGU,[17] where it accounts for more than one-third of the cases, strongly suggesting that *M. genitalium* and *C. trachomatis* act as separate causes of the condition.

Chronic Non-gonococcal Urethritis
M. genitalium is found in up to 40% of men with persistent or recurrent NGU after treatment with doxycycline,[26,27] probably due to the inefficiency of tetracyclines in eradicating *M. genitalium*.

Chronic Prostatitis
Despite *M. genitalium* being involved in chronic NGU, there is only limited evidence suggesting that it is associated with chronic prostatitis.

Acute Epididymitis
Clinical experience as well as the detection of *M. genitalium* in a few patients during an antibiotic trial[28] suggests that *M. genitalium* may be a cause of acute epididymitis in some patients. In a study from Japan it was detected in 9% of men <40 years of age with epididymitis,[29] but often together with *C. trachomatis*.

Proctitis
M. genitalium has been detected in 2–11% of rectal swabs from men who have sex with men (MSM), but the relation to symptoms is not clear.[30] Whether a rectal infection with *M. genitalium* can be transmitted, remains to be determined.

DISEASE IN WOMEN
Non-gonococcal Urethritis
M. genitalium has been associated with urethritis in women attending STD clinics.[31,32] It is unclear if *M. genitalium* explains a proportion of sterile pyuria.

Bacterial Vaginosis (BV) and Vaginitis
The association of *M. genitalium* with BV is controversial; most studies have not shown an association; *M. genitalium* has not been associated with vaginitis.

Cervicitis
M. genitalium is generally detected in 10–20% of women with cervicitis, and in the majority of studies, significantly more often in cases than in controls.[30] The association between *M. genitalium* and cervicitis is less strong than that seen for male NGU with pooled odds-ratios around 2.2.[17]

Pelvic Inflammatory Disease (PID)
PID is an inflammation of the upper genital tract and comprises endometritis and/or salpingitis. For all NAAT-based studies, *M. genitalium* has been associated with PID.[17,30] Odds-ratios for the association have been from 2.1 to 6.3, and symptom severity has been comparable to

that experienced in chlamydial PID, but milder than for gonococcal PID.[33] In most studies, 5–15% of PID could be attributed to *M. genitalium*, suggesting that in many settings it would significantly outnumber cases caused by *N. gonorrhoeae*.

Importantly, *M. genitalium* was also strongly associated with PID after termination of pregnancy, an observation that calls for further studies, as screening before the procedure as for *C. trachomatis* might be important.[34]

Infertility

Serological studies have shown an association with tubal factor infertility with around 20% of women having *M. genitalium* antibodies compared to 5% with normal tubes.[35,36] The association was statistically significant, also when controlling for *C. trachomatis*.

DISEASE IN BOTH MEN AND WOMEN

Sexually Acquired Reactive Arthritis

There are no systematic studies of the role of *M. genitalium* in reactive arthritis and Reiter's syndrome, but clinical experience suggests that it may have a role. *M. genitalium* has been detected by PCR in the knees of a patient with Reiter's syndrome.[37]

HIV and Immunosuppression

According to a meta-analysis, individuals infected with *M. genitalium* are twice as likely to be infected with human immunodeficiency virus (HIV).[38–40] *M. genitalium* is also associated with HIV shedding in women.[41]

Management

Antimicrobial treatment of *M. genitalium* has become a complicated issue. Although tetracyclines are active *in vitro*,[42] they only eradicate the infection from less than a third of infected patients. Azithromycin in a 1 g single dose commonly used for *C. trachomatis* infection had cure rates around 85% in clinical trials.[43,44] Azithromycin 500 mg day one followed by 250 mg days 2–5 as used for *M. pneumoniae* infections had a cure rate of 95%.[44] Unfortunately, an increasing proportion of *M. genitalium* strains have developed resistance to macrolides through mutations in region V of the 23S ribosomal RNA gene.[45] Rates of macrolide resistance around 40% have been reported both in Australia and Europe,[19,46,47] but in selected populations, resistance as high as 100% has been reported.[48] If azithromycin treatment fails, moxifloxacin (400 mg once daily for 7 days) can be used,[49] but this agent is not recommended as first-line therapy. Unfortunately, increasing quinolone resistance is seen, with emergence of strains resistant to both azithromycin and moxifloxacin.[42] Such strains may be extremely difficult to eradicate, but limited clinical experience suggests that pristinamycin may be effective.

Mycoplasma hominis and *Ureaplasma* spp.

Introduction

In this section, *M. hominis* and the ureaplasmas will be described together, as they are involved in the same disease conditions. The ureaplasmas have been reclassified from the original name *U. urealyticum* to now comprise two separate species, *U. urealyticum* and *U. parvum*.[50] The two species cannot be distinguished by culture methods so species names will be used only where such distinction has been possible. In studies based on undifferentiated culture findings, the bacteria will be referred to as ureaplasmas.

Nature

M. hominis and ureaplasmas are opportunistic pathogens, occasionally causing infections relating primarily to the urogenital tract.

Epidemiology

Ureaplasmas and *M. hominis* can be transmitted to about 40% of babies born to infected mothers.[51] Infants above 3 months of age are rarely colonized.[52]

In adults, the rate of colonization increases with the number of different sexual partners.[53] *M. hominis* and ureaplasmas can be found in the cervix or vagina of 20–50% and 40–80% of sexually active, asymptomatic women, respectively. The colonization rate is somewhat lower in the urethra of healthy males. It is important to note that colonization is strongly linked to BV in women. This may lead to an overestimation of the importance of *M. hominis* and ureaplasmas in diseases where BV is a risk factor.

Pathogenicity

Although *M. hominis* adheres to cells and possesses several adhesins, many of which are immunogenic in the host, and subject to variation in the bacterium,[54] the adhesion is less strong than that seen in *M. pneumoniae* and *M. genitalium*. *M. hominis* metabolizes arginine, and releases ammonia, which may cause local tissue damage. Similarly, the ureaplasmas adhere to cells[55] and also produce ammonia from the degradation of urea.

Diagnostic Microbiology

M. hominis and ureaplasmas are so commonly found in the lower genital tract of healthy men and women that detection from these sites is rarely relevant. Ureaplasmas and *M. hominis* usually show evidence of growth in special culture media within 1–5 days. *M. hominis* may grow on ordinary blood agar where it produces pinpoint colonies after extended incubation. NAAT assays for detection of *M. hominis* and *U. urealyticum/U. parvum* are available in some laboratories, and the ability to distinguish the two *Ureaplasma* species is important. Quantitative assays are recommended over qualitative assays. Serology cannot be recommended for diagnostic purposes.

Clinical Manifestations

DISEASE IN MEN

Non-gonococcal Urethritis

The role of ureaplasmas in NGU is less clear than for *M. genitalium*. Human inoculation studies[56,57] support a causal role for ureaplasmas in NGU, particularly chronic disease.[58] The role of *U. urealyticum* is still controversial, but an increasing number of studies have associated this species with NGU,[59] in particular when present in high titers.[60,61] *U. parvum* is detected more often from the control group, suggesting that this species has a lower pathogenic potential. There is no evidence supporting a role for *M. hominis* as a cause of urethritis.[62]

Prostatitis

Ureaplasmas have been isolated from expressed prostatic secretions after prostatic massage more often and in higher titers in men with chronic prostatitis than in controls.[63,64] However, there is not much evidence to support a role in acute or in chronic bacterial prostatitis, and *M. hominis* has not been associated with prostatitis of any kind.

Epididymitis

Ureaplasmas have been recovered from the urethra and directly from epididymal aspirate fluid, accompanied by a specific antibody response in a patient with acute epididymitis.[65] However, further studies are required to establish a causal role.

DISEASE IN WOMEN

Bacterial Vaginosis (BV)

BV affects 5–25% of women[66] and is characterized by a loss of *Lactobacillus* species and an increase in gram-variable coccobacilli, anaerobic organisms, as well as *M. hominis* and ureaplasmas.[67] Both ureaplasmas and *M. hominis* are found in higher titers in the vagina of women with BV than in healthy women, but they are not the cause of the condition.[68]

BV is a strong predictor of infectious complications in women, thus, the strong association between ureaplasmas, *M. hominis*, and BV leads to significant problems in defining the roles of these species, as BV has not been controlled for in most studies.

Cervicitis

The role of ureaplasmas and *M. hominis* in cervicitis has not been studied in great detail. Mucopurulent cervicitis has been associated with isolation of ureaplasmas,[69] although the role of bacterial vaginosis as a confounder was not assessed.

PID and Sequelae

PID is caused by microbes in the lower genital tract invading the upper genital tract. *C. trachomatis* and *Neisseria gonorrhoeae* are well established etiological agents, but the mixed bacterial flora associated with BV is also a cause of PID,[70] and the role of ureaplasmas and *M. hominis* should be considered in that context. *M. hominis* has been recovered more frequently from lower tract specimens from women with PID than from healthy women.[71,72] *M. hominis* has been isolated apparently in pure culture from the fallopian tubes of women with salpingitis diagnosed by laparoscopy, but not from women without lesions.[73] In several studies, a fourfold rise in antibody titer to *M. hominis* has been found more often among women who had PID than among controls, but no control for BV was reported.[71,74] Although ureaplasmas have also been isolated occasionally from the fallopian tubes of patients with PID,[75,76] they have usually been found in association with other known pathogens and are not thought to play a major role.

In conclusion, there is some evidence that *M. hominis* may be a cause of PID, possibly as part of the BV-associated flora, but there is very little evidence that ureaplasmas have a similar role.

Pregnancy-Related Complications

Infertility. Although ureaplasmas and *M. hominis* have been associated with both male-factor and female-factor infertility in some studies, no convincing evidence has been obtained.

Adverse Pregnancy Outcome. Isolation of ureaplasmas and *M. hominis* from the lower genital tract have shown a only a weak association with spontaneous abortion compared to studies based on detection from the endometrium or placenta but they may just be markers of concomitant BV, and BV in itself has been associated with both pre-term labor and stillbirth.[77,78]

Ureaplasmas have been isolated more frequently from spontaneously aborted fetuses and stillborn or premature infants than from induced abortions or normal full-term infants. Ureaplasmas have been isolated from lungs, brain, heart and viscera, suggesting that it was not merely superficial contamination.[79,80]

Chorioamnionitis and mycoplasma infection are significantly associated, even when corrected for the duration of rupture of the membranes. Both ureaplasmas and *M. hominis* can invade the amniotic sac before 20 weeks of gestation in the presence of intact fetal membranes. Detection in mid-trimester amniotic fluid was associated with preterm premature rupture of the membranes with subsequent preterm birth.[81,82] However, not all infected women delivered preterm.

Neonatal Infections. Ureaplasmas can be isolated from the respiratory tract of neonates. The isolation rate correlates strongly with birth-weight and infants below 1000 g are infected much more often than full-term infants.[83] A meta-analysis has shown that *Ureaplasma* colonization of the lower respiratory tract of infants <1500 g increases the risk of development of chronic lung disease.[84] *M. hominis* has very

rarely been implicated in pneumonia soon after birth, but both *M. hominis* and ureaplasmas have been isolated from the cerebrospinal fluid of neonates with meningitis or brain abscess and should be considered in culture-negative neonatal meningitis.[85]

Postpartum and Postabortal Fever. *M. hominis* is considered to be responsible for some cases of maternal fever after a normal delivery or abortion, accounting for almost 10% of positive cultures.[86] It is important to note that most commercially available blood culture media contain sodium polyanetholesulfonate (SPS), which inhibits the growth of mycoplasmas;[87] consequently, special media should be employed when mycoplasma infection is suspected.

DISEASE IN MEN AND WOMEN
Urinary Tract Disease

Pyelonephritis and Urinary Tract Infection. *M. hominis* does not appear to play an important role in acute cystitis.[88] However, ureaplasmas have been associated with symptoms of cystitis and with the acute urethral syndrome in women without significant bacteriuria, and have been isolated from up to 25% of suprapubic aspirates from such women.[89,90]

Despite the lack of evidence for *M. hominis* causing acute cystitis, it has been found in up to 10% of cases of acute pyelonephritis.[91] There is no evidence suggesting a similar role for ureaplasmas.

Urinary Calculi and Catheter Encrustations. Infection stones and catheter encrustations may be caused by urea-hydrolyzing bacteria and ureaplasmas have been detected in 12–27% of infection stones,[92] more often in the urine and stones of patients with infection stones, compared to those with metabolic stones.[93]

Infections in Immunodeficient Patients

Patients with antibody deficiencies such as hypo- or agammaglobulinemia are particularly susceptible to extragenital mycoplasma infections. *M. hominis* and ureaplasmas have been found in septic arthritis, osteomyelitis, subcutaneous abscesses and cellulitis.[94] Cystitis and chronic urethritis is common and it is often very difficult to eradicate the mycoplasmas.[95,96] Patients undergoing organ transplantation are also susceptible to both wound and systemic mycoplasma infections; patients having kidney, lung, heart and liver transplantations appear to be at high risk.

Prolonged intravenous and combination therapy with high doses of antibiotics should be considered to avoid development of antimicrobial resistance. In general, fluoroquinolones with extended gram-positive spectrum such as moxifloxacin are recommended due to their bactericidal effect and potency against a broad spectrum of mollicutes, but always in combination with another antibiotic class such as tetracyclines.

Management

Before treating *M. hominis* or ureaplasmas, the first consideration is whether to treat or not. The high carriage rate among healthy adults should always be kept in mind.

The main antibiotics are the tetracyclines, the macrolides, quinolones and clindamycin. *M. hominis* is intrinsically resistant to macrolides but most strains are susceptible to tetracyclines, quinolones and clindamycin. Ureaplasmas are susceptible to tetracyclines, quinolones and macrolides, whereas clindamycin is mostly inactive.

References available online at expertconsult.com.

KEY REFERENCES

Cassell G.H., Waites K.B., Crouse D.T., et al.: Association of *Ureaplasma urealyticum* infection of the lower respiratory tract with chronic lung disease and death in very-low-birth-weight infants. *Lancet* 1988; 2:240-245.

Eschenbach D.A., Buchanan T.M., Pollock H.M., et al.: Polymicrobial etiology of acute pelvic inflammatory disease. *N Engl J Med* 1975; 293:166-171.

Foy H.M., Grayston J.T., Kenny G.E., et al.: Epidemiology of *Mycoplasma pneumoniae* infection in families. *JAMA* 1966; 197:859-866.

Hay P.E., Lamont R.F., Taylor-Robinson D., et al.: Abnormal bacterial colonisation of the genital tract and subsequent preterm delivery and late miscarriage. *BMJ* 1994; 308(6924):295-298.

Jensen J.S., Bradshaw C.S., Tabrizi S.N., et al.: Azithromycin treatment failure in *Mycoplasma genitalium*-positive patients with non-gonococcal urethritis is associated with induced macrolide resistance. *Clin Infect Dis* 2008; 47(12):1546-1553.

Manhart L.E.: *Mycoplasma genitalium*: an emergent sexually transmitted disease? *Infect Dis Clin North Am* 2013; 27(4):779-792.

McCormack W.M., Almeida P.C., Bailey P.E., et al.: Sexual activity and vaginal colonization with genital mycoplasmas. *JAMA* 1972; 221:1375-1377.

Napierala Mavedzenge S., Weiss H.A.: Association of *Mycoplasma genitalium* and HIV infection: a systematic review and meta-analysis. *AIDS* 2009; 23(5):611-620.

Taylor-Robinson D., Csonka G.W., Prentice M.J.: Human intra-urethral inoculation of ureaplasmas. *Q J Med* 1977; 46:309-326.

Taylor-Robinson D., Jensen J.S.: *Mycoplasma genitalium*: from chrysalis to multicolored butterfly. *Clin Microbiol Rev* 2011; 24(3):498-514.

Taylor-Robinson D., Lamont R.F.: Mycoplasmas in pregnancy. *BJOG* 2011; 118(2):164-174.

Waites K.B., Katz B., Schelonka R.L.: Mycoplasmas and ureaplasmas as neonatal pathogens. *Clin Microbiol Rev* 2005; 18(4):757-789.

Waites K.B., Talkington D.F.: *Mycoplasma pneumoniae* and its role as a human pathogen. *Clin Microbiol Rev* 2004; 17(4):697-728, table.

187

Rickettsia and Rickettsia-Like Organisms

EMMANOUIL ANGELAKIS | DIDIER RAOULT

KEY CONCEPTS

- Molecular techniques have unveiled the great diversity of *Rickettsia* and rickettsia-like organisms.

- Globalization and warming trends are important factors that influence rickettsial transmission by arthropods.

- Murine typhus is most prevalent in warm countries and sporadic cases are reported in travelers who visited endemic areas.

- Scrub typhus is a re-emerging disease with more than a million cases annually in Asia.

- Infective endocarditis is a serious complication of Q fever and can be fatal without treatment.

- The approach to treatment of *Bartonella* infections must be adapted to each species and clinical situation.

Introduction

Rickettsia and rickettsia-like organisms are fastidious, obligate intracellular, coccobacilli that are transmitted to vertebrate hosts by arthropods. Traditional methods to classify bacteria are not useful for strict intracellular organisms as they have few phenotypes. The advent of molecular methods has enabled very accurate determinations of phylogenetic relationships between intracellular bacteria, and the order Rickettsiales has been reclassified to contain the genera *Anaplasma*, *Ehrlichia*, *Neorickettsia*, *Orientia*, *Rickettsia* and *Wolbachia*.[1] Phylogenetic studies have shown that several bacteria previously classified in the order Rickettsiales did not belong to the α subgroup of the Proteobacteria phylum;[1] the genus *Bartonella* was moved to the α$_2$ subgroup and the genus *Coxiella* to the γ subgroup (see Figure 187-1).

Molecular studies have also greatly facilitated the detection and description of new organisms and the *Rickettsia* genus now contains 24 recognized species classified into three groups based on their genomic, antigenic, morphologic and ecologic patterns: the spotted fever group (SFG), the typhus group and the *R. bellii* group.[1] Similarly, the number of *Bartonella* spp. and the clinical syndromes caused by these organisms have increased rapidly. While infections with *Anaplasma* and *Ehrlichia* spp. were previously considered only of veterinary importance, studies over the past two decades have revealed several new species or strains that are pathogenic in both people and animals. In this chapter we describe the infections caused by rickettsiae and rickettsia-like organisms.

Spotted Fever Group Rickettsiae

Nature

The SFG rickettsiae are obligate, intracellular, gram-negative, coccobacilli ($1.0–2.0 \times 0.3–0.7\,\mu m$) that can infect vertebrate (endothelium, vascular smooth muscle and macrophages) and invertebrate cells (hemocytes and salivary gland epithelium). The SFG rickettsiae have a high content of lipopolysaccharides which are highly immunogenic and are responsible for the considerable serologic cross-reactivity

between the different species within the group. There are, however, also species-specific antigens and these include the rickettsial outer membrane proteins A and B, rOmpA and rOmpB, respectively.[2] Prior to 1984, six pathogenic SFG rickettsial species were recognized, including *R. rickettsii*, *R. conorii conorii*, *R. conorii israelensis*, *R. sibirica sibirica* and *R. akari*.[3] The discovery of other SFG rickettioses during recent years was greatly facilitated by the extensive use of cell culture systems and the development of specific and sensitive molecular tools. As a result, since 1998 more species or subspecies of tick-borne SFG rickettsiae were identified as emerging pathogens.

R. felis is also a newly described pathogenic SFG rickettsia and has pili, which are probably involved in cell attachment and conjugation.[4]

The structure and the genome of *R. akari* is similar to that of other *Rickettsia* species.[5]

Epidemiology

Most SFG rickettsiae are found in only one or a limited number of species of ticks and hence the distribution of the various tick species determines the risk areas for SFG rickettsioses.[6] People are not considered good reservoirs for SFG rickettsiae as they are seldom infested with ticks for long periods and rickettsemia is normally of only short duration, especially with antibiotic intervention.

The reservoir and vector of *R. felis* may be cat fleas (*Ctenocephalides felis*) which transmits the organism transovarially. It appears that *R. felis* is transmitted to people by flea bites.[7]

R. akari is found in the mouse mite (*Liponyssoides sanguineus*), which is the vector and reservoir of infection. Transmission might also occur with the use of contaminated needles in intravenous drug users.[7] *R. akari* has been also isolated from various commensal and wild rodent species. In the laboratory, *Liponyssus bacoti*, the tropical rat mite, can become infected with *R. akari* and transmit transovarially to its progeny, but is not an efficient vector.

Pathogenicity

Ticks inject virulent SFG rickettsiae in their saliva while feeding and these adhere to endothelial cells, the most important target cells. Adherence is receptor-mediated and results in changes to the actin cytoskeletal structure and phagocytosis of organisms into the cell.[8] The resultant phagosome lyses very rapidly and organisms are released into the cytoplasm. Some organisms escape from infected endothelial cells at the tick attachment site and spread via lymphatics to regional lymph nodes causing enlargement of lymph nodes. They also enter the bloodstream and infect endothelial cells throughout the body.

Prevention

There are no vaccines against the SFG rickettsiae and prevention depends on reducing exposure to vectors by avoiding infested areas and controlling ticks and fleas on domestic animals. People living in endemic areas and travelers to these areas should use effective tick repellants on their clothing, such as DEET (*N*,*N*-diethyl-*m*-toluamide) or permethrins. Wearing light-colored clothes facilitates early tick detection and removal before they can attach. Prevention of rickettsial pox depends on rodent and mite control. In recent years, with the increase in international travel to increasingly distant locations and with recent measures to protect wild fauna in combination with land rehabilitation and management practices, particularly forestry, the potential exposure to arthropods has increased along with the consequent risk of rickettsial transmission. For example, among travelers returning from sub-Saharan Africa, rickettsial infections, primarily tick-borne spotted fever, occurred more frequently than typhoid or dengue.

Diagnostic Microbiology

The typical clinical picture of the SFG rickettsioses is high fever (39.5–40°C/103–104°F), headache and characteristic rash. Common non-specific laboratory abnormalities include mild leukopenia, anemia and thrombocytopenia.[9] Interestingly, recent studies have shown that testing ticks by matrix-assisted laser desorption/ionization time-of-flight (MALDI-TOF) technology makes it possible to identify the species in minutes. This technique, together with knowledge of the common pathogens found in the identified tick, has improved understanding of tick-transmitted agents.[10]

DIRECT DIAGNOSIS

Rickettsia spp. can be isolated from blood or tissue samples in cell cultures (Vero, L929, HEL, XTC-2 or MRC5 cells) in biosafety level 3 laboratories.[9] Direct immunofluorescence techniques on tissues have moderate sensitivity (53–75%) but are nearly 100% specific.[11] Greater sensitivity may be achieved with polymerase chain reaction (PCR) assays amplifying sequences of several genes, including 16S rDNA, *rOmpA*, *rOmpB*, *gltA* (citrate synthase) and gene D.[9] Swabbing of eschar or vesicular lesions for PCR has been recently found to be the most sensitive diagnostic tool.

INDIRECT DIAGNOSIS

Currently, the indirect microimmunofluorescence assay (IFA) is the most commonly used technique for the diagnosis of SFG rickettsioses.[12] Infection with the various SFG rickettsiae cannot always be differentiated by comparing IFA titers against the different members of the group. If differences in IFA assay titers between SFG rickettsiae are less than two serum dilutions, Western blot assays targeting two high-molecular-weight proteins (*rOmpA* and *rOmpB*)[13] and cross-absorption studies are needed to determine the SFG rickettsiae causing infection.[9]

Clinical Manifestations

Currently, there are 14 SFG rickettsiae that are pathogenic in people (Table 187-1).

R. africae is the etiologic agent of African tick-bite fever (ATBF), which is probably the most prevalent tick-borne SFG rickettsiosis in the world. It is transmitted by *Amblyomma hebraeum* and probably also by *A. variegatum* (Figure 187-1), with the majority of these ticks being infected and hence vectors of *R. africae* in sub-Saharan Africa. Fever is common (88%) and accompanying clinical signs are generally mild and include regional enlargement of lymph nodes (57%). A rash is seen in 49% of the patients and may be vesicular. To date, no deaths or severe manifestations have been reported in patients with ATBF.[9]

R. rickettsii is the agent of Rocky Mountain spotted fever (RMSF), which is the most severe of the SFG rickettsioses. In the USA the major vectors are *Dermacentor andersonii* (wood tick) and *D. variabilis* (American dog tick) while in Central and South America the major vector is *A. cajennense* (Cayenne tick). The incubation period of RMSF

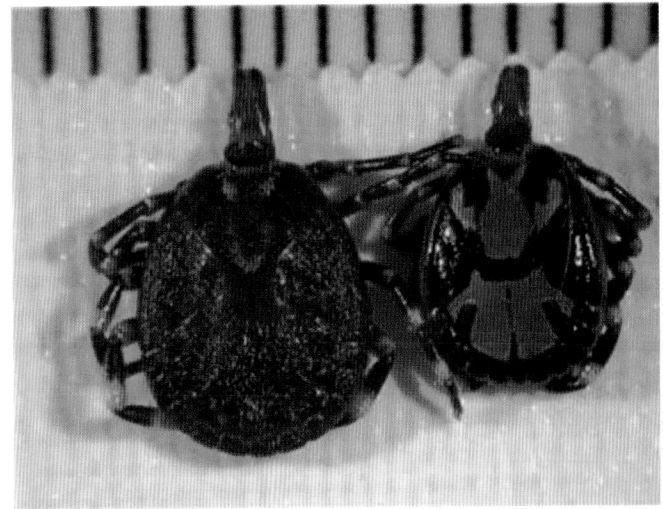

Figure 187-1 Female (left) and male (right) adult *Amblyomma variegatum*, vector and reservoir of *Rickettsia africae*.

TABLE 187-1	Prevalence of Signs and Prognoses for the More Common Spotted Fever Group Rickettsioses				
Spotted Fever Group	**Fever**	**Rash**	**Eschar**	**Regional Lymphadenopathy**	**Fatality Rate without Treatment**
African tick bite fever	88%	49%	53–98%	49–57%	None
Rocky Mountain spotted fever	Yes	90%	Rare	None	20–25%
Mediterranean spotted fever	100%	87%	53%	Rare	1–2.5%
Israeli spotted fever	Yes	100%	90%	None	0–3.5%
Astrakhan fever	Yes	94%	23%	Rare	None
Japanese spotted fever	Yes	100%	91%	None	None
Queensland tick typhus	Yes	100%	65%	70%	Two fatal cases
Flinders Island spotted fever	Yes	100%	25–55%	55%	None
Siberian tick typhus	Yes	Common	62–77%	Uncommon	None
Lymphangitis-associated rickettsiosis	Yes	Common	75%	100%	None
SENLAT	45%	Uncommon	100%	100%	None
Far Eastern spotted fever	Yes	Common but often faint	Yes	20%	None
Flea-borne spotted fever	Common	Rare	Rare	Rare	None
Rickettsialpox	Common	Common	Common	None	None

SENLAT-scalp eschar and neck lymphadenopathy.

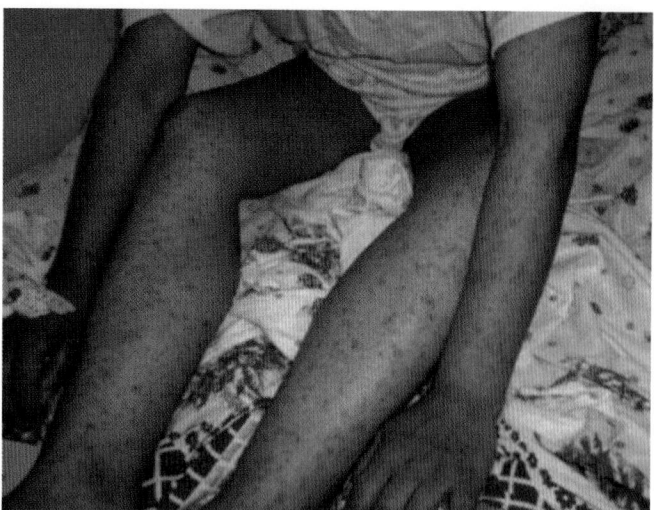

Figure 187-2   Maculopapular rash in a patient with Mediterranean spotted fever from Algeria. (*Courtesy Dr Nadjet Mouffok.*)

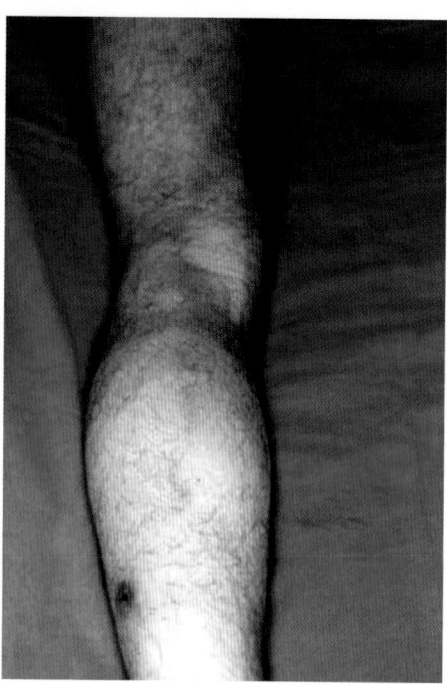

Figure 187-3   Lymphangitis expanding from the inoculation eschar on the left leg to an enlarged, painful lymph node in the left groin of a patient with *Rickettsia mongolotimonae* infection. (*From Fournier P.-E., et al. Rickettsia mongolotimonae: a rare pathogen in France. Emerg Infect Dis 2000; 6:290-332.*)

is 2–14 days and initial signs include high fever (>39°C/102°F) and headache. Although a macular rash, which appears first on the wrists and ankles before generalizing, is a characteristic feature of RMSF, it occurs in fewer than 50% of patients in the first 3 days of illness. In untreated patients, signs progress with the development of the vasculitis.

R. conorii has recently been shown to comprise three subspecies.[9]

- *R. conorii* subsp. *conorii* is the agent of Mediterranean spotted fever (MSF). After an incubation period of about 6 days, there is an abrupt onset of high fever (>39°C/102°F) and flu-like symptoms.[14] Typically, an eschar or tache noire (black spot) develops at the site of tick attachment. After about 4 days, a generalized maculopapular rash develops that also involves the palms and soles but spares the face (Figure 187-2). Most patients will recover over 10 days without treatment but the rash may still be visible for 10–20 days after remission of clinical symptoms. Severe forms of MSF are seen in 5–6% of patients and the mortality rate is around 2%.
- *R. conorii* subsp. *israelensis* is transmitted by *R. sanguineus* and causes Israeli spotted fever.[9] This disease has similar clinical features to MSF. Although Israeli spotted fever is typically milder and of shorter duration than classic MSF, several fatal cases and severe forms have been described.
- *R. conorii* subsp. *caspia* causes Astrakhan fever in the Caspian Sea area in Russia, and Chad.[9] The disease is similar to MSF but eschars are seen in relatively few patients (23%).

R. japonica causes Japanese or Oriental spotted fever, which occurs particularly along the coast of south-western and central Japan. The rash is usually found on the palms of the hands and the soles of the feet and may become petechial after a few days before it disappears over about 2 weeks. Up to 20% of patients may have severe disease, with encephalitis, disseminated intravascular coagulopathy, multiorgan failure and acute respiratory distress syndrome having been reported.[9]

R. australis is the agent of Queensland tick typhus and is transmitted principally by *Ixodes holocyclus* in Australia.[9] An eschar at the site of tick attachment and lymphadenopathy are found in 65% and 70% of cases, respectively.

R. honei causes Flinders Island spotted fever. The organism might be the most widely distributed of the SFG rickettsiae as it has recently been identified in Thailand and Texas.[9] Patients with Flinders Island spotted fever have a sudden onset of fever, headache, myalgia, joint swelling and pain, and a slight cough in some patients.

R. sibirica subsp. *sibirica* is the agent of Siberian or North Asian tick typhus, which occurs in Asiatic Russia and is transmitted by

Dermacentor spp.[9] The disease is usually mild and there are seldom severe complications.

R. sibirica subsp. *mongolotimonae* infections have now been described in 11 patients.[15] Infections cause a 'lymphangitis-associated rickettsiosis' with signs including fever, maculopapular rash, eschar, enlarged regional lymph nodes and rope-like lymphangitis (Figure 187-3).

R. massiliae was recently isolated from a patient with a maculopapular rash, eschar and slight hepatomegaly. The organism is transmitted by *Rhipicephalus* spp. in Europe and Central Africa.[16]

R. slovaca is transmitted by *D. marginatus* and *D. reticulatus*. Long considered nonpathogenic, *R. slovaca* has recently been found to be the agent of the SENLAT (Scalp Eschar and Neck LymphAdenopaThy) syndrome which is characterized by the presence of inoculation eschar on the scalp that is associated with cervical lymphadenopathy.[17]

R. heilongjiangensis is the agent of Far Eastern spotted fever and is found in *D. silvarum* in China and *Haemaphysalis* spp. from Siberia and the Russian Far East.[18] Infections result in fever, headache, rash, eschar, regional lymphadenopathy and conjunctivitis (Figure 187-4).

R. aeschlimannii occurs in *Hyalomma* spp. in Africa and Europe. Two patients have been described with *R. aeschlimannii* infections but there is evidence that these may be more widespread in southern Europe.[9]

R. parkeri occurs in *A. maculatum* in the southern USA. Although the organism has been known for over 60 years, it has only recently been recognized as a pathogen in two patients.[19]

R. felis, previously known as the ELB agent, is the recently described agent of 'flea-borne spotted fever'.[20] The vertical and horizontal transmission of *R. felis* in cat fleas is well documented and supports the role of this host as both vector and reservoir. Clinical signs are nonspecific, most commonly including fever, headache and rash. Other signs that have been reported are marked fatigue, myalgia, photophobia, conjunctivitis, abdominal pain, vomiting and diarrhea, and solitary black crusted skin lesions surrounded by a livid halo. This rickettsia has recently been shown to be extremely prevalent in tropical areas such as Africa, South East Asia and the South Pacific.[21] It may presents as an eruptive fever and can be associated with a vesicular localized lesion.[22] It may presented as isolated fever with cough and evidence of mosquito vector has been provided.[23]

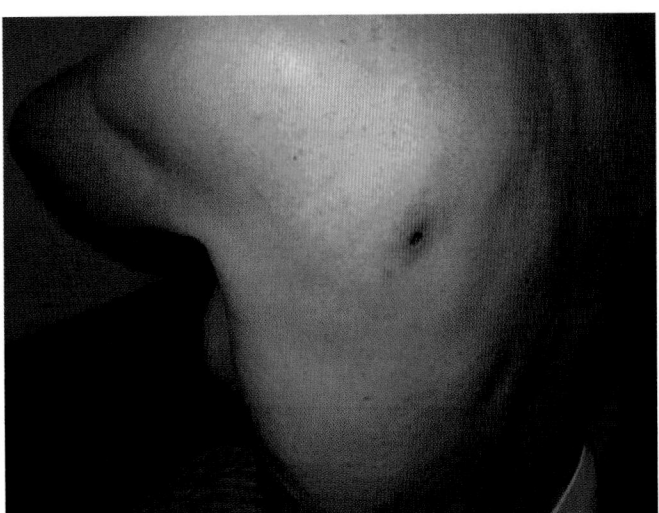

Figure 187-4 Eschar and faint macular rash in a patient with *Rickettsia heilongjiangensis* infection. *(From Mediannikov O.Y., et al. Acute tick-borne rickettsiosis caused by Rickettsia heilongjiangensis in Russian Far East. Emerg Infect Dis 2004; 10(5):810-817.)*

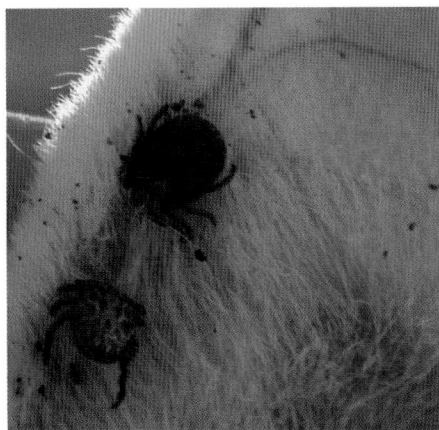

Figure 187-5 Ticks feeding on a rabbit.

R. akari causes rickettsial pox which is transmitted by the mouse mite and has been reported in the USA, Ukraine, Slovenia and Korea. The incubation period is about 10 days and clinical signs include fever, headache and myalgia. There is usually an inoculation eschar and regional lymphadenopathy. About 4 days after the first clinical signs, a rash appears which has macular then papular and then vesicular lesions. The disease is usually mild and self-limiting.

Management

In practice, doxycycline (200 mg/day) is the drug of choice and may be used for 3–14 days, depending on the severity of the infection. It should be given for at least 3 days after clinical defervescence and resolution of signs.[9] When doxycycline cannot be used, chloramphenicol (50–75 mg/kg) can be effective but there are treatment failures and side effects. Josamycin has been used successfully in pregnant women and children,[12] but children treated with azithromycin or clarithromycin required shorter courses of therapy and defervescence occurred in less than 7 days.

Typhus Group Rickettsiae

Nature

Both *R. prowazekii* and *R. typhi* are gram-negative, obligate intracellular bacilli and, as with other members of the genus *Rickettsia*, their outer walls have an inner leaflet that is thicker than the outer. *R. prowazekii* is a category B bioterrorism agent and has a genome of 1.1 Mb with a single circular chromosome and a high proportion of noncoding DNA (24%).[24] The genome of *R. typhi* is nearly identical to that of *R. conorii* and other SFG rickettsiae.

Epidemiology

The human body louse, which lives in clothing, is the only established vector of *R. prowazekii* (Figure 187-5). People are usually infected when feces from infected lice contaminate skin that has been scarified due to pruritus caused by the lice. Infections may also occur when conjunctivae or mucous membranes are exposed to the crushed bodies or feces of infected lice. Further, transmission might occur with inhalation of infected feces and through aerosols of feces-infected dust.

Murine typhus is one of the most prevalent rickettsial diseases throughout the world. The principal vectors are the rat flea (*Xenopsylla cheopis*) and the rat louse (*Polyplax spinulosa*). The primary reservoirs are commensal rats, mainly *Rattus rattus* and *Rattus norvegicus*, but various rodents and other wild and domestic animals, including domestic cats and opossums, have also been reported to act as hosts. Other possible vectors are the cat flea (*C. felis*) and the mouse flea (*Leptopsyllia segnis*).[25]

Pathogenicity

After local infection by *R. prowazekii* at the site of the louse bite, the organism infects the endothelial cells of capillaries and small blood vessels, producing a vasculitis. Tissue biopsies reveal perivascular infiltration with lymphocytes, plasma cells, polymorphonuclear leukocytes and histiocytes, with or without necrosis of the vessel.[26] Unlike SFG rickettsiae, *R. prowazekii* multiplies to large numbers within cells but does not cause significant injury to cells before they lyse. Infection of endothelial cells and the resultant vascular inflammation and hemostatic alterations are the principal pathogenic features of *R. typhi*.[26]

Prevention

Preventing epidemic typhus depends on eliminating human body lice with insecticides such as permethrin powder (1%) at doses of 30–50 g for an adult and 15–25 g for a child as the prescription of ivermectin orally.[27] Doxycycline can be used for chemoprophylaxis in visitors to high-risk areas. Vaccines using crude antigen and/or inactivated rickettsiae are partially protective against epidemic typhus but have undesirable toxic reactions and are difficult to standardize.[7]

Control of murine typhus depends on elimination of flea vectors and their mammalian reservoirs.

Diagnostic Microbiology

Epidemic typhus should be considered in patients with body lice and in poor people living in unhygienic conditions. Murine typhus should be considered in patients who are exposed to rodents and their fleas and who have prolonged fever and rash with or without lymphadenopathy.

DIRECT DIAGNOSIS

R. typhi can be isolated in shell vials containing Vero or L929 cells,[11] while *R. prowazekii* can be isolated in shell vials with human embryonic lung (HEL) fibroblasts in a biosafety level 3 containment laboratory. Direct immunodetection of organisms in tissues enables diagnosis before seroconversion and facilitates early and appropriate treatment. PCR and sequencing methods are useful, sensitive and rapid tools to detect and identify typhus group rickettsiae in blood and skin biopsies. Recently a 'suicide' PCR has been reported.[28]

INDIRECT DIAGNOSIS

The indirect immunofluorescence antibody assay is the reference method for diagnosing typhus group rickettsioses,[11] although an immunoperoxidase assay has been developed as an alternative for *R. typhi*.[11] Cross-adsorption followed by IFA and western blotting can differentiate antibodies to the organisms, but the expense of the technique limits its use.

Clinical Manifestations

Epidemic typhus occurs in two clinical forms: the primary febrile illness and the recrudescence of infection (Brill–Zinsser disease). After an incubation period of 10–14 days, patients may develop malaise and vague symptoms before the abrupt onset of fever (100%), headache (100%) and myalgia (70–100%). A rash is seen in 20–60% of patients[7] and typically begins in the axillary folds and upper trunk on about the fifth day of illness. In uncomplicated epidemic typhus, fever usually resolves after 2 weeks of illness if untreated, but full recovery usually takes 2–3 months. Without treatment, the disease is fatal in 13–30% of patients.[12] People who survive epidemic typhus remain infected with *R. prowazekii* for life. When stressed, they may experience a recrudescence, known as Brill–Zinsser disease, and they may become the source of a new epidemic if they become infested with body lice.[12]

Murine typhus is usually mild and many cases may be overlooked. Usually, after an incubation period of 6–14 days, patients present with an abrupt onset of symptoms like fever, rash, cough, headaches, maculopapular exanthema on the trunk, chills, as well as with myalgias and hepatomegaly. Complications of the central nervous system have been noted to occur from 10 days to 3 weeks after the initial onset of febrile illness, with patients presenting with headache, fever and stiff neck. The fatality rate may reach 4%.[12]

Management

Doxycycline (200 mg/day) is the recommended treatment and a single oral dose of doxycycline (200 mg) usually leads to defervescence within 48–72 hours. Treatment, however, is recommended for 7–15 days, or for at least 2 days after fever resolves. Chloramphenicol (2 g/day) can be given to patients who cannot be given tetracyclines and is the drug of choice in pregnancy, except near parturition when gray baby syndrome may develop.[25]

Scrub Typhus

Nature

Orientia tsutsugamushi, the causative agent of scrub typhus, is an obligate, intracellular, gram-negative bacterium (0.5 × 1.2–3.0 μm) that has a different cell wall structure and genetic makeup to other rickettsiae.[29] Although the species is genetically stable, there is enormous genetic and antigenic variability between strains of *O. tsutsugamushi*. There are three antigenically distinct prototype strains: Karp, Kato and Gilliam, originally isolated from New Guinea, Japan and Burma, respectively.[30]

Epidemiology

O. tsutsugamushi causes scrub typhus in the 'tsutsugamushi triangle' because of its vector, which is bounded to the north by Siberia and the Kamchatka Peninsula, to the south by Australia, to the east by Japan and to the west by Afghanistan and India[30] (Figure 187-6). The disease is transmitted by the bites of larval trombiculid mites (chiggers) of the genus *Leptotrombidium*. *L. deliense* is the most important vector species in South East Asia and southern China, whereas *L. akamushi*, *L. scutellare* and *L. pallidum* are the main vectors in Korea and Japan, and *L. chiangraiensis* is the likely vector in Thailand.[29]

Pathogenicity

Target cells of the bacteria are mainly endothelial cells but macrophages and polymorphonuclear leukocytes are also infected. The bacteria can induce apoptosis in a variety of host cells by retarding the release of intracellular calcium.[31] In murine macrophages, *O.*

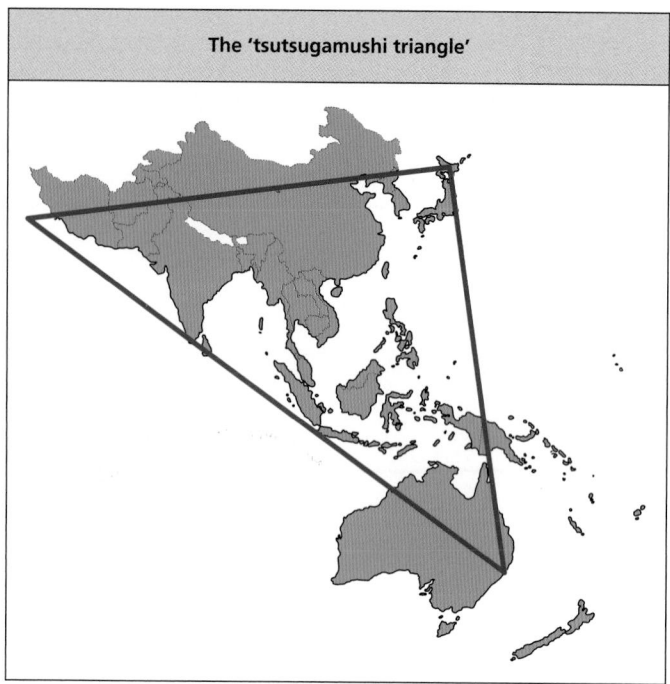

Figure 187-6   The 'tsutsugamushi triangle'.

tsutsugamushi produces inflammatory cytokines such as tumor necrosis factor (TNF) and interleukin (IL)-6. Tumor necrosis factor production appears to be inhibited by the production of IL-10.[29]

Prevention

Weekly doses of 200 mg doxycycline can prevent scrub typhus, but the efficacy of the daily 100 mg doxycycline dose regimen commonly used for malaria chemoprophylaxis has not been evaluated. Topical DEET applied to exposed skin and to the tops of boots and socks will prevent chiggers from feeding.

Diagnostic Microbiology

The eschar is the single most useful diagnostic clue. Concurrent leptospirosis and scrub typhus should be considered in patients who are at risk and who have atypical clinical features of either disease.

DIRECT DIAGNOSIS

O. tsutsugamushi can be isolated from blood or tissues injected into white mice, chicken embryos and various cell lines such as HeLa, Vero, BHK, McCoy and L929.[32] Detection of organisms by PCR of peripheral blood and skin biopsy or swabbing is a sensitive test but should be performed before antibiotic treatment or seroconversion.[29] Recently, a real-time PCR assay was described that can be used to diagnose scrub typhus by detecting major outer membrane antigen genes.[33]

INDIRECT DIAGNOSIS

The indirect microimmunofluorescence antibody assay has become the gold standard method for the diagnosis of scrub typhus. An immunoperoxidase assay has been developed as an alternative to the indirect microimmunofluorescence antibody assay; it has the advantages of being read with a conventional microscope and providing a permanent record of results.[11] Western blot assays differentiate true-positive from false-positive reactions with cross-reacting antibodies.

Clinical Manifestations

After an incubation period of 5–20 days, infections can be mild and unapparent or fulminant and rapidly fatal (up to 30%) depending on the susceptibility of the host and/or the virulence of the strain.[7] An eschar is common but may not be seen, as the chigger bite is painless and often occurs in areas not routinely examined such as the anogenital region, axilla and between skin folds. Generalized lymphadenopathy and the maculopapular rash may appear after 2–3 days. Gastrointestinal signs are common, and in 30% of patients the spleen and liver are moderately enlarged.[7] Coinfection with the HIV-1 virus does not increase the severity of scrub typhus, rather HIV-1 viral replication is suppressed in both *in vivo* and *in vitro O. tsutsugamushi* infections.[7]

Management

Chloramphenicol (2 g/day) was the first recommended treatment of scrub typhus as it is a cheaper alternative to the tetracyclines. Currently, however, a 1-week course of oral doxycycline (200 mg/daily) is the treatment of choice for uncomplicated cases. Chloramphenicol- and doxycycline-resistant strains of *O. tsutsugamushi* have been reported in Thailand and azithromycin has been shown to be an alternative antimicrobial treatment in areas where doxycycline-resistant scrub typhus is prevalent.[34] Recently, a patient with leptospirosis and scrub typhus was successfully treated by early plasma exchange and a 7-day course of moxifloxacin therapy.[35]

Ehrlichioses

Nature

Ehrlichia are obligate, intracellular, gram-negative bacteria that survive in phagosomal vacuoles within the host cell. With Romanowsky stains they appear as mulberry-like structures, known as morulae, in monocytes or neutrophils. Two forms can be differentiated by electron microscopy, dense-cored cells and reticulate cells, both of which are capable of binary fission.

Epidemiology

Ehrlichia chaffeensis is the agent of human monocytic ehrlichiosis while *E. ewingii* causes human granulocytic ehrlichiosis. The principal vector of both organisms is *Amblyomma americanum*, the Lone Star tick. Organisms are transmitted transstadially (larva to nymph to adult) but not transovarially (adult to larva). To date white-tailed deer (*Odocoileus virginianus*) appear to be the major reservoir of both *E. chaffeensis* and *E. ewingii*.[9,36] 'Candidatus Ehrlichia walkeri' also named 'Candidatus Neoehrlichia mikurensis' has not been cultured yet but is prevalent worldwide.

Pathogenicity

Ehrlichia chaffeensis preferentially infects mononuclear leukocytes while *E. ewingii* infects neutrophils. Within the cell the organism remains in the phagosome and inhibits its fusion with lysosomes. Ehrlichiae spread from the site of tick attachment via the lymphatics and bloodstream and infect cells around the body.[37]

Prevention

Avoidance of tick-infested areas is the first line of defense in preventing cases of human ehrlichiosis. If the use of protective clothing is not practical, insect repellents containing DEET can be used.

Diagnostic Microbiology

In endemic areas, the disease should be suspected in all patients presenting with fever, headache, elevated liver transaminases, thrombocytopenia and leukopenia, even if there is no history of tick attachment.

DIRECT DIAGNOSIS

Occasionally, diagnoses can be made when morulae are seen in monocytes in Romanowsky-stained peripheral blood smears, buffy coat preparations or cerebrospinal fluid (CSF). Various cell lines have been used for isolation, including a canine hysticocytic line (DH82), a human monocytic leukemia line (THP-1), HEL-22 cells (fibroblast-like cells), Vero cells and a human promyelocytic leukemia cell line (HL-60).[36] Detection of ehrlichial DNA/RNA in peripheral blood is probably the best method to diagnose human monocytic ehrlichiosis (HME) in the acute phase. Most often this is with primers that amplify a section of the 16S rRNA gene.[36] PCR is currently the only way to diagnose 'Candidatus Neoehrlichia'.

INDIRECT DIAGNOSIS

Most diagnoses are made using the indirect microimmunofluorescence antibody assay. Many diagnoses are made retrospectively with convalescent phase sera as relatively few patients (30%) seen in the acute phase of HME have reactive antibodies.[38] Immunoblotting procedures have higher specificity than the indirect microimmunofluorescence antibody assay but are generally available only in research laboratories.

Clinical Manifestations

The main clinical signs reported are fever (98%), malaise (30–80%), headache (77%), myalgias (65%), vomiting (36%), cough (25%) and neurologic signs with changes in mental status (20%).[37] A skin rash that involves the trunk and extremities, and less commonly the face, occurs in 12–36% of patients and is more common in children (67%). Although age (>60 years) is an independent risk factor for severe or fatal HME in some studies, many severe or fatal cases have been described in apparently healthy children or young adults. These also occur in immunocompromised patients.[37]

Human infections with *E. ewingii* were first reported in 1999. This organism appears to be less virulent than *E. chaffeensis* and most of the reported patients have been immunosuppressed.[39]

Management

Doxycycline (4 mg/kg q12h; maximum 100 mg/dose) has become the antimicrobial agent of choice, even in children.[36] In patients allergic to doxycycline, rifampin (rifampicin; 20 mg/kg q12h; maximum 600 mg) is an acceptable alternative.[36] Antimicrobial therapy should be continued for at least 3 days after the patient becomes afebrile with the minimum course being between 5 and 10 days.

Anaplasmosis

Nature

Anaplasma spp. are small, often pleomorphic or coccoid, gram-negative, nonmotile cells ranging from 0.3 to 0.4 μm in diameter. Lipopolysaccharides and lipo-oligosaccharides have not been detected in the cell wall of *Anaplasma* and it is unknown if they contain peptidoglycan.[40]

Epidemiology

Anaplasma phagocytophilum is the agent of human granulocytic anaplasmosis which is transmitted by *Ixodes* spp.: *I. scapularis* is the most important vector in North America, *I. ricinus* in Europe and *I. persulatus* in Eastern Europe and Asia.[40] Human granulocytic anaplasmosis is seasonal, with most cases occurring between May and October when tick vectors are most active, particularly the nymphs, which are difficult to detect because of their small size.[39]

Pathogenicity

The bacteria presumably infect neutrophils migrating to the site of tick attachment and disseminate as these cells migrate further. Infections might also spread if the organisms replicate locally in macrophages or endothelial cells and drain to local lymph nodes and the systemic bloodstream.[41]

Prevention

Vaccines against *A. phagocytophilum* are not currently available. People at risk should be informed of measures to prevent exposure to vectors, including the use of insect repellants such as DEET or permethrin on clothes and shoes.

Diagnostic Microbiology

Clinical signs are not specific; laboratory abnormalities can include leukopenia, a left shift, thrombocytopenia and elevated hepatic transaminases.

DIRECT DIAGNOSIS

The diagnosis can be confirmed by using Romanowsky stains to identify typical clusters of organisms.[42] *A. phagocytophilum* can be isolated in tissue cultures of a promyelocytic leukemia (HL-60) cell line or primary bone marrow cells. Several primer sets have been used to amplify different target sequences of *A. phagocytophilum* in clinical samples as well as in ticks.[43]

INDIRECT DIAGNOSIS

The indirect microimmunofluorescence antibody assay has been used most frequently. There is serologic cross-reactivity in indirect microimmunofluorescence antibody assays between *E. chaffeensis* and *A. phagocytophilum* as these organisms are related and have common antigens such as the heat shock proteins. Enzyme immunoassays have also been used to detect antibodies to *A. phagocytophilum*.[44]

Clinical Manifestations

The incubation period after tick attachment is 7–10 days and, although the majority of patients recall tick attachment or exposure, other routes of transmission such as exposure to deer blood, blood transfusion or perinatal infection have been reported.[41] Clinical signs include high fever, rigors, generalized myalgias, severe headache, arthralgia, nausea and a nonproductive cough. Rash is rare (<11%) and patients may present with atypical pneumonitis and Sweet's syndrome.[41] Fatal cases have been reported in the USA and the case fatality rate is estimated to be about 1%.[45]

Management

The recommended therapy for adults is oral doxycycline (200 mg/day).[42] Children older than 8 years should also be treated with doxycycline given in divided doses with dosage adjusted to the patient's weight (4.4 mg/kg q24h; maximum 100 mg/dose).[42] Rifamycin has excellent activity and can be used in cases of tetracycline allergy or pregnancy.[42]

Q Fever

Nature

Morphologically, *Coxiella burnetii* is a gram-negative, strictly intracellular, pleomorphic coccobacillus 0.2–1.0 μm in diameter. The organism may occur as either a small-cell or large-cell variant.[46] The small-cell variant is a compact, small rod with a very electron-dense center of condensed nucleoid filaments. The large-cell variant is larger and less electron-dense and is the metabolically active intracellular form of *C. burnetii*.

Antigenic variation or phase variation is an important characteristic of *C. burnetii* and is associated with changes in the lipopolysaccharide of the outer membrane. Organisms isolated from acutely infected animals express the phase I antigen and are very infectious. After serial passage in eggs or tissue culture, the lipopolysaccharide is modified and there is an antigenic shift to phase II organisms which are minimally infectious. Phase II organisms revert to phase I following passage in a vertebrate host. There are no distinct morphologic changes associated with this phase variation.

Epidemiology

C. burnetii has been found worldwide, with the notable exception of New Zealand. A wide variety of ticks, rodents, birds and wild and domestic mammals can be infected, but domestic ruminants are the major reservoirs for *C. burnetii* infections in humans. Although cattle, sheep and goats may remain chronically infected for weeks to years, the majority of infections are subclinical. Infected animals can shed large numbers of organisms in birth products (>10^9/g), feces and urine, and a major risk factor for people developing Q fever is contact with infected domestic livestock. Most human cases occur sporadically but outbreaks occur with high-risk occupations (farmers, hunters, workers in meat, milk or hide and fleece processing plants, slaughterhouses, veterinary schools, etc.).[46] Between 2007 and 2009 a very large outbreak linked to goats and caused by a single strain was observed in the Netherlands, and involved more than 3500 human cases.

Infections occur principally by inhalation of infected aerosols, with just a single organism being sufficient to cause infection. The organisms may remain infective in aerosols for up to 2 weeks and in the soil for as long as 5 months. In some outbreaks, however, there is no direct contact with infected farms or animals and their products. In these outbreaks the source has been ascribed to wind-borne spread of *C. burnetii* from infected areas in the vicinity.[46]

Pathogenicity

The target cells of *C. burnetii* are monocytes and macrophages. Most infections occur via the respiratory route and involve the alveolar macrophages.[46] The Kupffer cells of the liver are involved in infections that take place via the digestive tract. Attachment to the host cell is followed by passive entry into the phagolysosome, where production of a potent acid phosphatase protects the organism from enzyme attack. Disturbance of cytokine regulatory processes, allowing survival and replication of *C. burnetii* within host cells, is also important in establishing infection. Subsequently, there is a bacteremia, which in overt clinical cases in humans coincides with fever.

Prevention

Appropriate tick control strategies and good hygiene practices can decrease environmental contamination. Infected fetal fluids and membranes, aborted fetuses and contaminated bedding should be incinerated or buried. Vaccination of people in high-risk occupations should be considered. In Australia, a formalin-inactivated, whole cell *C. burnetii* (Henzerling strain, Phase I) vaccine (Q-Vax®, CSL) has proven highly effective in reducing Q fever in abattoir workers.[47]

Diagnostic Microbiology

While Q fever should be considered in patients who have close contact with domestic ruminants and cats, exposure to animals may not be reported as organisms persist in the environment for many years.

DIRECT DIAGNOSIS

Although *C. burnetii* does not grow on artificial media, it may be isolated in embryonated eggs, laboratory animals such as guinea pigs and mice, and in a number of tissue culture cell lines.[46] The shell vial assay may improve recovery of organisms from patients with endocarditis. A number of PCR assays have been described which detect various DNA sequences in *C. burnetii* and these have been shown to detect organisms in around 65% of patients with acute and chronic Q fever.[48]

INDIRECT DIAGNOSIS

The indirect microimmunofluorescence antibody assay has become the reference technique. Immunoglobulin M antibodies reactive with phase II *C. burnetii* appear rapidly, reach high titers within 14 days and persist for 10–12 weeks. Immunoglobulin M antibodies reactive with phase I antigens are usually at a much lower titer during acute infection. Immunoglobulin G antibodies reactive with phase II antigens reach peak titers about 8 weeks after the onset of symptoms, while those reactive with phase I antigens develop only very slowly and remain at lower titers than antibodies to phase II antigens, even after a year. In chronic Q fever, for instance in Q fever endocarditis where there is persistence of organisms, the IgG titers to phase I and phase II antigens may both be high, and the presence of IgA antibody to phase I antigen is usually, although not exclusively, associated with chronic infection.

Clinical Manifestations

The incubation period depends on the route of exposure, the inoculum dose and the age of the patient, but is usually about 3–4 weeks. Around 38% develop a mild, flu-like, self-limiting illness with low fever, headache, chills, sweating, cough, nausea and bradycardia relative to body temperature.[46] There is an inverse relationship between severity of disease and age, and infections in children may go unnoticed. Other frequently occurring signs include pneumonia which is found in almost 40% of patients and may be the only sign in 17%.

Women infected before they are pregnant do not have increased risks of abortion or premature delivery. When infections occur during pregnancy, however, fetal death or premature delivery is seen in almost every patient.[49] Chronic infections of the uterus develop in about 50% of patients and this may lead to abortions in subsequent pregnancies.

Chronic Q fever is seen in around 0.5% of patients and occurs months to years after infection. Endocarditis and vascular infections are the major clinical presentation of chronic Q fever and particularly involves the mitral and aortic valves but also vascular prosthesis and aneurysms. In other patients with chronic Q fever there may be osteo-articular infections, chronic hepatitis, chronic pulmonary infections and a chronic fatigue syndrome.

A PET scan may be helpful in establishing the diagnosis and localization of chronic Q fever.[50]

Management

Prompt treatment of acute Q fever with oral doxycycline, 100 mg twice a day for 14–21 days, is the treatment of choice. Trimethoprim-sulfamethoxazole (TMP–SMX) for the duration of pregnancy is recommended for pregnant women as it might decrease the possibility of abortion and premature delivery. In patients with endocarditis, treatment with hydroxychloroquine (600 mg/day initial dose and titration to achieve a plasma level of 1 mg/mL) and doxycycline (200 mg/day) for 18 months to 3 years is required before serology shows cure. In patients with predisposing lesions for endocarditis, prophylaxis with doxycycline and chloroquine have been shown to be efficient in avoiding endocarditis.

Bartonellosis

Nature

The *Bartonella* are gram-negative bacilli or coccobacilli that belong in the α_2 subgroup of the class Proteobacteria.[51] The principal human pathogens are *B. bacilliformis*, *B. quintana* and *B. henselae*, but eight other species have been implicated in human disease: *B. elizabethae*, *B. koehlerae*, *B. alsatica* and *B. vinsonii* subsp. *berkhoffii* in endocarditis, *B. vinsonii* subsp. *arupensis* in bacteremia and heart valve disease, *B. grahamii* in neuroretinitis, *B. clarridgeiae* in cat-scratch disease and *B. washoensis* in myocarditis (Table 187-2). Currently, there are more than 30 *Bartonella* species, and several 'Candidatus' species that have been isolated from humans and wild and domestic animals globally.

Epidemiology

Each *Bartonella* species is adapted to a mammalian reservoir host where organisms occur within erythrocytes and endothelial cells and cause a long-lasting bacteremia. They are transmitted between hosts by arthropod vectors, mainly sandflies, body lice, fleas and ticks.

Bartonella bacilliformis occurs only in remote Andean valleys of Peru, Ecuador and Columbia and humans are the main reservoir of infection. The sandfly *Lutzomyia verrucarum* is the most important vector.[52]

Humans are the only known reservoir of *B. quintana* and the body louse (*Pediculus humanus corporis*) is recognized as its major vector. Recent studies have implicated the cat flea *C. felis* in the transmission of *B. quintana*.[53]

The major vector of *B. henselae* is the cat flea *Felis domesticus* and large numbers of viable organisms can be found in flea feces. Contaminated cats' claws and teeth enable transmission of organisms by bites or scratches or when cats lick open wounds.[54]

Pathogenicity

In humans, the infection cycle of *Bartonella* spp. is initiated by the colonization of the so-called primary niche.[55] In this stage, infection is usually controlled by the immune system and the clinical manifestations are characterized by a local lymphadenopathy (*B. henselae*, *B. quintana* and *B. alsatica*).

In some cases, the commensal relationship of reservoir-adapted *Bartonella* spp. to the host is imperfect, resulting in a stealth pathogen strategy.[56] *Bartonella* are rapidly cleared from the blood into a primary niche, most likely endothelial cells.[57] At about 5-day intervals, further waves of erythrocyte infection occur from the primary niche, perhaps reflecting the duration of the infection cycle in these cells. *Bartonella* in erythrocytes do not cause clinical signs in most reservoir hosts; the exception is *B. bacilliformis*, which is associated with severe hemolytic anemia and Oroya fever.

In endothelial cells, *B. bacilliformis*, *B. quintana* and *B. henselae* have the unique ability to cause vasculoproliferative lesions (verruga peruana, bacillary angiomatosis and bacillary peliosis) by stimulating angiogenesis and the formation of new capillaries from old ones. Recently 'Candidatus Bartonella ancashi' was also associated with angioproliferative lesions in a patient from Peru.[58]

Prevention

Control of the arthropod vectors is most important. Cat fleas live on both cats and dogs and are best controlled by fumigating areas where cats and dogs live. People infested with body lice should bathe and use a pediculicide such as permethrin lotion, shampoo or powder on the hair-covered areas of the body. Sandflies can be controlled by spraying the environment with long-acting insecticides. Individual protection depends on avoiding high-risk environments at night and the use of insect repellents (DEET) or mosquito nets treated with permethrin/deltamethrin.

Diagnostic Microbiology

There are no pathognomonic clinical features in patients with bartonelloses and definitive diagnoses can only be made using laboratory testing.

DIRECT DIAGNOSIS

Bartonella grow on most blood-enriched media when incubated at 37 °C (99 °F) in an atmosphere containing 5% carbon dioxide. *Bartonella* can also be isolated in various cell lines in tissue culture with a shell-vial culture technique increasing the recovery rate.[59] Recently, pre-enrichment culture in *Bartonella* α Proteobacteria growth medium before subinoculation of agar plates has been reported to improve the isolation of *Bartonella* from clinical specimens.[60] Isolates are best identified using PCR-based methods which have also been shown to be more sensitive than culture in detecting organisms in tissues and blood.[51]

INDIRECT DIAGNOSIS

The most commonly used technique is the indirect microimmunofluorescence antibody assay although enzyme-linked immunosorbent assays have also been described. Care should be taken in interpreting

TABLE 187-2	Bartonella Species Reported to Date: Epidemiologic and Clinical Data			
Bartonella spp.	**Reservoir Host**	**Vector-Detection in Arthropods**	**Disease in Humans**	**First Cultivation**
B. bacilliformis	Human	Sandfly (Lutzomia spp.)	CD, END	1919
B. talpae	Mole	Unknown	Unknown	1911
B. peromysci	Unknown	Unknown	Unknown	1942
B. vinsonii subsp. vinsonii	Rodents	Unknown	Unknown	1946
B. quintana	Human, cats	Human body lice/fleas	TF, BA, BAC, END	1961
B. henselae	Cats, rats, dogs	Fleas (Ctenocephalides felis)	CSD, BA, BAC, LMF, END, PH, RET	1990
B. elizabethae	Rodents, dogs	Fleas	END (1 case)	1993
B. grahamii	Voles, rodents	Fleas?	RET (1 case)	1995
B. taylorii	Rats	Fleas?	Unknown	1995
B. doshiae	Voles	Fleas?	Unknown	1995
B. clarridgeiae	Cats, dogs	C. felis	Unknown	1995
B. vinsonii subsp. berkhoffii	Dogs, coyotes, gray foxes	Fleas and ticks	END	1995
B. vinsonii subsp. arupensis	Rodents, cattle	Deer ticks	BAC (1 case)	1999
B. tribocorum	Rats	Unknown	Unknown	1998
B. koehlerae	Cats	Fleas	END (1 case)	1999
B. alsatica	Rabbit	Fleas or ticks	END (1 case)	1999
B. bovis (weissii)	Cows, cats	Unknown	Unknown	1999
B. washoensis	Rodents, dogs	Unknown	MYOC (1 case)	2000
B. birtlesii	Rats	Unknown	Unknown	2000
B. schoenbuchensis	Wild roe deer	Unknown	Unknown	2001
B. capreoli	Wild roe deer	Unknown	Unknown	2002
B. chomelii	Cows	Unknown	Unknown	2004
B. rattimasilliensis	Rats	Unknown	Unknown	2004
B. phoceensis	Rats	Unknown	Unknown	2004
B. australis (Macropus giganteus)	Gray kangaroo	Unknown	Unknown	2007
B. coopersplainsensis	Rattus leucopus	Unknown	Unknown	2008
B. durdenii	Squirrel	Unknown	Unknown	2007
B. rattiaustraliensis	Tunney's rat	Unknown	Unknown	2008
B. tamiae	Human	Unknown	Fever	2008
B. rochalimea	Human	Unknown	Bacteremia, fever, splenomegaly	2007

BA, bacillary angiomatosis; BAC, bacteremia; CSD, cat-scratch disease; END, endocarditis; LMF, lymphadenopathy; MYOC, myocarditis; PH, peliosis hepatitis; RET, retinitis; TF, trench fever.

serology results from immunocompromised patients who might not mount significant antibody responses. Also, serology should be interpreted with caution in endocarditis patients as there are significant cross-reactions with other agents causing 'culture-negative' endocarditis such as C. burnetii and Chlamydia spp. Western blot analysis after cross-adsorption study has been shown to be a powerful tool for the identification of Bartonella at the species level in endocarditis (Figure 187-7).

Clinical Manifestations

A number of different clinical conditions have been associated with Bartonella infections.

CARRION'S DISEASE (ALSO KNOWN AS OROYA FEVER)

Carrion's disease is caused by B. bacilliformis. Clinical signs are seen mostly in children and teenagers and include fever, malaise, anorexia, nausea and vomiting, hepatomegaly, lymphadenopathy, pallor and a systolic murmur. Mortality rates can be high in untreated patients, reaching 90%, especially if infections are complicated with other diseases.[51] Approximately one-third of patients present with opportunistic infections due to nontyphoid salmonellas, sepsis by Shigella dysenteriae, Enterobacter, Pseudomonas aeruginosa, Staphylococcus aureus, pneumonia by Pneumocystis jirovecii or reactivation of tuberculosis, toxoplasmosis, and histoplasmosis.

TRENCH FEVER

The etiologic agent is B. quintana. After an incubation period of 2–3 weeks there is a sudden onset of fever, retro-orbital headache and intense pain in the long bones of the legs, in particular the tibias.[51] While fatal cases have not been reported, the disease may persist for 4–6 weeks and result in prolonged disability. Relapses may occur years later and in some cases there may be bacteremia with no clinical signs.

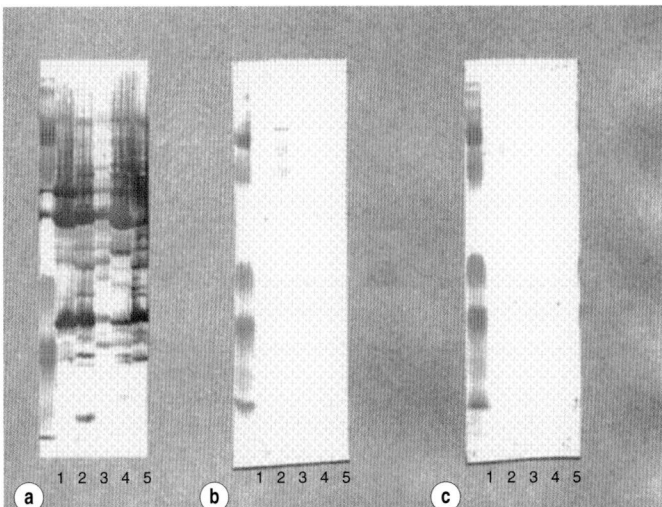

Figure 187-7 Western blot of a patient with *Bartonella henselae* before (a) and after cross-adsorption with (b) *B. quintana* or (c) *B. henselae*. Line 1: *B. quintana*; Line 2: *B. henselae*; Line 3: *B. elizabethae*; Line 4: *B. vinsonii* subsp. *berkhoffii*; Line 5: *B. alsatica*.

CAT-SCRATCH DISEASE

Bartonella henselae is the major etiologic agent of cat-scratch disease which is now generally recognized to be the most common cause of chronic benign lymphadenopathy. In 75% of patients the lymphadenopathy can be accompanied by mild systemic signs including fever, malaise, fatigue, headache, anorexia, weight loss and emesis that usually resolve within 2 weeks. Most cases are self-limiting, with the lymphadenopathy resolving spontaneously in 2 weeks to 4 months.[51]

Atypical manifestations of cat-scratch disease occur in about 15% of patients. The most common is Parinaud's oculoglandular syndrome where there is unilateral conjunctivitis with preauricular lymphadenopathy that probably results from inoculation into the conjunctiva rather than the skin.

BACILLARY ANGIOMATOSIS

Bacillary angiomatosis is a vascular proliferative disease caused by *B. henselae* or *B. quintana*.[51] It was first described in HIV-infected patients but also occurs in organ transplant recipients and in immunocompetent patients. Lesions most often involve the skin but can occur at other sites including bone marrow, spleen, liver and lymph nodes.

BACILLARY PELIOSIS

This rare condition is caused by *B. henselae* infections of the parenchymal vasculature which results in the development of cystic, blood-filled spaces, particularly in the liver (peliosis hepatis) but also in the spleen, bone marrow or lymph nodes.[51]

BACTEREMIA

Persistent bacteremia is now one of the most frequently reported manifestations of re-emergent *B. quintana* infections among homeless people and alcoholics.[51] Prolonged bacteremia can also occur with *B. henselae* in HIV-infected patients. Other *Bartonella* spp. have been isolated from individual patients with bacteremia including *B. koehlerae*, *B. tamiae*, *B. rochalimae*, *B. vinsonii* subsp. *arupensis*, *B. vinsonii* subsp. *berkhoffii* and '*Candidatus* Bartonella melophagi'. These infections may be asymptomatic or associated with an insidiously developing, prolonged symptom complex of malaise, fatigue, weight loss and recurring high-grade fevers.

ENDOCARDITIS

Bartonella endocarditis occurs in immunocompetent and immunocompromised patients and infections with these organisms should be suspected in all patients with endocarditis that is 'culture-negative' by routine blood culture techniques.[51] The most commonly identified agents of *Bartonella* endocarditis are *B. quintana*, followed by *B. henselae*. However, sporadic cases of endocarditis have been also associated by *B. koehlerae*, *B. vinsonii* subsp. *berkoffii*, *B. vinsonii* subsp. *arupensis*, *B. elizabethae* and *B. alsatica*.

Bartonella endocarditis causes significant destruction of the valvular cusps, which is characterized by mononuclear cell inflammation, extensive fibrosis, large calcification and small vegetations.

Management

Traditionally, patients with Oroya fever without complications were treated with ciprofloxacin (500 mg). However, *in vitro* evidence suggests that ciprofloxacin is inadequate for the treatment of *B. bacilliformis* bacteremia and it was proposed that it should be removed from the current guidelines. Chloramphenicol (50 mg/kg/day) during the first 3 days and then 25 mg/kg/day until completing 14 days of treatment should be used for the treatment of Oroya fever.[61] Patients with *Bartonella* sp. bacteremia should be treated with gentamicin (3 mg/kg of body weight once daily for 2 weeks), in combination with doxycycline (200 mg daily for 4 weeks). *B. quintana* bacteremia may result in occult endocarditis in people with existing heart valve abnormalities. The available data do not support the use of antibiotics for the treatment of CSD. It remains unclear whether the antibiotic treatment of localized CSD reduces the risk of the development of a systemic disease. In patients with suppurative lymph nodes, needle aspiration is an appropriate treatment.[61] Erythromycin (500 mg four times daily) for 3 months is the first-line antibiotic therapy for the treatment of angioproliferative lesions.

References available online at expertconsult.com.

KEY REFERENCES

Bakken J.S., Dumler J.S.: Human granulocytic ehrlichiosis. *Clin Infect Dis* 2000; 31:554-560.

Fenollar F., Fournier P.E., Raoult D.: Molecular detection of *Coxiella burnetii* in the sera of patients with Q fever endocarditis or vascular infection. *J Clin Microbiol* 2004; 42:4919-4924.

Fournier P.E., Gouriet F., Brouqui P., et al.: Lymphangitis-associated rickettsiosis, a new rickettsiosis caused by *Rickettsia sibirica mongolotimonae*: seven new cases and review of the literature. *Clin Infect Dis* 2005; 40:1435-1444.

Fournier P.E., Raoult D.: Suicide PCR on skin biopsy specimens for diagnosis of rickettsioses. *J Clin Microbiol* 2004; 42:3428-3434.

Gouriet F., Fenollar F., Patrice J.Y., et al.: Use of shell-vial cell culture assay for isolation of bacteria from clinical specimens: 13 years of experience. *J Clin Microbiol* 2005; 43:4993-5002.

La Scola B., Raoult D.: Laboratory diagnosis of rickettsioses: current approaches to the diagnosis of old and new rickettsial diseases. *J Clin Microbiol* 1997; 35:2715-2727.

Maurin M., Raoult D.: Q fever. *Clin Microbiol Rev* 1999; 12:518-553.

Parola P., Paddock C.D., Raoult D.: Tick-borne rickettsioses around the world: emerging diseases challenging old concepts. *Clin Microbiol Rev* 2005; 18(4):719-756.

Raoult D., Roux V.: Rickettsioses as paradigms of new or emerging infectious diseases. *Clin Microbiol Rev* 1997; 10:694-719.

Rolain J.M., Brouqui P., Koehler J.E., et al.: Recommendations for treatment of human infections caused by *Bartonella* species. *Antimicrob Agents Chemother* 2004; 48:1921-1933.

188

Chlamydia

MIRJA PUOLAKKAINEN | PEKKA A.I. SAIKKU

KEY CONCEPTS

- Chlamydiae are important human pathogens and inflammation is an essential component of the infection pathogenesis.

- Nucleic acid amplification tests are the recommended test method for genital *Chlamydia trachomatis* infections.

- *Chlamydia pneumoniae* seropositivity rate is high, suggesting that infections and re-infections are common.

- Single-dose azithromycin treatment was a major breakthrough in treatment of *C. trachomatis* infections, while the optimal treatment for *C. pneumoniae* infections and chronic forms of chlamydial infection remains unknown.

- Chlamydiae have a previously underestimated host range.

Introduction

Chlamydiae have a common tendency to cause infections with minimal or no symptoms, long-lasting infections, repeated infections and infections with inflammatory complications, especially in the absence of treatment.[1] Despite increased awareness, screening possibilities, improved diagnostics and prompt treatment, the number of reported sexually transmitted *Chlamydia trachomatis* infections is not decreasing.

Nature

The classification of chlamydial species has been evolving.[2] The Chlamydiaceae family now consists of the single genus *Chlamydia*.[3] *C. trachomatis* is a human pathogen with its closest relatives found in the mouse (*C. muridarum*) and pig (*C. suis*). *C. pneumoniae* is a human pathogen with strains isolated in the horse, marsupials and amphibians. *C. psittaci* is a pathogen of birds, *C. abortus* and *C. pecorum* are pathogens of ruminants, *C. felis* is a pathogen of cats and *C. caviae* is found in guinea-pigs. Chlamydial diversity started to widen in the 1990s when numerous bacteria resembling Chlamydiae were detected (by electron microscopy and 16S rRNA analysis) in environmental samples and also as symbionts of, e.g., amebae, fish and insects. These recently identified bacteria are now recognized as novel families (Criblamydiaceae, Parachlamydiaceae, Simkaniaceae, Rhabdochlamydiaceae and Waddliaceae) in the order Chlamydiales and collectively called environmental Chlamydiae or *Chlamydia*-related organisms.[2]

Epidemiology

C. trachomatis is the most common bacterial sexually transmitted infection (STI). The incidence is greatest in young sexually active people and varies widely among different areas. In trachoma-endemic areas, *C. trachomatis* is transmitted by direct contact, excretions and vectors such as flies and contaminated towels.

C. pneumoniae is a common respiratory pathogen worldwide. In tropical countries, infections are common during the first years of life. In industrialized countries, children begin to seroconvert at school age at the rate of 10% each year. The rate seems to depend on population density. At the age of 15, 25–50% of populations and nearly all elderly people have measurable antibodies. Because antibodies are lost by a

few years after an acute infection, this steady increase points to repeated infections during life and to possible chronic infections. Asymptomatic carriers are also found. In relatively sparsely inhabited areas in high latitudes, *C. pneumoniae* has caused epidemics at intervals of 5–7 years.

Avian *C. psittaci* is contagious in dried droppings of diseased birds and is typically transmitted by the inhalation of aerosolized bacteria. Patients are usually turkey or duck farmers, plant processors or persons who have contact with diseased caged or wild birds. Person-to-person transmission occasionally occurs. Ovine abortion strain *C. abortus* is known to cause septic abortions in pregnant women who are in contact with affected farm cattle. Pet cats can be a source of *C. felis* infections. *Chlamydia*-related organisms are identified in many environmental sources but their epidemiology is so far rather unknown.

Pathogenicity

Chlamydiae are small, gram-negative, obligatory intracellular bacteria (general properties are outlined in Box 188-1). They parasitize only living, metabolically active cells, and are not cultivable on synthetic media. They exist in two forms: a spherical, non-replicating, infectious dense particle (300 nm) called the elementary body (EB) and a loose, larger, intracellular form, the reticulate body (RB), which is able to multiply by binary fission but is noninfectious (0.8–1 μm) (Figure 188-1).[1] Chlamydiae have a double layer membrane of gram-negative bacteria with a periplasmic space. They harbor genes for peptidoglycan

---

BOX 188-1 GENERAL PROPERTIES OF CHLAMYDIA

- Obligatory intracellular gram-negative bacteria with distinct developmental cycle (elementary body–reticulate body)
- Common group antigen (lipopolysaccharide)
- Tendency to cause persistent infections
- Immunogenetic factors contribute to susceptibility to the infection and its inflammatory complications

---

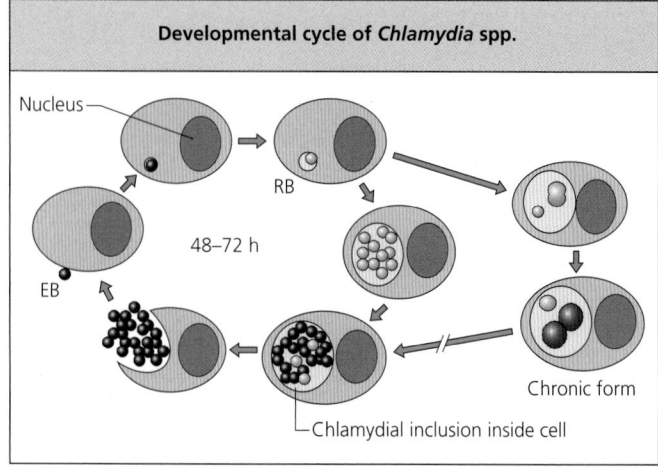

Developmental cycle of *Chlamydia* spp.

Nucleus

RB

48–72 h

EB

Chronic form

Chlamydial inclusion inside cell

Figure 188-1 Developmental cycle of *Chlamydia* spp.

synthesis and peptidoglycan has recently been demonstrated in the septum of dividing RBs,[4] but not in EBs. The circular genomes of *C. pneumoniae* and *C. trachomatis* contain 1 230 000 and 1 040 000 base pairs, with 1100 and 900 predicted coding sequences, respectively.[1] Because of their obligatory intracellular life, opportunities for horizontal gene transfer and recombination were considered unlikely. However, during mixed infection, Chlamydiae can recombine, and this might not be a rare event.[5] Species-specific plasmid is present in 10 copies in *C. trachomatis*,[1] but is not found in the human type of *C. pneumoniae*. The plasmid has a role in glycogen accumulation into the inclusion and it can modulate chlamydia transcription, but its eight ORFs do not encode for antibiotic resistance genes. Plasmid-free isolates of *C. trachomatis* exist and they might be associated with reduced infectivity and virulence.[6]

The major outer membrane protein (OmpA) forms the outer membrane of the particle with other outer membrane proteins of which two are rich in cysteine (OmcB, OmcC).[1] The OmpA of *C. trachomatis* contains four variable regions, which divide it into about 20 immunotypes denoted alphabetically.[1] The OmpA of *C. pneumoniae* is more homogeneous. *C. trachomatis* has nine and *C. pneumoniae* 21 genes for putative membrane proteins (pmps).[7] Chlamydial lipopolysaccharide (LPS) is of rough type, weakly endotoxic and situated in the outer membrane. It contains three KDO-residues, in which the α-2-8 bond is specific for *Chlamydia*. On electron microscopy, the surface consists of a hexagonal pattern with substructures made up of a few rosettes with short spikes (Figure 188-2).[8]

Electrostatic interactions and interactions between several chlamydial potential adhesins (including LPS, OmpA, high-mannose oligosaccharides, OmcB, hsp60, hsp70 and pmps) with various host cell receptors (including heparin sulphate receptor, mannose receptor, mannose 6-P/IGF2 receptor, growth factor receptors, estrogen receptor complex and Lox-1 receptor as well as apolipoprotein E4 and lipid rafts) play a role in chlamydial adhesion.[1] After attachment, the EBs inject via type three secretion system (TTSS) a translocated actin recruiting phosphoprotein (TARP) across the plasma membrane.[9] TARP mediates host cells cytoskeletal rearrangements and together with initiation of signaling cascades promotes internalization of EBs. Several cellular signaling pathways and trafficking pathways are activated. The chlamydial vacuole, termed inclusion, is modified and does not fuse with lysosomes. The inclusion travels on microtubules to a perinuclear region where many secretory organelles reside.[1] Inside the inclusion, the EB transforms into the RB, the disulfide bridges are reduced and OmpA acts as a porin. DNA, RNA and proteins are synthesized within the RB, which divides successively by binary fission.

The inclusion membrane acts as an important interface between the cell and the inclusion, and a variety of strategies contribute to amino acid, lipid (including glycerophospholipids, sphingolipids, and cholesterol), nucleotide and energy acquisition to the chlamydial inclusion.[1] Recycling endosomes, Golgi apparatus ministacks, lipid droplets, multivesicular bodies, mitochondria and the ER are observed in close association with the inclusions. Chlamydiae use their TTSS to modulate the host cell and interfere with cellular immune defense mechanisms. The early effectors obviously help to avoid lysosomal degradation and the mid-late effectors limit detection by immune surveillance and ensure bacterial replication and development.[1] Several TTSS substrates, including a cytotoxin and proteolytic enzymes, have been demonstrated.[10,11] Eventually, the inclusion may contain thousands of chlamydial RBs that start to condense into EBs (Figure 188-3), and apoptosis as well as proteolysis are promoted to liberate the new infectious particles. Sometimes the mature inclusion is expelled by exocytosis. The developmental cycle takes 2–3 days. *In vitro*, depletion of tryptophan or iron or the presence of penicillin or interferon-gamma (IFN-γ) at subinhibitory concentrations induces an aberrant form of RB, which can persist for long periods and produces proteins such as heat shock proteins (hsps) but not antigens of mature EBs.[12] In chronic infections this may be the dominant form of *Chlamydia*.[13] *Chlamydia*-related bacteria have a similar intracellular developmental cycle[2] that can take place in free-living amebae and possibly also in phagocytic cells.

The innate immune response of the infected epithelial cells initiates, and together with acquired immunity, sustains an inflammatory response which plays a role in tissue damage seen in complications of genital *C. trachomatis* infection[14] and trachoma.[15] Chlamydiae are potent inducers of proinflammatory cytokines, such as IFN-γ, interleukin (IL)-8 and IL-1.[1] In repeated chlamydial infections[16] there is a hypersensitivity component, apparently caused by common cross-reactive proteins, including hsp60.[17] It is related to the host's hsp60 and may initiate autoimmune reactions. Additionally, matrix metalloproteinase activity is important in the development of tissue injury. Interaction between *C. trachomatis* and viruses (HPV, HHV) might promote development of persistent infection,[18] chronic inflammation and even long-term complications especially among genetically susceptible individuals.

C. pneumoniae is able to disseminate inside circulating white blood cells. This explains why *C. pneumoniae* has been associated with a wide variety of diseases. Most important is the association with atherosclerosis.[19] Over 70 seroepidemiologic surveys have repeatedly demonstrated that the presence of elevated antibodies against *C. pneumoniae* is associated with an increased risk of a cardiac event. This is further supported by the presence of circulating immune complexes containing *C. pneumoniae* antibodies and antigens in sera, pointing to an access route of chlamydial components into the circulation. Human and chlamydial hsp60 co-localize in atherosclerotic plaques. Final demonstration of the common presence of the agent in the atherosclerotic lesion has been obtained by immunoelectron microscopy, immunohistochemistry, nucleic acid demonstration by polymerase chain

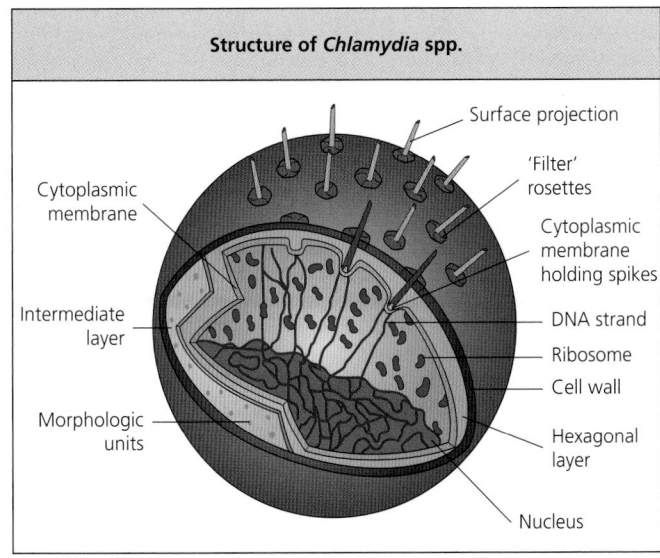

Structure of *Chlamydia* spp.

Surface projection

'Filter' rosettes

Cytoplasmic membrane

Cytoplasmic membrane holding spikes

Intermediate layer

DNA strand

Ribosome

Cell wall

Morphologic units

Hexagonal layer

Nucleus

Figure 188-2 Structure of *Chlamydia* spp. *(Courtesy of Dr A Matsumoto.)*

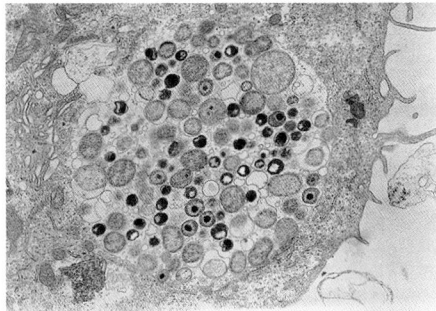

Figure 188-3 Electron microscopy of chlamydial inclusion. Reticulate bodies and transition stages to dense elementary bodies are shown. *Chlamydia pneumoniae* cultured in HL cells. *(Courtesy of Dr CH von Bonsdorff.)*

reaction (PCR), *in situ* hybridization and even isolation of the agent from lesions. The important question is, does this presence have an effect on the atherosclerotic process? *C. pneumoniae* may simply be an innocent bystander. However, it is an intracellular pathogen, able to multiply in macrophages, endothelial cells and smooth muscle cells. This multiplication is accompanied by induction of cytokines, adhesion molecules, growth factors and proteases. Oxidative substances appear as the host defense mechanisms against chlamydial infection. Chlamydial LPS induces foam cell formation in macrophages, the characteristic pathologic feature of the atherosclerotic plaque.[20] Several well-known risk factors for coronary heart disease are also associated with a chronic *C. pneumoniae* infection, such as smoking, elevated cholesterol levels, lowered levels of high-density cholesterol and elevated blood pressure. Animal experiments point to the possibility that it could even initiate the process. Also, young children with persistent *C. pneumoniae* infection show early signs of atherosclerosis including intimal thickening of their aortas.[21] *Chlamydia* can also be found in the vessel walls at the age of 14 years, decades before the complications of atherosclerosis, myocardial and cerebral infarctions start to appear. Finally, it should be noted that *C. pneumoniae* is only one of several infective agents that have been linked to the development of atherosclerosis, and the precise role of infections in the pathogenesis of this disease remains controversial.

The association of *C. pneumoniae* with childhood and adult asthma is established[22] and the association of *Chlamydia* with some forms of cancer (*C. trachomatis* with cervical cancer,[14] *C. pneumoniae* with lung cancer, *C. psittaci* with ocular adnexal MALT lymphoma) is suggested.[23]

Prevention

Vaccine development against human infections due to *Chlamydia* spp. is particularly challenging due to the lack of sterilizing immunity after natural infection. Chlamydial immunity is relatively short-lived, immunotype-specific and re-infections are common. Vaccines have been under development for 50 years in the shadow of concern that vaccine may make the outcome upon challenge worse. Limited understanding of the protective immune response mechanisms has delayed vaccine development. Knowledge of the complete genome and progress in immunology may alter this situation in the future.[1] It might be sufficient if a vaccine prevented disease rather than infection as a strategy for reducing long-term complications such as infertility in women. Even a therapeutic vaccine or some other immunomodulatory approach might prevent long-term complications. The advent of nucleic acid amplification tests (NAATs) has led some countries to introduce screening programs in order to eradicate *C. trachomatis* from the population. No vaccine is available for *C. pneumoniae* either, whereas vaccines are implemented in prevention of animal chlamydial infections.

In 1998 the World Health Organization (WHO) started a project to eradicate trachoma. It is based on SAFE strategy (lid Surgery, Antibiotic mass treatment, Facial cleanliness and Environmental hygiene). Mass medication campaigns, washing the face every second day with clear water and wiping it with a towel that is not shared with other people, is effective. Latrine hygiene is effective in controlling flies that spread trachoma.

Diagnostic Microbiology

The clinical features of chlamydial infections, such as their slow onset, long periods of asymptomaticity, the low numbers of infectious agents present and the potential cross-reactions seen in serology, challenge the diagnostic methods and testing strategies.[24–26]

CHLAMYDIA TRACHOMATIS INFECTIONS
Nucleic Acid Amplification Tests (NAATs)

For a number of compelling reasons, the NAATs have altered the former concept of culture as the 'gold standard' of *C. trachomatis* diagnosis. The NAATs have indeed replaced culture as the method of

choice for diagnosis.[24] *C. trachomatis* NAATs are usually based on the plasmid DNA, but can also amplify 16S rRNA or chromosomal DNA. The NAATs can detect a small amount of *C. trachomatis* nucleic acid in the samples. Transport and storage of the specimen is less stringent. Several test systems with corresponding specimen collection kits are commercially available and testing can be fully automated. A great advantage of NAATs is the possibility of using first void urine (especially for males) and self-collected vaginal samples for detection. Based on their superior sensitivity, NAATs are also recommended for detection of rectal and oropharyngeal *C. trachomatis* infections. Another advantage is that the NAATs can detect both *C. trachomatis* and *Neisseria gonorrhoeae* in the same specimen. Results from analytical studies suggest that there are no false-positive *C. trachomatis* NAAT results and the sensitivity is better than that of any other test available. But the NAATs are not without problems. There have been occasional reports of plasmid-free variants and, in 2006, a plasmid variant (not detectable by tests used widely at that time) caused an epidemic in Sweden.[27] There is no consensus as to whether the success of therapy should be monitored, and whether young females should be retested after 3–12 months.

Culture and Antigen Detection

Culture has low sensitivity (80% at best) in diagnosis of *C. trachomatis*. Although it is recommended in certain legal cases (samples from sexually abused boys and extragenital samples from prepubertal individuals), and to test antibiotic sensitivity, laboratories performing *Chlamydia* culture are nowadays rare.[24] The capability should, however, be maintained to enable monitoring of potential future changes in antibiotic resistance and for the surveillance of, e.g., potential mutated *C. trachomatis*.

The enzyme immunoassay (EIA) kits for the diagnosis of *C. trachomatis* measure the common LPS antigen present in all Chlamydiae. The antigen EIAs lack sensitivity and specificity compared to NAATs and their use is not encouraged. Direct fluorescent antibody (DFA) staining has been successfully used in diagnosis. The quality of the sample can be controlled in the stained smear. However, the interpretation demands expertise and is labor-intensive. The DFA test is only recommended for detection of ocular *C. trachomatis* infections.

Serology

Serology has been important in epidemiologic and disease-association studies. *C. trachomatis* antibodies start to appear at the sexually active age and peak at about 30 years of age. They are more often found in females than in males. In individual *C. trachomatis* infections, however, serologic tests lack precision in detecting acute infections and are of questionable value. The infection is often superficial without detectable systemic immune response (seroconversion). Proper antibiotic therapy can delay or even prevent antibody formation. Microimmunofluorescence (MIF) testing can differentiate between species and even immunotypes. It is, however, technically demanding and can be performed in few laboratories. MIF testing is usable in lymphogranuloma venereum, perihepatitis and infant pneumonitis, and it can also give a clue to the etiology of infertility and the triggering agent in reactive arthritis.

Enzyme immunoassays (EIA) based on purified chlamydial EBs, chlamydial LPS (group antigen) or peptides are commercially available but have not gained wide popularity. Their use in infertility studies can suggest tubal occlusions. The use of the complement fixation (CF) test in *C. trachomatis* infections is limited to lymphogranuloma venereum.

CHLAMYDIA PNEUMONIAE INFECTIONS
Culture

Samples for culture should contain live bacteria from the diseased area and this can be problematic if the pathogen has invaded deeper tissues. *C. pneumoniae* can be detected by immunofluorescence staining using *C. pneumoniae*- or LPS-specific monoclonal antibody. The consensus is that serology in acute infections is more sensitive than culture.[26]

Nucleic Acid Amplification Tests and Antigen Detection

In theory, NAATs should be as good for *C. pneumoniae* as for *C. trachomatis*. So far, most studies have been done with in-house kits and commercial kits have slowly appeared on the market. In acute infections, NAATs are more sensitive than culture. One difficulty is to get representative samples from the pneumonic area because upper respiratory tract specimens can remain negative. Direct fluorescent antibody staining from respiratory samples is difficult and used only occasionally. Since EIA detection tests are based on common chlamydial LPS they can be used in respiratory samples or even blood samples to obtain a presumptive diagnosis. This possibility has been used in only a few studies.

Serology

Serology has been the method most commonly used for diagnosis of *C. pneumoniae* infections. The need for paired samples to show seroconversion or titer rise considerably diminishes the value of serology in acute situations. Microimmunofluorescence (MIF) testing has been the most appropriate test for the serologic diagnosis of an acute *C. pneumoniae* infection.[26] In primary infections, the diagnosis can be obtained from the first sample that contains IgM antibodies specific for *C. pneumoniae*. The possibility of a false-positive reaction due to IgM rheumatoid factor should always be kept in mind. In patients undergoing re-infections, the potentially rapid serologic IgG response can be missed if the first serum sample is not collected early enough after the onset of disease. In MIF testing, strains of *C. pneumoniae* react much more uniformly than do those of *C. trachomatis*. EIA tests for chlamydial species-specific serology are currently replacing MIF due to their easy laboratory performance. They seem to be more sensitive than MIF, especially in acute infections of children. In *C. pneumoniae*

infections, the CF test shows sensitivity only in primary infections of young adults.

OTHER *CHLAMYDIA* AND *CHLAMYDIA*-LIKE ORGANISMS

Serology by CF test has been traditionally used in diagnosis of psittacosis. Isolation in cell cultures can only be attempted in biosafety level 3 facilities. NAATs are not currently commercially available for *C. psittaci*. A wide-spectrum pan-*Chlamydia* PCR assay that can detect chlamydial species and representatives of other families in Chlamydiales has recently been introduced.[28] The *Chlamydia*-related organisms can be isolated from different sources (water, soil) in co-cultures with amebae.[29] Simkaniaceae, Waddliaceae and Parachlamydiaceae can also be grown in cell culture. Commercial assays are not on the market and antigens of these *Chlamydia*-related organisms are not widely available, which limits diagnostic activities. Both acute and convalescent sera are desirable for serologic evaluation, but potential antigenic cross-reactions between the members of different families remain to be elucidated.

DIAGNOSIS OF CHRONIC CHLAMYDIAL INFECTIONS

Diagnosis of chronic chlamydial infections is problematic.[30] The number of infective organisms can be small and the site of infection can be difficult to reach. Culture often remains negative, especially from a peripheral site. Antibody responses can be quite variable or even lacking. However, persistently elevated antibody titers, especially of IgA type, have been suggested as a marker of chronic infection. Their value in individual diagnosis is, however, doubtful, especially if only a single sample is collected. EIAs have been inferior when compared to the MIF test in chronic infections. Measurements of local antibodies in asthma

TABLE 188-1	Diseases Associated with *Chlamydia* spp. and Novel *Chlamydia*-Related Organisms, or in Which a Possible Association Has Been Proposed			
Species	**Infection**	**Distribution**	**Disease**	**Incidence**
Chlamydia trachomatis	Acute	Female	Cervicitis	About 30%
			Endometritis	Common
			PID	10–70%
			Perihepatitis, splenitis, appendicitis	Isolated case reports
			Bartholinitis	Rare
		Male	Urethritis	10–30%
			Epididymitis	Rare
		Both sexes	Conjunctivitis	Uncommon
			Reactive arthritis	Common cause
		Neonates	Conjunctivitis	10%
			Infant pneumonitis	By definition
	Chronic	Female	Chronic PID	Common
		Both sexes	Trachoma	By definition
Chlamydia pneumoniae	Acute	Both sexes	Pneumonia, endemic	10%
			Pneumonia, epidemic	Up to 50%
			Acute bronchitis	5%
			Sinusitis	5%
			Otitis media	Case reports
			Common cold, subclinical	10% of school children annually
			Carditis	Case reports
			Reactive arthritis	Case reports
	Chronic	Both sexes	COPD, asthma	10–50% (?)
			Atherosclerosis	50–80% (?)
			Alzheimer's disease	?
			Multiple sclerosis	?
Chlamydia psittaci	Acute	Both sexes	Psittacosis–ornithosis	By definition
Chlamydia abortus	Acute	Female	Infectious abortion	Rare
Chlamydia felis	Acute	Both sexes	Conjunctivitis	Rare
Waddlia chondrophila	Acute	Female	Miscarriage	?
Parachlamydia acanthamoebae	Acute	Both sexes	Respiratory infection	?

COPD, chronic obstructive pulmonary disease; PID, pelvic inflammatory disease.

patients and antibodies to chlamydial hsp60, with or without inflammation markers such as C-reactive protein (CRP), have been used with success in some studies. Antigen detection in tissues by immunohistochemistry and nucleic acid by hybridization or PCR are sensitive, but currently used in research laboratories only. *C. pneumoniae* DNA can be detected by PCR in circulating white blood cells. The value of demonstrating circulating immune complexes that contain chlamydial antigens has been proposed, but the technique is quite demanding. A newly described method is to measure the presence of chlamydial LPS in the circulation. However, none of the serum-based approaches indicate the site of the infection. The above-mentioned markers are affected by age and season, and can also be found in otherwise healthy persons, perhaps suggesting common prevalence of chronic chlamydial infections. Novel biomarkers for detection of chronic chlamydial infection are needed. Chlamydial whole genome proteome arrays are available and identification of chlamydial antigens differentially expressed between acute infection and chronic infection is now within reach.

Clinical Manifestations

The diseases associated with chlamydial infection are listed in Table 188-1 and discussed in relevant chapters. *C. trachomatis* is worldwide a frequent cause of sexually transmitted infections, many of which remain asymptomatic. Besides respiratory infections, *Chlamydia pneumoniae* has been associated with a wide variety of diseases. The association with asthma and cardiovascular diseases is the strongest. The disease associations of *Chlamydia*-related organisms are currently being explored. PCR positivity without serologic response does suggest mere colonization and coinfections with established pathogens seem prevalent. *Waddlia chondrophila* is associated with miscarriages in humans, and *Parachlamydia acanthamoebae* with pneumonia and other respiratory infections.[1]

Management (see Chapters 28 and 66)

Chlamydiae are sensitive to tetracyclines, macrolides, azalides and newer fluoroquinolones. An antimicrobial effect is also seen with rifampin (rifampicin), clindamycin and chloramphenicol. Chlamydiae are resistant to aminoglycosides, vancomycin and cephalosporins. Uncomplicated urogenital *C. trachomatis* infections are widely treated with single-dose azithromycin. Although prompt treatment is aimed to prevent transmission and the development of immunopathology, it could also lead to arrested immunity.[31]

Chronic chlamydial forms seem very resistant to treatment and in intervention trials even 1-year courses of monotherapy have not led to eradication.[32] Recent controlled clinical trials have suggested that combination antibiotic therapy (either doxycycline and rifampin or azithromycin and rifampin) can improve clinical symptoms and promote microbiologic cure.[33] Treatment of infections due to *Chlamydia*-related bacteria is not established. Currently, novel antichlamydial compounds are actively sought.

References available online at expertconsult.com.

KEY REFERENCES

Carter J.D., Espinoza L.R., Inman R.D., et al.: Combination antibiotics as a treatment for chronic *Chlamydia*-induced reactive arthritis: a double-blind, placebo-controlled, prospective trial. *Arthritis Rheum* 2010; 62:1298-1307.

Deka S., Vanover J., Sun J., et al.: An early event in the herpes simplex virus type-2 replication cycle is sufficient to induce *Chlamydia trachomatis* persistence. *Cell Microbiol* 2007; 9:725-737.

Harris S.R., Clarke I.N., Seth-Smith H.M., et al.: Whole-genome analysis of diverse *Chlamydia trachomatis* strains identifies phylogenetic relationships masked by current clinical typing. *Nat Genet* 2012; 44:413-419, S1.

Hu V.H., Holland M.J., Burton M.J.: Trachoma: protective and pathogenic ocular immune responses to *Chlamydia trachomatis*. *PLoS Negl Trop Dis* 2013; 7(2):e2020.

Kuo C.C., Kaltenboek B., Bavoil P.M., et al.: Genus I. Chlamydia. In: Krieg N.R., Staley J.T., Brown D.R., et al., eds. *Bergey's manual of systematic bacteriology*, vol. 4. New York: Springer Press; 2010:846-865.

Papp J.R., Schachter J., Gaydos C.A., et al.: Recommendations for the laboratory-based detection of *Chlamydia trachomatis* and *Neisseria gonorrhoeae* – 2014. *MMWR Recomm Rep* 2014; 63:1-19.

Rosenfeld M.E., Campbell L.A.: Pathogens and atherosclerosis: update on the potential contribution of multiple infectious organisms to the pathogenesis of atherosclerosis. *Thromb Haemost* 2011; 1065:858-867.

Tan M., Bavoil P.: eds. *Intracellular pathogens I: Chlamydiales*. Washington, DC: American Society for Microbiology; 2012.

189

Opportunistic and Systemic Fungi

CHRIS KOSMIDIS | DAVID W. DENNING

KEY CONCEPTS

* Invasive fungal infections are becoming more common worldwide because of the increase in the number of susceptible hosts.

* Candidemia and deep organ infection carry a high mortality risk; early diagnosis with newer tests and prompt treatment with echinocandins can improve survival.

* *Aspergillus* causes a spectrum of clinical illness, ranging from allergic to chronic to invasive disease, depending on the interaction between pathogen and host. Azole resistance in *Aspergillus* is emerging and can lead to severely reduced options for treatment. Cryptococcal meningitis is a leading cause of mortality in patients with HIV infection, with the highest burden in sub-Saharan Africa.

* Systemic fungal infections due to organisms such as *Talaromyces (Penicillium) marneffei*, *Histoplasma* or *Coccidioides* were previously limited to well-described ecologic niches, but their epidemiology has changed as they have become implicated as opportunistic infections in patients with HIV.

* Newer diagnostic techniques are slowly replacing many of the slow and cumbersome methods of conventional mycologic microscopy and culture.

* The much wider range of antifungal drugs and the availability of susceptibility testing have greatly improved treatment options, but they have also created a much more complex treatment landscape.

Opportunistic Fungi

Introduction

Fungal infections are particularly important causes of death in immunocompromised patients and have increased in incidence, except in settings where they have been prevented with prophylaxis. The challenge for the clinician is that the clinical features of invasive fungal infections are usually subtle or non-existent in the early stages, and late diagnosis often results in death. Most of the affected patients have highly complex disease with many medical disciplines contributing to their care, even before a fungal diagnosis is entertained. An untreated opportunistic fungal infection almost always results in death, and invasive aspergillosis in particular is the most common missed infection at autopsy in hospitalized patients.

Some fungi cause disease worldwide, notably *Candida* spp., *Aspergillus* spp., *Pneumocystis jirovecii* and the Mucorales. Others are rare or non-existent in certain areas, notably *Histoplasma* in Europe, *Cryptococcus* spp. in northern Europe, *Coccidioides* spp. outside the Americas, *Talaromyces* (formerly *Penicillium*) *marneffeii* outside South East Asia and *Basidiobolus ranarum* outside the Middle East. Some species of *Aspergillus* and *Candida* are more common in certain institutions or locales. Emerging fungal pathogens are increasingly reported as causes of invasive infections.[1,2]

Moreover, the use of current antimicrobial prophylactic strategies has likely contributed to the changing epidemiology of invasive mycoses. Table 189-1 lists medically important fungi that can cause disseminated infection in humans. Table 189-2 shows the variables that likely account for the current trends in the epidemiology of opportunistic fungal infections. Table 189-3 lists the main techniques used for diagnosis of fungal infections.

Candidiasis

Nature

Candida spp. are yeasts that can form true hyphae as well as pseudohyphae. They are ubiquitous in soil and food and can be found as normal commensals on skin and mucosal membranes of the human gastrointestinal, genitourinary and respiratory tracts. They can cause localized infection, as well as disseminated infection in the immunocompromised host or when mucosal barriers are breached.

There are more than 350 *Candida* species, of which *C. albicans*, *C. glabrata*, *C. krusei*, *C. parapsilosis*, *C. tropicalis*, *C. guilliermondii*, *C. kefyr*, *C. lusitaniae*, *C. rugosa*, *C. norvegiensis* and *C. dubliniensis* are

TABLE 189-1	Numerically Most Important Fungi Causing Life-Threatening and/or Disseminated Infection in Humans in Approximate Order of Frequency	
Fungi	**Medically Important Species and Complexes**
Candida	C. albicans, C. tropicalis, C. glabrata, C. parapsilosis, C. guilliermondii, C. krusei, C. lusitaniae and many others
Aspergillus	A. fumigatus, A. flavus, A. niger, A. terreus, A. nidulans and some others
Cryptococcus	C. neoformans var. neoformans, C. neoformans var. grubii, C. gattii and other rarer species
Pneumocystis	Pneumocystis jirovecii
Histoplasma	H. capsulatum, H. duboisii
Mucorales	Rhizopus arrhizus, R. rhizopodiformis, Rhizomucor pusillus, Lichtheimia corymbifera, L. ramosa, Mucor spp., Cunninghamella bertholletiae, Apophysomyces elegans
Coccidioides	C. immitis, C. posadasii
Blastomyces	B. dermatitidis
Sporothrix	S. schenckii
Paracoccidioides	Paracoccidioides brasiliensis
Talaromyces	Talaromyces (Penicillium) marneffei
Fusarium	F. solani, F. oxysporum, F. moniliforme, F. dimerum
Rare yeasts	Trichosporon asahii, Geotrichum candidum, Rhodatorula rubra, Saccharomyces spp., Malassezia spp., Saprochaete capitata, Kodamaea (Pichia) ohmeri, Sporobolomyces spp., Pseudozyma spp.
Rare molds (both hyaline and dematiaceous)	Scedosporium apiospermum, Scedosporium prolificans, Paecilomyces spp., Bipolaris spp., Alternaria alternata and many others

clinically important. Some cryptic species exist and so clinical laboratories may choose to report some isolates as part of a complex if not fully identified – *Candida orthopsilosis* and *C. metapsilosis* being similar to *C. parapsilosis*, and *C. bracarensis* and *C. nivariensis* being similar to *C. glabrata*.

Epidemiology

The immunocompromised and patients in intensive care units are the groups of patients most at risk for invasive candidal infection. Among patients with cancer, those with hematologic malignancy and hematopoietic stem cell transplant (HSCT) have the highest incidence of candidemia (1.55%, compared to 0.23% in patients with solid tumors), as reported in a study by the European Organization for Research and Treatment of Cancer (EORTC).[3] The main causes for the greatly increased risk of candidemia in these patients are prolonged neutropenia, central venous catheters and breaks in mucosal integrity caused by chemotherapy.

Patients in intensive care account for many of the cases of candidemia in hospitals. Previous surgery is another predisposing factor; among patients in surgical intensive care units with candidemia, the majority had abdominal surgery (51.5%), whereas some patients had thoracic or neurosurgery.[4] Presence of central venous catheters, organ

transplant (mainly liver, pancreas and small intestinal), renal failure, broad-spectrum antibiotics, total parenteral nutrition and previous *Candida* colonization also predispose to candidal bloodstream infection. 'Hospital at home' practices are resulting in an increasing number of 'community-acquired' cases of candidemia.

Neonates, and especially very low birth-weight infants, are at very high risk of invasive candidal infection. The risk is directly related to birth-weight; incidence was 3.51 per 1000 patient-days for a birth-weight of less than 1000 g vs. 0.9 per 1000 patient days for a weight of 1001 to 1500 g in a study from the USA.[5] Immaturity of the immune system, broad-spectrum antibiotics, need for parenteral nutrition and invasive procedures account for the increased risk.

Small intestine, pancreas and liver transplant are linked with the highest rates of *Candida* infection, although all patients with solid organ transplant are at increased risk. *Candida* infection usually occurs within 3 months of transplant, as a postoperative infection. Other than the usual risk factors, the surgical anastomosis technique is relevant, e.g. in liver transplant, choledocho-jejunostomy is associated with a higher risk compared to choledocho-choledochostomy.[6] Prophylactic azoles are indicated in solid organ transplant patients at high risk. The American Society of Transplantation recommends fluconazole prophylaxis for 4 weeks in patients at high risk, e.g. prolonged operation, re-transplantation, renal failure or *Candida* colonization.[7]

C. albicans has been by far the most common clinically important species, followed by *C. glabrata*, *C. parapsilosis* and *C. tropicalis*. In a 1990s study by the EORTC in Europe, 92% of 270 episodes of candidemia in patients with solid tumors or hematologic malignancies were caused by *C. albicans*.[8] However, in recent years, the frequency of non-*albicans Candida* spp. has increased. *C. albicans* was seen in 45.6% of patients with invasive fungal infections in an American prospective study.[9] In a 2015 EORTC study focusing on cancer patients, the frequency of *C. albicans* was only 40%, followed by *C. tropicalis* (13%), *C. glabrata* (10%), *C. parapsilosis* (9%) and *C. krusei* (8%). The proportion of *C. albicans* was even smaller in patients with hematologic malignancies and/or HSCT (22%).[3] Although widespread azole use for prophylaxis has reduced the incidence and mortality from invasive candidal infection, it has resulted in an increase in the proportion of non-*albicans* isolates that may be fluconazole-resistant. In Asia and some tropical countries, there are many significant differences in species distributions, with a much higher rate of *C. tropicalis* infection (25%), especially in hemato-oncology wards.[10]

Molecular typing has shown that in the majority of cases, candidemia arises from an endogenous origin after previous colonization.

TABLE 189-2	**Variables That Likely Account for the Current Trends in the Epidemiology of Opportunistic Fungal Infections**

- Increasing number of susceptible hosts, including diabetes mellitus cases
- Greater laboratory expertise in the detection and identification of fungi
- Use of new transplantation modalities for hematopoietic stem cell transplantation (e.g. CD34+ selected autografts and peripheral blood stem cell transplantation)
- Evolution in organ transplantation practices
- Advances in surgical technology
- Use of corticosteroid-sparing regimens and an overall conservative approach to immunosuppression
- Use of novel immunosuppressive agents, notably selective immunosuppressive monoclonal antibody therapies
- Use of antimicrobial prophylactic practices (e.g. use of fluconazole for antifungal prophylaxis, ganciclovir for cytomegalovirus prophylaxis, quinolones for gram-negative bacterial prophylaxis)
- Organ dysfunction, notably renal and hepatic, but also cardiac and respiratory for pulmonary aspergillosis
- Excess antibiotic usage

TABLE 189-3	**Detection of Fungal Infections**			
Diagnostic Technique	**Major Features**	**Useful**	**Not Useful**	
Microscopy/histopathology	Rapid Relies on distinctive appearance of organism Not very sensitive	Histopathologic identification of: *Cryptococcus* *Blastomyces* *Histoplasma* *Coccidioides*	Cannot give a specific species classification for: *Aspergillus* *Candida*	
Culture-based methods Traditional culture	Inexpensive, insensitive	*Cryptococcus* grows rapidly *Aspergillus* – respiratory or tissue sample	Slow growth for most endemics Poor sensitivity for *Candida* in blood samples No value for *Aspergillus* in blood	
Automated blood culture methods	Early detection of growth Capital expense	*Candida* and bloodstream infection *Cryptococcus* and *Histoplasma*		
Non-culture methods Antigen	Sensitive and specific Blood, urine, CSF and BAL	*Cryptococcus* and *Histoplasma* *Aspergillus* galactomannan	No reliable tests for other mycoses	
Beta 1,3-D-Glucan	Moderately sensitive screen, better as a rule out test	*Candida* and *Aspergillus*	Negative for mucormycosis and other rarer pathogens	
Antibody	Moderately sensitive and specific	Endemic mycoses Key test for chronic pulmonary and allergic aspergillosis	No reliable tests for opportunistic fungi	
PCR	More sensitive than culture	*Aspergillus* in blood and sputum, *Candida* in blood	May also be useful combined with sequencing for identification of unusual fungi and histopathology	

This holds true for *C. albicans* and most non-*albicans Candida* spp. except for infections with *C. parapsilosis*, which are thought to arise mainly from infected biomaterials, intravenous fluids or the hands of healthcare workers. Also, human-to-human transmission (patient-to-patient, nurse-to-patient and between sexual partners) has become increasingly important. Recurrence of oropharyngeal candidiasis in patients who have an HIV infection with a low CD4+ cell count and recurrent vulvovaginal candidiasis has been shown to be mostly due to recurrence of the same strain (relapse), although infection with a new strain also occurs.

Pathogenicity

Intact barrier function is an essential feature of host defense against candidiasis. The virulence of *Candida* spp. has been shown to correlate with its ability to adhere to epithelial cells (especially *C. albicans*) or plastic polymers such as intravascular or urethral catheters (*C. tropicalis*). Adhesion to the epithelium via the *C. albicans* protein ALS3 is an integral part of the invasive process and constitutes the target for a candidiasis vaccine.[11] The fungus is capable of secreting proteinases and lipases that can assist invasion, although the clinical importance of these enzymes is not clear.[12]

After candidal invasion of the dermis or bloodstream, neutrophils constitute the first line of defense, followed by monocytes and eosinophils, which can kill *Candida* spp. via oxidative and nonoxidative pathways. Patients with neutropenia are particularly at risk of developing candidiasis, which underscores the importance of neutrophils in host defense against this fungus. The clinical outcome of infection is primarily determined by the host defense status. Clinical and experimental data suggest that:
- an impairment of T-cell immunity (e.g. in HIV infection) or STAT1 genetic defect predisposes mainly to mucocutaneous candidiasis (gastrointestinal and vaginal); and
- impaired phagocytosis, especially neutrophil function, with or without impaired T-lymphocyte function, is the major risk factor for the development of systemic candidiasis.

Humoral-acquired immunity is probably not key to the body's defense against candidal infection, whereas innate immunity is critical to the host defense against *Candida*.[13]

Biofilm formation is an important mechanism of *Candida* pathogenicity, implicated in infections of prosthetic materials and intravenous catheters. It has mainly been studied in *C. albicans*. Biofilm cells are more resistant to antifungal agents than planktonic cells, mainly because of drug sequestration by matrix beta-1,3-glucan, and may form mixed biofilms with bacteria.[14]

Diagnostic Microbiology

In culture, *Candida* spp. grow rapidly at 25–37 °C on simple media. On special culture media, hyphae or elongating pseudohyphae are formed. *Candida* spp. grow in routine aerobic blood culture bottles and on agar plates as smooth creamy-white colonies. A differential culture medium (CHROMagar Candida) can distinguish between *C. albicans* and certain non-*albicans Candida* spp. *C. glabrata* may appear first in an anaerobic blood culture bottle.

Specimens for microscopic evaluation give a better diagnostic yield after treatment with 10% potassium hydroxide, which lyses epithelial cells. The demonstration of blastoconidia (budding yeast), hyphae and pseudohyphae are highly suggestive but not diagnostic for tissue invasion. Staining with optical brighteners such as calcofluor white or Blankophor P is a sensitive method for the detection of fungi, but requires a fluorescent microscope. Although in the routine clinical microbiology laboratory the Gram stain is commonly used to detect yeast in blood culture slides (yeasts commonly stain gram-positive), morphologic details are more difficult to detect compared to staining with an optical brightener. Spores from molds in blood culture, which might be present in invasive fusariosis or scedosporiosis, might then be misinterpreted as yeast infection. *Candida* species identification can be achieved by the germ tube test, which enables identification of *C.*

albicans and *C. dubliniensis* (but not most non-*albicans Candida* spp.) by showing the formation of hyphal elements within 90 minutes.

Blood cultures should be sent promptly whenever disseminated *Candida* infection is suspected. Routine blood culture systems can detect yeasts, however blood cultures are positive only 40–70% of the time, with a reduced yield in those on fluconazole or if less than 20 mL of blood is cultured. This may reflect the absence of viable *Candida* cells in the circulation, or the intermittent nature of fungemia. *C. parapsilosis*, which has been linked to catheter-related infections in neonates, may be associated with higher burdens, whereas *C. glabrata*, which often originates in the gastrointestinal tract, may have lower bloodstream concentrations. Yeasts seen on Gram stain from positive blood culture bottles can be identified to the species level by peptide nucleic acid fluorescent in situ hybridization (PNA-FISH), which can detect up to five different *Candida* spp. in 90 minutes. Matrix-assisted laser desorption/ionization time-of-flight mass spectrometry (MALDI-TOF) is less sensitive for the detection of yeast in blood culture bottles.

The long time to positivity of blood cultures means that they cannot be used as an early marker in order to initiate antifungal therapy. Because of the high mortality of disseminated infection and the proven benefit of early initiation of antifungal therapy, more rapid, molecular detection methods have been introduced. Commercially available methods detect cell wall components such as (1,3)-β-D glucan (BDG) (Fungitell®), mannan antigen/antimannan antibody (Platelia®) and anti-*C. albicans* antibody detection (CAGTA®) (Vircell Microbiologist).

BDG is present in the cell wall of different fungal species, including *Candida*, *Aspergillus* and *Pneumocystis jirovecii*, and can be detected in the blood during systemic infection. BDG assay results are available much sooner than blood cultures, and its clinical utility lies mainly in its high negative predictive value. A negative BDG test excludes *Candida* systemic infection with good reliability, however a positive test may be due to infection by other fungi, some bacteria, or other causes. The sensitivity and specificity of the assay vary with different cutoffs. This assay can be useful for the diagnosis of deep-seated infection, when blood cultures are less likely to be positive.[15]

While the BDG assay is the most widely used, other molecular tests are also available. Detection of mannan antigen has been found to be less sensitive but more specific than the BDG assay.[16] Combination of mannan antigen and anti-mannan antibody improves sensitivity considerably. The newly marketed CAGTA® is also useful in ruling out infection, especially if used in combination with the BDG test (97% negative predictive value) in critically ill patients.[17]

Molecular diagnosis by polymerase chain reaction (PCR) is substantially more sensitive than blood culture, particularly for invasive candidiasis, and has recently been commercialized in a magnetic resonance PCR format, reducing processing effort and time and providing species-specific information.[18–20]

SUSCEPTIBILITY TESTING AND ANTIFUNGAL RESISTANCE

All *Candida* isolates from sterile sites should at a minimum have their fluconazole MIC determined.[21] In addition, *Candida* isolates from non-invasive infections that fail to respond to treatment should also have the MIC determined. The European Committee on Antimicrobial Susceptibility Testing (EUCAST) and the Clinical and Laboratory Standards Institute (CLSI) have determined breakpoints for *Candida* species, although the methods differ, and the CLSI updated their breakpoints in 2012. Both CLSI and EUCAST methods allow reading after 24 hours of incubation which provides clinicians with useful susceptibility information.

Fluconazole is not uniformly active against all *Candida* species. *C. albicans*, *C. tropicalis* and *C. parapsilosis* have the lowest MIC, whereas *C. glabrata* has higher MICs, and *C. krusei* is inherently resistant. Voriconazole and posaconazole are more active than fluconazole, although no breakpoints exist for *C. glabrata* or *C. krusei*.

Recently, breakpoints have been established for amphotericin B, micafungin and anidulafungin. EUCAST has not determined caspofungin breakpoints due to significant inter-laboratory variability in MIC determinations. Although the echinocandins are very active against all *Candida* species, the highest echinocandin MICs are seen with *C. parapsilosis* and *C. guillermondii*. Molecular confirmation of echinocandin resistance is important, as MICs are less reliable than target sequence data.

Fluconazole resistance remains uncommon in *C. albicans* but is more common in non-*albicans* species. A global antifungal resistance surveillance programme in 2012 detected no fluconazole-resistant *C. albicans* isolates from North America, 0.3% in Europe and 1.2% in Latin America. Fluconazole resistance ranged between 0 and 13.5% for *C. glabrata*, 1.8–7.3% for *C. parapsilosis*, and 0–9.1% for *C. tropicalis*. Resistance rates were generally higher in North America compared to Europe.[22] Several resistance mechanisms have been described, including modifications in the ergosterol synthesis pathway and efflux pump overexpression.

Rarely, elevated MIC values of echinocandins with occasional treatment failure have been reported for strains of *Candida*, and resistance was associated with amino acid substitutions in two 'hot-spot' regions of Fks1, the major subunit of glucan synthase.[23] This Fks1-mediated resistance mechanism probably accounts for intrinsic reduced susceptibility in *C. parapsilosis* and *C. guillermondii*.

Clinical Manifestations

The clinical manifestations of candidal infection can be divided into mucocutaneous infections and deep-seated infections. Mucocutaneous infections include thrush, *Candida* esophagitis, *Candida* vulvovaginitis and cutaneous candidiasis syndromes. Deep-seated infections include chronic disseminated candidiasis (hepatosplenic candidiasis), candidemia and candidiasis of various organ systems.

MUCOCUTANEOUS CANDIDIASIS

The most common clinical manifestation of candidal infection is oral thrush (oropharyngeal candidiasis), which presents as curd-like plaques on examination. Diagnosis is usually made clinically, but can be confirmed by demonstrating yeast in a Gram-stained direct smear, 10% potassium hydroxide preparation, calcofluor preparation or culture of scrapings. Oral thrush most often affects patients on broad-spectrum antibiotics, corticosteroids, including inhaled steroids used for asthma, or the immunocompromised. In the latter group, esophagitis may coexist, even with minimal symptoms.

Candida esophagitis presents with pain on swallowing, with or without thrush. It is frequently associated with HIV infection, lymphoma or leukemia, although it can occur in people who are not immunocompromised. Differential diagnosis in patients with HIV includes herpes and cytomegalovirus infection. Unlike *Candida* esophagitis, the latter two conditions may cause fever. Diagnosis is usually based on symptoms, and treatment with oral antifungals is given, particularly if oral thrush coexists, without confirming a diagnosis.

Candida vulvovaginitis presents mainly with pruritus, pain, dysuria or dyspareunia. Examination reveals redness; discharge may or may not be present. Risk factors include antibiotic use, diabetes, oral contraceptive use and immunosuppression, although no risk factor is apparent for a substantial subset of patients. Diagnosis is made on the basis of the combination of clinical symptoms, microscopy with 10% potassium hydroxide (including a wet preparation to exclude *Trichomonas vaginalis* and clue cells) and/or culture. The vaginal pH in candidiasis should be in the normal range (4.0–4.5); a pH higher than 4.7 indicates bacterial vaginosis or trichomoniasis. Recurrent infection can be particularly bothersome, may not have identifiable risk factors and is usually associated with the same strain of *Candida*.[24]

Chronic mucocutaneous candidiasis is a relatively rare genetic disease characterized by protracted and persistent infections with *Candida* spp. of skin, mucous membranes, hair and nails, and is frequently associated with endocrinopathies or autoimmune disorders.[25,26] The acronym APECED (autoimmune polyendocrinopathy, candidiasis, ectodermal dystrophy) is used for patients with this constellation of symptoms. Severe disease may prove fatal, usually due to bacterial sepsis. Disseminated candidiasis is a rare complication.

INVASIVE CANDIDIASIS

Invasive candidiasis comprises both candidemia and deep organ infection.[27] Clinical presentation of candidemia is nonspecific, and ranges from low-grade fever to septic shock. Examination is usually not revealing, except for characteristic skin lesions or eye involvement (chorioretinitis with or without vitritis), which are present in only 10% of cases of disseminated candidiasis (see Chapter 18). The source of infection may or may not be evident (e.g. line infection, intra-abdominal infection).

C. parapsilosis often causes line-related infections in neonates. Virtually every organ can be infected by *Candida* spp. *Candida* meningitis and encephalitis usually occur as a complication of disseminated candidiasis. *Candida* myocarditis may also develop, with electrocardiographic changes mimicking infarction and supraventricular tachycardias. *Candida* spp. are the major cause of fungal endocarditis, with up to 41% of cases caused by non-*albicans* spp. In most cases, blood cultures are positive. *Candida* pneumonia is usually associated with disseminated candidiasis and is very rare. Diagnosis is based on transbronchial biopsy.

In abdominal surgery, heavy growth of *Candida* spp. in the first culture (intraoperative or from abdominal drain) or an increasing fungal load in serial cultures has been shown to be highly predictive of the development of candidiasis. Pancreatitis represents a particularly well-recognised risk.[28,29]

Infection of the urinary tract with *Candida* spp. is difficult to discriminate from colonization or from disseminated candidiasis. Microscopic urine analysis does not discriminate, unless renal casts containing yeasts are found, and quantitation of candiduria (such as is used for bacterial urinary infections) is not a reliable indicator of deep infection.[30] Any patient who has persistent candiduria without a recent history of urinary tract instrumentation should be evaluated for diabetes mellitus, renal insufficiency or genitourinary tract abnormalities.[31]

Chronic disseminated (hepatosplenic) candidiasis is a syndrome seen almost exclusively in patients recovering from neutropenia following chemotherapy for hematologic malignancy. It presents with persistent fever, abdominal discomfort and elevated liver enzymes. Characteristic lesions are seen on imaging (with PET scans, lesions can remain active up to 6 months), and biopsy is not always undertaken. This condition is now less common because of the widespread use of antifungal prophylaxis.

Management

The drugs approved for treatment of systemic fungal diseases are listed in Table 189-4. Their mechanism of action is shown in Figure 189-1.

MUCOCUTANEOUS CANDIDIASIS

Oropharyngeal candidiasis

Mild disease can be treated with clotrimazole troches (one 10 mg troche five times daily) or nystatin suspension (400 000–600 000 units 4 times daily). Oral fluconazole (100–200 mg/day for 7–14 days orally) is recommended for moderate-to-severe disease. It has been shown that a single dose of fluconazole of 750 mg was as efficacious as a full 2-week course of 150 mg daily for the treatment of oropharyngeal candidiasis.[32] Recommended therapy for refractory disease includes itraconazole solution (200 mg/day for 7–14 days orally); voriconazole (200 mg/day orally); posaconazole (400 mg/day orally) or amphotericin B oral suspension.[33] Intravenous echinocandin or amphotericin B deoxycholate at 0.3 mg/kg per day were also shown to be effective and may be used as last-resort therapy in patients with refractory disease.

TABLE 189-4 **Drugs Approved for Treatment of Systemic Fungal Diseases**

Class	Generic Name	Available Formulation(s)	Year First Approved	Indications
Polyene	Amphotericin B	Intravenous, oral solution In lipid form or aqueous	1958	Broad spectrum; cryptococcal meningitis, invasive *Candida* infections, mucor, *Fusarium* fungemia, intrathecal for coccidioidal meningitis. Resistant pathogens include *A. terreus, A. nidulans, Scedosporium* spp., *Paecilomyces* spp. and others
Pyrimidine	Flucytosine	Oral tablet, intravenous	1972	Cryptococcal meningitis, CNS infections and *Candida* endocarditis or urinary tract infections especially
Azole	Ketoconazole	Oral tablet, shampoo	1981	Now withdrawn, except for shampoo
Azole	Fluconazole	Intravenous, oral tablet, oral suspension	1990	*Candida* infections, cryptococcal disease, other yeast infection, coccidioidomycosis. All filamentous fungi resistant
Azole	Itraconazole	Intravenous, oral capsule, oral solution	1992	Aspergillosis especially allergic and chronic infections, histoplasmosis, blastomycosis, paracoccidioidomycosis, sporotrichosis, coccidioidomycosis, dermatophyte infections
Azole	Voriconazole	Intravenous, oral tablet, oral suspension	2002	*Candida, Aspergillus, Scedosporium, Fusarium*
Azole	Posaconazole	Intravenous, oral tablet, oral solution	2006	*Candida, Aspergillus,* mucormycosis, *Fusarium*
Azole	Isavuconazole	Intravenous, oral tablet	2015	*Candida, Aspergillus,* mucormycosis
Allylamine	Terbinafine	Oral tablet	1992	Dermatophyte infections. May be useful in combination with flucytosine for *Scedosporium prolificans* infections. *Candida* spp.-resistant. Antagonistic with amphotericin B for invasive aspergillosis
Echinocandin	Micafungin	Intravenous	2002	*Candida, Aspergillus*
Echinocandin	Caspofungin	Intravenous	2002	*Candida, Aspergillus*
Echinocandin	Anidulafungin	Intravenous	2006	*Candida, Aspergillus*

CNS, central nervous system.

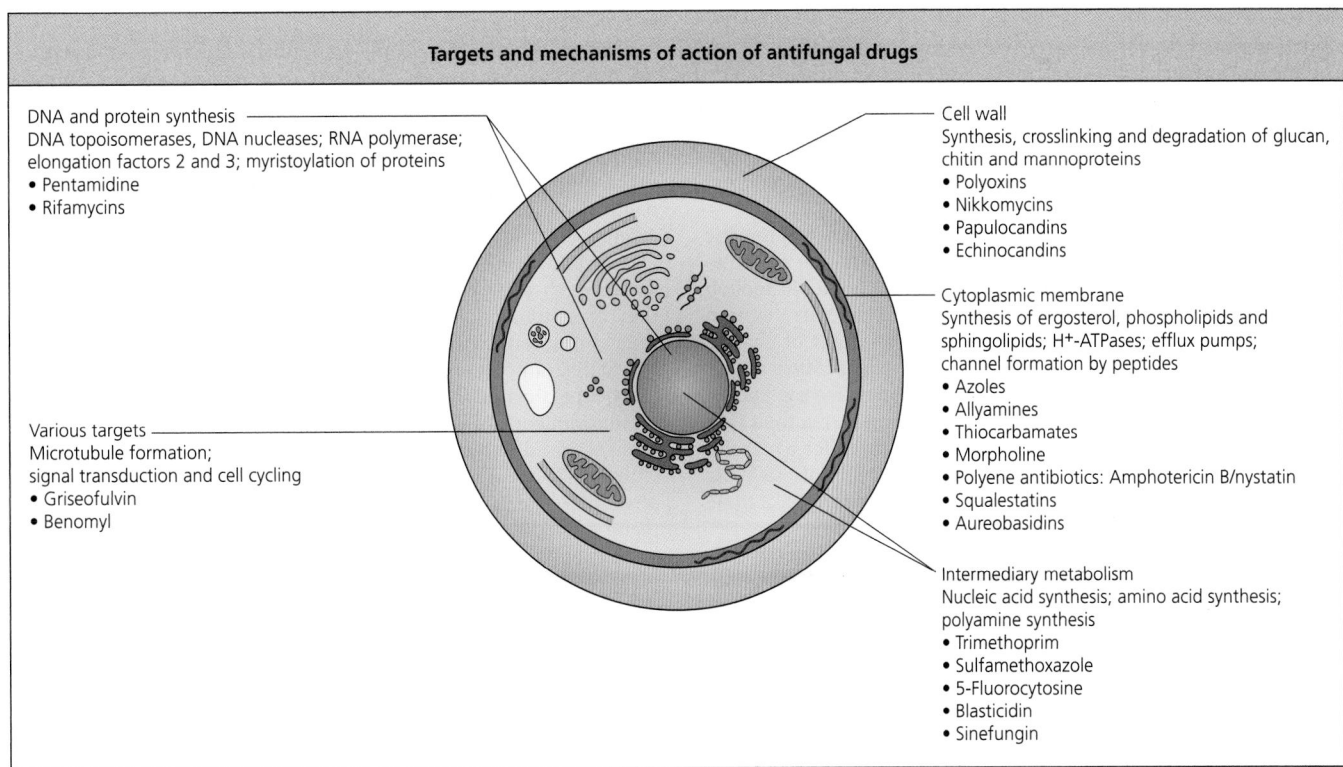

Figure 189-1 Targets and mechanisms of action of antifungal drugs.

Although suppressive therapy is effective for the prevention of recurrent infections, to reduce the likelihood of development of antifungal resistance it should be used only if the recurrences are frequent or disabling. Denture-related disease may require thorough disinfection of the denture for definitive cure. Oral thrush caused by inhaled steroids can be prevented by rinsing with saline after use.

Esophageal Candidiasis

Systemic therapy is required for effective treatment of esophageal candidiasis. Although symptoms of esophageal candidiasis may be mimicked by other pathogens, a diagnostic trial of antifungal therapy is often appropriate before endoscopy to search for other causes of esophagitis. A 14- to 21-day course of fluconazole (200–400 mg/day orally) is preferred. For patients who are unable to tolerate an oral agent, fluconazole may be administered intravenously, or an echinocandin or amphotericin B deoxycholate at a dose of ~0.7 mg/kg daily may be used. Suppressive therapy should be used occasionally in patients with disabling recurrent infections. Patients with refractory esophageal candidiasis should be treated with itraconazole oral solution (200 mg/day) or posaconazole 400 mg twice daily or voriconazole 200 mg twice daily. Intravenous amphotericin B (0.3–0.7 mg/kg per day as needed to produce a response) or an echinocandin may be used in patients with otherwise refractory disease.[33]

Vulvovaginal Candidiasis (VVC)

Around 70% of women suffer from VVC at some time in their life, often in pregnancy. This may be classified into complicated (severe, resistant species, impaired host defenses) and uncomplicated forms. Uncomplicated Candida VVC is seen in 90% of patients and responds readily to short-course oral or topical treatment with any of the therapies listed above, including a single dose of fluconazole, two doses of itraconazole or topical therapy. In contrast, the recurrent complicated vaginitis seen in 10% of patients is defined as severe or recurrent disease, with infection due to Candida spp. other than C. albicans and/or VVC in an abnormal host. Laboratories should be prepared to identify the infecting yeast to species level and susceptibility test isolates taken in patients on antifungal therapy. Complicated VVC requires topical therapy administered intravaginally daily for 7 days or multiple doses of fluconazole (150 mg every 72 hours for three doses).[34] C. glabrata usually fails to respond to azole therapy and may respond to topical boric acid 600 mg/day for 14 days, topical nystatin, topical 17% flucytosine cream alone or in combination with 3% amphotericin B cream, administered daily for 14 days. Azole-resistant C. albicans infections are rare.[35]

Recurrent VVC is defined as four or more episodes of symptomatic vulvovaginal candidiasis within 1 year and is usually due to azole-susceptible C. albicans. Around 6–9% of women (about 140 million worldwide) suffer from recurrent VVC at any one time. Its duration may be only 1 or 2 years, but is often longer. A variant of chronic Candida vaginitis has recently been described, which often evades culture-based diagnosis.[36] After control of causal factors (e.g. uncontrolled diabetes, HIV), induction therapy with 2 weeks of a topical or oral azole should be followed by a maintenance regimen for 6 months. If fluconazole therapy is not feasible, topical clotrimazole (500 mg vaginal suppository once weekly) or other intermittent topical azole treatments are recommended.[33]

The persistent immunologic defect of chronic mucocutaneous candidiasis (which may be due to an AIRE mutation, STAT1 mutation, dectin1 mutation or type 1 interferon antibody production)[37] requires a long-term approach. Systemic therapy is needed and all of the azole antifungal agents have been used successfully. The dosages required are similar to those used for other forms of mucocutaneous candidiasis. As with HIV-infected patients, development of resistance to these agents has also been described.

SYSTEMIC CANDIDIASIS

All patients with a positive blood culture should be treated, even if the sample is drawn from a catheter. Additionally, indwelling intravascular catheters should be removed or changed, preferably without using a wire for replacement. The evidence for this recommendation is strongest in the non-neutropenic patient population. In neutropenic patients, the role of the gastrointestinal tract as a source for disseminated candidiasis is evident from autopsy studies, but in an individual patient it is difficult to determine the primary source of fungemia. An exception is fungemia due to C. parapsilosis, which is very frequently associated with catheters.

Echinocandins are preferred for initial empiric or targeted treatment of candidemia, as they have a broader spectrum including C. glabrata and C. krusei, and are fungicidal. Infectious Diseases Society of America guidelines suggest either fluconazole or an echinocandin, with the latter preferred for moderate to severe disease. ESCMID guidelines recommend an echinocandin as first choice for all cases of confirmed candidemia. This recommendation is based on a comparative trial that showed better outcomes with anidulafungin over fluconazole.[38] An echinocandin is also recommended for treatment in neutropenic patients. Stepdown to oral fluconazole can be considered in stable patients, with fluconazole-sensitive isolates. The European Society of Clinical Microbiology and Infectious Diseases (ESCMID) recommend a 10-day course of intravenous therapy before switching to oral agents. However, a recent open-label study showed equivalent outcomes with earlier (5 days) stepdown to oral fluconazole.[39]

The recommended antifungal doses are: fluconazole, loading dose of 12 mg/kg (800 mg), then daily maintenance dose of 6 mg/kg (400 mg) or an echinocandin (caspofungin: loading dose of 70 mg, then 50 mg/day; micafungin: 100 mg/day; anidulafungin: loading dose of 200 mg, then 100 mg/day). For infection with C. glabrata, an echinocandin is preferred. Voriconazole is effective for candidemia, but offers little advantage over fluconazole. Polyenes, such as lipid-formulations of amphotericin B or amphotericin B deoxycholate, are alternatives if there is intolerance or in resource-limited situations.

Antifungal treatment should be continued for 2 weeks after the first negative blood culture, and patients should be followed for 3–6 months to detect long-term sequelae due to hematogenous seeding. Persistent candidemia despite antifungal therapy is found in up to 10% of candidemia cases.

Timely initiation of adequate antifungal therapy is important to improve clinical outcome[40,41] and empiric therapy should be considered in critically ill patients with risk factors for invasive candidiasis but with no known cause for the fever. For suspected candidiasis in non-neutropenic patients, empiric therapy is similar to proven candidiasis with either fluconazole or an echinocandin as initial therapy. In neutropenic patients, lipid-formulations of amphotericin B, echinocandins or voriconazole are recommended.

Candida chorioretinitis without vitritis can be treated with fluconazole, which achieves good local concentrations if the isolate is sensitive, or amphotericin B preferably with flucytosine, for resistant isolates or if sensitivities are unknown. Presence of vitritis necessitates intravitreal amphotericin B instillation with or without vitrectomy. Treatment is continued until resolution of all lesions.

Recommended treatment of central nervous system (CNS) candidiasis is a lipid formulation of amphotericin B (3–5 mg/kg) preferably with flucytosine. The flucytosine dose should be adjusted to produce serum levels of 40–60 µg/mL. Fluconazole can be used as step-down therapy at a dose of 400–800 mg/day (6–12 mg/kg). Treatment should be continued until all signs and symptoms, cerebrospinal fluid abnormalities and radiologic abnormalities have resolved. Intraventricular devices should be removed. The occurrence of a brain abscess worsens the prognosis considerably. The indication for surgery remains to be determined but surgical drainage, if feasible, is probably advisable. Neonates with Candida meningoencephalitis often suffer long-term neurologic sequelae.[42]

Native valve Candida endocarditis should be treated with an echinocandin as first-line therapy.[34] Amphotericin B, preferably with flucytosine, is an alternative therapy. Without surgical intervention, the mortality is high (90%); with combined surgical and medical treatment, the mortality has dropped to 45%. Fluconazole therapy (400–800 mg/day) can be considered as step-down therapy in patients with susceptible isolates who are clinically stable and who have cleared *Candida* from the bloodstream. Treatment should continue for at least 6 weeks after valve replacement, but a longer duration is recommended in patients with perivalvular abscesses and other complications. Because recurrences have occurred years later patients should be followed up for at least 2 years.

In *Candida* urinary tract infection, the clinical circumstances dictate the management because candiduria can represent colonization, cystitis, pyelonephritis, disseminated candidemia or a fungus ball. Treatment is not recommended for asymptomatic candiduria unless the patient belongs to a group at high risk of dissemination: neutropenic patients, low birth-weight infants and patients who will undergo urologic manipulations. Neutropenic patients and neonates with *Candida* urinary tract infection should be managed as described for invasive candidiasis, while those undergoing urologic procedures should receive fluconazole at a dosage of 200–400 mg/day or amphotericin B deoxycholate at a dosage of 0.3–0.6 mg/kg per day for several days before and after the procedure.

For cystitis, oral fluconazole at a dosage of 200 mg/day (3 mg/kg) for 2 weeks is recommended if the infection is due to a fluconazole-susceptible *Candida* spp. For fluconazole-resistant isolates, amphotericin B deoxycholate (0.3–0.6 mg/kg per day) for 1–7 days or oral flucytosine (25 mg/kg four times daily) for 7–10 days is recommended. There is no role for echinocandins, voriconazole or posaconazole as these drugs do not achieve clinically useful levels in the urine. Bladder irrigation with amphotericin B (50 mg/1000 mL of sterile water administered continuously over a three-way Foley catheter for 5–7 days) is not recommended as it only has a transient effect. If there is a fungus ball in the urinary tract, the treatment is surgical.

Chronic disseminated candidiasis (hepatosplenic candidiasis) is difficult to treat; this syndrome is not acutely life-threatening but does require prolonged therapy to produce a cure. Fluconazole at 6 mg/kg per day is generally preferred in clinically stable patients. Lipid formulations of amphotericin B at a dosage of 3–5 mg/kg per day or amphotericin B deoxycholate at 0.5–0.7 mg/kg per day may be used in acutely ill patients or patients with refractory disease. Some but not all experts recommend an initial 1–2 week course of amphotericin B for all patients, followed by a prolonged course of fluconazole. The echinocandins are alternatives for initial therapy. Therapy should be continued until calcification or resolution of lesions, particularly in patients receiving continued chemotherapy or immunosuppression. Premature discontinuation of antifungal therapy may lead to recurrence. Timing of the re-institution of chemotherapy for underlying leukemia is often a difficult decision, requiring expert input.

Prophylaxis

Antifungal prophylaxis is highly controversial because the relationship between candidal colonization and dissemination is often not clear and azole prophylaxis may select for *Candida* spp. that are resistant to azoles. Postoperative prophylaxis is recommended for high-risk liver, pancreas and small bowel transplant recipients with fluconazole at a dosage of 200–400 mg (3–6 mg/kg per day) or with liposomal amphotericin B at a dosage of 1–2 mg/kg per day. Patients with recent abdominal surgery and recurrent perforations or leakage are at high risk and should be offered prophylaxis. In cancer patients, strong evidence for antifungal prophylaxis exists only for the allogeneic HSCT patients.[43,44] Evidence is much weaker for patients with neutropenia due to chemotherapy (outside of HSCT) and for autologous HSCT.[45] There are several studies, some randomized, showing that premature infants weighing less than 1 kg benefit from fluconazole prophylaxis and other measures to reduce the risk of disseminated candidiasis.[46–48]

Aspergillosis

Nature

Aspergillus is a filamentous fungus genus that causes various clinical syndromes, including invasive, allergic and saprophytic disease. Aspergilli are ubiquitous in organic matter such as hay, decaying vegetation,

soil and in construction sites. Inhalation of conidia is frequent, but only a minority of exposed persons will develop disease. The genus *Aspergillus* contains over 260 species, although only a few are associated with disease. *Aspergillus fumigatus* is by far the most common cause of human disease, followed by *A. flavus*, *A. niger*, *A. terreus* and *A. nidulans*. Reports of cryptic species such as *A. lentulus* or *A. pseudofischeri*, which can be misidentified as *A. fumigatus*, but may have differing resistance profiles, are increasing in the literature. Invasive aspergillosis in immunocompromised patients may be acquired in the hospital or community. Recent reports of invasive aspergillosis in newly hospitalized chronic obstructive pulmonary disease (COPD) patients, many of whom, but not all, were treated with corticosteroids, emphasizes the high frequency of *Aspergillus* acquisition in the community.[49,50] Virtually all cases of allergic bronchopulmonary aspergillosis (ABPA), *Aspergillus* bronchitis and chronic pulmonary aspergillosis (CPA) are, or are presumed to be, acquired out of hospital. This is hardly surprising given the ubiquitous nature of *Aspergillus fumigatus* and other species.[51] Reports of community-acquired *Aspergillus* pneumonia and/or pneumonitis in non-immunocompromised patients are uncommon.

Epidemiology

Worldwide, aspergillosis is the most common invasive mold infection. It is estimated that over 200 000 patients develop invasive aspergillosis (IA) annually, with a mortality rate of around 50%. IA may affect around 10% of new acute myeloid leukemia diagnoses, and other at-risk groups include stem-cell and solid organ transplant recipients (particularly lung and heart) and patients with chronic obstructive lung disease.[50,52,53] The latter group may account for an increasing proportion of cases that may remain unrecognized. Mold infection was observed in 2.9% of patients with hematologic malignancies in a large cohort, with *Aspergillus* spp. being responsible for almost 90% of cases.[54] Autopsy studies indicate that approximately 15% of patients have a mixed fungal infection that is not diagnosed during life in the majority of patients. In hematology patients with invasive aspergillosis the survival at 12 weeks was 52.2%.[55] In most centers *Aspergillus fumigatus* is the most prevalent species and the lungs and the brain are the most common sites of infection.

The global burden of allergic *Aspergillus* diseases is also significant. Prevalence studies from various countries define the prevalence of ABPA from 0.7 to 3.5%, leading to the estimate of approximately 4.8 million adults worldwide having ABPA among the 193 million with asthma.[56] In addition, around 15% of patients with cystic fibrosis will develop ABPA.[57] *Aspergillus* and other molds are also increasingly recognized as causes of asthma exacerbation after occupational, indoor or outdoor exposure, and patients with severe asthma are more likely to have *Aspergillus* sensitization.[58]

Chronic pulmonary aspergillosis (CPA) complicates tuberculosis (TB) and other chronic lung diseases. Cavities persisted 6 months after completion of TB treatment in 21% of South African miners, and aspergillomas were detected in 22% of patients 4 years after treatment.[59] The global prevalence of CPA following TB is estimated to be around 1.2 million cases.[60] The proportion of patients with CPA as a consequence of treated TB varies by country, from 15.3% in the UK to 93% in Korea.[61,62]

Pathogenicity

Aspergillus conidia enter the body by inhalation after environmental exposure and settle in lungs or sinuses, but healthy subjects are able to rapidly remove inhaled conidia. In vulnerable individuals, conidia germinate into hyphae which cause allergic or invasive disease. Other uncommon routes of infection are traumatized skin, especially due to burns, laparostomy wounds, through indwelling intravenous catheters and intravenous drug use. Patient-to-patient transmission is exceptionally rare but has been reported via transplantation of an infected organ and from patients with cutaneous and bronchial aspergillosis.[63]

Neutrophils are the main line of defense against *Aspergillus*, supported by monocytes, tissue macrophages and platelets. Therefore, neutropenia, especially when prolonged and severe, and chronic granulomatous disease are the most well-recognized risk factors for IA. Other risk factors include organ transplant, particularly lung and heart transplant, high-dose corticosteroids or other immunosuppressive agents and HIV infection with a CD4+ lymphocyte count below 50/μL. Recently, IA has been increasingly described in COPD, in the setting of intensive care admission, in patients with high cumulative steroid doses, and in patients with liver disease.[49] IA has complicated influenza and patients on extracorporeal membrane oxygenation (ECMO). Rarely, IA can develop in previously healthy individuals after massive exposure to fungal conidia, e.g. in tree bark chippings or in dug wells. The hallmark of IA, in contrast to other forms of aspergillosis, is angioinvasion.[64] This occurs when hyphae are not contained by local defense mechanisms, and metastatic infections occur, such as brain and skin involvement.

In CPA, hyphae grow in abnormal areas of lung, including pre-existing cavities, e.g. in patients with previous TB, sarcoidosis or bullae, which may have been manifest by a prior pneumothorax. The interior of this cavity supports hyphal growth producing an irregular bumpy surface and mats of mycelia. Months or years later an aspergilloma forms from layers of fungal growth, and often the cavity expands or new cavities are formed. The course of CPA is much more indolent than IA. Other than the structural lung disease, patients with CPA do not usually have a major immune defect, although subtle defects such as gamma-interferon deficiency and vascular endothelial growth factor A (VEGFA) polymorphisms may play a role.[65] Use of immunosuppressive medications, especially corticosteroids, may modulate the course of CPA, leading to a more invasive form, termed semi-invasive aspergillosis, similar to IA but usually more indolent.

Patients with asthma or cystic fibrosis exhibit defective clearance of conidia from the airways, allowing germination, allergen production and stimulation of the production of pro-inflammatory cytokines that lead to the development of symptoms of ABPA.

The fungus secretes various metabolic products (gliotoxin), siderophores and enzymes, such as phospholipases and proteases, which may play a role in virulence, and some are key allergens, involved in setting up long-term allergic responses.[66] Multiple cell surface components resist phagocytic attack, including Rodlet proteins on conidia (which are also immunologically inert) and melanin. A recently discovered key adhesin in *A. fumigatus* is galactosaminogalactan (or GAG) and its epithelial surface-binding protein galectin-3.[67]

Diagnostic Microbiology

Aspergillus is a mold that grows in tissue with dichotomously branching and regular septate hyphae (Figure 189-2). Tissue samples showing microscopic evidence of fungal hyphae are more informative than culture alone, as a positive stain is a strong indicator of infection rather than colonization. Microscopy can also differentiate *Aspergillus* from non-septate molds such as Mucorales, but other molds such as *Fusarium* or *Scedosporium* have similar microscopic morphology. Optical brighteners, such as blankophor P or calcofluor, can improve sensitivity and are recommended especially for samples from immunocompromised patients.

Identification to the species level can be achieved only by culture or molecular testing. *Aspergillus* spp. readily grow on standard bacteriologic media, although mycologic media will give a higher yield and are therefore recommended. Identification to the complex level should always be performed with clinically relevant isolates, as *Aspergillus* spp. differ in their susceptibility to antifungal agents. The many cryptic species now identified in different *Aspergillus* genera prevent routine diagnostic laboratories from identifying each isolate to species level with certainty, so the terminology *A. niger* complex, for example, is used to indicate that sophisticated molecular identification has not been done.[68]

Examples of intrinsically resistant *Aspergillus* species include *A. terreus*, *A. alabamensis*, *A. alliaceus* (*A. flavus* complex) and *A. nidulans* (amphotericin B resistant), *A. ustus* complex (*A. calidoustus*, *A. insuetus* and *A. keveii*), panazole resistant, *A. lentulus* (*A. fumigatus* complex) amphotericin B, itraconazole and voriconazole resistant. *A viridinutans* and *A. fumigatiaffiinis* (*A. fumigatus* complex) itraconazole and voriconazole resistant, and both *A. niger* and *A. tubingensis* (*A. niger* complex) itraconazole and sometimes resistant to other azoles.[69] Therefore correct complex and species identification is important in clinical practice. Clinically significant *Aspergillus* isolates, even those from patients with ABPA, should be tested for antifungal resistance against the agents used for treatment (e.g. itraconazole or voriconazole). Previously rare, azole-resistant aspergillosis is increasingly being described. In a multicenter study, acquired *Aspergillus* resistance was documented in 11 of 17 European centers, with an overall prevalence of 3.2%; among patients with IA, the prevalence of resistance was 5.1%.[70] Resistance may develop on therapy as well, especially in those with a high load of organisms as in aspergilloma and in those with suboptimal concentrations of azole antifungal.[71] Isolates obtained from patients on antifungal therapy should be susceptibility tested.[21]

The diagnostic yield of cultures is low and a negative culture does not rule out the presence of disease. Therefore, at least three respiratory samples should be sent for culture when aspergillosis is suspected. Recent data indicate that culture of larger volumes and direct plating without pretreatment increases yield.[72] Sensitivity of BAL culture is around 30% in hematologic patients with IA, and probably in most other patient groups.[73]

Because of the poor sensitivity of cultures, non-culture-based molecular methods with higher sensitivity are relied upon for diagnosis, both in IA and CPA. The detection of circulating galactomannan (GM) by Enzyme Immuno Assay (Platelia Aspergillus, BioRad Laboratories, France) has become an important tool in the management of neutropenic patients with hematologic malignancy, although significant heterogeneity has been reported between centers using this assay. Serum GM is rarely positive in CPA or ABPA, is not as useful diagnostically in non-neutropenic patients with IA such as solid organ transplant recipients and its sensitivity is drastically reduced in neutropenic patients given mold-active prophylaxis.[74] Falsely positive serum GM has been reported in patients treated with certain antibiotics such as piperacillin–tazobactam (although this may not be an issue any more). The antigen can also be detected in bronchoalveolar lavage (BAL) fluid or CSF.[56] The optimal cutoff for BAL GM is between 1 and 3 arbitrary units. So a BAL GM <1.0 has a high negative predictive value for ruling out IA, especially if *Aspergillus* PCR is also negative, and a value of >3.0 is highly suggestive of an *Aspergillus* infection, which may be IA, CPA or ABPA, depending on the patient context.

(1,3)-β-D glucan (BG) antigen is released by *Aspergillus* and other fungi, and therefore is not a specific test. Its value as a screening assay during neutropenia has not been established, but it has diagnostic value in many settings. In addition, PCR is increasingly being used as an adjunctive diagnostic tool. Its value has been mainly documented

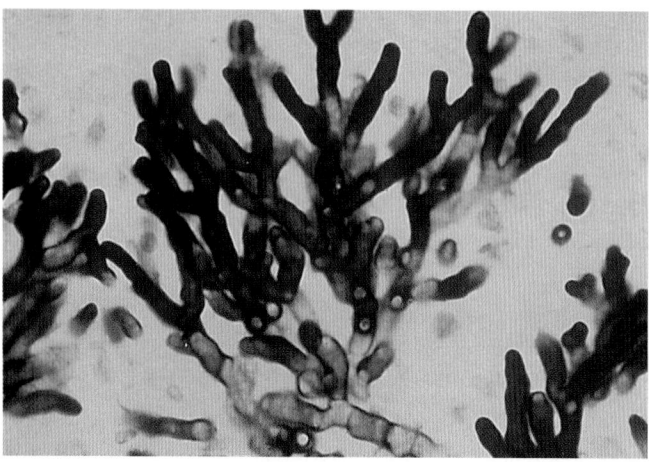

Figure 189-2 *Aspergillus* hyphae.

in blood samples from immunocompromised patients, but is also helpful in BAL or sputum samples. A negative *Aspergillus* PCR in serum has a high negative predictive value and can help rule out IA in high-risk patients. In order to increase sensitivity, culture, GM and PCR can all be sent, without compromising specificity.

Clinical Manifestations

The spectrum of disease caused by *Aspergillus* spp. includes:
- Allergic bronchopulmonary aspergillosis in patients with asthma or cystic fibrosis
- Invasive aspergillosis with pulmonary involvement, or extrapulmonary extension to, CNS, skin, bone and heart
- Chronic pulmonary aspergillosis in patients with underlying lung disease
- Invasive or chronic rhinosinusitis
- Bronchitis
- Superficial disease (external otitis, onychomycosis, keratitis).

ALLERGIC BRONCHOPULMONARY ASPERGILLOSIS

ABPA presents as poorly controlled asthma, with exacerbations consisting of increased amounts of sputum, with mucous plugs, and systemic symptoms like malaise and weight loss. The prerequisite is the presence of immediate-type skin reaction to *Aspergillus* (or *Aspergillus*-specific IgE); absence of the above rules out ABPA. An elevated total IgE (>1000 IU) was required for the diagnosis of ABPA, although the criteria are being revised and lower levels may be acceptable.[75] Peripheral eosinophilia and elevated *Aspergillus* IgG may also be present. Chest imaging may reveal mucous plugging, and, in later stages, central bronchiectasis.

CHRONIC PULMONARY ASPERGILLOSIS

Patients with CPA are more often middle-aged, male and present with long-standing constitutional symptoms (malaise, sweats, anorexia, weight loss) as well as productive cough, chest pain and dyspnea on exertion. Hemoptysis of varying severity is common. Diagnosis is suggested by positive microbiologic (culture, PCR, galactomannan) along with compatible radiologic findings. The confirmatory test is detection of *Aspergillus* IgG/precipitins. Various patterns of progression over time are recognized: patients with a higher degree of immunosuppression (e.g. steroids, diabetes mellitus or HIV) have a more rapid progression over time (usually within weeks), and radiology reveals nodules, infiltrates and cavities, usually with thin walls. This pattern is termed subacute invasive aspergillosis (or chronic necrotizing pulmonary aspergillosis). The majority of patients present with more indolent symptoms, over months or years, and multiple, usually thick-walled cavities on imaging, often with associated aspergillomas, and concomitant pleural fibrosis (termed chronic cavitary pulmonary aspergillosis). Rarely, imaging or lung biopsy show extensive parenchymal fibrosis, typically involving the entire lung (chronic fibrosing pulmonary aspergillosis).[76]

Aspergillomas are conglomerates of fungal material, fibrin and mucus and cellular debris that develop within pulmonary cavities. If there is a single cavity with aspergilloma, no symptoms and imaging is stable over a long period of follow up, a simple aspergilloma is diagnosed, and can be managed conservatively. Aspergillomas that present in the context of CPA require treatment. The most important complication of aspergillomas is hemoptysis, which can be life-threatening.

Finally, CPA may present as a pulmonary nodule, demonstrated incidentally on imaging. This usually raises concerns for malignancy, with evidence of *Aspergillus* found only after computed tomography (CT)-guided or excisional biopsy. If not resected, *Aspergillus* nodules can be followed up with serial imaging and with *Aspergillus* serology. Resection is curative, although monitoring for recurrence of *Aspergillus* disease is warranted. CT scans of various forms of pulmonary *Aspergillus* disease are shown in Figure 189-3.

INVASIVE ASPERGILLOSIS

Invasive aspergillosis may present with nonspecific symptoms, like chest pain, breathlessness, cough and fatigue; fever is often absent. As a result, diagnosis is frequently not suspected, especially in groups not considered high-risk, like ICU patients with COPD. Patients with lower degrees of immunosuppression, such as those on long-term steroids, may present with a more indolent course, termed subacute invasive aspergillosis (or chronic necrotizing pulmonary aspergillosis; see above). High-resolution CT has proved to be a more sensitive and specific tool than conventional chest radiograph in neutropenic patients to diagnose invasive aspergillosis. Findings associated with invasive aspergillosis, although nonspecific, include single or multiple nodules, consolidation, the halo sign and the air crescent sign. *Aspergillus* tracheobronchitis is often seen early in the course of IA, and characteristically affects lung transplant patients. Wheezing, increased secretions and dyspnea are the main features. Diagnosis may be made during surveillance endoscopy; typical features include pseudomembranes or ulcerations.

Invasive aspergillosis is classified according to the revised consensus definitions in the categories proven, probable or possible disease.[77] For definite proof of invasive aspergillosis, a biopsy is required which shows tissue invasion by hyphae in combination with identification of an *Aspergillus* species. CT-guided lung biopsy is a feasible tool in those with peripheral lesions, with negative or conflicting biomarker results, with a good diagnostic yield.[78] For example, in a recent pediatric study, biopsies from deep subcutaneous tissue, visceral organs, or the sinonasal cavity grew a fungus in 27 of 40 cultures submitted (68%). Communication of histology results prompted changes in antifungal therapy in 64% of patients, including initiation of antifungal therapy in 13; surgical excision was done in 15 patients.[79]

EXTRAPULMONARY ASPERGILLOSIS

Extrapulmonary dissemination of pulmonary aspergillosis, especially to the brain, is a well-known complication in the immunocompromised host. Meningitis due to *Aspergillus* spp. can occur, but is rare. Definitive diagnosis is made by biopsy, although the detection of GM in CSF is also highly indicative of CNS aspergillosis.

Virtually any organ can be infected by *Aspergillus* spp. The fungus may cause local infection in the ear or eye (endophthalmitis, keratomycosis). Direct bony invasion or hematogenous spread can occur, causing osteomyelitis. In the gastrointestinal tract, aspergillosis can lead to fatal perforation. Necrotizing skin lesions, similar to those of ecthyma gangrenosum, can be a sign of disseminated aspergillosis. As in candidiasis, aspergilli can form fungal balls in the urinary tract, which present as renal colic.

ASPERGILLUS RHINOSINUSITIS

Aspergillus causes an invasive rhinosinusitis in severely immunocompromised patients, a more chronic rhinosinusitis in patients with milder immunosuppression such as diabetes or steroid use, and allergic rhinosinusitis. Clinical features and predisposing conditions of fungal rhinosinusitis are listed in Table 189-5.[80] It is important to distinguish between noninvasive and invasive rhinosinusitis because the latter can progress through invasion into soft tissue, cartilage and bone into the palate and nose or it can invade cerebral blood vessels, resulting in ischemic infarction and direct infection of the brain.

Chronic indolent invasive sinonasal infections occur in immunocompetent hosts in regions with high levels of environmental spores, such as tropical or desert areas, and occasionally in patients with diabetes in other locales. *A. flavus* is the most common causative agent of these infections, in contrast to the frequent isolation of *A. fumigatus* from sites of infection in immunocompromised hosts. These infections have a progressive clinical course over months to years, with invasion of the surrounding tissues involving the ethmoid sinuses, orbit and subsequently cranial osteomyelitis and intracranial extension.

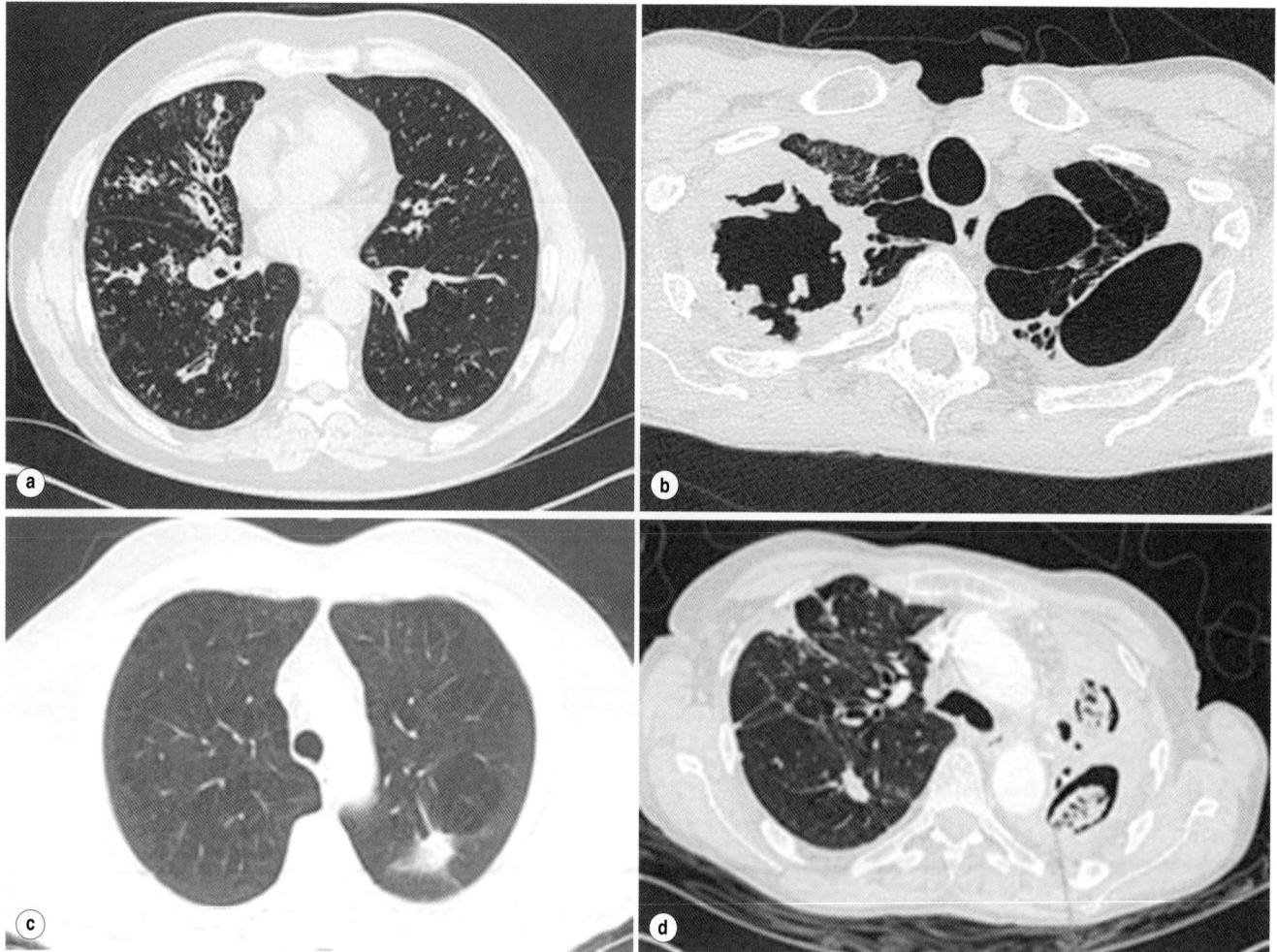

Figure 189-3   CT scan images of various forms of pulmonary *Aspergillus* disease. (a) Allergic bronchopulmonary aspergillosis; (b) chronic cavitary pulmonary aspergillosis; (c) *Aspergillus* nodule; (d) chronic fibrosing pulmonary aspergillosis.

TABLE 189-5	**Key Clinical Points in the Diagnosis and Treatment of Fungal Sinusitis**			
Type	**Clinical Clues**	**Most Common Causes**	**Diagnosis**	**Initial Management**
Noninvasive fungal sinusitis	Immunocompetent patient; intractable symptoms despite adequate treatment for bacterial sinusitis; allergic rhinitis, asthma, nasal polyps. Calcifications in sinus on CT; propoptosis in children	Hyaline molds, *Aspergillus* spp., *Fusarium* spp., dematiaceous molds, *Bipolaris* spp., *Curvularia lunata*, *Scedosporium apiospermum*	Aspiration of sinus contents should be followed by silver impregnation staining and culture of aspirate; sinus contents often have the consistency of peanut butter or cottage cheese; in patients who have diabetes mellitus or other conditions involving immunocompromised hosts, biopsy of healthy and diseased mucosa and bone should be considered to rule out tissue invasion	Surgery is necessary to establish drainage and to remove impacted mucus, polyps or fungus ball
Invasive fungal sinusitis	Fever, headache, epistaxis and cough in an immunocompromised patient; diabetes mellitus; hemochromatosis; protein-calorie malnutrition; leukemia; neutropenia; nasal mucosal ulcer or eschar; calcifications in sinus on CT; orbital apex syndrome; propoptosis in adults	Hyaline molds, mucormycosis *Aspergillus* spp., *Fusarium* spp., dematiaceous molds, *S. apiospermum*	Early endoscopic evaluation should be followed by biopsy of healthy and diseased mucosa and bone; sinus contents should be followed by silver impregnation staining culture of aspirate; if the results of endoscopic evaluation are negative, open biopsy should be performed immediately	Emergency surgery is necessary to remove necrotic and devitalized tissue; treatment with amphotericin B should be initiated on demonstration of tissue invasion and before culture results become available; immunosuppression should be reversed including discontinuation of corticosteroids and treatment of iatrogenic neutropenia

Adapted from DeShazo et al.[80]

Radiologic findings associated with fungal sinusitis are calcifications and loss of bony sinus margins, as well as features that are common in bacterial sinusitis, such as air–fluid levels of more than 8 mm of mucoperiosteal thickening.

To distinguish between invasive and noninvasive fungal sinusitis, adequate tissue biopsies as described in Table 189-5 are necessary. In superficial fungal disease, hyphae are found only in mucopurulent material within the sinus. In invasive fungal infection, hyphae penetrate into the sinus submucosa, blood vessels or bone. The main differential diagnosis is zygomycosis.

ASPERGILLUS BRONCHITIS

A subset of patients with no underlying immunosuppression, usually with bronchiectasis or cystic fibrosis but no other findings on chest imaging, may present with frequent infections not responding to antibiotics, recurrent isolation of *Aspergillus* or positive *Aspergillus* PCR from sputum, along with positive *Aspergillus* serology. For these patients, the term *Aspergillus* bronchitis has been used, and may respond to treatment with antifungals.[81]

ASPERGILLOSIS AND HIV

Aspergillosis and HIV is discussed in Chapter 94.

Management

A high index of suspicion and institution of appropriate antifungal treatment is crucial for survival in IA. Empiric treatment is warranted while awaiting results of investigations. Voriconazole is the first-line treatment for IA, based on a randomized multicenter study that showed a survival advantage over amphotericin B deoxycholate.[82] At week 12, a complete or partial response was noted in 53% of the patients treated with voriconazole compared to 32% of those receiving amphotericin B deoxycholate. Treatment should be started intravenously, at a dose of 6 mg/kg every 12 hours for 1 day followed by 4 mg/kg every 12 hours, and a switch to oral voriconazole (200 mg twice daily) can be considered when the patient is stable. Although use of intravenous voriconazole is not advised in patients with renal failure because of accumulation of the cyclodextrin component, many clinicians would still use it in IA because of the improved outcomes. Multiple observational studies support the preference for voriconazole over all other agents, with an improved survival at 12 weeks of 15–20%.[55,83,84]

Amphotericin B formulations, posaconazole, echinocandins and isavuconazole are all suggested as alternative agents in case voriconazole cannot be used. Isavuconazole has been approved by the FDA for use in IA, based on a non-inferiority trial comparing with voriconazole.[85] Posaconazole has good activity against *Aspergillus*; however not enough data exist on its use in IA. Amphotericin B formulations are not preferred as initial therapy because of the high incidence of nephrotoxicity, and poorer outcomes. The echinocandins are not recommended as initial treatment, except as part of combination regimens, especially in the most immunocompromised patients.

It is highly desirable to monitor azole blood levels, to avoid underexposure due to poor bioavailability, drug interactions with accelerated metabolism and poor compliance, and to minimize adverse events with high blood concentrations. Guidelines for therapeutic drug monitoring of antifungals have been published.[86]

The use of combination therapy for IA has been assessed, both as initial and as salvage therapy. A recent randomized trial of voriconazole vs. voriconazole with anidulafungin in patients with hematologic malignancy or HSCT showed a nonsignificant trend towards improved mortality risk at 6 weeks for the combination regimen (19% vs 28%; $p = 0.087$). Statistical significance was reached for the subgroup of patients with IA diagnosed with CT scan findings and maximum galactomannan positivity and in non-neutropenic patients.[87] In an earlier study, voriconazole plus caspofungin as salvage therapy was compared to historical controls who had received voriconazole monotherapy. Combination therapy resulted in significantly lower mortality at 3

months.[88] Therefore, the use of combination as initial therapy in IA may be considered, especially for the group of patients with proven or probable aspergillosis. Combination therapy without voriconazole cannot be recommended, as it has not been compared to voriconazole monotherapy. Amphotericin B/azole combinations would in theory be antagonistic. Salvage therapy in IA has disappointing results, stressing the importance of early appropriate therapy with voriconazole.[89]

Another issue that remains unresolved is the choice of antifungal in patients who have breakthrough infection during mold-active prophylaxis. Azoles, especially posaconazole, are increasingly used to prevent invasive fungal infection in high-risk patients. There are no studies that address the optimal choice of antifungal drug; breakthrough on itraconazole or posaconazole is usually related to low serum concentrations and intravenous voriconazole overcomes this issue.

Duration of treatment for IA is continued until resolution of clinical and radiologic signs of infection, in general around 6–12 weeks. Duration depends on the extent of disease, the response to therapy and the patient's underlying disease(s) or immune status. Continuation of antifungal therapy through re-induction cancer chemotherapy, or resumption of antifungal therapy in patients with apparently resolved fungal infection who are about to receive re-induction chemotherapy, is worthy of consideration. The ultimate response of these patients to antifungal therapy is largely related to host factors, such as the resolution of neutropenia and the return of neutrophil function, lessening immunosuppression and the return of graft function from a bone marrow or organ transplant, as well as the extent of aspergillosis when diagnosed.

Exacerbations of ABPA are treated with systemic corticosteroids. Various dosing regimens have been used; a regimen equivalent to 0.5 mg/kg of prednisolone, tapered over several weeks, may be used. Patients who respond to steroids are classified as being in remission. Those with recurrent and frequent exacerbations are treated with antifungals, mainly itraconazole. The efficacy of itraconazole in ABPA has been proven in several trials. Itraconazole reduces the fungal, and therefore the allergic, burden, and this can be documented by a reduction in *Aspergillus*-specific and total IgE. It also acts as a steroid-sparing agent and reduces the frequency of exacerbations. The marked interaction of itraconazole with some inhaled corticosteroids requires minimization of inhaled steroid dose, with attention to underlying adrenal reserve to avoid adrenal crises. The duration of treatment is not clear, but withdrawing the antifungal treatment may lead to recurrence.

For patients intolerant or nonresponsive to the azoles, or for azole-resistant disease, there are no satisfactory alternatives. Nebulized amphotericin B can be used, although ~50% of patients may not tolerate it because of bronchospasm, and only 14.3% had a benefit, as evaluated by quality of life questionnaires and FEV_1.[90]

Triazoles are the mainstay of treatment of CPA. Itraconazole is preferred because of cost, followed by voriconazole and posaconazole. Response is assessed by clinical symptoms and quality-of-life scores, *Aspergillus* microbiology and serology, lung function tests and imaging. Prolonged courses are necessary, although benefit is variable; 35% of patients on itraconazole for 6 months improved, 41% remained stable and 23% deteriorated. Relapses are common after discontinuation of antifungals, and some patients may have to be treated for prolonged periods, often lifelong.

For patients who do not respond to oral antifungals, amphotericin B or echinocandins can be used in the form of 3- or 4-week courses that can be repeated according to response or, exceptionally, long term.

Patients with simple aspergilloma can be followed clinically without therapy and preferably have the lesion resected. Aspergillus nodules can be treated with antifungals, although a conservative approach may also be adopted, as the natural history is not clear. Surgical excision may be appropriate for limited disease, with otherwise preserved lung function. Tranexamic acid and bronchial artery embolization can be offered as a temporary measure before surgery in life-threatening hemoptysis, or to avoid surgery in high-risk patients.

Prevention

Preventive measures against IA in high-risk populations include reduction of environmental exposure and antifungal prophylaxis. Specialized air-handling systems capable of excluding *Aspergillus* spores, such as high-efficiency particulate air (HEPA) filtration with or without laminar air flow ventilation, have proven to be very effective in reducing spore counts. However, there is evidence that 50–70% of patients acquire *Aspergillus* infection in the community and go on to develop clinical disease during admission. In those patients air-handling measures will not be effective. The alternative approach is universal or targeted antifungal prophylaxis for patients who are at high risk for developing invasive fungal infections.

The benefit of *Aspergillus* prophylaxis in patients with hematologic malignancy or allogeneic HSCT has been documented. Posaconazole improved survival compared to fluconazole or itraconazole in patients with acute myelogenous leukemia or myelodysplastic syndrome undergoing induction chemotherapy.[91] In allogeneic HSCT recipients, the usefulness of anti-mold prophylaxis has been demonstrated in the setting of graft-versus-host disease (GVHD) requiring high doses of steroids.[92] Different strategies are employed by various centers: the usual approach is to switch from fluconazole to voriconazole or posaconazole when grade II to IV GVHD develops.

In lung transplant recipients, either universal prophylaxis or targeted prophylaxis in patients at high risk (with pre- or post-transplant *Aspergillus* colonization) is used. Nebulized amphotericin B offers the advantage of lack of systemic side effects; however it may not be well tolerated and it is delivered preferentially to the allograft in single lung transplants.[93]

Prevention of allergic *Aspergillus* disease involves avoidance of exposure to fungi, such as in moldy or damp areas at home, or outdoors when handling compost or tree bark chippings. Face masks can be helpful during activities leading to inhalation of large numbers of fungi. Good and regular aeration of rooms is important; HEPA filters may also have a role.

Cryptococcosis

Nature

Cryptococcosis is a pulmonary and usually systemic infection caused by the encapsulated yeast-like fungus *Cryptococcus neoformans*. As early as 1894, Otto Busse described 'corpuscular' tumor-like lesions caused by 'coccidia species'. Since then *C. neoformans* has been known by a variety of names, including *Saccharomyces neoformans* and *Torula histolytica*. Recently common pathogenic species of *Cryptococcus* have been grouped in species complexes – *C. neoformans*, which includes *C. neoformans* var. *grubii* and *C. gattii*, and there are a number of rarer species that occasionally cause disease including *C. terreus*, *C. luteolus*, *C. laurentii*, *C. albidus* and *C. uniguttulatus*. Following from this are proposals that *C. grubii* and *C. neoformans* be recognized as separate species and that with *C. gattii*, there are five separate species.[94]

Cryptococcus neoformans or *C. gattii* commonly cause pulmonary infection, which most likely starts with inhalation of infectious basidiospores. Inhaled basidiospores may cause infection in mice and are more effective than yeast cells in causing cryptococcosis. Humans probably come into contact with *C. neoformans* frequently as the majority of children have been exposed to *C. neoformans* before they reach the age of 5 years, and antibodies are present in adults without a history of disease.[95] In the vast majority of apparently immunocompetent individuals *C. neoformans* infection is either cleared or remains dormant. In immunocompromised individuals, however, *C. neoformans* can cause several pulmonary manifestations and may disseminate, most notably to the CNS causing meningoencephalitis. *Cryptococcus gattii* primarily infects otherwise healthy individuals, with the exception of serotype C isolates of *C. gattii* that were found to be implicated in HIV-associated infections.

Epidemiology

Cryptococcus neoformans var. *grubii* occurs throughout the world and causes 99% of the cryptococcal infections in persons with HIV. *Cryptococcus neoformans* var. *neoformans* also occurs worldwide, but appears to be a more common cause of infection in Europe. *Cryptococcus gattii* infections have been geographically restricted to tropical and subtropical climates, until recently when autochthonous cases have been recognized in Europe and the NW of the USA. *C. gattii* has its main ecologic niche in eucalyptus trees. An outbreak initially detected in Vancouver Island (British Columbia, Canada), which has a temperate climate, has extended southwards over the last decade.[96] This incidence is significantly higher than areas where *C. gattii* is typically observed, such as Australia. The peak incidence of disease coincides with the flowering season of the eucalyptus tree, namely November through February.

Cryptococcal meningitis is one of the most common life-threatening fungal infections in people who have HIV infection.[97] The global burden of disease has been re-estimated using published studies.[98] The annual incidence is highest in sub-Saharan Africa. In HIV, the annual burden is estimated to be 230 100 cases (range 198 000 to 288 000) infections globally, with 169 900 (71%) cases occurring in sub-Saharan Africa. The annual mortality is estimated at 178 900 (126 000 to 236 000) globally. In sub-Saharan Africa, *Cryptococcus* is thought to be responsible for 14.2% of HIV-related deaths. The countries with the highest burdens are Nigeria, South Africa, India, Mozambique, Tanzania, Uganda, Kenya, Ethiopia and Thailand. Cryptococcal pneumonia is also probably common, but underdiagnosed.[99]

With the declining incidence of *C. neoformans* infection in HIV-infected patients treated with highly active antiretroviral therapy (HAART) in high-income countries, organ transplant recipients have re-emerged as one of the leading groups of immunocompromised patients at risk for cryptococcal infections.[100] Cryptococcosis is the third most commonly occurring invasive fungal infection in solid organ transplant (SOT) recipients, representing approximately 8% of invasive fungal infections.[100] Additional risk groups include patients with lymphoma, or receiving high-dose therapeutic steroids, e.g. in the context of sarcoidosis or systemic lupus erythematosus.

Pathogenicity

Cryptococcus neoformans is a facultative intracellular organism. Its pathogenicity depends upon the immune status of the host, virulence factors of the *C. neoformans* strain and the size of the inoculum.

The main fungal virulence factors consist of its ability to grow at body temperature, polysaccharide capsule, phospholipases and production of melanin and extracellular vesicles.[101] The polysaccharide capsule is known to interfere with phagocytosis, antigen presentation and leukocyte migration, and it can activate immunosuppressive T lymphocytes. Most clinical cryptococcal strains develop large capsules during infection. The cryptococcal metabolic products melanin and mannitol can function as antioxidants that can protect the yeast against oxidative attacks of phagocytes. A recent discovery is the recognition that the organism is able to undergo a morphogenetic change resulting in extremely large cells, so-called Titan cells, which appear to have a role in evading host defenses and perhaps in promoting dissemination to the CNS (Figure 189-4).[102] *C. neoformans* also survives macrophage ingestion by promoting what has been called 'vomocytosis' – causing the macrophage to 'spit out' live fungal cells from the phagosome, instead of killing them.[103]

The first line of host defense consists of alveolar macrophages. T lymphocytes are a critical component of the defense against cryptococcal infection, and neutrophils appear to play a minor role.

Diagnostic Microbiology

Cryptococcus neoformans grows on routine laboratory media such as Sabouraud's agar, producing white to cream-colored mucoid colonies, which develop within 36–72 hours. Unlike nonpathogenic cryptococci, *C. neoformans* replicates at 37°C. For blood cultures, the lysis–centrifugation (Isolator) method has been recommended, but more modern automated blood culture systems are also capable of supporting growth. Because *C. neoformans* is susceptible to cycloheximide, media containing cycloheximide should not be used. A rapid test to identify *C. neoformans* is the urease test because cryptococci

produce large amounts of urease in the presence of urea (as do all basidiomycetous yeasts). To distinguish *C. gattii* from *C. neoformans* var. *neoformans*, glycine-L-canavanine-bromothymol blue agar can be used.

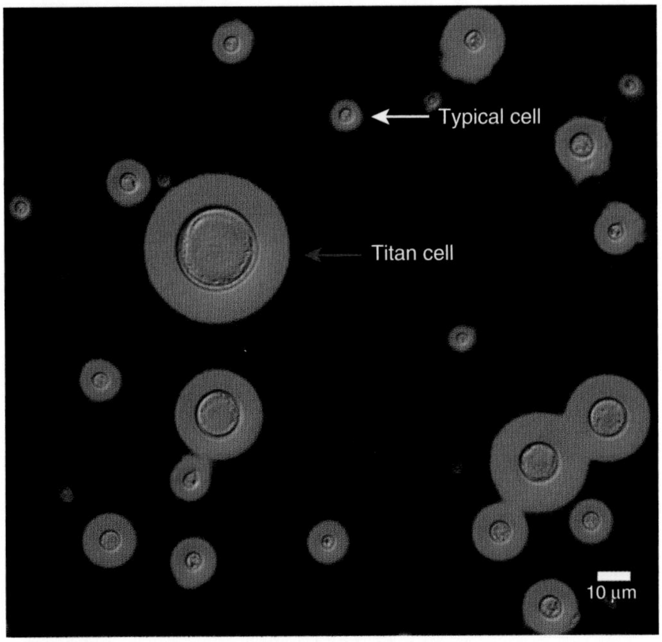

Microscopically, *C. neoformans* can be distinguished from other yeasts by its capsule, which is visualized by an India ink preparation (Figure 189-5). The preparation is made by mixing equal volumes of sample fluid and ink, and ideally one should be barely able to read a newspaper through the preparation. The preparation typically shows budding yeast with a double refractive wall, distinctly outlined capsule and refractive inclusions in the cytoplasm. Occasionally, short hyphal yeast forms can be seen. Unfortunately the India ink preparation is substantially less sensitive than direct detection of cryptococcal antigen in CSF or other fluids and really is only useful if antigen tests are unavailable or very slow to report.[104]

The laboratory diagnosis of cryptococcosis is rather straightforward compared with that of other fungal infections (see Table 189-3).

Cryptococcal antigen may be detected in many body fluids using a lateral flow antigen kit (LFA), latex agglutination tests or ELISA.[104] All species and serotypes are detectable. The LFA is usually used as a screening simple assay, and is suitable for CSF, serum, plasma, finger-prick whole blood samples and urine.[105] It is possible to generate a titer with the LFA, but requires multiple dilutions and LFA devices. As different commercial latex agglutination and ELISA kits vary, absolute titer values are not interchangeable. Low-level positives in non-HIV patients can be difficult to interpret. False-positive results can be caused by rheumatoid factor or (rarely) through cross-reaction with other micro-organisms such as *Trichosporon beigelii* and the bacterium *Capnocytophaga canimorsus* or contamination of the specimen with agar or agarose in the laboratory. Conversely, serum antigen is only detectable in ~70% of patients with cryptococcal meningoencephalitis without HIV, whereas >99% have CSF antigen detectable. False-negative results in blood can be caused by either very low or high antigen titers (prozone effect, especially in patients who have HIV) or because of immune complex formation. Pronase pre-treatment of

Figure 189-4 Cryptococcal 'titan' cell from bronchoalveolar lavage specimen in experimental infection. Red arrow: Titan cell; white arrow: typical cell. Bar = 10 μm. *(Courtesy of Zhongming Li and Kirsten Nielsen.)*

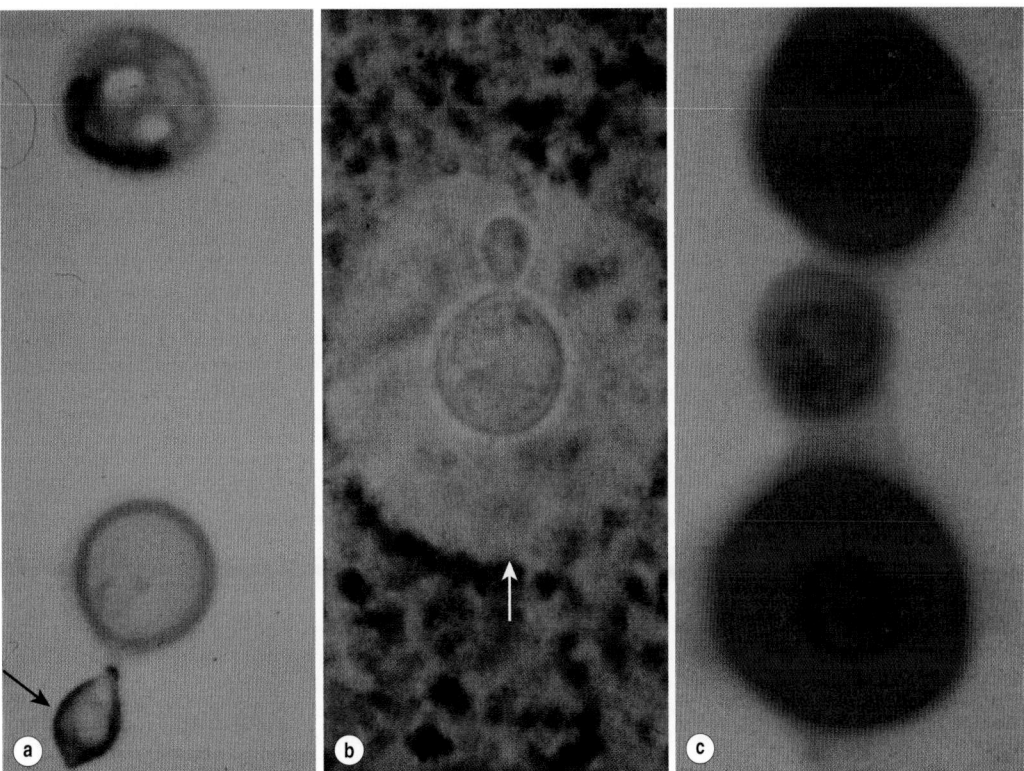

Figure 189-5 *Cryptococcus neoformans.* (a) Cytologic preparation of CSF, narrowly budding yeast (arrow); (b) India ink preparation, cryptococcal capsule shown as translucent halo (arrow); (c) Mayer's mucicarmine stain. *(With permission from Jaster J and Malecha MJ. Cryptococcal meningitis, New England Journal of Medicine 1996; 335:1962. Copyright 1996 Massachusetts Medical Society. All rights reserved.)*

the sample reduces both prozone reactions and rheumatoid factor interactions. Antigen testing in CSF is more sensitive than either India ink preparation or culture. In patients who have pulmonary cryptococcosis without dissemination, serum samples may test negative for cryptococcal antigen. However, in these cases, *C. neoformans* antigen is likely to be positive in BAL fluid. Cryptococci are occasionally isolated from the sputum, although colonies can resemble *Candida* on Sabouraud agar, and be missed. In patients who are not immunocompromised, it is safe to keep the patient under close observation without starting treatment. In all other cases, a careful search for infection of other sites should be made (including CSF examination) and there should be a low threshold for initiating therapy. The value of BAL and/ or sputum analysis for cryptococccal antigen has not been evaluated properly. Antibodies to *C. neoformans* have no diagnostic value and are found in healthy people as well as in those with cryptococcosis.

Susceptibility testing of isolates of *Cyptococcus* spp. is commonly done, but is of unproven value. *C. neoformans* exhibits a phenomenon of heteroresistance to fluconazole related to chromosomal changes and resistance. Isolates from patients with persistent infection or relapse should be checked for changes in the MIC from the original isolate. A fluconazole MIC of ≥16 mg/L or ≥32 mg/L for flucytosine is considered resistant. Amphotericin B resistance is exceptionally rare.

Clinical Manifestations

Although *C. neoformans* usually enters the body through the lungs, the main site of infection is the CNS. However, any other organ can be involved, mainly skin, bone, prostate and eye. The clinical picture of cryptococcosis in patients who have HIV resembles that in severely immunocompromised patients who do not have HIV infection. In SOT recipients the use of calcineurin inhibitors such as tacrolimus and ciclosporin may affect the clinical presentation of cryptococcal disease, but appears to have no influence on the incidence.[100]

In the immunocompetent host, disease is usually more focal, with cryptococcoma formation (especially with *C. gattii*), and disease is more often confined to the lungs.[106] Although survival is higher for infection with *C. gattii*, it causes more neurologic complications, residual disease and relapses than *C. neoformans* var. *neoformans* and *grubii*.[106]

PULMONARY INVOLVEMENT

The clinical picture of pulmonary cryptococcosis depends upon the immune status of the host. In the immunocompetent host, one-third of patients are asymptomatic and in some cases isolation of *C. neoformans* may represent colonization. The majority of patients present with pulmonary symptoms such as cough (54%), chest pain (46%) and sputum production (32%). If cryptococcosis is confined to the lungs, cultures and antigen titers in CSF, blood and urine can be negative.

Compared with the immunocompetent host, cryptococcosis in the immunocompromised patient without HIV infection has a more rapid course with early dissemination. In SOT recipients, 54% of patients had pulmonary disease. Patients receiving a calcineurin inhibitor-based regimen were less likely to have disseminated disease and more likely to have cryptococcosis limited to the lungs.[87] This is thought to be due to the anticryptococcal activity of these compounds.[107] In SOT recipients, pulmonary cryptococcosis may be asymptomatic, present with pneumonia or cavitating nodule and even as acute respiratory failure, which is associated with a grave prognosis.

Patients with HIV infection and pulmonary cryptococcosis are almost invariably symptomatic, presenting with fever (84%), cough (63%), dyspnea (50%), weight loss (47%) and headache (41%). They have disseminated disease, as shown by positive cultures and antigen testing in CSF, blood and urine. Most patients have low CD4+ lymphocyte counts, often less than 100/μL.

Pulmonary cryptococcosis is diagnosed through serum antigen detection or culture of expectorated sputum, BAL, transbronchial lung biopsy (Figure 189-6) or needle aspiration. In all cases, serum and CSF

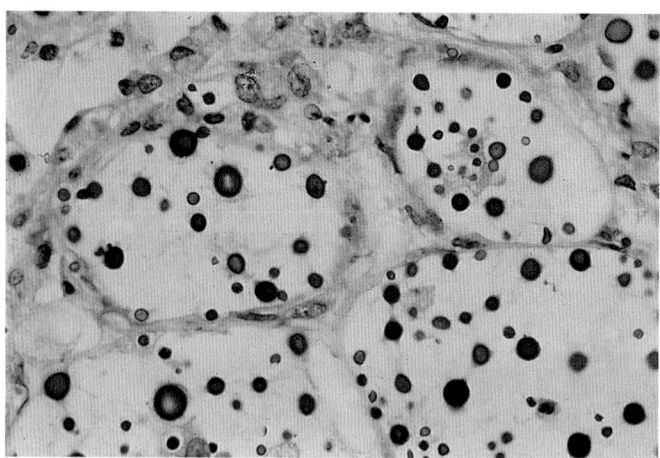

Figure 189-6 Histology of pulmonary cryptococcosis.

analysis for antigen and cryptococcal culture should be performed to assess dissemination.

CENTRAL NERVOUS SYSTEM INVOLVEMENT

If the CNS is involved in cryptococcosis, both the brain and the meninges are usually diffusely affected. In the immunocompromised patient, focal signs of disease are rare. Approximately 70–90% of patients present with signs of subacute meningitis or meningoencephalitis: headache, fever, irritability, dizziness, memory loss, personality change, somnolence, confusion or obtundation.

Classic signs of meningitis such as nuchal rigidity are often absent. Papilledema is seen in one-third and cranial nerve palsies in one-fifth of cases. Symptoms may wax and wane over weeks to months and are often nonspecific. As focal neurologic symptoms due to cryptococcosis occur in only 10% of patients with HIV, these symptoms should alert the physician to alternative pathologies.

Cryptococcal meningoencephalitis in immunocompromised patients who do not have HIV infection resembles the clinical picture in patients who do have HIV infection, with four exceptions:

- the duration of symptoms is usually shorter in patients who have HIV, due to paucity of the inflammatory response and high fungal burden;
- patients who have HIV tend to present earlier in the disease with additional sites of infection such as lungs, skin or blood;
- concomitant infection or malignancies are more likely in HIV;
- raised intracranial pressure is usually seen in patients with HIV, as measured by opening pressure on lumbar puncture.

Patients who improve and then deteriorate while being treated for cryptococcosis with insidious mental impairment, ataxia or other neurologic signs should be evaluated for hydrocephalus by CT. Shunting is indicated for hydrocephalus, without fear of shunt cryptococcal infection.

Cryptococcoma in the brain is rare, usually single and appears as a rounded mass on CT or MR scanning. It is much more common in non-immunocompromised patients, and may be mistaken for a brain tumor. It is problematic to manage. Surgical excision is rarely possible (but desirable if it is possible), and long-term antifungal therapy is usually necessary.

The CSF in cryptococcal meningitis may have glucose and protein levels that are normal, or low and high respectively.

Usually, the CSF contains remarkably few cells, usually all lymphocytes with lower counts in those with HIV and lower CD4+ counts. Cryptococci can be cultured or identified directly through staining with India ink (see Diagnostic microbiology, above); cryptococcal antigen levels in CSF and serum are almost always positive. Semiquantitative CSF cultures showed baseline CSF colony-forming units (cfu) to be an important prognostic factor, with a high burden associated with high mortality, and rate of cfu decline correlating with improved response.[108]

Brain CT is normal in 50% of patients who have cryptococcal meningitis, regardless of whether they have HIV infection. In patients without HIV, the CT may reveal hydrocephalus, gyral enhancement and/or multiple focal nodules with or without contrast enhancement. In patients with HIV, diffuse cortical atrophy is more common. Cerebral MRI appears to be more sensitive than CT in cryptococcal meningoencephalitis. The finding of pseudocysts and choroidal ependymal granulomas (cryptococcomas) is thought to be relatively specific for cryptococcosis. Lesions due to *C. neoformans* var. *gattii* tend to be fewer in number, bigger in size and surrounded by edema as compared to those caused by *C. neoformans* var. *neoformans* and *grubii*.

OTHER SITES OF INFECTION

About 10–15% of patients will develop skin manifestations, which can present in many forms, including papular, nodular or ulcerative lesions, or rarely as cellulitis. In patients without HIV, skin lesions can be the sole site of infection; however, in patients with HIV, cryptococcal skin lesions are almost always a sign of disseminated disease. A diagnosis of cryptococcal skin disease is confirmed by biopsy.

The eye may be affected by cryptococcosis. Visual loss may be due to optic neuritis, occipital lobe infarction or elevated intracranial pressure. Early diagnosis by ophthalmoscopy is important and prompt reduction in CSF pressure is required if elevated to preserve sight. Endophthalmitis occasionally occurs.

From 5% to 10% of patients have bone lesions, especially in those with sarcoidosis, which are mostly osteolytic and have to be distinguished from tuberculosis, other fungi or malignancy. Many other body sites can be affected by *C. neoformans*. In men, the prostate gland is thought to serve as an extraneural reservoir and source of relapse.

Management

In isolated pulmonary cryptococcosis and other non-CNS disease in patients who do not have HIV infection, patients can be treated according to their risk and disease severity. In the immunocompetent asymptomatic patient who has minor lesions on the chest radiograph and no extrapulmonary dissemination, careful observation or fluconazole monotherapy (200–400 mg/day for 3–6 months) is justified because many undergo spontaneous regression. Every patient who has symptomatic or disseminated disease or a compromised immune system should be treated with antifungal medication. In all cases, lumbar puncture should be performed to exclude meningeal involvement.

There is no consensus about the treatment schedule for pulmonary cryptococcosis and other non-CNS disease.[109] For patients who have extensive lobar consolidation or mass lesions (more frequent with *C. gattii*), surgical resection of the lesions can be warranted.

All patients who have cryptococcal meningitis should be treated, regardless of their immune status, because 10–20% will either die or develop serious neurologic sequelae. For patients who have cryptococcal meningitis and HIV, the antifungal regimen of choice is amphotericin B (1.0 mg/kg/day) plus flucytosine (100 mg/kg/day) for 2 weeks, followed by consolidation therapy with fluconazole 400 mg/day for 8–10 weeks, and subsequent maintenance therapy at 200 mg/day, until reconstitution of CD4 cell count (>100 cells/μL and undetectable viral load).[108] Combination therapy with amphotericin B and flucytosine will sterilize CSF within 2 weeks of treatment in 60–90% of patients. The addition of flucytosine to amphotericin B was independently associated with earlier CSF sterilization, and flucytosine prevents early relapse.[110,111] In patients treated with amphotericin B and flucytosine, factors independently associated with mycologic failure at 2 weeks were high serum antigen titer and abnormal brain imaging at baseline.[91] Hematologic malignancy, abnormal neurology at baseline and prescription of flucytosine for less than 14 days were independently associated with treatment failure at 3 months.[112] Recently a

randomized, open-label, phase II trial showed that amphotericin B combined with fluconazole at a dosage of 800 mg/day was safe and slightly more effective than amphotericin B alone, but less effective than amphotericin B and flucytosine, as judged by the rate of CSF clearance of cryptococci. An all-oral regimen of fluconazole 1200 mg and flucytosine 100 mg/kg daily was also more effective than fluconazole alone in reducing mortality.[113] The addition of gamma-interferon subcutaneously may also improve outcome, but has not yet been evaluated with the most active antifungal regimen.[114]

HIV patients with cryptococcal meningitis should have initiation of antiretroviral therapy (ART) deferred for at least 5 weeks to allow improvement in cryptococcosis – mortality is higher in those receiving therapy earlier due to an immune reconstitution syndrome (IRIS). A low CSF leukocyte count was associated with increased death in those given ART early.[115]

For patients with elevated baseline opening pressure, lumbar drainage should remove enough CSF to reduce the opening pressure by 50%. Prior teaching was that those with pressure >25 cm H_2O should have a repeat lumbar puncture every second or third day until the pressure falls into the normal range <19 cmH_2O. Recent data from HIV patients with cryptococcal meningitis suggest that survival is better if a second lumbar puncture is done regardless of the pressure, and if this observation is confirmed, should become standard practice.[116] Mannitol, corticosteroids and acetazolamide are not of value in reducing raised intracranial pressure. Those with persistently elevated pressures benefit from insertion of a lumbar drain, a problem that is more common in non-immunocompromised patients and those with *C. gattii* infections. Occasionally an intraventricular drain is required for persistently raised intracranial pressure. There are no data to support the routine use of direct intraventricular therapy (e.g. via an Ommaya reservoir).

For patients who have cryptococcal meningitis (Table 189-6),[117] but who do not have HIV infection, the regimen of choice is less well defined. In SOT recipients the use of the lipid formulations of amphotericin B (liposomal amphotericin B at a dosage of 3–4 mg/kg/day or amphotericin B lipid complex at a dosage of 5 mg/kg/day) is favored over amphotericin B deoxycholate, because many transplant recipients receiving calcineurin inhibitors have renal function impairment and any further worsening of organ dysfunction should be avoided.[109] A total treatment duration of 4–6 weeks has been successful, but the relapse rate may be lower with longer treatment courses or azole consolidation therapy.

TABLE 189-6	Preferred Treatment Options for Cryptococcal Disease in HIV-Negative Patients

Pulmonary and Other Non-CNS Disease

Mild-to-moderate symptoms or culture-positive specimen from this site
- Fluconazole, 200–400 mg q24h for 6–12 months
- Itraconazole, 200–400 mg q24h for 6–12 months
- Amphotericin B, 0.5–1 mg/kg q24h (total 1000–2000 mg)

Severe symptoms and immunocompromised hosts
Treat like CNS disease

CNS

Induction/consolidation: amphotericin B 0.7–1 mg/kg q24h plus flucytosine 100 mg/kg q24h for 2 weeks, then fluconazole 400 mg q24h for a minimum of 10 weeks

Amphotericin B 0.7–1 mg/kg q24h plus flucytosine 100 mg/kg q24h for 6–10 weeks

Amphotericin B 0.7–1 mg/kg q24h for 6–10 weeks

Lipid formulation of amphotericin B 3–6 mg/kg q24h for 6–10 weeks

The clinician must determine whether to follow lung therapeutic regimen or CNS (disseminated) regimen for treatment of infection in other body sites (e.g. skin). When other disseminated sites of infection are noted or the patient is at risk for disseminated infection it is important to rule out CNS disease. Duration of therapy is based on resolution of disease. *C. gattii* CNS infection may need longer therapy and flucytosine is advised.
Adapted from Saag et al.[117]

For consolidation therapy, it is unlikely that there is any added benefit to routine substitution of fluconazole with extended-spectrum azoles, such as itraconazole, voriconazole or posaconazole. Itraconazole (400 mg/day) was inferior to fluconazole during the consolidation and clearance phases, but may be useful if coexistent aspergillosis, histoplasmosis or fluconazole resistance is present, although monitoring of serum levels is strongly advised. Voriconazole and posaconazole are also alternative agents for similar reasons.

It has been shown that maintenance therapy can be safely discontinued if the CD4 cell count is ≥200/μL for 3 months. The latest guidelines from AIDSinfo (https://aidsinfo.nih.gov/guidelines) state that maintenance therapy can be discontinued when the CD4 cell count has risen to >100 cells/μL and viral load has been undetectable for at least three months, after at least one year of chronic suppressive therapy.

The immune reconstitution inflammatory syndrome (IRIS) is a particular problem in those with HIV, after birth should cryptococcal meningitis occur in pregnancy, and in transplant recipients in whom immunosuppressive medications are rapidly tapered.[118,119] In HIV, the rise in CD4 cell counts in response to antiretroviral therapy (ART) causes the problem. Once ART is started, IRIS develops in up to 20% of patients, days or weeks after starting antifungal therapy. The clinical features are similar to the initial presentation of cryptococcal meningitis, or in body sites not recognized as infected previously, notably lymph node enlargement. Distinguishing failure or relapse of meningitis from IRIS can be difficult, but a declining CSF antigen titer and a marked CSF inflammatory response (protein and leukocyte count) are more consistent with IRIS. No specific treatment is indicated, although a short course of corticosteroids may be helpful if headache and inflammation is marked. Antifungal therapy should continue.[119]

It is advisable to follow patients closely over the first 6–12 months because most relapses occur in the first year after treatment. A persistent CSF antigen titer ≥1:8 is associated with a higher relapse rate, especially in the non-HIV patient. Azole and/or flucytosine resistance may be responsible for relapse of persistent infection.

Prognosis

For patients who have HIV, the mortality rate during initial therapy has been 10–25%, and 30–60% of patients die within 12 months. The relapse rate without maintenance treatment is 50–60%. Currently, the prognosis is mainly determined by the response to HAART. The prognosis for patients who have a malignancy is worse than for patients who have HIV, but this probably reflects the course of the underlying disease rather than the cryptococcosis.

For patients who do not have HIV or cancer, the mortality rate due to cryptococcal infections is about 25–30%. After initial curative treatment, 20–25% of patients relapse. Among cured patients, 40% have significant neurologic deficits such as visual loss, cranial nerve palsy, motor dysfunction, personality change and decreased mental function due to chronic increased intracranial pressure or hydrocephalus. Mortality in patients after SOT is 33–49%.[100]

Adverse prognostic clinical features in patients who do not have HIV infection are listed in Table 189-7.[120]

Mucormycosis (Zygomycosis)

Nature

Agents of mucormycosis cause severe invasive infection in the immunocompromised and patients with diabetes, with high mortality, as well as superficial infection. Mucormycosis refers to disease caused by fungi belonging to the subphylum Mucormycotina, order Mucorales. Recent phylogenetic studies have redistributed the members of the class Zygomycetes to other groups, and therefore the term zygomycosis is no longer relevant. Members of the subphylum Entomophtoromycotina, which is closely related to the subphylum Mucormycotina,

TABLE 189-7	Adverse Prognostic Clinical Features in Cryptococcal Meningitis in Patients Who Do Not Have HIV Infection

- Initial positive India ink examination of CSF
- High CSF opening pressure
- Low CSF glucose
- Low CSF leukocyte count (<20/μL)
- Cryptococci isolated from extraneural sites
- Initial CSF (or serum) antigen titer >1:32
- Corticosteroid treatment or lymphoreticular malignancy

Recurrent cryptococcal disease
- Abnormal CSF glucose concentration after ≥4 weeks of therapy
- Absence of anticryptococcal antibodies
- Post-treatment CSF (or serum) cryptococcal antigen titer of ≥8
- No decrease in antigen titers during therapy
- Daily corticosteroid treatment ≥20 mg prednisone after completion of antifungal therapy

Adapted from Diamond and Bennett.[120]

TABLE 189-8	Risk Factors for Mucormycosis

- Diabetes mellitus, especially with ketoacidosis
- Immunosuppression, especially corticosteroid treatment
- Iron overload with or without deferoxamine treatment (e.g. hemodialysis, hemochromatosis)
- Hematologic disease, especially neutropenia
- Intravenous drug use (CNS mucormycosis)
- Sustained skin trauma/burns/bomb blast injury/tornado or tsunami injury (cutaneous mucormycosis)
- Kwashiorkor, adult malnutrition or acidosis (gastrointestinal mucormycosis)

From Sugar[122] and Yohai et al.[123]

are rare causes of superficial skin infections, mainly in immunocompetent children.

The major forms of mucormycosis include rhinocerebral, pulmonary, cutaneous, gastrointestinal and disseminated disease. The most common organisms that cause mucormycosis in humans are *Rhizopus, Mucor, Rhizomucor, Lichtheimia* (*Absidia*), *Cunninghamella, Saksenaea* and *Apophysomyces*.

Epidemiology

Although these organisms are ubiquitous and grow in decaying organic material, mucormycosis is uncommon and occurs almost exclusively in patients who have an underlying disease, like hematologic malignancy, diabetes with ketoacidosis or iron overload, although it can present in immunocompetent hosts after extensive trauma or burns. It has been reported in metabolicacidosis without diabetes.[121] Risk factors for mucormycosis are listed in Table 189-8.[122,123] Healthcare-associated cases have been linked to contaminated gauze, tongue depressors or intravascular catheters, e.g. in neonatal intensive care units. Multiple cases may occur following natural disasters, i.e. tornados or tsunamis, or after blast injuries in soldiers. Some investigators report an increase in the prevalence of mucormycosis, which might be associated with the increased use of voriconazole that has no activity against these fungi.[125] A comprehensive review of 929 cases of mucormycosis, however, indicated that the increase in cases occurred before the clinical use of voriconazole, especially in bone marrow transplant recipients.[125]

Pathogenicity

Infection usually occurs through inhalation of spores or deposition of spores in the nasal turbinates. Cutaneous mucormycosis is the primary presentation in immunocompetent patients, and results from direct inoculation on abraded skin.

After pulmonary infection, the first line of defense is provided by alveolar macrophages. In animal studies, alveolar macrophages from healthy mice have been shown to inhibit germination of

Rhizopus oryzae spores. In contrast, alveolar macrophages from corticosteroid-treated mice or diabetic mice fail to inhibit spore germination and the mice are rapidly killed by pulmonary and disseminated disease.

Neutrophils play an important role in the second line of host defense. Normal human serum can inhibit the growth of *Rhizopus* spp., unlike serum from patients who have diabetic ketoacidosis, which enhances fungal growth. The presence of elevated available serum iron, e.g. in iron overload states, predisposes the host to mucormycosis, and the iron chelator deferoxamine acts as a siderophore to *Rhizopus*. Although iron chelation with the oral agent deferasirox was beneficial in an experimental model of invasive mucormycosis and enhanced the host inflammatory response to the infection, a randomized combination study of the oral iron chelator with liposomal amphotericin B showed a higher mortality in the combination, compared with amphotericin alone.[126,127]

As in aspergillosis, a hallmark of mucormycosis is angioinvasion, resulting in thrombosis and tissue necrosis. The fungus has a predilection for veins over arteries.

Diagnostic Microbiology

On light microscopy, Mucorales have irregularly shaped, nonseptate, broad (10–20 mm in diameter) hyphae with right-angle branching, visualized with hematoxylin and eosin staining, periodic acid–Schiff (PAS) reaction or Grocott–Gomori methenamine silver nitrate stains (Figure 189-7).

Mucorales grow at temperatures of 25–55 °C with an optimal temperature of 30 °C. Clinical isolates will grow at 37 °C in the laboratory 2–5 days after incubation under aerobic conditions. Cycloheximide inhibits their growth, so culture media containing cycloheximide should not be used. Recovery in culture from clinical specimens is reduced by refrigeration of the sample, vigorous homogenization of the specimen and exposure to antifungal drugs.

As sensitivity of culture is poor, diagnosis is usually made by histology, visualizing the characteristic hyphae invading tissue in samples obtained from biopsy. If culture remains negative, further identification of the species with PCR on the histology sample can be used.

Clinical Manifestations

The clinical manifestations of mucormycosis can be divided into seven syndromes:
- rhinocerebral
- pulmonary
- cutaneous
- gastrointestinal
- CNS
- disseminated
- miscellaneous (e.g. bones, kidney, heart or mediastinum).

The clinical manifestations depend upon the underlying disease.[128] In patients who have diabetic ketoacidosis, rhinocerebral disease is the most common manifestation. Leukemic patients who have neutropenia are susceptible to rhinocerebral, pulmonary and disseminated disease. Children who have kwashiorkor (protein–calorie malnutrition) are especially at risk of developing gastrointestinal mucormycosis. Patients treated with deferoxamine because of iron or aluminum overload mainly present with disseminated mucormycosis.

In general, clues to the diagnosis of mucormycosis are signs of vasculitis with tissue necrosis, such as a black discharge or eschar on the skin, palate or nasal mucosa (Figure 189-8). Also, any radiographic imaging that reveals a lesion that surrounds vessels without a mass effect in an immunocompromised patient is suggestive of mucormycosis. However, no radiologic feature is specific of mucormycosis.

About 60% of rhinocerebral mucormycosis cases occur in diabetic patients. It is a rapidly fulminant disease, presenting with fever, nasal mucosal ulceration or necrosis, sinusitis (in 26% as an early sign), headache and facial pain or orbital involvement. It should be suspected in a diabetic patient presenting with ketoacidosis, who fails to improve or deteriorates after correction of the metabolic abnormality. Thorough physical examination including ear, nose and throat

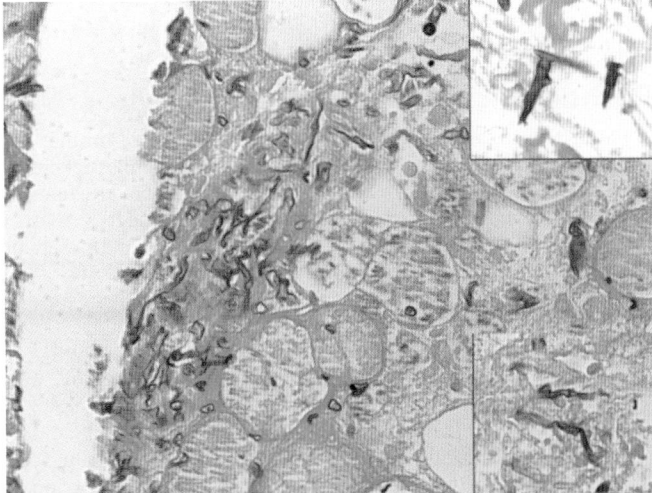

Figure 189-7 Pathology from CT-guided biopsy of lung mass demonstrating mucor. Upper right and lower right insets demonstrate higher magnification of image. *(From Pulmonary mucormycosis: empiricism backfires. Respiratory Medicine Extra 3(2):86–88. Figure 3. Elsevier; 2007.)*

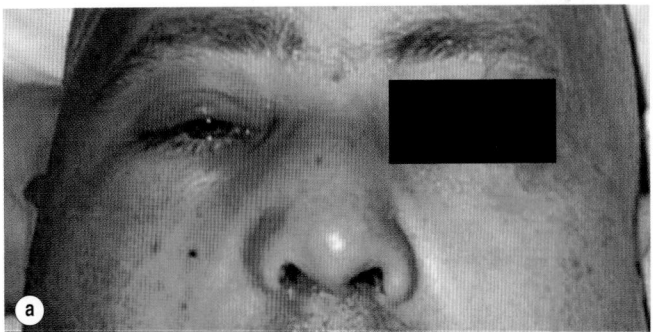
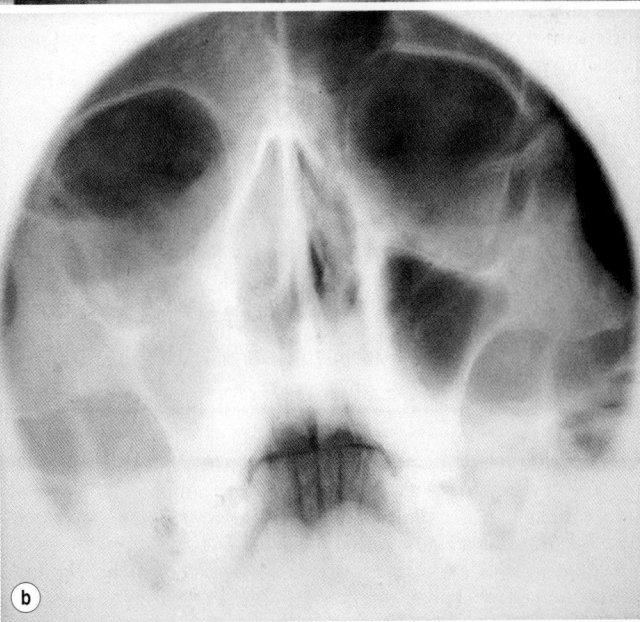

Figure 189-8 An HSCT patient with profound neutropenia who developed invasive mucormycosis. (a) Clinical image: note the altered anatomy over the right cheek as well as orbital swelling. (b) Sinus radiograph of the same patient demonstrating complete opacity of the right maxillary sinus and destruction of the lower bony orbit. *(Courtesy of Prof. J Cohen.)*

examination may reveal the presence of necrotic eschars in the palate or nasal cavity. In rare cases, rhinocerebral disease may follow a chronic course.

The pulmonary form of mucormycosis occurs predominantly in severely neutropenic hematologic patients or those who have diabetes mellitus. It presents with cough, fever, chest pain and dyspnea and progresses rapidly. The diagnosis of pulmonary mucormycosis is difficult to make as the clinical presentation is very similar to that of invasive aspergillosis in patients with cancer. However, concomitant sinusitis and voriconazole prophylaxis were significantly associated with mucormycosis.[129] CT images such as masses, halo sign, air crescent sign and cavities did not discriminate between aspergillosis and mucormycosis. The presence of 10 or more nodules and pleural effusion on the initial CT were associated with mucormycosis, as is the so-called reverse halo sign.[130]

Cutaneous mucormycosis usually occurs after extensive injuries, after exposure to soil or water in immunocompetent patients, but can occur after minor wounds in the diabetic or immunocompromised. It presents initially as cellulitis, with gradual evolution into a necrotic process causing tissue infarction. It has been described in patients on neonatal and critical care units who develop necrotizing infections under gauze dressings. Occasionally, cutaneous mucormycosis is a manifestation of systemic disease. Gastrointestinal mucormycosis is primarily found in patients who have extreme malnutrition. All segments of the gastrointestinal tract can be involved. The clinical symptomatology mimics an intra-abdominal abscess.

CNS mucormycosis is rare and occurs most frequently as a direct extension from the nose or paranasal sinuses, or is associated with intravenous drug use. Cerebral lesions appear on CT scanning as low-density masses with variable peripheral enhancement. Gadolinium-contrast MRI can suggest cavernous sinus thrombosis and thrombosis of other vessels as indirect signs of infection, or ocular muscle involvement may be demonstrated.

In India, a distinctive syndrome of renal mucormycosis is seen usually in non-immunocompromised previously healthy males.[131] Patients present with fever (88%), flank pain (70%) and hematuria or pyuria (70%), usually with concomitant bacterial urinary tract infection. An enlarged non-hydronephrotic kidney on contrast-enhanced CT, with hypodensities (infarctions) and perinephric stranding are typical, usually with the 'cortical rim sign'. Hypodense infarcts need to be distinguished from abscesses. Without early diagnosis and immediate antifungal therapy with amphotericin B and nephrectomy, renal mucormycosis is almost universally fatal.

Management

Mucormycosis is a rapidly progressive disease that warrants immediate aggressive combined surgical and medical treatment.[132] All devitalized tissue should be removed, if necessary repeatedly, followed by reconstructive surgery in a later phase. Optimal treatment of the underlying disease is vital, including rapid correction of ketoacidosis. Intravenous lipid formulation of amphotericin B in high (initial) doses of 5 mg/kg per day is the treatment of choice, and doses up to 10 mg/kg have been used. In a case series of 41 patients, it was shown that the combination of a polyene with caspofungin was more effective than amphotericin B alone for the treatment of invasive mucormycosis.[133] Patients treated with polyene–caspofungin therapy (six evaluable patients) had better survival (100% vs 45%, p=0.02), compared with patients treated with polyene monotherapy. Patients treated with amphotericin B lipid complex had a higher clinical failure rate (45% vs 21%, p=0.04), compared with patients who received other polyenes.

Posaconazole can be used as step-down treatment or as salvage therapy in patients failing amphotericin B. Posaconazole tablets rather the oral suspension should be used because of the uncertain absorption of the oral suspension. Isavuconazole may have a role, although there are no direct comparisons with other agents. A loading dose should be used for posaconazole and isavuconazole. Duration of treatment is prolonged, and depends on ongoing immunosuppression. In diabetic patients, treatment should continue until resolution of all signs of infection.

Prognosis

A high index of suspicion and early diagnosis remains the most important predictor of mortality. A combination of aggressive debridement and antifungal therapy offer the best chance of survival. In neutropenic patients, resolution of neutropenia is crucial. In general, the prognosis is better for those who have diabetes mellitus compared to patients with hematologic malignancy. In the review of 929 cases of invasive mucormycosis, analysis of survival by decade revealed that overall mortality fell from 84% in the 1950s to 47% in the 1990s.[125] However, mortality has remained essentially unchanged since the 1960s, when amphotericin B deoxycholate was introduced. Survival was 3% for cases that were not treated, 61% for cases treated with amphotericin B deoxycholate, 57% for cases treated with surgery alone and 70% for cases treated with antifungal therapy and surgery. By multivariate analysis, infection due to *Cunninghamella* species and disseminated disease were independently associated with increased rates of death. Adverse prognostic factors in rhinocerebral disease include hemiparesis or hemiplegia, bilateral infections, non-diabetic co-morbidity and extensive facial necrosis. Cutaneous disease usually has a better prognosis with aggressive debridement. Gastrointestinal mucormycosis has a high mortality rate and is usually diagnosed at autopsy.

Talaromyces (Penicillium) marneffei

Nature

The fungus *Talaromyces (Penicillium) marneffei* is a dimorphic mold with yeast-like growth in tissue. It came to prominence with the HIV epidemic. The fungus is endemic in South East Asia and was originally isolated from the bamboo rat *Rhizomys sinensis*. It causes deep-seated infections in humans and rodents. Its filamentous appearance is very similar to many species of *Penicillium*, and only recent taxonomy work has placed this dimorphic fungus in the *Talaromyces* genus.

Epidemiology

Before the HIV era, most patients in endemic regions (tropical Asia, especially Thailand, north-eastern India, China, Hong Kong, Vietnam and Taiwan) affected with *T. marneffei* had no known underlying disease. Now, the infection mainly affects patients who have HIV infection and is recognized as an HIV-defining opportunistic infection. In Thailand's Chiang Mai province it is the third most common HIV-related opportunistic infection (after tuberculosis and cryptococcosis).[134].

Pathogenicity

T. marneffei is a facultative intracellular yeast-like organism that can survive and replicate in macrophages. It was also shown that deficiency of CD4+ T-cell-dependent immunity contributes to the development of fatal disseminated infection in HIV-infected patients. Whether infection occurs as a consequence of zoonotic (animal) or saprophytic (environmental) transmission remains unknown.[135] The fungus can be cultured from the internal organs of four species of rodents but has also been recovered from soil specimens.

T. marneffei evokes three patterns of tissue response:
- in the immunocompetent host, granuloma formation with central necrosis;
- suppurative abscesses are found in various organs; and
- in the immunocompromised host, an anergic necrotizing reaction in lung, liver and skin is seen, with diffuse infiltration of macrophages in tissues with proliferating yeast.

Antibody-mediated immunity does not seem to play a major role in host defense, although the host–fungus interaction is poorly understood.[135]

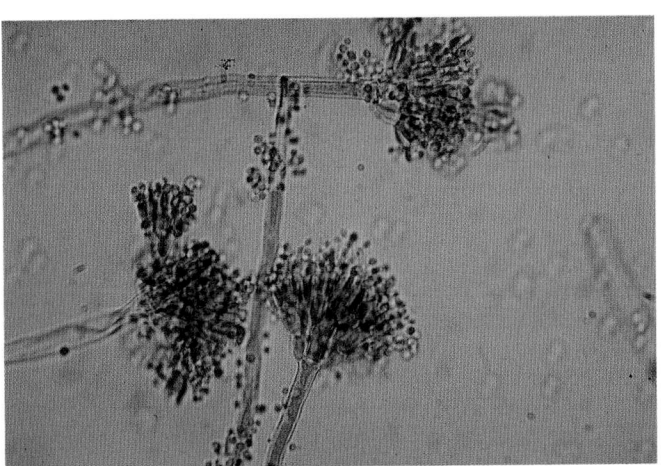

Figure 189-9 Lactophenol cotton blue preparation of *Talaromyces brevi compactum*.

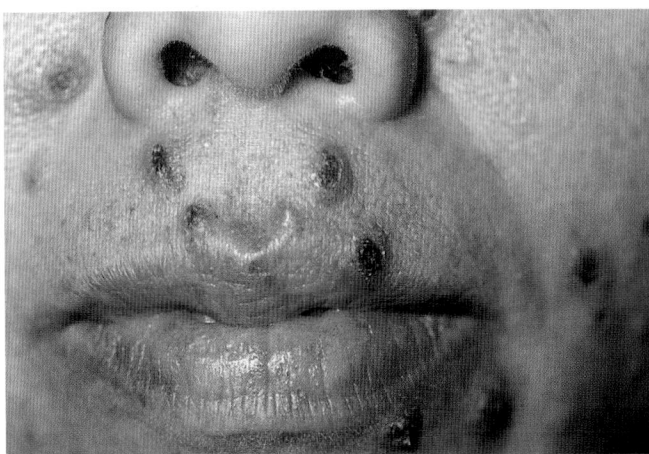

Figure 189-10 HIV-infected patient with *Talaromyces marneffei* infection with molluscum contagiosum-like lesions.

All ages and both sexes may be affected, although 90% of the cases reported in the English literature are male.[136]

Diagnostic Microbiology

In culture, *T. marneffei* exhibits temperature-dependent dimorphic growth. The fungus grows as a mold at 25 °C and looks grayish and downy. It produces a distinctive red diffusible pigment, which is visible on agar media. At 37 °C it grows as a yeast on Sabouraud's glucose agar with cerebriform colonies that do not produce the red pigment.

On microscopic examination (Figure 189-9) *T. marneffei* spp. appear as short, septate, branching hyphae as well as sausage-shaped cells that divide by fission instead of budding, and may show a central septum, which distinguishes it from *Histoplasma capsulatum*. *T. marneffei* can be identified both inside macrophages and extracellularly when tissue preparations are stained with PAS, Wright or Giemsa stain. An elongated yeast cell with a central dividing septum is highly characteristic. Clinical specimens that are commonly used for microscopy and culture include bone marrow aspirate, blood, lymph node biopsies, skin biopsies, skin scrapings, sputum, BAL pellet, pleural fluid, liver biopsies, CSF, pharyngeal ulcer scrapings, palatal papule scrapings, urine, stool samples, and kidney, pericardium, stomach or intestine specimens. Several non-culture-based methods have been developed and evaluated for rapid diagnosis of *T. marneffei* infection using the detection of circulating fungal antigens and fungal DNA. Assays that detect *Aspergillus* galactomannan cross-react with *T. marneffei* antigen.

Clinical Manifestations

In patients who are not immunocompromised, the clinical picture may strongly resemble that of tuberculosis or histoplasmosis (e.g. generalized lymphadenopathy, fever, weight loss, anemia and a nonproductive cough). In patients who have HIV infection, the disease is usually disseminated, affecting skin, reticuloendothelial system, lung and gut. Other tissues that may be involved are liver and spleen, kidney, bone, joints and pericardium. In contrast to histoplasmosis and tuberculosis, adrenal involvement and CNS infections are rare. The molluscum contagiosum-like lesions of skin and mucosa indicate disseminated disease (Figure 189-10).[136] Most patients acquire skin lesions on the face and neck.

Chest radiographs show patchy infiltration and sometimes abscess formation. Abdominal CT scanning often demonstrates hepatomegaly or hepatosplenomegaly, but the diffuse microabscesses that cause the hepatomegaly are usually indistinguishable.

The diagnosis is made by culturing *T. marneffei* from blood, bone marrow, skin scrapings or liver biopsy specimen or by identifying the organism microscopically in a touch smear of a skin biopsy or bone marrow aspirate.

Management

In vitro susceptibility testing shows that the fungus is highly susceptible to itraconazole, voriconazole and flucytosine, moderately susceptible to amphotericin B and not susceptible to fluconazole, whereas micafungin has *in vitro* activity. Recommended treatment of *T. marneffei* infection is amphotericin B (0.5–1.0 mg/kg/day for 2 weeks), followed by itraconazole 200–400 mg/day for 6 weeks for people who do not have HIV infection, and until CD4 count improves in patients with HIV.[137] Secondary itraconazole prophylaxis in advanced HIV disease is partially effective, with long-term survival benefit if combined with antiretroviral therapy.[138,139]

Fusariosis

Fusarium spp. are found in soil with a worldwide distribution and are important plant pathogens. Infections with *Fusarium* spp. are uncommon and are most frequently caused by *Fusarium solani* (50%) followed by *F. oxysporum* (approximately 20% of cases). In humans *Fusarium* spp. may cause a wide range of infections, including superficial (keratitis and onychomycosis), locally invasive and disseminated infections. There have been many well-documented oubreaks of keratitis associated with contaminated contact lens solutions.[140] *Fusarium* spp. may also cause allergic diseases (sinusitis) in immunocompetent individuals and mycotoxicosis in humans and animals following ingestion of food contaminated by toxin-producing *Fusarium* spp.[141] Immunocompromised patients at high risk for fusariosis are those with prolonged and profound neutropenia and/or severe T-cell immunodeficiency. Infections in these patient groups are characterized by rapid dissemination. Fusariosis may be acquired through inhalation of airborne conidia, but skin breakdown (trauma, burns, onychomycosis or cellulitis at toes and fingers) has also been shown to lead to disseminated infection. *Fusarium* spp. may also be recovered from hospital water, and water-related activities and showering appears to be a mechanism for transmission to the immunocompromised host.[142] Most patients have prolonged and severe neutropenia. The disease partially mimics aspergillosis and presents with an abrupt onset of fever, often combined with sinusitis, painful ecthyma gangrenosum-like skin lesions, pulmonary involvement and myalgia.

Histopathologic tissue examination with PAS or Gomori methenamine silver staining reveals vascular invasion by septate branching hyaline hyphae with infarction and necrosis. Contrary to aspergillosis,

50–70% of cases with disseminated fusariosis have positive blood cultures. *Fusarium* spp. grow rapidly on agar media but growth is inhibited by cycloheximide.

Localized infection is likely to benefit from surgical debridement, while systemic antifungal agents are required in disseminated disease. Different species may exhibit different susceptibility to antifungal agents, with *F. solani* commonly being resistant to azoles and with high MICs to amphotericin B, and *F. oxysporum* showing susceptibility to voriconazole and posaconazole. High-dose amphotericin B is therefore recommended for *F. solani* and *F. verticilloides*, and high-dose amphotericin B or voriconazole for other species. Performing *in vitro* susceptibility testing may help to guide antifungal therapy. Response rates are below 50% and depend on the underlying condition of the patient and the possibility of immune reconstitution. Successfully treated disseminated fusariosis tends to recur with repeated bone marrow suppression. Guidelines for the management of *Fusarium* infection are available.[143]

Systemic Fungi

Infections with systemic fungi are acquired by inhaling the airborne conidia (asexual spores) of dimorphic, exogenous fungi. In the lungs, these fungi convert to tissue forms that may disseminate to other internal organs as well as the skin. The etiologic agents, and consequently the prevalence and geographic distribution of their respective mycoses, tend to be restricted to certain geographic areas. The classification as systemic or endemic mycoses is not exclusive, as many opportunistic and subcutaneous mycoses often exhibit systemic clinical manifestations as well as discrete areas of endemicity.

This section will focus on four common systemic and endemic mycoses: blastomycosis, coccidioidomycosis, histoplasmosis and paracoccidioidomycosis. All are caused by dimorphic fungi. The fungi that cause coccidioidomycosis and histoplasmosis can be cultured from dry soil or soil mixed with guano. The habitats of the agents of blastomycosis and paracoccidioidomycosis have not been clearly defined in the environment. Inhalation of conidia of any of these fungi can lead to pulmonary infection, which may or may not be symptomatic. If symptoms are not transient, self-resolving or otherwise immediately manifested, the organism may become dormant and enter a latent phase with the potential to produce active disease in the future. Alternatively, progressive pulmonary disease may develop as may dissemination to other parts of the body. Except for a few extremely rare cases, these infections are not contagious, and there is scant evidence of transmission among humans or animals.

Although most symptomatic cases of blastomycosis, coccidioidomycosis, histoplasmosis and paracoccidioidomycosis occur in patients without significant pre-existing and predisposing disease, individuals with defects of cell-mediated immunity have long been recognized to be at risk for these mycoses if they are exposed by residence or travel in the appropriate endemic areas. In recent years, these infections have increasingly emerged as opportunistic mycoses in patients with HIV/AIDS, due either to new exposure or reactivation of previously latent infections. As described earlier in this chapter, the HIV pandemic has revealed another endemic and systemic, dimorphic, opportunistic pathogen, *Talaromyces marneffei*, which is prevalent in South East Asia.

Blastomycosis, coccidioidomycosis, histoplasmosis and paracoccidioidomycosis are caused respectively by the following dimorphic fungi: *Blastomyces dermatitidis*, *Coccidioides immitis* or *Coccidioides posadasii*, *Histoplasma capsulatum* and *Paracoccidioides brasiliensis*. Each species grows as a mold in nature or the laboratory at temperatures below 37 °C. On routine fungal culture media at 25–30 °C, they produce mycelial colonies that vary in texture, pigment and growth rate, but may be indistinguishable from each other or many saprophytic molds. The ecology and geographic distribution of these fungi is summarized in Table 189-9. Microscopically, the hyphae are uniform in width, hyaline (not pigmented), branched, septate and similar in appearance except for the production of asexual spores or conidia, which are helpful aids to their identification. In the host, or under the appropriate growth conditions *in vitro*, they convert to a distinctive form of growth that is found in tissue: *B. dermatitidis*, *H. capsulatum* and *P. brasiliensis* produce characteristic budding yeast cells, and *C. immitis* and *C. posadasii* produce spherules.

Genetic and molecular research on these fungi in recent years has identified specific genes and signal transduction pathways that trigger host recognition and morphogenetic conversion, which are essential for their pathogenicity.[144] Molecular phylogenetic studies have determined that these pathogenic fungi are closely related and classified

TABLE 189-9	Summary of Systemic Mycoses				
Mycosis	**Etiology**	**Ecology**	**Geographic Distribution**	**Mycelial Form***	**Tissue Form**
Blastomycosis	*Blastomyces dermatitidis*	Unknown (riverbanks?)	Endemic along Mississippi, Ohio and St Lawrence River valleys and southeastern USA	Slow to moderate growth rate. Colonies are white to tan, flat, velvety or cottony. Hyaline septate hyphae and short conidiophores bearing single globose to pyriform conidia, 2–10 μm	Thick-walled yeasts with broad-based, usually single, buds, 8–15 μm
Coccidioidomycosis	*Coccidioides immitis* and *C. posadasii*	Soil	Semiarid regions of southwestern USA, Mexico, Central and South America	Moderate to rapid growth rate. Colonies are white to brown, flat to woolly. Hyaline septate hyphae and arthroconidia, 3 × 6 μm	Spherules, 10–80 μm or larger, containing endospores, 2–4 μm
Histoplasmosis	*Histoplasma capsulatum* var. *capsulatum* and *H. capsulatum* var. *duboisii*	Bat and avian habitats (guano); alkaline soil	Global; endemic in Ohio, Missouri and Mississippi River valleys, central Africa (var. *duboisii*)	Slow growth rate. Colonies are white to brown, flat to woolly. Hyaline septate hyphae and arthroconidia, 3 × 6 μm	Oval yeasts, 2 × 4 μm, intracellular in macrophages
Paracoccidioidomycosis	*Paracoccidioides brasiliensis*	Unknown (soil?)	Central and South America	Slow growth rate. Colonies are flat to velvety, white to brown. Hyaline septate hyphae and rare globose conidia and chlamydospores	Large, multiple budding yeasts, 15–30 μm or larger

*Colony descriptions are for typical isolates grown at 25 °C on Sabouraud's glucose agar.

within the same family of the phylum Ascomycota. All four of these infections begin in the lungs and Chapter 33 provides detailed descriptions of pulmonary blastomycosis, coccidioidomycosis, histoplasmosis and paracoccidioidomycosis.

Blastomycosis

Blastomycosis is a chronic infection characterized by granulomatous and suppurative lesions, but the clinical manifestations may be protean. Following inhalation of airborne conidia, dissemination may occur to any organ, but preferentially to the skin and bones. Although the prevalence of blastomycosis is greatest on the North American continent, autochthonous cases have been documented in Africa, South America and Asia. It is endemic for humans and dogs in the eastern United States and south-eastern Canada. Early histopathologic evidence confirmed that both cutaneous and systemic manifestations originated in the lung; however, the respiratory episode may be completely asymptomatic.

Mycology

At temperatures below 35°C, B. dermatitidis grows as a mold, producing a colony of uniform, hyaline, septate hyphae and conidia. Isolates vary in their rate of growth, colony appearance, and degree and type of conidiation. Many strains produce a white, cottony mycelium that becomes tan to brown with age (Table 189-9). On enriched media at 37°C, B. dermatitidis converts to growth in the yeast form and produces colonies that are folded, pasty and moist.

The mycelia produce abundant conidia from short lateral conidiophores on the aerial hyphae. The conidia are spherical, ovoid or pyriform in shape, smooth-walled and up to 10μm in diameter. Because the colony and conidia of B. dermatitidis may be confused with many other fungi, identification must be confirmed by conversion to the characteristic yeast form. This conversion can be accomplished by in vitro cultivation on rich medium (e.g. brain–heart infusion, chocolate agar or Kelly's medium) at 37°C. Under these conditions or in tissue, B. dermatitidis grows as a thick-walled, spherical yeast that usually produces single buds (Figure 189-11). The bud and parent yeast have a characteristically wide base of attachment and the bud often enlarges to a size equal to that of the parent cell before they separate. Yeast cells are multinucleated and normally range in size from 8μm to 15μm, although some cells reach a diameter of 30μm.

The sexual or teleomorphic form is Ajellomyces dermatitidis. Sexual reproduction may be stimulated in vitro with appropriate tester mating strains, but patients are infected only with haploid strains of one mating type, which reproduce asexually.

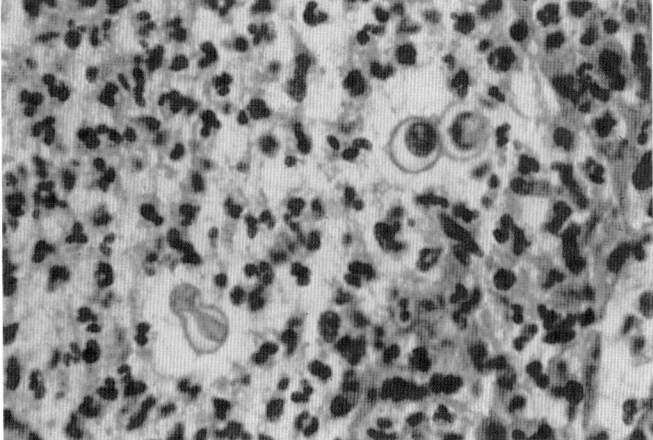

Figure 189-11 *Blastomyces dermatitidis*, yeast form in hematoxylin- and eosin-stained section of microabscess from a cutaneous lesion. This shows large spherical yeasts characterized by thick, highly refractile cell walls, single budding and a broad attachment between the parent yeast cell and bud.

Ecology and Epidemiology

The natural habitat of B. dermatitidis has not been resolved. Over the years, B. dermatitidis has been isolated, but never repeatedly, from soil samples collected in rural environments, including a chicken house, a cattle crossing and several river banks. Positive samples were collected in Wisconsin from a beaver dam associated with a large outbreak of blastomycosis and from a fishing site involved in another outbreak. Several clusters of cases, with or without recovery of B. dermatitidis from environmental samples, have implicated river banks, fresh water and soil.[145]

Dogs are commonly infected and there are numerous reports of isolated cases in other animal species, including indoor cats, but there is no evidence that an animal reservoir perpetuates B. dermatitidis. It probably resides in nature in a protected and dormant condition during most of the year, until it is stimulated by a suitable climatic or other specific but transient event to propagate and produce conidia that become airborne and infectious.

Because B. dermatitidis is not readily recoverable from nature and an adequate skin test antigen is not available for conducting population surveys of exposure, the geographic distribution of blastomycosis has been estimated from reports of human and canine cases. The endemic area extends broadly eastward from states that border the Mississippi River. Blastomycosis is endemic in southern Canada east of Manitoba and, in the USA, in Illinois, Wisconsin, Minnesota, Ohio, the Atlantic Coastal states and the south-eastern states with the exception of Florida. Blastomycosis is rare in the New England and western states. The highest incidence occurs in Arkansas, Kentucky, Illinois, Louisiana, Mississippi, North Carolina, Tennessee and Wisconsin. Within these areas, local pockets of high endemicity have been identified. Canine cases exhibit the same endemic pattern as those of humans. Indeed, blastomycosis may occur more frequently in dogs than in humans. Clinical reports have also documented autochthonous cases in both northern and southern Africa, as well as India, Israel, Mexico and Venezuela. Reports of the infection occurring elsewhere are dubious because the diagnosis was questionable or the patients had a history of travel to an endemic area.

The data from large clinical reviews indicate that blastomycosis occurs more frequently during middle age and in males. Although the disease can occur at any age, 60% of patients were between the ages of 30 and 60 years. Among the hundreds of cases compiled in several reviews, less than 4% of the patients were under 20 years of age and blastomycosis was rarely reported in children. However, in more recent studies, especially involving outbreaks, blastomycosis occurred equally in both sexes and two-thirds of the patients associated with outbreaks have been children (<16 years old).[145]

The male to female ratios reported in several surveys involving hundreds of patients vary from 6:1 to 15:1, but lower ratios have been reported in smaller studies and the overall sex ratio of outbreak cases is approximately 1. Perhaps both sexes are equally susceptible to acute blastomycosis, but males are more inclined to develop chronic or disseminated disease. The other systemic mycoses also occur more often in males (Table 189-10), and male animals are more susceptible (or less resistant) than females to challenge with B. dermatitidis. Blastomycosis may be similar to histoplasmosis in that children are equally susceptible to infection and disease, but the sex-related differences are manifested after puberty.

Genetic or racial differences in prevalence have not been confirmed. Socioeconomic and occupational data have associated blastomycosis with poverty, malnutrition, manual labor, agriculture, construction work and exposure to dust and wood. The incidence of blastomycosis among immunocompromised patients, including patients with HIV, is comparatively lower than that observed with other systemic mycoses.

Pathogenicity

Evidence has linked experimental virulence of strains of B. dermatitidis with the amount of α-1,3-glucan in the cell walls. However, the

TABLE 189-10	Summary of Serologic Tests for Antibodies to Systemic Dimorphic Fungal Pathogens in Patients Without HIV				
			SENSITIVITY AND VALUE		
Mycosis	**Test**	**Antigen**	**Diagnosis**	**Prognosis**	**Limitation/Specificity**
Blastomycosis	CF	By	Less than 50% of cases positive; reaction to homologous antigen only is diagnostic	Fourfold change in titer	Highly cross-reactive
	ID	Bcf	Up to 80% of cases positive, i.e. A band	Loss of A band	More specific than CF test
	EIA	A	Up to 90% of cases positive (titer ≥1:16)	Change in titer	92% specificity
Coccidioidomycosis	TP	C	Early primary infection; 90% cases positive	None	None
	CF	C	Titer ≥1:32 secondary disease	Titer reflects severity (except in meningeal disease)	Rarely cross-reactive with H
	ID	C	More than 90% cases positive, i.e. F and/or HL band		More specific than CF test
Histoplasmosis	CF	H	Up to 83% of cases positive (titer ≥1:8)	Fourfold change in titer	Cross-reactions in patients with blastomycosis, coccidioidomycosis, cryptococcosis, aspergillosis; titer may be boosted by skin test with H
		Y	Up to 94% of cases positive (titer ≥1:8)	Fourfold change in titer	Less cross-reactivity than with H
	ID	H(10X)	Up to 85% of cases positive, i.e. m or m and h bands	Loss of h	Skin test with H may boost m band; more specific than CF test
Paracoccidioidomycosis	CF	P	80–95% of cases positive (titer ≥1:8)	Fourfold change in titer	Some cross-reactions at low titer with aspergillosis and candidiasis sera
	ID	P	98% of cases positive (bands 1, 2 and/or 3)	Loss of bands	Band 3 and band m (to H) are identical

A, antigen A of *B. dermatitidis*; Bcf, culture filtrate of *B. dermatitidis* yeast phase; By, yeast phase of *B. dermatitidis*; C, coccidioidin; CF, complement fixation; EIA, enzyme immunoassay; H, histoplasmin; ID, immunodiffusion; P, culture filtrate of *P. brasiliensis* yeast phase; TP, tube precipitin; Y, yeast phase of *H. capsulatum*.

best characterized virulence factor is BAD1, a cell wall adhesin and immunodominant antigen. This protein contains multiple copies of a 25-amino acid tandem repeat, which binds to CR3 complement receptors and elicits both antibodies and cell-mediated immune responses.[146,147] Compared with less virulent mutants, the wild type contains less surface-bound BAD1. Although the mechanisms whereby BAD1, as well as α-1,3-glucan, contribute to virulence have not been fully elucidated, Klein and associates have postulated that shedding of BAD1 by virulent strains may neutralize macrophage defenses by occupying receptors, diminishing their ability to bind yeast cells.[146] In the alveoli, *B. dermatitidis* induces an inflammatory response characterized by the infiltration of both macrophages and neutrophils and leading to the subsequent formation of granulomata. Both conidia and yeast cells are susceptible to the killing mechanisms of neutrophils and macrophages.[147]

If the pathogenesis of blastomycosis resembles that of histoplasmosis and coccidioidomycosis, most infections may be subclinical and resolve spontaneously. However, because specific and sensitive skin test antigens are lacking, the extent of exposure to *B. dermatitidis* in the general population has not been determined. In addition, calcification is uncommon and there is little radiologic or histopathologic evidence of residual blastomycotic lesions. The best evidence for the existence of subclinical blastomycosis derives from the reported outbreaks, where specific serologic and skin test reactions documented exposure to *B. dermatitidis* in the absence of symptoms.[145]

Diagnostic Microbiology
MICROSCOPIC EXAMINATION
Blastomycosis is best diagnosed by direct examination or positive culture of sputa, skin lesions or other specimens. In calcofluor white

or KOH preparations of pus, exudate, sputum, BAL fluid or other specimens, a diagnosis can be established detecting the characteristic yeast cells of *B. dermatitidis* (see Table 189-9 and description above). In tissue stained with hematoxylin and eosin, the yeast cytoplasm stains darkly and the cell wall appears colorless (Figure 189-11). The multinucleated yeast cells are often abundant in cutaneous lesions. If the yeasts are sparse, fungal cell wall stains, such as PAS or methenamine silver, are helpful.

CULTURE
On most routine culture media, *B. dermatitidis* produces a mold with variable macroscopic features and conidia. Cultures should be incubated at 30°C or room temperature for at least 4 weeks. Their identification is confirmed by growth on a rich medium at 37°C and conversion to the characteristic yeast form. Alternatively, the identity of a culture may be established by an immunodiffusion test to detect a *B. dermatitidis*-specific antigen (antigen A). In addition, DNA probes are commercially available to identify cultures of *B. dermatitidis*, as well as other agents of systemic mycoses.

SEROLOGY
Since the tests for complement fixing antibodies and delayed-type skin reactivity lack specificity and sensitivity, they are not helpful unless the patient is negative to heterologous fungal antigens; even then, positive, monospecific serologic tests to *B. dermatitidis* may not indicate active infection. Serologic tests for antibodies to the specific antigen A, which can be detected by the immunodiffusion test or an enzyme immunoassay (EIA), are more suggestive of infection, but negative tests do not exclude blastomycosis. Table 189-10 summarizes the conventional serologic tests for antibodies to *B. dermatitidis* and other systemic fungi. The most useful serologic procedure is an EIA for antibodies to

antigen A, and EIA titers reflect the severity of disease. False-positive results may occur with sera from patients with histoplasmosis.

Clinical Manifestations

Two classic forms of blastomycosis are recognized: pulmonary, often with dissemination, and chronic cutaneous blastomycosis. Up to 50% of cases may be asymptomatic. A wide variety of symptoms, pathology and radiographic appearances may be observed in blastomycosis. The most common symptoms include cough, weight loss, chest pain, skin lesions, fever, hemoptysis and localized swelling. After the lung, the most frequently involved organs are the skin, bones and genitourinary tract, followed by the central nervous system, liver or spleen.

Primary pulmonary blastomycosis may be asymptomatic or present as acute or subacute pneumonia, ranging from mild to severe (see Chapter 33 for a detailed clinical description). In chronic cutaneous blastomycosis, lesions initially occur as one or more subcutaneous nodules that eventually ulcerate. Lesions are more common on exposed skin surfaces, such as the face or extremities. Spread may occur by extension to contiguous areas and require weeks or months for the ulcerative process to evolve. If untreated, elevated granulomatous lesions with advancing borders will develop. The yeast cells can be observed in microabscesses near the dermis. Extensive, often verrucous, epithelial hyperplasia overlying the abscesses may develop and resemble carcinoma. These extensive cutaneous lesions are characteristically discolored and crusty, and tend to heal and scar in the central, older areas. The active microabscesses found at the leading edge of the lesion can be aspirated or biopsied, and the typical yeast cells of *B. dermatitidis* can be observed on direct microscopic examination.

Dissemination may be widespread and unpredictable in blastomycosis and include the genitourinary tract, CNS and spleen, as well as the skin and bones. Less frequently, the liver, lymph nodes, heart and other viscera are infected. The progressive systemic form of blastomycosis develops in patients with unresolving pulmonary infection, but the degree of pulmonary involvement is not related to the extent of dissemination. This infection may be chronic, with few organisms present, or multiple pulmonary foci may be demonstrable at the time generalized systemic disease develops.

In fulminant cases, the dermal lesions may be more severe than those of chronic cutaneous blastomycosis and are seen in about 75% of cases. Overall, skeletal involvement occurs in approximately a third of patients. Osteomyelitis and, in some cases, draining sinuses to the skin develop, and should be examined for the presence of characteristic yeast cells. Because of the frequency of bone involvement and because almost any bone can be affected, whenever blastomycosis is diagnosed a complete radiographic examination is advisable. Arthritis may develop by extension from infected bone or by direct dissemination from the lung without bone infection. In up to 22% of patients the urogenital tract is involved, especially the prostate, male genitalia, kidney and adrenals. Dissemination to the CNS, resulting in meningitis or brain abscess, occurs in up to 10% of patients.

Primary cutaneous blastomycosis is initiated by traumatic autoinoculation or contamination of an open wound with infectious material. The lymphatics and regional lymph nodes are involved, but the infection remains localized and often resolves without treatment. The natural history and pathology are similar to subcutaneous mycoses (see Chapter 190) and systemic dissemination is rare in the immunocompetent host.

There are well-documented series of patients with HIV/AIDS and blastomycosis. However, the incidence of blastomycosis in HIV-positive patients is not as high as coinfection with other endemic mycoses. Because of the presumed rural reservoir of *B. dermatitidis* or its low census in nature, patients with HIV may be exposed less often than similar patients in the endemic areas for coccidioidomycosis or histoplasmosis. Alternatively, the host defenses against *B. dermatitidis* may be less dependent upon cell-mediated immunity. Cases of blastomycosis and HIV have presented with acute miliary pneumonia and a relatively higher frequency of CNS disease. The management of blastomycosis in immunocompromised patients is more difficult and the prognosis is worse.

Management

As demonstrated by several outbreak cases, primary blastomycosis in immunocompetent individuals may not require therapy. Patients with protracted, severe or progressive primary infection, chronic pulmonary or disseminated blastomycosis require treatment. Mortality is higher in patients with HIV and other immunocompromising conditions.

Itraconazole can be used for mild to moderate disease with success rates higher than 90%, although occasional relapses can occur.[148] Fluconazole was found to be only moderately effective in a pilot study.[149] Voriconazole has also been used successfully. Amphotericin B is recommended for severe disease, with step down to an oral azole after clinical improvement (Chapter 33).[150]

Involvement of the CNS may be treated with liposomal amphotericin B for 4–6 weeks, followed by an azole for 12 months; voriconazole would be preferred because of better CNS penetration.[151] Blastomycosis in patients with HIV may require suppressive therapy with itraconazole until immune reconstitution, similar to the management of cryptococcosis and histoplasmosis. There are no data on the use of echinocandins.

Surgery may be necessary as an adjunct to antibiotic treatment. Because of the occurrence of relapse or reactivation blastomycosis, patients should be observed for years after treatment and resolution of disease.

Prevention

There are no clear guidelines for the prevention of blastomycosis. However, the BAD1 antigen may be an excellent vaccine candidate for future study.

Coccidioidomycosis

Coccidioidomycosis is caused by either of two phenotypically indistinguishable species, *Coccidioides immitis* or *Coccidioides posadasii*, dimorphic fungi that normally live in well-defined geographic areas. Both agents are almost entirely limited to these endemic regions. It was recognized quite early that coccidioidomycosis is confined to the southwestern USA, contiguous regions of northern Mexico and specific areas of Central and South America. The natural reservoir was established by isolating *Coccidioides* species from soil samples collected throughout the endemic areas, and the environmental conditions under which the fungus was propagated have been described. From mycelial culture filtrates, the skin test antigen coccidioidin was developed to detect exposure to *C. immitis* or *C. posadasii* and used to conduct population surveys of skin reactivity. The more common primary form is a mild respiratory ailment, also called valley fever or San Joaquin Valley fever.

Mycology

C. posadasii was described by Fisher et al.[152] They compared the genotypes of isolates of '*C. immitis*' from different geographic regions and, based on their phylogenetic analyses of these populations, determined that the majority of isolates outside California belong to a different species, which they named *C. posadasii*. Although the two species differ in their geographic distribution and genotype, differences in their phenotypes or pathogenicity have yet to be delineated. Because they cannot be distinguished by simple laboratory tests, the more familiar name, *C. immitis*, will be used here.

The life cycle of *C. immitis* (or *C. posadasii*) encompasses several distinct morphologic structures that are produced under different conditions. In nature and in the laboratory, either species grows as a mold, producing hyaline, branching, septate hyphae. As the culture ages, characteristic arthroconidia are formed, usually, but not invariably, in alternate hyphal cells. With time, the arthroconidial chains fragment

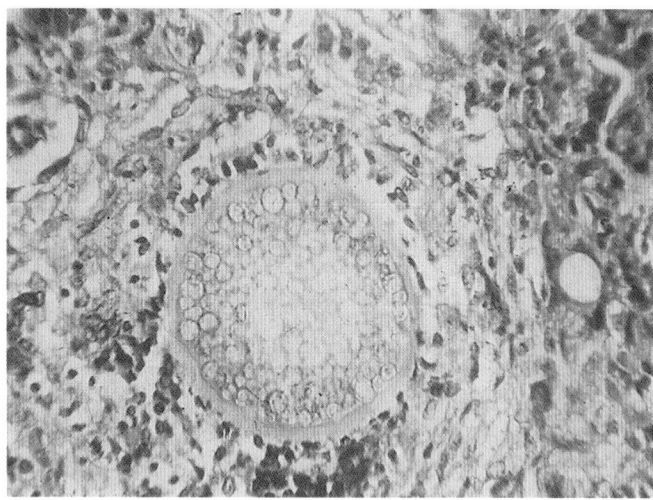

Figure 189-12 *Coccidioides immitis,* spherule in hematoxylin- and eosin-stained section of lung lesion. This shows refractile cell wall and internal endospores.

TABLE 189-11	Risk Factors for Disseminated Coccidioidomycosis
Age	Infants and elderly
Sex	Male
Genetics	Filipino > African American > Native American > Hispanic > Asian
Serum CF antibody titer	>1:32
Pregnancy	Late pregnancy and postpartum
Delayed-type hypersensitivity skin test	Negative
Depressed cell-mediated immunity	Malignancy, chemotherapy, steroid treatment, HIV infection

to release the unicellular, barrel-shaped arthroconidia, which are approximately 3×6 µm in size, easily airborne and small enough to be inhaled into the alveoli. They are highly resistant to desiccation, temperature extremes and deprivation of nutrients, and may remain viable for years. Under appropriate growth conditions the arthroconidia will germinate to recycle the saprophytic mycelial form.

It is likely that a single arthroconidium is capable of causing disease if inhaled. Following their inhalation, the arthroconidia become spherical. In the infected host, *C. immitis* exists as spherules (spherical thick-walled structures, 15–80 µm in diameter) that are filled with a few to several hundred endospores (see Figure 189-12). As a spherule enlarges, the nuclei undergo mitosis, the cytoplasm condenses around these nuclei and a cell wall forms around each developing endospore. At maturation, the spherule ruptures to release its endospores (2–5 µm in size), which may enlarge to form mature spherules. Short hyphae as well as spherules may be observed in the tissues and sputum of patients with coccidioidal cavities of the lungs.

On routine mycologic media, at the usual incubation temperature of 25–30 °C, different isolates of *C. immitis* produce a wide variety of colony types. Because numerous infectious arthroconidia are produced in culture and can be readily aerosolized in the dry state, cultures should be examined only under a safety cabinet that protects both the laboratory worker and the environment. Advice is available about the management of the potentially exposed laboratory worker.[153] Spherules can be produced in the laboratory on a complex medium at 40 °C under 20% CO_2.

Ecology and Epidemiology

In the USA, the geographic areas endemic for coccidioidomycosis and from which *C. immitis* can be isolated from the environment correspond to the Lower Sonoran life zone. These areas are characterized by a semiarid climate, alkaline soil and characteristic indigenous desert plants and rodents. The endemic foci in Mexico, Argentina and other areas of Central and South America are associated with ecologically similar environments. The mycelia, which can be found several inches beneath the soil surface, can be recovered at the surface after the spring rains. As the weather becomes hot and dry, the mycelia convert to infectious arthroconidia, accounting for the peak infection rate during the summer. In the endemic areas, natural infections also occur among indigenous fauna, such as desert rodents, dogs and cattle, as well as companion animals.

In the USA, about 60% of cases of coccidioidomycosis occur in Arizona. Rates have been increasing in many locations. In Arizona the incidence of coccidioidomycosis increased from 30.5 cases per 100 000 in 1998 to 248 cases per 100 000 in 2011.[154] Missouri, not a recognized

endemic area for coccidioidomycosis, had an increased incidence of reported cases from 0.05 per 100 000 population in 2004 to 0.28 per 100 000 in 2013.[155] Autochthonous cases have now been recognized in southern Washington State, and are likely to be found in Oregon.[156]

Inhalation of the arthroconidia of *C. immitis* leads to infection and acquisition of a positive delayed-type hypersensitivity response to coccidioidin. More than half of these infections are benign and most of the others are symptomatic but self-limited, with progressive pulmonary disease and/or dissemination in 1–4%. Some individuals have an increased risk of developing disseminated disease following primary infection (Table 189-11). These include persons in certain ethnic groups, notably Filipinos and African Americans, as well as those with immunosuppression, in receipt of anti-tumor necrosis factor (TNF) therapy and women in the third trimester of pregnancy (Table 189-11).[157] In addition, risks for severe pulmonary disease include diabetes, cigarette smoking, low income and old age.

The areas of endemicity defined by case reports and by isolation of *C. immitis* from soil have been confirmed by skin test surveys with coccidioidin in the USA. Within the endemic areas, which include portions of the southwestern USA (California, Arizona, New Mexico, Nevada, Utah and Texas) and northwestern Mexico, the percent reactivity varies; some of the highest rates are found in Phoenix and Tucson, Arizona, and Kern County, California. Isolated cases of coccidioidomycosis occurring outside the established areas of endemicity have been attributed to fomite transmission of the arthroconidia or to patient travel through the endemic area.

Numerous outbreaks of primary infection have been reported among individuals simultaneously exposed to a heavy aerosol of arthroconidia, notably construction workers, military personnel and archeology students. Prisoners in endemic areas appear to be at particular risk.

Pathogenicity

In vivo, potent cell wall antigens are released when the arthroconidia develop into spherules. Although arthroconidia and endospores are readily engulfed by alveolar macrophages, killing is enhanced by activation of macrophages with the appropriate T cells or cytokines.[158] When stimulated by spherules, leukocytes from both patients and skin test-positive subjects secrete potentially protective cytokines, such as interferon-gamma (IFN-γ) and IL-12 and TNF-alpha. Spherules are resistant to killing by neutrophils.

Investigators have identified several potential virulence factors. For example, *C. immitis* produces a serine proteinase with broad specificity for host substrates, such as elastin, collagen, IgG and IgA. Other proteinases have also been detected and are thought to contribute to the development of spherules and release of endospores.[158]

Many of the patients who develop disseminated coccidioidomycosis have depressed cell-mediated immunity. There is a marked inverse relationship between the antibody titer (see below) and specific cell-mediated immunity, as measured by skin test and, *in vitro,* by the numbers of CD4$^+$ and CD8$^+$ T lymphocytes, the responsiveness of T cells to mitogens or antigens, and the production of cytokines. In severe coccidioidomycosis, patients have elevated antibody titers, circulating immune complexes and depressed cellular immunity. This condition has been related to increased antigen burden, populations of suppressor cells, immune complexes and impaired lymphocyte circulation. Immune complexes are detected in serum of patients with coccidioidomycosis and correlate with the severity of disease.

In the mouse model of experimental coccidioidomycosis, specific anergy is correlated with the amount of coccidioidal antigen present. Recovery often leads to restoration of immune functions. However, the impaired cellular immune responses are likely governed by whether T-helper 1 (Th1) or Th2 responses predominate early in infection.[158] In strains of mice that differ in susceptibility to *C. immitis*, protective responses are correlated with the secretion of IFN-γ, which is a Th1-associated cytokine and potent activator of macrophages. Conversely, much of the immunopathology may be attributable to excess production of TNF. Perhaps the genetic predisposition to disseminated coccidioidomycosis is related to genetic control of the T-cell response to *C. immitis*.

Diagnostic Microbiology

MICROSCOPIC EXAMINATION

A definitive diagnosis of coccidioidomycosis requires the finding of spherules of *C. immitis* in sputum, draining sinuses or tissue specimens (see Figure 189-12). Clinical exudates should be examined directly in 10% or 20% KOH, with or without calcofluor white, and tissue obtained from biopsy can be stained with hematoxylin and eosin or special fungal stains, such as Gomori methenamine silver or the PAS stain, which stain fungal cell walls black or reddish, respectively. Direct microscopic examination of cutaneous or deep tissue specimens, either in calcofluor/KOH preparations or histologic sections, yields positive results in approximately 85% of proved cases. However, sputum specimens are positive by direct examination or culture in less than half of the cases.

CULTURE

C. immitis will grow on Sabouraud's agar or other routine fungal medium at 25–30°C, but not media most suited for bacterial growth. Colonies of *C. immitis* develop within 1 or 2 weeks and are examined for the production of characteristic arthroconidia. Microscopic preparations of mycelia should always be prepared under a biosafety hood. The identification of *C. immitis* can be readily confirmed by demonstrating the production of exoantigen F. Alternatively, DNA-based identification is available with commercial kits.

With the exception of tissue scrapings, biopsies and surgical specimens, cultures are more often positive than microscopic examinations of clinical material. However, use of both procedures will optimize the opportunity to establish a diagnosis. Between 25% and 50% of sputa, bronchial washes, spinal fluids and urine specimens yield positive cultures. Positive blood cultures are infrequent but significantly associated with acute, disseminated coccidioidomycosis and a poor prognosis. Notably, *C. immitis* is cultured from CSF in only approximately 10% of patients with coccidioidal meningitis.

SEROLOGY

Tube precipitins (TP) or latex agglutinins measure specific IgM antibodies. They assist in the diagnosis of primary infections because these antibodies are detected in 90% of patients within 2 weeks after the appearance of symptoms and disappear in most cases by 4 months.

The complement fixation (CF) test, which measures IgG antibodies to coccidioidin, is a useful diagnostic and prognostic tool. The CF titer correlates with the severity of disease, and falls with successful therapy. Most patients with extrapulmonary sites of coccidioidomycosis develop a titer of 1:16 or higher, whereas in pulmonary cases the titer is almost invariably lower, unless chronic cavitary disease is present. While a titer of 1:32 or higher reflects active, disseminated disease, a lower titer does not exclude disseminated disease, because many patients, such as those with single extrapulmonary lesions, notably coccidioidal meningitis, do not develop high titers. Multiple serum specimens are helpful because a change in the CF titer reflects the prognosis. The CF titer declines with recovery and eventually disappears, while a rising titer indicates active, uncontrolled infection and a poor prognosis.

The immunodiffusion (ID) method can be used to detect both TP and CF antibodies by using reference antisera and heated (TP only) and unheated antigen. Antibodies to two specific heat-labile antigens, termed F (or CF) and HL, may be detected.

SKIN TESTS

A positive test for delayed-type hypersensitivity to coccidioidin is denoted by induration exceeding 5 mm in diameter. Skin testing does not induce or boost an immune response. The skin test becomes positive within 2 weeks after the onset of symptoms and before the appearance of antibodies and often remains positive indefinitely. A positive reaction has no diagnostic significance without a history of conversion, but a negative test can be used to exclude coccidioidomycosis, except in patients with severe disseminated coccidioidomycosis who may have become anergic. Indeed, a negative skin test in confirmed cases is associated with a grave prognosis. Conversely, a positive skin test in healthy subjects implies immunity to symptomatic reinfection.

Clinical Manifestations

Following inhalation of arthroconidia, the primary infection in most individuals (around 60%) is asymptomatic. Others may develop flu-like symptoms, sometimes associated with erythema nodosum or erythema multiforme (especially in women), otherwise known as 'Valley Fever'. Primary pulmonary coccidioidomycosis is detailed in Chapter 33.

Primary infection may progress to secondary or disseminated coccidioidomycosis. The numerous manifestations of secondary coccidioidomycosis include chronic and progressive pulmonary disease, single or multiple extrapulmonary dissemination or generalized systemic infection. Dissemination may be fulminant or chronic, with periods of remission and exacerbation. Extrapulmonary lesions most frequently involve the meninges, skin or bone. Chronic cutaneous coccidioidomycosis develops from initial lesions that usually appear on the face or neck and that, over a period of years, evolve into thick, raised, verrucous lesions with extensive epithelial hyperplasia. Bone involvement may accompany generalized systemic disease. Osteomyelitis of long bones, vertebrae and other bones and arthritis may occur. Draining sinus tracts may evolve from subcutaneous and osseous lesions.

Coccidioidomycosis is the HIV-defining illness for many patients, who commonly present with fever and chills, weight loss and night sweats. After pulmonary disease, coccidioidal meningitis is a frequent complication. Serology is often negative in HIV patients and the mortality rate is high. Diffuse pulmonary disease and a low CD4$^+$ lymphocyte count (<50/µL) carry a poor prognosis.

Management

Symptomatic treatment is usually adequate for the patient with primary coccidioidomycosis, although itraconazole or fluconazole may reduce the symptoms. However, if the primary infection is persistent or severe, or if there is evidence of dissemination, fluconazole or itraconazole should be administered for 2–6 months. In an observational study of primary coccidioidomycosis, patients with more severe symptoms were treated; rates of relapse were higher in patients who received antifungals, suggesting that the severity of disease rather than antifungal treatment is the main determinant of relapse.[159]

The chronicity of the disseminated disease usually requires prolonged therapy. Successful treatment may require continuous administration for more than a year. Chronic coccidioidal meningitis is often treated with fluconazole, which has excellent penetration across the blood–brain barrier. Some cases may require the intrathecal administration of chemotherapy. Severe disease is treated with amphotericin B. For patients with HIV, the total dose of amphotericin B should be at least 1.0 g, after which a maintenance regimen of itraconazole or fluconazole may be started. Patients treated with amphotericin B or azoles are more likely to relapse if the delayed skin test becomes negative and the CF antibody titers equal or exceed 1 : 256.

Prevention

Coccidioides immitis cannot be eliminated from the soil, but public health efforts to reduce the dust associated with dispersion of the arthroconidia are helpful in areas of high endemicity. Another approach has focused on the development of a vaccine for persons at risk. In mice and humans, cell-mediated immunity to *C. immitis* confers excellent protection against disease. Spherule-derived vaccines in the past were not successful, but several new approaches to identify specific candidate epitopes are currently under investigation.[158]

Histoplasmosis

Histoplasmosis is caused by the thermally dimorphic fungus *Histoplasma capsulatum*. The infection occurs worldwide and is initiated by inhalation of microconidia produced by the mold form (see Table 189-9). The incidence varies considerably, being negligible in many parts of the world but significant in local regions of endemicity where most of the native population has been infected. Ninety-five percent of these infections are subclinical and detected only by the manifestation of residual lung calcification(s), a delayed hypersensitivity skin test reaction to histoplasmin, or both. The skin test antigen, histoplasmin, is a standardized culture extract similar to coccidioidin.

Mycology

There are three varieties of *H. capsulatum*, but most human cases are caused by *H. capsulatum* var. *capsulatum*, while *H. capsulatum* var. *duboisii* is found in Africa (see below), and *H. capsulatum* var. *farciminosum* causes infection in horses. Although *H. capsulatum* can undergo sexual reproduction with a compatible mating strain, clinical isolates reproduce asexually, being haploid and clonal. *H. capsulatum* and *B. dermatitidis* are closely related ascomycetous fungi and members of the same teleomorphic or sexual genus, *Ajellomyces*.

H. capsulatum is a thermally dimorphic fungus. At temperatures below 35 °C it grows as a mold, often white or brown in color, and at 37 °C it grows as a yeast with small, heaped and pasty colonies. *H. capsulatum* characteristically grows slowly. Under optimal conditions, the mold colony develops after 1 or 2 weeks and conidia are produced shortly thereafter. However, cultures of clinical specimens sometimes require incubation periods of 8–12 weeks before there is detectable growth. Primary isolates are often brown and become white with prolonged cultivation.

Microconidia and macroconidia are produced directly by the aerial hyphae at temperatures below 35 °C. The microconidia are globose and 1–5 μm in diameter. Upon dehydration, they are easily dislodged by the wind and become airborne. Their small size enables the microconidia to be inhaled into the alveoli. The macroconidia are larger and more distinctive. At 37 °C the mold converts to growth as a small, budding yeast. Conversion is often difficult to effect *in vitro* but is enhanced by a rich, complex medium, such as brain–heart infusion agar. The yeast cells are small, ellipsoidal, approximately 1–3 μm × 3–5 μm in size, and virtually identical to the yeasts observed *in vivo* within phagocytes (see Table 189-9 and Figure 189-13).

Ecology and Epidemiology

In nature, *H. capsulatum* lives in soil with a high nitrogen content and is associated with bat and avian habitats. *H. capsulatum* has been isolated many times from bird roosts, chicken houses, bat caves and

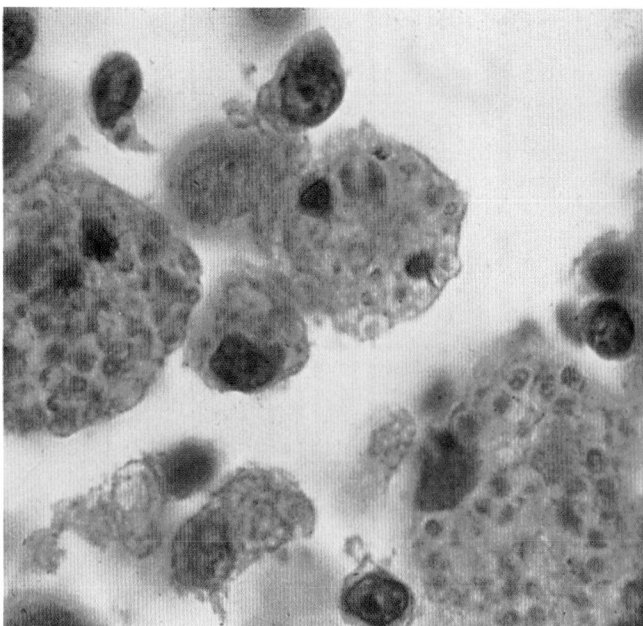

Figure 189-13   *Histoplasma capsulatum*. Small yeast cells packed inside macrophages in a Giemsa-stained smear of bone marrow aspirate.

similar environments. Conidia, when dry, are easily airborne and spread by wind currents, as well as by birds and bats. *H. capsulatum* is most prevalent in the environment where the infection is most endemic, namely in the Ohio–Mississippi Valley: in Missouri, Kentucky, Tennessee, Indiana, Ohio and southern Illinois. This region also has the highest population of starlings, which tend to congregate in large numbers. The excrement from these birds provides an ideal medium for the enrichment of *H. capsulatum*. In South America, the chief reservoir appears to be chicken coops and bat caves.

In cases of histoplasmosis from Africa, both *H. capsulatum* var. *capsulatum* and *H. capsulatum* var. *duboisii* have been isolated. Infections elsewhere are due to the global variety, *H. capsulatum* var. *capsulatum*. *H. capsulatum* var. *duboisii* causes African histoplasmosis, which is distinguished from the usual infection by:

- a greater frequency of skin and bone lesions;
- diminished pulmonary involvement;
- pronounced giant cell formation; and
- larger, thick-walled yeast cells in tissue.

Although these features are characteristic and reproducible, *H. capsulatum* var. *duboisii* cannot be reliably differentiated *in vitro* from the type species on the basis of morphology, physiology and antigenic composition.

Much of the knowledge concerning the prevalence of histoplasmosis has been derived from global skin test surveys with histoplasmin. The region with the highest level of reactivity is the central USA, along the river valleys of Ohio, Mississippi, St Lawrence and Rio Grande, where in some locales 80–90% of the population may be skin-test-positive by the age of 20 years. Foci of high reactivity exist elsewhere in the world, such as southern Mexico, Indonesia, the Philippines and Turkey. In the USA alone, projections based on skin test surveys have led to estimations that more than 40 million people have been exposed with 500 000 new infections every year. Of these, perhaps 55 000–200 000 cases will be symptomatic, 1500–4000 will require hospitalization annually and 25–100 deaths will occur. These projections were made prior to 1980 and do not reflect the increasing incidence of opportunistic histoplasmosis in patients with HIV. Histoplasmosis is the most common endemic mycosis in HIV patients.

Outbreaks or epidemics of acute respiratory histoplasmosis result from the simultaneous exposure of a large number of people. These epidemics are not caused by direct spread among humans or animals.

Rather, the sudden release leads to multiple exposure of a heavy inoculum that has accumulated in a dormant environment. Silos, air-conditioning units contaminated with bird droppings, and accumulations of guano in caves, attics or parks have all been implicated as reservoirs for *H. capsulatum* in outbreaks of this type.

Males develop symptomatic histoplasmosis more often than females and approximately 75% of cases occur in males. Before puberty, the attack rate for males and females is identical and the percentage of positive skin test reactors is the same for both sexes at all ages. These epidemiologic data suggest that either adult males are inherently more susceptible to the disease or females are more resistant. Severity of disease and mortality are greater at the age extremes, in infancy and after the age of 50.

In addition to humans, many wild and domestic animals are susceptible to histoplasmosis. Some animals, including bats, may act as vectors to disseminate the organism in nature.

Pathogenicity

All clinical forms are believed to evolve from the same natural history. Microconidia are inhaled from an exogenous source and penetrate to the alveoli, where they convert to small, budding yeast cells. The conversion of *H. capsulatum* to the yeast form at 37°C is essential for pathogenicity, and expression of yeast-specific genes has been correlated with virulence and thermal tolerance.[160] The yeast cells are readily phagocytized by alveolar macrophages. At this stage, the yeast-laden macrophages may be cleared through the upper respiratory tract. They may also disseminate through the circulation, spreading the yeasts to other reticuloendothelial organs, and/or they may invoke a tissue response *in situ*. The tissue reaction may involve an early influx of neutrophils and lymphocytes, but the pyogenic inflammatory response gives way to epithelioid cell tubercle formation. In the course of these various possible reactions, the intracellular yeasts may or may not be inactivated by the phagocytes, depending upon the immune status of the host.

The phagocytized yeast cells of *H. capsulatum* are able to survive intracellularly by a calcium-dependent process, block acidification within the phagolysosome and multiply within macrophages.[161] However, macrophages from immunized animals, as well as normal macrophages activated by immune lymphocytes or cytokines, restrict the growth of intracellular yeasts. In experimental, self-limited murine histoplasmosis, various parameters of cell-mediated immunity are depressed during the height of antigen (yeast) burden, suppressor T cells and macrophage-like suppressor cells are detected, and production of IL-1 and IL-2 is impaired. Concomitant with resolution of the infection, the number of suppressor cells in the spleen diminishes and T-helper cells increase.[147] These correlations of competent cell-mediated immune responses with resistance to infection are supported by the clinical data. Similar to coccidioidomycosis, there is an inverse relationship between the magnitude of the cell-mediated immune response, as measured by delayed-type hypersensitivity or *in vitro* lymphoblastogenesis and high levels of specific antibody, which correlate with the severity of the disease. Additional evidence suggests that TNF may be crucial in the induction of protective T-cell responses.[147]

Diagnostic Microbiology
MICROSCOPIC EXAMINATION

Histoplasmosis can be diagnosed on finding the yeast cells in clinical material. Suitable specimens include sputum, tissue from biopsy or surgical specimens, spinal fluid and blood. The buffy coat of a blood specimen may reveal yeast-filled macrophages. Bone marrow obtained when patients are febrile may contain yeast cells. Smears of infected sputum, blood, bone marrow or tissue that have been fixed with methanol and stained with the Wright or Giemsa stain will reveal the characteristically small, ellipsoidal yeast cells (approximately 2 × 4 μm) inside macrophages. With either stain, the larger end of the yeast cell contains an eccentric, red-staining mass (see Figure 189-13).

CULTURE

Sputum specimens should be collected early in the morning and purulent or sanguineous portions should be selected for culture. A bronchial wash is even more likely to be positive. Because *H. capsulatum* may grow very slowly, cultures should be incubated for up to 12 weeks, if possible, before discarding as negative. If a sporulating mold develops, *H. capsulatum* can be identified by the presence of its characteristic macroconidia (see Table 189-9) and by conversion to the yeast form by growth on an enriched medium at 37°C, by the detection of *H. capsulatum*-specific exoantigens or by using a specific DNA probe. Lysis-centrifugation is the most sensitive and rapid method to recover dimorphic fungi from blood, especially *H. capsulatum*.

SKIN TEST

The antigen, histoplasmin, is a standardized culture filtrate preparation and 0.1 mL is injected intradermally. A positive reaction is indicated by induration of >5 mm diameter after 48 hours. As with coccidioidin, a positive test, if specific, denotes previous sensitization to *H. capsulatum*. Without a history of prior negativity, the positive test has no diagnostic significance. Histoplasmin is a polyvalent mixture of antigens, only some of which are specific for *H. capsulatum*. Because some antigenic determinants are shared by other pathogenic fungi, cross-reactions can occur. The histoplasmin skin test is rarely used in clinical practice.

SEROLOGY

Antigen testing in blood, urine, BAL or CSF is sensitive, offers rapid diagnosis, and is particularly useful in the immunocompromised with disseminated infection or early in infection when serology is unlikely to be positive. Antigenuria was detected in 92% and antigenemia in 100% of patients with disseminated histoplasmosis, whereas antigenuria was detected in 87% of cases of chronic pulmonary histoplasmosis.[162] Antigen can be used to monitor response to therapy, and to detect relapse. False-positive results with other endemic fungi and rarely with aspergillus have been reported.

Specific antibodies to *H. capsulatum* antigens can be detected during infection. Two serologic tests are now widely accepted because of their convenience, availability and utility: the measurement of antibodies by complement fixation (CF) and the immunodiffusion (ID) test for precipitins. Both tests may be helpful in the diagnosis and prognosis of histoplasmosis, provided the results are properly interpreted (see Table 189-10).

CF tests detect antibodies to two antigens of *H. capsulatum*: histoplasmin and a standardized suspension of killed yeast cells. Because of the possibility of cross-reactivity, patient sera are tested concomitantly against other fungal antigens, such as coccidioidin, spherulin, *B. dermatitidis* or *Paracoccidioides brasiliensis*. Serum antibodies specific for *H. capsulatum* antigens can be detected by the CF test 2–4 weeks following exposure. Most laboratories perform the CF test on twofold dilutions of patient serum, beginning with a dilution of 1:8. With resolution of the infection, the antibody titer gradually declines and disappears (i.e. titer <1:8), in most cases by 9 months. The CF test with either *H. capsulatum* yeast or mycelial (histoplasmin) antigen is very sensitive and 90% of patients are positive (i.e. titer >1:8). A titer of 1:32 that persists or rises over the course of several weeks indicates active disease in patients with an established diagnosis of histoplasmosis. Unfortunately, in sensitive patients, the skin test antigen may boost the CF antibody titer to histoplasmin and the elevated titer may remain for as long as 3 months. If a patient's serum is reactive to more than one antigen or if it is anticomplementary, the ID test should be conducted.

Precipitins can be detected by immunodiffusion (ID) of serum and antigen in agarose. The ID test becomes positive in up to 80% of patients with histoplasmosis by the third or fourth week of infection. This test, while less sensitive and requiring a longer time to become positive, is more specific than the CF test. There are two specific precipitin bands, m and h. The m line, which is observed more frequently, appears soon after infection and may persist in the serum up to 3 years following recovery. The h band is more transient. Because it disappears soon after the disease, the presence of serum antibodies to the h antigen is better correlated with active infection. As with the CF titer, the m band may be boosted by the administration of the histoplasmin skin test.

Clinical Manifestations

Histoplasmosis presents as pulmonary disease in the immunocompetent and as disseminated disease in the immunocompromised. The initial pulmonary episode may be acute or chronic, or dissemination may occur by hematogenous or lymphatic spread from the lungs to other organs. Most individuals are able to contain the infection. The granulomata that form may undergo fibrosis and residual scars may remain in the lungs or spleen. Resolution appears to confer some immunity to re-infection. This process occurs without symptoms in 95% of all persons with acute, primary histoplasmosis, whether disseminated or confined to the lung. For a description of the pneumonic forms of histoplasmosis, see Chapter 33.

The gamut of clinical forms and pathology observed in pulmonary histoplasmosis can also occur in any other part of the body. The yeast cells are probably disseminated throughout the body while inside macrophages. The most common sites of involvement, after the lung, are the reticuloendothelial tissues of the spleen, liver, lymph nodes and bone marrow. However, lesions have been documented in almost every organ. Dissemination may be completely benign and unapparent except for the presence of calcified lesions, usually in organs of the reticuloendothelial system.

In the immunocompromised, disseminated histoplasmosis may be acute and progressive. In such cases, the pulmonary symptoms may not be prominent, and patients may have splenomegaly and hepatomegaly, weight loss, anemia and leukopenia. Skin and mucosal lesions are common. Granulomatous lesions and macrophages packed with yeast cells can be observed throughout the liver, spleen, marrow and, quite often, the adrenals. Acute progressive histoplasmosis is often fulminant and rapidly fatal; ultimately every organ can become diseased. This form of histoplasmosis is an opportunistic disease associated with compromised cell-mediated immunity, such as patients with HIV or those receiving immunosuppressive drugs, transplant patients and those with underlying lymphomatous neoplasia. In most cases, the compromising condition served to reactivate a quiescent lesion that was originally acquired years earlier. Within the endemic area, infants with histiocytosis may develop disseminated histoplasmosis that is characteristically fulminant. Chronic disseminated histoplasmosis may evolve from protraction of the acute disease.

Within endemic regions, histoplasmosis is often the initial HIV-defining condition. Histoplasmosis tends to occur late in the course of HIV; risk factors include environmental exposure to likely sources of *H. capsulatum* and a CD4[+] lymphocyte count of <100/μL.[133]

Management

Itraconazole is the first-line treatment for mild to moderate histoplasmosis, although voriconazole and posaconazole have also been used as salvage therapy. Fluconazole has inferior activity. Amphotericin B is active and is used in severe forms of disease. The echinocandins are ineffective.

Most primary pulmonary infections with *H. capsulatum* go undetected and require no treatment. Mild to moderate acute pulmonary histoplasmosis not requiring admission can be treated with itraconazole. More severe forms are treated with amphotericin B, and steroids are often used concurrently.[163] Management of pulmonary forms of histoplasmosis is discussed in Chapter 33. Recovery following treatment with amphotericin B is generally faster and fewer relapses occur than are experienced with blastomycosis and coccidioidomycosis. Chronic pulmonary lesions may be removed surgically. Cases of meningitis due to *H. capsulatum* are treated with an amphotericin B preparation followed by fluconazole. As noted earlier, voriconazole has been used successfully in a limited number of patients with endemic mycoses.

Prevention

Several approaches are currently underway to develop an effective vaccine for histoplasmosis.[124]

Paracoccidioidomycosis

Paracoccidioidomycosis (South American blastomycosis) is caused by the thermally dimorphic fungus, *Paracoccidioides brasiliensis*. The infection is restricted to endemic areas of Central and South America. It is a chronic, granulomatous disease that begins with a primary, pulmonary, usually inapparent infection that disseminates to produce ulcerative granulomata in the mucosal surfaces of the nose, mouth and gastrointestinal tract. In addition to the skin and lymph nodes, the infection may spread to the internal organs.

Mycology

Colonies of *P. brasiliensis* grow very slowly and the macroscopic features of the mold colony are variable and nonspecific. Various asexual reproductive structures are produced by *P. brasiliensis*, including chlamydospores, arthroconidia and singly borne conidia. In the absence of conidia, which may not be produced for 10 weeks in culture, the mycelia and colony may be indistinguishable from *B. dermatitidis* or many saprophytic molds. The yeast cells, which can be induced by cultivation on a rich medium at 35–37 °C, are readily identified by their unique appearance. As shown in Figure 189-14, the yeasts produce multiple buds, each attached to the parent yeast by a narrow base. The yeast cells are large, up to 30 μm in diameter, and have thinner walls than the yeasts of *B. dermatitidis*. These forms have been described as 'pilot wheels'.

Ecology and Epidemiology

The natural habitat of *P. brasiliensis* has not been proven, but is presumed to be soil. The organism has been recovered only sporadically and not repeatedly from soil in Venezuela and Argentina. Like *B.*

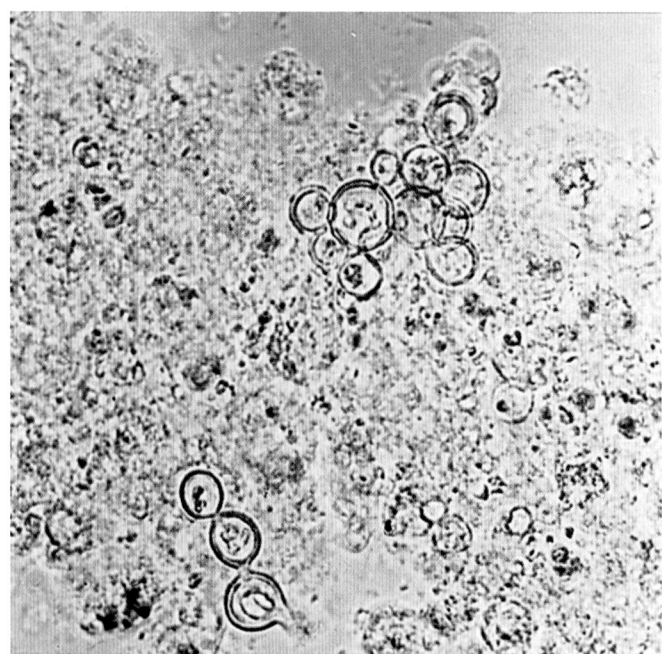

Figure 189-14 *Paracoccidioides brasiliensis*. Large multiply budding yeast cells in a potassium hydroxide preparation of a scraping of cutaneous paracoccidioidomycosis.

dermatitidis, its environmental niche and life cycle in nature are unknown. There is no evidence of an animal vector or transmission of the infection. Human infections are presumed to follow exposure to the organisms from an exogenous source. Most patients are males (>90%), agricultural workers, often malnourished, and usually 30–60 years of age.

Thousands of cases of paracoccidioidomycosis have been reported from Brazil, Venezuela and Colombia, and fewer cases from Argentina, Ecuador and other South and Central American countries, with the exception of Chile and the Caribbean nations. Discrete endemic foci exist within this broad area of geographic distribution. However, all cases are isolated and outbreaks have not been observed. The endemic zones are associated with moderate temperatures (14–30°C) and rainfall, elevation of 150–2000 meters, subtropical forests and river valleys, but not all areas fitting this description have paracoccidioidomycosis.

Skin test surveys have been conducted with various antigens derived from *P. brasiliensis*. These paracoccidioidins exhibit cross-reactivity with histoplasmin and it is difficult to interpret double reactions of equal size in the same individual. As with the skin test antigens of the other dimorphic, systemic pathogens, paracoccidioidin elicits a delayed, indurative reaction that indicates previous exposure. The percentage of reactivity in the endemic areas varies up to 75% and occurs equally in both men and women. Significant risk factors for infection (i.e. positive skin test) include agricultural occupations, association with certain aquatic environments and contact with bats. Many patients with paracoccidioidomycosis are malnourished and exhibit depressed cell-mediated immune responses.

Pathogenicity

P. brasiliensis, like the other systemic fungi, causes disease in males more frequently than females, although skin test surveys have revealed comparable reactivity between the sexes, implying equal exposure. Estrogen binds a regulatory protein in *P. brasiliensis* which blocks conversion of the mycelium to yeast at 37°C and explains the resistance of menstruating females to paracoccidioidomycosis.[164] Once yeast cells of *P. brasiliensis* have developed in the lung, yeast cell wall polysaccharides, such as α-glucan, are associated with virulence and the ability to stimulate granulomata.

Diagnostic Microbiology

Sputum, tissue or scrapings of mucocutaneous lesions may reveal the multiply budding yeast cells that are pathognomonic for *P. brasiliensis* (see Figure 189-14). Specimens should be cultured at 25–30°C on mycologic media. The yeast form often grows better at 35°C or 36°C than at 37°C.

The immunodiffusion (ID) test is extremely useful. As indicated in Table 189-10, nearly all patients have at least one of three specific precipitin lines, which are detected by identity with reference serum. The ID test also has prognostic value, as the bands disappear with clearing of the infection, and the number of bands is somewhat correlated with the severity of the disease. The complement fixation test is quantitative and useful for assessing prognosis, but cross-reactions occur with other fungi.

Clinical Manifestations

More than 90% of cases have a chronic illness which develops from activation of latent cells, usually after several years. In contrast, patients under 30 years of age may develop an acute, progressive 'juvenile' infection characterized by lymphonodular lesions in the lung, with secondary dissemination. The clinical features of paracoccidioidomycosis are discussed in Chapter 33. A rapid, progressive form of disease may occur in patients infected with HIV or other immunocompromised patients. Many patients with pulmonary paracoccidioidomycosis have co-existent pulmonary tuberculosis, regardless of their HIV status. The main sequelae of paracoccidioidomycosis include worsening breathlessness due to pulmonary fibrosis and cavitation, adrenal gland dysfunction (~30%), dysphonia and/or laryngeal obstruction, reduced mouth opening (facial fibrosis) and epilepsy and/or hydrocephalus (~15%).

Management

Since many of the antifungal drugs are effective against *P. brasiliensis*, the initial treatment choice may reflect the expense and local availability of antifungal agents. Itraconazole is currently the drug of choice and a clinical cure rate approaching 100% is achievable with a daily dose of 100 mg for 6 months. Relapses are rare. Fluconazole is also effective, producing cures in about 90% of patients who received 200–400 mg/day for 6 months. Although amphotericin B is highly effective against paracoccidioidomycosis, it should be reserved for patients with severe disease, who fail to respond or cannot tolerate one of the azoles. Trimethoprim–sulfamethoxazole (TMP–SMZ) is also effective against *P. brasiliensis*, although may be less well tolerated and more prolonged courses are needed in order to prevent relapse. After initiating therapy, serologic testing by ID is repeated every few months to document response. Treatment is continued for up to 2 years. Some clinicians recommend a maintenance regimen of TMP–SMZ or itraconazole for up to 1 year after serologic tests become negative or indefinitely for patients with HIV.

References available online at expertconsult.com.

KEY REFERENCES

Agarwal R., Chakrabarti A., Shah A., et al.: Allergic bronchopulmonary aspergillosis: review of literature and proposal of new diagnostic and classification criteria. *Clin Exp Allergy* 2013; 43(8):850-873.

Boulware D.R., Meya D.B., Muzoora C., et al.: Timing of antiretroviral therapy after diagnosis of cryptococcal meningitis. *N Engl J Med* 2014; 370(26):2487-2498.

Cornely O.A., Gachot B., Akan H., et al.: Epidemiology and outcome of fungemia in a cancer cohort of the Infectious Diseases Group (IDG) of the European Organization for Research and Treatment of Cancer (EORTC 65031). *Clin Infect Dis* 2015; 61(3):324-331.

Day J.N., Chau T.T., Wolbers M., et al.: Combination antifungal therapy for cryptococcal meningitis. *N Engl J Med* 2013; 368(14):1291-1302.

Held J., Kohlberger I., Rappold E., et al.: Comparison of (1->3)-beta-D-glucan, mannan/anti-mannan antibodies,

and Cand-Tec *Candida* antigen as serum biomarkers for candidemia. *J Clin Microbiol* 2013; 51(4):1158-1164.

Herbrecht R., Denning D.W., Patterson T.F., et al.: Voriconazole versus amphotericin B for primary therapy of invasive aspergillosis. *N Engl J Med* 2002; 347(6):408-415.

Hope W.W., Walsh T.J., Denning D.W.: The invasive and saprophytic syndromes due to *Aspergillus* spp. *Med Mycol* 2005; 43(Suppl.1):S207-S238.

Marr K.A., Schlamm H.T., Herbrecht R., et al.: Combination antifungal therapy for invasive aspergillosis: a randomized trial. *Ann Intern Med* 2015; 162(2):81-89.

Nguyen M.H., Wissel M.C., Shields R.K., et al.: Performance of *Candida* real-time polymerase chain reaction, beta-D-glucan assay, and blood cultures in the diagnosis of invasive candidiasis. *Clin Infect Dis* 2012; 54(9):1240-1248.

Reboli A.C., Rotstein C., Pappas P.G., et al.: Anidulafungin versus fluconazole for invasive candidiasis. *N Engl J Med* 2007; 356(24):2472-2482.

Roden M.M., Zaoutis T.E., Buchanan W.L., et al.: Epidemiology and outcome of zygomycosis: a review of 929 reported cases. *Clin Infect Dis* 2005; 41(5):634-653.

Schelenz S., Barnes R.A., Barton R.C., et al.: British Society for Medical Mycology best practice recommendations for the diagnosis of serious fungal diseases. *Lancet Infect Dis* 2015; 15(4):461-474.

van der Linden J.W., Arendrup M.C., Warris A., et al.: Prospective multicenter international surveillance of azole resistance in *Aspergillus fumigatus*. *Emerg Infect Dis* 2015; 21(6):1041-1044.

190

Superficial and Subcutaneous Fungal Pathogens

MALCOLM D. RICHARDSON | CAROLINE B. MOORE

KEY CONCEPTS

- Superficial fungal infections (dermatophytoses) are caused by dermatophytes and yeasts, and are among the most common of all communicable diseases.

- Subcutaneous fungal infections (mycoses of implantation) are caused by a large group of heterogeneous environmental fungi.

- Diagnosis is achieved by direct microscopy, culture and in certain infections using molecular tools.

- Superficial infections are treated with terbinafine and azole antifungals.

- Subcutaneous infections are treated with a combination of surgery and antifungal drugs.

Superficial Fungal Pathogens

The majority of superficial fungal infections are caused by three groups of fungi: dermatophytes, *Candida albicans* and *Malassezia* spp.[1] Other pathogens include: *Trichosporon inkin, Piedraia hortae, Neoscytalidium dimidiatum, Alternaria* spp. and non-dermatophyte species causing onychomycosis (for example: *Scopulariopsis brevicaulis*).

Nature

The dermatophytes are limited to the epidermis, hair and nail. Most are unable to survive as free-living saprophytes in competition with other keratinophilic organisms in the environment and thus are dependent on passage from host to host for survival. In general, these organisms have become well adapted to humans, evoking little or no inflammatory reaction from the host. Only dermatophyte infections are truly contagious. *Candida albicans* is the principal agent of candidosis. *Malassezia* spp. are lipophilic (lipid-requiring) yeasts found on the body surface as commensals and are agents of the skin disease tinea versicolor (pityriasis versicolor). In addition, they may be causal in seborrheic dermatitis.

Other fungi cause less common types of superficial disease. *Trichosporon* may cause white piedra, superficial colonizations of the scalp, and axillary and pubic hair shafts. The melanized yeast-like organism *Hortaea werneckii* causes the dark skin lesions of tinea nigra. The rare hair shaft colonization black piedra is caused by *Piedraia hortae*. Finally, approximately 35 nondermatophytic filamentous fungi and a few yeasts have been authenticated as causing onychomycosis. Most prominent among these are members of the genera *Scytalidium, Aspergillus, Scopulariopsis, Fusarium* and *Onychocola*.

Epidemiology

Many cases of dermatophytoses are never brought to medical attention, therefore fully reliable incidence figures do not exist. Onychomycosis, in which the great majority of cases are dermatophytic, may account for 10–30% of all superficial mycoses. An increase in onychomycosis is being seen in patients with diabetes. Tinea pedis has been found to affect 1.5% of pediatric patients, 5.9% of 11–15-year-olds and up to 45% of adult marathon runners. There is a significant age-dependent association between sporting activities and pedal dermatophytosis. Many of the most prevalent dermatophytes are cosmopolitan, but certain species, especially agents of tinea capitis, have defined endemic regions.

Superficial candidosis is in the majority of cases derived from the individual's own endogenous reservoir in the mouth, gastrointestinal tract, lower genital tract, or skin. Cutaneous candidosis is particularly common in infants, at least 10% of whom have candidal skin colonizations. Fifty percent of this colonized group go on to become symptomatic, usually with candidal diaper dermatitis. Many adults harbor an indigenous strain of *C. albicans*; up to 30% of healthy women, for example, are culture-positive for this species in vaginal swab samples, at least when pregnant or taking oral contraceptives. The lower gut may serve as a reservoir when other body sites are free of *C. albicans*. Normal skin only rarely yields *C. albicans* but the yeast may rapidly colonize chronically moist or damaged skin, including moist dermatophyte lesions. Chronic mucocutaneous candidosis (CMC) is a group of rare conditions (autosomal recessive autoimmune polyendocrinopathy candidiasis with ectodermal dystrophy (APECED), autosomal dominant CMC with or without thyroid disease, and autosomal recessive, isolated CMC) that occurs in individuals with underlying endocrinologic disorders or inherited defects in the cell-mediated immunologic responses.

Malassezia spp. have been found as skin commensals in over 90% of humans surveyed.[1] In the temperate zone they only occasionally proliferate to the point of causing the finely scaly maculae of tinea versicolor, but in the tropics the prevalence may reach 50% of the population. In patients who have human immunodeficiency virus (HIV) and other immunocompromised patients, *Malassezia* spp. may cause pustular hair follicle inflammations referred to as *Malassezia* folliculitis, and may be associated with an increased prevalence of seborrheic dermatitis.[1] In atopic individuals, *Malassezia* spp. growing commensally on skin may serve as a triggering allergen in atopic dermatitis.[1]

White piedra is found worldwide, but is now uncommon because of modern hygiene.[1] Black piedra is native to South East Asia, the Pacific and South America. Tinea nigra is of tropical or subtropical origin. *Neoscytalidium* infections of nails, soles or palms are usually acquired in the tropics. Most other agents of nondermatophytic onychomycosis are cosmopolitan saprophytic molds and, despite their opportunistic potential, are more frequently seen as insignificant contaminants of body surfaces than as etiologic agents.[1]

Pathogenicity

Dermatophytes normally infect only the keratinized stratum corneum of the epithelial skin layers.[1] They are restricted to the stratum corneum by cellular immune components. An indication of the relative importance of lymphocytes in host defense is seen in HIV infection, in which helper T-cell counts below 100 cells/mL correlate with a marked increase in onychomycosis, including the unusual 'proximal white' form.

Dermatophytes differ in their host interactions.[1] Anthropophilic dermatophytes, specific to human disease, are distinguished from zoophilic dermatophytes, which have specific animal associations but may be transmitted to humans, and from geophilic dermatophytes, which are occasionally pathogenic to humans or animals but primarily grow on decaying keratinous material. Infection of humans by zoophilic dermatophytes usually elicits a pronounced inflammatory response. Such inflamed lesions may resolve spontaneously, unlike the often chronic lesions of anthropophilic dermatophytoses.

The common anthropophilic dermatophytes include lower body dermatophytes associated with sites other than the scalp, and dermatophytes strongly adapted for tinea capitis, less commonly causing other tineas. *Trichophyton rubrum*, *T. mentagrophytes* complex and *Epidermophyton floccosum* are the common lower body species.[1] Tinea capitis dermatophytes consist of two major groups distinguished by their colonization of hair.

Tinea capitis agents primarily cause new infections in children, and may cause dramatic outbreaks.[1] *Microsporum audouinii* infections spontaneously resolve at 15–19 years of age, but most endothrix agents cause lifelong asymptomatic infections in some adult carriers.[2] New anthropophilic tinea capitis infections are usually acquired via shared headgear, bedding or grooming and haircutting instruments. Adults who acquire new infections caused by endothrix species usually have intimate contact with infected children. Anthropophilic lower body dermatophytoses are often acquired via the feet, either from family members or in communal aquatic or exercise facilities. After infecting the feet, these fungi may go on to infect other body sites.

Zoophilic dermatophytes usually cause tinea corporis or tinea capitis in humans.[1] They may be transmitted directly from infected animals or from fomites, such as fence posts in farm yards. *Microsporum canis* may cause limited outbreaks among humans before virulence is attenuated.

C. albicans is often acquired in the birth canal or in infancy from caregivers.[1] Generally, an individual harbors only one or two strains. Cutaneous candidosis is predisposed to by warm, moist conditions with abrasion, especially in the diaper rash of infancy but also in adult occupations that involve wet hands. In the latter cases, paronychia or interdigital erosion frequently results. Intertriginous candidosis occurs in moist body folds and is exacerbated by diabetes mellitus or obesity. Chronic mucocutaneous candidosis (CMC), in which skin and mucosa are extensively colonized by *C. albicans*, results from inherited defects in cellular immunity[1] (see also Chapter 78).

Malassezia spp. are also generally acquired as commensal surface flora in early infancy. They primarily use fatty acids secreted by the skin. Corticosteroid use, Cushing's disease, malnutrition and immunosuppression may contribute to an increased frequency of tinea versicolor.

Prevention

Details regarding the prevention of infection caused by agents of superficial fungal infection, diagnosis, clinical manifestations and management can be found in Chapters 14 and 79.

Diagnostic Microbiology

Additional details regarding diagnosis of superficial fungal infections can be found in Chapter 14.

DIRECT MICROSCOPY AND FUNGAL CULTURE

Superficial mycotic infections are best diagnosed by the combination of two techniques: direct microscopy to detect fungal elements in potassium hydroxide (KOH) slides, and fungal culture.[3] Direct microscopy may be facilitated by the use of fluorescent fungal cell wall dyes such as Calcofluor White or Congo Red. Histopathology performed with fungal stains has been suggested as an alternative to 'KOH and culture' for onychomycosis.[3]

The characteristics and criteria used in identifying dermatophytes are well illustrated in a recently published identification manual.[4] Since most dermatophyte species are susceptible to similar therapies (although duration of therapy may vary, e.g. between *Microsporum* spp. and the more rapidly inhibited endothrix *Trichophyton* spp. in

tinea capitis), species identification is salient primarily to recognize situations in which animal hosts or familial or institutional carriers constitute potential sources of re-infection and continuation of outbreaks. Zoophilic dermatophyte species and the endothrix tinea capitis agents are most notorious in these situations, but unusual outbreaks of anthropophilic lower body dermatophytoses may also be detected and controlled through species identification.

Candidosis in skin and nails is recognized in direct microscopy by the presence of budding yeast cells and candidal-type filaments; the yeast cells bud through a narrow constriction, unlike *Malassezia* yeasts, and the filaments give rise to budding cells on side branches, unlike dermatophyte filaments.[4] Although filaments indicate an invasive condition in cutaneous candidosis, and are usually found in any genuine case of infection, masses of budding cells alone may be seen in some nail specimens. In fingernails, this often indicates nearby paronychia that was not sampled directly. In some cases, however, especially with toenails, yeast cells merely indicate harmless growth of *Candida* spp. (other than *C. albicans*) of the normal skin flora in crevices in onychomycotic or traumatized nails. *C. albicans* should normally be identified when isolated from skin; there are a number of inexpensive, specific, rapid tests for this species such as inoculation of Czapek-dox agar for formation of chlamydospores under a cover slip. *Candida* spp. other than *C. albicans* need not be identified to species level from superficial sites except in rare cases in which they are isolated from material with conclusive evidence of invasive yeast infection (e.g. formation of filaments with lateral budding cells) in direct microscopy. Because *C. albicans* commonly contaminates moist dermatophyte lesions without significantly exacerbating symptoms, and because normal flora yeasts may proliferate harmlessly in nail crevices, the laboratory gold standard for any diagnosis of cutaneous yeast infection is the specific presence of yeast-type filamentous elements within cutaneous tissue in direct microscopy.

Tinea versicolor is recognized in direct microscopy by the rounded yeast cells and short, curved hyphal fragments ('spaghetti and meatballs') of *Malassezia* spp. Culture is normally unnecessary and may be problematic when attempted since the organism is unlikely to grow on routine culture media. Although there is considerable research interest in quantitative cultural analysis of *Malassezia* spp. in seborrheic dermatitis, clinical diagnosis based on symptoms remains the gold standard.

Other purely microscopic diagnoses not requiring culture include black and white piedra. Tinea nigra has distinctive dark filaments in direct microscopy, but is also readily cultured to yield the etiologic agent, *Hortaea werneckii* (formerly *Phaeoannellomyces werneckii* or *Exophiala werneckii*). No other organism shows melanized, two-celled yeasts budding from annellidic apertures heavily fringed with collarette remnants. All intertriginous skin samples should be stained with methylene blue preparations to detect erythrasma. In specimens from this infection, methylene blue deeply stains delicate branching filaments less than 1 μm in diameter, often seen breaking up into smaller bacillary or coccoid forms.

The correct diagnosis of onychomycosis caused by nondermatophyte molds can be especially challenging. These nondermatophyte filamentous fungi can easily be ascertained as causing onychomycosis if distinctive morphologic elements such as conidiophores are seen in addition to filaments in direct microscopy of nail specimen, or if a fungus from warm latitudes, such as a *Neoscytalidium*, is isolated in an area in which only such fungi occur in infected patients. Most cases are more ambiguous. A fungal species such as *Aspergillus sydowii* may be isolated either as a contaminant or as an etiologic agent, and filaments seen in direct microscopy may be either nonviable dermatophyte elements or genuine nondermatophyte elements. Therefore, even exclusive and heavy isolation of such a nondermatophyte from a specimen positive for fungal filaments does not guarantee that the nail is infected by the same nondermatophyte.[1] The current gold standard, which may not be easy to attain in practice, is:

- first, to demonstrate fungal elements in direct microscopy compatible with the suspected agent; and

- second, in culture, to show, through correlating the results of two nail samples collected at least 1 week apart, that the nondermatophyte in question consistently grows from the diseased nail.

True mixed infection by a dermatophyte and a nondermatophyte may occur, but again can only be demonstrated scientifically by showing a consistent presence of the latter in more than one serial sample.

SEROLOGY

No serologic tests are available for diagnosis of superficial fungal infections.

MOLECULAR IDENTIFICATION AND DETECTION

The development of molecular testing for diagnosis of dermatophyte and *Candida* infections, as well as culture identification, has received attention for a number of years, with abundant studies reported in the literature. Furthermore, commercial kits, based on polymerase chain reaction (PCR) methodology, for dermatophyte detection in nail specimens exist, although more costly than conventional diagnostic methods.[5]

Clinical Manifestations and Management

Details regarding clinical manifestations and management of superficial fungal infections can be found in Chapter 14.

Subcutaneous Fungal Pathogens (Mycoses of Implantation)

Although subcutaneous fungal infections exhibit extraordinary heterogeneity, they have certain features in common – infection is usually acquired from nature and not from infected humans or animals, and the endemic areas are delineated by an ecosystem that consists of altitude, temperature, rainfall, type of soil and type of vegetation. Most patients belong to low socioeconomic groups or live in rural areas. Subcutaneous mycoses arise from inoculation of soil or vegetation into the skin by minor trauma, and most patients have an occupation connected either with agriculture or an outdoor activity and do not use appropriate footwear. A wide variety of saprophytic fungi are implicated, belonging to very different taxa. It should be noted that many of the causative agents of subcutaneous mycoses may also cause systemic infection. These opportunistic infections usually occur in immunocompromised hosts and are acquired through the respiratory route.

The group of fungi that cause the majority of subcutaneous infections in humans are termed black molds.[1,6] Black molds are a heterogeneous group of darkly pigmented (dematiaceous) fungi, widely distributed in the environment, that occasionally cause infection in humans. The taxonomy and terminology of dematiaceous fungal infections is baffling. The term chromoblastomycosis was introduced in 1922 and was later modified in 1935 to a broader term 'chromomycosis'. More recently, the term 'phaeohyphomycosis' was proposed to cover 'all infections of cutaneous, subcutaneous and systemic nature caused by hyphomycetous fungi that develop in the host tissues in the form of dark walled dematiaceous septate mycelial elements'. In 1981, the term was further expanded to include deuteromycota and ascomycota whose tissue forms are filamentous and dematiaceous. This certainly excludes infections by fungi that produce thick-walled 'sclerotic bodies' in the tissues and are classically labeled as chromoblastomycosis. The line of demarcation is, however, only histopathologic and very thin because some of the fungi (e.g. *Exophiala dermatidis*), in addition to mycelial forms, produce rounded structures closely resembling sclerotic bodies. Thus, there has been plenty of overlap in the nomenclature of these cases, especially during the 1970s and 1980s.

The clinical spectrum of infection includes mycetomas, chromoblastomycosis, sinusitis and superficial, cutaneous, subcutaneous and systemic phaeohyphomycosis.[1] During the past few years, there have been reports of infections caused by black molds in previously healthy individuals and in immunocompromised patients.[5] Molecular studies have contributed to our understanding of the epidemiology of these infections. In addition, data on antifungal susceptibility tests have become available. Surgical excision and antifungal therapy (usually itraconazole) remain the standard treatment for these infections.

There are many extensive reviews of all the infections described here.[1,2]

Nature

CHROMOBLASTOMYCOSIS

Chromoblastomycosis (also known as chromomycosis, Carrión mycosis, Lane–Pedroso mycosis, verrucoid dermatitis and black blastomycosis) is a term that describes a group of chronic localized infections of the skin and subcutaneous tissue, most often involving the limbs.[1,7] It is characterized by raised crusted lesions as a result of excessive proliferation of host tissue. It is caused by traumatic inoculation of the skin with a number of brown pigmented (dematiaceous) molds. In tissue, the fungi basically occur as large, muriform, thick-walled dematiaceous cells.

ENTOMOPHTHOROMYCOSIS

The term entomophthoromycosis is now used to describe a group of fungal infections caused by molds belonging to the order Entomophthorales.[1] Traditionally, this order was assigned to the phylum Zygomycota together with the order Mucorales, which contains the etiologic agents of mucromycosis. However, following molecular analysis, the phylum Zygomycota is no longer accepted due to its polyphyletic nature. The subphylum Mucormycotina has been proposed to accommodate the Mucorales and the subphylum Entomophthoromycosis has been created for the Entomophthorales. Two distinct clinical forms of entomophthoromycosis are recognized: basidiobolomycosis and conidiobolomycosis. These diseases are usually slowly progressive subcutaneous infections that affect immunocompetent individuals and are transmitted through traumatic implantation of plant debris in tropical environments.

Rhinofacial conidiobolomycosis is a chronic mycosis affecting the subcutaneous tissues.[8] It originates in the nasal sinuses and spreads to the adjacent subcutaneous tissue of the face, causing disfigurement. Basidiobolomycosis is a chronic subcutaneous infection of the trunk and limbs.

LACAZIOSIS (LOBOMYCOSIS)

Lacaziosis (Lobomycosis), also known as keloidal blastomycosis or Lobo disease, is an uncommon and chronic subcutaneous mycosis of the skin and subcutaneous tissue.[1,9,10] The disease is a chronic dermal infection that presents a wide spectrum of dermatologic manifestations, mainly characterized by the development of keloid lesions as well as nodular, verrucoid and sometimes ulcerous forms. The etiologic agent at an international level, according to the consensus nomenclature, has been called *Loboa loboi*, even though recently it has been accommodated as *Lacazia loboi*.[1] *L. loboi* has never been isolated in culture. The disease is characterized by slowly developing, variably sized cutaneous nodules after a traumatic event. The dermal nodules manifest as smooth, verrucose or ulcerated surfaces that can attain the size of a small cauliflower-like keloid. The increase in size or number of lesions is a slow process, progressing over a period of 40–50 years. The lesions are composed of granulomatous inflammatory tissue containing numerous globose or subglobose to lemon-shaped, yeast-like fungal cells singly or in simple and branched chains.

A new monotypic genus, *Lacazia*, with *Lacazia loboi* as the type species, was recently proposed to accommodate the obligate etiologic agent of lobomycosis in mammals.[1] The continued placement of *L. loboi* in the genus *Paracoccidioides* as *Paracoccidioides loboi* was found to be taxonomically inappropriate. The older name *Loboa loboi* was considered to be a synonym of *P. brasiliensis*.

MYCETOMA

The term mycetoma is used to describe a slowly progressive, suppurative disease that affects the skin, the underlying subcutaneous tissue and sometimes adjacent muscle, connective tissue and bone.[1] The term 'mycetoma' has been concisely defined as an infection of humans and animals caused by one of a number of different fungi and actinomycetes and classically characterised by draining sinuses, granules and tumefaction.

The disease usually involves the feet or hands and may be caused by various species of fungi (eumycetoma) or aerobic actinomycetes (actinomycetoma) which have been inoculated into subcutaneous tissue as a result of traumatic implantation.[1] A characteristic feature of mycetoma is the production in infected tissue of abscesses which contain large compact masses of fungal or actinomycete filaments termed 'grains'. These are discharged to the outside through sinus tracts.

PHAEOHYPHOMYCOSIS

The term phaeohyphomycosis is used to describe infections caused by brown-pigmented (dematiaceous) molds that appear in tissue as septate hyphae, as pseudohyphal cells, as catenulate cells (toruloid hyphae), as yeast-like cells, or as any combination of these forms.[1,2,11] As with hyalohyphomycosis, the term phaeohyphomycosis was introduced in an attempt to stem the proliferation of new disease names each time an organism belonging to a new fungal genus was identified as the cause of human infection. This term was also created to segregate a heterogeneous group of infections caused by dematiaceous fungi from two specific pathologic conditions associated with these molds. In chromoblastomycosis, characteristic thick-walled muriform cells are formed in subcutaneous tissue, while mycetoma is characterized by the formation of grains that consist of compact masses of fungal filaments. However, it is now clear that several organisms can cause both chromoblastomycosis and phaeohyphomycosis, and others can cause both mycetoma and phaeohyphomycosis. Mycetoma and phaeohyphomycosis result in tissue necrosis, whereas chromoblastomycosis infections lead to excessive proliferation of host tissue.

RHINOSPORIDIOSIS

The term rhinosporidiosis is used to refer to an unusual infection of the nasal and other mucosal surfaces and ocular conjunctiva.[1,12] It is characterized by the development of large vegetative outgrowths. The causal agent is *Rhinosporidium seeberi*, an anomalous organism that has at different times been classified as a protozoan and a fungus. Because it resists culture, for more than 100 years true taxonomic identity of *R. seeberi* has been controversial.[13] Three hypotheses have been recently introduced: (1) that it is a prokaryote cyanobacterium in the genus *Microcystis*; (2) *R. seeberi* is a eukaryote pathogen in the Mesomycetozoa; and (3) *R. seeberi* is a fungus.[13] The reviewed literature on the electron microscopic, the histopathologic and more recently the data from several molecular studies strongly support the view that *R. seeberi* is a eukaryote pathogen, but not a fungus. The suggested morphologic resemblance of *R. seeberi* with the genera *Microcystis* (bacteria), *Synchytrium* and *Colletotrichum* (fungi) by different teams is merely hypothetical and lacked the scientific rigor needed to validate the proposed systems. A fundamental aspect against the prokaryote theory is the presence of nuclei reported by numerous authors and updated in a recent review.[13] Moreover, ultrastructural and key cell cycle traits exhibited by *Microcystis* and *Synchytrium* cannot be found in *R. seeberi* parasitic phase. These authors maintain that the placement of *R. seeberi* within the fungi is scientifically untenable. Further studies are needed to validate acquisition by *R. seeberi* of prokaryote plastids and other issues that still need careful scrutiny.

SPOROTRICHOSIS

The term sporotrichosis is used to refer to subacute or chronic infections caused by the dimorphic fungus, *Sporothrix schenckii*.[1,14–16] Following traumatic implantation, this organism can cause cutaneous or subcutaneous infection which commonly shows lymphatic spread.

Occasionally, infection of the lungs, joints, bones or other sites occurs in predisposed individuals.

Epidemiology
CHROMOBLASTOMYCOSIS

Chromoblastomycosis is encountered mainly in arid parts of tropical and subtropical regions.[1] Most cases occur in Central and South America, but chromoblastomycosis has also been reported in South Africa, Asia and Australia. Another major focus appears to be Madagascar. Although common in rural areas, the disease lacks epidemic potential.

Chromoblastomycosis is caused by various brown-pigmented (dematiaceous) molds, the most common of which are *Fonsecaea pedrosoi* and *Cladophialophora carrionii*.[1] *F. pedrosoi* is the most common etiologic agent of chromoblastomycosis worldwide, causing infections in both tropical rainforests such as the Amazon region of Brazil and Northern Madagascar, as well as in temperate regions of Latin America. *C. carrionii* is the predominant agent in arid or semi-desert regions such as Australia and South Africa. Other important agents are *Phialophora verrucosa*, *Fonsecaea compacta* and *Rhinocladiella acquaspersa*. However, sporadic cases of the disease have also been attributed to a number of other dematiaceous molds, including *Exophiala jeanselmei* and *E. spinifera*. It should be noted that several of these organisms (including *F. pedrosoi* and *P. verrucosa*) have also been incriminated as etiologic agents of phaeohyphomycosis. More recently, molecular analysis has indicated that *F. compacta* is a morphologic variant of *F. pedrosoi*.

The etiologic agents of chromoblastomycosis are widespread in the environment, being found in soil, wood and decomposing plant matter. Human infection usually follows the traumatic inoculation of the fungus into the skin. Minor trauma, such as cuts or wounds due to thorns or wood splinters, is often sufficient. The disease is most prevalent in rural parts of warmer climates where people go barefoot. There is no human-to-human transmission.

Chromoblastomycosis is unusual in children and adolescents. Men contract the disease much more frequently than women, reflecting the importance of occupational exposure. Men have a greater opportunity for soil contact and predisposition to injury while working in the fields. The majority are aged 30–50 years. The rarity of the disease in children exposed to the same environmental conditions as adults suggests a long period of latency.

ENTOMOPHTHOROMYCOSIS

Entomophthoromycosis occurs mainly in the tropical rain forests of East and West Africa, South and Central America, and South East Asia.[1,17]

Conidiobolus coronatus (*Entomophthora coronata*), the causative organism of rhinofacial conidiobolomycosis, lives as a saprophyte in soil and on decomposing plant matter in moist, warm climates. It can also parasitize certain insects.

The most widely held view is that *Basidiobolus ranarum* is the sole agent causing basidiobolomycosis, and that *B. meristosporus* and *B. haptosporus* are synonyms of the former; not all authors are of this opinion, however. *B. ranarum* has been recovered from soil and decaying vegetation; it has also been isolated from the gut of frogs, toads and lizards that had apparently swallowed infected insects. It is still uncertain how the disease is acquired and what is the length of incubation. Inoculation through a thorn prick or an insect bite has been suggested, as has contamination of a wound or other abrasion. The infection is most common in children.

LACAZIOSIS (LOBOMYCOSIS)

In lobomycosis, the onset of the disease is generally insidious and difficult to document.[1,10,11] The increase in size and number of lesions is a slow process; it can take 40–50 years. This latency period often makes it important to note the patient's history of travel or stay in areas of endemicity to arrive at a proper diagnosis. The history often reveals the cause being a trauma, for example an arthropod sting, a snake bite, a cut from an instrument, or a wound acquired while cutting vegetation. The causal agent of lobomycosis appears to be saprobic in aquatic environments, which probably plays an extremely significant part in its life cycle. Recent reports have substantiated the Amazon basin as an endemic area for the disease.

The human disease is endemic in the tropical zone of the New World. There have been isolated cases reported in Holland. Identification of the disease in dolphins widened the geographic distribution of the disease. Seven cases of lobomycosis involving two species of dolphins, namely marine dolphins (*Tursiops truncatus*) and marine freshwater dolphins (*Sotalia fluviatilis*), have been reported in Florida, the Texas coast, the Spanish–French coast, the South Brazilian coast and the Surinam River estuary. Although lobomycosis in dolphins has been reported in the USA, few human cases have been reported from there. Although identification of the disease in dolphins has widened its known geographic distribution, the source of the organism is still unknown

All attempts to isolate the fungus from lesions of infected people have failed. In the dermis it appears as spheric or elliptic budding cells. Although it is accepted that the infection is exogenous in origin, the natural habitat of the causal fungus remains unknown.

The organism gains entry through the skin; it develops *in situ* for an unspecified period (several years) and then reaches the subcutaneous tissue. The disease is most prevalent in men aged 30–40 years; it is much less common in women and children.

MYCETOMA

Mycetomas are most common in arid tropical and subtropical regions of Africa and Central America, particularly those areas bordering the great deserts.[1,18] However, sporadic cases have been reported from many parts of the world. The countries surrounding the Saharan and Arabian deserts form the most important endemic area, not only because of the number of new cases occurring each year, but also because of the diversity of causal organisms. Mycetoma is also endemic in certain regions of India and in Central and South America.

More than 20 species of fungi and actinomycetes have been implicated as etiologic agents of mycetoma. Many of these organisms have been isolated from the soil or from plants or trees, or from decomposing vegetation. About six species of fungi are common causes of eumycetoma and five aerobic actinomycetes are common etiologic agents of actinomycetoma.

The fungi involved include *Madurella mycetomatis* (about 70% of reported cases), *Scedosporium apiospermum* (about 10% of reported cases), *Leptosphaeria senegalensis*, *M. grisea*, *Neotestudina rosatii* and *Pyrenochaeta romeroi*. Other fungi that have sometimes been implicated as causes of eumycetoma include *Acremonium* spp. and *Aspergillus nidulans*. Actinomycetomas are caused by aerobic, gram-positive filamentous actinomycetes belonging to the genera *Actinomadura*, *Nocardia* and *Streptomyces*, including *A. madurae*, *A. pelletieri*, *N. asteroides*, *N. brasiliensis* (the most common organism) and *S. somaliensis*.

The predominant causes of mycetoma differ from one part of the world to another. The most important factor responsible for this variation is believed to be the climate, particularly the annual amount of rainfall. Worldwide, the prevalence rates of eumycetoma and actinomycetoma are similar. However, eumycetomas are the predominant form of the disease in Africa and southern Asia, while actinomycetomas are more common in Latin America.

Adults aged between 20 and 50 years are the most commonly affected, although cases in children have also been reported. Most patients come from rural districts in the tropics and subtropics, but cases often occur in some countries with a temperate climate, such as Romania.

Trauma is a critical factor in acquisition of the infection. The organisms may be implanted at the time of injury, or later as a result of secondary contamination of the wound. Traumas are often due to vegetable matter (grasses, wisps of straw, hay). In the tropics and subtropics thorny trees such as the acacia are abundant and are often used for fuel. Wounds caused by the thorns may facilitate the entry of soil organisms, or the causative agents may grow on the thorns and be implanted directly into the subcutaneous tissue. It is not surprising, therefore, that mycetomas affect mainly the feet of country-dwellers who walk barefoot.

PHAEOHYPHOMYCOSIS

Black molds are widely encountered in soil and wood.[1,11] Typically, the infection is acquired by the inoculation of the fungus through a penetrating injury. In addition, other possible portals of entry have been suggested, including the inhalation of spores with lung or sinus invasion, the ingestion of contaminated food or water with subsequent penetration through the gastrointestinal tract, contamination of the skin at the insertion of a vascular catheter, and contamination of the catheter itself. Some cases of systemic infection have no apparent portal of entry.

Phaeohyphomycosis has a worldwide distribution, but subcutaneous infection is most often seen in the rural population of tropical parts of Central and South America. Most cases of cerebral or paranasal sinus infection have been reported from the USA. There is little information on the incidence of phaeohyphomycosis. The number of organisms implicated as etiologic agents of phaeohyphomycosis is increasing. More than 80 different molds, classified in 40 different genera, have been incriminated. These fungi have often been given different names at different times, and there is therefore a great deal of confusion in the nomenclature used in different reports.

Among the more important etiologic agents, *Alternaria*, *Bipolaris*, *Curvularia*, *Exophiala*, *Exserohilum* and *Phialophora* spp. and *Xylohypha bantiana* can be included. Many of these organisms are found in soil or decomposing plant debris; others are plant pathogens. The most important predisposing factor for cutaneous and subcutaneous infection is exposure to contaminated material present in the environment (decaying wood, plants).

Human infection follows inhalation or traumatic implantation of the fungus. In addition to these agents of phaeohyphomycosis, others are being reported. For example, *Colletotrichum* spp., which are common plant pathogens, have been reported as a cause of subcutaneous phaeohyphomycosis in patients undergoing chemotherapy for hematologic malignancies and may cause life-threatening phaeohyphomycosis in immunosuppressed patients.

RHINOSPORIDIOSIS

Rhinosporidiosis is endemic in India and Sri Lanka, where the incidence is estimated at 1.4% of the pediatric population, as well as in South America and Africa.[1] Occasional cases have been reported from the USA, South East Asia and other parts of the world. Some arid countries of the Middle East also show a high incidence of the disease. Little is known about the natural habitat of *R. seeberi*, but it is believed that stagnant pools of water may be the source of human infection. The most prevalent location of the disease is the nasal cavity.

The disease is most prevalent in rural districts, particularly among people working or bathing in stagnant water (such as rice fields). Men are more commonly affected than women. In arid countries most infections are ocular and dust is postulated to be a vector.

The disease affects mostly males (70–90%) and the incidence is greater in those aged between 20 and 40 years. Ocular infection is more prevalent in women, while nasal and nasopharyngeal infection preferentially affects males.

SPOROTRICHOSIS

Sporotrichosis is worldwide in distribution, but occurs most frequently in temperate humid climatic regions.[1,14,15] At present, the largest number of reported cases comes from the North American continent. Other regions where the infection is endemic include South America, South Africa and South East Asia.

It is not clear whether the infection is more common among men than women. Incidence in the different age groups is also variously assessed, but children are less often affected than adults. Classically, infection is caused by traumatic inoculation of soil, plants and organic matter contaminated with the fungus, occasionally by inhalation. Some leisure and occupational activities such as agriculture and floriculture have been associated with transmission of the disease. To date, the largest epidemic of sporotrichosis occurred in Witwatersrand, South Africa, in the 1940s when about 3000 miners were infected from wood timbers in the mines. However, the literature about epidemics is scant and usually related to a common source of infection.

Although the main clinical characteristics of human and feline sporotrichosis have been described elsewhere, many questions related to the mechanism of zoonotic transmission and to the context in which this transmission occurs remain unanswered.

Recently, the role of felines in the transmission of sporotrichosis to humans has gained importance.[1] In Rio de Janeiro from 1998 to 2004, 759 humans, 64 dogs and 1503 cats were diagnosed with sporotrichosis. Of them, 85% of dogs and 83.4% of patients were reported to have had contact with cats with sporotrichosis, and 55.8% of the latter reported cat bites or scratches. Unusual manifestations were diagnosed in humans. Canine sporotrichosis presented as a self-limited mycosis. Feline sporotrichosis varied from subclinical infection to severe systemic disease with hematogenous dissemination of *Sporothrix schenckii*. The zoonotic potential of cats was demonstrated by the isolation of *S. schenckii* from skin lesion fragments and from material collected from their nasal and oral cavities.

Pathogenicity

CHROMOBLASTOMYCOSIS

The potential pathogenicity of a causative species of chromoblastomycosis is determined partly by its natural habitat.[19] Most agents are found in the domestic and man-made environment as saprobes colonizing inert surfaces, or in hydrocarbon- or heavy-metal-polluted habitats. The causative fungi require implantation through the skin into subcutaneous tissue. The lesion appears at the site of skin trauma or puncture wound. However, the inoculation may have occurred so long before that no history of injury can be elicited. In general, the disease remains localized to the area surrounding the initial infection. In rare cases, hematogenous spread to the brain, lymph nodes, liver, lungs and other organs is observed. The pathogenicity and virulence of the causative agents of chromoblastomycosis may differ significantly between closely related species.[19] The factors that are probably of significance for pathogenicity include the presence of melanin and carotene, formation of thick cell walls, presence of yeast-like phases, thermo- and perhaps also osmotolerance, adhesion, hydrophobicity, assimilation of aromatic hydrocarbons and production of siderophores. Host defense in chromoblastomycosis has been shown to rely mainly on the ingestion and elimination of fungal cells by neutrophils and macrophages. However, there is increasing evidence supporting a role of T-cell-mediated immune responses.[19]

ENTOMOPHTHOROMYCOSIS

Pathogenicity of the causal organisms is a reflection of inoculum size and frequency of exposure in endemic areas.[1] Basidiobolomycosis mainly involves the thigh, buttocks or trunk. There is a suggestion that the use of 'toilet leaves' to clean after defecation might explain the observed distribution of lesions and source of infection. *Conidiobolus* spp. typically cause a chronic, indolent infection of the face, typified by a progressive swelling mass over the nasal mucosa, nose, eyelids, and over the malar and frontal regions of the face. The Entomophthorales do not cause angioinvasive disease. For an exhaustive review of the pathogenicity of the agents causing entomophthoramycosis, refer to Prabhu and Patel.[17]

LACAZIOSIS (LOBOMYCOSIS)

Lobomycosis develops following trauma to the skin, but in most clinical histories the event is so minimal that it is not remembered.[1,9,10] The disease runs an extremely slow course and years may elapse before the patient seeks medical advice. The organism has been transmitted successfully to an armadillo and to tortoises. In addition, the infection has been maintained through nine generations in the footpads of mice. Most of our knowledge of the etiologic agent of lobomycosis is derived from histopathologic and electron microscopy studies. Lobomycosis is sometimes referred to as a zoonotic disease because it affects only specific delphinidae and humans; however, the evidence that it can be transferred directly to humans from dolphins is weak.[9,10] Dolphins have also been postulated to be responsible for an apparent geographic expansion of the disease in humans. Morphologic and molecular differences between the human and dolphin organisms, differences in geographic distribution of the diseases between dolphins and humans, the existence of only a single documented case of presumed zoonotic transmission, and anecdotal evidence of lack of transmission to humans following accidental inoculation of tissue from infected dolphins do not support the hypothesis that dolphins infected with *L. loboi* represent a zoonotic hazard for humans. In addition, the lack of human cases in communities adjacent to coastal estuaries with a high prevalence of lobomycosis in dolphins, such as the Indian River Lagoon in Florida, suggests that direct or indirect transmission of *L. loboi* from dolphins to humans occurs rarely, if at all. Nonetheless, attention to personal hygiene and general principals of infection control are always appropriate when handling tissues from an animal with a presumptive diagnosis of a mycotic or fungal disease.

The fungus is abundant in lobomycotic skin lesions. It is a strikingly homogeneous, spherical intracellular yeast, 5–12 μm in diameter. *L. loboi* is predominantly an intracellular pathogen. Organisms, singly or in chains, reside predominantly in macrophage vacuoles. They probably reproduce by budding; linear or radiating chains of as many as 20 organisms linked by tubules have been observed.

MYCETOMA AND PHAEOHYPHOMYCOSIS

The organisms causing these conditions are not regarded as being pathogenic. Typically, the infection is acquired by the inoculation of the fungus through a penetrating injury. The route of infection of systemic and disseminated cases is still a mystery for many of the black yeasts and their filamentous relatives.[19]

RHINOSPORIDIOSIS

Studies on the virulence of *R. seeberi* have not been carried out.[13] Nothing is known about the mode of infection. It is most likely that trauma is an essential factor in the initiation of disease. Spores of *R. seeberi* are not able to penetrate intact epithelium. Because the nose and eyes are the most common sites of the disease it is suggested that the organisms are transmitted in dust and water.

SPOROTRICHOSIS

Sporothrix schenckii usually enters the body through traumatic implantation of soil, plants and organic matter contaminated with the fungus.[1,14] Occasionally the fungus is introduced through inhalation of the conidia. Zoonotic transmission has been described in isolated cases or in small outbreaks. Several factors, such as inoculum load, immune status of the host, virulence of the inoculated strain, and depth of traumatic inoculation, influence the different forms of sporotrichosis. Because the infection can also be hematogenously disseminated, it may be that the yeast cells are able to resist phagocytosis and intracellular killing by host effector cells, although *in vitro* data suggest that the yeast cells are readily killed in the presence of human serum. Host defense mechanisms in response to *S. schenckii* have not been extensively studied.

Prevention

Avoidance of skin penetration is the best means of preventing chromoblastomycosis, entomophthoromycosis and phaeohyphomycosis. Suitable footwear will help to prevent chromoblastomycosis.

Very little is known about the ecology of *L. loboi*. However, the agent is probably introduced directly into the dermis through a penetrating injury, such as a thorn prick or an insect bite, or close, abrasive contact with a dolphin. In areas where infections have been reported it would be advisable to avoid penetrating injuries.

The causative agents of mycetoma normally live as saprophytes in the soil. Because the most common site for mycetoma is the foot it is reasonable to assume that the wearing of appropriate footwear would prevent infection. Avoidance of trauma to the hands and other areas is difficult to encourage because most infections seem to be related to outdoor activities.

Rhinosporidiosis can be prevented by avoiding eye and nose contact with contaminated dust and water.

Occupations that predispose persons to sporotrichosis include gardening, farming, masonry, floral work, outdoor labor and other activities involving exposure to contaminated soil or vegetation such as sphagnum moss or roses. Wearing gloves and protective clothing while carrying out these activities may therefore prevent traumatic implantation of the fungus through the skin.

Diagnostic Microbiology
CHROMOBLASTOMYCOSIS
Direct Microscopy and Fungal Culture

Microscopic examination of 10% KOH preparations of pus, scrapings or crusts from lesions can permit the diagnosis of chromoblastomycosis if clusters of the characteristic small, round, thick-walled, brown-pigmented sclerotic cells are seen (Figure 190-1). These cells are often divided by longitudinal and transverse septa. Dark wide hyphae are also seen on occasion. Detection of sclerotic bodies in tissue confirms the diagnosis of chromoblastomycosis, rather than phaeohyphomycosis, where hyphae will be observed.

The definitive diagnosis of chromoblastomycosis depends on the isolation of the etiologic agent in culture. Sabouraud agar may be used, with incubation at 25–28 °C for at least 4 weeks, due to the slow growth rate of the organisms involved. Natural culture media using tree fruit have been shown to decrease the time required for induction of sclerotic cells.[7] Identification of the individual etiologic agents by microscopy is difficult, due to their simple morphologies. Molecular sequencing may be required for speciation.

Serology

Serologic tests for detection of antibodies against *F. pedrosoi* have been developed, but suffer from low sensitivity.[20] Another study reported that *F. pedrosoi* metabolic antigen, chromomycin, was able to detect delayed hypersensitivity in patients with chromoblastomycosis and this antigen may be helpful as an additional diagnostic test.[7]

Detection of β-(1,3)-D-glucan, a cell wall constituent of many fungi, has been used to diagnose *Fonsecaea* infection where systemic infection had occurred.[7]

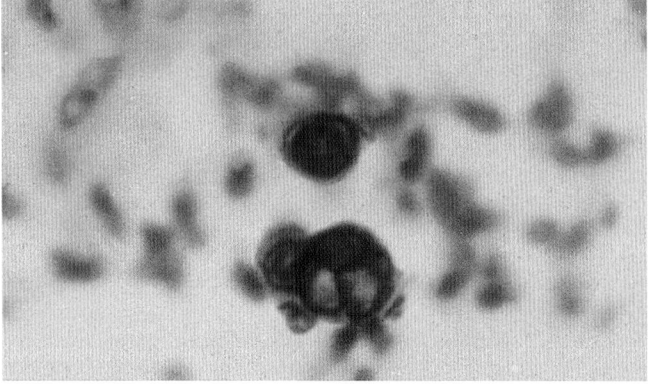

Figure 190-1 Chromoblastomycosis. Thick-walled, septate, dematiaceous muriform cells. (*With permission from Richardson MD, et al. Slide atlas of fungal infection: subcutaneous and unusual fungal infections. Oxford: Blackwell; 1995.*)

Molecular Detection and Identification

The loop-mediated isothermal amplification technique has been reported as a rapid specific diagnostic technique for *Fonsecaea* species.[7]

Sequencing of ITS regions of the rDNA gene has been used successfully for speciation of *Rhinocladiella* and *Fonsecaea*.[2]

ENTOMOPHTHOROMYCOSIS
Direct Microscopy and Fungal Culture

Microscopic examination of smears or tissue from the nasal mucosa will reveal broad, poorly septated (although more septate than the Mucorales), thin-walled mycelial filaments.[21]

The causal organisms of entomophthoramycosis are able to grow on standard mycologic media, including Sabouraud agar. Regardless, culture of both *Conidiobolus* and *Basidiobolus* is difficult. To optimize the recovery of fungus from clinical material, specimens must be transferred to the laboratory as quickly as possible, without refrigeration. Tissue should be carefully teased apart into small pieces with as little manipulation as possible and inoculated on the largest possible number of media.

Serology

Immunodiffusion tests for the detection of antibodies have been helpful in the diagnosis of conidiobolomycosis and basidiobolomycosis, although these are not available commercially.[22]

Molecular Detection and Identification

PCR techniques have been described both for identification of *Basidiobolus* directly from clinical specimens and for identification of culture growth. Again, these are not commercialized.[23]

LACAZIOSIS (LOBOMYCOSIS)
Direct Microscopy and Fungal Culture

The etiologic agent of lobomycosis is an obligate pathogen of humans and lower mammals that has yet to be isolated and grown *in vitro*; therefore, nothing is known of its basic cultural characteristics and growth.[11] Diagnosis is based on demonstrating the presence of globose, thick-walled, yeast-like cells ranging from 5 to 12 μm in diameter in lesion exudate or tissue sections.[21] The organism multiplies by budding and thus mother cells with single buds are often observed. However, characteristic sequential budding leads to the production of chains of cells that are linked to each other by a tubular connection, or isthmus. Budding may occur at more than one point on a cell, giving rise to branched or radiating chains of cells. In fresh lesions, numerous granules (five to eight) can be seen in the center. In older lesions, only one large inert granule may be evident. Hyphae are never observed. These thick-walled, hyaline, spherical cells with chains of cells interconnected by tubular connections are the basis on which a diagnosis of lobomycosis rests. These structures can be readily observed in tissue smears or exudates mounted in 10% KOH or in calcofluor white preparations. Tissue sections can be stained with the use of periodic acid–Schiff digest, Grocott–Gomori methenamine-silver nitrate or Gram stains. Newer techniques such as vinyl adhesive tape preparations or exfoliative cytology have been described.[10] These avoid the use of KOH or stains, and may provide simple rapid and inexpensive alternatives for diagnosis. Such microscopical examination of specimens of pathologic material will reveal numerous hyaline, round or ovoid cells with an average diameter of 9 μm (Figure 190-2). These cells closely resemble the yeast forms of *Paracoccidioides brasiliensis* or *Histoplasma duboisii*. The cells are enclosed in a double-contoured membrane and are capable of budding. They often form chains and appear to be joined together by bridge-like structures within the chain. If the individual elements show multiple budding, the chains are divided into branches.

L. loboi has never been successfully cultured *in vitro*. This distinguishes it from *P. brasiliensis*, which it closely resembles morphologically. *P. brasiliensis* can be grown in artificial culture and is known to be a dimorphic pathogen. The globose and subglobose budding cells of *L. loboi* resemble budding cells of *P. brasiliensis* in tissue.[21] However,

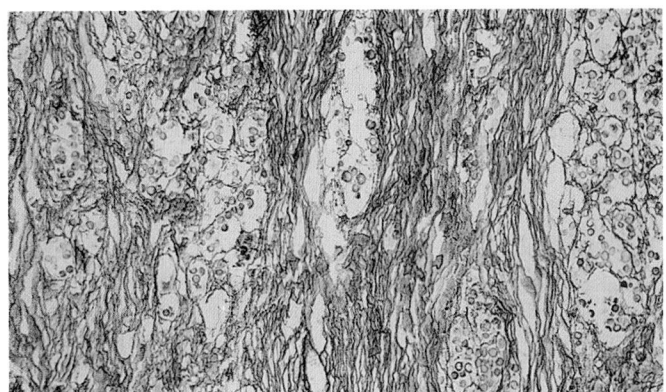

Figure 190-2 Lobomycosis. Yeast cells are attached to each other in short chains. Nonbudding and single-budding cells are also present.

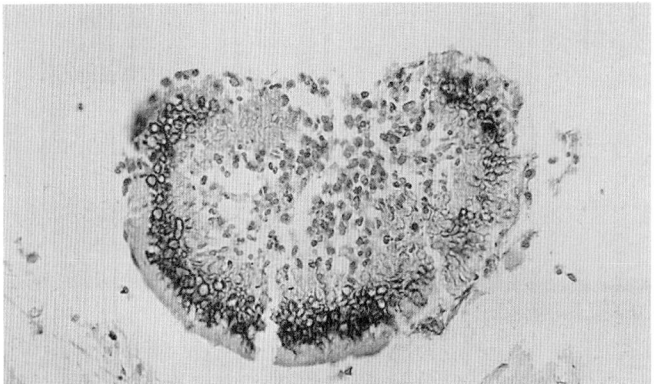

Figure 190-3 Granule of *Madurella mycetomatis*. The granules have a deeply pigmented periphery of compact hyphae. Randomly oriented, poorly pigmented fungal elements in the interior of the granule are less compact.

the central mother cells of *P. brasiliensis* become large and thick-walled compared to the daughter cells, which remain smaller. In contrast, yeast cells of *L. loboi* remain consistent in diameter, giving rise to branching chains of blastoconidia. In addition, the cell wall of *L. loboi* contains constitutive melanin which can be detected by the use of the Fontana–Masson histologic stain. The walls of cells of *P. brasiliensis* are not known to contain melanin.

Serology

Serologic tests have high sensitivity but lack specificity because of antigenic cross-reactivity with fungi from the genus *Paracoccidioides*.

Molecular Detection and Identification

Molecular methods have been used in an attempt to characterize the causative agent of lobomycosis.[10] Fungal-specific primers targeted for highly conserved genomic nucleic acid sequences were used in a PCR to amplify DNA from lobomycosis lesions in a bottlenose dolphin. Sequence alignments of this DNA possessed high homology to fungal ribosomal DNA sequences found in the genus *Cladosporium*. When used for *in situ* hybridization, the riboprobe transcribed from a cloned PCR-generated fragment bound to *L. loboi* cells. These results support the hypothesis that *L. loboi* in dolphin tissue is a fungus.

MYCETOMA

Direct Microscopy and Fungal Culture

The diagnosis of mycetoma depends on the identification of grains. These should, if possible, be obtained by puncture from a softened, but not ulcerated, nodule. Fine needle aspiration cytology, where a fine needle is attached to a syringe and inserted into the lesion using negative pressure, reportedly has diagnostic sensitivity in excess of 85% for both eumycetoma and actinomycetoma.[24]

Grains can also be obtained with a dissecting needle or by aspiration from the secretion flowing from a sinus. If there is no pus flowing from the lesion, small fragments of tissue should be removed. If possible, between 20 and 30 grains should be obtained; these should be rinsed in sterile saline before being cultured.

Gross examination of the grains may give a clue to the etiologic diagnosis. Black grains suggest a fungal infection, minute white grains often indicate a *Nocardia* infection, and larger white grains the size of a pinhead may be of either fungal or actinomycotic origin. Small, red grains are specific to *Actinomadura pelletieri*, but yellowish-white grains may be actinomycotic or fungal in origin. Their shape, consistency and structure must be carefully determined.

Direct microscopic examination will confirm the diagnosis of mycetoma and will also reveal whether the causative organism is a fungus or an actinomycete.[21,24] Actinomycotic grains contain very fine filaments (<1 μm diameter), whereas fungal grains contain short hyphae (2–4 μm diameter), which are sometimes swollen. This can be seen by direct microscopic examination of crushed grains in 10% KOH, Gram stain or, in the case of fungal elements, Calcofluor white,

but it is much more readily observed in stained histologic sections (Figure 190-3). For a detailed algorithm of histologic identification, the reader is referred to van de Sande *et al.*[24]

Although the identification of the causal agents of mycetoma can often be deduced from the morphologic characteristics of the grains, species identification is not definitive; therefore it is also important to isolate the organism in culture. Agar plates should be inoculated with several grains (or with secretion or tissue fragments). Primary isolation media should include blood, brain–heart infusion, Sabouraud and Löwenstein-Jensen agars. Agars containing antibiotics or cyclohexamide should not be used, especially if actinomycetoma is suspected. If sufficient material is available, two plates of each agar should be inoculated and incubated at 25°C and 37°C. Cultures should be retained for up to 6–8 weeks before being discarded. The actinomycetes grow much more slowly than the fungi. Furthermore, grains aspirated from draining sinuses may no longer be viable and are more prone to bacterial contamination.[24] Positive cultures can be identified by macro- and microscopic investigations. In addition, biochemical methods may be helpful in the identification of actinomycetes. However, definitive identification can be difficult, and molecular methods may be required.

Serology

Serologic tests have been developed for the diagnosis of mycetoma, based on antibody detection, although none is available commercially.[24] Such methods include immunodiffusion (ID), counterimmunoelectrophoresis (CIE), ELISA, indirect hemagglutination assay, dot blot and western blot, with ID and CIE most widely used. Varying figures for sensitivity and specificity have been reported, primarily depending on antigen used.[24]

In attempting to improve the identification of agents of mycetoma and, consequently, its diagnosis, molecular tests have been developed. PCR and sequencing of the 16S rRNA gene has been successful in reliable identification of *Actinomadura*, *Nocardia* and *Streptomyces* to the genus level. However, definitive species identification requires further investigation. Eumycetoma agents have been identified primarily based on sequencing of the internal transcribed spacer (ITS) region located between the 18S and 28S genes. This approach was used to develop a PCR for *Madurella mycetomatis*, which appears to be specific.[24]

ITS sequencing for identification of various agents of black-grain mycetomas has also been reported.[24] In contrast, molecular assays for identification of *Pseudallescheria boydii* have centered mainly on the β-tubulin gene which appears more specific than the ITS gene. This target was also used in the loop-mediated isothermal amplification method, developed as a more accessible alternative to PCR for the identification of *P. boydii* in endemic countries.[24] Currently, no commercial molecular test for any agent of mycetoma is available.

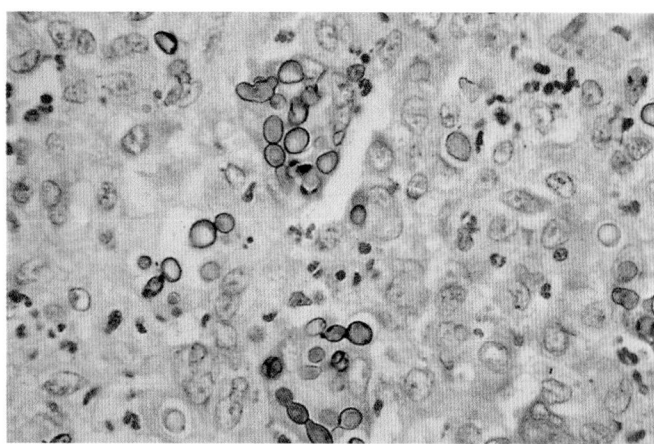

Figure 190-4 Subcutaneous phaeohyphomycosis caused by *Bipolaris spicifera*. The fungal elements are stained with Fontana–Masson, which accentuates and confirms the presence of melanin or melanin-like pigment in the fungal cell walls.

PHAEOHYPHOMYCOSIS
Direct Microscopy and Fungal Culture

One common factor among these fungi is their melanin formation in the cell wall in culture and, in most cases, in human tissue. Microscopic examination of stained histopathologic sections or wet preparations of clinical material, such as pus or skin scrapings, can permit the diagnosis of phaeohyphomycosis if brown-pigmented septate mycelium with occasional branching is seen (Figure 190-4).[21] Fontana–Masson stain may be utilized to confirm the presence of melanin in the fungal cell wall.

Since black molds may be environmental contaminants, positive cultures from non-sterile sites must be interpreted with caution. Diagnosis of phaeohyphomycosis can be made conclusively only by direct demonstration of organisms in tissue. Identification of the etiologic agent is essential for correct management. This generally cannot be accomplished from staining alone and depends on its isolation in culture. This may prove challenging as some species grow poorly *in vitro*. Specimens should be plated on conventional isolation media and incubated at 25°C for at least 4 weeks. If volume of material permits, it may also be useful to culture at higher temperatures. Brain–heart infusion agar may be useful for some species.[2]

Serology

No serologic tests are commercially available for any of the agents of phaeohyphomycosis.

Molecular Detection and Identification

Identification by PCR and sequencing, generally of the ITS and/or D1/D2 regions of rDNA, is often required for definitive identification of the black molds.

Methods for molecular detection of many genera have been reported, including *Bipolaris*, *Exophiala* and *Exserohilum*. None of these is commercially available, sometimes developed as a result of urgent clinical need in outbreak situations.[2]

RHINOSPORIDIOSIS
Direct Microscopy and Fungal Culture

Scrapings of accessible lesions, aspirated cells and biopsied or resected tissues can be used for diagnostic testing.[21,25] Microscopy using 10% KOH of such clinical material reveals round or ovoid organisms that, depending on age, vary in diameter with a prominent wall.[21] These mature forms are known as sporangia. Sporangia measure up to 350 μm in diameter and have a cell wall measuring about 5 mm. The sporangia may be filled with up to 12 000 endospores, 7–15 μm in diameter (Figure 190-5). The immature forms of the organism are known as trophocytes; they are smaller than sporangia, have a

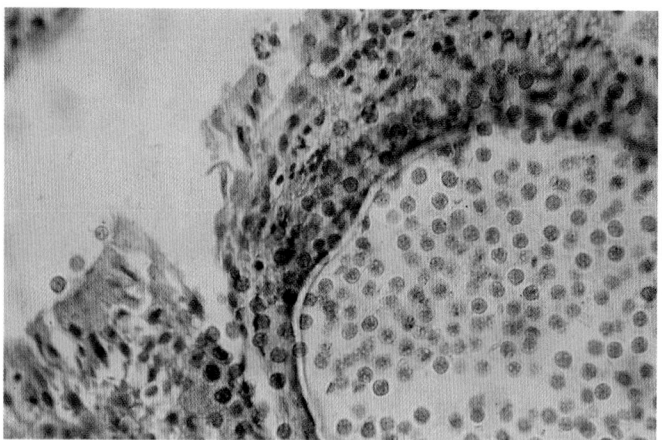

Figure 190-5 Rhinosporidiosis.

relatively thinner wall and do not contain endospores. Trophocytes mature into sporangia. Endospores develop within sporangia. Endospores are released upon maturity and thereafter develop into trophocytes. The organisms are abundant and appear in various sizes and stages of development. It is not necessary to perform special staining because of the size of the agent. However, mucicarmine stain may be helpful in differentiation from *Coccidioides immitis*, which has similar morphology. The sporangial walls of *R. seeberi* stain positively with mucicarmine, unlike those of *C. immitis*.[21]

Serology

Immunologic methods have been used to identify the causal agent of rhinosporidiosis *in situ* where the immunolocalization of *R. seeberi* antigens using sera from individuals infected with *R. seeberi* and tissue from Sri Lankan patients with rhinosporidiosis was determined by electron microscopy. This study found that the expression of this antigen occurs only in the final developmental stages of *R. seeberi* mature sporangia. The data may explain why circulating antibodies to *R. seeberi* were not detected previously in studies that used endospores as antigen in immunoassays. Furthermore, this has been suggested as a mechanism for evading the host immune system, similar to that seen in trypanosomal infection. Further evidence of immune evasion was suggested by studies showing the binding of human immunoglobulins to rhinosporidial antigens. No commercial serologic tests are available for diagnosis.

Molecular Identification and Detection

A multiplex PCR has been reported as useful in the direct detection of *R. seeberi* from clinical specimens, however no commercial molecular diagnostic tests are available.[26]

SPOROTRICHOSIS
Direct Microscopy and Fungal Culture

Direct examination of clinical material, such as pus or biopsied tissue, can be performed using 10% KOH. However, such examination is often disappointing because the organism is small (2–6 μm) and seldom abundant. However, examination can be of value if conducted with painstaking care. Gram or Giemsa stain can be used, although sensitivity may still be low. Detection of yeast cells alone is not conclusive for sporotrichosis; yeast cells of *Histoplasma capsulatum* or *Candida glabrata* can be misinterpreted.[14] The detection of typical ovoid or cigar-shaped cells (2 × 3 to 3 × 10 μm) or asteroid bodies of *S. schenckii* species complex is required to confirm the diagnosis (Figure 190-6).[21] Fluorescent-antibody staining often increases sensitivity, but is less likely to be available. Immunohistochemistry has been used in the diagnosis of sporotrichosis in dogs.[27]

Histopathologic sections can be stained with hematoxylin and eosin (H&E), or special stains such as periodic acid–Schiff (PAS) or Gomori methenamine silver (GMS), although detecting yeasts may

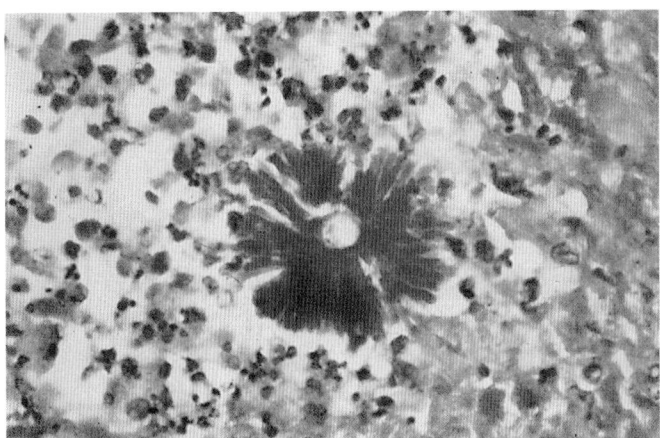

Figure 190-6 Asteroid body in cutaneous sporotrichosis. A yeast-like cell of *Sporothrix schenckii* with faintly basophilic, retracted cytoplasm is intimately surrounded by elongated spicules of Splendore–Hoeppli material.

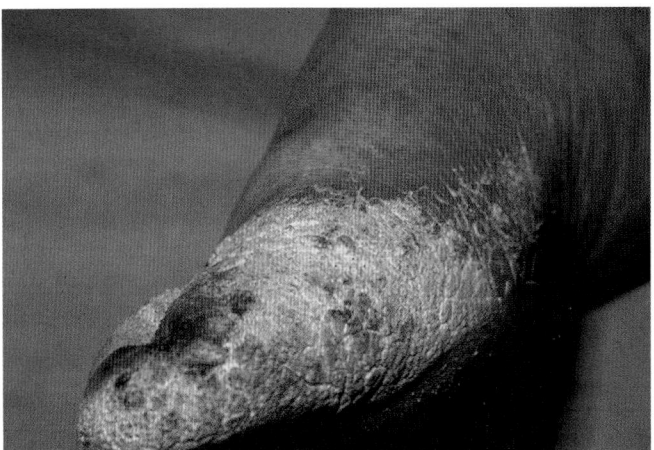

Figure 190-7 Cutaneous features of chromoblastomycosis. *(Reprinted from Dermatopathology: High-yield pathology. Elsevier Saunders; 2011: 256–257, Figure 1, with permission.)*

again be difficult due to low fungal burden in lesions.[21] The definitive diagnosis of sporotrichosis depends on the isolation of the etiologic agent in culture. Routine fungal media such as Sabouraud or mycobiotic agar can be used. Identifiable mycelial colonies will appear in 2–5 days at 25 °C. The color usually changes from cream or light brown to dark brown or black with age, particularly in the center of colonies. *S. schenckii* species complex is a dimorphic pathogen and confirmation of the identification depends on the morphologic characteristics of the mycelial form and its conversion to the yeast form. Conversion can be demonstrated by subculturing the organism onto enriched media such as brain–heart infusion, blood or chocolate agars with incubation at 35°–37 °C for 5–7 days.[14]

Serology
Over the years, numerous serologic tests have been described for the diagnosis of sporotrichosis; nevertheless none is currently available commercially. Based on antibody detection, methods include immunodiffusion (ID), immunoelectrophoresis, agglutination, immunoblot and, more recently, ELISA techniques. Varying reports of cross-reactivity, sensitivity and specificity have been noted, ultimately limiting the usefulness of such testing.[14,28]

Molecular Identification and Detection
Molecular techniques have been described both for direct detection of *S. schenckii* species complex DNA in clinical specimens and for the identification of cultured organisms.[29] Challenges surrounding efficiency of DNA extraction techniques and primer specificity warrant further investigation. Such tests have yet to reach standardization.

Clinical Manifestations
CHROMOBLASTOMYCOSIS
The clinical manifestations of chromoblastomycosis are similar, regardless of the organism causing it.[1,7] Lesions are usually unilateral and occur mainly on the exposed parts of the body, particularly the feet and lower legs (about 50% of cases). Other less common sites include the hands, arms, shoulders and neck. The initial lesion is a painless papule or nodule on an erythematous and occasionally verrucous base. The condition may also present as an abscess surrounded by infiltration or as a psoriasiform lesion with erythema and scaling. As the disease develops, the affected limb becomes enlarged. Small satellite nodules may occur at the edge of the original lesion. Itching often occurs and may be severe.

The primary lesion develops very slowly, its diameter increasing by only 1–2 mm per year. It is firm and elastic in consistency and colored red or violet verging on gray. There is a warty, papillomatous margin surrounding a center that may be flat, smooth or scaly, with areas of scarring (Figure 190-7).

Later in the disease, the lesion may become pedunculated or ulcerated (if bacterial superinfection occurs). However, the lesions usually retain a warty, dry character.

Secondary lesions may appear, especially along the lymphatics draining the site of infection; here again, development is slow and symptoms are few. The lymph nodes are only involved if there is superimposed bacterial infection.

In endemic areas the unilateral development of vegetative, atrophic and scarred lesions on a lower limb is suggestive of chromoblastomycosis. The condition must be distinguished from a number of other fungal infections, including blastomycosis, lobomycosis, paracoccidioidomycosis, phaeohyphomycosis, rhinosporidiosis and sporotrichosis. It must also be differentiated from protothecosis, leishmaniasis, verrucous tuberculosis, certain leprous lesions and syphilis. On the upper limbs the erythematosquamous lesions can be confused with psoriasis or subacute or discoid lupus erythematosus. Mycologic and histologic investigations are indispensable for confirmation of the diagnosis.

ENTOMOPHTHOROMYCOSIS
Two distinct clinical forms of entomophthoromycosis are recognized: basidiobolomycosis and conidiobolomycosis.[1,17] These diseases are usually slowly progressive subcutaneous infections that affect immunocompetent individuals.

Basidiobolomycosis is a chronic subcutaneous infection of the trunk and limbs. The subcutaneous swelling that characterizes this disease is usually localized to the buttock and thighs, but may also be found on the arm, leg or shoulder.

The initial swelling may be rapid or slow in onset and is hard and painless. The spread is slow but relentless, and a large mass is formed that is attached to the skin but not to the underlying tissue (unlike *Conidiobolus* infection). This is a disfiguring infection, but the skin covering the lesions does not ulcerate. Lymphatic obstruction may occur and can result in massive lymphedema. There is no functional impairment as long as the joints are not blocked by the volume of the swellings. The underlying bone and joints are not affected by the disease.

The disease is most common among adult males, particularly those living or working in tropical rain forests. Infection is acquired through inhalation of spores or their introduction into the nasal cavities by soiled hands. Very rarely, *B. ranarum* can cause gastrointestinal basidiobolomycosis.

Conidiobolus infection generally begins with unilateral involvement of the nasal mucosa. The most common nasal symptom is obstruction, but frequent nose bleeding can occur and is evidence of the development of a nasal polyp in the anterior region of the inferior turbinate.

Subcutaneous nodules then develop in the nasal and perinasal regions and may be associated with epidermal lesions.

The spread of the infection is slow but relentless. It is usually confined to the face, and the development of gross facial swelling involving the forehead, periorbital region and upper lip is very distinctive. As a rule, the lesions are firmly attached to the underlying tissue, although the bone is spared. The skin remains intact. Spread to the lymph nodes has been reported. Even if, in advanced cases, the diagnosis is obvious from the appearance, mycologic and histologic examinations are essential for its confirmation.

The disease can be diagnosed with confidence on the basis of appearance and the results of the mycologic and (in particular) the histologic examination. Specimens must be taken from the subcutaneous tissue where the infection develops.

LACAZIOSIS (LOBOMYCOSIS)

Lacaziosis is an indolent infection that first manifests as a papule or small nodule of normal pink skin color or with a grayish tinge.[1,10] The nodule then proliferates and, by partial or total coalescence, may form extensive multilobar lesions. The disease spreads by peripheral extension or autoinoculation from scratching, or it may follow the draining lymphatics, especially in elderly people. Because of the slow growth of lacaziosis lesions, patients do not present themselves for treatment until many years have passed and usually after the lesions have become large.

The lesions are located in the dermis and subcutis and may form massive tumors, which are firm and resistant to pressure at the outset, but which later become hard and fibrous and resemble a keloid. The typical keloid-like skin lesions appear only after several months. If there is ulceration, depressed scars may remain; their surface is smooth and shiny in places, owing to atrophy of the underlying epidermis, and wrinkled and fissured elsewhere.

The disease may be symptomless or cause itching and burning, and trauma to the affected area may be especially painful. The most common sites of infection are the coolest parts of the body – the limbs, face, ears and buttocks. Differentiation of keloidiform lesions on the ears from lepromatous leprosy is difficult, but in lacaziosis the presentation is unilateral. The lesions may cover a whole limb. If the head is involved, the patient may be so grossly disfigured as to be completely excluded from social life. With a few exceptions there are no adenopathies. No deaths from lacaziosis have been reported.

Lesions may be keloid scars or irregular fibrous changes of the skin without secretion. Leprosy, leishmaniasis and chromoblastomycosis can produce similar lesions. Mycologic and histologic examination will confirm the diagnosis.

MYCETOMA

Mycetoma is a chronic, suppurative infection of the subcutaneous tissue and contiguous bones.[1] The lesion appears to begin at a site of minor trauma and continues to spread locally over the ensuing months and years.

The clinical features of the disease are fairly uniform, regardless of the type of organism causing it. Eumycetoma follows a slower and generally less destructive course than actinomycetoma. Spread to the internal organs and involvement of the regional lymph nodes is rare, occurring in no more than 2–5% of cases.

The feet are by far the most common site of involvement and account for two-thirds or more of cases. Other sites include the lower legs, hands, head, neck, chest, shoulder, arms and abdomen.

In most cases, the first sign of the disease is a small, hard, usually painless, subcutaneous nodule that is not attached to the underlying tissue. It is covered by taut thinned skin, which is reddish-violet in color. A number of small nodules may coalesce to form a larger and frequently multilobar nodule (Figure 190-8).

Over the ensuing months the nodule begins to soften on the surface, caves in, ulcerates and partly empties, discharging a viscous, purulent fluid containing grains. If there is little fluid, the grains may not escape. The lesion then broadens out at the surface and also

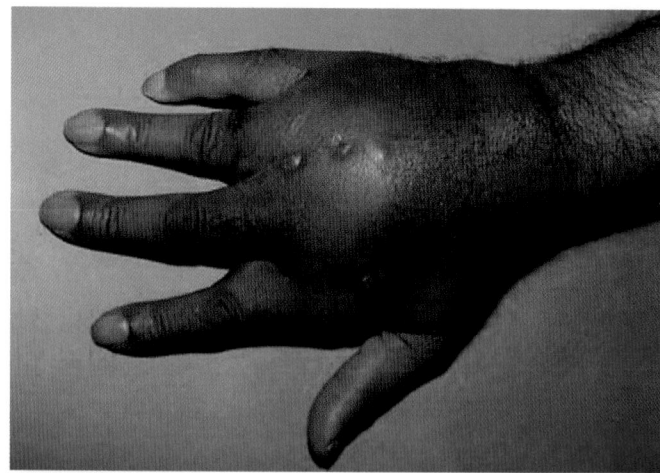

Figure 190-8 Cutaneous features of mycetoma – early lesions. *(Reprinted from Clinics in Dermatology: Fungal infections. Elsevier; 2006: Figure 3, with permission.)*

spreads inward to infect muscles and bones. The lesions, which are covered with depigmented and scarred skin, present as swellings, which are often covered with a crust. Later, the lesions develop sinus tracts that discharge pus and blood containing the characteristic grains (Figure 190-9).

The infection slowly spreads to adjacent tissue, including bone; this often causes considerable deformity. Mycetomas of the feet make the arches convex, thus preventing the toes from touching the ground. However, the general health of the patient is not affected. Pain, burning and pruritus may occur but are usually mild. Depending on the location and size of the lesion, and also on whether there is any bone involvement, limb function may be impaired.

Radiologic examination is useful in determining the extent of bone destruction. Abnormalities include periosteal reactions, sclerosis, endosteal reactions, cortical erosions and joint destruction. CT scanning is also helpful in delineating the extent of lesions.

Bacterial superinfection is not uncommon and is largely responsible for adenopathies and impairment of the general health. Visceral and especially cerebral metastases are the most serious complications; they cause cachexia and are often fatal. Fortunately, they are rare.

In most cases, the diagnosis of mycetoma of the feet presents no problems, but it may be difficult if other body sites are involved, particularly in regions where the disease is not endemic and if no grains have been discharged at the time of examination.

The characteristic feature of mycetoma is the presence in a fistulated swelling of grains that are found to contain actinomycotic or fungal filaments. This finding distinguishes mycetoma from chromoblastomycosis, cutaneous tuberculosis, certain syphilitic or leprous lesions, botryomycosis and other conditions.

PHAEOHYPHOMYCOSIS

Phaeohyphomycosis can be divided into a number of distinct clinical forms, including cutaneous and subcutaneous infection, paranasal sinus infection, cerebral infection and invasive and systemic disease.[1,11] The disease spectrum of noncutaneous phaeohyphomycosis includes sinusitis, pulmonary disease, CNS infection, ocular disease, arthritis, osteomyelitis, fungemia, endocarditis, peritonitis and gastrointestinal disease.

Subcutaneous Phaeohyphomycosis

Subcutaneous phaeohyphomycosis usually follows the traumatic implantation of the fungus into the subcutaneous tissue.[1] Minor trauma, such as cuts or wounds from thorns or wood splinters, is often sufficient. The principal etiologic agents include *E. jeanselmei*, *Exophiala spinifera*, *Exophiala dermatitidis* (*Wangiella dermatitidis*), *Phialophora richardsiae* and *Phialophora parasitica*.

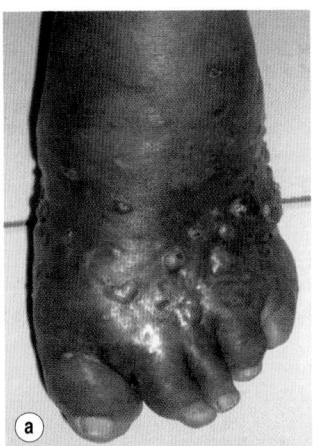

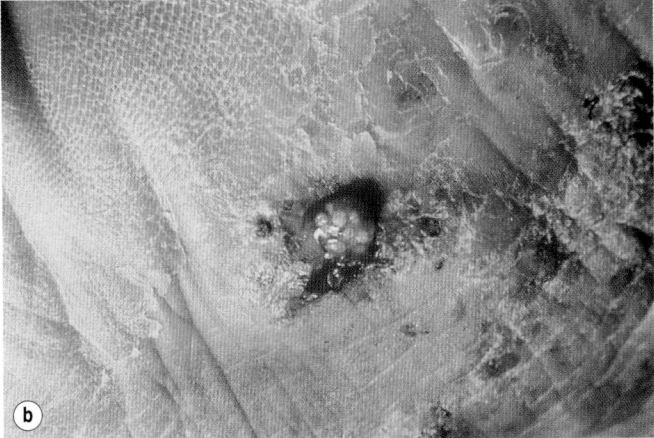

Figure 190-9 Mycetoma – late features: sinuses (a) and grains (b). *(Panel (a) with permission from Asly M., Rafaoui A., Bouyermane H., et al. Mycetoma (Madura foot): a case report. Annals of Physical and Rehabilitation Medicine 53 (2010). Elsevier Masson 2010: 650–654, Figure 1. Panel (b) Courtesy of Professor Oscar Romero. Reprinted from Pediatric dermatology, Elsevier Mosby; 2011: 1470-1534, Figure 26.20.)*

The lesions occur mainly on the arms and legs. Other less common sites include the buttocks, neck and face. The initial lesion is a firm, sometimes tender, subcutaneous nodule that may enlarge slowly to form a painless cystic abscess. Lesions are attached to the skin but not to the underlying tissue or bone. Unless the cyst ruptures, the overlying skin remains unaffected. In immunosuppressed patients with subcutaneous phaeohyphomycosis, the lesions are more likely to drain through sinuses.

Phaeohyphomycosis in Transplant Recipients
Infection of subcutaneous tissue by black fungi has only been reported in a few transplant patients, all of whom were solid organ recipients.[1] These patients presented with indolent, localized infections at least one year after transplant, while on maintenance immunosuppressive regimens. They were cured by surgical resection, either alone or in conjunction with antifungal agents. Local recurrence of subcutaneous phaeohyphomycosis in transplant recipients after medication or surgical treatment is also seen.

Paranasal Sinus Infection
This form of phaeohyphomycosis is becoming more common.[1] The principal etiologic agents include *Alternaria* spp., *Bipolaris spicifera*, *Bipolaris hawaiiensis*, *Curvularia lunata* and *Exserohilum rostratum*.

It is a slowly progressive condition that may remain confined to the sinuses or spread to contiguous structures. Affected people usually complain of longstanding symptoms of allergic rhinitis, nasal polyps

or intermittent sinus pain. Patients present with nasal obstruction and facial pain, with or without proptosis. The sinuses are filled with a thick, dark, tenacious, inspissated mucus.

CT scanning is the best method for evaluating the extent of the infection. The typical finding is a large mass filling one or more of the sinuses.

Alternaria and *Curvularia* spp. occasionally cause necrotic lesions of the nasal septum in patients with leukemia or AIDS.

Cutaneous Infection
Alternaria spp. and *Exophiala spinifera* have been seen in and isolated from crusted, ulcerated or scaling skin lesions. Many of these infections have followed traumatic implantation and a substantial proportion have occurred in leukemic patients or transplant recipients. The arms and legs are the more common sites of infection.

Other Forms of Phaeohyphomycosis
Dematiaceous molds have caused endocarditis after valve insertion or replacement, and peritonitis in patients on continuous peritoneal dialysis.[1] Fungemia due to black fungi is unusual. Fever without a clear source of infection is the most frequent presentation. In a series of 23 cases occurring in a tertiary hospital, fever was the most frequent clinical manifestation, and only one patient developed signs of deep-seated infection, with a clinical picture of necrotizing pneumonia similar to that caused by *Aspergillus* spp.

The lesions of subcutaneous phaeohyphomycosis can be confused with the small initial lesions of chromoblastomycosis, sporotrichosis, blastomycosis, coccidioidomycosis and paracoccidioidomycosis, as well as with cutaneous leishmaniasis. Lymphangitic spread of sporotrichosis and the development of verrucous lesions in the other conditions makes the distinction easier.

RHINOSPORIDIOSIS
Rhinosporidium seeberi causes the production of large polyps or wart-like lesions that occur predominantly on the mucous membranes.[1] The nasal mucosa is affected in more than 70% of cases. The onset of the disease in the nose is insidious and the patient remains unaware of its presence until symptoms of obstruction develop. In some cases, the patient complains of itching and unilateral coryza. Rhinoscopic examination will reveal papular or nodular smooth-surfaced lesions that gradually become pedunculated and acquire a papillomatous or proliferative appearance. They are pink, red or violet in color. The polyps may obstruct the nasal passages, particularly in the event of even slight trauma. If located low in the nostril, they may protrude and hang onto the upper lips. If they are sited in the posterior part of the fossa, they may partially obstruct the pharynx or larynx and cause dysphagia or dysphonia and dyspnea.

In some cases the eyes are affected, the lesions being located on the conjunctiva. Initially these are small, flat granulations that may grow to form multilobed polyps of a pale pink color. At the same time there is diffuse vascular dilation, photophobia and lacrimation, which is often due to involvement of the lacrimal sac and duct.

The ears may also become involved; depending on their size and location, these polyps may impair hearing.

Lesions may also develop on the male genital organs (the penis and, in exceptional cases, the urethra) and on the vulva and vagina in women. They may resemble flat or acuminate condylomas; lesions in the anus present as polyps and may sometimes be mistaken for hemorrhoids.

Dissemination to the internal organs or bones is rare. In most cases the general health of the patient is unimpaired.

The appearance of pedunculated or unpedunculated polyps or nodules covered with white dots on the nasal mucosa or the conjunctiva should suggest the diagnosis of rhinosporidiosis. The condition must be distinguished from cryptococcosis, cutaneous tuberculosis, leprous lesions, leishmaniasis, treponematoses and myospherulosis, an iatrogenic condition related to the application of nasal substances.

SPOROTRICHOSIS

The clinical manifestations of sporotrichosis are rather variable, which helps to explain the large number of different classification schemes that have been proposed.[1,16] The most common clinical presentation is a localized cutaneous or subcutaneous lesion. Lymphatic spread may then lead to the development of further cutaneous lesions. Much less commonly, the fungus may cause infection of the lungs, joints, bones, eyes and meninges. Widespread disseminated infection has been reported in patients with diabetes, alcoholics, drug abusers and patients with acquired immunodeficiency syndrome (AIDS) but will not be discussed here.

Cutaneous sporotrichosis tends to affect exposed sites, mainly the limbs and especially the hands and fingers. The right hand is affected more frequently than the left. The initial lesion develops at the site of implantation of the fungus. It is a painless nodule that is movable at first but that later becomes attached to the neighboring tissue. The skin turns red then violaceous, and the nodule breaks down to form an ulcer, which discharges a serous or purulent fluid. The edge of the ulcer is often irregular and it may become edematous, vegetative and crusted (Figure 190-10).

After a period of a few days to several weeks, the primary lesion may become surrounded by satellite lesions, or further nodules along the course of the draining lymphatics may develop. These soon become palpable and ulcerate through to the skin. In most cases, however, the lymphangitis heals or remains static for a long time without ulcers forming. In most cases the regional lymph nodes are not involved. However, this is not an invariable rule. Any involvement of these lymph nodes is evidence of a superimposed bacterial infection and they may ulcerate in turn.

Apart from these very typical lesions, sporotrichosis may present a different clinical picture. Extension over large areas of skin, often described as the disseminated cutaneous form, may occur. Flat, infiltrated or papulopustular or nodulopustular lesions may develop. Whether oozing, proliferative, papillomatous or verrucous, the lesions of sporotrichosis are generally painless but often pruritic. Several ulcers may be interconnected by subcutaneous fistular passages. Confluent lesions may form a purulent and warty plaque with a continually expanding margin, whereas the center becomes atrophied, smooth and shiny.

Primary cutaneous lesions may heal spontaneously, leaving behind unsightly and even disfiguring scars, which may be a functional impediment. However, secondary lesions may persist for several years.

The development of a cutaneous lesion on the limbs following trauma is suggestive of sporotrichosis, particularly if the patient is resident in an endemic region. The development of multiple ulcers along lymphatics is also suspicious. At a later stage of development sporotrichosis must be distinguished from mycoses such as blastomycosis, chromoblastomycosis and paracoccidioidomycosis, and from leishmaniasis, verrucous tuberculosis and tertiary syphilis. The diagnosis ultimately depends on mycologic and histologic examination.

Management

There are no trials comparing different strategies for the treatment of infection caused by black fungi.[1,2] Treatment depends on the clinical form of the disease. Cutaneous and subcutaneous phaeohyphomycosis are usually treated with complete surgical excision of the lesion, resulting in complete cure in the majority of cases.[1,2] In addition, various antifungal agents have been used. Itraconazole is considered the drug of choice, and the dose has ranged from 200 to 600 mg daily. The duration of treatment is not established. Although unusual, progression or recurrence of disease, even with adequate itraconazole serum levels, has been observed. Whenever possible, surgical resection is also recommended for lesions in other organs, in association with an antifungal agent. Voriconazole and posaconazole also demonstrate *in vitro* activities against black yeasts and molds. Importantly, due to the large variability in the spectrum of dematiaceous fungi, it is important to obtain *in vitro* susceptibilities of individual patient's fungal isolates. Culture and *in vitro* antifungal susceptibility testing provide useful information for selecting appropriate treatment protocols.

CHROMOBLASTOMYCOSIS

Chromoblastomycosis is a difficult condition to treat.[1] Successful management requires long-term antifungals, surgery, thermotherapy, chemotherapy, or combinations of these (reviewed by Seyedmousavi and colleagues[19]). Surgical excision should be reserved for small lesions; it carries a high risk of local dissemination and should be attempted only in conjunction with antifungal treatment.

There is no ideal antifungal treatment for chromoblastomycosis.[19] The most commonly used drug is flucytosine (150–200 mg/kg per day given as four divided doses), but resistance is a frequent problem during long-term treatment. Amphotericin B is not effective as monotherapy but appears to be effective in combination with 5-fluorocytosine (5-FC). Ketoconazole is effective in combination with 5-FC. Fluconazole is reported to be successful. Given extensive clinical experience, itraconazole and terbinafine, alone or in combination, are the currently recommended treatments for chromoblastomycosis.[1] The best option appears to be terbinafine, due to its high degree of effectiveness and tolerability.

Itraconazole is particularly effective when combined with liquid nitrogen cryotherapy.[1] The local application of heat to the lesions may be beneficial.

ENTOMOPHOROMYCOSIS

Conidiobolomycosis

There is no standard treatment for all forms of this disease.[1] Patients often respond to itraconazole (200-400 mg/day), ketoconazole (200–400 mg/day) or fluconazole (200 mg/day). Treatment should be continued for at least 1 month after the lesions have cleared. Surgical resection of infected tissue is seldom successful and may hasten the spread of infection. The condition can be treated with saturated potassium iodide solution (up to 10 mL q8h as tolerated). Long-term results

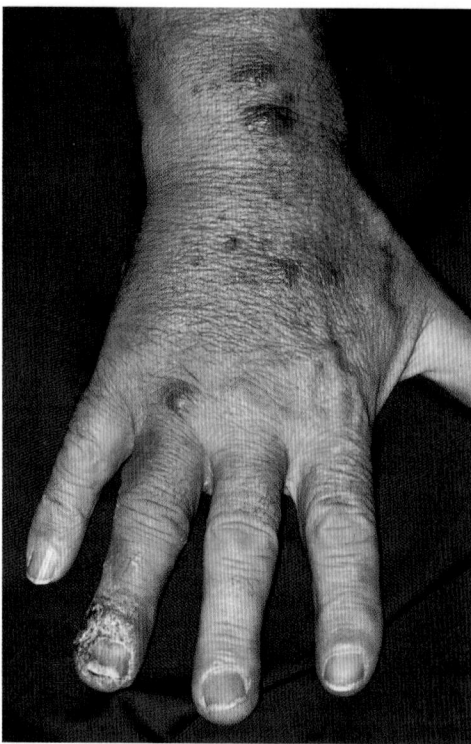

Figure 190-10 Sporotrichosis – cutaneous features. *(Reprinted from Andrews' diseases of the skin: clinical dermatology. Elsevier Saunders; 2011: 287–321, Figure 15-25, with permission.)*

are poor. Allergic reactions and gastrointestinal intolerance are common complications, and relapse is common even long after successful treatment.

Patients with rhinofacial conidiobolomycosis treated with fluconazole (200 mg/day for 4 months) have been completely cured or have exhibited considerable improvement. Some patients have responded to combination treatment with amphotericin B and terbinafine, or a combination of itraconazole and fluconazole.

Trimethoprim–sulfamethoxazole, amphotericin B and fluconazole are useful in the treatment of *C. incongruus* infection, but clinical failure has been reported during treatment with amphotericin B and flucytosine.

Basidiobolomycosis

The treatment of choice appears to be oral itraconazole (100–200 mg/day), which should be given for several months.[1] Oral ketoconazole (400 mg/day) has sometimes been successful, but amphotericin B has seldom been helpful. Saturated potassium iodide is another alternative. The starting dose is 1 mL three times daily and this is increased up to 4–6 mL three times daily as tolerated. In some cases, trimethoprim-sulfamethoxazole (TMP–SMX) has been found to be more effective than potassium iodide. The recommended dose is two tablets three times daily (each tablet contains 80 mg trimethoprim, and 400 mg sulfamethoxazole). As with potassium iodide solution, treatment should be continued for one month after the lesions have cleared.

Should a patient have an enlarged, useless limb resistant to medical treatment, amputation should be considered, to forestall bacterial superinfection.

LACAZIOSIS (LOBOMYCOSIS)

Antifungal drugs are ineffective.[1] Amphotericin B, griseofulvin, sulfonamides and ketoconazole have been employed without adequate clinical responses.

Cure can only be achieved by surgical excision, the extent of the lesions permitting. Care must be taken during surgery of lobomycosis to avoid contaminating healthy tissue. Cryosurgery has also been used. Unfortunately, however, recurrence after excision is common. In advanced cases, the extensive excision required to remove the lesion may not be justified if the infection is not life-threatening. In cases involving larger areas of infection, treatment with clofazimine (300 mg/day) is recommended. The drug must be used, after initial clinical improvement, for at least two years at 100 mg/day. At present, the disease does not have a satisfactory medical treatment. The course of the disease is slow and chronic and the prognosis is poor. Lacaziosis never heals spontaneously and is never fatal, but it may be a very serious impediment.

MYCETOMA

Early actinomycetomas (and some late and advanced cases) respond well to treatment.[1,30,31] The drug of choice is streptomycin sulfate (1000 mg/day intramuscularly). This should be combined with TMP–SMX 960 mg q12h in cases caused by *S. somaliensis*, *A. pelletieri* or *N. brasiliensis*. Other regimens include TMP–SMX and amikacin, and streptomycin combined with either dapsone or TMP–SMX. If no response is seen after 3 weeks of treatment, other regimens can be substituted. These include streptomycin and rifampin (rifampicin), or streptomycin and sulfadoxine plus pyrimethamine. Therapy must be continued for months or even years. In favorable cases, edema and tenderness regress, discharge of secretion and grains diminishes, and sinuses dry up and close.

Even after symptoms and clinical signs have disappeared, the disease has become clinically silent and laboratory tests have become normal, it is recommended that treatment be continued for the same period of time as was required to achieve these results.

The response of eumycetoma to antifungal treatment is challenging, and disappointing and requires a combination of medical and surgical treatment.[1] The fungal agents causing mycetoma are resistant to amphotericin B and 5-FC. The most effective drugs for eumycetoma are itraconazole (200–400 mg/day) and terbinafine (500–1000 mg/day) given for 18–24 months or longer, preferably at higher doses if tolerated. Ketoconazole (400–800 mg/day) has been useful in some cases, but it requires regular follow-ups to prevent hepatic and gonadal dysfunction. Mycetoma due to *Acremonium* spp. and *P. boydii* appears to respond to fluconazole (200 mg daily for 10–12 weeks).

Voriconazole (400–600 mg once daily) and posaconazole (400 mg twice daily) are other options, but experience with these drugs is limited. In the EU, posaconazole has been licensed for the salvage treatment of eumycetoma. Even with the new azoles, long-term treatment is still required.

Surgical excision is the method of choice if the eumycotic lesions are small enough for total removal to be possible.[1] Amputation is often required in advanced cases with bone involvement, particularly when there is no response to drug treatment. Prostheses and rehabilitation are indispensable in every case of mutilating surgery.

PHAEOHYPHOMYCOSIS

Subcutaneous Phaeohyphomycosis

Complete surgical excision of the entire lesion is usually curative and antifungal treatment is not required.[1,2] Incomplete removal of involved tissues, or incision and drainage procedures will result in recurrence. Lesions that cannot be resected can be treated with an azole or terbinafine, but later relapse after discontinuation of treatment has been common, particularly if the patient remains immunosuppressed. Combination treatment with itraconazole and terbinafine has been found to produce a good response in some cases. The optimum duration of antifungal treatment that should be given has not been defined, but several months' treatment is usually required, and close follow-up is recommended.

Paranasal Sinus Infection

Complete surgical debridement combined with amphotericin B treatment is essential to halt the progression of this form of phaeohyphomycosis.[1,2] Even so, it is not uncommon for the condition to recur. The need for repeated debridement is most evident in patients with disabling symptoms or erosion of the bone separating the paranasal sinus from the brain.

Oral treatment with itraconazole (100–400 mg/day) appears promising, although the optimum dosage and duration of treatment have not been defined. The role of the newer triazole antifungal agents, such as voriconazole and posaconazole, is unclear but promising. In *in vitro* tests the new azole antifungals, including voriconazole, appear to be as active as itraconazole against a number of agents of phaeohyphomycosis.

Necrotic nasal septum lesions due to *Alternaria* spp. or *Curvularia* spp. have been cured after surgical excision.

Cerebral Phaeohyphomycosis

In no case has a patient survived without surgical resection of the lesion.[1,2] Treatment with amphotericin B on its own is ineffective. Lesions that have not been completely removed have usually proved fatal. Combination treatment is recommended: terbinafine plus an azole; and echinocandin (caspofungin, micafungin and anidulafungin) plus amphotericin B or an azole; and flucytosine with combinations of amphotericin B, itraconazole or posaconazole, or an echinocandin. Nearly all successfully treated cases were treated with combination therapy; monotherapy might seem effective initially, but it almost always results in treatment failure. As new antifungals like voriconazole and posaconazole become available, however, monotherapy may become more successful because these agents have high efficiency, improved bioavailability and are well tolerated.

Cutaneous Infection

Surgical debridement of cutaneous lesions combined with parenteral amphotericin B is the most effective method of treatment. Topical antifungal treatment is seldom helpful.

RHINOSPORIDIOSIS

Spontaneous remission is unusual.[1] The treatment of choice is surgical excision, with or without cauterization. No drug treatment has proved effective. If left untreated, the polyps will continue to enlarge slowly. Local injection of amphotericin B may be used as an adjunct treatment to prevent re-infection and spread of the disease. In very rare cases, widely disseminated or deep-seated visceral lesions may develop.

SPOROTRICHOSIS

Oral itraconazole is the drug of choice for patients with cutaneous and lymphocutaneous forms of sporotrichosis.[1,14] Adults should be treated with a dosage of 200 mg/day or 5 mg/kg per day for 3–6 months. Children should receive a dosage of 6–10 mg/kg to a maximum of 400 mg/day. Treatment should be continued for 2–4 weeks after the lesions have cleared. Patients who fail to respond should be treated with a higher dosage of itraconazole (200 mg twice daily), or with terbinafine (500 mg twice daily). For patients in low- and middle-income countries who contract cutaneous sporotrichosis, saturated potassium iodide solution remains the treatment of choice, owing to its ease of administration and low cost.[32] The starting dose is 1 mL q8h, and this is increased to 4–6 mL q8h. Treatment should be continued for at least 1 month after clinical cure is obtained, which may take 2–4 months. Intolerance (iodism) is frequent and consequently therapy is often stopped.

Local heat, on its own or in combination with drug treatment, has been shown to improve cutaneous lesions. Besides thermotherapy, the simple warming of diseased limbs in winter months has proved helpful.

Amphotericin B has cured some patients with extracutaneous forms of sporotrichosis, but failures are common. In cases of arthritis or osteomyelitis, better results have been obtained when the drug has been combined with surgical debridement.

Itraconazole (400 mg/day) has given good results in patients with extracutaneous infection, especially in those who have not responded to fluconazole.

References available online at expertconsult.com.

KEY REFERENCES

Chowdhary A., Meis J.F., Guarro J., et al.: ESCMID and ECMM joint clinical guidelines for the diagnosis and management of systemic phaeohyphomycosis: Diseases caused by black fungi. *Clin Microbiol Infect* 2014; 20(Suppl. 3):47-75.

Ramos E., Silva M., Aquiar Santos Viela F., et al.: Lobomycosis: literature review and future perspectives. *Actas Dermosilifiliogr* 2009; 100(Suppl.1):92-100.

Richardson M.D., Warnock D.W.: *Fungal infection: diagnosis and management.* 4th ed. Chichester: Wiley–Blackwell; 2012.

Seyedmousavi S., Netea M.G., Mouton J.W., et al.: Black yeasts and their filamentous relatives: principles of pathogenesis and host defence. *Clin Microbiol Rev* 2014; 27:527-542.

Torres-Guerrero E., Isa-Isa R., Isa M., et al.: Chromoblastomycosis. *Clin Dermatol* 2012; 30:403-408.

Van de Sande W.W.J., Fahal A.H., Goodfellow M., et al.: Merits and pitfalls of currently used diagnostic tools in mycetoma. *PLoS Negl Trop Dis* 2014; 8:e2918.

Vilela R., Mendoza L.: The taxonomy and phylogenetics of the human and animal pathogen *Rhinosporidium seeberi*: a critical review. *Rev Iberoam Micol* 2012; 29:185-199.

191

Protozoa: Intestinal and Urogenital Amebae, Flagellates and Ciliates

LYNNE S. GARCIA

KEY CONCEPTS

- Pathogens discussed in this chapter include: *Entamoeba histolytica*, *Blastocystis* spp., *Giardia lamblia* (*G. duodenalis, G. intestinalis*), *Dientamoeba fragilis*, *Balantidium coli*, and the urogenital flagellate *Trichomonas vaginalis*.

- The true pathogen, *Entamoeba histolytica*, is morphologically identical to nonpathogenic protozoa (example: *Entamoeba dispar*); unless ingested red blood cells are seen in the trophozoite, immunoassays for specific *E. histolytica* are positive, or molecular methods confirm pathogenic *E. histolytica*, the report must indicate *Entamoeba histolytica/E. dispar* or *Entamoeba histolytica/E. dispar* group.

- *Blastocystis* spp. (formerly *Blastocystis hominis*) is comprised of a number of morphologically identical subtypes/species, some of which are pathogenic for humans and some are nonpathogenic. This is the most common protozoan seen in human fecal specimens throughout the world and should always be reported when seen.

- A *Giardia lamblia* (*G. duodenalis, G. intestinalis*) name change has not been formally recognized by the International Code of Zoological Nomenclature; thus the name *G. lamblia* will be maintained for this edition. Three designations for *Giardia* causing human infections are: *G. lamblia* (*G. duodenalis, G. intestinalis*).

- Recently, precyst and cyst forms of *Dientamoeba fragilis* have been described and documented in an animal model and in human stool specimens. However, they are very difficult to identify and occur infrequently. In many areas of the world, *D. fragilis* is as common as *G. lamblia* and causes symptoms in adults, as well as children.

- Molecular test kits and/or instruments are under development, in clinical trials, or US Food and Drug Administration (FDA) approved for the detection and identification of select gastrointestinal and urogenital protozoa.

This chapter discusses the amebae, flagellates and ciliates that parasitize the intestinal and urogenital systems of humans (Table 191-1). With the exception of *Trichomonas vaginalis*, all of the organisms live in the intestinal tract. Intestinal protozoa vary in pathogenicity and prevalence, but, with rare exceptions, all have a worldwide distribution.

Nature

Amebae, flagellates and ciliates are single-celled eukaryotic organisms belonging to the subkingdom or phylum Protozoa. In general, the organisms related to human infection change their form and function from the active, feeding trophozoites to the resting cyst form. All protozoa contain a nucleus, often with a karyosome near its center. The cytoplasm is composed of the endoplasm, which immediately surrounds the nucleus, and the ectoplasm, which functions as the locomotion apparatus. Reproduction is relatively simple and is accomplished through repeated asexual multiplication by binary fission. Although its classification is under review, *Blastocystis* spp. is a unicel-

lular, anaerobic, eukaryotic protist currently discussed with the intestinal protozoa and will be covered in this chapter.

Epidemiology

Intestinal amebae, flagellates and ciliates are transmitted through fecally contaminated food, water or other materials. Prevalence is correlated with socioeconomic conditions, and higher infection rates

TABLE 191-1	Amebae, Flagellates and the Ciliates that Parasitize the Intestinal and Urogenital Systems of Humans	
Type	**Species**	**Pathogenicity***
Amebae	*Entamoeba histolytica*	+
	Entamoeba dispar	−
	Entamoeba moshkovskii	± Pathogenicity remains controversial; possibly pathogenic in children
	Entamoeba bangladeshi	± Pathogenicity remains controversial; rare, not discussed in text; *like E. moshkovskii, E. bangladeshi* resembles *E. histolytica* and *E. dispar*
	Entamoeba hartmanni	−
	Entamoeba coli	−
	Entamoeba polecki	−
	Entamoeba gingivalis[†]	−
	Endolimax nana	−
	Iodamoeba bütschlii	−
	Blastocystis spp.	± Depends on the subtype(s) present; classification under review
Flagellates	*Dientamoeba fragilis*	+
	Giardia lamblia (*duodenalis, intestinalis*)	+
	Trichomonas vaginalis[‡]	+
	Pentatrichomonas (*Trichomonas*) *hominis*	−
	Trichomonas tenax[†]	−
	Chilomastix mesnili	−
	Enteromonas hominis	−
	Retortamonas intestinalis	−
Ciliate	*Balantidium coli*	+

*Pathogenicity: +, pathogenic; −, nonpathogenic; ±, pathogenicity controversial.
[†]Body site: mouth.
[‡]Body site: urogenital system.

occur in people who have poor personal hygiene, who live in areas with poor sanitation, or men who have sex with men.[1] Contaminated water supplies are a particular problem because the usual levels of chlorination may not kill cysts.[2] Filtration is required. Endemic and epidemic disease has been traced to water supplies that use surface water that is not filtered or has been improperly filtered.

These organisms generally have a cystic stage that develops when conditions in the environment are unfavorable for continued multiplication. The cyst wall is thicker than the trophozoite membrane, and thus provides protection. Once these cysts have been transferred to a new host, usually by fecal–oral contamination from person to person, the organisms excyst. Excystation factors include osmotic changes in the environment, enzymatic action of the enclosed organism on the inner surface of the cyst wall and, among the parasitic protozoa, favorable pH and enzymatic action of the host tissues. Transmission of those protozoa with no identified cyst stage has not been totally explained.

ENTAMOEBA HISTOLYTICA

Infections with *E. histolytica* are seen worldwide and are more prevalent in the tropics. Over 500 million people have been estimated to be infected with *E. histolytica*, of whom 50 million had extensive symptoms, including colitis or extraintestinal abscesses, and there were 110 000 deaths.[3] For every case of invasive disease diagnosed, there are at least 10–20 asymptomatic individuals excreting infective cysts. Population groups with a higher incidence of amebiasis include people from low- and middle-income countries (LMIC) or recent immigrants from there to industrialized nations.

Social changes seen in the late 1960s – wider acceptance of men having sex with men (MSM), increased sexual contacts, increased frequency of sexual activities and anonymity of sexual partners – contributed to dramatic increases in sexually transmitted organisms, including *E. histolytica*. Clinical presentations within the homosexual community often differ from those seen in the heterosexual population and almost 50% of all homosexual men found to be infected with *E. histolytica* were asymptomatic.[4] However, it is an accepted fact that the ameba morphologically identified as *E. histolytica* is actually two separate and distinct species. *E. histolytica* is the pathogenic species and is considered the etiologic agent of amebic colitis and extraintestinal amebiasis, while *E. dispar* is the nonpathogenic species and does not invade tissue or cause intestinal symptoms. Therefore, in epidemiologic studies prior to the development of specific reagents for the identification of true *E. histolytica*, those organisms identified as *E. histolytica* were actually in the *E. histolytica/E. dispar* group.

E. moshkovskii, which is morphologically identical to *E. histolytica* and *E. dispar* but biochemically and genetically different, has been considered until recently to be primarily a free-living (nonpathogenic) ameba. However, human isolates have now been detected in North America, Italy, South Africa, Bangladesh, India, Iran and Australia.[1] Recent studies suggest that infection with this species can cause diarrhea and other intestinal disorders.[1] Since *E. moshkovskii* is indistinguishable in its cyst and trophozoite forms from *E. histolytica* and *E. dispar*, it is not possible to differentiate the three species on the basis of traditional microscopic examination. Therefore, past studies on the prevalence of *E. histolytica* may be flawed if the possible presence of *E. dispar* and *E. moshkovskii* was not considered.

Epidemiologic evidence of sexual transmission of *E. histolytica* has grown significantly since the early 1970s, particularly in New York City and San Francisco. In San Francisco, the incidence of reported symptomatic intestinal amebiasis increased by over 1000% from 1978 to 1988 among MSM between 20 and 39 years of age.[4] Direct oral–anal contact (anilingus) leads to fecal exposure and oral contact with a variety of intestinal pathogens. Transmission can also occur during oral–genital sex after anal intercourse has occurred. Active heterosexuals can acquire infection with *E. histolytica* through sexual activities that provide an opportunity for fecal–oral contamination. The key factor is not necessarily homosexuality, but the frequency of sexual activity and potential for fecal–oral contact. In a study from Japan, symptomatic amebiasis is a disease that predominantly afflicts males,

and the high rates of patients who engaged in male homosexual or bisexual practices suggest that amebiasis is likely to be a sexually transmitted disease in homosexual or bisexual men. Invasive amebic diseases caused by *E. histolytica* are increasing among men who have sex with men and coinfection of ameba and HIV-1 remains an emerging problem in higher-income East Asian countries.[5]

With the advent of acquired immunodeficiency syndrome (AIDS), and the subsequent modifications in sexual practices within MSM, the incidence of *E. histolytica* infection has decreased. In recent years, the increased incidence of disease caused by coccidian parasites, *Cystoisospora belli* and *Cryptosporidium* spp. and the microsporidia *Enterocytozoon bieneusi* and *Encephalitozoon intestinalis*, has become much more of a problem in patients who have AIDS.

In certain urban areas (Mexico City, Mexico; Medellin, Colombia; and Durban, South Africa), the incidence of invasive disease is considerably higher than in the rest of the world. Contributing factors may include poor nutrition, tropical climate, decreased immunologic competence of the host, stress, altered bacterial flora in the colon, traumatic injuries to the colonic mucosa, alcoholism and genetic factors.

The human is the reservoir host for *E. histolytica/E. dispar* and can transmit the infection to other humans, primates, dogs, cats and possibly pigs. The cyst stages are very resistant to environmental conditions and remain viable in the soil for days. The asymptomatic cyst passer who is a food handler is thought to play the most important role in transmission.

It has been postulated that a colonization-blocking vaccine could eliminate *E. histolytica* as a cause of human disease, particularly as humans serve as the only significant reservoir host, and a number of potential protective antigens are being investigated.[6,7]

BLASTOCYSTIS SPECIES

Blastocystis spp. (formerly *Blastocystis hominis*) are transmitted via the fecal–oral route through contaminated food or water; the cysts survive in water for up to 19 days at normal temperatures.[2,8] Although other modes of transmission are not defined, the incidence and apparent worldwide distribution suggest the traditional route of infection. When genotypic results from animal isolates were compared with the diversity of genotypes of human *Blastocystis* spp. isolates, the human isolates were defined as the same as the subtypes of the pet isolates, as well as the tapwater isolates. Thus, the possibility of zoonotic transmission appears to be very likely.[9]

There are a number of different subtypes/strains/species included in this complex, some of which are considered pathogenic and some are nonpathogenic. Prevention would involve improved personal hygiene and sanitary conditions.

GIARDIA LAMBLIA (G. DUODENALIS, G. INTESTINALIS)

Although a number of papers on the nomenclature of *Giardia duodenalis* replacing *G. lamblia* or *G. intestinalis* have been published, apparently this change has not been formally recognized by the International Code of Zoological Nomenclature. Therefore, we will maintain the name *G. lamblia* for this edition.

Transmission is by ingestion of viable cysts, and contaminated food and drink are the usual sources. These zoonotic protozoa are responsible for disease in a broad range of hosts, including humans, have a low infectious dose enhancing the possibility of transmission, have transmission stages that are small and environmentally resistant, and are insensitive to the disinfectants commonly used in the water industry.[10] This infection is found in children or in groups that live in close quarters.[11,12] Also, there may be outbreaks caused by poor sanitation facilities or breakdowns; travelers and campers often experience such outbreaks.[13] There is also an increase in the prevalence of giardiasis in the male homosexual population, probably as a result of anal and/or oral sexual practices.[14]

Decreased gastric acid production may predispose people to infection with *G. lamblia*. Normal gastric acidity may act as a barrier to infection; patients who have had a gastrectomy are prone to infection with *G. lamblia*. Reduction in gastric acid also occurs as a result of malnutrition; and both factors may, as a group, increase susceptibility to infection with this organism. Impairment of the host's humoral immune system may also play a role.

Lower incidence of giardiasis in infants up to 6 months of age may be associated with breast-feeding and some protection against infection via secretory IgA; however, lower incidence may also be related to a decreased exposure to *G. lamblia* in breast-fed infants.

Giardiasis is one of the common causes of travelers' diarrhea and is worldwide in distribution. Visitors in areas endemic for *Giardia* spp. are more likely to become symptomatic than the inhabitants of that area; this is probably because the latter have developed immunity from previous, and possibly continued, exposure to the organism. A number of outbreaks in the USA have been attributed to resort or municipal water supplies, such as Oregon, Colorado, Utah, Washington, New Hampshire and New York.[2] High infection rates were also reported from hikers and campers who drank stream water. Because some of these areas were remote from human habitation, infected wild animals, especially the beaver, were suspected of being the source.[13,15-21] Surveys show human infection rates of 2-15% in various parts of the world.

Because of potential wild animal reservoirs and possibly domestic animal reservoir hosts, measures in addition to personal hygiene and improved sanitation have to be considered.[22,23] Iodine is recommended as an effective disinfectant for drinking water, but it must be used according to directions.[24] Filtration systems have also been recommended, although they have certain drawbacks, such as clogging.

Isoenzyme studies, used for parasite identification and classification, have provided information related to organism pathogenicity, possible implication in water-borne outbreaks and the potential cause of human disease. The examination of isoenzyme patterns of *G. lamblia* (*G. duodenalis*, *G. intestinalis*) obtained from humans and animals showed no obvious correlation between clinical symptoms and isoenzyme patterns. These studies also demonstrated significant differences between isolates from within a single region and those from other distant geographic locations.[25,26]

DIENTAMOEBA FRAGILIS

Infection with *D. fragilis* is commonly associated with enterobiasis, and it has been suggested that *D. fragilis* may infect *Enterobius* spp. eggs and thus bypass gastric acidity. However, recently a cyst form has been proposed, which implies a life cycle similar to those of other intestinal protozoa.[27-29] Although clinical infections with *D. fragilis* occur, they are not universally reported. This is probably because the infection is self-limiting, stool examination is not requested and laboratory identification is difficult. However, there exists a growing body of case reports from numerous countries around the world that have linked this protozoal parasite to clinical manifestations such as diarrhea, abdominal pain, flatulence and anorexia. A number of studies have incriminated *D. fragilis* as a cause of irritable bowel syndrome, allergic colitis and diarrhea in human immunodeficiency virus patients.[30-32] The incubation period for clinical disease is not clearly defined.

TRICHOMONAS VAGINALIS

Infection with *T. vaginalis* is acquired primarily through sexual intercourse; asymptomatic men therefore need to be diagnosed and treated. The infection sometimes expresses itself through sterile pyuria. The organism can survive for some time in a moist environment such as damp towels and underclothes; however, this mode of transmission is thought to be very rare.

BALANTIDIUM COLI

Domestic pigs are probably the most important reservoir host for human infection with *B. coli*. In areas in which pigs are the main domestic animal, the incidence of human infection can be quite high (e.g. New Guinea). Human infection is fairly rare in temperate areas, although once the infection is established it can develop into an epidemic, particularly when environmental sanitation and personal hygiene are poor. This situation has been seen in mental hospitals in

the USA. Preventive measures involve increased attention to personal hygiene and sanitation, as the mode of transmission is ingestion of infective cysts through contaminated food or water.

Prevention

Transmission of the majority of the intestinal protozoa occurs through ingestion of infective cysts, which can be acquired from food, water and person-to-person by the fecal–oral route. These infections tend to be found more frequently in groups that live in close quarters or in certain population groups. There may be outbreaks due to poor sanitation facilities or breakdowns as evidenced by infections in travelers and campers; certainly this has been found for giardiasis. Although amebiasis is usually associated with poor sanitation and LMIC, sexual transmission has also been documented, mainly among urban homosexual men. Prevention in this group is directly related to limiting sexual practices that provide an opportunity for fecal–oral contamination. The single most effective practice that prevents the spread of infections with intestinal protozoa, particularly in the childcare setting, is thorough hand washing by the children, staff and visitors. In the case of *D. fragilis*, it has been suggested that the trophozoites may infect *Enterobius* spp. eggs, thus allowing protection from gastric acidity; however, under most circumstances total prevention of enterobiasis and/or infection with *D. fragilis* is neither realistic nor possible, and a cyst stage has recently been documented. *T. vaginalis* is acquired primarily through sexual intercourse, hence the need to diagnose and treat asymptomatic males. The organism can also survive for some time in a moist environment such as damp towels and underclothes; however, this manner of transmission is considered rare.

Although incomplete epidemiologic investigation and reporting make it difficult to determine the significance of the water-borne transmission of giardiasis accurately, the water-borne route seems to be more important for this protozoan than for other more commonly recognized water-borne pathogens, with the possible exception of *Cryptosporidium* spp. Iodine has been recommended as an effective disinfectant for drinking water, but it must be used according to directions. Because of the potential for wild animal and possibly domestic animal reservoir hosts related to *Giardia* spp., measures in addition to personal hygiene and improved sanitary measures have to be considered and implemented. If appropriate procedures are followed, conventional water filtration should trap most protozoan parasites, including *Giardia* spp. One should avoid swallowing water when in lakes, rivers, pools, or hot tubs; and also not drink directly from lakes, rivers, streams, or springs. Filtration devices for hikers and campers are also available; however, one should look for 'reverse osmosis', 'absolute 1 micron', 'Standard 53', and the words 'cyst reduction' or 'cyst removal'. Boiling water, at a rolling boil, for 1 minute is sufficient to kill organisms, including *Giardia* spp. and *Cryptosporidium* spp. It is also important to thoroughly wash all fruits and vegetables if eating them uncooked, use safe water for washing food, peel fruit and avoid unpasteurized milk or dairy products.

Pathogenicity

Some of the intestinal protozoa are nonpathogenic and produce no disease; however, microscopists must be able to distinguish pathogenic from nonpathogenic species. The presence of nonpathogenic species indicates that the person has been exposed to fecal contamination.

Several species can cause mild to severe gastrointestinal symptoms, and *E. histolytica* may produce extraintestinal lesions. However, pathogenic or potentially pathogenic protozoa do not always produce symptoms or they may remain after symptoms have resolved. Asymptomatic individuals may serve as reservoirs for the infection. Detection of a potentially pathogenic protozoan does not necessarily prove that the organism is causing the illness. Patients may have diarrhea caused by other organisms, such as *Salmonella* spp., *Shigella* spp., *Escherichia coli* or rotavirus. Current intestinal protozoan pathogens included in this chapter are: *Entamoeba histolytica*, *Blastocystis* spp., *Giardia lamblia*, *Dientamoeba fragilis* and *Balantidium coli*. *Trichomonas vaginalis*, a urogenital flagellate, is also considered pathogenic, and may cause mild to severe vaginitis and other urogenital problems.

ENTAMOEBA HISTOLYTICA

Although many people worldwide are infected with *E. histolytica*, only a small percentage develop clinical symptoms. Morbidity and mortality caused by *E. histolytica* vary, depending on geographic area, organism species (*E. histolytica* vs *E. dispar*) and the immune status of the patient.

During the 1980s and 1990s several publications reviewed the issues regarding pathogenic *E. histolytica* vs nonpathogenic *E. dispar*. On the basis of current knowledge, pathogenic *E. histolytica* is considered to be the etiologic agent of amebic colitis and extraintestinal disease, whereas nonpathogenic *E. dispar* produces no intestinal symptoms and is not invasive in humans.[33-35] Diamond and Clark[36] redescribed the two species as *E. histolytica* (Schaudinn 1903), which is the invasive human pathogen, and *E. dispar* (Brumpt 1925), which is noninvasive and does not cause disease. During the past several years, extensive work has been published related to the pathogenesis of *E. histolytica*.[37,38]

BLASTOCYSTIS SPECIES

Currently, it is estimated that over 1 billion humans worldwide could be colonized with *Blastocystis* spp. The true role of this organism in terms of colonization or disease and the relevance of organism numbers require additional clarification. In studies of patients with irritable bowel syndrome, there are patients in whom the presence of *B. hominis* did not appear to be incidental.[39,40] The first report of a possible relationship between intestinal obstruction and a concomitant *B. hominis* infection has also been published.[41] In patients with other underlying conditions, the symptoms may be more pronounced.[42] There is evidence to indicate there are several subtypes/strains/species, and there may be a relationship between subtype and pathogenicity, only some of which will be responsible for increased intestinal permeability and symptoms.[43,44]

GIARDIA LAMBLIA (G. DUODENALIS, G. INTESTINALIS)

The majority of individuals infected with *G. lamblia* are asymptomatic. Preliminary studies indicate that there may be two different strains of *G. lamblia*, Group A and Group B, associated with different degrees of virulence. Group A appears to be more pathogenic and is associated with symptomatic infection. Isoenzyme and molecular studies also support the differences between these two groups.[45-49]

DIENTAMOEBA FRAGILIS

During the past several years, the pathogenicity of *D. fragilis* has been associated with a wide range of symptoms.[30-32] However, it appears there may be both pathogenic and nonpathogenic variants. Evidence for two genetically distinct forms has been obtained using polymerase chain reaction (PCR)-restriction fragment length polymorphism analysis of ribosomal genes.[50,51]

TRICHOMONAS VAGINALIS

T. vaginalis is site-specific and usually cannot survive outside the urogenital system. After introduction, proliferation begins, with resulting inflammation and large numbers of trophozoites in the tissues and the secretions. Nutrient acquisition and cytoadherence, immune system evasion and regulation of virulence genes are virulence factors associated with pathogenesis.[52] It appears that interference with trichomonads' mucin receptors and proteinases may form a strategy to prevent colonization with this pathogenic flagellate.[53]

BALANTIDIUM COLI

Some infections with *B. coli* produce no symptoms, while others cause symptoms with severe dysentery similar to that seen in patients with amebiasis. Symptoms usually include diarrhea or dysentery, tenesmus, nausea, vomiting, anorexia and headache. Insomnia, muscular weakness and weight loss have also been reported. Diarrhea may persist for weeks to months prior to the onset of dysentery. There may be tremendous fluid loss, with a type of diarrhea similar to that seen in cholera or in some coccidial or microsporidial infections.

On contact with the mucosa, *B. coli* may penetrate the mucosa with cellular infiltration in the area of the developing ulcer, which may extend to the muscular layer. The ulcers may vary in shape, and the ulcer bed may be full of pus and necrotic debris. Although the number of cases is small, extraintestinal disease has been reported (peritonitis, urinary tract, inflammatory vaginitis).[54]

Diagnostic Microbiology

Because intestinal symptoms are nonspecific, diagnosis requires laboratory identification of the organisms present. Immunodiagnostic methods for antibody detection are useful for the diagnosis of extraintestinal amebiasis, but their utility is limited for intestinal disease.

Organism morphology varies and species characteristics often overlap. For reliable identification, microscopists must be able to differentiate all species regardless of their potential for causing disease. Special attention will be given to the clinically significant intestinal pathogens, especially *E. histolytica*, *Blastocystis* spp., *G. lamblia*, *D. fragilis* and *B. coli*.

IDENTIFICATION OF AMEBAE IN FECAL SPECIMENS

Trophozoites and cysts are diagnostic stages of the amebae, and either or both stages can be detected in feces. Microscopists must be able to distinguish trophozoites and cysts from epithelial cells, polymorphonuclear leukocytes and macrophages, as well as from pus cells, yeasts, pollen, moulds, and vegetable and crystalline artifacts.

Trophozoite motility in physiologic saline mounts of fresh material and cytoplasmic inclusions, such as erythrocytes in trophozoites and chromatoid bodies in cysts, can be observed. Iodine solutions are used for temporary cyst stains of fresh or fixed specimens. Cyst characteristics are less variable than those of trophozoites, and species of cysts can often be identified in iodine-stained wet mounts. However, examination of permanent stained smears using oil immersion (x1000) is recommended for definitive identification of trophozoites and cysts. Size is not a reliable feature for species differentiation of either trophozoites or cysts except when separating the *E. histolytica*/*E. dispar* group from the nonpathogenic *Entamoeba hartmanni*.

The microscopist must observe the cytoplasmic and the nuclear characteristics of several organisms before making a final identification. Although cysts are more easily identified than trophozoites, several cysts (particularly if they are immature) should be observed to ensure that the identification is reliable. If two species are identified, there should be distinct populations of each.

Sometimes, although amebic organisms are seen, species cannot be identified. In these instances, the laboratory should report 'unidentified ameba trophozoites (or cysts)'; if the genus can be determined but the species cannot, 'unidentified *Entamoeba* trophozoites or cysts' should be reported, and another specimen should be requested.

Entamoeba histolytica

Intestinal infection is usually diagnosed by the microscopic identification of organisms in feces or in sigmoidoscopic material from ulcerations (Figure 191-1). Nonpathogenic amebae can be confused with pathogens (Figures 191-2 to 191-5). Only trophozoites are found in tissue lesions, but both trophozoites and cysts may be found in the intestinal lumen. Some patients who have invasive disease may have only trophozoites in fecal specimens, and examination of permanent stained smears may be required to establish the diagnosis. It is important to remember that unless trophozoites containing ingested red blood cells (confirmation of the true pathogen, *E. histolytica*) or positive results from an immunoassay specific for the pathogen, *E. histolytica*, are obtained, the laboratory report must indicate *E. histolytica*/*E. dispar* group.[54,55]

Suspected amebic abscesses are often diagnosed by positive serologic tests. Aspirates of abscesses or intestinal lesions may contain amebic trophozoites, sometimes with ingested erythrocytes seen in direct wet mounts or in permanent stains such as trichrome or iron-hematoxylin stains.[54,55] Other species of intestinal amebae are not pathogenic but must be differentiated from *E. histolytica*. *E. polecki* is seen occasionally in refugees from South East Asia and may be confused with *E. histolytica*, as can *E. moshkovskii*.[54] *Entamoeba gingivalis* is a common inhabitant of the oral cavity, particularly in patients who have poor oral hygiene. It resembles *E. histolytica* but has no known cyst stage. As a result, trophozoites of *E. gingivalis* may lead to the misdiagnosis of amebic lung abscess by morphologic examination of pulmonary material, especially sputum.

Currently, there are several immunoassays that can be used to identify organisms in the genus *Entamoeba* (*E. histolytica*/*E. dispar* group) and other reagents that can differentiate pathogenic *E. histolytica* from nonpathogenic *E. dispar*. The antigen detection enzyme-linked immunosorbent assay (ELISA) kits are based on specific amebic adhesin molecules found in the feces of people infected by either *E. histolytica* or *E. dispar*. The second ELISA reagent is able to detect the adhesin produced by *E. histolytica* in feces. Another immunoassay product is available for the detection of *E. histolytica* and *E. dispar* in fecal specimens; however, this kit does not differentiate between the two organisms, but is specific for the *E. histolytica*/*E. dispar* group.[56] These procedures are simple, sensitive and specific. It is important to remember that these kits require fresh stool specimens; specimens preserved in any of the routine stool collection fixatives are not acceptable. PCR

methods are also being developed for the differentiation of *E. histolytica* from *E. dispar*.[57]

Serologic testing for intestinal disease is not recommended unless the patient has true dysentery; even in these patients, the titer (e.g. indirect hemagglutination) may be low and difficult to interpret. The definitive diagnosis of intestinal amebiasis should not be made without demonstrating the organisms. When extraintestinal disease is suspected, serologic tests are much more relevant. Indirect hemagglutination and indirect fluorescent antibody tests (FAs) have been reported positive with titers of ≥1:256 and ≥1:200, respectively, in almost 100% of cases of amebic liver abscess.[54] Positive serologic results, in addition to clinical findings, make the diagnosis highly probable. In the absence of rapid serologic tests for amebiasis (tests with very rapid turnaround times for results), the decision as to causative agent often must be made on clinical grounds and on results of other diagnostic tests, such as scans.

Histologic diagnosis of amebiasis can be made when trophozoites within the tissue are identified and differentiated from host cells, particularly histiocytes and ganglion cells. Periodic acid-Schiff staining is often used; the organisms will appear bright pink with a green–blue background (depending on the counterstain used). Hematoxylin and eosin staining will also allow typical morphology to be seen. As a result of sectioning, some organisms will exhibit the evenly arranged nuclear chromatin with the central karyosome, and some will no longer contain the nucleus.

Blastocystis spp.

In many areas of the world, *Blastocystis* is the most common parasite found in stool specimens. The characteristic form of *B. hominis* that is usually seen in human fecal specimens varies in size from 6 to 40 μm and contains a large central body resembling a vacuole, which may be involved with carbohydrate and lipid storage. The amebic form can occasionally be seen in diarrheal fluid but may be difficult to recognize.[58] Generally, *B. hominis* will be identified on the basis of the typical round form containing the central body.[54] Routine stool examinations are very effective in recovering and identifying *B. hominis* (Figure 191-6), although the permanent stained smear is the procedure of choice because the examination of wet preparations may not easily reveal the organism. The organisms should be quantitated on the report form, that is, as rare, few, moderate, or many. It is also important to remember that other possible pathogens may be present and should be ruled out before a patient is treated for *Blastocystis* spp.

IDENTIFICATION OF FLAGELLATES IN FECAL SPECIMENS

The flagellates are a more diverse group than the amebae. The type of motility, shape, number of nuclei and other characteristics, such as an

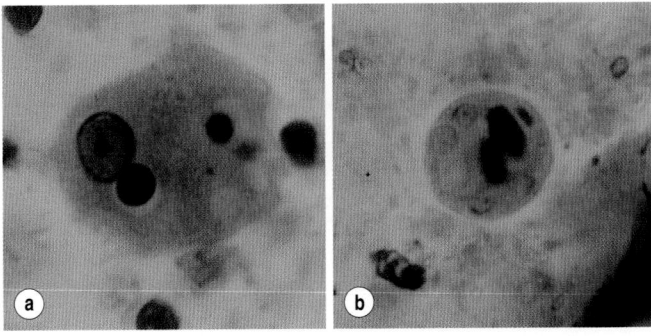

Figure 191-1 (a) *Entamoeba histolytica*, trophozoite containing ingested red blood cells (the presence of red blood cells confirms the organism is the true pathogen, *E. histolytica*). (b) *E. histolytica*/*E. dispar*, cyst containing four nuclei and chromatoidal bars with smooth, rounded edges (Trichrome stain). Note: from the cyst morphology, it is not possible to differentiate pathogenic *E. histolytica* from nonpathogenic *E. dispar*.

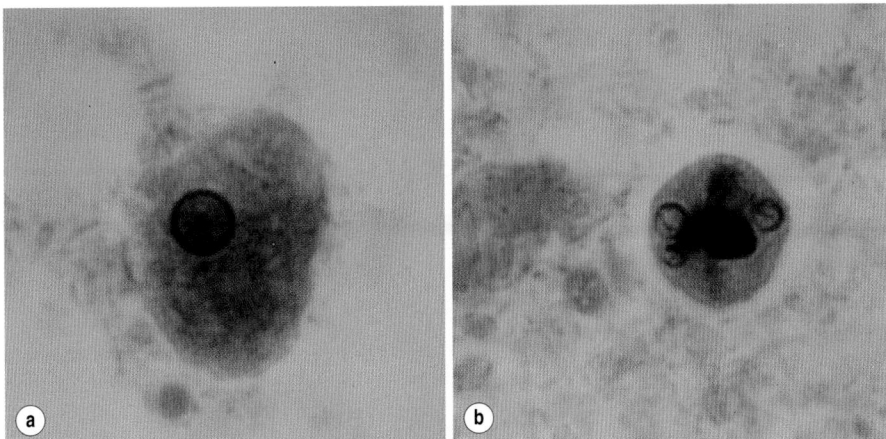

Figure 191-2 *Entamoeba hartmanni*. (a) Trophozoite. (b) Cyst containing up to four nuclei and chromatoidal bars with smooth, rounded edges (Trichrome stain). Note: *E. hartmanni* measures smaller than *E. histolytica*/*E. dispar*; the trophozoite is <12 μm and the cyst is <10 μm).

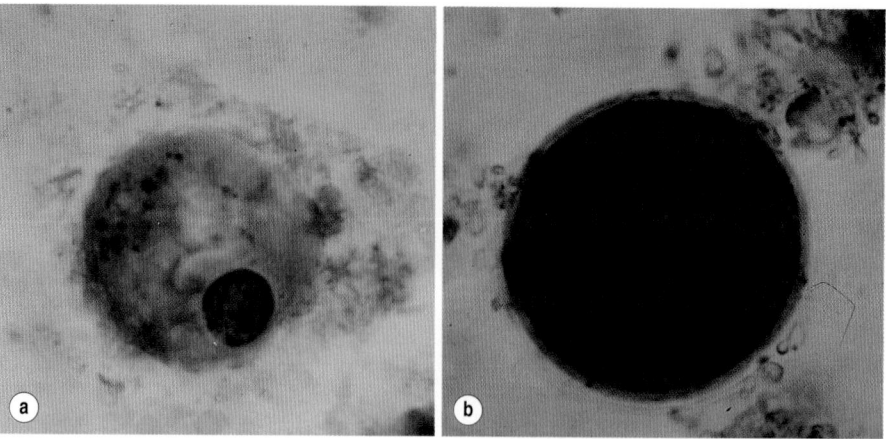

Figure 191-3 *Entamoeba coli.* (a) Trophozoite containing a single nucleus in which the karyosome is eccentric (tends to be centrally located in *E. histolytica/E. dispar*). (b) Cyst contains more than five nuclei (D'Antoni's iodine).

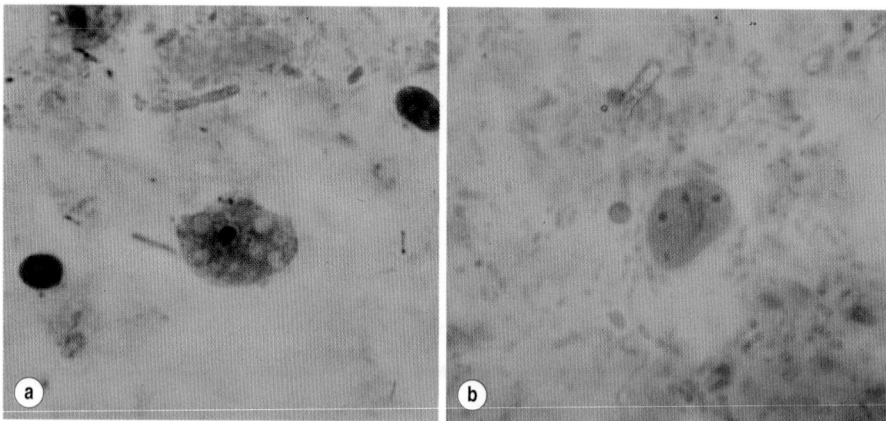

Figure 191-4 *Endolimax nana.* (a) Trophozoite containing a single nucleus with no peripheral chromatin (large karyosome only) and vacuolated cytoplasm. (b) Cyst containing four nuclei (three easily visible) (Trichrome stain).

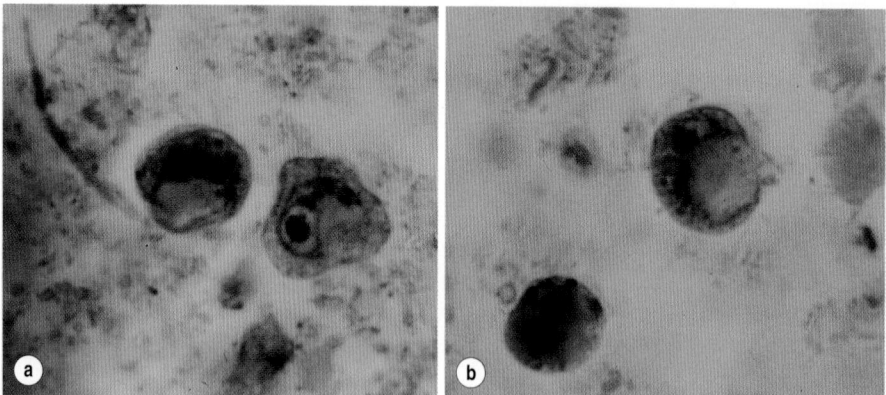

Figure 191-5 *Iodamoeba bütschlii.* (a) Trophozoite containing a single nucleus with a large karyosome and cyst containing a single nucleus and a large glycogen vacuole. (b) Cyst containing a single nucleus and a large glycogen vacuole – note the size of the karyosome (Trichrome stain). There is also a *Blastocystis* spp. central body form present at the lower left of the image.

undulating membrane, sucking disk, cytostome, spiral groove, and the number and location of flagellae, are important characteristics used to identify flagellate trophozoites. The organism shape and size, number and position of nuclei, and absence or arrangement of fibrils are used to identify flagellate cysts.

In some cases, species can be determined by the examination of either direct or concentrated wet mounts. Species of cysts may be identified in iodine-stained mounts. However, permanent stains are always recommended for every stool specimen submitted; organisms

identified in wet preparations may not represent all types of organisms present.

Giardia lamblia (G. duodenalis, G. intestinalis)

Diagnosis is usually established by the demonstration of cysts or, occasionally, trophozoites in feces (Figure 191-7). Nonpathogenic flagellates can be seen in Figure 191-8. Because of the variable shedding of organisms, several stool specimens should be examined before the infection is ruled out. In some cases, a series of stools can be examined

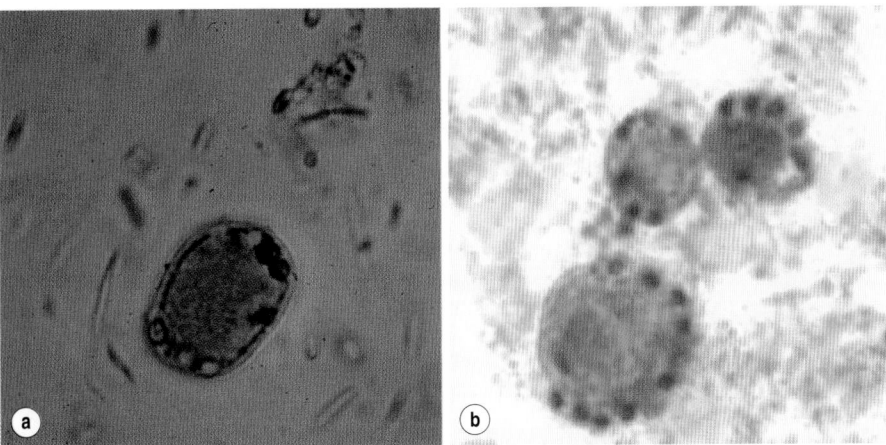

Figure 191-6 *Blastocystis* spp. (a) Central body form with large 'empty' area (appears like a vacuole) with multiple nuclei around the edges (D'Antoni's iodine). (b) Three central body forms with the large empty area surrounded by nuclei (Trichrome stain).

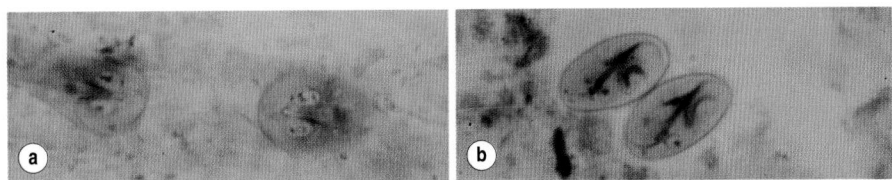

Figure 191-7 *Giardia lamblia*. (a) Trophozoites in mucus – note the sucking disk area, linear axonemes, curved median bodies and two nuclei (Trichrome stain). (b) Cysts containing multiple nuclei, linear axonemes and curved median bodies (iron-hematoxylin stain).

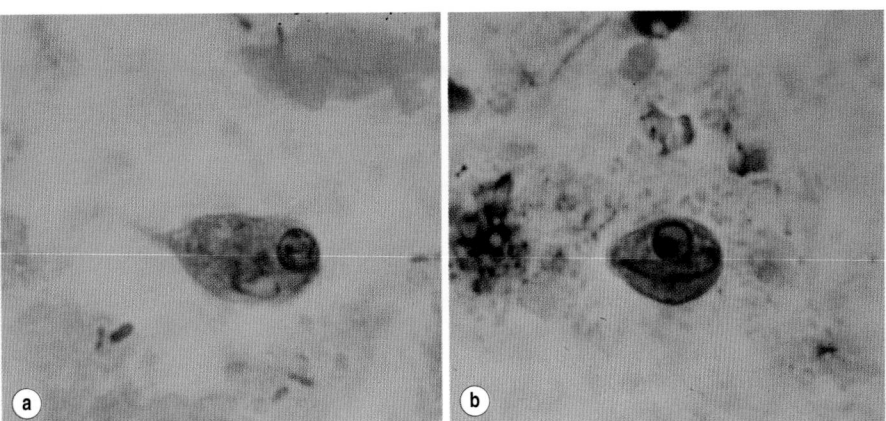

Figure 191-8 *Chilomastix mesnili*. (a) Trophozoite with single nucleus and clear feeding groove/cytostome. (b) Cyst containing single nucleus and curved fibril called the 'Shepherd's Crook' (Trichrome stain).

and be negative, and yet a successful therapeutic trial suggests that the patient did indeed have giardiasis. It is important for the laboratory and the clinician to recognize this fact. Permanent stains are recommended for the definitive diagnosis of this infection.

When *G. lamblia* organisms are not found in stool specimens, duodenal aspirates, string test mucus or biopsied mucosal tissue can be examined. The string test[54] is used to collect mucus from the duodenal area and its use may be less traumatic for the patient than other methods. Materials obtained by drainage, aspiration or the string test can be examined by simple, direct wet mounts. Biopsy tissue may be processed and stained by the usual histopathologic methods; however, before preservation, a fresh imprint smear of the mucosal surface on a slide can be made and stained with trichrome or Giemsa stain.

Immunoassay methods (enzyme immunoassay, FA, immunochromatographic lateral membrane flow assay) are available and may be appropriate. Education of the medical staff will be mandatory to ensure that tests are appropriately ordered and that there is complete understanding of the limits of the information generated (test results limited to absence or presence of *G. lamblia*). Industrial companies and municipalities have shown a great deal of interest in these reagents. This is particularly relevant when the water sources are used for drinking and/or recreational purposes.[54]

Dientamoeba fragilis

Permanent stains are required to diagnose this infection, and multiple specimens may be required because shedding varies from day to day. The delicately staining trophozoites are often binucleate, although the nuclei may be in different planes of focus (Figure 191-9). Trophozoites containing a single nucleus are also seen. The nuclei tend to be fragmented and the nuclear chromatin can often be seen in a 'tetrad' formation. These organisms must be differentiated from the trophozoites of *Endolimax nana*, *Iodamoeba bütschlii* and *Entamoeba hartmanni*. Nuclear characteristics, the presence of binucleate forms, tremendous size variation and the very rare number of cysts will aid in identification of this organism. Precysts and cysts are extremely difficult to

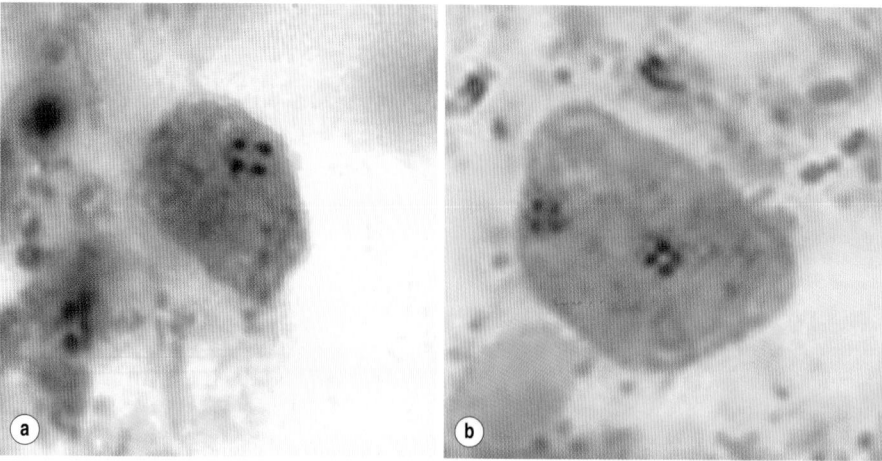

Figure 191-9 *Dientamoeba fragilis.* (a) Trophozoite with single nucleus fragmented into a 'tetrad' configuration. (b) Trophozoite containing two nuclei, each showing fragmented chromatin (Trichrome stain). A cyst form has recently been confirmed, although they are extremely rare in clinical specimens.

identify and tend to be quite rare when compared with cyst numbers of other protozoa.

A permanent stained smear should be examined for every stool specimen submitted to the laboratory for an ova and parasite examination.[54,55] If this approach is not used, then many infections with this organism can be missed. If a laboratory periodically finds and identifies *G. lamblia*, but never sees *D. fragilis*, then collection and diagnostic methods should be reviewed.

IDENTIFICATION OF FLAGELLATES IN UROGENITAL SPECIMENS

Trichomonas vaginalis

Infections with *T. vaginalis* are usually detected by finding the motile trophozoites in wet mounts of vaginal fluid, prostatic fluid or sediments of freshly passed urine. In wet mounts, the trophozoites move with a nervous, jerky motion and possess an undulating membrane, which extends only one-half the length of the organism (Figure 191-10). In old urine specimens, the organisms may be dead or badly distorted and thus cannot be identified or may be confused with host cells.

Specimens include vaginal fluid, scrapings or washings. They may be examined in a saline wet mount or as a stained smear, or the material can be cultured. Although some consider that wet-mount examinations are as efficient as cultures in revealing infections, current evidence suggests that cultivation methods are superior.[52] Immunofluorescent, ELISA and molecular methods have also been described. Organisms may be difficult to recognize in permanent stains; however, if a dry smear is submitted to the laboratory, Giemsa or Papanicolaou (Pap) stain can be used. Chronic *T. vaginalis* infections may cause atypical cellular changes that can be misinterpreted, particularly on the Pap smear. Organisms are routinely missed on Gram stains. The number of false-positive and false-negative results reported on the basis of stained smears strongly suggests that identification should be confirmed by observation of motile organisms, either from the direct wet mount or from appropriate culture media.

For culture, it is mandatory that the specimen be collected correctly, immediately inoculated into the proper medium and properly incubated. Excellent methods are available using plastic envelopes containing appropriate media. This envelope approach allows both immediate examination and culture in one self-contained envelope. These systems are commercially available and serve as the specimen transport container, the growth chamber during incubation and the 'slide' during microscopy.[54,59–61]

Monoclonal antibodies and DNA probe procedures for the detection of *T. vaginalis* have been reported as being very effective.[62,63] An enzyme immunoassay has been developed for the detection of the *T. vaginalis* antigen from vaginal swabs.[64,65] The predictive value of a positive test was 82% and that of a negative test was 99.3%. Commercial products based on these methodologies should be very helpful in diagnosing this infection. Serologic tests have been tried; however, none is commercially available.

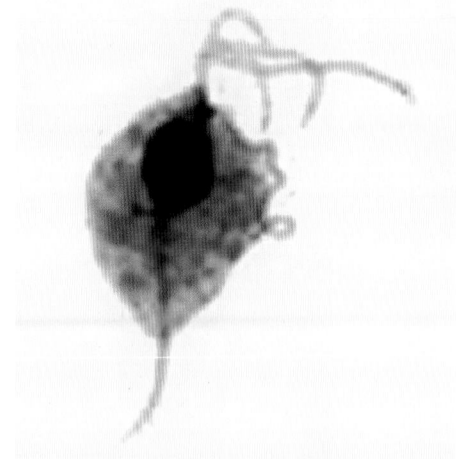

Figure 191-10 *Trichomonas vaginalis.* Trophozoites showing axostyle, flagella and part of the undulating membrane (smaller organism) (Giemsa stain). There is no known cyst form for this organism.

IDENTIFICATION OF CILIATES IN FECAL SPECIMENS

Balantidium coli

In human feces, *B. coli* trophozoites are readily recognized by their large size, their shape and their rapid, rotating motion. Cysts are less easily identified, but they usually cause few diagnostic problems. The morphology of trophozoites and cysts is seen in Figure 191-11.

Examination of direct saline mounts is the most practical method of detecting these protozoa. Cysts can be recovered by concentration, but in human infections trophozoites are usually more numerous than cysts. Iodine-stained mounts and permanent stains are of little value because the organisms tend to overstain and may resemble helminth eggs and/or debris.

MOLECULAR TESTING OF INTESTINAL AND UROGENITAL PROTOZOA

In 2013, the FDA approved the first test that can simultaneously detect 11 common viral, bacterial and parasitic (*Cryptosporidium*, *Giardia*, *Entamoeba histolytica*) causes of infectious gastroenteritis from a single

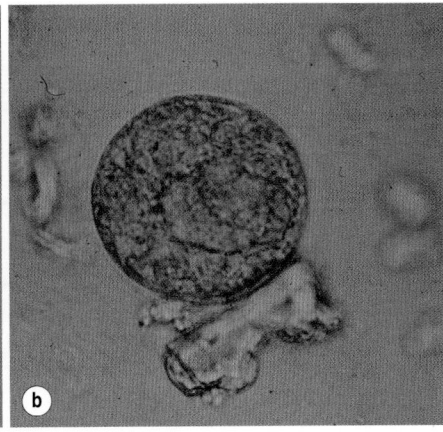

Figure 191-11 *Balantidium coli.* (a) Trophozoite – note the cilia around the edges ('fuzzy football'). (b) Cyst – note the cilia are difficult to see within the cyst wall (D'Antoni's iodine – light preparation, pale color).

patient sample (xTAG Gastrointestinal Pathogen Panel, Luminex, Inc, Austin, TX).[66,67] Another FDA-approved molecular diagnostic test for parasites is the APTIMA *Trichomonas vaginalis* Assay (GenProbe, San Diego, CA). This assay utilizes the same amplification technology that has been used for years to detect *Neisseria gonorrheae* and *Chlamydia trachomatis*,[68] It also uses the same specimen types (i.e. clinician-collected vaginal and endocervical swabs, female urine and PreservCyt solution). It has reported high sensitivity and specificity, and does not require organism viability or motility. It, as well as other antigen-based assays, represents advances in the detection of this parasite. The Affirm VPIII molecular test (Becton Dickinson, Burlington, NC) is used to detect and identify *Candida* species, *T. vaginalis* and *Gardnerella vaginalis*.[69]

There are also several molecular tests that are under development or in clinical trials for the detection of select gastrointestinal parasites. These tests are molecular gastrointestinal panels and target the most commonly occurring bacterial, viral and parasitic stool pathogens. Although there are laboratory developed tests for most parasites, these are not commercially available or available only in specialized testing centers. When such tests are used, there should be attention given to the use of internal amplification controls to detect inhibition, since common specimens, such as stool, contain PCR inhibitors. Thorough validation is required before these are implemented for clinical testing.

Clinical Manifestations and Management

The clinical manifestations and management of infections caused by these organisms are discussed in Chapters 53, 114 and 116.

References available online at expertconsult.com.

KEY REFERENCES

Baldursson S., Karanis P.: Waterborne transmission of protozoan parasites: review of worldwide outbreaks – an update 2004–2010. *Water Res* 2011; 45:6603-6614.

Barratt J.L., Harkness J., Marriott D., et al.: A review of *Dientamoeba fragilis* carriage in humans: several reasons why this organism should be considered in the diagnosis of gastrointestinal illness. *Gut Microbes* 2011; 2:3-12.

Barroso L., Abhyankar M., Noor Z., et al.: Expression, purification, and evaluation of recombinant LecA as a candidate for an amebic colitis vaccine. *Vaccine* 2014; 32: 1218-1224.

Clark C.G., Roser D., Stensvold C.R.: Transmission of *Dientamoeba fragilis*: pinworm or cysts? *Trends Parasitol* 2014; 30:136-140.

Eroglu F., Koltas I.S.: Evaluation of the transmission mode of *B. hominis* by using PCR method. *Parasitol Res* 2010; 107:841-845.

Garcia L.S.: *Diagnostic medical parasitology*, 5th ed. Washington, DC: ASM Press; 2007.

Johnson E.H., Windsor J.J., Clark C.G.: Emerging from obscurity: biological, clinical, and diagnostic aspects of *Dientamoeba fragilis*. *Clin Microbiol Rev* 2004; 17:553-570.

Khairnar K., Parija S.C.: A novel nested multiplex polymerase chain reaction (PCR) assay for differential detection of *Entamoeba histolytica*, *E. moshkovskii* and *E. dispar* DNA in stool samples. *BMC Microbiol* 2007; 6:47.

Munasinghe V.S., Vella N.G., Ellis J.T., et al.: Cyst formation and faecal–oral transmission of *Dientamoeba fragilis* – the missing link in the life cycle of an emerging pathogen. *Int J Parasitol* 2013; 43:879-883.

Rughooputh S., Greenwell P.: *Trichomonas vaginalis*: paradigm of a successful sexually transmitted organism. *Br J Biomed Sci* 2005; 62:193-200.

Schwebke J.R., Hobbs M.M.N., Taylor S.N., et al.: Molecular testing for *Trichomonas vaginalis* in women: results from a prospective U.S. clinical trial. *J Clin Microbiol* 2011; 49:4106-4111.

Stark D., van Hal S., Marriott D., et al.: Irritable bowel syndrome: a review on the role of intestinal protozoa and the importance of their detection and diagnosis. *Int J Parasitol* 2007; 37:11-20.

Stark D., Garcia L.S., Barratt J.L., et al.: Description of *Dientamoeba fragilis* cyst and precystic forms from human samples. *J Clin Microbiol* 2014; 52:2680-2683.

Vandenberg O., Peek R., Souayah H., et al.: Clinical and microbiological features of dientamoebiasis in patients suspected of suffering from a parasitic gastrointestinal illness: a comparison of *Dientamoeba fragilis* and *Giardia lamblia* infections. *Int J Infect Dis* 2006; 10: 255-261.

Wessels E., Rusman L.G., van Bussel M.S., et al.: Added value of multiplex Luminex Gastrointestinal Pathogen Panel (xTAG(®) GPP) testing in the diagnosis of infectious gastroenteritis. *Clin Microbiol Infect* 2014; 30:O182-O187.

Yoder J.S., Gargano J.W., Wallace R.M., et al.: Giardiasis surveillance – United States, 2009–2010. *MMWR Surveill Summ* 2012; 61:13-23.

192 Intestinal Coccidia and Microsporidia

RAINER WEBER

Intestinal coccidia and microsporidia have primarily gained attention as etiologic agents of HIV-associated diarrhea and intestinal disease among persons with other cellular immunodeficiencies, including organ transplant recipients or patients undergoing chemotherapy. These organisms, however, are not only opportunistic pathogens, but are also the cause of common, worldwide intestinal infections in immunocompetent children and adults. Also, newly described microsporidia are recognized as causing a wide range of organ or systemic infections in immunocompromised patients.

Nature

INTESTINAL COCCIDIA

The intestinal coccidia are obligate intracellular protozoa that belong to the phylum Apicomplexa, subphylum Sporozoa, and infect small intestinal enterocytes. Species of four genera (*Cryptosporidium*, *Cyclospora*, *Cystoisospora* [previously termed *Isospora*], and *Sarcocystis*) are pathogenic in humans.[1–5]

Among the 30 currently named *Cryptosporidium* species, 14 species have been detected in humans so far.[6] The most frequent species of human cryptosporidiosis are *C. hominis*[7] and the bovine species *C. pestis* (also known as the bovine genotype of the *C. parvum* species complex), which is the principal zoonotic species worldwide. Also, other zoonotic cryptosporidia have been identified in stools of patients with human immunodeficiency virus (HIV) infection and in HIV-seronegative persons, particularly children living in resource-poor countries, including species of moderate public health significance (*C. meleagridis*, *C. cuniculus*, *C. felis* and *C. viatorum*), species of minor public health significance (*C. muris*, *C. parvum*, *C. andersoni*, *C. canis*, *C. suis*, *C. fayeri* and *C. ubiquitum* [previously known as the cervine genotype]), and the *Cryptosporidium* monkey, horse, skunk, hedgehog and chipmunk genotypes.[6,8,9]

Cyclospora cayetanensis are intestinal organisms that previously were termed blue–green algae, cyanobacterium-like bodies or coccidia-like bodies.[2] *Cystoisopora belli* (formerly termed *Isospora belli*) has been identified as the only accepted cause of human cystoisosporiasis.[4] *Sarcocystis hominis* and *S. suihominis* are acquired by eating raw meat from infected cattle and pigs, respectively, but intestinal sarcocystosis in humans is infrequent, and is only rarely associated with diarrhea.[5] Other zoonotic *Sarcocystis* spp. may cause human disease. The zoonotic origin of a recent human outbreak in Malaysia due to *Sarcocystis nesbitti* infection, associated with febrile myositis, is unknown at present.[10–12]

MICROSPORIDIA

The term 'microsporidia' is a nontaxonomic designation commonly used to describe a group of obligate intracellular, spore-forming eukaryotes belonging to the phylum Microsporidia. Genome-wide sequence and synteny analyses suggest that Microsporidia belong to the kingdom of the Fungi,[13] being derived from an endoparasitic chytrid ancestor on the earliest diverging branch of the fungal phylogenetic tree.[14] Approximately 1400 species have been identified that are parasitic in every major animal group, and 16 of these can infect humans (Table 192-1). To date, nine genera (*Anncaliia*, *Encephalitozoon*, *Endoreticulatus*, *Enterocytozoon*, *Nosema*, *Pleistophora*, *Trachipleistophora*, *Tubulinosema* and *Vittaforma*) and unclassified microsporidia (referred to collectively as *Microsporidium*) have been implicated in human infections.[15–20]

Epidemiology

CRYPTOSPORIDIUM SPECIES

Cryptosporidial infections have been detected on all continents. Cumulative prevalence rates are between 1% and 3% in industrialized nations and between 5% and 10% in low- and middle-income countries (LMIC).[21] Children, particularly those under 2 years of age, have a higher prevalence of infection than adults.[22] Seroepidemiologic studies indicate that cryptosporidiosis may be more common than is estimated based upon surveys of fecal oocyst shedding. Seroprevalence rates in higher-income countries range between 25% and 35%, and in LMIC they are up to 65%. In severely immunodeficient patients with

TABLE 192-1	**Microsporidial Species Pathogenic in Humans, and Clinical Manifestations**	
	CLINICAL MANIFESTATIONS	
Microsporidial Species	**Immunocompromised Patients**	**Immunocompetent Persons**
Anncaliia algerae (formerly *Brachiola algerae* and *Nosema algerae*)	Myositis Nodular cutaneous lesions Vocal cord infection	Keratitis
Anncaliia connori (formerly *Brachiola connori* and *Nosema connori*)	Systemic infection	Not described
Anncaliia vesicularum (formerly *Brachiola vesicularum*)	Myositis	Not described
Encephalitozoon cuniculi	Systemic infection Keratoconjunctivitis Sinusitis, pneumonitis Urinary tract infection, nephritis Hepatitis Peritonitis Intestinal infections Encephalitis Endocarditis	Seizures, encephalitis, brain abscess
Encephalitozoon hellem	Systemic infection Keratoconjunctivitis Sinusitis, bronchitis, pneumonia Nephritis, ureteritis, cystitis, prostatitis, urethritis	Possibly diarrhea
Encephalitozoon intestinalis (formerly *Septata intestinalis*)	Diarrhea Cholangiopathy, cholangitis, acalculous cholecystitis Sinusitis, bronchitis, pneumonitis Urinary tract infection, nephritis Bone lesions Nodular cutaneous lesions	Self-limiting diarrhea, asymptomatic carriers
Endoreticulatus spp.	Not described	Myositis, systemic infection
Enterocytozoon bieneusi	Diarrhea, wasting syndrome Cholangiopathy, cholangitis, acalculous cholecystitis Sinusitis, bronchitis, pneumonitis	Self-limiting diarrhea in adults and children, travelers' diarrhea, asymptomatic carriers
Microsporidium africanum	Not described	Corneal ulcer, keratitis
Microsporidium ceylonensis	Not described	Corneal ulcer, keratitis
Nosema ocularum	Not described	Keratitis
Pleistophora ronneafiei	Myositis	Not described
Trachipleistophora anthropophthera	Systemic infection including brain, heart, kidney, eye	Not described
Trachipleistophora hominis	Myositis Keratoconjunctivitis Sinusitis	Keratitis
Tubulinosema acridophagus	Disseminated infection, including hepatitis, pulmonary and peritoneal infection Myositis Skin lesions	Not described
Vittaforma corneae (formerly *Nosema corneum*)	Systemic infection Urinary tract infection	Keratoconjunctivitis

HIV infection, cryptosporidiosis is among the most important causes of chronic diarrhea, accounting for 10–20% of diarrheal episodes.[23]

Sources of infectious cryptosporidial oocysts are humans and animals. Oocysts are transmitted by the fecal–oral route and infection may be acquired from contaminated surfaces, ground and recreational water, pets, farm animals (particularly cattle and sheep), contaminated foods and person-to-person contact, including transmission between household members, sexual partners, children in daycare centers and nosocomial infections involving both medical care staff and patients.[24–26] An increasing number of outbreaks of cryptosporidial infections attributed to drinking water have been reported, including an outbreak in Milwaukee, USA in 1993 that affected over 400 000 persons.[27] Ingestion of as few as 10 oocysts may cause diarrhea.

CYCLOSPORA SPECIES

Cyclospora spp. have been identified worldwide in stool specimens of immunocompromised and immunocompetent patients, including travelers, but the source of infection appears to be restricted to tropical and subtropical areas. The parasite is transmitted by the fecal–oral route and infection is most probably acquired from contaminated water or food (particularly raspberries and green leafy vegetables) from tropical or subtropical countries.[28,29] It is not known whether animals can be infected and serve as sources for human infection. Direct person-to-person transmission is unlikely because excreted oocysts require days to weeks to become infectious. Warm temperatures and high humidity facilitate sporulation.

CYSTOISOSPORA SPECIES

Cystoisospora belli is endemic in many parts of Africa, Asia and South America, and is particularly common in patients from developing countries who have acquired immunodeficiency syndrome (AIDS) and chronic diarrhea; for example, it occurs in 10–20% of such patients in Haiti or Africa. Modes of transmission are not known but it is assumed that they comprise water or food that contains oocysts.[3]

MICROSPORIDIA

Reported human infections are globally dispersed. Although microsporidiosis appears to occur most frequently in persons infected with HIV, it is emerging as an infection in otherwise immunocompromised hosts, such as organ transplant recipients or patients undergoing chemotherapy, and in immunocompetent individuals, including travelers, the elderly and children.[15,17]

The sources of microsporidia infecting humans and modes of transmission are uncertain. Because microsporidial spores are released into the environment via stool, urine and respiratory secretions, possible sources of infection may be persons or animals infected with microsporidia as well as contaminated water, food and soil.[16,30–32] Ingestion of microsporidial spores is the most probable mode of transmission. Transmission by the aerosol route has also been considered because spores have been found in respiratory specimens of patients who have *Encephalitozoon* spp. infection.[33] Recently, transplant-associated transmissions of *E. cuniculi* were documented.[34]

Pathogenicity

CRYPTOSPORIDIUM SPECIES

Cryptosporidium spp. develop intracellularly at the microvillous border of enterocytes (Figure 192-1). Infected cells lack microvilli at the site of parasite attachment and the mucosal surface appears disrupted. In immunocompetent individuals, infection is usually limited to the intestine. In immunocompromised patients, organisms are found throughout the entire gastrointestinal tract and within epithelial cells of the biliary tree, the pancreatic ducts and the airways. In the intestines, cryptosporidial infection induces atrophy, blunting or loss of villi, crypt hyperplasia and infiltration of lymphocytes, neutrophils, plasma cells and macrophages into the lamina propria. Cryptosporidial infection has been associated with marked reduction in the brush border enzyme activities, including sucrase, lactase and maltase deficiency, with impaired absorption of vitamin B12 and D-xylose, and with increased permeability of the intestinal epithelium to organic molecules. Malabsorption and intestinal injury appear to correlate with the number of organisms infecting the intestine. No specific virulence determinants of the parasite have been clearly linked to direct or indirect damage of intestinal host tissues. Putative virulence factors include molecules that are involved in parasite attachment to host cells and host cell membrane disruption.[26]

The immune response to cryptosporidial infection involves both innate and adaptive immune responses.[35] CD4+ lymphocytes and interferon-gamma (IFN-γ) play key roles in the memory response.[36]

Severe or persistent cryptosporidiosis has primarily been observed in HIV-infected patients with marked CD4+ cell immunodeficiency,[23] and rarely in persons with IFN-γ deficiency or with X-linked hyper-IgM syndrome which leads to secondary hypogammaglobulinemia and impaired cellular immune function.

CYSTOISOSPORA SPECIES

Cystoisospora belli develop within parasitophorous vacuoles deep in the cytoplasm of the enterocyte. Histologic abnormalities associated with cystoisosporiasis range from minimal changes of the small intestinal architecture to marked villous atrophy, crypt hyperplasia and inflammatory infiltrates in the lamina propria consisting of eosinophils, neutrophils, lymphocytes and plasma cells. The mechanisms by which these changes occur are unknown. As a result of the intestinal injury, malabsorption and steatorrhea have been documented.[3]

CYCLOSPORA SPECIES

Cyclosporiasis is associated with villous atrophy, crypt hyperplasia and inflammatory infiltrates. The mechanisms that lead to the clinical features are unknown.[29]

MICROSPORIDIA

Microsporidiosis has been associated with abnormalities in structure and function of infected organs but how the different microsporidial species cause disease is not sufficiently understood.[15,17]

Enterocytozoon bieneusi infection generally appears to be limited to intestinal enterocytes (Figure 192-2) and biliary epithelium. Patients who have severe cellular immunodeficiency appear at highest risk of developing microsporidial disease but little is known about immunity to *E. bieneusi* infection due to the lack of tissue culture or small animal models. It is not understood whether microsporidial infection in these patients is primarily a reactivation of latent infection acquired before the state of suppressed immunity or whether microsporidial disease is caused by recently acquired infection.

Encephalitozoon cuniculi and *E. hellem* infect a variety of cells, including epithelial and endothelial cells, fibroblasts, kidney tubule cells, macrophages and possibly other cell types in numerous mammalian hosts, for example rabbits, rodents, carnivores, monkeys and humans.[16] In mammals, they usually cause latent asymptomatic or chronic mildly symptomatic infection, but interstitial nephritis and severe neurologic disease caused by central nervous system vasculitis and granulomatous encephalitis may occur. The parasites are able to

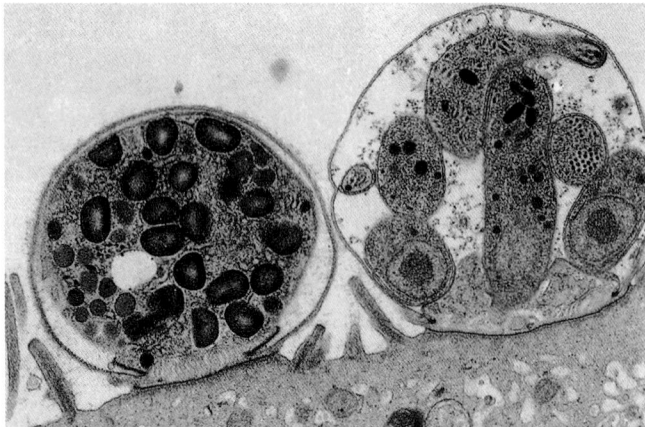

Figure 192-1 Intestinal cryptosporidial infection. Transmission electron micrograph of duodenal tissue of a patient with HIV infection showing two different developmental stages of *Cryptosporidium* spp. on the brush border of the mucosal surface: mature schizont with merozoites (right), undifferentiated zygote (left). *Cryptosporidium* spp. develop intracellularly just under the plasma membrane of the host cell. *(Courtesy of M.A. Spycher.)*

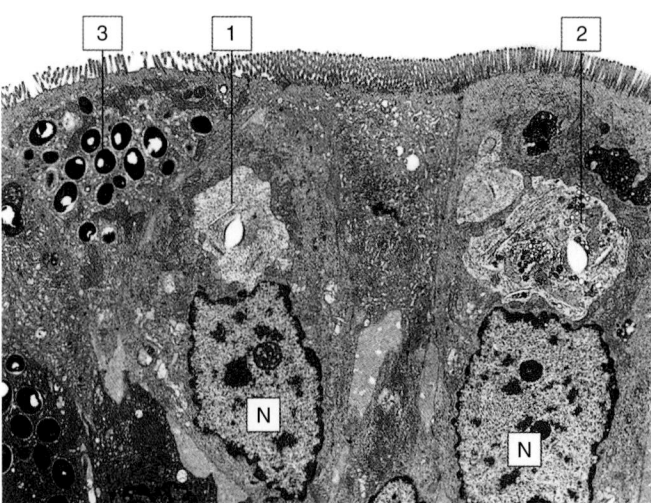

Figure 192-2 Intestinal *Enterocytozoon bieneusi* infection. Transmission electron micrograph showing duodenal epithelium of a patient with HIV infection who has *E. bieneusi* infection. The different developmental stages between the enterocyte nuclei (N) and the microvillous border include: (1) a proliferative plasmodium; (2) late sporogonial plasmodia; and (3) mature spores. *(Courtesy of M.A. Spycher.)*

persist in their animal hosts despite an active immune response. Microsporidial infection activates antibody production, although antibodies alone do not appear to yield protection. Gut-associated lymphoid tissues have been found to be important for the control of experimental oral infection.[37] The role of a competent cellular immune response in suppressing microsporidial multiplication is suggested by epidemiologic studies in humans, and has been established experimentally.[37–39] *In vitro* studies demonstrated the importance of IFN-γ and tumor necrosis factor in resistance to *Encephalitozoon* spp.[37,40] The pathogenesis of human *Encephalitozoon* infection has yet to be defined. Rare histologic and clinical investigations in immunodeficient patients have indicated that *E. cuniculi* and *E. hellem* usually cause disseminated infection in this patient group.[33]

Prevention

CRYPTOSPORIDIOSIS

No vaccine is available to prevent cryptosporidiosis. Cryptosporidial oocysts are remarkably resistant to many common disinfectants, including chlorine-based compounds. Therefore, the water industry has studied alternative methods to inactivate water-borne oocysts, including a water disinfection device delivering germicidal ultraviolet (UV) light that yielded promising results. However, control of surface-water contamination and adequate filter systems are required to guarantee the complete removal of cryptosporidia from water supplies.

CYCLOSPORIASIS, CYSTOISOSPORIASIS

Avoiding food or water that may be contaminated with feces may prevent cyclosporiasis and cystoisosporiasis, but details of the sources of infection and the modes of transmission often remain unknown. Molecular diagnostic tools may allow for surveillance of recognized vehicles of transmission, such as produce, fruits and water,[41] but whether such measures will reduce the burden of human infections is not proven.

MICROSPORIDIOSIS

Laboratory experiments indicate that the thick-walled spores may survive in the environment for months or years depending on the temperature and humidity. Exposure to recommended working concentrations of most disinfectants, boiling and autoclaving seem to kill *Encephalitozoon* spp. spores but no data are available for *Enterocytozoon* spp. Successful disinfection of *Encephalitozoon* spp. in water using chlorine and ozone disinfection has been demonstrated.[42]

Diagnostic Microbiology

Stool examination by light microscopy is the most important test to diagnose intestinal coccidia and intestinal microsporidia (Table 192-2). There are no culture methods for diagnostic purposes. In many laboratories, tests for *Cryptosporidium* spp., *Cystoisospora* spp., *Cyclospora* spp. and microsporidia must be specifically requested because the general request of 'stool for O & P' (ova and parasites) often does not mean that the specific methods to detect these organisms are applied. Microsporidial species that cause systemic infection are often detected in urine sediments.

CRYPTOSPORIDIUM SPECIES

Examination of Stool Specimens by Light Microscopy

To visualize cryptosporidial oocysts in fecal smears, acid-fast staining (e.g. modified cold Kinyoun technique; Figure 192-3) and the immunofluorescence (IF) technique are among the most sensitive, specific and widely used methods. The IF detection procedure is more sensitive than acid-fast staining, but the difference in sensitivity may not be of clinical relevance in clinical routine.[43] The oocysts should be measured in order to distinguish the coccidia (Table 192-2). Enhanced sensitivity of stool examination can be obtained by concentrating oocysts, preferably with the formalin-ethyl acetate (FEA) technique.

The exact sensitivity of the coprodiagnostic techniques is not known but some data raise questions about the widely held belief that these techniques are sufficient to meet the needs of clinicians and epidemiologists. Examination of multiple specimens may be necessary, because clinical studies have shown that examination of single stool specimens may have an insufficient diagnostic yield. Furthermore, in a prospective analysis of jejunal biopsies in patients who have AIDS, *Cryptosporidium* spp. were present in more than 10% of patients whose

---

TABLE 192-2	**Diagnosis of Intestinal Coccidia and Microsporidia**				
	INTESTINAL COCCIDIA			**MICROSPORIDIA**	
Microsporidial Species	*Cryptosporidia*	*Cyclospora*	*Cystoisospora*	Intestinal	Systemic
Routine Diagnostic Tests					
Light microscopy, stool	+	+	+	+	(+)
Light microscopy, urine and possibly other body fluids	–	–	–	–	+
Antigen detection, stool	+	–	–	–	–
Molecular detection	+	+	–	+	+
Culture	–	–	–	–	–
Serology	–	–	–	–	–
Biopsy	Intestinal	Intestinal	Intestinal	Intestinal	Infected organ
Morphology of Pathogen					
Staining	AF, IF	AF	AF	Chromotrope, calcofluor	Chromotrope, calcofluor, special tissue stains
Size of coccidial oocysts/ microsporidial spores	4–6 μm	8–10 μm	23–33 μm long, 10–19 μm wide	1–3.5 μm	1–3.5 μm
Species identification	Molecular analysis	Molecular analysis	Molecular analysis	Electron microscopy; molecular analysis	Electron microscopy; molecular analysis
Stool Concentration Techniques	FEA	FEA	FEA	–	–

Abbreviations: +, available or applicable; –, not available or not applicable; AF, acid-fast staining (e.g. modified cold Kinyoun technique); FEA, formalin-ethyl acetate technique; IF, immunofluorescence.

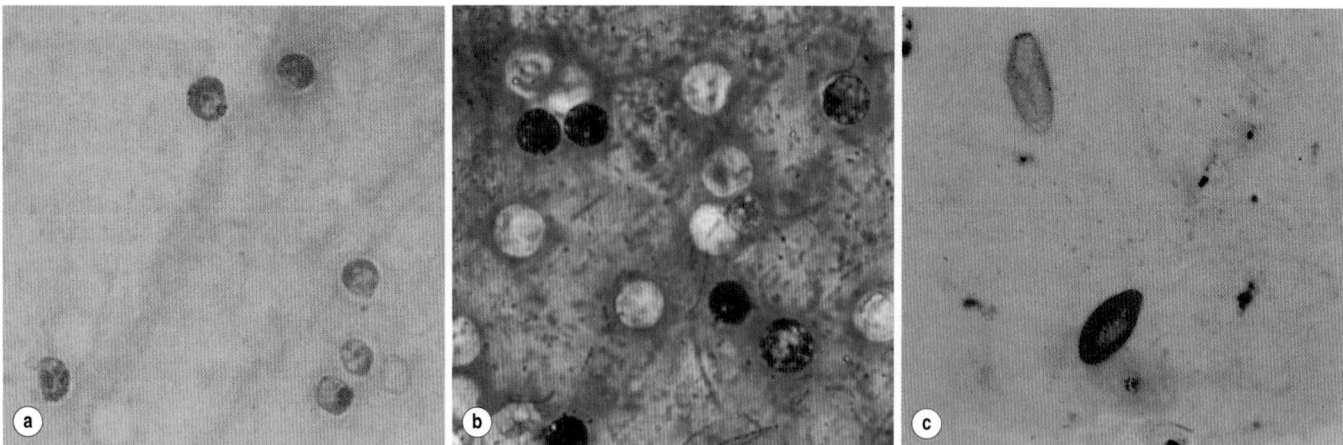

Figure 192-3 Acid-fast stained smears of fecal specimens showing intestinal coccidia. (a) *Cryptosporidium* spp., round, 4–6 μm diameter. (b) *Cyclospora* spp., round, 8–10 μm diameter. (c) *Cystoisospora belli*, elliptical, 23–33 μm long and 10–19 μm wide. Modified Kinyoun stain. *(Panel b, Courtesy of E.G. Long.)*

stool examinations were negative. Stool antigen detection techniques,[44] and molecular diagnostic methods, including multiplex polymerase chain reaction (PCR) techniques to detect multiple intestinal pathogens, have improved diagnostic yields but currently are not widely available in routine laboratories.[45]

Cytologic Diagnosis

Aspiration of duodenal fluid or small intestinal brushing can be used for diagnosis when upper endoscopy is performed. Examination of centrifuged duodenal aspirates under the microscope may be the most sensitive diagnostic procedure.

Histologic Examinations

Cryptosporidia appear basophilic by examination under the light microscope of small intestinal tissue sections stained with hematoxylin and eosin. The intracellular organisms seem to project into the intestinal lumen because of their apical extracytoplasmic localization. Under electron microscopy the unique ultrastructural features of different developmental stages of the parasite can be seen (Figure 192-1), but this is rarely necessary for diagnostic purposes.

Serology

Specific IgM or IgG antibodies to cryptosporidia can be detected within 2 weeks of onset of symptoms in most patients. In the majority of patients IgG titers may persist for long periods. Serologic testing is mainly used as an epidemiologic tool and has no diagnostic application, particularly because antibody persistence limits its use in the diagnosis of acute infection.

CYCLOSPORA SPECIES

Diagnosis of *Cyclospora* is dependent on detection by light microscopy of the refractile oocysts in wet mounts of fresh stool specimens or in acid-fast stained smears prepared from stool concentrated by the FEA sedimentation.[46] Acid-fast stained oocysts vary in appearance from faint pink to deep red, and many organisms remain as unstained spheres (Figure 192-3). The sensitivity of the coprodiagnostic techniques is unknown. In many patients' specimens, however, the number of oocysts detected per slide is low, indicating that not all symptomatic patients excrete a large enough number of oocysts for laboratory detection to be assured. Examination of small intestinal tissue of patients who have *Cyclospora* infection often did not reveal any parasites. The presence of intracellular parasites has rarely been documented in aspirated duodenal or jejunal fluid and on duodenal and jejunal biopsy (Figure 192-4). Molecular techniques including multiplex PCR methods to detect multiple parasites in stool samples have been described.[47]

CYSTOISOSPORA SPECIES

Diagnosis of *C. belli* is usually achieved by detection under the light microscope of the parasite oocysts in wet preparations or acid-fast

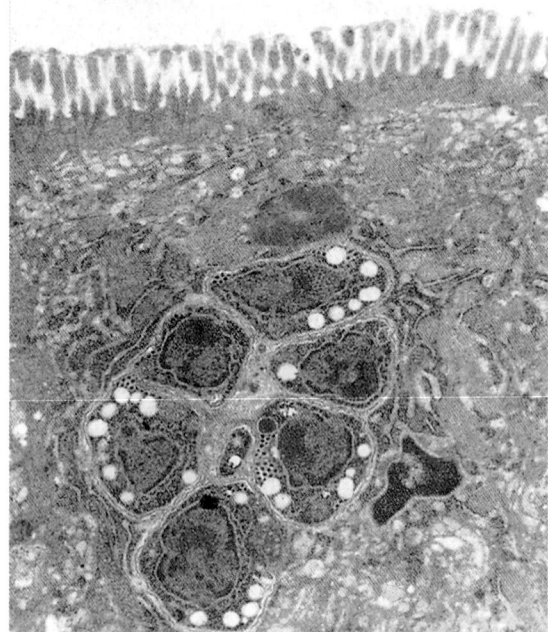

Figure 192-4 Intestinal *Cyclospora* infection. Transmission electron micrograph of duodenal epithelium obtained from a patient with HIV infection who has *Cyclospora cayetanensis* infection. A mature schizont filled with numerous merozoites is shown. *(Courtesy of A.M. Deloul and F.P. Chatelet.)*

stained smears of concentrated stool specimens (Figure 192-3). Repetitive stool examinations may be necessary because the parasite may be excreted intermittently or in low numbers. Histologic examination of small intestinal tissue sections may reveal the parasite within enterocytes.[29]

MICROSPORIDIA

Diagnosis of microsporidial infection is dependent on morphologic demonstration of the organisms themselves. This can be difficult because of the organisms' small size and staining properties which hamper visualization of the spores and developing stages using routine staining techniques. The spores, the stages by which microsporidia are usually identified, are small, ranging in size from 1 to 3.5 μm in diameter.

Evaluation of patients who have suspected microsporidiosis should begin with examination of body fluids by light microscopy using special staining techniques. Definitive species identification of microsporidia is made using electron microscopy, antigenic analysis and molecular analysis. Collection of fresh material (without fixative) may be useful for cell culture and for future molecular analysis.[15]

Examination of Stool Specimens

In patients who have suspected enteric microsporidiosis, examination of stool specimens by light microscopy is the first step. It is at least as sensitive as examination of biopsy specimens. Detection of microsporidial spores requires adequate illumination and magnification (i.e. ×630 or ×1000 magnification [oil immersion]), and special staining methods. The two most commonly used stains are the chromotrope stain, which appears to be the most specific (Figure 192-5),[48] and chemofluorescent agents, which might be more sensitive but may produce false-positive results.[49]

The differences in spore size between *Enterocytozoon* (1–1.5 μm in diameter) and *Encephalitozoon* spp. (2–3 μm in diameter) often permit a tentative diagnosis of the genus from examination of stool under the light microscope. The microsporidian should be identified to the level of genus by electron microscopy or molecular analysis because *Encephalitozoon* spp. have a propensity for dissemination, and have a different drug sensitivity pattern compared with *Enterocytozoon bieneusi*.

Immunofluorescent procedures for diagnosis of *Encephalitozoon*-like microsporidial spores are promising but not widely available. Diagnostic application of polyclonal antibodies in fecal samples has been hampered by background staining, cross-reactions with yeast and bacteria, and low sensitivity. Monoclonal antibodies against *Encephalitozoon* spp.[50] and against spores of *Enterocytozoon bieneusi* have been generated.[51]

Histologic Examination

Among patients with HIV infection who suffered from chronic diarrhea, stool examinations proved as sensitive as endoscopic evaluation.[23] Examination of duodenal and terminal ileal tissue has resulted in detection of microsporidia but the parasites are rarely found in colonic tissue sections. Only experienced pathologists have reliably and consistently identified microsporidia in tissue sections using routine techniques such as hematoxylin and eosin stain. In our experience, tissue Gram stains (such as Brown–Brenn or Brown–Hopps) have proved to be the most useful for the rapid and reliable identification of HIV-associated microsporidia in routine paraffin-embedded tissue sections

(Figure 192-6). Others prefer a silver stain (Warthin–Starry stain) or the chromotrope-based staining technique.

Cytologic Diagnosis

Microsporidial spores have been detected in sediments of duodenal aspirate, bile or biliary aspirates, urine (Figure 192-7), bronchoalveolar lavage fluid, cerebrospinal fluid (CSF) and in smears of conjunctival swabs, sputum and nasal discharge.[15] Because microsporidial infection often involves multiple organs, detection of microsporidia in virtually any tissue or bodily fluid should prompt a thorough search of other sites. In particular, urine specimens of patients suspected of having disseminated microsporidiosis should be examined.

Electron Microscopy

Microsporidial ultrastructure is unique and pathognomonic for the phylum and, with rare exceptions, ultrastructural features can distinguish between most genera of microsporidia (Figure 192-2 and 192-8).

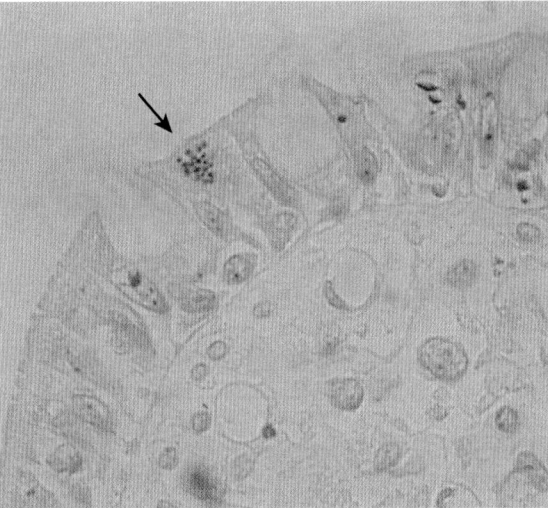

Figure 192-6 Intestinal *Enterocytozoon bieneusi* infection. Terminal ileal tissue obtained by ileocolonoscopy in a patient who has AIDS and chronic diarrhea caused by *E. bieneusi* infection. Gram-positive or gram-labile microsporidial spores (arrow) are found in supranuclear location within small intestinal enterocytes. Brown–Brenn stain.

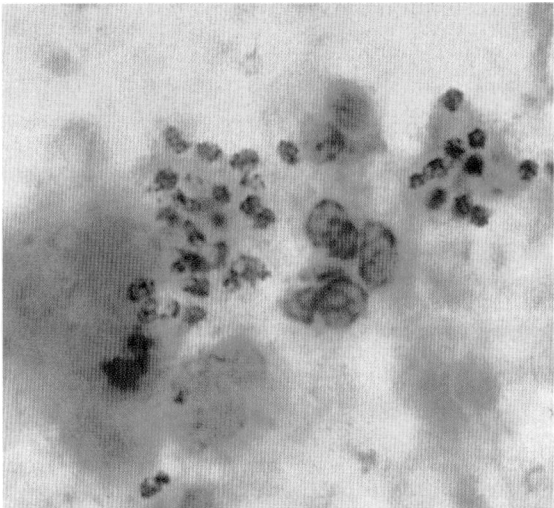

Figure 192-7 Detection of microsporidia in urine sediment. Urine sediment from a patient who has AIDS and disseminated *Encephalitozoon hellem* infection, showing gram-labile intracellular and extracellular microsporidial spores. Gram stain (oil immersion).

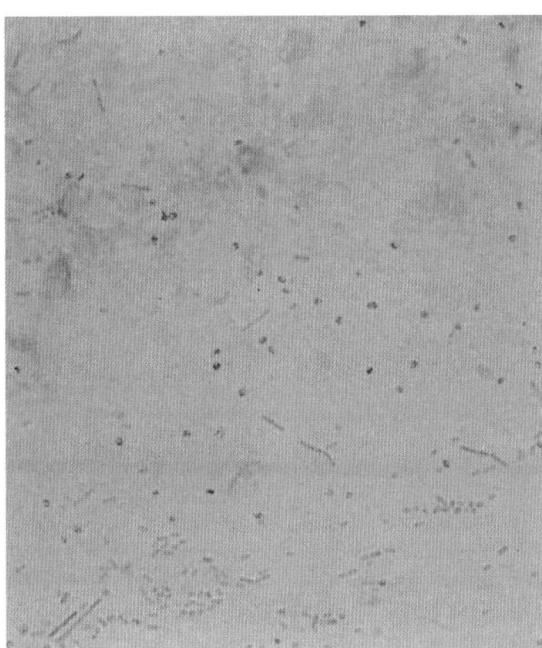

Figure 192-5 Detection of microsporidia in stool samples. Smear of a formalin-fixed, unconcentrated stool specimen of a patient who has AIDS and chronic diarrhea, showing pinkish-red-stained spores of *Enterocytozoon bieneusi*. Chromotrope staining (oil immersion).

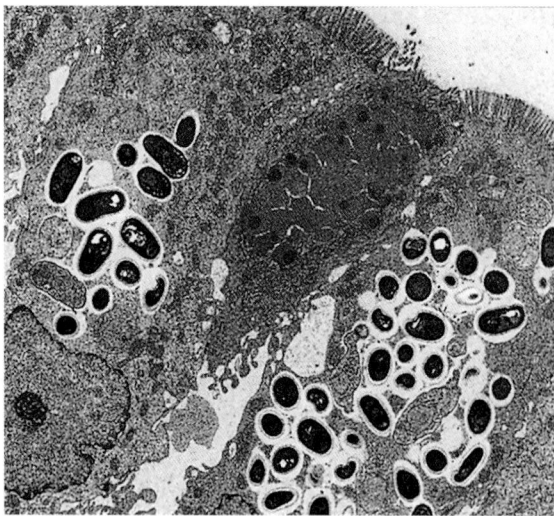

Figure 192-8 *Encephalitozoon intestinalis* (formerly *Septata intestinalis*): developing spores within enterocytes separated by a fibrillar matrix. *E. intestinalis* develop within parasitophorous vacuoles, unlike *Enterocytozoon bieneusi*, which develop in direct contact with enterocyte cytoplasm. *(Courtesy of M.A. Spycher.)*

Serology

Serologic assays (including carbon immunoassay, indirect IF test, enzyme-linked immunosorbent assay and Western blot immunodetection) have been useful in detecting antibodies to *E. cuniculi* in several species of animals, but reliable serologic tests for diagnosis of human microsporidiosis are lacking.

Cell Culture

Encephalitozoon spp., *Trachipleistophora* spp., *Vittaforma corneae* and *Anncaliia algerae* have been isolated using cell culture systems, but these tests are fastidious and costly, and the most common human species, *E. bieneusi*, has not been continuously propagated.

Molecular Techniques

Universal panmicrosporidian and species-specific primer pairs that amplify the short regions of the small subunit rRNA gene have been developed.[52,53] Simultaneous detection of four human pathogenic microsporidia from patients' specimens by oligonucleotide microarray has been described.[54] Molecular diagnosis and identification of microsporidia have been successfully performed with fresh stool specimens, formalin-fixed stool specimens, intestinal tissue obtained by endoscopic biopsy, urine specimens and other body fluids.[15] *In situ* hybridization to visualize *E. bieneusi* in tissue sections has been developed.

Clinical Manifestations

CRYPTOSPORIDIOSIS

For cryptosporidiosis the mean incubation period between infection and onset of symptoms is approximately 7–14 days (range 5–28 days). The severity and duration of illness vary depending on the age, nutritional status and immune status of the hosts. Children, the elderly and individuals with nutritional deficiencies may suffer from a more severe and prolonged disease, as is observed in immunodeficient patients.

Immunocompetent Patients

In immunocompetent patients, cryptosporidia cause a self-limiting, usually watery, diarrhea lasting 10–14 days (range 2–28 days), but the clinical presentation varies from asymptomatic shedding of oocysts to severe disease that may last up to 3 months.[27,55] Patients often complain of abdominal pain, flatulence, loss of appetite, nausea and vomiting, and may suffer from low-grade fever, anorexia, malaise, weakness, fatigue, myalgias and headaches. The diarrhea and abdominal pain are often made worse by eating. Cough appears significantly more frequent in children with cryptosporidiosis than in children with diarrhea of another etiology, but the parasite has rarely been documented in the airways of immunocompetent individuals. Single case reports of pancreatitis associated with cryptosporidiosis and reactive arthritis have been described. Poorly understood lasting adverse effects of infection in children may include deficits of linear growth and cognitive sequelae, even if cryptosporidial infection is otherwise symptomless.[56]

Immunocompromised Patients

In immunocompromised patients, particularly individuals with HIV infection and severe immunodeficiency, cryptosporidiosis is a more severe, often chronic and incurable illness that can be life-threatening. The main clinical presentation is watery diarrhea that can lead to severe dehydration, electrolyte depletion, malnutrition and weight loss. In addition, infection of the biliary tract and the gallbladder, resulting in acalculous cholecystitis, sclerosing cholangitis ('AIDS cholangiopathy') and stenosis of the papilla of Vater, frequently occurs. Infection of the epithelial cells of the respiratory tract, including sinuses, has been described, but it is not clear whether this finding is of clinical relevance because most of these patients have a concomitant respiratory infection. Systemic cryptosporidiosis has not been described.

The severity of HIV-associated cryptosporidiosis is highly variable, and it is related to the CD4 cell count. Four clinical patterns of disease have been identified:

- asymptomatic shedding of oocysts
- transient diarrhea with transient or chronic shedding of oocysts
- chronic diarrhea
- fulminant disease that leads to cachexia and death within months.

Most patients who have severe illness have $CD4^+$ lymphocyte counts below 50 cells/μL. Spontaneous clinical recovery may occur and is mainly correlated with higher $CD4^+$ lymphocyte counts, but a benign course of the diarrhea may also occur in severely immunodeficient patients. Clinical observations suggest that cryptosporidial disease is more severe if coinfections caused by other enteropathogens are present. Concurrent dual or multiple intestinal infection is found in up to 50% of patients who have HIV-associated cryptosporidiosis.

CYCLOSPORIASIS

The spectrum of *Cyclospora*-associated illness is not yet fully defined but it may range from asymptomatic carriage of the organism to severe and prolonged diarrhea in immunocompetent and immunocompromised patients. Patients who have AIDS tend to have a more prolonged and severe illness, and *Cyclospora*-associated cholangiopathy has been described in this group.[28,29]

The incubation period between infection and onset of symptoms ranges between 2 and 11 days and is usually about 7 days. In symptomatic infections the main clinical manifestation is mild to severe watery diarrhea, accompanied by abdominal cramps, bloating, increased flatus, nausea, anorexia, substantial weight loss and fatigue. Vomiting is less common and about 25% of the patients report fever and myalgias.

If not treated, diarrhea is self-limiting but may last for several weeks (range 2–107 days), and remissions and relapses may occur during gradual resolution of the illness. *Cyclospora* infection does not appear to provide lasting immunity.

CYSTOISOSPORIASIS

In immunocompetent persons, *C. belli* infection causes self-limited watery diarrhea accompanied by malaise, anorexia, cramping abdominal pain, weight loss and, less frequently, low-grade fever. In immunocompromised patients, the illness is more severe and prolonged, or chronic if untreated. Also, acalculous cholecystitis and cases of dissemination into mesenteric lymph nodes, liver and spleen, in patients with AIDS, have been reported.

MICROSPORIDIOSIS IN IMMUNOCOMPROMISED PATIENTS

The most frequent microsporidial disease is HIV-associated chronic diarrhea,[23] but the clinical spectrum of microsporidiosis is diverse and includes intestinal, ocular, muscular, cerebral, respiratory, urinary tract and systemic infections (Table 192-1). In addition to HIV-associated disease, microsporidiosis is also prevalent in otherwise immunocompromised patients, including organ transplant recipients, patients with hematologic malignancies receiving monoclonal antibody therapy, patients with rheumatic disease undergoing antitumor necrosis factor therapy, the elderly and malnourished children.[17]

Diarrhea, Cholangitis, Acalculous Cholecystitis

Two microsporidial species – *Enterocytozoon bieneusi* and *Encephalitozoon intestinalis* – cause chronic diarrhea and wasting, cholangiopathy and acalculous cholecystitis in patients who have HIV infection or who are otherwise immunodeficient, particularly when CD4+ lymphocyte counts drop below 50–100/μL.[23]

Enterocytozoon bieneusi is estimated to be one of the most important HIV-associated intestinal pathogens, present in 5–30% of those with otherwise unexplained diarrhea. The main symptoms are chronic nonbloody diarrhea, anorexia, weight loss and bloating. Some patients experience intermittent diarrhea, and a few excrete microsporidial spores without having diarrhea. The stool is watery or soft, and diarrhea seems to be worsened by most foods. Some of the patients report abdominal pain or nausea and vomiting. Laboratory evidence for intestinal malabsorption is common. *E. bieneusi* itself is not immediately life-threatening, but diarrhea is debilitating, and weight loss may lead to cachexia, which is a significant cause or cofactor in the deaths of many patients. Up to one-third of patients who have intestinal microsporidiosis have dual or multiple coinfection with other intestinal pathogens. The parasite has also been detected in the biliary tree and/or gallbladder of patients who have cholangitis and acalculous cholecystitis. Imaging procedures often reveal dilatation of both intrahepatic and common bile ducts, irregularities of the bile duct wall and gallbladder abnormalities such as wall thickening, distention or the presence of sludge.[15,23]

Encephalitozoon intestinalis primarily causes diarrhea, and the parasite may also spread into the biliary tract and gallbladder, causing cholangitis and cholecystitis. In contrast to *Enterocytozoon bieneusi*, systemic dissemination to kidneys and other sites may occur.[57]

Systemic Microsporidiosis

There are five microsporidial genera, *Anncaliia* spp., *Encephalitozoon* spp., *Trachipleistophora* spp., *Tubulinosema acridophagus* and *Vittaforma corneae*, which have been found to disseminate in severely immunodeficient patients with HIV infection or other immunodeficiency.[18,20,52,58-60]

Encephalitozoon spp. were initially identified in patients who had AIDS and keratoconjunctivitis.[61] Subsequently, the spectrum of recognized *Encephalitozoon*-associated disease has expanded to include keratoconjunctivitis, bronchiolitis, sinusitis, pneumonitis, nephritis, ureteritis, cystitis, prostatitis, hepatitis, peritonitis, diarrhea, encephalitis and endocarditis.[33,52,62] Clinical manifestations may vary substantially, ranging from an asymptomatic carrier state to organ failure. *Trachipleistophora anthropophthera* was identified at autopsy in cerebral, cardiac, renal, pancreatic, thyroid, hepatic, splenic, lymphoid and bone marrow tissue of two patients who had AIDS and initially presented with seizures.[59]

Urinary Tract Infection. Predominant genitourinary signs and symptoms caused by Encephalitozoon infections have been observed. Clinical manifestations included asymptomatic microhematuria, urethritis, prostatitis, acute cystitis and interstitial nephritis, associated with dysuria, gross hematuria and progressive renal insufficiency.[33]

Respiratory Tract Infection. In most patients who have respiratory tract microsporidial infection – including bronchiolitis, pneumonia and progressive respiratory failure – intestinal or systemic microsporidiosis was also present. Single cases of patients have been reported in whom sinusitis causing nasal obstruction and persistent mucopurulent nasal discharge was a predominant manifestation of systemic *Encephalitozoon* infection.

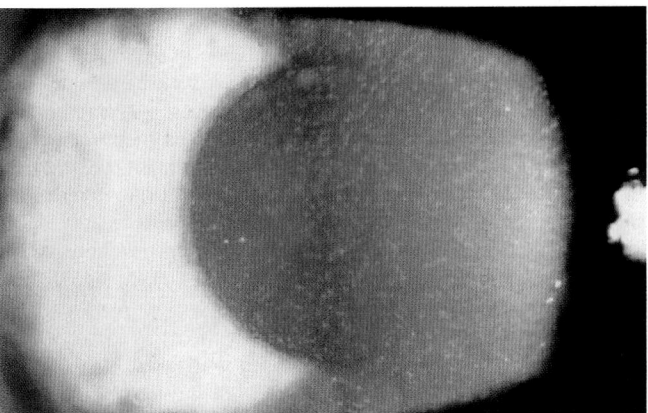

Figure 192-9 Keratopathy caused by *Encephalitozoon hellem*. Slit-lamp demonstration of punctate epithelial keratopathy in a patient who has AIDS and keratoconjunctivitis caused by *Encephalitozoon hellem*. Ocular microsporidiosis can often be diagnosed by examination under the light microscope of a smear obtained by a nontraumatic conjunctival swab. *(Courtesy of M. Diesenhouse and D.A. Schwartz.)*

Keratoconjunctivitis. HIV-associated ocular microsporidiosis caused by *Encephalitozoon* spp. is restricted to the superficial epithelium of the cornea and conjunctiva. Most patients exhibit bilateral coarse punctate epithelial keratopathy (Figure 192-9), conjunctival inflammation resulting in redness and foreign body sensation, decreased visual acuity and photophobia. In patients who initially present with symptomatic keratoconjunctival microsporidiosis, dissemination of the parasite may be common, but clinical manifestations other than keratoconjunctivitis may be mild or absent.[63]

Cerebral Microsporidiosis. Microsporidia were first reported in 1959 and 1984 as the etiologic agent of a neurologic disorder in two children with unknown immune status, who both presented with seizures. *Encephalitozoon cuniculi* and *Trachipleistophora anthropophthera* were detected in CSF or brain tissue of patients with HIV infection who presented with fever and somnolence or seizures and mental decline. MRI (magnetic resonance imaging) disclosed multiple small, contrast-enhancing, mostly ring-like lesions localized to the hippocampus, mesencephalon and cerebral cortex (Figure 192-10).[59,64]

Myositis. Myositis caused by different microsporidia, including *Anncaliia vesicularum*, *Endoreticulatus* spp., *Pleistophora* spp., *Trachipleistophora* spp. and *Tubulinosema acridophagus*, has been described in HIV-infected persons, otherwise immunocompromised patients and persons with no manifest immunodeficiency.[18,20,58,65]

MICROSPORIDIOSIS IN IMMUNOCOMPETENT PERSONS

Enterocytozoon bieneusi and *Encephalitozoon* spp. are associated with self-limiting watery diarrhea in immunocompetent adults as well as in children, particularly among persons who reside or have traveled in tropical countries.[66] An unexpectedly high prevalence (17%) of intestinal microsporidiosis due to *Enterocytozoon bieneusi* was found in HIV-seronegative elderly patients in Spain.[67]

Deep stromal infections of the cornea caused by different microsporidial species have been described in otherwise healthy persons who presented with severe keratitis or a corneal ulcer, or who were contact lens wearers (Table 192-1).[68]

Management

CRYPTOSPORIDIOSIS

The efficacy of antiparasitic therapy of cryptosporidiosis remains unclear.[69,70] Among immunocompetent patients, diarrhea due to cryptosporidial infection is usually self-limiting, but chronic infection may cause malnutrition in children in LMIC. Nitazoxanide may be useful in immunocompetent individuals with cryptosporidiosis. In a

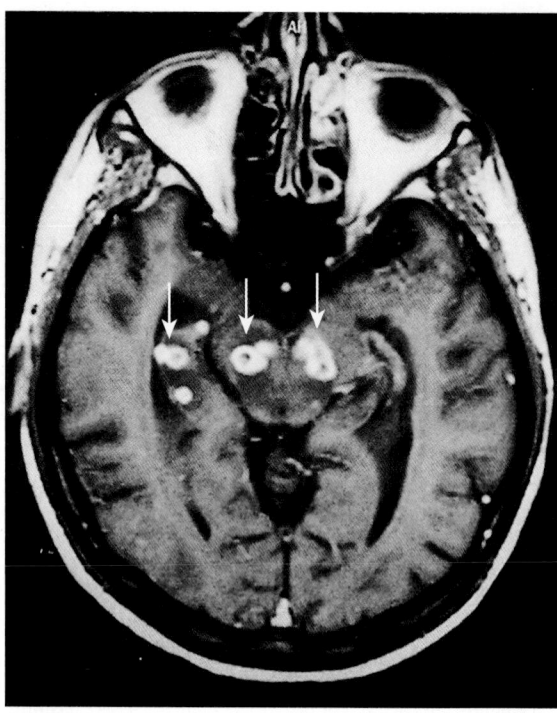

Figure 192-10 Cerebral microsporidiosis caused by *Encephalitozoon cuniculi* in a patient with HIV infection. The MRI shows multiple small contrast-enhancing, mostly ring-like, partly micronodular, lesions in hippocampal, mesencephal and intracortical regions (arrows), partly accompanied by slight edema, and congestion of the right ethmoid sinus. *E. cuniculi* was isolated from cerebrospinal fluid. (From Weber R., Deplazes P., Flepp M., et al. N Engl J Med 1997;336:474-8, with permission from Massachusetts Medical Society.)

randomized, placebo-controlled trial in apparently immunocompetent children and adults in Egypt, nitazoxanide (500 mg q12h for 3 days in adults, 100–200 mg q12h in children) decreased the duration of diarrhea and cryptosporidial oocyst shedding.[71]

In contrast, in patients who have AIDS no agent has proven effective in the absence of treatment of HIV infection. A randomized trial in HIV-infected persons with cryptosporidiosis in Mexico suggested a shorter duration of diarrhea and oocyst clearance with nitazoxanide treatment among patients with CD4[+] lymphocyte counts above 50/μL but no effect was found among patients with CD4[+] cell counts below 50/μL.[72] A randomized clinical trial in HIV-infected Zambian children with cryptosporidiosis with nitazoxanide showed no effect.[73] Case series and a randomized controlled trial suggested that treatment with oral paromomycin (500 mg q6h for at least 4 weeks) may result in decreased oocyst shedding and improved intestinal function and morphology,[74] but other investigators have not found any clinical benefit.[75] *In vitro* studies have indicated that nitazoxanide activity may be enhanced by the co-administration of azithromycin or rifabutin,[76] but clinical experience of such combinations is lacking. Uncontrolled studies showed resolution of cryptosporidia-associated diarrhea after treatment with rifaximin.[77] *In vitro* effects of hyperimmune bovine colostrum could not be reproduced in human studies.

Symptomatic treatment of diarrhea may include drugs that affect gut motility such as loperamide, diphenoxylate, opiates, somatostatin and octreotide. Immune reconstitution following initiation of potent antiretroviral therapy of patients who have HIV infection results in cessation of oocyst shedding and diarrhea, but cryptosporidial infection is controlled rather than cured because failure of antiretroviral therapy often results in relapse of cryptosporidiosis.

CYCLOSPORIASIS

A placebo-controlled trial showed that trimethoprim–sulfamethoxazole (TMP–SMX [co-trimoxazole]; double-strength TMP 160 mg/SMX 800 mg q12h for 7 days) was clinically successful and shortened oocyst shedding in immunocompetent patients who have cyclosporiasis.[78] In this study, 3 days of treatment with TMP–SMX was not sufficient to eradicate *Cyclospora*. Trimethoprim 160 mg/SMX 800 mg q6h for 10 days cured HIV-associated cyclosporiasis but the relapse rate was high (43%). Maintenance therapy with double-strength TMP–SMX three times per week did prevent relapses in these patients. For patients who cannot tolerate sulfonamides, a 1-week course of ciprofloxacin (500 mg q12h) may be an alternative although it was not as effective as TMP–SMX in a randomized trial.[79]

CYSTOISOSPORIASIS

Immunocompetent and immunocompromised patients respond promptly to therapy with TMP–SMX (double-strength TMP 160 mg/SMX 800 mg q6h for 10 days).[80] In patients with sulfonamide allergies, pyrimethamine 75 mg/day plus folinic acid 10 mg/day may be successful. To prevent the high rate of relapses in patients who have AIDS, maintenance therapy with double-strength TMP–SMX, three times per week, or pyrimethamine 25 mg/day plus folinic acid 5 mg/day, is recommended. In case of sulfonamide intolerance, a 1-week course of ciprofloxacin (500 mg q12h) may be an alternative although it was not as effective as TMP–SMX in a randomized trial among HIV-infected Haitians.[79]

MICROSPORIDIOSIS

Albendazole, fumagillin, its analog TNP-470, and nikkomycin Z have been found to inhibit completely or partially the replication or spore germination *in vitro* of *Encephalitozoon* spp. and *Vittaforma corneae*, but did not destroy mature microsporidial spores, so that these may sustain infection.[81] Numerous other antimicrobials have been tested *in vitro*, with negative findings. *In vitro* systems to investigate *E. bieneusi* are not available.

Among HIV-infected persons with access to antiretroviral therapy and immune reconstitution, the occurrence of microsporidiosis has been substantially reduced. Little information on clinical experience in the therapy of human microsporidiosis is available, and only two controlled treatment trials have been conducted,[82,83] confirming previous case observations which indicated that albendazole can result in clinical cure of HIV-associated encephalitozoonosis in parallel with the cessation of spore excretion. In contrast, albendazole is not effective for the treatment of *E. bieneusi* infection. Oral purified fumagillin, used in pilot studies and a small randomized trial to treat HIV-associated diarrhea due to *E. bieneusi*, appeared to eradicate the parasite, but serious adverse events and parasitic relapse were observed.[84]

Microsporidial keratoconjunctivits may be a self-limiting disease,[85] may be cleared by repeated corneal swabbing,[86] or may respond to systemic albendazole,[87] or topical voriconazole application.[88]

References available online at expertconsult.com.

KEY REFERENCES

Didier E.S., Weiss L.M.: Microsporidiosis: not just in AIDS patients. *Curr Opin Infect Dis* 2011; 24:490-495.

Fayer R.: *Sarcocystis* spp. in human infections. *Clin Microbiol Rev* 2004; 17:894-902.

Fayer R.: Taxonomy and species delimitation in *Cryptosporidium*. *Exp Parasitol* 2010; 124:90-97.

Herwaldt B.L.: *Cyclospora cayetanensis*: a review, focusing on the outbreaks of cyclosporiasis in the 1990s. *Clin Infect Dis* 2000; 31:1040-1057.

Legua P., Seas C.: *Cystoisospora* and *Cyclospora*. *Curr Opin Infect Dis* 2013; 26:479-483.

Lindsay D.S., Dubey J.P., Blagburn B.L.: Biology of *Isospora* spp. from humans, nonhuman primates, and domestic animals. *Clin Microbiol Rev* 1997; 10:19-34.

Mathis A., Weber R., Deplazes P.: Zoonotic potential of the microsporidia. *Clin Microbiol Rev* 2005; 18:423-445.

Ortega Y.R., Sanchez R.: Update on *Cyclospora cayetanensis*, a food-borne and waterborne parasite. *Clin Microbiol Rev* 2010; 23:218-234.

Ortega Y.R., Sterling C.R., Gilman R.H., et al.: *Cyclospora* species–a new protozoan pathogen of humans. *N Engl J Med* 1993; 328:1308-1312.

Shirley D.A., Moonah S.N., Kotloff K.L.: Burden of disease from cryptosporidiosis. *Curr Opin Infect Dis* 2012; 25:555-563.

Slapeta J.: Cryptosporidiosis and *Cryptosporidium* species in animals and humans: a thirty colour rainbow? *Int J Parasitol* 2013; 43:957-970.

Tzipori S., Widmer G.: A hundred-year retrospective on cryptosporidiosis. *Trends Parasitol* 2008; 24:184-189.

Weber R., Bryan R.T., Owen R.L., et al.: Improved light-microscopical detection of microsporidia spores in stool and duodenal aspirates. The Enteric Opportunistic Infections Working Group. *N Engl J Med* 1992; 326:161-166.

Weber R., Bryan R.T., Schwartz D.A., et al.: Human microsporidial infections. *Clin Microbiol Rev* 1994; 7:426-461.

Weber R., Ledergerber B., Zbinden R., et al.: Enteric infections and diarrhea in human immunodeficiency virus-infected persons: prospective community-based cohort study. Swiss HIV Cohort Study. *Arch Intern Med* 1999; 159:1473-1480.

193

Protozoa: Free-Living Amebae

JENNIFER RITTENHOUSE COPE | JONATHAN S. YODER |
GOVINDA S. VISVESVARA

KEY CONCEPTS

- The free-living amebae *Naegleria, Acanthamoeba* and *Balamuthia* are considered amphizoic, meaning they have the ability to exist as free-living in nature and as parasites within host tissue.

- *Naegleria fowleri* is a thermophilic ameba found in warm fresh water throughout the world and causes primary amebic meningoencephalitis when water containing the ameba enters the nose, allowing the ameba to invade the brain.

- *Acanthamoeba* spp. are found in both water and soil and cause skin and central nervous system disease predominantly in immunocompromised patients.

- *Balamuthia mandrillaris* has been isolated from soil and causes central nervous system disease in both immunocompromised and immunocompetent patients.

- *Acanthamoeba* spp. can also cause a sight-threatening infection of the cornea called *Acanthamoeba* keratitis that predominantly affects contact lens wearers with poor contact lens hygiene practices.

- Mortality is high (>90%) for central nervous system infections caused by the free-living amebae; treatment recommendations are based on a few case reports of survivors.

Nature

The concept that small free-living amebae, particularly *Acanthamoeba* spp., have the potential to cause disease in humans was developed by C.G. Culbertson of the Indiana University School of Medicine and the Eli Lilly Laboratories in 1958. The basis of this observation was a chance discovery of an ameba growing in a batch of monkey kidney cell cultures that were to be used for growing polio virus for the development of polio vaccine. This ameba, described as *Acanthamoeba* sp. (Lilly A-1), was found to produce, on intracerebral, intraspinal and intranasal inoculations, meningoencephalitis in cortisone-treated monkeys and mice.[1-3] This isolate is now called *Acanthamoeba culbertsoni*.

The first case of amebic meningoencephalitis in humans, attributed initially to *Acanthamoeba* although later the causative organism was identified as a species of *Naegleria*, was described in Australia in 1962. It is now known that besides *Acanthamoeba* spp., two other free-living amebae, *Naegleria fowleri* and *Balamuthia mandrillaris*, also cause central nervous system (CNS) disease in humans and other animals.[1-4] Recently, however, *Sappinia diploidea*, now re-identified as *Sappinia pedata*, a saprophytic ameba that has been previously isolated from the fecal specimens of lizards, elks and bisons, was identified in a brain biopsy specimen of a previously healthy 38-year-old man who developed visual disturbances, headache and a seizure.[5,6] This suggests that there are cases of human infections caused by free-living amebae other than *Acanthamoeba*, *Balamuthia* and *Naegleria* spp. that may have been either misdiagnosed or unrecognized.

TAXONOMY

The free-living amebae, according to the classic taxonomic system, were classified under the subphylum Sarcodina and superclass Rhizopodea.[3] The International Society of Protistologists abandoned the older hierarchical system and recently replaced it with a new classification system emphasizing modern morphologic approaches, biochemical pathways and molecular phylogenetics. According to this new schema the Eukaryotes have been classified into six clusters or 'Super Groups', namely Amoebozoa, Opisthokonta, Rhizaria, Archaeplastida, Chromalveolata and Excavata. *Acanthamoeba* and *Balamuthia* are included under Super Group Amoebozoa (Acanthamoebidae), along with *Sappinia* (Flabellinea: Thecamoebidae), and *Naegleria fowleri* under Super Group Excavata (Heterolobosia: Vahlkampfiidae).[7]

The free-living amebae (*Acanthamoeba, Naegleria, Balamuthia*) and the parasitic amebae (e.g. *Entamoeba histolytica*) move by producing cytoplasmic bulges, the lobopodia, from the surface of the body. In contrast to *E. histolytica*, which is a mitochondria-lacking ameba that causes gastrointestinal disease, *Naegleria, Acanthamoeba* and *Balamuthia* are mitochondria-bearing amebae that cause diseases of the CNS of humans and animals, which almost always lead to death. The term amphizoic amebae indicates the ability of these amebae to exist as free-living in nature and as parasites within host tissue; this differentiates them from the truly parasitic *E. histolytica*.[8]

Although several species of *Naegleria* have been described, so far only one species, *N. fowleri* (*N. aerobia* and *N. invadens* are non-valid synonyms), is known to infect the human CNS. Several of the more than 24 species of *Acanthamoeba* that have been described so far cause not only a chronic granulomatous CNS disease in humans and other animals, but also infect the cornea (*Acanthamoeba* keratitis), the skin, the nasal sinuses and pulmonary tissues. The disease caused by *Acanthamoeba* spp. has been described as granulomatous amebic encephalitis (GAE). *B. mandrillaris*, the only known species of *Balamuthia*, causes GAE and skin infections in humans and other animals.[1-3]

Naegleria fowleri

Naegleria fowleri is also described as an ameboflagellate because it has a transient flagellate stage in its life cycle in addition to a feeding and dividing form, the trophozoite, and a resistant cyst stage (Figure 193-1). The trophozoite, measuring 10–25 μm, normally feeds on bacteria and multiplies by binary fission. However, it is able to differentiate into a pear-shaped biflagellate stage in response to sudden changes in the ionic concentration of its environment. When the conditions

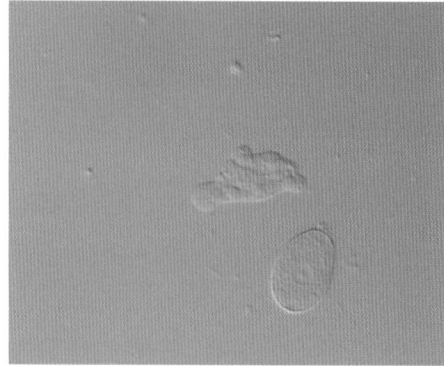

Figure 193-1 *Naegleria fowleri*. The trophozoite can be differentiated from the cyst by its characteristic lobopodial locomotion; both are taken from culture. Differential interference contrast.

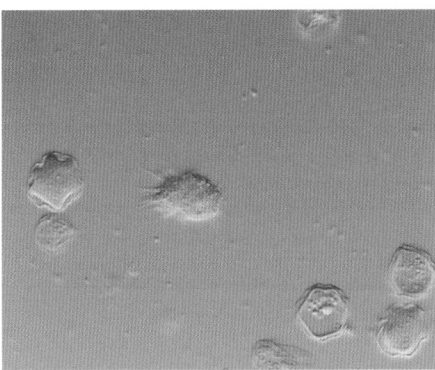

Figure 193-2 *Acanthamoeba castellanii*. The trophozoite has spiny acanthopodia whereas the cyst has an outer wrinkled ectocyst and a stellate endocyst; both are taken from culture. Differential interference contrast.

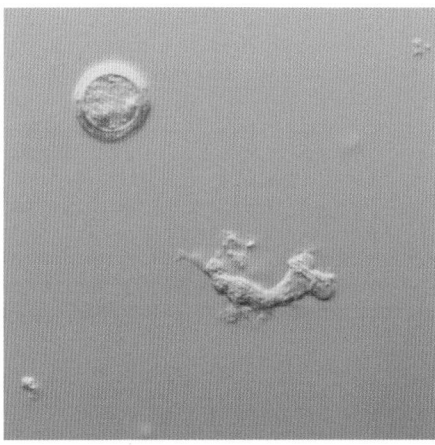

Figure 193-3 *Balamuthia mandrillaris*. The trophozoite is irregularly shaped whereas the cyst is spherical; both are taken from culture. Differential interference contrast.

become unfavorable the trophozoite differentiates into a resistant cyst stage. The trophozoite is usually uninucleate; the nucleus is spherical and contains a large, centrally placed, dense nucleolus. Additionally, numerous dumbbell-shaped mitochondria, vacuoles, lysosomes and ribosomes are present within the cytoplasm. Cysts are round and contain a single nucleus with a central dense nucleolus; the dense cyst walls are plugged with one or more flat pores. The cysts are 7–14 μm in diameter, with a mean of 10 μm.[3,8]

Acanthamoeba spp.

In 1930 Aldo Castellani isolated an ameba from a yeast culture; it was later named as *Acanthamoeba castellanii*.[1–3] Currently, more than 24 species have been identified in the genus *Acanthamoeba* based on morphologic criteria such as size of the trophozoites and cysts as well as differences in the cyst wall configuration. The various species are included in three different groups:

- Group I comprises those species that have large trophozoites with cysts that range in size from 16 to 35 μm (e.g. *A. astronyxis*, *A. comandoni*, *A. tubiashi*, *A. byersi*).
- Group II includes by far the largest number of species, with cysts measuring around 18 μm or less (e.g. *A. castellanii*, *A. polyphaga*, *A. rhysodes*, *A. hatchetti*).
- Group III consists of species with subtle differences in cyst morphology, also measuring 18 μm or less (e.g. *A. culbertsoni*, *A. royreba*, *A. lenticulata*).

Currently, identification of species based on morphologic criteria such as size are considered unreliable and hence sequencing of the 18S rDNA is being used not only to differentiate isolates but also to understand the phylogeny of *Acanthamoeba*. Based on sequence differences, 18 genotypes (T1–T18) of *Acanthamoeba* have been established.[1–4,9]

The life cycle of *Acanthamoeba* spp. consists of two stages: a feeding and reproducing trophozoite stage and a resistant cyst stage (Figure 193-2). The trophozoites are uninucleate and feed on bacteria and detritus present in the milieu and multiply by binary fission. The trophozoites of Group I measure from 30 to 125 μm; those of Group II and III are 15–45 μm in size. The nucleus has a centrally placed, large, densely staining nucleolus. The cytoplasm is finely granular and contains numerous mitochondria, ribosomes and lysosomes. Cysts of Group I are large and measure 16–35 μm; those of Group II and III are 10–25 μm in size. Cysts are double-walled: the outer wall (the ectocyst) is wrinkled and contains protein; the inner wall (the endocyst) is usually stellate, polygonal, oval or spherical and contains cellulose. Pores covered by opercula are present at the point of contact between the ectocyst and the endocyst. Cysts are uninucleate.

Balamuthia mandrillaris

Balamuthia mandrillaris, previously called leptomyxid ameba, is the only species included under the genus *Balamuthia*. Based on molecular analysis, all isolates studied so far appear to be homogeneous and belong to one genotype. *B. mandrillaris* has two stages in its life cycle

(Figure 193-3). The trophozoite is irregular in shape and measures from 12 to 60 μm with a mean size of about 30 μm. Although usually uninucleate, binucleate forms are occasionally seen. The nucleus contains a large centrally placed nucleolus. Occasionally, in infected human tissues, trophic stages containing a large nucleus with two or three nucleolar bodies have been observed. Cysts are also uninucleate, more or less spherical, and range in size from 12 to 30 μm with a mean of 15 μm. Cysts appear to be double-walled with a wavy ectocyst and a spherical endocyst when viewed under the light microscope. However, ultrastructurally the cysts are tripartite with an outer thin and irregular ectocyst, an inner thick endocyst and a middle amorphous fibrillar mesocyst.[1,2]

CULTIVATION

Acanthamoeba spp. and *N. fowleri*, but not *B. mandrillaris*, can be cultivated on non-nutrient agar plates coated with suitable gram-negative bacteria such as *Escherichia coli* or *Enterobacter aerogenes*. The amebae will feed on the bacteria, multiply and differentiate into cysts within a few days. They can be easily subcultured by transplanting a small piece of agar containing trophozoites and/or cysts onto a fresh agar plate coated with bacteria as before. *N. fowleri* and *Acanthamoeba* spp. can also be grown successfully on mammalian cell cultures. *B. mandrillaris* will not grow on bacteria-coated agar plates. However, it can be isolated from infected human or animal tissue by inoculating monkey kidney or human lung fibroblasts with the triturated tissue and from which a continuous culture can be established by periodic transfers.

N. fowleri and *Acanthamoeba* spp. can be grown axenically (bacteria-free) in a complex chemical medium containing fetal bovine serum. Although several different formulations are available, in our laboratory we use a modified version of Nelson's medium that contains a 0.5% solution of liver digest, 0.5% glucose and a low osmolarity buffered salt solution supplemented with 3–5% fetal bovine serum. *Acanthamoeba* spp. can also be easily grown in a medium composed of 2% proteose peptone, 0.5% yeast extract and 0.1% glucose made up in a low osmotic buffered salt solution with or without serum. Additionally, *N. fowleri* and several species of *Acanthamoeba* have also been grown in a chemically defined medium consisting of several different amino acids, vitamins, hemin and salts. *B. mandrillaris* has also been grown in a highly complex axenic medium, thus facilitating the screening of various pharmaceutical agents.[8]

Epidemiology

N. fowleri is widely distributed throughout the world and has been isolated from fresh water, thermal discharges of power plants, heated poorly disinfected swimming pools, hot springs, aquariums, soil, dust in air, sewage and even from nasal passages of children. *N. fowleri* is thermophilic and grows well, even at temperatures of up to 45°C (113°F). It is therefore not surprising that primary amebic meningo-encephalitis (PAM) cases have occurred in the hot summer months when many people engage in aquatic activities in lakes, ponds and poorly disinfected swimming pools that may harbor these amebae in large numbers. Most infections in the USA are in children (median age 11 years) and >75% of infections have been in males. Infected people were often reported to have participated in water-related activities such as swimming underwater, diving and head dunking that could have caused water to go up the nose.[10] In colder climates these amebae will probably encyst and remain dormant in the sediments of freshwater lakes, ponds, and rivers.[1–3,11] In the USA the ameba's predilection for warmer temperatures has led to a geographic distribution that is pre-dominantly in the southern tier states. However, in recent years cases have been reported from northern states.[12] Additionally, recent US cases have been associated with different exposure routes including use of neti pots (a small pot used at home to inhale water as a treatment for sinusitis or nasal allergies) and ritual ablution.[13,14]

Acanthamoeba spp. have been isolated from soil; sewage; fresh, brackish and sea water; bottled mineral water; cooling towers of elec-tric and nuclear power plants; physiotherapy pools; jacuzzis; heating, ventilating and air conditioning units; eye wash stations; dialysis machines; dust in the air; bacterial, fungal and mammalian cell cul-tures; contact lens paraphernalia; the nose and throat of patients who have respiratory complaints and healthy individuals; and biopsy or autopsy specimens of cornea, lungs, nasal sinuses, skin and CNS tissue of humans and animals. *Acanthamoeba* GAE occurs primarily among immunocompromised persons. Acanthamoebae have generated con-siderable interest in recent years because they act, under laboratory conditions, as hosts for pathogenic bacteria such as *Legionella* spp., *Mycobacterium avium*, *Listeria monocytogenes*, *Burkholderia pseud-omallei*, *Vibrio cholerae*, *Escherichia coli* serotype O157, *Francisella tula-rensis*, *Helicobacter pylori* and *Afipia felis*. They colonize the biofilm of water distribution and building plumbing systems, creating microbial environments that are difficult to control with chemical disinfection.[15] *Acanthamoeba* is therefore of great public health importance. Cases of GAE may occur at any time of the year and therefore transmission has no relation to seasonal changes.[1–3]

B. mandrillaris has been isolated from soil. A serologic study in the southwestern USA demonstrated evidence of seropositivity among 3% of asymptomatic persons suggesting that exposure is much more common than disease.[16] Infections appear to be more common among persons of Hispanic ethnicity.[17] Outbreaks have occurred following transplantation of organs received from a donor infected with *Bala-muthia*.[18,19] *B. mandrillaris* has also been isolated from biopsy and autopsy specimens of humans and other animals.[1,3]

Pathogenicity
NAEGLERIA FOWLERI
Primary amebic meningoencephalitis most often occurs in active healthy children and young adults with no known history of immune disorder, although it can occur at any age. Most patients who have PAM have a history of swimming, diving or playing under water; the ameba enters through the nasal passages. The route of invasion into the brain is through the fila olfactoria of the olfactory nerves. The trophozoites cross the cribriform plate and reach the subarachnoid space, which is richly vascularized and bathed in cerebrospinal fluid (CSF), thus constituting an ideal medium for their proliferation and subsequent dissemination into the brain parenchyma and other areas of the CNS.[1–3]

N. fowleri is a highly pathogenic and virulent ameba. However, the minimum number of amebae required to cause infection and death in humans is not known. Experiments with infection have shown that mice, when just a few amebae are instilled intranasally, die of PAM in a similar fashion to humans. However, different isolates of *N. fowleri* vary in their degree of virulence: some are highly virulent whereas

other isolates are only moderately virulent. Furthermore, any isolate can become avirulent on prolonged cultivation in an axenic medium. It is believed that the probability of infection in nature may depend upon the number and virulence of the amebae.[3,20]

The trophozoite of *N. fowleri* is highly phagocytic and induces necrosis of the CNS tissue. It is believed to ingest human tissue directly by producing a food cup or amebostome and by producing lysosomal hydrolases and phospholipases that degrade myelin. It has also been shown experimentally that the amebae exert a contact-dependent cytolysis mediated possibly by a multicomponent system that consists of a heat-stable hemolytic protein, heat-labile cytolysin and/or phos-pholipase A enzyme.[1–3,11,21]

The incubation period of PAM varies from 2 to 15 days depending on the size of the inoculum and the virulence of the amebae. In experi-mental infections with a mildly virulent *N. fowleri*, the incubation period has been as long as 3–4 weeks.[1–3] In a review of US cases, the mean incubation period was 5 days.[10]

ACANTHAMOEBA SPP. AND *B. MANDRILLARIS*
Granulomatous amebic encephalitis, caused by *Acanthamoeba* spp., usually occurs in chronically ill, debilitated individuals, in immuno-suppressed patients including those who have AIDS, or in those who have received broad-spectrum antibiotics or chemotherapeutic medications.[1–3] *B. mandrillaris* causes infection in both immunodefi-cient and immunocompetent individuals. The pathogenesis of GAE is complex and poorly understood. It is believed that the immunity is predominantly T-cell-mediated and therefore depletion of CD4+ and T-helper lymphocytes permits the growth and development of the amebae. The incubation period is unknown and several weeks or months may elapse before the disease becomes apparent. However, in three clusters of solid organ transplant-transmitted *Balamuthia* infec-tions in the USA, the incubation period ranged from 18 to 24 days, perhaps as a result of direct inoculation and the immunocompromised status of the patients. The respiratory tract or the skin may act as the portal of entry. One hypothesis is that ulceration of the skin may enable the amebae to enter.[1] The route of invasion to the brain must be via the bloodstream because there are no lymphatic channels within the brain.[1,22] Furthermore, trophozoites and cysts are often seen around blood vessels and within necrotic CNS tissue. The acanth-amoebae are known to secrete enzymes such as lysosomal hydrolases, aminopeptidases and phospholipases, which may contribute to CNS damage.[1,2]

According to more recent studies, the initial process of invasion, in the case of *Acanthamoeba*, occurs when a 136-kDa mannose-binding protein (MBP), a lectin, expressed on the surface of the ameba, adheres to mannose glycoproteins on the surface of the epithelial cells and causes destruction of the epithelial cells. *Acanthamoeba* may also produce food cups on its surface and ingest the epithelial cells.[23] *Balamuthia*, like *Acanthamoeba*, probably invades human tissue by interacting with the host connective tissue and ingesting bits and pieces of host tissue as well as by producing enzymes that will degrade the tissue.[24]

Acanthamoeba Keratitis
Acanthamoeba keratitis (AK) is a sight-threatening infection of the cornea typically associated with contact lens wear. *Acanthamoeba* spp. may adhere to the corneal epithelial cells as well as secrete proteolytic and collagenolytic enzymes that may damage the corneal epithelium and thus contribute to the pathogenesis of AK. If proper treatment is not provided, AK may lead to a vascularized scar within a thin cornea, causing impaired vision or perforation of the cornea and loss of the eye.[1–4,25]

Prevention
PRIMARY AMEBIC MENINGOENCEPHALITIS
The trophic and the cyst forms of *N. fowleri* are susceptible to chlorine at levels recommended for a properly maintained swimming pool. It

is therefore important for swimming pools to be maintained with adequate chlorination at all times. As it is not possible to disinfect natural bodies of water such as lakes and ponds in which *N. fowleri* may be found, swimmers in natural bodies of water should assume that *N. fowleri* is present, particularly during the hot summer months, and take appropriate actions to prevent or reduce water going up the nose.[1,2] These actions may include holding the nose shut, using nose clips, or keeping the head above water when taking part in water-related activities in bodies of warm fresh water. Water that is used for nasal and/or sinus rinsing should be boiled, filtered, labeled as distilled or sterile, or disinfected with chlorine bleach. More specific details on prevention measures can be found at: www.cdc.gov/parasites/naegleria/prevention.html.

GRANULOMATOUS AMEBIC ENCEPHALITIS

Since little is known about when and where exposure to *Acanthamoeba* and *Balamuthia* occurs in patients, steps to take for prevention of disease are largely unknown. Those who are immunocompromised should follow general guidance to avoid unsafe water and environmental exposures.[1-3]

ACANTHAMOEBA KERATITIS

It is recommended that eyecare professionals educate patients about the proper care and use of contact lenses. Contact lens wearers should follow the directions and recommendations of the manufacturers and eyecare professionals. Contact lens wearers should practice healthy habits such as replacing contact lens cases every 3 months and always using fresh solution (never tap water) to store their lenses. Additionally, contact lens wearers should remove their lenses before showering, swimming, or using a hot tub to minimize exposure to water. For more detailed prevention messages, see: www.cdc.gov/contactlenses.

Diagnostic Microbiology

PRIMARY AMEBIC MENINGOENCEPHALITIS

In individuals who have PAM, the CSF is characterized by pleocytosis, with predominance of polymorphonuclear leukocytes but without bacteria. The CSF pressure is elevated (100–600 mmHg). Glucose concentration may be low or normal, but the protein content is elevated, ranging from 100 mg/100 mL to 1000 mg/100 mL. CT scans may show obliteration of the cisterns around the midbrain and the subarachnoid space over the cerebral hemispheres. Early diagnosis of PAM and differentiating it from bacterial meningitis is dependent upon the detection of motile amebae in the CSF under a microscope. Smears of CSF should also be stained with Giemsa or trichrome stains for the delineation of the characteristic nuclear morphology. Gram stain is not useful. Care must be taken to differentiate amebic trophozoites from macrophages. Most cases have been diagnosed retrospectively based on examination of hematoxylin and eosin-stained sections or immuno-histochemical tests.[1-3]

A real-time multiplex polymerase chain reaction (PCR) assay has been developed which identifies *N. fowleri* DNA in the CSF within hours of receipt of the specimen, thus greatly facilitating a quick diagnosis so that anti-*N. fowleri* therapy can be initiated promptly.[26] Serologic tests are of no value in the diagnosis of PAM because most patients die too early (within 3–7 days) in the disease process to mount a detectable immune response.[1-3]

GRANULOMATOUS AMEBIC ENCEPHALITIS

Examination of the CSF in patients who have GAE reveals lymphocytic pleocytosis with mild elevation of proteins and normal levels of glucose. Visual detection of *Acanthamoeba* spp. and *B. mandrillaris* trophozoites in the CSF has rarely been reported. However, *Acanthamoeba* spp. have been identified in brain biopsies from several patients. Molecular techniques such as PCR and real-time PCR have also been developed to identify *Acanthamoeba* and *Balamuthia* in the CSF, brain and corneal tissue as well as in tear fluid.[1-3,26] CT scans and MRI findings are nonspecific and may show single or multiple heterogeneous, hypodense, non-enhancing, space-occupying lesions that involve the basal ganglia, cerebral cortex, subcortical white matter, cerebellum and pons, suggesting a brain abscess, brain tumor or intracerebral hematoma.

Brain and skin biopsies are important diagnostic procedures. *Acanthamoeba* spp. can be easily cultured from the brain, skin, lung and corneal tissue by placing a portion of the tissue that has been minced on non-nutrient agar plates coated with a layer of gram-negative bacteria. Specimens for culture should be processed as quickly as possible. The incubation temperature depends upon the source of the samples. The agar plate should be incubated at 30°C (86°F) if the specimens originate from cornea or skin, but at 37°C (98.6°F) if the specimens are from the brain, the lung or any other internal organ. Amebae, if present in the samples, will feed on bacteria and multiply by binary fission. If the plates are examined under the light microscope, distinctive track marks with an ameba at the end of each track may be seen. The amebae will differentiate into cysts after a few days of incubation. Amebae can be identified to the level of genus on the basis of the characteristic morphology of trophozoites and cysts. Additionally, *Naegleria* spp. can be identified if flagellates appear within 2–4 hours of taking a loopful of amebae from the agar plate and suspending in distilled water. Identification to the species level, however, is difficult on the basis of morphology alone; nonmorphologic methods such as serology, isoenzyme analysis or DNA profiles therefore need to be used.[1-3]

B. mandrillaris will not grow on bacteria-coated agar plates. However, *B. mandrillaris* can be isolated from the CNS by inoculating monkey kidney cell culture with brain extract and subsequently growing the amebae in an axenic medium.[8]

ACANTHAMOEBA KERATITIS

For the diagnosis of AK, deep corneal scraping and biopsy is recommended. Unfixed specimens should be processed for culture. Smears should also be prepared and fixed with methanol, Schaudinn's fixative or a spray-on fixative, and stained with Giemsa–Wright or Hemacolor, or with Wheatly's or Masson's trichrome stain. Hemacolor staining is quick and stains the distinctive cyst wall pinkish-red. The trichrome stains the nucleolus of the trophozoite reddish-pink and the cytoplasm greenish-purple and is therefore useful in differentiating trophozoites of *Acanthamoeba* spp. from the host cells.[1-3] Confocal microscopy is also used to diagnose AK.[27]

Clinical Manifestations

PRIMARY AMEBIC MENINGOENCEPHALITIS

The first case of PAM was reported in 1962.[1-3] Although at that time the case was thought to be caused by *Acanthamoeba* spp., it is now considered to be caused by *N. fowleri*. It is believed that more than 200 cases of PAM have occurred worldwide. Further, as of May 2015, there have been 133 cases reported in the USA alone since 1962. PAM has also been described in a South American tapir and in cattle.[1]

PAM is an acute, fulminant and usually fatal CNS disease that occurs mainly in healthy young adults and children with a recent history of water activities. PAM has a rapid onset and a short incubation period that lasts from 3 to 7 days. It is characterized by the sudden onset of headache, fever, nausea, vomiting and stiff neck. Nuchal rigidity usually occurs with positive Kernig's and Brudzinski's signs. Abnormalities in taste or smell, cerebellar ataxia and photophobia may also be seen early. An increase in intracranial pressure has been reported in most patients. Generalized seizures leading to lethargy, confusion, coma and death within 48–72 hours have been reported in a number of patients.[1]

Pathologic Features

At autopsy the cerebral hemispheres are swollen and edematous. The olfactory bulbs and the orbitofrontal cortices are necrotic and hemorrhagic. Because of increased intracranial pressure, uncal and cerebellar tonsillar herniations are usually seen. The arachnoid membrane is

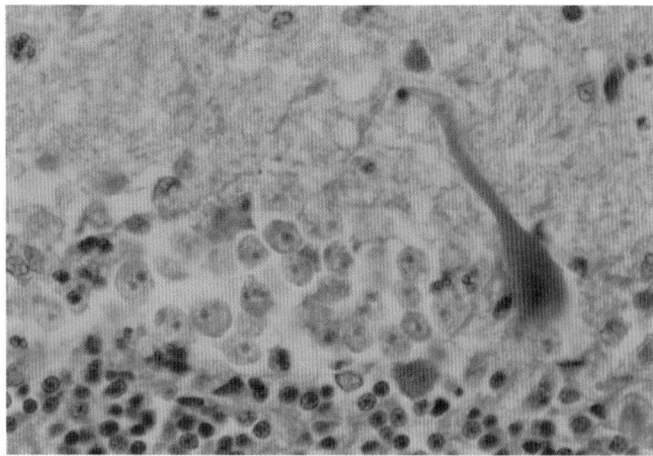

Figure 193-4 CNS section demonstrating numerous trophozoites of *Naegleria fowleri*. Note the absence of cysts. (H & E.)

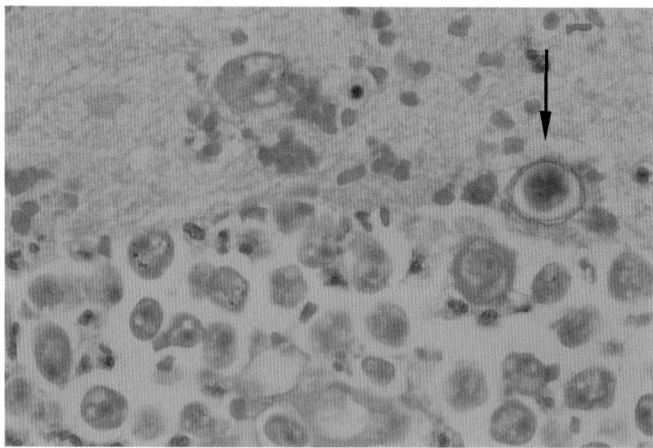

Figure 193-5 Brain section showing numerous trophozoites and a cyst (arrow) with typical features of *Acanthamoeba culbertsoni*. (Masson's trichrome.)

severely congested with scant purulent exudate. Amebic trophozoites are usually seen within the Virchow–Robin spaces with minimal or no inflammatory reaction (Figure 193-4). Cysts are not seen within the CNS lesions. Necrotizing angiitis may occasionally be seen.[1,2]

GRANULOMATOUS AMEBIC ENCEPHALITIS PRODUCED BY *ACANTHAMOEBA* SPP. AND *B. MANDRILLARIS*

Granulomatous amebic encephalitis caused by *Acanthamoeba* spp. occurs principally in individuals who are immunosuppressed (either iatrogenically or because of AIDS) and GAE caused by *B. mandrillaris* occurs in both immunosuppressed and immunocompetent individuals of all ages. Additionally, several cases of GAE caused by *Acanthamoeba* spp. have been described in gorillas, monkeys, dogs, sheep and cows, and *B. mandrillaris* in baboons and other primates.[1,3,28]

The clinical manifestations and pathologic features of GAE are similar regardless of which of these two organisms is the cause. It is an insidious disease and usually has a long and protracted clinical course of weeks to months. Some patients may have a persistent skin lesion for months prior to development of GAE symptoms. Clinical signs include personality changes, headache, low-grade fever, nausea, vomiting, lethargy, hemiparesis, seizures, depressed levels of consciousness and coma. Third and sixth cranial nerve palsies may be seen in some patients. Clinically, GAE may mimic bacterial leptomeningitis, tuberculous or viral meningitis, or single or multiple space-occupying lesions. Cerebellar ataxia and diplopia have been described in some patients. Pneumonitis with the presence of trophozoites and cysts within pulmonary alveoli has also been described.[1] In most cases of GAE, however, final diagnosis is made at autopsy.

Pathologic Features

The cerebral hemispheres are edematous. Encephalomalacia with multifocal areas of cortical softening and hemorrhagic necrosis may be seen. Multifocal necrotic lesions may also be seen in the posterior fossa structures, midbrain, thalamus, brain stem and cerebellum. Trophozoites and cysts of the infecting organisms are seen, most often in the necrotic lesions in basal ganglia, midbrain, brain stem and cerebral hemispheres (Figure 193-5). Microglial nodules may be seen within the necrotic tissues. Occasionally, angiitis may be seen with perivascular cuffing by inflammatory cells, chiefly lymphocytes, a few plasma cells and macrophages. In patients who have advanced AIDS there is very little inflammation. Trophozoites and cysts can easily be identified by light microscopic examination of the tissue sections. Also in patients who have AIDS, multiple ulcerations of the skin with acute and chronic inflammation may be seen and the ulcers may contain trophozoites and cysts of the infecting ameba (Figure 193-6). The kidneys, prostate gland, adrenal glands, lungs and liver may also be involved, suggesting

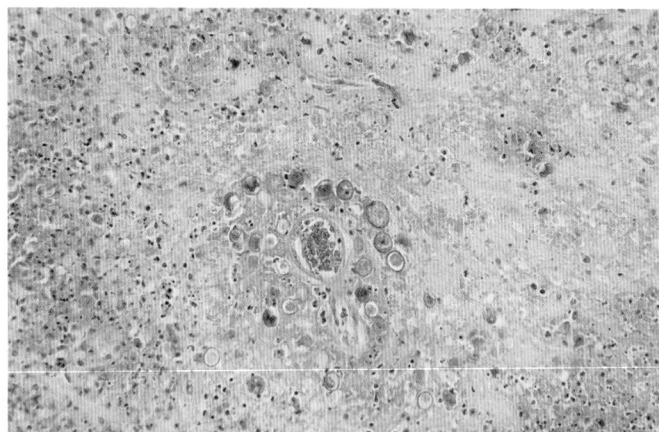

Figure 193-6 Trophozoites and cysts of *Acanthamoeba* spp. surrounding a blood vessel in a skin biopsy of a patient who has AIDS. A diffuse but modest inflammatory reaction is seen.

hematogenous dissemination. The ulcerated skin may serve as a portal of entry for the amebae in some patients. Several cases of skin and nasal infection without dissemination into the CNS have also been reported.[1,29–32]

In general, the trophic and cyst stages of *Acanthamoeba* spp. and *B. mandrillaris* look similar in formalin-fixed and hematoxylin and eosin-stained sections under the light microscope. In some patients, however, differential identification of *B. mandrillaris* can be made if the nuclei of the amebae in the sections possess two or three nucleolar elements because these are not seen in *Acanthamoeba* spp. (Figure 193-7). A definitive identification may be arrived at by carrying out immunohistochemical analysis of the tissue sections using rabbit anti-*Acanthamoeba* spp. or anti-*B. mandrillaris* sera or testing brain tissue with a multiplex PCR. The cyst wall of *B. mandrillaris* is characteristically tripartite and hence can be identified definitively by electron microscopy analysis of brain sections.[1–3]

ACANTHAMOEBA KERATITIS

Acanthamoeba keratitis is associated with contact lens wear, corneal abrasion or trauma. The first case of AK in the USA was reported in a farmer from south Texas with ocular trauma of the right eye. However, the first documented AK outbreak during 1985–1996, estimated to have included more than 700 infections, was associated with wearing contact lenses and using nonsterile homemade saline.[1–3,25] An increase in AK cases in the USA during 2003–2006[33,34] and the subsequent investigation linked cases to use of a particular multipurpose contact

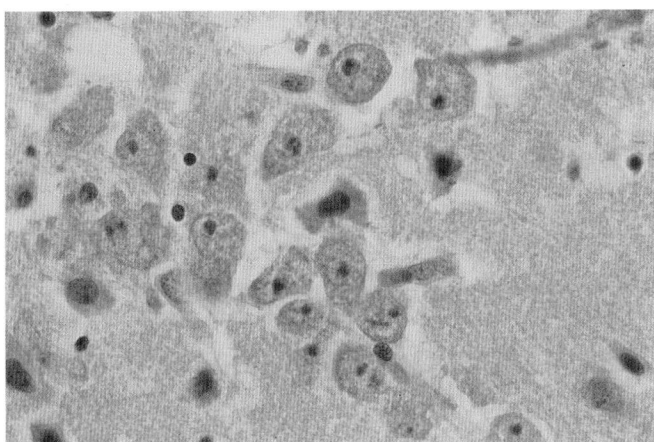

Figure 193-7 CNS section showing many trophozoites of *Balamuthia mandrillaris*. More than one nucleoli can be seen within the nuclei of the trophozoite.

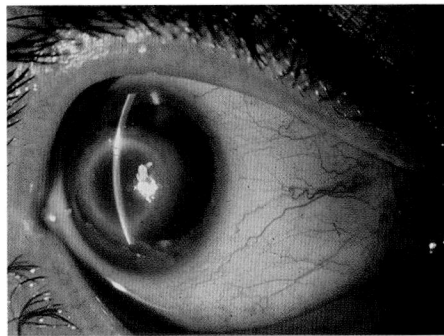

Figure 193-8 *Acanthamoeba keratitis*. Note the typical central or paracentral ring infiltrate. *(Courtesy of Dr Theodore.)*

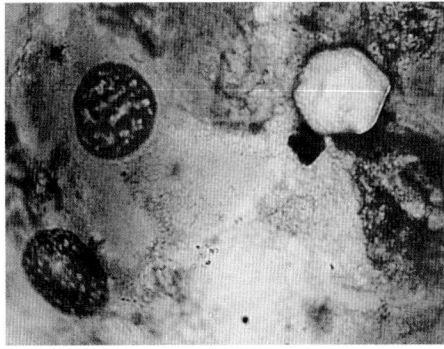

Figure 193-9 Characteristic star-shaped morphology of the cyst of *Acanthamoeba* spp. demonstrated by a corneal scraping stained with Hemacolor. *(Courtesy of Dr Theodore.)*

lens solution, leading to an international recall by the manufacturer.[35] Additionally, another study revealed that most contact lens solutions marketed in the USA do not have sufficient disinfection activity against *Acanthamoeba* spp.[36]

The hallmark of AK is severe ocular pain, photophobia, a central or paracentral 360° stromal ring infiltrate (Figure 193-8), recurrent breakdown of corneal epithelium with a waxing and waning clinical course and a corneal lesion refractory to the usual antibacterial, antiviral and antimycotic medications.[1–3]

When examined under the light microscope, corneal scrapings and/or sections of biopsied corneal tissue reveal trophozoites and cysts of *Acanthamoeba* spp. infiltrated between the lamellae of the cornea (Figure 193-9). Polymorphonuclear leukocytes, eosinophils, lymphocytes, macrophages and plasma cells have also been seen occasionally.

Ulceration, descemetocele formation and perforation are often seen in the later stages of AK.[1–3]

Management

PRIMARY AMEBIC MENINGOENCEPHALITIS

Primary amebic meningoencephalitis has almost always resulted in death. Treatment recommendations rely on a few case reports of survival, notably a 9-year-old girl from California, USA and a 10-year-old boy from Mexico and more recently, a 12-year-old girl from Arkansas, USA.[37–39] Based on these case reports as well as *in vitro* drug studies, the following drug regimen is recommended:

- intravenous amphotericin B (conventional formulation, i.e. not liposomal or lipid complex formulations)[40] 1.5 mg/kg body weight per day in two divided doses for 3 days and then 1 mg/kg
- intrathecal amphotericin B 1.5 mg/day for 2 days followed by 1 mg/day
- intravenous or oral fluconazole 10 mg/kg/day
- oral rifampin 10 mg/kg per day
- intravenous or oral azithromycin 10 mg/kg/day once daily
- oral miltefosine 50 mg three times a day for weight >45 kg, 50 mg twice a day for weight <45 kg.

The above drugs were given for a range of 9–30 days. Azithromycin has both *in vitro* and *in vivo* (mouse model) efficacy against *N. fowleri* and appears to be synergistic when administered with amphotericin B.[41] Miltefosine, a drug used to treat leishmaniasis, has *in vitro* activity against *N. fowleri* and has been used to successfully treat *Acanthamoeba* and *Balamuthia* infections.[42–44] For US patients, miltefosine is available through the US Centers for Disease Control and Prevention (CDC). Aggressive medical (steroids, therapeutic hypothermia) and neurosurgical interventions (extraventricular drain placement) should also be used as indicated to manage elevated intracranial pressure. The most up-to-date clinical guidance from the CDC can be found at: www.cdc.gov/parasites/naegleria/treatment-hcp.html.

GRANULOMATOUS AMEBIC ENCEPHALITIS

Although it is known from *in vitro* experiments that several drugs, including pentamidine, propamidine, dibromopropamidine, miconazole, paromomycin, neomycin, ketoconazole and 5-fluorocytosine, have inhibitory effects on several isolates of *Acanthamoeba*, there is as yet no effective treatment for GAE and therefore the prognosis is poor.[1–3] This is partly due to the difficulty in the diagnosis of GAE because of a lack of clear-cut symptoms, lack of a reliable noninvasive diagnostic test and lack of knowledge among clinicians; diagnosis is often made at the time of postmortem. However, several patients with GAE caused by *Acanthamoeba* spp., as well as *Acanthamoeba* cutaneous infections without CNS involvement, have been successfully treated with a combination of pharmaceuticals including pentamidine isethionate, sulfadiazine, flucytosine and fluconazole or itraconazole.[29,32,45] Several cases have been treated successfully with a combination of trimethoprim-sulfamethoxazole and rifampin.[46,47] Another drug, miltefosine, a hexadecylphosphocholine, has also been shown to have amebicidal potential and miltefosine has been successfully used to treat GAE patients.[43,48] For US patients, miltefosine is available through the US CDC. For *Acanthamoeba* cutaneous infection without CNS involvement, topical applications of chlorhexidine gluconate and ketoconazole cream in addition to the above have resulted in therapeutic success.[1–3,29]

Although the majority of patients with *Balamuthia* GAE have died, a few patients have survived the infection. For example, four patients – a 64-year-old man, a 5-year-old girl from California, a 72-year-old woman from New York and a 2-year-old male from Kentucky – survived *Balamuthia* GAE after treatment with a combination of pentamidine isethionate, sulfadiazine, macrolide antibiotics (azithromycin–clarithromycin), fluconazole and flucytosine (5-fluorocytosine).[49–51] Two Peruvian patients with cutaneous lesions recovered after prolonged therapy with albendazole and itraconazole.

One of the Peruvian patients had a large lesion on the chest wall that was surgically removed. Surgical excision of the lesion may have reduced the ameba load, thus helping in the recovery process.[52] A more recent Peruvian survivor had a prolonged course of cutaneous and neurologic disease and ultimately recovered with treatment that included albendazole, itraconazole and miltefosine.[44] One of the most recent survivors of *Balamuthia* GAE was a 27-year-old kidney transplant recipient who acquired infection via the donated kidney and was treated with pentamidine, sulfadiazine, flucytosine, fluconazole, azithromycin and miltefosine.[18,53]

ACANTHAMOEBA KERATITIS

Treatment of AK with topical application of polyhexamethylene biguanide or chlorhexidine gluconate in combination with propamidine isethionate appears to be the treatment of choice, as several patients have been treated successfully in this way.[1-3] Many patients have also been treated with topical application of propamidine isethionate 0.1% and dibromopropamidine, in conjunction with neosporin. Ketoconazole and clotrimazole appear to be effective *in vitro* and *in vivo*. Other reports of successful treatment with 0.1% hexamidine di-isethionate eye drops have been reported. Some patients have also been treated successfully with combinations of topical propamidine and miconazole and systemic ketoconazole, or topical clotrimazole or oral itraconazole with topical miconazole.[54] Medical cure has been achieved with the administration topically of polyhexamethylene biguanide[55] or chlorhexidine with or without propamidine.[56,57] Debridement of the cornea, penetrating keratoplasty and corneal grafting have also been performed with good results in some patients. Recurrence of AK has been reported after corneal transplantation, probably caused by cysts of *Acanthamoeba* spp. still present in the corneal stroma.

DISCLAIMER

The findings and conclusions in this report are those of the authors and do not necessarily represent the views of the US Centers for Disease Control and Prevention.

References available online at expertconsult.com.

KEY REFERENCES

Aichelburg A.C., Walochnik J., Assadian O., et al.: Successful treatment of disseminated *Acanthamoeba* sp. infection with miltefosine. *Emerg Infect Dis* 2008; 14:1743-1746.

Bravo F.G., Seas C.: *Balamuthia mandrillaris* amoebic encephalitis: an emerging parasitic infection. *Curr Infect Dis Rep* 2012; 14:391-396.

Centers for Disease Control and Prevention: *Balamuthia mandrillaris* transmitted through organ transplantation – Mississippi, 2009. *MMWR Morb Mortal Wkly Rep* 2010; 59:1165-1170.

Martinez A.J., Visvesvara G.S.: Free-living, amphizoic and opportunistic amebas. *Brain Pathol* 1997; 7:583-598.

Schuster F.L., Visvesvara G.S.: Free-living amoebae as opportunistic and non-opportunistic pathogens of humans and animals. *Int J Parasitol* 2004; 34:1001-1027.

Seidel J.S., Harmatz P., Visvesvara G.S., et al.: Successful treatment of primary amebic meningoencephalitis. *N Engl J Med* 1982; 306:346-348.

Stehr-Green J.K., Bailey T.M., Visvesvara G.S.: The epidemiology of *Acanthamoeba* keratitis in the United States. *Am J Ophthalmol* 1989; 107:331-336.

Verani J.R., Lorick S.A., Yoder J.S., et al.: National outbreak of *Acanthamoeba* keratitis associated with use of a contact lens solution, United States. *Emerg Infect Dis* 2009; 15:1236-1242.

Visvesvara G.S., Moura H., Schuster F.L.: Pathogenic and opportunistic free-living amoebae: *Acanthamoeba* spp., *Balamuthia mandrillaris*, *Naegleria fowleri*, and *Sappinia diploidea*. *FEMS Immunol Microbiol* 2007; 50:1-26.

Yoder J.S., Eddy B.A., Visvesvara G.S., et al.: The epidemiology of primary amoebic meningoencephalitis in the USA, 1962-2008. *Epidemiol Infect* 2010; 138:968-975.

194

Blood and Tissue Protozoa

MARÍA-JESÚS PINAZO | EDELWEISS ALDASORO |
ANTONIA CALVO-CANO | ALBERT PICADO | JOSE MUÑOZ |
JOAQUIM GASCON

KEY CONCEPTS

- Organisms of the genera *Plasmodium, Babesia, Toxoplasma, Leishmania* and *Trypanosoma* are the most prevalent protozoa able to invade blood and human tissues.

- For clinicians, knowing the geographical distribution of the parasites is essential, in order to make an accurate diagnosis and appropriate management of patients.

- Toxoplasmosis acquired during pregnancy or reactivated during immunosuppression could be associated with severe organ manifestations, such as severe neurologic or ophthalmic disease.

- Innate and adaptive immune responses help control *Leishmania* spp. infection.

- Chagas disease is currently a global emerging disease, and a public health problem in countries in which it was not endemic.

- In human African trypanosomiasis, the correct management of the patient is based on the infection diagnosis (by microbiologic methods) and the determination of the disease stage.

- Prevention methods of blood and tissue protozoa infections vary with the transmission routes of each parasite, vectors and human behavior.

- The individual immunologic characteristics may lead to different disease evolution, and may develop different clinical forms of parasitic infection.

Organisms of the genera *Plasmodium, Babesia, Toxoplasma, Leishmania* and *Trypanosoma* are the most prevalent protozoa able to invade blood and human tissues. They cause diseases of immense socioeconomic impact, most of them having a limited (although extensive) geographic distribution.

Malaria is considered separately in Chapter 117.

Babesiosis

Human babesiosis is a tick-borne parasitic malaria-like zoonotic disease that was first described by Victor Babes in Rumanian cattle in 1888. It was not reported as a human disease until 1957. Currently it is considered an emerging disease.

Nature

The genus *Babesia* belongs to the family Babesiidae, order Piroplasmida (phylum Apicomplexa) and is closely related to *Plasmodium, Theileria* and *Cytauxzoon*. *Babesia* comprises over 100 species that parasitize domestic and wild mammals and birds. Infection in cattle is widespread and it is an economically important disease. Piroplasms can be divided into five groups: (1) small *Babesia* (archaeopiroplasmids or *microti* group); (2) parasites from cervids (e.g. deer), dogs, and people (*duncani* group or prototheilerids); (3) primarily canine, bovine and cervine babesid species; (4) primarily bovine, equine and ovine species (unguilibabesids); (5) the *Theileria* and *Cytauxzoon* spp. (theilerids).

Epidemiology

Babesiosis cases have been described in North America, Europe and Asia, but the highest incidence in humans has been reported in the eastern USA.

In the USA, *B. microti* is the primary cause of human babesiosis and cases have been described in New York, Massachusetts, Rhode Island, focal areas in Connecticut, New Jersey, Wisconsin, Minnesota and recently in southern New England. Serologic surveys indicate that in highly endemic areas the prevalence is 9–21% (incidence of 900 cases/100 000 residents per year in new areas). The main vector is *Ixodes dammini* (a variant of *Ixodes scapularis*).[1] Cases of babesiosis can be acquired from blood products (asymptomatically infected donors), and one case of vertically transmitted infection has been also described. In the USA, at least four other species are associated with human infections: *B. duncani* (Washington and California, seroprevalence around 3.5–16%); *B. sp. CA-type* (California); *B. sp. MO1* (Missouri, Kentucky and Washington); and *Babesia sp.* from a patient in Tennessee. In Canada, transfusion cases by *B. microti* have been reported.

In Europe, *B. divergens* is the most common cause of human babesiosis in cattle-raising regions during summer months when *Ixodes ricinus* is most active and the incidence of red water fever in cattle is greatest. Other zoonotic species include a *B. divergens*-like species from the Canary Islands, *Babesia* sp. EU1 (also called *B. venatorum*), and a *B.microti*-like species. Cases from France, Ireland and Great Britain were reported, with fewer cases from Sweden, Switzerland, Spain, Portugal and Croatia.[2]

At least four species or genotypes of zoonotic *Babesia* have been detected in Asia (Japan, Taiwan, Korea, India, and China).[3] Isolated cases have been described in South and West Africa and Latin America.

Pathogenicity

After infectious blood is digested by the tick vector, *Babesia* replicates in the intestinal epithelium of the tick and develops in the salivary glands, ovaries and other tissues maturing as sporozoites, that are deposited in the skin of a vertebrate host during the tick's blood meal. There is no pre-erythrocytic phase. Following entry into the erythrocyte, the pear-shaped trophozoites replicate by asynchronous budding. During replication, double-membraned segments develop, resulting in both asexually reproducing merozoites and 'accordion'-like nonreplicating sexual parasites (gametocytes). Asexual forms appear as simple rings, pairs or tetrads and are difficult to distinguish from sexual stages by light microscopy.

Lysis of parasitized erythrocytes leads to anemia, hemoglobinemia, hyperbilirubinemia and, in severe cases, intense jaundice, massive hemoglobinuria and renal shutdown due, in severe cases, to acute tubular necrosis. Even in cases of parasite clearance secondary to treatment, ischemic necrosis of several organs has been described.

Cytokine-mediated shock syndrome has been described in several cases, as well as tumor necrosis factor-alpha (TNF-α) and interferon-gamma (IFN-γ) overproduction. Humoral immunity appears to be less important than cellular immunity in controlling human infection that may last more than one year, even in the absence of underlying illness.

Prevention

General recommendations include avoidance of known endemic areas in the warm months of the year. Spraying acaricides can reduce numbers of vector ticks, also in presumed cattle reservoirs for *B. divergens*. Reducing the density of rodent reservoirs seems impractical (*B. microti* transmission).

Public health strategies may be followed to protect human populations against babesial infection. Clothes should be sprayed with tick repellents (permethrin-based) before commencing outdoor activities and on return the skin should be thoroughly examined for the presence of ticks.

Diagnostic Microbiology

During the acute stage of the disease the number of parasites inside the erythrocytes is high, and they can be detected microscopically: thin and thick blood smears, brain smears (sample of grey matter of the cortex, by brain capillaries observation), and hemolymph smears (by tick tissues hemolymph cells observation).[4]

To perform thin blood smears, after collecting blood and staining it with Giemsa, intraerythrocytic parasites are observed under a microscope using a 100× objective. The diameter of the different *Babesia* species is: *B. bigemina*, paired merozoites measure 2.5–3.5 μm, *B. bovis* merozoites 1.5–2 μm and *B. divergens* merozoites 1.5–0.4 μm (detection for up to one infected erythrocyte/10 000 cells).

Thick smear technique was developed to detect lower levels of parasitemia, especially in cases of *B. bovis* suspicion. The small nucleus of *Babesia* can be difficult to identify on thick films. Sequential blood smears may be required when the level of parasitemia is low.

Babesia is distinguished on blood smear from *Plasmodium falciparum* by a combination of criteria, including the demonstration of basket-shaped and frequently extracellular merozoites, red blood cells containing four or more parasites, and the presence of tetrad forms (Maltese crosses, Figure 194-1). The absence of hemozoin (malarial pigment) is considered diagnostic for the piroplasms. *B. divergens* may be identified by the presence of paired divergent pyriforms, occupying 20–25% of the erythrocyte area, along with small single oval/round merozoites.[4]

In chronically infected individuals, immunologic methods searching for antibodies against proteins of blood stages are the best method to identify infected people. These methods are indirect immunofluorescent antibody test (IFAT), enzyme-linked immunosorbent assay (ELISA) and immunochromatography test (ICT). Absence or low titers of specific antibodies against *Babesia* when blood smears contain

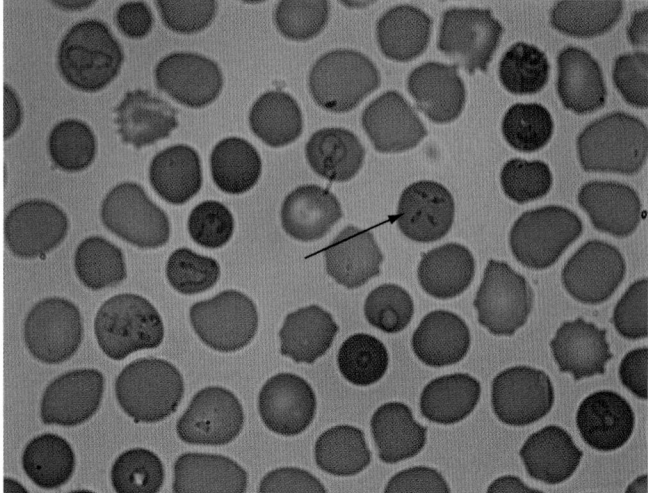

Figure 194-1 *Babesia* spp. heavy infection. Single and multiple intraerythrocytic parasites can be seen. The arrow marks a typical Maltese cross arrangement.

parasites suggest an infection by another *Babesia* sp. or an immunocompromised patient. Serologic tests are useful, particularly in chronic *B. microti* and WA-1 infections with low parasitemia that is not detectable in some cases.[4] Recent ELISA methods include the use of recombinant antigens and monoclonal antibodies, increasing specificity.

The ICT is a rapid diagnostic device that detects antibodies against a specific antigen in a small amount of serum that can be implemented in the field. It has been developed for several *Babesia* species, and the concordances compared with standard methods like ELISA and IFAT have been evaluated for *B. bovis* (92.5 and 90.3%), *B. bigemina* (96.8 and 92.5%) and *B. gibsoni* (100 and 85.7%). Nonetheless, ICTs are not yet commercially available in any country.[4]

Molecular methods have also been described to detect *Babesia* parasites in both acute and chronic stage of the disease. Among them, polymerase chain reaction (PCR), real-time PCR (RT-PCR), reverse line blot hybridization (RLB), and loop mediated isothermal amplification (LAMP) are being developed in order to improve diagnosis of *Babesia* spp., but their use in clinical settings is still limited.

Clinical Manifestations

The clinical forms of babesiosis vary widely depending upon the immune status of the host and the species of *Babesia* involved. Infection can be subclinical, cause a self-limited febrile illness, produce a moderate to severe illness resembling malaria, or progress rapidly to death.

The symptoms of *B. microti* infection (Nantucket fever) range from a nonspecific flu-like self-limited febrile illness to severe hemolytic anemia, or multiorgan failure. Most infections with *B. microti* are subclinical, and available data suggest the same for babesiosis due to WA-1 or CA-1. It is most severe in those who are older or asplenic (immunosuppressed host).

The incubation period is 1–4 weeks (4–9 after transfusion), during which people suffering babesiosis might experience malaise and discomfort. The onset of symptoms is gradual with nonspecific symptoms (fatigue, anorexia, headache, emotional lability and jaundice), followed within 1 week by sustained or intermittent high fever, sweats, and myalgia, with dark urine. Mild splenomegaly and hepatomegaly can be present.

Most patients have mild to moderate anemia, thrombocytopenia, and normal or depressed white blood cell count. Frequent findings are elevated hepatic enzymes, hyperbilirubinemia, elevated serum lactic dehydrogenase and decreased haptoglobin levels (secondary to hemolysis). After several days to several weeks, fever and more intense symptoms may resolve spontaneously, but weakness, malaise and fatigue persist for months. People with *B. microti* infection who are coinfected with *Borrelia burgdorferi* experience more symptoms and longer duration of illness.[5]

In asplenic or immunosuppressed people illness can be severe, with intense hemolysis leading to jaundice, severe anemia and renal failure. Parasitemia can reach 85% in asplenic patients, and severe pancytopenia could be due to hemophagocytosis. Disseminated intravascular coagulation, hypotension, and adult respiratory distress syndrome, has been described, along with noncardiac pulmonary edema. Recurrences can be prevented by treatment.

The European clinical cases, due mainly to *B. divergens*, occur mainly in immunosuppressed patients who present with a high fever and severe hemolytic anemia, and the infection is usually fatal. After an incubation period of 1–4 weeks, patients become acutely ill with high fever, prostration, rigors, diaphoresis, headache, myalgia, jaundice and hemogloblinuria. Nausea, vomiting and diarrhea are prominent symptoms, and the liver may be enlarged and painful. Most patients develop acute respiratory distress. Renal failure induced by intravascular hemolysis and hypotension ensues and is followed by coma and death, usually within 1 week of onset of symptoms.[6]

The differential diagnosis for babesiosis includes Lyme disease, ehrlichiosis, typhoidal tularemia and Rocky Mountain spotted fever, all of them endemic in regions in which *Babesia* is also endemic. Other diseases, such as viral hepatitis, bacterial sepsis, infectious mononucleosis, leptospirosis, malaria and relapsing fever, should be ruled out.

Management

Early treatment is recommended for all diagnosed cases to prevent long-term sequelae and potential transmission through blood donation.[4]

In non-immunosuppressed patients, atovaquone 750 mg q12h plus azithromycin (500–1000 mg on day 1, then 250–1000 mg/day orally for a total of 7–10 days). An alternate regime is quinine sulfate 1 g q12h intravenously or 650 mg q8h orally (25 mg/kg/day in children divided in three doses) plus clindamycin 1200 mg intravenously twice daily or 600 mg orally three times a day (20–40 mg/kg/day in children, divided in three doses), for 7–10 days. In immunosuppressed patients, at least a 6-week regimen at the same doses is recommended.[7]

Chloroquine is not recommended. Blood transfusion and general supportive treatment may be needed for severe disease. Exchange transfusion has been used in an attempt to decrease parasite load, but its usefulness has not been demonstrated. Coinfection by *Borrelia burgdorferi* and other tick-transmitted micro-organisms should be ruled out, but in case of suspicion, doxycycline 200 mg q12h is recommended.

Toxoplasmosis

Toxoplasmosis is a widespread zoonosis, caused by the coccidian parasite *Toxoplasma gondii*. Humans are usually infected orally, developing few, if any, symptoms of infection. The infection persists for life without signs of disease. However, if acquired during pregnancy or reactivated during immunosuppression, it results in organ manifestations such as severe neurologic or ophthalmic disease. Diagnosis usually requires a panel of tests and treatment may be adjusted to the different clinical forms.

Nature

T. gondii is a member of the Apicomplexa protozoan parasites, as are *Plasmodium* spp. and *Cryptosporidium* spp. They possess a unique apical complex structure involved in host cell invasion. It is a parasite of many species of mammals and birds, and its definitive hosts are felines (including domestic cats). The main forms of the parasite life cycle are oocysts (product of the sexual multiplication), tachyzoites (rapidly replicating intracellular form) and bradyzoites, the slowly replicating or dormant form, encysted in tissues.[8]

Epidemiology

Human disease caused by *T. gondii* is generally a consequence of either intrauterine acquisition or an immunocompromised state, and is much more restricted than the infection itself. It has been estimated that one-third of mankind is infected.[9] Seroprevalence varies widely between countries and the highest rates of infection with *T. gondii* have been reported in Brazil, Central America and Central Africa (50–80%), followed by Central and South Europe (30–50%).[10] Variability in infection rates in humans depends upon environmental factors and eating habits. Warm and humid climates are ideal for perpetuating the parasite life cycle. In resource-poor settings, the main transmission route of *Toxoplasma* infection is ingestion of oocysts (non-filtered water supply, contaminated soil where children play). In other settings, transmission occurs primarily through the ingestion on undercooked meat or by a mixed pattern. Increased socioeconomic levels, together with an improvement of hygienic conditions, changes in farming systems, the consumption of frozen meat and the feeding of cats with sterilized food[11] have led to a continuous decrease of the seroprevalence in most industrialized countries over the past decades.

Pathogenicity and Immunity

The life cycle of *Toxoplasma* is biphasic: a sexual cycle, which occurs exclusively in felines, and an asexual cycle, that occurs in noncarnivorous animals, including humans. Cats usually acquire the infection by ingesting tissue cysts from small prey. Replication occurs in the intestinal epithelium of felines, forming oocysts that are later excreted in feces, being environmentally resistant. The asexual phase begins when secondary hosts ingest uncooked meat containing tissue cysts or some water contaminated from oocysts. The parasite adopts tachyzoite stage, to infect nucleated cells that act as Trojan horses to disseminate *T. gondii* through the blood flow. Inside the cells, it multiplies until rupture. Tissue destruction activates inflammatory response and induces clinical symptoms. Once the immune system controls the infection, tachyzoites are sequestered in tissue cysts and form bradyzoites. Bradyzoites are indicative of the chronic stage of infection and can persist for the life of the individual, usually in muscle and brain. In humans, *Toxoplasma* infection also can be transmitted by the transplacental route and by hematopoietic or solid organ transplantation (especially heart, due to tropism for muscle). In an immunocompetent host, both humoral and cellular immune responses are important to control the infection. Strain virulence is also a determinant: there are three known clonal lineages (I, II and III), and the most virulent genotype has been found in South America, which is a recombinant among them.[12] Tachyzoites secrete signaling molecules to induce several mechanisms: (a) generation of specific antibodies; (b) attraction of macrophages, neutrophils and dendritic cells; (c) IFN-γ and interleukin (IL)-12 production provoking a potent T helper-1 (Th-1) response; and (d) stimulation of CD8+ lymphocytes that destroy both parasite and infected cell.

To avoid a severe inflammation, downregulation is performed by IL-10 and transforming growth factor-beta (TGF-β), which modulate macrophage activation.[13] Only strains type I and III are able to promote this downregulation. Toxoplasma can also inhibit apoptotic mechanisms of the infected cell, ensuring long-term survival of the parasite.[14] The occasional rupture of individual cysts containing bradyzoites can reactivate the infection in immunocompromised individuals, maintaining high titers of antibodies in immunocompetent hosts.

Prevention

Toxoplasmosis can be prevented at three different levels:
- prevention of primary infection
- prevention of vertical transmission and congenital disease
- prevention of disease in infected immunocompromised individuals.

To prevent primary infection, the exposure to parasite can be reduced by health education (Box 194-1). No vaccine is presently available.

BOX 194-1   TOXOPLASMOSIS PRIMARY PREVENTIVE MEASURES

- Do not eat undercooked or raw red meat or eggs. Cook meat until it is no longer pink in the center
- While handling raw meat avoid touching your mouth or contaminating other food. Normal hygienic washing of hands and utensils will suffice
- Cured or smoked meat is generally considered safe from *Toxoplasma*. Freeze it at –20°C (–4°F) for at least 24 hours as an additional precaution
- Consume only pasteurized or ultra-heat-treated (UHT) sterilized milk and dairy products
- Wash or peel all fruits and vegetables to be eaten uncooked
- Control insect pests and their access to foodstuffs
- Avoid living with cats or kittens. If unfeasible, take special care: change the cat litter box daily and rinse it with nearly boiling water. Wear gloves and wash your hands well with soap and water immediately after. Prevent your cat from hunting birds and rodents or eating raw meat
- Use gloves and wash your hands well after gardening and other outdoor activities with soil contact

Maternal immunity due to toxoplasmosis passed before conception protects the fetus from the infection. Immunodeficient patients receiving trimethoprim–sulfamethoxazole (TMP–SMX) as prophylaxis for *Pneumocystis* infection are substantially protected from toxoplasmosis.

To prevent vertical transmission, maternal antibodies of latent infection protect the fetus. Seronegative women should avoid exposure to sources of infection and seek medical attention if they experience mononucleosis-like syndrome during pregnancy. Maternal routine serologic screening during pregnancy remains controversial.[15] Whenever a pregnant woman is diagnosed with acute *Toxoplasma* infection, anti-*T. gondii* treatment is immediately offered to prevent maternal–fetal transmission and further evaluation of fetal and newborn infection is recommended. Therapies from diagnosis to delivery are spiramycin 3 g/day (1g q8h) orally and, if fetal infection is proven, sulfadiazine (3 g/day q12) plus pyrimethamine (200 mg orally once on the first day, then 50 mg once per day orally or 25 mg q12h) and folinic acid (5–20 mg 3×/week).

T. gondii IgG serology should be included in the initial workup of pre-transplant patients and transplantation of a solid organ from an IgM-seropositive donor to a seronegative recipient should be avoided.[16] In the case of a transplant performed in a recipient with negative antibodies for *Toxoplasma*, one possibility is to administer TMP–SMX for the first 6 months, being aware of the possibility of toxoplasmosis after discontinuation. Physicians should apply preventive measures, with hygienic measures during the post-transplant period, and be aware of symptoms compatible with *Toxoplasma* infection. The strategy for preventing toxoplasmosis in donor/recipient serology mismatch for non-heart solid organ transplantation in areas of high seroprevalence of *Toxoplasma* remains undetermined.[16]

HIV-positive individuals who are seronegative for *T. gondii* should also avoid being exposed to the parasite and receive primary prophylaxis if CD4 counts are less than 100 cells/μL. Once they have developed the disease due to reactivation, secondary prophylaxis is mandatory, being also discontinued in patients who achieve immune reconstitution with antiretroviral therapy.

Diagnostic Microbiology

The diagnosis of *T. gondii* infection is usually made indirectly by a panel of serologic tests interpreted within the clinical context.[17] IgM antibodies usually appear within one week and can remain positive for more than 12 months. IgG antibodies appear after the second week of primary infection and generally persist for life. Diagnosis of an acute infection in a patient with typical symptoms is easy if there is a positive result for IgM with a non-reactive IgG antibody. However, the most common situation is to find a positive result for both IgM and IgG. In this case, additional testing should be performed for confirmation (ELISA, avidity or agglutination testing). A positive IgG titer in an immunocompromised host does not distinguish reactivation disease from latent infection. Usually the patient may fit suggestive clinical history and typical radiographic findings. A negative IgG titer is strongly suggestive of an alternative diagnosis.

Diagnosis of maternal acute infection should be based on a minimum of two blood samples separated by 2 weeks showing seroconversion for IgG or IgM. For fetal infection polymerase chain reaction (PCR) for *T. gondii* DNA in amniotic fluid is the best method, with high sensitivity (92.2%) if seroconversion is after the first trimester.[18] Indirect diagnosis by fetal ultrasonography may show intracranial calcification or hydrocephalia only in cases of poor prognosis and after 21 weeks of gestation. For congenital infection newborn screening should include physical examination, serial serology, ophthalmologic and neurologic tests.

PCR of tissue or body fluids is the most specific diagnostic tool for active infection in an immunosuppressed host with suspected disseminated disease, but it is usually difficult to obtain a sample for testing (e.g. lumbar puncture is often contraindicated).

Examination of stained tissue or fluid smears with visualization of tachyzoites or cysts, growth in tissue cultures and experimental animal inoculation may be used. The most sensitive method to diagnose chorioretinitis is intraocular sampling for supportive evidence of antibody production against *Toxoplasma*.[19]

Clinical Manifestations

There are three different forms of toxoplasmosis: congenital infection, acute extrauterine infection and toxoplasmosis of the immunocompromised host.

CONGENITAL TOXOPLASMOSIS

Toxoplasmosis acquired *in utero* is mostly asymptomatic. The infection may produce signs of disease that can be present at birth or later in life. The risk of congenital toxoplasmosis depends upon the time of acquisition of acute maternal infection.[20] Vertical transmission of *T. gondii* increases with gestational age (15% in the first trimester of pregnancy, 44% in the second and 71% in the third).[21] Conversely, the severity of congenital disease is increased when infection occurs in early pregnancy. Signs of infection at delivery are present in less than 10–30% of newborns with congenital toxoplasmosis on routine physical examination. Specific tests are needed to assess central nervous system (CNS) or retinal abnormalities (Figure 194-2).[22]

Clinical manifestations of congenital toxoplasmosis include chorioretinitis, intracranial calcifications, seizures, hepatosplenomegaly, jaundice, anemia and thrombocytopenia. The characteristic triad of hydrocephalus, cerebral calcifications and chorioretinitis resulting in mental retardation, epilepsy and impaired vision is the most severe and extreme form of the disease. If there are late manifestations of untreated congenital infection, expected findings are mainly chorioretinitis and neurologic abnormalities (motor or intellectual disability, deafness).

ACQUIRED TOXOPLASMOSIS

In 90% of cases, no clinical symptoms are apparent during acute infection. Symptomatic patients present with bilateral, nontender cervical lymphadenopathy; malaise and low-grade fever are present in less than 50% of symptomatic cases. Differential diagnosis includes primary human immunodeficiency virus (HIV) infection, acute Epstein-Barr virus (EBV) or cytomegalovirus (CMV), and lymphoma. The histologic picture of acute *T. gondii* lymphadenopathy usually provides an indirect diagnosis, but biopsy is rarely performed.

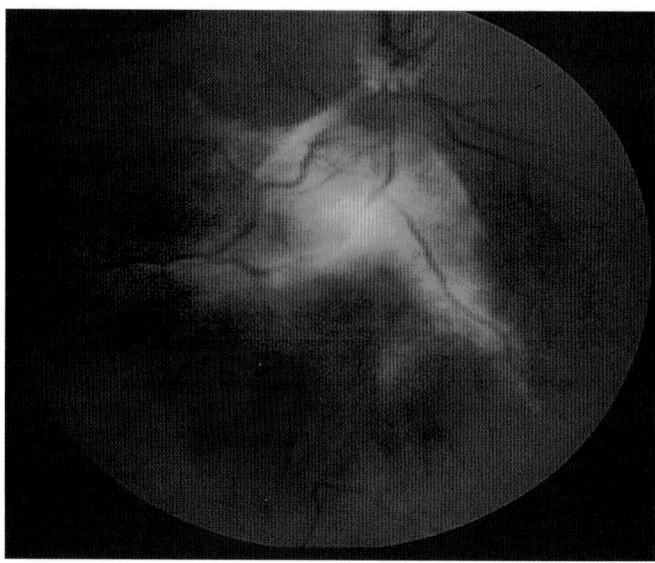

Figure 194-2 Fundoscopic image of toxoplasmic chorioretinitis. Most cases presenting in adults represent a late manifestation of congenitally acquired toxoplasmosis.

TOXOPLASMOSIS IN THE IMMUNOCOMPROMISED HOST

Toxoplasmosis is a serious disease in patients who have profound immunosuppression, such as those who have had a transplant or who have an HIV infection.

In transplant patients, the incidence and severity of the disease depends upon: (a) previous exposure to the parasite of the donor and recipient; (b) the type of transplanted organ (tropism of tissue cysts for striated muscle in heart transplantation); and (c) the lack of prophylaxis: at least 75% of the cases occur in patients who have not received prophylaxis.[23]

The disease can be due to reactivation of a chronic silent infection or an acute primary infection acquired from the transplanted organ, and it usually manifests within the first 3 months after transplantation, as a systemic disease with diverse degrees of multiorgan involvement, including pneumonitis, myocarditis or encephalitis.[23]

In patients who have an HIV infection, encephalitis is the usual presentation, especially if the CD4 count is less than 50–100 cells/μL. Ocular lesions and other extracranial symptoms have been described.[24]

The onset of *T. gondii* encephalitis is usually subacute and starts typically with headache. Focal neurologic deficits, seizures and fever are also common. Nausea, vomiting and mental status changes usually indicate elevated intracranial pressure. Chorioretinitis in HIV provokes eye pain and decreased visual acuity, not distinguishable from other ocular infections in HIV, such as cytomegalovirus retinitis.

Diagnosis is based upon: a compatible clinical syndrome; identification of multiple lesions by brain imaging (Figure 194-3); <100 CD4 cells/μL, a positive IgG titer (without prophylaxis against either toxoplasmosis or pneumocystis); and detection of the organism in a biopsy specimen. Biopsy is performed only when no improvement is achieved after anti-*T. gondii* treatment.

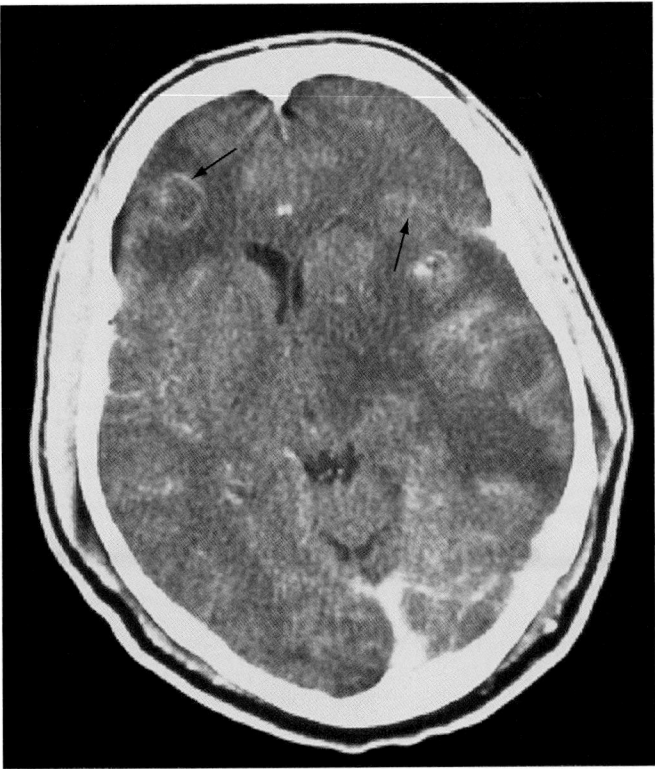

Figure 194-3 Toxoplasmic encephalitis in a person who has AIDS. A cranial CT scan shows bilateral contrast-enhanced ring lesions (arrows) with peripheral edema and mass effect.

Management

CONGENITAL TOXOPLASMOSIS

The majority of newborns with untreated (symptomatic or subclinical) congenital toxoplasmosis develop serious neurologic long-term sequelae. Therefore, it is recommended to give therapy for:

- infants with prenatal diagnosis (regardless of whether their mothers received chemotherapy)
- infants with infection confirmed by serology or PCR
- infants with recent maternal *T. gondii* infection and clinical triad (chorioretinitis, intracranial calcifications and/or hydrocephalus).

First-line regimen is pyrimethamine plus sulfadiazine and folinic acid usually for one year, because it has been demonstrated to improve long-term neurologic, cognitive and auditory outcomes and prevention of new ocular lesions. Blood count monitoring is recommended during treatment of drug-induced neutropenia and hemolysis, and clinical monitoring years after treatment for detecting late manifestations (ophthalmologic and neurologic).

All infected newborns should have anti-*T. gondii* treatment (sulfadiazine 10–25 mg/kg q12h plus pyrimethamine 1 mg/kg/day and folinic acid 5 mg/kg/day for at least 6 months).

A small proportion of women have their pregnancies terminated because of toxoplasmosis. Termination of pregnancy is offered in many countries to women who seroconvert in the first 8 weeks of pregnancy and to those infected in the first 22 weeks of pregnancy when fetal infection is confirmed. Most infected babies have a good prognosis. However, fetuses with ultrasound evidence of intracranial lesions are at high risk of serious neurologic damage or death, without evidence for prenatal treatment to reduce these risks.

ACQUIRED TOXOPLASMOSIS

Symptomatic *T. gondii* infection in nonpregnant immunocompetent individuals does not need to be treated since most resolve spontaneously.

TOXOPLASMOSIS IN THE IMMUNOSUPPRESSED HOST

Due to a lower incidence of relapse compared with others and despite high incidence of cutaneous adverse effects, the preferred first-line regimen for cerebral and extracerebral toxoplasmosis is a 6-week regimen with sulfadiazine 1000 mg q6h for weight <60 kg (1500 mg q6h for >60 kg) plus pyrimethamine as a first 200 mg loading dose followed by 50 mg/day for <60 kg (75 mg daily if >60 kg) plus folinic acid 10–25 mg/day (to prevent drug-induced hematologic toxicity). This regimen is followed by secondary prophylaxis.[25,26]

If there is intolerance to sulfadiazine, alternative therapies are pyrimethamine plus clindamycin (600 mg intravenously or orally q6h) and TMP–SMX (TMP 10 mg/kg/day + SMX 50 mg/kg/day; 50% if extracerebral).

In case of brain edema, corticosteroids should be given, but it should be considered that the clinical response to anti-*T. gondii* therapy may be masked by the unspecific improvement due to the reduction of edema (e.g. in lymphoma). To establish effective therapy a control computed tomography or magnetic resonance scan should be repeated after 2 weeks, and if no improvement is seen a biopsy should be performed to exclude lymphoma. A repeat scan can be carried out after completing treatment. If initiation of antiretroviral therapy (ART) is needed, expert recommendation is to wait for the second or third week under treatment for toxoplasmosis to avoid immune reconstitution syndrome.

SECONDARY PREVENTION

Approximately 80% of HIV-infected patients relapse after an initial episode of toxoplasmosis. Hence, 6 weeks' post-induction therapy is indicated to maintain a chronic suppressive therapy. The regimen of first choice is daily treatment with pyrimethamine (25–50 mg orally q24h) plus sulfadiazine (2–4 g orally divided in 2–4 doses/day) and folinic acid (10–25 mg daily). TMP–SMX (5–25 mg/kg/day) is widely used to reduce pill burden and achieve better adherence. Preventive treatment can be safely discontinued if immune system function is restored with ART (CD4 count >200 cells/μL for 6 months), ensuring the patient is aware of the importance of seeking medical attention if symptoms appear.

Leishmaniasis

Leishmaniasis is the term used to describe a group of chronic parasitic diseases caused by a number of species of the genus *Leishmania*. Three syndromes are usually identified – visceral leishmaniasis (VL), mucocutaneous leishmaniasis (MCL) and cutaneous leishmaniasis (CL) – but other secondary clinical forms exist. It is usually a zoonosis transmitted by Phlebotominae sand flies, which are endemic in areas of Southern Europe, Asia, Africa and the Americas (see Chapter 123).

Nature

The genus *Leishmania*, along with the genus *Trypanosoma*, belongs to the order Kinetoplastida, which comprises flagellated protozoa that possess a characteristic extranuclear DNA mass called the kinetoplast.

There are up to 20 species of the genus *Leishmania* that are pathogenic to humans. *Leishmania* parasites are often classified by their geographical origin into two broad groups:
- New World *Leishmania* spp. (Americas)
- Old World *Leishmania* spp. (Africa, Europe and Asia).

Closely related species are grouped into subgenera and complexes (Table 194-1).

Sand flies are small (3–4 mm), hairy mosquito-like insects, which transmit the *Leishmania* parasites. Old World sand flies belong to the genus *Phlebotomus*; New World species belong to the genera *Lutzomyia*.

Epidemiology

Leishmaniasis is endemic in 98 countries on five continents (see Chapter 123, Figure 123-1). According to recent estimates there are between 0.2 and 0.4 million, and 0.7 and 1.2 million VL and CL cases, respectively, per year.[27]

The vast majority of patients are infected by sand flies, but rare cases in which infection is transmitted by blood transfusion, organ transplant or needle sharing among drug users have been reported.

Pathogenicity

Leishmania species vary in pathogenicity and cause a variety of syndromes in different human populations. The infecting species, the parasite–host interaction and immunologic factors determine the clinical outcomes that range from asymptomatic to life-threatening systemic infection. Innate and adaptive immune responses help control the infection.

Sand fly vectors become infected when taking a blood meal containing infected macrophages, which are present in blood or skin. *Leishmania* live in the digestive tract of the insect as flagellated parasites (the promastigote form). The parasites divide in the midgut of the insect, except for the *Viannia* group, which multiply in the hindgut. The highly motile promastigotes migrate to the buccal cavity of the insect, which regurgitates them on biting, thereby infecting a vertebrate host. Promastigotes rapidly penetrate macrophages and transform into an aflagellated oval body measuring 2–3.5 mm across and called an amastigote (literally, 'without whip'). Amastigotes live as obligate intracellular parasites inside the macrophages where they multiply and are phagocytized by other mononuclear cells when the host cell ruptures. Depending on the tropism of the parasites – viscerotropic, dermotropic or mucotropic (Table 194-1) – the infection may disseminate to internal organs, persist as a chronic skin lesion or spread locally to mucous membranes causing one of the main clinical syndromes: VL, CL and MCL respectively. Some species have mixed tropisms and can cause different syndromes.

Prevention

Methods to prevent leishmaniasis vary with the type of cycle, vector and human behavior. As there is currently no vaccine that will prevent *Leishmania* infection, leishmaniasis control measures are directed toward vectors (e.g. indoor residual spraying of insecticides) and reservoir hosts. In anthroponotic leishmaniasis (*L. donovani* and *L. tropica*), early diagnosis and treatment of cases reduces the risk of transmission between people.

Diagnostic Microbiology

Each of the clinical syndromes poses its own diagnostic challenges. Demonstration of amastigotes in tissue samples remains the standard

TABLE 194-1	Taxonomy, Reservoirs, Distribution and Principal Tropism of Major *Leishmania* Parasites Affecting Humans				
Subgenus	**Complex**	**Main Pathogenic Species**	**Main Reservoir**	**Geographic Distribution**	**Principal Tropism**
LEISHMANIA	L. donovani	L. donovani L. infantum L. chagasi (infantum)	Humans Dogs Dogs	Indian subcontinent Mediterranean Basin and China Central and South America	Viscerotropic Viscerotropic Viscerotropic
	L. tropica	L. tropica	Humans	Towns in East Mediterranean countries, Middle East and central Asia	Dermotropic
	L. major	L. major	Birds, gerbils and other rodents	North and West Africa, the Middle East and central Asia	Dermotropic
	L. aethiopica	L. aethiopica	Hyraxes	East Africa	Dermotropic
	L. mexicana	L. mexicana L. amazonensis	Forest rodents and marsupials	North, Central and South America	Dermotropic
VIANNIA	L. braziliensis	L. braziliensis	Edentates, opossums, rodents and also dogs	South and Central America	Mucotropic
		L. peruviana	Dogs, wild marsupials and rodents	Peru	Dermotropic
	L. guyanensis	L. guyanensis L. panamensis	Sloths and arboreal ant-eaters Sloths	South America Central America and Colombia	Dermotropic Mucotropic

for leishmaniasis diagnosis. However, this method has, in general, poor sensitivity, requires invasive methods (e.g. bone marrow aspirates) and qualified personnel. Alternative methods such as molecular or serologic tests are available but their use is sometimes limited (e.g. technical requirements for PCR or lack of sensitivity for serologic tests in CL cases).

To study skin lesions in CL and MCL cases, smears can be prepared from the tissue fluid of the raised edge of an ulcer. The sample can be aspirated with a needle or scraped with a blade. Parasites can be detected by microscopy in 50% of cases of mucocutaneous leishmaniasis and 70% of cases of cutaneous leishmaniasis. In cases of visceral leishmaniasis sternal bone marrow and splenic fluid aspirates are the sample of choice for parasitologic diagnosis. Spleen aspirate has a higher sensitivity (93–99%) than bone marrow (53–86%) but splenic rupture may complicate the procedure. Other samples such as lymph node aspirates may be of value. The sensitivity can be increased by culture of the collected samples.

Molecular techniques (e.g. PCR) show higher sensitivity than standard parasitologic methods and, in some cases, species identification can be accomplished by molecular methods on tissue, smears and EDTA blood samples. However, in low- and middle-income countries these techniques remain restricted to referral hospitals and research centers.

Serologic tests such as indirect fluorescent antibody test (IFAT), direct agglutination test (DAT) or ELISA are useful in the diagnosis of VL. There are a number of commercial kits available but their implementation still requires trained personnel and laboratory facilities, restricting their use to hospitals. The sensitivity of these tests is low for HIV coinfected patients. New rapid diagnostic tests (RDT) are now available. These tests detect antibodies against recombinant kinesin proteins (e.g. rK39). RDTs are easy to perform, quick, cheap, give reproducible results, and can therefore be used for early diagnosis in peripheral health centers.[28] However the diagnostic accuracy of commercial RDTs may vary between endemic regions and they tend to have a reduced sensitivity in South America and East Africa.[29]

Clinical Manifestations

Most cases of leishmanial infection are probably subclinical. The three main clinical syndromes associated with *Leishmania* spp. infection are cutaneous, mucocutaneous and visceral leishmaniasis. There are, however, other secondary forms such as post kala-azar dermal leishmaniasis (PKDL) related to VL or diffuse cutaneous leishmaniasis (DCL) and leishmaniasis recidivans (LC) related to CL. Immunocompromised patients (e.g. leishmania–HIV coinfections) also require attention. The clinical forms are often classified by their clinical form and their location (i.e. Old or New World leishmaniasis).

VISCERAL LEISHMANIASIS

VL, also called kala-azar, is the most severe form of leishmaniasis and is fatal if not treated. VL is caused by *L. donovani* complex parasites: *L. infantum* (chagasi) in the Mediterranean basin, South America and China and *L. donovani* in the Indian subcontinent and East Africa. The incubation period is long and variable (2–8 months). The symptom triad of enlarged spleen, fever and pancytopenia is often present but other less specific symptoms (fatigue, weakness, loss of appetite and weight) are also common. In advanced disease, massive spleen enlargement, emaciation, ascites, subcutaneous edema, diarrhea, bleeding and severe anemia develop. PKDL is a secondary dermatosis that usually develops following treatment in *L. donovani* infected patients. PKDL due to *L. infantum* is rare. PKDL lesions range from hypopigmented macules to papules and nodules. Immunosuppressed patients (e.g. HIV-positive or transplant recipients) have an increased risk of developing the disease.[30] In Southern Europe, the prevalence of leishmaniasis among HIV-infected patients is 2–9%. This represents 10 000 times the rate in the general population. Some patients may develop manifestations in atypical locations or localized on bony prominences (Figure 194-4), tongue, larynx, intestinal tract and lung.

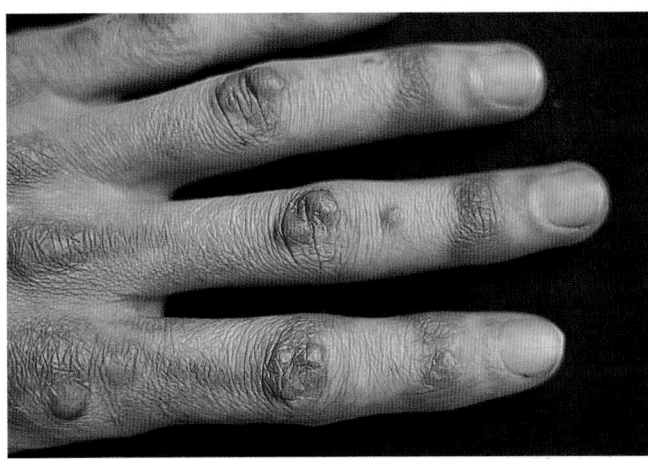

Figure 194-4   Cutaneous manifestation of kala-azar in HIV.

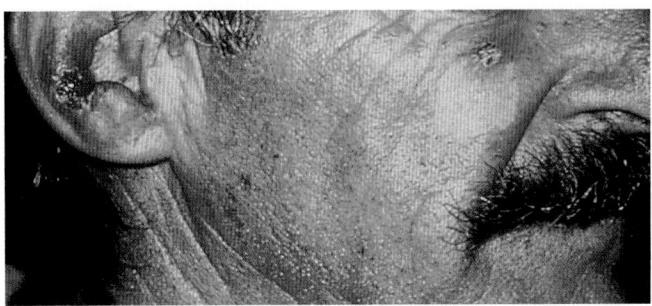

Figure 194-5   New World cutaneous leishmaniasis (Chiclero ulcer).

In immunocompromised patients relapse after treatment occurs frequently.[31]

CUTANEOUS LEISHMANIASIS

CL is the most common clinical form and it has the wider distribution. While sharing common elements, the clinical forms of CL vary by geographic area, the parasite and the type of transmission cycle. These elements are used for classification and diagnosis of CL.

Old World Cutaneous Leishmaniasis

Five species of *Leishmania* cause CL in the Old World. *L. infantum*, which also causes VL, is the most common cause of LC in Southern Europe. Lesions are usually a single node, which in some cases may ulcerate and tend to heal spontaneously. CL caused by *L. tropica* can be found from India to Morocco and it is characterized by the appearance of multiple painless ulcerative lesions that heal spontaneously leaving a scar. *L. major* CL is endemic in rural areas in North Africa, the Middle East and Central Asia. The lesion at the site of inoculation tends to evolve quickly to a large ulcerated lesion. Bacterial infection is common and the lesions tend to result in a significant scar. Finally, in East Africa *L. aethiopica* causes localized nodular lesions.

New World Cutaneous Leishmaniasis

In the USA, CL is caused by various species of *Leishmania* with variable clinical manifestations (see Table 194-1). In general, the CL caused by species of the *L. mexicana* complex develops *L. major*-like lesions that usually heal in 3–4 months. There are some characteristic clinical forms. For example, the 'Chiclero' ulcer, a destructive ulcer of the pinna of the ear or the face (Figure 194-5), is the name given in the Yucatan Peninsula (Mexico) to the lesions caused by *L. mexicana* when seated in the ear. Lesions associated with the subgenus *Viannia* may take longer to heal (6 months). The 'Uta', the typical CL form of the Andean valleys, is caused by *L. peruviana* and affects mainly children. The skin ulcer heals in 3–6 months leaving a disfiguring scar, usually on the face.

MUCOCUTANEOUS LEISHMANIASIS

Mucocutaneous leishmaniasis is caused by *L. braziliensis* and *L. guyanensis* in the Americas and is characterized by chronic and very destructive lesions in mouth and nose. MCL is a markedly disfiguring, life-threatening disease appearing during the first 10 years after resolution of cutaneous disease. It consists of a pseudotumoral destructive lesion. It usually starts in the nasal mucosa and spreads to the oropharyngeal mucosa, larynx and skin of the lips and nose. Death may be due to pneumonia, laryngeal obstruction, secondary sepsis or starvation. Spontaneous cure is rare and response to therapy is poor.

Management

Leishmaniasis treatment depends upon the clinical syndrome, the etiologic agent and the severity of the disease. Pentavalent antimonials (Sbv) have been the main antileishmanial drug since the 1920s. They still remain the first line of treatment for several forms of leishmaniasis but new drugs such as miltefosine, paromomycin or amphotericin B (or its lipid forms) are now available. The main antileishmanial treatments for the different clinical forms are summarized below.[32]

For VL caused by *L. donovani* in the Indian subcontinent, liposomal amphotericin B (3–5 mg/kg per day over 3–5 days up to a total dose of 15 mg/kg or 10 mg/kg as a single dose) is the preferred therapeutic option but is expensive. Miltefosine, the first antileishmanial oral drug, can also be used as monotherapy (2.5 mg/kg per day for 28 days) or in combination with liposomal amphotericin B or paromomycin. In East Africa pentavalent antimonials remain effective as monotherapy (20 mg Sbv/kg per day for 30 days) or combined with paromomycin. In the Mediterranean basin and South America where VL is caused by *L. infantum*, liposomal amphotericin B (3–5 mg/kg per day over a 3–6 days period) and pentavalent antimonials (20 mg Sbv/kg per day for 28 days) are used. A short course liposomal amphotericin B regimen (10 mg/kg per day for 2 days) is the recommended treatment for pediatric VL in France.[33] Liposomal amphotericin B (3–5 mg/kg daily or intermittently for 10 doses up to a total of 40 mg/kg) is recommended for HIV coinfected patients.

As cutaneous leishmaniasis is not a life-threatening condition and some cutaneous sores may resolve spontaneously (self-cure rate >50% at 6 months in *L. major*), in most instances local treatment is preferred. The local treatment options are: (1) intralesional pentavalent antimonials (0.5–5 ml injected into the base and margins of the lesion until healing); (2) cryotherapy; (3) thermotherapy; and (4) paromomycin ointment.[34] Combining treatment options (e.g. cryotherapy and intralesional injections of antimony) can be more effective than each technique alone. Local treatment should be proposed if the following criteria are fulfilled: *L. major* CL, fewer than four lesions, lesions <5 cm in diameter, no risk of disfiguring or disabling lesions and immunocompetent. Systemic treatments, mainly antimonials (20 mg/kg Sbv per day intramuscularly or intravenously for 10–20 days) are used in complicated Old World CL and in most New World CL. Two oral treatments – ketoconazole (600 mg daily for 28 days) and miltefosine (2.5 mg/kg per day for 28 days) – are an alternative systemic treatment for CL caused by *L. mexicana*.

MCL cases always require systemic treatments: pentavalent antimonials (20 mg/kg per day for 30 days) alone or in combination with pentoxifylline (400 mg/8h for 30 days) are used. Miltefosine (2.5–3.3 mg/kg per day for 28 days) have shown promising results for *L. braziliensis* MCL in Bolivia.

Trypanosomiasis

Trypanosomes produce two clinically and epidemiologically different diseases that are presented separately:

- American trypanosomiasis or Chagas disease, due to *Trypanosoma cruzi* infection
- African trypanosomiasis or sleeping sickness (*Trypanosoma brucei gambiense* and *Trypanosoma brucei rhodesiense*).

When a human host is infected, the organisms multiply in the inoculation area, then pass into the blood; in a third phase they localize in some internal organs, causing chronic disease.

Trypanosomes pass through the morphologic stages of amastigote and trypomastigote. The differences between the main species that can be found in humans are summarized in Table 194-2.

Chagas Disease (American Trypanosomiasis)

Chagas disease is a zoonosis that has been traditionally endemic in Latin America, caused by *T. cruzi*. It has been defined as a neglected disease by the World Health Organization (WHO), owing to the lack of knowledge of some aspects of the disease (pathogenesis, the lack of new and safe drugs, the lack of tools to assess early response to treatment, the lack of markers of the progression of the disease).

Nature

Chagas disease is caused by the hemoflagellate protozoan of *T. cruzi* species belonging to class Kinetoplastida, order Trypanosomatidae and *Trypanosoma* genus. *T. cruzi* has been classified into a series of strains by discrete typing units (DTUs). An expert committee established a new nomenclature, defining six strains of *T. cruzi* (TcI to TC VI).[35] The variety of *T. cruzi* strains has been related to the different clinical manifestations and natural history that shows the infection and/or disease in different geographical regions (see Chapter 124).

Epidemiology

Chagas disease is endemic in 21 Latin American countries. Eight to ten million people are infected by *T. cruzi* and 12 500 deaths a year are

TABLE 194-2	Taxonomy and Differences in Distribution and Principal Clinical Features of *Trypanosoma* Species Affecting Humans						
Human Pathogenic Species	Human Pathogenic Subspecies	Geographic Distribution	Transmission Routes	Clinical Disease	Organ Involvement	Main Course of the Disease
T. cruzi	–	America (mainly Central and South) Europe Australia Asia (sporadic cases)	Vectorial: Reduviidae (kissing bugs) Vertical Oral Transfusion Transplantation	Chagas disease	Heart Gastrointestinal (colon and esophagus) Nervous system (central and peripheric)	Chronic
T. brucei	*T. brucei gambiense*	West Africa	Vectorial: *Glossina* (tsetse flies)	Sleeping sickness	Nervous system (central)	Chronic
	T. brucei rhodesiense	East Africa	Vectorial	Sleeping sickness	Nervous system (central)	Acute

caused by this disease. The global economic burden of Chagas disease is calculated to be $7.19 billion per year, and it is estimated to be responsible for the loss of 806 170 disability-adjusted life years (DALYs) annually.[36]

In endemic areas, the main transmission route is due to hemipterous insects of the Reduviidae family (kissing bugs). Among them, five have major epidemiologic importance (*Triatoma infestans*, *Rhodnius prolixus*, *Triatoma dimidiata*, *Panstrongylus megistus* and *Triatoma brasiliensis*). Other transmission routes are vertical transmission (which occurs in approximately in 4–7% of children of infected mothers), blood transfusion, organ transplant and oral transmission.[37]

The epidemiology of Chagas disease has changed, due mainly to migration flows (rural to urban areas and endemic to non-endemic countries), programs of vector control and blood bank and maternity screening. Regarding non-endemic countries, one study in Europe estimated between 68 000 and 123 000 expected infections with *T. cruzi*, compared with 4,290 cases reported up to 2009.[38] In the USA, in 2011 there were about 300 000 people reported infected with *T. cruzi*.[39]

Pathogenicity

T. cruzi has a complex life cycle with different developmental stages in mammalian host and insect vectors. Triatomine species take circulating trypomastigotes from infected blood of mammals and humans, but they don't have the capability to develop the disease. Inside the vectors, trypomastigotes transform into flagellate epimastigotes with the capability of multiplying extracellularly, and migrating to hindgut, turning into metacyclic trypomastigotes. These circulating metacyclic trypomastigotes with infective capability can be transmitted to humans and other mammals: they could be injected by vector feces, and if they reach a tissue to enter through (broken skin, mucous, gastric surface), they invade local cells, and in some cases turn into amastigote forms that multiply intracellularly, breaking the host cell and spreading systemically as trypomastigotes via the hematogenous route. The passage of the parasite by peripheral blood is called parasitemia, which allows the parasite to reach distant organs and tissues, causing organ damage.

Different forms of the parasite in the host stimulate different immune response mechanisms, which can imply both humoral and cellular responses. The efficacy of the immune response depends on the parasite and the phase of the infection.

The way the parasite produces lesions in the host follows the sequence: cell lysis, inflammatory response, fibrosis. Fibrosis is a poorly vascularized neoformation, that does not return to normal tissue. This process occurs mainly in the heart and the digestive tract. In the two initial phases, macrophages, lymphocytes and polymorphonuclear cells are predominant, owing to the release of a large number of pro-inflammatory molecules, mainly in the acute phase. Afterwards, cellular lesions primarily affect muscle cells (myocytolysis) and nerve cells (autonomic neuronal denervation), being the result of direct destruction caused by intracellular parasitism and of necrosis due to the inflammation triggered by parasites.[40] Fibrosis gradually replaces normal tissue resulting in chronic loss of organ function.

Prevention

In endemic countries, continuous insecticide application together with hygiene education with community participation have been introduced in order to better control vector-borne reinfestation and transmission, including measures to prevent oral transmission. Strategies to screen blood donors and control vertical transmission are the second step in the prevention of new cases.

In non endemic countries, the screening of pregnant women and early treatment in newborns has been shown to be highly efficient. Screening of blood donors at risk of infection is carried out only in some European countries and in the USA. In the context of transplantation, preventing the transmission of the infection, and reactivations, should be reinforced.

Diagnostic Microbiology

The confirmatory microbiologic diagnosis of Chagas disease is based on two criteria:[41]
- History compatible with the epidemiology of the disease, i.e. possibility of having acquired the infection.
- Laboratory diagnosis, when people potentially infected by *T. cruzi* have a positive result in parasitology or at least two positive results with two serologic techniques based on different antigens.

With regard to the laboratory diagnosis of *T. cruzi* infection, there are two well-defined phases that should be managed in different ways.

ACUTE STAGE CHAGAS DISEASE

At this stage the parasite is easy to find in peripheral blood. The most used direct method is the fresh blood smear, but the main concentration methods are microhematocrit and Strout.

Fresh blood smear: an amount of around 10 μL of peripheral blood is deposited on a smear and covered by a cover slip. The parasite can be observed by the direct microscope technique.

Concentration methods: to perform a Strout, 3–5 mL of peripheral blood is collected and left to clot for 15–60 minutes, and after spinning, the supernatant is centrifuged. A clear supernatant for serology is obtained, and the remaining is taken and applied to a glass slide covered by a covering slip, and observed under the microscope in order to find the parasites. The microhematocrit technique is very useful to detect *T. cruzi* congenital transmission (high sensitivity with a small amount of blood [100 μL]). The sample is collected in four heparinized capillaries, which are spun down. The interface between sera and cells, where leukocytes and *T. cruzi* are, is observed on the microscope (it is important to discriminate platelets of *T. cruzi*). In case of suspicion of congenital *T. cruzi* infection, infants should be tested at 6–9 months to detect IgG by serology tests (they will have already lost maternal antibodies).

T cruzi DNA amplification techniques by PCR are currently being validated for its use in both the acute and chronic stage of the disease.

CHRONIC STAGE CHAGAS DISEASE

After the parasites multiply during the first 2 months in the host, antibody response starts and the number of circulating parasites decreases. The diagnosis in the chronic stage of the disease is based on serologic techniques, detecting IgG antibodies against *T. cruzi*.

Among serologic methods, ELISA has higher sensitivity but in some cases limited specificity.[42] It is a technique in which there is an objective reading of the results (spectrophotometer) and the possibility of automated handling of hundreds of samples at a time. ELISA cutoff should be calculated by the technical instructions of each kit, but a curve with negative, low-positive and high-positive controls is useful for the range of responses. Samples should be considered positive when optical densities are at least 10% higher than the cutoff.

Clinical Manifestations

The infection evolves through three different clinical stages: acute infection, asymptomatic period and chronic disease.

The acute phase of *T. cruzi* infection is asymptomatic or presents no specific symptoms due to the low parasite burden at the beginning of the infection. When symptoms appear, moderate but prolonged fever is the most frequent symptom (8–10 days after the parasite invasion). General symptoms like malaise, asthenia, anorexia and headache could be present. It is possible to observe painless and smooth liver and spleen enlargement, and/or lymph node involvement, and localized or generalized edema. A non-pruriginous, painless maculonodular erythematous lesion called 'chagoma' could be observed at the entry site of the parasite through the skin, and in some cases nearby lymph nodes could be enlarged, sometimes ulcerated, but this is an uncommon finding.[43] A pathognomonic but not frequent sign of acute Chagas disease can also be observed: the Romaña's sign (unilateral palpebral edema, conjunctivitis and ipsilateral regional

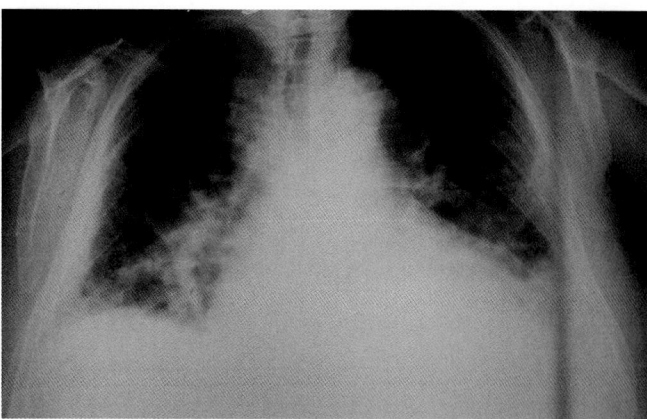

Figure 194-6 Chest radiograph of a patient with dilated cardiomyopathy in CCC patient. *(Courtesy of Dr Jareth Sánchez, Manuel Ascencio Villarroel Hospital, Cochabamba, Bolivia.)*

lymphadenopathy, usually in the preauricular region). Meningoencephalitis and/or myocarditis could be severe clinical manifestations of the acute stage of the disease. Both clinical pictures are also described in reactivations of the chronic disease, in the presence of immunosuppression.[44]

The chronic stage of Chagas disease presents a wide range of manifestations: from the absence of signs and symptoms (70% of people with *T. cruzi* infection, called indeterminate or asymptomatic stage) to sudden death in some cases (the cause of death in two out of three patients with chronic chagasic cardiomyopathy). It is estimated that 1–2% per year of *T. cruzi*-infected people in the indeterminate stage of the disease start with organ involvement.[37]

Chagas organ involvement (symptomatic chronic stage) is mainly of the heart, digestive tract, a combination of both (cardiodigestive form) and neurologic involvement.

Chagasic cardiomyopathy (CCC) is the most severe and frequent manifestation of the chronic stage of the disease (20–30% of *T. cruzi*-infected individuals). In advanced stages, it is irreversible. Nonspecific heart alterations typical of CCC are abnormalities of the conduction system (right bundle branch block or any of these conditions with epidemiologic data strongly suggestive of *T. cruzi* infection), apical aneurysms, cardiac failure, thromboembolism (mainly in brain, but also limbs and lung), and sudden death. Left heart failure can be present even in early stages of heart involvement, but the congestive failure is a late manifestation. Heart failure is associated with higher mortality in Chagas disease patients.[44] For the diagnosis of CCC, a 12-lead electrocardiogram, thoracic radiograph and echocardiography are recommended (Figure 194-6).

The digestive form of Chagas disease is diagnosed in 10–20% of patients with *T. cruzi* infection. Digestive symptoms related to Chagas disease are unspecific, but some of them are more frequent in people with *T. cruzi* infection. Esophagus and colon are the most commonly affected segments, but any of the organs of the digestive tract may be affected. Esophagus involvement usually produces dysphagia, but other symptoms could be present, such as odynophagia, epigastric pain, regurgitation, ptyalism, aerophagia, nocturnal cough, sialorrhoea and malnutrition in severe cases.

Regarding colonic involvement, the sigmoid segment is the most often affected, followed by rectum or descending colon, and the main symptom associated with colon involvement is chronic constipation, but other symptoms, like changes in bowel habit, straining at stool and incomplete evacuation sensation, could be present.

Symptoms such as dyspepsia, pyrosis, bloating and satiety sensation could be present if there are gastric and/or duodenal alterations.[45]

Barium swallow and barium enema are indicated to rule out gastrointestinal involvement in chronic Chagas disease (Figure 194-7).

Up to 10% of people with *T. cruzi* infection may present with neurologic involvement, but it is not only due to embolism sec-

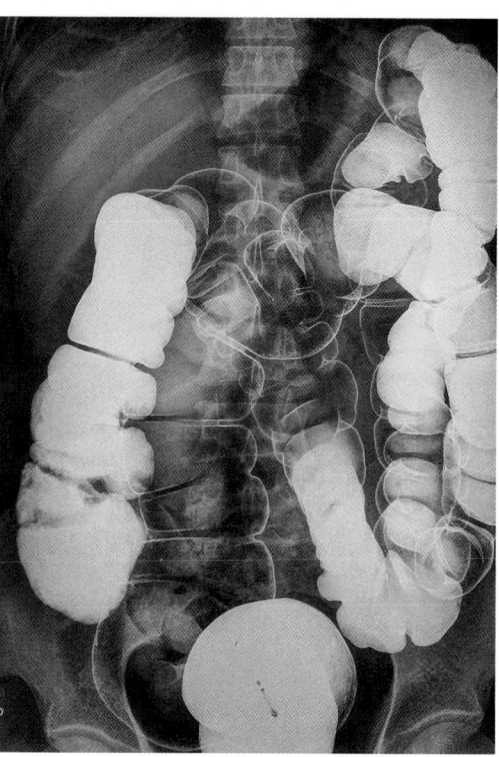

Figure 194-7 Megacolon in a patient with chronic Chagas disease. *(Courtesy of Dr Jareth Sánchez, Manuel Ascencio Villarroel Hospital, Cochabamba, Bolivia.)*

ondary to cardiac involvement. Infected individuals without cardiomyopathy can also present with stroke and peripheral neurologic involvement.[46]

In immunosuppressed patients (HIV infection, post transplantation, drugs, systemic diseases) with *T. cruzi* infection a reactivation in the chronic stage of the disease can appear, which is clinically similar to the acute stage of the disease. The management of these patients is an urgent matter.

Management

The treatment of Chagas disease should be focused on two aspects:
- The antiparasitic treatment in order to eradicate the parasite.
- The management of organ involvement due to the disease, following international recommendations similar to other etiologies.

Antitrypanosomal treatment is recommended where *T. cruzi* infection is diagnosed in the absence of contraindications (pregnancy, hepatic and or renal failure, breast-feeding and advanced cardiological and/or digestive involvement). It is strongly recommended in the acute stage of the disease and in case of reactivations in immunosuppressed patients, as well as in children up to 18 years old with chronic infection (with special attention to children <1 year old), and immunosuppressed patients without reactivations. It should be offered to adults in the chronic stage of the disease.[47]

Treatment regimens for *T. cruzi* infection are:
- Benznidazole (BZD): 10 mg/kg/day q12h for 60 days in children, and 5–7 mg/kg/day for adults × 60 days.
- Nifurtimox (NFX): 15–20 mg/kg/day q8h for 60–90 days for children, and 8–10 mg/kg/day in adults for 90–120 days.
- Treatment with these drugs provides cure rates of almost 100% in children under 12 months, around 60% in people with chronic recent infection and the efficacy in later chronic stages of the disease is unclear.[37] Even if BZD and NFX have shown high efficacy in some stages of the disease, they have a poor tolerance profile, and currently some clinical trials are underway to test new drugs for treatment of Chagas disease.

African Trypanosomiasis

There are two forms of human African trypanosomiasis (HAT), which are caused by:

- *Trypanosoma brucei gambiense*: the most common, located in West Africa and usually produces chronic infections
- *Trypanosoma brucei rhodesiense*: less frequent, present in East Africa and tends to produce a more acute disease.

In the initial stage the parasite is spread in hemolymphatic organs, whereas in the late stage the central nervous system (CNS) is affected by meningoencephalitis. One of its most striking symptoms is sleep abnormalities and the dysregulation of the circadian rhythm of the sleep/wake cycle, after which the disease was named 'sleeping sickness'.

Nature

African trypanosomiasis is caused by the hemoflagellate protozoan of the *T. brucei* species of class Kinetoplastida, order Trypanosomatidae and genus *Trypanosoma*; the subspecies *T.b. gambiense* and *T.b. rhodesiense* are pathogens for humans (see Chapter 110).

Epidemiology

The vector of *T. brucei* subspecies is a fly of the genus *Glossina* (tsetse fly), which is geographically confined to sub-Saharan Africa. Up to 70% of cases occur in the Democratic Republic of the Congo.[48] Transmission of the disease is usually related to outdoor activities such as agriculture, hunting, fishing or clothes-washing in rivers.[49]

Disease surveillance and control programs were successfully implemented and the prevalence and incidence of the disease dropped dramatically. All the measures taken were reinforced from the last decade of the 20th century.[48] Currently more than 250 active foci of infection are known and it is considered that there are 21 million people living in areas at moderate or high risk of infection.[50] The current estimation is that there are 20 000 cases and the population at risk is around 70 million people, being one of the leading causes of death in some areas.[48]

T. b. gambiense is endemic in West Africa and it is the main form of HAT (up to 97% of cases).[51] Humans are considered to be the main reservoir. Transmission usually occurs in the shaded riverine areas where *Glossina palpalis* and *Glossina tachinoides* live.

T. b. rhodesiense is responsible for less than 3% of all HAT cases, even though it is the main HAT form in travelers, usually related to safaris in East Africa.[51] It is transmitted by *Glossina morsitans*. This fly lives in the dry savannas of East Africa, feeding chiefly on the wild ungulates, which represent the main reservoir.

Pathogenicity

The vector fly is infected when taking a blood meal containing trypanosomes. The ingested parasites transform and multiply in the insect midgut and migrate to the salivary glands from where new hosts are infected by biting. It takes about 2–3 weeks to complete the cycle in the fly. Once infected, the fly remains infective throughout its lifetime (3 months).[49] In the human host the parasite multiplies asexually in the interstitial space and spreads through the lymphatic vessels to the lymph nodes and blood (Figure 194-8). In the late stage of the disease the parasite invades the CNS. The transition to the late stage can last from months to years in the *T. b. gambiense* infection, whereas in the infection by *T. b. rhodesiense* this progression takes only a few weeks or months.

Sequencing of the trypanosome genome has shown that 10% of the 9000 genes encode variant surface glycoproteins,[51] that enables it to elude the host immune response. Large amounts of IgM are produced in the serum and cerebrospinal fluid (CSF) and characteristic plasmacytic morular cells can be seen in tissues, blood, bone marrow and CSF, known as Mott cells. Autoimmune phenomena, circulating immune

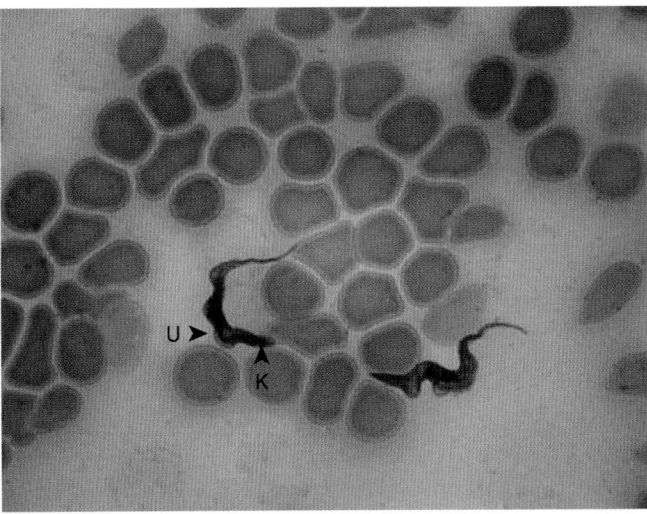

Figure 194-8 *Trypanosoma brucei* in a Giemsa-stained blood smear. Note the central nucleus on an undulating (U) membrane and a clump of mitochondrial DNA called a kinetoplast (K).

complex deposition and increased vessel permeability play an important role in pathogenesis.

Prevention

Prevention measures and methods are based in two complementary strategies: decrease of the reservoir of infection and vector control. Vector control strategies have been used successfully in the past: massive clearance of *Glossina* spp. habitats, insecticide spraying, destruction of wild game, periodic mass treatment or relocation of entire populations, and recently the use of *Glossina* spp.-attracting traps. Active surveillance is recommended periodically in areas of *T. b. gambiense* and during epidemics in *T. b. rhodesiense* areas. Regarding reservoir control, active surveillance programs in chronic asymptomatic/paucisymptomatic humans as the main *T.b. gambiense* reservoir should be useful. *T.b. rhodesiense* reservoir control is nearly impossible since infection is maintained by the wild animal reservoir.

There is no vaccine or chemoprophylaxis available, so travelers visiting should be advised of the types of activity that may increase the risk of acquiring HAT. Mosquito repellents and avoiding wearing dark clothes may be useful.

Diagnostic Microbiology

The correct assessment of the patient is based on the infection diagnosis and the determination of the disease stage.

Diagnosis can be made by parasitologic, serologic or molecular methods. The definitive diagnosis method is parasitologic which essentially depends upon the careful repeated microscopic examination of blood, CSF, lymph node or bone marrow samples. The probability of parasite detection is higher in the *T.b. rhodesiense* form and in the acute phase of infection. Lately new concentration methods such as the mAETC (miniature Anion-Exchange Centrifugation Technique) have been developed to increase sensitivity.[52]

Serologic screening can be carried out with the card agglutination test (CATT) for *T.b. gambiense* which has high negative predictive value, but confirmatory tests are needed,[51] and it is not useful in *T.b. rhodesiense* cases or in travellers.

PCR testing is available in some reference laboratories, which is helpful for diagnosis but not for follow-up.

The second step in diagnosis is the accurate staging of early and late HAT stage. Late-stage treatment can be very toxic so correct staging is critical. The established diagnosis method is the analysis of the CSF by lumbar puncture. The presence of the trypanosoma parasite or/and a white blood cell count above 5 cells per µL in CSF are the diagnosis criteria for late-stage based on WHO criteria.[51] However, it is under discussion whether the white blood cell criterion should be redefined to 10 or 20 white blood cells.[53] Increased intrathecal synthesis of IgM is a useful and sensitive marker of CNS involvement.

Clinical Manifestations

In African trypanosomiasis, the disease develops in two stages:

- hemolymphatic stage, which spares the nervous system
- meningoencephalic stage, defined by CNS involvement.

The disease produced by *T. b. gambiense* usually develops chronically in months or years whereas in *T. b. rhodesiense* infection the disease tends to be more acute, weeks to months, without a clear distinction between stages.

An infective bite by a *Glossina* spp. fly may produce an inoculation chancre, rarely in *T.b. gambiense* cases and in about 20% in *T.b. rhodesiense* infections.[49,51] Within days or weeks, the parasite disseminates to the blood and lymph systems. In the *gambiense* form of the disease, the patient may remain asymptomatic for years whereas in the *rhodesiense* infection this stage lasts from a few weeks to months. In the hemolymphatic stage, the symptoms may be few and nonspecific: intermittent fever, headache, malaise, weight loss, facial edema, arthralgia, diarrhea and pruritus. In *T.b. gambiense* infection enlarged posterior auricular lymph nodes may be present (Winterbottom's sign).

On physical examination there may be erythematous circinate papules on the trunk, disproportionate pain to soft tissue pressure (Kerandel's sign) and discrete enlargement of lymph nodes, liver and spleen. Pancarditis is common in the more acute forms, when it constitutes a major cause of death. Some degree of anemia, thrombocytopenia, leukocytosis, hypogonadism, renal disease and thymus atrophy may be seen. Characteristically, cardiac and hormonal involvement is more frequent and severe in *T.b. rhodesiense* infection.

The CNS manifestation that gave the disease its name is the disappearance of the circadian distribution of sleep and wakefulness, which are therefore fragmented throughout the day and night. Other CNS manifestations include altered reflexes, paresthesia, pareses, tremor, dyskinesia, choreoathetosis, epilepsy, slurred speech, mood changes, lethargy, delirium and psychosis. Psychiatric manifestations are common and it can be the leading and main symptom.[51] Without treatment, nearly all patients will develop neural involvement and die.

Management

The choice of antiparasitic drug will depend upon the HAT form and whether the CNS is infected or not. Pentamidine in *T.b. gambiense* or suramin in *T.b. rhodesiense* can be used when the CNS is spared from infection. Pentamidine dosage is 4 mg/kg/day, intramuscular or intravenous, for 7 days.[52] *T. b. rhodesiense* and some strains of *T. b.*

gambiense do not respond to pentamidine. Suramin dosage is 20 mg/kg/day (maximum 1500 mg), one intravenous injection every 5 days for 25 days (five total doses).

Melarsoprol and eflornithine are effective for both hemolymphatic and neural stages but because of their toxicity or administration requirements they are mostly used in the late-stage of the disease, where the CNS is involved.

Both drugs can be used in *T.b. gambiense* infection, but only melarsoprol is useful in *T.b. rhodesiense* infection because it is innately resistant to eflornithine.

Melarsoprol, a trivalent arsenical derivative, has been the treatment of choice for patients who have had CNS involvement for five decades. Arsenic-related encephalopathy syndrome occurs in 5–8% of cases and the mortality rate of this complication is up to 50%.[52,54] The treatment of this adverse effect is corticoids (dexamethasone 0.5–0.6 mg/kg/day, q12h or q8h), symptomatic treatment and supportive care. Melarsoprol dosage is 2.2 mg/kg/day intravenous injection for 10 days. Relapse after treatment occurs in 6% of cases.[54]

Eflornithine has been available since 2001 and being safer than melarsoprol it is preferred in the treatment of the late stage of *T.b. gambiense* infection. When eflornithine is administrated alone, its dosage is 100 mg, one intravenous injection q6h for 14 days.[52] Being much less toxic, intravenous eflornithine (400 mg/kg/day q12h for 7 days) plus nifurtimox (15 mg/kg/day given orally q8h for 10 days) appears to be a promising first-line therapy for second-stage sleeping sickness.[55,56]

General supportive treatment, anticonvulsant preventive therapy and early recognition and treatment of associated parasitic and bacterial infections are essential.

Infection by Other *Trypanosoma* Species

Trypanosoma rangeli is an American parasite transmitted by triatomids. In some areas of Central America human parasitization by *T. rangeli* is more frequent than that by *T. cruzi*. Although regarded as nonpathogenic to humans, it is medically important as a source of misdiagnosis of Chagas disease.

Animal pathogenic trypanosomes are lysed by apolipoprotein L-I, a component of human high-density lipoprotein (HDL). Patients with very low levels of high-density lipoproteins (such as those with Tangier's disease) may be susceptible to those trypanosomes. Two human cases on infection by *T. evansi* in India and *T. lewisi* from Thailand have been recently reported. Trypanosoma from rodents as potential source of infection in human-shaped landscapes of South East Asia.[57]

References available online at expertconsult.com.

KEY REFERENCES

Alvar J., Velez I.D., Bern C., et al.: Leishmaniasis worldwide and global estimates of its incidence. *PLoS ONE* 2012; 7(5):e35671.

Bern C., Montgomery S.P., Herwaldt B.L., et al.: Evaluation and treatment of Chagas disease in the United States: a systematic review. *JAMA* 2007; 298(18):2171-2181.

Buffet P.A., Rosenthal E., Gangneux J.P., et al.: Traitement des leishmanioses en France: proposition d'un référentiel consensuel. *Presse Méd* 2011; 40:173-184.

Kennedy P.G.: Clinical features, diagnosis, and treatment of human African trypanosomiasis (sleeping sickness). *Lancet Neurol* 2013; 12(2):186-194.

Miller C.M., Boulter N.R., Ikin R.J., et al.: The immunobiology of the innate response to *Toxoplasma gondii*. *Int J Parasitol* 2009; 39(1):23-39.

Montoya J.G., Liesenfeld O.: Toxoplasmosis. *Lancet* 2004; 363(9425):1965-1976.

Mosqueda J., Olvera-Ramirez A., Aguilar-Tipacamu G., et al.: Current advances in detection and treatment of babesiosis. *Curr Med Chem* 2012; 19(10):1504-1518.

Rassi A. Jr, Rassi A., Marin-Neto J.A.: Chagas disease. *Lancet* 2010; 375(9723):1388-1402.

Thiebaut R., Leproust S., Chene G., et al.: Effectiveness of prenatal treatment for congenital toxoplasmosis: a meta-analysis of individual patients' data. *Lancet* 2007; 369(9556):115-122.

Wallon M., Peyron F., Cornu C., et al.: Congenital toxoplasma infection: monthly prenatal screening decreases transmission rate and improves clinical outcome at age 3 years. *Clin Infect Dis* 2013; 56(9):1223-1231.

195

Helminths

H.D. ALAN LINDQUIST | JOHN H. CROSS[†]

Helminths are the most common parasites infecting humans. The world's population numbers approximately 7 billion, with probably a similar number of human helminth infections. Helminths are transmitted to humans through food, water and soil, arthropod and molluscan vectors. Helminths can infect every organ and organ system. Prevalent in the intestines, they are found in the liver, lungs, blood and occasionally the brain and other organs. This chapter describes some human parasitic worms, their biology, epidemiology, pathogenicity, clinical aspects of helminth infection, diagnosis and prevention.

Nature

The word helminth derives from a Greek word meaning worm. Helminths include both free living and parasitic worms. Most parasitic worms are in two phyla, the Nematoda or roundworms, and Platyhelminthes or flatworms. The main parasitic flatworms are Trematoda or flukes, and Cestoda or tapeworms (Table 195-1).

The helminths have an outer covering called a cuticle or tegument. This tegument may be tough or delicate, and protects the worm from such things as digestion in the host intestinal tract. This structure may possess spines, hooks, cutting plates or stylets, used for attachment or to aid in penetration. Some species have acetabula or suckers for attachment and some have lytic glands near the mouth that secrete enzymes to digest host tissue for food or to aid in migration.

Helminths have various digestive systems, excretory secretory systems and generally have massive reproductive systems. Most trematodes are hermaphroditic, with one organism having both male and female reproductive organs. Schistosomes are trematodes with separate sexes. In tapeworms, each segment has both male and female sex organs, whereas nematodes have separate sexes. Some worms produce larvae, most produce eggs that pass out of the host in the excrement,

or occasionally urine. Some worms that inhabit the circulatory system produce larvae that are ingested by blood-sucking arthropods and transmitted to other hosts via the bite from an infected vector. The life cycles of the helminths vary from direct transmission of eggs passed in the feces and eaten by a host, to complex life cycles involving one or more intermediate hosts (see Figures 195-1 to 195-5).

Epidemiology

Helminth infections are the most common parasitic infections in humans. The highest prevalence occurs in tropical countries with poor or inadequate food supplies, where insects, molluscs and other invertebrate vectors abound, and unsanitary conditions permit contamination of food with parasite eggs.

NEMATODES

Intestinal Nematodes

Perhaps 1.2 billion people are infected with *Ascaris lumbricoides*. Worldwide, about 740 million people are infected with the hookworms *Necator americanus, Ancylostoma duodenale* or both. The former has a worldwide distribution, the latter is only found in parts of Africa, China, India and Japan. About 795 million people are infected with *Trichuris trichiura*, and all age groups may be infected. These 2.7 billion infections do not represent the number of individuals, as many people have more than one type of nematode. These four parasites are often grouped as 'soil transmitted helminths' (STH) or nematodes. Infection is acquired by consumption or by exposure to contaminated soils. The differences in distributions of these worms is based on their biology, life cycle and the interaction between the parasite and the local environment and population. Significant factors include climate, soil type, customs and sanitation. For instance, in school-age children in Honduras, *A. lumbricoides* was found in 30%, hookworms in 16% and *T. trichuria* in 67%,[1] whereas a tribal population of Tamil Nadu, India had *A. lumbricoides* in 1.5% of the population, hookworm in 38% and no *T. trichuria* infections.[2]

Strongyloides stercoralis, like other soil transmitted helminths, is endemic in areas with high humidity, warm temperatures and poor sanitation. Prevalence of this parasite varies from 10% to 40% and up to 60% in areas of Africa, South America and Asia.[3]

Enterobius vermicularis, or pinworm, is a common nematode in the temperate regions with an estimated 200 million infections worldwide with a prevalence of 38% in one study of school children aged 5–7 years.[4] Most individuals acquire this parasite in childhood, but it is not uncommon in adults in families with infected children. It is common in the USA. A high prevalence of pinworms is reported in men who have sex with men.

Tissue Nematodes

Larva migrans is caused primarily by nematode parasites of lower animals. Larvae of dog hookworms, such as *Ancylostoma braziliensis* and *A. caninum*, penetrate human skin, migrating through the skin and causing creeping eruption or cutaneous larva migrans. This occurs worldwide, but mostly in warm, moist climates. *Ancylostoma caninum* can cause enteritis in humans, and is perhaps most common in Australia. The larvae of dog and cat *Toxocara* spp. ascarids cause visceral larva migrans in children, when embryonated eggs are ingested. England and France have high seroprevalence rates for *Toxocara* spp. antibodies. The prevalence of cutaneous larva migrans certainly

TABLE 195-1	The Major Parasitic Worms		
Nematodes (Roundworms)	**Intestinal**		
	Ascaris lumbricoides	Necator americanus	Trichuris trichiura
	Enterobius vermicularis	Strongyloides stercoralis	Capillaria philippinensis
	Ancylostoma duodenale	Trichostrongylus spp.	
	Tissue		
	Trichinella spiralis	Angiostrongylus cantonensis	Phocanema spp. (larvae from saltwater fish)
	Visceral larva migrans (Toxocara canis or Toxocara cati)	Angiostrongylus costaricensis	Contracaecum spp. (larvae from saltwater fish)
	Ocular larva migrans (Toxocara canis or Toxocara cati)	Gnathostoma spinigerum	Capillaria hepatica
	Cutaneous larva migrans (Ancylostoma braziliensis or Ancylostoma caninum)	Anisakis spp. (larvae from saltwater fish)	Thelazia spp.
	Dracunculus medinensis		
	Neural larva migrans (Baylisascaris procyonis)		
	Blood and tissues (filarial worms)		
	Wuchereria bancrofti	Onchocerca volvulus	Dirofilaria immitis (usually lung lesion; in dogs, heartworm)
	Brugia malayi	Mansonella ozzardi	
	Brugia timori	Mansonella streptocerca	Dirofilaria spp. (may be found in subcutaneous nodules)
	Loa loa	Mansonella perstans	
Platyhelminthes (Flatworms) Cestodes (Tapeworms)	**Intestinal**		
	Diphyllobothrium latum	Hymenolepis nana	Taenia solium
	Dipylidium caninum	Hymenolepis diminuta	Taenia saginata
	Tissue (larval forms)		
	Taenia solium	Echinococcus multilocularis	Spirometra mansonoides
	Echinococcus granulosus	Multiceps multiceps	Diphyllobothrium spp.
		Taenia multiceps	
Trematodes (Flukes)	**Intestinal**		
	Fasciolopsis buski	Heterophyes heterophyes	
	Echinostoma ilocanum	Metagonimus yokogawai	
	Liver/lung		
	Clonorchis (opisthorchis) sinensis	Paragonimus westermani	Paragonimus skrjabini
	Opisthorchis viverrini	Paragonimus mexicanus	Paragonimus spp.
	Fasciola hepatica	Paragonimus heterotremus	
	Blood		
	Schistosoma mansoni	Schistosoma japonicum	Schistosoma mekongi
	Schistosoma haematobium	Schistosoma intercalatum	

Adapted from Garcia L.S.: Classification of human parasites. Clin Infect Dis 1997;25:21–3

depends on factors including the presence of infected dogs or cats and contact with soil. In a study of participants in a religious celebration involving rolling the body in damp earth or sand, 58.2% showed signs of infection.[5] *Baylisascaris procyonis*, a roundworm of raccoons, can also be ingested and cause neural larva migrans resulting in severe encephalitis, usually in children, and ocular infections in adults.

The only species of *Trichinella* that is important to human health is *T. spiralis*. This species has a worldwide distribution in temperate regions, whereas other species are reported from animals in Africa (*T. nelson*), Arctic (*T. native*), Palearctic and Nearctic regions (*T. psuedospiralis, T. britovi, T. murrelli*), and the Australian region (*T. papuae*). Transmission occurs among animals by the ingestion of infected meat. All types of carnivorous mammals and birds are susceptible to infection. Most human infections are from eating infected pigs and wild animals. Trichinosis reports are sporadic, usually among participants in communal meals.

Dracunculus medinensis, the 'fiery serpent of medina', or 'Guinea worm', was reported from 17 African nations, Yemen, Saudi Arabia, India and Pakistan. The gender distribution is variable, with most infections in those aged 15–40 years. Several decades ago there were 17 million cases worldwide. In 1994 there were reportedly 168 334 cases, and in 2013, 148 cases were reported. Transmission is seasonal and related to rainfall, when the copepod vectors (*Cyclops* spp.) are abundant. When male and female larvae are swallowed in infected

copepods, they produce a gravid female which emerges from a wound in the leg. The female bears live larvae when the host contacts water, and these larvae infect subsequent copepods. The female survives for a single year. If there is no transmission in any year, the cycle is broken. Nations where the disease disappeared without human intervention indicate that transmission can be interrupted and the disease eradicated without specific vaccine or drug treatment.[6] Programs to educate and provide better access to safe water have led to near eradication of this disease. There are several challenges remaining to eradication, including political and civil unrest and a newly found animal reservoir, dogs in Chad.[7] Eradication of dracunculiasis would be a remarkable achievement.

Angiostrongyliasis or parastrongyliasis is caused by the molluscan-borne nematode *Angiostrongylus cantonensis*, the rat lung worm, and *Angiostrongylus costaricensis*. The former is endemic in rats (*Rattus* spp.) in Asia, the Pacific Islands, Australia, India, Africa, the Caribbean and Louisiana and Florida, and recently Hawaii in the USA.[8] *A. costaricensis* is reported in Latin America and Texas, but most human infections are from Costa Rica. Human infection with *A. cantonensis* is reported primarily from Taiwan and Thailand, with infection acquired from eating the snails *Achatina fulica* in Taiwan, and *Pila ampullacae* in Thailand. In Taiwan, most infections are in children of both sexes, while in Thailand, it is seen mostly in adult males. While most prevalent in these two countries, human infections have been reported in many areas. *Angiostrongylus costaricensis* is usually found in children who accidentally ingest the slug *Vaginulus plebeius* on vegetation. Rats (*Rattus* spp.), cotton rats (*Sigmodon* spp.) and rice rats (*Oryzomys* spp.) are natural hosts for *A. costaricensis*.

Anisakiasis is caused by third-stage larvae of *Anisakis simplex* and *Pseudoterranova decipiens*, acquired by eating raw marine fish and squid. The adult worms, related to *Ascaris* spp., are found in marine mammals worldwide. Most human infections have occurred in Japan and other countries with high consumption of uncooked marine fish and squid.

Gnathostoma spp. larvae can invade human tissue and most infections are reported from Thailand and Japan, and occasionally Mexico. *Gnathostoma spinigerum* is the most common species reported. *Gnathostoma hispidium* has also been found in humans. Dogs and cats are the natural hosts for adult worms. Copepods serve as the first intermediate host, while fish, frogs, snakes and chicken are the second intermediate hosts. Infections are more common in adults of both sexes.

Blood and Tissue Nematodes (see Chapter 121)

The filarids are nematodes that infect the lymphatic, subcutaneous and cutaneous tissues. There are seven major filarids of humans transmitted by arthropods in tropical and subtropical parts of the world.

Wuchereria bancrofti is the most widespread, being endemic in Asia, Africa, Central and South America and the Pacific Islands. Prevalence rates are highly variable depending upon the vector mosquito, temperature, humidity, a susceptible human population and environmental sanitation. There are different vectors in different endemic areas; the most extensive is *Culex quinquefasciatus*, whereas *Aedes polynesiensis* is important in the Pacific Islands. Nocturnal periodicity is associated with the feeding habits of the mosquitoes, except in the Pacific where there is diurnal periodicity of microfilariae and the mosquito vector feeds in the daytime. Although a limited number of monkeys have been experimentally infected with *W. bancrofti*,[9] there are no known natural animal reservoirs.

Brugia malayi is found only in rural Asia and infects approximately 12 million people.[10] Many islands of Indonesia are endemic, one study showing transmigrants having a 40% prevalence, 4 years after moving to an endemic area. The major mosquito vectors are *Mansonia*, *Anopheles*, and *Aedes* spp. Cats and *Macaca* and *Presbytis* spp. monkeys are known reservoir hosts.

Brugia timori is found only in the Lesser Sunda Islands of Indonesia. Prevalence can reach 10%. *Anopheles barbirostris* is a major mosquito vector and although no naturally infected reservoirs have been found, cats and Mongolian gerbils have been experimentally infected.

An estimated 120 million people worldwide may be infected with these three lymphatic filarial species,[11] with 50 million in Africa, 62 million in Asia, 2 million in the Pacific Islands and fewer than 1 million in Latin America.

Onchocerca volvulus is endemic in 26 countries in Africa and six in Central and South America. Approximately 18 million people may be infected and as a result, 270 000 are blind and 500 000 severely disabled,[12] with local seropositivity rates reaching 82%. Although this disease may not be eradicable by current technology,[13] there are local instances where transmission has been interrupted. Infections are more common in males than females, reflecting male occupational exposures to the fly vector. Prevalence is higher in areas close to running water where the blackfly *Simulium damnosum* and related species breed. In the Americas, infections are more common in the highlands, from about 300 to 1200 meters (1000–4000 feet) above sea level. In Africa, infection is more common lower than 300 meters (1000 feet) above sea level. Infections decrease with distance from rivers and streams. There are no animal reservoirs and no microfilarial periodicity.

Loa loa, the African eye worm, is endemic in West and Central Africa where *Chrysops* spp. are present. Prevalence rates vary from 8% to 40% with infections increasing with age; 20 to 30 million people live in endemic areas.[14] Transmission by the day-biting female deerflies is highest during wet seasons. Monkeys serve as reservoir hosts. The microfilaria are diurnal.

A unique feature of filarids is the dependency upon *Wolbachia* spp., an intracellular bacterial symbiont associated with pathogenesis and fertility.[15]

TREMATODES

Over 10 million people worldwide are infected with food-borne trematodes. The most important infect the liver, lungs, blood and intestines.

Liver/Lung Trematodes

The Chinese liver fluke, *Chlonorchis sinensis*, is reported from China, South Korea, Vietnam and the far east of Russia. Infections are highest in older males and females with a tendency toward familial aggregation. An estimated 7 million people are infected, with prevalence rates in China of up to 57% and up to 40% in Korea.[16] Infections in the snail and fish intermediate hosts are highest in the warmer months. Snails in the families Hydrobiidae, Melaniidae, Assimineidae and Thiaridae are first intermediate hosts, and fish, primarily of the family Cyprinidae, are second intermediate hosts.

Opisthorchis viverrini is endemic in South East Asia. An estimated 10 million people of both genders and all age groups are infected, increasing from children to adults. Prevalence varies from 2% to 71% in Thailand. *Bithynia* spp. are important snail hosts and *Cyclocheilichthys* spp. freshwater fish are important second intermediate hosts. Dogs, cats and other fish-eating mammals are reservoir hosts. *Opisthorchis felinus* infects more than 1.2 million people in Europe and Siberia.[17]

Fasciola hepatica, the sheep liver fluke, is endemic in most sheep-raising areas of the world. Human infections are increasing and are most common in parts of Europe, South America and the Middle East. Approximately 2.4 to 17 million people are infected with *F. hepatica* and the closely related *F. gigantica*.[18] Sheep, goats and cattle are the natural hosts, with infection rates varying. The prevalence in humans reaches 67% in Bolivia. Infections are more common in adults who acquire infection from eating watercress salads.

From more than 40 described species of *Paragonimus*, only a few infect humans, the Oriental lung fluke, *Paragonimus westermani*, being responsible for the most serious disease. It has been reported from China, Japan, Korea, the Philippines and Thailand. Other species occur in China, Thailand, Mexico, Ecuador, Peru and parts of Africa. Infection is acquired by eating metacercariae-laden crabs and crayfish. The juice from crabs, used for seasoning and traditional medicine, may contain metacercaria. Suspected prevalence is 1.7% in China, 16.8% in Nigeria and 12.7% in Vietnam. There are many snail hosts, with *Semisulcospira* spp. being the major vectors in China and Korea. The crabs *Eriocheir* and *Potamon* spp. and the crayfish *Cambaroides* spp. are important second intermediate hosts. Dogs, cats and other carnivorous mammals are reservoir hosts.

Intestinal Trematodes

There are a very large number (approximately 70) of intestinal flukes reported, mostly from Asia, where infections are acquired by eating raw food. *Fasciolopsis buski*, the giant intestinal fluke, is reported from China, Thailand, Bangladesh and India and occasionally from Indonesia. A survey in Thailand reported prevalence of 7.1%.[19] Pigs are the reservoir host, and snails such as *Segmentina*, *Hippeutis* and *Gyraulus* spp. are important vectors. Cercariae from snails encyst on water plants such as water caltrop, watercress, water bamboo and water chestnut, and cause infection when eaten uncooked.

Other important intestinal flukes include *Echinostoma*, *Heterophyes* and *Metagonimus* spp. There are an estimated 150 000 cases of echinostomiasis, 240 000 cases of heterophyiasis, and 650 000 cases of metagonimiasis, mostly in China, Korea and Japan. Echinostome metacercaria are acquired from snails, fish and other aquatic animals, whereas *Heterophyes*, and *Metagonimus* infective stages occur in fish. All ages and both genders are infected as a result of eating the second intermediate hosts uncooked.

Blood Trematodes (see Chapter 118)

Schistosomiasis is endemic to many tropical areas of the world:

- *Schistosoma japonicum* is found in Asia
- *S. hematobium* and *S. mansoni* are found in Africa and the Middle East
- *S. mansoni* is found in South America, and some islands in the Caribbean.

Other species of less importance are *S. mekongi* and *S. intercalatum*, which are found in foci located in South East Asia and Africa, respectively.

It is estimated that there are over 200 million infections, with the prevalence and intensity of infections highest in children aged 5–15 years. Infection rates depend upon water contact in endemic areas. Despite the widespread distribution of snails and frequent opportunities for water contact, high transmission occurs at only a few sites. It is important to identify these sites. Snail vectors are of the genera *Bulimus* spp. for *S. hematobium*, *Biomphalaria* spp. for *S. mansoni* and *Oncomelania* spp. for *S. japonicum*. Although *S. japonicum* is endemic on Taiwan, the strain of parasite will not infect humans and is considered to be zoophilic.[20]

CESTODES (see Chapter 119)

Cestode, or tapeworm, infections are acquired by ingestion of intermediate hosts containing infective larval stages:

- The beef tapeworm, *Tanea saginata*, and pork tapeworm *T. solium*, are acquired by ingesting the cysticercus stage in beef or pork.
- The fish tapeworm, *Dipyllobothrium latum*, is acquired by eating raw fish infected with the plerocercoid or sparganum stage.
- *Hymenolepis nana* and *H. diminuta* are acquired by ingesting eggs in contaminated food, or accidental consumption of insect intermediate hosts.

T. saginata is worldwide, with high infection rates in Africa and Asia. Most infections occur in adults. The cysticercus is found only in bovids; however, in parts of Asia, especially in Taiwan, pigs are a recognized source of infection for a strain of the parasite, known as *T. saginata (asiatica)*.[21]

T. solium is found sporadically in pigs worldwide with many human cases reported from Mexico and Central and South America, South West Asia and Africa. Human cysticercosis is present in these areas. Certain areas of Irian Jaya in Indonesia report many cases of cysticercosis due to consumption of uncooked pork.

H. nana is the most common tapeworm in North America and is particularly reported in children worldwide. *H. diminuta* is not common but is reported occasionally in South East Asia.

The incidence of *D. latum* in humans in Scandinavia, Finland, Alaska, Canada and the northern USA has probably diminished in recent years, although accurate epidemiological data are lacking. *D. dendriticum* has recently been identified as a potential emerging pathogen in Europe [22] and other species of *Diphyllobothrium* are reported from Japan and South America.[23]

Sparganosis, or infections with the larval stage of *Spirometra* spp., is reported occasionally from many parts of the world. Infection is acquired by ingesting copepods or second intermediate hosts (frogs, toads or other aquatic animals). Infections in southern Asia are attributed to the use of fresh animal tissues as poultices.

Echinococcus granulosus and *E. multilocularis* are associated with human hydatid disease, whereas *E. vogeli* and *E. oligarthus* rarely cause disease in humans. *E. granulosus* is the most important and found primarily in sheep-raising areas. Strains of the parasite are found in goats, swine, cattle, horses and camels. The parasitoses are worldwide, with canines the definitive host and animals such as sheep intermediate hosts. Humans acquire infection by ingesting eggs from dogs, whereas dogs acquire infection by eating sheep liver and organs containing cysts with large numbers of scolices. Infections usually occur in the young and the cysts develop over a period of years.

E. multilocularis has a limited distribution in dogs, foxes, wolves and cats as the reservoir hosts and larval stages in wild rodents, especially voles. The parasite is reported to be moving southward in the USA. Rare human infections are acquired by the ingestion of eggs passed by canines. Infection with any of the *Echinococcus* spp. is related to poor sanitary conditions in populations with low levels of education and closely associated with canine reservoir hosts.

Pathogenicity

Helminths seem to live in peaceful coexistence with their hosts and usually cause few problems. However, if there are many worms, there may be severe disease. Parasites, especially in the intestines, can cause obstruction and possibly perforation. The worms also secrete or excrete toxic substances, which affect tissues. Lytic substances, such as those secreted by hookworms to obtain blood, can induce inflammation and there may be changes due to malabsorption and competition for nutrients. Larval stages may be more pathogenic, secreting antigenic substances that cause hypersensitivity, while the antigens promote antibody production and cellular immune responses. Worms in the wrong place can be highly pathogenic.

Helminths have intricate life cycles and disease is usually associated with the larval migratory pathways and the final habitat of adult worms in the host. The amount of pathology and disease varies with the parasitosis.

NEMATODES LIVING IN THE INTESTINES (see Chapter 114)

Enterobius vermicularis

The life cycle of *Enterobius vermicularis* is presented in Figure 195-1. Adult pinworms reside in the large bowel, where mating occurs. Gravid females migrate out of the anus and deposit eggs on the perianal skin. Eggs under the fingernails in children lead to re-infection when the fingers are placed in the mouth. Eggs can be released onto the bedsheets and become disseminated throughout the household when the sheets are shaken. The eggs will survive for 2 weeks in a humid and cool environment. When eggs are ingested, they hatch in the intestine and the larvae migrate to the large intestine to mature in 6 weeks.

Ascaris lumbricoides

Infection with *Ascaris lumbricoides* can occasionally be highly pathogenic. The life cycle is presented in Figure 195-1. The adult male worm may measure 15–31 cm by 2–4 mm and the female 20–35 cm by 3–6 mm. The female can live for a year or more and produce 240 000 eggs/day. The eggs pass in the feces and embryonate in the soil in 10–14 days. Upon ingestion the egg hatches in the intestine. The liberated larva penetrates the mucosa, passes to the liver via the portal vessels and then moves to the lungs. After a few weeks, the larva penetrates the alveolar air sac, passes up the pulmonary tree, is coughed up, swallowed and becomes sexually mature in the small intestine in 60–75 days.

Trichuris trichiuria

Trichuris trichiuria has a direct life cycle (see Figure 195-1). Adult females in the large intestine deposit eggs in the fecal stream, which embryonate after a few weeks in the soil. When eggs are swallowed, they hatch in the intestine and larvae migrate to the colon. The worms bury their narrow anterior end into the mucosa with the wider posterior end extended freely into the lumen of the colon. The females lay eggs after 3 months and produce 3000–10 000 ova/day. The females measure 35–55 mm and the males 30–45 mm; in both sexes the slender anterior is about 0.1 mm, and the posterior thicker, about 0.5 mm.

Hookworms

Several hookworm species can infect humans, but most parasitize nonhuman animals (i.e. zoonotic parasites). Hookworms from other animals usually cause creeping eruption or cutaneous larva migrans. Only two hookworms are considered to be important human species:

- *Necator americanus*
- *Ancylstoma duodenale*

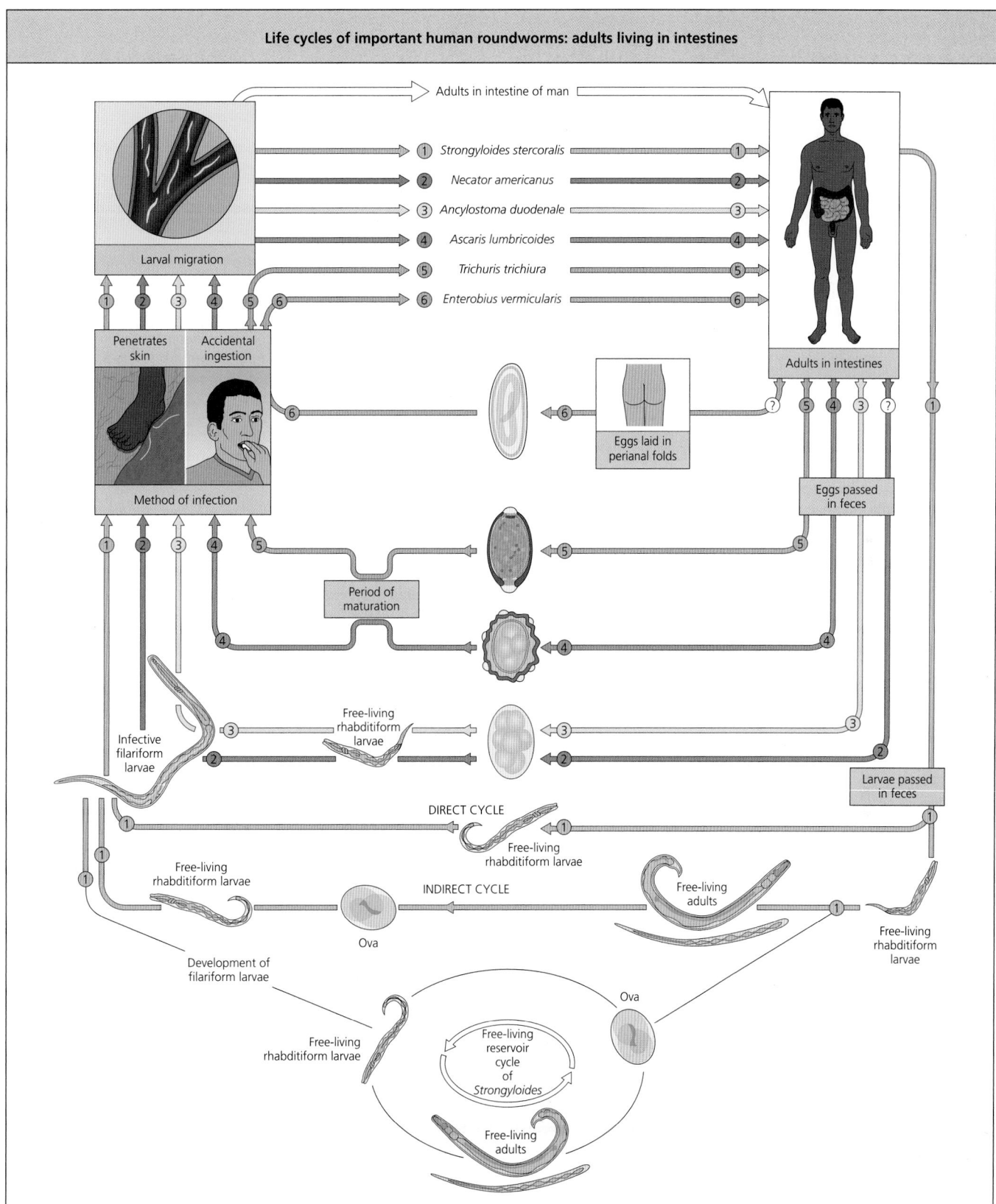

Figure 195-1 Life cycles of important human roundworms: adults living in intestines.

Both species measure about 10–13 mm for females and 6–11 mm for males and can be 0.4–0.6 mm in width. The anterior mouths have cutting plates or teeth and males have bell-shaped bursal rays at the posterior end that hold females during copulation. The vulva is mid-central and eggs pass from the females into the fecal stream and out with the host feces onto the soil. Female worms pass 5000–10 000 (*N. americanus*) and 10 000–20 000 (*A. duodenale*) eggs/day. In warm, moist environments the eggs embryonate in the soil and rhabditiform larvae are released. Within a few days the larvae molt and develop into the filariform larval infective stage. Filariform larvae climb to the top of the soil or grass, cling together and wait for a human host to come by. They penetrate the skin between the toes or other body surfaces. Some *A. duodenale* larvae may be ingested in water and enter the oral mucosa. The larvae are carried by the blood to the heart and then the lungs where they remain for a period, then break out into the alveoli, pass up the pulmonary tree and are swallowed. The parasite matures in the small intestine, copulates and produces eggs in about 5 weeks (see Figure 195-1).

Hookworm infections can remain active for as long as 13 years. The attachment of adult worms can cause small erosive lesions, hemorrhage, tissue cytolysis and neutrophilic infiltration. The worms change attachment sites regularly leaving old sites oozing blood and plasma. Iron deficiency anemia and blood loss result from long-term infection with a large number of worms.

Pathologic changes occur in the bone marrow due to blood loss. Liver function may change as a result of anemia, as well as reduced capacity for albumen synthesis. Hookworm disease with iron deficiency anemia, hypoproteinemia and hepatosplenomegaly may contribute to thousands of deaths each year.

Strongyloides stercoralis

Strongyloides stercoralis is a unique nematode having both parasitic and free-living cycles, with males and females present in the free-living cycle (see Figure 195-1) and only females present in the parasitic cycle. Parasitic females measure 1.5–2.5 mm and have a long cylindrical esophagus. The vulva is in the posterior third of the body and the paired uteri contain thin-shelled eggs.

Eggs are deposited in the small intestinal epithelium and hatch soon after release. The first-stage larva passes in the feces and develops into a second-stage and then a third or infective-stage filariform larva after a few days. The third-stage larvae penetrate the skin and migrate through the body and via the blood to the lungs; after several days they migrate up the respiratory tree and are swallowed. The larvae enter the intestinal mucosa and mature, and the female worms produce eggs parthenogenetically. Some rhabditiform larvae in soil transform into free-living male and female adults in the soil and reproduce. The eggs hatch, releasing rhabditiform larvae, which develop into filariform larvae that can enter the skin of a host.

Some larvae transform into infective forms in the bowel, penetrate the mucosa, migrate and develop into adults. This internal autoinfection can lead to hyperinfection in the immunocompromised host. Cellular immunity is responsible for keeping infections under control, but when affected by disease or immunosuppression, the parasite multiplies, leading to hyperinfection and dissemination (see also Chapter 94).

Capillaria philippinensis

In intestinal capillariasis the parasite can multiply in the digestive tract. *Capillaria philippinensis* is a tiny worm; females measure 2.5–5.3 mm and males 1.3–3.9 mm. The anterior body is narrow and the posterior is slightly wider and contains reproductive organs and the digestive tract. Females deposit eggs, which must reach water where they embryonate. When embryonated eggs are eaten by small freshwater fish, the eggs hatch and the larvae develop into infective stages in 3 weeks. When humans eat infected fish, the larvae mature in 2 weeks. After mating, the females first produce larvae that will mature in the gut. Second-generation worms produce thick-shelled eggs, which pass out in the feces. The parasites can multiply rapidly, producing thousands of

progeny.[24] If the patient is not treated, the disease can be fatal. Over 200 000 worms were recovered from 1 liter of bowel fluid at one autopsy. The worms enter the crypts and cause atrophy, the villi are flattened and denuded, the mucosal glands are denuded and the lamina propria is infiltrated with inflammatory cells. Other organs are also affected by malnutrition and hypokalemia. Most of the pathology is in the jejunum.[25]

NEMATODES LIVING IN TISSUES

Trichinella spiralis

Trichinella spiralis is related to other trichiurids having a slender anterior and a wider posterior end. Female worms measure 2–4 mm and males 1–1.5 mm. Infections are acquired by eating uncooked muscle containing encysted larvae from infected animals, usually pigs.

The larvae are digested from the cyst, pass to the small intestine and burrow beneath the epithelium where they develop into adults, re-enter the gut lumen and reproduce. The larvae enter the gut wall, are picked up by the blood and carried throughout the body to striated muscle where they become encysted. The larvae entering the muscle cell cause alterations in morphology, resulting in the characteristic 'nurse cell'. Morphologic and molecular changes occur in the cell until it becomes calcified. The larvae can remain alive for many years in the cell. Chronic inflammatory cells may surround the parasitized muscle cell.

Filarial Nematodes

The filarial nematodes are long and slender and are found in the lymphatics, tissues and body cavities. The life cycles of some of the filarids are presented in Figure 195-2. Microfilariae are produced by female worms and arthropods are the vectors (see Chapter 121).

***Wuchereria bancrofti, Brugia malayi* and *B. timori*.** The lymphatic filarids *Wuchereria bancrofti*, *Brugia malayi* and *B. timori* produce microfilariae that usually appear in the blood between 2200 and 0200 hours (nocturnal periodicity). *W. bancrofti* found in some Pacific Islands produce microfilariae that appear in the blood in the daytime (diurnal periodicity). Mosquitoes obtain blood at night and the larvae develop into the infective stage in 10–14 days. At the next feeding, infective larvae migrate from the thoracic muscles of the mosquito to the proboscis and crawl into the hole made by the bite. The larvae migrate in the host until they reach the definitive habitat and develop into adults. The worms copulate and females produce microfilariae; the life cycle of *W. bancrofti* is a few months longer than that of *B. malayi*. Infections may persist for several years.

The pathogenesis of lymphatic filariasis is unresolved. *Wolbachia* spp., a filariad endosymbiont, may be associated with the pathogenesis.[26] On the other hand, the pathology of lymphatic filariasis may be associated with the immunologic responsiveness. Some infected people are microfilaremic but without antibodies or disease, whereas others are amicrofilaremic and have antibodies. There is an inflammatory stage with lymph channel irritation. Adult worms can be found in the lymph vessels, primarily the axillary, epitrochlear, inguinal and pelvic nodes as well as those in the testis, epididymis and spermatic cord.

***Onchocerca volvulus*.** *Onchocerca volvulus* adults are coiled in fibrous tissue nodules in the subcutaneous tissue. The females reach 50 cm in length and 0.5 mm in diameter producing microfilariae that are released into the interstitium of the skin. Males are smaller, being 5 cm in length. Microfilaria are picked up by biting flies or blackflies of the genus *Simulium* spp., develop to the infective stage larvae and are introduced into a host at the next feeding. Larvae migrate through tissue and after many months settle down, usually in pairs, and become encapsulated (see Figure 195-2).

The microfilariae leave the nodule and migrate through the dermis provoking dermatitis and blindness.

***Loa loa*.** The African eye worm, *Loa loa*, moves through the subcutaneous tissue and often traverses the conjunctiva. The males are 3–4 cm and the females 4–7 cm in length and 3–5 mm wide. Microfilariae have a diurnal periodicity and are ingested by *Chrysops* spp. at the time of a blood meal. The larvae develop to the infective stage in

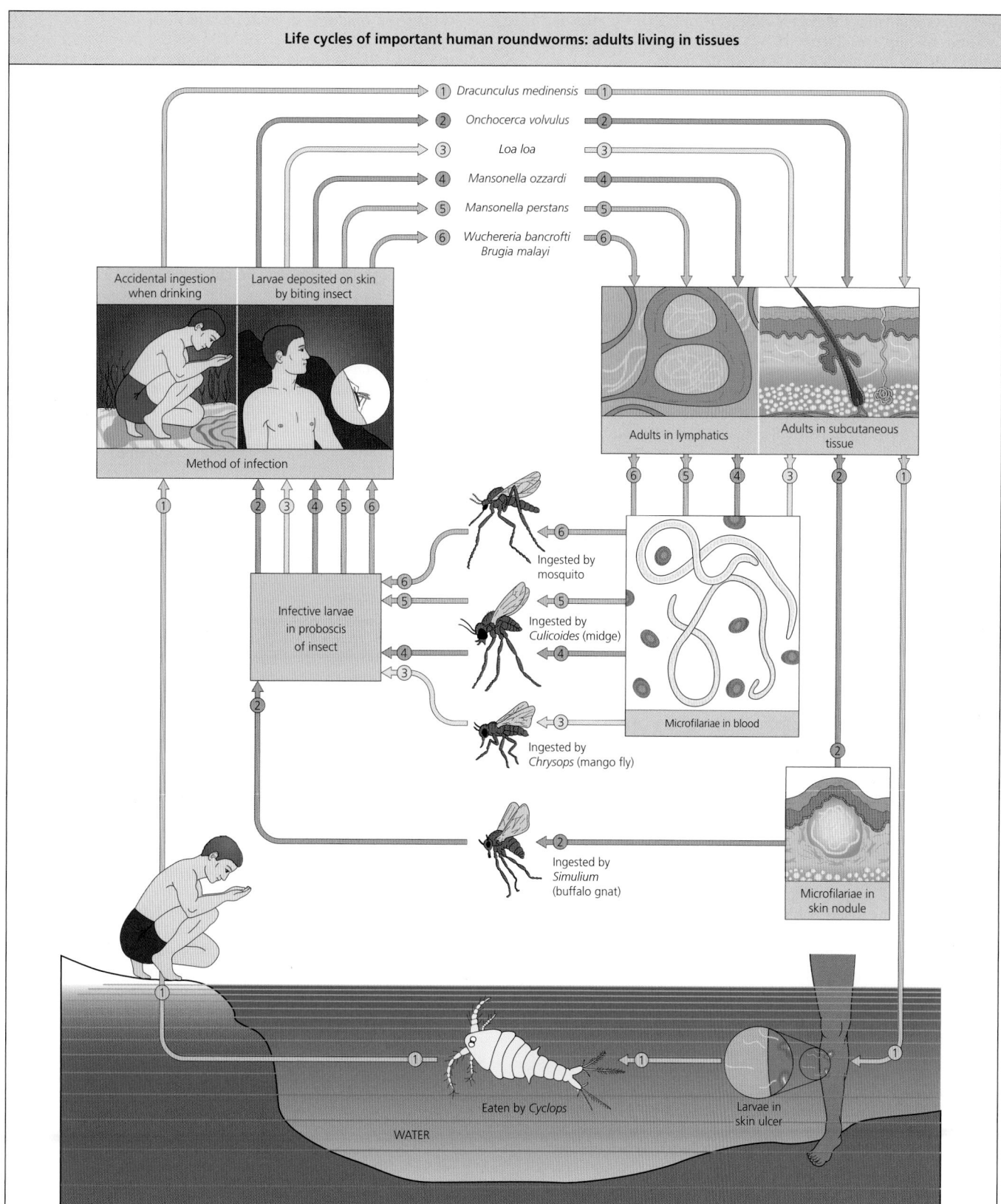

Figure 195-2 Life cycles of important human roundworms: adults living in tissues.

10–13 days and enter the host through the hole made by the bite at the next feeding (see Figure 195-2). The adult worms cause little damage as they migrate quickly through the tissue.

Dracunculus medinensis. *Dracunculus medinensis* is similar to the filarids. The females measure up to 120 cm long and 2 mm wide and the males 2 cm. The worms mature in the connective tissue; gravid females then migrate to the subcutaneous tissue where they cause ulcers through which larvae are released when the lesion is immersed in water. Larvae are ingested by copepods and develop into infective larvae in 2 weeks. When the copepods are ingested in drinking water, the larvae are liberated, penetrate the digestive tract and develop into adults in the connective tissue in a year (see Figure 195-2).

Angiostrongylus cantonensis

Angiostrongylus cantonensis is found naturally in the lungs of rats. Larvae produced by females move up the pulmonary tree, are swallowed and pass out in the rat feces. Molluscs (snails and slugs) serve as intermediate hosts and, when eaten by rats, the larvae are digested out of the snail, migrate from the gut to the brain, and after 3 weeks migrate to the lungs. Larvae are produced by adult females a few weeks later. Humans who eat snails or slugs acquire the infective larvae, which migrate to the central nervous system (CNS) and cause eosinophilic meningitis. The females reach 2–3 cm and the males 1–2 cm in length and 0.2–0.3 mm in width. In most human infections the larvae die in the brain and spinal cord and elicit an inflammatory reaction in the meninges. Eosinophils, monocytes and foreign body giant cells infiltrate around the dead worms. Tissue necrosis is also evident. Larvae are reported in the eye and are often recovered from cerebrospinal fluid (CSF). Adult worms have been found on a few occasions in the pulmonary artery.

Anisakis simplex and Pseudoterranova dicepiens

Anisakis simplex larvae measure 2–3 cm by 0.3–0.6 mm and *Pseudoterranova dicepiens* 2–3 cm by 0.3–1.2 mm. They are found in the muscle and body cavity of marine fish and squid. When eaten by marine mammals (e.g. whales, seals) the worms mature in the stomach and the females deposit eggs in the feces. In the ocean, a larva hatches from the egg and is eaten by a small marine crustacean. When the crustacean with a third-stage larva is eaten by fish, the freed larva migrates to the abdominal cavity. When infected fish are eaten raw by humans the liberated larvae penetrate the stomach or small intestine and provoke a foreign body reaction around the worm.

Gnathostoma spinigerum

Gnathostoma spinigerum is a robust nematode with a large globose head surrounded by rows of spines. The females measure 1–1.5 cm by 1–2.5 mm and the males 1–2.5 cm by 1–2 mm. The adults are coiled in the wall of the digestive tract of dogs and cats. Eggs pass in the feces, embryonate in fresh water and are ingested by copepods. The larvae hatch and develop into a second larval stage. When the copepod is eaten by a second intermediate host (for example fish or frogs), the third-stage larva develops and when this is eaten by a dog or cat, the worm penetrates the gut wall and matures. Humans who eat infected fish, frogs, or other aquatic food, raw or fermented, acquire the infection. The larvae migrate through tissues in a fashion similar to that of cutaneous larva migrans. The CNS may be invaded, resulting in an eosinophilic myeloencephalitis with eosinophilic pleocytosis and bloody xanthochromic CSF. The eye may also be invaded, causing palpebral edema, exophthalmos and subconjunctival hemorrhage.

Larva Migrans

Cutaneous larva migrans is caused by dog or cat hookworm larvae that enter the skin and cannot complete their life cycle. They either migrate through or encyst in subcutaneous tissue causing serpinginous erythematous tracts. These tracts eventually become dry and encrusted.

Visceral larva migrans is caused by dog and cat ascarid larvae (*Toxocara* spp.) that hatch from accidentally swallowed eggs. These larvae migrate through the tissue and encyst as second-stage larvae. The migrating larvae produce tracts with hemorrhagic necrosis.

Neural larva migrans, a severe encephalitis, may be caused by consuming the eggs of the raccoon nematode *B. procyonis*. Eggs are ingested, and hatched larvae migrate through the brain causing an eosinophilic encephalitis, or cause ocular larva migrans in adults. Most of these cases occur in children although it is unknown whether this is due to their increased exposure, or some biological factor that makes children more susceptible to disease.

TREMATODES LIVING IN LIVER, LUNGS, INTESTINES AND BLOOD

Although many trematodes infect humans, few are considered important pathogens. These flat worms are found in all organs, especially the intestines, with a few found in the liver, lungs and blood. The life cycles of the important trematodes are presented in Figure 195-3.

Opisthorchid Liver Flukes

Chlonorchis sinensis, *Opisthorchis viverini* and *Opisthorchis felineus* are found in the bile ducts. The worms are hermaphroditic and about 1.5 cm long and tapered at both ends. Eggs pass down the bile ducts to the intestine and out with the feces. In water, several species of snails (*Parafossarulus*, *Thiara* and *Bithenia*) serve as the first intermediate host; the snail ingests an egg and the miracidium is released. After reproducing by polyembryony, cercariae are produced that leave the snail and encyst as metacercariae in freshwater fish (cyprinids or carp). When infected fish is eaten raw or improperly cooked, the metacercariae are digested out of the fish and migrate down the bowel and into the bile passages. Cholangiocarcinoma is a possible complication. There may be an association with infection and consumption of carcinogenic nitrosamines found in Asian foods.[27]

Fasciolopsis buski

Fasciolopsis busci is the largest intestinal trematode of humans, measuring 5–7 cm by 8–20 mm by 1–3 mm. It has oral and ventral suckers, two large ceca, two branched testes and a central coiled uterus. Eggs pass in the feces into water and the hatched miracidium enters a specific planorbid snail. Cercariae released from the snail attach to aquatic vegetation and form metacercariae. When eaten, the metacercariae excyst and attach to the mucosa of the small intestine.

Fasciola hepatica

Fasciola hepatica is acquired by eating aquatic vegetation on which metacercariae are attached. Upon ingestion the metacercariae are released, penetrate the gut wall, traverse the peritoneal cavity, pass through the liver capsule into the liver parenchyma and enter the bile duct. Worms may re-enter the liver parenchyma. The worms are large, 4 cm in length, and 1.5 cm wide, with a large cephalic cone at the anterior end. The egg passes down the bile duct to the intestines and out with the feces. It hatches in the water and the miracidium enters into snails of the genus *Lymnea*. Cercariae are released and encyst on all varieties of aquatic vegetation.

Paragonimus westermani

Paragonimus westermani usually reside in pairs in the lung. They are reddish brown, plump bodied and shaped like coffee beans. They measure about 1.2 cm long, 0.6 cm wide and 0.4 cm thick. They have two large branching testes in the posterior half of the body. Eggs enter the alveoli, are coughed up and swallowed and pass out in the feces or in the sputum. The egg hatches in water, enters a specific snail and multiplies; released cercariae enter crabs and crayfish where the metacercariae encyst. When the infected crustacean is eaten the metacercariae are released from the cyst, penetrate the gut wall and enter into the peritoneum, diaphragm and lung.

Young migrating worms produce local hemorrhage and cellular infiltration. These worms may settle in ectopic locations and evoke a pronounced tissue reaction. In the lung and other locations a leukocytic infiltration develops around the worm and fibrous tissue infiltrates to form a cyst wall. Eggs may migrate into pulmonary tissue and other locations, evoking granulomatous reactions. Cerebral paragonimiasis often develops with hemorrhage, eosinophils, a yellowish

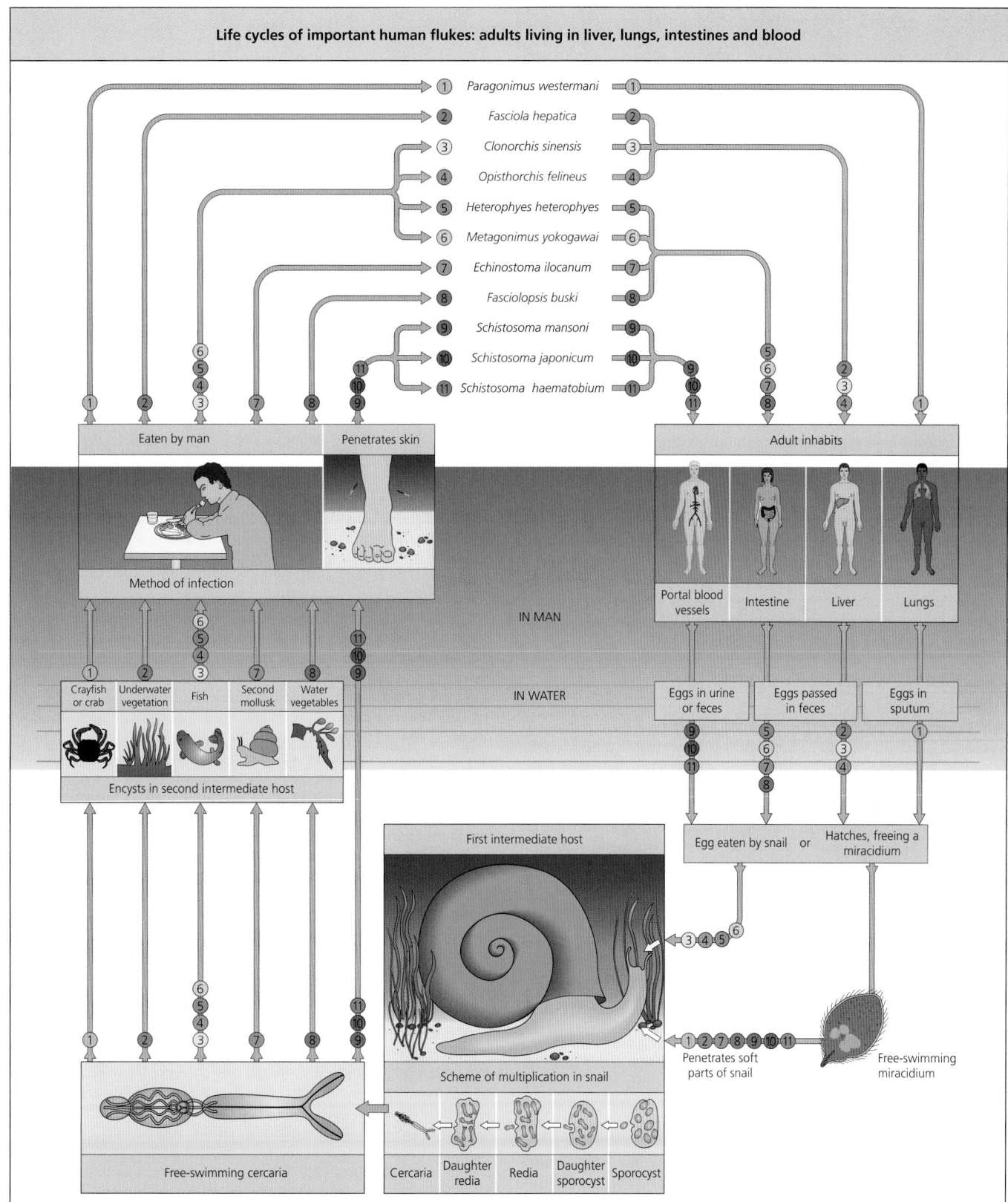

Figure 195-3   Life cycles of important human flukes: adults living in the liver, lungs, intestines and blood.

exudate and Charcot–Leyden crystals. Some lesions may eventually calcify.

Other species of *Paragonimus* can also infect humans and invade subcutaneous tissue and the abdominal cavity.

Other Intestinal Fluke Infections

Most intestinal fluke infections are innocuous unless there are a large number of worms. The eggs of the heterophyids are tiny and may be carried by the lymphatics and venules to ectopic locations such as the heart and evoke granulomas. Eggs of the intestinal flukes pass in the feces and hatch in water and the miracidia enter snails. Cercariae emerging from the snails enter fish and other aquatic animal life; when these animals are eaten the metacercariae excyst and develop into adults in the small intestine.

Human Schistosomes

Human schistosomes are found in the venous bloodstream. Eggs are passed into water and the miracidia search out specific snails in which to continue the life cycle. Cercariae released from the snails penetrate the host's skin and larval schistosomulae migrate to the lungs and then to the mesenteric and vesical veins. Eggs carried back through the mesenteric veins to the liver are responsible for granuloma formation.

The schistosomes are the only trematodes with separate sexes. They have oral and ventral suckers. The females are 1.5–2.5 cm in length and 0.2–0.3 mm in diameter. The male is 0.5–2 cm and, although flat, usually curls up to form the gynecophoral canal in which the female lies. The female leaves the male, crawls to the small venules close to the lumen of the gut or urinary bladder and deposits eggs. The miracidium in the egg releases enzymes to work with the spines on the *S. mansoni* and *S. haematobium* eggs to digest tissue and enter the lumen of the intestine or bladder. Some eggs are carried via the venules and veins to the liver. Infections persist for months[28] to years.[29] The life cycles of the human schistosomes are presented in Figure 195-3.

CESTODES LIVING IN THE INTESTINES AND TISSUES

Adult tapeworms residing in the intestines do not cause serious disease, but larval stages of two species are highly pathogenic. The adults in the intestines pass eggs, which are taken up by an intermediate host (see Figure 195-4).

Eggs of *T. saginata* and *T. solium* are ingested by bovids and swine, and larval or cysticercus stages develop in muscles. When insufficiently cooked meat is eaten, cysticerci are released and develop into adults in the small intestine. The life cycles of the fish tapeworm *D. latum* and related species involves two intermediate hosts. The egg hatches in water and the coricidium is taken in by a copepod and develops into a procercoid larva. When eaten by a fish, the larva develops into a plerocercoid larva. When the fish is eaten, the larva becomes an adult in the intestine.

Hymenolepid cestodes often require an insect (beetles and fleas) as an intermediate host. *H. nana* can also be acquired by ingestion of the egg. Some strains of *H. nana* are capable of internal autoinfection.

Morphologically, tapeworms have a scolex, neck and immature, mature and gravid proglottids. The scolex of *D. latum* has a sucking groove as a hold-fast organ, whereas other tapeworms have a scolex with four suckers. *T. solium* and *H. nana* have a rostellum on the scolex with rows of hooklets. Each mature proglottid is hermaphroditic with both male and female sex organs. The length and width of each species varies, with the longest being *D. latum* (2–15 m), followed by the taeniids (1–4 m), *H. nana* (1.5–4 cm) and *H. diminuta* (1–6 cm).

Larval stages of tapeworms also infect humans (Figure 195-5). Infection with the plerocercoid larva of diphyllobothriid species such as *Spirometra* is the cause of sparganosis. The larvae acquired from eating aquatic animals or drinking copepods in water penetrate the gut wall and migrate through the tissue. Animal poultices used in Asia are another source of infection. The larvae cause painful inflammatory swellings or transient lesions. The parasite may invade the eye causing periorbital edema.

Humans who become infected with the eggs of *T. solium* may develop cysticercosis. The larvae invade the muscles, brain, eye and skin. Although the cyst may remain intact and dormant for years, it may eventually rupture and the released fluids cause granulomas and calcification.

Echinococcosis or hydatid disease develops in humans who accidentally ingest the eggs of the dog tapeworms, *E. granulosa* or *E. multilocularis*. The egg hatches in the duodenum and the onchosphere penetrates the gut and becomes established in the liver or other organs. A cyst develops brood capsules and protoscolices proliferate from the inner germinal epithelium of the brood capsule. An outer laminated acellular limiting membrane forms and the cyst develops over many years. Unilocular cysts develop with *E. granulosus* and multilocular alveolar cysts with *E. multilocularis*. Cysts develop in many organs. The adult worms are parasites of canines and the intermediate host can be any animal, but is most often sheep for *E. granulosus* and rodents for *E. multilocularis*.

Prevention

Most parasitic infections can be prevented by following good sanitary practices. Soil-transmitted nematodes can be controlled and possibly eradicated with proper disposal of feces. Disposal of fecal matter into water bodies containing molluscan intermediate hosts perpetuates trematode infections. The construction and use of sanitary privies will go a long way toward preventing infections of all types, but in endemic areas indiscriminate defecation is the trend. Infection with skin-penetrating helminths, such as hookworm and *Strongyloides* spp., can be prevented by wearing shoes and protective clothing. Avoiding areas contaminated by raccoon feces can help avoid *B. procyonis*.

Arthropod-borne helminthiasis, such as filariasis, can be prevented by using insecticides in houses, including insecticide-treated bed nets. Breeding areas of vectors can be treated with insecticides, or environmental modifications, such as releasing larvivorous fish. The use of repellants will help as will sleeping under insecticide-impregnated bed nets, and wearing long clothing during vector biting hours.

The best example of preventive measures providing relief from disease is control of dracunculiasis. Education, monitoring and provision of sanitary water supplies has resulted in the near eradication of this disease.

The avoidance of waters known to harbor snail vectors will prevent schistosome infections. The destruction of snail breeding areas and the use of molluscicides will help to control infections.

Eating raw foods should be restricted in endemic areas. Eating raw fish is a practice in many countries, and discouraging this would prevent certain trematode and cestode infections. Cooking marine fish would prevent anisakiasis. Similarly, cooking aquatic vegetation would prevent trematode infections such as fascioliasis and fasciolopsiasis. Undercooked beef and pork are responsible for trichinosis and tapeworm infections, and thorough cooking will destroy these parasites. Freezing foods will kill most parasites and irradiation can make foods safe.[30] Microwave treatment is not considered adequate for destroying parasites.

Anthelmintics can be used to help control helminth infections. Mebendazole, albendazole, praziquantel and Diethylcarbamazine (DEC) have been used in mass treatment campaigns for various nematode and trematode infections, including widespread administration of DEC in table salt. Reduction of infections in a population will be of significant benefit and will augment control and eventual eradication programs (see Chapter 121). Use of drugs that **rapidly** destroy microfilaria may be contraindicated in areas with a high prevalence of *Loa loa*. In these areas drugs such as doxycycline that target the *Wolbachia* spp. endosymbiont may be particularly useful.

Diagnosis

Diagnosis of helminth infections depends upon the location of the parasite in the body. The majority of worms are in the digestive tract, and diagnosis is made by stool examination. Blood is examined for

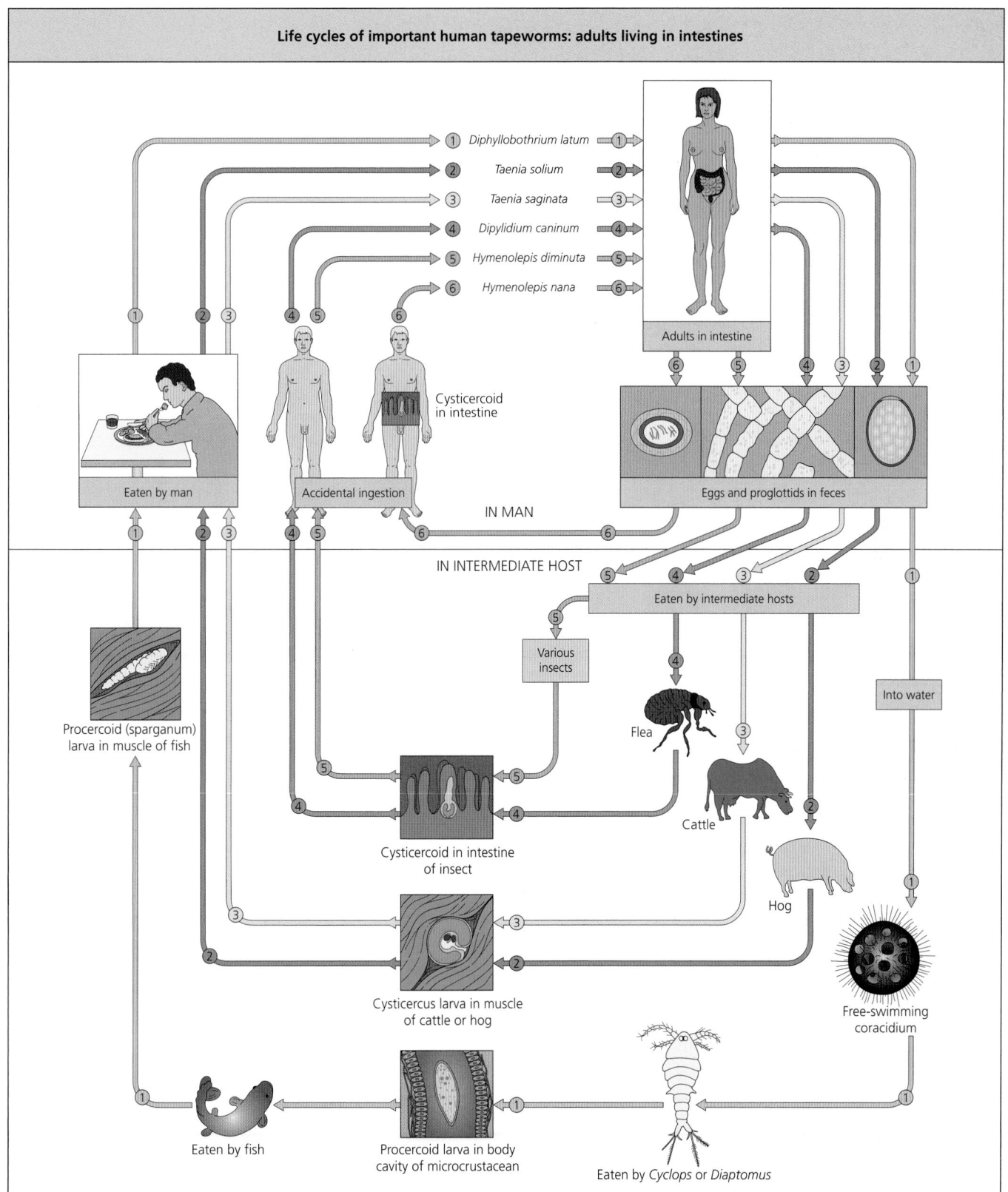

Figure 195-4   Life cycles of important human tapeworms: adults living in intestines.

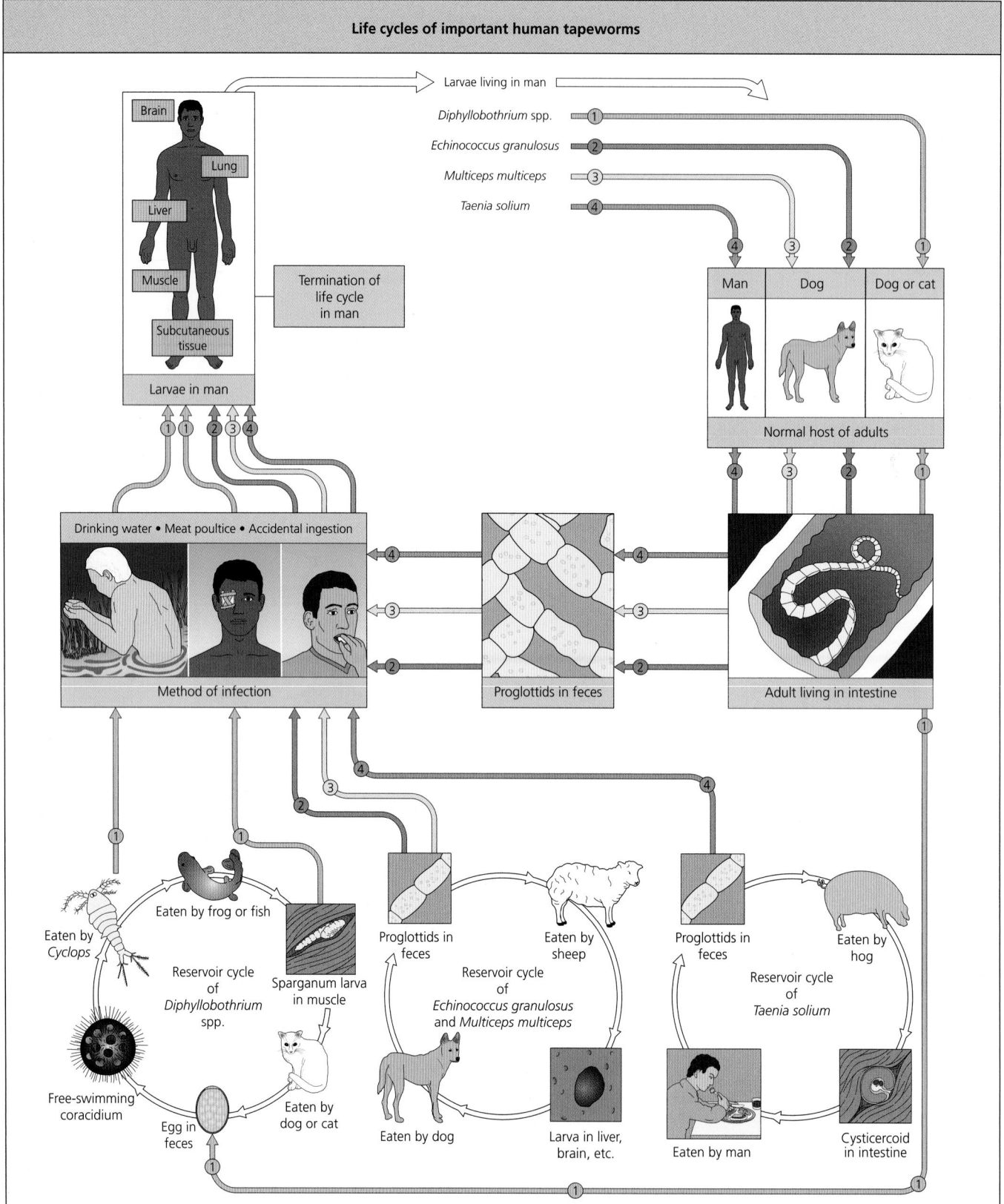

Figure 195-5 Life cycles of important human tapeworms; adults living in tissues and intestines and blood: humans are accidental hosts.

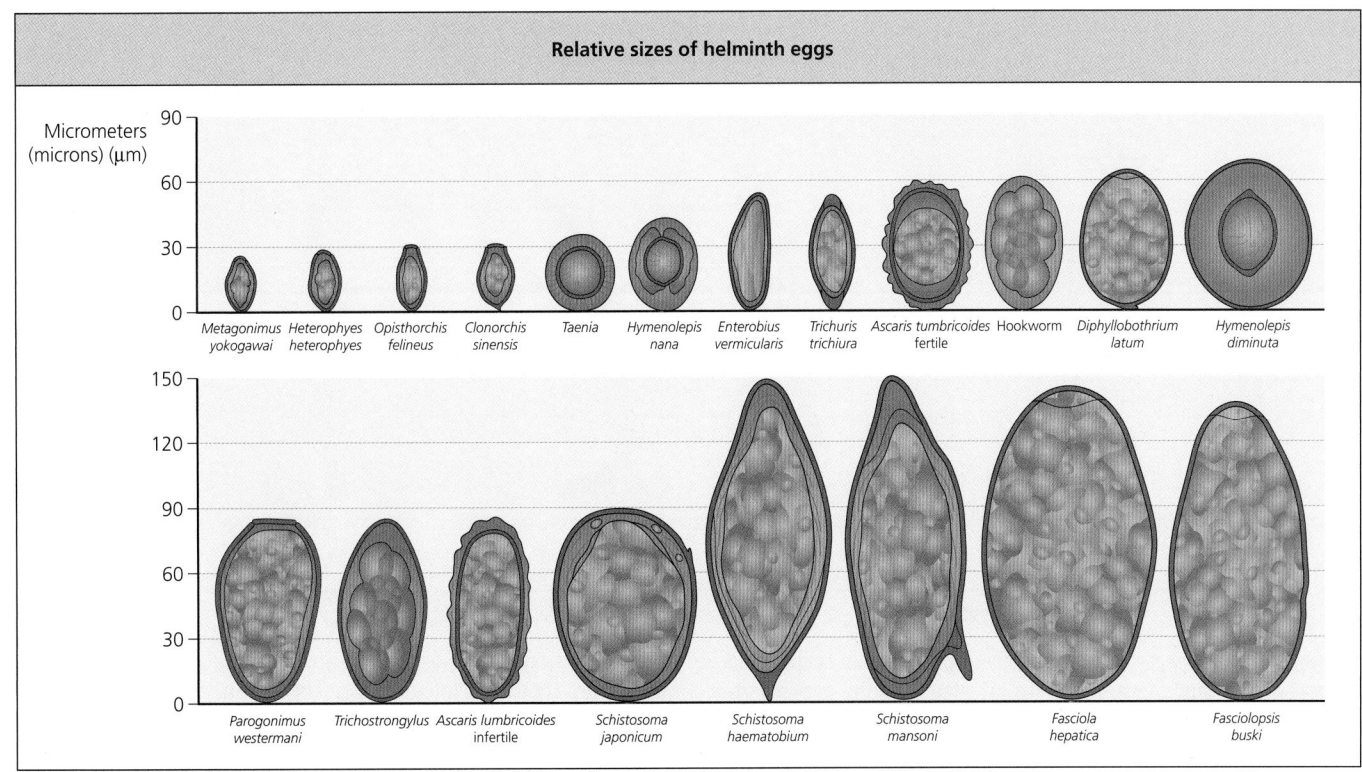

Figure 195-6 Relative sizes of helminth eggs. *(HHS Publication No. CDC 89–8116.)*

parasites in the circulatory system, and urine and sputum are examined for worms in the genitourinary systems and respiratory passages, respectively. Tissue parasites are diagnosed by biopsies and by immunologic methods. Many techniques have been developed to aid in the diagnosis and most of these have been presented in detail.[31] A variety of molecular and antibody techniques have been developed, however the availability of these may be limited to referral laboratories.

STOOL SPECIMENS

Intestinal parasites are detected by microscopic examination of preferably more than one stool specimen.[32] Stools should be collected in clean, dry containers and examined as soon as possible after being passed. Direct examination is made by making wet films on a clean microscope slide. A small portion of feces is mixed with a drop of saline on the slide and examined under low power (100×) and high power (450×) magnification if needed. The preparation should be thin enough to read newsprint through. Iodine stain preparations can also be used, but are more valuable for the examination of specimens for protozoa, and may obscure observations of the morphological details of helminth eggs and larvae. If a stool specimen cannot be examined within a few hours after passage, it should be placed in 10% v/v formalin or another preservative and the examination undertaken at a more convenient time.

Concentration techniques are available. The simplest is sedimentation of feces in a tube or sedimentation flask with the sediment examined microscopically. The formalin-ethyl acetate technique, in which stool is mixed with saline and passed through a gauze or screen, is also widely used. Sieved material is collected and centrifuged several times in saline, and finally in formalin. Ethyl acetate is added and the preparation centrifuged slowly. The detritus layer and supernatant are poured off and the sediment examined microscopically. The zinc sulfate flotation method is another technique in which small samples of feces are mixed thoroughly with zinc sulfate (made to a specific gravity of 1.18 for fresh, or 1.2 for formalinized stools). This is centrifuged or permitted to stand for a time and the surface fluid examined for eggs. This method is unsatisfactory for operculated eggs, however.

Eggs from various helminths as well as larvae of hookworms and the *Strongyloides* spp. are depicted in Figures 195-6 and 195-7.

The Kato–Katz technique is used to estimate the number of eggs in feces. Screened feces are placed into a small hole on a template which delivers 41.7 mg of feces onto a microscope slide. A Cellophane square soaked in glycerine-malachite green dye is placed over the feces and the preparation is incubated for 30–60 minutes. The glycerine clears the fecal material, and eggs can be seen against a green background. This technique is especially good for thick-shelled eggs such as *A. lumbricoides*, *T. trichiura* and *S. mansoni*. The preparation should be examined within 30 minutes for thin-shelled eggs like hookworms, which may dissolve if they stand for too long. The number of eggs is multiplied by 24 to obtain the number of eggs/g of feces. The Kato method uses only the glycerine soaked Cellophane and is not quantitative.

Fecal cultures can be used to recover nematode larvae, especially hookworms and *Strongyloides* spp. Feces are mixed with moist charcoal and placed into a Petri dish with moist filter paper lining the bottom and incubated at room temperature for several days. Larvae migrate to the surface of the charcoal. The culture is placed into a Baermann apparatus, a funnel with rubber tubing attached to the stem and a pinch clamp closing the tube. A sieve is placed in the top of the funnel and lined with gauze. The funnel is filled with warm water, and the culture placed into the gauze, the apparatus is incubated at room temperature for 10–12 hours and fluid drawn off through the tubing. Larvae can be collected from the fluid and examined microscopically to determine the species.

The Harada–Mori technique is used to culture feces and recover larvae. Filter paper strips are coated on one side with feces and placed into a tube containing a small amount of water. The tube is kept upright so the filter paper is kept moist by capillary action. After 4–10 days, the filter paper is removed and the water examined for larvae.

Agar plate culture is available for *Strongyloides* spp.[33] A few grams of feces are placed into the center of the agar and the plate incubated at room temperature for 48 hours. Tracks are made by the larvae in the agar and larvae can be recovered by a Pasteur pipette for microscopic identification.

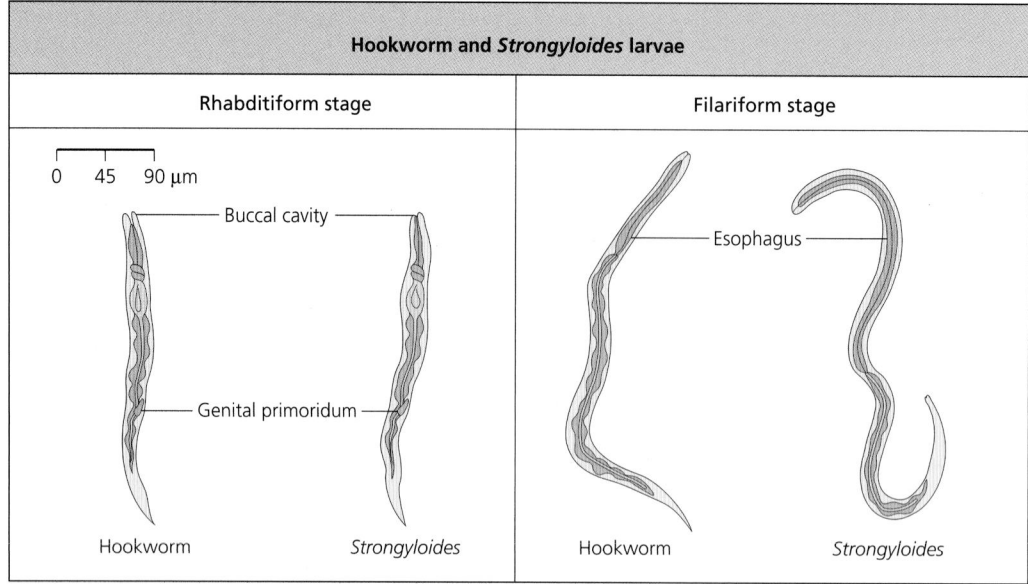

Figure 195-7 Hookworm and *Strongyloides* larvae. (HHS Publication No. CDC 89–8116.)

Some parasites' eggs can be picked up on perianal swabs. Swabs such as Scotch tape or paddle swabs are placed on the perianal area and then examined under a microscope. Pinworm, tapeworm and *A. lumbricoides* eggs can be recovered in this manner.

Schistosome eggs can be found in feces using some of the above-mentioned examination techniques. An egg-hatching technique can also be used in which feces are placed into a sidearm flask and water added until it reaches a level just below the sidearm. When the suspension settles, more water is added until the level is above the sidearm. A dark cloth or bag is placed over the flask without covering the sidearm. The sidearm is then placed into the light, and hatching miracidia from the schistosome eggs will be attracted to the light. They can be examined microscopically.

Material collected by duodenal aspiration can be examined microscopically for *Strongyloides* spp., *Ascaris* spp. and flukes. The Entero-Test or string capsule is a device for examining duodenal specimens. A gelatin capsule containing a string is swallowed and the end of the string taped to the cheek. The weighted string carries down the duodenum after the capsule dissolves. After 4 hours the string is pulled up and the mucus adhering to the string is examined microscopically.

Flatworms in the stool, tapeworm proglottids and adult trematodes should be collected, washed in water and placed between two microscope slides. The slides are tied together with string and specimens placed into a fixative – alcohol, formalin, acetic acid (AFA). After fixation the worms can be stained and examined for identification. India ink can be injected into the uterine pore of tapeworm proglottids to enhance visualization. Tapeworm proglottids with rosette-shaped uterine branches, are identified as a diphyllabothriid. Counting the uterine branches of *Taenia* spp. will identify *T. solium* (6–11 branches) and *T. saginata* (15–20 branches). Trematodes may be stained for examination.

SPUTUM SPECIMENS

Sputum to be examined for eggs or larvae should be mixed with 3% v/v sodium hydroxide, centrifuged, and the sediment examined.

URINE SPECIMENS

Urine specimens will sometimes help in the diagnosis of *S. haematobium* eggs or microfilariae of *W. bancrofti* and *O. volvulus*. The urine specimen is centrifuged and the sediment examined.

BLOOD SAMPLES

Several of the filarial infections can be diagnosed by the examination of drops of blood from the finger or ear lobe. The blood is placed onto a microscope slide covered with a coverglass and examined under low power for thrashing microfilariae. For specific identification, thick blood smears are made with several drops of blood, dried for several hours, and stained with Giemsa stain. Identifications are based upon, for example, microfilarial sizes, cephalic space and tail nuclei. Microfilariae of *W. bancrofti*, *B. malayi*, *B. timori* and *L. loa* are present in the blood. *O. volvulus* microfilariae are found in skin snips.

Blood should be obtained at night for most lymphatic filariae and in the daytime for *L. loa*. Microfilariae can be recovered from the blood by membrane filtration, or by quantitative buffy coat analysis tubes containing a fluorescent dye. In some cases of lymphatic filariasis adult worms may be seen by ultrasound and the worms can be seen 'dancing' in the lymph channels.[34]

CEREBROSPINAL FLUID

Cerebrospinal fluid is examined for evidence of helminth infections. Eosinophilic pleocystosis is suggestive of angiostrongyliasis, paragonimiasis, cysticercosis, gnathostomiasis and schistosomiasis. Larvae of *A. cantonensis* are reported in CSF, especially in children, and *T. spiralis* larvae can be found in the CSF in very heavy infections. The CSF is centrifuged and the sediment examined for evidence of a helminth infection.

TISSUE SPECIMENS

Tissue specimens may be taken and examined for helminth infections. Muscle biopsies can be sectioned and stained, or pressed between two microscope slides and examined microscopically for *T. spiralis* larvae. Rectal and bladder biopsy specimens can be examined for schistosome eggs. Skin biopsies may reveal microfilariae of *O. volvulus*. Fluid from suspected hydatid cysts, although dangerous to obtain, may reveal scolices of *E. granulosus*. Biopsies can be made when anticipating a diagnosis of migrating helminths, including gnathostomiasis and sparganosis.

IMMUNODIAGNOSTIC AND MOLECULAR TESTS

There are a myriad of immunodiagnostic and molecular tests available to aid in diagnosis of helminth infections. Some are presumptive, and in many cases finding worms, eggs or larvae provides the definitive diagnosis. Immunodiagnostic and molecular tests are particularly useful when the parasite is not demonstrated, such as in cases of toxocariasis, baylisascariasis, cysticercosis and echinococcosis. Immunodiagnostic and molecular techniques are promising tools for the diagnosis of helminth diseases but often have not been commercialized, are experimental, or are limited to laboratory, rather than field use.[35]

There are immunodiagnostic tests to detect antibodies and parasite antigens. Tests such as complement fixation are still of value in the diagnosis of cysticercosis, paragonimiasis and schistosomiasis, especially for indication of active infections. Gel diffusion has been used in fascioliasis and the circumoval precipitation test (COPT) is used to detect antibodies in schistosomiasis. In the latter, precipitates develop around the eggs of schistosomes in the presence of antibody-positive sera.

The enzyme-linked immunosorbent assay (ELISA) has been widely used for many parasitoses. Indirect immunofluorescent antibody staining is also helpful for microscopic identification, especially in tissue sections to detect antigens of the parasites. Indirect hemagglutination along with enzyme immunoassay (EIA) is used for hydatid disease, and EIA tests are used for many parasites. Lateral flow chromatographic assays have also been developed for a variety of nematodes.

Molecular analyses have been developed for almost all helminths of human disease significance, including polymerase chain reaction (PCR) assays, quantitative 'qPCR' assays, fluorescent in-situ hybridization tests (FISH) to facilitate visualization in microscopic specimens, and other types of assay. There are, for instance, multiple DNA-based assays for *B. malayi*.[36]

Clinical Manifestations

An intestinal helminthiasis is usually unnoticed unless a large worm is found by the patient in the feces.

PINWORMS

Pinworms generally cause little disease. In children infections lead to perianal itching, eczema, nose picking, pica and loss of sleep. Pinworms can be responsible for recurrent urinary tract infections in young girls when worms migrate into the vagina, uterus and fallopian tubes and peritoneal cavity.

ASCARIASIS

The migration of worms, for example *Ascaris* spp., through the lung during the developmental cycle causes Loeffler's syndrome (simple pulmonary eosinophilia, with wheezing, coughing, and other pulmonary symptoms).

Ascariasis is innocuous unless the worms become erratic and migrate into vital organs, or pass through one of the orifices – nose, mouth or anus. Erratic ascariasis may be caused by anesthesia, trauma or medication. A bolus of a large number of worms can cause volvulus or intussusception, blockage of the bile ducts, cholangitis, intestinal perforation, abdominal distress, pneumonitis and cough. Infection is often associated with malnutrition and decreased growth.

TRICHURIASIS

Severe trichuriasis can lead to abdominal discomfort, dysentery, colitis, anemia and bloody stools. There may be nutritional loss, weight loss and malnutrition. Rectal prolapse occurs with some infections.

HOOKWORM

Hookworm larvae entering the skin may provoke a ground itch, secondary bacterial infections and Loeffler's syndrome when larvae migrate through the lungs. Worms in the intestines can cause abdominal pain, nausea, vomiting and diarrhea. Large numbers of worms sucking blood cause iron deficiency anemia, hypoproteinemia and hepatosplenomegaly, and in children, impaired mental, physical and sexual development. Severe malnutrition develops, especially with concomitant infections with *A. lumbricoides*, and *T. trichiura*.

TOXOCARIASIS

Toxocariasis (visceral larva migrans) causes hypereosinophilia, hepatomegaly and symptoms of chronic pulmonary inflammation with cough. There may also be visual difficulties due to retinochoroiditis or peripheral retinitis.

BAYLISASCARIASIS

Baylisascariasis generally presents as acute fulminant eosinophilic meningoencephalitis, or less often, as an acute retinitis. The disease is often fatal or has severe sequelae, such as neurological deficit, blindness, or other severe symptoms of neurological trauma.

STRONGYLOIDIASIS

Early infections with *S. stercoralis* are similar to hookworm, causing ground itch and pneumonitis. Loeffler's syndrome may be present when larvae migrate through the lungs. Worms in the intestines cause inflammation, irritation, diarrhea, intestinal bleeding and melena. Sprue-like symptoms may develop, along with malabsorption, weight loss and eosinophilia. Dermal lesions may occur with urticarial eruptions on the buttocks, termed larva currens. Immunocompromised people, especially those with human T-cell leukemia virus 1 (HTLV-1) associated lymphoma, are at risk of developing disseminated strongyloidiasis and present with severe enteritis, a protein-losing enteropathy, bronchitis, pneumonia, pleural effusion, cough and a blood-tinged sputum with rhabditiform larvae; this is often referred to as the 'hyperinfection syndrome'. Eosinophilia is usually absent in these cases. Death may result. Disseminated strongyloidiasis may present as gram-negative pneumonia or meningitis, or as a polymicrobial bacteremia, with bacteria spread by worms migrating from the bowel.

CAPILLARIASIS

Capillariasis leads to a protein-losing enteropathy, malabsorption, electrolyte imbalance, weight loss, wasting and death. Patients initially present with abdominal pain, borborygmi and diarrhea. Untreated infections usually lead to death.[24]

TRICHINOSIS

Trichinosis is asymptomatic except when a large number of trichina larvae are ingested. Adult worms in the small intestine cause symptoms of gastroenteritis, nausea, abdominal pain, anorexia, diarrhea, fever and weight loss. During the migratory phase, muscle and joint pain develop, followed by periorbital edema and eosinophilia. Larvae can cause cell destruction, acute inflammatory changes and interstitial myocarditis. The infection can also cause neurologic and pulmonary complications.

LYMPHATIC FILARIASIS (see Chapter 121)

Symptoms associated with lymphatic filariasis are associated with the host's immune status; little immunity is associated with more severe disease. Early symptoms are fever, lymphangitis, lymphedema and lymphadenitis, which may be transitory and occur periodically. Scrotal involvement leads to orchitis, hydrocele and chyluria. Worms may block the lymph flow leading to lymphatic varicoses and eventual skin fibrosis, thickening and elephantiasis. Renal lesions may occur, with microfilariae in the urine and chyluria. There may be enlargement of the legs, arms, scrotum, mammary glands and vulva. Tropical pulmonary eosinophilia with fever, splenomegaly, pulmonary infiltrates and hypereosinophilia (Weingarten's syndrome) is associated with *W. bancrofti* and *B. malayi* infections. Microfilariae are absent in chronic infections.

Subcutaneous migration of *L. loa* may cause transient Calabar swellings, a local reaction to the worm and its secretory products. It is characterized by fever, eosinophilia and urticarial swellings, which are more common in Caucasians. Migrating adult worms may pass over the bridge of the nose or through the conjunctiva across the eyeball. Migration of the worms in abnormal locations can cause symptoms in the scrotum, bowel, kidney and heart, but not usually in natives living in the African endemic areas. Visitors suffer more than indigenous populations.

Onchocercomas due to *O. volvulus* develop over bony prominences. Some nodules develop in deeper tissue and are unnoticeable. Dermatitis and blindness are caused by the microfilariae. The inflammatory response in the eye may be induced by the endosymbiotic bacteria

Wolbachia spp. released by dead microfilariae.[37] Lymph nodes in the groin may show lymphocyte depletion and fibrosis, followed by 'hanging groin', especially in Africans from endemic areas. In the Americas, nodules commonly develop on the upper part of the body, whereas in Africa the nodules develop on the lower parts of the body.

GUINEA WORM/DRACUNCULIASIS

Guinea worm in the subcutaneous tissue elicits allergic manifestations such as itching. When the female worms get close to the skin there is a localized erythema followed by pruritus, nausea, vomiting, diarrhea, or asthmatic symptoms. The worm will secrete a toxic substance that causes a blister, which breaks when the area comes in contact with water and the female releases larvae when the lesion opens up. The area becomes painful. The worm dies and is resorbed or becomes calcified.

ANGIOSTRONGYLIASIS

Migrating third-stage larvae of *A. cantonensis* may cause vague symptoms of gastroenteritis, vomiting, headache and fever. Once the worms reach the CNS they cause headache, nausea, vomiting, stiff neck, myalgia, pain and paresthesia. Coma may be a feature of heavy infections. Worms have been seen in the eyes of some patients. There may be paralysis of eye muscles. Frequent signs are abnormal tendon reflexes including abnormal Achilles' reflex, a positive Kernig's sign (a sign of meningitis, pain when extending the knee if the hip is bent) and impaired sensorium and vision. Infections with a large number of worms may be fatal.[38]

Abdominal angiostrongyliasis due to *A. costaricensis* resembles acute appendicitis. A tumor-like mass is palpable in the right lower quadrant. There may be fever, diarrhea or vomiting along with eosinophilia.[39]

GNATHOSTOME AND ANISAKID LARVAE

Shortly after ingestion of gnathostome larvae there is nausea, vomiting, pruritus and urticaria, and at times upper abdominal pain. Larval invasion into the liver will cause right upper quadrant tenderness and changes in liver function. In the lung there is a pulmonary infiltration and pneumothorax in patients with pleural effusion. Larvae migrating through the subcutaneous tissue and skin cause a rash along with red pruritic painless swellings. Invasion of the CNS often leads to death.

Anisakid larvae in the throat may lead to a 'tickle-throat', causing cough, but when they invade the mucosa of the intestinal tract they provoke eosinophilic granuloma formation, severe abdominal pain, nausea, vomiting and diarrhea. Usually, only a single worm is involved and the symptoms disappear when it is removed.

TREMATODES

The trematodes, like the nematodes, cause little disease unless a large number of worms are involved. Liver flukes (*C. sinensis, O. viverini, O. felineus*) in the bile ducts may cause symptoms early in the infection such as hepatomegaly, jaundice, diarrhea, anorexia, epigastric pain and fever. Repeated infection over a period of years may lead to ductal fibrosis, obstruction, cholangitis, cholecystitis and cirrhosis, and in some patients cholangiocarcinoma.[40]

The sheep liver fluke *F. hepatica*, because of its large size, may block the bile ducts and cause cholangitis. Toxic secretions cause fever, chills, jaundice, an enlarged tender liver, cough, vomiting, abdominal symptoms and eosinophilia. Young worms may attack the pharyngeal mucosa, causing bleeding and edema. This occurs after eating raw sheep liver containing the parasite. This condition has been called halzoun.

Large numbers of the large intestinal fluke *F. buski* may cause intestinal blockage and toxemia. Eosinophilia is common and ulcers may develop, which often hemorrhage. It causes abdominal distention, hunger pangs and increased appetite, diarrhea and a foul-smelling yellowish stool. Allergic manifestations, nausea, vomiting, ascites and cachexia develop as a result of toxins secreted by the worms. Other intestinal flukes cause little disease, but tiny eggs of the heterophyids may enter the mucosa and be carried to ectopic locations such as the brain and heart provoking granuloma formation. Echinostomes may produce inflammation and ulceration with diarrhea and abdominal pain.

The young lung fluke of *P. westermani* produces little disease during migration, but once established in the lung may cause fever, dyspnea, cough, chest pain and the production of a rusty sputum. At first the disease is often thought to be tuberculosis. Worms may enter the cranial cavity and invade the brain causing fever, headache, nausea, vomiting and visual disturbances, convulsions and meningeal signs.

SCHISTOSOME INFECTIONS (see Chapter 118)

There may be petechial hemorrhages at the site of penetration where schistosome cercariae enter the skin. There will be localized edema and pruritus. After a few weeks there are toxic or allergic reactions and symptoms including fever, nausea, abdominal pain, rigor, urticarial rashes and eosinophilia. This acute stage is known as Katayama syndrome. In the chronic stage, granulomas have formed around the eggs, hepatomegaly develops and the spleen becomes enlarged. This is followed by esophageal varices and finally ascites. Intestinal disease, usually with *S. mansoni* and *S. japonicum*, may involve the entire intestine or more often the large bowel. There may be abdominal cramps, tenderness and bloody mucoid stools. A protein-losing enteropathy, weight loss and anemia may also develop.

Features of *S. haematobium* infection are dysuria, urinary frequency and hematuria. Eosinophils in the urine are not uncommon. Heavy infections, with the deposition of many eggs in the bladder tissue, can lead to squamous cell carcinoma. Pulmonary involvement can be a feature of all schistosome infections, and causes cor pulmonale with dyspnea, cough and hemoptysis.

Cerebral manifestations are common in oriental schistosomiasis (*S. japonicum* and *S. hematobium*), with symptoms of lethargy and confusion followed by speech difficulties and optical field defects. *Schistosoma mansoni* occasionally causes the spinal cord symptoms of transverse myelitis, usually in the lumbar region. Flaccid paralysis of the lower limbs is also reported.

TAPEWORM (see Chapter 119)

Tapeworms, even the larger ones, in the small intestine provoke few symptoms. A patient usually becomes aware of being infected when worm segments are passed in the feces. If *D. latum* attaches to the proximal portion of the jejunum, vitamin B12 deficiency may result leading to pernicious anemia, but this is now an exceptionally rare clinical presentation. Sparganosis associated with other diphyllobothriid species causes painful inflammatory swellings, which may be transient. The rare species of *Spirometra proliferium* causes proliferative sparganosis which is usually fatal. Spargana in the eyes cause intense reactions and periorbital edema.

Intestinal *Taenia* spp. are asymptomatic in most patients, but some have hunger pangs, abdominal discomfort and indigestion. Patients usually become symptomatic when proglottids are found in the feces or passing from the anus. Eosinophilia is not uncommon. Cysticercosis, or infection with *T. solium* larvae, is a serious disease, especially if cysticerci are in the CNS. Cysticerci in muscle are asymptomatic, but can give rise to myositis, fever and eosinophilia. Cysticerci usually die and become calcified. Cysticerci in the eye cause visual symptoms such as a decrease in visual acuity, retinal edema and hemorrhage. Neurocysticercosis results in arachnoiditis with CSF pleocytosis and an increase in CSF pressure. Obstructive hydrocephalus, cerebral infarction, epilepsy, papilledema, vomiting, headache, a toxic gait and cognitive deterioration may also develop. Dead or dying parasites may exacerbate symptoms. The location of the parasite in the CNS is responsible for a variety of CNS symptoms.

Hyperinfections with *H. nana* may cause diarrhea, loss of appetite, abdominal pain, headache, weakness, and at times epileptoid convulsion, dizziness and eosinophilia. *H. diminuta* may cause diarrhea.

Hydatid Disease

There are usually no symptoms with hydatid disease until, after years, the cysts are large and in vital organs. Cysts in the liver may put pressure on bile ducts and blood vessels. Large cysts in the lung can cause coughing, shortness of breath and chest pains. Involvement of the CNS results in symptoms depending upon the location of the cyst. Leaks of hydatid fluid sensitize the patient and can cause anaphylactic shock. A cyst in the eye causes proptosis.

Management (see Chapters 119, 121 and 157)

Management of helminth infection is variable and depends upon the specific parasite, the location in the host and the number of worms involved.

References available online at expertconsult.com.

KEY REFERENCES

Ash L.R., Orihel T.C.: *Ash and Orhiel's atlas of human parasitology*, 5th ed. Chicago, IL: ASCP; 2007.

Cairncross S., Tayeh A., Korkor A.S.: Why is dracunculiasis eradication taking so long? *Trends Parasitol* 2012; 28(6):225-230.

Cross J.H.: Intestinal capillariasis. *Clin Microbiol Rev* 1992; 5(2):120-129.

Cross J.H.: Angyostrongyliasis. In: Murrell K.D., Fried B., eds. *Food-borne parasitic zoonoses: fish and plant-borne parasites. World Class Parasites Series*, vol. II. New York: Springer; 2007.

Dadzie Y., Neira M., Hopkins D.: Final report of the conference on the eradicability of onchocerciasis. *Filaria J* 2003; 2(1):2.

Enserink M.: Infectious diseases. Guinea worm eradication at risk in South Sudanese war. *Science* 2014; 343(6168):236.

Hung N.M., Madsen H., Fried B.: Global status of fish-borne zoonotic trematodiasis in humans. *Acta Parasitol* 2013; 58(3):231-258.

McCarthy J.S., Lustigman S., Yang G.J., et al.: A research agenda for helminth diseases of humans: diagnostics for control and elimination programmes. *PLoS Neglect Trop D* 2012; 6(4):1601.

Schar F., Trostdorf U., Giardina F., et al.: *Strongyloides stercoralis*: global distribution and risk factors. *PLoS Negl Trop Dis* 2013; 7(7):2288.

Sithithaworn P., Yongvanit P., Duenngai K., et al.: Roles of liver fluke infection as risk factor for cholangio-carcinoma. *J Hepatobiliary Pancreat Sci* 2014; 21(5):301-308.

Taylor M.J., Hoerauf A.: *Wolbachia* bacteria of filarial nematodes. *Parasitol Today* 1999; 15(11):437-442.

World Health Organization: *Control of foodborne trematode infections. Report of a WHO Study Group. World Health Organization Technical Report Series, No. 849*. Geneva: WHO; 1995:1-157.

World Health Organization: *Progress report 2008–2009 and strategic plan 2010–2020 of the global program to eliminate lymphatic filariasis*. Geneva: WHO; 2010.

Zoure H.G., Wanji S., Noma M., et al.: The geographic distribution of *Loa loa* in Africa: results of large-scale implementation of the Rapid Assessment Procedure for Loiasis (RAPLOA). *PLoS Neglect Trop D* 2011; 5(6):e1210.

INDEX

Page numbers followed by "*f*" indicate figures, "*b*" indicate boxes, and "*t*" indicate tables.

A

A-B toxins, 19, 19*t*
Abacavir, 1148*t*, 1299
  adverse reactions of, 921, 1299
  antiretroviral drugs, 920–921, 936–937
  chemical structure of, 1296*f*
  description of, 1299
  dosage of, 1299
    in special circumstances, 1297*t*, 1299
  drug interactions of, 1299
  indications of, 1299
  perinatal HIV transmission prevention, 909*t*
  pharmacokinetics and distribution of, 1299
  resistance to, 1299
  route of administration of, 1299
Abacavir hypersensitivity syndrome, 886–887
Abatacept, 798*t*–799*t*, 801
Abdominal abscess, fever of unknown origin, 611
Abdominal compartment syndrome, 358
Abdominal disease, in immune reconstitution
    inflammatory syndrome, 863
Abdominal infection
  anaerobic bacteria in, 1632*f*
  antimicrobial therapy for, 1641*t*
  following abdominal surgery, 690
  in intestinal transplant patients, 757
Abdominal lymphadenopathy, 145
Abdominal surgery, *Candida* spp. and, 1684
Abdominal symptoms, in schistosomiasis, 1029
Abiotrophia, 457
Abortion, spontaneous. *see* Spontaneous abortion.
Abscesses, 84–94, 85*t*
  abdominal, 611
  aerobic actinomycetes and, 1549
  amebic, 1729
  brain. *see* Brain abscesses
  buccal space, 313, 313*f*
  cutaneous, in HIV/AIDS, 858
  deep neck, 1636*t*
  epidemiology of, 84
  and fever of unknown origin, 611
  formation of, anaerobic bacteria in, 1633
  in HIV, 882–883
  in immunologically mediated diseases, 772,
    772*f*
  for laboratory diagnosis of mycobacteria, 1651*t*
  liver. *see* Liver abscess
  lung. *see* Lung abscesses
  paraspinal, 1099, 1100*f*
  pelvic, 497
  peritonsillar, 235, 1636*t*
  pleural, 263–270
  prostatic, 533, 535
  pyogenic liver, 361
  renal. *see* Renal abscess
  retropharyngeal, 314–315, 315*f*, 1636*t*
  soft tissue, in immune reconstitution inflammatory
    syndrome, 862
  specimen collection of, 1634*t*
  splenic, 361
  from *Stenotrophomonas maltophilia*, 1597
  submandibular, 313, 313*f*
  tubo-ovarian, 493–494
  vaginal cuff, 497
  vestibular, 313, 313*f*
Absidia, 1696
Acanthamoeba
  cultivation of, 1745
  diagnostic microbiology of, 1747
  epidemiology of, 1746
  granulomatous amebic encephalitis and, 1746
  life cycle of, 1745
  nature of, 1744–1745
  pathogenicity of, 1746

Acanthamoeba (Continued)
  prevention of, 1747
  and recreational infections, 645
  taxonomy of, 1745
  treatment of, 1345*t*–1351*t*
Acanthamoeba castellanii, 1745, 1745*f*
Acanthamoeba culbertsoni, 1748*f*
Acanthamoeba keratitis, 155
  diagnostic microbiology of, 1747
  features of, 1748–1749, 1749*f*
  management of, 1750
  pathogenicity of, 1746
  prevention of, 1747
  treatment of, 1345*t*–1351*t*
Accessory gene regulator *(agr)*, 1515
'Accessory' genes, 12
Acclimatization, 951–952
AccuProbe culture confirmation test, 1654
Acetamide, in *Pseudomonas* isolation, 1580
Acetaminophen, antipyretic action, 609
Acetazolamide, for altitude acclimatization, 951–952
Acetylcholine release inhibition, 209–210
Acetyltransferases, 1185, 1185*t*
Achlorhydria, 328
Achromobacter, 1581*t*–1582*t*, 1597
Achromobacter xylosoxidans, nosocomial infections from,
  1588*t*
Aciclovir, 1146*t*–1147*t*, 1309–1312
  adverse reactions of, 1311
  dosage of, 1309–1310, 1310*t*
    in special circumstances, 1311, 1311*t*
  indications of, 1310–1311
    acute retinal necrosis syndrome, 172
    cercopithecine herpesvirus-1 (B virus), 1311
    chronic meningitis, 187*t*
    cytomegalovirus, 1311
    encephalitis, 197
    Epstein-Barr virus, 1311
    genital herpes, 569–570, 572–573, 573*t*, 1310*t*
    herpes simplex virus, 515
    herpes zoster ophthalmicus, 154
    herpesvirus, 1433
    herpetic gingivostomatitis, 317
    HSV infections, 1310, 1310*t*
    varicella zoster virus, 515, 1310–1311
  in liver transplant patients, 754*t*
  mechanism of action, 1309, 1309*f*
  pharmacokinetics and distribution of, 1309
  resistance to, 1311–1312
  route of administration, 1309–1310
  in vitro activity, 1309
Acid-fast bacilli (AFB), in leprosy, 958
Acid-fast stain, for laboratory diagnosis, of mycobacteria,
  1652, 1652*f*
Acidaminococcus, 1631
Acidosis
  metabolic. *see* Metabolic acidosis
  in severe malaria, 1019, 1020*t*
Acidovorax, 1598
  nomenclature of, 1581*t*–1582*t*
  prevalence of, 1579
Acinetobacter, 1593–1595
  clinical manifestations of, 1594–1595
  diagnostic microbiology of, 1594, 1594*f*
  epidemiology of, 1590*t*, 1593–1595
  hospital-acquired pneumonia and, 258, 259*t*
  management and resistance of, 1595
  molecular epidemiology of, 1593–1594
  nature and taxonomy of, 1593, 1593*f*
  nomenclature of, 1581*t*–1582*t*
  pathogenicity and pathogenesis of, 1590*t*, 1594–1595
  resistance
    in burns, 698
    to carbapenems, 1184
    to polymyxin, 1193
  tigecycline susceptibility, decreased, 1190

Acinetobacter baumannii
  in burn wounds, 698
  carbapenem-resistant, 1196
  epidemiologic markers for, 1583*t*–1584*t*
  epidemiology of, 1590*t*
  nature and taxonomy of, 1593, 1593*f*
  nosocomial infections from, 1588*t*
  pathogenicity of, 1590*t*
  prevalence of, 1579
  resistance
    antimicrobial, 1592*t*
    intrinsic, 1182*t*
    to β-lactam, 1184
    to tigecycline, 1190
  virulence-associated factors of, 1585*t*
Acinetobacter calcoaceticus, 1593
Acinetobacter calcoaceticus-Acinetobacter baumannii (Acb)
  complex, 1593
Acinetobacter genomic species 6, 1594
Acinetobacter genomic species 15BJ, 1593
Acinetobacter genomic species 15TU, 1593
Acinetobacter johnsonii, 1593
Acinetobacter junii, 1593
Acinetobacter lwoffii, 1593
Acinetobacter radioresistens, 1593
Acitretin, for psoriasis, 880, 880*f*
Acquired epidermodysplasia verruciformis, 881
Acquired immunity
  defects of, in cancer patients, 725, 725*f*
  see also Immunity
Acquired immunodeficiency syndrome. *see* AIDS.
Acremonium spp., 159
Acridine, prion infection and, 220
Acridine orange leukocyte cytospin (AOLC), 433–434
Acrodermatitis chronicum atrophicans, 409
Acropapulovesicular syndrome, 81, 81*f*
Actin-based intracellular motility, of microbial pathogens,
  16–17, 18*f*
Actinomadura, 1550*t*
  in cutaneous and soft tissue infection, 1551
  diagnostic microbiology of, 1549
Actinomadura pelletieri, 1717
Actinomyces, 1630
  brain abscess and, 199
  in chronic meningitis, 186*t*
  hospital-acquired pneumonia and, 259*t*
  in human bites, 683*t*
  in normal flora, 312, 1632, 1632*t*
  susceptibility to antimicrobial agents, 1642*f*
Actinomyces israelii, 315, 490, 1630
Actinomyces naeslundii, 315, 1630
Actinomyces odontolyticus, 315
Actinomyces viscosis, 315
Actinomycetes
  aerobic, 1547–1552
  mycetoma and, 1714
  taxonomy of, 1547*t*
Actinomycineae, 1547*t*
Actinomycosis, 315–316, 316*f*
Activation-induced cytidine deaminase deficiency,
  720–721
Acute bacterial skin and skin structure infections
  (ABSSSI), 1382–1383
Acute chest syndrome, sickle cell anemia and, 1056
Acute disseminated encephalomyelitis (ADEM), 194
Acute exacerbations, of chronic obstructive pulmonary
  disease, antibiotics for, 310–311
Acute flaccid paralysis, 1411
Acute hepatitis B, 1421–1422
Acute hepatitis E, 1419–1420
Acute miliary tuberculosis, 117–118
Acute mountain sickness (AMS), 951–952
Acute osteomyelitis, 388–398
  clinical features of, 391
  management of, 395–396
    antibiotic therapy for, 395, 395*t*

Acute osteomyelitis *(Continued)*
  initial actions for, 395
  prognosis of, 396
  surgery in, 395–396
Acute-phase proteins, 608–609, 608*t*
Acute pneumonia, chronic pulmonary infections, 254*t*
Acute renal failure, as rifampin adverse effect, 1269
Acute respiratory distress syndrome (ARDS)
  blastomycosis in, 294, 294*f*
  coccidioidomycosis in, 296
  histoplasmosis in, 292
  in severe malaria, 1021
Acute response to injury, 684
Acute retinal necrosis (ARN) syndrome, 166–167, 173
Acute retroviral syndrome, 143
Adalimumab, 797, 798*t*–799*t*
  immunosuppression and, 1380*t*
Adaptive immunity, 26, 27*f*, 32–39
  antibodies, 34–37
  cellular immune responses, 32–34, 32*f*
  complement, 37–39
  versus innate immunity, 26*t*
Adefovir, 1146*t*–1147*t*
  for chronic hepatitis B, 1329
Adenoidectomy, 237
Adenosine deaminase (ADA), 718
  deficiency in, 718
  in tuberculosis, 277
Adenoviridae, 1396
Adenovirus vector vaccine, 832
Adenoviruses, 6, 1472–1474
  apoptosis, 19
  and bioterrorism, 671*t*
  bronchitis and, 244*t*
  causing lymphadenopathy, 137*t*–138*t*
  causing retinitis and uveitis, 168*t*
  clinical manifestations, 1473–1474
  croup and, 233
  cytopathic effect, 1473*f*
  diagnosis of, 339
  diagnostic microbiology, 1472–1473
  encephalitis/myelitis and, 194*t*
  enteric. see Enteric adenoviruses
  epidemiology, 1472
  in hematopoietic stem cell transplantation, 743, 743*t*
  hospital-acquired pneumonia and, 259*t*
  in intestinal transplant patient, 760
  management, 1474
  nature, 1472
  and occupational infections, 657*t*
  pathogenicity, 1472
  in pericarditis, 450
  prevention, 1472
  subgroup, serotype and major site of infection, 1472*t*
  in thoracic transplantation patients, 749
Adenylate cyclase toxin (ACT), 1612, 1613*t*
Adhesin A, 323
Adhesins
  afimbrial, 14
  bacterial, 13–14, 14*f*
Adjunctive treatment, community-acquired pneumonia and, 256
Administration sets, in catheter-related bloodstream infection (CRBSI), 432
Adrenal glands, 279
Adrenaline, nebulized, 230–231
Adult respiratory distress syndrome, in cancer patients, 727
Adult T-lymphocyte leukemia, and human T-lymphocyte leukemia virus-1, 1491
Adults
  conjunctivitis in, 150–151
  immunocompetent, uveitis in, 167–172
  lower respiratory tract infection in, 264*f*
Advenella spp., 1597
Adverse pregnancy outcome, *Mycoplasma hominis* in, 1664
Aedes aegypti
  distribution of, 1119, 1119*f*
  spread of, 943
Aedes albopictus, 110*f*, 943, 945
Aedes polynesiensis, 1765
Aerobic actinomycetes, 1547–1552, 1550*t*
  clinical manifestations and management of, 1551–1552
  diagnostic microbiology of, 1549–1551
  epidemiology of, 1549

Aerobic actinomycetes *(Continued)*
  nature of, 1547–1549
  pathogenicity of, 1549
Aerobic bacteria
  in cancer patients, 723*b*
  from cat bites, 659
  gram-positive bacilli, 1537–1552, 1537*f*
  in human bites, 682, 683*t*
  necrotizing fasciitis and, 96
  in pelvic inflammatory disease, 492*t*
Aerobic cultures, intraoperative, in prosthetic joint infection (PJI), 401
Aerobic infections, from dog bites, 656
Aeromonas
  bacterial enteritis, 336
  diagnosis of, 339
  diarrhea, 331, 335
  and drowning-associated infections, 680
Aeromonas hydrophila
  alligator bites, 663
  cellulitis and, 91
  primary (spontaneous) peritonitis, 359
Aeromonas veronii, 336
Afimbrial adhesins, 14
African tick bite fever (ATBF)
  clinical manifestations of, 1667, 1667*t*
  location of, 1092*t*–1093*t*
African trypanosomiasis, 119, 1761–1762
  clinical manifestations of, 1762
  diagnostic microbiology of, 1761–1762
  epidemiology of, 1761
  human, 966–970
    clinical features of, 968
    diagnosis of, 968–969
    differential diagnosis of, 969
    epidemiology of, 966, 966*f*–968*f*, 967*t*
    laboratory methods of, 969
    management of, 969–970, 969*t*
    meningoencephalitis and, 968
    parasitologic, 969
    pathogenesis of, 966
    post-treatment follow-up of, 970
    prevention of, 966–967
  lymphadenopathy and, 137*t*–138*t*, 142
  management of, 1762
  nature of, 1761
  pathogenicity of, 1761, 1761*f*
  prevention of, 1761
Agammaglobulinemia
  autosomal recessive, 720
  X-linked, 719–720, 719*b*
Agar, antioxidant-supplemented, 1386
Agar proportion method, for mycobacteria, 1656
Age
  and endemic treponematoses, 961
  β-lactam antibiotics dosage and, 1212
  role of, in lymphadenopathy, 144
Aggregatibacter actinomycetemcomitans, 1622
Aggregatibacter aphrophilus, 1622
Aging HIV-positive patient, issues in, 927–930
  additional management considerations in, 930
  cancer in, 929–930
  cardiovascular disease in, 927–929
  fractures in, 929, 929*t*
  morbidity in, 927, 928*f*
  neurocognitive dysfunction in, 930
  osteoporosis in, 929
  percentage of, 928*f*
  renal dysfunction in, 930
Agriculture, parasites and, 990
Agrobacterium, 1581*t*–1582*t*, 1599
Aichi virus, 338
AIDS
  blastomycosis and, 1703
  burden of disease, 940
  Candida infection and, 444
  cryptosporidiosis in, 1742
  deep cervical space infection, 315
  geographic distribution of, 815–819
    Asia and the Pacific, 817–819, 818*f*
    Europe and Central Asia, 816–817, 817*f*
    Latin America and the Caribbean, 819
    Middle East and North Africa, 819, 819*f*
    North America, Australia, and New Zealand, 815–816, 816*f*

AIDS *(Continued)*
    sub-Saharan Africa, 817
  global response to, 819–823
    antiretroviral therapy for prevention among HIV-positives, 820
    HIV testing and counseling, 821–823, 822*f*
    pre-exposure prophylaxis for HIV-negatives, 820–821
    prevention of mother-to-child transmission in, 821, 821*f*
    treatment scale-up in, 819–820, 819*f*–820*f*
    voluntary medical male circumcision, 821, 822*f*
  histoplasmosis and, 292
  human papillomavirus and, 579
  in low and middle-income countries, 888–895
    clinical features of, 888–893, 889*f*
  lymphadenopathy and, 137*t*–138*t*
  myocarditis and, 448–449
  nocardiosis incidence in, 1549
  pericarditis and, 452
  progressive outer retinal necrosis, 173
  seborrheic dermatitis and, 128
  superficial fungal infections in, 126
  toxoplasmosis in, 1755*f*
  uveitis and, 173
  varicella-zoster epithelial keratitis, 154
  in women, 905
AIDS dementia complex, 227
AIDSVAX trials, 832
Airborne precautions, 59–60, 59*b*
Airway devices, hospital-acquired pneumonia and, 262
Alanine aminotransferase (ALT), for viral hemorrhagic fevers, 1116–1117
Albendazole
  for cysticercosis, 1035
  for echinococcosis, 1045
  for eosinophilia, 988
  for filariasis, 1050–1051
  for gastrointestinal helminth, 1000, 1001*t*
  for gastrointestinal protozoa, 1000*t*
  for helminths, 1772
  for liver flukes, 1036
  for microsporidiosis, 1742
  for parasitic infections, 1345*t*–1362*t*, 1370
  for schistosomiasis, 1029
Alberta Medical Association guideline, 231*f*
Albumin, in sepsis, 420
Alcaligenes, 1597
  nomenclature of, 1581*t*–1582*t*
  nosocomial infections from, 1588*t*
  prevalence of, 1579
Alcaligenes faecalis, 1597
Alcaligenes xylosoxidans, 1597
Alcoholic cirrhosis, and fever of unknown origin, 614–618
Alemtuzumab, 725, 1380*t*
'Algid malaria', 1021
Alginate, 1586
Alkylaminocyclines, 1168–1169
  bacterial targeting, 1168, 1171*f*
  chemical structure of, 1168, 1170*f*
  mode of action of, 1168
  pharmacodynamics of, 1169
  resistance to, 1168–1169
Alkylating agents, 1379
Allergic bronchopulmonary aspergillosis (ABPA), 245*t*, 1687, 1689, 1690*f*
Allergic conditions, eosinophilia and, 984*t*
Allergic reactions, 658–659
  diffuse folliculitis, 91
  of folate inhibitors, 1283
  β-lactam antibiotics, 1212–1215
  in vaginitis, 489
Alligator bites, 663
Alloimmune neonatal neutropenia, 706
Alpha toxin, 1633
Alphaviruses
  and bioterrorism, 671*t*
  infections caused by, 1495*t*
  viral exanthems, 75*t*
Alternaria, 1721
Alveolar septa, necrosis of, 1586*f*, 1587
Amantadine, 1146*t*–1147*t*, 1318
  adverse reactions and interactions of, 1318
  indications of, 1318
  pharmacokinetics and distribution of, 1318, 1320*t*
  resistance to, 1318
  route of administration and dosage of, 1318

Amblyomma americanum tick, 408
Amblyomma variegatum
  female, 105*f*
  male, 105*f*
Amebae
  epidemiology of, 1725–1727
  free-living, 1744–1750
  gastrointestinal, 989*t*
  identification in fecal specimens, 1728–1729
  intestinal and urogenital, 1725–1733, 1725*t*
  nature of, 1725
Amebiasis
  chronic diarrhea and, 348
  clinical features of, 995
  diagnostic microbiology of, 1729
  extraintestinal, clinical features of, 995–996
  intestinal, 1010, 1010*f*, 1010*t. see also* Amebic colitis;
      Amebic dysentery; Amebic peritonitis
    clinical features of, 995
    pathogenesis and pathology of, 990–991
  management of, 1000*t*, 1345*t*–1351*t*
  prevention of, 1727
Amebic abscesses, 1729
  see also specific locations
Amebic colitis, 1008*f*
  clinical features of, 1010, 1010*t*
  diagnosis of, 1011, 1011*f*–1012*f*
  Entamoeba histolytica in, 1726
  fulminant, 1012
  pathogenicity of, 1728
Amebic dysentery, 1008
  clinical features of, 1010
  treatment of, 997
Amebic infections, 1008–1013, 1008*f*–1009*f*
  clinical features of, 1009–1011
  diagnosis of, 1011–1012
  epidemiology of, 1009
  management of, 1012–1013
  pathogenesis of, 1009
  transmission and prevention of, 1009
Amebic meningoencephalitis, treatment of, 1345*t*–1351*t*
Amebic peritonitis, 1010
Amebicides, 1012
Ameboma, 1012
American Society of Anesthesiologists (ASA), physical
      status score, 686*t*, 687
American trypanosomiasis. *see* Chagas disease.
Amikacin
  background of, 1233
  for cancer patients, 734–735
  against carbapenemase-resistant gram-negative bacilli,
      1290*t*
  for catheter-related bloodstream infection (CRBSI),
      436*t*
  clinical use of, 1234
  for complicated urinary tract infection, 545*t*
  endophthalmitis and, 162
  hospital-acquired pneumonia and, 261
  for mycetoma, 1723
  for nocardiosis, 1551
  pharmacokinetic parameters for, 1234*t*
  resistance, 1185–1186
Amikacin-kanamycin, resistance to, mycobacterial, 1656*t*
Aminoglycoside-modifying enzymes, 1168, 1170*f*
Aminoglycosides, 1168, 1233–1238
  for *Acinetobacter baumannii*, 1590*t*
  adverse reactions of, 1153
  for *Alcaligenes* spp., 1597
  in antibiotic-impregnated cement, 1237
  as antituberculosis agents, 1270
  for *Bacillus cereus*, 1542
  for bacteremia, 1236–1237
  bacterial targeting, 1168
  for brucellosis, 1100
  for cancer patients, 735
  chemical structure of, 1168, 1169*f*
  clinical indications of, 1236–1237
  clinical pharmacology of, 1234–1236
  clinical use of, 1234
  for cystic fibrosis, 301, 1237
  dosing regimens, 1234–1235, 1235*t*
  endophthalmitis and, 162
  for gynecologic infections, 497

Aminoglycosides *(Continued)*
  for intra-abdominal infections, 1237
  intra-abdominal sepsis, 357–358
  keratitis and, 152
  for *Listeria monocytogenes*, 1540
  for lung abscess, 269*f*
  mechanism of action, 1233
  microbiologic activity, 1233–1234
  mode of action of, 1168
  for mycobacterial infections, 1237
  for *Mycobacterium avium* complex, 856
  for pelvic inflammatory disease, 493–494
  pharmacodynamics of, 1168
  for pneumonia, 1237
  for postpartum endometritis, 495
  in prophylaxis, 1237
  for prostatitis, 535
  for prosthetic joint infection (PJI), 402
  for *Pseudomonas aeruginosa*, 1589, 1590*t*
  for pyelonephritis, 552
  resistance to, 1168, 1185–1186, 1185*t*, 1234, 1592*t*
      Erysipelothrix rhusiopathiae, 1542
  for *Rhodococcus equi*, 1551
  for special populations, 1235
  spectrum of activity, 1233–1234
  for *Staphylococcus aureus*, 1520–1521
  toxicity of, 1235–1236, 1235*t*
  for tularemia, 1089, 1617
  for urinary tract infections, 1237
  see also individual drugs
Aminopenicillins
  antimicrobial spectrum, generic names, routes of
      administration and dosages, 1206*t*–1207*t*
  for staphylococcal infections, 1209
  use of, 1203
Aminopeptidase *N* (APN), 1474
Aminosidine. *see* Paromomycin.
Amodiaquine
  for falciparum malaria, 1022
  for malaria in pregnancy, 1143*t*
  for protozoal infections, 1352*t*–1362*t*, 1364
Amoebal keratitis, 175
Amoebozoa, 1744
Amorolfine, 128
Amoxicillin
  for actinomycosis, 316
  for anaerobic bacteria, 1642
  antimicrobial spectrum, routes of administration and
      dosages, 1206*t*–1207*t*
  for bronchitis, 248
  for cholera, 1607
  for complicated urinary tract infection, 544*t*
  for cystitis, 528*t*
  dosage in renal failure, 1213*t*–1214*t*
  for *Helicobacter pylori*, 326–327
  for leptospirosis, 1609
  for lung abscess, 269*f*
  for Lyme disease, 412
  for otitis media, 237
  for pharyngitis, 235
  for pneumococcal infections, 1209
  prophylaxis with, for postsplenectomy sepsis, 777
  in rheumatic fever, 476
    prophylaxis of, 475*t*
  for sinusitis, 241
  susceptibilities of selected bacteria to, 1208*t*–1209*t*
Amoxicillin-clavulanate
  for complicated urinary tract infection, 544*t*
  for cystitis, 528*t*
  for dog bites, 657*t*
  dosage in renal failure, 1213*t*–1214*t*
  for foot ulcers, 131*t*
  for human bites, 683
  for lung abscess, 269*f*
  otitis media and, 237
  pharmacokinetics of, 1205*t*
  susceptibilities of selected bacteria to, 1208*t*–1209*t*
Amoxicillin-clavulanic acid
  antimicrobial spectrum, routes of administration and
      dosages, 1206*t*–1207*t*
  bronchitis and, 244
  for cancer patients, 735–736
  intra-abdominal sepsis, 357

Amphibians, infections from, 661–662, 669
Amphotericin, for leishmaniasis, 1064
Amphotericin B
  for aspergillosis, 1691
  for basidiobolomycosis, 1723
  for blastomycosis, 295, 1703
  for *Candida* infection, 444–445
  for catheter-related bloodstream infection (CRBSI),
      436*t*
  for chromoblastomycosis, 1722
  for chronic meningitis, 187*t*
  for coccidioidomycosis, 1705–1706
  for conidiobolomycosis, 1723
  for cryptococcosis, 1695, 1695*t*
  for endophthalmitis, 162–163
  for fungal infections in HIV/AIDS, 855
  for fungal urinary tract infection, 545*t*
  for fusariosis, 1700
  for histoplasmosis, 294, 1708
  for keratitis, 154
  for leishmaniasis, 1758
  in liver transplant patients, 754*t*
  for mucormycosis, 1698
  for oropharyngeal candidiasis, 1684
  for paracoccidioidomycosis, 1709
  for parasitic infections, 1345*t*–1362*t*
  for penicilliosis, 299
  for phaeohyphomycosis, 1723
  for primary amebic meningoencephalitis, 1749
  prophylaxis with
    in cancer patients, 730
    for *Candida* spp., 1687
  for protozoal infections, 1364
  for rhinosporidiosis, 1724
  for sporotrichosis, 298, 1724
  for systemic candidiasis, 1686
  for *Talaromyces marneffei*, 1699
Amphotericin B deoxycholate, 1333–1335
  adverse effects of, 1334–1335
  for aspergillosis, 1691
  for blastomycosis, 295
  for cancer patients, 737
  chemical structure of, 1333*f*
  for coccidioidomycosis, 296
  dosage of, 1334
    in special circumstances, 1334
  drug interactions of, 1334–1335
  for esophageal candidiasis, 1686
  for histoplasmosis, 294
  indications of, 1334
  mechanism of action, 1333, 1333*f*
  for mucormycosis, 1698
  for oropharyngeal candidiasis, 1684
  overview of, 1333
  for paracoccidioidomycosis, 297
  pharmacodynamics of, 1334
  pharmacokinetics and distribution of, 1333–1334
  route of administration, 1334
  for sporotrichosis, 298
  for systemic candidiasis, 1686
Ampicillin
  for actinomycosis, 316
  for anaerobic bacteria, 1642
  antimicrobial spectrum, routes of administration and
      dosages, 1206*t*–1207*t*
  for complicated urinary tract infection, 545*t*
  for dog bites, 657*t*
  dosage in renal failure, 1213*t*–1214*t*
  drug interactions, 1216
  for enteric fevers, 1006
  for Fournier's gangrene, 98
  for gastrointestinal protozoa, 999, 1000*t*
  for gram-positive bacilli, 1210
  for *Haemophilus* spp., 1621
  infectious mononucleosis and, 377
  for infective arthritis, 386*t*
  for intrapartum prophylaxis, 1209
  for leptospirosis, 1609
  for *Listeria monocytogenes*, 1540
  for lung abscess, 269*f*
  for meningitis, 180
  prophylaxis, 1158*t*
  for pyelonephritis, 552

Ampicillin (Continued)
  resistance to
    in enteric fevers, 1005
    enterococci, 1526–1527
    in epiglottitis, 233
  susceptibilities of selected bacteria to, 1208t–1209t
Ampicillin-sulbactam
  antimicrobial spectrum, routes of administration and
    dosages, 1206t–1207t
  for community-acquired pneumonia, 255t
  for dog bites, 657t
  dosage in renal failure, 1213t–1214t
  for foot ulcers, 131t
  hospital-acquired pneumonia and, 260t
  for human bites, 683
  for intra-abdominal sepsis, 357
  for lung abscess, 269f
  pharmacokinetics of, 1205t
  prophylaxis, 1158t
  susceptibilities of selected bacteria to, 1208t–1209t
Amplicor Mycobacterium tuberculosis polymerase chain
  reaction assay, 1654
Amplified fragment length polymorphism (AFLP), for
  Acinetobacter baumannii, 1583t–1584t
Amplified Mycobacterium tuberculosis direct (MTD) test,
  268, 1654
Amprenavir, 1304
Amyloid, lymphadenopathy and, 137t–138t
Anaerobic bacteria, 1628–1644
  ability to tolerate oxygen, 1633
  antimicrobial susceptibility testing for, 1635, 1635b
  appropriate and inappropriate specimens of, 1634t
  associated with pleuropulmonary infections, 264t
  in bacterial arthritis, 383t, 384
  in cancer patients, 723b
  capsular polysaccharides in, 1633
  clinical manifestations of, 1635–1644
    bacteremia as, 1640–1641
    central nervous system infections as, 1635–1636
    female genital tract infection as, 1639
    head and neck and upper respiratory tract infections
      as, 1636–1638, 1636t
    intra-abdominal infections as, 1638–1639
    osteomyelitis and septic arthritis as, 1640
    pleuropulmonary infections as, 1638, 1638t
    skin and soft-tissue infections as, 1639–1640,
      1639f–1640f
  collection of specimens for, 1634–1635, 1634t
  empyema and, 266t
  epidemiology of, 1628
  hospital-acquired pneumonia and, 259t
  in human bites, 683t
  laboratory diagnosis for, 1635, 1635b
  lincosamides, 1224
  linezolid, 1230
  lipopolysaccharides in, 1633
  lymphadenitis and, 139
  macrolides, 1219, 1221
  management of, 1641–1644
    antimicrobial therapy for, 1641–1642, 1641t–1642t,
      1642f
    hyperbaric oxygen for, 1641
    surgical therapy for, 1641
  microbiology of, 1628–1631, 1628t–1629t, 1629f
    Fusobacterium spp., 1631
    gram-negative bacilli, 1631
    gram-negative cocci, 1631
    gram-positive cocci, 1631
    gram-positive nonspore-forming bacilli, 1630
    gram-positive spore-forming bacilli, 1628t,
      1629–1630
  necrotizing fasciitis and, 96
  in osteomyelitis, 390
  pathogenicity of, 1631–1634
    anaerobes as part of the normal flora in, 1631–1632,
      1632f, 1632t
    conditions predisposing to anaerobic infection in,
      1632–1633, 1633b
    virulence factors in, 1633–1634
  in pelvic inflammatory disease, 492t
  prevention of, 1634
  in prostatitis, 533t
  susceptibility to antimicrobial agents, 1642f
  synergistic capabilities of, 1633
  toxins in, 1633

Anaerobic bacteria (Continued)
  transportation of specimens for, 1634–1635
  volatile fatty acids in, 1633
Anaerobic cultures
  for Clostridium difficile, 1630
  intraoperative, in prosthetic joint infection, 401
Anaerobic infections
  clinical signs of, 1633b
  conditions predisposing to, 1632–1633
  from dog bites, 656
  β-lactam antibiotics for, 1210
Anaerobiospirillum thomasii, 660
Anaerococcus, lung abscess and, 264–265
Anakinra, 798t–799t, 801
Anal cancer, human papillomavirus and, 579
Anal carcinoma, 877–878
  clinical features of, 878
  management of, 878
  pathogenesis of, 877–878
Anal intercourse, and HIV transmission, 825
Anal intraepithelial neoplasia (AIN), 877–878
Anaphylaxis, β-lactam antibiotics, 1215
Anaplasma, 1671
  infection, diagnosis of, 195
Anaplasma phagocytophilum, 1671
Anaplasmosis, 1671–1672
Anatomic-physiologic staging system, in osteomyelitis,
  390, 390f
Ancylostoma braziliense, from dogs, 658
Ancylostoma braziliensis, 1763–1764
Ancylostoma caninum
  diffuse unilateral subacute neuroretinitis, 172
  from dogs, 658
  epidemiology of, 1763–1764
  treatment of, 1345t–1351t
Ancylostoma duodenale
  clinical features of, 996
  diagnosis of, 998t–999t
  epidemiology of, 1763
  life cycle of, 1767f
  pathogenesis and pathology of, 991
  pathogenicity of, 1768
  treatment of, 1001t, 1345t–1351t
Andes virus, 667, 1110, 1503t
Anemia
  Helicobacter pylori, 323
  and lymphadenopathy and splenomegaly, 1139–1140,
    1140b
  in severe malaria, 1019–1020, 1020t, 1022, 1025
Aneurysms, in syphilis, 562
Angioimmunoblastic lymphadenopathy, 137t–138t
Angiomatosis, bacillary. see Bacillary angiomatosis.
Angiostrongyliasis, 1764–1765
  abdominal, 1778
  treatment of, 1345t–1351t
Angiostrongyloidosis, 971, 973f
Angiostrongylus cantonensis, 971
  clinical manifestations of, 1778
  epidemiology of, 1764–1765
  life cycle of, 973f
  pathogenicity of, 1770
  treatment of, 1345t–1351t
Angiostrongylus costaricensis
  clinical manifestations of, 1778
  epidemiology of, 1764–1765
  treatment of, 1345t–1351t
Angiostrongylus spp., 186t
Angiotensin-converting enzyme (ACE), for myocarditis,
  449
Angular stomatitis, 963–964, 964f
Anidulafungin, 1341–1343
  adverse effects of, 1343
  for cancer patients, 737–738
  in Candida spp., 442
  in children, 1343
  dosing and administration, 1341
  drug interactions of, 1343
  indications for, 1341–1342
  mechanism of action, 1341
  pharmacodynamics of, 1341
  pharmacokinetics and distribution of, 1341
  structures of, 1342f
  for systemic candidiasis, 1686
Animal bites, Pasteurella infections from, 1625
Animal handlers, occupational infections, 648t–649t

Animal rabies, 1458, 1459t
Anisakiasis, 1765
  clinical features of, 997
  pathogenesis and pathology of, 991
  treatment of, 1345t–1351t
Anisakid larvae, 1778
Anisakis simplex
  epidemiology of, 1765
  pathogenicity of, 1770
Ann Arbor classification, of non-Hodgkin lymphoma,
  876t
Anncaliia spp., in systemic microsporidiosis, 1741
Anogenital cancers, papillomaviruses in, 1443
Anogenital infection, human papillomavirus, 575
Anopheles spp., 1014
  epidemiology of, 1016
  geographic distribution of, 1015–1016
  pathogenesis and pathology of, 1016
  see also Malaria
Anophelinae, 110
Anorectal gonorrhea, 1563
Anorectal syndrome, 141
Ansamycins, 1177
  chemical structure of, 1177
  mode of action of, 1177, 1177f
  pharmacodynamics of, 1177
Antenatal care
  absence of, perinatal infections and, 515, 516t
  diagnosis, of congenital infection, 511
Anterior uveitis, 175–176, 175t, 176f
  clinical features of, 166
  definition of, 165, 166t
Anthelmintic agents, 1370–1372, 1772
Anthrax, 1123–1128, 1541
  and bioterrorism, 670, 671t–673t, 673–675
  clinical features of, 1124–1126
  clinical manifestations of, 674–675, 675f
  cutaneous
    and bioterrorism, 672t–673t, 674f
    clinical features of, 1124–1125, 1125f, 1126t
    management of, 1127
    transmission of, 663–664
  diagnosis of, 1126–1127, 1126f
  differential diagnoses, 674
  epidemiology of, 1123, 1124f
  gastrointestinal
    clinical features of, 1125–1126
    transmission of, 663–664
  inhalational
    and bioterrorism, 672t–673t, 674f
    clinical features of, 1126
    clinical manifestations of, 674
    diagnosis of, 675
    recognition and treatment of, 675
    transmission of, 663–664
  lymphadenopathy and, 137t–138t
  management of, 1127, 1127t
  meningitis, 1126
  and occupational infections, 649, 651t–654t, 657t
    immunization, 650t–651t
  pathogenesis and pathology of, 1123–1124
  prevention of, 1124
  quinolones for, 1246
  risk factors for, 1123t
  sepsis, 1126
  skin ulceration and, 92f
  systemic, 1126
  transmission, 663–664
Anthrax vaccine adsorbed (AVA), 675
Anti-HBV nucleos(t)ides, in liver transplant patients, 754t
Anti-infective therapy
  choice of, 1145–1147
  combined drug regimens and, 1153
  dose selections of, 1147
  frequency of administration of, 1147
  pharmacodynamic parameters of, 1151–1153, 1151f,
    1153t
  pharmacokinetic parameters of, 1151–1153, 1151f,
    1153t
  pharmacokinetics of, 1147–1151
  prescribing, 1145–1154
  principles of, 1145–1161
  safety of, 1153
Anti-inflammatory agents, in rheumatic fever, 476
Anti-inflammatory response, 685, 685f

Anti-TB therapy, 556
Antiarrhythmic agent, for myocarditis, 449
Antibacterial drugs, 1382–1385
    bactericidal or bacteriostatic effects of, 1147, 1151t
Antibioprophylaxis, hospital-acquired pneumonia, 261
Antibiotic agents/therapy
    for *Acinetobacter baumannii*, 1590t–1591t
    acting on ATP synthase, 1180
    acting on cell wall, 1162–1167
    acting on membrane, 1178–1180
    acting on protein synthesis, 1167–1174
    active efflux of, 1194
    for acute exacerbations of chronic obstructive
        pulmonary disease, 310–311
    for acute osteomyelitis, 395, 395t
    antimetabolites, 1177–1178
    for bacterial arthritis, 385, 386t
    for bacterial infections, 1152t
    for catheter-related bloodstream infection (CRBSI), 435,
        436t
    for cellulitis, 91–92
    for chlamydia, 600–601, 600t–601t
    for cholera, 1607
    for chronic osteomyelitis, 396–398
    in *Clostridium difficile* infection (CDI), 352–353
    for cystic fibrosis, 301
    development of
        business models in, 1384
        strategies for, 1383, 1383f
    for diphtheria, 1546
    for drowning-associated infections, 681
    empiric
        for cancer patients, 734–735, 734f–735f
        for CAPD peritonitis, 380, 380t
    for endocarditis, 465–469, 466t–467t
    and fever of unknown origin, 624
    for food-borne diarrheal illness, 333–334
    late stage pipeline of, 1384, 1385t
    for leptospirosis, 1609
    for Lyme disease, 411–413, 412t
    malaria in pregnancy, 1143t–1144t
    mechanisms of action of, 1162–1180
    for meningitis, 180–181, 182t
    for nonfermenting gram-negative bacilli, 1579–1580
    oral, for cancer patients, 735
    otitis media and, 238t
    for pelvic inflammatory disease, 493–494
    pharmacodynamic parameters of, 1151–1153, 1151f,
        1153t
    pharmacokinetic parameters of, 1151–1153, 1151f,
        1153t
    for pleural effusion, 304
    for pregnancy, 504
    principles of, 691
    for prosthetic joint infection (PJI), 402–403
    for *Pseudomonas aeruginosa*, 1590t–1591t
    for recurrent cellulitis, 135
    regulatory environment for, 1382–1384
    for relapsing fevers, 1608
    safety of, 1153
    for sepsis, 426
    spectrum of, 1147
    systemic, endophthalmitis, 162–163
    topical
        endophthalmitis, 159, 162
        for selective decontamination of the digestive tract,
            694–697
        for surgical site infection prevention, 688–689
    for traveler's diarrhea, 950
Antibiotic-associated diarrhea, probiotics for, 1373–1375,
    1374t
Antibiotic-impregnated cement, aminoglycosides in, 1237
Antibiotic line locks treatment (ALT), for catheter-related
    bloodstream infection (CRBSI), 432, 432f, 435–436,
    436t
Antibiotic prophylaxis
    for cancer patients, 729–730, 732t
    choice of antibiotic in, 687, 1155
    dose of, 1155, 1158t
    duration of, 1156
    general principles of, 1155–1156
    for human bites, 682–683
    indications for, 687, 1154–1155

Antibiotic prophylaxis *(Continued)*
    less invasive procedures in, 1159–1161
        dental procedures, 1159, 1160t
        esophageal procedures, 1160t
        oral procedures, 1160t
        respiratory tract procedures, 1160t
    meningitis and, 181, 183t
    methicillin-resistant *Staphylococcus aureus*, 1156
    nonsystemic agents of, 1156
    in post-treatment Lyme disease syndrome (PTLDS), 414
    postoperative, 689
    in preterm delivery, 502
    principles of, 691
    in prosthetic joint infection (PJI), 403
    recommendations for specific procedures, 1156–1159
        cardiothoracic surgery, 1156, 1157t–1158t
        dose of, 1158t
        gastrointestinal surgery, 1156–1158, 1157t–1158t
        head/neck surgery, 1157t–1158t, 1158
        neurosurgery, 1157t–1158t, 1159
        obstetric/gynecologic surgery, 1157t–1158t, 1159
        ophthalmic surgery, 1157t–1158t
        orthopedic surgery, 1157t–1158t, 1159
        transplantation, 1157t–1158t
        urologic surgery, 1157t–1158t, 1159
        vascular surgery, 1157t–1158t, 1159
    in rheumatic fever, 475–476, 475t
    and the risk of surgical site infection, 686–688, 687t
    for streptococcal infections, 1535
    stress-ulcer, 261
    timing and duration of, 687–688, 688t, 1155–1156
    trauma-related infections, 688
Antibiotic resistance
    of *Acinetobacter* spp., 1595
    acquired, genetic bases of, 1194–1196
    of *Burkholderia* spp., 1596
    cholera, 1607
    detection of, 1387
    mechanisms of, 1181–1196
    multidrug, 1194
Antibiotic susceptibility testing
    for *Bacillus anthracis*, 1541
    for *Corynebacterium* spp., 1547
    for *Nocardia* spp., 1551
Antibodies, 34–37
    classes of, 34–35
    functions of, 36–37, 36b
    generation of diversity, 35–36, 36f
    isotype switching, 35–36
    response of, to HIV-1 infection, 841–842
    structure, 34, 34f
    testing of, in fever of unknown origin, 623
Antibody-dependent cellular cytotoxicity, 37
Antibody-dependent enhancement (ADE), 1120
Anticonvulsants, for convulsions, 1025
Anticytokine autoantibodies, 808, 810t
Antidiarrheal agents, for food-borne diarrheal illness,
    333
Antiemetics, malaria in pregnancy, 1143t–1144t
Antifungal agents/therapy, 689, 1149t
    for *Candida* spp., 441–442, 445
    empirical and pre-emptive, 737–738
    in hematopoietic stem cell transplantation, 744
    keratitis, 154
    polyene, 1333–1340
    systemic, 1333–1344
    triazoles, 1336
        second-generation, 1339
    for vulvovaginal candidiasis, 488
Antifungal prophylaxis
    absence of, in hepatosplenic candidiasis, 444
    in cancer patients, 730, 732t
    for *Candida* spp., 1687
    in kidney transplant patients, 763t
    in liver transplant patients, 755
Antifungal resistance, 440, 441t
    of *Candida*, 1683–1684
Antigen detection
    of *Chlamydia pneumoniae*, 1679
    of *Chlamydia trachomatis*, 1678
    for chronic chlamydial infections, 1679–1680
    in food-borne diarrheal illness, 333
    in histoplasmosis, 293

Antigen detection *(Continued)*
    for lymphatic filariasis, 1050
    for schistosomiasis, 1031
Antigen presentation, defects in, 718–719
Antigen-presenting cells (APCs), 33–34
    activation of T cells by, 801
Antigenic drift, 1466
    in influenza A, 25
Antigenic shift, 1466
    in influenza A, 25
Antigenic variations
    examples of, 24t
    in *Neisseria gonorrhoeae*, 24–25, 24f
    in *Trypanosoma brucei*, 25
Antiglomerular basement disease, immunologically
    mediated diseases, 772f
Antilatency drug, for HIV infection, 932–933, 932t
Antileprosy drugs, 959
Antimalarial drugs
    prophylactic use of, 1017–1018
    resistance, 1022
    for severe malaria, 1024, 1024t
Antimetabolites, 1177–1178
    immunosuppression and, 1379, 1380t
Antimicrobial agents/therapy
    for anaerobic bacteria, 1641–1643, 1641t–1642t, 1642f
        choice of, 1643–1644
    for bacterial arthritis, 385, 386t
    for brain abscess, 1636
    broad-spectrum *versus* narrow-spectrum, 1145–1147
    for cholera, 1607
    for complicated urinary tract infection, 544–545, 544t
        bacteriologic outcome in, 543t
    for cystic fibrosis, 301
    for ehrlichioses, 1671
    empiric, hospital-acquired pneumonia, 260t
    failure of, 1154
    for foot ulcers, 131
    for gonorrhea, 595
    for human bites, 683
    for hydrocephalus shunts, 223
    for intra-abdominal sepsis, 357–358
    optimizing use of, 1197–1202
    for pertussis, 1614
    prevalence and characteristics of use and misuse of,
        1197
    for *Pseudomonas aeruginosa*, 1589–1593, 1590t–1591t
    for pyelonephritis, 552, 552t
    for *Staphylococcus aureus*, 1520t–1521t
    subconjunctival, 159
Antimicrobial peptides (AMPs), 23–24, 24t, 1512
Antimicrobial prophylaxis
    in complicated urinary tract infection, 541, 542t
    in kidney transplant patients, 763t
    β-lactam antibiotics, 1206
    for plague, 1084
    for postsplenectomy sepsis, 777–778
    in pyelonephritis, 548–549
    in surgery, 1206
Antimicrobial resistance
    of *Acinetobacter baumannii*, 1592t
    of *Chryseobacterium* spp., 1598
    of *Elizabethkingia meningoseptica*, 1598
    enteric fevers, 1005
    of Enterobacteriaceae, 1576–1577
    for gonorrhea, 594
    of mycobacteria, 1655–1656, 1655f, 1656t
    of *Nocardia* spp., 1549
    of nonfermenting gram-negative bacilli, 1579–1580
    of *Pseudomonas aeruginosa*, 1589–1593, 1592t
    of *Stenotrophomonas maltophilia*, 1597
Antimicrobial stewardship, 54–61, 1197–1200, 1198t
    clinical decision support systems, 1199–1200
    dose optimization, 1199
    education, 1199
    formulary restriction and preauthorization, 1198
    guidelines and clinical pathways, 1199
    parenteral to oral conversion, 1199
    program, implementation and monitoring of, 1200
    prospective audit with intervention and feedback,
        1198–1199
    in settings other than acute care hospital, 1200
    streamlining or de-escalation of therapy, 1199

Antimicrobial susceptibility testing
  for anaerobic bacteria, 1635, 1635b
  for *Listeria monocytogenes*, 1539
Antimonials, for leishmaniasis, 1758
Antimycotics, for vulvovaginal candidiasis, 488
Antioxidant-supplemented agar, 1386
Antiparasitic agents, 1150t, 1345–1372
  dosage of, 1345t–1362t
Antiprotozoal agents, 1364–1370
Antipyretic therapy, 609–610
  endogenous, 609
  risks of, 609
Antipyretics
  and fever of unknown origin, 624
  and malaria in pregnancy, 1143t–1144t
Antiretroviral drugs
  and antituberculous therapy, 926
  baseline resistance testing in, 918–919
  drug interactions, 907t
    with antituberculosis agents, 1275
  in HIV
    adherence, 923
    co-morbidities, 920
    coinfections, 919–920
    currently licensed, 919t
    drug-drug interactions, 925–926
    drug interactions, 920
    monitoring of, 923
    new strategies, 923
    principles of second- and third-line treatments of,
      925
    recommended regimens, 920t
    resistance, 924
    starting of, 918–920, 920t
    tuberculosis and, 926
    virologic and immunologic responses, 923
    virologic failure, 923–924
  need for, 925
  for prevention of HIV transmission, 825–826
  viral load blips and, 925
Antiretroviral therapy (ART)
  benefits of, 870
  in developing co-morbid conditions, 927
  effects of, 859
  and fever of unknown origin, 615
  for HIV, 819–820, 820f, 912, 927
    autoimmune disease, 864
    changing, 916
    in children, 903b
    choice of regimen, 915
    general principles of, 914–915
    immune-mediated inflammatory disease, 864
    initiation of, 914
    in low- and middle-income countries, 895,
      936–937
    monitoring patients
      after regimen change, 916
      initial, 915–916
    objective of, 914
    to prevent perinatal transmission, 908–910,
      909t
    special considerations, 915
    toxicity, 916
    treatment failure, 916
  and HIV-associated TB, 868, 868f, 870–872
  and immune reconstitution disorders, 859
  influence of, on HIV-1 pathogenesis, 845
  initiation of, 936
  in occupational exposure, to HIV infection, 835
  optimal timing of initiation, 871–872, 872t
  pharmacokinetic interactions, 870–871, 871t
  for prevention among HIV positives, 820
  resistance, 1489
  second-line, 937
  and skin manifestations of HIV, 885–886
  third-line, 937
  tolerance, after exposure in utero, in HIV, 901–902
  treatment failure of, 937
  use of, during management of acute opportunistic
    infections, 850–851
  viral load in, 937
Antiseptic, choice of, for catheter-related bloodstream
    infection (CRBSI), 428
Antithrombin, 423
Antitoxin, diphtheria, 1546, 1546t

Antituberculosis agents, 1264–1276
  adverse reactions of, 1268t–1269t
  classification of, 1264, 1265t
  doses of, 1272t
  drug interactions, 1275, 1275b
    with antiretroviral agents, 1275
  drug-resistant tuberculosis and, 1273–1274
  drug toxicity of, 1265, 1267f, 1269f
  first-line drugs, 1265–1270, 1265t
  metabolic products and excretion of, 1267t
  mode of action of, 1264–1265
  new TB drugs development pipeline of, 1271–1272,
    1271f
  pharmacokinetics, 1264–1265, 1266t
  second-line drugs, 1270–1271
  in special circumstances, 1274–1275
  targets of, 1265f, 1266t
  therapeutic regimens of, basis and design of, 1272–1273,
    1273t
Antituberculosis therapy, abnormal liver enzymes and,
    308, 309f
Antituberculous therapy, ARV and, 926
Antiviral agents
  for HIV, 1148t
  for human bites, 682
  for influenza viruses, 1471, 1471t
  for non-HIV, 1146t–1147t
  against respiratory viruses, 1318–1326, 1322t–1323t
  strategies, for hematopoietic stem cell transplantation,
    741
  for viral hemorrhagic fevers, 1117
Antiviral prophylaxis
  for cancer patients, 732
  in kidney transplant patients, 763t
Antiviral therapy, 918–926
  for encephalitis, 197
  in genital herpes, 569, 573–574, 573t
  in HIV. *see* Antiretroviral drugs, in HIV
  for varicella management, 76
  see also Antiretroviral therapy
Aortitis, 562
APECED, 1684
Aphthous stomatitis, 234, 318
  in HIV/AIDS, 880
Aphthous ulcers, 586t–587t
Apolactoferrin (ALF), 1531–1532
Apophysomyces, 1696
Apoptosis, 19
Appendicitis, in pregnancy, 503
Aprons, 58
Arachnia propionica, 315
Arachnida, 104–107
  Acarina, 105–107
  Argasida-Argasidae, 104–105
  Ixodida-Ixodidae, 104
Arachnids, 104
Arboviruses, 1493, 1493f–1494f, 1495t
  and recreational infections, 644
Arcanobacterium, 1547, 1548t, 1630
Arcanobacterium haemolyticum, 234–235
Archaeologist, and occupational infections, 648t–649t
Archaeplastida, 1744
Arcobacter, 338, 1601t
Arcobacter butzleri, 338
Arcobacter cryaerophilus, 338
Arenaviridae, 1499–1501
  clinical manifestations of, 1501
  diagnostic microbiology of, 1501
  epidemiology of, 1500–1501
  management of, 1501
  nature, 1499–1500
  pathogenicity of, 1500
  prevention, 1501
Arenaviruses, 1110
  and bioterrorism, 671t
  causing human disease, 1500t
  classification, 1499
  clinical features of, 1114t–1115t
  clinical manifestations, 1501
  complexes, 1499
  epidemiology of, 1112t, 1500–1501, 1500f
  New World, 1499
  prevention, 1501
  from rodents, 667
  virions, 1499

Argentine hemorrhagic fever
  clinical manifestations of, 1501
  epidemiology of, 1500
  management of, 1117
  treatment of, 1501
Arginine vasopressin (AVP), 609
Argyll Robertson pupil, 563
Armadillos, infections from, 668
Arrhythmias, in myocarditis, 448–449
Artemether
  for parasitic infections, 1345t–1362t
  for severe malaria, 1024, 1024t
Artemether-lumefantrine, 1023, 1023t
Artemis deficiency, 718
Artemisinin
  adverse reactions, 1365
  dosage of, 1365
  and its derivatives, 1365
  for malaria in pregnancy, 1143t
  for parasitic infections, 1352t–1362t
  route of administration, 1365
  for schistosomiasis, 1031
Artemisinin combination therapy (ACT)
  for falciparum malaria, 1022–1023
  for vivax malaria, 1024
Arterial blood gas analysis, in sepsis, 420
Arterial blood gases, in melioidosis, 1077
Arterial graft infections, 436–438
  clinical features of, 437
  diagnosis of, 437, 437f–438f
  epidemiology of, 436
  management of, 437–438
  pathogenesis of, 436
  prevention of, 431t, 436–437
Artesunate
  and amodiaquine, 1022, 1023t
  and mefloquine, 1022, 1023t
  for parasitic infections, 1345t–1362t
  plus sulfadoxine-pyrimethamine, 1022, 1023t
  and pyronaridine, 1022
  for severe malaria, 1024, 1024t
Arthritis, 382–387
  bacterial, 382–385
    clinical features of, 384
    diagnosis of, 384–385
    epidemiology of, 382
    gonococcal, 384
    management of, 385, 385f, 386t
    nongonococcal, 384
    pathogenesis of, 382–383, 383t
    prevention of, 383
    radiology in, 385, 385f
    risk factors for, 382, 383t
  blastomycosis and, 1703
  from *Campylobacter* spp., 1602
  Lyme disease
    antibiotic regimens for, 412t
    clinical features of, 409
    diagnosis of, 411
    management of, 413
  post-streptococcal reactive, 473
  Pseudomonas spp. in, 1589
  reactive, 386–387, 386b
  rheumatic fever and, 471–473
  tuberculosis, 279
  viral, 385–386, 387t
Arthrocentesis, in bacterial arthritis, 384
Arthroconidia, of *Paracoccidioides brasiliensis*,
    1708
Arthropathy
  in human T-lymphocyte leukemia virus 1 (HTLV-1),
    1491
  as quinolones adverse effects, 1247
Arthroplasty, for prosthetic joint infection (PJI),
    402
Arthropods, 104
  arboviruses, 1493–1494
  causing encephalitis/myelitis, 191t
  and recreational infections, 644
  vectors of medical importance, 104–112
Artificial nails, 58
Ascariasis, 1777
  clinical features of, 996
  pathogenesis and pathology of, 991, 992f
  treatment of, 1345t–1351t

Ascaris
  clinical manifestations of, 1777
  epidemiology of, 989–990
  in myocarditis, 447
  prevention of, 994
Ascaris lumbricoides
  clinical features of, 996
  diagnosis of, 998t–999t
  epidemiology of, 1763
  life cycle of, 1767f
  pathogenesis and pathology of, 991, 992f
  pathogenicity of, 1766
  in population density and urbanization, 990
  prevention of, 994
  treatment of, 1000, 1001t, 1345t–1351t
Ascaris suum, 666
Aschoff body, 471
Ascites, culture-negative, 359
Ascomycota, 1712
Aspartate aminotransferase (AST), for viral hemorrhagic
    fevers, 1116–1117
Aspergillomas, 1689
Aspergillosis, 1687–1692
  allergic bronchopulmonary, 1687, 1690f
  in cancer patients, 730f
  clinical manifestations of, 1689–1691, 1690f, 1690t
  diagnostic microbiology of, 1688–1689, 1688f
  epidemiology of, 1687
  extrapulmonary, 1689
  in hematopoietic stem cell transplantation, 744
  in HIV/AIDS, 855–856
  invasive, 1689
  in kidney transplant patients, 768, 768f
  in liver transplant patients, 753
  management of, 1691
  nature of, 1687
  pathogenicity of, 1687–1688
  prevention of, 1692
  risk in T-cell depletion, 739
  in thoracic transplantation patients, 749, 750f
Aspergillus, 1681t
  in abscesses, 772
  in bacterial arthritis, 383t
  brain abscess and, 200
  in burn wounds, 699–700
  in cancer patients, 724, 728f, 737
  and chronic granulomatous disease, 708
  in chronic meningitis, 186t
  and drowning-associated infections, 680
  endophthalmitis and, 159
  epidemiology of, 1687
  in HIV/AIDS, 855
  hospital-acquired pneumonia and, 259t
  in infective endocarditis, 748
  keratitis and, 154
  nature of, 1687
  in thoracic transplantation patients, 747t, 749–750
  transmission of, 806
Aspergillus flavus, 1689
  in skin manifestation of HIV, 884t
Aspergillus fumigatus, 1689
  in hematopoietic stem cell transplantation, 744
  in skin manifestation of HIV, 884t
Aspergillus sydowii, diagnostic microbiology of,
    1711–1712
Aspiration cytology, of echinococcosis, 1043
Aspiration pneumonia
  and empyema, 263
  lung and pleural abscesses, 263
  risk factors for, 264t
Aspirin
  antipyretic action, 609
  for leprosy reactions, 959–960
  for pericardial effusion, 480
  for pericarditis, 454
Asplenia, functional, 775, 775t
Assisted ventilation, in malaria in pregnancy,
    1143t–1144t
Asthma
  Chlamydia pneumoniae and, 1678
  Mycoplasma pneumoniae in, 1661
Astrakhan fever, 1667t, 1668
Astroviridae, 1396

Astroviruses, 1396, 1396f
  clinical characteristics of, 1391t
  epidemiological characteristics of, 1391t
  structure and morphological characteristics of, 1391f,
    1391t
  viral enteritis and, 338
Asymmetric periflexural exanthem, 75t
Asymptomatic bacteriuria, 557
  management of, 558
Asymptomatic candiduria, 558
Asymptomatic infections, enteroviruses and, 1410
Atacicept, 798t–799t, 800
Ataxia telangiectasia, 721
Ataxia telangiectasia-like syndrome, 721
Atazanavir, 1148t, 1304
  adverse reactions of, 1304
  description of, 1304
  dosage of, 1304
    in special circumstances, 1304
  drug interactions of, 1304
  effect on oral contraceptives, 907t
  indications of, 1304
  perinatal HIV transmission prevention, 909t
  pharmacokinetics and distribution of, 1304
  resistance to, 1304
  and ritonavir, 922
  route of administration of, 1304
Atherosclerosis, *Chlamydia pneumoniae* and, 1677–1678
Atopobium, 1630
Atovaquone
  for babesiosis, 1753
  for parasitic infections, 1345t–1362t, 1365
  for *Pneumocystis jirovecii* pneumonia, 852
  for toxoplasmosis, in HIV/AIDS, 857
Atovaquone-proguanil, 1022
  for malaria in pregnancy, 1143t
  for malaria prophylaxis, 951
  for parasitic infections, 1345t–1362t, 1365
ATP-binding cassette (ABC), 1189, 1194f
Atrophic vaginitis, 489
Aureolysin, 1512, 1513t–1514t
Australian bat Lyssavirus, 1463
Australian Safety and Compensation Council (ASCC), 647
Auto-agglutination, malaria and, 1017
Autoimmune disease, in HIV patients receiving
    antiretroviral therapy, 864
Autoimmune lymphoproliferative syndrome, 721–722
Autoimmune neutropenia
  primary, 706
  secondary, 706
Autoimmunity, 21
Autonomic nervous system, abnormalities of, in chronic
    fatigue syndrome, 634
Autosomal recessive agammaglobulinemia, 720
Avian chlamydiosis, and occupational infections,
    651t–654t
Avian influenza, 651t–654t, 661, 668
  H5N1, 1470
  spread of, 945
  transmission of, to humans, 1466–1467
Axenfeld's chronic follicular conjunctivitis, 981t
Axillary lymphadenopathy, 145
Azalides, 1171
  classification, 1217
  definitions, 1217
Azathioprine, immunosuppression and, 1379
Azithromycin
  accumulation ratio of, 1222t
  for anaerobic bacteria, 1643
  for babesiosis, 1753
  for bronchitis, 248
  for *Campylobacter* spp., 1602
  for cat-scratch disease, 659
  for chancroid, 590
  characteristics of, 1218t
  chemoprophylaxis, for meningococcal disease, 1560
  community-acquired pneumonia and, 255t
  for cryptosporidiosis, 1742
  for dog bites, 657t
  for endemic treponematoses, 965
  for enteric fevers, 1006
  for food-borne diarrheal illness, 333–334
  for granuloma inguinale, 591

Azithromycin (Continued)
  for *Haemophilus ducreyi*, 1621
  for leptospirosis, 1609
  for lung abscess, 269f
  for Lyme disease, 412
  for lymphogranuloma venereum, 589
  for *Mycobacterium avium* complex (MAC) in HIV,
    856
  for parasitic infections, 1345t–1351t
  pharmacokinetics, 1222, 1223t–1224t
  for pharyngitis, 235
  in pregnancy, 910
  for primary amebic meningoencephalitis, 1749
  prophylaxis of, in rheumatic fever, 475t
  for renal insufficiency, 1222
  for scrub typhus, 1097, 1671
  stability in acidic medium, 1218, 1219f
  for syphilis, 560, 565
  tissue distribution, 1224t
  for trachoma, 981
  for travelers' diarrhea, 376, 950
  in vitro activity, 1219–1220, 1220t
Azithromycin-clarithromycin, resistance to, mycobacterial,
    1656t
Azlocillin, pharmacokinetics of, 1205t
Azoles
  for aspergillosis, 1691
  for chronic granulomatous disease, 709
  for cryptococcosis, 1696
  in hematopoietic stem cell transplantation, 744
  intra-abdominal candidiasis, 358
  for keratitis, 155
  for paracoccidioidomycosis, 1709
  for phaeohyphomycosis, 1723
  prophylaxis with, in cancer patients, 730, 737
  for vulvovaginal candidiasis, 488
Aztreonam
  antimicrobial spectrum, routes of administration and
    dosages, 1206t–1207t
  bronchiectasis and, 249
  against carbapenamase-resistant gram-negative bacilli,
    1290t
  dosage in renal failure, 1213t–1214t
  for *P. aeruginosa* infection, 1210
  pharmacokinetics of, 1205t
  prophylaxis, 1158t
  susceptibilities of selected bacteria to, 1208t–1209t
Aztreonam lysine (Cayston®), for cystic fibrosis, 301
Aztreonam lysine for inhalation (AZLI), bronchiectasis
    and, 249

B
B-cell-depleting therapies, infectious risk associated with,
    800
B-cell lymphocyte stimulator, 800
B-cell response, to enteroviruses, 1409–1410
B cells
  antibody diversity, 35
  differentiation of, 719f
B lymphocytes, and immunodeficiencies, 713
B virus, 661
  encephalitis/myelitis caused by, 193t–194t
  occupational infections, 648t–649t
Babesia
  diagnostic microbiology of, 1752, 1752f
  nature of, 1751
Babesia divergens, 1751
Babesia duncani, 1751
Babesia microti, 667
  clinical manifestations of, 1752
  epidemiology of, 1751
  nature of, 1751
  postsplenectomy sepsis, 778t
  treatment of, 1365, 1369
Babesiosis, 1751–1753
  clinical manifestations of, 1752–1753
  diagnostic microbiology of, 1752, 1752f
  epidemiology of, 1751
  and fever of unknown origin, 613
  management of, 1753
  nature of, 1751
  occupational infections, 648t–649t

Babesiosis *(Continued)*
pathogenicity of, 1751
postsplenectomy, prevention of, 776–777
prevention of, 1752
in transfusion-related infections, 704*t*
treatment of, 1345*t*–1351*t*
Bacampicillin
antimicrobial spectrum, routes of administration and
dosages, 1206*t*–1207*t*
pharmacokinetics of, 1205*t*
Bacillary angiomatosis, 93, 113, 113*f*, 659–660, 1675
in HIV/AIDS, 858, 858*f*
in skin manifestation of HIV, 883, 883*f*
Bacillary peliosis, 1675
Bacille Calmette-Guérin (BCG) vaccination
for leprosy, 956
lymphadenopathy, 145
for newborns of HIV-infected mothers, 901
and occupational infections, 651*t*
Bacilli
curved and spiral, 1600–1610
gram-negative. *see* Gram-negative bacilli
gram-positive. *see* Gram-positive bacilli
Bacillus, 1540
endophthalmitis and, 159
Bacillus anthracis, 1123, 1537, 1541
and bioterrorism, 671*t*, 673, 675*f*
clinical manifestations of, 1541
culture of, 1541
cycle of, 1124*f*
diagnostic microbiology of, 1541
direct examination of, 1541
epidemiology of, 1541
identification of, 1541
ketolides, 1220
lincosamides, 1224–1225
macrolides, 1220
pathogenesis and pathology of, 1123
pathogenicity of, 1541
see also Anthrax
Bacillus cereus, 1541–1542
characteristics of, in food-borne diarrheal illness, 330*t*
clinical manifestations of, 1542
diagnostic microbiology of, 1542, 1543*f*
endophthalmitis and, 159
epidemiology of, 1541
food poisoning from, 1542
management of, 1542
nature of, 1541
pathogenicity of, 1541–1542
Bacitracin, 1167
for anaerobic bacteria, 1643
for conjunctivitis, 152
for folliculitis/furunculosis prevention, 86
micrococci and, 1522
prophylaxis, endophthalmitis, 159
BacT/ALERT®, for mycobacteria, 1653
BACTEC 13A blood culture, for mycobacteria, 1653
BACTEC 460 TB System, for mycobacteria, 1656–1657
BACTEC MGIT 960 System, for mycobacteria, 1656–1657
Bacteremia
aerobic actinomycetes and, 1551–1552
aminoglycosides for, 1236–1237
anaerobic bacteria in, 1632*f*
antimicrobial therapy for, 1641*t*
from *Bartonella*, 1675
from *Campylobacter* spp., 1602
definition of, 415
Enterobacteriaceae in, 1576
group B streptococci and, 1533
in intestinal transplant patients, 757
linezolid, 1231*t*
Listeria monocytogenes and, 1539
melioidosis and, 1074
meningococcal, 1564
postoperative, 691
Pseudomonas aeruginosa in, 1586
Pseudomonas spp. in, 1589
in pyelonephritis, 547, 549–550
Rhodococcus equi and, 1551
Staphylococcus aureus, 1519
Stenotrophomonas maltophilia in, 1597
transient, in endocarditis, 459
vancomycin for, 1251
from *Vibrio alginolyticus*, 1607

Bacteria
adhesins, 13–14, 14*f*
anaerobic. *see* Anaerobic bacteria
antibiotic-resistant, controlling transmission of, 693–697
apoptosis, 19
cell walls, 11*f*
in chronic meningitis, 186*t*
colonization
of burn wounds, 699
in postoperative period, 688–689
comparison of fungi and, 5*t*
in complicated urinary tract infection, 540*t*
in congenital infection, 505*b*
decontamination of, in intensive care unit, 694–697
definition of, 4
diarrhea and, 328, 330–331, 333
adherence of, 329
dichotomy, 10
gene expression of, 10
general properties and classification of, 8–10
genetic information in, 19
genome, 62–67
analysis of genome sequences, 63–65
sequencing strategies, 62*f*, 63, 63*t*
using genome sequences, 65–66
in infectious diseases transmitted by grafts, 805
in infective arthritis, 383*t*
invasion, community-acquired pneumonia and, 252
motility, 10
in myocarditis, 446–447
organization of cell, 10
in pericarditis, 450, 451*t*–452*t*
proliferation of, 702–703
provoking immune reconstitution disorder, 860*t*
resistance, 1194. *see also* Antibiotic resistance
in sepsis, 419, 419*t*
transcription in, 10, 11*f*
translation in, 10, 11*f*
Bacterial arthritis, 382–385
clinical features of, 384
diagnosis of, 384–385
epidemiology of, 382
etiologic agents of, 383*t*
gonococcal, 384
management of, 385
antimicrobial therapy for, 385, 386*t*
debridement for, 385, 385*f*
synovial fluid drainage for, 385
nongonococcal, 384
pathogenesis of, 382–383
prevention of, 383
radiology in, 385, 385*f*
risk factors for, 382, 383*t*
Bacterial enteritis, 336–338
Bacterial infections
associated with erythema multiforme, 120*t*
associated with erythema nodosum, 121*t*
in cancer patients, 723–724, 723*b*
causing retinitis and uveitis, 169*t*
chronic diarrhea, 341–346, 345*t*
community-acquired pneumonia and, 255
dermatologic manifestations, 113–118, 114*t*–115*t*
from domesticated herbivores, 663–666
encephalitis/myelitis, 192*t*
erythema multiforme, 120
in eye involvement in tropical, 982
follicular conjunctivitis, 981*t*
in hematopoietic stem cell transplantation, 740–741,
741*t*, 743*t*
jaundice, 1135*t*
in kidney transplant patients, 762–765
lymphadenopathy and, 137*t*–138*t*
nitroimidazoles for, 1262
opportunistic, in HIV, 857–858
in pancreas transplant patients, 765
as skin manifestations of HIV, 882–883
in thoracic transplant patients, 749
from tumor necrosis factor inhibitors, 797–799
in varicella, 75–76
Bacterial toxins, 18–21, 19*t*
apoptosis, 19, 20*f*
damage resulting from cytotoxic lymphocytes, 21
diphtheria toxin, 19, 20*f*
infection and cancer, 21
virus-induced cytopathic effect, 19–21, 21*f*

Bacterial vaginosis, 483–485, 1374*t*, 1375
anaerobic bacteria in, 1639
clinical features of, 484
diagnosis of, 484, 484*t*
epidemiology of, 483
etiology of, 1138*t*
and HIV, 844
transmission, 905
management of, 484–485
Mycoplasma genitalium in, 1662
Mycoplasma hominis in, 1663–1664
pathogenesis and pathology of, 483–484
in pregnancy, 500–501, 500*t*
prevention of, 484
Bactericidal activity, 1147, 1151*t*
Bacteriospermia, 533
Bacteriostatic activity, 1147, 1151*t*
Bacteriuria
asymptomatic, 523–524, 528–529, 530*f*, 541–542, 544
detection of, 527
in kidney transplant patients, 763
in pregnancy, 500, 502–503
preoperative treatment of, 541
prevalence of, 523, 524*t*
symptomatic, 524, 526
Bacteroides
antimicrobial drugs of choice for, 1642*t*
in bacterial vaginosis, 483
empyema and, 266*t*
hospital-acquired pneumonia and, 259*t*
in human bites, 683*t*
in normal flora, 1632
in osteomyelitis, 395*t*
Bacteroides fragilis, 1631, 1632*f*
antimicrobial resistance in, 357
brain abscess and, 199
capsular polysaccharides of, 1633
enterotoxin of, 1633
in human bites, 682
identification of, 1635
intra-abdominal infections, 690
lipopolysaccharide of, 1633
lung abscess and, 264–265
microflora, 355–356
in normal flora, 1632, 1632*t*
susceptibility to antimicrobial agents, 1642*f*
BAD1, 1701–1702
Bairnsdale ulcer, 1648
Balamuthia, 1744
Balamuthia mandrillaris, 193*t*–194*t*, 196
cultivation of, 1745
diagnostic microbiology of, 1747
epidemiology of, 1746
granulomatous amebic encephalitis and, 1746
nature of, 1744
pathogenicity of, 1746
taxonomy of, 1745, 1745*f*
treatment of, 1345*t*–1351*t*
Balanitis, candidal, 586*t*–587*t*
Balantidiasis
chronic diarrhea and, 349
clinical features of, 996
treatment of, 1345*t*–1351*t*
Balantidium coli, 1725*t*
in chronic diarrhea, 347*t*, 349
clinical features of, 996
diagnosis of, 998*t*–999*t*
distribution of, 990
epidemiology of, 1727
identification in fecal specimens, 1732, 1733*f*
pathogenesis and pathology of, 991
pathogenicity of, 1728
treatment of, 999, 1000*t*, 1345*t*–1351*t*
Bannwarth's syndrome, 409
Barmah Forest virus, in infective arthritis, 387*t*
Barrier functions of the innate immune response,
26–27
Barrier precautions, 58
Bartonella, 1673
bacillary angiomatosis, 883
causing endocarditis, 461*t*
causing retinitis and uveitis, 169*t*
encephalopathy and, 190
infection, 648*t*–649*t*
ketolides, 1221

Bartonella (Continued)
  macrolides, 1221
  uveitis and, 175–176
Bartonella bacilliformis
  clinical manifestations of, 1674
  epidemiology of, 1673
  pathogenicity of, 1673
Bartonella henselae
  in bacillary angiomatosis, 93, 858
  cat-scratch disease, 659–660
  clinical manifestations of, 1675
  epidemiology of, 1673
  lymphadenopathy and, 139
  pathogenicity of, 1673
  uveitis and, 168
Bartonella quintana
  bacillary angiomatosis and, 93, 858
  clinical manifestations of, 1674
  endocarditis due to, 659
  epidemiology of, 1673
  pathogenicity of, 1673
Bartonellosis, 1673–1675
  clinical manifestations of, 1674–1675
  dermatologic manifestations of, 113, 114t–115t
  diagnostic microbiology of, 1673–1674, 1675f
  epidemiology of, 1673, 1674t
  management of, 1675
  nature of, 1673
  pathogenicity of, 1673
  prevention of, 1673
Basal cell carcinoma, in skin manifestation of HIV,
    884–885
Baseline resistance testing, 918–919
Basidiobolomycosis, 1712
  gastrointestinal, 1719
  management of, 1723
Basidiobolus ranarum, 1713, 1719
Bathing, and recreational infections, 645
Bats, 191t, 666
Baylisascariasis, 972, 975f, 1777
  clinical features of, 974
  treatment of, 1345t–1351t
Baylisascariasis meningoencephalitis, anthelmintic
    treatment of, 976
Baylisascaris procyonis, 193t–194t, 667
  diffuse unilateral subacute neuroretinitis, 172
  epidemiology of, 1763–1764
  life cycle of, 972, 975f
  treatment of, 1345t–1351t
Bayou (BAY) virus, 1503t
BDG assay, for *Candida* spp., 1682t, 1683
BDProbeTec SDA, 1654
Bears, infections from, 669
Bed bugs, 106t, 109f
Bedaquiline, 1271
  recommended regimen, 1274
Bednets, for malaria, 1056
Behavior, of travelers, 952
Behavior changes, and emerging infectious diseases, 45
Behçet's syndrome, 586t–587t
Bejel, dermatologic manifestations of, 114t–115t
Belatacept, 1380t
Belimumab, 798t–799t, 800
Bell's palsy, in Lyme disease, 411–412
Benchtop sequencers, genome sequencing, 63
Bengal strain, 1604–1605
Benzathine penicillin G
  for endemic treponematoses, 965
  pharmacokinetics of, 1204
  prophylaxis of, in rheumatic fever, 475t
  for syphilis, 560, 565
Benzimidazole, 1045
Benznidazole
  for Chagas disease, 1072, 1760
  for parasitic infections, 1345t–1362t, 1365
Benzodiazepines, 212
Benzoic acid, 128
Benzylpenicillin, neurologic effects of, 1215
Bergeyella, 1581t–1582t, 1597
'Berlin patient,' HIV cure for, 931, 932f
Bifidobacterium, 1630
  microflora, 355
  in normal flora, 1632, 1632t

Bigyra, gastrointestinal, 989t
Biliary sepsis, 360
Biliary surgery, high-risk, 687
Biliary system infections, β-lactam antibiotics for,
    1211
Bilophila wadsworthia, 355, 1631
Bilophilia, 1632
Binary toxin, *Clostridium difficile* infection (CDI), 351
Biocreep, 1382
Biodefense, 670–679
Biofilms
  in cystitis, 524–525, 525f
  in prosthetic joint infection (PJI), 399
Biologics
  immunosuppression and, 1377, 1377t, 1380t
  infections associated with, 1377–1381, 1377t
Biopsy
  and fever of unknown origin, 623
  in myocarditis, 448–449
  in osteomyelitis, 394–395
  in pericarditis, 452–453
  prostate, 532–534
  in syphilis, 563
Biopsy urease test, for *Helicobacter pylori*, 325
Bioterrorism, 670–679
  advantages of, 670
  agents of concern for use in, 671t
  associated issues and sequelae of, 678–679
  Bacillus anthracis in, 1541
  effectiveness of, 670
  Francisella tularensis and, 1085
  and management of special patient populations,
    678–679
  preparedness, 58
  and psychosocial morbidity, 679
  quarantine, 678
  recognition of, 672
  surveillance, 678
  threat agents, 672–678, 672t
  threat assessment, 670–671
Biotyping
  for *Acinetobacter baumannii*, 1583t–1584t
  for *Pseudomonas aeruginosa*, 1583t–1584t
Birds
  infections from, 191t, 668
  infectious diseases associated with, 660–661
    enteric, 661
    inhalation, 660–661
    viral, 661
Bismuth subsalicylate
  for food-borne diarrheal illness, 333
  for travelers' diarrhea, 376
Bites
  treatment of, 1462
  see also specific animal
Bithionol, for parasitic infections, 1345t–1362t, 1370
Bithynia spp., 1765
Biting midges, 106t, 112
BK polyomavirus (BKPyV), 1445
BK viruria, 1447
BK virus
  in hematopoietic stem cell transplantation, 743,
    743t
  in kidney transplant patients, 767, 767f
  quinolones for, 1246
BK virus nephropathy (BKVN), in kidney transplant
    recipients, 1447, 1447f
Black Creek Canal (BCC) virus, 1503t
Black flies, 106t, 111
Black molds, 1712
Black piedra
  epidemiology of, 1710
  nature of, 1710
Blackwater fever, 1020t, 1021, 1021f
Bladder
  cancer and *Schistosoma haematobium*, 21
  emptying of, by flow rate measurement, in prostatitis,
    534
Blastocystis, 1725t
  diagnostic microbiology of, 1729, 1731f
  epidemiology of, 1726
  infection, clinical features of, 996
  pathogenicity of, 1728

Blastocystis hominis
  clinical features of, 996
  diagnosis of, 998t–999t
  management of, 997
  treatment of, 1345t–1351t
Blastomyces, 1681t
Blastomyces dermatitidis, 1700
  in bacterial arthritis, 383t
  clinical features of, 294, 294f
  culture of, 1702
  diagnosis of, 294–295, 295f
  ecology of, 1701
  epidemiology of, 1701
  in lower respiratory tract infections, 264f
  management of, 295
  microscopic examination of, 1702
  mycology and epidemiology of, 294
  mycology of, 1701, 1701f
  pathogenesis and pathology of, 294
  pathogenicity of, 1701–1702
  in prostatitis, 533t
  serology of, 1702–1703, 1702t
  in skin manifestation of HIV, 884t
Blastomycosis, 294–295, 294f–295f, 648t–649t, 1700t,
    1701–1703
  clinical manifestations of, 1703
  cutaneous, 1703
  dermatologic manifestations of, 114t–115t, 118
  diagnostic microbiology of, 1702–1703, 1702t
  dissemination in, 1703
  ecology of, 1701
  epidemiology of, 1701, 1702t
  management of, 1703
  mycology of, 1701, 1701f
  pathogenicity of, 1701–1702
  prevention of, 1703
  pulmonary, 1703
  in skin manifestation of HIV, 883–884
Bleeding, abnormal, in severe malaria, 1020t, 1021
Blindness, in tropical eye infections, 979–982
Blistering distal dactylitis, 88–89
α-blockers, for prostatitis, 536
Blood
  contaminated, HIV transmission by, 814
  of infant, microbiologic investigation of, in congenital
    infection, 512t
  for laboratory diagnosis, of mycobacteria, 1651,
    1651t
  lower respiratory tract infections, 268
  transmission by, and recreational infections, 645
Blood-borne infections, in hemoglobin disorders,
    1057
Blood-brain barrier
  meningitis, 178–179
  in severe malaria, 1017
Blood culture-negative endocarditis (BCNE), 460
  intracellular bacteria causing, 461t
  treatment of, 469
Blood cultures
  of aerobic actinomycetes, 1549
  in arterial graft infections, 437
  for brucellosis, 1099–1100, 1615
  for burns, 699
  from cancer patients, 733
  of *Candida* spp., 441–442, 444, 1682t, 1683
  in catheter-related bloodstream infection (CRBSI), 434,
    434f
  in endocarditis, 460–461
  and fever of unknown origin, 620
  in food-borne diarrheal illness, 332
  in hospital-acquired pneumonia, 259–260
  in intra-abdominal sepsis, 357
  of *Listeria monocytogenes*, 1540
  meningitis and, 180
  and postoperative infection, 690
  in prosthetic joint infection (PJI), 401
  in pyelonephritis, 553
  of scrub typhus, 1096–1097
  in sepsis, 420
  splenic infection, 362
  of staphylococci, 1517f
  in Whipple's disease, 344
Blood films, for relapsing fevers, 1108, 1108f

Blood flukes, 1032, 1764t
epidemiology of, 1766
pathogenicity of, 1770–1772
see also Schistosoma; Schistosomiasis
Blood groups, cholera risk and, 1604–1605
Blood products, in transfusion-related infections, 702–703, 704t
Blood protozoa, 1751–1762
Blood samples
Clostridium difficile infection, 352
for helminths diagnosis, 1776
Blood smear, in malaria diagnosis, 1022
Blood sugar, and postoperative infection risk, 689–690
Blood tests
in melioidosis, 1077
in osteomyelitis, 393
Blood transfusion
Chagas disease transmission and, 1070, 1071t
for malaria in pregnancy, 1143t–1144t
risk factors for infection after, 686, 689
Bloodland Lake (BLL) virus, 1503t
Bloodstream infections, 1290
Acinetobacter baumannii in, 1587t
Acinetobacter spp. in, 1595
Alcaligenes xylosoxidans in, 1597
in cancer patients, 723–724, 724f, 726–727
Candida, 440–442
central line-associated, 60
Chryseobacterium indologenes in, 1598
Elizabethkingia meningoseptica in, 1598
in intestinal transplant patients, 756
postoperative, 691, 691t
Pseudomonas aeruginosa in, 1586, 1587t
see also Bacteremia
'Blueberry muffin spots', 77
Bocaparvovirus, 1449
Boceprevir (BCV), for hepatitis C, 1331
Body, washing of, with chlorhexidine, 694
Body cavity
specimen collection in, 1634t
see also specific cavities
Body lice, 108, 1669
Body temperature
measuring, 605
normal, 606, 606f
Bolivian hemorrhagic fever
clinical manifestations of, 1501
epidemiology of, 1501
Bone
biopsy, in osteomyelitis, 394–395
blastomycosis in, 1703
coccidioidomycosis in, 1705
for laboratory diagnosis, of mycobacteria, 1651t
specimen collection in, 1634t
Bone infections
antimicrobial therapy for, 1641t
Pseudomonas aeruginosa in, 1589
Bone lesions, cryptococcosis, 1695
Bone marrow
biopsy of, in fever of unknown origin, 623, 623t
cultures in brucellosis, 1615
hematopoietic stem cell transplantation, 739
for laboratory diagnosis, of mycobacteria, 1651, 1651t
transplant recipients, hemorrhagic cystitis in, 1447
transplantation
for HIV infection, 931, 932f, 932t, 1490
in X-linked severe combined immune deficiency, 715
Borderline-tuberculoid leprosy, 955–956, 956f
Bordetella, 1611–1614
clinical manifestations of, 1613–1614
diagnostic microbiology of, 1612–1613, 1613f
epidemiology of, 1611, 1612f
management of, 1614
nature of, 1611
pathogenicity of, 1612, 1613t
prevention of, 1612
Bordetella ansorpii, 1611
Bordetella avium, 1611
Bordetella bronchiseptica, 667
in cats, 660
diagnostic microbiology of, 1612
nature of, 1611
pathogenicity of, 1612
Bordetella hinzii, 1611
Bordetella holmesii, 1611

Bordetella parapertussis
bronchitis and, 244t
diagnostic microbiology of, 1612
nature of, 1611
pathogenicity of, 1612
Bordetella pertussis
bronchiectasis and, 243
bronchitis and, 244t
clindamycin, 1225
clinical manifestations of, 1613–1614
diagnostic microbiology of, 1612–1613, 1613f
epidemiology of, 1611
macrolides, 1221
management of, 1614
nature of, 1611
pathogenicity of, 1612
prevention of, 1612
Bordetella petrii, 1611
Bordetella trematum, 1611
Borrelia, 1600
geographic distribution of, 1105t
infections, 648t–649t
relapsing fevers and, 1105, 1105t, 1607–1608, 1608f
uveitis and, 175–176
Borrelia burgdorferi
in bacterial arthritis, 383t
biology of, 406–407
causing retinitis and uveitis, 169t
in chronic meningitis, 186t, 187
diagnosis of, 410, 410f
encephalitis/myelitis caused by, 193t–194t
enzootic cycles of, 405–406, 406f
genetic factors in, 407
history of, 405
host immune response in, 407
joint effusion in, 413
ketolides, 1221
macrolides, 1221
in myocarditis, 447
in pregnancy, 413
Borrelia duttonii, 1607–1608
Borrelia hermisii, 1607–1608
Borrelia hispanica, 1607–1608
Borrelia miyamotoi, 1607–1608
Borrelia persica, 1607–1608
Borrelia recurrentis, 1607–1608
Borrelia turicatae, 1607–1608
Borreliosis (Lyme), dermatologic manifestations of, 114t–115t
Botulinum toxin, 208f
of anaerobic bacteria, 1633
in food-borne diarrheal illness, 330
pathogenesis and pathology of, 209–210
Botulism, 208–213
and bioterrorism, 671t–673t, 677
clinical features of, 211, 677
diagnosis of, 212, 677
differential diagnosis of, 212
epidemiology of, 208–209
food-borne, 209, 212t
clinical features of, 211
from marine mammals, 667
infant, 210
management of, 212–213
pathogenesis and pathology of, 209–210
prevention of, 210
Boutonneuse fever, 137t–138t
Bovine papular stomatitis virus, 665
Bovine spongiform encephalopathy (BSE), 214, 215t, 665
epidemiology of, 215
molecular strain typing of, 218–219
Bowel decontamination, in liver transplant patients, 754, 754t
Bowel preparation, and surgical site infections, antibiotic prophylaxis for, 687
Brain
biopsy
encephalitis/myelitis, 196
granulomatous amebic encephalitis and, 1747
cryptococcoma in, 1694
in cystic echinococcosis, 1042
parenchyma inflammation in immune reconstitution inflammatory syndrome, 861–862, 861f

Brain abscesses, 198–203
anaerobic bacteria in, 1635–1636
clinical features of, 201
definition of, 198
diagnosis of, 201–202
epidemiology of, 199
Listeria monocytogenes and, 1540
management of, 202–203
nocardiosis and, 1551
pathophysiology of, 199–201
prevention of, 201
Pseudomonas aeruginosa in, 1589
Pseudomonas spp. in, 1589
site, based on predisposing condition, 199t
Brainerd diarrhea, 349
Branhamella spp., 151
Brazilian purpuric fever, 150
Breast-feeding
congenital infection in, 516
HIV transmission through, 901, 908
Brevibacterium, 1547, 1548t
Brevundimonas
nomenclature of, 1581t–1582t
prevalence of, 1579
Brill-Zinsser disease, 2, 1670
Brivudin, 1312–1313
adverse reactions of, 1313
dosage of, 1313
in special circumstances, 1313
indications of, 1313
mechanism of action, 1313
pharmacokinetics and distribution of, 1313
route of administration, 1313
in vitro activity of, 1313
Brodalumab, 802
Bronchial washing, for laboratory diagnosis of mycobacteria, 1651t
Bronchiectasis, 244–250
approach to diagnosis of, 246–247, 247f, 248t
bacteriology of, 246
clinical findings of, 246
definition of, 244–245
pathophysiology of, 245, 245t
prevention of exacerbations of, 247–249
principles of management of, 247
treatment of acute exacerbations of, 249
Bronchiolitis obliterans, 749
Bronchitis, 243–244
acute, 244t
antibiotics for, 1152t
approach to diagnosis of, 243–244
from Aspergillus, 1691
chronic, 243
quinolones for, 1243
definition of, 243
epidemiology of, 243
from Moraxella catarrhalis, 1624
pathogens of, 243
pathophysiology of, 243
principles of management of, 244
Bronchoalveolar lavage
Aspergillus in, 1688
fluid, microsporidia in, 1739
hospital-acquired pneumonia, 260
in immunologically mediated diseases, 771
for laboratory diagnosis of mycobacteria, 1651t
lower respiratory tract infections, 267–268
Bronchopneumonia, definition of, 253
Bronchoscopy
in immunologically mediated diseases, 771
in lower respiratory tract infections, 267–268
Brown adipose tissue, 606
Brucella, 1098, 1611, 1614–1616
and bioterrorism, 671t
causing endocarditis, 461t
in chronic meningitis, 186t
clinical manifestations of, 1616
diagnostic microbiology of, 1615–1616
epidemiology of, 1614
in jaundice, 1135t
management of, 1616
nature of, 1614, 1614t
in osteomyelitis, 390
pathogenesis of, 1614–1615, 1615f
prevention of, 1615

Brucella (Continued)
in prostatitis, 533t
transmission of, 665t
Brucella abortus, 1098, 1614t
nature of, 1614
transmission of, 663
Brucella canis, 1614t
from dog urine, 658
Brucella cetaceae, 1614t
Brucella inonimata, 1614t
Brucella melitensis, 1098, 1614t
nature of, 1614
transmission of, 663
Brucella microti, 1614t
Brucella neotomeae, 1614t
Brucella ovis, 1614t
Brucella pinnipediae, 1614t
Brucella suis, 1098, 1614t
nature of, 1614
transmission of, 663
Brucellosis, 1098–1101
and bioterrorism, 672t
chronic, 1098
clinical features of, 1098–1099
clinical manifestations of, 1616
complications of, 1099–1100, 1099t
dermatologic manifestations of, 113, 114t–115t
diagnosis of, 1099–1100
diagnostic microbiology of, 1615–1616
from dog urine, 658
epidemiology of, 1098, 1614
eye involvement in, 982
and fever of unknown origin, 613
management of, 1100, 1100t–1101t, 1616
myocarditis and, 446–447
and occupational infections, 648t–649t, 651t–654t
pathogenesis of, 1098, 1615f
prevention of, 1098, 1615
and recreational infections, 644
Brugia malayi
clinical manifestations of, 1777
epidemiology of, 1765
life cycle of, 1769f
pathogenicity of, 1768
treatment of, 1345t–1351t
Brugia timori
epidemiology of, 1765
pathogenicity of, 1768
Buboes, 1078, 1081
aspiration of, 1083
in bubonic plague, 1081–1082, 1082f
in chancroid, 590, 590f
in lymphogranuloma venereum, 587, 587f
management of, 1084
Bubonic plague, 140f, 1078
clinical features of, 1081–1082, 1082f
management of, 1083
Buccal space abscess, 313, 313f
Budesonide, 230
Buffalopox, 665
Bugs, 106t
see also specific types
Building cleaning worker, occupational infections, 648t–649t
Bullous impetigo, 88
Bunyaviruses, 1110
and bioterrorism, 671t
clinical features of, 1114t–1115t
epidemiology of, 1112t
Burkholderia, 1595–1596
clinical manifestations of, 1596
diagnostic microbiology of, 1596
epidemiology of, 1595–1596
management and resistance of, 1596
nature and taxonomy of, 1595
nomenclature of, 1581t–1582t
pathogenicity and pathogenesis of, 1596
Burkholderia cepacia
and chronic granulomatous disease, 708
clinical manifestations of, 1596
epidemiology of, 1595
hospital-acquired pneumonia and, 259t
nature and taxonomy of, 1595

Burkholderia cepacia (Continued)
nosocomial infections from, 1588t
prevalence of, 1579
virulence factors of, 1596
Burkholderia gladioli, 1595
Burkholderia mallei, 1595
and bioterrorism, 671t
glanders, 665
Burkholderia pickettii, 1595
Burkholderia pseudomallei, 1073, 1595
and bioterrorism, 671t
and drowning-associated infections, 680
pathogenesis and pathology of, 1073
prevention of, 1073
see also Melioidosis
Burkholderia thailandiensis, 1596
Burkitt-like lymphoma, 876
Burkitt's lymphoma, 626, 876
Burn wound, sepsis, Pseudomonas aeruginosa in, 1588, 1588f, 1592, 1593f
Burns, infection in, 698–700, 700f
classification of, 700t
guidelines for diagnosis of sepsis in, 698b
primary sites of, 698
Buruli ulcer, 92, 287, 1648, 1648f
Butcher, and occupational infections, 648t–649t
Butoconazole, for vulvovaginal candidiasis, 488t

C
C-reactive protein (CRP), 608–609
in chronic chlamydial infections, 1679–1680
in osteomyelitis, 393
in prosthetic joint infection (PJI), 400
in sepsis, 420
C-type lectin receptors (CLRs), 31
C5a peptidase, 1528
Calabar swellings, 1047, 1777
Calcineurin inhibitors, 1378–1379
Caliciviridae, 1393, 1394t
Caliciviruses, 1393–1396, 1394t
clinical manifestations of, 1396
diagnostic microbiology of, 1396
epidemiology of, 1394
nature of, 1393–1394
pathogenicity of, 1395
viral enteritis and, 338
Calymmatobacterium granulomatis, 1565
lymphadenopathy and, 141
Camels, 663–666
bites, 665
Brucella melitensis, 663
CAMP test, for Listeria monocytogenes, 1539
Camping, and recreational infections, 643–644
Campylobacter, 1600–1602, 1601t
bacterial enteritis and, 336
cellulitis and, 92
clinical features of, 1602
in contaminated food, 1600
diagnosis of, 339
diagnostic microbiology of, 1601–1602
enterocolitis, in HIV/AIDS, 858
epidemiology of, 1600
for food-borne diarrheal illness, 328
doses of, 329t
in human bites, 683t
management of, 339, 1602
microbiology of, 1600
and occupational infections, 648t–649t
pathogenesis of, 1600–1601
prevention of, 1601
quinolones for, 1246
in reactive arthritis, 386
travelers' diarrhea and, 375, 375t, 950
Campylobacter coli, 1600
bacterial enteritis and, 336
clinical features of, 1602
diagnosis of, 339
diagnostic microbiology of, 1602
Campylobacter fetus, 1600
bacterial enteritis and, 336
clinical features of, 1602

Campylobacter fetus (Continued)
diagnostic microbiology of, 1602
erysipelas and, 89
pathogenesis of, 1601
transmission of, 665t
Campylobacter hyointestinalis, 1601–1602
Campylobacter jejuni, 1600
bacterial enteritis and, 336
and bioterrorism, 671t
in cats, 660
characteristics of, in food-borne diarrheal illness, 330t
clindamycin, 1225
clinical features of, 1602
diagnosis of, 339
diagnostic microbiology of, 1602
diarrhea, 331
erysipelas and, 89
pathogenesis of, 1600–1601
Campylobacter laridis, transmission of, 665t
Campylobacter rectus, 1601–1602
Campylobacter upsaliensis, bacterial enteritis and, 336
Canakinumab, 798t–799t, 801
Canale Smith syndrome, 721–722
Duncan's syndrome, 721
Canaliculitis, 157
Canarypox vector prime, 833
Cancer
in aging HIV-positive patient, 929–930
in cryptococcosis prognosis, 1696
infections in, 723–738
clinical features of, 725–728
fever, 725–726
sites of infection in, 726–728, 726f
types of infection in, 726
diagnosis of, 733
medical history in, 733
microbiology, radiology, and histopathology in, 733
physical examination in, 733
epidemiology of, 723–724
bacterial infections in, 723–724, 723b, 724f
fungal infections in, 724
management of, 733–738
empiric antibiotic therapy in, 734–735, 734f–735f
reassessment of therapy in, 735–738
risk assessment in, 734, 734b
supportive care in, 738
pathogenesis of, 724–725
defects of innate and acquired immunity in, 725, 725f
underlying conditions in, 724–725
prevention of, 728–733
antimicrobial prophylaxis in, 729–732, 732t
environmental measures for, 728–729
immunoglobulins in, 732
vaccinations in, 732–733
oral lesions in, 318
Candida, 1681t
antifungal resistance of, 1683–1684
in bacterial arthritis, 383t
in bloodstream infection, 440–442
in burn wounds, 699–700
in cancer patients, 724, 737
in catheter-related bloodstream infection (CRBSI), 435
causing retinitis and uveitis, 170t
in central nervous system, 444
in chronic meningitis, 186t
in complicated urinary tract infection, 540
in cystitis, 530
distribution of, 439
endocarditis, 442
endophthalmitis and, 159
epidemiology of, 1682
fluconazole-resistant, 744
hospital-acquired pneumonia and, 259t
in human bites, 683t
infections caused by, in hematopoietic stem cell transplantation, 744
interaction of, 440
intra-abdominal, 358
microflora, 355
nature of, 1681
in organ transplantation, 806

Candida (Continued)
in pancreas transplant patients, 768
in pericarditis, 450
prophylaxis for, 689
in prostatitis, 533t
and secukinumab, 802
in sepsis, 419
and skin manifestations of HIV, 883
susceptibility testing of, 1683–1684
susceptibility to antifungals, 440
uveitis and, 169
Candida albicans, 854
antifungals in, 440, 441t
diagnosis of, 127
diagnostic microbiology of, 1683, 1711
endophthalmitis and, 159
epidemiology of, 122, 439, 1682, 1710
in hematopoietic stem cell transplantation, 744
in intestinal transplant patients, 760
in mouth, 318
nature of, 1710
in neurocandidiasis, 444
in ocular candidiasis, 445
paronychia and, 89
pathogenicity of, 1683, 1711
pharyngitis and, 234–235
resistance of, 1683
risk factors for, 439–440
uveitis and, 169
in vulvovaginal candidiasis, 486, 488–489, 1686
Candida dubliniensis, 854
diagnostic microbiology of, 1683
Candida glabrata, 854
antifungals and, 440, 441t
diagnostic microbiology of, 1683
endocarditis, 442
epidemiology of, 439, 1682
management of, 441–442
resistance of, 1683
in vulvovaginal candidiasis, 486, 488–489, 1686
Candida krusei
antifungals in, 440, 441t
epidemiology of, 439
management of, 441–442
resistance of, 1683
Candida parapsilosis, 854
antifungals in, 440, 441t
diagnostic microbiology of, 1683
epidemiology of, 122, 439, 1682
in intravenous catheters, 1686
Candida paronychia, and occupational infections, 648t–649t
Candida tropicalis
antifungals in, 440, 441t
epidemiology of, 439, 1682
pathogenicity of, 1683
in vulvovaginal candidiasis, 486
Candidemia, 439–442, 443t, 444–445, 1684
dermatologic manifestations of, 114t–115t, 118
Candidiasis, 1681–1687
chronic
disseminated, 1684, 1687
mucocutaneous, 125
clinical features of, 125–126
clinical manifestations of, 440–445, 1684
cutaneous, 123
diagnosis of, 127
epidemiology of, 122
and deep-seated infections, 1684
diagnostic microbiology of, 1683–1684
disseminated, 443t, 1684
epidemiology of, 1682–1683
esophageal, 1686
of fingernails, 123
hepatosplenic, 442–444, 728
in HIV/AIDS, 854
oral, 854, 854f
in intestinal transplant patients, 760
intra-abdominal, 358
invasive, 1684
in kidney transplant patients, 768
management of, 128, 1684–1687, 1685f, 1685t
mucocutaneous, 440, 444, 1684
nature of, 1681–1682
ocular, 445

Candidiasis (Continued)
oral, 318
oropharyngeal, 854
pathogenesis of, 440
pathogenicity of, 1683
pathogens and epidemiology of, 439–440
risk factors for, 439–440, 440b
as skin manifestation of HIV, 883, 884f
systemic, 439–445, 1686–1687
treatment of, 443t
vulvovaginal, 486–489, 1686
in HIV/AIDS, 854
Candiduria, in kidney transplant patients, 768
Cannibalism, 215–216
Capillaria philippinensis
in chronic diarrhea, 349
pathogenicity of, 1768
treatment of, 1345t–1351t
Capillariasis, 1777
chronic diarrhea and, 349
treatment of, 1345t–1351t
Capnocytophaga canimorsus
cellulitis and, 90
occupational infections, 648t–649t
postsplenectomy sepsis, 778, 778t
Capreomycin, as antituberculosis agent, 1270
Capsomere vaccines, 1441–1442
Capsular polysaccharides, of anaerobic bacteria, 1633
Capsules, *Neisseria*, 1558–1559, 1558f
Carbamazepine, 476
Carbapenamase-resistant gram-negative bacteria (CR GNB), 1289
antimicrobial agents used against, 1290t
Carbapenem-resistant *A. baumannii* isolates (CRAB), 1595
Carbapenem-resistant Enterobacteriaceae (CRE)
polymyxins for, 1287
in thoracic transplantation patients, 749
Carbapenemases, 1181
Carbapenems, 1162, 1203–1204, 1289
for *Alcaligenes* spp., 1597
for anaerobic bacteria, 1643
antimicrobial spectrum, generic names, routes of administration and dosages, 1206t–1207t
for cystic fibrosis, 301
dosage in renal failure, 1213t–1214t
drug interactions, 1216
for gram-negative organisms, 1210
for intra-abdominal sepsis, 357
in kidney transplant patients, 763
for *P. aeruginosa* infection, 1210
pharmacokinetics of, 1205t
for *Pseudomonas aeruginosa*, 1589
resistance to, 1184
Enterobacteriaceae, 1576–1577
gram-negative organisms, 1210
for staphylococcal infections, 1209
for *Staphylococcus aureus*, 1520
Stenotrophomonas maltophilia and, 1597
susceptibilities of selected bacteria to, 1208t–1209t
see also individual drugs
Carbenicillin
for *P. aeruginosa* infection, 1210
pharmacokinetics of, 1205t
susceptibilities of selected bacteria to, 1208t–1209t
Carboxypenicillins, antimicrobial spectrum, generic names, routes of administration and dosages, 1206t–1207t
Carbuncles, 86–87, 86f
Carcinoma, hepatocellular, and fever of unknown origin, 614
Carcinoma *in situ*, 580–581, 581f
Card agglutination test for trypanosomiasis (CATT), 142
Cardiac magnetic resonance imaging (CMR), in myocarditis, 448
Cardiac tamponade, 279
Cardiobacterium hominis, 1622
Cardiobacterium valvarum, 1622
Cardiomegaly, in pericarditis, 452, 452f
Cardiothoracic surgery, antibiotic prophylaxis and, 1156, 1157t–1158t
Cardiotoxicity, as quinolones adverse effect, 1247
Cardiovascular disease (CVD), in aging HIV-positive patient, 927–929
Cardiovascular imaging, 478
Cardiovascular syphilis, 562

Cardiovascular system
brucellosis complications in, 1099
Candida infection of, 443t
Mycoplasma pneumoniae in, 1662t
Cardioverter-defibrillator implantation, antibiotic prophylaxis and, 1160
Cardiovirus, 338
Carditis
diagnosis of, 474t
heart block caused by, 412
Lyme disease and, 408, 412, 412t
management of, 476
rheumatic fever and, 472–473, 473f
Carey Coombs murmur, 473
Carotenoids, 1646
Carrion's disease, 1674
Caspase-associated recruitment domains (CARD), 31–32
Caspofungin, 1341–1343
adverse effects of, 1343
for aspergillosis, 1691
for cancer patients, 737–738
for catheter-related bloodstream infection (CRBSI), 436t
in children, 1343
dosing and administration, 1341
drug interactions of, 1343
indications of, 1341–1342
mechanism of action, 1341
for mucormycosis, 1698
pharmacodynamics of, 1341
pharmacokinetics and distribution of, 1341
structures of, 1342f
Castleman's disease
lymphadenopathy vs, 137t–138t
multicentric, 877
clinical features of, 877
diagnosis of, 877
management of, 877–878
pathogenesis of, 877
Cat(s)
bites, 659, 659t
components of care for, 658t
infections from, 191t
infectious diseases associated with, 659–660, 659t
direct contact, 660
enteric, 660
inhalation, 660
mites, 660
rabies from, 659
sporotrichosis in, 1715
Cat flea, 1669, 1673
Cat-scratch disease, 659–660, 1675
encephalopathy and, 190
and fever of unknown origin, 613
lymphadenopathy and, 137t–138t, 139–140
Cat-scratch fever, occupational infections, 648t–649t
Catalase, 23, 1513t–1514t
Cathelicidins, 1512
Catheter encrustations, *Mycoplasma hominis* in, 1664
Catheter-related bloodstream infection (CRBSI), 427
and burn infections, 698
clinical features of, 427–428
coagulase-negative staphylococci and, 1511–1512
definitions for, 430t
diagnosis of, 433–434
epidemiology of, 427
local, 427, 430f
management of, 434–436
pathogenesis of, 427, 429f
prevention of, 428–433
rates of, 428t
risk factors for, 429t
systemic, 427–428
see also Central line-associated bloodstream infections (CLABSI)
Catheter-related infections
aerobic actinomycetes and, 1551–1552
in intestinal transplant patients, 756
Catheters
antimicrobial, 433
cuffs and, 433
in outpatient parenteral antimicrobial therapy, 1201
replacement, 433
risk of infection from, 689
site of, 428–430

Catheters (Continued)
  specimens in, for urine culture, 527
  tip of, 434
  see also specific sites
Cationic antiseptics, 155
Cattle
  bites, 665
  Brucella abortus, 663
  Escherichia coli O157:H7, 665
  variant Creutzfeldt-Jakob disease, 665
Cavernous sinus thrombosis, 313–314, 314f
CCR5, 1485
CCR5 inhibitors, antiretroviral drugs, 925
CCR5Δ32 mutation, of CCR5 gene, and HIV-1 infection, 844
CD3/T-cell receptor (CD3/TCR) complex, 716, 717f
CD4 cells
  in HIV-associated TB, 868
  as HIV prognostic marker, 912, 913t
  mycobacteria and, 1649–1650
CD4+ cells
  and opportunistic infection in HIV, 850
  in pregnancy, 501
CD4 lymphocytes, in rheumatic fever, 471–472
CD4+ T-cells
  cellular immune responses, 32–33
  in hematopoietic stem cell transplantation, 739
  in HIV patients receiving antiretroviral therapy, 864
  human T-lymphocyte leukemia virus-1, 1491
  in immune reconstitution disorder, 860–861, 863
CD4 T-cells
  response to HIV-1, 842
  roles of, in immune deficiency, 842–843
  in tuberculosis, 273
CD8 cells, mycobacteria and, 1649–1650
CD8 lymphocytes, in rheumatic fever, 471–472
CD8+ T-cell, cellular immune responses, 33
CD8 T-cell, response to HIV-1 of, 841
CD25 deficiency, 716
CD36, 1017
CD40, 33
CD40 deficiency, 720
CD40L deficiency, 720
CD45 deficiency, 716
CD127 deficiency, 716
CD154 deficiency, 720
Cefaclor
  antimicrobial spectrum, routes of administration and dosages, 1206t–1207t
  dosage in renal failure, 1213t–1214t
  pharmacokinetics of, 1205t
  susceptibilities of selected bacteria to, 1208t–1209t
Cefadroxil
  antimicrobial spectrum, routes of administration and dosages, 1206t–1207t
  dosage in renal failure, 1213t–1214t
  pharmacokinetics of, 1205t
  susceptibilities of selected bacteria to, 1208t–1209t
Cefamandole, prophylaxis, 1158t
Cefazolin
  for anaerobic infection, 1634
  antimicrobial spectrum, routes of administration and dosages, 1206t–1207t
  for catheter-related bloodstream infection (CRBSI), 436t
  for cellulitis, 92
  for complicated urinary tract infection, 545t
  dosage in renal failure, 1213t–1214t
  for endophthalmitis, 163t
  for infective arthritis, 386t
  for lung abscess, 269f
  neurologic effects of, 1215
  pharmacokinetics of, 1205t
  prophylaxis, 1158t
  susceptibilities of selected bacteria to, 1208t–1209t
Cefdinir
  antimicrobial spectrum, routes of administration and dosages, 1206t–1207t
  dosage in renal failure, 1213t–1214t
  otitis media and, 238t
  pharmacokinetics of, 1205t
  susceptibilities of selected bacteria to, 1208t–1209t

Cefditoren
  antimicrobial spectrum, routes of administration and dosages, 1206t–1207t
  dosage in renal failure, 1213t–1214t
  pharmacokinetics of, 1205t
  susceptibilities of selected bacteria to, 1208t–1209t
Cefepime
  antimicrobial spectrum, routes of administration and dosages, 1206t–1207t
  for complicated urinary tract infection, 545t
  dosage in renal failure, 1213t–1214t
  for hospital-acquired pneumonia, 260t
  indication, brain abscess, 202–203
  for lung abscess, 269f
  for P. aeruginosa infection, 1210
  pharmacokinetics of, 1205t
  susceptibilities of selected bacteria to, 1208t–1209t
Cefixime
  antimicrobial spectrum, routes of administration and dosages, 1206t–1207t
  for complicated urinary tract infection, 544t
  dosage in renal failure, 1213t–1214t
  for enteric fevers, 1006
  for gonorrhea, 595
  pharmacokinetics of, 1205t
  susceptibilities of selected bacteria to, 1208t–1209t
Cefmetazole, for anaerobic bacteria, 1643
Cefoperazone
  antimicrobial spectrum, routes of administration and dosages, 1206t–1207t
  dosage in renal failure, 1213t–1214t
  for P. aeruginosa infection, 1210
  pharmacokinetics of, 1204, 1205t
  susceptibilities of selected bacteria to, 1208t–1209t
Cefotaxime
  antimicrobial spectrum, routes of administration and dosages, 1206t–1207t
  for complicated urinary tract infection, 545t
  dosage in renal failure, 1213t–1214t
  for epiglottitis, 233
  for leptospirosis, 1103
  in liver transplant patients, 754t
  for lung abscess, 269f
  for meningitis, 180
  pharmacokinetics of, 1205t
  prophylaxis, 1158t
  susceptibilities of selected bacteria to, 1208t–1209t
Cefotetan
  for anaerobic bacteria, 1634, 1643
  antimicrobial spectrum, routes of administration and dosages, 1206t–1207t
  dosage in renal failure, 1213t–1214t
  indications, lung abscess, 269f
  pharmacokinetics of, 1204, 1205t
  susceptibilities of selected bacteria to, 1208t–1209t
Cefoxitin
  for anaerobic bacteria, 1634, 1643
  antimicrobial spectrum, routes of administration and dosages, 1206t–1207t
  for dog bites, 657t
  dosage in renal failure, 1213t–1214t
  for foot ulcers, 131t
  for lung abscess, 269f
  pharmacokinetics of, 1205t
  susceptibilities of selected bacteria to, 1208t–1209t
Cefpodoxime
  indication, otitis media, 238t
  indications, lung abscess, 269f
  susceptibilities of selected bacteria to, 1208t–1209t
Cefpodoxime proxetil
  antimicrobial spectrum, routes of administration and dosages, 1206t–1207t
  for complicated urinary tract infection, 544t
  for cystitis, 528t
  dosage in renal failure, 1213t–1214t
  pharmacokinetics of, 1205t
Cefprozil
  antimicrobial spectrum, routes of administration and dosages, 1206t–1207t
  dosage in renal failure, 1213t–1214t
  pharmacokinetics of, 1205t
  susceptibilities of selected bacteria to, 1208t–1209t

Ceftaroline
  antimicrobial spectrum, routes of administration and dosages, 1206t–1207t
  for complicated urinary tract infection, 545t
  dosage in renal failure, 1213t–1214t
  for lung abscess, 269f
  pharmacokinetics of, 1205t
  susceptibilities of selected bacteria to, 1208t–1209t
Ceftazidime
  antimicrobial spectrum, routes of administration and dosages, 1206t–1207t
  for brain abscess, 202–203
  for cancer patients, 734–735
  for catheter-related bloodstream infection (CRBSI), 436t
  for complicated urinary tract infection, 545t
  dosage in renal failure, 1213t–1214t
  for drowning-associated infections, 681
  for endophthalmitis, 162
  for hospital-acquired pneumonia, 260t
  for lung abscess, 269f
  for melioidosis, 1077t
  for P. aeruginosa infection, 1210
  pharmacokinetics of, 1205t
  susceptibilities of selected bacteria to, 1208t–1209t
Ceftazidime-avibactim, for complicated urinary tract infection, 545t
Ceftibuten
  antimicrobial spectrum, routes of administration and dosages, 1206t–1207t
  for complicated urinary tract infection, 544t
  dosage in renal failure, 1213t–1214t
  pharmacokinetics of, 1205t
  susceptibilities of selected bacteria to, 1208t–1209t
Ceftizoxime
  antimicrobial spectrum, routes of administration and dosages, 1206t–1207t
  dosage in renal failure, 1213t–1214t
  for lung abscess, 269f
  pharmacokinetics of, 1205t
  susceptibilities of selected bacteria to, 1208t–1209t
Ceftobiprole
  antimicrobial spectrum, routes of administration and dosages, 1206t–1207t
  dosage in renal failure, 1213t–1214t
  for P. aeruginosa infection, 1210
  pharmacokinetics of, 1205t
  susceptibilities of selected bacteria to, 1208t–1209t
Ceftolozane-tazobactam
  antimicrobial spectrum, routes of administration and dosages, 1206t–1207t
  dosage in renal failure, 1213t–1214t
  for P. aeruginosa infection, 1210
  pharmacokinetics of, 1205t
  susceptibilities of selected bacteria to, 1208t–1209t
Ceftriaxone
  antimicrobial spectrum, routes of administration and dosages, 1206t–1207t
  for cancer patients, 734–735
  for cellulitis, 92
  chemoprophylaxis, for meningococcal disease, 1560
  for community-acquired pneumonia, 255t
  for complicated urinary tract infection, 545t
  dosage in renal failure, 1213t–1214t
  for enteric fevers, 1006
  for epididymitis and orchitis, 538
  for epiglottitis, 233
  for foot ulcers, 131t
  for gonorrhea, 595
  for Haemophilus ducreyi, 1621
  for hospital-acquired pneumonia, 260t
  for infective arthritis, 386t
  for lung abscess, 269f
  for Lyme disease, 412
  for meningitis, 187t
  for otitis media, 238t
  in outpatient parenteral antimicrobial therapy, 1201
  pharmacokinetics of, 1204, 1205t
  susceptibilities of selected bacteria to, 1208t–1209t
  for syphilis, 565

Cefuroxime
  antimicrobial spectrum, routes of administration and
      dosages, 1206t–1207t
  for cellulitis, 92
  for dog bites, 657t
  dosage in renal failure, 1213t–1214t
  for epiglottitis, 233
  for keratitis, 152
  for lung abscess, 269f
  for Lyme disease, 412, 414
  prophylaxis, 1158t
  susceptibilities of selected bacteria to, 1208t–1209t
Cefuroxime axetil
  antimicrobial spectrum, routes of administration and
      dosages, 1206t–1207t
  for complicated urinary tract infection, 544t
  dosage in renal failure, 1213t–1214t
  pharmacokinetics of, 1205t
Cell culture, of microsporidia, 1740
Cell culture cytotoxicity neutralization assays (CCNAs),
    for Clostridium difficile, 1629–1630
Cell-mediated immunity, 32
Cellulitis, 84–94, 85t, 90f
  antibiotics for, 91–92, 1152t
  associated with bites, 90–91
  associated with predisposing conditions, 90
  from cat bites, 659
  caused by Staphylococcus aureus and Streptococcus
      pyogenes, 89
  clinical features, diagnosis and management, 86–93
  clostridial, 99
  differential diagnosis of, 91
  epidemiology of, 84
  exposure to fish, 91
  in HIV, 882–883
  lymphadenopathy, 140
  nonclostridial anaerobic, 99
  orbital, 313
  periorbital, 156–157
  prevention of, 86
  recurrent, 90, 91f, 133, 133f–134f
    assessment and diagnosis of, 135
    management of, 135
    microbiology of, 133–134
    prevention of, 135
  from Stenotrophomonas maltophilia, 1597
  types of, 92
  vaginal cuff, 497
  water exposure, 91
Centers for Disease Control and Prevention (CDC)
  in AIDS, 579
  and catheter insertion, 691
  for epididymitis and orchitis, 538
  guidelines for preventing healthcare workplace
      transmission of infectious diseases, 647
  vaccinations, 891
  webpages of, 952
Centipeda periodontii, 1631
Central European encephalitis, 1495t
Central fatigue, in chronic fatigue syndrome,
    633–634
Central line-associated bloodstream infections (CLABSI),
    60, 691, 691t
Central nervous system
  adverse reactions to
    of folate inhibitors, 1283
    of β-lactam antibiotics, 1215t
    of M2 inhibitors, 1318
  Candida infection in, 444
  candidiasis and, 1686
  cryptococcosis and, 1694–1695, 1695t
  cytomegalovirus disease of, 853
  focal pyogenic infections of, 198–207, 198f
  infections of
    in cancer patients, 728
    congenital, 510
  influenza virus and, 1470
  Lyme disease in, 408
  mucormycosis and, 1698
  Mycoplasma pneumoniae in, 1661
Central nervous system disease, in immune reconstitution
    inflammatory syndrome, 861
Central nervous system infections, 1290
  anaerobic bacteria in, 1632f, 1635–1636
  β-lactam antibiotics for, 1210–1211

Central nervous system infections (Continued)
    from Listeria monocytogenes, 1539–1540
    Pseudomonas aeruginosa in, 1589, 1592
Central nervous system reactions, of quinolones, 1247
Central venous catheterization, prolonged, risk of
    infection from, 689
Central venous catheters (CVCs)
  non-tunneled, 427, 435
  tunneled, 427–430
Cephalexin
  antimicrobial spectrum, routes of administration and
      dosages, 1206t–1207t
  for complicated urinary tract infection, 544t
  for cystitis, 528t
  for dog bites, 657t
  dosage in renal failure, 1213t–1214t
  for foot ulcers, 131t
  for lung abscess, 269f
  pharmacokinetics of, 1205t
  susceptibilities of selected bacteria to, 1208t–1209t
Cephalosporins, 1203
  adverse effects, 1215–1216
  adverse reactions of, 1153
  for Alcaligenes spp., 1597
  for anaerobic bacteria, 1210, 1643
  antimicrobial spectrum, generic names, routes of
      administration and dosages, 1206t–1207t
  for brain abscess, 206–207
  for cancer patients, 734–735
  for coagulase-negative staphylococcal infections,
      1521–1522
  discovery of, 1217
  dosage in renal failure, 1213t–1214t
  drug interactions, 1216
  endophthalmitis, 162
  for enteric fevers, 1006
  for Erysipelothrix rhusiopathiae, 1542
  for gonorrhea, 595
  for gram-negative organisms, 1210
  for Haemophilus spp., 1621
  for intra-abdominal sepsis, 357
  for leptospirosis, 1609
  meningitis and, 180
  for pelvic inflammatory disease, 493
  pharmacokinetics of, 1205t
  for pneumococcal infections, 1209
  for postpartum endometritis, 495
  in pregnancy, 504
  prophylaxis, 437
    of rheumatic fever, 475t
    and surgical site infections, 687
    for trauma-related infections, 688
  for Pseudomonas aeruginosa, 1589
  for pyelonephritis, 552
  resistance to, Bacillus cereus, 1542
  for staphylococcal infections, 1209
  for Staphylococcus aureus, 1520
  susceptibilities of selected bacteria to, 1208t–1209t
Cephalothin
  antimicrobial spectrum, routes of administration and
      dosages, 1206t–1207t
  indications for, 92
  pharmacokinetics of, 1205t
  susceptibilities of selected bacteria to, 1208t–1209t
Cephems, 1162
Cercarial dermatitis, 1028–1029
Cercopithecine herpesvirus-1, 666
Cerebellum abscess, 199
Cerebral angiostrongyliasis, treatment of, 975
Cerebral malaria
  clinical features of, 1019, 1021f
  immunologic factors and cytokines for, 1017
Cerebral microabscesses, Candida infections, 444
Cerebral microsporidiosis, 1741, 1742f
Cerebral phaeohyphomycosis, 1723
Cerebral vasculitis, 772–773
Cerebrospinal fluid (CSF)
  African trypanosomiasis and, 969
  analysis, meningitis and, 180
  Creutzfeldt-Jakob disease and, 217
  cryptococcosis and, 1694–1695
  Cryptococcus in, 1693–1694
  examination of, in syphilis, 564
  granulomatous amebic encephalitis and, 1747
  for helminths diagnosis, 1776

Cerebrospinal fluid (CSF) (Continued)
  hydrocephalus shunts and, 221
  for laboratory diagnosis, of mycobacteria, 1651, 1651t
  lumbar puncture. see Lumbar puncture
  Lyme disease in, 408
  meningitis, 177
  microbiologic investigation of, in congenital infection,
      512t
  microsporidia in, 1739
  penetration of aminoglycosides into, 1234
  primary amebic meningoencephalitis and, 1747
  West Nile virus, 1498
Certolizumab, 797
Certolizumab pegol, 798t–799t
Cervarix®, 1441
Cervical cancer
  clinical manifestations of, 1443, 1443t
  human papillomavirus and, 575, 576f–578f, 577, 579,
      582
  improved screening for, 1441
  prophylactic vaccines for, 1441–1442
  screening, for women with HIV, 906, 906t
Cervical intraepithelial neoplasia (CIN), 580–581
  diagnosis of, 582
  in HIV infection, 906
  management of, 583
Cervical lymphadenitis
  anaerobic bacteria in, 1636t, 1637
  Mycobacterium avium complex in, 1649
Cervical necrotizing fasciitis, 315
Cervical tuberculosis, 278f
Cervicitis, 490
  Mycoplasma genitalium in, 1662
  Mycoplasma hominis in, 1664
  from Neisseria gonorrhoeae, 1562
  nongonococcal, quinolones for, 1243
Cervicovaginal dysplasia, 906
Cesarean section
  closure of, 504
  perinatal HIV transmission prevention, 910
  postpartum endometritis and, 494–495, 495t
Cestoda, nature of, 1763
Cestodes, 989–990, 989f, 989t
  clinical manifestations of, 1778–1779
  description of, 1032
  epidemiology of, 1766
  importance of physical environment in, 990
  infections of, 1033–1036
    diagnosis of, 1033–1034
    management of, 1033–1034
  intestinal, 1764t, 1772
  life cycles of, 1773f–1774f
  pathogenesis and pathology of, 994
  pathogenicity of, 1772
  prevention of, 1772
  tissue, 1764t, 1772
  treatment of, 1001t
  zoonotic, 1033
  see also specific genera
Cethromycin
  peptidyltransferase center, 1221
  pharmacokinetics, 1222
  in vitro activity, 1219
Cetrimide, in Pseudomonas isolation, 1580
Chagas disease, 119, 1065–1072, 1758–1760
  acute phase of, 1067, 1069f, 1759
  chronic indeterminate phase of, 1067
  chronic stage of, 1759
  chronic symptomatic phase of, 1067–1070, 1069f–1070f
  clinical manifestations of, 1759–1760, 1760f
  congenital infection in, 1070
  diagnosis of, 1070–1071
  diagnostic microbiology of, 1759
  digestive form of, 1760
  epidemiology of, 1065–1067, 1758–1759
  etiologic agent of, 1065–1067
  geographic distribution of, 1065, 1066f
  in immunocompromised patients, 1070
  lymphadenopathy and, 137t–138t, 142
  management of, 1071–1072, 1760
  in myocarditis, 447
  nature of, 1758
  oral infection in, 1070
  pathogenicity of, 1759
  post-transfusion in, 1070

Chagas disease (Continued)
prevention of, 1071, 1759
in transfusion-related infections, 704, 704t
transmission of, 1065–1067
Chagasic cardiomyopathy (CCC), 1760
Chagoma, 1759–1760
Chancre, 561, 561f
African trypanosomiasis and, 968
soft, 589
tuberculous, 117
Chancroid, 561, 586t–587t, 589–590, 1137f, 1621
clinical features of, 589–590, 589f–590f
diagnosis of, 590
epidemiology of, 589
lymphadenopathy and, 137t–138t, 140–141
management of, 590
pathogenesis and pathology of, 589
quinolones for, 1243
Checklist Individual Strength, 631–632
Chediak-Higashi syndrome, 705t, 706
Chemokines, in phagocytes, 31
Chemoprophylaxis
for cystitis, 525–526, 526t
for Haemophilus influenzae, 1619
for HIV-associated TB, 868
for influenza viruses, 1469
for leprosy, 956
for meningococcal disease, 1560
quinolones in, 1246
for tuberculosis, 275, 275t
Chemotaxis, 10
Chemotaxis inhibitory protein of Staph. aureus (CHIPS), 1513t–1514t, 1514
Chemotherapy
for amebic liver abscess, 1012–1013
for Chagas disease, 1072
for gastrointestinal parasites, 995
and HIV-associated Kaposi's sarcoma, 875
for non-Hodgkin lymphoma, 875
for schistosomiasis prevention, 1028
Chest radiography
of blastomycosis, 294
of cancer patients, 733
of coccidioidomycosis, 296
of cystic fibrosis, 300
for drowning-associated infections, 681
of histoplasmosis, 292–293, 293f
hospital-acquired, 259
lung diseases in AIDs, 851, 851f
of melioidosis, 1075f, 1077
of paracoccidioidomycosis, 297, 297f
of penicilliosis, 298
for pleural discharge/fluid, 303, 303f
of pulmonary cytomegalovirus, 853
of pulmonary tuberculosis, 556
respiratory viruses, 743, 743f
of sporotrichosis, 298, 298f
in vasculitis, 771
Chest tube drainage
empyema and, 270
for pleural effusion, 304
Cheyletiella
cats, 660
from dogs, 658–659
Chicken, infections from, 191t
Chickenpox, dermatologic manifestations of, 114t–115t
Chiclero ulcer, 1757, 1757f
Chiggers, 1091, 1670
Chiggers mites, 106t
Chikungunya, 80, 1119–1122, 1495t
clinical features of, 1121–1122
diagnosis of, 1122
epidemiology of, 1119
management of, 1122
prevention of, 1120
Chikungunya fever, dermatologic manifestations of, 114t–115t
Chikungunya virus
in infective arthritis, 385–386, 387t
spread of, 944
Children
conjunctivitis in, 150
echinocandin lipopeptides in, 1343

Children (Continued)
fever of unknown origin in, 615
gonorrhea in, 1563
immunocompetent, uveitis in, 167–172
subdural empyema/intracranial epidural abscess in, 204, 205t
tuberculosis in, 275–276
see also Infants; Neonates
Chilomastix mesnili, 1725t, 1731f
Chinese-letter appearance, 1544
Chinese liver fluke, treatment of, 1345t–1351t
Chlamydia, 1676–1680
clinical manifestations of, 1679t, 1680
clinical syndromes caused by, 599t
diagnostic microbiology of, 1678–1680
encephalitis/myelitis and, 194t
epidemiology of, 597, 1676
jaundice, 1135t
life cycle of, 1676f
management of, 600–602, 600t–601t, 1680
nature of, 1676
oropharyngeal, 599–600
pathogenesis and immunity of, 597–598
pathogenicity of, 1676–1678, 1676b, 1677f
prevention of, 602, 1678
rates of, by sex, 598f
in reactive arthritis, 386–387
rectal, 599–600
structure of, 1677f
Chlamydia abortus, 1676, 1679t
Chlamydia caviae, 1676
Chlamydia felis, 1676, 1679t
Chlamydia-like organisms, 1679
Chlamydia muridarum, 1676
Chlamydia pecorum, 1676
Chlamydia pneumoniae
bronchitis and, 244t
diagnostic microbiology of, 1678–1679
diseases associated with, 1679t
epidemiology of, 1676
hospital-acquired pneumonia and, 259t
lower respiratory tract infections, 264f
nature of, 1676
pathogenicity of, 1676–1677
pharyngitis, 234–235
prevention of, 1678
Chlamydia psittaci, 660–661
and bioterrorism, 671t
diseases associated with, 1679t
epidemiology of, 1676
nature of, 1676
Chlamydia suis, 1676
Chlamydia trachomatis
in cervicitis, 490
clindamycin, 1225
clinical features of, 598–600, 599t, 980
conjunctivitis from, 150, 175
diagnosis of, 600
diagnostic microbiology of, 1678
diseases associated with, 1679t
epidemiology of, 597, 598f, 1676
in epididymitis, 537
etiology of, 1138t
in females, 598–599, 599f
in human papillomavirus, 577
immunity in, 597–598
infection, 597–602
ketolides, 1221
life cycle of, 597–598, 598f
lymphadenopathy and, 141
in lymphogranuloma venereum, 587, 589
macrolides, 1221
in males, 599, 599f
management of, 600–602
nature of, 1676
in neonatal infectious conjunctivitis, 594
pathogenesis and pathology of, 597–598
pathogenicity of, 979, 1676–1677
in pelvic inflammatory disease, 492
in postpartum endometritis, 494–495
in pregnancy, 500t
prevention of, 602, 1678
in prostatitis, 533

Chlamydia trachomatis (Continued)
in reactive arthritis, 386–387
trachoma and, 979
Chlamydial infections
chronic, 1679–1680
lymphadenopathy and, 137t–138t
Chlamydophila, in lymph node enlargement, 147t–148t
Chlamydophila pneumoniae
ketolides, 1221
macrolides, 1221
Chlamydospores, 1708
Chlonorchis sinensis
epidemiology of, 1765
pathogenicity of, 1770
Chloramphenicol, 1173, 1260
for actinomycosis, 316
adverse reactions, 1260
for Alcaligenes spp., 1597
for anaerobic bacteria, 1643
bacterial targeting, 1173
for bartonellosis, 1675
chemical structure of, 1173
for conjunctivitis, 152
drug-drug interactions, 1260
for Erysipelothrix rhusiopathiae, 1542
indications, 1260
for lung abscess, 269f
mode of action and spectrum, 1260
mode of action of, 1173
pharmacodynamics of, 1173
pharmacokinetics and distribution, 1260
for plague, 1083–1084, 1083t
prophylaxis, 159
for relapsing fevers, 1109
resistance to, 1173, 1190–1191, 1592t
by decreased drug uptake, 1190–1191
by drug inactivation, 1190
enteric fevers, 1005
route of administration and dosage, 1260
for scrub typhus, 1097, 1671
for spotted fever group rickettsiae, 1669
for syphilis, 565
for tularemia, 1089
for typhus group rickettsiae, 1670
Chlorhexidine
body washing with, 694
in cutaneous antiseptic, 428
indications, folliculitis/furunculosis prevention, 86
mouthwash, postoperative infection prevention with, 689
Chlorhexidine gluconate, 1156
for Acanthamoeba keratitis, 1750
keratitis and, 155
Chloroquine, 1365–1366
adverse reactions, 1366
for amebic infections, 1012
for babesiosis, 1753
dosage of, 1366
indications of, for parasitic infections, 1352t–1362t
for malaria, 1022–1023
for malaria prophylaxis, 951
pharmacokinetics and distribution of, 1366
resistance to, Plasmodium falciparum, 1022, 1366
route of administration, 1366
Chloroquine phosphate
for malaria in pregnancy, 1143t
for parasitic infections, 1345t–1351t
Chlorpromazine, prion infection and, 220
Cholangitis
microsporidiosis in immunocompromised patients and, 1741
sclerosing, 1044
Cholecystectomy, laparoscopic, 1161
Cholecystitis
acalculous
microsporidiosis in immunocompromised patients and, 1741
surgery complications in, 690
antibiotics for, 1152t
Cholera
antibiotic resistance, 1607
clinical features of, 1606–1607
diarrhea and, 335–337, 339

Cholera *(Continued)*
eye involvement in, 982
immunization for, and occupational infections, 650t–651t
management of, 1607
pandemics, 1604–1605
quinolones for, 1246
spread of, 944
tetracyclines for, 1259
trimethoprim-sulfamethoxazole for, 1282
vaccine for travelers, 949
see also Vibrio cholerae
Cholera gravis, 1606–1607
Cholera toxin, 18
Chondroitin sulfate A (CSA), 1017
CHOP regimen, for non-Hodgkin lymphoma, 875–876, 876t
Chorea
diagnosis of, 474t
management of, 476
rheumatic fever and, 472–473
streptococci and, 1533
Chorioamnionitis, *Mycoplasma hominis* in, 1664
Chorioretinitis
from *Candida*, 1686
subacute sclerosing panencephalitis and, 167
from *Toxoplasma gondii*, 1754, 1754f
Chromalveolata, 1744
Chromoblastomycosis
clinical manifestations of, 1719, 1719f
diagnostic microbiology of, 1716, 1716f
epidemiology of, 1713
management of, 1722
nature of, 1712
pathogenicity of, 1715
prevention of, 1715
Chromomycosis, 1712
Chronic ambulatory peritoneal dialysis (CAPD)
infections associated with, quinolones for, 1246
peritonitis and, 359
Chronic disseminated (hepatosplenic) candidiasis, 1684, 1687
Chronic fatigue syndrome, 631–635
abnormalities of the autonomic nervous system, 634
case definition and diagnostic approach, 631–632, 631b, 632t
central fatigue in, 633–634
diagnostic criteria for, 631b
disturbed perception of fatigue in, 634, 634f
epidemiology of, 632
etiology and pathogenesis of, 632–633
perpetuating factors, 633, 633f
precipitating factors, 632–633
predisposing factors, 632
prognosis and treatment of, 634–635
systematic differential diagnosis of, 632t
Chronic granulomatous disease, 705t, 707–709
granulomatous manifestations of, 708, 708f
Chronic hepatitis, in HIV, 926
Chronic hepatitis B, 1421–1422, 1422t
Chronic hepatitis E, 1420
Chronic inflammatory, autoimmune, or malignant diseases (CIAMD), 781
systematic approach to vaccinating patients with, 781–787
Chronic leg ulcers, thalassemia and, 1057, 1057f
Chronic mucocutaneous candidiasis (CMC), 125, 1711
Chronic obstructive pulmonary disease (COPD), 243
acute exacerbations of, 310–311, 310f
Chronic osteomyelitis, 388–398
clinical features of, 391, 391f
management of, 396–398
adjunctive factors in, 398
antibiotic therapy for, 396–398
initial actions for, 396, 396f–397f
soft-tissue, 398
surgery in, 396
Chronic pelvic pain syndrome (CPPS), 532
diagnosis of, 534
management of, 536
Chronic pulmonary aspergillosis (CPA), 1689, 1690f
Chronic relapsing multifocal osteomyelitis (CRMO), 393
Chronic skin involvement, in Lyme disease, 409
Chronic wasting disease (CWD), 215, 215t

Chryseobacterium, 1597–1598
clinical manifestations of, 1598
management of, 1598
microbiology of, 1598
nomenclature of, 1581t–1582t
nosocomial infections from, 1588t
prevalence of, 1579
Chrysops spp., 1765
Chyluria
in filariasis, 1049, 1051
management of, 1051
Ciclopirox, 128
Cidofovir, 759t, 1146t–1147t, 1316
adverse reactions of, 1316
dosage of, 1316
in special circumstances, 1316
indications of, 1316
cytomegalovirus retinitis, 1314t
in kidney transplant patients, 767
mechanism of action, 1316
pharmacokinetics and distribution of, 1316
resistance to, 1316
route of administration, 1316
in vitro activity of, 1316
Ciguatera, characteristics of, in food-borne diarrheal illness, 330t
Ciguatoxin poisoning, 331
Cilastatin, 1204
Ciliates
epidemiology of, 1725–1727
gastrointestinal, 989t
identification in fecal specimens, 1732, 1733f
intestinal and urogenital, 1725–1733, 1725t
nature of, 1725
Cimex lectularius, 109f
Cimicidae, 108–109
Cinchonism, 1370
Ciprofloxacin
for anaerobic bacteria, 1643
for anthrax, 1127
for *Bacillus cereus*, 1542
for bartonellosis, 1675
bronchitis and, 248
for *Campylobacter* spp., 1602
for cancer patients, 735–736
for catheter-related bloodstream infection (CRBSI), 436t
for chancroid, 590
for complicated urinary tract infection, 544t–545t
for cystic fibrosis, 301
for cystitis, 528t
for cystoisosporiasis, 1742
dissociation constants of, 535t
for endophthalmitis, 162
for foot ulcers, 131t
for gastrointestinal protozoa, 999, 1000t
for granuloma inguinale, 591
for *Haemophilus ducreyi*, 1621
for hospital-acquired pneumonia, 260t
for infective arthritis, 386t
for keratitis, 152
for lung abscess, 269f
for plague, 1083–1084
prophylaxis, 1158t
for prostatitis, 536t–537t
for tularemia, 1089, 1617
Circulatory shock, in severe malaria, 1020t
Circumoval precipitation test (COPT), for helminths diagnosis, 1777
Cirrhosis, 1422
alcoholic, and fever of unknown origin, 614–618
in hepatitis B virus (HBV), in HIV, 896
Citrobacter
in complicated urinary tract infection, 540t
diagnostic microbiology of, 1568t
endophthalmitis and, 159
microflora, 355–356
Citrobacter freundii, intrinsic resistance of, 1182t
Citrobacter koseri, 1575
Clarithromycin
accumulation ratio of, 1222t
for anaerobic bacteria, 1643
for anthrax, 1127
characteristics of, 1218t
classification, 1217

Clarithromycin *(Continued)*
for community-acquired pneumonia, 255t
for dog bites, 657t
for *Helicobacter pylori*, 326–327
for leprosy, 959
for lung abscess, 269f
for *Mycobacterium avium* complex (MAC) in HIV, 856
for parasitic infections, 1345t–1351t
pharmacokinetics, 1222, 1223t–1224t
prophylaxis
in HIV infected women, 910
in rheumatic fever, 475t
for renal insufficiency, 1222
stability in acidic medium, 1218
in vitro activity, 1219, 1220t
Classic lobar pneumonia, pathologic phases of, 253t
Clavams, 1162
Clean-contaminated operations
and antibiotic prophylaxis, 687
common pathogens in, 687
Climate
and emerging infectious diseases, 46–48, 46f
health consequences of changing, 40–48
Clinafloxacin, for anaerobic bacteria, 1643
Clindamycin
for actinomycosis, 316
activity against *Toxoplasma gondii*, 1226
for anaerobic bacteria, 1643
for anthrax, 1127
antibacterial activity, 1225
antiparasitic activity, 1226
for babesiosis, 1753
for *Bacillus cereus*, 1542
for bacterial vaginosis, 485
cellulitis and, 92
chemical structure, 1223
for dog bites, 657t
for drowning-associated infections, 681
in elderly patients, 1227
for *Erysipelothrix rhusiopathiae*, 1542
for foot ulcers, 131t
in hepatic impaired patients, 1227
for human bites, 683
intramuscular form, 1226
intraphagocytic concentration, 1227
intravenous form, 1226
for lung abscess, 269f
for malaria in pregnancy, 1143t
metabolism, 1227
for *Mycoplasma hominis*, 1664
for necrotizing fasciitis, 96–97
oral form, 1226–1227
for parasitic infections, 1345t–1362t, 1366
for pelvic inflammatory disease, 493–494
pharmacokinetics, 1226–1227
for pharyngitis, 235
for *Pneumocystis jirovecii* pneumonia, 851
in pregnancy, 504, 1227
prophylaxis, 1158t
for rheumatic fever, 475t
for surgical site infections, 687
in renal impaired patients, 1227
safety, 1227
for *Staphylococcus aureus*, 1520
for toxoplasmosis, in HIV/AIDS, 857
in vitro activity, 1225t
Clindamycin susceptibility testing, 1518, 1518t
Clinical pulmonary infection score, hospital-acquired pneumonia and, 259t
Clinically documented infections (CDI), in cancer patients, 726, 726f
Clofazimine
for leprosy, 959
for leprosy reactions, 959–960
for lobomycosis, 1723
Clonorchis sinensis
epidemiology of, 1036
life cycle of, 1771f
treatment of, 1345t–1351t
Clostridial cellulitis, 99
Clostridial gas gangrene, 99–102
Clostridium, 208, 351, 1629
antimicrobial drugs of choice for, 1642t
in bacterial arthritis, 382
brain abscess and, 199

Clostridium (Continued)
  endophthalmitis and, 159
  in human bites, 682
  microflora, 355
  in normal flora, 1632, 1632*t*
  susceptibility to antimicrobial agents, 1642*f*
  treatment, 1210
Clostridium botulinum, 1629
  diagnosis of, 212
  prevention of, 210
  toxins, 208*f*, 208*t*
    and bioterrorism, 671*t*, 677
    transmission, 665*t*
Clostridium difficile, 1629
  antimicrobial drugs of choice for, 1642*t*
  bacterial enteritis and, 338
  in burn wounds, 698
  in cancer patients, 727–728
  chronic diarrhea and, 341, 343
  clindamycin, 1225
  diagnosis of, 339
  diarrhea, 335
  in emerging infectious diseases, 45
  endoscopy for, 1630
  enterocolitis, in HIV/AIDS, 858
  fusidic acid for, 1277
  identification of, 1635
  laboratory diagnosis of, 1629–1630
  miscellaneous bacteria, 338
  in normal flora, 1632
  O27 outbreak, 1389
  probiotics for, 1374*t*, 1375
  toxin A and B, 1633
  travelers' diarrhea and, 375, 375*t*
Clostridium difficile-associated disease (CDAD), 688
  risk in graft-*versus*-host disease, 740–741
Clostridium difficile colitis, bronchiectasis and, 249
Clostridium difficile infection (CDI), 351–354
  clinical syndromes of, 352, 352*f*
  community-acquired, 353
  diagnosis of, 352
  hospital-acquired, 352–353
  microbiology of, 351
  pathogenesis of, 351–352
  prevention of, 353
  treatment of, 353
Clostridium histolyticum, 95*f*
Clostridium perfringens, 1629
  characteristics of, in food-borne diarrheal illness, 330*t*
  clindamycin, 1225
  diarrhea, 331
  epsilon toxin, and bioterrorism, 671*t*
  gas gangrene and, 95*f*, 101*f*
  susceptibility to antimicrobial agents, 1642*f*
  toxins of, 1633
  traumatic gas gangrene, 100*f*
Clostridium septicum, 1629
Clostridium sordellii, 1629
  infections, 102
Clostridium tertium, infections, 102
Clostridium tetani, 210*f*, 645, 1629
  clindamycin, 1225
  epidemiology of, 208
  pathogenesis and pathology of, 209
Clotrimazole
  for *Acanthamoeba* keratitis, 1750
  candidiasis, 128
  keratitis and, 155
  for oropharyngeal candidiasis, 1684
  for vulvovaginal candidiasis, 488*t*, 1686
Cloxacillin
  pharmacokinetics of, 1205*t*
  susceptibilities of selected bacteria to, 1208*t*–1209*t*
Clumping factor, 1513*t*–1514*t*, 1516–1517
Clutton's joints, 563
Co-morbid illnesses, exacerbation of, community-acquired pneumonia and, 256
Co-receptor targeting, in HIV, 1491
Co-trimoxazole, for pertussis, 1614
Coagulase-negative staphylococci
  in bacterial arthritis, 382*t*–383, 383*t*
  in catheter-related bloodstream infection (CRBSI), 435
  in complicated urinary tract infection, 540*t*

Coagulase-negative staphylococci *(Continued)*
  in endocarditis, 456–457
  epidemiology and infections of, 1511–1512
  fusidic acid for, 1277
  hospital-acquired pneumonia and, 259*t*
  lincosamides, 1224–1225
  management of, 1521–1522
  in osteomyelitis, 390
  in prosthetic joint infection (PJI), 400
Coagulase/von Willebrand binding protein, 1513*t*–1514*t*
Coagulation system, *Staphylococcus aureus* interactions with, 1515
Coats' disease, 172
Cobicistat
  effect on oral contraceptives, 907*t*
  for perinatal HIV transmission prevention, 909*t*
Coccidia
  gastrointestinal, 989*t*
  intestinal, 1734–1743
    diagnosis of, 1737*t*
    nature of, 1734
Coccidioides, 1681*t*
  in chronic meningitis, 186*t*
  clinical features of, 296, 296*f*
  diagnosis of, 296, 296*f*
  in liver transplant patients, 751
  management of, 296
  mycology and epidemiology of, 295
  pathogenesis and pathology of, 295
  transmission of, 806–807
Coccidioides immitis, 1700
  in bacterial arthritis, 383*t*
  in chronic meningitis, 188
  culture of, 1705
  ecology and epidemiology of, 1704
  geographic distribution of, 939
  in HIV/AIDS, 855
  lower respiratory tract infections, 264*f*
  microscopic examination of, 1705
  mycology and epidemiology of, 295
  mycology of, 1703
  pathogenicity of, 1704
  prevention of, 1706
  in prostatitis, 533*t*
  in skin manifestation of HIV, 884*t*
Coccidioides posadasii, 1700
  mycology and epidemiology of, 295
  mycology of, 1703
Coccidioidin, 1705
Coccidioidomas, 296
Coccidioidomycosis, 118, 295–296, 296*f*, 855, 1700*t*, 1703–1706
  clinical manifestations of, 1705
  cutaneous, 1705
  dermatologic manifestations of, 114*t*–115*t*
  diagnostic microbiology of, 1702*t*, 1705
  ecology of, 1704
  epidemiology of, 1704, 1704*t*
  geographic distribution of, 939
  lymphadenopathy and, 137*t*–138*t*
  management of, 1705–1706
  meningitis and, 1705–1706
  mycology of, 1703–1704, 1704*f*
  pathogenicity of, 1704–1705
  prevention of, 1706
  pulmonary, 1705
Cocoon strategy, 787
Coenurosis, 1035–1036
Cognitive behavioral therapy (CBT), in chronic fatigue syndrome, 635
Cognitive deficits, in Lyme disease, 409
Coinfections, in immune response, 843–844
Cold agglutinins, 1660–1661
Cold-sensitive neurons, 609
Colistimethate (CMS), 1286
Colistin sulfate, 1286
Colistins, 1178–1180
  against carbapenamase-resistant gram-negative bacilli, 1290*t*
  chemical structure of, 1178, 1285
  distribution of, 1286
  mode of action of, 1178, 1179*f*

Colistins *(Continued)*
  non-antibiotic pharmacologic and toxicologic properties related to chemical structure of, 1180
  pharmacodynamics of, 1180
  resistance to, 1180
  for *Stenotrophomonas maltophilia*, 1597
  for thoracic transplantation patients, 749
Colitis
  Clostridium difficile infection (CDI), 352
  in hematopoietic stem cell transplantation, 740–741
  pseudomembranous, vancomycin for, 1251
Collagen-binding protein, 1513*t*–1514*t*
Collagen shields, 162
Collagen vascular diseases, 450
Colomycin, 1286
Colon surgery, and surgical site infections, antibiotic prophylaxis for, 687
Colorado tick fever, 667
Colorado tick fever virus, 1495*t*
Coltivirus, 1495*t*
Coly-Mycin M, 1286
Coma, in severe malaria, 1020*t*
Comamonas, 1598
  nomenclature of, 1581*t*–1582*t*
  prevalence of, 1579
Combination antiretroviral therapy (cART), suppression of HIV infection using, 931
Combination therapy
  for hepatitis B, 1329–1330
  for hepatitis C, 1332
  of polymyxins, 1287
Common antigen testing, for *Clostridium difficile*, 1630
Common variable immunodeficiency (CVID), 720, 808, 810*t*
Community-acquired *Clostridium difficile* infection (CDI), 353
Community-acquired infections
  intra-abdominal, 689
  see also specific infections
Community-acquired MRSA (CA-MRSA), 1511, 1511*f*
  osteomyelitis and, 388–390
  trimethoprim-sulfamethoxazole for, 1282
Community-acquired MRSA CAP, 254
Community-acquired pneumonia (CAP), 251–257
  Acinetobacter spp. in, 1594–1595
  antibiotics for, 1152*t*
  clinical features of, 255*t*
  clinical manifestations of, 253
  common etiologies of, 254*t*
  determination of etiology of, 254–255
  diagnosis of, 251–252
  diagnostic testing in, 255*t*
  differential diagnosis of, 251*t*
    cavitary, 252*t*
  disposition of, 256, 256*t*
  duration of treatment, 255
  epidemiology of, 253, 253*t*
  etiology of, 253–255
  immunocompromise of, 253
  linezolid, 1231*t*
  meningococci in, 1564
  pathology of, 253
  pathophysiology of, 252–253
  prevention of, 256
  Pseudomonas aeruginosa in, 1588
  Pseudomonas spp. in, 1589
  quinolones for, 1245
  radiology and, 251–252
  treatment of, 255–256
Community-onset pneumonia syndromes, 254*t*
Compartmental model of influenza, 51–52, 51*f*
Complement, 37–39
  activation, 36–37
  alternate pathway, 37
  classic pathway, 37
  disorders of, 39
  evasion, of *Staphylococcus aureus*, 1512–1514, 1514*f*
  formation of membrane attack complex, 37
  initiation of the cascade, 37, 38*f*
  lectin pathway, 37
Complement fixation
  for helminths diagnosis, 1777
  in histoplasmosis, 293

Complement fixation *(Continued)*
　for lymphogranuloma venereum, 589
　test
　　for *Chlamydia trachomatis*, 1678
　　for coccidioidomycosis, 1705
　　for histoplasmosis, 1707
Complement system, in sepsis, 423
Computed tomography (CT)
　in arterial graft infection, 437, 437*f*
　in bacterial arthritis, 385
　brain abscess, 201*f*–204*f*
　in cancer patients, 733
　deep cervical space infection, 315
　of echinococcosis, 1043
　in endocarditis, 462–463, 463*f*
　of eosinophilic meningitis, 975, 978*f*
　and fever of unknown origin, 623
　in immunologically mediated diseases, 771
　for intra-abdominal infections, 690
　intra-abdominal sepsis, 356–357, 356*f*–357*f*
　lower respiratory tract infections, 267
　of melioidosis, 1077
　necrotizing fasciitis, 95–96, 96*f*
　of neurocysticercosis, 1035, 1035*f*
　in osteomyelitis, 394
　in pancreas transplant patients, 764
　pancreatic necrosis, 360, 360*f*
　of pericarditis, 454, 454*f*
　for pleural discharge/fluid, 303, 303*f*
　in pyelonephritis, 550, 550*f*–552*f*
　single photon emission. *see* Single photon emission CT
　　(SPECT)
　sinusitis, 240
　of urogenital tract tuberculosis, 556
Condoms
　in genital herpes, 569
　HIV transmission and, 906–907
　in syphilis, 560
　use of, in HIV, 826
Condylomata acuminatum, in pregnancy, 500*t*
Condylomata lata, 561–562
Congenital disease, in myocarditis, 448
Congenital heart disease
　brain abscess and, 199
　in endocarditis, 456, 459
Congenital infection
　active and passive immunization in, 507
　in Chagas disease, 1070
　clinical features of, 508–510, 509*t*
　clinical findings in, 509*t*
　diagnosis of, 511–513, 511*t*–512*t*
　education and exposure avoidance in, 507
　epidemiology of, 505–506, 505*b*
　factors affecting, 506–507, 506*t*
　fetal abnormalities, 508
　fetus, 507
　geography of, 505–506
　intervention, 508
　management of, 513–516, 514*t*, 516*t*
　maternal history relevant to, 511*b*
　maternal immunity in, 506–507
　monitoring for, 508
　pathogen in, 506
　pathogenesis and pathology of, 506–507
　placenta, 507
　prevention of, 507–508
　screening for, 507–508, 508*t*
　spontaneous abortion and stillbirth, 509
　syndromes of, 509–510
　syphilis. *see* Syphilis, congenital
　toxoplasmosis as, 1754–1755
Congenital rubella syndrome (CRS), 77, 78*f*
Congenital syphilis
　clinical features of, 563, 563*f*
　definitions of, 565*t*
　evaluation of neonates for, 564–565
　treatment of, 565
Congestive heart failure (CHF), 447–449
Congestive otitis (CO), 237
Conidia, 1706, 1708
Conidiobolomycosis
　management of, 1722–1723
　rhinofacial, 1712, 1723
Conidiobolus coronatus, 1713
Conidiobolus infection, 1719–1720

Conjugative plasmids, 1194–1195
　carrying antibiotic resistance genes, structure of, 1195*f*
Conjunctival filtering bleb, 161
Conjunctival suffusion, 1103
Conjunctivitis, 150–152
　in adults, 150–152
　in children, 150–152
　community-acquired infections, 150–151
　follicular, 981*t*
　gonococcal, 150, 1563
　infectious
　　diagnosis of, 151
　　management of, 152
　　prevention of, 151–152
　measles causing, 167
　in neonates, 150–151
　red eye and, 175, 175*t*
　treatment of, 596*t*
　viral, 151
Connective tissue disorders, lymphadenopathy and,
　137*t*–138*t*
Consciousness level decline, in meningitis, 183
Consolidation therapy, for cryptococcosis, 1696
Construction worker, and occupational infections,
　648*t*–649*t*
Contact dermatitis, 585, 586*t*–587*t*
Contact lens-related keratitis, 155–156
Contact precautions, 58–59
Contaminated operations, and antibiotic prophylaxis, 687
Contaminated specimens, of mycobacteria, 1652
Contamination, 13
Continuous ambulatory peritoneal dialysis (CAPD)
　aminoglycoside dosage in, 1235
　peritonitis associated with, 380–381
　　Staphylococcus aureus in, 1516
　vancomycin in, 1250
　see also Chronic ambulatory peritoneal dialysis (CAPD)
Contraception, in HIV infection, 906–908
Convulsions
　in cerebral malaria, 1019
　in severe malaria, 1025
Coprococcus, 1631
Cord blood transplantation, 739
Core temperature, 606
Corona veneris, 561
Corona viruses, bronchitis and, 244*t*
Coronary artery bypass graft (CABG), 687*t*
Coronavirus, 338, 1474–1475
　clinical manifestations, 1475
　diagnostic microbiology, 1475
　epidemiology, 1474
　management, 1475
　nature, 1474
　pathogenicity, 1474
　prevention, 1475
Correlates of protection, 781*t*
Cortical vein thrombosis, 205
Corticosteroids
　for acute exacerbations of chronic obstructive
　　pulmonary disease, 311
　for acute retinal necrosis syndrome, 172
　adjunctive, in tuberculosis and HIV infection, 306, 307*t*
　for aspergillosis, 1691
　for brain abscess, 203
　for croup, 229–230
　for cysticercosis, 1035
　for encephalitis, 197
　for endophthalmitis, 163
　in keratitis, 157
　for leprosy reactions, 959
　for *Mycobacterium tuberculosis*-associated immune
　　reconstitution inflammatory syndrome, 864
　for noncentral nervous system tuberculosis, 306
　for pericardial effusion, 480
　for pericarditis, 454
　for pertussis, 1614
　for *Pneumocystis jirovecii* pneumonia, 851–852
　respiratory syncytial virus, 1476–1477
　for rheumatic fever, 476
Corynebacterineae, 1547*t*
Corynebacterium, 1537, 1546–1547, 1548*t*
　clinical manifestations of, 1547
　diagnostic microbiology of, 1547, 1549*b*
　endophthalmitis and, 159
　epidemiology of, 1547

Corynebacterium (Continued)
　hospital-acquired pneumonia and, 259*t*
　in human bites, 683*t*
　management of, 1547
　nature of, 1546–1547
　pathogenicity of, 1547
Corynebacterium amycolatum, 1547
Corynebacterium diphtheriae, 1220, 1544–1546
　clinical manifestations of, 1545–1546
　conjunctivitis, 151
　diagnostic microbiology of, 1544–1545
　epidemiology of, 1544
　lincosamides, 1224–1225
　management of, 1546, 1546*t*
　nature of, 1544
　pathogenicity of, 1544, 1545*f*
　pharyngitis, 234
　prevention of, 1546
　transmission, 665*t*
Corynebacterium jeikeium, 1546–1547
　macrolides, 1220
Corynebacterium ulcerans, 1544–1546
　clinical manifestations of, 1545–1546
　diagnostic microbiology of, 1544–1545
　epidemiology of, 1544
　management of, 1546, 1546*t*
　nature of, 1544
　pathogenicity of, 1544, 1545*f*
　prevention of, 1546
　transmission, 665*t*
Corynebacterium urealyticum, 1547
　in complicated urinary tract infection, 540, 542
　macrolides, 1220
Coryneforms, 1546–1547
Cough
　bronchitis and, 243
　community-acquired pneumonia, 251
　croup and, 229
　whooping. *see* Pertussis
Councilman bodies, 1494
Counseling, in HIV infection, 913
Cow pox, dermatologic manifestations of, 114*t*–115*t*
Cowpox virus, 75*t*
　diagnosis of, 1456
　in rodents, 667
　transmission of, 1456
Coxiella burnetii, 1091, 1672
　causing endocarditis, 461*t*
　encephalitis/myelitis caused by, 193*t*–194*t*
　in myocarditis, 447
Coxiella burnetti
　and bioterrorism, 671*t*
　in camels, 663
　jaundice, 1135*t*
Coxsackieviruses
　in myocarditis, 446
　in pericarditis, 450, 452–453
　in pharyngitis, 233
Crabs, infections from, 191*t*
Cranberry juice, 526
Cranial nerve, eighth, streptomycin adverse reaction to,
　1270
Craniotomy
　brain abscess, 203
　subdural empyema/intracranial epidural abscess,
　　204
Creatinine phosphokinase (CPK), 448
Creutzfeldt-Jakob disease (CJD), 214
　clinical features of, 217
　iatrogenic, 215, 215*t*
　molecular strain typing of, 217
　pathology of, 219
　prevention of, 220
　transfusion-related infections and, 704
　transmission, 216, 220
　variant. *see* Variant Creutzfeldt-Jakob disease (vCJD)
Crimean-Congo hemorrhagic fever, 1495*t*
　and bioterrorism, 671*t*
Crimean-Congo hemorrhagic fever virus, 1110
　clinical features of, 1114*t*–1115*t*, 1116*f*
　epidemiology of, 1112*t*
　management of, 1117
Crohn's disease
　fever of unknown origin, 614
　in genital lesions, 586*t*–587*t*

Crohn's disease *(Continued)*
  lymphadenopathy, 145
  pathogenesis of, 626
Cronobacter sakazakii, 1576, 1577*t*
Croup, 229, 1544
  clinical features of, 229, 230*t*
  diagnosis of, 230
  epidemiology of, 232
Crowding, and emerging infectious diseases, 45–46
Cruise ships, and respiratory and gastrointestinal infections, 643
Cryopyrin-associated periodic syndrome (CAPS), 801
Cryosurgery, for human papillomavirus, 582–583
Cryotherapy, for human papillomavirus, 583
Cryptococcal meningitis, 1692
  in HIV/AIDS, 851
Cryptococcoma, 1694
Cryptococcosis, 118, 119*f*, 753, 1692–1696
  from birds, 661
  clinical manifestations of, 1694–1695, 1694*f*
  dermatologic manifestations of, 114*t*–115*t*
  diagnostic microbiology of, 1692–1694, 1693*f*
  epidemiology of, 1692
  in HIV/AIDS, in low- and middle-income countries, 893
  lymphadenopathy and, 137*t*–138*t*
  management of, 1695–1696, 1695*t*
  nature of, 1692
  opportunistic infection in HIV/AIDS, 854–855
  pathogenicity of, 1692, 1693*f*
  prognosis of, 1696, 1696*t*
  risk for, 1692
Cryptococcus, 1681*t*
  in chronic meningitis, 186*t*
Cryptococcus gattii
  diagnostic microbiology of, 1692–1693
  epidemiology of, 1692
  nature of, 1692
Cryptococcus neoformans
  from birds, 661
  brain abscess and, 200
  in cats, 660
  clinical manifestations of, 1694
  diagnostic microbiology of, 1692–1693, 1693*f*
  endophthalmitis and, 159
  epidemiology of, 1692
  in HIV in low- and middle-income countries, 893
  in myocarditis, 448
  nature of, 1692
  opportunistic infection of, in HIV/AIDS, 854–855
  pathogenicity of, 1692
  pulmonary involvement of, 1694
  in skin manifestation of HIV, 884*t*
Cryptosporidiosis, 1740
  chronic diarrhea and, 347–348
  clinical features of, 996
  in HIV/AIDS, 857
  human, species of, 1734
  in immunocompetent patients, 1740
  in immunocompromised patients, 1740
  intestinal, pathogenesis and pathology of, 991
  in kidney transplant patients, 768–769
  management of, 1741–1742
  and occupational infections, 648*t*–649*t*
  prevention of, 1737
  transmission of, 666
  treatment of, 1345*t*–1351*t*
Cryptosporidium
  chronic diarrhea and, 346–348
  diagnostic microbiology of, 1737–1738, 1738*f*
  diarrhea, 335
  epidemiology of, 989, 1734–1735
  life cycle of, 992*f*
  pathogenicity of, 1736, 1736*f*
  in population density and urbanization, 990
  prevention of, 994, 1727
  treatment of, 999
Cryptosporidium andersoni, 1734
Cryptosporidium canis, 991, 1734
Cryptosporidium cuniculus, 1734
Cryptosporidium felis, 991, 1734

Cryptosporidium hominis
  clinical features of, 996
  diagnosis of, 998*t*–999*t*
  nature of, 1734
  pathogenesis and pathology of, 991
Cryptosporidium meleagridis, 991, 1734
Cryptosporidium muris, 991, 1734
Cryptosporidium parvum
  and bioterrorism, 671*t*
  in chronic diarrhea, 347–348, 347*t*
  clinical features of, 996
  diagnosis of, 998*t*–999*t*
  doses of, in diarrheal illness, 329*t*
  in HIV/AIDS, 332, 857
  nature of, 1734
  parasite infections and, 73
  pathogenesis and pathology of, 991
  treatment of, 1345*t*–1351*t*
Cryptosporidium viatorum, 1734
Crystalluria, as quinolones adverse effect, 1248
Culex quinquefasciatus, 1765
Culicidae, 110
Culicinae, 110
Culture-independent sequence-based taxonomic and functional profiling of microbiome, 69–71
Culture-independent techniques to detect novel pathogens, 627–629, 627*t*, 628*f*
Culture-negative ascites, 359
Culture-negative peritonitis, 381
Cultures
  of anthrax, 1126
  of *Aspergillus*, 1688
  of *Bacillus anthracis*, 1541
  of blastomycosis, 1702
  for brucellosis, 1099–1100, 1615
  of *Candida* spp., 441–442, 444–445, 1682*t*, 1683
  in catheter-related bloodstream infection (CRBSI), 433–434
  in Chagas disease, 1071
  of *Chlamydia pneumoniae*, 1678
  of *Chlamydia trachomatis*, 600, 1678
  for chromoblastomycosis, 1716
  for coccidioidomycosis, 1705
  development of specific media, 66
  for diagnosis of superficial fungal infections, 127
  for diphtheria, 1545
  in food-borne diarrheal illness, 332
  for *Francisella tularensis*, 1617
  in genital herpes, 572
  in gonorrhea, 594
  for *Haemophilus influenzae*, 1620
  Helicobacter pylori, 325
  of histoplasmosis, 1707
  in HIV-associated TB, 870
  hydrocephalus shunts and, 223
  for *Legionella* spp., 1623, 1623*f*
  of *Listeria monocytogenes*, 1538–1539
  in Lyme disease, 409
  of melioidosis, 1075–1076, 1076*f*
  of microsporidia, 1740
  of mycobacteria, 1653
  renewal of, 1386
  of staphylococci, 1516, 1517*f*
  of superficial fungal pathogens, 1711–1712
  of tularemia, 1089
  in vulvovaginal candidiasis, 487
  see also specific micro-organisms
Cunninghamella, 1696
Cupriavidus, 1581*t*–1582*t*, 1598–1599
CURB-65 score, 256
Curvularia spp., 1721
Cutaneous candidosis
  diagnostic microbiology of, 1711
  epidemiology of, 1710
  pathogenicity of, 1711
Cutaneous disease, diphtheria and, 1545–1546
Cutaneous gnathostomiasis, treatment of, 975–976
Cutaneous human papillomaviruses, 1440
Cutaneous infection, aerobic actinomycetes and, 1551
Cutaneous involvement, brucellosis complications, 1099
Cutaneous larva migrans, treatment of, 1345*t*–1351*t*

Cutaneous leishmaniasis, 85*t*, 1757, 1757*f*
  clinical features of, 1062, 1062*f*
  epidemiology of, 1059–1060
  monitoring response to treatment for, 1064
Cutaneous lupus, in HIV patients receiving antiretroviral therapy, 864
Cutaneous malignancies, in HIV, 884–885
CVD103-HgR, 1606
CVID. *see* Common variable immunodeficiency (CVID).
CXCR4, 1485
Cyclic AMP, in food-borne diarrheal illness, 329
Cyclic hematopoiesis, 706
Cyclic neutropenia, 706
  and fever of unknown origin, 614
Cyclic polypeptides, 1178–1180
  chemical structure of, 1178
  mode of action of, 1178, 1179*f*
  non-antibiotic pharmacologic and toxicologic properties related to chemical structure of, 1180
  pharmacodynamics of, 1180
  resistance to, 1180
Cyclocheilichthys, 1765
Cyclooxygenase, 610
Cyclophosphamide, 1379
Cyclophosphamide/doxorubicin/etoposide (CDE), 875–876
D-cycloserine, 1167
Cycloserine, as antituberculosis agent, 1270–1271
Cyclospora
  diagnostic microbiology of, 1738, 1738*f*
  epidemiology of, 1735
  pathogenicity of, 1736
  spread of, 944–945
Cyclospora cayetanensis
  chronic diarrhea and, 347*t*, 348
  clinical features of, 996
  diagnosis of, 998*t*–999*t*
  nature of, 1734
  pathogenesis and pathology of, 991
  in population density and urbanization, 990
  treatment for, 999, 1000*t*, 1345*t*–1351*t*
  in diarrhea, 334
Cyclosporiasis, 1740
  chronic diarrhea and, 348
  clinical features of, 996
  management of, 1742
  prevention of, 1737
  treatment of, 1345*t*–1351*t*
  trimethoprim-sulfamethoxazole for, 1365
Cyclosporine, 1378
Cystectomy, for cystic echinococcosis, 1044
Cystic bronchiectasis post-tuberculosis, 246*f*
Cystic fibrosis (CF), 300–302
  acute exacerbations of
    management of, 301, 301*b*
    signs and symptoms of, 300, 300*b*
  Alcaligenes xylosoxidans in, 1597
  aminoglycosides for, 1237
  case of, 300
  definition of, 300
  diagnosis of, 300
  lung/heart transplantation, 746
  management of, 300–301
  quinolones for, 1245
Cystic fibrosis transmembrane conductance regulator (CFTR), 1584–1585
Cysticercosis, 1034–1035, 1778
  clinical features of, 1034, 1034*f*
  dermatologic manifestations of, 114*t*–115*t*
  diagnosis of, 1035, 1035*f*
  epidemiology of, 1034
  extraneural, 1034
  management of, 1035
  ophthalmic, 1034
  pathogenesis of, 1034, 1034*f*
  prevention of, 1034
Cystitis
  acute, 523–530
    bacterial, 527, 529*f*
    clinical features of, 526
    diagnosis of, 526–527, 526*t*–527*t*
    epidemiology of, 523
    management of, 527–530, 528*t*, 529*f*

Cystitis (Continued)
  pathogenesis of, 523–525, 524f–525f
  prevention of, 525–526, 526t
  ascent of, 523
  colonization of, 523
  complicated, 528
  hemorrhagic, Bk polyomavirus and, 1447
  invasive procedures in, 529
  in male, 529
  mechanisms of, 523–525
  organisms associated with, 523, 524t
  recurrent, 527–528, 530f
  risk factors for, 524t
  symptomatic, treatment of, 443t
  treatment for, 1687
    in the presence of renal failure, 529
Cystoisospora
  diagnostic microbiology of, 1738, 1738f
  epidemiology of, 1735
  pathogenicity of, 1736
Cystoisospora belli, 1734
  epidemiology of, 1735
  pathogenicity of, 1736
Cystoisosporiasis, 1740
  management of, 1742
  prevention of, 1737
  treatment of, 1345t–1351t
Cystourethritis, in pregnancy, 503
Cystourethrogram, 534
Cysts, 586t–587t
Cytidine deaminase deficiency, activation-induced, 720–721
Cytoadherence, in Plasmodium species, 1016–1017
Cytochrome P450, 609, 870–871
  antifungal triazoles, 1336
Cytochrome P450 CYP3A4, substrates, inhibitors, and inducers, 1301t
Cytokines
  in malaria, 1017
  in phagocytes, 31
  pyrogenic, 607, 608f
  in sepsis, 420, 422–423, 423t
  skin infections and, 86
Cytolethal distending toxin (CDT), of Campylobacter jejuni, 1601
Cytolytic T lymphocytes, 33
Cytolytic toxins, 1514–1515
Cytomegalovirus (CMV), 75t, 79, 703t
  acute, 79
  in cancer patients, 724
  in cervicitis, 490
  chronic diarrhea and, 345t, 349
  in chronic meningitis, 186t
  clinical features of, 79
  clinical manifestations of, 1437
  complications of, 79
  congenital
    in breast-feeding, 516
    clinical features of, 510
    diagnosis of, 511–512, 512t
    epidemiology of, 506
    management of, 513
    and perinatal infections, 1437
    screening for, during pregnancy, 507, 508t
  dermatologic manifestations of, 114t–115t
  drugs for treatment of, 1313–1316
  encephalitis, 773
  enteritis, 773
  eye involvement in, 982–983
  febrile transaminitis in, 377
  and fever of unknown origin, 613
  in hematopoietic stem cell transplantation, 741, 743t
  and HIV-1, 843–844
  in HIV/AIDS, 881
  hospital-acquired pneumonia and, 259t
  in immunocompromised patients, 1437
  in infectious mononucleosis, 377
  in intestinal transplant patients, 757–759
    clinical presentation of, 757–758
    diagnosis of, 758, 758t
    epidemiology of, 757–758
    prevention of, 758–759, 758t
    treatment of, 759, 759t
  jaundice, 1135t
  in kidney transplant patients, 762, 766, 766f

Cytomegalovirus (CMV) (Continued)
  late infection of, 748
  in liver transplant patients, 751, 751t
    prevention of, 754–755
    screening for, 754
  lymphadenopathy and, 137t–138t
  management of, 749
  in myocarditis, 447–449
  opportunistic infections of, in HIV/AIDS, 852–853
    of the central nervous system, 853
    gastrointestinal disease, 852
    management of, 853
    pulmonary disease of, 853
    retinitis, 852, 853f
  pathogenicity of, molecular and cellular basis of, 1431
  and pneumonia in thoracic transplant patient, 746–747
  in pregnant women, 910
  prevention and treatment of, in thoracic transplantation patients, 748
  retinitis, 172–173, 173f, 1314t
  risk for
    in hematopoietic stem cell transplantation, 739
    in T-cell depletion, 739
    in thoracic transplantation patients, 748
  salivary gland swelling, 319–320
  in thoracic transplantation patients, 747t, 748
  and tumor necrosis factor inhibitor, 800
Cytopathic effect, virus-induced, 19–21, 21f
Cytosine, chemical structure of, 1335f
Cytotoxic agents, immunosuppression and, 1379, 1380t
Cytotoxic lymphocytes, damage resulting from, 21
Cytotoxic T-lymphocyte-associated antigen 4 (CTLA4), 801
Cytotoxicity neutralization assays, cell culture, for Clostridium difficile, 1629–1630
Cytotoxin-associated gene (cag gene), 323
Cytotoxins
  in food-borne diarrheal illness, 330
  of Staphylococcus aureus, 1514–1515

D

Daclatasvir (DCV), for hepatitis C, 1332
Daclizumab, 1380t
Dacryoadenitis, 157
Dacryocystitis, 157
Dairy products, agents transmitted via, 664, 665t
Dalbavancin, 1253, 1254t
  mode of action of, 1164
  in outpatient parenteral antimicrobial therapy, 1201
Dalfopristin-quinupristin, 1229
  antibacterial activities, 1228t, 1229
  pharmacokinetics, 1229
Dallas criteria, 448–449
Damage-associated molecular patterns (DAMPs), 685
Dams, parasites from, 990
Dapsone
  folate inhibitor interactions, 1283
  immunosuppression and, 1380t
  for leprosy, 959
  for mycetoma, 1723
  for Pneumocystis jirovecii pneumonia, 852
  in pregnancy, 910
Daptomycin
  for catheter-related bloodstream infection (CRBSI), 436t
  for foot ulcers, 131t
  in outpatient parenteral antimicrobial therapy, 1201
  for prosthetic joint infection (PJI), 402–403
  for Staphylococcus aureus, 1520
Darkfield microscopy, in syphilis, 563
Darunavir, 1148t, 1304–1305
  adverse reactions of, 1305
  description of, 1304
  dosage of, 1305
    in special circumstances, 1305
  drug interactions of, 1305
  effect on oral contraceptives, 907t
  indications of, 1305
  perinatal HIV transmission prevention, 909t
  pharmacokinetics and distribution of, 1304
  resistance to, 1305
  and ritonavir, 922
  route of administration of, 1305

Dasabuvir, for hepatitis C, 1332
Data
  analysis, genome sequencing, 63
  metagenomic sequence, 69f
Data collection on Adverse events of anti-HIV Drugs (D:A:D) study, 928
Davercin, 1217
DC-SIGN, 31, 839–840, 1487
Deafness, congenital infection and, 510
Debridement
  for bacterial arthritis, 385, 385f
  for prosthetic joint infection (PJI), 402
Decay-accelerating factor, 1408
Decolonization
  of hospital-acquired Staphylococcal infections, 1516
  mupirocin, 694
Decontamination, of bacteria, in intensive care unit, 694–697
Decubitus ulcers, osteomyelitis complicating, 392–393
Deep cervical space infection, 314–315, 315f
Deep neck abscesses, anaerobic bacteria in, 1636t
Deep venous thrombosis (DVT), in travelers, 952
Deer flies, 106t
DEET, 951
  for anaplasmosis, 1672
  for bartonellosis, 1673
  for scrub typhus, 1670
  for tropical rickettsioses, 1094–1095
  for tularemia prevention, 1087
Defensins, 1512
Definitive treatment, for prosthetic joint infection (PJI), 402
Dehydration
  cholera and, 1606–1607
  in diarrhea, 338
  food-borne diarrheal illness and, 333
Dehydroemetine, 1012
Delamanid, 1271
  recommended regimen of, 1274
Delavirdine, 1148t, 1301
Delayed flap closure, for mediastinitis and sternal osteomyelitis, 482
Delftia, 1581t–1582t, 1598
Deltavirus (HDV), 703t
Dematiaceous molds, 1681t, 1721
Dementia, HIV-associated, 227
Dendritic cells (DCs)
  cellular immune response, 32
  in HIV-1 progression, 839–840
  maturation, 30f
  in phagocytes, 31
Dengue, 1119–1122, 1495t
  and bioterrorism, 671t
  clinical features of, 1120–1121, 1121f
  diagnosis of, 1122
  epidemiology of, 1119, 1119f
  lymphadenopathy and, 137t–138t
  management of, 1122
  pathogenesis and pathology of, 1120, 1120f
  prevention of, 1120
  transmission of, 1119
Dengue fever
  epidemiology of, 1110
  spread of, 943–944, 944f
  in travelers, 952
'Dengue hemorrhagic fever (DHF)', 1120
Dengue shock syndrome (DSS), 1120
Dengue virus infection, dermatologic manifestations, 114t–115t
Dental caries, 312–313
Dental infections, 312–314
  anaerobic bacteria in, 1636
  antimicrobial therapy for, 1641t
  brain abscess and, 200t
  clinical features of, 313
  complications of, 313, 313f–314f
  epidemiology of, 312
  management of, 313–314
  pathogenesis and pathology of, 312, 312f
  prevention of, 312–313
  subdural empyema/intracranial epidural abscess, 205t
Dental procedures, prevention of infective endocarditis, 1159, 1159b, 1160t
Dental pulp infections, 312f, 313
Dental worker, and occupational infections, 648t–649t

Dependoparvovirus, 1449
Depression, brucellosis complications, 1099
Dermacentor andersoni, 664
Dermatitis
    cercarial, 1028–1029
    contact, 585, 586t–587t
    seborrheic. see Seborrheic dermatitis
Dermatitis-arthritis-tenosynovitis syndrome, 1563
Dermatologic reactions, of quinolones, 1247
Dermatological system, *Mycoplasma pneumoniae* in, 1662t
Dermatophilus congolensis, 660
Dermatophytes
    anthropophilic, 1710–1711
    diagnostic microbiology of, 1711–1712
    infection, from domesticated herbivores, 666
    nature of, 1710
    pathogenicity of, 1710–1711
    zoophilic, 1711
Dermatophytosis
    from cats, 660
    clinical features of, 123
    epidemiology of, 122, 1710
    immune response to, 123
    in immunocompromised patients, 126
    pathogenesis and pathology of, 123
    pedal, 1710
    prevention of, 123
    superficial, and skin manifestations of HIV, 883
Dermonecrotic toxin (DNT), 1612, 1613t
Deuteromycota, 1712
Device-associated infections, 60
Dexamethasone
    croup and, 230
    meningitis and, 184
    for typhoid fever, 1007
Dextrans, 1527
dfrA gene, 1193
dfrB gene, 1193
Diabetes, rhinocerebral mucormycosis in, 1697–1698
Diabetes mellitus
    brain abscess and, 199
    cervical necrotizing fasciitis in, 315
Diabetic foot
    osteomyelitis, 392, 393f, 396f
    ulcers, 130–132
Diabetic ulcer, 1639f
Diagnosis, *Candida* spp., 441–442, 444
Diagnostic microbiology
    of *Acanthamoeba* keratitis, 1747
    of *Acinetobacter* spp., 1594, 1594f
    adenovirus, 1472–1473
    advances in, 1386–1389
    of aerobic actinomycetes, 1549–1551
    of African trypanosomiasis, 1761–1762
    of *Alcaligenes* spp., 1597
    of anaplasmosis, 1672
    arenavirus, 1501
    of aspergillosis, 1688–1689, 1688f
    of babesiosis, 1752, 1752f
    of *Bacillus anthracis*, 1541
    of bartonellosis, 1673–1674, 1675f
    of blastomycosis, 1702–1703
    of *Bordetella* spp., 1612–1613, 1613f
    of *Brucella* spp., 1615–1616
    of *Burkholderia* spp., 1596
    of caliciviruses, 1396
    of *Campylobacter* spp., 1601–1602
    of candidiasis, 1683–1684
    of Chagas disease, 1759
    of *Chlamydia*, 1678–1680
    of coccidioidomycosis, 1705
    coronavirus, 1475
    of *Corynebacterium*, 1547, 1549b
    of *Corynebacterium diphtheriae*, 1544–1545
    of cryptococcosis, 1692–1694, 1693f
    of *Cryptosporidium* spp., 1737–1738, 1738f
    of *Cyclospora* spp., 1738, 1738f
    of *Cystoisospora* spp., 1738, 1738f
    of ehrlichioses, 1671
    of Enterobacteriaceae, 1566–1569, 1568t
    of *Erysipelothrix rhusiopathiae*, 1542
    Filoviridae, 1506
    of *Francisella*, 1617

Diagnostic microbiology *(Continued)*
    of granulomatous amebic encephalitis, 1747
    of HACEK group, 1622
    of *Haemophilus*, 1619–1620, 1620f
    of *Haemophilus ducreyi*, 1621
    hantaviruses, 1504
    of *Helicobacter pylori*, 1603
    of histoplasmosis, 1706f, 1707–1708
    hospital-acquired pneumonia, 260b
    human bocavirus, 1481
    human metapneumovirus (hMPV), 1480
    human T-lymphocyte leukemia viruses, 1491
    influenza viruses, 1469
    of *Legionella* spp., 1623–1624, 1623f
    of leishmaniasis, 1756–1757
    of leptospirosis, 1609
    of *Listeria monocytogenes*, 1538–1539, 1539f
    of measles, 1399–1400
    of microsporidia, 1737t, 1738–1740, 1739f–1740f
    of molluscum contagiosum virus, 1456–1457
    of *Moraxella* spp., 1624
    of mucormycosis, 1697, 1697f
    of mumps, 1405
    of *Mycoplasma genitalium*, 1662
    of *Mycoplasma hominis*, 1663
    of *Mycoplasma pneumoniae*, 1660–1661
    of *Neisseria*, 1560–1562, 1560f, 1561t
    of orthopoxviruses, 1457
    papillomaviruses, 1442–1443
    of paracoccidioidomycosis, 1709
    parainfluenza virus, 1478
    of parapoxviruses, 1457
    of parvoviruses, 1451
    of *Pasteurella* spp., 1625
    of plague, 1627
    of polyomaviruses, 1446
    of primary amebic meningoencephalitis, 1747
    of protozoa, 1728–1733
    of *Pseudomonas* spp., 1580, 1580f, 1585f
    of Q fever, 1672–1673
    respiratory syncytial virus (RSV), 1476
    rhinovirus, 1477
    of rotaviruses, 1393
    of rubella, 1402–1403, 1403f
    of scrub typhus, 1670
    of spotted fever group rickettsiae, 1667
    of staphylococci, 1516–1519
    of *Stenotrophomonas maltophilia*, 1596
    of subcutaneous fungal pathogen, 1716–1719
    of superficial fungal pathogens, 1711–1712
    of *Talaromyces marneffei*, 1699, 1699f
    of toxoplasmosis, 1754
    tuberculosis, 280
    of typhus group rickettsiae, 1669–1670
    of ureaplasmas, 1663
    of *Vibrio cholerae*, 1606
    West Nile virus, 1498
    of yatapoxvirus, 1457
    yellow fever, 1494
    of yersiniosis, 1626–1627
Dialysis
    of kidney transplant patients, 762
    see also specific types
Diamidines, 155
Diaminopyrimidines, 1177–1178
    chemical structure of, 1177–1178, 1178f
    mode of action of, 1178
    pharmacodynamics of, 1178
    resistance to, 1178
Diarrhea
    within 1-2 days after eating, 331
    within 24 hours of eating, 331
    acute, 335–341
    antibiotic-associated, probiotics for, 1373–1375, 1374t
    from *Bacillus cereus*, 1542
    bloody, several days after eating, 331, 331f
    from *Campylobacter* spp., 1602
    chronic, 331, 341–350
        Brainerd, 349
        causes, 341b
            bacterial, 341–346
            parasitic, 346–349, 347t
            viral, 349

Diarrhea *(Continued)*
    evaluation of, 342f
    management of, 342f–343f
    tropical sprue, 349
    clinical features of, 336–338
        bacterial enteritis, 336–338
        viral enteritis, 338
    diagnosis of, 339
    empiric antibiotics for, 334
    epidemiology of, 335
    food-borne, 328–334
        bacterial cause of, 328
        clinical features of, 330–331
        diagnosis of, 332
        epidemiology of, 328, 329f
        host susceptibility in, 328–329
        infectious agents in, doses of, 329t
        management of, 333–334, 333f, 333t
        non-infective food poisoning, 331–332
        pathogenesis of, 329–330
        prevention of, 334
        public health management of, 334
        special clinical syndromes, 332
    gastrointestinal parasites associated with, 995t
    in hematopoietic stem cell transplantation, 740–741
    in HIV in low- and middle-income countries, 891–892
    in immunocompromised, 332
    in kidney transplant patients, 768
    management of, 339
    microsporidiosis in immunocompromised patients and, 1741
    osmotic, 336
    pathogenesis and pathology of, 335–336
    in pregnancy, 503
    prevention of, 338–339
    secretory, 336
    sources of pathogens, 335
    surveillance, 335
    travelers'. see Travelers' diarrhea (TD)
    from *Vibrio cholerae*, 1606–1607
    with vomiting, early onset, 331
Diarrheal disease, and occupational infections, 651t–654t
Diarrheal infections, burden of disease, 940
Diarylquinolines, 1180
Diazepam, 1025
Dibromopropamidine, for *Acanthamoeba* keratitis, 1750
Dichlorodiphenyltrichloroethane (DDT), 1017
Dicloxacillin
    for dog bites, 657t
    dosage in renal failure, 1213t–1214t
    for foot ulcers, 131t
    for lung abscess, 269f
    pharmacokinetics of, 1205t
    for *Staphylococcus aureus*, 87
    susceptibilities of selected bacteria to, 1208t–1209t
Didanosine, 1148t, 1295–1298
    adverse reactions of, 1298
    antiretroviral drugs, 921
    chemical structure of, 1296f
    description, 1295
    dosage of, 1295
        in special circumstance, 1295–1298, 1297t
    drug interactions of, 1298
    indications of, 1295
    perinatal HIV transmission prevention, 909t
    pharmacokinetics and distribution of, 1295
    resistance to, 1295
    route of administration of, 1295
Dientamoeba fragilis, 1725t
    epidemiology of, 1727
    identification in fecal specimens, 1731–1732, 1732f
    infection
        clinical features of, 996
        diagnosis of, 998t–999t
        management of, 1367
        treatment of, 999, 1345t–1351t
    pathogenicity of, 1728
    prevention of, 1727
Diethylcarbamazine
    for filariasis, 1050–1051
    for helminths, 1772
    for loiasis, 1051

Diethylcarbamazine (Continued)
for onchocerciasis, 1051
for parasitic infections, 1345t–1362t, 1370–1371
Diffuse cutaneous leishmaniasis (DCL), 1757
Diffusely adherent Escherichia coli (DAEC)
in intestinal infections, 1574
virulence factors of, 1572t
Difluoromethylornithine, 1352t–1362t, 1366
DiGeorge anomaly, and live vaccines, 795
DiGeorge syndrome, 721
Dihydroartemisinin, 1352t–1362t, 1365
Dihydroartemisinin-piperaquine, 1022
Dihydropteroate synthase (DHPS), 1192
Dihydrorhodamine (DHR) assay, 708
Diloxanide furoate
for amebic infections, 1012
for gastrointestinal protozoa, 997, 1000t
for parasitic infections, 1345t–1362t, 1366
for prevention of amebic infections, 1009
Diphtheria, 648t–649t, 1544
burden of disease, 941
clinical manifestations of, 1545–1546
cutaneous, 92
diagnostic microbiology of, 1544–1545
epidemiology of, 1544
eye involvement in, 982
laryngeal, 229
lymphadenopathy and, 137t–138t
management of, 1546, 1546t
nature of, 1544
pathogenicity of, 1544, 1545f
pharyngitis, 235f
prevention of, 1546
vaccination against, 782t–783t
Diphtheria toxin, 19
synthesis, 20f
Diphyllobothriasis, 1033
Diphyllobothrium latum, 1033
clinical features of, 997
clinical manifestations of, 1778
diagnosis of, 998t–999t, 1033–1034
epidemiology of, 1766
life cycle of, 1773f
pathogenesis and pathology of, 994
pathogenicity of, 1772
treatment of, 1001, 1001t, 1345t–1351t
Diphyllobothrium spp., life cycle of, 1774f
Dipstick assay, for plague, 1083
Dipstick test, for leishmaniasis, 1063
Dipylidium caninum, 660, 1033
life cycle of, 1773f
treatment of, 1345t–1351t
Direct-acting antivirals (DAAs)
combination therapy of, 1332
for hepatitis C, 371, 1330–1331
Direct agglutination test (DAT), 1060, 1063
for leishmaniasis, 1757
Direct contact, and recreational infections, 645–646
Direct fluorescent antibody (DFA)
for Bacillus anthracis, 1541
for Chlamydia pneumoniae, 1679
for Chlamydia trachomatis, 1678
Direct fluorescent antibody staining, of tularemia, 1089
Direct immunofluorescence
for plague, 1083
in syphilis, 563
Direct microscopy
for chromoblastomycosis, 1716
in diarrhea, 339
superficial fungal infections of, 127
of superficial fungal pathogens, 1711–1712
Direct stool toxin assays, for Clostridium difficile,
1629–1630
Directly observed therapy, short course (DOTS), for
HIV-associated TB, 869
Dirithromycin
accumulation ratio of, 1222t
characteristics of, 1218t
classification, 1217
pharmacokinetics, 1222, 1223t–1224t
tissue distribution, 1224t
in vitro activity, 1219
Dirty surgical incisions, 687
Disaster preparedness, 58
Disease, causation of, Evans' principles of, 1b

Diseases of unknown etiology, 625–630
alternative views of microbial causation of human
disease, 625–626, 626t–627t
culture-independent techniques to detect novel
pathogens, 627–629, 627t, 628f
definition of disease causation and etiologic agents,
625
hygiene hypothesis, 626–627
Koch's postulates, redefined, 627t
pathogenesis of inflammatory diseases, 626–627, 629t
role of human endogenous retroviruses (HERVS) in
health and disease, 628–629, 629t
Disinfection, 57
Disseminated candidiasis, treatment of, 443t
Disseminated disease, nontuberculous mycobacteria
(NTM), 287–288, 288f
treatment of, 290–291
Disseminated gonococcal infection (DGI), 1563
gonorrhea and, 594
treatment of, 596t
Disseminated infections
nocardiosis, 1551
see also specific infections
Disseminated intravascular coagulation (DIC)
in plague, 1081, 1082f
in sepsis, 423, 423f
Dithiothreitol (DTT), 1652
Diverticulitis, antibiotics for, 1152t
DNA
drugs affecting, 1174–1177
microarrays, 65
repair defects in, 717, 721
sequencing of, 628
targeted metagenomic sequencing, 69
viruses, 6t
DNA Data Bank of Japan, 62–63
DNA fingerprinting, for mycobacteria, 1655
DNA gyrase, 1186
DNA prime and adenovirus vector boost, 833
DNA sequencing, for lymphogranuloma venereum, 589
DNA subtraction, 628
DNAse, 1513t–1514t, 1516–1517
Dobrava/Belgrade (DOBV) virus, 1502, 1502t
Dobrava virus, 667
n-Docosanol, 1313
Dogs
bites, 656
components of care for, 658t
enteric diseases from, 656–658
fleas, 658
infections from, 191t
infectious diseases associated with, 656–658
acquired from direct contact with, 658–659
contact from dog urine, 658–659
rabies from, 656
sporotrichosis in, 1715
tick/flea-borne infectious diseases associated with, 658
Dolphins, lobomycosis from, 1714
Dolutegravir, 1307
adverse reactions of, 1307–1308
antiretroviral drugs, 922–923
description of, 1307
dosage of, 1307
in special circumstances, 1307
drug interactions, 1307–1308
effect on oral contraceptives, 907t
indications of, 1307
perinatal HIV transmission prevention, 910t
pharmacokinetics and distribution of, 1307–1308
resistance of, 1307
route of administration, 1307
Donor screening, for infectious diseases, transmitted by
grafts, 806t, 807
Donor-transmitted pathogens, 805t
Donovan bodies, 590–591
Donovanosis, 1576
Doripenem
for anaerobic bacteria, 1643
antimicrobial spectrum, routes of administration and
dosages, 1206t–1207t
against carbapenemase-resistant gram-negative bacilli,
1290f
for complicated urinary tract infection, 545t
dosage in renal failure, 1213t–1214t
for P. aeruginosa infection, 1210

Doripenem (Continued)
pharmacokinetics of, 1205t
susceptibilities of selected bacteria to, 1208t–1209t
Dornase alfa (Pulmozyme®), for cystic fibrosis, 301
DOTS. see Directly observed therapy, short course
(DOTS).
Doxorubicin/bleomycin/vinblastine/dacarbazine (ABVD),
877, 877t
Doxycycline
absorption of, 1257
for anaerobic bacteria, 1644
for anaplasmosis, 1672
for anthrax, 1127
background in, 1256
for bartonellosis, 1675
bronchitis and, 248
for brucellosis, 1100, 1616
for cat-scratch disease, 659
for cholera, 334
for ehrlichioses, 1671
for foot ulcers, 131t
for gastrointestinal protozoa, 999
for granuloma inguinale, 591
for leptospirosis, 1103, 1609
for Lyme disease, 412
for lymphogranuloma venereum, 589
for malaria prophylaxis, 951
for onchocerciasis, 1051
for parasitic infections, 1345t–1362t
for pelvic inflammatory disease, 493
for plague, 1083–1084, 1083t
for Q fever, 1673
for relapsing fevers, 1109, 1608
for respiratory infections, 1259
route of administration of, 1258
for scrub typhus, 1097, 1671
for spotted fever group rickettsiae, 1669
structure of, 1257f
for syphilis, 565
for tularemia, 1617
for typhus group rickettsiae, 1670
for Whipple's disease, 345
Dracunculiasis, 1778
treatment of, 1345t–1351t
Dracunculus medinensis, 1764
life cycle of, 1769f
pathogenicity of, 1770
treatment of, 1345t–1351t, 1368
Drains, risk of infection from, 689
Dressings, in catheter-related bloodstream infection
(CRBSI), 430
Droplet precautions, 59
Drowning, infections associated with, 680–681
antibiotics for, 681
clinical features and diagnosis of, 681
management of, 681
microbiology in, 680–681, 680b
pathogenesis and epidemiology of infection,
680
Drug
combined regimens of, 1153
efflux, 1168
eruption, 586t–587t
and fever of unknown origin, 614–618
hypersensitivity, lymphadenopathy, 137t–138t
pharmacokinetics of, 1147–1148
resistance assays, HIV, 1489
safety of, 1153
testing, nonradiometric broth-based methods for,
1656–1657
see also specific drugs
Drug delivery systems, outpatient parenteral antimicrobial
therapy, 1201
Drug-induced hypersensitivity syndrome (DISH), and
skin manifestations of HIV, 886–887
Drug interactions
of antituberculosis agents, 1275, 1275b
of chloramphenicol, 1260
of folate inhibitors, 1283, 1284t
in kidney transplant patients, 762
β-lactam antibiotics, 1216
of tetracyclines, 1259, 1259t
see also specific drugs
Drug-resistant infections, management strategies for,
1289–1292

Drug-resistant tuberculosis, 1273–1274
  causes of, 1273
Drug-susceptibility testing, 1275–1276
  methods of, 1276, 1276t
Duke criteria, modified, for endocarditis, 459, 460b
Dukoral, 376
Duodenal fluid aspirate
  Cryptosporidium spp. in, 1738
  microsporidia in, 1739
Duodenal ulceration, 321, 321f
  causes of, 322, 322t
  from *Helicobacter pylori*, 1604
  pathogenesis and pathology of, 324
Duvenhage virus, 1463
Dysglycemia, as quinolones adverse effect, 1247
Dysgonomonas capnocytophagoides, 338
Dyspepsia
  functional, 324
  uninvestigated, 325
Dysrhythmias, in Chagas disease, 1072
Dysuria, in cystitis, 526

E
E-cadherin, 1538
Ear, specimen collection in, 1634t
Ear infections
  Pseudomonas aeruginosa in, 1589
  quinolones for, 1243
  rhinosporidiosis in, 1721
Early localized disease, management of, 412
Eastern equine encephalitis virus, 193t–194t,
  1495t
Eaton-Lambert myasthenic syndrome, 212
Ebola-Marburg viral infection, 648t–649t
Ebola virus, 666, 1111f, 1113f
  and bioterrorism, 671t
  clinical features of, 1114t–1115t
  clinical manifestations of, 1506
  diagnosis, 1506
  epidemiology of, 1110, 1112t, 1506
  geographic distribution of, 939–940
  nature, 1505
  prevention, 1506
Echinocandin lipopeptides, 1341–1343
  adverse effects of, 1343
  in children, 1343
  dosing and administration, 1341
  drug interactions of, 1343
  indications of, 1341–1342
  mechanism of action, 1341, 1341f
  pharmacodynamics of, 1341
  pharmacokinetics and distribution of, 1341
  structures of, 1342f
Echinocandins
  for aspergillosis, 1691
  for cancer patients, 737–738
  for *Candida* infection, 439–440
  for candidemia, 441–442, 1686
  for esophageal candidiasis, 1686
  for intra-abdominal candidiasis, 358
  for oropharyngeal candidiasis, 1684
Echinococcal disease, 666
Echinococcosis, 1038–1045, 1772
  clinical features of, 1041–1042
  diagnosis of, 1043–1044
  epidemiology of, 1038–1039
  hepatic alveolar, 1042
  management of, 1044–1045
  pathogenesis and pathology of, 1039–1041
  prevention of, 1041
Echinococcus, 1038
  occupational infections, 648t–649t
Echinococcus granulosus
  diagnosis of, 1043
  from dogs, 656–658
  epidemiology of, 1038, 1039f, 1766
  life cycle of, 1038, 1039f, 1774f
  management of, 1044–1045
  pathogenesis and pathology of, 1039–1040,
    1041f
  pathogenicity of, 1772
  treatment of, 1345t–1351t

Echinococcus multilocularis
  diagnosis of, 1043–1044
  from dogs, 658
  epidemiology of, 1038–1039, 1040f, 1766
  life cycle of, 1038, 1040f
  management of, 1045
  pathogenesis and pathology of, 1040–1041, 1041f–1043f
  pathogenicity of, 1772
  treatment of, 1345t–1351t
Echinococcus oligarthus, epidemiology of, 1766
Echinococcus vogeli, from dogs, 658
Echinostoma, 1037, 1765
Echinostoma ilocanum, life cycle of, 1771f
Echinostomiasis
  clinical features of, 997
  pathogenesis and pathology of, 994
Echocardiography
  in endocarditis, 462, 463f
  in fever of unknown origin, 622
  of pericardial effusion, 478
  in pericarditis, 449, 454
  in rheumatic fever, 475
Echovirus
  in chronic meningitis, 186t
  in pericarditis, 450
Ecological parameters, 70
Econazole
  keratitis, 155
  for vulvovaginal candidiasis, 488t
Ecthyma, 85t, 88–89
Ecthyma gangrenosum, 113–116, 116f
  Pseudomonas aeruginosa in, 1586
  Stenotrophomonas maltophilia in, 1597
Ectocervicitis, 490
Ectodermal dysplasia with immunodeficiency, 720
Ectoparasites, 107
  skin, 107
Eculizumab, 798t–799t
Eczema, in HIV/AIDS, 879–880
Eczema vaccinatum, dermatologic manifestations of,
  114t–115t
Edwardsiella tarda, 1577t
Efavirenz, 1148t, 1301–1302
  adverse reactions of, 1302
  antiretroviral drugs, 921–922
  description of, 1301
  dosage of, 1301
    in special circumstances, 1302
  drug interactions of, 1302
  effect on oral contraceptives, 907t
  indications of, 1301–1302
  in occupational exposure, to HIV infection, 835
  perinatal HIV transmission prevention, 908–909, 909t
  pharmacokinetics and distribution of, 1301
  during pregnancy, 922
  resistance to, 1302
  route of administration of, 1301
  teratogenicity of, 901–902
Effector functions of the innate immune response, 27–32
Efflux, drug, 1168
Effusive pericarditis, 478
Eflornithine
  for African trypanosomiasis, 969t, 970, 1762
  for parasitic infections, 1345t–1362t, 1366
Eh-adherence lectin, 1009
Ehrlichia, 1671
  diagnosis of, 195
Ehrlichia chaffeensis, 1671
Ehrlichia ewingii, 1671
Ehrlichioses, 1671
  canine, 658
  and occupational infections, 648t–649t
  tetracyclines for, 1259
Eikenella corrodens, 1622
  in bacterial arthritis, 383t
  cellulitis and, 92
  in human bites, 682, 683t
El Moro Canyon (ELMC) virus, 1503t
Elbasvir, for hepatitis C, 1332
Elderly patients
  fever of unknown origin in, 615
  quinolones for, 1246
  tetracyclines for, 1259

Electrocardiography (ECG)
  in myocarditis, 447–448
  in pericarditis, 452, 453f
  in rheumatic fever, 473, 474f
Electrocautery, for anal carcinoma, 878
Electroencephalography (EEG)
  Creutzfeldt-Jakob disease and, 217
  encephalitis, 195
Electrolyte, in severe malaria, 1020t
Electron microscopy, of microsporidia, 1739, 1740f
Electrophysiologic studies, botulism diagnosis, 212
Electrospray ionization mass spectrometry (ESI-MS), 1388
  for *Acinetobacter baumannii*, 1583t–1584t
Elementary body (EB), of *Chlamydia trachomatis*, 597
Elephantiasis, 1047, 1048f, 1049
Elephants, infections from, 669
ELISPOT T-SPOT.TB, 1657–1658, 1658t
Elizabethkingia, 1597–1598
  clinical manifestations of, 1598
  management of, 1598
  microbiology of, 1598
  nomenclature of, 1581t–1582t
Elizabethkingia meningosepticum, nosocomial infections
  from, 1588t
Elvitegravir, 1307
  adverse reactions and interactions of, 1307
  antiretroviral drugs, 922
  description of, 1307
  dosage of, 1307
    in special circumstances, 1307
  effect on oral contraceptives, 907t
  indications of, 1307
  perinatal HIV transmission prevention, 910t
  pharmacokinetics and distribution of, 1307
  resistance to, 1307
  route of administration, 1307
Elvitegravir/cobicistat/tenofovir/emtricitabine, perinatal
  HIV transmission prevention, 910t
Embalmer, and occupational infections, 648t–649t
Emerging diseases and pathogens, 40–48, 41t
  examples of, 943–945
Emerging infectious diseases
  behavior changes and, 45
  climate, weather, natural disasters and, 46–48, 46f
  crowding, population density and, 45–46
  detecting pathogens and outbreaks, 48
  drivers of, 41b
  governmental and geopolitical factors associated with,
    43–45
  human ecosystem interactions and, 42–43
  medical technology and, 46
  poverty and, 43
  short history of, 41–42
  travel and, 43
Emetics, botulism, 212
Emetine hydrochloride, 1012
Emphysematous pyelonephritis, 547–548, 549f
Empiric antibiotic therapy, for cancer patients, 734–735,
  734f–735f
  reassessment of, 735–738
  therapeutic modifications
    based on culture results, 735, 736f
    based on initial response to, 735–738
Empiric treatment
  in intestinal transplant patients, 757
  for prosthetic joint infection (PJI), 402
Empyema, 263
  causes of, 265t
  clinical features of, 266
  epidemiology of, 263
  frequency of organisms, 266t
  management of, 270
  pathogenesis and pathology of, 265
  prevention of, 265–266
Emtricitabine, 1148t, 1299–1300
  adverse reactions of, 1300
  antiretroviral drugs, 921
  chemical structure of, 1296f
  for chronic hepatitis B, 1329
  description of, 1299
  dosage of, 1299–1300
    in special circumstances, 1297t, 1300
  drug interactions of, 1300

Emtricitabine (Continued)
  effect on oral contraceptives, 907t
  for hepatitis B virus (HBV), in HIV, 896–897
  indications of, 1300
  in occupational exposure, to HIV infection, 835
  perinatal HIV transmission prevention, 909t
  pharmacokinetics and distribution of, 1299
  resistance to, 1300
  route of administration, 1299–1300
Encephalitis, 189–197
  acute viral, 195
  anaerobic bacteria in, 1636
  from Candida, 1684
  clinical features of, 190–194, 195f
  cysticercosis and, 1034–1035
  definition of, 189
  diagnosis of, 195–197, 195t, 196f
  enteroviruses and, 1411
  epidemiology of, 189, 190f, 191t
  exposures associated with agents causing, 191t
  herpes simplex, 227, 227f
  from human immunodeficiency virus, 227
  from immune reconstitution inflammatory syndrome,
    861–862
  in immunologically mediated diseases, 772–773
  limbic, 227–228
  Listeria, 1540
  management of, 197
  microbiology of, 189–190
  pathogens anecdotally associated with, 194t
  pathology and pathogenesis of, 194–195
  psychiatric manifestations of, 227–228
  Toxoplasma gondii in, 1755
  toxoplasmic, 856–857
Encephalitozoon cuniculi, pathogenicity of, 1736–1737
Encephalitozoon hellem, pathogenicity of, 1736–1737
Encephalitozoon intestinalis
  chronic diarrhea, 348
  diagnostic microbiology of, 1740f
  in immunocompromised patients, 1741
Encephalitozoon spp.
  diagnostic microbiology of, 1739
  epidemiology of, 1736
  in immunocompetent persons, 1741
  pathogenicity of, 1736–1737
  prevention of, 1737
  in systemic microsporidiosis, 1741
Encephalomyelitis
  acute disseminated, 194
  postinflammatory, 194
Encephalopathy
  causes of, 190
  definition of, 190
  fulminant hepatic failure and, 363
  in HIV-infected children, 902–903
  influenza-associated, 1470
  JC polyomavirus and, 1447
  Lyme disease and, 409
  typhoid fever and, 1004
Endemic treponematoses, dermatologic manifestations of,
  114t–115t
Endocarditis, 456–470
  Alcaligenes xylosoxidans in, 1597
  aminoglycosides for, 1236–1237
  antibiotics for, 1152t
  from Bartonella, 1675
  Bartonella quintana, 659
  brucellosis complications, 1099
  in cancer patients, 728
  Candida, 442, 1684, 1686–1687
  causes of, 457b
  culture-negative, 457, 458t, 460, 462f, 466
  definitions of, 456, 456b
  diagnosis of, 459–464, 460b–461b, 461t, 462f–465f
  enterococci and, 1533
  epidemiology of, 456–457
  Erysipelothrix rhusiopathiae and, 1542
  etiologies of, 457, 458t
  host defenses in, 458t, 459
  β-lactam antibiotics for, 1211–1212
  management of, 464–469, 466t–467t, 469t
  micro-organisms in, 458–459, 458t
  native valve, 457, 458t, 462, 465, 466t, 468t
  from Neisseria gonorrhoeae, 1563
  nonpyogenic streptococci and, 1532

Endocarditis (Continued)
  pathogenesis of, 457–459
  phaeohyphomycosis and, 1721
  predisposing host factors, 457–458
  in pregnancy, 500–501
  prevention of, 459, 460t, 1535, 1536t
  prophylaxis, β-lactam antibiotics, 1206–1209
  prosthetic valves, 456–457, 458t, 463–465, 468t–469t,
    469
  Pseudomonas aeruginosa in, 1586, 1587t
  Stenotrophomonas maltophilia in, 1597
  transient bacteremia in, 459
  vancomycin for, 1251
Endocarditis stigmata, 120
Endocervicitis, 490
Endogenous infections, 12
Endolimax nana, 1725t, 1730f, 1731–1732
Endoluminal brush, in catheter, 433–434
Endometrial biopsy, for pelvic inflammatory disease,
  493
Endometritis
  from Neisseria gonorrhoeae, 1562–1563
  postpartum, 494–495
  in pregnancy, 503–504
Endomyocardial biopsy (EMB), in myocarditis, 446,
  448–449
Endophthalmitis, 158–164
  acute, 158–159
  adjunctive therapy of, 163
  antibiotic chemotherapy for, 162–163
  Candida, 445
    treatment of, 443t
  clinical features of, 160–161
  conjunctival filtering bleb associated, 158, 161
  definition and nomenclature, 158
  delayed onset, 158–159
  diagnosis of, 161–162
  differential diagnosis of, 161
  endogenous, 158t, 159, 161
  epidemiology of, 158, 158t
  filtering bleb, 161
  fungal, 159
  incidence and prevalence of, 158
  intraoperative precautions for, 160
  management of, 162–163
  metastatic, 169
    causing retinitis and uveitis, 169t
  microbial etiology of, 158t
  microbiologic investigations in, 161–162
  outcome of, 163
  pathogenesis and pathology of, 158–159
  post-traumatic, 158t, 159, 161, 161f
  postoperative, 158–159, 158t
    acute, 160, 160f
    delayed-onset, 160–161, 160f–161f
  preoperative precautions for, 159–160
  prevention of, 159–160
  Pseudomonas aeruginosa in, 1589
  Pseudomonas spp. in, 1589
Endophthalmitis Vitrectomy Study (EVS), 162
Endoscopic drainage, lung abscess, 270
Endoscopic retrograde cholangiopancreatography
  (ERCP)
  antibiotic prophylaxis and, 1160
  biliary sepsis, 360
Endoscopic tests, for Helicobacter pylori, 325
Endoscopic ultrasound-fine needle aspiration, 1160
Endoscopy
  for Clostridium difficile, 1630
  in food-borne diarrheal illness, 332
Endospores, 1718
Endovascular infections, β-lactam antibiotics for,
  1211–1212
Enfuvirtide, 887, 1148t, 1305
  adverse reactions of, 1305
  antiretroviral drugs, 925
  description of, 1305
  dosage of, 1305
    in special circumstances, 1305
  drug interactions of, 1305
  indications of, 1305
  perinatal HIV transmission prevention, 910t
  pharmacokinetics and distribution of, 1305
  resistance to, 1305
  route of administration of, 1305

Enoxacin
  dissociation constants of, 535t
  for prostatitis, 536t
Entamoeba, 1008
  chronic diarrhea, 348
  diarrhea, 332–333
Entamoeba bangladeshi, 1725t
Entamoeba coli, 1725t, 1730f
Entamoeba dispar, 1008, 1725t
  chronic diarrhea, 348
  diagnosis of, 1011
  epidemiology of, 1009, 1726
  pathogenicity of, 1728
Entamoeba gingivalis, 1725t, 1729
Entamoeba hartmanni, 1725t, 1729f, 1731–1732
Entamoeba histolytica, 1008, 1725t
  amebic liver abscess, 360–361
  amebicides in, 1012
  of chronic diarrhea, 347t, 348
  clinical features of, 995
  diagnosis of, 998t–999t, 1011, 1011f–1012f
  epidemiology of, 989–990, 1009, 1726
  food-borne diarrheal illness, characteristics of, 330
  identification in fecal specimens, 1728–1729,
    1729f–1730f
  jaundice, 1135t
  management of, 997, 1345t–1351t
  parasite infections and, 73
  pathogenicity of, 1728
  prevention of, 995
  transmission of, 1009
Entamoeba moshkovskii, 1008, 1725t
  diagnosis of, 1011
  diagnostic microbiology of, 1729
  epidemiology of, 1009, 1726
Entamoeba polecki, 1725t
  diagnostic microbiology of, 1729
Entecavir, 1146t–1147t
  for chronic hepatitis B, 1329
  for hepatitis B virus (HBV), in HIV, 896–897
Enteral nutrition, hospital-acquired pneumonia,
  261–262
Enteric adenoviruses, 1396
  clinical characteristics of, 1391t
  epidemiological characteristics of, 1391t
  structure and morphological characteristics of, 1391f,
    1391t
  viral enteritis and, 338
Enteric bacteria, polymicrobial peritonitis and, 381
Enteric fevers, 1002–1007
  acute shedding and chronic carriage and, 1004–1005
  antimicrobial drug resistance for, 1005
  case fatality of, 1005
  clinical features of, 1003–1005
  complications of, 1004, 1004b
  diagnosis of, 1005
  differential diagnosis of, 1005
  epidemiology of, 1002–1003, 1002f–1003f
  jaundice, 1135
  management of, 1005–1007, 1006t
  pathogenesis and pathology of, 1003
  prevention of, 1003
  relapse in, 1004
  vaccines for, 1003
  see also Paratyphoid fever; Typhoid fever
Enteric infections, trimethoprim-sulfamethoxazole for,
  1281–1282
Enteritis
  bacterial, 336–338
  from Campylobacter spp., 1602
  diagnosis of, 339
  viral, 338
Entero-Test, for helminths diagnosis, 1776
Enteroaggregative Escherichia coli (EAEC), 336
  in intestinal infections, 1573–1574
  virulence factors of, 1572t
Enterobacter
  in complicated urinary tract infection, 540t
  diagnostic microbiology of, 1568t
  hospital-acquired pneumonia and, 259t
  microflora, 355–356
Enterobacter cloacae
  in human bites, 683t
  intrinsic resistance of, 1182t
  in respiratory tract infections, 1575

Enterobacter hormaechei, 1577t
Enterobacteriaceae, 1565–1578
  aminopenicillins and, 1203
  antibiotic therapy for, in infective arthritis,
    386t
  brain abscess and, 199
  clinical manifestations of, 1569–1576
    bacteremia, 1576
    extraintestinal infections, 1575–1576
    intestinal infections, 1569–1575, 1572t
    meningitis, 1575
    neurologic infections, 1575
    other infections, 1576
    respiratory tract infections, 1575
    urinary tract infections, 1575
  clonal relationships of, 1565–1566
  diagnostic microbiology of, 1566–1569,
    1568t
  efflux systems in, 1186–1187
  emerging pathogens of, 1576, 1577t
  empyema and, 266t
  endophthalmitis and, 159
  in foot ulcers, 130–131
  general pathophysiologic considerations for, 1569,
    1569f–1570f
  and intra-abdominal infections, 690
  ketolides, 1220
  lower respiratory tract infections, 264f
  lung abscess and, 263–264
  macrolides, 1220
  microflora, 355–356
  in osteomyelitis, 389–390
  phylogeny of, 1565–1566, 1565f
  prevention, management and control of,
    1576–1578
  in prostatitis, 536
  resistance
    to carbapenems, 1185
    to β-lactam, 1184
    to polymyxin, 1193
    to tigecycline, 1190
  in skull-base osteomyelitis, 393
  taxonomy of, 1565–1566
  in vertebral osteomyelitis, 391–392
  virulence factors of, 1569, 1571t
Enterobiasis
  clinical features of, 996
  Dientamoeba fragilis and, 1727
  treatment of, 1345t–1351t
Enterobius vermicularis
  clinical features of, 996
  diagnosis of, 998t–999t
  epidemiology of, 1763
  life cycle of, 1767f
  pathogenicity of, 1766
  in population density and urbanization, 990
  prevention of, 995
  treatment of, 1000, 1001t, 1345t–1351t
Enterococci, 1523–1536
  aminoglycosides for, 1234
  antibiotic therapy for, in infective arthritis, 386t
  biliary sepsis, 360
  clinical manifestations of, 1533–1534
  in complicated urinary tract infection, 540t
  in dog bites, 656
  in endocarditis, 457, 458t
  epidemiology of, 1526–1527
  glycopeptide resistance in, 1191
  linezolid, 1230
  macrolides, 1220
  management of, 1534–1535
  microflora, 356
  molecular characterization and population structure of,
    1524–1525
  multidrug-resistant, 467
  in osteomyelitis, 390, 395t
  pathogenesis of, 1530–1531
  and postsplenectomy sepsis, 778t
  reduced susceptibility to sulfonamides and
    trimethoprim, 1192
  taxonomy and identification of, 1523–1524, 1523f
  vancomycin-resistant. see Vancomycin-resistant
    enterococci (VRE)

Enterococcus
  molecular characterization and population structure of,
    1525
  peritonitis and, 381
  in pyelonephritis, 547
Enterococcus faecalis
  genome sequence for, 1525
  intrinsic resistance of, 1182t
  microflora, 355–356
  and surgical site infections, 687
Enterococcus faecium
  management of, 1534
  resistance
    to ampicillin, 1184
    to glycopeptides, 1191
    intrinsic, 1182t
Enterocolitis
  in cancer patients, 727–728, 731f
  in HIV/AIDS, 858
  necrotizing, probiotics for, 1373, 1374t
  yersiniosis and, 1627
Enterocytozoon bieneusi
  chronic diarrhea, 348
  diagnostic microbiology of, 1739, 1739f
  in immunocompetent persons, 1741
  in immunocompromised patients, 1741
  pathogenicity of, 1736, 1736f
Enterocytozoon spp.
  diagnostic microbiology of, 1739
  prevention of, 1737
Enterohemorrhagic Escherichia coli (EHEC), 336
  cytotoxins, 330
  in intestinal infections, 1572–1573
  virulence factors of, 1572t
Enteroinvasive Escherichia coli (EIEC), 336
  in intestinal infections, 1573
  virulence factors of, 1572t
Enteromonas pathogens, 15–16
Enteromonas hominis, 1725t
Enteropathogen-M cell interactions, 17f
Enteropathogenic Escherichia coli (EPEC), 336, 1570–1572
  virulence factors of, 1572t
Enterotoxigenic Escherichia coli (ETEC)
  characteristics of, in food-borne diarrheal illness, 330t
  doses of, in diarrheal illness, 329t
  enterotoxins, 329–330
  in intestinal infections, 1570
  mechanism of, 331f
  travelers' diarrhea and, 950
  virulence factors of, 1572t
Enterotoxins
  of Bacteroides fragilis, 1633
  in food-borne diarrheal illness, 329–330
  Staphylococcus aureus and, 1513t–1514t
Enteroviruses, 75t, 80, 189
  assembly and release of, 1409
  attachment of, 1407–1408
  causing meningitis, 225, 772
  cell receptors of, 1408, 1409t
  circulation and geographic spread of, 1410
  classification of, 1406–1407, 1407t
  clinical manifestations of, 1410–1411, 1410t
  clinical syndromes of, 1410–1411
  congenital infection and
    diagnosis of, 512t
    in perinatal infections, 514–515, 514t
  control of infection, 1411–1412
  cytopathic effects of, 1409, 1412f–1413f
  D68 (EV-D68), 1410
  diagnosis of, 1412
    classic techniques for, 1412–1416
    isolation of, 1412f–1413f, 1413
    molecular techniques for, 1414f–1415f, 1416
    nonmolecular direct detection for, 1412, 1412f
    serologic analysis of, 1413–1416
    serotyping for, 1413, 1413f
    specimens for, 1412
  encephalitis/myelitis caused by, 192t
  entry and uncoating of, 1408
  epidemiology of, 1409–1410
  genera of, 1406–1407, 1406t
  history of, 1406
  hosts of, 1409

Enteroviruses (Continued)
  human, 1406–1416
  immune response to, 1409–1410
  infection, 1407–1416
    dermatologic manifestations of, 114t–115t
  in myocarditis, 447
  pathogenicity of, 1407–1409
  in pericarditis, 450
  physical and chemical properties of, 1406, 1406t
  routes of transmission, 1409, 1410t
  structure and genome organization of, 1407,
    1408f
  translation of viral genome and viral RNA synthesis,
    1408–1409
  treatment and prevention of, 1412
  vaccines for, 1411
Entomophthoromycosis
  clinical manifestations of, 1719–1720
  diagnostic microbiology of, 1716
  epidemiology of, 1713
  management of, 1722–1723
  nature of, 1712
  pathogenicity of, 1715
  prevention of, 1715
Entry inhibitors, 1305–1306
  perinatal HIV transmission prevention, 910t
  resistance to, 924
env genes, 1483, 1484f
Environment-derived risk factors, and infection following
  surgery and trauma, 686
Environmental health and safety, 57
Environmental services, 57
Enzyme immunoassays (EIAs)
  for Aspergillus, 1688
  for blastomycosis, 295, 1702–1703
  for caliciviruses, 1396
  for Chlamydia pneumoniae, 1679
  for Chlamydia trachomatis, 1678
  for chronic chlamydial infections, 1679–1680
  for Clostridium difficile, 352, 1630
  for hantavirus, 1504
  for helminths diagnosis, 1777
  for Lyme disease, 410b
  for rotaviruses, 1393
  treponemal, 564
Enzyme-linked immunosorbent assay (ELISA)
  for Babesia, 1752
  for brucellosis, 1100, 1615
  for Campylobacter spp., 1602
  for Entamoeba spp., 1729
  for gastrointestinal parasites, 997
  in genital herpes, 572–573
  for giardiasis, 347
  hantavirus, 1504
  for Helicobacter pylori, 1603
  for helminths diagnosis, 1777
  for HIV, 1487
    in low- and middle-income countries,
      893–894
  for leishmaniasis, 1063, 1757
  for Lyme disease, 409–410
  for mycobacteria, 1657–1658
  for papillomaviruses, 1443
  for plague, 1083
  for polyomaviruses, 1446
  in tuberculosis, 275
  uveitis and retinitis and, 167
  for viral hemorrhagic fevers, 1116
  in yellow fever, 1494
Enzyme-linked immunospot (ELISpot), 275
Enzymes, in sepsis, 419t
Eosinophilia
  approach to, in traveler from tropics, 984–988
  causes of, 984t
  clinical features of, 985, 986t
  diagnosis of, 985–986, 987t
  epidemiology of, 984, 984t
  helminth causes of, 986t
  management of, 986–988, 987f
  pathogenesis and pathology of, 984–985
  prevention of, 985
  tropical pulmonary, 1049
Eosinophilic folliculitis, in HIV/AIDS, 880–881

Eosinophilic meningitis, 971–978
  causes of, 971b
  clinical features of, 973–974
  diagnosis of, 974–975, 978f
  epidemiology of, 972–973, 976f–977f
  main sources of infection for, 974t
  management of, 975–976
  noninfective causes of, 978
  pathogenesis and pathology of, 971–972, 971b, 972f
  prevention of, 973, 974t
  uncommon infective causes of, 976
Eosinophils, 984
Epidemic keratoconjunctivitis, lymphadenopathy and,
    137t–138t
Epidemic typhus, 1670
  and bioterrorism, 671t
  location of, 1092t–1093t
Epidemics, 50
  typical, 49–50
Epidemiologic data, 50
  see also specific subjects
Epidermophyton, 122
Epidermophyton floccosum, 660
  clinical features of, 124
  pathogenicity of, 1711
Epididymitis, 537–538, 537t
  gonorrhea and, 594
  Mycoplasma genitalium in, 1662
  Mycoplasma hominis in, 1663
  from Neisseria gonorrhoeae, 1562–1563
  treatment of, 596t
Epididymo-orchitis, 537, 1099
Epidural empyema, 1589
Epiglottitis, 231–233, 1620
  clinical features of, 232
  diagnosis of, 232–233, 232f
  differential diagnosis of, 233
  epidemiology of, 232
  management of, 233
  physiology of, 232
  prevention of, 232
Episiotomy incisions, 504
Episiotomy infections, 495–496
Epitrochlear lymph adenopathy, 149
Epsilonproteobacteria, 1600, 1601t
Epstein-Barr virus (EBV), 703t
  causing retinitis and uveitis, 168t
  and chronic fatigue syndrome, 632–633
  encephalitis/myelitis caused by, 192t
  in hematopoietic stem cell transplantation, 741, 743t
  in HIV/AIDS, 882
  in immunocompetent host, 1437
  in immunocompromised host, 1437
  infection, 75t, 79
    clinical features of, 79
    complications of, 79
    dermatologic manifestations, 114t–115t
    management of, 79
  in infectious mononucleosis, 143–144, 377
    and fever of unknown origin, 613
  in intestinal transplant patients, 756, 759–760
    clinical presentation of, 759–760
    diagnosis of, 760
    epidemiology of, 759–760
    prevention of, 760
    treatment of, 759t, 760
  jaundice, 1135t
  in liver transplant patients, 751, 751t
  in malignant lymphomas, 875
  pathogenicity of, molecular and cellular basis of, 1431,
    1432f
  in thoracic transplant patients, 748
  vaccination, 1433
Ergosterol, 1333, 1333f
ERIC-PCR, 1583t–1584t
erm genes, 1189
Erosive lichen planus, 586t–587t
Ertapenem
  for anaerobic bacteria, 1634, 1643
  antimicrobial spectrum, routes of administration and
    dosages, 1206t–1207t
  for complicated urinary tract infection, 545t
  dosage in renal failure, 1213t–1214t
  for foot ulcers, 131t
  for hospital-acquired pneumonia, 260t

Ertapenem (Continued)
  for human bites, 683
  for lung abscess, 269f
  in outpatient parenteral antimicrobial therapy,
    1201
  pharmacokinetics of, 1205t
  susceptibilities of selected bacteria to, 1208t–1209t
Erysipelas, 89, 89f
Erysipeloid, 648t–649t, 1542
Erysipelothrix, 1537
Erysipelothrix rhusiopathiae, 1542
  from birds, 668
  from cat bites, 659
  cellulitis and, 91
  clindamycin, 1225
  clinical manifestations of, 1542
  diagnostic microbiology of, 1542
  epidemiology of, 1542
  ketolides, 1220
  macrolides, 1220
  management of, 1542
  from marine mammals, 668
  nature of, 1542
  pathogenicity of, 1542
  transmission of, 664
Erythema induratum, 118
Erythema infectiosum, 78–79
  clinical features of, 78
  dermatologic manifestations of, 114t–115t
Erythema marginatum, 472–473, 474f
Erythema migrans
  diagnosis of, 409–410
  Lyme disease and, 405, 407f–408f
Erythema multiforme, 586t–587t
  dermatologic manifestations of, 120, 120f
Erythema nodosum, 120–121, 121f, 121t
Erythema nodosum leprosum (ENL), 955, 958,
    958f
Erythematous maculopapulous exanthems, 75t
Erythrocyte sedimentation rate (ESR)
  in bacterial arthritis, 384
  and fever of unknown origin, 620
  in osteomyelitis, 393
  in prosthetic joint infection (PJI), 400
Erythromycin
  for actinomycosis, 316
  for anaerobic bacteria, 1643
  for anthrax, 1127
  for Bacillus cereus, 1542
  cellulitis and, 92
  for chancroid, 590
  chemical structure of, 1171
  conjunctivitis, 152
  for diphtheria, 1546
  for dog bites, 657t
  for Erysipelothrix rhusiopathiae, 1542
  for food-borne diarrheal illness, 333
  for granuloma inguinale, 591
  for leptospirosis, 1609
  for lung abscess, 269f
  for lymphogranuloma venereum, 589
  in pregnancy, 503
  for relapsing fevers, 1109, 1608
  for rheumatic fever, 476
  for Rhodococcus equi, 1551
  for syphilis, 565
  tissue distribution, 1224t
Erythromycin A, 1217, 1218f
  accumulation ratio of, 1222t
  characteristics of, 1218t
  classification, 1217
  intra-bacterial penetration, 1221
  peptidyltransferase center, 1221
  resistance, 1221–1222
  stability in acidic medium, 1217, 1219f
  in vitro activity, 1219, 1220t
Erythromycylamine, characteristics of, 1218t
Erythroparvovirus, 1449
Erythropoietin, 689
Erythrovirus B19, in infective arthritis, 385, 387t
Eschar, 698
Escherichia, taxonomy of, 1566
Escherichia albertii, 1577t
  diarrhea and, 336
  taxonomy of, 1565

Escherichia coli
  active efflux in, 1186
  azithromycin, 1220
  bacterial enteritis, 336
  biofilm in, 525f
  brain abscess and, 199
  in cancer patients, 723–724
  in complicated urinary tract infection, 540,
    540f
  in cystitis, 523, 527
  diagnosis of, 339
  diagnostic microbiology of, 1568, 1568t
  in diarrhea, 328–330, 333, 335
    characteristics of, 330t
    doses of, 329t
    invasive, 331
  diffusely adherent. see Diffusely adherent Escherichia
    coli (DAEC)
  in dog bites, 656
  in endocarditis, 468
  enteroaggregative. see Enteroaggregative Escherichia coli
    (EAEC)
  enterohemorrhagic. see Enterohemorrhagic Escherichia
    coli (EHEC)
  enteroinvasive. see Enteroinvasive Escherichia coli
    (EIEC)
  enteropathogenic. see Enteropathogenic Escherichia coli
    (EPEC)
  enterotoxigenic. see Enterotoxigenic Escherichia coli
    (ETEC)
  hospital-acquired pneumonia and, 258,
    259t
  in intestinal infections, 1569–1574, 1572t
  lipopolysaccharide of, 1633
  management, 339
  MAR system of, 1194, 1194f
  meningitis and, 177
  microflora, 355–356
  in neonatal meningitis, 1575
  O157:H7
    and bioterrorism, 671t
    transmission of, 665, 665t
  and occupational infections, 648t–649t
  in osteomyelitis, 395t
  primary (spontaneous) peritonitis, 359
  in prostatitis, 533, 536
  in pyelonephritis, 547, 548f
  pyogenic liver abscess, 361
  resistance
    multidrug, 1194
    to quinolones, 1186
    to tigecycline, 1190
  serotyping for, 1570
  Shiga-toxin producing, 336
  and surgical site infections, 687
  taxonomy of, 1566, 1567f
  in urinary tract infection, in pregnancy, 500
  uropathogenic. see Uropathogenic Escherichia coli
    (UPEC)
  virulence factors of, 1571t–1572t
Escherichia fergusonii
  diarrhea and, 336
  taxonomy of, 1566
Esophageal candidiasis, 1686
Esophagitis
  in cancer patients, 727–728
  from Candida, 1684
Etanercept, 797, 798t–799t
  immunosuppression and, 1380t
Ethambutol, 1269–1270
  adverse reactions of, 1268t–1269t
  hepatotoxicity and, 308, 309f
  for meningitis, 186–187, 187t
  for Mycobacterium avium complex, 856
  resistance to, 1194
    mycobacterial, 1656t
  for tuberculosis, 281, 283t
  for urogenital tract tuberculosis, 556
Ethionamide
  as antituberculosis agent, 1270
  for meningitis, 186–187
  resistance to, mycobacterial, 1656t
Ethmoiditis, purulent acute, 240, 240f–241f
Etoposide/prednisone/vincristine/cyclophosphamide/
    doxorubicin (EPOCH), 875–876

Etravirine, 1148t, 1302
  adverse reactions of, 1302
  description of, 1302
  dosage of, 1302
    in special circumstances, 1302
  drug interactions of, 1302
  effect on oral contraceptives, 907t
  indications of, 1302
  perinatal HIV transmission prevention, 909t
  pharmacokinetics and distribution of, 1302
  resistance to, 1302
  route of administration of, 1302
Eubacterium, 1630
  brain abscess and, 199
  halitosis, 319
  in human bites, 683t
  microflora, 355
  in normal flora, 1632, 1632t
Eukaryotes
  comparison of prokaryotes and, 5t
  definition of, 4
Eukaryotic virome, 73
European bat lyssaviruses, 1463
European Bioinformatics Institute (EBI), 62–63
European Committee on Antimicrobial Susceptibility
    Testing (EUCAST), for *Candida*, 1683
Evans' principles, of causation of disease, 1b
Exacerbations
  acute, quinolones for, 1243
  of cystic fibrosis
    management of, 301, 301b
    signs and symptoms of, 300, 300b
  prevention of, 311
Exanthema subitum, 79
  dermatologic manifestations of, 114t–115t
Exanthems
  of primary HIV
    acute, 879
    morbilliform, 886
  viral
    classic, 75–79
    nonclassic, 79–83
Excavata, 1744
Exfoliatin, toxin, 87
Exfoliative toxins, 1513t–1514t, 1515
Exogenous acquisition, 693
Exogenous infections, 12–13
Exotic ungulate encephalopathy, 215t
Exotoxin A, 1580, 1585
Exotoxins, 18–19
  of anaerobic bacteria, 1633
  in sepsis, 419, 419t
Expatriates, 1050
Expressed prostatic secretions (EPS), 532–534, 534f, 536
Extended-spectrum β-lactamases (ESBLs), 1181, 1210,
    1576
  multidrug-resistant gram-negative bacteria producing,
    1289
Extensively drug-resistant tuberculosis, 866
  treatment, 281
Extracellular adherence protein (Eap), 1513t–1514t
Extracellular complement binding protein (Ecb),
    1513t–1514t
Extracellular fibrinogen-binding protein (Efb),
    1513t–1514t
Extracellular matrix (ECM), 13
Extrapulmonary aspergillosis, 1689
Extrapulmonary disease, nontuberculous mycobacteria
    (NTM), 287–288, 288f
  treatment of, 290–291
Extrapulmonary manifestations, of *Mycoplasma
    pneumoniae*, 1661, 1662t
Extrapulmonary tuberculosis, 278–279
Eye
  involvement in leprosy, 958
  protection, 58
Eye damage, onchocerciasis and, 1049
Eye disease, in immune reconstitution inflammatory
    syndrome, 862
Eye infections
  cryptococcosis in, 1695
  Pseudomonas aeruginosa in, 1582–1584, 1588–1589
  rhinosporidiosis in, 1721

Eye infections *(Continued)*
  in tropics, 979–983
    bacterial, 982
    blinding, 979–982
    parasitic, 982
    viral, 982–983
  see also specific infections
'Eye worm', 1050

F

Face shields, 58
Factitious fever, 636–637
  characteristics of, 637b
  criteria for, 636
  diagnosis of, 637
  differential diagnosis of, 637b
  epidemiology, 636
  and fever of unknown origin, 614
  fraudulent, 636, 636t
  investigations, 637
  management of, 637
  mechanism of, 636t
  medicolegal issues, 637
  pathophysiology of, 636
  presentation of, 637
  prevalence of, 636t
  prognosis/outcome, 637
  self-induced, 636, 636t
Faget's sign, 1494–1496
Falciparum spp., jaundice, 1135t
Famciclovir, 1146t–1147t, 1312
  adverse reactions of, 1312
  dosage of, 1312
    in special circumstances, 1312
  for genital herpes, 573, 573t
  indications of, 1312
    Epstein-Barr virus, 1312
    genital herpes, 1310t, 1312
    hepatitis B, 1312
    herpes labialis, 1312
    herpes zoster, 1312
    herpesvirus, 1433
  mechanism of action, 1312
  resistance to, 1312
  route of administration, 1312
  in vitro activity, 1312
Familial hemophagocytic lymphohistiocytosis,
    638
Familial Mediterranean fever (FMF), and fever of
    unknown origin, 614
Far Eastern spotted fever, 1667t, 1668
Far-Eastern tick borne rickettsiosis, 1092t–1093t
Farm animals, infections from, 191t
Farm worker, and occupational infections, 648t–649t
'Farmyard-pox' diseases, 1454
Faropenem, 1162
Fas/FasL, apoptosis to delivery to, 721, 722f
Fasciola gigantica, 1036–1037
  jaundice, 1135t
Fasciola hepatica, 1036–1037, 1037f
  clinical manifestations of, 1778
  epidemiology of, 1765
  jaundice, 1135t
  life cycle of, 1771f
  pathogenicity of, 1770
  treatment of, 1345t–1351t
Fascioliasis, 1036–1037
  dermatologic manifestations of, 114t–115t
Fasciolopsis buski, 1037
  clinical features of, 997
  clinical manifestations of, 1778
  diagnosis of, 998t–999t
  epidemiology of, 1765
  life cycle of, 1771f
  pathogenesis and pathology of, 993–994
  pathogenicity of, 1770
  prevention of, 995
  treatment of, 1001, 1001t, 1345t–1351t
Fatal familial insomnia (FFI), 217
Fatigue, chronic fatigue syndrome. *see* Chronic fatigue
    syndrome.
Fatty acids, volatile. *see* Volatile fatty acids.

Favus, 124
FDG PET. *see* 2-Fluorodeoxyglucose-positron emission
    tomography (FDG PET).
Febrile neutropenia, and fever of unknown origin, 615
Febrile neutropenic patients, aminoglycosides for, 1236
Febrile transaminitis
  in immunocompromised patients, 377–378
  of viral etiology, 377–379, 377t–378t, 378f
Fecal specimens
  amebae identification in, 1728–1729
  ciliate identification in, 1732, 1733f
  flagellate identification in, 1729–1732
Feces, for laboratory diagnosis, of mycobacteria, 1652
Feline spongiform encephalopathy, 215t
Female genital schistosomiasis, 1030
Female genital tract
  anaerobic infection in, 1638t, 1639
  normal flora of, 1632, 1632t
  specimen collection in, 1634t
Females, *Chlamydia trachomatis* infection in, 598–599,
    599f
Fenticonazole, for vulvovaginal candidiasis, 488t
Fernandez reaction, 955
Ferripyochelin, 1585
Fetal distress, malaria in pregnancy, 1143t–1144t
Fetus
  abnormalities in, clinical features of, 508, 509t
  disease in, factors affecting, 506–507
  implications of maternal infections. *see* Congenital
    infection
  tolerance of antiretroviral prophylaxis by, 901–902
  ultrasound in, 508
Fever
  acute-phase response, 608–609
  in cancer patients, 725–726
    persistence of, 736–737
    prolonged, after empirical therapy, 737
    resolution of, 736
  common infections by region, 1130
  differential diagnosis of, 1129t
  factitious. *see* Factitious fever
  generation, 607–608
  and immunologically mediated disease, 771, 771t, 772f
  in malaria, 1018
  Mycoplasma hominis in, 1664
  pathogenesis of, 605–610
    antipyretics, 609–610
    clinical thermometry, 606
    historical considerations, 605
    versus hyperthermia, 605–606
    normal body temperature, 606, 606f
    thermoregulation, 606–607
  patient returning from tropics with, 1129–1131
  in pregnancy, 498
  seven questions to ask, 1129–1130, 1129t
  spotting danger signs, and outcomes, 1130
  viral hemorrhagic, 80
Fever of unknown origin (FUO), 611–624
  in cancer patients, 726, 726f
  category of
    determining, 615–618, 616t–617t
    diagnostic fever patterns by, 623t
    usual diagnostic fever ranges by, 622t
  classic causes of, 612t
  clinical approach to, 615–623
  clinical categories, 611–615
  clinical perspective for, 615
  criteria for, by Petersdorf and Beeson, 611
  diagnostic approach to
    focused, 623
    with localizing signs, 618–622
    without localizing signs, 622–623, 622t
  diagnostic significance
    of nonspecific laboratory test clues, 620, 620t–621t
    of physical examination clues in, 618, 618t–619t
  empiric therapy of, 624
  fever curves, diagnostic, 622
  imaging studies in, 620
  infectious disorders to consider with, 611–613
  invasive diagnostic tests for, 623, 623t
  malignant/neoplastic, 611
  miscellaneous disorders, 615–618, 624
  nonspecific tests

Fever of unknown origin (FUO) (Continued)
  additional, with relevance, 622
  key, 622–623
  and patient age, 615
  recurrent, 615, 624
  rheumatologic/inflammatory disorders, 613–614
  in specific populations, 615
  and travel history, 615
  unusual causes of, 623t
  by bone marrow biopsy or culture, 623t
Fibrillae, 14
Fibrinogen, 13
Fibrinogen-binding protein, 1516
Fibrinolysins, 1513t–1514t
Fibrinolytics, pleural, 304
Fibromyalgia, 632
Fibronectin, 13
Fibronectin-binding protein (fnb), 1513t–1514t
Fibrosing cholestatic hepatitis, 768
Fidaxomicin, 1262–1263
Filamentous fungi, in hematopoietic stem cell
     transplantation, 744–745
Filamentous hemagglutinin (FHA), 1612, 1613t
Filarial infections, 1046–1052, 1046f
  clinical features of, 1049–1050
  diagnosis of, 1050
  epidemiology of, 1046–1047
  loiasis. see Loiasis
  management of, 1050–1051
  onchocerciasis. see Onchocerciasis
  pathogenesis and pathology of, 1047–1048
  prevention of, 1048–1049
Filariasis
  lymphadenopathy and, 137t–138t, 142
  lymphatic. see Lymphatic filariasis
  treatment of, 1345t–1351t
Filarids, 1765
  pathogenicity of, 1768–1770
Filoviridae, 1505–1507
  clinical manifestations, 1506–1507
  diagnostic microbiology, 1506
  epidemiology, 1505–1506
  management, 1507
  nature, 1505
  pathogenesis, 1505
  prevention, 1506
Filoviruses, 1110
  and bioterrorism, 671t
  clinical features of, 1114t–1115t
  epidemiology of, 1112t, 1505f
  management of, 1117
Fimbriae, 14, 1613t
  in bacteriuria, 524
Fine needle aspiration biopsy (FNA-B)
  for echinococcosis, 1043
  for lymphadenopathy in HIV patients, 143
Finegoldia, lung abscess and, 264–265
Fish, infections from, 661–662, 668, 669t
Fish tank granuloma, 287
Fixed drug eruption, 586t–587t
Flaccid paralysis, acute, 1411
Flagella, 10, 1584–1585
Flagellates
  epidemiology of, 1725–1727
  identification of
    in fecal specimens, 1729–1732
    in urogenital specimens, 1732, 1732f
  intestinal, 989t
    and urogenital, 1725–1733, 1725t
  nature of, 1725
Flagellin, 28–29
Flavivirus encephalitis, 195
Flavivirus infection, dermatologic manifestations,
     114t–115t
Flaviviruses, 75t, 1110, 1495t
  and bioterrorism, 671t
  clinical features of, 1114t–1115t
  epidemiology of, 1112t
Flavobacterium spp., 1597–1598
Flea-borne spotted fever, 1092t–1093t, 1667t, 1668
Fleas, 106t, 108
  cat, 1669, 1673
  dogs, 658
  mouse, 1669
  plague and, 1078, 1081

Fleas (Continued)
  rats, 660, 1669
  for tropical rickettsioses, 1091, 1092t–1093t
Fleroxacin
  dissociation constants of, 535t
  for prostatitis, 536t
Flies, 106t
  tularemia and, 1086, 1087f
  see also specific types
Flight travel paths, in emerging infectious diseases, 44f
Flinders Island spotted fever, 1092t–1093t, 1667t, 1668
Flora
  normal, anaerobes of, 1631–1632, 1632f, 1632t
  see also Microflora; specific anatomical area
Florists, and occupational infections, 648t–649t
FLPR1 inhibitory proteins, 1513t–1514t
Flubendazole, 1352t–1362t, 1371
Flucloxacillin, 223–224
  dosage in renal failure, 1213t–1214t
  for foot ulcers, 131t
  pharmacokinetics of, 1205t
  susceptibilities of selected bacteria to, 1208t–1209t
Fluconazole, 1337–1338
  adverse effects of, 1338
  for blastomycosis, 295, 1703
  for Candida, 440, 442, 444–445, 744
  for candidemia, 1686
  for candidiasis, 128
  chemical structure of, 1337f
  for coccidioidomycosis, 296, 1705–1706
  for conidiobolomycosis, 1723
  for cryptococcosis, 1695, 1695t
  dosage of, 1337
    in special circumstances, 1338
  drug interactions of, 1338
  for endophthalmitis, 162–163
  for esophageal candidiasis, 1686
  for fungal urinary tract infection, 545t
  for histoplasmosis, 294, 1708
  indications, 1337–1338
  intra-abdominal candidiasis, 358
  keratitis and, 155
  in liver transplant patients, 754t
  for meningitis, 180
  for mycetoma, 1723
  for oropharyngeal candidiasis, 1684
  for paracoccidioidomycosis, 1709
  for parasitic infections, 1345t–1351t
  pharmacodynamics of, 1337
  pharmacokinetics and distribution of, 1337
  for primary amebic meningoencephalitis, 1749
  prophylaxis with, 689
    for cancer patients, 730, 737
    for Candida spp., 1687
    for candidiasis in HIV, 854–855
    for coccidioidomycosis, in HIV/AIDS, 855
  resistance to, Candida spp., 1683
  route of administration, 1337
  for sporotrichosis, 298
  for Talaromyces marneffei, 1699
  for vulvovaginal candidiasis, 488, 1686
Flucytosine, 1335–1336
  adverse effects of, 1336
  for Candida endocarditis, 442
  for Candida meningitis, 444
  chemical structure of, 1335f
  for chromoblastomycosis, 1722
  for cryptococcosis, 1695
  dosage of, 1335
    in special circumstances, 1336
  drug interactions of, 1336
  indications of, 1335–1336
  for keratitis, 154
  for parasitic infections, 1345t–1351t
  pharmacodynamics of, 1335
  pharmacokinetics and distribution of, 1335
  route of administration, 1335
  for systemic candidiasis, 1686
  for Talaromyces marneffei, 1699
5-Flucytosine, for fungal urinary tract infection, 545t
Fludarabine, 725
Fluid administration, for dengue, 1122
Fluid imbalances, in severe malaria, 1020t
Fluid replacement, for cholera, 1607
Flukes. see Trematodes.

Fluorescence in situ hybridization (FISH), 1580
Fluorescent microscopy, keratitis and, 155
Fluorescent polarization immunoassay (FPA), for
     brucellosis, 1616
Fluorescent treponemal antibody absorption (FTA-ABS)
     test, 964–965
  in syphilis, 564, 564t
5-Fluorocytosine (5-FC)
  for Candida endophthalmitis, 445
  for chromoblastomycosis, 1722
2-Fluorodeoxyglucose-positron emission tomography
     (FDG PET), 280f
Fluoroquinolones, 1174–1175
  absorption of, 1242
    interactions affecting, 1248
  activity of, 1240
  for Alcaligenes spp., 1597
  for anaerobic bacteria, 1643
  as antituberculosis agents, 1270
  bacterial targeting, 1174
  chemical structures of, 1174, 1175f
  for complicated urinary tract infection, 544
  for conjunctivitis, 176
  for cystitis, 529
  distribution of, 1242–1243
  for endophthalmitis, 162
  excretion of, 1243
  hepatotoxicity and, 308, 309f
  for human bites, 683
  for intra-abdominal sepsis, 357
  for keratitis, 152
  for leprosy, 959
  market withdrawal of, 1239, 1239t
  mode of action of, 1174, 1176f
  pediatric use of, 1246
  for pertussis, 1614
  pharmacodynamics of, 1174–1175
  for plague, 1083–1084
  prophylaxis with, in cancer patients, 731f,
     736
  for prostatitis, 535–536, 535t–537t
  for Pseudomonas aeruginosa, 1589
  for pyelonephritis, 552
  resistance to, 1174, 1186
    mycobacterial, 1656t
  for Rhodococcus equi, 1551
  for Stenotrophomonas maltophilia, 1597
  for travelers' diarrhea, 376, 950
  for tularemia, 1617
  for typhoid fever, 1005–1006
  see also individual drugs
Fluorouracil, chemical structure of, 1335f
Flurithromycin
  characteristics of, 1218t
  classification, 1217
  pharmacokinetics of, 1223t
Focal lesions, in Chagas disease, 1070
Focal neurologic abnormalities, 183–184
Focal pyogenic infections of the central nervous system,
     198–207, 198f
  see also specific infections
Folate inhibitors, 1280–1284
  adverse reactions and interactions of, 1283,
     1283t–1284t
  alone, use of, 1282
  dosage of, 1280, 1281t
    in special circumstances, 1282, 1282t
  indications of, 1281–1282
  kinetics in children, 1280, 1280t
  pharmacokinetics, 1280
  route of administration of, 1280
Folinic acid
  for cystoisosporiasis, 1742
  for toxoplasmosis, 1755
  in toxoplasmosis, in HIV/AIDS, 856–857
Folliculitis, 86–87, 86f
  diffuse, 87
  eosinophilic, in HIV/AIDS, 880–881
  in HIV, 882–883
  hot tub, 87
  Malassezia, 126, 1710
  prevention of, 86–87
  recurrent, 87
Folliculitis barbae, 87
Folliculosis, 981t

Food, contaminated
  Campylobacter spp. in, 1600
  Salmonella in, 1574
Food-borne illness
  definition of, 328
  diarrheal, 328–334
    characteristics of, 330*t*
    clinical features of, 330–331
    diagnosis of, 332–333
    epidemiology of, 328, 329*f*
    host susceptibility in, 328–329
    infectious agents in, doses of, 329*t*
    management of, 333–334, 333*f*, 333*t*
    non-infective food poisoning, 331–332
    pathogenesis of, 329–330
    prevention of, 334
    public health management of, 334
    special clinical syndromes, 332
  prevalence of, 335
Food-borne infections
  burden of disease, 941–942
  spread of, 944–945
Food hygiene, for prevention of food-borne diarrheal
  illness, 334
Food poisoning
  from airline food, 643
  from *Bacillus cereus*, 1542
  Campylobacter, 328
  from *Clostridium botulinum*, 1629
  epidemiology of, 328
  from *Listeria monocytogenes*, 1538
  non-infective, 331–332
  Salmonella, 328
Foot ulcers
  clinical features of, 130, 130*t*
  diagnostic tests for, 130
  infected, 130–132
  microbiology of, 130–131
  therapy for, 131–132, 131*t*
  see also Diabetic foot, ulcers
Forced expiratory volume of air in 1 second (FEV$_1$),
  247
Fordyce spots, 586*t*–587*t*
Forestry worker, and occupational infections, 648*t*–649*t*
Forkhead box P3 (Foxp3), 33
Formalin-ethyl acetate technique, 1775
Fosamprenavir, 1148*t*, 1304
  effect on oral contraceptives, 907*t*
  perinatal HIV transmission prevention, 909*t*
Foscarnet, 1146*t*–1147*t*, 1315–1316
  adverse reactions of, 1315
  for cytomegalovirus, 759*t*
    in HIV prophylaxis, 853
  dosage of, 1315
    in special circumstances, 1315
  drug interactions of, 1315
  in genital herpes, 573–574
  indications of, 1315
    cytomegalovirus retinitis, 1314*t*
  mechanism of action, 1315
  pharmacokinetics and distribution of, 1315
  resistance to, 1315–1316
  route of administration, 1315
  in vitro activity of, 1315
Fosfomycin, 1167, 1278–1279
  adverse reactions to, 1278*t*, 1279
  against carbapenamase-resistant gram-negative bacilli,
    1290*t*
  dosage of, 1279
  indications of, 1279
  mechanism of action, 1279
  mechanisms of resistance, 1279
  pharmacokinetics of, 1279
  resistance to, 1193, 1592*t*
  route of administration, 1279
  spectrum of activity, 1279
  structure of, 1168*f*
Fosfomycin trometamol, for cystitis, 528*t*
Fournier's gangrene, 98
Fractures
  in aging HIV-positive patient, 929, 929*t*
  as principal clinical consequence of osteoporosis,
    929

Francisella, 1611, 1616–1617
  clinical manifestations of, 1617
  diagnostic microbiology of, 1617
  epidemiology of, 1616
  management of, 1617
  nature of, 1616, 1616*t*
  pathogenicity of, 1617
  prevention of, 1617
Francisella tularensis, 1085
  and bioterrorism, 671*t*, 678
  clinical manifestations of, 1617
  diagnostic microbiology of, 1617
  epidemiology of, 1616
  life cycle of, 1085, 1085*f*
  management of, 1617
  nature of, 1616, 1616*t*
  pathogenesis and pathology of, 1087
  pathogenicity of, 1617
  prevention of, 1617
Free coagulase, 1516–1517
Free intraperitoneal air, 356–358, 356*f*
Fresh water, infections from, 191*t*
Friction rub, pericardial, 452
Friedländer's pneumonia, 1575
Frogs, infections from, 191*t*
Frogs' legs, 669
Frontal lobe abscess, 199
Fully suppressed virus, changes in treatment with, 923
Fulminant hepatitis, 363
Fumagillin
  for microsporidiosis, 1742
  for parasitic infections, 1345*t*–1362*t*, 1366
Functional cure, for HIV infection, 931
Functional dyspepsia, 324
Fungal infections
  associated with erythema multiforme, 120*t*
  associated with erythema nodosum, 121*t*
  in burn wounds, 699–700
  in cancer patients, 724
  chronic diarrhea and, 345*t*, 349
  in complicated urinary tract infection, 545, 545*t*
  dermatologic manifestations of, 114*t*–115*t*, 118–119
  detection of, 1682*t*
  from dogs, 657*t*
  endophthalmitis and, 160–161
  in hematopoietic stem cell transplantation, 741*t*, 743*t*,
    744–745, 744*f*
  in intestinal transplant patients, 760
  keratitis and, 154–155
  in kidney transplant patients, 768
  microbiome and, 73
  in myocarditis, 448
  opportunistic, 1681, 1682*t*
    in HIV/AIDS, 854–856
  oral, 318
  prophylaxis of, 689
  and skin manifestation of HIV, 883–884
    disseminated, 883–884, 884*t*
  superficial, 122–129
    clinical features of, 123–127
    diagnosis of, 127
    epidemiology of, 122–123
    immunocompromised patients, 126–127
    management of, 127–129
    pathogenesis and pathology of, 123–129
    prevention of, 123
  systemic, 1700–1701, 1700*t*
  in thoracic transplantation patients, 749–750
  and tumor necrosis factor inhibitor, 799–800
  see also specific fungi; specific infections
Fungal pathogens, 1710–1724
  in infectious diseases, transmitted by grafts, 806–807
  subcutaneous, 1712–1724
    clinical manifestations of, 1719–1722
    diagnostic microbiology of, 1716–1719
    epidemiology of, 1713–1715
    management of, 1722–1724
    nature of, 1712–1713
    pathogenicity of, 1715
    prevention of, 1715–1716
  superficial, 1710–1712
    clinical manifestations of, 1712
    diagnostic microbiology of, 1711–1712

Fungal pathogens (*Continued*)
    epidemiology of, 1710
    management of, 1712
    nature of, 1710
    pathogenicity of, 1710–1711
    prevention of, 1711
Fungal pneumonias, 292–299
Fungal sinusitis, 1689, 1690*t*
Fungemia, prophylaxis of, 689
Fungi
  brain abscess, 199
  causes of uveitis, 169–170, 170*f*
  in chronic meningitis, 186*t*
  comparison of bacteria and, 5*t*
  in congenital infection, 505*b*
  in endocarditis, 457, 458*t*
  hospital-acquired pneumonia and, 259*t*
  in infective arthritis, 383*t*
  lung abscess and, 263
  in lymph node enlargement, 147*t*–148*t*
  in pericarditis, 452
  provoking immune reconstitution disorder, 860*t*
  in sepsis, 419
  see also specific fungi
Funisitis, 563
Furazolidone
  for gastrointestinal protozoa, 1000*t*
  for parasitic infections, 1345*t*–1362*t*, 1366
Furuncles, 86–87, 86*f*
Furunculosis
  prevention of, 86
  recurrent, 87, 87*f*
fusA gene, 1193
Fusariosis, 1699–1700
Fusarium, 1681*t*, 1699
  endophthalmitis and, 159
  in hematopoietic stem cell transplantation, 744
  paronychia and, 89
Fusarium oxysporum, 1699
Fusarium solani, 1699
fusB gene, 1193
fusC gene, 1193
Fusidic acid, 1169, 1277–1278
  adverse reactions and interactions of, 1277–1278,
    1278*t*
  chemical structure of, 1169
  dosage of, 1277
  indications of, 1277
  mechanism of action, 1277
  mechanisms of resistance, 1277
  mode of action of, 1169
  pharmacodynamics of, 1169
  pharmacokinetics of, 1277
  resistance to, 1169, 1193
  route of administration, 1277
  spectrum of activity, 1277
  for *Staphylococcus aureus*, 1521
Fusin. *see* CXCR4.
Fusion inhibitors, 925
Fusobacterium, 1631, 1632*f*
  antimicrobial drugs of choice for, 1642*t*
  brain abscess and, 199
  empyema and, 266*t*
  hospital-acquired pneumonia and, 259*t*
  in human bites, 682, 683*t*
  microflora, 355
  in normal flora, 1632, 1632*t*
  penicillin resistance, 1210
  in sinusitis, 1637
  susceptibility to antimicrobial agents, 1642*f*
  treatment, 1210
Fusobacterium mortiferum, 1631
Fusobacterium necrophorum, 314, 1631
Fusobacterium nucleatum, 1631
  halitosis, 319
  lipopolysaccharide of, 1633
  lung abscess and, 264–265
Fusobacterium varium, 1631

G

gag genes, 1483, 1484*f*
Gallicola, lung abscess and, 264–265

Gallium scan, in fever of unknown origin, 620
Gamma chain deficiency, 714
Gammaproteobacteria, 1565
Ganciclovir, 1146t–1147t, 1313–1315
    adverse reactions of, 1314–1315
    for cytomegalovirus, 748, 759t, 1314
        in HIV prophylaxis, 853
    for cytomegalovirus retinitis, 1314t
    dosage of, 1313–1314
        in special circumstances, 1314, 1314t
    for Epstein-Barr virus, 759t
    for herpesvirus, 1433
    indications of, 1314
    for kidney transplant patients, 766
    in liver transplant patients, 754t
    mechanism of action, 1313
    in myocarditis, 448
    pharmacokinetics and distribution of, 1313
    prophylaxis with
        cytomegalovirus, 1314
        in intestinal transplant patients, 758–759, 758t–759t
    resistance to, 1315
    route of administration, 1313–1314
    in vitro activity, 1313
'Gangosa', 963, 964f
Gangrenous stomatitis, 316, 316f–317f
Gardasil®, 579, 1441
Gardening, and tetanus, 645
Gardnerella vaginalis
    in bacterial vaginosis, 483–484
    clindamycin, 1225
Garin-Bujadoux-Bannwarth (MPN-GBB), 409
Gas gangrene, 95–103
    clinical clues and differential diagnosis of, 95–96
    clostridial, 99–102
        epidemiology of, 99
        morbidity and mortality, 100
        recurrent, 99
        spontaneous/nontraumatic, 101–102
            clinical features of, 101, 102f
            diagnosis of, 101
            management of, 101
            pathogenesis of, 101
            prognosis of, 102, 102f
        traumatic, 99–101
            clinical findings of, 100, 100f
            diagnosis of, 100
            management of, 100–101
            pathogenesis, 99–100
            prevention of, 100
            prognosis of, 101
Gas-liquid chromatography, for anaerobic bacteria, 1635
Gastric adenocarcinoma, 321–322
    and Helicobacter pylori, 21
    pathogenesis and pathology of, 324
Gastric carcinoma, from Helicobacter pylori, 1604
Gastric lavage
    botulism, 212
    for laboratory diagnosis, of mycobacteria, 1651, 1651t
Gastric lymphoma
    from Helicobacter pylori, 1604
    pathogenesis of, 324
Gastric ulceration, 321, 321f
    causes of, 322, 322t
    from Helicobacter pylori, 323, 1604
    pathogenesis of, 324
Gastritis, 321–327
    atrophic, 323
    classification of, 321, 321t
    definition of, 321
Gastroenteritis
    antibiotics for, 1152t
    and bioterrorism, 671t
    from Listeria monocytogenes, 1538, 1540
    miscellaneous viruses, 338
    prevalence of, 335
    rotavirus in, 338
    from Salmonella, 1574
    Yersinia in, 337–338
    yersiniosis and, 1627
Gastroenteritis viruses, acute, 1390–1398
    clinical characteristics of, 1391t
    epidemiological characteristics of, 1391t
    management of, 1397
    prevention of, 1397–1398

Gastroenteritis viruses, acute (Continued)
    structure and morphological characteristics of, 1391f, 1391t
Gastroesophageal reflux disease (GERD), 324
Gastrointestinal adverse reactions, of folate inhibitors, 1283
Gastrointestinal anthrax, 1125–1126
Gastrointestinal bleeding, typhoid fever and, 1004
Gastrointestinal cytomegalovirus disease, 852
Gastrointestinal disease, probiotics for, 1373–1375, 1375f
Gastrointestinal effects, β-lactam antibiotics, 1215t, 1216
Gastrointestinal endoscopy, 1160
Gastrointestinal infections
    adenovirus in, 1473
    in cancer patients, 727–728, 731f
    in pregnancy, 500, 503–504
    quinolones for, 1245–1246
    see also specific infections
Gastrointestinal microbiota, 355
Gastrointestinal mucormycosis, 1697
Gastrointestinal parasites, 989–1001, 989t
    anatomic location of, 991t
    clinical features of, 995–997
    diagnosis of, 997, 998t–999t
    domestic environment and, 990
    epidemiology of, 989–990
    geographic distribution of, 990
        biologic environment, 990
        human behavior, 990
        physical environment, 990
    helminths, 989t, 991–994, 996–997, 1000–1001, 1001t
    host susceptibility and, 990
    human factors in, 990
    management of, 997–1001
    pathogenesis and pathology of, 990–994
    prevention of, 994–995
    protozoa, 989t, 990–991, 995, 997–1000, 1000t
    see also specific parasites
Gastrointestinal problems, in immunologically mediated diseases, 773, 773f
Gastrointestinal reactions, of quinolones, 1247
Gastrointestinal source, brain abscess and, 199
Gastrointestinal surgery, antibiotic prophylaxis and, 1156–1158, 1157t–1158t
Gastrointestinal tract
    basidiobolomycosis in, 1719
    brucellosis complications in, 1099
    colonization of, Pseudomonas aeruginosa in, 1586
    and HIV-associated TB, 868
    mucositis following hematopoietic stem cell transplantation, 740
    normal flora, 12, 1631–1632, 1632t
    parasitic infections of. see Gastrointestinal parasites
    role of, in HIV-1 infection, 840–841, 841f
Gastrointestinal tuberculosis, 341–343
Gatifloxacin
    dissociation constants of, 535t
    for enteric fevers, 1006
    for prostatitis, 536t
Gel diffusion, for helminths diagnosis, 1777
Gemella haemolysans, 156
Gemella morbiliform, in human bites, 683t
Gemella morbillorum, 1631
Gene cassettes, 1195–1196, 1196f
    resistance and mechanism of resistance for, 1196t
Gene expression
    bacteria, 10
    viral, 8
Gene sequencing, for mycobacteria, 1654
Gene therapy, for HIV infection, 932t, 934, 934f
Genes
    'accessory', 12
    'virulence', 12
Genetic diversity, 66
Genetic factors, in Lyme disease, 407
Genetic mutations, in nontuberculous mycobacteria (NTM) lung disease, 286
GeneXpert MTB/RIF assay, for Mycobacterium tuberculosis, 1654
Genital dysplasia, in HIV infection, 906
Genital herpes, 567–574
    clinical features of, 570–572
        first-episode, 571
        nonprimary first-episode, 571
        primary, 571, 571f

Genital herpes (Continued)
        recurrent, 571, 571f
    diagnosis of, 572–573
    differential diagnosis of, 572
    epidemiology of, 567, 568f
    lymphadenopathy and, 137t–138t, 141
    management of, 573–574, 573t
    pathogenesis of, 567–568, 569f–570f
    in pregnancy, 572
    prevention of, 568–570, 568t
Genital infection, herpes simplex virus and, 1436
Genital lesions, cutaneous, 585, 586t–587t
    see also specific lesions
Genital tract
    female
        normal flora of, 1632, 1632t
        specimen collection in, 1634t
    infection of, in pregnancy, 498–500
Genital ulcer syndrome (GUS)
    nonhealing, 1138t
    sexually transmitted infections, 1138
Genital warts, 586t–587t
    clinical features of, 580
    management of, 583
    papillomaviruses in, 1443, 1444f
    prevention of, 579–580
Genitourinary surgery, prophylactic antimicrobial therapy in, 541, 542t
Genitourinary system, Mycoplasma pneumoniae in, 1662t
Genitourinary tract
    adverse reactions to β-lactam antibiotics, 1215t
    brucellosis complications in, 1099
Genitourinary tract infections
    adenovirus in, 1473
    quinolones for, 1243
Genome analysis, 62
Genomic DNA, for Pseudomonas aeruginosa, 1583t–1584t
Genomics, advances in, 1388–1389
GenoType kits, 1654
Genotypes, hepatitis B virus, 364, 365f
Genotypic analyses, for herpesvirus, 1435
Genotypic tests, of HIV-1 drug resistance, 1489
Genotypic typing method, for Acinetobacter baumannii, 1583t–1584t
Genotyping, 1388
Gentamicin
    for bartonellosis, 1675
    for brucellosis, 1100
    against carbapenamase-resistant gram-negative bacilli, 1290t
    for catheter-related bloodstream infection (CRBSI), 436t
    clinical use of, 1234
    for complicated urinary tract infection, 545t
    for conjunctivitis, 152
    for drowning-associated infections, 681
    for endophthalmitis, 162
    for hospital-acquired pneumonia, 260t
    for keratitis, 152
    for Listeria monocytogenes, 1540
    pharmacokinetic parameters for, 1234t
    for plague, 1083, 1083t
    in pregnancy, 504
    prophylaxis, 1158t
    resistance, 1185–1186
    for tularemia, 1089
Geographic exposure, eosinophilia by, 986, 986t
Geography of infectious disease, 938–947
    factors influencing burden of disease, 940–943
    factors influencing emergence of disease, 943–945
    factors influencing geographic distribution of, 939–940
    geographic influences on differential diagnosis, 945
GeoSentinel Surveillance Network, 984
Germ theory, 625
Gianotti-Crosti syndrome, 75t, 81t, 82f
Giant cell arteritis, 613
Giardia
    diarrhea, 332–333
    doses of, in diarrheal illness, 329t
    pathogenesis and pathology of, 991
    prevention of, 1727
Giardia duodenalis
    of chronic diarrhea, 346–347, 347t
    parasite infections and, 73

Giardia intestinalis
  clinical features of, 996
  diagnosis of, 998t–999t
  epidemiology of, 989
  prevention of, 995
  treatment of, 997
Giardia lamblia, 1725t
  from birds, 661
  from dogs, 656
  epidemiology of, 1726–1727
  in food-borne diarrheal illness
    characteristics of, 330t
    mechanism of, 330
  identification in fecal specimens, 1730–1731, 1731f
  pathogenicity of, 1728
  treatment of, 1345t–1351t
Giardiasis
  chronic diarrhea and, 346–347
  from dogs, 656
  epidemiology of, 1726
  intestinal
    clinical features of, 996
    pathogenesis and pathology of, 991
  treatment of, 334, 1000t, 1345t–1351t
Gingivitis
  clinical features of, 313
  epidemiology of, 312
  necrotizing ulcerative, acute, 316, 316f–317f
  pathogenesis and pathology of, 312
Gingivostomatitis, primary herpetic, 317, 317f
Glanders
  and bioterrorism, 671t–672t
  from *Burkholderia mallei*, 1595–1596
  lymphadenopathy and, 137t–138t
  and occupational infections, 648t–649t, 650
  transmission of, 665
Glandular tularemia, 1088
Glaucoma, acute angle-closure, 175t
Glomerulonephritis
  acute, 1532–1533
  hepatitis C virus and, 370
  poststreptococcal, 1532–1533
Glossina, 1762
  African trypanosomiasis, 966
  lymphadenopathy, 142
Gloves, 58
Glucocorticoids
  immunosuppression and, 1377–1378, 1377t
  increased infection risk with, 796
  see also Corticosteroids
Glucose, malaria in pregnancy, 1143t–1144t
Glutamate dehydrogenase (GDH) antigen, 1630
Glycocalyx, 15
Glycopeptide-intermediate *Staph. aureus* (GISA), 1192
Glycopeptides, 1164–1167, 1249–1255
  for anaerobic bacteria, 1643
  in arterial graft infection, 437
  for *Bacillus cereus*, 1542
  for cancer patients, 733
  chemical structure of, 1164
  mode of action of, 1164
  pharmacodynamics of, 1167
  resistance to, 1164–1167, 1191–1192, 1191t
  for *Rhodococcus equi*, 1551
  Staphylococcus aureus and, 1518–1519
  see also specific drugs
Glycophosphatidylinositol anchor, 214, 214f
Glycosylphosphatidylinositol (GPI), 1017
Glycylcyclines
  for anaerobic bacteria, 1643
  origin of, 1256
  resistance to, 1592t
Gnathostoma spinigerum
  life cycle of, 971–972, 974f
  pathogenicity of, 1770
  treatment of, 1345t–1351t
Gnathostoma spp, 1765
Gnathostome, 1778
Gnathostomiasis, 971–972, 974f
  clinical features of, 974
  dermatologic manifestations of, 114t–115t
  prevention of, 973
  treatment of, 975–976, 1345t–1351t

Goats
  Brucella melitensis, 663
  infections from, 191t
Golimumab, 797, 798t–799t
Gonococcal arthritis, 384
Gonococcal infection
  dermatologic manifestations of, 114t–115t
  diagnostic microbiology of, 1560–1561, 1560f
  disseminated, 1563
  eye involvement in, 982
  localized, outside the urogenital tract, 1563
  prevention of, 1560
  urogenital, 1562–1563
Gonococcal Isolate Surveillance Project (GISP), 595
Gonococcal ophthalmia neonatorum, 594
Gonococci, in cystitis, 525
Gonorrhea, 592–596, 1553
  in children, 1563
  clinical features of, 594
  clinical manifestations of, 1562–1563
  diagnosis of, 594
  epidemiology of, 592, 593f, 1556
  management of, 595, 595t–596t, 1564, 1564t
  pathogenesis and pathology of, 592
  pathogenesis of, 1557
  prevention of, 592–594
  quinolones for, 1243
  tests for, number of, 593f
Good's syndrome, 809
Gordonia, 1550t, 1552
Gowns, 58
gP120 Envelope protein boost, 833
gP120 Envelope protein vaccine, 832
Graded exercise therapy (GET), 635
Graft-*versus*-host disease (GVHD), 713
  and hematopoietic stem cell transplantation, 739–741
Gram-negative bacilli, 1579–1599, 1628t, 1631
  antibiotic therapy for, 1579–1580
  catheter-related bloodstream infection (CRBSI), 427, 435
  drug-resistant, 1210
  endophthalmitis and, 160
  epidemiology of, 1579
  hospital-acquired pneumonia and, 259t
  infection sites of, 1629t
  lung abscess and, 263–264
  macrolides, 1219
  nomenclature of, 1581t–1582t
  nonfermenting, 1597–1599
  nosocomial infections due to, 1588t
  pathogenic role of, 1579, 1579t
  in pericarditis, 450
  in recurrent cellulitis, 134
  urinary tract infection with, 527t
Gram-negative bacteria
  in cancer patients, 723–724, 723b
  carbapenemase-resistant, 1290t
  cephalosporins and, 1203
  in endocarditis, 457, 459, 468
  enteric
    hospital-acquired pneumonia, 258
    peritonitis and, 381
  fosfomycin for, 1279
  in hematopoietic stem cell transplantation, 740
  β-lactam antibiotics for, 1210
  β-lactam antibiotics resistance, 1181, 1184f
  multidrug-resistant, 1289
  in sepsis, 419
  XDR, algorithm for management of, 1291f
Gram-negative cocci, 1631
  hospital-acquired pneumonia and, 259t
  macrolides, 1219
Gram-negative coccobacilli, 1611–1627
  see also specific pathogens
Gram-negative pathogens, aminoglycosides for, 1234
Gram-positive bacilli, 1629t
  aerobic, 1537–1552, 1537f
  hospital-acquired pneumonia and, 259t
  infection sites of, 1629t
  β-lactam antibiotics for, 1210
  nonspore-forming, 1628t, 1630
  spore-forming, 1628t, 1629–1630
  telithromycin, 1219

Gram-positive bacteria
  in cancer patients, 723b
  of endocarditis, 459
  fosfomycin for, 1279
  in hematopoietic stem cell transplantation, 740
  linezolid, 1230
  macrolides, 1219
  multidrug-resistant, 1289–1292
    Enterococci, 1290–1292
    Staphylococcus aureus, 1289–1290
  in sepsis, 419
Gram-positive cocci, 1628t, 1631
  aerobic
    in foot ulcers, 130–131
    in recurrent cellulitis, 133
  cephalosporins and, 1203
  in foot ulcers, 130–131
  hospital-acquired pneumonia and, 259t
  infection sites of, 1629t
  lincosamides, 1224
  lymphadenopathy, 144
  and surgical site infections, 687
Gram-positive pathogens, aminoglycosides for, 1235
Gram staining, in gonorrhea, 594
Granule Cell neuronopathy, JC polyomavirus and, 1447
Granulocyte colony-stimulating factor (G-CSF), 706
  for cancer patients, 738
  for melioidosis, 1076–1077
Granulocyte-monocyte colony-stimulating factor
    (GM-CSF), for cancer patients, 738
Granulocyte transfusions, for cancer patients, 738
Granuloma formation, nontuberculous mycobacteria
    (NTM) and, 286
Granuloma inguinale, 586t–587t, 590–591, 1576
  clinical features of, 591, 591f
  diagnosis of, 591
  epidemiology of, 590
  lymphadenopathy, 141
  management of, 591
  pathogenesis and pathology of, 590–591
Granulomas
  mycobacteria and, 1650
  pyogenic, 586t–587t
  in schistosomiasis, 1028, 1028f
  in tuberculosis, 273, 274f
Granulomatous amebic encephalitis
  diagnostic microbiology of, 1747
  management of, 1749–1750
  pathogenicity of, 1746
  pathologic features of, 1748, 1748f–1749f
  prevention of, 1747
Granulomatous disease
  chronic, aspergillosis and, 1687–1688
  histoplasmosis and, 1708
  paracoccidioidomycosis and, 1708
Graves' disease, 864
Gray matter, diminished volumes of, in chronic fatigue
    syndrome, 634, 634f
Grazoprevir, for hepatitis C, 1331
Grimontia (Vibrio) hollisae, 337
Griseofulvin, 1343
  adverse effects of, 1343
  dosage of, 1343
    in special circumstances, 1343
  drug interactions of, 1343
  indications of, 1343
  mechanism of action, 1343
  onychomycosis management, 128
  pharmacokinetics and distribution of, 1343
  route of administration, 1343
  tinea capitis, 127
Groove sign, 141f
Group A β-hemolytic streptococcal endometritis, 494–495
Group A β-hemolytic streptococci, in osteomyelitis, 395t
Group A streptococci
  autoimmune sequelae of, 1532–1533
  cellulitis and, 91f
  clinical manifestations of, 1532–1533
  epidemiology of, 1525–1526
  hyaluronic acid capsule and, 1528
  impetigo and, 88
  invasive infections from, 1532
  lincosamides, 1224–1225

Group A streptococci (Continued)
  management of, 1534
  molecular characterization and population structure of,
      1524–1525
  in myocarditis, 447
  necrotizing fasciitis and, 96, 98f
  pathogenesis of, 1528–1529, 1530f
  pharyngitis, 233
  prevention of, 1535
  proteases and, 1528–1529
  in rheumatic fever, 471
  scarlet fever, 116
  superficial infections from, 1532
  surface antigens and, 1528
  tonsillitis, 234f
  uncomplicated infections from, 1532
Group B streptococcal disease
  epidemiology of, 520
  management of, 521–522, 521t, 522f
  microbiology of, 520
  pregnant patient with previous pregnancy complicated
      by, 520–522
  prevention of, 520–521, 521f
  screening of, 520
Group B streptococci, 520
  adult disease from, 1533
  in breast-feeding, 516
  cellulitis and, 91f
  clinical manifestations of, 1533
  in complicated urinary tract infection, 540t
  epidemiology of, 1526, 1527f, 1529–1530
  lincosamides, 1224–1225
  management of, 1534
  meningitis and, 180
  microbiology of, 520
  molecular characterization and population structure of,
      1525
  neonatal disease from, 1533
  perinatal infections and, 498, 515
  in pregnancy, 500, 502–503, 502t
  prevention of, 1535
  treatment, 180
Group C streptococci
  autoimmune sequelae of, 1532–1533
  cellulitis and, 91f
  clinical manifestations of, 1532–1533
  epidemiology of, 1525–1526
  invasive infections from, 1532
  management of, 1534
  pathogenesis of, 1529
  uncomplicated infections from, 1532
Group D streptococci, in endocarditis, 457
Group G streptococci
  autoimmune sequelae of, 1532–1533
  cellulitis and, 91f
  clinical manifestations of, 1532–1533
  epidemiology of, 1525–1526
  invasive infections from, 1532
  management of, 1534
  pathogenesis of, 1529
  uncomplicated infections from, 1532
Growth hormone pathway, 633
Guanarito virus, 1110, 1112t, 1500t
Guillain-Barré syndrome, 212
  and Campylobacter jejuni, 1601
  differential diagnosis of, 212
Guinea worm, 1778
Gummas, 560, 562, 562f
  tuberculous, 118
Gut, in HIV-1 infection, 840–841, 840f
Gynecologic infections, postoperative,
    496–497
Gynecologic manifestations, of HIV, 906
Gynecologic surgery, antibiotic prophylaxis and,
    1157t–1158t, 1159
Gyrase, 1174, 1176f, 1186

H
H1N1 virus, influenza, 1466
  pdm09, 1467–1468, 1471
H2 antagonists, 328
H2N2 viruses, 1466
HAART. see Highly active antiretroviral therapy
    (HAART).

HACEK group, 1622
  clinical manifestations of, 1622
  diagnostic microbiology of, 1622
  in endocarditis, 457, 458t, 468
  management of, 1622
  nature of, 1622
  prevention of, 1622
HACEK organisms, and fever of unknown origin, 611
Haemophilus, 1611, 1617–1621
  clinical manifestations of, 1620–1621, 1620t
  diagnostic microbiology of, 1619–1620, 1620f
  epidemiology of, 1618
  in human bites, 682, 683t
  keratitis and, 152
  management of, 1621
  nature of, 1617–1618, 1618t
  pathogenicity of, 1618
  prevention of, 1618–1619, 1619f
Haemophilus aegyptius, 1618t
Haemophilus aphrophilus, 1617
Haemophilus ducreyi, 1618t, 1621
  in chancroid, 589
  diagnosis of, 590
  diagnostic microbiology of, 1621
  epidemiology of, 1621
  etiology of, 1138t
  infections, trimethoprim-sulfamethoxazole for, 1281
  lymphadenopathy, 140–141
  macrolides, 1221
  management of, 1621
  nature of, 1617
  pathogenicity of, 1621
  prevention of, 1621
Haemophilus haemolyticus, 1618t
Haemophilus influenzae, 1618t
  in bacterial arthritis, 383
  bronchiectasis and, 246
  bronchitis and, 243
  cellulitis and, 90
  in chronic obstructive pulmonary disease, 310
  conjunctivitis, 150
  diagnostic microbiology of, 1619–1620
  empyema and, 266t
  endophthalmitis and, 159
  epidemiology of, 1618
  genome, 62
  group b, in thoracic transplantation patients, 749
  in HIV in low- and middle-income countries, 891
  hospital-acquired pneumonia and, 259t
  invasive infections of, 1620
  β-lactam resistance in, 1184
  lower respiratory tract infections, 264f, 1221
  lung abscess and, 263–264
  meningitis and, 177
  nature of, 1617
  noninvasive infections of, 1621
  nontypeable, 1618, 1619t
  in osteomyelitis, 395t
  otitis media and, 236
  pathogenicity of, 1618
  pneumonia in HIV/AIDS, 857
  in postsplenectomy sepsis, 778t
  in prostatitis, 533t
  in sinusitis, 1637
  subdural empyema/intracranial epidural abscess,
      203–204
  in thoracic transplantation patients, 747t
Haemophilus influenzae type b, 177
  conjugate vaccine, 777
  epiglottitis and, 231–232
  incidence of, 1619f
  nature of, 1617
  pharyngitis, 232
  spectrum of infections caused by, 1620t
Haemophilus influenzae type b vaccination, 782t–783t,
    1618–1619
Haemophilus parahaemolyticus, 1618t
Haemophilus parainfluenzae, 1618t
  clinical manifestations of, 1620
  epidemiology of, 1618
  nature of, 1617
Haemophilus paraphrohaemolyticus, 1618t
Haemophilus paraphrophilus, 1617
Haemophilus pittmaniae, 1617, 1618t
Haemophilus sputorum, 1618t

Hafnia, microflora, 355–356
Hafnia alvei, 1577t
Halitosis, 319
Halofantrine, 1366–1367
Hand, foot and mouth disease, 80–81
  clinical features of, 80, 80f–81f
  management of, 81
  oral mucosa and, 317–318
Hand hygiene, 58
  in intensive care unit, 694
Hansen's disease. see Leprosy.
Hantaan virus, 667, 1110, 1502t
Hantavirus pulmonary syndrome (HPS), 667, 1110, 1502
  characteristics, 1502t
Hantaviruses, 1110, 1501–1505
  and bioterrorism, 671t
  characteristics, 1504t
  clinical features of, 1114t–1115t
  clinical manifestations, 1504–1505
  diagnostic microbiology, 1504
  epidemiology of, 1112t, 1502–1503
  management, 1505–1507
  nature, 1501–1502
  in North and South America, 1503t
  pathogenicity, 1503
  prevention, 1503–1504
Harada-Mori technique, for helminths diagnosis, 1775
Hard ticks, 104, 106t
Hares, infections from, 667
Haverhill fever, 661
Head and neck infections
  anaerobic bacteria in, 1632f, 1636–1638
  lymphadenopathy, 145
Head and neck surgery
  antibiotic prophylaxis and, 1157t–1158t, 1158
  infections after, anaerobic bacteria in, 1637
Health, occupational and employee, 57
Health beliefs models, and HIV transmission, 826
Health care, impact of HIV and AIDS on, in low- and
    middle-income countries, 895
Health-care associated pneumonia (HCAP), 258–262
Health consequences of changing climate, 40–48
Healthcare-associated infections (HAIs), 54, 60
  device-related, 60
  host factors contributing to, 684t
  procedure-related, 60
Healthcare-associated MRSA (HC-MRSA), 467
Healthcare-associated pneumonia (HCAP)
  community-acquired pneumonia and, 254
  criteria for, 254t
Healthcare worker, and occupational infections, 648t–649t
'Healthy microbiome', 71–72, 72f, 72t
Heart
  congenital infection in, 510
  in cystic echinococcosis, 1042
  disease, endocarditis, 456, 459
Heart-lung transplantation, 746–750
  cardiovascular infections in, 748
  and CMV prevention and treatment, 748
  considerations related to micro-organisms in, 748–750
    bacterial infections, 749
    fungal infections, 749–750
    viral infections, 748–749
  epidemiology of, 746
  for pneumonia, 746–747
  for postsurgical mediastinitis, 747
  risk factors for infection, 746, 747b
  specific clinical syndromes, 746–748
  for sternum osteomyelitis, 747
Heart transplantation, 746–750
  cardiovascular infections in, 748
  and CMV prevention and treatment, 748
  common indication for, 746
  considerations related to micro-organisms in, 748–750
    bacterial infections, 749
    fungal infections, 749–750
    viral infections, 748–749
  epidemiology of, 746
  pneumonia, 746–747
  for postsurgical mediastinitis, 747
  risk factors for infection, 746, 747b
  specific clinical syndromes, 746–748
  for sternum osteomyelitis, 747
Heat-labile toxin (LT), 329–330
Heat-stable toxin, 331

Heat stroke, 605–606
Helicobacter, 1600, 1601*t*
Helicobacter bizzozeronii, 660
Helicobacter felis, 321–322, 660
Helicobacter pylori, 321–322, 1602–1604
 acute, 325
 associations, 323
 in cats, 660
 chronic, 325
 clindamycin, 1225
 clinical features of, 325, 1603–1604
 diagnosis, 325
 diagnostic microbiology of, 1603
 endoscopic tests for, 325
 epidemiology of, 1602–1603
 and gastric adenocarcinoma, 21
 histology of, 325, 325*f*
 management of, 326–327, 1604
 nature of, 1602
 non-endoscopic tests for, 325
 pathogenesis of, 323–324, 1603
 pathology and disease associations of, 323, 323*f*
 prevalence and incidence of, 322–323, 322*f*
 prevention of, 324, 1603
 probiotics for, 1373, 1374*t*
 resistance, to metronidazole, 1193
 transmission of, 323
 treatment regimens, 326–327, 327*t*
Helminths, 1763–1779
 causes of eosinophilia by geographical exposure and
  symptomatology, 986*t*
 causing encephalitis/myelitis caused by, 193*t*–194*t*
 chronic diarrhea and, 347*t*, 349
 clinical manifestations of, 1777–1779
 diagnosis of, 1772–1777, 1775*f*–1776*f*
 epidemiology of, 1763–1766
 gastrointestinal, 989*t*, 991–994, 996–997, 1000–1001,
  1001*t*
 infections, 984
  dermatologic manifestations of, 114*t*–115*t*
  main available initial diagnostics for, 987*t*
 in lymph node enlargement, 147*t*–148*t*
 lymphadenopathy and, 137*t*–138*t*
 management of, 1779
 nature of, 1763, 1764*t*
 pathogenicity of, 1766–1772
 prevention of, 1772
 provoking immune reconstitution disorder, 860*t*
 relative size of eggs, 1775*f*
 see also Cestodes; Nematodes; Trematodes
Helper T cells
 cellular immune response, 32
 follicular, in HIV-1 infection, 841
 in HIV-1 infection, 842
Hemagglutination inhibition, yellow fever, 1494
Hemagglutinin-neuraminidase (HN), 1478
Hematocrit, 1122
Hematogenous osteomyelitis, 388, 388*f*
Hematologic conditions, eosinophilia and, 984*t*
Hematologic effects, of β-lactam antibiotics, 1215, 1215*t*
Hematologic evaluation, in sepsis, 420
Hematologic malignancies, 723
Hematologic reactions, of folate inhibitors, 1283
Hematologic toxicity
 ganciclovir, 1314
 valganciclovir, 1314
Hematological system, *Mycoplasma pneumoniae* in, 1662*t*
Hematology
 in cancer patients, 733
 see also specific tests
Hematophagous mites, 105–107, 106*t*
Hematopoiesis, cyclic, 706
Hematopoietic growth factors, 738
Hematopoietic stem cell transplantation, 739–745
 allogeneic, 791
 autologous, 791
 background and current practices, 739
 bacterial infections in, 740–741, 741*t*
 conditioning therapy, 740–741
 fungal infections in, 744–745
  Candida species, 744
  filamentous fungi, 744–745, 744*f*
  pneumocystis infections, 745

Hematopoietic stem cell transplantation (*Continued*)
 prevention strategies commonly employed in, 743*t*
 primary risk periods after, 742*f*
 revaccination schedules suggested after, 792*t*–793*t*
 risk for infections, 739–740
  graft and type of transplant, 739–740
  host factors, 740
  transplant complications, 740, 741*t*
 systematic approach to vaccinating patients with,
  790–791
 viral infections in, 741–744
  BK virus, 743
  community-acquired respiratory viruses in, 742–743,
   743*f*
  hepatitis viruses, 743–744
  herpes virus infections in, 741–742
Hematuria
 in schistosomiasis, 1031
 in urinary schistosomiasis, 1029, 1029*f*
Hemodialysis
 aminoglycoside dosage in, 1235
 Staphylococcus aureus in, 1516
Hemodynamic shock, in severe malaria, 1025
Hemoglobin (Hb), forms of, 1053
Hemoglobin-binding proteins, 1557*t*
Hemoglobin electrophoresis, for inherited hemoglobin
 disorders, 1055–1056
Hemoglobinopathies, 1016
α-Hemolysin (hla), 1513*t*–1514*t*
β-Hemolysin (hlb), 1513*t*–1514*t*
δ-Hemolysin (hld), 1513*t*–1514*t*
γ-Hemolysin, 1513*t*–1514*t*
Hemolytic-uremic syndrome (HUS), 1572
Hemophagocytic syndromes, 638–639
 clinical approach to, 639*t*
 diagnostic criteria for, 638
 infection-related, 638–639
  background on, 638, 638*f*
Hemoptysis, massive, in cystic fibrosis, 300
Hemorrhagic cystitis, Bk polyomavirus and, 1447
Hemorrhagic fever with renal syndrome (HFRS), 1110,
 1501–1502
 characteristics, 1502*t*, 1504
Hemorrhagic fevers. *see* Viral hemorrhagic fevers (VHF).
Hendra viral disease, and occupational infections,
 648*t*–649*t*
Hendra virus, 1507–1508
 clinical manifestations, 1507–1508
 diagnostic microbiology, 1508
 encephalitis/myelitis caused by, 193*t*–194*t*
 epidemiology, 1507
 management, 1508
 nature, 1507
 transmission of, 665
Henle, Friedrich, 1
Henle-Koch's postulates, 1
Heparin, in catheter-related bloodstream infection
 (CRBSI), 432
Heparin-related polysaccharides, 13
Hepatic alveolar echinococcosis, 1042
Hepatic disease
 antituberculosis agents in, 1274
 folate inhibitors for, 1282
Hepatic failure, fulminant, 363
 in liver transplant patients, 752
Hepatic impairment
 β-lactam antibiotics dosage in, 1212
 quinolones for, 1246
Hepatic infection, 360–361
Hepatic schistosomiasis, 1029–1030, 1030*f*
Hepatic side effects, of folate inhibitors, 1283
Hepatic system, adverse reactions to β-lactam antibiotics,
 1215*t*
Hepatitis, 363–374
 adverse reactions to β-lactam antibiotics, 1216
 coinfection with, in HIV-infected people, 915
 congenital infection and, 509
 fibrosing cholestatic, 768
 in hematopoietic stem cell transplantation, 743–744
 viral
  dosage regimens in, 1328*t*
  drugs to treat, 1327–1332
  features of, 1417*t*

Hepatitis A vaccination, 782*t*–783*t*
 for travelers, 949
Hepatitis A virus (HAV), 363–364, 364*f*, 701, 703*t*,
 1417–1419
 at-risk groups for, 1418
 burden of disease, 942
 diagnostic virology of, 1418–1419, 1419*b*
 epidemiology of, 1418
 genetic diversity of, 1418
 incidence and prevalence of, 1418
 in infective arthritis, 387*t*
 jaundice, 1135, 1135*t*
 life cycle of, 1417–1418
 in liver transplant patients, 751, 751*t*
 and occupational infections, 650, 651*t*–654*t*
  immunization for, 650*t*–651*t*
 pathogenicity of, 1418
 routes of transmission of, 1418
 virology of, 1417–1418
Hepatitis B e antigen (HBeAg), 365–366, 1327
Hepatitis B immunoglobulin, in liver transplant patients,
 754*t*
Hepatitis B surface antigen (HBsAg), 364, 366*f*
 screening for, before biologic therapy, 802–803
 vaccine of, 366
Hepatitis B vaccination, 782*t*–783*t*
Hepatitis B virus (HBV), 75*t*, 701, 703*t*, 805, 1420–1423
 acute, 1421
 at-risk groups for, 1421
 burden of disease, 940
 chronic, 364–367, 1421–1422, 1422*t*
  epidemiology of, 364, 365*f*
  genotypes of, 364, 365*f*
  hepatocellular carcinoma (HCC) and, development
   of, 366, 366*f*
  passive immunity in, 366
  serologic testing in, 364–366, 366*f*
  treatment of, 366–367
  vaccination for, 366
 dermatologic manifestations, 114*t*–115*t*
 diagnostic virology of, 1422–1423
 epidemiology of, 1421
 genetic diversity of, 1421
 in HIV, 896–897, 915, 926
  treatment of, 896–897, 897*f*
   assessment of, 897*f*
 and HIV-1, 843
 in immune reconstitution inflammatory syndrome, 863
 immunizations for, in travelers, 949
 incidence and prevalence of, 1421
 in infective arthritis, 385, 387*t*
 interferon-alpha for, 366
 jaundice, 1135, 1135*t*
 in kidney transplant patients, 767–768
 life cycle of, 1420–1421
 in liver transplant patients, 751, 751*t*
 prevention of, 755
 and occupational infections, 648*t*–649*t*, 650, 651*t*–654*t*
  immunization for, 650*t*
  vaccination for, 651*t*
 pathogenicity of, 1421–1422
 in perinatal infections, 514*t*, 515
 polymerase inhibitors of, 1327–1329
 and rituximab, 800
 routes of transmission, 1421
 screening for, during pregnancy, 508*t*
 treatment of chronic infection, 1327–1330
  adefovir for, 1329
  combination therapies for, 1329–1330
  emtricitabine, 1329
  entecavir, 1329
  interferons for, 1327
  nucleos(t)ide analogs for, 1327–1329
  telbivudine for, 1329
  tenofovir alafenamide for, 1329
  tenofovir disoproxil fumarate for, 1329
 and tumor necrosis factor inhibitor, 800
 virology of, 1420–1421
Hepatitis C virus (HCV), 701, 703*t*, 805, 1424–1425
 at-risk groups of, 1424–1425
 chronic, 367–371
  clinical manifestation of, 369–370, 369*f*
  diagnostic testing of, 369–370, 369*f*

Hepatitis C virus (HCV) (Continued)
  epidemiology of, 367–369, 368f
    modes of transmission, 368–369
    progression of, 370–371, 370f
    treatment of, 371
  combined drug regimens for, 1153
  diagnostic virology of, 1425, 1425t
  encephalitis/myelitis and, 194t
  epidemiology of, 1424–1425
  genetic diversity of, 1424
  genome of, 1330f
  in HIV, 898–899, 915, 926
    treatment for, 898–899, 899t
  and HIV-1, 843
  in immune reconstitution inflammatory syndrome, 863
  incidence and prevalence of, 1424
  in infective arthritis, 387t
  jaundice, 1135, 1135t
  in kidney transplant patients, 767–768
  life cycle of, 1424
  in liver transplant patients, 751–753, 751t
    prevention of, 755
  and occupational infections, 648t–649t, 650, 651t–654t
  pathogenicity of, 1425
  perinatal infections and, 515
  route of transmission of, 1424–1425
  treatment of chronic infection, 1330–1332
    combination therapy for, 1332
    direct-acting antiviral (DAAs), 1330–1331
    interferons for, 1330
    non-nucleos(t)ide polymerase inhibitors for, 1332
    NS5A inhibitors for, 1332
    nucleos(t)ide analog polymerase inhibitors for, 1331
    ribavirin, 1330
  virology of, 1424
Hepatitis D virus (HDV), 703t, 1423–1424
  chronic, 371–372
  diagnostic virology of, 1423–1424
  epidemiology of, 1423
  genetic diversity of, 1423
  jaundice, 1135t
  life cycle of, 1423
  pathogenicity of, 1423
  virology of, 1423
Hepatitis E virus (HEV), 1419–1420
  acute, 1419–1420
  chronic, 372–374, 1420
    clinical manifestations of, 372–373, 373f
    epidemiology of, 372, 373f
    prevention of, 373–374
  diagnostic virology of, 1419b, 1420, 1420t
  epidemiology of, 1419
  genetic diversity of, 1419
  jaundice, 1135, 1135t
  life cycle of, 1419
  pathogenicity of, 1419–1420
  virology of, 1419
Hepatitis viruses, 1417–1425, 1417t
  infections, in kidney transplant patients, 767–768
  surveillance for, in liver transplant patients, 754
Hepatocellular carcinoma (HCC), 1422
  development of, 366, 366f
  and fever of unknown origin, 614
  hepatitis B virus and, 364
  hepatitis C virus and, 371
Hepatosplenic candidiasis, 442–444, 728, 1684, 1687
Hepatosplenomegaly, in brucellosis, 1098
Hepatotoxicity, in tetracyclines, 1258–1259
'Herbert's pits', 980–981, 980f
Herbivores, infections from
  domesticated, 663–666
  large, 669
  see also specific animals
Herpangina, 317, 317f
Herpes B virus, 1438
Herpes gladiatorum, 645
Herpes simplex, dermatologic manifestations, 114t–115t
Herpes simplex encephalitis (HSE), 195, 773
Herpes simplex keratitis, 153, 176
Herpes simplex virus (HSV), 75t
  aciclovir for, 1310, 1310t
  in cancer patients, 723–724
  causing meningitis, 225
  in cervicitis, 490
  chronic diarrhea and, 345t, 349

Herpes simplex virus (HSV) (Continued)
  clinical manifestations of, 1435–1436, 1436f
  in congenital infection
    in breast-feeding, 516
    clinical features of, 510
    diagnosis of, 512t
    pathogenesis and pathology of, 506
    perinatal infections, 514t, 515
    screening for, during pregnancy, 508t
  cutaneous infections and, 93
  eye involvement in, 982–983, 983f
  febrile transaminitis in, 377–378
  genital infection and, 1436
  in genital lesions, 586t–587t
  in hematopoietic stem cell transplantation, 741, 743t
  in HIV/AIDS, 881, 882f
  hospital-acquired pneumonia and, 259t
  human papillomavirus and, 577
  in immune reconstitution inflammatory syndrome, 862
  infection
    opportunistic, in HIV, 853
    uveitis and, 168
  in liver transplant patients, 751–752, 751t
    prevention of, 754–755
  and natalizumab, 802
  oropharyngeal infection and, 1435–1436
  pathogenesis of, 567, 569f–570f
  pathogenicity of, molecular and cellular basis of, 1431
  pharyngitis, 233–234
  in pregnancy, 500t
  and recreational infections, 645
  in thoracic transplantation patients, 748
  and tumor necrosis factor inhibitor, 800
  vaccination, 1432–1433
Herpes simplex virus 1 (HSV-1)
  encephalitis from, 227, 227f
  encephalitis/myelitis caused by, 192t
  genital
    clinical features of, 572
    prevention of, 570
  gingivostomatitis and, 317
  keratitis and, 153–154
  in kidney transplant patients, 765–766
  in liver transplant patients, 751, 751t
Herpes simplex virus 2 (HSV-2)
  encephalitis/myelitis caused by, 192t
  etiology of, 1138t
  genital, disclosure of, 569
  gingivostomatitis and, 317
  and HIV transmission, 826
  keratitis and, 153–154
  in kidney transplant patients, 765–766
  in liver transplant patients, 751, 751t
Herpes simplex virus (HSV) antibody, 569–571, 573
Herpes zoster, 1436–1437
  antiviral therapy for, 1311b
  clinical features of, 75, 76f
  dermatologic manifestations of, 114t–115t
  in HIV infection, 853
  in immune reconstitution inflammatory syndrome, 862–863
  management of, 76
  and tumor necrosis factor inhibitor, 800
Herpes zoster ophthalmicus, 154, 154f
α–Herpesvirinae, in kidney transplant patients, 765–766
β–Herpesvirinae, in kidney transplant patients, 766, 766f
γ–Herpesvirinae, in kidney transplant patients, 766–767
Herpesvirus, 805, 1426–1438
  active immunization for, 1432–1433
  antiviral chemotherapy for, 1433–1434, 1433t–1434t
  cell transformation of, 1432
  cercopithecine, 661, 666
  for chronic meningitis, 187t
  clinical manifestations of, 1435–1438
  determinants of infection, 1428t, 1429–1430
  diagnostic virology of, 1434–1435, 1434t
  epidemiology of, 1426–1430
  genome of, 1426, 1428t, 1429f
  genotypic analyses for, 1435
  geographic aspects of, 1428
  in hematopoietic stem cell transplantation, 741–742
  infections
    drugs for, 1309–1317
    in kidney transplant patients, 765–767
  latency of, 1431, 1431t

Herpesvirus (Continued)
  management of, 1438
  nature of, 1426
  passive immunization for, 1433
  pathogenicity of, 1430–1432
  periodicity of, 1429
  prevalence of, 1427–1428
  prevention of, 1432–1434
  replication of, 1430–1431, 1430f
  structure of, 1426, 1427f–1428f
  taxonomy of, 1426, 1426t–1427t
  test specimens for, 1434–1435
  transmission pathways of, 1426–1427
  virion polypeptides of, 1430
  virus culture for, 1435
  virus serology for, 1435
  see also specific viruses
Herpetic gingivostomatitis, 317, 317f
Herpetic whitlow, 93
  and occupational infections, 648t–649t
Herxheimer-like reactions, 412
Heterophyes, 1037, 1765
Heterophyes heterophyes
  clinical features of, 997
  diagnosis of, 998t–999t
  life cycle of, 1771f
  pathogenesis and pathology of, 994
  prevention of, 995
  treatment of, 1001, 1001t, 1345t–1351t
Heterosexual individuals
  and HIV transmission, 905
  prevention trials, 827
Hidradenitis suppurativa, 87, 586t–587t
High-altitude cerebral edema (HACE), 951–952
High-altitude pulmonary edema (HAPE), 951–952
High-grade squamous intraepithelial lesion (HSIL), 580–581, 580f
High performance liquid chromatography (HPLC), for inherited hemoglobin disorders, 1055–1056
Highly active antiretroviral therapy (HAART)
  access to, 829
  chronic diarrhea and, 341, 348
  for HIV, in low- and middle-income countries, 895
  and HIV-1 infections, 845
Highly pathogenic avian influenza (HPAI) viruses, 1466–1467
Hiking, and recreational infections, 643–644
Hip arthroplasty, infection in, 399
Histamine fish poisoning (scombroid), 330t
Histiocytosis, malignant, 137t–138t
Histopathology, for cancer patients, 733
Histoplasma, 1681t
  in chronic meningitis, 186t, 188
  uveitis of, 169
Histoplasma capsulatum, 1700
  from bats, 666
  in birds, 661
  causing retinitis and uveitis, 170t–171t, 173
  clinical features of, 292–293
  clinical manifestations of, 1708
  culture of, 1707
  diagnosis of, 293, 293f
  ecology of, 1706
  epidemiology of, 292, 1706
  in HIV/AIDS, 855
  lower respiratory tract infections, 264f
  management of, 294, 1708
  mycology of, 292, 1706, 1706f
  oral fungal infections, 318
  pathogenesis and pathology of, 292
  pathogenicity of, 1707
  in pericarditis, 450
  in prostatitis, 533t
  serology for, 1707
  in skin manifestation of HIV, 884t, 885f
  skin test for, 1707
  and tumor necrosis factor inhibitor, 799–800
Histoplasmin, 1707
Histoplasmosis, 118, 119f, 292–294, 1700t, 1706–1708
  from bats, 666
  from birds, 661, 668
  chronic diarrhea, 345t, 349
  clinical features of, 292–293, 293f
  clinical manifestations of, 1708
  dermatologic manifestations of, 114t–115t

Histoplasmosis (*Continued*)
diagnosis of, 293, 293*f*
diagnostic microbiology of, 1702*t*, 1706*f*, 1707–1708
disseminated, 1708
and skin manifestations of HIV, 885*f*
ecology of, 1706–1707
epidemiology of, 292, 1706–1707
and fever of unknown origin, 613
lymphadenopathy and, 137*t*–138*t*
management of, 294, 1708
mycology of, 292, 1706, 1706*f*
and occupational infections, 648*t*–649*t*
opportunistic infection in HIV, 855
pathogenesis and pathology of, 292
pathogenicity of, 1707
prevention of, 1708
and tumor necrosis factor inhibitor, 799–800
uveitis and, 169–170
Hit and run hypothesis, 626, 627*t*
HIV-1
and bioterrorism, 671*t*
in children, 902*b*
chronic asymptomatic phase of, 837
and cytomegalovirus, 843–844
dissemination of, 840, 840*f*
systemic, 841
DNA polymerase chain reaction, 1488
early pathogenic events after entry into the body, 839–840
encephalitis from, 227
epidemiology of, 905
gastrointestinal pathology of, 840–841, 841*f*
genotypic tests of drug resistance, 1489
gynecologic manifestations of, 906
and hepatitis B virus, 843
and hepatitis C virus, 843
immune evasion of, 842
immunopathogenesis of, 837–845
infection
patient differences in timeline of, 837, 839*f*
primary, 837, 838*f*
life cycle, 1486*f*
long-term nonprogressors, 838, 839*f*
mechanism of immune deficiency in, 842–844
in monkeys, 666
mother-to-child transmission of, 900
natural course of, 838–839
nature, 1483
overt AIDS, 837
pathogenesis of, influence of antiretroviral therapy on, 845
and pelvic inflammatory disease, 906
in perinatal infections, 514*t*
phenotypic tests of drug resistance, 1489–1490, 1490*f*
rapid progressors, 838, 839*f*
role of gut and lymph nodes in infection, 840–841
role of immune response in determining set points for chronic asymptomatic infection of, 841–842
slow progressors, 838, 839*f*
and syphilis, 843
testing for, in women, 908
transmission
and local spread of, 839–841, 840*f*
male-to-female, 905
transmitted virus, features of, 839
and tuberculosis, 843
typical progressors, 837–838, 839*f*
untreated infection of, clinical course of, 837–839, 838*f*
uveitis and, 173, 173*f*
viral reservoirs of, 841
virion structure, 1485*f*
virus, scrub typhus and, 1670–1671
vs. HIV-2, 1484*t*
Western blot, 1487, 1487*f*
HIV-2
genomic organization, 1484*f*
in monkeys, 666
mother-to-child transmission of, 900
nature, 1483
vs. HIV-1, 1484*t*
Western blot, 1487
HIV-infected patients, travelers immunizations for, 950

HIV infection, 75*t*, 703*t*, 805–806, 1483–1491
acute, 79–80
clinical features of, 79, 80*f*
management of, 80
starting antiviral drugs, 918
acute exanthem of, 879
adjunctive corticosteroids for, 306, 307*t*
in aging patient, 927
Alcaligenes xylosoxidans in, 1597
antilatency drug approaches for, 932–933, 932*t*
aspergillosis in, 855–856
autoimmune disease in, 864
bacterial infections in, 857–858
baseline resistance testing in, 918–919
blastomycosis and, 1703
bone marrow transplantation for, 931, 932*f*, 932*t*
brain abscess and, 200*t*
candidiasis in, 854
CCR5, 1485
in children, 900–904
clinical patterns, 902–903
diagnosis in, 901
follow-up of, 901
mother-to-child transmission, 900
prognostic markers, 903
risk of transmission through breast-feeding in, 901
tolerance of antiretroviral drugs after exposure in utero of, 901–902
and transition to adult care, 904
treatment of, 903–904
uninfected, HIV-exposed, health of, 901–902
WHO classification for, 902*b*, 903*t*
chronic diarrhea in, 341, 343*f*, 349
in chronic meningitis, 186*t*
coccidioidomycosis in, 855, 1705
combined drug regimens for, 1153
cryptococcal meningitis and, 1696*t*
cryptococcosis in, 854–855, 1694
in low- and middle-income countries, 893
cryptosporidiosis in, 348, 857, 1742
CXCR4, 1485
cyclosporiasis in, 348
cytomegalovirus infections in, 852–853, 853*f*
DC-SIGN, 1487
dermatologic manifestations of, 114*t*–115*t*
cutaneous malignancies in, 884–885
infectious dermatoses, 881–884
inflammatory dermatoses, 879–881
treatment associated dermatoses in, 885–887
dermatophytes and, 1710
diagnosis of, 1487, 1488*t*
in children, 901
diarrhea and, 332
discovery of, 829
drug resistance, 1489, 1489*t*–1490*t*
drugs for, 1293–1308, 1294*t*, 1295*f*
entry inhibitors (EI), 1305–1306
integrase strand transfer inhibitors (INSTI), 1306–1308
non-nucleoside reverse transcriptase inhibitors (NNRTI), 1300–1303
nucleoside analog reverse transcriptase inhibitors (NRTI), 1293–1300. see also Nucleoside analog reverse transcriptase inhibitors (NRTI)
protease inhibitors (PIs), 1303–1305. see also Protease inhibitors (PIs)
toxicities of, 1298*t*
early treatment of, 931–932, 932*t*, 933*f*
emergence of disease, 943
and endemic treponematoses, 964
enterocolitis in, 858
epidemiology of, 812–823, 813*f*–814*f*
eradication and cure of, 931–935
eye involvement in, 982–983
and fever of unknown origin, 615
fungal infections in, 854–856
gag protein, 1483–1485
gastrointestinal parasites in, 996–997
gene therapy approaches for, 932*t*, 934, 934*f*
genital ulcer disease and, 585
genome organization and life cycle, 1483–1486
geographic distribution of, 815–819
Asia and the Pacific, 817–819, 818*f*

HIV infection (*Continued*)
Europe and Central Asia, 816–817, 817*f*
Latin America and the Caribbean, 819
Middle East and North Africa, 819, 819*f*
North America, Australia, and New Zealand, 815–816, 816*f*
sub-Saharan Africa, 817
global response to, 819–823
antiretroviral therapy for prevention among HIV-positives, 820
HIV testing and counseling, 821–823, 822*f*
pre-exposure prophylaxis for HIV-negatives, 820–821
prevention of mother-to-child transmission in, 821, 821*f*
treatment scale-up in, 819–820, 819*f*–820*f*
voluntary medical male circumcision, 821, 822*f*
gynecologic manifestations of, 906
hepatitis B virus (HBV) in, 896–897
treatment of, 896–897, 897*f*
assessment of, 897*f*
hepatitis C virus (HCV) in, 898–899
treatment for, 898–899, 899*t*
herpes simplex virus infections in, 853
histoplasmosis and, 855, 1708
human papillomavirus and, 576
immune manipulation for, 932*t*, 933–934, 933*f*
immune-mediated inflammatory disease in, 864
immune reconstitution disorders in, 859–864
infectious mononucleosis and, 377
in infective arthritis, 387*t*
isolation and resistance testing, 1487–1490
isosporiasis in, 348
jaundice, 1135*t*
Kaposi's sarcoma in, 874–875, 885, 885*f*
clinical features of, 874
diagnosis of, 874
management of, 874–875, 875*t*
oral cavity in, 874
pathogenesis of, 874
latency and prospects for cure, 1490–1491
life cycle of, 919*f*
in low and middle-income countries, 888–895
clinical features of, 888–893
epidemiology of, 888, 889*f*
impact on healthcare systems in, 895
prevention of opportunistic infections in, 894–895
testing in, 893–894
treatment in, 895
lymphadenopathy and, 137*t*–138*t*, 143
causes of, 143*t*
malignant lymphoma in, 875–877
management of, 912–917
baseline evaluation, 912–913, 913*t*
counseling, 913
history and physical examination, 912
metabolic testing, 913
prognostic laboratory markers, 912–913
prophylaxis, 914, 914*t*
resistance testing and evaluation of HLA-B*5701 allele status, 913
tuberculin skin test, 913
vaccinations, 913–914
microsporidiosis in, 348
modes of transmission, 813–815
contaminated blood, 814
injection drug use, 815, 815*f*
perinatal and postnatal, 814, 815*f*
sexual, 813–814
Mycobacterium avium complex in, 1649, 1649*f*
Mycoplasma genitalium in, 1663
in myocarditis, 448
nature, 1483
neoplastic disease in, 874–878
in newborns, to HIV-infected mothers, 900–902
choice of postnatal prophylaxis in, 900–901
immunizations in, 901
nutrition in, 901
perinatal care in, 900
nocardiosis in, 1551
non-AIDS-defining, 877–878
nonoccupational exposure, 835–836
nontuberculous mycobacterial infections in, 856
occupational exposure, 835

HIV infection (Continued)
and occupational infections, 651t–654t
opportunistic infections. see also specific infections
bacterial, 857–858
duration of prophylaxis for, 851
fungal, 854–856
level of immunosuppression in, 850
in low and middle-income countries, 888–889
management of, 850–858
nontuberculous mycobacterial, 856
parasitic, 856–857, 857f
prevention of, 850–858
in low- and middle-income countries, 894–895
prophylaxis of, 850–851
use of antiretroviral therapy during management of, 850–851
viral, 852–854
oropharyngeal candidiasis in, 1682–1683
parasitic infections in, 856–857, 857f
penicilliosis, 855
in pericarditis, 450
photodermatitis in, 881, 882f
Pneumocystis jirovecii pneumonia in, 851–852, 851f–852f
pol protein, 1483–1485
postexposure prophylaxis, 835–836
efficacy of, 835
guidelines for, 835–836, 836b
in pregnancy, 908–910
clinical syndrome, 499–500
epidemiology of, 498
implications of, 500t
prevention of
intravenous drug users, 828
in low- and middle-income countries, 894
outcome of large-scale and high-impact studies in the US, 827–828
psychosocial models of risk behavior, 826
screening as modality of, 826
trials delivered to heterosexual individuals in STI and Primary care clinics, 827
trials for men who have sex with men, 827
trials for women, 827–828
primary, 846–849
clinical features of, 846–848, 847f, 847t
diagnosis of, 848, 848f–849f
differential diagnosis of, 848, 848t
epidemiology, 846
features predicting the subsequent course toward AIDS, 848–849
management of, 848–849
pathogenesis and pathology, 846
treatment of, and long-term outcome, 849
progression of, 832
progressive multifocal leukoencephalopathy, 853–854, 854f
prophylaxis, 914, 914t
recommended initial antiretroviral regimens for, 1297t
resistance testing, 913
in women, 909
retinopathy, 173
Rhodococcus equi in, 1552
with salivary gland swelling, 319–320
screening
in low- and middle-income countries, 893
during pregnancy, 507
as prevention modality, 826
skin manifestations of, 879–887
splenic infection, 361–362
spread of, 943
strongyloidiasis in, 349
surveillance of, 812–813
syphilis and, 563
treatment of, 566
testing and counseling for, 821–823, 822f
toxoplasmosis in, 856–857, 857f, 1755
in low- and middle-income countries, 892
transmission of, 1487
antiretrovirals for, 825–826
approaches to preventing, 825f
behavioral approaches to, 826
bio-behavioral interventions to prevent, 824–828
biologic issues related to, 824–825
dynamics of, 824, 824t
epidemiologic issues related to, 825

HIV infection (Continued)
female-to-male, 905
heterosexual, 905
male-to-female, 905
maternal-infant, 908t
modifiers of efficiency of, 824t
perinatal, 908
prevention of, 906–910
risk of, 835, 836t
treating sexually transmitted infections, 826
treatment for, in low- and middle-income countries, 895
tuberculosis in. see Tuberculosis, in HIV
varicella-zoster virus infections in, 853
vif gene, 1486
viral infections in, 852–854
viral life cycle in, 1293, 1293f
virus, structure of, 830f
visceral leishmaniasis in, 1061, 1757
vpr gene, 1486
in women. see Women, HIV in
HIV-positive patients, with tuberculosis, 1274
HIV vaccines, 829–834
candidates for, possible outcome scenarios for, 830f
challenge to development of, 829
clinical trials to date, 832–833
correlates of immunity in, 833
definition of successful, 829, 829b
difficulties in, 829b
future, 833–834
natural history of HIV progression, 832
need for, 829
'novel' approaches, 833
starting point, 829–830
strategies for development of, 830–832
induction of neutralizing antibodies in, 830–831, 831b, 831f
induction of T-cell responses in, 831–832
mucosal vaccines in, 832
Prime-boost strategy, 832
HLA. see Human leukocyte antigen (HLA).
HLA-DR4, 414
HMGB1, in sepsis, 423
Hodgkin's lymphoma, 876–877
clinical features of, 877
diagnosis of, 877
management of, 877
pathogenesis of, 876
Homosexuality
amebiasis and, 1727
Entamoeba histolytica and, 1726
'Hong Kong' influenza pandemic, 1466
Hookworms
clinical features of, 996
clinical manifestations of, 1777
diagnosis of, 1776f
epidemiology of, 989–990
larvae of, 1776f
and occupational infections, 648t–649t
pathogenesis and pathology of, 991, 992f
pathogenicity of, 1766
treatment of, 1000, 1345t–1351t
Horizontal gene transfer, neisserial genome instability and, 1555
Hormonal contraceptives, in HIV infection, 907
Horse flies, 106t, 111, 111f
Horses
bites, 665
Brucella abortus, 663
Burkholderia spp. in, 1595–1596
Hendra virus, 665
infections from, 191t
Rhodococcus equi, 664
Hortaea werneckii
diagnostic microbiology of, 1711
epidemiology of, 122
nature of, 1710
Hospital-acquired *Clostridium difficile* infection (CDI), 352–353
Hospital-acquired MRSA (HA-MRSA), 1509
decolonization of, 1516
Hospital-acquired pneumonia (HAP), 258–262
bundles and prevention programs of, 262
definition of, 258
diagnosis of, 259–260

Hospital-acquired pneumonia (HAP) (Continued)
directed respiratory samples of, 260
early-onset, 691
epidemiology of, 258
incidence of, 690–691
late-onset, 691
mortality rate, 261
nondirected respiratory samples of, 260
nonrespiratory microbiologic samples of, 259–260
pathophysiology of, 258–259
prevention of, 261–262
prognosis of, 261
sampling strategy in clinical practice and, 260
treatment of, 260–261, 261t
Host defenses
community-acquired pneumonia and, 252–253
in endocarditis, 458t, 459
how micro-organisms escape, 22–24, 22t
Staphylococcus aureus and, 1512–1514
Host factors
genetic, in HIV-1 infection, 844
in vulvovaginal candidiasis, 486–487
Host responses
to infection, 26–39
in sepsis, 420–424
House mouse mite, in tropical rickettsioses, 1092t–1093t
Howell-Jolly bodies, 775
HSV. see Herpes simplex virus (HSV).
Human bite wound, 1639f
Human bites
antibiotic prophylaxis for, 688
antimicrobial therapy for, 683
antiviral agents for, 682
epidemiology of, 682
forensics, 683
management of, 682–683
mechanism of injury, 682
microbiology of, 682, 683t
prophylaxis for, 682–683, 683t
wound care for, 682
Human bocavirus, 1481
clinical manifestations, 1481
diagnostic microbiology, 1481
epidemiology, 1481
management, 1481
nature, 1481
pathogenicity, 1481
prevention, 1481
Human bocavirus 1 (HBoV1), bronchitis and, 244t
Human body, complex ecosystems in, 72
Human body louse, 1106
Human endogenous retroviruses (HERVs), 628–629, 629t, 1483
Human enteroviruses, 1406–1416
Human herpesvirus 6 (HHV-6), 75t, 1432
clinical manifestation of, 1437
encephalitis/myelitis and, 194t
in hematopoietic stem cell transplantation, 742
in kidney transplant patients, 766
in myocarditis, 447
in pericarditis, 450
Human herpesvirus 7 (HHV-7), 75t, 1432
clinical manifestation of, 1438
infection, dermatologic manifestations of, 114t–115t
in kidney transplant patients, 766
Human herpesvirus 8 (HHV-8), 1432
clinical manifestation of, 1438
in Kaposi's sarcoma, 874
in kidney transplant patients, 766–767
in multicentric Castleman's disease, 877
in thoracic transplantation patients, 748
Human herpesviruses (HHV), 702
Human immunodeficiency virus. see HIV infection.
Human leukocyte antigen (HLA)
class I, 719
in HIV-1 infection, 844
Human metapneumovirus (hMPV), 1480–1481
bronchitis and, 244t
clinical manifestations, 1480–1481
diagnostic microbiology, 1480
encephalitis/myelitis and, 194t
epidemiology, 1480
in hematopoietic stem cell transplantation, 743, 743f
management, 1481
nature, 1480

Human metapneumovirus (hMPV) (Continued)
  pathogenicity, 1480
  prevention, 1480
Human microbiota, 68
Human monocytic ehrlichiosis (HME), 408
Human papillomavirus (HPV) infections, 575–584
  chemoprevention of, 583
  clinical features of, 580–581, 580f–581f
  diagnosis of, 582–583, 582f
  epidemiology of, 575–579
  genitourinary and nongenital cancers, 579
  management of, 583
  oncogenesis of, co-factors for, 577–579
  pathogenesis and pathology of, 575–579
  prevention of, 579–580
  vaccination against, 579–580
Human papillomaviruses (HPVs)
  and anal carcinoma, 877–878
  cutaneous, 1440
  in HIV/AIDS, 881
  mucosal, 1439
  vaccination against, 782t–783t
Human-pathogen interface, 42f
Human pathogens
  factors influencing probability of exposure to, 942b
  life cycles of, 939f
  origins and conveyors of, 938t
Human rabies, 1458
Human retroviruses, 701
Human T-cell lymphotropic virus 1 (HTLV-1), 805–806
  in breast-feeding, 516
  infection, 702, 703t
Human T-cell lymphotropic virus 2 (HTLV-2)
  in breast-feeding, 516
  infection, 702, 703t
Human T-lymphocyte leukemia virus 1 (HTLV-1)
  clinical features, 1491
  diagnostic microbiology, 1491
  epidemiology, 1491
  lymphadenopathy and, 143
  nature, 1491
  pathogenesis, 1491
Human T-lymphocyte leukemia virus 2 (HTLV-2)
  diagnostic microbiology, 1491
  nature, 1491
Human T-lymphocyte leukemia viruses, 1491
  clinical features, 1491
  diagnostic microbiology, 1491
  epidemiology, 1491
  nature, 1491
  pathogenesis, 1491
Humoral immune response, 32f, 34
Hutchinson's teeth, 563
HVTN 505, 833
Hyaline molds, 1681t
Hyaluronic acid capsule, group A streptococci and, 1528
Hyaluronidase, 1513t–1514t
'Hydatid cyst,' pathogenesis and pathology of, 1039
Hydatid disease, 1772, 1779
  from dogs, 658
Hydrocele, in filariasis, 1049, 1051
Hydrocephalus, cysticercosis and, 1034
Hydrocephalus shunts
  clinical features of, 222t, 223
  diagnosis of, 223
  epidemiology of, 221
  infections in, 221–224, 221f
  management of, 223–224
  pathogenesis and pathology of, 221–222, 222f, 222t
  prevention of, 222
Hydrolyzing enzymes, 19
Hydropic fetus, parvovirus B19 in, 513
Hydroxychloroquine
  immunosuppression and, 1380t
  for Q fever, 1673
  for Whipple's disease, 345
Hygiene hypothesis, 626–627
Hymenolepis diminuta, 1033
  clinical manifestations of, 1778
  epidemiology of, 1766
  life cycle of, 1773f
  pathogenicity of, 1772

Hymenolepis nana, 1033
  clinical features of, 997
  clinical manifestations of, 1778
  diagnosis of, 998t–999t, 1033–1034
  epidemiology of, 1766
  life cycle of, 1773f
  pathogenesis and pathology of, 994
  pathogenicity of, 1772
  in population density and urbanization, 990
  treatment of, 1001, 1001t, 1345t–1351t
Hyper IgE-Job's syndrome, 87
Hyper-IgE syndrome, 705t, 707f, 713f, 713t
  recurrent, 711–712
Hyper-IgM syndrome, 720–721
Hyperbaric oxygen, for anaerobic bacteria, 1641
Hyperglycemia, and postoperative infection risk, 689–690
Hyperimmunoglobulinemia D (HIDS), 614
Hypermutation, neisserial genome instability and, 1555
Hypernatremia, in meningitis, 182–183
Hyperparasitemia, in severe malaria, 1020t
Hypersensitivity
  of drugs, 1153
  from β-lactam antibiotics, 1215t
  as quinolones adverse effect, 1248
Hypersensitivity pneumonitis, 287, 287f
Hypersensitivity reactions, 21–22
  type I (immediate), 21
  type II (cytotoxic), 21–22
  type III (immune complex-mediated), 22
  type IV (delayed-type), 22
Hyperthermia
  fever versus, 605–606
  malignant, 606
Hypertrophic pulmonary osteoarthropathy, 279
Hypervirulent Clostridium difficile strains, 351
Hypogammaglobulinemia, and rituximab, 800
Hypoglycemia
  quinine-induced hyperinsulinemic, 1024–1025
  in severe malaria, 1020–1021, 1020t, 1024–1025
Hypokalemia, 335–336
Hyponatremia, 182–183
Hypopigmentation, postinflammatory, 585, 586t–587t
Hypopyon, 166, 166f
Hypothalamic-pituitary-adrenal (HPA) axis, 633
Hypothalamus, and thermoregulation, 606–607
Hypoxic wound, protection of, 686
Hysterectomy, in postoperative gynecologic infections, 496–497

I

Ibuprofen, bronchitis and, 244
ICAM-1 (intercellular adhesion molecule 1), 1017
ICAMs (intercellular adhesion molecules), 709
Iclaprim, 1178f
ICU-acquired pneumonia, 1594–1595
Idiopathic CD4+ lymphocytopenia (ICL), 808, 810t
'Idiopathic' dilated cardiomyopathy, 446
Idiopathic thrombocytopenic purpura (ITP), 323–324
IgA1 protease, 1618
  Neisseria, 1557t
IgG antibodies, for coccidioidomycosis, 1705
IgG titer, 517–518
  initial or subsequent positive, 518
  negative, 518
IgM antibodies, for coccidioidomycosis, 1705
IgM antibody capture ELISA (MAC-ELISA), 1498
IgM titer
  equivocal, 518
  positive, 518
IL-12/IL-23 cytokine family, inhibition of, 801–802
IL-17, inhibition of, 802
Il-17/TH17 pathway, inhibition of, 801–802
Ileocecal tuberculosis, 279
Imaging. see specific techniques.
Imidazoles
  for endophthalmitis, 162–163
  for tinea nigra, 128
  for tinea pedis, 128
Imipenem, 1204
  for Alcaligenes spp., 1597
  for anaerobic bacteria, 1643

Imipenem (Continued)
  for complicated urinary tract infection, 545t
  hospital-acquired pneumonia and, 260t
  for lung abscess, 269f
  neurologic effects, 1215
  for nocardiosis, 1551
  for P. aeruginosa infection, 1210
  for Rhodococcus equi, 1551
  susceptibilities of selected bacteria to, 1208t–1209t
Imipenem-cilastatin
  antimicrobial spectrum, routes of administration and dosages, 1206t–1207t
  dosage in renal failure, 1213t–1214t
  for foot ulcers, 131t
  pharmacokinetics of, 1205t
Imiquimod, for anal carcinoma, 878
Immune activation, 843
Immune deficiency, mechanism of, in HIV-1 infection, 842–844
  and changes in the microbiome, 844
  immune exhaustion during chronic infections, 843
  role of CD4+ T cells in, 842–843
  role of inflammation in, 843
Immune deficit, children with, vaccination of, 791–795
  with congenital HIV infection, 794t, 795
  inherited, systematic approach to, 791–795, 794t
Immune exhaustion, 843
Immune manipulation, in reducing latent reservoir, 932t, 933–934, 933f
Immune-mediated inflammatory disease (IMID), 864
Immune-mediated neutropenia, 706
Immune reconstitution disorders, 859–864
Immune reconstitution inflammatory syndrome (IRIS), 859–864, 881, 1696
  clinical presentation of, 861–863, 861f–862f
  comparison of, with opportunistic infections in patients with HIV infection, 860t
  diagnostic features of, 859b
  and HIV-associated TB, 871, 872f
  management of, 864
  pathogenesis, 863
  progressive multifocal leukoencephalopathy in, 1447
  and skin manifestations of HIV, 886, 886t
Immune recovery uveitis (IRU), 862
Immune response
  and coinfections, 843–844
  in cystitis, 525
  genital herpes in, 567–568
  harmful, 21–22
  hepatitis C virus, 370
  HIV-1 escape from, 842
  host genetic factors, 844
  humoral. see Humoral immune response
  innate. see Innate immune response
  in Lyme disease, 407
  modulation of, 37
  role of, in determining set points for chronic asymptomatic infection, 841–842
  against Staphylococcus aureus, 1512
Immune senescence, 927
Immune suppression, in sepsis, 424
Immune system, response of, to thermal injury, 698, 699t
Immunity
  natural or vaccine-induced, accelerated decay of, in immunocompromised patient, 780
  in pregnancy, 501
Immunization
  in congenital infections, 507
  for herpesvirus, 1432–1433
  for laboratory and pathology staff, 651, 651t
  in newborns, and HIV infection, 901
  for occupational infections, 650, 650t
  passive. see Passive immunization
  to prevent postsplenectomy sepsis, 777–778
  response to, assessment of, in immunocompromised patients, 787
  see also Vaccination; Vaccines
Immunoassay methods, for Giardia lamblia, 1731
Immunobiologics
  general aspects of, 796, 797f
  infections associated with, 796–804
    B-cell-depleting therapies, 800
    inhibition of IL-1 pathway, 801

Immunobiologics (Continued)
  inhibition of IL-12/IL-23 cytokine family, 801–802
  inhibition of IL-17, 802
  inhibition of Il-17/TH17 pathway, 801–802
  inhibitors of tumor necrosis factor, 797–800
  selective adhesion molecule inhibitors, 802
  T-cell co-stimulatory blocker, 801
  targeting immunoglobulin E (IgE), 802
  infectious risk associated with, 796–802, 798t–799t
  screening for, 802–803, 803t
  targeting the interleukin-6 pathway, 801
  and vaccination, 803, 803t
Immunoblots
  in genital herpes, 572–573
  see also Western blot
Immunochromatographic strip test, 1606
Immunochromatography test (ICT), for Babesia, 1752
Immunocompetent hosts
  cryptosporidiosis, 347–348
  isosporiasis, 348
  microsporidiosis, 348
Immunocompetent patients
  cryptosporidiosis in, 1740
  microsporidiosis in, 1741
Immunocompromised hosts
  fever of unknown origin in, 615
  genital herpes in, 572
  toxoplasmosis in, 1755, 1755f
  travelers immunization and, 950
Immunocompromised patients
  adenovirus diseases in, 1473–1474
  chronic diarrhea in, 341
  cryptococcosis in, 1694
  cryptosporidiosis in, 1740
  fusariosis in, 1699
  microsporidiosis in, 1740–1741
  myocarditis in, 448, 448t
  parainfluenza virus in, 1479–1480
  recurrent cellulitis in, 135
  rhinovirus in, 1477–1478
  superficial fungal infections in, 126–127
  vaccination of, 780–795
    characteristics common in, 780–781
      accelerated decay of any previous vaccine-induced or natural immunity, 780
      need to assess vaccine-induced or natural immunity, 781
      need to catch up with vaccination protocols, 781, 782t–783t
    clinical conditions with specific additional vaccine indications, 783t
    correlates of protection in, 781t
    delay in cessation of therapy and administration of vaccines in, 788t
    dissimilarities in, 781–791
      systematic approach to vaccinating CIAMD patients in, 781–787
      systematic approach to vaccinating hematopoietic stem cell transplant patients, 790–791, 792t–793t
      systematic approach to vaccinating solid organ transplant patients, 787, 789t–790t
    impact of vaccinations on timing of planned therapy in, 783, 784t
    with inactivated vaccines, 783–785
    list of vaccines and formulations of, 785t
Immunodeficiencies, 705–722
  adult with suspected, 808–811
    algorithm for, 809f
    clinical evaluation of, 809–811
    differential diagnosis of, 808–809
    history of, 809, 810t
    laboratory evaluation of, 811
    microbiology of, 809–811
    radiology in, 811
  cyclic neutropenia/cyclic hematopoiesis and, 706
  defects in antigen presentation, 718–719
  defects of granule formation and content, 706–707
  defects of granulocyte production, 705–706
    severe congenital neutropenia, 705–706
  defects of oxidative metabolism in, 707–709, 707f
  immune defects with predominant immunoglobulin deficiency, 719–721
  immune-mediated neutropenia, 706
  interferon-γ/IL-12 pathway defects in, 710, 711f–712f

Immunodeficiencies (Continued)
  Kostmann syndrome, 706
  leukocyte adhesion deficiency, 709–710, 709f
  lymphocyte immune deficiencies, 712–718, 714f
  myeloid cells and defects, 705, 705t
  nuclear factor Kappa B pathway defects in, 710–711
  purine nucleoside phosphorylase deficiency, 718
  syndrome-associated immune deficiencies, 721–722
Immunodeficient patients, Mycoplasma hominis in, 1664
Immunodiagnostic tests
  for helminths diagnosis, 1776–1777
  for tuberculosis, 1657–1658, 1658t
Immunodiffusion (ID) test
  for blastomycosis, 1702–1703
  for coccidioidomycosis, 1705
  for histoplasmosis, 293, 1707
  for paracoccidioidomycosis, 1709
Immunofluorescence
  assay
    for Lyme disease, 410b
    for scrub typhus, 1096
  keratitis and, 156
  in melioidosis, 1076
  technique, for Cryptosporidium spp., 1737
Immunofluorescence microscopy, for influenza viruses, 1469
Immunofluorescent antibody (IFA)
  filovirus, 1506
  hantavirus, 1504
  test, for leishmaniasis, 1063
Immunoglobulin A (IgA), 34
  selective deficiency in, 720
Immunoglobulin D (IgD), 34
Immunoglobulin E (IgE), 34
  hyper-IgE syndrome, 705t, 707f, 711–712, 713f, 713t
Immunoglobulin G (IgG), 34
  antibodies, for Q fever, 1672–1673
Immunoglobulin M (IgM), 34
  anti-HAV, 364
  antibodies, for Q fever, 1672–1673
  hyper-IgM syndromes, 720–721
  Toxoplasma gondii-specific, 507–508
Immunoglobulins
  administration of, and live vaccine administration, 795
  in cancer patients, 732
  classes, 34–35, 34f
  deficiency in, 719–721
  innate immune response, 26–27
  see also specific immunoglobulins
Immunologic assays, for papillomaviruses, 1443
Immunologic conditions, eosinophilia and, 984t
Immunologic responses, of antiretroviral treatment, 923
Immunologically mediated disease
  clinical features and management of, 771–774
    abscesses, 772, 772f
    acute neurologic problems in, 771–773
    encephalitis, 772–773
    fever and pulmonary infiltrates in, 771, 771t, 772f
    gastrointestinal problems in, 773, 773f
    meningitis, 772
    skin, soft tissue and joints, 773–774, 774f
  pathogenesis, 770
  prevention of, 770–771
Immunoperoxidase assay
  for scrub typhus, 1096, 1670
  for typhus group rickettsiae, 1669–1670
Immunoproliferative small intestinal disease (IPSID), 1602
Immunostimulatory molecules, 1515, 1515f
Immunosuppressed patients
  blastomycosis, 294
  Chagas disease in, 1760
  coccidioidomycosis, 296
  histoplasmosis, 292
  uveitis and retinitis in, 172–173
  visceral leishmaniasis in, 1061, 1757
Immunosuppression, 25
  in human papillomavirus, 579
  in intestinal transplant patients, 756
  level of, and opportunistic infection in HIV, 850
  Mycoplasma genitalium in, 1663
  net state of, in liver transplant patients, 752
Immunosuppressive drugs, 1379, 1380t
Immunosuppressive therapy, for myocarditis, 449
Impetigo, 88, 89f
  bullous, 88

Implant retention, for prosthetic joint infection (PJI), 402
Inactivated vaccines
  for children with congenital HIV infection, 795
  and children with inherited immune deficiency syndrome, 795
  immunogenicity of, and patient's state of immunocompetency, 785–787
  post-transplantation revaccination process with, timing of, 791
  use of, in immunocompromised patients, 783–785
Incidence, definition, 49
Indian tick typhus, 1092t–1093t
Indinavir, 1148t, 1303
  effect on oral contraceptives, 907t
  perinatal HIV transmission prevention, 909t
Indirect fluorescent antibody test (IFAT), for Legionella spp., 1624
Indirect hemagglutination
  for helminths diagnosis, 1777
  test, of melioidosis, 1076
Indirect immunofluorescence antibody assay, for typhus group rickettsiae, 1669–1670
Indirect immunofluorescent antibody staining, for helminths diagnosis, 1777
Indirect immunofluorescent antibody test (IFAT)
  for Babesia, 1752
  for leishmaniasis, 1757
Indirect microimmunofluorescence antibody assay
  for anaplasmosis, 1672
  for bartonellosis, 1673–1674
  for ehrlichioses, 1671
  for Q fever, 1672–1673
  for scrub typhus, 1670
Indium scan, in fever of unknown origin, 620
Indoor residual insecticide spraying (IRS), 1017
Industrial Injuries Disablement Benefit (IIDB), 649
Infants, subdural empyema/intracranial epidural abscess in, 201, 205t
Infection(s)
  bacterial, 72–73
  control, in neonatal nursery, 521
  endogenous, 12
  eosinophilia and, 984t
  for eosinophilic meningitis, 974t
  exogenous, 13
  factors restricting introduction and spread of, 943b
  and fever of unknown origin, 611–613
  fungal, microbiome and, 73
  host responses to, 26–39
  micro-eukaryotic, microbiome and, 73–74
  parasite, microbiome and, 73–74
  process of, 13–15
    adherence, 13
    attachment to host cells, 13
    bacterial adhesins, 13–14, 14f
    ubiquitous receptors, 13
    viral adhesion, 14–15
  viral, 73
Infection prevention and control, 54–61
  collaboration with other programs, 57–58
  flow diagram of the detection, evaluation and implementation, 56f
  health-care and device-associated infections, 60
  isolation precautions, 58–60
  manage critical data and information, 54–55
  organization of, 54–58, 55b
  outbreak investigation, 55–56, 56b
  role of the microbiology laboratory, 56–57
  trends and complexity of current healthcare in developed countries, 54
Infectious agents, definition and comparison of, 4–5
Infectious (mycotic) aneurysms, imaging of, 464
Infectious diseases, 72–74
  dog-associated, 656–658
  dynamics of transmission, 49–50
    insights from, 50
  epidemiology, mathematical models in, 49–53
  geography of, 938–947
  microbiome in, 68–74
  models, structure of, 51–52
  pathogenesis of, 10–15
  transmitted by grafts, 805–807
    bacterial pathogens in, 805
    donor screening in, 807
    donor-transmitted pathogens, 805t

Infectious diseases (Continued)
    fungal pathogens in, 806–807
    parasitic pathogens, 807
    reporting of, 807
    viral pathogens in, 805–806
    see also specific diseases
Infectious inguinal lymphadenopathy, differential
    diagnosis of, 140t
Infectious keratitis, diagnosis of, 155–156, 156f
Infectious mononucleosis, 79, 143–144
    and chronic fatigue syndrome, 632–633
    clinical features of, 79
    complications of, 79
    and fever of unknown origin, 613
    lymphadenopathy and, 137t–138t
    management of, 79
    as mild febrile transaminitis, 377
    primary HIV infection resembling, 846
Infective endocarditis
    Candida, 442
    and fever of unknown origin, 611
    HACEK group in, 1622
    in heart transplant recipients, 748
    prevention of, in dental procedures, 1159, 1159b, 1160t
    in thoracic transplant patients, 748
Infertility
    Mycoplasma genitalium in, 1663
    Mycoplasma hominis in, 1664
Inflammation
    pathogenesis of, 684–686, 685f
    role of, in immune deficiency, 843
Inflammatory disease, pathogenesis of, 627t, 629t
Infliximab, 797, 798t–799t
Influenza
    avian. see Avian influenza
    and bioterrorism, 671t, 673t
    causing retinitis and uveitis, 168t
    compartmental models of, 51–52, 51f
    croup and, 229
    in hematopoietic stem cell transplantation, 742–743
    hospital-acquired pneumonia and, 259t
    human seasonal, 651t–654t
    and occupational infections, 648t–649t
    immunization for, 650t–651t
    pandemic, 52, 651t–654t
    replication, 1320f
    in thoracic transplantation patients, 747t, 749
    treatment of, 1319t
        community-acquired pneumonia and, 255–256
        M2 inhibitors, 1318
        neuraminidase inhibitors, 1319–1326
    vaccination, community-acquired pneumonia and, 256
Influenza A, 1466
    antigenic variation of, 1466
    from birds, 668
    from ducks, 661
    from marine mammals, 668
    from mustelids, 666
    shift and drift, 25
Influenza C, 1470
Influenza vaccine, 749
    in HIV infection, 913–914
Influenza viruses, 1465–1471
    antigenic variation of, 1466
    bronchitis and, 244t
    chemoprophylaxis for, 1469
    clinical manifestations of, 1470–1471
    diagnostic microbiology of, 1469–1470
    encephalitis/myelitis and, 194t
    epidemiology of, 1465–1466
    immunofluorescence microscopy for, 1469
    infection, in kidney transplant patients, 768
    life cycle of, 1467f
    management of, 1471, 1471t
    molecular detection for, 1469–1470
    natural reservoirs of, 1465
    nature of, 1465
    pandemics, 1466
    pathogenesis of, 1468
    pharyngitis, 233
    prevention of, 1468–1469
    rapid antigen testing for, 1469
    replication of, 1465

Influenza viruses (Continued)
    serology for, 1469
    structure of, 1465, 1466f
    use of cocoon strategy on, 787
    vaccination against, 782t–783t
Inguinal lymphadenopathy, 140–141, 140t, 145
Inhalation, and occupational infections, 648t–649t
Inhalation anthrax, 1126
Inhaled administration, of polymyxins, 1287–1288
Inherited hemoglobin disorders
    classification of, 1053, 1053b
    clinical features of, 1056–1057
    common, infections and, 1053–1058
    diagnosis of, 1057
    epidemiology of, 1053, 1053b, 1054f–1056f
    pathogenesis and pathology of, 1053–1058
    prevention of, 1055–1056
    treatment of, 1057–1058
Injection-site reactions, in skin manifestations of HIV, 887
Innate immune response
    barrier functions of, 26–27
    effector functions of, 27–32
    enteroviruses and, 1409
    immunoglobulins, 26–27
    macrophages, 31
    monocytes, 31
    mononuclear cells, 31
    phagocytes, 31–32
    phagocytosis, 31
    in respiratory tract, 28f
Innate immunity, 26–32, 27f
    barrier functions of, 26–27
    defects of, in cancer patients, 725, 725f
    recognition and effector functions of, 27–32
    in respiratory tract, 28f
    vs. adaptive immunity, 26t
INNO-LiPA multiplex probe assay, 1654
Insect repellents, 1017
Insecta, 107–112
    Anoploura, 107–108
    Diptera, 109–112
    Heteroptera, 108–109
    Siphonaptera, 108
Insecticides (ITNs), impregnated with, 1017
Insectivores, infections from, 668
Integrase inhibitors
    antiretroviral drugs, 925
    of antiretroviral therapy, 937
    perinatal HIV transmission prevention, 910t
    resistance to, 924
Integrase strand transfer inhibitors, 1306–1308
    antiretroviral drugs, 922–923
Integrins, 1408
Integrons, 1195–1196, 1196f
Intensive care unit (ICU)
    antibiotic-resistant bacteria in, controlling transmission
      of, 693–697
        interventions for, 695t–696t
    chlorhexidine body washing and mupirocin
      decolonization in, 694
    decontamination of bacteria in, 694–697
    hand hygiene in, 694
    hospital-acquired pneumonia and, 258
    meningitis management, 182–183
    screening of patients in, 693–694
    sepsis in, 415–416, 419
    and ventilator-associated pneumonia, 690–691
Intercellular adhesion molecule 1 (ICAM-1), 1017
Intercellular adhesion molecules (ICAMs), 709
Interdigital candidiasis, 126f
Interferon-α, 1146t–1147t
Interferon-α 2a, 875t
Interferon-γ/IL-12 pathway, 705t
    defects of, 710, 711f–712f
Interferon-gamma (IFN-γ), chronic granulomatous
    disease prophylaxis, 709
Interferon gamma release assays, 275, 1657
Interferons
    combination therapy based on, 1332
    for HRV colds, 1478
    indications for
      hepatitis B, 1327
      hepatitis C, 1330

Interferons (Continued)
    pegylated. see Pegylated interferons
    see also specific interferons
Interleukin-1
    in pneumonia, 253
    in sepsis, 420
Interleukin-1 pathway, inhibition of, 801
Interleukin-1 receptor antagonist (IL-1Ra), 801
Interleukin-2Rα deficiency, 716
Interleukin-6 pathway, immunobiologics targeting, 801
Interleukin-7 (IL-7), 716
Interleukin-7Rα deficiency, 716
Interleukin-10 (IL-10), 609
Interleukin-12 (IL-12), 705t
    defects in, 710, 710f–712f
Internalin A (InIA), 1538
Internalin B (InIB), 1538
Interstitial pneumonitis, 1099
Intertrigo, 125
Intestinal anthrax, 1125–1126
Intestinal capillariasis
    clinical features of, 996
    pathogenesis and pathology of, 991
Intestinal flukes, 989t, 1032, 1037, 1764t
    clinical manifestations of, 1778
    distribution of, 990
    epidemiology of, 1765
    pathogenicity of, 1770–1772
    treatment of, 1345t–1351t
Intestinal infections, Enterobacteriaceae in, 1569–1575
Intestinal perforation, typhoid fever and, 1004, 1004f
Intestinal schistosomiasis, 1029–1031, 1030f
Intestinal transplantation, 756–761
    epidemiology of, 756
    infectious complications in, timing and pattern of, 757,
      757t
    infectious syndromes in, 757–760
      abdominal infections, 757
      adenovirus, 760
      bacteremia, 757
      cytomegalovirus, 757–759
      Epstein-Barr virus, 759–760
    pathogenesis and pathology of, 756
    prophylactic strategies for, 758t
    rejection of, 756
    treatment strategies for, 759t
Intra-abdominal infections
    aminoglycosides for, 1237
    anaerobic bacteria in, 1638–1639, 1638t
    β-lactam antibiotics for, 1211
    in pancreas transplant recipients, 763–764
      diagnosis of, 763–764
        impact of surgical technique on risk of, 764, 765f
        prophylaxis and management of, 764, 764f
      risk factors for, 764
      timing and type of, 764
    postoperative, 690
    source control, 690
Intra-abdominal organs, infection of, in cancer patients,
    727–728
Intra-abdominal sepsis, 355–362
    clinical presentation of, 356
    investigations of, 356–357, 356f–357f
    microbiology of, 355–356
    pathophysiology of, 356
Intra-amniotic infection, 500, 503
Intracellular killing, Staphylococcus aureus and, 1514
Intracellular micro-organisms, hospital-acquired
    pneumonia and, 259t
Intracranial epidural abscess, 203–204
    clinical features of, 204
    diagnosis of, 204
    epidemiology of, 203
    management of, 204
    pathogenesis and pathophysiology of, 203–204
Intracranial infections, antimicrobial therapy for, 1641t
Intracranial pressure, in severe malaria, 1017
Intradermal vaccine regimens, for rabies, 1462–1463
Intramuscular vaccine regimens, for rabies, 1462
Intraocular aspirate, endophthalmitis, 161–162
Intraocular lens management, endophthalmitis, 163
Intrapartum antimicrobial prophylaxis (IAP), 520–521
    newborn management following, 521, 522f

Intrapartum prophylaxis, β-lactam antibiotics, 1209
Intrathecal administration, of polymyxins, 1287–1288
Intravascular access devices, infection from, in cancer
    patients, 727
Intravascular lines, infections with, 427–438
    see also catheter-related bloodstream infection (CRBSI)
Intravenous administration, Clostridium difficile infection
    (CDI), 353
Intravenous drug users
    in endocarditis, 457, 468–469
    HIV prevention interventions, 828
Intravenous formulations, of polymyxins, 1287
Intravenous immunoglobulin (IVIG), in intestinal
    transplant patients, 758–759, 758t
    for cytomegalovirus, 759t
    for Epstein-Barr virus, 759t
Intravenous infusions, malaria in pregnancy, 1143t–1144t
Intravenous pyelogram (IVP), 556
Intravitreal antibiotics, endophthalmitis, 162
Invasion, 15–25
    actin-based intracellular motility microbial pathogens,
        16–17, 18f
    antigenic and phase variations, 24–25
    bacterial toxins, 18–21
        apoptosis, 19, 20f
        cell and tissue damage induced by micro-organisms,
            18, 18t
        damage resulting from cytotoxic lymphocytes, 21
        diphtheria toxin, 19, 20f
        hydrolyzing enzymes, 19
        infection and cancer, 21
        virus-induced cytopathic effect, 19–21, 21f
    enteroinvasive pathogens and the membranous cell
        gateway, 15–16
    harmful immune responses, 21–22
    how micro-organisms escape host defense, 22–24
    invasive and noninvasive micro-organisms, 15–16, 15t,
        16f
    subepithelial, 17–18
        example of measles virus, 18
        infection of distant target organs, 17–18
    surviving phagocyte, 22
        avoiding ingestion, 23
        inactivation of reactive oxygen species, 23
        inhibition of the mobilization of phagocytes, 22
        killing the phagocyte before being ingested, 22–23
        'professional' phagocytes as vectors or refuges, 23
        resistance to antimicrobial peptides, 23
        survival within phagocytes, 23
Invasive aspergillosis, 1689
Invasive candidiasis, 118
Iodamoeba bütschlii, 1725t, 1730f, 1731–1732
Iodochlorhydroxyquin, 1367
Iodoquinol, for parasitic infections treatment, 1345t–
    1351t, 1367
IPEX, 722
'Iris pearls', 982
Iritis, red eye and, 175–176
Iron-binding proteins, Neisseria, 1557t
Iron deficiency anemia, Helicobacter pylori, 323–324,
    326
Irrigation, parasites from, 990
Irritable bowel syndrome (IBS), 341
    Blastocystis spp. in, 1728
    from Campylobacter jejuni, 1602
    Rome II criteria for, 375, 375b
IS6110 restriction fragment length polymorphism, for
    mycobacteria, 1655
Isavuconazole, 1340
    adverse effects of, 1340
    for aspergillosis, 1691
    chemical structure of, 1337f
    dosage of, 1340
        in special circumstances, 1340
    drug interactions of, 1340
    indications of, 1340
    for mucormycosis, 1698
    pharmacokinetics and distribution of, 1340
    route of administration, 1340
Ischemia, of gut, 686
Ischemic colitis, surgery complications, 690
Ischemic enteropathies
    surgery complications, 690
    see also specific conditions
Isla Vista (ISLA) virus, 1503t

Isolation precautions, 58–60
    standard, 58–60
    transmission-based, 58–60
Isolator System, for mycobacteria, 1653
Isoniazid, 1265–1267
    adverse reactions of, 1268t–1269t
    hepatotoxicity and, 308, 309f
    for meningitis, 187t
    for pericarditis, 454
    resistance to, 1193
        mycobacterial, 1656t
        tuberculosis, 866
    side effect of, 280–281
    for tuberculosis, 280–281, 283t
    for urogenital tract tuberculosis, 556
Isoniazid preventive therapy (IPT), for HIV-associated TB,
    868
Isospora, from dogs, 658
Isospora belli
    of chronic diarrhea, 347t, 348
    clinical features of, 996
    diagnosis of, 998t–999t
    pathogenesis and pathology of, 991
    treatment of, 999–1000, 1000t
        in diarrhea, 334
    see also Cystoisospora belli
Isosporiasis
    chronic diarrhea and, 348
    clinical features of, 996
Isotope scanning, in osteomyelitis, 394, 394f,
    394t
Isotype switching, antibody, 35–36
Isoxazolyl penicillins
    for coagulase-negative staphylococcal infections,
        1521–1522
    staphylococci and, 1518
    for Staphylococcus aureus, 1520
Israeli spotted fever, 1667t, 1668
Itraconazole, 1338–1339
    for Acanthamoeba keratitis, 1750
    adverse effects of, 1338–1339
    for aspergillosis, 1691
    for black fungi, 1722
    for blastomycosis, 295, 1703
    for candidiasis, 128
    chemical structure of, 1337f
    for chromoblastomycosis, 1722
    for coccidioidomycosis, 296, 1705–1706
    for conidiobolomycosis, 1722–1723
    for cryptococcosis, 1695t, 1696
    dosage of, 1338
        in special circumstances, 1338
    drug interactions of, 1338–1339
    for endophthalmitis, 162–163
    for esophageal candidiasis, 1686
    for histoplasmosis, 294, 1708
    indications of, 1338
    for keratitis, 154
    for mycetoma, 1723
    for onychomycosis, 128
    for oropharyngeal candidiasis, 1684
    for paracoccidioidomycosis, 297, 1709
    for parasitic infections, 1345t–1351t
    for penicilliosis, 299
    for phaeohyphomycosis, 1723
    pharmacodynamics of, 1338
    pharmacokinetics and distribution of, 1338
    prophylaxis with
        in cancer patients, 730, 737
        for chronic granulomatous disease, 709
    route of administration, 1338
    for sporotrichosis, 298, 1724
    for Talaromyces marneffei, 1699
    for tinea corporis and tinea cruris, 128
    for tinea manuum, 128
    for tinea pedis, 128
Ivermectin
    for filariasis, 1051
    for gastrointestinal helminth, 1000–1001,
        1001t
    for loiasis, 1051
    for onchocerciasis, 1051
    for parasitic infections, 1345t–1351t, 1371
    Strongyloides stercoralis, 773, 773f
Ixodes nymphs, epidemiology of, 405

Ixodes scapularis
    life cycle of, 405, 406f
    in Lyme disease, 407

J

Jacuzzis, infections from, 644–645
JAK3, 714
    deficiency in, 715–716
    pathway, 716f
    signaling, 716f
Janus associated kinase (JAK), 714
Japan, hepatitis C virus in, 367
Japanese B encephalitis, vaccination for, in travelers,
    950
Japanese encephalitis, 1495t
    immunization for, and occupational infections,
        650t–651t
Japanese encephalitis virus (JEV), 189
    encephalitis/myelitis caused by, 192t
Japanese spotted fever, 1092t–1093t, 1667t, 1668
Jarisch-Herxheimer reaction, 1107–1108, 1108f,
    1608
    for syphilis, 565
Jaundice
    acute hepatitis and, 363
    comparative health indicators, 1134t
    infectious causes of, 1134–1136
    in leptospirosis, 1103
    noninfectious causes of, 1134
    relapsing fevers and, 1106–1107, 1107f
    in severe malaria, 1020t, 1022
    in traveler returning from Nepal, 1134–1136, 1134f,
        1135t
JC polyomavirus (JCPyV), 1445
    associated syndromes, 1447
JC virus
    in HIV/AIDS, 853–854
    in kidney transplant patients, 767
Jet lag, 952
Joint excision, for prosthetic joint infection (PJI), 402
Joint infections
    antimicrobial therapy for, 1641t
    in immunologically mediated diseases, 773–774,
        774f
    Pseudomonas aeruginosa in, 1589
Jones criteria, 1533t
    in rheumatic fever, 472, 472t, 474–475
Josamycin
    accumulation ratio of, 1222t
    characteristics of, 1218t
    pharmacokinetics, 1223t–1224t
    for spotted fever group rickettsiae, 1669
    stability in acidic medium, 1217
    tissue distribution, 1224t
Junin viruses, 1500t
    epidemiology of, 1110–1113, 1112t, 1500
    vaccine, 1501

K

Kala-azar, 119
    see also Visceral leishmaniasis
Kaposi's sarcoma, 586t–587t, 874–875
    clinical features of, 874
    diagnosis of, 874
    in HIV infection, in low- and middle-income countries,
        893
    in immune reconstitution inflammatory syndrome,
        863
    in kidney transplant patients, 767
    management of, 874–875, 875t
        immunotherapy in, 875
        local therapy in, 875
        new therapeutic approaches in, 875
    oral cavity in, 874
    pathogenesis of, 874
    in skin manifestations of HIV, 885, 885f
    in thoracic transplantation patients, 748, 749f
Kaposi's sarcoma-associated herpesvirus (KSHV), 703t
Katayama fever, 1028
Kato-Katz technique, for helminths diagnosis, 1775
Kato-Katz thick smear, of schistosomiasis, 1031
Kato method, for helminths diagnosis, 1775
Kauffman-White scheme, 1568

Kawasaki disease, 640–642
    clinical and laboratory features, 641t
    clinical manifestations of, 640, 641f
    differential diagnosis of, 640t
    epidemiology of, 640
    long-term care, 642
    lymphadenopathy and, 137t–138t
    management of, 640–642
    pharyngitis, 234
Keloidal blastomycosis. see Lobomycosis.
Keratitis, 152–156
    Acanthamoeba. see Acanthamoeba keratitis
    amoebal, 175
    bacterial, 152–153
    community-acquired, 152–155, 152f
    contact lens-related, 155–156
    diagnosis of, 153f
    following ocular surgery, 156
    fungal, 154–155, 154f
    herpes simplex, 176
    herpes simplex virus dendritic, 156f
    herpes zoster ophthalmicus, 154, 154f
    infectious, diagnosis of, 155–156, 156f
    measles causing, 167
    microbial, 983, 983f
    Pseudomonas aeruginosa in, 1588
    Pseudomonas spp. in, 1589
    punctate or 'snowflake', 981
    red eye and, 175, 175t
    sclerosing, 981
    varicella-zoster epithelial, 154
Keratoconjunctivitis
    epidemic, lymphadenopathy and, 137t–138t
    systemic microsporidiosis in, 1741, 1741f
Keratoplasty, 156
Kerion, 124
Kerstersia, 1597
    nomenclature of, 1581t–1582t
Ketek scandal, 1382
Ketoconazole
    for *Acanthamoeba* keratitis, 1750
    for basidiobolomycosis, 1723
    for chromoblastomycosis, 1722
    keratitis and, 154–155
    for leishmaniasis, 1064
    for mycetoma, 1723
    for paracoccidioidomycosis, 297
    prophylaxis with, in cancer patients, 730
    seborrheic dermatitis, 128
Ketolides, 1171, 1172f, 1217–1222
    advantages, 1222
    adverse reactions and interactions, 1222
    characteristics of, 1218t
    classification, 1217
    clinical studies, 1222
    definitions, 1217
    exit tunnel, 1221
    intra-bacterial penetration, 1221
    intracellular concentrations, 1221
    mechanism of action, 1221
    mechanism of resistance, 1221–1222
    versus other antibacterials, 1222
    peptidyltransferase center, 1221
    pharmacodynamic properties, 1222
    pharmacokinetic properties, 1222, 1223t
    physicochemical characteristics, 1217–1218
    stability in acidic medium, 1217–1218
    in vitro activity, 1219–1221, 1220t
Khabarovsk (KHB) virus, 1502t
Kidney, adverse reactions to β-lactam antibiotics, 1215
Kidney disease, β-lactam antibiotics dosage in, 1212
Kidney injury, in immune reconstitution inflammatory syndrome, 863
Kidney-pancreas transplant recipients, in urinary tract infections, 558
Kidney transplant
    bacterial infections in, 762–765
    BK virus nephropathy in, 1447, 1447f
    drug interactions in, 762
    fungal infections in, 768
    parasitic infections in, 768–769
    preventive strategies for, 769
    urinary tract infection in, 762–763

Kidney transplant *(Continued)*
    vaccinations in, 769, 769t
    viral infections in, 765–768
        cytomegalovirus infection, 762, 766, 766f
        hepatitis virus infections, 767–768
        herpesvirus infections, 765–767
        polyomavirus infections, 767
Kidney transplant recipients, 762–769
    interferon-alpha in, 768
    urinary tract infections in, 557–558
Kikuchi's disease
    and fever of unknown origin, 614
    lymph node enlargement and, 146, 146f
    lymphadenopathy and, 137t–138t
Kinetoplastida, 1065, 1756
Kingella, 1622
Kingella kingae, 390
Kinyoun stain, for mycobacteria, 1652
Kissing bugs, 1759
Klebsiella
    antimicrobial resistance of, 1576
    in cancer patients, 723–724
    diagnostic microbiology of, 1568, 1568t
    hospital-acquired pneumonia and, 259t
    intrinsic resistance of, 1182t
    microflora, 355–356
    virulence factors of, 1571t
Klebsiella granulomatis, 590–591, 1576, 1577t
    etiology of, 1138t
Klebsiella oxytoca, 1576
    bacterial enteritis and, 338
    diagnosis of, 339
Klebsiella planticola, 1576
Klebsiella pneumoniae
    brain abscess and, 199–200
    in burn wounds, 698
    in complicated urinary tract infection, 540t
    hospital-acquired pneumonia and, 259t
    in liver abscess, 1576
    in osteomyelitis, 395t
    pneumonia in HIV/AIDS, 857
    primary (spontaneous) peritonitis, 359
    pyogenic liver abscess, 361
    in respiratory tract infections, 1575
    subspecies, 1576, 1577t
    in urinary tract infections, 1575
Klebsiella terrigena, 1576
Kluyvera ascorbata, 1577t
Knee arthroplasty, infection in, 399
Koch, Robert, 1
Koch's postulates, 1b, 625
    evolution of, 1–3
        historical perspective of, 1–2
    limitations of, 2, 2t
    microorganisms and chronic disease, 3, 3t
    'molecular', 2b
    note of caution, 3
    redefined, 627t
    virulence, pathogenicity and causation, 2–3
Koilocytotic dysplasia, 580–581
Koplik's spots, 76–77, 1400, 1401f
Kostmann syndrome, 706
Kuceria, 1509
Kuru, 215t
    clinical features of, 217
    pathology of, 219
    prevention of, 220
Kyasanur forest disease virus, 666

L

La Crosse virus, encephalitis/myelitis caused by, 192t
Laboratory-based diagnostics, in sepsis, 419–420
Laboratory diagnosis, of mycobacteria, 1650–1655
Laboratory worker, and occupational infections, 648t–649t
Lacazia loboi, 1712
Lacaziosis. see Lobomycosis.
Lacrymal system infections, 157
β-lactam antibiotics, 1162–1164, 1203–1216
    absorption of, 1204
    adverse reactions and interactions, 1153, 1212–1216, 1215t

β-lactam antibiotics *(Continued)*
    aminoglycosides and, 1236
    for cancer patients, 735
    chemical structure of, 1162, 1162f
    clinical use of, 1203t
    distribution of, 1204
    dosage in special circumstances, 1212, 1213t–1214t
    drug interactions, 1216
    for gonorrhea, 595
    indications for, 1206–1212
        anaerobic infections, 1210
        biliary system infections, 1211
        central nervous system infections, 1210–1211
        endovascular infections, 1211–1212
        gram-negative organisms, 1210
        gram-positive bacilli, 1210
        intra-abdominal infections, 1211
        Lyme disease, 1212
        neutropenic fever, 1212
        pancreatitis, 1211
        pneumococcal infections, 1209
        spontaneous bacterial peritonitis, 1211
        staphylococcal infections, 1209
        syphilis, 1212
    mechanism of action of, 1204
    mode of action of, 1162–1163, 1163f–1164f
    pharmacodynamics of, 1164
    pharmacokinetics and distribution, 1204, 1204f, 1205t
    for postsplenectomy sepsis, 777
    prophylaxis, 1206–1209
    for prostatitis, 535
    resistance to, 1163–1164, 1165f, 1166t, 1181–1185, 1184f, 1204
        β-lactamase-mediated, 1181–1184
        mediated by altered PBPs, 1184
        mediated by impermeability or efflux, 1184–1185
    route of administration and dosage, 1206
    spectrum of activity, generic names, routes of administration and dosages, 1206–1207t
    for *Staphylococcus aureus*, 1520
    susceptibilities of selected bacteria to, 1208t–1209t
    for tularemia, 1089
    in urinary tract infections, 763
    see also specific drugs
β-lactamase inhibitors, anaerobic bacteria and, 1643
β-lactamases, 1163–1164
    for *Acinetobacter baumannii*, 1590t
    for *Alcaligenes* spp., 1597
    anaerobic bacteria and, 1634, 1634b, 1642
    classification based on relevant functional properties and molecular class, 1183t
    extended-spectrum, 1210, 1576
    functional classification of, 1166t
    multidrug-resistant gram-negative bacteria producing extended-spectrum, 1289
    Neisseria, 1557t
    for *Pseudomonas aeruginosa*, 1590, 1590t
    resistance to, 1592t
    Stenotrophomonas maltophilia and, 1597
Lactate, plasma, 420
Lactation, quinolones in, 1246
Lactic acid bacteria (LAB), 1523
Lactic acidosis
    linezolid complications, 1231–1232
    nucleoside analogue reverse transcriptase inhibitor, 910
    zidovudine and stavudine causing, 920
Lactobacillus, 1630
    in atrophic vaginitis, 489
    in bacterial vaginosis, 483, 485
    in human bites, 683t
    microflora, 355
    in normal flora, 1632
    in vulvovaginal candidiasis, 486–487
Lactoferrin, 332–333
Lactoferrin-binding proteins, 1557t, 1559
Lady Windermere syndrome, 1649
Lagovirus
    nature of, 1393
    taxonomy of, 1394t
Lamivudine, 1146t–1148t, 1298–1299
    adverse reactions of, 1299
    antiretroviral drugs, 921
    chemical structure of, 1296f

Lamivudine *(Continued)*
for chronic hepatitis B, 1327–1329
description of, 1298
dosage of, 1298
in special circumstances, 1297t, 1299
drug interactions of, 1299
for hepatitis B virus, 366
in HIV, 896–897
for hepatitis D virus, 372
indications of, 1298–1299
perinatal HIV transmission prevention, 909, 909t
pharmacokinetics and distribution of, 1298
resistance to, 1299
route of administration, 1298
Lancefield grouping, 1523
Laninamivir, 1321
adverse reactions and interactions of, 1321
dosage of, 1321
in special circumstances, 1321
indications of, 1321
pharmacokinetics and distribution of, 1320t, 1321
prophylaxis, 1321
route of administration, 1321
treatment with, 1321
Lanosterol 14-α-demethylase, inhibition of, 1336
Laparoscopic surgery, clean-contaminated operations, 687
Laparoscopy
in diagnosis, of pelvic inflammatory disease, 493
intra-abdominal sepsis, peritonitis and, 356–357
Laparotomy, and surgical site infection, percentage rate of, 687t
Laribacter hongkongensis, 338
Larva migrans, 1763–1764
cutaneous, and occupational infections, 648t–649t
pathogenicity of, 1770
visceral, 1770
treatment of, 1345t–1351t
Laryngeal diphtheria, 229
Laryngitis, 229–231
clinical features of, 229–230
diagnosis of, 230, 230f
differential diagnosis of, 230, 230b
epidemiology of, 229
management and treatment of, 230–231
physiopathology of, 229
prevention of, 229
Laryngotracheobronchitis, 233
Lassa fever, 1500t
and bioterrorism, 671t
clinical manifestations, 1501
diagnostic microbiology, 1501
epidemiology, 1500
lymphadenopathy and, 137t–138t
management, 1501
prevention, 1501
Lassa virus, 1499
clinical features of, 1114t–1115t
epidemiology of, 1110–1113, 1112t
management of, 1117
Late stage antibacterial pipeline, 1384, 1385t
Latency reversing agents (LRAS), 1491
Lateral flow antigen kit (LFA), for *Cryptococcus*, 1693–1694
Lateral flow assay (LFA), for brucellosis, 1616
Latex agglutination, meningitis and, 187–188
Latex agglutination assays, for *Staphylococcus aureus*, 1516–1517
Latex agglutination tests
for coccidioidomycosis, 1705
for *Cryptococcus*, 1693–1694
for rotaviruses, 1393
Latin America, infections in, 1130
Leclercia adecarboxylata, 1577t
Lectin, 1009
Lectin pathway, complement, 37
Ledipasvir (LDV), for hepatitis C, 1332
Leflunomide, 1379
Legionella, 1611, 1622–1624
causing endocarditis, 461t
clinical manifestations of, 1624
diagnostic microbiology of, 1623–1624, 1623f
epidemiology of, 1622–1623
hospital-acquired pneumonia and, 259t
management of, 1624
nature of, 1622, 1622t

Legionella (Continued)
pathogenicity of, 1623
prevention of, 1623
and tumor necrosis factor inhibitor, 797–799
Legionella anisa, 1622t
Legionella bozemanii, 1622t
Legionella cincinnatiensis, 1622t
Legionella dumoffii, 1622t
Legionella feeleii, 1622t
Legionella gormanii, 1622t
Legionella hackeliae, 1622t
Legionella jordanis, 1622t
Legionella lansingensis, 1622t
Legionella longbeachae, 1622t
Legionella lytica, 1622t
Legionella maceachernii, 1622t
Legionella micdadei, 1622t
Legionella oakridgensis, 1622t
Legionella parisiensis, 1622t
Legionella pneumophila, 1622t
diagnostic microbiology of, 1623
epidemiology of, 1623
fusidic acid for, 1277
ketolides, 1221
macrolides, 1217, 1221
pathogenicity of, 1623
Legionella sainthelensi, 1622t
Legionella tucsonensis, 1622t
Legionella wadsworthii, 1622t
Legionellaceae, lower respiratory tract infections, 264f
Legionnaires' disease, 645, 1624
Leiomyoma, in HIV-infected children, 902–903
Leiomyosarcoma, in HIV-infected children, 902–903
Leishmania
in HIV in low- and middle-income countries, 892
jaundice, 1135t
nature of, 1756
New World, 1757
Old World, 1757
pathogenesis and pathology of, 1060
pathogenicity of, 1756
Leishmania aethiopica, 1059, 1756t
Leishmania braziliensis, 1756t
epidemiology of, 1059–1060
management of, 1758
mucocutaneous leishmaniasis caused by, 1758
Leishmania chagasi, 1059
in HIV in low- and middle-income countries, 892
Leishmania donovani, 1059, 1756t
in HIV in low- and middle-income countries, 892
Leishmania guyanensis, 1756t
Leishmania infantum, 1059
in HIV in low- and middle-income countries, 892
Leishmania major, 142, 1059, 1756t
Leishmania mexicana, 1059–1060, 1756t
Leishmania tropica, 1060, 1756t
epidemiology of, 1059
Leishmaniasis, 1059–1064, 1756–1758
clinical features of, 1060–1062
clinical manifestations of, 1757–1758
cutaneous. *see* Cutaneous leishmaniasis
dermatologic manifestations of, 114t–115t
diagnosis of, 1062–1063, 1062f–1063f
diagnostic microbiology of, 1756–1757
epidemiology of, 1059–1060, 1059f–1060f, 1756
lymphadenopathy and, 137t–138t, 142
management of, 1063–1064, 1758
mucocutaneous. *see* Mucocutaneous leishmaniasis
nature of, 1756, 1756t
New World, 1757, 1757f
Old World, 1757
pathogenesis and pathology of, 1060
pathogenicity of, 1756
post-kala-azar dermal, 1062
prevention of, 1060, 1756
in transfusion-related infections, 704
treatment of, 1345t–1351t, 1368–1369
and tumor necrosis factor inhibitor, 800
visceral. *see* Visceral leishmaniasis
Leishmaniasis recidivans (LC), 1757
Lemierre's syndrome, 314
anaerobic bacteria in, 1636, 1637f
Lenalidomide, 1379

Lepromatous leprosy, 955, 1648
borderline, 955–956
clinical features of, 956–957, 957f
mid-borderline, 955–956, 957f
Lepromin testing, 958
Leprosy, 954–960
from armadillos, 668
clinical features of, 956–958, 982
dermatologic manifestations of, 114t–115t
diagnosis of, 958
epidemiology of, 954, 1648
eye involvement in, 982
in HIV, in low- and middle-income countries, 891
indeterminate, 956
lepromatous. *see* Lepromatous leprosy
management of, 959–960
multidrug therapy for, 954–956, 959
multibacillary, 959
paucibacillary, 959
pathogenesis and pathology of, 955, 955f, 982
peripheral nerve involvement in, 957
prevention of, 955–956
pure neural, 957
quinolones for, 1245
reactions, 955, 957–960
tuberculoid. *see* Tuberculoid leprosy
Leptospira, 1102, 1102f, 1600, 1608–1610, 1610b
in chronic meningitis, 186t
jaundice, 1135t
lincomycin, 1225
Leptospira biflexa, 1608–1609
Leptospira interrogans, 1608–1609
ketolides, 1221
macrolides, 1221
Leptospirosis, 645, 1102–1104
from bears, 669
clinical features of, 1103
clinical manifestations of, 1609
definitions of, 1610b
diagnosis of, 1103
diagnostic microbiology of, 1609
from dog urine, 658
epidemiology of, 1102, 1609
eye involvement in, 982
from insectivores, 668
jaundice and, 1135–1136
management of, 1103–1104, 1609–1610
from marine mammals, 668
from mongooses, 667–668
and occupational infections, 648t–649t, 650, 651t–654t
pathogenesis and pathology of, 1102–1103, 1102f, 1609
prevention of, 1103, 1609
from rodents, 667
transmission of, 664
Leptotrombidium, 1091
Leuconostoc spp., intrinsic resistance of, 1182t
Leukemias
and fever of unknown origin, 611
lymphadenopathy and, 137t–138t
Leukocidin, 1585
Leukocidin E/D (LukED), 1513t–1514t
Leukocyte adhesion deficiency, 709–710
type 1, 705t, 709–710, 710f
type 2, 710
Leukoencephalopathy, progressive multifocal, 1446–1447
Leukotoxins, group A streptococci and, 1529
Levamisole, 1000, 1001t
Levofloxacin
for anaerobic bacteria, 1643
for community-acquired pneumonia and, 255t
for complicated urinary tract infection, 544t–545t
dissociation constants of, 535t
for foot ulcers, 131t
for hospital-acquired pneumonia, 260t
for infective arthritis, 386t
prophylaxis with, 1158t
in cancer patients, 729–730
for prostatitis, 536t
Lice, 106t, 107–108
relapsing fever from, 1607–1608
tropical rickettsioses, 1091, 1092t–1093t
see also specific types
Lichen planus, 585, 586t–587t
erosive, 586t–587t
Lichen sclerosis, 585, 586t–587t

Lichtheimia, 1696
Licks, treatment of, 1462
Lifestyle, in HIV infection risk, 927
Ligation-based genome sequencing, 63t
Light microscopy, examination by, of *Cryptosporidium* spp., 1737–1738
Limb inflammation, in filariasis, 1049
Limbal follicles, 980
Lincomycin, 1171, 1222
  antibacterial activity, 1224–1225
  chemical structure, 1223–1224
  in hepatic impaired patients, 1226
  intramuscular form, 1226
  intravenous form, 1226
  metabolism, 1226
  oral form, 1226
  pharmacokinetics, 1226
  rectal form, 1226
  in renal impaired patients, 1226
  safety, 1226
Lincosamides, 1171, 1222–1227
  antibacterial activity, 1224–1225, 1225t
  chemical structure of, 1171, 1223–1224
  exit tunnel, 1221
  mode of action of, 1171
    and resistance, 1225–1226
  pharmacokinetics, 1226–1227
  resistance to, 1171, 1187–1189, 1188t
    by efflux, 1189
    by enzymatic modification, 1189
    by target modification, 1187–1189
Line probe assay, for mycobacteria, 1654
Linezolid, 1230
  adverse reactions and interactions, 1231–1232
  for anaerobic bacteria, 1643
  for catheter-related bloodstream infection (CRBSI), 436t
  chemical structure of, 1173–1174, 1173f
  distribution, 1230
  dosage, 1230–1231
  for foot ulcers, 131t
  for hospital-acquired pneumonia, 260t
  for hydrocephalus shunts, 223
  indications for, 1230–1231, 1231t
  for infective arthritis, 386t
  for lung abscess, 269f
  pharmacokinetics, 1230
  resistance to, 1193, 1231
  route, 1230
  Staphylococcus aureus and, 1519
  in vitro antimicrobial susceptibility for, against common gram-positive pathogens, 1231t
Linopristin-flopristin, antibacterial activities, 1228t
Lipase, 1513t–1514t
Lipiarmycins, 1177
  chemical structure of, 1177
  mode of action of, 1177, 1177f
  pharmacodynamics of, 1177
Lipid A, 19t
Lipid abnormalities, in HIV infection, 913–914
Lipid formulation amphotericin B
  for blastomycosis, 295
  for coccidioidomycosis, 296
  for histoplasmosis, 294
  for paracoccidioidomycosis, 297
  for sporotrichosis, 298
Lipid formulations, amphotericin B deoxycholate and, 1333–1335
Lipid storage disease, lymphadenopathy and, 137t–138t
Lipo-oligosaccharide (LOS)
  and *Haemophilus influenzae*, 1618
  Neisseria, 1557t, 1559
Lipoarabinomannan (LAM), 870
Lipoatrophy, in skin manifestations of HIV, 886
Lipodystrophy, antiretroviral-associated, in skin manifestations of HIV, 886
Lipoglycopeptides, 1164–1167
  chemical structure of, 1164
  mode of action of, 1164, 1167f
  resistance to, 1164–1167
Lipohypertrophy, in skin manifestations of HIV, 886

Lipopeptides, 1178
  chemical structure of, 1178
  mode of action of, 1178
  pharmacodynamics of, 1178
  resistance to, 1178
Lipopolysaccharide, 12, 608
  of anaerobic bacteria, 1633
  in *Brucella* spp., 1614–1615
  chlamydial, 1677
  innate immunity, 28–29
  intra-abdominal sepsis, pancreatitis and, 356
  Neisseria, 1557t
  in pertussis, 1613t
  Pseudomonas aeruginosa and, 1584–1585
  in sepsis, 419, 419f, 422f
Liposomal AmB (L-AmB), for catheter-related bloodstream infection (CRBSI), 436t
Liposomal amphotericin, for leishmaniasis, 1064
Liposomal daunorubicin, 875t
Lipoteichoic acid, 14
Listeria
  keratitis and, 152
  treatment with β-lactam antibiotics, 1204
Listeria grayi, 1537–1538
Listeria innocua, 1537–1538
Listeria ivanovii, 1537–1538
Listeria monocytogenes, 1537–1540
  actin-based intracellular motility, 16–17, 18f
  bacterial enteritis and, 338
  and bioterrorism, 671t
  clinical manifestations of, 1539–1540
  in contaminated food, 1538
  culture of, 1538–1539
  diagnosis of, 339
  diagnostic microbiology for, 1538–1539
  diarrhea and, 331, 335
  direct examination of, 1538
  epidemiology of, 1538
  hospital-acquired pneumonia and, 259t
  identification of, 1539, 1539f
  intrinsic resistance of, 1182t
  jaundice, 1135t
  ketolides, 1220
  macrolides, 1220
  meningitis and, 177
  nature of, 1537–1538
  pathogenicity of, 1538
  prevention of, 1540
  in thoracic transplantation patients, 749
  transmission of, 664, 665t
  treatment of, 1540
Listeria seeligeri, 1537–1538
Listeria welshimeri, 1537–1538
Listeriolysin O (LLO), 16–17, 1538
Listeriosis
  annual incidence of, 1538
  encephalitis, 773
  neonatal, 1540, 1540t
  in pregnancy, 499t, 1540
Live attenuated vaccines, for kidney transplant patients, 769
Live vaccines
  for children with congenital HIV infection, 795
  for children with inherited immune deficiency syndrome, 791
  in cocoon strategy, 787
  immunogenicity of, and patient's state of immunocompetency, 787
  and immunoglobulin administration, 795
  for immunosuppressed patients, 785, 786t
  for solid organ transplant patients, 787
  timing of, in hematopoietic stem cell transplant, 791
Liver abscess
  amebic, 360–361
    clinical features of, 1010–1011, 1010f, 1010t
    complications of, 1011
    diagnosis of, 1011
    diagnostic microbiology of, 1729
    differential diagnosis of, 1012
    percutaneous drainage for, 1013
    surgical drainage for, 1013
    treatment of, 997, 1012–1013

Liver abscess *(Continued)*
  brain abscess and, 199
  in cancer patients, 728
  Klebsiella pneumoniae in, 1576
  in melioidosis, 1074
Liver disease
  HBV and HCV associated, 768
  in immune reconstitution inflammatory syndrome, 863
  β-lactam antibiotics dosage in, 1212
Liver enzymes, abnormal, on anti-TB therapy, 308, 309f
Liver failure, symptoms of, 363
Liver flukes, 1032, 1764t
  clinical features of, 1036
  clinical manifestations of, 1778
  diagnosis of, 1036
  epidemiology of, 1036, 1036f, 1765
  infections of, 1036
  management of, 1036
  pathogenesis and pathology of, 1036
  pathogenicity of, 1770–1772
Liver tests, monitoring, 308, 309f
Liver transplantation, 751–755
  clinical presentation of, 752–753, 753f
    beyond sixth month, 753
    in first month, 752
    in second to sixth month, 752–753
  diagnosis and surveillance, 753–754
    bacterial surveillance, 753–754
    diagnostic methodologies in, 754
    hepatitis virus surveillance in, 754
    screening for CMV in, 754
  management of, 754–755, 754t
    prevention in, 754–755, 754t
    therapy of established infection in, 755
  pre-transplant infectious disease evaluation, 751, 751t
  risk factors, 751–752, 752t
    epidemiologic exposures, underlying disease, and patient characteristics, 751–752
    net state of immunosuppression, 752
    surgical factors and the hospital environment, 752
Loa loa
  clinical manifestations of, 1777
  epidemiology of, 1046, 1765
  life cycle of, 1769f
  lymphadenopathy and, 137t–138t
  pathogenicity of, 1768–1770
  treatment of, 1345t–1351t
Lobo disease. *see* Lobomycosis.
Loboa loboi, 1712, 1715
  diagnostic microbiology of, 1716–1717
  prevention of, 1715–1716
Lobomycosis
  clinical manifestations of, 1720
  diagnostic microbiology of, 1716–1717, 1717f
  epidemiology of, 1713–1714
  management of, 1723
  nature of, 1712
  pathogenicity of, 1715
  prevention of, 1715–1716
Loiasis, 1047t
  clinical features of, 1050
  dermatologic manifestations of, 114t–115t
  diagnosis of, 1050
  epidemiology of, 1046
  management of, 1051
  pathogenesis and pathology of, 1047, 1048f
  prevention of, 1049
Lomefloxacin
  for anaerobic bacteria, 1643
  dissociation constants of, 535t
  for prostatitis, 536t–537t
Lone Star tick, 1671
Long-term acute care hospitals, antimicrobial stewardship in, 1200
Long-term antibiotic suppression, for prosthetic joint infection (PJI), 402
Long-term care facilities, antimicrobial stewardship in, 1200
Loop electrosurgical excision procedure (LEEP), 583
Loperamide, for food-borne diarrheal illness, 333
Lopinavir, 1148t
  effect on oral contraceptives, 907t
  perinatal HIV transmission prevention, 909t

Lopinavir-ritonavir, 1303–1304
  adverse reactions of, 1304
  antiretroviral drugs, 922
  description of, 1303
  dosage of, 1302
    in special circumstances, 1304
  drug interactions of, 1304
  indications of, 1303
  pharmacokinetics and distribution of, 1303
  resistance to, 1303–1304
  route of administration of, 1303
Loracarbef
  antimicrobial spectrum, routes of administration and
    dosages, 1206t–1207t
  dosage in renal failure, 1213t–1214t
  pharmacokinetics of, 1205t
  susceptibilities of selected bacteria to, 1208t–1209t
Lorazepam, for convulsions, 1025
Louse-borne relapsing fever, 1106, 1109
Low bone mineral density (BMD), osteoporosis and, 929
Low-grade squamous intraepithelial lesion (LSIL),
    580–581, 580f
Lower respiratory tract
  disease, in hematopoietic stem cell transplantation, 743
  secretions, 267
  special investigations and techniques, 258
Lower respiratory tract infections, 266t, 267f
  bacteria responsible for, 1221
  causes in adults, 264f
  macrolides and ketolides for, 1221
  in pregnancy, 503
  Pseudomonas aeruginosa in, 1587–1588
Ludwig's angina, 96, 96f, 313–314, 314f
  anaerobic bacteria in, 1636
  lymphadenopathy and, 137t–138t
Lujo virus, 1500t
Lumbar puncture
  brain abscess and, 201
  encephalitis/myelitis of, 196
  meningitis and, 184
Lumefantrine
  for falciparum malaria, 1022
  for parasitic infections, 1345t–1351t, 1367
Lumens, in catheter-related bloodstream infection
    (CRBSI), 430
Luminal amebicides, 1012
Lung abscesses, 263–270, 265f, 267f
  clinical features of, 266
  diagnosis of, 266–268
  epidemiology of, 263
  investigations of, 267–268
  management of, 268–270
  in melioidosis, 1074
  pathogenesis and pathology of, 263–265
  prevention of, 265–266
  risk factors for, 264t
Lung disease, in immune reconstitution inflammatory
    syndrome, 863
Lung flukes, 1032, 1764t
  clinical features of, 1037
  clinical manifestations of, 1778
  diagnosis of, 1037
  epidemiology of, 1037, 1765
  infections of, 1037
  management of, 1037
  pathogenesis and pathology of, 1037
  pathogenicity of, 1770–1772
  treatment of, 1345t–1351t
Lung infection, Rhodococcus equi and, 1551
Lung transplantation, 746–750
  cardiovascular infections in, 748
  and CMV prevention and treatment, 748
  considerations related to micro-organisms in, 748–750
    bacterial infections, 749
    fungal infections, 749–750
    viral infections, 748–749
  epidemiology of, 746
  indications for, 746
  for pneumonia, 746–747
  for postsurgical mediastinitis, 747
  risk factors for infection of, 746, 747b
  specific clinical syndromes, 746–748
  for sternum osteomyelitis, 747
Lungs, specimen collection in, 1634t
Lupus vulgaris, 117, 118f

Lyme disease, 405–414
  arthritis
    clinical features of, 409
    diagnosis of, 411
    management of, 413
  in chronic meningitis, 186t
  clinical features of, 407–409
  diagnostic investigations of, 409–411, 410b
  early
    clinical features of, 407–408, 407f–408f
    diagnosis of, 410–411
    management of, 412
  early disseminated disease
    clinical features of, 408–409
    diagnosis of, 411
    management of, 412
  epidemiology of, 405
  history of, 405
  β-lactam antibiotics for, 1212
  management of, 411–413, 412t
  in myocarditis, 447
  neurologic, 411
  persistent/late, clinical features of, 409
  post-Lyme disease syndrome, 413–414
  in pregnancy, 413, 499t
  prognosis of, 413–414
  and recreational infections, 644
  serologic response in, 410f
  tetracyclines for, 1259
  two-tiered testing for, 410f
Lymph node(s), 139f
  aspirates, in syphilis, 563
  blastomycosis and, 1703
  in bubonic plague, 1081–1082, 1082f
  disease, in tuberculosis, 278
  enlarged, 146–149
    clinical manifestations of, 146–149
    immune reconstitution and, 148f
    infectious etiologies of, 147t–148t
    investigations for, 149
    management of, 149
  in HIV infection, 840–841, 840f
  for laboratory diagnosis, of mycobacteria, 1651t
  lymphogranuloma venereum in, 587–588
  normal, 136, 136f
  physical characteristics of enlarged, 144
  regions, 136
Lymphadenitis
  acute cervical, 139
  acute suppurative, 139
  cervical. see Cervical lymphadenitis
  and HIV-associated TB, 868
  in immune reconstitution inflammatory syndrome, 862,
    862f
  mycobacterial, 140
  nontuberculous mycobacteria (NTM), 287
  pathogenesis and pathology of, 136–138
  tuberculosis, 278, 869
Lymphadenopathy, 136–145
  abdominal, 145
  axillary, 145, 149
  causes of, 1140b
  cervical, 149
  clinical features of, 139–144
  differential diagnosis of, 137t–138t
  disease progression of, 144
  epidemiology of, 138–139
  epitrochlear, 149
  head and neck, 145
  infectious, 137t–138t
  inguinal, 140t, 145, 149
  location of, 144–145, 144t
  in lymphogranuloma venereum, 587
  management, 144–145
  mode of presentation, 144
  noninfectious, 137t–138t, 147t
  parasitic, 141–143
  pathogenesis and pathology of, 136–138
  physical characteristics of enlarged lymph node, 144
  regional, 139–140
  role of age, 144
  and splenomegaly and anemia, 1139–1140
  suppurative, 149
  supraclavicular, 149
  in syphilis, 561–562

Lymphadenopathy (Continued)
    thoracic, 145
    viral, 143–144
    in visceral leishmaniasis, 1060–1061
Lymphangitis
    from cat bites, 659
    cellulitis and, 90f
    in filarial infections, 1050
    sclerosing, 586t–587t
Lymphangitis-associated rickettsiosis, 1667t, 1668, 1668f
    location of, 1092t–1093t
Lymphatic filariasis, 1047t, 1768, 1777–1778
    clinical features of, 1049
    diagnosis of, 1050
    epidemiology of, 1046
    management of, 1050–1051
    pathogenesis and pathology of, 1047, 1048f
    prevention of, 1048
Lymphedema, in Kaposi's sarcoma, 874
Lymphocyte immune deficiencies, 712–718, 714f
Lymphocytes
    changes in, during primary HIV infection, 848, 849f
    in tuberculosis, 273
    see also B lymphocytes; T lymphocytes
Lymphocytic choriomeningitis virus (LCMV), 661, 806,
    1499, 1500t
    in chronic meningitis, 186t
    clinical manifestations, 1501
    diagnostic microbiology, 1501
    encephalitis/myelitis caused by, 193t–194t
    epidemiology, 1500
Lymphogranuloma venereum (LGV), 141, 585–589,
    586t–587t
    Chlamydia trachomatis and, 597, 1678
    clinical features of, 587–589, 587f–588f
    diagnosis of, 589
    epidemiology of, 585–587
    and fever of unknown origin, 613
    lymphadenopathy and, 137t–138t
    management of, 589
    pathogenesis and pathology of, 587
Lymphohistiocytosis, familial, hemophagocytic, 721
Lymphoid follicles, 980
Lymphoid interstitial pneumonitis, 902–903, 903f
Lymphoma
    and fever of unknown origin, 611
    lymphadenopathy and, 137t–138t
    see also Hodgkin's lymphoma; Non-Hodgkin's
      lymphoma
Lymphomatoid granulomatosis, 137t–138t
Lymphophagous mites, 105
Lymphoproliferative syndrome, X-linked, 721
Lysis-centrifugation, for histoplasmosis, 1707
Lysozyme, 1522
Lyssaviruses, 666, 1458
    in Africa, 1463
    in Australia, 1463
    in China and Asia, 1463
    in Europe, 1463

M
M protein, 471–472, 475
M2 inhibitors, 1318
    adverse reactions and interactions of, 1318
    indications of, 1318
    pharmacokinetics and distribution of, 1318
    resistance to, 1318
    route of administration and dosage of, 1318
Machupo virus, 1110, 1112t, 1500t
Macroconidia, 1706
Macrolide antibiotics, 1367
Macrolide antimicrobials, for postsplenectomy sepsis,
    777
Macrolides, 1171, 1217–1222
    accumulation ratio of, 1222t
    advantages, 1222
    adverse reactions and interactions, 1222
    for anaerobic bacteria, 1643
    as antituberculosis agents, 1271
    bacterial targeting, 1171
    characteristics of, 1218t
    chemical structure of, 1171, 1172f
    classification, 1217, 1218f
    clinical studies, 1222

Macrolides (Continued)
definitions, 1217
exit tunnel, 1221
indications, community-acquired pneumonia, 255
intra-bacterial penetration, 1221
intracellular concentrations, 1221
for Legionella spp., 1624
mechanism of action, 1221
mode of action of, 1171, 1173f
for Mycoplasma hominis, 1664
versus other antibacterials, 1222
peptidyltransferase center, 1221
for pertussis, 1614
pharmacodynamic properties, 1222
pharmacodynamics of, 1171
pharmacokinetic properties, 1222, 1223t–1224t
physicochemical characteristics, 1217–1218
for prostatitis, 535–536
resistance to, 1171, 1187–1189, 1188t
by efflux, 1189
by enzymatic modification, 1189
mechanism of, 1221–1222
by target modification, 1187–1189
selection of drugs whose metabolism may interfere
with, 1225t
stability in acidic medium, 1217–1218, 1219f
tissue distribution, 1224t
in vitro activity, 1219–1221, 1220t
Macrophage activation syndrome (MAS), 638
Macrophages
cryptococcosis and, 1692
Histoplasma capsulatum and, 1707
innate immune response, 31, 31f
mycobacteria and, 1649, 1650f
polarization of, 638
in tuberculosis, 273
Macular retinitis, 168f
Macular star, 168, 169f
Maculopapular rash, 846, 847f
Madurella grisea, 1714
Madurella mycetomatis, 1717f
MagicPlex™ sepsis system, 1388
Magnetic resonance cholangiogram (MRC), biliary sepsis,
360
Magnetic resonance imaging (MRI)
in bacterial arthritis, 385, 385f
in cancer patients, 733
deep cervical space infection, 315
of echinococcosis, 1043–1044
encephalitis/myelitis of, 195
in endocarditis, 463
of herpes simplex encephalitis, 227f
for infected foot ulcers, 130
intra-abdominal sepsis, peritonitis and, 356–357
of melioidosis, 1077
necrotizing fasciitis, 95–96
of neurocysticercosis, 1035
in osteomyelitis, 394, 395f
spinal epidural abscess and, 206, 206f
studies, in chronic fatigue syndrome, 634
subdural empyema/intracranial epidural abscess, 205f
Major facilitator superfamily (MFS), 1194f
Major histocompatibility complex (MHC)
class II deficiency, 718–719
Listeria monocytogenes and, 1538
molecules, 32
mycobacteria and, 1649–1650
Malabsorption, lactose, in viral gastroenteritis, 1397
Malakoplakia, 1549
Malaria, 1014–1025
airport, 945
algid, 1021
bite avoidance measures of, 951
cerebral. see Cerebral malaria
chemoprophylaxis for, 951
clinical features of, 1018–1021
cerebral malaria, 1019, 1021f
severe, 1019–1021, 1019f, 1020t
abnormal bleeding, 1020t, 1021
acidosis, 1019, 1020t
acute renal failure, 1020t
anemia, 1019–1020, 1020t
blackwater fever, 1020t, 1021, 1021f

Malaria (Continued)
circulatory shock, 1020t, 1021
coma, 1020t
fluid/electrolyte imbalances, 1020t
hyperparasitemia, 1020t
hypoglycemia, 1020, 1020t
renal impairment, 1020–1021
respiratory distress, 1020t, 1021
severe jaundice, 1020t
uncomplicated, 1018
combined drug regimens for, 1153
diagnosis of, 1022
in pregnancy, 1142
differential diagnosis of, 1022
elimination and eradication of, 1018
epidemiology of, 1014–1016
epidemiologic factors, 1014
geographic distribution of, 1014–1016, 1015f
eye involvement in, 982
geographic distribution of, 939, 940f, 946f–947f
in geographic influences on differential diagnosis, 945
in HIV, in low- and middle-income countries, 892–893
jaundice and, 1136
management of, 1022–1025
in pregnancy, 1142
severe malaria, 1024–1025
acute renal failure, 1025
anemia, 1025
antimalarial treatment, 1024, 1024t
artesunate and artemether, 1024
convulsions, 1025
hemodynamic shock, 1025
quinine, 1024–1025
supportive treatment, 1025
uncomplicated
caused by P. vivax, P. ovale and P. malariae,
1023–1024, 1024b
caused by Plasmodium falciparum, 1022–1023,
1023t–1024t
pathogenesis and pathology of, 1016–1017
cytoadherence, 1016–1017
immunologic factors and cytokines, 1017
parasite, 1016, 1016f
permeability and intracranial pressure, 1017
red cell, resetting and auto-agglutination, 1017
postsplenectomy, prevention of, 776–777
in pregnancy, 498, 501, 503–504, 1141–1144, 1141t,
1143t–1144t
classification of, 1142t
treatment of, 1143t
prevention and control of, 950–951, 1017–1018
minimizing contact between vector and human host,
1017
prophylactic use of antimalarial drugs, 1017–1018,
1023t
vaccine development, 1018
severe
clinical cases, 1141–1142, 1142t
clinical features of, 1019–1021, 1019f, 1020t
abnormal bleeding, 1020t, 1021
acidosis, 1019, 1020t
acute renal failure, 1020t
anemia, 1019–1020, 1020t
blackwater fever, 1020t, 1021, 1021f
circulatory shock, 1020t, 1021
coma, 1020t
fluid/electrolyte imbalances, 1020t
hyperparasitemia, 1020t
hypoglycemia, 1020, 1020t
renal impairment, 1020–1021
respiratory distress, 1020t, 1021
severe jaundice, 1020t
management of, 1024–1025
acute renal failure, 1025
anemia, 1025
antimalarial treatment, 1024, 1024t
artesunate and artemether, 1024
convulsions, 1025
hemodynamic shock, 1025
quinine, 1024–1025
supportive treatment, 1025
tetracyclines for, 1259
in transfusion-related infections, 703, 704t

Malaria (Continued)
uncomplicated
clinical cases, 1142, 1142t
clinical features of, 1018
management of
caused by P. vivax, P. ovale and P. malariae,
1023–1024, 1024b
caused by Plasmodium falciparum, 1022–1023,
1023t–1024t
Malassezia
diagnostic microbiology of, 1711
epidemiology of, 122, 1710
nature of, 1710
normal skin flora, 127
pathogenicity of, 1711
Malassezia folliculitis
clinical features of, 126
management of, 128
Malassezia furfur, in HIV/AIDS, 879
Male circumcision
and HIV prevention, in low- and middle-income
countries, 894
voluntary, for HIV prevention, 821, 822f
Male genital tract, rhinosporidiosis in, 1721
Males, Chlamydia trachomatis infection in, 599, 599f–600f
Malignant histiocytosis, 137t–138t
Malignant lymphomas, 875–877
Malignant (necrotizing) otitis externa, 1589, 1592
Malta fever, 1616
Mandibular osteomyelitis, 393
Mange, 658–659
Mannitol, 203
Mansonella infections
clinical features of, 1050
dermatologic manifestations of, 114t–115t
epidemiology of, 1046–1047
management of, 1051
pathogenesis and pathology of, 1047–1048
prevention of, 1049
Mansonella ozzardi
life cycle of, 1769f
treatment of, 1345t–1351t
Mansonella perstans
life cycle of, 1769f
treatment of, 1345t–1351t
Mansonella streptocerca, treatment of, 1345t–1351t
Mansonellosis
clinical features of, 1050
epidemiology of, 1046
management of, 1051
pathogenesis and pathology of, 1047
Mantoux test, 274
MAR (multiple antibiotic resistance) system, 1194,
1194f
Maraviroc, 1148t, 1305–1306
adverse reactions of, 1306
antiretroviral drugs, 925
description of, 1305
dosage of, 1305–1306
in special circumstances, 1306
drug interactions of, 1306
effect on oral contraceptives, 907t
indications of, 1306
perinatal HIV transmission prevention, 910t
pharmacokinetics and distribution of, 1305
resistance to, 1306
route of administration of, 1305–1306
Marburg virus, 666
and bioterrorism, 671t
clinical features of, 1114t–1115t
clinical manifestations, 1506
diagnosis, 1506
epidemiology of, 1110–1113, 1112t, 1505–1506
geographic distribution of, 939–940
nature, 1505
prevention, 1506
Marine mammals, infections from, 668
Marshall's syndrome, pharyngitis, 234
Masks, 58
Mass gatherings, and recreational infections, 645–646
Mass spectrometry, 1387
matrix-assisted laser desorption/ionization-time of
flight (MALDI-TOF), 1580

Mastitis
pathogenesis of, 501
prevention of, 502
puerperal, 503
sporadic, 503
therapy of, 504
Mastoiditis
anaerobic bacteria in, 1636t
brain abscess and, 199, 200t
in otitis media, 238
subdural empyema/intracranial epidural abscess and, 203, 205t
Maternal immunity, 506–507
Maternal infections
fetal implications of, in pregnancy, 505–516. see also Congenital infection
serologic testing and, 511, 511b
Mathematical models in infectious disease epidemiology, 49–53
compartmental model of influenza, 51–52, 51f
dynamics of transmission, 50
emergency preparedness and response of, 52–53
epidemiologic data, 50
future research, 53
Matrix-assisted laser desorption/ionization-time of flight (MALDI-TOF) mass spectrometry, 156, 1386, 1388f, 1580
Mazzotti reaction, 1051
Meares and Stamey localization technique, 533, 534f
Measles, 1399–1402
acute, rash of, 77f
burden of disease, 940
clinical features of, 76–77, 982
clinical manifestations of, 1400–1401, 1401f, 1401t
croup and, 234–235
dermatologic manifestations of, 114t–115t
diagnostic microbiology of, 1399–1400
epidemiology of, 1399, 1400f
eye involvement in, 981–982
lymphadenopathy and, 137t–138t
management of, 1401–1402
nature of, 1399
and occupational infections, 648t–649t
immunization for, 650t
pathogenesis of, 981–982
pathogenicity of, 1399
pharyngitis, 234–235
in pregnancy, 499t
prevention of, 1399
secondary infections complicating, 77f
uveitis, 167
vaccination against, 782t–783t
in children with congenital HIV infection, 795
in children with inherited immune deficiency syndrome, 795
virus
actin-based intracellular motility, 18
encephalitis/myelitis caused by, 193t–194t
Measles, mumps and rubella (MMR) vaccination, for parotitis, 319
Measles, mumps and rubella viruses, 1399–1405
Mebendazole
for Echinococcus multilocularis, 1045
for gastrointestinal helminth, 1000, 1001t
for helminths, 1772
for parasitic infections, 1345t–1351t, 1371
mecA gene, 1181, 1184
Mechanical bowel preparation, 687
Median sternotomy, 481
Mediastinal fibrosis, 293–294
Mediastinal granuloma, 293–294
Mediastinitis, 481–482
classification of, 481t
diagnosis and treatment of, 481–482, 481f
Medical Outcomes Survey Short Form-36 (MOS SF-36), 631–632
Medical technology, emerging infectious diseases and, 46
Medicolegal issues, factitious fever, 637
Mediterranean spotted fever (MSF), 1667t, 1668, 1668f
location of, 1092t–1093t
Mefloquine
for falciparum malaria, 1022
for malaria prophylaxis, 951
Megacolon, chagasic, 1069, 1069f, 1072
Megaesophagus, chagasic, 1069, 1069f, 1072

Megasphaera spp., 1631
Meglumine antimoniate, for parasitic infections, 1345t–1362t, 1369
Melanin, 1716–1717
α-melanocyte stimulating hormone (αMSH), 609
Melanoma, in skin manifestation of HIV, 884–885
Melarsoprol
for African trypanosomiasis, 969–970, 969t, 1762
for parasitic infections, 1345t–1362t
Meleney's synergistic gangrene, 99
Melioidosis, 1073–1077, 1595
and bioterrorism, 671t
clinical features of, 1074–1075, 1075f–1076f
dermatologic manifestations of, 114t–115t
diagnosis of, 1075–1076, 1076f
epidemiology of, 1073, 1073t, 1074f
lymphadenopathy and, 137t–138t
management of, 1076–1077, 1077t
neurologic, 1077
pathogenesis and pathology of, 1073
prevention of, 1073, 1074b
Membrane, antibiotics acting on, 1178–1180
Membrane attack complex, 37
Membrane-disrupting toxins, 19t
Membranous cell gateway, 15–16
Menangle virus, 75t, 666
Mendelian disorders, late-onset, 809
Meningitis
Acinetobacter baumannii, 1595
acute bacterial, 177–185
adjunctive dexamethasone treatment of, 181–182, 184f
antibiotic prophylaxis of, 181, 183t
antibiotic treatment of, 180–181, 182t
clinical features of, 180
CSF analysis, 180
decline in consciousness of, 183
diagnosis and management of, 180–184
epidemiology of, 177
focal neurologic abnormalities of, 183–184
intensive care management of, 182–183
outcome of, 184–185
pathophysiology and pathology of, 177–180, 178f–179f, 181f
post-traumatic, 185
recurrent, 184
repeating a lumbar puncture, 184
skin biopsy, 180
vaccination, 177
Alcaligenes xylosoxidans in, 1597
anaerobic bacteria in, 1635
anthrax, 1126
antibiotics for, 1152t
in cancer patients, 728
from Candida, 444, 1684
chronic, 186–188, 186t
clinical features of, 186
cryptococcal, 1692, 1694, 1696t
in HIV, in low- and middle-income countries, 893
cryptococcosis in HIV/AIDS, 854–855
due to Aspergillus spp., 1689
due to Histoplasma capsulatum, 1708
Elizabethkingia meningoseptica in, 1598
Enterobacteriaceae in, 1575
eosinophilic, 971–978
causes of, 971b
clinical features of, 973–974
diagnosis of, 974–975, 978f
epidemiology of, 972–973, 976f–977f
main sources of infection for, 974t
management of, 975–976
noninfective causes of, 978
pathogenesis and pathology of, 971–972, 971b, 972f
prevention of, 973, 974t
uncommon infective causes of, 976
genital herpes and, 572
gonococcal, 1563
group B streptococci and, 1533
in immune reconstitution inflammatory syndrome, 861
in immunologically mediated diseases, 772
JC polyomavirus, 1447
β-lactam antibiotics for, 1210–1211
Leptospira spp. and, 1609
Listeria monocytogenes and, 1539
Lyme disease and, 409, 411–412, 412t

Meningitis (Continued)
meningococcal, 1563
permanent brain injury in, 179
plague, 1083
polymicrobial, 772
in pregnancy, 500, 503
Pseudomonas aeruginosa in, 1589
quinolones for, 1246
Stenotrophomonas maltophilia in, 1597
tuberculous, 186–187
viral
adaptation to local epidemiology and, 226
development and expansion of techniques for, 225–226
laboratory techniques for documentation of, 225–226
rapid viral detection in, 225–226
viruses causing, 225
Meningitis belt, 942f
Meningococcal carriage, 1564
Meningococcal disease
clinical manifestations of, 1563–1564, 1563f
diagnostic microbiology of, 1561
epidemiology of, 1556–1557, 1556f
management of, 1564
pathogenesis of, 1557–1558, 1558f
prevention of, 1560
Meningococcal infection, and occupational infections, 651t–654t
Meningococcal meningitis, 1553, 1563
eye involvement in, 982
Meningococcal vaccine
and occupational infections, 651t
for travelers, 950
Meningococcemia, 1563f, 1564
Meningococci, vaccination against, 782t–783t
Meningoencephalitis, 667
anthrax, 1127
in Chagas disease, 1072
cryptococcal, 1694
cryptococcosis in HIV/AIDS, 854–855
in melioidosis, 1074
mumps, 319
in primary HIV infection, 847
tuberculous, 279
Menopause, and HIV infection, 906
Menstrual cycle, and HIV infection, 906
Mepacrine, 1000t
Merkel cell cancer (MCC), 1447
Merkel cell polyomavirus (MCPyV), 1445
Meropenem
for anaerobic bacteria, 1643
antimicrobial spectrum, routes of administration and dosages, 1206t–1207t
against carbapenemase-resistant gram-negative bacilli, 1290t
for complicated urinary tract infection, 545t
dosage in renal failure, 1213t–1214t
for drowning-associated infections, 681
hospital-acquired pneumonia and, 260t
for melioidosis, 1077t
for P. aeruginosa infection, 1210
pharmacokinetics of, 1205t
for pneumococcal infections, 1209
susceptibilities of selected bacteria to, 1208t–1209t
Mesenteric adenitis, yersiniosis and, 1627
Metabolic acidosis, 1019, 1020t, 1021
Metabolic testing, in HIV infection, 915–916
Metagenomic sequence
data, 69f
shotgun, 70–71, 70f–71f
Metagenomics, 65
advances in, 1388–1389
Metagonimus spp., 1765
Metagonimus yokogawai
life cycle of, 1771f
treatment of, 1345t–1351t
Metapneumovirus. see Human metapneumovirus (hMPV).
Metastatic carcinoma, 137t–138t
Metastatic endophthalmitis, 169
causing retinitis and uveitis, 169t
Metastatic melanoma, lymphadenopathy and, 137t–138t
Metastatic tuberculous abscesses, 118

Methicillin
  pharmacokinetics of, 1205t
  susceptibilities of selected bacteria to, 1208t–1209t
Methicillin-resistant *Staphylococcus aureus* (MRSA), 254,
    1156, 1289–1290
  antimicrobials for, 1292f
  in arterial graft infection, 437
  in bacterial arthritis, 382–383
  Clostridium difficile infection (CDI), 352
  community-acquired, 1511, 1511f
  cutaneous abscesses in HIV/AIDS, 858
  in dog bites, 656
  endocarditis and, 467
  epidemiology of, 1509
  in foot ulcers, 130–131
  fusidic acid for, 1277
  in HIV/AIDS, 882–883
  identification of, 1518
  linezolid, 1231
  and occupational infections, 651t–654t
  in osteomyelitis, 395t
  prevention of, 1516
  pyomyositis and, 102–103
  screening for, 693–694
  and surgical site infections, 687
  treatment of, 691
  trimethoprim-sulfamethoxazole for, 1282
Methicillin-susceptible *Staphylococcus aureus* (MSSA),
    1509
  aminoglycosides for, 1233
Methotrexate, immunosuppression and, 1379
Metrifonate, 1352t–1362t, 1371
Metronidazole, 1261–1263
  for acute necrotizing ulcerative gingivitis, 316
  for amebic infections, 1012
  for anaerobic bacteria, 1262t, 1643
  for bacterial vaginosis, 484–485
  dosages of, 1261t
  for drowning-associated infections, 681
  for gastrointestinal protozoa, 997, 999, 1000t
  for giardiasis, 334
  for *Helicobacter pylori*, 326–327
  for intra-abdominal sepsis, 357
  for lung abscess, 269f
  for parasitic infections, 1345t–1362t, 1368
  prophylaxis, 1158t
  resistance to, 1193, 1261
  tetanus and, 212
  for trichomoniasis, 486
  for typhoid fever, 1007
Mezlocillin
  for anaerobic bacteria, 1210, 1643
  antimicrobial spectrum, routes of administration and
    dosages, 1206t–1207t
  dosage in renal failure, 1213t–1214t
  pharmacokinetics of, 1205t
  susceptibilities of selected bacteria to, 1208t–1209t
Micafungin, 1341–1343
  adverse effects of, 1343
  for cancer patients, 737–738
  for candidemia, 1686
  in children, 1343
  dosing and administration, 1341
  drug interactions of, 1343
  indications of, 1341–1342
  mechanism of action, 1341
  pharmacodynamics of, 1341
  pharmacokinetics and distribution of, 1341
  prophylaxis with, in cancer patients, 730
  structures of, 1342f
Michaelis-Gutmann bodies, 1549
Miconazole
  keratitis and, 154–155
  for primary amebic meningoencephalitis, 1749
  for vulvovaginal candidiasis, 488t
Micro-eukaryotic infections, microbiome and, 73–74
Micro-organisms, identification of, 1386–1387
Microabscesses, cerebral, *Candida* infections, 444
Microaerophilic bacteria, in human bites, 683t
Microagglutination test (MAT), 1103
Microbes, factors influencing types and abundance of,
    942b
Microbial-associated molecular patterns (MAMPs), 26

Microbial pathogenesis, important steps in, 11b
Microbial surface components recognizing adhesive
    matrix molecules (MSCRAMMs), 1512, 1513t–1514t
  enterococci and, 1530–1531
Microbial therapy, *Clostridium difficile* infection (CDI),
    353
Microbiologic diagnosis, of endocarditis, 460–461
Microbiologically documented infections (MDI), in cancer
    patients, 726, 726f
Microbiology
  in diagnosis, for cancer patients, 733
  intra-abdominal sepsis, 355–356
  in osteomyelitis, 389–390
Microbiology laboratory
  applications of genomics to, 64f
  see also Diagnostic microbiology
Microbiome, 72–74, 1373
  and bacterial infections, 72–73
  changes in, and immune response, 844
  Clostridium difficile infection (CDI), 351–352
  and fungal infections, 73
  in infectious diseases, 68–74
    culture-independent sequence-based taxonomic and
      functional profiling of, 69–71
    healthy, 71–72, 72f, 72t
    and micro-eukaryotic infections, 73–74
    and parasite infections, 73–74
    and viral infections, 73
Microbiota, human, 68
  micro-organisms in, 68f
Micrococcaceae, 1509
Micrococci, 1522
  diagnostic microbiology of, 1522
  management of, 1522
  nature of, 1509
Micrococcineae, 1547t
Microconidia, 1706
Microfilariae, detection of, 1050
Microflora
  anaerobes, 1631, 1632t
  normal, 12
  of human host, 4
Microhemagglutination assay for antibodies to *Treponema
    pallidum* (MHA-TP), in syphilis, 564, 564t
Microhematocrit centrifugation, African trypanosomiasis
    and, 969
Microimmunofluorescence (MIF) testing
  for *Chlamydia pneumoniae*, 1679
  for *Chlamydia trachomatis*, 1678
  for chronic chlamydial infections, 1679–1680
Microscopic agglutination test (MAT), 1609
Microscopic examination
  of blastomycosis, 1701f, 1702
  of coccidioidomycosis, 1705
  of histoplasmosis, 1707
Microscopy
  for Chagas disease, 1070–1071
  in diarrhea, 339
  for malaria diagnosis, 1022
Microsporidia
  of chronic diarrhea, 347t, 348
  diagnostic microbiology of, 1737t, 1738–1740,
    1739f–1740f
  epidemiology of, 1736
  intestinal, 1734–1743
  nature of, 1734, 1735t
  pathogenicity of, 1736–1737, 1736f
Microsporidiosis
  cerebral, 1741, 1742f
  chronic diarrhea and, 348
  in immunocompetent persons, 1741
  in immunocompromised patients, 1740–1741
  management of, 1742
  prevention of, 1737
  systemic, 1741
  treatment of, 1345t–1351t
Microsporum, 122
  diagnostic microbiology of, 1711
Microsporum audouinii
  clinical features of, 123–124, 123t
  epidemiology of, 122
  pathogenicity of, 1711
  prevention of, 123

Microsporum canis
  in cats, 660
  clinical features of, 123–124, 123t
  pathogenicity of, 1711
Mid-diastolic murmur, in rheumatic fever, 473
Middle East, infections in, 1130
Middle East respiratory syndrome coronavirus
    (MERS-CoV), 53, 1318, 1474
  infections, 1132
Midecamycin
  characteristics of, 1218t
  pharmacokinetics, 1223t
Midges, arboviruses, 1493
Midstream urine specimens, 527
Migration inhibitory factor, 422–423
Miliary tuberculosis, 277–278, 278f
Milk, agents transmitted via, 664, 665t
Miller-Fisher syndrome, 212
Miltefosine
  granulomatous amebic encephalitis, 1749–1750
  for leishmaniasis, 1064, 1758
  for parasitic infections, 1345t–1362t
  for primary amebic meningoencephalitis, 1749
Minimum inhibitory concentrations (MICs), 1590–1591
Minocycline
  background in, 1256
  for catheter-related bloodstream infection (CRBSI),
    436t
  for foot ulcers, 131t
  impregnated catheters, 433
  for leprosy, 959
  route of administration of, 1258
  for *Stenotrophomonas maltophilia*, 1597
  structure of, 1257f
Miocamycin
  characteristics of, 1218t
  pharmacokinetics, 1222, 1223t–1224t
  tissue distribution, 1224t
MiSeq platform, 69–70
'Mississippi baby,' HIV cure for, 931, 933f
Mites, 105–107, 107f
  scrub typhus and, 1091
  tropical rickettsioses and, 1091
  see also specific mites
Mitral valve prolapse, 459
Mitsuda reaction, 955
Mobiluncus, 1630
  in bacterial vaginosis, 483
  diagnosis of, 484
'Moccasin tinea pedis', 125, 125f
Models, 49
Molecular assays
  for detection of bacterial pathogens, 65
  in food-borne diarrheal illness, 333
Molecular detection, 1388
Molecular genotyping, 65
Molecular identification
  for chromoblastomycosis, 1716
  for lobomycosis, 1717
  of superficial fungal pathogens, 1712
'Molecular' Koch's postulates, 2b
Molecular methods
  for Chagas disease, 1071
  for microsporidia, 1740
  for mycobacteria identification, 1654
Molecular tests
  for helminths diagnosis, 1776–1777
  protozoa, intestinal and urogenital, 1732–1733
Molecular typing, of *Neisseria*, 1561–1562
Mollicutes, 1660
Molluscum contagiosum virus, 586t–587t, 1452f, 1454t
  clinical manifestations of, 1453–1454
  diagnosis and differential diagnosis of, 1454
  diagnostic microbiology of, 1456–1457
  epidemiology of, 1452
  geographic range of, 1452
  gross lesion pathology of, 1454, 1454f
  in HIV/AIDS, 882
  lesion histopathology of, 1453, 1453f
  management of, 1457
  pathogenicity of, 1452–1453
  prevalence and incidence of, 1452
  transmission of, 1452–1453

Mongooses, infections for, 667–668
Moniliformis moniliformis, treatment of, 1345t–1351t
Monkeypox virus, 75t, 1452, 1456
  dermatologic manifestations of, 114t–115t
  and occupational infections, 648t–649t
  transmission of, 661
Monkeys, infections from, 661
Monoarticular septic arthritis, 1563
Monobactams, 1162, 1203
  antimicrobial spectrum, generic names, routes of
    administration and dosages, 1206t–1207t
  dosage in renal failure, 1213t–1214t
  drug interactions, 1216
  pharmacokinetics of, 1205t
  for *Pseudomonas aeruginosa*, 1589
  susceptibilities of selected bacteria to, 1208t–1209t
Monoclonal antibodies, 773
  anti-prion, 220
  development, genome sequencing, 63
  immunosuppression and, 1379
Monocytes
  innate immune response, 31, 31f
  in tuberculosis, 272
Mononuclear cells, 31
Monte Carlo simulation, 1251–1252
Moraxella, 1611, 1624–1625
  clinical manifestations of, 1624
  conjunctivitis, 151
  diagnostic microbiology of, 1624
  endophthalmitis and, 161
  epidemiology of, 1624
  hospital-acquired pneumonia and, 259t
  management of, 1624–1625
  nature of, 1624
  pathogenicity of, 1624
  prevention of, 1624, 1624t
Moraxella atlantae, 1624
Moraxella catarrhalis
  bronchitis and, 243
  candidate vaccine antigens of, 1624t
  clinical manifestations of, 1624
  diagnostic microbiology of, 1624
  epidemiology of, 1624
  lower respiratory tract infections, 1221
  management of, 1624–1625
  nature of, 1624
  otitis media and, 236
  pathogenicity of, 1624
  pneumonia in HIV/AIDS, 857
  prevention of, 1624
  in sinusitis, 1637
  sinusitis and, 239
Moraxella lacunata, 1624
Moraxella nonliquefaciens, 1624
Moraxella osloensis, 1624
Morbilli, 76–77
  clinical features of, 76–77
  complications of, 77
  management of, 77
Morbilliform exanthems, and skin manifestations of HIV,
  886
Morbilliform rashes, late-onset, adverse reactions to
  β-lactam antibiotics, 1216
Morbillivirus, 75t
Morganella, microflora, 355–356
Morganella morganii
  in complicated urinary tract infection, 540
  diagnostic microbiology of, 1568t
Mosquitoes, 106t, 110
  arboviruses, 1493, 1495t
  avoidance of, 951
  bites
    cellulitis, 91
    infections from, 191t
    tularemia and, 1086
    West Nile virus, 1497
    yellow fever, 1494–1496
'Moth-eaten' calyces, 556
Mouse flea, 1669
Mouth
  infections of, in cancer patients, 727
  normal flora of, 1632t
Moxifloxacin
  for anaerobic bacteria, 1643
  for community-acquired pneumonia and, 255t

Moxifloxacin *(Continued)*
  dissociation constants of, 535t
  for dog bites, 657t
  for foot ulcers, 131t
  hospital-acquired pneumonia and, 260t
  for lung abscess, 269f
  for prostatitis, 536t
  for scrub typhus, 1671
Mpowerment Project, 827
MRSA. *see* Methicillin-resistant *Staphylococcus aureus*
  (MRSA).
MSCRAMMs, 458
mTOR inhibitors, 1378–1379
Mucocutaneous candidiasis, 440, 444, 1684
Mucocutaneous disease, immune reconstitution
  inflammatory syndrome, 862–863
Mucocutaneous effects, of folate inhibitors, 1283
Mucocutaneous leishmaniasis (MCL), 1758
  clinical features of, 1062, 1062f
  epidemiology of, 1059
  monitoring response to treatment for, 1064
Mucoid *Pseudomonas aeruginosa*, 1585f–1586f, 1586
Mucor, 1696
  in burn wounds, 699–700
Mucorales, 1681t
Mucormycosis, 1696–1698
  clinical manifestations of, 1697–1698, 1697f
  diagnostic microbiology of, 1697, 1697f
  epidemiology of, 1696, 1696t
  management of, 1698
  nature of, 1696
  pathogenicity of, 1696–1697
  prognosis of, 1698
Mucosa, *Pseudomonas aeruginosa* and, 1582–1584
Mucosal human papillomaviruses, 1439
Mucosal ulcerations, in primary HIV infection, 846, 847t
Mucosal vaccines, for HIV, 832
Mucositis, following hematopoietic stem cell
  transplantation, 740
Mucous membranes
  in exposure to HIV, 835
  polyps in, 1721
Multi-locus sequence typing (MLST), 1388
Multi-locus variable number of tandem repeats analysis
  (MLVA/VNTR), for mycobacteria, 1655
Multi-slice computed tomography, in endocarditis,
  462–463, 463f
Multiceps multiceps, 1774f
Multidrug and toxic compound extrusion (MATE), 1194f
Multidrug resistance, 1194
  of Enterobacteriaceae, 1576–1577
Multidrug-resistant bacteria
  in hematopoietic stem cell transplantation, 740
  hospital-acquired pneumonia and, 259b
Multidrug-resistant organisms, 60–61
Multidrug resistant (MDR) *S. Typhi*, enteric fevers and,
  1005
Multidrug-resistant tuberculosis (MDR-TB), 866
  prevalence of, 1264, 1273
  therapy for, 1273–1274, 1273b–1274b
  treatment, 283f
Multilocus enzyme electrophoresis (MLEE), 1566
Multilocus sequence analysis (MLSA)
  Enterococcus and, 1523
  Streptococcus and, 1523
Multilocus sequence typing (MLST), 65
  for *Acinetobacter baumannii*, 1583t–1584t
  enterococci and, 1524
  for *Escherichia coli*, 1566
  for *Pseudomonas aeruginosa*, 1583t–1584t
  staphylococci and, 1519
  streptococci and, 1524
Multinational Association for Supportive Care in Cancer
  (MASCC) score, 734
Multiple locus variable number tandem repeat analysis
  (MLVA), staphylococci and, 1519
Multiple organ dysfunction syndrome (MODS), 684, 685f
  clinical manifestations of, 686
Multiplexed RT-PCR, 1388
Multispacer typing (MST), 65
Mumps, 1404–1405
  causing meningitis, 225
  clinical manifestations of, 1405
  diagnostic microbiology of, 1405
  epidemiology of, 1404

Mumps *(Continued)*
  management of, 1405
  meningoencephalitis, 319
  nature of, 1404, 1404f
  occupational infections, 648t–649t
    immunization for, 650t
  orchitis, 537
  parotitis, 319–320
  pathogenicity of, 1404–1405
  prevention of, 1405
  vaccination against, 782t–783t
Mumps virus
  causing retinitis and uveitis, 168t
  in chronic meningitis, 186t
  encephalitis/myelitis caused by, 193t–194t
Mupirocin, 1156, 1170
  chemical structure of, 1170
  decolonization, 694
  mode of action of, 1170
  pharmacodynamics of, 1170
  prophylactic, folliculitis/furunculosis, 86
  resistance to, 1170, 1193
    micrococci, 1522
  Staphylococcus aureus eradication, 87, 1516
  and surgical site infections, 688
Murine typhus, 1669
  location of, 1092t–1093t
Murmur, in rheumatic fever, 473
Murray Valley encephalitis, 1495t
  virus, 193t–194t
Musculoskeletal effects, of quinolones, 1247
Musculoskeletal system, *Mycoplasma pneumoniae* in,
  1662t
Mushroom poisoning, 331–332
Mustelids, infections from, 666–667
Mutations, molecular detection of, in mycobacteria, 1657
Myalgia, 1609
Myasthenia gravis, 212
Mycetoma, 1551
  clinical manifestations of, 1720, 1720f–1721f
  diagnostic microbiology of, 1717, 1717f
  epidemiology of, 1714
  management of, 1723
  nature of, 1713
  pathogenicity of, 1715
  prevention of, 1716
Mycobacteria, 1645–1659
  antimicrobial resistance and susceptibility testing of,
    1655–1657, 1655f, 1656t
  cell envelope of, 1645, 1645f
  epidemiology and clinical manifestations of, 1647–1648
  general characteristics of, 1645–1647, 1645f–1647f,
    1647f
  immunodiagnostic tests for tuberculosis, 1657–1658,
    1658t
  in infective arthritis, 383t
  laboratory diagnosis of, 1650–1655
    acid-fast stain and smear microscopy for, 1652,
      1652f
    culture for, 1653
    general remarks in, 1650
    identification in, 1653–1654, 1653f–1654f
      conventional biochemical tests for, 1654
      immunochromatography methods for, 1654
      molecular methods for, 1654
    processing specimens for, 1652
    serodiagnosis, urine based diagnosis and pleural fluid
      chemistry in, 1654
    direct detection of *M. tuberculosis* complex by
      nucleic acid amplification for, 1654
    DNA fingerprinting for, 1655
    specimen collection for, 1650–1652, 1651t
  lower respiratory tract infections, 264f
  lung abscesses and, 263
  in lymph node enlargement, 147t–148t
  macrolides, 1219
  nontuberculous, 1648–1649, 1648t
  parotitis caused by, 320
  pathogenicity of, 1649–1650, 1650f
  in pericarditis, 450, 452, 453t
  and pneumonia in thoracic transplant patient, 747
  provoking immune reconstitution disorder, 860t
  rapid growers, 1649
    susceptibility testing for, 1657
Mycobacteria Growth Indicator Tube, 1653

Mycobacterial diseases, nontuberculous, 285–291
  clinical features of, 286–288
  diagnosis of, 288–289, 288b
  epidemiology of, 285–286
  management of, 289–291, 289t
    drug susceptibility testing in, 291
  pathogenesis of, 286
  pathology of, 286
Mycobacterial infections, 1649
  aminoglycosides for, 1237
  in hematopoietic stem cell transplantation, 741t
  in HIV in low- and middle-income countries, 890–891, 893
  linezolid, 1231
  in pancreas transplant patients, 765, 765f
  quinolones for, 1245
  and tumor necrosis factor inhibitors, 799
Mycobacterial interspersed repetitive units (MIRUs), 1655
Mycobacterial lymphadenitis, 140
Mycobacterium abscessus, 285t, 1648t
  antimicrobial resistance of, 1656t
  epidemiology of, 285
  rapidly growing mycobacteria, 287
  tenosynovitis, 288, 288f
  treatment of, 289t, 290
Mycobacterium africanum, general characteristics of, 1647t
Mycobacterium avium
  antimicrobial resistance of, 1656t
  and tumor necrosis factor inhibitor, 799
Mycobacterium avium complex (MAC), 285t, 1646–1649, 1648t
  and antiretroviral therapy, 860t
  bronchiectasis and, 246
  in cervical lymphadenitis, 1649
  epidemiology of, 285
  in extrapulmonary and disseminated disease, 287–288
  general characteristics of, 1646f
  in HIV/AIDS, 1649, 1649f
    in low- and middle-income countries, 891
    prophylaxis, 914
  identification of, 1653–1654, 1654f
  in opportunistic infections in HIV, 850, 856
    clinical features of, 856
    treatment of, 856
  pathogenesis and pathology of, 286
  prophylaxis, in HIV infected women, 910
  in pulmonary disease, 287
  susceptibility testing of, 1657
  treatment of, 289–290, 289t
    drug susceptibility testing in, 291
Mycobacterium avium-intracellulare
  in bacterial arthritis, 383t
  chronic diarrhea, 341–343, 345t
Mycobacterium bovis
  general characteristics of, 1647t
  from mustelids, 666–667
  transmission of, 664, 665t
Mycobacterium bovis BCG, 1647t
Mycobacterium canettii, 1647t
Mycobacterium caprae, 1647t
Mycobacterium chelonae, 285t, 1648t
  antimicrobial resistance of, 1656t
  rapidly growing mycobacteria, 287
Mycobacterium fortuitum, 285t, 1648t
  draining sinus associated with, 288f
  epidemiology of, 286
  general characteristics of, 1647f
  in HIV/AIDS, treatment of, 856
Mycobacterium genavense, in HIV/AIDS, treatment of, 856
Mycobacterium haemophilum, 1648t
  in HIV/AIDS, treatment of, 856
  susceptibility testing of, 1657
Mycobacterium intracellulare, 285t, 1656t
  epidemiology of, 285
  pulmonary disease, 286f
Mycobacterium kansasii, 285t, 1648t, 1649
  epidemiology of, 285
  in extrapulmonary and disseminated disease, 288
  general characteristics of, 1646f
  in HIV/AIDS, treatment of, 856
  pathogenesis and pathology of, 286
  susceptibility testing of, 1657

Mycobacterium kansasii (Continued)
  treatment of, 289, 289t
    drug susceptibility testing in, 291
Mycobacterium leprae
  antimicrobial resistance of, 1656t
  in bacterial arthritis, 383t
  epidemiology of, 954
  general characteristics of, 1645–1647
  in HIV, in low- and middle-income countries, 891
  pathogenesis and pathology of, 955
Mycobacterium malmoense, 285t, 1648t
  in extrapulmonary and disseminated disease, 288
  pathogenesis and pathology of, 286
  in pulmonary disease, 287
  treatment of, 289t, 290
    drug susceptibility testing in, 291
Mycobacterium marinum, 285t, 662, 1648t
  in bacterial arthritis, 383t
  cellulitis and, 91
  epidemiology of, 285
  fish tank granuloma, 287
  in HIV/AIDS, treatment of, 856
  and occupational infections, 648t–649t
  susceptibility testing of, 1657
  treatment of, 290
    drug susceptibility testing in, 291
Mycobacterium microti, 1647t
Mycobacterium mungi, 1647t
Mycobacterium orygis, 1647t
Mycobacterium pinnipedii, 1647t
Mycobacterium scrofulaceum
  general characteristics of, 1646f
  in HIV/AIDS, treatment of, 856
Mycobacterium simiae, 285t, 1648t
  epidemiology of, 285–286
  in HIV/AIDS, treatment of, 856
  susceptibility testing of, 1657
  treatment of, 289t, 290
Mycobacterium smegmatis, antimicrobial resistance of, 1656t
Mycobacterium szulgai
  general characteristics of, 1646f
  pulmonary disease, 286f
  treatment of, 289t
Mycobacterium tuberculae, jaundice, 1135t
Mycobacterium tuberculosis, 805, 1264
  antimicrobial resistance in, 1655, 1656t
  and antiretroviral therapy, 860t
  in bacterial arthritis, 383t
  and bioterrorism, 671t
  causing retinitis/uveitis, 171t
  in cervicitis, 490
  chronic diarrhea, 345t
  in chronic meningitis, 186t
  DNA fingerprinting of, 1655
  general characteristics of, 1645–1647, 1646f, 1647t
  genome sequence of, 1646
  growth of, 1386
  hospital-acquired pneumonia and, 259t
  host response to, 272–273, 274f
    innate, 272
  identification of, 1653, 1653f
  impaired immune responses to, 868
  indication, chronic meningitis, 186, 187t
  keratitis and, 152
  in liver transplant patients, 751
  nucleic acid amplification for, 1654
  in osteomyelitis, 390
  pathology and pathogenicity of, 272
  in prostatitis, 533t
  resistance in, 1193–1194
  spinal epidural abscess and, 206
  susceptibility testing of, 1656–1657
  in thoracic transplantation patients, 747t, 749
  and tumor necrosis factor inhibitor, 799
  urogenital tract tuberculosis and, 555
  uveitis and, 169
  worldwide incidence and prevalence, 271
Mycobacterium tuberculosis complex, antimicrobial resistance of, 1656t
Mycobacterium ulcerans, 285t, 1645, 1648t
  Buruli ulcer/Bairnsdale ulcer from, 92, 1648, 1648f
  Buruli ulcer disease, 287

Mycobacterium ulcerans (Continued)
  drug susceptibility testing in, 291
  treatment of, 291
Mycobacterium xenopi, 285t, 1648t
  pathogenesis and pathology of, 286
  in pulmonary disease, 287
  treatment of, 289t, 290
    drug susceptibility testing, 291
Mycophenolate mofetil, 1378–1379
Mycoplasma, 1660–1665, 1661t
  in bacterial arthritis, 383t
  in bacterial vaginosis, 483
  causing endocarditis, 461t
  and occupational infections, 648t–649t
  in pelvic inflammatory disease, 492t
  in pericarditis, 450, 453t
Mycoplasma genitalium, 1661–1663
  in cervicitis, 490
  clinical manifestations of, 1662–1663
  diagnostic microbiology of, 1662
  epidemiology of, 1662
  etiology of, 1138t
  management of, 1663
  nature of, 1661–1662
  pathogenicity of, 1662
  in pelvic inflammatory disease, 492
  prevention of, 1662
Mycoplasma hominis, 1663–1664
  in bacterial vaginosis, 484
  clindamycin, 1225
  clinical manifestations of, 1663–1664
  diagnostic microbiology of, 1663
  epidemiology of, 1663
  macrolides, 1221
  management of, 1664
  nature of, 1663
  pathogenicity of, 1663
  in postpartum endometritis, 494–495
Mycoplasma pneumoniae, 1660–1661
  bronchitis, 243, 244t
  clinical manifestations of, 1661, 1662t
  diagnostic microbiology of, 1660–1661
  encephalitis/myelitis and, 190, 194t
  epidemiology of, 1660
  hospital-acquired pneumonia and, 259t
  lower respiratory tract infections, 264f, 1221
  macrolides and ketolides, 1221
  management of, 1661
  nature of, 1660
  pathogenicity of, 1660
  pharyngitis, 234–235
  prevention of, 1660
  testing, 196–197
Mycoses
  of implantation, 1712–1724
  see also specific mycoses
Mycotic infection, lymphadenopathy and, 137t–138t
Myelitis, 189–197
  clinical features of, 190–194, 195f
  definition of, 189
  diagnosis of, 195–197, 195t, 196f
  epidemiology of, 189, 190f, 191t
  exposures associated with agents causing, 191t
  in immune reconstitution inflammatory syndrome, 862
  management of, 197
  microbiology of, 189–190
  pathogens anecdotally associated with, 194t
  pathology and pathogenesis of, 194–195
  transverse, 191
Myeloablative therapy, in hematopoietic stem cell transplant, 790–791
Myeloid cells and defects, 705, 705t
Myeloperoxidase deficiency, 705t, 709
Myocardial disease, diphtheria and, 1546
Myocarditis, 446–449
  bacteria in, 446–447
  from Candida, 1684
  causes of, 447t–448t
  clinical features of, 448
  diagnosis of, 448–449
  epidemiology of, 446
  in immunocompromised patients, 448
  influenza virus and, 1470

Myocarditis (Continued)
management of, 449
parasites in, 447
pathogenesis and pathology of, 446–448, 446f
spirochetes in, 447
toxoplasmic, 856–857
treatment of, 443t
viruses in, 447
Myonecrosis, 95–103
clinical clues and differential diagnosis of, 95–96
Myopathy, influenza virus and, 1470
Myositis, 95–103
clinical clues and differential diagnosis of,
95–96
influenza virus and, 1470
streptococcal. see Streptococcal myositis
systemic microsporidiosis in, 1741
Myroides, 1597–1598
clinical manifestations of, 1598
management of, 1598
microbiology of, 1598
nomenclature of, 1581t–1582t

N

N-acetyl-L-cysteine (NALC), 1652
Naegleria
nature of, 1744
and recreational infections, 645
taxonomy of, 1744
treatment of, 1345t–1351t
Naegleria fowleri, 193t–194t, 194–195
cultivation of, 1745
diagnostic microbiology of, 1747
epidemiology of, 1745–1746
nature of, 1744, 1744f
pathogenicity of, 1746
prevention of, 1746–1747
taxonomy of, 1744–1745
Nafcillin
for anaerobic bacteria, 1210
cellulitis and, 92
dosage in renal failure, 1213t–1214t
for infective arthritis, 386t
for lung abscess, 269f
pharmacokinetics of, 1204, 1205t
prophylaxis, 1158t
Staphylococcus aureus eradication, 87
susceptibilities of selected bacteria to,
1208t–1209t
Nairovirus, 1495t
Nalidixic acid
in Pseudomonas isolation, 1580
resistance to enteric fevers, 1005
Nanophyetus salmincola, treatment of, 1345t–1351t
Nantucket fever, 1752
Naprosyn test, 622
Narrow-spectrum cephalosporin, prophylaxis of, in
rheumatic fever, 475t
Natalizumab, 798t–799t, 802
Natamycin, 154
National Center for Biotechnology Information (NCBI),
62–63
National Health and Nutrition Examination Survey
(NHANES)
hepatitis C virus, 367–368
hepatitis E virus, 372
National Nosocomial Infections Surveillance Program, risk
factors, 687, 687t
National Nosocomial Infections Surveillance (NNIS)
score, 399
Native valve infective endocarditis, 457, 458t, 462, 465,
466t, 468t
Natural disasters, and emerging infectious diseases, 46–48,
46f
Natural immunity
accelerated decay of, in immunocompromised patient,
780
need to assess, 780
Natural killer (NK) cells, 1649–1650
Nature of micro-organisms, 4–25
see also specific micro-organisms
Nebovirus
nature of, 1393
taxonomy of, 1394t

Necator americanus
clinical features of, 996
diagnosis of, 998t–999t
epidemiology of, 1763
life cycle of, 1767f
parasite infections and, 74
pathogenesis and pathology of, 991
pathogenicity of, 1768
treatment of, 1001t, 1345t–1351t
Necrotizing bronchopneumonia, 1587
Necrotizing enterocolitis (NEC), probiotics for, 1373,
1374t
Necrotizing fasciitis, 96–98
in cancer patients, 727–728
cervical, 315
clinical features of, 96–97, 96f
diagnosis of, 97–98, 98f
diagnostic tests for, 96
histopathologic examination of, 96f
management of, 98
morbidity and mortality, 100
pathogenesis of, 97
streptococci and, 1532
treatment of, 96–97
type I, 95f, 96–97, 98f
type II, 97–98, 97f
from Vibrio vulnificus, 1607
Necrotizing infections, 96–99
Necrotizing otitis externa, 1589
Necrotizing retinitis, 862
Necrotizing ulcerative gingivitis, acute, 316, 316f–317f
Needles, sharing of, and HIV, 825
Needlestick injuries, and HIV transmission, 825
Negative anti-Toxoplasma gondii IgG, 517
Negative anti-Toxoplasma gondii IgM, 517
Negative-pressure wound therapy (NPWT), for
mediastinitis and sternal osteomyelitis, 482
Neisseria, 1553–1564, 1553t
clinical manifestations of
gonorrhea, 1562–1563
meningococcal infection, 1563–1564, 1563f
diagnostic microbiology of
gonococcal infection, 1560–1561, 1560f
meningococcal infection, 1561
epidemiology of, 1556–1557
gonorrhea, 1556
meningococcal disease, 1556–1557, 1556f
genome dynamics of, 1555–1556, 1555f
growth characteristics of, 1554–1555
hospital-acquired pneumonia and, 259t
in human bites, 683t
jaundice, 1135t
management of
gonorrhea, 1564, 1564t
meningococcal disease, 1564
mechanisms contributing to genetic instability of, 1555f
nature of, 1553–1556
nonpathogenic, 1562, 1562t
pathogenic, 1562t
pathogenicity of, 1557–1560, 1557f–1558f
gonococcal, 1557
meningococcal, 1557–1558
prevention of
gonococcal infection, 1560
meningococcal disease, 1560
structure and virulence factors of, 1557t, 1558–1560,
1558f
capsules, 1558–1559
lipo-oligosaccharide, 1559
peptidoglycan, 1559
pili, 1559
secreted factors, 1559–1560
surface proteins, 1559
taxonomy of, 1553, 1554f
Neisseria elongata, 1553
Neisseria gonorrhoeae, 1553
antigenic variations in, 24–25, 24f
azithromycin, 1221
in bacterial arthritis, 382, 383t, 384–385, 386t
capsules of, 1559
in cervicitis, 490
clinical features of, 594
clinical manifestations of, 1562–1563
in conjunctivitis, 150, 175
diagnosis of, 594

Neisseria gonorrhoeae (Continued)
epidemiology of, 1556
in epididymitis, 537
etiology of, 1138t
genome dynamics of, 1555
in gonorrhea, 592
growth characteristics of, 1554–1555
isolation of, 1561t
keratitis and, 152
β-lactam resistance in, 1184
management of, 595, 1564, 1564t
syndromes associated with, 596t
molecular typing of, 1561–1562
pathogenesis of, 592, 1557
pathology of, 592
in pelvic inflammatory disease, 492
pharyngitis, 234–235
pili of, 1559
in pregnancy, 500t
prevention of, 1560
in prostatitis, 533t
susceptibility testing of, 1137
Neisseria lactamica, genome dynamics of, 1555
Neisseria meningitidis, 1553
avoiding ingestion, 23
in bacterial arthritis, 383t
burden of disease, 942–943, 942f
capsules of, 1558–1559
conjunctivitis and, 151
genome dynamics of, 1555
growth characteristics of, 1554–1555
isolation of, 1561t
β-lactam resistance in, 1184
macrolides, 1220
meningitis and, 177
molecular typing of, 1561–1562
pili of, 1559
and postsplenectomy sepsis, 777, 778t
surface proteins of, 1559
Neisseria sicca, 1554–1555
Neisseria subflava, growth characteristics of, 1554–1555
Neisseria weaveri, 1553
Nelfinavir, 1148t, 1303
effect on oral contraceptives, 907t
perinatal HIV transmission prevention, 909t
Nematoda, nature of, 1763
Nematodes, 989t
blood and tissue, 1764t, 1765
epidemiology of, 1763–1765
intestinal, 1764t
epidemiology of, 1763
pathogenicity of, 1766–1768
life cycle of, 1767f
pathogenesis and pathology of, 991–993
pathogenicity of, 1766–1772
prevention of, 1772
tissue, 1764t
epidemiology of, 1763–1765
pathogenicity of, 1768–1770
treatment of, 1001t
see also specific genera
Neomycin
conjunctivitis treatment, 152
prophylaxis, 159
Neonatal candidiasis, treatment of, 443t
Neonatal herpes, 570
Neonatal infections
Mycoplasma hominis in, 1664
Ureaplasma in, 1664
Neonatal meningitis Escherichia coli (NMEC), 1575
Neonatal nursery, infection control in, 521
Neonates
evaluation of, for congenital syphilis, 564–565, 565t
group B streptococci in, 1533
infectious conjunctivitis in, 594
intra-amniotic infection in, 500
listeriosis in, 1540, 1540t
retinitis in, 166
sepsis in, 1598
subdural empyema/intracranial epidural abscess in, 205t
testing in, 509t, 511–513, 511t–512t
tetanus and, 208
tolerance of antiretroviral prophylaxis by, 901–902
Neoplasia, in pericarditis, 452–453
Neoplastic conditions, eosinophilia and, 984t

Neoplastic disease, 874–878
microbial disease associations with, 626t
Neoscytalidium infections, 1710
Neosporin, for *Acanthamoeba* keratitis, 1750
Nephritis, as quinolones adverse effect, 1248
Nephropathia epidemica, 1502
Nephropathy
Bk polyomavirus and, 1447, 1447f
BK virus-associated, 767, 767f
JC virus-associated, 767
Nephrotoxicity
of aminoglycosides, 357, 1235, 1235t
of foscarnet, 1315
polymyxins, 1288
of vancomycin, 1252
Nervous tissue, vaccines from, 1462
Netilmicin, pharmacokinetic parameters for, 1234t
Neuraminidase inhibitors, 1319–1326
resistance to, 1325
Neurocognitive dysfunction, in aging HIV-positive patient, 930
Neurocysticercosis, 1034, 1778
in chronic meningitis, 188
diagnosis of, 1035, 1035f
management of, 1035
Neurologic complications, of brucellosis, 1099
Neurologic disease
diphtheria and, 1546
Lyme disease, 407–409, 411–413, 412t
Neurologic effects, of β-lactam antibiotics, 1215
Neurologic infections, Enterobacteriaceae in, 1575
Neurologic problems, in immunologically mediated diseases, 771–773
Neurologic schistosomiasis, 1030
Neurologic syndromes
in primary HIV infection, 847
streptococci and, 1533
Neurological system, *Mycoplasma pneumoniae* in, 1662t
Neuromuscular blockade, of aminoglycosides, 1236
Neuroretinitis
diffuse unilateral, 172
stellate, 168
Neurosurgery, antibiotic prophylaxis and, 1157t–1158t, 1159
Neurosyphilis, 562–563
asymptomatic, 562
gummatous, 563
meningeal, 562–563
treatment of, 565t
Neurotoxicity, polymyxins, 1288
Neurotoxins, in food-borne diarrheal illness, 330
Neurotropic Macacine herpesvirus-1, 666
Neutralization, 36
Neutralizing antibodies, 829–830
for HIV-1 infection, 842
induction of, 830–831, 831b, 831f
Neutropenia
after hematopoietic stem cell transplantation, 740, 743t
alloimmune neonatal, 706
autoimmune
primary, 706
secondary, 706
brain abscess and, 199
candidiasis and, 439–440, 442, 444, 1683
treatment of, 443t
cyclic, 706
and fever of unknown origin, 614
definition of, 705, 725
immune-mediated, 706
and rituximab, 800
and secukinumab, 802
severe congenital, 705–706
Neutropenic fever, β-lactam antibiotics for, 1212
Neutropenic patients
quinolones for, 1246
trimethoprim-sulfamethoxazole for, 1282
Neutrophil extracellular traps (NETs), 1528–1529
Neutrophils, 705
in Chediak-Higashi syndrome, 706, 707f
cryptococcosis and, 1692
granule deficiency specific to, 706–707
Histoplasma capsulatum and, 1707

Neutrophils *(Continued)*
inhibition of recruitment of, *Staphylococcus aureus* and, 1514
mucormycosis and, 1697
Nevi, pigmented, 586t–587t
Nevirapine, 1148t, 1300–1301
adverse reactions of, 1301, 1301t
antiretroviral drugs, 921–922
description of, 1300
dosage of, 1301
in special circumstances, 1301
drug interactions of, 1301
effect on oral contraceptives, 907t
indications of, 1301
in newborns of HIV infected mothers, 900–901
patient monitoring, 910
perinatal HIV transmission prevention, 908, 909t
pharmacokinetics and distribution of, 1301
resistance to, 1301
route of administration of, 1301
New World arenaviruses, 1114t–1115t
New York (NY) virus, 1503t
Newborns, to HIV-infected mothers, 900–902
choice of postnatal prophylaxis in, 900–901
perinatal care in, 900
Newcastle disease, and occupational infections, 648t–649t
Niamey protocols, 1031
Niclosamide, 1352t–1362t, 1371
for gastrointestinal helminth, 1001, 1001t
Nicotinamide-adenine dinucleotide phosphate (NADPH)
oxidation, 707–708, 707f
Nifurtimox
for African trypanosomiasis, 969t, 970
for Chagas disease, 1072, 1760
for parasitic infections, 1345t–1362t
Nifurtimox-eflornithine combination therapy (NECT), for
African trypanosomiasis, 969
Nijmegen breakage syndrome, 721
Nikkomycin Z, for microsporidiosis, 1742
Nikolsky's sign, 87, 88f
Nipah viral disease, and occupational infections,
648t–649t
Nipah virus, 1507–1508
and bioterrorism, 671t
clinical manifestations, 1507–1508
diagnostic microbiology, 1508
encephalitis/myelitis caused by, 193t–194t
epidemiology, 1507
management, 1508
nature, 1507
transmission of, 666
Nitazoxanide
for cryptosporidiosis, 1741–1742
for *Cryptosporidium*, 334
for gastrointestinal protozoa, 999–1000, 1000t
for parasitic infections, 1345t–1362t
Nitric oxide (NO), in malaria, 1017
Nitrofurans, 1175–1177
chemical structure of, 1175, 1176f
mode and spectrum of action of, 1175–1177
pharmacodynamics of, 1177
resistance to, 1177
Nitrofurantoin, 1278
adverse reactions to, 1278, 1278t
for complicated urinary tract infection, 544t
for cystitis, 525–526, 528t, 529
dosage of, 1278
for enterococci, 1534
indications of, 1278
mechanism of action, 1278
mechanisms of resistance, 1278
pharmacokinetics of, 1278
in *Pseudomonas* isolation, 1580
route of administration, 1278
spectrum of activity, 1278
Nitrofurantoin monohydrate, for complicated urinary
tract infection, 544t
Nitroimidazoles, 1175–1177, 1261–1263
for anaerobic bacteria, 1643
chemical structure of, 1175, 1176f
mode and spectrum of action of, 1175–1177
pharmacodynamics of, 1177
resistance to, 1177

Nocardia, 1550t
abscesses, 772
bacteremia and, 1551–1552
and chronic granulomatous disease, 708
in chronic meningitis, 186t
in cutaneous and soft tissue infection, 1551
diagnostic microbiology of, 1549, 1717
endophthalmitis and, 161
hospital-acquired pneumonia and, 259t
keratitis and, 152
lincosamides, 1224–1225
in thoracic transplant patients, 749
uveitis and, 170, 170f
Nocardia brasiliensis, 1714
Nocardia farcinica, 1549
Nocardiosis
cell-mediated immunity in, 1549
disseminated infections and, 1551
incidence in AIDS patients, 1549
pulmonary infections and, 1551
Nod-like receptors (NLRs), 27, 30
in sepsis, 421, 422t
Noma, 316, 317f
Non-endemic countries, African trypanosomiasis and, 968
Non-HACEK species, in endocarditis, 468
Non-Hodgkin's lymphoma, 875–876
clinical features of, 875
diagnosis of, 875
fever of unknown origin, 611
management of, 875–876
staging of, 876t
Non-melanoma skin cancer (NMSC), in skin
manifestations of HIV, 884–885
Non-nucleos(t)ide polymerase inhibitors, for hepatitis C, 1332
Non-nucleoside reverse transcriptase inhibitors (NNRTIs),
1300–1303
antiretroviral regimens, 870–871, 871t, 925, 936–937
choosing, 921
resistance to, 924
Non-shivering thermogenesis, 606
Nonclostridial anaerobic cellulitis, 99
Nongonococcal infective arthritis, 384
etiologic agents of, 383t
Nongonococcal urethritis (NGU)
diagnosis of, 603
etiology of, 603
Mycoplasma genitalium in, 1662
Mycoplasma hominis in, 1663
persistent and recurrent, 603–604
treatment of, 603–604
Nonhuman primates, infections from, 661, 666
Noninfluenza respiratory viruses, 1472–1482
Noninvasive micro-organisms, 15–16, 15t, 16f
Nonpolio enterovirus, 1410–1411
Nonpyogenic/other streptococci, 1523
clinical manifestations of, 1534
epidemiology of, 1527
management of, 1535
pathogenesis of, 1532
Nonradiometric broth-based methods, for susceptibility
testing, 1656–1657
Nonsteroidal anti-inflammatory drugs (NSAIDs)
antipyretic action, 609
bronchitis and, 244
for leprosy reactions, 959–960
for pericardial effusion, 480
for pericarditis, 452–454
Nontuberculous mycobacterial (NTM) diseases, and
tumor necrosis factor inhibitor, 799
Nonulcer dyspepsia, from *Helicobacter pylori*, 1604
Norfloxacin
for complicated urinary tract infection, 544t
dissociation constants of, 535t
for prostatitis, 536t–537t
Noroviruses, 1393–1396
characteristics of, in food-borne diarrheal illness, 330t
clinical characteristics of, 1391t
clinical manifestations of, 1396
diarrhea, 335
electron micrograph of, 332f
epidemiological characteristics of, 1391t
epidemiology of, 1394

Noroviruses *(Continued)*
  life cycle of, 1395*f*
  and occupational infections, 648*t*–649*t*
  pathogenicity of, 1395
  prevalence of, 335
  structure and morphological characteristics of, 1391*f*,
    1391*t*
  taxonomy of, 1394*t*
  in travelers' diarrhea, 332
  viral enteritis, 338
North Africa, infections in, 1130
North Asian tick typhus, 1092*t*–1093*t*, 1668
Norwalk-like virus, doses of, in diarrheal illness, 329*t*
Norwalk virus (NV), 1393
Norwalk virus-like particle, 1393*f*
Nosocomial infections
  from aerobic gram-negative bacilli, 1588*t*
  from *Alcaligenes* spp., 1597
  Staphylococcus aureus, 1509–1511
  see also specific infections
Nosocomial meningitis, 177
Nosocomial pneumonia
  linezolid for, 1231*t*
  quinolones for, 1245
Notifiable diseases, 50
  occupational infections, 649
NS5A inhibitors, for hepatitis C, 1332
Nuclear factor Kappa B pathway, defects in, 710–711
Nuclease gene *(nuc)*, 1519
Nucleic acid amplification, for *Mycobacterium tuberculosis*,
    1654
Nucleic acid amplification tests (NAATs)
  for *Chlamydia pneumoniae*, 1679
  for *Chlamydia trachomatis*, 600, 1678
  in lymphogranuloma venereum, 589
  for *Mycoplasma pneumoniae*, 1660
Nucleic acid detection, for papillomaviruses, 1442
Nucleic acid hybridization tests, in gonorrhea, 594
Nucleic acid probes, for mycobacteria, 1654
Nucleic acids
  drugs affecting, 1174–1177
  transmissible spongiform encephalopathies, 214
  see also DNA; RNA
Nucleoside analog reverse transcriptase inhibitors (NRTI),
    1293–1300
  chemical structure of, 1296*f*
  mechanism of action of, 1293, 1296*f*
  in patients with renal dysfunction, 1297*t*
  toxicities of, 1298*t*
Nucleos(t)ide analogs
  for hepatitis B, 1327–1329
  for hepatitis C, 1331
Nucleos(t)ide-based therapy, for hepatitis B virus,
    366–367
Nucleos(t)ide reverse transcriptase inhibitors (NRTIs)
  antiretroviral drugs, 920–921
  resistance to, 924
Nucleotide oligomerization domains (NOD), 31–32
Nucleotidyltransferases (ANT), 1185, 1185*t*
Nutrition
  for food-borne diarrheal illness, 333
  and susceptibility to disease, 943
Nystatin
  for oropharyngeal candidiasis, 1684
  for vulvovaginal candidiasis, 488*t*

O

Obstetric gynecologic infection, anaerobic bacteria in,
    1632*f*
Obstetric surgery, antibiotic prophylaxis and, 1157*t*–1158*t*,
    1159
Occipital lobe, brain abscess and, 199
Occupational infections, 647–655
  classification of, 647, 648*t*–649*t*
  importance of, 647
  mode of transmission, 648*t*–649*t*
  prevention and control of, 650–651, 650*t*
  surveillance of, 647–650
  see also specific infections
Ochrobactrum, 1581*t*–1582*t*, 1597–1598
Ocrelizumab, 800
Ocular infections
  adenovirus in, 1473
  quinolones for, 1246

Ocular tuberculosis, 279
Oculoglandular syndrome, 139*t*
  follicular conjunctivitis, 981*t*
Oculoglandular tularemia, 1088
Odontogenic complications, anaerobic bacteria in, 1636*t*
Oerskovia, 1547, 1548*t*
Oesophagostomum bifurcum, treatment of, 1345*t*–1351*t*
Ofloxacin, 735
  for anaerobic bacteria, 1643
  for complicated urinary tract infection, 544*t*–545*t*
  dissociation constants of, 535*t*
  for infective arthritis, 386*t*
  for keratitis, 152
  for lung abscess, 269*f*
  for prostatitis, 536*t*–537*t*
Old World arenaviruses, 1114*t*–1115*t*
Old-world monkeys, infections from, 191*t*
Oleandomycin
  characteristics of, 1218*t*
  classification, 1217
  pharmacokinetics, 1223*t*
  tissue distribution, 1224*t*
Olecranon bursitis, 93, 93*f*
Oligella, 1581*t*–1582*t*, 1598
Omalizumab, 798*t*–799*t*, 802
Ombitasvir, for hepatitis C, 1332
Omenn syndrome, 717–718, 718*f*
Omsk hemorrhagic fever, 1495*t*
Onchocerca volvulus, 981
  clinical manifestations of, 1777–1778
  epidemiology of, 1046, 1765
  life cycle of, 1769*f*
  pathogenicity of, 1768
  treatment of, 1345*t*–1351*t*
Onchocerciasis, 981, 1047*t*
  clinical features of, 981, 1049
  diagnosis of, 1050
  epidemiology of, 1046
  geographic distribution of, 939
  lymphadenopathy and, 137*t*–138*t*, 142–143
  management of, 1051
  pathogenesis of, 981, 1047, 1048*f*
  pathology of, 1047, 1048*f*
  prevention of, 1048–1049
Onchocercomas, 1777–1778
OncoE6 Test®, 1442–1443
One exchange, in surgery, for prosthetic joint infection
    (PJI), 402
Onychomycosis
  clinical features of, 126
  diagnostic microbiology of, 1711–1712
  epidemiology of, 122–123, 1710
  management of, 128–129
  nature of, 1710
  nondermatophytic, 1711–1712
  superficial white, 125
  total dystrophic, 125
O'nyong-nyong, in infective arthritis, 387*t*
Opa genes, 1559
Opa protein, 1559
Open reduction and internal fixation of fractures, 687*t*
Ophthalmia neonatorum
  chlamydial, 982
  gonococcal, 982
Ophthalmic surgery, antibiotic prophylaxis and,
    1157*t*–1158*t*
Ophthalmologic abnormalities, congenital infection and,
    510
Opisthokonta, 1744
Opisthorchis felineus, 660
  epidemiology of, 1036
  life cycle of, 1771*f*
  pathogenicity of, 1770
Opisthorchis viverrini
  epidemiology of, 1036, 1765
  pathogenesis and pathology of, 1036
  pathogenicity of, 1770
  treatment of, 1345*t*–1351*t*
Opportunistic fungi, 1681, 1682*t*
Opportunistic infections, and rituximab, 800
Opsonization, 37
Optic neuritis, as ethambutol adverse effect, 1270
Optic neuropathy, linezolid and, 1231–1232
OqxAB, 1186–1187
Oral decontamination, hospital-acquired pneumonia, 261

Oral intercourse, and HIV transmission, 825
Oral lesions, in cancer, 318
Oral mucosa, infections of
  aphthous stomatitis, 318
  gangrenous stomatitis, 316, 316*f*–317*f*
  hand, foot, and mouth disease, 317–318
  herpangina, 317, 317*f*
  primary herpetic gingivostomatitis, 317, 317*f*
  primary syphilis, 318
Oral rehydration
  for cholera, 1605–1606
  of diarrhea, 339
  for food-borne diarrheal illness, 333
Oral selective bowel decontamination, in liver transplant
    patients, 754, 754*t*
Oral thrush, 1684
Orbital cellulitis, 156, 313
Orchitis, 537–538, 537*t*
  brucellosis complications, 1099
  gonorrhea and, 594
  treatment of, 596*t*
Orf, and occupational infections, 648*t*–649*t*, 651*t*–654*t*
Organ dysfunction
  pathogenesis of, 684–686, 685*f*
  in sepsis, 424
  see also Multiple organ dysfunction syndrome (MODS)
Organ transplantation, phaeohyphomycosis in, 1721
Organism detection assays, for *Clostridium difficile*, 1630
Organum vasculosum of the lamina terminalis (OVLT),
    608
Oriental spotted fever, 1092*t*–1093*t*
Orientia tsutsugamushi, 1091, 1670
Oritavancin, 1253–1254, 1254*t*
  mode of action of, 1164
  in outpatient parenteral antimicrobial therapy, 1201
  resistance to, 1164–1167
Ornidazole, 1261–1263
  dosage for, 1261–1262
  for parasitic infections, 1352*t*–1362*t*, 1368
  for trichomoniasis, 486
Ornithodoros
  geographic distribution of, 1105*t*
  relapsing fevers and, 1105
Ornithonyssus bacoti, 107*t*
Ornythodoros sonrai, 105*f*
Orocervical infection, 312–320
Oropharyngeal anthrax, 1125
Oropharyngeal candidiasis, 1682–1683
Oropharyngeal chlamydia, 599–600
Oropharyngeal infection, herpes simplex virus and,
    1435–1436
Oropharyngeal streptococci, lower respiratory tract
    infections, 264*f*
Oropharyngeal/tonsillar cancer, papillomaviruses in, 1443
Oropharyngeal tularemia, 1088–1089
Oroya fever, 1675
Orthopedic surgery, antibiotic prophylaxis and,
    1157*t*–1158*t*, 1159
Orthopoxviruses, 1454*t*, 1455–1457
  diagnostic microbiology of, 1457
  management of, 1457
  transmission of, 665
Oseltamivir, 742–743, 1146*t*–1147*t*, 1321–1324
  adverse reactions and interactions of, 1324
  dosage of, 1321
    in special circumstances, 1324
  indications of, 1321–1324
  pharmacokinetics and distribution of, 1320*t*, 1321
  prophylaxis, 1321
  route of administration, 1321
  treatment with, 1321–1324
Osler-Weber-Rendu disease, 199
Osmotic diarrhea, 336
Osteoarticular complications, of brucellosis, 1099,
    1099*f*–1100*f*
Osteoarticular infections, 1289–1290
  Candida infections, 443*t*
Osteochondritis, 1589
Osteomyelitis, 388–398
  acute
    clinical features of, 391
    management of, 395–396
  Alcaligenes xylosoxidans in, 1597
  anaerobic bacteria in, 1640
  antibiotics for, 1152*t*

Osteomyelitis (Continued)
blastomycosis and, 1703
chronic
clinical features of, 391, 391f
management of, 396–398, 396f–397f
chronic relapsing multifocal, 393
chronicity of, establishment of, 389
classification of, 390, 390f
clinical features of, 391–393
complicating decubitus ulcers, 392–393
diabetic foot, 392, 393f
diagnosis of, 393–395
epidemiology of, 388
foot ulcers and, 130
hematogenous, 388, 388f
host factors of, 389
management of, 395–396, 395t
mandibular, 393
microbial factors of, 388–389, 389f
microbiology of, 389–390
pathogenesis of, 388–390
pathology of, 390
periarticular, 382, 385
prevention of, 390
Pseudomonas aeruginosa in, 1589
sickle cell anemia and, 1056
skull-base, 393
in specific anatomic situations, 391–393
sternum, in thoracic transplantation patients, 747
subacute, 391
tests for, 394t
treatment of, 443t
tuberculosis, 278–279
vancomycin for, 1251
vertebral, 391–392, 392f
Osteopenia, 916
Osteoporosis, 916
in aging HIV-positive patient, 929
Otitis, 236–239
bacteriology of, 236–237
complications of, 237–238, 238f
congestive, 237
diagnosis of, 237, 239b
epidemiology of, 236
physiopathology of, 236
prevention of, 237
purulent, 237, 237f
treatment of, 238–239
vaccination of, 237
Otitis externa, malignant (necrotizing), 1589, 1592
Otitis media, 236
anaerobic bacteria in, 1636t, 1637
brain abscess and, 199, 200t
chronic, 237
epidemiology of, 236
from *Moraxella catarrhalis*, 1624
physiopathology of, 236
prevention of, 237
subdural empyema/intracranial epidural abscess and, 203, 205t
vaccination of, 237
Ototoxicity
of aminoglycosides, 1235t, 1236
irreversible, 357
of vancomycin, 1252
Outer membrane proteins (OMPs), *Neisseria*, 1557t
Outer membrane vesicle (OMV), vaccines, 1560
Outpatient medical practices, antimicrobial stewardship in, 1200
Outpatient parenteral antimicrobial therapy (OPAT), 1200–1201
indications, prescribing and monitoring, 1201, 1201t
patient selection, 1201
team, development of, 1200–1201
vascular access and drug delivery systems, 1201
Overwhelming post-splenectomy infection (OPSI), 775
clinical features of, 778, 778t
diagnosis of, 778, 778f–779f
management of, 778–779
Ovine chlamydiosis, and occupational infections, 651t–654t
Oxacephems, 1162

Oxacillin
dosage in renal failure, 1213t–1214t
for infective arthritis, 386t
pharmacokinetics of, 1205t
prophylaxis, 1158t
susceptibilities of selected bacteria to, 1208t–1209t
for treatment of hydrocephalus shunts, 223–224
Oxamniquine, for parasitic infections, 1345t–1362t, 1371
Oxazolidinones, 1173–1174, 1230–1232
adverse reactions and interactions, 1231–1232
as antituberculosis agents, 1271
chemical structure of, 1173–1174
dosage, 1230–1231
for enterococci, 1534
indications, 1230–1231
mode of action of, 1173f, 1174
pharmacodynamics of, 1174
pharmacokinetics and distribution, 1230
resistance to, 1174
route, 1230
Oxidative metabolism, defects of, 707–709, 707f
Oxolides, 1217
Oxygen, ability to tolerate, of anaerobic bacteria, 1633

P
P-selectin glycoprotein ligand-1 (PSGL-1), 1514
p24 antigen test, 848
p56lck/ZAP-70 pathway, defects of, 716
PA-824, 1271–1272
Pacemaker implantation, antibiotic prophylaxis and, 1160
Paclitaxel, 875t
Paecilomyces spp., 159
PAIR, 1044
Palivizumab
in hematopoietic stem cell transplantation, 742–743
respiratory syncytial virus, 1476–1477
Pan troglodytes troglodytes, 666
Pancreas
transplant recipients, 762–769
bacterial infections in, 765
intra-abdominal infections in, 763–764
diagnosis of, 763–764
impact of surgical technique on risk of, 764, 765f
prophylaxis and management of, 764, 764f
risk factors for, 764
timing and type of, 764
tuberculosis, 279
Pancreatitis, 355–362, 360f
acute, surgery complications, 690
β-lactam antibiotics for, 1211
Pancytopenia, 658
Pandemic influenza, 1471
Pandoraea, 1598
nomenclature of, 1581t–1582t
prevalence of, 1579
Pangenomics, genome sequencing, 63–65
Panophthalmitis, 158
Panstrongylus megistus, 1066
Pansystolic murmur, in rheumatic fever, 473
Pantoea agglomerans, 1577t
Panton-Valentine leukocidin, 1513t–1514t, 1514–1515
Panton-Valentine leukocidin toxin (PVL), in recurrent cellulitis, 133
Pap smear, 580, 582
Pap smear screening program, 1441, 1443
Papillary necrosis, 547–548, 549f
Papilloma, yaws and, 963, 963f
Papillomatosis, recurrent respiratory, 1443
Papillomaviruses, 1439–1444
clinical manifestations of, 1443
diagnostic microbiology for, 1442–1443
epidemiology of, 1439–1440
immunologic assays for, 1443
infection, 575–584
management of, 1443–1444
nature of, 1439, 1439f–1440f
nucleic acid detection for, 1442
pathogenicity of, 1440, 1440f, 1441f
prevention of, 1440–1442
prophylactic vaccine and screening of, 1442, 1442f

Papillomaviruses (Continued)
protein biomarkers for, 1442–1443
therapeutic vaccines for, 1442
Papular-purpuric gloves and socks syndrome (PPGSS), 75t, 82–83, 82f
clinical features of, 82–83
complications of, 83
management of, 83
Papulonecrotic tuberculid, 118
Papulovesiculous exanthems, 75t
Para-aminosalicylic acid, as antituberculosis agent, 1271
Parachlamydia, 1221
Parachlamydia acanthamoebae, 1679t
Paracoccidioides brasiliensis, in skin manifestation of HIV, 884t
Paracoccidioides, 1681t
Paracoccidioides brasiliensis, 1700, 1708
clinical manifestations of, 1709
diagnosis of, 297, 297f
diagnostic microbiology of, 1709
ecology and epidemiology of, 1708–1709
epidemiology of, 296
management of, 297, 1709
mycology of, 296, 1708, 1708f
oral fungal infections, 318
pathogenesis and pathology of, 297
pathogenicity of, 1709
Paracoccidioidins, 1709
Paracoccidioidomycosis, 119, 296–297, 297f, 1700t, 1708–1709
clinical manifestations of, 1709
dermatologic manifestations of, 114t–115t
diagnostic microbiology of, 1702t, 1709
ecology of, 1708–1709
epidemiology of, 1708–1709
lymphadenopathy and, 137t–138t
management of, 1709
mycology of, 1708, 1708f
and occupational infections, 648t–649t
pathogenicity of, 1709
Paragonimus
epidemiology of, 1765
pathogenicity of, 1770–1772
Paragonimus westermani
clinical features of, 1037
clinical manifestations of, 1778
epidemiology of, 1037, 1765
life cycle of, 1771f
pathogenesis and pathology of, 1037
pathogenicity of, 1770–1772
treatment of, 1345t–1351t
Parainfluenza
croup and, 229
in hematopoietic stem cell transplantation, 743
hospital-acquired pneumonia and, 259t
pharyngitis, 234–235
in thoracic transplantation patients, 749
Parainfluenza virus, 1478–1480
bronchitis and, 244t
clinical manifestations, 1478–1480
diagnostic microbiology, 1478, 1479f
epidemiology, 1478
management, 1480
nature, 1478
pathogenicity, 1478
prevention, 1478
Paraldehyde, 1025
Paramyxoviridae, 1480
Paranasal sinus infection, phaeohyphomycosis in, 1721, 1723
Parapoxviruses, 1454–1455, 1454t
clinical manifestations of, 1455, 1455f
diagnosis and differential diagnosis of, 1455
diagnostic microbiology of, 1457
epidemiology of, 1455
management of, 1457
pathogenicity of, 1455
transmission of, 665
Parasites
causes of uveitis, 170–172, 171f, 171t
in chronic meningitis, 186t
in myocarditis, 447
in pericarditis, 451t–452t

Parasites *(Continued)*
in transfusion-related infections, 703–704, 704*t*
see also specific parasites
Parasitic infections
associated with erythema nodosum, 121*t*
in cancer patients, 723*b*
causing jaundice, 1135*t*
chronic diarrhea, 346–349, 347*t*
from dogs, 657*t*
from domesticated herbivores, 666
enteric, in HIV, in low- and middle-income countries, 893
eye involvement in tropical, 982, 983*f*
in hematopoietic stem cell transplantation, 741*t*
in HIV/AIDS, 856–857, 857*f*
in kidney transplant patients, 768–769
microbiome and, 73–74
Parasitic pathogens, in infectious diseases, transmitted by grafts, 807
Paraspinal abscesses, 1099, 1100*f*
Parastrongyliasis, 1764–1765
Paratyphoid diseases, vaccination for travelers, 949
Paratyphoid fever
epidemiology of, 1002
and occupational infections, 648*t*–649*t*
prevention of, 1003
quinolones for, 1245
Parechovirus, perinatal infections and, 514–515
Parenteral antimicrobial agents, for melioidosis, 1076–1077
Parenteral penicillin G, for syphilis, 565
Parenteral therapy
for complicated urinary tract infection, 544
lung abscess and, 268
Pari passu, 2
Paritaprevir, for hepatitis C, 1331
Paromomycin
for amebic infections, 1012
for gastrointestinal protozoa, 999, 1000*t*
for leishmaniasis, 1064, 1758
for parasitic infections, 1345*t*–1362*t*, 1368
for prevention of amebic infections, 1009
Paronychia, 88–89
Parotitis, 319–320
anaerobic bacteria in, 1637
caused by *Mycobacteria* species, 320
in melioidosis, 1075
suppurative, 319*f*
Parturient animals, infections from, 191*t*
Parvoviridae, 78, 1449
Parvovirus B19, 75*t*, 702, 703*t*, 1449–1450, 1449*f*
clinical features of, 78
complications of, 78
in congenital infection
clinical features of, 510
diagnosis of, 512, 512*t*
management of, 513
pathogenesis and pathology of, 506
screening of, during pregnancy, 508*t*
encephalitis/myelitis and, 194*t*
infections, 78*f*
management of, 79
myocarditis and, 447
Parvoviruses, 1449–1451
clinical manifestation of, 1451, 1451*f*
diagnostic microbiology of, 1451
epidemiology of, 1450
management of, 1451
nature of, 1449–1450
and occupational infections, 648*t*–649*t*
pathogenicity of, 1450, 1450*f*
prevention of, 1450–1451
Passive hemagglutination assay (PHA), 1083
Passive immunization
for hepatitis A virus, 364
for hepatitis B virus, 366
with rabies immune globulin, 1463
Passive immunotherapy, for postsplenectomy sepsis, 779
Pasteurella, 1611, 1625
from cat bites, 659
clinical manifestations of, 1625
diagnostic microbiology of, 1625
epidemiology of, 1625
management of, 1625
nature of, 1625

Pasteurella (Continued)
pathogenicity of, 1625
prevention of, 1625
Pasteurella aerogenes, 665
Pasteurella multocida, 1625
in bacterial arthritis, 383*t*
cellulitis and, 90
Pasteurellosis, 648*t*–649*t*
Pastia's lines, 116
Pathogen-associated molecular patterns (PAMPs), 419, 421, 422*f*, 685, 842
Pathogen recognition receptors (PRRs), 26, 29*f*
collaborative interactions between, 31
Pathogenesis of infectious disease, 10–15
see also specific micro-organisms
Pathogenetic classifications, in osteomyelitis, 390
Pathogenicity islands (PAIs), 1569
Pathognomonic periportal fibrosis, 1030
Patient exposure history, selected historical points in, 664*t*
Patient posture, hospital-acquired pneumonia, 262
Patient safety, 58
PCR-restriction enzyme analysis (PRA), for mycobacteria, 1654
PD-1, 843
Pearly penile papules, 586*t*–587*t*
Pedal dermatophytosis, 1710
Pediatric autoimmune neuropsychiatric disorders associated with streptococci, 473–474
Pediatrics, quinolones for, 1246
Pediculus humanus capitis, 107*f*–108*f*
Pediculus humanus corporis, 107*f*
Pediococcus spp., intrinsic resistance of, 1182*t*
PEDIS Classification, on diabetic foot infection, 130*t*
Pedobacter, 1581*t*–1582*t*
Pefloxacin
for anaerobic bacteria, 1643
dissociation constants of, 535*t*
Pegylated interferon-α 2b, 875*t*
Pegylated interferons, 1327
in kidney transplant patients, 768
Pegylated liposomal doxorubicin, 875*t*
Peliosis, bacillary, 1675
Pelvic abscesses, 497
Pelvic infection, antimicrobial therapy for, 1641*t*
Pelvic inflammatory disease (PID), 492–494
antibiotics for, 1152*t*
clinical features of, 493
diagnosis of, 493
epidemiology of, 492
in gonorrhea, 592, 594
and HIV infection, 906
management of, 493–494, 494*t*
Mycoplasma genitalium in, 1662–1663
Mycoplasma hominis in, 1664
from *Neisseria gonorrhoeae*, 1562
pathogenesis and pathology of, 492, 492*t*
prevention of, 492
quinolones for, 1243
treatment of, 596*t*
Penams, 1162
Penciclovir, 1146*t*–1147*t*, 1312
adverse reactions of, 1312
dosage of, 1312
in special circumstances, 1312
for genital herpes, 573
indications of, 1312
genital herpes, 573, 1312
herpes labialis, 1312
herpes zoster, 1312
for herpesvirus, 1433
mechanism of action, 1312
resistance to, 1312
route of administration, 1312
in vitro activity, 1312
Penicillary arterioles, 775, 776*f*
Penicillin-binding proteins (PBPs), 1162–1163, 1181
Penicillin G
for anaerobic bacteria, 1642
for anthrax, 1127
dosage in renal failure, 1213*t*–1214*t*
for gram-positive bacilli, 1210
for lung abscess, 269*f*–270*f*
meningitis and, 187*t*
pharmacokinetics of, 1205*t*
prophylaxis

Penicillin G *(Continued)*
intrapartum, 1209
rheumatic fever, 1209
for syphilis, 565
for *Treponema pallidum*, 513
Penicillin-resistant *Streptococcus pneumonia*, prevalence of, 1529*f*
Penicillin V
for actinomycosis, 316
for acute necrotizing ulcerative gingivitis, 316
dosage in renal failure, 1213*t*–1214*t*
pharmacokinetics of, 1205*t*
in rheumatic fever, 476
prophylaxis of, 475*t*
Penicillinase-resistant penicillins, 1203
antimicrobial spectrum, generic names, routes of administration and dosages, 1206*t*–1207*t*
for lymph node enlargement, 149
for staphylococcal infections, 1209
Penicillins, 1181, 1203–1204
adverse reactions of, 1153
for anaerobic bacteria, 1210, 1642–1643
for anthrax, 1127
antimicrobial spectrum, generic names, routes of administration and dosages, 1206*t*–1207*t*
for brain abscess, 202–203
for cancer patients, 734–735
cellulitis and, 92
for croup, 235
for diphtheria, 1546
for dog bites, 657*t*
dosage in renal failure, 1213*t*–1214*t*
drug interactions, 1216
for endemic treponematoses, 965
in endocarditis, 466–467
for *Erysipelothrix rhusiopathiae*, 1542
for gas gangrene, 100–101
for gonorrhea, 595
for infective arthritis, 386*t*
for intra-abdominal sepsis, 357–358
for leptospirosis, 1103, 1609
for *Listeria monocytogenes*, 1540
in Lyme disease, 412
for mastitis, 504
for meningitis, 180
for necrotizing fasciitis, 97
pharmacokinetics of, 1205*t*
for pneumococcal infections, 1209
prophylaxis
for postsplenectomy sepsis, 778
for streptococcal infections, 1535
for *Pseudomonas aeruginosa*, 1589
for recurrent pharyngotonsillitis, 1637–1638
for relapsing fevers, 1109
resistance to, 1184
anaerobic bacteria, 1210
Bacillus cereus, 1542
meningitis and, 180
Streptococcus pneumoniae, 1535
in rheumatic fever, 476
prophylaxis of, 475, 475*t*
semisynthetic, discovery of, 1217
for staphylococcal infections, 1209
for *Staphylococcus aureus*, 1520
for streptococcal infections, 1534
for *Streptococcus pneumoniae*, 1535
susceptibilities of selected bacteria to, 1208*t*–1209*t*
for *Treponema pallidum*, 513
Penicilliosis, 298–299
in HIV/AIDS, 855
Penicillium, 1681*t*, 1698–1699
Penicillium marneffei
clinical features of, 298
diagnosis of, 298
in HIV/AIDS, 855
in low- and middle-income countries, 893
mycology and epidemiology of, 298
pathogenesis and pathology of, 298
in skin manifestation of HIV, 884*t*
Penis
cancer in, human papillomavirus and, 579
ulcers of, in primary HIV infection, 846, 847*f*
Pentamidine
for African trypanosomiasis, 969, 969*t*, 1762
for leishmaniasis, 1064

Pentamidine (Continued)
for parasitic infections, 1345t–1351t
Pneumocystis jirovecii pneumonia associated with, 851
in pregnancy, 910
Pentamidine isethionate
adverse reactions of, 1369
dosage of, 1368–1369
indications of, for parasitic infections, 1345t–1362t, 1368–1369
route of administration, 1368–1369
Pentatrichomonas (Trichomonas) hominis, 1725t
Pentavalent antimonial compounds, 1352t–1362t, 1369
Pentavalent antimonials
intralesional administration of, 1063
for leishmaniasis, 1063
toxicity of, 1063
Pentosan polysulphate, 220
Peptic ulceration, 321–327
discovery of infectious cause of, 625
management of, 326, 326f
see also Duodenal ulceration; Gastric ulceration
Peptidoglycan
biosynthesis, 1192f
neisserial, 1559
Staphylococcus aureus and, 1514f, 1516
synthesis inhibition of, 1163f, 1164
Peptidyltransferase center, 1221
Peptococcus, 1631
Peptoniphilus, lung abscess and, 264–265
Peptostreptococcus
antimicrobial drugs of choice for, 1642t
hospital-acquired pneumonia and, 259t
in human bites, 682, 683t
lung abscess and, 264–265
in normal flora, 1632, 1632t
in otitis media, 1637
susceptibility to antimicrobial agents, 1642f
Peptostreptococcus anaerobius, 1631
Peptostreptococcus asaccharolyticus, 1631
Peptostreptococcus magnus, 1631
Peptostreptococcus micros, 1631
Peptostreptococcus prevotii, 1631
Peramivir, 1324
adverse reactions and interactions of, 1324
dosage of, 1324
in special circumstances, 1324
indications of, 1324
pharmacokinetics and distribution of, 1320t, 1324
route of administration, 1324
Percutaneous drainage
for amebic liver abscess, 1013
procedures, for peritonitis, 359
Percutaneous endoscopic gastrostomy, antibiotic prophylaxis and, 1160
Percutaneous exposure, to HIV infection, 835
Percutaneous transhepatic cholangiography (PTC), biliary sepsis, 360
Pericardial effusion
clinical features of, 478, 478f
diagnosis of, 478–480, 479f
etiology of, 478–480
management of, 478–480
management therapy for, 480
in pericarditis, 450, 452, 453t
Pericardial friction rub, 452
Pericardiectomy, 454
Pericardiocentesis, 454, 478–480
Pericarditis, 449–454
in AIDS, 452
bacteria in, 450
causes of, 450b, 451t–452t
clinical features of, 452, 452f–453f
diagnosis of, 452–454, 453t, 454f
epidemiology of, 449
infectious agents in, 450
management of, 454
noninfectious agents in, 449–450
pathogenesis and pathology of, 449–452, 450f
treatment of, 443t
tuberculosis and, 279
viruses in, 450
Pericystectomy, for echinococcosis, 1044
Perihepatitis, 1563

Perinatal infections, 513–515, 514t
see also Congenital infection; Neonates
Perinatal transmission, HIV, 814
Periodontal infection, 312–314
clinical features of, 313
complications of, 313, 313f–314f
epidemiology of, 312
management of, 313–314
pathogenesis and pathology of, 312, 312f
prevention of, 312–313
Periorbital cellulitis, 156–157
Periorbital structures, 150–157
infections of, 156–157
Peripheral blood mononuclear cells (PBMC), 1657–1658
Peripheral blood stem cells (PBSCs), 739
Peripheral nerve involvement, in leprosy, 957
Peripheral neuropathy
in African trypanosomiasis, 969
linezolid and, 1231–1232
Peripherally inserted central catheters (PICCs)
catheter-related bloodstream infection (CRBSI) and, 428–430
in outpatient parenteral antimicrobial therapy, 1201
Peritoneum, 356
Peritonitis, 355–362
Alcaligenes xylosoxidans in, 1597
antibiotics for, 1152t
associated with chronic ambulatory peritoneal dialysis, 380–381
chronic ambulatory peritoneal dialysis (CAPD), 359
clinical presentation of, 356
culture-negative, 381
diffuse, 690
investigations of, 356–357
microbiology of, 355–356
pathophysiology of, 356, 356f
polymicrobial, with enteric bacteria, 381
postoperative, 358, 690
primary (spontaneous), 359
Pseudomonas aeruginosa and, 381
refractory, 380
spontaneous bacterial. see Spontaneous bacterial peritonitis (SBP)
tertiary, 690
tuberculous, 359–360
Peritonsillar abscess, 235, 1636t
Permethrin, for anaplasmosis, 1672
Persistent generalized lymphadenopathy (PGL) syndrome, 143
Persistent nongonococcal urethritis, 603–604
diagnosis of, 603
etiology of, 603
treatment of, 603–604
Personal hygiene measures, in gastrointestinal parasites, 995
Personal protective equipment (PPE), 58
Perstans filariasis
clinical features of, 1050
epidemiology of, 1046
management of, 1051
pathogenesis and pathology of, 1047
Pertactin (PRN), 1612, 1613t
Pertussis
complications of, 1613–1614
diagnostic microbiology of, 1612–1613
epidemiology of, 1611
management of, 1614
and occupational infections, 648t–649t
pathogenicity of, 1612
prevention of, 1612
vaccination, 782t–783t, 1611
Pertussis toxin (PT), 1612, 1613t
Pest control worker, and occupational infections, 648t–649t
Petechiae, conjunctival, 982
Petechial exanthems, 75t
Petechial hemorrhages, 1106–1107, 1107f
Pets, infections from, 656–662
see also specific animals
*Pf*EMP1, 1017
Phaeohyphomycosis
cerebral, 1723
clinical manifestations of, 1720–1721

Phaeohyphomycosis (Continued)
cutaneous, 1721, 1723
diagnostic microbiology of, 1718, 1718f
epidemiology of, 1714
management of, 1723
nature of, 1713
other forms of, 1721
in paranasal sinus infection, 1721, 1723
pathogenicity of, 1715
prevention of, 1715
subcutaneous, 1720–1721, 1723
in transplant recipients, 1721
Phage typing
for *Acinetobacter baumannii*, 1583t–1584t
for *Pseudomonas aeruginosa*, 1583t–1584t
Phagocytes
inhibition of the mobilization of, 22
innate immune response, 31–32
killing before being ingested, 22–23
professional, 23
surviving, 22–23
Phagocytosis, 23f
cryptococcosis and, 1692
innate immune response, 31
of mycobacteria, 1649, 1650f
resistance of *Staphylococcus aureus* to, 1514, 1515f
in tuberculosis, 272
Phagolysosome
Histoplasma capsulatum and, 1707
of mycobacteria, 1649
Phagosome, 1649
Phambili trials, 832
Pharmacokinetic (PK) enhancer, perinatal HIV transmission prevention, 909t
Pharmacokinetics, 1147–1151
see also specific class of drugs; specific drugs
Pharmacy, disease prevention and control, 57–58
Pharyngeal gonorrhea, 1563
Pharyngeal infections, 594–595
Pharyngitis, 233–235
clinical features of, 234–235, 234b, 235f
diagnosis of, 235
epidemiology of, 233
genital herpes and, 572
management of, 235
meningococcal, 1564
physiology of, 233–234
plague, 1083
prevention of, 234
Pharyngoconjunctival fever, 139t
lymphadenopathy and, 137t–138t
Pharyngotonsillitis, 1637–1638
Pharynx, infections of, in cancer patients, 727
Phase variation, 24–25
neisserial genome instability and, 1555
Phenothiazine
adverse reactions, 212
prion infection and, 220
Phenotype prediction, genome sequencing, 66
Phenotypic classification, of *Neisseria*, 1561–1562
Phenotypic identification, of *Acinetobacter* spp., 1594
Phenotypic tests, of HIV-1 drug resistance, 1489–1490, 1490f
Phenotypic typing method, for *Pseudomonas* spp., 1583t–1584t
Phlebitis, suppurative, 691
Phlebotomus perniciosus, 111f
Phlebovirus, 1495t
Phospholipase A2, 501
Phosphorylcholine (ChoP), pneumococcal cell wall, 1531–1532
Phosphotransferases (APH), 1185, 1185t
Photodermatitis, in HIV/AIDS, 881, 882f
'Phylodynamics', 53
Physical contact, and recreational infections, 645
Physiotherapy, for leprosy, 960
Picobirnaviruses, diarrhea and, 338
Picornavirales, causing meningitis, 225
Picornaviridae, 1477
Picornavirus, 1407
Piedra
black. see Black piedra
clinical features of, 126

Piedra (Continued)
   epidemiology of, 122
   management of, 128
   white. *see* White piedra
Piedraia hortae
   epidemiology of, 122
   nature of, 1710
Pigmentary alteration, and skin manifestations of HIV, 886
Pigs
   Brucella suis, 663
   Pasteurella aerogenes, 665
   Streptococcus suis, 664
   xenotransplantation of tissues from, 665
   Yersinia enterocolitica, 664
Pili, 14
   Neisseria, 1557t, 1559
   of *Pseudomonas aeruginosa*, 1584–1585
Pinta, 961
   clinical features of, 964
   dermatologic manifestations of, 114t–115t
   pathology of, 963
Pinworms, 1777
Piperacillin
   for anaerobic bacteria, 1210, 1643
   antimicrobial spectrum, routes of administration and
      dosages, 1206t–1207t
   for complicated urinary tract infection, 545t
   dosage in renal failure, 1213t–1214t
   drug interactions, 1216
   for lung abscess, 269f
   for *P. aeruginosa* infection, 1210
   susceptibilities of selected bacteria to, 1208t–1209t
Piperacillin-tazobactam
   antimicrobial spectrum, routes of administration and
      dosages, 1206t–1207t
   for complicated urinary tract infection, 545t
   dosage in renal failure, 1213t–1214t
   for foot ulcers, 131t
   hospital-acquired pneumonia and, 260t
   for lung abscess, 269f
   pharmacokinetics of, 1205t
   susceptibilities of selected bacteria to, 1208t–1209t
Piperaquine, 1352t–1362t, 1369
   for falciparum malaria, 1022
Piperazine, 1352t–1362t
Piperazine hydrate, 1000, 1001t
Piperazine phosphate, 1000, 1001t
Pirlimycin, 1223
Piroplasmida, 1751
Pityriasis versicolor
   clinical features of, 126, 126f
   management of, 128
Pivmecillinam, for cystitis, 528t
PK enhancer, perinatal HIV transmission prevention, 909t
Placenta, congenital infections in, 507
Plague, 1078–1084, 1575, 1627
   and bioterrorism, 671t, 677–678
      bubonic, and bioterrorism, 672t
      primary pneumonic, and bioterrorism, 672t–673t,
         677, 678f
      septicemic, and bioterrorism, 673t
   bubonic. *see* Bubonic plague
   clinical features of, 1081–1083
   diagnosis of, 1083
   disease incidence of, 1080
   epidemiology of, 1078–1081, 1079f, 1079t
   geographic distribution of, 1080, 1080f
   lymphadenopathy and, 137t–138t, 140
   management of, 1083–1084, 1083t
   and occupational infections, 648t–649t
   pathogenesis and pathology of, 1081
   pneumonic. *see* Pneumonic plague
   populations affected by, 1080
   prevention and control of, 1081
   risks for humans of, 1081
   seasonality of, 1081
   sepsis, 1081
   septicemic. *see* Septicemic plague
   sources of infection of, 1081
   transmission of, 1078, 1079f, 1079t, 1081
Plain radiography
   for infected foot ulcers, 130
   in osteomyelitis, 393
   in prosthetic joint infection (PJI), 401–402
   pulmonary tuberculosis, 276–277

Plaque, in dental and periodontal infections, 312
Plaque-reduction neutralization tests
   West Nile virus, 1498
   yellow fever, 1494
Plasma cell (Zoon's) balanitis, 586t–587t
Plasma HIV viral load, 912–913
Plasma kinetics, of sulfonamides, 1280
Plasmablastic lymphomas, 876
Plasmapheresis, 770
Plasmidotyping
   for *Acinetobacter baumannii*, 1583t–1584t
   for *Pseudomonas aeruginosa*, 1583t–1584t
Plasmids, of mycobacteria, 1646
Plasmodium
   life cycle of, 1014f
   in postsplenectomy sepsis, 778t
   transmission of, 807
   see also Malaria
Plasmodium falciparum, 1014, 1014f
   amodiaquine for, 1364
   chloroqine-resistant, 1345t–1351t, 1366
   cytoadherence and, 1016–1017
   epidemiology of, 1016
   geographic distribution of, 1015f, 1016
   glycosylphosphatidylinositol anchor of, 1017
   in HIV in low- and middle-income countries, 894–895
   incubation period of, 1018
   management of, 1022–1023, 1023t–1024t, 1345t–1351t
      in pregnancy, 1024t
   pathogenesis and pathology of, 1016, 1016f
   prevention of, 950–951
   vaccine against, 1018
Plasmodium knowlesi, 1014
Plasmodium malariae, 1014, 1014f
   geographic distribution of, 1016
   management of, 1023–1024
   pathogenesis and pathology of, 1016
Plasmodium ovale, 1014, 1014f
   geographic distribution of, 1016
   management of, 1023–1024, 1024b, 1345t–1351t
   pathogenesis and pathology of, 1016
Plasmodium vivax, 1014, 1014f
   epidemiology of, 1016
   geographic distribution of, 1016
   incubation period of, 1018
   management of, 1023–1024, 1024b, 1345t–1351t
   pathogenesis and pathology of, 1016
Platelet microbicidal proteins (PMPs), 459
Platinum coordination complexes, 1379
Platyhelminthes, nature of, 1763
plcHR, 1585
Pleconaril, in chronic meningitis, 185–186
Plesiomonas shigelloides, 1567–1568, 1577t
   diarrhea, 331
Pleural discharge/fluid
   analysis, 303–304, 304t
   imaging of, 303, 303f
   investigation of, 303–305
   lower respiratory tract infections, 268
   microbiology of, 303
   pathophysiology of, 303
Pleural effusion, 263
   community-acquired pneumonia and, 256
   HIV-associated TB, 869, 869f
   in immune reconstitution inflammatory syndrome, 863
   management of, 304, 305f
   thoracic surgery for, 304
Pleural fibrinolytics, 304
Pleuropulmonary infections, anaerobic bacteria in, 1638,
      1638t
PML-immune reconstitution inflammatory syndrome
      (IRIS), 1447
Pneumococcal capsule, 1531
Pneumococcal infections
   in HIV/AIDS, 857
   β-lactam antibiotics for, 1209
Pneumococcal meningitis, pathophysiology, 179
Pneumococcal polysaccharide vaccine (PPV23),
      community-acquired pneumonia and, 256
Pneumococcal vaccine, community-acquired pneumonia
      and, 256
Pneumococci
   antibiotic therapy for, in infective arthritis, 386t
   jaundice, 1135t
   vaccination against, 782t–783t

Pneumocystis, 1681t
   infections, in hematopoietic stem cell transplantation,
      745
Pneumocystis jirovecii
   hospital-acquired pneumonia and, 259t
   prevention n newborns born of HIV-infected mothers,
      901
   prophylaxis against, in cancer patients, 732
   splenic infection, 362
   in thoracic transplantation patients, 747t, 750
   and tumor necrosis factor inhibitor, 799–800
Pneumocystis jirovecii pneumonia (PJP)
   clinical features of, 851, 851f–852f
   in hematopoietic stem cell transplantation, 745
   in HIV/AIDS
      in low- and middle-income countries, 891
      opportunistic infection in, 850–852, 851f
   management of, 851–852
   prevention of, 852
   prophylaxis, 771
      in HIV-infected patients, 914
      in HIV-infected women, 910
   in thoracic transplantation patients, 750
Pneumonia, 1290
   Acinetobacter spp. in, 1594–1595
   Alcaligenes xylosoxidans in, 1597
   aminoglycosides for, 1237
   aspiration. *see* Aspiration pneumonia
   bacterial, in HIV/AIDS, 857
      in low- and middle-income countries, 891
   and bioterrorism, 673t
   Burkholderia spp. in, 1596
   in cancer patients, 727
   from *Candida*, 1684
   cavitary, 252f
   classic lobar, pathologic phases of, 253t
   community-acquired. *see* Community-acquired
      pneumonia (CAP)
   cryptococcal, 1692
   and drowning-associated infections, 680
   fungal, 292–299
   in hematopoietic stem cell transplantation, 742–743
   hospital-acquired. *see* Hospital-acquired pneumonia
      (HAP)
   ICU-acquired. *see* ICU-acquired pneumonia
   influenza virus and, 1470
   Mycoplasma pneumoniae in, 1661
   nosocomial, quinolones for, 1245
   pathogens, 691
   Pneumocystis jirovecii pneumonia (PJP). *see*
      Pneumocystis jirovecii pneumonia (PJP)
   postoperative, 690–691, 690t
   in pregnancy, 500–501
   Pseudomonas aeruginosa, 1592–1593
   respiratory syncytial virus, 1475–1476
   and smoke inhalation injury, 698
   and thoracic transplantation patients, 746–747
   vancomycin for, 1251
   ventilator-associated, 60, 1375
Pneumonia Severity Index (PSI), 256
Pneumonic plague, 672t–673t, 1078
   clinical features of, 1082–1083, 1082f
   diagnosis of, 677
   differential diagnosis of, 677
   management of, 1083
   presentation of, 677, 678f
   transmission of, 677–678, 1081
Pneumonic tularemia, 1089
Pneumonitis, toxoplasmic, 856–857
Point-of-care laboratories (POCLs), 1389
pol genes, 1483, 1484f
Poliomyelitis
   eradication of, 1411–1412, 1411t
   vaccination against, 782t–783t
Poliovirus
   electron microscopy for, 1412, 1412f
   paralysis in, 1411
   receptor, 1407
   serotyping for, 1412
   vaccines, 1411, 1411t
      endgame of, 1411–1412, 1411t
Polyarteritis nodosa (PAN), 614
Polyene, with caspofungin, 1698
Polyene antifungal agents, 1333–1340
   chemical structure of, 1333f

Polyhexamethylene biguanide, for *Acanthamoeba* keratitis, 1750
Polymerase chain reaction (PCR)
    adenovirus, 1472–1473
    for African trypanosomiasis, 1761
    in bacterial arthritis, 384–385
    for bartonellosis, 1673
    for *Bordetella pertussis*, 1613
    for brucellosis, 1100, 1615
    for *Campylobacter* spp., 1602
    in cancer patients, 733
    for *Candida* spp., 442, 1682t, 1683
    for Chagas disease, 1071
    for *Clostridium difficile*, 1630
    in endocarditis, 461
    endophthalmitis and, 162
    for *Entamoeba* spp., 1729
    for *Francisella tularensis*, 1617
    in genital herpes, 572
    for giardiasis, 347
    for *Helicobacter pylori*, 1603
    for helminths diagnosis, 1777
    for herpesvirus, 1435
    HIV-1, 1488
    in human papillomavirus, 576, 579
    for leishmaniasis, 1757
    for leprosy, 958
    for *Leptospira* spp., 1609
    in liver transplant patients, 753–754
    for lobomycosis, 1717
    in Lyme arthritis, 411
    in Lyme disease, 405
    in lymphogranuloma venereum, 588
    of melioidosis, 1076
    for *Moraxella catarrhalis*, 1624
    for mycobacteria, 1654
    for *Mycoplasma pneumoniae*, 1660
    in myocarditis, 448
    in newborns born of HIV-infected mothers, 901
    for plague, 1083
    for primary amebic meningoencephalitis, 1747
    for *Rhinosporidium seeberi*, 1718
    ribotyping, 351
    for *Rickettsia* spp., 1667
    for scrub typhus, 1670
    of scrub typhus, 1096–1097
    in syphilis, 563
    for *Toxoplasma gondii*, 1754
    of tularemia, 1089
    uveitis, 167
    for viral hemorrhagic fevers, 1116
    for Whipple's disease, 345
    yellow fever, 1494
Polymicrobial meningitis, 772
Polymicrobial peritonitis, with enteric bacteria, 381
Polymorphonuclear leukocytes (PMNLs)
    in pyelonephritis, 548f
    staphylococcal lesions and, 1516
    toll-like receptors (TLRs) in, 356
    in trichomoniasis, 485
Polymyxin B, 1286
    against carbapenamase-resistant gram-negative bacilli, 1290t
    chemical structure, 1285
Polymyxins, 1178–1180, 1285–1288
    adverse reactions of, 1288
    for *Alcaligenes* spp., 1597
    available preparations of, 1286
    chemical structure of, 1178, 1285
    clinical use of, 1287–1288
        for special circumstances, 1288
    drug-drug interactions of, 1288
    mechanism(s) of activity, 1285
    mode of action of, 1178, 1179f
    non-antibiotic pharmacologic and toxicologic
        properties related to chemical structure of, 1180
    pharmacodynamics of, 1180
    pharmacokinetics and distribution, 1286–1287, 1286t
    for *Pseudomonas aeruginosa*, 1589
    resistance to, 1180, 1193
    spectrum of activity, 1285–1286, 1286t
    in vitro susceptibility testing, 1286

Polyomaviruses, 1445–1448
    clinical manifestations of, 1446–1447
    diagnostic microbiology of, 1446
    epidemiology of, 1445
    in human malignancies, 1447
    in kidney transplant patients, 767
    management of, 1447–1448
    nature of, 1445, 1446t
    pathogenicity of, 1445
    prevention of, 1445–1446
Polypeptides, as antituberculosis agents, 1270
Polyps, in mucous membranes, 1721
Polyradiculopathy, cytomegalovirus, 853
Polysaccharide, 10, 12
Polysaccharide capsule, 1513t–1514t
    Neisseria, 1557t
Polysaccharide intercellular adhesin (PIA), 1513t–1514t
Polysaccharide meningococcal vaccines, 1560
Polyvalent pneumococcal vaccine, 688
Pontiac fever, 645, 1624
Population density, and emerging infectious diseases, 45–46
Population-level effects, 50
Population movements, parasites and, 990
Porins, *Neisseria*, 1558
Pork, infections from, 191t
Porphyromonas, 1631, 1632f
    and brain abscess, 199
    halitosis, 319
    in human bites, 682
    in normal flora, 1632, 1632t
    susceptibility to antimicrobial agents, 1642f
Posaconazole, 1340
    adverse effects of, 1340
    for aspergillosis, 1691
    for blastomycosis, 295
    for cancer patients, 737–738
    for *Candida* infection, 440
    chemical structure of, 1337f
    dosage of, 1340
        in special circumstances, 1340
    drug interactions of, 1340
    for esophageal candidiasis, 1686
    for fusariosis, 1700
    for histoplasmosis, 294
    indications of, 1340
    for mucormycosis, 1698
    for mycetoma, 1723
    for oropharyngeal candidiasis, 1684
    pharmacokinetics and distribution of, 1340
    prophylaxis with, in cancer patients, 730
    route of administration, 1340
Positron emission tomography (PET)
    in arterial graft infection, 437, 438f
    for echinococcosis, 1044
    for fever of unknown origin, 620
    2-fluorodeoxyglucose. *see* 2-Fluorodeoxyglucose-positron emission tomography (FDG PET)
Post-kala-azar dermal leishmaniasis, 1062, 1757
Post kala-azar dermatitis, 119
Post-Lyme disease syndrome (PLTDS), 413–414
Post-neurosurgery, brain abscess and, 199
Post-streptococcal reactive arthritis, 473
Post-transplant acute limbic encephalitis (PALE), 742
Post-transplant lymphoproliferative disease (PTLD)
    EBV-associated, 756
        diagnosis of, 760
        prevention of, 760
        treatment of, 759t, 760
    in thoracic transplantation patients, 748
Post-traumatic stress disorder (PTSD), 679
Postabortal fever, *Mycoplasma hominis* in, 1664
Postabortion sepsis, 496
Postantibiotic effect, 1233
Postexposure prophylaxis
    of HIV, 835–836, 836b
    for rabies, 1462
Postherpetic neuralgia, 76
Postinflammatory encephalomyelitis, 194
Postnatal transmission, HIV, 814
Postoperative infection
    bloodstream infection, 691, 691t
    diagnosis of, 690

Postoperative infection *(Continued)*
    intra-abdominal, 690
    pneumonia, 690–691, 690t. see also Pneumonia
    prophylaxis of, 689
Postoperative period, 688–691
    and blood transfusion, 689
    hyperglycemia and control of blood sugar, 689–690
    prophylaxis in, 689
Postpartum endometritis, 494–495, 495t, 500, 503
Postpartum fever, *Mycoplasma hominis* in, 1664
Postpartum infections, 500
Postpartum period, tuberculosis in, 1275
Postsplenectomy sepsis
    antimicrobial prophylaxis for, 777–778
    epidemiology of, 775
    immunizations to prevent, 777–778
    immunologic defects and factors predisposing to, 775, 776t
    predisposing factors to, 776
    prevention of, 776–778, 777t
    prophylaxis of, 688
    risk factors for, 776t
Poststreptococcal autoimmune neuropsychiatric disorder associated with streptococci, 1533
Potassium iodide solution
    for basidiobolomycosis, 1723
    for conidiobolomycosis, 1722–1723
    for sporotrichosis, 1724
Pott's disease, 278–279
Pott's puffy tumor, 204
Poultry worker, and occupational infections, 648t–649t
Poverty, and emerging infectious diseases, 43
Povidone-iodine, in cutaneous antiseptic, 428
Powassan, 1495t
Powassan virus, 193t–194t
Poxviruses, 1452–1457
    nature of, 1452, 1452f
    pathogenic for humans, 1452, 1454t
    prevention of, 1452
    replication cycle of, 1453f
Prawns, infections from, 191t
Praziquantel
    for cysticercosis, 1035
    for gastrointestinal helminth, 1001, 1001t
    for helminths, 1772
    for liver flukes, 1036
    for lung flukes, 1037
    for parasitic infections, 1345t–1362t, 1371–1372
    for schistosomiasis management, 1031
    for schistosomiasis prevention, 1029
Pre- and post-massage test (PPMT), 533
Pre-conception counseling, for HIV infection, 907–908
Pre-exposure prophylaxis (PrEP), for HIV, 825–826, 907–908
Pre-term premature rupture of membranes (pPROM)
    epidemiology of, 498
    in intra-amniotic infection, 500
Precipitins, 1707–1708
Preconception immunity, maternal immunity and, 506
Prednisone, for leprosy reactions, 959
Pregnancy
    African trypanosomiasis treatment in, 970
    brucellosis complications in, 1099
    complications of, 498–504, 499f
        antibiotics in, 504
        burden of disease, morbidity and mortality in, 500
        clinical features of, 503
        clinical syndrome of, 499–500
        diagnosis of, 503
        epidemiology of, 498–501
        immunity of, 501
        implications of
            sexually transmitted diseases on, 500t
            specific infections on, 499t
        incidence and prevalence of, 498–499
        management of, 503–504
        pathogenesis and pathology of, 501, 502t
        prevention of, 501–503
        risk factors of, 500–501
    drugs in
        clindamycin, 1227
        β-lactam antibiotics, 1212

Pregnancy (Continued)
    herpes in, 572
    HIV infection in. see HIV infection, in pregnancy
    listeriosis during, 1540
    Lyme disease in, 412t, 413
    malaria in, 1021, 1141–1144, 1141t, 1143t–1144t
        classification of, 1142t
        prevention of, 951
        treatment of, 951, 1143t
    maternal immunity in, 507
    Mycoplasma hominis during, 1664
    in occupational exposure, to HIV infection, 835
    quinolones in, 1246
    studies diagnostic of or consistent with acute infection
        in, 518
    termination of, 519
    toxoplasmosis in, 1755
    travelers immunization and, 950
    treatment of falciparum malaria in, 1024t
    treatment of positive Toxoplasma titer in, 517–519
    tuberculosis in, 1275
    typhoid fever in, 1004
    urinary tract infection in, 528, 528t, 530f
    viral hemorrhagic fevers in, 1117
Preseptal cellulitis, 156
Preterm birth, in pregnancy, 498, 500
Pretransplantation stage, periods of, 787
Prevalence, definition, 49
Prevertebral space, 314
Prevotella, 1631, 1632f
    and brain abscess, 204
    empyema and, 266t
    hospital-acquired pneumonia and, 259t
    in human bites, 682, 683t
    lung abscess and, 264–265
    in normal flora, 312, 1632, 1632t
    in sinusitis, 1637
    susceptibility to antimicrobial agents, 1642f
Prevotella bivia, 1631, 1632f, 1632t
Prevotella disiens, 1631, 1632f, 1632t
Prevotella intermedia, 319
Primaquine
    for malaria prophylaxis, 951
    for ovale malaria, 1024b
    for parasitic infections, 1345t–1362t, 1369
    for vivax malaria, 1024, 1024b
Primaquine phosphate, for parasitic infections,
        1345t–1351t, 1369
Primary amebic meningoencephalitis (PAM),
        1745–1746
    diagnostic microbiology of, 1747
    management of, 1749
    pathogenicity of, 1746
    pathologic features of, 1747–1748, 1748f
    prevention of, 1746–1747
Primary CNS lymphomas (PCNSL), 876
    clinical features of, 876
    diagnosis of, 876
    management of, 876
Primary effusion lymphoma, 876
Primary eosinophilia, 985
Primary flap closure, for mediastinitis and sternal
        osteomyelitis, 482
Primary inoculation, tuberculosis, 117
Primary reclosure, with suction, for mediastinitis and
        sternal osteomyelitis, 482
Primates, infections from, 661
Prime-boost strategy, 832
Prion, definition of, 4
Prion diseases
    animal, 215t
        epidemiology of, 214–215
    human, 215t
        clinical features of, 217
        epidemiology of, 215–217, 216f
    inherited, 215t
    pathogenesis of, 219
Prion protein (PrP), 214
Pristinamycin, 1228–1229
    antibacterial activities, 1227, 1228t
    interactions, 1229
    mechanism of action, 1228
    pharmacokinetics, 1229
    properties, 1227
    resistance, 1228–1229

Probenecid, interactions with β-lactam antibiotics,
        1216
Probiotics, 12, 1373–1376, 1374f, 1374t
Procaine penicillin G, pharmacokinetics of, 1204
Procalcitonin
    in cancer patients, 733
    in sepsis, 420
Proctitis
    gonococcal, 1563
    Mycoplasma genitalium in, 1662
Progressive multifocal leukoencephalopathy, 1446–1447
    in HIV/AIDS, 854f
        immune reconstitution inflammatory syndrome
            associated with, 859–860
        and natalizumab, 802
        and rituximab, 800
Progressive outer retinal necrosis (PORN), 173
Proguanil
    as antifolate agent, 1364
    for malaria prophylaxis, 951
    for parasitic infection, 1345t–1362t
Proinflammatory response, 685, 685f
Project EXPLORE, 827
Project RESPECT, 827
Prokaryotes, comparison of eukaryotes and, 5t
Prominent sebaceous glands, 586t–587t
Prontosil, 1177
Propamidine isethionate, for Acanthamoeba keratitis,
        1750
Prophylaxis
    aminoglycosides in, 1237
    in arterial graft infections, 436
    for Candida spp., 1687
    for gastrointestinal parasites, 995
    for malaria, 1056
Propionibacterineae, 1547t
Propionibacterium, 1630
    and brain abscess, 199, 204
    microflora, 355
    in normal flora, 1632
Propionibacterium acnes, 1630
    in normal flora, 1632t
    in prosthetic joint infection (PJI), 400
Propionibacterium propionicum, 1630
Prostaglandin E₂ (PGE₂), 608
Prostatic abscesses, 533, 535
Prostatic calculi, 533–534, 536
Prostatitis, 532–536
    acute, management of, 535
    antibiotics for, 1152t
    chronic
        diagnostic criteria of, 534f
        diagnostic management in, 535f
        management of, 535–536, 535t–537t, 536f
        symptoms in, 533t
    classification of, 532t
    clinical features and diagnosis of, 533–535, 533t,
        534f
    definition and nomenclature of, 532
    epidemiology of, 532–533
    in gonorrhea, 594
    incidence and prevalence of, 532–533
    management of, 535–536
    Mycoplasma genitalium in, 1662
    Mycoplasma hominis in, 1663
    quinolones for, 1243
    risk factors for, 533
Prosthetic joints infections (PJI), 399–404
    classification of, 400, 401f
    clinical features of, 400
    diagnosis of, 400–402
        differential, 402
    epidemiology of, 399
    laboratory for, 400–401
    management of, 402–403
        medical, 402–403
        surgical, 402
    microbiology of, 400
    pathogenesis of, 399
    pathology of, 399
    prevention of, 403
    radiology in, 401–402
    time to presentation, 400
Prosthetic valve infective endocarditis, 456–457, 458t,
        463–465, 468t–469t, 469

Protease inhibitors (PIs), 1303–1305
    antiretroviral drugs, 870–871, 871t, 922, 925, 936
    choosing, 921
    for hepatitis C, 1330–1331
        in HIV, 898–899
    perinatal HIV transmission prevention, 909t
    and prematurity, 901–902
    resistance to, 924
Proteases, 1514–1515
    group A streptococci and, 1528–1529
Protected specimen brush (PSB), hospital-acquired
        pneumonia and, 260
Protein A, 1513t–1514t, 1516–1517
Protein biomarkers, for papillomaviruses, 1442–1443
Protein C, in sepsis, 423–424
Protein conjugate vaccine (PCV13), community-acquired
        pneumonia and, 256
Protein synthesis, antibiotics acting on, 1167–1174
Proteobacteria, 1565
    and HIV-1, 844
Proteome prediction, genome sequencing, 66
Proteus
    brain abscess and, 199–200
    diagnostic microbiology of, 1568t
    endophthalmitis and, 159
    hospital-acquired pneumonia and, 259t
    microflora, 355–356
    virulence factors of, 1571t
Proteus mirabilis
    in complicated urinary tract infection, 540, 540t, 542
    intrinsic resistance of, 1182t
    in urinary tract infections, 1575
Prothionamide, as antituberculosis agent, 1270
Proton pump inhibitors (PPIs)
    Clostridium difficile infection (CDI), 352
    food-borne diarrheal illness, 328
    for Helicobacter pylori, 325
Protoscolices, 1039
Protozoa
    amebae, 1725–1733
        free-living, 1744–1750
    blood and tissue, 1751–1762
    causing encephalitis/myelitis caused by, 193t–194t
    in chronic diarrhea, 346–349, 347t
    ciliates, 1725–1733
    clinical manifestations and management of, 1733
    in congenital infection, 505b
    diagnostic microbiology of, 1728–1733
    in diarrhea, 330, 332–333
        treatment for, 334
    epidemiology of, 1725–1727
    flagellates, 1725–1733
    gastrointestinal, 989t, 990–991, 995, 997–1000, 1000t
    intestinal and urogenital, 1725–1733, 1725t
        molecular testing of, 1732–1733
    in lymph node enlargement, 147t–148t
    lymphadenopathy and, 137t–138t
    nature of, 1725
    pathogenicity of, 1727–1728
    prevention of, 1727
    provoking immune reconstitution disorder, 860t
    travelers' diarrhea and, 950
Protozoal infections
    dermatologic manifestations of, 114t–115t, 119
    in HIV in low- and middle-income countries,
        892–893
    nitroimidazoles for, 1262
Providencia spp.
    in complicated urinary tract infection, 540t
    diagnostic microbiology of, 1568t
Providencia stuartii, in complicated urinary tract infection,
        540
Proviruses, excision of, 1491
Prozone phenomenon, 564
Pruritic papular eruption (PPE), in HIV/AIDS, 880
Pruritus, in HIV/AIDS, 879–880
Pseudallescheria boydii, diagnostic microbiology of, 1717
Pseudallescheria spp., in chronic meningitis, 186t
Pseudobuboes, 141
Pseudoclarithromycin, 1219f
Pseudocowpox virus, 665
Pseudolymphoma, and fever of unknown origin, 614
Pseudomembranous colitis
    Clostridium difficile infection (CDI), 352, 352f
    vancomycin for, 1251

Pseudomonas, 1579–1599
  bacteriology of, 1580, 1580*f*, 1585*f*
  brain abscess and, 199–200
  bronchiectasis and, 246
  in catheter-related bloodstream infection (CRBSI), 434–435
  clinical manifestations of, 1589
  conjunctivitis and, 176
  diagnostic microbiology of, 1580, 1580*f*
  empyema and, 266*t*
  epidemiology of, 1580, 1583*t*–1584*t*, 1590*t*
  in foot ulcers, 130–131
  infection, keratitis and, 152
  isolation of, 1580
  nature and taxonomy of, 1580
  nomenclature of, 1581*t*–1582*t*
  pathogenicity of, 1589, 1590*t*
  prevention of, 1593
Pseudomonas aeruginosa, 1580–1593
  active efflux in, 1186
  antimicrobial therapy for, 1589–1593, 1590*t*–1591*t*
  in bacterial arthritis, 383*t*, 386*t*
  brain abscess and, 202–203
  bronchiectasis and, 246
  in burn wounds, 698
  in burns, 698
  in cancer patients, 723–724
  cellulitis and, 86
  clinical manifestations of, 1586–1589, 1587*t*
    bacteremia/bloodstream infections as, 1586
    ear infections as, 1589
    endocarditis as, 1586
    eye infections as, 1588–1589
    lower respiratory tract infections as, 1587–1588, 1588*t*
    miscellaneous, 1589
    skin and soft tissue infections as, 1588, 1588*f*, 1593*f*
    urinary tract infections as, 1589
  in complicated urinary tract infection, 540*t*
  in cystitis, 523
  dermatologic manifestations of, 113–116, 116*f*
  diagnostic microbiology of, 1580
  drug-resistant, 1210
  in endocarditis, 468
  epidemiologic markers of, 1580, 1583*t*–1584*t*
  epidemiology of, 1580
  in hematopoietic stem cell transplantation, 740
  hospital-acquired pneumonia and, 259*t*
  isolation of, 1580
  keratitis and, 155
  β-lactam antibiotics for, 1210
  lower respiratory tract infections, 264*f*
  microflora, 355
  mucoid, 1586, 1586*f*
  nature and taxonomy of, 1580
  nosocomial infections from, 1588*t*
  in osteomyelitis, 389–390, 395*t*
  in otitis media, 236–237, 1637
  pathogenicity and pathogenesis of, 1582–1586, 1585*t*
    bacterial factors in, 1584–1586
    host-related factors in, 1582–1584
    mucoid *Pseudomonas aeruginosa* in, 1586
    virulence-associated factors in, 1585*t*
  peritonitis and, 381
  pneumonia in HIV/AIDS, 857
  prevalence of, 1579
  prevention of, 1593
  pyogenic liver abscess, 361
  resistance
    aminoglycoside, 1186
    antimicrobial, 1589–1593, 1592*t*
    β-lactam, 1184
    to fluoroquinolones, 1186
    intrinsic, 1182*t*
    multidrug, 1194
    polymyxin, 1193
    trimethoprim, 1192
  in respiratory tract infections, 1575
  in sepsis, 419
  in skull-base osteomyelitis, 393
  and tumor necrosis factor inhibitor, 797–799
Pseudomonas alcaligenes, 1590*t*

Pseudomonas fluorescens
  antimicrobial resistance of, 1591
  epidemiology and pathogenicity of, 1590*t*
  nature and taxonomy of, 1580
  nosocomial infections from, 1588*t*
Pseudomonas oryzihabitans, 1591
Pseudomonas pseudoalcaligenes, 1590*t*
Pseudomonas putida
  antimicrobial resistance of, 1591
  epidemiology and pathogenicity of, 1590*t*
  nosocomial infections from, 1588*t*
Pseudomonas stutzeri
  antimicrobial resistance of, 1591
  epidemiology and pathogenicity of, 1590*t*
Pseudomoniasis, dermatologic manifestations of, 114*t*–115*t*
Pseudoramibacter, 1630
Pseudoterranova decipiens
  epidemiology of, 1765
  pathogenicity of, 1770
Psittacosis, 660–661, 668
  and bioterrorism, 671*t*
  and occupational infections, 648*t*–649*t*, 651*t*–654*t*
Psoriasis, 586*t*–587*t*
  in HIV/AIDS, 880, 880*f*
PspA, 1531–1532
PspC, 1531–1532
Psychiatric disorders, encephalitis and, 227
Psyrobacter, 1598
  nomenclature of, 1581*t*–1582*t*
Public health hygiene measures, in gastrointestinal parasites, 994–995
Public health measures, in tuberculosis, 273–274
Public health programs, for gonorrhea, 592–594
Public reporting, 58
Puerperal infections, prevention of, in pregnancy, 503
Puerperal mastitis, 503
Pulmonary disease
  in HIV-associated TB, 869
  Mycobacterium abscessus, 289*t*, 290
  Mycobacterium avium complex, 289–290, 289*t*, 1649
  Mycobacterium intracellulare, 286*f*
  Mycobacterium kansasii, 289, 289*t*
  Mycobacterium malmoense, 289*t*, 290
  Mycobacterium szulgai, 286*f*, 289*t*
  Mycobacterium xenopi, 289*t*, 290
  nontuberculous mycobacteria (NTM), 286–287
    issues in, 290
  treatment for, 289–290
  surgery in, 290
Pulmonary edema
  and drowning-associated infections, 681
  Pseudomonas aeruginosa in, 1587
  in severe malaria, 1020*t*
Pulmonary infection
  antimicrobial therapy for, 1641*t*
  blastomycosis in, 1703
  coccidioidomycosis in, 1705
  cryptococcosis in, 1694, 1694*f*, 1695*t*
  histoplasmosis in, 1708
  mucormycosis in, 1698
  nocardiosis, 1551
  paracoccidioidomycosis in, 1709
Pulmonary infiltrates, 771, 771*t*, 772*f*
Pulmonary involvement, in primary HIV infection, 847
Pulpitis, 1636
Pulsed-field gel electrophoresis (PFGE)
  for *Acinetobacter baumannii*, 1583*t*–1584*t*
  for *Listeria monocytogenes*, 1539
  for *Pseudomonas aeruginosa*, 1583*t*–1584*t*
  staphylococci and, 1519
Punctate keratitis, 981
Purified protein derivative (PPD) skin test, 751*t*
Purified tissue culture vaccines, 1462
Purine metabolic defects, 718
Purine nucleoside phosphorylase deficiency, 718
Purpura fulminans, 121, 121*f*
Purpuric exanthems, 75*t*
Purulent acute ethmoiditis, 240, 241*f*
Purulent otitis, 237, 237*f*
'Push incentive', 1384
Puumala virus, 667, 1502, 1502*t*, 1504

Pyelonephritis, 547–554
  acute, 548*f*
  antibiotics for, 1152*t*
  clinical features of, 549–550
  complicated *versus* uncomplicated, 547, 547*b*
  diagnosis of, 550–551, 550*f*–552*f*
  management of, 551–553
    antimicrobial selection, 552, 552*t*
    clinical guide for, 554*f*
    complications, 553
    expected clinical course, 552–553
    follow up, 553
  Mycoplasma hominis in, 1664
  pathogenesis of, 547–548, 548*f*–549*f*
  in pregnancy, 502–503
  prevention of, 548–549
  risk factors for, 548
  treatment of, 443*t*
Pyocin typing, for *Pseudomonas aeruginosa*, 1583*t*–1584*t*
Pyocyanin
  in *Pseudomonas aeruginosa*, 1585
  in *Pseudomonas* spp., 1580
Pyoderma, 84–94, 85*t*
Pyogenic abscess of liver, differential diagnosis of, 1012
Pyogenic bacteria, in lymph node enlargement, 147*t*–148*t*
Pyogenic granulomas, 586*t*–587*t*
Pyogenic infections, lymphadenitis, 139
Pyogenic liver abscess, 361
Pyogenic lung disease, brain abscess and, 199
Pyomelanin, in *Pseudomonas* spp., 1580
Pyomyositis, 102–103
Pyorubin, in *Pseudomonas* spp., 1580
Pyoverdin, in *Pseudomonas* spp., 1580
Pyrantel pamoate
  for gastrointestinal helminth, 1000, 1001*t*
  for parasitic infections, 1345*t*–1362*t*, 1372
Pyrazinamide, 1269
  adverse reactions of, 1268*t*–1269*t*, 1269
  hepatotoxicity and, 308, 309*f*
  indications
    meningitis, 187*t*
    tuberculosis, 281, 283*t*
  resistance to, 1194
    mycobacterial, 1656*t*
  for urogenital tract tuberculosis, 556
Pyrethroids, 1017
Pyrimethamine, 1280
  for cystoisosporiasis, 1742
  elimination of, 1280
  for mycetoma, 1723
  for parasitic infections, 1345*t*–1362*t*
  for protozoal infections, 1364
  for toxoplasmosis, 513, 1755
    in HIV/AIDS, 856–857
Pyrimethamine-sulfadiazine, use of, 1282
Pyrimethamine-sulfadoxine, use of, 1282
Pyrimethamine-sulfonamide, for gastrointestinal protozoa management, 999–1000
Pyrogenic cytokines, 607
Pyrogenic toxins, streptococcal, 1529
Pyronaridine, artesunate with, 1022
Pyrosequencing, genome, 63*t*
Pyuria
  in complicated urinary tract infection, 543
  diagnosis of, 526, 526*t*
  'sterile,' urogenital tract tuberculosis and, 556

Q
Q fever, 1091, 1672–1673
  and bioterrorism, 671*t*–672*t*
  clinical manifestations of, 1673
  diagnostic microbiology of, 1672–1673
  epidemiology of, 1672
  and fever of unknown origin, 613
  management of, 1673
  nature of, 1672
  and occupational infections, 648*t*–649*t*, 651*t*–654*t*
  pathogenicity of, 1672
  prevention of, 1672
  quinolones for, 1246
  and recreational infections, 644

QepA, 1186–1187
Quality of care, 58
QuantiFERON®-TB Gold In-Tube (QFNG-IT), 1657, 1658t
Quantitative bacteriology, in complicated urinary tract infection, 543
Quantitative buffy coat analysis (QBC), for malaria diagnosis, 1022
Quantitative 'qPCR' assays, for helminths diagnosis, 1777
Quarantine, and bioterrorism, 678
Queensland tick typhus, 1092t–1093t, 1667t, 1668
Quinacrine, 1345t–1351t, 1369
  prion infection and, 220
Quinidine, 1352t–1362t, 1369
Quinidine gluconate, 1345t–1351t
Quinine
  adverse reactions, 1370
  dosage of, 1370
  for malaria in pregnancy, 1143t
  for parasitic infections, 1345t–1362t, 1369–1370
  pharmacokinetics and distribution, 1369–1370
  route of administration, 1370
  for severe malaria, 1024–1025, 1024t
Quinine dihydrochloride, 1345t–1351t
Quinine sulfate, 1345t–1351t
Quinolones, 1239–1248
  for Acinetobacter baumannii, 1590t
  adverse reactions of, 1246–1248
  for anaerobic bacteria, 1643
  antibacterial spectrum and potency of, 1239–1240, 1241t
  bacterial resistance to, 1240–1242
  chemoprophylaxis, for meningococcal disease, 1560
  for cystitis, 528t
  dosage of, 1243, 1244t
    in special circumstances, 1246
  drug interactions of, 1248
  drug metabolism of, interactions affecting, 1248
  elimination of, 1243
  for food-borne diarrheal illness, 333
  indications of, 1243–1246
    BK virus infection and prevention, 1246
    chemoprophylaxis as, 1246
    gastrointestinal infections, 1245–1246
    genitourinary tract infections, 1243
    infections associated with chronic ambulatory peritoneal dialysis, 1246
    mycobacterial infections, 1245
    other, 1246
    respiratory tract infections, 1243–1245
    skeletal infections, 1245
    skin and soft tissue infections, 1245
  keratitis and, 152
  mode of action of, 1240
  for Mycobacterium avium complex (MAC) in HIV, 856
  for Mycoplasma hominis, 1664
  for pelvic inflammatory disease, 493
  pharmacokinetics and distribution of, 1242–1243, 1242t
  for Pseudomonas aeruginosa, 1590t
  resistance to, 1186–1187, 1592t
    Campylobacter spp., 1602
    by decreased uptake/active efflux, 1186–1187
    by drug inactivation, 1187
    enterococci, 1526–1527
    by target modification, 1186
    by target protection, 1187
  route of administration of, 1243
  structure of, 1240f
  for tularemia, 1089
Quinupristin-dalfopristin, 1171
  for anaerobic bacteria, 1643
Quorum-sensing
  systems, in Pseudomonas aeruginosa, 1586
  of Vibrio cholerae, 1605

R
Rabbit, infection from, 1086, 1087f
'Rabbit fever', 1086
Rabies, 1458–1464
  from bats, 666
  from cats, 659
  clinical features of, 1460–1461
  control for, 1460
Rabies (Continued)
  diagnosis of, 1461–1462, 1461t
  differential diagnosis of, 1460–1461
  from dogs, 656
  epidemiology of, 1458, 1459t
  immunology of, 1460
  lyssaviruses known to infect humans, 1464t
  management of, 1462
  from mustelids, 666–667
  nature of, 1458
  from nonhuman primates, 666
  and occupational infections, 648t–649t
    immunization for, 650t–651t
  passive immunization of, 1463
  pathogenesis of, 1458–1460, 1459f–1460f
  pathogenicity of, 1458–1460
  postexposure boosting for, 1463
  postexposure prophylaxis for, 1462
  postexposure vaccine regimens in, 1462–1463
  pre-exposure prophylaxis of, 1463
  prevention of, 1462–1463
  prognosis and recovery in, 1461
  structure of, 1458
  transmission of, 1458
  vaccination for, in travelers, 950
  vaccines, 1462
Rabies-related viruses, 1458–1464
  infecting humans, 1463, 1464t
Rabies virus
  actin-based intracellular motility, 16–17
  encephalitis/myelitis caused by, 192t
Raccoon-contaminated soil, avoidance of, 973
Raccoons, infections from, 191t, 667
Radiation-sensitive severe combined immune deficiency, 718
Radiculitis, in immune reconstitution inflammatory syndrome, 862
Radiculoneuropathy, 409, 411
Radiography
  anthrax, 1126
  of blastomycosis, 294
  chest. see Chest radiography
  of coccidioidomycosis, 296
  community-acquired pneumonia and, 251–252
  of cystic fibrosis, 300
  empyema and, 266–267
  of histoplasmosis, 292–293, 293f
  in immunologically mediated diseases, 771
  intra-abdominal sepsis, peritonitis and, 356–357, 356f
  lung abscess and, 266–267
  of paracoccidioidomycosis, 297, 297f
  of penicilliosis, 298
  in pericarditis, 452, 452f
  plain. see Plain radiography
  of pulmonary tuberculosis, 556
  of sporotrichosis, 298, 298f
  see also specific diseases; specific techniques
Radiology
  in adult, with suspected immunodeficiency, 811
  in bacterial arthritis, 385
  for cancer patients, 733
  in food-borne diarrheal illness, 332
  interventional, antibiotic prophylaxis and, 1160–1161
  in osteomyelitis, 393–394
  in prosthetic joint infection (PJI), 401–402
  see also specific diseases
RAG1/RAG2 deficiency, 717
Ralstonia, 1598–1599
  nomenclature of, 1581t–1582t
  prevalence of, 1579
Raltegravir, 1148t, 1306
  adverse reactions of, 1306
  antiretroviral drugs, 922
  description of, 1306
  dosage of, 1306
    in special circumstances, 1306
  drug interactions of, 1306
  effect on oral contraceptives, 907t
  indications, 1306
  perinatal HIV transmission prevention, 910t
  pharmacokinetics and distribution of, 1306
  resistance to, 1306
  route of administration of, 1306
Raman spectrometry, 1386–1387
Random amplified polymorphic DNA (RAPD) polymerase chain reaction (PCR)
  for Acinetobacter baumannii, 1583t–1584t
  for Pseudomonas aeruginosa, 1583t–1584t
Randomized controlled trials
  community
    for MSM, 827
    for women, 828
  individually
    for MSM, 827
    for women, 827–828
Rapid antigen testing, for influenza viruses, 1469
Rapid diagnosis, definition of, 225
Rapid diagnostic tests (RDT), for leishmaniasis, 1757
Rapid enzymatic test, for anaerobic bacteria, 1635
Rapid one-step immunoassays, for Helicobacter pylori, 1603
Rapid plasma reagin (RPR) test, 564, 564t, 751t
  for endemic treponematoses, 964–965
Rapid tests
  HIV, 1487
  see also specific tests
Rapid viral detection, in meningitis, 225–226
Rare molds, 1681t
Rare yeasts, 1681t
Rat-bite fever, 661
  lymphadenopathy and, 137t–138t
  from mustelids, 667
  and occupational infections, 648t–649t
Rat fleas, 660, 1669
Rat louse, 1669
Re-emerging infectious diseases, drivers of, 41b
Re-emerging pathogens and diseases, 40–48, 41t
Reactive arthritis, 386–387
  genital chlamydia and, 600
  micro-organisms associated with, 386, 386b
  yersiniosis and, 1627
Reactive oxygen species, 23
Real-time genomics, 65
Real-time PCR, 1387
Receptor antagonists, immunosuppression and, 1379
Recognition functions of the innate immune response, 27–32
Recombinant human activated protein C, 423
Recombinant IL-1 receptor antagonist, 801
Recombination, neisserial genome instability and, 1555
Recreational infections, 643–646, 643t
  caused by exposure to water, 644–645, 644t
  spread by direct contact, 645–646
  travel, 643
  zoonoses, 643–644
Rectal chlamydia, 599–600
Rectal infection, in gonorrhea, 594
Rectal swabs
  in diarrhea, 339
  in lymphogranuloma venereum, 589
Recurrent nongonococcal urethritis, 603–604
  diagnosis of, 603
  etiology of, 603
  treatment of, 603–604
Recurrent pericarditis, 478
Recurrent pharyngotonsillitis, 1637–1638
Recurrent respiratory papillomatosis (RRP), 1443
Recurrent tonsillitis, 1636t
Red eye, 175–176
  acute angle-closure glaucoma and, 175t
  anterior uveitis and, 175–176, 175t, 176f
  anti-infectious treatment for, 176
  conjunctivitis and, 175, 175t
  keratitis and, 175, 175t
  microbiologic sampling for, 176
  referral to ophthalmologist, 175, 175b
'Red man syndrome', 1252
Reed-Sternberg (RS) cells, 876
Refractory peritonitis, 380
Regulatory T cells, 33
  effect of HIV-1 on, 843
Rehydration
  of diarrhea, 339
  for Enterobacteriaceae infections, 1576
  for food-borne diarrheal illness, 333, 333f
    composition of, 333t
Reiter's syndrome, 586t–587t
Relaparotomy, peritonitis, 358
Relapsing disease, 876

Relapsing fevers, 1105–1109
  Borrelia, 1607–1608, 1608*f*
  clinical features of, 1106, 1107*f*
  diagnosis of, 1108
  differential diagnosis of, 1108
  epidemiology of, 1105–1106
  Jarisch-Herxheimer reaction, 1107–1108
  laboratory findings of, 1108
  louse-borne, 1106
  management of, 1108–1109
  pathogenesis and pathology of, 1106
  prevention of, 1106
  prognosis of, 1108
  spontaneous crisis and, 1107–1108
  supportive treatment of, 1109
  tick-borne, 1105–1106, 1105*t*
Renal abscess
  clinical features of, 549–550
  diagnosis of, 550, 551*f*
  management of, 553, 554*f*
Renal cell carcinoma, and fever of unknown origin, 611
Renal disease
  antituberculosis agents in, 1274
  with hepatitis C virus, 370
  in immune reconstitution inflammatory syndrome, 863
Renal dysfunction
  in aging HIV-positive patient, 930
  nucleoside analog reverse transcriptase inhibitors (NRTI) in, 1297*t*
Renal effects, β-lactam antibiotics, 1215, 1215*t*
Renal failure
  acute, in severe malaria, 1020–1022, 1020*t*, 1025
  presence of, in treatment of cystitis, 529
  treatment of, in complicated urinary tract infection, 545
Renal function, tenofovir and, 921
Renal impairment
  aciclovir in, 1311*t*
  ganciclovir in, 1314*t*
  β-lactam antibiotics dosage in, 1212
  quinolones in, 1246, 1247*t*
  valganciclovir in, 1314*t*
Renal insufficiency
  macrolides and ketolides, 1222
  polymyxins for, 1287, 1287*t*
Renal safety, of folate inhibitors, 1283
Reoviridae, 1390
Repetitive extragenic palindromic (REP) polymerase chain reaction (PCR), for *Acinetobacter baumannii*, 1583*t*–1584*t*
Reproduction number, 50–51
Reptiles, infections from, 661–662
Resistance, of antiretroviral drugs, 924
  by drug class, 924
  measuring, 924–925
  rates of, 925
Resistance integrons, 1195–1196
Resistance-nodulation-division (RND), 1194*f*
Resistance phenotype
  for *Acinetobacter baumannii*, 1583*t*–1584*t*
  for *Pseudomonas aeruginosa*, 1583*t*–1584*t*
Respiratory distress, in severe malaria, 1020*t*, 1021
Respiratory infections
  in hematopoietic stem cell transplantation, 743*f*, 743*t*
  probiotics for, 1374*t*, 1375
  tetracyclines for, 1259
Respiratory specimens
  for laboratory diagnosis, of mycobacteria, 1650–1651
  see also specific specimens
Respiratory syncytial virus (RSV), 1475–1477
  bronchitis and, 244*t*
  clinical manifestations, 1476
  cytopathic effect, 1476*f*
  diagnostic microbiology, 1476
  epidemiology, 1475–1476
  in hematopoietic stem cell transplantation, 742–743
  hospital-acquired pneumonia and, 259*t*
  nature and pathogenicity, 1475
  in thoracic transplantation patients, 749
  treatment and prevention, 1476–1477
Respiratory tract, innate immune responses in, 28*f*
Respiratory tract disease, diphtheria and, 1545

Respiratory tract infections
  Acinetobacter baumannii in, 1587*t*
  adenovirus in, 1473
  burden of disease, 940–942
  Burkholderia spp. in, 1596
  in cancer patients, 727–728, 729*f*–731*f*
  Enterobacteriaceae in, 1575
  Pseudomonas aeruginosa in, 1587*t*
  quinolones for, 1243–1245
  Stenotrophomonas maltophilia in, 1597
  systemic microsporidiosis in, 1741
  in traveler returning from Hajj, 1132–1133
  trimethoprim-sulfamethoxazole for, 1282
Respiratory-transmitted diseases, preventive measures against, 1132–1133
Respiratory viruses
  antiviral agents against, 1318–1326, 1322*t*–1323*t*
  community-acquired, in hematopoietic stem cell transplantation, 742–743, 743*t*
  in intestinal transplant patients, 760
  noninfluenza, 1472–1482
  in otitis media, 237
Restriction fragment length polymorphism (RFLP), 65
  in lymphogranuloma venereum, 589
  for *Pseudomonas aeruginosa*, 1583*t*–1584*t*
  tuberculosis, 272
Retapamulin, 1170
Reticulate body (RB), of *Chlamydia trachomatis*, 597
Retinal detachment, as quinolones adverse effect, 1247
Retinal vasculitis, 166
Retinitis
  bacterial causes of, 169*t*
  cytomegalovirus, 852, 853*f*
  epidemiology of, 165–166
  in immunosuppressed patients, 172–173
  infectious, 165–174
  necrotizing. *see* Necrotizing retinitis
  parasitic causes of, 171*t*
  toxoplasmic, 856–857
Retinoblastoma, 172
Retinoid-like effects, in skin manifestations of HIV, 887
Retortamonas intestinalis, 1725*t*
Retropharyngeal abscess, 314–315, 315*f*, 1636*t*
Retropharyngeal space, 314
Retroviral infection, 1483–1492
Retroviridae, 1483
Retroviruses, 805–806, 1483–1492
  electron microscopic view, 1484*f*
  env genes, 1483, 1484*f*
  gag genes, 1483, 1484*f*
  myelitis, 190–191
  nature, 1483
  pol genes, 1483, 1484*f*
  role of human endogenous, in health and disease, 628–629, 629*t*
  structure, 1483, 1484*f*
  see also specific retroviruses
rev protein, 1485
Reversal reactions (RR), of leprosy, 957–958, 958*f*
Reverse transcriptase polymerase chain reaction (RT-PCR)
  for caliciviruses, 1396
  for enteric adenoviruses, 1396
  Lassa fever, 1501
  for rotaviruses, 1393
rex protein, 1484*f*, 1491
Rhagades, 563
Rhamnolipids, 1585
Rheumatic fever, 471–477
  clinical features of, 472–474, 473*f*–474*f*
  dermatologic manifestations of, 116
  diagnosis of, 472*t*, 474*t*
  epidemiology and history of, 471, 472*f*
  management of, 476
  in myocarditis, 447
  pathogenesis of, 471–472
  pharyngitis and, 233
  prevention of, 475–476, 475*t*–476*t*
  prognosis and follow-up of, 476
  prophylaxis, β-lactam antibiotics, 1209
  from streptococcal, 1532, 1533*t*
Rheumatic heart disease (RHD), 456, 471
  prevalence of, 472*f*, 1526*f*
Rheumatic pneumonia, 473

Rheumatoid-like polyarthritis, 1451
Rheumatologic conditions, eosinophilia and, 984*t*
Rheumatologic disorders, and fever of unknown origin, 613–614
Rhinocerebral mucormycosis, 1697–1698
Rhinoceroses, infections from, 669
Rhinofacial conidiobolomycosis, 1712, 1723
Rhinosinusitis, from *Aspergillus*, 1689–1691
Rhinosporidiosis
  clinical manifestations of, 1721
  diagnostic microbiology of, 1718, 1718*f*
  epidemiology of, 1714
  management of, 1724
  nature of, 1713
  pathogenicity of, 1715
  prevention of, 1716
Rhinosporidium seeberi, 1713
  clinical manifestations of, 1721
  diagnostic microbiology of, 1718
  pathogenicity of, 1715
Rhinovirus, 1477–1478
  bronchitis and, 244*t*
  clinical manifestations, 1477–1478
  cytopathic effect, 1477*f*
  diagnostic microbiology, 1477
  epidemiology, 1477
  management, 1478
  nature, 1477
  pharyngitis, 233
  prevention, 1477
Rhizaria, 1744
Rhizobium, 1581*t*–1582*t*, 1599
Rhizomucor, 1696
Rhizopus, 1696
Rhizopus oryzae, 1696–1697
Rhodnius prolixus, 109*f*, 1066
Rhodococcus, 1550*t*
Rhodococcus equi
  bacteremia and, 1552
  clinical manifestations and management of, 1551
  diagnostic microbiology of, 1549
  epidemiology of, 1549
  pathogenicity of, 1549
  in thoracic transplantation patients, 749
  transmission of, 664
Rhombencephalitis, 1540
Ribavirin, 1146*f*–1147*t*, 1325–1326
  adverse reactions and interactions of, 1326
  arenaviruses, 1501
  dosage of, 1325–1326
    in special circumstances, 1326
  in hematopoietic stem cell transplantation, 742–743
  for hepatitis C, 1330
  indications of, 1326
  pharmacokinetics and distribution of, 1325
  respiratory syncytial virus, 1476–1477
  route of administration, 1325–1326
  for viral hemorrhagic fevers, 1117
Ribotyping
  for *Acinetobacter baumannii*, 1583*t*–1584*t*
  for *Pseudomonas aeruginosa*, 1583*t*–1584*t*
Ricinus communis toxin, and bioterrorism, 671*t*
Rickettsia
  actin-based intracellular motility, 16–17
  diagnosis of, 1667
  in lymph node enlargement, 147*t*–148*t*
  and rickettsia-like organisms, 1666–1675
    anaplasmosis, 1671–1672
    bartonellosis, 1673–1675
    ehrlichioses, 1671
    Q fever, 1672–1673
    scrub typhus, 1670–1671
    spotted fever group, 1666–1669
    typhus group, 1669–1670
Rickettsia aeschlimannii, 1668
Rickettsia africae, 1667
Rickettsia akari, 1091, 1666, 1669
Rickettsia australis, 1668
Rickettsia conori, jaundice, 1135*t*
Rickettsia felis, 1091, 1666, 1668
Rickettsia heilongjiangensis, 1668, 1669*f*
Rickettsia honei, 1668
Rickettsia japonica, 1668

Rickettsia massiliae, 1668
Rickettsia parkeri, 1668
Rickettsia prowazekii, 1091, 1096–1097, 1669
    and bioterrorism, 671*t*
Rickettsia rickettsii, 1667–1668
    in myocarditis, 447
Rickettsia sibirica, 1668
Rickettsia slovaca, 1668
Rickettsia tsutsugamushi, in myocarditis, 447
Rickettsia typhi, 1091, 1669
Rickettsiaceae, 1091
Rickettsiae, in myocarditis, 447
Rickettsial disease, jaundice and, 1136
Rickettsial infections
    lymphadenopathy and, 137*t*–138*t*
    tetracyclines for, 1259
    tick-borne, and occupational infections, 648*t*–649*t*
Rickettsialpox, 1667*t*
    location of, 1092*t*–1093*t*
    lymphadenopathy and, 137*t*–138*t*
    from rodents, 667
Rickettsiosis, dermatologic manifestations of, 114*t*–115*t*
Ridley-Jopling classification scheme, 1648
Rifabutin, 1269
    for cryptosporidiosis, 1742
    induced uveitis in HIV patients, 173
    for *Mycobacterium avium* complex (MAC) in HIV, 856
Rifampicin
    for brucellosis, 1100
    fusidic acid and, 1277
    impregnated catheters, 433
    for meningitis, 183*t*, 187*t*
Rifampin, 1267–1269
    adverse reactions of, 1268*t*–1269*t*
    for brucellosis, 1616
    for cat-scratch disease, 659
    chemical structure of, 1177
    chemoprophylaxis, for meningococcal disease, 1560
    for ehrlichioses, 1671
    hepatotoxicity and, 308, 309*f*
    indications
        gas gangrene, 100–101
        hydrocephalus shunts, 223
        meningitis, 183*t*, 187*t*
        for parasitic infections, 1345*t*–1351*t*
        tuberculosis, 281, 281*t*, 283*t*
    for leprosy, 959
    for mycetoma, 1723
    for pericarditis, 454
    for primary amebic meningoencephalitis, 1749
    for prosthetic joint infection (PJI), 403
    resistance to, 1592*t*
        mycobacterial, 1656*t*
        of tuberculosis, 866
    for *Rhodococcus equi*, 1551
    for scrub typhus, 1097
    side effect, 281
    for *Staphylococcus aureus*, 1521
    for tuberculosis, in thoracic transplantation patients, 749
    for urogenital tract tuberculosis, 556
Rifamycin, 1267–1269
    for anaplasmosis, 1672
    antiretroviral regimens, 870–871, 871*t*
    pharmacodynamics of, 1177
Rifapentine, 1269
Rifaximin, for travelers' diarrhea, 376
Rift Valley fever, 1495*t*
    and bioterrorism, 671*t*
    transmission of, 665
Rift Valley fever virus, 1110
    clinical features of, 1114*t*–1115*t*
    epidemiology of, 1112*t*
Rilpivirine, 1302–1303
    adverse reactions of, 1303
    antiretroviral drugs, 921–922
    description of, 1302
    dosage of, 1302
        in special circumstances, 1303
    drug interactions of, 1303
    effect on oral contraceptives, 907*t*
    indications of, 1302
    perinatal HIV transmission prevention, 909*t*
    pharmacokinetics and distribution of, 1302
    resistance to, 1303
    route of administration of, 1302

Rimantadine, 1146*t*–1147*t*, 1318
    adverse reactions and interactions of, 1318
    indications of, 1318
    pharmacokinetics and distribution of, 1318, 1320*t*
    resistance to, 1318
    route of administration and dosage of, 1318
'Ring vaccination' strategy, for smallpox, 677
Rio Mamoré (RIOM) virus, 1503*t*
Rio Segundo (RIOS) virus, 1503*t*
Risk behavior, psychosocial models of, in HIV
    transmission, 826
Risus sardonicus, 211, 211*f*
Ritonavir, 1148*t*, 1303
    antiretroviral drugs, 921
    effect on oral contraceptives, 907*t*
    perinatal HIV transmission prevention, 909*t*
Rituximab, 725, 798*t*–799*t*, 800
    for Epstein-Barr virus, 759*t*
    immunosuppression and, 1380*t*
    for multicentric Castleman's disease, 877
    for non-Hodgkin's lymphoma, 876
    and opportunistic infections, 800
RNA
    drugs affecting, 1174–1177
    viruses, 6*t*, 12
RNA assays, 1488–1489
RNA polymerase, 10
Rocky Mountain spotted fever, 644, 1667–1668, 1667*t*
    location of, 1092*t*–1093*t*
    in myocarditis, 447
Rodents
    arenavirus, 1500
    hantavirus, 1502
    infections from, 191*t*
    infectious diseases from, 667
    tularemia and, 1086
Rokitamycin
    accumulation ratio of, 1222*t*
    characteristics of, 1218*t*
    pharmacokinetics, 1222, 1223*t*
Romaña's sign, 982, 1067, 1069*f*
Romanowsky stains, for anaplasmosis, 1672
Rosai-Dorfman disease, 137*t*–138*t*
Roseola, in primary HIV infection, 846, 847*f*
Roseola infantum, 79
    clinical features of, 79
    complications of, 79
    dermatologic manifestations of, 114*t*–115*t*
    management of, 79
Ross River, 1495*t*
    in infective arthritis, 387*t*
Rotarix®, 1397, 1397*t*
RotaShield®, 1397
RotaTeq®, 1397, 1397*t*
Rotaviruses, 1390–1393
    and bioterrorism, 671*t*
    clinical characteristics of, 1391*t*
    clinical manifestations of, 1393
    diagnosis of, 339
    diagnostic microbiology of, 1393
    diarrhea and, 336
    encephalitis/myelitis and, 194*t*
    epidemiological characteristics of, 1391*t*
    epidemiology of, 1390
    in food-borne diarrheal illness, 334
    genome segments of, 1392*f*, 1392*t*
    nature of, 1390
    pathogenicity, 1390–1393
    prevention of, 338
    structure and morphological characteristics of, 1391*f*,
        1391*t*
    vaccines for, 1397, 1397*t*
    viral enteritis and, 338
Rothia, 1509, 1547, 1548*t*
Roundworms. *see* Nematodes.
Roxithromycin
    accumulation ratio of, 1222*t*
    characteristics of, 1218*t*
    classification, 1217
    for gastrointestinal protozoa management, 999–1000
    pharmacokinetics, 1222, 1223*t*–1224*t*
    for scrub typhus, 1097
    stability in acidic medium, 1218, 1219*f*
    tissue distribution, 1224*t*
    in vitro activity, 1219, 1220*t*

16S rRNA gene, 69–70
18S rRNA gene, 70
RT-PCR. *see* Reverse transcriptase polymerase chain
    reaction (RT-PCR).
RTS,S, 1018
Rubella, 75*t*, 77–78, 1402–1404
    clinical features of, 77, 78*f*
    clinical manifestations of, 1403–1404, 1403*f*, 1404*b*
    dermatologic manifestations of, 114*t*–115*t*
    diagnostic microbiology of, 1402–1403, 1403*f*
    epidemiology of, 1402
    lymphadenopathy and, 137*t*–138*t*
    management of, 78, 1404
    nature of, 1402
    and occupational infections, 648*t*–649*t*
        immunization for, 650*t*
    pathogenicity of, 1402
    prevention of, 1402, 1402*f*
Rubella vaccination, 78, 782*t*–783*t*
Rubella virus, 77
    in congenital infection, 505–506
        in breast-feeding, 516
        clinical features of, 510
        diagnosis of, 512*t*
        immunization for, 507
        management of, 513
        pathogenesis and pathology of, 506
        screening for, during pregnancy, 507, 508*t*
    encephalitis/myelitis caused by, 193*t*–194*t*
    in infective arthritis, 385, 387*t*
Ruminococcus sarcina, 1631
Russian spring-summer encephalitis, 1495*t*
RV144, 833

S
Sabia virus, 1110, 1112*t*, 1500*t*
Saccharomyces boulardii, 12
Sacroiliitis, 1099, 1099*f*
Safety, of probiotics, 1375
Safety profile, general, of folate inhibitors, 1283
Saksenaea, 1696
Salivary glands, infections of, 319–320, 319*f*
Salmonella
    from amphibians, 661
    azithromycin, 1220
    in bacteremia, 1576
    bacterial enteritis and, 336–337
    and bioterrorism, 671*t*
    from birds, 661
    blood cultures in, 332
    in breast-feeding, 516
    in cats, 660
    characteristics of, in food-borne diarrheal illness,
        330*t*
    in contaminated food, 1574
    diagnosis of, 339
    diarrhea, 331
    doses of, in diarrheal illness, 329*t*
    enterocolitis, in HIV/AIDS, 858
    from fish, 661
    food poisoning, 328
    in intestinal infections, 1574–1575
    management of, 333–334
    myocarditis and, 446–447
    and occupational infections, 648*t*–649*t*
    in osteomyelitis, 390, 395*t*
    in postsplenectomy sepsis, 778*t*
    from reptiles, 661
    resistance, to antimicrobial peptides, 24*f*
    from rodents, 667
    serotyping for, 1568
    spread of, 944
    taxonomy of, 1566, 1566*f*
    transmission of, 665, 665*t*
    travelers' diarrhea and, 332, 375, 375*t*, 950
    treatment with β-lactam antibiotics, 1204
    and tumor necrosis factor inhibitor, 797–799
    virulence factors of, 1571*t*
Salmonella bongori, taxonomy of, 1566
Salmonella-containing vacuole (SCV), 1574–1575
Salmonella enterica
    bacterial enteritis, 336
    diagnosis of, 339
    diagnostic microbiology of, 1568*t*

Salmonella enterica (Continued)
  in intestinal infections, 1574
  jaundice, 1135t
  management of, 339
  non-typhoidal, 336–337
  subspecies of, 1003
  taxonomy of, 1566
Salmonella paratyphi
  epidemiology of, 1002
  pathogenesis and pathology of, 1003
Salmonella typhi
  epidemiology of, 1002
  in osteomyelitis, 390
  pathogenesis and pathology of, 1003
Salmonellosis
  from birds, 668
  from frog's legs, 669
  from insectivores, 668
  from marine mammals, 668
  quinolones for, 1245
  transmission of, 665, 669
Salpingitis, from *Neisseria gonorrhoeae*, 1562–1563
Salt-and-pepper fundus, 168f
Sand flies, 106t, 111, 1673, 1756
  arboviruses, 1493, 1495t
  infections from, 191t
  leishmaniasis and, 1059
Sand fly fever Naples, 1495t
Sand fly fever Sicilian, 1495t
Sanger sequencing, 63, 63t
Sanitation, for prevention of food-borne diarrheal illness, 334
SAPHO syndrome, 393
Sapovirus, 1393–1396
  clinical characteristics of, 1391t
  clinical manifestations of, 1396
  diarrhea and, 335, 338
  epidemiological characteristics of, 1391t
  epidemiology of, 1394
  structure and morphological characteristics of, 1391f, 1391t
  taxonomy of, 1394t
Sappinia, 1744
Sappinia diploidea
  nature of, 1744
  treatment of, 1345t–1351t
Saquinavir, 1148t, 1303
  effect on oral contraceptives, 907t
  perinatal HIV transmission prevention, 909t
Sarcocystis hominis, 1734
Sarcocystis nesbitti, 1734
Sarcocystis suihominis, 1734
Sarcoidosis, 626
  in HIV patients receiving antiretroviral therapy, 864
  lymphadenopathy and, 137t–138t
Sarcoptes scabiei
  from cats, 660
  from dogs, 658–659
SARS. *see* Severe acute respiratory syndrome (SARS).
Scabies, 107, 586t–587t
  from cats, 660
  from dogs, 658–659
  and occupational infections, 648t–649t
Scalp, infection, 123t
Scarlet fever
  epidemiology of, 1525
  lymphadenopathy and, 137t–138t
  manifestations of systemic diseases, 116
  rash, 234
SCC*mec*, 1184
Schistosoma, 1026
  in myocarditis, 447
  in travelers, 952
Schistosoma haematobium, 1026
  and bladder cancer, 21
  clinical manifestations of, 1778
  diagnosis of, 1031
  epidemiology of, 1026, 1766
  female genital schistosomiasis and, 1030
  life cycle of, 1771f
  pathogenicity of, 1772
  treatment of, 1345t–1351t
  urinary schistosomiasis and, 1029, 1029f

Schistosoma intercalatum, 1026
  epidemiology of, 1026, 1766
  intestinal/hepatic schistosomiasis and, 1029–1030
Schistosoma japonicum, 1026
  clinical manifestations of, 1778
  epidemiology of, 1026, 1766
  intestinal/hepatic schistosomiasis and, 1029–1030
  life cycle of, 1771f
  neurologic schistosomiasis and, 1030
  pathogenesis and pathology of, 1028
  treatment of, 1345t–1351t
Schistosoma mansoni, 1026
  avoiding ingestion, 23
  chronic diarrhea, 349
  clinical manifestations of, 1778
  epidemiology of, 1026, 1766
  intestinal/hepatic schistosomiasis and, 1029–1030, 1030f
  life cycle of, 1771f
  parasite infections and, 73–74
  pathogenesis and pathology of, 1028
  pathogenicity of, 1772
  treatment of, 1345t–1351t
Schistosoma mekongi, 1026
  epidemiology of, 1026, 1766
  intestinal/hepatic schistosomiasis and, 1029–1030
  treatment of, 1345t–1351t
Schistosomes, 1772
Schistosomiasis, 645, 1026–1031, 1766, 1778
  chronic, 1029
  chronic diarrhea and, 349
  clinical features of, 1029–1030
    intestinal/hepatic schistosomiasis, 1029–1030, 1030f
    unusual consequences of, 1030
    urinary schistosomiasis, 1029, 1029f
  diagnosis of, 1030–1031
  epidemiology of, 1026–1028, 1027f
  female genital, 1030
  geographic distribution of, 939, 941f
  intestinal/hepatic, 1029–1030
  life cycle of, 1026f
  management of, 1031
  neurologic, 1030
  pathogenesis and pathology of, 1028, 1028f
  prevention of, 1028–1029, 1028f
  transmission of, 1031
  treatment of, 1345t–1351t
  urinary, 1029, 1029f
Schistosomiasis Control Initiative (SCI), 1029
Schnitzler's syndrome, 614
Sclerosing keratitis, 981
Sclerosing lymphangitis, 586t–587t
Scombroid poisoning, 331, 332f
Scopulariopsis brevicaulis, 122–123
Scrapie, 215t
  epidemiology of, 214–215
  pathology, 219–220
Scratches, treatment of, 1462
Screening, as prevention modality, in HIV, 826
Scrofuloderma, 117, 117f
Scrotum inflammation, in filariasis, 1049
Scrub typhus, 644, 1091–1097, 1670–1671
  clinical features of, 1095–1096, 1096f
  clinical manifestations of, 1670–1671
  diagnosis of, 1096–1097
  diagnostic microbiology of, 1670
  distribution of, 1094f
  epidemiology of, 1091–1094, 1094f–1095f, 1670, 1670f
  location of, 1092t–1093t
  lymphadenopathy and, 137t–138t
  management of, 1097, 1671
  in myocarditis, 447
  nature of, 1670
  and occupational infections, 648t–649t
  pathogenesis and pathology of, 1094
  pathogenicity of, 1670
  prevention of, 1094–1095, 1670
Scrumpox, 645
Scytalidium, 1710
Scytalidium dimidiatum, clinical features of, 126, 127f
Sea bathing, and recreational infections, 645
Seafood, in non-infective food poisoning, 331
Seal finger, 668
Seasonal influenza, 1470

Seborrheic dermatitis, 127, 586t–587t
  in HIV/AIDS, 879
  from *Malassezia*, 1710
  management of, 128
Seborrheic keratosis, 586t–587t
'Second genome', 68
Secondary eosinophilia, 985
Secreted factors, *Neisseria*, 1559–1560
Secretory diarrhea, 336
Secukinumab, 798t–799t, 802
Seizures
  adverse reactions to β-lactam antibiotics, 1215
  encephalitis/myelitis and, 190
  febrile, 609
  in meningitis, 183
Selective adhesion molecule inhibitors, 802
Selective decontamination of the digestive tract (SDD), 694–697
Selective IgA deficiency, 720
Selective oropharyngeal decontamination (SOD), 694–697
Selenium sulfide, 128
Semisulcospira spp., 1765
Seoul virus, 667, 1502t, 1504
Sepsis, 415–426
  anthrax, 1126
  anti-inflammatory mechanisms in, 424
  biliary, 360
  biochemical evaluation of, 420
  biomarkers for, 420
  burn wound. *see* Burn wound, sepsis
  campaign bundles, 426b
  causative agents in, 419, 419f–420f, 419t
  clinical signs and symptoms of, 415–416
  coagulation and, activation of, 423–424
  complications of, 418f
  definition of, 415
  dermatologic manifestations of, 119
  diagnostic criteria for, 415–416, 416b
  faces of, 417f
  gene polymorphisms in, 424, 425t
  guidelines for, 425b
  hematologic evaluation of, 420
  historical perspective of, 420
  host response in, 420–424, 421f
    deregulated, potential types of, 421–424
  immune suppression in, 424
  incidence of, 416
  intra-abdominal. *see* Intra-abdominal sepsis
  laboratory-based diagnostics in, 419–420
  mortality in, 416
  organ dysfunction and, 424
  pathogen recognition systems in, 421, 422f, 422t
  pathogens in, identification of, 420
  pathophysiology of, 420–424, 422t
  perspectives in, 426
  plague and, 1081
  postabortion, 496
  prevention of, 424
  pro-inflammatory mediators in, 422–423
  risk factors for, 416–419, 416b
  source of, 420
  therapy for, 424–426
  vascular endothelium and, malfunction of, 423–424
  virulence factors in, 419, 419f–420f, 419t
Sepsis-like illness, 509
Septic arthritis
  anaerobic bacteria in, 1640
  monoarticular, 1563
  treatment of, 443t
Septic shock
  in cancer patients, 727–728
  definition of, 415
  superantigens and bacterial components associated with, 22
  typhoid fever in, 1004
Septic thrombophlebitis, 500
Septicemia
  central line-associated, 60
  Erysipelothrix rhusiopathiae and, 1542
Septicemic plague, 1078
  clinical features of, 1082, 1082f
  pathogenesis and pathology of, 1081
Seroconversion, for *Leptospira* spp., 1609

'Seroconversion illness', 234–235
Serologic assays
  for filariasis, 1050
  HIV, 1487
  of melioidosis, 1076
Serologic tests
  for amebic colitis, 1011
  for anthrax, 1127
  for *Babesia*, 1752
  for brucellosis, 1100
  for endemic treponematoses, 964–965
  for *Entamoeba* spp., 1729
  for leishmaniasis, 1757
  for schistosomiasis, 1031
Serologic tools, development of, 66
Serological cross-reactivity, of eosinophilia, 986
Serological methods, for African trypanosomiasis,
    968–969
Serology
  for blastomycosis, 1702–1703
  for *Bordetella pertussis*, 1613
  for brucellosis, 1615
  for *Campylobacter* spp., 1602
  in cancer patients, 732
  of Chagas disease, 1071
  for *Chlamydia pneumoniae*, 1679
  for *Chlamydia trachomatis*, 1678
  in *Chlamydia trachomatis*, 597
  for chromoblastomycosis, 1716
  for coccidioidomycosis, 296, 1705
  for *Cryptosporidium* spp., 1738
  for echinococcosis, 1043
  in endocarditis, 461, 461*t*, 462*f*
  for enteric fevers, 1005
  in genital herpes, 572–573
  in hepatitis B virus, 364–366
  for histoplasmosis, 293, 1707–1708
  in human papillomavirus, 582–583
  for influenza viruses, 1469
  for *Legionella* spp., 1623
  for leishmaniasis, 1063
  for leprosy, 958
  for lobomycosis, 1717
  for Lyme disease, 409–410, 410*f*
  for lymphogranuloma venereum, 589
  maternal symptoms and, in congenital infections, 511,
      511*b*
  of microsporidia, 1740
  for *Mycoplasma pneumoniae*, 1660–1661
  in neonatal testing, 511
  in pregnancy, 507, 508*t*
  in rheumatic fever, 474, 476
  of superficial fungal pathogens, 1712
  in syphilis, 563–564, 564*t*
Serotonin pathway, in chronic fatigue syndrome, 633
Serotyping
  for *Acinetobacter baumannii*, 1583*t*–1584*t*
  for Enterobacteriaceae, 1568
  for *Escherichia coli*, 1570
  for *Listeria monocytogenes*, 1539
  for *Neisseria*, 1561
  for *Pseudomonas aeruginosa*, 1583*t*–1584*t*
  for *Vibrio cholerae*, 1606
Serous effusions, in immune reconstitution inflammatory
    syndrome, 863
Serratia
  diagnostic microbiology of, 1568*t*
  microflora, 355–356
Serratia marcescens
  and chronic granulomatous disease, 708
  intrinsic resistance of, 1182*t*
  keratitis and, 152
  in osteomyelitis, 395*t*
Serum agglutination test (SAT), for brucellosis, 1100,
    1615–1616
Serum resistance factor, 1613*t*
Serum sickness, adverse reactions to β-lactam antibiotics,
    1216
Serum sickness-like illness, 363
Severe acute respiratory syndrome (SARS), 42, 52–53
  and occupational infections, 648*t*–649*t*
  spread of, 943
Severe acute respiratory syndrome-associated coronavirus
    (SARS-CoV), 1474
  and bioterrorism, 671*t*

Severe combined immunodeficiency, 713–718
  CD45 deficiency, 716
  clinical features of, 713, 714*f*
  defects of p56lck/ZAP-70 pathway, 716
  diagnosis of, 715*f*
  DNA repair defects, 717
  IL-2Rα deficiency, 716
  IL-7Rα deficiency, 716
  JAK3 deficiency, 715–716, 716*f*
  Omenn syndrome, 717–718, 718*f*
  purine metabolic defects, 718
  radiation-sensitive, 718
  RAG1/RAG2 deficiency, 717
  vaccination for, 713
  X-linked, 714–715
Severe congenital neutropenia, 705–706
Severe malaria, clinical cases, 1141–1142
Sewage worker, and occupational infections, 648*t*–649*t*
Sex, and endemic treponematoses, 961
Sex partners, management of, 601
Sexual intercourse, in pregnancy, 502
Sexually acquired reactive arthritis, *Mycoplasma genitalium*
    in, 1663
Sexually transmitted diseases
  amebiasis as, 1727
  bacteria involved in, 1221
  Entamoeba histolytica in, 1726
  eye involvement in, 982
  macrolides and ketolides, 1221
  on pregnancy, 499, 500*t*, 501
  tetracyclines for, 1259
  tropical, 982
  see also specific diseases
Sexually transmitted infection
  etiology of, 1138*t*
  and HIV transmission, 826
  laboratory tests for, 1137*t*
  management of, 1138
  in traveler
      background information and, 1137
      returning from South Africa, 1137–1138
Shark bites, 663, 668–669
Sheep
  Brucella melitensis, 663
  infections from, 191*t*
  tularemia, 664
Sheep liver fluke, treatment of, 1345*t*–1351*t*
Shewanella, 1581*t*–1582*t*, 1599
Shiga toxin, 330
Shiga-toxin *Escherichia coli*
  antibiotic therapy of, 334
  doses of, in diarrheal illness, 329*t*
Shigella
  actin-based intracellular motility, 16–17
  azithromycin, 1220
  bacterial enteritis, 337
  characteristics of, in food-borne diarrheal illness, 330*t*
  diagnosis of, 339
  diagnostic microbiology of, 1568, 1568*t*
  diarrhea, 336
  doses of, in diarrheal illness, 329*t*
  in intestinal infections, 1573*f*, 1574
  management of, 339
  membranous cell gateway, 15
  taxonomy of, 1566, 1567*f*
  travelers' diarrhea and, 375, 375*t*, 950
  virulence factors of, 1571*t*
Shigella boydii
  diarrhea and, 337
  in intestinal infections, 1574
Shigella dysenteriae
  and bioterrorism, 671*t*
  cytotoxins in, 330
  diarrhea and, 337
  in intestinal infections, 1574
Shigella flexneri
  apoptosis, 19
  diarrhea and, 337
  enterocolitis, in HIV/AIDS, 858
  in intestinal infections, 1574
Shigella sonnei
  diarrhea and, 337
  in intestinal infections, 1574
Shigellosis, 1574
  quinolones for, 1246

Shivering, 606
Shock
  circulatory, 1020*t*
  hemodynamic, 1025
  septic. see Septic shock
  in severe malaria, 1021, 1025
  see also Toxic shock syndrome (TSS)
Shotgun metagenomic sequence, 70–71, 70*f*–71*f*
SHV-1, 1183
Siberian tick typhus, 1667*t*, 1668
Sickle cell anemia
  clinical features of, 1056
  pathogenesis and pathology of, 1053–1054
Sickness Impact Profile (SIP-8), 631–632
Signal regulatory proteins (SIRP's), 31–32
Silicone breast implant, lymphadenopathy, 137*t*–138*t*
Silver nitrate eye drops, 151
Simeprevir (SMV), for hepatitis C, 1331
Simian immunodeficiency virus (SIV), 666, 839
  pathogenesis and pathology, 846
  studies in, 846
Simkania, 1221
Simulium damnosum, 1765
Sin Nombre virus (SNV), 12, 1110, 1502, 1503*t*
Sindbis virus, in infective arthritis, 387*t*
Sine qua non, in wound evaluation, in burns, 699
Single cell genome sequencing, 63
Single nucleotide polymorphisms (SNPs), 65
Single photon emission CT (SPECT), brain abscess and,
    201
Sinuses, specimen collection in, 1634*t*
Sinusitis, 239–242
  anaerobic bacteria in, 1636*t*, 1637
  antibiotics for, 1152*t*
  bacterial, 239
  brain abscess and, 200*t*
  chronic, 239
  clinical features of, 240
  complications of, 240
  definition of, 239
  of dental origin, 239
  diagnosis of, 240–241, 241*b*, 241*f*
  epidemiology of, 239
  ethmoidal, 240
  frontal, 240
  fungal, 242, 1689, 1690*t*
      in cancer patients, 727, 729*f*
  management of, 241–242, 242*t*
  maxillary, 240
  from *Moraxella catarrhalis*, 1624
  pathogenesis of, 239–240
  prevention of, 240
  quinolones for, 1243
  sphenoid, 240
  subdural empyema/intracranial epidural abscess, 203,
      205*t*
Sirolimus, 1378
Sitafloxacin, for anaerobic bacteria, 1643
Sixth disease, 79
Skeletal infections, quinolones for, 1245
Skin
  folate inhibitors on, adverse reactions of, 1283
  insertion site, in culture of, 433
  manifestations of systemic diseases, 113
  normal flora of, 12–13, 1632, 1632*t*
Skin biopsy
  granulomatous amebic encephalitis and, 1747
  for laboratory diagnosis, of mycobacteria, 1651*t*
  for leprosy, 958
  meningitis and, 180
Skin damage, onchocerciasis and, 1049
Skin disease, nontuberculous mycobacteria (NTM),
    localized, 287
Skin infections, 85*t*
  anaerobic bacteria in, 1632*f*, 1638*t*, 1639–1640,
      1639*f*–1640*f*
  antimicrobial therapy for, 1641*t*
  blastomycosis in, 1703
  in cancer patients, 727, 727*f*
  candidosis in, 1710
  cryptococcosis in, 1695
  differential diagnosis of, 85*t*
  from groups A, C and G streptococci, 1532
  in HIV/AIDS, 858
  immunologically mediated diseases, 773–774, 774*f*

Skin infections (*Continued*)
linezolid, 1231, 1231*t*
in melioidosis, 1075
mucormycosis in, 1698
Mycoplasma pneumoniae in, 1661
nomenclature of, 85*t*
Pseudomonas aeruginosa in, 1582, 1587*t*, 1588, 1588*f*, 1593*f*
quinolones for, 1245
recurring, 133–135
Skin lesions
and bioterrorism, 673*t*
bullous, 85*t*
crusted, 85*t*
in genital herpes, 572
microbiologic investigation of, in congenital infection, 512*t*
ulceration, differential diagnosis of, 91*t*
see also specific lesions
Skin manifestations, of acute CMV, 79
Skin tests
adverse reactions to penicillins, 1215
for coccidioidomycosis, 1705
for histoplasmosis, 1707
for paracoccidioidomycosis, 1709
Skull-base osteomyelitis, 393
Skunks, infections from, 191*t*
'Slapped cheek,' in parvovirus infection, 1451, 1451*f*
Slaughterer, and occupational infections, 648*t*–649*t*
Slide coagulase test, for staphylococci, 1517*f*
Slime-associated antigen (SAA), 1516
Slit skin smears, for leishmaniasis, 1063, 1063*f*
Slugs, infections from, 191*t*
Small intestinal bacterial overgrowth (SIBO), 346
Small mammal pets, diseases associated with, 657*t*, 661
Small multidrug resistance (SMR), 1194*f*
Smallpox
and bioterrorism, 671*t*–673*t*, 675–677
clinical features of, 676, 676*f*
differential diagnosis of, 676
rash of, 676, 677*f*
transmission of, 676–677
dermatologic manifestations of, 114*t*–115*t*
immunization for, and occupational infections, 650*t*–651*t*
Smear microscopy, for laboratory diagnosis, of mycobacteria, 1652
Smoke inhalation injury, and pneumonia, 698
Snails
infections from, 191*t*
in schistosomiasis, 1026
'Snowflake' keratitis, 981
Social cognitive models, and HIV transmission, 826
Sodium absorption, 335–336
Sodium stibogluconate, for parasitic infections, 1345*t*–1362*t*, 1369
Sofosbuvir (SOF), for hepatitis C, 1331
Soft chancre, 589
Soft ticks, 104–105
Soft tissue, deep, 95
Soft tissue infections
aerobic actinomycetes and, 1551
anaerobic bacteria in, 1632*f*, 1638*t*, 1639–1640, 1639*f*–1640*f*
antimicrobial therapy for, 1641*t*
in cancer patients, 727, 729*f*
clinical features, diagnosis and management of, 86–93
etiology of, 85*t*
immunologically mediated diseases, 773–774, 774*f*
linezolid, 1231, 1231*t*
in melioidosis, 1075, 1076*f*
Pseudomonas aeruginosa in, 1587*t*, 1588, 1588*f*, 1593*f*
quinolones for, 1245
see also Skin infections; Subcutaneous infections; specific infections
Soil, infections from, 191*t*
Solid organ transplant (SOT), 781
candidates of, vaccination follow-up of, 789*t*
patients having, fever of unknown origin in, 615
recipients of, vaccinal follow-up of, 790*t*
systematic approach to vaccinating patients with, 787
see also Organ transplantation; specific organs
Sonication, in prosthetic joint infection (PJI), 401

Sore throat, streptococcal, 472
South American hemorrhagic fever, and bioterrorism, 671*t*
South Asia, infections in, 1130
South East Asia, infections in, 1130
Southern tick-associated rash illness (STARI), 408
Spa baths, and recreational infections, 644–645
Spa typing, staphylococci and, 1519
'Spanish influenza' pandemic, 1466
Sparfloxacin, dissociation constants of, 535*t*
Sparganosis, 1036, 1036*f*, 1766, 1772, 1778
from amphibians, 669
Specific granule deficiency, 705*t*
Specimen collection
in anaerobic bacteria, 1634–1635, 1634*t*
for laboratory diagnosis, of mycobacteria, 1650–1652, 1651*t*
for viral hemorrhagic fevers, 1116
see also Diagnostic microbiology; specific specimens
Sphingobacterium, 1581*t*–1582*t*, 1599
Sphingomonas, 1581*t*–1582*t*
Spinal cord, transverse myelitis and, 191
Spinal cord abscess, 207
Spinal cord injury, in complicated urinary tract infection, 541–542
Spinal epidural abscess, 206–207
clinical features of, 206
diagnosis of, 206
epidemiology of, 206
management of, 206–207
pathogenesis and pathophysiology of, 206
Spiramycin
accumulation ratio of, 1222*t*
for parasitic infections, 1345*t*–1351*t*, 1367
pharmacokinetics, 1223*t*
stability in acidic medium, 1218
tissue distribution, 1224*t*
for toxoplasmosis, 513
Spiramycin adipate, pharmacokinetics, 1224*t*
Spiramycin I, characteristics of, 1218*t*
Spirillum minus, rat-bite fever, 661
Spirochaetales, 1600, 1608–1609
Spirochetes, in myocarditis, 447
Spirometra, 1036, 1036*f*, 1772
Splanchnic bed, ischemia of, 686
Spleen
abscesses, in melioidosis, 1074
aspiration in leishmaniasis, 1063, 1063*f*
dysfunction of, 775–779
structure-function relationships in, 775
in visceral leishmaniasis, 1060–1061
Splenectomy, 775–779
babesiosis and malaria after, prevention of, 776–777
postsplenectomy sepsis, 775
antimicrobial prophylaxis for, 777–778
clinical features of, 778, 778*t*
diagnosis of, 778, 778*f*–779*f*
epidemiology of, 775
immunizations to prevent, 777–778
immunologic defects and factors predisposing to, 775, 776*t*
management of, 778–779
pathogenesis and pathology, 775–776
predisposing factors to, 776
prevention of, 688, 776–778, 777*t*
risk factors for, 776*t*
splenic salvage method, 777
Splenic infection, 355–362
Splenomegaly
causes of, 1140*b*
and lymphadenopathy and anemia, 1139–1140
splenic infection, 361
Spondylitis, 1099, 1100*f*
Spontaneous abortion
congenital infection and, 509
in pregnancy, 501
Spontaneous bacterial peritonitis (SBP), 359
β-lactam antibiotics for, 1211
Sporadic Creutzfeldt-Jakob disease (CJD), 215*t*
Sporangia, 1718
Sporothrix, 1681*t*
in chronic meningitis, 186*t*

Sporothrix schenckii
in bacterial arthritis, 383*t*
diagnostic microbiology of, 1719*f*
epidemiology of, 1715
mycology and epidemiology of, 297
pathogenesis and pathology of, 298
pathogenicity of, 1715
Sporotrichosis, 297–298, 298*f*, 645
clinical manifestations of, 1722, 1722*f*
cutaneous, 1722, 1722*f*
diagnostic microbiology of, 1718–1719, 1719*f*
epidemiology of, 1714–1715
management of, 1724
nature of, 1713
and occupational infections, 648*t*–649*t*
pathogenicity of, 1715
prevention of, 1716
Sporotrichosis schenckii, in skin manifestation of HIV, 884*t*
Sports, and recreational infections, 645
Spotted fever group rickettsiae, 1091, 1666–1669
clinical manifestations of, 1667–1669, 1667*f*–1669*f*, 1667*t*
diagnostic microbiology of, 1667
epidemiology of, 1666
management of, 1669
nature of, 1666
pathogenicity of, 1666
prevention of, 1666–1667
see also specific diseases
Sputum
Aspergillus in, 1688–1689
in bronchiectasis, 246
cultures, in sepsis, 420
histoplasmosis and, 1707
for laboratory diagnosis, of mycobacteria, 1650–1651, 1651*t*
paracoccidioidomycosis and, 1709
specimens
helminths in, 1776
tuberculosis, 280*f*–281*f*
Squamous cell carcinoma, 577, 579, 581*f*, 586*t*–587*t*
in skin manifestation of HIV, 884–885
Squamous cell carcinoma in situ, 586*t*–587*t*
Squamous cells, 580–581, 580*f*
Squamous intraepithelial lesion, 580*f*
SSSS. *see* Staphylococcal scalded skin syndrome (SSSS).
St Louis encephalitis, 1493*f*, 1495*t*
St Louis encephalitis virus (SLE), encephalitis/myelitis caused by, 192*t*
St Vitus' dance, 473, 1533
Standard non-treponemal (reaginic) tests, 563–564, 564*t*, 566
Staphopain A, 1513*t*–1514*t*
Staphylococcal complement inhibitor (SCIN), 1513*t*–1514*t*
Staphylococcal enterotoxin B, and bioterrorism, 671*t*
Staphylococcal immunoglobulin-binding protein (SBI), 1513*t*–1514*t*
Staphylococcal infection
dermatologic manifestations of, 114*t*–115*t*
lymphadenopathy and, 137*t*–138*t*
Staphylococcal scalded skin syndrome (SSSS), 87–88, 88*f*, 116, 116*f*
Staphylococcal superantigen-like 3, 1513*t*–1514*t*
Staphylococcal superantigen-like 5 (SSL5), 1513*t*–1514*t*, 1514
Staphylococcal superantigen-like 7 (SSL7), 1513*t*–1514*t*
Staphylococcal superantigen-like 10, 1513*t*–1514*t*
Staphylococci, 1509–1522
arterial graft infections, 436
brain abscess and, 202–203
catheter-related bloodstream infection (CRBSI), 427
cellulitis, 92
classification of, 1509
coagulase-negative. *see* Coagulase-negative staphylococci
dermatologic manifestations of, 116
diagnostic microbiology of, 1516–1519
differentiation from other Gram-positive cocci, 1517*t*
and drowning-associated infections, 680
in endocarditis, 457, 458*t*, 467–468
endophthalmitis and, 158
fusidic acid for, 1277
in human bites, 683*t*

Staphylococci *(Continued)*
  lincosamides, 1224–1225
  linezolid, 1230
  nature of, 1509, 1510*f*
  osteomyelitis and, 388–389, 389*f*
  paronychia, 89
  in pericarditis, 450
  peritonitis and, 380–381
  prevention of, 1516
  resistance
    aminoglycoside, 1185
    fusidic acid, 1193
    glycopeptides, 1191–1192
    methicillin, 1184
  in skull-base osteomyelitis, 393
  spinal epidural abscess, 206
  subdural empyema/intracranial epidural abscess, 204
  susceptibility testing for, 1517–1519, 1517*t*
  treatment
    β-lactam antibiotics for, 1209
    penicillins, 1203
  typing methods for, 1519
Staphylococcus aureus
  active efflux in, 1186
  adherence to host cells and tissues, 1512, 1512*f*
  aminoglycosides for, 1233
  in arterial graft infections, 436
  in bacterial arthritis, 382–385, 383*t*, 385*f*, 386*t*
  blistering distal dactylitis and, 89
  blocking host defenses, 1512–1514
  brain abscess and, 199
  in breast-feeding, 516
  in burn wounds, 698
  in catheter-related bloodstream infection (CRBSI), 435
  cellulitis and, 90*f*
  characteristics of, in food-borne diarrheal illness, 330*t*
  and chronic granulomatous disease, 708
  clinical manifestations of, 1519
  complement evasion of, 1512–1514, 1514*f*
  in complicated urinary tract infection, 540*t*
  cytolytic toxins and, 1514–1515
  cytotoxins and, 1514–1515
  decolonization of, 1516
  dermatologic manifestations of, 116
  diagnostic microbiology of, 1516–1519
  in diarrhea, with vomiting, 331
  ecthyma and, 88–89
  emerging and re-emerging pathogens and diseases, 40
  empyema and, 266*t*
  in endocarditis, 456–458, 458*t*
  endophthalmitis and, 159
  epidemiology of, 1509–1512
    community-acquired MRSA, 1511, 1511*f*
    nosocomial, 1509–1511
  folliculitis and, 86–87
  in foot ulcers, 130–131
  furunculosis and, 87, 87*f*
  fusidic acid for, 1277
  genetic location of, 1515
  hospital-acquired pneumonia and, 259*t*
  in human bites, 682, 683*t*
  hydrocephalus shunts and, 221
  immunostimulatory molecules of, 1515, 1515*f*
  impetigo and, 88
  infective endocarditis, 748
  inhibition of neutrophil recruitment and activation, 1514
  interactions with the coagulation system, 1515
  isolation and determination of, 1516–1517, 1516*f*–1517*f*
  lincosamides, 1224–1225
  linezolid, 1230
  lower respiratory tract infections, 264*f*, 1221
  management of, 1520–1521, 1520*t*–1521*t*
  in mastitis, 501
  methicillin-resistant. *see* Methicillin-resistant *Staphylococcus aureus* (MRSA)
  methicillin-susceptible. *see* Methicillin-susceptible *Staphylococcus aureus* (MSSA)
  multidrug-resistant gram-positive bacteria, 1289–1290
  myocarditis and, 446–447
  in osteomyelitis, 388–390, 389*f*, 394*f*, 395, 395*t*
  in otitis media, 236, 1637
  pathogenicity of, 1512–1515
  peritonitis and, 380–381
  pneumonia in HIV/AIDS, 857

Staphylococcus aureus (Continued)
  pristinamycin, 1228
  in prosthetic joint infection (PJI), 400
  proteases and, 1514–1515
  pyomyositis, 102*f*
  in recurrent cellulitis, 133
  resistance
    to antimicrobial peptides, 1512
    to glycopeptides, 1191
    intrinsic, 1182*t*
    to phagocytosis and intracellular killing, 1514
    to quinolones, 1186
  in respiratory tract infections, 1575
  sinusitis and, 240
  skin lesions and, 84
  spinal epidural abscess and, 206
  superantigens, 419
  and surgical site infections, 687
  susceptibility testing for
    genotypic, 1519
    phenotypic, 1517–1519, 1517*t*
  transmission of, 665*t*
  and tumor necrosis factor inhibitor, 797–799
  vancomycin-resistant. *see* Vancomycin-resistant *Staphylococcus aureus* (VRSA)
  vancomycin susceptibility for, 1249, 1249*t*
  in vertebral osteomyelitis, 391–392
  virulence factors of, 1513*t*–1514*t*, 1515
  wound infections with, 1509
Staphylococcus epidermidis
  endophthalmitis and, 159
  in human bites, 683*t*
  hydrocephalus shunts and, 222*f*, 223*b*
  in mastitis, 501
  pathogenicity of, 1515–1516
  and surgical site infections, 687
Staphylococcus hyicus, 1509
Staphylococcus intermedius, 1509
  cellulitis and, 90
Staphylococcus saccharolyticus, 1631
Staphylococcus saprophyticus, in cystitis, 523
Staphylokinase (SAK), 1512, 1513*t*–1514*t*
Staphylolysin, 1522
Staphyloxantin (golden pigment), 1513*t*–1514*t*
Starlings, 1706
Stavudine, 1148*t*, 1298
  adverse reactions of, 1298
  antiretroviral drugs, 920
  cause and, 920
  chemical structure of, 1296*f*
  description, 1298
  dosage of, 1298
    in special circumstances, 1297*t*, 1298
  drug interactions of, 1298
  indication for, 1298
  perinatal HIV transmission prevention, 909*t*
  pharmacokinetics and distribution of, 1298
  resistance to, 1298
  route of administration of, 1298
Stellate neuroretinitis, 168
Stem cell transplantation, 715
  see also Hematopoietic stem cell transplantation
Stenotrophomonas, nomenclature of, 1581*t*–1582*t*
Stenotrophomonas maltophilia, 1596–1597
  cellulitis and, 91
  clinical manifestations of, 1597
  diagnostic microbiology of, 1596
  epidemiology of, 1596
  hospital-acquired pneumonia and, 259*t*
  intrinsic resistance of, 1182*t*
  management and resistance of, 1597
  nature and taxonomy of, 1596
  nosocomial infections from, 1588*t*
  pathogenicity and pathogenesis of, 1596–1597
  prevalence of, 1579
STEP trial, 832
Sterilization, 57
Sterilizing cure, for HIV infection, 931
Sternal osteomyelitis, 481–482
  diagnosis and treatment of, 481–482, 481*f*
Steroids
  and chronic granulomatous disease, 708
  in chronic meningitis, 187
  in tuberculosis, 284

Stevens-Johnson syndrome, *Mycoplasma pneumoniae* in, 1661
Stillbirth, congenital infection and, 509
Still's disease, adult onset, and fever of unknown origin, 613, 622
Stomach, microbiology of, 355
Stomatitis
  aphthous, 318
    in HIV/AIDS, 880, 881*f*
  gangrenous, 316, 316*f*–317*f*
  in hand, foot and mouth disease, 81
Stool
  examination, in food-borne diarrheal illness, 332–333
  for laboratory diagnosis, of mycobacteria, 1651*t*
  microbiologic investigation of, in congenital infection, 512*t*
  schistosomiasis and, 1031
Stool antigen tests, for *Helicobacter pylori*, 325
Stool cultures
  of travelers' diarrhea, 375
  for *Vibrio cholerae*, 1606
Stool samples
  amebiasis, 348
  cryptosporidiosis, 347–348
  isosporiasis, 348
  microsporidiosis, 348
  parasites, 346
Stool specimens
  of *Cryptosporidium* spp., 1737–1738
  of *Cystoisospora belli*, 1738
  in diarrhea, 339
  for helminths diagnosis, 1775–1776
  of microsporidia, 1739, 1739*f*
Streptobacillus moniliformis
  in bacterial arthritis, 383*t*
  rat-bite fever, 661
  transmission of, 665*t*
Streptocerciasis
  clinical features of, 1050
  epidemiology of, 1047
  management of, 1051
  pathogenesis and pathology of, 1047–1048
Streptococcaceae, 1523
Streptococcal infection
  dermatologic manifestations of, 114*t*–115*t*
  lymphadenopathy and, 137*t*–138*t*
Streptococcal myositis, 1640*f*
Streptococcal sore throat, 472
Streptococcal toxic shock syndrome, 116
Streptococci, 1523–1536
  aminoglycosides for, 1234
  antibiotic therapy for, in infective arthritis, 386*t*
  associated with erythema nodosum, 121*t*
  brain abscess and, 199
  classification of, 1523
  dermatologic manifestations of, 116
  empyema and, 266*t*
  in endocarditis, 456–458, 458*t*
  endophthalmitis and, 159
  group A. *see* Group A streptococci
  group B. *see* Group B streptococci
  group C. *see* Group C streptococci
  group G. *see* Group G streptococci
  β-hemolytic
    epidemiology of, 1525–1526
    in foot ulcers, 130–131
    in human bites, 682
  intrinsic resistance of, 1182*t*
  lung abscess and, 264–265, 264*f*
  molecular characterization and population structure of, 1524–1525
  normal flora, 312
  penicillin-resistant, 467
  in pericarditis, 450
  peritonitis and, 381
  postsplenectomy sepsis, 778*t*
  in prosthetic joint infection (PJI), 400
  in recurrent cellulitis, 134
  subdural empyema/intracranial epidural abscess, 203–204
  taxonomy and identification of, 1523–1524, 1523*f*–1524*f*
  telithromycin, 1219
  typing of, 1524*t*
  vaccines for, 1536

Streptococci (Continued)
  viridans
    in mastitis, 501
    microflora, 355
Streptococcus agalactiae, meningitis and, 182t
Streptococcus anginosus, 1532, 1631
  in human bites, 683t
  pyogenic liver abscess, 361
Streptococcus constellatus, in human bites, 683t
Streptococcus gallolyticus
  clinical manifestations of, 1534
  management of, 1534–1535
Streptococcus iniae, 91
Streptococcus intermedius, in human bites, 683t
Streptococcus mutans
  clinical manifestations of, 1534
  dental caries with, 312
Streptococcus oralis, in human bites, 683t
Streptococcus pneumoniae
  avoiding ingestion, 23
  in bacterial arthritis, 383
  bronchiectasis and, 246
  bronchitis and, 243
  in chronic obstructive pulmonary disease, 310
  clinical manifestations of, 1534
  community-acquired pneumonia and, 253
  in conjunctivitis, 150
  empyema and, 266t
  epidemiology of, 1527
  in HIV in low- and middle-income countries, 891
  hospital-acquired pneumonia and, 259t
  ketolides, 1219
  lower respiratory tract infections, 264f, 1221
  management of, 1535
  meningitis and, 177
  molecular characterization and population structure of,
    1525
  opportunistic infection in HIV, 857
  in osteomyelitis, 395t
  otitis media of, 236
  pathogenesis of, 1531–1532, 1531f
  pneumonia in HIV/AIDS, 857
  in postsplenectomy sepsis, 777, 778t
  prevention of, 1535
  primary (spontaneous) peritonitis, 359
  resistance
    to penicillin, 1184
    to quinolones, 1186
  respiratory tract infection, 1132
  in sinusitis, 1637
  in thoracic transplantation patients, 747t
  treatment, β-lactam antibiotics, 1209
  see also Pneumococcal infections
Streptococcus pyogenes, 2
  avoiding ingestion, 23
  blistering distal dactylitis and, 89
  in burn wounds, 698
  cell wall of, 14f
  cellulitis and, 89, 92
  endophthalmitis and, 160
  erysipelas and, 89
  in human bites, 683t
  otitis media and, 237
  in recurrent cellulitis, 133
  skin lesions and, 84
  superantigens, 419
Streptococcus pyogenes cell envelope proteinase (SpyCEP),
    1528
Streptococcus suis
  and occupational infections, 648t–649t
  transmission of, 664
Streptococcus zooepidemicus, transmission of, 665t
Streptogramins, 1171–1173, 1227–1229
  antibacterial activities of, 1227, 1228t
  antibiotic combinations, 1227
  breakpoints, 1227
  chemical structure of, 1171
  for enterococci, 1534
  exit tunnel, 1221
  mode of action of, 1173
  pharmacodynamics of, 1173
  properties of natural, 1227
  resistance to, 1173, 1187–1189, 1188t

Streptogramins (Continued)
  by efflux, 1189
  by enzymatic modification, 1189
  by target modification, 1187–1189
  synergy between components A and B, 1227
Streptolysin O (SLO), 1529
Streptomyces, 1550t
  in cutaneous and soft tissue infection, 1551
  diagnostic microbiology of, 1549
  fosfomycin for, 1278
Streptomyces aureofaciens, 1256
Streptomycin, 1185, 1270
  adverse reactions of, 1268t–1269t
  chemical structure of, 1168
  in chronic meningitis, 186–187
  clinical use of, 1234
  for infective arthritis, 386t
  for meningitis, 186–187
  for mycetoma, 1723
  for mycobacterial infections, 1237
  for plague, 1083–1084, 1083t
  resistance to, 1186
    mycobacterial, 1656t
  for tuberculosis, 281, 283t
  for tularemia, 1089
Streptomycineae, 1547t
Streptosporangineae, 1547t
Stress-ulcer prophylaxis, hospital-acquired pneumonia, 261
String capsule, for helminths diagnosis, 1776
Strongyloides stercoralis, 773, 773f
  of chronic diarrhea, 347t, 349
  clinical features of, 996–997
  clinical manifestations of, 1777
  diagnosis of, 998t–999t, 1776f
  epidemiology of, 1763
  hospital-acquired pneumonia and, 259t
  larvae of, 1776f
  life cycle of, 993f, 1767f
  pathogenesis and pathology of, 991–993
  pathogenicity of, 1768
  prevention of, 994
  treatment of, 1000–1001, 1001t, 1345t–1351t
Strongyloidiasis, 1777
  chronic diarrhea and, 349
  clinical features of, 996–997
  pathogenesis and pathology of, 991–993, 993f–994f
  treatment of, 1345t–1351t
Strychnine poisoning, 212
Sub-Saharan Africa, infections in, 1130
Subacute osteomyelitis, 391
Subacute sclerosing panencephalitis (SSPE), 167
  measles and, 1400
Subconjunctival antibiotics, endophthalmitis, 162
Subconjunctival antimicrobials, 159
Subconjunctival hemorrhage, 1106–1107, 1107f
Subcutaneous infections, 84–94, 85t
  clinical features, diagnosis and management, 86–93
  epidemiology of, 84
  pathogenesis of, 84–86
  prevention of, 86
Subcutaneous nodules, in rheumatic fever, 473
Subdural empyema, 203–204
  clinical features of, 204
  diagnosis of, 204
  epidemiology of, 203
  management of, 204
  pathogenesis and pathophysiology of, 203–204
  Pseudomonas aeruginosa in, 1589
Subepithelial invasion, 17–18
Subglottic secretion drainage (SSD), hospital-acquired
    pneumonia and, 262
Submandibular abscess, 313, 313f
Submandibular spaces, 313
Suction, primary reclosure with, for mediastinitis and
    sternal osteomyelitis, 482
Sulbactam, against carbapenemase-resistant gram-negative
    bacilli, 1290t
Sulfadiazine
  impregnated catheters, 433
  for parasitic infections, 1345t–1362t
  for protozoal infections, 1364
  for toxoplasmosis, 513, 1755
    in HIV/AIDS, 857

Sulfadoxine
  for mycetoma, 1723
  for protozoal infections, 1352t–1362t, 1364
Sulfadoxine-pyrimethamine
  as antifolate agent, 1364
  artesunate plus, 1022, 1023t
  for Plasmodium falciparum malaria, 1022
Sulfamethoxazole
  chemical structure of, 1178f
  for parasitic infections treatment, 1352t–1362t,
    1364
Sulfonamides, 1177–1178, 1280
  chemical structure of, 1177–1178, 1178f
  elimination of, 1280
  mode of action of, 1178
  pharmacodynamics of, 1178
  pharmacokinetics of, 1280
  plasma kinetics of, 1280
  for protozoal infections, 1352t–1362t, 1364
  resistance to, 1178, 1192–1193
    Erysipelothrix rhusiopathiae, 1542
  side effects of, 1364
Sulfur granules, 316
Superantigens, 22, 1513t–1514t, 1515, 1515f
  in sepsis, 419, 419t
Superficial fungal infections, 122–129
Superinfection, from β-lactam antibiotics, 1215t
Superintegrons, 1195–1196
'Superiority trial,' in antibiotic development, 1383
Superoxide dismutase (SOD), 23
Suppurative intracranial phlebitis, 204–205
  clinical features of, 205
  diagnosis of, 205
  epidemiology of, 204–205
  management of, 205
  pathogenesis of, 204–205
  pathophysiology of, 204–205
Suppurative phlebitis, 691
Suppurative thyroiditis, 1636t
Suprapubic aspiration, in cystitis, 527
Suramin
  for African trypanosomiasis, 969, 969t, 1762
  dosage of, 1370
  for parasitic infections, 1345t–1362t, 1370
  route of administration, 1370
Surface antigens, group A streptococci and, 1528
Surface protein A (SpA), 1514
Surface proteins, 1559
Surgery
  for acute osteomyelitis, 395–396
  antimicrobial prophylaxis in, 1206
  for arterial graft infection, 437–438
  brain abscess and, 205
  for chronic osteomyelitis, 396
  for Echinococcus granulosus, 1044
  for Echinococcus multilocularis, 1045
  for endocarditis, 469, 469t
  infections following, 684–692
    antibiotic prophylaxis, 686–688, 687t
    antibiotic therapy principles for, 691
    environment-derived risk factors, 686
    pathogenesis of inflammation and organ dysfunction,
      684–686, 685f
    postoperative period, 688–691
    treatment-derived risk factors, 686
  peritonitis, 358–359
  in prosthetic joint infection (PJI), 402
Surgical drainage
  for amebic liver abscess, 1013
  for liver abscess, 1013
Surgical infections, quinolones for, 1246
Surgical prophylaxis, 1154
Surgical site infections (SSIs), 1154
  antibiotic prophylaxis and the risk of, 686–688
  pathogenesis of, 1154
  percentage rates for selected procedures, 687t
  prosthetic joint infection as, 403
  risk classification systems and risk factors, 1154,
    1155t
  staphylococci and streptococci carriers, 686
  surveillance for, 1154
Surgical therapy, for anaerobic bacteria, 1641
Surveillance, and bioterrorism, 678

Susceptibility testing
  of *Candida*, 1683–1684
  of mycobacteria, 1656–1657
  for staphylococci, 1517–1519, 1517*t*
Susceptible-Infected-Recovered (SIR) model, 51, 52*f*
Sutezolid, as antituberculosis agent, 1271
'Sweaty tennis shoe syndrome', 91
Swimmer's itch, 87, 88*f*, 645, 1029
Swimming pools, and recreational infections, 645
Swine, infections from, 191*t*
Swine erysipelas, 1542
Swine influenza (H1N1V) pandemic 2009, 1467–1468, 1468*f*
Swineherd's disease, 664
Sycosis barbae, 86
Sydenham's chorea, 471, 473, 1533
Symmer's pipe-stem fibrosis, 1030
Symptomatic cystitis, treatment of, 443*t*
Syndrome-based sampling, 1386, 1387*f*
Syndrome of inappropriate antidiuretic hormone secretion (SIADH), 279
Synergistic capabilities, of anaerobic bacteria, 1633
Synovial fluid, in bacterial arthritis, 384
  drainage, 385
Synthesis, genome sequencing by, 63*t*
Syphilis, 559–566, 586*t*–587*t*
  cardiovascular, 562
  clinical features of, 561–563, 561*f*
  congenital
    clinical features of, 563, 563*f*
    definitions of, 565*t*
    management of, 513
    neonatal testing for, 511–512
    neonates, evaluation of, 564–565
    pathogenesis and pathology of, 506
    screening for, 507
    treatment of, 565
  dermatologic manifestations of, 114*t*–115*t*
  diagnosis of, 563–565, 564*t*
  endemic, 961
    clinical features of, 963–964, 964*f*
    pathology of, 963
  epidemiology of, 559
  histologic appearances of, 560
  history of, 560*f*
  and HIV-1, 843
  HIV infection and, 563
  incubation period of, 561
  β-lactam antibiotics for, 1212
  late meningovascular, 563
  latent, 562
  lymphadenopathy and, 137*t*–138*t*, 141
  management of, 565–566, 565*t*
    sexual contacts, 566
  in myocarditis, 447
  neurosyphilis, 562–563
    asymptomatic, 562
    gummatous, 563
    meningeal, 562–563
  parenchymatous, 563
  pathogenesis and pathology of, 559–560
  prevention of, 560
  primary, 561, 561*f*
    oral mucosa and, 318
  prognosis of, 566
  secondary, 561–562, 561*f*–562*f*
    in chronic meningitis, 187
  and skin manifestations of HIV, 884
  tertiary gummatous, 562–563, 562*f*
  transmission of, 559
  uveitis and, 168–169
Syphilis condylomata lata, 586*t*–587*t*
Systemic antifungal agents, 1333–1344
Systemic candidiasis, 439–445, 1686–1687
Systemic disease, diphtheria and, 1546
Systemic fungi, 1700–1701, 1700*t*
Systemic infections, dermatologic manifestations of, 113–121
Systemic inflammatory response syndrome (SIRS)
  definition of, 415
  pathogenesis of, 684–685, 685*f*
Systemic lupus erythematosus (SLE), and fever of unknown origin, 613

T

T. pallidum hemagglutination assay (TPHA), 964–965
T-cell deficiency, brain abscess and, 199
T-cell depletion (TCD), in hematopoietic stem cell transplantation, 739
T-cell vaccines, against HIV, 831
T-cells
  activation of, by antigen-presenting cells, 801
  function defect of, and live vaccines, 795
T-helper cell subsets, 33*f*
T lymphocytes
  cellular immune responses, 32
  cryptococcosis and, 1692
  cytolytic, 33
  and immunodeficiencies, 713
  regulatory, 32–33
T-SPOT.TB assay, 1657–1658, 1658*t*
Tabes dorsalis, 563
Tacrolimus, 1378
Taenia, 1033–1034, 1033*f*
  clinical manifestations of, 1778
Taenia brauni, 1035–1036
Taenia multiceps, 1035–1036
Taenia saginata, 989*f*, 1033, 1033*f*
  cattle raising and, 990
  clinical features of, 997
  diagnosis of, 998*t*–999*t*
  epidemiology of, 989–990, 1766
  life cycle of, 1773*f*
  pathogenesis and pathology of, 994
  pathogenicity of, 1772
  transmission of, 666
  treatment of, 1001, 1001*t*, 1345*t*–1351*t*
Taenia serialis, 1035–1036
Taenia solium, 666, 1032, 1032*f*
  in chronic meningitis, 186*t*
  clinical features of, 997
  clinical manifestations of, 1778
  diagnosis of, 998*t*–999*t*
  epidemiology of, 1034, 1766
  life cycle of, 1773*f*–1774*f*
  in myocarditis, 447
  pathogenesis of, 994, 1034, 1034*f*
  pathogenicity of, 1772
  pathology of, 994
  treatment of, 1001, 1001*t*, 1345*t*–1351*t*
Taeniasis, 1033
Takayasu's arteritis, and fever of unknown origin, 614
Talaromyces, 1681*t*
Talaromyces marneffei, 1698–1699
  clinical manifestations of, 1699, 1699*f*
  diagnostic microbiology of, 1699, 1699*f*
  epidemiology of, 1698
  management of, 1699
  nature of, 1698
  pathogenicity of, 1698–1699
Tanapox, 666
Tannerella forsythensis, 319
Tap deficiency, 719
Tapeworms. *see* Cestodes.
Targeted metagenomic sequencing, 69–70
tat protein, 1485
tax protein, 1484*f*, 1491
Taxono-genomics, 65–66
Teacher, and occupational infections, 648*t*–649*t*
Tedizolid, 1230
Tegument, 1763
Teichoic acids, 1512, 1516
Teicoplanin, 1191, 1254, 1254*t*
  for anaerobic bacteria, 1643
  mode of action of, 1164
  pharmacodynamics of, 1167
Telaprevir (TVR), for hepatitis C, 1331
Telavancin, 1252–1253, 1254*t*
  mode of action of, 1164
  resistance to, 1164–1167
Telbivudine (LDT), for chronic hepatitis B, 1329
Telithromycin
  accumulation ratio of, 1222*t*
  characteristics of, 1218*t*
  concentration in lung tissues, 1224*t*
  controversies on, 1382
  peptidyltransferase center, 1221
  pharmacokinetics, 1222, 1223*t*–1224*t*

Telithromycin (*Continued*)
  for scrub typhus, 1097
  in vitro activity, 1219–1220, 1220*t*
TEM-1, 1183
TEM-2, 1183
Temozolomide, 725
Temporal arteritis, 613
Temporal classifications, in osteomyelitis, 390
Temporal lobe, brain abscess, 199
Tendinitis, in quinolones adverse effects, 1247
Tenofovir, 1148*t*, 1300
  adverse reactions of, 1300
  antiretroviral drugs, 920–921
  chemical structure of, 1296*f*
  description of, 1300
  dosage of, 1300
    in special circumstances, 1297*t*, 1300
  drug interactions of, 1300
  effect on oral contraceptives, 907*t*
  for hepatitis B virus (HBV), in HIV, 896–897
  for HIV, 825–826
  indications of, 1300
  in occupational exposure, to HIV infection, 835
  perinatal HIV transmission prevention, 909*t*
  pharmacokinetics and distribution of, 1300
  and renal function, 921
  resistance of, 1300
  route of administration, 1300
Tenofovir alafenamide (TAF), for chronic hepatitis B, 1329
Tenofovir disoproxil fumarate (TDF), for chronic hepatitis B, 1329
Tenosynovitis, 288
Terbinafine, 1343
  adverse effects of, 1343
  for candidiasis, 128
  for chromoblastomycosis, 1722
  for conidiobolomycosis, 1723
  dosage of, 1343
  drug interactions of, 1343
  indications of, 1343
  mechanism of action, 1343
  for mycetoma, 1723
  for onychomycosis, 128
  pharmacokinetics and distribution of, 1343
  for pityriasis versicolor, 128
  route of administration, 1343
  for seborrheic dermatitis, 128
  for tinea corporis and tinea cruris, 128
  for tinea manuum, 128
  for tinea pedis, 128
Terconazole, for vulvovaginal candidiasis, 488*t*
Testing algorithm, in HIV diagnosis, 1487, 1488*f*
Tetanospasmin (TS), 208
Tetanus, 208–213, 645
  cephalic, 211
  clinical features of, 211
  diagnosis of, 211–212
  differential diagnosis of, 212
  epidemiology of, 208, 209*f*
  forms of, 211
  generalized, 211, 211*f*
  in human bites, 682, 683*t*
  localized, 211
  management of, 212
  neonatal, 211
  and occupational infections, 648*t*–649*t*
  pathogenesis and pathology of, 209–210
  prevention of, 210
  prophylaxis, 210*t*, 688
  rating scale for, 211*t*
  toxin, of anaerobic bacteria, 1633
  vaccination against, 782*t*–783*t*
Tetracyclines, 1168–1169, 1256–1259
  absorption of, 1257
  for actinomycosis, 316
  adverse reactions and interactions of, 1259, 1259*t*
  for *Alcaligenes* spp., 1597
  for anaerobic bacteria, 1643
  for anthrax, 1127
  antimicrobial spectrum, 1256, 1258*t*
  bacterial targeting, 1168, 1171*f*
  chemical structure of, 1168, 1170*f*
  for cholera, 334, 1259, 1607
  distribution of, 1257
  for dog bites, 657*t*

Tetracyclines *(Continued)*
  dosage of, 1258, 1258*t*
    in special circumstances, 1258–1259
  efflux systems, 1189–1190
  for ehrlichiosis, 1259
  elimination of, 1257–1258
  for *Erysipelothrix rhusiopathiae*, 1542
  for gas gangrene, 100–101
  for gastrointestinal protozoa, 999
  indications for, 1259
  for lung abscess, 269*f*
  for Lyme disease, 412, 1259
  for malaria, 1259
  mode of action of, 1168
  for multidrug-resistant organisms, 1259
  for *Mycoplasma hominis*, 1664
  for parasitic infections, 1345*t*–1362*t*, 1370
  pharmacodynamics of, 1169
  pharmacokinetics of, 1257–1258, 1258*t*
  for plague, 1083–1084, 1083*t*
  for relapsing fevers, 1109
  resistance to, 1168–1169, 1189–1190, 1190*t*, 1256–1257, 1592*t*
    by ribosomal protection, 1189
  for respiratory infections, 1259
  for rickettsial infections, 1259
  route of administration of, 1258
  for scrub typhus, 1097
  for sexually transmitted diseases, 1259
  structure of, 1257*f*
  for syphilis, 565
  for trachoma, 981
  for tularemia, 1089, 1617
Tetraparvovirus, 1449
Th17 cells, 801
Thailand (THAI) virus, 1502*t*
Thalassemias
  clinical features of, 1056–1057, 1057*f*
  pathogenesis and pathology of, 1054–1055
α-Thalassemias, 1054
β-Thalassemias, 1054
Thalidomide, 960, 1379
Theory of reasoned action, and HIV, 826
Therapeutic drug monitoring (TDM), 916, 1153
Therapeutics, disease prevention and control, 57–58
Thermal injury, 698
  immune system response to, 698, 699*t*
Thermometry, clinical, 606
Thermonuclease, 1513*t*–1514*t*
Thermoregulation, 606–607, 607*f*
  acute-phase response, 608–609
  endogenous antipyretics, 609
Theta toxin, 1633
Thiabendazole, 1352*t*–1362*t*, 1372
  for gastrointestinal helminth, 1000–1001, 1001*t*
Thiacetazone, as antituberculosis agent, 1271
Thiamphenicol, 1173
  bacterial targeting, 1173
  chemical structure of, 1173
  mode of action of, 1173
  pharmacodynamics of, 1173
  resistance to, 1173
Thioamides, as antituberculosis agent, 1270
Thoracic infection, anaerobic bacteria in, 1632*f*
Thoracic lymphadenopathy, 145
Thoracic surgery, for pleural effusion, 304
Thoracoscopy, tuberculosis, 279–280
Thottapalayam (TMP) virus, 1502*t*
Throat swabs, for diphtheria, 1544
Thrombocytopenia
  linezolid complications, 1231
  X-linked, 721
Thrombophlebitis
  adverse reactions to β-lactam antibiotics, 1216
  septic, 500
Thrombosis
  catheter-related, 432
  cavernous sinus, 313–314, 314*f*
Thumb sign, in epiglottitis, 232–233, 233*f*
Thymoma, 809, 810*t*
Thyroiditis
  subacute, and fever of unknown origin, 614
  suppurative. *see* Suppurative thyroiditis

TIBOLA-DEBONEL-SENLAT, 1667*t*
Ticarcillin
  for anaerobic bacteria, 1210, 1643
  antimicrobial spectrum, routes of administration and dosages, 1206*t*–1207*t*
  dosage in renal failure, 1213*t*–1214*t*
  drug interactions, 1216
  for lung abscess, 269*f*
  for *P. aeruginosa* infection, 1210
  susceptibilities of selected bacteria to, 1208*t*–1209*t*
Ticarcillin-clavulanate
  for complicated urinary tract infection, 545*t*
  for cystic fibrosis, 301
  dosage in renal failure, 1213*t*–1214*t*
  for lung abscess, 269*f*
  pharmacokinetics of, 1205*t*
  susceptibilities of selected bacteria to, 1208*t*–1209*t*
Ticarcillin-clavulanic acid
  for *Alcaligenes* spp., 1597
  antimicrobial spectrum, routes of administration and dosages, 1206*t*–1207*t*
  for *Stenotrophomonas maltophilia*, 1597
Tick bite, infections from, 191*t*
Tick-borne diseases
  anaplasmosis, 1671
  ehrlichioses, 1671
  infections from, 658
  Q fever, 1672
  spotted fever group rickettsiae, 1667, 1667*f*
Tick-borne encephalitis
  central European, transmission of, 665*t*
  immunization for, and occupational infections, 650*t*–651*t*
  and recreational infections, 644
  vaccination, for travelers, 950
Tick-borne encephalitis virus, encephalitis/myelitis caused by, 192*t*
Tick-borne lymphadenopathy, 1092*t*–1093*t*
Tick-borne relapsing fever, 1105, 1105*t*, 1109
Tick-borne rickettsiae, and recreational infections, 644
Tick-borne rickettsial infections, and occupational infections, 648*t*–649*t*
Ticks
  arboviruses, 1493, 1495*t*
  relapsing fever from, 1607–1608
  topical rickettsioses and, 1091, 1092*t*–1093*t*
  tularemia and, 1086, 1087*f*
Tigecycline
  for anaerobic bacteria, 1643
  background in, 1256
  against carbapenamase-resistant gram-negative bacilli, 1290*t*
  chemical structure of, 1168
  for chronic obstructive pulmonary disease, 1259
  distribution of, 1257
  resistance to, 1169, 1257
  route of administration of, 1258
  for *Stenotrophomonas maltophilia*, 1597
  structure of, 1257*f*
Tinea barbae, clinical features of, 124, 124*f*
Tinea capitis, 1710
  anthropophilic, 123, 1711
  clinical features of, 123–124
  diagnostic microbiology of, 1711
  epidemiology of, 122
  management of, 127
  prevention of, 123
Tinea corporis
  clinical features of, 124, 124*f*
  management of, 128
Tinea cruris, 586*t*–587*t*
  clinical features of, 124
  management of, 128
Tinea faciei, 124
  clinical features of, 124
Tinea imbricata, 124
  clinical features of, 124
Tinea manuum
  clinical features of, 125
  management of, 128
Tinea nigra
  clinical features of, 126
  diagnostic microbiology of, 1711

Tinea nigra *(Continued)*
  epidemiology of, 122, 1710
  management of, 128
  nature of, 1710
Tinea pedis, 1710
  clinical features of, 125
  management of, 128
  moccasin, 125
  prevention of, 123
Tinea unguium, clinical features of, 125
Tinea versicolor, 1711
Tinidazole, 1261–1263
  for anaerobic bacteria, 1643
  for bacterial vaginosis, 484
  dosage for, 1261–1262
  for gastrointestinal protozoa, 997, 1000*t*
  for giardiasis, 334
  for parasitic infections, 1345*t*–1362*t*, 1368
  for trichomoniasis, 486
Tioconazole
  onychomycosis management, 128
  for vulvovaginal candidiasis, 488*t*
Tipranavir, 1148*t*, 1304
  antiretroviral drugs, 925
  effect on oral contraceptives, 907*t*
  perinatal HIV transmission prevention, 909*t*
Tissue
  biopsy. *see* Tissue biopsy
  damage induced by micro-organisms, 18, 18*t*
  see also specific tissues
Tissue amebicides, 1012
Tissue biopsy, for laboratory diagnosis, of mycobacteria, 1651–1652, 1651*t*
Tissue culture vaccines, side effects of, 1463
Tissue factor pathway inhibitor (TFPI), 423
Tissue-helminth infections, eosinophilia and, 985
Tissue protozoa, 1751–1762
Tissue specimen
  collection, 1634*t*
  for helminths diagnosis, 1776
TLRs. *see* Toll-like receptors (TLRs).
TMP-SMX. *see* Trimethoprim-sulfamethoxazole (TMP-SMX).
TNF receptor-associated periodic syndrome (TRAPS), 614
Tobramycin
  clinical use of, 1234
  for complicated urinary tract infection, 545*t*
  for conjunctivitis, 152
  for cystic fibrosis, 301
  for hospital-acquired pneumonia, 260*t*
  pharmacokinetic parameters for, 1234*t*
  resistance, 1185–1186
Tocilizumab, 798*t*–799*t*, 801
Tocolytic therapy, malaria in pregnancy, 1143*t*–1144*t*
Toll-like receptors (TLRs), 27–30, 30*t*
  in rheumatic fever, 472
  in sepsis, 421, 422*t*
Tongue coating, halitosis, 319
Tonsillitis, anaerobic bacteria in, 1636*t*, 1637–1638
Topical antiseptics
  endophthalmitis prevention, 159–160
  and surgical site infection prevention, 688–689
Topical therapies, for psoriasis, 880
Topografov (TOP) virus, 1502*t*
Topoisomerase IV, 1174, 1176*f*, 1186
Topoisomerases, inhibition of, 1174
TORCH syndrome, 166
Torovirus, diarrhea and, 338
Toscana, 1495*t*
Total dystrophic onychomycosis, 125, 125*f*
Total parenteral nutrition, in intestinal transplant patients, 756
Tourette's syndrome, in rheumatic fever, 473–474
Toxic epidermal necrolysis, 88, 88*f*
'Toxic' follicular conjunctivitis, 981*t*
Toxic shock syndrome (TSS)
  dermatologic manifestations of, 116
  group A streptococci and, 1529, 1530*f*
  influenza virus and, 1470
  streptococcal, 1532, 1532*b*
  superantigens, 419, 1515
    and bacterial components associated with, 22

Toxic shock syndrome toxin (TSST), 1513t–1514t, 1515
Toxin A (TcdA), *Clostridium difficile* infection (CDI), 351
Toxin B (TcdB), *Clostridium difficile* infection (CDI), 351–352
Toxin-coregulated pilus (TCP), 1605
Toxins
    alpha, 1633
    of anaerobic bacteria, 1633
    bacterial. *see* Bacterial toxins
    exotoxins. *see* Exotoxins
    group A streptococci and, 1529, 1530f
    theta, 1633
Toxocara canis
    causing retinitis and uveitis, 171t
    from dogs, 658
Toxocara cati, 660
    uveitis and, 172
Toxocariasis, 1777
    dermatologic manifestations of, 114t–115t
    treatment of, 1345t–1351t
    uveitis and, 172
Toxoplasma, in abscesses, 772, 772f
Toxoplasma gondii, 1753
    in cats, 660
    causing retinitis and uveitis, 171t
    clinical manifestations of, 1754–1755
    in congenital infection
        clinical features of, 510
        diagnosis of, 512t
        management of, 513
        pathogenesis and pathology of, 506
        preconception, in maternal immunity, 506–507
        screening for, during pregnancy, 507–508, 508t
    diagnostic microbiology of, 1754
    epidemiology of, 1753
    in HIV, in low- and middle-income countries, 892
    immunity of, 1753
    lincosamide, 1226
    lymphadenopathy, 142
    management of, 1755–1756
    in myocarditis, 448
    nature of, 1753
    opportunistic infection in HIV of, 856–857
    pathogenicity of, 1753
    prevention of, 1753–1754, 1753b
    transmission of, 665t, 807
    treatment of, 1345t–1351t
Toxoplasma titer
    difficulties in interpretation of serologic results of, 517, 518t
    history and examination of mother in, 518
    investigation of, 517–518
    management of, 518–519
    other considerations in, 519
    pathogenesis of, 517
    serologic studies in mother, 518
    treatment of, 518–519
        in pregnancy, 517–519
Toxoplasmosis, 1753–1756
    acquired, 1754–1755
    from bears, 669
    from cats, 660
    clinical manifestations of, 1754–1755
    congenital, 1754–1755, 1754f
    in congenital infection, 505–506
        clinical features of, 509
        diagnosis of, 511
        management of, 513, 514t
        pathogenesis of, 506
        screening for, during pregnancy, 507–508
    diagnostic microbiology of, 1754
    encephalitis, 773
    epidemiology of, 1753
    eye involvement in, 982
    and fever of unknown origin, 613
    in hematopoietic stem cell transplantation, 743t, 745f
    in HIV/AIDS, 856–857, 857f
        in low- and middle-income countries, 892
        primary prophylaxis for, 857
    immunity, 1753
    in the immunocompromised host, 1755, 1755f
    in kidney transplant patients, 768–769
    lymphadenopathy and, 137t–138t
    management of, 1755–1756
    nature of, 1753

Toxoplasmosis *(Continued)*
    pathogenicity of, 1753
    prevention of, 1753–1754, 1753b
    prophylaxis
        in HIV-infected patients, 914
        in HIV-infected pregnant women, 910
    secondary prevention of, 1755–1756
    in thoracic transplantation patients, 747t
    in transfusion-related infections, 704t
    treatment of, 1345t–1351t
    uveitis and, 166, 175–176
Tracheal colonization factor (TCF-A), 1613t
Tracheal cytotoxin (TCT), 1612, 1613t
Tracheobronchitis, in thoracic transplantation patients, 749
Trachipleistophora anthropophthera, in systemic microsporidiosis, 1741
Trachipleistophora spp., 1741
Trachoma, 151, 979–981, 1678
    in *Chlamydia trachomatis* infection, 597
    clinical features of, 980–981, 980f
    diagnosis of, 981
    epidemiology of, 979
    follicular conjunctivitis and, 981t
    management of, 981
    pathogenesis of, 979
    prevention of, 980
Traditional pricing model, 1384
Trans-theoretical model of change, in HIV, 826
Transaminase
    in hepatitis A virus, 364
    in hepatitis C virus, 369–370, 369f
    in hepatitis E virus, 372
Transcytosis, 15
Transesophageal (TEE) echocardiography, for infectious endocarditis, 611
Transferrin-binding proteins, 1557t, 1559
Transfusion-related infections, 701–704
    blood products as, bacterial contamination of, 702–703, 704t
    Creutzfeldt-Jakob disease (CJD) and, 704
    parasites in, 703–704, 704t
    risk of, 701t
        reducing, methods for, 702t
    viral pathogens in, 701–702, 703t
Transmissible mink encephalopathy, 215t
Transmissible spongiform encephalopathies (TSE), 214–220
    clinical features of, 217, 218f
    development of therapies for, 220
    epidemiology of, 214–215
    molecular strain typing of, 217–219
    pathogenesis and pathology of, 217–220, 219f
    prevention of, 220
Transmission
    based precautions, 58–60, 59b–60b
    dynamic, 50
    see also specific infections
'Transplant tourism', 806
Transplantation
    in antibiotic prophylaxis, 1157t–1158t
    bone marrow, Bk polyomavirus in, 1447
    brain abscess and, 199
    kidney, BK virus nephropathy in, 1447, 1447f
Transportation, of specimens, 1634–1635
Transposons, 1195
    carrying resistance genes, structure of, 1195f
Transthoracic (TTE) echocardiography, for infectious endocarditis, 611
Transtracheal aspiration, lower respiratory tract infections, 268
Trauma, 586t–587t
    brain abscess and, 199
    infections following, 684–692
        antibiotic therapy principles for, 691
        environment-derived risk factors, 686
        pathogenesis of inflammation and organ dysfunction, 684–686, 685f
        postoperative period, 688–691
        treatment-derived risk factors, 686
    mycetoma and, 1714
    subdural empyema/intracranial epidural abscess, 205t
Travel, and emerging infectious diseases, 43
Travel history, and fever of unknown origin, 615

Travel medicine, 948–953
    immunizations, 948–950
        recommended because of risk, 949
        required, 949
        for routine health maintenance, 948–949
    in special groups, 950
Travelers
    approach to eosinophilia in, from tropics, 984–988
    behavioral factors of, 952
    burden of disease, 941–942
    diarrhea. *see* Travelers' diarrhea (TD)
    environmental hazards in, 951–952
    jaundice in, 1134–1136, 1135t
    lymphadenopathy, splenomegaly and anemia, 1139–1140, 1140b
    other diseases and considerations in, 952
    post-travel illness in, 952
    and recreational infections, 643, 643t
    sexually transmitted diseases in, 952
    sexually transmitted infection in, 1137–1138
    sources of information and, 952
Travelers' diarrhea (TD), 332, 332f, 375–376, 950, 1727
    burden of disease, 941–942
    chronic complication of, 375
    clinical presentation of, 375, 375t
    epidemiology of, 375–376
    management of, 334, 376
    prevention of, 376, 950
    quinolones for, 1246
    risk factors for, 375–376
    treatment of, 950
Treatment-derived risk factors, infection following surgery and trauma, 686
Trematoda, nature of, 1763
Trematodes, 989t, 1764t
    blood. *see* Blood flukes
    clinical manifestations of, 1778
    description of, 1032
    epidemiology of, 1765–1766
    importance of physical environment in, 990
    infections of, 1032, 1036–1037
    intestinal. *see* Intestinal flukes
    liver. *see* Liver flukes
    lung. *see* Lung flukes
    pathogenesis and pathology of, 993–994
    pathogenicity of, 1770–1772
    prevention of, 1772
    treatment of, 1001t
    see also specific genera
Trench fever, 1674
Treponema, 1600
    in lymph node enlargement, 147t–148t
Treponema denticola, 319
Treponema pallidum, 559, 961
    causing retinitis and uveitis, 169t, 171t
    in chronic meningitis, 186t
    in congenital infection
        clinical features of, 510
        diagnosis of, 512, 512t
        management of, 513
        pathogenesis and pathology of, 506–507
        screening for, during pregnancy, 508t
    diagnosis of, 563–564
    encephalitis/myelitis caused by, 193t–194t
    etiology of, 1138t
    jaundice, 1135t
    in liver transplant patients, 751
    macrolides, 1221
    pathogenesis and pathology of, 559–560
    uveitis and, 168–169
Treponemal antibody tests, 564, 564t
Treponemal infections, 962t
Treponematoses, endemic, 961–965
    attenuated, 964
    clinical features of, 963–964
    diagnosis of, 964–965
    differential diagnosis of, 964
    epidemiology of, 961
    geographic distribution of, 961, 962f
    historic perspective of, 961
    HIV infection and, 964
    incidence and prevalence of, 961–963
    management of, 965
        contacts of, 965
        prognosis and follow-up of, 965

Treponematoses, endemic (Continued)
  pathology of, 963
  prevention of, 963
  transmission of, 963
Triatoma brasiliensis, 1066
Triatoma dimidiata, 1066
Triatoma infestans, 110f, 1066, 1068f
Triatoma rubrofasciata, 109
Triatominae, 106t, 109
Triazoles
  antifungal, 1336
    second-generation, 1339
  for aspergillosis, 1691
Trichiasis, 980–981, 980f
Trichinella, 1764
Trichinella spiralis
  chronic diarrhea, 349
  epidemiology of, 1764
  in myocarditis, 447
  pathogenicity of, 1768
  transmission of, 666
  treatment of, 1345t–1351t
Trichinellosis
  from bears, 669
  from marine mammals, 668
  from rodents, 667
Trichinosis, 1777
  chronic diarrhea and, 349
  and fever of unknown origin, 613
  treatment of, 1345t–1351t
Trichodysplasia spinulosa, 1447
Trichomonas tenax, 1725t
Trichomonas vaginalis, 1725t
  in cervicitis, 490
  epidemiology of, 1727
  etiology of, 1138t
  identification in urogenital specimens, 1732, 1732f
  parasite infections and, 73
  pathogenesis and pathology of, 485
  pathogenicity of, 1728
  in pregnancy, 500t
  prevention of, 1727
  in prostatitis, 533t
  treatment of, 1345t–1351t
Trichomoniasis, 485–486
  clinical features of, 485
  diagnosis of, 484t, 485–486
  epidemiology of, 485
  management of, 486
  pathogenesis and pathology of, 485
  prevention of, 485
  treatment of, 1345t–1351t
Trichophyton
  in cats, 660
  diagnostic microbiology of, 1711
Trichophyton concentricum, 124
Trichophyton mentagrophytes, 667
  clinical features of, 123t, 124f
  pathogenicity of, 1711
Trichophyton rubrum
  clinical features of, 124
  epidemiology of, 122–123
  pathogenicity of, 1711
Trichophyton schoenleinii, clinical features of, 124
Trichophyton soudanense
  clinical features of, 123t
  epidemiology of, 122
Trichophyton tonsurans
  clinical features of, 123t, 124
  epidemiology of, 122
  prevention of, 123
Trichophyton verrucosum
  clinical features of, 123t
  epidemiology of, 122
  prevention of, 123
Trichophyton violaceum, 123t
Trichosporon
  epidemiology of, 122
  nature of, 1710
Trichostrongyliasis, treatment of, 1345t–1351t
Trichuriasis, 1777
  chronic diarrhea and, 349
  clinical features of, 996

Trichuriasis (Continued)
  pathogenesis and pathology of, 991
  treatment of, 1345t–1351t
Trichuris muris, parasite infections and, 74
Trichuris trichiura
  of chronic diarrhea, 347t, 349
  clinical features of, 996
  clinical manifestations of, 1777
  diagnosis of, 998t–999t
  from dogs, 658
  epidemiology of, 1763
  life cycle of, 1767f
  pathogenesis and pathology of, 991
  pathogenicity of, 1766
  in population density and urbanization, 990
  prevention of, 994
  treatment of, 1000, 1001t, 1345t–1351t
Trichuris vulpis, from dogs, 658
Triclabendazole, for parasitic infections treatment, 1345t–1362t, 1372
Trifluridine, 1313
Trimethoprim, 1280
  chemical structure of, 1178, 1178f
  for complicated urinary tract infection, 544t
  for cystitis, 528t, 529
  distribution of, 1280
  elimination of, 1280
  for hydrocephalus shunts, 223
  in pregnancy, 503
  for prostatitis, 535
  for protozoal infections, 1352t–1362t, 1364
  for renal impairment, 1282t
  resistance to, 1192–1193
  use of, 1282
Trimethoprim-sulfamethoxazole (TMP-SMX)
  for Acinetobacter baumannii, 1591t
  for Alcaligenes spp., 1597
  for basidiobolomycosis, 1723
  for brucellosis, 1100
  in cancer patients, 732
  for complicated urinary tract infection, 544t–545t
  for conidiobolomycosis, 1723
  for cyclosporiasis, 1742
  for cystic fibrosis, 301
  for cystitis, 525–526, 528t
  for cystoisosporiasis, 1742
  for dog bites, 657t
  for food-borne diarrheal illness, 334
  for foot ulcers, 131t
  for gastrointestinal protozoa, 999, 1000t
  for granuloma inguinale, 591
  in hematopoietic stem cell transplantation, 745
  in HIV-infected children, 903–904
  for human bites, 683
  in immunologically mediated diseases, 771
  for Listeria monocytogenes, 1540
  for lung abscess, 269f
  for melioidosis, 1077t
  for mycetoma, 1723
  nitrofurantoin and, 1278
  for nocardiosis, 1551
  and opportunistic infections in HIV, in low- and middle-income countries, 894–895
  for paracoccidioidomycosis, 1709
  for parasitic infections, 1345t–1351t
  for plague, 1084
  for Pneumocystis jirovecii, in opportunistic infection in HIV, 851–852
  in pregnancy, 503, 910
  prophylaxis with
    for chronic granulomatous disease, 709
    and HIV-associated TB, 865, 870
    in liver transplant patients, 754t
  for protozoal infections, 1364
  for Pseudomonas aeruginosa, 1591t
  for pyelonephritis, 552
  for Q fever, 1673
  for renal impairment, 1282t
  resistance to, 1592t
    enteric fevers, 1005
    Erysipelothrix rhusiopathiae, 1542
  for Staphylococcus aureus, 1520
  for Stenotrophomonas maltophilia, 1597

Trimethoprim-sulfamethoxazole (TMP-SMX) (Continued)
  for thoracic transplantation patients, 749
  use of, 1281–1282, 1281t
  uveitis, 171–172
  for Whipple's disease, 345
Trimethoprim-sulfamethoxazole plus gentamicin, indication, meningitis, 187t
Trimethylamine, 483–484
Trimetrexate, 1352t–1362t, 1365
Trismus, lateral pharyngeal space infection, 314
Trombiculid mites, 105, 1670
  scrub typhus and, 1091
Tropheryma whipplei
  in bacterial arthritis, 383t
  bacterial enteritis and, 337
  causing endocarditis, 461t
  in chronic diarrhea, 344–345
  in chronic meningitis, 186t, 187
  encephalitis/myelitis caused by, 193t–194t
  lower respiratory tract infections, 1221
  uveitis and, 169
Trophocytes, 1718
Tropical pulmonary eosinophilia, 1049
  treatment of, 1345t–1351t
Tropical rickettsioses, 1091–1097, 1092t–1093t
Tropical spastic paresis, 1491
Tropical sprue, chronic diarrhea, 349
'Tropism', 15
Troponin T, 448
Trueperella, 1548t
Trypanosoma brucei
  antigenic variations in, 25
  epidemiology of, 1761
  lymphadenopathy, 142
  nature of, 1761
  pathogenicity of, 1761f
Trypanosoma brucei gambiense, 1761
  African trypanosomiasis, 966, 967f
  clinical features of, 968, 968f
  epidemiology of, 967t
  management of, 969t, 1345t–1351t
  prevention of, 967
Trypanosoma brucei rhodesiense, 1761
  African trypanosomiasis, 966
  clinical features of, 968
  epidemiology of, 967t
  management of, 969t, 1345t–1351t
  pathogenesis of, 966
Trypanosoma cruzi, 109, 1065, 1758
  in HIV in low- and middle-income countries, 892
  life cycle of, 1065–1066, 1067f
  in liver transplant patients, 751
  in myocarditis, 447
  transmission of, 807, 1065–1066, 1068f
  treatment of, 1345t–1351t
Trypanosoma rangeli, 1762
Trypanosomiasis, 119, 1758, 1758t
  African. see African trypanosomiasis
  American. see Chagas disease
  dermatologic manifestations of, 114t–115t
  in HIV in low- and middle-income countries, 892
  treatment of, 1345t–1351t
Tsetse flies, 106t, 111–112, 112f
  infections from, 191t
Tsukamurella, 1550t, 1552
Tsutsugamushi triangle, 1670, 1670f
Tuberculids, 118
Tuberculin skin test (TST), 274–275, 802, 1657, 1658t
  in HIV infection, 913
Tuberculoid leprosy, 955, 1648
  borderline, 955–956, 956f
  clinical features of, 956, 956f
Tuberculosis, 271–284, 1645
  adjunctive corticosteroids for, 306, 307t
  burden of disease, 940, 941f, 941t
  childhood infection, 275–276
  clinical features of, 275–279
    extrapulmonary tuberculosis, 278–279
    HIV-positive patients, 279
    noninfectious complications, 279
    pleural tuberculosis, 277

Tuberculosis *(Continued)*
    primary and childhood infection, 275–276
    pulmonary infection, 276–277
  clinical presentation of, 276–277, 276f–277f
  complications of, 277
  dermatologic manifestations, 114t–115t, 116–118
  diagnosis of, 279–280
  drug-resistant, 283–284, 872, 1273–1274
    endobronchial, 276
    in low- and middle-income countries, 891
  due to *Mycobacterium bovis*, 664
  epidemiology of, 271–272, 272f, 1647–1648
  extrapulmonary, 773, 869
    abdominal infection, 279
    central nervous system, 279
    dermatologic disease, 279
    eye disease, 279
    lymph node disease, 278
    musculoskeletal, 278–279
    pericardial infection, 279
  extremely drug-resistant, 1273
  eye involvement in, 982
  and fever of unknown origin, 611–613
  gastrointestinal, 341–343
  of the head and neck, 279
  in HIV, 865–873, 936
    clinical features of, 867f, 869–870
    diagnosis of, 870
    epidemiology of, 865–866, 866f
    global burden of, 865, 867f
    impact of, 271, 273f
    infection control, 868–869
    in low- and middle-income countries, 890–891,
      894–895
    management of, 870–872, 871t
    mortality of, and transmission risk, 865–866
    multidrug-resistant TB, 866
    pathogenesis of, 866–868
    prevention of, 868–869
    risk of, 865
  and HIV-1, 843
  HIV-positive patients with, 1274
  host response to, 272–273, 274f
  immunodiagnostic tests for, 1657–1658, 1658t
  immunotherapy and future, 284
  impact of HIV on, 271, 273f
  lymphadenopathy and, 137t–138t
  management of, 280–284
    first-line antimycobacterial drugs, 280–281
    in HIV, 870–872
    second-line drugs and, 281–282, 282t
    steroids, 284
    treatment regimens, 282–284, 283t
  from marine mammals, 668
  miliary, 277–278, 278f, 611–613
  multidrug-resistant
    prevalence of, 1264, 1273
    spread of, 943
    therapy for, 1273–1274, 1273b–1274b
  and occupational infections, 648t–649t,
    651t–654t
    immunization for, 650t
  in pancreas transplant patients, 765, 765f
  pathogen and, 272
  pathogenesis and pathology of, 272–273
  pleural, 277
  in pregnancy, 284
  prevention of, 273–275
  primary, 275
  prophylaxis, in HIV-infected pregnant women,
    910
  pulmonary, 276–277
    in breast-feeding, 516
    corticosteroids for, 306
  screening for, before biologic therapy, 802
  second stage-adaptive immunity to, 273
  spread of infection of, 271–272
  surgery for, 284
  in thoracic transplantation patients, 749
  transmission, in closed institutions, 271–272
  and tumor necrosis factor inhibitor, 799
  of urogenital tract. *see* Urogenital tract tuberculosis
  vaccination, for travelers, 950
  vaccines, 275
  worldwide incidence and prevalence, 271, 272f

Tuberculosis-associated immune reconstitution
    inflammatory syndrome (TB-IRIS), 859–860,
    861f–862f, 862
  common and important manifestations of, 861b
  corticosteroid therapy for, 864
Tuberculosis cutis orificialis, 117
Tuberculosis verrucosa cutis, 117
Tuberculous lymphadenitis, of axilla, 140f
Tuberculous meningitis, 186–187
Tuberculous pericarditis, 450, 454
  corticosteroids for, 480
Tuberculous peritonitis, 359–360
Tubo-ovarian abscesses, 493–494
Tubulinosema acridophagus, 1741
Tula (TUL) virus, 1502t
Tularemia, 1085–1090
  agent of, 1085
  and bioterrorism, 671t–673t, 678
  from birds, 668
  from cat bites, 659
  clinical features of, 1088–1089
  cutaneous, 92
  diagnosis of, 1089
  differential diagnostic possibilities of, 1089
  epidemiology of, 1085–1086
  geographic distribution of, 1085–1086, 1086f
  glandular, 1088
  incidence of, 1086, 1087f
  life cycle of, 1085, 1085f
  lymphadenopathy and, 137t–138t, 140
  management of, 1089
  and occupational infections, 648t–649t
  oculoglandular, 1088
  oropharyngeal, 1088–1089
  pathogenesis and pathology of, 1086–1088
  pneumonic, 1089
  populations affected, 1088
  prevention of, 1087–1088
  from rabbits, 667
  seasonality of, 1086
  in sheep, 664
  sources of human infection in, 1086
  typhoidal, 1089
  ulceroglandular, 1088, 1088f
Tumor necrosis factor (TNF), 797
  interferon γ/IL-12 pathway defects, 710
  in malaria, 1017
  mycobacteria and, 1649–1650
  in pneumonia, 253
  in sepsis, 420
Tumor necrosis factor (TNF) inhibitors, infectious risk
    associated with, 797–800
  bacterial infections, 797–799
  fungal infections, 799–800
  mycobacterial infections, 799
  protozoa, 800
  viral infections, 800
Tumors
  solid, 723
  see also Cancer; Neoplasia; specific tumors
Tunga penetrans, 108
Two-stage exchange, in surgery, for prosthetic joint
    infection (PJI), 402
Tympanostomy tubes, otitis media, 237
Typhlitis, in cancer patients, 727–728
Typhoid diseases, vaccination for travelers, 949
Typhoid fever, 1002–1007, 1574
  acute shedding and chronic carriage and, 1004–1005
  antimicrobial drug resistance for, 1005
  burden of disease, 941–942
  carriers, 1007
  case fatality of, 1005
  clinical features of, 1003–1005
  complications of, 1004, 1004b
  diagnosis of, 1005
  differential diagnosis of, 1005
  epidemiology of, 1002–1003, 1002f–1003f
  eye involvement in, 982
  and fever of unknown origin, 613
  lymphadenopathy and, 137t–138t
  management of, 1005–1007, 1006t
  and occupational infections, 648t–649t
    immunization for, 651t
  pathogenesis and pathology of, 1003
  prevention of, 1003

Typhoid fever *(Continued)*
  quinolones for, 1245
  severe, 1004, 1006–1007
Typhoid rose spots, 1004f
Typhoidal tularemia, 1089
Typhus
  epidemic. *see* Epidemic typhus
  eye involvement in, 982
  jaundice and, 1136
  murine. *see* Murine typhus
  and occupational infections, 648t–649t
  scrub. *see* Scrub typhus
Typhus group (TG), 1091
Typhus group rickettsiae, 1669–1670
  clinical manifestations of, 1670
  diagnostic microbiology of, 1669–1670
  epidemiology of, 1669, 1669f
  management of, 1670
  nature of, 1669
  pathogenicity of, 1669
  prevention of, 1669

U
Ubiquitous receptors, 13
Ulceration, 92
  bacillary angiomatosis, 93
  Buruli ulcer, 92
  cutaneous anthrax, 92, 92f
  cutaneous diphtheria, 92
  cutaneous manifestations of infections of deep soft
    tissues, 93, 93f–94f
  cutaneous tularemia, 92
  differential diagnosis of, 91t
  leishmaniasis, 92, 93f
  ulceroglandular tularemia, 92
Ulceroglandular tularemia, 1088, 1088f
Ultrasonography
  biliary sepsis, 360
  for echinococcosis, 1043–1044
  fetal, 508
  of intestinal/hepatic schistosomiasis, 1030, 1030f
  intra-abdominal sepsis, peritonitis and, 356–357
  of melioidosis, 1077
  in osteomyelitis, 393–394
  for pleural effusion, 303, 304f
  in pyelonephritis, 550
  for schistosomiasis diagnosis, 1031
  of urinary schistosomiasis, 1029, 1029f
  of urogenital tract tuberculosis, 556
Uncomplicated malaria, clinical cases, 1142
Uncontaminated specimens, of mycobacteria, 1652
Undercooked freshwater fish, infections from, 191t
Unilateral laterothoracic exanthem of childhood,
  82
  clinical features of, 82
  management of, 82
Unpasteurized milk, infections from, 191t
Upper respiratory tract, normal flora of, 1632t
Upper respiratory tract infection (URTI)
  anaerobic bacteria in, 1636–1638, 1636t
  antimicrobial therapy for, 1641t
  Mycoplasma pneumoniae in, 1660
  in pregnancy, 500
  sinusitis and, 240
  see also specific infections
Urea breath test, 1603
  for *Helicobacter pylori*, 325
Urea paste, onychomycosis management, 129
Urease test, 1603
  for *Cryptococcus neoformans*, 1692–1693
Ureaplasma, 1660–1665, 1661t
Ureaplasma parvum, 1663
Ureaplasma urealyticum, 1663
  in complicated urinary tract infection, 540
  macrolides and ketolides, 1221
  in postpartum endometritis, 494–495
  in prostatitis, 533
Ureidopenicillins
  for *Alcaligenes* spp., 1597
  antimicrobial spectrum, generic names, routes of
    administration and dosages, 1206t–1207t
  for biliary system infections, 1211
  pharmacokinetics of, 1204
Uremic pericarditis, 450

Urethra, cancer in, human papillomavirus and, 579
Urethral infection, in gonorrhea, 594
Urethral syndromes, 530
Urethritis, 526
　antibiotics for, 1152t
　gonorrhea and, 594
　male, 1138, 1138t
　from *Neisseria gonorrhoeae*, 1562–1563
　nongonococcal
　　Mycoplasma genitalium in, 1662
　　Mycoplasma hominis in, 1663
　　quinolones for, 1243
Urethrocystoscopy, for prostatitis, 534
Urinalysis, in pyelonephritis, 549–550
Urinary calculi, *Mycoplasma hominis* in, 1664
Urinary catheter, in complicated urinary tract infection, 539, 541, 541t
Urinary catheterization, prolonged, risk of infection from, 689
Urinary schistosomiasis, 1029, 1029f
Urinary tract
　abnormal, 526
　brain abscess and, 200t
　imaging of, 527
　specimen collection in, 1634t
Urinary tract infections (UTIs)
　Acinetobacter baumannii in, 1587t
　Acinetobacter in, 1595
　Alcaligenes xylosoxidans in, 1597
　aminoglycosides for, 1237
　antibiotics for, 1152t
　ascending, complicated, quinolones for, 1243
　in cancer patients, 728
　Candida, 443t, 1684, 1687
　clinical presentation of, 557
　complicated, 539–546
　　clinical features of, 541–542
　　diagnosis of, 542–543, 543t
　　epidemiology of, 539, 539t
　　indications for investigation, 546
　　management of, 543–546, 544t–545t, 546f
　　microbiology of, 540, 540t
　　pathogenesis of, 539–540, 540t
　　prevention of, 540–541, 541t
　Enterobacteriaceae in, 1575
　epidemiology of, 557
　health-care-associated infections, 60
　in kidney transplant patients, 762–763
　in kidney transplant recipients, 557–558
　lower, uncomplicated, quinolones for, 1243
　microbiology of, 557
　morbidity, 557
　Mycoplasma hominis in, 1664
　nitrofurantoin for, 1278
　polymyxins for, 1287
　in pregnancy, 500–501, 503, 528, 528t, 530f
　prevention of, 558
　in prostatitis, 533
　Pseudomonas aeruginosa in, 1587t, 1589
　in pyelonephritis, 548
　Stenotrophomonas maltophilia in, 1597
　symptomatic, 557
　　diagnosis and treatment of, 557–558
　systemic microsporidiosis in, 1741
　see also specific infections
Urine
　of infant, microbiologic investigation of, in congenital infection, 512t
　for laboratory diagnosis, of mycobacteria, 1651, 1651t
　schistosomiasis and, 1031
　uropathogens in, 525
Urine after prostatic massage (VB3), in prostatitis, 532–534, 534f
Urine cultures
　in pyelonephritis, 550
　in sepsis, 420
Urine specimens
　in complicated urinary tract infection, 542–543
　in cystitis, 527
　for helminths diagnosis, 1776
　for *Legionella* spp., 1623–1624
　microsporidia in, 1739, 1739f
Urodynamics, in cystitis, 525

Urogenital gonococcal infection, 1562–1563
Urogenital infections, trimethoprim-sulfamethoxazole for, 1281
Urogenital specimens, identification of flagellates in, 1732, 1732f
Urogenital tract infections, probiotics for, 1375
Urogenital tract tuberculosis, 555–556
　clinical features of, 555–556, 555t
　definition of, 555
　diagnosis of, 556
　pathogenesis of, 555
Urologic surgery, antibiotic prophylaxis and, 1157t–1158t, 1159
Uropathogenic *Escherichia coli* (UPEC), 524, 547, 548f, 1575
US Food and Drug Administration (FDA), evolution of, 1383, 1383t
US National Institute of Mental Health's Multisite HIV Prevention Trial, 827
Ustekinumab, 798t–799t, 801–802
Uta, 1757
Uveitis, 165f
　acute retinal necrosis syndrome, 172, 172f
　anterior. *see* Anterior uveitis
　bacterial causes of, 168–169, 169t
　classification of, 165f
　clinical features of, 166, 166f
　in community-based and tertiary ophthalmologists centers, 167t
　definition of, 165
　epidemiology of, 165–166
　fungal causes of, 169–170, 170f
　immune recovery, 862
　in immunocompetent adults and children, 167–172
　in immunosuppressed patients, 172–173
　infectious, 165–174
　intermediate of, 165, 166t
　laboratory diagnostics of, 167
　management of, 167–173
　in neonates, 166
　parasitic causes of, 170–172, 171f, 171t
　pathogenesis and pathology of, 166–167
　posterior, 166t
　　definition of, 165, 166t
　viral causes of, 167–168

V

Vaccination
　adenovirus, 1472
　in cancer patients, 732–733
　of children with inherited or congenital immune deficit, 791–795, 794t
　croup and, 232
　for diphtheria, 1546
　for Enterobacteriaceae, 1577–1578
　for group B streptococcus, 520
　for hepatitis A virus, 364
　for hepatitis B virus, 366
　for hepatitis E virus, 373–374
　in HIV infection, 913–914
　against human papillomavirus, 579–580
　and immunobiologics, 803, 803t
　in the immunocompromised patient, 780–795
　　characteristics common in, 780–781
　　clinical conditions with specific additional vaccine indications, 783t
　　correlates of protection in, 781t
　　delay in cessation of therapy and administration of vaccines in, 788t
　　dissimilarities in, 781–791
　　impact of vaccinations on timing of planned therapy in, 783, 784t
　　list of vaccines and formulations of, 785t
　immunological response to, 1462
　for influenza viruses, 1468–1469
　for inherited hemoglobin disorders, 1055–1056
　in kidney transplant patients, 769, 769t
　for leptospirosis, 1103
　in liver transplant patients, 754
　for measles, 1399
　meningitis and, 177

Vaccination *(Continued)*
　for mumps, 1405
　for otitis media, 237
　for papillomaviruses
　　prophylactic, 1441–1442
　　therapeutic, 1442
　for Q fever, 1672
　for rotaviruses, 1397, 1397t
　for sepsis, 424
Vaccine-induced immunity
　accelerated decay of, in immunocompromised patient, 780
　need to assess, 780
Vaccines
　associated with erythema multiforme, 120t
　for *Brucella* spp., 1615
　for *Campylobacter* spp. infections, 1601
　for *Chlamydia*, 1678
　in cystitis, 526
　design, 66
　for diarrhea, 339
　for enteric fevers, 1003
　for *Francisella tularensis*, 1617
　for gastrointestinal parasites, 995
　for genital herpes, 570
　for *Haemophilus influenzae*, 1618–1619, 1619t
　for hepatitis B virus, 515
　HIV. *see* HIV vaccines
　influenza, 749
　for *Leptospira* spp., 1609
　live attenuated, 829–830, 830t
　for malaria, 1018
　mucosal, 832
　outer membrane vesicle, 1560
　for pertussis, 1611
　polysaccharide, 1560
　for prevention, of food-borne diarrheal illness, 334
　rabies, 1462
　recombinant proteins, 829–830, 830t
　for rheumatic fever, 475
　streptococcal, 1536
　T-cell, 831
　in tuberculosis, 275
　for tularemia, 1087–1088
　for *Vibrio cholerae*, 1606
　whole inactivated, 829–830, 830t
Vaccinia virus, 75t, 1456
　encephalitis/myelitis caused by, 193t–194t
Vacuolating cytotoxin (VacA), 323–324
Vagina, rhinosporidiosis in, 1721
Vaginal cancer, human papillomavirus and, 579
Vaginal cuff, in postoperative gynecologic infection, 497
Vaginal discharge, sexually transmitted infection, 1138
Vaginal flora, 483, 548
Vaginitis, 483, 526
　atrophic, 489
　causes of, 483t
　diagnosis of, 484t
　Mycoplasma genitalium in, 1662
　noninfectious, 489, 489f
Vaginosis, bacterial. *see* Bacterial vaginosis.
Valaciclovir, 1146t–1147t, 1309–1312
　adverse reactions of, 1311
　in cancer patients, 732
　dosage of, 1309–1310
　　special circumstances, 1311
　for genital herpes, 569, 573, 573t
　indications of, 1310–1311
　　cercopithecine herpesvirus-1 (B virus), 1311
　　cytomegalovirus, 1311
　　Epstein-Barr virus (EBV), 1311
　　genital herpes, 1310t
　　HSV infections, 1310, 1310t
　　other viral infections, 1311
　　varicella zoster virus, 1310–1311
　mechanism of action, 1309
　pharmacokinetics and distribution of, 1309
　resistance to, 1311–1312
　route of administration, 1309–1310
　in vitro activity, 1309
Valganciclovir, 1146t–1147t, 1313–1315
　adverse reactions of, 1314–1315
　for cytomegalovirus, 748

Valganciclovir *(Continued)*
  congenital, 513
  in HIV prophylaxis, 853
  dosage of, 1313–1314
    in special circumstances, 1314, 1314t
  indications of, 1314
    cytomegalovirus, 1314
    cytomegalovirus retinitis, 1314t
  in intestinal transplant patients, 758–759
  for kidney transplant patients, 766
  mechanism of action, 1313
  pharmacokinetics and distribution of, 1313
  prophylaxis with
    in cytomegalovirus, 1314
    in liver transplant patients, 754t, 755
  resistance to, 1315
  route of administration, 1313–1314
  in vitro activity, 1313
'Vallecula sign,' in epiglottitis, 232–233
Valproate, 476
Valve culture, in endocarditis, 461
Valve lesions, degenerative, 457–458
Valve surgery, 476
van genes, 1191
VanA-type resistance, to glycopeptides, 1191, 1192f
Vancomycin, 1191, 1249–1252
  adverse reactions and interactions of, 1252
  for anaerobic bacteria, 1643
  for *Bacillus cereus*, 1542
  for cancer patients, 735
  for catheter-related bloodstream infection (CRBSI), 436t
  cellulitis and, 92
  for coagulase-negative staphylococcal infections, 1521–1522
  discovery of, 1217
  distributions of, 1249–1250, 1250t
  dosage of, 1250
    in special circumstances, 1251–1252, 1254t
  for foot ulcers, 131t
  indications, 1251
    bacteremia, 1251
    brain abscess, 206–207
    for CAPD peritonitis, 380, 380t
    endocarditis, 1251
    endophthalmitis, 162, 163t
    hospital-acquired pneumonia, 260t
    hydrocephalus shunts, 224
    lung abscess, 269f
    meningitis, 180
    osteomyelitis, 1251
    pneumonia, 1251
    pseudomembranous colitis, 1251
    skin and soft tissue, 1251
  for infective arthritis, 386t
  for intra-abdominal sepsis, 357–358
  β-lactam resistance, 1292
  mode of action of, 1164
  monitoring of, 1251
  in outpatient parenteral antimicrobial therapy, 1201
  pharmacodynamics of, 1167, 1250, 1251t
  pharmacokinetics of, 1249–1250, 1251t
  for pneumococcal infections, 1209
  prophylaxis with, 159, 1158t
    and surgical site infections, 687
  resistance to, *Erysipelothrix rhusiopathiae*, 1542
  route of administration of, 1250
  for *Staphylococcus aureus*, 1520
Vancomycin-intermediate *Staphylococcus aureus* (VISA), 468, 1192, 1249, 1249t
Vancomycin-resistant enterococci (VRE), 1249, 1249t
  epidemiology of, 1526–1527, 1528f
  resistance, 1191
Vancomycin-resistant staphylococci, 467–468
Vancomycin-resistant *Staphylococcus aureus* (VRSA), 1249, 1249t, 1519
VanX protein, 1191
VanY protein, 1191
Variant Creutzfeldt-Jakob disease (vCJD), 215t
  clinical features of, 217
  epidemiology of, 216
  iatrogenic, 216–217
  molecular strain typing of, 217–218
  pathology of, 218f, 219
  prevention of, 220
  transmission of, 665

Varicella, 1436
  in liver transplant patients, 751t
  and occupational infections, 648t–649t, 651t–654t
    immunization for, 651t
  vaccination against, 782t–783t
    in children with congenital HIV infection, 795
    in children with inherited immune deficiency syndrome, 795
Varicella syndrome, 510
Varicella-zoster virus, 75–76, 75t, 76f
  acute retinal necrosis syndrome, 173
  in cancer patients, 724
  causing meningitis, 225
  causing retinitis and uveitis, 168t
  clinical features of, 75
  clinical manifestations of, 1436–1437
  complications of, 75–76
  in congenital infection
    clinical features of, 510
    diagnosis of, 512t
    pathogenesis and pathology of, 506
    in perinatal infections, 514t, 515
    screening for, during pregnancy, 508t
  encephalitis/myelitis caused by, 192t
  epithelial keratitis, 154
  in hematopoietic stem cell transplantation, 741–742
  in HIV/AIDS, 881–882, 883f
  hyperimmune globulin, 1433
  in immunosuppressed patients, 1432
  in kidney transplant patients, 766
  management of, 76
  and natalizumab, 802
  opportunistic infection in HIV of, 853
  pathogenicity of, molecular and cellular basis of, 1431
  in pregnancy, 499t
  reactivation of, in liver transplant patients, 753
  in thoracic transplantation patients, 748
  vaccine, Oka-derived strain of, 1432
Variola virus, 75t
  and bioterrorism, 671t
Vascular access, outpatient parenteral antimicrobial therapy, 1201
Vascular cell adhesion molecule 1 (VCAM-1), 1017
Vascular surgery, antibiotic prophylaxis and, 1157t–1158t, 1159
Vasculitis, 770–774
  cerebral, 772–773
  clinical features and management of, 771–774
    abscesses, 772, 772f
    acute neurologic problems in, 771–773
    encephalitis, 772–773
    fever and pulmonary infiltrates in, 771, 771t, 772f
    gastrointestinal problems in, 773, 773f
    meningitis, 772
    skin, soft tissue and joints, 773–774, 774f
  epidemiology, 770
  pathogenesis, 770
  prevention, 770–771
  retinal, 166
Vasogenic cerebral edema, 179
Vasopressors, 426
VDRL slide test, 564, 564t
Vector-borne transmission, 693
Vector-borne zoonotic bacterial infection, 13
Vectors
  control of, 967
  geographic distribution of, 939–940, 940b
  movement of, 945
Vecuronium, 1216
Vedolizumab, 798t–799t
Veillonella, 1631
  brain abscess and, 199
  hospital-acquired pneumonia and, 259t
  in human bites, 682, 683t
  microflora, 355
Velocardiofacial syndrome, 721
Venezuelan equine encephalitis, 1495t
Venezuelan equine encephalitis virus, 193t–194t
Venous stasis, chronic, 90, 91f
Ventilator-associated pneumonia (VAP), 60, 258–262, 259t, 1375
  and burn infections, 698
  community-acquired pneumonia and, 254
  incidence of, 690–691, 690t
  Pseudomonas aeruginosa in, 1587

Ventriculoatrial shunts, 221f
Ventriculoencephalitis, cytomegalovirus, 853
Ventriculoperitoneal shunts, 221f
Vernal catarrh, 981t
Vero/SLAM cell line, 1399
Verruga peruana, 113
VersaTrek®, for mycobacteria, 1653
Vertebral osteomyelitis, 391–392, 392f, 1589
Vesicoureteral reflux, in pyelonephritis, 548
Vesiculobullous exanthems, 75t
Vesivirus
  nature of, 1393
  taxonomy of, 1394t
Vestibular abscess, 313, 313f
Vestibular toxicity, of aminoglycosides, 1235t, 1236
Veterinarians, and occupational infections, 648t–649t
Vibrio
  bacterial enteritis and, 337
  diagnosis of, 339
  from sharks, 663, 668–669
Vibrio alginolyticus, 337, 1607
Vibrio cholerae, 1604–1607
  and bioterrorism, 671t
  characteristics of, in food-borne diarrheal illness, 330t
  clinical features of, 1606–1607
  diagnostic microbiology of, 1606
  diarrhea and, 337, 339
  doses of, in diarrheal illness, 329t
  El Tor, 337
  epidemiology of, 1604–1605
  management of, 1607
  microbiology of, 1604
  pathogenesis of, 1605
  prevention of, 1605–1606
  spread of, 944
  variant O139, 1604–1605
Vibrio cholerae non-O1, 337
Vibrio cholerae O1, 337
Vibrio cholerae O139, 337
Vibrio cholerae O139 (Bengal), 337
Vibrio damselae, 1607
Vibrio fluvialis, 337, 1607
Vibrio furnisii, 337
Vibrio hollisae, 1607
Vibrio mimicus, 337, 1607
Vibrio parahaemolyticus, 1607
  characteristics of, in food-borne diarrheal illness, 330t
  diarrhea, 337
Vibrio PI (VPI), 1605
Vibrio vulnificus, 337, 662, 1607
  cellulitis and, 91
  and occupational infections, 648t–649t
Video-assisted thoracic surgery (VATS), for pleural effusion, 304, 305f
Vincent's angina, 316
  anaerobic bacteria in, 1636
Vincent's disease, 316, 316f
Vincent's infection, 316
Vincristine, immunosuppression and, 1380t
Viomycin, as antituberculosis agent, 1270
Viral arthritis, 385–386, 387t
Viral budding, 1486
Viral culture, in genital herpes, 572
Viral encephalitides, and bioterrorism, 672t
Viral enteritis, 338
Viral exanthems, 75–83, 75t
  classic, 75–79
  nonclassic, 79–83
  see also specific viral exanthems
Viral hemorrhagic fevers (VHF), 75t, 80, 1110–1118
  and bioterrorism, 671t–673t, 678
  diagnosis and clinical features of, 1113–1117, 1114t–1116t, 1116f
  epidemiology of, 1112t
  with hepatic involvement, 378–379
  management of, 1117, 1117t
  pathogenesis of, 1113
  prevention of, 1117–1118
  in travelers, 952
  virology of, 1110, 1111f
Viral hepatitis
  dosage regimens in, 1328t
  drugs to treat, 1327–1332

Viral infections, 73
  associated with erythema multiforme, 120t
  associated with erythema nodosum, 121t
  in cancer patients, 723b
  causing jaundice, 1135t
  dermatologic manifestations, 114t–115t
  from dogs, 657t
  from domesticated herbivores, 665
  eye involvement in tropical, 982–983
  follicular conjunctivitis, 981t
  in hematopoietic stem cell transplantation, 741t
  in intestinal transplant patients, 758, 758t
  lymphadenopathy and, 137t–138t
  opportunistic, in HIV/AIDS, 852–854
  as skin manifestations of HIV, 881–882
  in thoracic transplantation patients, 748–749
  and tumor necrosis factor inhibitor, 800
Viral 'lifestyles', 9f
Viral meningitis, 185–186
  antiviral treatment of, 185–186
  clinical features of, 185
  epidemiology of, 185
  laboratory findings of, 185
  pathophysiology and pathology of, 185
  supportive therapy of, 186
Viral pathogens
  in infectious diseases, transmitted by grafts, 805–806
  in transfusion-related infections, 701–702, 703t
Virginiamycin, 1227
Viridans group, 1523
  clinical manifestations of, 1534
  epidemiology of, 1527
  management of, 1535
  pathogenesis of, 1532
Virions, 5, 7f
Virulence factors identification, genome sequencing, 66
'Virulence' genes, 12
Virulent mycobacteria, 273
Viruria, BK polyomavirus, 1447
Virus-induced cytopathic effect, 19–21, 21f
Virus isolation, influenza viruses, 1469–1470
Virus-like particles, 832
Viruses
  adhesion, 14–15
  causing encephalitis/myelitis, 192t
  causing meningitis, 225
  causing retinitis and uveitis, 168t
  of chronic diarrhea, 345t, 349
  in chronic meningitis, 186t
  classification of, 6t
  in congenital infection, 505b
  definition of, 4
  in diarrhea, 331
  general properties and classification of, 5–8
  hospital-acquired pneumonia and, 259t
  lower respiratory tract infections, 264f
  in lymph node enlargement, 147t–148t
  in myocarditis, 447, 447t
  in pericarditis, 450, 451t–452t
  provoking immune reconstitution disorder, 860t
  replication, common steps in, 5
  respiratory, in chronic obstructive pulmonary disease, 310
  structure of, 5–8
    capsid, 5–8
    envelope, 8
    viral genome, 6
  taxonomy of, 5
  travelers' diarrhea and, 950
  viral gene expression strategies, 8
Visceral larva migrans, treatment of, 1345t–1351t
Visceral leishmaniasis, 1757, 1757f
  amphotericin B for, 1364
  clinical features of, 1060–1062, 1061f, 1061t
  dermatologic manifestations of, 119
  epidemiology of, 1059
  and fever of unknown origin, 613
  in HIV in low- and middle-income countries, 892
  lymphadenopathy and, 137t–138t
  monitoring response to treatment for, 1064
  post-kala-azar dermal, 1062
  spread of, 945
Visual inspection with acetic acid (VIA), 582, 582f

Vitamin A, deficiency, keratitis, 152
Vitamin D, for bone health, 929
Vitiligo, 586t–587t
Vitrectomy, endophthalmitis, 162
Vitreous specimens, endophthalmitis, 161–162
Vittaforma corneae, 1741
Volatile fatty acids, of anaerobic bacteria, 1633
Vomiting
  bacteria in, 330t
  early onset diarrhea with, 331
Voriconazole, 1339–1340
  adverse effects of, 1339–1340
  for aspergillosis, 1691
  for blastomycosis, 295, 1703
  for cancer patients, 737
  for Candida infection, 440
  for candidemia, 1686
  chemical structure of, 1337f
  for coccidioidomycosis, 296
  dosage of, 1339
    in special circumstances, 1339
  drug interactions of, 1339–1340
  for endophthalmitis, 162–163
  for esophageal candidiasis, 1686
  for fusariosis, 1700
  for histoplasmosis, 294
  indications of, 1339
  for mycetoma, 1723
  for oropharyngeal candidiasis, 1684
  for paracoccidioidomycosis, 297
  pharmacodynamics of, 1339
  pharmacokinetics and distribution of, 1339
  route of administration, 1339
  for sporotrichosis, 298
  for Talaromyces marneffei, 1699
  in thoracic transplantation patients, 750
Vulva, rhinosporidiosis in, 1721
Vulvar cancer, human papillomavirus and, 579
Vulvitis, 489–490, 526
Vulvovaginal candidiasis (VVC), 486–489, 1686
  chronic, 487
  classification of, 488t
  clinical features of, 487–488, 487f–488f
  diagnosis of, 484t, 488
  epidemiology of, 486
  management of, 488–489
  pathogenesis and pathology of, 486–487
  prevention of, 487
  recurrent, 487, 487f
    treatment of, 489
  systemic agents for, 488–489
  topical agents for, 488, 488t
Vulvovaginitis, from Candida, 1684

W

Waddlia chondrophila, 1679t
Walking dandruff, 658–659
Warts
  anogenital, 881
  in HIV, 881
  and occupational infections, 648t–649t
Water, exposure to, and recreational infections, 644–645
Water-borne infections
  burden of disease, 941–942
  see also specific infections
'Water bottle' heart, 452, 452f
Waterhouse-Friderichsen syndrome, 179–180
Weapons of mass destruction (WMD), 670
  see also Bioterrorism
Weather, and emerging infectious diseases, 46–48, 46f
Weeksella, 1581t–1582t, 1597
Weil-Felix test, for scrub typhus, 1096
Weil's disease, 1609
  in myocarditis, 447
West Nile fever, lymphadenopathy and, 137t–138t
West Nile virus (WNV), 189, 702, 806, 1495t, 1496–1499
  and bioterrorism, 671t
  from birds, 668
  clinical manifestations, 1498
  diagnostic microbiology, 1498
  encephalitis/myelitis, 42, 47f, 192t

West Nile virus (WNV) (Continued)
  epidemiology, 1496–1497, 1499f
  management, 1499
  and recreational infections, 644
Western blot
  assays
    for bartonellosis, 1673–1674, 1675f
    for Rickettsia spp., 1667
  HIV, 1487, 1487f
  in Lyme disease, 409–410, 410b
  for primary HIV infection, 848f
Western equine encephalitis, 1493f, 1495t
  virus, 193t–194t
Westley croup score, 230t
Whip worm infection, pathogenesis and pathology of, 991
Whipple's disease
  chronic diarrhea and, 344–345
    clinical features of, 344, 346b
    diagnosis of, 344–345
      strategy, 344f
    duodenal biopsies of, 346f
    epidemiology of, 344
    treatment of, 345
  in chronic meningitis, 187
  and fever of unknown origin, 613
  myocarditis and, 446–447
  uveitis of, 169
Whirlpools, and recreational infections, 644–645
White piedra
  clinical features of, 126
  epidemiology of, 1710
  nature of, 1710
Whitlow, herpetic, 93
  and occupational infections, 648t–649t
Whole genome sequencing (WGS), 1388
  for mycobacteria, 1655
  staphylococci and, 1519
Whooping cough. see Pertussis.
Widal tube agglutination test, 1005
'Wild bugs', 106t
Wild card patent exclusivity, 1384
Winterbottom's sign, 142f
Wiskott-Aldrich syndrome, 721
Wolbachia spp., 1768, 1777–1778
Women, HIV in, 905–911
  contraception in, 906–908
  disease manifestations and progression, 905
  epidemiology, 905
  gynecologic manifestations, 906
  prevention of, 906–910
    trials, 827–828
  transmission, 905
Wool and leather worker, and occupational infections, 648t–649t
World Health Organization (WHO), 952
Wound care, for human bites, 682
Wound closure, in surgery, of peritonitis, 358
Wound infections
  Acinetobacter spp. in, 1595
  in pregnancy, 501
  from Staphylococcus aureus, 1509
Wound management, tetanus prophylaxis, 210t
Wound surface cultures, for burns, 699
Wuchereria bancrofti
  clinical manifestations of, 1777
  epidemiology of, 1765
  life cycle of, 1769f
  lymphadenopathy and, 143
  pathogenicity of, 1768
  treatment of, 1345t–1351t

X

X-linked agammaglobulinemia, 719–720, 719b
X-linked lymphoproliferative syndrome, 721
X-linked severe combined immunodeficiency, 714–715
  diagnosis of, 714–715
  treatment o, 715
X-linked thrombocytopenia, 721
Xenodiagnosis, in Chagas disease, 1070–1071
Xenopsylla cheopis, 108f, 667

Xerosis, in HIV/AIDS, 879–880
Xpert Flu Enterovirus test, 225–226

Y

Yatapoxvirus, 1454*t*
  diagnostic microbiology of, 1457
  management of, 1457
Yaws, 961
  clinical features of, 963, 963*f*–964*f*
  dermatologic manifestations of, 114*t*–115*t*
  pathology of, 963
Yeast cells, 1709
Yeasts
  in complicated urinary tract infection, 540*t*
  provoking immune reconstitution disorder,
    860*t*
Yellow fever, 1494–1496
  and bioterrorism, 671*t*
  clinical manifestations, 1494–1496
  diagnostic microbiology, 1494
  epidemiology, 1494, 1496*f*–1498*f*
  jungle (sylvatic) cycle, 1494
  management, 1496
  nature, 1494
  pathogenicity, 1494
  prevention, 1494
  and recreational infections, 644
  urban (or epidemic) cycle, 1494
  vaccination for, 651*t*, 949, 1494
Yellow fever virus
  clinical features of, 1114*t*–1115*t*
  epidemiology of, 1112*t*
Yersinia, 1611, 1625–1627
  bacterial enteritis and, 337–338
  diagnostic microbiology of, 1568*t*
  erythema nodosum, 121*t*
  in intestinal infections, 1575
  nature of, 1625
  and occupational infections, 648*t*–649*t*
  plague from, 1627
  virulence factors of, 1571*t*, 1626*t*
  yersiniosis from, 1625–1627

Yersinia enterocolitica, 1625
  and bioterrorism, 671*t*
  diarrhea and, 331, 337–338
  epidemiology of, 1625–1626
  in intestinal infections, 1575
  pathogenicity of, 1626
  transmission of, 664, 665*t*
  virulence factors of, 1626*t*
Yersinia pestis, 1078, 1565, 1575, 1625
  and bioterrorism, 671*t*, 677
  in cats, 660
  geography of, 938
  life cycle of, 1078–1080
  multidrug-resistant, 1084
  pathogenesis and pathology of, 1081
  pneumonic, 678*f*
  in rodents, 667
  transmission of, 1078, 1079*f*, 1079*t*
  virulence factors of, 1626*t*
  see also Plague
Yersinia pseudotuberculosis, 1575, 1625
  in cats, 660
  diarrhea and, 337–338
  management of, 1627
  pathogenicity of, 1626
  virulence factors of, 1626*t*
Yersiniosis, 1575, 1625–1627
  clinical manifestations of, 1627
  diagnostic microbiology of, 1626–1627
  epidemiology of, 1625–1626
  management of, 1627
  pathogenicity of, 1626
  prevention of, 1626

Z

Zalcitabine, 1298
  chemical structure of, 1296*f*
Zanamivir, 1146*t*–1147*t*, 1324–1325
  adverse reactions and interactions of,
    1325
  dosage of, 1325
    in special circumstances, 1325

Zanamivir (*Continued*)
  indications of, 1325
  pharmacokinetics and distribution of, 1320*t*,
    1324–1325
  prophylaxis, 1325
  route of administration, 1325
  treatment with, 1325
ZAP70, defects in, 716
Zidovudine, 1148*t*, 1293–1295
  adverse reactions of, 1294–1295
  antiretroviral drugs, 920
  in antiretroviral therapy, 936
  chemical structure of, 1296*f*
  description of, 1293
  dosage of, 1294
    in special circumstances, 1294, 1297*t*
  drug interactions of, 1294–1295
  in HIV postexposure prophylaxis, 835
  indications of, 1294
  perinatal HIV transmission prevention, 908–910, 909*t*
  pharmacokinetics and distribution of, 1293
  resistance of, 1294
  route of administration, 1294
Zidovudine-associated hyperpigmentation, 886
Zidovudine monotherapy
  for postnatal prophylaxis of HIV, 900–901
  toxicity of, 901–902
Ziehl-Neelsen stain, for mycobacteria, 1652, 1652*f*
Zoo worker, and occupational infections, 648*t*–649*t*
Zoonoses, 13
  acquired, examples of routes, 664*f*
  acquired by ingestion, 644
  acquired by inhalation, 644
  arthropod-borne, 644
  and recreational infections, 643–644
  tapeworms, 1033
  see also specific animals
Zoonotic viruses, 1493–1508
  see also specific viruses
Zoon's balanitis, 586*t*–587*t*
Zygomycetes, 1696
  in hematopoietic stem cell transplantation, 744
Zygomycosis. see Mucormycosis.